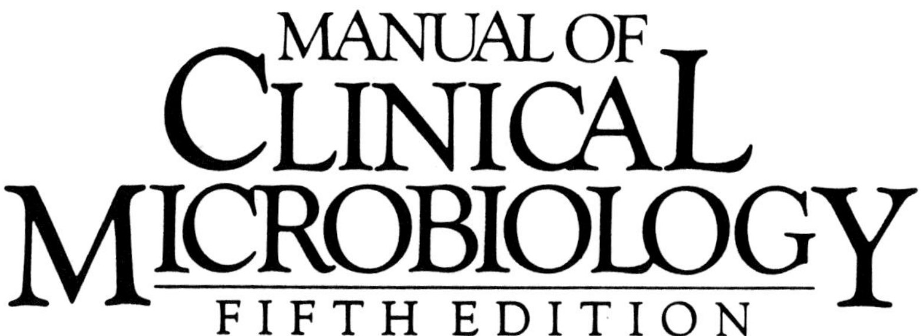
MANUAL OF
CLINICAL
MICROBIOLOGY
FIFTH EDITION

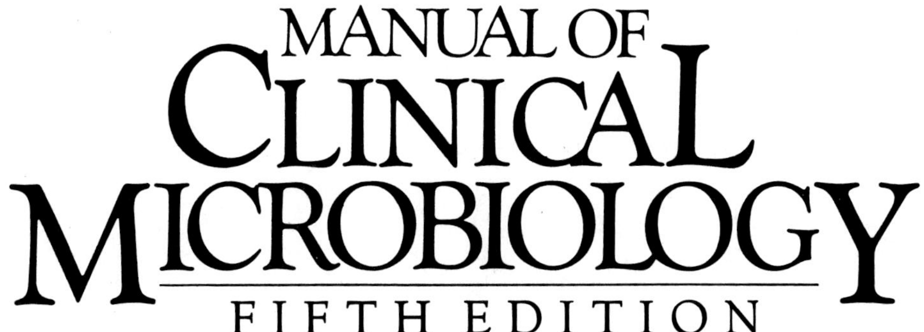

EDITOR IN CHIEF

ALBERT BALOWS

Emory University School of Medicine, Atlanta, Georgia

EDITORS

WILLIAM J. HAUSLER, JR.

University of Iowa Hygienic Laboratory, Iowa City, Iowa

KENNETH L. HERRMANN

Centers for Disease Control, Atlanta, Georgia

HENRY D. ISENBERG

Long Island Jewish Medical Center,
Long Island Campus for Albert Einstein College of Medicine, New Hyde Park, New York

H. JEAN SHADOMY

Virginia Commonwealth University, Richmond, Virginia

AMERICAN SOCIETY FOR MICROBIOLOGY

Washington, D.C.

1325 Massachusetts Ave., N.W.
Washington, DC 20005

Library of Congress Cataloging-in-Publication Data

Manual of clinical microbiology.—5th ed., : editor in chief, Albert Balows; editors, William J. Hausler, Jr. . . . [et al.]
p. cm.
Includes bibliographical references and indexes.
ISBN 1-55581-029-2 (hardcover).—ISBN 1-55581-030-6 (softcover)
1. Diagnostic microbiology—Handbooks, manuals, etc. 2. Medical microbiology—Handbooks, manuals, etc. I. Balows, Albert. II. American Society for Microbiology.
[DNLM: 1. Microbiology. QW 4 M294]
QR67.M36 1991
616'.01—dc20
DNLM/DLC
for Library of Congress

90-14499
CIP

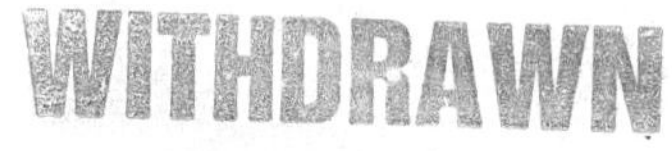

Contents

Section I. GENERAL ISSUES IN CLINICAL MICROBIOLOGY

Section Editor: Gary V. Doern

Section II. DIAGNOSTIC TECHNOLOGIES IN CLINICAL MICROBIOLOGY

Section Editors: Daniel Amsterdam, Roy W. Stevens, and Edward J. Bottone

Section III. NOSOCOMIAL AND COMMUNITY INFECTIONS: THE ROLE OF THE CLINICAL MICROBIOLOGY LABORATORY

Section Editor: Richard P. Wenzel

Section IV. BACTERIA

Section Editors: Richard F. D'Amato, Ellen Jo Baron, Russell C. Johnson, Patrick R. Murray, Frank G. Rodgers, and Alexander von Graevenitz

Section V. FUNGI

Section Editor: Robert A. Fromtling

Section VI. PARASITES

Section Editor: James W. Smith

Section VII. VIRUSES

Section Editors: David A. Lennette, C. George Ray, and Marilyn A. Menegus

Section VIII. RICKETTSIAE AND CHLAMYDIAE
Section Editor: Joseph E. McDade

Section IX. ANTIMICROBIAL AGENTS AND SUSCEPTIBILITY TESTS
Section Editor: Clyde Thornsberry

Section X. QUALITY CONTROL, MEDIA, REAGENTS, AND STAINS
Section Editor: Peter Nash

Editorial Board

Contributors

Sharon L. Abbott
Microbial Diseases Laboratory, California Department of Health Services, Berkeley, California 94704

Libero Ajello
Division of Mycotic Diseases, Centers for Disease Control, Atlanta, Georgia 30333

Aaron D. Alexander
Department of Microbiology, Chicago College of Osteopathic Medicine, Chicago, Illinois 60615

Stephen D. Allen
Department of Pathology, University Hospital, Indiana University School of Medicine, Indianapolis, Indiana 46202

Martin Altwegg
Department of Medical Microbiology, University of Zurich, CH-8028 Zurich, Switzerland

Daniel Amsterdam
Departments of Microbiology and Medicine, School of Medicine, SUNY at Buffalo, and Division of Clinical Microbiology and Immunology, Erie County Medical Center, Buffalo, New York 14215

John P. Anhalt
Section of Microbiology, Mayo Clinic, Rochester, Minnesota 55905

Ray R. Arthur
Department of Immunology and Infectious Diseases, Johns Hopkins School of Public Health, Baltimore, Maryland 21205

Ann M. Arvin
Department of Pediatrics, Stanford University School of Medicine, Stanford, California 94305

Lawrence R. Ash
Department of Epidemiology, School of Public Health, University of California at Los Angeles, Los Angeles, California 90024

David M. Asher
Laboratory of Central Nervous System Studies, National Institute of Neurological Disorders and Stroke, Bethesda, Maryland 20892

Albert Balows
Department of Pathology and Laboratory Medicine, Emory University School of Medicine, Atlanta, Georgia 30303

Susan W. Barnett
Cancer Research Institute, School of Medicine, University of California, San Francisco, California 94143

Ellen Jo Baron
Department of Medicine, UCLA School of Medicine, Los Angeles, California 90024, and VA Medical Center Research Service, Los Angeles, California 90073

Arthur L. Barry
The Clinical Microbiology Institute Inc., Tualatin, Oregon 97062

Marilyn S. Bartlett
Department of Pathology, Indiana University School of Medicine, Indianapolis, Indiana 46202

Raymond C. Bartlett
Division of Microbiology, Department of Pathology, Hartford Hospital, Hartford, Connecticut 06115

Jacques Bille
Clinical Bacteriology Laboratory, University Hospital, Centre Hospitalier Universitaire Vaudois, BH19-1011 Lausanne, Switzerland

Walter W. Bond
Hospital Infections Program, Centers for Disease Control, Atlanta, Georgia 30333

Edward J. Bottone
Department of Microbiology, Mt. Sinai Hospital, New York, New York 10029

Don J. Brenner
Division of Bacterial Diseases, Centers for Disease Control, Atlanta, Georgia 30333

Barbara A. Brown
Department of Microbiology, University of Texas Health Center at Tyler, Tyler, Texas 75710

Willy Burgdorfer
Rocky Mountain Laboratories, National Institute of Allergy and Infectious Diseases, Hamilton, Montana 59840

Kimberle Chapin-Robertson
Clinical Microbiology Laboratory, Yale-New Haven Hospital, and Department of Laboratory Medicine, Yale University School of Medicine, New Haven, Connecticut 06510

Max A. Chernesky
Regional Virology Laboratory, St. Joseph's Hospital, Hamilton, Ontario L8N 4A6, Canada

Mary L. Christensen
Department of Pathology, Northwestern University Medical School, Chicago, Illinois 60611, and Virology Laboratory, Department of Pathology, Children's Memorial Hospital, Chicago, Illinois 60614

Diane M. Citron
R. M. Alden Research Laboratory, Santa Monica Hospital Medical Center, Santa Monica, California 90404

James M. Conroy
Wadsworth Center for Laboratories and Research, New York State Department of Health, Albany, New York 12201

Robert C. Cooksey
Hospital Infections Program, Centers for Disease Control, Atlanta, Georgia 30333

Richard F. D'Amato
Division of Microbiology, The Catholic Medical Center of Brooklyn and Queens, Inc., Jamaica, New York 11432

Jacqueline E. Dawson
Division of Viral and Rickettsial Diseases, Centers for Disease Control, Atlanta, Georgia 30333

Edward P. Desmond
Doctor's Hospital, Pinole, California 94564

Dennis M. Dixon
Laboratories for Mycology, Wadsworth Center for Laboratories and Research, New York State Department of Health, Albany, New York 12201-0509

Gary V. Doern
Department of Clinical Microbiology, University of Massachusetts Medical Center, Worcester, Massachusetts 01655

Michael P. Doyle
Department of Food Microbiology and Toxicology, University of Wisconsin—Madison, Madison, Wisconsin 53706

Stephen C. Edberg
Clinical Microbiology Laboratory, Yale-New Haven Hospital, and Department of Laboratory Medicine, Yale University School of Medicine, New Haven, Connecticut 06510

M. Nixon Ellis
Wellcome Research Laboratories, Burroughs Wellcome Co., Research Triangle Park, North Carolina 27709

Mario R. Escobar
Department of Pathology, Medical College of Virginia, Richmond, Virginia 23298

Joseph J. Esposito
Division of Viral and Rickettsial Diseases, Centers for Disease Control, Atlanta, Georgia 30333

Richard R. Facklam
Division of Bacterial Diseases, Centers for Disease Control, Atlanta, Georgia 30333

J. J. Farmer III
Division of Bacterial Diseases, Centers for Disease Control, Atlanta, Georgia 30333

Martin S. Favero
Hospital Infections Program, Centers for Disease Control, Atlanta, Georgia 30333

Sydney M. Finegold
Research and Medical Services, VA Wadsworth Medical Center, Los Angeles, California 90073, and Departments of Medicine and Microbiology and Immunology, UCLA School of Medicine, Los Angeles, California 90024

Daniel B. Fishbein
Division of Viral and Rickettsial Diseases, Centers for Disease Control, Atlanta, Georgia 30333

Thomas J. Fitzgerald
Department of Medical Microbiology and Immunology, University of Minnesota—Duluth, Duluth, Minnesota 55812
Thomas M. Folks
Division of Viral and Rickettsial Diseases, Centers for Disease Control, Atlanta, Georgia 30333
Harvey M. Friedman
Department of Medicine, Hospital of the University of Pennsylvania, Philadelphia, Pennsylvania 19104
Robert A. Fromtling
Project Planning and Management: Infectious Diseases, Merck Institute for Therapeutic Research, Rahway, New Jersey 07065
Alice Gatson
Department of Pathology, University of Texas Medical Branch, Galveston, Texas 77550
Anne A. Gershon
Department of Pediatrics, Columbia Presbyterian Medical Center, New York, New York 10032
Gerald L. Gilardi
Department of Laboratories, North General Hospital, New York, New York 10035
Mary J. R. Gilchrist
Clinical Microbiology, VA Medical Center, Cincinnati, Ohio 45220
Norman L. Goodman
Department of Pathology, College of Medicine, University of Kentucky, Lexington, Kentucky 40536
Michael B. Gregg
Epidemiology Program Office, Centers for Disease Control, Atlanta, Georgia 30333
Dieter H. M. Gröschel
Department of Pathology, University of Virginia Medical Center, Charlottesville, Virginia 22908
Maurice W. Harmon
Division of Viral and Rickettsial Diseases, Centers for Disease Control, Atlanta, Georgia 30333
W. J. Hausler, Jr.
University of Iowa Hygienic Laboratory, Iowa City, Iowa 52242
Jean E. Hawkins
Reference Laboratory, VA Medical Center, West Haven, Connecticut 06516
George R. Healy
905 Vistavia Circle, Decatur, Georgia 30033 (U.S. Public Health Service [retired])
Karim E. Hechemy
Wadsworth Center for Laboratories and Research, New York State Department of Health, Albany, New York 12201
Donald A. Hendrickson
Department of Biology, Ball State University, Muncie, Indiana 47306
F. W. Hickman-Brenner
Division of Bacterial Diseases, Centers for Disease Control, Atlanta, Georgia 30333
John C. Hierholzer
Division of Viral and Rickettsial Diseases, Centers for Disease Control, Atlanta, Georgia 30333
Edgar L. Hill
Wellcome Research Laboratories, Burroughs Wellcome Co., Research Triangle Park, North Carolina 27709
Sharon Hillier
Department of Obstetrics and Gynecology, University of Washington, Seattle, Washington 98195
Richard L. Hodinka
Clinical Virology, Children's Hospital of Philadelphia, Philadelphia, Pennsylvania 19104
L. A. Holcomb
University of Iowa Hygienic Laboratory, Iowa City, Iowa 52242
Dannie G. Hollis
Division of Bacterial Diseases, Centers for Disease Control, Atlanta, Georgia 30333
Cynthia Howard
Virology Laboratory, Department of Pathology, Children's Memorial Hospital, Chicago, Illinois 60614

Henry D. Isenberg
Long Island Jewish Medical Center, Long Island Campus for Albert Einstein College of Medicine, New Hyde Park, New York 11042
Peter B. Jahrling
United States Army Medical Research Institute of Infectious Diseases, Fort Detrick, Frederick, Maryland 21701
J. Michael Janda
Microbial Diseases Laboratory, California Department of Health Services, Berkeley, California 94704
William M. Janda
Department of Pathology, University of Illinois at Chicago, Chicago, Illinois 60612
Russell C. Johnson
Department of Microbiology, University of Minnesota, Minneapolis, Minnesota 55455
Ronald N. Jones
Department of Pathology, University of Iowa Hospitals and Clinics, Iowa City, Iowa 52242
James H. Jorgensen
Department of Pathology, University of Texas Health Science Center, San Antonio, Texas 78284
Hannele R. Jousimies-Somer
Anaerobe Reference Unit, National Public Health Institute, Helsinki, Finland
Julius Kane
St. Joseph Health Center, Toronto, Ontario M6R 1B5, Canada
Michael T. Kelly
Division of Medical Microbiology, University Hospital-Shaughnessy Site, Vancouver, British Columbia V6H 3N1, Canada
Alan P. Kendal
Division of Viral and Rickettsial Diseases, Centers for Disease Control, Atlanta, Georgia 30333
Michael J. Kennedy
Microbiology and Nutrition Research, The Upjohn Company, Kalamazoo, Michigan 49001
George E. Kenny
Department of Pathobiology, University of Washington, Seattle, Washington 98195
Rima F. Khabbaz
Division of Viral and Rickettsial Diseases, Centers for Disease Control, Atlanta, Georgia 30333
Mogens Kilian
Department of Oral Biology, The Royal Dental College, DK-8000 Arhus C, Denmark
Yoo K. Kim
Department of Laboratory Medicine and Pathology, Mayo Clinic and Mayo Foundation, Rochester, Minnesota 55905
W. E. Kloos
Department of Genetics, North Carolina State University, Raleigh, North Carolina 27695
Elmer W. Koneman
Clinical Microbiology Laboratory, Denver Veterans Administration Hospital, Denver, Colorado 80220
J. M. Kramer
Food Hygiene Laboratory, Central Public Health Laboratory, London NW9 5HT, United Kingdom
T. Krech
Risch Medical Laboratories, FL-9494 Schaan, Liechtenstein
Michelle M. Krenz
R&D Systems, Inc., Minneapolis, Minnesota 55413
Donald J. Krogstad
Departments of Pathology and Internal Medicine, Washington University School of Medicine, St. Louis, Missouri 63110
Michael D. Lairmore
Division of Viral and Rickettsial Diseases, Centers for Disease Control, Atlanta, Georgia 30333
D. W. Lambe, Jr.
Department of Microbiology, East Tennessee State University, Johnson City, Tennessee 27614

Geoffrey Land
Department of Microbiology and Immunology, Methodist Medical Center, Dallas, Texas 75222

Marie L. Landry
Virology Reference Laboratory, Veterans Administration Medical Center, West Haven, Connecticut 06516

Francis K. Lee
Department of Pediatrics, Emory University School of Medicine, Atlanta, Georgia 30303

David A. Lennette
Virolab, Inc., Berkeley, California 94710

Evelyne T. Lennette
Virolab, Inc., Berkeley, California 94710

Jay A. Levy
Cancer Research Institute, School of Medicine, University of California, San Francisco, California 94143

James B. Mahony
Regional Virology Laboratory, St. Joseph's Hospital, Hamilton, Ontario L8N 4A6, Canada

Dennis J. McCance
Department of Microbiology and Immunology, University of Rochester, Rochester, New York 14642

Joseph E. McDade
Center for Infectious Diseases, Centers for Disease Control, Atlanta, Georgia 30333

Michael R. McGinnis
Department of Pathology, University of Texas Medical Branch, Galveston, Texas 77550

John E. McGowan, Jr.
Clinical Microbiology, Grady Memorial Hospital, Atlanta, Georgia 30335

Kenneth McIntosh
Department of Pediatrics, Children's Hospital, Boston, Massachusetts 02115

Joseph L. Melnick
Division of Molecular Virology, Baylor College of Medicine, Houston, Texas 77030

Marilyn A. Menegus
Clinical Microbiology Laboratories, University of Rochester Medical Center, Rochester, New York 14642

William G. Merz
Department of Laboratory Medicine (Pathology), Johns Hopkins University, Baltimore, Maryland 21205

J. Michael Miller
Hospital Infections Program, Centers for Disease Control, Atlanta, Georgia 30333

Thomas G. Mitchell
Department of Microbiology and Immunology, Duke University Medical Center, Durham, North Carolina 27710

Robert C. Moellering, Jr.
Department of Medicine, New England Deaconess Hospital, Boston, Massachusetts 02215

Bernard J. Moncla
Department of Oral Biology and Department of Periodontics, University of Washington, Seattle, Washington 98195

Josephine A. Morello
Departments of Pathology, Medicine, and Molecular Genetics and Cell Biology, University of Chicago, Chicago, Illinois 60637

N. P. Moyer
University of Iowa Hygienic Laboratory, Iowa City, Iowa 52242

Patrick R. Murray
Departments of Pathology and Medicine, Washington University School of Medicine, St. Louis, Missouri 63110

James H. Nakano
Division of Viral and Rickettsial Diseases, Centers for Disease Control, Atlanta, Georgia 30333 (deceased)

Peter Nash
Camas Diagnostic Company, Minneapolis, Minnesota 55414

Phuc Nguyen-Dinh
Division of Parasitic Diseases, Centers for Disease Control, Atlanta, Georgia 30333

David E. Normansell
Department of Pathology, University of Virginia Health Sciences Center, Charlottesville, Virginia 22908
Thomas C. Orihel
School of Public Health and Tropical Medicine, Tulane University, New Orleans, Louisiana 70122
Arvind A. Padhye
Division of Mycotic Diseases, Centers for Disease Control, Atlanta, Georgia 30333
Lester Pasarell
Department of Pathology, University of Texas Medical Branch, Galveston, Texas 77550
A. William Pasculle
Presbyterian-University Hospital, University of Pittsburgh School of Medicine, Pittsburgh, Pennsylvania 15216
J. R. Pattison
Department of Medical Microbiology, University College, London WC1E 6JJ, United Kingdom
John L. Penner
Department of Microbiology, Faculty of Medicine, Banting Institute, Toronto, Ontario M5G 1L5, Canada
Michael A. Pfaller
Department of Pathology, University of Iowa College of Medicine, and Veterans Administration Medical Center, Iowa City, Iowa 52242
M. John Pickett
Department of Microbiology, University of California, Los Angeles, California 90024
Peter Piot
Department of Microbiology, Institute of Tropical Medicine, B-2000 Antwerp, Belgium
Harry D. Pratt
879 Glen Arden Way, N.E., Atlanta, Georgia 30306
Charles G. Prober
Department of Pediatrics, Stanford University School of Medicine, Stanford, California 94305
C. George Ray
Department of Pathology, University of Arizona College of Medicine, Tucson, Arizona 85724
Michael G. Rinaldi
Department of Pathology, University of Texas Health Science Center at San Antonio, and Mycology Reference Laboratory, Audie L. Murphy Memorial Veterans' Hospital, San Antonio, Texas 78274
Glenn D. Roberts
Department of Laboratory Medicine and Pathology, Mayo Clinic and Mayo Foundation, Rochester, Minnesota 55905
Frank G. Rodgers
Department of Microbiology, University of New Hampshire, Durham, New Hampshire 03824
Alvin L. Rogers
Departments of Botany and Plant Pathology, Microbiology and Public Health, and Medical Technology, Michigan State University, East Lansing, Michigan 48824
Joseph A. Rosebrock
Zeus Scientific Inc., Raritan, New Jersey 08869
Daniel F. Sahm
University of Chicago Medical Center, Chicago, Illinois 60637
Ira F. Salkin
Wadsworth Center for Laboratories and Research, New York State Department of Health, Albany, New York 12201
Aimo A. Salmi
Department of Virology, University of Turku, SF-20520 Turku, Finland
Myron Sasser
Microbial Identification System, Newark, Delaware 19711
Julius Schachter
Chlamydia Laboratory, San Francisco General Hospital, San Francisco, California 94110
Peter Schantz
Division of Parasitic Diseases, Centers for Disease Control, Atlanta, Georgia 30333
Wiley A. Schell
Department of Hospital Laboratories, Duke University Medical Center, Durham, North Carolina 27710

Nathalie J. Schmidt
Viral and Rickettsial Disease Laboratory, California Department of Health Services, Berkeley, California 94704 (deceased)

Tom G. Schwan
Rocky Mountain Laboratories, National Institute of Allergy and Infectious Diseases, Hamilton, Montana 59840

H. Jean Shadomy
Department of Microbiology and Immunology, Virginia Commonwealth University, Richmond, Virginia 23298

Smith Shadomy
Department of Internal Medicine, Medical College of Virginia, Virginia Commonwealth University, Richmond, Virginia 23248

Keerti V. Shah
Department of Immunology and Infectious Diseases, Johns Hopkins School of Public Health, Baltimore, Maryland 21205

Robert E. Shope
Yale Arbovirus Research Unit, Yale University School of Medicine, New Haven, Connecticut 06510

Robert M. Smibert
Department of Anaerobic Microbiology, Virginia Polytechnic Institute and State University, Blacksburg, Virginia 24061

James W. Smith
Department of Pathology, Indiana University School of Medicine, Indianapolis, Indiana 46202

Jean S. Smith
Division of Viral and Rickettsial Diseases, Centers for Disease Control, Atlanta, Georgia 30333

Joseph Staneck
Department of Pathology, University Hospital, University of Cincinnati Medical Center, Cincinnati, Ohio 45267

Sharon P. Steinberg
Columbia Presbyterian Medical Center, New York, New York 10032

Roy W. Stevens
Wadsworth Center for Laboratories and Research, New York State Department of Health, Albany, New York 12201

John A. Stewart
Division of Viral and Rickettsial Diseases, Centers for Disease Control, Atlanta, Georgia 30333

Scott J. Stewart
Rocky Mountain Laboratories, National Institute of Allergy and Infectious Diseases, Hamilton, Montana 59840

Barbara A. Strain
Department of Pathology, University of Virginia Health Sciences Center, School of Medicine, Charlottesville, Virginia 22908

Charles W. Stratton
Vanderbilt University School of Medicine, Nashville, Tennessee 37232

Paul D. Swenson
Division of Laboratories, Seattle-King County Department of Public Health, Seattle, Washington 98104

Ella M. Swierkosz
Department of Pediatrics, School of Medicine, St. Louis University Medical Center, St. Louis, Missouri 63104

Andrea Talis
Division of Infectious Diseases, Department of Pediatrics, Children's Hospital, Boston, Massachusetts 02115

Fred C. Tenover
Hospital Infections Program, Centers for Disease Control, Atlanta, Georgia 30333

Clyde Thornsberry
Institutes for Microbiology Research, Franklin, Tennessee 37064

Thomas J. Tinghitella
Department of Pathology, Bridgeport Hospital, Bridgeport, Connecticut 06610

P. C. B. Turnbull
Public Health Laboratory Service Centre for Applied Microbiology and Research, Porton Down, Salisbury, Wiltshire SP4 0JG, England

Govinda S. Visvesvara
Division of Parasitic Diseases, Centers for Disease Control, Atlanta, Georgia 30333

Alexander von Graevenitz
Department of Medical Microbiology, University of Zurich, CH-8028 Zurich, Switzerland
Richard J. Wallace, Jr.
Department of Microbiology, University of Texas Health Center at Tyler, Tyler, Texas 75710
Kenneth W. Walls
4006 Northlake Creek Court, Tucker, Georgia 30084 (U.S. Public Health Service [retired])
Thomas J. Walsh
Infectious Diseases Section, National Cancer Institute, Bethesda, Maryland 20892
Joseh L. Waner
Pediatric Infectious Diseases, University of Oklahoma Health Sciences Center, Oklahoma City, Oklahoma 73190
Nancy G. Warren
Commonwealth of Virginia Division of Consolidated Laboratory Services, Richmond, Virginia 23219
John A. Washington II
Department of Microbiology, Cleveland Clinic Foundation, Cleveland, Ohio 44106
Emilio Weiss
Naval Medical Research Institute, Bethesda, Maryland 20014
Irene Weitzman
Mycology Laboratory, City of New York Department of Health, Bureau of Laboratories, New York, New York 10016
Richard P. Wenzel
Division of General Medicine, Clinical Epidemiology, and Health Services Research, Department of Internal Medicine, University of Iowa College of Medicine, and Program of Epidemiology, University of Iowa Hospitals and Clinics, Iowa City, Iowa 52242
Hannah M. Wexler
Research Service, VA Wadsworth Medical Center, and Department of Medicine, UCLA School of Medicine, Los Angeles, California 90073
Michael D. Wichman
University of Iowa Hygienic Laboratory, Iowa City, Iowa 52242
Marianna Wilson
Division of Parasitic Diseases, Centers for Disease Control, Atlanta, Georgia 30333
Joseph D. C. Yao
Calgary General Hospital, Calgary, Alberta, Canada T2E 0A1

Preface

In the past two decades we have witnessed a remarkable growth in the breadth and depth of clinical microbiology. Documentation of the increasing scope of technological advances during the past 20 years is evidenced in the first four editions of the *Manual of Clinical Microbiology* (MCM). This edition, MCM5, proudly joins its predecessors in documenting currently accepted practices in clinical microbiology as we enter the last decade of the 20th century. The excitement and challenges associated with MCM5 were evident from the beginning and have resulted in a remarkable collaborative effort among editors, authors, and the publisher. The result is a totally revised version that we hope retains a mark of distinction, as did the earlier editions.

The first edition of MCM, published in 1970 with 76 chapters in 727 pages, set the pace and was warmly welcomed by clinical microbiologists, infectious disease specialists, pathologists, medical technologists, clinicians, and students and their teachers as a useful and practical source of information on the detection, isolation, and identification of virtually all important agents of infectious diseases. MCM5, published 21 years later, has 122 chapters in approximately 1,400 pages and documents the dynamic changes that have occurred in all aspects of clinical microbiology.

Innovation is evident throughout MCM5. The number of volume and section editors was increased to accommodate the growth in size and scope. In the early planning stages of this edition, the decision was made to retain the flavor and style of previous editions and to involve and indoctrinate as many young scientists as possible to serve as editorial board members and chapter authors. As a result, at least 107 individuals served as first-time editors and authors for MCM5. The total effort of editors, authors, and an energetic ASM publications staff has resulted in a revised edition that we believe will be user friendly and helpful.

We express our thanks to the many secretaries who diligently produced the drafts and ultimately the final version of each chapter. Similarly, we thank the unsung support staff who did so many different but necessary tasks that contributed to the published manuscript and the successful book. We are appreciative of the efforts of the editorial board, who recruited authors, pressed them to adhere to schedules, and reviewed drafts and final versions of chapters until each chapter was at its scientific prime. Special thanks are due to the staff of the ASM Publications Department, who did everything and anything to assist the editors, editorial board, authors, and others connected with MCM5 in bringing it to fruition. We especially wish to recognize Kirk Jensen, Dennis Burke, and Susan Birch at ASM Publications, who worked patiently with editors and authors to resolve problems as they surfaced and to ensure timely publication.

We also wish to express our appreciation to Helen Whiteley, who was chairman of the ASM Publications Board when MCM5 was embryonic. The wisdom of her leadership and her dedication to ASM publications were of benefit to us. In a different vein, we also acknowledge and express our gratitude for the exemplary contributions of Edwin H. Lennette, whose imprimatur is evident in each of the first four editions of MCM and who set the tone for MCM5.

Finally, and with equal, if not greater, appreciation, we are grateful to the dedicated authors who tolerated the push for producing manuscripts that conformed to style, format, and design. They gave of their time, wisdom, and knowledge to make MCM5 the success that we believe it will be.

Albert Balows
William J. Hausler, Jr.
Kenneth L. Herrmann
Henry D. Isenberg
H. Jean Shadomy

Chapter 1

Introduction to the Fifth Edition of the *Manual of Clinical Microbiology*

ALBERT BALOWS

Clinical microbiology gained visibility in the 1950s and 1960s, when many new and different pathogenic agents were encountered and resistance to the available antibiotics was increasing. Recognition of clinical microbiology as a distinct discipline came during the late 1960s and early 1970s. Perhaps not coincidentally, the first edition of the *Manual of Clinical Microbiology* (MCM) was published in 1970. The fifth edition, MCM5, is strikingly different from its predecessors and, among other things, serves as strong evidence that recent advances in clinical microbiology have been dynamic and remarkable.

The editors and authors, who are listed in the front part of this volume, constitute a multidisciplinary group of well-qualified individuals who have combined their talents to produce a book that reflects the current practice of clinical microbiology. The primary purpose of MCM5 is to guide clinical microbiologists in selecting and performing laboratory procedures that lead to the establishment of the etiology of infectious diseases of humans and the determination, in vitro, of potentially effective therapeutic agents.

Some will view MCM5 as a reference book, and in some respects this is understandable. Others may regard MCM5 as a textbook, and still others may consider it a laboratory procedure manual. There are elements of all of these in MCM5. However, it lacks the in-depth presentation of fundamentals and theoretical considerations usually found in textbooks, and while segments of this book may be quoted or otherwise incorporated into the procedure manual of a given laboratory, MCM5 cannot and should not substitute for the comprehensive procedure manuals desirable, and in some instances required, in clinical microbiology laboratories.

Changes in how we define clinical microbiology continually occur. These changes parallel those that are taking place in the provision of medical care and health maintenance in the United States and other countries. Laboratories that provide clinical microbiology services now exist in physician offices, clinics, complex medical centers, general and specialty hospitals of all sizes, private, local, and regional reference laboratories, and local, state, and federal public health laboratories. Technological advances in molecular biology, protein and nucleic acid chemistry, immunology, microbial pathogenicity, and general microbiology have yielded something for everyone. One of the consequences of these advances is the almost overwhelming number of new reagents, diagnostic kits, semiautomated and automated instruments, and nucleic acid probes with which the clinical microbiologist is now confronted. These represent tangible evidence of the growing body of knowledge that extends the boundary of clinical microbiology in all directions and, in so doing, encompasses all of the types of laboratories and institutions described above.

With such divergence of laboratories, who are the intended users of MCM5? Is the book organized to facilitate its use by the users? How is MCM5 best utilized? Answers to these questions are general rather than specific. The intended users are those who work in any of the laboratory settings listed above and whose job responsibilities include clinical microbiology in any or all of its ramifications. There is one caveat: users must have knowledge of the fundamentals of microbiology and possess basic laboratory skills. With this background, each user can determine how MCM5 best fits his or her needs. Organizationally, the ten sections of MCM5 fall into three major groups. Sections I, II, III, and X are operational and organizational in content and contain chapters that address topics ranging from how to collect and safely manage clinical specimens in the laboratory to what methodologic approach is best for identifying a significant isolate or determining the strain identity or dissimilarity of multiple clinical isolates of the same species in the investigation of nosocomial infections. Sections IV through VIII contain chapters dealing with specific microorganisms as etiologic agents. Descriptions of important characteristics of the microorganisms, how they are isolated and identified, and their relevance to a patient's disease are presented. The chapters in section IX discuss how the clinical microbiology laboratory functions in the selection of antimicrobial agents for treating infectious diseases, performs tests related to defining the mode of antibiotic action or mechanisms of resistance, and conducts assays for antibiotics in blood and other body fluids.

How MCM5 will ultimately be used is up to the individual. Each user, however, is urged to become familiar with the organization and content of the book by reading all of the chapters in section I. These seven chapters not only set the tone for MCM5 but, more important, describe the fundamentals for the day-to-day operation of a clinical microbiology laboratory. As users gain familiarity with this book, they will find that MCM5 has kept pace with the new developments and technology in clinical microbiology. As a result, this enlarged and restructured edition serves as a definitive yet practical guide to clinical microbiology.

Chapter 2

Indigenous and Pathogenic Microorganisms of Humans

HENRY D. ISENBERG AND RICHARD F. D'AMATO

CHANGING CONCEPTS OF INFECTIOUS DISEASE

Traditionally, clinical microbiologists have been responsible for identifying microorganisms in a clinical specimen as accurately and quickly as possible. There is also a tacit agreement between clinicians and microbiologists that the microorganisms of interest are the so-called pathogens. This attitude suggests that a very small number of microorganisms incite infectious disease processes regardless of their quantity, their portal of entry, or the presence of other microorganisms. Most significantly, this view neglects the determinative roles of the host and the environment in the clinically overt manifestations of infectious disease, placing the onus for the disease squarely on the microorganism.

Dubos (7) and Burnet (2) have expanded the appraisal by Theobald Smith (20) of the numerous host and parasite interactions that culminate in clinically overt infectious disease. The studies of these investigators showed that the general health of the host, his or her previous contact with particular microorganisms, past medical history, and a variety of toxic, traumatic, or iatrogenic insults are significant determinants of infectious disease. Implied is the understanding that indigenous microflora, given the opportunity by an unrelated lowering of host resistance, may become involved in infectious disease. The numerous factors and conditions of microbial and host origins that must be considered in infection have been reviewed recently (12, 13).

The dilemma of the clinical microbiologist is deciding which of the microorganisms isolated from a clinical specimen are involved in disease. There are very few microorganisms to which the term "pathogenic" can be applied invariably, if "pathogenic" is defined as causing infectious disease at all times (16), yet the clinical microbiologist is expected to decide the causal relationship between a microorganism and a disease even though most of the organisms from clinical material are at best only sometimes pathogenic. All that can be presented here is a very limited discussion and outline of some of the factors that affect the categorizing of microorganisms as harmless, potentially hazardous, or actively involved in the observed pathology.

Microorganisms, i.e., bacteria, yeasts, fungi, protozoa, and viruses, are ubiquitous in and on the human body (17). From birth, people live in a microbial biosphere composed of innumerable microorganisms representing types, variants, strains, species, genera, etc. The composition of this microbial environment is dynamic. Numerous additions and deletions, both qualitative and quantitative, constantly take place. Many populated and sterile areas are found in and on the human body, as are sparsely populated areas or regions that harbor transient microbiota. These temporary habitats of microorganisms include the larynx, trachea, bronchi, accessory nasal sinuses, esophagus, stomach and upper portions of the small intestine, upper urinary tract (including the posterior urethra), and the corresponding distal areas of the male and female genital organs. The persistent finding of numerous microorganisms in these temporarily inhabited areas or in blood or other sterile body sites provides, according to Rosebury (16), as reliable a marker as can be found for the imaginary line that divides health from disease. Conclusions concerning the significance of a microorganism isolated from usually sterile areas must be based on properly obtained specimens that were properly handled and transported, that were examined promptly, and that yielded a large number of microorganisms unusual in a particular locale or present there occasionally in very small numbers.

One other aspect of microbiology cannot be ignored. Not all of the microorganisms that may be present in a given specimen can be cultivated; others have not yet been cultivated or are very difficult to cultivate. In most instances, the clinical microbiologist insists on examining stained preparations from clinical material, especially when the specimen is obtained directly from a pathological lesion or from suspect areas usually populated by a mixed microbiota. Innovative techniques of molecular biology and immunochemistry are now being developed for direct application to specimens, considerably augmenting the diagnostic capabilities of clinical microbiologists.

No hard and fast rule divides the human microbiota into clear-cut categories of harmless, commensal organisms and pathogenic species. The microbial species encountered are listed in the various tables of this chapter, along with their general anatomical locales and involvement in disease. The frequency of their presence and their role in infectious processes are graded in the tables as a guide. The clinical presentation of each patient must be considered in the interpretation of findings based on these tables, which are not exhaustive.

BODY AREAS

The indigenous and the pathogenic microorganisms of the various body areas have been compiled previously (4), but the list is constantly growing. All of the organisms listed in reference 4 were isolated from lesions or other appropriate specimen, although many times the causal relationship between the microbe recovered and the disease was tenuous at best. Despite the dearth of basic information and the cautious presentation of these listings, they have been accepted as authoritative. Organisms not mentioned as either indigenous or pathogenic are treated with an extreme degree of suspicion or, worse, ignored entirely. This practice still prevails despite considerable improvement in cultural technology and a changed approach to the basic tenets of infectious disease. Therefore, it must be stated categorically that the following compilations are not exhaustive; the omission or inclusion of a microbial species in any category does not imply that it cannot be isolated from a particular or any other body area or that it cannot incite disease, complicate underlying disease, or colonize anatomical abnormalities of congenital, traumatic, or iatrogenic origin. In the communities and especially in the hospitals of developed countries, antimicrobial drugs exert selective pressures that permit the entry of drug-resistant microorganisms into the intimate human biosphere from an inexhaustible pool in nature.

RESPIRATORY TRACT

See also references 4, 9, 11, and 16.

Areas that usually harbor microorganisms

Mouth. The mouth consists of the buccal cavity, teeth, tongue, gingivae, palates, and saliva. The following organisms are commonly found in this region. Various pigmented micrococci, *Staphylococcus epidermidis, Staphylococcus aureus,* and *Staphylococcus*-like anaerobic varieties are especially numerous in the saliva and on tooth surfaces, but they are not usually encountered in gingival crevices of healthy individuals. *S. aureus* and the anaerobic cocci are rare in the predentulous mouth. The viridans streptococci, including both the mitis and salivarius groups, are ubiquitously distributed on all surfaces of the mouth, with certain species favoring specific sites (10). Enterococci may be present. *Streptococcus pyogenes* is present in a small percentage (5 to 10%) of normal mouths, usually from throat cultures of asymptomatic individuals. The finding of group A streptococci in healthy individuals is restricted to the saliva or tooth surfaces of adults; peptostreptococci are also commonly found. *Streptococcus pneumoniae* may be present in the predentulous mouth and has been recovered from saliva and tooth surfaces of as many as 25% of healthy adults. Pigmented *Neisseria* spp., *Branhamella* (*Moraxella*) *catarrhalis, Veillonella* spp., and aerobic corynebacteria are very common in saliva and in gingival crevices. Several *Actinomyces* spp. can be isolated from the mouth. The lactobacilli are found in saliva, whereas the leptotrichiae are more frequently encountered on tooth surfaces. The family *Enterobacteriaceae* is well represented; *Escherichia coli* and the *Klebsiella-Enterobacter* group are among the most common enteric organisms isolated, especially in saliva and on teeth after the initiation of broad-spectrum antimicrobial therapy. At times, these enteric bacteria may be joined by oxidase-producing or nonfermenting gram-negative rods. *Haemophilus influenzae* and *Haemophilus parainfluenzae* are often recovered from normal mouths, as are *Bacteroides* and *Fusobacterium* spp., *Campylobacter sputorum,* and a variety of spirochetes, especially *Treponema denticola* and *Treponema refringens. Capnocytophaga* spp. are common colonizers. Several mycoplasmata have been isolated from the saliva of healthy individuals. *Candida albicans* and occasionally other *Candida* spp. exist in the oral cavity without disease production. The protozoa *Entamoeba gingivalis* and *Trichomonas tenax* are examples of ameba and flagellates found in the gingival crevices of some healthy adults.

This large array of microorganisms found in healthy mouths makes it inevitable that an even greater number of microorganisms will be found when infection is present; undoubtedly, some appear in lesions accidentally. Findings from gum lesions, root canals, caries, etc., reflect this state. Debilitated patients or those on prolonged chemotherapy often have lesions of the tongue from which fungi are isolated; other patients with nutritional deficiencies or possibly hygienic neglect may have membranous lesions involving the entire oral cavity. Numerous bacteria can be demonstrated in this disease picture, which is often referred to as Vincent's angina. Only very few of the component bacteria have been cultivated, and the causal relationship between the microbes and the disease is not clear. *Candida* spp., especially *C. albicans,* may take advantage of debilitation, various degrees of immunosuppression, chemotherapy, and malnutrition to produce lesions in the oropharynx commonly designated as thrush. Viruses involved in respiratory and other disease may be found in the mouth and in saliva (Table 1). In immunocompromised patients, filamentous fungi, particularly the zygomycetes, may cause disease.

Throat, including the nasopharynx, oropharynx, and tonsils. Micrococci are among the organisms usually found in the throat, nasopharynx, oropharynx, and tonsils. Coagulase-negative staphylococci may be found in the nasopharynx and on the tonsillar area of children older than infants. *S. aureus* is frequently present in the nasopharynx, the oropharynx, and the tonsils. The tonsils may harbor anaerobic cocci. Viridans streptococci are almost always present in the throat. Various hemolytic streptococci, among them *S. pyogenes,* can be found in the nasopharynx and especially in the tonsillar region of normal, healthy individuals but in small numbers. Enterococci may be present on tonsils. *Streptococcus pneumoniae* and the neisseriae that tolerate 20 to 25°C are present in the healthy throat, sometimes accompanied in the nasopharynx by *Neisseria meningitidis,* usually without any evidence of a disease process or contact with individuals ill with meningococcemia or meningococcal meningitis. *Veillonella* spp., corynebacteria, and *Actinomyces* spp. are present, especially on the tonsils. *E. coli,* the *Klebsiella-Enterobacter* group, and *Proteus* spp. can be found with varying frequency in different areas of the throat. A large number of healthy throats harbor *H. influenzae* or *H. parainfluenzae,* and the tonsils especially contain various *Bacteroides* spp., *Fusobacterium* spp., vibrios, and spirochetes. In addition, throat cultures from healthy individuals may indicate the presence of *Bacteroides pneumosintes,* very minute gram-negative rods capable of passing most bacterial filters, mycoplasmata, *C. albicans, Candida* spp., and the same protozoa described for the mouth.

Infectious disease of the throat can be caused by several microorganisms. Some lesions may be initiated by different viruses, only to be followed quickly by bacteria and fungi. In most geographical areas, *Streptococcus pyogenes* remains the major bacterial pathogenic bac-

TABLE 1. Microorganisms encountered in respiratory tract specimens

Organism	Frequency of isolation[a]	Disease involvement[b]
Absidia spp.	C	2
Acinetobacter spp.	B	2
Actinomyces spp.	A	2
Adenoviruses	B	3
Arachnia propionica	B	1
Ascaris lumbricoides larvae	C	3
Aspergillus spp.	B	2
Bacillus anthracis	C	3
Bacillus spp.	B	1
Bacteroides spp.	A	2
Bifidobacterium spp.	B	1
Blastomyces dermatitidis	C	3
Bordetella pertussis	B	3
Borrelia spp.	B	1
Branhamella (*Moraxella*) *catarrhalis*	B	2
Brucella spp.	C	3
Campylobacter spp.	B	1
Candida spp.	B	2
Capnocytophaga spp.	B	2
Cardiobacterium hominis	B	1
Chlamydia spp.	B	3
Clostridium spp.	B	2
Coccidioides immitis	B	3
Coronavirus	B	2
Corynebacterium diphtheriae (toxigenic)	C	3
Corynebacterium spp.	B	1
Coxiella burnetii	C	3
Cryptococcus neoformans	C	3
Cryptosporidium spp.	C	3
Cytomegalovirus	B	2
Echinococcus spp., protoscolices or hooklets	C	3
Eikenella corrodens	B	2
Entamoeba gingivalis	B	1
Entamoeba histolytica trophozoites	C	3
Enterobacteriaceae	B	2
Enterococcus spp.	C	1
Enteroviruses	B	2
Epstein-Barr virus	C	2
Flavobacterium spp.	C	2
Francisella tularensis	C	3
Fusobacterium spp.	A	2
Haemophilus spp.	A	2
Herpes simplex virus	B	3
Histoplasma capsulatum	B	3
Human immunodeficiency virus	C	2

Organism	Frequency of isolation[a]	Disease involvement[b]
Influenza viruses	B	3
Kingella spp.	C	2
Lactobacillus spp.	B	1
Legionella spp.	B	2
Leptotrichia buccalis	B	1
Measles virus	B	3
Micrococcus spp.	A	1
Moraxella spp.	B	1
Mucor spp.	C	2
Mumps virus	B	3
Mycobacterium spp.	B	2
Mycobacterium tuberculosis group	B	3
Mycoplasma spp.	B	2
Necator americanus	C	3
Neisseria gonorrhoeae	C	3
Neisseria meningitidis	B	2
Neisseria spp.	A	1
Nocardia spp.	B	2
Papillomaviruses	C	2
Paracoccidioides brasiliensis	C	3
Paragonimus spp. ova	C	3
Parainfluenza viruses	B	2
Pasteurella spp.	C	2
Penicillium spp.	C	1
Peptostreptococcus spp.	A	2
Petrilidium boydii	C	2
Pneumocystis carinii	B	2
Pseudomonas spp.	B	2
Respiratory syncytial virus	B	3
Rhinoviruses	B	2
Rhizomucor spp.	C	2
Rhizopus spp.	C	2
Rothia dentocariosa	B	1
Rubella virus	B	3
Selenomonas spp.	C	1
Sporothrix schenckii	C	3
Staphylococcus spp.	A	2
Streptococcus pneumoniae	B	2
Streptococcus pyogenes	B	2
Streptococcus spp.	A	2
Strongyloides stercoralis larvae	C	3
Treponema spp.	B	2
Trichomonas tenax	B	1
Varicella-zoster virus	B	3
Veillonella spp.	A	1
Vibrio spp.	B	1
Wollinella recta	B	1

[a] A, Commonly encountered in clinical specimens; B, occasionally encountered in clinical specimens; C, rarely encountered in clinical specimens.
[b] 1, When present, it is rarely if ever involved in disease production; 2, when present, it is occasionally involved in disease production; 3, when present, it is commonly involved in disease production.

terium involved in throat disease. Its detection is imperative to initiate therapy and prevent sequelae. Pneumococci do not contribute to pathological processes in the throat and indeed constitute part of the normal flora of many healthy adults. Although some hemophiline bacteria are normally present in the throat, *H. influenzae* serogroup b has been involved in epiglottitis, a disease of young children and, rarely, of young adults, with a grave prognosis. *S. aureus* may be involved in a variety of disease processes in the throat. Its presence is probably the most difficult to interpret. Repeated isolation of this bacterium in large numbers from a carefully cultured lesion diminishes such doubts. As a rule, *S. aureus* is present in small numbers in the normal throat. Thrush, already described for the mouth, may also involve the throat and esophagus. Candidal lesions may be found in the throat accompanying a variety of drug regimens, as well as in patients with debilitating and neoplastic diseases and immunosuppression and in neonatal infants. The throat, and especially the tonsils, may be a site for primary lesions of syphilis. *Neisseria gonorrhoeae* may also be detected in the throat and may give rise to a local disease in this area which can rapidly disseminate (8). Viral pharyngitis may be caused by adenovirus, type A coxsackieviruses, other enteroviruses, herpes simplex viruses, Epstein-Barr virus, rhinoviruses, and parainfluenza and influenza viruses (3, 6).

Nose. The nares are the usual habitat of the staphylococci. *S. epidermidis, S. aureus,* and other species are recovered with great frequency from this site. Although both organisms may not be present at all times in any one individual, their recovery from the nares is to be expected. On rare occasions, viridans streptococci can be isolated from the nasal passages. In children, and especially in infants, enterococci and other bacteria reflecting the fecal microbiota are not uncommon. On occasion, the nares of healthy persons have also yielded *S. pyogenes* and *S. pneumoniae.* The nonpathogenic neisseriae are transients in this location as well. Healthy contacts of patients with meningococcal disease may harbor *N. meningitidis.* Additional residents of the nose are various corynebacteria and occasionally *Moraxella lacunata.* Upper respiratory tract viruses may be found in this site (Table 1).

Actual disease of the nasal passages must be differentiated carefully from disease of adjacent areas, including the skin, nasopharynx, oropharynx, tonsils, and sinuses. In premature and newborn infants, lesions due to hemolytic *E. coli, Pseudomonas aeruginosa,* and *C. albicans* may be encountered, but these usually represent more generalized disease, as is indicated by the isolation of *Acinetobacter calcoaceticus* var. *lwoffii, Moraxella* spp., *Acinetobacter calcoaceticus* var. *anitratus,* and various flavobacteria. Ozaena, a disease characterized by atrophy of the nasal mucosa (22), is caused by gram-negative rods. An infective granuloma, rhinoscleroma, most often involves the nose, although the pharynx and the remaining upper respiratory tract may be involved as well. *Klebsiella pneumoniae* subsp. *rhinoscleromatis* is regarded by most investigators as the etiological agent. The disease is uncommon in the United States. Filamentous fungi such as the zygomycetes may be involved in serious disease process of the nasal sinuses.

Usually sterile areas. The larynx, trachea, bronchi, bronchioles, alveoli, and accessory nasal sinuses are usually sterile. Contamination by occasional microorganisms is usual, but the various defense mechanisms of these organs remove such offenders quickly and efficiently. The usual specimen submitted to the clinical microbiology laboratory for establishing infectious disease of the lower respiratory tract is the sputum specimen. Bronchial washings, bronchoalveolar lavage, and bronchoscopy specimens, thoracentesis fluid, and aspirates from tracheostomies or lung lesion biopsies are now frequently submitted for microbiological analysis. Sputum and some aspirates are invariably contaminated by the microbiota of the throat, nose, and mouth. Rapid processing, including examination of smears to evaluate leukocytes and epithelial cells, is imperative to prevent these contaminating microorganisms from obscuring etiological agents. The most commonly encountered bacteria in the sputum are various viridans streptococci, *Neisseria* spp., staphylococci, corynebacteria, the *Enterobacteriaceae, B. catarrhalis, P. aeruginosa,* and *C. albicans.* These organisms may be involved in infectious processes, they may be contaminants, or they may reflect superinfection after therapy.

Acute infectious bronchitis, most frequently seen during winter in children and the aged and associated with adenoviruses, influenza viruses, and parainfluenza viruses, may be complicated by *S. aureus, S. pneumoniae, S. pyogenes, H. influenzae,* and *Mycoplasma pneumoniae* (and *Bordetella pertussis* when whooping cough is present). Chronic bronchitis, of unknown etiology and associated frequently with pulmonary emphysema, is assuming increasing importance. Sputum from such patients displays a variety of microorganisms, not necessarily the same species on repeat examination. The presence of bacteria associated with pathology of the respiratory tract, such as *B. catarrhalis,* pneumococci, group A streptococci, *H. influenzae, M. pneumoniae,* and staphylococci, may be significant.

Acute mediastinitis is usually the result of perforation of the esophagus in conjunction with instrumentation, obstruction, external wounds, downward propagation of deep cellulitis of the neck, forceful vomiting, and occasionally the extension of infectious disease of the lungs, pleural cavity, or pericardium. The bacteria that contribute most frequently to the disease picture are the peptostreptococci, *Bacteroides* spp., fusobacteria, and occasionally clostridia. Pneumonia may be caused by *S. pneumoniae, S. pyogenes, H. influenzae, S. aureus, Enterobacteriaceae, Francisella tularensis, C. albicans, P. aeruginosa, Proteus* spp., *Legionella* spp., *Pneumocystis carinii, M. pneumoniae,* and *Chlamydia pneumoniae* (15). In newborn or very young infants, chlamydiae and respiratory syncytial virus should be ruled out as etiological agents.

Pulmonary abscesses may result from staphylococcal or *K. pneumoniae* pneumonias or the aspiration of particulate matter contaminated with oropharyngeal flora. The organisms most commonly cultured from such lesions are *Bacteroides* spp., *Fusobacterium* spp., peptostreptococci, staphylococci, clostridia, klebsiellae, escherichiae, and pseudomonads. The examination of such abscesses should include a search for acid-fast organisms, aerobic and anaerobic actinomycetes, and the fungi associated with pulmonary lesions. Empyema is usually a secondary disease, i.e., an extension of the primary disease. Special attention must be accorded certain clinical variants of empyema, especially empyema of infants, usually caused by *S. aureus,* and empyema caused by *Entamoeba histolytica, Actinomyces* spp., or *Nocardia* spp.

GASTROINTESTINAL TRACT

See also references 3, 4, 6, 9, and 11.

Areas that usually harbor microorganisms

The part of the gastrointestinal tract that invariably harbors microorganisms is the large intestine, although fecal organisms are recovered in aspirates of the lower ileum of normal individuals (16). Past the ileoccal valve, the contents of the large intestine reflect the fecal flora. It is surprising that information on normal fecal microflora is comparatively meager (5, 16). It seems almost superfluous to list the organisms that can be encountered; most are ignored in the search for enteric pathogens. The presence of viruses in the intestinal tract of healthy individuals has not been explored sufficiently to allow one to make definitive statements. Rosebury (16) lists the following microorganisms as indigenous: *S. epidermidis, S. aureus,* viridans streptococci, enterococci, occasionally *S. pyogenes* and related serogroups, peptostreptococci, lactobacilli (especially in infants), corynebacteria, mycobacteria, clostridia, actinomycetes, the *Enterobacteriaceae, P. aeruginosa, Alcaligenes faecalis, Flavobacterium* spp., *Bacteroides* spp., *Fusobacterium* spp., *Eubacterium* spp., *Propionibacterium* spp., *Bifidobacterium* spp., yeasts, filamentous fungi, and a large variety of protozoa such as *Entamoeba coli, Endolimax nana, Iodamoeba bütschlii, Trichomonas hominis,* and *Chilomastix mesnili.* Not all microbial groups are present in each individual at all times. Undoubtedly, many other genera can be found with some frequency. The dominance of the anaerobic bacteria in the normal adult colon must be emphasized even though these bacteria are not sought during routine stool cultures. Geographical distribution and dietary and sanitary habits are also influential in the selection of a resident microflora. A role of the normal intestinal microbiota in the production of quantities of carcinogens has been advocated. These microbial activities may bring new dimensions to clinical microbiology and our understanding of neoplasia (5).

Acute diarrheal diseases are a major cause of morbidity throughout the world. While some diarrheal disease is caused by bacterial and parasitic agents, a significant proportion, particularly in children, is caused by or associated with a number of fastidious or noncultivatable viral agents. The most important of these viral gastroenteritis agents are the rotaviruses, the Norwalk-like viruses, and the "enteric" adenoviruses (types 40 and 41). In addition, the astroviruses and caliciviruses are important causes of diarrhea in infants and children under age 2 years.

The most readily recognized bacterial agents of gastroenteritis are salmonellae, shigellae, campylobacters, and *Helicobacter pylori.* All members of the genus *Salmonella* are capable of evoking the various clinical symptoms of salmonellosis and its complications. The various shigellae can cause diarrhea or the syndrome known as bacillary dysentery. *Campylobacter jejuni* is a major cause of diarrhea; *C. laridis* and *C. coli* have also been involved in gastroenteritis. *H. pylori* may be involved in ulcer production in the stomach or duodenum (18). *Vibrio* spp. and the attendant disease are encountered increasingly in many parts of the world. Enteropathogenic, enterotoxigenic, enteroinvasive, and enterohemorrhagic *E. coli* are known to cause pathology in the human intestine. *Bacillus cereus* and staphylococcal food poisonings also affect the gastrointestinal tract, as do food poisoning due to clostridial toxins and botulism and pseudomembranous enterocolitis caused by *Clostridium difficile.* The toxins, rather than the microorganisms, cause the symptoms and should be the object of analytical efforts; the bacteria need not be demonstrated in feces or vomitus. Acute diarrhea may at times be associated with *P. aeruginosa, Proteus* spp., *Aeromonas* spp., *Plesiomonas shigelloides,* or *C. albicans. Entamoeba histolytica* is the etiological agent of amebic dysentery and its complications. Large numbers of *Giardia lamblia* may cause an infectious colitis. Localized pathology of the large intestine may involve *Aeromonas* spp., *Plesiomonas shigelloides,* or *Yersinia enterocolitica,* the latter causing not only occasional gastroenteritis but also the symptoms of appendicitis. Anal carriage of *S. pyogenes* in the nosocomial spread of the disease and of the gonococcus in clinical or cryptic disease must not be overlooked in specific investigations of these infections. A large number and variety of protozoa and helminths cause pathology in the gastrointestinal tract (Table 2).

Usually sterile areas

The esophagus and the stomach are contaminated with bacteria whenever food is ingested. The microbial population does not survive well in these two sections of the gastrointestinal tract. Similarly, the small intestine (except the distal ileum), the liver, and the gallbladder usually are free from microbial contamination or harbor transient microbial populations. This also applies to the peritoneum. When microorganisms are present in these areas, they are secondary to underlying diseases such as carcinoma or reach these sites because the large intestine has been punctured or ruptured. Peritonitis, regardless of its initial cause, can be incited by any of the fecal organisms listed in Table 2. A mixture of aerobic and anaerobic, gram-positive and gram-negative microorganisms participate. Peritonitis may give rise to intra-abdominal abscesses, especially pelvic, paracolic, intermesenteric, subphrenic, and retroperitoneal. All may show a mixed microbial population or single causative agents such as *S. aureus, Bacteroides* spp., enterococci, *P. aeruginosa,* and *E. coli.* Bacteria have been isolated in several cholecystitis cases, possibly as secondary opportunists. *E. coli,* enterococci, peptostreptococci, and clostridia are the most frequently encountered bacteria, but many other common and uncommon representatives of the fecal microflora in health and disease may be found. Bacterial cholangitis usually is secondary to intra- or extrahepatic obstruction in the area of the bile duct. Cholangitis caused by salmonellae, staphylococci, and streptococci may be accompanied by septicemia caused by these bacteria (3). Again, the organisms usually recovered reflect the microbiota of the intestinal tract. Amebic abscesses of the liver constitute a complication of primary amebic dysentery. Pyogenic hepatic abscesses in the antibiotic era yield *E. coli* most frequently. Pancreatic abscess formation is a secondary complication of pancreatitis. The microorganisms most frequently found are *S. aureus* and *E. coli.* Clostridial diseases are uncommon but not rare (3). They include acute gaseous cholecystitis caused by *Clostridium perfringens,* but other clostridia, *Enterobacteriaceae,* and aerobic and anaerobic streptococci have been associated with this entity. Invasion of the bile ducts from the intestinal tract results in clostridial choledochitis, from which *C. perfringens* has been isolated exclusively. Enteritis necroticans is caused by heat-resistant *C. perfringens* type C. Clostridial cellulitis of the abdominal wall is a complication of perforation by intestinal neoplasms with local peritonitis or of colon or biliary tract surgery (Table 2).

GENITOURINARY TRACT

See Table 3. See also references 3, 4, 6, 9, and 11.

Areas that usually harbor microorganisms

External genitalia. Rosebury (16) and Skinner and Carr (17) have listed the following organisms as present on the surface of genitalia: *S. epidermidis,* viridans streptococci, enterococci, peptostreptococci, corynebacteria, mycobacteria, various members of the *En-*

TABLE 2. Microorganisms encountered in gastrointestinal tract specimens[a]

Organism	Frequency of isolation[b]	Disease involvement[c]
Absidia spp.	C	1
Acidaminococcus fermentans	C	1
Acinetobacter calcoaceticus	B	1
Adenoviruses	B	2
Aeromonas spp.	B	2
Alcaligenes spp.	B	2
Ancylostoma duodenale	B	3
Angiostrongylus costaricensis	C	3
Anisakis spp. larvae	C	3
Ascaris lumbricoides	B	3
Astroviruses	C	2
Bacillus spp.	B	1
Bacteroides spp.	A	2
Balantidium coli	C	3
Bifidobacterium spp.	B	1
Blastocystis hominis	B	2
Caliciviruses	C	2
Campylobacter spp.	B	3
Candida spp.	B	2
Capillaria spp.	C	3
Chilomastix mesnili	B	1
Clonorchis sinensis	C	3
Clostridium spp.	A	2
Coronaviruses	C	2
Corynebacterium spp.	B	1
Cryptosporidium spp.	C	3
Dicrocoelium dentriticum ova	C	1
Dientamoeba fragilis	B	2
Diphyllobothrium latum	B	3
Dipylidium caninum	C	3
Endolimax nana	B	1
Entamoeba coli	B	1
Entamoeba hartmanii	B	1
Entamoeba histolytica	B	2
Enterobacteriaceae	A	2
Enterobius vermicularis	B	2
Enterococcus spp.	A	2
Enteromonas hominis	C	1
Enteroviruses	A	1
Eubacterium spp.	A	1
Fasciola hepatica	C	3
Fasciolopsis buski	C	3
Fusobacterium spp.	A	2
Gastrodiscoides hominis	C	3
Geotrichum candidum	C	1
Giardia lamblia	B	3
Heterophyes heterophyes	C	3
Histoplasma capsulatum	C	3
Hymenolepis spp.	C	3
Iodamoeba bütschlii	B	1
Isospora belli	C	2
Lactobacillus spp.	B	1
Metagonimus yokogawai	C	3
Microsporidian genera (several)	C	3
Mucor spp.	C	2
Mycobacterium spp.	B	2
Mycoplasma spp.	C	1
Necator americanus	B	3
Neisseria gonorrhoeae	C	3
Neisseria spp.	B	1
Norwalk and Norwalk-like viruses	B	3
Opisthorchis viverrini	C	3
Paracoccidioides brasiliensis	C	3
Paragonimus spp.	C	3
Peptococcus spp.	B	2
Peptostreptococcus spp.	B	2
Plesiomonas shigelloides	C	2
Pseudomonas spp.	B	2
Retortamonas intestinalis	C	1
Rhizomucor spp.	C	1
Rhizopus spp.	C	1
Rhodotorula spp.	C	1
Rotavirus	B	3
Ruminococcus bromii	C	1
Saccharomyces spp.	B	3
Sapporo agent	B	2
Sarcocystis spp.	C	2
Schistosoma spp.	B	3
Selenomonas spp.	B	1
Staphylococcus spp.	B	2
Streptococcus spp.	B	2
Strongyloides stercoralis	B	3
Succinimonas spp.	B	1
Succinivibrio spp.	B	1
Taenia spp.	C	3
Trichinella spiralis larvae	C	3
Trichomonas hominis	B	1
Trichosporon beigelii	C	1
Trichostrongylus spp.	C	2
Trichuris trichiura	B	2
Veillonella spp.	B	2
Vibrio spp.	B	2

[a] Diseases other than gastroenteritis may be caused by organisms listed. Several species of the genera listed may be found; not all of the species are involved in disease processes.

[b] A, Commonly encountered in clinical specimens; B, occasionally encountered in clinical specimens; C, rarely encountered in clinical specimens.

[c] 1, When present, it is rarely if ever involved in disease production; 2, when present, it is occasionally involved in disease production; 3, when present, it is commonly involved in disease production.

terobacteriaceae, Bacteroides spp., *Fusobacterium* spp., mycoplasmata, and *C. albicans* and other yeasts.

The external genitalia are subject to the same infectious diseases as are other skin areas. The special lesions of the external genitalia are venereal in nature and include the lesions of syphilis, chancroid or soft chancre, granuloma inguinale, which is primarily seen in the tropics and subtropics and is caused by *Calymmatobacterium granulomatis*, lymphogranuloma venereum resulting from infection with certain serogroups of *Chlamydia trachomatis*, herpes genitalis, and condylomata acuminata (venereal warts) caused by papillomaviruses.

Anterior urethra. An appreciable number and variety of microorganisms can usually be recovered from the anterior urethra in normal healthy individuals of both sexes: coagulase-negative and occasionally coagulase-positive staphylococci, enterococci, various nonpathogenic neisseriae, corynebacteria, rarely certain mycobacteria, the various enteric gram-negative rods, chlamydiae, *A. calcoaceticus, Gardnerella vaginalis*, mycoplasmata, and yeasts, including *C. albicans*. *Trichomonas vaginalis* may on occasion gain access to this part of the urethra without overt disease.

It is difficult to delineate exactly where the anterior

TABLE 3. Microorganisms encountered in genitourinary tract specimens

Organism	Frequency of isolation[a]	Disease involvement[b]	Organism	Frequency of isolation[a]	Disease involvement[b]
Acinetobacter spp.	B	2	*Histoplasma capsulatum*	C	3
Actinomyces spp.	B	2	Human immunodeficiency virus	B	2
Adenoviruses	B	1	*Lactobacillus* spp.	A	1
Alcaligenes spp.	C	2	*Leptospira interrogans*	C	3
Aspergillus spp.	C	1	*Listeria* spp.	C	2
Bacillus spp.	C	1	*Mobiluncus* spp.	B	2
Bacteroides spp.	A	2	Molluscum contagiosum virus	C	2
Bifidobacterium spp.	C	1	*Moraxella* spp.	B	1
Blastomyces dermatitidis	C	3	Mumps virus	C	3
Branhamella (*Moraxella*) *catarrhalis*	B	1	*Mycobacterium* spp.	B	2
Brugia malayi	C	3	*Mycoplasma hominis*	B	2
Calymmatobacterium granulomatis	C	3	*Neisseria gonorrhoeae*	B	3
Campylobacter spp.	C	2	*Neisseria meningitidis*	C	3
Candida spp.	B	2	*Neisseria* spp.	B	1
Chlamydia spp.	B	2	Papillomaviruses	C	2
Clostridium spp.	A	2	*Penicillium* spp.	C	1
Corynebacterium spp.	B	1	*Peptococcus* spp.	B	1
Cryptococcus spp.	C	2	*Peptostreptococcus* spp.	B	1
Cytomegalovirus	B	2	*Propionibacterium* spp.	B	1
Dioctophyma renale	C	3	*Pseudomonas* spp.	B	2
Entamoeba histolytica	C	3	*Rhodotorula* spp.	C	1
Enterobacteriaceae	A	2	*Saccharomyces* spp.	C	1
Enterobius vermicularis	B	2	*Schistosoma haematobium*	C	3
Enterococcus spp.	B	2	*Staphylococcus* spp.	A	2
Flavobacterium spp.	C	2	*Streptococcus* spp.	B	2
Fusobacterium spp.	B	1	*Torulopsis glabrata*	B	2
Gardnerella vaginalis	B	2	*Treponema pallidum*	B	3
Geotrichum candidum	C	1	*Trichomonas vaginalis*	B	3
Haemophilus ducreyi	B	3	*Ureoplasma urealyticum*	B	1
Hepatitis A and B viruses	B	2	*Wuchereria bancroftii*	C	3
Herpes simplex virus	B	3	Zygomycetes	C	1

[a] A, Commonly encountered in clinical specimens; B, occasionally encountered in clinical specimens; C, rarely encountered in clinical specimens.
[b] 1, When present, it is rarely if ever involved in disease production; 2, when present, it is occasionally involved in disease production; 3, when present, it is commonly involved in disease production.

portion of the urethra ends, especially when disease is present. Urethritis may be caused specifically by the gonococcus or nonspecifically by a variety of bacteria, including the staphylococci, chlamydiae, mycoplasmata, fecal gram-negative rods, and *Listeria* spp. In the female, contamination by vaginolabial microbiota of the anterior portion of the urethra is unavoidable. It is appropriate to emphasize that *N. gonorrhoeae* can be recovered from the anterior urethra of the female and from males with cryptic disease. Bacteriuria of young women caused by *Staphylococcus saprophyticus* is reported with increasing frequency.

Vagina. The usual microbiota of the vagina from menarche to menopause is dominated by lactobacilli, designated as Döderlein bacillus and constituted by glycogen-fermenting *Lactobacillus acidophilus* and related species. Prepubescent females from shortly after birth and postmenopausal women harbor skin microbiota in this region. Despite the control over the vaginal environment exerted by the lactobacilli, many other microorganisms can be cultivated from vaginal samples of healthy women: *S. aureus* and *S. epidermidis*, viridans streptococci, enterococci, peptostreptococci, group B streptococci, the low-temperature-tolerant neisseriae, corynebacteria, some actinomycetes, members of the family *Enterobacteriaceae*, acinetobacters, chlamydiae, *G. vaginalis*, occasionally clostridia and other anaerobic rods, mycoplasmas, *C. albicans*, other yeasts, and *T. vaginalis*.

The major infectious diseases of the female pudenda are the sexually transmitted diseases: chlamydiosis, syphilis, gonorrhea, and herpes simplex virus infections as well as candidiasis, trichomoniasis, and vaginosis caused by a variety of organisms that may act at times as opportunistic secondary invaders reflecting disturbances in the microbiological balance as a complication of disease elsewhere and its treatment. *G. vaginalis* and *Mobiluncus* spp. rank high among the so-called nonspecific vaginitides, but fecal and skin organisms, including staphylococci, enterococci, and *Listeria* spp., may contribute to clinically overt disease (16). *Campylobacter fetus* and related unclassified organisms have been isolated from the vaginas of women who have aborted repeatedly. The vaginal microflora, especially the anaerobic bacteria, may contribute to the complications of septic abortions. Postpartum sepsis and salpingitis, frequently caused by facultatively and obligately anaerobic gram-negative rods and to a lesser degree by clostridia and staphylococci, probably reflect the microbiota of the vagina. Similarly, colonization and infectious disease of the newborn reflect the microbial population of the vagina. Among the viruses, herpes simplex virus and papillomaviruses rank as significant causes of pathology.

Usually sterile areas. As a rule, the remaining structures of the genitourinary tract are without permanent microbiota. Infectious disease of the kidneys is still not completely understood, with two major theories advanced to explain the seeding of this organ by infectious organisms either by hematogenous or ascending routes. There are many predisposing factors for pyelonephritis, especially host factors and underlying diseases, which appear mandatory for the establishment of infection. The major bacterial offenders are the gram-negative rods, especially *E. coli, Proteus* spp., *P. aeruginosa,* and the *Klebsiella-Enterobacter* group; enterococci are not uncommon and can be demonstrated in adequate numbers repeatedly in untreated acute pyelonephritis. *Mycobacterium tuberculosis* may infect the kidney and be demonstrated in urine. Perinephric abscesses usually caused by *S. aureus* are not detected in urine unless the abscess ruptures into the kidney. The prostate in the male may become a secondary focus of gonorrheal disease. However, other microorganisms, including staphylococci, enterococci, listeriae, *E. coli,* mycoplasmata, pseudomonads, achromobacters, and rarely trichomonads, may lodge in this organ, especially in middle-aged and older males. Some viruses, notably cytomegalovirus, are commonly found in urine of persons acutely or chronically infected with these agents. Similarly, some viruses, including human immunodeficiency virus, hepatitis B virus, and cytomegalovirus, may be found in semen of chronically infected persons.

SKIN, WOUNDS, AND BURNS

See also references 3, 4, 6, 9, 11, and 16.

The outermost border of the body is constantly populated with microorganisms that reflect the contacts, habits, profession, and environment of the individual. Table 4 lists numerous microorganisms, but those usually found consist mostly of *Staphylococcus* spp., *Corynebacterium* spp., *Propionibacterium* spp., *Mycobacterium* spp., and various yeasts. Certain areas, especially those adjoining the various body openings, reflect the microbiota of these adjacent sites.

The most common and most obvious skin diseases are caused by the staphylococci. *S. aureus* is involved most frequently in boils and furuncles, and *S. epidermidis* is found in pimples and acne, often accompanied by *Propionibacterium acnes.* Pustulosis, especially of the newborn, is also caused by *S. aureus.* The agents of impetigo are *S. pyogenes* and *S. aureus.* Coagulase-positive staphylococci are also involved in superficial folliculitis and sycosis barbae. Although streptococci and other oral bacteria may also be found, *S. aureus* is the major etiological agent of acute suppurative parotitis. Actinomycosis is usually caused by aerobic and anaerobic members of the order *Actinomycetales* and represents a chronic suppurative or granulomatous disease culminating in abscesses. Deep cellulitis of the neck is most frequently caused by streptococci, both aerobic and anaerobic, as well as staphylococci. *S. aureus* is responsible for hydradenitis suppurativa, a disease more common in women and usually involving the axillae, and it is the most frequent disease-producing agent in acute mastitis and breast abscess. Paronychia most often involve staphylococci and streptococci and less commonly *C. albicans.* The former organisms are also frequently recovered from tenosynovitis. Clostridia are usually responsible for anaerobic cellulitis, mixtures of bacteria are responsible for crepitant cellulitis, and *S. pyogenes* is involved in necrotizing fascitis or hemolytic streptococcal gangrene. Erysipelas is a subcutaneous form of streptococcal cellulitis. Erysipeloid, an acute cutaneous, bluish-red inflammation of the hands and wrists that is usually seen in males in certain vocations, is caused by *Erysipelothrix* spp. Other microorganisms occasionally or rarely involved in skin and wound infections are also listed in Table 4. Many viral diseases are accompanied by exanthems and a variety of other skin lesions, some of which are typical for a specific etiological agent. Some of these lesions may yield the etiological agent. The dermatophytic fungi present skin lesions most of which yield the causative agent from properly obtained specimens; laboratorians must be aware of the special lipid requirements of certain fungi such as *Malassezia furfur.*

The microbiota of wounds reflects their anatomical site, the mode of infliction (i.e., traumatic or surgical), the environment, and the degree of microbial contamination of adjacent areas that were perforated in the process. These considerations supplement rather than substitute for the general considerations which maintain an adequate host-parasite equilibrium. Traumatic wounds are usually complicated by aerobic indigenous microorganisms, especially *S. aureus,* group A streptococci, enterococci, *P. aeruginosa, E. coli, Proteus* spp., flavobacteria, and *Acinetobacter* spp. Among the anaerobic bacteria associated with traumatic wounds, the histotoxic and neurotoxic clostridia are most prominent, leading, under proper conditions, to gas gangrene or tetanus. The most common clostridia of gas gangrene are *Clostridium perfringens* type A, *C. septicum,* and *C. novyii,* but these organisms may be harmless contaminants of wounds. The diagnosis of gas gangrene is strictly a clinical one; the isolation of clostridia may alert a clinician but does not constitute the diagnosis of clostridial cellulitis or clostridial myonecrosis. *Clostridium tetani* should not present a problem in properly immunized individuals but should not be ignored in deep puncture wounds when the immunization history is not known. Criminally inflicted stab wounds, often intentionally contaminated with feces, require not only expert surgical but also exquisite microbiological attention.

Infections complicating surgery may be of two kinds. One, the so-called wound infection, usually denotes a complication of a clean surgical procedure, a procedure performed under the best available aseptic conditions on tissues usually sterile and not found grossly contaminated during surgery. These wounds may yield *S. aureus,* enterococci, or gram-negative rods and rarely microorganisms such as *S. pyogenes,* corynebacteria, pneumococci, and *Bacillus subtilis.* The second kind of infection occurs when the surgeon performs all or part of the surgical procedures in a contaminated area, resulting in infectious disease complications in a certain percentage and often reflecting the state of health of the patient. The microorganisms mirror the microbiota of the particular anatomic site, but frequently minority members of the microflora attain a majority in the usually sterile tissue subjected to surgery and may gravely complicate the recovery of the patient. Among the bacteria involved in this complication are *E. coli, P. aeruginosa, Proteus* spp., *Providencia* spp., the *Klebsiella-*

TABLE 4. Microorganisms encountered in skin, wound, and burn specimens

Organism	Frequency of isolation[a]	Disease involvement[b]	Organism	Frequency of isolation[a]	Disease involvement[b]
Absidia spp.	A	1	*Listeria* spp.	C	2
Acinetobacter calcoaceticus	B	2	*Madurella* spp.	C	2
			Mansonella streptocerca	C	3
Actinomadura madurae	C	2	*Micrococcus* spp.	A	1
Actinomyces spp.	B	2	*Microsporum* spp.	B	3
Aeromonas spp.	B	2	*Moraxella* spp.	B	2
Ancylostoma spp.	C	3	*Mucor* spp.	A	1
Aspergillus spp.	B	1	*Mycobacterium* spp.	B	2
Bacillus anthracis	C	3	*Neisseria* spp.	B	2
Bacillus spp.	B	1	*Nocardia* spp.	B	2
Bacteroides spp.	B	2	*Oerskovia* spp.	C	2
Bartonella bacilliformis	C	3	*Onchocerca volvulus*	C	3
Bifidobacterium spp.	B	2	*Paracoccidioides brasiliensis*	C	3
Blastomyces dermatitidis	B	3			
Brugia spp.	C	3	Papillomaviruses	B	3
Candida spp.	A	2	*Pasteurella* spp.	C	2
Cephalosporium spp.	B	2	*Penicillium* spp.	B	1
Cladosporium carrionii	C	2	*Peptococcus* spp.	B	2
Clostridium spp.	B	2	*Peptostreptococcus* spp.	B	2
Coccidioides immitis	B	3	*Plesiomonas shigelloides*	C	2
Corynebacterium diphtheriae	C	3	Poxviruses	B	3
			Propionibacterium spp.	B	2
Corynebacterium spp.	B	2	*Pseudomonas* spp.	B	2
Cryptococcus neoformans	C	3	*Rhizomucor* spp.	B	1
			Rhizopus spp.	B	1
Cryptococcus spp.	C	1	*Rhodotorula* spp.	B	1
Dematiaceous fungi	B	2	*Rickettsia* spp.	B	3
Dirofilaria spp.	C	3	*Scopulariopsis brevicaulis*	B	2
Dracunculus medinensis	C	3			
Entamoeba histolytica trophozoites	C	3	*Spirillum minus*	C	3
			Sporothrix schenckii	B	2
Enterobacteriaceae	B	2	*Staphylococcus* spp.	A	2
Enterococcus spp.	B	2	*Streptobacillus moniliformis*	C	2
Epidermophyton floccosum	B	3			
			Streptococcus spp.	B	2
Erysipelothrix spp.	C	3	*Streptomyces somaliensis*	C	2
Eubacterium spp.	B	2			
Flavobacterium spp.	B	2	*Strongyloides* spp.	C	3
Fusarium spp.	B	2	*Taenia solium* cysticerci	C	3
Fusobacterium spp.	B	2	*Treponema* spp.	B	3
Geotrichum candidum	B	1	*Trichophyton* spp.	B	3
Herpes simplex virus	A	3	Varicella-zoster virus	B	3
Histoplasma capsulatum	B	3	*Veillonella* spp.	B	2
Leishmania spp.	C	3	*Vibrio* spp.	B	2
Leptospira spp.	C	3			

[a] A, Commonly encountered in clinical specimens; B, occasionally encountered in clinical specimens; C, rarely encountered in clinical specimens.
[b] 1, When present, it is rarely if ever involved in disease production; 2, when present, it is occasionally involved in disease production; 3, when present, it is commonly involved in disease production.

Enterobacter-Serratia group, flavobacteria, *Acinetobacter* spp., and *Bacteroides* spp.

Microbial contamination of severe burns can be a life-threatening complication. The organism most commonly encountered and most difficult to control is *P. aeruginosa*, often in conjunction with flavobacteria and other gram-negative rods and staphylococci, which abound in the institutional environment or on the uninvolved skin of the patient. Early microbiological analysis of burns usually shows a large number of a great variety of microorganisms, many of which are eventually supplemented by the bacteria cited above.

EYE

See also references 3, 4, 6, 9, 11, and 16.

The healthy conjunctiva of the eye may harbor a number of skin organisms. Among those most frequently recovered from the healthy eye are the staphylococci; viridans streptococci, *S. pyogenes*, the pneumococcus, neisseriae, and corynebacteria are recovered rarely. The fecal gram-negative rods have been isolated even less frequently from this site, but *H. influenzae* has an incidence second only to that of the coagulase-negative staphylococci. Conjunctival cultures have also yielded *C. albicans* and other yeasts. Eye disease has been caused by *S. aureus* and *P. aeruginosa* (very often iatrogenically) and occasionally by *S. pneumoniae*. More often, infectious diseases peculiar to the eye have yielded *M. lacunata*. *H. influenzae*, *Haemophilus aegyptius* (*H. influenzae* biotype III) and, on rare occasions, *Bacillus* spp. Still rarer etiological agents of eye infections and occasional commensal organisms are listed in Table 5.

TABLE 5. Microorganisms encountered in eye specimens

Organism	Frequency of isolation[a]	Disease involvement[b]
Absidia spp.	C	2
Acanthamoeba spp.	C	3
Achromobacter xylosoxidans	C	1
Acinetobacter spp.	B	2
Acromonium spp.	B	2
Actinobacillus actinomycetemcomitans	C	2
Actinomyces spp.	C	2
Adenoviruses	B	2
Aeromonas hydrophila	B	2
Alternaria spp.	B	2
Arachnia spp.	B	2
Aspergillus spp.	B	2
Aureobasidium spp.	C	1
Azotobacter spp.	C	1
Bacillus spp.	B	2
Bacteroides spp.	C	2
Bifidobacterium spp.	C	2
Blastomyces dermatitidis	B	3
Branhamella (*Moraxella*) *catarrhalis*	B	1
Brucella spp.	C	3
Candida spp.	B	2
Chlamydia trachomatis	B	3
Cladosporium spp.	B	1
Clostridium spp.	C	2
Coccidioides immitis	C	3
Corynebacterium diphtheriae	C	3
Corynebacterium spp.	B	2
Cryptococcus neoformans	C	3
Curvularia spp.	B	1
Cytomegalovirus	B	3
Drechlera spp.	B	1
Enterobacteriaceae	B	2
Epstein-Barr virus	C	3
Exophiala jeanselmei	C	1
Francisella tularensis	C	3
Fusarium spp.	B	2
Fusobacterium spp.	C	2
Haemophilus influenzae biotype III (*H. aegyptius*)	B	3
Herpes simplex virus	B	3
Lactobacillus spp.	C	2
Leptospira spp.	C	3
Loa loa	C	3
Measles virus	B	3
Moraxella spp.	B	2
Mucor spp.	B	2
Mumps virus	B	3
Mycobacterium spp.	C	2
Mycobacterium tuberculosis group	C	3
Neisseria gonorrhoeae	B	3
Neisseria meningitidis	B	3
Neisseria spp.	B	1
Nocardia spp.	C	3
Nosema spp.	C	3
Onchocerca volvulus	C	3
Paecilomyces spp.	B	1
Peptococcus spp.	C	2
Peptostreptococcus spp.	C	2
Poxvirus	C	3
Propionibacterium spp.	B	2
Pseudallescheria boydii	C	3
Pseudomonas spp.	B	2
Rhizomucor spp.	B	2
Rhizopus spp.	B	2
Rubella virus	B	3
Sporothrix schenckii	C	3
Staphylococcus spp.	A	2
Streptococcus spp.	B	2
Taenia solium larvae	C	3
Toxocara spp.	C	3
Toxoplasma gondii	B	3
Treponema pallidum	B	3
Varicella-zoster virus	B	3
Veillonella spp.	C	2

[a] A, Commonly encountered in clinical specimens; B, occasionally encountered in clinical specimens; C, rarely encountered in clinical specimens.
[b] 1, When present, it is rarely if ever involved in disease production; 2, when present, it is occasionally involved in disease production; 3, when present, it is commonly involved in disease production.

EAR

See also references 3, 4, 6, 9, 11, and 16.

The external auditory canal usually reflects the microbiota of skin. Perhaps *S. pneumoniae* and the gram-negative rods, including *P. aeruginosa*, have been recovered with greater frequency from this site than from other skin areas. The middle and inner ear are usually sterile. Diseases of the outer ear reflect the disorders of the skin. Other parts of the auditory organ may be involved during generalized disease or may be affected only locally by *S. aureus*, *S. pneumoniae*, *S. pyogenes*, *P. aeruginosa*, *H. influenzae*, and occasionally other microorganisms (Table 6).

BLOOD, CEREBROSPINAL FLUID, EXUDATES, AND TRANSUDATES

See also references 3, 4, 6, 9, 11, and 16.

The blood and spinal fluid of healthy individuals are usually sterile. Occasionally, microorganisms may be isolated from blood cultures of normal, asymptomatic individuals. Often they represent low-level contamination of the circulation from inapparent skin lesions or other sources. Such findings complicate the interpretation of laboratory results but are usually of no consequence. However, during several infectious diseases or during infectious complications of a primary disease, microorganisms may be recovered from blood. They may be present transiently or persistently. Positive blood cultures reflect a variety of conditions and diseases and encompass a large array of microorganisms. Positive blood cultures may result from traumatic and surgical wounds as well as from burns, injury to bones and joints, brain abscesses, furunculosis, cellulitis, meningitis, pneumonia, lung abscesses, empyema, mucoviscidosis, mycotic aneurysm, cardiac anomalies, peritonitis, intestinal or biliary obstruction, cholangitis, carcinoma, urinary obstruction, nephropathies, postpartum endometritis, and septic abortion. Immunosuppressive, cytotoxic, or radiation therapies and conditions such as arteriosclerosis, chronic debility, diabetic acidosis, hematological diseases, hepatic in-

TABLE 6. Microorganisms encountered in ear specimens

Organism	Frequency of isolation[a]	Disease involvement[b]
Achromobacter xylosoxidans	C	2
Adenoviruses	B	2
Aspergillus spp.	B	2
Bacteroides spp.	C	2
Bifidobacterium spp.	C	2
Branhamella (Moraxella) catarrhalis	B	2
Candida spp.	B	2
Chlamydia trachomatis	C	2
Clostridium spp.	C	2
Corynebacterium diphtheriae	C	3
Corynebacterium spp.	C	1
Coxsackievirus	B	2
Enterobacteriaceae	B	2
Enteroviruses	B	2
Eubacterium spp.	C	1
Fusobacterium spp.	C	2
Haemophilus influenzae	B	3
Herpes simplex virus	C	2
Influenza viruses	B	2
Mycobacterium spp.	C	2
Parainfluenza viruses	B	2
Peptococcus spp.	C	2
Peptostreptococcus spp.	C	2
Propionibacterium spp.	B	2
Pseudomonas aeruginosa	B	2
Respiratory syncytial virus	B	2
Staphylococcus spp.	B	2
Streptococcus pneumoniae	B	3
Streptococcus spp.	B	2
Varicella-zoster virus	B	2
Veillonella spp.	C	2
Vibrio spp.	C	2

[a] A, Commonly encountered in clinical specimens; B, occasionally encountered in clinical specimens; C, rarely encountered in clinical specimens.

[b] 1, When present, it is rarely if ever involved in disease production; 2, when present, it is occasionally involved in disease production; 3, when present, it is commonly involved in disease production.

sufficiency, and malignancies of all types may lead to positive blood cultures. No rule concerning the types of microorganisms of significance can be stated. Certainly staphylococci, not only *S. aureus* but also coagulase-negative staphylococci, have been recovered repeatedly. The latter can be involved in bacterial endocarditis and have complicated cardiac catheterization and prosthesis procedures. The gram-negative rods, especially *E. coli*, the obligately anaerobic bacteria of the colon, *Klebsiella-Enterobacter* organisms, *P. aeruginosa*, *Proteus* spp., and *Providencia* spp., have been recovered after trauma or surgery of contaminated body areas or as acquired microorganisms complicating protracted hospitalization of patients with a variety of diseases. Recovery of salmonellae from the blood of individuals with systemic salmonellosis is not uncommon. Other fevers of unknown origin may yield brucellae, pasteurellae, pneumococci, *N. meningitidis*, *Listeria monocytogenes*, fungi, and parasites. Bacterial endocarditis patients may harbor viridans streptococci, staphylococci, enterococci, corynebacteria, *Bacteroides* spp., and yeasts. Fungi have been found in blood cultures from patients with lung abscesses, mycotic aneurysms, and hematological disorders. Clostridia have been recovered in the blood of accident victims and from patients with cholangitis and postpartum complications. In the newborn with bacteremia or septicemia during the first week of life, the organisms most often responsible are *Streptococcus agalactiae* (21) and *S. aureus*.

Some viruses, including human immunodeficiency virus, hepatitis B virus, hepatitis C virus (formerly called hepatitis non-A non-B virus), and cytomegalovirus, have been shown to persist in circulating blood and blood cells of individuals in the absence of clinical disease. The potential risk of transmitting these agents via transfusion of or exposure to blood products from these chronically infected persons is well recognized.

Positive cultures obtained from cerebrospinal fluids also reflect a variety of conditions. Several conditions besides meningitis, including trauma, infectious complications of surgery, cranial and spinal epidural abscesses, subdural abscess, septic thrombophlebitis of the venous sinuses, and brain abscesses, contribute to positive findings. There are systemic infectious diseases that may afflict the meninges, including severe pneumococcal pneumonia, salmonellosis, *H. influenzae* pneumonia and bacteremia, tuberculosis, listeriosis, *A. calcoaceticus* var. *lwoffi* septicemia of the newborn, generalized candidiasis, and advanced sepsis with every type of gram-negative rod, especially *E. coli* and *P. aeruginosa*. Neonatal meningitis is most commonly caused by *S. agalactiae*, gram-negative rods, and listeriae. Meningitis is caused primarily by *H. influenzae* serotype b in children and by the meningococcus and pneumococcus in most adults; the aged are most frequently infected with the latter organism. *S. aureus*, *Enterobacteriaceae*, *P. aeruginosa*, and *L. monocytogenes* are sometimes recovered. *Flavobacterium meningosepticum* has been isolated occasionally. Viruses regularly associated with aseptic meningitis and easily recovered from cerebrospinal fluid include members of the enteroviruses (coxsackieviruses and echoviruses) and mumps virus. Viruses associated with true encephalitis (herpes simplex virus, the arboviruses, and rabies virus) are rarely recovered. Traumatic or surgical injury may be complicated by any one of many microorganisms, but the staphylococci, enterococci, and gram-negative rods predominate. In intracranial abscesses, anaerobic microorganisms are most common. These include peptostreptococci, *Bacteroides* spp., *Actinomyces* spp., *P. acnes*, and less frequently *Veillonella* spp. Cranial epidural abscesses have yielded staphylococci, streptococci, pneumococci, and occasionally gram-negative rods. Spinal epidural abscesses have involved *S. aureus* and *P. aeruginosa*. Other gram-positive cocci have been isolated, as have *Salmonella* spp., which have caused epidural abscesses while infecting vertebrae (3). Subdural abscess is a comparatively rare complication of *H. influenzae* meningitis in children. *Mycobacterium tuberculosis* infection and leptospiral disease of the meninges must also be considered. *Cryptococcus neoformans* and *Toxoplasma gondii* have assumed an important infectious role in AIDS patients.

Transudates and exudates accompany a large variety of clinical conditions. They may be sterile or contain a varied microflora. Any microorganisms that involve the afflicted organs may be recovered. The organisms found reflect the anatomical site of the disease nidus or adjacent areas. The organisms outlined in the foregoing sections may also be encountered. These include the anaerobic bacteria, fungi, *M. tuberculosis*, and legionellae.

SURGICAL SPECIMENS

See also references 3, 4, 6, 9, 11, and 16.

The microbiology of surgical specimens depends on the anatomic site and the underlying disease, the care exercised at the time of excision and during subsequent handling, and the available information that will help to narrow the number of etiological agents. The usual pyogenic organisms may be recovered, often as single components. Systemic fungi, nocardiae, actinomycetes, and various mycobacteria, including, of course, *M. tuberculosis*, as well as mixtures of anaerobic bacteria, have been found. In addition to yielding *S. aureus*, primary osteomyelitis has yielded peptostreptococci, *Salmonella* spp. (especially in children with sickle cell disease), gonococci, *Veillonella* spp., representatives of the fecal gram-negative rods, and rarely actinomycetes and *Blastomyces dermatitidis*. Foreign bodies, including prostheses, old sutures, and indwelling catheters, have been sources of many species of organisms, among them staphylococci, *P. aeruginosa*, and *Enterobacteriaceae*.

AUTOPSY SPECIMENS

Autopsy specimens can yield invaluable information when the examination is performed promptly and aseptically and when cultures are plated immediately and accompanied by smears. Routinely, the kidney, spleen, liver, and lung are negative unless distinct lesions are cultured or an appreciable portion of the organ is diseased. If more than 6 h has elapsed between death and the examination, heart blood cultures and the tissues will reflect postmortem or perimortem contamination by organisms from the large bowel. An experienced and interested prosector will culture the areas of tissues possibly involved in an infectious disease process. A large variety of suspected and totally unexpected microorganisms can be recovered and demonstrated subsequently in tissue sections. The microorganisms range from the usual bacteria to lesions populated by brucellae, nocardiae, penicillia, aspergilli, zygomycetes, pneumococci, group A streptococci, clostridia, salmonellae, and shigellae, to name but a few.

MICROBIAL NUMBERS AND CLINICAL DISEASE

The preceding considerations underline the lack of understanding, in quantitative terms, of the many factors that contribute to overt symptoms of infectious disease in any particular person. The notion that disease production in the host resides solely in the pathogenic and virulent properties of the microorganisms can no longer be accepted. The application of molecular biology has initiated a better understanding of the mechanisms of microbial attachment to host cells, the advantages of certain plasmids and episomes in the expression of filaments, fimbriae, and fibrillae, the utility of some lipoteichoic acids, and the protection of colonizing microorganisms by exopolysaccharides (1). However, the specific and nonspecific defense mechanisms of a host, the general health of the individual, and the various stresses to which he or she has been subjected have considerable influence, if not the determinant role, in the initiation and progression of an infectious disease. These roles are as multifarious as the genera and species of microorganisms that constitute the microbial ecosystem of the person. The understanding of microbial ecological relationships among the constituents of this large pool of microbes is lacking, especially with regard to the health of the host. We know very little about the selectivity exercised by the tissues and organs of the host in the establishment of a local, autochthonous microbiota. There are but a few indications that age, physical environment, and nutrition may affect the minimal infective dose of some microorganisms with more pronounced pathogenic proclivities. As with other areas of human biology, it is the abnormal condition that permits an intimation of understanding. Microorganisms of nosocomial significance are widely distributed in nature but are usually involved in disease complications only in medical facilities. They may be minority members of an individual's microbiota or they may reside in the hospital environment, where in some instances they are concentrated as a result of antimicrobial agent-associated selective pressures (14).

Although it is obvious that much must be learned before a clear understanding of infectious disease is established (19), it is equally clear that the concern and responsibility of the clinical microbiologist must transcend the narrow borders of microbial identification and encompass aspects of the history and condition, the treatment, and the present and past environment and community of the patient. This broader view is required to allow the proper distinction of significant microorganisms isolated from pathological specimens. Without such information, the unclear lines of separation between the indigenous and pathogenic microbiota of humans will be confused still more, depriving clinicians of information and the capability to intercede effectively against microorganisms for the benefit of their patients (13).

We gratefully acknowledge the thoughtful review of this chapter by Lynne S. Garcia and Kenneth L. Herrmann.

LITERATURE CITED

1. **Beachey, E. H.** 1980. Bacterial adherence. Chapman & Hall, Ltd., London.
2. **Burnet, F. M.** 1962. Natural history of infectious disease, 3rd ed. Cambridge University Press, Cambridge.
3. **Dalton, H. P., and H. C. Nottebart, Jr.** 1986. Interpretive medical microbiology. Churchill Livingstone, New York.
4. **D'Amato, R. F., M. F. Sierra, and M. R. McGinnis.** 1977. Infectious diseases and etiologic or associated bacterial/fungal agents, p. 11–38. *In* D. Seligson (ed.), CRC handbook series in clinical laboratory science. CRC Press, Inc., Cleveland.
5. **Drasar, B. S., and M. J. Hill.** 1974. Human intestinal flora. Academic Press, Inc. (London), Ltd., London.
6. **Drew, W. L.** 1986. Laboratory methods in basic virology, p. 632–677. *In* S. M. Finegold and E. J. Baron (ed.), Bailey and Scott's diagnostic microbiology. The C. V. Mosby Co., St. Louis.
7. **Dubos, R. J.** 1958. The evolution and the ecology of microbial diseases, p. 4–27. *In* R. J. Dubos (ed.), Bacterial

and mycotic infections of man, 3rd ed. J. B. Lippincott Co., Philadelphia.
8. **Fiumara, N. J., H. M. Wise, Jr., and M. Many.** 1967. Gonorrheal pharyngitis. N. Engl. J. Med. **276:**1248–1250.
9. **Garcia, L. S., and D. A. Bruckner.** 1988. Diagnostic medical parasitology. Elsevier, New York.
10. **Gibbons, R. J.** 1975. Attachment of oral streptococci to mucosal surfaces, p. 127–131. *In* D. Schlessinger (ed.), Microbiology—1975. American Society for Microbiology, Washington, D.C.
11. **Holt, J. G. (editor-in-chief).** 1989. Bergey's manual of systematic bacteriology, vol. 1 to 4. The Williams & Wilkins, Co., Baltimore.
12. **Isenberg, H. D.** 1988. Pathogenicity and virulence: another view. Clin. Microbiol. Rev. **1:**40–53.
13. **Isenberg, H. D., and A. Balows.** 1981. Bacterial pathogenicity in man and animals, p. 8–122. *In* M. P. Starr, H. Stolp, H. G. Truper, A. Balows, and H. G. Schlegel (ed.), The prokaryotes. Springer-Verlag, New York.
14. **Isenberg, H. D., and J. I. Berkman.** 1971. The role of drug-resistant and drug-selected bacteria in nosocomial disease. Ann. N.Y. Acad. Sci. **182:**52–58.
15. **Jones, G. L., and G. A. Hébert.** 1979. "Legionnaires": the disease, the bacterium and methodology. Center for Disease Control, Atlanta.
16. **Rosebury, T.** 1961. Microorganisms indigenous to man. McGraw-Hill Book Co., Inc. New York.
17. **Skinner, F. A., and J. G. Carr.** 1974. The normal microflora of man. Academic Press, Inc. (London), Ltd., London.
18. **Smibert, R. M.** 1978. The genus *Campylobacter.* Annu. Rev. Microbiol. **32:**673–709.
19. **Smith, H.** 1972. The little-known determinants of microbial pathogenicity, p. 1–24. *In* H. Smith and J. H. Pearce (ed.), Microbial pathogenicity in man and animals. Cambridge University Press, Cambridge.
20. **Smith, T.** 1934. Parasitism and disease. Princeton University Press, Princeton, N.J.
21. **Wilkinson, H. W.** 1978. Group B streptococcal infections. Annu. Rev. Microbiol. **32:**41–57.
22. **Wilson, G., A. Miles, and M. T. Parker.** 1982. Topley and Wilson's principles of bacteriology, virology and immunology, vol. 1 to 4. The Williams & Williams Co., Baltimore.

Chapter 3

Specimen Collection and Handling

HENRY D. ISENBERG, JOHN A. WASHINGTON II, GARY V. DOERN, AND DANIEL AMSTERDAM

SPECIMEN COLLECTION

The usefulness of analytical procedures performed on clinical specimens in the microbiology laboratory is directly influenced by the quality of the specimens themselves. Specimen quality is, in turn, largely a product of the nature of the clinical specimen (i.e., is it representative of the infectious disease problem and how was it collected?) and the manner in which it is transported to the laboratory. The intent of this chapter is to provide practical guidelines for the proper collection and handling of specimens destined for analysis in the clinical microbiology laboratory.

Blood cultures

The prompt and accurate isolation and identification of the etiological agents of bacteremia and fungemia remain among the most important functions performed by the clinical microbiology laboratory. Indications for obtaining blood cultures are a sudden relative increase in the pulse rate and temperature of a patient, a change in sensorium and the onset of chills, prostration, and hypotension, or a prolonged, mild, and intermittent fever in association with a heart murmur. Bacteremia is continuous in endocarditis and endarteritis, uncontrolled infections, and the early stages of typhoid fever and brucellosis; it is usually intermittent in other infections. Timing and the collection of the cultures in infective endocarditis, for example, may not be critical; in other diseases, however, timing of the collection is important because intermittent bacteremia may precede the onset of fever or chills by as much as 1 h.

In patients with suspected bacterial endocarditis, three blood cultures are sufficient to isolate the etiological agent in nearly all instances. These should be collected separately and, the condition of the patient permitting, at no less than hourly intervals within a 24-h period. In patients who have received antimicrobial agents between 1 and 2 weeks before culture, it is advisable to consider obtaining an additional two to three blood culture sets a day later, since culture-negative endocarditis today is most frequently associated with prior antimicrobial therapy and may require as many as five to six separate cultures for isolation of the etiological agent. A solitary blood culture is rarely if ever sufficient (1). At least two blood culture sets are necessary to rule out or establish a diagnosis of bacteremia when the anticipated pathogen is different from the usual contaminating flora and when the pretest probability of bacteremia is low to moderate. More blood cultures may be indicated when the pretest probability of bacteremia is high and the anticipated pathogens are common contaminants or the patient has received antimicrobial therapy within 1 or 2 weeks before culture. In such instances, the time interval between cultures is frequently determined by clinical circumstances and the urgency to initiate antimicrobial therapy. One may also consider techniques to absorb or inactivate any antimicrobial agents that may be present (see below). Patients with culture-negative endocarditis may have endocarditis caused by *Legionella* spp., fungi, or *Coxiella* spp.

It is essential that blood for culture be collected aseptically, first by cleansing the skin with 80 to 95% alcohol and then by applying 2% iodine in a concentric fashion to the venipuncture site. Because of the lower incidence of skin hypersensitivity to iodophors, they may be used in lieu of iodine. Instant antisepsis never occurs, and the disinfectant should remain intact on the skin for at least 1 min. The intended venipuncture site should not then be touched unless the gloved fingers used for palpation are similarly disinfected. After the venipuncture, any residual iodine should be removed with an alcohol sponge or pad.

Since the volume of blood per culture is the major determinant of yield, regardless of the blood culture system used, in adults it is recommended that at least 20 ml of blood be collected for each culture. Culture of a lesser volume results in lower recovery rates because of the relative paucity of microorganisms in most bacteremias, at least those occurring in adults. In infants and children, collection of 1 to 5 ml seems to be satisfactory. Optimally, the blood is inoculated directly into culture media at the bedside of the patient with the syringe and needle or a transfer set. Alternatively, the blood may be transported to the laboratory in a sterile evacuated test tube containing sodium polyanetholesulfonate (SPS) and then inoculated into culture media (79). Most available blood culture systems are based on growth of microorganisms in broth or broth-agar combinations and their detection by visual examination, microscopic examination, subculture, or the evolution of carbon dioxide from the metabolism of carbohydrates or amino acids in the medium. Broth-based approaches, regardless of the detection method, have a long-established record for the isolation of aerobic, facultatively anaerobic, and anaerobic bacteria and yeasts. The use of liquid medium containing isotopic carbon-labeled substrates has greatly accelerated the detection of mycobacteremia. Lysis-centrifugation has proved to be another useful approach for the detection of bacteria, mycobacteria, and fungi in blood (33, 34). Routine subculture has been greatly facilitated by the attachment of chambers containing differential solid media to the tops of blood culture bottles, thereby allowing a subculture to be performed by simply transiently inverting the bottle containing the blood-broth mixture. Because each system has its particular strengths and weaknesses and because culture of 20 ml of blood from adults is recommended, it may be advisable to use a combination of blood culture systems on a routine basis. For example, a 20-ml blood culture specimen could be divided equally between a broth-based system and a lysis-centrifugation system.

It has generally been recommended that blood specimens be diluted in broth on a 1:10 basis to help neutralize the bactericidal properties of blood and the presence of any antimicrobial agents in the sample. Any residual bactericidal effects remaining after this dilution of blood in the culture media have been shown to be abolished by the presence of 0.05 or 0.025% SPS, a polyanionic anticoagulant that is also anticomplementary and antiphagocytic. Preliminary data suggest that a lesser dilution of blood than 1:10 be used when the broth medium contains not only SPS but also resins.

Any general-purpose, commercially available nutrient broth medium may be used for the culture of blood. Soybean and casein digests such as tryptic soy broth (Difco Laboratories, Detroit, Mich.), Trypticase soy broth (BBL Microbiology Systems, Cockeysville, Md.), Columbia broth, and brain heart infusion broth are satisfactory. Strict reliance on fluid thioglycolate, Thiol (Difco), or supplemented, prereduced anaerobically sterilized media is not recommended because of lower isolation rates of aerobic or facultatively anaerobic bacteria, as well as yeasts, in these media. Commercially available liquid media are generally bottled under vacuum with CO_2 and contain 0.025% SPS. As such, they are satisfactory for cultivation of anaerobes from blood. Chapter 49 may be consulted for more details about anaerobic blood cultures. Bottles containing 50 or 100 ml of medium should be used.

A new blood culture system (BACTEC Plus; Johnston Laboratories, Inc., Towson, Md.) has recently been introduced; this system recommends culture of 10-ml blood samples in 30 ml of blood culture broth, resulting in only a 1:3 dilution of blood specimen. The broth contains antimicrobial absorbing resins; detection is instrument assisted and predicated on infrared spectroscopic analysis of headspace air from blood culture bottles for the presence of evolved CO_2. The utility of BACTEC Plus cannot be assessed at this time since no clinical laboratory evaluations of the system have been published.

The mutually exclusive atmospheric requirements of different microorganisms make the use of two bottles, one maintained under anaerobic conditions and the other vented, desirable. Venting is performed by aseptically inserting a sterile, cotton-blocked needle through the rubber stopper of the bottle and withdrawing the needle after the vacuum has been released. If the venting unit is left in place, the bottle should be incubated in an atmosphere containing 10% CO_2.

Cultures are incubated at 35°C and are examined macroscopically for evidence of growth or by use of an instrument for the detection of evolved CO_2 later on the day of collection and daily thereafter for at least 7 days. Clinically significant bacteria are recovered within this period in at least 95% of instances; however, longer incubation times may be necessary for specimens from seriously ill patients who are receiving and not responding to antimicrobial agents or from patients with endocarditis or endarteritis presumably due to fastidious microorganisms. Recovery of such bacteria beyond the first 7 days of incubation may provide the opportunity for administration of more specific and effective antimicrobial agents.

The efficacy of hypertonic media in the recovery of cell wall-deficient bacteria or L forms has never been substantiated.

Gram- or acridine orange-stained smears and aerobic and anaerobic subcultures of obvious or suspected positive cultures should be prepared immediately, and the results of the microscopic examination of the smear, if positive, should be reported at once by phone and in writing or via computer to the physician of record. Subcultures for direct antimicrobial susceptibility testing may be performed; however, these results should be considered tentative. They require confirmation by retesting of the isolate with a standardized method.

The issue of routine blind subculture of broth-based blood culture bottles remains controversial. Routine subculture is not required but may be helpful in systems in which growth detection is based on the evolution of carbon dioxide. Routine subculture of the vented or aerobic bottle of a pair of blood culture bottles is advised at an interval of between 6 and 18 h of incubation. Routine subcultures of the nonvented bottle of a pair of blood culture bottles is recommended when the blood culture has been obtained from a child in whom infection with *Haemophilus influenzae* is a possibility. Earlier subculture (6 to 18 h) is also advised in such cases. No further routine subcultures are indicated. Subcultures are inoculated onto quadrants of chocolate agar plates that are incubated in 3 to 6% carbon dioxide for 48 h. In the case of blood culture systems having an agar slide attachment, the agar slide should be attached to only one of the pair of bottles, and the bottle containing the agar slide attachment should be inverted immediately after the agar slide has been attached, after the initial visual examination of the bottle, and daily thereafter. Appropriate agar plates inoculated with the centrifugate of the lysis-centrifugation technique should be handled in biological safety cabinets, incubated under 5 to 10% CO_2, and inspected daily for 4 days for the presence of aerobic and facultatively anaerobic bacteria and yeasts. If prereduced agar plates have been inoculated, they must be held for 6 days. Some laboratories prefer to inoculate a sample of the centrifugate into suitable anaerobic broth media and hold these broths for a 7-day period. Agar plates inoculated from lysis-centrifugation-treated blood specimens for fungi should be incubated at appropriate temperatures for 6 days. Suspected *Histoplasma capsulatum* fungemia requires at least 3 weeks of incubation.

Routine anaerobic subcultures of the nonvented or anaerobic broth bottle are unnecessary. In some instances, a routine Gram- or acridine orange-stained smear (60) made within 24 h after blood collection has been helpful. The recovery of aerobic or anaerobic diphtheroids, *Bacillus* spp., or coagulase-negative staphylococci usually signifies contamination unless they are present in large numbers and in multiple cultures. Nonhemolytic streptococci, excluding group D streptococci, and alpha-hemolytic streptococci in single cultures are of uncertain significance. *Bacteroidaceae, Enterobacteriaceae, Pseudomonas aeruginosa, Haemophilus* spp., *Staphylococcus aureus,* pneumococci, and yeasts are nearly always clinically significant.

Polymicrobial bacteremia has been reported in as many as 21% of microbiologically proven septic episodes and is associated with a higher mortality than is monomicrobic infection (11, 77).

In cases of suspected mycobacteremia, blood may be inoculated directly into Middlebrook 7H9 broth medium containing radiolabeled substrates for radiometric detection of mycobacteria or, alternatively, after processing by lysis-centrifugation. In addition, the agar or semisolid egg media used for the cultivation of mycobacteria as a routine in each laboratory may be inoculated with the sediment of lysed and centrifuged blood.

Neutralization of antimicrobial agents present in blood at the time of blood culture can be accomplished in several ways. The customary 1:10 dilution of blood in broth will often reduce the concentration of the drugs to subinhibitory levels. Nearly all commercially available blood culture systems contain SPS, which, in addition to having anticomplement and antiphagocytic activity, inhibits aminoglycoside activity. Resins are commercially available that nonspecifically absorb antimicrobial agents that might be present in the blood specimen. Finally, lysis-centrifugation has been shown to enhance rates of bacteremia detection in patients receiving antimicrobial agents at the time blood cultures are performed.

Lysis-centrifugation has also been found to be useful in the isolation of various intracellular pathogens; in addition to mycobacteria, organisms such as *Brucella* and *Legionella* species have been isolated in this manner. In such instances, the lysed sediment should be inoculated onto media appropriate for the isolation of these microorganisms. Currently, lysis-centrifugation is a preferred method for the isolation of fungi from blood.

Leptospiremia is usually present only during the first week of illness. One to three drops of freshly drawn blood are inoculated into each of several tubes containing 5 ml of a suitable semisolid medium such as Fletcher or Ellinghausen medium (see chapter 121), and the cultures are incubated in the dark at 30°C for 28 days. A portion of each culture obtained from a site approximately 1 inch (ca. 2.54 cm) beneath the surface is examined weekly by dark-field microscopy for the presence of organisms morphologically compatible with leptospires.

Intravascular catheters

Intravascular catheters are an important potential source of bacteremia and fungemia as well as local infectious complications at sites of catheter insertion. Quantitative culturing of catheter tips is useful in assessing the relationship between catheters and sepsis (32, 49). A 2-inch (ca. 5-cm) distal segment of catheter should be submitted to the laboratory by aseptically clipping off the end of the catheter directly into a screw-cap, large-mouth sterile container at the time the catheter is removed. The specimen should be transported directly to the laboratory to prevent excessive drying. In the laboratory, the catheter segment is rolled over the surface of a sheep blood agar plate four times. The catheter segment may then be dropped into a tube of broth medium. The plate and tube are incubated for 48 h, and the number of colonies of individual colony types on the plate is counted. The presence of ≥15 CFU of a single organism per catheter is consistent with that organism as an etiological agent of bacteremia and perhaps septic thrombophlebitis (49). The presence of organisms in the broth culture does not permit quantitation and implies only that the catheter harbored the organism(s) at the time it was removed, possibly on the internal surfaces of the device (32).

Alternative or additional approaches for catheter assessment in the microbiology laboratory include Gram stains of catheters either in toto or cut longitudinally (17), culture and/or Gram stain of the proximal skin insertion segment of the catheter (52), and culture of catheter hubs (43). The ultimate merit of these approaches remains to be determined. A completely different approach to defining the presence of catheter-associated sepsis is based on quantitative cultures of blood aspirated through indwelling vascular catheters versus blood collected concomitantly by traditional venipuncture techniques. Colony counts, preferably obtained after lysis-centrifugation processing of the two blood samples, are compared. The presence of 5- to 10-times-higher colony counts in the catheter sample implies colonization of the catheter and a probable etiological role in bacteremia (58). However, the clinical utility of this approach has been questioned (56).

Wounds, tissue, abscesses, aspirates, and drainage specimens

Microbiological analysis of specimens such as these often provides the only definitive information on the etiology of a given infectious disease process. There are several rules that usually apply to these types of specimens. Tissue or fluid obtained from a site presumed to be involved on the basis of clinical grounds is always superior to swab specimens. Swab specimens should be discouraged when more representative specimens can be obtained. In general, the more specimen the better. There are circumstances, however, when only a swab specimen can be obtained. In such cases, the swabs should be used to extensively sample as representative a portion of the lesion as possible. Finally, it is usually desirable to perform both smear and culture procedures routinely on these types of specimens.

The microbiological examination of surgically obtained tissue debridement or biopsy specimens is of considerable importance because the specimen may represent the entire pathological process. Surgical specimens are obtained at considerable expense and some risk to the patient. Further surgery to obtain more material is costly and may be contraindicated or refused. In these instances, the microbiologist must be prepared to do whatever is necessary to establish a diagnosis, frequently in collaboration with a pathologist.

Numerous procedures have been described for processing tissue and biopsy specimens (66, 74–76). Selecting the proper specimen and collecting an adequate sample for examination are essential. Tissue and biopsy specimens should be placed in toto into sterile, wide-mouth, screw-cap containers and transported immediately to the laboratory. When the specimen is small, it should be bathed in sterile isotonic saline to prevent drying. When the lesions are large or numerous, multiple specimens from different sites should be obtained. In cases of osteomyelitis, bone biopsy often represents the only definitive means for establishing an etiological diagnosis (47). There are two exceptions. In patients with clinical and radiological evidence strongly suggestive of osteomyelitis, blood cultures yielding an organism compatible with the disease are probably sufficient to define the etiology. Also, in patients with a draining sinus overlying the area of bony involvement, recovery of *S. aureus* from the sinus tract is very strongly associated with identification of this organism as a cause of the underlying osteomyelitis (72). In these two instances, it may not be necessary to obtain specimens of bone for microbiological analysis.

Gross surgical specimens submitted for histopathological examination are ideal for microbiological study if they have been handled aseptically. Portions of the specimen should be carefully selected for analysis before the tissue is placed in fixative. Close rapport between microbiologists and surgical pathologists is invaluable. Histological examination may reveal whether a lesion is malignant, inflammatory, granulomatous, or suppurative. If it is malignant, cultures may not be necessary. If it is inflammatory, the nature of tissue reactivity may indicate the type of cultures needed. Histopathological diagnosis of infection depends on visualization of a sufficient number of organisms in characteristic form. Tissue stains for acid-fast bacilli provide positive results in only 30 to 40% of those specimens with positive cultures; special stains for fungi often reveal organisms not recovered in cultures (75). Inclusion bodies may be detected in lung tissue in only about 25% of cases from which cytomegalovirus is isolated (46). Cultures, therefore, are imperative to establish or confirm the diagnosis of an infectious process.

A gross surgical specimen may be bisected aseptically by the surgeon. One half is submitted to surgical pathology, and the other half is sent to the microbiology laboratory. Lung biopsy specimens from immunocompromised patients require processing that includes prompt microscopic examination of the specimen for bacteria, mycobacteria, fungi, and *Pneumocystis carinii* and cultures for bacteria, mycobacteria, fungi, and viruses (7). The tissue should be finely minced aseptically with sterile scissors and then ground with a sterile pestle and mortar, with 60-mesh aluminum oxide (Alundum) serving as an abrasive. Alternatively, the tissue may be homogenized in a sealed plastic bag by using a Stomacher Lab Blender (Spiral Systems Instruments, Inc., Bethesda, Md.). The homogenate should then be centrifuged and the sediment used to prepare smears. This procedure yields better detection of *P. carinii* cysts than do impression smears (70). Slides for Gram and special stains, prepared from the homogenate, help to determine the presence of microorganisms and guide the culture approach. Antigen detection methods may be used if appropriate and if reagents are available. A 20% suspension of the homogenate is prepared, using sterile broth and appropriate culture media inoculated with a sterile Pasteur pipette. Histological examinations suggestive of additional microbiological studies may take several days. Therefore, it is advisable to store any residual tissue emulsion at 5°C for 1 or 2 weeks before discarding. It is recommended that as much material as possible be examined microbiologically by the inoculation of multiple plates or tubes containing appropriate media. Inoculation of appropriate cell cultures for virus isolation should be done if indicated. Portions of the specimen can be stored at −70°C for delayed viral isolation. If electron microscopic study of the tissue for viruses is required, a portion of the involved tissue should be preserved appropriately (see chapter 4).

The value of postmortem microbiology remains controversial. In some institutions, heart blood is routinely cultured; in others, cultures are limited to specific organs in which infection is suspected. In recent years, attempts have been made to correlate clinical and autopsy evidence of infection to establish a basis for limiting sampling to involved tissues or organs and to establish a correlation between postmortem and antemortem cultures (23, 39, 79). These studies demonstrated significant information only with single etiological agents in overwhelming infections and in well-established disease entities.

When postmortem cultures are necessary, the prosecutor should aseptically obtain a generous portion of tissue with at least one serosal or capsular surface intact. This specimen should be processed immediately or stored at 5°C. Procedures useful in processing postmortem specimens have been described by Dolan (22). In the laboratory, the capsular or serosal surface is thoroughly seared with a soldering iron and incised with a sterile instrument. A 1-cm^3 portion of tissue is removed aseptically from the core of the tissue block; it is used to prepare impression smears and is then ground as described above to provide a 10 to 20% emulsion. This emulsion is used to inoculate appropriate culture media. When a specimen too small to be treated as described above is received, it may be immersed in boiling water for 3 to 5 s to decontaminate the surface. Any residual specimen should be retained at 4°C until it is established that there is no longer a need to retain the tissue.

Cultures of embalmed tissue are considered useless. Weed and Bagenstoss, however, were able to isolate tubercle bacilli, *Histoplasma capsulatum, Nocardia asteroides,* and various species of bacteria from tissues that had been embalmed for 24 to 48 h (76). Embalming will diminish considerably the probability of recovering an organism. In certain cases, however, when nothing else is available and the area of the embalmed tissue selected for culture is centrally located, cultures of tissues embalmed for as long as 48 h may be worthwhile.

Quantitative biopsy cultures may be performed in an attempt to define the presence of infection versus colonization or contamination and with the aim of providing information relevant to issues of wound closure or grafting. In general, a bacterial load of $\geq 10^5$ CFU/g of tissue has been used to distinguish an infected wound from one that is merely colonized or contaminated, particularly when the organisms isolated include *S. aureus,* streptococci, and the *Enterobacteriaceae* (42, 48, 51, 62). With biopsy specimens from burn wounds, quantitative cultures yielding *S. aureus* or *Pseudomonas aeruginosa* in quantities of $\geq 10^4$ CFU/g of tissue indicate that the burn wound is not amenable to permanent grafting (45).

Punch biopsies should be obtained from lesions that on clinical grounds appear to be infected. With respect to burn wounds for which there is often no clinical clue indicating a specific area of infection, punch biopsies are indicated. In lesions with eschars, the eschar should be removed or transposed before the biopsy is performed. At least 1 g of tissue should be collected.

Specimens obtained from abscesses should include a sample of the internal fluid contents of the abscess as well as a portion of the abscess wall whenever possible. Fluid is best collected by needle aspiration; swab specimens are inferior. Specimens obtained from abscesses likely to contain anaerobic bacteria should be transported in transport devices capable of maintaining the viability of anaerobes. Fluid specimens from lesions for which anaerobes are not a consideration can be transported in a leakproof sterile container. Swab specimens from such lesions can be transported in any suitable swab transport medium. A convenient means for transporting fluid specimens that have been collected into a syringe by needle aspiration is to aseptically plug the needle with a rubber stopper and then submit the needle and syringe in toto. However, given the potential for needle stick injuries, this technique should probably be avoided.

The diagnosis of soft tissue infections is often delayed until the lesion becomes sufficiently fluctuant to allow incision and drainage or to permit needle aspiration. The combination of Gram-stained smears and cultures facilitates the etiological diagnosis of soft tissue infections (71). Microbiologists are urged to consider the need to examine such specimens for agents other than the usual bacteria (i.e., viruses, *Chlamydia* spp., mycobacteria, and fungi) when appropriate. In this regard, close interaction between the clinician and the microbiologist is essential.

Superficial wounds, ulcers, sinus tracts, and drainage material may all harbor microorganisms responsible for infection. In addition, however, these lesions are frequently colonized or contaminated with microorganisms unrelated to a specific disease. A challenge to the clinician and microbiologist when working with specimens obtained from these lesions is to distinguish organisms that are clinically significant from those that are contaminants. To meet this challenge, one approach with wounds is to perform quantitative biopsy cultures as noted above. Further, it should be recognized that commensal organisms of the skin, such as staphylococci other than *S. aureus*, aerobic and anaerobic diphtheroids, and in many instances yeasts, are most commonly found as contaminants. Environmental organisms such as *Bacillus* and *Clostridium* spp. and selected saprophytic filamentous fungi may cause significant infection but are also often observed as contaminants. In reality, it is often difficult to define with certainty the clinical significance of microorganisms recovered from such lesions. This problem is further complicated by the fact that multiple organisms are often recovered.

At the very least, care must be exercised in collecting the most representative specimens while avoiding as much as possible contamination with endogenous or exogenous microorganisms. Again, tissue or fluid specimens are always preferred. Swab specimens should be used only as a last resort. Specimens from sinus tracts warrant special mention. Material draining from the sinus tract should be sampled directly. The tract itself is best sampled by first thoroughly cleaning the opening with a suitable antiseptic. Curettings of the lining of the tract should then be taken as close to the base of the tract as possible.

Ear

Streptococcus pneumoniae, *H. influenzae* and *Branhamella (Moraxella) catarrhalis* account for the large majority of cases of acute otitis media in childhood. *Streptococcus pyogenes* and *Staphylococcus aureus* may also cause this disease but are recovered far less frequently. *P. aeruginosa*, *Escherichia coli*, *Klebsiella pneumoniae*, and *S. aureus* may be isolated from middle ear effusions of infants (9, 55, 67) and in therapeutic failures when *S. aureus* and *P. aeruginosa* are predominant (9). The bacteriological findings from children with acute otitis media have been sufficiently consistent in reported studies that there is little justification for routinely performing tympanocentesis as a means of defining the specific cause of a child's infection. Furthermore, as tympanocentesis has become a less common procedure, physician familiarity and expertise with it have diminished. For these reasons, tympanocentesis is now usually reserved for patients with complicated middle ear infections such as recurrent otitis media and chronic persistent otitis. Tympanocentesis may also be considered in neonates and the elderly, since the etiology of otitis media in these populations is unpredictable. Finally, it should be emphasized that cultures of the nasopharynx or pharynx are not useful for establishing the etiology of middle ear infections and should not be done for this purpose.

Eye

Patients with ocular infections present special problems with respect to specimen collection and processing. Swabs are often inadequate because of the small sample size. In addition, the antimicrobial activity of topical anesthetics used when procuring eye specimens may interfere with culture (65). Microorganisms responsible for keratoconjunctivitis include aerobic and anaerobic bacteria, fungi, viruses, and amebae. It is therefore recommended that swabs for culture be taken before topical anesthetics are applied and that corneal scrapings be taken after they are applied. Examination of Gram- and Giemsa-stained smears of corneal scrapings may provide preliminary clues to the nature of the disease. As necessary, smears for acid-fast bacteria or fungi should be prepared and examined. Because of the limited amount of material available, it is recommended that scrapings be inoculated at the time of procurement directly onto each of the following media: chocolate agar, brain heart infusion agar with 5% sheep blood, inhibitory mold agar, and, if mycobacteria are suspected, Lowenstein-Jensen medium. Swab cultures may be inoculated onto one half of each agar plate and the scrapings onto the other half. Specimens suitable for culture of *Chlamydia* spp. are described in chapter 105.

Wearers of contact lenses may develop ocular infections due to *Acanthamoeba* spp. Scrapings from infected eyes should be cultured on nonnutrient agar with Page ameba saline and nourished with 18- to 24-h-old slant cultures of *E. coli* J12, *E. coli* U5-41, or *Enterobacter aerogenes*. The plates should be inoculated with 2 to 3 drops of the bacterial suspension on warmed agar before inoculation of the plate with the scrapings from the cornea. A more detailed description of procedures pertinent to the microbiological analysis of ocular specimens is found in *Cumitech 13* (36).

Feces

Collection and preservation of feces is a frequently neglected but important requirement for the isolation of microorganisms responsible for intestinal infections. Unless the specimen can be transported immediately to the laboratory and properly handled upon receipt, a number of important organisms such as *Shigella* spp. may not survive the changes in pH that occur in stool specimens with a drop in temperature. When delays are unavoidable, it should be a standard rule that stool specimens be submitted in a suitable preservative such as 0.033 M phosphate buffer mixed with equal volumes of glycerol and a pH indicator. If diarrhea is suspected to be caused by *Campylobacter* spp., Cary-Blair transport medium should be used unless the specimen can be cultured on appropriate media within 2 h. Cary-Blair transport medium may be stored at refrigerator temperatures after inoculation until processing. Deterioration of ova and parasites in stool may be prevented by the use of appropriate fixatives that preserve the morphology of the protozoa and prevent development or deterioration of helminth adults, eggs, or larvae. Care must be taken to ensure appropriate proportions of specimen and fixative. The usually recommended mixture consists of 1 part feces plus 3 parts fixative. It is also recommended that a two-vial system for the preservation of feces be used. One vial should contain polyvinyl alcohol preservative for the preparation of permanent-stained slides, and the second should contain 5 to 10% Formalin for concentration procedures (2). When viruses such as rotaviruses or enteric adenoviruses are sought, detection tests should be performed as quickly as possible.

Swabs may be used to obtain rectal specimens in selected circumstances. They should be passed beyond the anal sphincter, carefully rotated, and withdrawn. These swabs should be placed in a screw-cap tube containing preservative such as Cary-Blair medium and transported to the laboratory for culture. Patients or personnel responsible for obtaining stool specimens for laboratory analysis should be instructed explicitly to choose portions of the specimen that are most likely to reveal the infectious agent(s) (mucous, blood, pus, etc.) when present.

The isolation and identification of *Clostridium difficile* from stool specimens obtained from patients with antibiotic-associated pseudomembranous colitis is not as pathognomonic as the demonstration of the toxins produced by this organism. The demonstration of these toxins by immunological or cytological methods is the only acceptable proof that *C. difficile* is the cause of the observed clinical disease.

When a patient's history, clinical presentation, or initial laboratory findings are suggestive of *Clostridium* spp., *Bacillus* spp., staphylococci, *Vibrio cholerae*, *V. parahaemolyticus*, and other vibrios, or enterotoxigenic, enteroinvasive, enteropathogenic, or enterohemorrhagic *E. coli* as a potential cause of disease, media suitable for the recovery of these pathogens should be used. These media are discussed and described elsewhere in this Manual. It is important that the microbiologist become familiar with these media and their appropriate use.

A single negative stool culture or examination for ova and parasites cannot be regarded as sufficient for ruling out a particular gastrointestinal pathogen. Most infectious diarrheas will be diagnosed with careful and extensive evaluation of three stool specimens. Similarly, after an etiological diagnosis has been made, microbiological surveillance of the convalescent individual and of contacts who may have become carriers should be conducted at regular intervals until at least three consecutive negative specimens have been obtained.

When gastrointestinal mycobacteriosis is suspected, the clinical microbiology laboratory should refer to chapter 34. Specimens collected for the demonstration of intestinal parasites are discussed in section VI. Gram-stained smears for the demonstration of bacteria have not been used frequently in recent times. The presence of large number of neutrophils or mononuclear cells is helpful in guiding the detection of intestinal pathogens. For further details, refer to *Cumitech 12* (64). Readers should consult the chapters of this Manual that discuss individual organisms for additional information.

Cerebrospinal fluid

Cerebrospinal fluid (CSF) from patients suspected of having meningitis should be examined immediately by skilled personnel in the clinical microbiology laboratory. Bacterial meningitis is a rapidly fatal disease if untreated or inadequately treated, and appropriate antimicrobial therapy often requires prompt identification of the etiologic agent. Lumbar puncture and examination of CSF should be undertaken whenever meningitis is suspected. It must be remembered that the typical symptoms of meningeal irritation in the adult such as fever, headache, vomiting, nuchal rigidity, and hyperreflexia are usually absent in infants and neonates, in whom the clinical manifestation of meningitis are often vague and nonspecific. An unexplained febrile illness in an irritable infant who is doing poorly should lead one to suspect meningitis. Meningitides due to mycobacteria, fungi, leptospires, or protozoa are generally insidious in onset. The diagnosis of viral meningoencephalitis is frequently established by exclusion and by serological means. Although some viruses may be isolated from CSF, viral isolates are more likely to be obtained from other anatomic sources.

Lumbar puncture must be performed under conditions of strict asepsis, since contamination of the specimen can occur readily and confuse the identification of the etiological agent. The skin should be disinfected with povidone-iodine. Specimens should be collected in sterile containers that can be sealed with a screw cap to preclude leakage and loss or contamination of the contents. Cotton plugs or rubber-stoppered tubes should not be used; snap-top containers should be checked carefully to ensure that a tight seal does occur and that the contents are not aerosolized on opening.

Antigen detection methods for the diagnosis of *H. influenzae* serotype b, *Neisseria meningitidis*, *Streptococcus pneumoniae*, and *Streptococcus agalactiae* meningitis are available commercially. Such tests are particularly useful with Gram smear-negative CSF specimens from patients who have been previously treated with antimicrobial agents but have signs and symptoms suggestive of bacterial meningitis. In general, antigen detection tests for bacteria should not be performed when CSF indices such as leukocyte count, glucose, and protein determinations are normal. The detection of cryptococcal antigen in suspected cases of cryptococcal meningitis is also most helpful.

In meningitis, the risk of serious neurological sequelae or death is great, and clinicians often initiate empiric therapy before the results of microbiological analyses are known. Rapid transport of CSF specimens to the laboratory is mandatory, since fastidious organisms such as *H. influenzae*, pneumococci, and *N. meningitidis* may not survive storage or variation in temperature. To facilitate optimum collection and fast transport of CSF specimens to the laboratory, the clinical microbiologist should (i) examine the lumbar puncture tray routinely used in the hospital to ensure that the CSF containers are satisfactory (not all commercially available trays have airtight specimen containers), (ii) establish a standardized skin preparation procedure, and (iii) develop a system whereby the specimen can be transported expeditiously to the laboratory. An adequate sample (as much as possible) of CSF should be available for microbiological examination, particularly when the diagnosis of tuberculous or fungal meningitis is considered, since the numbers of these microorganisms present are often small. If several tubes of CSF are collected sequentially, the first tube should not be used for microbiological analysis. If only one specimen container is obtained, it should be submitted to the microbiology laboratory first so that it can be opened aseptically and samples for chemical and cytological studies can be removed at the time cultures are inoculated. The microbiology laboratory should process the fluid immediately by preparing Gram-stained smears and inoculating the appropriate culture media. Physicians should be encouraged to always perform blood cultures from patients suspected of having meningitis.

In most instances, some procedure for the concentration of any organism present in CSF should be performed. For smears and cultures, centrifugation of the specimen at 1,500 × *g* for 15 min is advocated (59). The supernatant fluid is removed for chemical or serological studies, and the sediment is used to prepare smears and to inoculate media. Even after concentration, the numbers of organisms present in CSF may be small. As a result, smears should be examined thoroughly before being considered negative, particularly when CSF leukocytosis has been noted. Another convenient and effective approach to concentrating CSF fluid for Gram smear examination is to process specimens in a cytocentrifuge. Although the Gram stain has generally been regarded as the smear of choice for CSF specimens, the acridine orange (41) and Wayson (19) stains have also proven very effective and may be more sensitive than the Gram stain.

The inflammatory and noninflammatory responses of the host may be helpful in the differential diagnosis of meningitis. Whereas the leukocyte response in CSF in acute bacterial meningitis is usually polymorphonuclear, that in viral, tuberculous, and fungal meningitis is usually lymphocytic and less intense. Although polymorphonuclear leukocytes may be predominant in the CSF early in the course of viral meningitis, there is usually a clear shift to mononuclear cells within 8 h (26). The CSF glucose is usually depressed in cases of acute bacterial or tuberculous meningitis and normal in the other meningitides; CSF protein is usually elevated. Cytological and chemical changes in the CSF may occur in patients with brain abscess and other perimeningeal foci of infection; however, smears and cultures of the CSF are typically negative in these cases.

It should be emphasized that in partially treated cases of bacterial meningitis, cellular and chemical findings and the recovery rates of bacteria in cultures may be altered (16, 18). Furthermore, gram-positive organisms tend to appear gram negative in such cases; hence, findings in a Gram-stained smear must be interpreted cautiously (16).

When cryptococcal meningitis is suspected, a drop of the CSF sediment should be mixed with a drop of India ink (Pelikan, Gunther and Wagner, Hanover, Federal Republic of Germany) or nigrosin (Harleco; Harman-Leddon Co., Philadelphia, Pa.) solution on a clean glass slide covered with a cover slip and examined with decreased intensity of light. Nigrosin is preferable to India ink because it is free from discernible particulate manner. The presence of round, encapsulated, budding, yeastlike cells of various sizes in such preparations is virtually diagnostic of cryptococcal meningitis. Excluding patients with AIDS, India ink or nigrosin preparations of CSF will be positive in 30 to 50% of patients with cryptococcal meningitis (61). In AIDS patients, these tests will be positive in approximately 80% of cases (21). Cryptococcal antigen may be detected in a much higher percentage of CSF specimens obtained from patients with cryptococcal meningitis by use of latex particle agglutination tests. These tests will be positive in approximately 90% of cases (20). As a result, they should be applied routinely to all CSF specimens obtained from patients in whom cryptococcal meningitis is a possibility.

The development of meningoencephalitis of obscure etiology in patients with a recent history of swimming in fresh water before the onset of symptoms is consistent with infection due to *Naegleria fowleri* and should lead to the prompt examination of CSF for motile amebae (24, 59).

Normally sterile body fluids other than CSF

Included in this category are pleural, peritoneal, pericardial, and synovial fluids. Specimens such as these are usually collected via percutaneous needle aspiration. It is essential that the overlying skin be disinfected thoroughly before the aspiration is performed and that the collection procedure itself be done by strict aseptic technique. The same specimen transport instructions described above for aspirates of abscesses and cellulitis fluid apply to the transport of normally sterile body fluids. The presence of microorganisms in normally sterile body fluid specimens may be representative of life-threatening infections. Furthermore, the concentration of microorganisms in such specimens may be low largely as a result of the excessive volume of fluid that may be present in a given site. These observations underscore the absolute need to collect and submit as large a specimen sample as possible, to transport body fluid specimens immediately to the laboratory, and to process such specimens expeditiously in the laboratory, using techniques designed to detect small numbers of organisms in large volumes of fluid specimens.

Grossly purulent body fluid specimens should be examined directly by Gram smear or acridine orange stain for bacteria and by other specialized stains as indicated by the attending physician's diagnostic workup. Specimens that are macroscopically clear should be centrifuged at 1,500 × *g* for 15 min, and the pellet should be stained before microscopic analysis. Alternatively, cytocentrifuge preparations may be used for microscopic analysis. Supernatant fluid from a centrifuged specimen may be used to perform direct soluble-antigen detection tests.

Culture of normally sterile body fluid specimens should include inoculation of suitable agar and broth media. As noted previously, the larger the volume of specimen cultured the better. For this reason, inoculation of large-volume fluid specimens into blood culture bottles (63), processing of specimens via lysis-centrifugation (80), and concentration by filtration (50) have all been used effectively to enhance recovery of microorganisms from these specimens. The use of at least one of these culture approaches is particularly relevant to peritoneal dialysate specimens. Because of dilution of peritoneal fluid in dialysate, organism concentrations in dialysate in patients with infections are usually extremely low. For this reason, at least 50 ml of specimen must be cultured (12), thus necessitating use of one of the high-volume culture techniques mentioned above.

Upper respiratory tract

Cultures of the upper respiratory tract (3, 5, 7, 73) must be interpreted cautiously because of the microorganisms normally present in the upper respiratory tract and in view of the frequency of nosocomial acquisition of potentially pathogenic microorganisms by seriously ill patients on antibiotic therapy. Since potential pathogens such as *S. aureus, H. influenzae, Streptococcus pneumoniae, B. catarrhalis, P. aeruginosa, Enterobacteriaceae,* and yeasts may be present in the oropharynx, their isolation from cultures of respiratory secretions does not represent a priori evidence of an etiological role in respiratory infections.

Nasopharyngeal swab cultures can be performed to detect carriers of *N. meningitidis, Corynebacterium diphtheriae,* and *Streptococcus pyogenes.* In addition, such cultures aid in the diagnosis of pertussis and croup. Nasopharyngeal specimens should be obtained with a Dacron, cotton, or calcium alginate swab on a flexible wire that is gently passed through the nose into the nasopharynx, rotated, removed, and placed into a suitable transport medium for shipment to the laboratory.

H. influenzae serotype b may cause acute epiglottitis. The rapidly progressive and fulminating course, which may lead to death within 24 h, demands prompt initiation of therapy. Blood cultures should be performed immediately. Once an airway has been established, a swab specimen of the upper respiratory tract should be obtained, preferably by sampling the mucosa of the epiglottis, and cultured for *H. influenzae.*

Laryngeal involvement is not uncommon in both acute and chronic disseminated forms of histoplasmosis and blastomycosis (7), tuberculosis, and leishmaniasis. Cultures for these agents and biopsy with histological demonstration of the organisms are necessary to establish the correct diagnosis. Nasopharyngeal swabs are also useful for the isolation of viral agents causing respiratory disease, such as the rhinoviruses. Nasopharyngeal washings, however, are superior for the diagnosis of respiratory syncytial virus infection. Throat swabs have been useful for the diagnosis of *Chlamydia trachomatis* pneumonia in infants and for the diagnosis of *Mycoplasma pneumoniae* in young adults. Throat swabs are adequate for the recovery of enteroviruses and adenoviruses. They may also be used for the demonstration of herpes simplex virus, but calcium alginate swabs should not be used for this purpose since they may inactivate the virus. Nasopharyngeal specimens are superior for the recovery of respiratory syncytial virus and probably parainfluenza virus (28).

Throat cultures are obtained for diagnosis of streptococcal pharyngitis and, as indicated clinically, for other diagnoses such as gonococcal pharyngitis and pharyngeal diphtheria. There is no need to identify other microorganisms in routinely submitted throat cultures, since there is little or no evidence to document their role in producing pharyngitis. Exudative pharyngitis and enlarged cervical lymph nodes, headache, nausea, vomiting, and abdominal pain are commonly associated with streptococcal pharyngitis, whereas cough, rhinorrhea, and hoarseness are commonly found in cases of viral pharyngitis (29). Many viral infections, however, can be confused clinically with streptococcal pharyngitis. Acute tonsillar pharyngitis with vesicles or shallow ulcers on the anterior fauces, palate, and buccal mucosa is usually due to herpes simplex virus or coxsackievirus A. In the absence of a prior history of immunization, the clinician should alert the microbiologist concerning *C. diphtheriae,* particularly when a peritonsillar pseudomembrane is present. Gonococcal pharyngitis should be suspected in patients with a suggestive epidemiologic history of gonococcal infections in other sites, especially among those practicing fellatio (78).

Requisitions for culture of specimens from the upper respiratory tract should specify the suspected etiological agent or the disease whenever possible. Throat cultures should be obtained by direct visualization with a Dacron, cotton, or calcium alginate swab (except as noted above). Both tonsillar areas, the posterior pharynx, and any areas of inflammation, ulceration, or exudation should be sampled. When present, a portion of a pseudomembrane should be dislodged and submitted for culture. The tongue should be depressed with a tongue blade or spoon to minimize contamination of the swab with oral secretions detrimental to the quality of the specimen. Swabs should be inoculated immediately onto sheep blood agar for the isolation of group A streptococci; however, if transport is delayed for longer than 2 h, a transport medium such as Stuart or Amies should be used. A transport medium suitable for viruses should be used with swab specimens for these agents. Swabs for culture of *Chlamydia* or *Mycoplasma* spp. should be placed into sucrose-phosphate medium. In general, swabs for viral cultures should be refrigerated but not frozen if delay is anticipated. Swabs for the culture of *Chlamydia* and *Mycoplasma* spp. should be refrigerated during transport and storage. If prolonged storage is anticipated, swabs in sucrose-phosphate medium should be frozen at −65 to −70°C.

Lower respiratory tract

Cultures of expectorated sputum for bacteria are fraught with error, and clear-cut results are seldom obtained. Specimens are frequently collected haphazardly by paramedical personnel who are not aware of the need for a fresh, clean specimen resulting from a deep cough. They also fail to transport the specimen to the laboratory promptly. Expectorated sputum is frequently contaminated with oropharyngeal flora, which makes it difficult to determine which of the organisms isolated is responsible for pulmonary infection. Rarely, a potential pathogen is isolated in pure culture and may be presumed to represent an etiological agent. To quote Barrett-Connor (4), who found no pneumococci in 45% of the sputum and nasopharyngeal cultures examined from patients with pneumococcal bacteremia, "The routine sputum culture for the diagnosis of acute bacterial pneumonia may be a sacred cow. Not only can the results lead to serious mismanagement of the patient, but also sputum cultures represent one of the largest workloads and expenses for the hospital bacteriology laboratory." Perhaps not surprisingly, correlation between results of cultures of transtracheal aspirates and results of qualitative and quantitative cultures of the sputum has been poor (30).

These problems underscore the need for sputum screening by Gram stain as a means of assessing specimen quality. Expectorated sputum specimens with ≥10 (53) and ≥25 (8) squamous epithelial cells per ×100 field have been judged as unsatisfactory because of the high probability of such specimens being significantly contaminated with oropharyngeal flora. Such specimens probably should not be cultured. In addition, screening of sputa by Gram stain can provide a basis for determining the extent to which identification and susceptibility testing of organisms recovered from specimens should be performed (27).

Lower respiratory tract secretions collected by aspiration through a nasotracheal or endotracheal catheter may be contaminated with oropharyngeal flora. This is also true to some extent of specimens collected with fiberoptic bronchoscopy and bronchoalveolar lavage. It has generally been held that transtracheal aspiration, performed with local anesthesia, is the specimen collection method most likely to yield lower respiratory secretions free of oropharyngeal flora (6).

Specimens obtained via bronchoscopy should be considered in one of two categories (7). In the first category are specimens obtained to detect microorganisms that do not pose a problem in interpretation since their presence is almost uniformly associated with disease (for example, mycobacteria, *Legionella* spp., dimorphic fungi, and *Pneumocystis carinii*). Contamination of bronchoscopy specimens by oropharyngeal flora in such instances is usually unimportant. Diagnosis is enhanced by aspiration of bronchial secretions and by transbronchial biopsy. In recent years, sampling of involved segments of lung, particularly in immunosuppressed patients, has been performed by the technique of bronchoalveolar lavage. The tip of the bronchoscope is wedged into the lingular or right middle lobe bronchus or into the involved segment if the infiltrate is localized and the segment is lavaged with isotonic saline in 20- to 40-ml samples. These samples are then aspirated and submitted to the laboratory for cytological and microbiological examinations. This procedure has been proved extremely valuable in the diagnosis of cytomegalovirus, mycobacterial, fungal, and *Pneumocystis* pneumonia. Quantitative culture of lavage fluids is helpful in distinguishing between pathogenic and contaminating bacteria. In general, the isolation of at least 100,000 CFU of a particular bacterial species per ml is considered clinically significant.

The second approach to the diagnosis of lower respiratory tract infection is through the use of the protected bronchial brush catheter. After specimen procurement and disinfection of the outer catheter surface, the brush is extended past the end of the catheter and transected with sterile scissors for transport to the laboratory, usually in 1.0 ml of lactated Ringer solution. Before culture, the container is mechanically agitated and 0.1-ml samples are dispensed to a series of culture media. Some authors have recommended cultures of 1:10 and 1:1,000 dilutions (10). Recovery of $\geq 10^3$ CFU of a particular microorganism per ml is considered indicative of that organism playing an etiological role in the patient's illness (15). Whereas bronchoalveolar lavage is generally used for the diagnosis of lower respiratory infections in immunosuppressed patients, including those with human immunodeficiency virus infection, the protected brush catheter is used for the diagnosis of lower respiratory infection in patients who are at risk for unusual bacterial infections, including alcohol abusers, diabetics, and seriously ill, intubated patients in an intensive-care unit setting; patients whose chest X-ray examinations indicate extensive disease or the presence of a necrotizing infection; and patients with bronchoectasis who are unresponsive to the usual antimicrobial therapy or in whom recurrent pneumonia develops (10).

Culture of early-morning freshly expectorated sputum or of expectorated sputum induced by heated aerosol of 10% glycerol and 15% sodium chloride, followed in about 1 h by gastric washing (13), is useful for recovery of mycobacteria and fungi. Gastric washings obtained after induced coughing may have more mycobacteria. A series of such collections may be desirable. However, the use of pooled specimens for the culture of mycobacteria is discouraged, since overgrowth by bacteria other than mycobacteria often ensues, resulting in the need for rigorous decontamination procedures that may lead to the loss of viability of the mycobacteria.

In some instances, the etiology of pulmonary infections may be diagnosed by percutaneous transfer needle biopsy of the lung, thoracentesis, needle aspiration of an abscess or empyema cavity, or open lung biopsy. When open biopsy is performed, multiple specimens should be obtained from different sites if the lesion is large or if multiple lesions are present. In addition, a portion of an abscess wall should be removed, as well as a sample of the pus within (57). In experienced hands, the diagnosis of pneumocystosis may be made rapidly from appropriately stained material obtained by bronchoalveolar lavage or transbronchial brush biopsy (14). The need for open lung biopsy has been substantially reduced by the advent of bronchoalveolar lavage. Moreover, the diagnosis of pneumocystosis can often be made in patients with human immunodeficiency virus infections by examining induced sputum.

Urine

Urinary tract infections may involve the kidneys, ureters, bladder, and urethra, with the urethra and bladder being most commonly affected. Infections are classified as uncomplicated when there are no anatomical or neurological abnormalities present and as complicated when residual inflammatory changes, obstructive uropathy, calculi, or neurological deficits are present (40). Infections usually arise via the urethra by the ascending route and, less commonly, hematogenously. In most hospitals, urinary tract infections represent the most common form of nosocomial infection (68).

Women with acute dysuria usually have acute cystitis but may also have occult pyelonephritis or acute urethral syndrome. Dysuria may also be due to urethritis caused by gonococci, chlamydiae, or herpes simplex virus. Vaginitis may be caused by *Trichomonas vaginalis*, *Candida albicans*, or mixed aerobic-anaerobic bacteria (69). Acute bacterial cystitis may be associated with the presence of low or high levels of bacteriuria, i.e., 10^2 to 10^6 CFU/ml.

Proper instruction of women regarding the collection of clean-catch, midstream specimens is critical to ensure the accuracy of results from culture. Instruction of nursing personnel in the proper methods for obtaining urine specimens from bedridden patients is likewise important. It has been shown in prospective studies of outpatients that neither meatal cleansing nor midstream sampling is usually necessary for obtaining urine specimens from men (44). It has also been shown that accurate cultures can be obtained from incontinent males if a new but nonsterile external catheter and drainage system are applied after the glans penis is cleaned with a povidone-iodine solution and the first voided specimen is collected from the drainage bag.

It should be remembered that urine is an excellent growth medium for microorganisms. Specimens should be cultured within 1 h of collection unless they are refrigerated. Urine should always be cultured quantitatively for bacteria, since the number of CFU per milliliter is of major importance in the interpretation of urine cultures. A similar correlation between yeast CFU per milliliter has not been established. Since the urethra is normally colonized with a variety of anaerobic bacteria, urine obtained by suprapubic aspiration is the only acceptable specimen for anaerobic culture.

According to Kunin (40), "The concept of 'significant bacteriuria' and the criterion of 100,000 or more CFU/ml is a useful, but not absolute criterion that stood well the test of time." There are certain exceptions to the criterion of 100,000 CFU/ml. As noted above, women with acute bacterial cystitis may have as few as a 100 CFU/ml in clean-catch, midstream voided urine. Studies of ambulatory men found that growth equal to or greater than 1,000 CFU of a single or a predominant species per ml from a voided urine specimen most accurately reflected true bacteriuria determined with urine obtained by suprapubic aspiration (36). These exceptions require notification of the laboratory to use methods that permit isolation of low levels of bacteriuria. Any number of bacteria in a suprapubic aspirate must be considered significant except for skin contaminants such as diphtheroids and coagulase-negative staphylococci, which may require repetition of the procedure to confirm or rule out their presence in the urine. The number of bacteria in urine can be low on a diurnal basis when the patient is well hydrated, if the urine pH is below 5.0 or its specific gravity is less than 1.003, in the presence of antimicrobial agents, in patients with complete ureteral obstruction, and in chronic inactive pyelonephritis.

There are numerous rapid detection methods for bacteriuria. Microscopy based on the examination of a methanol-fixed Gram-stained smear of a drop of uncentrifuged, well-mixed urine provides 95% sensitivity in detecting the presence of 100,000 CFU/ml. The use of leukocyte esterase and bacterial nitrite provides approximately 85% sensitivity in detecting 100,000 CFU/ml if the patients are not neutropenic and the bacteria produce nitrate reductase. Filtration, bioluminescence, and photometric methods provide at least 95% sensitivity in detecting 100,000 CFU/ml (57). The sensitivities of these procedures decline for the delineation of 10,000 CFU/ml but may be 90% for the bioluminescence and photometric procedures. The application of rapid screening methods must be carefully considered, especially when cultures are to be performed only because the rapid screening method is positive.

Contamination of the urine by urethral or introital bacterial flora may be avoided by suprapubic aspiration. This is a rapid, safe, and simple technique when performed by a qualified physician. It is indicated for patients with clinical evidence of urinary tract infection but in whom bacterial counts in clean-voided specimens are low and therefore indeterminate, in neonates and in young infants, in patients in whom catheterization may be contraindicated, and in those with suspected anaerobic bacteriuria. The patient should have a full bladder at the time the procedure is performed. After the skin has been properly disinfected, a 19- or 20-gauge needle attached to a syringe is passed through in the midline at the point approximately one-third the distance from the symphysis pubis to the umbilicus. Urine is aspirated into the syringe.

In patients with chronic indwelling urethral catheters attached to a closed drainage system, urine is collected for culture by disinfecting, with a suitable agent, the wall of the catheter at its juncture with the drainage tube and puncturing it with a 21-gauge needle attached to a syringe for urine aspiration. It is possible to puncture such a catheter repeatedly. The connection between the catheter and the drainage tube should not be broken for specimen collection, nor should material for culture be taken from the drainage bag.

During the course of cystoscopy, ureteral catheterization, or retrograde pyelography, urine may be collected for culture. In the case of an obstructed ureter, bladder urine may be sterile whereas the urine proximal to the obstruction may be infected; hence, the urologist will often collect several specimens and request that each be handled separately. Such localization studies require enumeration of any bacteria present in cultures.

Candiduria is abnormal. Its quantitation is of little importance and may even be misleading if standards applicable to bacteriuria are applied.

Pyuria without bacteriuria indicates the possibility of renal tuberculosis. There may be gross or microscopic hematuria, and secondary bladder involvement may produce symptoms of cystitis. Three consecutive clean-voided, early-morning specimens should be collected for culture. Twenty-four-hour urine collections are undesirable because of the frequent overgrowth of bacteria other than mycobacteria. A urinary calculus should be split to obtain cultures of its interior and of its surface, since one can isolate bacteria from the interior different from those present on the surface (54).

Sexually transmitted disease

Until recently, concern for gonorrhea has dominated the field of venereal disease (38, 73). The demonstration and culture of gonococci in the various exudates and lesions present in persons with the disease remains the definitive means for establishing an etiological diagnosis. In males, the microscopic observation of intracellular diplococci resembling gonococci in a Gram-stained smear of a urethral discharge is diagnostic. There is excellent correlation between the results of microscopy and culture. Direct inoculation of *Neisseria* selective medium, i.e., Thayer-Martin (TM) medium or its modifications, is advisable when inoculated agar can be transported to the laboratory immediately. If the history and symptoms suggest exposure but only scant urethral discharge is present, urethral scrapings should be procured by the clinician with a small swab or a smooth, small wire loop. The specimen should be cultured appropriately, and a smear should be examined. If it is known or suspected that the patient is homosexual, oropharyngeal and rectal cultures are indicated. TM agar or its modification should be inoculated directly. Recent reports of cryptic carriage of gonococci in the distal urethra of clinically asymptomatic men exposed to infected women make the cultures of small bacteriological loops inserted into the urethra for a short distance a significant test.

Obtaining an adequate specimen in female patients may present greater problems (25). The presence of a cervical discharge is helpful in the diagnosis. However, the Gram-stained smear obtained from such discharge cannot be considered pathognomonic for gonorrhea, and cultures must be performed. A cervical culture and, when possible, an anal culture are recommended. If pelvic examination suggests involvement of the vaginal glands or the urethra, swabs from this area should be cultured for gonococci on modified TM medium.

The use of *Neisseria* selective medium requires a caveat. Vancomycin-susceptible gonococci that are unable to grow on *Neisseria* selective media have been observed. These vancomycin-susceptible organisms may account for some Gram-stained smear-positive, culture-negative cases of gonorrhea and require the use of a vancomycin-free medium for their isolation. The existence of vancomycin-susceptible strains of *Neisseria gonorrhoeae* probably justifies the routine use of enriched chocolate agar any time *Neisseria* selective media are used.

Gonococcal skin lesions, especially in the female, have been observed with increasing frequency. Cultures of scrapings from the base of such lesions, however, are positive only infrequently. Careful abrading of the skin lesion with a sterile needle should be used to obtain specimens from these sites. Staining of smears of material from such sites with gonococcal fluorescent-antibody conjugate may help in establishing a rapid presumptive diagnosis.

In patients suspected of having gonococcal arthritis, synovial fluid aspirates of the involved joint(s) should be cultured on blood and chocolate agar plates. Caution must be exercised before such joints are needled, with particular emphasis on adequate skin preparation. It is advisable that smears be made from the aspirated material and that it also be cultured for organisms other than *N. gonorrhoeae*. Finally, when gonococcemia is suspected, the blood culture bottle should be subcultured minimally at 1-, 2-, and 4-day intervals on chocolate agar.

Nonselective enriched chocolate agar, TM medium, or modified TM medium is advocated for cultures of the exudate in ophthalmia neonatorum. Endocervical cultures of the mother should also be obtained immediately.

Dark-field or direct fluorescent-antibody demonstration of *Treponema pallidum* may be attempted from primary and secondary lesions of patients thought to have syphilis. Patients with such lesions must be examined within the vicinity of a dark-field microscope. Proper preparation of lesions and slides and the recognition of treponemes are discussed in chapter 55. However, because of the infrequency with which this examination is performed in the routine clinical microbiology laboratory, only very experienced personnel should be assigned the task of identifying *T. pallidum* in dark-field preparations. Patients should be sent to a laboratory where the test is performed routinely.

The incidence of chancroid has increased in recent years. *Haemophilus ducreyi* can be cultured on solid medium, using an enriched chocolate agar made selective by the addition of vancomycin. Proper attention to incubation is necessary (31; see chapter 45). The great variability in presentation of genital ulcers due to *T. pallidum*, herpes simplex virus, and *H. ducreyi* may make it difficult to clinically diagnose these diseases without laboratory confirmation. Specimens for culture of *H. ducreyi* should be taken from the usually purulent ulcer base without extensive cleaning.

The most common cause of sexually transmitted disease in the United States today is *Chlamydia trachomatis*. This organism typically causes nongonococcal urethritis in men and mucopurulent cervicitis and pelvic inflammatory disease in women. In many instances, infected women are asymptomatic. *C. trachomatis* is most accurately detected by culture of specimens in cycloheximide-treated McCoy cells. The specimen is inoculated by centrifugation onto the cell line either in shell vials or in microdilution trays. The culture method involves numerous variables, including the centrifugal force applied during inoculation, whether specimens are sonicated and vortexed, and whether serial passage of cell culture is performed at 48 to 72 h (37). Variations in the culture method have made evaluation of the sensitivity of direct immunofluorescence, enzyme immunoassays, and molecular probes difficult to assess (see chapters 12 and 17).

Genital herpesvirus infection, somewhat overshadowed by human immunodeficiency virus infection, causes a significant amount of morbidity in sexually active people. Although primary genital herpesvirus infection may be due to either herpes simplex virus type 1 or type 2, most genital infections in the United States are caused by type 2. Primary herpes simplex virus infections may also involve the pharynx and rectum. The laboratory diagnosis is based on the isolation of the virus in tissue culture or by direct detection of viral antigen, by direct immunofluorescence or enzyme immunoassay. Cytological examinations may also be helpful. Isolation of the virus or detection of its antigen is most successful during the vesicular stage of the disease. Isolation is less frequent during the ulcerative stage and is further diminished during the crusted stages of infection. Evaluation of the literature on direct detection methods has been complicated by frequent lack of definition of the stage of the disease at which specimens are taken (see chapter 75).

Bacterial vaginosis is associated with a thin, watery vaginal discharge, vaginal fluid pH of greater than 4.5, the presence of aromatic amines in vaginal secretions, and the appearance of clue cells in the vaginal discharge. The bacterial etiology of this condition remains somewhat uncertain but appears to be related to a shift in the vaginal flora from a predominance of lactobacilli to a predominance of anaerobic gram-negative bacilli and *Mobiluncus* species. In most cases, vaginal secretions also contain *Gardnerella vaginalis;* however, this organism can be isolated from up to 50% of asymptomatic, sexually active women. The diagnosis of bacterial vaginosis should be based on the character of the discharge, i.e., an elevated vaginal fluid pH, the evolution of aminelike odor on addition of KOH to vaginal secretions, the absence of lactobacilli, and the presence of clue cells. Cultures are of little value.

TRANSPORT OF SPECIMENS TO THE LABORATORY

The clinical microbiology laboratory may not always be responsible for the transport of specimens to the laboratory. Nevertheless, efforts should be made to educate personnel responsible for this service and their supervisors in the importance of prompt delivery of all specimens intended for microbiological analysis. Of equal importance is the need to instruct personnel who collect specimens to note the time of collection, thus enabling laboratory personnel to determine transit time. Laboratories should note the time of arrival of specimens in the laboratory. Specimens that have been in transit for an inordinate period of time may not be acceptable for microbiologic analysis. It is imperative that all specimens be transported to the microbiology laboratory in the appropriate containers. Continuing education in the proper method of collecting and transporting specimens is an important responsibility of the laboratory. The medical staff, house officers, and nursing personnel should be reminded as often as required that prompt and proper transport of specimens from clinics or patient floors to the microbiology laboratory is important. Many laboratories have established policies of refusing to process specimens that have been handled improperly.

Specimens come to the laboratory in essentially three forms: solid (e.g., tissue, biopsies, and formed stool), liquid (e.g., blood, CSF, other normally sterile body fluids, urine, sputum, diarrheal stool, and aspirates), and on swabs. The manner in which a specimen is transported is predicated on the nature of the specimen and the analyses to be performed. A comprehensive discussion of all issues pertaining to transport of clinical specimens for microbiological analysis is beyond the scope of this chapter. For detailed instructions beyond those provided in the first section of this chapter, readers are encouraged to consult *Cumitech 9* (35).

A few general statements are, however, appropriate. The intent of transport is simply to get specimens to the laboratory in a state precisely equivalent to the form in which they existed at the time they were collected. The qualitative and quantitative characteristics of any microorganisms present in the specimen should remain unchanged, and no exogenous contaminants should be introduced. Submitting specimens as they are at the time of collection, without the use of maintenance transport medium or preservatives, is always preferred, assuming that such specimens can be transported expeditiously without compromising their integrity. This is often, if not usually, impossible. Therefore, the transport devices used must provide conditions for stabilizing the specimen and the microorganisms in it. Specific recommendations for the transport of various types of specimens are provided above. All personnel who collect or handle specimens should understand that this activity may involve the risk of acquiring an infectious disease. Continual diligence must be exercised to minimize these risks by use of suitably safe procedures for collecting specimens and appropriate containment when transporting specimens to the laboratory. This last issue is discussed in greater detail in chapter 7.

LITERATURE CITED

1. **Aronson, M. D., and D. H. Bor.** 1987. Blood cultures. Ann. Intern. Med. **106**:246–253.
2. **Ash, L. R., and T. C. Orihel.** 1986. Parasites, a guide to laboratory procedures and identification. American Society of Clinical Pathologists, Chicago.
3. **Bannatyne, R. M., C. Clausen, and L. R. McCarthy.** 1979. Cumitech 10, Laboratory diagnosis of upper respiratory tract infections. Coordinating ed., I. B. R. Duncan. American Society for Microbiology, Washington, D.C.
4. **Barrett-Connor, E.** 1971. The nonvalue of sputum culture in the diagnosis of pneumococcal pneumonia. Am. Rev. Respir. Dis. **103**:845–848.
5. **Bartlett, J. G., N. S. Brewer, and K. J. Ryan.** 1978. Cumitech 7, Laboratory diagnosis of lower respiratory tract infections. Coordinating ed., J. A. Washington II. American Society for Microbiology, Washington, D.C.
6. **Bartlett, J. G., J. E. Rosenblatt, and S. M. Finegold.** 1979. Percutaneous transtracheal aspiration in the diagnosis of anaerobic pulmonary infection. Ann. Intern. Med. **79**:535–540.
7. **Bartlett, J. G., K. J. Ryan, T. F. Smith, and W. R. Wilson.** 1987. Cumitech 7A, Laboratory diagnosis of lower respiratory tract infections. Coordinating ed., J. A. Washington II. American Society for Microbiology, Washington, D.C.
8. **Bartlett, R. C.** 1974. A plea for clinical relevance in medical microbiology. Am. J. Clin. Pathol. **61**:867–872.
9. **Bland, R. D.** 1972. Otitis media in the first six weeks of life: diagnosis, bacteriology and management. Pediatrics **49**:187–197.
10. **Broughton, W. A., J. B. Bass, and N. B. Kirkpatrick.** 1987. The technique of protected brush catheter bronchoscopy and how to obtain lower airway secretions. J. Crit. Illness **2**:263–270.
11. **Bryant, J. K., and J. A. Washington II.** 1988. Polymicrobial septicemia. Lab. Med. **1988**:9–21.
12. **Buggy, B. P.** 1986. Culture methods for continuous ambulatory peritoneal dialysis-associated peritonitis. Clin. Microbiol. Newsl. **8**:12–14.
13. **Carr, D. T., A. G. Karlson, and G. G. Stillwell.** 1967. A comparison of cultures of induced sputum and gastric washings in the diagnosis of tuberculosis. Mayo Clin. Proc. **42**:23–25.
14. **Chalvardjian, A. M., and L. A. Grawe.** 1963. A new procedure for the identification of *Pneumocystis carinii* cysts in tissue sections and smears. J. Clin. Pathol. **16**:383–384.
15. **Chastre, J., J. Y. Fagan, P. Soler, and M. Bornet.** 1988. Diagnosis of nosocomial bacterial pneumonia in intubated patients undergoing ventilation: comparison of the usefulness of bronchoalveolar lavage and the protected specimen brush. Am. J. Med. **85**:499–506.
16. **Converse, G. M., J. M. Gewaltney, D. A. Strassburg, and J. Q. Hendley.** 1973. Alteration of CSF findings by partial treatment of bacterial meningitis. Clin. Res. **21**:120.
17. **Cooper, G. L., and C. C. Hopkins.** 1987. Rapid diagnosis of intravascular catheter-associated infection by direct gram staining of catheter segments. N. Engl. J. Med. **312:** 1142–1147.
18. **Dalton, H. P., and M. J. Allison.** 1968. Modification of laboratory results by partial treatment of bacterial meningitis. Am. J. Clin. Pathol. **49**:410–413.
19. **Daly, J. A., W. M. Gooch III, and J. M. Matsen.** 1985.

Evaluation of the Wayson variation of a methylene blue staining procedure for the detection of microorganisms in cerebrospinal fluid. J. Clin. Microbiol. **21:**919–921.

20. **Diamond, R.** 1985. The immunologic diagnosis of cryptococcus. Lab. Man. **March:**35–41.
21. **Dismukes, W. E.** 1988. Cryptococcal meningitis in patients with AIDS. J. Infect. Dis. **157:**624–628.
22. **Dolan, C. T.** 1979. Postmortem microbiology, p. 138–145. *In* J. Ludwig (ed.), Current methods of autopsy practice, 2nd ed. The W. B. Saunders Co., Philadelphia.
23. **Dolan, C. T., A. L. Brown, and R. E. Ritts, Jr.** 1971. Microbiological examination of postmortem tissues. Arch. Pathol. **92:**206–211.
24. **Duma, R. J., H. W. Ferrell, C. Nelson, and M. Jones.** 1969. Primary amebic meningoencephalitis. N. Engl. J. Med. **24:**1315–1323.
25. **Eschenbach, D., H. M. Pollock, and J. Schachter.** 1983. Cumitech 17, Laboratory diagnosis of female genital tract infections. Coordinating ed., S. J. Rubin. American Society for Microbiology, Washington, D.C.
26. **Feigin, R. D., and P. G. Shackelford.** 1973. Value of repeat lumbar puncture in the differential diagnosis of meningitis. N. Engl. J. Med. **289:**571–574.
27. **Geckler, R. W., D. H. Gremillion, C. K. McAllister, and C. Ellenbogen.** 1977. Microscopic and bacteriological comparison of paired sputa and transtracheal aspirates in the initial management of pneumonia. Chest **87:**631–635.
28. **Greenberg, S. B., and L. R. Krilow.** 1986. Cumitech 12, Laboratory diagnosis of viral respiratory disease. Coordinating ed., S. J. Rubin. American Society for Microbiology, Washington, D.C.
29. **Hable, K. A., J. A. Washington II, and E. C. Hermann, Jr.** 1971. Bacterial and viral throat flora: comparison of findings in children with acute upper respiratory tract disease and in healthy controls during winter. Clin. Pediatr. **10:**199–203.
30. **Hahn, H. H., and H. N. Beaty.** 1970. Transtracheal aspiration in the evaluation of patients with pneumonia. Ann. Intern. Med. **72:**183–187.
31. **Hammon, G. W., C. J. Lian, L. C. Wilt, and A. R. Ronald.** 1978. Comparison of specimen collection and laboratory techniques for isolation of *Haemophilus ducreyi*. J. Clin. Microbiol. **7:**39–43.
32. **Haslett, T. M., H. D. Isenberg, V. Tucci, B. Kaya, and E. M. Vellozzi.** 1988. Microbiology of in-dwelling central intravascular catheters. J. Clin. Microbiol. **26:**696–701.
33. **Isenberg, H. D.** 1983. The detection of small numbers of microorganisms in seeded blood samples using lysis-centrifugation, p. 19–30. *In* A. Balows and A. C. Sonnenwirth (ed.), Bacteremia: laboratory and clinical aspects. Charles C Thomas, Publisher, Springfield, Ill.
34. **Isenberg, H. D.** 1983. Clinical laboratory comparison of the lysis-centrifugation blood culture technique with radiometric and broth approaches, p. 38–54. *In* A. Balows and A. C. Sonnenwirth (ed.), Bacteremia: laboratory and clinical aspects. Charles C Thomas, Publisher, Springfield, Ill.
35. **Isenberg, H. D., F. D. Schoenknecht, and A. von Graevenitz.** 1979. Cumitech 9, Collection and processing of bacteriological specimens. Coordinating ed., S. J. Rubin. American Society for Microbiology, Washington, D.C.
36. **Jones, D. B., T. J. Liesegang, and N. M. Robinson.** 1981. Cumitech 13, Laboratory diagnosis of ocular infections. Coordinating ed., J. A. Washington II. American Society for Microbiology, Washington, D.C.
37. **Jones, R. B., A. van der Pol, and P. B. Katz.** 1989. Differences in specimen processing and passage technique by recovery of *Chlamydia trachomatis*. J. Clin. Microbiol. **271:**894–898.
38. **Kellogg, D. S., Jr., K. K. Holmes, and G. A. Hill.** 1976. Cumitech 4, Laboratory diagnosis of gonorrhea. Coordinating ed., S. Marcus and J. C. Sherris. American Society for Microbiology, Washington, D.C.
39. **Koneman, E. W., T. M. Minckler, D. B. Shires, and D. S. deJongh.** 1971. Postmortem bacteriology. II. Selection of cases for culture. Am. J. Clin. Pathol. **55:**17–33.
40. **Kunin, C. N.** 1987. Detection, prevention and management of urinary tract infections, 4th ed. Lea & Febiger, Philadelphia.
41. **Lauer, B. A., L. B. Reller, and S. Mirrett.** 1981. Comparison of acridine orange and Gram stain for detection of microorganisms in cerebrospinal fluid and other clinical specimens. J. Clin. Microbiol. **14:**201–205.
42. **Laurence, R. M., P. D. Hoeprich, A. C. Houston, and D. B. Benson.** 1978. Quantitative microbiology of traumatic orthopedic wounds. J. Clin. Microbiol. **8:**673–675.
43. **Linares, J., A. Sitges-Serra, J. Garan, J. L. Perez, and R. Martin.** 1985. Pathogenesis of catheter sepsis: a prospective study with qualitative and semiquantitative cultures of catheter hub and segments. J. Clin. Microbiol. **21:** 357–360.
44. **Lipsky, B. A.** 1989. Urinary tract infections in men: epidemiology, pathophysiology, diagnosis and treatment. Ann. Intern. Med. **110:**138–150.
45. **Loebl, E. C., J. A. Marvin, E. L. Heck, P. W. Curreri, and C. R. Baxter.** 1974. The method of quantitative burn-wound biopsy cultures and its routine use in the care of the burned patient. Am. J. Clin. Pathol. **61:**20–24.
46. **Macaset, F. F., K. E. Holley, T. F. Smith, and T. F. Keys.** 1975. Cytomegalovirus studies in autopsy tissue. II. Incidence of inclusion bodies and related pathological data. Am. J. Clin. Pathol. **63:**859–865.
47. **Mackowiak, P. A., S. R. Jones, and J. W. Smith.** 1978. Diagnostic value of sinus tract cultures in chronic osteomyelitis. J. Am. Med. Assoc. **239:**2772–2775.
48. **Magee, C., B. Haury, G. Rodeheaver, and J. Fox.** 1977. A rapid technique for quantitative wound bacterial count. Am. J. Surg. **133:**760–762.
49. **Maki, D. G., C. E. Wiese, and H. W. Sarafin.** 1977. A semiquantitative culture method for identifying intravenous catheter-related infection. N. Engl. J. Med. **296:**1305–1309.
50. **Males, B. M., J. J. Walshe, L. Garringer, D. Koscinski, and D. Amsterdam.** 1986. Addi-Chek filtration, BACTEC, and 10-ml culture methods for recovery of microorganisms from dialysis effluent during episodes of peritonitis. J. Clin. Microbiol. **23:**350–353.
51. **Marshall, K. A., M. T. Edgerton, and G. T. Rodeheaver.** 1976. Quantitative microbiology. Its application to hand injuries. Am. J. Surg. **131:**730–733.
52. **McGeer, A., and J. Righter.** 1987. Improving our ability to diagnose infections associated with central venous catheters: value of Gram staining and culture of entry site swabs. Intens. Care Med. **14:**227–231.
53. **Murray, P. R., and J. A. Washington II.** 1975. Microscopic and bacteriologic analysis of expectorated sputum. Mayo Clin. Proc. **50:**339–346.
54. **Nemoy, N. J., and T. A. Stamey.** 1971. Surgical, bacteriological and biochemical management of "infection" stones. J. Am. Med. Assoc. **215:**1470–1476.
55. **Ostfeld, E., M. Harrell, D. Michaeli, and E. Rubinstein.** 1978. Acute gram-negative bacillary otitis media. Am. J. Dis. Child. **132:**721–722.
56. **Paya, C. V., L. Guerra, H. M. Marsh, M. B. Farnell, J. A. Washington II, and R. L. Thompson.** 1989. Limited usefulness of quantitative culture of blood drawn through the device for diagnosis of intravascular device-related bacteremia. J. Clin. Microbiol. **27:**1431–1433.
57. **Pezzlo, M.** 1988. Detection of urinary tract infection by rapid methods. Clin. Microbiol. Rev. **1:**268–280.
58. **Raucher, H. S., A. C. Hyatt, and A. Barzilai.** 1984. Quantitative blood cultures in the elevation of septicemia in children with Broviac catheters. J. Pediatr. **104:**29–33.
59. **Ray, C. G., B. L. Wasilauskas, and R. Zabransky.** 1982. Cumitech 14, Laboratory diagnosis of central nervous system infections. Coordinating ed., L. R. McCarthy. American

Society for Microbiology, Washington, D.C.
60. **Reller, L. B.** 1983. Recent and innovative methods for detection of bacteremia and fungemia. Am. J. Med. **75**(Suppl. 1B):26–30.
61. **Rinaldi, M. G.** 1982. Cryptococcosis. Lab. Med. **13:**11–19.
62. **Robson, M. C., and J. P. Heggers.** 1969. Bacterial qualification of open wounds. Mil. Med. **134:**19–24.
63. **Runyon, B. A., E. T. Umland, and T. Merlin.** 1987. Inoculation of blood culture bottles with ascitic fluid. Arch. Intern. Med. **147:**73–75.
64. **Sack, R. B., R. C. Tilton, and A. S. Weissfeld.** 1980. Cumitech 12, Laboratory diagnosis of bacterial diarrhea. Coordinating ed., S. J. Rubin. American Society for Microbiology, Washington, D.C.
65. **Schmidt, R. M., and H. S. Rosenkranz.** 1970. Antimicrobial activity of local anesthetics: lidocaine and procaine. J. Infect. Dis. **121:**597–607.
66. **Segal, E. L., G. E. Starr, and L. A. Weed.** 1959. Study of surgically excised pulmonary granulomas. J. Am. Med. Assoc. **170:**515–522.
67. **Shurin, P. A., V. M. Howle, S. I. Pelton, J. H. Ploussard, and J. O. Klein.** 1978. Bacterial etiology of otitis media during the first six weeks of life. J. Pediatr. **92:**893–896.
68. **Stamm, W. E.** 1983. Measurement of pyuria and its relation to bacteriuria. Am. J. Med. **75**(Suppl. 1B):53–58.
69. **Stamm, W. E., M. H. Thomas, J. R. Johnson, C. Johnson, A. Stapleton, and S. D. Fihn.** 1989. The etiologic agents of vaginitis. J. Infect. Dis. **159:**400–406.
70. **Thomson, R. B., Jr., T. F. Smith, and W. R. Wilson.** 1982. Comparison of two methods used to prepare smears of mouse lung tissue for detection of *Pneumocystis carinii*. J. Clin. Microbiol. **16:**303–306.
71. **Uman, S. J., and C. M. Kunin.** 1975. Needle aspiration in the diagnosis of soft tissue infection. Arch. Intern. Med. **135:**954–961.
72. **Waldvogel, F. A.** 1985. *Staphylococcus aureus*, p. 1114–1117. *In* G. L. Mandell, R. G. Douglas, and J. E. Bennett (ed.), Principles and practice of infectious disease, 2nd ed. John Wiley & Sons, Inc., New York.
73. **Washington, J. A., II.** 1985. Laboratory procedures in clinical microbiology, 2nd ed. Springer-Verlag, New York.
74. **Weed, L. A.** 1954. Microbiological methods in surgical pathology. Mayo Clin. Proc. **29:**393–399.
75. **Weed, L. A.** 1958. Technics for the isolation of fungi from tissues obtained at operation and necroscopy. Am. J. Clin. Pathol. **29:**496–502.
76. **Weed, L. A., and A. H. Bagenstoss.** 1951. The isolation of pathogens from tissues of embalmed human bodies. Am. J. Clin. Pathol. **23:**114–1120.
77. **Weinstein, M. P., J. R. Murphy, L. B. Reller, and K. A. Lichtenstein.** 1983. The clinical significance of positive blood cultures: a comprehensive analysis of 500 episodes of bacteremia and fungemia in adults. II. Clinical observations with special reference to factors influencing prognosis. Rev. Infect. Dis. **5:**54–70.
78. **Weisner, P. J., E. Tronca, T. Bonin, A. H. B. Pedersen, and K. K. Holmes.** 1973. Clinical spectrum of pharyngeal gonococcal infection. N. Engl. J. Med. **268:**181–185.
79. **Wilson, W. R., C. T. Dolan, J. A. Washington II, A. L. Brown, and R. E. Ritts, Jr.** 1972. Clinical significance of postmortem cultures. Arch. Pathol. **94:**244–249.
80. **Woods, G. L., and J. A. Washington II.** 1987. Comparison of methods for processing dialysate in suspected continuous ambulatory peritoneal dialysis-associated peritonitis. Diagn. Microbiol. Infect. Dis. **7:**155–157.

Chapter 4

Microscopy

KIMBERLE CHAPIN-ROBERTSON AND STEPHEN C. EDBERG

MICROSCOPY AND CLINICAL MICROBIOLOGY

In a general sense, the field of clinical microbiology is defined by the microscope. Because most pathogenic microorganisms are considerably smaller than erythrocytes, their very presence escaped detection for several millennia as people intensively searched for the causes of acute, life-threatening, epidemic diseases. The first application of the microscope to the study of microorganisms occurred only in the late 1600s, when Antonie van Leeuwenhoek, a merchant, made simple, single-lens microscopes as a hobby. His clear, concise descriptions of the "little animalcules" he observed from teeth, throat, pond water, and other matter defined the major classes of microorganisms known to this day. Schwan, in the early 1800s, first used the microscope as a "clinical" tool. Having available reasonably well constructed compound microscopes, he engaged in a lifetime work of the systemic observation of the pathogenesis of disease. In early work funded by the brewery industry, he found that successful production of beer was always associated with globule elements, whereas unsuccessful production was always accompanied by the absence of these elements. He also found that he could bring about successful fermentation if he transferred these globules from a fermented to a nonfermented batch. These observations later became known as the Koch-Henle postulates to establish an organism as a causative agent of an infectious disease.

The microscopic examination of a clinical specimen is essential for establishing (i) whether the specimen represents a site of inflammation and (ii) which is the likely causative agent(s) of disease. Careful examination and quantification of stained preparations of clinical material can be as important as culture in both establishing a diagnosis and directing therapy. Accordingly, this chapter will discuss the tools (i.e., microscopes) and their utility in the clinical laboratory.

PURPOSE OF MICROSCOPES

The objectives of microscopy today are not appreciably different from those of van Leeuwenhoek. First, one wishes to magnify the image. Second, one must maximize resolution of the cellular and microbiological elements. Third, one must achieve contrast sufficient to differentiate microorganisms, cellular elements, and background. To achieve these goals, different types of microscopes have been developed, each applicable to certain kinds of microorganisms and clinical situations (9).

BRIGHT-FIELD MICROSCOPY

Virtually all bright-field light microscopes utilized in the clinical laboratory use white light as their source of illumination and direct this light to pass through the specimen. These microscopes possess at least two lens systems (objectives and eyepieces) and are therefore compound microscopes.

Magnification

Objective lenses are located on the nosepiece of the microscope and directly magnify the specimen to produce a real image. Generally, clinical microscopes have three to four objective lenses; each laboratory should have at least one to two microscopes with low-power (10×), high-dry (43×), and oil immersion (97×) objective lenses. The objective lenses gather light coming from each point of the specimen, unite the light in an image, and magnify that image. Because all objective lenses are biconvex disks, they will not produce a uniformly sharp image with white light. The image will be surrounded by color halos that can interfere with the visual observation of the specimen. This minidistortion is known as chromatic aberration. Chromatic aberration usually is corrected by using lenses made of two or more glass or mineral materials. Most clinical microscopes utilize simple achromatic lenses. However, for clinical photomicrography, greater correction is necessary. Lenses are available that can correct for three or more different wavelengths. Known as apochromatic lenses, they are composed of fluorite in combination with glass.

The objective lenses produce a real image that is remagnified by the ocular lenses to produce a virtual image. Ocular lenses generally magnify the real image either 10 or 15 times. In addition to magnifying the real image, the ocular lenses also correct some of the defects produced by the objective lenses. The total magnification of the specimen is the product of the magnification imparted by the objective lens times the magnification imparted by the ocular lens times the distance from the specimen to the eye piece in inches divided by 10.

Resolving power

Although the magnification of a specimen is obviously important, critical to a microscope's performance is its resolving power. Resolving power is the ability of the lens system of the microscope to distinguish two objects as separate rather than one. The resolving power is directly related to the wavelength (λ) of light used to illuminate the specimen and the numerical aperture of the system. Because the wavelength of light observed in bright-field microscopy is fixed within narrow limits, one may increase resolving power only through improved numerical aperture. Numerical aperture is a measure of the angle of the maximum cone of light that can enter the objective lens. Figure 1 demonstrates the salient features governing numerical aperture. Numer-

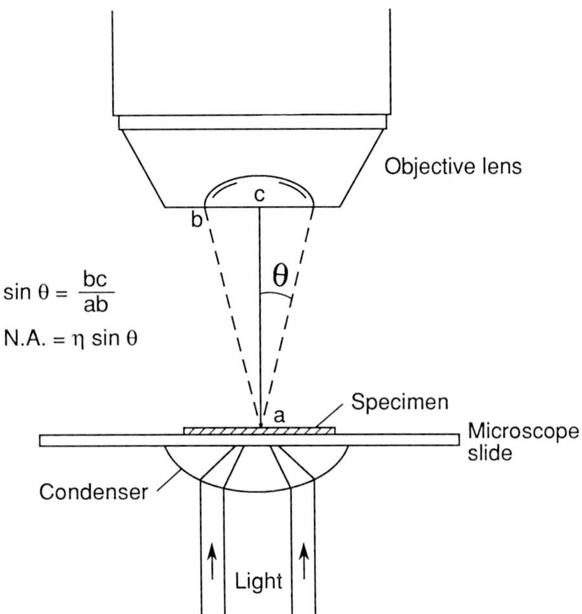

FIG. 1. Critical parts of the bright-field light microscope affecting resolution. Of greatest importance is the refractive index of the medium through which light passes and the angle of the cone of light from the specimen to the objective lens. N.A., Numerical aperture.

ical aperture = $\eta \sin \theta$, where η is the refractive index of the menstruum light passes through and $\sin \theta$ is one-half the angle of the cone of light produced between the specimen and the objective lens. The refractive index is determined by the simple equation, η = speed of light in a vacuum/speed of light in the material between the specimen and the objective lens.

Because the resolving power of a microscope is so essential to the ability of the clinical laboratory to properly interpret the various elements in a specimen, those parts of the microscope that can directly affect this parameter must be properly adjusted. Most critical in maximizing the resolving power is the proper use of the condenser. The condenser focuses light onto the plane of the specimen. There are several condensers available for clinical microscopes. The most commonly used is the Abbé condenser, which utilizes two lenses and produces a numerical aperture of 1.25. The Abbé condenser is suitable for most general clinical applications. Also available are variable-focus condensers, which also have numerical apertures of 1.25, and achromatic condensers, which have numerical apertures of 1.4. These condensers are primarily used for special purposes such as research microscopy or color photomicrography.

A second means of increasing resolving power is adjusting the menstruum through which light must pass between the objective lens and specimen. The refractive indices of special oils such as cedarwood, sandalwood, and balsam oils and the refractive index of glass are similar. The coincidence of these refractive indices permits more light to be gathered (thereby decreasing $\sin \theta$ and increasing the numerical aperture and resolving power).

Although the spectrum of light available to the bright-field microscope is narrow, the shorter the wavelength observed, the greater the resolving power of the system. Most microscopes use light generated by tungsten filaments, which produce wavelengths throughout the visible spectrum. Use of a blue filter permits primarily blue light to pass through the specimen. Because blue light is of shorter wavelength than the rest of the visible spectrum (yellow-green-red), the resolving power of the microscope may be somewhat increased.

Finally, the microscope has an iris to adjust the amount of light allowed to enter the system. Although the iris does not directly affect the resolving power of the microscope, it should be used in the same way that our eye uses its iris: to maximize the amount of effective light in conjunction with the other parameters of the optical system.

Overall, the resolving power of a well-adjusted light microscope should be approximately 0.2 μm at a magnification of approximately 970 with an oil immersion objective lens. At this level of resolving power, one is able to distinguish rods of the size of *Escherichia coli* from spheres of the size of staphylococci. However, the size of smaller rods, such as acinetobacters, may be somewhat below this resolving power, and therefore the microscope may not be able to distinguish a particular isolate as being either a rod or coccus (11).

Contrast

After maximizing the resolving power and magnification of the system, one must still be able to distinguish the various elements in the field. Because the refractive indices of microbes and the surrounding environment are approximately equal, unstained bacteria and yeasts are difficult to visualize. In unstained material, one may adjust the iris to decrease light and increase contrast, which is commonly done when one attempts to observe certain biological structures such as capsules.

Practically, contrast is enhanced by using dyes. The surfaces of microorganisms are negatively charged. Therefore, basically charged dyes will be naturally drawn to these negatively charged surfaces. We commonly use basic dyes to stain microbes and thus impart greater contrast to the organisms and their components. All stains used in the clinical microbiology laboratory can functionally be divided into four categories: primary stain, mordant, decolorizer, and secondary stain or counterstain.

The primary stain is generally a basic, positively charged dye. Common primary stains include carbolfuchsin, crystal violet, methylene blue, and safranin. These primary dyes will stain not only the target microorganism but also many non-target microorganisms and background material (Fig. 2 and 3). In the clinical microbiology laboratory, dyes are used in several ways: for direct staining of specimens to make microscopic objects more clearly visible than they would be unstained and to increase the usefulness of the optical microscope; as constituents of culture media, where they are used as indicators of pH changes or for their bacteriostatic action; and as oxidation-reduction indicators to demonstrate the presence or lack of anaerobic conditions.

Dyes are natural or artificial organic compounds that consist of three basic components: (i) a benzene or aromatic ring with (ii) chromophoric and (iii) auxo-

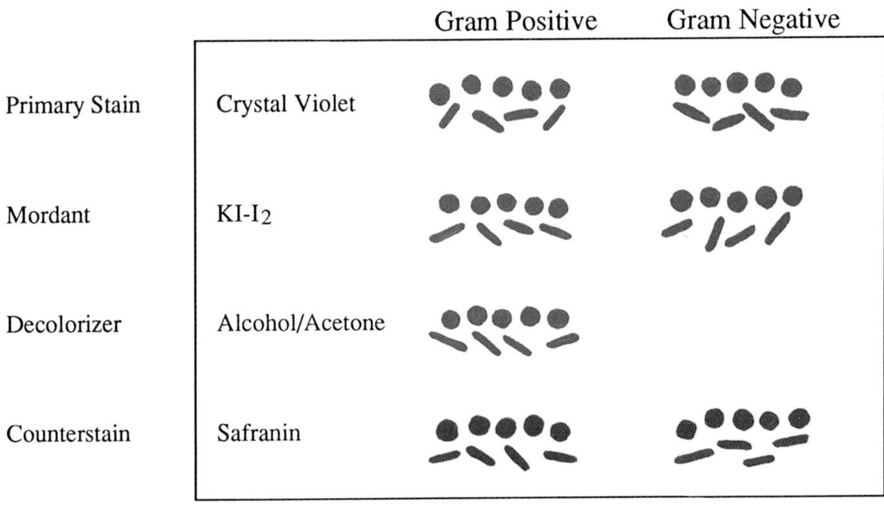

FIG. 2. Steps and results observed in performance of the Gram stain.

chromic groups. Most biologically useful dyes are derivatives of coal tar, with the fundamental structure being the aromatic benzene ring. Specific atomic groupings, known as chromophores, are associated with color. These specific chromophores are C=C, C=O, C=S, C=N, N=N, N=O, and NO_2. The more chromophores occurring in the benzene ring, the more pronounced the transmission of color. These chemical radicals absorb light of different wavelengths and act as chemical prisms. The benzene ring with chromophoric radicals is considered a chromogen and is colored, but by itself it is not a dye since it cannot bind to organisms or tissues. The auxochromic groups furnish the combining properties for the dye, usually by forming electrostatic salt linkages with ionizable radicals on proteins, glycoproteins, and lipoproteins on tissue or organism wall components. This process can occur either directly or through the chelating action of a mordant. Dyes are amphoteric; that is, they can act either as an acid or base, depending on whether the significant part of the dye is anionic (acidic) or cationic (basic). Practically, basic dyes stain structures that are acidic, such as nuclear chromatin, and acidic dyes react with basic substances, such as cytoplasmic and cell wall structures (3).

A mordant is a chemical or physical process that fixes the primary stain to the target microorganism. Common mordants include the iodine complex used in the Gram stain and heat or phenol used in the acid-fast stain.

A decolorizer is a chemical that removes unbound stain from the target microorganism. After the decolorizing step, the target microorganisms are the color of the primary stain and non-target organisms and background should be colorless. Common decolorizers include acetone or alcohol for the Gram stain and a mixture of acid and alcohol for the acid-fast stain.

Most biological staining systems employ a secondary or counterstain to provide color to non-target micro-

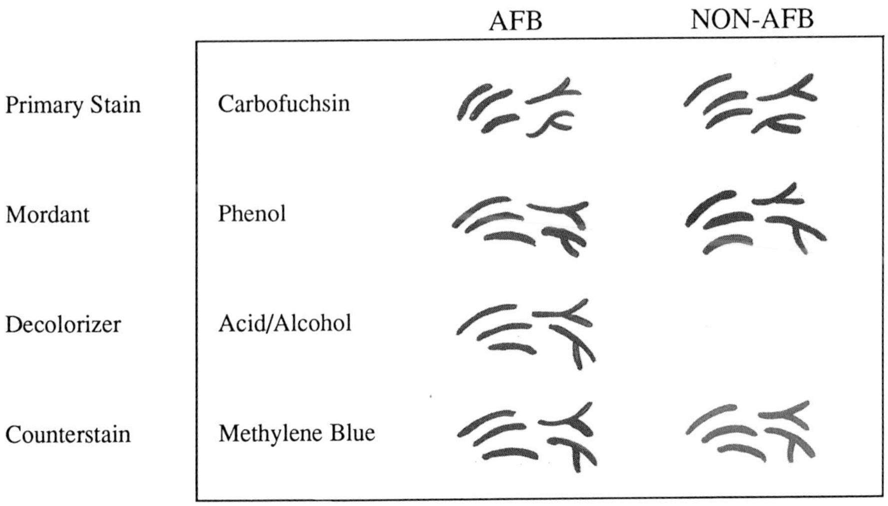

AFB
NON-AFB
Primary Stain
Carbofuchsin
Mordant
Phenol
Decolorizer
Acid/Alcohol
Counterstain
Methylene Blue

FIG. 3. Steps and results observed in performance of the acid-fast stain.

organisms. Generally, the counterstain is in a different part of the visible spectrum from the primary stain. Some counterstains are additive with the primary stains. For example, the red counterstain (safranin) of the Gram stain is additive with the blue primary stain (crystal violet) of the Gram stain to produce a purple target microbe. In other cases, the counterstain does not stain the target microorganism at all. For example, the blue counterstain (methylene blue) of the acid-fast stain does not penetrate into the target microbe (*Mycobacterium* sp.) to affect the red color of the target. Therefore, the target is red and the background is blue (10).

VARIATIONS ON BRIGHT-FIELD MICROSCOPY

Dark-field microscopy

The purpose of a dark-field microscope is to increase the apparent resolving power of the light microscope below 0.2 μm. In a normal bright-field microscope, the condenser focuses light directly onto a plane. In dark-field microscopy, this condenser is replaced by a special dark-field condenser. Light reaching the object is only from the circumference or periphery of the objective; all light from the center of the condenser has been blocked. Accordingly, the object within the specimen appears self-luminous or glowing. Cells such as spirochetes, which have diameters in the order of 0.1 to 0.15 μm, may now be distinguished as separate objects. They appear as bright halos in a dark background. There is no real increase in resolution, since the wavelength of light and the numerical aperture remain unchanged.

Three types of condensers are used for dark-field illumination. First, there is the standard Abbé condenser used in bright-field microscopy. It is modified for dark-field microscopy by insertion of a dark-field stop or disk between the light source and condenser. This type of dark-field condenser is most commonly used in routine diagnostic microbiology. Paraboloid dark-field condensers are used with high-power oil immersion objectives, and intensely concentrated light sources and cardioid condensers are used with arc lamp light sources. These last two condensers are primarily utilized for research and photomicrographic purposes.

Dark-field microscopy has primarily been limited to a very narrow range of microorganisms: those with diameters of between 0.1 and 0.2 μm. These include spirochetes, with direct dark-field examination of secondary syphilitic lesions for *Treponema pallidum*, cerebrospinal fluid for the agent of Lyme disease (*Borrelia burgdorfii*), and *Leptospira* spp. When specimens are collected and transported to the clinical laboratory for dark-field microscopy, it is imperative that they remain warm and be observed within 30 min of collection. If necessary, specimens can be diluted with tissue culture fluid without antibiotics (11, 13).

Phase-contrast microscopy

Phase-contrast microscopy, like dark-field microscopy, is a modification of bright-field microscopy. Here, advantage is taken of the change, or retardation, of light waves as they pass through biological structures of different densities. In a bright-field microscope equipped with a tungsten filament, light waves travel with the same amplitude and frequency so that their peaks and troughs pass a particular plane at the same time. They may be considered in phase. If these two parallel light waves strike two objects of differing density near each other, the light wave striking the denser object is retarded and its peaks and troughs are no longer coincident with the peaks and troughs of its formerly companion light wave. A special condenser takes advantage of these phase differences and makes them visible to the observer. This condenser has an annular diaphragm and permits only an outer ring of light to pass through the condenser and strike the specimen. The objective lens also has a phase-shifting filter. In combination, the phase-shifting filter and annular ring result in an amplification of the differences in density between objects. In a phase-contrast microscope, the less dense or transparent parts of the cell, such as the protoplasm, appear virtually the same as they would in a bright-field microscope—not distinguishable from background. The denser parts of the microbe, such as large organelles or the cell wall, appear as distinct dark entities in a light background.

In the clinical microbiology laboratory, phase-contrast microscopy is primarily used to enumerate yeasts and molds directly from specimens. They appear in bright-phase microscopy as typical molds or yeasts in a light background (4, 5, 12, 14).

FLUORESCENCE MICROSCOPY

Principle

Fluorescence occurs when a molecule is struck by a given wavelength of light and emits a wavelength longer than the one to which it was exposed. Therefore, fluorescence is described by the parameters maximum absorbency and maximum emission. Maximum absorbency is that wavelength of light for a particular substrate, or fluorochrome, that will optimally cause the substrate to resonate. Maximum emission is the longest wavelength of light that a fluorochrome emits after the resonating electrons return to their normal configuration. The fluorescence microscope uses filters in the light pathway to create monochromatic light for absorbency and to maximize monochromatic light for emission.

Fluorescence microscopy

The fluorescence microscope utilizes light of high energy under very restricted conditions. Therefore, unlike dark-field or phase-contrast microscopy, which are modifications of bright-field microscopy, fluorescent microscopy requires its own dedicated microscope system. The fluorescence microscope utilizes a mercury vapor lamp to generate the shorter wavelength of light required. This light source generates high-intensity UV, violet, and blue light. The mercury vapor lamp is considerably more costly and has a much shorter life expectancy than bright-field tungsten lamps. One should always obtain the highest wattage available in the best-quality bulb. The initial cost may be higher, but overall costs will be less. It is essential that the clinical laboratory properly maintain and quality control the mercury vapor lamp in strict accordance with the manufacturer's instructions.

The mercury vapor lamp is housed in a special compartment to guard against damage and aid in heat exchange. The light generated from this lamp is first directed through a filter that removes heat and infrared rays. Next, the light is passed through an excitation (or absorbency) filter to remove long wavelengths and other extraneous light. This excitation filter directs a narrow-range wavelength of light to the specimen. This narrow-range short-wavelength light is then directed through a special dark-field condenser to produce a dark background and achieve the maximum resolving power. This dark-field-directed short-wavelength light passes through the specimen. If there is a fluorochrome present in the specimen, this short-wavelength light is absorbed and long-wavelength light is emitted. An absorbency filter removes all short-wavelength light and permits the long wavelength fluorescence light to reach the eyepiece. Therefore, a "positive" is the observation of a typical wavelength of light (yellow-green for fluorescein; yellow for auramine O), and a "negative" is observation of a dark background (12).

Direct fluorescent stains

Auramine-rhodamine dye. The auramine-rhodamine combination of fluorescent dyes is used to directly visualize mycobacteria in clinical specimens. Their use is described in chapter 122.

Acridine orange. Acridine orange is similar to ethidium bromide in that it can intercalate into nucleic acid. At a low pH, bacterial nucleic acid fluoresces orange whereas mammalian nucleic acid fluoresces green. As described below, this differentiation is extremely useful in determining the presence or absence of bacteria in a specimen.

Fluorescent-antibody techniques

Direct fluorescent-antibody techniques are used to detect antigens in specimens. Indirect fluorescent-antibody methods are used to determine the presence of antibody, generally from a patient's serum or cerebrospinal fluid. Their use in the clinical laboratory is described in chapter 11.

NONFLUORESCENCE ANTIGEN-ANTIBODY MICROSCOPY

In an attempt to take advantage of the benefits offered by fluorescence microscopy while using the less expensive, easier-to-use bright-field microscopy, nonfluorescence antigen-antibody microscopy techniques have been developed. The first and most widely used employs an antibody molecule labeled with horseradish peroxidase instead of fluorescein isothiocyanate. Performance of the test is virtually the same as for fluorescent-antibody methods. Instead of observing the end product fluorescence, one floods a slide with a peroxidase substrate and observes the development of color where the antibody molecule fixes to the antigen. Peroxidase tests have been most extensively used for examination of tissue specimens in the pathology laboratory. A variation of the peroxidase system is the use of biotin-labeled antibody. An avidin molecule to which a signal such as a fluorochrome or an enzyme is attached is used to produce a signal (1, 6).

ELECTRON MICROSCOPY

Principle

As previously discussed, the resolving power of a microscope is directly related to the wavelength of light passing through the specimen. It was obvious throughout the 20th century that to improve on the performance of the light microscope, one could use a beam of electrons as the source of illumination. The wavelength produced by the electron beam would be on the order of 10^4 to 10^5 shorter than UV light and therefore decrease the resolution from 0.2 μm in the light microscope to 0.0005 μm in the electron microscope. In the late 1940s the first electron microscopes were constructed, and by the 1960s their availability was widespread. In the 1970s, techniques amenable to clinical laboratory testing, especially in the diagnosis of viral infections, became available. Along with the major advantage of the marked increase in resolution came one disadvantage: the electron microscope cannot examine living cells. Moreover, the preparation process creates artifacts that may make certain specimen types difficult to assess.

Electron microscopy

Figure 4 presents a comparison of bright-field and electron microscopy. In principle, the two types are similar. The illumination source in the electron microscope is a tungsten filament that is heated in a vacuum (similar to a light bulb), and electrons are emitted. Rather than having lenses to focus light, the electron microscope has magnetic coils to direct the electron beam. Analogous to a condenser, the electron microscope has a set of magnetic coils near the tungsten filament to capture and focus the electron beam onto the specimen. This focused electron beam passes through the specimen just as light passes through a specimen in bright-field microscopy. Dense areas of the specimen absorb and retard the electron beam, whereas less dense material permits the beam to pass unmodified. After passing through the specimen, the beam is refocused through a second series of magnetic coils, analogous to the function of objective lenses in the light microscope. After this refocusing, the beam is magnified by a third series of magnetic coils (projector coils) and directed to a screen, where the image can be observed visually and transferred to film. The screen is coated with a phosphorous compound that fluoresces upon contact with the electron beam.

There are two types of electron microscopes: transmission and scanning. Transmission electron microscopy utilizes an electron beam traveling directly through the specimen. A two-dimensional image of the specimen results. A scanning electron microscope uses modified electron beams to generate a three-dimensional image of the specimen. Only transmission electron microscopy currently is useful clinically.

Because the electron microscope utilizes differences in electron density of the specimen to create images, specimen preparation is unlike that for bright-field microscopy. In electron microscopy, contrast is created by treating specimens with chemicals to accentuate electron density differential. There are three basic means of preparing specimens for the electron microscope. First, one can negatively stain the specimen. In

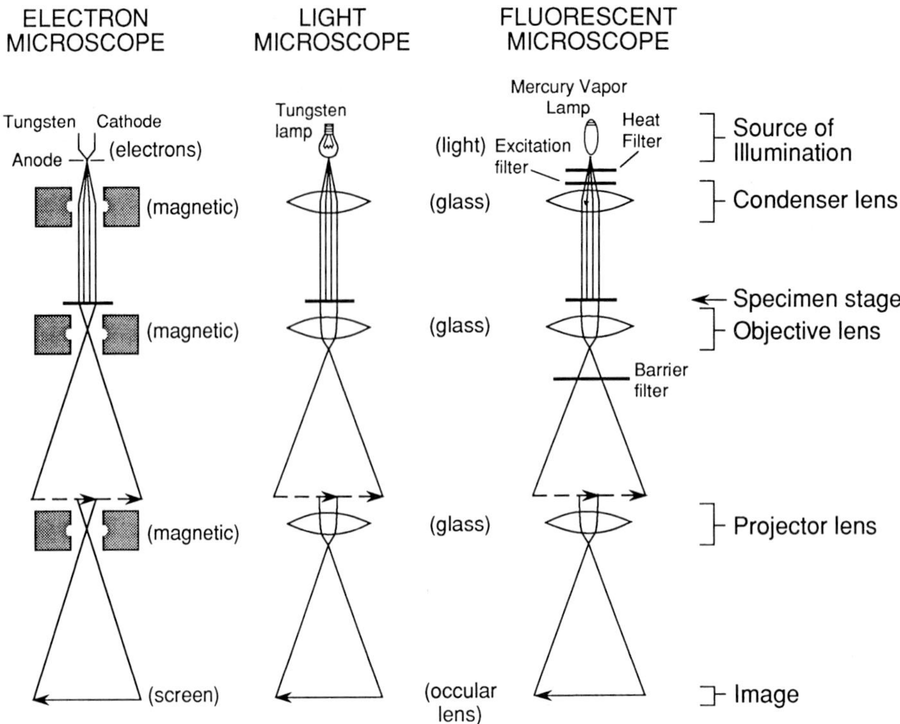

FIG. 4. Comparison of the essential components of the major types of microscopes: electron, light, and fluorescence.

this process, the background is stained with a heavy metal such as uranium or gold, leaving the actual target free of the metal. When an electron beam is directed through the negatively stained specimen, the target microbe appears light and the background appears dark. The second means of preparing specimens for the electron microscope involves freeze-etching. Here, the specimen is quickly frozen. This supercooling results in fractures along the lines of planes within the specimen. These planes separate when fractured, usually by physical impact. The third means of preparing specimens utilizes thin-sectioning techniques in which the specimen is treated with fixative material such as osmium tetroxide or glutaraldehyde, put through a dehydration process, and finally impregnated with epoxy resins so that sections as thin as 0.03 μm can be prepared. These thin sections can be further treated with a heavy metal such as uranium or lead to increase the contrast between the dense and less dense areas (7, 8).

Clinical utility

The clinical utility of the electron microscope has generally been confined to the diagnosis of viral infections (see section VII).

DIRECT EXAMINATION OF SPECIMENS

The first step in processing virtually all clinical material is microscopic examination of the specimen. Direct examination is a rapid, cost-effective diagnostic aid. Methods for direct examination are aimed at identifying microorganisms, enumerating the human cellular elements present, or observing certain biochemical, physiologic, or serologic characteristics. Visible microorganisms may indicate the presumptive etiologic agent, guiding the laboratory in selecting appropriate isolation media and the physician in empirical antibiotic therapy. The quality of the specimen and extent of the inflammatory response can also be evaluated (2).

We express our appreciation to Christine Kontnick and Linda Post for review of the manuscript and to Shirley Neill for its preparation.

LITERATURE CITED

1. **Balows, A., and W. Hausler.** 1988. Diagnostic procedures for bacterial, mycotic and parasitic infection, 7th ed. American Public Health Association, Washington, D.C.
2. **Bartlett, J., N. Brewer, and K. Ryan.** 1978. Cumitech 7, Laboratory diagnosis of lower respiratory tract infections. Coordinating ed., J. A. Washington II. American Society for Microbiology, Washington, D.C.
3. **Bloom, W., and D. Fawcett.** 1975. A textbook of histology, 10th ed. The W. B. Saunders Co., Philadelphia.
4. **Campbell, M., and J. Stewart.** 1980. The medical mycology handbook. John Wiley & Sons, Inc., New York.
5. **Emmons, C., C. Binford, K. J. Kwon-Chung, and J. Utz.** 1977. Medical mycology, 3rd ed. Lea & Febiger, Philadelphia.
6. **Finegold, S., and E. J. Baron.** 1986. Bailey and Scott's diagnostic microbiology, 7th ed. The C. V. Mosby Co. St. Louis, Mo.
7. **Glauert, A. M. (ed.).** 1975. Practice methods in electron microscopy. North-Holland Publishing Co., Amsterdam.

8. **Holt, S. C., and T. J. Beveridge.** 1982. Electron microscopy: its development and application to microbiology. Can. J. Microbiol. **28:**1–53.
9. **Koneman, E., S. Allen, V. R. Dowell, Jr., W. Janda, H. Sommers, and W. Winn, Jr.** 1988. Color atlas and textbook of diagnostic microbiology, 3rd ed. J. B. Lippincott Co. Philadelphia.
10. **Lillie, R. D.** 1977. H. J. Conn's biological stains, 9th ed. The Williams & Wilkins Co. Baltimore.
11. **Quesnel, L. B.** 1971. Microscopy and microtomy, p. 2–103. *In* J. R. Norris and D. W. Ribbons (ed.), Methods in microbiology, vol. 5a. Academic Press, Inc. (London), Ltd., London.
12. **Slayter, E. M.** 1970. Optical methods in biology. John Wiley & Sons, Inc., New York.
13. **Spencer, M.** 1982. Fundamentals of light microscopy. Cambridge University Press, New York.
14. **Wren, L. A.** 1963. Understanding and using the phase microscope. Unitron Instrument Co., Newton Highlands, Mass.

Chapter 5

Quality Assurance in the Clinical Microbiology Laboratory

RAYMOND C. BARTLETT

Passage of the Clinical Laboratory Improvement Act in 1967 focused attention on control of error in the testing of laboratory specimens. Supporting federal regulations developed by the Centers for Disease Control and adopted by the Health Care Financing Administration (HCFA) have required many procedures and materials to be closely monitored over the past 20 years (42 CFR part 74, 1968; 42 CFR part 74, 1979). Agencies such as the College of American Pathologists (CAP), the Joint Commission on Accreditation of Healthcare Organizations (JCAHO), the American Association of Bioanalysts, and others were required to follow the federal regulations in their inspection and accreditation of laboratories. Increasingly, questions arose in the minds of many laboratory scientists regarding the usefulness of some of the required procedures.

In 1982, a study of the cost effectiveness of such monitoring activities was reported which proposed changes that would reduce the cost of internal quality control in microbiology (2). Appendix C of the interpretive guidelines written by HCFA to provide details of expected quality control activity were repeatedly revised, and the frequency of required monitoring of many items was gradually reduced. Simultaneously, CAP, JCAHO, and other inspecting and accrediting agencies revised their standards to conform to the HCFA revisions. Recently, HCFA published proposed revisions of regulations (42 CFR part 74, 1988) which reflected the changes that have occurred in their interpretive guidelines. The proposal included use of recommendations of the National Committee for Clinical Laboratory Standards (NCCLS) for monitoring of culture media and antimicrobial susceptibility tests (21–23). Laboratory directors should obtain copies of the federal regulations, the NCCLS publications, and appendix C of the HCFA interpretive guidelines.

DEFINITION OF QUALITY

During the last 5 years, the application of quality control principles has shifted to a much broader aspect of health care than the monitoring and correction of deficiencies detected in processing and analyzing specimens. This has led to the use of a new term, "quality assurance." "Quality" is an elusive term. Donabedian has been the major contributor to a modern appreciation of quality assurance in health care (8–15). He stated, "The balance of health benefits and harms is the essential core of a definition of quality" (10). Much quibbling over semantics can be applied to the terms "control," "assurance," and "assessment." "Control" implies that we have the authority to establish the level of quality that will be provided. "Assurance" suggests that we will guarantee that quality (presumably the best that we can achieve) will be provided. Either will be true only within the limits of available laboratory resources. "Assessment" suggests only that we will measure the level of quality. It will be a separate process, often involving hospital administration, representatives of clinical departments, and perhaps government to determine how resources will be redistributed to ensure a uniform standard of quality throughout the institution or health care system.

INDUSTRIAL APPROACHES TO QUALITY

National and international competition has led industry to critically reexamine how products are manufactured, the waste that errors and deficiencies introduce into production, and how customer satisfaction with quality and price affects them. Crosby has defined quality as "conformance to the requirements" of customers (7). Harrington stated that quality is "meeting or exceeding customer expectations at a cost that represents value to them" (18). Feigenbaum (17) divided the cost for attaining quality performance between (i) the cost for prevention of error and (ii) the cost for appraisal of error rates and corrective action. The costs of not conforming to a competitive standard of quality are (i) internal, resulting from repeating work on a product before it is released, and (ii) external, resulting from complaints of failure of the product from customers requiring replacement and loss of marketing position and sales. These authors and others, including Juran (20) and Deming (27), have emphasized prevention of error rather than dependence on monitoring and corrective action for control of error. Quality control activity in clinical laboratories over the last 30 years has focused primarily on monitoring and corrective action. These authors have shown in industrial settings that a program that emphasizes prevention is less costly. As more time and effort are spent on prevention, the number of errors decreases and the cost of monitoring and corrective action decreases.

How can we introduce prevention as a quality assurance strategy? The key is participative management. Before tests are offered, the laboratory director should establish a quality council, or team, to ensure that the procedure is understood by persons responsible for the entire spectrum of activity related to the test, beginning with (i) ordering of the test by physicians, (ii) collection and transport, (iii) analysis, (iv) reporting and interpretation of results, and (v) the impact on diagnosis and treatment. This process should include establishing criteria for the clinical necessity for the test and the times that it will be available. Although the director must take the initiative to establish such teams, he or she must not dominate the discussion or suppress the free flow of ideas offered by the group. Such teams will be more successful if they are led by someone with some training in facilitation of group discussion; the director need not be the facilitator. The goal should be to establish error-free performance. Such a systematic approach should be applied over a reasonable period of time to all services and procedures offered.

QUALITY AND COST

As discussed above, industry has found that cost is inextricably related to quality. Donabedian has described optimally effective care as care that results from the maximum achievement of benefits at the least increase in cost (15). Physicians and almost everyone else in the health care field over the last 50 years assumed that expenditure on new technology would always improve the quality of care. It was considered difficult or impossible to determine the point at which progressive increase in cost and declining relative benefit would be reached, dictating the limit at which additional expenditure should be allowed. Now we are in an intense climate of cost containment that will tighten further, requiring that increasing scrutiny be applied to how resources can be redistributed to ensure that a relatively uniform level of quality is provided throughout the range of services offered. It is no longer a question of ensuring that we offer the maximum that technology can provide; we must determine that the cost of laboratory service provides a benefit for patient care that is commensurate with the costs and benefits of other services.

COMPETITION, COST, AND QUALITY: GOVERNMENT VERSUS THE PRIVATE ESTABLISHMENT

Attention to quality is being intensified by cost containment and competition. Provision of health care services may be directed more toward private enterprise than toward government. This redirection offers major opportunities to preserve quality while achieving maximum efficiency through competition. But as commercial organizations enter into the provision of health care, including laboratory services, there is great danger that quality will decline as a result of overzealous effort to reduce cost. Contrary to the impulsive negative reactions of many clinicians and laboratory scientists toward quality assurance activity, this is no time to abhor the trend toward introduction of programs for prevention of error as well as systematic and objective measurement of quality. The quality of our contribution to care of the patients of the future may become significantly compromised without a means to provide objective evidence of its deterioration.

STRUCTURE, PROCESS, AND OUTCOME

Donabedian has classified the basic elements of quality assurance into three classes of activities: structure, process, and outcome (8–15).

Structure

"Structure" constitutes the human and physical resources of a health service facility, including personnel, space, equipment, and standards of practice. Systematic monitoring of all aspects of structure must be conducted to detect deficiencies and apply corrective action. This monitoring encompasses recruitment of personnel, basic educational programs, forms of participative management designed to prevent error, continuing education programs, and the status of licensure of all personnel. It is important to monitor the workloads and productivity of personnel to ensure that staffing is adequate by comparison with peer institutions. Such comparison is afforded by participation in the Workload Recording Program of CAP (6). Calculation of available space and comparison with peer institutions may be accomplished with reference to the *Manual for Laboratory Planning and Design* published by CAP or the excellent analyses of space and personnel requirements reported by Elin and co-workers (5, 16). Failure to plan for future space requirements will compromise any other attempts to improve the quality of services provided. An inventory of all equipment should be maintained, with a detailed history of maintenance and repair to provide supporting justification for replacement. A schedule for regular replacement of capital equipment should be established.

The standards of practice include (i) the availability of services, especially those provided during evenings and weekends and on a stat basis, and (ii) the procedure manuals that define the full spectrum of collection, transport, and processing of specimens and the reporting and posting of information. The assessment of the adequacy of these functions will determine both licensure and accreditation and thus constitutes a solid basis for the capability of the institution to render a quality product. Thus, quality assurance has its basis in ensuring an appropriate structure for the institution.

An important element of structure is the reimbursement status of the institution. Periodic reassessment of the modes of reimbursement and the extent of discounts being rendered to various third-party payers must be regularly assessed to ensure the economic health of the institution. Loss of reimbursement through poor planning, errors in billing, and failure to take advantage of all reimbursement mechanisms will undermine the institution and compromise quality.

Process

"Process" is defined as the activities conducted by physicians and other health care workers to provide care for patients. With respect to the laboratory (Fig. 1), process includes (i) the criteria supporting test requests by physicians, (ii) collection, labeling, and transport of specimens, (iii) evaluation of the specimens and subsequent testing in the laboratory, (iv) the extent of work performed on specimens, (v) the procedures conducted to verify the accuracy and reproducibility of results, (vi) reporting of information in an organized and legible manner to the physician, and (vii) appropriate use of the information by the physician for diagnosis and treatment. This is a much broader concept of process than was applied in the 1960s and 1970s, when quality "control" focused almost exclusively on testing of specimens in the laboratory. I will return to process after considering outcome in some detail.

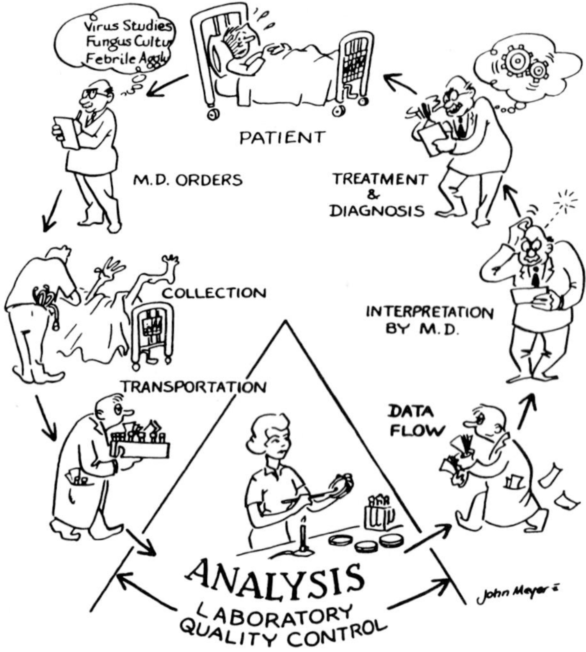

FIG. 1. Process in the laboratory. Quality assurance requires monitoring and corrective action throughout the full cycle of health care process conducted by a wide range of workers, including physicians and laboratory scientists.

Outcome

The ultimate outcome of a health care service is the length and quality of life that is provided for the patient. (It could be argued that the ultimate outcome is the beneficial impact on society, generally, nationally, or internationally. Extraordinary expenditure of health care resources may provide a superior outcome for individuals but may threaten the welfare of the whole by limiting the access of others to the system [19].) After treatment, does the patient enjoy a productive and satisfying existence, or are there repeated hospitalizations, chronic illness, discomfort, and despair? We are being told that quality assurance must focus on outcome. It would be extremely difficult to measure the degree to which clinical laboratory services in general or any particular laboratory test influences the ultimate outcome. To provide an extreme example, let us propose that all hospital admissions be randomized according to history number. Microbiology specimens from patients with even numbers would be handled very differently from those of patients with odd numbers. Only one variable could be studied simultaneously. For microbiology, this variable could represent a comparison of the rapid turnaround time made possible by new, rapid techniques with that obtained by using conventional, slower methods. Other variables could be omission of Gram-stained direct smear reports, reporting of very abbreviated culture information, or substantial differences in reporting of antimicrobial susceptibility data. After about 5 years of follow-up, a careful statistical comparison of patients matched for diagnosis, sex, and age might determine significant differences in the ultimate outcome resulting from differences in the laboratory practice applied to the two groups. Clearly, such studies would take years to perform, and it would be considered unethical to deprive some patients of information and service that is generally considered state of the art for patient care. Instead, we can address a more immediate outcome in terms of the morbidity, length of stay, and mortality of a recent hospitalization. Also, the effect that variables in process might have on immediate outcome could be assessed more quickly. Another aspect of outcome that can be assessed is the patient's satisfaction with laboratory services.

THE PATIENT'S PERCEPTION OF QUALITY AS AN ELEMENT OF OUTCOME

The perception of patients of the quality of care is viewed by some as an expression of outcome. This is more obvious in the outpatient environment. Here the attractiveness of the collection site, free parking, speed of specimen collection, and the courtesy they receive are important. Certainly with respect to marketing health care as a product, the satisfaction of the patient would be considered an important outcome. The relevance of such satisfaction to the true outcome may be uncertain. The fact that a patient views more convenient parking as a superior service may not mean that choosing a laboratory on that basis will ensure a superior health care outcome. Physicians who receive frequent complaints from their patients about laboratory collection facilities may send their patients elsewhere. Laboratories should consider providing explanatory information in lay language to assist patients in understanding the significance of microbiologic tests, as is often provided to help patients understand lipid profiles. In the near future, it may be expected that patients will be offered the option of ordering tests on themselves without having to go through a physician. Laboratories also should consider providing home testing kits and instruments for use by patients rather than lose this business to pharmacies and other providers of laboratory test kits. We must be cautious about the effect on the ultimate outcome of focusing too much attention on patient satisfaction. We must educate both the care giver and the patient with respect to the approach to testing that ensures a superior health care outcome, even though both may consider the convenience and rapid access to kits and tests to be of greater immediate interest.

INDICATORS OF OUTCOME

We need to consider the use of indicators of outcome rather than outcome itself to assess the quality of service because it is so difficult to measure both immediate and ultimate outcome. Indicators represent selected activities (aspects of process) that appear to have a conspicuous bearing on outcome. Turnaround time is one example. Could we assume, for example, that erroneous biochemical or serologic tests resulting in misidentification of *Shigella sonnei* as *Shigella boydii* would have less impact on patient care than would a system that requires an extra 2 days to put any report of the isolation of *Shigella* sp. on the medical record? This does not mean that we can ignore monitoring of internal laboratory process. Outcome does depend on the quality of internal laboratory process, but a favorable outcome cannot be ensured only by the monitoring and correction of errors in internal laboratory process.

An indicator that may bear a close relationship to the health care outcome is the perception of patient care givers of the quality of laboratory service. In the past, most pathologists and laboratorians tended to focus on the accuracy and reproducibility of tests performed, taking a rather indifferent attitude toward complaints and reports of inconveniences experienced by patient care givers. Laboratories providing services for outpatients and physician offices have long focused on the need to provide services that satisfy users because of a competitive environment. Laboratory scientists should appreciate that commercial laboratories are providing laboratory services in some hospitals in many parts of the United States, and this trend may continue. Laboratorians who neglect their users may find themselves without the support of those users when a representative from an aggressive commercial laboratory organization approaches the hospital administration, offering to provide the services at less cost and create greater user satisfaction.

As a general principle, we should operate our laboratories as though we were in competition with another laboratory within the same hospital or community. It may be useful to conduct a survey of care giver perception of services such as are available from professional management consultants who perform attitude surveys within hospitals. Items that invoke a consistently negative reaction among care givers should result in corrective action, and a subsequent survey should be conducted to determine whether the action was effective.

ELEMENTS OF PROCESS ASSOCIATED WITH ORDERING, COLLECTION, AND TRANSPORT AS INDICATORS OF OUTCOME

Process associated with ordering, collection, and transport of specimens involves accurate transcription of orders, ordering rationale, site selection for specimen collection, site preparation, use of proper containers, labeling of slips and containers, and transport within the specified time. These components probably influence outcome more than components of internal laboratory process. A standard of JCAHO states, "As a part of the hospital's quality assurance program the quality and appropriateness of pathology and medical laboratory services are monitored and evaluated, and identified problems are resolved." This requirement has created much controversy. Many laboratorians do not believe that it is their responsibility to monitor the rationale behind physician ordering practices. It becomes increasingly apparent that some mechanism must be developed to examine the rationale behind laboratory utilization. Although it may not be practical for microbiologists to undertake this effort by themselves, clearly a cooperative approach with clinical services is needed to identify conspicuous abusers. It is likely that third-party payers will threaten to disallow, and later will deny, reimbursement for laboratory utilization that departs from standards established by examination of the use patterns of peer groups. Criteria were developed in Connecticut by the Connecticut Peer Review Organization, operating under contract with Medicare, to provide a rational clinical basis for ordering urine cultures (Table 1). Random monitoring of urine culture requests was conducted in a number of hospitals, and in 50% of instances the patients' charts did not contain the minimum criteria agreed upon for justifying a urine culture. Consideration should be given to developing such criteria within hospitals through agreement between laboratory and clinical staffs. Subsequent monitoring could detect departures from these standards, which could be reported to department heads for corrective action. Other logical candidates for such surveys are sputum and blood cultures. Collection of more than three blood cultures for detection of bacteremia in association with any single septic episode should require a consultation between the ordering physician and the microbiologist. Conversely, single blood culture collections are not useful. An effective monitoring activity is detection of orders for single blood culture collections and query of physicians for the rationale for such requests. Physicians who order submission of any type of bacteriologic specimen on more than 2 consecutive days should be queried for the appropriateness of the request. Table 2 lists potential outcome indicators that could be usefully monitored.

The CAP checklist now places responsibility on the laboratory for accurate transcription of doctors' orders onto requisition slips.

The establishment of standards for specimen collection and transport are basic elements of structure. Failure to monitor adherence to these standards is a common deficit leading to compromise in the quality of specimens and their potential to produce useful information. Factors included are proper preparation and selection of a body site, use of the proper containers, proper labeling, and provision of necessary information as well as prompt transport. Transport that exceeds established time limits (usually 2 to 4 h) should result in a request for recollection or a request that the ordering physician consult with the microbiologist regarding processing.

These aspects of process probably are better indicators of the contribution of laboratory service to the outcome of health care than are many of the internal lab-

TABLE 1. Criteria for a urine culture

I. Symptoms or signs of urinary tract infection (UTI)
   A. On admission: one culture within the first 72 h
   B. Developing later: one culture when symptoms or signs appear
   C. One culture 48 h after beginning antibiotic therapy if fever persists
   D. After antibiotics have been discontinued in patients predisposed to UTI

II. Without symptoms of UTI
   A. One culture for female children previously uncultured
   B. One culture for other patients:
      1. With bacteriuria, pyuria, albuminuria, hematuria, or nitrites in urine
      2. With unexplained fever and no local signs or symptoms
      3. 48 h before genitourinary surgery if predisposed to UTI
      4. With fever within 48 h of genitourinary instrumentation
      5. With neurogenic bladder

TABLE 2. Errors in ordering rationale: potential outcome indicators

Blood cultures
Only one collection
More than three collections
Urine culture
Clean catch (see criteria in Table 1)
Closed catheter, frequency of collection
Wound and respiratory exudate contaminated with squamous cells and indigenous and colonizing bacteria; frequency of collection
Repeated consecutive daily submission of most types of specimens for culture
Material collected from inanimate objects or surfaces
Other specimens not likely to produce useful information
Mouth exudate (except for specific requests for Vincent's angina, *Candida* sp., herpesvirus, or *Treponema pallidum*)
Bowel content
Perirectal abscess
Colostomy drainage
Decubitus exudate
Pilonidal abscess
Foley catheter tip

TABLE 3. Laboratory process potentially related to outcome

Equipment
Daily monitoring of temperature-controlled devices and laboratory work areas
Centrifuge calibration
Rotator calibration
Preventive maintenance
Reagents
Follow NCCLS standards for media and antimicrobial susceptibility test materials (21–23)
Test all reagents when prepared or received
Test each day of use, using positive and negative controls: catalase, oxidase, coagulase; stains other than acid-fast bacillus and Gram stains; immunologic procedures except bacterial agglutinations
Test once a week: bacitracin, *o*-nitrophenylgalactoside, X-V disks, acid-fast bacillus stain, and Gram stain
Test once a month: antisera for bacterial agglutination

oratory process controls that we have preoccupied ourselves with for the last 20 years. CAP has introduced a program for distribution of "Q-probes," which will address the turnaround time for specific tests and other indicators of outcome. These indicators will need to be field tested to verify their importance as outcome indicators. JCAHO is now field testing indicators that have been proposed for monitoring the quality of clinical care in obstetrics and gynecology, anesthesiology, and emergency medicine.

PROCESS WITHIN THE LABORATORY

The rapid evolution of quality assurance has rendered most textbooks that address the microbiologic aspects of the subject moderately obsolete, with isolated exceptions (27). The following paragraphs emphasize aspects of laboratory process that may be important indicators of outcome (Table 3). Evaluation of specimens and control of the extent of work performed on them is important for optimizing the usefulness of information and minimizing cost (1). A mechanism must be established for notifying nursing care units, and physicians who order tests, of the need for consultation when processing of the type of specimen submitted will probably not produce useful information such as bowel content, exudate from decubiti, perirectal and pilonidal abscesses, specimens grossly contaminated with feces, Foley catheter tips, mouth specimens for bacterial culture, and inanimate objects not approved for culture by the Infection Control Committee. These specimens should be held in the laboratory at 4°C for some length of time that is agreed upon with the medical staff (5 to 7 days should be adequate) pending consultation. If consultation is not initiated during that time, specimens may be discarded.

Specimens from the throat should be cultured for group A beta-hemolytic streptococci only unless a specific search for other organisms such as *Corynebacterium diphtheriae* or *Neisseria gonorrhoeae* is requested. Exceptions to such guidelines can be made. Some of us have established programs in cooperation with clinical staff for monitoring colonization of the throat and other body sites of immunocompromised patients. In the hands of specialists, this information can be of prognostic value and enable prompt, effective treatment when symptoms of infection develop. Otherwise, some kind of control is needed to prevent reporting of information in settings where it may lead to inappropriate therapy. Use of the Gram stain will detect specimens of lower respiratory secretions and wound exudate that are excessively contaminated with squamous epithelial cells. These specimens are unlikely to produce useful information and will incur excessive expense for processing. Similarly, wound exudates that display on direct smear large numbers and mixtures of organisms suggesting gross contamination with fecal, oral, or vaginal flora should be considered inappropriate for culture unless isolation of specific organisms is requested. A more rapid and useful report may be rendered that indicates the Gram-stained smear findings and requests a consultation from the physician to discuss diagnosis and management of the patient.

Experience has dictated that the frequency of monitoring of equipment, reagents, and other materials originally specified in the federal regulations published in 1968 and 1979 is not cost effective for some procedures (2, 8, 25, 27). The recently proposed federal regulations (see above) contain revisions that agree quite well with the current requirements or recommendations of JCAHO, CAP, and NCCLS. These revisions include decreases in the frequency of monitoring of stable types of reagents and media and of antimicrobial agents incorporated in susceptibility testing systems (15, 23). A current unresolved problem is that of breakpoint susceptibility methods. These methods require use of a large number of control organisms or assay of the content of wells in trays or cards to verify accuracy. It is likely that new recommendations will place greater emphasis on manufacturer quality assurance of these procedures and deemphasize user quality assurance. A systematic procedure must be established for monitoring process, including such components as recording of delays or omissions in monitoring, numbers of deficiencies detected, appropriateness of corrective action, and recurrent deficiencies resulting from ineffective corrective action. Trends in these phenomena may be monitored and graphically displayed to show whether they are increasing or decreasing (Fig. 2). Personnel should receive acclaim when trends are downward. A corrective action program must be introduced when trends are upward.

Criteria should be established to limit the extent of work performed on certain kinds of specimens, at which point a consultation with the patient's physician will help to establish the clinical value of further microbiology effort. Such criteria are as follows: identification and antimicrobial susceptibility testing (ID/AST) of more than three pathogens without consultation; repeat ID/AST of same pathogens in daily sequential specimens; and selective reporting of AST results. It is unlikely that complete identification and testing of susceptibilities of more than three isolates will be more useful than empirical treatment of mixed infections. Unusual isolates that are difficult to identify and are of questionable pathogenicity from superficial body sites should be reported with limited identification, with request for consultation for further identification. Such isolates include most types of nonfermentative bacteria except *Pseudomonas aeruginosa* and *Acinetobacter calcoaceticus* from superficial body sites. Repeat complete identification and susceptibility testing need not be performed on isolates having the same gross colonial morphology in specimens received on consecutive days. As stated earlier, it would be useful to identify physicians who submit specimens on 3 or more consecutive days and request consultation for processing of any subsequent daily sequential submission. Reporting of susceptibility test results should be limited to drugs representing classes of antimicrobial agents as recommended by NCCLS (22, 23). Although multiple antibiotics may be tested in a panel, only those drugs useful for the treatment of the organism, or group of organisms, isolated should be reported. This will avoid confusing physicians with results of no clinical value and will avoid the potential reporting of an erroneous false-sensitive result such as *Klebsiella pneumoniae* susceptible to ampicillin (which has been described as a problem with some automated systems), resulting in potential improper use of this drug.

REPORTING

The importance of reporting laboratory data has been neglected. Reporting problems involving indicators potentially related to outcome include the following: organization, legibility, and format of reports; proper flagging of abnormal results; telephone calls for results; delay in posting results in medical record; reporting on or after the day of discharge; turnaround time, statistics, and routine matters (no preliminary report in 2 days; no final report in 5 days); and revisions.

The legibility and format of all laboratory reports should be reviewed with medical staff to ensure that they are optimum. The review should include the organization of reports in the medical record and the removal of outdated computer summary reports. As previously noted, the turnaround time between laboratory receiving and reporting of information is viewed as of considerable relevance to outcome. The average turnaround time may be calculated, but for bacteriology, a more important indicator may be the numbers of specimens for which no preliminary report has been rendered after 2 days and the number for which no final report has been rendered after 5 days (Fig. 3). In the Hartford Hospital laboratory, less than 2% of bacteriology specimens fall in these categories.

The number of telephone calls received for reports should be monitored, and the proportion that address information contained in reports that have been sent out should be determined. Points of delay in collation and transmission of reports should be studied to identify bottlenecks within the laboratory system. Other bottlenecks may occur in delivery of reports to patient care units or physician offices and the posting of the results in the medical record. It should be the responsibility of the laboratory to ensure that this latter process occurs in a timely manner.

There should be standards for critical values that must be flagged in a conspicuous manner. Physicians should

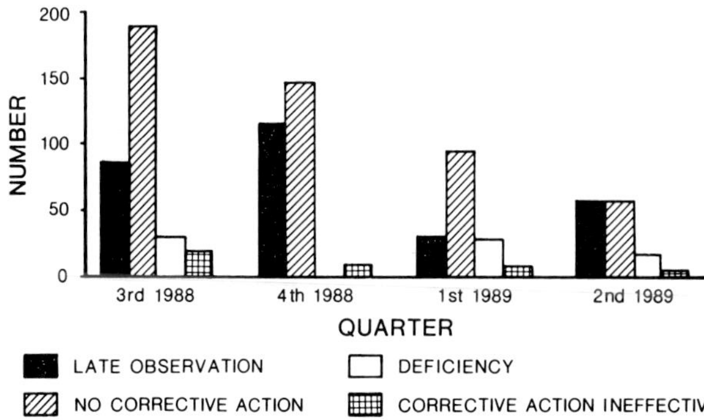

FIG. 2. Microbiology testing: total deficiencies. Trends in delays or omission in conducting surveillance (late observation), numbers of deficiencies found, failure to take appropriate corrective action, and recurrent deficiencies resulting from ineffective corrective action are ways of monitoring errors in process within the laboratory. (Data from the Hartford Hospital laboratory.)

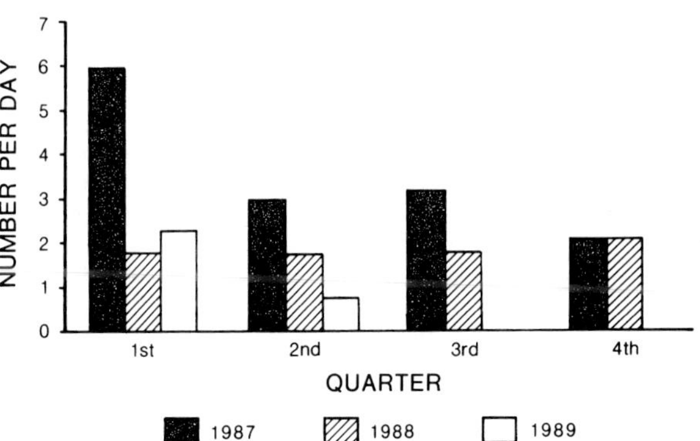

FIG. 3. Bacteriology reporting: no final report in 5 days. A downward trend reflects corrective action in numbers of bacteriology reports for which no final report is rendered in 5 days. This is a useful outcome indicator. (Data from the Hartford Hospital laboratory.)

be queried with regard to the conspicuousness of the technique used and whether they have actually observed specific critical values that have been reported.

Increase in effort to discharge patients earlier is increasing the frequency with which abnormal laboratory test results are reported on or after the day of discharge and are never seen by the physician. Some computer reporting systems detect this and report the information directly to the physician. An account should be taken of the number of reports that are received by the medical records department from patient care units after patients have been discharged. A procedure must be established to ensure that patients are not discharged when certain specified critical types of results are reported until they are reviewed by the responsible physician.

Revision of reports should be monitored (Fig. 4). A revision that involves updating of information, such as a change from *Pseudomonas* species to *Pseudomonas stutzeri*, is a desirable and acceptable revision. However, a change from a blood culture report indicating viridans streptococcus to *Streptococcus pneumoniae*, in which process the original reporting of the viridans streptococcus is obliterated, should never be permitted and constitutes falsification of the medical record. Correction fluid should never be used on laboratory reports. Revisions that represent improper use of computer reporting systems resulting in nonsense or unintended results should be monitored, and corrective action should be taken.

INCIDENT REPORTS

Useful indicators of outcome are the numbers and types of reports of departures that occur from expected performance, i.e., commendable performance, errors in performance, performance of care givers (collection, labeling, and transport), performance of laboratory (collection, labeling, and transport), laboratory processing, and laboratory reporting. These are usually called incident reports and are generally tabulated for both incidents connected with laboratory personnel and those associated with personnel outside the laboratory (Fig. 5). Typically, such incidents relate to labeling and handling of specimens, failure to follow procedures, safety violations, and uncooperative behavior. Unfortunately, little attention is given to commendable performance in most institutions. Recently, Berwick has drawn attention to the need to take a positive approach to improving performance instead of the prevalent use of inspection to find fault (3). In the Hartford Hospital laboratory, we have encouraged all personnel to submit reports of the commendable performance of others. The intent is to generate more commendable performance reports than incident reports indicating unsatisfactory performance. All commendable performance and incident reports should be reviewed by the microbiologist, who should acknowledge persons who exhibit exceptional performance as soon as possible, following the example of *The One Minute Manager* (4). Supervisors should discuss incident reports of unsatisfactory performance promptly with all involved personnel.

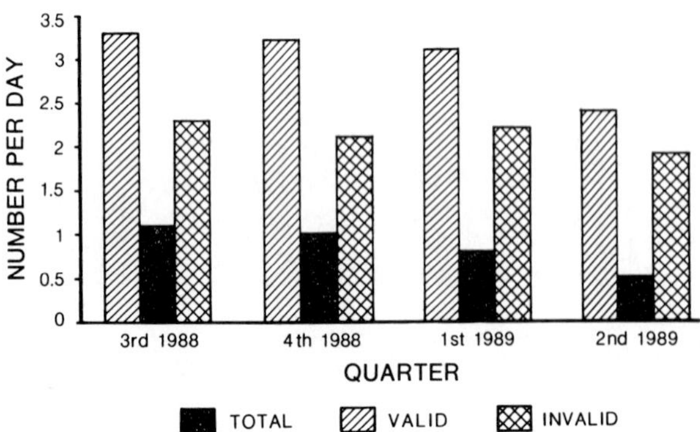

FIG. 4. Bacteriology reporting: revisions and validity. A decrease in the number of both acceptable and unacceptable revisions of reports is a favorable outcome indicator. (Data from the Hartford Hospital laboratory.)

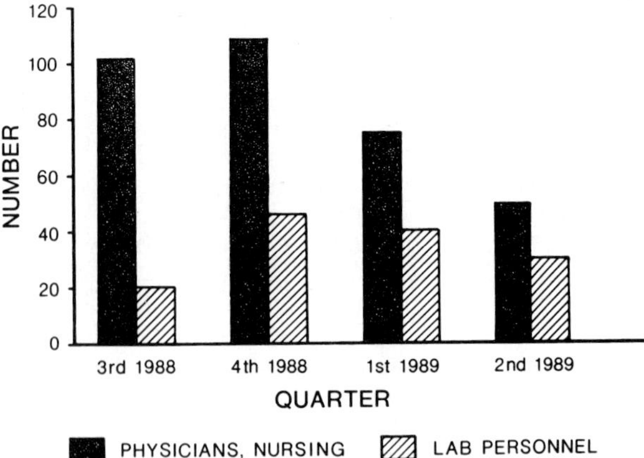

FIG. 5. Reporting of total incidents. Downward trends in incidents reflecting improper ordering, collection, and submission of specimens by physicians and nurses and a decrease in mistakes in processing by laboratory personnel are favorable outcome indicators. (Data from the Hartford Hospital laboratory.)

In summary, microbiologists should look on current trends in quality assurance as a means of ensuring adequate support for provision of services that will continue to produce high-quality health care. We must learn from the experience of industry, which has shown that placing the focus on quality rather than purely on cost ultimately reduces error and results in a more efficient and cost-effective operation. Attention also should be given to the outcome of providing health care; in practice, this will be accomplished by monitoring indicators of outcome. These indicators will represent aspects of process that include ordering, collection, and transport of specimens and the evaluation of their potential to produce useful information when received in the laboratory. The extent of work performed and the information reported should be controlled, with frequent requests for consultation from physicians when the usefulness of processing is in question. Monitoring of reagents, equipment, and testing procedures should be viewed as a small component of the full spectrum of activities that contribute to a high-quality health care outcome. The turnaround time and other aspects of the reporting of results should be monitored. More attention should be given to the perception of care givers of the quality of laboratory services.

LITERATURE CITED

1. **Bartlett, R. C.** 1985. Cost containment in microbiology. Clin. Lab. Med. **5:**761–791.
2. **Bartlett, R. C., C. A. Rutz, and N. Konopacki.** 1982. Cost effectiveness of quality control in bacteriology. Am. J. Clin. Pathol. **72:**184–190.
3. **Berwick, D. M.** 1989. Continuous improvement as an ideal in health care. J. Am. Med. Assoc. **320:**53–563.
4. **Blanchard, K., and S. Johnson.** 1982. The one minute manager. William Morrow and Co., Inc., New York.
5. **College of American Pathologists.** 1985. Medical laboratory planning and design. College of American Pathologists, Skokie, Ill.
6. **College of American Pathologists.** 1988. Manual for laboratory workload recording method. College of American Pathologists, Skokie, Ill.
7. **Crosby, P. B.** 1979. Quality is free. New American Library, New York.
8. **Donabedian, A.** 1966. Evaluating the quality of medical care. Milbank Q. **44:**166–203.
9. **Donabedian, A.** 1972. Models for organizing the delivery of health services and criteria for evaluating them. Milbank Q. **50:**103–154.
10. **Donabedian, A.** 1980. The definition of quality and approaches to its management, vol. 1. Explorations in quality assessment and monitoring. Health Administration Press, Ann Arbor, Mich.
11. **Donabedian, A.** 1982. The criteria and standards of quality, vol. 2. Explorations in quality assessment and monitoring. Health Administration Press, Ann Arbor, Mich.
12. **Donabedian, A.** 1983. Quality, cost, and clinical decisions. Ann. Am. Acad. Polit. Soc. Sci. **468:**196–204.
13. **Donabedian, A.** 1985. The epidemiology of quality. Inquiry **22:**282–292.
14. **Donabedian, A.** 1986. Criteria and standards for quality assessment and monitoring. Qual. Rev. Bull. **12:**99–108.
15. **Donabedian, A.** 1988. The quality of care. J. Am. Med. Assoc. **260:**1743–1748.
16. **Elin, R. J., E. A. Robertson, and G. A. Sever.** 1984. Workload, space, and personnel of microbiology laboratories in teaching hospitals. Am. J. Clin. Pathol. **82:**78–84.
17. **Feigenbaum, A. V.** 1987. ROI: how long before quality improvement pays off? Qual. Prog. **47:**32–35.
18. **Harrington, H. J.** 1987. The improvement process. The McGraw-Hill Book Co., New York.
19. **Hiatt, H. H.** 1975. Protecting the medical commons: who is responsible? N. Engl. J. Med. **293:**235–241.
20. **Juran, J. M.** 1988. Juran on planning for quality. The Free Press, New York.
21. **National Committee for Clinical Laboratory Standards.** 1987. Tentative standard M22-T. Quality assurance for commercially prepared microbiological culture media. National Committee for Clinical Laboratory Standards, Villanova, Pa.
22. **National Committee for Clinical Laboratory Standards.** 1988. Tentative standard M7-T2. Methods for dilution antimicrobial susceptibility tests for bacteria that grow aerobically, 2nd ed. National Committee for Clinical Laboratory Standards, Villanova, Pa.
23. **National Committee for Clinical Laboratory Standards.** 1988. Tentative standard M2-T4. Performance standards for antimicrobial disk susceptibility tests, 4th ed. National Committee for Clinical Laboratory Standards, Villanova, Pa.
24. **Smith, J. W. (ed.).** 1984. The role of clinical microbiology in cost-effective health care, CAP conference. College of American Pathologists, Skokie, Ill.
25. **Sommers, H. (ed.).** 1979. Clinical relevance in microbiology, CAP conference. College of American Pathologists, Skokie, Ill.
26. **Walton, M.** 1986. The Deming management approach. Dodd, Mead & Co., New York.
27. **Weissfeld, A., and R. C. Bartlett.** 1987. Quality control, p. 35–65. *In* B. J. Howard (ed.), Quality control in clinical pathogenic microbiology, vol. 3. The C. V. Mosby Co., St. Louis.

Chapter 6

Assessment of New Technology

JOHN A. WASHINGTON II AND GARY V. DOERN

The intent of this chapter is to present a discussion of those issues that should be taken into account when assessing new technology in the clinical microbiology laboratory. The first section addresses the general question, What factors are important when considering a new technique for implementation in the laboratory? Stated another way, when confronted with either a new and potentially useful technology or the perception of a previously unrecognized and therefore unaddressed clinical need, how does the clinical microbiologist decide whether to implement a new technique and if so, which one? The second section provides guidelines on how to design, conduct, and interpret the results of clinical laboratory investigations of a new technology. Emphasis will be placed on laboratory evaluations performed to assess the utility of a particular technology for implementation in the laboratory and, if desirable, to submit the findings for publication in an appropriate journal.

IMPLEMENTATION OF NEW TECHNOLOGIES

Arguably the single most important issue when considering implementation of a new technique in the laboratory is clinical justification; i.e., will the new technique have a desirable impact on patient care? Unfortunately, it is precisely this issue that is usually most difficult to define, quantitate, and address in an objective manner. The first step in considering any new technology should be an attempt to systematically examine its clinical impact. In some cases, soliciting the consensus views of clinicians likely to be affected by a new procedure is sufficient. In other instances, considerable data gathering is necessary. In either case, it is essential that clinical need first be defined as clearly as possible.

Having determined that a new procedure is clinically justified, it then is often important to assess which of several available techniques best satisfies the clinical need. Assume that it is determined that *Legionella* cultures are clinically warranted in a given care setting. The approach to this problem is relatively straightforward, since there exists a clear consensus as to how best to perform *Legionella* cultures. Nonselective media are inoculated with specimens unlikely to be contaminated with commensal bacterial flora, while both selective and nonselective media are used with contaminated specimens. Admittedly, decisions regarding sources of media, methods for identifying *Legionella* spp., and acceptable specimens have to be made, but selecting the basic culture technique is straightforward.

By contrast, consider the question of adopting a technique for detecting group A beta-hemolytic streptococci in upper respiratory tract secretions. Assume that a decision has been made to implement a direct streptococcal test. There are now over 30 commercially available direct streptococcal tests. Which one do you use? The most important consideration in answering this question is the ability of a particular test to meet a defined clinical need. In effect, what is the accuracy of the laboratory procedure? All laboratory procedures have inherent sensitivity and specificity. Test sensitivity is defined as the percentage of true positives that will be detected as being positive by the test or, stated another way, the probability that the test will be positive when the disease is present. Test specificity is defined as the percentage of true negatives that will be detected as being negative by the test or the probability that the test will be negative when the disease is not present. These parameters are largely a product of the test and will not vary greatly according to the population tested. They bear only indirectly, however, on the clinical utility of a given procedure.

The usefulness of a test in practice is a product of the predictive value of positive and negative results obtained through use of the test (3). With respect to disease diagnosis, the predictive value of a test is often used to determine how good a test is at confirming or ruling out a disease. The positive predictive value (PPV) of a test refers to the percentage of all positive test results that are truly positive or the probability that the disease is present when the test is positive. PPV is certainly influenced by test specificity, since the higher the specificity of a procedure (i.e., a low probability of false-positive results), the less likely it is that a positive test result will represent a false positive. The major determinant in the PPV, however, is the prevalence of what is being tested for in the population exposed to the test. The higher the prevalence, the higher the PPV, since there exist lower probabilities of false-positive test results in populations which have fewer true negatives.

Conversely, the negative predictive value (NPV) of a test refers to the percentage of all negative test results that are true negatives when a given population is examined or the probability that the disease is absent when the test is negative. The NPV of a test is influenced by test sensitivity. However, just as was the case with PPV, prevalence becomes the most important determinant; the lower the prevalence, the greater the likelihood of high NPVs. In effect, any test can be made to look good simply by changing the prevalence of the factor being assessed by the test in a given population. If a high PPV is desired, perform the test on a high-prevalence population (12). If a high NPV is sought, use a low-prevalence population.

Test accuracy is defined as the percentage of positive and negative results obtained with a test that are correct (3). As a result, a knowledge of the PPV and NPV of a test is essential in estimating the accuracy of a test. Since, as stated previously, predictive values are significantly influenced by prevalence, knowledge of prevalence becomes a central consideration. Furthermore, it should be clear from the foregoing discussion that use of predictive values to compare two different procedures is valid only when the predictive values of the two procedures have been calculated from studies performed on precisely the same populations or, at the very least, populations with the same prevalence of whatever is being measured by the test.

In general, procedures with high PPVs are desirable with conditions in which a false diagnosis can have profound consequences either because therapeutic modalities are not benign or because of the psychosocial or medical implications associated with a particular diagnosis. A good example of the last issue is the concern that must be brought to bear on new diagnostic tests for selected agents of sexually transmitted diseases. Obviously, the psychosocial and medical ramifications of a false-positive diagnostic test result can be profound.

By contrast, tests with high NPVs are desirable when you do not want to miss any positives. In this circumstance, one needs to be certain that the large majority of negative test results are truly negative. This would be the case, for example, with diseases that are readily treated but which could have fatal outcomes if not diagnosed and therefore not treated because of a false-negative test result. Similarly, screening tests, by definition, should have high NPVs.

The foregoing discussion of predictive value statistics has focused largely on procedures or tests that are used to achieve a diagnosis of a given infectious disease. It must be emphasized that the same logic and arithmetic can and should be applied to all procedures being considered for use in the clinical microbiology laboratory, irrespective of what their results are used for. This statistical analysis applies equally to an isolated biochemical parameter, an individual susceptibility test result, a general culture technique, or a specific direct detection assay. Any new procedure should be exposed to predictive value statistics as a means of defining its accuracy.

A third consideration when selecting a procedure or method for implementation in the laboratory is logistics. A great many factors must be taken into account when assessing test logistics: How technically demanding is the test? Does the laboratory have sufficient expertise to adapt easily and use the new procedure? Is the procedure similar to or compatible with an existing technique or technology? Does the new technique require instrumentation, and if so, what is the laboratory's capability of dealing with the required form of instrumentation? Does the instrument work, how reliable is it, and what are the nature and scope of maintenance arrangements that may need to be developed to ensure continued acceptable performance? If a commercial vendor is involved with the supplies or equipment necessitated by a new procedure, what is the quality of their product and how effectively do they provide service? What new quality control or quality assurance routines will have to be implemented as a consequence of a new procedure? What impact will a new technique have on work flow within the laboratory and on utilization of personnel resources? What are the biosafety ramifications of the new test? What effect will the new procedure have on existing laboratory procedures, both directly and indirectly? On what basis will the new procedure be implemented (will tests be performed individually or in batches)? If batch processing is selected, batch sizes and times of testing need to be addressed. Will the procedure be performed on a STAT basis? Does the laboratory have sufficient space with which to conveniently perform the new procedure? Finally, for those new procedures that generate patient results, consideration must be given to the issues of results reporting, i.e., when, how, and to whom will the results be conveyed.

A fourth major consideration is cost. At the very least, both direct costs (materials, personnel, instrumentation, service contracts, etc.) and indirect costs (institutional overhead, billing, space, etc.) should be taken into account. In addition, where possible, it is prudent to attempt to define what might be referred to as "ancillary" costs: what effect will a new technology or procedure have on other, apparently unrelated costs such as those associated with direct patient care, other departments within an institution (clinical pharmacy, other laboratory sections, etc.), or other activities within the microbiology laboratory? In this era of cost constraints in the health care industry, cost often becomes the primary determinant in decision making as it relates to new procedures.

For procedures that are billable and thus income generating upon implementation, revenue predictions are an important consideration in care settings where revenue remains a defined and desirable objective. The best example of such an environment is the private, independent, profit-making laboratory. When revenue is a motive, a major factor becomes profit margin (the difference between revenue and cost). It remains, however, that as the health care business in the United States has become increasingly influenced by prospective payment plans, revenue ceilings, and health maintenance organizations, expense rather than revenue has become an increasingly important consideration in adopting new technology in the laboratory.

A fifth factor to be taken into account when considering a new procedure for adoption in the laboratory is the requisite training of personnel before implementation. In some cases, the extent of personnel training necessitated by a particular procedure may be a determinant in the final decision as to which procedure to choose. In all cases, having finally selected a new test, a carefully constructed plan of action should be developed to ensure that personnel are adequately trained before the procedure is introduced.

Finally, once a new test has been selected and implemented, it is always appropriate to reexamine that test at defined intervals in the future from the perspective of the same factors used to make the original decision. Was the test, in reality, clinically relevant? Did the procedure selected effectively meet the perceived need? What were the real logistical impacts of the test? What were the real costs incurred by the test, and were revenue projections realistic? Finally, was the training undertaken when implementing the test adequate? The issue of initial training relates in turn to the question of the need for subsequent ongoing training and continuing education, perhaps as part of a quality assurance program. In short, it is not sufficient to select a new procedure, implement it, and then forget about it. Some effective means for ongoing monitoring of the test is essential.

The foregoing has been a brief discussion of the factors that should be taken into account when selecting and implementing a new procedure in the clinical microbiology laboratory. The issues that have been raised, although presented separately and in a particular order, are not mutually exclusive. Indeed, the relative weight given a particular issue will be determined by the specific procedure under consideration and the nature of the laboratory in which the procedure is being considered.

EVALUATION OF NEW IN VITRO DIAGNOSTIC TEST PROCEDURES

New and developing in vitro diagnostic techniques offer the potential of simplicity and speed, particularly for detection of microorganisms that have fastidious growth requirements or are simply not cultivable with currently available methods. In some instances, such procedures may obviate the need for culture of more common microorganisms and may therefore be suitable for tests performed in physician offices and perhaps ultimately in the home.

Regardless of where the test is performed, there are certain basic features of any new test that must be considered. As discussed above, it is first necessary to define how the test is to be used—as a screening test or as a confirmatory test. A screening test usually must be highly sensitive but may not have to be highly specific unless there is no confirmatory test available. On the other hand, a confirmatory test usually must be highly specific and may not have to be highly sensitive unless a screening test is not available. It is not always clear in the promotion of a new procedure whether its intended use is as a screening test or as a confirmatory test, and a decision to implement the test cannot be made on a rational basis without this knowledge.

Although their publication on test evaluation, performance, and use applied to human immunodeficiency virus (HIV) antibody tests, Schwartz et al. (10) proposed a number of components for test evaluation that have broad application to other tests. They categorized methodological problems with test evaluations as follows: (i) spectrum bias, (ii) use of an inadequate reference standard, (iii) failure in the case of immunoassays to use different cutoff points, (iv) referral bias, and (v) inadequate sample size.

Spectrum bias refers to the failure to consider the heterogeneity of diseased and nondiseased populations in assessing test performance (9). Accordingly, test sensitivity may vary according to the stage of disease at which the test is performed. In the case of HIV infection, these stages include recent infection, chronic asymptomatic infection, AIDS, and AIDS-related complex. As pointed out by Schwartz et al. (10), evaluation of an HIV test in patients with AIDS results in an overestimation of the sensitivity of the test.

An analogous situation may occur in the evaluation of rapid antigen tests for group A streptococci. If the test is used only with throat swabs from school-age children with sore throat, fever, enlarged tonsils with purulent exudate, and anterior cervical lymphadenopathy, it is likely that the sensitivity of the test will be overestimated, particularly if negative tests in which concurrent cultures yielding few colonies of group A streptococci are ignored. This last issue merits further comment. Negative results are often obtained with direct antigen tests for group A streptococci when tests are performed on individuals who yield small numbers of colonies on concomitant throat cultures. Manufacturers of direct antigen tests often imply that negative results in this setting represent true-negative and not false-negative results because patients with small numbers of group A streptococci in the throat, even though they may be symptomatic, are really only streptococcus carriers. That is, their symptoms are due to some other microorganism (e.g., viral); they just happen also to be colonized with group A streptococci. This logic, of course, will have the effect of increasing the sensitivity of the direct streptococcal test rather than decreasing its specificity. This logic is flawed for the following reasons. Although it is true that children with serologically confirmed (by anti-streptolysin O or anti-DNase B) streptococcal pharyngitis usually have more group A streptococcal colonies in throat cultures than those who do not have serologically confirmed group A streptococcal pharyngitis, it is also true that the seroconversion rates are equivalent (40 to 50%) when one compares groups of children and adults whose throat cultures yield light growth with those whose cultures yield heavy growth of group A streptococci (5, 6).

Additional variables affecting the sensitivity of rapid group A streptococcal tests are the populations studied, which often include nondiseased as well as diseased children and adults. Thus, technical factors aside, it should not be surprising that the reported sensitivities as such products vary from 45 to 100%. In most studies of group A streptococcal tests, it is not even possible to ascertain whether spectrum bias exists. In the case of HIV tests, Schwartz et al. (10) recommended that sensitivity be determined for the specific stages of the infection.

Spectrum bias may also affect the specificity of a test in that specificity may be overestimated if the test is not evaluated in noninfected patients with similar infections that are likely to be present in populations that are most likely to be tested (10). Although this has not proven to be the case with group A streptococcal tests, which have appeared to be highly specific in virtually all published studies, poor specificity has been described when antigen tests for meningococci and *Haemophilus influenzae* have been performed with concentrated urine and serum, particularly when such tests are performed with urine from patients without cerebrospinal fluid indices (polymorphonuclear leukocytes, decreased glucose, and elevated protein in the cerebrospinal fluid) suggestive of meningitis.

Reference standards are often problematic in clinical microbiology. Culture, whether it be for HIV, *Legionella* spp., or any other pathogenic microorganism, is often not 100% sensitive when compared with other test modalities such as serology. On the other hand, culture for certain pathogens, such as HIV and *Legionella* spp., is 100% specific. In contrast, culture is not very specific in the diagnosis of streptococcal pharyngitis since seroconversion (anti-streptolysin O or anti-DNase B) fails to occur in roughly one-half of culture-positive patients. Yet because of the lack of use of serology in the diagnosis of streptococcal pharyngitis, culture remains the reference standard for rapid group A streptococcal tests.

In this instance, however, the reference standard is far from perfect because there is still no consensus on what the standard method should be. Should the medium inoculated be nonselective or selective? Should incubation take place under room air, enhanced CO, or anaerobic conditions? Should cultures be incubated for 24 or 48 h? Is the identification of group A streptococci made presumptively (e.g., bacitracin susceptibility) or definitively by an extraction-serogrouping method? In general, however, the more selective and stringent the culture conditions, the greater the yield of positive cultures and the lower the sensitivity of the rapid antigen test. Moreover, the more vigorous the throat swabber, the more positive cultures and the more colonies per positive culture. Parallel issues exist with cultures for a variety of other pathogenic microorganisms.

Setting cutoff points can be problematic in immunoassays, since such assays are continuously scaled. Sensitivity and specificity are clearly affected by the definition of test reactivity so that in setting the cutoff point, it is necessary to weigh the benefits of true-positive and true-negative results against the costs of false-positive and false-negative errors (10). Selecting the arbitrary decision threshold as a function of various criteria for test reactivity and their effects on test sensitivity and specificity can be studied by receiver operating curve analysis (8, 11) and is illustrated in an evaluation by Lieu et al. (7) of a latex agglutination test for streptococcal pharyngitis. The best test may therefore be the one with the fewest false-positive results at any level of sensitivity, depending again on the objectives of the test, the prevalence of the disease, the cost of false-positive or -negative errors, and the availability of confirmatory testing.

An additional problem in assessing statistical parameters resulting from test evaluations is the extent to which the point estimates (i.e., sensitivity, specificity, and predictive values) that are derived from a particular study sample apply to the overall population. Confidence intervals give an estimate of the imprecision of the point estimates reported in a single study (4). The width of confidence intervals is markedly influenced by sample size as well as for percentages (proportions) near 0 or 100% (3). For example, for a test in which all of 15 samples tested (proportion or point estimate = 100%) are positive, the 95% confidence interval (CI) is 78 to 100%, in contrast with a test in which all of 245 samples tested (point estimate = 100%) are positive (95% CI = 99 to 100%). The 95% CI of 78 to 100% provides information on the precision of the test, which is that the true sensitivity falls within the range of 78 to 100% (3). In another example, if 152 of 245 (point estimate = 62%) samples tested are positive, the 95% CI is 56 to 68%, which is about 12 times greater than when 245 of 245 samples tested were positive, illustrating a characteristic of confidence intervals when percentages or proportions are near 50% (3). Thus, although a P value may demonstrate a statistically significant difference between point estimates of two tests, the 95% CI provides information regarding the (im)precision of each point estimate for the study sample.

Referral bias refers to the bias that may be introduced when an initially nonreactive or equivocally reactive specimen is retested with a different assay (10). In this instance, the sensitivity of the first test is underestimated, whereas that of the second is overestimated. Bias may also occur if equivocal or positive specimens assayed by one test are retested with a second test (10). In this instance, the specificity of the first assay is underestimated, whereas that of the second is overestimated.

One final consideration in assessing test performance is who did the evaluation. Most new kits or instruments are usually evaluated by skilled technical personnel who are motivated to carry out the evaluation as carefully as possible under optimum conditions. Once marketed, such tests are performed by people with a broad range of interests, training, skills, time, space, and responsibility. Use of the test may go beyond the indications listed in the package insert. Limitations listed for the test may be ignored. Who uses the test and how it is used are often unknown. Testing in the home raises additional issues. What level of credibility is accorded a disease-specific diagnostic test used in the home? Will therapy be instituted on the basis of the results of a disease-specific test used in the home, or will therapy be deferred until the test performed in the home is confirmed in the physician office laboratory or other laboratory? Although blood glucose monitoring is widely used in the home by diabetic patients, there is, according to an article in the *Wall Street Journal* (1), a very different perception among consumers between tests of a metabolic or physiologic function, such as glucose monitoring or pregnancy testing, and tests for presence of disease, such as those for occult blood or streptococcal pharyngitis.

In conclusion, many new in vitro diagnostic tests offer considerable potential for simplicity and speed in the diagnosis of certain infectious diseases. New technology is bringing more and more products to the market; however, new technology is not always synonymous with accurate technology when applied to the diagnosis of disease. Moreover, accurate technology may not always be cost-effective technology. Continued scrutiny of the performance characteristics of new products remains essential to their proper utilization.

Major portions of the second section of this chapter are from reference 13 and are reproduced with permission of the publisher.

LITERATURE CITED

1. **Agins, T.** 1988. Home test kits for serious ills fail to take off. Wall Street Journal, May 25, p. 25.
2. **Braitman, L. E.** 1988. Confidence intervals extract clinically useful information from data. Ann. Intern. Med. **108:** 296–298.
3. **Galen, R. S., and S. R. Gambino.** 1975. Beyond normality—the predictive value and efficiency of medical diagnosis. John Wiley & Sons, Inc., New York.
4. **Gardner, M. J., and D. G. Altman.** 1989. Statistics with confidence: confidence intervals and statistical guidelines. British Medical Journal, London.
5. **Gerber, M. A., M. F. Randolph, J. Chanatry, L. L. Wright, K. K. DeMeo, and L. R. Anderson.** 1986. Antigen detection for streptococcal pharyngitis: evaluation of sensitivity with respect to true infections. J. Pediatr. **108:**654–658.
6. **Komaroff, A. L., T. M. Pass, M. D. Aronson, C. T. Ervin, S. Cretin, R. N. Winickoff, and W. T. Branch.** 1986. The prediction of streptococcal pharyngitis in adults. J. Gen. Med. **1:**1–7.
7. **Lieu, T. A., G. R. Fleisher, and J. S. Schwartz.** 1988.

Clinical evaluation of a latex agglutination test for streptococcal pharyngitis: performance and impact on treatment rates. Pediatr. Infect. Dis. **7**:847–854.
8. **Metz, C. E.** 1978. Basic principles of ROC analysis. Semin. Nucl. Med. **8**:283–298.
9. **Rasohoff, D. F., and A. R. Feinstein.** 1978. Problems of spectrum bias in evaluating the efficacy of diagnostic tests. N. Engl. J. Med. **299**:926–931.
10. **Schwartz, J. S., P. E. Dans, and B. P. Kinosian.** 1988. Human immunodeficiency virus test evaluation, performance, and use: proposals to make good tests better. J. Am. Med. Assoc. **259**:2574–2579.
11. **Swets, J. A.** 1988. Measuring the accuracy of diagnostic systems. Science **240**:1285–1293.
12. **Vecchio, T. J.** 1966. Predictive value of a single diagnostic test in unselected populations. N. Engl. J. Med. **274**:1171–1173.
13. **Washington, J. A., II.** 1989. Evaluation of new in vitro diagnostic test procedures in clinical microbiology. Infect. Control Hosp. Epidemiol. **10**:77–79.

Chapter 7

Laboratory Safety in Clinical Microbiology

DIETER H. M. GRÖSCHEL AND BARBARA A. STRAIN

The safe operation of a clinical laboratory is one of the management responsibilities of the laboratory director and is ensured by compliance with the safety program by each laboratory worker. Heim, in one of the first textbooks on bacteriological investigation and diagnosis, published in 1894, advised laboratorians that burning, boiling, disinfecting, and cleaning of used materials must be done immediately after the completion of work and that the work environment must be kept clean (19). Despite such warnings, laboratory-associated infections have occurred, and some have resulted in death. Well-known examples are the physicians who lost their lives while studying rickettsial diseases: H. T. Ricketts (1910), S. J. M. von Prowazek (1915), and E. Weil (1922).

In 1949, Sulkin and Pike began to collect information on laboratory-associated infections from the literature and by mail surveys. By 1976, Pike had information on 3,921 cases (30). In 1979, he published a comprehensive review of the incidence, fatalities, causes, and prevention of laboratory-associated infections (31). These studies and the experiences in research laboratories, particularly those of the U.S. Army (29), led to the development of laboratory safety programs such as the one described in 1971 for what is now the Centers for Disease Control (CDC) (5) and the inclusion of chapters on biological safety in laboratory manuals such as the second edition of this Manual (22). These efforts resulted in an increased awareness of laboratory safety in microbiology laboratories but did not prevent all laboratory-associated infections. An example is the acquisition of typhoid fever from proficiency-testing specimens in Massachusetts (21). Increased concerns about laboratory-associated hepatitis B virus (HBV) infections enforced the safety concepts and extended them to blood banks and other specialties of laboratory medicine in the 1970s. A major revival of interest in laboratory safety was caused by the AIDS epidemic of the 1980s.

LEGISLATIVE AND REGULATORY CONCERNS

The risk of acquiring the human immunodeficiency virus (HIV) led to a series of recommendations by CDC beginning in 1982 (6). Universal precautions were introduced in 1987 (8), and the precautions were expanded to include other bloodborne pathogens in 1988 (9). The risk of HIV infection among laboratory workers was analyzed by Weiss et al. (40), and 25 cases of HIV infections associated with occupational exposure were summarized in the Occupational Safety and Health Administration (OSHA) proposed rules on occupational exposure to bloodborne pathogens (16). The interest of OSHA in bloodborne pathogens originated with the concerns of health care workers, especially in ancillary services, that precautions in health care institutions were insufficient for their protection. On the basis of the Occupational Safety and Health Act of 1970 (28), OSHA, together with the Department of Health and Human Services, first published an advisory notice on occupational exposure to HBV and HIV in October 1987 (12), which was followed by an advance notice of proposed rule making in November 1987 (14). A proposed rule and notice of hearing on occupational exposure to bloodborne pathogens was announced on 30 May 1989 (16). The proposed standard, to be added to 29 CFR part 1910, requires an employer of persons whose "reasonably anticipated duties may result in occupational exposure" to establish "a written infection-control plan designed to minimize or eliminate employee exposure." Universal precautions are to be observed, and engineering and work practice controls, including personal protective equipment, are to be examined and maintained. Policies for the handling of needles and other sharp instruments and adherence to good laboratory and housekeeping practices must be assured. Special requirements were set for HIV and HBV research laboratories and production facilities. Each employer is required to (i) make available to all employees at risk HBV vaccination and postexposure evaluation and follow-up, (ii) inform employees of the existence of hazards and provide appropriate training, and (iii) keep confidential medical and training records.

OSHA data (reference 16, p. 23085) show that current compliance with the basic requirements is high (around 90%) in dental and medical laboratories. One can assume that most clinical microbiology laboratories have had a high compliance rate for many years, especially since the training of microbiologists includes laboratory safety (1) and the voluntary inspection agencies such as the College of American Pathologists (4) and the Joint Commission for the Accreditation of Healthcare Organizations (24) include safety management in their inspection criteria and standards. Many states are also concerned about waste management of hospitals and laboratories (see chapter 25). Shipment of patient specimens and etiologic agents by mail and other carriers has been under scrutiny in recent years. Another aspect of federally mandated occupational safety and health plans is the Hazards Communication Act of 1984, which requires all employers to inform their employees about the potential dangers arising from exposure to chemicals and other hazardous materials (14).

Several recent publications can be consulted for additional details on establishment of a laboratory safety program (11, 17, 26, 27, 32–34, 38).

RISK ASSESSMENT

Our knowledge about the risk of laboratory-associated infections is rather limited, since there is no centralized state or federal reporting system. We base our risk assessment on data of Pike collected 10 years ago (31) and on data collected more recently, primarily by CDC and the National Institutes of Health (NIH), for HBV and HIV infections in the health care setting. Many procedures used today to prevent laboratory-associated infection were developed in the past 25 years, often in response to evaluations of laboratory accidents and subsequent recommendations by individuals or groups of laboratorians. Favero, discussing the changes in the education of laboratory workers in the past 10 to 20 years, the changes in laboratory technology and instrumentation, and the performance of laboratory testing outside of organized laboratories by untrained personnel, stated general concerns about laboratory safety and proposed a national program on surveillance of laboratory-associated infections (33). The proposed OSHA standard (16) will cover only bloodborne pathogens, not other bacteria, fungi, viruses, and parasites that present risk of infection to laboratory workers.

Epidemiologic considerations

Transmission of disease in clinical laboratories is not well understood, and a cause-effect analysis is often not possible. The methods of transmission and the routes of infection may be quite different from those known for an organism, and the infectious dose may be much higher than in a community-acquired infection (2). Nevertheless, epidemiologic principles apply, and risk assessment must be based on the classic factors of disease transmission: the host, the parasite, and the environment. According to recent OSHA statistics, there are 179,405 physician offices, 18,247 nursing homes, 5,983 hospitals, 4,916 medical laboratories, 29,706 outpatient care units, and 672 blood-plasma-tissue centers with about 250,000 laboratory workers (16). A previous OSHA profile of laboratories estimated a total of 370,000 employees in clinical laboratories (13). Among these personnel will be chronically ill persons with impaired immune defenses and persons with temporary systemic or local impairment. Some may be allergic to chemicals or microbial components. Although prudent employment practices usually require awareness of an employee's health and immune status, not all employers participate in employee health programs. In addition, laboratory tests are often performed by untrained personnel unfamiliar with the risks of laboratory-associated infections. Being unacquainted with basic safety measures, they are more prone to be exposed to and infected by pathogenic microorganisms.

In the clinical laboratory, a broad spectrum of infectious agents can be introduced with patient specimens. From the data of Pike (30, 31) and studies of pathogenesis, one can make a fair risk assessment for work with known pathogenic microorganisms, such as in research, teaching, or specialty laboratories. In the clinical laboratory, however, one is surprised to find different levels of safety consciousness during handling of the same patient sputum specimen in a mycobacteriology or a general bacteriology laboratory. Microbiologists are quite familiar with shigella infections occurring in laboratory technologists after they have handled a positive stool culture or with the skin test conversion of persons working with tuberculosis specimens or cultures, despite supposedly excellent precautions.

Information about infectious dose and route of transmission is available for many microorganisms encountered in clinical laboratories (16, 32, 39), yet the condition of pathogenic microorganisms in patient specimens, their ability to attach to tissue cells, their virulence, and their ability to multiply are usually unknown. Therefore, the general principles and methods of controlling laboratory-associated infections must be based on an assessment of probability of risk in the given environment.

In an organized laboratory service, much improvement has been realized in the past 20 years by preparing an environment that reduces the risk of disease transmission. Laboratory practices have been improved by providing biological safety cabinets and other equipment to safely handle patient specimens and cultures. Room ventilation, although not perfect in many laboratories, has been recognized as an important environmental factor, and sanitation has improved in response to the HBV infection scare. The greatest improvement was achieved by teaching personnel proper defensive behavior, the use of personal protective devices, and adherence to procedures that were developed with safety in mind. Laboratory organizations, voluntary accreditation programs, and federal regulations deserve recognition for their efforts in this area.

In devising appropriate control measures, the methods of disease transmission and the routes of infection must be analyzed. Direct contact with infectious material is possible at all stages of microbiological work. The use of protective devices, such as gloves and gowns, and hand decontamination interrupt this mode of transmission. Indirect contact usually occurs because surfaces of containers, work areas, or equipment are visibly or invisibly contaminated during transfer of a specimen or a culture and possibly also by the inadvertent use of a contaminated instrument or device. Although single exposure rarely causes transmission of disease, repeated exposure increases the risk and often indicates poor compliance with basic safety instructions. Good work habits and a decontamination-disposal program may interfere with this rather rare type of transmission. Common vehicles may be patient specimens, specimen containers, various liquids, grossly contaminated surfaces or instruments, and aerosols or airborne particles. Appropriate specimen procurement and handling criteria, plus environmental control and safety devices such as biological safety cabinets, closed centrifuge tubes, and facial masks, assist in prevention of transmission. Animal vectors can be animals used for diagnostic inoculations or serum production, or they can be nuisances present in the laboratory, such as mice, cockroaches, and insects. Adherence to protocols designed for the use of experimental animals and a good vermin and insect control program are necessary.

The classic routes of infection are still causes of laboratory-associated disease. Despite the rules about prohibiting eating, drinking, smoking, and application of cosmetics in the laboratory and the separation of food storage refrigerators from laboratory refrigerators, transmission by ingestion, probably by direct or indirect contact with the organisms, occurs. Twenty-three cases of typhoid fever were contracted from teaching or proficiency-testing specimens (21, 26). The number of cases of shigella infection acquired from patient or teaching cultures is unknown. Whereas *Salmonella typhi* requires an infectious dose of about 10^5 organisms, shigella can cause infection with 10^2 or fewer organisms (26, 39). Inhalation of infectious aerosols and airborne particles is generally considered a less likely route of acquiring laboratory-associated infections than is contact. However, one must consider the skin test conversion of workers in mycobacteriology laboratories, which occurs even in well-designed laboratories with appropriate containment facilities and air-handling equipment. Unfortunately, exact data are unavailable. The epidemiology of airborne laboratory infections is discussed in more detail by Mackel and Forney (25).

Much of our knowledge about transmission by inoculation comes from the CDC studies of HBV infections in health care workers (7, 26). Other bloodborne pathogens, especially HIV, are now of concern to laboratorians (6, 8–10) and regulators (12, 13, 15, 16). The risk of infection with HBV is still the highest of all laboratory-associated infections, possibly because patient blood can contain up to 10^8 virus particles per ml, whereas the concentration of HIV in blood is around 10^2/ml.

Penetration of intact skin by microorganisms is rare and usually involves organisms that can penetrate the skin in natural infection. Abraded, scratched, burned, or dermatitic skin, nasal and oral mucosa, and the conjunctiva, especially of contact lens wearers, are well-known portals of entry for a number of bacteria, fungi, and viruses. Mouth pipetting, aerosols, splashes, or hand-mucosa contact may bring organisms directly onto the mucous membranes. Today we are especially concerned about bloodborne viruses, such as HBV and HIV, that may be contained in human blood, serum, plasma, or other body fluids (10, 16).

Animal and insect bites are rare routes of infection, since animal inoculations are uncommon in modern diagnostic laboratories; in this country, exposure to infected insects may be limited to research laboratories.

RISK CATEGORIES

Guidelines, directives, and regulations are an important basis for risk assessment. However, day-to-day work cannot be governed by regulations and the like, since it is impractical to cover every situation. Songer's rules of reason (35) describe risk measurement by reasonableness:

1. Custom of usage or prevailing professional practice. The activities are generally recognized as safe but some of these formerly established activities may not be safe, for example, the practice of mouth pipetting.
2. Best available practice, highest practical protection, and lowest practical exposure.
3. Degree of necessity of benefit. Is the benefit worth the risk?
4. No detectable adverse effect. This could be an admission of uncertainty or ignorance.
5. Toxicologically (bacteriologically) insignificant levels. What may be insignificant today may be unsafe tomorrow.

When trying to establish reasonable safety measures and reach reasonable judgments, the microbiologist can consult the recently updated CDC-NIH publication on biosafety in microbiological laboratories (38). This document describes standard and special microbiological practices, safety equipment, and facilities at four biosafety levels. Statements are included for parasitic, fungal, bacterial, rickettsial, and viral (including arboviral) agents, and there is a special section on HIV. This informative guide, in combination with more detailed descriptions of hazards (26), enables clinical and public health microbiologists to assess the risks of laboratory operations.

Risk of laboratory infections with bloodborne pathogens

A recent document from CDC (10) summarizes the risk of virus transmission in the work place. The risk of HBV infection after exposure to blood by a needle stick or a cut is related to the probability that the blood contains HBV surface antigen, the immune status of the recipient, and the efficiency of transmission (infectious dose and route). The probability of HBV surface antigen positivity is 1 to 3 per 1,000 in the general population and increases to 5 to 15% in high-risk groups such as immigrants from certain parts of the world, patients of mental institutions, intravenous drug users, homosexual males, and household contacts of HBV carriers. Persons without prior HBV vaccination or postexposure prophylaxis have a 6 to 30% chance of being infected by a needle stick (7).

The risk of infection with HIV after needle stick exposure to blood of a person known to be infected with the virus is approximately 0.5% (8–10). The transmission rate is much lower than that for HBV, probably because of the lower virus concentration in the blood. OSHA estimates that approximately 4.7 million health care workers are at risk for HIV and that one- to two-thirds are at risk for HBV infection, depending on their immune status (16). The estimated frequency of exposure in this population is about 7,802/year. CDC (10) offers a hypothetical model for the risk of HIV infection after needle stick injury that may be useful for risk assessment (Table 1).

CDC estimates that 12,000 health care workers with occupational exposure to HBV will become infected each year, that 500 to 600 will be hospitalized, and that 700 to 1,200 will become HBV carriers. Approximately 250 will die from fulminant hepatitis, cirrhosis, and liver carcinoma. About 10 to 30% of medical and dental health care workers show serologic evidence of past or present infection (10).

As of September 1988, 3,182 health care employees were reported to CDC as having AIDS. In 5% (169 persons), the means of HIV infection was undetermined. Of the 44 investigated individuals, 18 reported exposure to blood or body fluids from patients in the 10 years before the diagnosis of AIDS, but none of the cases involved a patient with known AIDS or HIV infection. The case reports of 25 health care workers with HIV infection presumably acquired by occupational exposure are presented in a recent OSHA document (16), and a summary of the cases was published by CDC (10).

In the laboratory, blood droplets from splashes and aerosols can dry on work surfaces and instruments. HBV can survive in dried blood on environmental surfaces for several days. Drying high-titered HIV (10^7 tissue culture infectious doses per ml) causes a 1- to 2-log

TABLE 1. The risk of HIV infection after needle stick injury: hypothetical model[a]

Prevalence of HIV infection (A)	Probability of infection given needle stick injury with blood containing HIV (B)	Probability of infection given random needle stick (unknown serostatus) [A × B = (C)]	Probability of infection given 10 random needle sticks $[1 - (1 - C)^{10}]$	Probability of infection given 100 random needle sticks $[1 - (1 - C)^{100}]$
0.0001	0.001	0.0000001	0.000001	0.00001
0.0001	0.005	0.0000005	0.000005	0.00005
0.001	0.001	0.000001	0.00001	0.0001
0.001	0.005	0.000005	0.00005	0.005
0.01	0.001	0.00001	0.0001	0.001
0.01[b]	0.005	0.00005	0.0005	0.005
0.05	0.001	0.00005	0.0005	0.005
0.05	0.005	0.00025	0.0025	0.025

[a] From reference 10.

[b] For example, if the prevalence of infection in the population is 0.01 (i.e., 1 per 100) and the risk of a seroconversion after a needle stick injury with blood known to contain HIV is 0.005 (i.e., 1 in 200), then the probability of HIV infection given a random needle stick is 0.00005 (i.e., 5 in 100,000). If an individual sustains 10 needle stick injuries, the probability of acquiring HIV infection is 0.0005 (i.e., 1 in 2,000); if the individual sustains 100 needle stick injuries, the probability of acquiring HIV infection is 0.005 (i.e., 1 in 200).

reduction rapidly, but live virus can be detected for up to 15 days when left at room temperature and for up to 11 days when left at 37°C. Cell-associated HIV was recovered only up to 1 day (27). Experimental infection of simulated blood cultures showed that HIV can survive for 2 days in Middlebrook 7H12 broth and for 7 days in Columbia broth. HIV-infected cells without blood did not survive a holding time of 60 and 120 min in the Du Pont Isolator (20). If one considers the relatively low concentration of HIV in the blood of infected persons, one may assume that the risk of environmental transmission of HIV is low and that the housekeeping sanitation and disinfection routines now practiced are satisfactory (8, 9, 27).

For reviews of other bloodborne infections (e.g., cytomegaloviral and arboviral infections, viral hemorrhagic fever, syphilis, leptospirosis, borreliosis, brucellosis, malaria, and babesiosis) that may be hazardous to laboratory workers, the reader is referred to the OSHA proposed rule (16) and other literature (26).

SAFE HANDLING OF INFECTIOUS MATERIAL

Safe handling of patient specimens and microbiological cultures requires a personal attitude that is taught to every medical technology and microbiology student. Why do laboratory accidents still happen? An answer may be found in human behavior. Knowledge of behavioral factors helps to prevent unsafe acts and to make the work place safer. Two laboratory safety books (17, 26) contain chapters on human factors useful to laboratory supervisors and workers. An increase, actual or supposed, in the risk of laboratory-associated infection usually helps to heighten safety awareness.

Universal precautions

In 1987, CDC introduced the concept of "universal blood and body fluid precautions" or "universal precautions" to be applied consistently in the care of all patients and in the handling of blood and body fluid specimens (8). This approach, practiced for a number of years only for patients under blood and body fluid precautions (18), had been advocated for more than a decade as an effective way to reduce the risk of HBV transmission in clinical laboratories and blood banks. The arrival of AIDS, although the disease is rarely transmitted in the work place, was a strong motivating factor in revising existing safety programs and stimulated federal action such as the OSHA proposed rules (15). How do universal precautions affect the microbiologist? The National Committee for Clinical Laboratory Standards, in response to the CDC recommendations of 1987 (8), assembled a task force of experts in all areas of hospital laboratory sciences, who prepared a guideline for the protection of laboratory workers from infectious disease transmitted by blood and tissue (27). This document assists clinical laboratory scientists as well as anatomical pathologists in developing safety programs in accordance with universal precautions.

Blood collection

All blood specimens should be considered potentially infectious, and care must be taken not to spill blood in patient rooms, collection areas, and laboratories. Disposable paper covers in the work area help to absorb possible spills and are discarded as contaminated material in infectious waste containers. Gloves and protective garments (gown or apron) should be worn during venipuncture and the handling of blood. Needles and lancets must be dealt with carefully, especially with agitated patients, to avoid accidental self-injury (23). Great care must be taken when transferring blood from syringes to tubes or blood culture bottles because the chance of an accidental needle stick is very high. This precaution applies also to subculturing samples from incubated blood culture bottles. Blood and body fluids should not be forced from syringes into tubes or bottles in order to avoid popping of stoppers and spraying of contents. Needles should never be recapped by hand; needle recapping, removal, and protection devices are available commercially. Used needles and syringes must be discarded in needleproof containers for safe waste disposal. Many commercial designs are available, but one must ensure that they keep their integrity if they are to be decontaminated in a steam autoclave.

Bleeding of the venipuncture site should be controlled by exerting pressure with a sterile gauze pad; then the skin can be decontaminated with alcohol or iodophor, and an adhesive bandage can be applied. Before removing gloves, the venipuncturist should inspect the blood collection tubes for contamination on the outside. Any blood should be removed with an alcohol planchet before further processing.

Specimen handling

All patient specimens should be contained in a tightly closed, nonleaking solid container and placed in a secondary container such as a Zip-Lok bag for transport. The requisition should not be placed inside the bag so as to prevent contamination if leakage or breakage occurs.

The person collecting a specimen is responsible for removing any contamination of the outside of a primary specimen container with a disinfectant before sending it to the laboratory. Most laboratories will not accept containers with outside contamination.

Specimens stored on wards, in collection areas, or in the laboratory should be placed in a safe area (cupboard or refrigerator) that is clearly marked with the biohazard sign and identified as inaccessible to the public and not used for storage of food.

Specimens to be prepared for transport or divided in samples should be handled with gloved hands and on easily disinfected surfaces, possibly covered with a disposable mat.

Specimen transport

All specimens must be contained in a closed, leakproof primary container and a sealed secondary enclosure such as a plastic bag or cup. Transport personnel must be instructed in universal precautions and be familiar with spill cleanup procedures. When handling specimens, they should wear gloves and practice frequent hand washing. Transport carriers and carts should be routinely cleaned with a detergent-disinfectant. If mechanical devices such as pneumatic tubes or tote boxes are used for transport, the system must be tested to ensure that primary and secondary containers are not destroyed and do not leak. The receiver of transported specimens should inspect all primary and secondary containers for leakage or contamination before removing the specimen for further processing. The laboratory procedures should give clear instructions on how to handle contaminated or leaky specimens; usually, they are discarded.

Shipping of patient specimens and microbiological cultures

The shipping of specimens to reference laboratories by mail or other carriers has been under scrutiny for many years. Only recently, the U.S. Postal Service reviewed the "mailability of etiologic agents" (36, 37). Fortunately, the initial announcement prohibiting the mailing of etiologic agents was replaced by a proposed rule that "etiologic agents, etiologic agent preparations, clinical specimens and biological products" can be mailed "when their intended use is for medical use, research or laboratory certification related to public health" and when they are properly packaged. The amount of etiologic agents and etiologic agent preparations must not exceed 50 ml, and they must be packaged in a securely sealed and watertight primary container and a sealed and watertight durable secondary container with absorbent cushioning material. Several primary containers may be mailed in one secondary container as long as the liquid volume does not exceed 50 ml. These containers must then be enclosed in a shipping container of certain strength and must be labeled "etiologic agent/biomedical material" as required by 42 CFR part 72 (labels are available from label products companies; see also reference 35, p. 101 and 102). Clinical specimens and biological preparations may not exceed 1,000 ml per primary container, 2,000 ml per secondary container, and 4,000 ml per shipping container.

CDC is preparing a revised shipping regulation that should be available soon. For international shipment or importation of etiologic agents, one should consult with:

Centers for Disease Control
Office of Biosafety
1600 Clifton Road, N.E.
Atlanta, GA 30333
Telephone (404) 639-3883

Laboratory work practices

Each laboratory worker must be trained in safe working habits. The work place must be kept clean and uncluttered, and each employee must be responsible for disinfecting and cleaning the work area, for proper disposal of infectious material, for the use of personal protective devices, and for frequent hand washing. Eating, drinking, smoking, application of cosmetics, nail biting, and handling of contact lenses is not permitted in the work area. Pipetting is performed only with pipetting devices; centrifugation of specimens or cultures should be performed only in plastic or uncracked glass tubes with tightly fitting closures or in safety shields. Tissue grinding should be performed with approved, closed devices, preferably in a biological safety cabinet. Care must be taken when removing caps or stoppers from tubes or bottles; a plastic-backed paper wipe (Current Technologies, Inc., Crawfordsville, Ind.) placed over the top prevents splashes and aerosols.

Safety begins with the good laboratory practices of each laboratory worker. Initial orientation and training must be reinforced by continuing education and monitoring of compliance by the first-line supervisor. Unauthorized individuals, such as sales representatives and family members, should not be allowed in the work area of a microbiology laboratory. Authorized visitors, such as students and physicians, must be acquainted with basic laboratory safety rules.

SAFETY MANAGEMENT

The responsibility of management is to anticipate problems and to develop safety procedures and training programs based on present or potential hazards that may endanger personnel. Management must be committed to the goals of health and safety of the laboratory. Improved protection and promotion of employee health and safety are proportional to the participation of laboratory management in the planning and decision making related to laboratory safety (33). Employees must share the responsibility for their own safety and that of their co-workers once safety guidelines have been established.

Safety programs

Safety awareness should become habit and a way of life in the laboratory. Laboratorians must take the time to perform a procedure, no matter how urgent, in a safe manner, for it is as easy to work safely as it is to work dangerously.

Education is the keystone to effective safety programs. Educational activities should be provided to all persons who may become exposed to potential laboratory hazards. In addition to laboratory workers, these personnel include clerical support, maintenance, supply room, housekeeping, and other employees who may come into contact with laboratory operations.

All safety information should be in written form that is clearly understood and contained in a laboratory manual that is readily available at all times. The manual should include general information (emergency telephone numbers, proper apparel, personal hygiene, and first aid) as well as detailed policies and procedures based on the type of laboratory functions performed; it should be written according to established standards (4, 9, 27). The manual should also include specific guidelines about some of the following (26):

1. Universal precautions, with high-risk areas highlighted
2. Selection, preparation, and use of disinfectants for surfaces, spills, etc.
3. Spill cleanup
4. Location and permitted quantities of flammable compounds for daily use
5. Labeling and handling of flammable, caustic, toxic, carcinogenic, and radioactive materials
6. Storage and handling of compressed gas cylinders
7. Electrical safety
8. Control of aerosolization
9. Use and maintenance of chemical and biological safety cabinets
10. Use of steam autoclaves for both sterilization and decontamination

This list may be reduced or expanded, depending on the needs of the laboratory.

After policies and procedures have been written, they must be put into practice. Review of the safety manual and of the location and use of safety equipment should be done as part of the orientation program for new employees. If radioactive materials are used or stored in the laboratory, a radiation safety program should be included in the orientation. Further education should be an ongoing process on a regular basis to ensure that laboratory workers are always prepared and up to date. First-line supervisors must insist that safety procedures be consistently followed and should set good examples. Performance of work in a safe manner should be a part of each employee's job description, and failure to do so should result in a formal reprimand.

To help carry out safe practices and to keep all employees abreast of current regulations, a safety committee should be formed. Every laboratory, no matter what size, should have its own committee, and someone from the laboratory should be a member of an institution-wide committee. The committee should meet regularly to review accidents, perform inspections, and discuss other laboratory safety problems (22).

Each laboratory should appoint a safety officer who chairs or is a member of the institutional safety committee and helps to organize and update the safety policies and procedure manuals. The safety officer should regularly check eyewashes, safety showers, alarms, and gauges on fire extinguishers and should organize and conduct continuing safety education.

Although the effectiveness of safety programs is difficult to measure, one should compare the number of hours involved in training with the incident rate of laboratory accidents. Decreased rates may be influenced by other factors, but such a comparison would provide a rough approximation of their effectiveness (33).

Right to know

The hazard communication standard issued in 1984 by OSHA and published as a final rule in 1987 was developed to ensure the safety of employees who come or might come into contact with hazardous chemicals in the work place. Employers are responsible for disseminating information regarding the hazards of chemicals, using a comprehensive communication program. The program must include proper container labeling, manufacturer's material safety data sheets (MSDS), and an employee training program (14).

Employers must ensure that (i) labels on containers of hazardous chemicals are not removed or defaced, (ii) MSDS are kept on file and readily available to laboratory employees, and (iii) employees are made aware of chemical hazards through a training program.

The laboratory safety officer or other designated personnel should be responsible for the employees' right to know about hazardous chemicals. The officer should also be responsible for developing and implementing a training program that covers the necessary aspects of the hazard communication standard. The employee should be informed of the hazards during the initial orientation phase to the laboratory and yearly thereafter. There should be written documentation of training and review. Training could consist of a simple notebook containing examples of container labels and MSDS and how to interpret their information. The training notebook could also contain methods for detecting the presence of hazardous chemicals (e.g., by smell), where to find and how to use protective personal equipment, and a list of hazardous chemicals. The notebook could be combined with self-guided computer software or videotapes, both of which are commercially available. Training should also involve a tour of the laboratory, which could be part of the general safety orientation, to point out where chemicals are stored and used. The U.S. Department of Labor or the state occupational safety and health office can provide suggestions for setting up a training program.

Infection control and employee health programs

The hospital microbiology laboratory must establish an effective working relationship with the infection control officer. A system for notification of the presence of important nosocomial isolates and reportable communicable diseases to the infection control officer should be developed. The infection control officer should coordinate the monitoring of autoclaves used for sterilization of surgical instruments, contaminated waste, and other supplies and use the microbiology laboratory for consultation when necessary. The infection control officer is responsible for instruction of hospital staff on the proper use of patient isolation procedures. Such instruction should include the meaning of universal precautions and how they apply to the use of appropriate barrier protection during collection of patient samples.

All laboratory accidents should be reported to the supervisor. The employee involved should then be referred to the institution's employee health department. If the institution does not have such a department, then it must institute a mechanism for documentation of the laboratory accident and arrange for immediate and follow-up medical care by a medical practitioner, clinic, or hospital.

Forms for reporting accidents should be available. These forms should contain, in addition to the usual employee demographic data, written documentation of the nature of the accident, a statement as to whether the accident could have been prevented, and a description of measures that will be taken to prevent a recurrence. The reports should be reviewed by the safety committee at its regular meetings.

Among the basic functions of an employee health department are reducing the number of missed workdays and minimizing the number of on-the-job injuries and illnesses. In a hospital, the employee health department, in cooperation with the infection control officer, helps curb the spread of disease between patients and staff. The department also provides instructional programs, physical examinations, tuberculosis skin tests, vaccinations, and other services for the continued good health of employees. Under the proposed amendments to OSHA (29 CFR part 1910), employers must provide HBV vaccination to all employees who have potential occupational exposure to bloodborne pathogens (16). Most hospitals already have immunization programs in place. Laboratories not affiliated with a hospital or other medical facility must arrange with a licensed physician for an immunization program; this arrangement should include postexposure management. According to OSHA estimates (16), HBV vaccination of all health care workers would result in two fewer deaths and 18 to 28 fewer cases of hepatitis and its complications per 1,000 workers exposed over a lifetime.

Cooperation from all staff members is needed to prevent exposures to microbiological, chemical, and physical hazards and for prevention of occupational disease and injury.

CONTAINMENT DESIGN, EQUIPMENT, AND TECHNIQUES

Environmental safety and safety consciousness of employees are supported by appropriate design of clinical laboratories, the provision of safe equipment, and the adoption of appropriate containment techniques.

Design

The design of a clinical microbiology laboratory must be guided by the scope of its operations. Applying the CDC classification of etiologic agents and the concept of containment according to four levels of safety, CDC and NIH developed guidelines for microbiological laboratories that considered the potential hazard of microbial agents and laboratory function (38). Table 2 summarizes the recommended facilities, safety equipment, and practices.

The laboratory should be located away from patient care, visitor, and administrative areas and should have limited access. Ventilation and climate control systems should prevent airflow from laboratories into public corridors and nonlaboratory areas. Laboratories should be designed so that they can be easily cleaned, and the furniture should be of solid construction, with sufficient spacing to allow access for cleaning. Workbenches and equipment tables should be covered with water-impervious, heat- and chemical-resistant materials. Each lab-

TABLE 2. Summary of recommended biosafety levels for infectious agents[a]

Biosafety level	Practices and techniques	Safety equipment	Facilities
1	Standard microbiological practices	None; primary containment provided by adherence to standard laboratory practices during open bench operations	Basic
2	Level 1 practices plus laboratory coats, decontamination of all infectious wastes, limited access, protective gloves, and biohazard warning signs as indicated	Partial containment equipment (i.e., class I or II biological safety cabinets) used to conduct mechanical manipulative procedures that have high aerosol potential that may increase the risk of exposure to personnel	Basic
3	Level 2 practices plus special laboratory clothing and controlled access	Partial containment equipment used for all manipulations of infectious material	Containment
4	Level 3 practices plus entrance through change room where street clothing is removed and laboratory clothing is put on, shower before exit, and decontamination of all wastes upon exit	Maximum containment equipment (i.e., class III biological safety cabinet or partial containment equipment in combination with full-body, air-supplied, positive-pressure personnel suit) used for all procedures and activities	Maximum containment

[a] From reference 38.

oratory requires a sink for hand washing and an eyewash station. If laboratory windows open, they should be covered with insect screens. Most laboratory operations involving routine diagnostic patient care can be performed in a basic facility under biosafety level 2, using a biological safety cabinet and other partial containment for procedures that may increase the risk of exposure resulting from, for example, aerosol production. Specialty services such as the handling and identification of mycobacteria and certain biphasic fungi require biosafety level 3. Routine diagnostic procedures, however, may be performed in a biosafety level 2 laboratory, with strict adherence to the standard and special microbiological practices and the use of containment equipment as recommended for biosafety level 3. In level 3 laboratories, the interior surfaces of the rooms should be water resistant, the windows sealed, the access restricted, and a ducted exhaust air ventilation system provided.

In addition to complying with microbiological safety recommendations, the laboratories must adhere to the local fire and safety code by providing fire extinguishers, fire blankets, special storage of flammable materials, and compressed gases. Other safety requirements address the use and storage of chemicals and radioactive materials. The biohazard symbol must be displayed on laboratory doors and contain information about the type of hazard and names and telephone numbers of persons to be contacted in cases of emergency. An evacuation plan must be posted in each room.

Containment equipment

Containment equipment should allow the user to provide safe preparation and transfer of potentially hazardous materials without breaking the barrier, minimize exposure, and permit the safe decontamination of effluent and work area. The most important primary containment equipment in the clinical microbiology laboratory is the biological safety cabinet. Two types are commonly found in the microbiology laboratory: class 1, an open-fronted, negative-pressure ventilated cabinet with HEPA-filtered air exhaust; and class 2, a vertical laminar flow cabinet with HEPA-filtered recirculated airflow in the work area and HEPA-filtered air exhaust. With an inward face velocity of 75 ft/min (ca. 0.38 m/s), these cabinets are useful for partial containment of biosafety level 2 and 3 agents when used in conjunction with good laboratory practices. The National Sanitation Foundation has developed reference standards that are useful in the selection of such a cabinet. Class 1 cabinets protect the worker from contamination; class 2 cabinets protect the worker and the work area. Class 2 cabinets are most commonly used in microbiology laboratories, especially for virus and tissue culture work. All cabinets must be tested and certified after installation and after each move as well as at least annually thereafter. Laboratory workers must be trained in the proper use of the cabinets and be informed that containment, especially of aerosols, is not absolute, since interruption of the inward airflow by various means might lead to escape of particles from the work area. For a more detailed discussion of biological safety cabinets, the reader is referred to references 3 and 38.

Centrifugation has long been considered a particularly hazardous laboratory procedure. Of special concern is the centrifugation of digested sputum from tuberculosis patients. *Mycobacterium tuberculosis* has a 50% human infective dose of 10 organisms by the respiratory route (32). An early answer to the problem of centrifugation was the venting of centrifuge bowls to the outside, but now aerosol generation can be prevented to a very high degree by the use of special plug seal caps of disposable centrifuge tubes that provide a leakproof seal for the centrifugation of infectious material. Also, sealed centrifuge buckets and shields are available from all manufacturers as an additional safety feature. To reduce breakage of centrifuge tubes, only intact, unscratched glass tubes should be selected, but replacing all glass with plastic may be considered. Each laboratory must have a procedure addressing centrifuge accidents and tube breakage.

Blenders and homogenizers used to be known as aerosol producers, and even their use in a biological safety cabinet will not prevent potential worker exposure. Today, safe stainless steel containers, even for small volumes, are available for blenders (Eberbach Corp., Ann Arbor, Mich.; Waring Products Division, Hartford, Conn.). The Stomacher (Seward Laboratory, London, England) contains the material to be blended in a plastic bag that can be discarded after the operation. Chatigny (3) described other laboratory-made enclosures for hand-operated devices that could be adapted to motorized grinders and sonic disruptors. Even with such enclosures, these procedures should be performed in a biological safety cabinet when one is working with infectious agents or patient specimens.

For certain operations, especially in anaerobe and parasitology laboratories, explosionproof centrifuges and refrigerators are required. For work with toxic chemicals and solvents, a chemical hood must be available. Flammable and corrosive chemicals must be contained in safety containers and should be kept in a safety cabinet.

Stock cultures of microorganisms must be kept in containers that protect against breakage and should be stored in easily reached cabinets inaccessible to unauthorized persons.

For laboratory workers, the most important protection became the elimination of mouth pipetting and the introduction of pipetting devices. From small rubber bulbs to calibrated micropipettes with disposable, sterilizable tips and very sophisticated automated pipettes, users can select whatever is needed for the work at hand. When using automated pipettes, one should consider their potential contamination. Bacteriological inoculation loops need no longer be a source of aerosols during heat sterilization, since electrical incinerator loop sterilizers have virtually replaced the Bunsen burner. Disposable plastic loops and needles eliminate the need for heat sterilization devices.

Containment techniques

The best design and the optimal equipment cannot guarantee laboratory safety without the personal commitment of each worker and supervisor. Employers will soon be forced by law to provide employees with personal protection devices (16). These include barrier devices such as protective gowns and laboratory coats, aprons and other garments, gloves, goggles, and face shields.

Personnel should wear gowns and laboratory coats with long sleeves while working in the laboratory. A plastic disposable apron can protect against splashes of blood, body fluids, and liquid cultures. Other protective garments such as operating room gowns, scrub suits, or coveralls can be worn for special procedures. All contaminated garments should be decontaminated or sent to the laundry, as specified by established infection control protocols.

To prevent skin contamination with blood, body fluids, and other infectious materials, disposable gloves should be worn. Tightly fitted around the wrists, the gloves plus laboratory gowns protect the entire arm during work in biological safety cabinets. Disposable gloves are no absolute barrier for microorganisms and can lose their integrity, particularly after washing. After a task is performed (or if a tear occurs), the gloves should be removed immediately and the hands should be washed. Employees should be instructed that gloves protect only against contamination by contact and should remember that contaminated gloves can be a source of environmental transfer of infectious agents to themselves and their co-workers.

All laboratory procedures are performed in a way that minimizes the creation of aerosols (38). Procedures that have even the slightest potential of splashing, spurting, or aerosol formation should be performed only while the employee is wearing a mask and goggles or a face shield. The work performed may be the unprotected unstoppering of VACUTAINERs, the transfer of inocula from blood culture bottles with high internal gas pressure, the injection of materials through rubber stoppers, or the obtaining of an arterial blood sample from a patient. Needle sticks or other injuries from sharp instruments can be avoided by proper technique and provision of appropriate safety devices. All such injuries must be reported to the supervisor and to the person responsible for the employee health program for appropriate care and follow-up (23, 38).

Skin defects on hands, arms, neck, and face should be covered with a water-impermeable occlusive dressing (27). Under certain circumstances, the laboratory director or the employee health department may temporarily assign the employee to a nonrisk area.

Hand-washing sinks with nonirritating soap should be located in each laboratory. For accidental skin contamination with infectious agents, antiseptic soap should be available. In areas without hand-washing facilities, a waterless antiseptic preparation or alcohol planchets are useful for rapid skin decontamination after an accident. Thorough hand washing should follow.

Each work area should be disinfected after completion of work and after accidental contamination. The recommendations for disinfection presented in chapter 24 should be followed. Under no circumstances should antiseptics be used for disinfection. A procedure for the rapid treatment of spills and the appropriate materials should be available on all work stations.

Safety in the laboratory is based on strict adherence to standard microbiological practices and techniques, the provision and proper use of primary barrier equipment, and a facility that provides the laboratory with an environment adequate for its function. For the individual laboratory worker, safety is assured not by the employer but by a personal commitment to protect him- or herself and all co-workers.

LITERATURE CITED

1. **Barkley, W. E.** 1981. Containment and disinfection, p. 487–503. *In* P. Gephardt, R. G. E. Murray, R. N. Costilow, E. W. Nester, W. A. Wood, N. R. Krieg, and G. B. Phillips (ed.), Manual of methods for general bacteriology. American Society for Microbiology, Washington, D.C.
2. **Benenson, A. S. (ed.).** 1985. Control of communicable diseases in man, 14th ed. American Public Health Association, Washington, D.C.
3. **Chatigny, M.** 1986. Primary barriers, p. 144–163. *In* B. M. Miller, D. H. M. Gröschel, J. H. Richardson, D. Vesley, J. R. Songer, R. D. Housewright, and W. E. Barkley (ed.), Laboratory safety: principles and practices. American Society for Microbiology, Washington, D.C.
4. **Commission on Laboratory Accreditation.** 1988. Inspection checklist, section 1. Laboratory general. College of American Pathologists, Skokie, Ill.
5. **Center for Disease Control.** 1971. Laboratory safety at the Center for Disease Control, DHEW publication no. (HSM)72-8118. Public Health Service, U.S. Department of Health, Education, and Welfare, Atlanta.
6. **Centers for Disease Control.** 1982. Acquired immune deficiency syndrome (AIDS): precautions for clinical and laboratory staffs. Morbid. Mortal. Weekly Rep. **31:**577–580.
7. **Centers for Disease Control.** 1985. Recommendations for protection against viral hepatitis. Morbid. Mortal. Weekly Rep. **34:**313–324, 329–335.
8. **Centers for Disease Control.** 1987. Recommendations for prevention of HIV transmission in health-care settings. Morbid. Mortal. Weekly Rep. **36**(Suppl. 2):3S–18S.
9. **Centers for Disease Control.** 1988. Update: universal precautions for prevention of transmission of human immunodeficiency virus, hepatitis B virus, and other bloodborne pathogens in health-care settings. Morbid. Mortal. Weekly Rep. **37:**377–382, 387–388.
10. **Centers for Disease Control.** 1989. Guidelines for prevention of transmission of human immunodeficiency virus and hepatitis B virus to health-care and public-safety workers. Morbid. Mortal. Weekly Rep. **38**(Suppl. 6):1–37.
11. **Committee on Hazardous Substances in the Laboratory, National Research Council.** 1980. Prudent practices for handling hazardous chemicals in laboratories. National Academy Press, Washington, D.C.
12. **Department of Labor.** 1987. Department of Labor/Department of Health and Human Services joint advisory notice: protection against occupational exposure to hepatitis B virus (HBV) and human immunodeficiency virus (HIV). Fed. Regist. **52:**41818–41824.
13. **Department of Labor, Occupational Safety and Health Administration.** 1983. Profile of laboratories with the potential for exposure to toxic substances. U.S. Government Printing Office, Washington, D.C.
14. **Department of Labor, Occupational Safety and Health Administration.** 1987. 29 CFR part 1910.1200. Hazard communications, final rule. Fed. Regist. **52:**31852–31885.
15. **Department of Labor, Occupational Safety and Health Administration.** 1987. 29 CFR part 1910. Occupational exposure to hepatitis B virus and human immunodeficiency virus. Fed. Regist. **52:**45438–45441.
16. **Department of Labor, Occupational Safety and Health Administration.** 1989. 29 CFR 1910. Occupational exposure to bloodborne pathogens. Fed. Regist. **54:**23042–23139.
17. **Fuscaldo, A. A., B. J. Erlick, and B. Hindman.** 1980. Laboratory safety. Theory and practice. Academic Press, Inc., New York.
18. **Garner, J. S., and B. P. Simmons.** 1983. CDC guideline for isolation precautions in hospitals. Infect. Control **4:** 245–325.
19. **Heim, L.** 1894. Lehrbuch der bakteriologischen Untersuchung und Diagnostik, p. 488. F. Enke, Stuttgart, Germany.

20. **Hodinka, R. L., P. H. Gilligan, and M. L. Smiley.** 1988. Survival of human immunodeficiency virus in blood culture systems. Arch. Pathol. Lab. Med. **112:**1251–1254.
21. **Holmes, M. B., D. L. Johnson, N. J. Fiumara, and W. M. McCormack.** 1980. Acquisition of typhoid fever from proficiency-testing specimens. N. Engl. J. Med. **303:**519–521.
22. **Huffaker, R. H.** 1974. Biological safety in the clinical laboratory, p. 871–878. *In* E. H. Lennette, E. H. Spaulding, and J. P. Truant (ed.), Manual of clinical microbiology, 2nd ed. American Society for Microbiology, Washington, D.C.
23. **Jagger, J., E. H. Hunt, J. Brand-Elnaggar, and R. D. Pearson.** 1988. Rates of needle-stick injury caused by various devices in a university hospital. N. Engl. J. Med. **319:** 284–288.
24. **Joint Commission for the Accreditation of Healthcare Organizations.** 1988. Accreditation manual for hospitals, 1989. Joint Commission for the Accreditation of Healthcare Organizations, Chicago.
25. **Mackel, D. C., and J. E. Forney.** 1986. Overview of the epidemiology of laboratory-acquired infections, p. 37–42. *In* B. M. Miller, D. H. M. Gröschel, J. H. Richardson, D. Vesley, J. R. Songer, R. D. Housewright, and W. E. Barkley (ed.), Laboratory safety: principles and practices. American Society for Microbiology, Washington, D.C.
26. **Miller, B. M., D. H. M. Gröschel, J. H. Richardson, D. Vesley, J. R. Songer, R. D. Housewright, and W. E. Barkley (ed.).** 1986. Laboratory safety: principles and practices. American Society for Microbiology, Washington, D.C.
27. **National Committee for Clinical Laboratory Standards.** 1989. Tentative guideline M29-T. Protection of laboratory workers from infectious disease transmitted by blood and tissue. National Committee for Clinical Laboratory Standards, Villanova, Pa.
28. **Occupational Safety and Health Act.** 1970. 29 USC 651 et seq.
29. **Phillips, G. B.** 1961. Microbiological safety in U.S. and foreign laboratories, technical study 35. U.S. Army Chemical Corps Research and Development Command, U.S. Army Biological Laboratories, Fort Detrick, Md.
30. **Pike, R. M.** 1976. Laboratory associated infections: summary and analysis of 3,921 cases. Health Lab. Sci. **13:**105–114.
31. **Pike, R. M.** 1979. Laboratory-associated infections: incidence, fatalities, causes and prevention. Annu. Rev. Microbiol. **33:**41–66.
32. **Richardson, J. H., and W. E. Barkley.** 1985. Biological safety in the clinical laboratory, p. 138–142. *In* E. H. Lennette, A. Balows, W. J. Hausler, and H. J. Shadomy (ed.), Manual of clinical microbiology, 4th ed. American Society for Microbiology, Washington. D.C.
33. **Richardson, J. H., E. Schoenfeld, J. J. Tulis, and W. M. Wagner (ed.).** 1986. Proceedings of the 1985 Institute on Critical Issues in Health Laboratory Practice: safety management in the public health laboratory, p. 1–13. The DuPont Co., Wilmington, Del.
34. **Rose, S. L.** 1984. Clinical laboratory safety. J. B. Lippincott Co., Philadelphia.
35. **Songer, J. R.** 1986. Management and codification of risks in the laboratory, p. 120–122. *In* B. M. Miller, D. H. M. Gröschel, J. H. Richardson, D. Vesley, J. R. Songer, R. D. Housewright, and W. E. Barkley (ed.), Laboratory safety: principles and practices. American Society for Microbiology, Washington, D.C.
36. **U.S. Postal Service.** 1988. 39 CFR part III. Nonmailability of etiologic agents. Fed. Regist. **53:**23775–23776.
37. **U.S. Postal Service.** 1989. 39 CFR part III. Mailability of etiologic agents. Fed. Regist. **54:**11970–11972.
38. **U.S. Public Health Service, Centers for Disease Control, and National Institutes of Health.** 1988. Biosafety in microbiological and biomedical laboratories, 2nd ed., publication no. (NIH) 88-8395. Department of Health and Human Services, Washington, D.C.
39. **Wedum, A. G., W. E. Barkley, and A. Hellman.** 1972. Handling of infectious agents. J. Am. Vet. Assoc. **161:**1557–1567.
40. **Weiss, S. H., J. J. Goedert, S. Gartner, M. Popovic, D. Waters, P. Markham, F. di Marzo Veronese, M. H. Gail, W. E. Barkley, J. Gibbons, F. A. Gill, M. Leuther, G. M. Shaw, R. C. Gallo, and W. A. Blattner.** 1988. Risk of human immunodeficiency virus (HIV-1) infection among laboratory workers. Science **239:**58–71.

Chapter 8

Introduction and Overview

DANIEL AMSTERDAM, ROY W. STEVENS, AND EDWARD J. BOTTONE

The 11 chapters in this section describe general techniques that are used across the disciplines of bacteriology, mycology, mycobacteriology, virology, and diagnostic immunology. The last term deserves some definition in that it is recognized in the Clinical Laboratory Improvement Act of 1988 (CLIA 88) and includes all aspects of immunology (and serology) testing but not cellular immunology.

Over the past 150 years, since Koch first isolated the tubercle bacillus on heat-coagulated bovine serum albumin, microbiologists have endeavored to demonstrate the presence of pathogenic microorganisms associated with infectious diseases in clinical or pathologic specimens by cultural and subsequently noncultural techniques. Clinical microbiologists now have access to technologic advances of extraordinary efficiency for the detection and quantitation of markers of infectious disease. The most spectacular of these advances are those in molecular genetics achieved during the last two decades. Not to be outclassed are modern versions of techniques that were discovered early in the development of microbiology, such as assays based on agglutination of infectious agents or components and fixation of complement by antigen-antibody complexes. Other techniques, such as second-antibody procedures with enzyme substrate indicators and assays for quantitation of specific immunoglobulins, have matured only within the last decade but have already made major contributions to medical microbiology.

Although agglutination tests in one configuration or another are familiar to all microbiologists, the apparent simplicity of these reactions is deceptive. The complexities of these tests as they influence laboratory findings are described and discussed in chapter 9. This analysis of the principles of agglutination reactions provides an excellent understanding that may be translated into improved accuracy and precision of test performance. It is noteworthy that this earliest of microbiology techniques has been successfully adapted for an assay, used in many parts of the world as a screening test for human immunodeficiency virus infection.

Assays based on lysis of erythrocytes, like agglutination tests, are established techniques in the repertoire of clinical microbiologists. A reexamination of this science is timely, however, because of the vital contributions of these technologies to detection of antibody to particular viral and bacterial agents. Chapter 10 includes an innovative review of the principles of complement and enzyme-mediated hemolysis and an update on applications, as well as a primer on important principles of immunology best illustrated by immune-mediated (or immune-inhibited) hemolysis.

The combining (labeling) of antibodies with specific fluorescent dyes such as fluorescein or rhodamine enables the detection and localization of antigens in bacteria, tissues, and individual cells. Detection techniques can be direct and indirect. In the former, the antigen-specific antibody, usually a monoclonal antibody, is labeled and used to detect a specific antigen, e.g., *Legionella pneumophila* in bronchial secretions or herpes simplex virus-infected cells in scrapings of bullous lesions. With the indirect "sandwich" method, the antigen-specific antibody is devoid of a label and its binding to an antigen is detected with a second, labeled antibody which may be poly- or monoclonal. These techniques may be altered by the modification of the primary antibody label or detection system. For example, a popular technique is coupling of biotin (or dinitrophenol) to the antibody molecule, which can then be detected by labeled reagents such as a biotin-labeled enzyme of streptavidin (chapter 11).

Radioimmunoassay is used for the quantification of antigenic material in an otherwise heterogeneous mixture. The underlying principle in this technique is one of competitive inhibition of a reaction of specimen antibody with known amounts of radiolabeled antigen by a sample to be analyzed containing an unknown amount of antigen. The use of radiolabeled antigen greatly enhances test sensitivity.

A most important characteristic of second-antibody techniques with enzyme substrate indicators is sensitivity. This attribute, coupled with excellent specificity achieved by improved reagent chemistry and production, has clearly revolutionized the science of antigen and antibody detection. A description of the principles of enzyme-linked immunosorbent assays, a discussion of variations on the basic design, and illustrations of important diagnostic techniques are presented in chapter 12. The essentials of electrophoresis, transblot, and immunoenzyme detection (Western blot) of antigen-antibody markers are included in chapter 13. The description of blot chemistry is especially pertinent to serodiagnosis of human immunodeficiency virus and *Borrelia burgdorferi* infections.

Serologic precipitation reactions developed in an agar gel matrix are often used to analyze multiple reactants in which each specific antigen-antibody combination forms an independent precipitate. Antigen-antibody reactions occurring in a supporting matrix may be studied either as a simple gel diffusion or by the double-diffusion technique. As discussed in chapter 11, multiple precipitation patterns may be discerned which enable characterization of the reactants. However, this technology may have limited application when multiple antigen-antibody reactions with numerous precipitin lines are concurrently taking place in the agar matrix. To discriminate among such a heterogeneous mixture, a variety of electrophoretic separations may be necessary, followed by immunoprecipitation in agar (chapter 14).

Methods for the detection of specific immunoglobulins are described in chapter 15, with emphasis on the early diagnosis of infection in adults or infants. Detection of immunoglobulin M (IgM) prior to seroconversion mediated by IgG or detection of IgM or IgA in infants is diagnostic of exposure to the agent under study. For infants, these antibody techniques differentiate a specific and early response from passively transferred maternal antibody. Special applications of these techniques, with descriptions of recent advances in reagent characterization and technical improvements, are detailed.

An alternative approach to the analysis or identification of the genomic traits of bacteria and yeasts is presented in chapter 16. The techniques for chromatographic analysis of components of microorganisms and their metabolites are discussed. Also considered is the concept of multicomponent analysis, whereby whole cells of microorganisms are pyrolized by rapid heating and a diverse array of microbial biomolecules is analyzed. This technique is attractive in that the need for sample preparation is precluded.

Descriptions and approaches to the use of nucleic acid probes and other molecular biology techniques are presented in chapter 17; the chapter also discusses application of the polymerase chain reaction. Probes, at one time solely within the domain of molecular biologists, have crossed the research laboratory barrier and are part of the armamentarium of diagnostic reagents that are available to clinical microbiologists. Several probes are commercially available, and it is clear that the polymerase chain reaction technique will enhance the scope and increase the sensitivity of these assays.

The "kit" or, more properly, the system approach in diagnostic microbiology has been available and the mainstay of clinical microbiologists for several years. A number of these systems, originally conceived for the identification of gram-negative members of the family *Enterobacteriaceae*, have now been expanded and include application to nonfermenters, staphylococci, streptococci, *Branhamella*, *Haemophilus*, and *Neisseria* species, and yeasts. The concepts and details of the more commonly used systems are discussed in chapter 18.

Molecular biology techniques will play an ever-expanding role in the routine operation of the clinical microbiology laboratory, yet classic approaches are and will continue to be needed, as evidenced by the chapter on the use of animal and cell culture systems (chapter 19). For detecting viral agents and procaryotes with incomplete energy systems, cell cultures are still in order. The necessity for establishing lymphocyte cultures was crucial in preparing antigens for perfecting a test for the diagnosis of human immunodeficiency virus. Also, to elucidate one of the several potential roles of *Escherichia coli* (enteropathogenic, enterotoxigenic, enteroinvasive, or enterohemorrhagic) in human disease, what is required is reference and resort to the methodologies outlined in this chapter.

With the concept of species now more clearly defined at the molecular level, it is evident that in the next decade diagnostic approaches will be targeted to probe the identities of infective agents and the characteristics of disease processes at the genomic instead of the phenotypic level.

Chapter 9

Agglutination Tests and *Limulus* Assay for the Diagnosis of Infectious Diseases

THOMAS J. TINGHITELLA AND STEPHEN C. EDBERG

Agglutination tests have been part of the diagnostic laboratory since its institution. Within the last few years, agglutination procedures have become central in our ability to rapidly and specifically detect certain pathogens present in clinical specimens and to identify organisms isolated in culture. The overriding characteristic of agglutination tests is that the reaction can be easily observed. Their very nature makes them suitable for decentralized, uncomplicated application.

HISTORICAL DEVELOPMENT

In 1896, Gruber and Durham published their observations on the ability of antisera to clump bacterial cells and suggested that this phenomenon might be useful for identification purposes (75). In an extensive study of agglutination, Smith and Reogh demonstrated in 1903 that antisera to bacterial cell surface constituents appeared to be specific (37). Topley, Wilson, and Duncan extended this observation and developed the first diagnostic agglutination test (75). They made antisera against some of the major recognized groups of microorganisms (e.g., *Streptococcus pneumoniae* and *Salmonella typhi*); when one of these groups of bacteria was thought to be present in mixed culture, previously prepared antiserum against one species agglutinated only that species. They postulated that this phenomenon could be applied to the diagnosis of pulmonary and enteric infections even before the pathogen had been isolated in pure culture. Although they were overly enthusiastic, their supposition forms the basis for widespread use of agglutination tests today.

Stimulated by the clinical utility of agglutination and other serological tests, investigators began to explore the scientific basis for these tests. Paul Ehrlich, one of the early scientists interested in immunology, hypothesized that a cell had receptors on its surface that would recognize a foreign substance, i.e., antigen. When an antigen combined with the cell receptor, the cell produced and released more receptors, or antibody. This antibody could participate in serological reactions. Ehrlich's hypothesis was based on the observation that animals inoculated with a nonlethal dose of an intact bacterial pathogen produced antibody that had various characteristics: the serum containing antibody could be used to passively protect other animals from infection with the pathogen, could agglutinate or cause the bacteria to clump in vitro, could produce a precipitate in a filtrate from a broth culture of the pathogen, could increase phagocytosis (opsonization), and could activate (fix) complement. In what is now known as the unitary theory of antibody development, it is held that an antibody can participate in any of the different observed, or secondary, reactions, albeit various antibodies do so with differing abilities. Antibody efficiency is related to the type of immunoglobulin reacting, the physicochemical conditions of the mixture, and the valency of the reactants. Knowledge of the unitary theory is important for understanding under which conditions a given serological test can be used and why agglutination reactions are applicable in some circumstances but not others.

PRINCIPLES OF AGGLUTINATION

Reactions

Agglutination, like all serological reactions, occurs in two stages. The primary reaction is the combination of antigen with antibody. Bordet, in the first major exploration of the mechanism of agglutination, referred to this step as sensitization. A lower ionic strength favors the uptake of antibody. The primary reaction can be demonstrated only indirectly, through the decrease in one of the reactants (antigen or antibody) from solution. The primary reaction is independent of the type of test being performed.

The secondary, or visible, reaction is what is observed in the diagnostic laboratory as the "test." Each class of antibody has particular biological properties and participates with different efficiencies in the various serological tests. Two types of immunoglobulin are applicable to agglutination reactions: immunoglobulin M (IgM) and IgG. IgM appears in quantity within 1 or 2 days after infection. Its large (850,000-dalton) molecular size and circular arrangement make IgM most efficient in combining particles (e.g., bacteria and viruses) into clumps (agglutination) to facilitate their removal in vivo by the reticuloendothelial system. When antigen and antibody react, the IgM molecule is extremely efficient at activating complement. IgG appears later in the course of infection or exposure to an antigen. Unlike IgM, IgG antibody can be found in the serum for years and probably evolved as the "vaccine" or continuing-defense molecule. Its physical size and distribution make it most efficient at combining with the attachment site of an invading microbe, with resultant neutralization and opsonization, but less efficient at clumping and killing. Therefore, agglutination tests are much more efficient (approximately 750 times) (80) at measuring IgM than IgG antibody.

Agglutination versus precipitation

Agglutination is the clumping of particles by specific antibody or antigen under particular physicochemical conditions. It differs from precipitation in one major characteristic: in agglutination, one or both of the reactants (antigen and antibody) are adsorbed onto the surface of the particle carrier; in precipitation, both antigen and antibody are soluble. Although the basic theories governing the formation of an agglutinate or precipitate have much in common, this difference in the nature of the reactants permits agglutination to be a semiquantitative assay, yielding results that can be expressed only as relative units, such as titer. Precipitation can be used to determine the exact amount of antigen or antibody in solution; much of our understanding of the nature of antigen-antibody reactions came from the study of precipitation.

Lattice formation

The development of an observable in vitro secondary reaction in both precipitation and agglutination is governed by the lattice theory. Knowledge of the conditions leading to lattice formation is important in developing quality control parameters to govern the agglutination reaction. Bordet hypothesized that after the primary reaction, a second stage occurred that was responsible for the observation of agglutination. He felt that lattice formation was governed by physicochemical factors such as the nature of the surface of the particle and the ionic charge of the milieu. He had previously observed that clay particles in a river remained in suspension until they reached an estuary, where they agglutinated. He postulated that the salt caused the secondary reaction. Heidelberger believed that agglutination was similar to precipitation (75); the difference appeared to be the influence of charge by allowing the particles in agglutination to juxtapose and cross-link.

Factors affecting lattice formation

Heidelberger and Kendall described the parameters and quantified the factors governing lattice formation. The lattice theory stated that an observable reaction occurred when the concentrations of antigen and antibody were optimal to cross-link the particles. If there was too much antibody present in the reaction mixture, no visible reaction occurred because the particles coated with antigen were prevented from cross-linking and forming a lattice. Conversely, if there was too much antigen present, the antibody reacted with the antigen-coated particles but did not have sufficient antigen to cross-link the particles. Using *S. pneumoniae* type III polysaccharide antigen, lattice formation was found to occur in three phases: antibody excess (prozone); zone of equivalence (maximum secondary-reaction product); and antigen excess (postzone) (75). This observation governs the performance of tests in the clinical laboratory.

Two other conditions governing the ability of antibody and antigen to form an agglutinate are the number of binding sites (valency) available to participate in the reaction and the strength of the reaction, determined by avidity and affinity. IgM has 10 antigen-binding sites; in most functional situations, the valency is five. IgG has a maximum valency of two; if the antigen on a particle is repetitive, both binding sites may adhere to the same particle and not form a lattice (blocking antibody) (80). Polysaccharide antigens, which are the most commonly encountered in the clinical microbiology laboratory as the antigens of bacterial pathogens, tend to have repetitive sequences.

The strength of binding of antibody to antigen also significantly influences the formation of an agglutinate. Strength of binding can be considered to have two components: affinity and avidity. Affinity is the reaction constant (liters per mole) of a particular antibody for its antigen. Unless one is using a monoclonal antibody, there is an overall reaction constant resulting from closely related antibodies and antigens. Avidity can be considered the sum of the individual affinities of all antibodies and antigens in the reaction mixture. The avidity between antibody and antigen is governed by both the chemical nature of the antigen (e.g., hydrophobic or hydrophilic) and the conformational presentation of the antigen. The lattice is formed when the particles with the adsorbed reactant are cross-linked through soluble antigen or antibody to create a matrix that can no longer remain in suspension. (The appendix to this chapter provides the formulas and a description of the force that keeps particles in suspension.)

As discussed below, three factors hold cells apart.

1. Cells in solution have a negative charge surrounding them. One must decrease the diameter of this effective negative ionic layer in order for cells to come close enough for antibodies to form a lattice.

2. There is a layer of hydration around cells. Removal or blockage of hydrophilic groups leads to agglutination.

3. The cell membrane is in a steric conformation. The membranes of cells, especially those without cell walls, are not spherical. Therefore, antigens may be found in "valleys" and not be accessible to antibody. The steric conformation of cells may also be affected by the ionic charge matrix of the milieu.

Pollack described four main physicochemical parameters governing the formation of the lattice (37): ionic strength, pH, dielectric constant, and temperature. Probably most important in inhibiting the secondary reaction of particles is the electrostatic charge formed by the layer of charges surrounding the particle. The distance into the suspending solution where the effective electrostatic charge occurs is directly proportional to the ionic strength of the solution. The outer edge of the effect of the charge is known as the surface of shear. Between the surface of shear and the innate charge at the cell membrane (particle) is an electrostatic potential known as the zeta potential. The larger the zeta potential, the less likely cells can come into proximity so that antigen and antibody can combine to produce a secondary reaction.

The zeta potential, which is governed by the Smoluchowski equation (see the appendix to this chapter), must be controlled before this combination can occur.

Another major force governing agglutination, and the one that can be responsible for nonspecific clumping observed on slide agglutination tests, especially when one is identifying bacterial isolates, is the van der Waals forces, caused by hydrophobic interactions. This bond is permanent (e.g., van der Waals forces cause latex paint to stick to surfaces).

These physicochemical considerations must be controlled in the clinical laboratory; otherwise, false-positive (nonspecific agglutination) or false-negative (lack of agglutination in a positive test) results will be obtained. In the laboratory, it is most important to control the ionic strength of the buffer solution. As the ionic strength decreases, the radius of the effective zeta potential decreases. At the same time, the amount of antibody that can be adsorbed onto the surface of the particle increases. The optimum pH is between 6.7 and 7.2. Temperature also exerts an effect. As the temperature increases, the association constant between antibody and antigen decreases; at the same time, the dissociation constant decreases. The net results is an overall decrease in the reactivity of antigen and antibody with an increase in temperature; therefore, agglutination is less efficient at higher temperatures.

Using the physicochemical parameters governing lattice formation, one can take several actions to increase agglutination efficiency. It has been found that agglutination efficiency can be most easily increased by changing the dielectric constant. This modification is most directly effected by adding charge colloids and proteins, such as albumin and various enzymes and polymers. Also important is mechanical shaking, which overcomes the natural repulsive electrostatic charges.

Reading agglutination tests

The endpoint of agglutination is the clumping of the carrier particle. In an attempt to standardize the endpoint of clumping, a scheme to order the reading has been developed. For most laboratory purposes, it is not necessary to use such a discriminatory system; however, one must realize that a weak reaction may be more likely than complete clumping to represent nonspecific agglutination or a cross-reaction.

In an attempt to assign to agglutination reproducible units indicating the relative titer values, the agglutination unit was developed. Using this formula, manufacturers and research laboratories can generate a standardized measure to relate different lots of antisera to each other and dilute or concentrate them to ensure reproducible performance. Clinical laboratories can use the same formula when testing a patient serum over extended time points.

The agglutination unit can be defined as $U = Y + E/S$, where U is agglutination units per milliliter, Y is the concentration of antibody, S is the concentration of a standard agglutinogen (antigen if Y = antibody) expressed as titer, and E is the titer of the examined antiserum expressed as titer against S.

METHODS OF AGGLUTINATION TESTS

Particle agglutination tests come in several forms. The first type of routine particle agglutination diagnostic test contained latex particles in suspension in a test tube. The test serum was added, and a positive test was determined by the observation of clumps within the mixture. These tests are sensitive but difficult to standardize, and the particles are difficult to keep stable for periods of more than a few days. Most commonly used in the clinical laboratory is the slide agglutination procedure, in which the particle reagents are added to the surface of a slide. The slide generally has a color opposite that of the particles. Generally, the particles are white and the background slide is black; however, black latex particles are available on a white background, and there is no reason that other color combinations could not be produced. After the particle reagent coated with either antigen or antibody is added to the slide, the sample is placed next to it and the mixture is shaken. Clumping represents the combination of antigen and antibody.

Slide agglutination reactions have several major advantages: they are very easy to perform, their use in the laboratory can be decentralized so that they may be performed as needed without interference with the work flow, and they are cost efficient for the identification of microbes from cultures. Disadvantages of the slide test include the particular care needed to ensure that clumping is not due to nonspecific interactions or that neither antigen or antibody is missed because of a prozone effect.

NATURAL PARTICLE AGGLUTINATION

In the clinical microbiology laboratory, particle agglutination tests can be used to determine either antigen or antibody in a specimen. The first agglutination tests used a bacterial suspension as the reactant. These were known as direct tests because the antigen and antibody combined directly and became the interpreted endpoint. Some of the most useful tests included serological procedures for the diagnosis of rickettsial disease (the Weil-Felix test, which uses a *Proteus* species that has cross-reacting antigens on the cell surface), the Widal test for the diagnosis of typhoid fever, and Bang's test for the diagnosis of brucellosis. For many years, these tests were requested as a diagnostic panel called the febrile agglutinins or febrile agglutinations for patients with febrile illness. However, the panel yielded results that are difficult to interpret and are therefore misinterpreted; hence the febrile agglutination panel is not recommended as a useful screen to evaluate febrile patients.

The sensitivity of direct particle agglutination tests can be increased by manipulating the physicochemical environment in which the reaction occurred (26). The sensitivity of the direct agglutination reaction was found to be directly proportional to the avidity of the antiserum and the availability of the antigen to the antibody. Natural particles, including bacteria and erythrocytes, have irregular surfaces, with antigens not always accessible to the outside milieu. The antigen may be present on a peak or a valley on the cell surface. Furthermore, other structures may interfere with the ability of the antigen to find its corresponding antibody. IgM is much more efficient than IgG in agglutinating natural particles, presumably because it can span these irregularities more easily. The sensitivity of natural particle agglutination was found to be increased if the milieu was modified to decrease the distance between the particles as they were in suspension. Initial strategies concentrated on decreasing the zeta potential. Most efficient was a reduction in ionic strength by decreasing the sodium chloride concentration of the suspending medium. It was also found that the addition of colloids and charged proteins to the mixture increased sensitivity; albumin was commonly used. Although the exact mechanism for enhanced sensitivity of agglutination tests using albumin is not known, it appears to both reduce the zeta potential of cells and reduce the peaks and valleys of the cell surface, especially of erythrocytes. Increasing the viscosity of the milieu can increase the sensitivity of particle agglutination. Accordingly, long-chain polymers such as dextran and polyvinylpyrrolidone have been used in direct particle agglutination tests.

Another means to increase the sensitivity of direct agglutination tests with natural particles is enzymatic treatment of the cell surface. Trypsin, bromelin, and papain usually have been used. Again, although the mechanism of action of enzymes in increasing agglutination sensitivity is not known, it is felt that the treatment eliminates the peaks and valleys of cells by cleaving off irregularities. These lytic enzymes probably also remove the steric influence of structures that block the ability of antibody to combine with antigen.

INERT OR CARRIER PARTICLE AGGLUTINATION

The attractiveness of agglutination reactions soon motivated the development of techniques in which the reactant (either antigen or antibody) could be coated onto the surface of a particle that served as an inert carrier. This approach represents the indirect or passive type of agglutination. Many antigens will directly adsorb onto the surface of erythrocytes; this phenomenon is seen especially with polysaccharide antigens, although many proteins also attach. Until the 1970s, erythrocytes served as the major inert particle carrier. Unfortunately, erythrocytes are subject to degradation and must be treated to (i) provide stability and (ii) adsorb antigen onto the surface. Several chemical treatments were early found to be useful to satisfy both criteria. Formalin was used to increase the absorption of polysaccharides, proteins, and haptens (75). Other chemicals such as tannic acid and pyruvic aldehyde were found to stabilize the cell membrane through the tanning process.

Because many proteins do not readily adsorb onto the erythrocyte surface, means of chemical coupling have been developed. Among the agents commonly used are bisdiazobenzidine (which links protein to the surface of biological membranes through the diazo reaction), chromium chloride, carbodiimide, and 1,3-difluor-4,6-dinitrobenzene. Each protein or polysaccharide requires its own set of exacting conditions (80) in order to both adsorb onto the cell surface and produce a stabile end product. Chemical coupling has also been used for the attachment of antigens to the surfaces of other particles; latex and *Staphylococcus* sp. have certain properties that naturally adsorb large quantities of antibody onto their surfaces.

The search for particles that could adsorb antibody included the use of natural colloids as carriers. Colloidin was used first but was not stable for long periods in suspension. Kaolin, barium stearate, charcoal, glass beads, china clay, and bismuth oxygallate were tried and abandoned for the same reasons. Two natural particles did exhibit properties amenable to clinical laboratory usage and are still used for specific assays. Charcoal has the obvious advantage of being a black particle that can be easily read on a white background. It has a moderately hydrophobic surface that can adsorb lipophilic antigens (e.g., treponeme antigens). Once adsorbed, these antigens are quite stable, although the carbon particles themselves must be stabilized with detergents and continually mixed to prevent settling. The major disadvantages of charcoal particles are their propensity to come out of suspension and the narrow range of antigens that adsorb to their surfaces. Particles of bentonite (aluminum silicate), a naturally occurring clay, were commonly used as inert particles carriers in the 1950s and 1960s and are still used for several individual assays. Bentonite particles present a large surface area for adsorption of proteins. These particles are somewhat more stable than charcoal colloids but suffered from the narrow range of antigens that can adsorb to the particle surface and their lack of stability in suspension.

In 1955, Singer and Plotz, attempting to improve on the erythrocyte agglutination test for rheumatoid factor (Waaler-Rose test), examined a number of inert particle carriers. They found that the particles available at the time (bentonite, colloidin, and various clays) were quite irregular when examined under the electron microscope. While examining electron photomicrographs of the agglutination of various particles, they were struck by the uniformity of the particle used by the microscopist as a size standard—the 0.81-nm polystyrene latex particle. They obtained these particles and found that IgG naturally absorbed onto their surfaces. This fortuitous observation, plus the fact that the hydrophobic surface of polystyrene latex binds tightly to the Fc portion of IgG, led to the development of the diagnostic latex test that has been the mainstay of particle agglutination tests now in use. Once the Fc portion of IgG hydrophobically attaches to the polystyrene surface, the attachment is virtually irreversible. During their manufacture, detergents such as sodium lauryl sulfate are used to maintain the latex particles in their monodispersed state. Like natural particles, latex particles have a weak negative charge caused by sulfates used in the polymerization process. The negative cloud results in a zeta potential that helps keep the particles apart and stable. The nature of latex particles make them amenable for the assay of antigens. However, hydrophilic polysaccharide antigens and highly charged proteins do not naturally adsorb. As with erythrocytes, it is possible to couple these antigens to the surface of polystyrene latex through the sulfate groups, but the density is considerably lower than the amount of antibody adsorbed. Approximately 75,000 molecules of IgG adsorb onto the surface, whereas less than 10% of antigen can be chemically combined.

Latex particles offer many advantages to the clinical laboratory. They are inexpensive to manufacture, and they are readily coated with IgG and made more stable with proper concentrations of suitable detergents. However, because latex particle agglutination tests (LPA) are so widely used in the clinical laboratory, special note must be taken concerning performance characteristics that can lead to nonspecific agglutination. As mentioned, latex particles naturally absorb IgG. Therefore, when mixed with test serum, the patient's own IgG may adsorb onto the surface of the polystyrene latex, and when adsorbed through the Fc region, the rheumatoid factor- and complement-binding sites of IgG are exposed and activated. Therefore, virtually all LPA tests are natural rheumatoid factor agglutination tests. Accordingly, rheumatoid factor present in a patient serum specimen will cause a false-positive agglutination test result. It is imperative to always perform a rheumatoid factor control when performing any LPA (see below). Likewise, certain components of complement, particularly C1q and C3, are natural agglutinins. In the past, it was recommended that serum be heated to 56°C for 30 min to eliminate complement activity. This may not completely eliminate complement (especially C3) activity and may also increase the likelihood of nonspecific reactivity by polymerizing serum proteins. Various hydrophobic serum proteins may nonspecifically agglutinate latex particles. Although not common, spurious unexplainable false-positive tests occur in the diagnostic laboratory. Finally, nonspecific agglutination may be due to use of a diluent with incorrect ionic strength.

Latex particles are quite sensitive serological reagents but are subject to destabilization and nonspecific agglutination. In an effort to find a better particle, advantage was taken of a bacterium's own defense mechanism against the host. It had been observed that many isolates of *Staphylococcus aureus* have a protein outer coat (protein A) that could directly combine with the Fc portion of IgG, effectively negating the biological activity of this antibody. Serological reagents were constructed in which specific IgG antibody was adsorbed onto the surface of a designated culture of staphylococci and the bacterial spheres were monodispersed and stabilized with detergent. The name "coagglutination" was given to systems that used bacteria to which a ligand had been adsorbed as the inert carrier particle. The Fc portion of the IgG molecules is adsorbed, leaving the antigen-combining Fab portion facing the environment. Because the bond between Fc and protein A is one of high affinity, the reactivity of the particle carriers is long-lived. Coagglutination particles have the same basic advantages as latex particles. In addition, they are somewhat less susceptible to false-positive results due to complement and protein cross-linking. Because they can bind endogenous IgG present in serum, they may, however, be susceptible to false-positive results due to rheumatoid factor. They also exhibit somewhat greater stability than latex particles on storage and are more refractory to changes in ionic strength. Conversely, it appears that the price for this greater inherent stability may be a somewhat lower sensitivity than with latex particles, although it is difficult to compare the sensitivities of agglutination systems against a biological material such as an antigen. The data produced are semiquantitative, and in many instances there is no absolute standard. Another disadvantage of coagglutination compared with LPA is that bacterial carriers are not colored and may be somewhat more difficult to read. The latest development in particle carriers is the production of liposomes as carriers of antigen or antibody. Liposomes are artificially constructed biological membranes made by creating a typical cell membrane around an aqueous solution containing a particular indicator. During manufacture, the cell membranes trap in their interior a specific bioactive article, e.g., ions that change the electrical conductivity of the medium once released or enzymes such as β-galactosidase. In practice, an antigen or antibody is adsorbed or chemically combined onto the surface of the liposome membrane. When the corresponding ligand is present (e.g., antibody in patient serum or antigen in the cerebrospinal fluid [CSF]), a lattice is formed, linking the liposomes. The secondary reaction may be observable visually. However, the real strength of liposome technology lies in the ability of the liposomes to release their contents after antigen-antibody combination. One may then determine this secondary reaction by observing the release of dye or by measuring other chemicals released into the environment. The major advantage of liposomes is their great flexibility; liposomes can release a wide range of chemicals when antigen and antibody combine. They can also be constructed to suit the needs of a particular assay. Their disadvantages are that they are expensive to manufacture, their stability in suspension must be carefully controlled, and the reaction conditions are complex. To release the aqueous indicator from the lipid bilayer due to lysis after the combination of antigen and antibody, a narrow range zone of equivalence must be maintained.

A number of newer particles have been used in agglutination assays and are in development for use in the diagnostic laboratory. The bacteriophage immunoassay uses a constructed bacteriophage that is adsorbed with either antigen or antibody, generally antibody. The advantages of the bacteriophage assay are that it is quite sensitive and can be made very specific. The disadvantages are that the assay conditions are complex and must be very carefully controlled (10).

A number of systems have been developed to monitor the agglutination process by instrumentation. They are based on the principle that as particles combine, the ability of light to pass through the suspension increases. Latex particles have usually been used, but theoretically any monodispersed sphere can be used. The detection system measures light scattering at 180°. A photomultiplier tube detects the light passing through the reaction cell, and signals from it are interpreted in a computer. Although these automated systems show great promise for mechanizing and potentially quantifying the agglutination process, major practical problems remain to be solved. First, small amounts of spurious colloids present in the reaction mixture can cause major amounts of interference. Second, agglutination that may not be visible to the eye can be recorded and lead to false-positive results. A particular problem is the small amount of anti-IgG present in many animal species that can cause unwanted agglutination. Also, instrumented agglutination tests are quite susceptible to changes in ionic strength and other factors that decrease the zeta potential of the particles (41).

A recently introduced agglutination system uses the physical observation that colloidal gold forms a red suspension; when a lattice is formed, a blue to colorless suspension develops. The gold agglutination technique, also known as the sol particle assay, uses 40-nm-diameter colloidal gold particles. Antibody can be chemically attached to the surface of the particles. Gold agglutination tests are commonly used as passive procedures in which an antigen in a biological fluid is assayed. Colloid gold tests can be quite sensitive and are used to determine hormones (human choriogonadotropin or lactogen) from urine or serum. Modifications of the gold colloid test use disperse dyes as colloid carriers. Antibody is adsorbed onto the dye-colloid; a positive test is indicated when antigen present in the patient specimen causes a lattice to form with an observable colored agglutinate in the reaction vessel. Various dyes can be used in the same assay system, thereby allowing the simultaneous enumeration of multiple antigens (25, 48).

CONTROLLING AGGLUTINATION TESTS

Although each particle agglutination test has its own conditions for performance, certain quality control parameters are common to all. According to the lattice theory of secondary antibody-antigen reactions, quality control is divided into nonspecific agglutination, prozone, zone of equivalence, and postzone. Nonspecific agglutination occurs in direct tests using a bacterial isolate by naturally occurring lattices formed through hydrophobic interactions (e.g., autoagglutination of staphylococci). When inert particles are used as carriers, serum components are primarily involved. Quality control of nonspecific reactions is straightforward: the test particle suspension is added to diluent and the same biological fluid (e.g., serum or CSF) is added in another parallel assay, and the mixture is shaken. No agglutination should occur. Control of the prozone is more complex. If too much antigen is present in a specimen, lattice formation is inhibited. Because most clinical agglutination tests are performed according to preset dilution protocols, causes of antigen overload may be missed. The prozone phenomenon can be detected by two means. First, the specimen may be diluted (e.g., 1:10 or 1:100) and retested. Often this is difficult because little specimen remains. Second, antigen can be added to a negative agglutination test. If there is no antigen excess, one should observe agglutination. To quality control for the zone of equivalence, one should include antigen standards supplied by the manufacturer of the test. These known standards should be constructed to reflect the average amount of antigen present in the fluid under study. In addition, laboratories can maintain previously known positive fluids to be used as quality control biological agents in questionable assays. It is generally not necessary to quality control the postzone. For clinical particle agglutination tests, the postzone would be most commonly due to too many test particles in suspension. Commercially available tests generally control this parameter; homemade or outdated materials are subject to postzone inconsistencies.

LIMULUS TEST

In the 1960s, it was observed that when the horseshoe crab (*Limulus polyphemus*) became ill with gram-negative bacteria, it preserved body parts by a circulatory clotting that effectively walled off the limb. This observation led to the development of a means to diagnose the presence of small numbers of gram-negative bacteria in clinical specimens (and pharmaceuticals). The component of the gram-negative bacterium (gram-positive bacteria do not participate in the *Limulus* test) is the lipopolysaccharide (LPS) that arises from the outer membrane. The lipid part of the molecule is anchored into the cell membrane and is the biologically active pyrogen of the molecule. The complete LPS molecule is known as endotoxin. Endotoxin has considerable biological activity in the body, being responsible for disseminated intravascular coagulation. The physiological effects of endotoxin do not require living bacteria. Virtually all gram-negative bacteria contain biologically active LPS.

The *Limulus* test is based on the ability of LPS to activate *Limulus* amebocyte (the blood cell of the horseshoe crab) lysate (LAL) in the presence of calcium to active LAL enzyme. This enzyme acts as a serine protease that converts a soluble protein (coagulogen) to an insoluble complex (coagulin) by cleaving the LAL at the Arg-Lys and Arg-Gly linkage. The presence of endotoxin is detected by the observation of a gel, or clot, in the test mixture. For many years, the major difficulty in performing LAL assays was the small amount of spurious endotoxin present in the laboratory environment, including glassware and reagents. Use of disposable materials has largely eliminated this problem. A major variable with the assay was the reading of the gel endpoint. A problem occurred if the clot was partially formed: in the strict interpretation of the test, this phenomenon should be taken as negative; however, laboratories were uncomfortable with a quasi-endpoint.

In an attempt to develop a more specific endpoint indicator for the LAL assay, advantage was taken of the molecular nature of the reaction. Because it was known that the central chemical reaction involved the cleaving of Arg-Lys and Arg-Gly, the artificial hydrolyzable substrates Gly–Arg–*p*-nitroaniline and Arg–Lys–*p*-nitroaniline were constructed. In the presence of endotoxin, the substrate is cleaved and *p*-nitroaniline is released. When attached to the amino acids, *p*-nitroaniline is colorless; when cleaved, it is intensely yellow, with a maximum absorbancy at 405 nm. Although the production of the yellow end product offers several advantages over clot formation, it is still susceptible to the same nonspecific reactions as is the classic LAL test. In addition, the chromogenic substrate is more expensive.

The clinical utility of the LAL assay has generally been limited to the assay of endotoxin in CSF. A well-functioning LAL test should be able to detect approximately 1,000 gram-negative bacteria per ml. In untreated meningitis, one generally sees approximately 100,000 bacteria per ml (which coincides with about 1 bacterium per oil immersion field). Therefore, the sensitivity of the LAL test was found to be excellent in an untreated group (90% sensitive) but less so in patients who had been pretreated (65 to 75%). The test should not be performed using serum or urine specimens.

PRACTICAL CONSIDERATIONS IN THE USE OF AGGLUTINATION ASSAYS

Most clinical laboratories purchase agglutination kits from manufacturers who over the past 10 to 15 years have gained a great deal of experience in the production and marketing of these assays. The manufacturers of commercially available kits responsibly promote their products for use in a wide variety of clinical specimens and disease states. Nonetheless, the laboratory needs to understand the clinical value of these assays and know the technical controls that provide accurate and useful information to the referring clinician.

An extremely large and constantly expanding assortment of tests for the detection of antigens or antibodies is commercially available (5, 6, 8, 13, 45, 73, 78, 79). Many of these analytes can be detected by the agglutination assays discussed above (latex agglutination, hemagglutination, etc.). The literature of the past few years is replete with evaluations both of commercially available agglutination tests and of those used principally in research. Emphasis is placed on the assays that have been used extensively during the last few years and have found a place in clinical microbiology laboratories.

Commercially available agglutination kits are available for (i) detection of microbial antigen in body fluids (generally CSF, serum, or urine), (ii) serotyping and identification of bacterial colonies after growth on agar, (iii) identification of bacterial enzymes such as the coagulase of *S. aureus* (see chapter 28), (iv) detection of microbial antigens directly from swabs of particular body sites (group A and B streptococci), (v) screening for immune status to specific infectious agents, and (vi) semiquantitative assessment of antibody or antigen concentrations.

Although the assays have basic similarities, kits available from different manufacturers or even from the same manufacturer may have strikingly different protocols for performing the agglutination test. The quantity of body fluids or reagents, the number of microbial colonies needed for testing, and the need to concentrate, heat, or boil specimens vary from test to test and from manufacturer to manufacturer. Clinical microbiologists should strictly adhere to these protocols to achieve the sensitivity and specificity claimed by the manufacturer. These variations in protocols may be more or less useful to the work flow of an individual laboratory and may influence which manufacturers' kits are purchased.

SPECIFICITY AND SENSITIVITY

Knowledge of the sensitivity, specificity, and known cross-reactions is essential to the clinical microbiologist. The microbiology laboratory personnel must be familiar with each of these parameters for each assay performed in order to provide the clinician with appropriate information. These factors are inherently due to the properties of the antisera (polyclonal, monoclonal, avidity, affinity) or antigen from which the reagent is made; hence, these properties can conceivably change with new production materials.

A number of problems can plague the routine user of these commercial products. The possibility of a prozone can be a problem. Detection of *Haemophilus influenzae* type b has been observed on rare occasions to be in prozone when found in CSF, probably because of the greater sensitivity of most of the latex reagents used for this pathogen (1, 43, 46, 56). Gram stain results will generally be positive in such situations. Cryptococcal meningitis may be accompanied by large amounts of antigen in CSF, especially in patients with AIDS, and may be especially prone to the prozone.

A much greater problem to the routine user is the occurrence of nonspecific agglutination (i.e., false-positive result). Some of these reactions occur for unknown reasons, and others are due to cross-reactions with other organisms. A nonspecific reaction can be detected either as (i) reactivity occurring both with latex particles coated with specific antibody and with particles coated or attached to antibody to some irrelevant or unknown antigen or (ii) reactivity of more than one agglutination reagent. Neither approach is perfect. Both assume that the sensitivity to the nonspecific material is exactly the same for all components of testing. Clearly this is not the case, since false-positive results have been reported (5, 30, 57, 60, 65). The latter approach is also problematic because agglutination of multiple reagents can occur if there is a mixed infection (low probability) or multiple colonies (a problem that depends on the skill of the technologist). The clinical microbiologist must understand the use and limitations of the test components that detect nonspecific reactions.

Most manufacturers of agglutination tests intended principally for detecting antigen in body fluids recommend prior treatment of specimens to eliminate or decrease the likelihood of a nonspecific reaction. Again, the approaches vary with the manufacturer. One strategy is to heat the specimen to boiling so that coagulation and inactivation of protein (mostly albumin) take place. This procedure is useful when the antigen to be detected is a carbohydrate that is not affected by heating. Another approach is treatment of the specimen with a reducing agent or an enzyme such as pronase. Manufacturers often claim that these treatments have no effect on the sensitivity of their products; however, objective evidence using clinical specimens is lacking in the literature (18, 51, 65, 66). On the contrary, investigators who have detected cryptococcal antigen have shown that pretreatment can increase the observed titer of reactant (24).

QUALITY CONTROL

Commercial manufacturers follow quality control production procedures to ensure consistency of their products, and it is important that users follow the protocols in the package insert for obtaining quality results. Reagents should be stored appropriately and not used beyond the expiration date unless steps have been taken to ensure accuracy of results. In the daily performance of these tests, the laboratory protocol must allow for appropriate controls to be performed. Alongside each specific reagent (i.e., carrier with detecting antisera or antigen), the patient specimen (or colony) must be run with a nonspecific reagent, often called a control reagent (i.e., carrier with irrelevant antisera or antigen). Care must be taken to ensure that the control reagent used is similar in immunoglobulin components to the specific or test reagent (e.g., equine polyclonal antisera for both or mouse monoclonal IgG1 for both).

It is also important that both test and control reagents be tested with positive and negative controls. The laboratory can establish a protocol of doing these tests once each day or less frequently, as long as care has been taken to ensure kit integrity. If a manufacturer does not provide negative controls, the laboratory can easily provide and use its own. A negative control may be a pool of sera that has been repeatedly found to be negative and stored frozen at −70°C in appropriate sample sizes.

An additional potential problem is lot-to-lot variation in sensitivity and specificity. Again, it is good laboratory practice to make limited in-house evaluations of each new lot of materials. This can easily be done either by making serial dilutions of the positive control from each lot of reagent and running a comparison with both lots or by maintaining a laboratory-standardized pool of specimen and determining the titer of this pool with each new lot of reagent. This procedure addresses the sensitivity issue. Questions concerning specificity are more difficult to deal with on a routine basis, and the work and cost involved are generally beyond the scope of a busy microbiology laboratory.

Interpretation of the pattern of agglutination is subjective and hence an additional source of error. Most manufacturers provide instructions that use a 1+ to 4+ grading system as compared with either the positive or negative controls. Strict adherence to the labeling, package inserts, and recommendations of the manufacturer for interpretation is important for both accurate and consistent results. In laboratories in which more than one technologist performs these tests, each positive finding in body fluids should be confirmed by an additional reader. The reactions seen in serotyping or identifying from colonies or after growth of the microorganism has taken place are usually stronger, and additional confirmation may not be needed.

If an assay requires an endpoint determination, it is essential that the positive control be titered to beyond the endpoint for comparison with the results obtained with a patient specimen. A practical and cost-effective approach is to dispense the positive control (commercial or prepared in-house) and freeze it at −70°C at a dilution close to its endpoint. This provides for a greater quantity of positive control and a readily available comparison for endpoint reading which has been established by repeated past testing.

LABORATORY SAFETY

It is important to keep in mind the issue of transmission of infectious agents such as human immunodeficiency virus type 1, hepatitis B virus, or *Neisseria meningitis*. The degree of risk in performing these tests varies with the method used. Tests that require some extraction procedure (such as those for streptococcal organisms) release antigens and eliminate viable organisms. Tests that are performed on body fluids require additional care. Although tests that require a pretreatment step (pronase or boiling) reduce the risk of transmitting infectious agents, it is best to handle all of these specimens as potentially hazardous. Care should be taken to prevent aerosols from occurring. Pipette tips used to transfer patient specimens to the solid support should be discarded into a bag for autoclaving, as should disposable solid supports such as cardboard. Glass supports should be soaked in bleach (e.g., 1:10 chlorine bleach) solutions for 10 to 15 min and then washed, rinsed, and dried for further use. Autoclaving of these glass supports would precipitate protein, making their use in further testing questionable. Above all, it should be remembered that many of these agglutination assays do not destroy bacteria or viruses, and hence the specimens should be treated as potentially infectious material.

TECHNICAL ADVANTAGES AND DISADVANTAGES

Advantages

Agglutination tests for detection of antigens or antibody have considerable advantages to the clinical laboratory compared with many other methodologies. Sensitivity is greater than with the direct use of uncoupled antisera when one is serotyping organisms. Studies have generally found agglutination tests to be more sensitive than counterimmunoelectrophoresis (28, 53, 76). Some manipulations of these assays can approach or surpass the sensitivity of the enzyme-linked immunosorbent assay (4, 7, 22, 52, 64, 66, 70). In addition, latex agglutination appears to have greater sensitivity than coagglutination (19, 29, 40, 71), although most studies have not used identical antisera in preparation of the various reagents.

Testing time is generally 15 to 20 min, making agglutination tests faster than culture, biochemical identification, and most enzyme immunoassay and radioimmunoassay tests. Hence, the turnaround time for clinically critical information is considerably shortened.

The problems associated with transport and handling of specimens for culture are reduced. Since it is antigen that is being detected rather than viable organisms, positive findings can be obtained when handling and transporting conditions have resulted in loss of viability. There is little degradation of antigen unless extremes of heat or delays in testing take place.

While most of the earlier agglutination tests for the detection of antigen were designed either for use in body fluids, particularly CSF, or for serotyping of microbial colonies, researchers have extended their use by applying the same test kits for identification from blood culture bottles (e.g., the BACTEC system) when indications of growth are observed (42, 49, 50, 74). Each clinical microbiology laboratory can use these systems to develop protocols for quicker identification schemes much in the same way that biochemical or antibiotic sensitivities have been used in the past (36, 42, 58, 68). Each laboratory must evaluate the sensitivity, specificity, and predictive values for the protocol and the population for which the new protocol is designed.

Disadvantages

Cost has been one of the major disadvantages to the use of some of the commercially available agglutination tests. Traditionally, microbiologists have compared the cost of newer methodologies with the cost of culture media, the Gram stain, and the technologist's labor. The overall impression is that the agglutination tests are more expensive, particularly since one often is required to test not just for a single pathogen (antigen) but for a panel of suspected microorganisms, as is most often the case when one is dealing with suspected cases of bacterial meningitis.

In an era when the available resources are decreasing, each laboratory must make decisions based on the overall expense to the institution or the patient population. Agglutination tests for detection of group A streptococci from throat swabs might be cost-effective to a walk-in medical clinic but not to a large city hospital with a large mix of patient demographics. Each laboratory and associated medical staff must decide on the merits and the costs incurred for each assay on the basis of its primary need.

A more compelling disadvantage is the need for viable microorganisms when appropriate antimicrobial therapy must be formulated. In these instances, both agglutination tests and culture must be performed. Hence, parallel work is absolutely necessary when one is testing for the pathogens of bacterial meningitis but is not needed when one is screening for the presence of group A streptococci in throat swabs (3, 44, 54) or group B streptococci in vaginal swabs (21, 23, 44, 63, 68).

SPECIMEN TYPES AND ASSOCIATED PROBLEMS

Some commercially available kits used in clinical laboratories were originally designed for specific specimen types or anatomic sources, notably tests for the direct detection of group A streptococcal antigen after extraction from swabs. Other kits are designed to be used with a variety of body fluids, usually CSF, serum, or urine. Two aspects of this latter group need special consideration: (i) technical problems associated with each body fluid type and (ii) the clinical utility of each specimen type. CSF is the specimen with a minimum of associated technical problems. It has a relatively narrow and stable pH range, the concentration of protein even in the diseased state is low, and the prevalence of rheumatoid factor is negligible. For these reasons, the incidence of nonspecific findings is relatively low, although it varies among tests and among manufacturers. Conversely, when one uses serum, the incidence of nonspecific findings increases as a result of increased protein concentration and increased viscosity. Serum may also have high concentrations of rheumatoid factor, increasing the chances of false-positive results. Urine also becomes problematic because of significant fluctuation in pH as well as changes in electrolytes and the presence of cellular components. Manufacturers often provide buffer systems to control these conditions, but in clinical practice one rarely determines whether the buffer has provided the correct pH range for optimal test sensitivity and specificity.

CSF and urine specimens have an advantage over serum in that both can be concentrated if necessary to obtain an increase in antigen concentration and make the antigen detectable by the test system. This procedure has been found to be especially useful in the diagnosis of streptococcal group B meningitis or sepsis in newborns (17, 30, 55, 59).

Other clinical specimens that have been used for detecting pathogenic organisms are sputum and synovial fluid. These specimens also have associated problems due particularly to an increase in viscosity (both sputum and synovial fluid) or to the presence of cross-reacting bacteria (sputum). The use of mucolytic agents may make this testing possible. Unfortunately, the methods now available make it difficult to distinguish colonization of the oropharynx from infection when sputum is the specimen used. Examination of sputum (for example, for *S. pneumoniae*) appears to be more sensitive than Gram stain or culture (13, 16, 20, 29, 32, 40, 49, 77). However, the clinician may now be faced with the decision as to whether the patient is infected or colonized, particularly if the culture subsequently is negative. Investigations of whether semiquantitative antigen results can resolve this question need to be conducted.

Each specimen submitted by the clinician has its own predictive value in diagnosing infection with a particular pathogen. Direct comparisons are difficult to make because different researchers have used different commercially available tests. The results have as much to do with the severity or stage of disease as with the sensitivity of the assay; certain trends are observable. Reagents for detecting *H. influenzae* type b appear to have the greatest sensitivity and specificity (2, 4, 60, 62, 69, 77) regardless of the body fluid (1, 12, 40, 60), whereas detection of *S. pneumoniae* appears to be the most difficult in nearly all body fluids and tests used. Whether this difficulty is a function of the pathogenesis of pneumococcal disease or due to the inadequacy of antisera needed to detect so many serogroups is unclear. However, the clinical microbiologist should make the clinician aware that in systemic diseases the answer to the cause of infection may lie in the examination of several body fluids.

The predictive value of a test is directly related to the prevalence of the particular disease in a population. Therefore, antigen tests should not be used as screening procedures. In a low-prevalence population, false-positives often outnumber true-positives.

CLINICAL SIGNIFICANCE

Detection of antigen

The presence of antigen (assuming that it is not due to nonspecific agglutination) in otherwise sterile body fluids is a clinically significant finding. Whether it suggests active infection depends on the organism that the antigen is indicative of and, in some instances, the level of antigen in the body fluid. Detection of cryptococcal antigen in CSF, which has largely replaced the use of India ink wet mount and microscopy because of its greater sensitivity, indicates the presence of *Cryptococcus neoformans*. Levels of ≧1:8 are considered to indicate active infection (33a). On the other hand, detection of any quantity of an antigen representing an agent known to cause bacterial meningitis is indicative of active infection.

Determination of antigen concentration by twofold serial dilutions may also be used to monitor the response to therapy and has been found to be particularly useful in monitoring the course of cryptococcal meningitis (18, 31, 34). On the other hand, the presence of *H. influenzae* type b antigen may persist beyond the stage of active infection. Some studies have documented its persistence 4 to 5 weeks beyond the need for therapy (39).

Detection of antigen from sources other than sterile sites needs to be interpreted with care. As mentioned previously, detection of antigens in secretions that pass through contaminated areas such as the oropharynx may indicate colonization rather than active infection (13, 47, 56, 67). Conversely, the detection of group A streptococci from throat swabs should be considered significant because the sensitivity of commercially available tests has been generally adjusted to discount low-level colonization. Clinical interpretation also is important with respect to the detection of antigen in the urine of newborns; in particular, the finding of group B streptococcal antigen in the urine of newborn infants without any other clinical signs of disease should be regarded with suspicion (57). These specimens can easily be contaminated by skin or fecal flora, giving false-positive as well as nonspecific results (30, 35, 61).

Negative results should also be regarded carefully. Theoretically, a negative finding should not be used to rule out the absence of a particular pathogen (14, 27, 38, 47) or the absence of disease because the quantity of antigen could be below the sensitivity of reagents used. In addition, disease may be caused by a serotype not detected by the commonly available agglutination tests. Most but not all *H. influenzae* disease is caused by type b, although increasing numbers of other types or nontypable *H. influenzae* have been documented as pathogens. Since currently available kits detect only type b, the occasional disease caused by other serotypes will be missed. On the other hand, negative findings for the more common pathogens detected by these tests have a good predictive value because the tests are positive when disease occurs (14, 29, 60, 68).

Detection of antibody

When used to detect the presence of antibody, agglutination tests are actually screening tests; that is, they provide a yes or no answer to the presence of antibody. In some circumstances, this result can be interpreted as immune or susceptible (e.g., in determining immune status to rubella virus). When formulated in this way, agglutination tests cannot provide information as to the temporal sequence of current or past infection. Although IgM is a very good agglutinating agent, the methodology for determining this specific class of antibody is generally not performed for agglutination tests.

Serial dilutions of patient serum can, however, be used to obtain a semiquantitative concentration of antibody. This has some clinical value if one has performed epidemiological studies to determine normal limits. As with many other serological tests, demonstration of a change in titer can provide evidence for a recent infection. Clinicians and microbiologists must bear in mind that most of these tests are screening tests for antibody, and unless they are prepared by specific recombinant DNA procedures, the possibility for cross-reaction or nonspecific interaction exists. When more specific information (e.g., in human immunodeficiency virus type 1 infection) is required, methodologies such as immunofluorescence or Western immunoblotting are needed.

CRITERIA FOR TESTING

The decision to use most agglutination tests generally rests on the need for rapid results or the nature of a particular clinical setting. The issue of cost may at times also be decisive. Many investigations have repeatedly demonstrated that the CSF in patients with bacterial meningitis (other than neonates less than 6 weeks old [9, 11, 21]) demonstrates some abnormality of cell count or differential of the usual chemical analyses (9, 15). This appears to be true even when partial or ineffective antibiotic therapy has been initiated (33, 72). Hence, the laboratory should review as quickly as possible all of the CSF test results to determine whether bacterial antigen testing is still necessary. Direct antigen testing is usually without merit in CSF specimens normal by all established criteria.

Occasionally, the results of a Gram stain are inconclusive or difficult to interpret. In this situation, antigen testing may be performed to assist the laboratory in determining the etiology of disease.

When used appropriately as determined by clinical need, institutional setting, and disease state, agglutination tests can provide meaningful, rapid, and hence useful results for patient care.

APPENDIX

1. Particles in suspension are governed by

$$f = 6\pi \text{ (viscosity) (particle radius)}$$

The force (f) bringing the particle out of solution can be described by

$$f = \Delta d 4/3 \pi r^3 \text{ (gravity)}$$

where d is distance.

Therefore, the ability of a particle to leave solution is directly related to the r^2. Accordingly, agglutination would be much more efficient than precipitation in yielding an observable endpoint.

2. The zeta potential (z) or Smoluchowski equation is expressed by

$$z = \frac{4\pi \text{ (electrophoretic mobility)}}{\text{dielectric constant}}$$

which is applied to serological testing by

$$z = k_{1/D\mu} - k_{2/D \text{ volts}}$$

where D is the dielectric constant and μ is ionic strength. The constants are related to the individual electrolytes in solution.

3. The dipole interactions can be described by

$$f = \frac{\text{area (of the parts in juxtaposition)}}{\pi h^3}$$

where h is the distance between the particles. Therefore, the closer the particles approach, the greater the force of attraction cubed.

We express our appreciation to Shirley Neill for preparation of the manuscript.

LITERATURE CITED

1. **Ajello, G. W., G. A. Bolan, P. S. Hayes, D. Lehmann, J. Montgomery, J. C. Feeley, C. A. Perlino, and C. V. Broome.** 1987. Commercial latex agglutination tests for detection of *Haemophilus influenzae* type b and *Streptococcus pneumoniae* antigens in patients with bacteremic pneumonia. J. Clin. Microbiol. **25:**1388–1391.
2. **Ballard, T. L., M. H. Roe, R. C. Wheeler, J. K. Todd, and M. P. Glode.** 1987. Comparison of three latex agglutination kits and counterimmunoelectrophoresis for the detection of bacterial antigens in a pediatric population. Pediatr. Infect. Dis. J. **6:**630–634.
3. **Beach, P. S., L. C. Balfour, and H. L. Lucia.** 1989. Group A streptococcal rapid test. Antigen detection after 18–24 hours of penicillin therapy. Clin. Pediatr. **28:**6–10.
4. **Belmaaza, A., J. Hamel, S. Mousseau, S. Montplaisir, and B. R. Brodeur.** 1986. Rapid diagnosis of severe *Haemophilus influenzae* serotype b infections by monoclonal antibody enzyme immunoassay for outer membrane proteins. J. Clin. Microbiol. **24:**440–445.
5. **Benson, R. F., W. L. Thacker, B. B. Plikaytis, and H. W. Wilkinson.** 1987. Cross-reactions in *Legionella* antisera with *Bordetella pertussis* strains. J. Clin. Microbiol. **25:**594–596.
6. **Berke, A., and R. C. Tilton.** 1986. Evaluation of rapid coagulase methods for the identification of *Staphylococcus aureus*. J. Clin. Microbiol. **23:**916–919.
7. **Bevanger, L., J. A. Maeland, and A. I. Naess.** 1988. Agglutinins and antibodies to *Francisella tularensis* outer membrane antigens in the early diagnosis of disease during an outbreak of tularemia. J. Clin. Microbiol. **26:**433–437.
8. **Bibb, W. F., P. M. Arnow, L. Thacker, and R. M. McKinney.** 1984. Detection of soluble *Legionella pneumophila* antigens in serum and urine specimens by enzyme-linked immunosorbent assay with monoclonal and polyclonal antibodies. J. Clin. Microbiol. **20:**478–482.
9. **Blazer, S., and M. Berant.** 1983. Bacterial meningitis. Effect of antibiotic treatment on cerebrospinal fluid. Am. J. Clin. Pathol. **80:**386–387.
10. **Boguslaski, R. C.** 1987. Immunoassays monitored by virus, particle, and metal labels, p. 211–219. *In* R. C. Boguslaski, E. T. Maggio, and R. M. Nakamura (ed.), Clinical immunochemistry: principles of methods and applications. Little, Brown & Co., Boston.

11. **Bonadio, W. A.** 1989. How rapidly is cerebrospinal fluid pleocytosis manifested with bacterial meningitis? Pediatr. Infect. Dis. J. **8**:337–338. (Letter.)
12. **Boreland, P. C., S. H. Gillespie, and L. A. Ashworth.** 1988. Rapid diagnosis of whooping cough using monoclonal antibody. J. Clin. Pathol. **41**:573–575.
13. **Brogan, O., P. A. Garnett, C. C. Fox, and K. A. McCabe.** 1987. Evaluation of anaerobic culture and effect of culture medium supplementation with factor V on colonial morphology and efficacy of isolation of *Streptococcus pneumoniae* from sputum. J. Clin. Pathol. **40**:368–71.
14. **Bromberg, K., and M. R. Hammerschlag.** 1987. Rapid diagnosis of pneumonia in children [review]. Semin. Respir. Infect. **2**:159–165.
15. **Callaham, M.** 1989. Fulminant bacterial meningitis without meningeal signs. Ann. Emerg. Med. **18**:90–93.
16. **Congeni, B. L., H. J. Igel, and M. S. Platt.** 1984. Evaluation of a latex particle agglutination kit in pneumococcal disease. Pediatr. Infect. Dis. **3**:417–419.
17. **Coonrod, J. D.** 1983. Urine as an antigen reservoir for diagnosis of infectious diseases. Am. J. Med. **75**:85–92.
18. **Coovadia, Y. M., and Z. Solwa.** 1987. Sensitivity and specificity of a latex agglutination test for detection of cryptococcal antigen in meningitis. S. Afr. Med. J. **71**:510–512.
19. **Drow, D. L., and D. D. Manning.** 1983. Comparison of coagglutination, latex agglutination and enzyme-linked immunosorbent assay for detection of *Haemophilus influenzae* type b infection. Diagn. Microbiol. Infect. Dis. **1**: 317–322.
20. **Ericsson, C. H., H. O. Hallander, A. Rosen, A. M. Sjogren, and I. Sjogren.** 1986. Routine use of counterimmunoelectrophoresis for the detection of pneumococcal antigen in sputum. Med. Microbiol. Immunol. **175**:241–249.
21. **Facklam, R. R.** 1987. Specificity study of kits for detection of group A streptococci directly from throat swabs. J. Clin. Microbiol. **25**:504–508.
22. **Feng, C. S., I. B. Williams, R. S. Gohd, and A. P. Causey.** 1986. A comparison of four commercial test kits for detection of cytomegalovirus antibodies in blood donors. Transfusion **26**:203–204.
23. **Friedman, C. A., D. F. Wender, and J. E. Rawson.** 1984. Rapid diagnosis of group B streptococcal infection utilizing a commercially available latex agglutination assay. Pediatrics **73**:27–30.
24. **Gray, L. D., and G. D. Roberts.** 1988. Experience with the use of pronase to eliminate interference factors in the latex agglutination test for cryptococcal antigen. J. Clin. Microbiol. **26**:2450–2451.
25. **Gribnau, T., F. Roeles, J. V. Biezen, J. Leuvering, and A. Schuurs.** 1981. The applications of colloidal dye particles as labels in immunoassays: disperse(d) dye immunoassay (DIA). Anal. Chem. Symp. Ser. **9**:411–427.
26. **Halberstam, D., J. M. Singer, and E. G. Allen.** 1965. Influence of electrolytes on stability of 0.2 micron diameter polystyrene latex particles. Proc. Soc. Exp. Biol. Med. **118**: 319–323.
27. **Henne, G., F. W. Tiller, F. B. Spencker, W. Handrick, and G. Knoll.** 1989. Nonvalue of antigen quantitation in diagnosis of *Haemophilus* meningitis. Infection **17**:107–108.
28. **Hoban, D. J., E. Witwicki, and G. W. Hammond.** 1985. Bacterial antigen detection in cerebrospinal fluid of patients with meningitis. Diagn. Microbiol. Infect. Dis. **3**:373–379.
29. **Holmberg, H., and A. Krook.** 1986. Comparison of enzyme-linked immunosorbent assay with coagglutination and latex agglutination for rapid diagnosis of pneumococcal pneumonia by detecting antigen in sputa. Eur. J. Clin. Microbiol. **5**:282–286.
30. **Issacs, D.** 1989. Problems in determining the etiology of community-acquired childhood pneumonia. Pediatr. Infect. Dis. J. **8**:143–148.
31. **Kahn, F. W., and J. M. Jones.** 1986. Latex agglutination tests for detection of *Candida* antigens in sera of patients with invasive candidiasis. J. Infect. Dis. **153**:579–585.
32. **Kalin, M., and A. A. Lindberg.** 1983. Diagnosis of pneumococcal pneumonia: a comparison between microscopic examination of expectorate, antigen detection, and cultural procedures. Scand. J. Infect. Dis. **15**:247–255.
33. **Kaplan, S. L., E. O. Smith, C. Wills, and R. D. Feigin.** 1986. Association between preadmission oral antibiotic therapy and cerebrospinal fluid findings and sequelae caused by *Haemophilus influenzae* type b meningitis. Pediatr. Infect. Dis. **5**:626–632.

33a. **Kaufman, L., and E. Reiss.** 1986. Serodiagnosis of fungal diseases, p. 446–466. *In* N. R. Rose, H. Friedman, and J. L. Fahey (ed.), Manual of clinical laboratory immunology, 3rd ed. American Society for Microbiology, Washington, D.C.

34. **Koshi, G., A. Viswanathan, M. Chandy, and P. S. Jairaj.** 1987. Development of a coagglutination (COA) technic to detect *Candida* antigenemia. 1. COA versus *Candida* isolation. Am. J. Clin. Pathol. **88**:429–435.
35. **Krambovitis, E., M. B. McIllmurray, P. A. Lock, H. Holzel, M. R. Lifely, and C. Moreno.** 1987. Murine monoclonal antibodies for detection of antigens and culture identification of *Neisseria meningitidis* group B and *Escherichia coli* K-1. J. Clin. Microbiol. **25**:1641–1644.
36. **Krook, A., H. Holmberg, and A. M. Sjogren.** 1987. A new coagglutination test for detecting pneumococcal C-polysaccharide. Eur. J. Clin. Microbiol. **6**:68–69.
37. **Kwapinski, J. B.** 1972. Methodology of immunochemical and immunological research. John Wiley & Sons, Inc., New York.
38. **Lammier, C., K. Gurturk, and H. Blobel.** 1987. Streptococcal group B type antigen X in group L streptococci. J. Clin. Microbiol. **25**:1803–1804.
39. **La Scolea, L. J., Jr., S. V. Rosales, and P. L. Ogra.** 1985. *Haemophilus influenzae* type b infection in childhood history of bacteremia and antigenemia. Infect. Immun. **50**: 753–756.
40. **Lenthe-Eboa, S., G. Brighouse, R. Auckenthaler, D. Lew, A. Zwahlen, P. H. Lambert, and F. A. Waldvogel.** 1987. Comparison of immunological methods for diagnosis of pneumococcal pneumonia in biological fluids. Eur. J. Clin. Microbiol. **6**:28–34.
41. **Leuvering, J. H., P. J. Thal, M. Vander Waart, and A. H. Shuurs.** 1980. Sol particle immunoassay (SPIA). J. Immunoassay **1**:77–94.
42. **Lim, P. L., and Y. P. Fok.** 1987. Detection of group D salmonellae in blood culture broth and of soluble antigen by tube agglutination using an O-9 monoclonal antibody latex conjugate. J. Clin. Microbiol. **25**:1165–1168.
43. **Logan, S., J. Barbara, and I. Kovar.** 1988. Cytomegalovirus screened blood for neonatal intensive care units. Arch. Dis. Child. **63**(Spec. No. 7):753–755.
44. **Lotz-Nolan, L., T. Amato, J. Iltis, W. Wallen, and B. Packer.** 1989. Evaluation of a rapid latex agglutination test for detection of group B streptococci in vaginal specimens. Eur. J. Clin. Microbiol. Infect. Dis. **8**:289–293.
45. **Luo, Z., D. J. Smith, M. A. Taubman, and W. F. King.** 1988. Cross-sectional analysis of serum antibody to oral streptococcal antibody in children. J. Dent. Res. **67**:554–560.
46. **Marcon, M. J., A. C. Hamoudi, and H. J. Cannon.** 1984. Comparative laboratory evaluation of three antigen detection methods for diagnosis of *Haemophilus influenzae* type b disease. J. Clin. Microbiol. **19**:333–337.
47. **Martin, S. J., D. A. Hoganson, and E. T. Thomas.** 1987. Detection of *Streptococcus pneumoniae* and *Haemophilus influenzae* type b antigens in acute nonbacteremic pneumonia. J. Clin. Microbiol. **25**:248–250.
48. **Masson, P. L., C. L. Cambiaso, D. Collet-Cassart, C. G. M. Magnusson, C. B. Richards, and C. J. Sindic.**

1981. Particle counting immunoassay (PACIA). Methods Enzymol. **74:**106–139.

49. **Mayer, M. E., P. J. Geiseler, and B. Harris.** 1983. Coagglutination for detection and serotyping of bacterial antigens: usefulness in acute pneumonia. Diagn. Microbiol. Infect. Dis. **1:**277–285.
50. **Mayer, M. E., P. J. Geiseler, and B. Harris.** 1983. Rapid diagnosis of septic arthritis by coagglutination. J. Clin. Microbiol. **18:**1424–1426.
51. **Mittal, K. R., R. Higgins, S. Lariviere, and G. P. Martineau.** 1987. Effect of heat treatment on the surface antigens of *Haemophilus pleuropneumoniae*. Vet. Rec. **120:**62–65.
52. **Montie, T. C., and T. R. Anderson.** 1988. Enzyme-linked immunosorbent assay for detection of *Pseudomonas aeruginosa* H (flagellar) antigen. Eur. J. Clin. Microbiol. Infect. Dis. **7:**256–260.
53. **Moyer, N. P., G. M. Evins, N. E. Pigott, J. D. Hudson, C. E. Farshy, J. C. Feeley, and W. J. Hausler, Jr.** 1987. Comparison of serologic screening tests for brucellosis. J. Clin. Microbiol. **25:**1969–1972.
54. **Ogay, K., and J. Bille.** 1986. Rapid coagglutination test for the direct detection of group A streptococci from throat swabs. Eur. J. Clin. Microbiol. **5:**317–319.
55. **O'Neill, K. P., N. Lloyd-Evans, H. Campbell, I. M. Forgie, S. Sabally, and B. M. Greenwood.** 1989. Latex agglutination test for diagnosing pneumococcal pneumonia in children in developing countries. Br. Med. J. **298:**1061–1064.
56. **Platenkamp, G. J., A. M. VanDuin, J. C. Porsius, H. J. Schouten, P. E. Zondervan, and M. F. Michel.** 1987. Diagnosis of invasive candidiasis in patients with and without signs of immune deficiency: a comparison of six detection methods in human serum. J. Clin. Pathol. **40:**1162–1167.
57. **Rabalais, G. P., D. R. Bronfin, and R. S. Daum.** 1987. Evaluation of a commercially available latex agglutination test for rapid diagnosis of group B streptococcal infection. Pediatr. Infect. Dis. J. **6:**177–181.
58. **Rahman, M., D. A. Sack, S. Mahmood, and A. Hossain.** 1987. Rapid diagnosis of cholera by coagglutination test using 4-h fecal enrichment cultures. J. Clin. Microbiol. **25:** 2204–2206.
59. **Rench, M. A., T. G. Metzger, and C. J. Baker.** 1984. Detection of group B streptococcal antigen in body fluids by a latex-coupled monoclonal antibody assay. J. Clin. Microbiol. **20:**852–854.
60. **Rubin, L. J., and L. Carmody.** 1987. Pneumococcal and *Haemophilus influenzae* type b antigen detection in children at risk for occult bacteremia. Pediatrics **80:**92–96.
61. **Rubinstein, L. J., and K. E. Stein.** 1988. Murine immune response to the *Neisseria meningitidis* group C capsule polysaccharide. II. Specificity. J. Immunol. **141:**4357–4362.
62. **Rytel, M. W., and L. C. Preheim.** 1986. Antigen detection in the diagnosis and in the prognostic assessment of bacterial pneumonias. Diagn. Microbiol. Infect. Dis. **4**(Suppl. 3):35S–46S.
63. **Savoia, D., F. Cofano, and S. Landolfo.** 1986. A method for the rapid detection of streptococcal group A antigen by specific monoclonal antibody. Boll. 1st Sieroter. Milan **65:**69–72.
64. **Sekiguchi, S., H. Ikeda, T. Kato, R. Maeda, and K. Fukai.** 1988. An automated screening test for antibodies to human immunodeficiency virus-1. Transfusion **28:**581–585.
65. **Sippel, J. E., P. A. Hider, G. Contronі, K. D. Eisenach, H. R. Hill, M. W. Rytel, and B. L. Wasilauskas.** 1984. Use of the Directigen latex agglutination test for detection of *Haemophilus influenzae, Streptococcus pneumoniae,* and *Neisseria meningitidis* antigens in cerebrospinal fluid from meningitis patients. J. Clin. Microbiol. **20:**884–886.
66. **Sippel, J. E., C. M. Prato, N. I. Girgis, and E. A. Edwards.** 1984. Detection of *Neisseria meningitidis* group A, *Haemophilus influenzae* type b, and *Streptococcus pneumoniae* antigens in cerebrospinal fluid specimens by antigen capture enzyme-linked immunosorbent assays. J. Clin. Microbiol. **20:**259–265.
67. **Sofianou, D., and J. Doumboyas.** 1989. Detection of soluble *Pseudomonas aeruginosa* antigens in bronchial secretions by a coagglutination test. Eur. J. Clin. Microbiol. Infect. Dis. **8:**144–146.
68. **Stiller, R. J., E. Blair, P. Clark, and T. Tinghitella.** 1989. Rapid detection of vaginal colonization with group B streptococci by means of latex agglutination. Am. J. Obstet. Gynecol. **160:**566–568.
69. **Suwanagool, S., K. D. Eisenach, S. M. Smith, and R. H. Eng.** 1986. Detection of bacterial antigens in body fluids by the Phadebact system. Scand. J. Infect. Dis. **18:**347–352.
70. **Takimoto, T., E. Ono, T. Ito, and R. Yanagawa.** 1988. Affinity constants of anti-leptospira monoclonal antibodies, numbers of antigenic determinants on leptospiras, and their influence on the microscopic agglutination test and ELISA. Microbiol. Immunol. **32:**775–784.
71. **Tilton, R. C., F. Dias, and R. W. Ryan.** 1984. Comparative evaluation of three commercial products and counterimmunoelectrophoresis for the detection of antigens in cerebrospinal fluid. J. Clin. Microbiol. **20:**231–234.
72. **Valmari, P., H. Peltola, and M. Kataja.** 1986. Cerebrospinal fluid white cell glucose and protein changes during the treatment of *Haemophilus influenzae* meningitis. Scand. J. Infect. Dis. **18:**39–43.
73. **Van Der Auwera, P., A. Andre, G. Bulliard, J. C. Legrand, B. Gordts, H. Van Landuyt, and F. Schuyteneer.** 1983. Comparison of latex agglutination and counterimmunoelectrophoresis in the diagnosis of acute *Streptococcus pneumoniae* infections. Eur. J. Clin. Microbiol. **2:**534–540.
74. **Wetkowski, M. A., E. M. Peterson, and L. M. de la Maza.** 1981. Direct testing of blood cultures for detection of streptococcal antigens. J. Clin. Microbiol. **16:**86–91.
75. **Williams, C. A., and M. M. Chase (ed.).** 1970. Methods in immunology and immunochemistry, vol. 3, p. 1–125. Academic Press, Inc., New York.
76. **Wu, T. C., and S. Y. Koo.** 1983. Comparison of three commercial cryptococcal latex kits for detection of cryptococcal antigen. J. Clin. Microbiol. **18:**1127–1130.
77. **Zhang, X. P., K. E. Deng, Y. Q. Ye, and W. T. Luo.** 1988. Rapid detection pneumococcal antigens in sputa in patients with community-acquired pneumonia by coagglutination. Med. Microbiol. Immunol. **177:**333–338.
78. **Zhang, Y. H., W. F. Yu, J. Cai, D. Qian, T. X. Zhao, Z. Z. Xu, and M. X. Wan.** 1989. A rapid method for detection of flavivirus antigens: staphylococcal co-agglutination test using monoclonal antibodies to Japanese encephalitis virus. Acta Virol. **33:**24–31.
79. **Zhang, Y. H., D. N. Zhou, C. A. Wang, and T. Hung.** 1989. Rapid diagnosis of adult diarrhea rotavirus (ADRV): detection of viral antigens in faecal samples using staphylococcal co-agglutination test. Acta Virol. **33:**32–38.
80. **Zmijewski, C. M.** 1978. Immunohematology, 3rd ed., p. 149–180. Appleton-Century-Crofts, New York.

Chapter 10

Hemolytic Assays: Complement Fixation and Antistreptolysin O

MARIO R. ESCOBAR

The two hemolytic assays that are most widely used in clinical microbiology laboratories are complement fixation (CF) and antistreptolysin O (ASO). Although both assays have been selected for inclusion in this chapter, they differ substantially in terms of principle and breadth of application to the serodiagnosis of infectious diseases.

COMPLEMENT FIXATION

Background

Bordet and Gengou (2) devised the CF test in 1901 shortly after Ehrlich had coined the word "complement" (previously called "alexin" by Bordet and "cytase" by Metchnikoff) to identify the thermolabile constituent of serum that participated in cytolytic reactions. It is now known that complement is a system of at least 20 chemically and immunologically distinct plasma proteins capable of interacting with one another, with antibody, and with cell membranes. After activation of the system, these interactions lead to the generation of biologic activity which ranges from lysis of a number of different types of cells, bacteria, and viruses to direct mediation of inflammatory processes. Besides this function, complement is able to recruit and engage the participation of other humoral and cellular effector systems and induce histamine release from mast cells, chemotaxis of leukocytes, phagocytosis, and release of lysosomal constituents from phagocytes (4). For the purposes of this chapter, of all the functions of complement listed above, only that concerned with in vitro fixation of the components of complement that participate in the classical pathway of activation by antibody (immunoglobulin G [IgG] or IgM) and antigen is relevant to the CF test. IgM is more efficient than IgG in this regard, since only one IgM molecule is required for the fixation of the first complement component, whereas two IgG molecules in close proximity are needed for activation. In practice, however, many IgG molecules must be present in the reaction mixture in order to have two IgG molecules sufficiently close on the cell membrane to fix the first complement component in the indicator system (sheep erythrocytes [RBC] and hemolysin).

The CF test not only is one of the oldest serodiagnostic procedures but also has withstood the test of time. The CF test was used extensively in syphilis serology after its introduction by Wassermann in 1909. During the first third of this century, the CF test was widely used in the field of veterinary serology (e.g., study of vaccinia in calves, foot-and-mouth disease, psittacosis, and equine arthropod-borne encephalitides). During the second third of this century, however, the CF test was chosen as the routine laboratory procedure for the serodiagnosis of human infectious diseases. For a long time during the "serologic era," it was appropriately accepted as the standard against which the specificities of other methods were evaluated. This became possible because of (i) the advent of modern physicochemical procedures and advances in biotechnology that permitted the purification of reagents, leading to the refinement of the CF test; (ii) the establishment of host systems other than mice for the propagation of viruses that yielded high-titered type-specific antigens (e.g., embryonated chicken eggs and various kinds of cells in culture); and (iii) the development of a standardized CF test by the Communicable Disease Center (now the Centers for Disease Control), U.S. Department of Health and Human Services, Atlanta, Ga.

Since its introduction in the late 1950s and early 1960s, the CF test was adapted by Centers for Disease Control to the microtechnique methodology (4). This version, known as the Laboratory Branch complement fixation (LBCF) test, has been generally accepted as the standard. Over the years, the LBCF test has been revised twice, once in 1974 and again in 1981. With the availability of commercially prepared antigens and the standard LBCF test, results obtained by many laboratories are now comparable. Although there has been a definite trend in the last 15 years to replace the CF test with simpler as well as more direct, sensitive, and rapid methodologies, this technique is still an important constituent of the armentarium of viral, rickettsial, and fungal serologists (13, 14, 19).

Principle of the test

The CF test consists essentially of two antigen-antibody reactions, representing the test system and the indicator system, which occur in sequence (Fig. 1). The first reaction, between a known antigen and the patient serum or an unknown antigen (e.g., a virus isolate) and a specific antiserum, takes place in the presence of a predetermined amount of guinea pig complement. As this reaction proceeds in the presence of both specific antigen and antibody, complement is removed from solution (fixed) by becoming an integral part of the antigen-antibody complex. In the second antigen-antibody reaction, or indicator system, sheep RBC are coated (sensitized) with hemolysin (rabbit serum containing antibodies to sheep RBC). When this antigen-antibody complex is added to the components of the first reaction, the sensitized sheep RBC should fail to lyse because complement has been fixed by the antigen-antibody complex in the test system (Fig. 2). This is interpreted

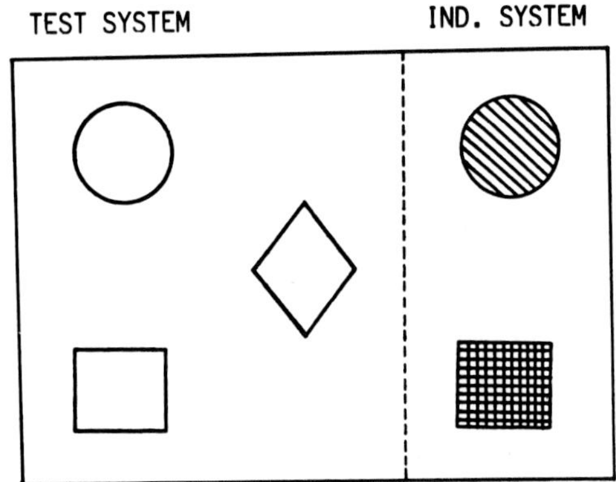

FIG. 1. Major components of the CF test. Symbols: ○, antigen; □, antibody; ◍, sheep RBC; ■, hemolysin; ◇, complement. Ind., Indicator.

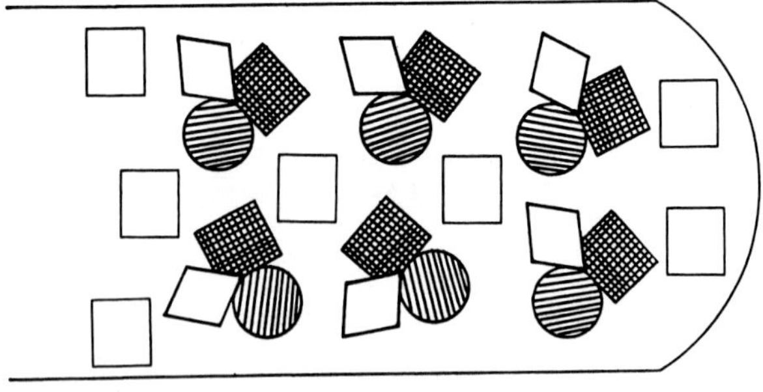

FIG. 3. Negative reaction showing the lysis of sheep RBC in the presence of complement that was not fixed in the test system because of the absence of antigen. See legend to Fig. 1 for explanation of symbols.

as a positive result indicating the presence of either antigen or antibody in the test system, depending on which of the two was being tested for. On the other hand, if either antigen (Fig. 3) or antibody (Fig. 4) is missing from the test system, complement should be free (unfixed) and will produce lysis of the sensitized sheep RBC in the indicator system. This is considered a negative result and indicates that either antigen or antibody is absent in the test system.

Test procedures

Although the CF test is regarded as relatively simple, it is a very exacting procedure involving five different components (derived from up to five different species). These include the antigen and antibody in each of the test and indicator systems in addition to complement for which the two systems compete. The hemolytic activity of complement depends on a number of factors besides complement concentration. Among the most important are concentration of sheep RBC, concentration of hemolysin, concentration of magnesium and calcium ions, ionic strength, reaction volume, reaction temperature, reaction time, and pH. The rigorous control of these factors will greatly reduce variations in complement titer that are not the result of variations in complement concentration alone (6). Therefore, the importance of accurate measurements cannot be overemphasized, particularly in the microtiter procedure because of the minute amount of each reagent used. This point is, however, also crucial with respect to complement for which the test and indicator systems compete in such a way that a suboptimal amount of complement would be responsible for an increase in sensitivity at the sacrifice of specificity, with concomitant false-positive results. Conversely, complement excess will produce false-negative results, with a decrease in sensitivity. Accordingly, the CF test design can be adapted to the particular laboratory setting by adjusting the sensitivity against the specificity of the test. Different versions of the CF test that are based on this principle have been described. For example, a CF test with a greater emphasis on sensitivity than specificity is more appropriate for screening purposes, whereas a CF test of high specificity is required for diagnostic purposes. In laboratories that test large numbers of specimens, use of an automatic microdiluting machine not only reduces the amount of time needed to perform the test but also increases accuracy.

The LBCF, which is a 50% endpoint method, is much more accurate than the 100% endpoint procedures. In the 50% endpoint method, the amount of complement is tightly controlled because the smallest variations in concentration around the 50% area of hemolysis (i.e., the steepest part of the sigmoid complement titration curve) will cause significant changes in hemolysis.

Standardization of reagents and quality control

Procedural details regarding the preparation of reagents and performance of the CF test are beyond the

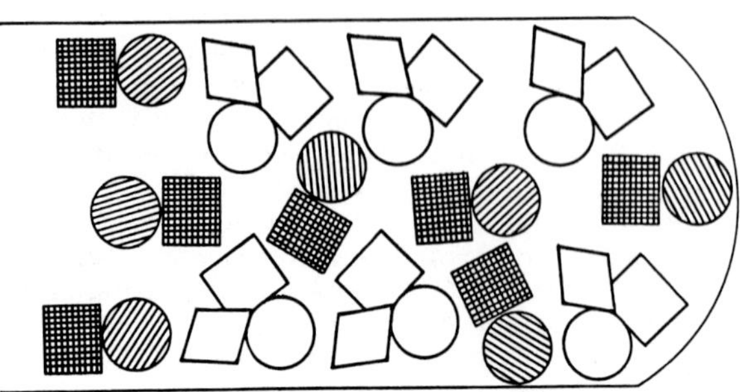

FIG. 2. Positive reaction indicating the presence of antibody or antigen in the test system. Sheep RBC are sensitized by hemolysin but do not lyse because of the lack of free complement. See legend to Fig. 1 for explanation of symbols.

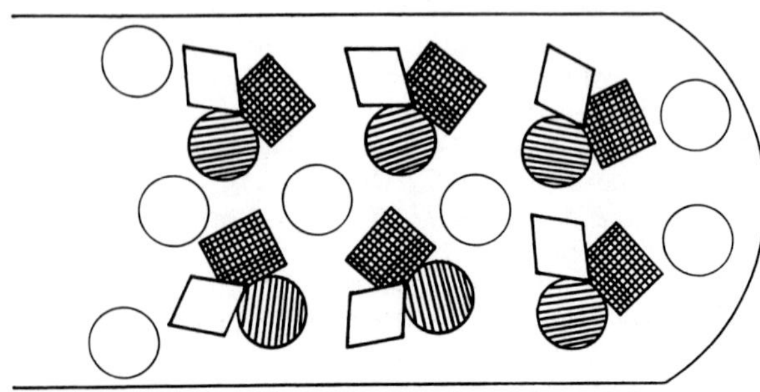

FIG. 4. Negative reaction showing the lysis of sheep RBC in the presence of complement that was not fixed in the test system because of the absence of antibody. See legend to Fig. 1 for explanation of symbols.

scope of this chapter. They have been well covered in other publications (3, 7, 14, 19), which the reader should consult if necessary. However, a few remarks concerning standardization and quality control are appropriate. Accuracy not only is vital in performance of the CF test but is equally important in standardization of the various components. Inaccuracies in the titrations of antigen (or antibody), complement, or hemolysin or in the standardization of sheep RBC may be compounded by errors during test performance. It is more accurate to perform the antigen or antibody titration by the checkerboard rather than the straight-line method. As previously mentioned, one must be certain that the complement concentration is precise. To ensure this, the LBCF was modified in our laboratory as follows: one further dilution (containing 0.625 complement hemolytic dose 50% endpoint [CH_{50}] unit) was added to the three conventional twofold dilutions (containing 5, 2.5, and 1.25 CH_{50} units) of the complement controls or back-titration. This modification provides for a more clear-cut and objective visualization of the correct amount of complement in the test, since the lowest dilution (containing 5 CH_{50} units) should yield 100% hemolysis and the highest dilution (containing 0.625 CH_{50} unit) should have no hemolysis. Although considered unnecessary by some laboratories, it is prudent to titrate complement in the presence of test antigen at the concentration to be used in the test, since different antigens vary in the ability to fix complement. Commercially prepared complement is usually obtained from fresh healthy guinea pig serum, which may contain antibody to the test antigen. Complement should therefore be tested for the presence of specific antibodies, particularly to certain viruses. Complement can be obtained commercially in a lyophilized preparation. After reconstitution, it should be divided into samples large enough for one run and kept frozen, preferably at −70°C. Each sample must be thawed only once just before use. Some manufacturers provide lyophilized complement containing a stabilizer, permitting the reconstituted material to be kept at 4 to 6°C for up to 4 weeks in tightly stoppered vials. If not handled properly, however, the reconstituted and stabilized complement will rapidly lose its activity. Sheep RBC should be obtained from a reliable source. Animals that are bled too frequently may produce abnormal RBC and must be avoided. Sheep RBC must be washed and standardized carefully to prevent cell lysis or enhanced sensitivity of the cell membrane to complement. Whether one uses the packed-cell or the spectrophotometric method for standardization, lysis of even a few RBC may produce inaccuracies in the test. A hemolysin titration should be performed each time a new lot of hemolysin is used. All of the necessary controls should be included in each run. For instance, for viral antigens one must include, in addition to the antigen control, a preparation from the uninfected cells in culture used to grow the virus. The patient serum control, complement controls (see above), and sheep RBC control, as well as positive and negative serum controls, must also be part of each run.

Specimen collection and preservation

Sera for CF tests must be collected in sterile tubes containing no preservatives or anticoagulants, mainly to avoid anticomplementary activity or false-positive reactions. Care must be taken to prevent hemolysis. If the laboratory is within reasonable distance from the collection point, serum is usually separated from the clot at the point of collection and stored at 4°C or frozen until dispatched. If no centrifuge is available at the collection point, settling of the sample overnight will usually provide a cell-free sample if care is exercised in removing the serum. All specimens for serology, which occasionally include cerebrospinal fluid or other body fluids, should be regarded as potentially infectious and treated accordingly in all phases of processing and testing. Whole blood should never be frozen since lysis of RBC will occur. Grossly hemolyzed serum must be treated to remove the hemoglobin if an accurate test is to be performed. Hemoglobin may be removed by molecular sieving through a Sephadex G-75 or G-100 column, a process that does not alter the antibody content of the serum. Nonetheless, these expensive and time-consuming treatments can be avoided by proper specimen collection and handling. If possible, two specimens of serum should be tested, the first taken as early as possible after the onset of symptoms and the second taken when the titer change is fourfold or higher. This interval may vary from 2 days to several weeks or even months, depending on the etiologic agent, but is usually 10 to 14 days. Occasionally, a third serum specimen may be helpful. On the other hand, testing of a single convalescent-phase specimen is not recommended for laboratory diagnosis of active infection except when a very high titer is obtained. In such cases, only a presumptive diagnosis may be warranted. When a differential titer rise or decline is to be established between specimens, the paired sera must be tested at the same time.

Anticomplementary activity

Anticomplementary activity is said to occur when complement is bound by either antigen or serum, but not both, before the addition of sensitized sheep RBC. This activity is considered to be nonspecific except when the patient serum contains immune complexes (e.g., during testing for hepatitis B surface antigen). Anticomplementary activity may be inherent in the patient as a result of chemotherapy or certain physiological changes. These are usually only transitory effects. Often this activity is destroyed during the heat inactivation step (30 min at 56°C) required before performance of the CF test. If heat inactivation is ineffective, 0.05 ml of undiluted complement is added to 0.15 ml of each serum pair, followed by incubation at 37°C for 30 min; 1.0 ml of Veronal buffer diluent is then added to yield a 1:8 dilution, and the sera are again inactivated by heating at 56°C for 30 min (7). If the serum continues to be anticomplementary, an additional serum specimen should be requested and tested. Generally, anticomplementary reactions occur in the lower serum dilutions (i.e., 1:8 to 1:16), which would not jeopardize test interpretation when the titer of the convalescent-phase serum is 64 or higher. Because of these problems, paired sera must be included in each CF test for the results to be valid. Anticomplementary activity may also occur during storage as a result of microbial contamination when the specimen was not collected aseptically or may occur as a result of the use of preservatives or anticoagulants.

Interpretation and clinical significance of test results

Similar to other laboratory test results, those generated by the CF test can serve to confirm the physician's provisional clinical diagnosis and should be considered within the larger context that includes the epidemiologic background (age, sex, travel history, and contacts of the patient, prevalence of the disease, etc.), past medical history, previous immunizations, pertinent laboratory data, and current physical examination findings. In addition, potential serological cross-reactions between the CF test antigens and those of related microorganisms must be recognized by the serologist. The reading and interpretation of the test results can be recorded only if all controls are within the acceptable range. According to the LBCF procedure (3), each dilution of patient serum yielding hemolysis of equal to or less than 30% is interpreted as positive for antibody. The titer should be equal to the reciprocal of the highest serum dilution yielding a positive result. Complement-fixing antibodies in many cases appear later than those detected by other tests (e.g., hemagglutination inhibition and neutralization) and are generally short-lived, becoming undetectable after a few years in most cases. This characteristic regarding the kinetics of CF antibodies can be useful in timing the activity of certain infections (e.g., rubella). Timing of infectious activity can also be ascertained by the use of different preparations of CF antigens. In mumps, for example, antibodies to the soluble antigens (i.e., mixture of virion components and virus-directed proteins released upon the disintegration of viral particles or infected cells) appear and disappear earlier than those produced against the viral antigens (i.e., intact virions), which rise later and persist for years (8). Another approach to determining the recent onset of a primary infection is the detection of IgM CF antibodies after the removal of IgG by a number of procedures (e.g., staphylococcal protein A or G). This approach does not always lead to conclusive results, since IgM antibodies may recur upon reactivation of a latent infection (e.g., cytomegalovirus), remain for more than a year (e.g., rubella virus), or persist at very low levels for many years in chronic carriers (e.g., hepatitis B virus).

ANTISTREPTOLYSIN O

Background

The beta-hemolytic group A streptococci elaborate two hemolysins, streptolysins O and S. Todd identified streptolysin O in 1932 (17) and differentiated it serologically from streptolysin S several years later (18). Streptolysin S is the factor responsible for the hemolytic zones surrounding streptococcal colonies on blood agar plates. Streptolysin S is not antigenic, but it may be inhibited by a nonspecific natural inhibitor (i.e., independent of past experience with streptococci) that is often present in human and animal sera.

Streptolysin O is a specific protein (molecular weight, 60,000) with enzymatic activity that is produced by almost all strains of Lancefield group A streptococci and a few strains of groups C and G. It has the ability to lyse RBC and leukocytes. It is destroyed at 55°C in 2 min and is reversibly inactivated by oxidizing substances, such as H_2O_2, iodine, cuprous oxide, iodoacetamide, and alloxan, and reinactivated by cysteine or dithionite.

Streptolysin O is prepared by growing any recently isolated strain of group A streptococci that does not produce hemolysis under aerobic conditions. The streptolysin O preparation can be used in liquid form as prepared, but it loses hemolytic activity after 7 to 60 days at 4°C. Lyophilized streptolysin O, however, has been found to be stable for 2 years.

Principle of the test

Streptolysin O combines quantitatively with ASO, an antibody that appears in humans after infection with any streptococci that produce streptolysin O. The basis of the ASO test is the neutralization of the hemolytic activity of the streptolysin O toxin for RBC by specific antibodies in serum.

Test procedures

The procedures for preparation of the reagents and performance of the ASO test have recently been described in detail (9). With regard to specimen collection and preservation, the information provided above for the CF test applies for the ASO test, including heat inactivation of the serum at 56°C for 30 min before performance of the test. Briefly, the principal steps in performing the test are the preparation of dilutions of the patient serum, addition of a fixed amount of streptolysin O to each dilution, and incubation of the mixture to permit neutralization of antigen by antibody if present, followed by the addition of a fixed volume of 2.5% human blood group O RBC (rabbit or sheep RBC may also be used), with reincubation of the sample. The presence of specific antibodies directed against streptolysin O is exhibited by the inhibition of RBC lysis. In most assays now used in various reference laboratories, the endpoint of the ASO neutralization test is the highest dilution of serum showing no hemolysis. The method recommended by most commercial suppliers for many years was that of Rantz and Randall (15), which was carried out in tubes. However, its major disadvantage was that the dilution intervals were not equally spaced on a logarithmic scale. The method of performing microtiter neutralization tests for ASO as described by Klein and co-workers (10, 12) has been widely used in the United States for the last 20 years and has a high degree of reproducibility, ranging between 95 and 98.1% (11). In this method, a serum dilution scheme is used in which the intervals are logarithmically spaced at 0.15-log intervals. The equal spacing of the intervals has advantages in the reporting and interpretation of significant results. Modifications of this scheme have also been used by others (5).

Another type of ASO test, used less frequently than the neutralization test, is the particle agglutination test (e.g., the Streptozyme test). In this type of test, the streptolysin O is coated onto particles such as latex, treated RBC, or certain bacterial cells. The coated particles are mixed with the diluted patient serum on a slide. The particles agglutinate in a few minutes if ASO is present in the serum. RBC can be used as a particle carrier for the streptolysin O in this type of test without being lysed because the streptolysin O is in the oxidized state and thus nonhemolytic. The main advantage of this type of test is that serum lipoproteins, bacterial growth products, or oxidized streptolysin O do not cause false-positive titers.

Standardization of reagents and quality control

All preparations of streptolysin O are tested by serological methods to measure their hemolytic and combining activities against standard antiserum. The standard ASO serum or Todd's standard serum is the equivalent of the World Health Organization international standard and contains 20,000 ASO units per ml. For the purposes of that standard, one minimal hemolytic dose was defined as the volume of streptolysin O preparation that completely hemolyzes 0.5 ml of a 5% suspension of rabbit RBC. One combining unit is the amount of streptolysin O that neutralizes 1 U of ASO. Since the combining unit is found to be more constant than the hemolytic unit, the strength of the streptolysin O preparation is usually expressed in terms of the combining units. Results are reported in Todd units (TU) or international units (IU), e.g., ASO titer = 240 TU or 240 IU. The number of units will be the same as the titer when streptolysin O produced in the United States is used. The titer should be expressed in Todd units if the potency of the streptolysin O used in the test has been adjusted against the Todd standard or international units if the World Health Organization international standard has been used. The units are equivalent for all practical purposes (16). There is a misconception that the Todd unit is associated with a particular dilution scheme or method such as the Rantz-Randall method. Instead, as pointed out above, the type of unit is determined by the standard used to adjust the potency of the streptolysin O included in the test.

Interpretation and clinical significance of laboratory results

None of the antibody tests discussed is considered diagnostic of a process such as acute rheumatic fever or acute glomerulonephritis. The specific antibody titers must be used only as serological aids in the diagnosis of streptococcal infection. No set normal ASO titer has been established, since many variables enter into the picture. Factors that determine the ASO titer include age, state of health, severity of the infection, amount of previous exposure to streptococcal infections, and the individual's ability to respond immunologically to streptolysin O by producing ASO. The ASO titer in fetuses, premature babies, and infants reflects approximately the ASO level in the mother's blood. A gradual decrease in ASO titer during the first 3 months of age has been reported. Between months 5 and 7, the ASO titer has been found to be as low as 5 TU. In month 8, it becomes equal to or perhaps higher than the ASO titer in the mother's blood. The ASO titer remains low during the early years of life. However, in the sera of children 8 to 12 years of age, the ASO titer is as high as in the sera of young adults of 20 years or more (1). Ideally, the limits of normal antibody titers for a normal population should be established in each laboratory servicing the population (5). A clinically significant titer is usually defined as a rise in titer of 2 or more dilution increments between the acute- and convalescent-phase sera, regardless of the height of the antibody titer (or 0.3 log or higher). Increased ASO titers develop as early as 1 week after the infection and reach a peak in 4 to 6 weeks; this peak usually occurs shortly after the onset of rheumatic fever. The antibody titers remain elevated for a variable period of time and gradually decrease over a period of several months. There is considerable variation among patients in the kinetics of decline of the ASO titer, and the specific titers may be altered by other intervening group A streptococcal infections. The upper limit of normal when only one specimen is available is usually defined as the highest titer that is exceeded by only 20% of a population (e.g., 240 or higher in a school-age patient). However, ASO titers must be interpreted with caution, since about 15% or more of patients with acute rheumatic fever may not have an elevated ASO titer or demonstrate a titer rise. In such cases, it is valuable to perform an alternative test such as the anti-DNase B or antihyalouronidase test after an acute group A streptococcal infection. Finally, the ASO test is not as useful as the anti-DNase B or antihyalouronidase tests in suspected cases of acute glomerulonephritis if the disease is a sequela of streptococcal pyoderma rather than pharyngitis. The advantage of the ASO test is that it has been the most widely used of the streptococcal antibody tests and thus is the most familiar. Some pitfalls of the ASO test are (i) the low titers associated with skin infections and their sequelae, (ii) false-positive titers associated with liver disease, (iii) false-positive titers caused by the growth of certain bacteria in the serum specimen, and (iv) false-positive titers caused by the oxidation of the streptolysin O reagent.

LITERATURE CITED

1. **Bennett, C. W.** 1968. Clinical serology, p. 136–143. Charles C Thomas, Publisher, Springfield, Ill.
2. **Bordet, J., and O. Gengou.** 1901. Sur l'existence de substances sensibilisatrices dans la plupart des serums antimicrobiens. Ann. Inst. Pasteur **15:**289–302.
3. **Casey, H. L.** 1965. Adaptation of LBCF method of microtechnique. *In* Microtest. Public Health monograph no. 74. Public Health Service publication no. 1228. U.S. Government Printing Office, Washington, D.C.
4. **Cooper, N. R.** 1987. The complement system, p. 114–127. *In* D. P. Stites, J. D. Stobo, and J. V. Wells (ed.), Basic and clinical immunology. Appleton and Lange, Norwalk, Conn.
5. **Ferrieri, P.** 1986. Immune responses to streptococcal infections, p. 336–341. *In* N. R. Rose, H. Friedman, and J. L. Fahey (ed.), Manual of clinical laboratory immunology, 3rd ed. American Society for Microbiology, Washington, D.C.
6. **Garvey, J. S., N. E. Cremer, and D. H. Sussdorf.** 1977. Methods in immunology, a laboratory text for instruction and research, 3rd ed., p. 379–410. W. A. Benjamin, Inc., Reading, Mass.
7. **Hawkes, R.** 1979. General principles underlying laboratory diagnosis of viral infections, p. 3–48. *In* E. H. Lennette and N. J. Schmidt (ed.), Diagnostic procedures for viral, rickettsial and chlamydial infections, 5th ed. American Public Health Association, Inc., Washington, D.C.
8. **Henle, G., S. Harris, and W. Henle.** 1948. The reactivity of various human sera with mumps complement fixation antigens. J. Exp. Med. **88:**133–147.
9. **Klein, G. C.** 1980. Immune response to streptococcal infection (antistreptolysin O, antideoxyribonuclease B), p. 431–440. *In* N. R. Rose and H. Friedman (ed.), Manual of clinical microbiology, 2nd ed. American Society for Microbiology, Washington, D.C.
10. **Klein, G. C., E. C. Hall, C. N. Baker, and B. V. Addison.** 1970. Antistreptolysin O test. Comparison of micro and macro techniques. Am. J. Clin. Pathol. **53:**159–162.

11. **Klein, G. C., and W. L. Jones.** 1971. Comparison of the streptozyme test with antistreptolysin O, antideoxyribonuclease B, and antihyalouronidase tests. Appl. Microbiol. **21:**257–259.
12. **Klein, G. C., M. D. Moody, C. N. Baker, and B. V. Addison.** 1968. Micro antistreptolysin O test. Appl. Microbiol. **16:**184.
13. **Palmer, D. F., L. Kaufman, W. Kaplan, and J. J. Cavallaro.** 1977. Serodiagnosis of mycotic disease. Charles C Thomas, Publisher, Springfield, Ill.
14. **Palmer, D. F., and S. D. Whaley.** 1986. Complement fixation test, p. 57–66. *In* N. R. Rose, H. Friedman, and J. L. Fahey (ed.), Manual of clinical laboratory immunology, 3rd ed. American Society for Microbiology, Washington, D.C.
15. **Rantz, L. A., and E. Randall.** 1945. A modification of the technique for determination of the antistreptolysin titer. Proc. Soc. Exp. Biol. Med. **59:**22–25.
16. **Spaun, J., M. M. Bentzon, S. O. Larsen, and L. F. Hewitt.** 1961. International standard for antistreptolysin O. Bull. WHO **24:**271–179.
17. **Todd, E. W.** 1932. Antigenic streptococcal hemolysin. J. Exp. Med. **55:**267–280.
18. **Todd, E. W.** 1938. The differentiation of two distinct serological varieties of streptolysin, streptolysin O and streptolysin S. J. Pathol. Bacteriol. **47:**423–445.
19. **Wellings, F. M., and A. L. Lewis.** 1986. Complement fixation test, p. 159–185. *In* S. Specter and G. J. Lancz (ed.), Clinical virology manual. Elsevier Science Publishing Co., New York.

Chapter 11

Labeled-Antibody Techniques: Fluorescent, Radioisotopic, Immunochemical

JOSEPH A. ROSEBROCK

The ability to detect and monitor the course of many infectious diseases has been enhanced by the development of immunoassays that use labeled antibodies. Coons et al. (2) reported the first use of fluorochrome-labeled antibodies to detect pneumococcal antigens in tissues in 1942. In 1954, an indirect fluorescent-antibody (IFA) technique useful for the detection of either antigen or antibody was described by Weller and Coons (27).

Radioisotopically labeled antibodies (and antigens) have been widely used for making quantitative analyte determinations since the introduction by Yalow and Berson in 1960 of a radioimmunoassay for the detection of insulin (29). Radioimmunoassays are still widely used for the detection of antigens and antibodies, especially in the assay of hepatitis B virus (5). In the early 1970s, the use of enzyme-labeled antibodies for making quantitative antibody and antigen determinations was introduced (4). The subsequent expansion and exploitation of enzyme immunoassay (EIA) or enzyme-linked immunosorbent assay (ELISA) technologies has resulted in a profusion of techniques that are widely used by the diagnostic community. These techniques are discussed elsewhere in this Manual.

A relatively recent labeled-antibody technology involves the use of lanthanide chelate-labeled antibodies and time-resolved fluorometry (13, 22). Time-resolved fluorescence immunoassays (FIA) represent a potential new generation of nonisotopic immunoassays with wide application.

In a broad sense, there are essentially two types of assays that utilize labeled antibodies: assays for the detection of antibodies and assays for the detection of antigens. These two basic types of assays may vary with respect to the choice of label (fluorochrome, radioisotope, enzyme, or rare earth metal) as well as specific steps within the assay procedure itself. The variations in assay procedure are generally reflected in the assay descriptions: indirect fluorescent-antibody test, direct antigen capture (sandwich) assay, etc. In some situations, crossover in methodologies can occur. For example, depending on the enzyme used to label the antibody preparation, the hydrolyzed substrate could be a fluorescent material (30), a radioactive material (11), a chemiluminescent material (17), or a chromogenic material (17). In each case the basic technique is an ELISA, but the method of detection can be quite varied, requiring different types of instrumentation. In many situations, practical considerations such as laboratory experience and preference, availability of commercial reagents, and instrumentation will ultimately dictate the final assay configuration.

A fundamental and sometimes neglected component of all labeled-antibody techniques is the immune response. Antibodies are elicited in response to a specific stimulation, whether natural (infection) or contrived (immunization); as a result, the cellular synthesis and secretion of a specific antibody molecule follow a logical progression which results in a population of antibodies exhibiting the appropriate functional characteristics of specificity, affinity, class, and anatomical location. If labeled antibodies are to be efficiently used for immunodiagnostic purposes, a fundamental understanding of antibody structure, function, and production is essential. This understanding has double implications since the immune response of some laboratory animals may need to be stimulated (manipulated) in a very specific manner for reagent production. By the same token, labeled antibodies are frequently used to measure the immune response in individuals and populations; therefore, assays must be designed to measure the appropriate component(s) of a complex response.

The primary purpose of this chapter is to present an overview of assay configurations that use labeled antibodies. Basic information on the elicitation of the immune response will be considered in the context of labeled-antibody techniques and supplemented by discussion relating the quality of labeled antibodies to assay performance.

IMMUNE RESPONSE

The basis of all immunochemical techniques is the interaction of an antibody with an antigen. While the production (synthesis and secretion) of antibody is the purview of B lymphocytes, accessory cells (macrophages and T lymphocytes) are required for the efficient and sustained production of antibodies of the appropriate specificity, affinity, and class. Although a detailed discussion of humoral immunity is not within the scope of this chapter, there are several aspects of antibody induction, production, structure, and function that directly influence the efficient use of labeled antibodies for immunodiagnostic purposes.

The production of specific antibodies is induced by exposure to foreign (non-self) molecules. In general terms, particulate antigens (microorganisms) are phagocytosed by macrophages, partially degraded, and reexpressed on the surface of the macrophage. B lymphocytes and helper T lymphocytes, all bearing the appropriate cell surface receptors for antigens on their respective membranes, bind to the antigen-presenting macrophages via the surface receptors. The resulting triumvirate of cells is responsible for the development of a specific and sustained immune response.

Specificity of the response is ensured by the preexposure expression of antigen receptors on the surfaces of the B cells and T cells. Since the surface receptor is structurally similar to secreted antibody, the interaction of macrophage-presented antigen with B-cell and T-cell surface receptors results in the selection of B-cell clones that will produce antibody with the same binding characteristics as the surface receptor. Through a series of complex feedback mechanisms involving several lymphokines, the antigen-specific B lymphocytes are stimulated to divide (clonal expansion) and begin to synthesize and secrete immunoglobulin M (IgM). The appearance of IgM marks the beginning of the primary immune response.

As the antigen-specific B-cell clones continue to expand by cell division, some cells continue down the differentiation pathway to become antibody (IgM)-producing cells, while other cells of the same lineage are arrested after several divisions. The arrested cells (memory cells) continue to express the incipient antigen receptors on their surface and are available to respond more rapidly (primed) to a subsequent exposure to the same antigen.

Antigenic stimulation of memory cells results in a secondary (anamnestic) response that is more rapid than the primary response and is characterized by further cell divisions, differentiation, and a class shift in antibody secretion (IgG). Therefore, the ability to differentiate antigen-specific IgM and IgG has important diagnostic implications.

In addition, and in response to the continued exposure to antigen, modifications occur in the antigen-binding site of the antibody. The net result of these modifications, which involve point mutations and genomic rearrangements, is a refinement of the antigen-binding site and a resultant increase in affinity. Since the refined antigen-binding site is also an integral part of the surface antigen receptor, it is easy to visualize how, in the continued presence of antigen, this process of affinity maturation results in the evolution of an immune response characterized by antibodies with greater specificity and affinity.

An important component of the interaction of an antibody with an antigen, and highly relevant to the use of labeled antibodies for immunodiagnostic purposes, is the strength of the antigen-antibody reaction. Affinity is a measure of the strength of this interaction. In general, high-affinity, specific antibodies will yield reagents with a higher overall level of performance in all immunochemical procedures, since increased antibody affinity ultimately results in the formation of a more stable antigen-antibody complex.

Antigen-antibody binding follows the basic thermodynamic principles of a bimolecular reaction. Under the same set of conditions (temperature, pH, and concentration), high- and low-affinity antibodies will diffuse at the same rate. Therefore, both high- and low-affinity antibodies will have comparable opportunities to encounter and interact with antigen. However, once binding has occurred, the antigen-antibody complex formed with the high-affinity antibody will be stable for a longer period of time.

Although this description is somewhat simplistic, antibody affinity has tremendous implications in situations in which equilibrium conditions are never fully attained (because of short incubation periods), are forced (reagent excess), or are rapidly modified (wash steps). For example, short-incubation, heterogeneous assays require several incubations and wash steps and use serum samples that contain populations of antibodies with different affinities, each at a different concentration. In addition, immunoassays measure binding activity, not mass. Therefore, comparable results (signals) can be obtained with use of one serum that contains a low concentration of high-affinity antibody and another serum that contains a high concentration of low-affinity antibody.

In a monoclonal antibody population, affinity can be readily determined. The situation is much more complex in a polyclonal antibody population, such as that which results from the antibody response to infection with a microorganism. In this case, avidity more readily describes the interaction of antigen with antibody.

Avidity is a measure of the overall stability of the antigen-antibody complex. In addition to the intrinsic affinity of an antibody for an antigenic determinant (epitope), there are two other factors that play a major role in describing avidity. One factor is the number of antigen-binding sites per antibody molecule and the number of epitopes per antigen. The other factor is the geometric arrangement of the interacting components. Therefore, the complete reaction, e.g., affinity, valence(s) of antibody and antigen, and geometry of the interaction, describes avidity.

Primary immune responses (predominantly IgM) are characterized as low affinity, high avidity because (i) affinity maturation has not yet occurred, (ii) specificity has not yet been refined, and (iii) each IgM contains 10 antigen-binding sites.

From a functional viewpoint, a high-avidity, primary immune response would appear to be a rapid, efficient mechanism for eliminating a microorganism. From a practical viewpoint, collection of antisera or production of hybridomas during the primary response for reagent production may not be as useful as after a boosting immunization.

The success of most immunochemical procedures is due, in large part, to the successful application of the principle of avidity. Most immunochemical procedures involve multivalent interactions, e.g., bivalent and/or decavalent antibody, and antigens with multiple epitopes (either identical repeating epitopes or multiple epitopes recognized by different antibodies). Therefore, low-affinity antibodies may often form stable antigen-antibody complexes through a process of cross-linking of antigen and, if sterically possible, binding of both antigen-binding sites to the antigen. In some immunochemical procedures, high-avidity binding is promoted by the application of a high concentration of antigen to a solid phase such as plastic or nitrocellulose; in the case of IFA, binding is promoted when there is a natural mechanism that results in the accumulation of concentrated antigen intracellularly.

There is an additional advantage to high, local concentrations of antigens. Since low-affinity antibodies tend to dissociate from antigen more rapidly than high-affinity antibodies, the high, local concentration of antigen promotes the rebinding of antibody before diffusion away from the antigen can occur. The impact of this phenomenon for different immunochemical procedures is important, since many procedures do not allow equilibrium to be established or, if equilibrium is established, conditions are rapidly changed by washing and subsequent incubations.

MONOCLONAL ANTIBODIES

Monoclonal antibodies have had a significant impact on the design of immunodiagnostic assays that use labeled antibodies for either antibody or antigen detection. Even though hybridoma technology is still labor intensive, complex, and equipment dependent, and the probability of success is not predictable, monoclonal antibodies are extremely useful for immunodiagnostic purposes. For example, after hybridomas are generated, large numbers of individual antibodies, which represent the individual components of the polyclonal response, can be screened and selected. The selected hybridoma(s) can then be expanded and stored, thus ensuring a steady and consistent supply of standardized reagents. The selection process, a luxury unavailable in the production of polyclonal antisera, allows precise control over antibody specificity and affinity.

The use of monoclonal antibodies is not without some restrictions. For example, since the specificity of a monoclonal antibody represents only a fraction of the reactivities present in a polyclonal antiserum, it may not be safe to assume that a monoclonal preparation and a polyclonal preparation can be interchanged for any given usage. In addition, whereas in some situations it may be desirable to select an antibody preparation of restricted specificity (for microbial differentiation or identification), there are other situations in which a somewhat broader specificity may be needed (detection of group-specific antigens, e.g., chlamydia antigens). The latter situation can be resolved in one of two ways with use of monoclonal antibodies: (i) attempt to develop and characterize a monoclonal antibody with the appropriate specificity by screening large numbers of hybridomas or (ii) identify and pool two or more monoclonal antibodies with more restricted specificities to produce a cocktail that will provide the desired range of specificities. It may be more expeditious to use the pooling concept, since monoclonal antibody generation is a no-guarantee prospect. In addition, whereas the affinity of any given monoclonal antibody may or may not be sufficient for the intended usage(s), a mixture of monoclonal antibodies may result in an immunoreagent of higher avidity and therefore be more useful. Finally, when one is attempting to incorporate monoclonal antibodies into immunoassays, it is important to screen the monoclonal antibodies by using a method that will be comparable to the final usage. This may seem like an obvious statement of fact; however, many monoclonal antibodies of the appropriate specificity that work will in one format (immunofluorescence) lack the affinity needed to function in a different immunoassay format (FIA or EIA).

LABELED-ANTIBODY TECHNIQUES

IFA test

The IFA test demonstrates the principle of antibody detection using fluorescein-labeled antibodies. The substrate consists of a mixture of virus-infected and uninfected cells (or a microorganism such as *Toxoplasma gondii*, *Treponema pallidum*, or *Borrelia burgdorferi*) that are fixed on a glass slide. The test sample is applied to the substrate, and specific antibody, if present, will bind to the appropriate antigen. Unreacted antibody is removed by washing, and bound antibody is detected by reacting the antibody-coated substrate with fluorescein isothiocyanate (FITC)-labeled anti-human immunoglobulin, followed by fluorescence microscopy evaluation (Table 1).

The IFA format is a time-proven method for detecting the presence of microorganism-specific antibody in a clinical specimen. An important advantage of the IFA test is that the observer can directly evaluate the quality of the result. For example, the subcellular fluorescence patterns that result from different viral infections are generally distinctive, usually a result of the infectious process and the accumulation of antigen within specific cellular organelles. Because of these microorganism-specific patterns, nonspecific staining reactions can be detected and interpreted as such. For example, it is not uncommon for serum samples to contain antinuclear antibody reactivities, which can be easily resolved by usual observation. Fc receptor expression is another nonspecific reaction, frequently encountered when herpesvirus (especially cytomegalovirus [CMV])-infected cells are used (6, 15, 18, 19).

The Fc receptor type of nonspecific reaction occurs as a result of Fc receptor induction by the infecting herpesvirus and the resultant binding of sample IgG via the Fc portion of the molecule, not the antigen-combining site. Fc receptor staining associated with CMV infection can appear to be very specific cytoplasmic staining since it appears in infected cells only, in association with the Golgi region. However, the staining pattern characteristic of CMV-infected cells is a distinctive bean-shaped nuclear inclusion. *T. gondii* serology can also be complicated by a nonspecific staining pattern referred to as polar staining, which is very characteristic in its distribution and easy to identify and interpret visually (1). Therefore, a skilled technician can quickly evaluate the quality of an IFA test and render an informed decision.

The IFA test not only is a time-proven and powerful diagnostic tool in its own right but also is used as a standard test to evaluate relative performance during the development of other types of tests (EIA, FIA, etc.). In fact, "transient" IFA tests are frequently developed in conjunction with other, more objective immunoassay procedures to assess the specificity of the reactive samples. At the other end of the spectrum, IFA tests can be used to confirm test results obtained by a different methodology, e.g., ELISA. For example, an ELISA-positive human immunodeficiency virus type 1 antibody result can be evaluated by IFA to assess the specificity of the result (7, 21).

The primary characteristic of IFA that makes this test so useful is the ability to visualize and discriminate various reactivities by evaluating the cellular and subcellular distribution of fluorescence. Therefore, the subjective nature of the evaluation step, which is frequently cited as a methodological liability, is actually an advantage that can lead to a better understanding of the reactivity of the clinical specimens and a more accurate diagnosis.

The substrate used for IFA testing frequently exhibits a self-contained mechanism that results in high sensitivity as well as specificity. For example, in the case of

TABLE 1. Antibody and antigen detection assays

Type	Solid phase	Test sample	Detection system
Antibody detection			
Indirect sandwich	1. Tissue culture cells, tissues, microorganisms 2. Purified preparations of infectious agents and/or synthetic or recombinant antigens	Human antibody	1. Fluorochrome-conjugated anti-human immunoglobulin 2. Enzyme-conjugated anti-human immunoglobulin 3. Lanthanide chelate-conjugated anti-human immunoglobulin
Competitive inhibition	Purified preparations of infectious agents and/or synthetic or recombinant antigens	Human antibody	1. Fluorochrome-conjugated species antiantigen 2. Enzyme-conjugated species antiantigen 3. Lanthanide chelate-conjugated species antiantigen 4. Radioisotope-conjugated species antiantigen
Indirect class capture	Species anti-human immunoglobulin (class specific)	Human antibody	1. Specific antigen plus fluorochrome-conjugated species antiantigen 2. Specific antigen plus enzyme-conjugated species antiantigen 3. Specific antigen plus lanthanide chelate-conjugated species antiantigen 4. Specific antigen plus radioisotope-conjugated species antiantigen
Direct sandwich	Purified preparations of infectious agents and/or synthetic or recombinant antigens	Human antibody	1. Fluorochrome-conjugated antigen 2. Enzyme-conjugated antigen 3. Lanthanide chelate-conjugated antigen 4. Radioisotope-conjugated antigen
Antigen detection			
Direct and indirect	Glass, plastic	Clinical specimen, smear (in transport medium)	1. Fluorochrome-conjugated antimicroorganism antibody 2. Enzyme-conjugated antimicroorganism antibody
Direct or indirect sandwich capture	Purified antimicroorganism antibody (polyclonal and/or monoclonal)	Clinical specimen (in transport medium)	1. Fluorochrome-conjugated antimicroorganism antibody 2. Enzyme-conjugated antimicroorganism antibody 3. Lanthanide chelate-conjugated antimicroorganism antibody 4. Radioisotope-conjugated antimicroorganism antibody

human immunodeficiency virus type 1-infected cells, viral component synthesis is concentrated in the cytoplasm, within the hilar region of the nucleus. The end result is a subcellular concentration of viral antigen in a specific region that facilitates the binding of antibody from the patient specimens and the subsequent concentration of fluorescent label. Other examples include the bean-shaped nuclear inclusions of CMV-infected cells and the larger cytoplasmic inclusions of chlamydia-infected cells.

Significantly, the close apposition of antigenic determinants allows antibodies to bind via both antigen-combining sites, resulting in a more stable antigen-antibody complex, and therefore withstand the subsequent washing and incubation steps which modify equilibrium and result in destabilization of antigen-antibody complexes.

IFA tests are useful for the detection of IgM (3) as well as IgG. As with any IgM test, IgG in the sample must be removed or neutralized to prevent false-negative results, since microorganism-specific IgG will effectively compete with specific IgM. Furthermore, the functional, if not physical, removal of IgG will also reduce the possibility of false-positive results due to the interaction of antigen-specific IgG and rheumatoid factor IgM (RF-IgM) (20). Several reagents and specimen treatment protocols are available for physically removing or functionally neutralizing total IgG (28). One of the most effective procedures uses anti-human IgG produced in goats or sheep. Depending on the titer of the anti-human IgG used, the human IgG in the sample can be precipitated (and removed by centrifugation) or neutralized in antibody (anti-human IgG) excess. In either case, human IgG–anti-human IgG immune complexes are formed, and RF-IgM will be absorbed by the immune complexes since RF-IgM molecules have a peculiar affinity for aggregated IgG.

Substitution of an enzyme label for the fluorochrome label, and the use of precipitable substrate, results in a methodology very similar to that for the IFA test which can also be used to detect microorganism-specific antibody (14). The precipitated reaction product is localized within the infected cells and can be detected by light microscopy, with or without the use of a counterstain. An advantage of this procedure is the substitution of a light microscope for a fluorescence microscope. There may be, however, a trade-off in overall resolution since the reaction product may not be as discretely localized as in the IFA test.

FIA

The basic format of the IFA test can be modified by changing the solid phase, and the form of the antigen on the solid phase, to produce an FIA. FIA (Table 1) are heterogeneous testing formats that use a plastic or membranous (nitrocellulose) solid phase and a purified antigen preparation (solubilized preparation of infected cells or microorganisms or synthetic or recombinant antigens). The test sample is applied to the solid phase, and specific antibody, if present, will bind to the antigenic substrate. Unreacted antibody is removed by washing. Antigen-specific antibody is detected by incubating the solid phase with fluorochrome-labeled anti-human immunoglobulin and evaluating the magnitude of the fluorescent signal by fluorometry (12, 23).

In principle, fluorescence measurement is very sensitive. Typically, anti-human immunoglobulins are coupled with FITC, which exhibits a very high fluorescence intensity. Unlike an EIA, which requires the conversion of substrate and the measurement of hydrolyzed product (indirect measure of bound antibody), FIA provides a direct measure of bound antibody. Furthermore, since the additional substrate incubation step is not needed, the complexity of the test is reduced.

Some problems can be encountered in the FIA since FITC has a very narrow Stokes shift (excitation and emission wavelengths) and can be sensitive to background interferences and light scattering from the sample or solid phase. In addition, some loss of fluorescence can occur as a direct result of the chemical coupling process. Fluorescence quenching can be a problem when FITC-labeled antibody nonspecifically binds to other proteins or when the close proximity of two fluorescent probes on a single antibody molecule leads to a diminution of fluorescence. Finally, continued exposure of FITC to the excitation source will result in bleaching and a total reduction of signal.

Time-resolved FIA

The principle and procedure for the time-resolved FIA are basically the same as for the FIA and EIA (Table 1), but the technique differs in the composition of the material used to prepare the anti-human immunoglobulin conjugate, a chelated form of a rare earth metal (lanthanide), and the instrumentation needed to measure the fluorescent signal (13, 22).

As mentioned in the section on FIA, assays that rely on the generation and measurement of fluorescent signals are subject to interference by light scattering and background fluorescence from the sample or solid phase, which can result in a loss of sensitivity. Fluorescence quenching will also contribute to a loss in sensitivity, since the specific fluorescence signal will be attenuated. Therefore, there are several general characteristics that a fluorescent probe should exhibit to maximize detection and minimize specific signal diminution: first, the probe should exhibit a high fluorescence intensity; second, the fluorescence signal must be distinguishable from the background fluorescence; and third, the binding of the fluorescent probe to an antibody or an antigen should not adversely affect the properties of the antibody, antigen, or probe. Lanthanide chelates (europium and terbium) meet the general requirements needed to be useful fluorescent probes.

Typically, lanthanide chelates exhibit a large Stokes shift (>250 nm, compared with about 50 nm for FITC) and a long fluorescence lifetime. Since the fluorescence lifetime of the probe is considerably longer than the delay of the background fluorescence, the temporal difference between these two signals can be used to increase the signal-to-noise ratio and therefore the sensitivity of the measurement. Time-resolved FIA can take advantage of the properties of the lanthanide chelates described above and provide an assay system of high sensitivity and specificity with a wide dynamic range.

Competitive antibody immunoassay

The solid phase that is used to detect and measure specific antibodies in an indirect assay format can also be used to measure specific antibodies in a competitive assay format (Table 1). For example, human antibody against a viral antigen(s) can be measured by combining the sample with a predetermined amount of conjugated antibody directed against the same viral antigen(s) and incubating the mixture with the antigen-coated solid phase. Specific antibody, if present in the sample, will compete with the conjugated antibody for binding sites on the solid phase and lead to a reduction in signal (25). Therefore, in the competitive assay format the signal generated will be inversely proportional to the amount of sample antibody.

The source of antibody for the conjugate can be varied. Antibodies against the antigens of interest can be prepared in animals. Alternatively, specific monoclonal antibodies can be developed or specific antibodies can be purified from human serum. Regardless of the source, the specific antibodies must be purified, conjugated with the appropriate label (fluorochrome, enzyme, lanthanide, or radioisotope), and rigorously evaluated before use.

An important aspect of conjugate evaluation involves the serial titration of the conjugate against serial dilutions of antigen to measure activity. The purpose of this exercise is to define the titration curve of the conjugate across several antigen concentrations. Each conjugate titration curve will exhibit a point at which the next dilution (or two) of conjugate will exhibit a substantial drop in signal. Several conjugate-antigen dilution pairs that meet the basic criteria listed above should be selected for further evaluation. The selected conjugate-antigen pairs are then further characterized with respect to sensitivity, using preparations containing known amounts of antigen-specific antibody. The ultimate goal in this part of the evaluation is to select the conjugate-antigen pair that contains the highest dilution of conjugate and antigen which will (i) permit the generation of high signal, (ii) exhibit a substantial reduction in signal in the presence of sample antibody, and (iii) allow the measurement of small amounts of sample antibody against all important antigenic determinants.

Unlike the indirect sandwich assays for antibody, which are reagent-excess types of assays, competitive assays are based on a limiting-reagent concept. In the case of indirect sandwich assays, solid-phase antigen is maximized and the system is more or less flooded with sample and conjugate. This procedure, in combination with incubation temperature and time, will drive the reaction to completion. In the case of competitive assays, however, solid-phase antigen and conjugate concentrations are minimized so that even small quantities of sample antibody can effectively block the binding of conjugate.

There are several advantages to using the competitive format for antibody measurement. One advantage is the relative ease with which highly specific antibodies, especially monoclonal antibodies, can be purified and conjugated. In general, antibodies are easier to purify than antigens, and since the specificity of the test is conveyed by the conjugate, relatively impure antigen can be used on the solid phase. Another advantage is a reduction in the number of procedural steps, since sample and conjugate can be incubated with the antigen on the solid phase.

Since the specificity of the competitive assay is conveyed by the conjugate, the quality of the antibody going into the conjugate must be scrupulously evaluated to avoid unwanted reactivities and false-positive results. Likewise, the range of specific antigenic determinants represented in the conjugate must be appropriate; otherwise, false-negative results will be obtained.

The direct competitive format can be easily modified to an indirect format. In this configuration, the microorganism-specific antibody (mouse antivirus, for example) is not conjugated but is directly mixed with the sample to be measured. The degree of sample antibody inhibition is measured by using an anti-mouse immunoglobulin conjugate.

Antibody class capture assay

The indirect antibody class capture assay is a useful test for evaluating patient specimens for the presence of antigen-specific antibodies of a specific class (Table 1). Traditionally, this assay configuration has been used to detect antigen-specific IgM and IgA. Modifications that permit the measurement of antigen-specific IgG as well are described below. Since the detection system can be varied (Table 1), the assay will be described for IgM with no regard to the detection system (8, 16).

For the indirect IgM capture assay to be successful, the solid phase must be coated with a purified, high-affinity, mu-chain-specific antibody preparation. The test sample is then incubated with the solid phase, and a representative sample of the total IgM population is captured. This step is followed by the addition of the purified antigen preparation of choice, e.g., *T. gondii* or CMV. If antigen-specific IgM molecules are present in the bound IgM sample, then antigen will bind during this incubation step. Bound antigen is then detected by using a labeled species antiantigen as described in Table 1.

One obvious advantage to this assay configuration is the elimination of a test sample pretreatment step to remove IgG, which must be performed when an indirect sandwich procedure for IgM detection is used (Table 1). Since only IgM molecules are captured, the sensitivity of the test is not compromised by the presence of antigen-specific IgG. In addition, false-positive results due to RF-IgM are minimized as well.

The sensitivity of the IgM class capture assay is directly affected by the quality of the capture antibody. The capture antibody must be of high affinity and mu-chain specific. Light-chain reactivities in the capture antibody preparation should be tested for, and preparations exhibiting light-chain reactivity should not be used. Since IgM antibodies are generally high-avidity antibodies, extreme care should be taken to ensure the purity of the antigen preparation and reduce the possibility of false-positive reactivity. The use of synthetic or recombinant antigen could be advantageous.

A modification of the procedure outlined in Table 1, and one that is not, strictly speaking, a labeled-antibody technique, is the substitution of labeled antigen for unlabeled antigen and conjugated antispecies antibody. This configuration has the advantage of one less step and reduces even more the possibility of a false-positive result due to RF-IgM. Again, the labeled antigen must be of high quality to avoid false-positive results. Variations in labeling from lot to lot could result in considerable variation in test results.

A further modification of the antibody class capture assay, and one that will permit the measurement of antigen-specific IgG, involves the use of labeled antigen and a solid phase coated with RF-IgM. A sample containing antigen-specific IgG is mixed with labeled conjugate and incubated with the solid phase coated with RF-IgM. Only antigen-specific IgG complexed with labeled antigen is bound by the RF-IgM; therefore, only a single incubation step is required. Again, antigen quality, as well as the quality of RF-IgM coating the solid phase, must be carefully assessed.

Direct sandwich antibody detection

An additional method for antibody detection, and one that is not actually a labeled-antibody technique, utilizes labeled antigen and is referred to as a direct sandwich assay for antibody (Table 1). In the interest of completeness, the technique is described here; some modifications of this technique do use labeled antibodies. The methodology is the same regardless of the label, and therefore the procedure will be discussed in generic terms (25).

The basis of the technique is the ability of specific antibody molecules to form immune complex bridges between soluble, labeled antigen and antigen coated on a solid phase. Carefully selected, high-quality antigens, which retain their antigenicity after labeling, are capable of forming extensive immune complexes with sample antibody. The resultant cross-linking of antibody to the solid phase imbues the assay with an exquisite sensitivity.

Modifications to this technique include biotin or fluorescein conjugation of the fluid-phase antigen. After incubation with the solid phase and a wash step, labeled avidin, labeled antibiotin, or labeled anti-FITC can be added to develop the reaction.

ANTIGEN DETECTION

The diagnosis of an infectious disease that must be based on the growth, isolation, and identification of the infecting microorganism in pure culture can be a difficult and time-consuming process. Many microorganisms require special techniques for growth that may not be generally available (and are therefore expensive). Some microorganisms are extremely fastidious or simply noncultivatable. And in some instances, clinical specimens that no longer contain viable organisms are received. Antigen detection based on labeled-antibody techniques therefore offers a useful alternative or adjunct to culture isolation.

Direct detection

One very useful antigen detection procedure involves the preparation of a smear from the clinical specimen on a glass slide (Table 1). After fixation, the slide may be stored or immediately reacted with an FITC-conjugated antibody preparation (polyclonal or monoclonal) directed against the antigen(s) of interest. After incubation with the antibody preparation, the slide is washed and examined by fluorescence microscopy (24, 26).

The direct fluorescent-antigen detection technique has proven to be useful for detection of chlamydia antigen and various viral infections (herpes simplex virus, respiratory syncytial virus, etc.). To be successful, the clinical specimen must be carefully taken and transferred to the slide such that elementary bodies (chlamydia) or infected cells (viral infections) are present in sufficient numbers for evaluation. Importantly, infectious material need not be present for the successful identification of the cause of the infection.

As in all antigen detection procedures using labeled antibodies, the specificity of the antibody is critical. The absolute level of specificity may vary depending on the intended usage (diagnosis versus typing); however, the production of the polyclonal antiserum or the screening process used for selecting monoclonal antibodies must be stringently controlled so that the antibody preparation is specific for the microorganism (or epitopes) of interest. To this end, reagent quality control should include testing against related and unrelated microorganisms that may be found in the same anatomical location. Also, use of the highest-affinity/avidity preparations with the appropriate specificity will yield the most useful immunoreagents.

In many situations, it may not be possible to use smears for the direct detection of microorganisms in clinical specimens and the sample must be cultured. Under these circumstances, labeled antibodies are frequently used to confirm the cause of the cytopathic effect (CPE); as has been shown with CMV (9), the presence of viral antigen can be demonstrated days before the appearance of CPE by using a fluorescein-conjugated monoclonal antibody against early antigen.

Culture confirmation using labeled antibodies combines the most advantageous components of culture isolation and direct detection. For example, culture is more or less an open system that has the potential to grow any number of microorganisms. Therefore, if a CPE is evident in a culture and the suspected microorganism is not confirmed by labeled-antibody staining, then the laboratory can begin a series of tests to identify the cause of the CPE. Since CPE alone may not be informative, and a negative result on a direct smear might not preclude infection with a different organism, the combination of the two technologies may offer the most appropriate investigative tool.

Culture confirmation need not be direct (unlabeled, microbe-specific antibodies can be used with an antispecies conjugate), and the conjugate does not need to be a fluorochrome. Enzyme-labeled conjugates and precipitable substrates are also commonly used (10, 31).

Antigen capture (sandwich) assay

One of the most versatile and frequently used antigen detection techniques that employs labeled antibodies is the capture assay (Table 1). The test design for this assay is as follows. The solid phase is coated with a purified preparation of high-affinity, antimicrobial antibody (polyclonal or monoclonal). After the nonabsorbed antibody is removed, the clinical specimen is incubated with the solid phase for some predetermined period of time, during which specific antigen, if present, will bind to the solid-phase antibody. After a wash step, labeled antibody, specific for the captured antigen, is added to complete the sandwich. Depending on the label used, antigen can be detected and quantitated if necessary (25).

It is easy to see why the antigen capture assay has been so widely accepted. The antibodies on either side of the sandwich may be any combination of polyclonal and monoclonal antibodies. The technique can be modified to an indirect form in which the detection system consists of an unlabeled antimicroorganism antibody and an antispecies conjugate. (The species used to produce the second antibody must not be the same as the species used to produce the capture antibody.) With use of the indirect method, a number of presentations are possible for the configuration of the second antibody and the detection system. For example, the second antibody can be biotinylated, in which case the conjugate can consist of labeled avidin or labeled antibiotin. Also, depending on the antibodies selected for capture and detection, labeled protein A can be used as the conjugate (25).

Competitive inhibition assay

Antigen detection can be readily performed by using a test design that results in the inhibition of labeled, specific antibody binding to a solid phase. The test design is similar to that for the indirect sandwich method for antibody detection in that the solid phase is coated with antigen. The unknown sample, suspected of containing the antigen of interest, is mixed with a well-defined preparation of labeled, high-affinity/avidity antiantigen antibodies (polyclonal or monoclonal). If antigen is present in the sample, it will bind to the conjugate and prevent the conjugate from binding to the solid phase (25).

As with all competitive-type assays, this is a limited-reagent assay and all of the components need to be carefully selected and balanced. Therefore, solid-phase antigen and labeled antibody need to be optimized concomitantly such that the assay is poised near the upper portion of a steep dose-response curve. If this is done and the labeled antibody is of sufficient avidity, then small amounts of antigen may be sufficient to reduce antibody binding to the solid phase, and a resultant decrease in signal will occur. In this type of assay, the decrease in signal is inversely proportional to the quantity of antigen present in the sample. Again, depending on preference, different labels and indirect methodologies can be used.

LITERATURE CITED

1. **Budzko, D. B., L. Tyler, and D. Armstrong.** 1989. Fc receptors on the surface of *Toxoplasma gondii* trophozoites: a confounding factor in testing for anti-*Toxoplasma* antibodies by indirect immunofluorescence. J. Clin. Microbiol. **27:**959–961.
2. **Coons, A. H., H. J. Creech, R. N. Jones, and E. Berliner.** 1942. The demonstration of pneumococcal antigen in tissues by the use of fluorescent antibody. J. Immunol. **45:** 159–170.
3. **Cremer, N. E., and J. L. Riggs.** 1979. Immunoglobulin classes and viral diagnosis, p. 191–208. *In* E. H. Lennette and N. J. Schmidt (ed.), Diagnostic procedures for viral, rickettsial and chlamydial infections, 5th ed. American Public Health Association, Washington, D.C.
4. **Engvall, E., and P. Perlmann.** 1971. Enzyme-linked immunosorbent assay (ELISA). Quantitative assay of immunoglobulin G. Immunochemistry **8:**871–874.
5. **Forghani, B.** 1979. Radio-immunoassay, p. 171–189. *In* E. H. Lennette and N. J. Schmidt (ed.), Diagnostic procedures for viral, rickettsial and chlamydial infections, 5th ed. American Public Health Association, Washington, D.C.
6. **Gallo, D.** 1986. Elimination of Fc receptor binding of human immunoglobulin G in immunofluorescence assays for herpes simplex virus antibodies. J. Clin. Microbiol. **24:** 672–674.
7. **Gallo, D., J. L. Diggs, G. R. Shell, P. J. Daily, M. N. Hoffman, and J. L. Riggs.** 1986. Comparison of detection of antibody to the acquired immune deficiency syndrome virus by enzyme immunoassay, immunofluorescence, and Western blot methods. J. Clin. Microbiol. **23:**1049–1051.
8. **Gat, J.-P., C. Speiss, S. Schmitt, and A. Kirn.** 1985. Rapid diagnosis of acute mumps infection by a direct immunoglobulin M antibody capture enzyme immunoassay with labeled antigen. J. Clin. Microbiol. **21:**346–352.
9. **Gleaves, C. A., T. F. Smith, E. A. Shuster, and G. R. Pearson.** 1984. Rapid detection of cytomegalovirus in MRC-5 cells inoculated with urine specimens by using low-speed centrifugation and monoclonal antibody to an early antigen. J. Clin. Microbiol. **19:**917–919.
10. **Gleaves, C. A., D. J. Wilson, A. D. Wold, and T. F. Smith.** 1985. Detection and serotyping of herpes simplex virus in MRC-5 cells by use of centrifugation and monoclonal antibodies 16 h postinoculation. J. Clin. Microbiol. **21:**29–32.
11. **Harris, C. C., R. H. Yolken, H. Krokan, and I. C. Hsu.** 1979. Ultrasensitive enzymatic radioimmune assay for detection of cholera toxin and rotavirus. Proc. Natl. Acad. Sci. **76:**5336–5339.
12. **Hechemy, K. E., H. L. Harris, J. A. Wethers, R. W. Stevens, B. R. Stock, A. A. Reilly, and J. L. Benach.** 1989. Fluoroimmunoassay studies with solubilized antigens from *Borrelia burgdorferi*. J. Clin. Microbiol. **27:**1854–1858.
13. **Hemmıla, I.** 1985. Fluoroimmunoassays and immunofluorometric assays. Clin. Chem. **31:**359–370.
14. **Karpas, A., W. Gillson, P. C. Bevan, and J. K. Oates.** 1985. Lytic infection by British AIDS virus and development of a rapid cell test for antiviral antibodies. Lancet **ii:** 675–677.
15. **Keller, R., R. Peitchel, J. N. Goldman, and M. Goldman.** 1976. An IgG-Fc receptor induced in cytomegalovirus-infected human fibroblasts. J. Immunol. **116:**772–777.
16. **Parry, J. V., K. R. Perry, and P. P. Mortimer.** 1987. Sensitive assays for viral antibodies in saliva: an alternative to test on serum. Lancet **ii:**72–75.
17. **Pronovost, A. D., A. Baumgarten, and W. A. Andiman.** 1982. Chemiluminescent immunoenzymatic assay for rapid diagnosis of viral infections. J. Clin. Microbiol. **16:** 345–349.
18. **Rahman, A. A., M. Teschner, K. K. Sethi, and H. Brandis.** 1976. Appearance of IgG (Fc) receptor(s) on cultured human fibroblasts infected with human cytomegalovirus. J. Immunol. **117:**253–258.
19. **Rand, K. H., H. J. Houck, and M. Dickinson.** 1986. False positive indirect fluorescent antibody (IFA) tests for antibody to herpes simplex 1. Am. J. Clin. Pathol. **86:**765–768.
20. **Rossier, E., H. R. Miller, and P. H. Phipps.** 1989. Rapid viral diagnosis by immunofluorescence—an atlas and practical guide, p. 7–32. University of Ottawa Press, Ottawa, Ontario, Canada.
21. **Sandstrom, E. G., R. T. Schooley, D. D. Ho, R. Byington, M. G. Sarngadharan, M. E. MacLane, M. Essex, R. C. Gallo, and M. S. Hirsch.** 1985. Detection of human anti-HTLV-III antibodies by indirect immunofluorescence using fixed cells. Transfusion **25:**308–312.
22. **Soini, E., and H. Kojola.** 1983. Time-resolved fluorometer for lanthanide chelates—a new generation of nonisotopic immunoassays. Clin. Chem. **29:**65–68.
23. **Stevens, R. W., and R. F. Schell.** 1982. Solid-phase fluoroimmunoassay for treponemal antibody. J. Clin. Microbiol. **15:**191–195.
24. **Treuhaft, M. W., J. M. Soukup, and B. S. Sullivan.** 1985. Practical recommendation for the detection of pediatric respiratory syncytial virus infections. J. Clin. Microbiol. **22:**270–273.
25. **Voller, A., and D. Bidwell.** 1986. Enzyme-linked immunosorbent assay, p. 99–109. *In* N. R. Rose, N. Friedman, and J. L. Fahey (ed.), Manual of clinical laboratory immunology, 3rd ed. American Society for Microbiology, Washington, D.C.
26. **Waner, J. L., N. J. Whitehurst, T. Downs, and D. G. Graves.** 1985. Production of monoclonal antibodies against parainfluenza 3 virus and their use in diagnosis by immunofluorescence. J. Clin. Microbiol. **22:**535–538.
27. **Weller, T. H., and A. H. Coons.** 1954. Fluorescent antibody studies with agents of varicella and herpes zoster propagated *in vitro*. Proc. Soc. Exp. Biol. Med. **86:**789–794.
28. **Wiedbrank, D. L., and H. Y. K. Chuang.** 1988. Managing IgM serologies: getting the IgG out. Lab. Manage. **24:**24–27.
29. **Yalow, R. S., and S. A. Berson.** 1960. Immunoassay of endogenous plasma insulin in man. J. Clin. Invest. **39:** 1137–1175.
30. **Yolken, R. H., and P. J. Stopa.** 1979. Enzyme-linked fluorescence assay: ultrasensitive solid-phase assay for detection of human rotavirus. J. Clin. Microbiol. **10:**317–321.
31. **Zhao, L., M. L. Landry, E. S. Balkovic, and G. D. Hsiung.** 1987. Impact of cell culture sensitivity and virus concentration on rapid detection of herpes simplex virus by cytopathic effects and immunoperoxidase staining. J. Clin. Microbiol. **25:**1401–1405.

Chapter 12

Enzyme Immunoassay

JAMES M. CONROY, ROY W. STEVENS, AND KARIM E. HECHEMY

PRINCIPLES AND HISTORICAL DEVELOPMENT

Enzyme immunoassay (EIA) is an outgrowth of earlier immunological procedures that used radioisotopes or fluorochromes as reporter molecules. Instead of relying on the disintegration of radioactive isotopes or fluorescence as a readout, EIA depends on the detection of colored products generated by enzyme-labeled molecules. In general, color intensity is proportional to the concentration of analyte in the specimen. Other variants of EIA use products that are fluorescent (13), bioluminescent (24), or chemiluminescent (1) to increase assay sensitivity. The initial EIA procedures described in the early 1970s (10, 22) were performed in individual polystyrene tubes. However, several assay formats are now in use. EIA performed in 96-well microplates allows the screening of large sample loads. Cassette and dot blot EIA protocols are also widely used. Western immunoblotting procedures (19) are used to detect specific antibodies directed against individual microbial constituents.

The widespread use of EIA in clinical microbiology is a result of not only format versatility but also the availability of enzyme-labeled reagents and substrates tailored for the assay variations. Alkaline phosphatase and horseradish peroxidase are most commonly used in EIA because of a large turnover number in generating colored products and the availability of substrates that yield soluble products for microplate assays or insoluble products needed to visualize cassette, dot blot, and Western blot procedures (Table 1).

MICROPLATE EIA

Commercial microplate EIA kits are available for several applications in clinical microbiology. These kits ordinarily contain plates that can be separated into individual strips of 8 or 12 wells. The plates can be used intact when large numbers of specimens are tested. Alternatively, a few strips can be used when only a few tests are required. The kits also include diluents for all reagents, concentrates for wash buffers, enzyme substrates, and solutions to stop color development.

Microplate EIA in clinical microbiology is performed in two test configurations to detect either microbial antigens (antigen capture) or specific antibodies directed against microbes (antibody capture). Microbial antigens are ordinarily detected by EIA procedures in which specific antibody is used to coat the microplate wells (Fig. 1A). The specific antibody adsorbed to the well is most often a monoclonal antibody directed against a single epitope of the antigen. Solutions suspected of containing the antigen are incubated in the microplate well. Capture of the antigen is then detected by using an enzyme-labeled monoclonal antibody that recognizes a different epitope of the antigen.

The antigen capture format can also be used to quantify microbial antigens in specimens (23). In this procedure, known amounts of antigen are added to several wells, and the color intensities of these wells are used to establish a standard curve. The color intensities of wells containing unknown samples are then related to the standard curve. Special care must be used in optimizing assay conditions to ensure that a linear relationship between color intensity and antigen concentration exists over a meaningful range.

In the antibody capture configuration (Fig. 1B), microbial antigens are used to coat the microplate wells. Serum or cerebrospinal fluid from individuals presumptively infected with the microbe is added to the wells. Detection of microbe-directed specific antibodies is then performed by using an enzyme-labeled antibody directed against immunoglobulin. A variation of antibody capture EIA is used to distinguish acute (immunoglobulin M [IgM] response) from chronic (IgG response) infections. In this variation, the enzyme-labeled antibody is specific for the heavy chain of a particular immunoglobulin isotype. Alternatively, an IgM capture method can be used to determine acute-phase responses (9). This procedure uses immobilized antibodies specific for IgM to trap antibodies of this isotype from serum. Antigen is then added to the plate, followed by an enzyme-labeled antibody that recognizes the antigen. Antibody capture methods can also be used to obtain semiquantitative estimates of antimicrobial antibody levels in sera. In this method, serial dilutions of sera are incubated with antigen-coated microplates. The highest dilution yielding color intensities above the cutoff is reported as the endpoint. This procedure is especially useful in monitoring the immune response to pathogens or the effectiveness of an immunization protocol.

Design of microplate EIA procedures

If commercial EIA kits are not available for a particular application, it may be necessary to design a microplate assay. The following paragraphs outline some of the parameters that must be considered in developing a microplate EIA procedure.

Choice of microplate. Microplates suitable for EIA are available from several manufacturers. Rigid polystyrene plates are most commonly used and are available in untreated, irradiated, and tissue culture-treated forms. Each form has different surface characteristics that may be more appropriate for binding an individual protein. Polyvinyl chloride plates are also used in EIA. As an early step in EIA design, several different types of plates should be evaluated to determine which is most

TABLE 1. Enzymes commonly used in EIA

Enzyme	Source	Soluble product(s)	Insoluble product(s)	Inhibitor
Peroxidase	Horseradish	*o*-Phenylenediamine 2,2-Azino-di(3-ethylbenzothiazoline-6-sulfonate) 5,5′-Tetramethylbenzidine hydrochloride 5-Aminosalicylic acid	4-Chloro-1-naphthol Diaminobenzidine	Azide
Alkaline phosphatase	Calf intestine	*p*-Nitrophenyl phosphate	Bromochloroindolyl phosphate-Nitro Blue Tetrazolium	Phosphate

suitable for a given assay.

Plate coating. The efficient adsorption of antigen or antibodies to the surface of plastic microplates depends on many factors. An initial consideration is the protein concentration of the coating solution. Because of the low binding capacity of plastic plates, protein concentrations of 10 μg/ml ensure an excess of the material to be adsorbed. Detailed studies of microplate binding characteristics (16) determined that plastic microplate wells are saturated with protein concentrations of 4 μg/ml. Typically, protein concentrations of 1 to 10 μg/ml are used. As a rule of thumb, the lowest concentration of coating material that gives maximal analyte binding is used.

Enzyme-antibody conjugation. Excellent enzyme-labeled antibodies of various specificities are available from several commercial sources. However, in some circumstances it may be necessary to label antibodies in the laboratory. The procedure begins with enrichment of the antibodies from serum or ascites fluid. This initial step is required so that proteins other than antibodies will not be labeled and give false-positive results. Antibody enrichment is conveniently performed by using ammonium sulfate fractionation, ion-exchange chromatography, or protein A columns. The second stage represents coupling of the enzyme to antibody. Several methods, including periodate oxidation (17) and glutaraldehyde procedures (2), are widely used. The conditions used ordinarily result in optimum labeling of the antibody.

Blocking and wash solutions. Blocking solutions and wash buffers containing detergent are required to decrease nonspecific color intensity in EIA procedures. When the concentration of protein in the coating solution is suboptimal for saturation of microwell binding sites, an immunologically irrelevant protein is used to occupy (block) the remaining plate surface. Buffers containing bovine serum albumin or gelatin are commonly used for this purpose.

To prevent nonimmunological interactions in the microwell plate wells, all subsequent reagents are added in buffers containing detergent (usually 0.1% Tween 20). In addition, all washing steps between reagent additions are also done in buffers with Tween 20.

Assay optimization. The aim of microplate EIA is to detect clinically relevant levels of analytes (antibody or microbial antigen). In antibody capture formats, the assay must detect levels of specific antibody found in persons infected by a microbe without high background color intensities. In practice, sera from known infected individuals must be tested in serial dilutions to define a single dilution useful in the assay. When antigen capture formats are used, known quantities of microbial antigens isolated from infected cells or cultures must be tested in the assay. This procedure serves to determine the sensitivity of the EIA. Assay optimization must also be performed with the enzyme-labeled antibody used in either format. Other important considerations are the time and temperature of incubation with each reagent as well as the period of color development.

Alternative recognition molecules

Proteins A and G. In the mid-1960s, Forsgren and Sjoquist (11) described a cell wall protein in Cowan strains of *Staphylococcus aureus* that bound to immunoglobulins from several species in a nonimmunological fashion. Each protein A molecule has four regions that bind to the Fc portion of immunoglobulins. The immunoglobulin-binding properties of protein A make this molecule useful as a developing reagent in enzyme immunoassays. Protein A covalently bound to enzymes is available from several commercial sources and can

A) ANTIGEN CAPTURE

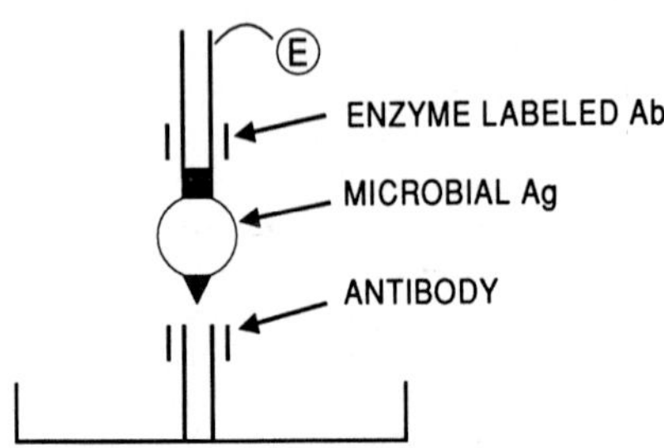

B) ANTIBODY CAPTURE

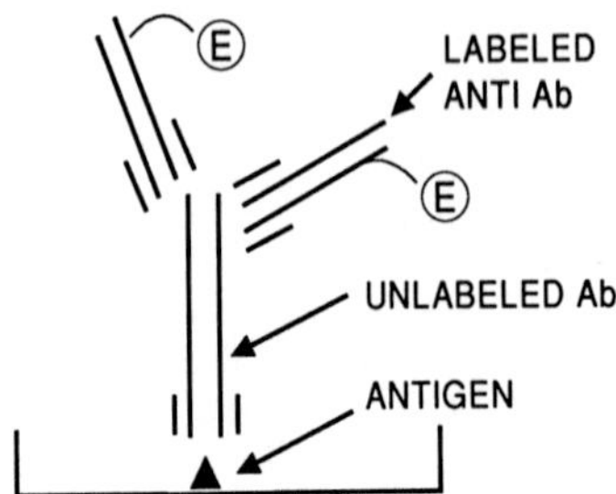

FIG. 1. Microplate EIA formats. Antigen capture formats (A) use immobilized monoclonal antibodies (Ab) to trap analytes. A second enzyme-labeled monoclonal antibody is used to detect the captured antigen (Ag). Antibody capture formats (B) use immobilized microbial antigens to bind specific antibody. An enzyme-labeled anti-immunoglobulin is used to detect the bound antibody.

substitute for enzyme-labeled second antibodies in EIA.

Although protein A has many desirable properties, it binds poorly to human IgG3 and some immunoglobulins from other mammals. Protein G, a cell wall constituent of some *Streptococcus* strains, exhibits high-affinity interactions with these immunoglobulins (5). Protein G is used in EIA much like protein A and is available in a genetically engineered form designed to reduce nonspecific interactions.

Protein G is now being used to detect IgA and IgM responses to microbial antigens (25). In this method, IgG is removed from sera by using protein G coupled to agarose. The residual antibodies are then incubated with the target antigen. The use of enzyme-labeled second antibodies that recognize the heavy chain of IgM or IgA allows a resolution of immune responses of these isotypes.

Avidin-biotin systems. The strong interaction between avidin, an egg white protein, and biotin, a low-molecular-weight vitamin, has been used to amplify the sensitivity of EIA. Each of the four subunits of avidin contains a site that interacts with the ureido ring of biotin. The remaining valeric acid side chain of the biotin molecule can be chemically modified to generate reactive groups without altering avidin interactions (4). The length of the spacer between the ureido group and the chemically reactive group is sufficient in several commercially available forms of biotin to allow attachment of the biotin to antibodies or enzyme and still permit interactions with avidin. Avidin itself may be covalently linked to enzyme reporter molecules by using several available methods.

Streptavidin from *Streptomyces avidinii* (7) is being used more widely than egg white avidin because of lower background intensity. Egg white avidin (pI 10.5) binds nonspecifically to proteins at physiological pH through charge-charge interactions. The lower isoelectric point of streptavidin reduces this background problem.

EIA using avidin-biotin interactions is performed in two major variations (Fig. 2). The first method makes use of a biotinylated second antibody (Fig. 2A). Avidin-enzyme conjugates are then used to detect bound biotinylated antibodies. The increase in sensitivity over standard EIA methods results from a pyramidlike enhancement of reporter group molecules. The other major format of avidin-biotin EIA (Fig. 2B) takes advantage of the multivalency of avidin. In this procedure, unconjugated avidin serves as a bridge between biotinylated antibody and biotin-enzyme conjugates. Alternatively, complexes of avidin and biotinylated enzyme can be used to detect the biotinylated antibody.

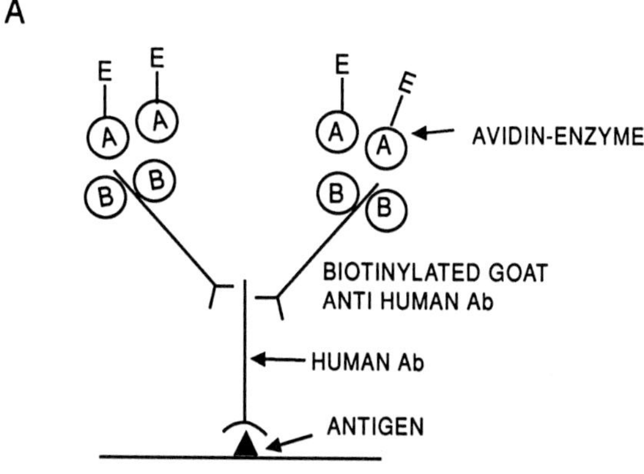

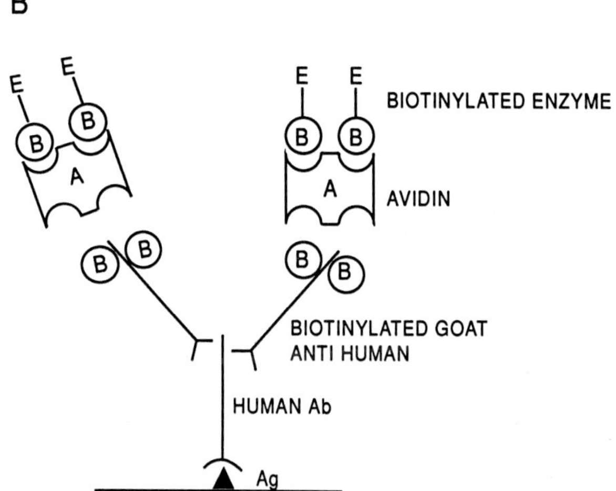

FIG. 2. Avidin-biotin EIA. Avidin-biotin EIA is performed in formats in which enzyme-labeled avidin is used to detect biotinylated antibodies (Ab) (A) or in which avidin is used to bridge biotinylated antibodies and enzyme (B). Ag, Antigen.

DOT AND SLOT BLOT ASSAYS

Dot blots (12) and the similar slot blot techniques are modifications of standard EIA assays. Both techniques are rapid means to screen a single serum specimen against a number of ligands or a number of sera against one or more ligands. The modification is that the whole ligand or a fraction thereof is directly applied onto, or filtered through, nitrocellulose or a comparable membrane. For direct application, the ligand, up to 2 μg in a 2-μl test dose, is pipetted carefully onto nitrocellulose or other sheets for a dot or applied with a pen for a slot blot (18). Alternatively, the ligand in the 200-μl sample is filtered into nitrocellulose or other suitable membranes. The filtration is carried out most often by means of a manifold apparatus having the shape of a microtiter plate. In dot blot filtration, the shape of the wells and the resultant dot is circular. With the slot blot, the configuration is a slot (Fig. 3). The geometric configuration of the ligand on the membrane is the major difference between the assays. The slot blot configuration is preferred if quantitation by densitometry is to be done.

After ligand application, the membrane is dried and blocked with a milk solution, and an immunoassay that is analogous to microplate EIA is conducted. The immunoassay can be performed by using the filtering manifold when large numbers of serum specimens are screened. The first antibody is allowed to percolate through the wells of the manifold. The wells are then washed with appropriate buffer, and the second antibody is allowed to filter through. After washing, the manifold is disassembled and the final reagent is added directly to the nitrocellulose sheets in a shallow dish. Alternatively, for screening a small number of serum specimens or for screening one specimen with a num-

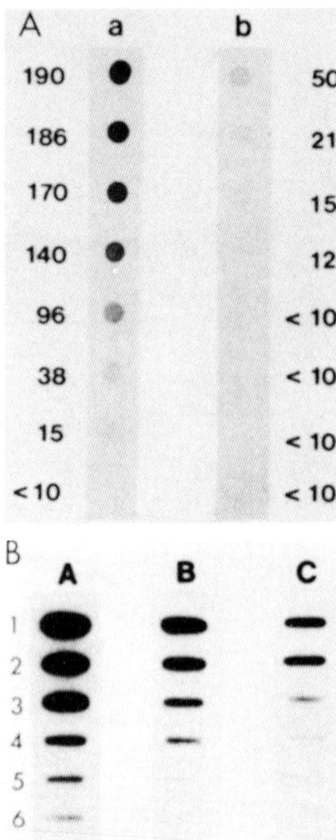

FIG. 3. Dot and slot blot assays. (A) Nitrocellulose strips with eight replicate dots of the same antigen concentration. Serial dilutions of reactive (a) and nonreactive (b) serum were applied to the dots. The numbers adjacent to the strips show the color intensities measured by an optical scanner. (Adapted from reference 20.) (B) A nitrocellulose sheet with panels of six antigen dilutions in the slots. Reactivities of antisera A, B, and C with the panel are shown.

ber of ligands, the manifold is disassembled, the sheet is cut to accommodate the number of ligands and specimens being tested, and the cut membrane pieces are placed in dishes and processed as described above.

CASSETTE EIA

Cassette EIAs provide an attractive alternative to microplate procedures when small numbers of specimens are tested. Since each clinical specimen is tested in a separate disposable cassette, the use of an entire strip of wells or microplate can be avoided when only a few assays are required. An additional benefit of cassette EIAs is that they can be performed more quickly than microplate tests. Typically, the entire procedure can be carried out in less than 10 min (8). Cassette assays use elevated concentrations of reactants to drive the assay to completion. The inherent low protein-binding capacity of plastic microplates prevents a useful elevation of reactant concentrations. As a result, microplate EIA procedures often require 2 to 4 h to complete. Finally, cassette EIA results are read visually. In laboratories with small specimen loads such as a physician's office, the expense and space required for microplate washers and readers are avoided.

Cassette EIA is performed in two basic formats. In the first, antigens are immobilized at a specific location on a membrane fixed in a disposable cassette. Nitrocellulose, which has high protein-binding capacity, is often used as the membrane. Sera to be tested are placed on the membrane and allowed to filter into absorbent material below the membrane in the cassette base. After washing to remove unbound antibody, a labeled antibody specific for the immunoglobulin of interest is used to flood the membrane. After additional washing, a substrate mixture that will generate insoluble enzyme products is added. Positive test results are indicated by a colored product at the spot where antigen was immobilized. An attractive feature of this method is that internal positive (e.g., human immunoglobulin) and negative (irrelevant protein) controls can be incorporated at additional sites on the membrane (Fig. 4). Simple visual inspection of the cassette membrane yields the test result and a validation of the procedure.

In the alternative format, the primary reaction between antigen and antibody occurs in solution outside the cassette. Typically, antigen is coupled to a particle such as agarose or latex and incubated with a serum specimen. After an incubation, the reaction mixture is applied to the cassette membrane. In this procedure, the membrane captures the particles by filtration. Subsequent assay steps are the same as for the other cassette format.

QUALITY CONTROL

Quality control is especially important in the performance of EIA tests, largely because of the complexity and sensitivity of the procedures. These factors tend to magnify errors in performance or materials, and exacting control standards are needed to ensure accurate and precise test results. Critical elements of a control program are standardization of the serochemistry, continuous monitoring of the test processes, and pretest inspection of test specimens (6, 14).

Determination of optimum antigen-antibody concentrations is a first requirement in the development of diagnostic EIA procedures. These optima are established by conventional block titrations with reference specimens. From these experiments, the test reagent concentrations for maximum specific reactivity and minimum nonspecific signal are established. Provisional test protocols are further validated by testing of known positive and presumed normal specimens from the target-diagnostic population. From these developmental studies, the test finding that correctly differentiates reactive-positive specimens from nonreactive-negative specimens is identified. This cutoff value is expressed as (i) a fixed absorbance value determined on the basis of the experience of the test developer, (ii) an absorbance value that is a multiplier or number of standard deviations above the negative population absorbance, (iii) a fraction or percentage of a known positive reference value, or (iv) a combination of these. In every instance, specimens with absorbance values greater than the cutoff are reactive or positive, and those with values less than the cutoff are nonreactive or negative.

The equipment manuals provided by manufacturers must be consulted for performance characteristics, calibration specifications, and operating procedures of all instruments used with EIA tests. As noted, EIA techniques are especially sensitive and therefore require

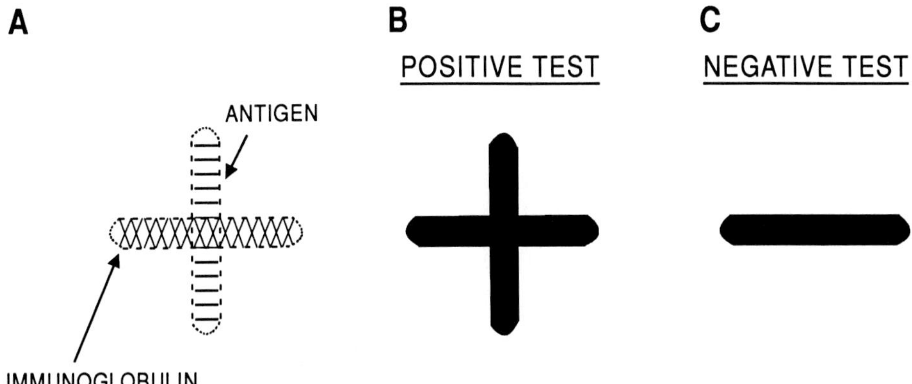

FIG. 4. Interpretation of cassette EIA results. The pattern of immobilized proteins on the cassette membrane (A) allows simple antibody capture EIA interpretation. The test antigen is immobilized in a vertical pattern while an immunoglobulin from the species of interest is placed horizontally. Positive results (B) are indicated by the plus pattern. Negative results (C) are indicated by a minus sign. Absence of the horizontal bar indicates an invalid test.

accurate fluid measurements. Pipetting devices, plate washers, and well readers must be calibrated, and schedules for calibration checks and routine maintenance must be established and recorded. However, records of calibrations, maintenance, and procedures must be kept in all laboratories. Special attention must be paid to pipetting devices. Accuracy for these devices is maximized by ensuring correct fit of the tips to the device barrel, by prewetting tips, and by delivery below a reagent level or against a vessel side wall. Washers, like reagent delivery devices, must perform exactly as specified. Vacuum and fluid delivery must be set for and matched to the plate test wells. A simple measure of wash efficiency is a plate-to-plate inspection for residual wash fluid. Either excess residual fluid or excessive aspiration in wash cycles, and thus excessive drying,

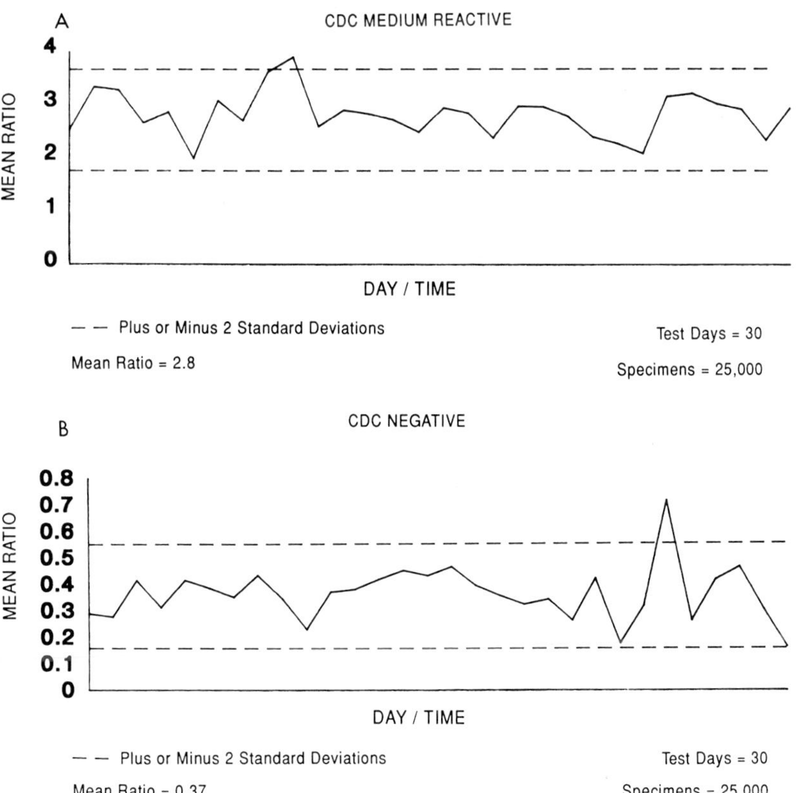

FIG. 5. Quality control chart of EIA tests on newborn dried blood spots showing chronological plots of the Centers for Disease Control (CDC) human immunodeficiency virus type 1 antibody blood spot controls. (A) Plot of mean absorbance/cutoff values for triplicates of mid-range virus antibody-reactive spots. (B) Plot of mean values for three antibody-negative control spots. The historic mean and 2 standard deviations above or below the historic mean are charted for each control.

may adversely affect test reactivity. Finally, since all EIA reactions are temperature and time sensitive, technical protocols must include clocks and thermometers as standard monitoring devices to ensure compliance with the parameters established for each test.

Each EIA run should include controls from the reagent manufacturer, a set prepared in-house or obtained from other sources (external or supplemental controls), as well as, whenever possible, a set of primary standards from a recognized reference laboratory, such as College of American Pathologists, Centers for Disease Control, or state health department laboratories (3). This last set is used initially, and at appropriate intervals, to ensure the optimum level of reactivity in consensus with other laboratories. The control set provided by the manufacturer describes the optimum performance characteristics of the test. The results of this control set, however, apply only to the potency of the reagent set in use. Variations in reagents, kit to kit or lot to lot, are monitored by the external control set, which should consist of multiple (duplicate or triplicate) high- and mid-range-reactive specimens or specimen pools and a nonreactive specimen or specimen pool. This external control thus serves not only to detect immediate failure but also to monitor both excessive run-to-run variation and long-term trends. Values obtained at each test run are efficiently monitored by charts that show, for example, nonreactive or background as well as levels of specific reactivity over time (Fig. 5).

Control oversight includes a critical inspection of test specimens. The established protocols for collection, transport, and storage of serum, plasma, cerebrospinal fluid, and dried blood spots should be followed (21). Serum and plasma are equally suitable for routine EIA tests. There are no adverse effects generally attributable to commonly used anticoagulants. Although hemolysis may not affect serum or plasma test results, it may be an indicator of improper handling that adversely affects antibody structure and activity and must be included in an interpretation of test results. For cerebrospinal fluid, color suggestive of hemolysis may indicate contamination with plasma proteins introduced during the spinal tap procedure; positive findings on fluid so contaminated may not be attributable solely to antigen or antibody within the cerebrospinal fluid compartment. Microbial contamination signals possible enzymatic degradation of specimen analyte and therefore loss of antigen or antibody reactivity. Urine and saliva have only recently been proposed as suitable for routine detection of IgG antibody. Although standards for handling and testing these specimens have not been established, the principles adopted for preservation of immunoglobulins in blood and cerebrospinal fluid apply.

LITERATURE CITED

1. **Arakawa, H., M. Maeda, and A. Tsuji.** 1979. Chemiluminescence enzyme immunoassay of cortisol using peroxidase as label. Anal. Biochem. **97:**248–254.
2. **Avrameas, S., T. Ternynck, and J. Guesdon.** 1978. Coupling of enzymes to antibodies and antigens. Scand. J. Immunol. **8**(Suppl. 7):7–24.
3. **Balfour, A. H., and J. P. Harford.** 1990. Quality control and standardization, p. 36–47. *In* T. G. Wreghitt and P. Morgan-Capner (ed.), ELISA in the clinical microbiology laboratory. Public Health Laboratory Service, London.
4. **Bayer, E., and M. Wilchek.** 1980. The use of the avidin-biotin complex as a tool in molecular biology. Methods Biochem. Anal. **26:**1–45.
5. **Bjork, L., and G. Kronvall.** 1984. Purification and some properties of streptococcal protein G, a novel IgG binding reagent. J. Immunol. **133:**969–974.
6. **Calamel, M., and M. Lambert.** 1988. E.L.IS.A. standardised technique. Laboratoire National de Pathologie, Paris.
7. **Chaiet, L., and F. Wolf.** 1964. The properties of streptavidin, a biotin-binding protein produced by Streptomyces. Arch. Biochem. Biophys. **106:**1–5.
8. **Cleveland, P., and D. Richman.** 1987. Enzyme immunofiltration staining assay for immediate diagnosis of herpes simplex virus and varicella zoster virus directly from clinical specimens. J. Clin. Microbiol. **25:**416–420.
9. **Duermeyer, W., and J. van der Veen.** 1978. Specific detection of IgM antibodies by ELISA as applied to hepatitis A. Lancet **ii:**684–685.
10. **Engvall, E., and P. Perlmann.** 1971. Enzyme-linked immunosorbent assay (ELISA). Quantitative assay of immunoglobulin G. Immunochemistry **8:**871–874.
11. **Forsgren, A., and J. Sjoquist.** 1966. "Protein A" from S. aureus. 1. Pseudo-immune reaction with human gamma globulin. J. Immunol. **97:**822–827.
12. **Hawkes, R., E. Niday, and J. Gordon.** 1982. A dot-immunobinding assay for monoclonal and other antibodies. Anal. Biochem. **119:**142–147.
13. **Ishikawa, E., and K. Kato.** 1978. Ultrasensitive enzyme immunoassay. Scand. J. Immunol. **8**(Suppl. 7):43–55.
14. **Kemeny, D. M., and S. J. Challacombe.** 1988. ELISA and other solid phase immunoassays. John Wiley & Sons, Inc., New York.
15. **Laemmli, U. K.** 1970. Cleavage of structural proteins during the assembly of the head of bacteriophage T4. Nature (London) **227:**680–685.
16. **Lovborg, U.** 1984. Guide to solid phase immunoassays. A/S Nunc, Denmark.
17. **Nakane, P., and A. Kawaoi.** 1974. Peroxidase-labeled antibody. A new method of conjugation. J. Histochem. Cytochem. **22:**1084–1091.
18. **Raoult, D., and G. Dasch.** 1989. An immunoassay for monoclonal and other antibodies. Its application to the serotyping of Gram negative bacteria. J. Immunol. Methods **125:**57–67.
19. **Towbin, H., T. Staehelin, and J. Gordon.** 1979. Electrophoretic transfer of proteins from polyacrylamide gels to nitrocellulose sheets: procedure and some applications. Proc. Natl. Acad. Sci. USA **76:**4350–4354.
20. **Urakami, H., S. Yamamoto, T. Tsuruhura, N. Ohashi, and A. Tamura.** 1989. Serodiagnosis of scrub typhus with antigens immobilized on nitrocellulose sheet. J. Clin. Microbiol. **27:**1841–1846.
21. **U.S. Public Health Service.** 1989. Serologic assays for human immunodeficiency virus antibody in dried-blood specimens collected on filter paper from neonates. Centers for Disease Control, Atlanta.
22. **Van Weemen, B., and A. Schuurs.** 1971. Immunoassay using antigen-enzyme conjugates. FEBS Lett. **15:**232–236.
23. **Voller, A., A. Bartlett, D. Bidwell, M. Clark, and A. Adams.** 1976. The detection of viruses by enzyme-linked immunosorbent assay. J. Gen. Virol. **33:**165–167.
24. **Wannlund, J., and M. Deluca.** 1982. A sensitive bioluminescent immunoassay for dinitrophenol and trinitrotoluene. Anal. Biochem. **122:**385–393.
25. **Weiblen, B., R. Schumacher, and R. Hoff.** 1990. Detection of IgM and IgA HIV antibodies after removal of IgG with recombinant protein G. J. Immunol. Methods **126:** 199–204.

Chapter 13

Immunoelectroblot Techniques

KARIM E. HECHEMY, ROY W. STEVENS, AND JAMES M. CONROY

Electroimmunoblot technology has been recognized as a powerful tool not only for research studies but also for the routine serodiagnosis of disease. At present, the immunoblot (Western blot) is the definitive test for the serodiagnosis of human immunodeficiency virus (HIV) infection (3) and is important in determining the specificity of screening tests for Lyme disease antibody (7). The technique is as sensitive as the standard enzyme immunoassays but is potentially more specific. The greater specificity is obtainable because of the direct visualization of antigen-antibody reactions with isolated known antigens of infectious agents. Electroimmunoblot (1, 2) is actually a combination of three powerful analytical techniques: (i) separation of ligand-antigen components by electrophoresis (10), (ii) electroblotting (electrotransfer) of the electrophoresed ligand (13), and (iii) immunoassay to identify reactivity with the target ligands (13).

The three techniques involve six essential steps:

1. Solubilization of the ligand.
2. Preparation of the gel.
3. Electrophoretic separation of the ligand in the gel.
4. Electrotransfer or electroblot of the electrophoresed ligand to an immobilizing support membrane.
5. Blocking of free protein-binding sites (membrane sites that are not occupied by the ligand) on the membrane.
6. Enzyme immunoassay or radioimmunoassay to (i) detect the antibodies in unknown serum specimens or (ii) probe with known antisera for a specific antigen band(s) separated by the electrophoresis.

The major advantages of using the immobilized, electrophoretically resolved ligand on the surface of the support membrane, instead of the ligands in the gel, are (i) the immobilized ligand(s) does not diffuse, (ii) the electrophoretic resolution of the ligand is retained by electroblotting, and (iii) the separated ligand is easily accessible to the probe. Ligands in gels do diffuse and are not readily accessible to the probe.

SOLUBILIZATION OF THE LIGAND

The reasons for solubilizing the ligand are twofold. The first is to breakdown the ligand into component polypeptides of different molecular weights. This breakdown is done in such a way that the epitopes on the polypeptides are not destroyed and antigenicity is retained. The second reason is to impart a uniformly negative charge to the polypeptides so that when the ligand preparation is subjected to an electric field, the movement of the peptides is dependent solely on molecular weight and not on both molecular weight and the various inherent ionic charges of the component peptides.

Optimum conditions for solubilization vary according to the complexity of the ligand to be studied. Most solubilization buffers are made according to the formula of Laemmli (10) or modifications thereof. The composition of the reagent used in our laboratory is either a 1× or 2× solubilizing buffer. The 1× formula is the following:

Component	Volume (ml)
10% sodium dodecyl sulfate (SDS)	2.0
2-Mercaptoethanol	0.4
Glycerol	1.0
1 M Tris, pH 6.8	0.62
Bromophenol blue dye	0.5 (tracking dye)
Distilled water to	10.0

Buffer concentration required will vary according to whether the ligand is in solution or in suspension. A 2× buffer may be required for ligand in suspension.

The incubation time required for solubilization must be established for each ligand. Also, the optimum temperature for solubilization may vary from 25 to 100°C. Thus, the time and temperature of incubation may vary from 2 min at 100°C to 30 min at 25°C. If parts of the ligand are still insoluble after the treatment, it is advisable to centrifuge the ligand in a microcentrifuge and use the supernatant for the gel electrophoresis. The use of suspended material may cause uneven separation of the polypeptides. Insoluble materials are seen as a smear in the high-molecular-weight region of a gel.

PREPARATION OF POLYACRYLAMIDE GELS

Polyacrylamide gels (4) are formed by copolymerization of the monomers acrylamide and bisacrylamide. The reaction is a vinyl addition polymerization initiated by *N,N,N′,N′*-tetramethylenediamine and ammonium persulfate. The elongating polymer chains are randomly cross-linked by bisacrylamide, resulting in a polymer with a characteristic porosity that depends on the polymerization conditions and monomer concentrations. Gels of appropriate porosity and stability may be purchased or prepared in the laboratory.

The proportions of the monomer reactants are important in gel preparation. Increasing the amount of the initiators results in a decrease in the average polymer chain length, an increase in gel turbidity, and a decrease in gel elasticity. In contrast, reducing the amount of the initiators results in longer polymerization chain length, greater elasticity of the gel, and slower polymerization. Too slow a polymerization may result in trapping of air, resulting in gels that are too porous and mechanically weak. As a precaution against air entrapment, the acrylamide solution should be degassed before the polymerization process.

The gel can be prepared as (i) a continuous system in which the concentration of the acrylamide is the same the whole length of the gel, (ii) a discontinuous system with two different gel concentrations, or (iii) a gradient system with various concentrations of gel over the length of the electrophoretic path. In general, the discontinuous gel system is most often used. In discontinuous systems, higher acrylamide concentrations are used to form resolving gels and lower concentrations are used to make stacking gels. The use of a relatively low gel concentration as the stacking gel will allow the various fractions to migrate at nearly the same rate in the stacking gel and be concentrated at the beginning of the resolving gel. Therefore, all fractions will move into the separating gel at the same time.

The composition of gels used in commercial assays is described in the instructions provided by the manufacturers, along with detailed instructions on the preparation and use of the apparatus and on the recommended electrophoretic conditions. A general outline of procedures for the preparation and running of gels is shown in Fig. 1 and described below. The resolving (lower) gel is poured between the two glass plates, water is carefully added to flatten the solution surface, and the gel is allowed to polymerize for 2 to 18 h. The water is removed, and the comb or block to define the electrophoretic lanes is placed between the glass plates. The comb will allow the ligand to move in lanes with empty spaces between them and to separate the ligand in one lane from a ligand in an adjacent lane. A comb is used when various ligands are electrophoresed in the same gel or only a section of the gel is needed. In the latter case, Laemmli buffer is added in the unused lanes. The block will allow the ligand to move as a solid mass. A block is used when one ligand is used with a full gel. The stacking (upper) gel is poured on top of the resolving gel, water is carefully added, and the gel is allowed to polymerize for 1 h. After polymerization, the overlay water is decanted; the gel is ready for sample application. Each well of the block is filled with electrode buffer. Samples and controls, mixed with an inert tracking dye and prestained molecular weight standards, are underlaid into appropriate wells by means of syringe and needle. Specimens should be concentrated so that, for example, 2 to 20 μg of protein is delivered in 20 μl per lane or 3 to 300 μg is contained in 1,000 μl per block. The tracking dye is used to monitor the progress of the electrophoresis run; the molecular weight standards indicate the relative molecular weights of the resolved polypeptides. For electrophoresis, the block or the comb is removed and the gel is placed into the chamber as instructed by the manufacturer. The power is turned on, and 30 mA per gel is applied until the tracking dye moves into the separating gel; the electric field is then increased to 60 mA per gel. The current

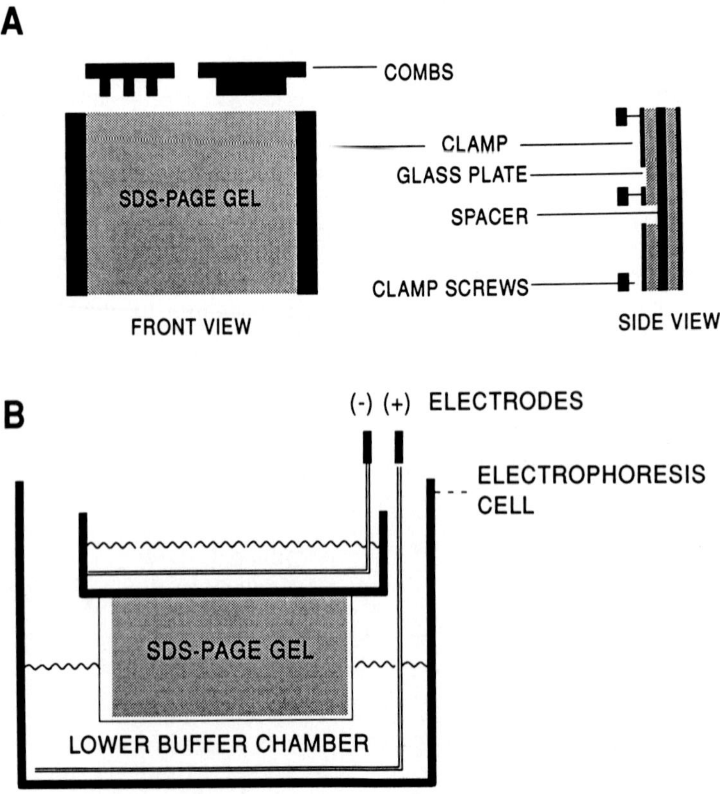

FIG. 1. Schematic representation of a gel cassette and electrophoresis cell. (A) Front and side views of the gel sandwich. The side view shows the layers that make up the sandwich. (B) The electrophoresis cell, showing the gel cassette in place, the upper and lower buffer chambers, and the electrode positions.

is turned off when the dye is driven to within 0.5 cm of the lower end of the gel. The gel is removed carefully by use of a gentle stream of distilled water. A lane containing electrophoresed antigen is cut from the gel, fixed overnight, treated with Coomassie blue, and destained. This lane serves as a control on the electrophoresis process. The remaining gel is electroblotted (see below) immediately after removal of the lane. Delay in electroblotting may cause the antigen to diffuse in the gel so as to reduce the resolution of the process and of the bands detected on immunoassay.

IMMOBILIZING MATRICES

The immobilizing matrices, or membranes, are classified according to the type of binding: hydrophobic (for example, nitrocellulose [13] or polyvinylidene fluoride [11]) or ionic (for example, a positively charged membrane [7]).

Nitrocellulose was the first material used and is still the immobilizing membrane of choice for most electroblot investigations. It has a comparatively high binding efficiency of approximately 80 μg of protein per cm^2, depending on the protein. The binding of proteins presumably involves hydrophobic forces. Blocking of free sites is easily achieved so that the color of the background after staining is minimal. Because they are brittle when dry, nitrocellulose sheets must be handled carefully.

Another type of hydrophobic support is the polyvinylidene fluoride membrane (11). This solid matrix offers a high capacity for adsorption of proteins. Its open, porous polymeric structure offers a large surface area that is entirely accessible for protein adsorption. It is critical to prewet the polyvinylidene fluoride membrane with methanol for a few seconds to allow the hydrophobic sites to become fully wet when the membrane is immersed in the aqueous solution. The membrane should remain wet at all times and can be used in the same fashion as nitrocellulose. If the membrane dries, it must be rewet before manipulation. This type of membrane is less brittle than nitrocellulose.

Positively charged nylon-based membranes are made by incorporating tertiary and quaternary amines into nylon. These membranes are also less brittle than nitrocellulose and have an especially high capacity for proteins (480 μg/cm^2). However, blocking of the free binding sites is more difficult. Therefore, high background after staining may occur if unoccupied sites on the membrane have not been properly blocked.

PROTOCOL FOR ELECTROBLOTTING

Determination of the optimum transfer time and selection of transfer buffer are important factors to consider in electroblotting. The transfer run can be overnight with low-field intensity at 250-mA constant current at 4°C with standard-size (16- by 14-cm) gels or for 3 to 5 h with high-field intensity. The latter is performed at 200 V (constant voltage) with standard gels or at 100 V with minigels (10 by 9 cm). A transfer buffer recommended for a low-field run is 25 mM phosphate buffer, pH 7.4. A buffer for a high-field run is 24 mM Tris with 192 mM glycine and 20% methanol (3.03 g, 14.4 g, and 200 ml, respectively, with distilled H_2O to 1 liter). The final pH is approximately 8.3 and need not be adjusted.

A general outline of the electroblotting procedure is described below.

1. Equilibrate the gel in 500 ml of electroblotting (transfer) buffer for 30 min.

2. Assemble the sandwich as described by the manufacturer of the electroblot apparatus. The apparatus (Fig. 2) essentially consists of the gel holder (clamps) in which are sequentially inserted the sponge, filter paper pads, the gel and the membrane (blotting matrix), another filter paper, and sponge pad. All are presaturated with cold transfer buffer. During presoaking, the nitrocellulose membrane should be touched to the buffer and allowed to be wet by capillary action. Abrupt immersion may result in entrapment of air bubbles in areas of the matrix, resulting in erratic or no transfer of the ligands in these areas. For other types of membranes, follow the instructions of the manufacturer. Place the gel holder in the half-filled tank (Fig. 1). Placement of the sandwich in the tank is very important. Be certain that the gel is placed such that the anions flow first through the gel containing the ligands and then through the membrane (Fig. 2). Failure to so orient the gel holder will result in transfer of the ligands to the buffer in the tank.

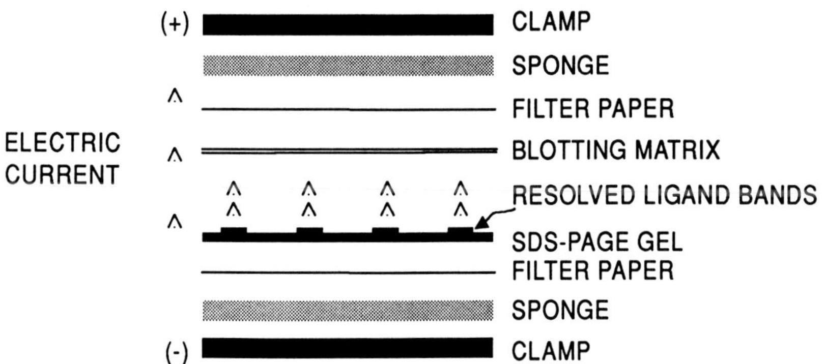

FIG. 2. Schematic representation of the transblot cassette. The essential layering of the components is shown. The flow of electric current (^) from the anode (−) through the apparatus toward the cathode (+) is illustrated. The bands of separated protein-ligand, depicted as protruding above the gel, move with the current from the SDS-polyacrylamide (SDS-PAGE) gel into the blotting matrix.

3. Electroblot the ligand as described above. Cooling may not be required for the low-intensity transfer but is required for the high-intensity transfer.

4. After the electroblotting is completed, wash the membrane in distilled water and dry it at 25°C. The gel is then processed for Coomassie blue staining (Fig. 3) to ensure that the ligands were in fact transferred from the gel as a quality control measure. An additional test is conducted by probing the electroblotted nitrocellulose membrane with colloidal gold (12) (Fig. 3) or India ink (8) to determine whether the ligands were transferred onto the nitrocellulose and not into the buffer. Perform the colloidal gold or the amido black tests as described by the manufacturer. Extra precautions should be used in handling the nitrocellulose (use gloves in handling the membrane).

Poor transfer of the ligands from the gel could be due to too high a gel concentration, too short a transfer time, low power settings, precipitation of the protein in the gel, or a power interruption. To address these problems, eliminate the methanol in the transfer buffer or decrease the percentage of the monomer or cross-linker in the gel. Alternatively, increase the electroblotting time or use the high-field-intensity protocol. Other remedies are to (i) add 0.1% SDS to the electroblotting buffer to prevent precipitation of protein in the gel and (ii) check the power circuitry.

MEMBRANE IMMUNOPROBE PROCEDURES

After transfer of the ligand bands onto the membrane is probed with colloidal gold, the antigenicity of the electroblotted ligand bands is checked with a reference antiserum or the reactivity of test specimen sera to the isolated proteins is determined (Fig. 4).

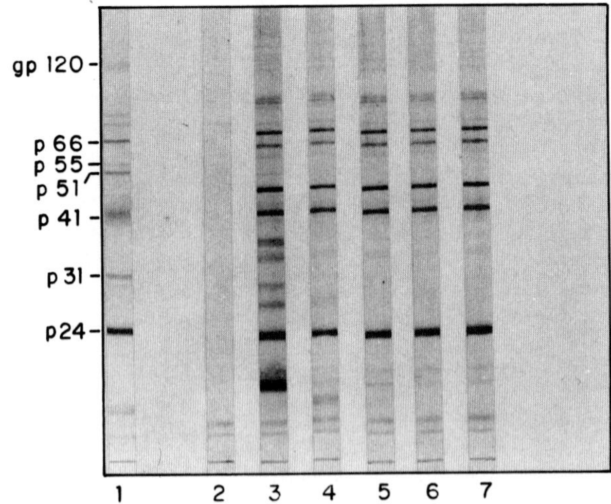

FIG. 4. Electroimmunoblot assay for confirmation of human T-cell lymphotropic virus types I and II (HTLV-I/II) enzyme-linked immunosorbent assay-reactive specimens. Serum specimens were examined for reactivity to HTLV-I/II isolated antigens in a blot procedure. For antigen-blot preparation, HIV-1 lysate was electrophoresed into the first lane of the polyacrylamide gel and HTLV-I/II lysate was electrophoresed into lanes 2 through 7. The separated proteins were transblotted to a nitrocellulose sheet. Results are shown with HIV-1-reactive reference serum added to lane 1, HTLV-I/II-negative serum added to lane 2, HTLV-I-reactive reference added to lane 3, and test specimens added to lanes 4 through 7. The positions of HIV-1 and HTLV-I reference sera define the molecular weights of HTLV-I/II specimen-reactive bands; densities of HIV-1 and HTLV-I/II reference bands ensure both test sensitivity and reproducibility. The test specimens have antibody to proteins at the 24-, 46-, and 61/68-kilodalton molecular mass positions and therefore are positive for HTLV-I/II.

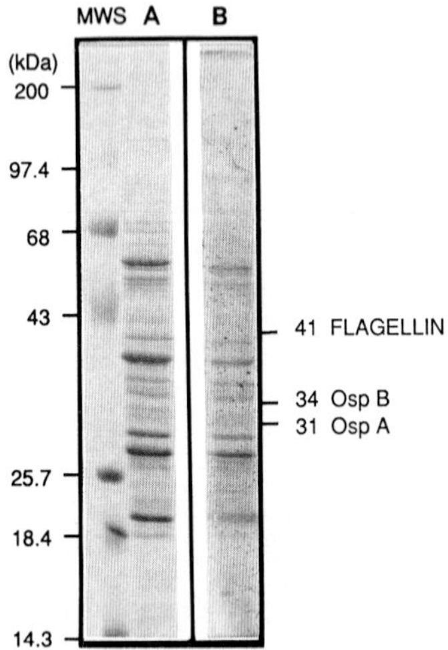

FIG. 3. Quality control lanes of an SDS-gel with electrophoresed and electroblotted molecular weight standards (MWS) and protein antigens of *Borrelia burgdorferi*. After electrophoresis, gel sections containing standards (MWS) and antigens were stained with Coomassie blue (A). After electroblotting, lanes from the nitrocellulose were treated with a colloidal gold probe to confirm the transfer of the bands (B). *B. burgdorferi*-specific antigens flagellin and outer surface proteins A (Osp A) and B (Osp B) are identified on the gold-probed nitrocellulose. kDa, Kilodaltons.

Any unoccupied sites on the membrane are first blocked with one of a number of blocking agents. The blocking agent most often used is 5 to 10% nonfat dry milk, 3% albumin, or 0.01% Tween 20. A mixture of albumin and Tween may also be used. The optimum time of exposure of the membrane to each blocking agent must be determined for each system. The most effective time may range from 30 min to 18 h. Prolonged incubations with milk should be performed at 5°C, since milk will coagulate on the membrane if incubation is at 37°C.

Probing is routinely done with enzyme immunoassay second-antibody systems. After incubation of the membrane with the first antibody (serum test specimen or polyclonal or monoclonal reference antiserum), a horseradish peroxidase-labeled anti-antibody (as the second antibody) is applied. The developer often used to visualize the immune reaction is the substrate 4-chloro-1-naphthol (9). Other substrates have been used. Some, however, are suspected or known to be carcinogens. Other enzyme-labeled second antibodies have also been used. See chapter 12 for a discussion of alternative conjugates and substrates.

Optimum incubation time with the first antibody must be established for each system. However, as a rule of thumb for monoclonal antibodies, the incubation is best performed overnight at 37°C. In contrast, polyclonal antibody incubation times vary between 1 and 4 h at

22°C. The serum containing the first antibodies is usually diluted 1:50 to 1:100 with a blocking buffer. Lower dilutions may lead to unacceptable background levels. After incubation with the first antibody, the membrane is washed at least three times for 10 min each with 0.01% Tween 20 in phosphate-buffered saline, pH 7.4. Sometimes a second 5-min soaking with the blocking buffer, before incubation with the second antibody, is necessary to obtain a clean background. The second antibody is diluted with the blocking buffer at an optimum concentration determined for each conjugate. The membrane is then incubated for 30 min to 2 h with the second antibody at 37°C, washed with phosphate-buffered saline–Tween as described above, and developed with the enzyme substrate as described by the manufacturer.

INTERPRETATION OF TEST RESULTS

Immunoblot is primarily a qualitative technique. Analysis of the immunoblot is made on the basis of at least two criteria: (i) the presence of a particular band, or of a specific set or pattern or of a minimum number of bands of given molecular weights, and (ii) the intensity of the staining of the band(s). Reading of the relative degree of staining of the bands is done visually or with a densitometer.

In serodiagnostic tests, a number of presumed normal subjects may react with some of the bands but give a lower intensity of staining as a result of the presence of cross-reacting antibodies to shared epitopes. Because of this cross-reactivity, a number of presumed normal control sera (50 to 100) should be first immunoblotted with a given electrophoresed and electroblotted antigen to establish nonspecific reactivity and the intensity of nonspecific staining of the bands. When the background levels of nonspecific reactivity in a population are established, the immunoblot is a very useful tool to confirm qualitatively (positive or negative) the test results obtained with the established quantitative serodiagnostic assays. This qualitative corroboration of the test result can be especially helpful in the interpretation of the "weakly reactive" quantitative test results obtained with standard diagnostic assays (5). This is because the immunoblot allows direct visualization of the specific antigen band(s) that reacts with the test sera. Thus, a determination is made of the specificity of the initial screening test reaction. However, one must keep in mind that a given band may have specific as well as shared epitopes. A study of the extent of the cross-reactivity of a test specimen or of known antiserum to ligand bands from different organisms that share common epitopes can be undertaken with the immunoblot assay (Fig. 5). The serum can be absorbed, if necessary, with the heterologous antigen. For quality control, it is retested for specificity to the homologous antigen (Fig. 6).

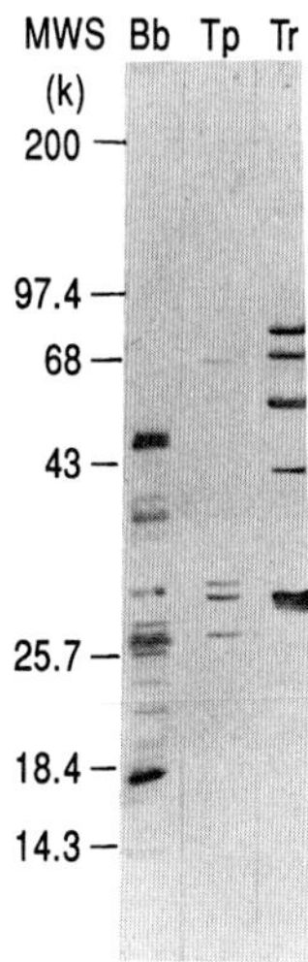

FIG. 5. Cross-reactivity pattern of a human serum from a patient with Lyme borreliosis immunoblotted with *Borrelia burgdorferi* antigens (Bb), *Treponema pallidum* antigens (Tp), and *Treponema phagedenis* (biotype Reiter) antigens (Tr). MWS, Molecular weight standards; k, kilodaltons.

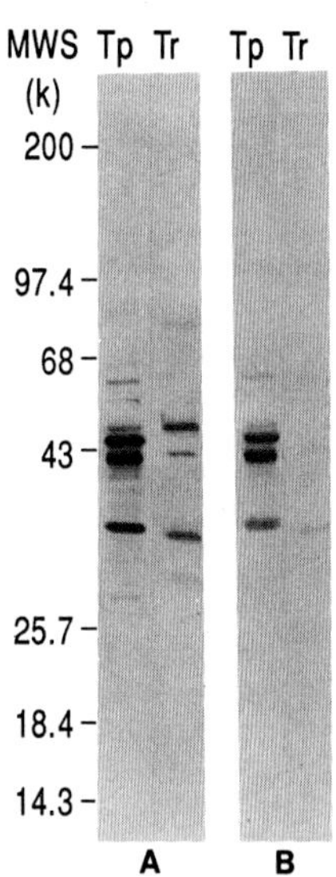

FIG. 6. Human syphilitic serum immunoblotted with *Treponema pallidum* (Tp) and *Treponema phagedenis* (biotype Reiter) (Tr) antigens before (A) and after (B) absorption with a *T. phagedenis* lysate. MWS, Molecular weight standards; k, kilodaltons.

LITERATURE CITED

1. **Baldo, B. A., and E. R. Tovey (ed.).** 1989. Protein blotting: methodology, research, and diagnostic applications. Kayer, Basel.
2. **Bjerrum, O. J., and H. H. Heegard (ed.).** 1988. CRC handbook of immunoblotting of proteins, vol. 1 and 2. CRC Press, Inc., Boca Raton, Fla.
3. **Centers for Disease Control.** 1987. Public Health Service guidelines for counseling and antibody testing to prevent HIV infection and AIDS. Morbid. Mortal. Weekly Rep. **36:** 502–510.
4. **Chrambach, A., T. M. Jouiun, P. J. Svendsen, and D. Rodbard.** 1976. Analytical and preparative polyacrylamide gel electrophoresis. An objectively defined fractionation route apparatus and procedures, p. 27, 144. *In* N. Catsinapoolas (ed.), Methods of protein separation, vol. 2. Plenum Publishing Corp., New York.
5. **Galen, R. S., and S. R. Gambino.** 1975. Beyond normality: the predictive value and efficiency of medical diagnoses, p. 1–49. John Wiley & Sons, Inc., New York.

6. **Gershoni, J. M., and G. E. Palade.** 1982. Electrophoretic transfer of proteins from sodium dodecyl sulfate-polyacrylamide gels to a positively charged membrane filter. Anal. Biochem. **174:**396–405.
7. **Grodzicki, L., and A. C. Steere.** 1988. Comparison of immunoblotting and indirect immunosorbent assay using different antigen preparations for diagnosing early Lyme disease. J. Infect. Dis. **157:**790–797.
8. **Hancock, K., and V. C. W. Tsay.** 1983. India ink staining of proteins on nitrocellulose paper. Anal. Biochem. **133:** 157–162.
9. **Hawkes, R., E. Niday, and J. Gordon.** 1982. A dot-immunobinding assay for monoclonal and other antibodies. Anal. Biochem. **119:**142–147.
10. **Laemmli, U. K.** 1970. Cleavage of structural proteins during the assembly of the head of bacteriophage T4. Nature (London) **227:**680–685.
11. **Product Information Bulletin.** 1984. Pall Biodyne immunoaffinity membrane, p. 1–4. Pall Ultrafine Corp., Glen Cove, N.Y.
12. **Surek, B., and E. Latzko.** 1984. Visualization of antigenic proteins blotted onto nitrocellulose using the immunogold-staining (IGS) method. Biochem. Biophys. Res. Commun. **121:**284–289.
13. **Towbin, H., T. Staehelin, and J. Gordon.** 1979. Electrophoretic transfer of proteins from polyacrylamide gels to nitrocellulose sheets: procedure and some applications. Proc. Natl. Acad. Sci. USA **76:**4350–4354.

Chapter 14

Immunoprecipitation: Passive Immunodiffusion, Electroimmunodiffusion

DAVID E. NORMANSELL

Immunoprecipitation is the formation of an antigen-antibody complex in solution followed by precipitation of the complex from solution. If the reaction occurs in aqueous solution within the matrix of a clear gel, such as in an agarose gel, the complex will form within the fluid spaces of the gel, will rapidly exceed the pore size of the gel, and will be trapped in position. Complexes of a sufficiently large size will be visible. The gel used must be clear, strong, inert, and of appropriate pore size; it must be easily prepared and must be solid at working temperatures. In immunodiffusion reactions, the formation of the antigen-antibody complex follows the diffusion of one or both of the reactants through the gel. Diffusion may be passive, resulting from lateral diffusion of the reactants, or it may be forced by an applied electric field.

Although immune reactions have been used diagnostically for nearly a century, it was 1946 before the technique of immunodiffusion was described in detail by Oudin (6). Double diffusion was described by Ouchterlony (4) and by Elek (1) in 1948, and many modifications since have been introduced. The use of agar for the gel matrix first was suggested by Frau Fannie Hesse, in 1881 (2); she suggested the use of the kitchen jellifying agent agar-agar as an alternative to gelatin or potatoes for bacteriological cultures.

Agar is a complex polysaccharide extracted from red algae seaweeds with hot acid. Many different purification schemes exist, and although the final product varies from manufacturer to manufacturer, the properties of agar gels are fairly standard. The pore size of the matrix varies with the concentration of the agar in the gel; concentrations of 0.5 to 1.0% offer very little hindrance to migration of most serum proteins. However, lower concentrations of agar cannot be used because they are physically too weak to maintain the structure of the matrix. Agar contains many ions, especially sulfate and carboxyl groups, and carries a net negative charge. As a result of this charge, some antigens and basic dyes react strongly with the agar matrix itself. In addition, the presence of these fixed charges on the gel matrix causes buffer ions to move to the cathode on application of an electric field. This is the electroendosmotic effect, which results in reduced mobility of anions. Agar is a mixture of two polymers, agarose and agaropectin. Most of the charge is on the agaropectin molecule, and the use of purified agarose provides a clearer and stronger gel that carries very little charge. Agarose is a polymer of alternating residues of 3,6-anhydro-α-L-galactopyranose and β-D-galactopyranose. The purification of agarose is a tedious procedure, but many commercial suppliers now carry agarose and it can be obtained with different gel characteristics, as needed.

Other materials have been proposed for the gel matrix, including polyacrylamide, cellulose acetate, gelatin, starch, and cross-linked dextrans. Polyacrylamide would seem to be superior to agarose in that it is chemically inert, it has no fixed charge, and the composition and pore size can be decided in advance. However, it is less convenient to use since it must be freshly prepared before each use and the chemicals involved are neurotoxic. The other supports are rarely if ever used because of problems with transparency (cellulose acetate, starch, and dextrans) or physical strength (gelatin). Agarose is the gel of choice for double diffusion and for techniques that do not need the electroendosmotic effect.

Agarose is best prepared in bulk and divided into smaller portions for storage at 4°C before use. For double diffusion, phosphate-buffered saline (PBS; 0.01 M phosphate plus 0.15 M sodium chloride, pH 7.4) containing either 0.01% sodium azide or 0.1% Merthiolate is used as the diluent. Five grams of agarose should be added to 500 ml of warm buffer, with stirring, and the mixture should be heated gently until the solution clarifies (95 to 98°C). Direct heating on a hot plate is satisfactory provided that the plate is not set on "high," the mixture is well stirred, and the mixture does not boil strongly. Excessive evaporation also should be avoided. Plates can be poured using hot gel except for applications in which antibodies are added to the gel; in that case, the agarose must be cooled to 45°C before the addition of antibody. The remainder of the mixture should be stored in 30-ml samples in 50-ml capped tubes (Fisher no. 14-932E or equivalent) and stored tightly capped at 4°C. For use, the gel is melted by heating the tube (loosen the cap first) in a boiling water bath. Care should be taken to remove any "skin" of unmelted agarose in the tube before dispensing the gel. The gels should be poured on glass or on clear plastic plates, which must be precoated with a dilute (0.1%) agarose solution in order to obtain a strong adherence of the agarose or agar gel to the plate. For most purposes, the agarose and agar gels are used at 1% concentration and with a thickness of 1.5 to 2.0 mm. For pouring, the plates are placed on a level, dust-free surface. The agarose is dispensed by using a warmed pipette held just above the plate at a 45° angle, and the agarose stream is directed to the edges of the plate. Surface tension will prevent the agarose solution from spilling over the edge. The flow should be controlled to prevent air bubbles in the gel; if bubbles form, they should be removed immediately by flaming the surface of the molten gel with a Bunsen flame. After pouring, the plate should be covered loosely until the gel has set. Plates can be used within 20 min of being poured or may be stored in a humid chamber for up to 1 week. Plates that have been stored for more than 1 day after pouring should be examined for bacterial growth before use. Wells should be punched with sharp clean punches, and the agarose should be removed with a Pasteur pipette attached to a vacuum. Any moisture in the wells or on top of the gel should be removed with a piece of rolled tissue.

THE PRECIPITIN CURVE

In the procedures discussed here, the formation of precipitating antigen-antibody complexes is described by the classical precipitin curve (Fig. 1). Antigen (multivalent) and antibody (di- or polyvalent) molecules interact to form a three-dimensional lattice. The fit between the combining sites of the antibody molecules and the complementary epitopes on the antigen molecules leads to expulsion of water molecules from the hydration layers between the apposed surfaces of the reactants. This expulsion of water molecules alters the net entropy of the complex and causes precipitation. For maximum precipitation, the reactants must be present in proportions such that there will be few spare valencies. If the reactants are not present in optimum proportions, so that either the antigen or antibody is in moderate excess, the lattice will not be as extensive and spare valencies will be common. Fewer water molecules will be expelled, and the tendency to precipitate will be reduced. A gross excess of either reactant will result in greatly decreased precipitate formation. In gross antigen excess, there will be no precipitate formation at all because the antibody valencies will be fully saturated with antigen and the amount of cross-linking will be very small or zero. In gross antibody excess, the situation is somewhat different because polyvalent antibody preparations have a range of affinity constants. This means that in gross antibody excess, the most avid antibody molecules will preferentially bind the antigen molecules present, resulting in small amounts of precipitate. Moreover, in the antibody excess zone, the amount of precipitate is proportional to the antigen concentration.

The equivalence zone is defined as the range of reactant ratios that results in maximum precipitation of both reactants. This zone is usually quite broad for most antigen-polyclonal antibody systems, although it is difficult to ensure total precipitation of both reactants. However, in the context of precipitation in a matrix, the reactants diffuse toward and into each other until the concentrations reach values appropriate for equivalence. Precipitation of the immune complexes prevents further migration.

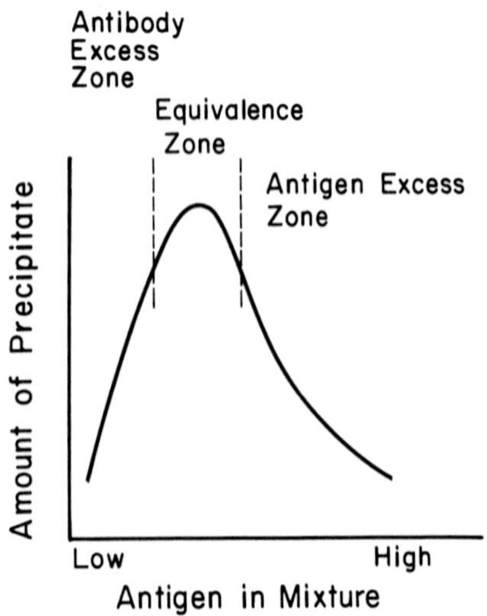

FIG. 1. Quantitative precipitin curve showing variation in the amount of precipitate formed between a constant amount of antibody and an increasing amount of antigen.

PASSIVE IMMUNODIFFUSION

Many different forms of passive immunodiffusion have been developed, but the most useful are double diffusion and radial immunodiffusion.

Double diffusion

In double diffusion, the two reagents diffuse toward each other through the gel. The concentration of each reagent decreases as it diffuses according to the square dilution law, $C = C_0 \cdot 1/r^2$, where C_0 is the initial concentration and C is the concentration after diffusion to the radius r from the origin. A precipitate will develop where antigen and antibody meet, provided that their concentrations are in the range for equivalence. As the advancing fronts meet and react, the reactant at higher concentration will diffuse into the weaker one, preventing the formation of large aggregates of complex until equivalence is reached and the precipitating complex is stable. If one reactant is at a much higher relative concentration than the other, the complex will form closer to the well containing the weaker reactant (Fig. 2). In cases of extreme concentration imbalance, a precipitate may not be seen at all.

The simple type of double diffusion (Fig. 2) is used to detect the presence of antigen or antibody in a monospecific system. This has a sensitivity of 1 to 10 mg/liter unless the precipitate is developed with a second reagent. The formation of an antigen-antibody precipitate in a gel results in the formation of an apparent barrier; the precipitate represents the area of equivalence, with

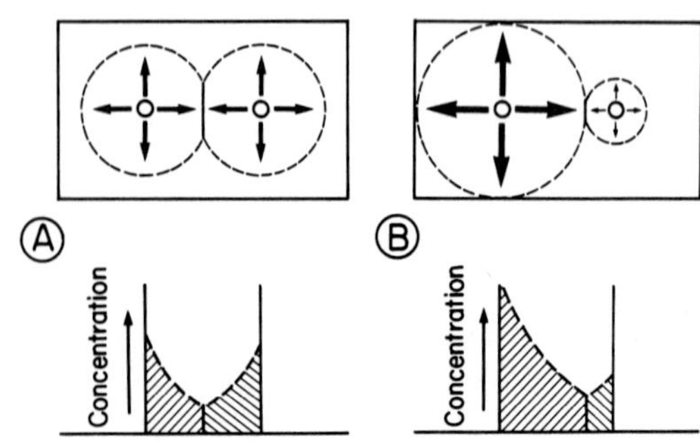

FIG. 2. Double diffusion in agarose. (A) Equivalent concentrations of antigen and antibody; (B) unequal concentrations of antigen and antibody.

one side being in antigen excess and the other being in antibody excess. Each reactant is free to diffuse into and through the precipitated complex, but when they do, they encounter an increasing amount of the other reactant and precipitate. Thus, for all intents and purposes, they do not penetrate through the precipitate. Figure 2A shows the result when both reactants are at similar concentrations, with similar diffusion coefficients; the precipitin line is straight. If one reactant is at a higher concentration than the other, the precipitin line will be displaced toward the well containing the reactant with the lower concentration, since the relative position will depend on the reactant concentrations required for equivalence. The precipitin line will still be straight, however, because the reactants have similar mobilities (Fig. 2B). When one of the reagents has a lower diffusion coefficient than the other, the precipitin line will be curved toward the component with the lower diffusion coefficient. This occurs because once equivalent concentrations have been achieved, lateral development of the precipitin line occurs between reactants with different mobilities. The more the precipitate develops laterally, the more the equivalence zone will be displaced toward the reactant with lower mobility. The precipitin line thus will become an arc, concave to the reactant of lower mobility. The relative position of this arc between the wells will reflect the relative concentrations of the two reactants.

Double diffusion often is used to compare antigens (Fig. 3). Usually, different antigens are compared by using a single antiserum. In Fig. 3A, antiserum to antigen a reacts with antigen a, which is in both of the antigen wells. A precipitin line will form between the antiserum well and each antigen well, and these lines will fuse to form a smooth junction, as shown. This is a reaction of identity, and the precipitin line follows the diffusion pattern of the antigen, as shown by the dashed lines. The shape and position of each line will depend on the diffusion coefficient and relative concentration of each reactant. In Fig. 3B, the antigen wells contain different antigens, a and b, whereas the antiserum well contains antibodies to both antigens. A precipitin line forms between each antigen and its homologous antibody, but since the antigens are not related to each other, the precipitin lines form independently and cross through each other, as shown. This is a reaction of nonidentity, and each system behaves as though the other one does not exist. Under normal circumstances, the lines cross sharply and these reactions are easy to see. However, problems arise when one of the antigens has a high diffusion coefficient so that its precipitin line bends toward the antiserum well; the resulting immunodiffusion

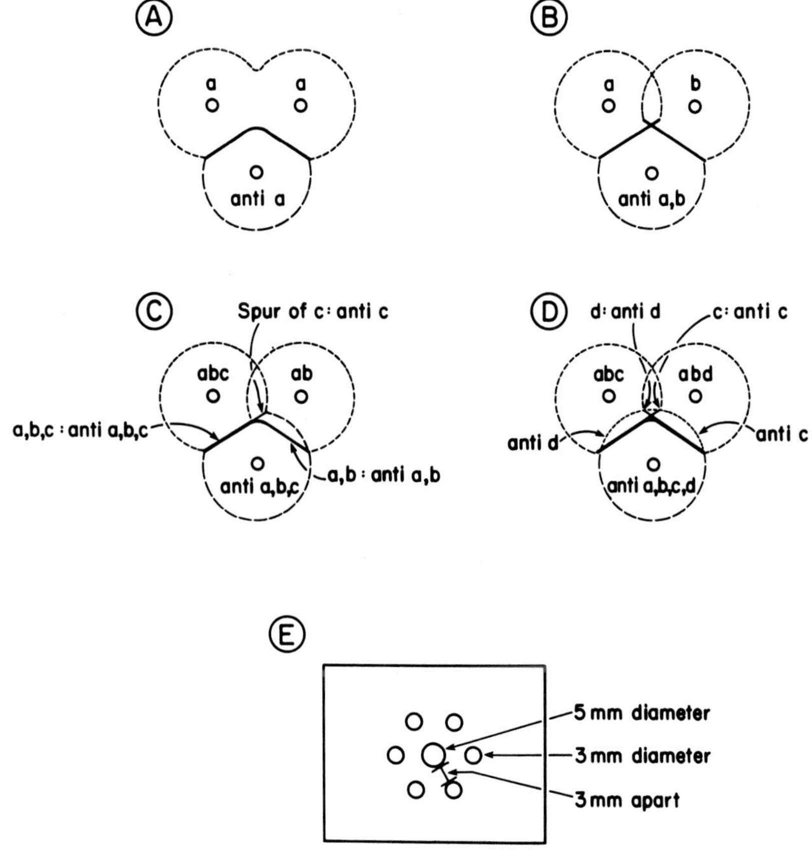

FIG. 3. Comparison of antigens in double diffusion. (A) Reaction of identity. Both antigen wells contain the same antigen. (B) Reaction of nonidentity. The antigen wells contain unrelated antigens. (C) Reaction of partial identity. The antigen wells contain related antigens, one of which is antigenically deficient with respect to the other. (D) Reaction of mixed identity. The antigen wells contain related antigens with common and unique determinants. (E) Double diffusion template.

pattern may resemble a reaction of partial identity and may mislead the observer.

Cross-reacting antigens produce a reaction of partial identity (Fig. 3C). In this example, one antigen well contains an antigen molecule with determinants a, b, and c, whereas the other antigen well contains a related but different antigen molecule that expresses only determinants a and b. The antiserum well contains antibodies to all three determinants. The antigen expressing all three determinants will form a stronger precipitin line with the antiserum than will the deficient antigen. Antibodies to determinants a and b will react with both antigens, but antibodies to determinant c will react only with the antigen expressing this determinant and will pass through the precipitin line formed with the deficient antigen and keep diffusing. Some of these antibodies will meet the complete antigen beyond the ab line of identity and will continue the abc precipitin line, as shown. It should be noted that the formation of a spur reflects relative antigenicity of the antigens and is not an absolute reference; it does not mean that the antigen with major reactivity must be the homologous antigen. In addition, it is important to realize that a single precipitin line may contain several antigen-antibody systems and that in such a complex system, a spur may be caused by overlapping precipitin lines, one of identity and one of nonidentity.

The final example (Fig. 3D) concerns double-spur formation. In this example, the two antigens share some determinants, a and b, but each has a unique determinant, c or d, respectively, and the antiserum well contains antibodies reactive with all four determinants. Note that each spur is weaker than the common precipitin line, and the intersection point is not sharp but rounded, indicating some identity.

Figure 3E shows a conventional template used for analysis of antigens. The well size and the distance apart are usually individual choices, but the dimensions shown in Fig. 3E have been found to be useful in many different situations. Reagents should be added gently with a volumetric pipette or with a Pasteur pipette or capillary tube and should just fill the well. Every care must be taken to avoid overfilling the wells. When full, the plate should be left undisturbed in a humidified atmosphere to develop. Glass plates are best put in a petri dish, resting on top of wooden sticks on moistened filter paper. Precipitin lines generally develop after overnight incubation at room temperature. If expected lines are not apparent at this time, the plate may be flushed by filling each well with PBS and allowing this to diffuse into the gel. Alternatively, the wells may be refilled with the original reactants to increase the amount of precipitate formed. However, in instances when increased sensitivity is needed, it is best to use secondary development procedures as discussed below. Occasionally, the systems do not react with sufficient affinity to permit extensive lattice formation to occur; only small complexes develop, which fail to form a visible precipitate. The addition of low concentrations of polyethylene glycol (PEG), such as 4% PEG 6000, to the gel often promotes precipitate formation in these situations, since the PEG reduces the hydration layer around the protein molecules.

Procedures available for enhancing faint precipitin lines include (i) staining the gel with a protein stain such as Coomassie brilliant blue or amido black, (ii) incubation with a second antibody, followed by protein staining, and (iii) incubation with a labeled second antibody or a reagent such as protein A. These procedures generally require an initial thorough washing of the gel with PBS to remove all nonprecipitated protein. For protein staining, the salt must be removed by washing the gel in deionized water, and the gel must be dried. This is most easily accomplished by covering the gel with moistened filter paper, removing air bubbles, and leaving the plate to dry. The dry paper can be peeled off once it has been moistened, and the plate can then be stained. A 0.5% solution of Coomassie brilliant blue (Fisher Scientific Co. or Sigma Chemical Co.) in 5% acetic acid–water usually is used, followed by destaining in acetic acid-methanol-water (20%, 30%, 50%). The sensitivity of this procedure can be increased by using a second antibody before protein staining. After diffusion, the plate is washed with PBS and then immersed in a solution of antibody to the primary antibody, such as goat anti-rabbit immunoglobulin G (IgG). After incubation overnight, the plate is washed again with PBS and then with deionized water and is dried and stained as before. As an alternative to the protein staining, the second antibody may be labeled with an enzyme or an isotope, and after incubation and washing, the labeled antibody can be detected by addition of substrate or by autoradiography, as appropriate. These procedures can lead to a sensitivity of the order of tens of nanograms per milliliter of reagents but may take several days for completion.

Other applications of double diffusion

Radial immunodiffusion. The procedure for radial immunodiffusion involves the diffusion of an antigen from a well into a gel containing antiserum. A ring of precipitation forms around the well, the diameter of the ring being directly proportional to the concentration of the antigen. This technique was introduced in 1932 by Petrie (7), who first described the rings of precipitation surrounding bacterial colonies growing on gels containing specific antiserum. Ouchterlony also noted, in 1949 (5), that when colonies of *Corynebacterium diphtheriae* were grown on agar that contained antibody, the diameter of the precipitin ring correlated directly with the amount of toxin produced by the cultures. This is a very useful procedure for quantitation of antigens in complex mixtures, but it is dependent on the availability of monospecific antisera and suitable standards.

Secondary diffusion. Double diffusion often is used as a second step to identify components separated by a primary procedure such as electrophoresis. For example, immunoelectrophoresis involves an initial separation of an antigen by electrophoresis on agar or agarose. After electrophoresis, a trough is cut parallel to the direction of separation and antiserum is added to the trough. The antiserum diffuses toward the separated antigens, leading to the formation of a set of precipitin arcs (Fig. 4A). The distance of the precipitin arc from the antiserum trough depends on the concentration of the antigen; high antigen concentration results in a precipitin arc closer to the antiserum trough than for low antigen concentration. This technique can be used for detecting multiple components, such as serum proteins in urine or cerebrospinal fluid, or for detecting single

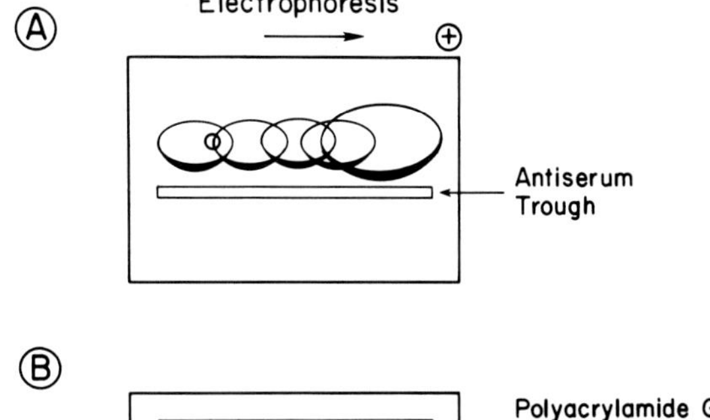

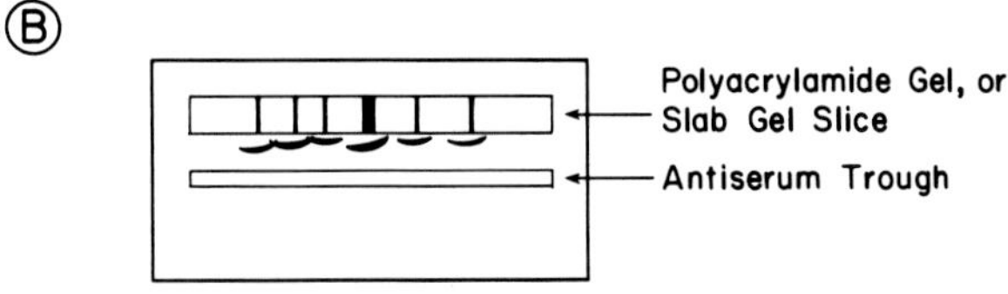

FIG. 4. Combined electrophoresis and double diffusion. (A) Immunoelectrophoresis; (B) detection of components in a polyacrylamide gel or slab gel slice.

components in a complex mixture, depending on the specificity of the antiserum. To detect components in polyacrylamide gel electrophoresis, the gel containing separated components is placed in an appropriate template, agarose at 45°C is poured around it, and then an antiserum well is cut parallel to the acrylamide gel (Fig. 4B).

ELECTROIMMUNODIFFUSION

Electroimmunodiffusion is similar to passive immunodiffusion except that the migration of one or both reactants is forced by an applied electric field. The advantage of this procedure is that the time taken for precipitation is decreased greatly. In addition, there is considerably less dilution of each reactant per unit distance traveled than in passive immunodiffusion, and this procedure is thus more sensitive than simple diffusion procedures.

The technique of electroimmunodiffusion was introduced by Macheboeuf et al. in 1953 (3) and developed by Ressler in the early 1960s (8). Several varieties of the procedure exist: single and double electroimmunodiffusion in one or two dimensions (Fig. 5). Single electroimmunodiffusion in one dimension, known as rocket electrophoresis, consists of an antigen that is forced to diffuse into an antiserum-containing gel by the electric field (Fig. 5A). This procedure is analogous to single radial diffusion for quantitation of antigens, but results can be obtained more rapidly. At pH 8.6, many antigens are negatively charged, whereas antibody molecules carry only a very small charge. Thus, in agarose at pH 8.6 containing antibody, a strongly negatively charged antigen will move rapidly into the gel and react with the antibody, and a rocket-shaped cone of precipitate will develop. For antigens that have the same charge range as IgG, it is necessary to alter the charge on the antibody molecules, for example by carbamy-

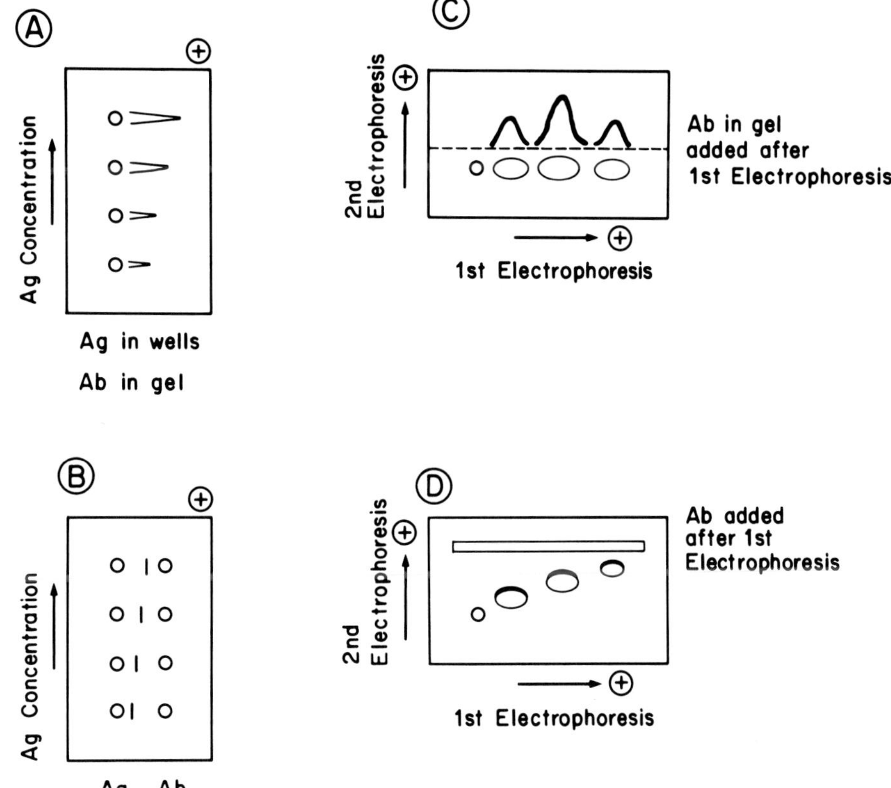

FIG. 5. Electroimmunodiffusion techniques. (A) Rocket electrophoresis; (B) counterimmunoelectrophoresis; (C) crossed immunoelectrophoresis; (D) two-dimensional counter immunoelectrophoresis. Ag, Antigen; Ab, Antibody.

lation, so that the analysis can be performed at a different pH.

Double electroimmunodiffusion in a single dimension (Fig. 5B) is known as counterimmunoelectrophoresis. In this technique, antigen and antibody are electrophoresed toward each other so that they interact and form a precipitate. This is accomplished by making use of the electroendosmotic effect of agar or by using special agarose that retains the electroendosmotic properties of agar. At pH 8.6, negatively charged antigens will have anodic mobility, whereas the electroendosmotic effect will give antibody molecules cathodic mobility. Thus, under the influence of the electric field, the antigen and antibody molecules will migrate toward each other. However, because the reactants are being forced to move, once they meet there will be little time available for the lattice to develop. Consequently, the antibodies used must be of high affinity. In addition, the ionic strength of the buffer should be low to promote precipitation (barbital buffer, pH 8.6, with ionic strength of 0.05 is appropriate). Since the reactants will be close to their original concentrations when they meet, they need to be at near equivalence ratio to begin with; the reactants cannot diffuse to achieve equivalence ratio as in double diffusion. Antigen excess can therefore be a serious problem; when the antigen concentration is unknown, several different antigen/antibody ratios should be used to try to bracket the equivalence ratio. The plate should be watched closely during electrophoresis. A precipitate may become visible within 10 min of the start; the power should then be switched off and the lattice allowed to build up. If no precipitate is seen, the electrophoresis should be continued for a limited time only, usually 30 min, and the plate should then be left for 10 to 20 min to permit any lattice to form. It is a mistake to continue electrophoresis beyond about 30 min, since the reactants will have moved through each other.

One application for which electroimmunodiffusion is especially useful is the rapid diagnosis of infectious disease, particularly bacterial meningitis. It is also an extremely efficient technique for the detection of anti-DNA antibodies in serum, since DNA is highly negatively charged. If standards with known antigen concentrations are used, the procedure can be made semiquantitative.

Electroimmunodiffusion also can be performed in two dimensions (Fig. 5C and 5D). Basically, these tests resemble immunoelectrophoresis and are useful for the rapid (30 to 60 min) analysis of complex antigen mixtures.

Double diffusion and electroimmunodiffusion differ in the effects of the separation of the antibody molecules. Antibody molecules, except for IgM, and surface IgA are homogeneous with respect to diffusion coefficient, whereas they are not homogeneous with respect to charge. Thus, a reaction that gives a single precipitin line by double diffusion may be quite complex by electroimmunodiffusion as a result of separation of the antibody molecules on the basis of charge.

LITERATURE CITED

1. **Elek, S. D.** 1948. The recognition of toxicogenic bacterial strains *in vitro*. Br. Med. J. **1:**493–496.
2. **Hitchens, A. P., and M. C. Leikind.** 1939. The introduction of agar-agar into bacteriology. J. Bacteriol. **37:**485–493.
3. **Macheboeuf, M., R. Rebeyrotte, J.-M. Dubert, and M. Brunerie.** 1953. Microélectrophorèse sur papier avec évaporation continue du soluent (électrorhéophorèse). Bull. Soc. Chim. Biol. **35:**334–345.
4. **Ouchterlony, O.** 1948. *In vitro* method for testing the toxin-producing capacity of diphtheria bacteria. Acta Pathol. Microbiol. Scand. **25:**186–191.
5. **Ouchterlony, O.** 1949. *In vitro* method for testing the toxin-producing capacity of diphtheria bacteria. Acta Pathol. Microbiol. Scand. **26:**516–524.
6. **Oudin, J.** 1946. Méthode d'analyse immunochimique par précipitation spécifique en milieu gélifié. C. R. Acad. Sci. **222:**115–116.
7. **Petrie, G. F.** 1932. A specific precipitin reaction associated with the growth on agar plates of meningococcus, pneumococcus and *B. dysenteria* (Shiga). Br. J. Exp. Pathol. **13:** 380–394.
8. **Ressler, N.** 1960. Two dimensional electrophoresis of protein antigens with an antibody containing buffer. Clin. Chim. Acta **5:**795–800.

Chapter 15

Detection and Quantitation of Specific Immunoglobulin Responses

FRANCIS K. LEE

Serologic testing is an important arm of laboratory diagnosis of infectious diseases. The technology of detecting antibody-antigen reactions has undergone significant improvements with the introduction of new methodologies such as solid-phase immunoassays and labeled antibodies. Moreover, recent advances in monoclonal antibody affinity chromatography, recombinant protein production, and peptide synthesis have led to the general availability of antigens of improved purity, suitable for the new generation of sensitive antibody assays. Many of the tests that once were special tools of research laboratories are now packaged in commercial kits that can readily be used by clinical laboratories. Descriptions of the various techniques and their applications to specific infectious agents have been presented in other chapters of this Manual. However, the optimal use of these assays for diagnostic purpose requires some basic knowledge of host immune responses, immunochemical reactions, and statistical inference. The purpose of this chapter is to review the general principles behind qualitative and quantitative antibody testing and the interpretation of results.

IMMUNOGLOBULIN ISOTYPES OF MICROBIAL ANTIBODIES

Five classes of immunoglobulin have been identified in human serum and external secretions (immunoglobulin M [IgM], IgG, IgA, IgD, and IgE). They are differentiated by molecular structure as well as by antigenic properties of the heavy chain. Most antimicrobial activity is associated with IgM, IgG, and IgA. In addition, specific reactivity to parasitic, viral, and fungal antigens has been demonstrated in the IgE isotype (25).

IgM is a large pentameric molecule (sedimentation coefficient 19S). It is mostly intravascular in distribution, constituting 15% of serum immunoglobulin content. A small amount of IgM is also synthesized locally in mucosal surfaces and can be found in external secretions. IgM does not cross the placenta, but a developing fetus, after the first trimester, is capable of mounting an antibody response of this isotype. It is the predominant immunoglobulin class produced during the neonatal period. Specific antibodies to most bacteria, viruses, fungi, and other protein antigens have been found in this immunoglobulin. In particular, most antibodies to self-antigens (autoantibodies) and blood group antigens belong to this class.

IgG (sedimentation coefficient 7S) represents approximately 75% of total serum immunoglobulins. It consists of four subclasses, IgG1 to IgG4, with antigenic and functional differences. Antibodies specific for viruses and other protein antigens usually are found predominantly in IgG1 and IgG3 (14); antibody reactive to bacterial polysaccharide often belongs to subclass IgG2 (8). IgG can also be detected in saliva, urine, and other body fluids. It is the principal class of antibodies detected in most immunoassays. Long-term immunity after natural infection or vaccination is generally associated with the persistence of IgG antibodies. IgG is actively transported across the placenta to the fetus and may confer some protection against infection in the infant.

Serum IgA is generally found as a 7S monomeric molecule. It recently has been demonstrated that after some viral infections, specific IgA first appears in polymeric forms (9, 18), later to be replaced by the monomers. IgA consists of two subclasses, IgA1 and IgA2. It constitutes only about 10% of the total serum immunoglobulin content, with 90% belonging to subclass 1. It is, however, the predominant immunoglobulin class in most secretions. Secretory IgA, found in mammary glands, the gastrointestinal and respiratory tracts, and ocular tissues, is a dimeric 11S molecule consisting of two 7S monomers, a J chain, and a secretory component. Approximately 50% of secretory IgA belongs to IgA subclass 2. Unlike IgG, IgA does not cross the placenta. The protective effect of secretory IgA in mucosal surfaces has been well documented (16). The function of serum IgA remains unclear.

IgD and IgE are present in serum in very low concentrations. Elevation of the serum IgE level (normal range, 0.6 to 320 ng/ml) is known to be associated with some parasitic or fungal infections. Specific IgE antibody to parasites is believed to facilitate the elimination of the parasites from the host (2). IgE-containing immune complexes can activate mast cells and cause inflammatory and allergic responses (19). Relatively little is known about specific serum IgD antibodies, although immunoglobulin of this isotype reactive to herpes simplex virus (HSV) has been detected (unpublished results). Their natural function is not yet understood.

Immunoglobulin isotypes vary markedly in the strength of reaction that they will produce. For example, complement fixation is restricted to IgM and IgG subclasses 1 to 3. IgM usually produces stronger signals in the agglutination and precipitation type of assays, mainly because of its multivalency and larger molecular size. These variations in antibody activity should be taken into consideration when serologic tests are selected.

ANTIBODY RESPONSES TO MICROBIAL AGENTS

After natural infection or immunization with microbial agents, the host humoral immune response involves the three major classes of immunoglobulin in a sequential manner. The initial response is characterized by the appearance of the IgM class of antibody, which is subsequently replaced by IgG and IgA. The observed time course of this progression varies with the microbial agents involved, the pathogenesis of the infection, and the method used to detect antibody. In general, IgM reaches a maximum within 1 to 2 weeks and declines to an undetectable level in 1 to 2 months. It has been demonstrated by radioimmunoassay that specific poliovirus IgM can be detected in the serum as early as 24 h after immunization (17). Low levels of IgG antibodies appear shortly after IgM but may remain undetectable in regular serologic assays, partly because of competitive binding of antigen from IgM. As the level of IgM declines, the level of IgG antibodies steadily increases for 3 weeks or longer. IgG constitutes the major bulk of serum antibody after 2 to 4 weeks and may persist for years. Serum IgA antibody appears within a few days to several weeks after the appearance of IgG but usually at a relatively low magnitude. Similar to the IgG response, the IgA response is long lasting.

Subsequent encounter with the antigen leads to renewed IgG antibody synthesis with reduced lag time (2 to 3 days) and at a greatly accelerated rate. This response is often reflected in an increase of serum antibody titer. Secondary response in the IgM class is less certain. No anamnestic response has been found in this immunoglobulin class. However, renewed IgM antibody production, approximately similar to the initial response in magnitude and duration, has been detected after booster immunization with poliovirus vaccine (17). In contrast, little or no secondary IgM response has been observed after measles virus vaccine booster (15). In the case of natural infections, HSV-specific IgM can sometimes be detected during recurrent or reactivated episodes (10).

The general progression of an immune response should be considered when serologic methods are to be used to establish a diagnosis. During the acute phase of infection, testing for specific IgM should be the first choice, provided a reliable test is available. A positive IgM test is considered diagnostic of current or recent infection. However, IgM antibody is present only for a limited time. Because of competitive binding for available antigens, it may also be difficult to detect specific IgM in the presence of a high level of IgG antibody. This competitive binding may occur after the first 2 to 3 weeks of a primary infection or in infants with maternal transplacental antibodies. In such cases, removal of IgG, by adsorption with protein G-conjugated Sepharose (24) or other methods, should increase the sensitivity of the assay. It should also prevent false-positive results due to rheumatoid factor of the IgM class which could be linked to the antigen through the specific IgG antibodies. Alternatively, a reverse solid-phase enzyme immunoassay would achieve the same effect (6). In such assays, solid-phase monoclonal antibody specific for human μ chain is used to capture IgM from the serum specimen. Reactivity to a specific microbial antigen is demonstrated by using antigens that have been labeled with radioisotopes or enzymes. Similar techniques can also be used to detect specific IgA for the diagnosis of infection in infants (24) in the presence of transplacental IgG of maternal origin.

Serodiagnosis by detection of antibody of the IgG class requires both acute- and convalescent-phase serum specimens. Specific IgG is usually undetectable during the acute phase of a primary infection; a positive IgG assay in convalescent-phase serum constitutes a seroconversion and is considered diagnostic. When IgG antibodies are present in the early serum, a fourfold or greater rise in antibody titer in the convalescent-phase serum must be demonstrated to confirm the diagnosis. If IgG antibody has already reached peak titer before the first specimen can be collected, serodiagnosis becomes very difficult. The importance of obtaining specimens early in the course of the disease and of collecting paired (acute- and convalescent-phase) specimens cannot be overemphasized.

ASSAYS FOR SPECIFIC ANTIBODIES

Specificity of antibody

The cornerstone of serology has been the unique specificity of a given antibody. The specificity of an antibody is genetically determined in antibody-producing cells and is effected by the amino acid sequence in the hypervariable portion of the molecule, which determines the idiotype. Recent reports describing some monoclonal antibodies that can react with two apparently dissimilar antigens (7) suggest that specificity is not always absolute. However, the majority of antigens involved in such reactions have as one partner either a cell surface antigen or an antigen present at high local concentrations with a repeating structure, such as bacterial lipopolysaccharide, DNA, or carrier proteins heavily substituted with haptens. The monoclonal antibodies involved were mostly of the IgM class, which generally have low affinity but high avidity as a result of their multivalence. Therefore, the phenomenon is likely due to a special type of low-affinity cross-reactivity rather than true multispecificity of the antibody. Moreover, this type of reaction is often reduced in solid-phase immunoassays involving multiple washing steps. Its practical impact on serodiagnosis may be insignificant except for the special class of antigens mentioned above. For practical purposes, it can be assumed that antibodies reacting to a microbial antigen arise from prior immunological stimulation by the same antigen. Thus, the detection of antibodies specific to a microbial agent indicates infection or immunization.

The binding of antibody to antigen is often described by the lock-and-key analogy. In fact, factors affecting binding specificity and strength include structural and spatial conformity of the antigen and antibody, hydrogen bonding, electrostatic attraction, van der Waals forces, and hydrophobic interactions (21). Therefore, it is possible to have more than one nonidentical antibody reactive to an antigenic site, each with a different affinity depending on the composition of the idiotype. Antigen-antibody reaction may be better viewed as a reversible chemical reaction, governed by the law of mass action, $[aby\text{-}ag] = [aby]\,[ag]\,K$, where aby represents antibody, ag represents antigen, [ ] represents the concentration of the reactants, and K is the intrinsic association constant of the reaction (a function of the affinity and avidity of the antibody). Since microbial antigens are polyvalent and antibody molecules have a valency of 2 (IgG and IgA), 4 (dimeric IgA), or 10 (IgM), multiple-bond binding may occur, which increases the total binding strength (avidity) by many orders of magnitude. Specific antibody-antigen reactions typically have K values of 10^7 or higher. It should be noted that according to the law of mass action, the concentration of an antigen-antibody complex is dependent on the concentration of the two other reactants. In a typical serology assay, the concentration of antigen in the system is fixed. Therefore, the concentration of the immune complex is proportional to the concentration of antibodies in the specimen. However, since the affinity and avidity of antibodies vary (and often rise during the course of an immune response), an increase in the immune complex may reflect an increase in antibody level, an increase in avidity, or both.

Detection of specific antibodies and interpretation of data

The essential element of serodiagnosis is the detection of antibodies reacting to specific microbial antigens. The differences in the various techniques lie primarily in the indicator system with which the basic phenomenon, i.e., the antibody-antigen reaction, is demonstrated. Antibody assays can be grouped into two basic categories. The first category depends on the inhibitory effect of an antibody on the specific biological function of the antigen, e.g., virus neutralization and hemagglutination inhibition tests. These assays detect only antibodies to special functional sites on the infectious agent. They tend to be very specific but of modest sensitivity. They are also more complex, requiring technical expertise special to the infectious agents being tested for. The second category consists of various techniques to detect formation of immune complexes in the test system. It includes the complement fixation test, agglutination, precipitation and nephelometry, as well as the new generation of solid-phase, labeled antibody-based immunoassays which are becoming very popular because of their sensitivity and simplicity. It should be pointed out that the specificity of assays in this category depends markedly on the overall purity of antigens used, since immune complex formation due to antibodies reactive to contaminating antigens (e.g., tissues used to propagate virus) will give signals indistinguishable from those formed by microbial agents. The current trend appears to favor the use of purified proteins produced by DNA recombinant technology and synthetic peptides. Affinity-purified proteins may also be used to increase the specificity of the assay. Indeed, the use of specific polypeptides, rather than whole microbial agents, as antigen has permitted the differentiation of antibody responses to closely related viruses such as HSV types 1 and 2 (11, 13). The methodologic details of these various assays are described elsewhere in this Manual.

All antibody detection systems depend on a conveniently measurable signal that the indicator system produces when antibody-antigen binding occurs. This signal may be based on visual appraisal, which gives binomial results (positive or negative), or it may be quantitative (e.g., optical density [OD]). In the latter case, a cutoff point is chosen based on measurements made on negative controls and other considerations. Test results are judged to be positive if the observed signal exceeds the cutoff point.

Since the primary goal of any serologic assay is to differentiate normal and infected individuals, an ideal test should have a cutoff point that separates these two populations 100% of the time. In practice, there is often an overlapping area where the measure signal (or titer) will be found in both normal and infected individuals. Raising the cutoff point would increase the specificity of the test but would also decrease the sensitivity. Lowering the cutoff point would produce the opposite effects. In test performance evaluations, specificity is defined as the proportion of subjects without the infection who have a negative assay, and sensitivity is the proportion of subjects with the disease who have a positive assay. A ROC (receiver operator characteristic) curve, which plots (1 − specificity) against sensitivity of the assay, is a graphic way of portraying the trade-offs involved between improving either a test's sensitivity or its specificity (22). The serologist must weigh the relative importance of the sensitivity and specificity of the test and set the cutoff point accordingly. Generally, a screening assay should favor sensitivity, whereas a confirmation assay requires high specificity.

Since no serologic test is 100% accurate, the practical value of a diagnostic test depends not only on its sensitivity and specificity but also on the prevalence of the disease in the population being tested. As the prevalence of a disease decreases, it becomes less likely that someone with a positive test actually has the disease and more likely that the test represents a false-positive. Conversely, in a high-risk population, a test must be very sensitive to be useful to clinicians; otherwise, a negative result is likely to represent a false-negative. The prevalence is also called the prior probability, which is the probability, based on demographic and clinical characteristics, that a particular patient has the disease, as estimated before performing the test. With these three parameters, the predictive value of a test can be evaluated. The predictive value of a positive test result (PV+) is the probability that a test-positive individual truly has been infected. It can be mathematically expressed as $PV+ = Se \times PB/(Se \times PB) + [(1 - Sp) \times (1 - PB)]$, where Se represents sensitivity, Sp represents specificity, and PB represents prior probability. Similarly, the predictive value of a negative test result (PV−) is the probability that a test-negative individual truly is not infected: $PV- = Sp \times (1 - PB)/[Sp \times (1 - PB)] + [(1 - Se) \times PB]$.

Because it incorporates information on both the test and the population being tested, predictive value is a good measure of the overall clinical usefulness of a test. Understanding the predictive value is very important for the proper interpretation of results obtained from a serologic assay.

QUANTITATION OF SPECIFIC ANTIBODIES

If the observed signal is binomial in nature (i.e., positive or negative), antibodies are measured by testing serial dilutions of the serum, and the result is expressed as the reciprocal of the highest dilution at which the test signal remains positive (titer). The process is termed antibody titration. For assays in which the primary signal is quantitative in nature (e.g., OD or radioactivity counts), the concentration of antibody can be expressed in various ways. A titration can be performed, and the antibody titer will be equal to the reciprocal of the serum dilution that produces a signal equal to the cutoff point, as determined by linear regression analyses (plotting OD versus dilution factor). Alternatively, the quantitative signal obtained by testing the serum at a single, fixed dilution may be reported directly or as a ratio of observed signal to cutoff value. Many clinicians prefer the titration method since they are more familiar with the concept of antibody titer, and the fourfold increase of titer is traditionally accepted as evidence of seroconversion. However, quantitation using a single serum dilution is an attractive alternative because it saves reagents and effort. In some instances, optical density generated by single-dilution testing in an enzyme immunoassay may be converted to titer, usually by using standard prediction curves. For example, one may perform titrations on 50 or more individual sera to obtain the antibody titer and then plot the OD produced by each serum at a fixed single dilution against the antibody titer of the serum to obtain a best-fit regression curve (prediction curve). Other sera to be analyzed are tested at the single dilution, and their predicted titer can be estimated by reading off the prediction curve. Since the prediction curve cannot be repeated with each test, very strict quality control, using multiple standard sera, must be observed to minimize intertest fluctuations. An alternative to this method is use of a standard serum pool consisting of 50 or more individual positive sera. A titration of this pool is performed in each assay run, with the unknown sera tested at a single dilution. Using the OD produced by the unknown serum, an equivalent dilution of the standard pool that would produce the same OD is read off the titration curve. The predicted titer of the unknown serum is obtained by multiplying the titer of the standard serum pool with the ratio of the equivalent dilution to the test serum dilution. For example, at a 1:50 dilution, the unknown serum produces an OD that is obtained by the standard pool at a 1:200 dilution. Therefore, it may be assumed that the standard pool is four times (200/50) as strong as the unknown serum. If the titer of the standard pool is 12,800 (as determined by the titration curve), the estimated titer of the unknown serum would be 12,800/4, or 3,200. Both of these methods have significant limitations. The major source of error in using prediction curves is the assumption that the titration curves of different sera have similar regression parameters. In fact, the slopes from different sera can vary significantly, depending on the avidity of the antibodies. As mentioned earlier, the average affinity and avidity of specific antibodies in the serum often increase in an infected individual as the immune response progresses. Therefore, the predicted titer is at best an imprecise measurement of the antibody concentration. It is nevertheless very useful for large-scale seroepidemiological studies.

DETECTION OF SPECIFIC ANTIBODIES IN OTHER BODY FLUIDS

Specific microbial antibodies have been demonstrated in other body fluids. Since most of the serologic assays have been developed and standardized for serum specimens, one should exercise caution when applying the assays for other body fluids. The concentration of immunoglobulins may vary greatly in these fluids because of natural dilution factors; it is advisable to measure the total immunoglobulin content in the same specimen used for specific antibody detection and interpret the test results accordingly. It has been demonstrated that human immunodeficiency virus (HIV) antibodies can be readily detected in urine (4) and saliva (1) specimens. This finding may prove valuable when a serum specimen is unavailable.

Of greater importance is the fact that antibody detection in other body fluids can, in special circumstances, provide serodiagnosis that is not possible by the examination of serum alone. Detection of locally produced specific antibodies in cerebrospinal fluid (CSF) or aqueous fluid of the eye indicates infections of the associated organs by the microbial agent in question, regardless of the systemic immune status. Special emphasis must be placed on establishing the local origin of these antibodies. Inflammation may lead to breakdown of the CSF-blood or aqueous fluid-blood barrier, and contamination of these fluids by serum antibodies can occur. To differentiate local antibodies from contaminants, it is necessary to prove that leakage from the vascular compartment cannot account for the titer observed in the local fluids. This may be accomplished by comparing the ratio of antibody titer specific to the suspected etiologic agent in the local fluid to serum and the ratio of another serum component, such as serum albumin. If the ratio for specific antibody is significantly higher than the ratio for serum albumin, then it is established that diffusion from blood cannot account for all of the antibody observed in the local fluid, suggesting local production. In some studies, quantitation of serum albumin has been replaced by measurement of total IgG to circumvent errors due to the different diffusion characteristics of immunoglobulin and albumin across the blood-brain barrier. This approach introduces another possible error by assuming that all IgG in the local fluid comes from serum, when in fact some may be the result of local production that the test is trying to establish. This method has been subsequently refined by use of CSF/serum ratios of specific antibodies to the suspected agent and that of specific antibodies to an irrelevant but common virus, adenovirus (ADV) (3), which is present in the serum of over 99% of the population. This modification takes advantage of the high sensitivity of the enzyme immunoassays for specific antibodies (aby) to these microbial agents and avoids the possible errors of the earlier methods. For example, in a test for HSV encephalitis, if $R1$ = CSF HSV aby/serum HSV aby and $R2$ = CSF ADV aby/serum ADV aby, then $R1 \gg R2$ indicates a positive test for intrathecal production of HSV antibodies.

DETECTION OF SPECIFIC ANTIBODY-SECRETING CELLS

A new approach for detection of humoral immune response is the demonstration and quantitation of specific circulating antibody-secreting cells (ASC). This method is particularly useful for the diagnosis of infection in neonates and infants, since it circumvents the problem in serologic diagnosis caused by the presence of maternally acquired transplacental antibodies, which can persist for up to 15 months (20). Studies in volunteers immunized with tetanus toxoid indicated that specific ASC were detectable in the peripheral blood from day 3 or 4 after antigenic stimulation and lasted for only 2 to 3 weeks (23). Therefore, presence of circulating ASC to a microbial agent would indicate current infection. In the case of a persistent infection such as with HIV, specific ASC are demonstrable as long as the viral antigen stimulus persists (12).

A simple method that can be used to detect ASC is a modification of the solid-phase enzyme immunoassay called the enzyme-linked immunospot assay (5). This method has been adopted for the diagnosis of HIV infection in infants born to seropositive mothers (12) but could be modified for other infectious agents. Briefly, microtiter wells with a nitrocellulose membrane bottom are coated with an HIV recombinant protein antigen. Peripheral blood mononuclear cells obtained from study subjects are isolated by Ficoll-Hypaque gradient centrifugation. Cell suspensions in tissue culture medium are incubated in antigen-coated wells overnight in 5% CO_2 at 37°C. During this short culture period, specific antibodies being secreted by the B lymphocytes react with the antigen on the solid phase in the immediate area surrounding the cell. The cells are then removed by washing with phosphate-buffered saline. The local zones of immune complex in the wells are visualized by sequential treatment (similar to the procedure for the Western immunoblot assay) with biotinylated goat anti-human IgG (2 h), avidin conjugated with horseradish peroxidase (1 h), and enzyme substrate solution containing 3-amino-9-ethylcarbazole and H_2O_2. The reaction is terminated after 30 min by washing with distilled water. The appearance of dark red circular foci or "spots" on the antigen-coated nitrocellulose membrane indicates the presence of specific ASC. The characteristic spots have a homogeneously stained center and a slightly diffuse periphery. The number of spots can be enumerated under low magnification to provide quantitative measurements. Our experiences indicate that over 75% of HIV-infected children have circulating HIV-specific ASC. False-negative results are caused partly by the inability to produce immunoglobulins in hypogammaglobulinemic or dysgammaglobulinemic patients.

STANDARDIZATION OF RESULTS

This is the best and the worst of times for serological diagnosis of infectious diseases. Modern clinical microbiology laboratories have the potential to test antibodies to a wide spectrum of microbial agents, and for each agent a multiple choice of assays is often available. However, little or no qualitative or quantitative standardization exists among different antibody assays for most infectious agents. As a result, comparison of serological data obtained from different laboratories is often difficult, particularly for quantitative assays. Antibody titers on a single specimen can deviate significantly when tested in different laboratories by similar assay systems. The old wisdom that antibody titer difference between specimens is of limited significance unless the specimens were tested simultaneously using the same assay by the same technician in the same laboratory still holds true. With new assays appearing on the market every year, the problem is unlikely to be resolved in the near future. It remains the responsibility of the practitioners as well as users of serologic assays to understand the strengths and limitations of the different assays so that appropriate information can be obtained.

LITERATURE CITED

1. **Archibald, D. W., L. I. Zon, J. E. Groopman, J. S. Allan, M. F. McLane, and M. E. Essex.** 1986. Salivary antibodies as a means of detecting human T cell lymphotropic virus type III/lymphadenopathy-associated virus infection. J. Clin. Microbiol. **24:**873–875.
2. **Capron, A., J. Dessaint, M. Capron, and H. Bazin.** 1975. Specific IgE antibodies in immune adherence of normal macrophages to *Schistosoma mansoni* schistosomules. Nature (London) **253:**474–475.
3. **Cerny, E., E. Hambie, F. K. Lee, C. Farshy, and S. Larsen.** 1985. Adenovirus ELISA for the evaluation of cerebrospinal fluid in patients with suspected neurosyphilis. Am. J. Clin. Pathol. **84:**505–507.
4. **Connell, J., J. Parry, P. Mortimer, J. Duncan, K. McLean, A. Johnson, M. Hambling, J. Barbara, and C. Farrington.** 1990. Accurate assays for anti-HIV in urine. Lancet **335:** 1366–1369.
5. **Czerkinsky, C., L. Nilsson, H. Nygren, O. Ouchterlony, and A. Tarkowski.** 1983. A solid phase enzyme-linked immunospot (ELISPOT) assay for enumeration of specific antibody-secreting cells. J. Immunol. Methods **65:**109–121.
6. **Frisk, G., E. Torfason, and H. Diderholm.** 1984. Reverse radioimmunoassays of IgM and IgG antibodies to coxsackie B viruses in patients with acute myopericarditis. J. Med. Virol. **14:**191–200.
7. **Ghosh, S., and A. Campbell.** 1986. Multispecific monoclonal antibodies. Immunol. Today **7:**217–222.
8. **Hammarstrom, L., and C. I. E. Smith.** 1986. IgG subclasses in bacterial infections. Monogr. Allergy **19:**122–133.
9. **Hashido, M., T. Kawana, and S. Inouye.** 1989. Differentiation of primary from nonprimary genital herpesvirus infections by detection of polymeric immunoglobulin A activity. J. Clin. Microbiol. **27:**2609–2611.
10. **Kimmel, N., M. G. Friedman, and I. Sarov.** 1982. Enzyme-linked immunosorbent assay (ELISA) for detection of herpes simplex virus-specific IgM antibodies. J. Virol. Methods **4:**219–227.
11. **Lee, F. K., R. M. Coleman, L. Pereira, P. D. Bailey, M. Tatsuno, and A. J. Nahmias.** 1985. Detection of herpes simplex virus type 2-specific antibody with glycoprotein G. J. Clin. Microbiol. **22:**641–644.
12. **Lee, F. K., A. J. Nahmias, S. Lowery, S. Reef, S. Thompson, J. Oleske, A. Vahlne, and C. Czerkinsky.** 1989. ELISPOT—a new approach to study the dynamics of virus-immune system interaction for diagnosis and monitoring of HIV infection. AIDS Res. Hum. Retroviruses **5:**503–509.
13. **Lee, F. K., L. Pereira, E. Reid, and A. J. Nahmias.** 1986. A novel glycoprotein (gG-1) for detection of herpes simplex virus type 1 specific antibodies. J. Virol. Methods **14:**111–116.
14. **Linde, A., V. Sundqvist, T. Mathiesen, and B. Wahren.** 1988. IgG subclasses to subviral components. Monogr. Allergy **23:**27–32.
15. **Linnemann, C., M. Hegg, M. Rotte, J. Phair, and G. Schiff.** 1973. Measles IgM response during reinfection of previously vaccinated children. J. Pediatr. **82:**798–801.
16. **McGhee, J., and J. Mestecky.** 1990. In defense of mucosal surfaces. Infect. Dis. Clin. North Am. **4:**315–341.
17. **Ogra, P., D. Karzon, F. Righthand, and M. MacGillivray.** 1968. Immunoglobulin response in serum and secretions after immunization with live and inactivated poliovaccine and natural infection. N. Engl. J. Med. **279:**893–900.
18. **Ponzi, A. N., C. Merlino, A. Angeretti, and R. Penna.** 1985. Virus-specific polymeric immunoglobulin A antibodies in serum from patients with rubella, measles, varicella, and herpes zoster virus infections. J. Clin. Microbiol. **22:**505–509.
19. **Rankin, J., M. Hitchcock, and W. Merrill.** 1982. IgE-de-

pendent release of leukotriene C4 from alveolar macrophages. Nature (London) **297**:329–331.

20. **Rubeinstein, A., and L. Bernstein.** 1986. The epidemiology of pediatric acquired immunodeficiency syndrome. Clin. Immunol. Immunopathol. **40**:115–121.
21. **Steward, M., and J. Steensgaard (ed.).** 1983. Antibody affinity: thermodynamic aspects and biological significance. CRC Press, Inc., Boca Raton, Fla.
22. **Swets, J.** 1988. Measuring the accuracy of diagnostic systems. Science **240**:1285–1290.
23. **Tarkowski, A., C. Czerkinsky, and L. Nilsson.** 1985. Simultaneous induction of rheumatoid factor- and antigen-specific antibody-secreting cells during the secondary immune response in man. Clin. Exp. Immunol. **61**:379–387.
24. **Weiblen, B., F. K. Lee, S. D. Landesman, K. McIntosh, A. J. Nahmias, S. Pelton, and R. Hoff.** 1990. Serodiagnosis of HIV infections in infants by detection of HIV IgA antibodies. Lancet **335**:988–990.
25. **Young, M., and R. Geha.** 1985. Ontogeny and control of human IgE synthesis. Clin. Immunol. Allergy **5**:339–350.

Chapter 16

Identification of Microorganisms through Use of Gas Chromatography and High-Performance Liquid Chromatography

MYRON SASSER AND MICHAEL D. WICHMAN

Identification of bacteria and yeasts traditionally has been through use of microscopically determined traits and use of positive/negative biochemical tests. Specific assays such as growth factor requirements, toxicity to selected animals, hemolysis, coagulase activity, phage or plasmid typing, smell, colony color and appearance, adherence to media, shape of cells, etc., have varying degrees of utility and may involve substantial subjectivity in interpretation. Since all these traits are genetically determined, the composite picture is essentially a reflection of the genome. Another set of genomic traits can be measured through chemical analysis of components of microorganisms by utilizing chromatographic techniques.

COMPOSITION OF MICROORGANISMS

Bacteria and yeasts are composed of four major classes of biomolecules: nucleic acids, proteins, carbohydrates, and lipids. The use of DNA methods, as well as immunodiagnostic and serological techniques, is covered in other chapters of the Manual. Though not widely utilized, electrophoretic analysis of proteins is a tool possessing considerable promise for identification of microorganisms. Chemotaxonomy or chemoidentification using these molecules will depend upon the ability to resolve them and to interpret the information carried in the biopolymers. Viewed from the standpoint of the monomers constituting these large biomolecules, the nucleic acids are composed of five bases, proteins are composed of 20 amino acids, and only a dozen sugars constitute most carbohydrate structures, but there are more than 300 known fatty acids (and their analogs) in microorganisms. These plus the quinones and a few metabolites constitute the basis for chemical analysis in the identification of microorganisms.

CHROMATOGRAPHY

Basic principles (12, 20, 48)

Chromatography is basically a method of separation based upon the varying extraction or partitioning properties of two mutually immiscible phases. All chromatographic methods involve a mobile phase and an immobile or stationary phase. Separations involving chromatography are dependent upon physical partitioning or adsorption of sample components between the mobile and stationary phase. The mobile phase may be a gas, liquid, or supercritical fluid, and the stationary phase may be a solid or liquid.

Generally, chromatographic methods are characterized according to the mobile phase utilized. Gas chromatography (GC) utilizes a gas as the mobile phase, liquid chromatography (LC) utilizes a liquid as the mobile phase, and supercritical fluid chromatography utilizes a supercritical fluid as the mobile phase. Chromatographic methods are further classified according to stationary phase and separation process. Thus gas-solid chromatography (GSC), gas-liquid chromatography (GLC), liquid-solid chromatography (LSC), and liquid-liquid chromatography (LLC) are characterized according to respective mobile and stationary phases. Paper chromatography and thin-layer chromatography (TLC) utilize a solid stationary phase. Size exclusion or gel permeation chromatography is a form of liquid chromatography that utilizes the stationary phase as a molecular sieve, and separations occur based on molecular size and weight. Ion-exchange chromatography utilizes a solid stationary phase, and separation is due to varying absorption of sample components.

GC (12, 17, 20, 21, 29, 39, 48, 49)

The analytical process involved in GC determination is shown schematically in Fig. 1. The basic components of a gas chromatograph are the carrier gas or mobile phase; the sample injection system; the analytical column, where sample component separation occurs; the detector; and some type of system for reading detector response. In most gas chromatographs, the injection system, column housing, and detector are all thermostated and heated independently. The sample must instantaneously vaporize without degradation upon injection; therefore, the sample components or their derivatives must have a relatively low boiling point in reference to the liquid stationary phase. Due to this boiling point restriction, GC determinations are limited to relatively low-molecular-weight compounds. Once the sample is volatilized in the injection system of the gas chromatograph, the sample components are carried onto the column by the mobile carrier gas. Typical carrier gases are hydrogen, helium, and nitrogen. Sample components are separated into individual compounds by partitioning between the liquid stationary phase and the carrier gas or adsorbing to the solid stationary support. Compounds with the least affinity for the liquid stationary phase, or which are adsorbed most weakly onto the support, are eluted from the column first. Compounds which have greater affinity or are adsorbed more strongly elute later, thus effecting separation of the injected sample into various components. The var-

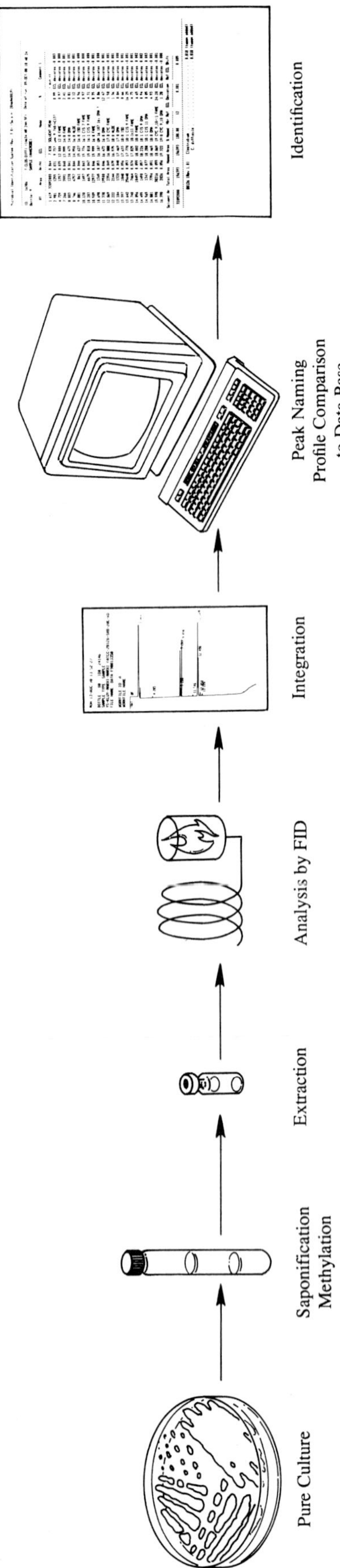

FIG. 1. GC analysis of microbial fatty acids. FID, Flame ionization detector.

ious components are detected after they are eluted from the column by any one or more of a multitude of detectors. The analog signal from the detector is recorded on a strip chart recorder. The analog signal from the detector can also be converted to a digital number for computer manipulation via an analog-to-digital converter. The time between sample injection and elution from the column for a particular compound is referred to as retention time (RT). The RT of an individual sample component will remain essentially constant for specific chromatographic conditions, injection temperature, column, column temperature, carrier gas, flow rate, detector, detector temperature, etc., and thus is used to identify specific compounds in a sample. Qualitative determination of sample components is made by comparing the RT of known standards determined with the same specific chromatographic conditions. Quantitation of sample components is accomplished by comparing peak heights or areas of individual components against respective peak heights or areas produced by known concentrations of standards at the same RT.

GC columns. GC columns are referred to typically as packed or capillary columns. Packed columns are generally constructed of stainless steel, aluminum, copper, or glass, range in diameter from 1.6 to 9.5 mm and in length from 1 to 3 m, and are packed with particles of an inert solid support (e.g., diatomaceous earths) with an average particle diameter of 160 μm, coated with a liquid mobile (e.g., Carbowax, etc.) phase for GLC. In GSC applications the stationary phase consists of particles of an adsorbent (e.g., silica gel, alumina, etc.) or an adsorbent chemically bonded to the solid support. Capillary columns are typically constructed of Pyrex glass or fused silica, having an internal diameter ranging from 0.25 to 0.75 mm, and ranging in length from 15 to 150 m. Capillary columns are being utilized more and more extensively due to the fact that these columns produce greater resolution between individual sample components in less time as compared with packed column counterparts.

GC detectors. The most commonly used detectors for GC determinations are the thermal conductivity detector, flame ionization detector, photoionization detector, and electron capture detector. Other detectors are used for specific applications, such as the Hall electrolytic conductivity detector for halogen containing compounds; the thermionic emission detector, which is more commonly referred to as the NP detector for the determination of nitrogen- and phosphorus-containing compounds; the flame photometric detector, which is used primarily for the determination of sulfur-containing compounds; and the recently introduced helium microwave-induced plasma atomic emission detector with photodiode array spectrometric detection for a variety of compounds.

The thermal conductivity detector is one of the most versatile developed for GC detection. Basically, the detector compares the resistance of heated wire filaments. Pure carrier gas is passed across one wire filament while carrier gas plus sample components is passed across another identical filament simultaneously. The difference in resistance and thus conductivity between the two filaments is measured by a Wheatstone bridge. The thermal conductivity detector responds to virtually all types of inorganic and organic compounds. The sensitivity of this detector can be as low as 0.3 ng, with a linear dynamic range of approximately 5 orders of magnitude. The flame ionization detector, however, is probably the most widely utilized detector for GC determinations due to its high sensitivity and dynamic range. Sample components eluting from the chromatographic column are burned in a hydrogen-air flame, producing ions and free electrons. The resulting current flow is measured by electrodes. The flame ionization detector is sensitive to virtually all organic compounds, yet is insensitive to water, CO, CO_2, and many other inorganic gases. The sensitivity of the flame ionization detector can be as low as 10^{-12} g/s for fairly high-molecular-weight compounds, with a linear dynamic range covering approximately 7 orders of magnitude. The photoionization detector utilizes a lamp that emits UV radiation causing ionization of certain organic compounds. The ions produced cause a current flow which is measured by a pair of electrodes. The photoionization detector responds to many aliphatic compounds, aromatic compounds, aldehydes, ketones, esters, many other organic compounds, and some inorganic compounds. This instrument has a linear dynamic range of approximately 7 orders of magnitude, with a sensitivity as low as 2×10^{-12} g/s. Another commonly used detector with extremely high sensitivity for halogen-containing compounds is the electron capture detector. Here, compounds eluting from the chromatographic column pass between two electrodes. One of the electrodes is treated with a radioactive source that generally emits beta particles, which ionizes the eluting carrier gas. The electrons produced from the ionization of the carrier gas are captured by compounds that have an affinity for electrons. Sample components eluting from the chromatograph capture electrons from the ionized carrier gas, resulting in a net decrease in current which is measured. The electron capture detector is sensitive to as low as 10^{-13} g/s for halogen-containing compounds, but the linear dynamic range is somewhat limited at approximately 4 orders of magnitude.

LC: HPLC (2, 8, 18, 22, 43, 50, 51)

High-performance (pressure) liquid chromatography (HPLC) was developed from column LC, and instruments have been commercially available since 1969 (49). HPLC methods are not limited by boiling point or stability of compounds to thermal degradation, which restrict GC methods. The analytical process involved in HPLC determinations is shown schematically in Fig. 2. The basic components of an HPLC apparatus are the mobile phase (solvent) reservoir(s), pump, injection valve, chromatographic column (which may or may not be thermostated), detector, recorder, and some type of data system to manipulate analytical data. As the name implies, HPLC separations utilize a liquid mobile phase at high pressure to carry the sample through a column where separation into various components occurs. As the individual sample components elute from the column, the compounds are detected by one or more of a variety of detectors. As discussed previously for GC determinations, qualitative identification of compounds is made by comparing the RT of known standards determined employing identical chromatographic conditions. Sample components are quantitated by comparing peak heights or areas of individual components against the area produced by known concentrations of calibration standards at the same RT.

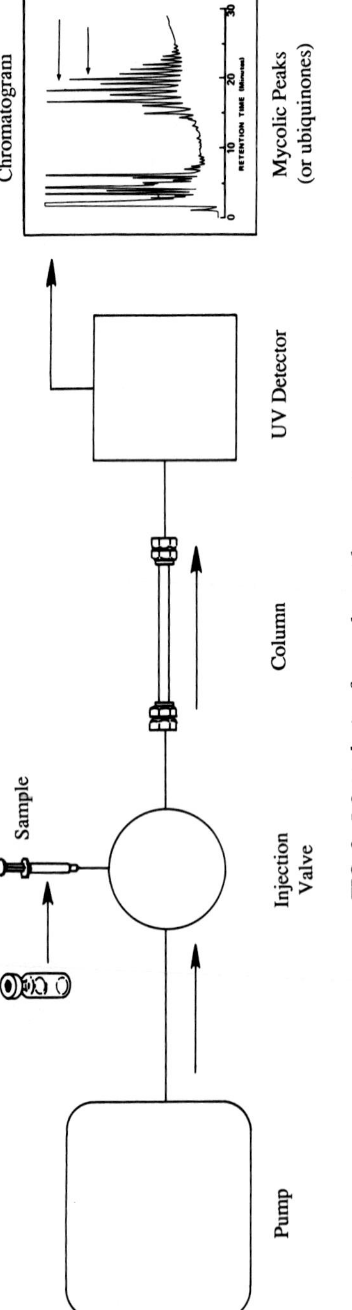

FIG. 2. LC analysis of mycolic acids or quinones.

The terms "normal phase" and "reverse phase" refer to the polarity of the mobile liquid phase and stationary phase utilized for a particular separation. Normal-phase chromatography is similar to the typical GLC separation in which the mobile phase is nonpolar (e.g., hexane) and the stationary phase is polar (e.g., silica gel). Conversely, reverse-phase separations utilize a polar mobile phase (e.g., methanol) and a nonpolar stationary phase (e.g., hexane or octadecane). Gradient elution techniques, in which the polarity of the mobile solvent phase is changed either continuously or in increments, are often employed for sample determinations to improve separation efficiency of closely related compounds. Gradient elution techniques are also employed to reduce analysis time required for separation of dissimilar compounds. Techniques utilizing "precolumn" and "postcolumn" derivatization are employed when the compound to be determined cannot be separated without derivatization or when the detector is insensitive to the underivatized compound.

HPLC columns. HPLC columns are typically constructed of stainless steel in order to withstand the high pressures necessary to force sample and mobile phase through the stationary phase. Columns range from 4 to 6 mm in diameter and from 5 to 25 cm in length. The primary stationary phases utilized for LSC are silicas and aluminas with particle diameters ranging from 1 to 10 μm. The liquid stationary phase utilized for LLC is either coated on a solid support or chemically bonded to the solid support, with typical particle diameters ranging from 3 to 10 μm.

HPLC detectors. The most commonly utilized detectors for HPLC determinations are the UV absorption detector, refractive index detector, and the fluorescence detector. There are a variety of other detectors which are utilized with limited applicability such as the photoconductivity detector, the flame photometric and emission detectors, and plasma emission detectors. The typical UV detector operates at fixed mercury line emission wavelengths of 254 and 280 nm. Variable-wavelength UV detectors utilize a deuterium lamp as the source and either interference filters or a grating for wavelength selection. These detectors are limited to compounds that absorb radiation at these wavelengths. Typical UV detectors are sensitive down to 2×10^{-10} g/ml with a linear dynamic range of approximately 5 orders of magnitude. Refractive index detectors differentiate the sample components from the mobile solvent phase based on differences in refractive index. Such detectors are sensitive to 10^{-7} g/ml with a maximum linear dynamic range of 4 orders of magnitude. Fluorescence detectors utilize a variety of sources such as tungsten-halide or xenon arc lamps to produce excitation wavelengths. Sample components absorb radiation at the excitation wavelength and fluoresce at a longer, lower-energy wavelength. Interference filters or gratings provide both excitation and fluorescence wavelength selectivity. A photomultiplier tube is utilized to detect the fluoresced radiation. Fluorescence detectors are sensitive to 10^{-11} g/ml with an approximate linear dynamic range of 3 orders of magnitude.

TLC (40)

TLC methods provide rapid, cost-effective analysis of sample mixtures. Commercial TLC plates with coated and bonded phases with fine particles in the range of 5 to 15 μm are available. Generally, TLC is used in conjunction with other techniques such as HPLC for method development or for qualitative determinations of sample components. Sample components are assessed qualitatively by comparing their R_f values with those of standards which are typically on the same TLC plate. Quantitative determinations can be performed utilizing scanning densitometers. Detection limits can be as low as 0.1 to 0.5 ng by absorbance and 5 to 10 pg by fluorescence.

Hyphenated techniques (3, 8, 15, 24, 46, 47)

There are a variety of so-called "hyphenated techniques" that combine various instrumental techniques for more definitive analytical determinations. GC-mass spectrometry (GC/MS) is probably the most developed of the hyphenated techniques. Several GC/MS instruments are now available commercially. GC/MS is currently used routinely for many types of analyses. GC-Fourier transform infrared (GC/FTIR) instruments are also commercially available. Extended hyphenated instruments such as GC/FTIR/MS have been reported and are also now commercially available. In this instance FTIR information is utilized to determine structural isomers. Currently there are instruments available commercially that link HPLC and MS. HPLC/MS is not as well developed as GC/MS due to difficulties encountered in interfacing the two instruments. The many other hyphenated techniques include HPLC/FTIR, supercritical fluid chromatography-MS, LC/GC, supercritical fluid extraction-GC, and supercritical fluid extraction-supercritical fluid chromatography. Many of these instruments are also available commercially.

MICROBIAL IDENTIFICATION: ROLE OF GC AND HPLC

Metabolites

A major role for GC analysis in identification has been in determination of short-chain acids produced by anaerobic bacteria (sometimes referred to as volatile fatty acids), other acids, and alcohols, with the data from these analyses used as qualitative additions to morphological and biochemical parameters (26, 27). The GC system used in analyzing acid and alcohol products is typically a packed column system using a thermal conductivity detector with helium as the carrier gas. The culture is grown in broth culture, 1 ml is pipetted into a clean tube and extracted with ethyl ether, and the extract is chromatographed for volatile fatty acids and alcohols. Another aliquot is methylated through addition of methanol and acid followed by heating. The methyl derivatives of pyruvic, lactic, fumaric, and succinic acids can then be extracted into chloroform and analyzed (26).

Fatty acids

While short-chain (volatile) fatty acids are used as adjuncts to biochemical identification, the fatty acids in the size range of 9 to 20 carbons in length are easily analyzed by GC and are used alone or with biochemical information. Very large fatty acid materials such as the mycolic acids may be analyzed by HPLC or TLC and used alone or in conjunction with biochemical tests to identify mycobacteria, *Nocardia* sp. and *Rhodococcus* sp. (9, 10, 14, 32).

A considerable mass of literature has accumulated on the utility of whole-cell fatty acid (9 to 20 carbons, chain length) analysis for identification of microorganisms (e.g., 1, 5, 16, 30). The lipids of bacteria are overwhelmingly structural in nature, occurring in the membrane and in the wall. In yeasts and other fungi, there is the possibility of storage lipids obscuring the fatty acid composition of the organism. This problem can be minimized by using cultures which are in an active growth stage in broth.

For comparison of unknown strains, it is necessary to standardize the growth conditions and the analysis. A procedure used in our laboratory (M.S.), which is modified from that of Miller (34), follows. Aerobic bacteria are grown on a designated agar medium (or in broth for anaerobes), at a specified temperature, and ca. 60 mg is harvested at a predesignated physiological growth stage (usually 24 h of culture, and selection from a quadrant streak area which is not heavily overgrown). The cells are placed in a culture tube (13 by 100 mm) and saponified by use of 1.5 ml of a 3.75 M sodium hydroxide solution containing 50% methanol. The tube is sealed with a Teflon-lined cap and is heated at 100°C for 30 min. Methylation is accomplished by addition of 2 ml of 3.25 M HCl in 50% methanol to bring the pH below 1.5, and the solution is heated for 10 ± 1 min at 80 ± 1°C in a sealed tube. Extraction into 1.25 ml of hexane-methyl *tert*-butyl ether (1:1) is followed by washing the extract with 3.0 ml of a 0.2 M NaOH solution to remove acid residues which may damage the GC column.

Analysis of the derived fatty acid methyl esters can be carried out using hydrogen as a carrier gas through a fused-silica capillary column having a cross-linked phenylmethyl silicone liquid phase. Oven temperatures may be programmed to rise from 170 to 270°C at a rate of 5°C per minute. Detection by a flame ionization detector will yield highly reproducible chromatograms. Peak identification can be a challenge, but may be accomplished by comparison with standards and by building a literature file of compositions of various species of bacteria which can then be used to identify peaks in runs of known strains which can be run preceding the strains in question. Thus, a suspected *Legionella* strain could be analyzed in sequence with a known strain of *Legionella* and, by comparison of the peaks, some degree of confidence could be developed that the peaks were, or were not, the same in each (30). Printed summaries of the fatty acid compositions of about 600 species and subspecies of bacteria can be obtained free of charge from the authors of this chapter.

The fatty acid profiling technique has been used for identification of gram-negative nonfermenters (11, 44, 45), mycobacteria (31, 33), and yeasts (5). If the data are used in multivariate analysis programs (16, 33, 36), tremendous information can be obtained from fatty acid analysis. Since part of current taxonomy is based on biochemical test data, the analyst should not expect all species in a genus to resemble each other. For example, the genus *Brevibacterium* has species in it that have a predominance of branched-chain fatty acids while others have only straight-chain compounds. In the same vein, since *Escherichia coli* and *Shigella* spp. exhibit more than 70% relatedness in DNA homology (4) it is not reasonable to expect to differentiate these organisms by fatty acid analysis.

Mycolic acids are 30 to 80 carbons in length and thus are more amenable to analysis by HPLC than by GLC. A typical protocol for analysis includes saponification, derivatization, and extraction similar to that of shorter-chain fatty acids. A synopsis of a typical procedure follows. Approximately 60 mg of bacterial cells is placed in an extraction tube with 2 ml of 0.9 M KOH containing 50% ethanol. The tubes are heated at 85°C for ca. 16 h, cooled to ambient temperature, and acidified with 0.5 ml of 6 N HCl. Extraction into 2 ml of chloroform is followed by taking to dryness under a stream of nitrogen gas and resuspension in a small amount of chloroform. The phenyl esters for UV visualization are formed using *p*-bromophenylacyl (Pierce, Rockford, Ill.) as the derivatizing agent. Analysis by HPLC can be performed using a UV detector adjusted to a wavelength of 254 nm, or through use of a diode array UV detector. Chromatography can be performed by utilizing a C18 reverse-phase column and a linear mobile-phase gradient (90: 10, acetonitrile-chloroform, going to 40:60) at a flow rate of 1.5 ml/min. Profiles of unknown strains of *Nocardia*, *Rhodococcus*, and *Mycobacterium* spp. have been found to be distinct and reproducible (9, 10).

Carbohydrates

Sugars and amino sugars which are structural in microorganisms have been less frequently used in bacterial identification. Some reasons for this are the difficulties in sample preparation and in interpretation of the results of the analysis. One problem is in the lack of a good derivatization procedure. The current procedures are lengthy and messy and can lead to degradation of some structures and the formation of multiple derivatives from others. Despite these technical problems, analysis of carbohydrates has been proven useful in several groups of organisms (23, 41).

Menaquinones and ubiquinones

The menaquinones and ubiquinones are ubiquitous in microorganisms and occur in several structural forms, and as such can be detected by routine procedures and utilized for identification of the microorganisms. These isoprenoid quinone compounds are found in microbial membranes and may act in electron transport mechanisms and in protection from free radical damage. Menaquinones and ubiquinones are soluble in lipid solvents and are commonly separated and identified by assay by TLC. These compounds are too large for easy GC analysis, but lend themselves to HPLC or to supercritical fluid chromatographic separations (25, 35, 37). Following HPLC separation, detection is usually by use of a UV detector (either diode array or variable wavelength). Even with the use of reverse-phase HPLC, not all components of these isoprenoid components are cleanly resolved, indicating the need for further research in this area. Moss (35) has published a concise protocol for assay of quinones by TLC or by HPLC, which can be used in "cookbook" fashion for analysis of these materials. An excellent review article by Collins and Jones (13) discusses the occurrence of the isoprenoid quinones in bacteria and their significance in bacterial taxonomy.

Multicomponent analysis

Pyrolysis GC is a technique whereby whole cells of microorganisms are decomposed by rapid heating of the sample (usually by applying the sample to a wire through which an electrical current is passed to cause great heat). The sample is then swept onto the column by a flow of the carrier gas and the chromatography is handled routinely. The identification of peaks may require a mass spectrometer, and there may be a considerable problem with the signal-to-noise ratio in the information due to the wide range of products generated by the somewhat nonreproducible cleavage of all the biomolecules of the microbe. Despite the technical difficulties in handling the data, pyrolysis GC is an attractive technique in that it does not require the sample preparation inherent in the other types of analysis. This technique has resulted in many papers (e.g., 19, 23) and a review article (42).

"DO-IT-YOURSELF" CHROMATOGRAPHY

Laboratory application of chromatography to identification of bacteria and yeasts can be as simple as TLC of quinones in comparison to those of known organisms (30), or as complex as the use of pattern recognition algorithms to complex fatty acid profiles derived by GLC (33). For a general introduction to the subject matter of chromatography, the review article by Novotny (37) is recommended. The chapter by Moss (35) in the fourth edition of the *Manual of Clinical Microbiology* provides an earlier overview of the use of chromatography in microbial identification, and the literature cited therein contains many useful references. The role of chromatography in "chemotaxonomy" is discussed in the section by Jones and Krieg in *Bergey's Manual* (28).

The application of any chromatographic technique to microbial identification involves several considerations: growth of the organisms in a manner to assure comparability; extraction (and derivatization) of the chemical compounds to be analyzed; chromatographic analysis of the material; identification (and quantitation) of the compounds; data processing to extract the information. The growth conditions, chemical extraction and derivatization, and chromatography are presented in the materials and methods sections of the literature cited and can usually be adopted by a beginner. Other matters such as peak naming are more difficult to duplicate (especially if the literature cites GC/MS as the peak identification technique), but may involve use of purchased standards, such as the Supelco (Supelco Inc., Bellefonte, Pa.) fatty acid mixture, individual quinones purchased from a supplier such as Sigma (Sigma Chemical Co., St. Louis, Mo.), or carbohydrates from Aldrich (Aldrich Chemical Co., Milwaukee, Wis.). Another approach is to duplicate analysis of a known strain of an organism under exactly the same conditions given in a scientific paper and use this information for peak naming purposes. Some researchers may also be willing to share extracts of organisms and the corresponding peak naming (and quantitation) information.

Reference papers are a good starting point for HPLC analysis of quinones (30), mycolic acids (9, 10), and sugars (41). Similarly, there are references for GLC techniques for volatile metabolites (26), fatty acids (30, 36), and sugars (23) and for pyrolysis GLC (19, 42). Data handling can be by finding signal peaks (6, 7, 38), by cluster analysis (36), or through pattern recognition (33). Suppliers of chromatographic equipment and supplies are often good sources of information and may have suggestions related to columns, detectors, and derivatization techniques. A telephone call to an author of a recent paper may elicit information about newly developed techniques which may not yet have been published, or suggestions as to alternate procedures.

SUMMARY

Chromatographic analysis of microbial components for use in identification may be used as a complement to biochemical tests or as a stand-alone identification technique. The disadvantages of the chromatographic techniques are high capital investment for equipment, some lack of acceptance of nontraditional approaches to identification, and the need for establishment of a data base with which unknowns can be compared. Advantages of the approach are objectivity of the results, low cost per sample, and the ability to handle organisms which do not have distinctive enzymatic profiles or are very difficult or slow to process using conventional tests. Improvements in chromatographic hardware and operating software promise to greatly increase speed, reproducibility, and sensitivity of the current procedures, possibly leading to direct-from-tissue assays, or at least identification from single colonies from primary isolation medium.

LITERATURE CITED

1. **Athalye, M., W. C. Noble, and D. E. Minnikin.** 1985. Analysis of cellular fatty-acids by gas chromatography as a tool in the identification of medically important coryneform bacteria. J. Appl. Bacteriol. **58:**507–512.
2. **Belton, K. B.** 1988. Advances in LC. Anal. Chem. **60:** 1045A–1047A.
3. **Borman, S.** 1987. Hyphenated MS at the Pittsburgh Conference. Anal. Chem. **59:**769A–774A.
4. **Brenner, D. J.** 1973. Deoxyribonucleic acid reassociation in the taxonomy of enteric bacteria. Int. J. Syst. Bacteriol. **23:**298–307.
5. **Brondz, I., I. Olsen, and M. Sjostrom.** 1989. Gas chromatographic assessment of alcoholized fatty acids from yeasts: a new taxonomic method. J. Clin. Microbiol. **27:** 2815–2819.
6. **Brooks, J. B., M. I. Daneshvar, D. M. Fast, and R. C. Good.** 1987. Selective procedures for detecting femtomole quantities of tuberculostearic acid in serum and cerebrospinal fluid by frequency-pulsed electron capture gas-liquid chromatography. J. Clin. Microbiol. **25:**1201–1206.
7. **Brooks, J. B., J. V. Kasin, D. M. Fast, and M. I. Daneshvar.** 1987. Detection of metabolites by frequency-pulsed electron capture gas-liquid chromatography in serum and cerebrospinal fluid of a patient with *Nocardia* infection. J. Clin. Microbiol. **25:**445–448.
8. **Brown, P. R.** 1990. High performance liquid chromatography, past developments, present status, and future trends. Anal. Chem. **62:**995A–1007A.
9. **Butler, W. R., and J. O. Kilburn.** 1988. Identification of major slowly growing pathogenic mycobacteria and *Mycobacterium gordonae* by high-performance liquid chromatography of their mycolic acids. J. Clin. Microbiol. **26:** 50–53.
10. **Butler, W. R., J. O. Kilburn, and G. P. Kubica.** 1987. High-performance liquid chromatography analysis of mycolic acids as an aid in laboratory identification of *Rhodococcus* and *Nocardia* species. J. Clin. Microbiol. **25:** 2126–2131.
11. **Canonica, F. P., and M. Pisano.** 1988. Gas-liquid chromatographic analysis of fatty acid methyl esters of *Aeromonas hydrophila*, *Aeromonas sobria*, and *Aeromonas caviae*. J. Clin. Microbiol. **26:**681–685.
12. **Christian, G. D.** 1971. Analytical chemistry, p. 104–140. Xerox College Publishing, Ginn and Co., Waltham, Mass.
13. **Collins, M. D., and D. Jones.** 1981. Distribution of iso-

prenoid quinone structural types in bacteria and their taxonomic implications. Microbiol. Rev. **45**:316–354.
14. **Damato, J. J., C. Kniseley, and M. T. Collins.** 1987. Characterization of *Mycobacterium paratuberculosis* by gas-liquid and thin-layer chromatography and rapid demonstration of mycobactin dependence using radiometric methods. J. Clin. Microbiol. **25**:2380–2383.
15. **Davies, I. A., M. W. Raynor, J. P. Kithinji, K. D. Bartle, P. T. Williams, and G. E. Andrews.** 1988. Interfacing LC/GC, SFC/GC, and SFE/GC. Anal. Chem. **60**:683A–702A.
16. **Eerola, E., and O.-P. Lehtonen.** 1988. Optimal data processing procedure for automatic bacterial identification by gas-liquid chromatography of cellular fatty acids. J. Clin. Microbiol. **26**:1745–1753.
17. **Ewing, G. W.** 1975. Instrumental methods of chemical analysis, 4th ed., p. 364–387. McGraw-Hill Book Company, New York.
18. **Ewing, G. W.** 1975. Instrumental methods of chemical analysis, 4th ed., p. 388–411. McGraw-Hill Book Company, New York.
19. **French, G. L., I. Phillips, and S. Chinn.** 1981. Reproducible pyrolysis gas chromatography of microorganisms with solid stationary phases and isothermal oven temperatures. J. Gen. Microbiol. **125**:347–356.
20. **Fritz, J. S., and G. H. Schenk.** 1974. Quantitative analytical chemistry, 3rd ed., p. 367–382. Allyn and Bacon, Inc., Boston.
21. **Fritz, J. S., and G. H. Schenk.** 1974. Quantitative analytical chemistry, 3rd ed., p. 383–402. Allyn and Bacon, Inc., Boston.
22. **Fritz, J. S., and G. H. Schenk.** 1974. Quantitative analytical chemistry, 3rd ed., p. 403–420. Allyn and Bacon, Inc., Boston.
23. **Gilbart, J., A. Fox, and S. L. Morgan.** 1987. Carbohydrate profiling of bacteria by gas chromatography-mass spectrometry: chemical derivatization and analytical pyrolysis. Eur. J. Clin. Microbiol. **6**:715–723.
24. **Gurka, D. F., L. D. Betowski, T. A. Hinners, E. M. Heithmar, R. Titus, and J. M. Henshaw.** 1988. Environmental applications of hyphenated quadrupole techniques. Anal. Chem. **60**:454A–467A.
25. **Harpold, D. J., and B. L. Wasilauskas.** 1987. Rapid identification of obligately anaerobic gram-positive cocci using high-performance liquid chromatography. J. Clin. Microbiol. **25**:996–1001.
26. **Holdeman, L. V., E. P. Cato, and W. E. C. Moore.** 1977. Anaerobe laboratory manual, 4th ed. Anaerobe Laboratory, Virginia Polytechnic Institute and State University, Blacksburg.
27. **Johnson, L. L., L. V. McFarland, P. Dearing, V. Raisys, and F. D. Schoenknecht.** 1989. Identification of *Clostridium difficile* in stool specimens by culture-enhanced gas-liquid chromatography. J. Clin. Microbiol. **27**:2218–2221.
28. **Jones, D., and N. R. Krieg.** 1984. Bacterial classification V: serology and chemotaxonomy, p. 15–18. *In* N. R. Krieg and J. G. Holt (ed.), Bergey's manual of systematic bacteriology. Williams & Wilkins, Baltimore.
29. **Kenner, C. T., and R. E. O'Brien.** 1971. Analytical separations and determinations, p. 272–294. The Macmillan Company, New York.
30. **Lambert, M. A., and C. W. Moss.** 1989. Cellular fatty acid compositions and isoprenoid quinone contents of 23 *Legionella* species. J. Clin. Microbiol. **27**:465–473.
31. **Larsson, L., J. Jiminez, A. Sonesson, and F. Portaels.** 1989. Two-dimensional gas chromatography with electron capture detection for the sensitive determination of specific mycobacterial lipid constituents. J. Clin. Microbiol. **27**:2230–2231.
32. **Levy-Frebault, V., K.-S. Goh, and H. L. David.** 1986. Mycolic acid analysis for clinical identification of *Mycobacterium avium* and related mycobacteria. J. Clin. Microbiol. **24**:835–839.
33. **Maliwan, N., R. W. Reid, S. R. Pliska, T. J. Bird, and J. R. Zvetina.** 1988. Identifying *Mycobacterium tuberculosis* cultures by gas-liquid chromatography and a computer-aided pattern recognition model. J. Clin. Microbiol. **26**:182–187.
34. **Miller, L. T.** 1982. Single derivatization method for routine analysis of bacterial whole-cell fatty acid methyl esters, including hydroxy acids. J. Clin. Microbiol. **16**:584–586.
35. **Moss, C. W.** 1985. Uses of gas-liquid chromatography and high-pressure liquid chromatography in clinical microbiology, p. 1029–1036. *In* E. H. Lennette, A. Balows, W. J. Hausler, Jr., and H. J. Shadomy (ed.), Manual of clinical microbiology, 4th ed. American Society for Microbiology, Washington, D.C.
36. **Mukwaya, G. M., and D. F. Welch.** 1989. Subgrouping of *Pseudomonas cepacia* by cellular fatty acid composition. J. Clin. Microbiol. **27**:2640–2646.
37. **Novotny, M. V.** 1989. Recent developments in analytical chromatography. Science **246**:51–77.
38. **Odham, G., A. Tunlid, G. Westerdahl, L. Larsson, J. B. Guckert, and D. C. White.** 1985. Determination of microbial fatty-acid profiles at femtomolar levels in human urine and the initial marine microfouling community by capillary gas chromatography-chemical ionization mass spectometry with negative ion detection. J. Microbiol. Methods **3**:331–344.
39. **Peters, D. G., J. M. Hayes, and G. M. Hieftje.** 1974. Chemical separations and measurements, p. 560–580. W. B. Saunders Company, Philadelphia.
40. **Poole, C. F., and S. K. Poole.** 1989. Modern thin-layer chromatography. Anal. Chem. **61**:1257A–1269A.
41. **Pritchard, D. G., J. E. Coligan, S. E. Speed, and B. M. Gray.** 1981. Carbohydrate fingerprints of streptococcal cells. J. Clin. Microbiol. **13**:89–92.
42. **Quinn, P. A.** 1976. Identification of microorganisms by pyrolysis: the state of the art, p. 178–186. *In* H. H. Johnson and S. W. B. Newsom (ed.), Proceedings of the Second International Symposium on Rapid Methods and Automation. Learned Information, Inc., Oxford.
43. **Snyder, L. R., and J. J. Kirkland.** 1979. Introduction to modern liquid chromatography, 2nd ed. John Wiley & Sons, Inc., New York.
44. **Veys, A., W. Callewaert, E. Waelkens, and K. van den Abbeele.** 1989. Application of gas-liquid chromatography to the routine identification of nonfermenting gram-negative bacteria in clinical specimens. J. Clin. Microbiol. **27**:1538–1542.
45. **Wallace, P. L., D. G. Hollis, R. E. Weaver, and C. W. Moss.** 1988. Cellular fatty acid composition of *Kingella* species, *Cardiobacterium hominis*, and *Eikenella corrodens*. J. Clin. Microbiol. **26**:1592–1594.
46. **Warner, M.** 1987. LC/MS and SFC/MS: will they replace GC/MS? Anal. Chem. **59**:855A–858A.
47. **Wilkins, C. L.** 1987. Linked gas chromatography infrared mass spectrometry. Anal. Chem. **59**:571A–581A.
48. **Willard, H. H., L. L. Merritt, Jr., J. A. Dean, and F. A. Settle, Jr.,** 1981. Instrumental methods of analysis, 6th ed., p. 430–453. Wadsworth Publishing Company, Belmont, Calif.
49. **Willard, H. H., L. L. Merritt, Jr., J. A. Dean, and F. A. Settle, Jr.,** 1981. Instrumental methods of chemical analysis, 6th ed., p. 454–494. Wadsworth Publishing Company, Belmont, Calif.
50. **Willard, H. H., L. L. Merritt, Jr., J. A. Dean, and F. A. Settle, Jr.,** 1981. Instrumental methods of chemical analysis, 6th ed., p. 495–528. Wadsworth Publishing Company, Belmont, Calif.
51. **Willard, H. H., L. L. Merritt, Jr., J. A. Dean, and F. A. Settle, Jr.,** 1981. Instrumental methods of chemical analysis, 6th ed., p. 529–564. Wadsworth Publishing Company, Belmont, Calif.

Chapter 17

Molecular Methods for the Clinical Microbiology Laboratory

FRED C. TENOVER

The acceptance of nucleic acid hybridization-based assays by microbiologists has steadily increased during the last several years. There are now a variety of DNA probe assays used routinely in many diagnostic laboratories both for culture confirmation and for the direct detection of pathogens in clinical samples (45). The drawbacks, such as the inability to perform antimicrobial susceptibility testing and strain-typing procedures concurrently with identifications, while important, have not caused microbiologists to shy away from these techniques (44). Nonetheless, solutions to these problems are continually being sought (35). Given the advances in hybridization technology, newer signal-generating systems, and particularly nucleic acid amplification technology, the use of probe-based assays in the diagnostic laboratory will continue to increase. The challenge to the laboratory will be to keep up with the new technology as it unfolds.

Because the role of hybridization technology in the diagnostic laboratory will continue to expand, clinical microbiologists must become fluent with the language of molecular biology. Whether they use these techniques in their own laboratories or not, nucleic acid hybridization-based tests and signal and target amplification methods will have an impact on our understanding of the epidemiology and pathogenesis of many infectious diseases, and it is important that microbiologists be able to assist clinicians in understanding the proper use and interpretation of these tests.

In this chapter, I will discuss hybridization reactions, the concept of stringency, and target and signal amplification schemes. I also will explore the role of nucleic acid probes in the laboratory. For those microbiologists who wish to prepare their own probes for identifying fastidious organisms or for strain typing, some direction as to how to proceed is provided. This chapter will not present an in-depth methods section. Those wishing to undertake serious hybridization projects should invest in the second edition of *Molecular Cloning: a Laboratory Manual* by Sambrook and co-workers (39). It is an excellent resource manual and contains a wealth of information regarding the development and use of nucleic acid probes.

DEFINITIONS

Nucleic acids

There are two types of nucleic acid commonly found in most organisms, DNA and RNA. Native DNA is a double-stranded molecule composed of two sugar phosphate strands with pairs of nucleotide bases held between them by hydrogen bonds (Fig. 1A). DNA is the major repository of genetic information in a cell, whereas RNA, which occurs in several forms in a cell, is involved in the intricate process of translating the information encoded in DNA into protein. DNA is composed of adenine, thymine, guanine, and cytosine; adenine molecules occur opposite thymine moieties, and guanine molecules occur opposite cytosine moieties. RNA is normally a single-stranded molecule, similar to DNA in chemical composition except that thymine molecules are replaced by uracil. Reoviruses, which contain several double-stranded RNA segments, are the exception to the single-stranded RNA rule.

Denaturation

The two strands of DNA can be separated, or denatured, by heating or by strong bases (Fig. 1B). This is the first step in hybridization reactions involving DNA and double-stranded RNA targets. Since DNA is most stable in double-stranded form, the two complementary molecules, when placed in proximity to one another, will recombine to form a duplex structure. Single-stranded DNA and RNA molecules also can form stable hybrids if they have complementary sequences (adenine will bind to uracil in this situation).

Nucleic acid probes

Nucleic acid probes consist of segments of DNA or RNA that can seek out and bind to their complementary sequences to form a novel duplex molecule (Fig. 1C). Probes are labeled with radioisotopes, enzymes, or chemiluminescent molecules, so that the formation of duplex molecules can be readily detected. Probes can be tailored to be genus, species, or even strain specific by varying the nucleotide sequence that is used. Virtually all microorganisms contain some unique nucleotide sequences in their genomes that can be exploited as fingerprints for rapid identification. The high specificity of probes and the rapid kinetics of hybridization reactions make this technology particularly appealing to laboratories trying to reduce the time required to generate results.

Stringency

A critical concept in understanding the process of hybridization is the stringency of the reaction. Stringency refers to the number of mismatched base pairs that can be tolerated between two strands of DNA, or a strand of DNA and a strand of RNA, and still form a stable double-stranded molecule. Stringency is determined by the temperature, ionic strength, length of the

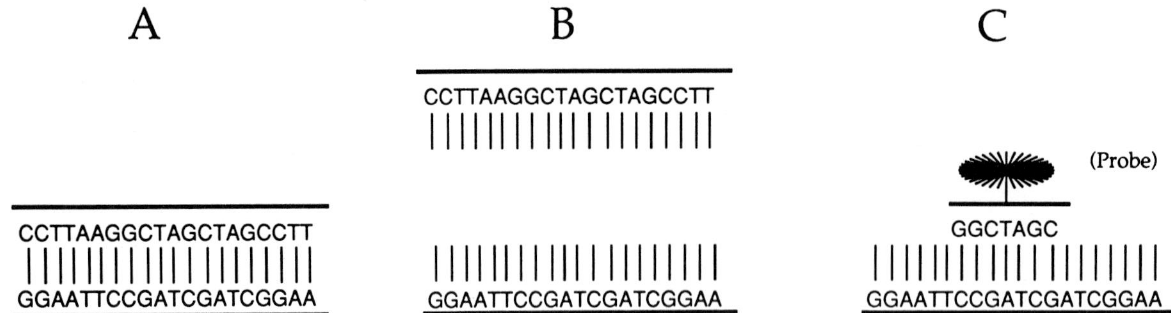

FIG. 1. (A) Native, double-stranded DNA showing pairing of nucleotide bases. (B) Denaturation of DNA segment. (C) Binding of probe DNA to target DNA. *, Reporter molecule on probe DNA.

probe, and presence of denaturants (such as formamide) in the buffers used in hybridization reactions. At low stringency, a probe that is only partially complementary to its target sequence can still bind and form a stable hybrid, whereas under conditions of high stringency, the probe would not form a stable double-stranded molecule. In practical terms, this means that a probe directed against the DNA of *Staphylococcus aureus* may bind at conditions of low stringency to DNA from *Staphylococcus epidermidis* or *Staphylococcus saprophyticus* and form a stable hybrid, whereas at high-stringency conditions, the probe would bind exclusively to *S. aureus* DNA and not to DNA of other staphylococcal species. Maintaining the appropriate reaction conditions to ensure the desired level of stringency is very important because the specificity of a probe can be altered significantly if the temperature and ionic strength of the hybridization buffers are not carefully controlled. For probes >150 base pairs in length, maximum stringency is achieved at 5°C below the melting temperature (T_m) of the probe. T_m is determined by the equation (48) $T_m = 81.5°C + 16.6 \log M + 41(\%G+C) - 500/L - 0.62(\%$ formamide), in which M is monovalent cations in moles per liter and L is the length of the probe in nucleotides; the pH of the reaction is between 5 and 9. For oligonucleotide probes (14 to 20 base pairs), the dissociation temperature, or T_d (which is similar to T_m) is defined by the equation T_d (°C) = 4(G+C) + 2(A+T), in which, G, C, A, and T are the numbers of each base in the probe. Stringency conditions are particularly critical for oligonucleotide probes since small changes in temperature can have a dramatic effect on the binding characteristics of the probe.

Restriction fragment length polymorphisms

Another concept that is important, particularly for laboratories that wish to use probes for strain identification, is the use of restriction fragment length polymorphisms. Most if not all organisms have regions of their genomes that are highly variable. That is, certain nucleotide sequences in parts of the chromosome tend to vary from strain to strain but not within a given strain. This variability can be seen when chromosomal DNA is purified and cleaved into thousands of pieces with restriction endonucleases (enzymes that cut DNA at specific stretches of nucleotides). If one cleaves DNA from two different strains and separates the fragments on an agarose gel, it is often possible to distinguish the differences in the banding patterns by visual examination. In some cases the differences may be subtle and difficult to discern. However, by choosing probes that specifically hybridize within these highly variable regions, the differences between strains can be accentuated and more readily recognized. For example, in Fig. 2A, DNA from four strains of *Xanthomonas maltophilia* has been purified and digested with the enzyme *Bgl*II (lane 4 is a control). The patterns are unique but difficult to discern. In Fig. 2B, the DNA from five strains of *X. maltophilia* has been digested with *Bgl*II, electrophoresed, transferred to a nylon filter, and hybridized with a plasmid containing cloned *Escherichia coli* rRNA genes (5). The banding pattern, which is unique for each strain, is produced as the probes hybridize to restriction fragments of different lengths (polymorphisms) created by the variability in the recognition sites of the enzymes around the rRNA genes (lane 4 is a control). This makes the presence of multiple strains much easier to discern. Thus, restriction fragment length polymorphism analysis, particularly using rRNA genes, can be a powerful tool for strain typing (43).

Hybridization conditions

It is important to emphasize that there is no universal set of hybridization conditions that can be used for all probes and all organisms. The optimal conditions for a hybridization reaction depend on the nucleotide content of both the probe and the target DNA (percent

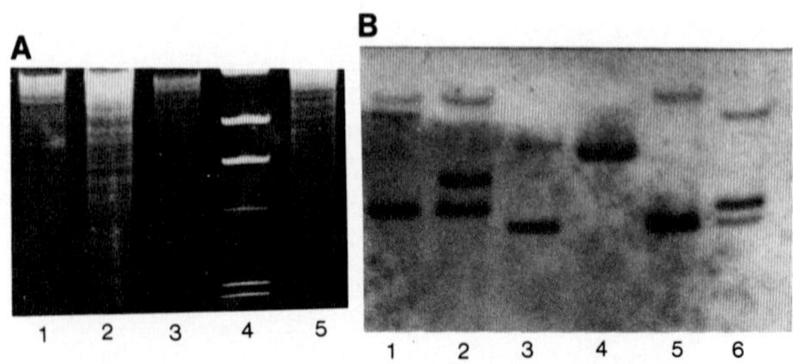

FIG. 2. (A) *Bgl*II restriction digests of chromosomal DNA from four strains of *X. maltophilia* (lane 4 contains molecular size standards). (B) Southern blot of chromosomal *Bgl*II restriction digests of DNA from five isolates of *X. maltophilia* probed with plasmid pKK3535 containing cloned rRNA genes from *E. coli* (lane 4 contains a positive control). The probe was labeled with digoxigenin, using the Genius kit from Boehringer Mannheim Biochemicals (Indianapolis, Ind.).

G+C), the length of the probe, and the stringency desired (see above). Hybridization conditions must be established for each probe and target DNA set. Those laboratories adapting probe procedures from the literature for organism identification or strain typing should pay close attention to the hybridization conditions outlined in the paper. Several excellent texts on the parameters of hybridization are available to aid investigators new to the field (19, 39, 48).

USES OF DIAGNOSTIC PROBES IN THE LABORATORY

Probes for identifying microorganisms can be used in two formats in the laboratory. The first format is culture confirmation, whereby probes are used to identify organisms already growing on a solid medium or in broth. A variety of commercially available probes have been produced for culture confirmation, and many more will follow. The second format is the direct detection of pathogens in clinical samples. This procedure has the advantage of speed and specificity, although one still must culture positive specimens for susceptibility testing and strain typing. Each of these formats will be explored in greater detail.

Culture confirmation

The primary use of probes in the clinical laboratory to date has been for the identification of mycobacteria growing on solid media. Probes for *Mycobacterium tuberculosis, M. avium, M. intracellulare,* and more recently *M. gordonae* have reduced the time required to identify these organisms from weeks to hours (12, 17, 22). Although there are some strains of the *M. avium* complex that do not react with these probes, they are relatively uncommon (17). It should be noted that the *M. tuberculosis* probe also recognizes the other members of the *M. tuberculosis* complex, including *M. bovis* and *M. africanum.*

All of the mycobacterial probes also have been used to identify organisms grown in BACTEC vials (8), although such identifications should be considered preliminary at this point and should be confirmed on colonies growing on solid media. Probes have been instrumental in demonstrating that mixed mycobacterial infections do occur (7). These probes are currently labeled with ^{125}I, which often has a practical shelf life of 1 month after receipt in the laboratory. These probes will be converted to a nonradioactive chemiluminescent reporter system sometime in the future. This system, which is more sensitive, also has a longer shelf life.

Additional assays for the confirmation of thermophilic campylobacters, *Neisseria gonorrhoeae,* group B betahemolytic streptococci, and other pathogens soon will be available from several manufacturers. There also are a number of kits available for the identification of viruses growing in cell culture (16). Probes to the herpes simplex viruses, cytomegalovirus, and adenovirus are commercially available.

Direct detection of organisms in clinical samples

The excitement over nucleic acid probes has focused on their ability to detect infectious agents directly in clinical samples, circumventing the need for culture. Probes to the sexually transmitted organisms *Chlamydia trachomatis* (25) and *N. gonorrhoeae* (18) and to the respiratory pathogens *Legionella pneumophila* (11, 34) and *Mycoplasma pneumoniae* (13, 46) are examples of commercially prepared probes for direct detection of pathogens in clinical samples. The probe kits for *C. trachomatis* and *N. gonorrhoeae* are usually sold as packages of 100 test kits and thus are intended for use by laboratories with high volumes of specimens. Both use acridinium ester chemiluminescent probes (2). The tests for *L. pneumophila* and *M. pneumoniae* currently use ^{125}I-labeled probes.

Probes for the STIa and STIb heat-stable toxins of *E. coli* also are available commercially (30). These are oligonucleotide probes that are directly conjugated to alkaline phosphatase and are particularly suited to filter hybridization formats. Probes to aid in the detection of human papillomavirus in genital warts are available, but only for research use at this point in time.

The necessity for susceptibility testing and strain typing depends on the organisms tested and has not presented a major problem to date. However, as probes for the detection of enteric pathogens such as salmonellae and shigellae and for sexually transmitted agents such as *N. gonorrhoeae* are used with increasing frequency, this question will need to be addressed.

Automated probe analysis

Robotics that can perform hybridization analysis of tissue sections mounted on glass slides have been developed (28). Probes to several viral pathogens have been used successfully in this system. There are as yet no automated analyzers that utilize hybridization technology that are designed for use in microbiology laboratories. However, such machines may be introduced in the near future.

DEVELOPING AND USING PROBES

Developing probes

Some microbiologists question whether they should develop their own probe assays for pathogens that are nonreactive in biochemical testing schemes or for organisms that cannot easily be typed by traditional methods. For such purposes, probes are indeed attractive. It should be noted, however, that developing new probes to pathogenic microorganisms requires considerable effort and resources and represents an investment in time and expense that few clinical laboratories should undertake independently. Those that do should pay particular attention to testing the specificity of their probes. Rigorous specificity testing of new probes must be undertaken before the probes can be field tested in the laboratory. Testing too few organisms to prove the specificity of a probe is a frequent mistake of those new to probe development.

Using probes described in the literature

There are a large number of probes to bacterial and fungal genes described in the literature that have utility for typing organisms that have proven refractory to other typing schemes. Probes such as the cloned exotoxin A and pilin genes of *Pseudomonas aeruginosa* (38), the nuclease gene of *S. aureus* (26), and the *toxB* and *attB* probes for *Corynebacterium* spp. (9), probes for differentiating among isolates of certain *Salmonella* serotypes (47), and probes for *Candida albicans* (6, 15) have all been described. Preparing and labeling probes such as these is within the scope of larger diagnostic laboratories and reference laboratories. Such techniques would be of considerable help in investigations of nosocomial and community outbreaks of infectious diseases.

PREPARING PROBES

The restriction endonuclease fragments that constitute many DNA probes are encoded on plasmids. These sequences can be extracted, labeled, and used to identify unknown isolates in dot blot or solution hybridization procedures or on Southern blots for differentiating among strains of the same species. The procedures for probe preparation have been greatly simplified during the last few years by the introduction of a wide variety of commercially prepared kits that facilitate isolation of plasmids, preparation of probes, and labeling of the nucleic acid. It is no longer necessary to prepare cesium chloride-ethidium bromide gradients. Rather, several column methods are now available to isolate and purify plasmids from bacteria. Specific DNA fragments can be isolated from low-melting-point agarose gels and labeled with a variety of nonisotopic detection systems. In addition, several companies have introduced inexpensive nucleic acid membrane transfer chambers that assist in the preparation of Southern blots. These new techniques have made probe preparation and Southern blotting practical for clinical and reference laboratories. This advance puts the latest molecular biology techniques for identifying and typing organisms within reach of many diagnostic laboratories.

Another major advance in molecular biology in recent years is the development of nucleic acid (oligonucleotide) synthesizers. These machines can prepare specific probes varying from 15 to 100 nucleotides in length. A single batch of oligonucleotides, which takes less than 24 h to prepare, is enough to last a laboratory for at least a year. Although purchasing and operating a DNA synthesizer are not practical for a clinical laboratory, the cost of purchasing commercially synthesized oligonucleotide probes is moderate enough to make their use economically feasible.

LABELING METHODS

Traditionally, probes were labeled with ^{32}P by nick translation, a process whereby DNase I was used to nick or break the DNA backbone while DNA polymerase I subsequently repaired the strands by placing new nucleotide bases into the damaged regions (36). At least one of four nucleotide bases used in the repair process was labeled with ^{32}P so that the repaired molecule became radioactive. Although effective for labeling long stretches of nucleotides, probes less than 200 bases in length were not efficiently labeled.

A newer method, called random priming, uses random hexanucleotide segments of DNA and DNA polymerase I to synthesize new stretches of DNA on a template strand, incorporating radioactive bases into the new DNA. This method is suitable for relatively short probes (<100 nucleotides) and long probes. Both nick translation and random priming can be used with nucleotides tagged with nonradioactive labels, such as sulfone groups or digoxigenin. Both of these substrates are antigenic and will react with enzyme-conjugated antibodies, thus serving as an effective alternative to radioisotopes.

DNA also can be labeled with biotin, which, after the hybridization reaction is completed, is reacted with avidin- or streptavidin-enzyme conjugates. One problem with biotin is that it is present naturally in many organisms, including bacteria. As a result, lengthy washing or deproteinizing procedures are required to rid cells of endogenous biotin before application of avidin or streptavidin conjugates (4). For the most part, all of the labeling methods mentioned above are easy to perform, use nontoxic reagents, and have long shelf lives.

Oligonucleotide probes, on the other hand, can be end labeled with polynucleotide kinase and various substrates, or enzymes such as alkaline phosphatase can be directly conjugated to probes via linker arms (20). This latter technology is available in some commercially prepared oligonucleotide probes and has proven very effective (30).

RESTRICTION ENZYME ANALYSIS OF CHROMOSOMAL DNA

Restriction enzyme analysis of chromosomal DNA has been used effectively to type many different species of bacteria. The key step in this procedure is the isolation of high-molecular-weight chromosomal DNA. Several new column techniques, and other rapid methods using glass or silicon beads, are now being produced to aid in this process. One such device has been used in my laboratory to isolate DNA from *Serratia marcescens, X. maltophilia, S. aureus,* and even *Acanthamoeba castellani* for analysis with restriction endonucleases.

Once obtained, the DNA is divided into aliquots and digested into a series of fragments, using a different restriction endonuclease in each aliquot. Then, the fragments of each individual digest are separated in an agarose gel by electrophoresis and visualized by staining the gel with ethidium bromide (Fig. 3A). The digests of the isolates are then examined for similarities. The technique is relatively crude and relies on the ability of the investigator to discern the often subtle differences between isolates, but it is still effective. However, with some additional effort, the laboratory can prepare a Southern blot and use a DNA probe to generate a hybridization pattern that is much easier to interpret.

SOUTHERN BLOTS

Southern blots are named after their inventor, Edwin Southern, who optimized the procedure of transferring DNA fragments from agarose gels to nitrocellulose paper (42). (The transfer of RNA in an analogous process is referred to as Northern blotting, and the transfer of proteins to nitrocellulose is referred to as Western blotting.) The procedure is outlined in Fig. 3. After digestion of the chromosomal DNA with restriction enzymes, the fragments are subjected to electrophoresis in an agarose gel. The gel is stained with ethidium bromide to reveal the DNA fragments, photographed, and treated successively with acidic and basic solutions to depurinate and denature the nucleic acid present. After neutralization,

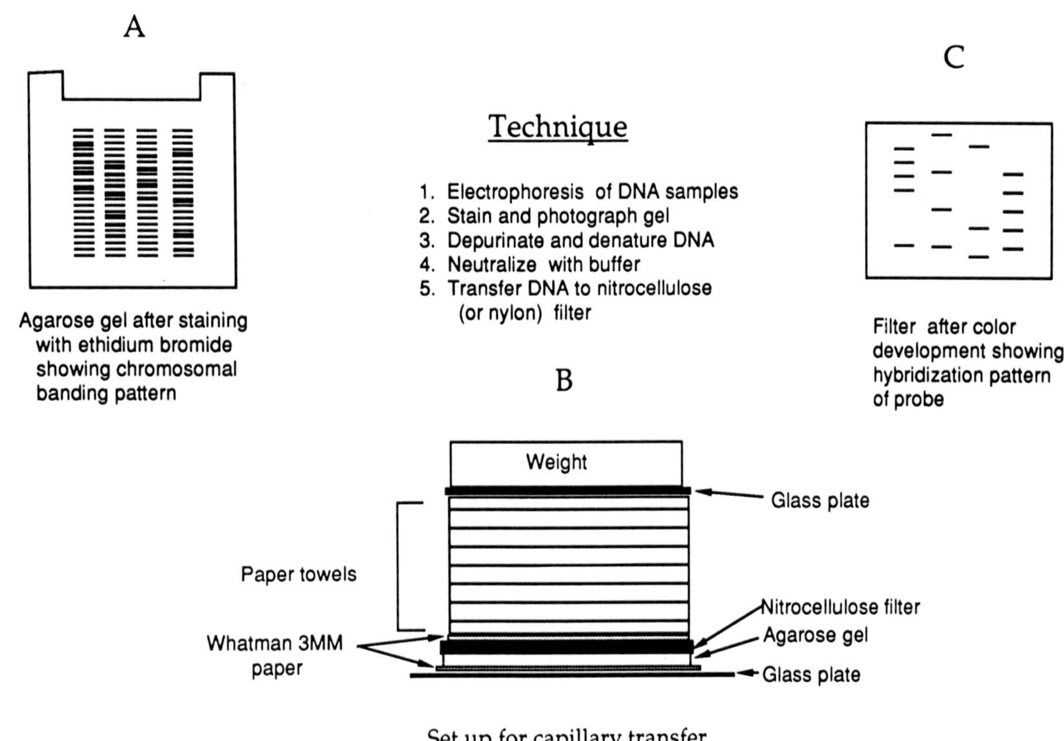

FIG. 3. Preparation of a Southern blot. (A) Agarose gel showing restriction digest of chromosomal DNA. Darker bands represent plasmid DNA contained with the isolates. (B) Method of preparing a Southern blot (42). (C) Nylon filter after color development showing restriction fragment length polymorphisms identified by the hybridization assay.

the gel is placed on several sheets of Whatman 3MM filter paper soaked in a sodium chloride-sodium citrate solution (SSC; 1× SSC is 0.15 M sodium chloride plus 0.015 M trisodium citrate, pH 7.0) (Fig. 3B). The filter paper usually is placed on a glass plate. The gel is placed on top of the filter paper, and a piece of nitrocellulose, wetted in 3× SSC, is placed on top of the gel, making sure that no bubbles are present. Another sheet of Whatman 3MM filter paper, also soaked in 3× SSC, is placed on top of the nitrocellulose filter, and plastic wrap (e.g., Saran Wrap) is used to ensure that the moisture in the filter paper reservoir can escape only through the agarose gel. A stack of paper towels is placed on top of the filter paper. Finally, a glass plate is placed on top of the towels, and a weight (such as the previous edition of this Manual) is added to the top of the paper towels (the glass plate distributes the weight evenly over the gel). As the SSC is drawn up from the filter paper through the gel by capillary action, the DNA is carried to the nitrocellulose filter, where it is retained by electrostatic charge. After overnight transfer of the DNA, the filter is air dried and heated to permanently bind the DNA to the filter membrane. The nitrocellulose now is ready for hybridization.

In recent years, several new membrane filters, including nylon and nylon-nitrocellulose mixtures, have been developed. Each has advantages and disadvantages, and the choice of filter depends on the hybridization procedure one wishes to use. Virtually all of the molecular biology supply houses have toll-free customer service numbers that are staffed by knowledgeable (and remarkably patient) representatives. They can assist in helping one choose the appropriate filter for the type of hybridization studies one wants to perform.

To facilitate the preparation of Southern blots, several companies have introduced vacuum-mediated or positive-pressure transfer devices that increase the efficiency of transfer of nucleic acids from gels to nylon or nitrocellulose filters. Solutions for depurination and denaturation are added directly to the chamber, and transfer can be completed in less than 3 h. These chambers cost less than $1,000 and simplify the entire procedure. Microbiologists in large clinical laboratories and reference laboratories that are involved in strain typing should consider adopting techniques such as plasmid fingerprinting and restriction enzyme analysis to aid smaller laboratories in investigations of outbreaks.

HYBRIDIZATION PROCEDURES

There are as many different hybridization procedures as there are probes. Each procedure, however, begins with a prehybridization step in which heterologous DNA, such as calf thymus DNA, is added to the Southern blot in a reagent mix similar to that used for hybridization. The DNA is used to saturate those sites that bind DNA nonspecifically before addition of the probe DNA. This process usually takes 1 h. After this time, the prehybridization cocktail containing the calf thymus DNA is drained from the filter and fresh hybridization buffer containing the labeled probe is added to the Southern blot. Some investigators prefer to perform the hybridization reactions in sealed freezer bags placed in slowly shaking water baths, whereas others simply place the filter in plastic wrap, distribute the probe over the filter carefully with a pipette, fold the plastic wrap, enclose it in aluminum foil, and place the entire unit in a stationary incubator. Hybridization chambers with roller bottles now are available to facilitate the process. All of these methods work well. The length of incubation for hybridization reactions varies from 0.5 to 18 h, depending on the length of the probe.

After hybridization is complete, the filters are washed in several solutions containing NaCl and sodium dodecyl sulfate at temperatures that again vary according to the desired stringency. After washing, the filters are air dried and autoradiographed (if ^{32}P was used as a label) or subjected to the color development process (if nonradioactive labels were used).

RIBOTYPING

Stull and co-workers were the first to report the utility of using rRNA from *E. coli* to probe chromosomal DNA in Southern blots for typing of bacterial strains (43). This method of strain typing, called ribotyping, exploits the fact that rRNA genes are scattered throughout the chromosome of most bacteria and produce polymorphic restriction endonuclease patterns when probed with rRNA. Cloned rRNA genes (5) have also been used as probes and produce similar banding patterns (1). Ribotyping has proven useful for differentiating among strains of *Haemophilus influenzae, Pseudomonas cepacia, E. coli* (43), *Providencia stuartii* (33), and *Salmonella typhi* (1). Figure 2B shows a ribotyping analysis of several strains of *X. maltophilia* collected from a single hospital. The results demonstrate that the isolates from this hospital did not represent an outbreak, since each isolate has a different banding pattern (lane 4 contains a control band).

POLYMERASE CHAIN REACTION

The polymerase chain reaction (PCR) is a technique that can be used to find very low quantities of an infectious agent present in clinical samples by increasing the quantity of a specific nucleotide sequence contained

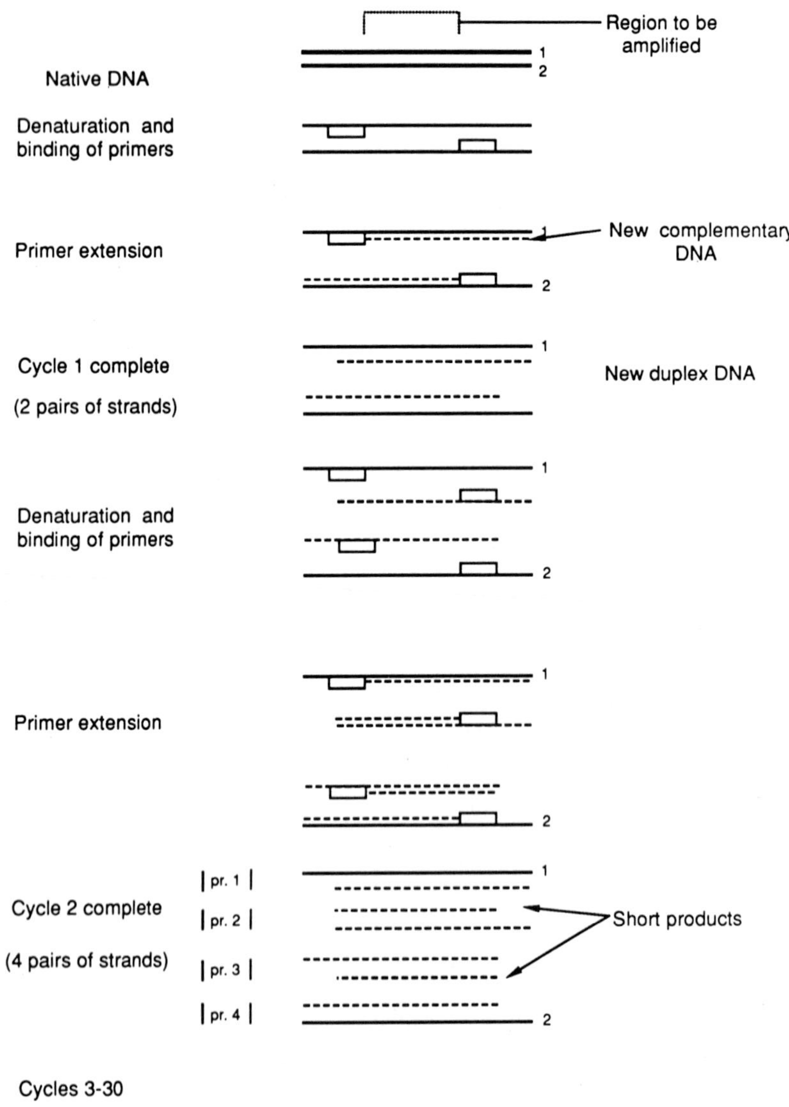

FIG. 4. Schematic presentation of PCR.

within the organism by a process of directed DNA synthesis. As described by Mullis and Faloona (29), PCR consists of three steps: denaturation of the DNA in the sample, binding of the primers (short segments of DNA complementary to the 5′ and 3′ ends of the sequence to be amplified), and extension of the primers by DNA polymerase to produce two DNA strands that are identical copies of the original target strand. Thus, the DNA located between the two primers is amplified (Fig. 4).

As each cycle of denaturation, binding, and extension is performed, the number of DNA copies increases by a factor of 2^n, where n is the number of cycles. Thus, after 30 cycles, approximately 10^6-fold amplification of a specific DNA segment can be achieved (14). Thus, theoretically, even a single copy of human immunodeficiency virus present in only 1 of every 10^6 T cells can be detected (24, 32). The majority of the DNA that is produced consists of short products representing only the area between the oligonucleotide primers. In the early cycles of PCR, longer strands of DNA are made as the polymerase moves down the primary target strands. These long strands represent <1% of the final product, and the amplification of sequences outside of the primers is minor.

The cycling process, which involves alternately heating the reaction mix to 95°C and then cooling it to 50°C, continues efficiently as a result of the use of a heat-stable DNA polymerase from *Thermus aquaticus*, an organism that usually lives in hot springs (37). The reaction continues in a sealed tube without the need to add more enzyme at each step, reducing the possibility of contamination. There are reports describing PCR assays for a wide variety of pathogens, including human immunodeficiency virus (24, 32), cytomegalovirus (10), hepatitis B virus (21), human papillomavirus (41), the polyomaviruses BK and JC (3), bacterial pathogens such as enterotoxigenic *E. coli* (31), and many other infectious agents (40). Thirty cycles can usually be completed within 4 h. Figure 5 demonstrates the specificity of the PCR procedure in detecting a 310-base-pair fragment of a unique aminoglycoside resistance gene when performed on plasmid DNA.

Three key points regarding the use of PCR must be emphasized. First, in order to use PCR to detect a microorganism in a sample, specific primers must be constructed, which means that nucleotide sequence data must be available for the organism in question. Second, PCR must be conducted under tightly controlled conditions of ionic strength, temperature, and primer and nucleotide concentration. Deviations can result in nonspecific amplification, which can lead to false-positive assay results. Figure 5, for example, demonstrates the nonspecific products that are formed when temperature conditions are below the optimal temperature (lanes H to J). Third, the assays must be conducted in such a way as to minimize the possibility of outside contamination of the sample. Contamination of assays by extraneous DNA has been a serious problem for investigators developing these assays and has led to the use of positive displacement pipettors, use of separate rooms for dividing all reagents into aliquots, and use of sealed containers. This need for such stringent conditions may well limit the utility of this technique in the routine clinical laboratory until adequate controls for contamination have been developed. It is important to note, however, that PCR is not the only amplification scheme available to aid in detection of infectious agents present in low quantities. Other amplification procedures, such as the transcription amplification system (23), which also has been shown to be highly effective for detecting low numbers of human immunodeficiency virus particles in clinical samples, also are being explored.

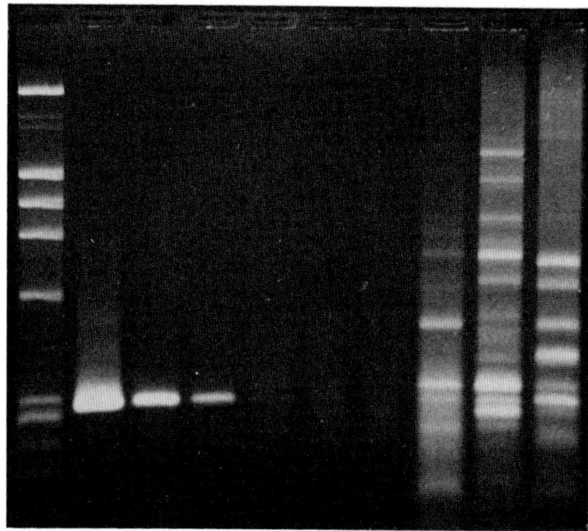

FIG. 5. PCR amplification of a specific DNA segment from the 2″-*O*-adenylyltransferase gene. Lanes: A, molecular size standards; B, amplification of 1 ng of pFCT3103 DNA for 30 cycles at optimum temperature and salt conditions; C, amplification of 10 pg of pFCT3103 DNA under optimum conditions; D, amplification of 1 pg of pFCT3103 DNA under optimal conditions; E to G, negative controls; H to J, amplification of DNA samples under nonoptimal temperature conditions. Many nonspecific fragments are seen. Amplifications were performed by using a temperature cycler from Coy Laboratory Instruments, Ann Arbor, Mich.

SIGNAL AMPLIFICATION

The final technique that will have an impact on clinical microbiology in the future is nucleic acid hybridization coupled with signal amplification instead of target amplification. The key example of this technique is the Qβ replicase and MDV-1 template RNA. The replicase, which is derived from a bacteriophage, will replicate only a very select group of RNA molecules that have a unique secondary structure (27). The replicase can use nascent strands of RNA that it has just produced as templates. Thus, the production of new RNA molecules increases geometrically. As many as 10^9 copies of the RNA template can be produced in as little as 30 min. Moreover, Lizardi and co-workers discovered that probes up to 100 base pairs in length can be incorporated into the MDV-1 RNA without affecting its secondary structure. Thus, after the probe (which is cloned into the RNA template) has hybridized to the appropriate target (27), the RNA can be amplified to enhance detection and can easily be recognized by fluorometry after ethidium bromide staining. Thus, one amplifies the signal after hybridization occurs instead of the target. This procedure can effectively eliminate the contamination problem of PCR whereby extraneous DNA that is not part of the clinical sample is amplified, giving a false-positive result. With the Qβ replicase system, hybridization occurs first, the bound probe that is incorporated into the highly unique MDV-1 RNA template molecule is separated from the rest of the sample, and the replicase amplifies the RNA at a geometric rate. This technology now is being incorporated into some diagnostic probe kits.

CONCLUSIONS

Nucleic acid probes will play a major role in both the detection and identification of pathogenic microorganisms in diagnostic laboratories in years to come. Probes will also find increased usage in strain-typing systems, particularly in Southern blotting procedures. Ribotyping in particular has proven to be a very powerful tool for differentiating among strains and will gain prominence in investigations of outbreaks of nosocomial and community-acquired infections.

I thank Cindy Fennell and Kathy Phillips for their technical assistance in the preparation of Fig. 2 and 5 and Dan Leong for providing the *X. maltophilia* strains cited herein.

LITERATURE CITED

1. **Altwegg, M., F. W. Hickman-Brenner, and J. J. Farmer III.** 1989. Ribosomal RNA gene restriction patterns provide increased sensitivity for typing *Salmonella typhi* strains. J. Infect. Dis. **160:**145–149.
2. **Arnold, L. J., Jr., P. W. Hammond, W. A. Wiese, and N. C. Nelson.** 1989. Assay formats involving acridinium-ester-labeled DNA probes. Clin. Chem. **35:**1588–1594.
3. **Arthur, R. R., S. Dagostin, and K. V. Shah.** 1989. Detection of BK virus and JC virus in urine and brain tissue by the polymerase chain reaction. J. Clin. Microbiol. **27:**1174–1179.
4. **Bialkowska-Hobrzanska, H.** 1987. Detection of enterotoxigenic *Escherichia coli* by dot blot hybridization with biotinylated DNA probes. J. Clin. Microbiol. **25:**338–343.
5. **Brosius, J., A. Ullrich, M. A. Raker, A. Gray, T. J. Dull, R. R. Gutell, and H. F. Noller.** 1981. Construction and fine mapping of recombinant plasmids containing the *rrnB* ribosomal RNA operon of *E. coli*. Plasmid **6:**112–118.
6. **Cheung, L. L., and J. B. Hudson.** 1988. Development of DNA probes for *Candida albicans*. Diagn. Microbiol. Infect. Dis. **10:**171–179.
7. **Conville, P. S., J. F. Keiser, and F. G. Witebsky.** 1989. Mycobacteremia caused by simultaneous infection with *Mycobacterium avium* and *Mycobacterium intracellulare* detected by analysis of a BACTEC 13A bottle with the Gen-Probe kit. Diagn. Microbiol. Infect. Dis. **12:**217–219.
8. **Conville, P. S., J. F. Keiser, and F. G. Witebsky.** 1989. Comparison of three techniques for concentrating positive BACTEC 13A bottles for mycobacterial DNA probe analysis. Diagn. Microbiol. Infect. Dis. **12:**309–313.
9. **Coyle, M. B., N. B. Groman, J. Q. Russell, J. P. Harnisch, M. Rabin, and K. K. Holmes.** 1989. The molecular epidemiology of three biotypes of *Corynebacterium diphtheriae* in the Seattle outbreak, 1972–1982. J. Infect. Dis. **159:**670–679.
10. **Demmler, G. J., G. J. Buffone, C. M. Schimbor, and R. A. May.** 1988. Detection of cytomegalovirus in urine from newborns by using polymerase chain reaction DNA amplification. J. Infect. Dis. **158:**1177–1184.
11. **Doebbling, B. N., M. J. Bale, F. P. Koontz, C. M. Helms, R. P. Wenzel, and M. A. Pfaller.** 1988. Prospective evaluation of the Gen-Probe assay for detection of *Legionellae* in respiratory specimens. Eur. J. Clin. Microbiol. Infect. Dis. **7:**748–752.
12. **Drake, T. A., J. A. Hindler, O. G. W. Berlin, and D. A. Bruckner.** 1987. Rapid identification of *Mycobacterium avium* complex in cultures using DNA probes. J. Clin. Microbiol. **25:**1442–1445.
13. **Dular, R., R. Kajioka, and S. Kasatiya.** 1988. Comparison of Gen-Probe commercial kit and culture technique for the diagnosis of *Mycoplasma pneumoniae* infection. J. Clin. Microbiol. **26:**1068–1069.
14. **Erlich, H. A., R. Gibbs, and H. H. Kazazian, Jr. (ed.).** 1989. Polymerase chain reaction. Cold Spring Harbor Laboratory, Cold Spring Harbor, N.Y.
15. **Fox, B. C., H. L. T. Mobley, and J. C. Wade.** 1989. The use of a DNA probe for epidemiological studies of candidiasis in immunocompromised hosts. J. Infect. Dis. **159:**488–494.
16. **Gleaves, C. A., D. A. Hursh, D. H. Rice, and J. D. Meyers.** 1989. Detection of cytomegalovirus from clinical specimens in centrifugation culture by in situ hybridization and monoclonal antibody staining. J. Clin. Microbiol. **27:**21–23.
17. **Gonzalez, R., and B. A. Hanna.** 1987. Evaluation of Gen-Probe DNA hybridization systems for the identification of *Mycobacterium tuberculosis* and *Mycobacterium avium-intracellulare*. Diagn. Microbiol. Infect. Dis. **8:**69–72.
18. **Granato, P. A., and M. R. Franz.** 1989. Evaluation of a prototype DNA probe test for noncultural diagnosis of gonorrhea. J. Clin. Microbiol. **27:**632–635.
19. **Hames, B. D., and S. J. Higgins.** 1985. Nucleic acid hybridization: a practical approach. IRL Press, Oxford.
20. **Jablonski, E., E. W. Moomaw, R. H. Tullis, and J. L. Ruth.** 1986. Preparation of oligodeoxynucleotide-alkaline phosphatase conjugates and their use as hybridization probes. Nucleic Acids Res. **14:**6115–6128.
21. **Kaneko, S., R. H. Miller, S. M. Feinstone, M. Unoura, K. Kobayashi, N. Hattori, and R. H. Purcell.** 1989. Detection of serum hepatitis B virus DNA in patients with chronic hepatitis using the polymerase chain reaction assay. Proc. Natl. Acad. Sci. USA **86:**312–316.
22. **Kiehn, T. E., and F. F. Edwards.** 1987. Rapid identification using a species specific DNA probe of *Mycobacterium avium* complex from patients with acquired immunodeficiency syndrome. J. Clin. Microbiol. **25:**1551–1552.
23. **Kwoh, D. Y., G. R. Davis, K. M. Whitfield, H. L. Chappelle, L. J. DiMichele, and T. R. Gingeras.** 1989. Transcription-based amplification system and detection of amplified human immunodeficiency virus type 1 with a bead-based sandwich hybridization format. Proc. Natl. Acad. Sci. USA **86:**1173–1177.
24. **Kwok, S., D. H. Mack, K. B. Mullis, B. Poiesz, H. Erlich, D. Blair, A. Friedman-Kien, and J. J. Sninsky.** 1987. Identification of human immunodeficiency virus sequences by *in vitro* enzymatic amplification and oligomer cleavage detection. J. Virol. **61:**1690–1694.
25. **LeBar, W., B. Herschman, C. Jemal, and J. Pierzchala.** 1989. Comparison of DNA probe, monoclonal antibody enzyme immunoassay, and cell culture for the detection of *Chlamydia trachomatis*. J. Clin. Microbiol. **27:**826–828.
26. **Liebl, W., R. Rosenstein, F. Gotz, and K. H. Schleifer.** 1987. Use of a staphylococcal nuclease gene as a probe for *Staphylococcus aureus*. FEMS Microbiol. Lett. **44:**179–184.
27. **Lizardi, P. M., C. E. Guerra, H. Lomeli, I. Tussie-Luna, and F. R. Kramer.** 1988. Exponential amplification of recombinant-RNA hybridization probes. Bio/Technology **6:**1197–1202.
28. **Montone, K. T., D. J. Brigati, and L. R. Budgeon.** 1989. Anatomic viral detection is automated: the application of a robotic molecular pathology system for detection of DNA viruses in anatomic pathology substrates using immunocytochemical and nucleic acid hybridization techniques. Yale J. Biol. Med. **62:**141–158.
29. **Mullis, K. B., and F. A. Faloona.** 1987. Specific synthesis of DNA *in vitro* via a polymerase catalyzed chain reaction. Methods Enzymol. **155:**335–350.

30. **Nishibuchi, M., M. Arita, T. Honda, and T. Miwatani.** 1988. Evaluation of a nonisotopically labeled oligonucleotide probe to detect the heat-stable enterotoxin gene of *Escherichia coli* by the colony hybridization test. J. Clin. Microbiol. **26:**784–786.
31. **Olive, D. M.** 1989. Detection of enterotoxigenic *Escherichia coli* after polymerase chain reaction amplification with a thermostable DNA polymerase. J. Clin. Microbiol. **27:**261–265.
32. **Ou, C.-Y., S. Kwok, S. W. Mitchell, D. H. Mack, J. J. Sninsky, J. W. Krebs, P. Feorino, D. Warfield, and G. Schochetman.** 1988. DNA amplification for direct detection of HIV-1 in DNA of peripheral blood mononuclear cells. Science **239:**295–297.
33. **Owen, R. J., A. Beck, P. A. Dayal, and C. Dawson.** 1988. Detection of genomic variation in *Providencia stuartii* clinical isolates by analysis of DNA restriction fragment length polymorphisms containing rRNA cistrons. J. Clin. Microbiol. **26:**2161–2166.
34. **Pasculle, A. W., G. E. Veto, S. Krystofiak, K. McKelvey, and K. Vrsalovic.** 1989. Laboratory and clinical evaluation of a commercial DNA probe for the detection of *Legionella* spp. J. Clin. Microbiol. **27:**2350–2358.
35. **Perine, P. L., P. A. Totten, K. K. Holmes, E. H. Sng, A. V. Ratnam, W. Widy-Wersky, H. Nsanze, E. Habtegabr, and W. G. Westbrook.** 1985. Evaluation of a DNA hybridization method for detection of African and Asian strains of *Neisseria gonorrhoeae* in men with urethritis. J. Infect. Dis. **152:**59–63.
36. **Rigby, P. W. J., M. Dieckmann, C. Rhodes, and P. Berg.** 1977. Labeling deoxyribonucleic acid to high specific activity *in vitro* by nick translation with DNA polymerase. J. Mol. Biol. **113:**237–251.
37. **Saiki, R. K., D. H. Gelfend, S. Stoffel, S. J. Scharf, R. Higuchi, G. T. Horn, K. B. Mullis, and H. A. Erlich.** 1988. Primer-directed enzymatic amplification of DNA with a thermostable DNA polymerase. Science **239:**487–491.
38. **Samadpour, M., S. L. Moseley, and S. Lory.** 1988. Biotinylated DNA probes for exotoxin A and pilin genes in the differentiation of *Pseudomonas aeruginosa* strains. J. Clin. Microbiol. **26:**2319–2323.
39. **Sambrook, J., E. F. Fritsch, and T. Maniatis.** 1989. Molecular cloning: a laboratory manual, 2nd ed. Cold Spring Harbor Laboratory, Cold Spring Harbor, N.Y.
40. **Schochetman, G., C. Y. Ou, and W. K. Jones.** 1988. Polymerase chain reaction. J. Infect. Dis. **158:**1154–1157.
41. **Shibata, D. K., N. Arnheim, and W. J. Martin.** 1988. Detection of human papilloma virus in paraffin-embedded tissue using the polymerase chain reaction. J. Exp. Med. **167:**225–230.
42. **Southern, E. M.** 1975. Detection of specific sequences among DNA fragments separated by gel electrophoresis. J. Mol. Biol. **98:**503–517.
43. **Stull, T. L., J. J. LiPuma, and T. D. Edlind.** 1988. A broad spectrum probe for molecular epidemiology of bacteria: ribosomal RNA. J. Infect. Dis. **157:**280–286.
44. **Tenover, F. C.** 1988. Diagnostic deoxyribonuclic acid probes for infectious diseases. Clin. Microbiol. Rev. **1:**82–101.
45. **Tenover, F. C.** 1989. DNA probes for infectious diseases. CRC Press, Inc., Boca Raton, Fla.
46. **Tilton, R. C., F. Dias, H. Kidd, and R. W. Ryan.** 1988. DNA probe versus culture for detection of *Mycoplasma pneumoniae* in clinical samples. Diagn. Microbiol. Infect. Dis. **10:**109–112.
47. **Tompkins, L. S., N. Troup, A. Labigne-Roussel, and M. L. Cohen.** 1986. Cloned, random chromosomal sequences as probes to identify *Salmonella* species. J. Infect. Dis. **154:**156–162.
48. **Wahl, G. M., S. L. Berger, and A. R. Kimmel.** 1987. Molecular hybridization of immobilized nucleic acids: theoretical concepts and practical considerations. Methods Enzymol. **152:**399–406.

Chapter 18

Substrate Profile Systems for the Identification of Bacteria and Yeasts by Rapid and Automated Approaches

RICHARD F. D'AMATO, EDWARD J. BOTTONE, AND DANIEL AMSTERDAM

Before the use of gelatin agar in 1881 by Robert Koch, the practice of microbial identification was limited to observing microorganisms after growth in a liquid medium and hence often in mixed culture. The use of agar-based growth media permitted, for the first time, the macroscopic observation and characterization of microorganisms in pure culture. This significant event was followed by Gram's description in 1884 of a staining reaction which permitted microbiologists to describe bacteria according to microscopic and tinctorial properties. These innovations provided the foundation for the identification of microorganisms.

The advent of the so-called classical or conventional approaches to microbial identification began with the introduction of tests that used various carbon sources and assays for metabolic end products. These advances were augmented by serological techniques that recognized characteristic microbial antigens, further supplemented by pathogenicity studies using animals.

Initially, the choice of biochemical test substrates, the method of substrate preparation, the reading of test results, and the interpretation schemes for microbial identification were highly individualistic, making laboratory-to-laboratory comparisons of individual test results and final identifications difficult at best. At least 24 h was required to read results. Quality control efforts, if exercised, were far below today's standards. In the 1940s and 1950s, some farsighted microbiologists, realizing the need for more rapid tests, approached the problem through the miniaturization of conventional procedures (13). They assumed that a sufficient concentration of preformed enzymes was present in bacterial cells after primary growth for rapid characterization. By using a concentrated inoculum and a small volume of sensitized (e.g., with limited buffering capacity for pH-dependent tests) substrates, these investigators developed rapid identification tests that required no additional bacterial growth beyond primary isolation. This approach to bacterial identification was subsequently exploited commercially in the form of reagent-impregnated strips. In the late 1960s, a transition from the classical, multistep procedures to contemporary, unistep methodologies with emphasis on speed, standardization, reproducibility, mechanization, and automation began. This transition was characterized by the commercial availability of miniaturized identification systems based on classical methods.

The first-generation systems, which addressed the family *Enterobacteriaceae,* included a series of miniaturized tubes containing individual substrates, multicompartment tubes or plates with multiple substrates, and paper strips or disks impregnated with dehydrated substrates. Tests included in the various identification systems were judiciously selected to ensure reproducibility and provide slightly more rapid results than did their classical counterparts. Reaction endpoints were reached after 18 h of incubation, and identifications were based on percentage tables published by Edwards and Ewing for *Enterobacteriaceae* (8). Although the initial systems were an improvement over their classical predecessors, they had a significant flaw. The formulations and volumes of the test substrates, the types of reaction indicators, and the incubation periods used in the commercial systems not only differed from each other but, more importantly, often were not the same as those used by Edwards and Ewing to establish their identification schemes. Therefore, each system had some inherent problems with accuracy of identification of particular genera or species. Almost exclusively through the efforts of the commercial manufacturers, this problem has been resolved in the second-generation systems by the incorporation of highly sophisticated, computer-generated identification data bases tailored for each system. Additional advantages of the second-generation systems include (i) expanded identification to include additional groups of microorganisms; (ii) reaction endpoints that can be reached after 4 h of incubation; (iii) mechanized or automated inoculation, test reading, and identification; and (iv) further miniaturization of test substrate containers. Not all of the current systems have all of the above-mentioned attributes. However, with any of these systems, each laboratory can identify an appreciable number of medically significant microorganisms with accuracy, alacrity, reproducibility, and a sense of security engendered by the knowledge that other laboratories performing the same test on the same isolate will arrive at the same identification. A review of the systems approach to microbial identification is presented by D'Amato et al. (5).

The literature contains numerous evaluations of the currently available commercial bacterial and yeast identification systems, all of which cannot be discussed in this chapter. Early evaluations of these systems compared the percentage agreement of individual biochemical reactions versus a "standard" method, followed by investigations that compared only final identifications. The many factors to consider in performing a comparison of one or more identification systems have been reviewed by D'Amato et al. (5) and

Edberg and Konowe (7). The general aspects of classification and taxonomy are presented in chapter 26.

MICROBIAL IDENTIFICATION SYSTEMS

A significant contribution of industry to the clinical microbiology laboratory was the development and introduction of the systems approach to microbial identification. An identification system consists of a series of tests judiciously selected and formulated to identify microorganisms to a desired level, accompanied by identification schemes, often computer based and developed for each system. The systems may be manual, mechanized, or automated; some systems are available in all three configurations. Regardless of its level of sophistication, each system consists of a complete package for the identification of a particular group of microorganisms, including the *Enterobacteriaceae*, nonfermenters and oxidase-positive fermenters, anaerobes, streptococci, *Neisseria* spp., *Moraxella catarrhalis*, *Haemophilus* spp., and certain yeasts. The salient characteristics of commonly used identification systems are outlined in the appendix.

The nature of the tests used in an identification system depends on numerous factors, such as level of selectivity (differentiation ability), reproducibility, time for reaction endpoints to be reached, readability (visually, photometrically, by video imaging, etc.), and ease and cost of manufacture. Many of the tests used in commercial identification systems are basically modifications of classical methods. Examples include tests for fermentation, assimilation, oxidation, degradation, and hydrolysis. Their incorporation in commercial systems is based on tradition and their ability to discriminate among genera and species in the shortest time interval. The inclusion of chromogen-linked enzyme substrates in the current generation of diagnostic systems or their exclusive use is based on their discriminatory powers, ability to be read by using instrumented approaches, and the reduced time to reach reaction endpoints. Both the classical and novel approaches exploit the vast array of enzymes that microbes use to metabolize various substrates. Species identification is based on the presence of a particular reaction pattern(s) established by an isolate's metabolism of the substrates included in the identification system.

It is beyond the scope of this chapter to describe all tests included in the numerous commercially available identification systems. Therefore, we will present the basic concepts of each test category.

Fermentation and oxidation reactions are among the tests most commonly used in identification systems. Fermentation tests exploit the ability of an isolate to metabolize carbohydrates in the absence of atmospheric oxygen. The substrates are incompletely metabolized, resulting in the formation of organic acids. In fermentation reactions, organic compounds serve as both electron donors and electron acceptors. Oxidation tests are based on the ability of an isolate to metabolize the aforementioned substrates with oxygen as the final electron acceptor. Both fermentation and oxidation test reactions are usually detected by the use of pH indicators incorporated in the test medium.

As mentioned above, systems now include the means of enzymatic profiling of microorganisms with test substrates that upon hydrolysis release a chromogen or fluorogen that can be detected chemically or fluorometrically (R. F. D'Amato, Clin. Microbiol. Newsl. **2**:1–4, 1980). These tests take advantage of the presence of preformed enzymes, obviating extended incubation before results are available. Enzymatic profiling of microorganisms by using chromogenic or fluorogenic substrates maximizes the advantage of assaying for preformed enzymes. The principle of the test is as follows: RS + enzyme → $R + S$, where R is the chromogen or fluorogen, S is the substrate, and RS is the chromogen/fluorogen-substrate complex that is colorless or nonfluorescent before hydrolysis. The substrate complex is hydrolyzed by the appropriate enzyme, and free chromogen or fluorogen is released. Special equipment is not required for the detection of enzymatic hydrolysis. The tests are sensitive, rapid (reaction endpoints are reached ≤4 h after inoculation), and reproducible, and they are easily miniaturized and automated. In most cases, a single well-isolated microbial colony will produce sufficient inoculum for a large battery of test substrates. The interpretation of test results is not complicated by side effects of multiple reactions that may occur when test substrates are incorporated in complex nutrient culture media.

Assimilation (utilization) tests play an important role in microbial identification, particularly with reference to yeasts and certain nonfermenting gram-negative rods. These tests are based on the ability of microorganisms to use select carbon and nitrogen sources for growth. A single carbon or nitrogen source is incorporated into a basal medium that contains all substances required for growth except a carbon or nitrogen source. Growth on an agar surface or in a broth medium constitutes a positive result. Examples of assimilation substrates commonly used for bacterial identification are citrate and acetate. Carbohydrate and nitrate assimilation tests represent the foundation for the biochemical identification of yeasts. Some yeast assimilation identification systems use a pH indicator to detect a positive reaction, which may be caused by assimilation or fermentation of the carbon source, with the production of an acid end product. Traditional yeast assimilation identification schemes are based on the presence of visible growth on or in the various test substrates (no pH indicator used) and should never be used with systems relying on changes in a pH indicator.

Tests for microbial identification also may use compounds that selectively inhibit metabolic pathways, providing the division of major groups of microorganisms into categories which can be further classified on the basis of biochemical activity on other test substrates. Historically, growth in the presence of potassium cyanide, which inhibits respiration in certain bacteria, divided the family *Enterobacteriaceae* into two categories. Other commonly used inhibitory compounds are bile, heavy metals, and sodium chloride. Today, compounds such as irgasan and *p*-coumaric acid, which interfere with glucose fermentation of some gram-negative bacteria, have aided in the recognition of specific genera and species.

Determination of the susceptibility of a microorganism to antimicrobial agents is of paramount importance for the selection of appropriate therapy. Microbiologists have long appreciated that determining susceptibility to various antimicrobial agents can be helpful in identification. For example, isolates of *Klebsiella pneumo-*

niae are usually susceptible to cephalothin and resistant to carbenicillin, *Proteus* spp. are usually resistant to polymyxin B and colistin, and *Pseudomonas aeruginosa* is usually resistant to kanamycin. Some of the identification systems listed in the appendix incorporate antimicrobial agents in their test panels for this purpose. However, because antimicrobial susceptibility can be influenced by many factors, such as the antimicrobial usage patterns at a particular institution, definitive identification cannot be based on susceptibility patterns. This is particularly true when antimicrobial agents that are commonly used therapeutically are also used for identification.

The classical degradative or dissimilation tests using primarily the amino acids lysine, ornithine, arginine, and phenylalanine are very useful for bacterial identification and have been adapted for use in commercial identification systems. The differential ability of bacteria to produce enzymes capable of decarboxylating lysine or ornithine or of hydrolyzing arginine, forming alkaline end products, can be detected with a basal medium containing the amino acid, glucose, and a pH indicator. Glucose permits bacterial growth with the production of acid. The decarboxylation of lysine and ornithine, resulting in cadaverine and putrescine, respectively, and the production of ammonia by arginine dihydrolase cause the pH indicator to shift to alkaline, indicating a positive reaction. The ability of certain bacteria to oxidatively degrade phenylalanine and tryptophan is also of taxonomic importance. The enzyme phenylalanine deaminase degrades phenylalanine to phenylpyruvic acid, which yields a blue-green color in the presence of ferric ions. The oxidative deamination of tryptophan produces indole pyruvic acid, which forms a cherry red complex with ferric ions. Other bacteria produce indole from tryptophan by means of enzymes collectively referred to as tryptophanases. Indole is detected by the addition of Ehrlich or Kovacs reagent.

The differential ability of microorganisms to hydrolyze various substrates continues to occupy an important role in identification systems. Commonly used hydrolysis tests include urea, gelatin, and esculin tests. Microorganisms producing the enzyme urease hydrolyze urea to ammonia, which causes a change in a pH indicator to the alkaline range. Gelatin hydrolysis or liquefaction is mediated by a gelatinase enzyme found in various bacteria. A positive reaction is evidenced by liquefaction of the gelatin substrate. Esculin, a β-glucoside, is hydrolyzed by microorganisms possessing this enzyme, resulting in esculetin, which reacts with ferric ions to produce a black precipitate.

APPLICATION OF SYSTEM DATA BASES FOR PROFILE ANALYSIS AND IDENTIFICATION OF MICROORGANISMS

Nungester (19) enumerated five objectives for identifying microorganisms: (i) determine rapidly the susceptibility to antimicrobial drugs; (ii) obtain information that may have prognostic value to clinicians; (iii) identify organisms in terms of their potential danger to individuals in contact with patients; (iv) aid epidemiologists in tracing sources of infections; and (v) accumulate data of interest to those studying infectious diseases. These objectives, enunciated more than 25 years ago, are pertinent today.

In an early paper, Steel (28) indicated that classification was an art and identification was a science. Developments during the last decade have diminished this disparity. The terms classification, identification, and diagnosis have been used interchangeably and differently, but here the terms profile analysis and identification will be used synonymously. It is generally agreed that one has to classify an isolate before an identification can be performed. Identification should be contrasted with taxonomy or systematics, which according to Simpson (24) includes classification, nomenclature, and identification. Identification is the pragmatic arm of taxonomy.

Clinical microbiologists may be surprised to learn that they think in mathematical sets and with symbolic logic, but this kind of reasoning occurs for every identification and the subsequent clinical correlation of bacterial diagnosis with laboratory data. These acts can be ascribed to exercises in deductive and inductive reasoning and can be described with appropriate mathematical diagrams and symbols. The branches of mathematics or philosophy used for these functions are called set theory and symbolic logic.

In identifying microorganisms, the clinical microbiologist arrives at an identification by taking the initial knowledge of the morphologic appearance of a single pure colony or a preliminary set of biochemical data and applying it to subsequent observations. From this initial data base, he or she draws tentative conclusions, acts on the basis of them, performs additional tests, observes what happens thereafter, and uses this additional information to confirm or refute the initial decisions. The clinical microbiologist then relates all of these events back to the original observations and uses the total outcome to integrate or augment his or her existing parameters. Some of these processes are performed by conscious discipline using specific data or by overt classifications and delineated reasoning processes. Some of these processes are accomplished so quickly and almost reflexively. The process becomes subconscious or intuitive, leaving the microbiologist unaware of exactly what he or she has done and how the store of background and experience has been used to form a new observation (1, 2).

In analogy to the rules of grammar, humans organize their thoughts for logical reason in a way that resembles their organization of words for proper speaking. The laws of rational thought have been studied and established by mathematicians and philosophers, who have constructed and illustrated the system of logic by which human reasoning is formed and communicated. The mathematical development of this kind of rational thought was named after its founder, George Boole (Boolean algebra). It deals with sets of collections (classes of objects) rather than single objects and contemplates the relations of the collection or classes. A set can be defined as a collection of objects or elements of which all possess some common defining property: the set of all bacteria of medical importance, the set of all gram-negative bacteria, etc. Every object contained in a set must have the characteristic property of the set in addition to many other properties. Different sets have different characteristic properties, but each set can contain many subdivisions, called subsets, each with its own characteristic property. Thus, the set of all gram-negative rods is composed of the set of fermenting and nonfermenting rods. The set of all fermentative gram-negative organisms contains such subsets as the phenylalanine deaminase-positive and phenylalanine-negative taxa. While it is evident that a particular gram-negative organism may belong to many sets, all gram-positive bacteria would be excluded from those particular sets and subsets. Several of the commercial system manufacturers (see appendix) have adapted this approach and designed system subsets suitable only for a particular class or group of microorganisms.

Identification processes depend on gathering adequate information for characterizing known organisms, and numerous ways have been proposed for handling that information. Some are based on the use of dichotomous keys (also known as decision trees, flow charts, and the sequence approach); others are based on diagnostic schemes and tables; and a third category utilizes the simultaneous or pattern method. Classically, microbiologists have depended on flow charts in making selections or identifications. The inherent problem with flow charts is that adherence must be absolute with regard to the presence or absence of a reaction to a particular substrate. If the unknown organism does not conform perfectly to the flow chart, an error will inevitably result. Since the decision tree bases the selection of each succeeding test on the previous test result, until the lowest branch is reached, each separating group becomes the weakest link, depending on the number of branches in the network, and is a potential source for possible breakdowns in the identification method. Furthermore, most flow charts do not allow for biologic variations to occur as expressed by differing biochemical reactions of the organism. Since a decision tree represents a model of a diagnostic process, it is also a "discrimination net" and therefore has holes.

Diagnostic keys and tables have a severe limitation in that the specimen must belong within the group of organisms for which the scheme was devised; otherwise, aberrant identification or failure to identify will result. Access to data processing systems could significantly expand the number of diagnostic characters. However, with keys and tables, investigators are restricted by memory to a limited number of indices for which they can recognize similarities and differences while making simultaneous comparisons. Because of these limitations, Cowan and Steel (4) constructed a mechanical device called the determinator for the compilation of suitable tables. Another mechanical approach for comparing characters of unknown and known microorganisms is the use of punched cards, by hand or by sorting methods as described by Schneierson and Amsterdam (23). The advantage of computers is that an almost limitness number of criteria that are part of the identification scheme can be stored in the core microbial memory of the computer. Therefore, these flow charts and schemes are suitable for examination purposes, but they do not represent the manner in which we actually deliberate; we think in terms of sets (16).

The simultaneous or pattern recognition approach to identification tests an organism for a large number of characters at one time. The simultaneous method has the advantage of speed and the decreased likelihood of gross error if a single test is read incorrectly. However, it lacks the inherent orderliness of the sequential method. Assisted by a computer, it can handle a vast number of test patterns. If 15 characters are included in the matrix (table) for identification, then 2^{15} or 32,768 combinations are possible, an unwieldy number for any microbiologist to sort and recognize. An unresolved issue is whether 32,768 combinations represent true taxa (16).

D'Amato et al. (5) have clearly set forth the elements for the development of a microbial identification system. They include the process of test selection and construction of the data base. Three elements should be considered before a test set is used in any approach to microbial identification: the probability of a positive or negative result for each test, the separation value of the test (8), and the reproducibility of the test.

The result of any test can be scored as either positive (1) or negative (0); therefore, the sum of the probabilities for a positive and a negative result for any given organism is equal to 1. Tests usually are not universally (100%) positive or negative for a taxon. As the ratio approaches one-half (0.5) of positive to negative, the usefulness of a particular test becomes nil. One can calculate the probability of a set of results by multiplying the probabilities of individual test results (17). However, this assumes that the tests are statistically independent—an assumption which cannot be strictly justified but which usually is necessary in this kind of approach. Usually, probabilities greater than or equal to 0.85 are classified as positive, whereas those equal to or less than 0.15 are considered negative.

Gyllenberg (11) described the concept of the "separation-figure," referred to as the S value. It is obtained by multiplying the number of taxa yielding a positive result in a given test by the number of pairs of taxa that can be separated by a particular test and represents the overall differentiating power of each test. It should be noted that although two tests rate high S values, they may separate only the same set of pairs. The S values of commonly used diagnostic tests for fermentative taxa can be ranked (1).

The third important characteristic of a test set is reproducibility. Test error is most readily estimated by analysis of variance of replicates (27). When the average probability of an incorrect test is greater than 10%, serious distortion of identification can result. This type of distortion must be judged against that due to sampling error, which predominates when the number of tests is small. Hence, numerical taxonomists advocate the use of as many tests as possible provided that the test error for any one is not too large (27). The upper limit to the permissible error on any one test is not defined.

It is necessary to know the reproducibility of any one test within the laboratory. Inattention to test error will explain unsatisfactory results between laboratories. Theoretically, replicates should yield identical results in the same laboratory, but differences often occur. Factors that impair intralaboratory reproducibility are reading intervals (overnight versus actual elapsed 18 or 24 h) and variations in incubation temperature due to inaccurate temperature setting or fluctuations in temperature that occur from shelf to shelf within air-convected incubators. Variation in the reproducibility of tests between laboratories is expected to be larger than variation within a laboratory because of factors other than those mentioned above. Variations can be due to batch or brand differences among culture media, differences in inoculation techniques, or discrepancies between observing and reading results. As with all variations, statistical errors tend to accumulate rather than cancel out one another.

Since the first suggestions (3, 25) of the use of computers in bacterial identification, numerous investigators have made significant contributions (6, 10, 11, 17, 18, 20–22, 26). Only two states exist in the algebra of logic under which computers operate: yes or no; true or untrue; present or not present. They are represented by 1 and 0, respectively. (Within the computer electronic logic, these states refer to different voltage levels.) Binary logic is also representational of the qualitative manner in which diagnostic tests are interpreted. Hence, computers seem ideally suited to diagnostic evaluation. (Computers could handle multistate reactions as well.) If an organism were tested for five biochemical attributes and the first three were positive and the last two were negative, then the binomial result would be 11100, and 32 (or 2^5) combinations are possible.

Diagnostic kits designed for the identification of microorganisms use anywhere from 6 to 95 tests and express test results in a binomial manner. Stringent adherence to the sequence position of each reaction as instructed by the manufacturer permits positive or negative results to be recorded as a coded number. A resulting number (in decimal format) encompasses the accumulated reactivity of the bacterium to the various biochemical substrates. Often the manufacturer supplies an abbreviated matrix (table) of all possible combinations. It is readily understandable that these tables would be abbreviated, because for 21 tests there would be 2^{21} (2,097,152) listings. In addition, the manufacturer usually offers a computer identification program based on a most likelihood or Bayes theorem identification approach. Once instructed with the decimal representation of the biochemical profile of an organism, the computer converts the data to the corresponding binomial index, searches the matrix program, and prints out an identification.

Although Bayes' theorem is readily derived from rules of mathematical theory of probability as a basic concept, detractors have not agreed with the controversial meaning of probability (29). Early application of Bayes theorem was suitable for clinical diagnosis but was considered inappropriate for bacterial identification (6). The major reason for disallowing its use in clinical microbiology was a paucity of quantitative data. Friedman et al. (9, 10) overcame this problem by using the considerable amount of test data derived from the *Enterobacteriaceae*.

Computer methods for identifying bacteria rely on a matrix that is similar in form to a diagnostic table but gives the probability of a positive result for each of the taxa for each of the tests. Compiling the matrix involves the testing of as many strains as possible of each taxon for all tests included in the matrix. The construction of the matrix is analogous to using a diagnostic table, such as those of Cowan and Steel (4), and substituting percentage positive values for "positive," "negative," and "delayed" results in the table.

The computer program can then calculate the likelihoods of all taxa on the pattern of test results given by the unknown strain. The likelihood that an unknown belongs to a particular taxon based on a set of test results is the probability of the results for the taxon, and this is calculated by multiplying together the probabilities of the individual results. (The probabilities stored in the matrix are the probabilities of obtaining positive results; the probability of a negative result is 1 minus the probability of obtaining a positive result.) The program described by Lapage et al. (18) can be used as an example. It converts the likelihoods to "identification scores" by dividing each likelihood by the sum of the likelihoods for all of the taxa, and the program suggests a definite identification only if the highest score exceeds 0.999 (identification threshold level). Other investigators dealing with computer identification of bacteria (6, 12) calculate likelihoods in the same way but use different methods of displaying the relative values obtained and making an identification decision. The multiplying together of the probabilities (obtained from the matrix) of individual test results represents the absolute likelihood; the conversion of these likelihoods by the normalization process described above yields the relative likelihood. Although the method of Lapage et al. (18) does not utilize the absolute likelihood in reaching an identification decision, other authors have done so but differ in the ways of displaying the values obtained and of reaching an identification decision. The relative and absolute likelihoods may be combined in concluding an identification decision, and such a method has been adopted by manufacturers. For example, Analytab Products has used the relative likelihood in making an identification decision even though only the absolute likelihood values are displayed. Micro-ID system comments are also given as to the level of acceptability of an identification (i.e., an identification decision is made). For the Enterotube II, the index used appears to display only the relative likelihood values and then only when additional tests are necessary to further the identification. The programs used by the manufacturers of identification systems have not been published, but the principles involved, as illustrated by the API 20E, are generally known and acceptable (5).

The threshold levels that likelihood values must exceed for various identification decisions as in the API 20E and other systems have not been published, but for any commercial identification system the problem is similar: a high identification threshold level reduces the risk of misidentifications but diminishes the rate of identification; a low identification threshold level increases the rate of identifications but carries a greater risk of misidentification (14, 15). Because of the limitation in number of tests used in some commercial identification systems, the identification threshold level will generally be lower than that accepted by a reference laboratory. However, various features, such as recommendation for serological confirmation of the suggested identifications, may be incorporated into the identification scheme in order to reduce the misidentification risk to an acceptable level. As noted above, sophisticated identification schemes must be used to overcome the deficiency in number of tests. That such schemes can be developed has been demonstrated in the evaluation of the API 20E system carried out by Holmes et al. (15): the identification rate for 206 strains, using the results of 50 conventional tests and analysis by use of a probability matrix, was 94% with no misidentifications; using the results of only the 20 API 20E tests in conjunction with the API Analytical Profile Index and Computer Service, the figures for these same 206 strains were 88% with 2% misidentified.

There are problems associated with identification using probability matrices. These include the limits on matrix entries mentioned above as well as (i) unknown matrix entries (i.e., there are incomplete data on the performance of some taxa in some tests); (ii) test linkage (for example, if growth at 37°C is negative, then motility at 37°C must be negative), since the probabilistic method assumes that the test results are independent; and (iii) multistate tests, such as pigment production, in which strains may be negative or produce one of several different colored pigments. Methods for overcoming these problems are described by Willcox et al. (29). A disadvantage of relying solely on the relative likelihood value to make an identification decision in the probabilistic approach is that if a strain belongs to a taxon not included in the matrix, it could be misidentified as a taxon in the matrix if the strain resembled that taxon much more closely than it did any other taxon in the matrix.

APPENDIX

SYSTEMS FOR *ENTEROBACTERIACEAE*, NONFERMENTERS, AND OTHER GRAM-NEGATIVE BACTERIA

Quantum II Microbiology System. *Manufacturer:* Abbott Diagnostics, Abbott Laboratories, Abbott Park, Ill. *Application:* Identification of *Enterobacteriaceae*, nonfermenters, and other gram-negative bacteria. *Packaging:* Cartridge of multicompartment wells containing dried substrates. *Storage:* 2 to 8°C. *Tests:* 20; fermentation/oxidation, degradation, inhibition. *Incubation period:* 4 to 5 h. *Susceptibility testing capabilities:* No. *Instrumentation:* Quantum II automated reader.

GN Microplate; ES Microplate. *Manufacturer:* Biolog, Hayward, Calif. *Application:* Identification of gram-negative bacteria. *Packaging:* Dehydrated microplates. *Storage:* 2 to 8°C. *Tests:* 95; utilization (assimilation). *Incubation period:* 4 to 24 h. *Susceptibility testing capabilities:* No. *Instrumentation:* Automated reader.

API 20E. *Manufacturer:* Analytab Products, Plainview, N.Y. *Application:* Identification of *Enterobacteriaceae*, nonfermenters, and other gram-negative bacteria. *Packaging:* Microtubes containing dehydrated substances on strips. *Storage:* 2 to 8°C. *Tests:* 20; fermentation/oxidation, degradation, hydrolysis. *Incubation period:* 24 to 48 h. *Susceptibility testing capabilities:* No. *Instrumentation:* No.

UniScept 20E. *Manufacturer:* Analytab Products, Plainview, N.Y. *Application:* Identification of *Enterobacteriaceae*, nonfermenters, and other gram-negative bacteria. *Packaging:* Strips of microtubes containing dried test substrates. *Storage:* 2 to 8°C. *Tests:* 23; fermentation/oxidation, degradation, assimilation, hydrolysis. *Incubation period:* 24 to 48 h. *Susceptibility testing capabilities:* MIC and Bauer-Kirby. *Instrumentation:* (i) Inoculation and spectrophotometric test reading and interpretation; (ii) ALADIN—this automatic inoculation, on-board incubation, video image-reading, reagent-adding, and interpretation device can be used with UniScept 20E.

Rapid E. *Manufacturer:* Analytab Products, Plainview, N.Y. *Application:* Identification of *Enterobacteriaceae*. *Packaging:* Strips of microtubes containing dried test substrates. *Storage:* 2 to 8°C. *Tests:* 21; fermentation/oxidation, degradation, hydrolysis, assimilation. *Incubation period:* 4 h. *Susceptibility testing capabilities:* No. *Instrumentation:* No.

Rapid NFT. *Manufacturer:* Analytab Products, Plainview, N.Y. *Application:* Identification of gram-negative nonfermentative bacteria and some fermentative bacteria not belonging to the family *Enterobacteriaceae*. *Packaging:* Strips of microtubes containing dried test substrates. *Storage:* 2 to 8°C. *Tests:* 20; assimilation, chromogenic, hydrolysis, degradation, fermentation/oxidation. *Incubation period:* 24 h. *Susceptibility testing capabilities:* No. *Instrumentation:* No.

Minitek. *Manufacturer:* BBL Microbiology Systems (Becton Dickinson), Cockeysville, Md. *Application:* Identification of *Enterobacteriaceae* and nonfermentative gram-negative bacteria. *Packaging:* Impregnated substrate disks, Minitek plate, enteric and nonfermenter broth. *Storage:* 2 to 25°C. *Tests:* 21; fermentation/oxidation, hydrolysis, degradation. *Incubation period:* 24 to 48 h. *Susceptibility testing capabilities:* No. *Instrumentation:* No.

Minitek. *Manufacturer:* BBL Microbiology Systems (Becton Dickinson), Cockeysville, Md. *Application:* Rapid (4-h) identification of *Enterobacteriaceae*. *Packaging:* Reagent-impregnated substrate disks, Minitek plate, Minitek enteric broth. *Storage:* 2 to 25°C. *Tests:* 21; fermentation/oxidation, hydrolysis, assimilation, degradation. *Incubation period:* 4 h. *Susceptibility testing capabilities:* No. *Instrumentation:* No.

Difco/Pasco Tri Panel. *Manufacturer:* Difco/Pasco Laboratories, Wheat Ridge, Colo. *Application:* Identification of gram-negative and gram-positive bacteria. *Packaging:* Hydrated microtiter plates. *Storage:* −20°C. *Tests:* 30; fermentation, degradation, hydrolysis, chromogenic, inhibition. *Incubation period:* 16 to 20 h, 40 to 44 h. *Susceptibility testing capabilities:* No. *Instrumentation:* Yes.

Enteric-Tek. *Manufacturer:* Flow Laboratories, Inc., McLean, Va. *Application:* Identification of *Enterobacteriaceae*. *Packaging:* Multicompartment plastic plate with 11 peripheral wells, and 1 center well containing solid media. *Storage:* 2 to 8°C. *Tests:* 14; fermentation, degradation, hydrolysis. *Incubation period:* 18 to 24 h. *Susceptibility testing capabilities:* No. *Instrumentation:* No.

Micro-ID System. *Manufacturer:* Organon Teknika, Durham, N.C. *Application:* Identification of *Enterobacteriaceae*. *Packaging:* Molded styrene tray containing 15 reaction chambers with individual test substrates incorporated into paper disks. *Storage:* 2 to 8°C. *Tests:* 15; fermentation, degradation, hydrolysis. *Incubation period:* 4 h. *Susceptibility testing capabilities:* No. *Instrumentation:* No.

RapID SS/U. *Manufacturer:* Innovative Diagnostic Systems, Inc., Atlanta, Ga. *Application:* Identification of commonly occurring urinary microorganisms: *E. coli*, *Klebsiella* spp., *Enterobacter* spp., *Proteus* spp., *Serratia* spp., *Citrobacter* spp., *Providencia* spp., *Morganella morganii*, *Pseudomonas* spp., *Enterococcus* spp., *Staphylococcus* spp., and *Candida albicans*. *Packaging:* Dehydrated panel. *Storage:* 2 to 8°C. *Tests:* 11; chromogenic, hydrolysis, inhibition. *Incubation period:* 2 h. *Susceptibility testing capabilities:* No. *Instrumentation:* No.

Frozen Gram-Negative Panel. *Manufacturer:* American MicroScan, Sacramento, Calif. *Application:* Identification of *Enterobacteriaceae*, nonfermenters, and other gram-negative bacteria. *Packaging:* Hydrated tray. *Storage:* −20°C. *Tests:* 34; fermentation/oxidation, degradation, hydrolysis, inhibition. *Incubation period:* 18 to 24 h. *Susceptibility testing capabilities:* Yes. *Instrumentation:* No.

Micro-Media Quad Enteric Panel. *Manufacturer:* Micro-Media Systems, Inc., San Jose, Calif. *Application:* Identification of *Enterobacteriaceae*. *Packaging:* 80-well plastic microtiter tray (four sets of 20 reactions). *Storage:* −20°C. *Tests:* 20; fermentation, degradation, chromogenic, hydrolysis. *Incubation period:* 18 to 24 h. *Susceptibility testing capabilities:* No. *Instrumentation:* No.

Sensititre. *Manufacturer:* Sensititre, Salem, N.H. *Application:* Identification of *Enterobacteriaceae*, nonfermenters, and other gram-negative bacteria. *Packaging:* Plastic microtiter tray. *Storage:* Room temperature. *Tests:* 32; fluorogenic substrates. *Incubation period:* 5 to 18 h. *Susceptibility testing capabilities:* Yes. *Instrumentation:* Fluorometer.

Enterotube II. *Manufacturer:* Roche Diagnostics, Nutley, N.J. *Application:* Identification of *Enterobacteriaceae. Packaging:* Compartmentalized plastic tube containing agar media. *Storage:* 2 to 8°C. *Tests:* 15; fermentation/oxidation, degradation, hydrolysis. *Incubation period:* 18 to 24 h. *Susceptibility testing capabilities:* No. *Instrumentation:* No.

Oxi-Ferm. *Manufacturer:* Roche Diagnostics, Nutley, N.J. *Application:* Identification of gram-negative, nonfermentative bacteria and of oxidase-positive fermentative bacteria. *Packaging:* Compartmentalized plastic tube containing agar media. *Storage:* 2 to 8°C. *Tests:* 9; fermentation/oxidation, degradation, hydrolysis. *Incubation period:* 24 and 48 h. *Susceptibility testing capabilities:* No. *Instrumentation:* No.

Cobas-Bact ID. *Manufacturer:* Roche Diagnostics, Basel, Switzerland. *Application:* Identification of *Enterobacteriaceae. Packaging:* Round disposable plastic rotor (ID-E rotor) with a central chamber and 16 peripheral cuvettes containing dehydrated biochemical substrates. *Storage:* 2 to 8°C. *Tests:* 16; fermentation, degradation, hydrolysis. *Incubation period:* 4 h. *Susceptibility testing capabilities:* No. *Instrumentation:* Spectrophotometer.

Gram Negative Identification Card (GNI). *Manufacturer:* Vitek Systems, Inc., Hazelwood, Mo. *Application:* Identification of *Enterobacteriaceae* and other gram-negative bacteria. *Packaging:* Cards with rows of wells containing dried test substrates. *Storage:* 2 to 8°C. *Tests:* 29; fermentation/oxidation, assimilation, degradation, inhibition. *Incubation period:* 4 to 13 h. *Susceptibility testing capabilities:* Yes. *Instrumentation:* Inoculation, incubation, turbidimetric/colorimetric test reading, test interpretation.

EPS (Enteric Pathogens Screen Card). *Manufacturer:* Vitek Systems, Inc., Hazelwood, Mo. *Application:* Identification of *Edwardsiella tarda, Salmonella* spp., *Salmonella typhi, Shigella* spp., and *Yersinia enterocolitica. Packaging:* See GNI above. *Storage:* 2 to 8°C. *Tests:* 10; fermentation, degradation, hydrolysis. *Incubation period:* 4 to 8 h, Vitek incubator. *Susceptibility testing capabilities:* No. *Instrumentation:* See GNI above.

Urine Identification 3 Card. *Manufacturer:* Vitek Systems, Inc., Hazelwood, Mo. *Application: Citrobacter freundii, Serratia* spp., *Klebsiella* and *Enterobacter* spp., *Proteus* spp., *E. coli, P. aeruginosa*, group D enterococci, *Staphylococcus* spp., and yeasts. *Packaging:* See GNI above. *Storage:* 2 to 8°C. *Tests:* Nine; fermentation, inhibition, chromogenic. *Incubation period:* 1 to 13 h. *Susceptibility testing capabilities:* No. *Instrumentation:* See GNI above.

SYSTEMS FOR STAPHYLOCOCCI, STREPTOCOCCI, AND OTHER GRAM-POSITIVE BACTERIA

API 20S. *Manufacturer:* Analytab Products, Plainview, N.Y. *Application:* Identification of streptococci and aerococci. *Packaging:* Strips of microcupules containing dried test substrates. *Storage:* 2 to 8°C. *Tests:* 20; fermentation/oxidation, degradation, hydrolysis, chromogenic. *Incubation period:* 4 h. *Susceptibility testing capabilities:* No. *Instrumentation:* No.

UniScept 20GP. *Manufacturer:* Analytab Products, Plainview, N.Y. *Application:* Identification of staphylococci and streptococci. *Packaging:* Strips of microtubes containing dried test substrates. *Storage:* 2 to 8°C. *Tests:* 20; fermentation/oxidation, degradation, hydrolysis, chromogenic. *Incubation period:* 18 to 24 h. *Susceptibility testing capabilities:* MIC and Bauer-Kirby. *Instrumentation:* (i) Incubation and spectrophotometric test reading and test interpretation; (ii) ALADIN—this automatic inoculation, on-board incubation, video image-reading, reagent-adding, and interpretation device can be used with the UniScept 20GP.

Staph-Ident. *Manufacturer:* Analytab Products, Plainview, N.Y. *Application:* Identification of staphylococci. *Packaging:* Strips of microtubes containing dried test substrates. *Storage:* 2 to 8°C. *Tests:* 10; fermentation/oxidation, chromogenic, degradation, hydrolysis. *Incubation period:* 5 h. *Susceptibility testing capabilities:* No. *Instrumentation:* No.

Rapid STREP. *Manufacturer:* Analytab Products, Plainview, N.Y. *Application:* Identification of streptococci. *Packaging:* Strips of microtubes containing dried test substrates. *Storage:* 2 to 8°C. *Tests:* 20; fermentation/oxidation, chromogenic, degradation, hydrolysis. *Incubation period:* 4 to 24 h. *Susceptibility testing capabilities:* No. *Instrumentation:* No.

Minitek. *Manufacturer:* BBL Microbiology Systems (Becton Dickinson), Cockeysville, Md. *Application:* Identification of gram-positive cocci. *Packaging:* Reagent-impregnated substrate paper disks, Minitek plate, Minitek gram-positive broth. *Storage:* 2 to 25°C. *Tests:* 20; fermentation, decarboxylation, hydrolysis. *Incubation period:* 24 h. *Susceptibility testing capabilities:* No. *Instrumentation:* No.

RapID STR System. *Manufacturer:* Innovative Diagnostic Systems, Atlanta, Ga. *Application:* Identification of Lancefield group A, B, C, and G streptococci, *Streptococcus anginosus, Enterococcus* spp., aerococci, and viridans streptococci. *Packaging:* Dehydrated panel. *Storage:* 2 to 8°C. *Tests:* 14; degradation, hydrolysis, inhibition. *Incubation period:* 4 h. *Susceptibility testing capabilities:* No. *Instrumentation:* No.

Gram Positive Identification Card (GPI). *Manufacturer:* Vitek Systems, Inc., Hazelwood, Mo. *Application:* Identification of streptococci, staphylococci, and certain gram-positive bacilli. *Packaging:* Cards with rows of wells containing dried test substrates. *Storage:* 2 to 8°C. *Tests:* 29; fermentation/oxidation, degradation, inhibition. *Incubation period:* 4 to 15 h. *Susceptibility testing capabilities:* MIC. *Instrumentation:* Inoculation, incubation, turbidimetric/colorimetric test reading, test interpretation.

Bacillus Biochemical Card. *Manufacturer:* Vitek Systems, Inc., Hazelwood, Mo. *Application:* Identification of *Bacillus* spp. *Packaging:* Dehydrated. *Storage:* 2 to 8°C. *Tests:* 29; substrates/inhibitors. *Incubation period:* 15 h. *Susceptibility testing capabilities:* No. *Instrumentation:* See GPI above.

SYSTEMS FOR *HAEMOPHILUS, NEISSERIA,* AND *BRANHAMELLA* SPECIES

Quad FERM +. *Manufacturer:* Analytab Products, Plainview, N.Y. *Application:* Identification of *Neisseria* spp. and *Branhamella catarrhalis. Packaging:* Strips of microcupules containing dried test substrates. *Storage:* 2 to 8°C. *Tests:* Four; carbohydrate utilization, β-lactamase production. *Incubation period:* 2 h. *Susceptibility testing capabilities:* No. *Instrumentation:* No.

RIM-N (Rapid Identification Method—Neisseria). *Manufacturer:* Austin Biological Laboratories, Inc., Austin, Tex. *Application:* Identification of *Neisseria* spp. and *Branhamella (Moraxella) catarrhalis. Packaging:* Kit containing tubes, four carbohydrate substrate solutions (2%), and a control. *Storage:* 2 to 8°C. *Tests:* Four; carbohydrate utilization. *Incubation period:* 30 to 60 min. *Susceptibility testing capabilities:* No. *Instrumentation:* No.

Minitek. *Manufacturer:* BBL Microbiology Systems (Becton Dickinson), Cockeysville, Md. *Application:* Identification of *Neisseria* spp. *Packaging:* Reagent-impregnated substrate disks, Minitek plate, neisseria broth. *Storage:* 2 to 25°C. *Tests:* Four; fermentation, hydrolysis. *Incubation period:* 4 h. *Susceptibility testing capabilities:* No. *Instrumentation:* No.

RapID NH System. *Manufacturer:* Innovative Diagnostic Systems, Atlanta, Ga. *Application:* Identification of *Neisseriaceae, Haemophilus* and other bacterial spp., and *Moraxella catarrhalis. Packaging:* Dehydrated. *Storage:* 2 to 8°C. *Tests:* 13; degradation, hydrolysis, inhibition. *Incubation period:* 1 to 4 h. *Susceptibility testing capabilities:* No. *Instrumentation:* No.

HNID Panel. *Manufacturer:* American MicroScan, Sacramento, Calif. *Application:* Rapid identification of and detection of β-lactamase production in *Neisseria, Haemophilus, Branhamella,* and *Gardnerella* spp.; biotyping of *Haemophilus influenzae* and *Haemophilus parainfluenzae. Packaging:* Dehydrated. *Storage:* 2 to 8°C. *Tests:* 18; fermentation, degradation, hydrolysis, chromogenic. *Incubation period:* 4 h. *Susceptibility testing capabilities:* No. *Instrumentation:* No.

NHI. *Manufacturer:* Vitek Systems, Inc., Hazelwood, Mo. *Application:* Identification of *Neisseria* and *Haemophilus* spp. *Packaging:* Cards with rows of wells containing dried test substrates. *Storage:* 2 to 8°C. *Tests:* 15; fermentation/oxidation, degradation, chromogenic. *Incubation period:* 4 h. *Instrumentation:* Tests are read manually, but identification is made with the Vitek computer.

SYSTEMS FOR ANAEROBES

API 20A. *Manufacturer:* Analytab Products, Plainview, N.Y. *Application:* Identification of anaerobes. *Packaging:* Microtubes containing dehydrated substrate strips. *Storage:* 2 to 8°C. *Tests:* 21; fermentation, hydrolysis. *Incubation period:* 24 h in anaerobic conditions. *Susceptibility testing capabilities:* No. *Instrumentation:* No.

An-Ident. *Manufacturer:* Analytab Products, Plainview, N.Y. *Application:* Identification of anaerobes. *Packaging:* Strips of microtubes containing dried test substrates. *Storage:* 2 to 8°C. *Tests:* 21; chromogenic, degradation. *Incubation period:* 4 h, aerobic. *Instrumentation:* No.

Minitek Anaerobe II. *Manufacturer:* BBL Microbiology Systems (Becton Dickinson), Cockeysville, Md. *Application:* Identification of anaerobes. *Packaging:* Reagent-impregnated paper disks, Minitek plate, Minitek anaerobe broth. *Storage:* 2 to 25°C. *Tests:* 20; fermentation, hydrolysis. *Incubation period:* 48 h, in anaerobic conditions. *Susceptibility testing capabilities:* No. *Instrumentation:* No.

Anaerobe-Tek (A/T). *Manufacturer:* Flow Laboratories, Inc., McLean, Va. *Application:* Identification of sporeforming and nonsporeforming anaerobic bacteria. *Packaging:* Multicompartment plastic plate containing 11 peripheral wells and one central well. *Storage:* 2 to 8°C. *Tests:* 12; fermentation, hydrolysis, inhibition. *Incubation period:* 48 h, in anaerobic conditions. *Susceptibility testing capabilities:* No. *Instrumentation:* No.

RapID ANA II System. *Manufacturer:* Innovative Diagnostic Systems, Atlanta, Ga. *Application:* Identification of anaerobic bacteria. *Packaging:* Dehydrated substrates. *Storage:* 2 to 8°C. *Tests:* 18; fermentation, assimilation, reduction, chromogenic. *Incubation period:* 4 to 6 h. *Susceptibility testing capabilities:* No. *Instrumentation:* No.

Rapid Anaerobe ID Panel. *Manufacturer:* American MicroScan, Sacramento, Calif. *Application:* Identification of anaerobes. *Packaging:* Dehydrated 96-well trays. *Storage:* 2 to 8°C. *Tests:* 24; fermentation, hydrolysis, inhibition. *Incubation period:* 4 h, in anaerobic conditions. *Susceptibility testing capabilities:* No. *Instrumentation:* Automated reader.

ANI. *Manufacturer:* Vitek Systems, Inc., Hazelwood, Mo. *Application:* Identification of anaerobes. *Packaging:* Cards with rows of wells containing dried test substrates. *Storage:* 2 to 8°C. *Tests:* 28; fermentation/oxidation, degradation, chromogenic. *Incubation period:* 4 h, aerobic. *Susceptibility testing capabilities:* No. *Instrumentation:* Tests are read manually, but identification is made with the Vitek computer.

SYSTEMS FOR YEASTS

Quantum II Microbiology System. *Manufacturer:* Abbott Diagnostics, Abbott Laboratories, Abbott Park, Ill. *Application:* Identification of yeasts. *Packaging:* Cartridge of multicompartment wells containing dried substrates. *Storage:* 2 to 8°C. *Tests:* 19; assimilation, hydrolysis. *Incubation period:* 22 to 26 h. *Susceptibility testing capabilities:* No. *Instrumentation:* Automated reading and interpretation.

Yeast-Ident. *Manufacturer:* Analytab Products, Plainview, N.Y. *Application:* Identification of yeasts. *Packaging:* Strips of microtubes containing dried test substrates. *Storage:* 2 to 8°C. *Tests:* 19; chromogenic, hydrolysis. *Incubation period:* 4 h. *Susceptibility testing capabilities:* No. *Instrumentation:* No.

API 20C. *Manufacturer:* Analytab Products, Plainview, N.Y. *Application:* Identification of yeasts. *Packaging:* Strips of microcupules containing dried test substrates. *Storage:* 2 to 8°C. *Tests:* 19; assimilation. *Incubation period:* 72 h. *Susceptibility testing capabilities:* No. *Instrumentation:* No.

Minitek. *Manufacturer:* BBL Microbiology Systems (Becton Dickinson), Cockeysville, Md. *Application:* Identification of yeasts. *Packaging:* Reagent-impregnated disks, yeast carbon assimilation agar, petri dish. *Storage:* 2 to 25°C. *Tests:* 12; assimilation. *Incubation period:* 48 to 72 h. *Susceptibility testing capabilities:* No. *Instrumentation:* No.

Uni-Yeast Tek. *Manufacturer:* Flow Laboratories, Inc., McLean, Va. *Application:* Identification of yeasts. *Packaging:* Multicompartment plastic plate with 11 peripheral wells and 1 center well containing solid media. *Storage:* 2 to 8°C. *Tests:* 11; germ tube, morphology on cornmeal agar, assimilation of carbohydrate and potassium nitrate, hydrolysis. *Incubation period:* up to 6 days. *Susceptibility testing capabilities:* No. *Instrumentation:* No.

VITEK Yeast Biochemical Card. *Manufacturer:* Vitek Systems, Inc., Hazelwood, Mo. *Application:* Identification of yeasts. *Packaging:* Cards with rows of wells containing dried test substrates. *Storage:* 2 to 8°C. *Tests:* 26; assimilation, inhibition, hydrolysis. *Incubation period:* 24 to 48 h. *Susceptibility testing capabilities:* No. *Instrumentation:* Inoculation, turbidimetric/colorimetric test reading, test interpretation.

LITERATURE CITED

1. **Amsterdam, D.** 1977. Computers and clinical microbiology: perspectives and applications. Mt. Sinai J. Med. **44:** 113–133.
2. **Amsterdam, D., and S. S. Schneierson.** 1969. Electronic data processing system for the clinical microbiology laboratory. Appl. Microbiol. **17:**93–97.

3. **Beers, R. J., and W. R. Lockhart.** 1962. Experimental methods in computer taxonomy. J. Gen. Microbiol. **28:** 633–640.
4. **Cowan, S. T., and K. J. Steel.** 1960. A device for the identification of microorganisms. Lancet **i:**1172–1173.
5. **D'Amato, R. F., B. Holmes, and E. J. Bottone.** 1981. The systems approach to diagnostic microbiology. Crit. Rev. Microbiol. **9:**1–44.
6. **Dybowski, W., and D. A. Franklin.** 1968. Conditional probability and the identification of a bacteria: a pilot study. J. Gen. Microbiol. **54:**215–229.
7. **Edberg, S. C., and L. S. Konowe.** 1982. A systematic means to conduct a microbiology evaluation, p. 268–299. *In* V. Lorian (ed.), Significance of medical microbiology in the care of patients, 2nd ed. The Williams & Wilkins Co., Baltimore.
8. **Edwards, P. R., and W. H. Ewing.** 1972. Identification of *Enterobacteriaceae*. Burgess Publishing Co., Minneapolis.
9. **Friedman, R., and J. MacLowry.** 1973. Computer identification of bacteria on the basis of their antibiotic susceptibility patterns. Appl. Microbiol. **26:**314–317.
10. **Friedman, R. B., D. Bruce, J. MacLowry, and V. Brenner.** 1973. Computer-assisted identification of bacteria. Am. J. Clin. Pathol. **60:**395–403.
11. **Gyllenberg, H. G.** 1965. Model for computer identification of microorganisms. J. Gen. Microbiol. **39:**401–405.
12. **Gyllenberg, H. G., and T. K. Niemela.** 1975. Basic principles in computer-assisted identification of microorganisms, p. 201–223. *In* C.-G. Heden and T. Ileni (ed.), New approaches to the identification of microorganisms. John Wiley & Sons, Inc., New York.
13. **Hartmen, P. A.** 1968. Miniaturized microbiological methods. Academic Press, Inc., New York.
14. **Holmes, B., J. Dowling, and S. P. Lapage.** 1979. Identification of gram-negative nonfermenters and oxidase-positive fermenters by the Oxi-Ferm tube. J. Clin. Pathol. **32:** 78–85.
15. **Holmes, B., W. R. Wilcox, and S. P. Lapage.** 1978. Identification of *Enterobacteriaceae* by the API 20E system. J. Clin. Pathol. **31:**22–30.
16. **Isenberg, H. D., and J. D. MacLowry.** 1976. Automated methods and data handling in bacteriology. Annu. Rev. Microbiol. **30:**483–505.
17. **Lapage, S. P., S. Bascomb, W. R. Willcox, and M. A. Curtis.** 1970. Computer identification of bacteria, p. 1–22. *In* A. Baillie and R. J. Gilbert (ed.), Automation, mechanization and data handling in microbiology. Academic Press, Inc., New York.
18. **Lapage, S. P., S. Bascomb, W. R. Willcox, and M. A. Curtis.** 1973. Identification of bacteria by computer: general aspects and perspectives. J. Gen. Microbiol. **77:**273–290.
19. **Nungester, W. F.** 1963. Contributions of microbiology and immunology to medicine and some unfinished business. Tex. Rep. Biol. Med. **21:**315–330.
20. **Payne, L. C.** 1963. Towards medical automation. World Med. Electronics **2:**6–11.
21. **Rypka, E. W., and R. Babb.** 1970. Automatic construction and use of an identification scheme. Med. Res. Eng. **9:**9–19.
22. **Rypka, E. W., W. E. Clapper, I. G. Bowen, and R. Babb.** 1967. A model for the identification of bacteria. J. Gen. Microbiol. **46:**407–424.
23. **Schneierson, S. S., and D. Amsterdam.** 1964. A punch card system for identification of bacteria. Am. J. Clin. Pathol. **42:**328–331.
24. **Simpson, G. C.** 1961. Principles of animal taxonomy. Columbia University Press, New York.
25. **Sneath, P. H. A.** 1957. The application of computers to taxonomy. J. Gen. Microbiol. **17:**201–221.
26. **Sneath, P. H. A.** 1964. New approaches to bacterial taxonomy: use of computers. Annu. Rev. Microbiol. **18:**335–346.
27. **Sneath, P. H. A., and R. Johnson.** 1972. The influence on numerical taxonomic similarities of errors in microbiological tests. J. Gen. Microbiol. **72:**377–392.
28. **Steel, K. J.** 1962. The practice of bacterial identification. Symp. Soc. Gen. Microbiol. **12:**405–432.
29. **Willcox, W. R., S. P. Lapage, S. Bascomb, and M. A. Curtis.** 1973. Identification of bacteria by computer: theory and programming. J. Gen. Microbiol. **77:**317–330.

Chapter 19

Animal and Animal Cell Culture Systems

J. MICHAEL JANDA, EDWARD P. DESMOND, AND SHARON L. ABBOTT

Over the past two decades, it has become increasingly apparent to microbiologists that many clinically significant infectious agents would not have been identified without the aid of animals and animal cell culture systems. This is particularly true for many of the viral agents and specific biotypes of pathogenic bacteria associated with a variety of enteric infections. The use of cell culture systems has expanded from the simple detection of viruses in its infancy to providing the laboratory with powerful tools for the detection of toxigenic, invasive, and adherent bacteria. In addition, cell culture has in many instances supplanted the need to use animal models to detect certain by-products (heat-labile enterotoxins [LT]), although the latter system is still needed in the detection of heat-stable enterotoxins (ST) and to fulfill Koch's postulates regarding the pathogenicity of newly described agents. This chapter presents an overview of the use of animals and cell culture systems for identification of microbial agents of clinical significance.

SAFETY

Practices to prevent infection of laboratory personnel working with animals and cell cultures should follow general guidelines for avoiding the hazards of aerosol use, needle sticks, pipetting accidents, and other risks that are known to be responsible for laboratory infections. Because working with animals and preparing primary cell cultures have been shown to be frequent causes of laboratory-associated infection (36), special precautions must be followed in performing these activities (1, 37). When animals are infected with hazardous agents, a physically separate facility with separate ventilation must be used. Contaminated food, feces, urine, and bedding must be carefully handled and sterilized. Laboratory-issued outerwear must be used; the garments should be worn only within the animal facility and changed often. Because primates may have latent infections transmissible to humans, similar precautions in their handling are required. Cell cultures derived from animals pose potential hazards, since they may harbor unrecognized viruses (20). Even established (continuous) cell lines may pose a similar threat (4). For further information on biological safety, see chapter 7.

ESTABLISHING AND MAINTAINING CELL CULTURE SYSTEMS

Cultured cells can be categorized on the basis of source, karyotype, and multiplication potential. Primary cell cultures are started from tissues taken directly from a human or lower animal. Once primary cells have been subcultured sufficiently, they develop into a cell line. Cell lines can be classified as diploid (having the same chromosome number as the somatic cells of the species from which they are derived) or heteroploid (with an altered chromosome number). Human fetal diploid cell lines cannot be subcultivated indefinitely but tend to suffer a reduction in growth rate (and a loss of ability to propagate viral infection) after 20 to 50 passages (see the section below on quality control). Continuous cell lines are those that have demonstrated the ability to be subcultured indefinitely in vitro (38).

The most commonly used cell cultures are monolayer cultures, with a single layer of cells attached to the surface of the culture vessel. Some cell types (called anchorage independent) do not require attachment for growth; they will grow, with agitation, in suspension cultures in a liquid medium. To grow cells in suspension culture, levels of calcium and magnesium in the medium are reduced to inhibit attachment, and higher levels of nutrients and buffers are required to support the high cell densities that are attained. Most established cell lines have been grown in suspension culture; failures have been reported for monkey kidney cell lines and the human fetal diploid line WI-38 (29).

CELL CULTURE MEDIA

Cultured cells differ in medium requirements, but all require sugars, essential amino acids, vitamins, and usually choline and inositol. These are the ingredients of "minimal" media. The medium must also have an acceptable pH, maintained by a buffer system, and osmolarity and redox potential must also be kept within acceptable limits. Many cell types require macromolecular growth factors or have other, often unique requirements.

Serum is an effective supplement to cell culture media because it contains multiple growth-promoting factors such as hormones, peptide growth factors, trace elements, proteins that bind toxins, attachment factors, and protease inhibitors. Fetal calf serum is widely used because of a lack of immunoglobulins, which could interfere with many applications for cell culture. Serum as a medium supplement has the disadvantages that it is not a defined component and therefore can vary from batch to batch, contains a multitude of extraneous proteins, and has many times been reported to be a source of bacterial, fungal, mycoplasmal, and viral contaminants. Serum-free media have been developed for specific cell types after laborious studies of their requirements. The serum-free media, with minimal protein content, are especially useful for cell cultures that yield products such as monoclonal antibodies or hormones.

The most widely used buffering system for cell culture media is the CO_2-bicarbonate system. This system requires keeping culture vessels sealed or incubating them in a CO_2 incubator to prevent loss of CO_2 and resultant increase in pH to an inhibitory or toxic level. Organic buffers such as HEPES (*N*-2-hydroxyethlpiperazine-*N*′-2-ethanesulfonic acid) are also widely used, often together with bicarbonate for cell types that require the bicarbonate ion (38). Formulations of specific media are listed in chapter 121 for commonly used cell types.

The quality of water used in preparing cell culture media and additives is critically important. Sterile, pyrogen-free water prepared for intravenous use in humans has been found to be satisfactory for most applications, although expensive. Water that has been deionized and then triple distilled in glass will usually be satisfactory, particularly if it is sterilized soon after distillation to prevent growth of bacteria and formation of pyrogens. Conductivity checks should show a resistance of at least 10^6 ohms.

QUALITY CONTROL

A program of quality control for cell culture should include detection of contamination by infectious agents or other mammalian cell types. Antibiotics in cell culture media can greatly reduce the incidence of contamination of cell cultures by bacteria or fungi. However, mycoplasmas, viruses, and antibiotic-resistant bacteria and fungi can infect cell cultures, often without visible effect, and can profoundly affect the metabolism of cultured cells.

Mycoplasma infection of continuous cell cultures occurs with an incidence of approximately 15% (27). These organisms have major effects on the metabolism of cultured cells, often interfering with their intended functions of propagating viruses or producing antibodies. Mycoplasma contamination of a cell culture may cause a visible cytopathic effect (CPE) or even turbidity, but it often is insidious, producing little or no observable effect.

The most practical methods for detection of mycoplasmas in cell cultures are direct culture or a DNA fluorochrome stain such as Hoechst 33258 (H stain; Hoechst-Roussel Pharmaceuticals Inc., Somerville, N.J.). Culture is the most sensitive method, provided that optimal media and incubation conditions are used. The H stain is rapid and sensitive and detects mycoplasmas such as *Mycoplasma hyorhinis* that are difficult to culture.

Mycoplasmas may be cultured in broth or on solid media. A large-specimen broth culture method is recommended for testing liquid specimens such as bovine sera (3). Various media may be used, and some are commercially available (23, 26). A recent study of mycoplasma culture methods showed that a fortified commercial medium was superior to others tested (M. D. Gabridge and D. J. Lundin, Zentralbl. Bakteriol. Hyg. A, in press). This complex medium is not available commercially but can be prepared from commercially available ingredients (23). Duplicate aerobic and anaerobic cultures are recommended and incubated for 2 to 3 weeks. For further information on mycoplasma culturing, see chapter 47.

The DNA fluorochrome H stain can be used directly on cell culture or after inoculation of the test cells into an indicator cell culture such as Vero cells (27). For mycoplasma DNA staining, H stain is prepared as a 50-μg/ml stock solution in Hanks basal salt solution (BSS) without $NaHCO_3$ or phenol red. A working solution is prepared by making a 1:500 dilution of stock solution in 0.01 M phosphate-buffered saline (PBS), pH 7.3.

For examination of stained cells, a polyvinyl alcohol or buffered glycerol mounting medium is used with a fluorescence microscope equipped with exciter and barrier filters appropriate for this fluorochrome (and usually different from those used for immunofluorescence). Usable filter combinations are a BG-12 exciter filter with a Zeiss 50 barrier filter or a UG-1 or UG-5 exciter filter with a 41 or 47 barrier filter. Control slides are available commercially (Bionique Laboratories, Saranac Lake, N.Y.), eliminating the need for working with mycoplasma stock cultures. Laboratories that are unable to test their own cell lines for mycoplasmas can send cell culture samples to a commercial laboratory for testing.

Contamination of cell lines with other cell types is also a concern. Cultured cells can be characterized by extraction of enzymes and comparison of the electrophoretic mobilities of sets of isoenzymes (20, 35). Commercial kits for isoenzyme characterization of cell cultures are available from Innovative Chemistry, Inc., Marshfield, Mass.

Suppliers of bovine serum can be asked to provide a sample bottle of each lot before purchase. The sample can then be tested for bacteria, fungi, mycoplasma, and the ability to promote growth of cell cultures.

Analysis of the ability of cell lines to support propagation of various viruses is usually performed only when the cell line is established. No clear guidelines exist for the regular checking of established cell lines to verify their sensitivity to viruses. Exceptions include the use of HEp-2 cells for respiratory syncytial virus and use of human fetal diploid fibroblasts for cytomegalovirus, which show strain- and passage-dependent variability in sensitivity to the viruses (28). Laboratories purchasing commercial cell cultures may wish to check with their suppliers to determine whether regular tests of the sensitivity of their cells to viruses are performed.

Tubes, flasks, and pipettes used for cell culture must be new or very thoroughly rinsed in distilled water after washing in detergent, with at least two final rinses in ultrapure water. Steam for autoclaving must be free of impurities, and uncovered cotton stoppers should be avoided since they can leach toxic oils into the cell culture apparatus.

COMMONLY USED CELL CULTURE TYPES AND APPROPRIATE METHODS FOR PROPAGATION

Many types of cell culture can be propagated with a growth medium of 90% Eagle minimal essential medium (MEM) in Hanks BSS with 10% fetal bovine serum (FBS). For example, in Table 1, which lists cell culture types useful in clinical virology, all but lymphocytes and MDCK cells can be grown in this medium and maintained in Eagle MEM in Earle BSS with 2% FBS. The medium requirements for MDCK cells and lymphocytes are described below in the discussions of continuous cell lines and lymphocyte culture, respectively. Formulas for the growth and maintenance media mentioned above are included in chapter 121.

TABLE 1. Cell types useful in virus isolation

Cell type	Animal and tissue source	Primary, diploid, or continuous	Useful for isolation of[a]:
Human fetal diploid fibroblast (e.g., WI-38 or MRC-5)	Human kidney, lung, foreskin, etc.	Diploid	HSV, CMV, VZ, entero, rhino, RSV, adeno
Primary monkey kidney	Rhesus or cynomolgus monkey kidney	Primary	Entero, influenza, parainfluenza, RSV, measles, mumps
African green monkey kidney	Monkey kidney	Primary	Rubella
BGMK	Monkey kidney	Continuous	Entero
HeLa	Human	Continuous	HSV, RSV, adeno
HEp-2	Human	Continuous	RSV, adeno
Human embryonic kidney	Human kidney	Primary	Adeno
MDCK	Canine kidney	Continuous	Influenza
Peipheral blood lymphocyte	Human lymphocyte	Primary	HIV
Primary rabbit kidney	Rabbit kidney	Primary	HSV
RD	Human rhabdomyosarcoma	Continuous	Entero
RK-13	Rabbit kidney	Continuous	Rubella
Vero	Monkey kidney	Continuous	Rubella

[a] adeno, Adenovirus; CMV, cytomegalovirus; entero, enteroviruses; HIV, human immunodeficiency virus; HSV, herpes simplex virus; rhino, rhinovirus; VZ, varicella-zoster virus; RSV, respiratory syncytial virus.

For subcultivation of a cell culture, confluent monolayers are removed from the cell culture vessel and dispersed by trypsinization. A trypsin-EDTA mixture with 0.5 g of trypsin (1:250) and 0.2 g of EDTA per liter in PBS may be used. This trypsin-EDTA mixture can be purchased at use dilution or made up as a 10× stock solution, divided into smaller samples, and frozen (38). For trypsinization, the cell culture medium is removed and replaced with enough of the trypsin-EDTA mixture to cover the cell sheet. After a brief period of contact with the cell sheet (30 s to 5 min, depending on cell type), all but a few drops of the trypsin-EDTA is removed, and the cells are incubated at 37°C until microscopic examination shows that they are dislodged and pulled apart. The cells are then suspended in an appropriate volume of growth medium for a 1:2 split and incubated at 37°C in a closed container or CO_2 incubator. If the cell sheet is not confluent after 2 days, the growth medium should be replaced with fresh growth medium. After confluency is reached, the growth medium is replaced with maintenance medium.

Primary monkey kidney cells

The preparation of primary monkey kidney cells from fresh tissue has been described elsewhere (5, 38). The cells may be maintained with the 98% Eagle MEM in Earle BSS with 2% FBS.

McCoy cells

McCoy cells are often used for culture of chlamydia in shell vials that enable the specimen to be centrifuged onto the cell sheet. Shell vials are prepared by trypsinizing a confluent monolayer of McCoy cells in a flask with trypsin-EDTA (see above). The trypsinized cells are suspended to a concentration of 1.25×10^5 to 2.5×10^5 cells per ml in a modified Eagle MEM (42). Cell concentrations can be determined by counting well-dispersed cells with a standard hemacytometer. The cells in 10 large squares are counted, and the sums are multiplied by 1,000 to give the number of cells per milliliter. One-dram shell vials are seeded with 1 ml of the cell suspension and incubated at 35°C. Confluency should be reached within 1 to 3 days (41). For passaging McCoy cells to 75-cm^2 flasks, approximately 2.5×10^6 to 5×10^6 cells should be suspended in 20 ml of growth medium and seeded into each flask.

Continuous cell lines

Many types of continuous cell lines can be propagated by using the growth and maintenance media described above. Others have been found to grow better with more complex media. For example, Y1 adrenal cells grow well in RPMI 1640 medium with added L-glutamine and antibiotics, CHO cells are grown in a 1:1 mixture of Ham F12 medium and medium 199 with antibiotics and 10% FBS, and MDCK cells are grown in Dulbecco modified Eagle MEM with 10% FBS.

Split ratios vary with the cell type, medium used, passage level, and other variables. Some experimentation may be required to determine the inoculation size and split ratios in each laboratory. A first approximation is made by suspending trypsinized cells to a density of approximately 10^5/ml in growth medium and seeding 1 ml into a 16- by 125-mm tube or 20 ml into a 75-cm^2 flask.

Lymphocyte culture

Cultured human lymphocytes are required for the isolation of retroviruses and for the production of retrovirus antigens and nucleic acids. Lymphocytes may be obtained from the buffy coat of centrifuged, freshly collected blood. They are banded on a Ficoll-Hypaque gradient by centrifugation.

Lymphocytes will not divide in cell culture unless stimulated by an antigen or mitogen such as phytohemagglutinin and grown in the presence of interleukin-2. Media and procedures for lymphocyte cultures have been described elsewhere (2, 25).

Cryopreservation of cell cultures

Cultured cells may be preserved in the frozen state if they are treated with a cryoprotective agent such as dimethyl sulfoxide and cooled slowly to allow water to migrate out of the cells. Trypsinized cells are suspended in a freezing medium consisting of the growth medium for the cell type, along with 10% FBS and 10% dimethyl sulfoxide. The cell suspension is then apportioned into vials that can be sealed airtight. A slow rate of freezing can be achieved by placing the vials in a styrofoam box at −70°C for 2 to 3 h. The vials are then rapidly transferred into canes and stored in liquid nitrogen. Cells may be preserved at −70°C for shorter periods of time.

When vials frozen in liquid nitrogen are thawed, there is a danger of explosion if liquid nitrogen has leaked into the vials. A face shield and protective gloves must be worn, and the vial should be placed in 37°C water in a covered pan to bring about the rapid thawing that is important in protecting the frozen cells. After thawing, the cells are suspended in an appropriate volume of growth medium and planted into cell culture vessels (7, 38).

CELL CULTURE SYSTEMS IN VIROLOGY

Table 1 shows the cell types most useful in the detection and propagation of viruses. Note that a dual cell culture system of primary monkey kidney and human fetal diploid fibroblast cells will be sensitive to a broad range of viruses. The chapters in section VII discuss optimal cell cultures for the various viruses.

Once a cell culture has been inoculated with a patient specimen, viruses can be detected by the development of visible CPE in cells infected by viruses that produce such effects. The appearance of the CPE and its timing will often give a clue to the identity of the infecting virus. Other methods for detecting and characterizing viruses in cell culture include:

1. Hemadsorption. Because of incorporation of viral hemagglutinins into the cell membrane, infected cells may be detected by adsorption of erythrocytes from various animal species.
2. Immunofluorescence and immunoperoxidase. Viral antigens may be detected in infected cells by the use of specific antibodies conjugated to fluorescein, horseradish peroxidase, or other compounds. Viral antigens may be detectable well before any visible CPE.
3. Nucleic acid probes. Viral nucleic acids may be detected by specific probes; several with radioactive or enzymatic labeling are available commercially.
4. Reverse transcriptase assay. Retroviruses growing in lymphocyte culture may be detected by means of their unique RNA-dependent DNA polymerase activity.

DETECTION OF BACTERIAL TOXINS

For purposes of this section, discussion of animal and cell culture assays is limited to bacterial exotoxins that are involved in human diarrheal disease and produced in the intestine after bacterial ingestion. Diarrheal exotoxins (products released during growth or at cell death that cause damage to or malfunction of host tissues) are listed in Table 2, along with bacteria known to produce toxins and assays used in their detection. LT and ST cause disease by stimulating natural biochemical processes of the host cell but cause little or no damage to the tissue. The other two toxin groups, however, bring about host cell death, cytotoxins by inhibiting cellular functions, notably protein synthesis, and cytolysins by damaging and lysing the host cell membrane. A toxin may be clearly, although not necessarily solely, responsible for disease production (i.e., *Vibrio cholerae* toxin). Conversely, the exact role of a toxin in pathogenesis may be unclear and therefore controversial; however, such toxins merit consideration since they are produced in vitro by a variety of disease-causing bacteria.

The discovery of diarrheal toxins and much of our subsequent knowledge of them are due in large part to the development of animal models and subsequently cell culture assays. Although quicker methods are available today, the biological activity of toxins or of the strains possessing toxin determinants can still be established only by tests using animals or cell culture cell lines. Before proceeding to a discussion of assays used to detect diarrheal toxins, it is appropriate to consider in vitro toxin production in bacterial culture supernatants, since it not only is a common feature of many tests but also is of primary concern.

To prepare test samples, bacteria are grown in one of several media, most commonly Casamino Acids (Difco Laboratories, Detroit, Mich.)-yeast extract (13) or syncase (15) broth; Penassay, tryptic soy (with or without 0.5% yeast extract), and brain heart infusion broths are also used. Although sometimes recommended, use of iron-depleted media for Shiga and Shiga-

TABLE 2. Selected bacterial toxins involved in diarrheal disease

Toxin	Implicated bacteria	Assay system[a]	Morphologic or biologic effect
Enterotoxin			
Heat labile	*V. cholerae* O1, non-O1, *V. mimicus*, *E. coli*	Y1 CHO RIL	Cytotonic rounding Cell elongation Fluid accumulation
Heat stable	*E. coli*, *Y. enterocolitica*, *Campylobacter* spp.	SM, RIL	Fluid accumulation
Cytotoxin	*Shigella* spp. *Clostridium difficile* *E. coli* (O157:H7)	Vero, HeLa Vero, CHO Vero, HeLa	Cell death, primarily without overt lysis
Cytolysin	Many species	HEp-2, HeLa	Cell death with lysis

[a] Y1, Y1 adrenal cells; CHO, Chinese hamster ovary cells; RIL, rabbit ileal loop; SM, suckling mice.

like toxins is not necessary for the high-level toxin-producing strains involved in disease. Aeration during incubation either is required for most toxins or gives increased yields; exceptions are *V. cholerae* El Tor strains, which produce increased levels of toxin in stationary cultures, and non-O1 *V. cholerae*, for which aeration appears to make little difference. Roller drums are best for aeration; however, rotary shakers are acceptable. Enterotoxin production in *V. cholerae*, both O1 and non-O1 strains, and in *Escherichia coli* is stimulated in culture broths supplemented with 300 μg of lincomycin per ml; however, many strains must be adapted to grow at that concentration of antibiotic. Cell-bound toxins of *E. coli* and shigellae may be released from periplasmic spaces by incubating pelleted cells in 0.1 mg of polymyxin B per ml for 30 min. Peak toxin production varies with the toxin, but generally incubation at 37°C for 18 h (cells in late log or stationary phase) works well. To prepare test samples, aliquots or bacterial cultures are centrifuged at 750 × *g* and the supernatants are filtered through 0.22- or 0.45-μm-pore-size filters. Filtrates ideally should be tested immediately, but they may be held refrigerated for several days or at −70°C for several weeks.

LT

Cholera toxin (CT) and several closely related *E. coli* LT similar in structure and mode of action to CT are clearly incriminated in diarrheal disease. CT and LT are high-molecular-weight proteins that are heat labile at 56°C for 30 min. Both CT and LT stimulate adenylate cyclase, leading to elevated cyclic AMP levels. Because host tissue remains intact and viable, CT and LT are considered cytotonic toxins.

No definite role in pathogenesis has yet been attributed to the cytotonic enterotoxins produced by *Vibrio*, *Aeromonas*, and *Salmonella* spp., nor have they been isolated in sufficient quantity or purity to allow determination of their structures. However, all are heat labile and act similarly to CT in animal or tissue culture assays.

The rabbit ileal loop (RIL [10]) test was the first assay developed to implicate *V. cholerae* or its toxic properties in disease; subsequently, it has been used to detect a wide variety of toxins. Filtrates or live organisms can be used as inoculum. For viable cells, doses range from 10^3 to 10^8; for filtrates or filtrate dilutions (1:2 to 1:256 in PBS), 0.5 ml per loop is used. Rabbits (2 to 2.5 kg), given access to water, are fasted for 48 h before being anesthetized. After laparotomy, the small intestine is ligated into 6- to 10-cm loops separated by 2-cm segments. First and last loops are not used, and occasionally only one test loop plus a blank and a positive control are used per rabbit. Animals are sutured and held 16 to 18 h to allow for the delayed onset of CT and LT activity before being sacrificed. Fluid accumulation ratios are based on fluid volume (in milliliters) per loop length (in centimeters). Values of ≥1.0 are positive, and values of ≤0.3 are negative; results in between are equivocal, and the test should be repeated. Positive, negative, and broth controls should be included for each rabbit, and every sample should be tested in two rabbits. Results from rabbits with inappropriate control responses should be discarded.

Other animal models include the infant rabbit assay, in which 16-day-old rabbits are inoculated intraintestinally with viable organisms and checked for diarrhea or death. The RITARD (removable intestinal tie-adult rabbit diarrhea) model is a variation of the RIL test that allows colonization by challenge organisms. The adult sealed mouse assay uses mice anorectally occluded with cyanoacrylamide ester glue to prevent fluid loss after oral inoculation with organisms or filtrates. In the ligated rat enterotoxin model, perfusion studies are performed by using filtrates.

Two nonintestinal cell lines, Y1 (a clone of a mouse adrenal tumor line) and CHO, have been used to elucidate the mechanism of action of LT and are still extensively employed in detection of these toxins. Both cell lines demonstrate morphologic changes in the presence of increased cyclic AMP, and assays using them have greater sensitivities for CT and LT than does the RIL test, detecting toxin levels as low as 5 pg as opposed to approximately 30 ng.

In the Y1 adrenal cell assay (12), CT and LT induce a morphologic change in the cell from flat to spherical. They also cause a steroidogenic effect, which is an increased production and secretion of steroids that can be quantitated and used to determine CT or LT activity. Maneval et al. (24) have published a standardized method for the Y1 assay. All incubations involving monolayers are at 37°C in 5% CO_2. Y1 cells (approximately 10^5 per well in flat-bottom, 96-well microdilution plates) are grown in RPMI 1640 medium with 10% FBS to 80% confluency in 24 h. Nonspecific rounding of 5% or less of cells is acceptable; greater rounding confuses reading of results. Twofold dilutions (1:2 to 1:256; final volume, 50 μl) of test and of positive and negative control filtrates are made in RPMI medium in an empty 96-well plate. Diluent and culture media (50 μl each) are included as controls. RPMI 1640 medium is aspirated from the cells by using a multichannel pipetter, and diluted filtrates and controls are transferred to the Y1 monolayers. Filtrates are removed after a 5-min incubation and replaced with 0.2 ml of fresh RPMI, and the monolayers are reincubated. After 24 h, Y1 cells are examined under an inverted phase-contrast scope for a refractile, spherical shape indicating CT or LT activity. To confirm the results, toxin-positive filtrates should be retested in the presence of cholera antitoxin (commercially available), GM_1 ganglioside, or choleragenoid, any of which will neutralize the toxigenic effects. Bacterial cytolysins such as hemolysins produce a CPE that may be mistaken for, or mask the effect of, CT or LT. Adding protease inhibitors to culture broths, checking Y1 cells for exclusion of trypan blue, a vital dye, or retesting toxins on cell lines that lack steroidogenic and cyclic AMP elevation responses (HeLa or HEp-2; human carcinoma) can be used to distinguish between cytotonic and cytolytic reactions.

In the CHO assay (19), after exposure to CT or LT, the CHO cell exhibits a distinctive elongation approximately three times that of a normal cell in response to increased cyclic AMP levels. By using Ham F12 medium with 10% FBS, trypsinized suspensions of cells (10^3/ml) are mixed with twofold dilutions of filtrates (final concentrations of 1:2 to 1:256), and 0.20 ml is delivered into a 96-well tissue culture plate. Monolayers are incubated at 37°C in 5% CO_2 and read at 24 h.

V. cholerae 569B (serotype INABA, biotype classical) and *E. coli* H10407 (serotype O78:H11) are used as positive controls for CT and LT, respectively.

Cytotonic enterotoxin production may be demonstrated by using B16 murine melanoma cells. The presence of toxin is determined by increased tyrosinase activity and accumulation of melanin in the B16 cells.

ST

ST are small peptides that withstand temperatures up to 100°C. They are produced by a variety of bacteria, most notably *E. coli*, in which there are two recognized types (however, since it is not involved in human disease, STb, or ST II, is not discussed). *E. coli* STa (or ST I) attaches to and stimulates a host membrane receptor protein that increases guanylate cyclase activity, resulting in elevated cyclic GMP levels and ultimately fluid loss.

The suckling mouse assay (11) specifically detects ST. It is reproducible and less cumbersome than the RIL test.

Four 1- to 4-day-old mice, not taken from the same litter, are used per filtrate. Since the mice are injected intragastrically, using a syringe and 27-gauge needle, they are removed from their mothers just before inoculation to ensure the presence of milk in their stomachs, which serves both to stretch the stomach taut and to make a clearly visible target. Each mouse receives 0.1 ml of toxin filtrate. To determine whether the stomach was injected, filtrates contain 1 drop of 2% Evans blue dye per ml. Mice are held for 4 h and then euthanized with CO_2 (dry ice) or ether. Intestines (not including the stomach) in one group of mice are removed, pooled, and weighed, as are the four carcasses. Mice with white stomachs or blue liquid in the peritoneal cavity were not properly injected and should be discarded. Gut-to-body-weight ratios of $\geq$0.08 are generally considered positive.

ST also give a fluid response in the RIL assay and are tested as for LT except that rabbits are sacrificed at 4 h to detect the rapid onset of fluid accumulation. Rat intestinal loops can also be used to test for ST. *E. coli* H10407 (ST^+ LT^+) is used as a positive control. Unfortunately, ST are not active in any tissue culture assay.

Cytotoxins

The Shiga toxin of shigellae, Shiga-like toxins (SLT) or verocytotoxins of *E. coli*, and toxins A and B of *Clostridium difficile* are all cytotoxins associated with disease. *Campylobacter* and *Salmonella* spp. also produce toxins with cytotoxic activity; however, the roles of these toxins have not been defined. Like CT or LT, the cytotoxins of shigellae and *E. coli* must traverse the cell membrane; they are, however, released intracellularly only after endocytosis of the bacterial cell into the host tissue. *E. coli* produces two cytotoxins (SLT I and II) involved in human disease and a third, porcine toxin similar or identical to SLT II, which will not be discussed. *E. coli* strains may produce either or both SLT I and II; SLT I alone is more common, but SLT II is a more active toxin. Both Shiga and Shiga-like toxins inactivate the 60S ribosomal subunits of ribosomes, terminating protein synthesis.

Shiga and Shiga-like toxin activity is restricted to cell lines of primate or human origin. HeLa or Vero (monkey kidney) cell lines, susceptible to exogenous toxin, have been used to elucidate mode of action, whereas Henle (human intestine) 407 or CHO cells, resistant to exogenous toxin, probably more closely resemble the action of these toxins in vivo.

For the Vero cell assay (21), monolayers are grown in medium 199E with 5% FBS or MEM with 10% FBS in flat-bottom, 96-well microdilution plates and incubated for 48 h in 5% CO_2 at 37°C. Then 50-µl volumes of twofold serial dilutions of test and of positive and negative control filtrates are added to 200 µl of medium 199E on the cell sheets; an uninoculated well and a well containing 50 µl of bacterial culture medium serve as controls. Monolayers are reincubated and read daily for 3 days for CPE (detached, floating cells). Polymyxin B-extracted filtrates are used to release cell-bound toxin. For screening, "sweeps" of colonies from isolation plates should be tested as for single colonies, since numbers of SLT-positive *E. coli* in a specimen may be too low to detect by random picking. To determine the presence of free SLT in feces, equal volumes of feces and PBS are vigorously vortexed, centrifuged, filtered, and tested as for cultures. CPE should be confirmed by neutralization, using specific antitoxin (not commercially available) to shiga toxin or SLT I and II. Karmali (21) has used convalescent patient serum mixed in equal volumes with filtrate and preincubated for 45 min before inoculation onto monolayers. Shiga antitoxin will neutralize SLT I but not SLT II; SLT I and II will not cross-neutralize one another. Retesting positive filtrates in a mutant Vero cell line specifically resistant to Shiga and Shiga-like toxins may be an additional method of confirmation.

Animal models that will detect SLT include RIL, rhesus monkey, and the infant rabbit. The RIL may be inoculated with filtrates or organisms; for the other assays, oral inoculation of organisms is used. *E. coli* H30 (serotype O26) can be used as a positive control.

Toxins A and B of *C. difficile* have been implicated in antibiotic-associated pseudomembranous colitis. In ligated RILs, toxin A causes bloody fluid secretion; in colonic loops, it causes a nonbloody, watery fluid accumulation. Toxin B exhibits little effect in animal assays except to act synergistically with toxin A after toxin A-induced trauma.

Both toxins are cytotoxic for a wide variety of cell lines (6). Toxin B is cytopathic in picogram amounts to all types of tissue culture cells from any species. Cell lines already present in the laboratory for detection of other toxins, such as Vero or CHO, are frequently used.

Toxin may be detected directly from stools by mixing equal volumes of stool and PBS and preparing specimens as for SLT. Monolayers of Vero cells in MEM with 10% FBS are grown to 10^3 cells per well in 24 multiwell tissue culture plates and incubated in 5% CO_2 at 37°C. Twofold dilutions of filtrate (final concentration, 1:100 to 1:2,000) are added to the cells, and the plate is reincubated. Cells are examined for rounding at 24 and 48 h under an inverted phase-contrast scope. Some cell lines will exhibit cytoplasmic projections or radiating processes as well as rounding. CPE should be neutralized by *Clostridium sordelii* antitoxin (commercially available). Preparation of crude filtrates from organisms requires $(NH_4)_2SO_4$ precipitation or passage through columns.

Cytolysins

Cytolysins are proteins that are active in many animal and cell culture assays and cause nonspecific fluid accumulation and cell death. They are commonly inactivated by heating at 56°C for 30 min and by glycophorin. *Aeromonas* and *Vibrio* spp. frequently produce such cytolysins, some of which have been shown to have enterotoxic activity.

ADHESION ASSAYS

Methods for studying the potential role of attachment structures or factors in the colonization of epithelial cell surfaces by gram-negative bacteria have been established for a number of years. Recently, however, these assays have taken on a new diagnostic significance, since recent investigations have shown that under specific conditions newly identified groups of diarrheagenic *E. coli* can be recognized by using cell culture methods; these adhesion assays now provide laboratories with a workable test that can screen for such agents in cases for which no satisfactory technique was formerly available.

In 1979, Cravioto and colleagues (8) described an HEp-2 adhesion assay that could detect members of the enteropathogenic *E. coli* group, previously recognized only by their specific serotypes and their association with sporadic cases and outbreaks of infantile gastroenteritis. Subsequent studies revealed that at least three distinct adherence patterns detectable on HEp-2 cells (localized, aggregative, and diffuse adherence) have been associated with potential diarrheagenic *E. coli* (33). For the first two patterns (localized and aggregative), strong epidemiologic data link these strains with gastroenteritis episodes in case-controlled studies.

Adhesion assays to detect such bacteria can be performed with either HEp-2 or HeLa cells. Generally, strains to be studied are grown overnight at 37°C in a tryptone-water broth containing 1% D-mannose to inhibit type 1 pili; other reported media suitable for similar purposes include L and tryptic soy broths. After overnight incubation, either small inocula (20 to 40 μl) of the original bacterial suspension or appropriate dilutions of that material in cell culture medium (without antibiotics) are added to the monolayer to initiate attachment. Although the confluency of monolayers varies among studies, cell concentrations covering between 25 and 50% of the surface area facilitate determinations of adherence patterns of individual cells. After appropriate incubation periods (3 to 6 h), cell monolayers are washed to remove unattached bacteria and are then fixed and stained. Stained slides are observed microscopically for the characteristic adherence pattern. Criteria used to determine such patterns include at least 40% of the cells displaying the definition adherence characteristic, with some isolates noted to simultaneously exhibit multiple adherence patterns (diffuse and localized). As always, known positive and negative control strains should be included in each run. Nonadherent strains normally attach to less than 10% of the monolayer cells. Finally, strains exhibiting a localized adherence pattern should be serotyped to determine whether they fall into traditionally recognized serogroups of enteropathogenic *E. coli,* since other isolates tested that are not associated with gastroenteritis (such as urinary isolates) may occasionally (15 to 30%) attach to HEp-2 cells also.

DETECTION OF INVASIVE BACTERIA

The ability of certain gram-negative microorganisms to penetrate and replicate in a variety of eucaryotic cells and subsequently infect surrounding host tissues, producing an observable pathologic effect, has been a recognized virulence trait of many pathogenic bacteria for a number of years (17). Bacteria possessing such invasive capabilities are referred to as containing invasion genes or determinants responsible for cell penetration; these genes may be chromosomally located or of plasmid origin. In some instances, particularly in the case of *Shigella* and *Yersinia* spp., multiple loci harboring invasion genes may be involved. In general, invasion of host cells by bacteria is an endocytic process (particle activated, cytochalasin sensitive); the molecular mechanisms and cellular processes involved in bacterial invasion are poorly understood (17, 18, 44).

Diagnostically, invasion assays have typically been used for several purposes: (i) to identify organisms capable of causing dysentery that cannot easily be detected by other conventional procedures (e.g., enteroinvasive *E. coli* [EIEC]); (ii) to assess the relative virulence of a given strain or species; (iii) to functionally confirm the presence of invasion genes that have been identified by some other method such as probe analysis; and (iv) as a clinical research tool to identify potentially new agents associated with unexplained cases of bloody diarrhea or colitis. Such invasive bacteria can be detected by a variety of techniques, including cell culture assays and animal models; each system has some inherent advantages and disadvantages.

The use of cell culture systems to screen for invasive bacteria is a widely used technology in reference, public health, and large clinical microbiology laboratories. The most common clinical use for this procedure is to screen relevant phenotypes of *E. coli* (lysine decarboxylase negative, motility negative) that resemble *Shigella* spp. for invasive characteristics, since studies have shown that only 50% of such strains will actually be confirmed as being EIEC (43). Most cell culture invasion assays have been performed with either HEp-2 (epidermoid carcinoma, larynx, human) or HeLa (epithelioid carcinoma, cervix, human) cell monolayers. However, other eucaryotic host cells, including Vero (African green monkey kidney), CHO (hamster ovary), and MDCK (canine kidney), can also be used in such tests; some of these lines have distinct advantages, such as enhanced resistance to the effects of bacterial cytotoxins or cytolysins or greater permissiveness to microbial invasion by a single species. However, they usually have counterbalancing disadvantages such as a decreased rate of penetration by most other invasive genera (16). Cell lines chosen for invasion studies can be propagated in a number of suitable vessels, including Leighton tubes (Costar, Cambridge, Mass.), cover slips placed in 24-well tissue culture plates, or chamber slides (Miles Scientific, Div. Miles Laboratories, Inc., Naperville, Ill.); the choice of a software system to screen for invasive organisms is usually based on reagent cost, number of strains to be screened, purpose and frequency of test to be performed, and number of manipulations and technical expertise required for each system.

Cell culture invasion assays are normally performed by growing the appropriate host cell in culture medium supplemented with serum and antibiotics in a CO_2 atmosphere; 24 h before infection, the cell culture medium is removed and replaced with growth medium lacking antibiotics. This step is important, since residual antimicrobial agents could affect the outcome of invasion assays by exerting inhibitory effects on the challenge organism. When monolayers are ready for invasion studies (semiconfluent to confluent), overnight broth-grown cultures of individual strains to be tested are appropriately diluted in cell culture medium (without antibiotics) such that the challenge inoculum ranges from 10^5 to 10^8 CFU, depending on the species to be evaluated and the type and size of cell culture apparatus used; prewashed monolayers are then challenged with the test strain, usually for 1 to 2 h at 35°C under CO_2. Once the infection process has ended, the residual inoculum is removed and the monolayer is extensively washed with PBS to remove as many adherent (but not invaded) bacteria as possible. After the postinfection washes, cell culture medium is placed on the cell sheet, which contains high concentrations (40 to 100 μg/ml) of an aminoglycoside (usually gentamicin); this solution may also contain lysozyme at a concentration of 300 μg/ml. The addition of an aminoglycoside to the cell culture medium effectively kills any external bacteria that were not removed by the PBS washes; since aminoglycosides cannot penetrate eucaryotic cell membranes, invasive bacteria that have penetrated the host cell are protected from its bactericidal effects. During this period (replication phase), which usually lasts 1 to 4 h, organisms that have penetrated host cells have the opportunity to replicate and multiply within the eucaryotic cytoplasm. When the replication period is over, monolayers are again washed with PBS before fixation (methanol) and staining (Giemsa) for direct microscopic observation; alternatively, cell sheets can be lysed to release invasive bacteria, which can be enumerated either qualitatively or quantitatively.

Criteria used to determine whether a given strain is truly invasive are somewhat arbitrary, and determinations can be based on either cytologic evidence of cellular penetration or qualitative or quantitative data on the number of gentamicin-resistant progeny recoverable after the replication period. Many studies cite the early investigations by Labrec et al. (22) on *Shigella flexneri* 2a and Mehlman and collaborators (30) on EIEC as guidelines for establishing such standards. Regardless of the criteria chosen, known positive (invasive) and negative (noninvasive) controls should be included with each run; strains of *Shigella* spp. or EIEC are excellent for the former purpose, and *E. coli* HB101 is a good choice for a noninvasive strain. In assessing cytologic evidence for invasion, Mehlman et al. (30) initially suggested that at least 1% of the cells in two of three independent trials contain five or more internalized bacteria. However, care should be exercised in using such values as the only evidence for invasion, since hydrophobic strains may stick to and be superimposed over host cells, thereby giving the untrained observer the appearance of invasiveness. This problem can be partially circumvented by ensuring that the bacteria and the nucleolus or cytoplasm are in the same focal plane. Another problem that can arise concerns the screening of hemolytic or cytotoxin-producing strains for invasive characteristics. In many instances, the toxic effects of these isolates completely destroy host cell monolayers before invasive properties can be properly studied. This problem can sometimes be circumvented by choosing cell lines for invasion assays that are relatively toxin resistant, by extensively washing the bacterial culture to remove residual toxin, or by adjusting the challenge concentration of the test strain.

Under microscopic observation, invaded cells usually exhibit large arrays of bacteria within the cytoplasm or nucleus (Fig. 1). Bacteria can often be seen arranged in parallel rows of replicating microorganisms within invaded cells; sometimes these numbers are so large that the cytoplasm is completely obliterated by internalized bacteria. Another cytologic approach to confirming the invasive nature of a given strain is to stain unfixed monolayers with acridine orange and then counterstain them with crystal violet (31). Cells stained in this manner can be observed under UV light for green fluorescing (viable) internalized bacteria as opposed to red (nonviable) cells. If a laboratory has the availability of Nomarski optics (differential interference contrast microscopy), internalized bacteria can readily be distinguished from adherent organisms overlying the cell surface. Finally, monolayers can be appropriately fixed, stained, and thin sectioned for transmission electron microscopy; invaded (internalized) bacteria can then be observed within the bacterial cytoplasm often enclosed in an endocytic vacuole.

Besides cytologic studies, the invasive characteristics of a given strain can be determined through semiquantitative or quantitative assays by taking advantage of the fact that invasive bacteria are protected from the deleterious effects of aminoglycosides that are added during the replication period (14). To assess the relative number of viable aminoglycoside-resistant progeny, a sample of the cell-free supernatant containing gentamicin is plated at the end of the replication period (control), after which the monolayer is washed and then lysed with a mild detergent to release internalized and replicated bacteria into the external environment, which is now devoid of antibiotics. Typical lysing agents used for this purpose include Triton X-100, deoxycholate, Tween 20, and *N*-laurylsarcosine, usually applied in final concentrations ranging between 0.5 and 1.0%. By lysing infected cells for a brief period (ca. 5 min), released bacteria can be recovered and appropriately diluted in PBS for plate counts; the number of CFU of gentamicin-resistant bacteria recovered in such a manner can then be expressed as a percentage of the initial

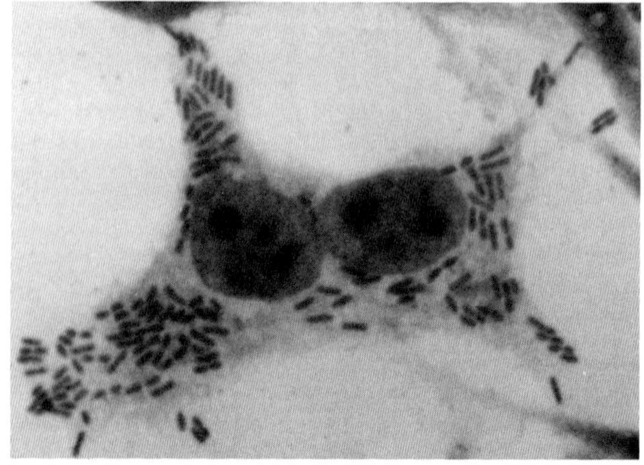

FIG. 1. Penetration of HEp-2 cells by EIEC.

standardized inoculum. Besides plate counts, certain bacterial isolates, such as *Shigella* spp., can be evaluated for invasion by plaque assays, performed as in diagnostic virology laboratories (34). At appropriate ratios of inoculum to host cells, virulent shigellae will infect monolayers, multiply, and then reinfect surrounding uninfected cells. When an overlay medium containing agarose is added to the maintenance medium, plaques result instead of complete monolayer destruction. This assay, while suitable for *Shigella* spp. because of their specific invasion and replication strategy, is not applicable for all invasive bacteria, and the procedure requires longer incubation periods and more media components than do other assays. Under ideal conditions, at least one cytologic and one quantitative assay should be performed in any studies investigating the invasive potential of any microbial species.

In the mid-1950s, Sereny described in a series of articles an animal model that faithfully reproduced the pathomorphologic lesions observed clinically associated with bacillary dysentery (39, 40). The model, termed the keratoconjunctivitis assay (also known as the Sereny test), involves the inoculation of small volumes (20 μl) of a dense bacterial suspension (10^8 to 10^9 CFU/ml) into the conjunctival sac of a guinea pig. When *Shigella* or *Shigella*-like (EIEC) organisms are introduced in such a manner into test animals, a fulminant keratoconjunctivitis ensues within 72 h postinoculation, characterized sequentially by edema, a mucopurulent exudate, and eventually inflammation of the cornea. Invading shigellae in these latter stages can be found multiplying within the corneal epithelium to produce this macroscopic effect. Although the keratoconjunctivitis will spontaneously heal with time (weeks), some pathologic effects (edema or corneal opacity) may ultimately remain as a consequence of the infection.

The classical Sereny test can be performed by using either guinea pigs or rabbits as the animal model; as always, known positive and negative controls should be included with each run. Recently, Murayama and others (32) have demonstrated that mice can also be used for this purpose, although macroscopic changes are not as pronounced as with the guinea pig and were more transient (disappearing within 3 to 7 days). Although the results of Sereny tests performed with rabbits or guinea pigs are typically easy to score, the cost of such animals, including the appropriate care and feeding, prohibits their use under most circumstances. Studies indicate that Sereny-positive organisms are almost invariably positive in HEp-2 or HeLa cell penetration assays (9); however, the converse statement is not true, since many bacteria that penetrate and replicate in eucaryotic cells fail to elicit keratoconjunctivitis in the appropriate animal model. Organisms included in this latter group are members of the genus *Salmonella* and some pathogenic serogroups of *Yersinia enterocolitica*.

The use of animals and animal cell culture systems has expanded over the past 30 to 40 years to take a preeminent place in large clinical or reference laboratories for the detection of infectious agents. Through improved methodologies for the maintenance, growth, and culture of animal cells, numerous cell lines have now been established, providing the microbiologist with an array of cell types to use in a variety of assays. Advances will continue to occur, since recent studies indicate that potentially new enteropathogenic groups of *E. coli*, *Citrobacter freundii*, and *Klebsiella oxytoca* may have been identified by using both cell culture and animal models. Besides the uses of animal models cited within this chapter, animals are continuing to be used on a research basis to establish relevant models for the study of meningitis, osteomyelitis, anaerobic abscesses, and wound infections. Studies using such systems not only will provide necessary information regarding the pathogenesis of specific groups of microbial agents but also will lead to development of methods for successful chemotherapeutic regimens for resolution of such infections and for eventual vaccine development. It therefore appears that the use of animal and animal cell culture systems in clinical microbiology will continue to benefit the field for the foreseeable future.

LITERATURE CITED

1. **Anonymous.** 1985. Guide for the care and use of laboratory animals. NIH publication no. 86-23. National Institutes of Health, Bethesda, Md.
2. **Ascher, M. S., D. Gallo, and D. P. Francis.** 1989. Human retroviruses, p. 1113–1139. *In* N. J. Schmidt and R. W. Emmons (ed.), Diagnostic procedures for viral, rickettsial, and chlamydial infections, 6th ed. American Public Health Association, Inc., Washington, D.C.
3. **Barile, M. F.** 1973. Mycoplasma contamination of cell cultures: mycoplasma-virus-cell interactions, p. 131–172. *In* J. Fogh (ed.), Contamination in tissue culture. Academic Press, Inc., New York.
4. **Barkley, W. E.** 1979. Safety considerations in the cell culture laboratory. Methods Enzymol. **58:**36–43.
5. **Bashor, M. M.** 1979. Dispersion and disruption of tissues. Methods Enzymol. **58:**119–131.
6. **Chang, T., M. Lauermann, and J. G. Bartlett.** 1979. Cytotoxicity assay in antibiotic-associated colitis. J. Infect. Dis. **140:**765–770.
7. **Coriell, L. L.** 1979. Preservation, storage, and shipment. Methods Enzymol. **58:**29–36.
8. **Cravioto, A., R. J. Gross, S. M. Scotland, and B. Rowe.** 1979. An adhesive factor found in strains of *Escherichia coli* belonging to the traditional infantile enteropathogenic serotypes. Curr. Microbiol. **3:**95–99.
9. **Day, N. P., S. M. Scotland, and B. Rowe.** 1981. Comparison of an HEp-2 tissue culture test with the Sereny test for detection of enteroinvasiveness in *Shigella* spp. and *Escherichia coli*. J. Clin. Microbiol. **13:**596–597.
10. **De, S. N., and D. N. Chattergee.** 1953. An experimental study of the mechanism of action of *Vibrio cholerae* on the intestinal mucous membrane. J. Pathol. Bacteriol. **66:** 559–562.
11. **Dean, A. G., Y. Ching, R. G. Williams, and L. B. Harden.** 1972. Test for *Escherichia coli* enterotoxin using infant mice: application in a study of diarrhea in children in Honolulu. J. Infect. Dis. **125:**407–411.
12. **Donta, S. T., and M. King.** 1973. Induction of steroidogenesis in tissue culture by cholera enterotoxin. Nature (London) New Biol. **243:**246–247.
13. **Evans, D. J., D. G. Evans, and S. L. Gorbach.** 1973. Production of vascular permeability factor by enterotoxigenic *Escherichia coli* isolated from man. Infect. Immun. **8:**725–730.
14. **Falkow, S., P. Small, R. Isberg, S. F. Hayes, and D. Corwin.** A molecular strategy for the study of bacterial invasion. Rev. Infect. Dis. **9:**S450–S455.
15. **Finkelstein, R. A., P. Atthasampunna, N. Chulasamaya, and P. Charunmethee.** 1966. Pathogenesis of experimental cholera: biologic activities of purified procholeragen A. J. Immunol. **96:**440–449.
16. **Finlay, B. B., and S. Falkow.** 1988. A comparison of microbial invasion strategies of *Salmonella*, *Shigella*, and

Yersinia species, p. 227–243. *In* M. A. Horowitz (ed.), Bacteria-host cell interaction. Alan R. Liss, Inc., New York.

17. **Finlay, B. B., and S. Falkow.** 1989. Common themes in microbial pathogenicity. Microbiol. Rev. **53:**210–230.
18. **Formal, S. B., T. L. Hale, and J. J. Sansonetti.** 1983. Invasive enteric pathogens. Rev. Infect. Dis. **5:**S702–S707.
19. **Guerrant, R. L., L. L. Brunton, T. C. Schnaitman, L. I. Rebhlin, and A. G. Gilman.** 1974. Cyclic adenosine monophosphate and alteration of Chinese hamster ovary cell morphology: a rapid, sensitive in vitro assay for the enterotoxins of *Vibrio cholerae* and *Escherichia coli.* Infect. Immun. **10:**320–327.
20. **Hay, R. J.** 1988. The seed stock concept and quality control for cell lines. Anal. Biochem. **171:**225–237.
21. **Karmali, M. A.** 1987. Laboratory diagnosis of verotoxin-producing *Escherichia coli* infections. Clin. Microbiol. Newsl. **9:**65–70.
22. **Labrec, E. H., H. Schneider, T. J. Magnani, and S. B. Formal.** 1964. Epithelial cell penetration as an essential step in the pathogenesis of bacillary dysentery. J. Bacteriol. **88:**1503–1518.
23. **Macy, M. L.** 1980. Tests for mycoplasma contamination of cultured cells as applied at the ATCC. *In* TCA manual 5, p. 1151–1155. American Type Culture Collection, Rockville, Md.
24. **Maneval, D. R., R. R. Colwell, S. W. Josephs, R. Grays, and S. T. Donta.** 1980. A tissue culture method for the detection of bacterial enterotoxins. J. Tissue Culture Methods **6:**85–90.
25. **Markham, P. D., and S. Z. Salahuddin.** 1987. *In vitro* cultivation of human leukocytes: methods for the expression and isolation of human viruses. BioTechniques **5:**432–443.
26. **McGarrity, G. J.** 1979. Detection of contamination. Methods Enzymol. **58:**18–29.
27. **McGarrity, G. J., J. Sarama, and V. Vanaman.** 1985. Cell culture techniques. ASM News **51:**170–183.
28. **McIntosh, K., and J. C. Clark.** 1985. Parainfluenza and respiratory syncytial viruses, p. 763–768. *In* E. H. Lennette, A. Balows, W. J. Hausler, Jr., and H. J. Shadomy (ed.), Manual of clinical microbiology, 4th ed. American Society for Microbiology, Washington, D.C.
29. **McLimans, W. F.** 1979. Mass culture of mammalian cells. Methods Enzymol. **58:**194–211.
30. **Mehlman, I. J., E. L. Eide, A. C. Sanders, M. Fishbein, and C. C. G. Aulisio.** 1977. Methodology for recognition of invasive potential of *Escherichia coli.* J. Assoc. Off. Anal. Chem. **60:**546–562.
31. **Miliotis, M. D., H. J. Koornhof, and J. I. Phillips.** 1989. Invasive potential of noncytotoxic enteropathogenic *Escherichia coli* in an in vitro Henle 407 cell model. Infect. Immun. **57:**1928–1935.
32. **Murayama, S. Y., T. Sakai, S. Makino, T. Kurata, C. Sasakawa, and M. Yoshikawa.** 1986. The use of mice in the Sereny test as a virulence assay of shigellae and enteroinvasive *Escherichia coli.* Infect. Immun. **51:**696–698.
33. **Nataro, J. P., J. B. Kaper, R. Robins-Browne, V. Prado, P. Vial, and M. M. Levine.** 1987. Patterns of adherence of diarrheagenic *Escherichia coli* to HEp-2 cells. Pediatr. Infect. Dis. J. **6:**829–831.
34. **Oaks, E. V., M. E. Wingfield, and S. B. Formal.** 1985. Plaque formation by virulent *Shigella flexneri.* Infect. Immun. **48:**124–129.
35. **Peterson, W. D., W. F. Simpson, and B. Hukku.** 1979. Cell culture characterization: monitoring for cell identification. Methods Enzymol. **58:**164–178.
36. **Pike, R. M.** 1976. Laboratory infections: summary and analysis of 3921 cases. Health Lab. Sci. **13:**105–114.
37. **Richardson, J. H., and W. E. Barkley, ed.** 1988. Biosafety in microbiological and biomedical laboratories. HHS publication no. (NIH) 88-8395. U.S. Government Printing Office, Washington, D.C.
38. **Schmidt, N. J.** 1989. Cell culture procedures for diagnostic virology, p. 51–100. *In* N. J. Schmidt and R. W. Emmons (ed.), Diagnostic procedures for viral, rickettsial, and chlamydial infections, 6th ed. American Public Health Association, Inc., Washington, D.C.
39. **Sereny, B.** 1955. Experimental *Shigella* keratoconjunctivitis. A preliminary report. Acta Microbiol. Acad. Sci. Hung. **2:**293–296.
40. **Sereny, B.** 1956. Experimental keratoconjunctivitis shigellosa. Acta Microbiol. Acad. Sci. Hung. **4:**367–377.
41. **Smith, T. F.** 1989. Chlamydia, p. 1165–1198. *In* N. J. Schmidt and R. W. Emmons (ed.), Diagnostic procedures for viral, rickettsial, and chlamydial infections, 6th ed. American Public Health Association, Inc., Washington, D.C.
42. **Smith, T. F., and B. B. Wentworth.** 1984. Chlamydial infections, p. 81–104. *In* B. B. Wentworth and F. N. Judson (ed.), Laboratory methods for the diagnosis of sexually transmitted diseases. American Public Health Association, Inc., Washington, D.C.
43. **Toledo, M. R. F., and L. R. Trabulsi.** 1983. Correlation between biochemical and serological characteristics of *Escherichia coli* and results of the Sereny test. J. Clin. Microbiol. **17:**419–421.
44. **Williams, P. H., M. Roberts, and G. Hinson.** 1988. Stages in bacterial invasion. J. Appl. Bacteriol. **65:**131S–147S.

Section III. Nosocomial and Community Infections: the Role of the Clinical Microbiology Laboratory

Chapter 20

Epidemiology of Hospital-Acquired Infection

RICHARD P. WENZEL

IMPACT OF INFECTIONS

At least 5 to 10% of patients entering U.S. hospitals acquire an infection that was not present or incubating on admission (16). Such hospital-acquired (nosocomial) infections add significantly to the morbidity, mortality, and economic burden expected from the underlying diseases alone (5, 9, 12, 13, 15, 18, 28, 30, 33, 35, 36, 41) (Table 1). As a result, it can be stated with confidence that these infections represent a leading cause of death (39) and an important health care cost (5, 30). Specifically, of the 40 million patients admitted to acute-care institutions, 2 million to 4 million will develop a nosocomial infection. If 100,000 to 400,000 episodes of nosocomial bloodstream infections alone occurred, there would be 40,000 to 160,000 deaths overall and 25,000 to 100,000 deaths directly attributable to the infections. By the same reasoning, there would be expected at least 20,000 deaths directly attributable to nosocomial pneumonias each year (25) (Table 1). Similarly, if infections added only an additional 5 days to the expected stay at an average cost of $750/day, the economic burden would be $7.5 billion to $15 billion dollars annually. Therefore, it is not surprising that in 1989 the National Foundation for Infectious Diseases targeted nosocomial infections as an important area needing major funding for research.

PREVENTABLE INFECTIONS

Not all infections are currently preventable. Data from the Study of the Efficacy of Nosocomial Infection Control (SENIC) performed by the Centers for Disease Control in the early and mid-1970s and published in 1985 (17) estimated that approximately one-third are preventable. It is unclear whether that figure is still accurate, since 15 to 20 years have elapsed since that study was performed. There is also a general consensus that the average severity of illness has increased since the introduction of the diagnosis-related groups as the system for reimbursement of hospital costs (22, 37), and it is likely that the practice of infection control has improved since the time of the SENIC. Nevertheless, a minority of infections are still preventable, and by definition all clusters and epidemics are preventable (38). An epidemic is defined statistically ($P \leq 0.05$) when the existing rates exceed those observed in the past. The term "cluster" is sometimes used for an elevated rate in which there are also strong epidemiological links between an organism and a certain event(s) but in which the statistical threshold for an epidemic is not reached. It is estimated that almost 5% of nosocomial infections occur as part of an epidemic and that a similar proportion occurs as part of a cluster (19, 40). Thus, at least 90% of infections are endemic in nature. Of the latter, perhaps 20% and maybe up to 33% (the estimate from the SENIC) are preventable.

MICROBIOLOGY

The organisms causing hospital-acquired infection can best be understood in terms of their selection on the basis of current antibiotic use and clinical practices (Fig. 1). In the preantibiotic era, streptococci (both *Streptococcus pyogenes* and *Streptococcus pneumoniae*) were the major nosocomial pathogens. Coincident with the introduction and use of penicillin and sulfonamides, *Staphylococcus aureus* emerged as the most common offending agent in the 1950s. Subsequently, associated with the use of first-generation cephalosporins and aminoglycosides, aerobic gram-negative rods accounted for 70% of nosocomial bloodstream pathogens in the 1970s. In the late 1970s and early 1980s, there was great usage of broad-spectrum cephalosporins and an associated exponential use of vascular catheters and other medical devices. Associated with these events, there was a major shift in pathogens from gram-negative to gram-positive species: coagulase-negative staphylococci, *S. aureus*, and the enterococci. Not only were there endemic problems with the new organisms, but also important epidemics of methicillin-resistant *S. aureus* occurred internationally in the 1980s (R. L. Thompson and R. P. Wenzel, Editorial, Ann. Intern. Med. **97**:925–926, 1982; R. P. Wenzel, Editorial, Ann. Intern. Med. **97**:440–442, 1982). As a result of both endemic and epidemic infections with gram-positive organisms frequently resistant to methicillin, the usage of vancomycin increased linearly in the mid-1980s in the United States. In most large hospitals, it became the major antibiotic prescribed and the most expensive item in the hospital pharmacy. Since vancomycin has been the mainstay of therapy for infections caused by coagulase-negative staphylococci, methicillin-resistant *S. aureus*, and often the enterococci, it is of some concern that reports of vancomycin resistance began to appear in the late 1980s (14, 34; L. Veach et al., unpublished data). The major pathogen has been *Staphylococcus haemolyticus*.

By 1990, it became obvious that *Candida* species represented important nosocomial pathogens, accounting for almost 10% of all hospital-acquired bloodstream infections in some institutions (21, 41). This organism is associated with an alarming crude case fatality rate and high attributable mortality (41) as well as an excess hospital stay, in large part because of the need for prolonged therapy with amphotericin B. What is obviously needed are newer drugs to prevent and treat infections caused by antibiotic-resistant staphylococci and more active

TABLE 1. Estimates of the impact of hospital-acquired infections

Anatomic site	Infection rate (no./100 admissions)	% of all hospital-acquired infections	Mortality (%)		Excess length of stay (days)
			Crude	Attributable[a]	
Urinary tract	2.6–3.0	35–40	?	?	2
Operative incision	1.9	25	?	?	7
Lungs	0.75	10	30–35	10[b]	7–9
Bloodstream	0.375–0.75	5–10	25–60[c]	14–38[d]	7–30
Other	1.5	20	?	?	?

[a] Difference between the crude or overall mortality in cases and the crude or overall mortality in matched controls without a nosocomial infection at that site (39).
[b] Approximately one-third of the deaths in patients with nosocomial pneumonia are due directly to the pneumonia (25).
[c] Crude mortality is 34 to 40% for gram-negative rod or enterococcal bloodstream infections, 30% for coagulase-negative bloodstream infections, and 60% for *Candida* bloodstream infections (28, 39, 41).
[d] Attributable mortality is approximately 25% for gram-negative rod or enterococcal bloodstream infections, 14% for coagulase-negative bloodstream infections, and approximately 38% for *Candida* bloodstream infections (28, 39, 41).

and effective drugs to prevent and treat serious *Candida* infections.

RESERVOIRS AND MODES OF TRANSMISSION

The term "reservoir" is used to designate the origin or niche of important pathogens. In modern hospitals, it is people—both health care personnel and patients—who represent the major reservoir of common hospital pathogens. Less commonly, the environment is important. For example, *Legionella* species and often certain other vegetative bacteria (e.g., *Pseudomonas* species) reside in water. Some *Pseudomonas* strains and other *Enterobacteriaceae* have also been described as bacteria found in foods (4, 23, 42). More recently, it has become obvious that contaminated enteral nutrition solutions can lead to nosocomial bloodstream infections (26), as can contaminated breast milk introduced by nasoduodenal feeding tubes (8); *Klebsiella* and *Enterobacter* species have been the primary pathogens implicated. Aspergillus spores are found residing in the air of hospitals and have on numerous occasions been implicated in serious infections of immunosuppressed hosts (31). *Clostridium difficile,* a human pathogen, has been found to contaminate the environment where such patients have resided and at times to remain viable as a secondary reservoir on inanimate surfaces (29).

In general, infections can be transmitted from the reservoir to patients by close contact, by vehicles, or by the airborne route. In the hospital, it is thought that most infections are spread by close contact and that hand washing and optimal techniques used for procedures are important preventive measures (24). Occasionally, gastrointestinal infections are a result of contaminated food (vehicle), and *Aspergillus* infections in immunosuppressed hosts are transmitted by the airborne route. The exact mode of transmission of legionnellosis is not known, but it can be spread by the airborne route also. Thus, providing uncontaminated water and filtered air are infection control measures required of hospitals in which the latter pathogens have been identified in important frequencies (2, 3, 6, 7, 10, 11, 20, 31).

It is likely that although the environment is not a common reservoir for infections, it will become increasingly important as more immunosuppressed patients are managed in hospitals. The goals of hospital administrators and hospital epidemiologists will be to maintain clean air and water as well as clean surfaces, which might occasionally be the reservoirs of hospital pathogens. Nevertheless, continued efforts need to be directed at improving hand-washing agents and hand-washing compliance (1) and improving protocols for the insertion and maintenance of medical devices (27), and while doing so to identify economically beneficial alternatives. In addition, since infection is a direct function not only of organism dose and virulence but also of host resistance, new agents to boost host immunity will be welcomed.

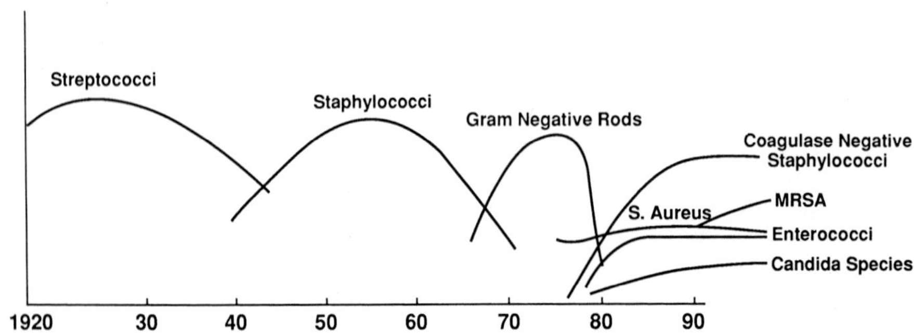

FIG. 1. Schematic representation of the relationship between time and usage of antibiotics and the emergence of "new" pathogens responsible for most nosocomial infections. MRSA, Methicillin-resistant *S. aureus.*

ROLE OF THE LABORATORY

It should become obvious that the laboratory plays a key role in the control of nosocomial infection by (i) accurately identifying the causative organisms, (ii) providing individual and annually trended institutional data on antibiograms of common hospital pathogens, (iii) assisting the infection control team in identifying the likely reservoir and mode of transmission of agents causing nosocomial infection, (iv) assisting the infection control team in accurately typing organisms (this is extremely important in identifying a point-source cluster or epidemic and distinguishing this situation from an unrelated number of endemic infections), and (v) working effectively with the clinical infectious diseases team and helping to differentiate a true epidemic from a pseudoepidemic (32, 38).

SUMMARY

Nosocomial infections affect at least 2 million to 4 million patients in the United States each year, add greatly to the cost of health care, and represent an important cause of death. Understanding the interaction of patient (and patient immune status), organism, and environment (including use of antibiotics and of medical devices) is essential to prevention and control. In that regard, the clinical microbiology laboratory plays an important role, working with the infection control team and infectious diseases clinicians. Chapters 21 to 25 elaborate on some of these points.

LITERATURE CITED

1. **Albert R., and F. Condi.** 1981. Handwashing patterns in medical intensive-care units. N. Engl. J. Med. **304:**1465–1466.
2. **Bartlett, C. L. R.** 1984. Potable water as reservoir and means of transmission, p. 210–215. *In* C. Thornsberry, A. Balows, J. C. Feeley, and W. Jakubowski (ed.), *Legionella:* Proceedings of the Second International Symposium. American Society for Microbiology, Washington, D.C.
3. **Best, M., J. Stout, R. R. Muder, V. L. Yu, A. Goetz, and F. Taylor.** 1983. *Legionellaceae* in the hospital water supply: epidemiological link with disease and evaluation of a method for control of nosocomial legionnaires' disease and Pittsburgh pneumonia. Lancet **ii:**307–310.
4. **Casewell, M., and I. Phillips.** 1978. Food as a source of *Klebsiella species* for colonization and infection of intensive care patients. J. Clin. Pathol. **31:**845–849.
5. **Dixon, R. E.** 1987. Costs of nosocomial infections and benefits of infection control programs, p. 19–25. *In* R. P. Wenzel (ed.), Prevention and control of nosocomial infections. The Williams & Wilkins Co., Baltimore.
6. **Doebbeling, B. N., M. A. Ishak, B. H. Wade, M. A. Pasquale, R. E. Gerszten, D. H. M. Groschel, R. J. Kadner, and R. P. Wenzel.** 1989. *Legionella micdadei* pneumonia: 10 years experience and a case-control study. J. Hosp. Infect. **129:**289–298.
7. **Doebbeling, B. N., and R. P. Wenzel.** 1987. The epidemiology of *Legionella pneumophila* infections. Semin. Respir. Infect. **2:**206–221.
8. **Donowitz, L. G., F. J. Marsik, K. A. Fisher, and R. P. Wenzel.** 1981. Contaminated breast milk: a source of klebsiella bacteremia in a newborn intensive care unit. Rev. Infect. Dis. **3:**716–720.
9. **Donowitz, L. G., and R. P. Wenzel.** 1980. Endometritis following cesarean section: a controlled study of the increased duration of hospital stay and direct cost of hospitalization. Am. J. Obstet. Gynecol. **137:**467–469.
10. **Edelstein, P. H., R. E. Whittaker, R. L. Kreiling, and C. L. Howell.** 1982. Efficacy of ozone in eradication of *Legionella pneumophila* from hospital plumbing fixtures. Appl. Environ. Microbiol. **44:**1330–1334.
11. **Fisher-Hoch, S. P., J. O'H. Tobin, A. M. Nelson, M. G. Smith, J. M. Talbot, C. L. R. Bartlett, M. G. Pritchard, R. A. Swann, and J. A. Thomas.** 1981. Investigation and control of an outbreak of Legionnaires' disease in a district general hospital. Lancet **ii:**932–936.
12. **Freeman, J., and J. E. McGowan, Jr.** 1978. Risk factors for nosocomial infection. J. Infect. Dis. **138:**811.
13. **Freeman, J., B. A. Rosner, and J. E. McGowan, Jr.** 1979. Adverse effects of nosocomial infection. J. Infect. Dis. **140:** 732–740.
14. **Froggat, J. W., J. L. Johnston, D. W. Galletto, and G. L. Archer.** 1989. Antimicrobial resistance in nosocomial isolation of *Staphylococcus haemolyticus*. Antimicrob. Agents Chemother. **33:**460–466.
15. **Green, J. W., and R. P. Wenzel.** 1977. Postoperative wound infection: a controlled study of the increased duration of hospital stay and direct cost of hospitalization. Ann. Surg. **185:**264–268.
16. **Haley, R. W., D. H. Culver, J. W. White, W. M. Morgan, and T. G. Emori.** 1985. The nationwide nosocomial infection rate: a new need for vital statistics. Am. J. Epidemiol. **121:**159–167.
17. **Haley, R. W., D. H. Culver, J. W. White, W. M. Morgan, T. G. Emori, V. P. Munn, and T. M. Hooton.** 1985. The SENIC. 3. The efficacy of infection surveillance and control programs in preventing nosocomial infections in United States hospitals. Am. J. Epidemiol. **121:**182–205.
18. **Haley, R. W., D. R. Schaberg, S. D. Von Allmen, and J. E. McGowan, Jr.** 1980. Estimating the extra charges and prolongation of hospitalization due to nosocomial infections: a comparison of methods. J. Infect. Dis. **141:**248–257.
19. **Haley, R. W., J. H. Tenney, J. O. Lindsey, J. S. Garner, and J. V. Bennett.** 1985. How frequent are outbreaks of nosocomial infection in community hospitals? Infect. Control **6:**233–236.
20. **Helms, C. M., R. M. Massanari, R. P. Wenzel, M. A. Pfaller, N. P. Moyer, and N. Hall.** 1988. Legionnaires' disease associated with a hospital water system: a five year progress report on continuous hyperchlorination. J. Am. Med. Assoc. **259:**2423–2427.
21. **Horan, T., D. Culver, W. Jarvis, G. Emori, S. Banerjee, W. Martone, and C. Thornsberry.** 1988. Pathogens causing nosocomial infections. Preliminary data from the National Nosocomial Infection Surveillance System. Antimicrob. Newsl. **5:**65–67.
22. **Iglehart, J. K.** 1982. The new era of prospective payment for hospitals. N. Engl. J. Med. **307:**1288–1292.
23. **Kominos, S. D., C. E. Copeland, B. Grosiak, and B. Postic.** 1972. Mode of transmission of *Pseudomonas aeruginosa* in a burn unit. Appl. Microbiol. **23:**567–572.
24. **Larson, E.** 1987. Skin cleansing, p. 250–256. *In* R. P. Wenzel (ed.), Prevention and control of nosocomial infections. The Williams & Wilkins Co., Baltimore.
25. **Leu, H. S., D. L. Kaiser, M. Mori, R. F. Woolson, and R. P. Wenzel.** 1989. Hospital-acquired pneumonia: attributable morbidity and mortality. Am. J. Epidemiol. **129:** 1258–1267.
26. **Levy J., Y. Van Laethem, C. Verhaegen, C. Perpete, J. P. Butzler, and R. P. Wenzel.** 1989. Enteral nutrition solutions as a cause of nosocomial sepsis. J. Parenter. Enteral Nutr. **13:**228–234.
27. **Maki, D.** 1989. Risk factors for nosocomial infection in intensive care—'devices vs nature' and goals for the next decade. Arch. Intern. Med. **149:**30–35.
28. **Martin, M. A., M. A. Pfaller, and R. P. Wenzel.** 1989. Mortality and hospital stay attributable to coagulase-negative staphylococcal bacteremia. Ann. Intern. Med. **110:** 9–16.

29. **McFarland, L. V., M. E. Mulligan, R. Y. Y. Kwok, and W. E. Stamm.** 1989. Nosocomial acquisition of *Clostridium difficile* infections. N. Engl. J. Med. **318:**204–209.

30. **McGowan, J. E., Jr.** 1981. Cost and benefit in control of nosocomial infection: methods for analysis. Rev. Infect. Dis. **3:**790–797.

31. **Rhame, F. S.** 1989. Nosocomial aspergillosis: how much protection for which patients? Infect. Control. Hosp. Epidemiol. **10:**296–298.

32. **Ristuccia, P. A., and B. A. Cunha.** 1987. Microbiologic aspects of infection control, p. 205–232. *In* R. P. Wenzel (ed.), Prevention and control of nosocomial infections. The Williams & Wilkins Co., Baltimore.

33. **Rose, R., K. J. Hunting, T. R. Townsend, and R. P. Wenzel.** 1977. Morbidity/mortality and economics of hospital-acquired bloodstream infections: a controlled study. South. Med. J. **70:**1267–1269.

34. **Schwalbe, R. S., J. T. Stapleton, and P. H. Gilligan.** 1987. Emergence of vancomycin resistance in coagulase-negative staphylococci. N. Engl. J. Med. **316:**927–931.

35. **Spengler, R. F., and W. E. Greenough III.** 1978. Hospital costs and mortality attributed to nosocomial bacteremias. J. Am. Med. Assoc. **240:**2455.

36. **Townsend, T. R., and R. P. Wenzel.** 1981. Nosocomial bloodstream infections in a newborn intensive care unit: a case-matched control study of morbidity, mortality, and risk. Am. J. Epidemiol. **114:**73–80.

37. **Wenzel, R. P.** 1985. Nosocomial infections, diagnosis-related groups, and study on the efficacy of nosocomial infection control. Economic implications for hospitals under the prospective payment system. Am. J. Med. **78**(Suppl. 6B):3–7.

38. **Wenzel, R. P.** 1987. Epidemics—identification and management, p. 94–108. *In* R. P. Wenzel (ed.), Prevention and control of nosocomial infections. The Williams & Wilkins Co., Baltimore.

39. **Wenzel, R. P.** 1988. The mortality of hospital-acquired bloodstream infections: need for a new vital statistic? Int. J. Epidemiol. **17:**225–227.

40. **Wenzel, R. P., R. L. Thompson, S. M. Landry, B. S. Russel, P. J. Miller, S. Ponce de Leon, and G. B. Miller.** 1983. Hospital-acquired infections in intensive care unit patients: an overview with emphasis on epidemics. Infect. Control **4:**371–375.

41. **Wey, S. B., M. Mori, M. A. Pfaller, R. F. Woolson, and R. P. Wenzel.** 1988. Hospital-acquired candidemia: attributable mortality and excess length of stay. Arch. Intern. Med. **148:**2642–2647.

42. **Wright, C., S. D. Kominos, and R. B. Yee.** 1976. Enterobacteriaceae and *Pseudomonas aeruginosa* recovered from vegetable salads. Appl. Environ. Microbiol. **31:**453–454.

Chapter 21

Communication with Hospital Staff

JOHN E. McGOWAN, JR.

The process of reporting bears more closely on the outcome of patient care than do intralaboratory activities (1), yet a recent paper labels our current age "the misinformation era" in health care (3). The hospital microbiology laboratory plays a major role in care of patients with infection. In addition, the laboratory has important responsibilities in the surveillance, control, and prevention of nosocomial infections. Neither of these missions can be carried out effectively without proper attention to communication with the medical staff who directly care for patients (24).

"Perhaps nowhere in medicine is the interface between clinician and microbiologist as critical or as logical as it is in the diagnosis and treatment of infectious diseases" (29). Several means of communication exist between laboratory and clinician. This chapter reviews these and discusses ancillary ways to "get the word out" from the laboratory.

REPORTING OF LABORATORY DATA ABOUT INDIVIDUAL PATIENTS

There are three major aspects to reporting of patient data: content of the report, speed of reporting, and degree of understanding by the patient's physician. Optimizing each requires several steps.

Monitoring the content of reports

Since microbiology reports tend to be more complex than other laboratory reports, they can benefit the most from clear format. The optimal reporting system would allow for reporting in simple, easily understood terms. It would enable highlighting results of significance and allow considerable free text to permit interpretations of unusual results (17). Few current systems, whether computerized or not, meet these goals.

The microbiologist must monitor legibility and format of all laboratory reports regularly and frequently to confirm that the intended information is presented. This is especially important in hospitals that use computerized reporting, as several formats may be used for reporting data. For example, the display of information on the ward cathode ray terminal (CRT) may vary from the format used for the printed report, or the printed interim report may be different in format from the final discharge summary. Designing of report format should involve consultation with the hospital staff to ensure that the reports are arranged for the convenience of care givers rather than for the convenience of computer programmers or laboratory workers (15).

Content of the report is as important as format; elimination of transcription errors has become a major focus of quality assurance review programs (1) and should be a major goal of every microbiologist. Flagging of abnormal results is more difficult for microbiology than in many other laboratory sections but is no less important (36).

Simplifying the way in which results are reported

The degree to which culture results are described plays a major role in determining how easy the results are to understand. For example, a listing of six organisms and their susceptibilities from an ear culture is probably of less value than reporting that the specimen is characteristic of endogenous flora from the site. When quantitative results are to be reported, use of Système International d'Unités (SI) units may or may not be a good way to present the results (35). Identification and testing of susceptibilities to more than three isolates has not been shown useful in therapy of mixed infections (1), and circumstances in which such processing will be cost effective are few. Thus, reporting of group results rather than full identification and susceptibility testing of all isolates is encouraged (1).

The results of susceptibility testing should be reported in the format in which they will provide the most meaningful information to physicians (22). Most susceptibility testing systems allow for reporting quantitative MIC results or categories of susceptibility (susceptible, intermediate, resistant, etc.). There is little proven, objective information that routine provision of MIC rather than susceptibility category is better for patient care (30). Thus, in the interest of simplicity, many hospitals choose to report susceptibility categories. The standard format for reporting of susceptibility results, and exceptions in which other formats will be used, should be decided through discussions between those who perform the tests and those who will use the data for patient management. If MIC reporting is chosen, consideration should be given to providing interpretative guides (inhibitory quotient, etc.) to assist understanding by the staff (8).

Regardless of the format, certain conventions of category and report must be observed for selected drug-organism test combinations (30). For example, zone diameters obtained when testing enterococci against either ampicillin or penicillin are interpreted as either resistant or moderately susceptible. Likewise, methicillin-resistant *Staphylococcus aureus* (MRSA) should not be reported as susceptible to any β-lactam antimicrobial agent, including all cephalosporins and imipenem, regardless of in vitro test results. Handling of special situations such as these may require variation from usual reporting practices, especially if usual reporting is done through interface between susceptibility test equipment and laboratory information system. Selective ability to report on the basis of predefined algorithms or to append interpretations may be essential to deal with these situations.

Improving hospital use of antimicrobial agents and implementing cost containment for hospital care have become major concerns (2, 22). The laboratory can assist in these two efforts by the way it reports results of susceptibility testing (22, 30). For example, reports of susceptibility testing against a defined routine battery of drugs for all organisms of a given type (gram-negative aerobic bacilli, etc.) can be the rule, with a second list of agents tested and reported only when the initial battery reveals unusual resistance of the organism or at the request of the patient's physician. In this example, resistance to certain drugs from the initial test battery can signal the testing of selected drugs from a backup battery, without further request from the patient's physician. Such systems work best in hospitals in which the great majority of organisms are susceptible to routinely tested drugs (30).

Monitoring turnaround time

Data from the clinical microbiology laboratory are most useful to a physician at the time a patient-related decision must be made (23). Thus, actual time that reports are available for physician review is a critical issue. One good way to review this aspect of reporting is to visit the wards at the time that reports should be available and see whether they have actually reached the charts (or CRT). Removing outdated information from the patient's record is as important as entering current information (1). The College of American Pathologists has made evaluation of turnaround time for certain microbiologic tests part of its new quality assurance review program (Q-Probes Program [32]). Calls to the laboratory for results that already should be available to the clinical staff can be used as another indicator of how well reports are reaching their targets (1).

Speeding up the reporting of results

One way in which many laboratories can improve communication with the medical staff is by decreasing the interval between completion of testing and receipt of the report by the patient's doctor. Recent articles differ in their assessment of the impact of rapid identification and susceptibility testing methods on patient care (4, 5, 33). Problems in selection of patients or randomization in studies to date prevent a definitive answer to the question. However, they make it clear that attempts to provide timely reports are worth pursuing.

As a first step, the interval between receipt of specimen and reporting of results (turnaround time) should be defined clearly. When this is done, relatively inexpensive steps that would markedly decrease this period may be apparent (25). Methods to monitor report interval and turnaround time have been suggested (1, 14, 34). Distinguishing between laboratory turnaround time (when the result is available in the laboratory) and total turnaround time (when the result is available to the patient's physician) may help in planning corrective action.

Once the actual turnaround times are known, a judgment can be made about their appropriateness. This requires a knowledge of the clinical patterns of care in the institution. For example, if the physicians on a given service make rounds at 7 a.m. and then at 4 p.m., culture results that are available before 4 p.m. will be used in patient care decisions that day, but results not available until 5 p.m. will have the same clinical impact as all further results reported before 7 a.m. rounds. Thus, changes in laboratory procedure that make results available at 3:30 rather than 4:30 p.m. may be worth pursing, but changes that make these results available at 5:30 instead of 6:30 p.m. may not be worth much effort. This concept makes it important to carefully evaluate equipment that is said to permit "rapid reporting" or "same-day reporting" to see if the shorter turnaround produced by the equipment would make any difference in the particular institution.

Many hospitals use a computerized laboratory reporting system to speed availability of results to the bedside (6, 19). At Grady Memorial Hospital (Atlanta, Ga.), the laboratory information system is linked to more than 200 CRT reporting stations throughout the hospital, in most wards and clinic areas (25). Patient reports from microbiology can be retrieved from this system for approximately 1 year after the tests are requested. This system operates in parallel with the system for printed reports, which are generated twice each day. Surveys in this hospital have shown that clinicians obtain most of their information on their patients by using the CRTs. Such information is available to practitioners as soon as it is recorded by the laboratory technologists, and technologists are encouraged to enter information as soon as possible after it is generated. This speed of entry can have a great effect on turnaround time, since clinicians have the ability to bypass the delivery of printed reports to the ward and the subsequent distribution of the reports to patient charts. Such a system minimizes the need for many tests that require special reporting of results. Turnaround can be facilitated especially in settings where the laboratory generating the microbiology data is not at the same site as the patient care institution. At the same time, several problems can arise. One cannot assume that the data have reached the medical staff just because they have been entered into the computer; this is not necessarily the case (7). In addition, the need for security of the system, to ensure that unauthorized persons do not have access to patient data, is a limiting factor in use of this mechanism (3). Finally, instant dissemination of information means that incorrect result reporting can have an immediate adverse effect on patient care, even if the error is detected soon after the results are entered (1).

One need not have a computer to speed result reporting to the hospital staff (26). Other mechanisms for speeding reporting of results include the technologist calling the physician or ward with results or the microbiologist speaking with the physician about interpretation of the results. These tactics are discussed below.

Adding information about test results to the written report

Communication with the patient's physician often is incomplete if it merely reports presence or absence of organisms. Interpretative information often is needed to guide physician decision making and patient management (23). For example, provision of information about MIC almost demands that an interpretation be provided, unless the medical staff of an institution is unusually sophisticated about the import of these data.

Also, results for specimens that are not collected or transported properly, even when handled as well as possible once they reach the laboratory, are likely to reflect contamination rather than true pathogens. To deal with this, the laboratory report must make clear to the patient's physician the individual specimens in which it appears likely that contaminants are present (diphtheroids recovered only from subculture of blood, etc.). Reporting of the microscopic review of Gram stain of sputum specimens exemplifies another excellent way to report whether or not specimens are contaminated (1). The laboratory must monitor overall specimen handling continually. Reports summarizing this surveillance should be made periodically to the Quality Assurance Committee, to the Infection Control Committee, and to the individual wards, clinics, and offices to ensure that the possibility of contaminated specimens or missed organisms is minimized.

Used correctly, the computer provides a mechanism for interpretative guidance to the patient's physician (23). For example, appending information to flag the information that the organism isolated was not susceptible to the antibiotic the patient was receiving or to indicate that the patient could be receiving less expensive antibiotics has helped one hospital change the pattern of antibiotic use (10). Appending pertinent organism-related information or possible therapy choices is another way to influence care. For example, at Grady Memorial Hospital, we append to each report of MRSA the comment that "cephalosporins are unreliable for MRSA—vancomycin is drug of choice." The clinical microbiologist must remain alert for such opportunities to guide as well as to inform.

Reporting directly to the physician or ward

Entry of information in the patient's medical record or in the laboratory information system does not ensure that the hospital staff has taken note of the results (7). However, when the attending physicians are contacted directly, it is certain that they have received the information. Nearly all laboratories have procedures for special reporting of critical results to the ward or to the physician. Such procedures in a given hospital should be modified as it becomes clear which specific tests influence care or length of hospital stay. For example, reports of positive blood cultures usually are called immediately to the clinician; however, this initial report may include only the Gram stain result and the morphologic appearance. Further identification of the organism may be equally important in determining whether or for how long the patient receives antibiotic therapy. In some hospitals, these additional tests might be added to the list whose results are to be reported to the patient's physician as soon as they are known, instead of by the routine reporting mechanism (25). For example, MRSA strains have increased in prevalence during the past decade. Because of this change, vancomycin is often used in therapy of staphylococcal infection until it is known whether the organism is methicillin susceptible or resistant. Vancomycin has a much greater potential for producing adverse effects in patients than do the β-lactam drugs that could be used when the *S. aureus* organism is methicillin susceptible. As a result, the potential for toxic effect of vancomycin therapy could be reduced considerably by more rapidly communicating whether the organism is methicillin susceptible or resistant.

Documentation of the time that the call was made and the person to whom the results were given is a key part of establishing that the task was completed (18), and review of these logs permits adjustment of the call-up mechanism when problems occur. Again, confidentiality of patient data remains a problem unless messages are called only to physicians or other designated hospital staff.

Communicating directly with the patient's physician

Clinicians depend on the clinical microbiologist for concise and lucid interpretations when necessary (29). The best way to achieve this quality of reporting in many cases is direct communication with the patient's physician by the clinical microbiologist (21). However, the laboratory staff usually does not have the time to employ this mechanism for many reports, and the hasty phone call or personal visit have a greater potential for misunderstanding of data than does the printed page. Therefore, the laboratory must establish certain guidelines by which the clinical microbiologist is alerted to the need to speak with the patient's physician. Whether by a formal consultation mechanism or by an informal contact (phone call, etc.), the communication must be specific and as brief as appropriate (12). The microbiologist must be willing to suggest further consultation or additional diagnostic testing, if this is appropriate for the patient, when dealing with medical staff who are not familiar with the specific infectious disease problem that has arisen. In this way, the microbiologist serves most effectively as a member of the team to improve patient care; this concept of team effort for the process of improving use of antimicrobial agents recently has been emphasized by the Infectious Diseases Society of America (22).

REPORTING OF LABORATORY DATA THAT INDIRECTLY AFFECT PATIENT CARE

The microbiologist should be available to discuss issues such as improving antimicrobial agent use, reducing unnecessary testing, and improving quality of care with colleagues from the medical, nursing, and administrative staffs as appropriate. In addition, the laboratory can provide several types of information to aid patient care.

Susceptibility patterns

In liaison with the Infection Control Committee, the laboratory should provide a summary of susceptibility patterns and make it available to the medical staff on at least an annual basis (22). Profiles showing the susceptibilities of frequently tested pathogens at a given hospital to the antimicrobial agents in the hospital formulary can be of considerable assistance in guiding therapy for sepsis of unclear cause and for other infections. Testing of other organisms (e.g., slow-growing bacteria or organisms requiring special test procedures) can be performed at intervals to develop profiles of their susceptibilities; as long as susceptibility patterns can be presumed to remain stable, such testing may be a useful substitute for testing each isolate at the time of recovery.

In the susceptibility summary for the medical staff, tabulations that may be of particular use include frequency of susceptibility to individual drugs by site of infection (to provide guidance for empiric therapy of infection before the causative organism has been identified) and frequency of susceptibility to individual antimicrobial agents by pathogen (to direct therapy after an organism has been identified but before susceptibility tests have been completed). The Infection Control Committee, a medical staff committee, the Quality Assurance Committee, or more than one of these may wish to receive such data to guide their review of antibiotic use (24).

Antimicrobial agent costs

Information on costs of antimicrobial agents can be helpful, since in some settings physicians "have no idea how expensive all the tests, medications, and procedures are that they are ordering" (27). The laboratory can assist in communicating these costs to the prescribers. A variety of ways can be used.

Figure 1 shows the main screen (index) for the supplementary information file (HELP file) maintained on the laboratory information system at Grady Memorial Hospital. Most of the information presented deals with antibiotic susceptibility. In addition, however, the relative costs of the currently used antimicrobial agents for parenteral and oral use are given from information provided periodically by the pharmacy. The information listed is available 24 h each day all week and can be retrieved directly by the medical personnel at any CRT. Such a data bank does not interfere with provision of patient results, since the supplementary information is consulted only when necessary and is not displayed at other times.

In other institutions, the laboratory staff have disseminated susceptibility or cost data by printing a publication (sometimes in a wallet-size reference form), by supplying pages in ward or nursing procedure manuals, by including the information as part of a laboratory, pharmacy, or infection control newsletter, or by several other means (25).

Specimens and their processing

Clinicians want to offer the best diagnostic procedures to their patients but do not necessarily know how to make optimum use of the resources available. Physicians depend on clinical microbiologists to advise them on selection and proper collection of the appropriate specimens (29). The laboratory must teach hospital staff about proper selection of specimens and appropriate collection methods (28). The HELP file of the Grady Memorial Hospital laboratory information system (Fig. 1) also provides information on specimen requirements for certain types of cultures and immunologic tests, as well as about procedures for susceptibility testing (which organisms are routinely tested, which are tested in special circumstances, and which cannot be tested). This information is also provided on the front and back of the microbiology test requisition form, in the *House Staff Manual*, and in the ward procedure manuals. In other institutions, the laboratory staff disseminate the data by printing them as a separate publication, by supplying pages for nursing or ward procedure manuals, by including the information as part of a laboratory, pharmacy, or infection control newsletter, or by several other means (25). Hospitals with computerized order entry systems have the ability to control this aspect of specimen quality by monitoring format and content of the order screens for each microbiologic test. The laboratory should remain alert to opportunities to discuss these issues with the medical staff and the other hospital personnel involved with specimen collection and transport. Information from the laboratory quality assurance program dealing with specimen adequacy can be used to improve the format, content, and method of communicating this important aspect of laboratory function (1).

```
          MICROBIOLOGY INFORMATION                                    PAGE 11
          (LAST UPDATED AUGUST 2, 1989)
ENTER PAGE YOU WISH TO VIEW:
  12-GUIDE TO SUSCEPTIBILITY PATTERNS
  13-CODES (ABBREVIATIONS) FOR ANTIBIOTICS AS OF JANUARY, 1989
  14-SUSCEPTIBILITY PATTERNS-ORGS. IN URINE CULTURE, JAN-JUNE, 1989
  15-SUSCEPTIBILITY OF RESISTANT ORGANISMS IN URINE, JAN-JUNE, 1989
  16-SUSCEPTIBILITY-ISOLATES IN STOOL CULTURE, JAN-JUNE 1989 VS 1988
  17-SUSCEPT: GRAM-NEG. BACILLI IN BLOOD CULTS., JAN-DEC, 1988
  18-SUSCEPT. OF STAPH. AUREUS FROM BLOOD CULTS., JAN-DEC, 1988
  19-''ANTIBIOTIC REPORT CARD'': GM-NEG RODS, ALL SITES, JAN-JUNE, 1989
  20-SUSCEPTIBILITY OF HEMOPHILUS INFLUENZAE ISOLATES, 1987-1989
  21-COST OF PARENTERAL ANTIBIOTICS AS OF AUGUST, 1988
  22-COST OF ORAL ANTIBIOTICS AS OF AUGUST, 1988
  23-AVAILABLE SUSCEPTIBILITY TESTS; WHAT SPECIMENS/DRUGS TESTED
  24-AVAILABLE SUSCEPTIBILITY TESTS; GRAM-POSITIVE COCCI
  25-AVAILABLE SUSCEPTIBILITY TESTS; GM-NEGATIVE AEROBIC BACILLI
  27-AVAILABLE SUSCEPTIBILITY TESTS; OTHER BACTERIA
  28-SUSCEPTIBILITY OF M. TUBERCULOSIS ISOLATES, 1988
  29-SPECIMEN COLLECTION AND HANDLING INSTRUCTIONS
(NOTE: ENTER X TO EXIT AT ANY TIME FROM THIS MATERIAL)
ENTER PAGE NUMBER, OR PAGE 1 FOR GENERAL INDEX, OR X TO EXIT>:
```

FIG. 1. Index screen from microbiology section of HELP file, laboratory information system, Grady Memorial Hospital.

```
PAGE          FUNCTION               DESCRIPTION                                    PAGE 1
----          --------               ---------------------
ENTER PAGE YOU WISH TO VIEW:
 1                                   REFERENCE INDEX (VIEWING NOW)
 2               --                  WHAT'S NEW IN THE LAB
 3               --                  WHAT'S NEW IN THE LAB (CONT'D)
 4               --                  WHAT'S NEW IN THE LAB (CONT'D)
 5               --                  WHAT'S NEW IN THE LAB (CONT'D)
 6               --                  GENERAL INFORMATION ABOUT COMPUTER FUNCTIONS
 7               TL                  TEST LIBRARY       -DISPLAYS INFORMATION ON A TEST
 7               TI                  TEST INQUIRY       -DISPLAYS TEST NUMBER
 8               PR                  PATIENT RESULTS    -DISPLAYS ALL LABORATORY DATA
 9               PS                  PATIENT STATUS     -DISPLAYS TODAY'S LABORATORY DATA
10               SC                  SIMULATED CALCULATOR-USE CRT LIKE A CALCULATOR
11               --                  MICROBIOLOGY INDEX-SUSCEPTIBILITY DATA,
                                            COST OF ANTIBIOTICS, AND AVAILABLE SUSCEPTIBILITY
                                            TESTS. (UPDATED 2 AUGUST 1989)
32               --                  PROPHYLAXIS PROCEDURES FOR HEPATITIS B VIRUS
34               -                   STEPS TO FOLLOW FOR EMPLOYEES AFTER NEEDLE STICK.
36               --                  GMH ISOLATION/PRECAUTION GUIDELINES

                *****FOR ADDITIONAL INFORMATION OR HELP, CALL 53832******
                  *****ENTER PAGE YOU WANT TO REVIEW OR X TO EXIT>******
```

FIG. 2. Main index screen from HELP file, laboratory information system, Grady Memorial Hospital.

Hospital infection control and employee health procedures

Another type of information that the laboratory can disseminate deals with hospital infection control and employee health. For example, the HELP file at Grady Memorial Hospital presents procedures for hospital employees to follow after needle stick (Fig. 2). This information is provided to the laboratory by the infection control team periodically and specifies both laboratory testing that is needed and other measures for the employee to take. We also present information on universal precautions, in a format similar to the way that disease-specific isolation guidelines were adapted to the hospital information system at a Utah medical center (16).

Access to and effective management of medical information have become increasingly important in the practice of medicine today (6). These examples illustrate the central role that the laboratory can play in communicating with the staff—the laboratory information system can provide ready access to more than laboratory data and thus further improve the approach to diagnosis and therapy of infectious diseases.

REPORTING OF LABORATORY DATA ABOUT NOSOCOMIAL INFECTION

The laboratory can make major contributions to infection control when the persons responsible for infection control efforts and those in charge of the clinical microbiology laboratory cooperate closely to attack this problem. About half of those who chair infection control committees are pathologists or other laboratory personnel, making communication between laboratory and infection control perfect (24, 31).

Routine reporting to the hospital infection control program

Laboratory records are an important tool for surveillance of nosocomial infection (31). More than 80% of infections defined as nosocomial by bedside review of each patient could be identified by review of positive cultures from the microbiology laboratory (11), and identification of nosocomial infection by laboratory-based surveillance was 92% as sensitive as identification by review of the nursing care plan (37). Laboratory data are an especially sensitive tool for detecting nosocomial cases of bloodstream or urinary tract infection (32). Thus, laboratory data form an important base for surveillance efforts (20), and review of laboratory records is the most common method for surveillance carried out by infection control practitioners in the United States (9).

Introduction of a laboratory information system often makes it possible to produce special reports for the infection control practitioner. At Grady Memorial Hospital, we generate such a report at the start of each day. The report lists positive cultures and immunologic tests from the previous day, sorted by ward in the order in which each practitioner makes daily rounds. The reports summarize for each ward the patient, time and source of specimen, and the results of study, both preliminary and final. The only test results selected for this report are those specified as a result of consultation between the laboratory and the epidemiology personnel. This approach maintains a relatively concise report while ensuring that the infection control officer has access to all relevant information of current interest. The list of results to be selected can be changed on a periodic basis to make sure that current needs are addressed, e.g., when the name of an organism has changed or when a new nosocomial pathogen has arisen at the institution. Flagging conditions that increase the risk of nosocomial infection (e.g., positive cultures from blood or surgical wounds in patients hospitalized ≥72 h) might increase the probability of identifying patients with nosocomial infection (37). Such programming would increase the ability of the laboratory summary to highlight likely hospital infections, but its effectiveness has not yet been demonstrated.

Test results from the microbiology laboratory are crucial data for successful infection control. Moreover, any information that permits the successful tracing of organism movement within the hospital can be of use to the infection control team. Thus, the ability of the laboratory to isolate and identify responsible microorganisms is as crucial to infection control as it is to the individual patient (24). This is true whether the positive cultures or immunologic tests represent episodes of infection or indicate colonization of the patient.

Provision of information from the laboratory can be made relatively swift and efficient. However, further data from clinical rounds must be added to obtain an accurate estimate of the occurrence of nosocomial infection in a given hospital (11). The laboratory can only indicate which organisms were present in culture; this screening procedure for identification of nosocomial infection will be ineffective if cultures or samples for immunologic testing are not submitted (31). In addition, the predictive value for presence of infection of positive cultures is relatively low, especially for wound or lower respiratory tract cultures (37). Thus, the epidemiologist must supplement laboratory data with clinical information to determine whether organisms found in culture indicate infection or colonization. In turn, the epidemiologic summary may be helpful to the microbiologist in determining the extent to which further cultures or immunologic test specimens from the same source will be processed. Communication here is a two-way street, and both laboratory and clinician can gain from exchanging this information.

The laboratory must communicate information in addition to that from patient specimens as a part of epidemiologic surveillance. For example, laboratory evaluation of the quality of specimens submitted for examination produces results that are pertinent to infection control as well as to the individual patient. These findings can improve the interpretation of infection surveillance data, which otherwise might be confounded by isolates of questionable significance.

Changes in laboratory procedures and techniques that affect the identification of nosocomial pathogens (for example, changes in the basic techniques for primary isolation, species identification, or antibiotic susceptibility testing) should be communicated by the microbiologist to the hospital epidemiologist on a regular basis.

Reporting results of special importance for infection control

To deal with individual problems of nosocomial infection in the hospital as they arise, control measures must be taken as quickly as possible and must be based on accurate assessment of the problem and its causes (13). Without rapid identification and reporting of the organisms involved, control measures cannot be efficiently and rationally designed and implemented.

Even in the absence of an outbreak, microbiologic and immunologic reports may be the starting point for further epidemiologic investigations (24). Often, these investigations also require information about the attributes of the patient, the personnel involved in care, or the diagnostic and therapeutic procedures that were provided to the patient. Obtaining these nonlaboratory data usually is easier when the patient is still present in the hospital, or at least is still fresh in the minds of the hospital personnel. Prompt reporting of pertinent laboratory results facilitates information retrieval of this type.

When isolates of special nosocomial significance are presumptively identified, prompt reporting to infection control personnel as well as to clinical staff is essential. Examples of such isolates include *Neisseria meningitidis; Salmonella* isolates (from nursery patients), *Clostridium difficile* toxin, or shigellae from stool; positive smears and cultures for *Mycobacterium tuberculosis* from any patient or employee; and organisms resistant to an unusually large number of antimicrobial agents. These and other situations require quicker action than a "final report" or daily infection control summary, since important epidemiologic investigations often can be triggered by preliminary data from the laboratory. At the same time, "early warning" must not be requested for so many situations that this becomes an unreasonable burden for the laboratory personnel (24).

Results can be brought to the attention of infection control colleagues by telephone or by page if the matter is urgent. Otherwise, a mention during the daily visits of the infection control staff to the laboratory usually suffices.

Retention of laboratory records for infection control purposes

In addition to instituting control measures, infection control workers often need to analyze laboratory data from various time periods to try to detect patterns of nosocomial infection (24). To assist this effort, it is helpful if the laboratory can archive summaries of pertinent results. The specific laboratory results that can aid epidemiologic analyses will vary from hospital to hospital; the data to be included, and the frequency with which such summaries are made, should be determined by the individuals providing (laboratory) and using (epidemiology) the information. As a general guide, the source of each specimen, date of collection, patient identification, hospital service, ward, and the organisms identified in the final report should be recorded. Records also should be kept of results of antibiotic susceptibility tests and of any special biochemical or typing studies.

All tests should be recorded so that results are readily available by date, by type of specimen, and by pathogens isolated. Computer storage and retrieval of all results is optimal, but noncomputerized rapid retrieval and sorting systems may also be useful. For example, in a smaller hospital, records could be maintained simply and inexpensively in bound logbooks kept chronologically for each major type of specimen (blood, wound, skin, cerebrospinal fluid, urine, stool, sputum, etc.). Sole reliance on a filing system of loose laboratory slips is not desirable.

The permanent records of the microbiology laboratory should include dates and other details of any major changes in culture or immunologic techniques or laboratory procedures. Dates of changes in the criteria for identification or of taxonomic designations applied to the isolates should be recorded as well.

The length of time such records can be maintained depends on hospital size, work volume of the laboratory, and available storage facilities. Thus, storage time should be determined by laboratory personnel after consultation with the hospital infection control staff. Six months is a desirable minimum (24).

For some nosocomial infection investigations, access to the organisms is important. The laboratory must retain strains that may relate to nosocomial infection for a given period, while it is determined whether further testing is needed or not. In cooperation with infection control personnel, the laboratory should subculture and save epidemiologically important isolates, whether such isolates are from outbreaks or from single cases of unusual or potentially epidemic diseases. How long a storage period is required for this purpose will vary from hospital to hospital and should be agreed upon between epidemiologist and clinical laboratory supervisor (24). A system for reviewing and periodically discarding these isolates also must be established by communication between laboratory and epidemiology personnel.

Infection Control Committee activities

A representative from the microbiology laboratory staff must be an active member of the hospital's Infection Control Committee, according to guidelines of several regulatory agencies (31). This participation contributes significantly to close cooperation between infection control and microbiology personnel.

In the typical hospital, most members of the Infection Control Committee do not have a background in microbiology (13). Thus, the laboratory's representative will provide needed microbiologic expertise for determining the significance of test data and for laboratory aspects of investigations undertaken by the group. In addition, the insights and methods that the microbiologist has developed in making cost-benefit decisions for the laboratory should be useful to the Infection Control Committee as well as to Quality Assurance operations at the hospital.

Microbiology and epidemiology cross-training

Since the key to success in infection control is communication, it is necessary that all members of the infection control team speak the same language and understand certain concepts. For this purpose, some training of epidemiology personnel in clinical microbiology is important. The goal of such teaching is not necessarily to make the infection control staff accomplished laboratory workers, but rather to familiarize them with the procedures and practices of the laboratory, with the microorganisms involved in nosocomial infection, with the validity of test procedures used in identifying these pathogens, and with the strengths and limitations of the resulting data (24). Similarly, it is important for the microbiologist to learn some of the concepts of the epidemiologist, since few laboratory directors or technologists have adequate grounding in epidemiology (13). Especially important is exposure to techniques used for measuring frequency of infection and to the concept of colonization versus infection.

Such joint efforts permit ready communication between the two groups of colleagues. Teaching of this type can be done formally or informally, as part of the day-to-day contacts between laboratory personnel and the infection control staff.

LITERATURE CITED

1. **Bartlett, R. C.** 1989. Quality assurance in clinical microbiology. ASCP check sample-microbiology, no. MB 89-5 (MB-186), p. 1–9. American Society of Clinical Pathologists, Skokie, Ill.
2. **Beam, T. R., Jr.** 1988. Recent advances in curtailing costs of antimicrobial agents. An update on antimicrobial cost containment programs. Antimicrob. Newsl. **3:**17–21.
3. **Burnum, J. F.** 1989. The misinformation era: the fall of the medical record. Ann. Intern. Med. **110:**482–484.
4. **Campo, L., and J. M. Mylotte.** 1988. Use of microbiology reports by physicians in prescribing antimicrobial agents. Am. J. Med. Sci. **296:**392–398.
5. **Dennehy, P. H., W. E. Tente, D. J. Fisher, B. A. Veloudis, and G. Peter.** 1989. Lack of impact of rapid identification of rotavirus-infected patients on nosocomial rotavirus infections. Pediatr. Infect. Dis. J. **8:**290–296.
6. **DeTore, A. W.** 1988. Medical informatics: an introduction to computer technology in medicine. Am. J. Med. **85:**399–403.
7. **Doern, G. V.** 1986. Clinically expedient reporting of rapid diagnostic test information. Diagn. Microbiol. Infect. Dis. **4:**151S–156S.
8. **Ellner, P. D., and H. C. Neu.** 1981. The inhibitory quotient. A method for interpreting minimum inhibitory concentration data. J. Am. Med. Assoc. **246:**1575–1578.
9. **Emori, T. G., R. W. Haley, and J. S. Garner.** 1981. Techniques and uses of nosocomial infection surveillance in U.S. hospitals, 1976–1977. Am. J. Med. **70:**933–940.
10. **Evans, R. S., R. A. Larsen, J. P. Burke, R. M. Gardner, F. A. Meier, J. A. Jacobson, M. T. Conti, J. T. Jacobson, and R. K. Hulse.** 1986. Computer surveillance of hospital-acquired infections and antibiotic use. J. Am. Med. Assoc. **256:**1007–1011.
11. **Freeman, J., and J. E. McGowan, Jr.** 1981. Methodologic issues in hospital epidemiology. I. Rates, case-finding, and interpretation. Rev. Infect. Dis. **3:**658–667.
12. **Goldman, L., T. Lee, and P. Rudd.** 1983. Ten commandments for effective consultations. Arch. Intern. Med. **143:** 1753–1755.
13. **Goldmann, D. A., and A. B. Macone.** 1980. A microbiologic approach to the investigation of bacterial nosocomial infection outbreaks. Infect. Control **1:**391–400.
14. **Hilborne, L. H., R. K. Oye, J. E. McArdle, J. A. Repinski, and D. O. Rodgerson.** 1989. Evaluation of stat and routine turnaround times as a component of laboratory quality. Am. J. Clin. Pathol. **91:**331–335.
15. **Hirschfeld, T.** 1989. Making laboratory reports easier to read. N. Engl. J. Med. **320:**321.
16. **Jacobson, J. T., D. S. Johnson, C. A. Ross, M. T. Conti, R. S. Evans, and J. P. Burke.** 1986. Adapting disease-specific isolation guidelines to a hospital information system. Infect. Control **7:**411–418.
17. **Jorgensen, J. H.** 1985. The choice between custom programming and purchasing a vendor-packaged system for computerization of a clinical microbiology laboratory, p. 523–528. *In* J. W. Smith (ed.), The role of clinical microbiology in cost-effective health care. CAP conference/1984. College of American Pathologists, Skokie, Ill.
18. **Koontz, F.** 1984. E.T.—call the floor (telephone laboratory results). Clin. Microbiol. Newsl. **6:**66–67.
19. **Korpman, R. A.** 1987. Using the computer to optimize human performance in health care delivery: the pathologist as medical information specialist. Arch. Pathol. Lab. Med. **111:**637–645.
20. **Laxson, L. B., M. J. Blaser, and S. M. Parkhurst.** 1984. Surveillance for the detection of nosocomial infections and the potential for nosocomial outbreaks. I. Microbiology culture surveillance is an effective method of detecting nosocomial infection. Am. J. Infect. Control **12:** 318–324.
21. **MacLowry, J. D.** 1985. The consultative role of the clinical microbiology laboratorian, p. 575–579. *In* J. W. Smith (ed.), The role of clinical microbiology in cost-effective health care. CAP conference/1984. College of American Pathologists, Skokie, Ill.

22. **Marr, J. J., H. L. Moffet, and C. M. Kunin.** 1988. Guidelines for improving the use of antimicrobial agents in hospitals: a statement by the Infectious Diseases Society of America. J. Infect. Dis. **157:**869–876.
23. **Matsen, J. M.** 1985. The potential use of computers for cost control in clinical microbiology, p. 505–513. *In* J. W. Smith (ed.), The role of clinical microbiology in cost-effective health care. CAP conference/1984. College of American Pathologists, Skokie, Ill.
24. **McGowan, J. E., Jr.** 1985. Role of the microbiology laboratory in prevention and control of nosocomial infections, p. 110–122. *In* E. H. Lennette, A. Balows, W. J. Hausler, Jr., and H. J. Shadomy (ed.), Manual of clinical microbiology, 4th ed. American Society for Microbiology, Washington, D.C.
25. **McGowan, J. E., Jr., and D. H. Vroon.** 1984. Decreasing turnaround time: critical steps to implementation, p. 489–494. *In* J. W. Smith (ed.), The role of clinical microbiology in cost-effective health care. CAP conference/1984. College of American Pathologists, Skokie, Ill.
26. **Murray, P. R.** 1985. Manual approaches to rapid microbiology results. Diagn. Microbiol. Infect. Dis. **3:**9S–14S.
27. **Petermann, C.** A suggestion for cost containment. N. Engl. J. Med. **320:**630.
28. **Reller, L. B.** 1985. Consultative role of the clinical microbiology laboratory: a clinician's viewpoint, p. 581–583. *In* J. W. Smith (ed.), The role of clinical microbiology in cost-effective health care. CAP conference/1984. College of American Pathologists, Skokie, Ill.
29. **Rosenblatt, J. E.** 1988. Maximizing the productive interface between the clinical microbiologist and the infectious disease clinician. Am. J. Clin. Pathol. **90:**355–357.
30. **Sahm, D. F., M. A. Neuman, C. Thornsberry, and J. E. McGowan, Jr.** 1988. Cumitech 25, Current concepts and approaches to antimicrobial agent susceptibility testing. Coordinating ed., J. E. McGowan, Jr. American Society for Microbiology, Washington, D.C.
31. **Schifman, R. B.** 1989. Surveillance for nosocomial infections: the laboratory component. ASCP check sample-microbiology, no. MB89-1 (MB-182), p. 1–10. American Society of Clinical Pathologists, Skokie, Ill.
32. **Steindel, S. J., P. J. Howanitz, R. B. Schifman, and G. Detweiler.** 1989. Development and evaluation of a quality assurance program based on an interlaboratory comparison. Clin. Chem. **35:**1160–1161.
33. **Trenholme, G. M., R. L. Kaplan, P. H. Karakusis, T. Stine, J. Fuhrer, W. Landau, and S. Levin.** 1989. Clinical impact of rapid identification and susceptibility testing of bacterial blood culture isolates. J. Clin. Microbiol. **27:**1342–1345.
34. **Valenstein, P. N., and K. Emancipator.** 1989. Sensitivity, specificity, and reproducibility of four measures of laboratory turnaround time. Am. J. Clin. Pathol. **91:**452–457.
35. **Washington, J. A., II.** 1989. Comment on SI units. Rev. Infect. Dis. **1:**127.
36. **Watts, N. B.** 1988. Medical relevance of laboratory tests. A clinical perspective. Arch. Pathol. Lab. Med. **112:**379–382.
37. **Wenzel, R. P., and S. A. Streed.** 1989. Surveillance and use of computers in hospital infection control. J. Hosp. Infect. **13:**217–229.

Chapter 22

Procedures for Investigating a Community Outbreak

MICHAEL B. GREGG

This chapter discusses the basic principles of epidemiology, the methods used, and the application of these methods to the investigation of an epidemic of an infectious disease in a mid-size community. The focus is on the practical aspects of an epidemiologic investigation of infectious diseases, with emphasis on surveillance techniques, investigative procedures in the field, and appropriate analytic methods. Although the discussion focuses on the use of epidemiology in relation to infectious diseases, the principles and methods apply equally to noninfectious diseases.

DEFINITION, PURPOSES, AND METHODOLOGY

The word "epidemiology," derived from the Greek "epi" (on or upon), "demos" (people), and "logia" (the study or knowledge of), has been defined many ways. However, all definitions include two basic elements: the study of human health events in groups of people. A usable definition of epidemiology, therefore, might be the study of the distribution and determinants of health events in human populations. Epidemiologists study groups of people rather than the single individual, yet like the practicing physician, they may need to examine patients and have laboratory tests performed. However, epidemiologists study populations by using special techniques, and their ultimate goal is prevention and control of disease rather than diagnosis and treatment of the patient.

Primarily, the epidemiologist tries to determine the etiology of disease, the source(s) of the agent(s) responsible, the mode(s) of transmission, who is at risk of becoming ill, and what exposures predispose to disease. The answers to one or more of these questions may provide a basis for prevention and control. In other words, epidemiologists attempt to explain disease occurrence by studying the character of the agent, the human host, and the nature of the environment in which they interact. Indeed, historically, extensive field and laboratory investigations of agents, host populations, and environmental determinants have successfully defined reservoirs, modes of spread, and human risk factors related to the occurrence of many infectious diseases.

To help define and understand the forces that produce disease in human populations, epidemiologists perform, in general, three very basic functions: they count cases (or health events), determine rates, and then compare rates. For instance, in an investigation of an epidemic of salmonellosis in a community, the epidemiologist would first determine the number of ill persons and then calculate illness rates in various subpopulations in the affected community. Finally, the investigator would compare rates of illness between certain exposed and nonexposed populations in hopes of explaining why salmonella infections occurred in some persons but not in others.

Although these functions represent in simplistic fashion exactly what epidemiologists do, they actually reflect two basic kinds of epidemiologic study: descriptive and analytic. In the first instance (with reference to the example presented above), information is collected that describes the setting in which the salmonella epidemic occurred, i.e., the time, the place, and the person. The duration of the salmonella epidemic, where disease was acquired or recognized, and the characteristics of the ill people are then the descriptive aspects of the epidemiologic investigation. Often, simply by knowing these facts and the diagnosis, one can determine the source, mode of spread of the agent, the group at greatest risk, and the specific exposure that caused disease. Common sense may provide this information, and little or no further investigation is required.

In some instances, however, the agent, its reservoir, its mode of spread, or the risk factors are obscure, and only by more refined analytic techniques will the true picture emerge. These analyses prove most useful for posing and testing hypotheses that may explain what places human populations at risk and what specific exposures predispose most frequently to infection. Epidemiologic analyses range from the most simple, almost intuitive procedures to highly complex functions requiring extensive knowledge of biostatistics as well.

TASKS OF THE EPIDEMIOLOGIST

Since the primary purposes of epidemiology are to prevent and control disease, what then are the primary tasks of the epidemiologist to achieve these goals? First, there must be an established system of continual data collection, specific and sensitive enough to provide rapid, reliable information. The system should be designed to define disease trends and to alert health officials to real or potential health problems. The word "surveillance" is used to describe this task. Next, having recognized an outbreak, an epidemic, or a need to analyze data more carefully or rapidly, the epidemiologist must examine further the circumstances surrounding this problem and may have to perform a field investigation. Finally (and as a part of any field investigation), the epidemiologist must perform appropriate analyses of the data, draw defensible inferences from them, and make recommendations for prevention and control of disease. The next sections of this chapter discuss each of these three tasks.

SURVEILLANCE

Although there is no universally agreed-upon definition of surveillance, for purposes of this discussion it can be defined as the systematic, continued, careful watchfulness over relevant health data, with appropriate analyses and inferences, and the rapid dissemination of this information to those who need to know (6). Intrinsic in the concept of surveillance is rapid and appropriate action for disease prevention and control. The basic functions of surveillance, namely, data collection, analyses, and dissemination, are included in the definition.

The purpose of surveillance is most broadly to provide a scientific data base for rational prevention and control of disease. However, there are more specific purposes that should be recognized. Surveillance provides essential data to recognize and to define health events, to determine specific objectives, to establish priorities, to determine strategies, to evaluate prevention and control methods, and to suggest areas for further research. Therefore, surveillance not only gives epidemiologists information regarding what the health problem is but in many ways serves as a management tool for prevention and control measures.

There are many sources of health-related data that epidemiologists may develop or use for any surveillance system. Following are brief descriptions of some basic data systems most useful and relevant to epidemiologists at a local or state level.

Mortality Data

Virtually all health jurisdictions in all countries have systems of counting deaths in their populations. Unfortunately, mortality statistics often suffer from lack of specificity, sensitivity, and particularly timeliness. Considerable variation may exist in the quality of mortality statistics from community to community and from country to country, making comparisons difficult if not impossible. Inherent delays in reporting, registration, analyses, and publication of mortality statistics limit their usefulness for rapid detection of infectious disease trends. However, perhaps the most useful, regular application of mortality statistics to infectious disease control has been in monitoring and assessing influenza epidemics. Counting deaths attributed to pneumonia and influenza has provided an index of the extent and impact of influenza A and B epidemics both regionally and nationally (2). This system has given useful epidemiological information on the periodicity of influenza epidemics and those at highest risk of death, both of which serve as a basis for vaccine recommendations.

Morbidity Data

Morbidity data can often provide much more useful, timely, and particularly sensitive systems of surveillance. Again, most health jurisdictions have at least rudimentary systems of morbidity reporting for communicable diseases. Depending on the degree of reporting by the physician or health care provider, such systems may give extremely important and useful information. Sources of morbidity data usually include city, county, state, or provincial data bases that list cases of selected communicable diseases reported often by week, sometimes biweekly, and occasionally by month. By careful, regular analyses of these data, the epidemiologist frequently can acquire the basic elements of descriptive epidemiology, namely, the time and place of occurrence of disease and perhaps the age and gender of patients. Other useful data sources include schools, factories, or large businesses where absentee data are routinely collected. In the developing world, fever clinics or dispensaries catering to special age groups or health care problems may be useful. Some countries have included in their reporting systems an "unusual event" category which encourages physicians to report any unusual case, cluster of disease, or death. Hospital- or clinic-based morbidity systems have been extremely useful and frequently help confirm and localize the existence of an epidemic.

Laboratory

Whether serving the interests of a single hospital, local or state health department, or national or international agency, the laboratory has proven an indispensable source of surveillance data for infectious disease epidemiologists. By reporting increases in microbial isolates, by similar recognition of rare or unusual sero- or biotypes, or simply by informing health officials of increasing demands on laboratory facilities, laboratories have played a pivotal role in detection and investigation of epidemics.

Single-Case Investigation

Because some infectious diseases have high ratios of inapparent to apparent disease, a single clinical case should be considered a sentinel health event and investigated immediately. A single case of paralytic poliomyelitis or aseptic meningitis represents 100 to 200 other cases of mild to subclinical disease elsewhere in the community. One full-blown case of classic arthropod-borne encephalitis or dengue represents tens if not hundreds of other cases as yet unrecognized or unreported and should stimulate an immediate field investigation.

Surveys

Among the most useful tools for epidemiologic assessment in infectious diseases are culture and serologic surveys. Most frequently performed during or after the recognition of an epidemic, these surveys may be the only way to confirm a diagnosis. Ongoing, yearly serologic studies of high-risk populations may also provide useful information, particularly by helping define the actual incidence of disease on a year-by-year basis.

Knowledge of Vertebrate and Arthropod Vector Species

An important adjunct to or surrogate for human disease surveillance is the monitoring of nonhuman vertebrate hosts and vector species. For example, in many arboviral infections, generally with high ratios of inapparent to apparent disease, humans represent an incidental or dead-end host and contribute insignificantly to the zoonotic cycle. Since illness and death among susceptible animal species frequently precede recognition of human disease, surveillance of appropriate zoonotic species should be strongly considered in areas where epizootics are likely to occur and where human surveillance is poor or nonexistent.

Demographic and Environmental Factors

As with all epidemiologic investigations, it is essential to know the basic demographic characteristics of the population at risk, i.e., number, age, and sex distribution. Without these data, no rates can be determined. That is to say, one must have a denominator to calculate rates of illness or exposure. In some instances, these data are not readily available and must be acquired during the field investigation itself. However time consuming and expensive to acquire, demographic data are indispensable; without them, valid comparisons of populations and exposures are impossible.

Characteristics such as heat, cold, air flow, humidity, rainfall, and other variables may be the essential environmental determinants that predispose to disease and consequently must be measured or assessed during a field investigation.

INVESTIGATIVE TECHNIQUES

This section describes how to perform a field investigation of an infectious disease outbreak and what important administrative and public health realities are faced by the investigative team. The scenario consists of a request for epidemiologic assistance from a local health jurisdiction to a state, provincial, or federal health department. The epidemic is a presumed, point-source (common-source) outbreak in a mid-size community.

Pace and Commitment

Underlying this discussion runs the current to act quickly, to establish operational priorities, and to perform responsibly. Every effort should be made to collect and analyze data in the field and make recommendations before departure to home base. With the recent availability of computers and easy data-handling equipment, there is a strong tendency to take the data home and perform the analyses there. Local health officials often view such action as a lack of commitment or interest or even as possessiveness. Equally important, premature departure makes any further collection of data or direct contact with study populations or local health officials difficult if not impossible. The total commitment to the field investigation, the urgency, and the impetus to investigate are lost once the investigating team has left the scene.

Recognition and Response to a Request for Assistance

The report

In most instances, a state or regional health officer will be informed of an unusual number of cases of an infectious disease from local health officials, hospitals, physicians, or occasionally the news media. The local health officer probably will have a working diagnosis, and the consultant epidemiologist should try to get as much information as possible with regard to the number of cases, the time and place of occurrence, and any demographic information that is available. Depending on the size and sophistication of the local health department, relatively extensive information may already have been collected which may be very useful in planning the field investigation.

The request

At this time, it is important to know why help is requested. Possibilities include simply a need for more professional help to perform or complete the investigation, to share the responsibility of the investigation with others more experienced and knowledgeable, or, quite often, to acquire added professional expertise. Sometimes legal and ethical issues may complicate the investigation, and the investigator should be alert to such possibilities. Rarely, a local health department will virtually declare the existence of an epidemic to awaken public concern or even to secure funds. No matter what the motivation behind the request for assistance, there must be an official basis for such a request and local permission for a field investigation. There is no greater embarrassment to the investigative team than to arrive in the field unannounced and unwelcome.

The response and responsibilities

Relationships between state and local health departments vary not only from state to state within countries but from country to country. In general, the larger health districts help serve the smaller, yet the sensitivities between the two are frequently delicate, particularly as they relate to competence, local jurisdiction, and final authority. Therefore, great care must be taken by the larger health department to provide the most appropriate response to its local constituency.

There are several reasons why requests for a field investigation should be answered, if not encouraged: (i) to control and prevent further disease; (ii) to provide agreed-upon or statutorily mandated services; (iii) to derive more information about interactions among the human host, the agent, and the environment; (iv) to assess the quality of surveillance at the local level; (vi) to maintain or improve such surveillance by personal and direct contact; (vi) to establish a new system of surveillance; and (vii) to provide training opportunities in practical field epidemiology.

If a health officer decides to provide field assistance, both he or she and the local health official should discuss and agree upon (i) what resources (including personnel) will be available locally; (ii) what resources will be provided by the team; (iii) who will direct the day-to-day investigation; (iv) who will provide overall supervision and ultimately be responsible for the investigation; (v) how the data will be shared and who will be responsible for their analysis; (vi) whether a report of the findings will be written, who will write it, to whom will it go; and (vii) who will be the senior author of a scientific paper, should one be written. These are extremely important issues, some of which cannot be totally resolved before the investigation. However, they must be addressed, discussed openly, and agreed upon as soon as possible.

Preparation for the field investigation

No attempt will be made to describe in detail what personnel or equipment should be used for the field investigation. These decisions will depend on the presumed cause, magnitude, and geographical extent of the epidemic and the resources available. Rather, the emphasis focuses on the necessary collaborative relationships between health professionals and key instructions to the investigating team before it departs.

Collaboration and Consultation

Virtually all investigations of infectious disease outbreaks require the support of a competent laboratory. Even though they are not likely to go into the field, microbiologists are an essential part of the investigative team and should be consulted immediately. They should be asked to recommend what kinds of specimens to collect and how they should be collected and processed. Also, there may be substantive basic or applied research questions that could be answered during the field investigation, and these issues should be discussed in detail with the microbiologists.

Advice on statistical methods may also be sought at this time. The same philosophy applies to contacting other health professionals, such as veterinarians, mammalogists, or entomologists, whose expertise can be crucial to a successful field investigation. Moreover, serious consideration should be given to including such professionals on the investigative team in the field. It is important to determine whether such scientists should be part of the initial team so that appropriate information and, particularly, specimens can be collected concomitantly with other relevant epidemiologic information. Other persons who can be extremely important in the overall management of a field investigation are information specialists. When the investigation involves large outbreaks of disease that will likely attract even moderate local or regional attention in the news media, the presence of an experienced and knowledgeable information officer who can respond to public inquiries and meet with the news media on a regular basis can be invaluable.

Basic Administrative Instructions

Once the field team has been formed, certain key instructions should be emphasized. (i) Identify the team leader and the person to whom he or she should report regularly at the central or home base. (ii) Specify when and how communications should be established for information exchange and guidance. Do not permit the investigating team to notify the supervisors of the progress of the investigation when it is convenient to the team. Establish within reason fixed times and places for regular communication regardless of whether new facts or findings have been uncovered. There may be just as important reasons for the home base to communicate with the field team as the reverse. (iii) Emphasize the need for the team to meet with appropriate local health officials immediately upon arriving in the field. If the local official has not already been identified, instruct the team leader to determine as soon as possible who at the local level will be in charge. Encourage the team to identify and meet with all persons from whom they may need cooperation in the investigation. Such persons include local health department directors or chiefs of epidemiology and personnel in laboratory services, vital statistics, nursing, and maternal and child health. Other important persons often include the mayor, the local medical society, and hospital administrators and staff. It is highly preferable to take the day or so needed to meet these persons initially, so that key doors will be opened, than to spend valuable time later in the investigation mending bridges. (iv) Have the team leader identify the appropriate local person to speak for the entire investigative team when necessary. In general, the visiting team should try to avoid direct contact with the news media and should always defer to local health officials. The investigative team is usually working at the request and under the aegis of the local health authorities. Therefore, it is the local officials who not only know and appreciate the local aspects of the epidemic but are the appropriate persons to comment on the findings of the investigation. In the most practical sense, the less the news media make contact with the investigative team, the more can be done at the pace and discretion of that team.

The Field Investigation

Ten essential steps of a typical field investigation are listed below. These tasks should not be considered fixed or binding but logical in terms of field operations and epidemiologic thinking. The epidemiologist may perform several of these functions simultaneously or in different order during the investigation. He or she may even institute control and prevention measures soon after beginning the investigation on the basis of intuitive reasoning or common sense. No two epidemiologists will take the same pathway of investigation, for each epidemic is unique. In general, however, the data they collect, the analyses they apply, and the control and prevention measures they recommend will likely be similar.

Since, by definition, the epidemic in question has resulted from a point source and may be continuing or nearly over before the field team arrives, the investigation will be retrospective in nature. This should alert the epidemiologist to some fundamental aspects of any investigation that occurs after the fact. First, because many illnesses and critical events have already occurred, much information acquired and related to the epidemic will be based on memory. Health officers, physicians, and patients are likely to have different recollections or perceptions of what transpired, what caused the disease, and even who or what was responsible for the epidemic. Information may conflict, may not be accurate, and certainly cannot be expected to reflect a precise account of past events. Yet just as the clinician may ask patients what they think is making them sick, the epidemiologist will do well to ask members of the affected community what they think caused the epidemic. For the young, inexperienced epidemiologist steeped in the tradition of molecule and millimole determinations, the "more-or-less" measurements in the field can initially be major hurdles to a successful field investigation. However lacking in accuracy these data may be, they are the only data available and must be collected, analyzed, and interpreted with care, imagination, and caution.

Determine the existence of an epidemic

In most instances, local health officials will know whether more cases of disease are occurring than would normally be expected. Since most local health departments have ongoing records of the occurrence of communicable diseases, comparisons by week, month, and year can be made to determine whether the observed numbers exceed the normally expected level. Although strict laboratory confirmation may be lacking at this time, an increase in the number of cases of a disease reasonably accurately reported by local physicians should stimulate further inquiry. However, the terms "epidemic" and "outbreak" are quite subjective, and their usage reflects not only how local health officials view the expected rises and falls in disease incidence but also whether such changes merit investigation. One must be acutely aware of artifactual causes of increases or decreases in numbers of reported cases, such as changes in local reporting practices, increased interest in certain diseases because of local or national awareness, or changes in methods of diagnosis. Even the presence of a new physician or clinic in the community may lead to a substantial increase in reported numbers of cases yet not represent a true increase above normal. In certain situations, however, it may be difficult to document the existence of an epidemic rapidly. One may need to acquire information from such sources as school or factory absentee records, outpatient clinic visits, hospitalizations, laboratory records, or death certificates. Sometimes a simple survey of practicing physicians will strongly support the existence of an epidemic, as would a similar rapid survey of households in the community. Frequently, such quick assessments entail asking about signs and symptoms rather than about specific diagnoses. For example, such inquiry might involve asking physicians or clinics whether they were seeing more people than usual with sore throats, gastroenteritis, fever with rash, etc., in order to obtain an index of disease incidence. Although not specific for any given disease, such surveys can often document the occurrence of an epidemic. Sometimes it is extremely difficult to establish satisfactorily the existence of an epidemic, yet because of local pressures, epidemiologists may be obliged to continue the investigation even if they believe that no significant health problem exists.

Confirm the diagnosis

Every effort possible should be made to confirm the clinical diagnosis by standard laboratory techniques such as serology or isolation and characterization of the agent. One should not attempt to apply newly introduced, experimental, or otherwise not broadly recognized confirmatory tests, at least not at this stage in the investigation. If possible, visit the laboratory and verify the laboratory findings in person. Not every reported case has to be confirmed. If most patients have the expected or similar clinical signs and symptoms and, perhaps, 15 to 20% of the cases are laboratory confirmed, one does not need more confirmation at this time; these data should be ample. One should try to examine or see several representative cases of the disease as well; clinical assumptions should not be made. The diagnosis should be verified by a physician member of the team. Nothing convinces epidemiologists and responsible health officers more than an eyewitness confirmation of clinical disease by the investigating team.

Create a case definition and determine the number of cases

Now the epidemiologist must create a workable case definition, decide how to find cases, and determine how to count them. The simplest and most objective criteria for a case definition are usually the best (for example, fever, X-ray evidence of pneumonia, leukocytes in the spinal fluid, number of bowel movements per day, blood in the stool, skin rash, etc.). However, be guided by the accepted, usual presentation of the disease, with or without standard laboratory confirmation, in the case definition. Where time may be a critical factor in a rapidly unfolding field investigation, a simple, easily applicable definition should be used, recognizing that some cases will be missed and that some noncases will be included. Some factors that can help determine the levels of sensitivity and specificity of the case definition are the following:

1. What is the usual apparent-to-inapparent clinical case ratio?
2. What are the important and obvious pathognomonic or strongly clinically suggestive signs and symptoms of the disease?
3. What isolation, identification, and serologic techniques are easy and reliable?
4. How accessible are the patients or those at risk; can they be recontacted after the initial investigation for follow-up questions, examination, or serology?
5. In the event that the investigation requires long-term follow-up, can the case definitions be applied easily, consistently, and objectively by individuals other than the current investigating team?
6. Is it absolutely necessary that all patients be identified during the initial investigation, or would only those seen by physicians or hospitalized suffice?

These considerations and others should help determine how cases will be defined and how intensive case investigation will be. However, no matter what criteria are used, the case definition must be applied equally and without bias to all persons under investigation.

Methods for finding cases will vary considerably according to the disease and the community setting. In many field investigations, the techniques for identifying cases will be relatively self-evident. Most outbreaks involve certain clearly identifiable groups at risk. It is simply a matter of intensifying reporting from physicians, hospitals, laboratories, or school and industrial contacts, or perhaps using some form of public announcement to identify most of the remaining, unreported cases. However, there may be times when more intensive efforts, such as physician, telephone, door-to-door, culture, or serologic surveys, may be necessary to find cases. Regardless of the method, some system(s) of case identification must be established for the duration of the investigation and perhaps afterwards.

In most instances, simply determining the number of cases does not provide adequate information. Control and prevention measures depend on knowledge of the source and mode of spread of an agent as well as certain characteristics of ill patients. Therefore, the process of case finding must include collecting pertinent information likely to provide leads to the natural history of the epidemic and, particularly, relevant characteristics of the ill. First, one should collect basic information about each patient's age, sex, residence, occupation, date of onset, etc., to define the simple and basic descriptive aspects of the epidemic. However, if the disease under investigation is usually water- or foodborne, one should ask questions about exposure to various water and food sources. If the disease is most frequently transmitted by person-to-person contact, one should seek information that will help determine the frequency, duration, and nature of personal contacts. If the nature of the disease is not known or cannot be comfortably presumed, the epidemiologist will need to ask a variety of questions covering all possible aspects of disease transmission and risk.

Orient the data with respect to time, place, and person

Having reasonably accurately determined the number of cases, the epidemiologist should now analyze the descriptive aspects of the investigation. The epidemic should be characterized with respect to when patients became ill, where patients resided or became ill, and what characteristics the patients possess. There may be a tendency to wait until the epidemic is over or until all likely cases have been reported before performing such an analysis. This tendency should be strongly resisted because the earlier one can develop ideas of why the epidemic started, the more pertinent and accurate data one can collect. Moreover, inclusion of a proportionately small number of cases will usually not affect the analysis or recommendations.

Time. In most instances, it will be valuable to describe the cases by time of onset by constructing a graph that depicts the occurrence of cases over an appropriate time interval (Fig. 1). This "epidemic curve," as it is frequently called, can give a considerably deeper appreciation for the magnitude of the outbreak, its possible mode of spread, and the possible duration of the epidemic than would a simple listing of cases. A remarkable amount of information can be inferred from a pictorial representation of times of onset of disease. If the incubation period of the disease is known, relatively firm inferences can be made regarding the likelihood of a point-source exposure, person-to-person spread, or a mixture of the two. Also, if the epidemic is in progress, one may be able to predict, using the epidemic curve, how many more cases are likely to occur. Finally, a pictorial representation of cases over time serves as an excellent way of communicating with nonepidemiologists, administrators, and others who need to grasp in some fashion the nature and magnitude of the epidemic. The epidemic curve in Fig. 1 portrays cases of campylobacter gastroenteritis that occurred in a small town in Kansas, May and June 1988, by day of onset (Centers for Disease Control, unpublished data). The epidemic was rapid in onset, suggesting (i) simultaneous common-source exposure of many persons, (ii) a disease with a short incubation period, and (iii) a continuing exposure spanning several weeks. Indeed, the source was contaminated raw milk, probably from a single dairy where *Campylobacter jejuni* of the same serotype as the epidemic strain was isolated from the milk filter.

Place. Exposures to microbial agents sometimes occur in unique locations in the community, which, if properly depicted and analyzed, may provide clues to the source of the agent or the nature of exposure. Water supplies, milk distribution routes, sewage disposal outflows, prevailing wind currents, airflow patterns in buildings, and ecologic habitats of animals may play important roles in disseminating microbial pathogens and thus in determining who is at risk of acquiring disease. If cases are plotted geographically, a pattern of distribution may emerge that approximates these known sources and routes of potential exposure, which may help identify the vehicle or mode of transmission. Figure 2 illustrates the usefulness of a "spot map" in the investigation of an outbreak of shigellosis in Dubuque, Iowa, in 1974 (4). Initially, the investigation revealed that cases were not clustered by area of residence or age or sex. A history of drinking water gave no useful clue as to a possible source and mode of transmission. However, it was later learned that some patients had been exposed to water by recent swimming in a camping park located on the Mississippi River. The river sites where 22 culture-positive patients swam within 3 days of onset of illness strongly suggested a common source of exposure (Fig. 2).

Ultimately, the epidemiologists incriminated the Mississippi River water by documenting gross contamination by the city's sewage treatment plant 5 miles up-

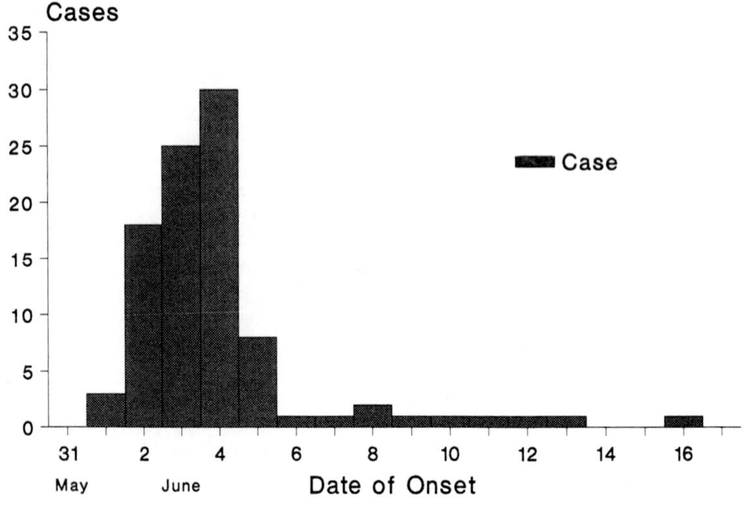

FIG. 1. Campylobacter gastroenteritis cases by date of onset, Kansas, 1988.

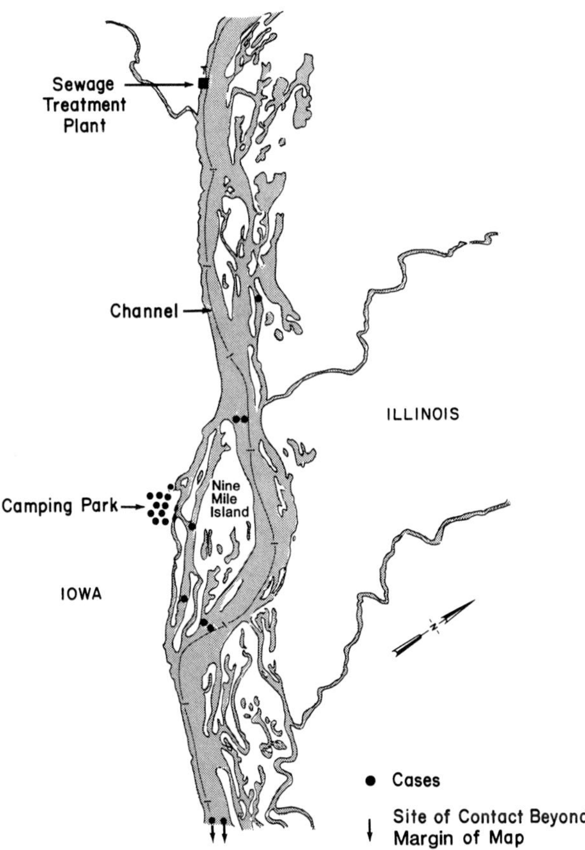

FIG. 2. Mississippi River sites where 22 culture-positive patients swam within 3 days of onset of illness.

stream and by isolating *Shigella sonnei* from a sample of river water near the camping area.

Person. Finally, the epidemiologist should examine the characteristics of the patients themselves with respect to age, sex, race, occupation, or virtually any other characteristic that may be useful in portraying the uniqueness of the case population. Some diseases primarily affect certain age groups or races; frequently, occupation is a key characteristic of people with certain infectious diseases. The list of human characteristics is nearly endless. However, the more the investigators know about the disease in question (the reservoir, mode[s] of spread, and persons usually at greatest risk), the more specific and pertinent information they should seek from the cases to determine whether any of these characteristics predispose to illness.

Determine who is at risk of becoming ill

Now the team knows the number of people ill, where they were when they became ill, when they were there, and what their general characteristics are. Usually, there will be a firm diagnosis or a good working diagnosis. These data frequently provide enough information to indicate who was at risk of becoming ill. For example, this information may strongly suggest that only people in a particular community supplied by a specific water system were at risk of getting sick, or that only certain students in a school or workers in a single factory became ill. Perhaps it was only a group of people who attended a local restaurant who reported illness. In other words, the simple descriptive aspects of the epidemic frequently identify those most likely at risk of disease. However, no matter how obvious it might appear that only a single group of persons was at risk, the epidemiologist may have to apply some analytic methods to support this conclusion. For example, if fever, abdominal cramps, and diarrhea occurred among 35 residents of housing subdivision A (presumably caused by water contaminated with shigella) and no similar illness was reported from subdivision B over the same time period, one would logically conclude that only subdivision A residents were at risk of developing disease. However, only after surveying the residents of subdivision B or even elsewhere in the community, looking for the same illness and comparing illness rates in such groups, can one legitimately infer that the at-risk population were all residents of subdivision A.

Develop a hypothesis that explains the specific exposure that caused disease and test this hypothesis by appropriate statistical methods

The next analytic step is often the most difficult one to perform. By now the epidemiologists should have an excellent grasp of the epidemic and an overall feel for the most likely source and mode of transmission. However, they must still determine the most likely exposure that caused disease. A classic example of what is meant here is an investigation of an outbreak of nausea, vomiting, and diarrhea among people who had attended a church supper presumedly caused by staphylococcal contamination of food eaten at the supper. Since the disease was most likely acquired by eating or drinking something (because of the signs and symptoms) and because no other cluster of similar disease had occurred elsewhere in the community, the investigators considered only those who attended the supper to be at greatest risk. The hypothesis posed was that the exposure necessary to develop nausea, vomiting, and diarrhea was consumption of some food contaminated with staphylococcal enterotoxin. Therefore, the ill people were asked what they had eaten at the church supper (i.e., what they had been exposed to), and their food histories were taken. To determine whether the exposures to certain foods among these ill persons (cases) were unique, these exposures were compared with exposures of people who had not become ill (controls) but had also attended the church supper. Comparisons of food histories (eating or exposure rates) between the ill and the well participants were made and statistically analyzed. The food exposure rates between the cases and controls were found to be similar for almost all foods served. But for one food, the exposure rates were very different and unlikely to be different simply by chance alone. Therefore, the inference was drawn that eating that specific food was the exposure that caused the illness and, therefore, the source of the enterotoxin.

Several specific examples of field investigations of infectious diseases may serve to illustrate how hypotheses are developed and tested.

In August 1980, a community hospital in Michigan recognized seven cases of group A streptococcal (GAS) postoperative wound infections that had occurred over the previous 4 months (1). This represented more cases than usual, and an investigation was started. Using a standard case definition, the epidemiologists ultimately identified 10 cases that had occurred over this time period, all of whom were patients on several surgical wards. The same streptococcal serotype common to all cases, the geographical clustering, plus the fact that the infections developed within 1 to 2 days after surgery suggested a common source of exposure, presumably in the operating rooms. Although streptococcal disease can rarely be transmitted by inanimate objects, within the hospital setting the most frequent sources of streptococci are humans and the most common mode of spread is from person to person. Therefore, the epidemiologists hypothesized that the probable risk factor unique to these patients was contact with or exposure to an infected or colonized member of the hospital's professional staff sometime during surgery. The investigators then compared GAS-infected patients (cases) with non-GAS-infected postsurgical patients (controls) with respect to what exposure they had had to a total of 38 surgeons, anesthesiologists, and nursing staff during surgery for the epidemic period. Rates of exposure to various hospital staff except for one nurse were not statistically different between cases and controls. This nurse was cultured and found to be an anal and vaginal carrier of a streptococcal strain identical to the epidemic strain. After appropriate treatment, this strain could no longer be cultured from her, so she returned to work. Six months later there were two more cases of postoperative GAS infection, caused by a different serotype. The same nurse was found to be a vaginal and anal carrier of this different strain. No further cases were reported after the nurse was relieved of her work in the hospital.

The following investigation of an epidemic of *Listeria monocytogenes* is a classic example of how the epidemiologic method, simple inferences, and persistent reexamination of data can point to a hitherto unknown source and mode of spread of disease. Thirty-four cases of perinatal listeriosis and seven cases of adult disease occurred between 1 March and 1 September 1981 in several maritime provinces of Canada (5). These cases represented a severalfold increase over the number of cases diagnosed in previous years, suggesting some common exposure. Although *L. monocytogenes* is a common cause of abortion and nervous system diseases in cattle, sheep, and goats, the source of human infection has been obscure. The epidemiologists, therefore, undertook an investigation to determine whether cases had had contact with one another or whether there had been a common environmental source that would explain their disease. Cases could not be linked together by person-to-person contact; they shared no common water source; and food exposures, as determined from a general food history, were not different between cases and controls. However, a second, more detailed food history and subsequent intensive interrogation revealed that there was a statistically significant difference between cases and controls regarding exposure to coleslaw. Even though this food had never been known as a source of *Listeria* spp., it was the only food item statistically incriminated and essentially the only lead the investigators had at the time. Armed with this association, the team subsequently found a specimen of coleslaw in the refrigerator of one of the patients which grew out the same *Listeria* serotype found in the epidemic-associated cases. No other food items in the refrigerator were positive for *Listeria* spp. The coleslaw had been prepared by a regional manufacturer who had obtained cabbages and carrots from several wholesale dealers and many local farmers. Although environmental cultures from the coleslaw plant failed to reveal *Listeria* organisms, two unopened packages of coleslaw from the plant subsequently grew *L. monocytogenes* of the same epidemic serotype. The sources of the vegetable ingredients were examined, and a single farmer who had grown cabbages and also maintained a flock of sheep was identified. Two of his sheep had died of listeriosis in 1979 and 1981. Also, he was in the habit of using sheep manure to fertilize his cabbage.

It cannot be proven that this particular farm was the source of the *Listeria* organisms that caused the epidemic. However, the hypothesis that coleslaw was the source and the statistical test that supported this hypothesis provided the necessary impetus to continue the investigation. Ultimately, a single highly suggestive source of the bacteria was discovered. These findings strongly implicated listeriosis as a zoonotic infection transmitted from infected animals via contaminated vegetables to humans.

A similar logic in a much more difficult situation was applied to the outbreak of Legionnaires disease among conventioneers attending meetings in Philadelphia, Pa., in July 1976 (3). From the beginning to the end of the field investigation, neither the clinical presentation nor laboratory results provided epidemiologists with a diagnosis. Although initially it appeared that disease was not transmitted from person to person, being a conventioneer who stayed at or visited the Bellevue Stratford Hotel in Philadelphia conferred an increased risk of disease. This conclusion, however, did not provide enough information about the source or mode of spread of the agent to be particularly useful. To put it another way, a person's mere presence in the Bellevue Stratford did not help explain what the specific exposure was or how the disease was acquired. A Legionnaire could easily have eaten a meal, consumed water from the hotel, or simply breathed in the air in the hotel—all possible exposures to the agent that could place him in the high-risk category of becoming ill. Therefore, a series of hypotheses was proposed to determine whether eating meals, drinking water, or simply being in the hotel conferred increased risk of developing illness among the Legionnaires. When the final analysis was done, there was no significant difference between ill and well Legionnaires with regard to eating or drinking at the hotel. However, spending at least 1 h in the hotel lobby conferred a much greater risk of disease than would have been expected by chance alone. Therefore, the investigators inferred that being in the lobby of the hotel was the necessary exposure for acquiring disease. This, coupled with the clinical features of the disease (pneumonia), implied that the agent was airborne and was transmitted through the air-conditioning system. Although the bacterium responsible for Legionnaires disease was not isolated from the Bellevue Stratford Hotel air-conditioning system at that time, it was later recovered from lung tissue of several diseased Legionnaires. Moreover, not only have subsequent investigations of similar epidemics of Legionnaires disease elsewhere confirmed the epidemiologic pattern of this disease, but *Legionella* bacteria have been isolated from similar air-conditioning systems.

Again, this phase of the investigation clearly poses the greatest challenge to epidemiologists. They must review their findings carefully, weigh the clinical, laboratory, and epidemiologic features of the disease, and hypothesize exposures that could plausibly cause disease. In other words, they must seek from the patients' histories exposures that could conceivably predispose to illness. If exposure histories for cases and controls are not significantly different, the epidemiologists must develop new hypotheses. This may require imagination, perseverance, and sometimes resurveying those at risk to obtain more pertinent information.

Compare the hypothesis with the established facts

Having determined by epidemiologic and statistical inference the probable exposure responsible for disease, the epidemiologist still must test the hypothesis against the clinical, laboratory, and other epidemiologic facts of the investigation. In other words, do the proposed exposure, mode of spread, and population affected fit well with the known facts of the disease? For example, if, in the staphyloccocal gastroenteritis outbreak referred to above, the analysis incriminated an uncooked food left at room temperature for 18 to 24 h and previously known to promote growth of staphylococci, the hypothesis would fit well with our understanding of staphylococcal food poisoning. However, if the analysis incriminated coffee or water—highly unlikely sources of staphylococcal enterotoxin—the epidemiologist would have had to reassess the findings, perhaps secure more information, reconsider the clinical diagnosis, and certainly pose and test new hypotheses. When the disease is undiagnosed, the epidemiologist will clearly find it very difficult to fit a hypothesis to the natural history of the disease in question. All that can be hoped is that the clinical, laboratory, and epidemiologic findings portray a coherent, plausible, and physiologically sound series of findings and events that make sense.

Plan a more systematic study

The actual field investigation and analyses may be completed by now, requiring only a written report (see below). However, because there may be a need to find more patients or to define better the extent of the epidemic or because a new laboratory method or case-finding technique needs to be evaluated, the epidemiologists may want to perform more detailed and carefully executed studies. With the pressure of the investigation somewhat removed, the field team can now consider surveying the population at risk in a variety of ways to help improve the quality of data and answer particular questions. Perhaps the most important reasons to perform such studies are to improve the sensitivity and specificity of the case definition and establish more accurately the true number of persons at risk, i.e., to improve the quality of numerators and denominators. For example, serosurveys coupled with a more complete clinical history can often sharpen the accuracy of the case count and define more clearly those truly at risk of developing disease. Moreover, repeat interviews of patients with confirmed disease may enable rough quantitation of degrees of exposure or dose responses, useful information in understanding the pathogenesis of certain diseases.

Prepare a written report

Frequently, the final responsibility of the investigative team is preparation of a written report to document the investigation, the findings, and the recommendations. It is beyond the scope of this chapter to provide a detailed set of guidelines on scientific report writing. However, in most instances there are several important reasons why a report should be written and as soon as possible.

Administrative or operational purposes. (i) A document for action. Control and prevention efforts sometimes are undertaken only when a report of all relevant findings has been written. This fact can and should place a heavy but necessary burden on epidemiologists to complete their work quickly. Even if all possible cases have not yet been found or some laboratory results are still pending, reasonable written assumptions and recommendation can usually be made without fear of retraction or subsequent major change.

(ii) A record of performance. In this day of input and output measurements, program planning, program justifications, and performance evaluations, there is often no better record of accomplishment than a well-written report of a completed field investigation. The number of investigations performed and the time and resources expended not only document the magnitude of health problems, changes in disease trends, and the results of control and prevention efforts but also serve as concrete evidence of program justification and needs.

(iii) A document for potential medical or legal issues. Presumably, epidemiologists investigate epidemics with objective, unbiased, and scientific purposes and similarly prepare written reports of their findings and conclusions objectively, honestly, and fairly. Such information may prove absolutely invaluable to consumer, physician, or local and state health department officials in any legal action regarding health responsibilities and jurisdictions. In the long run, the health of the public is best served by simple, careful, honest documentation of events and findings made generally available for interpretation and comment.

Scientific or epidemiologic purposes. (i) Enhancement of the quality of the investigation. Although not fully explained and rarely referred to, the actual process of writing and viewing data in written form often generates new and different thought processes and associations in the mind of the epidemiologist. The discipline of committing to paper the clinical, laboratory, and epidemiologic findings of an epidemic investigation almost always brings to light a better understanding not only of the natural unfolding of events but also of the importance of these events with respect to the natural history and development of the epidemic. The actual process of creating scientific prose, summarizing data, and making tables and figures representing the established facts forces one to view the entire series of events in a balanced, rational, and explainable way, considerably more so than does presenting an oral report to the local health department on the day of departure from the field. Occasionally, previously unrecognized associations emerge, and the exercise of writing what was done and what was found sometimes uncovers facts and events that were more or less assumed to be true but not specifically sought for during the investigation. This, in turn, may stimulate further inquiry and fact finding to verify these assumptions.

(ii) An instrument for teaching epidemiology. There would hardly be disagreement among epidemiologists that the exercise of writing the results of an investigation constitutes an essential building block in learning epidemiology. Much the way a lawyer prepares a brief, the epidemiologist should know how to organize and present in logical sequence the important and pertinent findings of an investigation, their quality and validity, and the scientific inferences that can be made by their written presentation. The simple, direct, and orderly array of facts and inferences will reflect not only on the quality of the investigation itself but on the writer's basic understanding and knowledge of the epidemiologic method.

Execute control and prevention measures

It is not the purpose of this chapter to elaborate on control and prevention measures. Nevertheless, the underlying purposes of all epidemic investigations are to control and prevent further disease.

ANALYTIC METHODS

This section describes some of the more common analytic tools used in field investigations of infectious diseases. These discussions cover only the highlights and key points for emphasis. Standard texts of epidemiology and biostatistics elaborate more fully and should be referred to for detailed methods and procedures.

Case Control and Cohort Studies

As already mentioned, the primary purpose of any epidemiologic study is to determine why certain individuals develop disease. To answer this question, hypotheses of exposure are generated and rates are compared. The epidemiologist selectively compares rates of disease in various populations in hopes of uncovering what risk factors and specific exposures may be responsible for illness.

Because of their practical application to investigation of infectious disease, two basic kinds of epidemiologic study are discussed below: case control studies and cohort studies. In this context, both kinds are called observational, meaning that no human intervention is involved in assigning persons to study groups. Cross-sectional studies, sometimes useful in infectious disease evaluation, will not be described, nor will experimental (randomized clinical trial) studies.

Case control studies

The kind of study most frequently performed in infectious disease investigations is the case control study. Conceptually, the study proceeds from disease to exposure. In this instance, the epidemiologist identifies cases of disease that have already occurred and compares their characteristics and exposure history with those of noncases, or controls. If the exposure rates of the two groups are different, statistical analyses are made to determine whether the difference was likely to have occurred by chance alone or whether it represents a likely causal association between exposure and illness. If the observed difference occurs, for example, only once in 200 similar analyses, the epidemiologist would likely conclude there is a probable causal relationship between that particular exposure and development of infection.

The logic of case control studies is applied frequently without regard to statistical tests when it is intuitively clear that study populations are ill and others are not after certain exposures. However, further analyses of specific exposures may be necessary to define more clearly the exact host or environmental factors responsible for disease. For example, in the previous section on investigative techniques, the analysis by Berkelman et al. (1) was a case control study. These investigators compared infected and noninfected persons with regard to specific exposures within the hospital and showed a statistically significant different exposure rate to a single nurse. The inference was then drawn that this specific exposure materially contributed to acquiring infection.

Case control studies are usually relatively simple and inexpensive to perform and frequently can be completed in several days to weeks. Also, they are ideally suited to study rare diseases because one can collect many cases that have occurred over a long time period and analyze them quite quickly.

However, in other studies, particularly ones involving large groups of people or entire communities, methodological problems arise, particularly as they relate to selection of control populations. Cases and controls should be as comparable as possible in all respects other than the risk or exposure factor under study. Studies performed on special groups such as hospital patients or particular occupational groups may not be suitable for extrapolation to the population at large. Case ascertainment, or the ability to recognize all cases, may also play an important role in performing valid objective case control studies. These and other methodological concerns must be considered when implementing a case control study. The epidemiology literature is replete with articles, even entire books, on the subject. Suffice it to say that carefully designed and well-performed case control studies have served and will continue to serve the epidemiologist well.

Cohort study

Conceptually, the cohort study proceeds from exposure to disease. The epidemiologist starts with exposed and nonexposed groups and monitors them to determine whether their disease rates differ.

Such studies may require long periods of observation, sometimes years, and considerable resources but are traditionally considered less biased and more scientifically appealing, since the approach or view of the data is prospective in nature and not after the fact. However, under certain circumstances a well-defined population may be studied by the cohort method after the fact, a so-called retrospective cohort study.

Yet there are still methodological problems that must be considered. Again, comparability of exposed and nonexposed groups may pose problems. Another important consideration is the expected frequency of disease in the exposed and nonexposed populations. With rare diseases, cohort studies may not detect enough cases to permit valid statistical comparisons at the end of observation. During prolonged prospective studies, members of both exposed and unexposed populations may be lost to follow-up, or diagnoses may not remain standardized. Successful cohort studies depend heavily on known specific exposure over time. For infectious diseases, such close observation may be very labor intensive and expensive.

The best examples of observational cohort studies in infectious diseases are determinations of vaccine efficacy in well-defined populations. Here, rates of illness are compared after natural exposure among immunized and nonimmunized populations.

Age-Adjusted Rates

Emphasis has been placed throughout this chapter on the concept of determining rates of illness or exposures as the most appropriate way of determining the impact of any given factor under study. Only by determining rates can the epidemiologist make fair and scientifically objective comparisons between study populations. Despite this need to determine rates for appropriate comparative purposes, sometimes comparison of disease or death rates between different populations reveals differences that are considerably misleading. For example, as part of a large field investigation, it may be necessary to compare two (or more) study populations. However, if these populations are dissimilar with respect to age, sex, race, vaccination status, or other factors, one may have to adjust these rates so that fair comparisons can be made. Most often, adjustments are made because of age differences in the study groups. This is particularly true when rates within the populations vary with age and when the study groups differ appreciably in age composition. An age-adjusted rate can be defined as an estimated overall rate that would have occurred in a selected standard population had the age-specific rates, which did occur in the study population, prevailed. The reader is directed to consult standard epidemiology texts for the exact methods of age adjustment.

Serosurveys

One of the most common epidemiologic tools applied in infectious disease investigations is the collection of blood specimens for antibody testing. Initially specimens are usually collected for diagnostic purposes, but subsequently serum may be collected to (i) define the cumulative infection experience of a population to a given agent, (ii) estimate the ratio of apparent to inapparent infection rates, (iii) define environmental and host-related factors underlying exposure, and (iv) estimate reinfection rates.

Detection of specific antibodies to a single infectious agent at a single point in time defines the prevalence of antibodies to that particular agent. This antibody prevalence reflects the cumulative experience, both past and present, with that specific agent, presuming lifelong presence of antibody. Testing of paired acute and convalescent sera for demonstration of a rise in antibody titer or the use of a serologic assay applied to single samples that measure only very recent infection (e.g., immunoglobulin M enzyme-linked immunosorbent assay or complement fixation tests) provide an estimate of the incidence of infection during the epidemic or study period. Coupled with good clinical histories from a field investigation, serologic tests for recent infection can provide information on ratios of inapparent to apparent infections and also materially supplement and refine acute morbidity reporting. Serum specimens collected before an anticipated epidemic or before contact with an agent may permit determination of protective antibody levels to that agent after challenge or relationships between previous infection and development of severe disease. Reinfection rates can also be determined by collecting paired sera before and after exposure. Regardless of purpose, rigorous standards of sampling must be applied to the test population. There are several basic sampling methods applicable to serosurveys that may be used, depending on the questions to be answered.

The random sample

Under ideal circumstances, a random sample of the population under study provides the most useful and statistically powerful results. However, simple random sampling of individuals is often highly impractical, expensive, and time consuming. The investigators, essentially by definition, have to know the location of the entire population under study for random sampling to be applied. On the other hand, a small population of perhaps up to 1,000 or 1,500 in a small village whose population has been or can easily be counted is very suitable for random sampling. By assigning a number to each individual and by selecting the numbers randomly, the serosurvey can be completed with relative ease.

Multistage sampling

When larger populations are to be studied, the sampling method most effectively is divided into several stages of selection. As an example, a city can be divided into census tracts or districts, blocks of housing units, and ultimately dwellings. Depending on the information to be obtained and the statistical confidence desired, random sampling of each of these clusters is applied. When the blocks have been identified, there can be a simple random selection of housing units in the blocks, and either all or a selected segment of each household may be interviewed and bled. Obviously, the more levels or groups there are to sample, the less statistical strength there is to the results. This fact is usually compensated for by increasing the number of census tracts or blocks to increase confidence in the results. In such a sampling scheme, a specific segment of the population, such as the very young or women in their reproductive years, can be targeted for serologic surveys. When such selectivity is applied to a household with more than one member present in that subset, random selection is preferred and strengthens the significance of the results.

Stratification sampling

When sampling of large and particularly diverse geographical areas is contemplated, it is highly desirable to subdivide the entire area into several strata by geographic, climatic, or meteorologic characteristics to ensure that these markedly different areas are represented in the survey. Then a sample can be selected from each stratum in proportion to its population size or other characteristic deemed important. This system of stratification guarantees representation from different geophysical areas of the entire population studied.

In all sampling of this kind, the essential point to bear

in mind is that there must be a probability of selection of geographical areas and individuals; i.e., no single geographical unit or individual should be excluded from the possibility of being selected.

LITERATURE CITED

1. **Berkelman, R. L., D. Martin, D. R. Graham, J. Mowry, R. Freisem, J. A. Weber, J. L. Ho, and J. R. Allen.** 1982. Streptococcal wound infections caused by a vaginal carrier. J. Am. Med. Assoc. **248:**2680–2682.
2. **Choi, K., and S. B. Thacker.** 1981. An evaluation of influenza mortality surveillance, 1962–1979. Am. J. Epidemiol. **113:**215–226.
3. **Fraser, D. W., T. F. Tsai, W. A. Orenstein, W. E. Parkin, H. J. Beecham, R. G. Sharrar, J. Harris, G. F. Mallison, S. M. Martin, J. E. McDade, C. C. Shepard, P. S. Brachman, and the investigative team.** 1977. Legionnaires disease. Description of an epidemic of pneumonia. N. Engl. J. Med. **297:**1189–1197.
4. **Rosenberg, M. D., K. K. Hazlet, J. Schaefer, J. G. Wells, and C. Pruneda.** 1976. Shigellosis from swimming. J. Am. Med. Assoc. **236:**1849–1852.
5. **Schlech, W. F., III, P. M. Lavigne, R. A. Bortobussi, A. C. Allen, E. V. Haldane, A. J. Wort, A. W. Hightower, S. E. Johnson, S. H. King, E. S. Nicholls, and C. V. Broome.** 1983. Epidemic listeriosis—evidence for transmission by food. N. Engl. J. Med. **308:**203–206.
6. **Thacker, S. B., and R. L. Berkelman.** 1988. Public health surveillance in the United States. Epidemiol. Rev. **10:**164–190.

Chapter 23

Typing Methods for Epidemiologic Investigation

MICHAEL A. PFALLER

Nosocomial infections are an important cause of morbidity and mortality among hospitalized patients. The investigation and control of nosocomial infections is a complex issue involving clinical, infection control, and laboratory personnel. The clinical microbiology laboratory clearly plays a key role in the diagnosis of nosocomial infections and frequently is called upon to assist in the epidemiologic investigation of clusters of nosocomial infections.

There are several essential prerequisites for an adequate workup of a nosocomial infection outbreak, including (i) good communication between the microbiology laboratory and the infection control team; (ii) timely reporting and access to laboratory records; (iii) routine antimicrobial susceptibility testing and identification of nosocomial pathogens to species level; and (iv) limited storage and access to bacterial (and fungal) strains. Epidemiologists frequently rely on the laboratory identification and typing of nosocomial pathogens to provide evidence for the biologic and genetic relatedness of these organisms as an aid in the epidemiologic investigation (1, 14, 27, 33, 40, 60, 63, 64, 82, 117). In many cases, just the species identification and antimicrobial susceptibility pattern (antibiogram) are sufficient to confirm the epidemiologic relationship between different isolates; however, there is an increasing need for more detailed subspecies delineation or typing of nosocomial pathogens. The rationale for such strain delineation is that repeated isolation of an organism with identical markers from one or more patients suggests that the organism may have originated from a single clone and therefore is more likely to represent infection (individual patient) or transmission from patient to patient from a common source or by a common mechanism. When a bacterial or fungal species that appears to be the cause of infection is a frequent or universal member of the normal flora or environment, simple species identification is no longer useful in distinguishing between infection and colonization or in tracing the source of the infecting organism. The ubiquitous nature of many important nosocomial pathogens such as *Staphylococcus epidermidis, Staphylococcus aureus, Enterococcus faecalis,* and *Pseudomonas aeruginosa* has necessitated the development of additional methods of strain delineation within species for use as epidemiologic and diagnostic tools.

REQUIREMENTS OF AN EPIDEMIOLOGIC TYPING SYSTEM

The intelligent, cost-effective application of epidemiologic typing methods requires that typing be performed only with clear objectives in mind. Most commonly, these objectives include (1, 33, 40, 60, 63, 64) (i) determination of the extent of an outbreak, (ii) determination of the mode of transmission and evaluation of preventive measures, and (iii) monitoring of infection in special areas where infection is a particular hazard. Each of these objectives places different demands on an epidemiologic typing system. For example, although the existence of multiple different strains of *P. aeruginosa* in a burn unit may not be cause for alarm, the detection of nosocomial spread of a single strain of this organism may have profound implications for infection control and patient care efforts.

The ideal typing system should (i) be standardized, (ii) have established precision and reproducibility, (iii) be stable over time, (iv) be sensitive enough to distinguish organisms that are similar but not identical, (v) be broadly applicable, available, and inexpensive, and (vi) be of proven value based on epidemiologic investigation (1). Critical appraisal of the available typing methods suggests that no one method is ideal and that most epidemiologic investigations require more than one typing method for optimal strain delineation (1, 4, 15, 21, 24, 26, 27, 31, 39, 40, 42, 44, 57, 64, 77). Regardless of the methods used, indiscriminate application of typing methods without sound epidemiologic guidance is generally wasteful and may provide conflicting and confusing information.

EPIDEMIOLOGIC TYPING METHODS

Several different epidemiologic typing methods have been applied in studies of nosocomial pathogens (Tables 1 and 2). These include antimicrobial susceptibility profiles (antibiogram), biochemical profiles (biotype), serological typing, bacteriocin typing, and bacteriophage susceptibility patterns (phage typing) (1, 9–12, 27, 28, 33–36, 64, 88, 90). More recently, molecular typing methods such as plasmid profiling, restriction endonuclease analysis of plasmid and genomic DNA, Southern hybridization analysis, immunoblotting, outer membrane protein profiling, and isoenzyme analysis have been used to type nosocomial pathogens (2–6, 14, 23, 26, 31, 37, 40, 42, 45, 51–57, 60, 67, 68).

Each of these typing methods has advantages and disadvantages when applied to a specific situation. A comparison of some important aspects of several of the more common typing methods is provided in Table 1. In addition to the ability to discriminate strains within species, of major importance to the clinical laboratory is the ease of performance and interpretation of the test and the availability of reagents. The usefulness of the typing systems may vary with the specific nosocomial pathogen of interest (Table 2); however, all of these typing systems have been helpful in understanding the epidemiology of nosocomial infections and in establishing

TABLE 1. Epidemiologic typing methods for the clinical microbiology laboratory[a]

Typing method	Score[b]			References
	Ease of performance and interpretation	Availability of reagents	Strain discrimination	
Antibiogram	++++	++++	++	35, 39, 42, 66, 77, 80
Biotyping	+++	++++	++	15, 35, 77, 80, 90
Serotyping	++	++	++	25, 82, 84, 90, 119
Bacteriocin typing	++	+	++	34, 82, 83, 118
Phage typing	+	+	+++	12, 42, 70, 80, 90, 105
Plasmid analysis	+++	++++	++++	39, 42, 60, 66, 77, 82, 84, 95, 96, 109, 117, 118, 119

[a] From M. A. Pfaller and R. J. Hollis (Clin. Microbiol. Newsl., **11**:137–141, 1989), with permission.
[b] ++++ better than +++ and so on.

the natural history of other, community-acquired infections.

Regardless of the typing system (or systems) used, one basic principle to keep in mind is that a valid comparison between two or more isolates cannot be made unless all typing procedures are performed in parallel, in the same laboratory, by the same personnel, on the same day, and using the same reagents. In addition, when typing isolates from a nosocomial outbreak, it is not sufficient to show that the outbreak isolates have identical epidemiologic markers. To make valid conclusions concerning the epidemic strain, it must be shown that control isolates from epidemiologically unrelated patients and environmental sources (where appropriate) are different from the outbreak strain (60). With this approach, the timely delineation of specific phenotypic (or genotypic) profiles of nosocomial pathogens by one or more of the above methods provides the basis for studies designed to answer important epidemiologic and pathogenetic questions, including (i) the site of origin (reservoir) of organisms causing nosocomial infections and (ii) the frequency and mechanism of patient-to-patient spread of nosocomial pathogens.

Antibiogram and resistotyping methods

The antibiogram or resistotyping method of epidemiologic typing is based on the determination of the pattern of susceptibility or resistance of an organism to a panel of antibiotics or other antimicrobial substances such as dyes or heavy metals. Most clinical microbiology laboratories routinely perform antibiotic susceptibility testing for clinical purposes, using either a broth dilution or disk diffusion method. Although resistotyping is less commonly performed, the technique is similar to the antibiogram except that organic and inorganic chemicals are used instead of antibiotics (1, 61, 64). The antibiogram is attractive as an epidemiologic typing method because it is readily available, easy to perform, broadly applicable to many different organism groups, and relatively inexpensive. Both disk diffusion and broth dilution antimicrobial susceptibility testing methods have been carefully standardized (8, 48, 70, 71) and, when performed in a standardized fashion, are reproducible within and between laboratories (8, 48). The sensitivity of the antibiogram for epidemiologic purposes is dependent on the organism, the number and type of antibiotics tested, and the manner in which the results are reported. The sensitivity is generally increased with increasing number of antibiotics tested and by including antibiotics or other antimicrobial agents (resistotyping) with epidemiologic as well as clinical value. Reporting the actual zone diameters (disk test) or MIC values (dilution test) rather than a category designation of "resistant" or "susceptible" may also be useful in differentiating strains within a given species of organism (28). The epidemiologic value of the antibiogram has been demonstrated for both gram-positive and gram-negative nosocomial pathogens (21, 27, 28, 32, 39, 41, 42, 55, 64, 67). Thus, the temporal and spatial clustering of aminoglycoside-resistant *Enterobacteriaceae* or methicillin-resistant *S. aureus* in a hospital where these strains are not known to be endemic is of major clinical and epidemiologic importance. Clearly, attention to the antibiogram of nosocomial pathogens should be included in routine infection control surveillance.

Disadvantages of the antibiogram as an epidemiologic typing method include limited sensitivity for both highly resistant (e.g., *P. aeruginosa*) and highly susceptible (e.g., streptococci) organisms and instability of the antibiotic susceptibility pattern because of antibiotic pressure, environmental factors, and the gain and loss of plasmids containing resistance factors (1, 30, 64, 66, 77, 78, 94). In addition, most antimicrobial susceptibility testing panels have been designed with clinical, not epidemiologic, purposes in mind, and there is no consen-

TABLE 2. Epidemiologic typing methods for the eight most frequently reported nosocomial bloodstream pathogens, National Nosocomial Infections Surveillance System, January 1985 to August 1988[a]

Rank	Pathogen	Typing methods[b]
1	Coagulase-negative staphylococci	PREA, AB, BT, PT, ST, BC
2	*Staphylococcus aureus*	PREA, PT, AB, BT, ST, BC
3	Enterococci	PREA, AB, BT
4	*Candida* spp.	REA, BT, KT, AB, ST
5	*Escherichia coli*	PREA, AB, ST, BT, PT, BC
6	*Enterobacter* spp.	AB, BT, BC, PREA, PT, ST
7	*Pseudomonas aeruginosa*	ST, BC, AB, BT, PT, PREA
8	*Klebsiella pneumoniae*	AB, ST, BT, PREA, PT, BC

[a] From T. Horan, D. Culver, W. Jarvis, G. Emori, S. Banerjee, W. Martone, and C. Thornsberry (Antimicrob. Newsl. **5**:65–67, 1988).
[b] PREA, Plasmid and restriction endonuclease analysis; AB, antibiogram; BT, biotype; PT, phage type; ST, serotype; BC, bacteriocin type; REA, restriction endonuclease analysis of genomic DNA; KT, killer toxin type. Typing methods are listed in decreasing order of usefulness.

sus as to how much difference between antibiograms is necessary to distinguish unrelated strains. This problem is compounded by the ever-increasing number of new antibiotics which compete for space on the test panels and for which there is little or no epidemiologic experience. The advantages of resistotyping, in which uncommonly used (clinically) antibiotics and chemicals are employed, are that the composition of the panel can be specifically selected for epidemiologic purposes and that the susceptibility patterns are less likely to change because there is little or no selective pressure in the hospital. Unfortunately, lack of standardization and reproducibility for methods other than routine antibiotic susceptibility testing limits the application of resistotyping in the clinical microbiology laboratory.

Biotyping

The use of biotyping to differentiate strains within species is based on properties such as differences in biochemical reactions, morphology, and environmental tolerances such as ability to grow at extremes of pH or temperature. The temporal and spatial clustering of a unique or unusual biotype such as an indole-negative *Escherichia coli* or a lactose-positive *Providencia rettgeri* (Table 3) may be all that is needed to provide microbiologic confirmation of cross-infection occurring on a given hospital unit. Biotyping may also be useful clinically. For example, Ruoff et al. (92) have found that bloodstream isolates of *Streptococcus bovis* biotype I are highly associated with both endocarditis and colonic neoplasm, whereas *S. bovis* biotype II is more commonly associated with a hepatobiliary source of bacteremia and rarely with endocarditis or colonic neoplasm.

Because most commercially available identification systems are based on biochemical reactions, a biochemical profile or biotype is automatically generated as part of the routine identification process. For purposes of analysis, the biochemical reactions in most commercial systems are reduced to a numerical code, thus providing a biotype number that can be used as a means of strain identification. The advantages of using a commercially available identification system as a means of biotyping nosocomial pathogens are that the methods are standardized, widely available, and relatively easy to perform. Unfortunately, the commercially available systems were designed for taxonomic rather than epidemiologic purposes and thus lack sensitivity and sufficient reproducibility of the individual test reactions to be of much use as epidemiologic typing systems (7, 18, 21, 27, 33, 41, 69). Selected organisms may be more precisely characterized by using a biotyping scheme developed specifically for the organism group being studied. Systems for biotyping *Candida albicans* (73), *Serratia marcescens* (36, 101), and *Staphylococcus epidermidis* (11, 21, 41, 77, 80) have been described and used successfully in epidemiologic investigations. In general, these noncommercial systems are tedious and difficult to control, and they lack standardization. Finally, regardless of the system used, the biotype is not a stable property and may be influenced by a variety of technical and environmental factors as well as the gain and loss of plasmids (1, 7, 11, 33, 36, 41, 64, 69, 87).

Despite the limitations of both the antibiogram and biotyping methods, it is occasionally useful to employ these two simple and routinely available typing methods in combination to produce a composite antimicrobial-biochemical profile. The ability of such a combined approach to more precisely define strains within a given species was described by Christensen et al. (21), who typed nosocomial isolates of *S. epidermidis* by using phage typing, a noncommercial biotyping system, the API Staph-Ident system (Analytab, Plainview, N.Y.), an antimicrobial susceptibility test panel (antibiogram, 10 antibiotics), and the presence or absence of slime production (Table 4). They analyzed the results of the typing systems alone and in combination and calculated the probability (assignment probability) under each typing system of assigning by chance alone two randomly selected isolates to a single phenotype. The results (Table 4) clearly demonstrate the advantage (decreased assignment probability) of combining a biotyping system (either API or noncommercial) with a second typing system such as phage typing or antibiogram (with or without determination of slime production) in discriminating strains among clinical isolates of *S. epidermidis*.

Serotyping

Serologic typing (serotyping) of microorganisms is based on the presence or absence of somatic, flagellar, capsular, or envelope antigenic determinants and their reaction with specific antisera. Serotyping is a common means of routine taxonomic grouping of some species, and its epidemiologic value in delineating strains within species is well documented, particularly with nosocomial pathogens such as *P. aeruginosa* and *Klebsiella* spp. (Table 2) (15, 24, 25, 64, 82, 84, 90, 119). Serotyping is broadly applicable to a wide range of nosocomial pathogens, and the serotype appears to be a stable marker for many microorganisms. The methods used to perform serotyping include a variety of agglutination, coagglutination, fluorescent-antibody, and enzyme im-

TABLE 3. Phenotypic characteristics (biotypes) that may be useful as epidemiologic markers[a]

Organism	Characteristic
Escherichia coli	Indole negative
Providencia rettgeri	Lactose positive
Salmonella group B	H_2S negative
Serratia marcescens	Pigmented
Pseudomonas aeruginosa	No blue-green pigment

[a] From reference 27.

TABLE 4. Comparison of the probability of assigning two random coagulase-negative staphylococci to the same type with various typing systems[a]

Typing system	Assignment probability (%)
Phage typing	35.6
Biotyping (11 tests)	24.0
Phage plus biotyping	8.5
API Staph-Ident	34.6
Antibiogram (10 antibiotics)	7.7
Antibiogram plus API	3.7
Antibiogram plus slime	4.9
Antibiogram plus API and slime	2.6

[a] From reference 21.

munoassay techniques. The technology necessary to perform serotyping is readily available in most clinical microbiology laboratories; however, the development of serotyping as an epidemiologic tool has been limited by poor sensitivity for some organism groups, lack of reproducibility, lack of standardized methods, and the limited availability of high-quality antisera. The problems with quality and availability of antisera may be at least partially addressed through the use of monoclonal antibody technology to provide a consistent source of reagent-grade antisera. Panels of monoclonal antibodies have been developed specifically to facilitate the epidemiologic typing of organisms such as *Legionella pneumophila* serogroup 1 (47, 57). Such reagents have been used successfully to type both clinical and environmental isolates of *L. pneumophila* serogroup 1 in several nosocomial outbreaks (26, 57, 81, 113). Expansion of this approach to other organism groups will improve both the diagnostic and epidemiologic utility of serotyping.

Bacteriocin typing

The differentiation of strains within species by bacteriocin typing is based on the differential sensitivity of the test strains to the bacteriocins or toxins produced by a set of selected producer strains (bacteriocin susceptibility). Alternatively, strains can be typed on the basis of the sensitivity of a panel of indicator strains to the bacteriocins produced by the strains being evaluated (bacteriocin production). Bacteriocin typing, by definition, is limited to bacteria; however, an analogous approach (killer toxin typing) has been developed for *Candida* spp., particularly *C. albicans* (85). Although not commonly employed, bacteriocin (or killer toxin typing) may be a sensitive means of typing certain organism groups (Table 2) and is especially useful in typing organisms not easily typed by other methods, such as *P. aeruginosa* (pyocin typing) and *Candida* spp. (killer toxin typing) (1, 9, 10, 15, 34, 64, 82, 84, 85, 88, 118). One of the major advantages of bacteriocin typing is that it may increase the sensitivity of epidemiologic typing when used in combination with other typing systems such as serotyping, antimicrobial susceptibility typing (antibiogram), or biotyping.

The combined use of bacteriocin (pyocin) typing and serotyping was helpful in investigating a cluster of infections caused by *P. aeruginosa* occurring in the Burn Treatment Center at the University of Iowa Hospitals and Clinics (Table 5). These techniques clearly defined a common strain of *P. aeruginosa* that was isolated from several environmental sources and was distinctly different from the patient isolates. Each patient appeared to be infected with his or her own unique strain of *P. aeruginosa*. In this example, the typing techniques used allowed the infection control team to determine that the patients were not becoming infected with the common environmental strain of *P. aeruginosa* and that although there was a cluster of infections due to *P. aeruginosa*, there was no evidence that this represented the spread of a single strain among patients. This information greatly simplified the recommendations of the infection control team and provided reassurance that proper infection control guidelines were being followed.

As with many of the typing systems described thus far, bacteriocin typing suffers from lack of standardization and poor reproducibility. In addition, because the stability of the indicator or producer strains is an issue of concern, the test must be extensively and carefully controlled, and loss or acquisition of new bacteriocin-producing (or susceptibility) properties may obscure the results of an epidemiologic investigation (1, 64, 88). The variability of the technique is such that only isolates in the same test run should be compared. Thus, bacteriocin typing is subject to considerable variation, is labor intensive, and should generally be limited to reference laboratories.

TABLE 5. Strain variation in clinical and environmental isolates of *P. aeruginosa* from a burn treatment center[a]

Culture source	Serotype	Pyocin type
Sink 1	10	751624
Sink 2	10	751824
Sink 3	10	751624
Toilet	10	751624
Faucet	10	751624
Air vent	10	751824
Patient 1 burn wound	4	781341
Patient 2 burn wound	6	888878
Patient 3 burn wound	6	273426
Patient 4 burn wound	11	431311

[a] All cultures were obtained on the same day. From M. A. Pfaller et al. (unpublished data).

Bacteriophage typing

The use of bacteriophage typing is based on the susceptibility of the test strain to lysis by a panel of bacteriophages selected to offer maximum sensitivity for differentiating strains within species. This method of typing has been applied to a number of bacteria associated with nosocomial infections (Table 2), and its epidemiologic utility is especially well documented for *S. aureus*, *P. aeruginosa*, and *Salmonella* spp. (1, 4, 12, 21, 42, 51, 64, 67, 77, 90, 105). As shown previously (Table 4), bacteriophage typing may be particularly useful in combination with other typing methods such as biotyping or serotyping to increase the sensitivity of typing.

Disadvantages of bacteriophage typing include lack of standardization, poor reproducibility, and limited availability. The stability of the method over time must be carefully documented and controlled, and the method is rather labor intensive. The bacteriophage type may be altered by changes in environmental conditions, serial passage on laboratory media, exposure to UV light, and introduction of plasmids. Finally, interpretation of the results may be difficult despite the availability of published guidelines (20). Bacteriophage typing remains a tool of the research and reference laboratory.

Molecular typing methods

Given the many limitations of the more established conventional typing methods, it is not surprising that microbiologists and epidemiologists have looked to the newer techniques of modern molecular biology as additional, and perhaps more definitive, means of typing nosocomial pathogens. Several techniques have been adapted for use as molecular epidemiologic typing methods (Table 6). In contrast to several of the conventional typing methods, many of these techniques are broadly applicable to a wide variety of nosocomial

TABLE 6. Molecular methods for epidemiologic typing

Method	References
Plasmid pattern analysis	2–5, 31, 39, 41, 42, 45, 46, 57, 60, 68, 78, 83, 84, 95, 96, 109
Restriction endonuclease analysis of plasmid and chromosomal DNA	26, 37, 40, 42, 51, 52, 60, 79, 89, 97, 113, 115, 116
Southern hybridization analysis (DNA probes)	29, 30, 56, 59, 74, 76, 98, 102, 103, 106, 112
Immunoblot fingerprints	17, 54, 62, 67, 68
Protein profiling by polyacrylamide gel electrophoresis	6, 16, 22, 23, 25, 50–52, 75, 100, 104, 107, 114
Multilocus enzyme electrophoresis	19, 26, 31, 72, 86, 99
Orthogonal field alternation gel electrophoresis	53, 65

pathogens without significant changes in equipment, reagents, or procedure. Several of these techniques offer the possibility of strain differentiation at the genomic level and thus are potentially very powerful epidemiologic tools.

Plasmid analysis. The application of plasmid pattern analysis and restriction endonuclease analysis of plasmid DNA is proving to be a promising means of identifying strains within a given species of bacteria (3, 5, 14, 39, 42, 45, 60, 68, 80, 81, 95, 96, 117). The principle underlying the use of plasmid profiling or fingerprinting is that isolates of the same strain contain the same number of plasmids with the same molecular weights and restriction digest patterns and are phenotypically similar, as judged by antibiotic susceptibility profile or biotype. In contrast, epidemiologically unrelated isolates have distinctly different plasmid fingerprints (60). Plasmid analysis is now available in a number of clinical microbiology laboratories and provides a rapid method of characterizing bacterial isolates. Several features of plasmid analysis make it especially appealing in the study of nosocomial pathogens in the clinical laboratory. (i) The ease with which plasmids can be detected by gel electrophoresis from crude bacterial lysates puts plasmid analysis well within the capabilities of many clinical laboratories (45, 60, 95, 96, 109, 117). (ii) In contrast to other typing methods such as biotyping, serotyping, bacteriocin typing, and phage typing, plasmid analysis may employ a single set of reagents and equipment in typing several different species of bacteria (60, 109). (iii) A high percentage of many of the commonly encountered gram-positive and gram-negative nosocomial pathogens have at least one and frequently multiple plasmids (Table 7). Therefore, each strain produces a characteristic profile made up of its distinct plasmids. (iv) Further identification of individual plasmids can be achieved by restriction endonuclease treatment of the plasmids before gel electrophoresis (14, 60, 109). (v) Studies of gram-negative and gram-positive nosocomial pathogens have demonstrated transfer of antibiotic resistance plasmids among these organisms (2, 30, 60, 91, 94, 96, 117). These studies suggest that in addition to being significant nosocomial pathogens, certain organisms (*Enterobacteriaceae* and coagulase-negative staphylococci) may also serve as reservoirs of antibiotic resistance factors for other organisms. (vi) Plasmid analysis has been shown to be a useful tool in evaluating a number of clinical situations, including septicemias (3, 39, 66, 77, 78), and in differentiating contaminants from organisms responsible for prosthetic valve endocarditis, intravenous catheter sepsis, urinary tract infections, and osteomyelitis (5, 40, 66, 78, 80).

TABLE 7. Frequency of plasmids in selected bacterial pathogens[a]

Organism	% of isolates reported to contain plasmids	Reference(s)
Staphylococcus epidermidis	74–97	3, 5, 66, 77, 78, 80
Staphylococcus aureus	80–90	32, 55
Pseudomonas aeruginosa	13–30	83, 84, 119
Escherichia coli	65–70	60
Klebsiella pneumoniae	100	118
Serratia marcescens	20–98	31, 46
Legionella pneumophila	57–63	57, 81, 113

[a] From Pfaller and Hollis (Clin. Microbiol. Newsl., **11**:137–141, 1989), with permission.

Despite the many advantages of plasmid profiling, the use of this technique is not without shortcomings (2, 40, 45, 60, 66, 77, 80, 109, 111, 117). (i) Technical factors such as variations in the plasmid extraction methods, which may convert one molecular form of the plasmid to another, or variations in the conditions of electrophoresis can all influence the final profile. (ii) Strains may lose antibiotic resistance plasmids or cryptic plasmids. (iii) The ability to distinguish between two isolates decreases directly with the number of bands present and the diminishing difference in molecular size between two bands. (iv) Conjugal transfer of plasmids within or between species can lead to differences in plasmid patterns. (v) An existing plasmid can undergo a molecular rearrangement or deletion, resulting in a difference in molecular size or restriction fragment pattern. These differences may erroneously be interpreted as strain differences between two isolates. Mickelsen et al. (66) observed that epidemiologically related strains of *S. epidermidis* may differ by as many as three plasmids. They found that despite the lack of complete identity of all isolates, a conserved core of several plasmids of identical molecular weight enabled them to recognize the relatedness of isolates from the same as well as from different patients. They suggested that additional experience is needed with isolates that are well defined epidemiologically, phenotypically, and genotypically to define the limitations of plasmid pattern analysis as an epidemiologic tool. Likewise, Parisi (77) and Parisi and Hecht (78) noted occasional minor differences in plasmid pattern among isolates of *S. epidermidis* that were otherwise identical by phenotypic and epidemiologic criteria.

The methodology necessary to perform plasmid profiling has become quite streamlined as the technique has been adapted for clinical and epidemiologic purposes. The first applications of plasmid profiling to clinical and epidemiologic investigation employed elaborate extraction, purification, and detection methods that were impractical for use in the clinical laboratory (93). To make this procedure more time efficient and clinically relevant, the various steps have been simplified, and now there are numerous "miniprep" protocols described in the literature (13, 40, 43, 49, 58, 60, 108, 111). Almost all miniprep protocols follow the same basic steps and can be completed in 12 to 24 h. The cost of performing these procedures is surprisingly low and comparable to that observed for many other procedures performed in the clinical laboratory. A complete system, including microcentrifuge, power supply, electrophoresis cell, UV light source, fixed-focal-length camera, hood, filters, agarose, film, micropipetters, and instruction manual, is available for between $3,000 and $4,000. Many clinical laboratories already have access to items such as a microcentrifuge and electrophoresis equipment and thus would have lower start-up costs. In general, the cost of performing plasmid analysis ranges from $6.00 to $25.00 per isolate, depending on the number of isolates included in the procedure.

All of the miniprep procedures are applicable for use in the clinical laboratory and generally start with a relatively small number of cells grown in broth (2 to 20 ml) or on agar plates. The cells are lysed after exposure to detergent with or without NaOH and enzymes such as lysozyme or lysostaphin. The lysate is treated with phenol, chloroform-isoamyl alcohol, or sodium dodecyl sulfate to remove proteins and with RNase to remove contaminating RNA. The plasmid DNA is extracted by precipitation in ethanol or isopropanol. The DNA extraction procedure takes advantage of the covalently closed supercoiled structure of plasmid DNA to provide a DNA extract enriched in plasmid DNA. However, because most procedures do not employ the expensive and time-consuming cesium chloride density centrifugation, the resulting DNA preparation always contains various amounts of fragmented chromosomal DNA as well as plasmid DNA. The chromosomal DNA rarely causes a problem in analysis, since it always migrates in the gel as a readily identifiable diffuse band at a position equivalent to a 12-megadalton plasmid. After extraction, the DNA is applied to agarose gels and electrophoretically separated. The gels are stained with ethidium bromide, and the plasmids are visualized under UV light. The rate of migration of plasmid DNA in a gel is inversely proportional to the molecular weight, and the different-size plasmids appear as distinct bands in the gel. The gels may be photographed to provide a permanent record. As many as 25 different DNA preparations plus molecular weight standards can be run on a single gel. This is important for comparison purposes, since the agarose concentrations and electrophoretic conditions as well as the plasmid isolation technique can affect the final plasmid profile.

The technique of restriction endonuclease analysis may be necessary to confirm the identity between plasmids with a high degree of confidence (14, 40, 60, 80, 109, 111, 117). Restriction endonucleases are enzymes that recognize specific, palindromic base sequences at a defined position. No two different plasmids should have the identical restriction sites at identical intervals along the plasmid DNA. Thus, two plasmids with identical products or fingerprints after digestion with these enzymes are likely to be identical. Demonstration that two (or more) plasmids have identical patterns after digestion with two or more enzymes with different specificities further confirms their identity. Cutting plasmids with these enzymes adds about 1 h (10 to 20 min of hands-on time) to the plasmid isolation procedure and only slightly increases the cost of the procedure.

The protocols for doing plasmid analysis can be adapted to a wide variety of bacteria (Tables 2 and 7) by simple modifications. Several complete protocols suitable for performance in the clinical microbiology laboratory have been published and include detailed procedures for plasmid isolation, restriction endonuclease analysis, electrophoresis, staining, and photography (13, 43, 49, 58, 60, 95, 108, 109, 111).

Examples of the clinical and epidemiologic applications of plasmid profiling with and without restriction endonuclease analysis are shown in Fig. 1 and 2. The example in Fig. 1 shows the recurrent isolation of the same strain of *S. epidermidis* from the bloodstream of a patient with presumed Hickman catheter-related bacteremia. The isolation of *S. epidermidis* with identical plasmid profiles both before (lanes A and C [10/26] and D [10/29]) and after (lane E [12/16]) appropriate antistaphylococcal therapy suggested therapeutic failure rather than reinfection or contamination with a new strain. Bloodstream isolates of *S. epidermidis* from epidemiologically unrelated patients had plasmid patterns distinctly different from those observed in lanes A, C, D, and E. The isolate in lane B was considered a contaminant. On the basis of this information the catheter was removed. Figure 2 documents the occurrence of a cluster of infections caused by a single strain of *S. aureus* in patients hospitalized in a neonatal intensive-care unit. In each case (lanes A to E), examples of both undigested (U) and *Eco*RI restriction enzyme-digested (R)

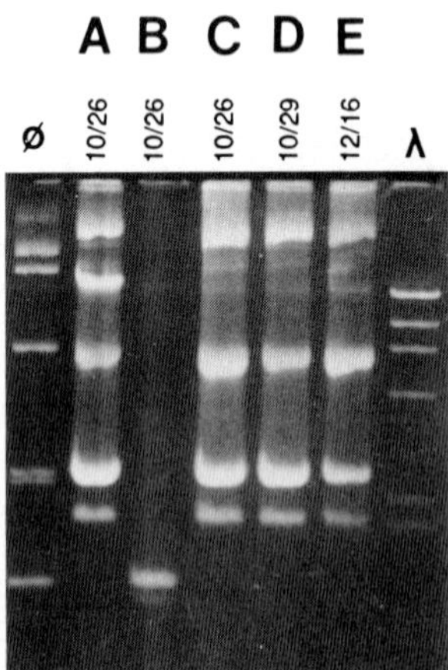

FIG. 1. Agarose gel electrophoresis of plasmid DNA from five bloodstream isolates (A to E) of *S. epidermidis* from a single patient. The date of isolation of each organism is shown above the respective lane. Lane ϕ (reference undigested plasmid DNA [Dupont, NEN Research Products, Boston, Mass.]) and lane λ (reference lambda phage DNA [*Hin*dIII digested]) contain standard molecular weight markers. The plasmid patterns of isolates in lanes A, C, D, and E are similar or identical, suggesting sustained infection with a single strain of *S. epidermidis*. The isolate in lane B has a different plasmid pattern and was considered a contaminant.

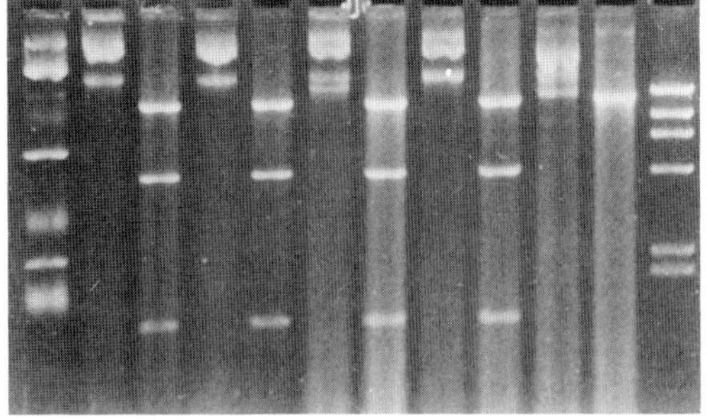

FIG. 2. Agarose gel electrophoresis of *Eco*RI-digested (R) and undigested (U) plasmid DNA from five clinical isolates (A to E) of *S. aureus* from individual patients hospitalized in the same bed unit. Lanes ϕ and λ contain the molecular weight standards described in the legend to Fig. 1. Isolates A to D are identical by restriction endonuclease analysis, suggesting the possibility of patient-to-patient transmission of a single strain of *S. aureus*.

preparations are shown. Four of the patients (A to D) were infected with the same strain of *S. aureus*. Patients hospitalized in other units during the same time period had unique strains of *S. aureus* that were different from the isolates in lanes A to D. This information suggested transmission of the infecting strain from patient to patient within the unit. The outbreak was controlled by appropriate infection control measures, including isolation and increased attention to hand washing. These examples illustrate the usefulness of plasmid profiling in both diagnostic and infection control efforts.

At present, it appears that although plasmid profiling is a powerful epidemiologic tool, plasmid profiles may be most useful when combined with another typing method such as serotyping, biotyping, antimicrobial susceptibility testing, or phage typing. Strains that have similar plasmid profiles but are grossly different by one of the other typing systems generally are not considered to be identical. It is important to remember that the use of plasmid profiling, as with other typing methods, should always be coupled with a sound epidemiologic investigation and with clear goals in mind (1, 33, 40, 60).

Restriction endonuclease analysis of chromosomal DNA. Restriction endonuclease analysis can also be used to type organisms not containing plasmids. Chromosomal DNA can be digested by restriction endonucleases, resulting in unique reproducible electrophoretic gel patterns. This technique has been useful in typing *Candida* spp. (Fig. 3) as well as a variety of bacteria and viruses causing both nosocomial and community-acquired infections (29, 37, 40, 51, 52, 60, 74, 76, 79, 89, 97, 98, 102, 103, 106, 112, 115–117). Visualization of DNA restriction fragment polymorphisms has been accomplished by ethidium bromide staining (Fig. 3) or by Southern hybridization analysis using DNA or RNA probes specific for mitochondrial DNA (74), ribosomal DNA (56, 76, 106), antibiotic resistance genes (30, 110), various toxin genes (40, 117), and cloned mid-repeat chromosomal sequences (29, 98, 102, 103, 112).

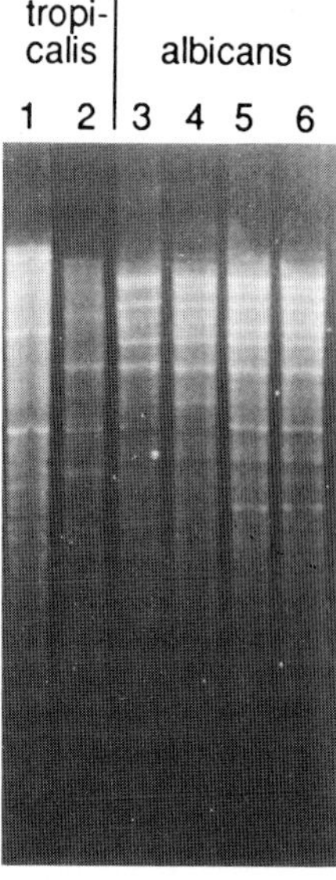

FIG. 3. Agarose gel electrophoresis of *Eco*RI-digested chromosomal DNA from clinical isolates of *Candida tropicalis* (lanes 1 and 2) and *C. albicans* (lanes 3 to 6). Two strains of *C. tropicalis* and three strains of *C. albicans* (patterns in lanes 5 and 6 are considered to be the same) are shown.

The simplest of these techniques is visualization of restriction fragment patterns by ethidium bromide staining (Fig. 3); however, the patterns may be quite complex and difficult to interpret. Because of the large number of bands present, small differences may be missed. The use of Southern hybridization analysis takes advantage of thc fidelity of DNA base pairings to examine specific areas of the genome. The patterns obtained after autoradiography or other means of visualization are generally much simpler than those obtained with ethidium bromide staining, and the polymorphisms observed serve as the basis for strain delineation. Depending on the probe used, one can study the epidemiology of specific genotypic traits such as antibiotic resistance or toxin production as well as determine strain distribution in a more general fashion. Additional work will be required to identify the probes that will be most useful as markers of strain variation for epidemiologic purposes. The patterns obtained with some mid-repeat-sequence probes have been shown to be highly variable over time, possibly because of frequent episodes of gene transposition or rearrangement, and therefore would not be useful for epidemiologic purposes (102, 103).

Clearly, the use of DNA probe technology to provide genotypic characterization of nosocomial pathogens is an extremely versatile and powerful means of typing organisms for epidemiologic purposes; however, additional work will be required to define the limitations, as well as the advantages, of this approach before it can be applied routinely in the clinical laboratory. Currently, the limitations of this technique for application in the clinical laboratory include (i) lack of standardization both in terms of methodology and limits of interpretation, (ii) the labor-intensive nature of the procedure, (iii) limited availability of probes, and (iv) the use of radioisotopes (autoradiography) as a means of visualization. Ongoing research efforts promise to address many of these problems and may soon provide a convenient means of genotyping nosocomial and community-acquired pathogens in the clinical laboratory.

Other molecular typing methods. Aside from the various DNA typing methods, a number of different techniques employing gel electrophoresis have been used as epidemiologic typing methods (Table 6). Immunoblot fingerprinting, using either pooled human serum or antisera specifically derived for the organism of interest, has been successfully applied in epidemiologic studies of *Clostridium difficile* (62, 68), *S. aureus* (67), and *Candida albicans* (17, 54). Immunoblot typing results generally correspond to phage typing results, susceptibility patterns, and plasmid fingerprints and may further define strains not readily separated by these techniques (67, 68). The methodology and reagents, particularly the antisera used, will require extensive standardization. Likewise, the limits of sensitivity and stability of immunoblot patterns must be defined before this method is widely applied as an epidemiologic tool.

Protein profiling by polyacrylamide gel electrophoresis has been used to subtype pathogenic organisms in a number of studies. Outer membrane profiling has been used to demonstrate strain variation in *Neisseria* spp. (16, 114), *Haemophilus influenzae* (6), and *E. coli* (75). This technique requires careful standardization and is not applicable to all gram-negative organisms, since epidemiologically unrelated isolates of *P. aeruginosa* show no major differences in their outer membrane protein profiles (38). Polyacrylamide gel electrophoresis analysis of cellular proteins, using either [^{35}S]methionine or various staining techniques to visualize the banding patterns, has been used to type a number of different organisms (23, 50–52), including coagulase-negative staphylococci (104), *S. aureus* (22, 67), *C. difficile* (25, 62, 68, 107), and *Candida* spp. (100). These methods require careful standardization, produce an excessive number of bands, and may be less sensitive than other typing methods in identifying strains within a given species (100).

Multilocus enzyme electrophoresis has been shown to be a useful epidemiologic tool as well as a powerful technique with which to study genetic diversity and structure in natural populations of a variety of bacteria (19, 26, 31, 72, 86, 99). The technique takes advantage of shifts in electrophoretic mobility of specific genetically controlled variants of bacterial enzymes (alloenzymes). The use of this technique as an epidemiologic tool is based on the analysis of the electrophoretic profile of a panel of enzymes for each organism. The alloenzymes are identified by comparing the relative mobilities of the enzyme variants on the gel after histochemical staining with specific substrates. The electrophoretic type for each organism is determined by the pattern of alloenzymes or electromorphs observed for the enzymes tested. This technique has been successfully applied in epidemiologic studies of *L. pneumophila* (26), *Serratia marcescens* (31), and *E. coli* (72). It appears to be an extremely powerful and versatile typing method; however, its usefulness in the clinical laboratory remains to be established.

Finally, the technique of orthogonal field alternation gel electrophoresis has been used to resolve chromosome-size DNA molecules into an electrophoretic karyotype for a number of organisms, including isolates of *C. albicans* (65) and *Candida stellatoidea* (53). Merz et al. (65) found that the electrophoretic karyotype of *C. albicans* exhibited dramatic variations among clinical isolates from different patients yet a relative stability of the karyotypes of isolates obtained from the same patient. Thus, most patients were colonized by only one genetic strain. Furthermore, isolates of *C. albicans* recovered from blood or deep tissue sites were identical to those obtained from colonization sites before deep infection developed. This technique appears to be sensitive and may be broadly applicable as an epidemiologic tool. Application to other groups of nosocomial pathogens is now under investigation.

SUMMARY AND CONCLUSIONS

The availability of an epidemiologic typing system that is broadly applicable, sensitive, rapid, inexpensive, and easy to perform would clearly be an advantage to the microbiologist and hospital epidemiologist in the ongoing struggle to detect and prevent the spread of nosocomial infection. This is particularly true given the increasing prominence of organisms such as coagulase-negative staphylococci, *S. aureus, Enterococcus* spp., and *Candida* spp., which are ubiquitous members of the normal flora yet are also the leading causes of nosocomial bloodstream infection (Table 2). Unfortunately, the ideal epidemiologic typing system does not yet exist. The newer techniques of molecular epidemiology are highly promising; however, given the limitations of the individual typing methods described in this chapter, the combined use of two or more methods may still be necessary to increase the sensitivity and usefulness of epidemiologic typing. Because epidemiologic typing requires the expenditure of precious hospital and laboratory resources, both the epidemiologist and the microbiologist must be aware of the advantages and limitations of the available typing methods and use these methods with clear epidemiologic objectives in mind. Whenever possible, all organisms to be typed should be typed by the same person on the same day, and typing should include unrelated as well as epidemiologically related isolates. The intelligent application of available technology will allow most clinical microbiology laboratories to provide useful typing information that can be effectively applied to the prevention and control of nosocomial infection.

LITERATURE CITED

1. **Aber, R. C., and D. C. Mackel.** 1981. Epidemiologic typing of nosocomial microorganisms. Am. J. Med. **70:**899–905.
2. **Archer, G. L., D. R. Dietrick, and J. L. Johnston.** 1985. Molecular epidemiology of transmissible gentamicin resistance among coagulase-negative staphylococci in a cardiac surgery unit. J. Infect. Dis. **151:**243–251.
3. **Archer, G. L., A. W. Karchmer, N. Vishniavsky, and H. G. Stiver.** 1984. Plasmid pattern analysis for the differentiation of infecting from noninfecting *Staphylococcus epidermidis*. J. Infect. Dis. **149:**913–920.
4. **Archer, G. L., and C. G. Mayhall.** 1983. Comparison of epidemiological markers used in the investigation of an outbreak of methicillin-resistant *Staphylococcus aureus* infections. J. Clin. Microbiol. **18:**395–399.
5. **Archer, G. L., N. Vishniavsky, and H. G. Stiver.** 1982. Plasmid pattern analysis of *Staphylococcus epidermidis* isolates from patients with prosthetic valve endocarditis. Infect. Immun. **35:**627–632.

6. **Barenkamp, S. J., R. S. Munson, Jr., and D. M. Granoff.** 1981. Subtyping isolates of *Haemophilus influenzae* type b by outer-membrane protein profiles. J. Infect. Dis. **143:** 668–676.
7. **Barry, A. L., R. E. Badal, and L. J. Effinger.** 1979. Reproducibility of three microdilution systems for identification of Enterobacteriaceae, compared with API 20E and Micro-ID systems. Curr. Microbiol. **3:**21–25.
8. **Barry, A. L., M. B. Coyle, C. Thornsberry, E. H. Gerlach, and R. W. Hawkinson.** 1979. Methods of measuring zones of inhibition with the Bauer-Kirby disk susceptibility test. J. Clin. Microbiol. **10:**885–889.
9. **Bauernfeind, A., and C. Petermüller.** 1984. Typing of *Enterobacter* spp. by bacteriocin susceptibility and its use in epidemiological analysis. J. Clin. Microbiol. **20:**70–73.
10. **Bauernfeind, A., C. Petermüller, and R. Schneider.** 1981. Bacteriocins as tools in analysis of nosocomial *Klebsiella pneumoniae* infections. J. Clin. Microbiol. **14:** 15–19.
11. **Bentley, D. W., R. Haque, R. A. Murphy, and M. H. Lepper.** 1968. Biotyping, an epidemiological tool for coagulase-negative staphylococci, p. 54–59. Antimicrob. Agents Chemother. 1967.
12. **Bergan, T.** 1978. Phage typing of *Pseudomonas aeruginosa*, p. 169–199. *In* T. Bergan and J. Norris (ed.), Methods in microbiology, vol. 10. Academic Press, Inc. (London), Ltd., London.
13. **Birnboim, H. C., and J. Doly.** 1979. A rapid alkaline extraction procedure for screening recombinant plasmid DNA. Nucleic Acids Res. **7:**1513–1523.
14. **Bjorvatn, B., and B. E. Kristiansen.** 1985. Molecular epidemiology of bacterial infections. Clin. Lab. Med. **5:** 437–445.
15. **Brokop, C. D., and J. J. Farmer.** 1979. Typing methods for *Pseudomonas aeruginosa*, p. 89–133. *In* R. G. Dogett (ed.), Clinical manifestations of infection and current therapy. Academic Press, Inc., New York.
16. **Buchanan, T. M., and J. F. Hildebrandt.** 1981. Antigen-specific serotyping of *Neisseria gonorrhoeae:* characterization based upon principal outer membrane protein. Infect. Immun. **32:**985–994.
17. **Burnie, J. P., R. Matthews, W. Lee, J. Philpott-Howard, R. Brown, N. Damani, J. Breuer, K. Honeywell, and Z. Jordan.** 1987. Four outbreaks of nosocomial systemic candidiasis. Epidemiol. Infect. **99:**201–211.
18. **Butler, D. A., C. M. Lobregat, and T. L. Gavan.** 1975. Reproducibility of the Analytab (API 20E) system. J. Clin. Microbiol. **2:**322–326.
19. **Caugant, D. A., K. Bovre, P. Gustad, K. Bryn, E. Holten, E. A. Hoiby, and L. O. Froholm.** 1986. Multilocus genotypes determined by enzyme electrophoresis of *Neisseria meningitidis* isolated from patients with systemic disease and from healthy carriers. J. Gen. Microbiol. **132:** 641–652.
20. **Centers for Disease Control.** 1981. National nosocomial infections study report, annual summary: 1978, p. 40–42. Centers for Disease Control, Atlanta, Ga.
21. **Christensen, G. D., J. T. Parisi, A. L. Bisno, W. A. Simpson, and E. H. Beachey.** 1983. Characterization of clinically significant strains of coagulase-negative staphylococci. J. Clin. Microbiol. **18:**258–269.
22. **Clink, J., and T. H. Pennington.** 1987. Staphylococcal whole-cell polypeptide analysis: evaluation as a taxonomic and typing tool. J. Med. Microbiol. **23:**41–44.
23. **Costas, M., B. Holmes, and L. L. Sloss.** 1987. Numerical analysis of electrophoretic protein patterns of *Providencia rustigianii* strains from human diarrhoea and other sources. J. Appl. Bacteriol. **63:**319–328.
24. **Crichton, P. B., and D. C. Old.** 1980. Differentiation of strains of *Escherichia coli:* multiple typing approach. J. Clin. Microbiol. **11:**635–640.
25. **Delmer, M., J. Laroche, V. Avesani, and G. Cornelis.** 1986. Comparison of serogrouping and polyacrylamide gel electrophoresis for typing *Clostridium difficile*. J. Clin. Microbiol. **24:**991–994.
26. **Edelstein, P. H., C. Nakahama, J. O. Tobin, K. Dalarco, K. B. Beer, J. R. Joly, and R. K. Selander.** 1986. Paeleoepidemiologic investigation of Legionnaires' disease at Wadsworth Veterans Administration Hospital by using three typing methods for comparison of legionellae from clinical and environmental sources. J. Clin. Microbiol. **23:**1121–1126.
27. **Farmer, J. J.** 1988. Conventional typing methods. J. Hosp. Infect. **11**(Suppl. A):309–314.
28. **Flournoy, D. J.** 1982. Quantitative antibiogram as a potential tool for epidemiological typing. Infect. Control **3:** 384–387.
29. **Fox, B. C., H. L. T. Mobley, and J. C. Wade.** 1989. The use of a DNA probe for epidemiological studies of candidiasis in immunocompromised hosts. J. Infect. Dis. **159:** 488–494.
30. **Galetto, D. W., J. L. Johnston, and G. L. Archer.** 1987. Molecular epidemiology of trimethoprim resistance among coagulase-negative staphylococci. Antimicrob. Agents Chemother. **31:**1683–1688.
31. **Gargallo-Viola, D.** 1989. Enzyme polymorphism, prodigiosin production, and plasmid fingerprints in clinical and naturally occurring isolates of *Serratia marcescens*. J. Clin. Microbiol. **27:**860–868.
32. **Gillespie, M. T., J. W. May, and R. W. Skurray.** 1984. Antibiotic susceptibilities and plasmid profiles of nosocomial methicillin-resistant *Staphylococcus aureus:* a retrospective study. J. Med. Microbiol. **17:**295–310.
33. **Goldman, D. A., and A. B. Macone.** 1980. A microbiologic approach to the investigation of bacterial nosocomial infection outbreaks. Infect. Control **1:**391–400.
34. **Govan, J. R. W.** 1978. Pyocin typing of *Pseudomonas aeruginosa*, p. 61–91. *In* T. Bergan and J. Norris (ed.), Methods in microbiology, vol. 10. Academic Press, Inc. (London), Ltd., London.
35. **Granato, P. A., E. A. Jurek, and L. B. Weiner.** 1983. Biotypes of *Haemophilus influenzae:* relationship to clinical source of isolation, serotype, and antibiotic susceptibility. Am. J. Clin. Pathol. **79:**73–77.
36. **Grimont, P. A. D., and F. Grimont.** 1978. Biotyping of *Serratia marcescens* and its use in epidemiological studies. J. Clin. Microbiol. **8:**73–83.
37. **Grothues, D., U. Koopmann, H. von der Hardt, and B. Tümmler.** 1988. Genome fingerprinting of *Pseudomonas aeruginosa* indicates colonization of cystic fibrosis siblings with closely related strains. J. Clin. Microbiol. **26:** 1973–1977.
38. **Hancock, R. E., and L. Chan.** 1988. Outer membranes of environmental isolates of *Pseudomonas aeruginosa*. J. Clin. Microbiol. **26:**2423–2424.
39. **Hartstein, A. I., M. A. Valvano, V. H. Morthland, P. C. Fuchs, S. A. Potter, and J. H. Crosa.** 1987. Antimicrobic susceptibility and plasmid profile analysis as identity tests for multiple isolates of coagulase-negative staphylococci. J. Clin. Microbiol. **25:**589–593.
40. **Hawkey, P. M.** 1987. Molecular methods for the investigation of bacterial cross-infection. J. Hosp. Infect. **9:** 211–218.
41. **Hébert, G. A., R. C. Cooksey, N. C. Clark, B. C. Hill, W. R. Jarvis, and C. Thornsberry.** 1988. Biotyping coagulase-negative staphylococci. J. Clin. Microbiol. **26:** 1950–1956.
42. **Holmberg, S. D., I. K. Wachsmuth, F. W. Hickman-Brenner, and M. L. Cohen.** 1984. Comparison of plasmid profile analysis, phage typing, and antimicrobial susceptibility testing in characterizing *Salmonella typhimurium* isolates from outbreaks. J. Clin. Microbiol. **19:**100–104.
43. **Holmes, D. S., and M. Quigley.** 1981. A rapid boiling method for the preparation of bacterial plasmids. Anal. Biochem. **114:**193–197.
44. **Hunter, P. R., and M. A. Gaston.** 1988. Numerical index

of the discriminatory ability of typing systems: an application of Simpson's index of diversity. J. Clin. Microbiol. **26:**2465–2466.

45. **John, J. F., and J. A. Twitty.** 1986. Plasmids as epidemiologic markers in nosocomial gram-negative bacilli: experience at a university and review of the literature. Rev. Infect. Dis. **8:**693–704.
46. **John, J. F., Jr., and W. F. McNeill.** 1981. Characteristics of *Serratia marcescens* containing a plasmid coding for gentamicin resistance in nosocomial infections. J. Infect. Dis. **143:**810–817.
47. **Joly, J. R., R. M. McKinney, J. O. Tobin, W. F. Bibb, I. D. Watkins, and D. Ramsay.** 1986. Development of a standardized subgrouping scheme for *Legionella pneumophila* serogroup 1 using monoclonal antibodies. J. Clin. Microbiol. **23:**768–771.
48. **Jones, R. N.** 1982. The antimicrobial susceptibility test: rapid and overnight, agar and broth, automated and conventional, interpretation and trend analysis, p. 341–369. *In* V. Lorian (ed.), Significance of medical microbiology in the care of patients, 2nd ed. The Williams & Wilkins Co., Baltimore.
49. **Kado, C. I., and S. T. Liu.** 1981. Rapid procedure for detection and isolation of large and small plasmids. J. Bacteriol. **145:**1365–1373.
50. **Kersters, K.** 1985. Numerical methods in the classification of bacteria by protein electrophoresis, p. 337–368. *In* M. Goodfellow, D. Jones, and F. G. Priest (ed.), Computer assisted bacterial systematics. Academic Press, Inc. (London), Ltd., London.
51. **Krech, T., J. de Chastonay, and E. Falsen.** 1988. Epidemiology of diphtheria: polypeptide and restriction enzyme analysis in comparison with conventional phage typing. Eur. J. Clin. Microbiol. Infect. Dis. **7:**232–237.
52. **Kuÿper, E. J., L. van Alphen, E. Leenders, and H. C. Zanen.** 1989. Typing of *Aeromonas* strains by DNA restriction endonuclease analysis and polyacrylamide gel electrophoresis of cell envelopes. J. Clin. Microbiol. **27:**1280–1285.
53. **Kwon-Chung, K. J., B. L. Wickes, and W. G. Merz.** 1988. Association of electrophoretic karyotype of *Candida stellatoidea* with virulence for mice. Infect. Immun. **56:**1814–1819.
54. **Lee, W., J. Burnie, and R. Matthews.** 1986. Fingerprinting *C. albicans*. J. Immunol. Methods **93:**177–182.
55. **Locksley, R. M., M. L. Cohen, T. C. Quinn, L. S. Tompkins, M. B. Coyle, J. M. Kirihara, and G. W. Counts.** 1982. Multiply antibiotic resistant *Staphylococcus aureus:* introduction, transmission, and evolution of nosocomial infection. Ann. Intern. Med. **97:**317–324.
56. **Magee, B. B., T. M. D'Souza, and P. T. Magee.** 1987. Strain and species identification by restriction fragment length polymorphisms in the ribosomal DNA repeat of *Candida* species. J. Bacteriol. **169:**1639–1643.
57. **Maher, W. E., M. F. Para, and J. F. Plouffe.** 1987. Subtyping of *Legionella pneumophila* serogroup 1 isolates by monoclonal antibody and plasmid techniques. J. Clin. Microbiol. **25:**2281–2284.
58. **Maniatis, T., E. F. Fritsch, and J. Sambrook.** 1982. Molecular cloning: a laboratory manual. Cold Spring Harbor Laboratory, Cold Spring Harbor, N.Y.
59. **Mason, M. M., B. A. Lasker, and W. S. Riggsby.** 1987. Molecular probe for identification of medically important *Candida* species and *Torulopsis glabrata*. J. Clin. Microbiol. **25:**563–566.
60. **Mayer, L. W.** 1988. Use of plasmid profiles in epidemiologic surveillance of disease outbreaks and in tracing the transmission of antibiotic resistance. Clin. Microbiol. Rev. **1:**228–243.
61. **McCreight, M. C., and D. W. Warnock.** 1982. Enhanced differentiation of isolates of *Candida albicans* using a modified resistogram method. Mykosen **25:**589–598.
62. **McFarland, L. V., M. E. Mulligan, R. Y. Y. Kwok, and W. E. Stamm.** 1989. Nosocomial acquisition of *Clostridium difficile* infection. N. Engl. J. Med. **320:**204–210.
63. **McGowan, J. E., Jr.** 1985. Role of the microbiology laboratory in prevention and control of nosocomial infections, p. 110–122. *In* E. H. Lennette, A. Balows, W. J. Hausler, Jr., and H. J. Shadomy (ed.), Manual of clinical microbiology, 4th ed. American Society for Microbiology, Washington, D.C.
64. **Meitert, T., and E. Meitert.** 1978. Usefulness, applications, and limitations of epidemiological typing methods to elucidate nosocomial infections and the spread of communicable diseases, p. 1–37. *In* T. Bergan and J. R. Norris (ed.), Methods in microbiology, vol. 10. Academic Press, Inc. (London), Ltd., London.
65. **Merz, W. G., C. Connelly, and P. Hieter.** 1988. Variation of electrophoretic karyotypes among clinical isolates of *Candida albicans*. J. Clin. Microbiol. **26:**842–845.
66. **Mickelsen, P. A., J. J. Plorde, K. P. Gordon, C. Hargiss, J. McClare, F. D. Schoenknect, F. Condie, F. C. Tenover, and L. S. Tompkins.** 1985. Instability of antibiotic resistance in a strain of *Staphylococcus epidermidis* isolated from an outbreak of prosthetic valve endocarditis. J. Infect. Dis. **152:**50–58.
67. **Mulligan, M. E., R. Y. Y. Kwok, D. M. Citron, J. F. John, Jr., and P. B. Smith.** 1988. Immunoblots, antimicrobial resistance, and bacteriophage typing of oxacillin-resistant *Staphylococcus aureus*. J. Clin. Microbiol. **26:**2395–2401.
68. **Mulligan, M. E., L. R. Peterson, R. Y. Y. Kwok, C. R. Clabots, and D. N. Gerding.** 1988. Immunoblots and plasmid fingerprints compared with serotyping and polyacrylamide gel electrophoresis for typing *Clostridium difficile*. J. Clin. Microbiol. **26:**41–46.
69. **Murray, P. R.** 1978. Standardization of the Analytab Enteric (API 20E) System to increase accuracy and reproducibility of the test for biotype characterization of bacteria. J. Clin. Microbiol. **8:**46–49.
70. **National Committee for Clinical Laboratory Standards.** 1984. Performance standards for antimicrobial disk susceptibility tests. Approved standard M2-A3. National Committee for Clinical Laboratory Standards, Villanova, Pa.
71. **National Committee for Clinical Laboratory Standards.** 1985. Standard methods for dilution antimicrobial susceptibility tests for bacteria which grow aerobically. Approved standard M7-A. National Committee for Clinical Laboratory Standards, Villanova, Pa.
72. **Ochman, M., T. S. Whittam, D. A. Caugant, and R. K. Selander.** 1983. Enzyme polymorphism and genetic population structure in *Escherichia coli* and *Shigella*. J. Gen. Microbiol. **129:**2715–2726.
73. **Odds, F. C., and A. B. Abbott.** 1980. A simple system for the presumptive identification of *Candida albicans* and differentiation of strains within the species. Sabouraudia **18:**301–317.
74. **Olivo, P. D., E. J. McManus, W. S. Riggsby, and J. M. Jones.** 1987. Mitochondrial DNA polymorphism in *Candida albicans*. J. Infect. Dis. **156:**214–215.
75. **Overbeeke, N., and B. Lagtenberg.** 1980. Major outer membrane proteins of *Escherichia coli* strains of human origin. J. Gen. Microbiol. **121:**373–380.
76. **Owen, R. J., A. Beck, P. A. Dayal, and C. Dawson.** 1988. Detection of genomic variation in *Providencia stuartii* clinical isolates by analysis of DNA restriction fragment length polymorphisms containing rRNA cistrons. J. Clin. Microbiol. **26:**2161–2166.
77. **Parisi, J. T.** 1985. Coagulase-negative staphylococci and the epidemiological typing of *Staphylococcus epidermidis*. Microbiol. Rev. **49:**126–139.
78. **Parisi, J. T., and D. W. Hecht.** 1980. Plasmid profiles in epidemiologic studies of infections by *Staphylococcus epidermidis*. J. Infect. Dis. **141:**637–643.
79. **Patterson, J. E., T. F. Patterson, P. Farrel, W. J. Hierholzer, Jr., and M. J. Zervos.** 1989. Evaluation of restric-

tion endonuclease analysis as an epidemiologic typing system for *Branhamella catarrhalis*. J. Clin. Microbiol. **27**:944–946.

80. **Pfaller, M. A., and L. A. Herwaldt.** 1988. Laboratory, clinical, and epidemiological aspects of coagulase-negative staphylococci. Clin. Microbiol. Rev. **1**:281–299.
81. **Pfaller, M., R. Hollis, W. Johnson, R. M. Massanari, C. Helms, R. Wenzel, N. Hall, N. Moyer, and J. Joly.** 1989. Application of molecular and immunologic techniques to study the epidemiology of *Legionella pneumophila* serogroup 1. Eur. J. Clin. Microbiol. Infect. Dis. **12**:295–302.
82. **Pitt, T. L.** 1988. Epidemiological typing of *Pseudomonas aeruginosa*. Eur. J. Clin. Microbiol. Infect. Dis. **7**:238–247.
83. **Plesiat, P., B. Alkhalof, and Y. Michael-Briand.** 1988. Prevalence and profiles of plasmids in *Pseudomonas aeruginosa*. Eur. J. Clin. Microbiol. Infect. Dis. **7**:261–264.
84. **Poh, C. L., E. H. Yap, L. Tay, and T. Bergan.** 1988. Plasmid profiles compared with serotyping and pyocin typing for epidemiological surveillance of *Pseudomonas aeruginosa*. J. Med. Microb. **25**:109–114.
85. **Polonelli, L., C. Archibusacci, M. Sestito, and G. Morace.** 1983. Killer system: a simple method for differentiating *Candida albicans* strains. J. Clin. Microbiol. **17**: 774–780.
86. **Porras, O., D. A. Caugant, T. Lagergard, and C. Svanborg-Eden.** 1986. Application of multilocus enzyme gel electrophoresis to *Haemophilus influenzae*. Infect. Immun. **53**:71–78.
87. **Reeve, E. C. R., and J. A. Braithwaite.** 1973. Lac$^+$ plasmids are responsible for the strong lactose-positive phenotype found in many strains of *Klebsiella* species. Genet. Res. **22**:329–333.
88. **Reeves, P.** 1965. Bacteriocins. Bacteriol. Rev. **29**:25–45.
89. **Renaud, F., J. Freney, J. Etienne, M. Bes, Y. Brun, O. Barsotti, S. Andre, and J. Fleurette.** 1988. Restriction endonuclease analysis of *Staphylococcus epidermidis* DNA may be a useful epidemiological marker. J. Clin. Microbiol. **26**:1729–1734.
90. **Rennie, R. P., C. E. Nord, L. Sjoberg, and I. B. R. Duncan.** 1978. Comparison of bacteriophage typing, serotyping, and biotyping as aids in epidemiological surveillance of *Klebsiella* infections. J. Clin. Microbiol. **8**:638–642.
91. **Rubens, C. E., W. E. Farrar, Z. A. McGee, and W. Schaffner.** 1981. Evolution of plasmid mediated resistance to multiple antimicrobial agents during a prolonged epidemic of nosocomial infection. J. Infect. Dis. **143**:170–181.
92. **Ruoff, K. L., S. I. Miller, C. V. Garner, M. J. Ferraro, and S. B. Calderwood.** 1989. Bacteremia with *Streptococcus bovis* and *Streptococcus salivarius*: clinical correlates of more accurate identification of isolates. J. Clin. Microbiol. **27**:305–308.
93. **Sadowski, P. L., B. C. Peterson, D. N. Gerding, and P. P. Cleary.** 1979. Physical characterization of ten R plasmids obtained from an outbreak of nosocomial *Klebsiella pneumoniae* infections. Antimicrob. Agents Chemother. **15**:616–624.
94. **Schaberg, D. R., C. E. Rubens, R. H. Alford, W. E. Farrar, W. Schaffner, and Z. A. McGee.** 1981. Evolution of antimicrobial resistance in nosocomial infection—lessons from the Vanderbilt experience. Am. J. Med. **70**: 445–448.
95. **Schaberg, D. R., L. S. Tompkins, and S. Falkow.** 1981. Use of agarose gel electrophoresis of plasmid deoxyribonucleic acid to fingerprint gram-negative bacilli. J. Clin. Microbiol. **13**:1105–1108.
96. **Schaberg, D. R., and M. Zervos.** 1986. Plasmid analysis in the study of the epidemiology of nosocomial gram-positive cocci. Rev. Infect. Dis. **8**:705–712.
97. **Scherer, S., and D. A. Stevens.** 1987. Application of DNA typing methods to epidemiology and taxonomy of *Candida* species. J. Clin. Microbiol. **25**:675–679.
98. **Scherer, S., and D. A. Stevens.** 1988. A *Candida albicans* dispersed, repeated gene family and its epidemiologic applications. Proc. Natl. Acad. Sci. USA **85**:1452–1456.
99. **Selander, R. K., D. A. Caugant, H. Ochman, J. M. Musser, M. N. Gilmour, and T. S. Whittam.** 1986. Methods of multilocus enzyme electrophoresis for bacterial population genetics and systematics. Appl. Environ. Microbiol. **51**:873–884.
100. **Shen, H. D., K. B. Choo, W. C. Tsai, T. M. Jen, J. Y. Yeh, and S. H. Han.** 1988. Differential identification of *Candida* species and other yeasts by analysis of [^{35}S] methionine-labeled polypeptide profiles. Anal. Biochem. **175**:548–551.
101. **Sifuentes-Osornio, J., G. M. Ruiz-Palacios, and D. H. M. Gröschel.** 1986. Analysis of epidemiologic markers of nosocomial *Serratia marcescens* isolates with special reference to the Grimont biotyping system. J. Clin. Microbiol. **23**:230–234.
102. **Soll, D. R., C. J. Langtimm, J. McDowell, J. Hicks, and R. Galask.** 1987. High-frequency switching in *Candida* strains isolated from vaginitis patients. J. Clin. Microbiol. **25**:1611–1622.
103. **Soll, D. R., M. Staebell, C. Langtimm, M. Pfaller, J. Hicks, and T. V. Gopala Rao.** 1988. Multiple *Candida* strains in the course of a single systemic infection. J. Clin. Microbiol. **26**:1448–1459.
104. **Stephenson, J. R., and S. Tabaqchali.** 1986. New method for typing coagulase-negative staphylococci. J. Clin. Pathol. **39**:1271–1275.
105. **Stringer, J.** 1984. Phage typing of *Streptococcus agalactiae*, p. 1–22. *In* T. Bergan (ed.), Methods in microbiology, vol. 16. Academic Press, Inc. (London), Ltd., London.
106. **Stull, T. L., J. J. LiPuma, and T. D. Edlind.** 1988. A broad spectrum probe for molecular epidemiology of bacteria:ribosomal RNA. J. Infect. Dis. **157**:280–286.
107. **Tabaqchali, S., D. Holland, S. O'Farrell, and R. Silman.** 1984. Typing scheme for *Clostridium difficile:* its application in clinical and epidemiological studies. Lancet **i**: 935–938.
108. **Takahashi, S., and Y. Nagano.** 1984. Rapid procedure of isolation of plasmid DNA and application to epidemiological analysis. J. Clin. Microbiol. **20**:608–613.
109. **Tenover, F. C.** 1985. Plasmid fingerprinting: a tool for bacterial strain identification and surveillance for nosocomial and community acquired infections. Clin. Lab. Med. **5**:413–436.
110. **Tenover, F. C.** 1986. Studies of antimicrobial resistance genes using DNA probes. Antimicrob. Agents Chemother. **29**:721–725.
111. **Tompkins, L. S.** 1985. DNA methods in clinical microbiology, p. 1023–1028. *In* E. H. Lennette, A. Balows, W. J. Hausler, Jr., and H. J. Shadomy (ed.), Manual of clinical microbiology, 4th ed. American Society for Microbiology, Washington, D.C.
112. **Tompkins, L. S., N. Troup, A. Labigne-Roussel, and M. L. Cohen.** 1986. Cloned, random chromosomal sequences as probes to identify *Salmonella* species. J. Infect. Dis. **154**:156–162.
113. **Tompkins, L. S., N. J. Troup, T. Woods, W. Bibb, and R. M. McKinney.** 1987. Molecular epidemiology of *Legionella* species by restriction endonuclease and alloenzyme analysis. J. Clin. Microbiol. **25**:1875–1880.
114. **Tsai, C.-M., C. E. Frasch, and L. F. Mocca.** 1981. Five structural classes of major outer membrane proteins in *Neisseria meningitidis*. J. Gen. Microbiol. **121**:373–380.
115. **van Ketel, R. J.** 1988. Similar DNA restriction endonuclease profiles in strains of *Legionella pneumophila* from different serogroups. J. Clin. Microbiol. **26**:1838–1841.
116. **van Ketel, R. J., and B. de Wever.** 1989. Genetic typing in a cluster of *Legionella pneumophila* infections. J. Clin. Microbiol. **27**:1105–1107.

117. **Wachsmuth, K.** 1986. Molecular epidemiology of bacterial infections: examples of methodology and of investigations of outbreaks. Rev. Infect. Dis. **88:**682–692.
118. **Walia, S., T. Madhaven, P. Reuman, R. Tewari, and D. Duckworth.** 1988. Plasmid profiles and klebocin types in epidemiologic studies of infections by *Klebsiella pneumoniae*. Eur. J. Clin. Microbiol. Infect. Dis. **7:**279–284.
119. **Walia, S., T. Madhaven, T. Williamson, A. Kaiser, and R. Tewari.** 1988. Protein patterns, serotyping, and plasmid DNA profiles in the epidemiologic fingerprinting of *Pseudomonas aeruginosa*. Eur. J. Clin. Microbiol. Infect. Dis. **7:**248–255.

Chapter 24

Sterilization, Disinfection, and Antisepsis in the Hospital

MARTIN S. FAVERO AND WALTER W. BOND

The effective use of antiseptics, disinfectants, and sterilization procedures is important in preventing nosocomial infections. Physical agents, such as moist or dry heat, play the major role in sterilization, and chemical germicides are used primarily for disinfection and antisepsis. In recent years, there continues to be a rapid increase in the number and variety of germicidal products available to hospitals in the United States. In 1973, the American Society for Microbiology Ad Hoc Committee on Microbiological Standards of Disinfection in Hospitals surveyed 16 U.S. hospitals with a combined bed capacity of more than 9,000. The survey showed that the average number of different formulations used per hospital was 14.5, with a range of 8 to 22. A total of 224 products was used in the 16 hospitals, and 125 of them were proprietary products.

The choice of agents and procedures to be used for hospital environmental disinfection, sanitization, and antisepsis depends on a variety of factors, and no single agent or procedure is adequate for all purposes. Factors to be considered in selection of procedures include the degree of microbial killing required, the nature of the item or surface to be treated, and the cost and ease of using the available agents. This chapter discusses each of these factors and practical methods for estimating the effectiveness of the various agents and procedures.

REGULATION OF CHEMICAL GERMICIDES IN THE UNITED STATES

Chemical germicides used in health care settings in the United States are regulated by two government agencies: the Environmental Protection Agency (EPA) and the Food and Drug Administration (FDA). Chemical germicides formulated as disinfectants or sterilants are initially regulated and registered by the Disinfectants Branch, Office of Pesticide Programs, EPA. The authority for this responsibility comes under the Federal Insecticide, Fungicide, and Rodenticide Act. The EPA requires manufacturers of chemical germicides formulated as sanitizers, as general disinfectants, or as disinfecting or sterilizing (sporicidal) products to test formulations by using specific protocols for microbicidal activity, stability, and toxicity to humans. Also, if a germicidal chemical is advertised and marketed for use on a specific medical device, e.g., a hemodialysis machine or a flexible fiberoptic endoscope, then the germicide falls under the additional regulatory control of the Center for Devices and Radiological Health, FDA, which is the federal agency that regulates medical devices. Under authority of the 1976 Medical Device Amendment to the Food, Drug and Cosmetic Act, a germicide that is marketed for use on a specific medical device is itself considered a medical device in a regulatory sense, and the manufacturer must, in addition to complying with EPA registration, contact FDA and submit a pre-market notification [510(k)] before the product can be legally marketed. Specific microbiological activity data or other data such as device or chemical compatibility may be requested from the manufacturer before completion of the pre-market notification process. Also, the FDA regulatory authority over a particular instrument or medical device dictates that the manufacturer is obligated to provide the user adequate instructions for the "safe and effective" use of that instrument or device. These instructions must include methods to clean and disinfect or sterilize the item if it is marketed as a reusable medical device. Manufacturers must provide the users of these germicides specific direction for use on the product label.

Currently, approximately 14,000 products have been registered with the EPA; approximately 300 active ingredients have been listed on the labels for these products. Of these 300 active ingredients, only 14 are in 92% of the registered products. Consequently, health care professionals who are in charge of obtaining germicides should keep in mind that this field is highly competitive and that exaggerated claims are often made about the germicidal efficacy of specific formulations that may be very similar in composition and activity to other products. As mentioned previously, the decision to register a disinfectant is based on data provided to the EPA by the manufacturer. A number of years ago, the EPA had the ability to independently test and verify formulations of chemical germicides for their claimed activity levels. Since the closing of the EPA laboratory in 1982, however, the registration of germicidal products has been based solely on manufacturer-supplied test data. This lack of independent verification has caused long-standing concern among health professionals who had previously considered the EPA test verification, particularly of sporicidal or sterilant claims, a significant factor in the selection of a chemical sterilant or high-level disinfectant. Therefore, new formulations of chemical germicides that become commercially available should be scrutinized by health care professionals, and it may also be necessary to consult with the Disinfectants Branch of the EPA or with the FDA Center for Devices and Radiological Health when questions regarding specific claims or patterns for use arise. Studies published in the scientific literature or presented at scientific meetings also provide important information on the capabilities or limitations of these formulations.

Chemical germicides that are formulated as antiseptics, preservatives, or drugs that are used on or in the human body or as preparations to be used to inhibit or kill microorganisms on the skin are regulated by the FDA. However, the FDA method of regulating these formulations differs significantly from the EPA method for disinfectants. The FDA has an advisory review panel on nonprescription, antimicrobial drug products. Manufacturers of such formulations voluntarily submit data to the panel, which in turn categorizes the products for their intended use, e.g., antimicrobial soaps, health care personal hand washes, patient preoperative preparations, skin antiseptics, skin wound cleansers, skin wound protectants, and surgical hand scrubs. Generic chemical germicides for each use are further divided into category I, safe and efficacious; category II, not safe or efficacious; and category III, insufficient data to categorize. Consequently, chemical germicides formulated as antiseptics and regulated by the FDA are categorized basically by use pattern and level of antimicrobial activity and are not regulated or registered in the same fashion that the EPA regulates and registers a disinfectant chemical for use on an inanimate surface. For more extensive discussions of these subjects, the reader is referred to publications by Bruch and Larson (28), Block (16), and Zanowiak and Jacobs (75).

The Centers for Disease Control (CDC) is not a regulatory agency and does not test, evaluate, or otherwise recommend specific brand name products of chemical germicides formulated as disinfectants or sterilants, as antiseptics, or as soaps for skin preparations. However, the Hospital Infections Program of CDC has published a guideline containing general considerations for methods and indications for hand washing and also strategies for disinfecting or sterilizing medical instruments as well as environmental surfaces (42). This guideline is updated periodically and is provided to all hospitals in the United States; it should be consulted for current information and CDC recommendations for disinfection and sterilization strategies, environmental microbiological control, and hand-washing strategies.

The choice of specific disinfectants in association with protocols for cleaning is a decision that is made broadly and at various levels of hospital and other health care facilities. No single chemical germicide procedure is adequate for all disinfection or sterilization purposes, and the realistic use of chemical germicides depends on a number of factors that should be considered in selecting among the available procedures. These include the degree of microbial killing required, the nature and composition of the surface item or device to be treated, and the cost, safety, and ease of use of the available agents. This chapter will deal with each of these factors, and practical methods for estimating the effectiveness of the various agents and procedures will be discussed.

ANTIMICROBIAL EFFECTIVENESS

Although the definitions of sterilization, disinfection, and antisepsis have been accepted generally (16, 68), it is quite common to see all three terms misused. Exact distinction among the three terms and basic knowledge of how to achieve and monitor each state are important if effective application of long-known principles is to be realized.

Sterilization

Sterilization is defined as the use of a physical or chemical procedure to destroy all microbial life, including large numbers of highly resistant bacterial endospores. In the hospital, this definition pertains specifically to microorganisms that may exist on inanimate objects. Moist heat by steam autoclaving, ethylene oxide gas, and dry heat are the major sterilizing agents used in hospitals. However, as will be discussed, there are a variety of chemical germicides that have been used for purposes of sterilization and appear to be effective when used appropriately. These same germicides (chemical sterilants) when used in a different manner may actually be part of a disinfection process. Unfortunately, some health professionals refer to disinfection as sterilization, which leads to a degree of confusion that often becomes magnified with routine use. A good example is the use of glutaraldehyde-based germicides for the disinfection of certain flexible fiberoptic endoscopes. Some practitioners refer to this as sterilization of endoscopes. For instance, a 2% glutaraldehyde solution is capable of sterilization, but only after extended contact time in the absence of extraneous organic material. Unfortunately, flexible fiberoptic endoscopes of recent "totally immersible" design are not physically capable of withstanding repeated immersion in fluid for 6 to 10 h; in fact, most manufacturers state that repeated prolonged immersion will damage the instruments and recommend that routine immersion times not exceed 20 to 30 min. Thus, the procedure used for most flexible endoscopes is one of disinfection and not sterilization, even though colloquially it is often referred to in the hospital as sterilization.

Disinfection

Disinfection is generally a less lethal process than sterilization. It eliminates virtually all recognized pathogenic microorganisms but not necessarily all microbial forms (e.g., bacterial endospores) on inanimate objects. As can be seen by this definition, disinfection does not ensure an overkill, and therefore disinfection processes lack the margin of safety achieved by sterilization procedures. The effectiveness of a disinfection procedure is controlled significantly by a number of factors, each of which may have a pronounced effect on the end result. Among these are the nature and number of contaminating microorganisms (especially the presence of bacterial endospores), the amount of organic matter (soil, feces, blood, etc.) present, the type and configuration of the medical and surgical materials to be disinfected, the type and concentration of the chemical germicide used, and the time and temperature of exposure. Accordingly, disinfection is a procedure that reduces the level of microbial contamination, but there is a broad range of activity that extends from sterility at one extreme to a minimal reduction in the number of microbial contaminants at the other. It is emphasized that the acceptance of such distinction is consistent with the abilities of certain nonsporicidal disinfectant solutions to completely destroy microbial contamination on medical and surgical materials. Indeed, this probably happens very often when spores are absent before the disinfection procedure and the numbers of other microbial contaminants are low. Nevertheless, these procedures should not be referred to as sterilization and, as will be discussed, not even as high-level disinfection.

By definition, chemical disinfection differs from sterilization by its lack of sporicidal power. This is an oversimplification of the actual situation, because a few chemical germicides used as disinfectants do, in fact, kill large numbers of spores even though high concentrations and several hours of exposure time may be required.

Nonsporicidal disinfectants may differ in their capacity to accomplish disinfection or decontamination. Some germicides rapidly kill only the ordinary vegetative forms of bacteria such as staphylococci and streptococci, some forms of fungi, and lipid-containing viruses, whereas others are effective against such relatively resistant organisms as *Mycobacterium tuberculosis* var. *bovis*, nonlipid viruses, and most forms of fungi. The latter group therefore represents a level of activity that is intermediate between those of sporicides and many commonly used germicides.

Absolute sterility is difficult to prove, and as a result it is common to define sterility in terms of the probability that a contaminating organism will survive treatment. For example, sterilizing processes are designed and often monitored by using a high number (10^6 to 10^7) of dried bacterial endospores, and sterilization is defined as that state in which the probability of any one spore surviving is 10^{-6} or lower. This rationale has been used to establish cycles for steam autoclaves, dry-air ovens, and ethylene oxide gas sterilizers, and it produces a great degree of overkill as well as a quantitative assurance of sterilization. It is virtually impossible to evaluate liquid chemical sterilization or disinfection processes by using these criteria. Procedures that use chemical germicides do not have the same reliability as sterilization procedures such as steam autoclaving.

Decontamination

Decontamination is a term used to describe a process or treatment that renders a medical device, instrument, or environmental surface safe to handle; in the case of medical instruments or devices, use of a decontamination process or treatment does not necessarily ensure that the item is safe for patient reuse. A decontamination procedure can range from a sterilization or disinfection procedure to simple cleaning with soap and water.

Antisepsis

An antiseptic is defined as a germicide that is used on skin or living tissue for the purpose of inhibiting or destroying microorganisms. However, the distinction between an antiseptic and a disinfectant quite often is not made. A disinfectant is a germicide that is used solely for destroying microorganisms on inanimate objects such as medical devices or environmental surfaces, whereas an antiseptic germicide is used on or in living tissue. Although some germicides contain active chemicals that are used for both purposes (i.e., iodophors or alcohols), adequacy for one purpose does not ensure adequacy for the other. Consequently, it is not good practice to use an antiseptic for the purpose of disinfection and vice versa, because manufacturers specifically formulate these germicides for their intended use.

DISINFECTANT ACTIVITY

Classification of chemical germicides in their respective concentrations according to level of microbicidal potency is important but arbitrary. We have decided to retain the system originally proposed by Spaulding (67, 68). He first categorized medical and surgical materials as critical, semicritical, and noncritical. He also proposed three levels of germicidal action to be recognized for properly carrying out strategies for disinfection in hospitals. The proposed levels of activity (high, intermediate, and low) are based on the fact that microorganisms can usually be categorized into several general groups according to their innate resistance levels to a spectrum of physical or chemical germicidal agents. These groups are shown in broad descending order of resistance is shown in Fig. 1; the examples of microorganisms listed in each group represent some of the test organisms used to qualify germicides for a particular EPA registration category. The relationship of these general levels of microbial resistances to the levels of germicidal activity are shown in Table 1.

High-level disinfection

Most critical instruments and devices are heat stable and are not adversely affected by repeated sterilizing cycles in a steam autoclave or dry-air oven. Other items

BACTERIAL SPORES
Bacillus subtilis
Clostridium sporogenes
↓
MYCOBACTERIA
Mycobacterium tuberculosis var. *bovis*
↓
NONLIPID OR SMALL VIRUSES
Poliovirus
Coxsackievirus
Rhinovirus
↓
FUNGI
Trichophyton sp.
Cryptococcus sp.
Candida sp.
↓
VEGETATIVE BACTERIA
Pseudomonas aeruginosa
Staphylococcus aureus
Salmonella choleraesuis
↓
LIPID OR MEDIUM-SIZE VIRUSES
Herpes simplex virus
Cytomegalovirus
Respiratory syncytial virus
Hepatitis B virus
Human immunodeficiency virus

FIG. 1. Descending order of resistance to germicidal chemicals.

TABLE 1. Levels of disinfectant action according to type of microorganism

Disinfectant level	Killing effect[a]					
	Bacteria			Fungi[b]	Virus	
	Spores	Tubercle bacillus	Vegetative cells		Nonlipid and small	Lipid and medium size
High	+[c]	+	+	+	+	+
Intermediate	−[d]	+	+	+	±[e]	+
Low	−	−	+	±	±	+

[a] +, Killing effect can be expected; −, little or no killing effect.
[b] Includes asexual spores but not necessarily chlamydospores or sexual spores.
[c] Only with extended exposure times are high-level disinfectants capable of killing high numbers of bacterial spores in laboratory tests; they are, however, capable of sporicidal activity (see text and Table 3).
[d] Some intermediate-level disinfectants (e.g., hypochlorites) may exhibit some sporicidal activity, whereas others (e.g., alcohols or phenolic compounds) have no demonstrated sporicidal activity.
[e] Some intermediate-level disinfectants, although tuberculocidal, may have limited virucidal activity (see text).

in this category, e.g., certain plastic or plastic-coated items, are not heat stable and must be sterilized by "cold" methods such as ethylene oxide gas or powerful, broad-spectrum liquid chemical germicides. There are relatively few critical instruments or devices in use today that are routinely processed between patients by methods less rigorous than a sterilizing treatment. Notable among this latter category are the "telescope" (optic-containing) portions of certain rigid endoscopic sets such as laparoscopes or arthroscopes. Although these instruments penetrate during use into normally sterile areas of the body, the widely accepted between-patient processing method of high-level disinfection has been successful, with no apparent adverse effect on patients (12, 47). CDC guidelines state that sterilization of laparoscopes and arthroscopes is preferable but, if sterilization is not feasible, then the minimum treatment should be high-level disinfection (42). It should be emphasized that the optic portions of these types of endoscopes are relatively fragile but are constructed of smooth, easily cleanable surfaces, with no internal channels and few surface irregularities. As a result, efficient precleaning of such items will ensure that little if any residual organic material and only low numbers of microorganisms will challenge the liquid chemical germicide in the subsequent disinfecting procedure.

High-level disinfection is the minimum treatment recommended by CDC in guidelines for the reprocessing of semicritical instruments or devices (42); an essential property of a high-level disinfectant is a demonstrated level of activity against bacterial endospores (Table 1). The capability of killing bacterial spores is an assurance of the relative power and activity spectrum of a germicide. Thus, if the contact time is long enough, this type of germicide can be used as a sterilant; it is important to recognize that contact time is the single variable between sterilization or high-level disinfection with a specific chemical germicide.

High-level disinfectants are often used to treat certain medical and surgical materials, and in the absence of bacterial spores they are rapidly effective. The absence of spores normally cannot be ensured, although it has been shown that the number of spores on items subjected to such treatments is generally low (65). The effective sporicidal activity of a high-level disinfectant depends on both the specific chemical agent and the manner in which it is used. Table 2 shows several disinfectants that are categorized as having high-level activity. These disinfectants include a number of glutaraldehyde-, chlorine dioxide-, hydrogen peroxide-, and peracetic acid-based formulations; they are commercially available germicides that have been approved by the EPA as sterilants or disinfectants. As will be pointed out later, the Association of Official Analytical Chemists (AOAC) sporicidal test is highly stringent (11); therefore, chemical germicides designated as sterilants according to this test methodology are most likely to be effective in killing all groups of microorganisms, including high numbers of bacterial spores. Some of these products combine various chemicals such as glutaraldehyde with formaldehyde and glutaraldehyde with phenol or phenolic compounds. Peracetic acid in liquid and vapor states has been described in the past as a sterilant or disinfectant, but its application in high concentrations presents major difficulties (45, 57), especially with medical and surgical items. However, germicidal products based on low concentration mixtures of hydrogen peroxide and peracetic acid have recently been approved by the EPA as sterilants or disinfectants.

Germicides classified as sporicides have been shown to kill large numbers of resistant bacterial endospores under stringent test conditions but may require as long as 24 h of contact time to do so (55). Although this type of germicide may qualify technically as a cold sterilant, it may receive very little use as such because of the exposure time necessary. In addition, most medical devices in actual practice are not contaminated with extraordinarily high levels of bacterial endospores; therefore, if a small number of spores constituted the initial population, sterilization may occur much more quickly than by 24 h. In other words, given the circumstances of relatively few bacterial spores present, sterilization could theoretically be achieved by a weaker germicide. However, since medical devices and items are not routinely monitored microbiologically, one cannot consistently ensure the absence of bacterial spores; with certain critical types of medical devices and items, it may be good practice to rely on germicides that either have been documented in the scientific literature as producing a sporicidal effect in a given amount of time or have been approved by the EPA as sterilants or disinfectants. In any event, these germicides can be expected to produce sterility if the exposure conditions of contact time, temperature, pH, and other factors are met. The assurance of sterilization is significantly less for a chemical germicide than for a physical process such as steam

TABLE 2. Methods of sterilization or disinfection; activity levels of selected liquid germicides[a]

Method	Concn or level[b]	Disinfectant activity
Sterilization		
Heat		
Moist heat (steam under pressure)	250°F (121°C) or 271°F (132°C) for various time intervals (see ref. 10)	
Dry heat	171°C for 1 h; 160°C for 2 h; 121°C for 16 h	
Gas		
Ethylene oxide	450–500 mg/liter at 55–60°C (see ref. 9)	
Liquid		
Glutaraldehyde	Variable[c]	
Hydrogen peroxide	6–30%	
Formaldehyde	6–8%[d]	
Chlorine dioxide	Variable[e]	
Peracetic acid	Variable[f]	
Disinfection		
Heat		
Moist heat (includes hot water pasteurization)	75–100°C	(High)
Liquid[g]		
Glutaraldehyde	Variable	High to intermediate
Hydrogen peroxide	3–6%	High to intermediate
Formaldehyde	1–8%	High to low
Chlorine dioxide	Variable	High
Peracetic acid	Variable	High
Chlorine compounds[h]	500–5,000 mg of free or available chlorine/liter	Intermediate
Alcohols (ethyl, isopropyl)[i]	70%	Intermediate
Phenolic compounds	0.5–3%	Intermediate to low
Iodophor compounds[j]	30–50 mg of free iodine/liter; up to 10,000 mg of available iodine/liter	Intermediate to low
Quaternary ammonium compounds	0.1–0.2%	Low
Antisepsis[k]		
Alcohols (ethyl, isopropyl)	70%	
Iodophors	1–2 mg of free iodine/liter; 1–2% available iodine (see ref. 38)	
Chlorhexidine	0.75–4.0%	
Hexachlorophene	1–3%	
Parachlorometaxylenol	0.5–4.0%	

[a] This list of chemical germicides centers on generic formulations. Several commercial products based on these generic components can be considered for use. Users should ensure that commercial formulations are registered with the EPA and, if used on medical instruments or devices, listed with the FDA. Information in the scientific literature or presented at symposia or scientific meetings can also be considered in determining the suitability of certain formulations; particular attention should be given to the instructions for use printed on the label of all EPA-registered products. Adequate precleaning of surfaces is the first prerequisite for any sterilizing or disinfecting procedure. The longer the exposure to a liquid chemical agent, the more likely that all pertinent microorganisms will be eliminated. The generally recommended exposure times of manufacturers may not be adequate to disinfect certain instruments or devices, especially those that are difficult to clean because of narrow channels or other areas that may harbor organic material as well as microorganisms; this fact is of particular importance when high-level disinfection is to be achieved.

[b] For sterilization or disinfection, refer to the instructions of the manufacturer for exposure times and conditions as well as recommendations for rinsing and subsequent handling of processed items.

[c] There are several glutaraldehyde-based proprietary formulations on the U.S. market, e.g., low-, neutral-, or high-pH products recommended for use at normal or elevated temperatures with or without ultrasonic energy. Some of the products are supplied as ready-to-use preparations, and other are sold in concentrated forms that require various dilutions to be made before a specific use; others may also require mixing of two or more components such as buffers or active ingredients (e.g., phenol or phenolic compounds). Therefore, it is imperative that the user closely follow the instructions of the manufacturer regarding use as a sterilant or disinfectant; some manufacturers supply test kits to aid in monitoring glutaraldehyde concentrations during the use life of the product.

[d] Because of the ongoing controversy over the role of formaldehyde as a potential occupational carcinogen, the use of formaldehyde is limited to certain specific circumstances under carefully controlled conditions, e.g., for the disinfection of certain hemodialysis equipment. There are no EPA-registered products designed for liquid chemical sterilizing or disinfecting that contain formaldehyde.

[e] Chlorine dioxide is claimed to be the active chemical resulting from mixing water, sodium chlorite, and lactic acid in various proportions, depending on the intended use as a sterilant or disinfectant. Similar to the case with other chlorine compounds, the spectrum of germicidal action is broad, but oxidative effects on metal or plastic surfaces may limit effective use.

[f] In recent years, a limited number of trade name products containing low concentrations (<0.1%) of peracetic (peroxyacetic) acid combined with low concentrations (<1.0%) of hydrogen peroxide at the in-use dilution have been registered with the EPA as sterilants or as sterilants or disinfectants. This combination of two powerful oxidizing chemicals at low concentration has made possible a rapid, broad spectrum of germicidal activity while minimizing negative effects such as corrosiveness at higher concentrations of peracetic acid.

[g] As of December 1988, there were approximately 85 proprietary formulations registered with the EPA as hospital disinfectants that are also tuberculocidal, virucidal, and fungicidal. Among this registration listing are formulations composed of a single category of active ingredients (e.g., glutaraldehyde, phenolic compound, or iodophor), but others may contain such an array of "active" chemical agents that the user may have difficulty in defining a generic classification. For this reason among others, the user is urged to pay particular attention to the information on the product label and accompanying package literature (spectrum of activity, approved use patterns, directions for use, safety precautions, etc.). At present, product information and claims in written or verbal advertising are not as closely regulated as information and claims on the product container label.

[h] Generic disinfectants containing chlorine are available in liquid or solid form, e.g., sodium or calcium hypochlorite. Although the indicated

(*Continued on next page*)

(Continued from previous page)
concentrations are rapid acting and broad spectrum (tuberculocidal, bactericidal, fungicidal, and virucidal), no proprietary hypochlorite formulations are formally registered with the EPA as such (common household bleach is an excellent and inexpensive source of sodium hypochlorite). Concentrations of between 500 and 1,000 mg of chlorine per liter are appropriate for the vast majority of uses requiring an intermediate level of germicidal activity; higher concentrations are extremely corrosive as well as irritating to personnel, and they should be used only on organic material that is difficult to clean (e.g., porous surfaces) or contains unusually high concentrations of microorganisms (e.g., spills of cultured material in the laboratory).

[i] The effectiveness of alcohols as intermediate-level germicides is limited, since they evaporate rapidly, resulting in very short contact times, and also lack the ability to penetrate residual organic material. They are rapidly tuberculocidal, bactericidal, and fungicidal but may vary in spectrum of virucidal activity (see text). Items to be disinfected with alcohols should be carefully precleaned and then totally submerged for an appropriate exposure time (e.g., 10 min).

[j] Only iodophors registered with the EPA as hard-surface disinfectants should be used, and the instructions of the manufacturer regarding proper dilution and product stability should be closely followed. Antiseptic iodophors are not suitable for disinfecting medical instruments or devices or for disinfecting environmental surfaces.

[k] This is not a complete listing of formulations categorized by the FDA, but it includes selected germicides that are commonly used as antiseptics in hospitals. For more detail, the reader is referred to papers by Zanowiak and Jacobs (75) and Bruch and Larson (28). Chemical germicides formulated specifically for use as antiseptics are not appropriate for use as disinfectants; the converse is also true.

autoclaving or dry heat. The latter procedures are much less prone to effects of human error than are those associated with chemical germicides.

One question that is worthy of consideration is whether high-level germicides (sporicidal chemicals) should be promoted as sterilizing agents. For example, a variety of glutaraldehyde-based products registered by the EPA as sterilants or disinfectants have been marketed for many years throughout the world. In recent years, however, the glutaraldehyde-based products in this EPA category have been joined by several other broad-spectrum germicide formulations containing active ingredients such as hydrogen peroxide, chlorine dioxide, and peracetic acid (Table 2). Although these formulations have been shown in laboratory tests to be capable of killing as many numbers and types of bacterial spores as, for instance, a steam autoclave cycle, their use in health care facilities is almost exclusively limited to disinfection rather than sterilization.

The question of how many of these products should be classified as sterilizing agents tends to be academic, because all of them require longer cycle times than does a steam autoclave. Although the AOAC sporicidal test is stringent and is a major criterion used by the EPA for designating a germicide as a sterilant, actual procedures associated with the use of chemical germicides demand much more in the way of microbiological verification because the potency of the chemicals is affected by the organic load of the device being processed, contact time, temperature, and the use history of the liquid product (e.g., age and dilution during use). The effort expended by the manufacturer in designing and verifying the effectiveness of a sterilization process is extensive and technically sophisticated. The same approach cannot be used in a modern-day hospital; in this setting, the use of biological indicators with steam and ethylene oxide sterilizers is about the only reliable monitoring procedure that can be carried out.

There is no direct way to verify microbiologically the sterility or the level of disinfection of a medical devices or item without sampling the item itself. With heat or gaseous chemical sterilization procedures, each process cycle can be monitored to verify that the exposure parameters are capable of inactivating 10^6 to 10^7 bacterial endospores by using commercial biological indicators. Liquid chemical sterilization or disinfection procedures cannot be monitored biologically; therefore, the existence of an established set of controls associated with the procedure as well as the liquid germicide itself takes on critical importance. A good example is the use of glutaraldehyde-based germicides which are capable of sterilization, but only after extended contact time and in the absence of extraneous organic material. Unfortunately, some materials are not physically able to withstand immersion in these fluids for 6 to 10 h. Even if prolonged contact time were possible, the treated materials would have to be retrieved from the germicide and handled with sterile implements, rinsed thoroughly with sterile water, dried with sterile towels or in a special cabinet with sterile air, and if not used immediately, stored in a sterile container to ensure that the materials remained sterile. However, it is common to observe staff members in hospitals and other settings soaking items in 2% glutaraldehyde germicides for 10 to 30 min, rinsing them in nonsterile water, and referring to the items as sterile. This particular situation indicates a misunderstanding of the terms "sterile" and "disinfected" as well overconfidence in a particular germicide and overestimation of the safety of the processed item.

Intermediate-level disinfection

Intermediate-level disinfectants are not necessarily capable of killing bacterial spores, but they do inactivate *M. tuberculosis* var. *bovis*, which is significantly more resistant to aqueous germicides than are ordinary vegetative bacteria (Table 1). These disinfectants are also effective against fungi (including asexual spores but not necessarily dried chlamydospores or sexual spores) as well as lipid and most nonlipid medium-size and small viruses. Examples of intermediate-level disinfectants include alcohols (70 to 90% ethanol or isopropanol), chlorine compounds (free chlorine, i.e., hypochlorus acids derived from sodium or calcium hypochlorite, gaseous chlorine or chlorine dioxide [500 mg/liter]), and certain phenolic or iodophor preparations, depending on formulation.

Although viruses and vegetative bacteria generally have similar susceptibilities to heat and other physical agents, Klein and Deforest (50) observed that viruses may differ significantly in susceptibility to disinfectant chemicals. Furthermore, they suggested that the presence or absence of lipid in the viral protein coat as well as the relative size of a virus may be useful guides in predicting viral susceptibility to a particular disinfectant. For instance, their data showed that small nonlipid viruses were significantly more resistant to a spectrum of germicides than were medium-size viruses or those with a lipid component in their protein coats. Some of the most widely used germicides (certain phenolic and quaternary ammonium compounds) failed to inactivate several small nonlipid viruses tested (e.g., picornaviruses such as enteroviruses and rhinoviruses). Conversely, the presence of a lipid component in viral composition was associated with a general susceptibility to all classes of germicides tested. Also, nonlipid viruses larger than picornaviruses (e.g., adenoviruses and reovirus) showed a susceptibility to the germicides similar to that of the lipid-containing viruses. Even though intermediate-level (tuberculocidal) disinfectants are generally considered effective against a wide range of viruses, they are not necessarily capable of destroying all viruses. When choosing a chemical agent for a particular situation, it would be prudent for the user to thoroughly examine the EPA-registered label claims for specific activity of brand name disinfectants and to consult the scientific literature for information on the virucidal spectra of generic chemicals such as alcohols and halogens. For example, the human hepatitis viruses (hepatitis B virus [HBV] and hepatitis C viruses) are of current importance and concern in hospital infection control strategies. These viruses have not been cultured in the laboratory, and this difficulty has prevented EPA in certain instances from allowing activity claims on the labels or in advertising of commercial products. However, there is no evidence that any of these viruses are unusually resistant to disinfectants (21, 25, 51, 54).

In 1977, we proposed that the resistance level of HBV be considered to be between that of the tubercle bacillus and bacterial spores but nearer that of the former (25). At that time, this type of rationale appeared reasonable, and it was felt that the most conservative approach would be to recommend at least high-level disinfecting procedures for all types of medical devices known or suspected of being contaminated with HBV. When considering sterilization or disinfection strategies for other hepatitis viruses that have not been studied extensively (hepatitis A and C viruses), a similar rationale has been proposed (40). Subsequently, two studies using direct chimpanzee inoculation with disinfectant-treated human serum with high titers of HBV showed that a variety of intermediate- to high-level disinfectant chemicals (two commercial glutaraldehyde-based products, 500 mg of free chlorine per liter from sodium hypochlorite, an iodophor product, 70% isopropanol, 80% ethanol, and dilutions of glutaraldehyde as low as 0.1%) were effective inactivators of the virus in relatively short exposure times and at low temperatures (21, 51).

Another virus of current importance and concern in health care settings is human immunodeficiency virus (HIV). Studies have shown that HIV is relatively unstable in the environment (59) and also is rapidly inactivated after being exposed to commonly used chemical germicides at concentrations much lower than are used in practice (52, 53, 69, 70). When considered in the context of environmental conditions in health care facilities, the demonstrated sensitivity of HIV in addition to low viral titers in blood of infected patients (ca. 100 HIV particles per ml) has resulted in no changes of currently recommended strategies for sterilization, disinfection, or housekeeping (31). Even though the EPA has recently approved specific HIV label claims for a large number of proprietary germicidal formulations (mostly germicides used for housekeeping purposes), the presence or absence of such a claim should not be the major criterion in the selection of germicidal products.

Some chemical germicides with good tuberculocidal activity can destroy small nonlipid viruses. Klein and Deforest (49) showed that, both 70% ethanol and isopropanol are rapidly virucidal, and alcohols are also known to be rapidly tuberculocidal (44, 66). Only ethanol, however, was found by Klein and Deforest to consistently destroy the small nonlipid viruses they studied, but Wright (74) reported that ethanol failed to kill a test virus that, on the basis of the study of Klein and Deforest, would be expected to be quite susceptible. At best, an intermediate-level (tuberculocidal) disinfectant may not necessarily be an effective broad-spectrum virucide.

The major exception to the rule of viral inactivation is the causative agent of Creutzfeldt-Jacob disease (CJD) or related infectious agents responsible for certain fatal degenerative diseases of the central nervous system in humans or lower animals. These diseases, collectively referred to as slow viral infections (e.g., CJD and kuru in humans and scrapie of sheep and goats) are caused by agents that are commonly referred to as unconventional viruses (5). As with the human hepatitis viruses, difficulties in determining the specific virucidal activities of disinfectants are complicated by the fact that precise assays require large numbers of experimental animals and extended periods of postinoculation observation. Limited studies to date on the physical and chemical inactivation kinetics of the scrapie agent have shown inconsistent results but have suggested that slow viruses as a group have rather unusual levels of resistance (7). These controversial data have led to rather unconventional recommendations for disinfection and sterilization (2), and the existing guidelines for terminal processing of CJD agent-contaminated medical devices and surfaces far exceed the levels of treatment with conventional sterilization cycles. However, until the CJD and related agents are studied further, it would be prudent for health care workers to follow published guidelines within reason to maintain a rational balance among infection transmission risk, personal safety from toxic chemicals, and physical integrity of medical devices and environmental surfaces (2, 5, 46).

The germicidal resistance of fungi is probably about the same as that of gram-positive vegetative bacteria (56, 58). However, experimental recognition of bacteriostasis may have been overlooked in many of the published reports, and there is now a reason to believe that some forms of pathogenic fungi may be considerably more resistant than most vegetative bacteria. Since it is likely that germicidal chemicals that are tuberculocidal and virucidal may not be capable of killing the more resistant fungi, intermediate-level germicides should be carefully examined with regard to demonstrated activity against specific groups or types of microorganisms.

Low-level disinfection

Low-level disinfectants are those that cannot be relied on to destroy, within a practical period of time, bacterial endospores, mycobacteria, all fungi, or all small or nonlipid viruses. These disinfectants may be useful in actual practice because they can kill rapidly vegetative forms of bacteria and most fungi as well as medium-size or lipid-containing viruses. Examples of low-level disinfectants are quaternary ammonium compounds and certain iodophors and phenolic compounds. In addition, the germicidal activity is flexible, depending on the concentration of the active ingredient. Disinfection levels of iodophors and phenolic compounds may be classified as intermediate or low, depending on the concentrations of the active ingredients. All germicidal chemicals do not have this capacity. For example, even a 5 to 10% concentration of a quaternary ammonium compound may fail to meet the tuberculocidal or virucidal criterion of intermediate-level disinfection (49). For the most part, germicides formulated and used as antiseptics have active ingredients that, if used as disinfectants, would be classified as low-level agents (Table 2).

SELECTION OF DISINFECTION LEVEL

Patient care instruments and devices have been categorized as critical, semicritical, and noncritical, and environmental surfaces have been categorized as medical equipment surfaces and housekeeping surfaces. The level of disinfection that should be used depends in part on the particular category and nature of the item and the manner in which it is to be used.

Critical instruments or devices

It would serve no useful purpose to name all of the critical instruments and devices and the large number of related medical and surgical materials in use in modern hospitals. The concept of a critical instrument is clear; the user must make his or her own list. All but a few articles in this category are either presterilized commercially or steam autoclaved by the user. A few important critical devices, however, are reused repeatedly and not steam autoclaved for one reason or another. Examples are transfer forceps and container, an increasing number of plastic parts on medical devices, hemodialyzers, and certain rigid endoscopic devices or accessories to flexible fiberoptic endoscopes. To sterilize or disinfect these items, one must rely on proper use of certain chemical germicides formulated as sterilants or disinfectants and classified in this chapter as high-level disinfectants. Thorough cleansing must always precede chemical disinfection of such items, because the mechanical action alone can remove a large proportion of contaminating microorganisms and a good deal of organic material which may tend to occlude microorganisms or inactivate the germicide. The number of bacterial spores is usually small, and they would not be expected to occur in relatively high numbers except when grossly contaminated objects have not been well cleansed; this fact should not be interpreted as a rationale to substitute chemical sterilization for autoclaving when autoclaving is a feasible procedure. To do so would lower safety standards; also, use of sterilant or disinfectant (high-level) chemical germicides is inconvenient because several hours must be allowed to ensure sterilization, and the exposed materials must be rinsed and dried or aired aseptically and kept in a sterile state before use.

One may debate the importance of an occasional bacterial endospore that may remain viable after a critical device has been disinfected. There have been no epidemiologic studies that can answer this question, but there are two points which deserve mention. First, critical instruments should be sterilized. If sterilization is not feasible, they should at a minimum receive high-level disinfection. The second point pertains to the view that most bacterial spores are nonpathogenic and thus may be ignored without incurring significant risk of infection. The distinction between pathogenic and nonpathogenic species is vague and relative rather than absolute, and in the modern hospital environment, the level of resistance of the host is the decisive factor in determining whether infection will develop. Classic nonpathogens such as *Bacillus subtilis* can produce serious and even fatal infections in immunosuppressed and immunocompromised hosts (32, 35, 71). But overriding the arguments regarding the possible consequences of infection with a bacterial spore is the fact that sterilizing or high-level disinfecting (sporicidal) procedures have the capability of killing all other groups of microorganisms that may cause infection. Thus, application of a germicide with such broad-spectrum capability will increase levels of assurance that no infection will be transmitted from patient to patient.

Certain critical items deserve special attention. Sterility is essential for hypodermic needles because they enter deep tissues. Use of liquid germicides cannot guarantee sterility for a number of reasons but primarily because of restricted access of the agent into the narrow lumen. Fortunately, the widespread use of presterilized disposable needles has almost eliminated the risky practice of reusing chemically sterilized needles. With the advent of disposable sterile items, there is an increasing practice, based on economic factors, of reusing these items. A good example is the artificial kidney. Hemodialyzers are manufactured and delivered to the user in a sterile state. Assurance that the item is sterile is dependent on the quality assurance and sterilization cycle verification programs of the manufacturer.

Approximately seventy percent of the chronic dialysis centers of the United States reuse hemodialyzers (1). This is a practice that has been followed for many years (33), and it appears that if the procedures of cleaning and disinfection are performed correctly and with the use of good protocols, there are no infectious disease problems among patients who are dialyzed on reused dialyzers. However, since these devices are not subjected to the same stringent sterilization cycles and controls that are performed by the manufacturer with new sterile dialyzers, the margin of safety is not as great as it would be with the manufacturer's processing. Consequently, there have been occasions when human error has caused a significant increase in pyrogenic reactions or infections associated with the reuse of dialyzers (37, 43).

Semicritical instruments or devices

Instruments or devices classified as semicritical are likewise diverse, and the health care worker should make his or her own listing unique to a particular medical practice. Basically, these are the items that make contact with mucous membranes during use but do not ordinarily penetrate the blood barrier or enter other normally sterile areas of the body. Examples in this category are flexible fiberoptic endoscopes, laryngoscopes, vaginal specula, anesthesia breathing circuits, a variety of dental equipment such as amalgum condensers, and a number of ophthalmic devices such as direct contact tonometers. Local host defense mechanisms can be expected to protect against challenges from small numbers of exogenous microorganisms, but these types of instruments should not be contaminated with a variety of vegetative bacteria, fungi, or viruses. Although sterilization is desirable and quite often the most economical procedure available (e.g., autoclaving), it is not absolutely essential as it is with critical items. For semicritical items that do not tolerate heat or cannot withstand repeated prolonged immersion in liquid chemical germicides or repeated exposures to ethylene oxide gas cycles, it is reasonable to use a high-level disinfection process. This is a procedure that is designed to destroy mycobacteria (e.g., *M. tuberculosis* var. *bovis*), small or nonlipid viruses, fungi, vegetative bacteria, and medium-size or lipid viruses and is accomplished with a high degree of assurance by using a germicide that is capable of killing large numbers of bacterial spores. It is important to note that the only variable between sterilization and high-level disinfection with a liquid germicide is contact time (Table 3); in this context, the reader should be aware of a potentially confusing situation in the current germicide marketplace. Several products currently registered with the EPA as sterilant or disinfectant products give instructions for sterilization with a concentrate or slightly diluted product and disinfection with higher dilutions that exceed the capacity of the chemical(s) to inactivate bacterial spores. In these instances, if a sterilant or disinfectant chemical is diluted beyond its ability to kill bacterial spores (either before or during use), then it no longer qualifies for Spaulding's or our designation of "high-level disinfectant." It is the responsibility of the user to read and interpret the EPA-approved product label to ensure this distinction of chemical potency as related to dilution, shelf life, and use patterns. Some products in this category of germicide often provide test kits designed to aid the user in monitoring effective levels of active ingredients during the use life of the product.

Noncritical instruments or devices

Noncritical instruments or devices include those instruments such as electrocardiogram electrodes, physical measurement devices, blood pressure cuffs, and stethoscopes that ordinarily touch only intact skin of the patient during routine use and seldom, if ever, become contaminated with patient material, in particular, blood. These items generally offer little risk of transmitting infectious agents; consequently, many individuals rely on detergent and water cleaning or the use of low-level disinfectants either alone or in addition to the cleansing. Chemical disinfection is also widely practiced with low-level disinfectants used either alone or in addition to the cleansing, depending on the nature and degree of contamination during use. Examples of these types of disinfectants are shown in Tables 2 and 3.

Environmental surfaces

We have elected to modify slightly and expand Spaulding's classification of the inanimate environment in health care facilities in order to present a more precise concept of infection transmission risk. Recent reviews of environmental issues and the role of inanimate surfaces in transmission of nosocomial infection (60, 63) suggest that direct patient contact with inadequately disinfected critical or semicritical medical instruments has been directly implicated in a wide variety of nosocomial infections but that environmental surfaces such as instrument knobs or handles, instrument carts, sinks, table tops, floors, or walls may play theoretical but certainly less significant roles in disease transmission than do medical instruments. Because of recent increases in levels of concern about transmission risks of a number of microbial agents, in particular, bloodborne viruses, it is not uncommon to observe a variety of health care professionals regarding and decontaminating environmental surfaces in manners appropriate for medical instruments. Certainly, microbiological assays of samples taken from many environmental sources have shown the presence of potentially pathogenic bacteria or fungi, but the direct relationship between the presence of these agents and the incidence of infection transmission has not been demonstrated. Other evidence, however, has suggested that innate microbial characteristics such as the ability of extremely high numbers of a particular pathogen to survive for ex-

TABLE 3. Comparison of EPA product terminology and CDC germicidal process terminology

EPA product classification	CDC process classification
Sterilant/disinfectant (e.g., glutaraldehyde-, chlorine dioxide-, hydrogen peroxide-, or peracetic acid-based products)	Sterilization[a] (sporicidal chemical, prolonged contact time) High-level disinfection[b] (sporicidal chemical, short contact time)
Hospital disinfectant[c] with label claim for tuberculocidal activity (e.g., phenolic compounds, iodophors, or chlorine compounds)	Intermediate-level disinfection[d]
Hospital disinfectant with no label claim for tuberculocidal activity; includes sanitizers (e.g., quaternary ammonium compounds, some iodophors, and some phenolic compounds)	Low-level disinfection[e]

[a] This type of sterilization procedure should be used only with instruments (critical or semicritical) that are not heat stable. As indicated in the text, sterilization with liquid chemical germicides is not a biologically monitorable procedure and requires many cumbersome postexposure manipulations such as rinsing with sterile water and drying with sterile towels before use on a patient.

[b] High-level disinfection, as defined above and in the text, is appropriate for semicritical instruments that are not heat stable and therefore cannot be sterilized by steam autoclaving between uses. As with liquid chemical sterilization, thorough rinsing with sterile water after the required exposure time is appropriate.

[c] This class of germicide includes a number of generic hypochlorite formulations that are EPA registered but do not have specific label designations of "hospital disinfectant" or "tuberculocidal."

[d] Intermediate-level disinfection is appropriate for between-patient processing of certain noncritical instruments or devices or for environmental surfaces, particularly after significant spills of blood in any area or spills of microbial cultures in the laboratory.

[e] Low-level disinfection is appropriate for between-patient processing of certain noncritical instruments or devices or for routine cleaning and housekeeping. The label information, particularly for EPA-approved patterns of use, should be closely followed.

tended periods of time in or on environmental surfaces may be related to an increased potential for environmentally mediated disease transmission. Several microorganisms having either one or both of these qualities are influenza or other upper respiratory tract viruses, *Clostridium difficile*, and HBV.

Since the early 1970s, it has been recognized that many instances of HBV infection among hemodialysis patients or clinical laboratory workers have not been accompanied by overt or recognized parenteral or mucous membrane contact. Subsequent studies have shown that a variety of environmental surfaces in areas such as hemodialysis units, clinical laboratories, and dental operatories where there is frequent contamination with blood may show the presence of hepatitis B surface antigen, even in the absence of visible or even chemically detectable blood. Other studies have shown that HBV occurs in extremely high numbers (between 10^8 and 10^9 particles per ml) in the blood and blood components of infected persons (64), that high numbers of HBV will survive for at least 1 week after drying and storage under typical ambient conditions (22), and that very small amounts of HBV-positive material placed on or splashed into the eyes (and presumably on broken skin) will result in infection (26, 48). For these reasons, HBV has come to be regarded by many infection control practitioners as a model "worst-case" scenario with respect to potential for bloodborne cross-contamination and disease transmission among patients and health care workers. Coupled with observations that HBV does not appear to be unusually resistant to germicidal chemicals (21, 51), a number of recent recommendations and strategies for employment of protective barriers (gloves, face protection, etc.), environmental controls or barriers (e.g., impervious coverings for frequently contaminated surfaces that are difficult to clean and disinfect), and general methods for cleaning and disinfecting have been based on this model.

Medical equipment surfaces. Examples of medical equipment surfaces are adjustment knobs, handles, buttons, or levers on a variety of medical equipment such as hemodialysis machines, X-ray machines, instrument trays and carts, or dental units. These surfaces almost never come into direct contact with the patient, but because of the nature of the treatment or the equipment design, they may frequently become contaminated with patient material, particularly blood, and are repeatedly touched by health care personnel during procedures involving parenteral or mucous membrane contact with patients. These surfaces have a distinct potential for secondary transmission of microorganisms from patient to patient or from patient to health care worker. A good example of this potential would be a dentist performing a surgical procedure and intermittently adjusting the dental unit light during progressive stages of the procedure; the light handle almost invariably becomes contaminated with blood and oral secretions, and if not adequately cleaned and disinfected after the procedure, it may allow cross-contamination in subsequent procedures. Equipment surfaces such as this should, at a minimum, be cleaned of visible material with soap and water. It may also be prudent to disinfect with a germicide having an intermediate level of activity (Table 2).

Housekeeping surfaces. Environmental surfaces such as floors, walls, sinks, table tops, and related objects are not associated with transmission of infections to patients or health care workers, and therefore extraordinary attempts to disinfect these surfaces are not necessary. However, general cleaning and removal of visible soil should be done routinely. The chemicals appropriate for this routine cleaning are low-level disinfectants (e.g., EPA-registered nontuberculocidal "hospital disinfectants"), but the actual removal of soil and microorganisms by scrubbing is probably at least as important as any germicidal activity of the cleaning agent used.

Special protocols to augment routine cleaning may be applicable if, in the judgment of responsible workers, specific sites within a health care facility have become significantly contaminated with blood or other patient material. Such a strategy is relatively conservative and requires common sense judgment in determining the relative levels of disease transmission risk involved, e.g., the nature, size, and location of the spill. In this instance of a significant spill, the visible material should first be cleaned from the surface and then the immediate vicinity disinfected with an intermediate-level germicide (Table 2); this strategy, often referred to as specific-site decontamination, can be done by moderately wetting the precleaned surface with germicide (wiping or spraying) and then allowing the surface to air dry.

Spills in certain clinical laboratory areas, however, may involve higher risks of disease transmission than in other areas of the health care facility. Serology areas usually process large volumes of blood, and microbiology procedures involve the culturing or concentrating of pathogenic microorganisms. Because of the volume of human source material and high numbers of microorganisms associated with diagnostic cultures or concentrates, the use of an intermediate-level germicide for routine decontamination in the laboratory might be prudent. Significant spills of human source material should be cleaned and disinfected in the usual manner, but spills of cultured material should first be confined (if necessary) with absorbent material and then flooded with a germicide of at least intermediate level; the germicide should then be given time to exert its effect (i.e., 10 min or as directed on the product label), followed by cleaning of the surface and reapplication of fresh germicide as described above.

FACTORS INFLUENCING GERMICIDAL PROCEDURES

Microorganisms vary widely in their responses to physical and chemical stresses. The most resistant to such stresses are bacterial endospores, and few if any other microorganisms approach this broad level of resistance. There are a number of factors, some associated with the microorganisms themselves and others associated with the surrounding physical and chemical environment, which influence the overall effectiveness of chemical germicides. Some factors are more important than others, but all of them should be considered when planning a strategy for the chemical disinfection of medical and surgical materials.

Nature of the item to be disinfected or sterilized

The easiest surface to disinfect or even sterilize chemically is one that is smooth, nonporous, and cleanable, such as a variety of unjointed retractors or probes. Crevices, joints, and pores in surfaces constitute barriers to the cleaning and subsequent penetration of liquid germicides and can result in prolonged contact times necessary to accomplish disinfection; in fact, it is highly likely that a disinfection procedure will fail under these circumstances. If microorganisms are entrapped in occluded spaces or within organic materials, even an ethylene oxide sterilization procedure may fail, especially when the level of contaminating microorganisms is high and composed, even in part, of bacterial spores. In the past 25 years, there have been a number of instruments or devices made of heat-sensitive materials which require that chemical germicides be used to accomplish sterilization or high-level disinfection. If sterilization is the objective of a treatment, contact times of 6 to 10 h are required, and this is often detrimental to material in the devices. For example, flexible fiberoptic endoscopes cannot be subjected routinely to long contact times in liquid germicides without risking the eventual degradation of lenses or other components. It is for this reason that if sterilization is to be accomplished, ethylene oxide gas may be the only feasible treatment; even this treatment will rapidly degrade certain components of the endoscopes, and it has the added negative factor that the instrument is out of service for the often lengthy period of time necessary for gas processing and aeration. Since these instruments are expensive and are used frequently, most practitioners have necessarily elected to routinely practice high-level disinfection rather than sterilization. Any alternative approach to reprocessing of this category of instrument will be difficult until the manufacturers of the instruments alter the designs and materials to allow more efficient cleaning as well as physical stability.

The size of a medical device also limits the types of germicides that can be used and whether sterilization or high-level disinfection will be the intended treatment. If an instrument is too large to be conveniently and adequately immersed in solutions or placed in an ethylene oxide chamber, then disinfection may be accomplished only by cleaning and then wiping with liquid. This procedure would include primarily noncritical devices.

Thus, the nature and use of a medical device or item may dictate the type and use of a chemical germicide. Practitioners should be aware of this fact; when medical devices are purchased, at least one criterion to be considered should be the ease with which the device can be efficiently cleaned and sterilized or disinfected.

Number of microorganisms present

Under a given set of circumstances, the higher the level of microbial contamination, the longer must be the exposure to the chemical germicide before the entire microbial population is killed. This factor does not stand alone, because the amount of time necessary to inactivate 100 bacterial spores would be significantly longer than the time required to inactivate 10^6 viruses or 10^4 cells of *Staphylococcus aureus* or most other vegetative bacteria. When one considers a natural microbial population composed of various types of microorganisms that have different degrees of resistance to physical or chemical stress, the survivor curve with all factors controlled would be parabolic and not straight as it might be if a pure culture of a particular microorganism were used (Fig. 2). Furthermore, the most resistant microbial subpopulation, even though it may be present in a relatively lower concentration than the entire microbial population, tends to control sterilization or disinfection time (24).

Innate resistance of microorganisms

As mentioned above, microorganisms vary widely in their resistance to chemical germicides, and thus the types that are present on medical items or surgical materials may have a significant effect on the time as well as the concentration of germicides necessary for sterilization or disinfection. The most resistant types of microorganisms are bacterial spores, some of which are significantly more resistant to both chemical and physical stresses than are a wide variety of other microorganisms (19, 23). In a broad descending order of relative resistance, considerably below bacterial endospores are the tubercle bacilli, small or nonlipid viruses, vegetative fungi and asexual fungal spores, vegetative bacteria, and medium-size or lipid-containing viruses (Fig. 1). Obviously, the biggest difference in resistance is between bacterial spores and lipid viruses such as herpesviruses, HBV, and HIV. Smaller but important differences exist between the tubercle bacillus and non-acid-fast bacteria and among fungi and certain groups of viruses.

The differences in resistance exhibited by various vegetative bacteria to chemical germicides are relatively minor except for the tubercle bacilli and other nontuberculous acid-fast mycobacteria (30), which presumably, because of their hydrophobic cell surfaces, are comparatively resistant to a variety of disinfectants, especially those in the low-level category. Among the ordinary vegetative bacteria, staphylococci and enterococci are somewhat more resistant to chemical germicides than are most other gram-positive bacteria. It is interesting that antibiotic-resistant "hospital" strains of staphylococci do not appear to be more re-

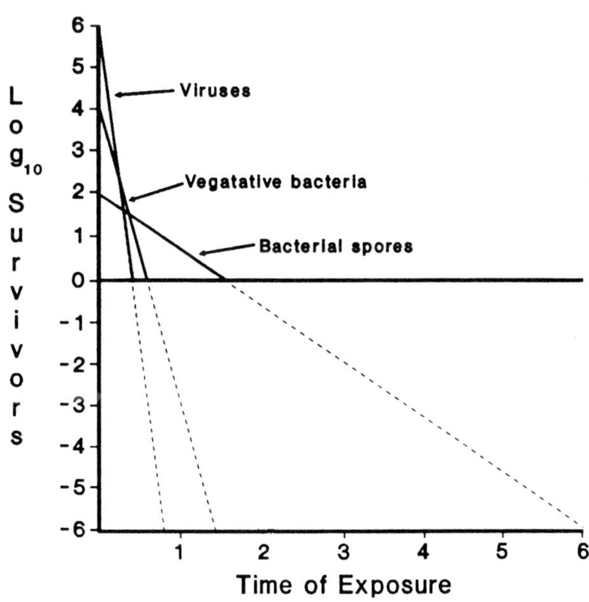

FIG. 2. Inactivation kinetics of a mixed microbial population.

sistant than ordinary isolates to chemical germicides. A number of gram-negative bacteria such as *Pseudomonas, Klebsiella, Enterobacter,* and *Serratia* spp. also may show somewhat greater resistance to some disinfectants than do other gram-negative bacteria. This finding may be significant because many of these gram-negative bacteria are frequently known to be responsible for outbreaks of hospital infections, especially in compromised hosts.

Gram-negative water bacteria that have the ability to grow well and achieve levels of 10^3 to 10^7 cells per ml in distilled, deionized, or reverse-osmosis water have been shown to be significantly more resistant to a variety of disinfectants in their naturally occurring state (i.e., isolated and grown in pure culture in water without subculturing on laboratory media) than are bacterial cells subcultured in the normal fashion (29, 41) (Fig. 3). This phenomenon also has been shown to occur with nontuberculous mycobacteria (30). These differences in resistance become important when low-level disinfectants are used, particularly at marginal or dilute concentrations, or when disinfectants having greater germicidal properties are used inappropriately (e.g., surfaces are not adequately cleaned before application of the germicide or significant organic loads are allowed to accumulate in the germicide container). The resistance of naturally occurring microorganisms also extends to bacterial spores, and it has been shown that naturally occurring bacterial spores in soil are significantly more resistant to dry heat than are those that are subcultured (23).

Amount of organic soil present

Blood, mucus, or feces, when present on items to be processed for reuse, may contribute to the failure of a given disinfection or sterilization procedure in three ways. The organic soil may contain large or diverse microbial populations, may occlude microorganisms and prevent penetration of chemical germicides, or may directly and rapidly inactivate certain germicidal chemicals such as chlorine- and iodine-based disinfectants or quaternary ammonium compounds. This effect is correspondingly greater with weak concentrations and with low-level germicides than with strong concentrations and high-level germicides. In addition, this factor underscores the importance of thoroughly cleaning a medical device before chemical disinfection; failure to do this may cause the disinfection or sterilization procedure to fail. In fact, physical cleaning is quite often the most important step in a disinfection process that by definition does not include the overkill factor of a sterilization process. Indeed, a report implicated a flexible fiberoptic endoscope in an outbreak of septicemia caused by *Serratia marcescens* (72); this instrument had been "sterilized" with ethylene oxide gas but had not been properly cleaned before the gassing cycle. Consequently, even a rigorous cycle capable of killing exposed bacterial spores may not kill even relatively delicate vegetative bacterial cells if these cells are protected by extraneous organic material. This factor also is intimately associated with the number of microorganisms present, so that effective cleaning procedures which remove organic soil simultaneously tend to lower significantly the general level of microbial contamination associated with the soil. More recent reports in the field of endoscopy have indicated that physically complex accessories to the endoscopic set such as suction valves or biopsy forceps may be extremely difficult or even impossible to clean and have been responsible for transmission of a variety of organisms such as *Mycobacterium* spp. (73) and *Salmonella newport* (34). After investigating and reporting episodes of disease transmission, some workers have suggested redesign of endoscopic equipment (15).

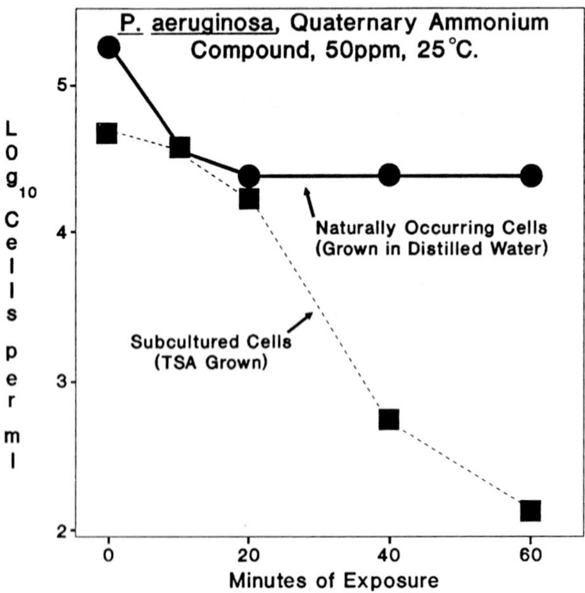

FIG. 3. Comparative survival of naturally occurring and subcultured cells of *P. aeruginosa* exposed to a quaternary ammonium compound.

Type and concentration of germicide used

Generally, with all other variables constant, the higher the concentration of a chemical agent, the greater its effectiveness and the shorter the length of time required to disinfect or sterilize an item. What is not generally recognized, however, are the wide differences in potency that exist among chemical germicides used for the same purpose. For example, Spaulding (67) compared the tuberculocidal activities of several proprietary phenolic and iodophor-based compounds with that of isopropanol and determined that there were significant differences in the amount of time to accomplish disinfection (Table 4).

Usually the disinfection time can be shortened significantly by increasing the use concentration. Some

TABLE 4. Tuberculocidal activity of alcohol, phenolic compounds, and an iodophor[a]

Compound	Disinfection time
Phenolic I, 3%	2–3 h
Phenolic II, 3%	45–60 min
Iodophor, 450 ppm (450 mg/liter)	2–3 h
Isopropanol, 70%	5 min

[a] From reference 67. Data are for a simultaneous mucin loop test. Number of *M. tuberculosis* per loop was approximately 10^4.

chemical germicides are appropriately used only at strong concentrations. This is true for many of the high-level chemical germicides such as glutaraldehyde-, hydrogen peroxide-, or chlorine dioxide-based products that are sporicides. It is also true of ethanol and isopropanol because a dilution with water beyond 50 to 60% would significantly reduce microbicidal activity. Some intermediate-level disinfectants may become useful sporicides when the concentration is increased significantly. This is probably true for hydrogen peroxide- or chlorine-based products but is not true for all intermediate-level disinfectants, in particular, phenolic compounds. In addition, complexed iodine solutions represent an instance of confusion between chemistry and strategies of use. Iodophor germicides are significantly affected by the amount of potassium iodide and water used in their formulations (6, 14, 36). Consequently, the label instructions describing a particular use dilution are much more critical than for other chemical germicides, because in the case of iodophors, use dilution is designed to yield the maximum possible amount of free iodine. Under- or overdiluting the disinfectant may significantly reduce the germicidal potency. In other words, if an iodophor disinfectant is meant to be diluted 1:213, an undiluted or 1:10 aqueous dilution may have less microbicidal activity than the recommended use dilution. Furthermore, it is not clear what iodine species should be used to gauge germicidal potency. Most iodophor disinfectants or antiseptics are formulated to contain a specific amount of complexed iodine yielding a certain percentage of available iodine with an unspecified amount of free iodine contained in the use dilution. Available iodine, which is simply the amount of iodine in solution that titrates with sodium thiosulfate, does not imply microbicidal effectiveness. Certainly, the amount of available iodine present is important because it can be converted to free iodine, depending on a number of other factors, including the amount of water present. Consequently, care should be taken to follow the label instructions for proprietary disinfectant iodophor preparations so that the proper use dilutions are made.

Duration and temperature of exposures

As expected, with all other variables constant, the longer the germicidal process is continued, the greater is its effectiveness. One possible exception is with some low-level disinfectants, for which there might be a minimum threshold concentration of the chemical that may have no killing effect on a microbial population no matter how long the contact time. For example, some quaternary ammonium disinfectants, used either in insufficient concentrations or in solutions that have deteriorated by age or by the presence of organic soil, not only may fail to kill some microbial populations (especially gram-negative bacteria) but may actually support their growth.

An increase in the temperature of a germicidal solution during the exposure time can significantly increase the efficacy of chemical germicides.

Directions for using commercially available chemical germicides

Another important factor that should be kept in mind when formulating a procedure for sterilization, disinfection, or antisepsis is the necessity to read and follow the manufacturer's directions for use. This applies to sterilization equipment, such as steam sterilizers and ethylene oxide gas sterilizers, as well as to commercially available chemical germicides. For disinfectants and antiseptics, general guidelines for use and contraindications, as well as a listing of the active ingredients, are found on labels and in the literature supplied with the products. When these directions are not taken into consideration, significant errors can be made in use dilutions as well as in applying certain chemical germicides. A good example is iodophors.

Iodophors are the combination of iodine and a solubilizing agent or carrier in which the resulting complex or combination acts as a reservoir of iodine and liberates small amounts of free iodine when diluted with water (38). Examples of carriers are quaternary ammonium compounds, detergents, and polyvinylpyrrolidone (povidone). Formulations containing iodophors usually list certain percentages of available iodine and do not specify the amount of free iodine, which is the chemical form responsible for killing microorganisms. Available iodine content often is used as an indicator of germicidal potency, but this approach is incorrect. Many aspects related to the physical and organic chemistry of iodine complexes are not fully understood. For example, a povidone-iodine germicide formulated as an antiseptic may contain 10% povidone-iodine and 1% available iodine. The term "available" when used with iodine refers to the amount of iodine that is titratable with sodium thiosulfate. When a solution contains 1% available iodine, almost all of it is in a complexed form and very little exists as free iodine, but during the chemical assay with sodium thiosulfate, both the complexed and free iodine titrate. The amount of free iodine in these types of solutions is approximately 1 mg/liter and is controlled significantly by the amount of potassium iodide present as well as by the amount of water. Concentrated solutions of iodophor contain less free iodine in undiluted solutions than do those diluted up to a specific point. It is virtually impossible to chemically assay free iodine in the presence of complexed iodine without resorting to an extraction technique using solvent. Thus, one can readily appreciate that the manufacturer's label direction for an iodophor disinfectant that calls for a 1:213 aqueous dilution of a concentrated formulation is designed to give the maximum degree of microbicidal efficiency that correlates with the amount of free iodine present.

The amount of available iodine noted on the label of a chemical germicide formulated as an antiseptic may be very similar to that listed on one formulated as a disinfectant. This does not alter the rationale for classifying disinfectants as having intermediate-level activity, but it does present a problem in defining the appropriate use concentration. Since it is complicated to assay for free iodine in the presence of iodophor solutions and since it is the current practice of manufacturers to include the amount of available iodine on product labels as an implication of potency, we have elected to retain the amount of available iodine to indicate strength (Table 2). With iodophors, label directions are much more critical with respect to actual use dilutions with water than most other disinfectants, and as mentioned previously, care should be taken to follow the directions closely. Furthermore, iodophors formulated as antiseptics contain significantly less free iodine than do those formulated as disinfectants; therefore, iodophor antiseptics should not be used as disinfectants and vice versa.

EVALUATING ACTUAL GERMICIDAL EFFECTIVENESS

Microbiological assays

A hospital can make a rational choice from the various sterilizing, disinfecting, and antiseptic processes that are available by considering the intended uses for the product (is sterility required, or may high-, intermediate-, or low-level disinfections be adequate?) and by understanding the factors that influence germicidal effectiveness discussed above. It is not practical for hospital laboratories to test the antimicrobial effectiveness of commercially available chemical germicides unless such testing is part of a well-designed research project. As mentioned in the first part of this chapter, in past years the hospital could rely on testing performed by the EPA for chemical germicides classified as sporicides. These types of formulations registered with the EPA were thought to meet standard test criteria for effectiveness. Currently, hospitals should rely on the scientific literature, papers presented at scientific meetings, scientific data provided by manufacturers, and guidelines of professional organizations (e.g., the Association for Practitioners for Infection Control [62]) and the CDC, in addition to EPA registration and FDA categorization. Testing of antiseptics (28) and disinfectants (11) is a complex and expensive process, and few clinical microbiology laboratories will devote their resources to such testing.

The actual effectiveness of a germicide is influenced only in part by the nature of the agent. Of equal or perhaps greater importance is the way it is used in the hospital. Many disinfectants, especially low- and intermediate-level disinfectants, have little margin of safety; a variety of misuses by hospital personnel such as the use of a product on a surface that has been inadequately precleaned may lead to failure of a germicidal process. Thus, a hospital infection control program may decide to use microbiological assays in a limited program to monitor the effectiveness of disinfection and sterilization. Routine or widespread environmental culturing is generally discouraged because it offers few data of use to an infection control program. Moreover, an environmental monitoring program must be well designed with a specific objective in mind. It makes little sense, for example, to evaluate items or areas that are unlikely to play a role in disease transmission. Thus, floors, furniture, or similar environmental surfaces should not be tested even to evaluate the effectiveness of hospital housekeeping personnel. Microbiological assays of the inanimate environment, to the extent that they are used, should be limited to high-risk items such as critical or semicritical medical instruments or devices. Even then, these assays should not take the place of scrupulous attention to the actual performance of the sterilization or disinfection procedures. With these cautions in mind, the following guidelines are offered for the microbiological monitoring of selected high-risk procedures.

Steam autoclaves

Steam sterilizers (autoclaves) are monitored for several physical parameters during the sterilization process. For example, autoclaves equipped with time and temperature recorders generally ensure an adequate sterilization cycle. However, assurance that the process actually sterilized objects and liquids can be inferred only after a number of factors have been controlled. These factors include properly loading the sterilizer, eliminating residual air, properly bleeding the autoclave so that superheating does not produce false readings, and properly operating physical gauges. Commercially prepared biological indicators, i.e., of *Bacillus stearothermophilus* spores, should be used at least once a week to confirm that a routine cycle achieves actual sterilization. Where the biological indicator is placed is important and depends on the type of load to be monitored. As a general rule, spore carriers should be placed in the center of the largest pack in the largest load or in an area of the load that is least likely to reach sterilizing temperature. The biological indicator should not be placed on an open shelf or on the peripheral exterior surface of a pack. The indicator should be processed as recommended by the manufacturer. For more extensive discussions of steam sterilization, the reader is referred to current guidelines of the Association for the Advancement of Medical Instrumentation (10).

Gas sterilizers

Gaseous ethylene oxide sterilization provides a much narrower margin of safety than does steam sterilization, and malfunctions that are not detectable by the physical gauges associated with the commercial units can occur. When ethylene oxide gas is used to treat implantable devices that require sterility, each load should be monitored; otherwise, the sterilizer should be monitored weekly. Biological indicators containing spores of *B. subtilis* var. *niger* (*globigii*), also commercially available, should be used. Here again, where the spore carrier is placed is important. It should be in the middle of the largest pack in an area of the pack that is least likely to receive adequate exposure to ethylene oxide. The specific assay procedure should be performed as instructed by the manufacturer. Guidelines for the evaluation and monitoring of ethylene oxide sterilizers are available (9).

Dry-heat sterilizers

Dry-heat sterilizers should be checked at least once weekly by the basic strategies described above and with biological indicators containing spores of *B. subtilis* var. *niger* (*globigii*).

Respiratory therapy and anesthesia breathing circuits

The most important part of an environmental control program to reduce infections transmitted directly or indirectly by respiratory therapy and anesthesia equipment breathing circuits is the use of proper cleaning and reprocessing procedures for reusable components. The most efficient and cost-effective way to accomplish these goals is to sterilize these devices with steam under pressure or with ethylene oxide. If this is not possible, the minimum procedure that should be used is one that achieves high-level disinfection. In this case, these items may be spot checked every few months or when disinfection or usage procedures change. Routine or scheduled bacteriological testing is not required. Although there is no adequate, well-supported microbiological guideline for this strategy, the most widely used criterion of acceptability is the absence of vegetative bacteria on components of the breathing circuits after the disinfection process (3, 38).

Hemodialysis systems

Gram-negative water bacteria have the ability to multiply rapidly in fluids associated with hemodialysis systems such as distilled, softened, deionized, and reverse-osmosis water as well as in the dialysis fluid itself. Although these fluids do not need to be sterile, excessive levels of gram-negative bacterial contamination pose a risk of pyrogenic reactions and septicemia. A quantitative microbiological guideline for levels of contamination has been proposed (8, 37, 39).

Dialysis fluids and water used to prepare dialysis fluids should be checked microbiologically at least once a month. Microbiological guidelines for these procedures include sampling the water used to prepare dialysis fluid at the point where it is mixed with concentrated dialysis fluid, and the level of bacterial contamination should not exceed 200 CFU/ml. Dialysis fluid should be sampled at the end of a dialysis treatment, and the level of bacterial contamination should not exceed 2,000 CFU/ml. In both instances, routine standard plate count or membrane filter assay procedures using appropriate culture media such as tryptic soy agar can be used. Hemodialysis systems are among the few medical devices for which periodic microbiological assays are recommended and for which the few microbiological quantitative guidelines are actually based on epidemiologic studies (37, 39, 42).

Arterial pressure transducers

Arterial pressure transducers have been incriminated in disease transmission, and the best means of control are adequate cleaning and sterilization as well as proper placement. Scheduled microbiological sampling is not required, but these items should then be assayed occasionally to determine whether they are being used properly. The criterion of acceptability is sterility (13).

Endoscopic equipment

In recent years, flexible and rigid endoscopic devices for use on patients have increased in both number and complexity of design. These devices have the advantage in many cases of eliminating surgical procedures for clinical or diagnostic purposes, but since they touch mucous membranes or are placed into normally sterile areas of the body, they are in the category of semicritical to critical instruments. Ideally, all endoscopes including flexible fiberoptics should be appropriately cleaned and then sterilized between uses. In practice, however, the vast majority of all flexible or rigid endoscopic procedures performed worldwide are done with disinfected rather than sterilized optic portions of the endoscopic set. The reasons for this practice are that almost all optic portions of endoscopic devices are very delicate and are, in varying degrees, degraded or destroyed by steam autoclaving; some endoscopes are damaged even by repeated ethylene oxide cycles, and this type of processing will remove the instruments from service for hours or sometimes even days because of process and aeration times. In these instances, the absolute minimum strategy should be the use of meticulous cleaning and high-level disinfection (4, 17, 18, 20, 27, 42, 61). A variety of chemical germicides that are classified as high-level disinfectants have already been discussed. When selecting a germicide for use with lensed instruments, one must consider not only the activity of the germicide but also the chemical compatibility after extended use with the instrument. Currently, the most widely used high-level disinfectants with endoscopic equipment are glutaraldehyde- or hydrogen peroxide-based germicides. As with other critical and semicritical items, the best method for ensuring success of the disinfection procedure is strict adherence to established cleaning and disinfection protocols. Because of the physical variety and complexity of endoscopic devices, particularly flexible endoscopes, the user is cautioned to pay particular attention to the instructions of the manufacturer for physical access and cleaning of all device surfaces; if patient material remains in or on instrument surfaces, virtually all germicidal procedures short of a steam autoclave cycle may fail in their intended purpose (34, 73). Scheduled microbiological sampling is not required, but if it is done periodically, the criterion of acceptability is the absence of vegetative bacteria.

Miscellaneous procedures and equipment

There are numerous items and patient care equipment that pose various degrees of infection risk associated with their use. They may make direct contact with skin and mucous membranes of body orifices or with the peritoneal cavity, but usually not with deep tissue. Items in this category, in addition to flexible fiberoptic and other endoscopic equipment, are hydrotherapy equipment, peritoneal dialysis equipment, and certain dental handpieces or tooth scalers. With these items, as with others mentioned above, the most important element in environmental control is not microbiological sampling but rather adherence to established protocols associated with their cleaning, preparation, disinfection or sterilization, length of use, and maintenance. Even spot checking these items and procedures is not recommended in most cases because of the absence of meaningful microbiological guidelines supported by epidemiologic criteria. One arbitrary guideline that can be used is the absence of recognized pathogens after a particular cleaning and disinfection procedure, which can be interpreted, from a practical standpoint, as the absence of vegetative bacteria.

Unnecessary microbiological assays

There are a number of items and procedures in hospitals and other health care facilities for which microbiological sampling on either a scheduled or periodic basis is not cost effective or rational. Included in this category are sterile intravenous solutions, injectable solutions, disposable syringes, disposable blood lines, artificial kidneys (even those that are reused), and all other items that are received in a sterile state. Equipment and solutions sterilized within the hospital need not be sampled microbiologically. Instead, quality assurance testing associated with sterilization procedures, such as appropriate biological indicator spores, should be used to ensure that the sterilization process per se is performing to specifications and that the associated personnel practices are being performed correctly.

It is recognized that inanimate surfaces and air associated with critical areas such as surgical suites and intensive-care areas may contain, to varying degrees, reservoirs of microorganisms. However, the chance for disease transmission in environments that are routinely cleaned and maintained is remote. Environmental control procedures associated with housekeeping and engineering services should adhere to established cleaning, disinfection, and maintenance protocols. Microbiological sampling on either a scheduled or periodic basis should not be done on floors, walls, intramural air, or other inanimate environmental surfaces. Conversely, appropriate sampling should be done when a disease outbreak appears to be associated with a certain part of the environment such as the air ventilation system.

Environmental microbiological sampling during outbreaks of disease

The strategy that should be used during an outbreak of disease with respect to environmental microbiological sampling depends on several factors. First, the infection control practitioner or epidemiologist must determine whether certain procedures, equipment, instruments, or other parts of the environment are contributing directly or indirectly to the outbreak. An outbreak of nosocomial disease does not necessarily mean that environmental microbiological sampling at any level is required. Second, if environmental microbiological sampling is believed to be necessary, the microbiologist and infection control practitioner or epidemiologist should coordinate the sampling scheme and determine the assay procedures as well as the items or parts of the environment that require microbiological assay.

The microbiological guideline applied in this context differs from one that is associated with scheduled or periodic sampling. During the investigation of an outbreak of nosocomial infection, environmental testing is usually directed toward the specific pathogenic microorganism. Consequently, if the outbreak is caused by *Pseudomonas aeurginosa,* this organism is sought in or on the various environmental items that are sampled. In this respect, the guideline tends to be more qualitative than quantitative, although in some instances one must rely on established guidelines. For example, if there is an outbreak of pyrogenic reactions in a hemodialysis center, established guidelines are available (8, 39). If water or ice in a hospital is incriminated in an outbreak of nosocomial salmonellosis, assays for determining fecal coliform bacteria and the total number of microorganisms, as well as a selective assay for salmonellae, should be used. Thus, the microbiological guideline in this situation is flexible and basically determined by the nature of the disease outbreak.

LITERATURE CITED

1. **Alter, M. J., M. S. Favero, J. K. Miller, L. A. Moyer, and L. A. Bland.** 1990. National surveillance of dialysis-associated diseases in the United States, 1988. Trans. Am. Soc. Artif. Intern. Organs **36:**107–118.
2. **American Neurological Association.** 1986. Committee on Health Care Issues: precautions in handling tissues, fluids, and other materials from patients with documented or suspected Creutzfeldt-Jacob disease. Ann. Neurol. **19:** 75–77.
3. **American Public Health Association.** 1978. Committee on Microbial Contamination of Surfaces: a proposed microbiologic guideline for respiratory therapy equipment and materials. Health Lab. Sci. **15:**177–179.
4. **American Society for Gastrointestinal Endoscopy.** 1988. Infection control during gastrointestinal endoscopy: guidelines for clinical application. Gastrointest. Endosc. **34**(Suppl.):37–40.
5. **Anderson, L. J., S. C. Hadler, C. Lopez, W. R. Jarvis, S. Fisher-Hoch, W. W. Bond, and D. B. Fishbein.** 1988. Nosocomial viral infections, p. 12–38. *In* E. H. Lennette, F. A. Murphy, and P. Halonen (ed.), Laboratory diagnosis of infectious diseases, vol. II. Viral, rickettsial and chlamydial diseases. Springer-Verlag, New York.
6. **Anderson, R. L.** 1989. Iodophor antiseptics: intrinsic microbial contamination with resistant bacteria. Infect. Control Hosp. Epidemiol. **10:**443–446.
7. **Asher, D. M., C. J. Gibbs, and D. C. Gajdusek.** 1986. Slow viral infections: safe handling of the agents of subacute spongiform encephalopathies, p. 59–71. *In* B. M. Miller, D. H. M. Gröschel, J. H. Richardson, D. Vesley, J. R. Songer, R. D. Housewright, and W. E. Barkley (ed.), Laboratory safety: principles and practices. American Society for Microbiology, Washington, D.C.
8. **Association for the Advancement of Medical Instrumentation.** 1982. American standard for hemodialysis systems. Association for the Advancement of Medical Instrumentation, Arlington, Va.
9. **Association for the Advancement of Medical Instrumentation.** 1985. Performance evaluation of ethylene oxide sterilizers of ethylene oxide test packs. Association for the Advancement of Medical Instrumentation, Arlington, Va.
10. **Association for the Advancement of Medical Instrumentation.** 1988. Steam sterilization and sterility assurance. Association for the Advancement of Medical Instrumentation, Arlington, Va.
11. **Association of Official Analytical Chemists.** 1984. Official methods of analysis, 14th ed. Association of Official Analytical Chemists, Arlington, Va.
12. **Association for Practitioners in Infection Control; Ad Hoc Committee on Infection Control in the Handling of Endoscopic Equipment.** 1980. Guidelines for preparation of laparoscopic instrumentation. AORN J. **32:**65–76.
13. **Beck-Sague, C., and W. R. Jarvis.** 1989. Epidemic bloodstream infections associated with pressure tranducers: a persistent problem. Infect. Control Hosp. Epidemiol. **10:** 54–59.
14. **Berkelman, R. L., B. W. Holland, and R. L. Anderson.** 1982. Increased bactericidal activity of dilute preparations of povidone-iodine solutions. J. Clin. Microbiol. **15:**635–639.
15. **Birnie, G. G., E. M. Quigley, G. B. Clements, E. A. C. Follett, and G. Watkinson.** 1983. Endoscopic transmission of hepatitis B virus. Gut **24:**171–174.
16. **Block, S. S. (ed.).** 1983. Disinfection, sterilization and preservation, 3rd ed. Lea & Febiger, Philadelphia.
17. **Bond, W. W.** 1987. Virus transmission via fiberoptic endoscope: recommended disinfection. J. Am. Med. Assoc. **257:**843–844.
18. **Bond, W. W.** 1987. Disinfecting and sterilizing of flexible fiberoptic endoscopes (FEE) and accessories. Endosc. Rev. **5:**55–58.
19. **Bond, W. W., and M. S. Favero.** 1977. *Bacillus xerothermodurans,* sp. nov., a species forming endospores extremely resistant to dry heat. Int. J. Syst. Bacteriol. **27:** 157–160.
20. **Bond, W. W., M. S. Favero, D. C. Mackel, and G. F. Mallison.** 1979. Sterilization or disinfection of flexible fiber-

optic endoscopes. AORN J. **30:**350–352.

21. **Bond, W. W., M. S. Favero, N. J. Petersen, and J. W. Ebert.** 1983. Inactivation of hepatitis B virus by intermediate- to high-level disinfectant chemicals. J. Clin. Microbiol. **18:**535–538.
22. **Bond, W. W., M. S. Favero, N. J. Petersen, C. R. Gravelle, J. W. Ebert, and J. E. Maynard.** 1981. Survival of hepatitis B-virus after drying and storage for one week. Lancet **i:** 550–551.
23. **Bond, W. W., M. S. Favero, N. J. Petersen, and J. H. Marshall.** 1970. Dry-heat inactivation kinetics of naturally occurring spore populations. Appl. Microbiol. **20:**573–578.
24. **Bond, W. W., M. S. Favero, N. J. Petersen, and J. H. Marshall.** 1971. Relative frequency distribution of D_{125C} values for spore isolates from the Mariner-Mars 1969 spacecraft. Appl. Microbiol. **21:**832–836.
25. **Bond, W. W., N. J. Petersen, and M. S. Favero.** 1977. Viral hepatitis B: aspects of environmental control. Health Lab. Sci. **14:**235–252.
26. **Bond, W. W., N. J. Petersen, and M. S. Favero.** 1982. Transmission of type B viral hepatitis via eye inoculation of a chimpanzee. J. Clin. Microbiol. **15:**533–534.
27. **British Society of Gastroenterology.** 1988. Cleaning and disinfection of equipment for gastrointestional flexible endoscopy: interim recommendations of a working party. Gut **29:**1134–1151.
28. **Bruch, M. K., and E. Larson.** 1989. Regulation of topical antimicrobials: history, status and future perspective. Infect. Control Hosp. Epidemiol. **10:**505–508.
29. **Carson, L. A., M. S. Favero, W. W. Bond, and N. J. Petersen.** 1972. Factors affecting comparative resistance of naturally occurring and subcultured *Pseudomonas aeruginosa* to disinfectants. Appl. Microbiol. **23:**863–869.
30. **Carson, L. A., N. J. Petersen, M. S. Favero, and S. M. Aguero.** 1978. Growth characteristics of atypical mycobacteria in water and their comparative resistance to disinfectants. Appl. Environ. Microbiol. **36:**839–846.
31. **Centers for Disease Control.** 1987. Recommendations for prevention of HIV transmission in health-care settings. Morbid. Mortal. Weekly Rep. **36:**1–18.
32. **Conrad, J. E., P. J. Leadley, and T. C. Eickhoff.** 1971. *Bacillus cereus* pneumonia and bacteremias. Am. Rev. Respir. Dis. **103:**711–714.
33. **Deane, N., C. Blagg, J. Bower, J. De Palma, C. Gutch, A. Kanter, D. Ogden, J. Sadler, A. Siemsen, B. Teehan, and A. Sosin.** 1978. A survey of dialyzer reuse practice in the United States. Dialysis Transplant. **7:**1128–1130.
34. **Dwyer, D. M., E. G. Klein, G. R. Istre, M. G. Robinson, D. A. Neumann, and G. A. McCoy.** 1987. *Salmonella newport* infections transmitted by fiberoptic colonoscopy. Gastrointest. Endosc. **33:**84–87.
35. **Farrer, W. E.** 1963. Serious infections due to "non-pathogenic" organisms of the genus *Bacillus*. Am. J. Med. **34:** 134–141.
36. **Favero, M. S.** 1982. Iodine: champagne in a tin cup. Infect. Control **3:**30–32.
37. **Favero, M. S.** 1985. Dialysis-associated diseases and their control, p. 267–284. *In* J. V. Bennett and P. S. Brachman (ed.), Hospital infections, 2nd ed. Little, Brown, and Co., Boston.
38. **Favero, M. S.** 1989. Principles of sterilization and disinfection. Anaesthesiol. Clin. North Am. **7:**941–949.
39. **Favero, M. S., and N. J. Petersen.** 1977. Microbiologic guidelines for hemodialysis systems. Dialysis Transplant. **6:**34–36.
40. **Favero, M. S., N. J. Petersen, and W. W. Bond.** 1986. Transmission and control of laboratory-acquired hepatitis infection, p. 49–58. *In* B. M. Miller, D. H. M. Gröschel, J. H. Richardson, D. Vesley, J. R. Songer, R. D. Housewright, and W. E. Barkley (ed.), Laboratory safety: principles and practices. American Society for Microbiology, Washington, D.C.
41. **Favero, M. S., N. J. Petersen, L. A. Carson, W. W. Bond, and S. H. Hindman.** 1975. Gram-negative water bacteria in hemodialysis systems. Health Lab. Sci. **12:**321–334.
42. **Garner, J. S., and M. S. Favero.** 1985. Guidelines for handwashing and hospital environmental control. HHS publication no. 99-1117. Centers for Disease Control, Atlanta.
43. **Gordon, S. M., M. A. Tipple, L. A. Bland, and W. R. Jarvis.** 1988. Pyrogenic reactions associated with the reuse of hollow-fiber hemodialyzers. J. Am. Med. Assoc. **260:**2077–2081.
44. **Heister, D., C. H. Shaffer, Jr., M. Hill, and L. F. Ortenzio.** 1986. Studies on the A.O.A.C. tuberculocidal test. J. Assoc. Off. Anal. Chem. **51:**3–6.
45. **Hoffman, R. K., and B. Warshowsky.** 1958. Beta-propiolactone vapor as a disinfectant. Appl. Microbiol. **6:**358–362.
46. **Jarvis, W. R.** 1982. Precautions for Creutzfeldt-Jacob disease. Infect. Control **3:**238–239.
47. **Johnson, L. L., D. A. Schneider, M. D. Austin, F. G. Goodman, J. M. Bullock, and J. A. DeBruin.** 1982. Two percent glutaraldehyde: a disinfectant in arthroscopy and arthroscopic surgery. J. Bone Joint Surg. **64A:**237–239.
48. **Kew, M. C.** 1973. Possible transmission of serum (Australia-antigen-positive) hepatitis via the conjunctiva. Infect. Immun. **7:**823–824.
49. **Klein, M., and A. Deforest.** 1963. Antiviral action of germicides. Soap Chem. Spec. **39:**70–72, 95–97.
50. **Klein, M., and A. Deforest.** 1983. Principles of viral inactivation, p. 422–434. *In* S. S. Block (ed.), Disinfection, sterilization and preservation. Lea & Febiger, Philadelphia.
51. **Kobayashi, H., M. Tsuzuki, K. Koshimizu, M. Toyama, N. Yoshihara, T. Shikata, K. Abe, K. Mizuno, N. Otomo, and T. Oda.** 1984. Susceptibility of hepatitis B virus to disinfectants and heat. J. Clin. Microbiol. **20:**214–216.
52. **Martin, L. S., J. S. McDougal, and S. L. Loskoski.** 1985. Disinfection and inactivation of the human T lymphotrophic virus type III lymphadenopathy-associated virus. J. Infect. Dis. **152:**400–403.
53. **McDougal, J. S., S. P. Cort, M. S. Kennedy, C. D. Cabridilla, P. M. Feorino, D. P. Francis, D. Hicks, V. S. Kalyanaraman, and L. S. Martin.** 1985. Immunoassay for the detection and quantitation of infectious human retrovirus, lymphadenopathy-associated virus (LAV). J. Immunol. Methods **76:**171–183.
54. **Miner, N. A.** 1978. Viral hepatitis: prevention and control. Postgrad. Med. **60:**19–22.
55. **Ortenzio, L. F.** 1966. Collaborative study of improved sporicidal test. J. Assoc. Off. Anal. Chem. **49:**721–726.
56. **Petrocci, A. N.** 1983. Surface-active agents: quaternary ammonium compounds, p. 309–329. *In* S. S. Block (ed.), Sterilization, disinfection, and preservation. Lea & Febiger, Philadelphia.
57. **Portner, D. W., and R. K. Hoffman.** 1968. Sporicidal effect of peracetic acid vapor. Appl. Microbiol. **16:**1782–1785.
58. **Prindle, R. F.** 1983. Phenolic compounds, p. 197–224. *In* S. S. Block (ed.), Sterilization, disinfection, and preservation. Lea & Febiger, Philadelphia.
59. **Resnik, L., K. Veren, S. F. Salahuddin, S. Tondreau, and P. D. Markham.** 1986. Stability and inactivation of HTLV-III/LAV under clinical and laboratory environments. J. Am. Med. Assoc. **255:**1887–1891.
60. **Rhame, F. S.** 1986. The inanimate environment, p. 223–249. *In* J. V. Bennett and P. S. Brachman (ed.), Hospital infections, 2nd ed. Little, Brown, and Co., Boston.
61. **Ridgway, G. L.** 1985. Decontamination of fiberoptic endoscopes. J. Hosp. Infect. **6:**363–368.
62. **Rutala, W. A.** 1990. Guideline for selection and use of disinfectants. Am. J. Infect. Control **18:**99–117.
63. **Rutala, W. A., and D. J. Weber.** 1987. Environmental issues and nosocomial infections, p. 131–171. *In* B. F. Farber (ed.), Clinics and critical care medicine: infection control in intensive care. Churchill Livingstone, New York.
64. **Shikata, T., T. Karasawa, K. Abe, T. Uzawa, H. Suzuki,**

T. Oda, M. Imai, M. Mayumi, and Y. Mortisugu. 1977. Hepatitis B e antigen and infectivity of hepatitis B virus. J. Infect. Dis. **136:**571–576.

65. **Spaulding, E. H.** 1939. Chemical sterilization of surgical instruments. Surg. Gynecol. Obstet. **69:**738–744.
66. **Spaulding, E. H.** 1964. Alcohol as a surgical disinfectant. AORN J. **2:**67–71.
67. **Spaulding, E. H.** 1971. Role of chemical disinfection in the prevention of nosocomial infections, p. 247–254. *In* P. S. Brachman and T. C. Eickoff (ed.), Proceedings of International Conference on Nosocomial Infections, 1970. American Hospital Association, Chicago.
68. **Spaulding, E. H.** 1972. Chemical disinfection and antisepsis in the hospital. J. Hosp. Res. **9:**5–31.
69. **Spire, B., F. Barre-Sinoussi, D. Dormont, L. Montagnier, and J. C. Chermann.** 1985. Inactivation of lymphadenopathy-associated virus by heat, gamma rays, and ultraviolet light. Lancet **i:**188–189.
70. **Spire, B., F. Barre-Sinoussi, L. Montagnier, and J. C. Chermann.** 1984. Inactivation of lymphadenopathy associated virus by chemical disinfectants. Lancet **ii:**899–901.
71. **Tuazon, C., H. Murray, C. Levy, M. Solny, J. Curtin, and J. Sheagren.** 1979. Serious infections from *Bacillus* sp. J. Am. Med. Assoc. **241:**1137–1140.
72. **Webb, S. F., and A. Vall-Spinosa.** 1975. Outbreak of *Serratia marcescens* associated with the flexible fiberbronchoscope. Chest **68:**703–708.
73. **Wheeler, P. W., D. Lancaster, and A. B. Kaiser.** 1989. Bronchopulmonary cross-colonization and infection related to mycobacterial contamination of suction values of bronchoscopes. J. Infect. Dis. **159:**954–958.
74. **Wright, H. S.** 1970. Test method for determining the virucidal activity of disinfectants against vesicular stomatitis virus. Appl. Microbiol. **19:**92–95.
75. **Zanowiak, P., and M. R. Jacobs.** 1982. Topical anti-infective products, p. 525–542. *In* Handbook of nonprescription drugs, 7th ed. American Pharmaceutical Association, Washington, D.C.

Chapter 25

Waste Management

DIETER H. M. GRÖSCHEL

BACKGROUND INFORMATION

Clinical microbiologists have been cognizant for many decades of the dangers of infectious waste generated in their laboratories and have instituted proper waste disposal procedures. Furthermore, with the rise and recognition of laboratory-acquired cases of hepatitis B and the arrival of serological testing for the "Australia antigen," during the 1960s and 1970s clinical laboratorians in other subspecialty areas have become aware of the potential dangers of laboratory waste. The first federal inspection and licensing act for clinical laboratories, the Clinical Laboratories Improvement Act of 1967 (29), did not specifically address the question of waste management but addressed "freedom from unnecessary chemical, radiological, biological, and other hazards which may contaminate or otherwise adversely affect examination of specimens" and stated, "where applicable, provision shall be made for sterilization of contaminated material." The document did not, however, specifically address the safety of personnel or the environment. The Hospital Infections Program of the Centers for Disease Control and the Joint Commission for the Accreditation of Hospitals recommended the designation of certain hospital solid waste as infectious and suggested appropriate disposal methods (12, 13, 34, 37). (The Joint Commission for the Accreditation of Hospitals listed infectious waste as one of the hazardous materials and wastes in 1986 but now addresses only the specific policies and procedures relating to the handling and disposal of biological waste [reference 17, p. 74].) These recommendations were used as guidelines by hospitals and laboratories and remained unchanged despite the concerns about the transmission of the human immunodeficiency virus (2) and the introduction of universal precautions (3, 4). The College of American Pathologists addresses waste disposal in its inspection checklist and refers to federal, state, and local regulations (6). A review by Odette and Rutala of 200 U.S. hospitals in 43 states showed that most had adequate infectious waste disposal programs in 1987, but many employed overly inclusive definitions (R. L. Odette and W. A. Rutala, Program Abstr. 28th Intersci. Conf. Antimicrob. Agents Chemother., abstr. no. 641, 1988).

In the summer of 1988, widespread stories in the lay press about beach pollution with medical waste (e.g., in the *Washington Post* [Health] of 23 August 1988) caused paniclike reactions by public and legislators and led to emergency legislation in a number of states. The Office of Technology Assessment reviewed for Congress the issues in medical waste management (26), and Congress passed the Medical Waste Tracking Act of 1988 (36).

REGULATION OF INFECTIOUS WASTE

In 1986 the Environmental Protection Agency (EPA) published a guide for infectious waste management (9) that addressed the question of infectious waste as a solid waste regulated by the Resource Conservation and Recovery Act of 1976. Infectious waste was not considered to be hazardous waste, but the federal agency felt that generators of such waste should be advised about proper management. In subsequent years several states, among them the Commonwealth of Massachusetts, published revised, new, or emergency regulations on infectious waste because waste haulers and landfill operators became greatly concerned about the possibility of acquired immunodeficiency syndrome spreading from hospitals into communities through hospital waste. Hospital waste, mainly due to several instances of mismanagement by hospitals or waste contractors, became a publicly discussed issue, complicated by decisions at the local and state levels by the NIMBY (not in my backyard) attitude forbidding landfill and incineration operations to accept and process medical waste. Since that time and in an accelerated pace since summer 1988, many states, 44 according to the Office of Technology Assessment (26), have issued or are in the process of issuing or preparing regulations on infectious waste (e.g., references 1, 7, 8, and 15). The waste management industry has reacted to the challenge and has established waste transportation, treatment, and disposal facilities, especially for those states with the strongest regulations. It should not be surprising that the National Solid Wastes Management Association produced a model state infectious waste regulation that is very broad in its scope and proposes severe penalties (24).

The EPA Office of Solid Waste invited comments from the public on five issues affecting medical waste management in 1988 (10) and held a public meeting in November 1988 to discuss the comments received as well as the Medical Waste Tracking Act of 1988 (36). In March 1989, EPA published the standards for the tracking and management of medical waste (11) and began the implementation of the act.

With regard to the regulation of medical infectious waste at the local level, microbiologists are advised to consult the local or state health or waste management departments. Since there is a tendency on the part of regulators and commercial waste managers to include many more categories of waste under the category infectious waste than is necessary for public health reasons, microbiologists should participate in the review of proposed waste regulations to prevent unscientific designations of waste categories.

INFECTIOUS WASTE MANAGEMENT IN HOSPITALS AND LABORATORIES

General information

U.S. hospitals produce about 13 to 14 lb (ca. 6 to 6.5 kg) of solid waste per bed per day (26) and about 10% is considered to be infectious waste according to the Centers for Disease Control definitions (12, 13). Whereas the disposal of general solid waste costs $0.01 to $0.25/lb, usually for transportation to a landfill, commercial off-site treatment such as steam sterilization or incineration costs $0.30 to $1.00 (16) and even more in some areas. Therefore, for fiscal reasons it is important that the generator of waste defines infectious and noninfectious waste clearly and conservatively and designs a program that will allow the personnel of hospitals and laboratories to separate all waste at the site of generation. Rutala (31) reported that the change of infectious waste designations from 13 to 4 saved a 600-bed university hospital more than $200,000 annually.

Definition of infectious waste

In contrast to radioactive or chemical waste, infectious waste cannot be identified objectively (32, 33). One could define it as waste that can cause infectious disease and consider it to be hazardous according to the Resource Conservation and Recovery Act of 1976 if it can "pose a substantial present or potential hazard to human health or the environment when improperly treated, stored, transported, or disposed of, or otherwise managed" (9). The basic epidemiologic factors required for the transmission of disease include dose, resistance of the host, portal of entry, presence of a pathogen, and its virulence. Grieble et al. (14) reported in 1974 that a chute-hydropulping waste disposal system caused airborne dissemination of bacteria into the patient care areas. Circumstantial evidence focused blame on the system for an increase in nosocomial gram-negative bacterial infections. This report, the established transmission of infectious disease from microbiological cultures, and documented injuries with sharp items such as needles, scalpels, or broken contaminated glass, with subsequent infection such as hepatitis B, are the only documented examples indicating that waste could transmit infection; but there is a lack of good data that waste other than microbiological cultures and "sharps" can transmit infectious disease. This is not surprising, since the risk is remote (30). There is no epidemiologic evidence that disposed-of hospital waste causes disease in the community (32) and there is no microbiological evidence that hospital waste is more infective than residential waste. Kalnowski et al. (20) showed that hospital waste is not more contaminated than household waste (Table 1).

Considering the potential public health impact of waste on co-workers and the community, one should classify as potential infectious waste only microbiological cultures and stocks (see the discussion in Public Health Service publication reference 5, p. 7–9) and used sharp instruments such as needles, lancets, and scalpels or contaminated broken glass (sharps). Complying with the concept of universal precautions for the protection of health care personnel, one can include blood, blood products, and body fluids as well as materials heavily contaminated with them in the designation "infectious waste." Pathological waste from operating rooms, surgical pathology, and autopsies is often treated like infectious waste but for aesthetic reasons and not because it is infectious per se. To include certain noninfectious waste in regulations, waste-containing infectious material may also be called biological, biomedical, medical, or hospital waste by regulators and lawyers. Table 2 shows the designation of infectious medical waste by several organizations. It is obvious that the original designations by the Centers for Disease Control in 1987 and 1988 (3, 4) are the most acceptable ones from a scientific point of view. They were also shown to be associated with considerable savings when an infectious waste management system was being designed for a hospital (31). When assisting in the designation of infectious waste, microbiologists should insist on scientific definitions supported by epidemiologic considerations. The lower the percentage of designated infectious waste, the cheaper will be the disposal cost for the institution. Obviously, local, state, and federal regulations must be respected.

Segregation of infectious from noninfectious waste

The organization of a successful waste management system begins with the segregation of infectious from noninfectious waste at the site of generation. Appropriate receptacles must be provided and laboratory and hospital employees must be instructed about the designations and the collection and disposal of waste. Receptacles for solid infectious waste should be used for that purpose only and not for the deposit of wastepaper or coffee cups.

Liquid infectious waste such as blood, body fluids, and suctioned fluids can be disposed of by the generator in a designated sink directly into the sanitary sewer system. Pathological waste may be ground and flushed into the sanitary sewer with the permission of the local sewer authority (2, 12). Laboratory liquid waste such as su-

TABLE 1. Microbial contamination of household and hospital waste[a]

Bacteria	Contamination (mean CFU/g)			
	Household waste	Hospital waste		
		General care	Intensive care	Operating suite
Aerobes	6.1×10^9	3.4×10^8	2.2×10^6	2.3×10^4
Gram-negative organisms	6.0×10^7	2.8×10^7	7.2×10^4	5.8×10^3
Group D streptococci	1.0×10^7	1.2×10^6	2.9×10^5	0

[a] Adapted from Kalnowski et al. (20).

TABLE 2. Definition of infectious waste by various organizations

Source/type	Definition by following organization[a] (reference):					
	CDC (12)	EPA I (9)	EPA II (11)	NSWMA (24)	MN (1)	VA (8)
Microbiological cultures/stocks	+	+	+	+	+	+
Human blood/blood products	+	+	+	+	+	+
Contaminated laboratory waste	−	(+)[b]	−	+	−	−
Body fluids	−	+	+	+	+	+
Communicable disease isolation	+	+[c]	+	+	−	−
Human pathology waste	+	+	+	+	+	+
Secretions/excretions	−	−	−	+	−	−
Used sharps	+	+	+	+	+	+
Surgical waste	−	(+)	−	+	−	−
Dialysis waste	−	(+)	−	+	−	−
Contaminated animal waste	−	+	+	+	+	+
Contaminated equipment	−	(+)	−	−	−	−
Spill cleanup waste	−	−	−	−	−	+
[Chemotherapy]	−	−	−	+	−	−
Contaminated and mixed waste	−	−	+	−	−	+
Unused sharps	−	−	+	−	−	−

[a] CDC, Centers for Disease Control; NSWMA, National Solid Wastes Management Association; MN, Minnesota; VA, Virginia.
[b] (+), Designated as optional category.
[c] Highly communicable diseases.

pernatants of body fluids, tissue suspensions, or liquefied sputum after centrifugation or fluids from feeding and washing of infected cell cultures is best collected in special leak-proof and unbreakable receptacles. Decanting should be performed in a biological safety cabinet because of the generation of droplets and aerosols. Most laboratorians keep a disinfectant in the receptacle at a concentration that considers the inactivation by proteins and the dilution by the liquids. Liquid laboratory waste, especially from mycobacteriology, mycology, and virology laboratories, is usually steam sterilized in the laboratory. If it is decontaminated at a site away from the laboratory, it must be contained in a closed, leak-proof, and unbreakable container (5) that may be placed in a contaminated material box for transport.

Convention and regulations have used the red color of bags or containers to designate infectious waste receptacles. Plastic bags should be leak proof and capable of passing the 125-lb (ca. 57-kg) drop weight test of the American Society for Testing and Materials (8). Usually, two plastic bags are used (and required) for sturdiness and as an infection control measure. The bags must be closed tightly with tape before transport. "Double bagging" was introduced in infection control practice to prevent the transport of bags potentially contaminated in an isolation room of a patient from being carried through the hospital. Maki et al. (22) showed that surface contamination is low and comparable whether one or two bags are used. The authors advocated a single heavy-duty bag for the collection of waste and linen and pointed out the potential savings.

Many institutions collect solid waste, including sharps, in double-walled corrugated fiber board boxes or equivalent rigid containers lined with a plastic bag (Fig. 1). The introduction of a new "contaminated materials container" in 1976 at a university hospital for the disposal of needles and syringes as well as other contaminated materials resulted in a drop in needle stick injuries from 11.1 per 1,000 in 1971 to 8.1 per 1,000 employees in 1973 (27). A recent report by Kennedy et al. (V. A. Kennedy, K. Getz, J. Duncan, and E. Paleologo, 28th ICAAC, abstr. no. 640, 1988) confirmed these findings. It is, however, advisable that if sharp items are disposed of in such boxes, one test for penetration through the box wall of needles and scalpels. Heavy materials must be supported in appropriate containers. Sharps should be deposited directly in puncture-proof rigid boxes at the site of use (laboratory bench, patient room, venipuncture tray, or cart). If these containers are steam sterilized on site, one should assure the continued integrity of the container after sterilization to avoid needle sticks occurring during the removal for disposal. These containers should not be placed in compactors.

Venipuncture personnel and medical technologists using needles for the transfer of specimens or for subculturing blood culture media must be provided with appropriate devices for the disposal of needles that do not require recapping or removal by hand.

The advantages of a lined rigid container over a plastic bag are realized by the personnel responsible for transporting the waste. Frequently, broken glass or needles penetrate the plastic bags, cause injuries, and may also lead to leakage of waste. Different sizes of lined containers and different openings in the lid allow their use in many areas of the health care institution such as patient rooms, laboratories, and hemodialysis units and also for the disposal of various components of larger equipment. Considerations about size should include the expected weight and the dimensions of steam autoclaves and incinerators used for the treatment of infectious waste.

Contaminated material containers should display the international biohazard sign and a reference to the content (infectious, medical, biomedical, biological, or hospital waste). If the containers are transported outside the premises of the generator, the name and telephone number of the responsible office (safety office, infection control office, administrator, laboratory director, etc.) should be printed on the box. The generator of the waste (laboratory, nursing unit, clinic) should indicate the ac-

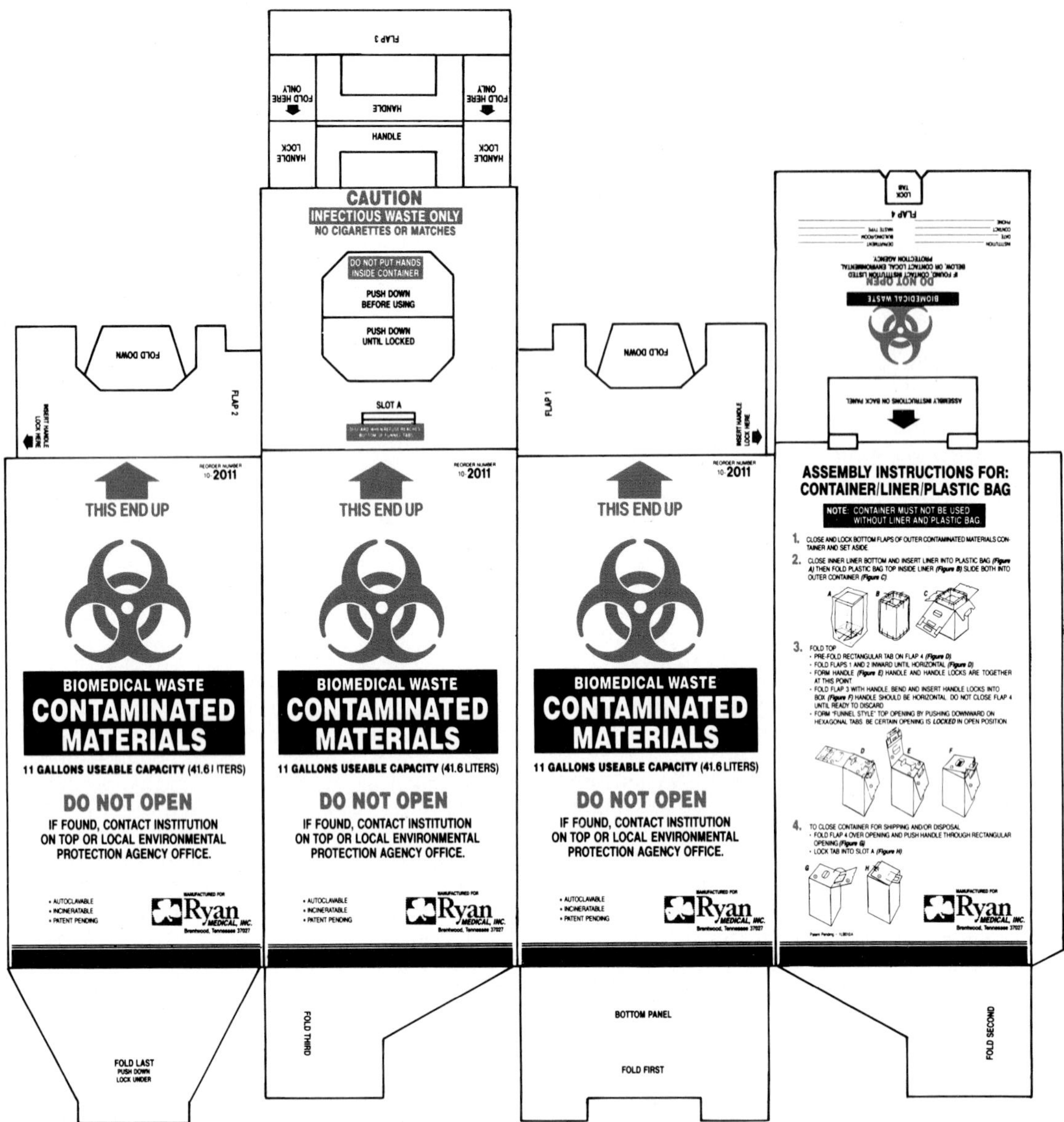

FIG. 1. Contaminated materials container. Original design by Osterman (27), Wenzel, and Loving, University of Virginia, distributed by Ryan Medical, Inc., Brentwood, Tenn. (patent pending).

tual content of the container (sharps, microbiological cultures, blood tubes, dialysis materials), the location, the name and telephone number of the responsible person, and the date of disposal. This permits safety and employee health personnel to assess infection risks after exposure or injury.

Storage

Areas for the storage of infectious waste must be clean and impervious to liquids. Floor drains should discharge into the sewer system, and ventilation should consider the potential exposure of humans and animals to the effluent. There should be an ongoing cleaning program as well as vermin and insect control. Access to the storage space must be limited to authorized personnel, and the doors must carry the biohazard sign with information about the content and the name and telephone number of the responsible person or office. If infectious waste is stored for longer periods, such as more than 72 h in Virginia (8) and up to 7 days in some states, or the geographic location is associated with high ambient temperatures that may allow bacteria and fungi to grow freely, the waste should be stored in refrigerated space at 2 to 7°C (35 to 45°F). Local regulations or ordinances may limit the storage time under refrigeration.

Transport

Transport of infectious waste in health care institutions usually occurs in two phases: collection within the institution and transport to the treatment facility. Waste containers are collected from nursing units, clinics, and laboratories by housekeeping personnel and brought either to the on-site treatment area or to the collection point for pickup for off-site treatment. Mechanical devices should not be used for the transfer of infectious waste containers (9). Carts used for the transport of waste should be designed for that purpose and be cleaned regularly with a detergent-germicide.

For off-site transport, closed, leak-proof dumpsters or trucks are recommended, displaying the biohazard symbol. Scattering and spilling of or leakage from the transported material must be prevented. EPA does not consider a truck to be a rigid containment system; therefore, all waste must be contained in rigid or semi-rigid, leak-proof containers before being loaded on a truck (9). Present regulations and policies of the U.S. Department of Transportation and the U.S. Department of Energy about displaying the biohazard sign are confusing to institutional and commercial waste haulers (reference 26, p. 10–11) and need to be standardized.

Under the proposed Occupational Safety and Health Administration regulations (25) employers must assure the protection of all employees against occupational exposure to blood-borne diseases, especially hepatitis B and human immunodeficiency viruses, and train employees in recognizing risks and in using protective measures. Health care workers and their unions or organizations have been concerned about the exposure in high-risk tasks such as transporting infectious waste. Of all of the needle stick or other sharps injuries reported to the employee health service of a university hospital, the incidence was highest in the employees of environmental services (16). All needle stick injuries listed in Table 3 were due to the negligent disposal of needles in bags for noninfectious hospital waste. In contrast, personnel transporting properly contained infectious waste to an off-site incinerator had very few sharps injuries over a 4-year period.

Another problem of concern to waste transporters is the spill of infectious material from broken containers. Policies and procedures for cleanup must be available and be part of training and continuing education.

Treatment

Until a few years ago certain localities permitted the disposal of infectious waste in landfills without prior treatment. Now EPA (9) recommends, and many states and localities require, appropriate treatment of infectious waste to reduce the potential hazard associated with infectious agents. Once infectious waste has been effectively treated, it may be handled and disposed of as noninfectious, general solid waste unless it is subject to other regulations as a radioactive or chemical hazard.

Incineration and steam sterilization are the most common treatment methods for infectious waste, but chemical and thermal disinfection is often practiced in clinical laboratories.

Incineration has the advantage of greatly reducing the volume of treated materials and thus was favored by many health care institutions for on-site treatment of both infectious and noninfectious waste. However, the high content of plastics, the location in densely populated areas, the often inadequate operation of the incinerators, the desire to incinerate ever increasing amounts of hospital waste, leading to overload, and the increased concerns of the public and environmental control agencies about high emission rates of pollutants due to plastics and metals have made on-site incineration less desirable. Many hospital-owned incinerators were closed down by authorities or were severely restricted as to waste categories. Regional cooperative or commercial incineration plants were developed to provide for the treatment of infectious waste according to the state of the art. In some states or regions it is presently prohibited to install new incinerators or to operate existing ones for treating infectious waste. This has caused considerable problems for hospitals in disposing of infectious waste and has increased the cost of waste handling.

Steam sterilization is mainly practiced in clinical laboratories and occasionally in central on-site plants of hospitals. Efficacy of the process depends on the type, volume, and density of materials, their packaging, and the presence of water. These factors influence steam penetration and heat conduction and, consequently, the degree of microbial killing as well as the time required to achieve sterility. Biological indicators are used to control the efficacy of the sterilizer. For the steam sterilization of clean instruments, dressings, and supplies, standard operating procedures were promulgated by hospital and professional organizations (28). In contrast, steam sterilization of waste is not standardized although one often finds that the same operating standards are applied to waste as to operating room packs. Experimental studies by Lauer et al. (21) and Rutala et al. (35) clearly demonstrated the need for different operating parameters of steam sterilizers for the treatment of laboratory waste. Some of these parameters were discussed by Vesley and Lauer (reference 23, p. 190–192). It is quite possible that the total processing time for waste may be 60 to 90 min, thereby greatly restricting the use

TABLE 3. Incidence of reported injuries with sharps[a]

Location/service	Dates	No. of employees	No. (%) of injuries[b]
700-bed university hospital	May 1986–April 1987		
Clinical laboratories		209	21 (10)
Nursing		1,640	282 (17)
Environmental		160	39 (24)
University-wide waste incineration service (pickup, transport, incineration)[d]	July 1984–July 1988	4	3[c]

[a] Personal communications from E. H. Hunt and J. Loving, University of Virginia.
[b] Among 2,009 employees at the hospital, there were 342 injuries (17%).
[c] Two injuries in the same person.
[d] Daily volume, 2 tons (ca. 1.8 metric tons): 1 ton from the university hospital; 1 ton from research laboratories, dialysis center, and animal quarters.

of the autoclave for other purposes. The question was raised by Rutala et al. (35), Vesley (personal communication), and others (reference 15, p. IV–23) whether it is necessary to achieve overkill, that is, sterilization of *Bacillus stearothermophilus* spores or even sterilization of the waste itself, when rendering infectious waste noninfectious. The setting of an arbitrary standard such as monitoring the efficacy of waste treatment with temperature-sensitive chemical indicators (8) or spore strips certainly is a less reliable control of successful treatment than the ongoing operation and process control of steam autoclaves by trained persons and their supervisors. Autoclave tape demonstrates only the attainment of a certain temperature, and spore strips require at least 24 h of incubation. The proper performance of a steam sterilizer is more reliably controlled by an ongoing quality control (inspection and maintenance) program and occasional testing with thermocouples.

Autoclaved waste must be distinguished from nontreated infectious waste if it is transported within the facility or transferred to a landfill. If material in red containers (bags or boxes) is transported, it should be placed in a regular waste bag or, preferably, in a neutral transport box. The generator is responsible for marking the container as containing waste rendered noninfectious by steam treatment. The Commonwealth of Virginia Department of Waste Management proposed placing infectious waste to be steam autoclaved in orange containers (8). Objections were raised to this proposal because red and orange colors are adjacent in the prism and may not be easily differentiated by some personnel. Some local and state regulations have strict requirements for record keeping, identification, and tracking of steam-sterilized waste.

Very large steam sterilizers are presently operated by cooperative or commercial waste disposal firms. They require special steam generators with specifications that surpass the capability of most hospital steam-generating plants.

Novel approaches to the treatment of infectious waste are grinding and decontamination with chlorine bleach (Medical SafeTEC, Indianapolis, Ind.) or with microwave irradiation (Vetco-Sanitec, Celle, Federal Republic of Germany).

Disposal of treated waste

After treatment, infectious waste should be noninfectious and can be disposed of like other solid waste. The need for labeling autoclaved infectious waste was mentioned earlier. Properly labeled autoclaved waste will be recognized as being noninfectious by waste haulers and landfill operators. Sometimes the waste is compacted together with regular trash and sent to the landfill. Since compacting may reexpose red plastic bags or containers, it is important that the generator assure the waste hauler and the landfill operator, preferably in writing, that the waste was treated in a steam autoclave and is now considered to be noninfectious (1, 15). Disinfected sharps should not be compacted (1), to prevent sharp injuries at the landfill.

The disposal of ashes in landfills has raised concerns from landfill operators and environmentalists. Heavy metals such as lead and cadmium are found not only in incineration emissions but also in ash from hospital incinerators. The Commonwealth of Virginia (8) requires that ash be analyzed frequently for the presence of toxic substances and the total organic carbon content. If ash is found to be hazardous on the basis of a sample and a confirmation sample, it must be disposed of as hazardous waste and the incineration unit will be closed.

INFECTIOUS WASTE MANAGEMENT PROGRAM

Each institution should have a plan for the proper management of infectious waste (19). The Joint Commission on Accreditation of Healthcare Organizations assigns the responsibility for assuring policies and procedures relating to the handling and disposal of biological waste in pathology and medical laboratory services as well as the evaluation of the hospital disposal systems for all liquid and solid wastes to the infection control committee (17, 18). Table 4 shows the waste treatment and disposal plan of a university hospital as it was developed by hospital epidemiology, microbiology, the safety committee, and the university office of environmental health and safety in compliance with proposed state regulations.

TABLE 4. Treatment and disposal of infectious waste in a university hospital

Source/type of infectious waste	Treatment/disposal[a,b]			
	Steam	Incineration	Chemical	Sewer
Microbiological waste	+	+	+	−
Human blood and blood products, body fluids	+	+	−	+
Dialysis waste, solid	−	+	−	−
Waste from strict isolation[c]	+	+	+	+
Pathological waste	−	+	−	+
Used sharps	+	+	−	−
Cleanup of infectious waste spill	+	+	−	−
Animal carcasses and waste	−	+	−	−
Animal carcasses and waste, infected with human pathogen	+	+	−	−

[a] Approved containers: sharps boxes, contaminated material containers (23), and double plastic bags (to be replaced with larger boxes).

[b] Treatment of waste: steam—sterilization with steam autoclave by generator or centrally, disposal by contractor; incineration—incineration in university incineration plant; chemical—disinfection with EPA-approved chemical disinfectant (also physical disinfection by boiling), incineration or disposal by contractor; sewer—disposal of liquid waste in sanitary sewer system.

[c] Includes waste from patients isolated because of infection with methicillin-resistant *Staphylococcus aureus*.

Laboratories and hospitals should have contingency plans for the treatment of infectious waste in case the established equipment fails.

All personnel generating, collecting, transporting, and storing infectious waste must be trained in infectious waste management, protective behavior and equipment, and procedures and policies regarding spills of liquid or solid infectious waste. Personnel specifically charged with waste handling must participate in employee health and continuing education programs. All personnel experiencing direct exposure to infectious waste must report this to their supervisor and to the employee health coordinator for appropriate immediate and follow-up care (25).

Although insufficient research data are available to support all recommendations in this chapter, basic safety and infection control measures as well as knowledge of microbiology and epidemiology allow the design of an infectious waste management system that should protect laboratory and hospital workers, waste haulers, employees of treatment facilities and landfills, and the public from infectious disease generated by medical waste.

LITERATURE CITED

1. **Attorney General.** 1988. Draft infectious waste legislation. State of Minnesota, St. Paul.
2. **Centers for Disease Control.** 1985. Recommendations for preventing transmission of infection with human T-lymphotropic virus type III/lymphaodenopathy-associated virus in the work place. Morbid. Mortal. Weekly Rep. **34:** 681–686, 691–695.
3. **Centers for Disease Control.** 1987. Recommendations for prevention of HIV transmission in health-care settings. Morbid. Mortal. Weekly Rep. **36:**3s–18s.
4. **Centers for Disease Control.** 1988. Update: universal precautions for prevention of transmission of human immunodeficiency virus, hepatitis B virus, and other bloodborne pathogens in health-care settings. Morbid. Mortal. Weekly Rep. **37:**377–382, 387–388.
5. **Centers for Disease Control/National Institutes of Health.** 1988. Biosafety in microbiological and biomedical laboratories, 2nd ed., HHS publication no. (NIH) 88-8395. U.S. Department of Health and Human Services, Public Health Service, Washington, D.C.
6. **College of American Pathologists.** 1988. Commission on Laboratory Accreditation inspection checklist, laboratory general, p. 23. College of American Pathologists, Skokie, Ill.
7. **Department of the Environment.** 1988. Title 26, subtitle 13, Disposal of controlled hazardous substances, chapter 11, special medical wastes. State of Maryland, Baltimore.
8. **Department of Waste Management.** 1988. Infectious waste management regulations. October 1, 1989. Commonwealth of Virginia, Richmond.
9. **Environmental Protection Agency.** 1986. EPA guide for infectious waste management, EPA 1530-SW-86-014. Office of Solid Waste, Washington, D.C.
10. **Environmental Protection Agency.** 1988. 40 CFR part 261. Hazardous waste management system; identification and listing of hazardous waste; infectious waste management. Fed. Regist. **53:**20140–20143.
11. **Environmental Protection Agency.** 1989. 40 CFR parts 22 and 259. Standards for the tracking and management of medical waste; interim final rule and request for comments. Fed. Regist. **54:**12326–12395.
12. **Garner, J. S., and M. S. Favero.** 1986. CDC guideline for handwashing and hospital environmental control, 1985. Infect. Control **7:**231–243.
13. **Garner, J. S., and B. P. Simmons.** 1983. CDC guideline for isolation precautions in hospitals. Infect. Control **4:** 245–325.
14. **Grieble, H. G., T. J. Bird, H. M. Midea, and C. A. Miller.** 1974. Chute-hydropulping waste disposal system; a reservoir of enteric bacteria and *Pseudomonas* in a modern hospital. J. Infect. Dis. **130:**602–607.
15. **Humphrey, H. H.** 1988. Report and recommendations on the regulation of infectious waste. Attorney General, State of Minnesota, St. Paul.
16. **Jagger, J., E. H. Hunt, J. Brand-Elnaggar, and R. D. Pearson.** 1988. Rates of needle-stick injury caused by various devices in a university hospital. N. Engl. J. Med. **319:** 284–288.
17. **Joint Commission on Accreditation of Healthcare Organizations.** 1988. Accreditation manual for hospitals, 1989, p. 68–79. Joint Commission on Accreditation of Healthcare Organizations, Chicago.
18. **Joint Commission on Accreditation of Healthcare Organizations.** 1988. Consolidated standards manual, 1989, p. 211. Joint Commission on Accreditation of Healthcare Organizations, Chicago.
19. **Jonsson, V.** 1986. The safe handling of infectious waste. Exec. Housekeep. Today **March:**6–7.
20. **Kalnowski, G., H. Weigand, and H. Rüden.** 1983. The microbial contamination of hospital waste. Zentrbl. Bakteriol. Mikrobiol. Hyg. Abt. 1 Orig. B **178:**364–379.
21. **Lauer, J. L., D. R. Battles, and D. Vesley.** 1982. Decontaminating infectious laboratory waste by autoclaving. Appl. Environ. Microbiol. **44:**690–694.
22. **Maki, D. G., C. Alvarado, and C. Hassemer.** 1986. Double-bagging of items from isolation rooms is unnecessary as an infection control measure: a comparative study of surface contamination with single- and double-bagging. Infect. Control **7:**535–537.
23. **Miller, B. M., D. H. M. Gröschel, J. H. Richardson, D. Vesley, J. R. Songer, R. D. Housewright, and W. E. Barkley (ed.).** 1986. Laboratory safety: principles and practice. American Society for Microbiology, Washington, D.C.
24. **National Solid Wastes Management Association.** 1988. Model state infectious waste regulation. Infectious Waste Council, Washington, D.C.
25. **Occupational Safety and Health Administration, Department of Labor.** 1989. 29 CFR part 1910. Occupational exposure to bloodborne pathogens; proposed rule and notice of hearing. Fed. Regist. **54:**23042–23138.
26. **Office of Technology Assessment.** 1988. Issues in medical waste management. Background paper, OTA-BP-0-49. U.S. Congress, Washington, D.C.
27. **Osterman, C. A.** 1975. Relation of new disposal unit to risk of needle puncture injuries. Hosp. Top. **March/April 1975.**
28. **Perkins, J. J.** 1969. Principles and methods of sterilization in health sciences. Charles C Thomas, Publisher, Springfield, Ill.
29. **Public Health Service, Department of Health, Education, and Welfare.** 1968. Clinical Laboratories Improvement Act of 1967. Fed. Regist. **33:**15297–15303.
30. **Rutala, W. A.** 1984. Infectious waste. Infect. Control **5:** 149–150.
31. **Rutala, W. A.** 1985. Cost-effective application of the Centers for Disease Control guidelines for handwashing and hospital environmental control. Am. J. Infect. Control **13:** 218–224.
32. **Rutala, W. A.** 1987. Infectious waste—a growing problem for infection control. Asepsis **9(4):**2–6.
33. **Rutala, W. A.** 1987. Disinfection, sterilization, and waste disposal, p. 257–282. *In* R. P. Wenzel (ed.), Prevention and control of nosocomial infections. The Williams & Wilkins Co., Baltimore.
34. **Rutala, W. A., and F. A. Sarubbi.** 1983. Management of infectious waste from hospitals. Infect. Control **4:**198–204.

35. **Rutala, W. A., M. M. Stiegel, and F. A. Sarubbi.** 1982. Decontamination of laboratory microbiological waste by steam sterilization. Appl. Environ. Microbiol. **43:**1311–1316.
36. **U.S. Congress.** 1988. 42 USC 6901. Medical Waste Tracking Act of 1988. Public law 100-582. U.S. Congress, Washington, D.C.
37. **Wenzel, R. P., and D. H. M. Gröschel.** 1985. Sterilization, disinfection, and disposal of hospital waste, p. 1609–1612. *In* G. L. Mandell, R. G. Douglas, and J. E. Bennett (ed.), Principles and practice of infectious diseases, 2nd ed. John Wiley & Sons, Inc., New York.

Chapter 26

Taxonomy, Classification, and Nomenclature of Bacteria

DON J. BRENNER

DEFINITIONS

Taxonomy is the science of classification. In practice, bacterial taxonomy consists of classification, identification, and nomenclature of microorganisms. Classification is simply an orderly arrangement of bacteria into groups. There is nothing inherently scientific about classification. Manley Mandel said that "like cigars, a good species and a good classification is one which satisfies." Sam Cowan correctly observed that classification is purpose oriented; thus, a successful classification is not necessarily a good one, and a good classification is not necessarily successful. Various subspecialty groups frequently classify the same organism with different criteria or to a different level (species, serotype, presence of a specific mutation or gene, and so forth).

Identification is the practical use of a classification scheme to isolate and distinguish desirable organisms from undesirable ones, to verify the authenticity or special properties of a culture, or to isolate and identify the causative agent of a disease. Nomenclature is the mechanism through which the characteristics of a taxonomic group are defined and communicated. It is essential that names, especially at the genus and species level, have the same meaning to all microbiologists, yet there are cases of one organism being classified in two different genera or having two species names.

As a science, taxonomy is dynamic and subject to change on the basis of available data. New findings often necessitate changes in taxonomy, frequently resulting in changes in the existing classification, in nomenclature, in criteria for identification, and in the recognition of new species.

The term "species" as applied to bacteria has been defined as a distinct group of organisms that have certain distinguishing features and generally bear a close resemblance to one another in the more essential features of organization. The problem with this definition is that it is subjective. What is "a close resemblance"? What are "more essential features"? How many "distinguishing features" are sufficient to create a species? Historically, these questions have been answered arbitrarily. Species were often defined solely on the basis of criteria such as the ability or inability to produce gas in fermentation of a given sugar and rapid or delayed fermentation of sugars. Since there was no way to devise a single definition of species that could be applied to all groups, criteria used to define species were heavily slanted toward the prejudices of the investigators who described the species. For example, Fritz Kauffmann defined a species as "a group of related serobiophagotypes" and believed that serology was the ultimate criterion in taxonomy. To him, each *Salmonella* serotype was a separate species. We now know that almost all *Salmonella* serotypes are genetically the same species. These practices probably led Cowan to state that "taxonomy . . . is the most subjective branch of any biological science, and in many ways is more of an art than a science."

Phil Edwards and Bill Ewing, in their monumental studies on members of the family *Enterobacteriaceae* (2), pioneered the principles for characterization, classification, and identification of bacteria:

1. Classification and identification of an organism should be based upon its overall morphological and biochemical pattern. A single characteristic (e.g., pathogenicity, host range, or biochemical reaction), regardless of its importance, is not a sufficient basis for classifying or identifying an organism.
2. To accurately determine the biochemical characteristics of a given species, one must test a large and diverse sample of strains. The reactions of these strains to any test should be expressed in percentages.
3. Atypical strains, when adequately studied, are often perfectly typical members of a given biogroup within an existing species, and sometimes they are typical members of a new species.

NUMERICAL TAXONOMY

In the 1960s, numerical taxonomy (also called computer taxonomy, phenetics, or taxometrics) became widely used, and this technique significantly improved the classification and identification of bacteria. In this method, 100 or more biochemical, morphological, and cultural characteristics are used to determine the degrees of similarity between organisms. Some laboratories recently have added susceptibility to antibiotics and to inorganic compounds to the characteristics used in numerical taxonomy. Many new and some previously ignored biochemical tests were assayed as possible aids in classification, and species- and genus-specific tests were identified. Clinical and applied laboratories could then use these tests to help separate specific species and groups of organisms.

In the numerical approach to taxonomy, investigators often calculate the coefficient of similarity or percentage of similarity between strains. (For this discussion, "strain" refers to a single isolate from a clinical or other specimen.) A dendrogram (phenogram or similarity matrix) is constructed that joins individual strains into groups and joins one group with other groups on the basis of their percentage of similarity. A hypothetical example of a dendrogram is shown in Fig. 1. In this figure, group 1 represents three strains that are about 95% similar, and these strains join with a fourth strain at the level of 90% similarity. Group 2 is composed of three strains that are 95% similar, and group 3 contains two strains that are 95% interrelated and a third strain to which they are 90% similar. Similarity between groups 1 and 2 occurs at the 70% level, and group 3 is about 50% similar to groups 1 and 2.

In some studies, all of the characteristics included in the similarity matrix are given equal weight; in others, certain characteristics are weighted. (For example, the presence of spores in a *Clostridium* isolate might be weighted more heavily than the ability to utilize a particular carbon source.) A given level of similarity may be equated to species-level, and sometimes to genus- and subspecies-level, relatedness. A taxospecies is one designated by numerical taxonomy, a genospecies is designated by DNA relatedness (see below), and a nomenspecies, is any group with a formal binomial name that may or may not constitute a taxospecies or a genospecies (13). Although there is no similarity value that equates a taxospecies with a genospecies, 80% similarity is commonly seen among strains in a given taxospecies. If 80% is used for species-level similarity and 60% is arbitrarily deemed to represent genus similarity, then the strains in groups 1, 2, and 3 in Fig. 1 would each represent a separate species. The species represented by groups 1 and 2 would be placed in the same genus, and the species represented by group 3 would be in a separate genus.

In designing numerical taxonomic studies, one must determine how many and which tests should be included, whether to weight certain tests, and if so, how. In drawing conclusions, it is important to decide what level of similarity is indicative of species- and perhaps genus-level relatedness in the groups under study, since there is no single value that applies to all bacteria.

The molecular weight of DNA in most bacteria is between 1×10^9 and 8×10^9, enough to specify some 1,500 to 6,000 average-size genes. Therefore, even a battery of 300 tests would assay only between 5 and 20% of the genetic potential of bacteria. It is almost certainly true that tests which are comparatively simple to carry out and assay, such as tests for carbohydrate utilization and for enzymes whose presence can be assayed colorimetrically, predominate over tests for structural genes, for genes involved in macromolecular synthesis, reproduction, or regulatory functions, and for other genes whose presence is difficult to assay. Potential sources of error must be considered when identifying species solely on the basis of phenotype:

1. Different enzymes specified by different genes may catalyze the same reaction.
2. Negative reactions can occur when the metabolic gene is present and functional through such mechanisms as the inability of the substrate to enter the cell and a regulatory or suppressor mutation.
3. A negative reaction can occur when the gene is present but not functional because of a mutation in a portion of the gene that is necessary for enzyme activity.
4. The correlation between a reaction and the number of genes (or enzymes) necessary to carry out that reaction is not necessarily 1 to 1. If one assays for the end product, a positive reaction may indicate the presence and function of as many as six or more enzymes in the pathway resulting in the observed reaction, whereas a negative reaction can mean that the pathway is absent or that one or more genes in the pathway are absent or nonfunctional.
5. Fastidious strains will not cluster with nonfastidious strains from the same species. This is often seen with *Escherichia coli* and *Klebsiella pneumoniae*. Other strain characteristics, such as slow growth rate, temperature of incubation (*Yersinia* and *Erwinia* species), salt requirement (marine *Vibrio* species), and pH (*Legionella* species), may drastically affect phenotypic characterization.
6. Plasmids carrying metabolic genes can enable strains to carry out reactions that are rarely if ever seen in the absence of the plasmid.

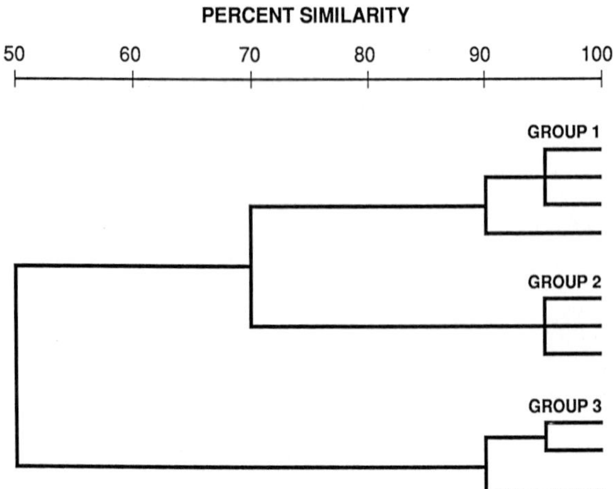

FIG. 1. Hypothetical example of a dendrogram.

The same set of "definitive" reactions cannot be used to classify all groups of organisms, and there is no definitive number of specific reactions that allows one to define a species. Taxospecies defined by numerical taxonomy usually correlate well with genospecies, but exceptions exist, and it is prudent to confirm numerical taxonomic groups by DNA relatedness. A more detailed discussion of numerical taxonomy is given by Sneath (13) and in the references he cites.

DNA HYBRIDIZATION

Ideally, one would like to classify bacteria and define species by comparing each gene sequence in a given strain with the gene sequences of every known species. At present, this is impossible. However, it is possible to compare the total DNA of one organism with that of any other organism. This method, pioneered by Marmur and Doty (8), Gillespie and Spiegelman (4), McCarthy and Bolton (9), and Britten and Kohne (1), is called nucleic acid hybridization or DNA hybridization. The method can be used to measure the amount of DNA sequences held in common between any two organisms and to estimate the percentage of divergence or unpaired nucleotide bases within related but not identical nucleotide sequences. DNA relatedness studies have been done in yeasts, viruses, bacteriophages, almost all major families of bacteria, and many groups of plants and animals. A partial list of the bacteria includes members of the family *Enterobacteriaceae* and strains of *Neisseria, Mycobacterium, Legionella, Haemophilus, Enterobacteriaceae, Pseudomonas, Flavobacterium, Vibrio, Aeromonas, Clostridium, Bacteroides, Brucella, Staphylococcus,* and *Streptococcus.*

DNA relatedness is determined by allowing single-stranded DNA from one strain to reassociate (hybridize) with single-stranded DNA from a second strain to form a double-stranded DNA molecule. DNA reassociation is a specific, temperature-dependent reaction. The optimal temperature for DNA reassociation is 25 to 30°C below the temperature at which native double-stranded DNA is denatured into single strands. Studies with numerous groups indicate that a bacterial species is composed of strains that are usually 70 to 100% related. Relatedness between species is most often 0% to about 60%. It is important to emphasize that the term "related" does not necessarily mean "identical" or "homologous." At optimal reassociation conditions nucleotide sequences that contain as many as 15% or more noncomplementary bases can hybridize.

It has been shown that each 1% of unpaired nucleotide bases in a double-stranded DNA sequence causes a 1% decrease in the thermal stability of that DNA duplex. By comparison of the thermal stability of a control double-stranded molecule in which both strands of DNA are from the same organism with a heteroduplex or DNA strands from two different organisms, differences in thermal stability can be assessed. Decreased thermal stability can be thought of as divergence in nucleotide sequences. In practice, strains that are 70% or more related show from 0% to about 5% divergence in related sequences, whereas sequences held in common between different species usually show 8 to 20% divergence.

When the incubation temperature used for DNA reassociation is changed from 25 to 30°C below the renaturation temperature to 10 to 15°C below the denaturation temperature, only DNA sequences that are very closely related, and therefore have high thermal stability, can reassociate. With this stringent (supraoptimal) criterion, strains from the same species prove to be 60 to 100% related, whereas relatedness between species is usually less than 50%. An in-depth discussion of DNA hybridization methods and applications has been presented by Johnson (6).

Experience with several hundred species led taxonomists to formulate a phylogenetic definition of a species or genospecies as "strains with approximately 70% or greater DNA-DNA relatedness and with 5°C or less ΔT_m" (divergence) (14). Occasionally, the 70% species relatedness rule has been ignored when the existing nomenclature is both deeply ingrained and useful. One such example is *E. coli* and the four species of *Shigella.* These organisms are all 70% or more related and should therefore be grouped into a single species instead of the present five species in two genera. This change has not been made primarily to avoid the confusion that would be created among members of the medical community. Other examples of single genospecies that have been split into two or more nomenspecies are *Yersinia pseudotuberculosis* and *Yersinia pestis, Neisseria meningitidis* and *Neisseria gonorrhoeae,* and species of *Brucella.*

DNA relatedness provides a single species definition that can be applied equally to all organisms and is not subject to phenotypic variation, mutations, or variations in metabolic or other plasmids. The major advantage of this process is that it measures overall relatedness, and therefore the effects of atypical biochemical reactions, mutations, and plasmids are minimal since they affect only a very small percentage of the total DNA. This point is illustrated by DNA relatedness data obtained from several biochemically atypical *E. coli* or *E. coli*-like strains (Table 1). Many of these biochemically atypical strains were shown to be genetically typical *E. coli.* The biochemical borders of *E. coli,* therefore, include all of these biogroups. Two groups of strains were shown not to belong to *E. coli.* These are KCN- and cellobiose-positive, yellow-pigmented strains, which proved to be a new species, *Escherichia hermannii,* and urea-, KCN-, citrate-, and cellobiose-positive strains that belonged in the genus *Citrobacter.*

G+C RATIO AND GENOME SIZE

G+C ratio and genome size are two other measurements of DNA that are often helpful in classifying organisms not fitting a known genus or family. The G+C content in bacterial DNA ranges from about 25 to 75%. The G+C percentage is specific for a given species but not unique for that species. For example, most *Legionella* species and species of *Proteus* and *Providencia* have G+C contents of 38 to 42 mol%. Therefore, two strains with similar G+C percentages may or may not belong to the same species. On the other hand, if the G+C contents are very different, the strains cannot be members of the same species. G+C content may be useful by indicating the need for appropriate further testing. A good example is a recently isolated organism that is biochemically between *Vibrio* and *Aeromonas.* It was placed in the genus *Vibrio* because its G+C content was 50%, which is within the range for *Vibrio* species and is significantly less than the 57 to 60% G+C found in *Aeromonas* species.

Genome size or the molecular mass of bacterial DNA

TABLE 1. Definition of the biochemical characteristics of *E. coli* on the basis of DNA relatedness

Biotype relatedness to typical *E. coli*	Characteristic
80% or more	Urea$^+$; KCN$^+$; mannitol$^-$; citrate$^+$; inositol$^+$; yellow pigment; H_2S^+; phenylalanine deaminase$^+$; triple decarboxylase$^-$; indole$^-$; adonitol$^+$; methyl red$^-$; urea$^+$, mannitol$^-$; H_2S^+, citrate$^+$; H_2S^+, citrate$^+$; anaerogenic, nonmotile, lactose$^-$; methyl red$^-$, mannitol$^-$
60% or less	KCN$^+$, yellow pigment, cellobiose$^+$ = *Escherichia hermannii*
	Urea$^+$, KCN$^+$, citrate$^+$, cellobiose$^+$ = *Citrobacter amalonaticus*

ranges between 1×10^9 and 8×10^9 daltons. Genome size determinations can, in certain circumstances, distinguish between groups that differ in this respect. Such determinations were used to distinguish *Legionella pneumophila* from *Rochalimaea* (*Rickettsia*) *quintana*. *L. pneumophila* has a genome size of about 3×10^9 daltons, whereas that of *R. quintana* is about 1×10^9.

INTEGRATION OF PHYLOGENETIC AND PHENOTYPIC CHARACTERISTICS

At present, genetic parameters are unrealistic for clinical laboratories. Therefore, practical biochemical tests must be correlated with the genetic data. For example, yellow-pigmented strains of *Enterobacter cloacae* were shown to be a separate species genetically but were not designated as such (*Enterobacter sakazakii*) until three practical tests were found that correlated with the genetic data. Taxonomists have recommended that genospecies not be named if they cannot be differentiated phenotypically. One example of this is in the genus *Hafnia*, in which a second genospecies has not been named because it cannot be phenotypically differentiated from *H. alvei*.

In practice, bacterial taxonomy should combine phenotypic and phylogenetic approaches. Unidentifiable and atypical strains should first be grouped by biochemical reactions and any other characteristics of interest. The phenotypic groups should then be tested for DNA relatedness to determine whether the observed phenotypic homogeneity is reflected phylogenetically. The final and, for most clinical microbiologists, the most important step is to reexamine the phenotypic characteristics of the genospecies (DNA relatedness groups and DNA hybridization groups). This procedure allows a determination of the biochemical borders of each group and of those reactions that are of diagnostic value for the group. For identifying a given organism, specific tests are weighted on the basis of their correlation with DNA results. Occasionally, the commonly used reactions will not totally distinguish between two distinct DNA relatedness groups. In these cases, other biochemical tests that are of diagnostic value are required. Heavily weighted tests are of great value for specific organisms (coagulase for *Staphylococcus aureus*, DNase for *Serratia* spp., etc.). It is often forgotten that before these weighted tests are of diagnostic value, the organism has been well characterized by growth on selective media, by colonial and cellular morphology, and by other biochemical tests.

The purpose of classification and identification is to provide the ability to distinguish one organism from another and to group similar organisms on the basis of criteria of interest either to all microbiologists or to specialty groups. The purpose of nomenclature is to provide a convenient system of communication that defines an organism without the necessity of listing its characteristics. This standardization is most important at the species level. A species name should mean the same thing to everyone, regardless of specialty. Nomenclature, and therefore effective communication, breaks down if strains of the same species are given different names on the basis of source of isolation, serotype, presence or absence of a converting bacteriophage, or the ability to perform specific functions, such as cause a disease or produce an antibiotic. Species have been created on the basis of these and many other criteria. Although these criteria may be extremely important for a specialty group, alone they are not a sufficient basis for naming a species. Rather, species should be established on the basis of sound phenotypic and phylogenetic criteria.

Clinical, plant, industrial, and other subspecialties in microbiology must frequently differentiate below the species level. Sometimes species are divided at the level of subspecies. Subspecies can be established on the basis of phenotypic or phylogenetic differences. The six subspecies in *Salmonella choleraesuis* reflect both biochemical and DNA relatedness differences. Three subspecies were recently proposed for *L. pneumophila* solely on the basis of phylogenetic differences, whereas subspecies of *Campylobacter* were defined by pathogenic host range or biochemical differences.

Special-interest groups of microbiologists need to communicate, but their needs can and should be met by designations below the species level as "groups" or "types" established on the basis of common serological or biochemical reactions, phage or bacteriocin sensitivity, pathogenicity, or other characteristics. For example, a bioserogroup or bioserotype is a group of strains of the same species with common biochemical and serological characteristics that set them apart from other members of the species. Many of these groupings are already commonly used and accepted: serotype, phage type, colicin type, biotype, bioserotype, and pathotype. The ending "var" (phagovar, etc.) can be substituted for "type." The designation "pathovar" can be used to describe differences in pathogenicity, but it appears to be used mainly for plant pathogens to designate host range, as for the six pathovars in *Erwinia chrysanthemi*. Pathovar may be a useful designation in human and animal diseases; after all, enteropathogenic, enterohemorrhagic, enterotoxigenic, enteroinvasive, and several other groups of *E. coli* strains are unnamed pathovars.

OTHER MOLECULAR APPROACHES

Several newer molecular methods are now in use for identifying and classifying pathogenic and other bacteria at and below the species level. Several of these methods are covered in detail elsewhere in this volume. Specific immunologic and nucleic acid probes are being used to detect a growing number of bacterial virulence factors, including *Vibrio cholerae* toxin, heat-labile and heat-stable toxins, invasiveness factors, cytotoxin, and adherence factors in *E. coli*, virulence-associated plasmid in *Yersinia enterocolitica*, and hemolysin in *Listeria monocytogenes*. Gene probes are available for detecting *N. gonorrhoeae*, legionellae, salmonellae, *L. monocytogenes*, *Mycobacterium tuberculosis*, *Mycobacterium avium*, *Mycobacterium intracellulare*, and other bacteria.

Molecular analysis of plasmids after electrophoretic separation has recently been used extensively to identify epidemic strains of bacteria. Plasmids of similar size can be specifically fragmented, by treatment with restriction endonucleases that cleave DNA at specific sites, to determine similarities precisely. For plasmid profile and restriction endonuclease analysis to be effective in monitoring epidemic strains, the strains must contain plasmids that are different from those of nonepidemic strains. Fortunately, these conditions are met in the majority of the *Enterobacteriaceae* and other bacteria found in outbreaks of nosocomial disease.

Several other methods have been used for epidemiologic subtyping (so-called fingerprinting) of strains of bacteria associated with disease outbreaks. Each of these methods is believed to be sufficiently sensitive to differentiate between clones (progeny of a single bacterial cell) of at least many bacterial species. Sodium dodecyl sulfate-polyacrylamide gel electrophoresis can be used to separate either whole-cell proteins or outer membrane proteins. A large number of protein bands are generated (usually 70 or more) that can be difficult to interpret, especially for comparing data from different experiments and for storing data. Restriction endonuclease analysis of chromosomal DNA has been used effectively to subtype strains of pathogenic bacteria, but again numerous DNA fragments are generated, and data comparisons are difficult. Gene restriction analysis of rRNA combines restriction endonuclease analysis with hybridization to rRNA. Only DNA fragments that contain a portion of the rRNA genes are visualized, thus decreasing the number of stained (or radiolabeled) fragments in the gel to 20 or less (5). Multilocus enzyme electrophoresis (enzyme typing) has been used extensively to determine clonal diversity in a variety of pathogenic bacteria (11). All of these methods have been useful in subtyping. No one method is best for all bacteria, and systematic comparisons have rarely been done on more than two methods with the same strains.

rRNA cataloging and sequencing is being used to determine evolutionary relationships among bacteria at taxonomic levels from kingdom through genus when total DNAs are essentially totally unrelated. This is possible because the genes for rRNA contain some sequences that have diverged only very slightly through the course of evolution, as well as moderately conserved sequences and some highly variable sequences (15).

rRNA sequencing is an extremely powerful tool, but most taxonomists feel that unless corroborative phenotypic data are available, it should not be used to designate families and genera (14). Similarly, total DNA relatedness data do not provide a practical genus definition. If they did, an ideal genus would be composed of species that are similar phenotypically and genetically (50 to 65% related). Some genera that contain phenotypically similar species (*Citrobacter*, *Yersinia*, and *Serratia*, to name a few) approach this genetic criterion. More often, the phenotypic similarity is present, but the genetic relatedness is not. For example, *Legionella* and *Campylobacter* (even without *Campylobacter pylori*) are good or at least well-accepted phenotypic genera in which DNA relatedness between several species is 0 to 5%. When both phenotypic similarity and genetic similarity are not present, phenotypic similarity should generally be given priority in establishing genera. The reason for phenotypic priority at the genus level is a practical one. When identifying organisms at the bench, it is desirable to have the most phenotypically similar species in the same genus. Primary consideration for a genus is that it contains biochemically similar species that are convenient or important to consider as a group and that must be separated from one another at the bench.

NAMING OF BACTERIA

Until 1 January 1980, priorities for names dated from 1 May 1753. This caused much confusion, since it was difficult to search the literature to ensure that a species had not been previously proposed. The early descriptions were often sketchy and based on fewer, often different tests than are now used. Furthermore, strains representing the species proposed in the 19th century often were not available, were of uncertain authenticity, or, when tested, did not exactly correspond to the published properties of the species. It was not unknown for a single species to have 30 or more known or presumed nomenclatural synonyms.

Priorities for bacterial names now start as of 1 January 1980. On that date, the Approved Lists of Bacterial Names were published in the *International Journal of Systematic Bacteriology* (IJSB) (12). The editors of the Approved Lists sought to include only species that were adequately described and for which a type or reference strain was available. Names not on those lists lost all standing ("*Arizona hinshawii*" is an example). It is now possible to determine whether a species has been previously published by consulting the Approved Lists and the lists of valid names published in each issue of IJSB. The Approved Lists and the requirement to search only to 1980 for prior species proposals will continue to remove much of the past confusion and will avert many future problems.

It is a common misconception that there has been an explosive increase in the number of bacterial genera and species since the application of DNA hybridization to taxonomy. When published in 1966, the *Index Bergeyana*, an alphabetical listing of bacterial names, included some 29,000 names. The *Supplement to Index Bergeyana*, published in 1981, contained an additional 5,700 species names and over 700 genus names. When published in 1980, the Approved Lists contained approximately 290 genera and 1,693 species. Additions through 1988 brought the number of genera to 494 (a yearly increase of 6.6%) and the number of species to 2,681 (a yearly increase of 5.6%), only a small fraction of the genus and species names that existed before 1980. Although a few synonyms exist, almost all current names uniquely represent a species. Almost all newly designated species are, in fact, new and usually well studied.

With the greatly enhanced armamentarium now available for taxonomic purposes, it is not surprising that the number of both medically important and other bacterial species has increased. Since 1974, the number of genera in the family *Enterobacteriaceae* has increased from 12 to 29 and the number of species has increased from 42 to 145 (about 30 of which have yet to be named). Similar increases occurred in *Vibrio* (5 to 38 species) and in *Campylobacter* (4 to 16 species). *Legionella*, which was not described until 1979, now has 28 named and 17 unnamed species. Virtually all of these new species are genetically unique. For some genera, the number of species has been substantially reduced. *Streptomyces*, in which most species were proposed solely on the basis of antibiotic production, contained 463 species and subspecies in 1974 but now contains 383 species. Continuing work is expected to further reduce this number by at least one-third.

Why should species be named, how are they named, and where are they named? According to the *Interna-*

tional Code of Nomenclature of Bacteria (7) (*Bacteriological Code*), "The primary purpose of giving a name to a taxon is to supply a means of referring to it." In other words, names are intended to foster communication and to ensure that the description of a given set of characteristics (by using a name to define them) has the same meaning to all scientists. An equivalent would be that it is more meaningful to say "Louis Pasteur" than "the man who disproved spontaneous generation" and "Judy Garland" rather than "the star of *Wizard of Oz*."

Species are named in accordance with principles and rules of nomenclature as set forth in the *Bacteriological Code* (7). The first principle of bacterial nomenclature is concerned with creating stability, avoiding or rejecting names that cause error or confusion, and avoiding the useless creation of names. Scientific names are usually taken from Latin or Greek and are treated as Latin regardless of their origin. The correct name of a species or higher taxonomic designation is determined by three criteria: valid publication, legitimacy of the name with regard to the rules of nomenclature, and priority of publication (it is the first validly published name for the taxon). "A name has no status under the rules and no claim to recognition unless it is validly published" (7).

To be validly published, a new species proposal must contain the species name, a description of the species, and the designation of a type strain for the species, and the name must be published in IJSB. The proposed name is automatically validly published if the proposal is published in IJSB. If the proposed name is published in another journal, it is not validly published until it appears in IJSB. It is the responsibility of the author to send reprints of such publications to the editor and to request publication of the new name(s) in IJSB. In this case, the date of valid publication is the date of publication in IJSB.

It is generally believed that once proposed, a name must go through some formal process leading to official acceptance. The opposite is true: a validly published name is assumed to be correct unless it is officially challenged. A challenge is made by publishing a request for an opinion to the Judicial Commission of the International Union of Microbiological Societies in IJSB. The Judicial Commission will then seek advice from appropriate experts and render an opinion. This is done only in cases in which the validity of a name is questioned with respect to compliance with the rules of the *Bacteriological Code*.

Generally, the existence of two names for one species results from two groups working independently. When it is subsequently shown that the two names represent the same organism, the name first published in IJSB has priority, and the other name is invalid. Two recent examples are *Providencia rustigianii* having priority over *Providencia fredericiana* and *Yokenella regensburgei* having priority over *Koserella trabulsii*.

A question of classification that is based on scientific data (for example, whether a species should, on the basis of biochemical or genetic characteristics or both, be placed in a new genus or an existing genus) is not settled by the Judicial Commission but by the preference and usage of the scientific community. This is why generic synonyms exist. Some more recent examples are *Citrobacter (Levinea) amalonaticus*, *Citrobacter diversus (Levinea malonatica)*, *Morganella (Proteus) morganii*, *Legionella (Tatlockia) micdadei*, and *Legionella (Fluoribacter) dumoffii*.

Changes in classification at the level of genus or family usually result from two types of studies. In one, an established group is reinvestigated, and the data obtained are interpreted to indicate errors in the original classification. An example is the genera *Proteus*, *Providencia*, and *Morganella*. These were once all in the single genus *Proteus*. Then "*Proteus inconstans*" was placed in a second genus, *Providencia*, as two species, *Providencia alcalifaciens* and *Providencia stuartii*. DNA relatedness studies indicated that *Proteus rettgeri* was more closely related to *Providencia* than to *Proteus* and that *Proteus morganii* was less related to *Proteus* and *Providencia* than to most other genera in the family *Enterobacteriaceae*. It was therefore proposed that *Proteus rettgeri* be transferred to *Providencia* and that *Proteus morganii* be transferred to a separate genus, *Morganella*. These changes appear to have gained wide acceptance by the scientific community.

In the second type of study, two groups of investigators look at essentially the same group of strains by similar techniques and interpret similar data differently. One research group interpreted their data for members of the family *Legionellaceae* as being most compatible with all species in the single genus *Legionella*. A second group classified the first five species in three genera, *Legionella*, *Tatlockia*, and *Fluoribacter*. At present the single genus concept is largely, but not exclusively, used.

Similarly, changes at the family and genus level were recently proposed for the family *Vibrionaceae* on the basis of rRNA cataloging and DNA-rRNA hybridization data. These proposals recommended placing *Aeromonas* in the new family *Aeromonadaceae*, removing *Plesiomonas* from the family, perhaps into *Enterobacteriaceae*, and dividing the genus *Vibrio* into three genera.

The reader is invited to consult the *Bacteriological Code*, the Approved Lists, and *Bergey's Manual of Systematic Bacteriology* for further details on bacterial nomenclature.

Taxonomy, albeit far from perfect, is not designed to create confusion in the lives of clinical or other microbiologists. The task of the taxonomist is to describe all species, using the best available scientific tools. Newly recognized species have sometimes been masquerading as members of well-known species. Such was the case with *Klebsiella oxytoca* (indole-positive *K. pneumoniae*), *Enterobacter sakazakii* (yellow-pigmented, sorbitol-negative, delayed DNase-positive *E. cloacae*), and *Vibrio mimicus* (sucrose-negative *V. cholerae*). Seven additional species were found in the *Y. enterocolitica* complex, and an equal number will probably be found within the *Citrobacter freundii* complex. Many other new species had not been previously recognized; these include *Borrelia burgdorferi*, all legionellae, the *Capnocytophaga* species associated with dog bites, and *Yersinia ruckeri*.

CONCLUSIONS

Clinical microbiologists should keep up with taxonomic changes to know which newly described species present potential clinical problems as pointed out by Farmer (3) and which are rarely, if ever, human pathogens. The most comprehensive treatment of bacterial classification, particularly for nomenclature, type strains, description of taxa, and references to pertinent literature, is *Bergey's Manual of Systematic Bacteriology*. The first two volumes, published in 1984 and 1986, contain almost all bacteria of medical importance. Volume 3 (published in 1989) contains gliding, fruiting, sheathed, budding and appendaged, chemolithotrophic, and photosynthetic bacteria, as well as cyanobacteria and archaeobacteria. Volume 4 (published in 1989) contains the streptomycetes and related bacteria. These are invaluable reference sources that should be at the desk of every microbiologist. The use of such volumes will ensure that clinical microbiologists are fully informed of taxonomic developments. Given that *Bergey's Manual* is never current, updated information can be obtained by searching IJSB. This journal, in which all new species must be described, also contains proposed name changes and all Requests for Opinions on changing or maintaining existing nomenclature. Many new species of clinical importance were described in the *Journal of Clinical Microbiology*, and some were described in *Systematic and Applied Microbiology, Research in Microbiology* (formerly *Annales de l'Institut Pasteur/Microbiology*), and *Zentralblatt für Bakteriologie Mikrobiologie und Hygiene* (International Journal of Medical Microbiology), journals which clinical microbiologists should already be reading for their clinical content.

A strong argument has been made for identifying species in the clinical laboratory. As previously stated, the probability of correctly identifying an organism, especially an atypical strain, is dependent upon the number of tests done. There is no absolute number of tests, because both the number and type of tests used vary from one group of organisms to another. How far one should go in identifying organisms and which organisms one should screen for are decisions that must be made in each laboratory on the basis of the type of population served and the function of the laboratory (primary or reference).

A final word of caution: a given organism will never be detected if appropriate isolation and enrichment media and proper identification tests are not used. Newly described biochemical tests should be done exactly as described in the literature. Modifications, shortcuts, or any change in media or reagents must not be attempted unless these changes have been published or shown to yield comparable results in well-controlled experiments by the laboratory.

LITERATURE CITED

1. **Britten, R. J., and D. E. Kohne.** 1966. Nucleotide sequence repetition in DNA. Carnegie Inst. Wash. Yearb. **65:**78–106.
2. **Ewing, W. H.** 1986. Edwards and Ewing's identification of *Enterobacteriaceae*, 4th ed. Elsevier, New York.
3. **Farmer, J. J., III.** 1981. Should clinical microbiology keep up with taxonomy—yes. Clin. Microbiol. Newsl. **1:**5–6.
4. **Gillespie, D., and S. Spiegelman.** 1965. A quantative assay for DNA/RNA hybrids with DNA immobilized on a membrane. J. Mol. Biol. **12:**829–843.
5. **Grimont, F., and P. A. D. Grimont.** 1986. Ribosomal ribonucleic acid gene restriction patterns as potential taxonomic tools. Ann. Inst. Pasteur Microbiol. (Paris) **137B:**165–175.
6. **Johnson, J. L.** 1981. Genetic characterization, p. 450–474. *In* P. Gerhardt, R. G. E. Murray, R. N. Costilow, E. W. Nester, W. A. Wood, N. R. Krieg, and G. B. Phillips (ed.), Manual of methods for general bacteriology. American Society for Microbiology, Washington, D.C.
7. **Lapage, S. P., P. H. A. Sneath, E. F. Lessel, V. B. D. Skerman, H. P. R. Seeliger, and W. A. Clark (ed.).** 1975. International code of nomenclature of bacteria, 1976 revision. American Society for Microbiology, Washington, D.C.
8. **Marmur, J., and P. Doty.** 1961. Thermal renaturation of DNA. J. Mol. Biol. **3:**585–594.
9. **McCarthy, B. J., and E. T. Bolton.** 1963. An approach to the measurement of genetic relatedness among organisms. Proc. Natl. Acad. Sci. USA **50:**156–164.
10. **Schildkraut, C. L., J. Marmur, and P. Doty.** 1961. The formation of hybrid DNA molecules and their use in studies of DNA homologies. J. Mol. Biol. **3:**595–617.
11. **Selander, R. K., D. A. Caugant, H. Ochman, J. M. Musser, M. N. Gilmour, and T. S. Whittam.** 1986. Methods of multilocus enzyme electrophoresis for bacterial population genetics and systematics. Appl. Environ. Microbiol. **51:**873–884.
12. **Skerman, V. B. D., V. McGowan, and P. H. A. Sneath (ed.).** 1980. Approved lists of bacterial names. Int. J. Syst. Bacteriol. **30:**225–420.
13. **Sneath, P. H. A.** 1984. Bacterial classification II. Numerical taxonomy, p. 5–7. *In* N. R. Krieg, and J. G. Holt (ed.). Bergey's manual of systematic bacteriology, vol. 1. The Williams & Wilkins Co., Baltimore.
14. **Wayne, L. G., D. J. Brenner, R. R. Colwell, P. A. D. Grimont, O. Kandler, M. I. Krichevsky, L. H. Moore, W. E. C. Moore, R. G. E. Murray, E. Stackebrandt, M. P. Starr, and H. G. Trüper.** 1987. Report of the Ad Hoc Committee on Reconciliation of Approaches to Bacterial Systematics. Int. J. Syst. Bacteriol. **37:**463–464.
15. **Woese, C. R.** Bacterial evolution. Microbiol. Rev. **51:**221–271.

Chapter 27

Recommendations for the Isolation of Bacteria from Clinical Specimens

HENRY D. ISENBERG, ELLEN JO BARON, RICHARD F. D'AMATO, RUSSELL C. JOHNSON, PATRICK R. MURRAY, FRANK G. RODGERS, AND ALEXANDER VON GRAEVENITZ

This chapter contains a number of recommendations to guide clinical microbiologists in their analytical tasks. We recognize that individual laboratories may have special needs and circumstances that dictate other approaches to specimen recording (accessioning) and processing. The vast array of commercially available media precludes commentary on all. The media listed are general examples; equivalent substitutions can be made with equally acceptable results in almost every instance.

These guidelines address only those bacteria considered within the routine of clinical bacteriology. For the isolation of anaerobic bacteria, mycobacteria, aerobic actinomycetes, spirochetes, and mycoplasmas and ureaplasmas, please consult chapters 49, 34, 35, 56, and 47, respectively. Recommendations for the transport of specimen to the laboratory are provided in chapter 3.

Suggestions for the accessioning of specimens are listed in Table 1; these suggestions are intended to ensure accurate recordkeeping and reporting of pertinent information.

Table 2 lists recommended primary media. We have listed these media generically where possible, but the reader should be aware of many modifications, variations, and substitutions in the formulation of most bacteriological media. These recommendations address general isolation procedures. Additional procedures, germane to the identification to the genus and species levels, are provided in the chapters of this section that deal with specific groups of bacteria.

Table 3 contains recommendations for using the media listed in Table 2 during processing of commonly submitted clinical specimens.

TABLE 1. Accessioning and initial processing of laboratory specimens

1. Each specimen must be accompanied by a correct and corresponding requisition that contains the minimal required information.
2. Minimal information required: last name; first name; middle initial; medical record or hospital number; exact location of patient; specimen source; name of physician who ordered the test; examination requested; special instructions; therapy administered, especially antibiotics; clinical or working diagnosis listed on chart.
3. An accession number consistent with laboratory protocol must be assigned to each specimen.
4. Each specimen must be cultured on media selected to facilitate growth of bacteria of etiological significance.
5. A Gram-stained smear of a clinical specimen is important and useful for rapid diagnostic information, for ascertaining the quality and acceptability of certain specimens, and as a control of cultural results. Certain specimens should always be accompanied by slides for staining. Examples are wounds, discharges, and others when only swabs representing the specimen rather than aspirates or tissues are submitted. Smears of sputum, cerebrospinal fluid, or normally sterile body fluids other than blood should always be prepared in the laboratory with appropriate stains.
6. Permanent records of all laboratory observations must be kept.

TABLE 2. Primary culture media

Medium	Incubation atmosphere[a]	Type[b]	Inhibitor or indicator[c]	Purpose
Blood agar (5% defibrinated sheep blood in a nutrient agar base)	CO_2 or ANO_2	N		Growth of most medically significant bacteria; determination of hemolysis depends on source of erythrocytes; will not support growth of *Haemophilus* spp., *Neisseria gonorrhoeae, Calymmatobacterium granulomatis,* mycobacteria, leptospires, mycoplasmas, borreliae, treponemes, rickettsiae, chlamydiae, *Bordetella pertussis, Francisella tularensis,* and legionellae.
Enteric agars				Selective agars for *Enterobacteriaceae;* support growth of some other gram-negative rods (i.e., *Pseudomonas* and *Acinetobacter* spp.); inhibitory for most gram-positive bacteria; differentiate lactose (and sucrose in eosin-methylene blue agar)-fermenting and nonfermenting gram-negative rods.
MacConkey agar	O_2	S, D	Bile salts, crystal violet, lactose, neutral red	Formula available without crystal violet supports growth of staphylococci and enterococci.
Deoxycholate	O_2	S, D	DC, lactose, neutral red	
Eosin-methylene blue agar	O_2	S, D	Eosin Y, methylene blue, lactose, sucrose	
Selective agars for streptococci and staphylococci				
Phenylethyl alcohol	CO_2	S	Phenylethyl alcohol (2.5 mg/ml)	Isolation of streptococci and staphylococci; inhibition of most gram-negative bacteria.
Blood agar (Columbia base) + colistin + nalidixic acid	CO_2	S	Colistin (10 μg/ml), nalidixic acid (15 μg/ml)	Supports gram-positive bacteria and inhibits most gram-negative organisms.
Mannitol salt	O_2	S, D	NaCl, mannitol, phenol red	Isolation of staphylococci; most other bacteria inhibited.
Selective enterococcus agar	O_2	S, D	Oxgall, esculin, sodium azide	Selection of enterococci.
Selective agars for enteric pathogens				Isolation of *Salmonella* spp. and in some cases *Shigella* spp. At least two types should be used, preferably one of moderate selectivity (M) and one of high selectivity (H).
Bismuth sulfite agar (H)	O_2	S, D	Brilliant green, bismuth sulfite, ferrous sulfate	Isolation of *Salmonella typhi* and other *Salmonella* spp. Inhibits most other *Enterobacteriaceae,* including *Shigella* spp.
Brilliant green agar (H)	O_2	S, D	Brilliant green, lactose, sucrose, phenol red	Isolation of *Salmonella* spp.; inhibits most other *Enterobacteriaceae,* including *Shigella* spp.

(*Continued on next page*)

TABLE 2—*Continued*

Medium	Incubation atmosphere[a]	Type[b]	Inhibitor or indicator[c]	Purpose
Hektoen enteric agar (M)	O_2	S, D	Bile salts, FAC, STS, lactose, sucrose, salicin, bromthymol blue, fuchsin	Isolation of most *Enterobacteriaceae*, including *Shigella* spp. and other gram-negative bacilli; differentiation of lactose and sucrose fermenters and nonfermenters and H_2S producers and nonproducers.
Deoxycholate-citrate agar (M)	O_2	S, D	DC, SC, FC, lactose, neutral red	Isolation of *Salmonella* spp. and some *Shigella* spp.
Salmonella-shigella agar (M)	O_2	S, D	Bile salts, brilliant green, FC, SC, STS, lactose, neutral red	Isolation of *Salmonella* spp., some *Shigella* spp., and some other gram-negative bacilli; differentiation of lactose fermenters.
Xylose-lysine-deoxycholate agar (M)	O_2	S, D	DC, STS, FAC, L-lysine, xylose, lactose, sucrose, phenol red	Similar to Hektoen enteric agar.
Enteric enrichment broths				
GN broth	O_2	E	DC, citrate	Enrichment for *Salmonella* and *Shigella* spp.
Selenite F broth	O_2	E	Selenium salts	Enrichment for *Salmonella* spp.
Tetrathionate broth	O_2	E	Bile salts, STS	Enrichment for *Salmonella* spp.; some *Shigella* spp. may also grow.
Campylobacter agar	5% O_2, 10% CO_2	S	Amphotericin (2 µg/ml), cephalothin (15 µg/ml), trimethoprim (5 µg/ml), vancomycin (10 µg/ml), polymyxin B (2.5 U/ml)	Isolation of *Campylobacter* spp. Other media may be substituted. Consult appropriate chapter for choice.
Chocolate agar (enriched)	CO_2	N		Growth of bacteria that grow on blood agar and *Haemophilus* spp. and *Neisseria gonorrhoeae*.
Selective agars for pathogenic neisseriae				
Thayer-Martin agar (modified)	CO_2	S	Vancomycin (3.0 µg/ml), colistin (7.5 µg/ml), nystatin (12.5 U/ml), trimethoprim lactate (5 µg/ml)	Isolation of *Neisseria meningitidis*, *N. gonorrhoeae*, and *N. lactamica*; most other bacteria will not grow.
Martin-Lewis agar	CO_2	S	Vancomycin (4 µg/ml), colistin (7.5 µg/ml), anisomycin (20 µg/ml), trimethoprim lactate (5 µg/ml)	As for Thayer-Martin agar.
New York City agar	CO_2	S	Vancomycin (2 µg/ml), colistin (5.5 µg/ml), amphotericin B (1.2 µg/ml), trimethoprim lactate (3 µg/ml)	As for Thayer-Martin agar; also supports select mycoplasmas.
Anaerobic agars				
Anaerobic blood agar	ANO_2	N		Growth of all anaerobic bacteria; should contain yeast extract, vitamin K, and hemin.
Anaerobic kanamycin-vancomycin laked blood agar	ANO_2	S	Kanamycin (100 µg/ml), vancomycin (7.5 µg/ml), menadione (0.5 µg/ml)	Isolation of *Bacteroides* spp.

(*Continued on next page*)

TABLE 2—*Continued*

Medium	Incubation atmosphere[a]	Type[b]	Inhibitor or indicator[c]	Purpose
Bacteroides bile-esculin agar	ANO_2	D, S	Gentamicin (100 μg/ml), oxgall (20 μg/ml), esculin, FAC	Isolation of *Bacteroides fragilis* group
Chopped meat-glucose	O_2	E	Supplemented with 0.5 μg of menadione per ml	
Thioglycolate broth	O_2	E	Various enrichments available	
Enrichment broths such as brain heart infusion broth and tryptic digest broth	O_2	E	Inhibitors and indicators may be added	Support growth of most bacteria.
Legionella medium	CO_2	S	Vancomycin (2 μg/ml), colistin (3.75 μg/ml), anisomycin (10 μg/ml)	Selects legionellae. Other media may be substituted. Consult chapter 42 for selection.

[a] O_2, Aerobic incubation; CO_2, incubation with 3 to 10% CO_2; ANO_2, incubation under anaerobic conditions.
[b] N, Nutrient; D, differential; S, selective; E, enrichment.
[c] DC, Deoxycholate; FAC, ferric ammonium citrate; STS, sodium thiosulfate; SC, sodium citrate; FC, ferric citrate.

TABLE 3. Suggested plating media for bacteriology specimens[a]

Specimen	Direct smear	Routine media	Suggested additional media	Comments
Abscess or pus (closed wound)	+	BA, EA, CA, SAGP, AM, EB	As smear indicates.	Wash any granules and "emulsify" in saline.
Autopsy (blood, tissue)			Follow procedure for specimen type.	
Blood (peripheral)		Blood culture set (O_2 and ANO_2)		Smear when evidence of growth.
Body fluids (except blood, CSF, urine)		Centrifuge fluids for 15 min at 2,500 rpm except when grossly purulent. Stain and culture sediment.		
Bile	+	BA, EA, AM, EB	As smear indicates.	
Hematoma	+	Treat as abscess.	As smear indicates.	
Joint	+	BA, CA, EB	As smear indicates.	
Pericardial, peritoneal	+	BA, EA, CA, AM, EB, SAGP		
Pleural empyema	+	BA, EA, CA, AM, EB, SAGP		
Bone marrow		EB, BA, CA, AM		
Catheters				
Central venous pressure lines, umbilical or intravenous catheters		BA, EB		Roll segment back and forth across agar with sterile forceps four times; may also be immersed in EB.
Foley		Do not culture.		

(*Continued on next page*)

TABLE 3—*Continued*

Specimen	Direct smear	Routine media	Suggested additional media	Comments
Central nervous system				
Brain tissue	+	Treat as abscess.		
CSF, shunt, meningomyelocele, ventricular fluid	+	Centrifuge for 15 min at 2,500 rpm, smear, and culture sediment. BA, CA, EB, AM	As smear indicates.	*Haemophilus influenzae* may not sediment at 2,500 rpm and may require 10,000 × *g* for 10 min. Alternatively, culture entire specimen.
Ear				
Internal	+	BA, CA, EA, EB, SAGP	As smear indicates.	
External	+	BA, EA, CA, SAGP	As smear indicates.	
Eye				
Conjunctiva	+	BA, CA	As smear indicates.	
Other	+	BA, EB, CA	As smear indicates.	
Genital tract (female)				
Amniotic fluid	+	BA, EA, CA, AM, SAGP	As smear indicates.	Should be collected without contamination by normal flora.
Cervix	+	BA or SAGP, SNA	As smear indicates.	*Gardnerella* and *Mobiluncus* spp.
Cul de sac	+	BA, EA, SNA, AM, EB, SAGP	As smear indicates.	
Urethra	+/−	SNA		
Uterine material (endometrium, products of conception, fetus, placenta, lochia, fallopian tubes, ovaries)	+	BA, EA, SNA, AM, EB, SAGP	As smear indicates.	Anaerobic culture is done on material collected without vaginal contamination.
Vagina (except cuff)	+/−	BA, SAGP, SNA	As smear indicates.	Vaginal cuff infections are treated as abscess or pus.
Vulva (Bartholin abscess)	+	BA, EA, SNA, AM, EB, SAGP	As smear indicates.	
Genital tract (male)				
Prostatic fluid	+	BA, EA, SNA, EB, SAGP		
Testes and epididymis (aspirate)	+	BA, EA, SNA		
Urethra	+	SNA, BA, CA		
Intestinal tract (colostomy, ileostomy, feces, rectal swab)		EA, ESA (2 types), EEB, CAMP		Special media may be required for isolation of *Vibrio* and *Yersinia* spp. If gonorrhoea is suspected, culture swab on SNA.

(*Continued on next page*)

TABLE 3—*Continued*

Specimen	Direct smear	Routine media	Suggested additional media	Comments
Plastic prostheses	–	EB, BA for catheters		
Pus (closed wound)		See abscess or pus		
Respiratory tract				
Bronchial secretions lavage	+	BA, EA, CA	As smear indicates.	If indicated, use legionella medium.
Epiglottis	–	BA, CA, EB		
Nasal sinus	+	BA, EA, CA, EB, AM		
Nasopharynx	–	BA, CA		
Nose	–	BA, SAGP		
Oral cavity	+			Culture for yeast.
Pleural fluid		See body fluids		
Sputum	+	BA, EA, CA	As smear indicates.	
Throat or pharynx	–	BA		Routine culture for group A streptococci only. Special media required for isolation of *Corynebacterium diphtheriae*, *Neisseria gonorrhoeae*, and *Bordetella pertussis*.
Tracheal aspirate	+	BA, EA, CA, SAGP	As smear indicates.	If indicated, use legionella medium.
Skin				
Deep wound (open)	+	BA, CA, EA, AM, EB, SAGP	As smear indicates.	
Superficial wound	+	BA, EA, SAGP	As smear indicates.	
Traumatized areas (burns, bites, decubitus ulcers)	+	BA, EA, EB, SAGP, AM	As smear indicates. Swab specimens of decubitus ulcers must not be examined; for this site, a biopsy specimen should be submitted.	
Tissue (surgical or biopsy)	+	Macerate aseptically; BA, EA, AM, SAGP	As smear or clinical impression indicates.	
Urine				
Clean voided, catheterized	+/–	BA, EA		
Suprapubic bladder tap, cystoscopy, or urostomy	+	BA, EA, AM		

[a] Abbreviations not given in Table 2, footnote *a*: CSF, cerebrospinal fluid; BA, blood agar; EA, enteric agars; CA, chocolate agar; SAGP, selective agars for streptococci and staphylococci; AM, anaerobic agars; EB, enrichment broths; SNA, selective agars for pathogenic neisseriae; ESA, selective agars for enteric pathogens; EEB, enteric enrichment broths; CAMP, campylobacter agar.

Chapter 28

Staphylococcus

W. E. KLOOS AND D. W. LAMBE, JR.

DESCRIPTION OF THE GENUS

Members of the genus *Staphylococcus* are gram-positive cocci (0.5 to 1.5 μm in diameter) that occur singly and in pairs, tetrads, short chains (three or four cells), and irregular "grape-like" clusters. Ogston (85) introduced the name "staphylococcus" (from *staphylé*, a bunch of grapes) for the group of micrococci causing inflammation and suppuration. Rosenbach (100) used the term in a taxonomic sense and provided the first description of the genus *Staphylococcus*. Staphylococci are nonmotile, nonsporeforming, and usually catalase positive, and they are usually unencapsulated or have limited capsule formation. Most species are facultative anaerobes. Except for *S. saccharolyticus* and *S. aureus* subsp. *anaerobius*, their growth is more rapid and abundant under aerobic conditions. These exceptional organisms are also catalase negative. Some uncommon strains of *S. aureus* may require the presence of CO_2 or other metabolites (hemin, menadione, etc.) for growth. Rare cell wall-deficient forms require a hypertonic environment.

The cell wall contains peptidoglycan and teichoic acid (102). The diamino acid present in the peptidoglycan is L-lysine. The interpeptide bridge of the peptidoglycan consists of oligoglycine peptides (susceptible to the action of lysostaphin). Depending on the species and relative amount of glycine present in the growth medium, some glycine residues may be substituted with L-serine or L-alanine. Cell wall teichoic acids of staphylococci may be poly(polyolphosphate), poly(glycerolphosphate-glycosylphosphate), or poly(glycosylphosphate), depending on the species. Glycerol or ribitol or both occur as typical components of poly(polyolphosphate) teichoic acids. Substituents of these teichoic acids may include *N*-acetylgalactosamine, glucose, and *N*-acetylglucosamine. Members of the gram-positive, catalase-positive genus *Micrococcus*, which have been confused in the past with staphylococci, have no glycine in the interpeptide bridge of the peptidoglycan and do not have teichoic acids. The respiratory chains of staphylococci and micrococci differ in cytochrome and menaquinone composition. Most staphylococci contain only *a*- and *b*-type cytochromes, whereas micrococci also have *c*- and *d*-type cytochromes. The exceptional species *S. caseolyticus*, *S. lentus*, and *S. sciuri* contain *a*-, *b*-, and two *c*-type cytochromes. Staphylococci contain unsaturated polyisoprenoid side chains in their menaquinones, whereas micrococci have hydrogenated menaquinones. In the clinical laboratory, staphylococci can be easily distinguished from micrococci on the basis of their resistance to bacitracin (0.04-U disk) and susceptibility to furazolidone (100-μg disk) (11). The main characteristics used for differentiating staphylococci from other gram-positive cocci encountered in the clinical laboratory are listed in Table 1.

The G+C content of DNA (63), DNA-DNA hybridization (63, 109), DNA-rRNA hybridization (53), comparative oligonucleotide cataloguing of 16S rRNA (76), and comparative immunology of catalases and fructose-1,6-biphosphate aldolases (101) have indicated that the genus *Staphylococcus* forms a coherent and well-defined natural group at the genetic and epigenetic levels. The genus *Staphylococcus* belongs to the broad *Bacillus-Lactobacillus-Streptococcus* cluster. The closest extant relatives of staphylococci appear to be *Planococcus*, *Bacillus*, *Enterococcus*, and *Brochothrix* species.

The genus *Staphylococcus* is currently composed of 27 species: *S. aureus* (100), *S. epidermidis*, *S. haemolyticus*, *S. saprophyticus*, *S. cohnii* and *S. xylosus* (107), *S. capitis*, *S. warneri*, *S. hominis*, and *S. simulans* (60), *S. caprae* and *S. gallinarum* (29), *S. saccharolyticus* (54), *S. lugdunensis* and *S. schleiferi* (35), *S. auricularis* (62), *S. kloosii*, *S. equorum*, and *S. arlettae* (105), *S. carnosus* (103), *S. intermedius* (42), *S. delphini* (113), *S. hyicus* (28), *S. chromogenes* (28, 43), *S. caseolyticus* (106), and *S. sciuri* and *S. lentus* (64, 104). Seven subspecies have been described, three of which have been given names. These subspecies are *S. aureus* subsp. *anaerobius* (25), *S. capitis* subsp. *ureolyticus* (T. L. Bannerman and W. E. Kloos, submitted for publication), *S. cohnii* subsp. *urealyticum* and *S. cohnii* subsp. 3 (67), and *S. haemolyticus* subsp. 2 and *S. warneri* subsp. 2 (65). *S. auricularis* subsp. 2 has been given only a brief mention (56). The named subspecies can be distinguished clearly on the basis of simple phenotypic characteristics. The remainder can be separated primarily on the basis of DNA divergence.

NATURAL HABITATS

Staphylococci are widespread in nature, though they are mainly found living on the skin, skin glands, and mucous membranes of mammals and birds. They are sometimes found in the mouth, blood, mammary glands, and intestinal, genitourinary, and upper respiratory tracts of these hosts.

Staphylococci found on humans include *S. aureus*, *S. epidermidis*, *S. capitis*, *S. capitis* subsp. *ureolyticus*, *S. saccharolyticus*, *S. warneri*, *S. haemolyticus*, *S. hominis*, *S. lugdunensis*, *S. schleiferi*, *S. auricularis*, *S. saprophyticus*, *S. cohnii*, *S. cohnii* subsp. *urealyticum*, *S. xylosus*, and *S. simulans* (35, 55, 56, 60, 62, 67). Other primates carry *S. aureus*, *S. capitis* subsp. *ureolyticus*, *S. warneri* subsp. 2, *S. haemolyticus* subsp. 2, *S. auricularis* subsp. 2, *S. saprophyticus*, *S. cohnii* subsp. *urealyticum*, *S. cohnii* subsp. 3, *S. xylosus*, and *S. simulans* (55, 65, 67). *S. aureus* is found on various other mammals and on some host species may be represented by different ecovars (82). *S. aureus* subsp. *anaerobius* has been isolated from sheep (25). *S. kloosii* has been found

TABLE 1. Differentiation of the genus *Staphylococcus* from some other gram-positive cocci[a]

Genus and exceptional species	Characteristic[b]																				
								Growth on:										Resistance to:			
	Mol% G+C of DNA	Strict aerobe	Facultative anaerobe or microaerophil	Strict anaerobe	Tetrad cell arrangement	Strong adherence on agar	Motility	5% NaCl agar	6.5% NaCl agar	12% NaCl agar	P agar in 18 h[c]	Catalase[d]	Benzidine test[e]	Modified oxidase test[f]	Anaerobic acid from glucose[g]	Aerobic acid from glycerol	Growth on Schleifer-Krämer agar[h]	Lysostaphin (200 μg/ml)	Erythromycin (0.04 μg/ml)	Bacitracin (0.04-U disk)[i]	Furazolidone (100-μg disk)[j]
Staphylococcus	30–39	–	d	–	d	–[k]	–	+	+	d	+	+	+	–	d	+	+	–	+	+	–
S. aureus subsp. *anaerobius*		–	±	±	–	–	–	+	+	d	–	–	–	–	+	+	ND	–	+	ND	–
S. saccharolyticus		–	±	±	+	–	–	+	+	±	–	–	±	–	+	+	ND	–	+	ND	–
S. hominis		±[l]	±	–	+	–	–	+	+	±	+	+	+	–	+	+	+	–	+	+	–
S. auricularis		–	+	–	+	–	–	+	+	±	–	+	+	–	+	+	ND	–	+	+	–
S. saprophyticus, S. cohnii, S. xylosus		d	d	–	–	–	–	+	+	±	+	+	+	–	–	+	+	–	+	+	–
S. kloosii, S. equorum, S. arlettae		±	±	–	–	–	–	+	+	±	d	+	+	–	–	+	+	–	+	+	–
S. intermedius		–	+	–	–	–	–	+	+	+	+	+	+	–	+	+	±	–	+	+	–
S. caseolyticus, S. sciuri, S. lentus		±	±	–	d	–	–	+	+	d	d	+	+	+	–	+	+	–	+	+	–
Enterococcus	34–42	–	+	–	–	–	d	+	+	(±)	±	–	–	–	+	d	(±)	+	+	+	–
Streptococcus	34–46	–	+	d	–	–	–	d	d	–	–	–	–	–	+	d	–	+	–	d	–
Aerococcus	35–40	–	+	–	+	–	–	+	+	+	–	–	–	–	(+)	ND	ND	+	ND	–	–
Planococcus	39–52	+	–	–	d	–	+	+	+	+	–	+	+	ND	–	–	ND	+	ND	ND	–
Stomatococcus	56–60	–	+	–	d	+	–	–	–	–	–	±	+	–	+	d	ND	+	ND	–	–
Micrococcus	66–75	+	–	–	+	–	–	+	+	d	–	+	+	+	–	–	–	+[m]	–[n]	–	+
M. kristinae		±	±	–	+	–	–	+	+	±	–	+	+	+	(+)	+	(±)	+	–	–	+
M. agilis		+	–	–	+	–	d	+	±	–	–	+	+	+	–	–	–	d	–	–	+

[a] The genera *Staphylococcus, Planococcus, Stomatococcus,* and *Micrococcus* are included in the family *Micrococcaceae* (Privot). The genera *Enterococcus, Streptococcus,* and *Aerococcus* are also included in the table, since they may be found together with staphylococci in clinical specimens and share certain properties with them. Exceptional species of these three genera have not been separated out for comparisons.

[b] Symbols (unless otherwise indicated): +, 90% or more species or strains positive; ±, 90% or more species or strains weakly positive; –, 90% or more species or strains negative; d, 11 to 89% of species or strains positive; ND, not determined; ( ), delayed reaction.

[c] Growth on P agar is under aerobic conditions and at 35 to 37°C. +, Detectable colony formation of at least 1 mm in diameter; ±, detectable colony formation of between 0.5 and 1 mm in diameter. Growth on sheep or bovine blood agar is slightly greater but less discriminating between staphylococci and other genera.

[d] Sometimes a weak catalase or pseudo-catalase reaction may be observed in certain strains of species designated as catalase negative (102). In some species, catalase activity may be activated by hemin supplementation.

[e] Detects the presence of cytochromes (24). Some strains of species that give negative results can synthesize cytochromes on aerobic media supplemented with hemin.

[f] Modified oxidase test of Faller and Schleifer (32) for the detection of cytochrome *c*.

[g] Standard oxidation-fermentation test (111).

[h] Growth on Schleifer-Krämer agar (KRAN agar supplemented with sodium azide, potassium thiocyanate, lithium chloride, and glycine) (108) is under aerobic conditions and at 35 to 37°C for 24 to 48 h. +, Number of CFU on the selective medium comparable to that on plate count agar and a colony size of 0.5-mm diameter; ±, significantly less CFU on the selective medium than on plate count agar; (±), colony diameter of pinpoint size to 0.5-mm diameter.

[i] +, Resistance and no zone of inhibition. *Micrococcus, Stomatococcus,* and *Aerococcus* species are susceptible and have an inhibition zone size of 10 to 25 mm in diameter (11, 31).

[j] +, Resistance and from no zone of inhibition to 9 mm. Susceptible species have an inhibition zone size of 15 to 35 mm (11).

[k] Some strains of *Staphylococcus epidermidis* adhere tenaciously to the surface of agar, and this property is correlated with heavy slime production.

[l] *S. hominis* does not demonstrate growth in the anaerobic portion of a thioglycolate medium (61) within 24 h and may produce only very poor growth in this portion after 3 to 5 days of incubation. However, it will grow and ferment glucose anaerobically (standard oxidation-fermentation test). Failure to grow anaerobically in thioglycolate may be due in part to inhibition by certain of the ingredients.

[m] Some strains of *Micrococcus luteus, M. roseus, M. agilis,* and *M. sedentarius* demonstrate susceptibility to lysostaphin, presumably because of contaminating levels of endo-β-*N*-acetylglucosaminidase activity.

[n] A few *Micrococcus* strains demonstrate high-level (MIC, ≥50 μg/ml) erythromycin resistance.

on a variety of mammals, including marsupials, rodents, carnivora, and pigs (105). *S. arlettae* has been isolated from poultry and goats (105), *S. equorum* has been isolated from horses (105), and *S. gallinarum* has been isolated from poultry (29). *S. carnosus* is being used as a starter culture in the processing of fermented meats, such as sausage and salami (103). The natural habitat of this species has not been adequately determined, although it is probably of animal origin. *S. intermedius* is found frequently on carnivora and has been isolated also from certain other mammals and birds (42, 55). *S. delphini* was isolated from dolphins (113). *S. hyicus* is found frequently on pigs, whereas *S. chromogenes* is found predominantly on cattle (28, 43). *S. caprae* has been isolated from goats (29), and *S. lentus* has been isolated from goats and sheep (64) and occasionally from other farm animals (26). *S. sciuri* is found on rodents and certain other mammals (64). *S. caseolyticus* has been isolated from milk and dairy products (106).

Some *Staphylococcus* species demonstrate habitat or niche preferences on their particular hosts. For example, *S. capitis* is found as large populations on the adult human head, especially the scalp and forehead, where sebaceous glands are numerous and well developed. *S. auricularis* has a strong preference for the external auditory meatus. *S. hominis* and *S. haemolyticus* generally produce larger populations in areas of the skin where apocrine glands are numerous, such as the axillae and pubic areas. *S. aureus* prefers the anterior nares as a habitat, especially in the adult human.

Certain *Staphylococcus* species are found frequently as etiologic agents of a variety of human and animal infections. In this chapter, we will be concerned primarily with the identification of *S. aureus, S. epidermidis, S. haemolyticus, S. lugdunensis,* and *S. saprophyticus,* species most commonly associated with human infections, and *S. intermedius* and *S. hyicus,* species of special veterinary interest. *S. schleiferi* has been considered to be a significant pathogen in some European countries but has been rarely isolated from infections in the United States.

CLINICAL SIGNIFICANCE

Skin infections caused by the coagulase-positive species *S. aureus* are the most common human staphylococcal infections. These include folliculitis, furuncles, carbuncles, cellulitis, impetigo, scalded skin syndrome, and postoperative wound infections of various sites. A common community-acquired disorder is food poisoning caused by thermostable enterotoxins elaborated in foods during growth of *S. aureus.* Serious processes such as bacteremia, endocarditis, meningitis, pneumonia, pyoarthrosis, and osteomyelitis continue to be seen as both community- and hospital-acquired infections.

In the late 1950s and early 1960s *S. aureus* caused considerable morbidity and mortality as a nosocomial pathogen of hospitalized patients. The advent and use of penicillinase-resistant, semisynthetic penicillins in the intervening years have provided successful therapy of serious *S. aureus* infections. However, methicillin-resistant *S. aureus* strains (MRSA) have emerged in the 1980s as a major clinical and epidemiological problem in hospitals. Although MRSA have most often been isolated from extremely ill patients in large, tertiary care hospitals, they have also been seen in patients in smaller community hospitals and rehabilitation facilities (2). The majority of these strains are resistant to several of the most commonly used antimicrobial agents, including macrolides, aminoglycosides, and β-lactam antibiotics. Serious infections caused by MRSA have most often been successfully treated with an older antibiotic, vancomycin.

A community-acquired disease of potentially serious consequence, toxic shock syndrome, also has been attributed to infection or colonization with *S. aureus* (110). Most of the patients with toxic shock syndrome have been young, menstruating females who use certain types of highly absorbent tampons during menses (86). However, the toxic shock syndrome toxin 1 (TSST-1) associated with the syndrome may also be elaborated by *S. aureus* present at sites other than the genital area in nonmenstruating women and in men. Although coagulase-negative staphylococci (CNS) that produce TSST-1 or a staphylococcal enterotoxin or both have been reported (20), other studies have found no TSST-1 or enterotoxin in CNS (33, 90). New methods for recognizing TSST-1 production include radioimmunoassay, enzyme-linked immunosorbent assay (ELISA), and reversed passive latex agglutination (RPLA) kits. Toxic shock toxin ELISA reagents are marketed by Toxin Technology, Inc., Madison, Wis., and an RPLA diagnostic kit (TST-RPLA) has been made commercially available by Oxoid, U.S.A., Columbia, Md. An evaluation of the TST-RPLA kit suggesting that it is reliable has been published (114). Strains of *S. aureus* positive by gel diffusion were also positive by RPLA, and nonspecific reactions were not observed. Both of these companies also offer kits for the identification of staphylococcal enterotoxins.

Since the CNS constitute a major component of our normal microflora, especially of the skin, these organisms formerly were considered to be saprophytes or of low pathogenicity for humans. However, several species of CNS are now documented as opportunistic human pathogens. There are currently 13 CNS species recognized from humans (see the foregoing discussion of natural habitats). Previously, some of these species were included in the species *S. epidermidis* and *S. albus* or as micrococci. In the last decade there has been a marked increase in documented infections caused by the CNS (33, 34, 88, 93, 97), especially with the use of invasive medical procedures and indwelling foreign bodies. A need exists for accurate identification of these bacteria in the clinical microbiology laboratory so that we can be precise in delineating the clinical diseases produced by the CNS (see qualifying statements below and in the section on identification). Clinicians and microbiologists must work together to define the clinical syndromes and determine the etiologic agent.

Of all of the species of CNS, *S. epidermidis* appears to have the greatest pathogenic potential and diversity. It is the major agent of nosocomial sepsis in oncological and neonatal services (12, 115). *S. epidermidis* has been isolated from 74 to 92% (79, 96) of hospital-acquired CNS bacteremias. Cardiac infections caused by *S. epidermidis* have occurred after procedures such as cardiac valve surgery, cardiovascular surgery, and cardiotomy (8, 68). These infections include mediastinitis (13), permanent pacemaker infections (16), infections of vascular grafts (75), endocarditis associated with prosthetic heart valves (99), and mitral valve prolapse (10). *S. epidermidis* is the primary pathogen in infections associated with cerebrospinal fluid shunt recipients, and with these patients bacteremia is frequently present (37). *S. epidermidis* is responsible for approximately 40% of all prosthetic joint infections (14). It is the most common isolate from infections of a variety of orthopedic devices (18) and has been associated with joint infections in which there were no predisposing factors (84). It rarely causes human osteomyelitis, but it has been reported from a few cases (87). *S. epidermidis* is the primary agent in peritonitis during continuous ambulatory peritoneal dialysis (69) and is a common isolate from urinary tract infections such as cystitis, urethritis, and pyelonephritis (33, 73).

Strains of CNS isolated from blood cultures in hospitalized patients show resistance of up to 56% to methicillin (79). Nosocomial methicillin-resistant *S. epidermidis* strains (MRSE) are a clinical problem, especially in patients with prosthetic heart valves (51) or those who have undergone other forms of cardiac surgery (8). Resistance to methicillin is heterogeneic and may extend to the cephalosporin antibiotics. Difficulties in performing in vitro tests that adequately recognize cephalosporin resistance of these strains continue to be a problem (112). Serious infections due to MRSE have been successfully treated with combination therapy that includes vancomycin plus rifampin or an aminoglycoside (51).

S. haemolyticus is the second most frequently encountered species of CNS in clinical infections and has been implicated in native valve endocarditis (G. M. Caputo et al., Program Abstr. 45th Intersci. Conf. Antimicrob. Agents Chemother., abstr. no. 898, 1985), septicemia, peritonitis, urinary tract infections, and wounds (34, 39, 73, 79, 96).

Two newly described species of CNS, *S. lugdunensis* and *S. schleiferi* (33, 35), appear to be significant opportunistic pathogens. They have been shown to colonize implanted materials such as catheters and drains. Both species are quite uncommon on normal human skin and when found are usually present in very small populations. They also may be found in hospitals. *S. lugdunensis* has been implicated in serious infections such as natural and prosthetic valve endocarditis, septicemia with shock, brain abscess, deep tissue infections, osteitis, chronic osteoarthritis, vascular prosthesis infections, wound and skin infections, soft tissue infections, peritoneal fluid infections, and infections from use of catheters (30, 33, 71a; T. E. Herchline and L. Ayers, Abstr. Annu. Meet. Am. Soc. Microbiol. 1989, C154, p. 419). Many of these patients had predisposing factors to infection, such as diabetes mellitus, surgery or trauma, renal failure, cancer, AIDS, eczema or psoriasis, or multiple underlying diseases. Approximately one-third of the isolates from these infections were considered to be pure cultures. The sources of infection in patients with diabetes mellitus include peritoneal fluid, finger, foot, and abdominal cellulitis, neck and pubic furuncles, foot bone, and gangrenous toes.

S. schleiferi occurs less frequently than *S. lugdunensis* in the hospital environment and in human infections. The organism has been isolated from brain empyema, wound infections, bacteremia with rachis osteitis, and a cranial drain and jugular catheter (33, 35).

S. saprophyticus has been clearly identified as one of the most common causes of urinary tract infections in young, sexually active females; it may be the second most common cause of such infections in this group. Some investigators propose that *S. saprophyticus* is an agent of nongonococcal urethritis in males or causes other sexually transmitted diseases (47) and prostatitis (3). *S. saprophyticus* has been isolated from wound infections and septicemia (34, 78).

Other staphylococcal species such as *S. hominis*, *S. warneri*, *S. simulans*, *S. cohnii*, *S. saccharolyticus*, *S. capitis*, and *S. xylosus* occur in low incidence in a variety of human infections (10, 34, 39, 73, 77–79, 93). In most cases, the presence of these species in clinical specimens requires considerable supporting evidence before causality can be established. *S. warneri* has been reported as the causative agent of vertebral osteomyelitis (52), and it has been associated with urinary tract infections in males and females (73).

The coagulase-positive species *S. intermedius* and the coagulase-variable species *S. hyicus* are of particular importance in veterinary medicine. These species and *S. aureus* are serious opportunistic pathogens of animals. *S. intermedius* has been implicated in a variety of canine infections such as otitis externa, pyoderma, abscesses, reproductive tract infections, mastitis, and wound infections (27, 95, 98). *S. hyicus* has been implicated in infectious exudative epidermitis and septic polyarthritis of pigs and is occasionally isolated from the milk of cows suffering from mastitis (27, 94, 95). *S. chromogenes* is commonly isolated from the milk of cows suffering from mastitis, although its role as an etiologic agent is questionable. *S. aureus* subsp. *anaerobius* is the etiologic agent of an abscess disease in sheep, an ailment symptomatically similar to caseous lymphadenitis (25).

Subcutaneous abscess formation in mouse models is useful for estimating the pathogenicity of microorganisms and the efficacy of treatment with various antibiotics (17, 72, 80). Compared with some other CNS species, *S. epidermidis*, *S. lugdunensis*, and *S. schleiferi* are the most pathogenic in a mouse model (71a). All three species cause a high percentage of abscess formation, and they can be recovered in culture from the implanted foreign body and from the abscess. The mouse subcutaneous abscess is characterized by infiltration of polymorphonuclear leukocytes and shares features with CNS abscesses and certain other infections in humans. CNS can induce abscess formation in the mouse in the absence of a foreign body, although it enhances the incidence of subcutaneous abscesses (72, 80). Similarly, a foreign body increases the likelihood of CNS infection in humans. In the mouse model, *S. epidermidis* grows on the surface of the foreign body in microcolonies composed of cocci and bacterial glycocalyx (72). The extracellular slime and organisms cover the surface of the foreign body as a bacterial biofilm. On polyethylene catheters immersed in sodium chloride containing *S. epidermidis*, a similar growth of a bacterial biofilm occurs in which *S. epidermidis* attaches preferentially to surface defects on the catheter surface (74). Catheters obtained from patients with *S. epidermidis* septicemia reveal a similar morphological picture, with biofilms up to 160 μm thick (92). Several other animal models have also indicated a pathogenic potential for *S. epidermidis* (1, 9, 49) and *S. saprophyticus* (46).

COLLECTION, TRANSPORT, AND STORAGE OF SPECIMENS

The general principles of collection, transport, and storage of specimens (chapter 3) are applicable to staphylococci. No special methods or precautions are usually required because staphylococci are easily obtained from clinical material of most infection sites and are relatively resistant to drying and to moderate temperature changes. Special hypertonic media may be required for the transport and growth of cell wall-deficient forms encountered under certain circumstances (50). Some strains may require anaerobic conditions or CO_2 supplementation for satisfactory growth, but these strains survive transport and limited storage in air.

DIRECT EXAMINATION

The direct microscopic examination of normally sterile fluids such as cerebrospinal fluid, joint aspirates, or pulmonary secretions collected by transtracheal aspiration can be of great value (58). Direct examination of certain nonsterile fluids may also be very useful if the microscopist carefully evaluates the specimen by noting the presence of inflammatory cells versus epithelial cells. Even if large numbers of gram-positive cocci are present, only a presumptive report of "gram-positive cocci resembling staphylococci" should be made. This report must be confirmed by culture and appropriate identification techniques. It must also be emphasized that microscopy by itself cannot adequately differentiate various species of staphylococci from one another or from micrococci, planococci, some streptococci, aerococci, or various anaerobic cocci.

CULTURE AND ISOLATION

The basic procedures for culture and isolation described in chapter 3 should be followed. Regardless of the source of the specimen, blood agar (preferably sheep blood agar) and a liquid medium such as thioglycolate broth should be inoculated. On blood agar, abundant growth of most staphylococcal species occurs within 18 to 24 h. By this time, colonies will be 1 to 3 mm in diameter, and they are usually circular, smooth, and raised, with a butyrous consistency. Only individual colonies should be picked for preliminary identification testing at this time (e.g., from acute infections). Since most species cannot be distinguished from one another on the basis of colony morphology within a 24-h incubation period, colonies should be allowed to grow for at least an additional 2 days before the primary isolation plate is confirmed for species or strain composition (60). This growth period is particularly important if it is necessary to sample more than one colony to obtain sufficient inocula and for determining the predominant organism or a pure culture. Failure to hold plates for 72 h can result in (i) selection of more than one species or strain if two or more colonies are sampled to produce an inoculum, (ii) selection of an organism(s) not producing the infection if the specimen contains two or more different species or strains, and (iii) incorrect labeling of a mixed culture as a pure culture. Colonies should be Gram stained, subcultured, and tested for genus, species, and, when applicable, strain properties. Most staphylococci of major medical interest produce growth in the upper as well as the lower anaerobic portions of thioglycolate broth or semisolid agar (61).

Specimens from heavily contaminated sources such as feces should be streaked also onto a selective medium: Schleifer-Krämer agar (108), mannitol-salt agar, Columbia CNA agar, lipase-salt-mannitol agar (Remel, Lenexa, Kans.), or phenylethyl alcohol agar (see chapter 121). These media inhibit the growth of gram-negative organisms but allow staphylococci and certain other gram-positive cocci to grow. On selective media, incubation should be extended to at least 48 to 72 h for discernible colony development.

IDENTIFICATION

Staphylococcus species can be identified on the basis of colony morphology, coagulase production, oxygen requirements, hemolysins, resistance to certain antibiotics, various enzyme activities, and aerobic acid production from certain carbohydrates (Table 2). Most clinically significant species can be identified on the basis of several key characteristics (Table 3).

Correct identification of the coagulase-positive species as etiologic agents or indicators of potential health risk is of prime importance in both human and veterinary clinical laboratories. Of the CNS, *S. epidermidis* and *S. saprophyticus* are the best-documented opportunistic pathogens, although evidence is accumulating that *S. haemolyticus*, *S. lugdunensis*, and *S. schleiferi* are clinically significant species. Until the clinical significance of other species can be clearly established, some laboratories may choose to restrict complete species identification to isolates from normally sterile sites such as blood, joint, or cerebrospinal fluid and to distinguish routinely (i) *S. saprophyticus* from other CNS isolated from urine, (ii) *S. epidermidis*, *S. lugdunensis*, and *S. schleiferi* isolated from colonized shunts, catheters, or prosthetic devices, and (iii) *S. epidermidis*, *S. lugdunensis*, and *S. haemolyticus* isolated from soft tissue infections or endocarditis. These species may be considered suspect if a particular strain has been isolated as the predominant organism or in pure culture. Multiple isolations of a large population of a strain (e.g., from blood or urine) strengthens the case for identifying it as an etiologic agent. These criteria apply also to other staphylococcal species found infrequently in infections.

Colonial appearance

On nonselective blood agar, nutrient agar, tryptic soy agar, brain heart infusion agar, or P agar (60, 107), isolated colonies of most staphylococci are 1 to 3 mm in diameter within 24 h and 3 to 10 mm in diameter by 5 days of incubation in air at 34 to 37°C, depending on the species. The exceptional species *S. aureus* subsp. *anaerobius*, *S. saccharolyticus*, *S. auricularis*, *S. equorum*, and *S. lentus* grow more slowly than other staphylococci and usually require 24 to 36 h for detectable colony development. Colony morphology can be a useful supplementary characteristic in the identification of species. Descriptions should be made for isolated colonies that have developed for several days at 34 to 35°C, followed by 2 days of growth at room temperature.

Colonies of *S. aureus* are usually large (6 to 8 mm in diameter), smooth, entire, slightly raised, and translucent. On P agar, they become nearly transparent by 3 to 5 days of incubation. The colonies of most strains are pigmented, ranging from cream yellow to orange. Some unusual strains of *S. aureus* produce dwarf colonies. Rare strains with relatively large capsules produce colonies that are smaller and more convex than those of unencapsulated strains and have a glistening, wet appearance. Upon storage, these colonies become slimy and run down the surface of agar under normal gravitational force. On selective mannitol-salt agar, *S. aureus* and some other mannitol-positive species produce yellow colonies and a yellow color in the surrounding medium as a result of acidification of mannitol in the presence of phenol red indicator. On lipase-salt-mannitol agar, most strains of *S. aureus* produce a yellow (acid) zone as a result of the acidification of mannitol and, in addition, produce an opaque zone around the colony as a result of the presence of lipovitellin-lipase activity. *S. epidermidis* colonies are relatively small and 2.5 to 6 mm in diameter. Pigment is not usually detected. Rare strains may produce colonies that are yellowish, brownish, or violet, the pigment being more intense in the center of the colony. With increasing age, elevated temperatures (above 35°C), or crowding, most colonies develop translucent to transparent dark centers and become more sticky in consistency. Some of the slime-producing strains are extremely sticky and adhere to the agar surface. Colonies of *S. haemolyticus* are usually larger than those of *S. epidermidis* and other related species and are 5 to 9 mm in diameter. They are smooth, butyrous, and opaque like those of the related species *S. hominis*, though much larger. Approximately one-half of the strains are pigmented, ranging from cream to yellow. Colonies of *S. lugdunensis* are usually 4 to 7 mm in diameter and cream to yellow-orange in color. Some strains are unpigmented. Colonies are smooth and glossy. The edge is entire and rather flat, while the center is slightly domed or acuminated. They are sometimes confused with colonies of *S. warneri*. *S. schleiferi* colonies are usually 3 to 5 mm in diameter and unpigmented. They are smooth and glossy and are slightly convex with entire edges. Colonies of *S. saprophyticus* are large (5 to 8 mm in diameter), entire, very glossy, opaque, smooth, butyrous, and more convex than the colonies of the aforementioned species. Approximately one-half of the strains are pigmented, ranging from cream to yellow-orange. Colonies of *S. intermedius* and *S. hyicus* are relatively large and usually 5 to 8 mm in diameter. They are slightly convex, entire, smooth, glossy, and usually unpigmented. Colonies of *S. intermedius* are translucent. Those of *S. hyicus* are more opaque, becoming translucent with prolonged incubation. On P agar, some strains of *S. intermedius* produce a faint violet pigment. On crystal violet agar, growth occurs as white colonies of the positive type E rather than as yellow or violet colonies typical for *S. aureus* of positive type A/B or C/D.

Coagulase production

The ability to clot plasma continues to be the most widely used and generally accepted criterion for the identification of pathogenic staphylococci associated with acute infections, i.e., *S. aureus* in humans and animals and *S. intermedius* and *S. hyicus* in animals (28, 42, 63). Two different coagulase tests can be performed: a tube test for free coagulase and a slide test for bound coagulase, or clumping factor (58). While the tube test is definitive, the slide test may be used as a rapid screening technique to identify *S. aureus*. The slide test may also be used to identify the new species *S. lugdunensis* and *S. schleiferi* (35) but not *S. intermedius* or *S. hyicus*. A variety of plasmas may be used for either test; however, dehydrated rabbit plasma containing citrate or EDTA is commercially available and most satisfactory for the identification of *S. aureus*, *S. intermedius*, and *S. hyicus*. Human plasma is somewhat more satisfactory for the identification of *S. lugdunensis* and *S. schleiferi*. Human plasma should not be used unless it has been carefully tested for clotting capability and for lack of inhibitors.

The tube coagulase test is best performed by mixing 0.1 ml of an overnight culture in brain heart infusion broth with 0.5 ml of reconstituted plasma, incubating the mixture at 37°C in a water bath or heat block for 4 h, and observing the tube for clot formation by slowly tilting the tube 90°. Alternatively, a large, well-isolated colony on a noninhibitory agar can be transferred into 0.5 ml of reconstituted plasma and incubated as described above. Any degree of clotting constitutes a positive test. However, a flocculent or fibrous precipitate is not a true clot and should be recorded as a negative result. Incubation of the test overnight has also been recommended for *S. aureus*, since a small number of strains may require longer than 4 h for clot formation. For veterinary clinical laboratories, it is important to note that some strains of *S. intermedius* and most coagulase-producing strains of *S. hyicus* require more than 4 h for a positive coagulase test. Clot formation by these species may require 12 to 24 h of incubation. If incubation exceeds 4 h, the following points must be considered: (i) staphylokinase produced by some strains may lyse the clot after prolonged incubation, yielding false-negative results; (ii) if the plasma used is not sterile (and some are not), either false-positive or false-negative results may occur; and (iii) an inoculum from an agar-grown colony may not be pure, and a contaminant may produce false results after prolonged incubation. In this regard, plasma containing EDTA is superior to citrated plasma because citrate-utilizing organisms (e.g., some streptococci) may produce clot formation by consuming the citrate. For those uncommon *S. aureus* strains requiring a longer clotting period, other characteristics (Table 3) should also be tested to confirm identity. Additional characteristics are required to identify rare coagulase-negative mutants and some encapsulated strains.

The slide coagulase test is performed by making a heavy uniform suspension of growth in distilled water, stirring the mixture to a homogeneous composition so as not to confuse clumping with autoagglutination, adding 1 drop of plasma, and observing for clumping within 10 s. The slide test is very rapid and more economical of plasma than the tube test. However, 10 to 15% of *S. aureus* strains may yield a negative result, which requires that the isolates be reexamined by the tube test. Slide tests must be read quickly because false-positive results may appear with reaction times longer than 10 s. In addition, colonies for testing must not be picked from media containing high concentrations of salt (e.g., mannitol-salt agar) because autoagglutination and false-positive results may occur. Some uncommon strains of *S. intermedius* may give a positive slide test result. Alternative methods for the slide test include

TABLE 2. Differentiation of *Staphylococcus* species

Species	Characteristic[a]																	
	Colony size (large)[b]	Colony pigment[c]	Anaerobic growth[d]	Aerobic growth[e]	Staphylocoagulase	Clumping factor[f]	Heat-stable nuclease	Hemolysins[g]	Catalase[h]	Oxidase[i]	Alkaline phosphatase	Arginine arylamidase	Pyrrolidonyl arylamidase[j]	Ornithine decarboxylase	Urease[j]	β-Glucosidase[j]	β-Glucuronidase[j]	β-Galactosidase[j]
S. aureus	+	+	+	+	+	+	+	+	+	−	+	−	−	−	d	+	−	−
S. aureus subsp. *anaerobius*	−	−	(+)	(±)	+	−	+	+	−	−	+	ND	ND	ND	ND	−	−	−
S. epidermidis	−	−	+	+	−	−	−	(d)	+	−	+[m]	−	−	(d)	+	(d)	−	−
S. capitis	−	−	(+)	+	−	−	−	(d)	+	−	−	−	−	−	−	−	−	−
S. capitis subsp. *ureolyticus*	−	(d)	(+)	+	−	−	−	(d)	+	−	−	−	(d)	−	+	−	−	−
S. caprae	d	−	(+)	+	−	−	−	(d)	+	−	(+)	−	d	−	+	−	−	−
S. saccharolyticus	−	−	+	(±)	−	−	−	−	−	−	d	−	ND	ND	ND	ND	ND	ND
S. warneri	d	d	+	+	−	−	−	(d)	+	−	−	−	−	−	+	+	d	−
S. haemolyticus	+	d	(+)	+	−	−	−	(+)	+	−	−	−	+	−	−	d	d	−
S. hominis	−	d	−	+	−	−	−	−	+	−	−	−	−	−	+	−	−	−
S. lugdunensis	d	d	+	+	−	(+)	−	(+)	+	−	−	−	+	+	d	+	−	−
S. schleiferi	−	−	+	+	−	+	+	(+)	+	−	+	−	+	−	−	−	−	(+)
S. auricularis	−	−	(±)	(+)	−	−	−	−	+	−	−	+	d	−	−	−	−	(d)
S. saprophyticus	+	d	(+)	+	−	−	−	−	+	−	−	−	−	−	+	d	−	+
S. cohnii	d	−	d	+	−	−	−	(d)	+	−	−	−	−	−	−	−	−	−
S. cohnii subsp. *urealyticum*	+	d	(+)	+	−	−	−	(d)	+	−	+	−	d	−	+	−	+	+
S. xylosus	+	d	d	+	−	−	−	−	+	−	d	−	d	−	+	+	+	+
S. kloosii	d	d	−	+	−	−	−	(d)	+	−	d	−	d	−	d	d	d	d
S. equorum	−	−	−	(+)	−	−	−	(d)	+	−	(+)	−	−	−	+	ND	+	d
S. arlettae	d	+	−	+	−	−	−	−	+	−	(+)	−	−	−	−	ND	+	d
S. gallinarum	+	d	(+)	+	−	−	−	(d)	+	−	(+)	−	−	−	+	+	d	d
S. simulans	+	−	+	+	−	−	−	(d)	+	−	(d)	−	+	−	+	−	d	+
S. carnosus	+	−	+	+	−	−	−	−	+	−	+	−	+	−	−	−	−	+
S. intermedius	+	−	(+)	+	+	d	+	d	+	−	+	−	+	−	+	d	−	+
S. delphini	+	−	(+)	+	+	−	−	+	+	−	+	ND	ND	ND	+	ND	ND	ND
S. hyicus	+	−	+	+	d	−	+	−	+	−	+	−	−	−	d	d	+	−
S. chromogenes	+	+	+	+	−	−	−	−	+	−	+	−	d	−	+	d	−	−
S. caseolyticus	−	d	(±)	+	−	−	ND	−	+	+	−	ND	+	−	−	−	−	−
S. sciuri	+	d	(+)	+	−	−	−	−	+	+	+	−	−	−	−	+	−	−
S. lentus	−	d	(±)	(+)	−	−	−	−	+	+	(±)	−	−	−	−	+	−	−

[a] Symbols (unless otherwise indicated): +, 90% or more strains positive; ±, 90% or more strains weakly positive; −, 90% or more strains negative; d, 11 to 89% of strains positive; ND, not determined; ( ), delayed reaction.

[b] Positive is defined as a colony diameter of ≥6 mm after incubation on P agar at 34 to 35°C for 3 days and at room temperature (ca. 25°C) for an additional 2 days (60).

[c] Positive is defined as the visual detection of carotenoid pigments (e.g., yellow, yellow-orange, or orange) during colony development at normal incubation or room temperatures. Pigments may be enhanced by the addition of milk, fat, glycerol monoacetate, or soaps to P agar.

[d] Anaerobic growth in a semisolid thioglycolate medium (61). Symbols: +, moderate or heavy growth down tube within 18 to 24 h; ±, heavier growth in the upper portion and weaker growth in the lower, anaerobic portion of tube; −, no visible growth within 48 h, but by 72 to 96 h very weak diffuse growth or a few scattered, small colonies may be observed in the lower portion of tube; ( ), delayed growth appearing within 24 to 72 h, sometimes noted as large discrete colonies in the lower portion of tube.

[e] On P agar or bovine, sheep, or human blood agar at 34 to 37°C. *S. equorum* grows slowly at 35 to 37°C; its optimum growth temperature is 30°C. The anaerobic species *S. saccharolyticus* and subspecies *S. aureus* subsp. *anaerobius* grow very slowly in the presence of air. Aerobic growth may be increased slightly by subculture in the presence of air. *S. aureus* subsp. *anaerobius* requires the addition of blood, serum, or egg yolk for growth on primary isolation medium. *S. auricularis* and *S. lentus* produce just detectable colonies on P agar or blood agar in 24 to 36 h, and these remain very small (1 to 2 mm in diameter).

commercial hemagglutination slide tests for clumping factor (BBL Microbiology Systems, Cockeysville, Md.; BioMerieux, Marcy l'Etiole, France) and commercial latex agglutination tests that detect both clumping factor and protein A (Scott Laboratories, Inc., Fiskeville, R.I.; I-M, Inc., Operating Unit of American Micro Scan, Lexington, Ky.; Carr-Scarborough Microbiologicals, Inc., Stone Mountain, Ga.; Wellcome Diagnostics, Dartford, England). Latex agglutination tests often have a higher specificity and sensitivity than the conventional slide

TABLE 2—*Continued*

	Characteristic[a]																	
							Acid (aerobically) from:											
	Arginine utilization[j]	Acetoin production	Nitrate reduction	Esculin hydrolysis	Novobiocin resistance[k]	Polymyxin B resistance[l]	D-Trehalose	D-Mannitol	D-Mannose	D-Turanose	D-Xylose	D-Cellobiose	L-Arabinose	Maltose	α-Lactose	Sucrose	*N*-Acetylglucosamine	Raffinose
S. aureus	+	+	+	−	−	+	+	+	+	+	−	−	−	+	+	+	+	−
S. aureus subsp. *anaerobius*	ND	−	−	−	−	ND	−	ND	−	ND	−	−	−	+	−	+	−	−
S. epidermidis	d	+	+	−	−	+	−	−	(+)	(d)	−	−	−	+	d	+	−	−
S. capitis	d	d	d	−	−	−	−	+	+	−	−	−	−	−	−	(+)	−	−
S. capitis subsp. *ureolyticus*	+	d	+	−	−	ND	−	+	+	−	−	−	−	+	(d)	+	−	−
S. caprae	+	+	+	−	−	−	(+)	d	+	−	−	−	−	(d)	+	−	−	−
S. saccharolyticus	+	ND	+	ND	−	ND	−	−	(+)	ND	−	−	−	−	−	−	ND	−
S. warneri	d	+	d	−	−	−	+	d	−	(d)	−	−	−	(+)	d	+	−	−
S. haemolyticus	+	+	+	−	−	−	+	d	−	(d)	−	−	−	+	d	+	+	−
S. hominis	d	d	d	−	−	−	d	−	−	+	−	−	−	+	d	(+)	d	−
S. lugdunensis	−	+	+	−	−	d	+	−	+	(d)	−	−	−	+	+	+	+	−
S. schleiferi	+	+	+	−	−	−	d	−	+	−	−	−	−	−	−	−	(+)	−
S. auricularis	d	−	(d)	−	−	−	(+)	−	−	(d)	−	−	−	(+)	−	d	−	−
S. saprophyticus	−	+	−	−	+	−	+	d	−	+	−	−	−	+	d	+	d	−
S. cohnii	−	d	−	−	+	−	+	d	(d)	−	−	−	−	(d)	−	−	−	−
S. cohnii subsp. *urealyticum*	−	d	−	−	+	−	+	+	+	−	−	−	−	(+)	+	−	d	−
S. xylosus	−	d	d	d	+	−	+	+	+	d	+	−	d	+	d	+	+	−
S. kloosii	−	d	−	d	+	−	+	+	−	−	(d)	−	d	d	(d)	(±)	−	−
S. equorum	−	−	+	d	+	ND	+	+	+	d	+	(d)	+	d	d	+	d	−
S. arlettae	−	−	−	−	+	ND	+	+	+	+	+	−	+	+	+	+	−	+
S. gallinarum	−	−	+	+	+	−	+	+	+	+	+	+	+	+	d	+	+	+
S. simulans	+	d	+	−	−	−	d	+	d	−	−	−	−	(±)	+	+	+	−
S. carnosus	+	+	+	−	−	−	d	+	+	−	−	−	−	−	d	−	ND	−
S. intermedius	d	−	+	−	−	−	+	(d)	+	d	−	−	−	(±)	d	+	+	−
S. delphini	+	−	+	ND	−	ND	−	(+)	+	ND	−	ND	−	+	+	+	ND	ND
S. hyicus	+	−	+	−	−	+	+	−	+	−	−	−	−	−	+	+	+	−
S. chromogenes	+	−	+	−	−	+	+	d	+	d	−	−	−	d	+	+	d	−
S. caseolyticus	d	−	+	ND	−	−	d	−	−	−	−	−	−	+	+	d	ND	ND
S. sciuri	−	−	+	+	+	−	+	+	(d)	(±)	(d)	+	d	(d)	(d)	+	d	−
S. lentus	−	−	+	+	+	−	+	+	(+)	(±)	(±)	+	d	d	d	+	d	+

[f] Detected in rabbit or human plasma (slide coagulase test). Human plasma is preferred for the detection of clumping factor with *S. lugdunensis* and *S. schleiferi*. Latex agglutination is somewhat less reliable for detection of clumping factor or fibrinogen affinity factor in *S. lugdunensis*.

[g] Hemolysis on bovine blood agar (58). Symbols: +, wide zone of hemolysis within 24 to 36 h; (+), delayed moderate to wide zone of hemolysis within 48 to 72 h; (d), no or delayed hemolysis; −, no or only very narrow zone (≤1 mm) of hemolysis within 72 h. Some of the strains designated negative may produce a slight greening or browning of blood agar.

[h] Catalase and cytochrome synthesis cannot be induced in *S. aureus* subsp. *anaerobius* by the addition of H_2O_2 or hemin to the culture medium. Catalase can be induced in *S. saccharolyticus* by hemin supplementation. In this species, cytochromes *a* and *b* are present in small quantities.

[i] Determined by the modified oxidase test of Faller and Schleifer (32) used to detect the presence of cytochrome *c*.

[j] Pyrrolidonyl arylamidase, urease, β-glucosidase, β-glucuronidase, β-galactosidase, and arginine utilization are characteristics that have been determined primarily by commercial rapid-identification test systems (e.g., API Staph-Ident, DMS Staph Trac, ATB 32 Staph, Baxter-MicroScan Pos Combo Type 5 panel and RAPID POS ID panel, Becton Dickinson Minitek Gram-Positive Set, and Vitek Systems Gram-Positive Identification Card).

[k] Positive is defined as an MIC of ≥1.6 μg/ml or a growth inhibition zone diameter of ≤16 mm with a 5-μg novobiocin disk.

[l] Positive is defined as a growth inhibition zone diameter of <10 mm with a 300-U polymyxin B disk.

[m] Alkaline phosphatase activity is negative for approximately 6 to 15% of strains of *S. epidermidis*, depending on the population sampled. A low but significant number of clinical isolates have been phosphatase negative.

test for the identification of *S. aureus*, though they are presently less reliable for the identification of *S. lugdunensis*. When the organism being tested is suspected of being *S. aureus*, negative slide tests should be confirmed by the tube coagulase test.

Heat-stable nuclease

A heat-stable staphylococcal nuclease (thermonuclease [TNase]) that has endo- and exonucleolytic properties and can cleave DNA or RNA is produced by

TABLE 3. Key tests for identification of the most clinically significant species

Species	Test[a]																			
													Acid (aerobically) from:							
	Colony pigment[b]	Staphylocoagulase	Clumping factor[b]	Heat-stable nuclease	Alkaline phosphatase	Pyrrolidonyl arylamidase[b]	Ornithine decarboxylase	Urease[b]	β-Galactosidase[b]	Acetoin production	Novobiocin resistance[b]	Polymyxin B resistance[b]	D-Trehalose	D-Mannitol	D-Mannose	D-Turanose	D-Xylose	D-Cellobiose	Maltose	Sucrose
S. aureus	+	+	+	+	+	−	−	d	−	+	−	+	+	+	+	+	−	−	+	+
S. epidermidis	−	−	−	−	+	−	(d)	+	−	+	−	+	−	−	(+)	(d)	−	−	+	+
S. haemolyticus	d	−	−	−	−	+	−	−	−	+	−	−	+	d	−	(d)	−	−	+	+
S. lugdunensis	d	−	(+)	−	−	+	+	d	−	+	−	d	+	−	+	(d)	−	−	+	+
S. schleiferi	−	−	+	+	+	+	−	−	(+)	+	−	−	d	−	+	−	−	−	−	−
S. saprophyticus	d	−	−	−	−	−	−	+	+	+	+	−	+	d	−	+	−	−	+	+
S. intermedius	−	+	d	+	+	+	−	+	+	−	−	−	+	(d)	+	d	−	−	(±)	+
S. hyicus	−	d	−	+	+	−	−	d	−	−	−	+	+	−	+	−	−	−	−	+

[a] Symbols: +, 90% or more strains positive; ±, 90% or more strains weakly positive; −, 90% or more strains negative; d, 11 to 89% of strains positive; ( ), delayed reaction.

[b] Descriptions are the same as for Table 2.

most strains of *S. aureus*, *S. schleiferi*, *S. intermedius*, and *S. hyicus*. Some strains of *S. epidermidis*, *S. simulans*, and *S. carnosus* demonstrate a weak TNase activity. TNase can be detected by using a metachromatic-agar diffusion procedure and DNA-toluidine blue agar (70) or buffered peptone-DNA agar (36). A seroinhibition test has been developed to distinguish *S. aureus* TNase from those of other species (71). A commercial TNase test with toluidine blue agar is available (Remel) and can be interpreted in 4 h.

Phosphatase activity

Phosphatase activity can be determined by using a modification of the technique of Pennock and Huddy (91), in which a 0.005 M solution of phenolphthalein diphosphate (sodium salt in 0.01 M citric acid-sodium citrate buffer, pH 5.8) is used as the substrate. Alternatively, 0.01 M disodium phenylphosphate or 0.005 M phenolphthalein monophosphate can be used, though a higher background or negative control color is observed with these substrates (61). Tubes containing 0.5 ml of this buffer should be inoculated with a loopful of an overnight culture to a density of approximately 10^9 CFU/ml. After incubation at 37°C for 4 h, the reaction is stopped by adding 0.5 ml of 0.5 N sodium hydroxide and 0.5 ml of 0.5 M sodium bicarbonate. Color is developed by adding 0.5 ml of 4-aminoantipyrine solution (0.6 g/100 ml) and 0.5 ml of potassium ferricyanide solution (2.4 g/100 ml). Phosphatase activity is indicated by the development of a deep red color. A newer, alternative method for determining phosphatase activity based on the hydrolysis of *p*-nitrophenylphosphate into P_i and *p*-nitrophenol by alkaline phosphatase has been incorporated into several of the commercial biochemical test systems for staphylococcal species identification. Phosphatase activity is indicated by the release of yellow *p*-nitrophenol from the colorless substrate.

Strains of *S. aureus*, *S. schleiferi*, *S. intermedius*, and *S. hyicus* and most strains of *S. epidermidis* are alkaline phosphatase positive. Approximately 10 to 15% of *S. epidermidis* strains isolated from clinical specimens are phosphatase negative. These can be distinguished from the related species *S. hominis*, which is also phosphatase negative, on the basis of their strong anaerobic growth in thioglycolate within 18 to 24 h or resistance to polymyxin B (300-U disk). *S. haemolyticus*, *S. lugdunensis*, and *S. saprophyticus* are phosphatase negative.

Pyrrolidonyl arylamidase activity

Pyrrolidonyl arylamidase (pyrrolidonase) activity can be determined by the hydrolysis of pyroglutamyl-β-naphthylamide (L-pyrrolidonyl-β-naphthylamide [PYR]) into L-pyrrolidone and β-naphthylamine, which combines with a PYR reagent (*p*-dimethylaminocinnamaldehyde) to produce a red color. A commercial kit containing PYR broth and PYR reagent (Carr-Scarborough) recommended for the identification of group A streptococci and enterococci is also useful for distinguishing certain staphylococcal species (45). A slight modification in the standard procedure is required. A loopful of a 24-h agar slant culture or several well-isolated colonies are dispersed in the PYR broth (containing 0.01% PYR) to a turbidity of a McFarland no. 2 standard. The suspension is incubated at 35°C for 2 h. After incubation, 2 drops of PYR reagent is added to each tube without mixing. The development of a dark purple-red color within 2 min is indicative of a positive activity. Yellow, orange, or pink color is considered a negative result. Alternatively, the basic features of the test have been incorporated into several of the commercial biochemical test panels for the identification of staphylococcal species. *S. haemolyticus, S. lugdunensis, S. schleiferi,* and *S. intermedius* are usually pyrrolidonase positive. *S. aureus, S. epidermidis, S. saprophyticus,* and *S. hyicus* are pyrrolidonase negative.

Ornithine decarboxylase activity

A positive ornithine decarboxylase activity can identify the species *S. lugdunensis* with considerable accuracy. To date, ornithine decarboxylase-negative strains of *S. lugdunensis* have not been reported. Some strains of *S. epidermidis* demonstrate a delayed activity; however, these strains are trehalose and pyrrolidonase negative and often phosphatase positive, opposite reactions from those of *S. lugdunensis.* Ornithine decarboxylase activity can be determined by a slight modification of the test described by Moeller (83). Decarboxylase basal medium (BBL; Difco Laboratories, Detroit, Mich.; GIBCO Laboratories, Grand Island, N.Y.) is prepared according to the instructions of the manufacturer, 1% (wt/vol) L-ornithine dihydrochloride is added, and the final medium is adjusted to pH 6 with 1 N sodium hydroxide before sterilization. The medium is dispensed in 3- to 4-ml amounts in small (13 by 100 mm) screw-cap tubes and autoclaved at 121°C for 10 min. A loopful of an overnight agar slant culture or several well-isolated colonies are dispersed in the test broth, followed by overlaying each tube with 4 to 5 mm of sterile mineral oil. Inoculated tubes should be incubated at 35 to 37°C for up to 24 h. They can be read initially as early as 8 h for the positive identification of most strains of *S. lugdunensis;* at this time, *S. epidermidis* will produce negative results. A positive reaction is indicated by alkalinization of the medium, with a change in the initial grayish color or slight yellowing (caused by the initial fermentation of glucose) to violet (caused by decarboxylation of L-ornithine). A yellow color at 24 h indicates a negative result. The basic features of this test have been incorporated into the ATB 32 Staph (API System, La Balme-les-Grottes, France) identification system.

Urease activity

A conventional urease test broth (Urea R broth; Difco) with a reduced buffer capacity can be used for detecting urease activity within 4 h in staphylococcal species. The test detects the release of ammonia from urea, resulting in an increase in pH which is shown by the phenol red indicator changing from yellow or orange to red or cerise. At present, comprehensive studies using this medium for the identification of staphylococcal species have not been reported. However, a miniaturization of this urease test has been incorporated into several of the commercial biochemical test systems for species identification of staphylococci and is represented by a large data base. *S. epidermidis, S. intermedius,* and most strains of *S. saprophyticus* are usually urease positive; *S. aureus, S. lugdunensis,* and *S. hyicus* are urease variable; and *S. haemolyticus* and *S. schleiferi* are urease negative.

β-Galactosidase activity

Detection of high levels of β-galactosidase activity for the differentiation of certain staphylococcal species can be accomplished by commercial biochemical test systems that use 2-naphthol-β-D-galactopyranoside as a substrate. Fast blue BB salt in 2-methoxyethanol is added to the test well after an appropriate incubation period to detect free β-naphthol released by β-galactosidase. A positive activity is indicated by a plum purple color. A negative test is indicated by an absence of color or yellow color. By this assay, *S. intermedius* and most strains of *S. saprophyticus* are β-galactosidase positive; *S. schleiferi* is delayed or weakly positive; and *S. aureus, S. epidermidis, S. haemolyticus, S. lugdunensis,* and *S. hyicus* are negative.

Acetoin production

Acetoin production from glucose or pyruvate is a useful alternative characteristic to distinguish *S. aureus* (positive) from another coagulase-positive species, *S. intermedius* (negative), and coagulase-positive strains of *S. hyicus* (negative) (28, 42). The rapid paper disk method of Davis and Hoyling (22) is recommended for this test. Cultures are inoculated as a patch or smear onto tryptone-yeast extract-glucose agar. After 48 h of incubation at 30°C, a 1-cm disk of Whatman 3M paper freshly soaked in 10% sodium pyruvate solution is placed on each growth patch, and the plates are reincubated for 3 h. Acetoin production is detected by spotting 1 drop each of 40% potassium hydroxide, 1% creatinine, and 1% α-naphthol (alcoholic) solution onto each disk and observing the development of a pink-red color within 1 h at room temperature. The accuracy of the disk test is comparable to that of conventional Voges-Proskauer tests requiring longer incubation. Alternatively, acetoin production can be determined by a miniaturized Voges-Proskauer test incorporated into several of the commercial biochemical test systems for staphylococcal species identification.

Novobiocin resistance

A simple disk diffusion test for estimating novobiocin susceptibility and distinguishing *S. saprophyticus* from other clinically important species can be performed by use of a 5-μg novobiocin disk on either P agar (61), Mueller-Hinton agar (4), or tryptic soy sheep blood agar (41). With an inoculum suspension equivalent in turbidity to a 0.5 McFarland opacity standard and incubation at 35 to 37°C for overnight to 24 h, novobiocin resistance is indicated by an inhibition zone diameter of ≤16 mm with any of these media. Rapid disk elution procedures using either manual or automated instrument interpretation have also been reported to predict reliably novobiocin resistance after only 4 to 5 h of incubation (5, 44). Novobiocin resistance is intrinsic to *S. saprophyticus* and several other species (Table 2), but it is uncommon in the other clinically important species.

Polymyxin B resistance

A simple disk diffusion test for estimating polymyxin B susceptibility to distinguish several of the clinically important species can be done by using a 300-U polymyxin B disk (45). The test can be performed on any of the media mentioned above for estimation of novobiocin resistance. However, the largest data base has been obtained with the use of tryptic soy sheep blood agar

(TSA II; BBL). Test conditions should be similar to those described above for novobiocin resistance. The 5-μg novobiocin disk and the 300-U polymyxin B disk can be tested on the same inoculated plate. Polymyxin B resistance is indicated by an inhibition zone diameter of <10 mm. *S. aureus, S. epidermidis, S. hyicus,* and *S. chromogenes* are usually resistant. Some strains of *S. lugdunensis* are also resistant. Other staphylococcal species are usually susceptible and demonstrate an inhibition zone diameter of 11 to 19 mm.

Acid production from carbohydrates

Acid production from carbohydrates can be easily detected by using an agar plate method (61). Carbohydrate agars are prepared by adding an appropriate amount of filter-sterilized carbohydrate stock solution to an autoclave-sterilized purple agar base medium (containing bromcresol purple indicator) to give a final carbohydrate concentration of 1%. Culture streaks to be tested are prepared by lightly inoculating a 0.5- to 1-cm-long streak on the surface of a partitioned quadrant agar plate containing the appropriate carbohydrate. Cultures are incubated at 34 to 37°C in air and examined at 24 and 72 h. Reactions are interpreted as follow: +, moderate to strong acid, yellow indicator color (pH ≤ 5.2) extends out from culture streak into the surrounding medium within 12 to 72 h; ±, weak acid, distinct yellow indicator color confined to under culture streak within 72 h; −, no acid, very faint or no yellow indicator color under the culture streak within 72 h. Carbohydrate reactions are also incorporated into several of the commercial biochemical test systems for staphylococcal species identification. These systems use a more acid-sensitive indicator than bromcresol purple described above; e.g., API Staph-Ident uses Cresol red, which turns yellow at pH 7.2, and Baxter-MicroScan Pos Combo Type 5 panel uses phenol red, which turns yellow at pH 6.8. For this and other reasons, results with conventional carbohydrate tests (Tables 2 and 3) may be slightly different from those obtained with rapid commercial biochemical test systems.

S. epidermidis can be distinguished from other novobiocin-susceptible species by its production of acid from maltose and sucrose and absence of acid production from trehalose and mannitol. Most strains of *S. epidermidis* produce acid from mannose slowly. Some rare strains of this species may produce acid from trehalose. These isolates can be distinguished from other species on the basis of phosphatase activity, anaerobic growth in thioglycolate, polymyxin B resistance, colony morphology, and absence of ornithine decarboxylase and pyrrolidonase activities. *S. lugdunensis* can be identified by its production of acid from trehalose, mannose, maltose, and sucrose and absence of acid production from mannitol. *S. schleiferi* produces acid from mannose and sometimes from trehalose but does not produce acid from mannitol, maltose, or sucrose. *S. saprophyticus* can be distinguished from other novobiocin-resistant species by its production of acid from sucrose and turanose and absence of acid production from mannose, xylose, cellobiose, arabinose, and raffinose. *S. intermedius* and *S. hyicus* can be distinguished from *S. aureus* by their weak and lack of acid production from maltose, respectively. Furthermore, *S. hyicus* does not produce acid from mannitol.

Identification of species by using commercial biochemical test systems

Some of the methods described in this chapter may not be suitable for routine use in certain clinical laboratories because a number of specialized media are required which must be prepared by the laboratory. Several manufacturers of commercial kit identification systems or automated instruments have released products that can identify a number of the *Staphylococcus* species with an accuracy of 70 to >90% with relative speed and simplicity (6, 21, 38, 48, 66). Since their introduction, systems have been improved and expanded to include more species. Their reliability will continue to increase as the result of a growing data base and development of more discriminating tests. *S. aureus, S. epidermidis, S. capitis, S. haemolyticus, S. saprophyticus, S. simulans,* and *S. intermedius* can be identified reliably by most of the commercial systems now available. For some systems, reliability depends on additional testing as suggested by the manufacturer or by published evaluations of the product (21, 38, 48, 66, 93). Additional testing might include determining coagulase, clumping factor, or ornithine decarboxylase activity, anaerobic growth in thioglycolate, or novobiocin resistance. If one or more of these key tests are not included in the particular manufacturer's product, identification could be uncertain with respect to some species. For example, in the API Staph-Ident system (Analytab Products, Plainview, N.Y.), phosphatase-negative *S. epidermidis* strains would be confused with *S. hominis* having an API profile of 2000 or 2040 (66). By determining the overnight anaerobic growth of such strains in a thioglycolate semisolid medium, one can then distinguish between these species (61). Identification systems now available include the following: API Staph-Ident and DMS Staph Trac (Analytab Products); Staph Trac and ATB 32 Staph (API System S.A.); MicroScan Pos Combo Type 5 panel and MicroScan RAPID POS ID panel, for use with the automated autoSCAN-W/A system (Baxter Healthcare Corp., MicroScan Division, West Sacramento, Calif.); Sceptor Staphylococcus MIC/ID panel (Becton Dickinson Diagnostic Instrument Systems, Towson, Md.); Minitek Gram-Positive Set (Becton Dickinson Microbiology Systems, Cockeysville, Md.); and Gram-Positive Identification Card for use with the automated Vitek system (Vitek Systems, Inc., Hazelwood, Mo.).

The kits marketed by Analytab Products, Baxter-MicroScan, and Becton Dickinson consist of strips or trays with microcupules or wells containing dehydrated substrates, biochemicals, and/or nutrient media which serve as a reaction vessel and support for tests. Depending on the system, 10 to 32 tests are included for identification of staphylococcal species. After inoculation, strips or trays are incubated for 5 to 24 h and then interpreted. Some tests require the addition of reagents before the interpretation of the results. Positive reactions are converted to profiles according to the instructions of the manufacturer and compared against a registry of profiles compiled from a data base.

The automated systems produced by Baxter-MicroScan and Vitek incubate inoculated trays or cards, respectively, read and interpret results, and with the aid of their programmed computer determine the identification of organisms. An identification report may be given after 2 h of incubation with the Baxter-MicroScan autoSCAN W/A system using the RAPID POS ID panels containing fluorogenic substrates or fluorometric indicators. The Vitek system using the Gram-Positive Identification Card can provide a preliminary identification report in as little as 4 h. The computer software for these systems converts results to profiles or biotype numbers that are compared against a data base and probability tables. These systems can perform rapid antibiotic susceptibility determinations, some in conjunction with species identification.

Methicillin-resistant staphylococci

For proper selection of antimicrobial agents for therapy and for hospital infection control, it is extremely important that methicillin-resistant staphylococci be quickly and accurately recognized. Methicillin resistance rates range from about 10 to 50% in hospitals throughout the United States, and rates are comparable in several other countries. Nosocomial methicillin-resistant staphylococci are usually resistant to several other antibiotics, such as erythromycin, clindamycin, tetracycline, chloramphenicol, and gentamicin, although the specific resistance pattern may vary among hospitals. These strains should also be considered resistant to all β-lactam antibiotics, regardless of in vitro susceptibility. The presence of the penicillin-binding protein 2a in MRSA, MRSE, and methicillin-resistant *S. haemolyticus* has been linked with therapeutic failure of β-lactam antibiotics of penicillin, cephalosporin, and penem classes, indicating cross-resistance to these antibiotics in vivo (15).

During the past several years, numerous reports have documented the technical difficulties of detecting MRSA and MRSE by conventional or instrument susceptibility test methods. These strains are mainly heteroresistant to β-lactam antibiotics in that two subpopulations (one susceptible and the other resistant) coexist within a culture. Each cell in the population may have the genetic information for resistance, but only a small fraction (usually 10^{-6} to 10^{-4}) can actually express the resistant phenotype under in vitro testing conditions. The resistant subpopulation usually grows much more slowly than the susceptible one and therefore may be missed when in vitro testing is performed. Successful detection of heteroresistant, methicillin-resistant staphylococci depends largely on promoting the growth of the more resistant subpopulation, which is favored by neutral pH (7.0 to 7.4), cooler temperatures (30 to 35°C), the presence of sodium chloride (NaCl, 2 to 4%), and, under certain conditions, prolonged incubation (up to 48 h) (19, 81). Reliable recognition of MRSA and MRSE can be made by using disk diffusion and broth microdilution susceptibility methods recommended by the National Committee for Clinical Laboratory Standards and described in chapter 115.

EPIDEMIOLOGICAL TYPING SYSTEMS

Because of the widespread occurrence of staphylococci in nature and medical facilities, it is sometimes desirable to identify specific strains, types, or groups of these organisms. The identification of strains of staphylococci may be important for a variety of reasons, such as in monitoring staphylococcal community structure of individual patients or facilities, in the course of determining an etiologic agent, and in tracing the source of infection. Strain identification is also necessary when one is monitoring the distribution of potential pathogens or antibiotic resistance reservoirs in a hospital or community. More attention is being given to strain identification as it is becoming clear that within opportunistic, pathogenic staphylococcal species there exists considerable strain variation with respect to virulence properties and antibiotic resistance, including the capacity to transfer or accept virulence or resistance genes. It follows that species identification alone provides only limited information when one is characterizing mixed populations of staphylococci from infections for which any one of the several species present could possibly be the etiologic agent. Under these circumstances, the persistence or reputation of a particular strain may offer a better clue of causality.

A variety of techniques can be used to identify different strains, including bacteriophage typing, colony morphology, biochemical reactions, antibiotic susceptibility patterns (antibiograms), plasmid composition, and restriction enzyme fragment patterns of plasmids and chromosomal DNA. Each of these techniques has practical limitations. The identification of strains should include at least two or more of the techniques described below for a reasonably accurate determination.

The most established system for epidemiological typing of *S. aureus* is bacteriophage typing. Since 1952 this technique has found widespread use, and an international system has been established to control both the typing phages and the procedures for typing human strains. Systems for typing various animal strains are in different stages of development. Bacteriophage typing is not a static system, as it must respond to the emergence of new strains of staphylococci that are nontypeable by the latest set of phages. Some large reference laboratories offer this service or can forward cultures to the Centers for Disease Control, Atlanta, Ga., where a reference center of *S. aureus* phages is maintained. Sets of phages for typing strains of *S. epidermidis* are available, but these have not received international approval or standardization. The normal variations existing in bacteriophage typing patterns of *S. epidermidis* are not well defined, and because this species is considerably less epidemic in character than *S. aureus,* typing it may be less productive. Phage typing of *S. saprophyticus* and *S. intermedius* is currently under investigation.

Colony morphology can be a very useful characteristic in strain identification. Colonies should be well isolated and allowed to develop on a suitable agar medium for several days at 34 to 35°C, followed by 2 days at room temperature (60, 63). This extended time for colony development definitely enhances individual strain characteristics. Colonies of the same strain demonstrate very similar features of size, consistency, profile, edge, luster, and color. Some strains exhibit specific sectoring patterns of two or more different forms of a colony characteristic(s), e.g., sectors of different pigments, light transmission (opaque versus translucent), or amount of growth. However, it is possible that a variant morphotype(s) may be produced by certain strains which if found would be misclassified as a different strain.

A combination of several biochemical characteristics

known to be variable within species can aid in the differentiation of strains. Characteristics most often analyzed include enzyme activities (e.g., alkaline phosphatase, urease, β-glucosidase, β-glucuronidase, arginine dihydrolase, esterase, nitrate reductase, pyrrolidonyl arylamidase, lipase, protease, and hemolysins) and acid production from various carbohydrates (e.g., α-lactose, D-mannitol, D-mannose, maltose, D-trehalose, sucrose, D-turanose, D-melezitose, D-ribose, D-xylose, and L-arabinose) (56, 57, 101). The choice of combination of characters depends on the particular species being examined. Many of the biochemical properties of strains can be determined by using the same commercial biochemical test systems for species identification of staphylococci. However, caution should be exercised in relying on biotyping alone, since some of the rapid tests are not always reproducible. Clonal variation is more prevalent for some characteristics than for others, and such variation tends to accumulate with successive subculture on laboratory media.

Antibiograms can be used epidemiologically since they are commonly determined in the laboratory, and highly standardized procedures have been established (57, 88). A unique susceptibility pattern can serve as a valuable marker for strain identity. The more common patterns will provide some support for identification if testing is confined to a small area or community. It must be recognized, however, that susceptibility patterns can be strongly influenced by the scope of antibiotic use within a given locale, so that results can vary considerably from one community to another. Susceptibility profiles may even change within an institution over time or at different locations within the institution. On occasion, a strain may demonstrate variation in pattern because of plasmid instability or high mutation rate, making strain identification more difficult.

Plasmid composition and the restriction endonuclease analysis of specific plasmids can serve as valuable molecular typing systems for strain and clone identification (7, 59, 89). For species carrying multiple plasmids, each strain has a reasonably good probability of having a characteristic profile. Species with most strains carrying several different plasmids include *S. epidermidis, S. haemolyticus, S. hominis, S. capitis, S. warneri, S. saprophyticus, S. cohnii,* and *S. xylosus.* On the other hand, some species, such as *S. lugdunensis, S. intermedius, S. auricularis, S. sciuri,* and *S. lentus,* rarely contain plasmids or carry only one or two. In most staphylococcal species there is a relationship between antibiotic resistance pattern and the presence of certain plasmids carrying resistance genes. In this regard, plasmid composition may not be entirely independent of the antibiogram. Restriction endonuclease fragment analysis of plasmids can be useful in distinguishing plasmids of identical size (as judged by their similar positions on an agarose gel after electrophoresis). Such plasmids are considered to be different if their fragment patterns are different. However, some common plasmids are highly conserved (e.g., small tetracycline [*tetA tetB*] resistance plasmids or small erythromycin [*ermC*] resistance plasmids) and often have identical fragment patterns irrespective of the strain or species carrying them. Some strains exhibit clonal variation in their plasmid profiles. This variation is most often represented by the addition or deletion of an entire plasmid or a restriction fragment within a plasmid, though occasionally different recombinant plasmids may be observed.

Chromosomal DNA can also be analyzed by restriction endonucleases, producing a manageable number of fragments which are also unique in different species and strains (23, 40). At present, this approach to strain identification is beyond the scope of most clinical laboratories but should show promise for the future as the technology becomes more simplified or automated.

LITERATURE CITED

1. **Adlam, C., J. C. Anderson, J. P. Arbuthnott, C. S. F. Easmon, and W. C. Noble.** 1983. Animal and human models of staphylococcal infection, p. 357–384. *In* C. S. F. Easmon and C. Adlam (ed.), Staphylococci and staphylococcal infections, vol. 1. Academic Press, Inc. (London), Ltd., London.
2. **Aeilts, G. D., F. L. Sapico, H. N. Canawati, G. M. Malik, and J. Z. Montgomerie.** 1982. Methicillin-resistant *Staphylococcus aureus* colonization and infection in a rehabilitation facility. J. Clin. Microbiol. **16:**218–233.
3. **Akatov, A. K., M. L. Khatenever, and L. A. Devriese.** 1981. Identification of coagulase-negative staphylococci isolated from clinical sources, p. 153–161. *In* J. Jeljaszewicz (ed.), Staphylococci and staphylococcal infections. Gustav Fischer Verlag, Stuttgart, Federal Republic of Germany.
4. **Almeida, R. J., and J. H. Jorgensen.** 1982. Use of Mueller-Hinton agar to determine novobiocin susceptibility of coagulase-negative staphylococci. J. Clin. Microbiol. **16:**1155–1156.
5. **Almeida, R. J., and J. H. Jorgensen.** 1983. Rapid determination of novobiocin resistance of coagulase-negative staphylococci with the MS-2 system. J. Clin. Microbiol. **17:**558–560.
6. **Almeida, R. J., J. H. Jorgensen, and J. E. Johnson.** 1983. Evaluation of the AutoMicrobic System Gram-Positive Identification Card for species identification of coagulase-negative staphylococci. J. Clin. Microbiol. **18:** 438–439.
7. **Archer, G. L., D. R. Dietrick, and J. L. Johnson.** 1985. Molecular epidemiology of transmissible gentamicin resistance among coagulase-negative staphylococci in a cardiac surgery unit. J. Infect. Dis. **151:**243–251.
8. **Archer, G. L., and M. J. Tenenbaum.** 1980. Antibiotic-resistant *Staphylococcus epidermidis* in patients undergoing cardiac surgery. Antimicrob. Agents Chemother. **17:**269–272.
9. **Baddour, L. M., G. D. Christensen, M. G. Hester, and A. L. Bisno.** 1984. Production of experimental endocarditis by coagulase-negative staphylococci: variability in species virulence. J. Infect. Dis. **150:**721–727.
10. **Baddour, L. M., T. N. Phillips, and A. L. Bisno.** 1986. Coagulase-negative staphylococcal endocarditis: occurrence in patients with mitral valve prolapse. Arch. Intern. Med. **146:**119–121.
11. **Baker, J. S.** 1984. Comparison of various methods for differentiation of staphylococci and micrococci. J. Clin. Microbiol. **19:**875–879.
12. **Baumgart, S., S. E. Hall, J. M. Campos, and R. A. Polin.** 1983. Sepsis with coagulase-negative staphylococci in critically ill newborns. Am. J. Dis. Child. **137:**461–463.
13. **Bor, D. H., R. M. Rose, J. F. Modlin, R. Weintraub, and G. H. Friedland.** 1983. Mediastinitis after cardiovascular surgery. Rev. Infect. Dis. **5:**885–897.
14. **Brause, B. D.** 1986. Infections associated with prosthetic joints. Clin. Rheum. Dis. **12:**523–535.
15. **Chambers, H. F.** 1987. Coagulase-negative staphylococci resistant to β-lactam antibiotics in vivo produce penicillin-binding protein 2a. Antimicrob. Agents Chemother. **31:** 1919–1924.

16. **Choo, M. H., D. R. Holmes, B. J. Gersh, J. D. Maloney, J. Meredith, J. R. Pluth, and J. Trusty.** 1981. Permanent pacemaker infections: characterization and management. Am. J. Cardiol. **48:**559–564.
17. **Christensen, G. D., W. A. Simpson, A. L. Bisno, and E. H. Beachey.** 1983. Experimental foreign body infections in mice challenged with slime-producing *Staphylococcus epidermidis.* Infect. Immun. **40:**407–410.
18. **Clarke, A. M.** 1979. Prophylactic antibiotics for total hip arthroplasty—the significance of *Staphylococcus epidermidis.* J. Antimicrob. Chemother. **5:**493–502.
19. **Coudron, P. E., D. L. Jones, H. P. Dalton, and G. L. Archer.** 1986. Evaluation of laboratory tests for detection of methicillin-resistant *Staphylococcus aureus* and *Staphylococcus epidermidis.* J. Clin. Microbiol. **24:**764–769.
20. **Crass, B. A., and M. S. Bergdoll.** 1986. Involvement of coagulase-negative staphylococci in toxic shock syndrome. J. Clin. Microbiol. **23:**43–45.
21. **Crouch, S. F., T. A. Pearson, and D. M. Parham.** 1987. Comparison of modified Minitek system with Staph-Ident system for species identification of coagulase-negative staphylococci. J. Clin. Microbiol. **25:**1626–1628.
22. **Davis, G. H. G., and B. Hoyling.** 1973. Use of a rapid acetoin test in the identification of staphylococci and micrococci. Int. J. Syst. Bacteriol. **23:**281–282.
23. **DeBuyser, M.-L., A. Morvan, F. Grimont, and N. El Solh.** 1989. Characterization of *Staphylococcus* species by ribosomal RNA gene restriction patterns. J. Gen. Microbiol. **135:**989–999.
24. **Deibel, R. H., and J. B. Evans.** 1960. Modified benzidine test for the detection of cytochrome-containing respiratory systems in microorganisms. J. Bacteriol. **79:**356–360.
25. **De La Fuente, R., G. Suarez, and K. H. Schleifer.** 1985. *Staphylococcus aureus* subsp. *anaerobius* subsp. nov., the causal agent of abscess disease of sheep. Int. J. Syst. Bacteriol. **35:**99–102.
26. **Devriese, L. A., and G. O. Adegoke.** 1985. Identification of coagulase-negative staphylococci from farm animals. J. Appl. Bacteriol. **55:**45–55.
27. **Devriese, L. A., and V. Hájek.** 1980. A review. Identification of pathogenic staphylococci isolated from animals and foods derived from animals. J. Appl. Bacteriol. **49:** 1–11.
28. **Devriese, L. A., V. Hájek, P. Oeding, S. A. Meyer, and K. H. Schleifer.** 1978. *Staphylococcus hyicus* (Sompolinsky 1953) comb. nov. and *Staphylococcus hyicus* subsp. *chromogenes* subsp. nov. Int. J. Syst. Bacteriol. **28:**482–490.
29. **Devriese, L. A., B. Poutrel, R. Kilpper-Bälz, and K. H. Schleifer.** 1983. *Staphylococcus gallinarum* and *Staphylococcus caprae,* two new species from animals. Int. J. Syst. Bacteriol. **33:**480–486.
30. **Etienne, J., B. Pangon, C. Leport, M. Wolff, B. Clair, C. Perronne, Y. Brun, and A. Bure.** 1989. *Staphylococcus lugdunensis* endocarditis. Lancet **i:**390.
31. **Falk, D., and S. J. Guering.** 1983. Differentiation of *Staphylococcus* and *Micrococcus* spp. with the Taxo A bacitracin disk. J. Clin. Microbiol. **18:**719–721.
32. **Faller, A., and K. H. Schleifer.** 1981. Modified oxidase and benzidine test for separation of staphylococci from micrococci. J. Clin. Microbiol. **13:**1031–1035.
33. **Fleurette, J., M. Bes, Y. Brun, J. Freney, F. Forey, M. Coulet, M. E. Reverdy, and J. Etienne.** 1989. Clinical isolates of *Staphylococcus lugdunensis* and *S. schleiferi:* bacteriological characteristics and susceptibility to antimicrobial agents. Res. Microbiol. **140:**107–118.
34. **Fleurette, J., Y. Brun, M. Bes, M. Coulet, and F. Forey.** 1987. Infections caused by coagulase-negative staphylococci other than *S. epidermidis* and *S. saprophyticus,* p. 195–208. *In* G. Pulverer, P. G. Quie, and G. Peters (ed.), Pathogenicity and clinical significance of coagulase-negative staphylococci. Gustav Fischer Verlag, Stuttgart, Federal Republic of Germany.
35. **Freney, J., Y. Brun, M. Bes, H. Meugneir, F. Grimont, P. A. D. Grimont, C. Nervi, and J. Fleurette.** 1988. *Staphylococcus lugdunensis* sp. nov. and *Staphylococcus schleiferi* sp. nov., two species from human clinical specimens. Int. J. Syst. Bacteriol. **38:**168–172.
36. **Gemmel, C. G., M. S. Huhssin, and A. F. McIntosh.** 1981. Development of a sensitive assay for the detection of nuclease (DNase) produced by *Staphylococcus aureus* and *Staphylococcus epidermidis,* p. 363–368. *In* J. Jeljaszewicz (ed.), Staphylococci and staphylococcal infections. Gustav Fischer Verlag, Stuttgart, Federal Republic of Germany.
37. **George, R., L. Leibrock, and M. Epstein.** 1979. Long term analysis of cerebrospinal fluid shunt infections: a 25-year experience. J. Neurosurg. **51:**804–811.
38. **Giger, O., C. C. Charilaou, and K. R. Cundy.** 1984. Comparison of API Staph-Ident and DMS Staph-Trac systems with conventional methods used for the identification of coagulase-negative staphylococci. J. Clin. Microbiol. **19:**68–72.
39. **Gill, V. J., S. T. Selepak, and E. C. Williams.** 1983. Species identification and antibiotic susceptibilities of coagulase-negative staphylococci isolated from clinical specimens. J. Clin. Microbiol. **18:**1314–1319.
40. **Goering, R. V., and T. D. Duensing.** 1990. Rapid field inversion gel electrophoresis in combination with a rRNA gene probe in the epidemiological evaluation of staphylococci. J. Clin. Microbiol. **28:**426–429.
41. **Goldstein, J., R. Schulman, E. Kelly, G. McKinley, and J. Fung.** 1983. Effect of different media on determination of novobiocin resistance for differentiation of coagulase-negative staphylococci. J. Clin. Microbiol. **18:**592–595.
42. **Hájek, V.** 1976. *Staphylococcus intermedius,* a new species isolated from animals. Int. J. Syst. Bacteriol. **26:**401–408.
43. **Hájek, V., L. A. Devriese, M. Mordarski, M. Goodfellow, G. Pulverer, and P. E. Varaldo.** 1986. Elevation of *Staphylococcus hyicus* subsp. *chromogenes* (Devriese et al., 1978) to species status: *Staphylococcus chromogenes* (Devriese et al., 1978) comb. nov. Syst. Appl. Microbiol. **8:**169–173.
44. **Harrington, B. J., and J. M. Gaydos.** 1984. Five-hour novobiocin test for differentiation of coagulase-negative staphylococci. J. Clin. Microbiol. **19:**279–280.
45. **Hébert, G. A., C. G. Crowder, G. A. Hancock, W. R. Jarvis, and C. Thornsberry.** 1988. Characteristics of coagulase-negative staphylococci that help differentiate these species and other members of the family *Micrococcaceae.* J. Clin. Microbiol. **26:**1939–1949.
46. **Hjelm, E., E. Larsson, and P.-A. Mårdh.** 1986. Experimental urinary tract infection in rats induced by *Staphylococcus saprophyticus,* p. 161–168. *In* P.-A. Mårdh and K. H. Schleifer (ed.), Coagulase-negative staphylococci. Almqvist and Wiksell International, Stockholm.
47. **Hovelius, B., I. Thelin, and P. A. Mårdh.** 1979. *Staphylococcus saprophyticus* in the aetiology of nongonococcal urethritis. Br. J. Vener. Dis. **55:**369–374.
48. **Hussain, Z., L. Stoakes, D. L. Stevens, B. C. Schieven, R. Lannigan, and C. Jones.** 1986. Comparison of the MicroScan system with the API Staph-Ident system for species identification of coagulase-negative staphylococci. J. Clin. Microbiol. **23:**126–128.
49. **Jonsson, P., O. Kinsman, O. Holmberg, and T. Wadstrom.** 1981. Virulence studies on coagulase-negative staphylococci in experimental infections: a preliminary report, p. 661–666. *In* J. Jeljaszewicz (ed.), Staphylococci and staphylococcal infections. Gustav Fischer Verlag, Stuttgart, Federal Republic of Germany.
50. **Kagan, B. M.** 1972. L-forms, p. 65–74. *In* J. O. Cohen (ed.), The staphylococci. John Wiley & Sons, Inc., New York.
51. **Karchmer, A. W., G. L. Archer, and W. E. Dismukes.**

1983. *Staphylococcus epidermidis* causing prosthetic valve endocarditis: microbiologic and clinical observations as guides to therapy. Ann. Intern. Med. **98:**447–455.

52. **Karthigasu, K. T., R. A. Bowman, and D. I. Grove.** 1986. Vertebral osteomyelitis due to *Staphylococcus warneri.* Ann. Rheum. Dis. **45:**1029–1030.
53. **Kilpper, R., U. Buhl, and K. H. Schleifer.** 1980. Nucleic acid homology studies between *Peptococcus saccharolyticus* and various anaerobic and facultative anaerobic Gram-positive cocci. FEMS Microbiol. Lett. **8:**205–210.
54. **Kilpper-Bälz, R., and K. H. Schleifer.** 1981. Transfer of *Peptococcus saccharolyticus* Foubert and Douglas to the genus *Staphylococcus: Staphylococcus saccharolyticus* (Foubert and Douglas) comb. nov. Zentralbl. Bakteriol. Parasitenkd. Infektionskr. Hyg. Abt. 1 Orig. Reihe C **2:** 324–331.
55. **Kloos, W. E.** 1980. Natural populations of the genus *Staphylococcus.* Annu. Rev. Microbiol. **34:**559–592.
56. **Kloos, W. E.** 1986. Ecology of human skin, p. 37–50. *In* P.-A. Mårdh and K. H. Schleifer (ed.), Coagulase-negative staphylococci. Almqvist and Wiksell International, Stockholm.
57. **Kloos, W. E.** 1986. Community structure of coagulase-negative staphylococci in humans, p. 132–138. *In* L. Leive (ed.), Microbiology—1986. American Society for Microbiology, Washington, D.C.
58. **Kloos, W. E., and J. H. Jorgensen.** 1985. Staphylococci, p. 143–153. *In* E. H. Lennette, A. Balows, W. J. Hausler, Jr., and H. J. Shadomy (ed.), Manual of clinical microbiology, 4th ed. American Society for Microbiology, Washington, D.C.
59. **Kloos, W. E., B. S. Orban, and D. D. Walker.** 1981. Plasmid composition of *Staphylococcus* species. Can. J. Microbiol. **27:**271–278.
60. **Kloos, W. E., and K. H. Schleifer.** 1975. Isolation and characterization of staphylococci from human skin. II. Descriptions of four new species: *Staphylococcus warneri, Staphylococcus capitis, Staphylococcus hominis,* and *Staphylococcus simulans.* Int. J. Syst. Bacteriol. **25:**62–79.
61. **Kloos, W. E., and K. H. Schleifer.** 1975. Simplified scheme for routine identification of human *Staphylococcus* species. J. Clin. Microbiol. **1:**82–88.
62. **Kloos, W. E., and K. H. Schleifer.** 1983. *Staphylococcus auricularis* sp. nov.: an inhabitant of the human external ear. Int. J. Syst. Bacteriol. **33:**9–14.
63. **Kloos, W. E., and K. H. Schleifer.** 1986. Genus IV. *Staphylococcus* Rosenbach 1884, p. 1013–1035. *In* J. G. Holt, P. H. A. Sneath, N. S. Mair, and M. S. Sharpe (ed.), Bergey's manual of systematic microbiology, vol. 2. The Williams & Wilkins Co., Baltimore.
64. **Kloos, W. E., K. H. Schleifer, and R. F. Smith.** 1976. Characterization of *Staphylococcus sciuri* sp. nov. and its subspecies. Int. J. Syst. Bacteriol. **26:**22–37.
65. **Kloos, W. E., and J. F. Wolfshohl.** 1979. Evidence for deoxyribonucleotide sequence divergence between staphylococci living on human and other primate skin. Curr. Microbiol. **3:**167–172.
66. **Kloos, W. E., and J. F. Wolfshohl.** 1982. Identification of *Staphylococcus* species with the API STAPH-IDENT system. J. Clin. Microbiol. **16:**509–516.
67. **Kloos, W. E., and J. F. Wolfshohl.** 1983. Deoxyribonucleotide sequence divergence between *Staphylococcus cohnii* subspecies populations living on primate skin. Curr. Microbiol. **8:**115–121.
68. **Kluge, R. M., F. M. Calia, J. S. McLaughlin, and R. B. Hornick.** 1974. Sources of contamination in open heart surgery. J. Am. Med. Assoc. **230:**1415–1418.
69. **Kraus, E. S., and D. A. Spector.** 1983. Characteristics and sequelae of peritonitis in diabetics and nondiabetics receiving chronic intermittent peritoneal dialysis. Medicine **62:**52–57.
70. **Lachica, R. V. F., P. D. Hoeprich, and C. Genigeorgis.** 1972. Metachromatic agar-diffusion microslide technique for detecting staphylococcal nuclease in foods. Appl. Microbiol. **23:**168–169.
71. **Lachica, R. V. F., S. S. Jang, and P. D. Hoeprich.** 1979. Thermonuclease seroinhibition test for distinguishing *Staphylococcus aureus* and other coagulase-positive staphylococci. J. Clin. Microbiol. **9:**141–143.

71a. **Lambe, D. W., Jr., K. P. Ferguson, J. L. Keplinger, C. G. Gemmell, and J. H. Kalbfleisch.** 1990. Pathogenicity of *Staphylococcus lugdunensis, Staphylococcus schleiferi,* and three other coagulase-negative staphylococci in a mouse model and possible virulence factors. Can. J. Microbiol. **36:**455–463.

72. **Lambe, D. W., Jr., K. J. Mayberry-Carson, B. Tober-Meyer, J. W. Costerton, and K. P. Ferguson.** 1987. A comparison of the effect of clindamycin and cefazolin on subcutaneous abscesses induced with *Staphylococcus epidermidis* and foreign body implant in the mouse, p. 275–286. *In* G. Pulverer, P. G. Quie, and G. Peters (ed.), Pathogenicity and clinical significance of coagulase-negative staphylococci. Gustav Fischer Verlag, Stuttgart, Federal Republic of Germany.
73. **Leighton, P. M., and J. A. Little.** 1986. Identification of coagulase-negative staphylococci isolated from urinary tract infections. Am. J. Clin. Pathol. **85:**92–95.
74. **Locci, R., G. Peters, and G. Pulverer.** 1981. Microbial colonization of prosthetic devices. I. Microtopographical characteristics of intravenous catheters as detected by scanning electron microscopy. Zentralbl. Bakteriol. Parasitenkd. Infektionskr. Hyg. Abt. 1 Orig. Reihe B **173:** 285–292.
75. **Lowy, F. D., and S. M. Hammer.** 1983. *Staphylococcus epidermidis* infections. Ann. Intern. Med. **99:**834–839.
76. **Ludwig, W., K. H. Schleifer, G. E. Fox, E. Seewaldt, and E. Stackebrandt.** 1981. A phylogenetic analysis of staphylococci, *Peptococcus saccharolyticus* and *Micrococcus mucilaginosus.* J. Gen. Microbiol. **125:**357–366.
77. **Males, B. M., W. R. Bartholomew, and D. Amsterdam.** 1985. *Staphylococcus simulans* septicemia in a patient with chronic osteomyelitis and pyarthrosis. J. Clin. Microbiol. **21:**255–257.
78. **Marsik, F. J., and S. Brake.** 1982. Species identification and susceptibility to 17 antibiotics of coagulase-negative staphylococci isolated from clinical specimens. J. Clin. Microbiol. **15:**640–645.
79. **Martin, M. A., M. A. Pfaller, and R. P. Wenzel.** 1989. Coagulase-negative staphylococcal bacteremia. Ann. Intern. Med. **110:**9–16.
80. **Mayberry-Carson, K. J., B. Tober-Meyer, L. R. Gill, D. W. Lambe, Jr., and W. R. Mayberry.** 1988. Effect on subcutaneous abscesses induced with *Staphylococcus epidermidis* and a foreign body implant in the mouse. Microbios **54:**45–59.
81. **McDougal, L. K., and C. Thornsberry.** 1984. New recommendations for disk diffusion antimicrobial susceptibility tests for methicillin-resistant (heteroresistant) staphylococci. J. Clin. Microbiol. **19:**482–488.
82. **Meyer, W.** 1967. A proposal for subdividing the species *Staphylococcus aureus.* Int. J. Syst. Bacteriol. **17:**387–389.
83. **Moeller, V.** 1955. Simplified tests for some amino acid decarboxylases and for the arginine dihydrolase system. Acta Pathol. Microbiol. Scand. **36:**158–172.
84. **Morris, I. M., P. C. Mattingly, and B. E. Gostelow.** 1986. Coagulase-negative *Staphylococcus* as a cause of joint infection. Br. J. Rheum. **25:**414–415.
85. **Ogston, A.** 1883. Micrococcus poisoning. J. Anat. Physiol. **17:**24–58.
86. **Osterholm, M. T., J. P. Davis, R. W. Gibson, J. S. Mandel, L. A. Wintermeyer, C. M. Helms, J. C. Forfang, J. Randeau, and J. M. Vergeront.** 1982. Tri-state toxic-shock syndrome study. I. Epidemiologic findings. J. Infect. Dis. **145:**431–440.

87. **Paley, D., C. F. Moseley, P. Armstrong, and C. G. Prober.** 1986. Primary osteomyelitis caused by coagulase-negative staphylococci. J. Pediatr. Orthop. **6:**622–626.
88. **Parisi, J. T.** 1985. Coagulase-negative staphylococci and the epidemiological typing of *Staphylococcus epidermidis.* Microbiol. Rev. **49:**126–139.
89. **Parisi, J. T., and D. W. Hecht.** 1980. Plasmid profiles in epidemiologic studies of infections of *Staphylococcus epidermidis.* J. Infect. Dis. **141:**637–643.
90. **Parsonnet, J., A. E. Harrison, S. E. Spencer, A. Reading, K. C. Parsonnet, and E. H. Kass.** 1987. Nonproduction of toxic shock syndrome toxin 1 by coagulase-negative staphylococci. J. Clin. Microbiol. **25:**1370–1372.
91. **Pennock, C. A., and R. B. Huddy.** 1967. Phosphatase reaction of coagulase-negative staphylococci and micrococci. J. Pathol. Bacteriol. **93:**685–688.
92. **Peters, G., R. Locci, and R. G. Pulverer.** 1981. Microbial colonization of prosthetic devices. II. Scanning electron microscopy of naturally infected intravenous catheters. Zentralbl. Bakteriol. Parasitenkd. Infektionskr. Hyg. Abt. 1 Orig. Reihe B **173:**293–299.
93. **Pfaller, M. A., and L. A. Herwaldt.** 1988. Laboratory, clinical, and epidemiological aspects of coagulase-negative staphylococci. Clin. Microbiol. Rev. **1:**281–299.
94. **Phillips, W. E., Jr., R. E. King, and W. E. Kloos.** 1980. Isolation of *Staphylococcus hyicus* subsp. *hyicus* from a pig with septic polyarthritis. Am. J. Vet. Res. **41:**274–276.
95. **Phillips, W. E., Jr., and W. E. Kloos.** 1981. Identification of coagulase-positive *Staphylococcus intermedius* and *Staphylococcus hyicus* subsp. *hyicus* isolates from veterinary clinical specimens. J. Clin. Microbiol. **14:**671–673.
96. **Ponce de Leon, S., S. H. Guenther, and R. P. Wenzel.** 1986. Microbiologic studies of coagulase-negative staphylococci isolated from patients with nosocomial bacteraemias. J. Hosp. Infect. **7:**121–129.
97. **Pulverer, G.** 1985. On the pathogenicity of coagulase-negative staphylococci, p. 1–9. *In* J. Jeljaszewicz (ed.), The staphylococci. Proceedings of the V International Symposium on Staphylococci and Staphylococcal Infections. Gustav Fischer Verlag, Stuttgart, Federal Republic of Germany.
98. **Raus, J., and D. N. Love.** 1983. Characterization of coagulase-positive *Staphylococcus intermedius* and *Staphylococcus aureus* isolated from veterinary clinical specimens. J. Clin. Microbiol. **18:**789–792.
99. **Richardson, J. V., R. B. Karp, J. W. Kirklin, and W. E. Dismukes.** 1978. Treatment of infective endocarditis: a 10 year comparative analysis. Circulation **58:**589–597.
100. **Rosenbach, F. J.** 1884. Mikro-organismen bei den Wund-Infections-Krakheiten des Menschen. J. F. Bergmann, Wiesbaden, Federal Republic of Germany.
101. **Schleifer, K. H.** 1986. Taxonomy of coagulase-negative staphylococci, p. 11–26. *In* P.-A. Mårdh and K. H. Schleifer (ed.), Coagulase-negative staphylococci. Almqvist and Wiksell International, Stockholm.
102. **Schleifer, K. H.** 1986. Gram-positive cocci, p. 999–1002. *In* J. G. Holt, P. H. A. Sneath, N. S. Mair, and M. S. Sharpe (ed.), Bergey's manual of systematic bacteriology, vol. 2. The Williams & Wilkins Co., Baltimore.
103. **Schleifer, K. H., and U. Fischer.** 1982. Description of a new species of the genus *Staphylococcus: Staphylococcus carnosus.* Int. J. Syst. Bacteriol. **32:**153–156.
104. **Schleifer, K. H., U. Geyer, R. Kilpper-Bälz, and L. A. Devriese.** 1983. Elevation of *Staphylococcus sciuri* subsp. *lentus* (Kloos *et al.*) to species status: *Staphylococcus lentus* (Kloos *et al.*) comb. nov. Syst. Appl. Microbiol. **4:** 382–387.
105. **Schleifer, K. H., R. Kilpper-Bälz, and L. A. Devriese.** 1984. *Staphylococcus arlettae* sp. nov., *S. equorum* sp. nov. and *S. kloosii* sp. nov.: three new coagulase-negative staphylococci from animals. Syst. Appl. Microbiol. **5:**501–509.
106. **Schleifer, K. H., R. Kilpper-Bälz, U. Fischer, A. Faller, and J. Endl.** 1982. Identification of *"Micrococcus candidus"* ATCC 14852 as a strain of *Staphylococcus epidermidis* and of *"Micrococcus caseolyticus"* ATCC 13548 and *Micrococcus varians* ATCC 29750 as members of a new species, *Staphylococcus caseolyticus.* Int. J. Syst. Bacteriol. **32:**15–20.
107. **Schleifer, K. H., and W. E. Kloos.** 1975. Isolation and characterization of staphylococci from human skin. I. Amended descriptions of *Staphylococcus epidermidis* and *Staphylococcus saprophyticus* and descriptions of three new species: *Staphylococcus cohnii, Staphylococcus haemolyticus* and *Staphylococcus xylosus.* Int. J. Syst. Bacteriol. **25:**50–61.
108. **Schleifer, K. H., and E. Krämer.** 1980. Selective medium for isolating staphylococci. Zentralbl. Bakteriol. Parasitenkd. Infektionskr. Hyg. Abt. 1 Orig. Reihe C **1:**270–280.
109. **Schleifer, K. H., S. A. Meyer, and M. Rupprecht.** 1979. Relatedness among coagulase-negative staphylococci. Deoxyribonucleic acid reassociation and comparative immunological studies. Arch. Microbiol. **122:**93–101.
110. **Schlievert, P. M., K. N. Shands, B. B. Dan, G. P. Schmid, and R. D. Nishimura.** 1981. Identification and characterization of an exotoxin from *Staphylococcus aureus* associated with toxic shock syndrome. J. Infect. Dis. **143:** 509–516.
111. **Subcommittee on Taxonomy of Staphylococci and Micrococci.** 1965. Recommendations. Int. Bull. Bacteriol. Nomencl. Taxon. **15:**107–110.
112. **Thornsberry, C., and L. K. McDougal.** 1983. Successful use of broth microdilution in susceptibility tests for methicillin-resistant (heteroresistant) staphylococci. J. Clin. Microbiol. **18:**1084–1091.
113. **Veraldo, P. E., R. Kilpper-Bälz, F. Biavasco, G. Satta, and K. H. Schleifer.** 1988. *Staphylococcus delphini* sp. nov., a coagulase-positive species isolated from dolphins. Int. J. Syst. Bacteriol. **38:**436–439.
114. **Wieneke, A. A.** 1988. The detection of enterotoxin and toxic shock syndrome toxin-1 production by strains of *Staphylococcus aureus* with commercial RPLA kits. Int. J. Food Microbiol. **7:**25–30.
115. **Winston, D. J., D. V. Dudnick, M. Chapin, W. G. Ho, R. P. Gale, and W. J. Martin.** 1983. Coagulase-negative staphylococcal bacteremia in patients receiving immunosuppressive therapy. Arch. Intern. Med. **143:**32–36.

Chapter 29

Streptococcus and Related Catalase-Negative Gram-Positive Cocci

RICHARD R. FACKLAM AND JOHN A. WASHINGTON II

DESCRIPTION

The latest edition of *Bergey's Manual of Systematic Bacteriology* lists seven genera of facultative anaerobic gram-positive cocci; two genera (*Staphylococcus* and *Stromatococcus*) contain cytochromes, and five genera (*Streptococcus, Leuconostoc, Pediococcus, Aerococcus,* and *Gemella*) do not. The bacteria that contain cytochrome enzymes are catalase positive, and those that do not are catalase negative (84). In previous editions of this Manual, it was stated that the taxonomic position of the pediococci and gemellas was uncertain and that *Leuconostoc* strains were not found in human infections (27). Recent reports, however, document the isolation of *Leuconostoc* (29, 82), *Pediococcus* (29, 82), and *Gemella* (13) species from human infections. In addition, it is now accepted that the genus *Streptococcus* has been divided into three genera, *Streptococcus, Enterococcus,* and *Lactococcus* (85–87).

The clinical microbiologist, then, is confronted with the problem of identifying seven different genera of catalase-negative, gram-positive cocci. Although the Gram stain characteristics of these genera are similar in many respects, this method must be used to aid in differentiating the genera as well as in identifying them as members of the catalase-negative, gram-positive cocci. When smears for Gram stains are prepared from agar growth, some *Leuconostoc* and *Streptococcus* strains may appear coccobacillary and even rod shaped and are confused with members of the genus *Lactobacillus,* which may also be catalase negative and gram positive. If Gram stains are not carefully done, some strains belonging to the genus *Gemella* may appear gram negative.

The most consistent Gram stains can be prepared from growth in thioglycolate broth. The catalase reaction resulting from flooding the growth of the bacteria on a blood-free medium with 3% hydrogen peroxide and observing for bubbling (positive reaction) is usually satisfactory for differentiating the staphylococci and stromatococci from the other gram-positive cocci. In some cases, however, weak positive catalase reactions may be observed with some strains of aerococci and streptococci, and negative reactions can be observed with some strains of staphylococci and stromatococci. In these instances, a modified benzidine test for cytochromes must also be done (104). Once it has been established that the bacteria are facultatively anaerobic, cytochrome-negative, gram-positive cocci, the characteristics listed in Table 1 can be used to identify the genus to which they belong.

CLINICAL SIGNIFICANCE AND ANTIBIOTIC SUSCEPTIBILITY

Group A streptococci (*S. pyogenes*)

Group A streptococci are the most common cause of bacterial pharyngitis in children 5 to 10 years of age. Infection occurs predominantly during a child's first few years of school but may also occur in epidemic form in military training camps and in college dormitories. Pharyngitis is typically characterized by fever, pharyngeal erythema and edema, tonsillar exudate, and anterior cervical lymphadenopathy. However, the presence of each of these physical findings varies such that the distinction between pharyngitis due to group A streptococci and that due to other etiologic agents (e.g., viral, mycoplasmal, or chlamydial) cannot be accurately made on clinical grounds alone.

Although suppurative complications of group A streptococcal pharyngeal infections occur infrequently, peritonsillar and retropharyngeal abscesses may result from spread of the infection to contiguous areas. Infection may also spread hematogenously to cause infection in other areas of the body (e.g., brain abscess, septic arthritis, acute bacterial endocarditis, or meningitis). Group A streptococci may secondarily infect traumatically acquired, operative, or burn wounds; however, streptococcal pyoderma or impetigo is presumed to result from the intradermal invasion following colonization of the skin of young children. Group A streptococci that elaborate erythrogenic toxin may produce scarlet fever that is characterized by a scarlatina-like rash that affects the trunk, neck, and extremities.

Of major concern are the nonsuppurative sequelae of group A streptococcal infection: acute rheumatic fever and acute glomerulonephritis. Both complications have been strongly associated with antecedent group A streptococcal infection. Although the frequency of scarlet fever and acute rheumatic fever in this country has declined substantially in the last few decades, there have been resurgences of these diseases, along with the appearance of a streptococcal toxic shock-like syndrome, in various geographic areas of the United States in the past few years (92).

Non-group A streptococci

The role of non-group A streptococci in causing pharyngitis has been the subject of some confusion and controversy (16). The pharyngeal carriage rate of group

TABLE 1. Identification of catalase-negative, gram-positive cocci

Genus	Test[a]										
	GS				VA	GG	PYR	LAP	NaCl	45	10
	Ch	P	T	Cl							
Streptococcus	+	+	−	−	S	−	−[b]	+	−	V	−
Enterococcus	+	+	−	−	S	−	+	+	+	+	+[c]
Lactococcus	+	+	−	−	S	−	−[b]	+	V	−	+
Aerococcus	−	+	+	+	S	−	+	−	+	−	−
Gemella	+	+	+	+	S	−	+	V	−	−	−
Pediococcus	−	+	+	+	R	−	−	+	V	+	−
Leuconostoc	+	+	−	−	R	+	−	−	V	−	+

[a] GS, Gram stain (Ch, chains; P, pairs; T, tetrads, Cl, clumps); VA, vancomycin (S, susceptible; R, resistant); GG, gas from glucose; PYR, pyrrolidonyl arylamidase; LAP, leucine aminopeptidase; NaCl, 6.5% NaCl broth; 45, growth at 45°C; 10, growth at 10°C; +, positive reaction; −, negative reaction; V, variable reactions (some strains +, others −).

[b] *S. pyogenes* (group A streptococcus) and *L. garviae* are the only species of *Streptococcus* and *Lactococcus*, respectively, that are positive for PYR.

[c] Occasional exception.

C streptococci, for example, is generally approximately 3%; however, carriage rates of up to 30% have been reported in children, especially in tropical areas (2). Although circumstantial data suggest an etiologic role for group C streptococci in cases of endemic pharyngitis, confirmatory evidence is lacking, either because of the absence of a serological response or because of the concurrent presence of another established pathogen (2, 47). Group C streptococci may, however, cause epidemic foodborne pharyngitis, which may be complicated by the development of acute glomerulonephritis (2). Recognition of such epidemics is obviously complicated by the frequent pharyngeal carriage rate of the organism. No cases of acute rheumatic fever have been recognized after group C streptococcal infection.

Epidemic pharyngitis and infrequently endemic pharyngitis have also been associated with group G streptococci (37, 47). As with group C streptococci, acute glomerulonephritis may follow pharyngeal infection, but there has been no reported association between group G streptococci and acute rheumatic fever. Both group C and group G streptococci are more frequently recognized as causes of bacteremia, endocarditis, meningitis, pneumonitis, bone and joint infections, soft tissue infections, and, in the case of group G streptococci, puerperal sepsis (2, 37, 69, 96, 100).

The roles of beta-hemolytic group F streptococci and of nongroupable beta-hemolytic *Streptococcus anginosus* ("*Streptococcus milleri*") in causing pharyngitis have not been clearly established (16); however, these organisms have been associated with bacteremia and endocarditis and often with polymicrobial suppurative infections of the central nervous system, abdomen, and pelvis (40, 65, 80).

Group B streptococci

In contrast with group A, C, and G streptococci, group B streptococci are most notable for their role in causing neonatal sepsis and meningitis. Two forms of neonatal infection have been recognized on clinical and epidemiologic grounds: early-onset disease, which usually occurs within the first 10 days after delivery, and late-onset disease, which usually, though not always, occurs 10 days after birth. Early-onset disease is thought to be due to acquisition, perhaps by aspiration, of the organism from the female genital tract at the time of delivery. Late-onset disease may be due to nosocomial acquisition of the organism. Bacteremia is common to both forms of the disease; however, involvement of the lung predominates in the early form, and meningitis is common in the late form. Mortality is higher in the early form.

Other infections caused by group B streptococci in children and adults include bacteremia, endocarditis, pneumonia, osteomyelitis, septic arthritis, and puerperal sepsis (4, 34, 35, 61, 64, 68, 98, 99). Although the presence of $\geq 10^5$ CFU of group B streptococci per ml of urine frequently is indicative of bacteriuria, the presence of the organism in urine, particularly in low numbers, may often represent urethral contamination (73).

All beta-hemolytic streptococci are susceptible to the β-lactam group of antibiotics. At least 95% of isolates in North America remain susceptible to erythromycin; however, susceptibility to the tetracyclines is variable. The failure of group A streptococcal pharyngitis to respond to penicillin has been ascribed to poor compliance on the part of patients receiving oral therapy, the presence of β-lactamase-producing bacteria (e.g., staphylococci, *Bacteroides* species, *Branhamella catarrhalis*, or *Haemophilus* species) in the oropharynx, or penicillin tolerance. The failure of penicillin in the therapy for invasive group B streptococcal infections has been ascribed to the large number of CFU per milliliter of cerebrospinal fluid in patients with meningitis or to infection with penicillin-tolerant bacteria. Since the demonstration of tolerance of streptococci and staphylococci to cell wall-active antibiotics is dependent on several factors (the type of medium used for the test, whether the inoculum is in the logarithmic or stationary phase of growth, exposure of the full inoculum to the antibiotic, or antibiotic carryover [45]), it is difficult to assess the clinical significance of tolerance, as defined by delayed killing, in group A or B streptococci (56). Since penicillin or ampicillin acts synergistically with aminoglycosides in vitro and in experimental models of endocarditis, invasive group B streptococcal infections, particularly meningitis, are usually treated with such combinations.

S. pneumoniae

S. pneumoniae is a common component of the indigenous flora of the oropharynx, although the carrier rate varies according to age, environment, season, and the presence of upper respiratory infection. Pneumococci are the leading cause of community-acquired pneumonia and a frequent cause of otitis media, sinusitis, and meningitis.

Although most pneumococci remain susceptible to penicillin (MIC, ≤0.06 μg/ml), relatively less susceptible strains (MIC, 0.12 to 1.0 μg/ml) and resistant strains (MIC, ≥2.0 μg/ml) have been recognized with increasing frequency throughout the world. Resistance to penicillins is due to alterations in penicillin-binding proteins. Such strains are uniformly susceptible to vancomycin.

Viridans streptococci

Although viridans streptococci are primarily known for their role in cariogenesis and infective endocarditis, viridans streptococcal bacteremia appears to be occurring with increasing frequency in patients with neutropenia (97). Cases of other infections, e.g., pulmonary infections, meningitis, bacteremia in children, empyema with pericarditis, mediastinitis, septic thrombophlebitis, osteomyelitis, and peritonitis due to viridans streptococci, have also been reported (15, 36, 38, 50, 76, 77). Viridans streptococci are usually susceptible to β-lactams, vancomycin, rifampin, macrolides, lincosamides, and aminoglycosides (7). Of particular interest, however, are the reports by Goldfarb et al. (38) and by Quinn et al. (77) of patients with serious infections caused by penicillin-resistant (MIC, ≥4 μg/ml) strains, which in one study (77) were found to have altered penicillin-binding proteins. Such strains are susceptible to vancomycin.

NVS

Nutritionally variant streptococci (NVS) account for approximately 5% of viridans streptococcal endocarditides and may infect either native or prosthetic valves. Infections are characterized by a prolonged, indolent course before diagnosis and by higher treatment failure and mortality rates than occur with other viridans streptococcal or enterococcal infections (91). Thus, although most patients with endocarditis caused by NVS have been treated with a combination of a penicillin and an aminoglycoside, both of which are usually effective in vitro against these organisms, treatment failure has been observed in 38% of reported cases (91).

S. bovis

An association between *S. bovis* bacteremia and gastrointestinal lesions, especially colonic cancer, has been well documented in the past decade. Particularly striking is the association between bacteremia due to *S. bovis* biotype I and colonic neoplasia (83). *S. bovis* has also been associated with neonatal septicemia and meningitis (1). Isolates of *S. bovis* are frequently resistant to penicillin (78) and may therefore warrant combination therapy with a penicillin and an aminoglycoside.

Enterococcus species

Enterococci are frequently associated with bacteriuria in patients who have an underlying structural abnormality or have had urologic manipulations: bacteremia following urologic, intra-abdominal, or hepatobiliary surgery; wound or intra-abdominal sepsis following intra-abdominal surgery; or subacute bacterial endocarditis (42, 67). Intra-abdominal wound and urinary enterococcal infections and bacteremias are frequently polymicrobial, typically with *Enterobacteriaceae* and *Bacteroidaceae*. Enterococcal bacteremia often occurs in elderly patients who have serious underlying medical problems, have had prolonged hospitalization, and have received prior antibiotic therapy, most frequently with an expanded-spectrum cephalosporin (42, 67). Enterococcal bacteremia may also occur perinatally (42).

One of the most important and often overlooked characteristics of the enterococci is that they are not killed by any single currently available antimicrobial agent at clinically attainable serum or tissue levels, although they usually appear to be susceptible to the penicillins and vancomycin. Since bactericidal therapy is required for the treatment of serious enterococcal infections such as endocarditis, treatment with a combination of a penicillin or vancomycin and an aminoglycoside is necessary for cure.

Synergism between penicillins or vancomycin and aminoglycosides can be predicted by the susceptibility of an isolate to 2,000 μg of streptomycin per ml or to 500 μg of gentamicin per ml, and the lack of synergy can be predicted by the resistance of an isolate to the same high concentrations of streptomycin and gentamicin. Although high-level plasmid-mediated resistance to streptomycin in one-third to one-half of isolates of enterococci has been widely recognized for nearly 20 years, and high-level plasmid-mediated resistance to gentamicin was first recognized about 10 years ago, the incidence of strains with high-level resistance to gentamicin was generally low until 1986 (105), and the first cases of endocarditis associated with high-level gentamicin-resistant enterococci were not reported until 1989 (66).

Enterococci have also recently acquired plasmid-mediated resistance to vancomycin and teicoplanin (63) and to penicillins (71). High-level penicillin resistance that is not due to β-lactamase has also been found among isolates of enterococci (11). The clinical significance of all of these novel resistance mechanisms is that except for β-lactamase, which can be inactivated, each reduces or eliminates the synergism that occurs between penicillins or vancomycin and aminoglycosides and thereby seriously compromises the efficacy of antibiotic therapy for serious enterococcal infections. Currently available incidence figures indicate that it is important for clinical laboratories to test enterococcal isolates routinely for high-level streptomycin and gentamicin resistance. If other medical centers confirm the observations of Bush et al. (11), testing for high-level penicillin resistance may also become warranted.

Leuconostoc and *Pediococcus* species

Vancomycin-resistant, gram-positive coccal and coccobacillary bacteria resembling viridans streptococci in colonial morphology have occasionally been isolated from various clinical sources (29, 82). Over a 28-month period at the Cleveland Clinic, the incidence of vancomycin-resistant, gram-positive cocci and coccobacilli among all isolates resembling viridans streptococci on initial isolation from blood agar was 0.3% (77a). Most such clinical isolates have been identified as *Leuconostoc* species; the remainder appear to be *Lactobacillus* and *Pediococcus* species. *Leuconostoc* species have been isolated from blood of both immunocompetent and immunosuppressed patients who were infected by intravascular catheters; however, since most isolations have been from single blood cultures, their clinical significance is often difficult to assess.

The clinical significance of lactobacilli and pediococci is likewise difficult to assess, since they are usually isolated in mixed cultures from intra-abdominal or fecally contaminated sites. An increased awareness of the existence of these microorganisms and of how to identify them will allow further clarification of their ecological niche in the indigenous flora of humans and of their role in causing infections. Vancomycin-resistant gram-positive cocci may also be resistant to teicoplanin but are generally susceptible to daptomycin, a new lipopeptide antibiotic, as well as to imipenem, minocycline, chloramphenicol, and gentamicin or tobramycin (93).

A. viridans

Aerococcus viridans is a rare cause of human infection, such as endocarditis, meningitis, and recently nosocomial infection in immunosuppressed patients (12). Buu-Hoi et al. (12) in France recently reported that *A. viridans* accounted for 3% of viridans streptococcus-like isolates in their laboratory. *A. viridans* is susceptible to β-lactams, vancomycin, macrolides, tetracycline, and chloramphenicol but is resistant to aminoglycosides (12).

Gemella species

G. haemolysans has been isolated from the upper respiratory tract but is a rare cause of infective endocarditis (13). The little information available on the gemellas suggests that they are susceptible to penicillins, cephalosporins, vancomycin, and aminoglycosides (13).

COLLECTION, TRANSPORT, AND STORAGE OF SPECIMENS

Methods of collection

Throat. The technique of swabbing the throat is as important in isolating streptococci as cultivation of the specimens that are obtained. The two most common mistakes that result in inadequate specimens are (i) swabbing the tongue or uvula tissues rather than the pharynx and (ii) inadequately exposing the pharynx. The pharynx must be adequately exposed and illuminated. The tonsils and pharynx should be rubbed with a cotton- or Dacron-tip applicator (swab), and the tongue and uvula tissues should be avoided. Any exudate should be touched with the swab.

Nose. Nasal cultures should be taken with a sterile cotton-tip flexible wire. The swab may be moistened with sterile water or saline before it is introduced into the nose. The tip of the nose is raised with one hand, and the swab is introduced gently along the floor of the nasal cavity, under the middle turbinate, until the pharyngeal wall is reached. Force should not be used; if any obstruction is encountered, the nasopharyngeal culture cannot be taken on that side.

Skin. Culture specimens are best obtained from skin lesions by removing the crusts of the pustule or vesicle cap. The sterile swab should be firmly rubbed into the lesion. This may cause the patient some discomfort, but the procedure is necessary to ensure maximum recovery of streptococci.

Wound. Wound cultures should be treated as described above for skin. If the lesions or wounds are dry, a moistened swab should be used.

Blood, cerebrospinal fluid, sputum, urine, and other body fluids. The methods used for collecting and processing these specimens are described in chapter 3.

Transport

Throat, nasopharyngeal, and skin swabs. The method of transporting the swab specimen to the microbiology laboratory depends on (i) the source of the specimen, (ii) the length of time the specimen is expected to be in transit, and (iii) the opinions of the physician submitting the specimen and of the laboratory director as to which bacteria they consider to be pathogens. Before laboratory procedures are begun, the submitting physician and the laboratory director should decide on the extent of bacteriological examination needed for each specimen from each source. Special procedures and media may be warranted in some situations but not in others. If the specimen is taken from the throat, only the beta-hemolytic streptococci and *Corynebacterium diphtheriae* are usually considered as bacterial pathogens. On occasion, *Haemophilus influenzae* is considered pathogenic, especially in young children, and some physicians request special bacteriological testing of specimens taken from patients at risk.

If no more than 2 h is expected to elapse between the time the swab specimen is collected and the time it is examined in the laboratory, no special precautions are necessary. The streptococci survive well in a dry environment, and the swab may be returned to the paper envelope or a sterile test tube for transit to the laboratory. If the swab is not to be processed until the next day, or if the specimen is to be tested for other pathogens such as those from wound infections, a holding medium (for example, Stuart or Amies medium) should be used. If the swab is to be in transit for more than 1 day, the silica gel or the dry filter paper transport system should be used. These systems can be used for both throat and skin swabs. The materials needed for these systems are available commercially (Carter, Rice, Storrs & Bement, Inc., East Hartford, Conn.). A modified silica gel transport system can be made by placing enough silica gel crystals in a 15- by 125-mm screw-cap tube to cover the cotton tip of the swab. The tube and crystals are then autoclaved and dried in a hot-air oven.

Blood, cerebrospinal fluid, sputum, urine, and other body fluids. Most evidence indicates that the gram-positive cocci will survive in these body fluids for the time required to transport the collected fluid from the patient to the microbiology laboratory. However, they should be transported as quickly as possible, preferably in less than 1 h.

Storage

Most specimens survive for several months on tightly capped blood agar slants stored at 4°C. The exceptions are the pneumococci and some viridans streptococci that do not survive more than a week. None of the gram-positive cocci survive well in broth cultures; some strains die after only 3 or 4 days. Gram-positive cocci survive 1 to 2 years frozen in blood at −70°C and 20 or more years if they are lyophilized.

DIRECT EXAMINATION

Gram stains

Direct examination of throat, nose, and skin specimens is of little value in identifying pathogenic streptococci. These areas are normally inhabited by nonpathogenic streptococci, which do not differ from the pathogenic streptococci in their staining characteristics or cellular morphology. However, Gram-stained smears of blood, cerebrospinal fluid, and other body fluids are of some help in identifying the pathogen as a gram-positive coccus. Gram-stained smears of sputum are of value in identifying pneumococci when increased numbers of polymorphonuclear leukocytes are also noted. The sputum should be gently homogenized with 1 to 2 ml of sterile saline. This can be done by refluxing the sputum saline mixture in a small syringe without a needle attached. Sputum treated in this way should be placed on a glass slide, air dried, heat fixed, and stained by the Gram technique. Gram-positive cocci found singly, in pairs, and in short chains are indicative of pneumococci.

Quellung test

Pneumococci can also be identified by directly examining body fluids with the Quellung test. Various body fluids (including cerebrospinal fluid, peritoneal fluid, transtracheal aspirates, or sputa) or cells from a single colony suspended in a drop of physiological saline can be examined with the Quellung test.

To perform the test, place a small drop of culture, cell suspension, or body fluid on a glass slide.

Add 1 loopful (1 mm) of antiserum and mix well.

Add a small loopful of saturated aqueous methylene blue dye and mix. Place a cover slip over the mixture; after 10 min, examine microscopically with an oil immersion lens.

To avoid antigen excess, which may cause negative reactions, prepare slides so that each microscopic field contains 50 to 100 cells.

To obtain the oblique illumination needed to examine the slide, adjust the iris diaphragm so that only about one-third of the light passes through the condenser at low power (×10).

Minor modifications of the Quellung test are given in detail by Austrian (3). A positive Quellung reaction is the result of the binding of pneumococcal capsular polysaccharide with type-specific antiserum. The corresponding change in refractive index causes the capsule to appear swollen; actually, it becomes more visible. The pneumococcal cell stains dark blue and is surrounded by a sharply demarcated halo, which represents the outer edge of the capsule. The light transmitted through the capsule appears brighter than either the pneumococcal cell or the background of the slide. Single cells, pairs, chains, and even clumps of organisms may have positive Quellung reactions.

In the Quellung test, pneumococci are identified by using a battery of antisera. The Statens Serum Institute, Copenhagen, Denmark, produces polyvalent antiserum (omniserum) with 83 different type-specific antibodies. They also produce polyvalent pooled antisera (nine pools, A through I). Each pool contains 7 to 11 type- or group-specific antisera, the latter containing one to four types. Other commercial type-specific, group-specific, and pooled antisera are available; however, the antibody compositions of the pools vary among the different sources. Therefore, instructions supplied with each antiserum must be followed. Unless typing is required for epidemiologic purposes, omnisera and pooled sera are used to identify pneumococci. The presence of cross-reactive antibodies in omnisera means that colonial and Gram stain morphology must also be relied on for identification.

Antigen detection

Direct antigen tests (DAT) for the detection of group A and group B streptococci are commercially available. When patients are available immediately after the DAT is performed, the test is useful in determining the method of treatment. There is no particular advantage of performing DAT on swab specimens that have been transported or when the patient is not immediately available for treatment.

Throat swabs. There are approximately 30 commercial kits for direct detection of group A antigen in throat swabs. These commercial kits contain materials for extraction of the group A streptococcus antigen from the swab by enzymatic or chemical means. Generally, the enzymatic extractions require longer times (30 to 60 min) than do chemical extractions (2 to 10 min). The DAT systems included in the kits are either enzyme-linked immunoabsorbent assays (ELISA) or agglutination reagents (latex or coagglutination). The agglutination tests are generally less complex and require less time to perform than the ELISA. For the microbiologist, all DAT are simple to perform, requiring less than 2 to 5 min of hands-on time.

Controversy exists over the sensitivity of the DAT compared with that of conventional throat culturing practices. Results of studies conducted in microbiology laboratories differ from those of studies conducted in office settings. The sensitivities of DAT ranged from 60 to 85% compared with those of conventional culture techniques when tests were performed by microbiologists. When testing was done in physician office laboratories, the reported sensitivities of DAT were about 90 to 95% compared with those of conventional culture techniques (49, 94). In physician offices, the results of DAT and conventional culture techniques for identifying group A streptococci were equivalent. However, most microbiology laboratories prefer to use a conventional culture technique if the DAT result is negative. The specificities of the DAT are very good (95 to 99%), ensuring the validity of positive results (26).

Urogenital swabs. Direct antigen testing of urogenital swabs for group B streptococci is performed in two different ways. One procedure involves testing the urogenital swab in the same manner as described for group A streptococcus antigen detection. The specimen is extracted with chemicals (21) or enzyme (9), and the extract is then tested for group B antigen by slide agglutination. Commercial versions of these tests are now available.

A second method involves placing the urogenital swab in an enrichment broth for several hours before testing the broth for group B antigen. The broth (Lim broth; GIBCO Laboratories, Grand Island, N.Y.) consists of Todd-Hewitt base with an additional 1% yeast extract and 10 μg of colistin and 15 μg of nalidixic acid per ml. The swab is placed in the medium and incubated for approximately 4 h; it is then tested for group B antigen by agglutination (48, 95). The use of heat may be necessary to remove nonspecific reactions (reactions in more than one antibody reagent) (48). The authors of the second procedure believe that this technique is sufficient to identify all or most of the patients at greatest risk for developing group B streptococcal disease.

Each of the DAT has advantages and disadvantages. Before adopting one of these methods, be sure to evaluate the complexity of the procedure and the turnaround time involved to ensure that the procedure will fit the needs of the laboratory and physicians. Obtain and study the package insert instructions for each product under consideration.

Blood, cerebrospinal, peritoneal, and pleural fluids. Direct antigen testing of these body fluids is described in chapter 9.

CULTURE AND ISOLATION

Recommendations for primary throat cultures

Streptococci are fastidious with respect to their nutritional requirements. Enriched infusion agar and broth, such as tryptic soy, heart infusion, Todd-Hewitt, or proteose peptone, should be used. These media are free of reducing sugars, i.e., substances that influence the expression of beta-hemolysis by streptococci. The pH of the medium should be 7.3 to 7.4. Because colonies of *Haemophilus haemolyticus* are indistinguishable from those of beta-hemolytic streptococci, sheep blood is recommended as a medium for throat cultures. This blood lacks sufficient amounts of pyridine nucleotides (V factor) to support the growth of *H. haemolyticus*. Different concentrations of blood affect the size of the area of erythrocyte (RBC) destruction (zone size) and may affect the decision as to the type of hemolysis that occurred. If streak plates are used, lower concentrations of blood may make it difficult to distinguish alpha- from beta-hemolysis. Higher concentrations of blood may cause beta-hemolytic strains to appear nonhemolytic unless the agar is cut or stabbed with inoculum. The best blood agar plates for primary isolation contain 5% defibrinated blood in agar approximately 4 mm deep.

Pour-streak plate

1. Place the throat swab in 1 ml of broth and incubate it at 37°C for 2 h. Specimens that are received in the laboratory within 2 to 4 h after they are taken may be cultured after 0 to 2 h of incubation in broth. Specimens that have been in transit for 4 to 8 h should be incubated in broth for a minimum of 2 h, whereas those in transit over 8 h should be incubated in broth for 4 to 5 h.
2. Remove the swab from the 1 ml of broth, drain it against the inside of the tube, and place it in a sterile tube.
3. Melt 15 to 20 ml of blood agar base in a tube and hold the tube in a water bath at 50°C.
4. Add 0.8 to 1.0 ml of sterile defibrinated blood to the melted and cooled agar.
5. Pick up a loopful of broth containing swab washings, drain the contents against the side of the broth tube, and transfer the drained loopful to the blood agar tube.
6. Mix the contents thoroughly, hold the tube lip to a flame, and pour the medium into a sterile petri dish.
7. When the agar is hard, rotate the specimen swab over a small section of the surface. Using an inoculating loop, spread the inoculum over half of the plate and crosshatch for isolation. Stab into the agar after each crosshatch series.

Overnight incubation in broth

1. Insert the specimen swab into a tube of broth, incubate the culture overnight, and then mix the broth tube to get an even suspension of organisms. Transfer 1 loopful of broth culture to 15 ml of sterile saline and mix well. (If growth is light, it may be necessary to use 2 to 3 loopfuls.)
2. Follow the procedure for steps 3 through 7 of the pour-streak plate method described above, except in step 5 use a loopful of the saline dilution, not a drained loopful.

Streak plate. Swabs may be cultured on blood agar plates immediately after collection or after enrichment or selective enrichment for any time period. If the swab has been enriched, press the swab against the wall of the tube to remove excess moisture before transferring the inoculum to the agar plate. Firmly roll the swab over one-sixth of the plate. Use a sterile wire loop to cross hatch the remainder of the plate. Stab the agar several times with the wire loop. Make two or three stabs in an area of the plate that has not been streaked. The wire loop does not have to be resterilized at any stage of the streaking or stabbing of the plate.

Recommendations for primary cultures other than throats

Sputum. The sputum should be homogenized as described above for direct examination. A loopful of the sputum should be streaked on the surface of a blood agar infusion base medium as described above for streak plates.

Other body fluids. Other body fluids may be processed by either the pour plate or streak plate method. Use a loopful of the body fluid and follow the directions outlined above for the method selected.

Incubation atmosphere and temperature

Pour plates. Incubate pour plates under any atmosphere. They are anaerobic by nature of their preparation.

Streak plates. Streak plates for pneumococci should be incubated in a candle extinction jar or a CO_2 incubator with 5 to 10% CO_2. Preferably, streak plates for streptococci should be incubated under anaerobic conditions with 5 to 10% CO_2 and 85 to 90% N_2. These plates can be incubated under normal aerobic conditions with very little loss of the recovery rates of group A streptococci. This procedure, however, has not been equally successful in all laboratories (23, 72, 75). Some non-group A streptococci may fail to grow in normal atmospheres. If stabs are made with a wire loop in the streak plates, these plates can be incubated in candle extinction jars or CO_2 incubators. If the latter method is used, the stabbed area of the plate must be used to determine streptococcal hemolysis as described below.

Incubation temperature. All plates and broths should be incubated at temperatures of between 35 and 37°C.

Other culture methods

When quantitative information is not being sought, enrichment, selection, or selective enrichment techniques may be used for primary isolation of streptococci. Opinions differ as to whether patients should be treated on the basis of the numbers of beta-hemolytic organisms present on blood agar plates. If colony counts on primary isolation plates are needed, enrichment should not be used. If, on the other hand, the objective is to detect even low numbers of streptococci, enrichment (incubation of the inoculum in broth), selection (incubation in an environment more conducive to the growth of streptococci than of unwanted organisms), or selective enrichment may be advantageous.

Enrichment. Any of the aforementioned infusion broths can be used for enrichment. Group A and B streptococci can be identified by immunofluorescence (IF) within 4 h, even in the presence of large numbers of contaminating organisms. Otherwise, specimens can be incubated in Todd-Hewitt broth overnight. Blood agar plates are then inoculated with the broth culture, and if contaminants overgrow the culture on nonselective medium, selective blood agar, i.e., Columbia colistin (10 μg/ml)-nalidixic acid (15 μg/ml), phenylethyl alcohol (0.25%), or colistin (10 μg/ml)-oxolinic (5 μg/ml), can be used for isolating the streptococci (22, 24, 74).

Selective techniques. The source of the specimen may dictate which selective agent to use. For example, inhibitors of gram-negative bacilli (neomycin [30 μg/ml] or nalidixic acid [15 μg/ml] and polymyxin [10 μg/ml]) are not usually necessary for throat swabs but are very useful for rectal, vaginal, or wound specimens. Conversely, crystal violet (1 μg/ml), an inhibitor of staphylococci which are often found in the throat, is useful in streptococcal throat swab cultures. Sulfamethoxazole (23.75 μg/ml)-trimethoprim (1.25 μg/ml) has also been used in tryptic soy agar (TSA) to inhibit staphylococci, viridans streptococci, and gram-negative bacilli (43). Sulfamethoxazole-trimethoprim has been used in primary blood agar plates with various degrees of success (23, 60). Investigators attempting to recover beta-hemolytic streptococci have usually reported higher isolation rates with gentamicin (5.5 μg/ml in Columbia or 5.0 μg/ml in TSA) than with nonselective media (6, 72). The improved recovery rate was due to better growth of non-group A rather than of group A streptococci. Selective agar (TSA) containing gentamicin (5.0 μg/ml) has been reported to substantially improve the recovery rates of pneumococci from the oropharynx (17).

Selective enrichment technique. As the name suggests, selective enrichment broths provide the advantages of both enrichment and selection by providing optimal conditions for streptococcal growth while inhibiting the growth of competitors. The most frequently used selective agents have been sodium azide (1:16,000) to inhibit gram-negative bacilli and crystal violet (1: 500,000) to inhibit staphylococci. Todd-Hewitt broth has been modified for the selection of group B streptococci (nalidixic acid [15 μg/ml] and gentamicin [8 μg/ml] or nalidixic acid [15 μg/ml], polymyxin [1 μg/ml], and crystal violet [0.1 μg/ml]). A common mistake made in preparing selective enrichment broths is using the same concentration of inhibitors for broth as for selective agar. The fact that some inhibitors diffuse more widely in broth may dictate that their concentrations be reduced (41). Regardless of whether enrichment, selection, or selective enrichment is used, there is no substitute for a well-prepared streak plate with stabs onto the agar or a pour plate for determining the type of hemolysis from the primary plates.

IDENTIFICATION

Recognition of the colonies

After 18 to 24 h of incubation on blood agar, the colonies of group A streptococci typically are about 0.5 mm in diameter, transparent or translucent, and domed; they have a smooth or semimatte surface and an entire edge. They are surrounded by a well-defined zone of complete hemolysis, usually two to four times the diameter of the colony; however, considerable variations occur. The appearance of the colonies depends greatly on the medium used and to some extent on the atmosphere of incubation. All colonial characteristics are not manifested on a single medium or atmosphere. Subsurface colonies also vary. Some colonies are lancet shaped, whereas others are oval or round. The appearance of surface or subsurface beta-hemolytic group C or group G streptococcal colonies does not differ sufficiently from that of group A colonies to be of any value in identification.

Group B streptococcal colonies may be somewhat larger than group A colonies, but both are smooth, with entire edges. The group B colonies are surrounded by a much smaller zone of complete hemolysis, and some strains do not lyse RBCs at all. Group D streptococcal colonies (*S. bovis*) are somewhat larger than other streptococcal colonies on the surface of blood agar (0.5 to 1.0 mm). They are less opaque, raised, and gray to gray-white. No hemolytic zone is present around *S. bovis* colonies. Group F streptococci (*S. anginosus*) generally form minute colonies. Zones of hemolysis similar in size to those produced by group A streptococci surround these minute colonies. This characteristic has little diagnostic value, however, since some strains of groups C and G and even some strains of group A also form minute colonies.

The viridans streptococcal colonies vary in size from pinpoint (0.1 mm) to a size equal to or larger than that of group A streptococci (0.5 mm). The colonies are usually considerably smaller than those of the pneumococci. They may appear mucoidal and translucent or glossy and nontranslucent. The colony size and appearance are affected by the composition of the medium and the atmosphere of incubation. The colonies may be surrounded by a small zone of alpha-hemolysis (partial destruction of RBCs) or have no zone of hemolysis. Under anaerobic incubation, viridans streptococci are usually nonhemolytic.

Pneumococcal colonies are round with entire edges, mucoid, and about 1 mm in diameter. When the culture has been incubated in candle extinction jars or CO_2 incubators, the colonies are surrounded by a fairly large zone of alpha-hemolysis. Microscopic examination (magnification of ×40 to ×50) of the colonies is a useful aid in differentiating the pneumococci from the viridans streptococci. Young pneumococcal colonies are raised (like viridans streptococci), but as the culture ages, the colonies become flattened and the central part of the colony may become depressed (unlike viridans streptococci).

The colonies of *Aerococcus, Gemella,* and *Pediococcus* species are similar to those of the viridans streptococci, although some strains may form larger colonies. The colonies are usually surrounded by a zone of alpha-hemolysis, although some strains are nonhemolytic.

The colonies of *Enterococcus, Lactococcus,* and *Leuconostoc* species are larger than those of the streptococci on blood agar (0.5 to 1.5 mm). The colonies are raised and white or gray-white. *Enterococcus faecalis* and *E. durans* may exhibit beta-hemolytic zones on blood agar. The hemolytic activity of *E. faecalis* may vary, depending on the species of blood used in the agar plate. Some *E. faecalis* strains may be beta-hemolytic on horse or rabbit blood but nonhemolytic on sheep blood. Most *Enterococcus, Lactococcus,* and *Leuconostoc* strains are nonhemolytic initially on blood agar; a weak alpha-hemolysis may develop upon continued incubation (48 to 72 h).

Hemolysis

Hemolysis is the most useful characteristic for identifying streptococci. The hemolytic action of streptococci on RBCs was described and defined by Brown in 1919 (9a) as follows:

1. Alpha-hemolysis—An indistinct zone of partial destruction of RBCs about the colony, often accompanied by a greenish to brownish discoloration of medium.
2. Beta-hemolysis—A clear, colorless zone around the streptococcal colonies in which the RBCs have undergone complete discoloration.
3. No hemolysis—No apparent hemolytic activity or discoloration produced by the colony.
4. Alpha-prime or wide-zone alpha-hemolysis—A small halo or envelope of intact or partially lysed RBCs lying adjacent to the bacterial colony, with a zone of complete hemolysis extending farther into the medium. When examined macroscopically, alpha-prime-hemolysis can be confused with beta-hemolysis.

Brown's observations were based on microscopic examination of subsurface colonies in blood agar pour plates. Through the years, these definitions have been used to characterize colonies growing on the surface of streaked blood plates. However, this extended application has not been made easily because of the characteristic of the hemolysins responsible for beta-hemolysis and because of the misinterpretation of alpha-prime-hemolysis as beta-hemolysis.

Among the streptococci, two distinct hemolysins are responsible for beta-hemolytic activity. The hemolysins of group A streptococci, streptolysin O and streptolysin S, are differentiated on the basis of antigenicity and susceptibility to inactivation by oxidation. Streptolysin O is antigenic and oxygen labile; streptolysin S is nonantigenic and oxygen stable. Oxygen-sensitive streptolysin O can be reactivated in the presence of reducing agents. Furthermore, streptolysin S is not produced in serum-free broth, and its production is inhibited in media rich in fermentable carbohydrate. When these restrictive properties are considered, it becomes obvious that aerobic incubation of streaked blood plates inhibits the hemolytic activity of streptolysin O and limits the characterization of beta-hemolytic streptococci to streptolysin S activity, which may vary from strain to strain.

When streaked blood plates are incubated in the presence of atmospheric oxygen, the investigator imposes limitations on the hemolytic expression of the organism, which could cause the beta-hemolytic characteristic to be overlooked. Peroxide-producing beta-hemolytic streptococci can appear alpha-hemolytic on the surface of blood agar plates incubated aerobically or in atmospheres of increased CO_2. In addition, peroxide-producing alpha-hemolytic streptococci may inhibit the expression of beta-hemolysis produced by group A streptococci on the surface of blood agar plates (46, 62). This phenomenon is especially important to consider when determining hemolysis on primary isolation plates from throat swabs, because alpha-hemolytic streptococci are part of the normal throat flora and may obscure the potentially pathogenic beta-hemolytic streptococci. If the streak plate method is used, the streaked plate should, at the very least, be stabbed with the inoculating loop to obtain subsurface growth and to permit detection of both streptolysins O and S. At a magnification of approximately ×60, beta-, alpha-, and alpha-prime-hemolysis can be differentiated around the subsurface growth in blood agar pour and stabbed plates.

Identification of genera

The tests listed in Table 1 can be used to differentiate the catalase-negative, gram-positive cocci. Catalase tests should be performed on all cultures that require definitive identification. If the catalase test is inconclusive, the porphyrin test described by Wong (104) should be used to detect cytochrome-containing enzymes. The species belonging to the genera *Streptococcus, Enterococcus, Lactococcus, Gemella, Pediococcus,* and *Leuconostoc* are catalase negative and do not contain cytochromes. Some aerococci may yield a weak catalase test result (effervescence of hydrogen peroxide), but they do not contain cytochrome-containing enzymes.

Gram stains. Cellular arrangement and Gram stain characteristics are seen most reliably if the smears are prepared from cultures grown in thioglycolate broth. The smear should be air dried on the slide and then fixed with methanol rather than heat. The air-dried smear is flooded with methanol and allowed to dry at room temperature. The application of mordant, decolorizer, and counterstain is done in the same manner as for the routine Gram stain procedure. If Gram stains are prepared from agar-grown cultures, some species may show elongated forms. *Streptococcus mutans,* in fact, will appear as a bacillus, and some *Leuoconostoc* strains will appear more coccobacillary than coccal in form. The streptococci, enterococci, lactococci, and leuconostocs will appear primarily in chains and diplococci, whereas the aerococci, pediococci, and gemellas will appear in tetrads and clumps. There is some overlapping in the cellular arrangement, but it is a useful guide in the overall identification.

Vancomycin susceptibility. To determine the susceptibility to vancomycin, 5 to 10 colonies or a drained swab of a broth culture should be spread over one-half of a TSA plate with a wire loop or cotton swab to achieve confluent growth. A 30-μg vancomycin disk is then placed in the center of the inoculated plate, and the plate is incubated in a candle extinction jar or a 5% CO_2 incubator overnight at 35°C. Strains with any zone of inhibition are considered susceptible, and strains that exhibit growth up to the disk are considered resistant. All *Pediococcus* and *Leuconostoc* species are resistant to vancomycin, whereas all *Streptococcus, Lactococcus, Aerococcus,* and *Gemella* species are susceptible. Most enterococci are also susceptible, but an occasional strain will have no zone of inhibition in this test. At this time, less than 1% of the enterococci are resistant to vancomycin (29).

Gas from glucose. Production of gas from glucose is determined by inoculating *Lactobacillus* Mann, Rogosa, and Sharpe (MRS) broth (29). A loopful of broth culture or a colony from a blood agar plate is used to inoculate the broth. The inoculated tube is overlaid with melted petrolatum and incubated for up to 7 days at 35°C. Gas production is indicated when the petrolatum plug is completely separated from the broth in the tube. Among the genera listed in Table 1, only the *Leuconostoc* species form gas in MRS broth.

PYR test. There are several versions of the pyrrolidonyl arylamidase (PYR) test (26, 39). Several commercial sources have complete packages of the reagents necessary for performing the test. These packages are recommended, since individually purchased reagents (L-pyroglutamic acid-β-naphthylamide and *p*-dimethylaminocinnamaldehyde; Sigma Chemical Co., St. Louis, Mo.) similar to those included in the packaged tests failed to produce a usable product (33). The commercially available tests are nearly all equal in specificity and sensitivity, and any of them can be used with good results. All of the species included in the genera *Enterococcus, Aerococcus,* and *Gemella* are PYR positive. All *Leuconostoc* and *Pediococcus* species react negatively in the PYR test. In the genera *Streptococcus* and *Lactococcus*, only *S. pyogenes* and *L. garviae*, respectively, are PYR positive. Users of the PYR test should examine the hands-on and turnaround times of the different tests and choose one that best suits the laboratory.

The PYR test is an excellent test for identifying group A streptococci. It is more specific than the bacitracin test for the presumptive identification of these bacteria. As few as one or two isolated colonies are all that is required for the PYR test. Some species of staphylococci and stromatococci are also PYR positive; therefore, only pure cultures should be tested (26). Instructions included in the package inserts of each PYR test should be followed.

LAP test. The leucine aminopeptidase (LAP) test is available only in the Rapid Strep identification system (Analytab Products, Plainview, N.Y.). Test kits similar to those for the PYR test will be available shortly from commercial suppliers. All *Streptococcus, Enterococcus, Lactococcus,* and *Pediococcus* species are LAP positive, whereas all *Aerococcus* and *Leuconostoc* species are LAP negative. Among the *Gemella* species, *G. morbillorum* is LAP positive and *G. haemolysans* is LAP negative. Instructions for performing the LAP test are included in the package insert instructions of each product.

Growth in 6.5% sodium chloride broth (NaCl test). The NaCl test is used primarily for identifying the non-beta-hemolytic strains of catalase-negative, gram-positive cocci. We have successfully used the formulation given in chapter 121 for several years. The test is performed by inoculating the broth with two or three colonies of the bacteria and incubating the broth at 35°C for up to 72 h. Most *Enterococcus* and *Aerococcus* species grow in the broth after 24 h. A positive test result is indicated by frank growth in the broth as evidenced by increased turbidity. A color change may occur, but it is not necessary for a positive result. Neither *Gemella* or non-beta-hemolytic *Streptococcus* species grow in NaCl broth. A negative result is indicated when no growth occurs (no increase in turbidity) after 72 h.

Previous editions of this Manual suggested that the NaCl test together with the bile esculin (BE) test could be used to identify presumptively the enterococci (27). With the isolation of *Pediococcus* and *Leuconostoc* species from human infections, it is now apparent that this presumptive identification could be erroneous because some strains of these two genera yield positive results with both the BE test and the NaCl test (29). For presumptive identification of enterococci, an alternative procedure is suggested later.

Growth at 10 and 45°C. We have used the broth formulation given in chapter 121 for several years. We found that several broth media (Todd-Hewitt, *Lactobacillus* MRS, and tryptic soy broths) did not improve the differentiation of the genera (R. Facklam, unpublished observations). We did note that the 45°C test performed with incubation in a water bath controlled at 45°C gave better results than use of a dry incubator controlled at 45°C.

The tests are performed by inoculating the broths with a single colony or a drop of broth culture (18 to 24 h old). The broths are then incubated at 10 or 45°C for up to 7 days. The time between inoculation and placement at the proper temperature should not be longer than 10 min. If the test cultures are inspected for growth during the incubation period, the tubes should be returned to the proper temperature without being allowed to warm or cool. A positive result is indicated by frank growth, which may be accompanied by a color change in the indicator. A color change is not necessary to determine a positive reaction; an increase in turbidity should be the indicator.

Be sure to rotate the tube vigorously after the 7-day incubation period. Some bacterial strains have a tendency to settle to the bottom of the tube, and turbidity will not be apparent until the contents of the tube are mixed. These tests are especially useful in identifying enterococci (positive growth at both 10 and 45°C), lactococci (growth at 10 but not 45°C), and *aerococci* and gemellas (no growth at either 10 or 45°C).

Identification of beta-hemolytic streptococci

Nearly all beta-hemolytic streptococci isolated from human infections possess specific carbohydrate antigens. These carbohydrate antigens are called streptococcal group antigens, and they can be demonstrated by a variety of techniques. Group-specific, precipitating, agglutinating, and fluorescent-antibody sera, which can be used with extracts, cell suspensions, and spent broth media, are commercially available. Attempts to extend these procedures to the non-beta-hemolytic streptococci have been unsuccessful. We recommend use of group A, B, C, F, and G antisera for identifying beta-hemolytic streptococci and the use of only group B and D antisera for identifying non-beta-hemolytic streptococci.

There are several procedures for extracting streptococcal antigens. These include the Lancefield hot HCl, hot formamide, autoclave, nitrous acid, *Streptomyces albus* enzyme, pronase B enzyme, and *S. albus*-lysozyme extraction procedures. Each extraction method has advantages and disadvantages. For example, the Lancefield hot acid technique is the standard for grouping and must be used for typing group A and B streptococci. It is the only technique available for extracting the protein type-specific antigens as well as the carbohydrate (groups A, B, C, F, and G) and teichoic acid (groups D and N) antigens. However, it is somewhat more complex and time consuming than other methods.

Lancefield extraction (hot HCl extract). Grow pure cultures in 30 ml of Todd-Hewitt or other suitable broth for 18 to 20 h at 35 to 37°C.

Pack the cells by centrifugation.

Discard the supernatant fluid and add 1 drop of 0.04% *m*-cresol purple and about 0.3 ml of 0.2 N HCl (in 0.85% NaCl) to the sedimented cells. Mix the fluids well and transfer the suspension to a small tube. If the suspension is not definitely pink (pH 2.0 to 2.4), add another drop of 0.2 N HCl.

Place the tube in a boiling-water bath for 10 min. Shake the tube several times.

Remove the tube from the water bath and centrifuge it.

Decant the supernatant fluid into a small clean tube.

Neutralize the contents by adding 0.2 N NaOH (in distilled water) drop by drop until the extract is slightly purple (pH 7.4 to 7.8). A deep purple color indicates that the pH is too high, a condition that may cause nonspecific cross-reactions. Although it is better not to add more salts or to increase the volume, a back-titration with 0.2 N HCl may be necessary.

Centrifuge the extract and decant the supernatant fluid into a small screw-cap vial. Add 1 drop of a 1:500 dilution of Merthiolate (1% in 1.4% sodium borate) and store the solution at 4 or −20°C.

Autoclave extraction. A satisfactory alternative to the Lancefield extraction technique is the autoclave extraction technique. It is relatively simple and can be used for extraction of the group carbohydrate of beta-hemolytic streptococci.

Grow cells in 30 ml of Todd-Hewitt or other suitable broth for 18 to 20 h at 35 to 37°C.

Pack the cells by centrifugation.

Discard the supernatant fluid, add 0.5 ml of 0.85% NaCl solution to the cells, and shake the contents to suspend the cells.

Autoclave the tube for 15 min at 121°C.

Centrifuge the tube.

Decant the supernatant fluid into a clean, sterile container.

Several other extraction techniques are outlined in the previous edition of this Manual (27).

Demonstrating that all strains of *Streptococcus bovis* and *Enterococcus* species possess group D antigen is difficult. Supplementing the 30 ml of Todd-Hewitt broth with 0.6 ml of filter-sterilized 50% dextrose improves the growth of non-beta-hemolytic streptococci and enterococci. The supplemented Todd-Hewitt broth is incubated for 48 h at 35°C rather than the 18 h suggested for growing the beta-hemolytic strains in unsupplemented broth.

Capillary precipitin test. The effectiveness of all extraction techniques depends largely on the quality of the antiserum used in the precipitin test. With potent, specific antiserum, all techniques work well within the limits of the extraction procedures described above. Control streptococcal strains should be used to test each new lot of commercial antiserum. Some are of notoriously poor quality. Cost, complexity, and efficiency of extraction are all factors that influence the choice of extraction technique. The recommended procedure for performing the capillary precipitin test for detecting streptococcal group antigens is as follows.

Dip a capillary tube (vaccine capillary tube with 1.2- to 1.5-mm outside diameter, Kimble borosilicate glass, both ends open, and lightly fire polished) into antiserum (in a screw-cap vial) until a column about 1 cm long has been drawn in by capillary action. (To maintain sterility of the serum, sterilize the capillary tubes and keep them sterile at the lower end until after the serum is taken up.)

Holding the tube carefully so that air does not enter it, wipe it with facial tissue.

Dip the tube into streptococcal extract until an amount equal to that in the serum column is drawn up. If an air bubble separates serum and extract, discard the tube and repeat the procedure.

Wipe the tube carefully. Fingerprints, serum, or extracts on the outside of the tube may simulate or obscure a positive reaction.

Plunge the lower end of the tube into plasticine until a small plug fills the opening. Do not let the reactants mix. The plasticine plug (at the same end of the tube as the reactants) will hold the reactants in place while the tube is inverted. Alternatively, hold a finger over the end of the tube until the next step is completed.

Invert the tube and insert it gently into the plasticine-filled groove of a capillary holding rack.

Examine the tube in bright light against a dark background. If a white precipitate appears within 5 min, the reaction is strongly positive; weaker reactions develop more slowly. Precipitates that appear after 30 min should be disregarded.

Slide agglutination tests. Two slide agglutination tests in which carrier particles for the group-specific antisera are used have been described. The reagents for these tests are now available from several commercial sources. In the coagglutination test, specially prepared protein A-rich staphylococcal cells conjugated to group-specific streptococcal antisera are used. Latex particles conjugated to group-specific streptococcal antisera are used in the latex agglutination test. The carrier particles in these tests (staphylococcal cells and latex particles) are so large that agglutination can be seen without the aid of magnification.

The most distinctive characteristic of these reagents is that they shorten the identification time over that of conventional extraction and capillary precipitation tests yet are equal in accuracy. These reagents can be used to detect streptococcal group antigens directly on cells in culture, in extracts, or from spent broth medium. To ensure accurate results, the package insert instructions that accompany each product should be strictly followed. These instructions are generally simple and often offer alternative procedures to ensure accurate identification. The slide agglutination tests have been used to identify beta-hemolytic colonies from primary throat culture blood agar plates. In some cases single colonies have been used (89), whereas other investigators have used four or five beta-hemolytic colonies per grouping reagent (10, 44, 90) or mixed flora (14). When these direct testing procedures fail to identify the beta-hemolytic colonies, 4-h and overnight broth cultures and culture supernatants have been used as antigens. Most of these reagents are of high quality, and the choice of which one to use is a matter of personal preference.

Identification of groups A and B by IF staining

Until the recent advances in direct antigen detection for group A and B streptococci from throat and vaginal swabs, IF had advantages over conventional identification techniques (70). These advantages included rapidity (several hours rather than several days), sensitivity (detection of small numbers of streptococci in mixed cultures), and detection of nonhemolytic group B streptococci (often missed with conventional techniques). The IF reagent, or conjugate, is composed of appropriate dilutions of anti-group carbohydrate immunoglobulin attached to fluorescein isothiocyanate. Nonspecific staining of *Staphylococcus aureus* or members of other streptococcal groups, which cannot be distinguished from group A streptococci morphologically, can be avoided by adding either unlabeled streptococcal group C antiserum or unlabeled nonimmune serum to the conjugate. The blocking of nonspecific staining is explained theoretically by the demonstrated nonimmune binding of unlabeled immunoglobulin (by the Fc portion) to staphylococcal protein A or certain streptococcal receptors (59), which can prevent the nonspecific binding of the IF reagent to these receptors (i.e., by the Fc portion of the conjugated antiserum).

The group B streptococcal IF procedure, described by Romero and Wilkinson (79), is less widely used because specific reagent is not commercially available. If all serotypes are to be stained, the group B conjugate must contain, in addition to unlabeled nonimmune serum (for the same reasons as stated above), both group B and type-specific fluorescein isothiocyanate-labeled antibodies. Specific group A and group B conjugates should not contain antibodies reactive with the several R-protein antigens found among many streptococcal groups. Detailed procedures for IF identification of group A and B streptococci are outlined in the previous edition of this Manual (27).

Identification of the beta-hemolytic streptococci by demonstrating that the strain possesses a group antigen is considered a definitive identification. Determination of the antigenic characteristic of the *Streptococcus* strain does not necessarily correlate with the *Streptococcus* species identification. Investigators have found that group C strains phenotypically resembling *S. dysgalactiae,* as well as *S. equisimilis* and groups G (large-colony form) and L, formed one DNA homology group (31, 52). This finding led to the proposal that this group of streptococci be referred to as *S. dysgalactiae. S. dysgalactiae* is an alpha-hemolytic strain and is rarely if ever found in human infections. The proposal that this group of strains be referred to as *S. dysgalactiae* did not consider the value of the serological group identification for clinicians. In our opinion, the identifications listed in Table 2 are of value to physicians in determining antibiotic therapies. We believe that these identifications should be considered as "working" species.

VP test. The Coblentz modification of the Voges-Proskauer (VP) test can be used to determine the production of acetylmethylcarbinol. The unknown strain is grown on an agar plate overnight at 35°C. With use of a swab, all of the growth on the plate is transferred to 2 ml of VP broth. The broth is incubated at 35°C for 6 h and then tested (reagents A and B are added). A positive reaction is indicated when a cherry red color develops within 30 min. The broth is vigorously shaken periodically during the 30-min period. Weak reactions (rust or pink colors) are interpreted as positive for streptococcal identification (33). Among the beta-hemolytic streptococci, only *S. anginosus* is positive.

PYR test. The PYR test is an excellent presumptive test for the identification of group A streptococci. It is more specific than and as sensitive as the bacitracin test for this purpose.

Carbohydrate fermentation test. The test for determining acid formation in various carbohydrate broths is described in chapter 121. Briefly, the carbohydrate broth is inoculated with a loopful of broth or several colonies from an agar plate. The carbohydrate broth is incubated at 35°C for up to 7 days. A positive reaction is recorded when the indicator turns yellow (if bromcresol purple is the indicator). Acid formation in broth containing trehalose or sorbitol is used to differentiate the beta-hemolytic group C streptococci (Table 2).

Identification of non-beta-hemolytic streptococci

The source of the clinical specimen determines the extent of the laboratory identification of non-beta-hemolytic streptococci. Since streptococci are ubiquitous, the non-beta-hemolytic strains are usually identified only if they are isolated from a normally sterile body fluid. However, some laboratories may identify some of the non-beta-hemolytic streptococci from nonsterile sources, e.g., *S. pneumoniae* from sputum. The tests

TABLE 2. Identification of beta-hemolytic streptococci

Species/group	Serological group	Test			
		VP	PYR	TRE	SORB
S. pyogenes	A	−	+	NA	NA
S. agalactiae	B	−	−	NA	NA
S. equi	C	−	−	−	−
S. equisimilis	C	−	−	+	−
S. zooepidemicus	C	−	−	−	+
Lancefield group G	G	−	−	NA	NA
S. anginosus[b]	A, C, F, G, or none	+	−	NA	NA

[a] VP, Voges-Proskauer; PYR, pyrrolidonyl arylamidase; TRE, trehalose; SORB, sorbitol; +, positive reaction; −, negative reaction; NA, not applicable.

[b] Some consider *S. milleri* a synonym for *S. anginosus*.

listed in Table 3 can be used to categorize the non-beta-hemolytic streptococci. It is not necessary to perform all of the tests for each strain in order to identify the isolate. Determining that an alpha-hemolytic streptococcus is susceptible to optochin is sufficient to identify presumptively the strain as a pneumococcus. A more confident identification that an optochin-susceptible, alpha-hemolytic streptococcus is a pneumococcus strain can be achieved by determining the bile solubility of the strain. Optochin-susceptible viridans streptococci are occasionally identified, but these strains are rarely if ever bile soluble.

To be certain that a strain is *S. bovis*, it should be demonstrated that the strain possesses the group D antigen and that the strain does not grow in 6.5% NaCl broth or is PYR negative. A presumptive identification can be achieved by demonstrating that the streptococcus strain is BE positive and does not grow in 6.5% NaCl broth or is PYR negative. This method will result in some erroneous identifications because some strains of viridans streptococci will have the same pattern of reactions. If precise identification of *S. bovis* is necessary, identification based on the presence of group D antigen, in addition to negative results on an NaCl tolerance or PYR test, must be demonstrated.

Ruoff et al. (81) have proposed a more elaborate scheme to identify *S. bovis* and its variant strain by physiological tests. Serological testing is not necessary with this procedure. In addition, two phenotypic strains of *S. bovis* can be identified by determining acid formation in mannitol and inulin, hydrolysis of starch and urea, and production of extracellular polysaccharide. The exact taxonomic status of *S. bovis*, *S. bovis* variant, and *S. equinus* is not certain. Three recent genetic studies have not resolved the different opinions on taxonomy or the exact phenotypic characteristics that will be useful for clinical microbiologists (19, 32, 57). The procedures proposed by Ruoff and colleagues are a satisfactory means of identifying the important clinical isolates of *S. bovis* (81, 83).

Some strains of group B streptococci are nonhemolytic. These strains possess the same potential for causing infections as do the beta-hemolytic strains. Therefore, it is not unusual to occasionally find a nonhemolytic group B streptococcus in clinical samples. If an unknown strain is shown by serological techniques to possess a group B antigen, this is considered a definitive identification. No other streptococci except *S. agalactiae* possess the group B antigen. Group B streptococci, nonhemolytic as well as beta-hemolytic strains, can be presumptively identified by the CAMP reaction. This test, described below, is also specific for the identification of group B streptococci if it is performed under controlled conditions.

The viridans streptococci are identified by exclusion; i.e., if all test results are negative (Table 3), the non-beta-hemolytic strain is a viridans streptococcus. Identification of the different viridans streptococcal species is discussed later.

The NVS can be identified either by demonstrating that the unknown strain requires pyridoxal or by performing the satellite test. Strains that fail to grow in broth or on agar (usually found in blood culture bottles) but that do grow when satellited or when pyridoxal is added to the medium are NVS. These strains, once thought to be variants of viridans streptococci, are now believed to be specific entities (8). Two species are proposed, *S. adjacens* and *S. defectivus;* differentiation of the two species is described in reference 8.

Optochin test. Suspect colonies (colonies with alpha-hemolytic zones and depressed centers) are streaked onto a quarter of a blood agar plate, and the optochin disk is placed in the upper third of the streaked area. The plate is incubated overnight at 35°C in a candle extinction jar or CO_2 incubator. Cultures do not grow as well in normal atmosphere, and larger zones of inhibition occur. If a 6-mm disk is used, a zone of inhibition of at least 14 mm in diameter is considered positive for pneumococci. A zone of inhibition of between 6 and 14 mm is questionable identification for pneumococci, and a strain is presumptively identified as a pneumococcus only if it is bile soluble. For 10-mm optochin disks, a zone of inhibition of at least 16 mm in diameter is positive, and strains with inhibition zones of between 10 and 16 mm should be tested for bile solubility.

Bile solubility test. The bile solubility test can be performed by making a saline suspension of cells from growth on an agar plate. A turbidity equal to that of a 0.5 to 1.0 McFarland density standard should be used. Place 0.5 ml of the suspension in each of two 13- by 100-mm test tubes. Add 0.5 ml of 2% sodium deoxycholate (bile) to one tube and 0.5 ml of saline to the other. Incubate the tubes at 35°C and examine them periodically for up to 2 h. A clearing of turbidity in the bile tube but not in the saline control tube indicates a positive result; i.e., the pneumococcal cells were lysed (solubilized).

The bile solubility test can be performed on cultures grown in broth as well, but caution should be used. Be sure to adjust the pH of the broth to 7.0 before adding the bile salts and saline suspensions. For broth cultures

TABLE 3. Identification of non-beta-hemolytic streptococci

Species/group	Test[a]							
	OPT	BS	BE	NaCl	PYR	SAT	CAMP	GRP
S. pneumoniae	+	+	−	−	−	−	−	−
S. bovis	−	−	+	−	−	−	−	D
S. agalactiae	−	−	−	±	−	−	+	B
Viridans streptococci	−	−	−[b]	−	−	−	−	−
Nutritionally variant streptococci	−	−	−	−	+	+	−	−

[a] OPT, Optochin; BS, bile solubility; BE, bile esculin; NaCl, 6.5% NaCl broth; PYR, pyrrolidonyl arylamidase; SAT, test for satellitism; CAMP, CAMP test; GRP, serogroup reaction; +, positive reaction; −, negative reaction.

[b] Occasional exception.

that have been incubated overnight, vortex the cultures, place 0.5 ml into two tubes, add an indicator, adjust the pH to 7.0 with 1 N NaOH, and proceed as described above for suspensions prepared from agar. Strains that are only partially lysed by this procedure either are mixed or the pH has not been properly adjusted.

BE test. The BE medium can be used in agar slants or agar plates. Inoculate the BE medium with one to three colonies and incubate it at 35°C in a normal atmosphere. Atmospheres with increased CO_2 will increase the number of viridans streptococci that give positive BE reactions; group D streptococci and the enterococci all grow well in atmospheres without increased CO_2. The BE test should be read after overnight incubation and after 48 h if the result is negative at 24 h. The BE test result is positive when a black color forms over one-half or more of the slant or when any blackening occurs on the agar plate. If no blackening occurs, the result is negative.

NaCl tolerance and PYR tests. The NaCl tolerance and PYR tests should be performed as previously described.

Satellitism test. To identify NVS strains, a test for satellitism can be easily performed. The unknown culture (from a source such as blood or other body fluid or from a strain that has grown poorly on chocolate agar) is streaked or smeared over the entire surface of a blood agar plate. A single streak of *Staphylococcus aureus* ATCC 25923 is made across the plate. The plate is incubated in a candle extinction jar or CO_2 incubator at 35°C for 24 h. If the NVS strain is not growing after that time, incubate the culture for another 24 h. Satellitism is demonstrated when growth of the NVS strain occurs only near the *Staphyloccus* streak, usually only 4 to 6 mm away from the streak.

An alternative procedure is to keep a stock solution of pyridoxal (0.01%) in the laboratory. The stock solution should be kept frozen. When needed, the pyridoxal can be added to the medium in (or on) which the NVS is to be grown. The final concentration of pyridoxal in the growth medium should be about 0.001%.

CAMP test. The CAMP test is used to identify presumptively group B streptococci. Two procedures are used to determine the CAMP reaction of streptococci: a conventional test in which a beta-lysin-producing *S. aureus* strain is used and a disk test in which a disk containing the staphylococcal beta-lysin is used. This test is performed on a sheep or bovine blood agar plate by making a single streak of the unknown *Streptococcus* strain perpendicular to, but not touching (3 to 4 mm apart), a streak of beta-lysin-producing *S. aureus* strain or the disk containing beta-lysin. Washed sheep RBCs that have been suspended in sterile physiological saline and TSA are recommended for the medium. Control strains of group A, B, C, and G streptococci should be used, especially when plates are obtained commercially.

The inoculated plates should be incubated in a candle extinction jar or in normal atmosphere but not anaerobically. Some group A streptococci are CAMP positive when incubated in the candle extinction jar, and even more strains are positive when incubated anaerobically. Group B streptococci produce a substance (CAMP factor) that enlarges the zone of lysis produced by the *Staphylococcus* beta-lysin to form a typical arrowhead or flame-shaped clearing at the juncture of the two organisms or a crescent-shaped clearing at the juncture of the beta-lysin-containing disk and the group B streptococci. PYR-negative, beta- or nonhemolytic streptococci can be reported as presumptive group B streptococci by a positive CAMP reaction (30).

Antigen testing. Testing the non-beta-hemolytic streptococci for group D and B antigens is performed as described above for determining the antigenic characteristics of the beta-hemolytic streptococci.

Identification of viridans streptococci

Perhaps no group of gram-positive cocci is more difficult to identify to the species level than the viridans streptococci. Recent genetic studies have not resolved this situation and, in fact, may have made the classification of this group confusing. Coykendall (18) confirmed this observation in a recent review of the status of DNA homology experiments as related to phenotypic identification by laboratory tests. Future studies in which genetic probes are used may resolve much of the confusion. Meanwhile, we cannot offer much hope for the clinical microbiologist who is asked to identify a viridans streptococcus to the species level. The wisest decision would be to avoid this type of identification altogether. If identification must be carried out, the tests listed in Table 4 can be used to place the strains to a species/group. The five species/groups listed in Table 4 include all of the strains commonly isolated from human infections. In most cases, there is more than one genospecies within each species/group. However, identification of the viridans streptococci to this level

TABLE 4. Identification of viridans streptococci

Species/group	Test[a]					
	MAN	SORB	VP	ARG	ESC	URE
S. mutans (includes *S. cricetus, S. downei, S. ferus, S. macace, S. rattus* [ARG+], *S. sobrinus*)	+	+	+	−	+	−
S. salivarius (includes *S. intestinalis, S. vestibularius*)	−	−	+	−	+	±
S. sanguis (includes *S. gordonii*, group H and W streptococci)	−	−[b]	−	+	+	−
S. mitis (includes *S. mitior, S. oralis, S. sanguis* biotype II)	−	−	−	−	−	−
S. anginosus (includes *S. intermedius, S. constellatus, S. milleri*, DNA groups I and III)	−[b]	−[b]	+[b]	+	+	−

[a] MAN, Mannitol; SORB, sorbitol; VP, Voges-Proskauer; ARG, arginine; ESC, esculin; URE, urease; +, positive reaction; −, negative reaction; ±, some strains positive, other strains negative.

[b] Occasional exception.

should provide enough information to physicians to aid in treating patients.

As previously mentioned, the viridans streptococci are identified by exclusion. The viridans streptococci yield negative reactions in most tests designed to identify the genus. They are gram-positive cocci, are not beta-hemolytic, are bile insoluble (most are also optochin negative), do not have group B or D antigen, do not tolerate 6.5% NaCl, are PYR negative, and do not grow at 10°C; most are BE negative and fail to grow at 45°C. All are susceptible to vancomyin and fail to produce gas in MRS broth. When these characteristics are known, the microbiologist can proceed to differentiate the species/group by using the tests listed in Table 4.

S. mutans species/group represents a collection of seven genospecies (18). These strains are characterized by the capacity to form acid in nearly all carbohydrate broths, including mannitol and sorbitol broths. Among the viridans streptococci, this property is unique to the *S. mutans* strains. Most *S. mutans* strains require atmospheres with increased CO_2 for growth on blood agar plates, and when the growth is Gram stained from solid medium, the cells appear rodlike rather than coccal. The procedures outline in references 18 and 103 can be used to differentiate the genospecies of *S. mutans*.

S. salivarius species/group represents at least three genospecies. *S. intestinalis* has not been documented from humans, but *S. vestibularius* has been isolated from the oral cavity (102). The three species have several characteristics in common. The majority of strains hydrolyze urea, and they are the only streptococci to do so. *S. salivarius* is often misidentified as *S. bovis* because 10 to 20% of the true *S. salivarius* strains give positive BE reactions. The morphology of *S. salivarius* on blood agar medium also resembles that of *S. bovis*, since the colonies are large and no hemolysis is present. In contrast, the morphology of *S. vestibularis* and *S. intestinalis* is characterized by colonies that are small, similar to *S. mitis* colonies, and surrounded by an alpha-hemolytic zone on blood agar medium. Procedures for differentiation of the three species have not been developed.

S. sanguis species/group contains at least two genospecies (18, 51). Group H strains are genetically and phenotyptically identical to *S. sanguis*. Group W strains have not been genetically tested, but phenotypically they closely resemble *S. sanguis*. The description of *S. gordonii* has not been published (18); thus, differentiation of the genospecies is not possible at this time. The colonies of *S. sanguis* are small and surrounded by an alpha-hemolytic zone on blood agar medium.

S. mitis species/group contains at least two genospecies. Most strains phenotypically identified as *S. mitis* are genetically identical to *S. mitior* and *S. oralis* (54). Strains previously identified as *S. sanguis* biotype II also genetically join this group (88). Additional confusion regarding the identification of *S. mitis* is due to an erroneously identified type strain (NCTC 3165), which phenotypically resembles *S. sanguis*. This error has led to the suggestion to reject NCTC 3165 as the type strain for *S. mitis* and accept the type strain for *S. oralis* (NCTC 11427) as the type strain. Since *S. oralis* is genetically identical to *S. mitis*, there would no longer be a need for the term *S. oralis* (18). *S. mitis* strains are identified by exclusion; the strains are negative in all tests listed in Table 4. The colonies of *S. mitis* are small and surrounded by a zone of alpha-hemolysis on blood agar plates. Strains of *S. mitis* grow better in CO_2-enriched incubation atmospheres.

No group of streptococcal strains has caused greater consternation than the species/group *S. anginosus*. At least five genospecies have been identified by two groups of investigators (55, 58). Two genospecies include beta-hemolytic varieties, *S. anginosus* and *S. constellatus* (*S. milleri* is genetically homologous to *S. constellatus*) (55). Genetic groups *S. intermedius*, homology group I, and homology group III do not include beta-hemolytic strains (58). Two other groups of investigators concluded that all strains of *S. anginosus* formed one homology group (20, 101). From these results, we can conclude that much needs to be done to clarify the current classification.

It is not clear how all five genospecies can be identified by using conventional tests. A positive reaction in VP, arginine, and esculin tests is unique to *S. anginosus* species/group. However, VP-negative strains (DNA group III) exist and may be misidentified as *S. sanguis* by the procedures outlined in Table 4. Most strains of *S. sanguis* form acid in inulin broth and produce extracellular polysaccharide on 5% sucrose agar, whereas the *S. anginosus* species/group strains do not. These tests should be incorporated into any scheme designed to categorize the viridans streptococci more than presumptively; the scheme outlined in Table 4 provides only a presumptive categorization.

Acid formation. Acid formation in mannitol and sorbitol broths and VP reaction are determined as described for acid formation for determining the species of group C streptococci. In tests for acid formation, the cultures should be incubated at 35°C for up to 7 days.

Arginine deamination. Deamination of arginine is determined in Moeller decarboxylase medium. The medium is inoculated with a fresh culture and is then overlaid with sterile mineral oil and incubated at 35°C for up to 7 days. A positive reaction is recorded when the indicator turns a deep purple, indicating an alkaline reaction. A yellow color or no color change indicates a negative reaction.

Esculin hydrolysis. Hydrolysis of esculin is determined on esculin agar slants. The medium is inoculated with a fresh culture and incubated at 35°C for up to 7 days. A positive reaction is recorded when the medium turns black. No change in the color of the agar indicates a negative reaction.

Urea hydrolysis. Hydrolysis of urea is determined on Christensen urea agar slants. The medium is inoculated and incubated in the same manner as the esculin slant. A positive reaction is recorded when a light or dark pink color develops in the agar slant. No change in color or a yellow color is a negative reaction.

Identification of *Enterococcus* species

The genus *Enterococcus* was established in 1984 (85). At that time only two species were included in the genus, *E. faecalis* and *E. faecium*. Several of the other streptococcal species informally termed enterococci, *S. durans*, *S. faecium* var. *S. casseliflavus*, and *S. avium*, as well as new species, have since been added (28, 86). There are now 12 *Enterococcus* species, and all but 2 have been isolated from human infections (28).

All members of the genus *Enterococcus* are PYR and LAP positive, tolerate 6.5% NaCl broth, are BE positive, grow at 10 and 45°C, and do not form gas from glucose (in MRS broth). Most strains are susceptible to vancomycin, and most have group D antigen.

Once it is established that the unknown isolate is an *Enterococcus* strain, the tests listed in Table 5 can be used to identify the species. It is best to separate the species into three groups on the bases of (i) acid formation in mannitol, sorbitol, and sorbose broths and (ii) hydrolysis of arginine. Group I species, *E. avium, E. malodoratus, E. raffinosus,* and *E. pseudoavium,* form acid in all three of the aforementioned carbohydrate broths but do not hydrolyze arginine. Group II species, *E. faecalis, E. solitarius, E. faecium, E. casseliflavus, E. mundtii,* and *E. gallinarum,* form acid in mannitol broth and hydrolyze arginine but fail to form acid in sorbose broth and give variable reactions in sorbitol broth. Group III species, *E. durans, E. hirae,* and *E. faecalis* variant, hydrolyze arginine but do not form acid in either carbohydrate broth.

The species within each group are then identified by specific reactions. The species in group I are identified by the reactions in arabinose and raffinose broths (Table 5). In group II, *E. faecalis* is the only member to tolerate tellurite and utilize pyruvate, and *E. solitarius* reacts negatively in both of these tests but similarly to *E. faecalis* in all other tests. *E. faecium* and *E. gallinarum* also have similar characteristics but can be differentiated by the motility test. *E. gallinarum* is motile, but *E. faecium* is not. *E. casseliflavus* and *E. mundtii* are pigmented (yellow) and similar in other characteristics as well; however, *E. casseliflavus* is motile, but *E. mundtii* is not. The members of group III are easily identified by their reactions in the pyruvate, raffinose, and sucrose tests. *E. durans* gives a negative reaction in all tests. *E. hirae* strains react positively in one or both raffinose and sucrose tests and negatively in the pyruvate test, and the *E. faecalis* variant strain is positive in the test for pyruvate utilization but not in that for acid formation in raffinose or sucrose broth (Table 5).

The majority of clinical isolates of enterococci will be *E. faecalis* (80 to 90%) and *E. faecium* (5 to 10%). *E. avium, E. raffinosus,* and *E. gallinarum* will be found infrequently, but clusters of infections with *E. raffinosus* have been reported. *E. solitarius, E. casseliflavus, E. mundtii, E. durans, E. hirae,* and *E. faecalis* variant strains have only rarely been isolated from human sources (28). *E. malodoratus* and *E. pseudoavium* have not been isolated from human infections.

Arginine hydrolysis and acid formation. The tests for arginine hydrolysis and acid formation in mannitol and sorbitol have been described previously. Acid formation in arabinose, raffinose, sorbose, and sucrose is determined as described for acid formation in trehalose.

Tellurite tolerance. Tolerance to tellurite is determined on agar medium containing 0.04% potassium tellurite. The agar may be contained in a tube or plate. The medium is inoculated with a fresh culture of the enterococcal strain and incubated at 35°C for up to 7 days. Tolerance (positive result) is indicated whenever black colonies form on the surface. *E. faecalis* and *E. faecalis* variant strains are usually positive after 2 days. Some *E. faecium* strains may form gray colonies; this should be read as a negative result.

Motility. Motility is determined in conventional motility medium (see chapter 121). The medium is inoculated with a single stab about 1 inch (2.54 cm) into the medium. The inoculated tube is incubated at 30°C for 2 days. Motility is indicated by the spread of growth to the bottom and sides of the tube. Growth along and slightly away from the stab indicates negative motility.

Pigmentation. Pigmentation is determined by examining a swab that has been smeared across growth on a TSA 5% sheep blood agar plate that has been incubated at 35°C for 24 h. Pigmentation is indicated by a yellow color of the growth. A cream, white, or gray color does not indicate pigmentation.

Pyruvate utilization. A fresh culture is used to inoculate a tube of pyruvate broth. The inoculated broth is incubated at 35°C for up to 7 days. A positive reaction is indicated by the development of a yellow color. If the broth remains green or greenish yellow, the test result is negative. A yellow color with a hint of green is usually a positive reaction. This latter reaction may be observed with some strains of *E. faecalis* and *E. faecalis* variant.

Identification by kits, aids, and devices

Have the changes in taxonomy of the genus *Streptococcus*, i.e., splitting the genus into three genera, *Strep-*

TABLE 5. Identification of *Enterococcus* species

Species	Test[a]										
	MAN	SORB	SOR	ARG	ARA	RAF	TEL	MOT	PIG	SUC	PYU
E. avium	+	+	+	−	+	−	−	−	−	+	+
E. malodoratus	+	+	+	−	−	+	−	−	−	+	+
E. raffinosus	+	+	+	−	+	+	−	−	−	+	+
E. pseudoavium	+	+	+	−	−	−	−	−	−	+	+
E. faecalis	+	+	−	+	−	−	+	−	−	+[b]	+
E. solitarius	+	+	−	+	−	−	−	−	−	+[b]	−
E. faecium	+	−[b]	−	+	+	−[b]	−	−	−	+[b]	−
E. casseliflavus	+	−[b]	−	+	−	+	−[b]	+	+	+	−[b]
E. mundtii	+	−[b]	−	+	−	+	−	−	+	+	−
E. gallinarum	+	−	−	+	+	+	−	+	−	+	−
E. durans	−	−	−	+	−	−	−	−	−	−	−
E. hirae	−	−	−	+	−	±	−	−	−	±	−
E. faecalis (variant)	−	−	−	+	−	−	+	−	−	−	±

[a] MAN, Mannitol; SORB, sorbitol; SOR, sorbose; ARG, arginine; ARA, arabinose; RAF, raffinose; TEL, 0.04% tellurite; MOT, motility; PIG, pigmentation; SUC, sucrose; PYU, pyruvate; +, >90% positive; −, <10% positive; ±, 60 to 90% positive.

[b] Occasional exception (≤5% of strains show aberrant reactions).

tococcus, *Enterococcus*, and *Lactococcus*, and the establishment of new species within some genera, affected the accuracy of identification of these bacteria by the rapid identification systems (e.g., Rapid Strep, API 20S, and RapID STR) or automated identification systems (e.g., AutoMicrobic Gram-Positive and MicroScan Gram Positive)? The answer to this question is not clear. In all probability, the identification of *E. faecalis* will be as correct as it was for *S. faecalis*, since the description of the species did not change; however, the identification of the remaining *Enterococcus* species by these systems is questionable. For example, *E. raffinosus* was split from *S. avium*, and *E. gallinarum* is separated from *E. faecium* only by motility. In all probability, *E. raffinosus* and *E. avium* would be identified as *S. avium*, and *E. gallinarum* and *E. faecium* would both be identified as *S. faecium* by these identification systems. Similar problems exist with the remaining enterococci.

The suggested changes in the procedures for identifying the viridans streptococcal species will require considerable changes in the data banks and decoding manuals by the commercial companies. It may be several years before the problems concerning classification and identification procedures for the viridans streptococci are resolved. The value of the kits, aids, and devices was questionable before the changes in the taxonomy of the viridans streptococci; these changes have not improved the likelihood of correct identification of these species with the current formats of the kits, aids, and devices.

Identification of *S. bovis* by these systems should be as correct as it was before the changes in taxonomy were made.

Identification of *Lactococcus* species

The transfer of the species of lactic streptococci (group N) to the genus *Lactococcus* was made in 1985 (87). The species included in this genus are thought to be nonpathogenic for humans. In fact, *L. lactis* (*S. lactis*) and *L. cremoris* (*S. cremoris*) are used in the dairy industries and are included in foodstuffs. We have isolated several strains of lactococci from human sources, but we have not established the clinical significance of these strains (29). These strains can be identified to the genus level by the tests listed in Table 1. The majority of lactococci that we have identified have resembled the enterococci in presumptive tests (BE, NaCl, and PYR). They differ from the enterococci by failing to grow at 45°C.

Identification of *Gemella* species

Streptococcus morbillorum has been transfered to the genus *Gemella*. (53). *G. morbillorum* and *G. haemolysans* make up the entire genus. The two species can be differentiated by the tests listed in Table 6. The acid formation tests using mannitol and sorbitol should be performed as described previously; however, the incubation period may have to be longer (up to 10 to 14 days). The inoculum for the PYR test may have to be taken from an entire blood agar plate or from a blood agar plate that has been incubated for 48 h at 35°C. A more detailed description of the two species is given in reference 5. Because of the slow growth on blood agar plates by the *Gemella* species, these strains may be confused with the NVS. In such cases, it is necessary to

TABLE 6. Identification of *Gemella* species

Species	Test[a]			Cellular arrangement in Gram stain
	PYR	MAN	SORB	
G. haemolysans	+	−	−	Pairs, tetrads, clusters
G. morbillorum	+w	+w	+w	Pairs, short chains

[a] PYR, Pyrrolidonyl arylamidase; MAN, mannitol; SORB, sorbitol; +, positive reaction; −, negative reaction; +w, weak positive reactions.

perform the satellitism test to confirm the identity of NVS.

Most strains that are identified by the characteristics listed in Tables 1 and 6 as gemellas would have been identified as *S. morbillorum* by previously recommended procedures (25, 27). Both *G. morbillorum* and *G. haemolysans* have been isolated from human sources and associated with infections, including endocarditis (13, 27).

Identification of *Aerococcus* species

The genus *Aerococcus* currently contains only one species, *A. viridans;* thus, identification of an unknown isolate as an *Aerococcus* strain constitutes complete identification. The aerococci resemble the enterococci in that growth in 6.5% NaCl broth and positive PYR tests are universal characteristics of both; in addition, some of the aerococcal strains are BE positive, which also is a characteristic of enterococci. However, aerococci do not grow at 10 or 45°C, which differentiates them from the enterococci. An independently packaged leucine aminopeptidase would be of considerable help in identifying the aerococci. All streptococci and enterococci are LAP positive, whereas the aerococci are LAP negative.

Identification of *Pediococcus* species

Identification of the pediococci is accomplished by demonstrating that the unknown strain is vancomycin resistant, is PYR negative, and does not form gas from glucose in MRS broth (Table 1). Only two species of pediococci have been isolated from humans, *P. acidilactici* and *P. pentosaceus* (29). Identification of the species is accomplished by performing the tests listed in Table 7. *P. pentosaceus* forms acid in maltose and arabinose broths, whereas *P. acidilactici* does not. All strains of pediococci isolated from humans have been BE and arginine positive, and most have demonstrated

TABLE 7. Identification of *Pediococcus* species[a]

Species	Test[b]				
	MAL	ARA	STR	SUC	NaCl
P. acidilactici	−	−	−	−	+
P. pentosaceus	+	+	−	−	+
P. damnosus	+	−	−	+	−
P. dextrinicus	+	−	+	+	−
P. urinequi	+	−	−	+	+
P. parvulus	−	−	−	−	+

[a] *P. halophilus* is not a pediococcus.
[b] MAL, Maltose; ARA, arabinose; STR, starch; SUC, sucrose; NaCl, 6.5% NaCl broth; +, positive reaction; −, negative reaction.

TABLE 8. Identification of *Leuconostoc* species

Species	Test[a]							
	ESC	LM	RAF	MEL	NaCl	ARA	TRE	5%SUC
L. citreum	+	−	−	−	±	+	+	+
L. lactis	−	+	+	+	−	−	−	−
L. mesenteroides	+	−[b]	+	+	+[b]	+	+	+
L. pseudomesenteroides	+	+	+[b]	+	−	+	+	+
L. paramesenteroides	+	?	+	+	+	+	+	−
L. cremoris	−	?	−	−	−	−	−	−
L. dextranicus	+	?	+	+	−	−	+	−

[a] ESC, Hydrolysis of esculin; LM, acid and clot in litmus milk; RAF, raffinose; MEL, melibiose; NaCl, 6.5% NaCl broth; ARA, arabinose; TRE, trehalose; 5%SUC, extracellular polysaccharide (slime) production; +, positive reaction; −, negative reaction; ?, unknown.

[b] Occasional exception.

group D antigen in Lancefield extracts. All strains have failed to form acid in lactose broth, and most have grown very slowly if at all in NaCl broth. These reactions led us to identify the strains as *Streptococcus constellatus* or *Streptococcus equinus* by previous methods. Incorporating the vancomycin screening test and including type strains of *Pediococcus* in the quality controls of our identification schemes have corrected these potential errors.

Acid formation and NaCl tests. Acid formation in maltose is determined as described for other carbohydrate broths. The NaCl test has been previously described.

Starch hydrolysis. Hydrolysis of starch is demonstrated by inoculating a starch agar plate with a single heavy streak of a fresh culture. The plate is placed in a candle extinction jar or CO_2 incubator at 35°C for 48 h. The plate is flooded with Gram iodine after incubation. A clear zone surrounding the growth indicates a positive result; i.e., the strain has hydrolyzed the starch. A deep purple to black or bluish color of the agar indicates that starch has not been hydrolyzed, and thus the result is negative. For negative results, the deep color develops in the agar right up to the growth.

Identification of *Leuconostoc* species

Identification of the leuconostocs is accomplished by demonstrating that the strains are vancomycin resistant, are PYR and LAP negative, and form gas from glucose in MRS broth (Table 1). Four species have been isolated from humans (29). The reactions listed in Table 8 can be used to identify the species. *L. citreum* hydrolyzes esculin, produces slime on 5% sucrose agar, and does not form acid in raffinose or melibiose broth. *L. lactis* does not hydrolyze esculin, does not form slime on 5% sucrose agar, but does form acid in raffinose and melibiose broths. This strain resembles *S. sanguis* biotype II phenotypically, with the exceptions of vancomycin susceptibility and production of gas from glucose in MRS broth. Both *L. mesenteroides* and *L. pseudomesenteroides* hydrolyze esculin, form slime on 5% sucrose agar, and form acid in raffinose and melibiose broths. The latter two species are differentiated by their tolerance to NaCl and reaction in litmus milk. *L. mesenteroides* grows in NaCl broth and does not form acid or clot in litmus milk. *L. pseudomesenteroides* gives the opposite reactions. *L. cremoris, L. dextranicus,* and *L. paramesenteroides* have not been isolated from human infections.

Litmus milk. Tubes containing litmus milk are inoculated with a fresh culture and incubated at 35°C for 7 days. The tubes are inspected for color change (from light blue to pink to white) and for clot solidification of the tube contents. A positive reaction is indicated by a white color and by partial or complete solidification of the tube contents. A negative reaction is indicated by no color change or a pink color and no solidification.

Acid formation. Acidification of raffinose, melibiose, arabinose, and trehalose is determined as previously described.

Slime formation on 5% sucrose agar. Production of slime on 5% sucrose agar is detected by inoculating 5% sucrose agar with a fresh culture and incubating the agar plate in a candle extinction jar or a CO_2 incubator at 35°C for 48 h. A positive reaction is shown by the production of extracellular slime, indicated by large amounts of mucoidal runny material or large "gumdrop" colonies. The capsular-like material appears similar to that produced by the *S. bovis* biotype I colonies. The reaction is considered negative if extracellular material is not apparent on the 5% sucrose agar by visual inspection.

It is difficult to judge the importance of identifying either the *Leuconotoc* or *Pediococcus* species. Very little information is available regarding the clinical significance of the different species of either genus. However, it is important to identify the genera because the antibiotic susceptibilities of these strains are different from those of the bacteria that they may be confused with, such as *Enterococcus* and *Streptococcus* species.

LITERATURE CITED

1. **Alexander, J. B., and G. P. Giacoia.** 1978. Early onset nonenterococcal group D streptococcal infection in the newborn infant. J. Pediatr. **93:**489–490.
2. **Arditi, M., S. T. Shulman, and A. T. Davis.** 1989. Group C β-hemolytic streptococcal infections in children: nine pediatric cases and review. Rev. Infect. Dis. **11:**34–45.
3. **Austrian, R.** 1976. The Quellung reaction, a neglected microbiologic technique. Mount Sinai J. Med. **43:**699–703.
4. **Bayer, A. S., A. W. Chow, B. F. Anthony, and L. B. Guze.** 1976. Serious infections in adults due to group B streptococci: clinical and serotypic characteristics. Am. J. Med. **61:**498–503.
5. **Berger, U., and A. Pervanidis.** 1986. Differentiation of *Gemella haemolysans* (Thjotta and Boe 1938) Berger 1960, from *Streptococcus morbillorum* (Prevot 1933)

Holdeman and Moore 1974. Zentralbl. Parasitenkd. Infektionskr. Bakteriol. Hyg. 1 Orig. Reihe A **261:**311–321.

6. **Black, W. A., and F. Van Buskirk.** 1973. Gentamicin blood agar as a general-purpose selective medium. Appl. Microbiol. **25:**905–907.
7. **Bourgault, A. M., W. R. Wilson, and J. A. Washington II.** 1979. Antimicrobial susceptibility of species of viridans streptococci. J. Infect. Dis. **140:**316–321.
8. **Bouvet, A., F. Grimont, P. A. D. Grimont.** 1989. *Streptococcus defectivus* sp. nov. and *Streptococcus adjacens* sp. nov., nutritionally variant streptococci from human clinical specimens. Int. J. Syst. Bacteriol. **39:**290–294.
9. **Brady, K., P. Duff, J. C. Schilhab, and M. Herd.** 1989. Reliability of a rapid latex fixation test for detecting group B streptococci in the genital tract of parturients at term. Obstet. Gynecol. **73:**678–681.

9a. **Brown, J. H.** 1919. The use of blood agar for the study of streptococci. Monograph no. 9. Rockefeller Institute for Medical Research.

10. **Burdash, N. M., N. E. West, R. T. Newell, and G. Teti.** 1981. Group identification of streptococci. Evaluation of three rapid agglutination methods. Am. J. Clin. Pathol. **76:**819–822.
11. **Bush, L. M., J. Calmon, C. L. Cherney, M. Wendeler, P. Pitsakis, J. Poupard, M. Levison, and C. C. Johnson.** 1989. High level penicillin resistance among isolates of enterococci: implications for treatment of enterococcal infections. Ann. Intern. Med. **110:**515–520.
12. **Buu-Hoi, A., C. LeBouguenec, and T. Houraud.** 1989. Genetic basis of antibiotic resistance in *Aerococcus viridans*. Antimicrob. Agents Chemother. **33:**529–534.
13. **Buu-Hoi, A., A. Sapoetra, C. Branger, and J. F. Acar.** 1982. Antimicrobial susceptibility of *Gemella haemolysans* isolated from patients with subacute endocarditis. Eur. J. Clin. Microbiol. **1:**101–106.
14. **Castle, D., S. Dessock-Philp, and C. S. F. Easmon.** 1982. Evaluation of an improved Streptex kit for the grouping of beta-haemolytic streptococci by agglutination. J. Clin. Pathol. **35:**819–822.
15. **Catto, B. A., M. R. Jacobs, and D. M. Shlaes.** 1987. *Streptococcus mitis:* a cause of serious infection in adults. Arch. Intern. Med. **147:**885–888.
16. **Cimolai, N., R. W. Elford, L. Bryan, C. Anand, and P. Berger.** 1988. Do the β-hemolytic non-group A streptococci cause pharyngitis? Rev. Infect. Dis. **10:**587–601.
17. **Converse, G. M., and H. C. Dillon.** 1977. Epidemiological studies of *Streptococcus pneumoniae* in infants. Methods of isolating pneumococci. J. Clin. Microbiol. **5:**293–296.
18. **Coykendall, A. L.** 1989. Classification and identification of the viridans streptococci. Clin. Microbiol. Rev. **2:**315–328.
19. **Coykendall, A. L., and K. B. Gustafson.** 1985. Deoxyribonucleic acid hybridizations among strains of *Streptococcus salivarius* and *Streptococcus bovis*. Int. J. Syst. Bacteriol. **35:**274–280.
20. **Coykendall, A. L., P. M. Wesbecher, and K. B. Gustafson.** 1987. *"Streptococcus milleri," Streptococcus constellatus*, and *Streptococcus intermedius* are later synonyms of *Streptococcus anginosus*. Int. J. Syst. Bacteriol. **37:**222–228.
21. **Dashefsky, B., E. R. Wald, and M. Green.** 1988. Prevention of early-onset group B streptococcal sepsis. J. Pediatr. **112:**1039–1042.
22. **Dayton, S. L., D. D. Chips, D. Blasi, and R. F. Smith.** 1974. Evaluation of three media for selective isolation of gram-positive bacteria from wounds. Appl. Microbiol. **27:** 420–422.
23. **Dykstra, M. A., J. C. McLaughlin, and R. C. Bartlett.** 1979. Comparison of media and techniques for detection of group A streptococci in throat swab specimens. J. Clin. Microbiol. **9:**236–238.
24. **Ellner, P. D., C. J. Stoessel, E. Drakeford, and F. Vasi.** 1966. A new culture medium for medical microbiology. Am. J. Clin. Pathol. **45:**502–504.
25. **Facklam, R. R.** 1977. Physiological differentiation of viridans streptococci. J. Clin. Microbiol. **5:**184–201.
26. **Facklam, R. R.** 1987. Specificity study of kits for detection of group A streptococci directly from throat swabs. J. Clin. Microbiol. **25:**504–508.
27. **Facklam, R. R., and R. B. Carey.** 1985. Streptococci and aerococci, p. 154–175. *In* E. H. Lennette, A. Balows, W. J. Hausler, Jr., and H. J. Shadomy (ed.), Manual of microbiology, 4th ed. American Society for Microbiology, Washington, D.C.
28. **Facklam, R. R., and M. D. Collins.** 1989. Identification of *Enterococcus* species isolated from human infections by a conventional test scheme. J. Clin. Microbiol. **27:**731–734.
29. **Facklam, R. R., D. Hollis, and M. D. Collins.** 1989. Identification of gram-positive coccal and coccobacillary vancomycin-resistant bacteria. J. Clin. Microbiol. **27:**724–730.
30. **Facklam, R. R., J. F. Padula, E. C. Wortham, R. C. Cooksey, and H. A. Rountree.** 1979. Presumptive identification of group A, B, and D streptococci on agar plate media. J. Clin. Microbiol. **9:**655–672.
31. **Farrow, J. A. E., and M. D. Collins.** 1984. Taxonomic studies on streptococci of serological groups C, G, and L and possibly related taxa. Syst. Appl. Microbiol. **5:**483–493.
32. **Farrow, J. A. E., J. Kruze, B. A. Phillips, A. J. Bramley, and M. D. Collins.** 1984. Taxonomic studies on *Streptococcus bovis* and *Streptococcus equinus:* description of *Streptococcus alactolyticus* sp. nov. and *Streptococcus saccharolyticus* sp. nov. Syst. Appl. Microbiol. **5:**467–482.
33. **Fertally, S. S., and R. Facklam.** 1987. Comparison of physiologic tests used to identify non-beta-hemolytic aerococci, enterococci, and streptococci. J. Clin. Microbiol. **25:**1845–1850.
34. **Fischel, K. D., and M. H. Weisman.** 1985. Unique features of group B streptococcal arthritis in adults. Arch. Intern. Med. **145:**97–102.
35. **Gallagher, P. G., and I. C. Watanakunakorn.** 1986. Group B streptococcal endocarditis: report of seven cases and review of the literature, 1982–1985. Rev. Infect. Dis. **8:**175–188.
36. **Gaudreau, C., J. Delage, D. Rousseau, and E. D. Cantor.** 1981. Bacteremia caused by viridans streptococci in 71 children. J. Can. Med. Assoc. **125:**1246–1249.
37. **Gaunt, P. N., and D. V. Seal.** 1987. Group G streptococcal infections. J. Infect. **15:**5–20.
38. **Goldfarb, J., G. P. Wormser, and J. H. Glaser.** 1984. Meningitis caused by multiple antibiotic resistant viridans streptococci. J. Pediatr. **105:**891–895.
39. **Gordon, D. B., P. C. DeGirolami, S. Bolivar, G. Karafotias, and K. Eichelberger.** 1988. A comparison of the identification of group A streptococci and enterococci by two rapid pyrrolidonyl aminopeptidase methods. Am. J. Clin. Pathol. **90:**210–212.
40. **Gossling, J.** 1988. Occurrence and pathogenicity of the *Streptococcus milleri* group. Rev. Infect. Dis. **10:**257–266.
41. **Gray, B. M., M. A. Pass, and H. C. Dillon, Jr.** 1979. Laboratory and field evaluation of selective media for isolation of group B streptococci. J. Clin. Microbiol. **9:**466–470.
42. **Gullberg, R. M., S. R. H. Gomann, and J. Phair.** 1989. Enterococcal bacteremia: an analysis of 75 episodes. Rev. Infect. Dis. **11:**74–85.
43. **Gunn, B. A., K. K. Ohashi, D. A. Gaydes, and E. S. Holt.** 1977. Selective and enhanced recovery of group A and B streptococci from throat cultures with sheep blood agar containing sulfamethoxazole and trimethoprim. J. Clin. Microbiol. **5:**650–655.
44. **Hamilton, J. R.** 1988. Comparison of Meritec-Strep with Streptex for direct colony grouping of beta-hemolytic streptococci from primary isolation and subculture

plates. J. Clin. Microbiol. **26:**692–695.

45. **Handwerger, S., and A. Tomasz.** 1985. Antibiotic tolerance among clinical isolates of bacteria. Rev. Infect. Dis. **7:**368–386.
46. **Holmberg, K., and H. O. Hallander.** 1973. Production of bactericidal concentrations of hydrogen peroxide by *Streptococcus sanguis*. Arch. Oral Biol. **18:**423–434.
47. **Huovinen, P., R. Lahtonen, T. Ziegler, O. Meurmanh, K. Hakkarainen, A. Mettinen, P. Arstila, J. Eckola, and P. Saikku.** 1989. Pharyngitis in adults: the presence and coexistence of viruses and bacterial organisms. Ann. Intern. Med. **110:**612–616.
48. **Jones, D. E., K. S. Kanarek, J. L. Angel, and D. V. Lim.** 1983. Elimination of multiple reactions of the Phadebact *Streptococcus* coagglutination test. J. Clin. Microbiol. **18:** 526–528.
49. **Kellogg, J. A., and J. P. Manzella.** 1986. Detection of group A streptococci in the laboratory or physician's office culture vs antibody methods. J. Am. Med. Assoc. **255:** 2638–2642.
50. **Kiddy, K., P. P. Brown, J. Michael, and D. Adu.** 1985. Peritonitis due to *Streptococcus viridans* in patients receiving continuous ambulatory peritoneal dialysis. Br. Med. J. **290:**969–970.
51. **Kilian, M., B. Nyvad, and L. Mikkelsen.** 1986. Taxonomic and ecological aspects of some oral streptococci, p. 391–400. *In* S. Hamada et al. (ed.), Molecular microbiology and immunobiology of *Streptococcus mutans*. Elsvier Science Publishers BV, Amsterdam.
52. **Kilpper-Bälz, R., and K. H. Schleifer.** 1984. Nucleic acid hybridization and cell wall composition studies of pyogenic streptococci. FEMS Microbiol. Lett. **24:**355–364.
53. **Kilpper-Bälz, R., and K. H. Schleifer.** 1988. Transfer of *Streptococcus morbillorum* to the *Gemella* genus, *Gemella morbillorum* comb. nov. Int. J. Syst. Bacteriol. **38:**442–443.
54. **Kilpper-Bälz, R., P. Wenzig, and K. H. Schleifer.** 1985. Molecular relationships and classification of some viridans streptococci as *Streptococcus oralis* and amended description of *Streptococcus oralis* (Bridge and Sneath 1982). Int. J. Syst. Bacteriol. **35:**482–488.
55. **Kilpper-Bälz, R., B. L. Williams, R. Lutticken, and K. H. Schleifer.** 1984. Relatedness of "*Streptococcus milleri*" with *Streptococcus anginosus* and *Streptococcus constellatus*. Syst. Appl. Microbiol. **5:**494–500.
56. **Kim, K. S., and B. F. Anthony.** 1981. Penicillin tolerance in group B streptococci isolated from infected neonates. J. Infect. Dis. **144:**411–419.
57. **Knight, R. G., and D. M. Shlaes.** 1985. Physiological characteristics and deoxyribonucleic acid relatedness of human isolates of *Streptococcus bovis* and *Streptococcus bovis* (var.). Int. J. Syst. Bacteriol. **35:**357–361.
58. **Knight, R. G., and D. M. Shlaes.** 1988. Physiological characteristics and deoxyribonucleic acid relatedness of *Streptococcus intermedius* strains. Int. J. Syst. Bacteriol. **38:**19–24.
59. **Kronvall, G.** 1973. A surface component in group A, C, and G streptococci with non-immune reactivity for immunoglobulin G. J. Immunol. **111:**1401–1406.
60. **Kurzynski, T. A., and C. M. Van Holten.** 1981. Evaluation of techniques for isolation of group A streptococci from throat cultures. J. Clin. Microbiol. **13:**891–894.
61. **Laster, A. J., and M. L. Michaels.** 1984. Group B streptococcal arthritis in adults. Am. J. Med. **76:**910–915.
62. **LeBien, T. W., and M. C. Bromel.** 1975. Antibacterial properties of a peroxidogenic strain of *Streptococcus mitior* (mitis). Can. J. Microbiol. **21:**101–103.
63. **Leclerq, R., E. Derlot, J. Duval, and P. Courvalin.** 1988. Plasmid-mediated resistance to vancomycin and teicoplanin in *Enterococcus faecium*. N. Engl. J. Med. **319:** 157–161.
64. **Lerner, P. I., K. V. Gopalakrishna, E. Wolinsky, M. C. McHenry, J. S. Tan, and M. Rosenthal.** 1977. Group B streptococcus (*S. agalactiae*) bacteremia in adults: analysis of 32 cases and review of the literature. Medicine **56:** 457–473.
65. **Libertin, C. R., P. E. Hermqans, and J. A. Washington II.** 1985. Beta-hemolytic group F streptococcal bacteremia: a study and review of the literature. Rev. Infect. **7:** 498–503.
66. **Lipman, M. L., and J. Silva, Jr.** 1989. Endocarditis due to *Streptococcus faecalis* with high-level resistance to gentamicin. Rev. Infect. Dis. **11:**325–328.
67. **Maki, D. G., and W. A. Agger.** 1988. Enterococcal bacteremia: clinical features, the risk of endocarditis, and management. Medicine **67:**248–269.
68. **Memon, I. A., N. M. Jacobs, and T. F. Yeh.** 1979. Group B streptococcal osteomyelitis, and septic arthritis. Am. J. Dis. Child. **133:**921–923.
69. **Mohr, D. N., D. J. Feist, J. A. Washington II, and P. E. Hermans.** 1979. Infections due to group C streptococci in man. Am. J. Med. **66:**450–456.
70. **Moody, M. D., A. C. Siegel, B. Pittman, and C. C. Winter.** 1963. Fluorescent-antibody identification of group A streptococci from throat swabs. Am. J. Public Health **53:** 1083–1092.
71. **Murray, B. E., and B. Mederski-Samaroj.** 1983. Transferable β-lactamase: a new mechanism for in vitro penicillin resistance in *Streptococcus faecalis*. J. Clin. Invest. **72:**1168–1171.
72. **Murray, P. R., A. D. Wold, C. A. Schreck, and J. A. Washington II.** 1976. Effects of selective media and atmosphere of incubation on the isolation of group A streptococci. J. Clin. Microbiol. **4:**503–560.
73. **Persson, C. M. S., M. Grabe, P. Kristiansen, and A. Farsgren.** 1988. Significance of group B streptococci in urine cultures from males and nonpregnant females. Scand. J. Infect. Dis. **10:**47–53.
74. **Petts, D.** 1984. Colistin-oxolinic acid blood agar: a new selective medium for streptococci. J. Clin. Microbiol. **19:** 4–7.
75. **Pien, F. D., C. L. Ow, N. S. Issacson, N. T. Goto, and R. C. Ruddy.** 1979. Evaluation of anaerobic incubation for recovery of group A streptococci from throat cultures. J. Clin. Microbiol. **10:**392–393.
76. **Pratter, M. R., and R. S. Irwin.** 1980. Viridans streptococcal pulmonary parenchymal infections. J. Am. Med. Assoc. **243:**2515–2517.
77. **Quinn, J. P., C. A. DiVincenzo, D. A. Lucks, R. L. Luskin, K. L. Shatzer, and S. A. Lerner.** 1988. Serious infections due to penicillin-resistant viridans streptococci with altered penicillin-binding proteins. J. Infect. Dis. **157:**764–769.

77a. **Riebel, W. J., and J. A. Washington.** 1990. Clinical and microbiological characteristics of pediococci. J. Clin. Microbiol. **28:**1348–1355.

78. **Roberts, R. B., A. G. Krieger, N. L. Schiller, and K. C. Gross.** 1979. Viridans streptococcal endocarditis: the role of various species, including pyridoxal-dependent streptococci. Rev. Infect. Dis. **1:**955–965.
79. **Romero, R., and H. W. Wilkinson.** 1974. Identification of group B streptococci by immunofluorescence staining. Appl. Microbiol. **28:**199–204.
80. **Ruoff, K. L.** 1988. *Streptococcus anginosus* ("*Streptococcus milleri*"): the unrecognized pathogen. Clin. Microbiol. Rev. **1:**102–108.
81. **Ruoff, K. L., M. J. Ferraro, J. Holden, and L. J. Kunz.** 1984. Identification of *Streptococcus bovis* and *Streptococcus salivarius* in clinical laboratories. J. Clin. Microbiol. **20:**223–226.
82. **Ruoff, K. L., D. R. Kuritzkes, J. S. Wolfson, and M. J. Ferraro.** 1988. Vancomycin-resistant gram-positive bacteria isolated from human sources. J. Clin. Microbiol. **26:** 2064–2068.
83. **Ruoff, K. L., S. I. Miller, C. V. Garner, M. J. Ferraro, and S. B. Calderwood.** 1989. Bacteremia with *Strepto-*

coccus bovis and *Streptococcus salivarius:* clinical correlates of more active identification of isolates. J. Clin. Microbiol. **27:**305–308.

84. **Schleifer, K. H.** 1986. Gram positive cocci, p. 999–1002. *In* P. H. A. Sneath, N. S. Mair, M. E. Sharpe, and J. G. Holt (ed.), Bergey's manual of systematic bacteriology, vol. 2. The Williams & Wilkins Co., Baltimore.
85. **Schleifer, K. H., and R. Kilpper-Bälz.** 1984. Transfer of *Streptococcus faecalis* and *Streptococcus faecium* to the genus *Enterococcus* nom. rev. as *Enterococcus faecalis* comb. nov. and *Enterococcus faecium* comb. nov. Int. J. Syst. Bacteriol. **34:**31–34.
86. **Schleifer, K. H., and R. Kilpper-Bälz.** 1987. Molecular and chemotaxonomic approaches to the classification of streptococci, enterococci, and lactococci: a review. Syst. Appl. Microbiol. **10:**1–19.
87. **Schleifer, K. H., J. Kraus, C. Dvorak, R. Kilpper-Bälz, M. D. Collins, and W. Fischer.** 1985. Transfer of *Streptococcus lactis* and related streptococci to the genus *Lactococcus* gen. nov. Syst. Appl. Microbiol. **6:**183–195.
88. **Schmidhuber, S., R. Kilpper-Bälz, and K. H. Schleifer.** 1987. A taxonomic study of *Streptococcus mitis, S. oralis,* and *S. sanguis.* System. Appl. Microbiol. **10:**74–77.
89. **Slifkin, M., and G. Intercal.** 1980. Serogrouping single colonies of beta-hemolytic streptococci from primary throat culture plates with nitrous acid extraction and Phadebact streptococcal reagents. J. Clin. Microbiol. **12:** 541–545.
90. **Slifkin, M., and G. R. Pouchet-Melvin.** 1980. Evaluation of three commercially available test products for serogrouping beta-hemolytic streptococci. J. Clin. Microbiol. **11:**249–255.
91. **Stein, D. S., and K. E. Nelson.** 1987. Endocarditis due to nutritionally deficient streptococci: therapeutic dilemma. Rev. Infect. Dis. **9:**908–916.
92. **Stevens, D. L., M. H. Tanner, J. Winship, R. Swarts, K. M. Ries, P. M. Schlievert, and E. Kaplan.** 1989. Severe group A streptococcal infections associated with a toxic shock-like syndrome and scarlet fever toxin A. N. Engl. J. Med. **321:**1–7.
93. **Swenson, J. M., R. R. Facklam, and C. Thornsberry.** 1990. Antimicrobial susceptibility of vancomycin-resistant *Leuconostoc, Pediococcus,* and *Lactobacillus* species. Antimicrob. Agents Chemother. **34:**543–549.
94. **Taubman, B., R. P. Barroway, and K. L. McGowan.** 1989. The diagnosis of group A, β-hemolytic streptococcal pharyngitis in the office setting: rapid latex test vs throat culture. Am. J. Dis. Child. **143:**102–104.
95. **Tuppurainen, N., and M. Hallman.** 1989. Prevention of neonatal group B streptococcal disease: intrapartum detection and chemoprophylaxis of heavily colonized parturients. Obstet. Gynecol. **73:**583–587.
96. **Vartian, C., P. I. Lerner, D. M. Shlaes, and K. V. Gopalakrishna.** 1985. Infections due to Lancefield group G streptococci. Medicine **64:**75–88.
97. **Venditti, M., P. Baiocchi, L. Santini, C. Brandimarte, P. Serra, G. Gentle, and C. Girmania.** 1989. Antimicrobial susceptibilities of *Streptococcus* species that cause septicemia in neutropenic patients. Antimicrob. Agents Chemother. **33:**580–582.
98. **Verghese, A., S. L. Berk, L. J. Boelin, and J. K. Smith.** 1982. Group B streptococcal pneumonia in the elderly. Arch. Intern. Med. **142:**1642–1645.
99. **Verghese, A., K. Mireault, and R. D. Arbeit.** 1986. Group B streptococcal bacteremia in men. Rev. Infect. Dis. **8:** 912–917.
100. **Watsky, K. L., N. Kollisch, and P. Densen.** 1985. Group G streptococcal bacteremia: the clinical experience at Boston University Medical Center and a critical review of the literature. Arch. Intern. Med. **145:**58–61.
101. **Welborn, P. P., W. K. Hadley, E. Newbrun, and D. M. Yajko.** 1983. Characterization of strains of viridans streptococci by deoxyribonucleic acid hybridization and physiologic tests. Int. J. Syst. Bacterol. **33:**293–299.
102. **Whiley, R. A., and J. M. Hardie.** 1988. *Streptococcus vestibularis* sp. nov. from the human oral cavity. Int. J. Syst. Bacteriol. **38:**335–339.
103. **Whiley, R. A., R. R. B. Russell, J. M. Hardie, and D. Beighton.** 1988. *Streptococcus downei* sp. nov. for strains previously described as *Streptococcus mutans* serotype h. Int. J. Syst. Bacteriol. **38:**25–29.
104. **Wong, J. D.** 1987. Porphyrin test as an alternative to benzidine test for detecting cytochromes in catalase-negative gram positive cocci. J. Clin. Microbiol. **25:**2006–2007.
105. **Zervos, M. J., S. Dembinski, T. Mikesell, and D. R. Shaberg.** 1986. High-level resistance to gentamicin in *Streptococcus faecalis:* risk factors and evidence for exogenous acquisition of infection. J. Infect. Dis. **153:**1075–1083.

Chapter 30

Neisseria and *Branhamella*

JOSEPHINE A. MORELLO, WILLIAM M. JANDA, AND GARY V. DOERN

CHARACTERIZATION

At present, *Neisseria* species are classified in the family *Neisseriaceae*, along with *Kingella*, *Moraxella*, and *Acinetobacter* species. Recent taxonomic studies have indicated that the neisseriae are more closely related to *Eikenella*, *Simonsiella*, and *Alysiella* species as well as CDC groups EF-4 and M-5. A proposal has been made to emend the family *Neisseriaceae* to include these organisms (which are found among the oral flora of humans and animals), along with *Kingella*, and to exclude *Moraxella* and *Acinetobacter* species (69). *Branhamella* species, once classified as *Neisseria* species, are more closely related to members of the genus *Moraxella;* therefore, branhamellae have been placed in a subgenus of *Moraxella*. The most common species found in humans is referred to as *Moraxella* (*Branhamella*) *catarrhalis* (5). For the sake of continuity with recent practice in clinical microbiology and infectious disease, the name *Branhamella catarrhalis* will be used in this chapter.

Species of *Neisseria* and *Branhamella* are alike with regard to morphology, limited metabolic activity, and usual habitat but differ in pathogenic potential and genetic relatedness (32). These organisms are gram-negative cocci that may be somewhat refractory to decolorization. The cells usually occur in pairs with flattened adjacent sides, a characteristic that is responsible for their kidney or coffee bean appearance in microscopic preparations. Cell division is in two planes at right angles, sometimes resulting in tetrad formation. Individual cells may vary in size from 0.6 to 1.5 μm, depending on the species, source of the isolate (clinical specimen or culture), and age of the culture. One species, *Neisseria elongata*, is a short rod, 0.5 μm wide, which often occurs as a diplobacillus (80). Older cells of some species tend to autolyze in culture, with resulting ballooning of the organisms. The cells produce no endospores and are nonmotile. Some species are encapsulated, and some produce a yellow-green carotenoid pigment.

Physiologically, most *Neisseria* and *Branhamella* strains have complex growth requirements, have an optimum growth temperature of 35 to 37°C, and degrade few or no carbohydrates. All species are aerobes that produce the enzymes cytochrome oxidase and, except for *N. elongata*, catalase.

The natural habitat of these organisms is the mucous membranes of warm-blooded animals. Only two species, *Neisseria gonorrhoeae* and *Neisseria meningitidis*, are considered to be primary pathogens, and both infect humans only. Although *N. gonorrhoeae* is isolated from many patients with asymptomatic infection, it is always considered to be a disease producer. On the other hand, *N. meningitidis* may be isolated from the nasopharynx and throat of a variable proportion of healthy humans as well as from patients with meningococcal disease. Most other *Neisseria* species and *B. catarrhalis* have been isolated from serious infections, but they are considered to be opportunistic pathogens.

Since the isolation and identification of *N. gonorrhoeae* and *N. meningitidis* are of primary interest in the clinical microbiology laboratory, the major portion of this chapter deals with the clinical and diagnostic features of these two organisms. The chapter concludes with a brief discussion of other *Neisseria* species and *B. catarrhalis*.

NEISSERIA GONORRHOEAE

Clinical significance

Despite estimates that perhaps only one-half of cases are reported, gonorrhea is the most commonly reported bacterial infection in the United States (14). In recent years, the reported incidence has become somewhat cyclical, having increased ca. 10% each year from 1964 to 1977 and then declining until 1985, when the incidence increased again. During 1988, ca. 700,000 cases were reported, a 22% decrease from the 1983–1987 median of 900,000 cases. Two important factors responsible for the high gonorrhea prevalence are the increasing resistance of *N. gonorrhoeae* to available antimicrobial agents and a large reservoir of asymptomatic females and males who unknowingly transmit the disease to their sexual partners.

N. gonorrhoeae is highly susceptible to adverse environmental influences such as temperature extremes and drying, and it does not survive long outside its natural host. Gonorrhea is transmitted between individuals by direct, close, usually sexual contact. In males, the most common manifestation of infection is acute urethritis, characterized by the abrupt onset of dysuria and a purulent urethral discharge. The incubation period is ca. 2 to 7 days. Complications such as prostatitis, epididymitis, and urethral stricture occur less frequently now than in the preantibiotic era, presumably because of successful therapy of initial uncomplicated infections. The overall incidence of asymptomatic gonorrhea in men has been estimated to be from 1 to 5% (14), although it may be higher in contacts of symptomatic females.

The primary site of urogenital gonorrhea in females is the endocervix. Infection may be accompanied by a purulent vaginal discharge, dysuria, and urinary frequency. Most women with uncomplicated gonorrhea, however, remain asymptomatic or do not develop severe enough symptoms to seek medical help. In some females with gonococcal cervicitis, the infection ascends, resulting in salpingitis, pelvic peritonitis, or both, complications referred to as pelvic inflammatory disease (PID). Although other organisms may cause PID, gonococci are isolated from the cervices of 10 to 70% of affected women (14), indicating that gonococci probably play a major role at least in initial episodes of this disease. Repeated episodes of PID commonly involve anaerobes from the vaginal flora. The inflammatory reaction of PID may cause tubal scarring and blockage, leading to infertility or ectopic pregnancies. Some women with gonococcal PID develop perihepatitis (Fitz-Hugh–Curtis syndrome), presumably by spread of gonococci through the peritoneal cavity. Gonococci from cervical secretions may also contaminate the female perineum, resulting in anorectal and periurethral gland infections.

Although anorectal and oropharyngeal gonorrhea can occur in women as a result of rectal intercourse and fellatio, infections at these sites are more common in homosexual males. The majority of cases of both anorectal and oropharyngeal gonorrhea are asymptomatic, but patients may present with proctitis or acute pharyngitis and tonsillitis (35).

In a small percentage of individuals with gonorrhea (0.5 to 3%), the organisms spread hematogenously to produce disseminated gonococcal infection (DGI). DGI is characterized by the presence of a sparse rash on the extremities and arthritis in one or more joints. At present, gonococci are the major cause of septic arthritis in young adults. Although *N. gonorrhoeae* may be isolated from the blood, skin lesions, or joint fluid of patients with DGI, often the organism is isolated only from genital, anorectal, or pharyngeal cultures of affected individuals with signs and symptoms of DGI. Disseminated infection occurs more commonly in females than males, perhaps because there is a greater tendency for the organisms to disseminate during menstruation and pregnancy. In rare instances, DGI may result in gonococcal endocarditis or meningitis.

In some areas of the United States, the unusual AHU strain of *N. gonorrhoeae*, which requires arginine, hypoxanthine, and uracil for growth on defined media, has been isolated from a disproportionate number of patients with DGI (61) and from males with asymptomatic urethral gonorrhea (13). The ability of these AHU strains to withstand the bactericidal action of human serum may be responsible, in part, for their increased tendency to disseminate (60).

Infants born to infected mothers may develop gonococcal ophthalmia (ophthalmia neonatorum) if the prophylactic eyedrops or ointment usually administered at birth are not used or, as happens rarely, are not effective. Gonococcal ophthalmia must be treated immediately, or blindness can result. Nonsexually transmitted infections may occur in very young children, usually after accidental contamination with discharges from an infected parent or relative. In older children, however, gonococcal infections are acquired primarily by precocious sexual activity or sexual molestation. The primary syndrome in prepubertal girls is vulvovaginitis; otherwise, the clinical picture is similar to that seen in adults.

Specimen collection

For diagnosing gonorrhea, appropriate sites for specimen collection depend to some extent on the age, sex, and sexual practices of the individual and the clinical features of the infection. When specimens are taken, lubricate any instruments used (vaginal speculums, anoscopes) with warm water only, as other lubricants may be toxic for gonococci. Specimens may be collected on swabs or, in some instances, with spurfree, platinum-iridium bacteriological loops. Some cotton swabs contain unsaturated fatty acids that are inhibitory for gonococci (44). Use these only if the specimen can be plated immediately onto culture medium or sent to the laboratory in transport medium containing activated charcoal to absorb the inhibitory substances. Swabs composed of synthetic material such as calcium alginate or Dacron are recommended, although one report suggests that some lots of calcium alginate swabs are toxic for gonococci (52). Collect material on separate swabs for Gram stain and for culture. Appropriate culture sites and collection techniques are described below and in Table 1.

Endocervix. For suspected gonorrhea or when screening for infection in women, always collect endocervical specimens because they most often yield gonococci in both symptomatic and asymptomatic infections. After inserting the speculum, wipe away cervical mucus with a cotton ball; then carefully swab the endocervical canal, moving the swab from side to side. Do not use any disinfectant before collecting the specimen, and avoid contaminating the swab with vaginal flora.

Urethra. Collect urethral specimens from symptomatic and asymptomatic males at least 1 h after the patients have urinated. Purulent discharge can be collected directly on a swab; if there is no discharge, obtain a specimen by gently scraping the mucosa of the an-

TABLE 1. Body sites to culture for *N. gonorrhoeae*

Patient	Site	
	Primary	Secondary
Female	Endocervix	Rectum, (urethra), pharynx[a]
Male		
Heterosexual	Urethra	
Homosexual	Urethra, rectum, pharynx	
DGI		
Female	Blood, endocervix, rectum	Pharynx,[a] skin lesions,[b] joint fluid,[b] urethra
Male	Blood, urethra	Pharynx,[a] skin lesions,[b] joint fluid,[b] rectum[c]

[a] If there is a history of oral-genital contact.
[b] If present.
[c] If there is a history of anal-genital contact.

terior urethra with a sterile loop. Preferably, insert a urethral or nasopharyngeal swab ca. 2 cm into the urethra and rotate the swab gently as it is withdrawn. Collect female urethral specimens in a similar matter from symptomatic patients with urethral exudate.

Anorectal specimens. Collect anorectal specimens from all patients who may have DGI, homosexual males, females with urogenital symptoms, and asymptomatic females likely to be infected (e.g., contacts of known or suspected infected males). In some instances, gonococci may be isolated from an anal canal culture when the endocervical culture is negative, especially after antimicrobial therapy (i.e., test of cure). Obtain the specimen by inserting a swab ca. 4 to 5 cm into the anal canal. Move the swab from side to side to sample the crypts. If fecal contamination occurs, discard the swab and use another to obtain the specimen. An anoscope may be used to visualize and collect mucopurulent material directly, but this procedure is not mandatory.

Oropharynx. When oropharyngeal infection is suspected, swab the posterior pharynx and the region of the tonsillar crypts.

Conjunctiva. In infants (and occasionally other age groups) with conjunctivitis, obtain swabs of conjunctival exudate for Gram stain and culture.

Bartholin's gland. Collect any draining pus on swabs, or aspirate material from closed abscesses with a syringe and needle. In the latter instance especially, infection with anaerobes as well as gonococci should be considered, and the specimens should be handled appropriately.

Blood. Obtain blood for culture from any patient with suspected DGI and inoculate it directly into a suitable culture medium. Blood may be sent to the laboratory in a sterile, evacuated blood collection tube containing sodium polyanetholsulfonate (SPS). SPS is toxic for some strains of gonococci (see blood culture section); therefore, if this method is used, the blood specimen should be inoculated into broth as soon as possible, preferably within 1 h after collection.

Joint fluid. In patients with DGI, aspirate material from possibly infected joints. Transport the material directly in a capped syringe or in a sterile specimen container to the laboratory for Gram stain and culture.

Skin lesions. A small punch biopsy is preferable to material aspirated from the lesion. Place the specimen on a chocolate agar plate or other sterile, moist container to prevent drying during transport. The positive culture rate is low.

Specimen transport

Gonococci are highly susceptible to adverse environmental conditions, and often only small numbers of organisms are present in clinical material. When specimens are sent to the laboratory, they must be transported in a manner that preserves organism viability. Appropriate transport conditions depend to some extent on the type of facility in which the specimen is obtained, for example, public health clinic, private physician office, hospital room or clinic, or emergency room. In each of these situations, the time elapsed between specimen collection and receipt at the laboratory differs and may be unpredictable.

Direct plating. The greatest number of gonococcal cultures are positive when specimens are inoculated in the patient care area directly onto a nutritive growth medium such as modified Thayer-Martin (MTM) (55), Martin-Lewis (ML) (56), or New York City (NYC) (26), incubated immediately at 35 to 37°C in an atmosphere of 3 to 10% CO_2, and examined within 48 h. This is the method of choice whenever an incubator and a candle extinction jar are available, and the jars can be transported readily to the laboratory after 24 to 48 h of incubation. These conditions seldom exist, however, and alternative transport methods are most commonly used.

Nonnutritive transport media. Buffered holding media such as that of Stuart and Amies (chapter 121) were originally devised to maintain gonococci during transit, although at present they are widely used to preserve a great variety of clinically significant bacteria. Gonococci survive well in these media for at least 6 to 12 h, provided that they are not exposed to temperature extremes. By 24 h, however, the numbers of gonococci decrease to an extent that may prevent their recovery, especially if small numbers were present initially in the specimen. Do not use this type of transport medium if the specimen cannot be delivered to the laboratory and plated onto growth medium within 12 h. The advantages of these holding media are that they are simple to use, require no special equipment, are relatively inexpensive, and have a long shelf life at room temperature.

Nutritive (growth) transport systems. When prolonged delays in transit are expected, systems that incorporate culture medium and a method for increasing CO_2 concentration are required. A commonly used approach is inoculation of a biological environment chamber such as the JEMBEC plate (57). This plate is a rectangular polystyrene dish with a removable cover and a molded inner well that holds a CO_2-generating tablet (composed of sodium bicarbonate and citric acid). The plates are prepared with one of the gonococcal selective media, such as MTM, ML, or NYC. For inoculation, roll the specimen swab over one-third to one-half of the agar surface; then cross-streak the remainder of the plate with a bacteriological loop or a fresh swab. Insert a CO_2-generating tablet in the well, replace the cover, and place the entire unit into a small plastic zip-locked bag. Moisture evaporated from the medium is sufficient to activate the tablet and provide a CO_2 atmosphere during incubation. For maximum recovery and survival of gonococci, incubate the inoculated plates for ca. 18 to 24 h at 35 to 37°C before delivering or mailing them to the laboratory. If the plates are preincubated, they may be inspected for the presence of gonococcal colonies immediately upon arrival, and negative cultures may be incubated for an additional 24 h. If further incubation in the laboratory is necessary, remove the plates from the plastic bag and incubate them under increased CO_2 tension. Colonies growing on media in the JEMBEC plates are easy to observe and subculture because the plates are handled exactly like petri plates.

In other nutritive transport systems, for example, the Bio-Bag and Gono-Pak Systems (Becton Dickinson Microbiology Systems, Cockeysville, Md.), conventional culture plates are inoculated and then placed into individual plastic zip-locked bags, each of which contains a CO_2-generating ampoule or tablet. These bags can be handled in the same manner as JEMBEC plates.

Transport containers for specimens not collected on swabs are discussed above in the section on specimen collection. All of these containers must be delivered to the laboratory as quickly as possible for proper plating and incubation.

Direct examination

Gram stain. The Gram stain is the method of choice for direct examination of genital specimens. When smears of urethral exudate from males are properly prepared and stained and correctly interpreted, correlation with culture results is greater than 95% (14). In many sexually transmitted disease clinics, such specimens are not cultured if the Gram-stained smear is positive. In females, however, smears of endocervical secretions detect only 50 to 70% of culture-positive specimens (54). Thus, both Gram-stained smears and cultures of endocervical secretions should be done. Examining Gram-stained smears of intraurethral specimens from asymptomatic males is not a sensitive diagnostic test; therefore, cultures are required as well. Smears prepared from blind rectal swabs are difficult to interpret, so smear examination is not recommended. Direct visualization of the rectal mucosa and sampling of purulent material through an anoscope frequently yield easily interpretable Gram-stained preparations (Fig. 1), but culture should also be performed. In our experience, smear examination has worked well for rapid diagnosis of symptomatic gonococcal proctitis in homosexual men. Gram-stained smears for detecting *N. gonorrhoeae* in oropharyngeal specimens are not recommended because other *Neisseria* and *Branhamella* species of the upper respiratory tract flora are morphologically indistinguishable from gonococci.

Smear preparation. For optimal results, smears should be prepared directly from the specimen immediately after collection. In smears prepared from swabs sent in an aqueous or semisolid transport medium, organisms may appear atypical. In addition, dilution of the specimen by the medium may affect the sensitivity of smear examination results, particularly if the discharge is scant. If both a culture and a smear are required, two swab specimens should be collected. The swab should be rolled gently over the surface of a glass microscope slide in one direction only. This method minimizes distortion and breakage of polymorphonuclear leukocytes (PMN) and preserves the characteristic appearance of the microorganisms. Three or four complete, nonoverlapping rolls of the swab on the slide are sufficient. Excessively thick smears do not decolorize properly during the Gram stain procedure and may decrease its diagnostic utility.

Smear interpretation and reporting. Gram-stained smears of the urethral discharge from men with gonococcal urethritis typically contain gram-negative diplococci located intracellulary in PMN. Usually, two or more pairs of organisms are observed within some PMN, whereas many other leukocytes contain no bacteria at all (Fig. 2). Few, if any, other bacteria are seen on the smear. Smears from men with early symptomatic disease frequently show rare intracellular gram-negative diplococci and many extracellular organisms trapped in stringy mucous material. In Gram-stained smears of rectal mucopurulent material collected under direct visualization through an anoscope, gram-negative intracellular diplococci are usually seen.

Gram-stained smears from properly collected cervical discharge may show intracellular gram-negative diplococci, but accurate smear interpretation may be complicated by the presence of normal female genital flora that resemble *Neisseria* species. The tendency to overinterpret endocervical and rectal smears, which usually contain gram-negative coccobacilli and bipolarly staining enteric bacilli, must be avoided. The observations should be considered presumptive until culture results are known.

Report the numbers, Gram stain properties, and morphology of all organisms present and the numbers and types of cells (PMN, squamous epithelial) seen in smears. Organisms resembling *Neisseria* species that are located within PMN should be quantified and reported as "gram-negative intracellular diplococci." The quantity may be described in words (few, moderate, many) or scored from 1+ to 4+ as described in *Cumitech 4* (44).

Gram stains prepared from conjunctival pus in ophthalmia and from petechial lesions and joint fluid

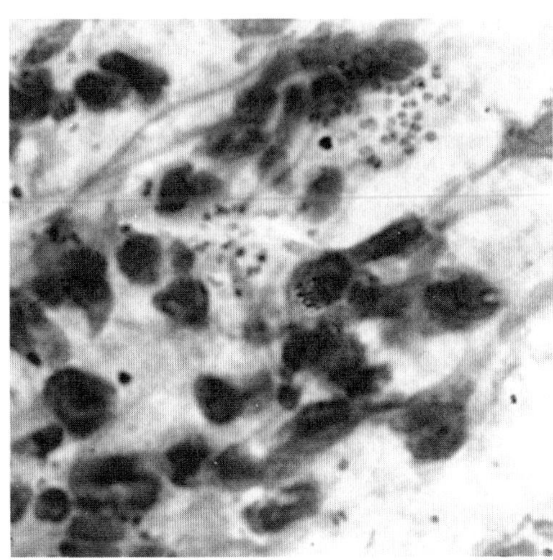

FIG. 1. Gram stain of mucopurulent rectal exudate showing many diplococci inside PMN. ×1,500.

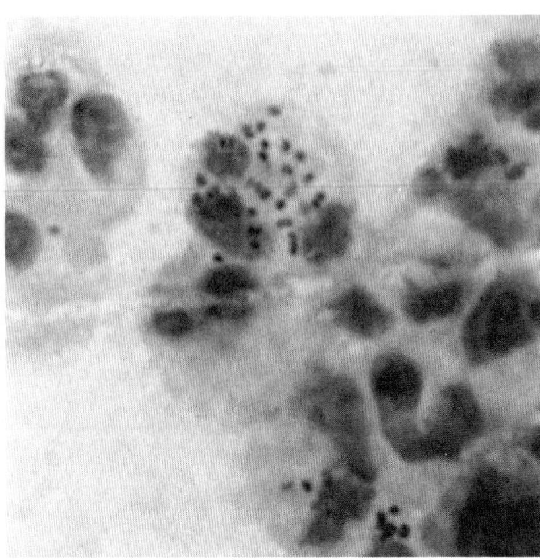

FIG. 2. Gram stain of male urethral exudate. Some PMN contain many diplococci; others contain none. ×1,500.

of patients with DGI may aid diagnosis. In the last two specimen types especially, organisms may not grow in culture even though they are seen in the smear.

Culture and isolation

Specimens transported on selective agar media. Many specimens arrive at the laboratory previously plated onto selective agar media such as MTM, ML, and NYC. Basically, MTM and ML media are chocolate agar with four antimicrobial agents added: vancomycin (MTM, 3 μg/ml; ML, 4 μg/ml) to inhibit gram-positive bacteria; colistin (7.5 μg/ml) to inhibit gram-negative bacteria, including commensal *Neisseria* species; trimethoprim lactate (5 μg/ml) to inhibit swarming *Proteus* species; and an antifungal agent to inhibit molds and some yeasts (MTM, 12.5 μg of nystatin per ml; ML, 20 μg of anisomycin per ml). If they are correctly prepared and used while fresh, these media afford excellent growth of most strains of pathogenic *Neisseria* species while inhibiting the growth of commensal *Neisseria* species and other commensals that are likely to contaminate oropharyngeal and anogenital specimens. NYC is a clear medium in which hemolyzed horse erythrocytes, horse plasma, and yeast dialysate are used in place of the hemoglobin and defined supplements present in chocolate, MTM, and ML media. Selectivity is provided by adding the following antimicrobial agents: vancomycin, 2 μg/ml; colistin, 5.5 μg/ml; amphotericin B, 1.2 μg/ml; and trimethoprim lactate, 3 μg/ml. NYC medium has also been prepared without the hemolyzed horse cells and used successfully for gonococcal isolation (30). NYC medium supports luxuriant growth of pathogenic *Neisseria* species, large-colony mycoplasma, and T-strain mycoplasma (*Ureaplasma urealyticum*).

If the cultures have been incubated at 35 to 37°C for 18 h or more before they arrive at the laboratory, examine them immediately to detect typical colonies of *N. gonorrhoeae*. If they have not been preincubated or if no growth is observed, incubate them in a CO_2 atmosphere and observe them daily for at least 2 but preferably 3 days.

From 3 to 10% or more of gonococci (usually AHU strain organisms) are susceptible to the concentrations of vancomycin used in the selective media and therefore will not be recovered (59). Some gonococcal strains are also susceptible to trimethoprim, but the concentrations used in these media do not appear to affect their recovery as much as vancomycin does. Nevertheless, because the normal flora of the pharynx, rectum, and female genital tract grows more rapidly than gonococci and in some instances inhibits gonococcal growth (70), antibiotic-containing media that suppress these commensals usually permit better isolation of gonococci than do nonselective media.

Other specimens. As soon as possible after their arrival in the laboratory, inoculate onto growth medium all specimens received in nonnutritive transport medium or sterile containers. Conjunctival swabs, skin biopsies, and joint fluids can be plated onto chocolate agar rather than a selective medium because they are not likely to be contaminated with commensal organisms. When possible, inoculate male and female genital exudate specimens onto chocolate agar as well as onto a selective medium to help detect vancomycin-susceptible organisms.

Inoculate chocolate agar by rolling the swab across one quadrant of the plate, making certain that all areas of the swab are sampled. Streak the remainder of the plate with an inoculating loop to obtain isolated colonies after incubation. Heavily inoculate selective media by rolling the swab across one-third to one-half of the plate surface; then streak to obtain isolated colonies.

Most of the commonly used blood culture broths (e.g., tryptic soy, Columbia, and brain heart infusion) support the growth of gonococci, provided that the broth is vented and incubated under increased CO_2 tension. SPS, a common blood culture broth additive, inhibits the growth of some gonococci and meningococci (24, 75). Gelatin neutralizes this inhibitory effect (24, 75) and can be added to the broth (in a 1% final concentration) when either of these organisms is suspected. Joint fluids may be inoculated into liquid as well as onto solid media. *N. gonorrhoeae* grow in and are detected by the BACTEC system (Becton Dickinson Diagnostic Instrument Systems, Towson, Md.).

Incubation conditions. Although not all gonococci have an absolute requirement for CO_2, their growth is stimulated by it. Therefore, always incubate specimens in a CO_2 incubator or candle extinction jar. Use unscented white wax candles because colored and scented candles may produce toxic substances while burning. The level of CO_2 in the jar is ca. 3% when the candle flame dies out. Alternatively, use commercially available CO_2-generating envelopes (similar to envelopes that produce an anaerobic environment) (Becton Dickinson Microbiology Systems) in a tightly closed chamber such as a candle jar or an anaerobic jar with the catalyst removed.

High humidity is also essential for good gonococcal growth. In a candle jar, humidity is provided by evaporated moisture from the culture medium. In CO_2 incubators that do not have built-in humidifiers, pans of water on the lower shelf can provide moisture during incubation. If the surface of a commercially prepared agar plate appears dry, add a few drops of sterile culture broth to the plate surface and allow it to soak in before the plate is streaked.

Incubate agar media at 35 to 37°C for at least 72 h before sending a negative culture report. For blood broths that do not show microbial growth after 24 to 48 h of incubation, make blind subcultures on chocolate agar. Hold blood cultures for at least 7 days before discarding them.

Identification

Gonococcal colonies are best observed with the aid of a magnifying glass or, preferably, a stereoscopic microscope. After 24 h of incubation, the colonies are ca. 0.5 to 1 mm in diameter and appear gray to white, opaque, raised, and glistening. Isolated colonies may increase in size to 3 mm with further incubation.

In culture, gonococci produce at least five different colony types, termed types 1 through 5 (T1 through T5) (8). T1 and T2 (sometimes referred to as P^+ because the organisms are piliated) colonies are small and raised and predominate in cultures of clinical material. When colonies growing on chocolate agar are viewed microscopically with incident light (striking their surface from above), T1 and T2 colonies reflect the light and appear to have bright highlights. Cultures can be maintained in this state by selectively subculturing T1 and T2 colonies. With nonselective subculture, however, these colony forms dissociate to types 3 to 5 (P^-), which are larger, flatter, and less opaque and do not reflect the light (Fig. 3). Even gross observation of gonococcal cultures, without a stereoscopic microscope, will reveal colonies that differ in size and morphology, especially if the culture has been transferred two or three times. This colony variation is sometimes mistaken for a mixed culture but can serve as a clue to the presence of *N. gonorrhoeae*. Most organisms that may be confused with gonococci produce colonies of uniform size.

So-called atypical or AHU strains of gonococci grow slowly, produce smaller than normal colonies on agar plates, and are often difficult to identify biochemically (61). Microbiologists must be aware of their existence because in certain areas of the United States they are isolated from a majority of patients with DGI and asymptomatic infections. AHU strains also produce several colony types in culture, but all forms are smaller than those produced by normal strains (Fig. 4).

Presumptive identification. Examine the culture plates daily for at least 72 h. Colonies of the slow-growing AHU strain may not be visible before 48 h. Flooding the plates with oxidase reagent after 48 to 72 h may help detect very small numbers of colonies, but these must be subcultured immediately because the reagent kills the organisms. Once plates have grown out, do not continue incubating them because gonococci autolyze as they age, and the culture becomes nonviable. If identification tests cannot be performed when the plates are removed from the incubator, place them in a candle extinction jar, light the candle, and store the closed jar at room temperature. Although further workup should be performed as soon as possible, the organisms will survive for 2 or 3 days under these conditions. If they are left this long, however, prepare a fresh subculture before proceeding with biochemical tests.

Before attempting further identification of gonococci, perform an oxidase test and Gram stain on all suspicious colonies. Place a few drops of oxidase reagent (1% solution of di- or tetramethyl-*p*-phenylenediamine dihydrochloride) on a piece of filter paper, pick up a portion of a colony with a platinum inoculating loop or straight wire, and rub the growth into the impregnated area of the filter paper. With the tetramethyl reagent, the dark purple of a positive test appears rapidly, usually within 10 s if the test culture is fresh. The dimethyl reagent is more toxic, and the color change, proceeding through pink and maroon to black, is slower. Use of Nichrome wire instead of platinum inoculating needles may cause false-positive reactions. Commercially available paper strips impregnated with oxidase reagent (Pathotec-CO; General Diagnostics, Warner-Lambert Co., Morris Plains, N.J.) are satisfactory for the test.

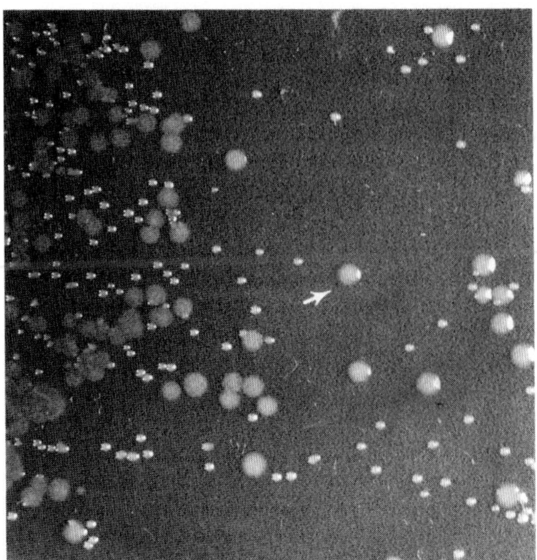

FIG. 3. *N. gonorrhoeae* on chocolate agar. Small colonies with bright highlights are types T1-T2; larger colonies (arrow) are types T3-T4. ×2.5.

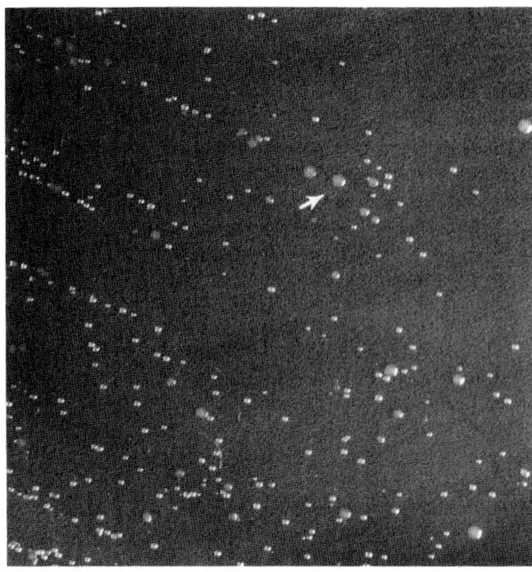

FIG. 4. AHU strain of *N. gonorrhoeae* on chocolate agar. Compare the sizes of types T1-T2 and T3-T4 (arrow) with the sizes shown in Fig. 3. ×2.5.

Even when the oxidase test is positive, a Gram stain is essential because certain oxidase-positive, gram-negative bacilli, such as *Kingella denitrificans*, grow on the selective media and produce colonies resembling those of gonococci (46). Oxidase-positive, gram-negative diplococci isolated from urogenital specimens may be identified presumptively as *N. gonorrhoeae*.

Confirmatory identification. Confirmatory tests are recommended for all isolates from urogenital sites and are required for isolates from other body sites. Methods available include assays for carbohydrate degradation that depend on growth or preformed enzymes; chromogenic enzyme substrate tests; and serological methods such as fluorescent-antibody and coagglutination tests.

Carbohydrate degradation tests in CTA base medium. The standard method for identifying *Neisseria* species is to determine their acid production from carbohydrates in a cystine-tryptic digest agar (CTA) base medium (81). Conventional CTA-carbohydrate media are semisolid agar deeps containing 1% filter-sterilized carbohydrate. The test battery includes glucose, maltose, sucrose, fructose, lactose, and a carbohydrate-free control tube. The test for enzymatic breakdown of *o*-nitrophenyl-β-D-galactopyranoside (ONPG) may be substituted for the lactose tube.

Many laboratory workers have difficulty obtaining satisfactory results with CTA media, but when the test is performed properly, an identification usually can be made within 24 h. The major pitfalls are failure to (i) use a heavy inoculum, (ii) work with pure cultures, and (iii) use reagent-grade carbohydrates. To avoid the first two problems, do not attempt to inoculate carbohydrate tubes with growth from the selective primary isolation plates, which may contain only a few colonies of gonococci as well as inhibited contaminants. Instead, first subculture several typical colonies onto one or two chocolate agar plates (not selective medium) and incubate them in CO_2 for up to 18 h. With longer incubation, the organisms begin to autolyze, the inoculum becomes gummy (related to released nucleoprotein from autolyzed gonococci), and biochemical reactions are delayed. AHU strains of gonococci, however, may require incubation for 24 h or longer to achieve sufficient growth on chocolate agar.

Examine the subculture plates carefully to ascertain that the cultures are pure, and then perform an oxidase test and Gram stain to confirm the presence of gram-negative diplococci. The carbohydrate medium may be inoculated by either of the following methods. (i) Prepare a dense suspension of the organisms in 0.5 ml of saline. With a capillary pipette, dispense 1 drop of suspension onto the surface of each agar deep; then stab the inoculum into the upper third of the medium. (ii) For each tube, scrape a full 3-mm loopful of growth from the surface of the chocolate agar plate and deposit this inoculum a few millimeters below the surface of the medium. In our experience, the latter method provides more rapid and reliable results. A change in the color of the phenol red indicator from orange-pink to yellow, signifying carbohydrate degradation, often occurs within 1 or 2 h.

A heavily inoculated modified CTA-carbohydrate medium consisting of CTA agar (1.5%) slants with 2% carbohydrates can also be used. The aerobic neisseriae prefer the larger surface area provided by the slant. Carbohydrate breakdown is detected first in the area of the slant directly under the inoculum, usually within 1 h and almost invariably by 4 h.

Incubate carbohydrate tubes at 35 to 37°C in a non-CO_2 incubator. Inspect the tubes at periodic intervals for 24 h. If the inoculum is sufficient, positive reactions should be seen within this time, and further incubation is unnecessary. A few strains may require more prolonged incubation. Characteristically, gonococci produce acid from glucose only (Table 2).

Problems that occur when CTA-carbohydrate media are used for gonococcal identification include: (i) no carbohydrate degradation observed, usually related to lack of sufficient inoculum or use of an old culture; (ii) degradation of both glucose and maltose, usually related to contamination of the maltose reagent with glucose or to the presence of a meningococcus rather than a gonococcus; and (iii) all carbohydrates appear degraded, related either to incubation of the tubes in a CO_2 atmosphere (faint color change) or to a contaminated inoculum (usually a bright yellow color throughout the medium). Any tube that appears bright yellow should be considered possibly contaminated, and a smear should be prepared for Gram stain.

When either of the first two problems listed above is encountered, it is best to confirm the identification with one of the alternative tests to be described. Until confirmatory identification is completed, suspected gonococci should be subcultured daily onto chocolate agar so that a viable culture is always available for repeat testing.

Rapid carbohydrate degradation test. A nongrowth carbohydrate degradation test may be used to detect acid production from carbohydrates (44). Small volumes (0.1 ml) of phosphate-buffered saline solution (pH 7.0) containing phenol red indicator are dispensed into nonsterile tubes to which single drops of 20% filter-sterilized carbohydrates (glucose, maltose, sucrose, lactose, fructose) are added. A dense suspension of the organism to be identified is prepared in 0.3 to 0.8 ml of the phosphate-buffered saline solution and mixed well to disperse clumps. One drop of the suspension is added to each of the carbohydrate-containing tubes; all tubes are incubated for 4 h at 35°C in a non-CO_2 incubator or a water bath and then observed for an indicator color change. This test is economical, the reagents are easy to prepare and inoculate, and the results are clear-cut. The ONPG test may be substituted for the lactose tube. Because high concentrations of both carbohydrate and organism are used to detect preformed enzymes, purified reagent-grade carbohydrates should be used to prevent false-positive results. If sufficient colonies are present and the growth is less than 24 h old, inocula may be obtained from the primary culture. Small numbers of contaminants present do not interfere with the results because bacterial growth does not occur in the test medium. Incubation cannot be continued overnight, however.

Commercial carbohydrate degradation tests. Several systems are commercially available for identifying *Neisseria* species and *B. catarrhalis.* The API QuadFERM+ (Analytab Products, Plainview, N.Y.) consists of a plastic strip with several cupules, seven of which contain dehydrated buffer and a phenol red indicator. Test cupules contain glucose, maltose, sucrose, and lactose, plus a control containing only the buffer-indicator solution. The sixth cupule contains phenol red and penicillin for acidometric determination of β-lactamase production by *N. gonorrhoeae* and *B. catarrhalis;* the seventh cupule contains an acidometric test for detecting DNase production by *B. catarrhalis.* After inoculation with a dense organism suspension (McFarland no. 3) and incubation for 2 h at 35°C, the reactions are interpreted. This method is comparable to use of CTA-carbohydrate media for determining carbohydrate degradation, and the additional tests allow simultaneous detection of β-lactamase and DNase activity (41).

In the RIM (rapid identification method)-*Neisseria* test (Austin Biological Laboratories, Austin, Tex.), vials of 2% carbohydrate-phenol red indicator solutions (glucose, maltose, sucrose, and lactose, plus a control lacking carbohydrate) are provided. Two to three drops of each solution are dispensed into five specially buffered microtubes. Inocula from a pure primary culture or subculture are delivered into each of the microtubes with disposable plastic loops. The tubes are incubated for 1 h at 35°C in air. Results are easily interpreted and often may be observed within 30 min of the 1-h incubation period. A DNase test is also available. Good agreement between results of this method and those of conventional tests has been reported (18, 40).

In the Minitek method (Becton Dickinson Microbiology Systems), paper disks impregnated with high concentrations of the appropriate carbohydrates are

TABLE 2. Characteristics of *Neisseria* species and *B. catarrhalis*[a]

Species	Colony morphology	Growth on:			Acid production from:					Reduction of:		Polysaccharide synthesis	DNase
		MTM, ML, or NYC medium	Chocolate or blood agar at 22°C	Nutrient agar at 35°C	Glucose	Maltose	Lactose	Sucrose	Fructose	NO_3	NO_2[b]		
N. gonorrhoeae	Gray to white, smooth, up to five colony types on primary cultures	+	0	0	+	0	0	0	0	0	0	0	0
N. meningitidis	Nonpigmented or gray to white, some yellowish, smooth, transparent, encapsulated strains mucoid	+	0	0	+	+	0	0	0	0	V	0	0
N. lactamica	Nonpigmented or yellowish, smooth, transparent	+	V	+	+	+	+	0	0	0	V	0	0
N. sicca	Nonpigmented, wrinkled, coarse and dry, adherent	0	+	+	+	+	0	+	+	0	+	+	0
N. subflava[c]	Greenish, yellow, smooth, often adherent	0	+	+	+	+	0	V	V	0	+	V	0
N. mucosa	Sometimes yellowish, mucoid appearance due to capsule	0	+	+	+	+	0	+	+	+	+	+	0
N. flavescens	Yellow, opaque, smooth	0	+	+	0	0	0	0	0	0	+	+	0
N. cinerea	Grayish white, slightly granular	V[d]	0	+	0	0	0	0	0	0	+	0	0
N. polysaccharea	Nonpigmented or yellowish, convex and shiny after growth on sucrose	V	0	+	+	+	0	0	0	0	V	+	0
N. elongata[e]	Grayish white, slight yellowish tinge, flat, glistening, dry, claylike consistency	0	+	+	0	0	0	0	0	0	+	0	0
B. catarrhalis	Nonpigmented or gray, opaque, smooth	V	V	+	0	0	0	0	0	+	+	0	+

[a] Symbols: +, strains typically positive, but genetic mutants lacking the requisite enzyme activity are occasionally encountered; 0, most strains negative; V, variable characteristic.
[b] Results listed are for 0.1% (wt/vol) nitrite; *N. gonorrhoeae* and some other species listed as negative can reduce 0.01% (wt/vol) (46).
[c] Includes biovars *subflava*, *flava*, and *perflava* (46).
[d] Some strains grow on selective media even though they are colistin susceptible. Colistin susceptibility is an important characteristic distinguishing *N. cinerea* from *N. gonorrheae*, which is colistin resistant (46).
[e] Weakly positive or negative catalase test, in contrast to other *Neisseria* species.

placed in individual wells of a plastic plate (62). A small volume (0.05 ml) of a heavy suspension of the organism prepared in a standard broth is pipetted into each disk-containing well. Plates are incubated without CO_2 and observed hourly. Most positive reactions occur within 4 h; the remainder are read after overnight incubation. Care must be exercised in interpreting Minitek reactions, particularly after overnight incubation. Weak positive glucose reactions have been noted for some strains of *Neisseria cinerea* and may result in misidentification of these strains as *N. gonorrhoeae* (6, 23). Other commercial modifications of the rapid carbohydrate degradation test are the Neisseria-Kwik test kit (Micro-BioLogics, St. Cloud, Minn.) and the Gonobio-Test (I.A.F. Production Inc., Laval, Quebec, Canada) (18).

When the test results are considered together with other characteristics such as colony morphology and growth on selective media, the commercial carbohydrate degradation systems generally suffice for identifying the pathogenic *Neisseria* species. Some fastidious gonococci, such as AHU auxotypes, may produce weak glucose reactions in both conventional (61) and commercial identification systems. In these instances, other characteristics, such as ability to grow on selective media, resistance to colistin, and reactions in monoclonal antibody systems are helpful for identifying these isolates.

Chromogenic enzyme substrate systems. Chromogenic enzyme substrate identification systems use specific biochemical reagents that, upon hydrolysis by bacterial enzymes, yield a colored end product that is detected either directly or after addition of a detection reagent. To avoid confusion with commensal *Neisseria* species that may give similar reactions, use of these systems is restricted to identifying only those species that grow on selective media, i.e., *N. gonorrhoeae*, *N. meningitidis*, and *N. lactamica*. These systems also provide presumptive identification of *B. catarrhalis*, which may also grow on selective media.

The enzymatic activities detected in commercial systems include β-galactosidase, γ-glutamylaminopeptidase, and hydroxyprolylaminopeptidase (Table 3). β-Galactosidase and γ-glutamylaminopeptidase are hydrolyzed specifically by *N. lactamica* and *N. meningitidis*, respectively. Absence of these activities but presence of prolylaminopeptidase identifies an organism as *N. gonorrhoeae*. *B. catarrhalis* lacks all three enzyme activities.

The commercially available systems that use this approach are Gonochek II (E. I. duPont de Nemours & Co., Inc., Wilmington, Del.) and Identicult-Neisseria (Scott Laboratories, Fiskeville, R.I.). In the Gonochek II system, all three chromogenic substrates are dehydrated in a single tube. The substrates are rehydrated with a phosphate buffer and then inoculated with growth from selective media or a suitable subculture. The presence of specific color reactions after 30 min of incubation provides the identification of the organism (18, 40). In the Identicult-Neisseria system, three individual filter paper circles impregnated with the enzyme substrates are moistened with a buffer, and growth from agar media is rubbed onto each. The isolate is identified after 10 to 15 min by the development of specific colors on the papers either directly or after addition of the developing reagent (39).

N. cinerea is hydroxyprolylaminopeptidase positive and, if inoculated into either the Gonochek II or Identicult-Neisseria system, may be misidentified as *N. gonorrhoeae* (39, 46). However, most strains of this organism do not grow well on selective media and are susceptible to colistin (50). Some *N. subflava* biovar *perflava* strains may also grow on selective media and may be hydroxyprolylaminopeptidase positive (39). Careful attention to colony morphology and other characteristics (e.g., pigmentation, colony size, and consistency) is necessary for selection and use of appropriate identification methods. Isolates that have atypical characteristics, are recovered from extragenital sites, or have medical-legal importance (suspected sexual abuse, isolates from children) require further testing with other methods (46, 85).

Multitest identification systems. Tests for identifying *Neisseria* species and *B. catarrhalis* have been incorporated into commercial systems that identify other fastidious bacteria as well. These systems use both modified conventional tests (e.g., rapid carbohydrate, ornithine decarboxylase, and nitrate reduction tests) and chromogenic enzyme substrates to identify *Neisseria* species, *B. catarrhalis*, *Haemophilus* species, and certain other microorganisms. The RapID NH panel (Innovative Diagnostics Systems, Inc., Decatur, Ga.), the *Haemophilus-Neisseria* identification (HNID) panel (American Micro Scan, Sacramento, Calif.), and the Vitek *Neisseria-Haemophilus* identification (NHI) card (Vitek Systems, Inc., Hazelwood, Mo.) are the multitest systems currently available. The RapID NH is a plastic cuvette containing dehydrated substrates for 12 tests. After inoculation and incubation, positive and negative tests are recorded, a code number is determined, and a computer-generated data base is consulted for the identification. This system has recently been reformatted to include a tributyrin esterase test and a nitrite reduction test for identifying *B. catarrhalis* and *N. cinerea*, respectively. The HNID panel contains 18 tests in a microdilution tray format. After inoculation and a 4-h incubation period, reactions are developed and in-

TABLE 3. Enzyme activities used in chromogenic substrate tests for identifying *Neisseria* species that grow on selective media and *B. catarrhalis*

Species	Activity		
	β-Galactosidase	γ-Glutamylaminopeptidase	Hydroxyprolylaminopeptidase[a]
N. gonorrhoeae	0	0	+
N. meningitidis	0	+	0
N. lactamica	+	0	+
B. catarrhalis	0	0	0

[a] *N. cinerea* and *K. denitrificans*, which may also grow on selective media, are positive for hydroxyprolylaminopeptidase and may be mistaken for *N. gonorrhoeae*.

terpreted, and a computer-assisted identification is made. The NHI card is used in conjunction with the automated Vitek identification-susceptibility test system. The 16-test card is inoculated with a saline suspension of the organism and incubated for 4 h, and the color reactions are read visually. Tests results are entered into the Vitek system computer, which provides an identification.

All three systems reliably identify the pathogenic *Neisseria* spp. and *B. catarrhalis*, although additional tests may be required for some isolates (36, 37, 67). The three systems also include acidometric tests for detecting β-lactamase production by *N. gonorrhoeae* and *B. catarrhalis*.

Immunologic procedures

Currently, immunologic identification tests are restricted to culture confirmation of *N. gonorrhoeae*. Methods include fluorescent-antibody (FA) and coagglutination procedures.

FA test. Older FA tests employed fluorescein-conjugated polyclonal antigonococcal antibodies raised in rabbits. Nongonococcal isolates often cross-reacted with these reagents and some gonococci reacted weakly or not at all (46). The FA procedure now commercially available (*Neisseria gonorrhoeae* Culture Confirmation Test; Syva Co., Palo Alto, Calif.) uses monoclonal antibodies that recognize epitopes on protein I, the principal outer membrane protein of *N. gonorrhoeae*. To perform the test, a light suspension of the organism is dried and heat fixed on an FA slide, overlaid with the FA reagent, and incubated for 15 min. After the smear is rinsed, dried, and mounted with a cover slip, it is examined with a fluorescence microscope. *N. gonorrhoeae* organisms appear as apple green fluorescent diplococci. This FA reagent is highly sensitive and specific (53, 83); however, some gonococcal strains may be weakly fluorescent or fail to fluoresce (82). The advantages of the test are that it is rapid, colonies can be tested directly from selective media, and only a small amount of growth is needed.

Coagglutination methods. Protein A-enriched *Staphylococcus aureus* cells sensitized with monoclonal antibodies against *N. gonorrhoeae* are used as the reagent for confirmatory identification. Three kits are commercially available: the GonoGen I test (New Horizons Diagnostics, Columbia, Md.), the Phadebact GC OMNI test (Pharmacia Diagnostics, Rahway, N.J.), and the Meritec GC test (Meridian Diagnostics, Cincinnati, Ohio). Test performance is similar for the three kits. A standardized suspension of the organism is prepared and boiled for 5 or 10 min. After cooling, the suspension is reacted with single drops of the test and the control reagents included in the kit. After the contents are mixed for a prescribed length of time, agglutination in the test reagent is compared with that in the control.

In general, the coagglutination tests are reliable for identifying *N. gonorrhoeae* (9, 18, 25). However, the instructions of the manufacturers must be followed exactly, and all materials used must be adequately quality controlled. For example, with the Phadebact GC OMNI test, testing of organism suspensions heavier than a 0.5 McFarland turbidity standard or use of saline with a pH of <7.2 has been reported to yield false-positive results when *N. lactamica* and other *Neisseria* species are tested (9, 25). Another confirmatory test (preferably a carbohydrate degradation test) should always be used when (i) isolates suspected of being gonococci produce weak or equivocal reactions with coagglutination procedures, (ii) positive tests are obtained with isolates from extragenital sites of persons at low risk for gonococcal infection, or (iii) positive tests are obtained with isolates from both genital and extragenital sites of children (i.e., sexual abuse is suspected).

Other technology. The GonoGen II is a new immunologic test that has not been extensively evaluated. In this test, a suspension of the test organism is prepared in a lysing solution, and then a drop of gonococcal protein I monoclonal antibodies conjugated to colloidal gold is added. After 2 to 10 min, 2 drops of the suspension are passed through a microfilter that retains antigen-antibody complexes. When *N. gonorrhoeae* is present, a red color is seen on the filter; with nongonococcal isolates, the filter remains white or becomes pale pink.

Comments. The choice of method(s) for identifying gonococci and other *Neisseria* species depends on the number of isolates to be identified, the desired turnaround time, and the frequency with which *Neisseria* species other than *N. gonorrhoeae* are isolated and need to be identified. Carbohydrate degradation tests are advantageous because they can be used to identify all *Neisseria* species encountered in the clinical laboratory. With most commerical systems, results are available in 1 to 4 h. Additional tests must be done to confirm the identification of some species, such as *N. cinerea* and *B. catarrhalis*. Chromogenic enzyme substrate tests are reliable only for those *Neisseria* species that grow well on selective media. Performing tests for *N. gonorrhoeae* only may be appropriate when confirming the identity of genital and extragenital isolates from high-risk or high-prevalence populations but is less desirable under other circumstances, such as suspected sexual abuse in children. If the immunologic tests are used for rapid identification of gonococci, a carbohydrate degradation test should be retained as backup. Products that use dehydrated substrates and thus have a longer shelf life (e.g., the API QuadFERM+) are more feasible for small laboratories that do only a few tests. The CTA-carbohydrate and rapid carbohydrate degradation tests are the most economical, provided personnel are available to prepare them; results can be obtained within 4 h when a heavy inoculum is used.

Direct detection methods

Two methods are available for the direct detection of *N. gonorrhoeae* in urogenital specimens: enzyme immunoassay and nucleic acid probes.

***N. gonorrhoeae* detection by enzyme immunoassay.** The Gonozyme test (Abbott Laboratories, North Chicago, Ill.) is an indirect enzyme immunoassay for detecting gonococci directly in male urethral specimens and in endocervical specimens. For male urethral specimens, Gonozyme has been reported to be equivalent to the Gram-stained smear in sensitivity and specificity. It has also been used successfully for detecting gonococci in first-catch urine specimens from males (68). The test is less sensitive and specific for detecting gonococci in endocervical specimens (72); a positive test is considered only a presumptive result that must be confirmed by culture. The predictive values of positive and negative Gonozyme test results also depend on the prevalence of gonococcal infection in the population being screened; therefore, the prevalence must be considered before the enzyme immunoassay procedure is instituted (72, 76). The use of Gonozyme precludes the performance of other assays that rely on the presence of viable organisms (e.g., antimicrobial susceptibility testing). In addition, expensive proprietary reagents and equipment are required.

Nucleic acid probe. The PACE (probe assay-chemiluminescence enhanced) system (Gen-Probe, San Diego, Calif.) for direct detection of gonococci in urogenital specimens is a 2-h method in which a nonisotopic DNA probe is used to hybridize specifically with gonococcal rRNA. To perform the test, specimens are collected as for culture and placed in a lysing-transport solution; then the hybridization and separation steps are performed. The system uses magnetic particles and a magnetized separation unit for these last steps. Upon addition of an alkaline hydrogen peroxide solution, a light reaction occurs (caused by hydrolysis of the ester bond of the acridinium ester-labeled probe-rRNA duplex) and is read in a chemiluminometer. The amount of light released is directly proportional to the amount of gonococcal rRNA in the specimen. The assay is completed in ca. 2 h. An evaluation of the prototype test in a clinic population having a 21% prevalence of gonococcal infection (29) showed sensitivity and specificity of 93 and 99%, respectively, in comparison with culture on ML medium. The predictive values of positive and negative PACE tests were 97 and 99%, respectively.

Antimicrobial susceptibility testing of *N. gonorrhoeae*

Before 1976, antimicrobial susceptibility testing of *N. gonorrhoeae* isolates was not routinely performed. At that time, however, strains of penicillinase-producing *N. gonorrhoeae* (PPNG) imported from Africa, Asia, and the Philippines were reported in the United States (43). These organisms contain a plasmid that codes for the production of a TEM-type β-lactamase. Between 1976 and 1979, PPNG were associated with sporadic gonorrhea outbreaks in the United States. These outbreaks were usually related to imported strains and were easily controlled. Between 1979 and 1982, however, the number of gonorrhea cases caused by PPNG strains increased 15-fold (34, 84). Large outbreaks occurred in several cities, including New York City, Los Angeles, and Miami. PPNG strains are now endemic in these and other metropolitan areas.

With the appearance of disease caused by PPNG strains, spectinomycin became the drug of choice for treating these infections. By 1981, however, four spectinomycin-resistant *N. gonorrhoeae* isolates had been reported; subsequently, spectinomycin-resistant PPNG strains also appeared (3, 86). Spectinomycin resistance is due to a single-step ribosomal mutation that results in high-level resistance (MIC, ≥256 μg/ml). Most spectinomycin-resistant strains encountered thus far have been linked to overseas sources, and many are also resistant to other antimicrobial agents.

In 1983, non-β-lactamase-producing gonococci resistant to penicillin were described. In these isolates, penicillin resistance is due to the additive effects of mutations at several chromosomal loci, hence their designation as chromosomally mediated resistant *N. gonorrhoeae* (64). Generally, these strains have penicillin MICs of >1 μg/ml, with 75% of these having MICs of >2 μg/ml. Most strains also show moderate resistance to tetracycline and decreased susceptibility to erythromycin and cefoxitin but usually are susceptible to both spectinomycin and ceftriaxone.

In 1985, strains that were penicillin susceptible but showed high-level resistance to tetracycline were isolated (51). These organisms had tetracycline MICs of 16 to 32 μg/ml. Tetracycline-resistant *N. gonorrhoeae* harbor a 25.2-megadalton plasmid resulting from the insertion of a tetracycline resistance determinant (*tetM*) into the 24.5-megadalton conjugative plasmid found in some gonococcal strains (63). The *tetM* determinant is believed to code for a protein(s) that interacts with the gonococcal ribosome to prevent inhibition of protein synthesis by tetracycline.

Because of increasing resistance of *N. gonorrhoeae* to previously useful antimicrobial agents, ceftriaxone is now recommended for therapy by the Public Health Service (12). While most strains are exquisitely susceptible to ceftriaxone, a few strains have been recovered that are less susceptible (MIC, 0.06 μg/ml) and tend to be chromosomally resistant to other agents as well.

For surveillance purposes, all gonococcal isolates should be tested for β-lactamase production. Rapid acidometric, iodometric, or chromogenic cephalosporin methods may be used (chapter 115). When possible, β-lactamase tests should be performed with growth from primary isolation media because the plasmid coding for the enzyme is unstable in some strains and may be lost on subculture. In some regions of the United States, the prevalence of resistant strains has increased to such an extent that antimicrobial susceptibility tests may need to be performed routinely, although primarily for surveillance of gonococcal resistance patterns rather than for individual patient management (12, 47). The recommended procedures for gonococcal antimicrobial susceptibility testing are described in chapter 112.

Gonococcal typing

Although several methods for differentiating strains of *N. gonorrhoeae* have been investigated, auxotyping (11) and serological tests (49) have received the most attention. Auxotyping separates gonococcal strains according to their requirement for one or more metabolites. The organisms are inoculated onto an array of synthetic media from which various substances (primarily amino acids and nitrogenous bases) have been individually omitted. If a strain cannot grow on medium from which arginine, for example, has been omitted, it requires arginine for growth. Auxotyping has permitted characterization of unusual strains of gonococci, such as the small-colony AHU strains that often cause DGI. Most gonococci belong to one of only three or four auxotypes, but they can be further separated by serological analysis.

Methods for serotyping gonococci have included coagglutination, microimmunofluorescence, and enzyme-linked immunosorbent assays. With these methods, the gonococcal outer membrane protein I has been characterized and two serogroups, termed IA and IB, have been distinguished (49). As has been found with the auxotyping method, specific gonococcal characteristics are associated with the serological groups. For example, one serogroup (IA) is highly correlated with DGI and resistance to the bactericidal action of normal human serum. In further epitope analyses using monoclonal antibody reagents, gonococci have been assigned to 18 IA and 28 IB serovars (49). A dual auxotype-serovar classification system has been used to describe gonococcal strain populations and determine epidemiologic correlates of infection (71). In addition, serovar analysis has shown a difference in the distribution of serovars among strains causing DGI and uncomplicated infection (60). Coagglutination reagents for gonococcal serotyping are available commercially (New Horizons Diagnostics, Inc., Columbia, Md.) (60).

NEISSERIA MENINGITIDIS

Clinical significance

Meningococci are isolated most commonly from the oropharynx or nasopharynx of asymptomatic persons who carry the organism for variable time periods, usually only a few weeks. The organism survives poorly in the environment and has no other host; therefore, human carriers are the major reservoir. Person-to-person transmission occurs by direct contact with respiratory secretions or by airborne droplets contaminated with the organism. The usual meningococcal carriage rate is ca. 5 to 15%, but it may rise to higher levels in confined populations, such as among military recruits. Homosexual men have a 40% or higher incidence of meningococcal oropharyngeal carriage (35).

In a small percentage of colonized individuals, the organisms disseminate from the nasopharynx through the bloodstream to produce meningococcemia, meningitis, or both. The disease may be mild, or it may progress extremely rapidly, resulting in the death of a previously healthy person within a few hours. The incidence of disease is highest in infants between 6 months and 1 year of age and in adolescents.

Meningococcemia usually is characterized by profound vascular effects, the most visible being a petechial or purpuric skin rash that occurs in about 75% of patients with the disease. In fulminant infection (Waterhouse-Friderichsen syndrome), there is widespread intravascular coagulation with resulting shock and usually death. The pathogenetic mechanism of these effects is not entirely clear, but presumably it is related to or initiated by endotoxin in the meningococcal outer membrane.

Although the symptoms of meningococcal meningitis are similar to those of other purulent meningitides, when the rash is present a presumptive diagnosis can be made, since this combination of findings is unusual in other infections. Meningococci have also been implicated as agents of arthritis, which is a relatively common complication of meningococcemia, and rarely of purulent conjunctivitis, sinusitis, endocarditis, and primary pneumonia. Persons with inherited deficiencies in their complement system are at greater risk for acquiring systemic meningococcal (and gonococcal) infections and are subject to recurrent episodes of these systemic infections (17).

Screening programs for gonococci have incidentally revealed that meningococci are found in the cervix and vagina, where they may cause serious pelvic disease (28), and they also have been isolated from the anal canal and male urethra (35). Although the clinical implications are not always clear, these findings emphasize the need for species identification of neisserial isolates from these sites.

Meningococci are subdivided into serological groups according to the presence of either capsular or outer membrane protein antigens. Currently, 13 serogroups are recognized (A, B, C, D, 29E, H, I, K, L, W135, X, Y, and Z) but A, B, C, Y, and W135 are most commonly implicated in systemic disease (87). Classically, group A is responsible for epidemic meningococcal disease, and groups B and C are responsible for infections during interepidemic periods, although the latter groups have also been implicated in epidemics. During outbreaks of disease, carriers tend to be colonized with the prevailing serogroup. Other serotypes are isolated sporadically from both carriers and patients with disease.

Specimen collection and transport

Meningococci are isolated most readily when specimens are obtained before antimicrobial therapy is initiated and are transported rapidly to the laboratory with protection from drying and temperature extremes, especially cold. Depending on the clinical presentation, appropriate specimens include blood, cerebrospinal fluid (CSF), petechial aspirates or biopsy, joint fluid, conjunctival swabs, sputum or transtracheal aspirates, and nasopharyngeal swabs. Consult chapter 3 for details of specimen collection and handling.

CSF. The first sample of CSF collected is most likely to be uncontaminated and is best for culture. Subsequent samples can be used for hematological and chemical determinations or for detecting meningococcal antigen by available methods, such as coagglutination or latex agglutination.

Blood. Inoculate blood directly into culture broth. Since there is evidence that the anticoagulant SPS is toxic for some strains of meningococci (24), evacuated blood collection tubes containing this substance probably should not be used when meningococcemia is suspected.

Skin lesions. For petechial cultures, a small amount of sterile saline may be injected into the lesion and then carefully aspirated with a fine hypodermic needle. If possible, appropriate media should be inoculated at the patient's bedside. Alternatively, because the volume of fluid collected is usually small, recap the end of the needle cautiously and deliver the syringe to the laboratory rather than transfer the fluid to another container. If petechial biopsy specimens are obtained, they must be kept moist by transporting them immediately to the laboratory on a chocolate agar plate or in a sterile, closed container with a few drops of saline inside.

Nasopharyngeal swabs. Send nasopharyngeal specimens and other material on swabs (e.g., conjunctival pus) to the laboratory in nonnutritive, semisolid medium such as Amies or Stuart medium. Alternatively, if the specimen must be sent through the mail, plant it directly onto medium in a JEMBEC plate or other CO_2-containing system. Whenever possible, incubate these cultures for 24 h before sending them to the laboratory. Incubated specimens must be shipped in accordance with U.S. postal regulations. Although meningococci can be isolated from the throat, a higher yield is obtained from the nasopharynx, which is the preferred site for specimens.

Direct examination

Gram stain: smear preparation. Because only a few meningococci may be present during the early stages of infection, concentrate CSF specimens by centrifugation or filtration as described in chapter 3. Decant all except 1 ml of the supernatant and save it for an antigen detection test or for culture. Suspend the sediment in the remaining fluid and prepare one or two smears for Gram stain. For noncloudy CSF specimens, it may be necessary to layer several drops to see any organisms after staining. During the staining procedure, rinse the slide on the back surface with gentle rocking to direct the stream of water over the stained area on the front surface. This maneuver prevents the smear from washing away. Little information is gained from Gram-stained smears of sputum or nasopharyngeal swabs because meningococci cannot be distinguished from commensal neisseriae and other morphologically similar bacteria of the upper respiratory tract.

Smear interpretation and reporting. In clinical specimens, meningococci are gram-negative, bean-shaped diplococci, ca. 0.8 by 0.6 μm in diameter. In some instances, they resist decolorization and may appear very deep pink, almost gram positive. The organisms are usually found both extracellularly and intracellularly in PMN (Fig. 5). The presence of PMN is correlated with a good host response and favorable prognosis; therefore, in addition to reporting the numbers, staining characteristics, and morphology of microorganisms present, report the type(s) of inflammatory cells seen and whether the organisms are located intra- or extracellularly. Smears may require examination for 10 min or longer before organisms are seen.

In patients with meningococcal pneumonia, Gram-stained smears of tracheal aspirate reveal PMN and a predominance of gram-negative diplococci. In contrast, in patients with aspiration pneumonia, myriad other organisms are seen along with gram-negative diplococci. The latter most likely are commensal *Neisseria* or *Veillonella* species rather than meningococci. This important distinction must be made because initial patient management is often based on the Gram-stained smear report. Interpretation of smears in meningococcal infections at unusual sites may be further complicated by the occurrence of gram-negative coccobacilli (*Acinetobacter* or *Moraxella* species) in fresh clinical specimens.

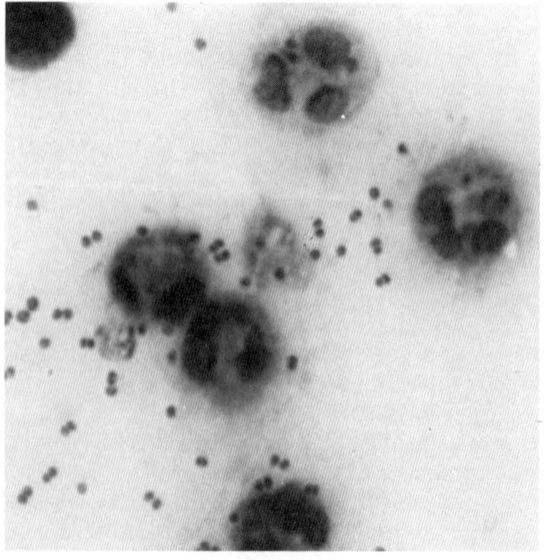

FIG. 5. Gram stain of CSF from a child with meningococcal meningitis. Many intra- and extracellular diplococci are present. ×1,500.

Latex agglutination and coagglutination tests. Both latex agglutination and coagglutination tests for detecting meningococcal antigens in body fluids are commercially available (latex agglutination tests from Becton Dickinson Microbiology Systems and from Wellcome Diagnostics, Research Triangle Park, N.C.; coagglutination test available from Pharmacia). The kits contain polyvalent reagent for serogroups A, C, Y, and W135, with a separate reagent for *N. meningitidis* serogroup B that also detects the cross-reacting *Escherichia coli* K1 antigen. In the clinical laboratory, antigen detection tests should always be used in conjunction with Gram stain and culture. Positive results provide a rapid, presumptive diagnosis and allow early administration of appropriate therapy. Negative results, however, do not exclude a bacterial etiology of the disease.

Culture and isolation

Meningococci are not as nutritionally fastidious as gonococci, but specimens from patients with suspected meningococcal disease must be cultured on enriched medium. Plate all specimens except those likely to contain mixed flora, e.g., nasopharyngeal swabs, onto blood and chocolate agar plates. Streak to obtain isolated colonies. Although meningococci (and gonococci) do not grow well in liquid medium, specimens from sterile sites should also be inoculated into aerobic and anaerobic broths such as tryptic soy broth with blood and supplemented thioglycolate broth to aid recovery of other organisms. Incubate all aerobic media at 35 to 37°C in a 3 to 10% CO_2 environment. Be certain that CO_2 incubators have 50% or higher humidity.

Plate nasopharyngeal swabs onto blood agar and MTM, ML, or NYC medium. Rub the swab over one-quarter of the area of the blood agar plate and one-half of the selective agar medium; then streak the remainder of the plate to obtain isolated colonies. The antimicrobial agents present in the selective media inhibit most, but not all, nasopharyngeal flora except *N. meningitidis*, *N. gonorrhoeae*, and *N. lactamica*. Coexistence of any of these three organisms in a single specimen may be difficult to determine unless the colonies are well separated by streaking. Incubate all media at 35 to 37°C under increased CO_2 and humidity.

Standard blood culture broths such as tryptic soy, Columbia, and brain heart infusion support the growth of meningococci. Commercially available blood culture bottles must be vented to establish appropriate atmospheric conditions. The concentration of SPS present in most commercial broths (0.02 to 0.05%) inhibits some strains of meningococci. As described for gonococci, the addition of gelatin to a final concentration of 1% neutralizes this adverse effect. Lysed blood also neutralizes the inhibitory effects of SPS on meningococci; therefore, cell lysis in the Du Pont Isolator system (E. I. du Pont de Nemours & Co., Inc.) overcomes the

SPS effect on these organisms (73). Meningococci grow and are detected in the BACTEC blood culture system.

Identification

Colony morphology. On agar media, well-isolated meningococcal colonies are much larger than gonococcal colonies, usually attaining a diameter of 1 mm or greater after 18 h of incubation (Fig. 6). The colonies are round and convex, with a smooth, moist, glistening surface and an entire edge. Encapsulated groups A and C may appear mucoid. Although meningococcal colonies are usually not described as being pigmented, on sheep blood agar they often appear gray, whereas some groups (notably 29E and W135) are creamy white in the area of heavy inoculum. In addition, the medium beneath and adjacent to the colonies exhibits a greenish cast. Young cultures have a butyrous consistency, and the colonies emulsify easily in saline. With continued incubation, however, the organisms autolyze, nucleoprotein is released from the cells, and the colonies become sticky and rubbery. At this point, most of the cells are nonviable. Close examination of the culture plate may reveal small daughter colonies growing from the edges of the larger colonies. Often, the culture can be recovered only by subculturing from these small colonies, which revert to normal size on fresh agar medium. Colony variation such as that found with *N. gonorrhoeae* strains is not seen.

Presumptive identification. Meningococcal isolates from CSF and skin lesions are usually present in pure culture. *N. gonorrhoeae* and *N. lactamica* may coexist with meningococci in the nasopharynx. They will grow on the selective ML, MTM, and NYC media commonly used for nasopharyngeal specimens, as may certain gram-negative bacilli that commonly inhabit the nasopharynx (strains of *Kingella*, *Moraxella*, and *Eikenella*). Therefore, carefully examine primary isolation plates, preferably with increased magnification, to determine whether all colonies appear similar. Screen all suspicious colonies with an oxidase test and a Gram stain, as described for the presumptive identification of gonococci. If the primary culture is not pure or is more than 36 h old, prepare a subculture of oxidase-positive, gram-negative diplococci on fresh blood or chocolate agar plates. Incubate for 18 to 24 h at 35°C under increased CO_2 tension; then perform a confirmatory test.

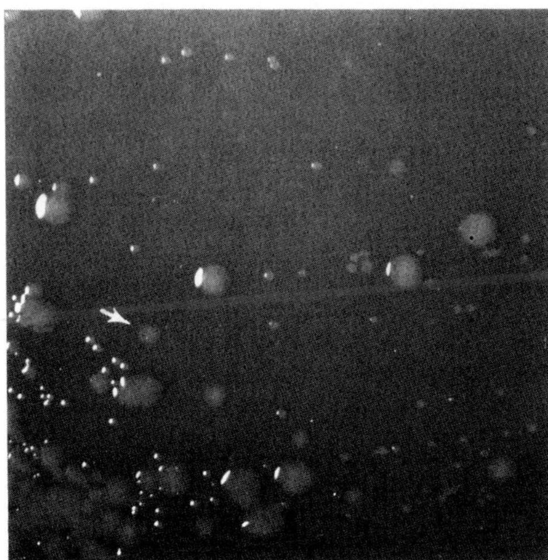

FIG. 6. *N. meningitidis* and *N. gonorrhoeae* on chocolate agar. Meningococcal colonies are larger than gonococcal T3-T4 colonies (arrow). ×2.5.

Confirmatory identification. Characteristically, meningococci degrade glucose and maltose, but not sucrose, fructose, or lactose (Table 2). For the most part, the methods described for the identification of gonococci are used to identify meningococci. Since meningococci grow more rapidly and luxuriantly, however, fewer problems arise.

Carbohydrate degradation tests. The CTA-carbohydrate media, rapid carbohydrate degradation test, and chromogenic substrate tests used for *Neisseria* identification are discussed above. When meningococci are heavily inoculated in the CTA-carbohydrate media, reactions generally are pronounced after 1 to 4 h. A bright yellow color signifies acid production, and negative reactions are indicated by an alkaline (pink) or neutral (orange) reaction. During growth, meningococci degrade peptones in the medium to yield alkaline products which, with prolonged incubation, may obscure the acid reactions in the glucose and maltose tubes. Therefore, examine reactions after 1, 4, and, if necessary, 24 h to detect acid production. If the inoculum was light, further incubation may be necessary.

On initial isolation, some strains of meningococci, primarily those that are resistant to sulfonamides, do not produce acid from maltose (45). Repeated subculture on noninhibitory medium often restores maltose-degrading capability; thus, suspected meningococcal strains that are maltose negative should be retested after several transfers on blood or chocolate agar. The occurrence of glucose-negative meningococci has also been reported. Whenever a suspicious organism is isolated that does not behave as expected biochemically, use an alternative identification system.

Antimicrobial susceptibility testing

In the clinical laboratory, routine antimicrobial susceptibility testing of meningococci is not required because most strains remain highly susceptible to penicillin. A meningococcus harboring the same β-lactamase plasmid as PPNG has been reported from Canada (19) and at least two additional β-lactamase-producing strains have been reported. Several isolates from an epidemic in Spain during the early 1980s showed relative resistance to penicillin (MICs of 0.1 to 0.7 μg/ml, as compared with $\leq$0.06 for susceptible strains) (58). The mechanism of resistance appeared related to reduced binding affinity of penicillin-binding protein 3. Although it is as yet an uncommon event, microbiologists should be alert to the possible occurrence of such penicillin-resistant organisms. Isolates from patients who are not responding well to antimicrobial therapy warrant an agar dilution susceptibility or β-lactamase test to detect possible resistance.

Physicians may request sulfadiazine susceptibility tests to determine whether this drug will be effective for prophylactic treatment of close contacts. The agar dilution method (chapter 110), performed with a limited series of concentrations, is satisfactory for this purpose. Plate 10^5 to 10^6 organisms on Mueller-Hinton agar plates containing 1, 5, or 10 μg of sulfadiazine per ml. Isolates growing at this last concentration are considered resistant. Control plates, including known susceptible and resistant meningococci, as well as an antimicrobial agent-free plate, must be run at the same time. For rifampin, growth on Mueller-Hinton agar plates containing 0.25 μg of rifampin is considered evidence of rifampin resistance.

Meningococcal grouping

Several serological methods have been used to group meningococci; however, agglutination is the most reliable and routinely used technique (79). In 0.5 ml of phosphate-buffered saline (pH 7.2), prepare a milky suspension of cells grown for 8 to 12 h on blood agar. Allow any clumps of organisms to settle for 1 min; then, with a Pasteur pipette, mix 1 drop of the suspension with 1 drop of antiserum on a slide or in the well of a plastic tray. Rotate the mixture for 2 to 4 min, observing the reaction with indirect lighting. High-titer, specific antiserum usually produces a strong reaction within 2 min. Almost all meningococci isolated from systemic infections are groupable by this technique. Nasopharyngeal isolates from carriers, however, may not be groupable; i.e., they agglutinate in all (autoagglutinable) or in none of the antisera. Rapid passage of the organism on blood agar or the use of pH 6.8 buffer for the agglutination test may resolve the problem. Meningococcal grouping sera are available commercially from Difco Laboratories and Wellcome Diagnostics. Other methods that have been used to type meningococci include antigenic analysis of outer membrane proteins and electrophoretic analysis of soluble cytoplasmic enzymes, or combinations of both (1).

The auxotyping technique is not useful for differentiating strains of meningococci because they are biosynthetically more competent than gonococci (see the section on gonococcal typing). All gonococci require cysteine (or cystine) for growth, whereas ca. 90% of meningococci do not. Because of this difference, a nutritionally complete medium lacking only cysteine can be used to differentiate gonococci from most strains of meningococci.

NEISSERIA SPECIES

Clinical significance

The primary habitats of other *Neisseria* species that colonize humans are the nasopharynx and oropharynx. These species include *N. lactamica, N. cinerea, N. polysaccharea, N. flavescens, N. subflava* (including biovars *subflava, flava,* and *perflava*), *N. sicca, N. mucosa,* and *N. elongata* (46, 80). Although they are considered to be of low virulence, on a few occasions several of these organisms have been implicated as the etiological agent of one or more of the following infections: meningitis, bacteremia, endocarditis, empyema, pericarditis, and pneumonia (33). *N. lactamica* has also been isolated from the urogenital tract (42). When they are isolated from blood, CSF, or other normally sterile body fluids and secretions, these organisms must be identified and distinguished from *N. meningitidis* or even *N. gonorrhoeae. N. lactamica* and *N. polysaccharea* are most often confused with *N. meningitidis* because they grow on gonococcal selective media and ferment both glucose and maltose (Table 2). Both are isolated primarily from the nasopharynges of young children (4, 65), in contrast to meningococci, which are more often carried by teenagers and young adults. Although *N. cinerea* usually does not grow on gonococcal selective media, it may be misidentified as *N. gonorrhoeae* in specimens plated on nonselective media (16). A strain referred to as *N. gonorrhoeae* subsp. *kochii* has been isolated in Egypt from patients with conjunctivitis and urethritis (46). This strain has the biochemical but not serological characteristics of *N. gonorrhoeae* and a colony morphology resembling that of *N. meningitidis* strains. Rarely, species that colonize animals may be isolated from humans, e.g., *Neisseria canis* from a cat bite wound (31).

Identification

Identification of *Neisseria* species other than *N. gonorrhoeae* and *N. meningitidis* generally is not necessary unless the organism is determined to be clinically significant or is isolated from a systemic site such as blood or CSF. Identification is based on colony morphology and pigmentation, presence or absence of growth on selective media and on nutrient agar at 35 and 22°C, acid production from carbohydrates, reduction of nitrate and nitrite, and synthesis of a starchlike polysaccharide from sucrose (Table 2). Acid production from fructose and sucrose is helpful for separating the three biovars of *N. subflava* and can be performed with the rapid carbohydrate degradation procedure described above (biovar *perflava* produces acid from both carbohydrates, biovar *flava* produces acid from fructose but not sucrose, and biovar *subflava* produces acid from neither). Nitrate and nitrite reduction are determined in tryptic soy or brain heart infusion broth containing 0.01% (wt/vol) nitrate and 0.01 or 0.001% (wt/vol) nitrite (potassium salts), respectively. Reactions are developed with standard nitrate test reagents after 48 h of incubation. To detect polysaccharide synthesis, inoculate the organism onto brain heart infusion agar plates with and without added 5% sucrose. After 48 h of incubation, flood the plates with Lugol iodine (1:4 dilution in water). In a positive test, the colonies on the sucrose plate turn deep blue in comparison with the control plate. We have observed positive reactions (deep blue color) when Gram iodine was added to inoculated and incubated (ca. 4 h) CTA-sucrose agar slants or the sucrose-containing tube of the rapid carbohydrate degradation test. Iodine added to any other carbohydrate-containing tube serves as a negative control (brown color).

Identification errors likely to be made in the clinical laboratory are illustrated by a report from the Centers for Disease Control (85) in which 14 isolates initially identified as *N. gonorrhoeae* were confirmed to be other species. These isolates, all from children, represented approximately one-third of the strains received over a 2-year period. The initial incorrect diagnosis led to investigations for suspected sexual abuse in almost all instances, even though it had not been suspected in 10 children. The sources of the isolates were as follows: throat, five; eye, four; vagina, two; CSF, one; rectum, one; and urethra, one. The confirmed identifications were the following: *N. cinerea*, four; *N. lactamica*, three; *B. catarrhalis*, three; *N. meningitidis*, two (including the CSF isolate); *K. denitrificans*, one; and unidentified *Neisseria* species, one. This report highlights the need to be suspicious of "gonococci" isolated from unusual sources or unlikely clinical situations and to perform more than one confirmatory test with them.

Coccobacillary gram-negative rods in the family *Neisseriaceae* closely resemble *Neisseria* species in Gram-stained smears and culture, but a simple test is available to determine their true bacillary morphology. Streak the organism in question on a blood agar plate and place a 10-U penicillin disk on the inoculated area. Incubate the plate for 18 to 24 h and then examine growth from the edge of the zone of inhibition by preparing a crystal violet-stained smear. Under the influence of subinhibitory concentrations of penicillin, bacilli form long, stringy cells, whereas cocci retain their coccal morphology (10) (Fig. 7). In this test, *N. elongata* forms long cells and must be differentiated from gram-negative bacilli in the family *Neisseriaceae* by additional tests (5).

BRANHAMELLA CATARRHALIS

B. catarrhalis has been recognized as a cause of human infections since the early 1900s; however, only during the past 10 to 15 years has there been a clear appreciation of the extent of disease in which it is involved (20). The genus *Branhamella* consists of three species in addition to *B. catarrhalis*: *B. caviae*, *B. ovis*, and *B. cuniculi*. These species are known to colonize various animals (e.g., guinea pigs, sheep, and rabbits) but have not been described in association with humans. They will not be described further here.

Clinical significance

B. catarrhalis causes a wide variety of human infections, ranging from systemic, life-threatening diseases such as endocarditis and meningitis to acute, localized processes such as acute otitis media, sinusitis, and bronchopulmonary infections. Among the diseases ascribed to *B. catarrhalis*, the last three are the most important in terms of incidence and morbidity. *B. catarrhalis* is the third most common bacterial cause of acute otitis media, accounting for 10 to 15% of cases (27). It occupies an equally important role in acute maxillary sinusitis. In certain epidemiologic settings, *B. catarrhalis* represents the second or third most common cause of bacterial infections of the lower respiratory tract. For example, among elderly patients with chronic obstructive pulmonary disease, *B. catarrhalis* is exceeded only by *Haemophilus influenzae*, and perhaps *Streptococcus pneumoniae*, as a cause of acute purulent exacerbations of chronic bronchitis (20); it is also associated with frank pneumonia.

B. catarrhalis is part of the commensal flora of the upper respiratory tract of healthy humans. Infections of the middle ears or maxillary sinuses arise after direct contiguous spread of the organism from its normal site. Similarly, bronchopulmonary infections result from endobronchial seeding of the lungs. Pathogenetic mechanisms that could explain the disease-causing potential of *B. catarrhalis* have not been elucidated.

Specimen selection and initial processing

The specimens of choice in patients with acute otitis media and maxillary sinusitis are tympanocentesis fluid and sinus aspirates, respectively. Such specimens are usually not forthcoming, however, because their collection requires invasive procedures, with the attendant risks of untoward side effects, patient discomfort, and cost. As a result, these diseases are usually treated empirically. When middle ear fluid or sinus aspirates are received in the laboratory for microbiological analysis, to recover *B. catarrhalis* they should be cultured in the same manner as described below for expectorated sputum.

Expectorated sputum is a satisfactory specimen from most patients with *B. catarrhalis* lower respiratory tract infections. In two investigations comparing paired expectorated sputa and transtracheal aspirates, equivalent Gram stain and culture findings were reported (2, 77). A Gram-stained smear should be performed initially. Gram stain typically reveals numerous PMN, abundant mucus strands, and large numbers of gram-negative diplococci, 0.5 to 1.5 μm in diameter. The organisms are almost always extracellular and often arranged in rows along strands of mucus. These Gram stain findings

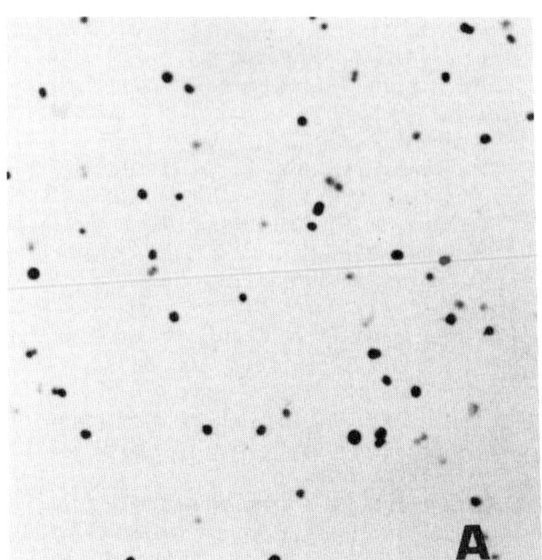

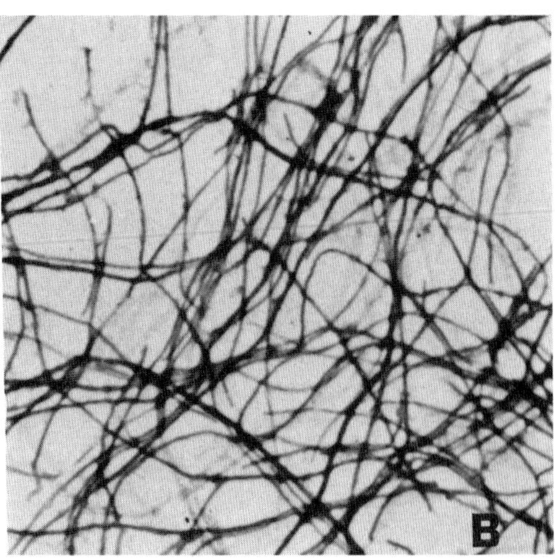

FIG. 7. Cocci (A) and bacilli (B) exposed to subinhibitory concentrations of penicillin. Some cocci are swollen but still coccoid; bacilli form long strings. ×1,000.

are nearly diagnostic for *B. catarrhalis* bronchopulmonary infection. *Neisseria* species, which could be confused with *B. catarrhalis* because of similar morphology, rarely cause lower respiratory tract infections. Furthermore, most patients with acute bronchitis or pneumonia due to *B. catarrhalis* produce sputum with this Gram stain appearance. As a diagnostic procedure, Gram stain of expectorated sputum has excellent sensitivity, as does Gram stain of middle ear fluid or sinus aspirates from patients with *B. catarrhalis* infections at those sites.

To recover *B. catarrhalis* in culture, inoculate specimens onto 5% sheep blood agar or chocolate agar or both. Incubate plates at 35°C in either ambient air or 5 to 7% CO_2 before examining them. A variable percent of *B. catarrhalis* strains also grow on media selective for gonococci and meningococci (21).

Identification

After overnight growth on sheep blood or chocolate agar, *B. catarrhalis* produces small, round, entire, whitish gray colonies approximately 3 to 5 mm in diameter. The colonies may be swept across the plate nearly intact with a bacteriological loop, a "hockey puck" characteristic that is very suggestive of *B. catarrhalis*. Gram-stained smears of colonies reveal kidney bean-shaped, gram-negative diplococci, 0.5 to 1.5 μm in diameter. The organisms are oxidase and catalase positive.

Identifying characteristics include failure to ferment glucose, maltose, sucrose, and lactose or to grow on nutrient agar at room temperature; DNase production; nitrate reduction (21) (Table 2); and production of butyrate esterase. Carbohydrate degradation may be determined over 72 h by using 1 to 2% concentrations of carbohydrates and a pH indicator in any of the following basal media: CTA (44), NYC fermentation medium (26), cysteine proteose peptone agar (67), or proteose peptone agar containing NaCl and K_2HPO_4 (48). Rapid, same-day determination of carbohydrate fermentation patterns based on detection of preformed enzymes in heavy inoculum suspensions can be performed by the methods described above for identifying *Neisseria* species (7, 36, 37, 44, 62, 66, 67).

B. catarrhalis is thought not to produce β-galactosidase, prolylaminopeptidase, and γ-glutamylaminopeptidase, the three enzymes used in the rapid chromogenic enzyme systems. However, false-positive reactions for both prolylaminopeptidase and γ-glutamylaminopeptidase may be obtained with some clinical isolates. Therefore, these systems must be used with care.

The two most useful identifying characteristics for *B. catarrhalis* are DNase and butyrate esterase production. Any test that has proven reliable with the *Enterobacteriaceae* may be used to detect DNase production (74). Butyrate esterase activity may be detected fluorometrically with methylumbelliferyl butyrate as the substrate (15, 78) or colorimetrically with tributyrin as the substrate (38).

Antimicrobial susceptibility testing of *B. catarrhalis* is discussed in chapter 112. All clinically significant isolates should be tested for β-lactamase production with a nitrocefin-based test. If positive, this test may also be used to identify presumptively *B. catarrhalis* if the isolate is an oxidase-positive, gram-negative diplococcus recovered from middle ear fluid, sinus aspirates, or representative specimens from the lower respiratory tract. At present, the only β-lactamase-producing, oxidase-positive, gram-negative diplococcus recovered from these three sites is *B. catarrhalis*. Furthermore, at least 85% of clinically significant isolates produce this enzyme (22).

LITERATURE CITED

1. **Achtman, M., B. A. Crowe, A. Olyhoek, W. Strittmatter, and G. Morelli.** 1988. Recent results on epidemic meningococcal meningitis. J. Med. Microbiol. **26:**172–177.
2. **Aitken, J. M., and P. E. Thornley.** 1983. Isolation of *Branhamella catarrhalis* from sputum and tracheal aspirates. J. Clin. Microbiol. **18:**1262–1266.
3. **Ashford, W. A., D. W. Potts, H. J. U. Adams, J. C. English, S. R. Johnson, J. W. Biddle, C. Thornsberry, and H. W. Jaffe.** 1981. Spectinomycin-resistant penicillinase-producing *Neisseria gonorrhoeae*. Lancet **ii:**1035–1037.
4. **Boquete, M. T., C. Marcos, and J. A. Sáez-Nieto.** 1986. Characterization of *Neisseria polysacchareae* sp. nov. (Riou, 1983) in previously identified noncapsular strains of *Neisseria meningitidis*. J. Clin. Microbiol. **24:**973–975.
5. **Bøvre, K.** 1984. *Moraxella*, p. 296–303. *In* N. R. Krieg (ed.), Bergey's manual of systematic bacteriology, vol. 2. The Williams & Wilkins Co., Baltimore.
6. **Boyce, J. M., and E. B. Mitchell, Jr.** 1985. Difficulties in differentiating *Neisseria cinerea* from *Neisseria gonorrhoeae* in rapid systems used for identifying pathogenic *Neisseria* species. J. Clin. Microbiol. **22:**731–734.
7. **Brown, W. J.** 1974. Modification of the rapid fermentation test for *Neisseria gonorrhoeae*. Appl. Microbiol. **27:**1027–1030.
8. **Brown, W. J., and S. J. Kraus.** 1974. Gonococcal colony types. J. Am. Med. Assoc. **228:**862–863.
9. **Carlson, B. L., M. B. Calnan, R. E. Goodman, and H. George.** 1987. Phadebact monoclonal GC OMNI test for confirmation of *Neisseria gonorrhoeae*. J. Clin. Microbiol. **25:**1982–1984.
10. **Catlin, B. W.** 1975. Cellular elongation under the influence of antibacterial agents: way to differentiate coccobacilli from cocci. J. Clin. Microbiol. **1:**102–105.
11. **Catlin, B. W.** 1978. Characteristics and auxotyping of *Neisseria gonorrhoeae*, p. 345–380. *In* T. Bergen and J. R. Norris (ed.), Methods in microbiology, vol. 10. Academic Press, Inc., New York.
12. **Centers for Disease Control.** 1987. Antibiotic resistant strains of *Neisseria gonorrhoeae:* policy guidelines for detection, management, and control. Morbid. Mortal. Weekly Rep. **36:**1S–18S.
13. **Crawford, G., J. S. Knapp, J. Hale, and K. K. Holmes.** 1977. Asymptomatic gonorrhea in men: caused by gonococci with unique nutritional requirements. Science **196:** 1352–1353.
14. **Dallabetta, G., and E. W. Hook III.** 1987. Gonococcal infections. Infect. Dis. Clin. N. Am. **1:**25–54.
15. **Dealler, S. F., M. Abbott, M. J. Croughan, and P. M. Hawkey.** 1989. Identification of *Branhamella catarrhalis* in 2.5 min with an indoxyl butyrate strip test. J. Clin. Microbiol. **27:**1390–1391.
16. **Denison, M. R., S. Perlman, and R. D. Andersen.** 1988. Misidentification of *Neisseria* species in a neonate with conjunctivitis. Pediatrics **81:**877–888.
17. **Densen, P.** 1989. Interaction of complement with *Neisseria meningitidis* and *Neisseria gonorrhoeae*. Clin. Microbiol. Rev. **2:**S11–S17.
18. **Dillon, J. R., M. Carballo, and M. Pauze.** 1988. Evaluation of eight methods for identification of pathogenic *Neisseria* species: Neisseria Kwik, RIM-N, Gonobio-Test, Minitek, Gonochek II, GonoGen, Phadebact Monoclonal GC OMNI test, and Syva Micro Trak test. J. Clin. Microbiol. **26:**493–497.

19. **Dillon, J. R., M. Pauze, and K.-H. Yeung.** 1983. Spread of penicillinase-producing and transfer plasmids from the gonococcus to *Neisseria meningitidis*. Lancet **i**:779–781.
20. **Doern, G. V.** 1986. *Branhamella catarrhalis*—an emerging human pathogen. Diagn. Microbiol. Infect. Dis. **4**:191–201.
21. **Doern, G. V., and S. A. Morse.** 1980. *Branhamella (Neisseria) catarrhalis:* criteria for laboratory identification. J. Clin. Microbiol. **11**:193–199.
22. **Doern, G. V., and T. A. Tubert.** 1987. Detection of β-lactamase activity among clinical isolates of *Branhamella catarrhalis* with six different β-lactamase assays. J. Clin. Microbiol. **25**:1380–1383.
23. **Dossett, J. H., P. C. Appelbaum, J. S. Knapp, and P. A. Totten.** 1985. Proctitis associated with *Neisseria cinerea* misidentified as *Neisseria gonorrhoeae* in a child. J. Clin. Microbiol. **21**:575–577.
24. **Eng, J., and E. Holten.** 1977. Gelatin neutralization of the inhibitory effect of sodium polyanethol sulfonate on *Neisseria meningitidis* in blood culture media. J. Clin. Microbiol. **6**:1–3.
25. **Evins, G. M., N. E. Pigot, J. S. Knapp, and W. E. DeWitt.** 1988. Panel of reference strains for evaluating serologic reagents used to identify gonococci. J. Clin. Microbiol. **26**:354–357.
26. **Faur, V. C., M. H. Weisburd, M. E. Wilson, and P. S. May.** 1973. A new medium for the isolation of pathogenic *Neisseria* (NYC medium). 1. Formulation and comparisons with standard media. Health Lab. Sci. **10**:44–52.
27. **Giebink, G. S.** 1989. The microbiology of otitis media. Pediatr. Infect. Dis. J. **8**:518–520.
28. **Givan, K. F., B. W. Thomas, and A. G. Johnston.** 1977. Isolation of *Neisseria meningitidis* from the urethra, cervix and anal canal: further observations. Br. J. Vener. Dis. **53**:109–112.
29. **Granato, P. A., and M. R. Franz.** 1989. Evaluation of a prototype DNA probe test for the noncultural diagnosis of gonorrhea. J. Clin. Microbiol. **27**:632–635.
30. **Granato, P. A., C. Schneible-Smith, and L. B. Weiner.** 1981. Primary isolation of *Neisseria gonorrhoeae* on hemoglobin-free New York City medium. J. Clin. Microbiol. **14**:206–209.
31. **Guibourdenche, M., T. Lambert, and J. Y. Riou.** 1989. Isolation of *Neisseria canis* in mixed culture from a patient after a cat bite. J. Clin. Microbiol. **27**:1673–1674.
32. **Henriksen, S. D.** 1976. *Moraxella, Neisseria, Branhamella,* and *Acinetobacter*. Annu. Rev. Microbiol. **30**:63–83.
33. **Herbert, D. A., and J. Ruskin.** 1981. Are the "nonpathogenic" neisseriae pathogenic? Am. J. Clin. Pathol. **75**:739–742.
34. **Hook, E. W., W. E. Brady, C. A. Reichert, D. M. Upchurch, L. A. Sherman, and J. N. Wasserheit.** 1989. Determinants of emergence of antibiotic-resistant *Neisseria gonorrhoeae*. J. Infect. Dis. **159**:900–907.
35. **Janda, W. M., M. Bohnhoff, J. A. Morello, and S. A. Lerner.** 1980. Prevalence and site-pathogen studies of *Neisseria meningitidis* and *N. gonorrhoeae* in homosexual men. J. Am. Med. Assoc. **244**:2060–2064.
36. **Janda, W. M., J. J. Bradna, and P. Ruther.** 1989. Identification of *Neisseria* spp., *Haemophilus* spp., and other fastidious gram-negative bacteria with the MicroScan *Haemophilus-Neisseria* identification panel. J. Clin. Microbiol. **27**:869–873.
37. **Janda, W. M., P. J. Malloy, and P. C. Schreckenberger.** 1987. Clinical evaluation of the Vitek *Neisseria-Haemophilus* identification card. J. Clin. Microbiol. **25**:37–41.
38. **Janda, W. M., and P. Ruther.** 1989. B. CAT CONFIRM, a rapid test for confirmation of *Branhamella catarrhalis*. J. Clin. Microbiol. **27**:1130–1131.
39. **Janda, W. M., and V. Sobieski.** 1988. Evaluation of a ten-minute chromogenic substrate test for identification of pathogenic *Neisseria* species and *Branhamella catarrhalis*. Eur. J. Clin. Microbiol. Infect. Dis. **7**:25–29.
40. **Janda, W. M., M. G. Ulanday, M. Bohnhoff, and L. J. LeBeau.** 1985. Evaluation of the RIM-N, Gonochek II, and Phadebact systems for the identification of the pathogenic *Neisseria* spp. and *Branhamella catarrhalis*. J. Clin. Microbiol. **21**:734–737.
41. **Janda, W. M., K. L. Zigler, and J. J. Bradna.** 1987. API QuadFERM+ with rapid DNase for identification of *Neisseria* spp. and *Branhamella catarrhalis*. J. Clin. Microbiol. **25**:203–206.
42. **Jephcott, A. E., and R. S. Morton.** 1972. Isolation of *Neisseria lactamica* from a genital site. Lancet **ii**:739–740.
43. **Johnson, S. R., and S. A. Morse.** 1988. Antibiotic resistance in *Neisseria gonorrhoeae:* genetics and mechanisms of resistance. Sex. Transm. Dis. **15**:217–224.
44. **Kellogg, D. S., Jr., K. K. Holmes, and G. A. Hill.** 1976. Cumitech 4, Laboratory diagnosis of gonorrhea. Coordinating ed., S. Marcus and J. C. Sherris. American Society for Microbiology, Washington, D.C.
45. **Kingsbury, D. T.** 1967. Relationship between sulfadiazine resistance and the failure to ferment maltose in *Neisseria meningitidis*. J. Bacteriol. **94**:557–561.
46. **Knapp, J. S.** 1988. Historical perspectives and identification of *Neisseria* and related species. Clin. Microbiol. Rev. **1**:415–431.
47. **Knapp, J. S.** 1988. Laboratory methods for the detection and phenotypic characterization of *Neisseria gonorrhoeae* strains resistant to antimicrobial agents. Sex. Transm. Dis. **15**:225–233.
48. **Knapp, J. S., and K. K. Holmes.** 1983. Modified oxidation-fermentation medium for detection of acid production from carbohydrates by *Neisseria* spp. and *Branhamella catarrhalis*. J. Clin. Microbiol. **18**:56–62.
49. **Knapp, J. S., M. R. Tam, R. C. Nowinski, K. K. Holmes, and E. G. Sandström.** 1984. Serological classification of *Neisseria gonorrhoeae* with use of monoclonal antibodies to gonococcal outer membrane protein I. J. Infect. Dis. **150**:44–48.
50. **Knapp, J. S., P. A. Totten, M. H. Mulks, and B. H. Minshew.** 1984. Characterization of *Neisseria cinerea,* a nonpathogenic species isolated on Martin-Lewis medium selective for pathogenic *Neisseria* spp. J. Clin. Microbiol. **19**:63–67.
51. **Knapp, J. S., J. M. Zenilman, J. W. Biddle, G. H. Perkins, W. E. DeWitt, M. L. Thomas, S. R. Johnson, and S. A. Morse.** 1987. Frequency and distribution in the United States of strains of *Neisseria gonorrhoeae* with plasmid-mediated, high-level resistance to tetracycline. J. Infect. Dis. **155**:819–822.
52. **Lauer, B. A., and H. B. Masters.** 1988. Toxic effect of calcium alginate swabs on *Neisseria gonorrhoeae*. J. Clin. Microbiol. **26**:54–56.
53. **Laughon, B. E., J. M. Ehret, T. T. Tanino, B. Van der Pol, H. H. Handsfield, R. B. Jones, F. N. Judson, and E. W. Hook.** 1987. Fluorescent monoclonal antibody for confirmation of *Neisseria gonorrhoeae* cultures. J. Clin. Microbiol. **25**:2388–2390.
54. **Lossick, J. G., M. P. Smeltzer, and J. W. Curran.** 1982. The value of the cervical Gram stain in the diagnosis and treatment of gonorrhea in women in a venereal disease clinic. Sex. Transm. Dis. **9**:124–127.
55. **Martin, J. E., J. H. Armstrong, and P. B. Smith.** 1974. New system for cultivation of *Neisseria gonorrhoeae*. Appl. Microbiol. **27**:802–805.
56. **Martin, J. E., and J. S. Lewis.** 1977. Anisomycin: improved antimycotic activity in modified Thayer-Martin medium. Public Health Lab. **35**:53–62.
57. **Martin, J. E., Jr., and R. L. Jackson.** 1975. A biological environment chamber for the culture of *Neisseria gonorrhoeae*. J. Am. Vener. Dis. Assoc. **2**:28–30.
58. **Mendelman, P. M., J. Campos, D. O. Chaffin, D. A. Serfass, A. L. Smith, and J. A. Sáez-Nieto.** 1988. Relative penicillin G resistance in *Neisseria meningitidis* and reduced affinity of penicillin-binding protein 3. Antimicrob. Agents Chemother. **32**:706–709.

59. **Mirrett, S., L. B. Reller, and J. S. Knapp.** 1981. *Neisseria gonorrhoeae* strains inhibited by vancomycin in selective media and correlation with auxotype. J. Clin. Microbiol. **14:**94–99.
60. **Morello, J. A., and M. Bohnhoff.** 1989. Serovars and serum resistance of *Neisseria gonorrhoeae* from disseminated and uncomplicated infections. J. Infect. Dis. **160:** 1012–1017.
61. **Morello, J. A., S. A. Lerner, and M. Bohnhoff.** 1976. Characteristics of atypical *Neisseria gonorrhoeae* from disseminated and localized infections. Infect. Immun. **13:** 1510–1516.
62. **Morse, S. A., and L. Bartenstein.** 1976. Adaptation of the Minitek system for the rapid identification of *Neisseria gonorrhoeae*. J. Clin. Microbiol. **2:**8–13.
63. **Morse, S. A., S. R. Johnson, J. W. Biddle, and M. C. Roberts.** 1986. High-level tetracycline resistance in *Neisseria gonorrhoeae* is result of acquisition of streptococcal *tetM* determinant. Antimicrob. Agents Chemother. **30:**664–670.
64. **Rice, S. J., J. W. Biddle, Y. A. JeanLouis, W. E. DeWitt, J. H. Blount, and S. A. Morse.** 1986. Chromosomally-mediated resistance in *Neisseria gonorrhoeae* in the United States: results of surveillance and reporting, 1983–1984. J. Infect. Dis. **153:**340–345.
65. **Riou, J.-Y., and M. Guibourdenche.** 1987. *Neisseria polysaccharea* sp. nov. Int. J. Syst. Bacteriol. **37:**163–165.
66. **Robinson, A., S. B. Griffith, D. G. Moore, and J. R. Carlson.** 1985. Evaluation of the RIM system and GonoGen test for identification of *Neisseria gonorrhoeae* from clinical specimens. Diagn. Microbiol. Infect. Dis. **3:**125–130.
67. **Robinson, M. J., and T. R. Oberhofer.** 1983. Identification of pathogenic *Neisseria* species with the RapID NH system. J. Clin. Microbiol. **17:**400–404.
68. **Roongpisuthipong, A., J. S. Lewis, S. J. Kraus, and S. A. Morse.** 1988. Gonococcal urethritis diagnosed from enzyme immunoassay of urine sediment. Sex. Transm. Dis. **15:**192–195.
69. **Rossau, R., G. Vandenbussche, S. Thielemans, P. Segers, H. Grosch, E. Göthe, W. Mannheim, and J. DeLey.** 1989. Ribosomal ribonucleic acid cistron similarities and deoxyribonucleic acid homologies of *Neisseria, Kingella, Eikenella, Simonsiella, Alysiella,* and Centers for Disease Control groups EF-4 and M-5 in the emended family *Neisseriaceae*. Int. J. Syst. Bacteriol. **39:**185–198.
70. **Saigh, J. H., C. C. Sanders, and W. E. Sanders, Jr.** 1978. Inhibition of *Neisseria gonorrhoeae* by aerobic and facultatively anaerobic components of the endocervical flora: evidence for a protective effect against infection. Infect. Immun. **19:**704–710.
71. **Sarafian, S. K., and J. S. Knapp.** 1989. Molecular epidemiology of gonorrhea. Clin. Microbiol. Rev. **2:**S49–S55.
72. **Schachter, J., W. M. McCormack, R. F. Smith, R. M. Parks, R. Bailey, and A. C. Ohlin.** 1984. Enzyme immunoassay for diagnosis of gonorrhea. J. Clin. Microbiol. **19:** 57–59.
73. **Scribner, R. K., and D. F. Welch.** 1984. Neutralization of the inhibitory effect of sodium polyanetholsulfonate on *Neisseria meningitidis* in blood cultures processed with the Du Pont Isolator system. J. Clin. Microbiol. **20:**40–42.
74. **Soto-Hernandez, J. L., D. Nunley, S. Holtsclaw-Berk, and S. L. Berk.** 1988. Selective medium with DNase test agar and a modified toluidine blue O technique for primary isolation of *Branhamella catarrhalis* in sputum. J. Clin. Microbiol. **26:**405–408.
75. **Staneck, J. L., and S. Vincent.** 1981. Inhibition of *Neisseria gonorrhoeae* by sodium polyanetholsulfonate. J. Clin. Microbiol. **13:**463–467.
76. **Thomason, J. L., S. M. Gelbart, V. J. Sobieski, R. J. Anderson, M. B. Schulien, and P. R. Hamilton.** 1989. Effectiveness of Gonozyme for detection of gonorrhea in low-risk pregnant and gynecologic populations. Sex. Transm. Dis. **16:**28–31.
77. **Thornley, P. E., J. Aitken, C. J. Drennan, J. MacVicar, and N. J. Sleven.** 1982. *Branhamella catarrhalis* infection of the lower respiratory tract: reliable diagnosis by sputum examination. Br. Med. J. **285:**1537–1542.
78. **Vaneechoutte, M., G. Verschraegen, G. Claeys, and P. Flamen.** 1988. Rapid identification of *Branhamella catarrhalis* with 4-methylumbelliferyl butyrate. J. Clin. Microbiol. **26:**1227–1228.
79. **Vedros, N. A.** 1978. Serology of the meningococcus, p. 293–314. *In* T. Bergen and J. R. Norris (ed.), Methods in microbiology, vol. 10. Academic Press, Inc., New York.
80. **Vedros, N. A.** 1984. *Neisseria*, p. 290–296. *In* N. R. Krieg (ed.), Bergey's manual of systematic bacteriology, vol. 1. The Williams & Wilkins Co., Baltimore.
81. **Vera, H. D.** 1948. A simple medium for identification and maintenance of the gonococcus and other bacteria. J. Bacteriol. **55:**531–536.
82. **Walton, D. T.** 1989. Fluorescent-antibody-negative penicillinase-producing *Neisseria gonorrhoeae*. J. Clin. Microbiol. **27:**1885–1886.
83. **Welch, W. D., and G. Cartwright.** 1988. Fluorescent monoclonal antibody compared with carbohydrate utilization for rapid identification of *Neisseria gonorrhoeae*. J. Clin. Microbiol. **26:**293–296.
84. **Whittington, W. L., and J. S. Knapp.** 1988. Trends in resistance of *Neisseria gonorrhoeae* to antimicrobial agents in the United States. Sex. Transm. Dis. **15:**202–210.
85. **Whittington, W. L., R. J. Rice, J. W. Biddle, and J. S. Knapp.** 1988. Incorrect identification of *Neisseria gonorrhoeae* from infants and children. Pediatr. Infect. Dis. J. **7:**3–10.
86. **Zenilman, J. M., L. J. Nims, M. A. Menegus, F. Nolte, and J. S. Knapp.** 1987. Spectinomycin-resistant gonococcal infections in the United States, 1985–1986. J. Infect. Dis. **156:**1002–1004.
87. **Zollinger, W. D., B. L. Brandt, and E. C. Tramont.** 1986. Immune response to *Neisseria meningitidis*, p. 346–352. *In* N. R. Rose, H. Friedman, and J. L. Fahey (ed.), Manual of clinical laboratory immunology, 3rd ed. American Society for Microbiology, Washington, D.C.

Chapter 31

Corynebacterium and Related Organisms

T. KRECH AND DANNIE G. HOLLIS

DESCRIPTION OF THE GENUS AND RELATED ORGANISMS

The genus *Corynebacterium* was originally created for the "Diphtherie-Bacillus" (12). Subsequently, further bacteria of human, animal, and plant origin were included in the genus on morphologic grounds until the genus encompassed a wide collection of gram-positive, nonsporeforming, non-acid-fast, aerobic or facultative anaerobic, catalase-positive, nonmotile, and slightly curved club-shaped rods. In *Bergey's Manual of Systematic Bacteriology* (12, 34), the genus is restricted to bacteria containing *meso*-diaminopimelic acid in their cell wall, as well as *arabino*-galactan polymer and short-chain (C_{22} to C_{36}) mycolic acids. Cellular fatty acids are predominantly straight-chain saturated and monounsaturated (12). Corynebacteria have a DNA G+C content of 51 to 65 mol%. On chemotaxonomic grounds, the genus *Corynebacterium* is most closely related to the genera *Rhodococcus, Nocardia,* and *Mycobacterium* (34).

The genus *Corynebacterium* includes obligate human pathogens and opportunistic species (Table 1). Disease in immunocompetent individuals is caused not only by *Corynebacterium diphtheriae* but also rarely by "*C. ulcerans*" (not approved as a species; 12) and *C. pseudotuberculosis* (formerly *C. ovis*) (45). The three pathogens, the only possible diphtheria toxin producers, also have some biochemical characteristics in common (12, 64). Therefore, they will be discussed together in this chapter.

The incidence of infections with *C. diphtheriae* has steadily declined in industrial countries since World War II (8, 9). However, in developing countries, diphtheria is still endemic. Travelers and refugees may bring diphtheria to Western countries, either as symptomatic patients or as healthy carriers. It is essential that clinical laboratories retain the capability of recognizing *C. diphtheriae,* since the mortality from diphtheria in Western countries ranges between 7 and 20%.

The term "diphtheroids" has been used in medical microbiology for coryneform bacteria, i.e., pleomorphic gram-positive rods that stain irregularly. In common with species of the genus *Corynebacterium,* they are usually aerobic or facultatively anaerobic, nonmotile, catalase positive, nonsporeforming, and non-acid fast, with little tendency to branch. However, if characterized further, many diphtheroids turn out not to belong to the genus *Corynebacterium.* Further investigations by chemical and genetic analyses will allow a better grouping of these bacteria.

Group JK represents a group of multiresistant coryneforms (37). Recent polyacrylamide gel electrophoresis of cell proteins and results of DNA-DNA hybridization studies indicate that the JK organisms represent a new species of the genus *Corynebacterium* (33); therefore, the name *Corynebacterium jeikeium* has been proposed for this species. However, recent DNA relatedness studies revealed that there is probably a core of closely related strains in group JK representing the species *C. jeikeium* as well as some more distant strains that cannot be included in this species (33; Centers for Disease Control [CDC], unpublished observations). Some types of "*C. genitalium*" and "*C. pseudogenitalium*" (19, 22) as well as "*C. bovis*" are very similar to the group JK organisms, including *C. jeikeium.* Group F-1 coryneforms are biochemically closely related to "*C. pseudogenitalium*" type C-5.

The genus *Rhodococcus* contains 16 species, most of which were formerly assigned to the genus or taxon *Nocardia, Mycobacterium, Rhodochrous,* or *Gordona* (13, 24, 69). The genus *Oerskovia* contains the two motile species *Oerskovia turbata* ("*Nocardia turbata*") and *O. xanthineolytica* ("*Arthrobacter luteus*"). Nonmotile *Oerskovia*-like strains have been isolated from humans. They represent a group of bacteria that should be placed taxonomically between the genera *Oerskovia* on one side and *Cellulomonas* and *Nocardia* on the other (43).

Although diphtheroids are normal inhabitants of mucosa and skin, the incidence of opportunistic infections caused by these organisms has steadily increased during the last 15 years (45). To obtain more information about their clinical relevance, it would be useful to regularly identify coryneform bacteria obtained from clinical material. In this chapter, we attempt to provide information on almost all of the coryneform bacteria that have been isolated from humans (Table 2). Nonapproved species names are in quotation marks.

NATURAL HABITAT AND CLINICAL SIGNIFICANCE

Corynebacteria of medical importance are mostly restricted to humans and animals (Table 1). *C. diphtheriae* may be found in diseased persons and in healthy throat carriers (28, 48). Diphtheric skin ulcers are an important source of infection in developing (28) and occasionally also in Western countries (30). Reservoirs other than human beings probably do not exist.

Although the clinical manifestations of diphtheria are caused by toxin-producing strains, nontoxigenic bacteria may also cause mild local symptoms, such as sore throat and enlarged tonsils (8, 48). In such cases, other possibilities must be considered. Toxin detection is not always reliable if only the agar diffusion (Elek) test is used (3, 66); furthermore, toxigenic and nontoxigenic variants of a single strain can be found in the same patient (65). Other pathogens mimicking diphtheritic membranes, such as Epstein-Barr virus, hemolytic

TABLE 1. Natural habitats and clinical significance of medically important corynebacteria and related organisms

Species or group[a]	Natural habitat	Proven or probable clinical significance in humans	Reference(s)
Corynebacterium diphtheriae	Humans	Diphtheria, endocarditis	48
"*C. ulcerans*"[b]	Cattle, horses	Sore throat, diphtherialike illness	45, 59
C. pseudotuberculosis	Sheep, goats, horses, etc.	Granulomatous lymphadenitis, pneumonia	45
C. xerosis	Humans (nasopharynx, skin, conjunctiva)	Endocarditis, pneumonia, arthritis, wound infection, septicemia	45, 54, 73
C. striatum	Humans (nasopharynx, skin), cattle	Pleuropneumonia, lung abscess	2
C. kutscheri	Rodents	Chorioamnionitis, septic arthritis	21, 49
C. renale group	Cattle	Abscesses (rectum, breast)	45
C. pseudodiphtheriticum	Humans (pharynx, skin)	Endocarditis, urinary tract infection, lymphadenitis, pneumonia, skin graft infection	42, 44, 45, 51
Group JK, including *C. jeikeium*	Humans (skin)	Wound infections, urinary tract infection, septicemia, endocarditis, meningitis, peritonitis, lung infections[c]	37, 75
C. minutissimum	Humans (skin)	Erythrasma, bacteremia, endocarditis and retinopathy	4, 26
C. mycetoides	Not known	Tropical ulcers, septicemia	12
"*C. aquaticum*"[b]	Distilled and natural fresh water	Endocarditis, meningitis, urinary tract infection, peritonitis in continuous ambulatory peritoneal dialysis, septicemia	36, 45, 71
"*C. genitalium*"[b]	Humans (skin)	Possibly urethritis	19, 22, 37
"*C. pseudogenitalium*"[b]	Humans (skin)	Not known	19, 22, 37
"*C. bovis*"[b]	Cows	Septicemia, eye infections, peritonitis	12, 45
C. matruchotii	Humans (oral cavity), primates	Eye infections	77
Arcanobacterium haemolyticum	Probably humans	Pharyngitis, sometimes diphtheria- or scarlet fever-like illness, skin ulcers, abscesses, septicemia	11, 45, 50
Rhodococcus spp.	Soil in association with livestock	Wound infections, meningitis, eye infection	18, 25, 61
Rhodococcus equi	Soil in association with livestock	Usually AIDS-related; tuberculosislike manifestations, primarily of the lung, septicemia, peritonitis, osteomyelitis, abscesses, endophthalmitis	16, 31, 35, 57, 58, 74
Oerskovia spp.	Soil, aluminum hydroxide gels	Endocarditis, pyonephrosis	15, 43
Group A-3	Not known	Not known	
Group A-4	Probably humans	Foreign body infection of vitreous humor	15, 29
Group A-5	Not known	Not known	
Group ANF	Not known	Not known	
Group B	Not known	Not known	
Group D-2	Probably humans (skin)	Wound infection, peritonitis, urinary tract infection, pneumonia, endocarditis(?), septicemia	41, 68
Group E	Not known	Pyelonephritis and septicemia, empyema	27
Group F	Not known	Not known	
Group G	Probably humans	Endocarditis	1
Group I	Humans	Endocarditis, wound infection	20, 63
Group 1	Probably humans	Endophthalmitis	56
Group 2	Probably humans	Not known	

[a] CDC coryneform group.
[b] Not recognized as a species of the genus *Corynebacterium* by *Bergey's Manual of Systematic Bacteriology* (12).
[c] CDC has received at least three group JK strains (one each from tibia, hip, and bone) isolated from patients with a diagnosis of osteomyelitis.

TABLE 2. Identification of medically significant corynebacteria and related organisms[a]

Species or group[b]	Catalase	Beta-hemolysis	Nitrate reduction	Urease	Gelatin hydrolysis	Motility	Esculin hydrolysis	Carbohydrate utilization: Glucose	Maltose	Sucrose	Mannitol	Xylose
Corynebacterium diphtheriae[c,d]	+	v[c]	+[c]	–	–	–	–	+	+	–[c]	–	–
"*C. ulcerans*"[d,e]	+	+	–	+	+ at 25°C	–	–	+	+	–	–	–
C. pseudotuberculosis[d,f]	+	+	v	+	–	–	–	+	+	–	–	–
C. xerosis	+	–	+	–	–	–	–	+	+	+	–	–
C. striatum	+	–	+	–	–	–	–	+	–	+	–	–
C. kutscheri	+	v	+	+	–	–	+	+	+	+	–	–
C. renale group	+	–	–	+	–	–	–	+	–	–	–	v
C. pseudodiphtheriticum	+	–	+	+	–	–	–	–	–	–	–	–
Group JK, including *C. jeikeium*	+	–	–	–	–	–	–	+	v	–	–	–
C. minutissimum	+	–	–	–	–	–	–	+	+	v	–	–
C. mycetoides	+	–	–	–	–	–	–	w	–	–	–	–
"*C. aquaticum*"	+	–	–	–	–	+	+	+	+	+	+	+
"*C. genitalium*"[g]	+	–	–	–	–	–	–	+	w	–	–	–
"*C. pseudogenitalium*"[h]	+	–	–	–	–	–	–	+	w	–	–	–
"*C. bovis*"	+	–	–	–	–	–	–	+	–	–	–	–
C. matruchotii	+	–	v	–	–	–	–	+	v	v	v	–
Rhodococcus spp.	+	–	v	v	–	–	v	+	v	+	–	v
Rhodococcus equi	+	–	v	v	–	–	–	v	v	–	–	–
Arcanobacterium haemolyticum	–	+	–	–	–	–	–	+	+	v	–	–
Actinomyces pyogenes	–	+	–	–	+	–	–	+	+	v	v	+
Oerskovia turbata	+	–	v	v	+	+	+	+	+	+	–	+
O. xanthineolytica	+	–	+	v	+	+	+	+	+	+	–	+
Group A-3	+	–	+	–	–	+	+	+	+	+	–	+
Group A-4	+	–	v	–	v	v	+	+	+	+	+	+
Group A-5	+	–	v	–	v	v	v	+	+	+	+	–
Group ANF	+	–	v	–	–	–	–	–	–	–	–	–
Group B	+	–	v	–	+	–	–	v	v	v	–	–
Group D-2	+	–	–	+	–	–	–	–	–	–	–	–
Group E	–	–	–	–	–	–	v	+	+	+	–	+
Group F-1	+	–	v	+	–	–	–	+	v	+	–	–
Group F-2	+	–	v	+	–	–	–	+	+	–	–	–
Group G-1	+	–	+	–	–	–	–	+ or (+)	v	+ or (+)	–	–
Group G-2	+	–	–	–	–	–	–	+ or (+)	v	+ or (+)	–	–
Group I	+	–	+	–	–	–	–	+	v	–	–	–
Group 1	+	–	+	–	–	–	–	+	+	+	+	+
Group 2	–	–	–	–	–	–	–	w	+	–	–	–

[a] Symbols: +, 90% or more positive within 2 days; –, 90% or more negative; + or (+), 90% or more positive [(+) indicates that some strains are positive only after 2 or more days]; v, more than 10% and less than 90% positive; w, weakly positive. Data are from records of the Special Bacteriology Reference Laboratory of CDC and may differ slightly from other sources.

[b] CDC coryneform group.

[c] Biotype *mitis* is weakly beta-hemolytic; it includes sucrose-positive strains that are rare in the United States and nitrate-negative strains that are of the variety *belfanti*. Biotype *gravis* attacks glycogen and starch and includes a few weakly hemolytic strains and rare isolates that are sucrose positive.

[d] Produces halos on Tinsdale medium and does not hydrolyze pyrazinamide.

[e] Also ferments glycogen and usually trehalose and starch.

[f] Does not attack glycogen or trehalose and usually does not attack starch.

[g] Reactions are those of biotypes 2 (ATCC 33031) and 4 (ATCC 33033).

[h] Reactions are those of biotypes C-1 (ATCC 33035) and C-2 (ATCC 33036).

streptococci, and the agents of Vincent's angina, must be excluded as well.

"C. ulcerans" may be isolated from humans with sore throats and from the nasopharynx of carriers. In rare instances it has caused mastitis in cows. It has been isolated from horses (64). Human infection is usually associated with consumption of raw milk and generally presents as a mild sore throat, although occasional infections indistinguishable from diphtheria with formation of pseudomembranes are seen. In contrast to *C. diphtheriae*, spread from person to person has not been documented (7, 12, 59, 64). *"C. ulcerans"* may produce a phospholipase D identical to the *C. pseudotuberculosis* toxin and a protein identical to diphtheria toxin (7, 79). Both diphtheria toxin producers and nonproducers can cause disease.

The natural habitats of *C. pseudotuberculosis* are animals (sheep and horses). Rarely, infection occurs in humans, either by ingestion of milk or by direct contact. The disease usually presents as granulomatous, necrotizing lymphadenitis of the axilla, groin, or cervical region. The pathogen is most prevalent in Australia, but human infections have been described from the United States and from France (45). Although it is capable of bacteriophage-induced diphtheria toxin production (64), not a single human isolate reported to date has been shown to be a diphtheria toxin producer.

The natural habitat and clinical significance of diphtheroids are summarized in Table 1. Their etiologic significance is not always clear, since they may be skin or mucous membrane contaminants. They cause disease predominantly in immunocompromised hosts.

COLLECTION, TRANSPORT, AND STORAGE OF SPECIMENS

The collection and storage of specimens for isolation of corynebacteria and related organisms are not different from general procedures outlined in chapter 27.

If diphtheria is suspected, collection of swabs depends on the site of infection. Most viable bacteria are in the deep layers of the pseudomembrane; thus, superficial swabs may not contain many corynebacteria. Nasal samples are best obtained with a flexible alginate swab that can reach deep into both posterior nares. If no lesions are present, the tonsillar fossae, posterior pharynx, and retrouvular areas as well as the nares should be sampled, since multisite sampling increases sensitivity (46). Additional samples must be collected to rule out other pathogens (see above). If cutaneous lesions, conjunctivitis, otitis, or vulvovaginitis is present, the involved site and the respiratory tract should be sampled.

Ordinary semisolid transport media such as Amies or Stuart should be satisfactory for transport, at least if the transport time is less than 24 h. If rapid processing is not possible, a silica gel transport medium (38) or a special liquid enrichment medium for *C. diphtheriae* containing tellurite (64) may be used. The latter may give better isolation rates in antibiotic-treated patients, since inhibiting substances are diluted. If this liquid transport medium is used alone, some strains may be missed because of tellurite sensitivity (14). The inoculated medium is kept either at room temperature or at 4°C. Since there may be some overgrowth even in tellurite-containing liquid enrichment media (e.g., by staphylococci and fungi), we recommend addition of fosfomycin and nystatin. In a survey of healthy carriers, *C. diphtheriae* as well as other *Corynebacterium* species were isolated by use of liquid enrichment medium (T. Krech, unpublished observation).

No systematic investigations have determined the optimal specimen transport medium for other corynebacteria.

CULTURE AND ISOLATION

Preparation of Gram-stained smears from clinical material is of little value for the diagnosis of diphtheria, since *C. diphtheriae* cannot reliably be differentiated from saprophytic corynebacteria. The method also lacks sensitivity.

Swabs suspected to contain corynebacteria are streaked onto a blood agar plate and on tellurite-containing media, e.g., cystine-tellurite agar (47) or modified Tinsdale medium (47, 64). Tinsdale medium reportedly has a shelf life of only 4 days, and *C. diphtheriae* may not grow on some batches (14). However, the laboratory of one of us (T. Krech) has stored it for up to 4 weeks with no ill effect on cultures. It also has the advantage of serving as an identification medium.

If selective media are not available, a fosfomycin disk may be placed on blood agar, selecting coryneforms in the surrounding zone (78). Additional inoculation of Loeffler or Pai slants may increase the sensitivity if no liquid enrichment medium was used for transport (64). Finally, the swab is transferred to a serum- or blood-containing liquid medium and can be subcultured on the media described above.

When silica gel is used for transportation, it is essential that desiccated swabs be incubated overnight in a broth supplemented with plasma or blood before they are plated on the routine media recommended (38). All media are incubated at 35 to 37°C.

Some diphtheroids may grow better in a CO_2-enriched atmosphere or under anaerobic conditions. Tween-containing media favor the growth of lipophilic cutaneous diphtheroids and are useful for colonization studies (76). As a rule, plates should be observed for at least 48 h before they are reported negative for coryneform bacteria.

IDENTIFICATION

C. diphtheriae, "C. ulcerans," and *C. pseudotuberculosis*

A presumptive diagnosis of coryneform bacteria is best done by Gram staining a few colonies taken from Loeffler or Pai slants. On blood agar, suspicious colonies are grayish and may be surrounded by a small zone of hemolysis. On media containing tellurium salts, corynebacteria form black or brownish colonies; however, other bacteria (e.g., streptococci and staphylococci) can also grow as black colonies. In addition to the black colonies, *C. diphtheriae, "C. ulcerans,"* and occasionally *C. pseudotuberculosis* produce gray-brown halos on Tinsdale agar (only rarely may streptococci, staphylococci, and some other bacteria show this phenomenon).

Suspicious colonies are subcultured to blood agar and, for storage, to Loeffler or Pai slants. Final identification of *C. diphtheriae, "C. ulcerans,"* and *C. pseudotuberculosis* is made from these media.

Three cultural types (commonly referred to as biotypes) of *C. diphtheriae,* namely, *gravis, intermedius,* and *mitis,* can be distinguished (64). A weak beta-hemolysis is observed with *mitis* strains and a few *gravis* strains. In general, colonies of the *intermedius* type are smaller than those of the other types. *Gravis* strains, but not *mitis* and *intermedius* strains, ferment starch and glycogen. *Intermedius* strains do not ferment dextrin, in contrast to the other types (64). For biochemical differentiation of biotype *gravis* from biotypes *mitis* and *intermedius,* the Special Bacteriology Reference Laboratory of CDC uses heart infusion broth medium with bromocresol purple indicator adjusted to a pH of 7.8. The differentiation is not easily done and might have lost its relevance, since a relationship between severity of the disease and biotype can no longer be recognized. It may have some importance for epidemiologic considerations, but phage typing (64) and newer techniques such as polypeptide analysis by sodium dodecyl sulfate-polyacrylamide gel electrophoresis (40) or DNA fingerprinting (62) have proved more useful.

C. diphtheriae shows metachromatic granules when stained with Loeffler or Neisser stain. For optimal expression, staining must be performed from colonies on Loeffler slants. Metachromatic phosphate deposits are reddish purple in Loeffler stain and black against the brownish cell body in Neisser stain, resulting in an appearance of scattered matches. Coryneforms with metaphosphate granules arranged in a V or X shape and growing with a halo on Tinsdale medium are highly suggestive of *C. diphtheriae.* The cultural types also have distinctive microscopic characteristics when grown on Loeffler (but not on Pai) slants. The type *mitis* meets the textbook description of *C. diphtheriae,* having long, pleomorphic, but rigid club-shaped rods. Type *intermedius* is highly pleomorphic, ranging from very long to very short rods. Cells of type *gravis* are usually short, coccoid or pyriform rods morphologically resembling *C. pseudodiphtheriticum* cells.

Final identification is obtained from biochemical reactions (Table 2). The enteric fermentation base containing Andrade indicator is satisfactory for biochemical testing of corynebacteria. One or two drops of rabbit serum may need to be added to each tube, since most *intermedius* strains, as well as occasional isolates of other biotypes and lipophilic coryneforms, will not grow well enough to change the pH in unsupplemented broth. Biochemical tests can be read in 24 h, but negative media should be held for 72 h. The most significant reactions of *C. diphtheriae* are the halo on Tinsdale medium (or the blackening of stabbed Pisu agar) due to production of H_2S by cystinase (64) and the failure to metabolize urea. The confirmation of *C. diphtheriae* should be done by an experienced laboratory.

C. diphtheriae, "C. ulcerans," and *C. pseudotuberculosis* can be distinguished from all other coryneform bacteria found in humans by a rapid pyrazine carboxylamidase test which is positive only in the latter (70). *"C. ulcerans"* differs from *C. pseudotuberculosis* in its ability to ferment glycogen and, usually, trehalose and starch (reactions should be read for 7 days). Gelatin hydrolysis by *"C. ulcerans"* is negative or weak at 37°C but positive at 25°C. For *C. pseudotuberculosis,* the gelatin reaction is reported to be positive at 30°C after 14 days; the nitrate reaction is usually negative in strains from sheep and goats and positive in strains from horses and cattle. Phospholipase D-producing strains will inhibit the hemolysis of beta-hemolysin-producing *Staphylococcus aureus* on blood agar in a test analogous to the CAMP test. Morphologically, *"C. ulcerans"* and *C. pseudotuberculosis* are pleomorphic with metachromatic granules. In *"C. ulcerans,"* coccoid forms may predominate.

Toxigenicity testing. Toxigenicity testing should be done on all isolates of *C. diphtheriae, "C. ulcerans,"* and *C. pseudotuberculosis.* At least 10 colonies should be tested because both toxigenic and nontoxigenic variants of the same strain may be found in one patient (65). Diphtheria toxin can be detected in vivo (in the guinea pig lethality test) or in vitro (in the Elek agar immunodiffusion test). For inexperienced investigators, the guinea pig test is the more reliable assay. The inoculum is prepared either from the entire growth of a 24-h Loeffler or Pai slant suspended in 12 ml of sterile broth (saline cannot be used, since *C. diphtheriae* rapidly loses viability in saline suspensions) or from a heavy 24- to 48-h broth culture (at least McFarland no. 3 density). One animal is injected intraperitoneally with 1,000 to 2,000 IU of diphtheria antitoxin. One to three hours later, this and another animal are inoculated with 2 to 3 ml of the culture suspension. A toxigenic strain will cause death in the test animal usually within 1 to 3 days, whereas the protected animal will survive. When toxigenicity of *"C. ulcerans"* or *C. pseudotuberculosis* is investigated, the protected animal may also die. In this case, the strain produces other toxins (such as phospholipase D), and it is difficult to decide whether diphtheria toxin is also produced. The adrenal glands, however, show hemorrhages only when diphtheria toxin is produced.

In contrast to the guinea pig test, there is no interference of *C. pseudotuberculosis* nondiphtheria toxin in the in vitro Elek test (3). Test strains are streaked at a right angle at a distance of 5 to 10 mm from an antitoxin-saturated filter paper strip laid on KL virulence agar (47). If toxin is produced, a precipitation line develops between growth and filter paper within 16 to 48 h of incubation at 35 to 37°C. The line is intensified by subsequent storage of the plates in a refrigerator. A positive and a negative control strain must be included. The specificity of the test depends greatly on the quality of the antiserum used. No additional lines should be formed, even after 48 h. Ready-to-use strips (KL virulence strips) from Difco Laboratories (Detroit, Mich.) may give nonspecific precipitates. Goat antitoxin (Berna, Bern, Switzerland) fulfills requirements for in-house preparation. Sterilized filter strips (Whatman no. 3; 1 by 6 cm) are dipped into a tube containing the diluted antitoxin (500 to 1,000 IU/ml). Excess fluid is drained off, and the strips are dried for 1 h in an incubator. They can be kept in a tube at 4°C for several months. Numerous reports of technical problems caused by variable reagents (3, 66) indicate that the Elek test should be done only in reference laboratories.

Diphtheria toxin can also reliably be detected in tissue culture cells. Several cell lines have proved useful (23, 52, 55). The following procedure gives reliable results in Buffalo green monkey cells and may be adapted to other cell lines. To cells suspended in 150 ml of tissue culture growth medium, 1 ml of 1 N NaOH is added to neutralize the acidity of the bacterial culture supernatant added later. A 175-μl volume of the cell suspension is placed in each well of a sterile, flat-bottom microtitration plate. In two of the wells, 50 µl of the supernatant from a heavily inoculated broth culture of the test strain incubated overnight on a shaker is added. In one of these wells, 50 µl of an antitoxin (approximately 1.0 IU/ml, diluted in minimum essential medium) is added. The plate is covered with a lid and incubated at 37°C in a CO_2-enriched (5%) atmosphere for 72 h. A cytotoxic effect may be seen under the microscope as early as after 24 h: most cells are rounded and are loosely attached to the plastic surface. In contrast, the antitoxin-protected cells grow out to an even monolayer.

Diphtheroids

Coryneform bacteria should be differentiated at least if they are isolated repeatedly or cultured pure or in high numbers (10) or if colonies are pigmented or surrounded by hemolysis. For biochemical testing, enteric fermentation base containing Andrade indicator can be used; however, certain organisms, e.g., group JK and *C. jeikeium*, *"C. bovis," "C. genitalium," "C. pseudogenitalium," Actinomyces pyogenes*, groups E, G, and 2, as well as some strains of *Corynebacterium* (formerly *Bacterionema*) *matruchotii* and group F, require the addition of 1 to 2 drops of sterile rabbit serum.

Rapid tests (32) and commercial systems for testing biochemical reactivities of corynebacteria have also been described. Most data have been obtained with the commercial galleries API 20 Strep (API BioMérieux, Lyon, France) and API 20 S (Analytab Products, Plainview, N.Y.), but sufficient information is available only for *C. jeikeium* and group D-2 coryneforms (72). API 20 Strep has also been used for identification of *Actinomyces pyogenes* (53). The inoculum must be heavy enough (McFarland no. 4), and supplementary tests for urease reactivity and nitrate reduction have to be performed (37, 72). Recently, results obtained with a novel gallery specially designed for corynebacteria have been reported (I. Caniaux, M. Doucet, D. Monget, M. Desmonceaux, and M. Guicherd, Abstr. Annu. Meet. Am. Soc. Microbiol. 1990, C308, p. 395).

C. xerosis may microscopically resemble *C. diphtheriae*, but there is a preponderance of barred forms over granular forms. It is grown readily on ordinary media; lipid does not enhance growth. Colonies may be yellow to tan. Distinctive biochemical features include the ability to reduce nitrate and to ferment several carbohydrates. Urease activity is absent, and no halo is produced on Tinsdale medium.

C. striatum, named after its microscopic appearance, shows short and thick gram-variable rods with a striped or barred coloration caused by the arrangement of metachromatic granules. The biochemical reactions (Table 2) reflect the reactions obtained with the type strain ATCC 6940 and with 65 human isolates that have been identified by CDC. A few similar strains have also reduced nitrite. The sucrose, maltose, and nitrate reactions differ from those given in *Bergey's Manual of Systematic Bacteriology* (12). Bovine strains are included in other collections and may account for different biochemical patterns described in other reports (45).

The morphology of *C. kutscheri* is not distinctive, consisting of small, gray-white to yellowish colonies with serrate edges and irregularly staining rods that are slender, clubbed, and in cuneiform arrangements and contain metachromatic granules. Esculin, nitrate, and urea reactions are positive.

Members of the *C. renale* group produce dry, white to pale yellow colonies and a lace doily-like pellicle on the surface of heart infusion broth culture after 1 to 2 days. The bacilli are relatively large, 0.7 by 3.0 µm or more, and contain metachromatic granules. Both *C. pilosum* and *C. cystitidis* can be distinguished from *C. renale*, since *C. cystitidis* produces acid from xylose in serum broth and *C. pilosum* reduces nitrate.

The colonial morphology of *C. pseudodiphtheriticum* (*C. hofmannii*) can mimic that of *C. diphtheriae*. It is inert in commonly used carbohydrate tests; nitrate and urease reactions are positive.

"C. aquaticum" is small, coccobacillary, and weakly gram positive. Its motility is due to a few peritrichous flagella, some of which may be curly (motility excludes it from the genus *Corynebacterium*). Growth is aerobic. After overnight incubation of 5% sheep blood agar, the lemon yellow colonies are convex and nonhemolytic. It does not attack starch. The reactions shown in Table 2 are those of type strain ATCC 14655.

C. minutissimum (Table 2) is a well-defined entity that presumably represents one of the eight different groups of coryneforms isolated from erythrasma (67). It can be distinguished from *C. xerosis*, another fluorescing diphtheroid, by its inability to reduce nitrate. Fluorescence of colonies can be demonstrated by illumination with UV light at 365 nm. The type strain of *C. minutissimum*, NCTC 1088, is sucrose positive, but another reference strain, ATCC 23346 (no longer in the ATCC catalog), is sucrose negative.

Microcolonies of *C. matruchotii* are flat, filamentous, and spiderlike. Macrocolonies vary in appearance; they are opaque and tough and adhere to the agar (12). Microscopically, cells are pleomorphic. Septate and nonseptate, branched filaments containing metachromatic granules are formed. A characteristic form of this species is a bacterial cell body attached to a filament ("whip handle"). Acid formation of sugars is variable and takes place under aerobic and anaerobic conditions. The type strain ATCC 14266 hydrolyzes esculin, hippurate, and starch (12). However, strains tested at CDC are usually esculin negative.

C. mycetoides cells are short to medium length, often contain metachromatic granules, and may arrange in a V shape. Growth is fastidious and enhanced by Tween. The shiny, yellow colonies are convex with entire margins and are 1 mm in diameter. The fructose reaction is negative.

"C. genitalium" and *"C. pseudogenitalium"* are lipophilic. They may be grown on Trypticase soy agar (BBL Microbiology Systems, Cockeysville, Md.) containing 0.1% Tween 80 or on blood agar plates that have been partially converted to chocolate agar by heat at 65°C for 30 to 40 min. Subcultures will grow on blood agar but not on commercially prepared chocolate agar (19, 22). The reactions of *"C. genitalium"* shown in Table 2 are those of biotypes 2 (ATCC 33031) and 4 (ATCC 33033). Fermentation of fructose is negative, in contrast to *"C. pseudogenitalium"* (biotypes C-1 [ATCC 33035] and C-2 [ATCC 33036]).

"C. bovis" is inert in tests with most sugars. It ferments glucose and sometimes lactose. The *o*-nitrophenyl-β-D-galactopyranoside (ONPG) test is positive.

Rhodococcus spp.

Most members of the genus *Rhodococcus* show a morphogenetic cycle that begins with a coccus or short-rod stage and is completed by filaments, in some cases with branching. Some strains are slightly acid fast. All strains grow aerobically on standard nutrient media. Several species have been isolated from respiratory secretions, but identification to the species level is difficult (24).

Rhodococcus (formerly *Corynebacterium*) *equi* produces large, mucoid to runny, pale pink or salmon pink colonies. The morphologic cycle from coccoid to rod (sometimes rudimentary branching) to coccoid takes about 24 h. It does not ferment carbohydrates; however, some strains slowly oxidize glucose and maltose. In the CAMP test with beta-hemolysin of *S. aureus*, a complete hemolysis of sheep erythrocytes is effected, similar to the reaction for *Streptococcus agalactiae* (60). *Tsukamurella paurometabolum* (formerly *Rhodococcus aurantiacus, Gordona aurantiaca, Corynebacterium paurometabolum*) (13) forms rough, cream to orange colonies. Acid is produced from glucose, galactose, mannitol, mannose, sorbitol, trehalose, and xylose but not from rhamnose. Nitrate is not reduced. *Rhodococcus rhodochrous* forms rough, orange to red colonies. Branched filaments undergo fragmentation into rods and cocci during the growth cycle. In contrast to the other above-mentioned *Rhodococcus* species, nitrate is reduced to nitrite.

Arcanobacterium haemolyticum

Arcanobacterium (formerly *Corynebacterium*) *haemolyticum* produces small colonies on sheep blood agar (0.1 mm at 24 h; 0.5 mm at 48 h), with a narrow zone of hemolysis that may not be present within the first 24 h of incubation. On rabbit and human blood agar, colonies are larger and zones of hemolysis are three to five times wider than the colony diameters. *A. haemolyticum* must be differentiated from *Actinomyces pyogenes* and beta-hemolytic streptococci. All three are negative for catalase by conventional methods, whereas corynebacteria are positive. The microscopic morphologic characteristics of *A. haemolyticum* grown on Loeffler medium are similar to those of *C. diphtheriae*. However, growth on tellurite medium is poor. The description of *A. haemolyticum* by Clarridge, which is based on conventional methods, is most useful for the clinical laboratory (11). Fermentation of glucose and maltose usually occurs within 24 to 48 h, but some strains require 5 days. The addition of serum stimulates growth in broth; however, serum addition is not recommended for fermentation tests, since false-positive reactions may occur. In contrast to *Actinomyces pyogenes*, beta-hemolysis of *S. aureus* is inhibited by *A. haemolyticum* in a reverse CAMP test.

Actinomyces pyogenes

Actinomyces (formerly *Corynebacterium*) *pyogenes* produces pinpoint, whitish, beta-hemolytic colonies on aerobic sheep blood agar; the zone of hemolysis is at least twice the diameter of the colony. In 3 to 7 days, the colonies develop a brick red color. Serum is required in carbohydrate broths for growth. The key reactions that distinguish *Actinomyces pyogenes* from *A. haemolyticum* are fermentation of xylose and inability to peptonize litmus milk. A detailed description of the microorganism is given in chapter 51.

Oerskovia spp.

Oerskovia species belong to the coryneform bacteria of CDC group A. This group comprises motile, yellow-pigmented organisms that have been divided into five subgroups, primarily on the basis of carbohydrate reactions (15, 43) (Table 2). Members of groups A-1 and A-2 can be assigned to the genus *Oerskovia*, characterized by colonies with a filamentous appearance that is observed with a light microscope under low power. The filaments break up into motile rods that are usually monotrichous when small and coccobacillary and peritrichous when longer. All *Oerskovia* species hydrolyze both gelatin and casein, whereas a majority of isolates in groups A-3, A-4, and A-5 react negatively in these tests. CDC has received at least 19 strains (10 of which were from blood) that were similar to group A-3 except for motility (−), nitrate reduction (−), and pigment (−). These strains may represent another coryneform group.

CDC groups of coryneforms

Group ANF (absolute nonfermenter) corynebacteria do not react with carbohydrates. The strains are urease negative and nonmotile. On the basis of nitrate reaction, they can be subdivided into two groups. Nitrate-positive strains are similar to *C. pseudodiphtheriticum* except for the lack of urease production. Inability to produce urease also distinguishes nitrate-negative strains from group D-2 corynebacteria.

Group B is a group of eugonic, nonfermentative strains that usually produce a brown soluble pigment, liquefy gelatin, and frequently utilize citrate and nitrate. This group has been subdivided into group B-1, which oxidizes glucose and sometimes sucrose and maltose, and group B-3, which is inert.

Group D-2 are lipophilic diphtheroids. Their growth is enhanced by Tween 80. Like most group JK corynebacteria, they are multiresistant to antibiotics. They can be distinguished from group JK by the ability to grow on triple sugar iron slant agar, by rapid urease activity, and by the inability to acidify sugars. They differ from *C. pseudodiphtheriticum* by the inability to reduce nitrate. Group D-2 is indistinguishable from "*C. genitalium*" biotype VI (ATCC 33798).

Coryneform group E is a heterogeneous group that includes some organisms that have been recently recognized as aerotolerant *Bifidobacterium adolescentis* strains (27). This group is fastidious, catalase and urease negative, and usually negative for nitrate reduction. In serum-supplemented broths, the members of this group attack all of the carbohydrates listed in Table 2 except mannitol. End products of carbohydrate metabolism are useful in distinguishing members of the genus *Bifidobacterium* from other group E coryneforms (14).

Group F contains fermentative, urease-positive organisms. The group has been divided into two subgroups on the basis of carbohydrate reactions. Some strains of group F-1 are fastidious. Group F-2 can be distinguished from "*C. ulcerans*" and *C. pseudotuberculosis* by the lack of beta-hemolysis, the inability to produce a halo on Tinsdale agar, and a negative phospholipase D test result. Nitrate-positive strains of group F-1 are indistinguishable from "*C. pseudogenitalium*" biotype C-5 (ATCC 33039).

Coryneform group G is a fastidious group of diphtheroids that is very similar to *C. matruchotii* and indistinguishable from it by the tests listed in Table 2; however, none of the isolates received in the Special Bacteriology Reference Laboratory at CDC have stained with the *C. matruchotii* fluorescent-antibody conjugate. The group was divided into two subgroups on the basis of the nitrate reaction.

Group JK corynebacteria are gram-positive coccobacillary or coccal short rods that resemble streptococci. Colonies are slow growing, small, gray to white, glistening, and usually nonhemolytic on sheep blood agar. Biochemical reactions that differentiate the group from other corynebacteria are the inability to produce urease, to reduce nitrate, and to ferment most carbohydrates (the reactions listed in Table 2 may represent the combined reactions of two or more as yet undefined species within group JK). Fermentation of sugars in serum-supplemented peptone broth occurs after prolonged incubation in glucose and galactose. Fermentation of starch, maltose, fructose, mannose, dextrin, and glycogen occurs variably, often after incubation for up to 3 weeks (45). Other distinguishing features in common with group D-2 are marked growth enhancement on Trypticase soy agar supplemented with Tween 80 (0.1%) and frequently multiresistance against antibiotics. Fructose-negative strains are indistinguishable from "*C. genitalium*" types II and IV.

Coryneform group I organisms are quite similar to *C. diphtheriae*. They can be distinguished from *C. diphtheriae* by the hydrolysis of pyrazinamide, the inability to produce a halo on Tinsdale medium, and sometimes the maltose reaction.

CDC fermentative coryneform group 1 organisms are similar to group A-4, the major differentiating characteristic being the inability to hydrolyze esculin (56). Also, the cellular fatty acid profile of group 1 is not consistent with that of A-4.

CDC fermentative coryneform group 2 contains fastidious small coryneform organisms. They are negative for catalase, urease, nitrate reduction, esculin hydrolysis, and motility. In serum-supplemented broths, they attack glucose (sometimes slowly and weakly) and maltose.

Other coryneform genera

Some coryneform isolates may not be identified by using the criteria given in Table 2. Such isolates may belong to other coryneform genera, such as *Caseobacter, Brevibacterium, Cellulomonas, Curtobacterium, Arthrobacter,* or *Microbacterium*. However, the available information does not enable clinical microbiologists to assign most coryneform isolates to a genus other than *Corynebacterium* without the benefit of cell wall or fatty acid analysis and, in some cases, G+C content of the DNA or DNA-DNA hybridization studies.

SEROLOGIC TESTING

Serologic tests are of minor importance for species or type identification of coryneforms (64). However, detection of antitoxic serum antibodies is useful for determining an individual's immune status (6, 39).

ANTIMICROBIAL SUSCEPTIBILITY

Antibiotics have little or no effect on the clinical course of diphtheria, but treatment of both patients and carriers is a major means of limiting the size of an outbreak. *C. diphtheriae* is susceptible to penicillin, vancomycin, and usually erythromycin and most of the other antibiotics commonly used against gram-positive organisms. The possibility of erythromycin resistance probably warrants susceptibility testing of all *C. diphtheriae* isolates (30).

Mueller-Hinton agar supplemented with 5% sheep blood may be used for standard disk diffusion tests or agar dilution tests of MICs, since some corynebacteria and coryneforms will not grow on plain Mueller-Hinton agar. Trypticase soy broth or brain heart infusion broth supplemented with 10% fetal calf serum or Tween 80 may be used for broth dilution tests. Strains of *C. jeikeium* and group D-2 isolated from patients are usually multiply resistant (37), but all isolates of the genus *Corynebacterium* and of diphtheroids have so far been susceptible to vancomycin.

LITERATURE CITED

1. **Austin, G. E., and E. O. Hill.** 1983. Endocarditis due to *Corynebacterium* CDC group G2. J. Infect. Dis. **147:**1106.
2. **Barr, J. G., and P. G. Murphy.** 1986. *Corynebacterium striatum:* an unusual organism isolated in pure culture from sputum [letter]. J. Infect. **13:**297–298.
3. **Bickham, S. T., and W. L. Jones.** 1972. Problems in the use of the *in vitro* toxigenicity test for *Corynebacterium diphtheriae*. Am. J. Clin. Pathol. **57:**244–246.
4. **Brian, H. J., and A. J. Brucker.** 1985. Embolic retinopathy due to *Corynebacterium minutissimum* endocarditis. Br. J. Ophthalmol. **69:**29–31.
5. **Broughton, R. A., H. D. Wilson, N. L. Goodman, and J. A. Hendrick.** 1981. Septic arthritis and osteomyelitis caused by an organism of the genus *Rhodococcus*. J. Clin. Microbiol. **13:**209–213.
6. **Camargo, M. E., L. Silveira, J. A. Furuta, E. P. T. Oliveira, and O. A. Germek.** 1984. Immunoenzymatic assay of antidiphtheric toxin antibodies in human serum. J. Clin. Microbiol. **20:**772–774.
7. **Carne, H. R., and E. O. Onon.** 1982. The exotoxins of *Corynebacterium ulcerans*. J. Hyg. **88:**173–191.
8. **Centers for Disease Control.** 1985. Diphtheria, tetanus, and pertussis: guidelines for vaccine prophylaxis and other preventive measures. Morbid. Mortal. Weekly Rep. **34:**405–426.
9. **Chen, R. T., C. V. Broome, R. A. Weinstein, R. Weaver, and T. F. Tsai.** 1985. Diphtheria in the United States 1971–1981. Am. J. Public Health **75:**1393–1397.
10. **Clarridge, J. E.** 1986. When, why, and how far should coryneforms be identified? Clin. Microbiol. Newsl. **8:**32–34.
11. **Clarridge, J. E.** 1989. The recognition and significance of *Arcanobacterium haemolyticum*. Clin. Microbiol. Newsl. **11:**41–45.
12. **Collins, M. D., and C. S. Cummins.** 1986. Genus *Corynebacterium* Lehmann and Neumann 1896, p. 1266–1276. *In* P. H. A. Sneath, N. S. Mair, M. E. Sharpe, and J. G. Holt (ed.), Bergey's manual of systematic bacteriology, vol. 2. The Williams & Wilkins Co., Baltimore.
13. **Collins, M. D., J. Smida, M. Dorsch, and E. Stackebrandt.** 1988. *Tsukamurella* gen. nov. harboring *Corynebacterium paurometabolum* and *Rhodococcus aurantiacus*. Int. J. Syst. Bacteriol. **38:**385–391.
14. **Coyle, M. B., D. G. Hollis, and N. B. Groman.** 1985. *Corynebacterium* spp. and other coryneform organisms, p. 193–204. *In* E. H. Lennette, A. Balows, W. J. Hausler, Jr., and

H. J. Shadomy (ed.), Manual of clinical microbiology, 4th ed. American Society for Microbiology, Washington, D.C.

15. **Cruickshank, J. G., A. H. Gawler, and C. Shaldon.** 1979. *Oerskovia* species: rare opportunistic pathogens. J. Med. Microbiol. **12:**513–515.
16. **Ebersole, L. L., and J. L. Paturzo.** 1988. Endophthalmitis caused by *Rhodococcus equi* Prescott serotype 4. J. Clin. Microbiol. **26:**1221–1222.
17. **Eliakim, R., P. Silkoff, G. Lugassy, and J. Michel.** 1983. *Corynebacterium xerosis* endocarditis. Arch. Intern. Med. **143:**1995.
18. **Ellis-Pegler, R. B., D. H. Parr, and V. A. Orchard.** 1983. Recurrent skin infection with *Rhodococcus* in an immunosuppressed patient. J. Infect. **6:**39–41.
19. **Evangelista, A. T., K. M. Coppola, and G. Furness.** 1984. Relationship between group JK corynebacteria and the biotypes of *Corynebacterium genitalium* and *Corynebacterium pseudogenitalium.* Can. J. Microbiol. **30:**1052–1057.
20. **Farrer, W.** 1987. Four-valve endocarditis caused by *Corynebacterium* CDC group I1. South. Med. J. **80:**923–925.
21. **Fitter, W. F., D. J. de Sa, and M. Richardson.** 1979. Chorioamnitis and funisitis due to *Corynebacterium kutscheri.* Arch. Dis. Child. **55:**710–712.
22. **Furness, G., M. H. Kamat, Z. Kaminski, and J. J. Seebode.** 1973. An investigation of the relationship of nonspecific urethritis corynebacteria to the other microorganisms found in the urogenital tract by means of a modified chocolate agar medium. Invest. Urol. **10:**387–391.
23. **Gabliks, J., and M. Solotorovsky.** 1962. Cell culture reactivity to diphtheria, staphylococcus, tetanus and *Escherichia coli* toxins. J. Immunol. **88:**505–512.
24. **Goodfellow, M.** 1986. Genus *Rhodococcus* Zopf 1891, p. 2362–2371. *In* S. T. Williams, M. E. Sharpe, and J. G. Holt (ed.), Bergey's manual of systematic bacteriology, vol. 4. The Williams & Wilkins Co., Baltimore.
25. **Gopaul, D., C. Ellis, A. Maki, and M. G. Joseph.** 1988. Isolation of *Rhodococcus rhodochrous* from a chronic corneal ulcer. Diagn. Microbiol. Infect. Dis. **10:**185–190.
26. **Guarderas, J., A. Karnad, S. Alvarez, and S. L. Berk.** 1986. *Corynebacterium minutissimum* bacteremia in a patient with chronic myeloid leukemia in blast crisis. Diagn. Microbiol. Infect. Dis. **5:**327–330.
27. **Guillard, F., P. C. Appelbaum, and F. B. Sparrow.** 1980. Pyelonephritis and septicemia due to Gram-positive rods similar to *Corynebacterium* group E (aerotolerant *Bifidobacterium adolescentis*). Ann. Intern. Med. **92:**635–636.
28. **Gunatillake, P. D., and G. Taylor.** 1968. The role of cutaneous diphtheria in the acquisition of immunity. J. Hyg. **66:**83–88.
29. **Hanscom, T., and W. A. Maxwell.** 1979. *Corynebacterium* endophthalmitis. Laboratory studies and report of a case treated by vitrectomy. Arch. Ophthalmol. **97:**500–502.
30. **Harnisch, J. P., E. Tronca, C. M. Nolan, M. Turck, and K. K. Holmes.** 1989. Diphtheria among alcoholic urban adults. A decade of experience in Seattle. Ann. Intern. Med. **111:**71–82.
31. **Hillerdal, G., I. Riesenfeldt-Örn, A. Pedersen, and E. Ivanicova.** 1988. Infection with *Rhodococcus equi* in a patient with sarcoidosis treated with corticosteroids. Scand. J. Infect. Dis. **20:**673–677.
32. **Hollis, D. G., F. O. Sottnek, W. J. Brown, and R. E. Weaver.** 1980. Use of the rapid fermentation test in determining carbohydrate reactions of fastidious bacteria in clinical laboratories. J. Clin. Microbiol. **12:**620–623.
33. **Jackman, P. J. H., D. G. Pitcher, S. Pelczynska, and P. Borman.** 1987. Classification of corynebacteria associated with endocarditis (group JK) as *Corynebacterium jeikeium* sp. nov. Syst. Appl. Microbiol. **9:**83–90.
34. **Jones, D., and M. D. Collins.** 1986. Irregular, nonsporing gram-positive rods, p. 1261–1434. *In* P. H. A. Sneath, N. S. Mair, M. E. Sharpe, and J. G. Holt (ed.), Bergey's manual of systematic bacteriology, vol. 2. The Williams & Wilkins Co., Baltimore.
35. **Jones, M. R., T. J. Neale, P. J. Say, and J. G. Horne.** 1989. *Rhodococcus equi*—an emerging opportunistic pathogen? Aust. N.Z. J. Med. **19:**103–107.
36. **Kaplan, A., and F. Israel.** 1988. *Corynebacterium aquaticum* infection in a patient with chronic granulomatous disease. Am. J. Med. Sci. **296:**57–58.
37. **Kerry-Williams, S. M., and W. C. Noble.** 1987. Group JK coryneform bacteria. J. Hosp. Infect. **9:**4–10.
38. **Kim-Farely, R. J., T. I. Soewarso, S. Rejeki, S. Soeharto, A. Karyadi, and S. Nurhayati.** 1987. Silica gel as transport medium for *Corynebacterium diphtheriae* under tropical conditions (Indonesia). J. Clin. Microbiol. **25:**964–965.
39. **Kjeldsen, K., O. Simmonsen, and I. Heron.** 1988. Immunity against diphtheria and tetanus in the age group 30–70 years. Scand. J. Infect. Dis. **20:**177–185.
40. **Krech, T., J. de Chastonay, and E. Falsen.** 1988. Epidemiology of diphtheria: polypeptide and restriction enzyme analysis in comparison with conventional phage typing. Eur. J. Clin. Microbiol. Infect. Dis. **7:**232–237.
41. **Langs, J. C., D. de Briel, C. Sauvage, J. F. Blickle, and H. Akel.** 1988. Endocardite à *Corynebacterium* du groupe D2 à point de depart urinaire. Med. Mal. Infect. **5:**293–295.
42. **LaRocco, M., C. Robinson, and A. Robinson.** 1987. *Corynebacterium pseudodiphtheriticum* associated with suppurative lymphadenitis [letter]. Eur. J. Microbiol. **6:**79.
43. **Lechevalier, H. A., and M. P. Lechevalier.** 1986. Genus *Oerskovia* Prauser, Lechevalier and Lechevalier 1970, emended Lechevalier 1972, p. 1489–1491. *In* P. H. A. Sneath, N. S. Mair, M. E. Sharpe, and J. G. Holt (ed.), Bergey's manual of systematic bacteriology, vol. 2. The Williams & Wilkins Co., Baltimore.
44. **Lindner, P. S., D. J. Hardy, and T. F. Murphy.** 1986. Endocarditis due to *Corynebacterium pseudodiphtheriticum.* N.Y. State J. Med. **86:**102–104.
45. **Lipsky, B. A., A. C. Goldberger, L. S. Tomkins, and J. J. Plorde.** 1982. Infections caused by nondiphtheria corynebacteria. Rev. Infect. Dis. **4:**1220–1235.
46. **Lyman, E. D., and J. A. Youngstrom.** 1956. Diphtheria cases and contacts: is it necessary to take cultures from both nose and throat? Nebr. State Med. J. **41:**361–362.
47. **MacFaddin, J. F.** 1985. Media for isolation-cultivation-identification-maintenance of medical bacteria, vol. 1. The Williams & Wilkins Co., Baltimore.
48. **McCloskey, R. V.** 1985. *Corynebacterium diphtheriae* (diphtheria), p. 1171–1174. *In* G. L. Mandell, R. G. Douglas, and J. E. Bennett (ed.), Principles and practice of infectious disease, 2nd ed. John Wiley & Sons, Inc., New York.
49. **Messina, O. D., J. A. Maldonado-Cocco, A. Pescio, A. Farinati, and O. Garcia-Morteo.** 1989. *Corynebacterium kutscheri* septic arthritis [letter]. Arthritis Rheum. **32:**1053.
50. **Miller, R. A., and F. Brancato.** 1984. Peritonsillar abscess associated with *Corynebacterium haemolyticum.* West. J. Med. **140:**449–451.
51. **Miller, R. A., A. Rompalo, and M. B. Coyle.** 1986. *Corynebacterium pseudodiphtheriticum* pneumonia in an immunologically intact host. Diagn. Microbiol. Infect. Dis. **4:**165–171.
52. **Miyamura, K., S. Nishio, A. Ito, R. Murata, and R. Kono.** 1974. Micro cell culture method for determination of diphtheria toxin and antitoxin titers using VERO cells. J. Biol. Stand. **2:**189–201.
53. **Morrison, J. R. A., and G. S. Tillotson.** 1988. Identification of *Actinomyces* (*Corynebacterium*) *pyogenes* with the API 20 Strep system. J. Clin. Microbiol. **26:**1865–1866.
54. **Munnelly, P., A. A. O'Brien, D. P. Moore, C. T. Keane, and J. A. Keogh.** 1988. *Corynebacterium xerosis* septicaemia in a haemodialysis patient. Nephrol. Dial. Transplant. **3:**87–88.
55. **Murphy, J. R., P. Bacha, and M. Teng.** 1978. Determination of *Corynebacterium diphtheriae* toxigenicity by a colorimetric tissue culture assay. J. Clin. Microbiol. **7:**91–96.

56. **Na'Was, T. E., D. G. Hollis, C. W. Moss, and R. E. Weaver.** 1987. Comparison of biochemical, morphologic, and chemical characteristics of Centers for Disease Control fermentative coryneform groups 1, 2, and A-4. J. Clin. Microbiol. **25:**1354–1358.
57. **Novak, R. M., E. L. Polisky, W. M. Janda, and C. R. Libertin.** 1988. Osteomyelitis caused by *Rhodococcus equi* in a renal transplant recipient. Infection **16:**186–188.
58. **Peloux, Y., J. M. Durand, and T. Fosse.** 1985. Péritonite à *Corynebacterium* (*Rhodococcus*) *equi* chez un cirrhotique. Sem. Hop. Paris **61:**2441–2442.
59. **Pers, C.** 1987. Infection due to "*Corynebacterium ulcerans*" producing diphtheria toxin. A case report from Denmark. Acta Pathol. Microbiol. Immunol. Scand. Sect. B **95:**361–362.
60. **Prescott, J. F., M. Lastra, and L. Barksdale.** 1982. Equi factors in the identification of *Corynebacterium equi* Magnusson. J. Clin. Microbiol. **16:**988–990.
61. **Prinz, G., E. Ban, S. Fekete, and Z. Szabo.** 1985. Meningitis caused by *Gordona aurantiaca* (*Rhodococcus aurantiacus*). J. Clin. Microbiol. **22:**472–474.
62. **Rappuoli, R., M. Perugini, and E. Falsen.** 1988. Molecular epidemiology of the 1984–1986 outbreak of diphtheria in Sweden. N. Engl. J. Med. **318:**12–14.
63. **Riche, O., V. Vernet, C. Rouger, and V. Erhardt.** 1989. Suppuration à *Corynebacterium* I_2. Presse Med. **18:**1033–1034.
64. **Saragea, A., P. Maximescu, and E. Meitert.** 1979. *Corynebacterium diphtheriae:* microbiological methods used in clinical and epidemiological investigations, p. 61–176. *In* T. Bergan and J. R. Norris (ed.), Methods in microbiology, vol. 13. Academic Press, Inc., New York.
65. **Simmons, L. E., J. D. Abbott, M. E. Macaulay, A. E. Jones, A. G. Ironside, B. K. Mandal, T. N. Stanbridge, and P. Maximescu.** 1980. Diphtheria carriers in Manchester: simultaneous infection with toxigenic and nontoxigenic *mitis* strains. Lancet **i:**304–305.
66. **Snell, J. J. S., J. V. Demello, P. S. Gardner, W. Kwantes, and R. Brooks.** 1984. Detection of toxin production by *Corynebacterium diphtheriae:* results of a trial organised as part of the United Kingdom National External Microbiological Quality Assessment Scheme. J. Clin. Pathol. **37:** 796–799.
67. **Somerville, D. A.** 1972. A quantitative study of erythrasma lesions. Br. J. Dermatol. **87:**130–137.
68. **Soriano, F., and R. Fernandez-Roblas.** 1988. Infections caused by antibiotic-resistant *Corynebacterium* group D2. Eur. J. Clin. Microbiol. Infect. Dis. **7:**337–341.
69. **Stackebrandt, E., J. Smida, and M. Collins.** 1988. Evidence of phylogenetic heterogeneity within the genus *Rhodococcus:* revival of the genus *Gordona* (Tsukamura). J. Gen. Appl. Microbiol. **34:**341–348.
70. **Sulea, I. T., M. C. Pollice, and L. Barksdale.** 1980. Pyrazine carboxylamidase activity in *Corynebacterium.* Int. J. Syst. Bacteriol. **30:**466–472.
71. **Tendler, C., and E. J. Bottone.** 1989. *Corynebacterium aquaticum* urinary tract infection in a neonate, and concepts regarding the role of the organism as a neonatal pathogen. J. Clin. Microbiol. **27:**343–345.
72. **Tillotson, G., M. Arora, M. Robbins, and J. Holton.** 1988. Identification of *Corynebacterium jeikeium* and *Corynebacterium* CDC group D 2 with the API 20 Strep system. Eur. J. Clin. Microbiol. Infect. Dis. **7:**675–678.
73. **Valenstein, P., A. Klein, C. Ballow, and W. Greene.** 1988. *Corynebacterium xerosis* septic arthritis. Am. J. Clin. Pathol. **89:**569–571.
74. **Van Etta, L. L., G. A. Filice, R. M. Ferguson, and D. N. Gerding.** 1983. *Corynebacterium equi:* a review of 12 cases of human infection. Rev. Infect. Dis. **5:**1012–1018.
75. **Waters, B. L.** 1989. Pathology of culture-proven JK *Corynebacterium* pneumonia. An autopsy case report. Am. J. Clin. Pathol. **91:**616–619.
76. **Wichmann, S., C. H. Wirsing von König, E. Becker-Boost, and H. Finger.** 1984. Isolation of *Corynebacterium* group JK from clinical specimens with a semiselective medium. J. Clin. Microbiol. **19:**204–206.
77. **Wilhelmus, K. R., N. M. Robinson, and D. B. Jones.** 1979. *Bacterionema matruchotii* ocular infections. Am. J. Ophthalmol. **87:**143–147.
78. **Wirsing von König, C. H., T. Krech, H. Finger, and M. Bergmann.** 1988. Use of fosfomycin disks for isolation of diphtheroids. Eur. J. Clin. Microbiol. Infect. Dis. **7:**190–193.
79. **Wong, T. P., and N. Groman.** 1984. Production of diphtheria toxin by selected isolates of *Corynebacterium ulcerans* and *Corynebacterium pseudotuberculosis.* Infect. Immun. **43:**1114–1116.

Chapter 32

Listeria and *Erysipelothrix*

JACQUES BILLE AND MICHAEL P. DOYLE

LISTERIA

On the basis of recent taxonomic studies, the genus *Listeria* is now classified in the group of regular nonsporeforming gram-positive rods and comprises seven species. Listeriae are widespread in the environment and are able to colonize many animal species as well as humans. The recent association of *Listeria monocytogenes* with food-borne outbreaks of high mortality has stimulated research on the taxonomy, pathogenicity, diagnosis, and epidemiology of the etiologic agent of listeriosis (3, 34).

Description of the Genus

Members of the genus *Listeria* are mesophilic, facultatively anaerobic, nonsporeforming, nonacid fast, gram-positive bacteria that appear microscopically as nonbranching, regular, short (0.4 to 0.5 µm in diameter by 0.5 to 2 µm in length) rods with rounded ends. They are motile by a few (one to five) peritrichous flagella and grow well in complex media at a wide range of temperature (3 to 42°C) and pH (from ≤5.5 to 9.5) and in the presence of high concentrations of sodium chloride (up to 10 to 12%). *Listeria* spp. are catalase positive and oxidase negative, hydrolyze esculin, and ferment glucose without production of gas. They are methyl red and Voges-Proskauer positive, do not produce indole or H_2S, and do not hydrolyze urea (27).

Previously classified in the family *Corynebacteriaceae*, the genus *Listeria* is now taxonomically included in the *Clostridium-Lactobacillus-Bacillus* branch of the gram-positive bacteria phylogeny, which also includes the staphylococci and streptococci (27). Common features of this group are a low G+C DNA content (<50%), lack of mycolic acids, and presence of lipoteichoic acids.

On the basis of recent DNA-DNA hybridization and 16S rRNA cataloging studies, the genus *Listeria* has been divided into seven species, with two genomically distinct groups (20). In one group are *L. murrayi* and *L. grayi*, which are rarely isolated and are presently considered to be nonpathogenic (22). The other five species are genomically closely related and include three hemolytic species (*L. monocytogenes*, *L. seeligeri*, and *L. ivanovii*) and two nonhemolytic species (*L. innocua* and *L. welshimeri*) (19, 25, 28). *L. denitrificans* has been transferred to a new genus (*Jonesia*), a member of the coryneform-actinomycetes group (23). Of these, only *L. monocytogenes* and rarely *L. ivanovii* are human pathogens. *L. ivanovii* is mostly pathogenic for animals. Because of its pathogenic potential, *L. monocytogenes* should be differentiated from the other *Listeria* species.

Habitat

Listeria spp. are widely distributed in the environment and often have been isolated from soil (believed to be the natural reservoir), plants, decaying vegetation, silage, water, and sewage. More recently, *L. monocytogenes* has been isolated, usually in low numbers, from raw or processed foods, including dairy products, meat, vegetables, and seafood, as well as from the food-processing environment.

Clinical Significance

Recent outbreaks suggest that listeriosis is a food-borne disease (see references 3 and 34 for reviews). Many wild and domestic animal species, including sheep, cattle, pigs, poultry, birds, and fish, are intestinal carriers of listeriae. *L. monocytogenes* is often present in the digestive tracts and feces of animals, probably after oral ingestion of contaminated feed.

In animals, *L. monocytogenes* principally affects the central nervous system, causing encephalitis (circling disease among cattle and goats), and the female reproductive tract, causing septic abortion. Sporadic cases as well as epidemic outbreaks can occur. In humans, *L. monocytogenes* mainly causes meningitis, encephalitis, or septicemia in nonpregnant adults (14). At particular risk are elderly patients or individuals with predisposing conditions that lower cell-mediated immunity such as transplants, lymphomas, and AIDS. A minority of patients have no known predisposing conditions. The tropism of *L. monocytogenes* for the central nervous system leads to severe disease requiring prompt recognition and therapy and often leads to high mortality (20 to 50%) or neurological sequelae among survivors. Diagnosis of listeriosis among individuals with listeric septicemia or central nervous system infection is based on the culture of cerebrospinal fluid (CSF) and blood. Often the number of organisms within the CSF is low, and direct examination of specimens by Gram stain is negative. In most cases, if clinical material has been cultured before the administration of antibiotics, *L. monocytogenes* will be detected within 1 to 2 days in cultures from CSF or from blood.

In pregnant women, *L. monocytogenes* often causes an influenzalike bacteremic illness which, if unrecognized and untreated, may after a few days or weeks lead to amnionitis and infection of the fetus, resulting in abortion, stillbirth, or premature birth of an infected infant. Diagnosis at the early bacteremic stage is made by detecting *L. monocytogenes* in maternal blood cultures; at birth, this diagnosis is made by detecting the organism in CSF, blood, amniotic fluid, respiratory secretions, placenta or cutaneous swabs, gastric aspirate, or meconium of the neonate. Detecting gram-positive rods in these various specimens by direct microscopic examination could be of particular value in early diagnosis and treatment of disease.

Focal infections occur rarely after an episode of bacteremia. However, primary cutaneous listeriosis with or without bacteremia has been reported among veterinarians or abbatoir workers who acquire the illness through contact with infected animal tissue. Infrequently, endocarditis, arthritis, osteomyelitis, intra-abdominal abscesses, endophthalmitis, and pleuropulmonary infections have been described.

The incubation period and the infective dose are not firmly established, although they may be inversely related. Reported incubation times vary from a few days to 2 to 3 months. Gastrointestinal symptoms such as diarrhea have been observed in some cases of listeriosis, but they are not commonly associated with ingestion of contaminated food. A transient carrier state varying from 2 to 20% exists in animals and humans.

Listeriosis can occur as sporadic cases or as epidemics. A few limited, non-food-related, nosocomial outbreaks have been described, mainly in nurseries. The number of sporadic cases of listeriosis in countries that report the illness is typically about five to eight cases per 10^6 general population per year (34), but in foodborne outbreaks this incidence may rise to 50 per 10^6 population. Foods implicated as vehicles of infection include coleslaw (cabbage), soft cheeses, poultry, turkey frankfurters, mushrooms, and milk. Large numbers ($>10^3$/g) of *L. monocytogenes* were detected in those foods quantitatively assayed for the organism.

The pathogenesis of *L. monocytogenes* in human infection is unclear. However, after the ingestion of contaminated food, an invasive infection develops in some people, depending on several factors (host susceptibility, gastric acidity, inoculum size, and virulence factor[s]). After penetrating the epithelial barrier of the intestinal tract, *L. monocytogenes* can grow within hepatic and splenic macrophages, which they destroy with hemolysin, a protein that binds to lipids of the host cell membrane. Immunity relies mainly on T-cell-mediated activation of macrophages by lymphokines, and the role of humoral defenses is not fully understood.

Collection, Transport, and Handling of Clinical Specimens

Clinical specimens from normally sterile sites such as CSF, blood, amniotic fluid, or tissue biopsy do not require special procedures for collection or transport. If processing is delayed, specimens should be held at 35°C in an incubator (but for no longer than 48 h). Specimens from unsterile sites such as meconium or feces, vaginal secretions, respiratory secretions, or skin or mucous swabs, as well as food and environmental specimens, require prompt handling and the addition of selective agents to the usual culture media. If processing of specimens is delayed, the material should be kept refrigerated at 4°C (or frozen at −20°C if testing is delayed more than 48 h) to prevent overgrowth by other microorganisms.

Detection and Isolation Procedures

Microscopic examination

A tentative diagnosis can be determined by direct examination of Gram-stained sediment of normally sterile fluids such as CSF or amniotic fluid. However, *Listeria* cells in smears of CSF may be confused with streptococci or corynebacteria and, if excessively decolorized, *Haemophilus influenzae*. Hence, culture is needed for confirmation.

Microscopic appearance of Gram-stained *Listeria* cells may differ according to culture conditions. Cells from colonies grown on solid media may appear as cocci, resembling streptococci or coccobacilli. In contrast, cells grown in broth are longer and more rod shaped and may resemble corynebacteria.

Culture conditions

Clinical specimens obtained from normally sterile sites such as CSF, blood, amniotic fluid, or tissue biopsy do not require special media for the primary inoculation. Blood agar (human, sheep, or horse) supports the growth of listeriae. Several broth formulations, e.g., Trypticase soy, brain heart infusion, or thioglycolate, can be used as liquid media. Inoculated media should be incubated at 35°C for 5 to 7 days and examined daily for growth. If growth occurs in broth, colonies should be isolated on blood agar; *L. monocytogenes* will generally grow in 1 to 2 days. Although additional isolations from clinical specimens may be made by cold enrichment, this is not suitable for rapid diagnosis but requires several weeks of culture. Generally too few isolations of clinically relevant listeriae are made to warrant use routinely by clinical laboratories.

After 24 h on primary blood agar, *Listeria* colonies are small (≤1 mm in diameter), round, smooth, and translucent. Colonies of *L. monocytogenes* are surrounded by a narrow zone of beta-hemolysis (Fig. 1) which is discrete and may be best observed by removing the colony.

Clinical specimens that are obtained from unsterile sites or may be contaminated with competing flora should be processed as for environmental and food specimens. These procedures involve an enrichment step and the use of selective media. Shortened (2-day) enrichment procedures at 30 to 37°C have been designed for isolating *Listeria* spp. from food. They rely on antimicrobial agents that are inhibitory to the competitive microflora but generally not to *Listeria* spp. Although these procedures have not been fully evaluated with clinical specimens, preliminary studies suggest that they increase rates of isolation of *L. monocytogenes* from clinical samples. One such procedure that has proven quite effective for *Listeria* isolation from food samples is the U.S. Department of Agriculture Food Safety and Inspection Service two-stage enrichment procedure, which relies on nalidixic acid and acriflavin as inhibitory agents to suppress growth of the competitive flora (11; see chapter 121 for media). Samples are incubated at 30°C for 24 h in a primary enrichment broth and then subcultured to a secondary enrichment medium at 30°C for 24 h. Subsequently, a portion of the enrichment culture is streaked onto lithium chloride-phenylethanol-moxalactam (LPM) agar (see chapter 121 for media), which is a highly selective medium that contains lithium chloride and moxalactam as inhibitory agents (9). Other selective media useful for isolating *L. monocytogenes* include Oxford agar, modified Oxford agar, and polymyxin-acriflavin-lithium chloride-ceftazidime-esculin-mannitol (PALCAM) agar (1, 11, 30).

LPM agar was developed as a modification of the McBride selective agar that has been used for isolating

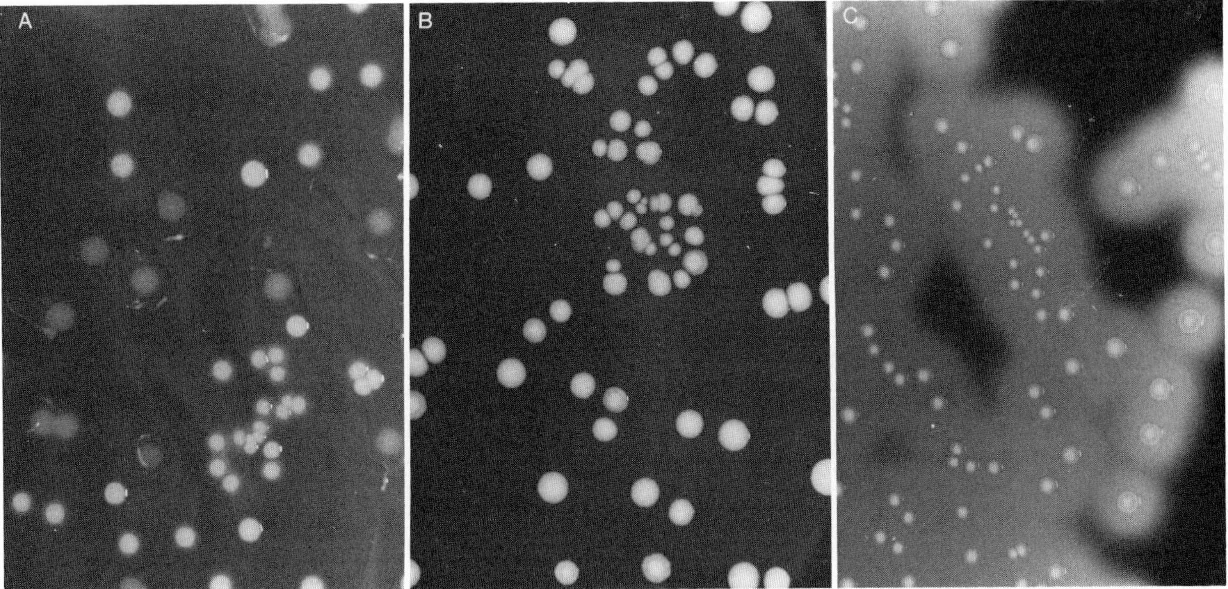

FIG. 1. Macroscopic view of colonies on 5% human blood agar plates after 24 h of incubation. (A) *L. monocytogenes* (discrete zone of beta-hemolysis under the removed colonies). (B) *L. innocua* (no hemolysis). (C) *L. ivanovii* (marked zone of beta-hemolysis around the colonies).

Listeria spp. *Listeria* colonies growing for 1 to 2 days on this medium or on other types of clear (blood-free), selective agar are best recognized with a dissecting microscope (×15 by ×25), using oblique lighting directed to the microscope stage by a concave mirror positioned at a 45° angle to the light source (Henry's technique). With this type of illumination, *Listeria* colonies on LPM agar appear blue (small, young colonies) to white (larger, older colonies), whereas non-*Listeria* colonies generally are yellowish or orange.

The recently developed Oxford, modified Oxford, and PALCAM agars are popular because of their differential as well as selective properties. *Listeria* colonies appear black with a black halo after 24 to 48 h at 35 to 37°C on Oxford or modified Oxford agar; this appearance is due to the hydrolysis of esculin and the formation of black iron phenolic compounds in the medium. *L. monocytogenes* appears as gray-green colonies with black background on PALCAM agar. The principal ingredients in PALCAM medium responsible for this differential reaction are esculin, ferric iron, D-mannitol, and phenol red.

New methodology for rapid detection

The direct examination of Gram-stained clinical specimens generally is of limited value because *L. monocytogenes* is often present in low numbers in clinical specimens such as CSF or because listeriae closely resemble other bacteria such as streptococci or corynebacteria. Hence, this technique often lacks sensitivity or specificity for detecting listeriae.

Other approaches for rapid detection have recently been described. A direct immunofluorescence test using specific *L. monocytogenes* monoclonal antibodies conjugated to fluorescein isothiocyanate has been applied to food specimens and used to presumptively identify *L. monocytogenes* isolates growing on agar media (12).

Monoclonal antibodies that specifically recognize a genus-specific heat-stable protein have been used in an enzyme-linked immunosorbent assay for the rapid detection of listeriae in broth enrichment cultures of foods (10). This procedure is accomplished within 48 h. A radiolabeled DNA probe hybridization test based on the detection of a specific sequence of the rRNA also has been developed for rapid detection of *Listeria* spp. in enrichment cultures of foods (8). Other DNA probes encoding β-hemolysin or a delayed hypersensitivity factor have been developed to specifically detect *L. monocytogenes* (rather than *Listeria* spp.) (2, 15).

Identification

Determination of *Listeria* spp.

A comprehensive protocol for identification of listeriae to the genus level includes the following steps.

Wet mount phase-contrast microscopy. *Listeria* cells appear as short rods with rotating or tumbling motility; motility is most pronounced when cells are grown at 25°C and may be absent at 37°C.

Gram stain of 16- to 24-h broth culture. *Listeria* cells appear as short, gram-positive rods; older cultures may appear gram variable.

Biochemical analysis. See Table 1.

Identification to the species level

The principal characteristics used to identify *Listeria* species are given in Table 2 (21, 27). Tests used include the following.

Hemolysis. Using an inoculating needle, colonies are stab inoculated in 5% sheep blood agar plates and incubated at 35°C for 48 h. Only three *Listeria* species, *L. monocytogenes*, *L. seeligeri*, and *L. ivanovii*, are beta-hemolytic. Both *L. monocytogenes* and *L. seeligeri* produce narrow, slight zones of hemolysis when growing on an agar surface, but hemolysis is marked in an agar

TABLE 1. Characteristics for identification of *Listeria* spp. and *Erysipelothrix* sp.

Test[a]	Reaction	
	Listeria spp.	*Erysipelothrix* sp.
Catalase	+	–
Hemolysis	Beta or no	Alpha or no
Nitrate reduction	– (*L. murrayi* +)	–
SIM motility at 25–30°C	+	–
MR-VP	+/+	–/–
TSI agar (slant/butt)	Acid/acid	Acid/acid
H_2S production	–	+
Carbohydrate fermentation (1 wk at 35°C)		
Glucose	+	+ (weak)
Mannitol	– (*L. murrayi*, *L. grayi* +)	–
Maltose	+	+
Lactose	V	+ (weak)
Sucrose	V	–
Additional tests		
Indole	–	–
Urease	–	–
Oxidase	–	–
Growth at 4°C	+	
Growth in 10% NaCl	+	–
Sodium hippurate hydrolysis	+	–
Tellurite reduction	+	
Gentamicin susceptibility	+	–

[a] SIM, Sulfide-indole-motility medium; MR-VP, methyl red–Voges-Proskauer test; TSI, triple sugar iron.

stab (Fig. 1). *L. ivanovii* produces a wide, clearly delineated zone of hemolysis on an agar surface or in an agar stab. The CAMP test is useful for verifying hemolytic activity of *Listeria* spp.; the CAMP test is done with *Staphylococcus aureus* for *L. monocytogenes* and *L. seeligeri* and with *Rhodococcus equi* for *L. ivanovii* (Fig. 2). The CAMP test is especially useful for differentiating *L. monocytogenes*, which may produce a slight zone of hemolysis, from *L. innocua*, which is nonhemolytic and avirulent but is often isolated on selective media from specimens with mixed flora. The hemolysin activity of *L. monocytogenes* is enhanced and easily observed in the CAMP test. This test is performed by streaking a beta-hemolytic *S. aureus* strain (ATCC 25923) and an *R. equi* strain (NCTC 1621) in parallel and diametrically opposite to each other on a freshly prepared sheep blood agar plate. Test strains are streaked as shown in Fig. 2.

After 24 to 48 h at 35°C, the plate is examined for hemolysis. Hemolysis by *L. monocytogenes* and *L. seeligeri* is enhanced near the growth of *S. aureus*, whereas *L. ivanovii* hemolysis is enhanced near the growth of *R. equi*, producing a typical arrowhead zone of complete hemolysis. Known strains of *L. monocytogenes*, *L. innocua*, and *L. ivanovii* should be included in the test as controls.

Nitrate reduction. The nitrate reduction test is used to differentiate *L. murrayi*, which can reduce nitrate, from the other *Listeria* spp., which cannot.

Carbohydrate fermentation. Fermentation patterns of L-rhamnose, D-xylose, α-methyl-D-mannoside, and mannitol are essential for identifying *Listeria* species.

Abbreviated protocol for identification of *L. monocytogenes*

Because *L. monocytogenes* is the species of principal concern in human infections, identification of this organism is of primary interest to the clinical laboratory. In many circumstances, comprehensive testing for definitive identification is unnecessary. The following tests are sufficient for presumptive identification of *L. monocytogenes*: tumbling, end-over-end motility of cells as

TABLE 2. Key characteristics of *Listeria* species[a]

Test	Reaction						
	L. monocytogenes	*L. ivanovii*	*L. seeligeri*	*L. innocua*	*L. welshimeri*	*L. murrayi*	*L. grayi*
Beta-hemolysis	+	++	+	–	–	–	–
CAMP test							
S. aureus	+	–	+	–	–	–	–
R. equi	–	+	–	–	–	–	–
Acid production from:							
L-Rhamnose	+	–	–	(+)V[b] (most)	(+)V	V	–
D-Xylose	–	+	+	–	+	–	–
α-Methyl-D-mannoside	+	–	– V	+	+		
Mannitol	–	–	–	–	–	+	+
Pathogenicity for mice	+	+	–	–	–	–	–
Serovar(s)	1/2a, 1/2b, 1/2c, 3a, 3b, 3c, 4a, 4ab, 4b, 4c, 4d, 4e, 7	5	1/2b, 4c, 4d, 6b, US[c]	4ab, 6a, 6b, US	6a, 6b		

[a] See reference 27.
[b] V, Variable.
[c] US, Undesignated serovar.

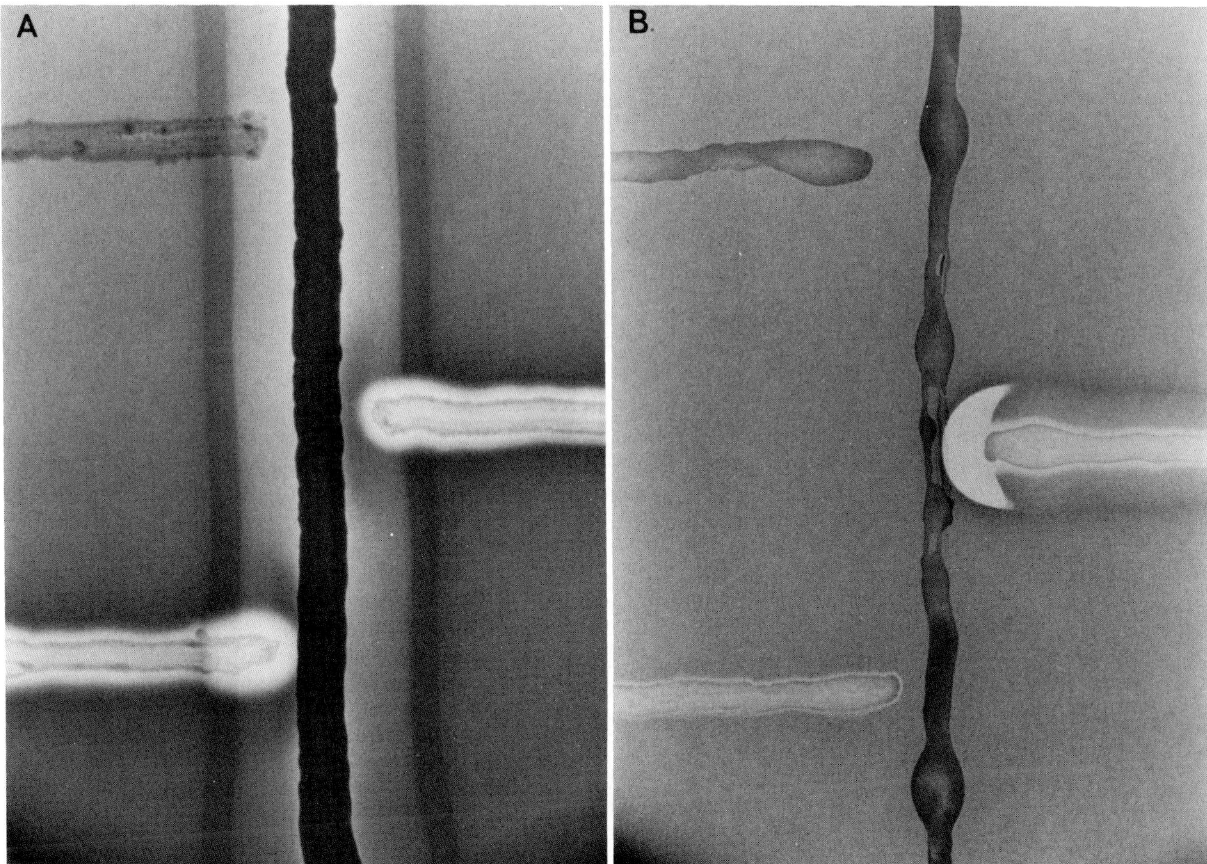

FIG. 2. CAMP test done with *S. aureus* (A) and with *R. equi* (B), read after 24 h of incubation. Upper left, *L. innocua;* lower left, *L. monocytogenes;* middle right, *L. ivanovii.*

determined by microscopic examination of a wet mount slide of a *Listeria*-like colony; gram-positive coccobacilli; catalase production; "umbrella"-type formation in the subsurface when cells are grown in semisolid motility medium incubated at 25 to 30°C; beta-hemolysis in sheep blood agar and the CAMP test with *S. aureus;* esculin hydrolysis; and acid production from rhamnose and α-methyl-D-mannoside but not from xylose.

Differentiation of *Listeria* from related genera

Bacteria of several genera have many characteristics common to *Listeria* spp.; hence, key distinguishing properties must be considered to avoid misidentification. Genera with properties in common include *Streptococcus, Erysipelothrix, Lactobacillus,* and *Corynebacterium,* as well as two nonclinically pathogenic genera (*Kurthia* and *Brochothrix*). *L. monocytogenes* is most frequently misidentified as *Streptococcus* sp. or may be discarded as a contaminating diphtheroid. The most practical tests for differentiating *Listeria* spp. from group B streptococci and enterococci are Gram stain morphology, motility, and catalase activity. Motility distinguishes *Listeria* spp. from *Erysipelothrix* sp. and *Corynebacterium* spp. *Corynebacterium aquaticum,* a motile species, can be differentiated from *L. monocytogenes* by the ability of the coryneform to produce acid from glucose aerobically only and a Voges-Proskauer-negative reaction. Major differences with other genera include the following: *Lactobacillus* spp. generally are nonmotile and catalase negative; *Kurthia* spp. are strictly aerobic, oxidase positive, and esculin negative and do not ferment glucose; and isolates of *Brochothrix,* the genus closest to *Listeria,* are nonmotile, are unable to grow at 37°C, and do not hydrolyze sodium hippurate.

Serology

Serology is of limited value both for diagnosing suspect cases of listeriosis and for broad-based screening for immunity. Instances of both false-negative and false-positive serology have been documented. *L. monocytogenes* is antigenically related to several other bacteria, including *S. aureus* and *Enterococcus faecalis.* Hence, serum samples from individuals who have no history of listeriosis but have been previously exposed to these organisms may have apparently high false-positive antibody titers to *L. monocytogenes.* In contrast, low antibody titers have been observed with serum samples of immunosuppressed patients and neonates who had confirmed listeriosis (5). Immunoglobulin M antibodies are principally involved in the immune response to *Listeria* infection, and elevated immunoglobulin M titers may persist for years in immunocompetent individuals exposed to *L. monocytogenes.*

Typing

Serotyping

The present serotyping scheme for *Listeria* spp. is based on 5 heat-labile flagellar antigens and 14 heat-stable somatic antigens. The scheme distinguishes 16 serovars; excluded are *L. grayi* and *L. murrayi*, which do not share major serological components with the other species (26). Except for serovar 5, which includes only *L. ivanovii*, the serovars are not species specific. Nonpathogenic species (*L. innocua* and *L. seeligeri*) share one or more common antigens with *L. monocytogenes;* hence, serotyping alone without complete species identification cannot reliably identify *L. monocytogenes*. The prevalence of serotypes of human, animal, food, and environmental isolates is highly variable; however, three serotypes (1/2a, 1/2b, and 4b) represent >90% of *L. monocytogenes* isolates from human and animal sources. Hence, serotyping is of limited epidemiologic value.

Other typing schemes

A standardized bacteriophage typing scheme using phage specific for *Listeria* spp. and *L. monocytogenes* serogroups is able to type between 50 and 80% of isolates. This scheme has proven valuable in identifying the vehicle or source of *L. monocytogenes* in several outbreaks of listeriosis (18). Only a few laboratories worldwide are equipped to phage type *Listeria* spp.

Other promising approaches that have been used recently for typing listeriae, in particular *L. monocytogenes*, include multilocus enzyme electrophoresis (16), DNA restriction enzyme analysis (D. A. Nocera, M. H. Fonjallaz, E. Bannerman, J. C. Piffaretti, J. Rocourt, and J. Bille, Abstr. Annu. Meet. Am. Soc. Microbiol. 1989, D-233, p. 121) and rRNA typing (B. Swaminathan, L. M. Graves, G. M. Carlone, and B. D. Plikaytis, Abstr. Annu. Meet. Am. Soc. Microbiol. 1988, D-61, p. 81). Both multilocus enzyme electrophoresis and rRNA typing schemes have been used successfully in epidemiologic investigations.

Pathogenicity Testing

Tests to evaluate virulence of *Listeria* spp. are available but generally are not used routinely. Those available include intraperitoneal inoculation of mice, inoculation of the chorioallantoic membrane of embryonated eggs, and inoculation of the conjunctiva of rabbits (Anton test). A sensitive immunocompromised mouse model (29) has been developed in which relatively low numbers of virulent listeriae cause death of these immunosuppressed animals.

Susceptibility to Antibiotics

The pattern of antimicrobial susceptibility and resistance of *L. monocytogenes* has been relatively stable for many years. In vitro, the organism is susceptible to penicillin, ampicillin, gentamicin, erythromycin, tetracycline, rifampin, and chloramphenicol (24, 32). However, many of these antibiotics are only bacteriostatic. Penicillin or ampicillin with or without an aminoglycoside is usually recommended for treatment of listeriosis. Studies in vitro and in an animal model have revealed that an aminoglycoside enhances the antimicrobial (bactericidal) activity of penicillin to *L. monocytogenes* (13). Cotrimoxazole and aminoglycosides are among the few anti-infective agents that are bactericidal to *L. monocytogenes*, and only cotrimoxazole has been used occasionally with success.

A good candidate for antibiotic treatment of *L. monocytogenes* infections should reach high concentrations within phagocytic cells, should cross the blood-brain barrier, and should be rapidly bactericidal. Cephalosporins, which are ineffective, should never be administered if a listerial infection is suspected.

ERYSIPELOTHRIX

Although *Erysipelothrix* sp. resembles actinomycetes and was at one time classified in the coryneform group, it is now classified within the regular, nonsporeforming gram-positive rods, a group that includes the genera *Listeria* and *Lactobacillus*. The genus *Erysipelothrix* has only one member, *E. rhusiopathiae*, which is widely distributed in nature and can be carried by a variety of animals. It has been recognized for more than 100 years as the agent of swine erysipelas and occasionally causes erysipeloid, a human cutaneous infection usually localized to the hands and fingers (17).

Description of the Genus

Erysipelothrix organisms are mesophilic, facultatively anaerobic, nonsporeforming, non-acid-fast, gram-positive bacteria that appear microscopically as short rods (0.2 to 0.5 μm in diameter by 0.8 to 2.5 μm in length) with rounded ends and occur singly, in short chains, or in long nonbranching filaments (60 μm or more in length). They are nonmotile and grow in complex media at a wide range of temperatures (5 to 42°C; optimum, 30 to 37°C) and at an alkaline pH (6.7 to 9.2; optimum, 7.2 to 7.6). They can grow in the presence of high concentrations of sodium chloride (up to 8.5%). Metabolically, *Erysipelothrix* organisms are catalase negative and oxidase negative, do not hydrolyze esculin, and weakly ferment glucose without the production of gas. They are methyl red and Voges-Proskauer negative, do not produce indole or hydrolyze urea, but do produce H_2S in triple sugar iron agar (6).

Habitat

E. rhusiopathiae is widespread in nature and is remarkably persistent in an environment with conditions such as low temperature, alkaline pH, and the presence of organic matter favoring survival. The organism is parasitic on mammals, birds, and fish but is most frequently associated with pigs, in which it causes erysipelas. Contamination of water and soil often occurs from the feces and urine of sick and asymptomatic animals.

Clinical Significance

Infection with *E. rhusiopathiae* is a zoonosis. Many animal species, especially turkeys and swine, carry the organism in their digestive tracts or tonsils. *E. rhusiopathiae* causes chronic or acute swine erysipelas. Symptoms include septicemia, endocarditis, arthritis, and urticarial or cutaneous forms of infection. Other domestic and wild animals and birds also can be affected, in particular sheep, rabbits, cattle, and turkeys. Infection is most likely acquired by ingestion of contaminated matter (33).

In humans, *E. rhusiopathiae* causes erysipeloid, a localized cellulitis developing within 2 to 7 days around the inoculation site. The disease is contracted through skin abrasion, injury, or a bite on the hands or arms of individuals handling animals or animal products. Erysipeloid is an occupational disease, occurring most frequently among veterinarians, butchers, and fish handlers. The lesion usually is violaceous and painful, indurated with edema and inflammation but without suppuration, and clearly delineated at the border. Regional lymphangitis may be present, as well as an adjacent arthritis. Dissemination and endocarditis can occur, especially in immunocompromised patients; their prognosis is generally poor (4). Healing usually takes 2 to 4 weeks, sometimes months, and relapses are common. No apparent immunity develops after an episode of erysipeloid.

Collection and Handling of Specimens

Biopsy specimens from erysilepoid lesions are the best source of *E. rhusiopathiae*. Care should be taken to cleanse and disinfect the skin before sampling. The organisms typically are located deep in the subcutaneous layer of the leading edge of the lesion; hence, a biopsy of the entire thickness of the dermis at the periphery of the lesion should be taken for Gram stain and culture. Swabs from the surface of the skin are not useful. In disseminated disease, the organism can be cultured from blood and infected organs (31).

Detection and Isolation

Microscopic examination

Generally, direct examination of Gram-stained biopsy specimens is of little value. However, the presence of long, slender, gram-positive rods in tissue from an individual with a consonant history is suggestive of erysipeloid.

Culture conditions

Biopsy specimens should be placed in Trypticase soy or Schaedler broth and incubated at 35°C aerobically or in 5% CO_2 for 7 days with daily examination. If growth occurs, the culture should be streaked onto blood agar plates and incubated as described above. *E. rhusiopathiae* colonies generally develop in 1 to 3 days. For chronic infections in which the number of organisms is likely to be low, enrichment culture may require 10 or more days. Blood from patients with septicemia or endocarditis can be plated directly onto blood agar plates for primary isolation.

Erysipelothrix colonies are pinpoint (<0.1 to 0.5 mm in diameter) on blood agar plates after 24 h of incubation; at 48 h, two distinct colony types can be observed. The smaller, smooth form are 0.3 to 1.5 mm in diameter, transparent, convex, and circular with entire edges. Larger rough colonies are flatter and more opaque and have a matt surface and an irregular, fimbriated edge. A zone of greenish discoloration frequently develops underneath the colonies on blood agar plates after 2 days of incubation (6).

Identification

Tests

Identification of *E. rhusiopathiae* should include the following tests.

Gram stain of colonies from a 24-h blood agar plate. Cells stain gram positive but can decolorize and appear gram negative, with gram-positive granules giving a beaded effect. Cells from smooth colonies appear as rods or coccobacilli, sometimes in short chains. Cells from rough colonies appear as long filaments, often more than 60 μm in length.

Biochemical analysis. See Table 1.

Differentiation of *Erysipelothrix* from related genera

Genera that have morphological and physiological characteristics in common with *Erysipelothrix* include *Lactobacillus*, *Listeria*, *Brochothrix*, and *Kurthia*. All are regular nonpigmented, nonsporing, gram-positive rods (7). A major discriminatory test is that *E. rhusiopathiae* produces H_2S in triple sugar iron, whereas species of the other genera do not. Furthermore, *Listeria*, *Brochothrix*, and *Kurthia* species are catalase positive. In addition, *Listeria* isolates are motile, are esculin-positive, and are not alpha-hemolytic. *Brochothrix* isolates strongly ferment carbohydrates, are Voges-Proskauer positive, and do not grow above 30°C. *Kurthia* species are strict aerobes, motile, and nonhemolytic. Corynebacteria and streptococci also can be confused with *E. rhusiopathiae*, but careful examination of cell morphology should facilitate the distinction.

The production of H_2S in triple sugar iron by a gram-positive bacterium is usually indicative of *E. rhusiopathiae* because very few gram-positive bacteria of clinical origin produce H_2S. Exceptions include some *Streptococcus* and *Bacillus* strains, but they are easily differentiated from *E. rhusiopathiae* by cellular morphology and spore formation, respectively. An additional trait highly characteristic of *E. rhusiopathiae* is its "pipe cleaner" pattern of growth in gelatin stab cultures incubated at 22°C (6, 31).

Serology

Immunoserological diagnosis

Since humans apparently do not develop immunity after an episode of erysipeloid, there are no serological tests for routine use to demonstrate antibodies to *E. rhusiopathiae*. Active immunization of animals with a live attenuated vaccine protects against erysipelas; however, a natural infection of erysipeloid in humans does not prevent relapses or reinfection from occurring.

Serotyping

Twenty-two serovars of *E. rhusiopathiae* have been identified on the basis of heat-stable somatic antigens. Although most isolates are serovars 1 or 2, no serotyping schemes are available for routine use in clinical laboratories (6).

Pathogenicity Testing

Most strains of *E. rhusiopathiae* are virulent for mice, and new isolates can be identified in a mouse protection test. This test involves injecting 0.1 ml of a 24-h broth culture subcutaneously into the loose skin of the flank of two or more mice, followed by 0.3 ml of commercial horse antierysipelothrix serum into the opposite flank. An additional group of two or more mice should be used as controls. If the organism is *E. rhusiopathiae*, mice receiving the culture and antiserum should survive, whereas those receiving only culture will die within 6 days (6, 31).

Susceptibility to Antibiotics

E. rhusiopathiae isolates are susceptible to penicillin, cephalosporins, tetracycline, chloramphenicol, and erythromycin and are usually resistant to aminoglycosides, sulfonamides, and vancomycin. Penicillin is the treatment of choice for both localized and systemic infections (4).

LITERATURE CITED

1. **Curtis, G. D. W., R. G. Mitchell, A. F. King, and E. J. Griffin.** 1989. A selective medium for the isolation of *Listeria monocytogenes*. Lett. Appl. Microbiol. **8:**95–98.
2. **Datta, A. R., B. A. Wentz, D. Shook, and M. W. Trucksess.** 1988. Synthetic oligodeoxyribonucleotide probes for detection of *Listeria monocytogenes*. Appl. Environ. Microbiol. **54:**2933–2937.
3. **Gellin, B. G., and C. V. Broome.** 1989. Listeriosis. J. Am. Med. Assoc. **261:**1313–1320.
4. **Gorby, G. L., and J. E. Peacock, Jr.** 1988. *Erysipelothrix rhusiopathiae* endocarditis: microbiologic, epidemiologic, and clinical features of an occupational disease. Rev. Infect. Dis. **10:**317–325.
5. **Hudak, A. P., S. H. Lee, A. C. Issekutz, and R. Bortolussi.** 1984. Comparison of three serological methods: enzyme-linked immunosorbent assay, complement fixation, and microagglutination in the diagnosis of human perinatal *Listeria monocytogenes* infection. Clin. Invest. Med. **7:**349–354.
6. **Jones, D.** 1986. Genus *Erysipelothrix* Rosenbach 1909, 367[AL], p. 1245–1249. *In* P. H. Sneath, N. S. Mair, M. E. Sharpe, and J. G. Holt (ed.), Bergey's manual of systematic bacteriology, vol. 2. The Williams & Wilkins Co., Baltimore.
7. **Kandler, O., and N. Weiss.** 1986. Regular, nonsporing Gram-positive rods, p. 1208–1209. *In* P. H. Sneath, N. S. Mair, M. E. Sharpe, and J. G. Holt (ed.), Bergey's manual of systematic bacteriology, vol. 2. The Williams & Wilkins Co., Baltimore.
8. **Klinger, J. D., A. Johnson, D. Croan, P. Flynn, K. Whipple, M. Kimball, J. Lawrie, and M. Curiale.** 1988. Comparative studies of a nucleic and hybridization assay for *Listeria* in foods. J. Assoc. Off. Anal. Chem. **71:**669–673.
9. **Lee, W. H., and D. McClain.** 1986. Improved *Listeria monocytogenes* selective agar. Appl. Environ. Microbiol. **52:**1215–1217.
10. **Mattingly, J. A., B. T. Butman, M. C. Plank, and R. J. Durham.** 1988. A rapid monoclonal antibody-based ELISA for the detection of *Listeria* in food products. J. Assoc. Off. Anal. Chem. **71:**679–681.
11. **McClain, D., and W. H. Lee.** 1988. Development of USDA-FSIS method for isolation of *Listeria monocytogenes* from raw meat and poultry. J. Assoc. Off. Anal. Chem. **71:**660–664.
12. **McLauchling, J., and P. N. Pini.** 1989. The rapid demonstration and presumptive identification of *Listeria monocytogenes* in food using monoclonal antibodies in a direct immunofluorescence test (DIFT). Lett. Appl. Microbiol. **8:**25–27.
13. **Moellering, R. C., G. Medoff, I. Leech, C. Wennersten, and L. J. Kunz.** 1972. Antibiotic synergism against *Listeria monocytogenes*. Antimicrob. Agents Chemother. **1:**30–34.
14. **Nieman, R. E., and B. Lorber.** 1980. Listeriosis in adults: a changing pattern: report of eight cases and review of the literature, 1968–1978. Rev. Infect. Dis. **2:**207–227.
15. **Notermans, S., T. Chakraborty, M. Leimeister-Wächter, J. Dufrenne, K. J. Heuvelman, H. Maas, W. Jansen, K. Wernars, and P. Guinee.** 1989. Specific gene probe for detection of biotyped and serotyped *Listeria* strains. Appl. Environ. Microbiol. **55:**902–906.
16. **Piffaretti, J. C., H. Kressebuch, M. Aeschbacher, J. Bille, E. Bannerman, J. M. Musser, R. K. Selander, and J. Rocourt.** 1989. Genetic characterization of clones of the bacterium *Listeria monocytogenes* causing epidemic disease. Proc. Natl. Acad. Sci. USA **86:**3818–3822.
17. **Reboli, A. C., and W. E. Farrar.** 1989. *Erysipelothrix rhusiopathiae:* an occupational pathogen. Clin. Microbiol. Rev. **2:**354–359.
18. **Rocourt, J., A. Audurier, A. L. Courtieu, J. Durst, S. Ortel, A. Schrettenbrunner, and A. G. Taylor.** 1985. A multi-centre study on the phage typing of *Listeria monocytogenes*. Zentralbl. Bakteriol. Parasitenkd. Infektionskr. Hyg. Abt. 1 Orig. Reihe A **259:**489–497.
19. **Rocourt, J., and P. A. D. Grimont.** 1983. *Listeria welshimeri* sp. nov. and *Listeria seeligeri* sp. nov. Int. J. Syst. Bacteriol. **33:**866–869.
20. **Rocourt, J., F. Grimont, P. A. D. Grimont, and H. P. R. Seeliger.** 1982. DNA relatedness among *Listeria monocytogenes* serovars. Curr. Microbiol. **7:**383–388.
21. **Rocourt, J., A. Schrettenbrunner, and H. P. R. Seeliger.** 1983. Différentiation biochimique des groupes génomiques de *Listeria monocytogenes sensu lato*. Ann. Microbiol. (Paris) **134A:**65–71.
22. **Rocourt, J., U. Wehmeyer, P. Cossart, and E. Stackebrandt.** 1987. Proposal to retain *Listeria murrayi* and *Listeria grayi* in the genus *Listeria*. Int. J. Syst. Bacteriol. **37:** 298–300.
23. **Rocourt, J., U. Wehmeyer, and E. Stackebrandt.** 1987. Transfer of *Listeria denitrificans* to a new genus *Jonesia* gen. nov. as *Jonesia denitrificans* comb. nov. Int. J. Syst. Bacteriol. **37:**266–270.
24. **Scheld, W. M.** 1983. Evaluation of rifampin and other antibiotics against *Listeria monocytogenes* in vitro and in vivo. Rev. Infect. Dis. **5**(Suppl. 3):S593–S599.
25. **Seeliger, H. P. R.** 1981. Apathogene Listerien. *Listeria innocua* sp. n. (*Seeliger* et *Schoofs*). Zentralbl. Bakteriol. Parasitenkd. Infectionskr. Hyg. Abt. 1 Orig. Reihe A **249:** 487–493.
26. **Seeliger, H. P. R., and K. Hohne.** 1979. Serotyping of *Listeria monocytogenes* and related species. Methods Microbiol. **13:**31–49.
27. **Seeliger, H. P. R., and D. Jones.** 1986. Genus *Listeria* Pirie, 1940, 383[AL], p. 1235–1245. *In* P. H. A. Sneath, H. S. Mair, M. E. Sharpe, and J. G. Holt (ed.), Bergey's manual of systematic bacteriology, vol. 2. The Williams & Wilkins Co., Baltimore.
28. **Seeliger, H. P. R., J. Rocourt, A. Schrettenbrunner, P. A. D. Grimont, and D. Jones.** 1984. *Listeria ivanovii* sp. nov. Int. J. Syst. Bacteriol. **34:**336–337.
29. **Stelma, G. N., A. L. Reyes, J. T. Peeler, D. W. Francis, J. M. Hunt, P. L. Spaulding, C. H. Johnson, and J. Lovett.** 1987. Pathogenicity test for *Listeria monocytogenes* using immunocompromised mice. J. Clin. Microbiol. **25:**2085–2089.
30. **Van Netten, P., I. Perales, A. van de Moosdijk, G. D. W. Curtis, and D. A. A. Mossel.** 1989. Liquid and solid selective differential media for the detection and enumeration of *L. monocytogenes* and other *Listeria* spp. Int. J. Food Microbiol. **8:**299–316.
31. **Weaver, R. E.** 1985. *Erysipelothrix*, p. 209–210. *In* E. H. Lennette, A. Balows, W. J. Hausler, Jr., and H. J. Shadomy (ed.), Manual of clinical microbiology, 4th ed. American Society for Microbiology, Washington, D.C.
32. **Wiggins, G. L., W. L. Albritton, and J. C. Feeley.** 1978.

Antibiotic susceptibility of clinical isolates of *Listeria monocytogenes*. Antimicrob. Agents Chemother. **13:**854–860.

33. **Wood, R. L.** 1975. Erysipelothrix infection, p. 271–281. *In* W. T. Hubbert, W. F. McCullough, and P. R. Schnurrenberger (ed.), Diseases transmitted from animals to man, 6th ed. Charles C Thomas, Publisher, Springfield, Ill.
34. **World Health Organization.** 1988. Report of a WHO Informal Working Group (Geneva, 15–19 Feb. 1988). WHO/EHE/FOS/88.5. World Health Organization, Geneva.

Chapter 33

Bacillus

P. C. B. TURNBULL AND J. M. KRAMER

DESCRIPTION OF THE GENUS

The family *Bacillaceae* comprises the rod-shaped bacteria that form endospores. The two principal members of the family are the anaerobic endospore-forming bacilli of the genus *Clostridium* (chapter 50) and the aerobic or facultatively anaerobic endospore-forming bacilli that make up the genus *Bacillus*.

Bacillus species, familiarly known as aerobic spore-bearing bacilli, are gram positive or gram variable, some species being clearly gram positive only in very young cultures. The vegetative cells are straight, round- or square-ended rods ranging from 0.5 × 1.2 μm to 2.5 × 10 μm in diameter (3), occurring singly or in chains that may range from a few to many cells in length. The endospores, formed one per mother cell (sporangium) in the presence of oxygen, are cylindrical, oval, round, or occasionally kidney shaped; depending on the species, they are centrally or terminally placed, characteristically swelling or not swelling the sporangium. Under appropriate conditions (the presence of HCO_3^- in an anaerobic or CO_2 atmosphere), *B. anthracis, B. subtilis, B. licheniformis*, and *B. megaterium* produce a polypeptide (poly-γ-D-glutamic acid) capsule visible when stained with polychrome methylene blue (M'Fadyean reaction). With the principal exceptions of *B. anthracis* and *B. cereus* var. *mycoides*, almost all *Bacillus* species are motile, although there is great strain-to-strain variation in the extent of motility in any one species.

Most strains are catalase positive. The G+C content of DNA is 32 to 69 mol%.

NATURAL HABITATS

Bacillus species are mostly saprophytes widely distributed in nature, particularly in soil, whence they are spread in dust, in water, and on materials of plant and animal origin. Survival during this distribution results from the resistance of the spores to adverse conditions. The broad range of physiological characteristics exhibited within the genus is reflected in a widely diverse range of facultative variants of mesophilic species, facultative and obligate thermophiles, psychrophiles, acidophiles, halophiles, and so on, capable of survival or growth at extremes of temperature, pH, or salinity that would inhibit or kill most other living organisms. As a result, members of the genus are encountered in almost every conceivable natural environment, from Arctic soil to thermal springs and from freshwater deposits to stagnant salt pond or marine sediments. The ecology of *Bacillus* species has been comprehensively reviewed elsewhere (17).

CLINICAL SIGNIFICANCE

The majority of *Bacillus* species apparently have little or no pathogenic potential and are rarely associated with disease in humans or lower animals. The best-known exception to this statement is *B. anthracis*, the agent of anthrax, but a number of other species, particularly *B. cereus*, have been implicated or incriminated to an increasing extent in recent years in food poisoning and in other human and animal infections. Several of the species, however, are of clinical importance in other capacities, such as antibiotic assays (*B. pumilus, B. cereus*, and *B. stearothermophilus*), assays of other organic compounds, such as aflatoxin (*B. megaterium* ATCC 25848), folic acid (*B. coagulans* ATCC 12245), and hexachlorophene (*B. subtilis* ATCC 6533), and tests for monitoring the efficacies of heat, chemical or radiation processes for sterilization or fumigation purposes or for preservation of pharmaceutical or food commodities (*B. stearothermophilus* and *B. subtilis* var. *globigii* NCTC 10073). Several species are producers of antibiotics such as bacitracin (*B. subtilis* and *B. licheniformis*), polymyxin (*B. polymyxa*), and gramicidin (*B. brevis*) and of numerous enzymes used by pharmaceutical and other industries. The resistance of the spores to heat, radiation, disinfectants, and desiccation also results in *Bacillus* species being troublesome contaminants in pharmaceutical products and foods, in the operating room, on surgical dressings, and so on.

Five *Bacillus* species, *B. thuringiensis, B. popilliae, B. sphaericus, B. larvae*, and *B. lentimorbus*, are insect pathogens. The first three are used in commercial insecticides for the control of crop-destroying and disease-carrying insects.

The clinical conditions associated with *Bacillus* species are summarized in Table 1. Recognition of the pathogenic potential of *Bacillus* species other than *B. anthracis* has been slow to develop, partly because of the lack of order in their taxonomy until quite recently and partly because of a tendency to dismiss them as contaminants when they are seen in laboratory cultures. These bacteria are now being taken more seriously in relation to infections of immunocompromised or otherwise debilitated hosts (e.g., alcoholics, diabetics, and drug abusers), in mixed infections, as secondary invaders, and particularly in the case of *B. cereus*, as occasional primary pathogens.

B. cereus has long been associated with food poisoning. To a lesser extent, *B. subtilis, B. licheniformis*, and occasionally other *Bacillus* species are also being incriminated increasingly in foodborne illness.

B. cereus is the etiological agent of two distinct food-poisoning syndromes: (i) the diarrheal type, characterized by abdominal pain with diarrhea 8 to 16 h after ingestion of the contaminated food and associated with a diversity of foods from meats and vegetable dishes to pastas, desserts, cakes, sauces, and milk (12), and (ii) the emetic type characterized by nausea and vomiting 1 to 5 h after eating the offending food (predominantly

TABLE 1. *Bacillus* infections reported since 1960

Species	Clinical condition(s)	Reports or occurrence[a]
B. alvei	Sepsis, meningitis	+
B. anthracis	Anthrax	++++
	Cutaneous (eschar, malignant pustule)	
	Intestinal	++
	Pulmonary	+
	Meningitis (secondary to cutaneous)	+
B. brevis	Bacteremia	+
B. cereus	Infected wounds, mild to severe, necrotic or gangrenous	++++
	Bovine mastitis	++++
	Bacteremia or septicemia, including drug abuse	+++
	Bovine abortion	+++
	Pneumonia, pleurisy, empyema, meningitis, endocarditis, osteomyelitis, panophthalmitis or endophthalmitis	++
	Other (burns, ear infection, peritonitis, urinary tract infection)	+
	Food poisoning	++++
B. circulans	Meningitis	+
B. coagulans	Bacteremia or septicemia	+
B. licheniformis	Bacteremia or septicemia	+++
	Other (peritonitis, ophthalmitis, bovine toxemia)	+
	Food poisoning	+++
B. macerans	Bacteremia or septicemia	+
B. pumilus	Rectal fistula	+
B. sphaericus	Bacteremia, endocarditis, meningitis, pseudotumor	+
	Food poisoning	+
B. subtilis	Bacteremia or septicemia, endocarditis, respiratory infections	++
	Food poisoning	++
B. thuringiensis	Wound, eye infection, bovine mastitis	+

[a] +, One or two reports (of each of the clinical entities shown); ++, a few reports; +++, several reports; ++++, many reports or frequent and regular occurrence now accepted. Most of the relevant reports can be found in references 1, 2, 6, 12, 17, 18, 20, 21, 22, 23, 25, 26, 28, and 29.

oriental rice dishes, although occasionally other foods such as pasteurized cream, milk pudding, pastas, and reconstituted infant formulas are implicated) (12). Both syndromes arise as a direct result of the fact that *B. cereus* spores can survive normal cooking procedures; under conditions (primarily temperature and type of food concerned) of improper storage after cooking, the spores germinate and the resulting vegetative cells multiply.

The toxin of *B. anthracis* is now well characterized (see later discussion of toxin detection). The toxigenic basis of *B. cereus* food poisoning and other infections has been partially elucidated (13, 23, 25, 26), but no toxins or other virulence factors have yet been identified to account for symptoms periodically associated with other *Bacillus* species.

ANTHRAX

Anthrax has been a scourge of animals and humans throughout history. It is primarily a disease of herbivores; before an effective veterinary vaccine became available in the late 1930s, anthrax was one of the foremost causes worldwide of mortality in cattle, sheep, goats, and horses. Humans almost invariably contract anthrax directly or indirectly from animals. The development and application of a successful veterinary vaccine (together with improvements in factory hygiene and sterilization procedures for imported animal products, increased use of man-made alternatives to animal hides or hair, and the availability of a vaccine for humans in at-risk occupations) has thus been reflected in the past four decades in a marked decline in the incidence of the disease in both animals and humans. Nevertheless, the disease is far from being eradicated and continues to be endemic in many countries, particularly those that lack an efficient vaccination policy. Even among developed countries, few are entirely free of the disease (9, 23a). Because anthrax spores remain viable in soil for many years and their persistence does not depend on animal reservoirs, *B. anthracis* is exceedingly difficult to eradicate from an endemic area; nonendemic regions must be constantly on the alert for the arrival of *B. anthracis* in imported products of animal origin.

In comparison with herbivores, humans are moderately resistant to anthrax. Human anthrax is traditionally classified as (i) nonindustrial, resulting from close contact with infected animals, or (ii) industrial, as acquired by those employed in processing wool, hair, hides, bones, or other animal products. Nonindustrial anthrax usually manifests itself as the cutaneous form of the disease or, far less frequently, as intestinal anthrax if infected meat is eaten. Industrial anthrax may be cutaneous but has a far higher probability of taking the pulmonary form from inhalation of spore-laden dust. There are a few reports of laboratory-acquired infections, and direct human-to-human transmission is exceedingly rare (23a).

In cutaneous anthrax, which accounts for 95 to 99% of human cases worldwide, infection occurs via a small cut or abrasion or possibly through an insect bite; exposed regions of the body are therefore most frequently affected. Probably no more than 20% of untreated cases of cutaneous anthrax are fatal, but when treatment is available, this figure falls almost to zero. The main dangers are obstruction of the airways by the accompanying extensive edema when the lesion is on the face or neck and sequela of secondary cellulitis or meningitis. The intestinal and pulmonary forms are more often fatal than the cutaneous type because they go unrecognized until it is too late for treatment to be effective.

The incubation period in cutaneous anthrax is 2 to 3 days, after which a small pimple or papule appears; over the next 24 h a ring of vesicles develops around the papule which ulcerates, dries, and blackens into the characteristic eschar. The eschar enlarges, becoming thick and adherent to underlying tissues over the ensuing week. The lesion is surrounded by edema, which may be very extensive. Pus and pain are present only if there is secondary infection by a pyogenic organism. Likewise, marked lymphangitis and fever probably indicate secondary infection.

Intestinal anthrax can be most simply explained as cutaneous anthrax occurring on the intestinal mucosa. Symptoms of gastroenteritis sometimes, but not invariably, occur. In pulmonary anthrax, the inhaled spores are carried from the lungs by macrophages to the lymphatic system, where they germinate and commence the multiplication that ultimately leads to fatal septicemia.

In fatal cases of any of the forms, generalized symptoms may be mild (fatigue, malaise, and slight fever) or absent before sudden onset of acute illness characterized by dyspnea, cyanosis, severe pyrexia, and disorientation, followed by circulatory failure, shock, coma, and death, all within a few hours. Depending somewhat on the host species, there is a rapid buildup of the bacteria in the blood over the last few hours to terminal levels of 10^9/ml. Behind these events is the toxin of *B. anthracis*, although the precise manner in which the toxin produces the signs and symptoms observed has yet to be elucidated. The topic is extensively reviewed elsewhere (23a, 26a).

COLLECTION, TRANSPORT, AND STORAGE OF SPECIMENS

Bacillus species are not regarded as fragile and can generally be expected to survive transport to the laboratory in a reasonable period of time either in the freshly collected specimen or in a standard transport medium; a transport medium is, in fact, unnecessary.

Swabs are appropriate for collecting wound exudates that may be infected with a *Bacillus* species or the vesicular exudate commonly found in early cutaneous anthrax lesions. In the absence of obvious vesicular exudate from the anthrax lesion, a topical swab may fail to pick up the bacilli. In this case, the edge of the eschar should be lifted with forceps, and fluid should be obtained by application of a capillary tube under the edge. Despite its frequently angry appearance, the lesion is not painful (unless secondarily infected), and this procedure does not cause the patient undue discomfort. In suspected anthrax, one swab or a portion of the collected fluid should be sent for culture; with a second swab or portion of the fluid, a M'Fadyean-stained smear should be prepared.

B. anthracis in infected tissues will not sporulate until exposed to the air, and the vegetative cells are susceptible to the metabolites of putrefactive bacteria, quickly dying off in an aging specimen or rotting carcass; hence, most countries require that anthrax carcasses be burned or buried unopened. The same may be true of other deep-seated *Bacillus* infections, and undue delay in bacteriologically processing a specimen should obviously be avoided. All specimens should be handled with caution, preferably in a biosafety level 3 safety cabinet, because of the risk of releasing dust carrying the spores during manipulation. If infected blood or other body fluids must be stored for prolonged periods, refrigeration is preferable to freezing. Specimens from anthrax-infected materials should be autoclaved and incinerated as soon as possible.

ISOLATION PROCEDURES

In blood or tissue specimens, *Bacillus* species responsible for infections are usually present in large numbers after overnight incubation of a direct blood or nutrient agar isolation plate. If the *Bacillus* species is mixed with other microflora, techniques may need to be more selective, e.g., examination of stools or foods in food-poisoning investigations, specimens from old animal carcasses, or environmental specimens in epidemiological, quality control, or sanitation-hygiene studies. *Bacillus* species in such specimens will mostly be present as spores, and heating the sample (solid samples usually mixed with preheated sterile deionized water, 1:1 [wt/vol]) at 62.5°C for 15 min will effectively destroy nonsporeforming contaminants. Alternatively, extraction in 50% (final concentration) filter-sterilized ethanol for 45 to 60 min may be a more gentle but equally effective technique. Direct plate cultures are made on blood, nutrient, or, as appropriate, selective agars from undilute and 10-, 100-, and 1,000-fold dilutions of the treated sample.

Generally speaking, the presence of a *Bacillus* species in a clinical specimen is insufficient grounds for incriminating it as the etiological agent of the clinical condition being investigated, and enrichment procedures are inappropriate. Exceptions are in searches for *B. anthracis* in old specimens or *B. cereus* in stools ≥ 3 days after a food-poisoning episode. In these circumstances, enrichment may be carried out by adding nutrient or tryptic soy broth with polymyxin to the heat- or ethanol-treated specimen.

The selective agar for *B. anthracis* that has stood the test of time is polymyxin-lysozyme EDTA-thallous acetate (PLET) agar (11). Our routine procedure for specimens in which detection of *B. anthracis* is likely to be difficult is to plate loopfuls of the undiluted and diluted heat- or alcohol-treated suspensions of the specimen onto blood agar (incubated overnight at 37°C) and to spread 0.25-ml volumes on PLET plates (incubated for 48 h at 37°C). Typical, gray-white, nonhemolytic colonies on the blood agar and circular white colonies, 1 to 3 mm diameter, with a ground-glass texture are subcultured on (i) blood agar plates to test for gamma phage and penicillin susceptibility and hemolysis and (ii) directly or subsequently in blood to look for capsule production. PLET performs better with some samples than others; *B. anthracis* may be hard to differentiate from other *Bacillus* species, particularly *B. cereus*, that are present in large numbers in calcareous soils and partially overcome the selectivity of the medium. Prespreading PLET plates with 0.25 ml of a solution containing 0.3% calcium phosphate and 0.3% calcium chloride enhances the growth of *B. anthracis;* some selectivity is lost, but this drawback may be outweighed by the enhanced growth of identifiable *B. anthracis* colonies.

Several selective agars have been designed for isolation, identification, and enumeration of *B. cereus* (12, 26a). The essential ingredients of all of these agars are egg yolk, mannitol, and a dye, exploiting the mannitol-negative, lecithin-hydrolyzing nature of *B. cereus*. Pyruvate is added in some formulas to reduce the size of colonies (important for plate counts, for example), and polymyxin is included in others to improve selectivity for specimens likely to contain gram-negative bacteria (stools or feces-contaminated specimens in particular). Three satisfactory formulations (MYP [16], PEMBA [8], and BCM [14]) are supplied in chapter 121.

In the case of other *Bacillus* species, need and demand have not merited the development of selective media.

IDENTIFICATION

Catalase production and aerobic endospore formation distinguish *Bacillus* species from clostridia. The few catalase-negative *Bacillus* species are unlikely to be encountered in a clinical laboratory.

Most *Bacillus* species form acid alone on carbohydrate media, but a few, such as *B. macerans* and *B. polymyxa*, also produce gas. Glucose, maltose, and sucrose are commonly fermented, mannitol and salicin are less commonly fermented, and lactose is rarely fermented. The end products of glucose fermentation vary greatly.

Many *Bacillus* species secrete proteolytic enzymes and hydrolyze casein and gelatin. *B. cereus, B. mycoides, B. thuringiensis*, and to a lesser extent *B. anthracis* synthesize lecithinases, forming opaque zones of precipitation around colonies on egg yolk agar. *B. laterosporus, B. macerans*, and *B. polymyxa* produce lecithinase more weakly, and on egg yolk agar the reaction is only visible beneath the colony when growth is scraped away.

Several *Bacillus* species, particularly those in morphological group 1 (see below), elaborate one or more hemolysins. Some species, in particular *B. subtilis, B. brevis, B. firmus, B. megaterium*, and *B. sphaericus*, are strict aerobes; others are facultative anaerobes. Nitrate reduction is a common property.

Parasporal bodies are characteristic of certain *Bacillus* species, and differentiation of *B. thuringiensis* from *B. cereus* is largely dependent on observation of the cuboid or diamond-shaped parasporal crystals of *B. thuringiensis* in sporulation agar or old (>2 days) nutrient agar cultures by phase-contrast microscopy or after staining with buffalo black or malachite green. These glycoprotein crystals are the active toxic principles in *B. thuringiensis* insecticides.

For the purposes of differentiation and identification of the many diverse members of this very large genus, Gordon et al. (7) divided the genus *Bacillus* into three morphological groups, based on spore and sporangium morphologies, as follows:

Group 1. Sporangia not swollen. Spores ellipsoidal or cylindrical, central or terminal. Gram positive. Subgroup A (large-cell group): bacillary body width, ≥1 μm; protoplasmic globules demonstrable. Subgroup B (small-cell group): width, <1 μm; protoplasmic globules not demonstrable.

Group 2. Sporangia swollen by ellipsoidal spores, central or terminal. Gram variable.

Group 3. Sporangia swollen. Spores spherical, subterminal or terminal. Gram variable.

The predominant species within these groups are shown in Table 2. *Bacillus* species that did not appear to belong to any of these groups were placed in a fourth group termed "unassigned strains." In the routine laboratory, the identification scheme of Gordon et al. still remains the simplest way to identify the commonly encountered isolates.

B. anthracis, B. cereus, B. cereus var. *mycoides* (sometimes referred to simply as *B. mycoides*), and *B. thuringiensis* are so closely related that some taxonomists consider them varieties of *B. cereus*. Basic distinguishing features for laboratory diagnosis are shown in Table 3. Contrary to the impression frequently given in textbooks, it is generally easy to distinguish *B. anthracis* from other members of the *B. cereus* group. For all practical purposes, an isolate with the correct colonial morphology, white or gray in color, nonhemolytic or only weakly hemolytic, nonmotile, gamma phage and penicillin susceptible, and able to produce the characteristic capsule is *B. anthracis*.

The capsule of *B. anthracis* can be demonstrated after culture on nutrient agar containing 0.7% sodium bicarbonate incubated overnight under CO_2 (a candle jar will do). Colonies of the capsulated *B. anthracis* appear mucoid, and the capsule can be visualized by staining smears with M'Fadyean polychrome methylene blue or India ink (30). Alternatively, 2 ml of blood (any source, but defibrinated horse blood appears to give most satisfactory results) can be inoculated with a pinhead quantity of growth from the initial suspect colony and incubated for 6 to 18 h at 37°C. The encapsulated *B. anthracis* can be observed in a M'Fadyean-stained smear of this blood. If any doubt remains as to the identity of the isolate as *B. anthracis*, subcutaneous inoculation of a light suspension of the bacteria in a mouse is necessary. A M'Fadyean-stained blood smear taken at death occurring after 48 h will reveal large numbers of the typical large capsulated square-end rods in chains of one to several bacilli.

The technology now exists to look in a routine manner for the anthrax toxin and the pXO1 and pXO2 plasmids which code, respectively, for the toxin and capsule. However, these tests are still confined to the specialist laboratory. Environmental isolates which may be *B. anthracis* organisms that have lost one or both plasmids are being observed, but without the ability to regain these very large plasmids naturally, it is academic to the clinical laboratory whether these isolates are recorded as *B. cereus*.

Identification of *Bacillus* isolates to species level has been greatly facilitated by the availability of the API 50 CH test strip (API Laboratory Products, Inc.; marketed by Analytab Products, Plainview, N.Y.), which is designed for use in conjunction with the API 20E test strip and the morphological characteristics described above to identify up to 38 *Bacillus* species and subspecies.

TABLE 2. Characteristics used for identification of selected *Bacillus* species

Morphological group[a]	Characteristic[b]															
				Spores												
	Gram reaction	Lipid globules in protoplasm	Catalase production	Ellipsoidal	Spherical	Central or paracentral	Terminal or subterminal	Swelling sporangium	Motility	Anaerobic growth	V-P reaction	pH in V-P broth of <6.0	Growth at 50°C	Growth at 60°C	Egg yolk reaction	Growth in 0.001% lysozyme
Group 1																
Subgroup A																
B. megaterium	+	+	+	+	−	+	−	−	+	−	−	v	−	−	−	−
B. cereus "group"[c]	+	+	+	+	−	+	−	−	v[c]	+	+	+	−	−	+	+
Subgroup B																
B. licheniformis	+	−	+	+	−	+	−	−	+	+	+	v	+	−	−	−
B. subtilis	+	−	+	+	−	+	−	−	+	−	+	v	+	−	−	b
B. pumilus	+	−	+	+	−	+	−	−	+	−	+	+	+	−	−	a
B. firmus	+	−	+	+	−	v	v	−	a	−	−	−	−	−	−	−
B. coagulans	+	−	+	+	−	v	v	v	+	+	a	+	+	v	−	−
Group 2																
B. polymyxa	v	−	+	+	−	v	v	+	+	+	+	v	−	−	−	a
B. macerans	v	−	+	+	−	−	+	+	+	+	−	−	+	−	−	−
B. circulans	v	−	+	+	−	v	v	+	a	a	−	v	+	−	−	b
B. stearothermophilus	v	−	v	+	−	−	+	+	+	−	−	+	+	+	−	−
B. alvei	v	−	+	+	−	v	v	+	+	+	+	+	−	−	−	+
B. laterosporus[d]	v	−	+	+	−	+	−	+	+	+	−	−	+	−	(+)	+
B. brevis	v	−	+	+	−	v	v	+	+	−	−	−	+	v	−	b
Group 3																
B. sphaericus	v	−	+	−	+	−	+	+	+	−	−	−	−	−	−	a

[a] From Gordon et al. (7).
[b] V-P, Voges-Proskauer; AS, ammonium salt; +, ≥85% of strains examined by Gordon et al. (7) positive; a, 50 to 84% positive; b, 15 to 49% positive; −, <15% positive; v, inconstant; n, not applicable; (+), under colony which needs to be scraped off for reaction to be seen.
[c] See Table 3.
[d] Spore in sporangium has characteristic canoe shape.

SEROLOGICAL TESTS

Species and strain differentiation

Although much work has been put into attempts at developing simple serological species and strain differentiation systems for *Bacillus* species over the past four decades, few of any real practical value have emerged, and none have become commercially viable. Because of numerous cross-reacting antigens and hydrophobic surface properties leading to autoagglutination, spores have not readily lent themselves to such systems; likewise cross-reacting antigens and the difficulties of obtaining vegetative cell material free of spore antigens have precluded serological systems based on vegetative cell antigens. Specific polysaccharide epitopes have been identified in the spore cortex and cell wall of *B. anthracis* (5), and monoclonal antibodies to these epitopes are used in routine identification of *B. anthracis* in the U.S. Army Medical Research Institute of Infectious Diseases, Fort Detrick, Md. However, these are species-specific antibodies and a strain differentiation system for *B. anthracis*, serological or other, has yet to be developed.

A strain differentiation system for *B. cereus* based on the recognition of more than 40 flagellar (H) antigens was developed in the Food Hygiene Laboratory, Central Public Health Laboratory, Colindale, London, England (12, 14). This system is used for investigations of food-poisoning outbreaks or other *B. cereus*-associated clinical problems. A similar system has been developed by the Tokyo Metropolitan Research Laboratory of Public Health, Tokyo, Japan.

B. thuringiensis strains are classified on the basis of their flagellar antigens; 14 serotypes have been recognized (4), with further subdivisions in some cases on the basis of H-antigenic subfactors.

Toxin and antitoxin detection

The three protein components of anthrax toxin, protective antigen, lethal factor, and edema factor, can now be purified on demand (19), and both the antigens and the antibodies to them have proved suitable for use in enzyme immunoassay systems (10, 24, 27). For routine confirmation of infection or monitoring vaccine response, protective antigen is usually used, but lethal factor is equally good. Experience has shown, however, that confirmatory serological analysis with human anthrax has limited use; either treatment initiated early

TABLE 2—*Continued*

	Characteristic[b]																
			Acid from:														
	Growth at pH 5.7	Growth in 7% NaCl	AS glucose	AS arabinose	AS xylose	AS mannitol	Acid + gas from AS glucose	Starch hydrolysis	Citrate utilization	Propionate utilization	Nitrate reduction	Dihydroxyacetone production	Indole production	Phenylalanine deamination	Casein decomposition	Tyrosine decomposition
Group 1																
Subgroup A																
B. megaterium	+	+	+	a	a	+	−	+	+	n	b	n	n	a	+	a
B. cereus "group"[c]	+	+	+	−	−	−	−	+	v[c]	n	+	n	n	−	+	v[c]
Subgroup B																
B. licheniformis	+	+	+	+	+	+	−	+	+	+	n	n	n	+	b	
B. subtilis	+	+	+	+	+	+	−	−	+	−	−	n	n	n	+	−
B. pumilus	−	+	+	b	b	+	−	+	−	−	+	n	n	n	+	b
B. firmus	+	−	+	a	a	b	−	+	b	−	b	n	n	n	b	−
B. coagulans	+	−	+	a	a	b	−	+	b	−	b	n	n	n	b	−
Group 2																
B. polymyxa	+	−	+	+	+	+	+	+	−	n	+	+	−	n	+	−
B. macerans	+	−	+	+	+	+	+	+	b	n	+	−	−	n	−	−
B. circulans	b	b	+	+	+	+	−	+	b	n	b	−	−	n	b	−
B. stearothermophilus	−	−	+	b	a	b	−	+	−	n	a	−	−	n	a	−
B. alvei	−	−	+	−	−	−	−	+	−	n	−	+	+	n	+	b
B. laterosporus[a]	−	b	+	−	−	+	−	−	−	n	+	−	a	−	+	+
B. brevis	b	−	+	−	−	a	−	−	b	n	a	−	−	−	+	+
Group 3																
B. sphaericus	b	b	−	−	−	−	−	−	b	n	−	−	−	+	a	−

TABLE 3. Distinguishing characteristics of *B. cereus* and closely related species

Species	Characteristic[a]											
	Colony on blood agar	Motility[b]	Hemolysis[c]	Lysis by gamma phage	Penicillin susceptibility	Crystalline parasporal inclusion	Citrate utilization	Growth in 7% NaCl	Tyrosine decomposition	Elaboration of anthrax toxin and capsule and possession of plasmids pXO1 and pXO2	Virulence in mice	M'Fadyean reaction in killed mice
B. cereus	Slight green tinge	+	+	−	−	−	+[b]	+[b]	+[b]	−	−	−
B. anthracis	Gray-white to white; generally smaller than *B. cereus*	−	−	+	+	−	b	+[b]	−[b]	+	+	+
B. thuringiensis	As *B. cereus*	+	+	−	−	+	+[b]	+[b]	+[b]	−	−	−
B. cereus var. *mycoides*	Spreading rhizoid colonies with marked tailing	−	(+)	−	−	−	a	a	a	−	−	−

[a] +, ≥85% of strains positive; a, 50 to 84% positive; b, <15 to 49% positive; −, 15% positive; (+), usually weakly positive.
[b] From Gordon et al. (7).
[c] On sheep or horse blood agar, at 24 h.

aborted the infection before it had the opportunity to induce adequate antibodies or the individual died. Serological testing has proved useful for epidemiological investigations in animals (24).

The toxin held responsible for the diarrheal type of *B. cereus* food poisoning has been partially purified and characterized. It appears to be a toxin complex and is the basis for systems designed to detect the toxin in foods and feces (Central Public Health Laboratory, London, England; U.S. Food and Drug Administration, Washington, D.C.).

ANTIBIOTIC SUSCEPTIBILITIES

B. anthracis is almost invariably susceptible to penicillin; only three resistant isolates have been reported. The basis of resistance in the rare exceptions is discussed elsewhere (15). It is also susceptible to gentamicin, erythromycin, chloramphenicol, tetracycline, and ciprofloxacin, mostly susceptible to streptomycin, and resistant to cefuroxime.

B. cereus and *B. thuringiensis* produce a broad-spectrum β-lactamase and are thus resistant to penicillin, ampicillin, and cephalosporins. They are also almost always susceptible to clindamycin, erythromycin, chloramphenicol, vancomycin, and aminoglycosides and usually to tetracycline and sulfonamides also but are resistant to trimethoprim (1, 21, 22, 26, 29).

LITERATURE CITED

1. **Anonymous.** 1983. *Bacillus cereus* as a systemic pathogen. Lancet **ii:**1469.
2. **Chastel, C., and O. Masure.** 1986. Bactériémies, septicémies et infections diverses à *Bacillus licheniformis*. Med. Mal. Infect. **4:**226.
3. **Claus, D., and R. C. W. Berkeley.** 1986. Genus *Bacillus* Cohn 1872, 174, p. 1105–1139. *In* P. H. A. Sneath, N. S. Mair, M. E. Sharpe, and J. G. Holt (ed.), Bergey's manual of systematic bacteriology, vol. 2. The Williams & Wilkins Co., Baltimore.
4. **de Barjac, H.** 1981. Insect pathogens in the genus *Bacillus*, p. 241–250. *In* R. C. W. Berkeley and M. Goodfellow (ed.), The aerobic endospore-forming bacteria: classification and identification. Academic Press, Inc. (London), Ltd., London.
5. **Ezzell, J. W.** 1990. Analyses of *Bacillus anthracis* vegetative cell surface antigens and of serum protease cleavage of protective antigen. Proceedings of the International Workshop on Anthrax. Salisbury Med. Bull. no. 68, Special Suppl., p. 43–44.
6. **Gilbert, R. J., P. C. B. Turnbull, J. M. Parry, and J. M. Kramer.** 1981. *Bacillus cereus* and other *Bacillus* species: their part in food poisoning and other clinical infections, p. 297–314. *In* R. C. W. Berkeley and M. Goodfellow (ed.), The aerobic endospore-forming bacteria. Academic Press, Inc. (London), Ltd., London.
7. **Gordon, R. E., W. C. Haynes, and C. H.-N. Pang.** 1973. The genus *Bacillus*. U.S. Department of Agriculture agricultural handbook no. 427. U.S. Department of Agriculture, Washington, D.C.
8. **Holbrook, R., and J. M. Anderson.** 1980. An improved selective and diagnostic medium for the isolation and enumeration of *Bacillus cereus* in foods. Can. J. Microbiol. **263:**753–759.
9. **Hugh-Jones, M.** 1990. Global trends in the incidence of anthrax in livestock. Proceedings of the International Workshop on Anthrax. Salisbury Med. Bull. no. 68, Special Suppl., p. 2–4.
10. **Ivins, B. E., and S. L. Welkos.** 1988. Recent advances in the development of an improved, human anthrax vaccine. Eur. J. Epidemiol. **4:**12–19.
11. **Knisely, R. F.** 1966. Selective medium for *Bacillus anthracis*. J. Bacteriol. **92:**784–786.
12. **Kramer, J. M., and R. J. Gilbert.** 1989. *Bacillus cereus* and other *Bacillus* species, p. 21–70. *In* M. P. Doyle (ed.), Foodborne bacterial pathogens. Marcel Dekker, Inc., New York.
13. **Kramer, J. M., P. C. B. Turnbull, K. Jørgensen, J. M. Parry, and R. J. Gilbert.** 1978. Separation of exponential growth exotoxins of *Bacillus cereus* and their preliminary characterization. J. Appl. Bacteriol. **45:**xix.
14. **Kramer, J. M., P. C. B. Turnbull, G. Munshi, and R. J. Gilbert.** 1982. Identification and characterization of *Bacillus cereus* and other *Bacillus* species associated with food poisoning, p. 261–286. *In* J. E. L. Corry, D. Roberts, and F. A. Skinner (ed.), Isolation and identification methods for food poisoning organisms. Society for Applied Bacteriology technical series no. 17. Academic Press, Inc. (London), Ltd., London.
15. **Lightfoot, N. F., R. J. D. Scott, and P. C. B. Turnbull.** 1990. Antimicrobial susceptibility of *Bacillus anthracis*. Proceedings of the International Workshop on Anthrax. Salisbury Med. Bull. no. 68, Special Suppl., p. 95–98.
16. **Mossel, D. A. A., M. J. Koopman, and E. Jongerius.** 1967. Enumeration of *Bacillus cereus* in foods. Appl. Microbiol. **15:**650–653.
17. **Norris, J. R., R. C. W. Berkeley, N. A. Logan, and A. G. O'Donnell.** 1981. The genera *Bacillus* and *Sporolactobacillus*, p. 1711–1742. *In* M. P. Starr, H. Stolp, H. G. Trüper, A. Balows, and H. G. Schlegel (ed.), The prokaryotes. A handbook on habitats, isolation, and identification of bacteria, vol. 2. Springer-Verlag, New York.
18. **Parry, J. M., P. C. B. Turnbull, and J. R. Gibson.** 1983. A colour atlas of *Bacillus* species. Wolfe Medical Atlas no. 19. Wolfe Medical Publications, London.
19. **Quinn, C. P., C. C. Shone, P. C. B. Turnbull, and J. Melling.** 1988. Purification of anthrax toxin components by high-performance anion-exchange, gel-filtration and hydrophobic-interaction chromatography. Biochem. J. **252:**753–758.
20. **Siegman-Igra, Y., J. Lavochkin, D. Schwartz, and N. Konforti.** 1983. Meningitis and bacteremia due to *Bacillus cereus*. A case report and review of *Bacillus* infections. Isr. J. Med. Sci. **19:**546–551.
21. **Sliman, R., S. Rehm, and D. M. Shlaes.** 1987. Serious infections caused by *Bacillus* species. Medicine **66:**218–223.
22. **Tuazon, C. U., H. W. Murray, C. Levy, M. N. Solny, J. A. Curtin, and J. N. Sheagren.** 1979. Serious infections from *Bacillus* sp. J. Am. Med. Assoc. **241:**1137–1140.
23. **Turnbull, P. C. B.** 1986. *Bacillus cereus* toxins, p. 397–448. *In* F. Dorner and J. Drews (ed.), Pharmacology of bacterial toxins. International encyclopedia of pharmacology and therapeutics, section 119. Pergamon Press, Oxford.

23a. **Turnbull, P. C. B.** 1990. Anthrax, p. 364–377. *In* G. R. Smith and C. R. Easmon (ed.), Topley and Wilson's principles of bacteriology, virology and immunity, 8th ed., vol. 3. Edward Arnold, Sevenoaks, Kent, United Kingdom.

24. **Turnbull, P. C. B., J. A. Carman, P. M. Lindeque, F. Joubert, O. J. B. Hubschle, and G. H. Snoeyenbos.** 1989. Further progress in understanding anthrax in the Etosha National Park. Madoqua **16:**93–104.
25. **Turnbull, P. C. B., K. Jørgensen, J. M. Kramer, R. J. Gilbert, and J. M. Parry.** 1979. Severe clinical conditions associated with *Bacillus cereus* and the apparent involvement of exotoxins. J. Clin. Pathol. **32:**289–293.

26. **Turnbull, P. C. B., and J. M. Kramer.** 1983. Non-gastrointestinal *Bacillus cereus* infections: an analysis of exotoxin production by strains isolated over a two-year period. J. Clin. Pathol. **36:**1091–1096.

26a. **Turnbull, P. C. B., J. M. Kramer, and J. Melling.** 1990. Bacillus, p. 187–210. *In* M. T. Parker and B. I. Duerden (ed.), Topley and Wilson's principles of bacteriology, virology and immunity, 8th ed., vol. 2. Edward Arnold, Sevenoaks, Kent, United Kingdom.

27. **Turnbull, P. C. B., S. H. Leppla, M. G. Broster, C. P. Quinn, and J. Melling.** 1988. Antibodies to anthrax toxin in humans and guinea pigs and their relevance to protective immunity. Med. Microbiol. Immunol. **177:**293–303.

28. **Warren, R. E., D. Rubenstein, D. J. Ellar, J. M. Kramer, and R. J. Gilbert.** 1984. *Bacillus thuringiensis* var. *israelensis:* protoxin activation and safety. Lancet **i:**678–679.

29. **Wiedermann, B. L.** 1987. Non-anthrax *Bacillus* infections in children. Pediatr. Infect. Dis. J. **6:**218–219.

30. **Williams, R. P.** 1981. *Bacillus anthracis* and other aerobic spore-forming bacilli, p. 315–326. *In* A. I. Braude (ed.), Medical microbiology and infectious diseases. The W. B. Saunders Co., Philadelphia.

Chapter 34

Mycobacterium

GLENN D. ROBERTS, ELMER W. KONEMAN, AND YOO K. KIM

The field of clinical mycobacteriology has changed more during the past 10 years than any other time during its history. The single event that appears to be responsible for this renewal of interest was the development and introduction of a rapid radiometric mycobacterial detection system. This method prompted the adaptation of the system to separate *Mycobacterium tuberculosis* from other mycobacteria and also to perform antimicrobial susceptibility testing of mycobacteria, particularly *M. tuberculosis*.

Separately, gas-liquid chromatography (GLC) was also introduced as a reliable and rapid method for the identification of species of clinically important mycobacteria and is now commercially available to all laboratories. The most recent development in the field of mycobacteriology is the use of nucleic acid probes for the identification of *M. tuberculosis, M. avium-intracellulare* (MAI), and *M. gordonae*. Newer methods and probes for other species are currently being evaluated and will be discussed in this chapter.

All of the above-mentioned methods may be used in a routine clinical laboratory setting and will be considered as standard methods available to those who choose to use them. Certainly conventional biochemical and cultural characteristics remain important in making the definitive identification of a mycobacterial species. However, with newer methods, these tests have become less important and are used on a much more selective basis than in the past; nevertheless, their role should not be underemphasized.

Using the methods described in this chapter, laboratories should be able to provide physicians with accurate and rapid culture results within a clinically relevant period of time. Many laboratories have followed the trend of sending specimens or cultures to reference laboratories much more suited for the recovery and definitive identification of the species. This trend will probably continue because of the emphasis on financial constraints and cost containment in clinical laboratories. However, this practice will not compromise patient care or cause a delay in the reporting of results to physicians, since all of the methods are available to laboratories of all sizes and are highly reliable.

GENERAL CHARACTERISTICS OF CLINICALLY IMPORTANT MYCOBACTERIA

The mycobacteria are acid-fast, aerobic, nonspore-forming, nonmotile bacteria. These bacteria are slightly curved or straight bacilli, 0.2 to 0.6 by 1.0 to 10.0 μm in size. They have cell walls rich in lipid content, which is responsible for the ability of the organisms to withstand staining by usual aniline dyes; therefore, stains like the Gram stain are relatively ineffective. Methods that promote the uptake of dyes are available; however, when mycobacteria are stained, they are not easily decolorized even with acid alcohol. Therefore, they are described as acid fast. They often stain irregularly and appear beaded or granular; during growth on certain culture media, some of the mycobacteria may appear to be non-acid fast. A computer-generated description of members of the family *Mycobacteriaceae* is available in *Bergey's Manual* (244).

In general, the growth rate for the mycobacteria is slow and requires 2 to 8 weeks or longer for detection by use of traditional mycobacteriology media. However, they may be detected much earlier with use of a radiometric system that detects the metabolism of a ^{14}C-labeled substrate and detection of the evolution of ^{14}C-labeled carbon dioxide as a metabolic by-product of the organism (147). The latter criterion is used as a basis for mycobacterial detection with the BACTEC TB system (see below). It is important to remember that the growth rate is dependent on the size of the inoculum present in the clinical specimen and the medium on which the specimen is inoculated for primary recovery. The term "rapidly growing mycobacteria" is a bit of a misnomer. On primary recovery media, they generally grow no more quickly than other mycobacteria; however, subculture of the organisms may require less than 5 days for growth to become apparent. Certain mycobacteria, including *M. ulcerans, M. haemophilum,* and *M. marinum,* require temperatures of 30 to 32°C for primary recovery; *M. xenopi* and MAI are best recovered at temperatures above 37°C. The colonial morphologic features of the mycobacteria vary with the species. Colonies may be rough, with the bacilli compacted into dense aggregates (e.g., *M. tuberculosis*); they may be smooth and transparent, with bacilli arranged in no definite pattern (e.g., MAI); or they may appear to be slightly rough in texture (e.g., *M. kansasii*). Colonies of some of the species (*M. xenopi* and some of the rapidly growing mycobacteria) form fragile, branching filamentous colonies on the surface of the culture media. Some isolates may have colonies that penetrate the medium or even project into the air. Pigmentation is unique to certain species of mycobacteria. Some species are photochromogenic (light is required for the formation of pigment), whereas others are scotochromogenic (pigment is formed in either the light or the dark) or have no or varied pigment production, depending on the species.

At least 25 species of mycobacteria are associated with human disease and produce usually slowly developing, destructive granulomas that may undergo necrosis with ulceration or cavitation. However, it is now common to find mycobacterial infections without granuloma formation in immunocompromised patients, particularly those having acquired immunodeficiency syndrome (AIDS). Disease may be confined to a cooler, more superficial part of the body, or it may invade the internal organs and cause disseminated disease. Tuberculosis of the lungs always disseminates to other parts of the body by way of the blood, lymphatics, or gastrointestinal tract. Certain mycobacterial infections are associated with occupation. For example, infection due to *M. marinum* is most common in patients who have tropical fish tanks or are around an aquatic environment.

GROUPING OF MYCOBACTERIA AS APPLICABLE TO THE CLINICAL LABORATORY

In 1959, Runyon established a grouping for mycobacteria other than *M. tuberculosis* or *M. bovis* that occurred in clinical specimens (188). The groups were not species; rather, each group consisted of several species. Group I consisted of the photochromogenic mycobacteria, group II consisted of scotochromogenic species, group III contained the nonphotochromogenic and often, at least initially, nonchromogenic, slowly growing mycobacteria, and group IV consisted of the rapidly growing species that required less than 1 week of incubation at 25 or at 37°C. The Runyon grouping was based on pigmentation, colonial morphology, and growth rate. After several years, it became apparent that all species of mycobacteria did not fit within the Runyon grouping and that many newly described species could not be categorized. For example, some isolates of MAI, a nonchromogen, appeared highly pigmented and could not be grouped into the Runyon scheme. *M. szulgai* is photochromogenic at 25°C and scotochromogenic at 37°C, demonstrating the failure of the Runyon grouping for the classification of the species of mycobacteria. It is now recommended that all mycobacteria be identified to the species level and that the Runyon grouping scheme not be used by clinical laboratories.

As other species of non-*M. tuberculosis* mycobacteria were described, they were placed in a general group of "atypical mycobacteria," because the species were not typical of *M. tuberculosis*. Since these mycobacteria are not atypical but are characteristic of their own species, the term "atypical mycobacteria" is also unsuitable for clinical laboratories. Terms such as "mycobacteria other than tuberculosis" or "nontuberculosis mycobacteria" have been used, but they are also inadequate for describing the species of mycobacteria. Again, it is important that the mycobacteria be referred to by species name because of the therapeutic implications of infections caused by the various species of clinically important mycobacteria.

Table 1 shows the classification of the mycobacteria other than *M. tuberculosis* originally proposed by Wolinski (252) and refined by Woods and Washington (255), which is based on human pathogenicity and has been offered as an approach that is more clinically relevant.

TABLE 1. Mycobacteria other than *M. tuberculosis*

Group	Species
Species pathogenic in humans	*M. leprae*
Species potentially pathogenic in humans	*M. avium-intracellulare*, *M. kansasii*, *M. fortuitum-chelonae* complex, *M. scrofulaceum*, *M. xenopi*, *M. szulgai*, *M. malmoense*, *M. simiae*, *M. marinum*, *M. ulcerans*, *M. haemophilum*
Saprophytic mycobacteria rarely causing disease in humans	
Slow growth rate	*M. gordonae*, *M. asiaticum*, *M. terrae-triviale* complex, *M. gastri*, *M. nonchromogenicum*, *M. paratuberculosis*
Intermediate growth rate	*M. flavescens*
Rapid growth rate	*M. thermoresistibile*, *M. smegmatis*, *M. vaccae*, *M. parafortuitum* complex, *M. phlei*

SAFETY PROCEDURES

It is necessary to implement and enforce certain safety procedures specific to the clinical microbiology laboratory because of the nature of the organisms and the mode of transmission. Common sense regarding minimization of the dispersal of mycobacteria into the air and avoidance of the inhalation of airborne bacilli is of utmost importance. Direct contact with mycobacteria is to be avoided if possible. Persons working with mycobacteria should be in overall general good health, and those who are immunocompromised should be discouraged from working in that area.

Persons working in the mycobacteriology laboratory should have a regularly scheduled annual skin test; if they have had a previously positive skin test, they should have a chest X-ray examination at yearly intervals. Physical examinations should be obtained when circumstances indicate that it is necessary.

All specimens suspected of containing mycobacteria should be treated appropriately. A separate room under negative pressure and equipped with a class I or IIA biological safety cabinet should be used. Some laboratory directors feel that employees should wear a mask, gloves, cap, gown, and shoe covers when working in the mycobacteriology laboratory. The use of gloves and laboratory coats or gowns is essential; however, this is probably all that is necessary. All work involving specimens or cultures, such as making smears, inoculating media, and adding reagents to biochemical tests, must be performed within a biological safety cabinet. The handling of all specimens suspected of containing mycobacteria (including specimens processed for other microorganisms), with the exception of centrifugation for concentration purposes, must be done within the laminar-flow type of biological safety cabinet. Specimens that are to be taken from under the hood to a decontamination area must be covered before transport. Towels soaked with a phenolic disinfectant can be used to cover the work surfaces, to line discard pans, and to wipe the edges of culture tubes to prevent dripping. The cabinet area and work area should be cleaned with disinfectant before and after work, and a UV light should radiate the work area when it is not in use. It is important that the UV lights be kept clean to maintain their effectiveness. To prevent aerosols, sealed centrifuge cups, electric incinerators, and splashproof discard containers must be used. The excess inoculum from inoculating loops, wires, or spades may be removed by placing them in a bottle containing 5% phenol in sand or in 95% ethanol. The former is preferred, since the abrasive action of the sand will remove most of the excess inoculum before flaming. It is important to reiterate that all activities associated with the handling of mycobacteria should be done within a laminar-flow biological safety cabinet. In general, safety measures observed in the clinical microbiology laboratory should be followed by those working in the mycobacteriology area.

DECONTAMINATION PROCEDURES

All persons leaving the mycobacteriology laboratory should wash their hands thoroughly with any good hand soap. There is no need for germicidal or tuberculocidal compounds to be used on the hands as long as adequate rinsing is used along with hand washing.

Suitable disinfectants for laboratory bench surfaces and biosafety cabinets are as follows:

1. Phenol-soap mixtures employing *o*-phenol or other phenol derivatives, with contact periods of 10 to 30 min. Examples of these products are Amphyl (Lehn and Fink, Toledo, Ohio), Osyl (National Laboratories, Toledo, Ohio), and Staphene and Vesphen (Vestal Laboratories, St. Louis, Mo).
2. Sodium hypochlorite, 1:200 or 1:1,000 concentration. Contact should be 10 to 30 min, and the solution should be made fresh daily.
3. Formaldehyde, 3 to 8%; alkaline glutaraldehyde, 2%. Contact time should be at least 30 min and preferably longer.
4. Phenol, 5%. A contact time of 10 to 30 min is adequate, and this compound is recommended for many clinical laboratories. It should be mentioned that phenol is irritating to the skin.

SPECIMEN COLLECTION

Laboratory personnel should provide guidance and consultation in the collection of specimens submitted for the recovery of mycobacteria. Decisions on how fresh samples are handled at the bedside, the type of holding medium, selection of transport containers, and the conditions under which specimens must be maintained should be made with appropriate input from clinical microbiologists. This team approach is currently even more urgent, since mycobacterial infections are frequently presenting as clinical syndromes other than the classic chronic pulmonary disease. For example, in patients with suspected AIDS, it is recommended that the laboratory receive stool specimens, blood, and urine samples for acid-fast smear and culture in addition to sputum or respiratory secretions (101, 104). Bone marrow cultures may be a valuable source of recovery for MAI if cultures of blood and other sites have been negative for acid-fast bacilli (172). Clinicians should consider the diagnosis of mycobacterial disease in patients with or at risk for human immunodeficiency virus infection even if the clinical presentation is unusual (82), and sputum samples should be collected even if results of chest X-ray examinations are negative (11).

In brief, for the diagnosis of classic cases of pulmonary tuberculosis, at least three successive first-morning, deep-cough sputum samples should be collected. Although sputum collection devices are commercially available, a sterile wide-mouth jar with a tightly fitted screw-cap lid is adequate. The patient should be instructed to press the rim of the container under the lower lip at the time of expectoration to minimize the chance of contaminating the outside of the container. Allen and Darrell (2) found that the outside of 3% of sputum sample containers in their study were contaminated with mycobacteria.

The material obtained from bronchial brushings and from fine-needle aspirates can be placed in a sterile vial or tube containing approximately 10 ml of Middlebrook 7H9 broth supplemented with bovine serum albumin (final concentration of 1 to 2%) and Tween 80 (0.5%). Bronchial washings and bronchoalveolar lavage fluid can usually be sent directly to the laboratory in the containers in which they were collected. Cerebrospinal fluid, urine, and other body fluids can also be sent directly in sterile containers. It may be necessary to add an anticoagulant to containers for collection of fluids that may contain fibrinogen (pericardial, pleural, and peritoneal effusions, for example). Gastric washings should be transported to the laboratory as quickly as possible and, if possible, should be neutralized before processing.

Stool specimens collected in clean containers may be sent directly to the laboratory as collected, or a sample transferred to a clean vial or tube containing 7H9 broth can be transported. In previous years, it would have been virtually impossible to detect or recover acid-fast bacilli from feces; however, the numbers of organisms found in the bowel in patients with AIDS is extremely high. Biopsies of the bowel often reveal large clusters of mycobacteria within macrophages of the lamina propria, with histological changes resembling Whipple's disease (77). Thus, acid-fast bacilli are often in sufficient concentration in the feces not only to be seen in acid-fast stains but also to be recovered in culture amid the heavy background of fecal flora.

Mycobacteremia is also common in patients with AIDS. The diagnosis is often not difficult to make in patients with the miliary form of the disease because organisms often circulate in high concentrations. Blood culture techniques are also vastly improved, making detection of even small concentrations of organisms possible (168, 262). The Isolator lysis-centrifugation system (Du Pont Co., Wilmington, Del.) is recommended for obtaining blood cultures to recover mycobacteria (101, 104), although the BACTEC 13A blood culture bottle, which also contains a lysing agent, has been found to be a viable method (102). These systems are discussed in more detail below.

SPECIMEN PROCESSING AND CULTURE

The laboratory diagnosis of mycobacterial diseases depends on the detection and recovery of acid-fast bacilli from clinical specimens. As indicated, microbiologists must be prepared to process and culture a variety of both respiratory and nonrespiratory specimens, some of which are contaminated and others not. Several steps are required to recover mycobacteria: bacterial flora must be eliminated or significantly reduced in number from contaminated specimens, mycobacterial cells trapped in mucin must be released, and when present in small numbers, mycobacterial cells must be concentrated to enable detection in stained smears and by culture. Appropriate culture media and conditions of incubation must be selected to facilitate optimal recovery of mycobacteria.

Liquefaction and Decontamination

Specimens submitted for the culture of mycobacteria should be processed as soon as possible. Since slow-growing species of mycobacteria can be easily overgrown by more rapidly proliferating bacteria, contaminated specimens must be decontaminated before inoculation onto culture media. The selection of a liquefaction-decontamination procedure that maintains the viability of the mycobacteria but eliminates all unwanted microorganisms is optimal. The mycobacteria are somewhat protected from the effects of various chemical digestants by the lipids contained within the cell wall. However, even under the best of conditions, most decontamination procedures eliminate all but about 10 to 20% of the mycobacteria contained in the specimen. Thus, the best yield of mycobacteria may be expected to result from the use of the mildest decontamination procedure that gives sufficient control over contaminants.

The presence of large quantities of mucin in the specimen may also compromise the recovery of mycobacteria. Mucin-trapped mycobacterial cells may not be available for culture; contaminating bacteria may be protected from action of the decontaminating agent. Therefore, liquefaction of certain specimens, particularly sputum, is often necessary. Sodium hydroxide, the most commonly used decontaminant, serves both functions but must be used cautiously because it is only somewhat less harmful to tubercle bacilli than to the contaminating organisms. The stronger the alkali, the higher its temperature during the time it acts on the specimen; the longer it is allowed to act, the greater will be the killing action on both contaminants and mycobacteria (114).

More commonly, a combination liquefaction-decontamination mixture is used. *N*-Acetyl-L-cysteine (NALC), dithiothreitol, and several other enzymes effectively liquefy sputum. These agents have no direct inhibitory effect on bacterial cells; however, their use permits treatment using lower concentrations of sodium hydroxide, thereby indirectly improving the recovery of mycobacteria. Cetylpyridinium chloride in specimens mailed from remote collection stations to a central processing station has shown a good recovery of *M. tuberculosis* without a significant overgrowth by contaminating oropharyngeal bacteria (203).

The three most widely used digestion methods are the NaOH method, the Zephiran-trisodium phosphate method, and the NALC-NaOH method. Trisodium phosphate liquefies sputum rapidly but requires a long exposure for decontamination of the specimen when used alone. Benzalkonium chloride (Zephiran) with trisodium phosphate as described below shortens the required period of exposure and selectively destroys many contaminants with little bactericidal action on tubercle bacilli. Many laboratories prefer the NALC-NaOH method for the following reasons: (i) a large number of specimens can be handled in a short time, (ii) concentrated smears can be ready to stain within a short time, and (iii) there is a high rate of recovery of mycobacteria. This technique utilizes a mucolytic agent, NALC, for digestion and sodium hydroxide for decontamination. The sodium citrate included in the mixture exerts a stabilizing effect on the NALC by chelating any heavy-metal ions that may be present in the specimen. Some of these methods are described below.

NALC-Alkali Decontamination Procedure

Reagents

Digestant. Combine 50 ml of 2.94% trisodium citrate · $3H_2O$ (=0.1 M) with 50 ml of 4% NaOH. To this solution add 0.5 g of powdered NALC just before use. Refrigerate the solution when it not in use. Discard the solution after 24 or 48 h.

Phosphate buffer. 0.067 M, pH 6.8.

Bovine serum albumin. Sterile 0.2% solution of bovine albumin fraction V adjusted to pH 6.8.

Procedure

1. Add an equal amount of the decontaminating agent to sputum in a sterile, aerosol-free, 50-ml screw-cap centrifuge tube (dispense solution with a fresh, sterile pipette for each specimen, taking every precaution to avoid contamination). If the amount received is more than 10 ml, select with a pipette about 10 ml of purulent-appearing material (final concentration of NaOH is 1%).
2. Stopper the tube tightly and mix the contents for approximately 20 s on a Vortex test tube mixer until liquefied. If liquefaction is not complete in this time, agitate the solution at intervals during the following decontamination period.
3. Allow the mixture to stand for 15 min at room temperature with occasional gentle shaking. Avoid the kind of movement that causes aeration of the specimen, since the NALC is readily inactivated by oxidation, and mucoid material may repolymerize. A small pinch of crystalline NALC may be added to especially viscous specimens to effect better liquefaction.
4. Centrifuge the solution for at least 15 min at 2,200 to 2,500 × *g* or higher relative centrifugal force (RCF) if suitable equipment is available.
5. Wipe the top of the tube with cotton or a sponge moistened with 5% phenol. Decant the supernatant fluid into a splashproof discard can containing 5% phenol solution or other germicide. Again, wipe the lip of the tube with phenol.
6. Using a sterile applicator stick or a flamed, 3-mm-diameter bacteriological loop, smear a portion of the sediment onto a microscope slide, covering an area approximately 1 by 2 cm for the acid-fast smear, which is discussed in chapter 122. If the quantity of sediment is very small, delay making smears until after the next step (addition of albumin).
7. Add to the sediment 1 ml of the sterile, 0.2% bovine serum albumin.
8. Prepare a 1:10 dilution of 0.5 ml of the albumin suspension in 4.5 ml of sterile water. Inoculate diluted and undiluted specimens onto appropriate solid culture media (Lowenstein-Jensen [L-J] slant, Middlebrook 7H11 medium, or Middlebrook selective 7H11 medium). If biplates are used, both diluted and undiluted suspensions may be in the same plate. Inoculation may be done with disposable capillary pipettes delivering 3 drops to each medium. Plates should be tilted or the

drops should be streaked to ensure isolated colonies and the detection of more than one colony type, if present. Diluting the resuspended sediment decreases the concentration of any toxic materials present which may be inhibitory to mycobacteria. The dilution schema may be applied to any decontamination method.

9. Incubate all cultures at 37°C for 8 weeks before discarding as negative. 7H11 plates should be placed into CO_2-permeable polyethylene bags to prevent drying and then placed into CO_2-enriched incubators. Candle jars are not acceptable as a source of CO_2 because the oxygen tension is reduced below that required for growth of mycobacteria.

Ratnam et al. (180) have found that the omission of the step of adding water or buffer to the treated specimen before centrifugation (step 4) as advocated in the initial procedure (117) did not have a significant effect on the growth or isolation rate of mycobacteria.

Sodium Hydroxide Decontamination Procedure

For the sodium hydroxide procedure, follow the steps described for the NALC-alkali method, substituting sodium hydroxide (≤2%) for the NALC-alkali digestant. In all NaOH procedures, timing must be rigidly controlled. If it is absolutely necessary to reduce excessive contamination, the NaOH concentration can be increased to 3 or 4% rather than increasing the time of exposure to the alkali. The procedure used at Mayo Clinic for freshly collected specimens is as follows.

1. Add an equal volume of 2% sodium hydroxide to the specimen.
2. Screw the cap on tightly, shake the specimen for 5 to 30 s on a Vortex mixer, and allow the mixture to react for the amount of time presented below:

Specimen type	Time (min)
Bronchial washings	15
Gastric washings	15
Urine	15
Sputum, induced sputum	20
Urine containing gram-positive organisms[a]	20
Specimens known to contain gram-negative organisms[a]	25
Cerebrospinal fluid, tissue, other uncontaminated body fluids	No treatment necessary

[a] Specimens of body fluids are cultured onto blood agar plates and read before mycobacterial culture is performed.

3. After the decontamination time is completed, specimens should be neutralized with 1.25 N HCl containing bromocresol purple. The tube must be thoroughly mixed and acid addition stopped when the solution becomes blue.

Zephiran-Trisodium Phosphate Decontamination Procedure

Reagents

Zephiran-trisodium phosphate digestant. Dissolve 1 kg of trisodium phosphate ($Na_3PO_4 \cdot 12H_2O$) in 4 liters of hot distilled water. To this solution add 7.5 ml of Zephiran concentrate (17% benzalkonium chloride; Winthrop Laboratories, New York, N.Y.) and mix.

Neutralizing buffer. The neutralizing buffer, pH 6.6, is prepared by adding 37.5 ml of 0.067 M disodium phosphate to 62.5 ml of 0.067 M monopotassium phosphate. The pH is measured after mixing.

Procedure

1. Add an equal volume of Zephiran-trisodium phosphate digestant to the specimen in a screw-cap jar or bottle. Agitate the mixture vigorously for 30 min on a mechanical shaker. Permit the material to stand, without shaking, for an additional 30 min.
2. In a safety hood, transfer all or a portion of the specimen to a screw-cap, 50-ml centrifuge tube.
3. Centrifuge the specimen and collect the sediment as specified in the description of the NALC-alkali method. Thoroughly suspend the sediment in 20 ml of neutralizing buffer and centrifuge the specimen again for 20 min (the neutralizing buffer serves to inactivate traces of Zephiran in the sediment).
4. Discard the supernatant fluids; there will be sufficient residual buffer to permit resuspension of the sediment. With a disposable capillary pipette, inoculate 3 drops of the sediment onto each medium to be used, and streak the drops to distribute the inoculum for isolated colonies.

The liquefaction-decontamination procedure should be monitored in each laboratory to determine whether the delicate balance between recovery of mycobacteria and suppression of contaminants is being maintained. A low rate of recovery of mycobacteria in the face of signs and symptoms of classical clinical disease may indicate that the treatment is too stringent. On the other hand, excessive contamination, defined as a rate exceeding 5% of all specimens cultured, indicates that the treatment of specimens is inadequate. If a high contamination rate occurs, one of the following measures may be used.

1. Cautiously increase the strength, duration, or temperature of the alkali treatment. Maximal limits are arbitrary, but 4% NaOH at 37°C for more than 60 min will probably kill most tubercle bacilli.
2. Use a selective medium (one that contains antibiotics in addition to the dye, malachite green) and a nonselective primary culture medium to inhibit growth of bacterial and fungal contaminants. Selective 7H11 agar (Mitchison medium), Mycobactosel agar (167) (BBL Microbiology Systems, Cockeysville, Md.), or the Gruft modification of L-J medium (which has penicillin [50 U/ml] and nalidixic acid [35 μg/ml] added to the regular formula) are viable options (see Tables 2 and 3).
3. The oxalic acid method of Corper and Uyei (38) is reported to be superior to alkali for the elimination of *Pseudomonas aeruginosa* and certain other contaminants. Liquefy the sputum with an equal volume of 5% oxalic acid. Agitate the solution on a mixer and then allow it to stand at room temperature for 30 min, with occasional shaking. Add sterile physiologic saline. Centrifuge the solution in a sealed cup, decant the supernatant fluid, and add a few drops of 4% NaOH to bring the pH to 7.
4. Liquefaction, including viscosity reduction, in the presence or even in the absence of a digestant is facil-

TABLE 2. Primary mycobacterial recovery media[a]

Middlebrook	Components	Malachite green[b] (g/100 ml)
American Thoracic Society	Fresh egg yolks, potato flour, glycerol	0.02
Lowenstein-Jensen	Fresh whole eggs, defined salts, glycerol, potato flour	0.025
Petragnani	Fresh whole eggs, egg yolks, whole milk, potato, potato flour, glycerol	0.052
Middlebrook 7H10	Defined salts, vitamins, cofactors, oleic acid, albumin, catalase, glycerol, glucose	0.00025
Middlebrook 7H11	Defined salts, vitamins, cofactors, oleic acid, albumin, catalase, glycerol, 0.1% casein hydrolysate	0.0025
Middlebrook 7H12	7H9 broth base, casein hydrolysate, bovine serum albumin, catalase, ^{14}C-labeled palmitic acid	

[a] Modified from H. M. Sommers, "Mycobacterial Diseases," *in* J. B. Henry (ed.), *Clinical Diagnosis and Management by Laboratory Methods,* 16th ed., The W. B. Saunders Co., Philadelphia, 1979.
[b] Inhibitory agent.

itated by the vigorous mixing of a solution in a sealed container with a Vortex-type mixer. If such mixers are properly used, aerosol production is minimized. The tube should be held on the vibrating base in such a way that churning, splashing, and foaming of the mixture are avoided. Homogenization should occur not by vibratory agitation but by centrifugal swirling, and this swirling should not be vigorous enough to permit material to rise to the cap. Wait at least 15 min after agitation before opening the tube to allow any fine aerosol droplets formed during the mixing to settle. All such procedures should be carried out in a biological safety hood, and disposable gloves should be worn.

Procedure for Blood Cultures

Most bacteriological blood culture systems are usually not suitable for the recovery of mycobacteria. Berlin et al. (14) devised a biphasic system using modified 7H11 oleic acid albumin agar as the solid phase and brain heart infusion broth as the liquid phase and reported recovery of MAI within 6 to 8 days. The ability to use colonies from the agar slant for biochemical identification and antimicrobial susceptibility testing is a distinct advantage over broth recovery systems. Currently, most laboratories are using the Isolator (lysis-centrifugation system) or the radiometric (BACTEC 13A) blood culture system, either separately or in combination. No prior processing is necessary, since both systems utilize a lysing agent to free mycobacteria from mononuclear cells.

The protocol for the use of the Isolator system has been outlined by Gill et al. (62) and by Kiehn et al. (104). The Isolator tube contains an anticoagulant and saponin, the lytic agent. Ten milliliters of blood should be collected into this tube. The tube should be inverted several times to ensure mixing and complete lysis of the cells. The tube is then centrifuged at 3,000 × *g* for 30 min. Approximately 1.6 ml of sediment is obtained, from which approximately 0.2-ml aliquots can be removed for inoculation onto appropriate culture media. An advantage of the use of the Isolator system is the capability of assessing semiquantitative blood cultures.

BACTEC vials can also be used in conjunction with Isolator tubes. In a study of 46 AIDS patients with positive blood cultures, Gill et al. (62) found a reduction of approximately 7 days in the mean detection time of mycobacteria recovered from the inocula from the Isolator when using BACTEC 12A (not available) vials versus conventional media (9.5 days versus 16.1 days, respectively). Detection times for MAI in the BACTEC 12A (not available) vials were as short as 4 to 6 days when more than 100 colonies were recovered on L-J slants, whereas up to 29 days was required in specimens with fewer than 10 colonies per slant. When the Isolator system is not used, Kiehn and Cammarata (102) advise that the blood obtained from Vacutainer tubes can be directly inoculated into a BACTEC 13A vial (current BACTEC product), with no difference in detection time in comparison with Isolator sediment-inoculated vials. Witebsky et al. (251) found the BACTEC 13A bottle to be a satisfactory alternative to the Isolator system, and they recommend its use.

Spark and Fried (207) reported that 98.8% of 343 isolates were detected with BACTEC within 5 weeks and advised that holding vials beyond 5 weeks was not cost

TABLE 3. Selective mycobacterial isolation media[a]

Medium	Components	Inhibitory agents
Gruft modification of Lowenstein-Jensen	Fresh whole eggs, defined salts, glycerol, potato flour, RNA (5 mg/100 ml)	Malachite green (0.025 g/100 ml), penicillin (50 U/ml), nalidixic acid (35 μg/ml)
Mycobactosel (BBL) Lowenstein-Jensen	Fresh whole eggs, defined salts, glycerol, potato flour	Malachite green (0.025 g/100 ml), cycloheximide (400 μg/ml), lincomycin (2 μg/ml), nalidixic acid (35 μg/ml)
Middlebrook 7H10	Defined salts, vitamins, cofactors, oleic acid, albumin, catalase, glycerol, glucose	Malachite green (0.0025 g/100 ml), cycloheximide (360 μg/ml), lincomycin (2 μg/ml), nalidixic acid (20 μg/ml)
Selective 7H11 (Mitchison medium)	Defined salts, vitamins, cofactors, oleic acid, albumin, catalase, glycerol, glucose, casein hydrolysate	Carbenicillin (50 μg/ml), amphotericin B (10 μg/ml), polymyxin B (200 U/ml), trimethoprim lactate (20 μg/ml)
Middlebrook 7H12	7H9 broth base, casein hydrolysate, bovine serum albumin, catalase, ^{14}C-labeled palmitic acid	Polymyxin B (50 U/ml), amphotericin B (5 μg/ml), nalidixic acid (20 μg/ml), trimethoprim (5 μg/ml), azlocillin (10 μg/ml)

[a] Modified from H. M. Sommers, Mycobacterial diseases, *in* J. B. Henry (ed.), *Clinical Diagnosis and Management by Laboratory Methods,* 16th ed., The W. B. Saunders Co., Philadephia, 1979.

effective; this finding needs further confirmation. Vannier et al. (231) cited three cases of false-positive BACTEC results from cross-contamination. Positive culture vials were positioned immediately after vials that were positive for *M. avium*. Investigation revealed a defective heating block used for needle sterilization. Obviously, rigid quality control procedures and constant vigil by microbiologists using any of these systems is necessary to avoid spurious results. The time for sterilization of needles on the BACTEC 460 has been extended to alleviate this problem and to prevent others.

Procedure for Decontamination of Urine

Urine specimens submitted for the recovery of mycobacteria can be processed without treatment by directly inoculating them onto appropriate culture media with portions of centrifuged sediment. However, it is recommended that cultures for bacteria be prepared to determine whether the specimen should be decontaminated, since many contain bacteria. To eliminate possible inhibitory factors, 10% calcium chloride solution can be added to 10 to 15 ml of urine until a precipitate is formed. The specimen is then transferred to 50-ml centrifuge tubes with a tightly fitting lid and centrifuged for 30 min at 2,500 × *g*. The supernatant is decanted, and portions of sediment are inoculated onto appropriate culture media.

Procedure for Decontamination of Fecal Material

The procedure reported by Kiehn et al. (104) is recommended. Acid-fast smears are made directly from unprocessed fecal material. If organisms are not seen, the specimen is not processed further. If acid-fast organisms are seen in the smear, a suspension of feces (1 g in 5 ml of Middlebrook 7H9 broth) is processed for culture by the NaOH sputum digestion method described previously. Contamination of media by intestinal bacteria rarely occurred in the experience of these workers, indicating that the decontamination procedure is adequate. The normal intestinal flora of the patients may be reduced because of their underlying disease and antibiotic therapy. Mycobacteria, primarily MAI, can be recovered from fecal specimens probably because large numbers of organisms are present.

Procedure for Handling Sterile Specimens

Some specimens may not need decontamination; these include aseptically obtained urine (for clean-catch specimens, the calcium chloride procedure described above should be used), surgical specimens, cerebrospinal, synovial, or other internal body fluids, and biopsies of deep visceral organs. Tissues are processed by cutting them into pieces with sterile scissors and reducing the pieces to pulp with mortar and pestle or with a tissue grinder. The addition of 10 parts of sterile water results in a soupy fluid that can be transferred to culture media with a pipette. It may be necessary to decontaminate autopsy tissue.

Tissues, bronchial washings, or needle aspiration material should be placed in Middlebrook 7H9 or 7H11 broth. Although collection of swab specimens should be discouraged, such specimens can be treated by placing the swabs in about 5.0 ml of Middlebrook 7H11 broth and extracting the inoculum on a Vortex mixer for about 30 s. After mixing, such specimens should be centrifuged at 2,500 × *g* for 15 min, and portions of the sediment should be transferred onto appropriate culture media, using a sterile pipette. Body fluids can be cultured by adding approximately 10 ml of specimen to approximately 100 ml of 7H11 broth and incubating the specimen at 37°C, preferably with gentle agitation for aeration. After 3 weeks of incubation, a small amount of fluid is removed from the flask and inoculated onto appropriate culture media. Direct transfer of 10 ml of fluid to a BACTEC 12B or 13A vial is an alternative.

For specimens that are difficult or impossible to duplicate, it is good practice to keep a sample in a freezer pending results on the first portion cultured. Whenever doubt concerning contamination of a specimen exists, a portion of the specimen may be inoculated without prior treatment into liquid medium (Dubos, Proskauer-Beck, or Middlebrook 7H9 medium) while the remainder is kept refrigerated. Inspect the liquid culture daily; if contamination develops, as shown by Gram and acid-fast stains, subject both this culture and a portion of the specimen to an appropriate decontamination procedure.

Concentration of Bacilli by Centrifugation

The concentration of mycobacteria by centrifugation is affected by the adequacy of prior homogenization to reduce the viscosity of the specimen, the relative specific gravity of the bacilli versus the suspending fluid, the RCF used, and the duration of centrifugation. Since the density of tubercle bacilli is only slightly greater than that of liquefied sputum, centrifugation should be at a high RCF and should be for as long as possible. In the previous edition of this manual, the work of Rickman and Moyer (181) was cited as showing a dramatic increase in the acid-fast smear–culture correlation as the RCF used for processing specimens increased from 1,260 to 3,800 × *g*. However, more recent experimental data reported by Ratnam and March (179) do not confirm this observation. In their studies (using a Beckman 7-6B refrigerated centrifuge fitted with a Beckman rotor model JS4.2 with a 24-place adapter), increasing the RCF from 2,074 to 3,895 × *g* did not result in an increase in fluorochrome smear positivity. Their findings support the observations of Lipsky et al. (133) that smear sensitivity is dependent on the type of patient population, the nature of the specimen and the number of organisms present, the species of mycobacteria present in the specimen, and the experience, alertness, and persistence of technologists in detecting small numbers of mycobacteria. Furthermore, Ratnam and March (179) found that the recovery rates of mycobacteria were not significantly lower with an RCF of 2,074 × *g* for 20 min (within the range of speed normally recommended) than with RCFs of 3,005 and 3,895 × *g* for 15 min.

If specimens are to be centrifuged at an RCF above 3,000 × *g*, care must be taken to ensure that the centrifuge tubes can withstand the centrifuge force and not collapse. Since centrifugation at high speeds may be associated with the generation of heat, there should be careful monitoring to ensure that no increase in temperature that could injure or decrease the viability of mycobacteria occurs in the clinical specimens. The decrease in time of exposure of mycobacteria to the

NALC-NaOH digestant at higher RCFs may still have an advantage over extended centrifugation times at lower RCFs. Refrigerated centrifuges are recommended when high RCFs are used. All centrifugation should be carried out in sealed safety cups (e.g., sealed dome shields, no. 1124; International Equipment Co., Div. Damon Corp., Needham Heights, Mass.).

Since acid-fast bacilli tend to be buoyant in centrifugation, some laboratories include inoculation onto culture media of a portion of the supernatant fluid as well as the sediment. Ratnam and March (179) report that as much as 30% of the mycobacteria were recovered from the supernatant after centrifugation at RCFs of 2,000 to 4,000 × *g*. They point out, however, that any advantage in culturing the supernatant in common practice may be negated by the dilution effect and the relatively small number of organisms in most clinical specimens. For some fluids, particularly cerebrospinal fluid, the use of a 0.45-μm filter may be an effective concentration procedure.

Culture Media for Recovery of Mycobacteria

Culture media for the recovery of mycobacteria should include both a primary, nonselective medium and a selective medium, the latter containing one or more antibiotics to prevent overgrowth by contaminating bacteria or fungi (Tables 2 and 3). Three general types of formulations may be used for both selective and nonselective media: BACTEC Middlebrook 7H12 liquid medium; an inspissated egg medium such as L-J, Petragnani, or American Thoracic Society (ATS) medium; and a semisynthetic agar medium (Middlebrook 7H10 and 7H11) containing defined salts, vitamins, cofactors, oleic acid and glucose (enrichment), catalase and biotin (stimulate revival of damaged bacilli), albumin (stimulates growth by binding toxic products), and glycerol. The most reliable and sensitive medium is Middlebrook 7H12 medium (Becton Dickinson Diagnostic Instruments Systems, Towson, Md.) prepared in 4-ml amounts of broth in vials. The sediment of the decontaminated specimen (0.5 ml) is added to the BACTEC 12B vial containing antibiotics supplied by the manufacturer and a ^{14}C-labeled substrate (palmitic acid). As the mycobacteria metabolize, $^{14}CO_2$ is liberated and is detected by the BACTEC 460 instrument. A growth index of ≥10 is considered significant; however, other bacteria (particularly gram-positive bacteria) commonly grow within the bottle, and it is necessary to perform an acid-fast smear from the culture vial and to subculture to recover the mycobacteria. Figure 1 presents a scheme for use of the BACTEC TB system. It is recommended that a biplate containing Middlebrook 7H10 and 7H11 selective agars (144) be used with the BACTEC TB system to ensure optimal recovery.

Recent studies have shown that the use of the radiometric (BACTEC) method has significantly improved the recovery rates and times of mycobacteria from respiratory secretions and other specimen sources (120). Roberts et al. (182), in a multicenter study of acid-fast smear-positive specimens, reported an average detection time of 8 days for *M. tuberculosis* with the BACTEC system versus 19.4 days for conventional media, and 5.2 days for mycobacteria other than *M. tuberculosis* by BACTEC versus 17.8 days for conventional media. Kirihara et al. (112) found essentially similar time reductions with the BACTEC system for smear-positive cases and for smear-negative cases of MAI; however, differences in the mean detection times of *M. tuberculosis* from smear-negative specimens were not as significant. Morgan et al. (153), using acid-fast smear-negative specimens, found that recovery times for *M. tuberculosis* were 13.7 and 26.3 days for the BACTEC system and conventional media, respectively. The BACTEC TB system has been proven to be the most rapid and sensitive detection system. It can identify members of the *M. tuberculosis* complex, but a subculture is necessary for identification of other species.

The BACTEC TB system may also be used for antimicrobial susceptibility testing of *M. tuberculosis* (182) as discussed in chapter 114.

The advantages of egg-based media are the long shelf life (1 year when refrigerated), which is ideal for laboratories that process only a few specimens, and the low cost for preparation. The disadvantages are the difficulty in discerning colonies from debris and the inability to achieve accurate and consistent drug concentrations for susceptibility testing because of binding of the antimicrobial agent. Egg media require heat for solidification, which, along with the presence of albumin, inactivates certain antituberculous drugs. In general, L-J medium recovers *M. tuberculosis* well but is not as reliable for the recovery of other species and is not used by many laboratories.

Conversely, agar-based media provide a ready means for detecting early growth of microscopic colonies that are easy to distinguish from inoculum debris (later in this chapter, the examination of microcolonies on clear agar is discussed further). Accurate drug concentrations may be achieved for susceptibility testing. However, the prepared plates are expensive to prepare (the oleic acid enrichment is a costly ingredient and often is difficult to obtain), and shelf life is relatively short (1 month in the refrigerator).

Some laboratories suggest that one egg-based medium, one agar medium, and one selective medium be used; the last is reserved for specimens in which contamination with other microorganisms is anticipated. Although the clear agar media permit earlier detection of mycobacteria, on prolonged incubation, L-J medium often yields a greater number of positive results (114). Of the egg-based media, L-J is most commonly used in clinical laboratories. This medium is commercially available from most reagent companies and has a standard formulation. Miomer and Olsson (150) have shown a 9.2% increase in isolation and early growth of mycobacteria other than *M. tuberculosis* with use of L-J medium containing isoniazid.

Petragnani medium, which contains about twice as much malachite green as does L-J medium, is more commonly used in public health laboratories than in clinical laboratories for the recovery of mycobacteria from heavily contaminated specimens. The increased concentration of malachite green can cause partial inhibition of some strains of mycobacteria. ATS medium, in contrast, contains a slightly smaller concentration of malachite green and thus is more easily overgrown by contaminants. ATS medium is best reserved for specimens that are only lightly contaminated or clean, such as cerebrospinal fluid and pleural fluid. Growth of mycobacteria will be less inhibited, resulting in the earlier growth of larger colonies.

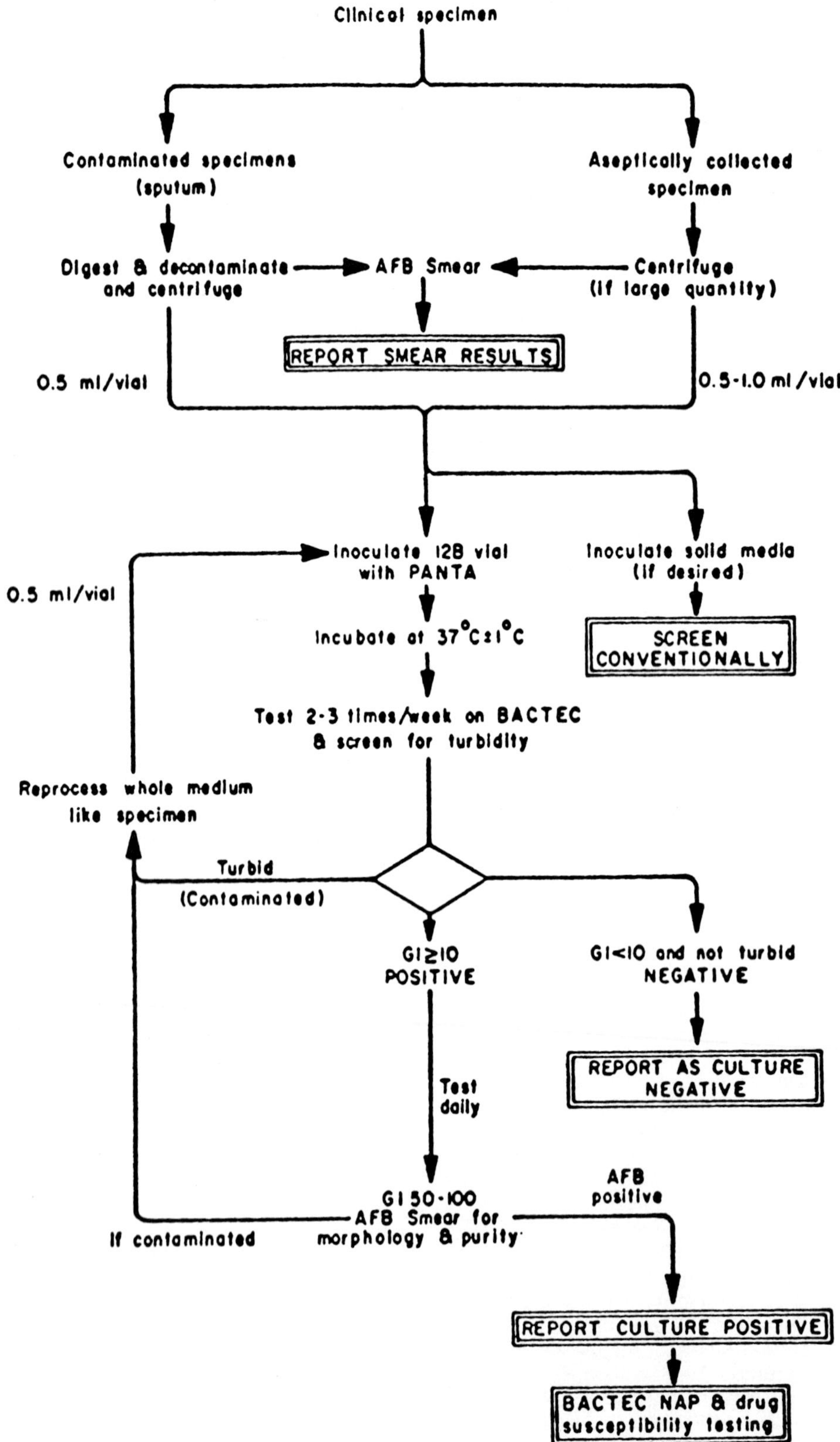

FIG. 1. Outline of the BACTEC primary isolation procedure. (From the 1986 BACTEC product and procedure manual; used with permission.)

Of the agar-based media, the Middlebrook 7H11 formula is preferred over 7H10. The addition of the 0.1% casein in the 7H11 formula (the only difference from 7H10) improves the recovery of isoniazid-resistant strains of *M. tuberculosis*. Additional supplements may be helpful for recovering mycobacteria in other situations. The addition of 0.2% pyruvic acid is recommended when *M. bovis* is suspected (44), and 0.25% L-asparagine or 0.1% potassium aspartate must be added to 7H10 agar for maximal production of niacin (108). Care should be exercised in the preparation, incubation, and storage of Middlebrook media because excessive heat or light exposure may result in the release of formaldehyde, which is toxic to mycobacteria (148).

Incubation and Reading of Cultures

An atmosphere of 5 to 10% CO_2 is stimulatory to the growth of all mycobacteria grown in tubes or culture dishes (12). However, it is necessary to incubate cultures under CO_2 only for the first 7 to 10 days after inoculation (the log phase of growth); subsequently, cultures can be removed to ambient air incubators if space is a problem. In the absence of a CO_2 incubator, CO_2-permeable bags with CO_2-generating tablets are commercially available.

Before inoculation, all BACTEC 12B vials should be tested on the BACTEC 460 instrument to eliminate bottles with high background counts and also to establish a carbon dioxide-enriched atmosphere within the vial. It should be mentioned that the BACTEC 13A blood culture vials should not be tested on the BACTEC 460 instrument before specimen inoculation. They normally have negative pressure within the vial so that 5 to 6 ml of blood is drawn into the system at the bedside. After inoculation, the bottle should be purged with carbon dioxide as previously described. Clinical specimens that contain cells, such as body fluids (including blood and tissues), often give false-positive results. Early after inoculation, the cells metabolize and utilize ^{14}C-labeled palmitic acid. If vials yield an elevated growth index shortly after the initial stage of incubation, it is prudent to examine these cultures at frequent intervals to determine whether metabolism is due to the cells themselves or to the mycobacteria. Most often, it is due to cellular metabolism.

BACTEC TB System

The reading schedule for BACTEC 12B vials varies according to the laboratory workload. Laboratories with a low volume may prefer to read cultures three times a week for the first 3 weeks of incubation and weekly thereafter for a total of 8 weeks. Laboratories with larger volumes may choose to read cultures twice a week for the first 2 weeks and then weekly thereafter for a total of 8 weeks. A growth index of ≥ 10 is considered positive. At this point, the vials should be removed and an acid-fast stain prepared to determine whether the culture contains mycobacteria. In addition, the vial should be subcultured onto a sheep blood agar plate to determine whether contamination is present. If bacterial growth is not evident after 24 h, the BACTEC vial should be read daily until a growth index of 50 is obtained so that additional tests and a subculture can be performed at that point.

Tube and Plate Cultures

Plates should be placed inverted in polyethylene, carbon dioxide-permeable bags and sealed. Tubes are placed in a horizontal position on a slant until the sediment has been absorbed; then they can be incubated in a vertical position with the caps ajar. Incubation is at 35 to 37°C in an atmosphere of 5 to 10% carbon dioxide for the first 3 weeks, followed by a tightening of the caps on the tubes and incubation of the tubes and plates at 35 to 37°C in an atmosphere of ambient air for an additional 5 weeks. All specimens with positive acid-fast smears but negative cultures at the end of 8 weeks are incubated for an additional 8 weeks. A duplicate set of media for cultures of skin lesions and environmental samples should be incubated at 30°C to enhance the recovery of *M. marinum* and *M. ulcerans*. Specimens from skin lesions should also be inoculated onto blood agar, chocolate agar, Middlebrook 7H10 agar with hemolyzed sheep erythrocytes, L-J medium containing 1% ferric ammonium citrate, or a plate of Middlebrook 7H10 medium containing an X-factor disk to enhance recovery of *M. haemophilum*, which requires hemin for growth. All cultures should be examined for presence of mycobacteria as well as fungi. Young cultures up to 4 weeks of age should be examined two times per week; older cultures should be examined at weekly intervals.

Acid-Fast Smear

Acid-fast smear examination has been routinely used in many clinical microbiology laboratories because of its simplicity, rapidity, and high specificity. The sensitivity of the acid-fast smear examination for the diagnosis of mycobacterial infection is lower than that of culture methods. The overall sensitivity has been reported to be from 22 to 43% (22, 27, 133, 142, 156, 212). The factors influencing sensitivity include types of specimen, concentrations of mycobacteria in specimens, and staining techniques (133, 223). Respiratory specimens yielded the highest smear positivity rate, followed by tissue specimens and cerebrospinal fluid (133). Other reports also supported the high yield of respiratory specimens (156, 171). Furthermore, if more than one respiratory tract specimen is submitted to the laboratory, 96% of patients with pulmonary tuberculosis may be detected by the acid-fast smear examination (133). It was also documented that the direct smear examination has less value detecting the presence of infection caused by mycobacteria other than *M. tuberculosis*.

Several reports have indicated that positivity is correlated with the number of colonies recovered on culture plates (133, 156, 171). If the number of colonies on culture plates were grouped into 1 to 10, 11 to 50, 51 to 100, and more than 100 colonies, the smear positivity rates were 13, 71, 78, and 92%, respectively.

The auramine-rhodamine stain is more sensitive than the carbol fuchsin stain (204). The carbol fuchsin stain failed to detect acid-fast bacilli in up to 18% of auramine-rhodamine stain-positive specimens. It has proven to be a very reliable and specific staining method (214).

The specificity of the direct smear examination is very high. False-positive results (specimens with positive acid-fast smears and negative culture results) ranging from 1 to 55% were reported (27, 53, 156, 171, 181). It

TABLE 4. Distinctive properties of cultivable mycobacteria encountered in clinical specimens[a]

Species	Growth rate at[b]:				Usual colony morphology[c]	Pigmentation[d]	Niacin	Susceptibility to T2H (5 μg/ml)	Nitrate reduction	Semiquantitative catalase (mm)
	45°C	37°C	31°C	24°C						
M. ulcerans	–	–	S	–	R	N	–	–	–	<45
M. tuberculosis	–	S	S	–	R	N (100)	+ (95)	–	+ (97)	<45 (89)
M. bovis	–	S		–	Rt	N (100)	– (4)	+	– (9)	<45 (69)
M. marinum		–/+	M	M	S/SR	P (100)	–/+ (21)	–	– (0)	<45 (98)
M. kansasii		S	S	S	SR/S	P (96)	– (4)	–	+ (99)	>45 (93)
M. simiae	–	S			S	P (90)	± (63)	–	– (28)	>45 (93)
M. asiaticum	–	S		S		P (86)	– (0)	–	– (5)	>45 (95)
M. scrofulaceum		S	S	S	S	S (97)	– (0)	–	– (5)	>45 (84)
M. szulgai		S	S	S	S or R	S/P (93)	– (0)	–	+ (100)	>45 (98)
M. gordonae		S		S	S	S (99)	– (0)	–	– (1)	>45 (90)
M. flavescens		M		M	S	S (100)[g]	– (0)	–	+ (92)	>45 (94)
M. xenopi	S	S			S[h]	S (21)	– (0)	–	– (7)	>45 (85)
M. avium-intracellulare complex	–/+	S		±	St/R	N (87)	– (0)	–	– (4)	<45 (98)
M. gastri		S		S	S/SR/R	N (100)	– (0)	–	– (0)	<45 (100)
M. malmoense		S	S	S	S	N (88)	– (0)	–	– (1)	<45 (99)
M. haemophilum	–	–	S[h]	S	R	N	–	–	–	<45
M. nonchromogenicum		S		S	SR	N	–	–	–	>45
M. terrae		S		S	SR	N (93)	– (1)	–	± (67)	>45 (93)
M. triviale		M		S	R	N (100)	– (0)	–	+ (89)	>45 (100)
M. fortuitum	–	R		R	Sf/Rf	N (100)	–/+	–	+ (100)	>45 (93)
M. chelonae	–	R		R	S/R	N (100)	–/+	–	– (1)	>45 (92)
M. phlei	R	R		R	R	S			+	>45
M. smegmatis	R	R		R	R/S	N			+	>45
M. vaccae		R		R	S	S			+	>45

[a] Modified from reference 157. Plus and minus signs indicate the presence and absence, respectively, of the feature; blank spaces indicate either that the information is not currently available or that the property is unimportant. V, Variable; ±, usually present; –/+, usually absent. Percentage of Centers for Disease Control-tested strains positive in each test (66) is given in parentheses, and test result is based on these percentages. MAIS group is scotochromogenic, Tween negative, nitrate negative, catalase = <45 mm, and urease positive (rarely); tellurite gives inconsistent results (78).

[b] S, Slow; M, moderate; R, rapid.

[c] R, Rough; S, smooth; SR, intermediate in roughness; t, thin or transparent; f, filamentous extensions.

[d] P, Photochromogenic; S, scotochromogenic; N, nonchromogenic. *M. szulgai* is scotochromogenic at 37°C and photochromogenic at 24°C.

[e] Urease test was performed by the method of Steadham (210).

[f] Arylsulfatase reaction at 14 days is positive.

[g] Young cultures may be nonchromogenic or possess only pale pigment that may intensify with age.

[h] Requires hemin as growth factor.

[i] *M. chelonae* subsp. *chelonae* is negative; *M. chelonae* subsp. *abscessus* is positive.

is worth noting that in one laboratory, if a strict protocol was applied, the elevated rate dropped from 55 to 1%. Excluding these two studies, the overall unexplained false-positivity rate was approximately 10 to 20%. Laboratory errors and patients on antimycobacterial drug therapy could explain part of the false-positive smears. Thirty percent of specimens from patients with pulmonary tuberculosis who received antimycobacterial drug therapy had a positive direct smear examination and a negative culture. This result is attributed to killing of mycobacterial cells by therapeutic agents; however, nonviable mycobacteria were present, as detected by the auramine-rhodamine stain. Conversely, the unexplained false-positivity rate dropped to 7.5% for patients not receiving treatment (171). Prolonged specimen decontamination and short incubation of cultures are also attributed to producing smear-positive and culture-negative results. Cross-contamination and the use of contaminated water during staining procedures are also responsible for true false-positive results (45, 156).

With use of strict procedures and experienced laboratory personnel, the direct smear examination is a very valuable diagnostic procedure for the detection of mycobacteria in clinical specimens. It is very helpful in developing countries that have a high prevalence of mycobacterial infections and where mycobacterial culture systems are not readily available (39).

Information regarding specific staining procedures and reporting is presented in chapter 122.

PROPERTIES USED FOR THE IDENTIFICATION OF MYCOBACTERIA

According to traditional methods, mycobacteria are usually identified by rate of growth, colonial morphology, pigmentation, and biochemical profiles. The identification should be based on as many observations as possible, and it is prudent to select only those biochemical tests which appear to be useful for the species suspected. Table 4 presents the characteristics of common species of mycobacteria recovered from clinical specimens. Many strains will have biochemical profiles and morphologic features compatible with the data in this table; however, it should be emphasized that variation occurs among strains and that properties may deviate from those presented in the table. In many instances, it is necessary to identify an organism based on a best-fit basis. With newer laboratory methods, such as GLC and nucleic acid probes, the reliance on bio-

TABLE 4—*Continued*

	68°C catalase	Tween hydrolysis	Tellurite reduction	Tolerance to 5% NaCl	Iron uptake	Arysulfatase, 3 days	MacConkey agar	Urease[e]	Pyrazinamidase, 4 days	Nucleic acid probes available
M. ulcerans	+	–		–	–	–		V	–	
M. tuberculosis	– (1)	± (68)	–/+ (36)	– (0)	–	– (0)	–	± (64)	+	+
M. bovis	– (2)	– (21)		– (0)	–	– (0)	–	± (50)	–	+
M. marinum	– (30)	+ (97)	–/+ (39)	– (0)	–	–/+ (41)[f]	–	+ (83)	+	–
M. kansasii	+ (91)	+ (99)	–/+ (31)	– (0)	–	– (0)	–	–/+ (49)	–	–
M. simiae	+ (95)	– (9)	+ (82)	– (0)	–	– (0)		± (69)	+	–
M. asiaticum	+ (95)	+ (95)	– (20)	– (0)	–	– (0)		– (10)	–	–
M. scrofulaceum	+ (94)	– (2)	± (64)	– (0)	–	V (0)	–	V (31)	±	–
M. szulgai	+ (93)	–/+ (49)	± (53)	– (0)	–	V (0)	–	+ (72)	+	–
M. gordonae	+ (96)	+ (100)	– (29)	– (0)	–	V (0)	–	V (31)	–/+	+
M. flavescens	+ (100)	+ (100)	–/+ (44)	± (62)	–	– (0)	–	+ (72)	+	
M. xenopi	± (31)	– (12)	± (65)	– (0)	–	± (36)	–	– (0)	V	–
M. avium-intracellulare complex	± (60)	– (2)	+ (81)	– (0)	–	– (1)	–/+	– (2)	+	+
M. gastri	– (11)	+ (100)	± (50)	– (0)	–	– (0)	–	–/+ (44)	–	–
M. malmoense	± (66)	+ (99)	+ (74)	– (0)	–	– (0)		– (9)	+	–
M. haemophilum	–	–	–	–	–	–	–	–	+	–
M. nonchromogenicum	+	+	–	–	–	–	V	–	V	–
M. terrae	+ (92)	+ (99)	–/+ (46)	– (2)	–	– (2)	V	– (13)	V	–
M. triviale	+ (100)	+ (100)	– (25)	+ (100)	–	± (56)	–	–/+ (33)	V	–
M. fortuitum	+ (90)	–/+ (43)	+ (92)	+ (85)	+	+ (97)	+	+ (70)	+	–
M. chelonae	± (53)	–/+ (39)	+ (89)	V[i]	–	+ (95)	+	+ (89)	+	–
M. phlei	+	+	+	+	+	–	–			
M. smegmatis	+	+	+	+	+	–	–			
M. vaccae	+	+	+	V	+	–	–			

chemical profiles and the above-mentioned characteristics appears to be of less importance than in the past. A complete description of each species is presented in the following sections.

Microscopy is the first observation needed for species identification. The examination of a smear made from the clinical specimen or its concentrate is as important as the observation of the stained preparation of the colonies of organisms recovered from the clinical specimen. This observation is to confirm that the growth is of mycobacterial origin and to determine whether the culture is contaminated with aerobic bacteria. Although certain morphologic features of mycobacteria have been associated with certain species, the microscopic morphologic features should not be the basis for the final species identification.

Growth Characteristics

With the BACTEC TB system, it is difficult to determine the growth rate of mycobacteria present in a clinical specimen. This determination is based somewhat on the number of organisms present as well as on the growth rate of the individual organism. The elevated growth index really gives no suggestion as to the identity of the organism present in the BACTEC vial. For example, a large number of cells of *M. tuberculosis* may produce an elevated growth index within 2 to 3 days, whereas very few cells of a rapidly growing species such as *M. fortuitum* may take substantially longer before the growth index becomes elevated beyond 10.

By using conventional culture methods, evidence of rapidly growing mycobacteria may be commonly seen at the first weekly inspection of the cultures, although some strains exhibit their characteristic growth rates only upon subculture. Isolates of *M. fortuitum* or *M. chelonae* are classified as rapidly growing mycobacteria but may require more than 5 days for growth to appear. Growth temperature relationships observed by using traditional culture media may provide useful information for cultures and their identification. The following relationships may be important: (i) if growth appears in <1 to 1 week at 24 or 35 to 37°C and appears also at 42°C, the strain will usually be other than *M. fortuitum* or *M. chelonae;* (ii) if growth is slow, requiring 2 or more weeks, and occurs at 35 to 37°C but not at 24 or 42°C, *M. tuberculosis* and *M. bovis* are suspected; (iii) if growth occurs at 35 to 37 and 42°C but not at 24°C, *M. xenopi* and some MAI strains are suspected; (iv) if growth appears at 35 to 37°C, is slower at 24°C, and is negative at 42°C, *M. kansasii* is suspected; (v) if growth appears at 32 and 24°C in 2 weeks and no growth occurs or is slower at 35 to 37°C, *M. marinum* is suspected; (vi) if growth occurs at 32°C in 2 to 4 weeks, occurs in double that time at 25 or 35°C, and does not occur at 37°C, *M. haemophilum* is suspected; and (vii) if growth occurs at 32°C in greater than 3 weeks but not at 24 or 35 to 37°C, *M. ulcerans* is suspected.

The growth relationships are important in identification of *M. marinum, M. ulcerans, M. haemophilum,* and *M. xenopi.* Since *M. szulgai* is both photochromogenic and scotochromogenic, it is necessary to incubate cultures at 25 and 35 to 37°C. The growth of *M. szulgai* will be considerably slower at 25°C.

Colonial Morphologic Features

Some microbiologists feel that a tentative identification of the species of mycobacteria can be made by microscopically observing young colonies, using a stereomicroscope and a 10× objective with transmitted light, according to the scheme developed by Runyon (190). This is best accomplished on a medium like Middlebrook 7H10 or 7H11 agar so that colonies are easily visualized. Specific colonial morphologic features will be described in the sections describing the individual species. Colonial morphologic features often provide a tentative identification and suggest which biochemical tests or nucleic acid probes to use for the final identification.

Pigment Production and Response to Light

Mycobacteria which have colonies that are definitely pigmented contain principally carotenoid pigments that range from yellow to red. Scotochromogenic strains form pigment in the presence or absence of light; commonly, more pigment is produced if growth occurs in a lighted incubator. Photochromogenic strains are stimulated to produce pigment by light exposure and ordinarily do not show yellow pigmentation unless exposed to light during the early phase of growth of cultures with good aeration of their surface (241). *M. kansasii* becomes definitely yellow 6 to 12 h after 1 h of exposure to bright light. *M. szulgai* is unique and is scotochromogenic when grown at 37°C but photochromogenic if grown at 25°C. During routine examination of cultures, if the first colonies appear to be nonpigmented, they should be left close to a bright incandescent or fluorescent light in the laboratory for 1 h or more. During this period, smears may be made and examined, and the cultures are returned to the incubator. Colonies should be examined the next morning for yellow pigmentation; often color changes are pale, and they can be questionable. When pigmentation due to light exposure is suspected, tubes of L-J or of Middlebrook 7H10 or 7H11 medium should be inoculated in duplicate; one tube should be covered with dark paper or with aluminum foil, and the other should be left exposed to any ambient light in the room. Cultures are incubated with the caps loosely ajar in an atmosphere of 5 to 10% carbon dioxide. As sufficient growth appears, the uncovered tube is exposed to light for 30 to 60 min. The uncovered tube is reincubated for an additional 24 h and is observed for yellow pigmentation of colonies. The covered tube is unwrapped and examined for the presence of pigmentation. If the culture exposed to light becomes pigmented compared with buff-colored colonies (in the uncovered tube), the organism is considered photochromogenic. If both tubes show pigmentation, the organism is considered scotochromogenic. If both tubes remain nonpigmented, the organism is considered nonchromogenic. Characteristic pigmentation profiles for these species are given in Table 4.

IDENTIFICATION OF CLINICALLY IMPORTANT SPECIES OF MYCOBACTERIA

As is well known, the detection and identification of mycobacteria in clinical specimens often requires several days to several weeks before results are available to clinicians. The trend during the last several years has been to develop methods that would make clinically useful information available sooner within a clinically relevant period of time, in contrast to the conventional identification methods used today. The most current and most promising innovation for the identification of mycobacteria is the use of the nucleic acid probe technology.

Isotopic Nucleic Acid Probes

In 1987, nucleic acid probes for the identification of *M. tuberculosis* complex (*M. tuberculosis, M. bovis, M. africanum*, and *M. microti*), *M. avium*, and *M. intracellulare* became available from Gen Probe, Inc., San Diego, Calif. The rapid diagnostic system kits utilized nucleic acid hybridization assays based on the ability of complementary nucleic acids strands to bond and form stable, double-stranded complexes under appropriate test conditions. An ^{125}I-labeled single-stranded DNA probe complementary to the rRNA of the target organisms was used. The rRNA was released from the test organism through the action of a lysing reagent, heat, and sonication. The ^{125}I-labeled DNA probe then hybridized with the rRNA of the target organism to form a stable DNA-RNA hybrid. A separation suspension separated the labeled complex from the unhybridized DNA. The radioactive labeled DNA-RNA hybrids were counted, and test results were calculated as a percentage of input probe hybridized. The early studies by Drake et al. (48), Gonzalez and Hanna (65), Kiehn and Edwards (103), and Musial et al. (158) demonstrated clearly that the nucleic acid probes used for the identification of *M. avium, M. intracellulare*, and *M. tuberculosis* complex were highly sensitive and specific. Furthermore, they could be used in a clinical microbiology laboratory with ease.

Kiehn and Edwards (103) demonstrated that *M. avium* could be identified directly from BACTEC 12B vials. This was accomplished by centrifuging 3 ml of the BACTEC 12B broth at 3,000 × *g* for 10 min if the growth index was ≥999. Ellner et al. (51) showed that the BACTEC TB system could be combined with the nucleic acid probe technology to provide for rapid identification of the mycobacteria. This was accomplished by using BACTEC 12B vials that had a growth index of ≥80. Two milliliters of the medium was removed and centrifuged at 2,000 × *g* for 10 min. The sediment was adjusted with sterile water to a turbidity of a McFarland no. 1 standard, and the sediment was tested by nucleic acid hybridization methods provided by the manufacturer.

Recently, Conville et al. (36) used nucleic acid probes for identifying mycobacteria in BACTEC 13A bottles that contained predominately MAI. The study was primarily based on seeded cultures containing *M. avium* and a few patient samples that contained the same organism. A growth index threshold of 86 was found necessary when the samples were concentrated directly and then tested with a probe. Further, a threshold growth index of 42 was established in instances when the concentration technique and a lysing and wash reagent were used as instructed by the manufacturer. Their study found that direct testing of concentrates from the BACTEC 13A bottles using the Gen Probe rapid diagnostic system for *M. avium* complex proved to be a rapid, sensitive, and specific procedure as long as the previous thresholds for the growth index were followed. Peterson et al. (166) also used nucleic acid probes to identify isolates of *M. tuberculosis* complex, *M. avium*, and *M. intracellulare*. When BACTEC 12B vials had a growth index of ≥100, 1 ml of Middlebrook 7H12 broth was placed in each of three microfuge tubes, which were centrifuged at 15,000 × *g* for 15 min, followed by testing with each of the previously mentioned probes. Results with the three probes used for the same sample were compared, and the highest percent hybridization was divided by the average of the two lower hybridization values. If the value was ≥3, the results were interpreted to be positive for the probe yielding the highest percent hybridization. Their study identified 83% of 64 isolates of *M. tuberculosis* complex, 92% of 61 isolates of *M. avium* isolates, and 86% of 14 isolates of *M. intracellulare*. Their recommendation was that conventional cultures should still be performed in parallel even when the BACTEC TB system is combined with the use of nucleic acid probes. On the basis of the limited number of studies available in the literature, it appeared that the Gen Probe rapid diagnostic system for mycobacteria could be used in combination with the BACTEC TB detection system. This procedure would allow a laboratory to detect and identify mycobacteria present in clinical samples within a relatively short period of time.

The major problems associated with the use of the isotopic nucleic acid probes included the inconvenience of handling radioactive materials, the instability of the reagents (stable for 1 month), and the cost of the nucleic acid probes. In general, the use of radioactive nucleic acid probes required special handling procedures and disposal methods for radioactive waste. Rapid decay of ^{125}I provided for only a short shelf life compared with most other reagents used in the laboratory. The nucleic acid probes available from Gen Probe included those for *M. tuberculosis* complex, *M. avium*, *M. intracellulare*, and *M. gordonae*. The use of nucleic acid probes was expensive, and in many laboratories the entire battery of probes was used. When the probes were used in this fashion, the cost was somewhat prohibitive to smaller laboratories. However, the use of nucleic acid probes for the identification of clinically important mycobacteria was still available to all laboratories. Their use in individual laboratories depended on the volume, incidence of mycobacterial infections, and type of clinical specimens received.

Nonisotopic Nucleic Acid Probes

Recently, nonisotopic nucleic acid probes for *M. tuberculosis* complex, *M. avium*, *M. intracellulare*, *M. avium* complex, and *M. gordonae* have become available and have replaced the isotopic probes. These probes use an acridinium ester-labeled single-stranded DNA probe complementary to the rRNA of the target organism. After rRNA is released from the organism, the labeled nucleic acid probe combines with the rRNA of the target organism to form a stable DNA-RNA hybrid. A differential hydrolysis reagent allows for the differentiation of nonhybridized and hybridized probe. The acridinium ester label associated with the hybrids is detected by using a luminometer.

The homogeneous, nonisotopic nucleic acid probe format uses a hybridization protection assay (6). In brief, the chemiluminescent acridinium ester is attached to the nucleic acid probe in such a manner that when hybrids are formed, the acridinium ester is oriented within the DNA-RNA hybrid so that it is protected from the hydrolysis process that is used to make the unbound acridinium nonchemiluminescent. Only the acridinium that is bound to the probe is detected by the chemiluminescence assay by using a luminometer. A summary of the procedure using a nonisotopic method is as follows:

1. A 100-μl sample of a specimen diluent and 100 μl of a probe diluent are added to a dry lysing tube (containing glass beads).
2. A portion of a colony of an unknown organism is transferred to the reconstituted lysing tube, which is sonicated in a water bath at room temperature for 15 min to lyse the organism.
3. The tube is removed, and the organism is killed by heat inactivation for 15 min at 95 ± 5°C.
4. A 100-μl amount of the lysate (lysed cells) is transferred to a lyophilized probe tube, which is incubated for 15 min at 60°C.
5. A 300-μl amount of the hydrolysis reagent (tetraborate buffer containing Triton X-100) is added to the tube, which is incubated for 5 min at 60°C.
6. The acridinium ester label associated with a hybrid is measured by using a luminometer that injects hydrogen peroxide and sodium hydroxide to elicit chemiluminescence. Results are expressed in relative light units and are based on a cutoff value of 50,000 relative light units.

At the time of this writing, a premarket evaluation of the nonisotopic nucleic acid probes shows that they are highly specific and sensitive for the identification of *M. tuberculosis* complex, *M. avium*, *M. intracellulare*, *M. avium* complex, and *M. gordonae* in culture. Preliminary data indicate they are also very useful for the identification of mycobacteria from BACTEC 12B vials, even when the growth index is at a low level. The nonisotopic nucleic acid probes have an extended shelf life of at least 6 months and are somewhat less costly than the isotopic probes already available; however, a price is currently unavailable. It is our opinion that nucleic acid probes will, and should be, used by clinical microbiology laboratories for the identification of most common clinically important mycobacteria. However, isolates for which probes are not available will require confirmation by conventional biochemical tests or GLC. Nucleic acid probes for the direct detection of mycobacteria in clinical specimens are on the horizon. In the future, perhaps only those specimens containing mycobacteria as detected by a genus probe will be cultured or tested further by nucleic acid probes. A combination of nucleic acid amplification in clinical specimens followed by detection using probes offers great promise.

GLC Analysis of Cell Wall Lipids

The chromatographic analysis of mycobacterial cell wall lipids has been of interest for several years. Methods used over the years include high-performance liquid chromatography (28), thin-layer chromatography (24), and GLC (93, 218, 219).

Tisdall et al. (218, 219) developed a method for the saponification of mycobacteria using methanol and sodium hydroxide, treatment with BF_3 in methanol, and extraction with a chloroform-hexane mixture. The hydrolysis products were analyzed by GLC. A decision tree (identification schema) was developed on the basis of the fatty acid profile for each species of mycobacteria. A high percentage of common mycobacterial species could be identified to the species level or could be separated into a group of two or three species which could be further separated by morphologic features or a minimal number of biochemical tests. As little as a 1-mm loopful of organism was used, and the total time for hydrolysis and analysis was less than 2 h. This system has been used in the Mayo Clinic mycobacteriology laboratory since 1982 and has been highly specific and reproducible.

A modification of the previously mentioned system is currently available from a commercial source (Microbial ID, Inc., Newark, Del.) as the Microbial Identification System. It consists of a gas chromatograph (HP 5890A; Hewlett-Packard Co., Palo Alto, Calif.) and a computer (HP series 310, HP 98561A). The latter utilizes software that contains a library of cell wall lipids for the species of clinically important mycobacteria. The library is composed of a collection of well-characterized species, including the American Type Culture Collection type culture and numerous clinical isolates (26 species). Profiles of unknown mycobacteria are compared with those contained within the library, and the unknown species are named. This method has been in routine use in the Mayo Clinic mycobacteriology laboratory and is considered rapid (<2 h) and highly reliable for the identification of mycobacteria in culture.

Another approach to the diagnosis of mycobacterial infections is detection of tuberculostearic acid in clinical specimens by selected-ion monitoring, using mass spectrometry (124). The system is not yet available for routine use in the clinical laboratory.

BIOCHEMICAL TESTS

Biochemical Test Used with the BACTEC TB System

p-Nitro-α-acetylamino-β-hydroxypropiophenone) (NAP) (125, 152, 209) is an intermediate compound in the synthesis of chloramphenicol and inhibits species of mycobacteria in the *M. tuberculosis* complex. Other species are not inhibited in the presence of this compound. With use of the BACTEC TB system, if mycobacteria are inhibited, they are unable to metabolize in the presence of NAP and are unable to produce $^{14}CO_2$.

Inoculum. After a BACTEC 12B vial becomes positive with a growth index of ≥10, it should be incubated at 37°C and read daily until the growth index reaches 50 to 100. When the vial has a growth index > 50, a portion is removed and added to a new 4-ml 12B vial (without antibiotics) as follows:

Growth index	Amt (ml) removed and added to 12B vial
50–100	No dilution made
101–200	0.8
201–400	0.6
401–600	0.4
601–800	0.3
801–999	0.2

Reagents. The NAP test vial contains a paper disk impregnated with 5 mg of NAP.

Procedure. If the growth index is 50 to 100, 1 ml of the medium in a 12B vial is added to the NAP vial. If the growth index is >100, a portion is added to an NAP vial. Both vials are read immediately after inoculation and are read daily for 2 to 5 days. The remaining medium in the original vial is used as the growth control.

The growth index of the control vial will increase as the culture metabolizes. However, the growth index of culture in the NAP vial will also increase if the organism is not a member of the *M. tuberculosis* complex. Mycobacteria other than *M. tuberculosis* may show a daily growth index increasing to >400 within 4 days or no increase or a slight decrease during the first 1 to 2 days after inoculation and then two consecutive daily increases after the second day. Members of the *M. tuberculosis* complex may show two consecutive decreases in growth index after inoculation or a slight but not significant increase during the first 1 to 2 days and then no increase or a decrease in the growth index. A significant increase or decrease implies a ≥20% change from one day to the next. The average time for completion of the test is 5 days. In some instances, *M. kansasii* may show a growth index of 5 to 10 after 5 days of testing, and the vials should be read for an additional 2 days.

Controls. Isolates of *M. tuberculosis* and MAI should be used as positive and negative controls, respectively.

Conventional Biochemical Tests

Traditionally, mycobacteria have been definitively identified by using biochemical tests, including niacin accumulation, nitrate reduction, Tween 80 hydrolysis, iron uptake, inhibition of growth by thiophene-2-carboxylic acid hydrazide (T2H), ability to grow on MacConkey agar, and production of the enzymes catalase, arylsulfatase, pyrazinamidase, and urease. Tables and schema for definitive identification of clinically important mycobacteria can be found in numerous textbooks of microbiology. Table 4 presents characteristic biochemical profiles for the most commonly encountered species.

Arylsulfatase

The 3-day arylsulfatase test (239) is used mainly to differentiate clinically significant rapid growers. With few exceptions, only *M. fortuitum* and *M. chelonae* split phenolphthalein from tripotassium phenolphthalein sulfate within 3 days. The 14-day test may be useful in the identification of slowly growing mycobacteria such as *M. marinum, M. szulgai, M. xenopi, M. triviale,* and *M. flavescens.* Two procedures for the determination of arylsulfatase production are available: (i) Wayne Arylsulfatase Agar (BBL) and (ii) the 3- and 14-day broth tests of Kubica and Rigdon (119). For most purposes, the 3-day test described below is adequate and easier to perform.

Inoculum. Prepare a slightly turbid suspension.

Reagents. (i) Substrate. Incorporate 1 ml of glycerol and 65 mg of tripotassium phenolphthalein disulfate (Nutritional Biochemicals Corp., Cleveland, Ohio) into 100 ml of melted Dubos oleic agar base (Wayne Arylsulfatase Agar). Dispense the mixture in 2-ml amounts into screw-cap vials (18 by 60 mm). Autoclave the vials. Permit the mixture to harden in an upright position. (ii) Na_2CO_3, 1 M (10.6 g in water to make 100 ml).

Procedure. Inoculate the medium with 1 drop of the bacillary suspension. Incubate the medium at 37°C for

3 days. Add 1 ml of Na_2CO_3 solution and observe the medium for pinkness, indicating free phenolphthalein and a positive test.

Controls. Use cultures of *M. fortuitum* and *M. avium* complex as positive and negative controls, respectively.

Catalase drop method

Essentially all mycobacteria are catalase positive. The only exceptions are some isoniazid-resistant mutants of *M. tuberculosis* and *M. gastri* and some nonpathogenic, isoniazid-resistant strains of *M. kansasii.* The catalase drop test is very useful for the quick and easy determination of significant isoniazid resistance of *M. tuberculosis,* which ordinarily reflects prior contact with this drug.

Cultures. Any mycobacterial culture may be tested, but the test is usually limited to those cultures suspected or known to be *M. tuberculosis.* Only colonies on media without drugs are tested.

Reagents. Use a 1:1 mixture of 10% Tween 80 and 30% hydrogen peroxide (Superoxol; Merck & Co., Inc., Rahway, N.J.). Prepare a fresh mixture for use each day.

Procedure. Add a drop of the reagent to growth on a slant or plate. Observe for the formation of bubbles (O_2) around the colonies. Note that some colonies may be positive and others negative.

Catalase after heating to 68°C

The test for catalase after heating the cells to 68°C (118) is valuable in conjunction with the niacin test for the recognition of tubercle bacilli. A positive test definitely indicates a species other than *M. bovis, M. tuberculosis, M. gastri,* or *M. haemophilum,* which are always negative. Strains of other species (Table 4) may be negative for this test.

Cultures. Well-developed, isolated colonies, preferably from egg-based culture medium, e.g., L-J, are tested.

Reagents. (i) A 1:1 mixture of 10% Tween 80 and 30% hydrogen peroxide (freshly prepared). (ii) Phosphate buffer, 0.067 M, pH 6; 1.1 ml of 0.067 M Na_2HPO_4 (9.47 g/liter); 38.9 ml of 0.067 M KH_2PO_4 (9.07 g/liter).

Procedure. Suspend several colonies in 0.5 ml of phosphate buffer (0.067 M), pH 7, in a screw-cap tube (16 by 125 mm). Place the tube in a water bath at 68°C for 20 min. Cool the suspension to room temperature and add 0.5 ml of the Tween-peroxide mixture. Observe the mixture for bubbling and record the result as positive or negative. Hold the tubes for 20 min before discarding them as negative.

Controls. Use cultures of *M. kansasii* and *M. tuberculosis* as positive and negative controls, respectively.

Semiquantitative catalase test

The semiquantitative test for catalase has proved valuable in the separation of some species of mycobacteria. Two subgroups of *M. kansasii* have been recognized; one produces <45 mm of bubbles, whereas those strains more commonly associated with disease produce >45 mm of bubbles. *M. tuberculosis, M. bovis, M. marinum,* the *M. avium* complex, *M. gastri, M. malmoense, M. xenopi,* and *M. haemophilum* produce a column of bubbles < 45 mm high, but other species usually produce a higher column.

Inoculum. Use a 7-day broth culture or a cell suspension of comparable turbidity.

Reagent and medium. (i) Freshly prepared 1:1 mixture of 10% Tween 80 and 30% hydrogen peroxide. (ii) L-J deep tubes (available commercially). Dispense 5 ml of L-J medium into screw-cap tubes (20 by 150 mm). Inspissate the medium with tubes in an upright position in a water bath at 85°C for 60 min. Do not substitute agar medium. Remove the tubes and incubate them at 35 to 37°C overnight to check for sterility.

Procedure. Inoculate an L-J medium deep tube with 0.2 ml of the bacterial suspension. Incubate the medium for 2 weeks at 35°C with the cap loosened. Add 1 ml of the Tween-peroxide mixture to the L-J culture and measure the column of bubbles in millimeters after the tube has stood for 5 min in an upright position at room temperature. Note the two categories: those that produce more and those that produce less than 45 mm of bubbles.

Controls. Use *M. tuberculosis* (which produces a column <45 mm high) and *M. kansasii* (which produces a column >45 mm high) as positive controls; use uninoculated medium as a negative control.

Inhibition tests for identification

Casal and Rodriguez (30) and Wallace et al. (235) have proposed disk susceptibility tests with pipemidic acid and polymyxin (Table 5), respectively, for the differentiation of *M. fortuitum* and *M. chelonae.* The value of the pipemidic acid test has been confirmed by Lévy-Frébault et al. (129).

Procedure. For pipemidic acid susceptibility tests, suspend the cells from a 7-day culture on Middlebrook 7H10 medium in saline or water to a turbidity equivalent to a McFarland no. 1 standard. Dilute the suspension 1:1,000 and evenly inoculate plates of Mueller-Hinton agar. Place a disk containing 20 μg of pipemidic acid on the plate and incubate the culture. Examine the plates after 2 and 5 days and measure the zone of inhibition. A zone of ≥10 mm is interpreted as inhibition. Strains of *M. chelonae* are resistant to pipemidic acid, whereas strains of *M. fortuitum* are susceptible.

For polymyxin susceptibility tests, dilute growth in Middlebrook 7H9 liquid medium to one-half the turbidity of the McFarland no. 1 standard. Swab the suspension onto a Mueller-Hinton agar plate that has been poured to a depth of 4 mm and previously swabbed on the surface with 10% Middlebrook OADC (oleic acid, albumin, dextrose, catalase; added to Middlebrook 7H10 and 7H11 agar after autoclaving). Place a disk containing 300 U of polymyxin on the surface of the agar and incubate the culture at 35°C for 72 h. Measure the zones of frank inhibition around the disks, but ignore a fine haze of growth that may appear. Strains of *M. fortuitum* are inhibited with zones of ≥9 mm, whereas strains of *M. chelonae* are completely resistant to the drug.

Iron uptake

In the iron uptake test (242), only rapid growers, such as *M. fortuitum* and *M. phlei,* are positive. *M. chelonae* does not take up iron except for the unnamed subspecies (see below and Table 4) detected by the alternate procedure.

Cultures. Inoculate L-J slants with 1 drop of barely turbid aqueous suspension of the strain to be tested.

TABLE 5. Distinctive characteristics of the *M. fortuitum-chelonae* complex

Species	Biovariant or subspecies	Tolerance to 5% NaCl (28°C)	Color after iron uptake		Utilization of:			Inhibition by:	
			Rust	Tan	Sodium citrate	Mannitol	Inositol	Pipemidic acid	Polymyxin B
M. fortuitum	Biovar *fortuitum*	+	+		−	−	−	+	+
	Biovar *peregrinum*	+	+		−	+	−	+	+
	Unnamed biovariant	+	+		−	+	+		
M. chelonae	Subsp. *chelonae*	−	−	−	+	−	−	−	−
	Subsp. *abscessus*	+	−	−	−	−	−	−	−
	Unnamed subspecies	−	−	+[a]	+	+	−		

[a] See the text for explanation.

Reagent. Use aqueous ferric ammonium citrate, 20%. Dispense the reagent into small containers. Autoclave the containers.

Procedure. Incubate the L-J slants at 37°C until definite growth appears. Add about 1 drop of the sterile citrate solution for each 1 ml of L-J medium. Incubate the culture at 35 to 37°C for a maximum of 21 days. Record the appearance of a rusty brown color in the colonies and a tan discoloration of the medium as positive.

Controls. Use *M. fortuitum* as a positive control and *M. chelonae* as a negative control.

Alternate procedure. See reference 199 also.

Prepare L-J medium and add 2.5% (wt/vol) ferric ammonium citrate. Inspissate the medium in a slanted position. Inoculate the medium with 1 drop of a barely turbid suspension of the culture to be tested; incubate the culture for 10 to 24 days at 28°C in a slanted position with the caps loosened. Colonies appear rusty brown if iron is taken up (a positive reaction). When a colony is tan and a rusty brown color appears around the edge of the slant, record the reaction as ±. Record a negative reaction if growth appears the same as in medium without added ferric ammonium citrate. Only the unnamed subspecies of *M. chelonae* has been found to give the ± reaction.

MacConkey agar growth test

Growth on MacConkey agar without crystal violet is used to distinguish the species of the *M. fortuitum-chelonae* complex from other species (96). Only species of this complex grow within 5 days.

Inoculum. Use Tween-albumin broth or 7H9 broth cultures 7 to 10 days old.

Medium. Prepare medium from dehydrated MacConkey agar without crystal violet (Difco Laboratories, Detroit, Mich.) base; pour about 15 ml into each plate. This medium is not commonly used for gram-negative bacteria. Since crystal violet inhibits mycobacteria, check to ensure that no crystal violet is present.

Procedure. Inoculate a plate of MacConkey agar without crystal violet with a 3-mm loopful of the broth culture, streaking to obtain isolated colonies (a spiral inoculation from the center outward is best). Examine for growth after 5 and 11 days. Only strains of the *M. fortuitum-chelonae* complex (Table 2) grow to the end of the streak. Other mycobacteria may show some growth where the inoculum is very heavy.

Controls. Use *M. fortuitum* as a positive control and *M. phlei* as a negative control.

Niacin test

The ability of *M. tuberculosis* to produce abundant niacin has been widely demonstrated. Niacin is secreted from bacilli into the medium; if the medium is not liquid, an aqueous extract of the medium around the colonies is tested. If the test is negative but other properties indicate *M. tuberculosis* (such as nitrate strongly reduced and catalase destroyed after heating at 68°C), the niacin test should be repeated. Cultures less than 3 weeks old or containing only small numbers of colonies may not yet have produced enough niacin to be detected, so they should be tested for up to 6 weeks. Niacin-negative *M. tuberculosis* strains are exceedingly rare. Positive niacin tests with strains of other *Mycobacterium* species are also rare except for *M. simiae* and some BCG (bacillus Calmette-Guérin) strains of *M. bovis*. Most of these strains may be immediately recognized as other than tubercle bacilli by rapid growth, pigmentation, or the clinical history. *M. simiae* cultures may produce niacin slowly and become positive after prolonged incubation. In a clinical laboratory, there is little advantage in doing niacin tests on strains that are scotochromogenic or rapidly growing. Photochromogenic isolates should be studied to exclude or establish *M. simiae*. The possibility of individual strains or nonpigmented slow growers other than *M. tuberculosis* being niacin positive must not be ignored.

Some laboratory workers avoid doing niacin tests because of the toxicity of one of the reagents, cyanogen bromide (CNBr; tear gas). Its easily recognized odor is a warning. The less obvious danger of pipetting tubercle bacilli is probably greater. Both dangers are well controlled by the use of a biological safety cabinet vented to the outside. A paper strip method for niacin determination has the advantages of simplicity and of reduced exposure to tear gas (no handling of CNBr). The paper strip method is fully dependable (105, 263).

Cultures. Luxuriant growth will occur on egg medium or on Middlebrook 7H10 or 7H11 medium enriched with 0.25% L-asparagine or 0.1% potassium aspartate (108).

Include a known culture of *M. tuberculosis* and an uninoculated medium control.

Reagents. (i) CNBr, 10%. Working in a chemical fume hood and wearing gloves, place about 2 tablespoons of pure CNBr in a tared Erlenmeyer flask. Weigh the flask. Add enough water to make a 10% solution. When the CNBr is fully dissolved, transfer it to a brown bottle and cap the bottle tightly. Include on the label the date prepared and a caution to avoid inhalation of fumes and contact with skin or mucous membranes. Keep both the solution and the stock bottle in a refrigerator. (ii) Aniline, 4%, in alcohol. Add 4 ml of aniline to 96 ml of 95% ethyl alcohol. Keep the mixture in a refrigerator in a brown bottle labeled with the contents and the date of preparation. If pure, this solution is clear and colorless. If it is brown or becomes so, discard it. Pure aniline may be obtained by redistillation.

Tube or spot plate test. See reference 191 also.

Working in a hood, layer 0.5 to 1.5 ml of sterile water over the medium around the colonies. If growth is confluent, scrape it to one side so that the water comes in direct contact with the underlying medium. Let the water stand at 36°C for 10 to 15 min (rarely, an extended extraction time of 60 min may be necessary), and then remove a portion of the water (0.5 ml or 2 drops) to a small test tube or to a porcelain spot plate. Add an equal volume of the aniline solution, and make note of any color; no yellow should be evident. Add cyanogen bromide in the same volume as that of aniline. An immediately developing yellow color indicates niacin is present. Add an excess of NaOH to eliminate toxicity before discarding the tests. The porcelain plate may be reconditioned by placing it in boiling water for a few minutes. Always discard CNBr in NaOH to prevent the unintentional formation of hydrogen cyanide.

Paper strip method. See references 105 and 263 also.

Niacin test strips are commercially available (Niacin Test Strips, TB, Difco; Remel, Lenexa, Kans.). Follow the directions provided with the strips. Some investigators have found that 2 h for the extraction of niacin (rather than the recommended 30 min) yields more strongly positive reactions for *M. tuberculosis* without causing false-positive reactions for other species.

Controls. Use *M. tuberculosis* as a positive control and the *M. avium* complex and uninoculated medium as negative controls.

Nitrate reduction

The nitrate reduction test (232) is valuable for the identification of *M. tuberculosis, M. kansasii, M. szulgai,* certain non-disease-associated strains of nonphotochromogens, and *M. fortuitum,* which are nitrate reductase positive. *M. bovis, M. marinum, M. simiae, M. avium* complex, *M. xenopi, M. gastri, M. malmoense,* and *M. chelonae* are negative or only very weakly positive.

Cultures. Cultures on solid medium should be 3 to 4 weeks old except for rapid growers, which may be 2 to 4 weeks old.

Reagents. (i) A 1:2 dilution of concentrated HCl. (ii) 0.2% aqueous solution of sulfanilamide. (iii) 0.1% aqueous *N*-(1-naphthyl)ethylenediamine dihydrochloride. (iv) 0.01 M solution of $NaNO_3$ in 0.022 M phosphate buffer, pH 7 (Difco nitrate broth may be substituted). (v) Powdered zinc.

Store the solutions at room temperature. They remain stable for several weeks. Record the date of preparation. If either reagent ii or iii changes color, discard it and prepare a fresh solution.

Procedure. Place a few drops of sterile distilled water in a screw-cap tube (16 by 125 mm). Grind in 1 loopful or one spadeful of mycobacterial growth. Add 2 ml of $NaNO_3$ solution. Shake the mixture and incubate it in a water bath at 37°C for 2 h. Add 1 drop of reagent i, 2 drops of reagent ii, and 2 drops of reagent iii. Examine the solution immediately for the development of a pink to red color contrasting with the reagent control. Color intensity should be related to separately prepared color standards, since only a definite red is considered positive. Add a pinch of powdered zinc to all of the negative tubes to reduce nitrate to nitrite. The formation of a red color indicates that the negative reading was valid. Recently, a nitrate reductase test that uses dry, crystalline reagents has been described (237). The initial response by laboratory workers using the procedure has been very favorable. The test is simple, easily performed, and thought to be more sensitive than the standard tube test (see above).

Paper strip method. See reference 177 also.

Commercially available paper strips (Nitrate Test Strips; Difco) also are satisfactory for the nitrate reduction test. Follow the directions provided with the strips. If a strip is negative and other procedures suggest that the test should be positive, the result should be confirmed by the tube test.

Controls. Use *M. tuberculosis* as a positive control and uninoculated medium as a negative control.

Pyrazinamidase

The deamidation of pyrazinamide to pyrazinoic acid in 4 days is useful for the differentiation of *M. marinum* (positive) from *M. kansasii* (negative) and of weakly niacin-positive *M. bovis* (negative) from *M. tuberculosis* (positive) and members of the *M. avium* complex (positive) (240).

Reagents. (i) Dubos broth base containing 0.1 g of pyrazinamide, 2.0 g of pyruvic acid, and 15.0 g of agar per liter. Dispense the base in 15-ml amounts into screw-cap tubes. Autoclave the tubes for 15 min at 121°C. Solidify the agar with tubes in an upright position. (ii) Aqueous ferrous ammonium sulfate, 1%, freshly prepared.

Procedure. Heavily inoculate the agar with growth from a 2- to 3-week-old culture. The inoculum should be visible. Incubate the culture at 37°C for 4 days. Add 1 ml of freshly prepared ferrous ammonium sulfate to the tubes and place them in a refrigerator for 4 h. Examine the tubes for a pink band in the agar.

Controls. Use *M. avium* complex and uninoculated medium as positive and negative controls, respectively.

Sodium chloride tolerance

Of the slowly growing mycobacteria, only *M. triviale* grows in the presence of 5% NaCl. Of the medically significant, rapidly growing mycobacteria, only *M. chelonae* subsp. *chelonae* and the unnamed subspecies fail to grow in the presence of 5% NaCl (100) (Table 5).

Inoculum. Use a barely turbid suspension.

Substrate. ATS or L-J medium containing 5% NaCl (Difco and Remel) is used. The same medium without salt should be used for controls.

Procedure. Inoculate the medium with 0.1 ml of the bacterial suspension. Incubate the culture at 37°C. Read the culture for growth or no growth at 4 weeks.

Controls. Inoculate the media both with and without 5% NaCl with *M. fortuitum* (positive) and *M. tuberculosis* (negative).

Substrate utilization

See reference 221 also.

It has been proposed that substrate utilization tests be used for the differentiation of biovariants and subspecies of strains in the *M. fortuitum* complex (199).

Inoculum. Use 7-day-old cultures incubated at 35°C in 5 ml of Middlebrook 7H9 liquid medium in screw-cap tubes. Dilute the cultures 1:10 in physiologic saline and inoculate slants of complete medium with 0.1 ml of the diluted suspension.

Media. Basal medium contains $(NH_4)_2SO_4$, 2.4 g; KH_2PO_4, 0.5 g; $MgSO_4 \cdot 7H_2O$, 0.5 g; and distilled water, 950 ml. This salt solution is adjusted to pH 7.0 with 10% KOH for tests with sodium citrate and to pH 7.2 for tests with mannitol, inositol, or control medium. Add 20 g of purified agar per 1,000 ml of salt solution. After sterilization at 121°C for 20 min, cool the solution to 56°C and add 50 ml of filter-sterilized substrate. Substrate solutions contain 5.0 g of mannitol or inositol or 5.6 g of sodium citrate per 50 ml of distilled water. Add sterile water without substrate for the control medium. Dispense the medium in 8-ml amounts into screw-cap tubes (20 by 150 mm) and allow the medium to solidify in a slanted position.

Procedure. Incubate the inoculated tubes at 25 to 28°C for 2 weeks. Growth on medium with substrate is interpreted as positive, whereas no growth, as on the control medium, is interpreted as negative.

Controls. Use *M. fortuitum* biovar *perigrinum* as a positive control for mannitol and *M. chelonae* subsp. *chelonae* as a positive control for citrate. Negative controls are media without substrate.

Tellurite reduction

The reduction of colorless potassium tellurite to black metallic tellurium within 3 to 4 days is a distinctive property of *M. avium* complex strains (107). Of other mycobacteria tested, only rapid growers are also positive within this period.

Cultures. Use 7-day-old cultures in 5 ml of Middlebrook 7H9 liquid medium in screw-cap tubes. The broth medium should be fairly turbid as an indication of active growth.

Reagent. Use a 0.2% aqueous solution (0.1 g in 50 ml of distilled water) of potassium tellurite. After the salt is dissolved in water, dispense the solution in 2- to 5-ml amounts and sterilize the tubes in an autoclave at 121°C for 10 min. To avoid contamination, use only one tube of tellurite solution for a series of tests performed on 1 day; discard the remainder of the solution.

Procedure. Add 2 drops of the tellurite solution to each culture and return the cultures to the incubator. Examine the cultures daily for 4 or more days. A positive test is reflected by a jet black precipitate.

Controls. Use *M. avium* complex as a positive control and *M. kansasii* as a negative control.

T2H susceptibility

The T2H test is used for distinguishing *M. bovis* from *M. tuberculosis* and other species. Only *M. bovis* is susceptible to low concentrations (5 μg/ml) of this compound (20). Some strains of *M. tuberculosis* are inhibited by 10 μg/ml, and some strains of *M. bovis* may show minimal growth at 1 μg/ml.

Substrate. Use Dubos oleic acid agar with albumin complex or Middlebrook 7H11 medium. Incorporate 5 μg of T2H (Aldrich Chemical Co., Inc., Milwaukee, Wis.) per ml into the agar. Dispense the substrate in 5-ml amounts onto slants or onto Felsen disposable plastic quadrant plates, alternating with the same medium without T2H.

Procedure. Prepare a barely turbid suspension of the organisms to be tested in sterile water. Dilute this suspension 1:1,000 with sterile water. Inoculate 3 drops of the 1:1,000 suspension onto the T2H-containing and control media and incubate the media at 37°C. Record the time when definite growth is observed on the control medium. Maintain the T2H-containing medium for an additional 3 weeks unless definite growth appears earlier. Record the organism as resistant if growth on the T2H medium is greater than 1% of the growth on the control. If the control plate has confluent growth, assume that this equals 10^4 organisms.

Controls. Use *M. tuberculosis* as a positive control and *M. bovis* as a negative control.

Tween 80 hydrolysis

The enzymatic hydrolysis of Tween 80 (a polyethylene derivative of sorbitan monooleate) releases complexed neutral red, resulting in a change in color of the test substrate (243). The change in color is not due to a pH shift from the formation of oleic acid but to the destruction (hydrolysis) of Tween 80. The test is helpful in the identification of scotochromogenic and nonphotochromogenic mycobacteria. Species of these two groups that hydrolyze Tween 80 readily are seldom of clinical significance. *M. scrofulaceum* strains are negative; *M. gordonae* and *M. malmoense* strains are positive. *M. avium* complex, *M. xenopi*, and *M. haemophilum* are negative; other nonphotochromogens are positive.

Inoculum. Use actively growing colonies obtained from solid medium.

Reagents. (i) Phosphate buffer, 0.067 M, pH 7, 100 ml. (ii) Tween 80, 0.5 ml. (iii) Neutral red stock solution, 2 ml: 0.1% aqueous solutions of actual dye content (e.g., if actual dye content is 85%, dissolve 0.1 g in 85 rather than 100 ml of water). Mix the three reagents and note that the color is amber as the dye is complexed. Dispense the mixture in 4-ml amounts in screw-cap tubes (16 by 125 mm) and autoclave the tubes at 121°C for 15 min. Incubate the mixture at 35 to 37°C overnight to ensure sterility. Store the mixture in a refrigerator and protect it from light. The substrate is not stable longer than 2 weeks at 4 to 10°C. A concentrate for the preparation of the test substrate can be obtained from Difco (106).

Procedure. Emulsify a 3-mm loopful of growth in a tube of substrate. Incubate the culture at 35 to 37°C. Observe the tubes for a color change from amber (straw) to red after 1, 5, and 10 days.

Interpretation. Record the number of days required for the first appearance of pink. If this time is less than 5 days, the test is positive; if the time is 5 to 10 days, the test is doubtful; if no change in color occurs by day 10, the test is negative.

Controls. Use *M. kansasii* as a positive control and *M. scrofulaceum* as a negative control.

Urease

The determination of the ability of an isolate to hydrolyze urea often helps in the characterization of mycobacterial strains aberrant in some other property. For example, *M. scrofulaceum* is urease positive, whereas members of the *M. avium* complex are urease negative. The urease test will help in the recognition of the occasionally encountered pigmented strain of *M. avium* complex. Similarly, *M. bovis* is urease positive, and this test helps distinguish a drug-resistant *M. bovis* strain from *M. avium* complex. The method described here is a modification of the procedure of Toda et al. (220).

Inoculum. Use actively growing colonies obtained from solid medium.

Reagents. Mix 1 part of urea agar-base concentrate (Difco or an equivalent product) with 9 parts of sterile water. Do not add agar. Dispense the mixture in 4-ml amounts into screw-cap tubes (16 by 125 mm) and store the tubes at 4°C.

Procedure. Emulsify the equivalent of a 3-mm loopful of growth in a tube of substrate. Incubate the culture at 35 to 37°C and observe the culture for a color change from amber to pink or red. Discard the culture after 3 days.

Interpretation. A change in the color of the medium to pink or red within 3 days is recorded as a positive reaction.

Disk test for urea

Murphy and Hawkins (155) have described a procedure to detect urease production with a urea-impregnated paper disk (available from Difco). This procedure has been reported to yield results more quickly than the test described above, with a more consistent separation into positive and negative responses by species.

Use *M. kansasii* as a positive control and *M. gordonae* as a negative control.

Steadham (210) has described a carefully buffered urea broth that is simple to prepare and reliable in test results obtained after 7 days of incubation.

SPECIES OF CLINICALLY IMPORTANT MYCOBACTERIA

Detailed descriptions of the species of clinically important mycobacteria are presented below, followed by a brief review of other mycobacterial species that have proven to be occasional pathogens in humans. Also included is a brief description of the uncultivatable organism *M. leprae* and leprosy. Wolinski (252) reviewed mycobacteria other than *M. tuberculosis* through 1979, and the review by Woods and Washington (255) brings the descriptions up to date. Because of the excess numbers of references available, only some are cited. Rather, the reader is encouraged to consult these papers for the vast amount of information they contain and so that the excellent work of so many investigators over the past few decades can be given proper credit.

Mycobacterium tuberculosis

The discovery of the tubercle bacillus as the cause of tuberculosis by Robert Koch had as great an impact on the consumption-ravaged world of that era as if someone today were to discover the cure for AIDS. The organism was initially named *Bacterium tuberculosis* by Zoppf in 1883, an epithet later changed to *Mycobacterium tuberculosis* by Lehmann and Neumann in 1886, presumably because the slow-growing nature of the organism and the rough appearance in culture made it look funguslike.

Volumes have been written on the clinical manifestations of tuberculosis, presenting in the initial infection, commonly in children, as a nonprogressive focal nidus of infection in the lung with an accompanying locus in a hilar lymph node, terminating in a healed Ghon complex. Disseminated or miliary spread of infection occurred in certain people, usually those with malnutrition, immunosuppression, or other chronic debilitating diseases. Reinfection or adult-type tuberculosis is a slowly progressive inflammatory process in the lungs characterized by intense chronic inflammation, necrosis, and caseation (a process colloquially called consumption), with the propensity of the process to break into bronchi whereby large numbers of tubercle bacilli are not only spread to fresh foci within the lung but coughed out to infect others in close contact. Cough, weight loss, low-grade fever, dyspnea, and chest pain are the usual clinical signs and symptoms of chronic progressive pulmonary tuberculosis. Tuberculosis has taken a new turn in patients with AIDS (16), with a greater tendency toward more rapid progression, less focal fibrosis, sometimes with no granuloma formation or caseation and miliary dissemination, including episodes of septicemia when blood cultures may be positive. *M. tuberculosis* has been recovered from cases of cervical adenitis (99), skin infection (194), pericarditis (230), synovitis (215), and numerous cases of meningitis.

The organism grows in culture as slowly developing, rough colonies with a characteristic buff color. The variations in hue and texture of colonies of tubercle bacilli on a given medium are readily learned but difficult to describe. On the most favorable culture media and without other optimal condition, colonies are recognizable in ≤3 weeks, but some strains, especially those resistant to isoniazid and those growing on suboptimal media after decontamination with harsh digestion agents, may require 4 to 6 weeks or longer. Characteristic microcolonies may be readily recognized in less than 1 week by the microscopic observation of growth on Middlebrook 7H11 plates (189, 190). Although a definitive identification cannot be made on the basis of microcolony morphology, the development of a colony with serpentine cord formations resulting from the production of cord factor is sufficient presumptive evidence to warrant initiation of drug therapy directed against *M. tuberculosis*. Rough variants of other *Mycobacterium* species may also produce similar stranding of bacilli; however, with some experience, the true cord formation of *M. tuberculosis* can usually be differentiated (see discussion on microcolony morphology later in this chapter).

The typical cell morphology of *M. tuberculosis* as seen in acid-fast stains is a thin, slightly curved bacillus measuring 0.3 to 0.6 by 1 to 4 μm, deeply red staining (strongly acid fast), with a distinct beaded appearance. In the preparation of smears from cultures, the individual cells are often difficult to disperse, appearing as irregular aggregates or in parallel strands, but the acid-fast stain cannot be used to make even a presumptive identification.

The key identifying characteristic for the identification of *M. tuberculosis* is the accumulation of niacin on appropriate medium because of the lack of an enzyme possessed by most *Mycobacterium* species that converts free niacin to niacin ribonucleotide. *M. simiae*, certain strains of *M. bovis*, and occasional strains of *M. marinum* and *M. chelonae* may also be niacin positive; therefore, this is not an absolute characteristic. The growth of *M. bovis* is inhibited by T2H, the one characteristic that will separate this species from *M. tuberculosis*. *M. simiae* is catalase positive at 68°C and does not produce pyrazinamide, characteristics opposite in reactivity from *M. tuberculosis*. *M. marinum* does not grow well at 35°C, does not reduce nitrates, and hydrolyzes Tween 80. *M. chelonae* grows rapidly (3 to 5 days), does not reduce nitrates, and is arylsulfatase positive. If the niacin test is negative, a number of other tests must be performed, including repeat of the niacin test after further incubation. If a strain of *M. tuberculosis* is isoniazid resistant, it may produce no catalase at all and have reduced or no virulence for guinea pigs. The NAP test used with the BACTEC TB system produces inhibition of the *M. tuberculosis* complex, resulting in a declining growth index when compared with other species. The test is specific and very reliable (70, 125, 152, 210). Of the newer antibiotics, *M. tuberculosis* is susceptible to some of the quinolones (ciprofloxacin and ofloxacin), clavulanic acid when combined with amoxicillin or ticarcillin, amikacin (or streptomycin), and some cephalosporins (ceftizoxime and cephapirin).

Mycobacterium bovis

M. bovis is the designation given in 1896 by T. Smith for the bovine tubercle bacillus. It produces tuberculosis typically in cattle but may also infect other animals, including dogs, cats, swine, rabbits, and possibly certain birds of prey. The human disease closely resembles that caused by *M. tuberculosis* and is treated similarly. Wilkins et al. (248) recently reported on 20 patients with pulmonary tuberculosis caused by *M. bovis*, representing less than 1% of all acid-fast isolates at the Liverpool (England) Public Health Laboratory. They reported, however, that in some areas in Scotland and in Czechoslovakia, where cattle and dairy farming is still the chief livelihood, *M. bovis* can make up as much as 39% of all cases of tuberculosis.

The human strains are generally niacin negative and have a very slow growth rate, producing "dysgonic"-appearing colonies on L-J medium. Growth of most strains is better on L-J medium than on Middlebrook 7H11 or equivalents. The medium most favorable for *M. bovis* contains 0.4% pyruvate, without glycerol (44). Colonies are buff, low, and small and may appear either smooth or rough on egg medium. On Middlebrook 7H11 agar, colonies are very thin and often show little or no stranding (referred to as water droplet-like). If pyruvate has been added to the medium, colonies may show serpentine cords similar to those of eugonic *M. tuberculosis*.

A problem in recognizing *M. bovis* may arise in laboratories where L-J cultures are discarded after 4 weeks, in that it takes 6 to 8 weeks for the small, clear, water droplet-like colonies to develop, almost appearing as imperfections on the surface of the slant. Once the organisms are recognized, a problem may still arise in differentiating these strains from dysgonic forms of MAI. The latter are catalase positive at 68°C, do not produce urease, and are pyrazinamidase positive.

The microscopic morphology in acid-fast-stained smears is not distinctive. *M. bovis* cells tend to be somewhat longer, less curved, and less beaded than *M. tuberculosis* cells. Serpentine cord formations may be seen, particularly in preparations made from cultures containing medium.

M. bovis, most strains of which are generally niacin negative and do not reduce nitrates or produce pyrazinamidase, can be distinguished from *M. tuberculosis*. *M. bovis* will not grow in medium containing T2H. In recent years, a unique problem has arisen with BCG strains of *M. bovis*. BCG strains or attenuated strains that have lost their original virulence after repeated laboratory subcultures and have been used as vaccines in areas of the world where the incidence of tuberculosis is high. In the laboratory, these strains differ from the usual strains of *M. bovis* by being eugonic, more rapidly growing (3 to 4 weeks on L-J medium), having a rough, buff appearance, and in some cases accumulating niacin. However, the T2H, nitrate reduction, and pyrazinamidase tests as mentioned above will serve to differentiate BCG strains from *M. tuberculosis;* however, bacteriophage typing is diagnostic.

Mycobacterium leprae

Mycobacterium leprae, the etiologic agent of leprosy (Hansen's disease), produces an infection of the skin, mucous membranes, and peripheral nerves. The organism has been recognized since the late 1800s and has been responsible for millions of infections in humans. The world prevalence rate is approximately 12 million cases.

The major endemic areas for leprosy include Southeast Asia, the Philippines, New Guinea, China, Korea, Africa, islands of the Pacific, and Latin America. Within the United States, most cases have been reported in areas with a warm climate, including California, Texas, Louisiana, Hawaii, Florida, Puerto Rico, and New York.

The clinical presentation varies a great deal, depending on the patient. Most cases can be categorized as lepromatous or tuberculoid. The former produces skin lesions; facial changes occur with lysis of nasal cartilage and bone; and with time, symmetrical nerve damage occurs and results in anesthesia. Tuberculoid leprosy produces few skin lesions in some patients. When present, they are raised and bilaterally asymmetrical, usually with severe peripheral nerve involvement.

M. leprae differs from all other mycobacteria in that it cannot be cultured in vitro. Like *M. tuberculosis* and *M. bovis*, it is transmissible from person to person. The natural reservoir has not been well documented; however, some association between *M. leprae* and the nine-banded armadillo found in Texas and Louisiana has been made.

The laboratory diagnosis depends on the demonstration of acid-fast bacilli in skin biopsy specimens. The diagnosis is presumptive and depends on the correlation of typical histopathological lesions with the presence of acid-fast organisms. The organism occurs in bunches in lepromatous leprosy and fails to grow on conventional mycobacteriological culture media (64). Lesions are abundant in patients with lepromatous leprosy and sparse in patients with tuberculoid leprosy (15). Numerous bacilli may also be found in discharge from the mouth and nose.

Current therapy usually includes clofazamine, dapsone (diamino, diphenyl sulfone), or rifampin.

Mycobacterium avium-intracellulare

M. avium was first found in the late 1800s to cause disease in chickens. Occasionally, chicken farmers were reported to have pulmonary disease due to this organism. In fact, Runyon later separated the virulent strains causing disease in chickens and rabbits (*M. avium*) from the avirulent strains that he called *M. intracellulare*. After further studies, Wolinski (252) stated, "I believe it is reasonable to call these strains *M. avium-intracellulare* or *M. avium* complex." In the late 1950s, this same organism caused an outbreak of pulmonary tuberculosis at the Battey State Hospital in Rome, Ga., and for some time carried the designation "Battey bacillus."

The organism is ubiquitous in the environment and has been recovered from soil, house dust, water, and other environmental sources. Gruft et al. (71) recovered the organism from 25% of 520 water samples taken from estuaries in South Carolina, Georgia, and other Gulf Coast states and also from air samples, the latter explaining the pulmonary route of infection in humans. MAI is also widely distributed in water, soil, dust, animals, and poultry in Japan (224). The organism is of low pathogenicity and until recently was considered a colonizer that rarely caused disease. However, during the past two decades, an increasing number of MAI infections have been reported; by 1980, only *M. tuberculosis* was recovered with more frequency than MAI (67). Currently, MAI is the most commonly enountered species of mycobacteria seen in most clinical laboratories.

Pulmonary manifestations of MAI infections are seen commonly (226) and are similar to those of *M. tuberculosis:* cough, fatigue, weight loss, low-grade fever, and night sweats. Cavitary disease can be demonstrated radiologically in most patients; in others, solitary nodules or more diffuse infiltrates may be observed. Occasionally, patients may be asymptomatic (35, 84, 90, 109, 162, 176, 208, 224). Recently, disseminated disease due to MAI has become more common. Horsburgh et al. (85) reviewed 37 patients with disseminated MAI infection, 20 of whom were immunocompromised; others had hematologic abnormalities. MAI organisms were recovered from sputum, bone, liver, and lymph nodes. Numerous other cases of disseminated disease have been reported (13, 49, 59, 89, 113, 131, 257).

The greatest upsurge in MAI infections during the past decade has been in patients with AIDS, to the point that in some settings MAI is more frequently recovered than *M. tuberculosis*. From the several papers linking MAI infections with AIDS as cited by Woods and Washington (255) and from our personal experience, certain features stand out. Often there is heavy gastrointestinal involvement, with the aggregation in some cases of large foamy macrophages reminiscent of Whipple's disease (63). Often the intramacrophage accumulation of mycobacteria is so dense as to simulate the lepra cells seen in *M. leprae* infections. This heavy gastrointestinal involvement suggests that ingestion of contaminated water or food may be the mode of transmission. Lesions also may be seen in other organs, notably the lungs, liver, spleen, and lymph nodes. In these patients, the normal cellular response to such a challenge does not always occur, and little inflammation may be seen at the time of death. Histologically, the lesions are more those of necrotizing inflammation, and granuloma formation and caseation necrosis are less common. Young et al. (261, 262), Hawkins et al. (77), and Pierce et al. (168), among others, also report on the high concentration of organisms seen in these patients and, with the increased sensitivity of mycobacterial blood culture systems as discussed above, point to the frequency with which MAI organisms can be recovered from blood cultures (137).

MAI organisms can also be recovered from the lymph nodes of children with scrofulalike cervical lymphadenitis (110, 122). Woods and Washington (255) cite several other MAI infections, including granulomatous synovitis (215), genitourinary tract disease, otomastoiditis (111), cutaneous lesions (59, 165), osteomyelitis (164), meningitis, arthritis (81), pericarditis (253), and colonic ulcers. In this regard, Hampson et al. (75) propose a possible link between MAI infection and Crohn's disease; however, a stronger correlation has been made with *M. paratuberculosis*.

M. avium complex organisms are characterized on primary isolation media by slowly growing, thin, transparent or opaque, homogeneous, smooth colonies, sometimes with "asteroid" margins. A small proportion of *M. intracellulare* colonies may be partially or completely rough; for *M. avium*, the proportion of rough colonies may often be greater. After subculture, a transformation to more eugonic-type colonies may occur, with the centers becoming prominently domed. Eventually all colonies may be hemispherical. Usually nonpigmented, the colonies, particularly the dome-shaped ones, may become yellow with age; rarely are colonies pigmented from the onset of detectable growth. Pathogenicity may be correlated with these colony variations.

The cells are typically short and coccobacillary, although early in culture and under certain conditions, long, thin bacilli may be seen. Staining is usually uniform without beading or banding.

In the laboratory, MAI organisms are best characterized by the battery of negative reactions. The organisms do produce heat-stable catalase and have the ability to grow on T2H; otherwise, they are biochemically inert. Another feature of the MAI organisms, and possibly related to their pathogenicity and lack of response to therapy in patients with AIDS, is the general resistance to antituberculous drugs. Thus, multidrug therapy using various combinations of rifampin, streptomycin, ethambutol, and ethionamide added to cycloserine or kanamycin have been used with little success. Rifabutin and clofazamine have been used with limited success. The quinolones have little activity against MAI; however, vancomycin, amikacin, and some cephalosporins may be efficacious.

Two groups of organisms that appear intermediate between *M. avium* complex and *M. scrofulaceum* have been recognized (78). Both are pigmented, but one group produces a column of foam greater than 45 mm in the semiquantitative catalase test and is urease negative; the second group produces less than 45 mm of foam and is urease positive. These organisms have been assigned the acronym MAIS complex. Those with the latter reactions are much less common than the first group.

Other species of slowly growing nonphotochromogens not known as pathogens but encountered in the clinical laboratory generally differ from members of the MAI complex in hydrolyzing Tween in 5 days or less. *M. triviale* colonies may resemble those of MAI complex and in some instances may be so rough as to be confused with tubercle bacilli; however, these strains are niacin negative. *M. triviale* is Tween positive, whereas MAI complex organisms are Tween negative. Strains of *M. triviale* are distinguished from other nonphotochromogenic bacteria by their ability to grow on media containing 5% NaCl. *M. gastri* and *M. terrae* complex are other nonphotochromogenic species that may require biochemical differentiation (Table 4). Although the organisms are usually nonpathogenic, case reports of pulmonary infection caused by *M. terrae* complex have appeared (115, 116).

Mycobacterium kansasii

M. kansasii is the current name given to the "yellow bacillus" first described in 1953 by Buhler and Pollak (25). Pulmonary infections resembling classical tuberculosis have been caused by this organism, with most cases reported from the southern United States (Texas, Louisiana, and Florida), Midwest (Illinois and Missouri), and California. A decline in incidence over the past decade has been reported in the United States (109); however, Tsukamura et al. (224) reported an increase in incidence in Japan, particularly in Tokyo and Osaka, possibly related to dust generated from new construction.

Chronic pulmonary disease is the most common manifestation, classically involving the upper lobes, with cavitation and scarring evident in most cases (35, 84, 90, 109, 208, 224). Occasional cases of extrapulmonary infections have been reported, including scrofulalike lymphadenitis in children (259), sporotrichosislike cutaneous infections (194), osteomyelitis (149), soft tissue infections and tenosynovitis (215), and prostatitis (127). *M. kansasii* rarely disseminates except in the presence of severe immunosuppression and most recently in patients with AIDS. Scherer et al. (196) reported a case of disseminated *M. kansasii* infection involving the bowel and mesenteric lymph nodes, with caseating granulomas and the accumulation of foamy histiocytes resembling Whipple's disease. Other cases of disseminated infection were reported by Bennett et al. (13) and Tempero and Smith (217).

M. kansasii occurs in several forms. It is found most commonly as photochromogenic, with high catalase production; less commonly encountered are photochromogenic, low-catalase-producing strains; rarely isolated are scotochromogenic and nonchromogenic strains. The distinctive feature is the dependence on light exposure for carotene formation, usually coupled with carotene crystal production. Other photochromogens include *M. marinum* (which grows optimally at 30°C), *M. simiae* (weakly photochromogenic), *M. szulgai* (which is variably photochromogenic at lower temperatures), and the saprobe *M. vaccae*, a rapidly growing nonpathogen. Thus, the recovery of a photochromogen from a clinical specimen having a growth rate similar to (or slightly more rapid than) that of *M. tuberculosis* at 37°C is presumptive evidence for reporting *M. kansasii*. However, *M. kansasii* can grow slowly at lower temperatures, and colony growth is more rapid when observed in subcultures. *M. kansasii* also differs from *M. marinum* by producing large amounts of nitroreductase.

Young cells observed in acid-fast smears are characteristically long and broad, with distinct cross-banding, presumed to be structural evidence of utilization of the fatty material of the medium; however, this feature is not diagnostic.

Colonies are characteristically intermediate between fully rough and fully smooth (certain strains are totally one or the other). The centers are elevated, and in the thinner margins, curving strands of bacilli may usually be seen with a low-power microscope. Upon prolonged light exposure, red β-carotene crystals typically appear.

In the laboratory, this organism is recognized by its strong photochromogenic properties when incubated at 37°C, ability to hydrolyze Tween in 3 days, and strong activity for nitroreductase, catalase, and pyrazinamidase. Most strains are susceptible to rifampin but are slightly resistant to isoniazid, ethambutol, and streptomycin. Treatment usually includes two or more antituberculous drugs, one of which is rifampin. Of the newer drugs, the quinolones appear to have some activity. Vancomycin, erythromycin, minocycline, and sulfonamides with trimethoprim may also be efficacious.

Mycobacterium fortuitum-chelonae complex

The rapidly growing mycobacterium currently designated *M. fortuitum* was first described in 1938 by daCosta Cruz and fully described by Gordon and Smith in 1955. Because another rapidly growing organism, designated *M. chelonae* since the 1923 edition of *Bergey's Manual*, shares a number of similar metabolic characteristics with the organism described by daCosta Cruz and because the two organisms are not infrequently found in the same types of infections, they have been referred to as the *M. fortuitum-chelonae* complex. As defined by Silcox et al. (199), any organism must be acid fast, be nonpigmented, grow in less than 7 days at its optimum temperature, have arylsulfatase activity at 3 days, and grow at 38°C on MacConkey agar without crystal violet to be placed in the *M. fortuitum-chelonae* complex. However, since these two species can be biochemically separated (*M. chelonae* does not reduce nitrates or take up iron, whereas *M. fortuitum* has these properties) and more importantly because recent studies have shown that most strains of *M. fortuitum* are more susceptible to antimicrobial agents than is *M. chelonae*, there are compelling reasons why the two species should be considered separately.

The taxonomy is yet more complex because *M. fortuitum* exists in three biovariants: biovariant *fortuitum*, biovariant *peregrinum*, and an unnamed biovariant designated "third group." Biovariant *peregrinum* cannot grow on medium containing mannitol as the only carbon source, whereas biovariant *fortuitum* can. *M. chelonae* also has three subspecies, subsp. *chelonae*, subsp. *abscessus*, and an unnamed subspecies known as *M. chelonae*-like organisms. *M. chelonae* subsp. *abscessus* can grow on L-J medium containing 5% NaCl at 28°C, whereas subsp. *chelonae* cannot. Steele and Wallace (211) suggest the use of differences in susceptibility to polymyxin B (*M. fortuitum* is resistant), pipemidic acid (*M. fortuitum* is susceptible), and the quinolone ciprofloxacin (*M. fortuitum* is susceptible) to differentiate between these species (Table 5). Although it may not be clinically necessary to make identifications beyond the species level in most cases of human infections, separation into the biovariants and subspecies may be required for certain epidemiological applications.

Both *M. fortuitum* and *M. chelonae* have been associated with a variety of infections, involving the lungs, skin, bone, central nervous system, and prosthetic heart valves, and also with disseminated disease (10, 29, 199, 255). Cutaneous lesions are particularly prevalent and often evolve into draining subcutaneous abscesses (76). Wallace et al. (236) recently reviewed 125 human infections due to rapidly growing mycobacteria in which *M. fortuitum* and *M. chelonae* were equal in frequency. Fifty-nine percent of the cases involved the skin (37, 69, 79, 194), most commonly secondary to postsurgical wound infections, accidental trauma, or needle injections (other outbreaks with *M. chelonae* have occurred after administration of diphtheria-pertussis-tetanus–polio vaccines and after histamine injections) (21). Fonseca et al. (56) reported several cases of disseminated cutaneous and soft tissue infections, usually following trauma or surgery and also from contaminated catheters and prostheses. Other entities include keratitis (145) and corneal ulcers (250, 258) (usually following trauma), bacteremia (168), cervical lymphadenitis, peritonitis during peritoneal dialysis (123, 146, 254), and rare cases of hepatitis and synovitis (255). Zabel et al. (264) reported a case of *M. chelonae* keratitis in a person wearing soft contact lenses. *M. chelonae* has also been the cause of osteomyelitis (80, 88), pulmonary infection (185, 206), mammoplasty infection (33, 193), sternotomy infection, endophthalmitis (187), intraoral infection (163), soft tissue infection (5, 19), arthritis (97), synovitis (215), orbital infection (202), pericarditis and mediastinitis (88), vasculitis (88), cervicofacial infection (17), endocarditis (3), and tenosynovitis (265). Lowry et al. (135) reported a recent outbreak of *M. chelonae* otitis media in an office clinic setting where transfer occurred between patients from contaminated instruments.

M. fortuitum has been recovered from water, soil, and dust. Laussuco et al. (126) reported a hospital ward outbreak of skin infections due to *M. fortuitum* from exposure to a contaminated ice machine. *M. fortuitum* has been reported to also be the cause of sternotomy infection (86, 183, 236), pulmonary infection (109, 185, 208, 224, 230), bacteremia (23, 86, 168), endocarditis (4), mammoplasty infections (33), pericarditis (230), osteomyelitis (161), infection of the spine (201), mastoiditis, disseminated infection (54), prostatitis (127), and endobronchitis (57).

After 2 to 4 days of incubation, the colonies appear smooth and hemispherical and may have a butyrous or waxy consistency. *M. fortuitum* characteristically has branching, filamentous extensions from 1- to 2-day-old colonies on cornmeal-glycerol or Middlebrook 7H11 agar, and short aerial hyphae from rough colonies may be seen with a stereomicroscope. *M. chelonae* lacks the filamentous extensions from colonies at 1 to 2 days that are typical of *M. fortuitum*. Colonies are nonchromogenic but may appear off-white or faintly cream colored.

In acid-fast-stained preparations, the organisms often show considerable pleomorphism, ranging from long filamentous forms to short, thick rods. At times the cells may appear beaded or swollen, and nonstaining ovoid bodies may be seen at one end. The biochemical characteristics of these organisms are listed in Table 4. Of the newer agents available, *M. fortuitum* appears to be susceptible to the quinolones (260), sulfonamides, doxycycline, and amikacin (260), and some isolates are susceptible to imipenem, vancomycin, and erythromycin.

M. chelonae is much more resistant to antibiotics but sometimes is susceptible to amikacin and a sulfonamide, but *M. chelonae* subsp. *chelonae* is resistant to amikacin and cefoxitin. Imipenem, tobramycin, and erythromycin may have some effect on some isolates.

Mycobacterium scrofulaceum

The species name *scrofulaceum* was derived from the term "scrofula," a word classically used to describe tuberculosis of the cervical lymph glands. This organism was named in 1956 by Prissik and Mason (174) from reports of mycobacterial cervical lymphadenitis in children, which is the most common form of disease caused by this organism. In a recent review of 16 children with lymphadenitis caused by atypical mycobacteria, Gill et al. (61) found that 6 were caused by *M. scrofulaceum*, 4 were caused by *M. tuberculosis*, and 4 were caused by *M. avium* complex.

The disease is usually unilateral, involving nodes adjacent to the mandible and high in the neck. The children usually are healthy and free of constitutional symptoms, and pain is either minimal or absent. Nodes often rupture and drain without sequelae. In the series reported by Gill et al. (see above), no portal of entry was found, an experience previously reported by others. Colonization of the organism in the mouth and throat is presumed to be the site of origin. *M. scrofulaceum* may also cause pulmonary infection (109, 227).

In the laboratory, colonies of *M. scrofulaceum* grow slowly (4 to 6 weeks) at various temperatures (25, 31, and 37°C). They are typically smooth, buttery in consistency, and globoid, with pigmentation ranging from light yellow to deep orange. Pigment is produced when cultures are incubated in the absence of light and may darken when the colonies are exposed to light.

In addition to the characteristics cited above, *M. scrofulaceum* fails to hydrolyze Tween, does not reduce nitrate, but does possess urease activity. Other slow-growing scotochromogens include certain strains of *M. avium* complex, *M. gordonae*, and *M. szulgai*. Differential characteristics include Tween hydrolysis (the latter two are positive [*M. szulgai* may require 7 days or more], whereas *M. scrofulaceum* is negative) and urease activity (*M. scrofulaceum* hydrolyzes urea, whereas the other species, including pigmented strains of *M. avium* complex, cannot).

M. scrofulaceum demonstrates in vitro resistance to isoniazid, streptomycin, ethambutol, and *p*-aminosalicylic acid. Treatment for cervical lymphadenitis is usually incision and drainage of the involved nodes; only rarely are antituberculous drugs necessary.

Mycobacterium xenopi

As the species name would suggest (*Xenopus* = frog genus), *M. xenopi* was first isolated from an African toad. The organism has been recovered from hot and cold water taps, including water storage tanks of hospitals, and until recently was considered nonpathogenic. However, by 1979, Wolinski (252) had listed 50 cases of human infections associated with *M. xenopi*, reported primarily in England, France, Denmark, Australia, and the United States. Birds that frequent the costal regions in Great Britain comprise an important reservoir.

Most human cases of *M. xenopi* infections have been pulmonary (18, 46, 83, 84, 90, 104, 169, 200, 216, 225, 256), usually in patients with preexistent lung disease or predisposing conditions (alcoholism, malignancy, or diabetes mellitus). Contreras et al. (35), in reviewing 89 adult patients with pulmonary infections, reported that *M. xenopi* was isolated in 38% of the cases in their institution, usually occurring in patients with preexistent pulmonary disease or in those with alcoholism. Clinically, the pulmonary infections resemble those seen in patients with *M. tuberculosis, M. kansasii,* or MAI infections, and radiographically multinodular densities, often showing cavitation and fibrosis, often are seen. Ausina et al. (9) report *M. xenopi* infections in eight patients with AIDS, thought to be nosocomial in nature and obtained from four hot water generators. In most instances intrapulmonary spread was evident, with *M. xenopi* recovered from sputa and bronchial washings. In disseminated cases (245), organisms were also recovered from bone marrow aspirates. Wolinski (252) also listed cases of extrapulmonary infection involving bone (140), lymph node, epididymis, sinus tract, and a prosthetic temporomandibular joint. Prosser (175) reports a case involving the lumbar spine in a 55-year-old female complaining of low back pain, nausea, and weight loss.

M. xenopi can be recognized in culture by its small, erect colonies, slow growth, characteristic yellow color (occasional strains are nonpigmented), more rapid growth at 42 than 37°C, and failure to grow at 25°C. Although this species has been placed with the nonphotochromogenic mycobacteria, observation of the brightly pigmented yellow colonies usually found on primary isolation suggests that the organism would be better considered with the scotochromogens. Persistent branching and filamentous extensions (as observed microscopically under low-power magnification) around the circular colonies on cornmeal-glycerol agar are very distinctive. Rough colonies usually exhibit aerial hyphae. Microscopic colonial morphology shows a distinctive "bird's nest" appearance with sticklike projections in young colonies on cornmeal agar.

Acid-fast-stained smears reveal long, filamentous rods that are tapered at both ends and arrange in palisades. The characteristics by which species identification can be made are optimum growth at 42°C, yellow scotochromogenic pigment, negative reactions for niacin accumulation, nitrate reduction, and positive reactions for heat stable catalase, arylsulfatase, and pyrazinamidase.

The quinolones (ciprofloxacin, fleroxacin, and ofloxacin) are highly active against *M. xenopi,* and some isolates are susceptible to vancomycin, erythromycin, or cefuroxime.

Mycobacterium szulgai

M. szulgai is named after the Polish microbiologist T. Szulga and was officially reported as a species in 1972 by Marks et al. (141), who were studying the thin-layer chromatography lipid patterns of scotochromogens. The chief characteristic of this organism is the taxonomic inconsistency shown in the laboratory: when grown at 37°C, the organism is scotochromogenic; when grown at room temperature (25°C), the colonies are photochromogenic.

Maloney et al. (139) presented three cases of human infections with *M. szulgai* and reviewed 24 previous cases reported in the literature before 1987. Pulmonary disease (two-thirds of cases) simulating *M. tuberculosis* was the most common type of disease, and chest roentgenograms commonly revealed unilateral or bilateral apical disease with cavitation. Fever, cough, hemoptysis, and weight loss were common symptoms. Dylewski et al. (50) also reported a case of pulmonary disease revealing clinical and radiologic manifestations similar to those described above. Additional cases of pulmonary infection were reported by Jenkins (90), Kim et al. (109), and Pocza (170). Other presentations reported by Maloney et al. (139) include olecranon bursitis, tenosynovitis (213) and carpal tunnel syndrome, osteomyelitis, and localized cutaneous disease. Three previous cases occurred in immunocompromised patients, two of whom were taking steroids. *M. szulgai* osteomyelitis at multiple sites was found in the third patient following *Salmonella paratyphi* D bacteremia. Smooth and rough colonies may be seen on egg medium in 2 weeks at 37°C. Orange pigment may be observed, intensifying with exposure to continuous light. Microscopically in smear preparations, moderately long rods with some cross-barring is characteristic.

Differentiating characteristics include slow hydrolysis of Tween, positive activity for nitroreductase and arylsulfatase activity, and intolerance to 5% NaCl (these latter two features distinguish *M. szulgai* from the scotochromogen *M. flavescens,* which has opposite reactions). *M. szulgai* is much more susceptible than *M. avium* complex to conventional antimycobacterial drugs, including amikacin in combination with cefoxitin.

Mycobacterium malmoense

The species name is derived from Malmo, Sweden, the origin of the strain used in the first case reported by Schröder and Juhlin in 1977 (197). The organism is nonchromogenic and associated with pulmonary disease in Sweden (197). France et al. (58) reported 20 cases occurring in Scotland. The disease was primarily pulmonary in nature, with roentgenograms indistinguishable from those for *M. tuberculosis.* Twelve strains of *M. malmoense* were isolated in the United States in 1980 (67). More recently, Jenkins (91) and Jenkins and Tsukamura (92) cite three papers reporting pulmonary infections and cervical adenitis (34, 128, 238). Alberts et al. (1) reported four patients with chronic lung disease from the United States. Two of their patients developed progressive disease. They make the point that *M. malmoense* infections may not be as rare as suspected and that cases may be underreported because 8 to 12 weeks is required to isolate some strains from clinical specimens, which is 2 to 6 weeks longer than cultures are held in most laboratories in the United States. A single report by Prince et al. (173) describes *M. malmoense* associated with carpal tunnel syndrome.

This organism grows slowly, being seen after 2 to 3 weeks of incubation at 37°C and after up to 7 weeks of incubation at 22°C. As mentioned above, some strains may require as long as 12 weeks before colonies become visible. The growth rate may be shortened by the addition of pyruvate to culture media and the use of a low pH (6.5).

Colonies are grayish white and appear smooth, glistening, opaque, colorless, domed, and circular, 0.5 to 1.5 mm in diameter. Exposure of the colonies to light does not produce pigment. On acid-fast smears, the organisms appear coccoid or as short bacilli without crossbands.

This species does not accumulate niacin, is nitrate negative, hydrolyzes Tween 80, and usually produces heat-labile catalase (Table 4). *M. malmoense* biochemically resembles *M. gastri* except that *M. malmoense* is urease negative and pyrazinamidase positive, reactions opposite those of *M. gastri.* Although resistant to isoniazid, streptomycin, *p*-aminosalicylic acid, and rifampin, it is susceptible to ethambutol and cycloserine.

Mycobacterium simiae

As suspected from the species name, the first *M. simiae* isolate was from monkeys, specifically recovered by Karassova et al. (98), from lymph nodes of *Macaca* rhesus monkeys imported into Hungary from India in 1965. The designation *M. simiae* was made by Weiszfeiler and Karczag (246) in 1971. Valdivia et al. (229), working in Cuba, recovered a niacin-producing strain of a nonchromogenic mycobacterium in 1971 from patients with pulmonary tuberculosis. This organism, which they named *M. habana,* was subsequently shown to be the same organism as *M. simiae* (246). The organism has been repeatedly recovered from tap water.

Reports of human infection from *M. simiae* are relatively few. Lévy-Frébault et al. (131) cited several reports from France, Israel, Thailand, and the United States pointing to *M. simiae* as a cause of pulmonary disease. A case reported by Lévy-Frébault et al. (131) involved a 43-year-old man with AIDS who developed disseminated mycobacterial infection, with organisms recovered from blood, jejunal fluid, and duodenal and rectal biopsies. *M. simiae* and *M. avium* complex were both involved.

Smooth colonies develop within 2 to 3 weeks on egg base media. Most strains are photochromogenic, although prolonged light exposure may be required, and then some isolates fail to produce pigment. The biochemical characterization includes a positive test for niacin accumulation, slow hydrolysis of Tween (more than 10 days), and high thermostable catalase activity. Identification of some strains is difficult because of poor reproducibility of test results, and *M. simiae* can be misidentified as members of the MAIS species. The definitive differentiation of *M. simiae* can be made by studying the mycolic acid composition (characteristic pattern including alpha, alpha-prime short nonoxygenated and keto mycolates) (131).

Mycobacterium marinum

The species name, meaning "of the sea," reflects the first encounter with *M. marinum* by Aronson (7) in 1926, when he was investigating disease of saltwater fish. The organism has also been called *M. platypoecilus,* from infections observed in Mexican platyfish, and also *M. balnei* (a name referring to bath or spas). All are the same organism. *M. marinum* was first implicated in human infections by Norden and Linell in Sweden (160); since then, there have been reports of several outbreaks of cutaneous infections resulting when traumatized skin came in contact with inadequately chlorinated fresh water or salt water (swimming pools, tropical fish aquariums, or water cooling towers) (94). Fisher (55) recently reported three cases of cutaneous skin infection in lifeguards, citing this infection as a hazard of the occupation. Included in the paper are good color photographs of the skin lesions.

The skin lesions may be of two types. One is a sporotrichosislike lesion in which the primary area of inoculation develops into an abscess, with secondary spread centrally along the lymphatics. The more typical presentation is a tender, red or blue-red subcutaneous nodule, usually involving the elbow, knee, toe, or finger ("swimming pool granuloma") (194). This nodule develops about 2 weeks after exposure and may progress to a wartlike lesion or ulcerate. Aubrey and Fam (8) report a case in which *M. marinum* infection was not suspected because the lesions simulated rheumatoid nodules. They cite other cases in which deeper structures are involved, including subcutaneous bursae, tendon sheaths (95), joints (121, 215), and bone.

Colonies appear in 8 to 14 days when incubated at 30 to 32°C. On subculture, there may be better tolerance for growth at 37°C. Early colonies, particularly those grown in the dark, may be nonpigmented; however, when the organism is exposed to light, a deep yellow color develops. The colonies may be wrinkled and rough but may also be smooth and hemispherical, particularly if grown on 7H10 and 7H11 agar (which contains oleic acid and albumin). Microscopically, the cells are relatively long bacilli with frequent cross-barring.

The photochromogenicity and preference for growth at 30°C are initial clues to the identification of *M. marinum.* Some strains may accumulate niacin; however, *M. marinum* does not reduce nitrates. Tween is hydrolyzed, and urease and pyrazinamidase are produced. Heat-stable catalase is not produced. Treatment is usually localized to the lesions (curettage, electrodesiccation, or excision). In more chronic cases or when lymphatic spread is evident, antituberculous therapy may be required. Most strains are susceptible to rifampin and ethambutol but resistant to isoniazid and streptomycin. The quinolones, amikacin, and minocycline all exhibit activity against *M. marinum.* Sulfonamides alone or with trimethoprim may be drugs of choice.

Mycobacterium ulcerans

Buruli ulcer is one of the designations given to the human disease caused by *M. ulcerans,* from the Australian town where the organism was first recognized by Alsop and Searls in the 1930s. Most cases have been seen in Central and West Africa (Zaire, Uganda, Cameroon, Nigeria, and Ghana), Malaysia, New Guinea, Guyana, Mexico, and Australia (178). Igo and Murthy (87) reviewed the clinical, histological, and microbiological features of 46 cases studied in several villages along the Sepik River in New Guinea, and Burchard and Bierther studied 23 patients in Lambarene, Gabon (26).

Typically, the disease begins as a painless "boil" or lump under the skin at the site of previous trauma. In a few weeks, a shallow ulcer with a necrotic base develops at the site of the lump. Some of the lesions studied by Igo and Murthy (87) were quite severe, with avascular coagulation necrosis extending deep into the subcutaneous fat. Satellite nodules that ulcerate may also develop. Constitutional or systemic symptoms rarely develop, and patients are rarely febrile unless bacterial superinfection occurs.

M. ulcerans grows optimally at 33°C and not at all at 37°C. Six to twelve weeks may be required for colonies to develop, which tend to resemble those of *M. tuberculosis:* rough, lightly buff or nonpigmented, and convex to flat, with irregular outline. Microscopically, the acid-fast cells are moderately long and rod shaped without banding or beading. *M. ulcerans* is biochemically inert, showing only heat-stable catalase activity among the several tests usually used to identify mycobacteria.

Mycobacterium haemophilum

M. haemophilum was first recovered in 1978 in Israel by Sompolinsky et al. (205) from a subcutaneous lesion of a patient with Hodgkin's disease. The organism has a low potential for pathogenicity, and infections occur primarily in immunosuppressed patients, particularly those who are lymphopenic (154). Most cases have been reported from Australia. Rogers et al. (184) reviewed 13 cases previously reported and added two cases of infections in patients with AIDS. The clinical presentation is that of subcutaneous nodules, painful swellings, and ulcers that can progress into abscesses and draining fistulas. In the AIDS patients described by Rogers et al. (184), the skin lesions were multiple, involving the upper arm, hands, and feet (excellent color photographs of these lesions are included in this paper). Males et al. (138) also reported isolation of *M. haemophilum* from the wrist and ankle at sites of tenosynovitis in a patient with AIDS. Gouby et al. (68) reported infections in two patients in a renal dialysis unit who were receiving corticosteroids and speculate on the possibility of human-to-human transmission; Dawson et al. (42) reported a case of submandibular lymphadenitis in a child.

The organism is unique in requiring hemoglobin or hemin for growth. Appropriate media for culture include chocolate agar, 5% sheep blood Columbia agar, Mueller-Hinton agar with Fildes supplement, and L-J medium containing 2% ferric ammonium citrate (255). Vadney and Hawkins (228) reported success in recovering *M. haemophilum* by placing an X-factor strip in the area of inoculation on 7H10 agar. Optimum growth occurs at 28 to 32°C; some strains grow at 20°C, and little or no growth occurs at 37°C. Growth is stimulated in the presence of 10% CO_2.

The colonies are nonpigmented and may be rough or smooth after 2 to 4 weeks of incubation at 32°C on egg medium or 7H10 agar (supplemented with hemoglobin or hemin as discussed above). Microscopically, the cells are short, curved, and strongly acid fast without banding or beading. This organism is also biochemically inert, with the production of pyrazinamidase the only positive reaction among the commonly used tests to identify mycobacteria.

Saprophytic *Mycobacterium* Species Rarely Causing Human Disease

Of the usually nonpathogenic mycobacteria listed above, only brief mention will be made of a few of the species that rarely cause human infections.

Mycobacterium gordonae

Of the usually nonpathogenic mycobacteria, perhaps *M. gordonae* is recovered in clinical laboratories with greatest frequency. The organism can be recovered from soil and water, the latter property leading to the alternate designation of *M. aquae* or the "tap water bacillus." Isolated reports of infections in the literature as cited by Woods and Washington (255) include meningitis secondary to ventriculoatrial shunts, hepatoperitoneal disease (120), endocarditis in a prosthetic aortic valve, synovitis (215), cutaneous lesions of the hand (60, 198), and possible cases of pulmonary involvement (47, 72, 208). London et al. (134) reported a case of peritonitis in a patient undergoing ongoing peritoneal dialysis, and Moore et al. (151) reported a case of keratitis. With *M. gordonae* being so prevalent in the aquatic environment and the increasing number of patients undergoing ambulatory dialysis, infections with this organism may emerge as a significant problem. The organism is a scotochromogen, readily recognized by the smooth, deeply yellow-orange pigmented colonies that develop after 7 days of incubation at 37°C. The organism hydrolyzes Tween 80 and produces heat-stable catalase. *M. gordonae* is resistant to isoniazid, streptomycin, and *p*-aminosalicylic acid but susceptible to rifampin and ethambutol.

Mycobacterium asiaticum

M. asiaticum was first isolated in Hungary from the lymph nodes and viscera of healthy monkeys. Rarely have cases of human infection appeared in the literature (67). *M. asiaticum* is photochromogenic but, in contrast to *M. simiae,* is negative for niacin production.

Mycobacterium thermoresistibile

M. thermoresistibile was originally encountered by Tsukamura in 1966 and given species designation in 1981 (222). The organism may grow slowly on primary isolation medium and may be mistaken for a slow-growing scotochromogen; however, on subculture to egg base medium it will produce smooth or rough yellow colonies within 3 to 5 days. This organism has the unique ability to grow at 52°C (130). In one human infection reported (247), the organism was recovered from bronchoscopy and lung specimens of an immunocompetent middle-aged woman. Histological examination of the lung tissue revealed numerous microabscesses and granulomata with giant cells of the Langhans type. Willemse et al. (249) reported the recovery of *M. thermoresistibile* from subcutaneous nodules and lymph nodes of a cat. This organism is potentially pathogenic; however, the infrequency of case reports indicates that either exposure is minimal or the organism is of very low virulence.

Mycobacterium terrae-triviale complex

M. terrae first was recovered from washings of a radish by Richmond and Cummings in 1950 (thus, the colloquial designation "radish bacillus"). *M. triviale* is now included with *M. terrae* in a common complex. Both species grow slowly at 25 and 37°C. Colonies of *M. terrae* tend to be smoother than the rough colonies of *M. triviale;* both are nonphotochromogens. Woods and Washington (255) cited a few reported cases of human infection: septic arthritis due to *M. triviale* in an infant (52), synovitis and osteomyelitis due to *M. terrae* in a young man with Fanconi's pancytopenia, and possible disseminated *M. terrae* infection in a young woman with previous miliary tuberculosis. Rougraff et al. (186) recently reported a case of osteomyelitis and septic arthritis in a normal host. Krisher et al. (116) reported a case of pulmonary infection caused by *M. terrae* complex (136) and cited six previous cases of respiratory infection. Kremer et al. (115) reported two cases of *M. terrae* tenosynovitis of the fingers in middle-aged fishermen who incurred puncture wounds while handling crappie fins in addition to three other reported cases involving the hand (43, 74, 143).

Other Species of Clinically Important Mycobacteria

Isolated reports of human infections associated with rarely encountered mycobacterial species have been reported in the recent literature. Three cases of primary lung disease due to *M. nonchromogenicum*, a nonphotochromogen, have been reported (223), and six cases were reported by Krisher et al. (116). *M. flavescens* was recovered from bronchial washings obtained to investigate a cavitation of the left lung in an elderly man with metastatic melanoma (31). Wallace et al. (234) reported 22 human isolates of *M. smegmatis* from Australia and the United States. Three of these patients had pulmonary disease; the remaining patients had skin, soft tissue, and, in one instance, bone infections. Wallace et al. (233) also described other rapidly growing mycobacteria as a cause of post-cardiac surgery infections. *M. paratuberculosis* is the causative agent of Johne's disease, an intestinal infection of cattle, sheep, goats, and other ruminants, manifesting as chronic diarrhea and intermittent fever. Chiodini et al. (32) isolated a *Mycobacterium* species, most closely resembling *M. paratuberculosis*, from samples taken from resected terminal ileum of three patients with Crohn's disease. Saxegaard (195) reported success in the recovery of this organism from the mesenteric lymph nodes of goats (a serious disease in Norway) by use of selective Dubos medium. Selective Dubos medium is conventional Dubos medium supplemented with carbenicillin, polymyxin, trimethoprim, and amphotericin B. This medium is highly recommended for the recovery of *M. paratuberculosis* from contaminated material. Davison et al. (41) reported the recovery of *M. neoaurum* from the blood of an immunocompromised patient with an indwelling Hickman catheter. *N. neoaurum* is a rapidly growing mycobacterium found in soil, dust, and water that previously had never been reported as a human pathogen. The organism closely resembles *M. aurum* and *M. parafortuitum*, and the differential characteristics are presented in the paper cited. Recently, Linton et al. (132) reported a case of peritonitis caused by *M. gastri* in a patient undergoing ambulatory peritoneal dialysis.

This brief review points to the importance of several old and new species of mycobacteria other than members of the *M. tuberculosis* complex that have emerged as human pathogens. Clinical microbiologists must be alert to the potential recovery of these organisms from clinical specimens, particularly from patients who are immunocompromised, who are receiving corticosteroid therapy, or who have chronic conditions, particularly old pulmonary disease, that are known to predispose to mycobacterial infections. Infections in patients with AIDS may present with more rapid and miliary forms of disease, and cultures of multiple sites may be necessary, including culture of the blood, to distinguish between local and disseminated disease.

SERODIAGNOSIS

The serological diagnostic approach in the diagnosis of mycobacterial infections has been studied for a long time, and its reproducibility and reliability have been reported (159). The main obstacles encountered in serodiagnosis of mycobacterial infection are its low specificity and nonstandardization. A variety of mycobacterial antigens, including crude mycobacterial antigens, tuberculin, and purified mycobacterial antigens, were used for the detection of antibody against mycobacteria. The sensitivity and specificity of serological tests depend on what types of antigens are used. Higher specificity is achieved with a purified antigen. Serodiagnosis can be applied for the diagnosis of tuberculous meningitis; in this case, it is very difficult to culture the causative mycobacterium, and the organism is rarely detected by direct smear examination. One study showed promising results for enzyme-linked immunosorbent assay (ELISA) detecting mycobacterial antigen (192). A large-scale study will be required to verify the results. The detection of antibody against mycobacteria in cerebrospinal fluid was rather disappointing. An ELISA test indicated less than 20% of tuberculosis meningitis cases were detected when a high sensitivity was needed (40). Further studies are required for the application of serology in the field of diagnostic microbiology.

QUALITY CONTROL

An ongoing, active quality control program is essential in the mycobacteriology laboratory. Control organisms are available through proficiency testing programs, the American Type Culture Collection, and the Trudeau Mycobacterial Culture Collection based at the National Jewish Hospital and Research Center in Denver, Colo. The Trudeau Mycobacterial Culture Collection has prepared a mycobacterial Standard Taxonomic Characters Kit that is available at no charge by writing on letterhead stationery to the Curator, Mycobacterial Culture Collection, National Jewish Hospital and Research Center, 3800 East Colfax Avenue, Denver, CO 80206.

Mycobacterial cultures can be maintained on egg-based medium slants at 4°C for up to 12 months. Alternatively, the growth from several slants can be suspended in skim milk, placed in small vials, rapidly frozen in a slurry of dry ice and alcohol, and stored at −20°C or preferably −70°C. More frequently needed mycobacterial species can be maintained in Middlebrook 7H9 broth at 37°C or room temperature and can be subcultured monthly or bimonthly.

Positive control smears should be included with each set of patient specimen slides to ensure that the stain, staining procedure, and microscope are functioning properly. Smears containing mycobacteria can be made from broth cultures. The best method is to prepare a large set of smears from concentrated sputum specimens collected from patients with active tuberculosis. The staining and morphologic features of these organisms are more characteristic of organisms causing disease than are the features of organisms grown in culture. Care should be exercised in the handling of such slides, as heat fixation at 65°C for 2 h does not always inactivate mycobacteria.

Upon preparation or receipt in the laboratory, each lot of culture medium should be inoculated with stock strains of *M. tuberculosis, M. kansasii, M. avium* complex, and *M. fortuitum*. In most instances, media can be stored for 10 to 14 days, after which quality control results are available. In the case of Middlebrook 7H10 and 7H11 agars, the media can be inoculated with clinical specimen concentrates within a week of the time at which quality control organisms are inoculated, as long as clinical specimen concentrates are maintained in the refrigerator for 2 to 3 weeks afterward. Should the quality control strain not perform well on the new medium, the refrigerated concentrates can be reinoculated to another lot or a different type of medium. Storage of Middlebrook 7H10 and 7H11 media for more than 5 weeks may be associated with poor growth characteristics, since formaldehyde may form after prolonged storage or direct exposure to light (148).

Appropriate positive and negative control organisms should be included when one is testing each identification characteristic. Similarly, a selection of resistant and susceptible organisms should be inoculated onto each lot of susceptibility test medium, including a strain of *M. tuberculosis* that is susceptible to all antimycobacterial agents and a select strain of *M. kansasii* that is known to be resistant to low concentrations of isoniazid but susceptible to high concentrations. Gutheritz et al. (73) caution that different lots of commercial components that constitute the basal medium used for susceptibility testing can vary significantly and can dramatically affect test results and susceptibility profiles. They used a grading system based on the sizes (large, medium, small, and pinpoint) and number of colonies in assessing the suitability of new batches of medium. In this way, the performance of new lots can be compared with that of old lots, and appropriate corrections can be made before spurious results are reported.

In addition to observing internal quality control measures, including the use of authenticated strains of *Mycobacterium* species, laboratories should participate in mycobacterial proficiency-testing surveys. Surveys are extremely helpful in providing feedback on the ability of a laboratory to isolate and identify mycobacteria and to test for susceptibility. The surveys also provide the opportunity to compare the capabilities of a laboratory with those of its peers. Proficiency surveys are usually designed for laboratories to participate to the extent or level of service that they normally offer. This flexibility provides an opportunity for small laboratories to improve their ability to work with different species and further develop their ability to offer more advanced services without placing them at risk of licensure during a training period. Such surveys also provide a good opportunity to obtain strains of mycobacteria showing specific characteristics, e.g., unusual species or those with highly selective drug resistance patterns. It is incumbent on the laboratory directors and supervisors to see that all information pertaining to the survey samples be distributed to and discussed with those actually performing the tests so that any discrepancies can be reconciled. These discussions can be incorporated into regularly scheduled rounds so that proficiency testing becomes a truly educational experience and not a punitive exercise.

LITERATURE CITED

1. **Alberts, W. M., K. W. Chandler, D. A. Solomon, and A. L. Goldman.** 1987. Pulmonary disease caused by *Mycobacterium malmoense*. Am. Rev. Respir. Dis. **135:**1375–1378.
2. **Allen, B. W., and J. H. Darrell.** 1983. Contamination of specimen container surfaces during collection. J. Clin. Pathol. **36:**479–481.
3. **Altmann, G., A. Horowitz, N. Kaplinsky, and O. Frankl.** 1975. Prosthetic valve endocarditis due to *Mycobacterium chelonei*. J. Clin. Microbiol. **1:**531–533.
4. **Alvarez-Elcoro, S., M. Mateos-Mora, and A. Zajarias.** 1985. *Mycobacterium fortuitum* endocarditis after mitral valve replacement with a bovine prosthesis. South. Med. J. **78:**865–866.
5. **Anouchi, Y. S., and I. Froimson.** 1988. Hand infections with *Mycobacterium chelonei:* a case report and review of the literature. J. Hand Surg. **13:**331–332.
6. **Arnold, L. J., P. W. Hammond, W. A. Wiese, and N. C. Nelson.** 1989. Assay formats involving acridinium-ester-labeled DNA probes. Clin. Chem. **35:**1588–1594.
7. **Aronson, J. D.** 1926. Spontaneous tuberculosis in salt water fish. J. Infect. Dis. **39:**313–320.
8. **Aubrey, M., and A. G. Fam.** 1987. A case of clinically unsuspected *Mycobacterium marinum* infection. Arthritis Rheum. **301:**1317–1318.
9. **Ausina, V., J. Barrio, M. Luguin, M. A. Sambeat, M. Gurgui, G. Verger, and G. Prats.** 1988. *Mycobacterial xenopi* infections in AIDS. Ann. Intern. Med. **109:**927–928.
10. **Azadian, B. S., A. Beck, J. R. Curtis, L. E. Cherrington, P. E. Gower, M. Phillips, J. B. Eastwood, and J. Nicholls.** 1981. Disseminated infection with *Mycobacterium chelonei* in a hemodialysis patient. Tubercle **62:**281–284.
11. **Barnes, P. F.** 1987. Six cases of *Mycobacterium tuberculosis* bacteremia. J. Infect. Dis. **156:**377–379.
12. **Beam, E. R., and G. P. Kubica.** 1968. Stimulatory effects of carbon dioxide on the primary isolation of tubercle bacilli on agar containing medium. Am. J. Clin. Pathol. **50:**395–397.
13. **Bennett, C., J. Vardiman, and H. Golomb.** 1986. Disseminated atypical mycobacterial infection in patients with hairy cell leukemia. Am. J. Med. **80:**891–896.
14. **Berlin, O. G., P. Zakowski, D. A. Bruckner, and B. L. Johnson, Jr.** 1984. New biphasic culture system for isolation of mycobacteria from blood cultures of patients with the acquired immunodeficiency syndrome. J. Clin. Microbiol. **20:**572–574.
15. **Binford, C. H.** 1985. Leprosy, p. 322–334. *In* W. A. D. Anderson and S. M. Kissave (ed.), Pathology, 8th ed. The C. V. Mosby Co., St. Louis.
16. **Bishburg, E., G. Sunderam, L. B. Reichman, and R. Kapila.** 1986. Central nervous system tuberculosis with the acquired immune deficiency syndrome and its related complex. Ann. Intern. Med. **105:**210–213.
17. **Blake, G. C., J. J. Murray, and K. W. Lee.** 1976. Cervicofacial infection with *Mycobacterium chelonei*—a case report. Br. J. Oral Surg. **13:**278–281.
18. **Bogaerts, Y., W. Elinck, D. van Renterghem, R. Pauwels, and M. van der Straeten.** 1982. Pulmonary disease due to *Mycobacterium xenopi*. Report of two cases. Eur. J. Respir. Dis. **63:**298–304.
19. **Bolan, G., A. L. Reingold, L. A. Carson, V. A. Silcox, C. L. Woodley, P. S. Hayes, A. W. Hightower, and L. McFarland.** 1985. Infections with *Mycobacterium chelonei* in patients receiving dialysis and using processed hemodialyzers. J. Infect. Dis. **152:**1013–1019.

20. **Bönicke, R.** 1958. Die Differenzierung humaner und boviner Tuberkelterien mit Hilfe von Thiophen-2-carbonsaure-hydrazid. Naturwissenschaften **46:**392–393.
21. **Borghans, J. G., and J. L. Stanford.** 1973. *Mycobacterium chelonei* in abscesses after injection of diphtheria-pertussis-tetanus-polio vaccine. Am. Rev. Respir. Dis. **107:** 1–8.
22. **Boyd, J. C., and J. J. Marr.** 1975. Decreasing reliability of acid-fast smear techniques for detection of tuberculosis. Ann. Intern. Med. **82:**489–492.
23. **Brannan, D. P., R. E. DuBois, M. J. Ramirez, M. J. Ravry, and E. O. Harrison.** 1984. Cefoxitin therapy for *Mycobacterium fortuitum* bacteremia with associated granulomatous hepatitis. South. Med. J. **77:**381–384.
24. **Brennan, P. J., M. Heifets, and B. P. Ullom.** 1982. Thin-layer chromatography of lipid antigens as a means of identifying nontuberculous mycobacteria. J. Clin. Microbiol. **15:**447–455.
25. **Buhler, V. B., and A. Pollak.** 1953. Human infection with atypical acid-fast organisms. Am. J. Clin. Pathol. **23:** 363–374.
26. **Burchard, G. D., and M. Bierther.** 1986. Buruli ulcer: clinical pathological study of 23 patients in Lambarene, Gabon. Trop. Med. Parasitol. **37:**1–8.
27. **Burdash, N. M., J. P. Manos, D. Ross, and E. R. Bannister.** 1976. Evaluation of the acid-fast smear. J. Clin. Microbiol. **4:**190–191.
28. **Butler, W. R., D. G. Ahearn, and J. O. Kilburn.** 1986. High-performance liquid chromatography of mycolic acids as a tool in the identification of *Corynebacterium, Nocardia, Rhodococcus,* and *Mycobacterium* species. J. Clin. Microbiol. **23:**182–185.
29. **Carpenter, J. L., M. Troxell, and R. J. Wallace, Jr.** 1984. Disseminated disease due to *Mycobacterium chelonei* treated with amikacin and cefoxitin. Abscess of killing with either agent and possible role of granulocytes in clinical response. Arch. Intern. Med. **144:**2063–2065.
30. **Casal, M. J., and F. C. Rodriguez.** 1981. Simple, new test for rapid differentiation of the *Mycobacterium fortuitum* complex. J. Clin. Microbiol. **13:**989–990.
31. **Casimir, M. T., V. Fainstein, and N. Papadopolous.** 1982. Cavitary lung infection caused by *Mycobacterium flavescens.* South. Med. J. **75:**253–254.
32. **Chiodini, R. J., H. J. VanKruiningen, R. S. Merkal, W. R. Thayer, Jr., and J. A. Couta.** 1984. Characteristics of an unclassified *Mycobacterium* species isolated from patients with Crohn's disease. J. Clin. Microbiol. **20:**966–971.
33. **Clegg, H. W., M. T. Foster, W. E. Sanders, Jr., and W. B. Baine.** 1983. Infection due to organisms of the *Mycobacterium fortuitum* complex after augmentation mammoplasty: clinical and epidemiologic features. J. Infect. Dis. **147:**427–433.
34. **Connolly, M. J., J. G. Magee, D. J. Hendrick, and P. A. Jenkins.** 1985. *Mycobacterium malmoense* in the north-east of England. Tubercle **66:**211–217.
35. **Contreras, M. A., O. T. Cheung, D. E. Sanders, and R. S. Goldstien.** 1988. Pulmonary infections with non-tuberculous mycobacteria. Am. Rev. Respir. Dis. **137:**149–152.
36. **Conville, P. S., J. F. Keiser, and F. G. Witebsky.** 1989. Comparison of three techniques for concentrating positive BACTEC 13A bottles for mycobacterial DNA probe analysis. Diagn. Microbiol. Infect. Dis. **12:**309–313.
37. **Cooper, J. F., M. J. Lichtenstein, B. S. Graham, and W. Schaffner.** 1989. *Mycobacterium chelonae:* a cause of nodular skin lesions with a proclivity for renal transplant recipients. Am. J. Med. **86:**173–177.
38. **Corper, H. J., and N. Uyei.** 1930. Oxalic acid as a reagent for isolating tubercle bacilli and a study of the growth of acid-fast nonpathogens on different mediums with their reactions to chemical reagents. J. Lab. Clin. Med. **15:**348–369.
39. **Daniel, T. M.** 1989. Rapid diagnosis of tuberculosis: laboratory techniques applicable in developing countries. Rev. Infect. Dis. **11**(Suppl.)**:**S471–S478.
40. **Daniel, T. M., and S. M. Debanne.** 1987. The serodiagnosis of tuberculosis and other mycobacterial diseases by enzyme-linked immunosorbant assay. Am. Rev. Respir. Dis. **135:**1137–1151.
41. **Davison, M. B., J. G. McCormack, Z. M. Blacklock, D. J. Dawson, M. H. Tilse, and F. B. Crimmins.** 1988. Bacteremia caused by *Mycobacterium neoaurum.* J. Clin. Microbiol. **26:**762–764.
42. **Dawson, D. J., Z. M. Blacklock, and D. W. Kane.** 1981. *Mycobacterium haemophilum* causing lymphadenitis in an otherwise healthy child. Med. J. Aust. **2:**289–290.
43. **Deenstra, W.** 1988. Synovial hand infection from *Mycobacterium terrae.* J. Hand Surg. **13:**335–336.
44. **Dixon, J. M. S., and E. H. Cuthbert.** 1967. Isolation of tubercle bacilli from uncentrifuged sputum on pyruvic acid medium. Am. Rev. Respir. Dis. **96:**119–122.
45. **Dizon, D., C. Mihailescu, and H. C. Bae.** 1976. Simple procedure for detection of *Mycobacterium gordonae* in water causing false-positive acid-fast smears. J. Clin. Microbiol. **3:**211.
46. **Dornetzhuber, V., R. Martis, B. Burjanova, K. Pavukova, M. Turzova, and M. Vincurova.** 1982. Pulmonary mycobacteriosis caused by *Mycobacterium xenopi.* Report of a case. Eur. J. Respir. Dis. **63:**293–297.
47. **Douglas, J. G., M. A. Calder, Y. F. Choo-Kang, and A. G. Leitch.** 1986. *Mycobacterium gordonae:* a new pathogen? Thorax **4:**152–153.
48. **Drake, T. A., J. A. Hindler, O. G. W. Berlin, and D. Bruckner.** 1987. Rapid identification of *Mycobacterium avium* complex in culture using DNA probes. J. Clin. Microbiol. **25:**1442–1445.
49. **Dugdale, D. C., D. Stevens, and L. L. Knight.** 1989. Mycotic aneurysm and disseminated *Mycobacterium avium-intracellulare* infection in a patient with hairy cell leukemia. West. J. Med. **150:**207–208.
50. **Dylewski, J. S., H. M. Zackon, A. H. Latour, and G. R. Berry.** 1987. *Mycobacterium szulgai:* an unusual pathogen. Rev. Infect. Dis. **9:**578–580.
51. **Ellner, P. D., T. E. Kiehn, R. Cammarata, and M. Hosmer.** 1988. Rapid detection and identification of pathogenic mycobacteria by combining radiometric and nucleic acid probe methods. J. Clin. Microbiol. **26:**1349–1352.
52. **Elting, J. J., and W. O. Southwick.** 1974. Acute infantile septic arthritis of the hip due to *Mycobacterium triviale.* A case report. J. Bone Joint Surg. **56:**184–186.
53. **Fierer, J., and R. Merino.** 1975. Acid-fast smears and tuberculosis. Ann. Intern. Med. **83:**430–431.
54. **Feinberg, K. A., and S. S. Schneierson.** 1969. Disseminated infection by *Mycobacterium fortuitum.* J. Mt. Sinai Hosp. N.Y. **36:**375–379.
55. **Fisher, A. A.** 1988. Swimming pool granulomas due to *Mycobacterium marinum:* an occupational hazard of lifeguards. Cutis **41:**397–398.
56. **Fonseca, E., C. Alzate, T. Cannedo, and F. Contreras.** 1987. Nodular lesions in disseminated *Mycobacterium fortuitum* infection. Arch. Dermatol. **123:**1603–1604.
57. **Foote, W. C., and B. F. Polk.** 1974. Endobronchitis and *Mycobacterium fortuitum.* Ann. Intern. Med. **80:**272–273.
58. **France, A. J., D. T. McLeod, M. A. Calder, and A. Seaton.** 1987. *Mycobacterium malmoense* infections in Scotland: an increasing problem. Thorax **42:**593–595.
59. **Gallo, J. H., G. A. Young, P. R. Forrest, P. C. Vincent, and F. Jennis.** 1983. Disseminated atypical mycobacterial infection in hairy cell leukemia. Pathology **15:**241–245.
60. **Gengoux, P., F. Portaels, J. M. Lachapelle, D. E. Minnikin, D. Tennstedt, and P. Tamigneau.** 1987. Skin granulomas due to *Mycobacterium gordonae.* Int. J. Dermatol. **26:**181–184.
61. **Gill, M. J., E. A. Fanning, and S. Chomyc.** 1987. Child-

hood lymphadenitis in a harsh northern climate due to atypical mycobacteria. Scand. J. Infect. Dis. **19:**77–83.

62. **Gill, V. J., C. H. Park, F. Stock, L. Gosey, F. G. Witebsky, and H. Masur.** 1985. Use of lysis-centrifugation (Isolator) and radiometric (BACTEC) blood culture systems for the detection of mycobacteria. J. Clin. Microbiol. **22:**543–546.
63. **Gillin, J. S., C. Urmacher, R. West, and M. Shike.** 1983. Disseminated *Mycobacterium avium-intracellulare* infection in acquired immunodeficiency syndrome mimicking Whipple's disease. Gastroenterology **85:**1187–1191.
64. **Godal, T., and L. Levy.** 1984. *Mycobacterium leprae,* p. 1083–1128. *In* G. P. Kubica and L. G. Wayne (ed.), The mycobacteria—a sourcebook. Marcel Dekker, Inc., New York.
65. **Gonzalez, R., and B. A. Hanna.** 1987. Evaluation of Gen-Probe DNA hybridization systems for the identification of *Mycobacteria tuberculosis* and *Mycobacterium avium-intracellulare.* Diagn. Microbiol. Infect. Dis. **8:**69–78.
66. **Good, R. C., V. A. Silcox, J. O. Kilburn, and B. D. Plikaytis.** 1985. Identification and drug susceptibility test results for *Mycobacterium* spp. Clin. Microbiol. Newsl. **7:** 133–135.
67. **Good, R. C., and D. E. Snider.** 1982. Isolation of nontuberculous mycobacteria in the United States. 1980. J. Infect. Dis. **146:**829–833.
68. **Gouby, A., B. Branger, R. Oules, and M. Ramuz.** 1988. Two cases of *Mycobacterium haemophilum* infection in a renal dialysis unit. J. Med. Microbiol. **25:**299–300.
69. **Gremillion, D. H., S. B. Mursch, and C. J. Lerner.** 1983. Injection site abscesses caused by *Mycobacterium chelonei.* Infect. Control **4:**25–28.
70. **Gross, W. M., and J. E. Hawkins.** 1985. Radiometric selective inhibition tests for differentiation of *Mycobacterium tuberculosis, Mycobacterium bovis* and other mycobacteria. J. Clin. Microbiol. **21:**565–568.
71. **Gruft, H., D. Blanchard, and J. Wheeler.** 1976. Ocean waters a source of *Mycobacterium intracellulare.* Am. Rev. Respir. Dis. **113**(no. 4, part 2):60.
72. **Guarderas, J., S. Alvarez, and S. L. Berk.** 1986. Progressive pulmonary disease caused by *Mycobacterium gordonae.* South. Med. J. **79:**505–507.
73. **Gutheritz, L. S., M. E. Griffith, E. G. Ford, J. M. Janda, and T. F. Midura.** 1988. Quality control of individual components used in Middlebrook 7H11 medium for mycobacterial susceptibility testing. J. Clin. Microbiol. **26:** 2338–2342.
74. **Halla, J. T., J. S. Gould, and J. G. Hardin.** 1979. Chronic tenosynovial hand infection from *Mycobacterium terrae.* Arthritis Rheum. **22:**1386–1390.
75. **Hampson, S. J., J. J. McFadden, and J. Hermon-Taylor.** 1988. Mycobacteria and Crohn's disease. Gut **29:**1017–1019.
76. **Hanson, P. J. V., J. M. Thomas, and J. V. Collins.** 1987. *Mycobacterium chelonei* and abscess formation in soft tissue. Tubercle **68:**297–299.
77. **Hawkins, C. C., J. W. M. Gold, E. Whimbey, T. E. Kiehn, P. Brannon, R. Cammarata, A. E. Brown, and D. Armstrong.** 1986. *Mycobacterium avium* complex infections in patients with the acquired immune deficiency syndrome. Ann. Intern. Med. **105:**184–188.
78. **Hawkins, J. E.** 1977. Scotochromogenic mycobacteria which appear intermediate between *Mycobacterium avium-intracellulare* and *Mycobacterium scrofulaceum.* Am. Rev. Respir. Dis. **116:**963–964.
79. **Hendrick, S. L., J. L. Jorizzo, and R. C. Newton.** 1986. Giant *Mycobacterium fortuitum* abscess associated with systemic lupus erythematosus. Arch. Dermatol. **122:**695–697.
80. **Hing, D. C., J. F. Delohery, and M. R. Abbott.** 1983. Multifocal osteomyelitis caused by *Mycobacterium chelonei.* A therapeutic dilemma. Med. J. Aust. **1:**529–531.
81. **Hoffman, G. S., R. L. Myers, F. R. Stark, and C. O. Thoen.** 1978. Septic arthritis associated with *Mycobacterium avium:* a case report and literature review. J. Rheumatol. **5:**199–209.
82. **Holzman, R. S., P. C. Hopewell, A. E. Pitchenik, L. B. Reichman, and R. L. Stoneburner.** 1987. Diagnosis and management of mycobacterial infection and disease in persons with human immune deficiency virus infection. Ann. Intern. Med. **106:**254–256.
83. **Horak, Z., H. Polakova, and M. Kralova.** 1986. Water-borne *Mycobacterium xenopi*—a possible cause of pulmonary mycobacteriosis in man. J. Hyg. Epidemiol. Microbiol. Immunol. **30:**405–409.
84. **Hornick, D. B., C. S. Dayton, G. N. Bedell, and R. B. Fick, Jr.** 1988. Nontuberculous mycobacterial lung disease. Substantiation of a less aggressive approach. Chest **93:**550–555.
85. **Horsburgh, C. R., Jr., U. G. Mason III, D. C. Farhi, and M. D. Iseman.** 1985. Disseminated infection with *Mycobacterium avium-intracellulare.* A report of 13 cases and review of the literature. Medicine **64:**36–48.
86. **Hoy, J. F., K. V. Rolston, R. L. Hopfer, and G. P. Bodey.** 1987. *Mycobacterium fortuitum* bacteremia in patients with cancer and long-term venous catheters. Am. J. Med. **83:**213–217.
87. **Igo, J. D., and D. P. Murthy.** 1988. *Mycobacterium ulcerans* infection in Papua New Guinea: correlation of clinical, histological and microbiologic features. Am. J. Trop. Med. Hyg. **38:**391–392.
88. **Jauregui, L., A. Arbulu, and F. Wilson.** 1977. Osteomyelitis, pericarditis, mediastinitis, and vasculitis due to *Mycobacterium chelonei.* Am. Rev. Respir. Dis. **115:**699–703.
89. **Jenkin, D. J., and G. Dall.** 1975. Lesions of bone in disseminated infection due to the *Mycobacterium avium-intracellulare* group. Report of case. J. Bone Joint Surg. **57:**373–375.
90. **Jenkins, P. A.** 1981. The epidemiology of opportunist mycobacterial infections in Wales, 1952–1978. Rev. Infect. Dis. **3:**1021–1023.
91. **Jenkins, P. A.** 1985. *Mycobacterium malmoense.* Tubercle **66:**193–195.
92. **Jenkins, P. A., and M. Tsukamura.** 1979. Infections with *Mycobacterium malmoense* in England and Wales. Tubercle **60:**71–76.
93. **Jiminez, J., and L. Larsson.** 1986. Heating cells in acid methanol for 30 minutes without freeze-drying provides adequate yields of fatty acids and alcohols for gas chromatographic characterization of mycobacteria. J. Clin. Microbiol. **24:**844–845.
94. **Johnston, J. M., and A. K. Izumi.** 1987. Cutaneous *Mycobacterium marinum* infection ("swimming pool granuloma"). Clin. Dermatol. **5:**68–75.
95. **Jones, M. W., I. A. Wahid, and L. P. Mattews.** 1988. Septic arthritis of the hand due to *Mycobacterium marinum.* J. Hand Surg. **13:**333–334.
96. **Jones, W. D., and G. P. Kubica.** 1964. The use of MacConkey's agar for differential typing of *Mycobacterium fortuitum.* Am. J. Med. Technol. **30:**187–195.
97. **Kaplinsky, N., A. Pines, A. Mazar, and G. Altman.** 1982. Gonarthritis due to *Mycobacterium chelonei.* Rheumatol. Rehabil. **21:**158–160.
98. **Karassova, V., J. Weiszfeiler, and Krasznay.** 1965. Occurrence of atypical mycobacteria in macacus rhesus. Acta Microbiol. Acad. Sci. Hung. **12:**275–282.
99. **Katila, M. L., E. Brander, and A. Backman.** 1987. Neonatal BCG vaccination and mycobacterial cervical adenitis in childhood. Tubercle **68:**291–296.
100. **Kestle, D. G., V. D. Abbott, and G. P. Kubica.** 1967. Differential identification of mycobacteria. II. Subgroups of groups II and II (Runyon) with different clinical significance. Am. Rev. Respir. Dis. **95:**1041–1052.
101. **Kiehn, T. E., and R. Cammarata.** 1986. Laboratory diagnosis of mycobacterial infections in patients with ac-

centrifugal force and centrifugation time on sedimentation of mycobacteria in clinical specimens. J. Clin. Microbiol. **23**:582–585.

180. **Ratnam, S., F. A. Stead, and M. Howes.** 1987. Simplified acetylcysteine-alkali digestion-decontamination procedure for isolation of mycobacteria from clinical specimens. J. Clin. Microbiol. **25**:1428–1432.
181. **Rickman, T. W., and N. P. Moyer.** 1980. Increased sensitivity of acid-fast smears. J. Clin. Microbiol. **11**:618–620.
182. **Roberts, G. D., N. L. Goodman, L. Heifets, H. W. Larsh, T. H. Lindner, J. K. McClatchy, M. R. McGinnis, S. H. Siddiqi, and P. Wright.** 1983. Evaluation of the BACTEC radiometric method for recovery of mycobacteria and drug susceptibility testing of *Mycobacterium tuberculosis* from acid-fast smear-positive specimens. J. Clin. Microbiol. **18**:689–696.
183. **Robicsek, F., H. K. Daugherty, J. W. Cook, J. G. Selle, and T. N. Masters.** 1978. *Mycobacterium fortuitum* epidemics after open-heart surgery. J. Thorac. Cardiovasc. Surg. **75**:91–96.
184. **Rogers, P. L., R. E. Walker, H. C. Lane, F. G. Witebsky, J. A. Kovacs, J. E. Parrillo, and H. Masur.** 1988. Disseminated *Mycobacterium haemophilum* infection in two patients with the acquired immunodeficiency syndrome. Am. J. Med. **84**:640–642.
185. **Rolston, K. V., P. G. Jones, V. Feinstein, and G. P. Bodey.** 1985. Pulmonary disease caused by rapidly growing mycobacteria in patients with cancer. Chest **87**: 503–506.
186. **Rougraff, B. T., C. C. Reeck, and T. G. Slama.** 1989. *Mycobacterium terrae* osteomyelitis and septic arthritis in a normal host. Clin. Orthop. **238**:308–310.
187. **Roussel, T. J., W. H. Stern, D. F. Goodman, and J. P. Whitcher.** 1989. Postoperative mycobacterial endophthalmitis. Am. J. Ophthalmol. **107**:403–406.
188. **Runyon, E. H.** 1959. Anonymous mycobacteria in pulmonary disease. Med. Clin. N. Am. **43**:273–290.
189. **Runyon, E. H.** 1970. Identification of mycobacterial pathogens using colony characteristics. Am. J. Clin. Pathol. **54**:578–586.
190. **Runyon, E. H.** 1972. Identification of acid-fast pathogens utilizing colony characteristics, 3rd ed. Veterans Administration, Salt Lake City, Utah.
191. **Runyon, E. H., M. J. Selin, and H. W. Harris.** 1959. Distinguishing mycobacteria by the niacin test. Am. Rev. Tuberc. Pulm. Dis. **79**:663–665.
192. **Sada, E., G. M. Ruiz-Palacios, Y. Lopez-Vidal, and S. Ponce de Leon.** 1983. Detection of mycobacterial antigens in cerebrospinal fluid of patients with tuberculous meningitis by enzyme-linked immunosorbent assay. Lancet **ii**:651–652.
193. **Safranek, T. J., W. R. Jarvis, L. A. Carson, L. B. Cusick, L. A. Bland, J. M. Swenson, and V. A. Silcox.** 1987. *Mycobacterium chelonae* wound infections after plastic surgery employing contaminated gentian violet skin-marking solution. N. Engl. J. Med. **317**:197–201.
194. **Santa-Cruz, D. J., and D. S. Strayer.** 1982. The histologic spectrum of the cutaneous mycobacterioses. Hum. Pathol. **13**:485–495.
195. **Saxegaard, F.** 1985. Isolation of *Mycobacterium paratuberculosis* from intestinal mucosa and mesenteric lymph nodes of goats by use of selective Dubos medium. J. Clin. Microbiol. **22**:312–313.
196. **Scherer, R., R. Sable, M. Sonnenberg, S. Cooper, P. Spencer, S. Schwimmer, F. Kocka, P. Muthuswamy, and C. Kallick.** 1986. Disseminated infection with *Mycobacterium kansasii* in the acquired immunodeficiency syndrome. Ann. Intern. Med. **105**:710–712.
197. **Schröder, K. H., and I. Juhlin.** 1977. *Mycobacterium malmoense* sp. nov. Int. J. Syst. Bacteriol. **27**:241–246.
198. **Shelley, W. B., and A. T. Folkens.** 1984. *Mycobacterium gordonae* infection of the hand. Arch. Dermatol. **120**: 1064–1065.
199. **Silcox, V. A., R. A. Good, and M. M. Floyd.** 1981. Identification of clinically significant *Mycobacterium fortuitum complex* isolates. J. Clin. Microbiol. **14**:686–691.
200. **Simor, A. E., I. E. Salit, and H. Vellend.** 1984. The role of *Mycobacterium xenopi* in human disease. Am. Rev. Respir. Dis. **129**:435–438.
201. **Smith, E. R.** 1976. *Mycobacterium fortuitum* spinal infection: case report. Pathology **8**:289–292.
202. **Smith, R. E., J. J. Salz, R. Moors, D. Silverstein, and W. Lewis.** 1980. *Mycobacterium chelonei* and orbital granuloma after tear duct probing. Am. J. Ophthalmol. **89**:139–141.
203. **Smithwick, R. W., C. B. Stratigos, and H. L. David.** 1975. Use of cetylpyridinium chloride and sodium chloride for the decontamination of sputum specimens that are transported to the laboratory for the isolation of *Mycobacterium tuberculosis*. J. Clin. Microbiol. **1**:411–413.
204. **Sommers, H. M., J. K. McClatchy, and J. A. Monella.** 1983. Cumitech 16, Laboratory diagnosis of the mycobacterioses. Coordinating ed., H. M. Sommers and J. K. McClatchy. American Society for Microbiology, Washington, D.C.
205. **Sompolinsky, D., A. Lagziel, D. Naveh, and T. Yankilevitz.** 1978. *Mycobacterium haemophilum* sp. nov., a new pathogen of humans. Int. J. Syst. Bacteriol. **28**:67–75.
206. **Sopko, J. A., J. Fieselmann, and J. E. Kasik.** 1980. Pulmonary disease due to *Mycobacterium chelonei* subspecies abscessus: a report of four cases. Tubercle **61**:165–169.
207. **Spark, R. P., and M. L. Fried.** 1988. Negative BACTEC 460 TB cultures: how long to incubate. Am. J. Clin. Pathol. **90**:213–215.
208. **Sriyabhaya, N., and S. Wongwatana.** 1981. Pulmonary infection caused by atypical mycobacteria: a report of 24 cases in Thailand. Rev. Infect. Dis. **3**:1085–1089.
209. **Stager, C. E., J. R. Davis, and S. H. Siddiqi.** 1988. Identification of *Mycobacterium tuberculosis* in sputum by direct inoculation of the BACTEC NAP vial. Diagn. Microbiol. Infect. Dis. **10**:67–73.
210. **Steadham, J. E.** 1979. Reliable urease test for identification of mycobacteria. J. Clin. Microbiol. **10**:134–137.
211. **Steele, L. C., and R. J. Wallace, Jr.** 1987. Ability of ciprofloxacin but not pipemidic acid to differentiate all three biovariants of *Mycobacterium fortuitum* from *Mycobacterium chelonae*. J. Clin. Microbiol. **25**:456–457.
212. **Stottmeier, K. D.** 1975. Acid-fast smears and tuberculosis. Ann. Intern. Med. **83**:429–430.
213. **Stratton, C. W., D. B. Phelps, and L. B. Reller.** 1978. Tuberculoid tenosynovitis and carpal tunnel syndrome caused by *Mycobacterium szulgai*. Am. J. Med. **65**:349–351.
214. **Strumpf, I. J., A. Y. Tsang, and J. W. Sayre.** 1979. Reevaluation of sputum staining for the diagnosis of pulmonary tuberculosis. Am. Rev. Respir. Dis. **119**:599–602.
215. **Sutker, W. L., L. L. Lankford, and R. Tompsett.** 1979. Granulomatous synovitis: the role of atypical mycobacteria. Rev. Infect. Dis. **1**:729–735.
216. **Tellis, C. J., C. R. Beechler, D. K. Ohashi, and S. A. Fuller.** 1977. Pulmonary disease caused by *Mycobacterium xenopi:* two case reports. Am. Rev. Respir. Dis. **116**: 779–783.
217. **Tempero, M. A., and P. W. Smith.** 1981. Disseminated *Mycobacterium kansasii* presenting with skin lesions in a patient with chronic lymphocytic leukemia. Med. Pediatr. Oncol. **9**:283–288.
218. **Tisdall, P. A., D. R. DeYoung, G. D. Roberts, and J. P. Anhalt.** 1982. Identification of clinical isolates of mycobacteria with gas-liquid chromatography: a 10-month follow-up study. J. Clin. Microbiol. **16**:400–402.
219. **Tisdall, P. A., G. D. Roberts, and J. P. Anhalt.** 1979. Identification of clinical isolates of mycobacteria with gas-liquid chromatography alone. J. Clin. Microbiol. **10**: 506–514.

220. **Toda, T., Y. Hagihara, and K. Takeya.** 1960. A simple urease test for the classification of mycobacteria. Am. Rev. Respir. Dis. **83:**757–761.
221. **Tsukamura, M.** 1966. Adasonian classification of mycobacteria. J. Gen. Microbiol. **45:**253–273.
222. **Tsukamura, M.** 1981. Numerical analysis of rapidly growing, nonphotochromogenic mycobacteria including *Mycobacterium agri* (Tsukamura 1972) Tsukamura sp. nov., nom. rev. Int. J. Syst. Bacteriol. **31:**247–258.
223. **Tsukamura, M., N. Kita, W. Otsuka, and H. Shimoide.** 1983. A study of the taxonomy of the *Mycobacterium nonchromogenicum* complex and report of six cases of lung infection due to *Mycobacterium nonchromogenicum*. Microbiol. Immunol. **27:**219–236.
224. **Tsukamura, M., N. Kita, H. Shimoide, H. Arakawa, and A. Kuze.** 1988. Studies on the epidemiology of nontuberculous mycobacteriosis in Japan. Am. Rev. Respir. Dis. **137:**1280–1284.
225. **Tsukamura, M., K. Sekine, A. Yokota, A. Kuze, M. Shibata, and K. Sato.** 1984. Lung infection due to *Mycobacterium xenopi:* report of the first case in Japan. Microbiol. Immunol. **28:**123–127.
226. **Tsukamura, M., H. Shimoide, N. Kita, K. Kawakami, T. Ito, N. Nakajima, N. Kondo, and Y. Yamamoto.** 1981. Epidemiologic studies of lung disease due to mycobacteria other than *Mycobacterium tuberculosis* in Japan. Rev. Infect. Dis. **3:**997–1007.
227. **Umeki, S.** 1989. A case of *Mycobacterium scrofulaceum* lung infection occurring in old lung tuberculosis lesion. Kekkaku **64:**31–35.
228. **Vadney, F. S., and J. E. Hawkins.** 1985. Evaluation of a simple method for growing *Mycobacterium haemophilum*. J. Clin. Microbiol. **22:**884–885.
229. **Valdivia, A., J. S. Mendez, and M. E. Font.** 1971. *Mycobacterium habana:* probable nueva especie dentro dellas microbacterias no classificadas. Bol. Hig. Epidemiol. **9:**65–73.
230. **Valliere, W. E., and J. T. Griffith.** 1979. Pericarditis due to *Mycobacterium tuberculosis* and *Mycobacterium fortuitum:* a case report. Am. J. Med. Technol. **45:**31–33.
231. **Vannier, A. M., J. J. Tarrand, and P. R. Murray.** 1988. Mycobacterial cross contamination during radiometric culturing. J. Clin. Microbiol. **26:**1867–1868.
232. **Virtanen, S.** 1960. A study of nitrate reduction by mycobacteria. Acta Tuberc. Scand. Suppl. **48:**1–119.
233. **Wallace, R. J., Jr., J. M. Musser, S. I. Hull, V. A. Silcox, L. C. Stelle, G. D. Forrester, A. Labidi, and R. K. Selander.** 1989. Diversity and sources of rapidly growing mycobacteria associated with infection following cardiac surgery. J. Infect. Dis. **159:**708–716.
234. **Wallace, R. J., Jr., D. R. Nash, M. Tsukamura, Z. M. Blacklock, and V. A. Silcox.** 1988. Human disease due to *Mycobacterium smegmatis*. J. Infect. Dis. **158:**52–59.
235. **Wallace, R. J., Jr., J. M. Swenson, V. A. Silcox, and R. C. Good.** 1982. Disk diffusion testing with polymyxin and amikacin for differentiation of *Mycobacterium fortuitum* and *Mycobacterium chelonei*. J. Clin. Microbiol. **16:**1003–1006.
236. **Wallace, R. J., Jr., J. M. Swenson, V. A. Silcox, R. C. Good, J. A. Tschen, and M. S. Stone.** 1983. Spectrum of disease due to rapidly growing mycobacteria. Rev. Infect. Dis. **5:**657–679.
237. **Warren, N. G., B. A. Body, and H. P. Dalton.** 1983. An improved reagent for mycobacterial nitrate reductase tests. J. Clin. Microbiol. **18:**546–549.
238. **Warren, N. G., B. A. Body, V. A. Silcox, and J. H. Mattews.** 1984. Pulmonary disease due to *Mycobacterium malmoense*. J. Clin. Microbiol. **20:**245–247.
239. **Wayne, L. G.** 1961. Recognition of *Mycobacterium fortuitum* by means of the three-day phenophthalein sulfatase test. Am. J. Clin. Pathol. **36:**185–187.
240. **Wayne, L. G.** 1974. Simple pyrazinamidase and urease tests for routine identification of mycobacteria. Am. Rev. Respir. Dis. **109:**147–151.
241. **Wayne, L. G., and J. R. Doubek.** 1964. The role of air in the photochromogenic behavior of *Mycobacterium kansasii*. Am. J. Clin. Pathol. **42:**431–435.
242. **Wayne, L. G., and J. R. Doubek.** 1968. Diagnostic key to mycobacteria encountered in clinical laboratories. Appl. Microbiol. **16:**925–931.
243. **Wayne, L. G., J. R. Doubek, and R. L. Russell.** 1964. Tests employing Tween 80 as substrate. Am. Rev. Respir. Dis. **90:**588–597.
244. **Wayne, L. G., and G. P. Kubica.** 1986. Family *Mycobacteriaceae* Chester, p. 1436–1457. *In* P. H. A. Sneath, N. S. Mair, M. E. Sharpe, and J. G. Holt (ed.), Bergey's manual of systematic bacteriology, vol. 2. The Williams & Wilkins Co., Baltimore.
245. **Weinberg, J. R., G. Dootson, D. Gertner, S. T. Chambers, and H. Smith.** 1985. Disseminated *Mycobacterium xenopi* infection. Lancet **i:**1033–1034.
246. **Weiszfeiler, J. G., and E. Karczag.** 1971. Synonymy of *Mycobacterium simiae* Karasseva et al., 1965 and *Mycobacterium habana* Valdivia et al. Int. J. Syst. Bacteriol. **26:**474–477.
247. **Weitzman, I., D. Osadczyi, M. L. Corrado, and D. Karp.** 1981. *Mycobacterium thermoresistibile:* a new pathogen for humans. J. Clin. Microbiol. **14:**593–595.
248. **Wilkins, E. G. L., R. J. Griffiths, and C. Roberts.** 1986. Pulmonary tuberculosis due to *Mycobacterium bovis*. Thorax **41:**685–687.
249. **Willemse, T., D. G. Groothuis, J. P. Koeman, and E. G. Beyer.** 1985. *Mycobacterium thermoresistibile:* extrapulmonary infection in a cat. J. Clin. Microbiol. **21:** 854–856.
250. **Willis, W. E., and P. R. Laibson.** 1971. Intractable *Mycobacterium fortuitum* corneal ulcer in man. Am. J. Ophthalmol. **7:**500–504.
251. **Witebsky, F. G., J. Keiser, P. Conville, R. Bryan, C. H. Park, R. Walker, and S. H. Siddiqi.** 1988. Comparison of BACTEC 13A medium and Du Pont Isolator for detection of mycobacteremia. J. Clin. Microbiol. **26:**1501–1505.
252. **Wolinski, E.** 1979. Nontuberculous mycobacteria and associated diseases. Am. Rev. Respir. Dis. **119:**107–159.
253. **Woods, G. L., and J. C. Goldsmith.** 1989. Fatal pericarditis due to *Mycobacterium avium-intracellulare* in acquired immunodeficiency syndrome. Chest **95:**1355–1357.
254. **Woods, G. L., G. S. Hall, and M. J. Schreiber.** 1986. *Mycobacterium fortuitum* peritonitis associated with continuous ambulatory peritoneal dialysis. J. Clin. Microbiol. **23:**786–788.
255. **Woods, G. L., and J. A. Washington II.** 1987. Mycobacteria other than *Mycobacterium tuberculosis:* review of microbiologic and clinical aspects. Rev. Infect. Dis. **9:** 275–294.
256. **Woolcock, W. J., and D. J. Dawson.** 1979. Pulmonary disease caused by *Mycobacterium xenopi* in an Australian man. Med. J. Aust. **25:**175–177.
257. **Wrzolek, M. A., C. Rao, P. B. Kozlowski, and J. H. Sher.** 1989. Muscle and nerve involvement in AIDS patient with disseminated *Mycobacterium avium intracellulare* infection. Muscle Nerve **12:**247–249.
258. **Wunsh, S. E., G. L. Byle, I. H. Leopold, and M. L. Littman.** 1969. *Mycobacterium fortuitum* infection of corneal graft. Arch. Ophthalmol. **82:**602–607.
259. **Yamauchi, T., P. Ferrieri, and B. F. Anthony.** 1980. The aetiology of acute cervical adenitis in children: serological and bacteriological studies. J. Med. Microbiol. **13:**37–43.
260. **Yew, W. W., S. Y. Kwan, W. K. Ma, M. Aung-Khin, and C. K. Mok.** 1989. Combination of ofloxacin and amikacin in the treatment of sternotomy wound infection. Chest **95:**1051–1055.
261. **Young, L. S.** 1987. *Mycobacterium avium* complex infection. J. Infect. Dis. **157:**863–867.

262. **Young, L. S., C. B. Interlied, O. G. Berlin, and M. S. Gottlieb.** 1986. Mycobacterial infections in AIDS patients with emphasis on the *Mycobacterium avium* complex. Rev. Infect. Dis. **8:**1024–1033.

263. **Young, W. D., Jr., A. Maslansky, M. S. Lefar, and D. P. Kronish.** 1970. Development of a paper strip test for detection of niacin produced by mycobacteria. Appl. Microbiol. **20:**939–945.

264. **Zabel, R. W., G. Mintsioulis, and I. MacConald.** 1988. *Mycobacterium chelonei* keratitis in a soft contact lens wearer. Can. J. Ophthalmol. **23:**315–317.

265. **Zachary, L. S., G. L. Clark, Jr., J. M. Kleinert, and C. O'Donovan.** 1988. *Mycobacterium chelonei* tenosynovitis. Ann. Plast. Surg. **20:**360–362.

Chapter 35

Aerobic Pathogenic *Actinomycetales*

GEOFFREY LAND, MICHAEL R. McGINNIS, JOSEPH STANECK, AND ALICE GATSON

INTRODUCTION

The aerobic actinomycetes are catalase-producing, diphtheroidlike to branched filamentous bacteria belonging to the order *Actinomycetales* (32, 52, 64, 66). They may aggregate as a rudimentary to well-developed mycelium with or without aerial hyphae (11, 86). Although the actinomycetes superficially resemble true fungi both microscopically and macroscopically, they exhibit cellular characteristics of bacteria, including the presence of enantiomers of diaminopimelic acid in their cell wall and procaryotic cellular organization (4, 19, 48). These organisms are ubiquitous, having been isolated from the skin, oropharynx, and gastrointestinal tract of humans and animals as well as from soil, plants, and compost (Table 1) (5, 47, 75, 109). Human infection results from inhalation of these bacteria and/or their contamination of an area of trauma (5, 57, 80, 109).

Characterization

The actinomycetes are considered to be related to mycobacteria on the basis of morphology, acid-fastness of some taxa, biochemical reactivity, the presence of mycolic acid derivatives, and the carbohydrate composition of their cell walls (33, 37, 42). They stain gram positive, although some of the more common pathogens stain with a characteristic irregularly beaded appearance. *Nocardia* spp. and *Rhodococcus* spp. are partially acid fast when decolorized with a mild mineral acid. This corresponds to a type IV cell wall carbohydrate composition as defined by Becker et al. (9) and to lysozyme resistance (40, 46). The cell walls of the other actinomycetes have been shown to be either type I, III, or IV (9, 33, 34). *Oerskovia* spp. differ from other actinomycetes in that they have a type VI cell wall. Because of this fact and other physicochemical differences, the classification of *Oerskovia* in this group of organisms remains questionable (32).

The morphology of the aerobic actinomycetes varies considerably between genera and within different strains of the same taxon (11, 57). Some species never develop beyond a typical bacteriumlike coccoid or bacillary form (*Rhodococcus* spp.), others form extensively branched filaments (*Nocardia, Streptomyces, Actinomadura,* and *Nocardiopsis* spp.), while others may form branched filaments and later fragment into motile flagellated cells (*Dermatophilus* and *Oerskovia* spp.; Table 1) (31, 32, 36, 37). Colonies may be bacteriumlike, i.e., butyrous to waxy and glabrous, or funguslike with heaped, leathery, and membranous colonies covered with aerial hyphae. Two groups of medically important actinomycetes, *Thermomonospora* and *Micropolyspora,* are true thermophiles and are capable of growing at temperatures up to 50°C (32; G. E. Hollick, Clin. Microbiol. Newsl. **8**[Mar.]:29–32, 1986).

MEDICALLY IMPORTANT SPECIES

The actinomycetes that are considered human pathogens include *Nocardia asteroides, N. brasiliensis, N. otitidiscaviarum* (syn. *N. caviae*), *Actinomadura madurae, A. pelletieri, Nocardiopsis dassonvillei, Streptomyces somaliensis, S. paraguayensis, Rhodococcus* spp., *Dermatophilus congolensis,* and *Oerskovia turbata* (Table 1) (5, 31, 39, 41, 43, 44, 52, 66). Although it is apparent that a variety of actinomycetous genera can cause human infection, *Nocardia* spp. represent the vast majority of reported systemic cases. Thus, the term "nocardiosis" is used as a synonym for pulmonary and disseminated infection caused by all of the aerobic actinomycetes (80). In 1976, Beaman and colleagues (6) estimated that there were between 500 and 1,000 cases of nocardiosis annually in the United States. Eighty-five percent of the cases were serious pulmonary and systemic infections. *N. asteroides* caused between 81 and 91% of these, and *N. brasiliensis* was a distant second. In contrast, *N. brasiliensis, S. somaliensis,* and *A. madurae* are the most common agents of actinomycotic mycetoma (65). *Rhodococcus* spp. infections have been reported from skin and open-space wounds (20, 69), abscessed nerve sheaths (103), and lungs (104), as well as bones and joints (15). *D. congolensis* is a worldwide cause of a pustular and exudative dermatitis in animals and, rarely, humans (16, 35, 37, 79). *O. turbata* has been isolated from a case of endocarditis and a kidney abscess (22, 37, 80).

SPECTRUM OF DISEASES

The diseases caused by the aerobic actinomycetes are worldwide in occurrence. The resulting pathology is attributed to a combination of organism type, affected tissue, and the immune state of the patient (5, 20, 80). In the immune-competent host, for example, two diseases predominate. One is a noninvasive, acute to chronic allergic respiratory syndrome colloquially referred to as "farmer's lung," while the other is a subcutaneous tumefaction of muscle, fascia, and bone called a mycetoma (20, 57, 80). In the immunosuppressed patient, infection may begin as an acute to chronic suppurative process in the lung which can progress to cavitation and multilobular pulmonary disease (Fig. 1) (24, 70). Infection may spread and further involve other organ systems, showing a predilection for the central nervous system.

Diseases of immune-competent hosts

Allergic respiratory disease (farmer's lung) is a hypersensitivity reaction to repeated exposure to antigens produced by the actinomycetes, especially the thermophiles (20, 80). The most common actinomycetous

TABLE 1. Taxonomy of the common pathogenic aerobic actinomycetes (20, 31, 32, 37, 57, 80, 103, 109)

Aggregate group	Description	Organism	Disease	Habitat	Appearance in host tissue		Sabouraud dextrose agar culture (27 to 37°C)
					Exudate	Stained sections	
Nocardioforms	Diphtheroid to filamentous, true branching mycelial elements, commonly fragmented to give coccoid to bacillary spores. Some species are partially acid-fast and produce aerial hyphae.	*Nocardia asteroides*	Pulmonary: transient to chronic suppurative abscesses. Generalized systemic disease often with central nervous system involvement. Mycetoma rare.	Ubiquitous in soil, animals, and humans.	Granules are small (25 to 150 μm), soft, white to yellowish, lobulated, sometimes clubbed, occurring only rarely, generally in mycetomata; usually occurs as clumped or scattered, acid-fast, branched filaments, undergoing fragmentation.	Granules are rare, irregularly oval, staining lightly with hematoxylin, often with a distinct eosinophilic periphery (Fig. 2b), fringed, and sometimes clubbed. Gram stain gives similar patterns (Fig. 5); more commonly, colonies are either loose mycelium or scattered, fragmenting filaments (Fig. 4).	Colonies are orange, glabrous, heaped and folded, to white or pink, raised and chalky with aerial hyphae (Fig. 7, 8, 21, 22a, 22b), crumbly to leathery and adherent. Hyphae fragment into bacillary and coccoid elements (Fig. 17) or form chains of arthrospores; growth at 46°C (Fig. 19).
		Nocardia brasiliensis	Frequent agent of mycetoma and isolated sporotrichoid lesions. Pulmonary and generalized disease rare.	Ubiquitous in soil: predominantly North and South America, Central Plateau of Brazil, and India.	As above, but granules are common in mycetomata; branched filaments in cutaneous abscesses.	As above, but granules are common in mycetomata.	As above; no growth at 46°C.
		Nocardia otitidiscaviarum	Generalized systemic disease: mycetoma.	Ubiquitous in soil: predominantly Tunisia, Japan, India, Mexico, and United States.	As observed for *N. brasiliensis.*	As observed for *N. brasiliensis.*	As above; growth at 46°C variable.
		Rhodococcus spp.	Generalized granulomatous disease, central nervous system involvement, eczematous and granulomatous dermatitis, septicemia, and pericarditis.	Ubiquitous in soil and plant material.	Small, white to yellowish soft granules. May appear as loose colonies of coccobacilli. Some species are acid fast.	Granules are similar to those of botryomycosis: masses of gram-positive coccobacilli surrounded by suppuration. Also form granulomata with epithelial and giant cells.	Colonies are light pink-orange to coral red. Soft, creamy to butyrous colonies. No aerial hyphae; fragment into coccobacilli and diphtheroids. Most strains grow well at 30°C (Fig. 22d).

(*Continued on next page*)

TABLE 1—*Continued*

Aggregate group	Description	Organism	Disease	Habitat	Appearance in host tissue		Sabouraud dextrose agar culture (27 to 37°C)
					Exudate	Stained sections	
Maduromycetes	Filamentous with mycelial elements fragmenting to coccobacillary forms. Spores formed within a sheath on aerial or substrate mycelium.	*Actinomadura madurae*	Mycetoma.	Ubiquitous in soil, plants, thorns, and decaying vegetation.	Large (1 to 5 mm), soft, white to yellowish or reddish granules, irregularly oval, serpiginous, or lobulated.	H&E[a]: center of granule is hollow or tenuous, surrounded by denser network staining dark purple; wide, dense, pink border with long fringes and usually clubs.	Optimal temperature, 30 to 37°C; colonies are waxy, heaped and folded (Fig. 10), membranous and tough; white to tan; pale orange, pink, or red; nonfragmenting, but sparse aerial hyphae may form short chains of spores (Fig. 22f).
		Actinomadura pelletieri	Mycetoma.	Soil, thorns, plants, and decaying vegetation. Found in West Africa, Trans Africa Belt, and India.	Granules are soft, small (300 to 500 μm), deep red, smooth-edged or finely denticulate, irregularly spherical, sometimes with large lobes.	H&E: granules round, sharply delimited, characteristically fracturing into large segments; stain basophilic with a lighter purple peripheral band.	Optimal temperature, 30 to 37°C; colony resembles a crushed cranberry, with areas of bright and dark red; slow-growing, heaped, irregularly waxy and granular (Fig. 11); may have sparse aerial hyphae (Fig. 20); pigment soluble in mineral oil.
		Nocardiopsis dassonvillei	Mycetoma.	Ubiquitous in soil.	Insufficient information; granules not reported.	Insufficient information.	Densely filamentous colonies (Fig. 9) (*Streptomyces*-like) with abundant aerial mycelium and long aerial chains of spores (Fig. 18). Vegetative mycelium may fragment to some extent into rods; growth (80% of strains) at 40°C; no growth at 45°C.

Streptomycetes	Well-developed, branching aerial and substrate mycelium. Mycelial elements do not fragment. Spores borne in characteristic chains on extensive aerial mycelium.	*Streptomyces somaliensis*	Mycetoma.	Found in soil: South Africa, South America, United States, and Arabia.	Hard, yellow to brown, round to oval granules, 1 to 2 mm wide.	H&E: granules are both large and tiny, round, dense and homogeneous, but staining light purple and often partially pink in patches; tend to rupture into parallel strips; smooth, sharply defined, nonbanded border (Fig. 3).	Optimal temperature, 30°C; slow-growing, leathery, eventually heaped and folded (Fig. 13); cream colored to brown or black, glabrous. White aerial hyphae may form chains of spores characteristic of the genus.
		Streptomyces paraguayensis	Mycetoma.	Soil, thorns, plants, decaying vegetation of Mexico, Central America, and South America.	Black granules.	Insufficient information.	There is doubt as to the existence of this species as a distinct, pathogenic agent. Cultures designated *S. paraguayensis* resemble saprophytic *Streptomyces* spp. (white or cream to gray, tough colonies with raised center [Fig. 12], often bearing short aerial hyphae).
	Nonpathogenic.	*Streptomyces* spp.	Nonpathogenic.	Ubiquitous, common environmental isolates. Usually found in soil, manure, composts, plants, and air-conditioning ducts.	N/A	N/A	Colonies are tough, glabrous, velvety, or (most often) chalky, of various colors. Commonly white or grayish; often with earthy odor. Hyphae are nonfragmenting; specialized aerial hyphae may form medium to long, curved or spiral chains of spores.

(*Continued on next page*)

TABLE 1—*Continued*

Aggregate group	Description	Organism	Disease	Habitat	Appearance in host tissue		Sabouraud dextrose agar culture (27 to 37°C)
					Exudate	Stained sections	
Micropolysporas	Mycelial elements show slight to no fragmentation. Spores are formed singly in pairs or short chains on either aerial or substrate mycelium.	*Saccharomonospora viridis, S. internatus Micropolyspora faeni, M. caesis*	Restrictive allergic pulmonary disease.	Ubiquitous: ventilation ducts, manure, and compost.	N/A	N/A	N/A
Thermoactinomycetes	Mycelial elements do not fragment. Bacterial endospore is borne singly on aerial or substrate mycelium.	*Thermoactinomyces vulgaris, T. sacchari, T. candidus*	Restrictive allergic pulmonary disease.	Ubiquitous in ventilation ducts, manure, composts, humidifier water, hay, moldy sugar cane.	N/A	N/A	N/A
Multilocular sporangia forms	Mycelial elements divide transversely and in at least two longitudinal planes to form masses of motile coccoid cells. Aerial mycelium usually absent (Fig. 15, 23, 24).	*Dermatophilus congolensis*	Epidemic eczema.	Humans and animals: Australia, Africa, United States.	N/A	Pustules to intense suppurative dermatitis (Fig. 6).	No growth. Grows well on sheep blood agar or Loeffler medium (Fig. 14).

[a] H&E, Hematoxylin-eosin stain.

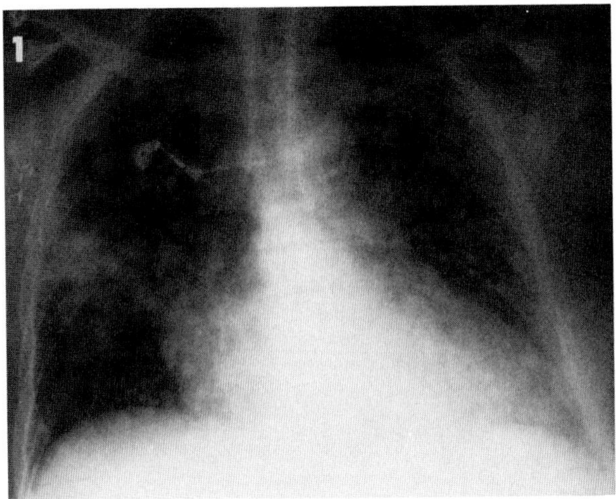

FIG. 1. Disseminated pulmonary nocardiosis (*N. asteroides*) in a 38-year-old woman on maintenance therapy for amyelotropic lateral sclerosis. Note the right mid-lung consolidation and the bilateral diffuse nodular and fluffy pattern of infiltrates.

causes of farmer's lung are *Micropolyspora faeni, Thermoactinomyces vulgaris,* and *T. viridis* (Hollick, Clin. Microbiol. Newsl. **8**[Mar.]:29–32, 1986). Although these organisms do not represent all of the possible etiologies of this syndrome, they are responsible for a large number of the reported cases. The thermophilic actinomycetes are usually found in closed barns, silos, grain mills, sugar cane waste (bagasse), air conditioning vents, and sorghum waste processing areas (109).

Although first reported in 1924 as an acute or chronic lung infection, it wasn't until 1958 that farmer's lung was identified as an allergic alveolitis, occurring in response to an exposure to antigens present in decaying vegetation. The pathologic mechanism is not totally understood. However, it is believed to be immune mediated and involves type III and/or type IV immune reactions in response to repeated host inhalation of actinomycete antigens, fungi, or other organic debris (20, 101). These responses eventually manifest themselves as granulomatous lung changes, eosinophilia, production of specific immunoglobulin E antibody, and pulmonary edema (80). Chronic exposure leads to increased edema and interstitial pulmonary fibrosis. Anaphylaxis has been described in more sensitive individuals.

Fixed cutaneous nocardiosis is a localized pustular cellulitis around an area of trauma containing soil or decaying plant material contaminated by actinomycetes (5, 24, 85). Cutaneous lesions may also be accompanied by pyoderma and lymphadenopathy that resembles sporotrichosis (47). Other primary cutaneous manifestations include keratitis (49) and primary granulomatous dermatitis (21). In immunocompromised patients lesions may not remain localized, but can spread as disseminated soft tissue abscesses that could eventually lead to other organ involvement as well (70, 80, 87).

Mycetoma, like hypersensitivity pneumonitis, has multiple etiologies that include true fungi (eumycetoma) and the *Actinomycetales* (actinomycotic mycetoma) (80). Actinomycotic mycetoma is typified as a chronic cutaneous and subcutaneous, suppurative, deforming tumefication of fascia, muscle, and bone (Fig. 2a) (65). Infection is a result of traumatic implantation of contaminated vegetation and/or soil containing the etiologic agent. Although mycetomata may occur anywhere on the human body, they are more commonly found on the extremities. Lesions appear as suppurating abscesses containing a characteristic granule, similar to the sulfur granule formed by *Actinomyces* spp. in tissue (Fig. 2b and 3). Abscesses can develop into burrowing, draining sinus tracts, and granules are surrounded by a dense layer of degenerating neutrophils, followed by a thick fibrotic capsule.

D. congolensis parasitizes the epidermis, manifesting itself as a pustular exudative dermatitis (10, 80). Called streptotrichosis, epidemic eczema, strawberry foot rot, or contagious dermatitis, it infects some herbivorous animals such as horses, goats, sheep, cows, and deer (62). Infection begins with a pustular stage and is followed by the appearance of scales, crusts, and exudates matting the hide of the animal. Eventually, healing occurs and the crusts fall off, leaving an area of alopecia and scarring. Humans have been incidentally infected by handling diseased animals, including four reported cases in hunters as a result of processing an infected deer (38). Human infection is characterized by the appearance of multiple, nonpainful pustules within a week of exposure or, in the immunocompromised patient, as white hyperkeratotic plaques resembling hairy leukoplakia (16). Pustules progress to reddish ulcers and furuncles, which become covered by brownish scabs (80). Scabs persist for several days and then the lesions heal spontaneously, leaving purplish-red scars.

Diseases in compromised hosts

Invasive pulmonary and disseminated nocardioses are true opportunistic infections, occurring as a result of a variety of clinical and therapeutic factors (56, 77, 95). Those individuals with a T-cellular immune deficiency appear most susceptible to actinomycotic infection (5, 7, 24, 51). T-cell depletion may be a direct result of hematologic malignancy and its treatment (5, 19, 23, 82), antirejection therapy for organ allografts (55, 83, 84, 110), intravenous drug abuse (105), or natural or acquired immunodeficiency (51, 58, 72, 95) as well as a variety of other clinical and therapeutic factors (56, 77, 95). Mycobacteria (99, 111) and fungi (27) associated with stagnant water, mud, or soil have been reported as causing severe peritonitis in home dialysis patients. Since the aerobic actinomycetes share similar habitats, it is not inconceivable that they may also emerge as pathogens in these individuals. The actinomycetes invade the lung parenchyma and form localized abscesses (97). Progressive infection is characterized by suppurative, necrotic inflammation with multiple fibrogenic, loculating abscesses which lead to burrowing sinus tracts throughout the soft tissues (5, 20, 80).

Systemic disease is a subsequent event of dissemination from a primary, usually pulmonary, infection. However, in the compromised patient, dissemination from a primary cutaneous site may occur (80, 92). Although dissemination may be to any organ, the brain appears to be the most common secondary site (51, 72, 82). Brain lesions appear as single to multiple abscesses, the latter coalescing to a single large abscess as the

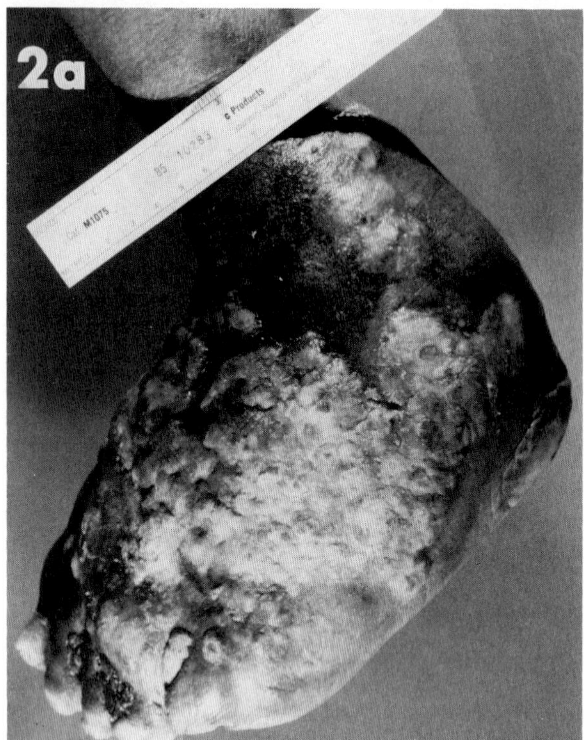

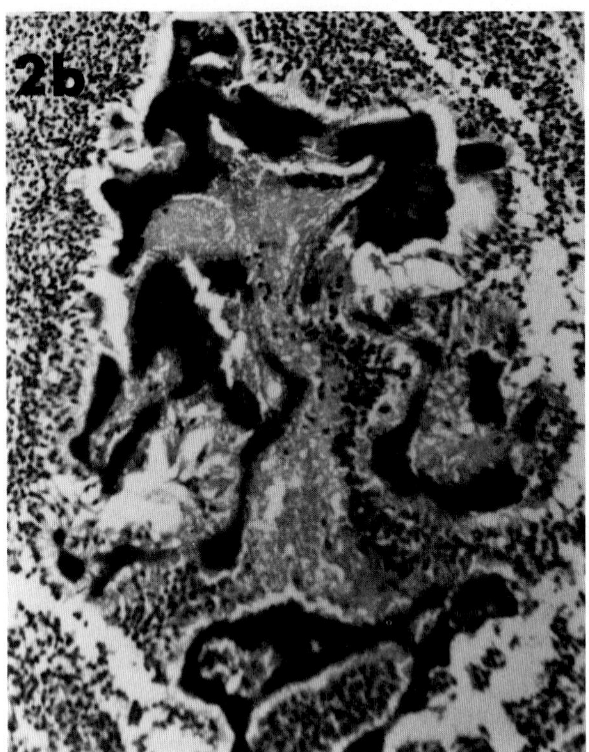

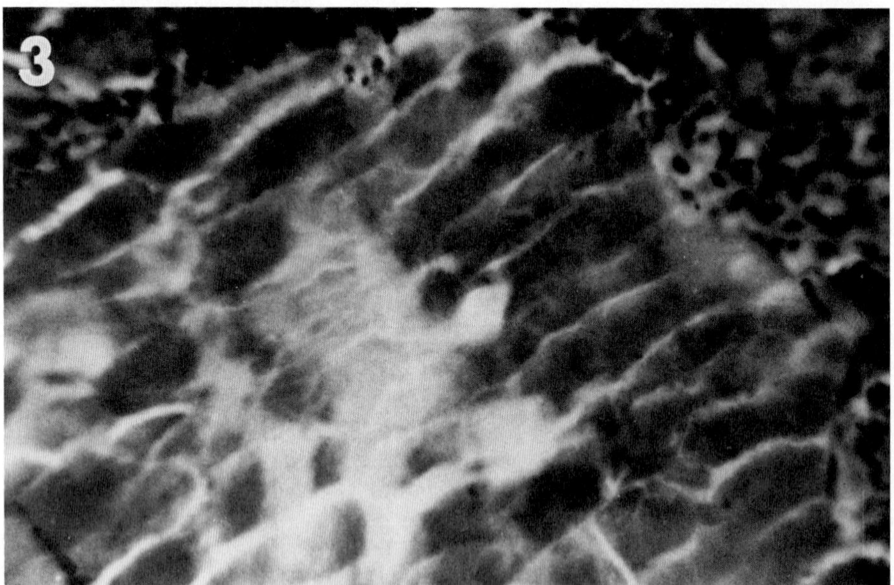

FIG. 2. (a) Actinomycotic mycetoma: left foot of a 78-year-old woman. Typical pustules and draining abscesses are apparent. (Reprinted with permission from reference 57). (b) *N. asteroides* granule from the patient depicted in panel a. The intense basophilic staining of the granule periphery, the lacy staining of the center, and the surrounding inflammatory response are typical. (Reprinted with permission from reference 57.)

FIG. 3. *S. somaliensis* in a section from a human mycetoma. Round, dense granule, lightly stained with hematoxylin, fracturing into strips. Hematoxylin and eosin stain. Magnification, ×378. Courtesy M. A. Gordon (37).

disease progresses (23, 24, 80). The meninges are rarely involved to the point that they cause diagnostic changes in the spinal fluid. Occasionally there may be some osteolytic changes in the vertebrae or cranium (15, 80, 112). The kidneys are the next most commonly infected organ, with heart, spleen, liver, and adrenal disease reported to a lesser extent (6, 82). Early manifestations of primary cutaneous dissemination are multiple soft tissue abscesses (85, 92). These may remain subcutaneous or may progress to other systems, primarily the central nervous system.

A form of nocardiosis which is opportunistic, but is

not necessarily related to underlying malignancy or immune deficiency, is that associated with pulmonary alveolar phospholipoproteinosis (76). Clinical features of this disease are similar to those of hypersensitivity pneumonitis, e.g., dyspnea, cough, fever, and pain. The disease is relatively uncommon (260 reported cases by 1980), and there appears to be some genetic predisposition to it as well as an association with inhalation of various dusts and chemicals. There has been, however, a striking association of superinfection with *Nocardia* spp. in patients with this underlying problem. Both pulmonary and disseminated nocardiosis have been described in these individuals.

Histopathology

Actinomycete invasion of humans results in an acute to chronic inflammatory reaction, associated with single to multiple abscess formation (20, 80). Abscesses may be loosely organized or encapsulated, but all are densely packed with polymorphonuclear leukocytes, plasma cells, lymphocytes, and fibrin. In patients with fixed cutaneous or systemic disease, the aerobic actinomycetes form a loosely arranged network of organisms called a pseudogranule (Fig. 4). In mycetoma, compact granules are formed, similar to those observed in anaerobic actinomycotic infections (Fig. 5) (65, 80). In either situation, the actinomycetes usually appear as long, incompletely staining filaments with true branching. *Rhodococcus* spp. and related organisms occur as coccobacillary forms arranged in palisades and typical diphtheroid configurations. *D. congoliensis* shows irregularly branched filaments that are divided longitudinally and transversely, forming packets of coccoid cells. The methenamine silver stain is an ideal stain for detecting these organisms in clinical specimens. Gram stain and acid-fast staining, although not always effective, can provide a means to make a provisional identification of the organism.

Microscopically, pulmonary alveolar phospholipoproteinosis is characterized by areas where large groups of alveoli become filled with a granular and floccular material composed of phospholipid and small amounts of protein (76). The normal architecture of the alveolar septae and interstitium remains normal. When *Nocardia* spp. or other microorganisms superinfect, acute inflammatory foci are found in the alveolar exudate.

CLINICAL SPECIMENS

Collection, transportation, and processing of specimens

Clinical specimens received for the isolation of aerobic actinomycetes typically include bronchial washings, sputa, tissue (biopsy, surgical, autopsy), exudates, blood, cerebrospinal fluid, urine, and scrapings from lesions. All specimens must be collected aseptically and transported to the laboratory in a prompt manner to prevent dehydration. If delays are anticipated and specimens cannot be processed immediately, they may be stored temporarily at 4°C. Skin scrapings and lesion material from *D. congolensis* infections should be kept in dry sterile containers at ambient temperature.

Sputa must be fresh and collected in the same manner as for *Mycobacterium* spp. (87, 88). Briefly, at least three consecutive, fresh, early morning specimens should be collected. Cumulative specimens are neither useful nor acceptable. Sputa and bronchial washings are collected in sterile screw-capped containers for direct microscopy and culture. Exudates, fluids, and pus should be aspirated into a syringe, the syringe should be capped or sealed, and the specimen should be transported immediately to the laboratory. Fluids are concentrated by centrifugation, tissues are homogenized prior to plating, and blood specimens are inoculated to standard blood culture systems. Swabs should be avoided when collecting specimens for the recovery of actinomycetes. If

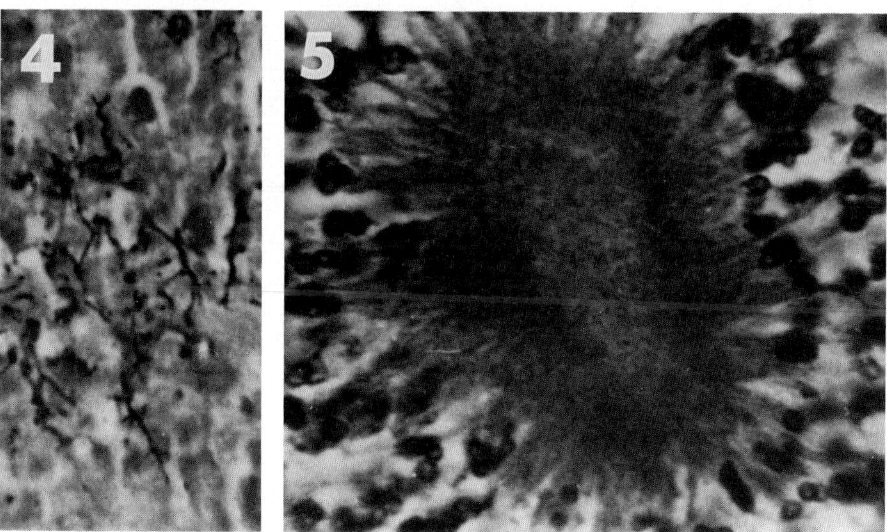

FIG. 4. *N. asteroides* in a section of human brain. Grocott stain. Magnification, ×850. Courtesy M. A. Gordon (37).

FIG. 5. *N. asteroides* granule in a section of abscessed omentum from an experimentally infected guinea pig. Gram-positive interior; fringed, clubbed, gram-negative border. Gram-Weigert stain. Magnification, ×850. Courtesy M. A. Gordon (37).

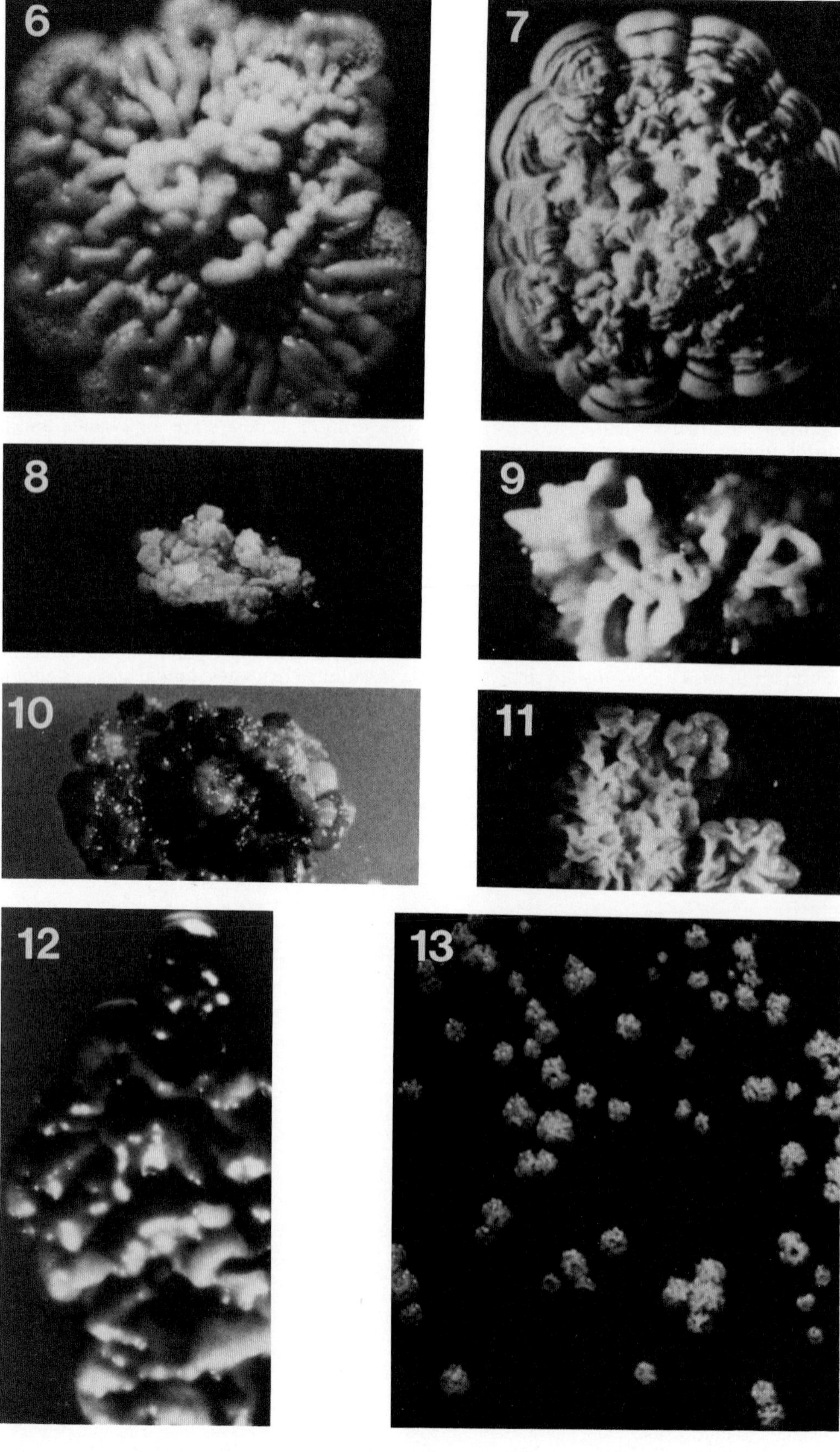
6
7
8
9
10
11
12
13

swabs are the only alternative, they should be placed in appropriate transport media and taken immediately to the laboratory.

Primary plating, incubation, and reading of cultures

There are no routine media specifically for the primary isolation of aerobic actinomycetes. It has been recommended that a clinical specimen be inoculated to three or four primary plates (87, 90). Since most of the time these bacteria are recovered without their presence being suspected, increasing the amount of specimen plated will improve yield. Blood specimens can be inoculated to either conventional two-bottle broth blood culture systems, biphasic blood culture bottles, or radiometric or nonradiometric automated systems (81). Blood specimens processed by lysis-centrifugation, fluids, or homogenized tissue specimens are plated directly onto media such as Sabouraud dextrose agar, Sabouraud dextrose agar with heart infusion supplementation (Sabhi), brain heart infusion (BHI) agar, sheep blood agar, or tryptic soy agar. For heavily contaminated specimens like sputa or bronchial washes, BHI agar containing cycloheximide and chloramphenicol or the paraffin baiting technique should be used (91). Selective recovery of nocardiae from contaminated specimens has been reported with a chemically defined agar containing paraffin and/or gelatin as the sole carbon source (90).

Nocardia spp. and some rhodococci often survive the concentration and decontamination steps used to isolate mycobacteria from respiratory specimens (50). Recommended procedures include alkali digestion with sodium hydroxide or treatment with dithiothreitol or with *N*-acetyl-L-cysteine. Digests may be inoculated onto standard mycobacterial isolation media such as Lowenstein-Jensen or 7H10 (oleic acid-albumin) agar. However, caution must be exercised when digestion-decontamination techniques are used, since many of these organisms are killed upon exposure to 0.5% *N*-acetyl-L-cysteine, 2% NaOH–*N*-acetyl-L-cysteine, or benzalkonium chloride in trisodium phosphate (71).

Cultures may be incubated at either 37°C or 25 to 30°C. Even though the thermophiles and *N. asteroides* and *N. brasiliensis* grow well at 37°C and above, other aerobic actinomycetes often grow best at lower temperatures (33, 37, 86, 87). For this reason, it is recommended that all specimens be incubated at 30°C. If *Nocardia* spp. are indicated to the exclusion of the other actinomycetes in a clinical specimen, then 37°C or greater should be used as a means of enhancing their growth. Any specimen for which the anaerobic actinomycetes have not been excluded must also be inoculated into thioglycolate broth, anaerobic blood plates, or chopped-meat glucose broth and incubated at 37°C (87).

The presence or absence of 5 to 20% CO_2 in the incubation atmosphere has little effect upon the initial isolation of aerobic actinomycetes. If petri plates are used instead of screw-capped tubes, they should contain twice the normal amount of medium and/or should be sealed with gas-permeable tape to prevent dehydration.

Material containing *D. congolensis* should be dried and streaked directly onto an enriched medium like BHI-blood agar (35, 37, 80, 87). Heavily contaminated specimens such as dry crusts, skin scales, or hair containing scales are ground to a fine powder, suspended in 2 ml of sterile distilled water, mixed, and allowed to settle for 15 min. Supernatants are streaked onto BHI-blood agar containing 1,000 IU of polymyxin B and incubated at 37°C. In an alternative procedure, emulsions of exudates and crusts are made in sterile saline. Emulsions are filtered through a 1.22-μm-pore-size sterile syringe filter, streaked over the surface of blood agar or BHI-blood agar, and incubated at 37°C.

All inoculated media must be examined periodically for the presence of actinomycete colonies; usually every 3 to 4 days will suffice. When cultures are being examined, activities that may cause aerosolization should be conducted in a biological safety cabinet (64). *Nocardia* spp., *Streptomyces* spp., and *D. congolensis* are fast growing and usually appear on plated media within 2 to 10 days, whereas slower-growing organisms like *Actinomadura* spp. may require up to 3 weeks for primary isolation (80, 87, 88).

Direct examination

Microscopic examination of clinical material submitted to the laboratory for culture is an important part of diagnosing actinomycotic infections. Specimens that may contain aerobic actinomycetes are usually heavily cellular, i.e., respiratory secretions, pus, skin crusts, scales, homogenized tissue, etc. For this reason, mounting clinical material in equal volumes of 10 to 20% potassium hydroxide, subsequent clearing, and direct microscopic examination may provide valuable preliminary information as to the identity of the invading organism. To facilitate specimen clearing, slides may be placed in a petri plate with some moistened gauze to prevent dehydration and gently warmed on a slide warmer for 10 to 15 min. For larger amounts of specimens, equal volumes of specimen and potassium hydroxide may be placed in a screw-capped test tube and incubated in a heating block (45 to 56°C) for 20 to 30 min. Specimens containing granules, like those from mycetoma, may be placed in a drop of saline and crushed between two microscope slides, aseptically placed in a sterile saline and minced, or sheared in a sterile tissue homogenizer and then used to make the appropriate smears.

In clinical specimens, the filamentous aerobic actinomycetes appear as they do in tissue, exhibiting in-

---

FIG. 6 to 11. "Giant" colonies of various species on Sabouraud dextrose agar plates, after 9 days at 27°C. Magnification, ×6. FIG. 6, *N. asteroides*, glabrous orange form. FIG. 7, *N. asteroides*, gypsoides (white, chalky) variety (*N. brasiliensis* and *N. otitidiscaviarum* are similar to *N. asteroides*). FIG. 8, *Nocardiopsis dassonvillei*. FIG. 9, *A. madurae*. FIG. 10, *A. pelletieri*. FIG. 11, *S. paraguayensis*. Courtesy M. A. Gordon (37).

FIG. 12. *S. somaliensis*, streaked heavily on blood agar slant, after 3 days at 17°C. Magnification, ×6. Courtesy M. A. Gordon (37).

FIG. 13. Colonies of *D. congolensis* on blood agar streak plate, after 3 days at 37°C. Magnification, ×3.6.

complete or beaded staining, with coccobacillary to diphtheroid forms taking up most of the stain (80). All morphologic forms, including bacterial and filamentous, are approximately 1 μm in diameter, in contrast to fungal hyphae which are approximately 3 to 5 μm in diameter. They all are gram positive, and two genera, *Nocardia* spp. and often *Rhodococcus* spp., are acid fast to partially acid fast when stained with a modified Kinyoun method using 2% H_2SO_4 as the decolorizing agent (46). Because of the faint staining properties of the more common aerobic actinomycetes, care must be taken when reviewing slides for their possible presence. It is advisable to stain several smears and then scan all of them before reporting microscopic results.

IDENTIFICATION

Purification of isolates

Pure cultures of the aerobic actinomycetes may be obtained in the same manner as other bacteria. Portions of well-isolated colonies or mycelial mats may be taken from primary plates and streaked for isolation on fresh media (BHI-blood agar, Sabhi agar, Sabouraud dextrose agar, blood agar, etc.). Since the aerobic actinomycetes as a whole are slower growing than common clinically important bacteria, care must be taken to find a colony well removed from other microbes for further purification.

Macroscopic characteristics

Colonies of the aerobic actinomycetes may appear initially as waxy to powdery (Fig. 6 and 7), and as they mature, they may become white, gray, buff, orange, red, or purple (Fig. 8 through 12) (46, 64, 80, 87). Some species may produce diffusible brown to black pigments, and most produce strong "earthy" or "new-mown hay"-like odors. *D. congolensis* appears as a grayish-white, sunken, adherent beta-hemolytic colony at 72 to 96 h, changing to yellow or orange upon aging (Fig. 13 and 14) (35, 36). Because colonial characteristics of the actinomycetes are influenced by cultivation conditions, there is no consistent relationship between them and specific taxa. However, these characteristics, in conjunction with microscopic morphology, staining characteristics, and evaluation of growth on tap water agar as described in subsequent sections of this chapter, may give a presumptive identification of the unknown organism.

Microscopic characteristics

Culture material may be prepared for microscopic examination by a variety of methods, including slide culture, tease mounts, smears, or wet mounts. Their appearance can be enhanced by the Gram stain, acid-fast stain, or histopathological stains such as methenimine-silver or periodic acid-Schiff (80). Care must be taken with tease mounts, wet mounts, smears, etc., so that one does not disrupt the delicate conidial structures or spontaneous sporelike fragments produced by some of these organisms which may be confused with fragments produced by shearing during the slide preparation technique.

Microscopic examination of all slide preparations (Fig. 15 through 21) must be done with an oil immersion objective. The aerobic actinomycetes are gram positive and appear as delicate branching filaments or as diphtheroidlike arrangements of coccobacilli approximately 1 μm in diameter (Fig. 15). *Nocardia* spp. and *Rhodococcus* spp., which generally manifest a partially acid-fast character, have a tendency to fragment into coccobacillary forms (Fig. 16). The non-acid-fast genera *Actinomadura* and *Streptomyces* remain as a mycelium and do not fragment. The aerial hyphae of the streptomycetes and *Nocardiopsis dassonvillei* characteristically form chains of conidia that are often arranged in spirals or whorls and may sometimes be acid fast (Fig. 17). Short chains of aerial spores which may spontaneously fragment occur in some pathogenic strains (Fig. 18 and 19); some of these may also stain as acid-fast structures. It is necessary that one be able to distinguish between acid-fast hyphae, which are of clinical importance, and these acid-fast spores, which are not. If acid-fast staining of primary culture is equivocal, staining may be enhanced by passing the organism through a high-lipid medium such as Middlebrook 7H10, Lowenstein-Jensen, casein, or litmus milk agars or passage through sterile milk (46).

Tap water agar morphology

Unknown organisms should be streaked in a straight line on a sterile medium consisting of 20 g of plain agar dissolved in 100 ml of tap water (11, 57). Inoculated plates are incubated at 25 to 30°C and examined daily for up to 7 days. Microscopic examination is done through the unopened plate by focusing a ×10 objective (×100 total magnification) on the agar surface. Contrast between bacteria and the agar surface may be enhanced by reducing the iris diaphragm and lowering the substage condenser of the microscope.

When viewed on this medium, the substrate and surface hyphae of *Nocardia* spp. appear as very fine, dichotomously branched filaments (Fig. 20 and 21a). Movement of the objective up and down through several planes of focus will also reveal aerial hyphae (Fig. 21b). The presence of aerial hyphae differentiates *Nocardia* from the other acid-fast genera like *Rhodococcus* and *Mycobacterium*. The rapidly growing mycobacteria, which phenotypically and biochemically resemble the nocardiae, have a simple frostlike to fir tree-like arrangement of substrate hyphae in contrast to the complex branching of the latter (Fig. 21c). Rhodococci grow only on the agar surface as coccobacilli arranged in a classic diphtheroid fashion (Fig. 21d). Neither demonstrates the presence of aerial hyphae.

Of the remaining medically important groups, *Nocardiopsis* spp., *Streptomyces* spp., and *Actinomadura* spp. have substrate, surface, and aerial hyphal morphology similar to those of the nocardiae. However, none of these is acid fast, and the latter two genera often show the presence of spores arranged in characteristic patterns. *Micromonospora* spp., for example, have only surface and substrate mycelium and produce subsurface spores which may occur singly or in grape-like clusters. In contrast, *Thermomonospora* spp. form aerial mycelium and produce single endospores on both subsurface and aerial hyphae. *O. turbata* and *D. congolensis* are non-acid-fast bacteria and have an extensively branched substrate and surface mycelium. Additionally, *Oerskovia* spp. produce mono- and polytrichous motile spores from fragmentation of the primary mycelium, while the family *Dermatophilaceae*

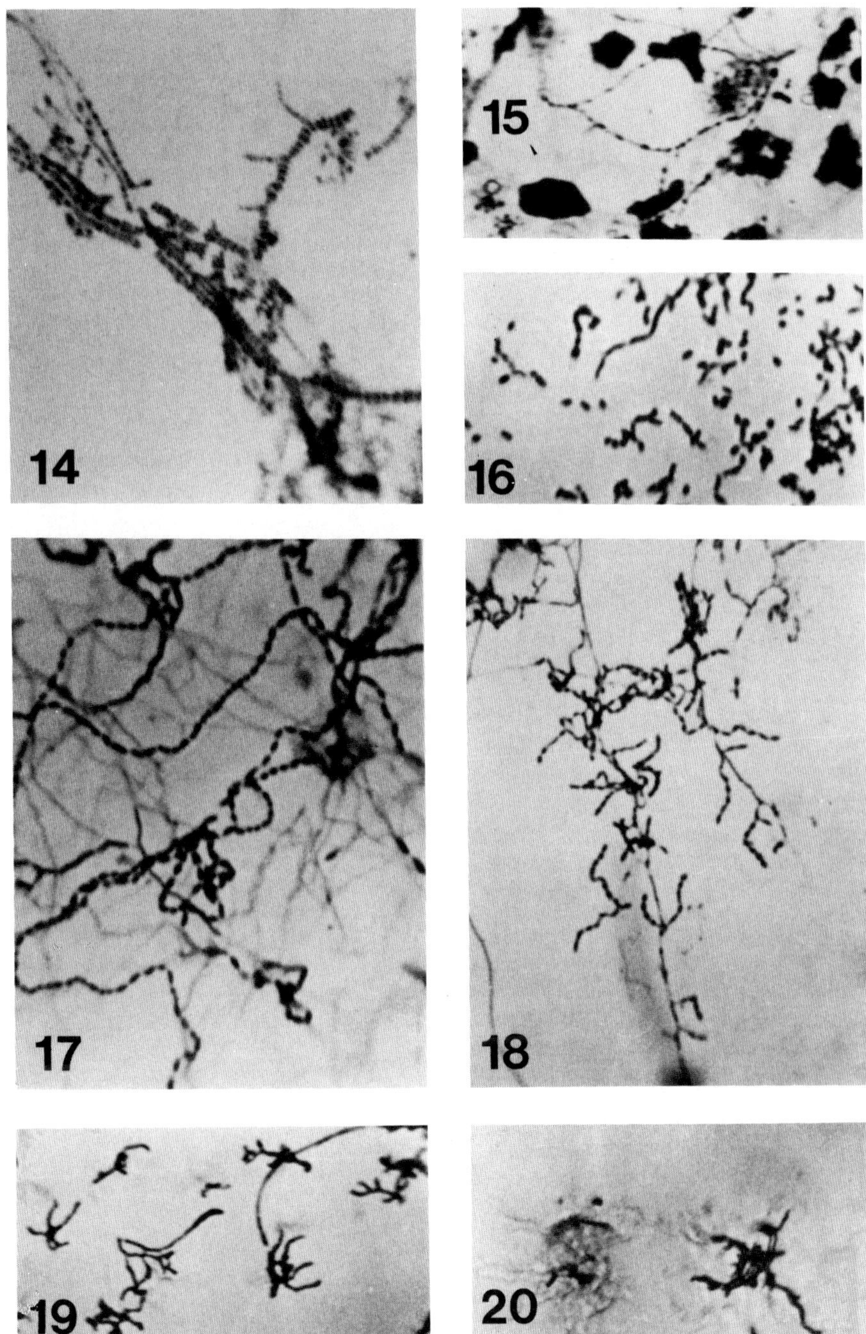

FIG. 14. *D. congolensis*, showing the early segmentation stage from BHI agar, after 3 days at 37°C. Methylene blue stain. Magnification, ×972.

FIG. 15. *N. asteroides* in a smear of abscessed omentum from an experimentally infected guinea pig. Modified Kinyoun acid-fast stain. Magnification, ×972. Courtesy M. A. Gordon (37).

FIG. 16. *N. asteroides* in a smear from a glabrous orange colony on Sabouraud dextrose agar, after 3 weeks at 27°C; extensive fragmentation. Gram stain. Magnification, ×972. Courtesy M. A. Gordon (37).

FIG. 17. *Nocardiopsis dassonvillei*, showing long chains of ovate spores. Slide culture on Hickey and Tresner medium, incubated for 10 days at 25°C. Giemsa stain. Magnification, ×972. Courtesy M. A. Gordon (37).

FIG. 18. *N. asteroides*, showing chains of aerial spores. Slide culture on Hickey and Tresner medium. Giemsa stain. Magnification, ×972. Courtesy M. A. Gordon (37).

FIG. 19. *A. pelletieri* smear from a colony on Sabouraud dextrose agar (27°C), prepared in the manner of a blood film, causing moderate traumatic fragmentation. Gram stain. Magnification, ×972. Courtesy M. A. Gordon (37).

FIG. 20. Pour-slide culture of *N. asteroides* on Hickey and Tresner medium after 3 days at 27°C; photographed in situ with a 43× objective to illustrate the contrast between aerial (darker) and substrate hyphae. Magnification, ×432. Courtesy M. A. Gordon (37).

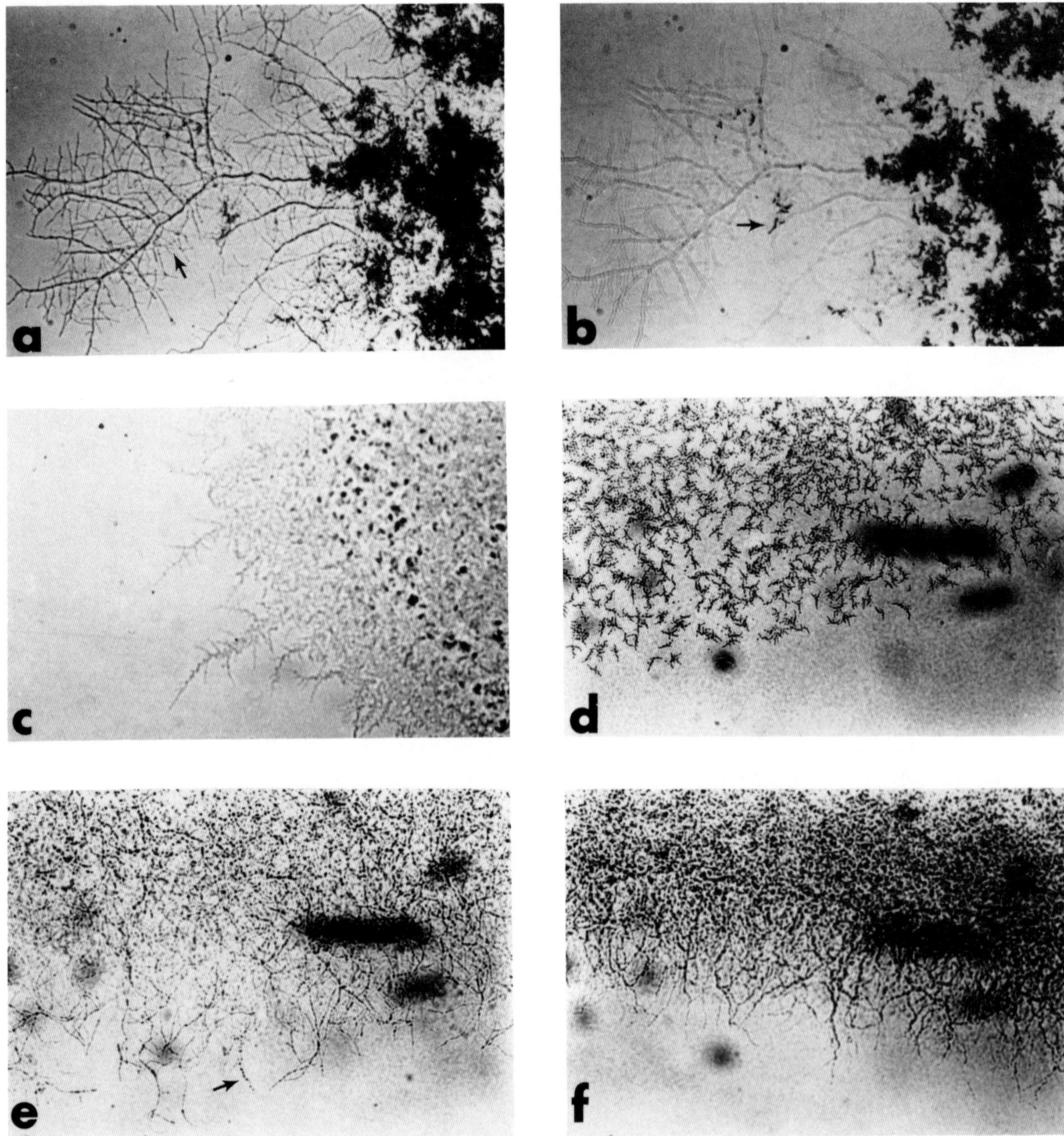

FIG. 21. Growth of aerobic actinomycetes on tap water agar; magnification, ×89. (a) *N. asteroides*, 72 h of incubation; arrow indicates substrate hyphae. (b) Same field as for panel a; altered plane of focus to illustrate aerial hyphae (arrow). (c) *M. fortuitum*, 48 h of incubation. (d) *Rhodococcus* spp., 72 h of incubation. (e) *Streptomyces* spp., 72 h of incubation; note chains of spores (arrow). (f) *A. madurae*, 72 h of incubation. Magnification, ×400. (Reprinted with permission from reference 57.)

produce motile zoospores from coccoid packets formed by longitudinal and transverse septation of hyphal branches (32, 80; Hollick, Clin. Microbiol. Newsl. **8**[Mar.]:29–32, 1986).

Physiological and biochemical characterization

Once the presence of an aerobic actinomycete has been deemed possible on the basis of the cultural, tinctorial, and morphological properties described above, a variety of simple physiological tests (Table 2) are useful in further delineating the genus and species of the organism. Performance of these tests is well within the scope of the routine clinical laboratory, and their results provide valuable information regarding the clinical relevance of an isolate. More definitive taxonomic classification than the above requires determining either an extensive array of physiological properties, such as those reported by Mishra et al. (67), or the presence of chemotaxonomic biochemical markers in the cell wall (32–34, 60, 68).

TABLE 2. Selected biochemical characteristics for presumptive identification of aerobic actinomycetes

Organism	Characteristics									
	Acid-fast stain or lysozyme resistance[a]	Hydrolysis of casein	Hydrolysis of xanthine	Hydrolysis of tyrosine	Urease activity	Gelatin liquification	Ethylene glycol degradation	Beta-D-galactosidase activity	Nitrate reductase (24 h)	Resistance to mitomycin C (≥5 μg/ml)
Nocardia asteroides	+	−	−	−	+	−	−	+	+	+
Nocardia brasiliensis	+	+	−	+	+	+	−	+	−	+
Nocardia otitidiscaviarum	+	−	+	−	+	−	−	+	+/−	+
Rhodococcus spp.	+/−[b]	−	−	+/−	+/−	+	+	−	+	−
Rhodococcus aurantiaca[c]	+	−	−	−	+	+	+	+	−	+
Rhodococcus equi[c]	−	−	−	−	−	+	+	−	+	−
Actinomadura spp.	−	+	−	+	−	+	−	−	+	+
Nocardiopsis spp.	−	+	+/−	+	+/−	+	−	+	+	+
Streptomyces somaliensis	−	+	+	+	+/−	+	−	+	−	+
Streptomyces spp.	−	+	+/−	+	+/−	+	−	+	−	+
Mycobacterium spp.[d]	+/−	−	−	−	+/−	−	−	−[e]	+[e]	−[e]

[a] Modified Kinyoun stain.
[b] Reactions variable, predominantly positive.
[c] *R. aurantiaca*, syn. *Gordona aurantiaca*; *R. equi*, syn. *Corynebacterium equi*.
[d] Rapidly growing mycobacteria.
[e] Except *M. fortuitum* (beta-D-galactosidase, nitrate), *M. smegmatis*, and *M. phlei* (mitomycin C).

Amino acid decomposition

The casein, tyrosine, and xanthine decomposition pattern and acid-fast qualities of an actinomycete can be used to differentiate the more commonly encountered nocardiae, *N. asteroides, N. brasiliensis,* and *N. otitidiscaviarum* (11, 59) (Table 2). Decomposition media may also be of limited use in species determination of the non-acid-fast genera *Actinomadura, Nocardiopsis,* and *Streptomyces*. Hydrolysis of a substrate is indicated by a clearing or dissolution of the suspended substrate around colonial growth. Recognition of decomposition reaction is technique dependent and is facilitated by incorporation of finely granular xanthine, tyrosine, or casein (dried skim milk) into the basal agar. Thus, it may be necessary to grind extremely coarse reagents via mortar and pestle to produce a good homogeneous medium. After autoclaving, the substrate is carefully and evenly suspended in medium cooled almost to the point of solidification. Plates are inoculated by cutting shallow wells into the agar and placing a large portion of mycelium or colony in the well. This allows for more complete and earlier recognition of substrate hydrolysis (46, 57, 64). Such tests should be incubated at either room temperature or 30°C for at least 14 days or until good growth occurs. *Streptomyces* spp. (capable of hydrolysis of all three) and *N. asteroides* (which hydrolyzes none of these three substrates) serve as positive and negative controls, respectively.

Additional biochemical parameters

Resistance to the enzyme lysozyme generally mimics the acid-fast nature of the organism. *Nocardia* spp., *Mycobacterium* spp., and the occasional *Rhodococcus* sp. are resistant to lysozyme, while *Streptomyces* spp., *Actinomadura* spp., *Nocardiopsis* spp., and the majority of rhodococci are lysozyme susceptible. The procedure can be performed either as a growth-dependent test (11) or as a direct lysis test (40). The former requires incubation in a lysozyme-glycerol broth for up to 2 weeks, whereas the latter uses dissolution of a suspension of the test organism in the presence of lysozyme as an endpoint. Known isolates of *N. asteroides* and *Streptomyces* spp. serve as respective positive and negative control organisms.

The production of urease as detected by growth on Christensen's urea agar is characteristic of *N. asteroides, N. brasiliensis,* and *N. otitidiscaviarum*, whereas it is not characteristic of *Actinomadura* spp. The urease reactions of *Streptomyces* spp., *Nocardiopsis* spp., or *Rhodococcus* spp. are variable and contribute little to their identification. Gelatin is liquified by most aerobic actinomycetes except *N. asteroides* and *N. otitidiscaviarum* and may be of some use in distinguishing these two species from others.

The majority of *Rhodococcus* spp. will degrade 1% ethylene glycol incorporated into solid 7H10 agar, whereas other aerobic actinomycetes will generally fail to show such activity (96). Inoculated plates with and without ethylene glycol are kept at 37°C for at least 5 to 10 days to allow confluent growth to occur. Degradation of substrate changes the initial granular appearance of the agar to a milky turbidity. Known *N. asteroides* and *Rhodococcus* spp. are recommended as negative and positive controls, respectively.

The occasional ethylene glycol-negative *Rhodococcus*

sp. and the rapidly growing mycobacteria may closely resemble *N. asteroides* in physiological parameters, and the rare *N. asteroides* isolate that degrades this substance will likewise cause confusion (26, 93, 96; R. J. Wallace, Antimicrob. Newsl. **2**:85–92, 1985). Several aids to further differentiate these taxa include colonial and morphological characteristics, beta-galactosidase activity, and resistance to mitomycin C. The nocardial colony is rough to membranous in texture and is composed of extensively branched filaments, with some forming aerial mycelium. This is in direct contrast to the creamy bacteriumlike colonies and the coccobacillary to diphtheroid morphology of the rhodococci and mycobacteria. *Nocardia* spp., *Streptomyces* spp., and *Nocardiopsis* spp. have beta-D-galactosidase activity (88), while *Nocardia* spp. and *Rhodococcus aurantiaca* are resistant to ≥5 μg of mitomycin C per ml in the growth medium (102). The remainder of the rhodococci and *Mycobacterium* spp. lack beta-D-galactosidase activity and are susceptible to mitomycin C. Reference laboratories and other interested parties may wish to pursue more defined species characterization of not only the clinically isolated actinomycetes but some that may be relevant to human or veterinary medicine as well. Toward that end, a dichotomous key has been developed which identifies 16 species of aerobic actinomycetes. Identifications are based upon biograms developed by an isolate through growth on 40 different substrates (67). A more rapid variation of this approach has been to determine an actinomycetes constitutive enzyme profile via a commercially prepared substrate panel (54).

Chemotaxonomic markers

Reference level identification of the aerobic actinomycetes may also be achieved by chemical evaluation of their cell wall structure (chemotaxonomy). Interest has focused principally on the lipid (33, 68), carbohydrate (11, 94), 2,6-diaminopimelic acid (DAP) isomer (11, 100), and mycolic acid (17, 48, 69) composition of the cell wall. Such determinations are generally made through hydrolysis of harvested whole cells with subsequent analysis of end products using paper (8, 9), thin-layer (94), and liquid (48, 100) chromatography. This permits organisms to be classified into a variety of cell wall "types" such as those proposed by Lechevalier and Lechevalier (60). Goodfellow and Cross (32) and Goodfellow and Minikin (34) offer excellent reviews on the use of cell wall chemistry for classification of the *Actinomycetales*. In the future, nucleic acid probes may also be a means for definitive identification of aerobic actinomycetes in culture or in a freshly submitted clinical specimen (63).

By combining information on chemotaxonomic markers with key physiological characteristics, differentiation can be made between closely related taxa. Certain markers unique to the more commonly encountered actinomycotic genera are described in Table 3. Note that the presence of LL-DAP is unique to and very specifically delineates the genus *Streptomyces* from all other closely related organisms, which contain the *meso* isomer of DAP. Although the DAP and carbohydrate characteristics are identical among *Nocardia* spp., *Mycobacterium* spp., and *Rhodococcus* spp. (cell wall type IV), mycobacteria do not contain the cell wall lipid consistent for *Nocardia* (LCN-A) characterized by Mordarska and Rethy (68). This marker has been useful in distinguishing between infection due to *N. asteroides* and rapidly growing mycobacteria such as *Mycobacterium fortuitum* (93). High-pressure liquid chromatographic analysis of mycolic acids is useful in differentiating *Rhodococcus* spp. and *Nocardia* spp. (17).

Failure to identify isolates by using the more easily determined properties of morphology, staining characteristics, and selected biochemical reactions should prompt consulting a referral laboratory capable of characterizing chemotaxonomic markers. The true value of chemotaxonomy may lie in its potential to directly detect one of the *Actinomycetales* in a clinical specimen. Metabolites of *Nocardia* have been detected in cerebrospinal fluid and serum by frequency-pulsed electron capture gas-liquid chromatography (14). However, it should be pointed out that taxonomic definition to this extent, given the time, expense, and energy required to complete such analyses, must be evaluated in light of the diagnostic and therapeutic value of the information it gives.

DIAGNOSTIC IMMUNOLOGY

Extrinsic alveolar pneumonitis

Agar gel immunodiffusion or gel immunodiffusion (GID) remains the technique of choice in the serodiagnosis of actinomycotic extrinsic alveolar pneumonitis, often referred to as hypersensitivity pneumonitis (80). Although counterimmunoelectrophoresis has proven to be a more rapid and sensitive technique, GID appears to be much more specific and reproducible in detecting extrinsic alveolar pneumonitis (87; Hollick, Clin. Microbiol. Newsl. **8**[Mar.]:29–32, 1986). Specific

TABLE 3. Chemotaxonomic markers useful for the identification of aerobic actinomycetes of clinical interest

Species	DAP	Diagnostic compound[a]	LCN-A[b]	Cell wall type
Streptomyces spp.	LL-	None	−	I
Nocardia asteroides	*meso-*	ARA + GAL	+	IV
Nocardia brasiliensis	*meso-*	ARA + GAL	+	IV
Nocardia otitidiscaviarum	*meso-*	ARA + GAL	+	IV
Rhodococcus spp.	*meso-*	ARA + GAL	+	IV
Mycobacterium spp.	*meso-*	ARA + GAL	−	IV
Actinomadura spp.	*meso-*	GAL + MAD	−	IIIB
Nocardiopsis spp.	*meso-*	GAL or none	−	IIIC

[a] ARA, Arabinose; GAL, galactose; MAD, madurose. Note: All actinomycetes are likely to contain glucosamine, muramic acid, ribose, alanine, and glutamic acid in various amounts.

[b] LCN-A, Lipid characteristic of *Nocardia* spp. type A.

precipitin antibodies are detected by GID when a patient's serum forms lines of identity with a control system consisting of antigens from one or more of the thermophilic actinomycetes and a specific antiserum (sera) directed against them. Diagnosis of extrinsic alveolar pneumonitis is made by a combination of a history of potential allergen inhalation, appropriate clinical and radiological results, and positive specific precipitin antibody. However, a negative precipitin test does not rule out hypersensitivity pneumonitis. Reagents for this test, including antigens and control sera for *M. faeni, T. vulgaris,* and *T. candidus,* are produced commercially by Greer Laboratories and Hollister-Stier Laboratory.

Nocardiosis

A variety of extracellular and whole-cell homogenate antigens have been produced for use in complement fixation and immunodiffusion tests. Pier and colleagues (74, 75) produced an extracellular antigen from *N. asteroides* which could be made subspecific for four antigenic types and was used extensively in diagnosing bovine nocardiosis. When tested for the serodiagnosis of human disease, the antigen cross-reacted with sera from patients with mycobacterial infections and did not detect antibody in some patients having nocardiosis (73, 89). Blumer and Kaufman (13) compared pooled culture filtrate antigens with whole-cell homogenates in a microimmunodiffusion test with similar results. The pooled filtrate antigen proved superior to the homogenate by detecting 70% versus 49% of the cases, respectively. However, the filtrate antigen had a higher number of false-positive reactions as well. The majority of these cross-reactions were nonidentical and were observed in patients with tuberculosis or nonnocardial forms of actinomycosis.

Recent advances have centered upon development of monoclonal antibodies directed to isolated epitopes of *Nocardia* spp. Sugar and colleagues (98) identified two immunodominant proteins in culture filtrates of the three commonly isolated nocardiae, and El-Zaatari et al. (28) produced two monoclonal antibodies specific to *N. asteroides* antigens. Both of these reagents may have the potential to be developed into a specific nocardial serodiagnostic test. Another approach has been to use whole-cell extracts of *N. asteroides* and *N. brasiliensis* to produce a library of monoclonal antibodies (53). Although these monoclonal antibodies exhibited various degrees of cross-reactivity with mycobacterial antigens in an enzyme-linked immunosorbent assay, they may serve as a point of departure for producing more specific diagnostic reagents.

Dermatophilosis

D. congolensis does not exhibit the antigenic heterogeneity characteristic of the nocardiae and mycobacteria (35, 37). Antigens for GID and complement fixation tests are prepared from the disruption of washed whole cells grown in serum broth cultures for 72 to 96 h at 37°C (79). Antibodies have been raised to these whole-cell antigens, conjugated with fluorescein, and used to detect the organism in smears of crusts and exudates. Chloroform extracts of partially purified cell walls have been used as antigens for GID and passive hemagglutination tests to detect antibodies in serum and milk from animals within the endemic region.

In summary, a great deal of effort is currently being expended in developing reagents and tests for the serodiagnosis of aerobic actinomycete infections. Some, like gel immunodiffusion for detecting antibodies to hypersensitivity pneumonitis (80; Hollick, Clin. Microbiol. Newsl. **8**[Mar.]:29–32, 1986), dermatophilosis (79), and mycetoma (65, 80), are fairly reliable. Others, especially those developed for the serodiagnosis of nocardiosis, remain unsatisfactory, and none of the reagents are available for routine testing. Consequently, the diagnosis of invasive actinomycete infection still must rely upon histopathology and culture until such time reagents are commercially produced and have the consistent sensitivity and specificity necessary for serodiagnostic testing.

ANTIMICROBIAL SUSCEPTIBILITY

Antimicrobic therapy

The treatment of choice for systemic nocardiosis in the immune-compromised patient is two or more sulfonamides (5, 7, 13, 29). In the past, the most common regimen has been dual therapy consisting of sulfadiazine and sulfamethoxazole. Recent attempts to use trimethoprim-sulfamethoxazole as a single therapy for nocardiosis have achieved considerable success, although there have been reports of resistant cases and relapses (1, 10, 92).

These results suggest that the effectiveness of trimethoprim-sulfamethoxazole is limited and that it should not be used singly but rather in combination with another sulfa, tetracycline, or aminoglycoside (7, 108). Mycetoma has also been effectively treated with trimethoprim-sulfamethoxazole, either singly or in combination (65, 80). The addition of streptomycin, rifampin, diaminodiphenylsulfone (Dapsone), or a combination of these to the regimen has been shown to improve these results. It is noteworthy that in the more severe cases of mycetoma and other forms of nocardiosis surgery is required in addition to antimicrobial therapy. Fixed cutaneous nocardiosis appears to be a relatively benign disease and may spontaneously heal or resolve with a short course of sulfa therapy.

Other antimicrobial agents which have shown in vitro and in vivo efficacy for nocardiosis are minocycline and amikacin, a tetracycline and aminoglycoside, respectively (3, 12, 25, 45, 111–113). Pulmonary nocardiosis has been treated with minocycline in combination with ampicillin and erythromycin (2). β-Lactam antibiotics which have shown limited in vitro effectiveness against the nocardiae are cefotaxime, cefmenoxime, ceftriaxone, cefuroxime, and *N*-formimidoyl thienamycin (imipenem) (30, 37, 107). However, there are no studies for any one of these antibiotics with enough patients to correlate laboratory findings with clinical response.

Treatment of the remaining diseases caused by the aerobic actinomycetes is much less stringent. Hypersensitivity pneumonitis is treated with glucocorticosteroids and bronchodilation (80). Dermatophilosis responds to a long course of either high-dose penicillin therapy or a combination of penicillin and streptomycin (35, 37, 80). For those patients with penicillin allergy, streptomycin, cholamphenicol, tetracycline, erythromycin, kanamycin, and the sulfonamides have all proven effective. *Rhodococcus* spp. have shown in vitro susceptibility to a variety of antibiotics, including vancomycin, erythromycin, the aminoglycosides, and chloramphenicol (15, 69). However, *R. aurantiacus* appears to be fairly resistant to these antibiotics, which is one of the reasons for considering placement of this organism in another genus, *Gordona* (78, 104). This disparity in susceptibility between species is borne out by the few clinical papers published, in which treatment of abscesses caused by *Rhodococcus equi* in noncompromised patients appears to be uncomplicated whereas abscesses caused by *R. aurantiacus* are quite resistant to therapy. Doxycycline has been used to successfully treat a primary granulomatous dermatitis that was unresponsive to minocycline as well as oral trimethoprim-sulfamethoxazole (21).

Susceptibility testing

The highly individualized in vitro response of the aerobic actinomycetes to antibiotics and their unpredictable clinical behavior emphasize the need for laboratory susceptibility testing. A variety of susceptibility tests have been tried and found to be successful, but none has achieved consensus as a standard method (5, 18, 61, 106–108; Wallace, Antimicrob. Newsl. **2**:85–92, 1985). Once a standard method has been determined, its clinical predictive capabilities may be hindered by two factors. The first, alluded to earlier, concerns the lack of statistically valid patient groups in any one series of cases to correlate in vitro with in vivo results. Second, there is the insurmountable problem of ascertaining how a single laboratory test can predict a "cure" when elimination of disease is due to a vast complex of therapeutic and physiological factors, the least of which is the antimicrobial agent used.

In light of those caveats, one can show with certain systems a consistent antibiogram for a given isolate against certain antibiotics. The most common organisms tested have been *Nocardia* spp. and *Rhodococcus* spp. The most frequently used testing methods have been a modified Kirby-Bauer disk diffusion or an agar dilution system using single or dual sulfas, aminoglycosides, second-generation and broad-spectrum cephalosporins, and imipenem. The success of either of these methods is contingent upon obtaining a homogeneous suspension of the test organism from which a standardized inoculum (0.5 McFarland) may be made. This is accomplished by one of two methods: agitating equal volumes of a broth culture and sterile glass beads or suspending growth from a plate in sterile saline with an equal volume of 0.5-μm glass beads and disrupting with a sterile, disposable tissue homogenizer. Homogeneous suspensions, free of large clumps, may then be diluted to a 0.5 McFarland standard. Mueller-Hinton agar plates are inoculated with the standardized suspension, commercially prepared antibiotic diffusion disks are applied, and cultures are incubated for 5 to 10 days with care being taken to prevent dehydration (106, 107; Wallace, Antimicrob. Newsl. **2**:85–92, 1985). Conventional zone diameters are used to define susceptibility or resistance.

MICs have been determined by conventional agar dilution testing. A standardized inoculum poses the biggest problem to testing, and this may be overcome as described above. Interpretive criteria are based upon the assumption that MICs below achievable serum levels of a particular antibiotic constitute susceptibility. Data on the correlation of such interpretations with clinical outcome, however, are lacking.

It is obvious that the use of any antimicrobial susceptibility testing system for the aerobic actinomycetes to predict clinical response must be questioned. As in the susceptibility testing for any organism, one should err towards the conservative side. Thus, the in vitro resistance of an actinomycete to a specific antibiotic under carefully controlled test conditions may be a reasonable predictor of negative clinical response. Used in this manner, susceptibility testing for the aerobic actinomycetes can play a valuable role in determining therapy.

SUMMARY

The aerobic *Actinomycetales* encompass a variety of organisms that are grouped together on the basis of similar cell wall chemistry, staining properties, and microscopic morphology. As a group they are gram positive and catalase producing and stain partially acid fast (*Nocardia* spp., mycobacteria, and some *Rhodococcus* spp.). They vary in form from coccobacillary diphtheroids to filaments that are dichotomously branched and 1 μm in diameter. Some genera further exhibit complex branching with or without the production of aerial hyphae (*Nocardia* spp., *Streptomyces* spp., *Actinomadura* spp., and *Nocardiopsis* spp.). *Nocardia* spp. differ from the remainder of the *Actinomycetales* by virtue of their partial acid-fastness, filaments with extensive branching, and leathery to membranous colonies. Both the nocardiae and mycobacteria have type IV cell wall chemistry, and while most species are partially acid fast and share resistance to lysozyme, only the nocardiae produce aerial hyphae.

Nocardia spp. are the most common agents of human infection and can be presumptively identified by staining properties, microscopic morphology, and substrate degradation. *Nocardia* spp. are variably acid fast when decolorized with a weak mineral acid (modified Kinyoun), and they produce complex branching filaments and aerial hyphae. *N. asteroides* fails to hydrolyze casein, L-tyrosine, and xanthine; *N. brasiliensis* hydrolyzes casein and L-tyrosine, and *N. otitidiscaviarum* hydrolyzes xanthine. The thermophilic actinomycetes grow at temperatures of greater than 42°C and may be further differentiated by a variety of biochemical tests. *D. congolensis* appears in clinical specimens as longitudinally and transversely sectioned branching filaments forming discrete packets of cells. They may be further differentiated by biochemical tests. Reference level identification of all members of the *Actinomycetales* may be done through extensive biochemical testing with conventional substrates and cellular chemistry via component extraction and analysis by thin-layer, high-pressure liquid, or gas-liquid chromatography.

We wish to dedicate this chapter to Morris A. Gordon on the occasion of his retirement and to thank him for his generous contribution of Fig. 3 through 20 to this chapter, as well as his efforts in producing the actinomycete chapter for earlier editions of the *Manual of Clinical Microbiology*. Dr. Gordon has had a profound influence on many generations of scientists, including the authors of this chapter, and leaves a rich legacy in medical mycology in general and actinomycotic biology in particular.

LITERATURE CITED

1. **Adams, H. G., B. A. Beeler, L. S. Wann, C. K. Chin, and G. F. Brooks.** 1984. Synergistic action of trimethoprim and sulfmethoxazole for *Nocardia asteroids:* efficacious therapy in five patients. Am. J. Med. Sci. **287:**8–12.
2. **Bach, M. C., A. P. Monaco, and M. Finland.** 1973. Pulmonary nocardiosis: therapy with minocycline and with erythromycin plus ampicillin. J. Am. Med. Assoc. **224:** 1378–1381.
3. **Bach, M. C., L. D. Sabath, and M. Finland.** 1973. Susceptibility of *Nocardia asteroides* to 45 antimicrobial agents in vitro. Antimicrob. Agents Chemother. **3:**1–8.
4. **Beadles, T. A., G. A. Land, and D. J. Knezek.** 1980. An ultrastructural comparison of the cell envelopes of selected strains of *Nocardia asteroides* and *Nocardia brasiliensis.* Mycopathologia **70:**25–32.
5. **Beaman, B. L.** 1984. Actinomycete pathogenesis, p. 457–459. *In* M. Goodfellow, M. Mordarski, and S. T. Williams (ed.), The biology of the actinomycetes. Academic Press, Inc. (London), Ltd., London.
6. **Beaman, B. L., J. Burnside, B. Edwards, and W. A. Causey.** 1976. Nocardial infections in the United States—1971–1974. J. Infect. Dis. **124:**286–289.
7. **Beaman, B. L., and A. M. Sugar.** 1983. *Nocardia* in naturally acquired and experimental infections in animals. J. Hyg. **91:**393–419.
8. **Becker, B., M. P. Lechevalier, R. E. Gordon, and H. A. Lechevalier.** 1964. Rapid differentiation between *Nocardia* and *Streptomyces* by paper chromatography of whole-cell hydrolysates. Appl. Microbiol. **12:**421–423.
9. **Becker, B., M. P. Lechevalier, and H. A. Lechevalier.** 1965. Chemical composition of cell-wall preparations from strains of various form-genera of aerobic actinomycetes. Appl. Microbiol. **13:**236–243.
10. **Bennett, J. E., and A. E. Jennings.** 1978. Factors influencing susceptibility of *Nocardia* species to trimethoprim-sulfamethoxazole. Antimicrob. Agents Chemother. **13:** 624–627.
11. **Berd, D.** 1973. Laboratory identification of clinically important aerobic actinomycetes. Appl. Microbiol. **25:**663–681.
12. **Black, W. A., and P. A. McNellis.** 1970. Susceptibility of *Nocardia* species to modern antimicrobials. Antimicrob. Agents Chemother. **10:**346–349.
13. **Blumer, S. O., and L. Kaufman.** 1979. Microimmunodiffusion test for nocardiosis. J. Clin. Microbiol. **10:**308–312.
14. **Brooks, J. B., J. V. Kaskin, D. M. Fast, and M. I. Daneshvar.** 1987. Detection of metabolites by frequency-pulsed electron capture gas-liquid chromatography in serum and cerebral spinal fluid of a patient with *Nocardia* infection. J. Clin. Microbiol. **25:**445–448.
15. **Broughton, R. A., H. D. Wilson, N. L. Goodman, and J. A. Hendrick.** 1981. Septic arthritis and osteomyelitis caused by an organism of the genus *Rhodococcus.* J. Clin. Microbiol. **25:**445–448.
16. **Bunker, M. L., L. Chewning, S. E. Wang, and M. A. Gordon.** 1988. *Dermatophilus congolensis* and "hairy" leukoplakia. Am. J. Clin. Pathol. **89:**683–687.
17. **Butler, W. R., J. O. Kilburn, and G. P. Kubica.** 1987. High performance liquid chromatography analysis of mycolic acids as an aid in laboratory identification of *Rhodococcus* and *Nocardia* species. J. Clin. Microbiol. **25:**2126–2131.
18. **Caroll, G. F., J. M. Brown, and L. D. Haley.** 1977. A method for determining *in vitro* drug susceptibilities of some *Nocardia* and *Actinomadurae.* Am. J. Clin. Pathol. **68:**279–283.
19. **Casale, T. B., A. M. Macher, and A. S. Fauci.** 1984. Concomitant pulmonary aspergillosis and nocardiosis in a patient with chronic granulomatous disease of childhood. South. Med. J. **77:**274–275.
20. **Cawson, R. A., A. W. McCracken, P. B. Marcus, and G. S. Zaatari.** 1989. Pathology: the mechanisms of disease, 2nd ed. C. V. Mosby, St. Louis, Mo.
21. **Chanda, J. J., and J. T. Headington.** 1983. Primary granulomatous dermatitis caused by *Rhodochrous.* Arch. Dermatol. **119:**994–997.
22. **Cruickshank, J. G., A. H. Gawler, and C. Shaldon.** 1979. *Oerskovia* species: rare opportunistic pathogens. J. Med. Microbiol. **12:**513–515.
23. **Curry, W. A.** 1974. *Nocardia caviae:* a report of 13 new isolations with clinical correlation. Appl. Microbiol. **28:** 193–198.
24. **Curry, W. A.** 1980. Human nocardiosis. Arch. Intern. Med. **140:**818–826.
25. **Dalovisio, J. R., and G. A. Pankey.** 1978. In vitro susceptibility of *Nocardia asteroides* to amikacin. Antimicrob. Agents Chemother. **13:**128–129.
26. **Damskey, B.** 1980. Nontuberculous *Mycobacteria* as an unsuspected agent of dermatological infections: diagnosis through microbiological parameters. J. Clin. Microbiol. **11:**569–572.
27. **Eisenberg, E. S., B. E. Alpert, R. A. Weiss, N. Mittman, and R. Soerio.** 1983. *Rhodotorula rubra* peritonitis in patients undergoing continuous ambulatory peritoneal dialysis. Am. J. Med. **75:**349–352.
28. **El-Zaatari, F. A., E. Reiss, A. M. Yakrus, S. D. Bragg, and L. Kaufman.** 1986. Monoclonal antibodies against isoelectrically focused *Nocardia asteroides* proteins characterized by the enzyme-linked immunoelectrotransfer blot method. Methods Diag. Immunol. **4:**97–106.
29. **Geiseler, P. J., and B. R. Anderson.** 1979. Results of therapy in systemic nocardiosis. Am. J. Clin. Med. Sci. **278:**188–194.
30. **Gombert, M. E., and T. M. Aulicino.** 1983. Synergism of imipenem and amikacin in combination with other antibiotics against *Nocardia asteroides.* Antimicrob. Agents Chemother. **24:**810–811.
31. **Goodfellow, M., and G. Alderson.** 1977. The actinomycete-genus *Rhodococcus:* a home for the *'rhodochrous'* complex. J. Gen. Microbiol. **100:**99–122.
32. **Goodfellow, M., and T. Cross.** 1984. Classification, p. 7–164. *In* M. Goodfellow, M. Mordarski, and S. T. Williams (ed.), Biology of the actinomycetes. Academic Press, Inc. (London), Ltd., London.
33. **Goodfellow, M., and T. Cross.** 1984. Characterization of *Mycobacterium, Nocardia, Corynebacterium* and related taxa. Ann. Soc. Belge Med. Trop. **53:**287–298.
34. **Goodfellow, M., and D. E. Minnikin.** 1977. Nocardioform bacteria. Annu. Rev. Microbiol. **31:**159–180.
35. **Gordon, M. A.** 1964. The genus *Dermatophilus.* J. Bacteriol. **88:**509–522.
36. **Gordon, M. A.** 1974. Family V. *Dermatophilaceae* Austwick 1958, 42, *emend. mut. char.* Gordon 1964, 521, p. 723–726. *In* P. E. Buchanan and N. E. Gibbons (ed.), Bergey's manual of determinative bacteriology, 8th ed. The Williams and Wilkins Co., Baltimore.
37. **Gordon, M. A.** 1985. Aerobic pathogenic *Actinomycetaceae,* p. 249–262. *In* E. H. Lennette, A. Balows, W. J. Hausler, and H. J. Shadomy (ed.), Manual of clinical microbiology, 4th ed. American Society for Microbiology, Washington, D.C.
38. **Gordon, M. A., I. F. Salkin, and W. B. Stone.** 1977. *Dermatophilus* dermatitis enzootic in deer in New York State and vicinity. J. Wild. Dis. **13:**184–190.
39. **Gordon, R. E.** 1966. Some criteria for the recognition of *Nocardia madurae* (Vincent) Blanchard. J. Gen. Microbiol. **45:**355–364.
40. **Gordon, R. E., and D. A. Barnett.** 1977. Resistance to rifampin and lysozyme of strains of some species of *Mycobacterium* and *Nocardia* as a taxonomic tool. Int. J. Syst. Bacteriol. **27:**176–178.
41. **Gordon, R. E., D. A. Barnett, J. E. Handerhan, and C. H.-N. Pang.** 1974. *Nocardia coeliaca, Nocardia auto-*

trophica, and the nocardin strain. Int. J. Syst. Bacteriol. **24:**54–63.
42. **Gordon, R. E., and W. A. Hagen.** 1936. A study of some acid fast actinomycetes from soil with special reference to pathogenicity to animals. J. Infect. Dis. **59:**200–206.
43. **Gordon, R. E., and J. M. Mihm.** 1959. A comparison of *Nocardia asteroides* and *Nocardia brasiliensis*. J. Gen. Microbiol. **20:**129–155.
44. **Gordon, R. E., and J. M. Mihm.** 1975. A comparative study of some strains received as nocardiae. J. Bacteriol. **73:**15–27.
45. **Gutmann, L., F. W. Goldstein, M. D. Kitzls, B. Hatefort, C. Darmon, and J. F. Acar.** 1983. Susceptibility of *Nocardia asteroides* to 46 antibiotics, including 22 β-lactams. Antimicrob. Agents Chemother. **23:**248–251.
46. **Haley, L. D., and C. S. Callaway.** 1978. Laboratory methods in medical mycology, p. 139–152. Laboratory Training and Consultation Division, Center for Disease Control, Atlanta, Ga.
47. **Hay, R. J.** 1983. Nocardial infection of the skin. J. Hyg. **91:**385–391.
48. **Hecht, S. T., and W. A. Causey.** 1976. Rapid method for the detection and identification of mycolic acids in aerobic actinomycetes and related bacteria. J. Clin. Microbiol. **4:**284–287.
49. **Hirst, L. W., G. K. Harrison, W. G. Merz, and W. J. Stark.** 1979. *Nocardia asteroides* keratitis. Br. J. Ophthalmol. **63:**449–454.
50. **Hosty, T. S., C. McDurmont, L. Ajello, L. K. George, G. L. Brumfield, and A. A. Colix.** 1961. Prevalence of *Nocardia asteroides* in sputa examined by a tuberculosis diagnostic laboratory. J. Lab. Clin. Med. **58:**107–114.
51. **Houang, E. T., I. S. Lovett, F. D. Thompson, A. R. Harrison, A. M. Doekes, and M. Goodfellow.** 1980. *Nocardia asteroides* infection—a transmissible disease. J. Hosp. Infect. **1:**31–40.
52. **Jensen, H. L.** 1953. The genus *Nocardia* (or *Proactinomyces*) and its separation from other *Actinomycetales*, with some reflections on the phylogeny of the actinomycetes, p. 61–68. *In* E. Baldacci and P. Redacelli (ed.), Proceedings of the Symposium on the *Actinomycetales*, 6th International Congress of Microbiology, Rome, Italy. Emanuele Paterna, Rome.
53. **Jimenez, T., A. M. Diaz, and H. Zlotnik.** 1990. Monoclonal antibodies to *Nocardia asteroides* and *Nocardia brasiliensis* antigens. J. Clin. Microbiol. **28:**87–91.
54. **Kilian, M.** 1978. Rapid identification of *Actinomycetaceae* and related bacteria. J. Clin. Microbiol. **8:**127–133.
55. **Krick, J. A., E. B. Stinson, and J. S. Remington.** 1975. Nocardia infection in heart transplant patients. Ann. Intern. Med. **82:**18–26.
56. **Land, G. A., and I. F. Salkin.** 1986. Opportunistic zoopathogenic yeasts and their identification. Mycopathologia **99:**155–171.
57. **Land, G. A., and J. Staneck.** 1988. The aerobic actinomycetes, p. 271–302. *In* B. B. Wentworth, M. S. Bartlett, B. E. Robinson, and I. F. Salkin (ed.), Diagnostic manual for mycotic and parasitic infections, 7th ed. American Public Health Association, Washington, D.C.
58. **Law, B. J., and M. I. Marks.** 1982. Pediatric nocardiosis. Pediatrics **70:**560–565.
59. **Lechevalier, M. P.** 1968. Identification of aerobic actinomycetes of clinical importance. J. Lab. Clin. Med. **71:** 934–944.
60. **Lechevalier, M. P., and H. L. Lechevalier.** 1970. Chemical composition as a criterion in the classification of aerobic actinomycetes. Int. J. Syst. Bacteriol. **20:**435–443.
61. **Lerner, P. I., and G. L. Baum.** 1973. Antimicrobial susceptibility of *Nocardia* species. Antimicrob. Agents Chemother. **4:**85–93.
62. **Lloyd, D. D., and K. C. Sellars (ed.).** 1976. *Dermatophilus* infection in animals and man. Academic Press, Inc. (London), Ltd., London.
63. **Loeffelholz, M. J., and D. R. Scholl.** 1989. Method for improved extraction of DNA from *Nocardia asteroides*. J. Clin. Microbiol. **27:**1880–1881.
64. **McGinnis, M. R., R. F. D'Amato, and G. A. Land.** 1982. Pictorial handbook of medically important fungi and aerobic actinomycetes. Praeger, New York.
65. **McGinnis, M. R., and R. C. Fader.** 1988. Mycetoma: a contemporary concept. Infect. Dis. Clin. North Am. **2:** 939–954.
66. **Meyer, J.** 1976. *Nocardiopsis*, a new genus of the order *Actinomycetales*. Int. J. Syst. Bacteriol. **26:**487–493.
67. **Mishra, S. K., R. E. Gordon, and D. A. Barnett.** 1980. Identification of nocardiae and streptomycetes of medical importance. J. Clin. Microbiol. **11:**728–736.
68. **Mordarska, H., and A. Rethy.** 1970. Preliminary studies on the chemical character of the lipid fraction in *Nocardia*. Arch. Immunol. Ther. Exp. **18:**455–459.
69. **Muller, F., K. P. Schaal, A. von Graevenitz, L. von Moos, J. B. Woolcock, J. Wust, and A. F. Yassin.** 1988. Characterization of a *Rhodococcus equi*-like bacterium isolated from a wound infection in a noncompromised host. J. Clin. Microbiol. **26:**618–620.
70. **Murray, J. F., S. M. Finegold, S. Froman, and D. W. Will.** 1961. The changing spectrum of nocardiosis. Am. Rev. Respir. Dis. **83:**351–330.
71. **Murray, P. R., R. L. Heeren, and A. C. Niles.** 1987. Effect of decontamination procedures on recovery of *Nocardia* spp. J. Clin. Microbiol. **25:**2010–2011.
72. **Palmer, D. L., R. L. Harvey, and J. K. Wheeler.** 1974. Diagnostic and therapeutic considerations in *Nocardia asteroides* infections. Medicine **53:**391–401.
73. **Pier, A. C., and R. E. Fichtner.** 1971. Serologic typing of *Nocardia asteroides* by immunodiffusion. Am. Rev. Respir. Dis. **103:**698–707.
74. **Pier, A. C., and R. E. Fichtner.** 1981. Distribution of serotypes of *Nocardia asteroides* from animal, human, and environmental sources. J. Clin. Microbiol. **13:**548–553.
75. **Pier, A. C., E. H. Willers, and M. J. Mejia.** 1961. *Nocardia asteroides* as a mammary pathogen of cattle. II. The sources of nocardial infection and experimental reproduction of the disease. Am. J. Vet. Res. **22:**698–703.
76. **Prakash, U. B., S. S. Barnham, H. A. Carpenter, D. E. Dines, and H. M. Marsh.** 1987. Pulmonary alveolar phospholipoproteinosis: experience with 34 cases and a review. Mayo Clin. Proc. **62:**499–518.
77. **Presant, C. A., P. H. Wiernik, and A. A. Serpick.** 1973. Factors affecting survival in nocardiosis. Am. Rev. Respir. Dis. **108:**1444–1448.
78. **Prinz, G., E. Ban, S. Fekete, and Z. Szabo.** 1985. Meningitis caused by *Gordona aurantiaca (Rhodococcus aurantiacus)*. J. Clin. Microbiol. **22:**472–473.
79. **Richard, J. L., J. R. Thurston, and A. C. Pier.** 1976. Comparison of antigens of *Dermatophilus congolensis* isolates and their use in serologic tests in experimental and natural infections, p. 216–227. *In* D. Lloyd and K. Sellars (ed.), *Dermatophilus* infections in animal and man. Academic Press, Inc., New York.
80. **Rippon, J. W.** 1988. Medical mycology: the pathogenic fungi and the pathogenic actinomycetes, 3rd ed. W. B. Saunders Co., Philadelphia.
81. **Roberts, G. D., N. S. Brewer, and P. E. Hermans.** 1974. Diagnosis of nocardiosis by blood culture. Mayo Clin. Proc. **49:**293–296.
82. **Rosett, W., and G. R. Hodges.** 1978. Recent experiences with *Nocardia* infections. Am. J. Sci. **276:**279–285.
83. **Ruebush, T. K., and J. S. Goodman.** 1975. *Nocardia asteroides* bacteremia in an immunosuppressed renal-transplant patient. Am. J. Clin. Pathol. **64:**537–539.
84. **Sack, K.** 1985. Nocardial infection in a renal transplant recipient—a case report. Scand. J. Urol. Nephrol. **92**(Suppl.):59–66.
85. **Satterwhite, T. K., and R. J. Wallace.** 1979. Primary

cutaneous nocardiosis. J. Am. Med. Assoc. **242:**333–336.

86. **Schneidau, J. D., and M. F. Shaffer.** 1957. Studies on *Nocardia* and other *Actinomycetales.* I. Cultural studies. Am. Rev. Tuberc. Pulm. Dis. **76:**770–788.
87. **Shaal, K. P.** 1984. Laboratory diagnosis of actinomycete diseases, p. 425–456. *In* M. Goodfellow, M. Mordarski, and S. T. Williams (ed.), The biology of the actinomycetes. Academic Press, Inc. (London), Ltd., London.
88. **Shadomy, H. J., and N. G. Warren.** 1988. Nocardiosis, p. 671–677. *In* A. Balows, W. J. Hausler, Jr., M. Ohashi, and A. Turano (ed.), Laboratory diagnosis of infectious diseases: principles and practices, vol. I. Springer-Verlag, New York.
89. **Shainhouse, J. Z., A. C. Pier, and D. A. Stevens.** 1978. Complement fixation antibody test for human nocardiosis. J. Clin. Microbiol. **8:**516–519.
90. **Shawar, R. M., D. G. Moore, and M. T. LaRocco.** 1990. Cultivation of *Nocardia* spp. on chemically defined media for selective recovery of isolates from clinical specimens. J. Clin. Microbiol. **28:**508–512.
91. **Singh, M., R. S. Sandhu, and H. S. Randhawa.** 1987. Comparison of paraffin baiting and conventional culture techniques for isolation of *Nocardia asteroides* from sputum. J. Clin. Microbiol. **25:**176–177.
92. **Smego, R. A., and H. A. Gallis.** 1984. The clinical spectrum of *Nocardia brasiliensis* infection in the United States. Rev. Infect. Dis. **6:**164–180.
93. **Staneck, J. L., P. T. Frame, W. A. Altemeier, and E. H. Miller.** 1981. Infection of bone by *Mycobacterium fortuitum* masquerading as *Nocardia asteroides.* Am. J. Clin. Pathol. **76:**216–222.
94. **Staneck, J. L., and G. D. Roberts.** 1974. Simplified approach to identification of aerobic actinomycetes by thin-layer chromotography. Appl. Microbiol. **28:**226–231.
95. **Stevens, D., A. Pier, B. Beaman, P. A. Morozum, I. S. Lovett, and E. T. Houang.** 1981. Laboratory evaluation of an outbreak of nocardiosis in immunocompromised hosts. Am. J. Med. **71:**928–934.
96. **Stottmeier, K. D., and M. E. Molloy.** 1973. Rapid identification of the taxon *Rhodochrous* in the clinical laboratory. Appl. Microbiol. **26:**213–214.
97. **Stropes, L., M. Bartlett, and A. White.** 1980. Multiple recurrences of nocardia pneumonia. Am. J. Med. Sci. **280:**119–122.
98. **Sugar, A. M., G. K. Schoolnik, and D. A. Stevens.** 1985. Antibody response in human nocardiosis: identification of two immunodominant culture-filtrate antigens derived from *Nocardia asteroides.* J. Infect. Dis. **151:**895–901.
99. **Svirbely, J. R., W. J. Buesching, L. W. Ayers, P. B. Baker, and A. J. Britton.** 1983. *Mycobacterium fortuitium* infection of a Hickman catheter site. Am. J. Clin. Pathol. **80:**733–735.
100. **Tisdall, P. A., and J. P. Anhalt.** 1979. Rapid differentiation of *Streptomyces* from *Nocardia* by liquid chromatography. J. Clin. Microbiol. **10:**503–505.
101. **Truehaft, M. W., and M. P. Arden-Jones.** 1982. Comparison of methods for isolation and enumeration of thermophilic actinomycetes from dust. J. Clin. Microbiol. **16:**995–999.
102. **Tsukamura, M.** 1981. Test for susceptibility to Mitomycin C as aids for differentiating the genus *Rhodococcus* from the genus *Nocardia,* and for differentiating *Mycobacterium fortuitum* and *Mycobacterium cheoni* from other rapidly growing mycobacteria. Microbiol. Immunol. **25:**1197–1199.
103. **Tsukamura, M., K. Hikosaka, K. Nishimura, and S. Hara.** 1982. Severe progressive subcutaneous abscesses and necrotizing tenosynovitis caused by *Rhodococcus aurantiacus.* J. Clin. Microbiol. **26:**201–205.
104. **Tsukamura, M., and K. Kawakami.** 1982. Lung infection caused by *Gordona aurantiaca (Rhodococcus aurantiacus).* J. Clin. Microbiol. **16:**604–607.
105. **Vanderstigel, M. V., R. Leclercq, C. Brun-Buisson, A. Schaeffer, and I. Duval.** 1986. Blood-borne pulmonary infections with *Nocardia asteroides* in a heroin addict. J. Clin. Microbiol. **23:**175–176.
106. **Wallace, R. J., E. J. Septimus, D. M. Musher, and R. R. Martin.** 1977. Disc diffusion susceptibility testing of *Nocardia* species. J. Infect. Dis. **135:**568–575.
107. **Wallace, R. J., K. Weiss, R. Curvey, P. H. Vance, and J. Steadham.** 1983. Differences among *Nocardia* spp: susceptibility to aminoglycosides and beta-lactam antibiotics and their potential use in taxonomy. Antimicrob. Agents Chemother. **23:**19–21.
108. **Wallace, R. J., Jr., E. J. Septimus, D. M. Musher, M. B. Berger, and R. R. Martin.** 1979. Treatment of experimental nocardiosis in mice: comparison of amikacin and sulfonamide. J. Infect. Dis. **140:**244–248.
109. **Williams, S. T., S. Lanning, and E. M. H. Wellington.** 1984. Ecology of actinomycetes, p. 480–528. *In* M. Goodfellow, M. Mordarski, and S. T. Williams (ed.), The biology of the actinomycetes. Academic Press, Inc. (London), Ltd., London.
110. **Wilson, J. P., H. R. Turner, K. A. Kirchner, and S. W. Chapman.** 1989. Nocardial infections in renal transplant patients. Medicine **68:**38–84.
111. **Woods, G. L., G. L. Hall, and M. J. Schreiber.** 1986. *Mycobacterium fortuitum* peritonitis associated with continuous ambulatory peritoneal dialysis. J. Clin. Microbiol. **23:**786–788.
112. **Wren, M. V., A. M. Savage, and R. H. Alford.** 1979. Apparent cure of intracranial *Nocardia asteroides* infection by minocycline. Arch. Intern. Med. **139:**249–250.
113. **Yogev, R., T. Greenslade, C. F. Firlit, and P. Lewy.** 1980. Successful treatment of *Nocardia asteroides* infection with amikacin. J. Pediatr. **96:**771–773.

Chapter 36

Enterobacteriaceae

J. J. FARMER III AND MICHAEL T. KELLY

It is becoming increasingly difficult to adequately cover the family *Enterobacteriaceae* in a single chapter. The family includes the plague bacillus *Yersinia pestis*, the typhoid bacillus *Salmonella typhi*, 4 species that often cause diarrhea and other intestinal infections, 7 species associated with nosocomial infections, many species that cause human or animal infections, and over 40 species that occasionally occur in human clinical specimens. This chapter covers all of the species in a six-part format: (i) the family *Enterobacteriaceae* as a group; (ii) *Escherichia coli;* (iii) *Shigella;* (iv) *Salmonella;* (v) *Yersinia enterocolitica;* and (vi) other organisms in the family (parts ii to v deal with the four important causes of intestinal infections). Owing to space limitations, it was not possible to include many primary references and coverage of many topics has necessarily been limited. Several other sources are recommended for additional information (9–11, 13, 16, 17, 20, 21, 23, 24, 26, 27, 29, 31, 32, 38, 41, 44, 46, 49, 54, 58, 61, 63, 67, 70, 73, 76).

NOMENCLATURE AND CLASSIFICATION OF *ENTEROBACTERIACEAE*

The nomenclature and classification of *Enterobacteriaceae* has always been a confusing subject (10, 12, 24, 29, 46, 49). Until recently, genera and species were defined by biochemical and antigenic analysis (46). Now, techniques such as nucleic acid hybridization that measure evolutionary distance have better defined the relationships of all organisms in the family (10, 29).

In this chapter, we use the nomenclature and classification used in the Enteric Bacteriology Laboratories, Centers for Disease Control (29, 31), which may differ from other familiar classifications (12, 24, 49, 70). Table 1 lists all of the genera, species, biogroups, and unnamed groups included in the family. Most of the newly described organisms in Table 1 are very rare in clinical specimens (29), and most clinically significant isolates belong to 20 to 25 species that have been well known for many years (24, 46). This pattern is illustrated by the lists of organisms that most often cause nosocomial infections (Table 2), bacteremia and meningitis (Table 3), and infections of the gastrointestinal tract (Tables 5 and 6). Tables 1, 4, and 7 to 24 summarize the properties of the organisms in the family.

DESCRIPTION OF THE FAMILY

Most organisms in the family *Enterobacteriaceae* share the following properties: are gram negative; are rod shaped; are motile by peritrichous flagella or nonmotile; do not form spores; grow on peptone or meat extract media without the addition of sodium chloride or other supplements; grow well on MacConkey agar; grow both aerobically and anaerobically; ferment (rather than oxidize) D-glucose, often with gas production; are catalase positive and oxidase negative; reduce nitrate to nitrite; and have a 39 to 59% G+C content of DNA (49, 70).

NATURAL HABITATS

Enterobacteriaceae are widely distributed on plants and in soil, water, and the intestines of humans and animals (49, 70). Some species occupy a very limited ecological niche. *S. typhi* causes typhoid fever and is found only in humans (24, 41, 46). In contrast, strains of *Klebsiella pneumoniae* are distributed widely in the environment and contribute to biochemical and geochemical processes (58). However, strains of *K. pneumoniae* also cause human disease ranging from asymptomatic colonization of the intestinal, urinary, or respiratory tracts to fatal septicemia.

HUMAN DISEASE

Strains of *Enterobacteriaceae* are associated with abscesses, pneumonia, meningitis, septicemia, and infections of wounds, the urinary tract, and the intestine. They are a major component of the normal intestinal flora of humans but are relatively uncommon on other body sites. Several species of *Enterobacteriaceae* are very important causes of nosocomial infections (Table 2). Of clinically significant isolates, *Enterobacteriaceae* may account for 80% of gram-negative bacilli and 50% of all clinically significant isolates in clinical microbiology laboratories. They account for nearly 50% of septicemia cases (Table 3), more than 70% of urinary tract infections (8), and a significant percentage of intestinal infections.

Human extraintestinal infections

Except for the species of *Shigella*, which rarely cause infections outside the gastrointestinal tract, many species of *Enterobacteriaceae* commonly cause extraintestinal infections. However, a small number of species, including *Escherichia coli*, *K. pneumoniae*, *K. oxytoca*, *Proteus mirabilis*, *Enterobacter aerogenes*, *Enterobacter cloacae*, and *Serratia marcescens*, account for most of these infections (Tables 2 and 3). Urinary tract infections, primarily cystitis, are the most common (8), followed by respiratory, wound, bloodstream, and central nervous system infections. Many of these infections, especially sepsis and meningitis, are life threatening and are often hospital acquired. Because of the severe nature of these infections, prompt isolation, identification, and susceptibility testing of *Enterobacteriaceae* isolates are essential.

TABLE 1. Biochemical reactions of the named species, biogroups, and enteric groups of the family *Enterobacteriaceae*[a]

Species	Indole production	Methyl red	Voges-Proskauer	Citrate (Simmons')	Hydrogen sulfide (TSI)	Urea hydrolysis	Phenylalanine deaminase	Lysine decarboxylase	Arginine dihydrolase	Ornithine decarboxylase	Motility (36°C)	Gelatin hydrolysis (22°C)	Growth in KCN	Malonate utilization	D-Glucose, acid	D-Glucose, gas	Lactose fermentation	Sucrose fermentation	D-Mannitol fermentation	Dulcitol fermentation	Salicin fermentation	Adonitol fermentation	*myo*-Inositol fermentation	D-Sorbitol fermentation	L-Arabinose fermentation	Raffinose fermentation	L-Rhamnose fermentation	Maltose fermentation	D-Xylose fermentation	Trehalose fermentation	Cellobiose fermentation	alpha-Methyl-D-glucoside fermentation	Erythritol fermentation	Esculin hydrolysis	Melibiose fermentation	D-Arabitol fermentation	Glycerol fermentation	Mucate fermentation	Tartrate, Jordan's	Acetate utilization	Lipase (corn oil)	DNase at 25°C	Nitrate → Nitrite	Oxidase, Kovacs	ONPG[c] test	Yellow pigment	D-Mannose fermentation
Budvicia																																														
B. aquatica[b]	0	93	0	0	80	33	0	0	0	0	27	0	0	0	100	53	87	0	60	0	0	0	0	0	80	0	100	0	93	0	0	0	0	0	0	27	0	20	27	0	0	0	100	0	93	0	0
Buttiauxella																																														
B. agrestis	0	100	0	100	0	0	0	0	0	100	100	0	80	60	100	100	100	0	100	0	100	0	0	0	100	100	100	100	100	100	100	0	0	100	100	0	60	100	60	0	0	0	100	0	100	0	100
Cedecea																																														
C. davisae[b]	0	100	50	95	0	0	0	0	50	95	95	0	86	91	100	70	19	100	100	0	99	0	0	0	0	10	0	100	100	100	100	5	0	45	0	100	0	0	0	0	91	0	100	0	90	0	100
C. lapagei[b]	0	40	80	99	0	0	0	0	80	0	80	0	100	99	100	100	60	0	100	0	100	0	0	0	0	0	0	100	0	100	100	0	0	100	0	100	0	0	0	60	100	0	100	0	99	0	100
C. neteri[b]	0	100	50	100	0	0	0	0	100	0	100	0	65	100	100	100	35	100	100	0	100	0	0	100	0	0	0	100	100	100	100	0	0	100	0	100	0	0	0	0	100	0	100	0	100	0	100
Cedecea sp. 3[b]	0	100	50	100	0	0	0	0	100	0	100	0	100	0	100	100	0	50	100	0	100	0	0	0	0	100	0	100	100	100	100	50	0	100	100	100	0	0	0	50	100	0	100	0	100	0	100
Cedecea sp. 5[b]	0	100	50	100	0	0	0	0	50	50	100	0	100	0	100	100	0	100	100	0	100	0	0	100	0	100	0	100	100	100	100	0	0	100	100	100	0	0	0	50	50	0	100	0	100	0	100
Citrobacter																																														
C. freundii[b]	5	100	0	95	80	70	0	0	65	20	95	0	96	15	100	95	50	30	99	55	5	0	3	98	100	30	99	99	99	99	55	5	0	0	50	0	98	95	90	80	0	0	99	0	95	0	100
C. diversus[b]	99	100	0	99	0	75	0	0	65	99	95	0	0	90	100	98	35	45	100	50	20	98	0	99	100	0	100	100	100	100	99	40	0	2	0	100	98	93	75	75	0	0	100	0	96	0	100
C. amalonaticus[b]	100	100	0	85	0	80	0	0	85	95	98	0	95	0	100	97	50	15	100	0	40	0	0	100	100	5	99	99	99	100	100	5	0	10	5	0	70	98	85	75	0	0	99	0	100	0	100
C. amalonaticus biogroup 1[b]	100	100	0	1	0	45	0	0	85	100	99	0	96	0	100	93	19	100	100	4	5	0	0	100	100	100	100	100	100	100	100	70	0	0	100	0	55	100	93	82	0	0	100	0	100	0	100
Edwardsiella																																														
E. tarda[b]	99	100	0	1	100	0	0	100	0	100	98	0	0	0	100	100	0	0	0	0	0	0	0	0	9	0	0	100	0	0	0	0	0	0	0	0	30	0	25	0	0	0	100	0	0	0	100
E. tarda biogroup 1[b]	100	100	0	0	0	0	0	100	0	100	100	0	0	0	100	50	0	100	100	0	0	0	0	0	100	0	0	100	0	0	0	0	0	0	0	0	0	0	0	0	0	0	100	0	0	0	100
E. hoshinae[b]	50	100	0	0	0	0	0	100	0	95	100	0	0	100	100	35	0	100	100	0	50	0	0	0	13	0	0	100	0	100	0	0	0	0	0	0	65	0	0	0	0	0	100	0	0	0	100
E. ictaluri	0	0	0	0	0	0	0	100	0	65	0	0	0	0	100	50	0	0	0	0	0	0	0	0	0	0	0	100	0	0	0	0	0	0	0	0	0	0	0	0	0	0	100	0	0	0	100
Enterobacter																																														
E. aerogenes[b]	0	5	98	95	0	2	0	98	0	98	97	0	98	95	100	100	95	100	100	5	100	98	95	100	100	96	99	99	100	100	100	95	0	98	99	100	98	90	95	50	0	0	100	0	100	0	95
E. cloacae[b]	0	5	100	100	0	65	0	0	97	96	95	0	98	75	100	100	93	97	100	15	75	25	15	95	100	97	92	100	99	100	99	85	0	30	90	15	40	75	30	75	0	0	99	0	99	0	100
E. agglomerans[b]	20	50	70	50	0	20	20	0	0	0	85	2	35	65	100	20	40	75	100	15	65	7	15	30	95	30	85	89	93	97	55	7	0	60	50	50	30	40	25	30	0	0	85	0	90	75	98
E. gergoviae[b]	0	5	100	99	0	93	0	90	0	100	90	0	0	96	100	98	55	98	99	0	99	0	0	0	99	97	99	100	99	100	99	2	0	97	97	97	100	2	97	93	0	0	99	0	97	0	100
E. sakazakii[b]	11	5	100	99	0	1	50	0	99	91	96	0	99	18	100	98	99	100	100	5	99	0	75	0	100	99	100	100	100	100	100	96	0	100	100	0	15	1	1	96	0	0	99	0	100	98	100
E. taylorae[b]	0	5	100	100	0	1	0	0	94	99	99	0	98	100	100	100	10	0	100	0	92	0	0	1	100	0	100	99	100	100	100	1	0	90	0	0	1	75	0	35	0	0	100	0	100	0	100
E. amnigenus biogroup 1[b]	0	7	100	70	0	0	0	0	9	55	92	0	100	91	100	100	70	100	100	0	91	0	0	9	100	100	100	100	100	100	100	55	0	91	100	0	0	35	9	0	0	0	100	0	91	0	100
E. amnigenus biogroup 2	0	65	100	100	0	0	0	0	35	100	100	0	100	100	100	100	35	0	100	0	100	0	0	100	100	0	100	100	100	100	100	100	0	100	100	0	0	100	0	0	0	0	100	0	100	0	100
E. intermedium	0	100	100	65	0	0	0	0	0	89	89	0	65	100	100	100	100	65	100	100	100	0	0	100	100	100	100	100	100	100	100	100	0	100	100	0	100	100	100	0	0	0	100	0	100	0	100
E. asburiae[b]	0	100	2	100	0	60	0	0	21	95	0	0	97	3	100	95	75	100	100	0	100	0	0	100	100	70	5	100	97	100	100	95	0	95	0	0	11	21	30	87	0	0	100	0	100	0	100
E. cancerogenus	0	0	100	100	0	0	0	0	100	100	100	0	100	100	100	100	0	0	100	0	100	0	0	0	100	0	100	100	100	100	100	0	0	100	0	0	0	100	0	33	0	0	100	0	100	0	100
E. dissolvens	0	0	100	100	0	100	0	0	100	100	0	0	100	100	100	100	0	100	100	0	100	0	0	100	100	100	100	100	100	100	100	100	0	100	100	0	0	100	0	100	0	0	100	0	100	0	100
E. nimipressuralis	0	100	100	0	0	0	0	0	0	100	0	0	100	100	100	100	0	0	100	0	100	0	0	100	100	0	100	100	100	100	100	100	0	100	100	0	0	100	0	0	0	0	100	0	100	0	100
Escherichia-Shigella																																														
E. coli[b]	98	99	0	1	1	1	0	90	17	65	95	0	3	0	100	95	95	50	98	60	40	5	1	94	99	50	80	95	95	98	2	0	0	35	75	5	75	95	95	90	0	0	100	0	95	0	98
E. coli, inactive[b]	80	95	0	1	1	1	0	40	3	20	5	0	1	0	100	5	25	15	93	40	10	3	1	75	85	15	65	80	70	90	2	0	0	5	40	5	65	30	85	40	0	0	98	0	45	0	97
Shigella, O groups A, B, C[b]	50	100	0	0	0	0	0	0	5	1	0	0	0	0	100	2	0	0	93	2	0	0	0	30	60	50	5	30	2	80	0	0	0	0	50	0	10	0	30	2	0	0	100	0	2	0	100
S. sonnei[b]	0	100	0	0	0	0	0	0	2	98	0	0	0	0	100	0	2	1	99	0	0	0	0	2	95	3	75	90	2	100	5	0	0	0	25	0	15	10	90	0	0	0	100	0	90	0	100
E. fergusonii[b]	98	100	0	17	0	0	0	95	5	100	93	0	0	35	100	95	0	0	98	60	65	98	0	0	98	0	92	96	96	96	96	0	0	46	0	100	20	0	96	96	0	0	100	0	83	0	100
E. hermannii[b]	99	100	0	1	0	0	0	6	0	100	99	0	94	0	100	97	45	45	100	19	40	0	0	0	100	40	97	100	100	100	97	0	0	40	0	8	3	97	35	78	0	0	100	0	98	98	100
E. vulneris[b]	0	100	0	0	0	0	0	85	30	0	100	0	15	85	100	97	15	8	100	0	30	0	0	1	100	99	93	100	100	100	100	25	0	20	100	0	25	78	2	30	0	0	100	0	100	50	100
E. blattae	0	100	0	50	0	0	0	100	0	100	0	0	0	100	100	100	0	0	0	0	0	0	0	0	100	0	100	100	100	75	0	0	0	0	0	0	100	50	50	0	0	0	100	0	0	0	100

(*Continued on next page*)

TABLE 1—*Continued*

Species	Indole production	Methyl red	Voges-Proskauer	Citrate (Simmons)	Hydrogen sulfide (TSI)	Urea hydrolysis	Phenylalanine deaminase	Lysine decarboxylase	Arginine dihydrolase	Ornithine decarboxylase	Motility (36°C)	Gelatin hydrolysis (22°C)	Growth in KCN	Malonate utilization	D-Glucose, acid	D-Glucose, gas	Lactose fermentation	Sucrose fermentation	D-Mannitol fermentation	Dulcitol fermentation	Salicin fermentation	Adonitol fermentation	*myo*-Inositol fermentation	D-Sorbitol fermentation	L-Arabinose fermentation	Raffinose fermentation	L-Rhamnose fermentation	Maltose fermentation	D-Xylose fermentation	Trehalose fermentation	Cellobiose fermentation	alpha-Methyl-D-glucoside fermentation	Erythritol fermentation	Esculin hydrolysis	Melibiose fermentation	D-Arabitol fermentation	Glycerol fermentation	Mucate fermentation	Tartrate, Jordan's	Acetate utilization	Lipase (corn oil)	DNase at 25°C	Nitrate → Nitrite	Oxidase, Kovacs	ONPG[c] test	Yellow pigment	D-Mannose fermentation
Ewingella																																														
E. americana[b]	0	84	95	95	0	0	0	0	0	0	60	0	5	0	100	0	70	0	100	0	80	0	0	0	0	0	23	16	13	99	10	0	0	50	0	99	24	0	35	10	0	0	97	0	85	0	99
Hafnia																																														
H. alvei[b]	0	40	85	10	0	4	0	100	6	98	85	0	95	50	100	98	5	10	99	0	13	0	0	0	95	2	97	100	98	95	15	0	0	7	0	0	95	0	70	15	0	0	100	0	90	0	100
H. alvei biogroup 1	0	85	70	0	0	0	0	100	0	45	0	0	0	45	100	0	0	0	55	0	55	0	0	0	0	0	0	0	0	70	0	0	0	0	0	0	0	0	30	0	0	0	100	0	30	0	100
Klebsiella																																														
K. pneumoniae[b]	0	10	98	98	0	95	0	98	0	0	0	0	98	93	100	97	98	99	99	30	99	90	95	99	99	99	99	98	99	99	98	90	0	99	99	98	97	90	95	75	0	0	99	0	99	0	99
K. oxytoca[b]	99	20	95	95	0	90	1	99	0	0	0	0	97	98	100	97	100	100	99	55	100	99	98	99	98	100	100	100	100	100	100	98	2	100	99	98	99	93	98	90	0	0	100	0	100	1	100
K. ornithinolytica[b]	100	96	70	100	0	100	0	100	0	100	0	0	100	100	100	100	100	100	100	10	100	100	95	100	100	100	100	100	100	100	100	100	0	100	100	100	100	96	100	95	0	0	100	0	100	0	100
K. planticola[b]	20	100	98	100	0	98	0	100	0	0	0	0	100	100	100	100	100	100	100	15	100	100	100	92	100	100	100	100	100	100	100	100	0	100	100	100	100	100	100	62	0	0	100	0	100	1	100
K. ozaenae[b]	0	98	0	30	0	10	0	40	6	3	0	0	88	3	100	50	30	20	100	2	97	97	55	65	98	90	55	95	95	98	92	70	0	80	97	95	65	25	50	2	0	0	80	0	80	0	100
K. rhinoscleromatis[b]	0	100	0	0	0	0	0	0	0	0	0	0	80	95	100	0	0	75	100	0	98	100	95	100	100	90	96	100	100	100	100	0	0	30	100	100	50	0	50	0	0	0	100	0	0	0	100
K. terrigena	0	60	100	40	0	0	0	100	0	20	0	0	100	100	100	80	100	100	100	20	100	100	80	100	100	100	100	100	100	100	100	100	0	100	100	100	100	100	100	20	0	0	100	0	100	0	100
Kluyvera																																														
K. ascorbata[b]	92	100	0	96	0	0	0	97	0	100	98	0	92	96	100	93	98	98	100	25	100	0	0	40	100	98	100	100	99	100	100	98	0	99	99	0	40	90	35	50	0	0	100	0	100	0	100
K. cryocrescens[b]	90	100	0	80	0	0	0	23	0	100	90	0	86	86	100	95	95	81	95	0	100	0	0	45	100	100	100	100	91	100	100	95	0	100	100	0	5	81	19	86	0	0	100	0	100	0	100
Koserella																																														
K. trabulsii[b]	0	100	0	92	0	0	0	100	8	100	100	0	92	0	100	100	0	0	100	0	8	0	0	0	100	25	100	100	100	100	100	0	0	67	92	0	0	0	0	25	0	0	100	0	100	0	100
Leclercia																																														
L. adecarboxylata[b]	100	100	0	0	0	48	0	0	0	0	79	0	97	93	100	97	93	66	100	86	100	93	0	0	100	66	100	100	100	100	100	0	0	100	100	96	3	93	83	28	0	0	100	0	100	37	100
Leminorella																																														
L. grimontii[b]	0	100	0	100	100	0	0	0	0	0	0	0	0	0	100	33	0	0	0	83	0	0	0	0	100	0	0	0	83	0	0	0	0	0	0	0	17	100	100	0	0	0	100	0	0	0	0
L. richardii[b]	0	0	0	0	100	0	0	0	0	0	0	0	0	0	100	0	0	0	0	0	0	0	0	0	100	0	0	0	100	0	0	0	0	0	0	0	0	50	100	0	0	0	100	0	0	0	0
Moellerella																																														
M. wisconsensis[b]	0	100	0	80	0	0	0	0	0	0	0	0	70	0	100	0	100	100	60	0	0	100	0	0	0	100	0	30	0	0	0	0	0	0	100	75	10	0	30	10	0	0	90	0	90	0	100
Morganella																																														
M. morganii[b]	98	97	0	0	5	98	95	0	0	98	95	0	98	1	100	90	1	0	0	0	0	0	0	0	0	0	0	0	0	10	0	0	0	0	0	0	5	0	95	0	0	0	90	0	5	0	98
M. morganii biogroup 1[b]	100	95	0	0	41	100	100	100	0	95	0	0	91	5	100	91	0	0	0	0	0	0	0	0	0	0	0	0	0	0	0	0	0	0	0	0	100	0	100	0	0	0	91	0	0	0	95
Obesumbacterium																																														
O. proteus biogroup 2	0	15	0	0	0	0	0	100	0	100	0	0	0	0	100	0	0	0	0	0	0	0	0	0	0	0	15	50	15	85	0	0	0	0	0	0	0	0	15	0	0	0	100	0	0	0	85
Pragia																																														
P. fontium	0	100	0	89	89	0	22	0	0	0	100	0	0	0	100	0	0	0	0	0	78	0	0	0	0	0	0	0	0	0	0	0	0	78	0	0	0	0	0	0	0	0	100	0	0	0	0
Proteus																																														
P. mirabilis[b]	2	97	50	65	98	98	98	0	0	99	95	90	98	2	100	96	2	15	0	0	0	0	0	0	0	1	1	0	98	98	1	0	0	0	0	0	70	0	87	20	92	50	95	0	0	0	0
P. vulgaris[b]	98	95	0	15	95	95	99	0	0	0	95	91	99	0	100	85	2	97	0	0	50	0	0	0	0	1	5	97	95	30	0	60	1	50	0	0	60	0	80	25	80	80	98	0	1	0	0
P. penneri[b]	0	100	0	0	30	100	99	0	0	0	85	50	99	0	100	45	1	100	0	0	0	0	0	0	0	1	0	100	100	55	0	80	0	0	0	0	55	0	85	5	45	40	90	0	1	0	0
P. myxofaciens	0	100	100	50	0	100	100	0	0	0	100	100	100	0	100	100	0	100	0	0	0	0	0	0	0	0	0	100	0	100	0	100	0	0	0	0	100	0	100	0	100	50	100	0	0	0	0
Providencia																																														
P. rettgeri[b]	99	93	0	95	0	98	98	0	0	0	94	0	97	0	100	10	5	15	100	0	50	100	90	1	0	5	70	2	10	0	3	2	75	35	5	100	60	0	95	60	0	0	100	0	5	0	100
P. stuartii[b]	98	100	0	93	0	30	95	0	0	0	85	0	100	0	100	0	2	50	10	0	2	5	95	1	1	7	0	1	7	98	5	0	0	0	0	0	50	0	90	75	0	10	100	0	10	0	100
P. alcalifaciens[b]	99	99	0	98	0	0	98	0	0	1	96	0	100	0	100	85	0	15	2	0	1	98	1	1	1	1	0	1	1	2	1	0	0	0	0	0	15	0	90	40	0	0	100	0	1	0	100
P. rustigianii[b]	98	65	0	15	0	0	100	0	0	0	30	0	100	0	100	35	0	35	0	0	0	0	0	0	0	0	0	0	0	0	0	0	0	0	0	0	5	0	50	25	0	0	100	0	0	0	100
P. heimbachae	0	85	0	0	0	0	100	0	0	0	46	0	8	0	100	0	0	0	0	0	0	92	46	0	0	0	100	54	8	0	0	0	0	0	0	92	0	0	69	0	0	0	100	0	0	0	100

Species	Indole production	Methyl red	Voges-Proskauer	Citrate (Simmons)	Hydrogen sulfide (TSI)	Urea hydrolysis	Phenylalanine deaminase	Lysine decarboxylase	Arginine dihydrolase	Ornithine decarboxylase	Motility (36°C)	Gelatin hydrolysis (22°C)	Growth in KCN	Malonate utilization	D-Glucose, acid	D-Glucose, gas	Lactose fermentation	Sucrose fermentation	D-Mannitol fermentation	Dulcitol fermentation	Salicin fermentation	Adonitol fermentation	*myo*-Inositol fermentation	D-Sorbitol fermentation	L-Arabinose fermentation	Raffinose fermentation	L-Rhamnose fermentation	Maltose fermentation	D-Xylose fermentation	Trehalose fermentation	Cellobiose fermentation	alpha-Methyl-D-glucoside fermentation	Erythritol fermentation	Esculin hydrolysis	Melibiose fermentation	D-Arabitol fermentation	Glycerol fermentation	Mucate fermentation	Tartrate, Jordan's	Acetate utilization	Lipase (corn oil)	DNase at 25°C	Nitrate → Nitrite	Oxidase, Kovacs	ONPG[c] test	Yellow pigment	D-Mannose fermentation
Rahnella																																															
R. aquatilis[b]	0	88	100	94	0	0	95	0	0	0	6	0	0	100	100	98	100	100	100	88	100	0	0	94	100	94	94	94	94	100	100	0	0	100	100	0	13	30	6	6	0	0	100	0	100	0	100
Salmonella																																															
Subgroup 1 strains[b]																																															
Most serotypes[b]	1	100	0	95	95	1	0	98	70	97	95	0	0	0	100	96	1	1	100	96	0	0	35	95	99	2	95	97	97	99	5	2	0	5	95	0	5	90	90	90	0	2	100	0	2	0	100
S. typhi[b]	0	100	0	0	97	0	0	98	3	0	97	0	0	0	100	0	1	0	100	0	0	0	0	99	2	0	0	97	82	100	0	0	0	0	100	0	20	0	100	0	0	0	100	0	0	0	100
S. choleraesuis[b]	0	100	0	25	50	0	0	95	55	100	95	0	0	0	100	95	0	0	98	5	0	0	0	90	0	1	100	95	98	0	0	0	1	0	45	1	0	0	85	1	0	0	98	0	0	0	95
S. paratyphi A[b]	0	100	0	0	10	0	0	0	15	95	95	0	0	0	100	99	0	0	100	90	0	0	0	95	100	0	100	95	0	100	5	0	0	0	95	0	10	0	0	0	0	0	100	0	0	0	100
S. gallinarum[b]	0	100	0	0	100	0	0	90	10	1	0	0	0	0	100	0	0	0	100	90	0	0	0	1	80	10	10	90	70	50	10	0	1	0	0	0	0	50	100	0	0	10	100	0	0	0	100
S. pullorum[b]	0	90	0	0	90	0	0	100	10	95	0	0	0	0	100	90	0	0	100	0	0	0	0	10	100	1	100	5	90	90	5	0	0	0	0	0	0	0	0	0	0	0	100	0	0	0	100
Subgroup 2 strains[b]	2	100	0	100	100	0	0	100	90	100	98	2	0	95	100	100	1	1	100	90	5	0	5	100	100	0	100	100	100	100	0	8	0	15	8	0	25	96	50	95	0	0	100	0	15	0	95
Subgroup 3a strains[b] (*Arizona*)	1	100	0	99	99	0	0	99	70	99	99	0	1	95	100	99	15	1	100	0	0	0	0	99	99	1	99	98	100	99	1	1	0	1	95	1	10	90	5	90	0	2	100	0	100	0	100
Subgroup 3b strains[b] (*Arizona*)	2	100	0	98	99	0	0	99	70	99	99	0	1	95	100	99	85	5	100	1	0	0	0	99	99	1	99	98	100	99	1	1	0	1	95	1	10	30	20	75	0	2	100	0	100	0	100
Subgroup 4 strains[b]	0	100	0	98	100	2	0	100	70	100	98	0	95	0	100	100	0	0	98	0	60	5	0	100	100	0	98	100	100	100	50	0	0	0	100	5	0	0	65	70	0	0	100	0	0	0	100
Subgroup 5 strains[b]	0	100	0	100	100	0	0	100	100	100	100	0	100	0	100	80	0	0	100	100	0	0	0	100	100	0	100	100	100	100	0	0	0	0	75	0	0	100	0	100	0	0	100	0	100	0	100
Subgroup 6 strains[b]	0	100	0	89	100	0	0	100	67	100	100	0	0	0	100	100	22	0	100	67	0	0	0	0	100	0	100	100	100	100	0	0	0	0	89	0	33	100	100	89	0	0	100	0	44	0	100
Serratia																																															
S. marcescens[b]	1	20	98	98	0	15	0	99	0	99	97	90	95	3	100	55	2	99	99	0	95	40	75	99	0	2	0	96	7	99	5	0	1	95	0	0	95	0	75	50	98	98	98	0	95	0	99
S. marcescens biogroup 1[b]	0	100	60	30	0	0	0	55	4	65	17	30	70	0	100	0	4	100	96	0	92	30	30	92	0	0	0	70	0	100	4	0	0	96	0	0	92	0	50	4	75	82	83	0	75	0	100
S. liquefaciens group[b]	1	93	93	90	0	3	0	95	0	95	95	90	90	2	100	75	10	98	100	0	97	5	60	95	98	85	15	98	100	100	5	5	0	97	75	0	95	0	75	40	85	85	100	0	93	0	100
S. rubidaea[b]	0	20	100	95	0	2	0	55	0	0	85	90	25	94	100	30	100	99	100	0	99	99	20	1	100	99	1	99	99	100	94	1	0	94	99	85	20	0	70	80	99	99	100	0	100	0	100
S. odorifera biogroup 1[b]	60	100	50	100	0	5	0	100	0	100	100	95	60	0	100	0	70	100	100	0	98	50	100	100	100	100	95	100	100	100	100	0	0	95	100	0	40	5	100	60	35	100	100	0	100	0	100
S. odorifera biogroup 2[b]	50	60	100	97	0	0	0	94	0	0	100	94	19	0	100	13	97	0	97	0	45	55	100	100	100	7	94	100	100	100	100	0	7	40	96	0	50	0	100	65	65	100	100	0	100	0	100
S. plymuthica[b]	0	94	80	75	0	0	0	0	0	0	50	60	30	0	100	40	80	100	100	0	94	0	50	65	100	94	0	94	94	100	88	70	0	81	93	0	50	0	100	55	70	100	100	0	70	0	100
S. ficaria[b]	0	75	75	100	0	0	0	0	0	0	100	100	55	0	100	0	15	100	100	0	100	0	55	100	100	70	35	100	100	100	100	8	0	100	40	100	0	0	17	40	77	100	92	8	100	0	100
S. entomophila	0	20	100	100	0	0	0	0	0	0	100	100	100	0	100	0	0	100	100	0	100	0	0	0	0	0	0	100	40	100	0	0	0	100	0	60	0	0	100	80	20	100	100	0	100	0	100
"*Serratia*" *fonticola*[b]	0	100	9	91	0	13	0	100	0	97	91	0	70	88	100	79	97	21	100	91	100	100	30	100	100	100	76	97	85	100	6	91	0	100	98	100	88	0	58	15	0	0	100	0	100	0	100
Tatumella																																															
T. ptyseos[b]	0	0	5	2	0	0	90	0	0	0	0	0	0	0	100	0	0	98	0	0	55	0	0	0	0	11	0	0	9	93	0	0	0	0	25	0	7	0	0	0	0	0	98	0	0	0	100
Yersinia																																															
Y. enterocolitica[b]	50	97	2	0	0	75	0	0	0	95	2	0	2	0	100	5	5	95	98	0	20	0	30	99	98	5	1	75	70	98	75	0	0	25	1	40	90	0	85	15	55	5	98	0	95	0	100
Y. frederiksenii[b]	100	100	0	15	0	70	0	0	0	95	5	0	0	0	100	40	40	100	100	0	92	0	20	100	100	30	99	100	100	100	100	0	0	85	0	100	85	5	55	15	55	0	100	0	100	0	100
Y. intermedia[b]	100	100	5	5	0	80	0	0	0	100	5	0	10	5	100	18	35	100	100	0	100	0	15	100	100	45	100	100	100	100	96	77	0	100	80	45	60	6	88	18	12	0	94	0	90	0	100
Y. kristensenii[b]	30	92	0	0	0	77	0	0	0	92	5	0	0	0	100	23	8	0	100	0	15	0	15	100	77	0	0	100	85	100	100	0	0	0	0	45	70	0	40	8	0	0	100	0	70	0	100
Y. rohdei[b]	0	62	0	0	0	62	0	0	0	25	0	0	0	0	100	0	0	100	100	0	0	0	0	100	100	62	0	0	38	100	25	0	0	0	50	0	38	0	100	0	0	0	88	0	50	0	100
Y. pestis[b]	0	80	0	0	0	5	0	0	0	0	0	0	0	0	100	0	0	0	97	0	70	0	0	50	100	0	1	80	90	100	0	0	0	50	20	0	50	0	0	0	0	0	85	0	50	0	100
Y. pseudotuberculosis[b]	0	100	0	0	0	95	0	0	0	0	0	0	0	0	100	0	0	0	100	0	25	0	0	0	50	15	70	95	100	100	0	0	0	95	70	0	50	0	50	0	0	0	95	0	70	0	100
Y. aldovae	0	80	0	0	0	60	0	0	0	40	0	0	0	0	100	0	0	20	80	0	0	0	0	60	60	0	0	0	40	80	0	0	0	0	0	0	0	0	100	0	0	0	100	0	0	0	100
Y. bercovieri[b]	0	100	0	0	0	60	0	0	0	80	0	0	0	0	100	0	20	100	100	0	20	0	0	100	100	0	0	100	100	100	100	0	0	20	0	0	0	0	100	0	0	0	100	0	80	0	100
Y. mollaretii[b]	0	100	0	0	0	20	0	0	0	80	0	0	0	0	100	0	40	100	100	0	20	0	0	100	100	0	0	60	60	100	100	0	0	0	0	0	20	0	100	0	0	0	100	0	20	0	100
"*Yersinia*" *ruckeri*[b]	0	97	10	0	0	0	0	50	5	100	0	30	15	0	100	5	0	0	100	0	0	0	0	50	5	5	0	95	0	95	5	0	0	0	0	0	30	0	30	0	30	0	75	0	50	0	100

(*Continued on next page*)

TABLE 1—*Continued*

Species	Indole production	Methyl red	Voges-Proskauer	Citrate (Simmons)	Hydrogen sulfide (TSI)	Urea hydrolysis	Phenylalanine deaminase	Lysine decarboxylase	Arginine dihydrolase	Ornithine decarboxylase	Motility (36°C)	Gelatin hydrolysis (22°C)	Growth in KCN	Malonate utilization	D-Glucose, acid	D-Glucose, gas	Lactose fermentation	Sucrose fermentation	D-Mannitol fermentation	Dulcitol fermentation	Salicin fermentation	Adonitol fermentation	*myo*-Inositol fermentation
Xenorhabdus																							
X. luminescens (25°C)	50	0	0	50	0	25	0	0	0	0	100	50	0	0	75	0	0	0	0	0	0	0	0
X. luminescens DNA group 5[b]	0	0	0	20	0	60	0	0	0	0	100	80	20	0	100	0	0	0	0	0	0	0	0
X. nematophilus (25°C)	40	0	0	0	0	0	0	0	0	0	100	80	0	0	80	0	0	0	0	0	0	0	0
Enteric Group 58[b]	0	100	0	85	0	70	0	100	0	85	100	0	100	85	100	85	30	0	100	85	100	0	0
Enteric Group 59[b]	10	100	0	100	0	0	30	0	60	0	100	0	80	90	100	100	80	0	100	0	100	0	0
Enteric Group 60[b]	0	100	0	0	0	50	0	0	0	100	75	0	0	100	100	100	0	0	50	0	0	0	0
Enteric Group 63	0	100	0	0	0	0	0	100	0	100	65	0	0	0	100	100	0	0	100	0	100	0	0
Enteric Group 64	0	100	0	50	0	0	0	0	50	0	100	0	100	100	100	50	100	0	100	0	100	100	0
Enteric Group 68[b]	0	100	50	0	0	0	0	0	0	0	0	0	100	0	100	0	0	100	100	0	50	0	0
Enteric Group 69	0	0	100	100	0	0	0	0	100	100	100	0	100	100	100	100	100	25	100	100	100	0	0
Enteric Group 90[b]	13	100	0	88	100	0	0	100	0	100	100	0	100	0	100	100	0	0	100	0	13	0	0

Species	D-Sorbitol fermentation	L-Arabinose fermentation	Raffinose fermentation	L-Rhamnose fermentation	Maltose fermentation	D-Xylose fermentation	Trehalose fermentation	Cellobiose fermentation	alpha-Methyl-D-glucoside fermentation	Erythritol fermentation	Esculin hydrolysis	Melibiose fermentation	D-Arabitol fermentation	Glycerol fermentation	Mucate fermentation	Tartrate, Jordan's	Acetate utilization	Lipase (corn oil)	DNase at 25°C	Nitrate → Nitrite	Oxidase, Kovacs	ONPG[c] test	Yellow pigment	D-Mannose fermentation
Xenorhabdus																								
X. luminescens (25°C)	0	0	0	0	25	0	0	0	0	0	0	0	0	0	0	50	0	0	0	0	0	0	50	100
X. luminescens DNA group 5[b]	0	0	0	0	0	0	0	0	0	0	0	0	0	0	0	60	20	0	0	0	0	0	60	100
X. nematophilus (25°C)	0	0	0	0	0	0	0	0	0	0	0	0	0	0	0	60	0	0	20	20	0	0	60	80
Enteric Group 58[b]	100	100	0	100	100	100	100	100	55	0	0	0	0	30	0	60	45	0	0	100	0	100	0	100
Enteric Group 59[b]	0	100	0	100	100	100	100	100	10	0	100	0	10	10	60	50	50	0	0	100	0	100	25	100
Enteric Group 60[b]	0	25	0	75	0	0	100	0	0	0	0	0	0	75	0	75	0	0	0	100	0	100	0	100
Enteric Group 63	100	100	0	100	100	100	100	100	65	0	100	0	0	0	65	0	0	0	0	100	0	100	0	100
Enteric Group 64	0	100	0	100	100	100	100	100	0	0	100	0	100	0	100	50	0	0	0	100	0	100	0	100
Enteric Group 68[b]	0	0	0	0	50	0	100	0	0	0	0	0	0	50	0	0	0	0	100	100	0	0	0	100
Enteric Group 69	100	100	100	100	100	100	100	100	100	0	100	100	0	0	100	0	25	0	0	100	0	100	100	100
Enteric Group 90[b]	100	100	0	100	100	100	100	100	0	0	13	0	0	0	100	50	88	0	0	100	0	100	0	100

[a] Each number gives the percentage of positive reactions after 2 days of incubation at 36°C (unless a different temperature is indicated). The vast majority of these positive reactions occur within 24 h. Reactions that become positive after 2 days are not considered.

[b] Known to occur in clinical specimens.

[c] ONPG, *o*-Nitrophenyl-β-D-galactopyranoside.

Human intestinal infections

Several organisms in the family *Enterobacteriaceae* are also important causes of intestinal infections of humans (see Tables 5 and 6) and animals in the United States and worldwide (5, 7, 9, 16, 45, 46, 68). Although many species in the family have been implicated as causes of diarrhea, only organisms in four genera, *Escherichia, Salmonella, Shigella,* and *Yersinia,* have been clearly documented as enteric pathogens. These four genera are discussed separately.

SPECIMEN COLLECTION, TRANSPORT, AND PROCESSING

Extraintestinal specimens

Enterobacteriaceae are recovered from infectious processes at many different body sites, and effective practices should be followed for collecting blood, body fluid, respiratory, wound, and other specimens. For urine specimens, the clean-catch, midstream technique, catheterization under aseptic conditions, and in certain instances suprapubic aspiration reduce the possibility of contaminating the specimens. Most *Enterobacteriaceae* multiply rapidly in fluids such as urine, so it is important to transport specimens to the laboratory as quickly as possible to avoid overgrowth, especially if quantitation is required. Specimens should be refrigerated unless they can be cultured within 2 h of collection. Alternatively, urine preservative systems may be used if specimen transportation will be delayed. The importance of rapid and correct specimen processing and collection cannot be overemphasized. Inadequate specimen delivery systems may reduce the quality of otherwise properly collected specimens.

Intestinal specimens

Collection and transport. Stool cultures are usually submitted to the laboratory with a request to isolate and identify the cause of a possible intestinal infection, usually manifested as diarrhea. The groups of *Enterobacteriaceae* usually associated with diarrhea in the United States are *Salmonella, Shigella,* and certain pathogenic strains of *E. coli* and *Yersinia enterocolitica.* Occasionally other *Enterobacteriaceae* such as strains of *Citrobacter, Proteus, Klebsiella, Enterobacter,* and *Serratia* have also been implicated. "Enterotoxin-producing strains" of these *Enterobacteriaceae* have been isolated from people with diarrhea (74), but their etiological role is not well established. Some laboratories issue reports for stool cultures such as "*Klebsiella pneumoniae* in pure culture (10 of 10 colonies tested)" to reflect this drastic change in stool flora. There is no evidence that these strains are important causes of diarrhea.

Stool specimens require special attention to both collection and transportation and should be taken early in the course of illness, when the causative agent is likely to be present on primary plates in largest numbers. At this stage, enrichment broths should be unnecessary. With the exception of typhoid fever, the isolation rate for enteric pathogens declines as the patient recovers. Freshly passed stool is better than rectal swabs since there is less chance for improper collection, and mucus- and blood-stained portions can be selected for culture.

TABLE 2. Important causes of nosocomial infections in the United States[a]

Organism	Proportion (%) of infections caused by each pathogen at given site						Total no. of isolates	%
	Urinary tract	Surgical wound	Lower respiratory	Primary bacteremia	Cutaneous	Other		
Enterobacteriaceae								
E. coli	30.7	11.5	6.4	10.1	7.0	7.4	5,266	17.8
Klebsiella spp.	8.0	5.2	11.6	7.8	3.8	4.6	2,193	7.4
Enterobacter spp.	4.8	7.0	9.4	6.3	4.5	3.9	1,748	5.9
Proteus spp.	7.4	5.2	4.2	0.8	3.3	2.1	1,522	5.1
Serratia spp.	1.2	2.1	5.8	3.0	2.2	1.5	691	2.3
Citrobacter spp.	1.8	1.4	1.4	0.7	0.7	0.9	414	1.4
Other organisms (for comparison)								
P. aeruginosa	12.7	8.9	16.9	7.6	9.2	6.7	3,366	11.4
Enterococcus spp.	14.7	12.1	1.5	7.1	8.8	7.0	3,063	10.4
Staphylococcus								
S. aureus	1.6	18.6	12.9	12.3	28.9	14.6	3,059	10.3
Coagulase negative	3.4	8.3	1.5	14.9	11.5	11.6	1,868	6.3
Candida spp.	5.4	1.7	4.0	5.6	5.8	14.1	1,620	5.5
Other fungi	2.2	0.4	1.4	1.3	0.9	2.8	496	1.7
Bacteroides spp.	0.0	3.7	0.2	3.4	1.2	1.4	355	1.2
Streptococcus spp., group B	0.9	1.3	0.7	2.3	1.1	1.9	348	1.2
Other anaerobes	0.0	1.7	0.1	1.8	0.8	4.4	300	1.0
All others[b]	5.2	10.9	22.0	15.0	10.3	15.1	3,253	11.1
No. of isolates	12,218	5,500	4,567	2,264	1,690	3,323	29,562	100.0

[a] Based on nosocomial infection surveillance for the United States in 1984.
[b] Other pathogens were combined, since none of them accounted for more than 3% of the isolates at any site.

Stool cultures should be plated within 2 h of collection in order to recover fastidious pathogens in the genus *Shigella*. If rapid processing is not possible, a small portion or a swab coated with feces should be placed in transport medium. Commonly used transport media include Stuart, Amies, Cary-Blair, and buffered glycerol-saline. Cary-Blair is probably the best overall transport medium for diarrheal stools. Specimens held in transport media should be refrigerated until examined. In certain circumstances rectal swab specimens, such as from infants or during mass screening in outbreak investigations, may be useful. Mucosa within the rectal vault must be sampled for these specimens to be of optimum value.

Many different procedures have been described for processing stool specimens (70). Some laboratories are content to isolate strains of *Salmonella* and *Shigella*, but isolation procedures for stools should be designed to include all possible pathogens (see other chapters in this Manual). In cases of chronic or severe diarrhea, rare pathogens should also be considered. More information about the isolation and identification of *Salmonella* and *Shigella* strains, *E. coli*, and *Y. enterocolitica* is given in subsequent sections.

Microscopic examination. Stool specimens should be examined visually for the presence of blood or mucus. They can also be examined microscopically for leukocytes (39, 62). Small flecks of mucus or stool are mixed with 0.1 ml of Loeffler methylene blue stain on a glass microscope slide. A cover slip is added, and the suspension is examined microscopically for leukocytes. Pickering et al. (62) found leukocytes more frequently in *Shigella*-positive stools than in stools that yielded other pathogens, no pathogen, or invasive *E. coli*. Examination for fecal leukocytes is not a substitute for culture and is not used routinely in most clinical laboratories. Definitive identification of *Enterobacteriaceae* is almost always based on biochemical reactions of pure cultures rather than on microscopic examination. Although identification by fluorescent-antibody staining is theoretically possible for all enteric pathogens, it has been of limited success because of serological cross-reactions among the species of *Enterobacteriaceae* (24, 59). This technique has been limited to detection of *Salmonella* strains (primarily by the food industry) and certain serogroups of *E. coli* and to investigations of outbreaks.

ISOLATION

Extraintestinal specimens

Most strains of *Enterobacteriaceae* grow readily on media commonly used in clinical microbiology laboratories. Specimens from a normally sterile body site are cultured on blood or chocolate agar. Specimens such as urine, respiratory, and wound that are likely to contain mixtures of organisms are almost always cultured on selective media to enhance recovery of *Enterobacteriaceae*. MacConkey agar, generally interchangeable with EMB (eosin methylene blue) agar, is usually used because it allows a preliminary grouping of enteric and other gram-negative bacteria. The most common isolates of *Enterobacteriaceae* have a characteristic appearance on blood agar and MacConkey agar which is useful for preliminary identification. Broth enrichment may be of value if small numbers of *Enterobacteriaceae* are present.

Intestinal specimens

Selective media that should be used routinely include a nonselective medium such as blood agar, a differential medium of low to moderate selectivity such as MacConkey agar, a more selective differential medium such as xylose-lysine-deoxycholate agar or Hektoen enteric

TABLE 3. Distribution of *Enterobacteriaceae, Vibrionaceae,* and other organisms in bacteremia and meningitis[a]

Organism	Distribution[b]	
	Blood	Spinal fluid
Family *Enterobacteriaceae*		
Escherichia coli	5,473 (568)†	58 (10)
Klebsiella, all species	1,233 (167)	16 (4)
K. pneumoniae	996 (142)	12 (4)
K. oxytoca	215 (23)	4
K. ozaenae	22 (2)	0
Proteus, all species	940 (120)	8 (1)
P. mirabilis	762 (85)	8 (1)
P. vulgaris	58 (13)	0
Enterobacter, all species	441 (61)	7 (1)
E. cloacae	326 (46)	6 (1)
E. aerogenes	75 (10)	1
E. agglomerans group	45 (5)	0
E. sakazakii	7 (1)	0
E. intermedium	6 (1)	0
Salmonella, all serotypes	343 (21)	5
S. typhi	94	0
S. typhimurium	60 (8)	0
S. paratyphi A	47	0
S. enteritidis	43 (5)	1
S. virchow	25	0
S. paratyphi B	10	0
S. panama	11	0
S. dublin	8	1
S. stanley	7	0
Morganella morganii	121 (21)	1 (1)
Citrobacter freundii	92 (11)	0
Serratia marcescens	82 (10)	2 (1)
Serratia liquefaciens group	42 (2)	1
Providencia stuartii	28 (3)	0
Citrobacter diversus	25 (1)	0
Yersinia enterocolitica	13 (2)	0
Hafnia alvei	7	0
Shigella flexneri	4	0
Providencia rettgeri	3	0
Serratia odorifera	2	0
Edwardsiella tarda	1	0
Serratia plymuthica	1	0
Yersinia pseudotuberculosis	1	0
Family *Vibrionaceae*		
Aeromonas spp.	31 (8)	0
Plesiomonas shigelloides	1	0
Other organisms (for comparison)		
Staphylococcus aureus	3,461 (420)	50 (12)
Streptococcus pneumoniae	2,210 (352)	369 (70)
Pseudomonas aeruginosa	685 (192)	13 (2)
Haemophilus influenzae	470 (37)	488 (17)
Streptococcus spp., group B	385 (38)	67 (14)
Neisseria meningitidis	223 (39)	651 (46)

[a] Data for bacteremia (blood, bone marrow, spleen, or heart) and meningitis are from the surveillance reports for England, Wales, and Ireland for 1986. These are not reportable diseases in the United States.

[b] The first number gives the number of cases, and the number in parentheses gives the number of these cases that were fatal.

agar, and a broth enrichment such as selenite. These media should be adequate for detection of strains of *Salmonella, Shigella, E. coli,* and perhaps also *Y. enterocolitica.* A highly selective medium for *Salmonella* strains such as brilliant green agar or bismuth sulfite agar can also be included. When *Y. enterocolitica* is suspected, a selective-differential medium such as CIN (cefsulodin-irgasan-novobiocin) agar (also called *Yersinia* selective agar) can be added if resources permit. A complete stool culture procedure should also include media for isolation of *Campylobacter* species and possibly *Vibrio* species in areas where cholera and other *Vibrio* infections are common.

IDENTIFICATION

There are many different approaches to identifying *Enterobacteriaceae* (4, 29, 70). Twenty years ago (46), this topic was less complex than it is today because the basic question concerned which and how many conventional biochemical tests are needed for identification.

Conventional biochemical tests in tubes

Tube testing was once used by clinical microbiology laboratories and is still widely used in reference and public health laboratories (24, 29, 46). Biochemical test media are prepared, dispensed into glass tubes, and sterilized. Although many laboratories prepare their own, most media are also available commercially. Growth from a single colony is inoculated into each tube, and the tests are read at 24 h and usually also at 48 h (and kept longer by reference laboratories). Unfortunately, the media and tests are not well standardized, and few laboratories use exactly the same procedures. Even with so many variables, this approach usually results in correct identification of the common species of *Enterobacteriaceae.* Table 1 gives the results for *Enterobacteriaceae* in 47 tests.

Kits for identification

A "kit" is defined as a series of miniaturized or standardized tests that are available commercially. This approach is similar to the conventional tube method, with the main differences being in the miniaturization, the number of tests available, and the method of reading results (sometimes by machine). Kits are now used by most American laboratories and are discussed in other chapters of this Manual.

Problem strains

Most strains of *Enterobacteriaceae* grow readily on plating media. A few grow poorly on blood agar but much better on chocolate agar incubated in a candle jar. This characteristic suggests a possible nutritional requirement or a mutation involving respiration. There are slow-growing strains of *E. coli, K. pneumoniae,* and *Serratia,* and typical biochemical reactions of these strains usually require extended incubation. A second type of problem organism is sometimes isolated from patients who are taking antimicrobial agents. Li et al. described such "pleiotropic" mutants of *Serratia marcescens* (52) and *Salmonella.* These strains react atypically in many of the standard biochemical tests and are difficult to identify.

Laboratories occasionally isolate strains that grow rapidly but whose biochemical reactions do not fit the described species of *Enterobacteriaceae.* At present, these cultures can only be reported as "unidentified." They may be named as new species or Enteric Groups (Table 1) which can then be routinely identified (29).

TABLE 4. Intrinsic antimicrobial resistance in *Enterobacteriaceae*

Species	Most strains resistant to:
Buttiauxella sp.	Cephalothin
Cedecea spp.	Polymyxins, ampicillin, cephalothin
Citrobacter amalonaticus	Ampicillin
C. freundii	Cephalothin
C. diversus	Ampicillin, carbenicillin
Edwardsiella tarda	Colistin
Enterobacter cloacae	Cephalothin
E. aerogenes	Cephalothin
Many other *Enterobacter* spp.	Cephalothin
Escherichia hermannii	Ampicillin, carbenicillin
Ewingella americana	Cephalothin
Hafnia alvei	Cephalothin
Klebsiella pneumoniae	Ampicillin, carbenicillin
Kluyvera ascorbata	Ampicillin
K. cryocrescens	Ampicillin
Proteus mirabilis	Polymyxins, tetracycline, nitrofurantoin
P. vulgaris	Polymyxins, ampicillin, cephlothin, nitrofurantoin
Morganella morganii	Polymyxins, ampicillin, cephalothin
Providencia rettgeri	Polymyxins, cephalothin, nitrofurantoin, tetracycline
Other *Providencia* spp.[a]	Polymyxins, nitrofurantoin
Serratia marcescens[b]	Polymyxins, cephalothin, nitrofurantoin
Serratia fonticola	Ampicillin, carbenicillin, cephalothin
Other *Serratia* spp.	Polymyxins,[c] cephalothin

[a] Most strains of *P. stuartii* are also resistant to cephalothin and tetracycline.

[b] *S. marcescens* can also have intrinsic resistance to ampicillin, carbenicillin, streptomycin, and tetracycline.

[c] Resistance to polymyxins is common in *Serratia* species, but some strains have zones of 10 to 12 mm or larger.

ANTIBIOTIC SUSCEPTIBILITY

Several methods are available for testing *Enterobacteriaceae*, but the most popular are disk diffusion and broth dilution, both of which are described in detail in other chapters. The reader should consult a current textbook or review on infectious diseases (54) for a description of antibiotic usage in clinical practice.

When antibiotics were first introduced, there was only slight resistance among the species of *Enterobacteriaceae*. Today, antibiotic resistance is much more common among strains isolated from human and animal diseases, and resistance patterns vary by species and geographical location (70).

Intrinsic resistance

Intrinsic resistance is a genetic property of most strains of a species and evolved long before the clinical use of antibiotics. This evolution can best be shown in strains isolated and stored before the antibiotic era or by studying strains from nature that presumably have not been exposed to antibiotics. A third way is to collect a large number of strains from a wide variety of sources and identify those that have the most susceptible patterns. For example, all strains of *S. marcescens* apparently have intrinsic resistance to penicillin G, colistin, and cephalothin (73). Table 4 lists some species of *Enterobacteriaceae* and their intrinsic resistance patterns.

Nonintrinsic resistance

Much of the antibiotic resistance occurring today is due to the selective pressure of antibiotic usage, and many strains of *Enterobacteriaceae* that cause disease have become highly antibiotic resistant through this evolutionary mechanism. Genetic studies have shown that this type of antibiotic resistance is usually plasmid mediated.

The antibiogram as a marker in epidemiological studies

Antibiotic susceptibility testing is usually done on isolates that are clinically significant and provides an antibiogram useful for comparing isolates in epidemiological studies. When the selective ecological pressure of antibiotics is changed, the resistance patterns of epidemic (or endemic) strains may also change. These changes have been documented in outbreaks that have lasted for several months or longer. Even with these limitations in genetic stability, antibiograms probably provides the most useful laboratory markers for comparing strains and recognizing infection problems.

ESCHERICHIA COLI

E. coli is the organism most commonly isolated in the clinical microbiology laboratory. It is an important cause of both intestinal (17, 20, 21, 23, 44, 47, 65, 67, 72) and extraintestinal (17, 59) infections (Tables 2 and 3), and different virulence factors appear to be involved in these diverse disease processes (20, 21, 44, 67). *E. coli* is usually present as normal flora in the intestines of humans and animals, but some strains can cause diarrhea. Although a variety of methods have been developed to differentiate the pathogenic strains of *E. coli*, most are too complicated to be widely used in clinical microbiology laboratories.

ESCHERICHIA COLI AS AN ENTERIC PATHOGEN

Four main groups of *E. coli* strains have been defined as enteric pathogens: the classical enteropathogenic strains or serotypes (EPEC); those that produce heat-labile or heat-stable enterotoxin(s) (ETEC); enteroinvasive strains (EIEC) that mimic *Shigella* strains in their ability to invade and multiply within intestinal epithelial cells; and strains that cause hemorrhagic colitis or produce Shiga-like toxin(s). Studies in different countries have shown that certain serotypes (based on both O and H antigens) are associated with these four groups (Table 5).

Strains of *E. coli* that cause intestinal infections resemble normal gut strains on common plating media and in biochemical test results. Unlike *Salmonella* and *Shigella* strains, pathogenic strains of *E. coli* can be lactose positive or negative; therefore, both red-pink and colorless colonies should be picked from MacConkey agar. After subculture, these strains can be serotyped or tested in specific virulence assays as described in the sections that follow. Most methods for detecting strains with the potential to cause diarrhea are too complicated for wide use in clinical microbiology laboratories. The exception is the simple methodology for *E. coli* O157:H7, which is now known to be an important enteric pathogen. A detailed description of methods for isola-

TABLE 5. Serotypes of *Escherichia coli* associated with human diarrhea and intestinal infections

Enterotoxigenic (ETEC)	Enteropathogenic (EPEC)	Enteroinvasive (EIEC)	Shiga-like toxin producers	
O6:H16	O26:NM	O28ac:NM	O1:NM	O113:H7
O8:NM	O26:H11	O29:NM	O2:H5	O113:H21
O8:H9	O55:NM	O112ac:NM	O2:H7	O114:H48
O11:H27	O55:H6	O115:NM	O4:NM	O115:H10
O15:H11	O86:NM	O124:NM	O4:H10	O117:H4
O20:NM	O86:H2	O124:H7	O5:NM	O118:H12
O25:NM	O86:H34	O124:H30	O5:H16	O118:H30
O25:H42	O111ab:NM	O135:NM	O6:H1	O121:NM
O27:H7	O111ab:H2	O136:NM	O18:NM	O121:H19
O27:H20	O111ab:H12	O143:NM	O18:H7	O125:NM
O63:H12	O111ab:H21	O144:NM	O25:NM	O125:H8
O78:H11	O114:H2	O152:NM	O26:NM	O126:NM
O78:H12	O119:H6	O164:NM	O26:H11	O126:H8
O85:H7	O125ac:H21	O167:NM	O26:H32	O128:NM
O114:H21	O127:NM		O38:H21	O128:H2
O115:H21	O127:H6		O39:H4	O128:H8
O126:H9	O127:H9		O45:H2	O128:H12
O128ac:H7	O127:H21		O50:H7	O128:H25
O128ac:H12	O128ab:H2		O55:H7	O145:NM
O128ac:H21	O142:H6		O55:H10	O145:H25
O148:H28	O158:H23		O82:H8	O146:H21
O149:H4			O84:H2	O153:H25
O159:H4			O91:NM	O157:NM
O159:H20			O91:H21	O157:H7
O166:H27			O103:H2	O163:H19
O167:H5			O111:NM	O165:NM
			O111:H8	O165:H19
			O111:H30	O165:H25
			O111:H34	

tion and identification will be given, since this pathogen has not been thoroughly discussed in previous editions of this Manual.

Enteropathogenic *E. coli* (EPEC)

Although many early investigators suspected that *E. coli* was an enteric pathogen, the classical enteropathogenic strains were the first group whose etiological role was conclusively shown. In the 1940s, strains of *E. coli* were isolated during many nursery outbreaks of severe diarrhea in which the death rate was as high as 70%. Studies by Kauffmann and DuPont (47) in Denmark, Taylor and co-workers in England, and Ewing and co-workers (23) in the United States firmly established that specific strains of *E. coli* serogroups O55 and O111 were important causes of infantile diarrhea worldwide (35, 59). These strains were identified serologically, and soon O55 and O111 antisera became commercially available and were included in the laboratory routine for the isolation and identification of enteric pathogens. Additional strains that caused diarrhea in infants were discovered, and the number of sera used for identifying these "enteropathogenic serotypes" was expanded. However, these particular strains of *E. coli* soon declined in industrialized countries, and over the years routine serotyping was discontinued in most laboratories (35). Enteropathogenic strains of *E. coli* are still important in developing countries (20, 21, 37, 56), and polyvalent sera for detecting these O groups are still commercially available. In industrialized countries, these sera probably do not have a place in the normal routine, but can be used in outbreaks and in severe or chronic cases of diarrhea. Strains that agglutinate in the serological screening test must be confirmed by titration (59) and should be submitted to a reference laboratory for confirmation and H-antigen determination. This precaution will avoid the false-positive results that have caused the technique to lose favor (35, 59).

Enterotoxin-producing *E. coli* (ETEC)

Characteristics. Enterotoxin-producing strains of *E. coli* belong to a few serotypes (Table 5) and cause diarrhea by colonizing the small intestine and producing enterotoxin(s) (20, 21, 22, 37, 67). They are common in developing countries but rare in industrialized countries such as the United States. They often cause diarrhea in travelers to Central America, Asia, and Africa (20, 37). These strains produce one or more enterotoxins. The heat-labile enterotoxin (LT) is structurally similar to cholera toxin, and immunological assays usually detect both toxins (33, 53, 66, 71, 77). The heat-stable enterotoxin (ST) (19) is now known to be a group of structurally similar small peptides that are also similar in chemical structure to the heat-stable enterotoxins produced by several other bacteria. The genes for LT and ST production and for colonization factors are usually plasmid borne (59, 67).

Detection of enterotoxins. Until recently, the assays for LT and ST were complicated and used primarily in reference and research laboratories (19, 22, 33, 53, 56, 66, 69, 71, 77). However, there are now two commercial products to assay for LT (see chapter 122 under Enterotoxin Testing Reagents for *E. coli*), but there are no commercial products for ST. Because enterotoxin-producing strains of *E. coli* are rare in the United States, laboratories that can do toxin testing usually choose to do it only in outbreaks or for severe or chronic cases of diarrhea.

Enteroinvasive *E. coli*

Characteristics. Enteroinvasive strains of *E. coli* were first isolated in Italy during World War II (24), but their pathogenic mechanism was not discovered until many years later (21, 48, 72). These strains belong to a few serotypes (15) (Table 5) and usually produce a self-limiting, watery diarrhea (40, 55, 72), often with mucus and polymorphonuclear leukocytes but seldom with frank blood. In most studies, enteroinvasive strains appear to be relatively rare in both developing and industrialized countries, although they have not always been adequately looked for and the methods have not been optimum for detection. Like strains of *Shigella*, these strains have both chromosomal and plasmid genes that are necessary for virulence (48, 72).

Isolation and identification. Invasive strains of *E. coli* are isolated on routine media and can be identified by the Sereny test, ELISA (enzyme-linked immunosorbent assay) (60), or DNA probe assays, none of which is commercially available. There is no easy way for the hospital clinical microbiology laboratory to detect these strains. However, unlike most *E. coli* strains found in the intestine, they are often lactose negative, lysine decarboxylase negative, and nonmotile. Strains sometimes cross-react with *Shigella* antisera.

Shiga-like toxin (verotoxin)-producing *E. coli*

It was recently discovered that some strains of *E. coli* (Table 5) produce one or both of two antigenically distinct toxins that are cytotoxic for HeLa and Vero cells in tissue culture. In the literature, these are referred to as verotoxins 1 and 2 and also as Shiga-like toxins I and II (44). Since no commercial products to assay for these toxins are yet available, testing is usually done in reference or research laboratories. Strains of *E. coli* that produce one or both of these toxins can apparently cause diarrhea that is often bloody; in its severe form this condition has been called hemorrhagic colitis (65). In addition, these toxin-producing strains are associated with two serious extraintestinal diseases known as hemolytic uremic syndrome and thrombotic thrombocytopenic purpura (44, 45). In the United States, *E. coli* O157:H7 is the most important serotype associated with hemorrhagic colitis and the extraintestinal diseases, and it is the only serotype that can easily be isolated and identified in the clinical microbiology laboratory.

E. coli O157:H7

In 1982, *E. coli* O157:H7 caused two outbreaks of an unusual enteric disease termed hemorrhagic colitis (65, 75), characterized by severe abdominal pain with cramps, watery diarrhea followed by grossly bloody diarrhea, and evidence of colonic inflammation but little or no fever. Since then, *E. coli* O157:H7 has become a very important enteric pathogen that is found more frequently than strains of *Salmonella* or *Shigella* in some locations (44).

Isolation. *E. coli* O157:H7 is not usually detected with the methods normally used for isolating and identifying traditional bacterial enteric pathogens (28, 75). Strains of *E. coli* O157:H7 ferment lactose rapidly and are indistinguishable from other *E. coli* strains on lactose-containing media (28), which could result in a report of "negative for enteric pathogens."

There are two main approaches to the isolation of *E. coli* O157:H7 (28, 75): to use MacConkey sorbitol agar or to screen colonies from MacConkey agar for sorbitol fermentation or agglutination with O157 serological reagents. In contrast to most *E. coli*, strains of serotype O157:H7 ferment D-sorbitol slowly or not at all (28). This finding led to the development (28) of MacConkey sorbitol agar (also known as sorbitol MacConkey agar, SMA, or SMac), which is now commercially available (see chapter 121). Stool specimens are plated on this medium and incubated at 35 to 37°C overnight. Sorbitol-negative colonies are colorless and considered "suspicious for *E. coli* O157:H7"; other *E. coli* colonies are pink to red. If MacConkey sorbitol agar cannot be used, 5 to 10 lactose-positive colonies from MacConkey agar can be screened serologically or tested for sorbitol fermentation (75). At least five colonies should be selected, since the organism is not always present in pure culture. Colonies that do not ferment sorbitol within 24 h should be screened for agglutination in *E. coli* O157 antiserum. The routine use of MacConkey sorbitol agar has led to a much higher isolation rate for *E. coli* O157:H7.

Identification. Strains of *E. coli* O157:H7 rapidly agglutinate in commercially available O157 and H7 antisera (28, 75), but it is essential to follow manufacturers' instructions. Two commercial companies, Oxoid (Columbia, Md.) and Pro-Lab (Round Rock, Tex.), recently introduced latex reagents for detecting *E. coli* O157 that can be used to screen colonies directly from MacConkey or MacConkey sorbitol agar plates. A control culture of *E. coli* O157:H7 should be used for quality control and to set up all routine serological screening procedures (see chapter 120 for list of control cultures). Laboratories that frequently encounter *E. coli* O157 may also want to do agglutination tests for H7 antigen (49) with commercially available serum (see chapter 122 for sources). This procedure would eliminate a few false-positive results because some strains of *E. coli* O157 that do not produce Shiga-like toxin have an H antigen other than H7. A few nonmotile strains of *E. coli* O157 that produce toxin have also been isolated. Laboratories that rarely isolate *E. coli* O157:H7 can refer cultures to reference laboratories for H-antigen determination or toxin testing.

For laboratories that examine a large number of specimens, it may be desirable to use a medium that combines sorbitol fermentation and immobilization with *E. coli* H7 antiserum (28). Colonies can be screened in this medium before O-antigen determination. If this test is done in 24-well plastic tissue culture plates, it is essential to dry the media in the plates to remove excess surface moisture. This step does not seem to be a problem if screw-cap tubes are used. A strain of *E. coli* O157: H7 (see chapter 120) should be included in each run as a positive quality control.

Reporting. *E. coli* O157:H7 should be reported as an enteric pathogen in a manner similar to that used for cultures of *Salmonella* or *Shigella*. It would be helpful to physicians to indicate on the report form that this organism causes diarrhea and hemorrhagic colitis and can sometimes cause serious extraintestinal illness such as hemolytic uremic syndrome and thrombotic thrombocytopenic purpura (44). Outbreaks or clusters of any of these illnesses should be reported to public health authorities.

Other serotypes involved. *E. coli* O157:H7 appears to be the main serotype that causes diarrhea and hemorrhagic colitis (44). However, several other *E. coli* serotypes (Table 5) are isolated from and apparently cause hemolytic uremic syndrome and thrombotic thrombocytopenic purpura (44). Unfortunately, there are no simple methods or commercial products to detect strains that produce Shiga-like toxin, but this test is done in several reference laboratories (44) and at least one commercial laboratory.

SHIGELLA

Shigella species cause classical bacillary dysentery characterized by severe cramping, abdominal pain, and diarrhea with blood and mucus (3, 16, 48, 51). These organisms invade mucosal cells, causing death and sloughing of the cells into the bowel lumen. However, they seldom invade beyond the mucosa. *Shigella* infections remain one of the most commonly recognized causes of bacterial diarrhea in the United States (14), and *S. sonnei* and *S. flexneri* are the most commonly isolated species (Table 6).

Nomenclature and classification

The four named groups of *Shigella* are *S. dysenteriae* (serological group A), *S. flexneri* (group B), *S. boydii* (group C), and *S. sonnei* (group D); commercial antisera are available to differentiate these four groups. Complete antigenic analysis which subdivides the species into epidemiologically useful serological types is usually limited to reference laboratories. There are 13 O-antigen groups in *S. dysenteriae*, 6 (13 including subfactors) in *S. flexneri*, 18 in *S. boydii*, and 1 in *S. sonnei*, which includes a smooth (form I) and a rough (form II) variant. Strains are also isolated from dysentery cases that are "biochemically *Shigella*" but cannot be serotyped. They are "provisional *Shigella* serotypes" and may be added to the *Shigella* schema as a new O group in one of the species. These strains are best reported as "*Shigella* species" until they can be further defined. The four species of *Shigella* could be considered one species on genetic grounds (10).

TABLE 6. *Salmonella* and *Shigella* serotypes reported in the United States for 1988

Serotype	No. of isolates
Salmonella typhimurium	9,611
Salmonella enteritidis	6,952
Salmonella heidelberg	4,950
Salmonella newport	2,628
Salmonella hadar	2,369
Salmonella agona	1,042
Salmonella infantis	958
Salmonella thompson	921
Salmonella montevideo	749
Salmonella braenderup	624
Subtotal	30,804
Salmonella typhi	443
Salmonella paratyphi A	77
Salmonella paratyphi B	121
Salmonella paratyphi C	2
Salmonella choleraesuis	57
Other *Salmonella* serotypes	8,697
Salmonella, not completely typed	3,524
Total *Salmonella* isolates	43,776
Shigella sonnei (group D)	15,254
Shigella flexneri (group B)	4,475
Shigella boydii (group C)	488
Shigella dysenteriae (group A)	218
Shigella, serotype not reported	2,377
Total *Shigella* isolates	22,812

Isolation

In the acute phase of illness, patients with dysentery due to *Shigella* infection typically have stools that contain blood and mucus (16, 48). A cotton swab can be used to pick bits of mucus- and blood-stained material for streaking onto enteric media. On MacConkey agar, *Shigella* isolates appear as lactose-negative colonies, and this medium should be useful even for strains that are inhibited on more selective media. Xylose-lysine-deoxycholate agar is a plating medium of intermediate selectivity and is excellent for isolating *Shigella* strains. It contains D-xylose as a differentiating agent, and since most *Shigella* strains do not ferment xylose (Table 1), they appear as red colonies on the plate. *Shigella* isolates that rapidly ferment xylose may be missed on this medium, but they should be detected on MacConkey agar. Many laboratories also use Hektoen enteric agar. Stool cultures taken late in the illness or specimens that have had less than optimum collection or processing can be enriched in GN broth. Selenite broth may be useful in isolating *S. sonnei.*

Identification

Suspect colonies can be identified in one of the many commercial systems, or they can be screened in an abbreviated schema. Colonies can be picked from each selective agar plate to triple sugar iron (TSI) or Kligler iron agar slants. Isolates whose TSI or Kligler iron agar reaction is alkaline/acid with no H_2S or gas can then be screened serologically with antisera to *Shigella* O groups A, B, C, and D. Occasional strains that are biochemically *Shigella* will not agglutinate in *Shigella* antisera. These cultures should be heated in a water bath at 100°C for 15 to 30 min and retested for agglutination.

Differentiation from *E. coli*

Differentiation of *Shigella* strains from *E. coli* can pose one of the most difficult problems for a laboratory and may reflect the fact that *E. coli* and all four *Shigella* species are really the "same species" on the basis of their close relatedness by DNA-DNA hybridization (10). The best approach is to do a complete set of biochemical reactions and compare the pattern with that of *E. coli* as well as the *Shigella* species (Tables 1 and 7). The following generalizations are suggested as guidelines for identifying shigellae:

1. Cultures are always nonmotile and lysine negative.
2. With the exception of a few strains of *S. flexneri* 6, *S. boydii* 13 and 14, and *S. dysenteriae* 3, gas is not produced during carbohydrate fermentation.
3. Cultures that ferment mucate or give an alkaline

TABLE 7. Tests helpful in differentiating strains of *Escherichia coli* from those of *Shigella*

Test or property	Reaction[a]						
	E. coli "normal"	*E. coli* inactive	*S. dysenteriae*	*S. flexneri* O1–5	*S. flexneri* O6	*S. boydii*	*S. sonnei*
Agglutination in *Shigella* group and type antisera	(+)	(+)	++++	++++	++++	++++	++++
Motility	85	0	0	0	0	0	0
D-Glucose, gas production	91	0	0	0	18	0	0
Lactose fermentation	90	0	0	0	0	1	2
Indole production	99	90	44	62	0	29	0
Mucate fermentation	94	25	0	0	0	0	16
Acetate utilization	84	59	0	0	0	0	0
Christensen citrate	24		0	0	0	0	0
Lysine decarboxylase	88	43	0	0	0	0	0
Arginine dihydrolase	17	2	2	0	49	18	1
Ornithine decarboxylase	63	18	0	0	0	3	99
Sucrose fermentation	51	11	0	2	0	0	0.1
Salicin fermentation	37	3	0	0	0	0	0

[a] Symbols: (+), only a few strains react; ++++, almost all strains react. Numbers indicate percent positive for the test after 48 h of incubation.

reaction on acetate agar or Christensen citrate agar are likely to be *E. coli.*

4. *S. boydii* and *S. dysenteriae* are very rare in the United States, and cultures identified as one of these species should be retested biochemically and serologically before a final report is made.
5. *Shigella* cultures should be sent to the state health department for confirmation and tabulation as part of the *Shigella* surveillance system.

No definitive rules on the identification of *Shigella* isolates can be made. Although most *Shigella* isolates agglutinate in a polyvalent *Shigella* serum and a specific serum, *E. coli* cultures frequently cross-react in these sera. Because it is essential to differentiate *E. coli* from *Shigella* strains, complete biochemical and serological typing should be done in each instance.

SALMONELLA

Salmonellosis is an important enteric diseases (1, 2, 5, 6, 7, 68) (Table 6). This point was reemphasized by the recent outbreak of *S. typhimurium* in Chicago that had an estimated 150,000 to 300,000 cases and by the recent outbreaks of *S. enteritidis* that have been associated with eggs. *Salmonella* strains cause a wide range of human enteric disease, from self-limited gastroenteritis with mild symptoms of short duration to severe gastroenteritis with or without bacteremia to typhoid fever, a severe, debilitating, and potentially life-threatening illness. *S. choleraesuis, S. paratyphi* A, and *S. typhi* are important because of their frequent association with severe disease and bacteremia. These serotypes are common in many developing countries but not in the United States (Table 6). Other *Salmonella* serotypes may also cause bacteremia, but they are more likely to cause uncomplicated gastroenteritis. *Salmonella* strains typically invade the bowel mucosa and multiply in the submucosa. Depending on the virulence of a particular strain and the host response, they may invade the bloodstream, lymphatic tissue, or both. Salmonellae are among the most common causes of bacterial diarrhea in the United States.

Nomenclature and classification

Strains in the *Salmonella-Arizona* group represent a continuum, so it is not surprising that *Salmonella* nomenclature and classification have changed over the years and caused confusion (18, 31). Over the years, there have been many changes in the nomenclature, classification, and reporting of this group of bacteria (24, 29, 31, 46). Most strains in the group are highly related in an evolutionary sense (18), and a recent classification lumped all *Salmonella* strains in a single species (50). However, there are seven distinct subgroups in the genus *Salmonella,* whose properties are summarized in Table 8. Although subspecies names for each of the seven subgroups were proposed (50), we prefer a simplified nomenclature for routine use that considers all of the named serotypes of *Salmonella* as species. Thus, *Salmonella* serotype Typhimurium is conveniently written as *Salmonella typhimurium.* This simple notation, although less correct in a phylogenetic sense, is widely accepted and will be used here. As indicated in Table 8, most *Salmonella* serotypes associated with human disease belong to subgroup 1, but strains in subgroups 3a and 3b ("*Arizona*") are occasionally isolated. Strains of *Salmonella* subgroups 2, 4, 5, and 6 are very rare in human clinical specimens.

Definition of serotypes

Serotypes of *Salmonella* are defined on the basis of their antigenic structure (46, 76) and occasionally by additional biochemical reactions. In antigenic formulas, the O antigen is listed first, followed by the H antigen. Major antigens are separated by colons, and the components of an antigen (also called serofactors) are separated by commas. Therefore, the formula "1,4,5,12:i:1,2" would indicate that the strain had O-antigen factors 1, 4, 5, and 12 (O factor 4 defines this as serogroup B), flagella phase one antigen i, and phase two antigens 1 and 2. Names have been given to most of the important *Salmonella* serotypes to avoid complex antigenic formulas; "*S. typhimurium*" is reported rather than "*Salmonella* 1,4,5,12:i:1,2." Although more than 2,000 *Salmonella* serotypes have been described (76), most are rarely isolated from human infections.

TABLE 8. Properties of the seven *Salmonella* subgroups[a]

Property or test	*Salmonella* subgroup						
	1	2	3a	3b	4	5	6
DNA hybridization group of Crosa et al. (18)	1	2	3	4	5	Not studied	Not studied
Genus according to Ewing (24)	*Salmonella*	*Salmonella*	*Arizona*	*Arizona*	*Salmonella*	*Salmonella*	*Salmonella*
Salmonella subgenus name formerly used	I	II	III	III	IV		
Subspecies according to Le Minor et al. (50)	*choleraesuis*	*salamae*	*arizonae*	*diarizonae*	*houtenae*	*bongori*	*indica*
Flagella are usually monophasic (Mono) or diphasic (Di)	Di	Di	Mono	Di	Mono	Mono	Di
Usually isolated from humans and warm-blooded animals	+	–	–	–	–	–	–
Usually isolated from cold-blooded animals and the environment	–	+	+	+	+	+	+
Pathogenic for humans	++++	+	+	+	+	+?	+?
Differential tests[b]							
Dulcitol fermentation	96	90	0	1	0	92	62
Lactose fermentation	1	1	15	85	0	0	25
ONPG[c] test	2	15	100	100	0	92	50
Malonate utilization	1	95	95	95	0	0	0
Growth in KCN medium	1	1	1	1	95	100	0
Mucate fermentation	90	96	90	30	0	85	100
Gelatin hydrolysis[d]	–	+	+	+	+	–	+
D-Galacturonic acid fermentation	–	+	–	+	+	100	100
Lysis by bacteriophage O1	+	+	–	+	–	46	88
D-Sorbitol fermentation	+	+	+	+	96	100	0

[a] Adapted from Le Minor et al. (references 93 and 94 in reference 29) and Farmer et al. (29).

[b] Numbers indicate percent positive after 2 days of incubation and are based on actual Centers for Disease Control data; symbols are based on the data of Le Minor et al.: +, 90% or more positive; –, 10% or fewer positive.

[c] ONPG, *o*-Nitrophenyl-β-D-galactopyranoside.

[d] Rapid film method at 37°C (almost all strains are negative by the tube method at 22°C within 2 days).

Clinical laboratories do "grouping" in commercial antisera to determine the O antigen and provide rapid reports such as "*Salmonella* serogroup B" or "*Salmonella* serogroup C." Most state and territorial health departments in the United States do complete analysis of both O and H antigens and report serotype names.

Isolation

Low-selectivity media (MacConkey, EMB, and deoxycholate agar) and intermediate-selectivity media (XLD [xylose-lysine-deoxycholate], deoxycholate citrate, SS [salmonella-shigella], and Hektoen enteric agars) are widely used by laboratories that screen for both *Salmonella* and *Shigella* isolates because they support the growth of both. However, if laboratory resources permit, a highly selective *Salmonella* medium such as brilliant green can be included. Bismuth sulfite agar is the preferred medium for isolating *S. typhi*, and it is also very useful for detecting strains of *Salmonella* that ferment lactose.

Although *Salmonella* colonies are usually found in high numbers on primary plates inoculated with feces from persons who are acutely ill with diarrhea, an enrichment broth is used in some laboratories to enhance isolation when the number of organisms is low. Most *Salmonella* enrichment broths are highly selective; the three most widely used are tetrathionate broth, tetrathionate broth with brilliant green, and selenite F broth.

Identification

"Suspicious *Salmonella* colonies" can be selected from the plating media and tested in a commercial identification system. An alternative is to inoculate suspicious colonies into tubes of screening media such as TSI and LIA (lysine iron agar). The latter medium indicates decarboxylation or deamination of lysine and the production of hydrogen sulfide. These two media are particularly helpful for the presumptive detection of *Salmonella* strains which typically have a TSI reaction of alkaline/acid, gas positive, and H_2S positive. Rare strains that are lactose or sucrose positive will have an acid slant but will often be H_2S negative. The usual reaction on LIA will be alkaline/alkaline and H_2S positive; however, lysine- and H_2S-negative strains occasionally occur (Table 1). Isolates with typical reactions on either TSI or LIA should be tested by slide agglutination with commercial polyvalent antisera specific for *Salmonella* O-group antigens A, B, C_1, C_2, D, E, and Vi. A positive reaction in polyvalent O antisera and a typical TSI and LIA reaction indicate a presumptive *Salmonella* isolate, which must then be confirmed with a complete set of biochemical tests. Some *Salmonella* strains have O antigens that are not represented in these commercial antisera and will not agglutinate. These strains can be detected only with a more complete set of biochemical reactions and antisera to the higher O groups. *Salmonella* isolates that have been confirmed with a complete set of biochemical tests should be forwarded to a reference laboratory for complete serotyping. In the United States, most state health departments do complete serotyping as part of the national *Salmonella* surveillance system.

Serodiagnosis

A serodiagnostic test known as the Widal reaction (5, 7) is sometimes used in diagnosing typhoid fever. This test measures agglutinating antibodies to O and H antigens of *S. typhi* and is usually used when typhoid fever is in the differential diagnosis but *S. typhi* cannot be isolated. There are many reagents commercially available for the serodiagnosis of typhoid and paratyphoid fevers as well as for some of the other *Salmonella* serotypes. It has also been shown that many typhoid carriers may have titers against the Vi antigen; this test is commercially available on a fee-for-services basis.

YERSINIA ENTEROCOLITICA

During the past few years, it has been clearly demonstrated that *Y. enterocolitica* is a significant enteric pathogen (9, 13, 43), particularly in Scandinavia. It has also been reported from Europe, Canada, and some parts of the United States. Although some strains apparently produce a heat-stable enterotoxin (57) that closely resembles that of *E. coli*, *Y. enterocolitica* is considered an invasive pathogen. Involvement of intestinal lymph nodes is common, and the condition is difficult to distinguish from acute appendicitis. As with *E. coli*, only strains of *Y. enterocolitica* that possess essential virulence factors are capable of causing human intestinal disease (9, 13, 43, 64).

Nomenclature and classification

Until the early 1970s, *Y. enterocolitica* was thought to be a single species with considerable variation in its properties (9). However, the "biochemically atypical strains" have now been classified as seven additional species within the *Y. enterocolitica* group: *Y. aldovae*, *Y. bercovieri*, *Y. frederiksenii*, *Y. intermedia*, *Y. mollaretii*, *Y. kristensenii*, and *Y. rohdei*. These species occasionally cause only extraintestinal infections and can easily be confused with *Y. enterocolitica* in routine identification (Tables 1, 9 and 10). Unless otherwise indicated, the remainder of this section is limited to *Y. enterocolitica*.

Isolation

Although strains of *Y. enterocolitica* grow faster at 37°C than at 25°C, the lower temperature is recommended for isolation. Strains of *Y. enterocolitica* grow well on MacConkey agar incubated at 37°C, but the colonies are much smaller than those of most other species of *Enterobacteriaceae*. Several serotypes of *Yersinia* may be inhibited on more selective media such as SS or Hektoen enteric agar. CIN agar, also known as *Yersinia* selective agar, was designed specifically for the isolation of *Yersinia* strains and, depending on resources, is used routinely in some laboratories for stool specimens. Plates of CIN agar are inoculated and incubated at 32°C for 24 h or at 22 to 25°C for 48 h. After 18 to 24 h, colonies of *Y. enterocolitica* are translucent with or without dark red centers; by 48 h, they are dark pink with translucent borders occasionally surrounded by a zone of precipated bile. Both pathogenic and nonpathogenic strains of *Y. enterocolitica* and other *Yersinia* species grow on CIN agar, but most other organisms are inhibited. Instead of using a dedicated plate

TABLE 9. Differentiation within the *Yersinia enterocolitica* group

Fermentation of:	Reaction[a]							
	Y. enterocolitica	*Y. kristensenii*	*Y. intermedia*	*Y. frederiksenii*	*Y. aldovae*	*Y. rohdei*	*Y. mollaretii*	*Y. bercovieri*
Sucrose	+	−	+	+	−	+	+	+
Raffinose	−	−	+	−	−	+	−	−
L-Rhamnose	−	−	+	+	+	−	−	−
Cellobiose	+	+	+	+	−	+	+	+
α-Methyl-D-glucoside	−	−	+	−	−	−	−	−
Melibiose	−	−	+	−	−	+	−	−

[a] These characteristic fermentation patterns occur rapidly at 25°C but are sometimes delayed at 37°C. Symbols: +, most strains positive; −, most strains negative.

for *Yersinia* isolation, some laboratories examine MacConkey agar plates (24 h of incubation at 35 to 37°C) for small colorless colonies that become much larger after an additional 24 h of incubation at room temperature. Strains of *Y. enterocolitica* are usually lactose negative, but lactose-positive strains occur; this is probably a plasmid-mediated reaction. Cold enrichment will probably increase the number of *Yersinia* isolates but is not a very practical method because of the long incubation time and because it also selects for nonpathogenic strains of *Y. enterocolitica* and other *Yersinia* species.

Identification

Suspicious colonies from CIN, MacConkey, or other enteric media should be picked for complete identification or screened in biochemical media such as TSI, urea, and motility. On TSI, strains of *Y. enterocolitica* typically produce an acid/acid reaction with no gas or H_2S. However, some strains may have an alkaline slant because of slow sucrose fermentation or the production of alkaline products from digestion of the peptone in the medium. Strains are urea positive (often at 24 h, but sometimes several days are required) and motile at 25 but not 37°C. Isolates with this typical pattern should be identified to species (Table 9).

Differentiation and reporting of pathogenic serotypes (strains)

Only certain strains of *Y. enterocolitica* appear to cause intestinal infections. Until recently, it has not been practical for clinical microbiology laboratories to identify these pathogenic strains (9, 13). However, there are now several simple tests (see chapters 121 and 122 for formulas and procedures) with an excellent correlation with pathogenicity (Table 10), and these should be incorporated into the normal laboratory routine for processing *Yersinia* cultures. Cultures of *Y. enterocolitica* are streaked onto CR-MOX agar (64; Fig. 1) and inoculated in media for determining pyrazinamidase (43), salicin fermentation, and esculin hydrolysis (Table 10).

Until recently, laboratory reports for stool cultures have read "positive for *Yersinia*" or "positive for *Y. enterocolitica*," implying that an enteric pathogen is present. Now it is possible to report only the pathogenic strains of *Y. enterocolitica*. Nonpathogenic strains can be discussed by telephone with an explanation that there is no convincing evidence that they are enteric pathogens. Some state health departments and reference laboratories may do additional virulence tests and serotyping.

Serodiagnosis

Yersiniosis is sometimes considered in the differential diagnosis of an illness in the absence of a positive culture. Antibody levels (34) to *Y. enterocolitica*, *Y. pseudotuberculosis*, or both are then requested. There are at least two commercial companies that test sera for *Yersinia* antibodies on a fee-for-services basis. Microbiology Reference Laboratory, 10703 Progress Way, Cypress, CA 90630-4714 [phone: (800) 445-0185], does a (micro)agglutination titration against whole cells of

TABLE 10. Simple laboratory tests for identifying pathogenic serotypes and virulent strains of *Yersinia enterocolitica*

Test	Reaction[a]		
	Y. enterocolitica		Other species in the *Y. enterocolitica* group[b]
	Pathogenic serotypes	Nonpathogenic serotypes	
Pyrazinamidase test (43)	−	+	(+)
Salicin fermentation	−	+	(+)
Esculin hydrolysis	−	+	(+)
Tiny red colonies on CR-MOX agar (64; Fig. 1)	+[c]	−	−

[a] Symbols: +, most strains (generally about 90 to 100%) positive; (+), many strains (generally about 75 to 90%) positive; −, most strains negative (generally about 0 to 10% positive).

[b] Includes *Y. aldovae*, *Y. bercovieri*, *Y. frederiksenii*, *Y. intermedia*, *Y. mollaretii*, *Y. kristensenii*, and *Y. rohdei*.

[c] Most freshly isolated strains of pathogenic serotypes will be positive; however, strains that have lost the *Yersinia* virulence plasmid will be negative.

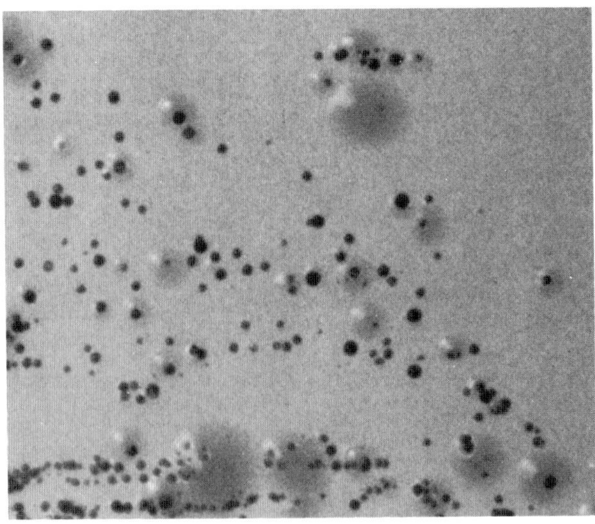

FIG. 1. A pathogenic serotype of *Yersinia enterocolitica* streaked onto CR-MOX agar. Small red colonies (that appear black in this photograph) still contain the *Yersinia* virulence plasmid; the large gray to colorless colonies have lost the plasmid.

Y. enterocolitica serotypes O3, O5, and O8 and against *Y. pseudotuberculosis*. Titers of greater than 1:160 are reported as positive. Specialty Laboratories, P.O. Box 92722, Los Angeles, CA 90009 [phone: (800) 421-7110], offers four enzyme immunoassays (EIA) for *Y. enterocolitica:* EIA Panel—immunoglobulin G (IgG), IgM, IgA; EIA—IgG; EIA—IgM; and EIA—IgA. Each of these detects antibodies to *Y. enterocolitica* O3, O4, O5, O6, and O8 (as a pooled antigen, not to each of the individual serotypes). In addition, they offer complement fixation tests for *Y. enterocolitica* serogroups O3, O8, and O9 and for *Y. pseudotuberculosis*.

Virion (U.S.) Inc., 4 Upperfield Road, Morristown, NJ 07960 [phone: (800) 524-2689 or (201) 993-8214], sells a reagent kit for complement fixation antibody titers for *Y. pseudotuberculosis* and three kits for *Y. enterocolitica* (types O3, O8, and O9). These kits may be useful for those who want to test for *Yersinia* antibodies; however, the reagents are not approved as "in vitro diagnostic reagents" in the United States.

OTHER GENERA

Several other genera of *Enterobacteriaceae* are frequently isolated in the clinical microbiology laboratory (Table 1). These include *Citrobacter, Enterobacter, Hafnia, Klebsiella, Morganella, Proteus, Providencia,* and *Serratia*. Several species in these genera are important opportunistic pathogens that have caused serious infections, many of which are hospital acquired (Table 2). Species in other genera are occasionally isolated in the clinical microbiology laboratory, but their clinical significance is unknown in many instances. However, many have been isolated from blood cultures, which suggests they should be considered as rare opportunistic pathogens. The biochemical properties, differential reactions, and properties of the other genera of *Enterobacteriaceae* are given in Tables 1, 7 to 9, and 11 to 24. These new genera and species were reviewed by Farmer et al. (29), who included all of the original literature citations.

The genus *Budvicia*

The genus *Budvicia* was described in 1985 and includes a single species, *B. aquatica*. Most strains have been isolated from water, but a few have been isolated from human feces. *B. aquatica* is one of the new H_2S-positive species in the family (Table 11).

The genus *Buttiauxella*

The genus *Buttiauxella* was described in 1981 and includes a single species, *B. agrestis*. Strains of *B. agrestis* are biochemically similar to *Kluyvera* strains and to Enteric Groups 63 and 64 (Table 12). To date all strains of *B. agrestis* have been from water, but the organism is included in this discussion because biochemically it is similar to and can be confused with *Kluyvera* species.

TABLE 11. Differentiation of the four new species that are H_2S positive

Test	Reaction[a]			
	Budvicia aquatica	*Leminorella grimontii*	*Leminorella richardii*	*Pragia fontium*
H_2S production (TSI)	(+)	+	+	(+)
Methyl red	+	+	−	+
Citrate (Simmons)	−	+	−	+
Motility	(−)	−	−	+
Gas production from D-glucose (7 days)	(+)	+	−	−
ONPG[b] test	+	−	−	−
Fermentation of:				
D-Mannitol (7 days)	+	−	−	−
L-Rhamnose	+	−	−	−
Dulcitol	−	(+)	−	−
L-Arabinose	(+)	+	+	−
D-Xylose	+	(+)	+	−

[a] Symbols: +, most strains (generally about 90 to 100% positive); (+), many strains (generally about 75 to 90% positive); (−), many strains negative (generally about 10 to 25% positive); −, most strains negative (generally about 0 to 10% positive).

[b] ONPG, *o*-Nitrophenyl-β-D-galactopyranoside.

TABLE 12. Differentiation of strains of *Kluyvera*, *Buttiauxella*, and two related enteric groups

Test or property	Reaction[a]				
	K. ascorbata	*K. cryocrescens*	*B. agrestis*	Enteric Group 63 (*Buttiauxella*-like)	Enteric Group 64 (*Buttiauxella*-like)
Ascorbate (7 days)	+	−	−	+	−
Growth at 4°C (14 days)	−	+			
Citrate utilization (Simmons)					
2 days	+	(+)		−	v
7 days	+	(+)	+	v	+
Lysine decarboxylase	+	(−)	−	+	−
Fermentation of:					
Sucrose					
2 days	+	(+)	−	−	−
7 days	+		v	−	−
D-Arabitol	−	−	−	−	+
Melibiose					
2 days	+	+	+	−	−
7 days	+	+	+	v	−
Raffinose	+	+	+	−	−
α-Methyl-D-glucoside					
2 days	+	+	−	v	−
7 days	+	+	−	+	+
Lactose	+	+	+	−	+

[a] Symbols (all data are for reactions within 2 days at 35 to 37°C unless otherwise specified): +, 90 to 100% positive; (+), 75 to 89.9% positive; v, 25.1 to 74.9% positive; (−), 10.1 to 25% positive; −, 0 to 10% positive.

The genus *Cedecea*

The genus *Cedecea* was described in 1981 and now includes *C. davisae*, *C. lapagei*, *C. neteri*, and two unnamed species (Table 13). Strains of *Cedecea* resemble the species of *Serratia* in many of the common tests used for identification, but they can be distinguished because they are negative for DNase. Strains of *Cedecea* are very rare in clinical specimens, but a case of bacteremia due to *C. neteri* has been reported.

The genus *Citrobacter* (26)

Citrobacter is an old genus that now includes three species and a biogroup (Table 14). *C. freundii* is isolated from both feces and extraintestinal specimens. Some strains of *C. freundii* agglutinate in *Salmonella* polyvalent O antiserum and can result in erroneous identifications unless the strains are biochemically confirmed. *C. diversus* (also known as *C. koserii* in England and as *Levinea malonatica* in France) is an important cause of neonatal meningitis, sepsis, and other extraintestinal infections. *C. amalonaticus* is isolated occasionally from feces but rarely from extraintestinal specimens.

The genus *Edwardsiella* (27)

The genus *Edwardsiella* was described in 1965, and until recently *E. tarda* was the only species. *E. tarda* is a well documented cause of extraintestinal infections, and its role as an enteric pathogen has been suggested but not firmly established (27). *E. tarda* is rarely isolated but is easily recognized because it is H_2S positive and ferments only a few sugars. *E. hoshinae*, *E. ictaluri*, and *E. tarda* biogroup 1 have been described recently but are extremely rare (Table 15).

The genus *Enterobacter* (11)

Enterobacter is an old genus. Two of its species, *E. cloacae* and *E. aerogenes*, are frequently isolated from clinical specimens (Table 16) and are important causes of nosocomial infections (Table 2). *E. agglomerans* (25, 36) is occasionally isolated from clinical specimens. *E. sakazakii* is a rare but important cause of life-threatening neonatal meningitis and sepsis. The other species of *Enterobacter* are rare, but their differentiation can be difficult (42) because of their biochemical similarities (Table 16).

TABLE 13. Differentiation within the genus *Cedecea*

Test or property	Reaction[a]				
	C. davisae	*C. lapagei*	*C. neteri*	*Cedecea* sp. 3	*Cedecea* sp. 5
Ornithine decarboxylase	+	−	−	−	v
Fermentation of:					
Sucrose	+	−	+	v	+
D-Sorbitol	−	−	+	−	+
Raffinose	−	−	−	+	+
D-Xylose	+	−	+	+	+
Melibiose	−	−	−	+	+
Malonate utilization	+	+	+	−	−

[a] For definition of symbols, see Table 12, footnote *a*.

TABLE 14. Differentiation within the genus *Citrobacter*

Test or property	Reaction[a]		
	C. amalonaticus	*C. freundii*	*C. diversus*
Biochemical tests			
Indole production	+	−	+
H_2S production (TSI)	−	+	−
Malonate utilization	−	(−)	+
KCN, growth in	+	+	−
Tyrosine clearing	−	−	+
Adonitol fermentation	−	−	+
Antibiogram			
Cephalothin, 30 μg[b]	18.0 (2.0)	10.9 (2.9)	23.5 (1.2)
Ampicillin, 10 μg	8.7 (2.4)	14.3 (3.1)	7.1 (1.2)
Carbenicillin, 100 μg	16.5 (2.4)	24.1 (0.9)	12.6 (1.6)

[a] For definition of symbols, see Table 12, footnote *a*. Where numbers are given, the first number is the mean zone size (in millimeters) and the number in parentheses is the standard deviation of the zones of inhibition. Data are based on 10 strains of each species. One strain was found to have multiple antibiotic resistance and was replaced with a sensitive strain.

[b] Numbers give the amount of antibiotic per disk.

The genus *Escherichia*

In addition to *E. coli*, the genus *Escherichia* includes *E. fergusonii, E. hermanii*, and *E. vulneris* (Table 17), which occasionally occur in human clinical specimens. Recently, it has been noticed that some strains of *E. hermanii* agglutinate in *E. coli* O157 antiserum. This reaction could lead to misidentification unless the strain is confirmed biochemically and serologically (H7 antigen).

The genus *Ewingella*

The genus *Ewingella*, described in 1983, includes a single species, *E. americana*. This organism is very rare in human clinical specimens but can cause bacteremia and nosocomial outbreaks.

The genus *Hafnia*

The genus *Hafnia* has a single species, *H. alvei*, that is occasionally isolated from a wide variety of extraintestinal specimens. Biochemically, *H. alvei* is somewhat similar to the species of *Enterobacter*, and it was once classified in this genus as *Enterobacter hafniae*.

The genus *Klebsiella* (58)

K. pneumoniae is an important cause of nosocomial and community-acquired infections (Table 2). This organism is easily recognized by the large mucoid colonies that it produces on MacConkey agar, its biochemical activity, and its characteristic resistance to ampicillin and carbenicillin. *K. oxytoca* is biochemically similar to *K. pneumoniae* but is indole positive (Table 18). *K. ozaenae* and *K. rhinoscleromatis*, which are associated with ozaena and rhinoscleroma, are rarely isolated in the United States. These diseases of the nose are found in the tropics and in a few other locations. *K. planticola, K. terrigena*, and *Klebsiella* group 47 (29), which is also known as *K. ornithinolytica*, are very rare in human clinical specimens but probably will be misidentified as *K. pneumoniae* unless special tests are done (Table 18).

The genus *Kluyvera*

The genus *Kluyvera* was described in 1981 and includes two species. Strains of *K. ascorbata* are occasionally isolated from clinical specimens, but *K. cryocrescens* is extremely rare. These two species are very similar biochemically (Table 12), and most clinical laboratories report them as "*Kluyvera* species."

The genus *Koserella (Yokenella)*

The genus *Koserella* was described in 1985 and includes a single species, *K. trabulsii*. It is biochemically similar to *H. alvei* (Table 1) and has been isolated from the respiratory tract, wounds, urine, and feces. *Yokenella regensburgei*, another new species, appears to be identical to *K. trabulsii*, so one of the names will eventually be dropped.

The genus *Leclercia*

The genus *Leclercia* was described in 1986 and includes a single species, *L. adecarboxylata*, which had previously been known as *Escherichia adecarboxylata*

TABLE 15. Differentiation within the genus *Edwardsiella*

Test or property	Reaction[a]			
	E. tarda		*E. hoshinae*	*E. ictaluria*
	Most strains	Biogroup 1		
Indole production	+	+	(−)	−
H_2S production (TSI)	+	−	−	−
Motility	+	+	+	−
Malonate utilization	−	−	+	−
Fermentation of:				
D-Mannitol	−	+	+	−
Sucrose	−	+	+	−
Trehalose	−	−	+	−
L-Arabinose	−	+	(−)	−
Tetrathionate reduction[b]	+	−	+	−
Present in human clinical specimens	+	−	−[c]	−

[a] For definition of symbols, see Table 12, footnote *a*.

[b] Data from Grimont et al. (reference 68 in reference 29).

[c] Two isolates from feces have been reported.

TABLE 16. Differentiation within the genus *Enterobacter*

Test or property	Reaction[a]								
	E. cloacae	*E. aerogenes*	*E. agglomerans*	*E. sakazakii*	*E. gergoviae*	*E. taylorae*	*E. asburiae*	*E. intermedium*	*E. amnigenus* biogroup	
									1	2
Lysine decarboxylase	–	+	–	–	+	–	–	–	–	–
Arginine dihydrolase	+	–	–	+	–	+	(–)	–	–	v
Ornithine decarboxylase	+	+	–	+	+	+	+	(+)	+	+
KCN, growth in	+	+	v	+	–	+	+	v	+	+
Fermentation of:										
Sucrose	+	+	(+)	+	+	–	+	v	+	–
Dulcitol	(–)	–	(–)	–	–	–	–	+	–	(–)
Adonitol	(–)	+	–	–	–	–	–	–	–	–
D-Sorbitol	+	+	v	–	–	–	+	+	–	+
Raffinose	+	+	v	+	+	–	v	+	+	–
α-Methyl-D-glucoside	(+)	+	–	+	–	v	+	+	v	+
D-Arabitol	(–)	+	–	–	+	–	–	–	–	–
Yellow pigment	–	–	(+)	+	–	–	–	–	–	–
Present in human clinical specimens	++++	+++	++	+	+	+	+	–	–	–

[a] For definition of symbols, see Table 12, footnote *a*.

and as Enteric Group 41 (29). *L. adecarboxylata* has been isolated from a variety of human clinical specimens, food, and water.

The genus *Leminorella*

The genus *Leminorella* was described in 1985 and includes two H_2S-positive species, *L. grimontii* and *L. richardii* (Table 11). Most isolates have been from feces, with a few from urine.

The genus *Moellerella*

The genus *Moellerella* was described in 1984 and includes one species, *M. wisconsensis*, which is biochemically inactive (Table 1). Most of the isolates have been from human feces.

The genus *Morganella*

The genus *Morganella* includes a single species, *M. morganii*, that was originally classified in the genus *Proteus* as *Proteus morganii* (61). *M. morganii* is a well-known cause of urinary tract and other extraintestinal infections. In the early literature, *M. morganii* is mentioned as a possible enteric pathogen, but its etiological role is doubtful. A group of *M. morganii* strains known as biogroup 1 are nonmotile, are lysine negative, and ferment glycerol within 24 h.

The genus *Pragia*

The genus *Pragia* was described in 1988 and includes a single species, *P. fontium*, which has been isolated only from water. It is another of the new H_2S-positive species in the family (Table 11).

The genus *Proteus*

Proteus is a well-established genus that is familiar to clinical microbiologists (61). Recently, the description of the genus has been restricted with the establishment of two additional genera, *Providencia* and *Morganella*, for some of the species formerly included in *Proteus*.

P. mirabilis and *P. vulgaris* are often isolated from urinary tract and other extraintestinal infections and are easily recognized on nonselective media such as blood agar because they swarm and have a characteristic odor. Strains of *P. mirabilis* are indole negative and ornithine positive (Table 19), traits that differentiate them from strains of *P. vulgaris*. *P. penneri* is a new species that is occasionally isolated from clinical specimens.

The genus *Providencia* (61)

The genus *Providencia* was originally established for urease-negative organisms that were biochemically similar to the species of *Proteus* (Tables 1, 20, and 21). *P. rettgeri* and *P. stuartii* are well-known causes of urinary tract and other extraintestinal infections and have caused many nosocomial outbreaks. *P. alcalifaciens* is usually isolated from feces and is rarely isolated in most clinical microbiology laboratories. *P. rustigianii* is a new species that is also rare. *P. heimbachae* has not been isolated from human clinical specimens.

The genus *Rahnella*

The genus *Rahnella*, described in 1979, includes a single species, *R. aquatilis*. Most of the strains have been

TABLE 17. Differentiation within the genus *Escherichia*

Test or property	Reaction[a]				
	E. blattae	*E. coli*	*E. fergusonii*	*E. hermannii*	*E. vulneris*
Indole production	−	+	+	+	−
Lysine decarboxylase	+	+	+	−	(+)
Ornithine decarboxylase	+	V	+	+	−
Motility	−	(+)	+	+	+
KCN, growth in	−	−	−	+	(−)
Fermentation of:					
D-Mannitol	−	+	+	+	+
Adonitol	−	−	+	−	−
D-Sorbitol	−	+	−	−	−
Cellobiose	−	−	+	+	+
D-Arabitol	−	−	+	−	−
Mucate	V	+	−	+	(+)
Yellow pigment	−	−	−	+	V
Present in human clinical specimens	−	+	+	+	+
Isolates from cockroaches	+	−	−	−	−

[a] For definition of symbols, see Table 12, footnote *a*.

TABLE 18. Differentiation within the genus *Klebsiella*

Test	Reaction[a]				
	K. pneumoniae	*K. oxytoca*	*K. terrigena*	*K. planticola*	*Klebsiella* group 47, Ind$^+$ Orn$^+$
Indole production[b]	−	+	−	(−)	+
Ornithine decarboxylase[b]	−	−	−	−	+
Growth at[c]:					
5°C	−	−	+	+	+
10°C	−	+	+	+	+
41°C	+	+	+	−	−
44.5°C	+	−	−	−	−

[a] For definition of symbols, see Table 12, footnote *a*.
[b] Based on data from our laboratory.
[c] Based on limited data from our laboratory; compiled from the literature (58, and reference 59 in reference 29); 44.5°C is the temperature used for the fecal coliform test.

TABLE 19. Differentiation within the genus *Proteus*

Test or property	Reaction[a]				
	P. mirabilis	*P. myxofaciens*	*P. penneri*	*P. vulgaris* biogroup 2	*P. vulgaris* biogroup 3
Indole production	−	−	−	+	+
Ornithine decarboxylase	+	−	−	−	−
Maltose fermentation	−	+	+	+	+
D-Xylose fermentation	+	−	+	+	+
Salicin fermentation	−	−	−	+	−
Esculin hydrolysis	−	−	−	+	−
Chloramphenicol susceptibility	S	S	R	V	S
Present in human clinical specimens	+	−	+	+	+
Occurs as a pathogen of gypsy moth larvae	−	+	−	−	−

[a] For definition of symbols, see Table 12, footnote *a*. S, Susceptible; R, resistant; V, variable (strain-to-strain variation in susceptibility).

TABLE 20. Differentiation of the three genera in the *Proteus* group

Test or property	Reaction[a]		
	Proteus	*Providencia*	*Morganella*
H_2S production (TSI)	+	−	−
Swarming[b]	+	−	−
D-Mannose fermentation	−	+	+
Gelatin liquefaction	+	−	−
Lipase (corn oil)	+	−	−
Citrate utilization	v	+	+
Ornithine decarboxylase	v	−	+

[a] For definition of symbols, see Table 12, footnote *a*.
[b] On sheep blood agar or Trypticase soy agar.

TABLE 21. Differentiation within the genus *Providencia*

Test	Reaction[a]			
	P. stuartii	*P. rettgeri*	*P. alcalifaciens*	*P. rustigianii*
Urea hydrolysis	v	+	−	−
Fermentation of:				
myo-Inositol[b]	+	+	−	−
Adonitol[b]	−	+	+	−
D-Arabitol	−	+	−	−
Trehalose	+	−	−	−
D-Galactose	+	+	−	+

[a] For definition of symbols, see Table 12, footnote *a*.
[b] Strains of *P. stuartii* biogroup 4 are inositol negative, and strains of biogroup 6 are adonitol positive; both of these biogroups are rare.

isolated from water, but one was from a human burn wound (29).

The genus *Serratia* (38, 73)

S. marcescens is an important cause of extraintestinal infections and has caused many nosocomial outbreaks. Several other *Serratia* species have recently been described (Table 22): *S. ficaria*, *S. fonticola*, *S. liquefaciens*, *S. odorifera*, and *S. plymuthica*. They occasionally occur in clinical specimens but have unclear clinical significance. *S. marcescens* does not ferment L-arabinose, which differentiates it from the other species except for the newly described *S. entomophila*, which does not occur in human clinical specimens.

The genus *Tatumella*

The genus *Tatumella* was first described in 1981 and has a single species, *T. ptyseos*, which is rare in clinical specimens. Most strains have been isolated from the respiratory tract and are of unknown clinical significance, but several isolates have been from blood.

The genus *Xenorhabdus*

The genus *Xenorhabdus* was described in 1979 and has two species, *X. nematophilus* and *X. luminescens*, which are pathogenic for nematodes and are important in insect control. Recently, several unusual strains isolated from human blood and wounds were identified as *X. luminescens* DNA hybridization group 5 (30). This unusual organism can be recognized by its unusual biochemical reactions (Table 1) and by the faint bioluminescence (up to 15 min in a totally dark room may be required) (Table 23).

The genus *Yersinia*

The genus *Yersinia* was formerly classified in the family *Pasteurellaceae*, but since strains of *Yersinia* contain the enterobacterial common antigen and are related to *E. coli* by DNA-DNA hybridization, the genus is now a well-accepted member of the family *Enterobacteriaceae*.

TABLE 22. Differentiation within the genus *Serratia*

Test or property	Reaction[a]						
	S. marcescens	*S. liquefaciens* group	*S. rubidaea*	*S. odorifera*	*S. plymuthica*	*S. ficaria*	*S. fonticola*
DNase (25°C)	+	(+)	+	+	+	+	−
Lipase (corn oil)	+	(+)	+	v	v	(+)	−
Gelatinase (22°C)	+	+	(+)	+	v	+	−
Lysine decarboxylase	+	+	v	+	−	−	+
Ornithine decarboxylase	+	+	−	v	−	−	+
Odor of *S. odorifera*	−	−	(−)	−	−	+	−
Red, pink, or orange pigment	v	−	v	−	v	−	−
Fermentation of:							
L-Arabinose	−	+	+	+	+	+	+
D-Arabitol	−	−	(+)	−	−	+	+
D-Sorbitol	+	+	−	+	v	+	+
Adonitol	v	−	+	v	−	−	+
Dulcitol	−	−	−	−	−	−	+
Frequency in human clinical specimens	++++	+	+	+	+	+	+

[a] For definition of symbols, see Table 12, footnote *a*.

TABLE 23. Differentiation of *Xenorhabdus luminescens* DNA hybridization group 5 from other species of *Enterobacteriaceae*

Test or property	Reaction[a]		
	X. luminescens DNA group 5	*X. nematophilus*	Most other *Enterobacteriaceae*
Bioluminescent	+	−	−
Catalase	+	−	+
Nitrate reduction to nitrite	−	−	+
Yellow pigment	+	−	−[b]

[a] Symbols: +, most strains positive; −, most strains negative.
[b] A few species produce yellow pigment.

The genus *Yersinia* has 11 named species (Tables 1, 9, and 24), all of which occur in clinical specimens. Those most important in human disease are *Y. pestis*, *Y. pseudotuberculosis*, and *Y. enterocolitica*. *Y. pestis* causes plague, which historically has been one of the most important infectious diseases and a scourge through the ages (13). *Y. pseudotuberculosis* is very similar biochemically to *Y. pestis* (Table 24) and causes infections that have a broad clinical picture that closely resembles that of *Y. enterocolitica*. Both *Y. pestis* and *Y. pseudotuberculosis* are rarely isolated in the United States (13).

Isolation and identification of *Y. pestis*. Infections due to *Y. pestis* are rare in the United States (63), with about 15 confirmed cases each year, usually in New Mexico, Arizona, and California. Although plague is rare, it is important to be aware of a possible plague case because the mortality in untreated individuals is about 60%. In the early phase of illness, there is an intermittent bacteremia; therefore, blood cultures are likely to be positive. Swollen lymph nodes (bubos) are also likely to contain abundant organisms.

Y. pestis is not a fastidious organism; it grows well on blood agar and many of the other enteric media. However, after 24 h the colonies are pinpoint, which is in marked contrast to other species of *Enterobacteriaceae*, whose colonies are typically 2 to 3 mm in diameter. After 48 h, the colonies of *Y. pestis* are 1 to 1.5 mm in diameter, are gray to grayish white, and may appear slightly mucoid.

Y. pestis is inactive in routine biochemical tests but has a typical pattern that closely resembles that of *Y. pseudotuberculosis* (Tables 1 and 24). Cultures of *Y. pestis* never produce a uniform turbidity in broth but have a characteristic "stalactite pattern" in which clumps of cells adhere to the side of the tube and settle to the bottom if the tube is jarred. Since many of the commercial identification systems do not include *Y. pestis*, it is important to suspect it from its characteristic appearance on primary plates and from clinical and epidemiological information furnished with the specimen. Strains suspected to be or presumptively identified as *Y. pestis* should be reported immediately by telephone to the state health department, which will request that the culture be sent immediately for identification or ask that it be sent to a plague reference laboratory. In the United States, the national plague reference laboratory identifies (Table 9) isolates with a number of specialized methods [contact Plague Branch, Division of Vector-Borne Infectious Diseases, Center for Infectious Diseases, Centers for Disease Control, Fort Collins, CO 80522-2087; phone: (303) 221-6450]. See reference 63 for more details on the microbiology of *Y. pestis*.

Other species of *Yersinia*. The other eight species of *Yersinia*, *Y. aldovae*, *Y. bercovieri*, *Y. frederiksenii*, *Y. intermedia*, *Y. kristensenii*, *Y. mollaretti*, *Y. rohdei*, and "*Y.*" *ruckeri*, occasionally occur in both intestinal and extraintestinal specimens and are very similar biochemically (Table 9). In extraintestinal specimens they can be regarded as opportunistic pathogens, since they apparently lack the tissue invasiveness genes found in *Y. pestis*, *Y. pseudotuberculosis*, and *Y. enterocolitica*. There is little evidence that they cause human intestinal infections, although they occur occasionally in feces. This occurrence is probably temporary intestinal colonization or passage through the gut of strains found in food, water, or the environment. These species can grow at 4°C and can multiply in refrigerated food, which is a likely source of transient strains found in feces. They also grow on CIN agar and must be differentiated from pathogenic serotypes of *Y. enterocolitica*.

TABLE 24. Properties and differentiation of *Yersinia pestis* and *Y. pseudotuberculosis*

Test or property	Reaction[a]	
	Y. pestis	*Y. pseudotuberculosis*
Motility		
37°C	−	−
20–25°C	−	+
Urea hydrolysis	−	+
Uniform turbidity in broth cultures	−	+
Fermentation of:		
Adonitol	−	+
L-Rhamnose	−	+
Melibiose	(−)	+
Phage susceptibility[b]		
37°C	+	v
20°C	+	−
Reaction with *Y. pestis* fraction 1 antiserum	+	−
Coagulase production	+	−
Fibrinolysin production	+	−
Pathogenic for:		
Mice	+	+
White rats	+	−
Guinea pigs	+	+
Gerbils	+	+
Hamsters	−	−

[a] For definition of symbols, see Table 12, footnote *a*. Strains that have lost the *Yersinia* virulence plasmid may be negative for some of the virulence tests. Occasional strains may take longer than 2 days to become positive in the biochemical tests.
[b] To the *Yersinia* phage useful in identification.

The genus *Yokenella*

See the section on *Koserella*.

Some of the material in this chapter was taken from or adapted from publications by authors from the Centers for Disease Control, including other chapters and reviews of the family (29, 32). Under the Copyright Act, these are considered "works of the United States Government" for which copyright protection under Title 17 of the United States Code is not available. We thank these authors for allowing us to use this material with a minimum of rewriting. We thank N. A. Strockbine, J. G. Wells, I. K. Wachsmuth, and P. A. Blake for their critical review of this chapter; we thank G. P. Carter and the entire staff of the Enteric Bacteriology Laboratories for their work on updating the data in Table 1, which will be described in more detail in a separate publication.

LITERATURE CITED

1. **Aserkoff, B. A., and J. V. Bennett.** 1969. Effect of antibiotic therapy in acute salmonellosis on the fecal excretion of Salmonellae. N. Engl. J. Med. **281:**636–640.
2. **Baine, W. B., E. J. Gangarosa, J. V. Bennett, and W. H. Barker.** 1973. Institutional salmonellosis. J. Infect. Dis. **128:**357–360.
3. **Barrett-Connor, E., and J. D. Connor.** 1970. Extraintestinal manifestations of shigellosis. Am. J. Gastroenterol. **53:**234–245.
4. **Bartlett, R. C.** 1977. Medical microbiology: how fast to go—how far to go, p. 15–35. *In* V. Lorian (ed.), Significance of medical microbiology in the care of patients. The Williams & Wilkins Co., Baltimore.
5. **Bennett, I. L., and E. W. Hook.** 1959. Infectious diseases (some aspects of salmonellosis). Annu. Rev. Med. **10:**1–20.
6. **Black, P. H., L. J. Kunz, and M. N. Swartz.** 1960. Salmonellosis—a review of some unusual aspects. N. Engl. J. Med. **262:**813–817.
7. **Blake, P. A., and R. A. Feldman.** 1986. Salmonellosis, p. 406–410. *In* J. M. Last (ed.), Maxey-Rosenau public health and preventive medicine, 19th ed. Appleton-Century-Crofts, Norwalk, Conn.
8. **Blazevic, D. J., and J. E. Stemper.** 1972. Organisms encountered in urine culture over a 10-year period. Appl. Microbiol. **23:**421–422.
9. **Bottone, E. J. (ed.).** 1981. *Yersinia enterocolitica.* CRC Press, Inc., Boca Raton, Fla.
10. **Brenner, D. J.** 1981. Introduction to the family *Enterobacteriaceae,* p. 1105–1127. *In* M. P. Starr, H. Stolp, H. G. Trüper, A. Balows, and H. G. Schlegel (ed.), The prokaryotes. Springer-Verlag KG, Berlin.
11. **Brenner, D. J.** 1981. The genus *Enterobacter,* p. 1173–1180. *In* M. P. Starr, H. Stolp, H. G. Trüper, A. Balows, and H. G. Schlegel (ed.), The prokaryotes. Springer-Verlag KG, Berlin.
12. **Buchanan, R. E., and N. E. Gibbons (ed.).** 1974. Bergey's manual of determinative bacteriology, 8th ed. The Williams & Wilkins Co, Baltimore.
13. **Butler, T.** 1983. Plague and other *Yersinia* infections. Plenium Medical Book Co., New York.
14. **Centers for Disease Control.** 1988. *Shigella,* annual tabulation 1988. Centers for Disease Control, Atlanta.
15. **Cheasty, T., and B. Rowe.** 1983. Antigenic relationships between the entero-invasive *Escherichia coli* O antigens O28ac, O112ac, O124, O136, O143, O144, O152, and O164 and *Shigella* O antigens. J. Clin. Microbiol. **17:**681–684.
16. **Christie, A. B.** 1974. Infectious diseases: epidemiology and clinical practice, 2nd ed., p. 122–147. Churchill Livingstone, London.
17. **Cooke, E. M.** 1973. *Escherichia coli* and man. Churchill Livingstone, London.
18. **Crosa, J. H., D. J. Brenner, W. H. Ewing, and S. Falkow.** 1973. Molecular relationships among the *Salmonelleae.* J. Bacteriol. **115:**307–315.
19. **Dean, A. G., C. Vi-Chuan, G. Williams, and B. Barden.** 1972. Test for *Escherichia coli* enterotoxin using infant mice: application in a study of diarrhoea in children in Honolulu. J. Infect. Dis. **125:**407–411.
20. **DuPont, H. L.** 1982. *Escherichia coli* diarrhea, p. 219–234. *In* A. S. Evans and H. A. Feldman (ed.), Bacterial infections of humans. Plenum Medical Book Co., New York.
21. **DuPont, H. L., S. B. Formal, R. B. Hornick, M. J. Snyder, J. P. Libonati, D. G. Sheahan, E. H. LaBrec, and J. P. Kalas.** 1971. Pathogenesis of *Escherichia coli* diarrhea. N. Engl. J. Med. **285:**1–9.
22. **Evans, D. G., R. P. Silver, D. J. Evans, Jr., D. G. Chase, and S. Gorbach.** 1975. Plasmid-controlled colonization factor associated with virulence in *Escherichia coli* enterotoxigenic for humans. Infect. Immun. **12:**656–667.
23. **Ewing, W. H.** 1963. Isolation and identification of *Escherichia coli* serotypes associated with diarrhea disease. Center for Disease Control, Atlanta.
24. **Ewing, W. H.** 1986. Edwards and Ewing's identification of *Enterobacteriaceae,* 4th ed. Elsevier Science Publishing Co., New York.
25. **Ewing, W. H., and M. A. Fife.** 1972. *Enterobacter agglomerans* (Beijerinck) comb. nov. (the *herbicola-lathyri* bacteria). Int. J. Syst. Bacteriol. **22:**4–11.
26. **Farmer, J. J., III.** 1981. The genus *Citrobacter,* p. 1140–1147. *In* M. P. Starr, H. Stolp, H. G. Trüper, A. Balows, and H. G. Schlegel (ed.), The prokaryotes. Springer-Verlag KG, Berlin.
27. **Farmer, J. J., III.** 1981. The genus *Edwardsiella,* p. 1135–1139. *In* M. P. Starr, H. Stolp, H. G. Trüper, A. Balows, and H. G. Schlegel (ed.), The prokaryotes. Springer-Verlag KG, Berlin.
28. **Farmer, J. J., III, and B. R. Davis.** 1985. H7 antiserum-sorbitol fermentation medium: a single tube screening medium for detecting *Escherichia coli* O157:H7 associated with hemorrhagic colitis. J. Clin. Microbiol. **22:**620–625. [PLEASE NOTE: This paper has a misprint in the formula for MacConkey sorbitol agar. The paper says to use 22.2 g of MacConkey agar base; the correct amount is 40 g, which is given in the instructions on the bottle.]
29. **Farmer, J. J., III, B. R. Davis, F. W. Hickman-Brenner, A. McWhorter, G. P. Huntley-Carter, M. A. Asbury, C. Riddle, H. G. Wathen, C. Elias, G. R. Fanning, A. G. Steigerwalt, C. M. O'Hara, G. K. Morris, P. B. Smith, and D. J. Brenner.** 1985. Biochemical identification of new species and biogroups of *Enterobacteriaceae* isolated from clinical specimens. J. Clin. Microbiol. **21:**46–76.
30. **Farmer, J. J., III, J. H. Jorgensen, P. A. D. Grimont, R. J. Akhurst, G. O. Poinar, Jr., E. Ageron, G. V. Pierce, J. A. Smith, G. P. Carter, K. L. Wilson, and F. W. Hickman-Brenner.** 1989. *Xenorhabdus luminescens* (DNA hybridization group 5) from human clinical specimens. J. Clin. Microbiol. **27:**1594–1600.
31. **Farmer, J. J., III, A. C. McWhorter, D. J. Brenner, and G. K. Morris.** 1984. The *Salmonella-Arizona* group of *Enterobacteriaceae:* nomenclature, classification and reporting. Clin. Microbiol. Newsl. **6:**63–66.
32. **Farmer, J. J., III, J. G. Wells, P. M. Griffin, and I. K. Wachsmuth.** 1987. *Enterobacteriaceae* infections, p. 233–296. *In* B. B. Wentworth (ed.), Diagnostic procedures for bacterial infections, 7th ed. American Public Health Association, Inc., Washington, D.C.
33. **Finkelstein, R. A., and Z. Zang.** 1983. Rapid test for identification of heat-labile enterotoxin-producing *Escherichia coli* colonies. J. Clin. Microbiol. **18:**23–28.
34. **Fowler, J. M., and R. R. Brubaker.** 1985. Immunology of yersiniae, p. 371–374. *In* N. R. Rose, H. Friedman, and J. L. Fahey (ed.), Manual of clinical laboratory immunology, 3rd ed. American Society for Microbiology, Washington, D.C.
35. **Gangarosa, E. J., and M. H. Merson.** 1977. Epidemiologic assessment of the relevance of the so-called enteropathogenic serogroups of *Escherichia coli* in diarrhea. N. Engl. J. Med. **296:**1210–1213.
36. **Gilardi, G. L., E. Bottone, and M. Birnbaum.** 1970. Unusual fermentative, gram-negative bacilli isolated from clinical specimens. I. Characterization of *Erwinia* strains of the "lathyri-herbicola group." Appl. Microbiol. **20:**151–155.
37. **Gorbach, S. L., B. H. Kean, D. G. Evans, D. J. Evans, Jr., and D. Bessudo.** 1975. Travelers' diarrhea and toxi-

genic *Escherichia coli*. N. Engl. J. Med. **292:**933–936.

38. **Grimont, P. A. D., and F. Grimont.** 1981. The genus *Serratia*, p. 1187–1203. *In* M. P. Starr, H. Stolp, H. G. Trüper, A. Balows, and H. G. Schlegel (ed.), The prokaryotes. Springer-Verlag KG, Berlin.
39. **Harris, J. C., H. L. DuPont, and R. B. Hornick.** 1971. Fecal leukocytes in diarrheal illness. Ann. Intern. Med. **76:**697–703.
40. **Harris, J. R., J. Mariano, J. G. Wells, B. J. Payne, H. D. Donnell, and M. L. Cohen.** 1985. Person-to-person transmission in an outbreak of enteroinvasive *Escherichia coli*. Am. J. Epidemiol. **122:**245–252.
41. **Hickman, F. W., and J. J. Farmer III.** 1978. *Salmonella typhi:* identification, antibiograms, serology, and bacteriophage typing. Am. J. Med. Technol. **44:**1149–1159.
42. **Izard, D., F. Gavini, P. A. Trinel, and H. Leclerc.** 1981. Deoxyribonucleic acid relatedness between *Enterobacter cloacae* and *Enterobacter amnigenus* sp. nov. Int. J. Syst. Bacteriol. **31:**35–42.
43. **Kandolo, K., and G. Wauters.** 1985. Pyrazinamidase activity in *Yersinia enterocolitica* and related organisms. J. Clin. Microbiol. **21:**980–982.
44. **Karmali, M. A.** 1989. Infection by verocytotoxin-producing *Escherichia coli*. Clin. Microbiol. Rev. **2:**15–38.
45. **Karmali, M. A., M. Petric, C. Lim, P. C. Fleming, and B. T. Steele.** 1983. *Escherichia coli* cytotoxin, hemolytic-uremic syndrome, and hemorrhagic colitis. Lancet **ii:** 1299–1300.
46. **Kauffmann, F.** 1966. The bacteriology of *Enterobacteriaceae*. The Williams & Wilkins Co., Baltimore.
47. **Kauffmann, F., and A. DuPont.** 1950. *Escherichia* strains from infantile gastro-enteritis. Acta Pathol. Microbiol. Scand. **27:**552–564.
48. **Kopecko, D. J., L. S. Baron, and J. Buysse.** 1985. Genetic determinants of virulence in *Shigella* and dysenteric strains of *Escherichia coli:* their involvement in the pathogenesis of dysentery. Curr. Top. Microbiol. Immunol. **118:**71–95.
49. **Krieg, N. R. (ed.).** 1984. Bergey's manual of systematic bacteriology, vol. 1. The Williams & Wilkins Co., Baltimore.
50. **Le Minor, L., M. Y. Popoff, B. Laurent, and D. Hermant.** 1986. Individualisation d'une septième sous-espèce de *Salmonella: S. choleraesuis* subsp. *indica* subsp. nov. Ann. Microbiol. (Paris) **137B:**211–217.
51. **Levin, M. M., H. L. DuPont, S. B. Formal, R. B. Hornick, A. Takeuchi, E. J. Gangarosa, M. J. Snyder, and J. P. Libonati.** 1973. Pathogenesis of *Shigella dysenteriae* 1 (Shiga) dysentery. J. Infect. Dis. **127:**261–270.
52. **Li, K., J. J. Farmer III, and A. Coppola.** 1974. A novel type of resistant bacteria induced by gentamicin. Trans. N.Y. Acad. Sci. **36:**369–396.
53. **Lockwood, D. E., and D. E. Robertson.** 1984. Development of a competitive enzyme-linked immunosorbent assay (ELISA) for *Escherichia coli* heat-stable enterotoxin (ST_a). J. Immunol. Methods **75:**295–307.
54. **Mandell, G. L., R. G. Douglas, Jr., and J. E. Bennett.** 1990. Principles and practice of infectious diseases, 3rd ed. Churchill Livingstone, New York.
55. **Marier, R., J. G. Wells, R. C. Swanson, W. Callahan, and I. J. Mehlman.** 1973. An outbreak of enteropathogenic *Escherichia coli* foodborne disease traced to imported French cheese. Lancet **ii:**1376–1378.
56. **Merson, M. H., B. Rowe, R. E. Black, I. Huq, R. J. Gross, and A. Eusof.** 1980. Use of antisera for identification of enterotoxigenic *Escherichia coli*. Lancet **ii:**222–224.
57. **Nunes, M. P., and I. D. Ricciardi.** 1981. Detection of *Yersinia enterocolitica* heat-stable enterotoxin by suckling mouse bioassay. J. Clin. Microbiol. **13:**783–786.
58. **Orskov, I.** 1984. Genus V. *Klebsiella* Trevisan 1885, 105^{AL}, p. 461–465. *In* N. R. Krieg (ed.), Bergey's manual of systematic bacteriology, vol. 1. The Williams & Wilkins Co., Baltimore.
59. **Orskov, I., F. Orskov, B. Jann, and K. Jann.** 1977. Serology, chemistry, and genetics of O and K antigens of *Escherichia coli*. Bacteriol. Rev. **41:**667–710.
60. **Pal, T., A. S. Pacsa, L. Emody, S. Voros, and E. Selley.** 1985. Modified enzyme-linked immunosorbent assay for detecting enteroinvasive *Escherichia coli* and virulent *Shigella* strains. J. Clin. Microbiol. **21:**415–418.
61. **Penner, J. L.** 1981. The tribe *Proteeae*, p. 1204–1224. *In* M. P. Starr, H. Stolp, H. G. Trüper, A. Balows, and H. G. Schlegel (ed.), The prokaryotes. Springer-Verlag KG, Berlin.
62. **Pickering, L. K., H. L. DuPont, J. Olarte, R. Conklin, and C. Ericsson.** 1977. Fecal leucocytes in enteric infections. Am. J. Clin. Pathol. **68:**562–565.
63. **Quan, T. J.** 1987. Plague, p. 445–453. *In* B. B. Wentworth (ed.), Diagnostic procedures for bacterial infections, 7th ed. America Public Health Association, Inc., Washington, D.C.
64. **Riley, G., and S. Toma.** 1989. Detection of pathogenic *Yersinia enterocolitica* by using congo red-magnesium oxalate agar medium. J. Clin. Microbiol. **27:**213–214.
65. **Riley, L. W., R. S. Remis, S. D. Helgerson, H. B. McGee, J. G. Wells, B. R. Davis, R. J. Hebert, E. S. Olcott, L. M. Johnson, N. T. Hargrett, P. A. Blake, and M. L. Cohen.** 1983. Hemorrhagic colitis associated with a rare *Escherichia coli* serotype. N. Engl. J. Med. **308:**681–685.
66. **Ronnberg, B., and T. Wadström.** 1983. Rapid detection by a coagglutination test of heat-labile enterotoxin in cell lysates from blood agar-grown *Escherichia coli*. J. Clin. Microbiol. **17:**1021–1025.
67. **Sack, R. B.** 1975. Human diarrheal disease caused by enterotoxigenic *Escherichia coli*. Annu. Rev. Microbiol. **29:** 333–353.
68. **Saphra, I., and J. W. Winter.** 1957. Clinical manifestations of salmonellosis in man. N. Engl. J. Med. **256:**1128–1134.
69. **Seriwatana, J., P. Echeverria, J. Escamilla, R. Glass, I. Huq, R. Rockhill, and B. J. Stoll.** 1983. Identification of enterotoxigenic *Escherichia coli* in patients with diarrhea in Asia with three enterotoxin gene probes. Infect. Immun. **42:**152–155.
70. **Starr, M. P., H. Stolp, H. G. Trüper, A. Balows, and H. C. Schlegel (ed.).** 1981. The prokaryotes. Springer-Verlag KG, Berlin.
71. **Svennerholm, A., and G. Wiklund.** 1983. Rapid GM 1-enzyme-linked immunosorbent assay with visual reading for identification of *Escherichia coli* heat-labile enterotoxin. J. Clin. Microbiol. **17:**596–600.
72. **Tullock, E. F., Jr., K. J. Ryan, S. B. Formal, and F. A. Franklin.** 1973. Invasive enteropathogenic *Escherichia coli* dysentery. Ann. Intern. Med. **78:**13–17.
73. **von Graevenitz, A., and S. J. Rubin (ed.).** 1980. The genus *Serratia*. CRC Press, Inc., Boca Raton, Fla.
74. **Wadström, T., A. Aust-Kettis, D. Habte, J. Holmgren, G. Meeuwisse, R. Mollby, and O. Soderlind.** 1976. Enterotoxin-producing bacteria and parasites in stool of Ethiopian children with diarrhoeal disease. Arch. Dis. Child. **51:**865–870.
75. **Wells, J. G., B. R. Davis, I. K. Wachsmuth, L. W. Riley, R. S. Remis, R. Sokolow, and G. K. Morris.** 1983. Laboratory investigation of hemorrhagic colitis outbreaks associated with a rare *Escherichia coli* serotype. J. Clin. Microbiol. **18:**512–520.
76. **World Health Organization, Centre for Reference and Research on *Salmonella*.** 1980. Antigenic formulae of the *Salmonella*. WHO International *Salmonella* Center, Institut Pasteur, Paris.
77. **Yolken, R. H., H. B. Greenberg, M. H. Herson, R. B. Sack, and A. Z. Kapikian.** 1977. Enzyme-linked immunosorbent assay for detection of *Escherichia coli* heat-labile enterotoxin. J. Clin. Microbiol. **6:**439–444.

Chapter 37

Vibrio

MICHAEL T. KELLY, F. W. HICKMAN-BRENNER, AND J. J. FARMER III

Organisms in the genus *Vibrio* constitute a major portion of the family *Vibrionaceae*. *Vibrio* species are thought to be rare in inland laboratories, but the increasing consumption of seafoods, especially uncooked seafoods, may increase the occurrence of the organisms even in areas remote from the ocean. In addition, travelers to coastal areas may return to their inland residences with *Vibrio* infections. Laboratories serving coastal areas in North America are likely to encounter *Vibrio* infections, especially during the summer months. *Vibrio* infections are more common in other areas of the world, and infections such as *Vibrio parahaemolyticus* diarrhea (Japan) and cholera (developing nations) are very important diseases. *Vibrio* species are natural inhabitants of aquatic environments, and most infections are acquired by exposure to such environments or to foods derived from them. Of the more than 30 *Vibrio* species currently recognized, 12 are known to be human pathogens; this chapter will focus on these organisms. For information on other members of the *Vibrionaceae*, the reader is referred to several excellent reviews (1, 2, 5, 28).

DESCRIPTION OF THE GENUS

Members of the genus *Vibrio* are facultatively anaerobic, asporogenous gram-negative rods that are motile by sheathed, polar flagella (unsheathed peritrichous flagella may also be produced on solid media). Vibrios require or growth is stimulated by NaCl, and they are capable of respiratory and fermentative metabolism. Of the *Vibrio* species capable of causing human infections, all except *V. metschnikovii* are oxidase positive and reduce nitrate. Growth of vibrios is inhibited by the compound O129 (2,4-diamino-6,7-diisopropylpteridine).

CLASSIFICATION

Vibrio isolates encountered in the clinical laboratory may initially resemble members of the family *Enterobacteriaceae* or *Pseudomonadaceae*, and the characteristics of these families (Table 1) may be useful for initial characterization of isolates. For clinical microbiology laboratories, isolation of a fermentative, oxidase-positive, gram-negative rod that requires NaCl for growth should prompt an investigation for *Vibrio* species.

The genus *Vibrio* is classified in the family *Vibrionaceae* along with three other genera: *Aeromonas, Photobacterium,* and *Plesiomonas* (28). *Photobacterium* organisms are not associated with human infections and are not likely to be encountered in clinical microbiology laboratories. The characteristics of *Aeromonas* and *Plesiomonas* species are presented in chapter 38; vibrios can be readily separated from these genera by biochemical tests. The NaCl requirement of many vibrios is particularly important in this regard.

Within the genus *Vibrio*, clinical laboratories can restrict their efforts to the identification of the 12 clinically significant species (Table 2). Isolates that resemble vibrios but do not fit any of the 12 species associated with human infections can be reported as marine vibrio species. Such organisms should be oxidase positive, ferment D-glucose, and require supplemental NaCl for growth in nutrient broth. They can be identified to the species level, but the identification methods required are not available in most clinical laboratories.

CLINICAL SIGNIFICANCE

Vibrio species are most widely recognized for their role in human intestinal infections, and cholera and *V. parahaemolyicus* diarrhea are important worldwide. However, vibrios also cause extraintestinal infections that range from simple wound infections to lethal septicemia; these infections are increasingly recognized. The types of human infections associated with each clinically significant *Vibrio* species are listed in Table 2 and will be discussed in more detail in the section on each species.

COLLECTION, TRANSPORT, AND STORAGE OF SPECIMENS

Extraintestinal specimens

The usual procedure for collecting and processing specimens is followed (there are no special procedures for vibrios). Pus, body fluids, or tissues rather than swabs should be submitted for culture whenever possible. When swabs must be used, they should be transported to the laboratory in suitable holding media to avoid desiccation.

Feces

Stool specimens should be collected early, preferably within the first 24 h of illness, and before the patient has received any antimicrobial agents. Fluid stool may be collected by inserting a petrolatum-lubricated soft rubber catheter into the rectum. Rectal swabs may also be used, but care must be exercised in collection of rectal swab specimens to ensure that mucus inside the rectal vault, not merely the anal surface, is sampled. Although highly efficient in the acute phase of illness, rectal swabs probably are less satisfactory for convalescent patients or transiently infected asymptomatic persons. Administration of purgatives has been reported to increase the detection of organisms in persons excreting small numbers of vibrios. Vomitus, if available, may also be collected for culture.

TABLE 1. Characteristics of the families *Enterobacteriaceae*, *Vibrionaceae*, and *Pseudomonadaceae*

Characteristic[a]	Property of family:		
	Enterobacteriaceae	*Vibrionaceae*	*Pseudomonadaceae*
Typical genus	*Escherichia*	*Vibrio*	*Pseudomonas*
Growth in the presence of oxygen	+[b]	+	+
Growth in the absence of oxygen	+	+	−[b]
Metabolism of D-glucose	Fermentation	Fermentation	Oxidation
Location of flagella	Peritrichous	Polar[c]	Polar
Oxidase production	−	+	+
Often bioluminescent	−	+	−
Na^+ required by many species	−	+	−
Inhibited by the vibriostatic compound O129	−	+[d]	−

[a] These data apply to most species in the families, but there are exceptions.
[b] Symbols (all data are for reactions within 2 days at 35 to 37°C unless otherwise specified): +, most strains (generally about 90 to 100%) positive; −, most strains negative (generally about 0 to 10% positive).
[c] Some *Vibrio* species have a sheathed polar flagellum when grown in a liquid medium but have peritrichous flagella when grown on a solid medium.
[d] Except *Aeromonas* species.

Transport

Whenever possible, stool or rectal swab specimens should be inoculated on isolation plates with minimal delay. Viability of *Vibrio* species is well maintained at the alkaline pH of rice water stool but is unpredictable in formed stools. Vibrios are very susceptible to desiccation; hence, specimens must not be allowed to dry.

When there will be a delay in plating a specimen (especially when it must be transported by courier), rectal swabs or fecal material should be placed in the semisolid transport medium of Cary and Blair, which maintains viability of *Vibrio* cultures for up to 4 weeks. Buffered glycerol-saline, often used in enteric bacteriology, is an unsatisfactory transport medium even for short periods. Tellurite-taurocholate-peptone broth has been extensively used with success as an enrichment transport medium at the Cholera Research Laboratory in Dacca, Bangladesh, where specimens collected in the field are generally plated within 12 to 24 h. In the absence of available suitable transport media, strips of blotting paper may be soaked in liquid stool and inserted into airtight plastic bags. Specimens collected in this way may remain viable for up to 5 weeks.

TABLE 2. *Vibrio* species that may be found in human clinical specimens

Species	Occurrence in human clinical specimens[a]	
	Intestinal	Extraintestinal
V. alginolyticus	+	++
V. carchariae	−	+
V. cholerae		
Serogroup O1	++++	+
Non-O1	++	++
V. cincinnatiensis	−	+
V. damsela	−	++
V. fluvialis	++	−
V. furnissii	++	−
V. hollisae	++	−
V. metschnikovii	−	+
V. mimicus	++	+
V. parahaemolyticus	++++	+
V. vulnificus	+	+++

[a] The symbols +, ++, +++, and ++++ give the relative frequency of each organism in the specimens. −, Not found.

Storage

Specimens in transport media should be shipped to the laboratory without refrigeration.

CULTURE AND ISOLATION

Extraintestinal specimens

Extraintestinal specimens are usually processed with no particular attention to vibrios. The *Vibrio* species of medical importance grow well on common plating media such as blood, chocolate, and Mueller-Hinton agars, and many also grow on MacConkey agar. However, a more thorough search for *Vibrio* isolates can be done with oxidase testing (see below) or by including a plate of thiosulfate-citrate-bile salts-sucrose (TCBS) medium.

Stool specimens

Stool specimens are usually plated on a variety of selective-differential and nonselective media (see discussion of specimen processing in chapter 27). *Vibrio*

TABLE 3. Growth and appearance of *Vibrio* species on TCBS agar

Organism	Colony appearance on TCBS (%)[a]		Growth-plating efficiency
	Green	Yellow	
V. cholerae	0	100	Good
V. mimicus	100	0	Good
V. metschnikovii	0	100	May be reduced
V. hollisae	100	0	Very poor
V. damsela	95	5	Reduced at 36°C
V. fluvialis	0	100	Good
V. furnissii	0	100	Good
V. alginolyticus	0	100	Good
V. parahaemolyticus	99	1	Good
V. vulnificus	90[b]	10[b]	Good
V. carchariae	0	100	Good
V. cincinnatiensis	0	100	Very poor
Marine vibrios	Variable	Variable	Variable

[a] Percentage of strains that produce colonies of the given color.
[b] The original report describing this species gave the percentage positive for sucrose fermentation as 3%. At the CDC *Vibrio* Laboratory, about 15% of the strains have been sucrose positive.

TABLE 4. Biochemical and other characteristics of the 12 *Vibrio* species that are found in human clinical specimens

Test[a]	% Positive[b] for:											
	V. cholerae	*V. mimicus*	*V. metschnikovii*	*V. cincinnatiensis*	*V. hollisae*	*V. damsela*	*V. fluvialis*	*V. furnissii*	*V. alginolyticus*	*V. parahaemolyticus*	*V. vulnificus*	*V. carchariae*
*Indole production (HIB, 1% NaCl)	99	98	20	8	97	0	13	11	85	98	97	100
Methyl red (1% NaCl)	99	99	96	93	0	100	96	100	75	80	80	100
*Voges-Proskauer (1% NaCl, Barritt)	75	9	96	0	0	95	0	0	95	0	0	50
Citrate, Simmons	97	99	75	21	0	0	93	100	1	3	75	0
H_2S on TSI	0	0	0	0	0	0	0	0	0	0	0	0
Urea hydrolysis	0	1	0	0	0	0	0	0	0	15	1	0
Phenylalanine deaminase	0	0	0	0	0	0	0	0	1	1	35	NG
*Arginine, Moeller (1% NaCl)	0	0	60	0	0	95	93	100	0	0	0	0
*Lysine, Moeller (1% NaCl)	99	100	35	57	0	50	0	0	99	100	99	100
*Ornithine, Moeller (1% NaCl)	99	99	0	0	0	0	0	0	50	95	55	0
Motility (36°C)	99	98	74	86	0	25	70	89	99	99	99	0
Gelatin hydrolysis (1% NaCl, 22°C)	90	65	65	0	0	6	85	86	90	95	75	0
KCN test (% that grow)	10	2	0	0	0	5	65	89	15	20	1	0
Malonate utilization	1	0	0	0	0	0	0	11	0	0	0	0
*D-Glucose, acid production	100	100	100	100	100	100	100	100	100	100	100	50
*D-Glucose, gas production	0	0	0	0	0	10	0	100	0	0	0	0
Acid production from:												
D-Adonitol	0	0	0	0	0	0	0	0	1	0	0	0
*L-Arabinose	0	1	0	100	97	0	93	100	1	80	0	0
*D-Arabitol	0	0	0	0	0	0	65	89	0	0	0	0
*Cellobiose	8	0	9	100	0	0	30	11	3	5	99	50
Dulcitol	0	0	0	0	0	0	0	0	0	3	0	0
Erythritol	0	0	0	0	0	0	0	0	0	0	0	0
D-Galactose	90	82	45	100	100	90	96	100	20	92	96	0
Glycerol	30	13	100	100	0	0	7	55	80	50	1	0
myo-Inositol	0	0	40	100	0	0	0	0	0	0	0	0
*Lactose	7	21	50	0	0	0	3	0	0	1	85	0
*Maltose	99	99	100	100	0	100	100	100	100	99	100	100
*D-Mannitol	99	99	96	100	0	0	97	100	100	100	45	50

Test												
D-Mannose	78	99	100	100	100	100	100	100	99	100	98	50
Melibiose	1	0	0	7	0	0	3	11	1	1	40	0
α-Methyl-D-glucoside	0	0	25	57	0	5	0	0	1	0	0	0
Raffinose	0	0	0	0	0	0	0	11	0	0	0	0
L-Rhamnose	0	0	0	0	0	0	0	45	0	1	0	0
*Salicin	1	0	9	100	0	0	0	0	4	1	95	0
D-Sorbitol	1	0	45	0	0	0	3	0	1	1	0	0
*Sucrose	100	0	100	100	0	5	100	100	99	1	15	50
Trehalose	99	94	100	100	0	86	100	100	100	99	100	50
D-Xylose	0	0	0	43	0	0	0	0	0	0	0	0
Mucate, acid production	1	0	0	0	0	0	0	0	0	0	0	0
Tartrate, Jordan	75	12	35	0	65	0	35	22	95	93	84	50
Esculin hydrolysis	0	0	60	0	0	0	8	0	3	1	40	0
Acetate utilization	92	78	25	14	0	0	70	65	0	1	7	0
*Nitrate → nitrite	99	100	0	100	100	100	100	100	100	100	100	100
*Oxidase	100	100	0	100	100	95	100	100	100	100	100	100
DNase, 25°C	93	55	50	79	0	75	100	100	95	92	50	100
*Lipase (corn oil)	92	17	100	36	0	0	90	89	85	90	92	0
*ONPG test	94	90	50	86	0	0	40	35	0	5	75	0
Yellow pigment at 25°C	0	0	0	0	0	0	0	0	0	0	0	0
Tyrosine clearing	13	30	5	0	3	0	65	45	70	77	75	0
Growth in nutrient broth with:												
*0% NaCl	100	100	0	0	0	0	0	0	0	0	0	0
*1% NaCl	100	100	100	100	99	100	99	99	99	100	99	100
6% NaCl	53	49	78	100	83	95	96	100	100	99	65	100
*8% NaCl	1	0	44	62	0	0	71	78	94	80	0	0
*10% NaCl	0	0	4	0	0	0	4	0	69	2	0	0
12% NaCl	0	0	0	0	0	0	0	0	17	1	0	0
Swarming (marine agar, 25°C)	–	–	–	+	–	–	–	–	+	+	–	100
String test	100	100	100	80	100	80	100	100	91	64	100	100
O129, zone of inhibition[c]	99	95	90	25	40	90	31	0	19	20	98	100
Polymyxin B, zone of inhibition	22	88	100	92	100	85	100	89	63	54	3	100

[a] *, Test is recommended as part of the routine set for *Vibrio* identification; HIB, heart infusion broth; 1% NaCl, 1% NaCl has been added to the standard medium to enhance growth; TSI, triple sugar iron agar.

[b] After 48 h of incubation at 36°C (unless other conditions are indicated). Most of the positive reactions occur during the first 24 h. NG, No growth (probably because NaCl concentration is too low); – and +, see Table 1, footnote *b*.

[c] Disk potency, 150 μg.

species do not grow well on many selective-differential plating media but do grow on blood agar, and most grow on MacConkey or sorbitol-MacConkey agar if they are incorporated into the plating battery. On blood agar, *Vibrio* colonies may be beta-, alpha-, or nonhemolytic, and on MacConkey agar they are lactose negative (with the possible exception of *Vibrio vulnificus*). Colonies growing on blood agar and lactose-negative colonies growing on MacConkey agar or other media can be tested for oxidase. However, lactose-positive colonies from selective-differential media may give false-negative oxidase reactions.

Reliance on blood or MacConkey agar for detection of vibrios may be sufficient for many laboratories in inland locations where vibrios are seldom encountered. In coastal regions, in areas where *Vibrio* infections are endemic, or when *Vibrio* infection is suspected, addition of a TCBS plate to the routine battery may be indicated. TCBS agar is a selective-differential plating medium that may enhance the recovery of *Vibrio* species. *Vibrio* species produce yellow or green colonies on this medium, which aids in their recognition (Table 3). However, routine use of TCBS is probably not cost effective for most laboratories. There is considerable lot-to-lot variation in performance of the medium for isolation of organisms such as *V. parahaemolyticus;* therefore, the medium should be quality controlled with known *Vibrio* strains when it is used. In addition, TCBS is not reliable for isolation of all clinically significant *Vibrio* species (Table 3). In North America, most cases of *Vibrio* diarrhea are seasonal, and a reasonable compromise for laboratories serving coastal areas may be to use a TCBS plate during the summer months on a trial basis for two seasons. Continued use of the medium could be based on the yield of organisms obtained during the trial period. Another method recommended by some authors for increasing the yield of vibrios from stool specimens is enrichment in alkaline peptone water incubated for 5 to 8 h (12, 32). The surface of the enrichment broth is then subcultured to TCBS agar. Use of this method may be indicated for areas where *Vibrio* infections are endemic but probably not for most laboratories in North America.

Screening for vibrios by oxidase testing

Since *Vibrio* species likely to be encountered in clinical specimens are oxidase positive, oxidase testing of colonies growing on blood agar is an alternative method for the detection of these organisms. Two different approaches to the detection of vibrios by oxidase testing have been used. One involves spot testing of suspect colonies on filter paper saturated with Kovacs reagent. The second involves placing a drop of Kovacs reagent on an area of the blood agar plate where the colonies are crowded but still separated. A recent comparison of these two methods in the laboratory of one of us (M.T.K.) indicated that the filter paper test is 15 to 20% more sensitive for detection of oxidase-positive colonies than the plate oxidase test. Oxidase-positive colonies detected by either method can be subcultured and identified as possible *Vibrio* species.

CHARACTERIZATION

Microscopic examination

Although rice water stool from patients with cholera often reveals curved gram-negative bacilli typical of vibrios, the morphology of the organisms is sufficiently variable that direct examination of stool specimens is not recommended. Gram-stained smears of broth cultures inoculated with clinical specimens containing *Vibrio* species (e.g., blood cultures) often reveal pleomorphic gram-negative bacilli, including typical curved forms as well as straight rods and large bulbous elements. *Vibrio* species should not be ruled out on the basis of microscopic morphology.

Biochemical identification

Vibrio species vary considerably in pathogenicity and epidemiological significance. Therefore, clinical *Vibrio* isolates should be identified to species, and biochemical testing is required for such identification. Classical biochemical tests commonly available for the *Enterobacteriaceae* work well for *Vibrio cholerae* and *V. mimicus* because they have only a slight requirement for Na^+, which is fulfilled by the amount of NaCl in the media. However, most of the halophilic *Vibrio* species require much more Na^+ for growth, and supplementation of biochemical test media with 1% NaCl is recommended (10). In addition, more *Vibrio* species are indole positive when heart infusion broth rather than peptone water is used. More strains are Voges-Proskauer positive when the reagent for detecting acetylmethylcarbinol contains α-naphthol. Table 4 gives the biochemical reactions for 12 *Vibrio* species that occur in clinical specimens. The vast majority of *Vibrio* cultures isolated from clinical specimens are easily identified as one of the species listed.

Vibrio species can be divided into six groups on the basis of requirement for Na^+, oxidase production, reduction of nitrate to nitrite, *myo*-inositol fermentation, and production of arginine dihydrolase, lysine decarboxylase, and ornithine decarboxylase (Table 5). Grouping of isolates in this way is a useful initial step in identification of *Vibrio* species. Additional biochemical tests are needed to differentiate the vibrios in the six groups (see below).

Commercial identification systems

Some commercially available systems intended for identification of gram-negative bacilli can be used for *Vibrio* identification provided that NaCl-supplemented solutions are used for preparing organism suspensions. One problem has been that some of these products confuse the identification of *Aeromonas* species with *Vibrio fluvialis*. These organisms can easily be differentiated with one additional test: *V. fluvialis* is a halophilic vibrio and does not grow in nutrient broth without added NaCl, but *Aeromonas* isolates grow in this medium. In summary, the kits have improved in their ability to identify *Vibrio* species, but misidentifications are still a problem. One of us (M.T.K.) with experience with several kits prefers conventional tube tests for *Vibrio* identification.

ANTIBIOTIC SUSCEPTIBILITY

Mueller-Hinton agar and broth contain sufficient salt to support the growth of *Vibrio* species likely to be encountered in clinical specimens, and standardized disk diffusion or dilution susceptibility testing methods can be applied to *Vibrio* isolates. The antimicrobial susceptibility of vibrios is variable, and testing of clinical isolates is indicated. Table 6 presents the susceptibility

TABLE 5. Eight key differential tests to divide the 12 clinically significant *Vibrio* species into six groups

Test	Reactions of the species in[a]:											
	Group 1		Group 2	Group 3	Group 4	Group 5			Group 6			
	V. cholerae	*V. mimicus*	*V. metschnikovii*	*V. cincinnatiensis*	*V. hollisae*	*V. damsela*	*V. fluvialis*	*V. furnissii*	*V. alginolyticus*	*V. parahaemolyticus*	*V. vulnificus*	*V. carchariae*
Growth in nutrient broth:												
With no NaCl added	+	+	−	−	−	−	−	−	−	−	−	−
With 1% NaCl added	+	+	+	+	+	+	+	+	+	+	+	+
Oxidase			−	+	+	+	+	+	+	+	+	+
Nitrate → nitrite			−	+	+	+	+	+	+	+	+	+
myo-Inositol fermentation	−	−	−	+	−	−	−	−	−	−	−	−
Arginine dihydrolase					−	+	+	+	−	−	−	−
Lysine decarboxylase					−				+	+	+	+
Ornithine decarboxylase					−							

[a] For symbols, see Table 1, footnote *b*. Key test results are boxed.

TABLE 6. Antibiotic susceptibility (disk diffusion method) of 1,025 strains of the clinically significant *Vibrio* species

Antibiotic	% of strains susceptible (no. of strains studied)[a]:											
	V. cholerae (480)	*V. mimicus* (75)	*V. metschnikovii* (22)	*V. cincinnatiensis* (14)	*V. hollisae* (34)	*V. damsela* (21)	*V. fluvialis* (25)	*V. furnissii* (9)	*V. alginolyticus* (69)	*V. parahaemolvticus* (144)	*V. vulnificus* (130)	*V. carchariae* (2)
Penicillin G (12–21)[b]	2	3	9	0	97	0	0	0	0	0	2	0
Ampicillin (12–13)	87	97	31	36	100	52	32	11	0	12	99	0
Carbenicillin (18–22)	64	8	27	7	100	14	16	0	0	1	54	0
Cephalothin (15–17)	98	100	100	100	100	76	40	0	32	17	65	100
Colistin (9–10)	4	61	91	93	100	76	100	100	25	11	2	0
Tetracycline (15–18)	98	100	73	93	97	86	88	89	94	98	99	100
Sulfadiazine (13–16)	26	17	5	36	56	71	36	11	16	3	28	50
Chloramphenicol (13–17)	99	100	100	100	100	10	88	100	100	100	100	100
Streptomycin (12–14)	60	61	32	86	100	24	84	100	54	17	42	50
Kanamycin (14–17)	92	89	14	79	100	43	88	100	62	37	53	100
Gentamicin (13–14)	98	99	100	100	100	100	100	100	100	97	100	100
Nalidixic acid (14–18)	99	99	100	100	100	100	100	100	97	99	99	100

[a] Studied at the CDC *Vibrio* Laboratory and done on Mueller-Hinton agar (with no added NaCl) at 35 to 37°C.

[b] Numbers give the zone size range for the category "intermediate." For example, (12–21) means that resistant strains have 6- to 11-mm zones, strains of intermediate susceptibility have zones that are 12 to 21 mm, and susceptible strains have zones of 22 mm or larger. These particular breakpoints are the ones established in the early 1970s for each antibiotic and have been used in our laboratory for over 15 years for taxonomic studies. They may differ slightly from current breakpoints.

patterns of *Vibrio* species referred to the Centers for Disease Control (CDC). We and others have found that most *Vibrio* isolates are also susceptible to trimethoprim-sulfamethoxazole and norfloxacin (25). Such information on the antimicrobial susceptibility profiles of vibrios can be used for initial selection of antimicrobial therapy while one is awaiting the results of susceptibility testing. In most cases, antimicrobial resistance of vibrios is probably intrinsic to the species rather than acquired through plasmid transfer or through antibiotic exposure. The one exception to this generalization is the antibiotic resistance found in some outbreaks of infections caused by *V. cholerae* strains that have become resistant through the acquisition of R factors. In the United States, strains of *V. cholerae* and other *Vibrio* species have rarely had this type of resistance. Resistance to polymyxin antibiotics (polymyxin B or colistin) can be useful in detecting a culture of the eltor biogroup of *V. cholerae* or in detecting a culture of *V. vulnificus*. Most other *Vibrio* species are more susceptible.

VIBRIO CHOLERAE

V. cholerae, the causative agent of cholera, was discovered by Robert Koch in 1884. Cholera has probably always existed in India, and spread of the disease outside of India in the form of pandemics has been known since at least 1816. Seven cholera pandemics have occurred in recorded history, and the seventh is still ongoing (19). Spread of cholera is mainly via contaminated water. Diagnosis of cholera is based primarily on isolation of the organism from stool specimens, although demonstration of a rising agglutinating, vibriocidal, or antitoxin titer in serum samples is also effective for retrospective diagnosis (11).

Identification

The key characteristics of *V. cholerae* are listed in Table 7. *V. cholerae* and *V. mimicus* are distinguished from other vibrios by growth in nutrient broth without added NaCl, and both are arginine dihydrolase negative but lysine and ornithine decarboxylase positive. Sucrose fermentation is the key characteristic for separating *V. cholerae* from *V. mimicus*. *V. cholerae* strains fall into two groups on the basis of serotyping. O group 1 strains (O1) are associated with epidemic cholera; non-O1 strains may cause choleralike and other illnesses (15, 26), but they are not involved in epidemics. *V. cholerae* O1 strains are divided into two or three subtypes (Table 7). *V. cholerae* O1 strains are further divided into two biogroups, classical and eltor (Table 8). Serotyping schemes are also available for non-O1 *V. cholerae*, but they are generally not applicable in clinical laboratories.

Because of the clinical and epidemiological importance of cholera, it is critical to determine as quickly as possible whether a *Vibrio*-like isolate from a patient with watery diarrhea is *V. cholerae*. Yellow colonies from TCBS agar or suspicious colonies from other media should be subcultured by heavy inoculation to blood or other nonselective media. After 5 to 8 h, good growth should be present, which can be used for oxidase testing and for agglutination in polyvalent antisera to *V. cholerae* serogroup O1 (9). Oxidase-positive organisms that agglutinate in the antisera can be reported presumptively as *V. cholerae* O1 to the requesting physician and public health authorities. The isolate should be forwarded to a public health reference laboratory for confirmatory biochemical and serological testing.

Significance

Isolation of *V. cholerae* O1 from human feces is always significant clinically or epidemiologically. Clinically, cholera may range from asymptomatic colonization to severe, life-threatening diarrhea. Many patients have mild diarrhea lasting 1 to 5 days, followed by spontaneous recovery without specific therapy. On the other extreme, patients may experience severe diarrhea with massive fluid loss, leading to dehydration, electrolyte disturbances, and death. *V. cholerae* causes this secretory diarrhea by colonization of the small intestine and production of a potent enterotoxin (cholera toxin). Each cholera toxin molecule is composed of five B subunits and one A subunit, and the A subunit has A1 and A2 components. The toxin binds to enterocytes via its five B subunits, the A2 subunit facilitates penetration of the cell, and the A1 subunit increases the level of cyclic AMP, which results in net secretion of fluid and electrolytes (19).

Cholera is often thought of as a severe life-threatening illness occurring in developing nations of the Indian subcontinent and the Middle East. However, the eltor

TABLE 7. Subtypes of *V. cholerae* serogroup O1

Serogroup O1 subtype	O factors present in culture	Agglutination in absorbed serum[a]:	
		Ogawa	Inaba
Ogawa	A, B	+	–
Inaba	A, C	–	+
Hikojima[b]	A, B, C	+	+

[a] The specific factor sera are prepared by absorption. For example, an Ogawa antiserum is prepared by injecting an Ogawa culture and then absorbing the resulting antiserum with an Inaba culture, which removes the antibodies to O-antigen factor A, leaving antibodies to O-factor B.

[b] Some authorities do not recognize subtype Hikojima and report cultures as Inaba or Ogawa, depending on which serum causes the first and strongest agglutination.

TABLE 8. Characteristics and differentiation of the classical and eltor biogroups of *V. cholerae* serogroup O1

Test or property	Biogroup[a]	
	Classical	Eltor
Isolated on the Indian subcontinent	Occasional[b]	Common
Isolated in the rest of the world	Very rare	Common
Differential tests		
Hemolysis of erythrocytes	–	+
Voges-Proskauer	–	+
Inhibition by polymyxin B (50-U disk)	+	–
Agglutination of chicken erythrocytes	–	+
Lysis by bacteriophage:		
classical IV	+	–
FK	+	–
Eltor 5	–	+

[a] For symbols, see Table 1, footnote *b*.

[b] The classical biotype reappeared several years ago on the Indian subcontinent and is being found in certain locations but not in others.

biogroup of *V. cholerae* O1 is currently predominant; with this biogroup, the milder form of illness is seven times more common than severe cholera. Also, in 1988, the World Health Organization reported 44,120 cases of cholera from 30 countries, reflecting the widespread nature of the current pandemic. An endemic focus of cholera has even been identified in the Gulf Coast region of the United States (3, 20) in association with a *V. cholerae* O1, eltor, Inaba strain that is distinct from the current pandemic strain.

Isolation of non-O1 *V. cholerae* from stool specimens is often significant, and the organism can cause diarrhea that is often related to consumption of raw shellfish (26). Non-O1 *V. cholerae* strains occasionally produce cholera toxin, and such isolates cause diarrhea that is clinically indistinguishable from cholera (20). Some strains may be associated with a milder form of secretory diarrhea, and others may cause invasive diarrhea with blood and mucus in the stool. Extraintestinal infections are also associated with non-O1 *V. cholerae;* we have isolated the organism, or isolates have been referred to us, from blood, wound, ear, respiratory tract, and other specimens. Non-O1 *V. cholerae* is commonly found in aquatic environments, and most infections due to the organism are apparently of environmental origin.

VIBRIO MIMICUS

V. mimicus is a relatively new species that was originally recognized as a sucrose-negative variant of *V. cholerae*. However, DNA hybridization studies revealed that these sucrose-negative variants were only 24 to 54% related to *V. cholerae*, and a new species was proposed (8). *V. mimicus* is associated with gastroenteritis, usually after consumption of seafood, especially raw oysters. The organism appears to have worldwide distribution, and its ecology may be similar to that of non-O1 *V. cholerae*.

Identification

V. mimicus does not require supplemental NaCl for growth and is otherwise phenotypically similar to *V. cholerae* except that it does not ferment sucrose. As a result of this characteristic, *V. mimicus* produces green colonies on TCBS agar (Table 3). Most strains are also Voges-Proskauer negative, whereas 95% of *V. cholerae* isolates are positive. In addition, 95% of *V. cholerae* isolates but only 10% of *V. mimicus* isolates are lipase positive. Serological identification is not required for *V. mimicus*.

Significance

V. mimicus has been associated with diarrhea and ear infections, although it appears to be a less common cause of infection than are other *Vibrio* species (30). Isolation of *V. mimicus* from a symptomatic patient should be regarded as potentially significant. Isolates from patients with diarrhea often are negative in assays for pathogenicity, but some strains have been found to produce heat-labile or heat-stable enterotoxins. Isolates of *V. mimicus* have antimicrobial susceptibility patterns similar to those of *V. cholerae*, but the role of antimicrobial therapy in *V. mimicus* infections is unclear.

VIBRIO PARAHAEMOLYTICUS

V. parahaemolyticus has been known as a cause of acute gastroenteritis since 1950, when a large outbreak of food poisoning in Japan led to the discovery of the organism. Food-borne outbreaks and sporadic cases occur worldwide and are usually associated with the consumption of contaminated seafood (18). The organism is a natural inhabitant of temperate marine environments around the world, and it is a well-recognized cause of seafood-related gastroenteritis worldwide. Although *V. parahaemolyticus* is an unusual cause of diarrhea in North America, it is a common cause of food-borne gastroenteritis in other countries (e.g., Japan) (18,29).

Isolation and identification

The fact that *V. parahaemolyticus* was not detected as a significant cause of diarrhea until 1950 emphasizes the unreliability of routine enteric plating media for detection of this organism. Use of TCBS agar or blood agar screened with oxidase may increase the yield of *V. parahaemolyticus* isolates from stool specimens. The organism produces green colonies on TCBS agar and nonhemolytic colonies on sheep blood agar.

V. parahaemolyticus is halophilic and a member of the lysine decarboxylase-positive, arginine dihydrolase-negative group (Table 5). It is distinguished from the other members of the group by negative reactions for sucrose, salicin, and cellobiose fermentation (Table 9). In addition, most *V. parahaemolyticus* isolates are positive for arabinose fermentation.

Significance

V. parahaemolyticus causes gastroenteritis with nausea, vomiting, abdominal cramps, low-grade fever, and chills. The diarrhea is usually watery but sometimes bloody. Most cases are mild and self-limiting, but severe or even fatal illness may also occur. Sporadic cases as well as outbreaks of *V. parahaemolyticus* diarrhea occur, and one of us has encountered 20 such cases over the past 5 years in the Pacific Northwest (21, 22). Outbreaks of *V. parahaemolyticus* diarrhea may be directly or indirectly associated with seafood. Direct infection results from ingestion of raw seafood contaminated with *V. parahaemolyticus*, and indirect infection results from ingestion of cooked foods that are subsequently contaminated with the organism. The latter mechanism accounts for large outbreaks that have occurred on cruise ships. Treatment of the milder forms of *V. parahaemolyticus* diarrhea requires only supportive care, but antimicrobial therapy may be beneficial in more severe or prolonged infections. Tetracycline appears to be the drug of choice for treatment of such infections.

V. parahaemolyticus also causes extraintestinal infections. Wound, ear, and eye infections may occur, and one of us has encountered eight such infections over a 5-year period in the Pacific Northwest (21, 22). All of the infections were acquired after exposure to marine environments harboring the organism, and all responded promptly to local therapy or antibiotics. *V. parahaemolyticus* has also been reported as a cause of severe, life-threatening infections, but subsequent examination of the isolates from these cases has indicated that they were actually *V. vulnificus*.

TABLE 9. Differentiation of the arginine dihydrolase-negative, lysine decarboxylase-positive *Vibrio* species

Test or property	Reaction[a]			
	V. alginolyticus	*V. parahaemolyticus*	*V. vulnificus*	*V. carchariae*
Voges-Proskauer	+	−	−	−
Growth in nutrient broth with:				
8% NaCl	+	(+)	−	−
10% NaCl	v	−	−	−
Fermentation of:				
Sucrose	+	−	(−)	+
Salicin	−	−	+	−
Cellobiose	−	−	+	−
Lactose	−	−	(+)	−
L-Arabinose	−	(+)	−	−
Swarming (marine agar, 25°C)	+	+	−	+
Zone of inhibition around:				
Colistin	Large	Large	Small	Small
Ampicillin	Small	Small	Large	Small
Carbenicillin	Small	Small	Large	Small

[a] + and −, See Table 1, footnote *b*; (+), many strains (generally about 75 to 90%) positive; v, strain-to-strain variation (generally about 25 to 75% positive); (−), many strains negative (generally about 10 to 25% positive).

A positive Kanagawa test, which detects lysis of human erythrocytes in a special medium (Wagatsuma agar), has been associated with the pathogenic potential of *V. parahaemolyticus* (29). This association is based on the observation that most clinical isolates of the organism are Kanagawa positive, whereas only 1% of environmental isolates are positive. However, the role of the Kanagawa hemolysin in pathogenesis has not been proven. Recent studies indicate that Kanagawa-negative strains can cause significant infections, and one study found that isolates from intestinal as well as extraintestinal infections in the Pacific Northwest were all Kanagawa negative, whereas isolates from patients with traveler's diarrhea were Kanagawa positive (22).

Until recently, *V. parahaemolyticus* isolates were considered to be urease negative. However, during the past 10 years, urease-positive but otherwise typical *V. parahaemolyticus* isolates have been increasingly recognized. At present, more than 50% of clinical isolates from the Pacific Coast of North America are urease positive. In the study cited above (22), extraintestinal isolates and traveler's diarrhea isolates were urease negative, whereas isolates from locally acquired intestinal infections were urease positive. It appears that Kanagawa-negative, urease-positive isolates may be emerging as the predominant strains of *V. parahaemolyticus* associated with diarrhea on the Pacific Coast of North America. Laboratories using a positive urease test to screen out potential enteric pathogens from stool cultures should exercise care so as not to miss urease-positive *V. parahaemolyticus.*

VIBRIO VULNIFICUS

V. vulnificus has been recognized as a species since 1976, when its association with virulent infections was noted (14). The organism was referred to previously as "lactose positive," "Lac$^+$," or "L$^+$" vibrio.

Isolation and identification

V. vulnificus can be recovered from blood or wound specimens, and it may rarely be recovered from other body sites as well. The organism grows well on blood and MacConkey agar, and it grows readily in blood culture broths.

V. vulnificus is a halophilic species that is lysine decarboxylase positive and arginine dihydrolase negative and is therefore in the same group as *V. parahaemolyticus* (Tables 5 and 9). It is differentiated from other organisms in the group by fermentation of salicin and cellobiose (Table 9). Most strains of *V. vulnificus* are also α-nitrophenyl-β-D-galactopyranoside (ONPG) positive and ferment lactose, whereas other organisms in the group yield mostly negative results in these tests. The disk diffusion antibiogram is also useful for differentiating *V. vulnificus* from other members of the lysine decarboxylase-positive, arginine dihydrolase-negative group. *V. vulnificus* is resistant to colistin but susceptible to ampicillin and carbenicillin (Table 9).

Significance

V. vulnificus is found in marine environments on the Gulf, Atlantic, and Pacific coasts of North America, and it has been associated with two categories of infection, primary septicemia and wound infections (4). Primary septicemia is a rapidly progressive and highly fatal (50% mortality rate) bloodstream infection that occurs most often in persons with preexisting liver disease and may be associated with the development of bullous skin lesions. The infection is often associated with consumption of raw oysters. *V. vulnificus* wound infections occur after exposure to marine environments. Although these infections have a lower mortality rate than does primary septicemia, they can progress rapidly, with the development of swelling and erythema followed by the appearance of bullae or vesicles and necrosis. The organism may rarely be associated with other infections, including pneumonia, endometritis, and diarrhea.

VIBRIO ALGINOLYTICUS

V. alginolyticus is a halophilic species in the lysine decarboxylase-positive, arginine dihydrolase-negative group of vibrios (Table 5). The organism is very common in the marine environment; it occasionally causes extraintestinal infections in humans exposed to such environments.

Identification

Characteristics useful in differentiating *V. alginolyticus* from related halophilic vibrios are shown in Table 9. *V. alginolyticus* is more halotolerant than other members of the group; all isolates grow in 8% NaCl, and most grow in 10% NaCl. *V. alginolyticus* is also Voges-Proskauer positive. In addition, *V. alginolyticus* ferments sucrose but not arabinose, lactose, salicin, or cellobiose.

Significance

V. alginolyticus has not been associated with diarrhea, but it is an often reported cause of soft tissue infections. Wound, ear, and eye infections have been reported most often, but we have also isolated the organism from sputum and burn infections. Most clinical isolates of *V. alginolyticus* come from infected wounds exposed to the marine environment.

VIBRIO CARCHARIAE

V. carchariae is the most recently recognized human pathogen in the genus *Vibrio*. This organism is a pathogen of sharks that has recently been isolated from human extraintestinal infections (27).

Identification

V. carchariae is a member of the halophilic, arginine dihydrolase-negative, lysine decarboxylase-positive *Vibrio* group (Tables 5 and 9). It ferments sucrose but not salicin, cellobiose, lactose, or arabinose (Table 6). *V. carchariae* is distinguished from *V. alginolyticus* by its lower salt tolerance and resistance to colistin.

Significance

V. carchariae causes lethal infections in sharks, but it was only recently recognized as a human pathogen. The organism was isolated from a leg wound resulting from a shark bite that occurred off the South Carolina coast. The isolate was resistant to ampicillin and carbenicillin but susceptible to cephalothin, and the wound healed after treatment with cephradine. This case suggests that *V. carchariae* may be a human pathogen, but additional experience with the organism will be required to assess its importance.

VIBRIO DAMSELA, VIBRIO FLUVIALIS, AND *VIBRIO FURNISSII*

V. damsela, V. fluvialis, and *V. furnissii* are recently recognized halophilic *Vibrio* species that have occasionally been reported in association with human infections. These organisms are natural inhabitants of marine environments. Our recent studies in the Pacific Northwest indicate that the three organisms may be isolated from marine environments and shellfish, but *V. fluvialis* is much more common than the others.

Identification

V. damsela, V. fluvialis, and *V. furnissii* comprise the arginine dihydrolase-positive group of vibrios (Table 5). *V. damsela* is differentiated from the other species in the group by a positive Voges-Proskauer reaction, negative citrate test, and negative tests for sucrose, mannitol, and arabinose fermentation (Table 10). *V. fluvialis* and *V. furnissii* have very similar biochemical reactions, but tests for gas production, esculin hydrolysis, and carbon source utilization can be used to differentiate them (Table 11) (7). Of greater importance is differentiation of these organisms from *Aeromonas* species. This can be done simply by performing a test for salt requirements; *V. fluvialis* and *V. furnissii* require supplemental NaCl for growth, whereas *Aeromonas* does not (Table 10).

Significance

V. fluvialis has been associated with sporadic cases of diarrhea worldwide (16, 23), and it may also be capable of causing outbreaks of diarrhea (31). The diarrhea is usually watery and may be associated with vomiting, abdominal pain, and occasionally severe dehydration. *V. furnissii* has also been isolated from patients with diarrhea, but the role of the organism as an enteric pathogen has not been firmly established (7). *V. damsela* has been isolated from wound infections in patients exposed to marine environments, but such infections appear to be rare (24).

TABLE 10. Differentiation of the arginine dihydrolase-positive *Vibrio* species and comparison with *Aeromonas* species

Test or property	Reaction[a]			
	V. damsela	*V. fluvialis*	*V. furnissii*	*Aeromonas* spp.
Growth in nutrient broth with:				
No added NaCl	−	−	−	+
1% NaCl	+	+	+	+
Voges-Proskauer	+	−	−	v
Citrate, Simmons	−	+	+	v
Fermentation of:				
D-Galacturonic acid	−	+	+	−
L-Arabinose	−	+	+	v
D-Mannitol	−	+	+	+
Sucrose	−	+	+	(+)
Gas production during fermentation	v	−	+	v

[a] See Table 9, footnote *a*.

TABLE 11. Differentiation of *V. fluvialis* and *V. furnissii*

Test or property	Reaction[a]	
	V. fluvialis	*V. furnissii*
Simple tests		
Gas production during fermentation	0	99
Esculin hydrolysis	12	0
Carbon source utilization,[b] growth on:		
Citrulline	97	4
D-Glucuronic acid	94	7
Putrescine	31	100
δ-Aminovalerate	0	63
Cellobiose	63	4
Glutaric acid	−	+

[a] Percent positive after 48 h of incubation at 35 to 37°C (unless other conditions are indicated). Most of the positive reactions occur during the first 24 h. − and +, See Table 1, footnote *b*.

[b] Data are from Lee et al. (23) except those for glutaric acid, which are from Baumann and Schubert (2). These carbon source utilization tests are usually done in research laboratories rather than in public health or clinical laboratories.

VIBRIO CINCINNATIENSIS, VIBRIO HOLLISAE, AND *VIBRIO METSCHNIKOVII*

V. cincinnatiensis, V. hollisae, and *V. metschnikovii* are halophilic vibrios that do not fall into the other major *Vibrio* groups on the basis of biochemical reactions (Table 5). *V. metschnikovii* has been recognized since 1884 (17), but *V. cincinnatiensis* and *V. hollisae* are recently named *Vibrio* species.

Identification

V. cincinnatiensis is distinguished from other clinically significant vibrios by its ability to ferment *myo*-inositol (Table 5). It also is oxidase and nitrate positive, sensitive to O129, and lysine decarboxylase positive but arginine dihydrolase negative (6). The organism ferments salicin, sucrose, mannose, arabinose, and arbutin but not indole, ornithine, or lactose; it does not produce gelatinase or urease. The distinctive feature of *V. hollisae* is a pattern of negative reactions for lysine and ornithine decarboxylases and arginine dihydrolase (Table 5). *V. metschnikovii* is the only clinically significant *Vibrio* that is oxidase and nitrate reductase negative (Table 5).

Significance

V. cincinnatiensis was initially reported as an isolate from the blood and spinal fluid of a patient in Cincinnati (6). Five other human clinical isolates have been identified in the CDC culture collection. Therefore, it appears that the organism can cause human infections, but such infections are very rare. Recognition of these organisms in clinical laboratories will help to clarify the role of *V. cincinnatiensis* as a human pathogen. *V. hollisae* is clearly a cause of diarrhea in humans (13), but these infections appear to be rare, and only 30 isolates have been referred to the CDC. However, increased awareness of the organism may reveal that *V. hollisae* infections are more common than currently recognized. *V. metschnikovii* has been recovered from blood, urine, and other human sources (17), but only seven isolates have been referred to the CDC. It appears that the organism may be able to cause human infections, but they occur very rarely.

We thank Betty Davis and other members of the CDC Enteric Reference Laboratories who did some of the biochemical testing and antibiograms included in the tables. We also thank numerous investigators and laboratories who sent interesting *Vibrio* cultures for identification.

LITERATURE CITED

1. **Baumann, P., A. L. Furniss, and J. V. Lee.** 1984. Genus I. *Vibrio* Pacini 1854, 411[AL], p. 518–538. *In* N. R. Krieg and J. G. Holt (ed.), Bergey's manual of systematic bacteriology, vol. 1. The Williams & Wilkins Co., Baltimore.
2. **Baumann, P., and R. H. W. Schubert.** 1984. Family II. *Vibrionaceae* Vernon 1965, 5245[AL], p. 516–517. *In* N. R. Krieg and J. G. Holt (ed.), Bergey's manual of systematic bacteriology, vol. 1. The Williams & Wilkins Co., Baltimore.
3. **Blake, P. A.** 1981. New information on the epidemiology of *Vibrio* infections, p. 107–117. *In* T. Holme, J. Holmgren, M. H. Merson, and R. Mollby (ed.), Acute enteric infections in children. New prospects for treatment and prevention. Elsevier-North Holland Biomedical Press, Amsterdam.
4. **Blake, P. A., M. H. Merson, H. E. Weaver, D. G. Hollis, and P. C. Heublein.** 1979. Disease caused by a marine vibrio: clinical characteristics and epidemiology. N. Engl. J. Med. **300:**1–5.
5. **Blake, P. A., R. E. Weaver, and D. G. Hollis.** 1980. Diseases of humans (other than cholera) caused by vibrios. Annu. Rev. Microbiol. **34:**341–367.
6. **Brayton, P. R., R. B. Bode, R. R. Colwell, M. T. MacDonell, H. L. Hall, D. J. Grimes, P. A. West, and T. N. Bryant.** 1986. *Vibrio cincinnatiensis* sp. nov., a new human pathogen. J. Clin. Microbiol. **23:**104–108.
7. **Brenner, D. J., F. W. Hickman-Brenner, J. V. Lee, A. G. Steigerwalt, G. R. Fanning, D. G. Hollis, J. J. Farmer III, R. E. Weaver, and R. J. Seidler.** 1983. *Vibrio furnissii* (formerly aerogenic biogroup of *Vibrio fluvialis*), a new species isolated from human feces and the environment. J. Clin. Microbiol. **18:**816–824.
8. **Davis, B. R., G. R. Fanning, J. M. Madden, A. G. Steigerwalt, H. B. Bradford, Jr., H. L. Smith, Jr., and D. J. Brenner.** 1981. Characterization of biochemically atypical *Vibrio cholerae* strains and designation of a new pathogenic species, *Vibrio mimicus*. J. Clin. Microbiol. **14:**631–639.
9. **Donovan, T. J., and J. V. Lee.** 1982. Quality of antisera used in the diagnosis of cholera. Lancet **ii:**866–868.
10. **Farmer, J. J., III, F. W. Hickman-Brenner, and M. T. Kelly.** 1985. *Vibrio*, p. 281–301. *In* E. H. Lennette, A. Balows, W. J. Hausler, Jr., and H. J. Shadomy (ed.), Manual of clinical microbiology, 4th ed. American Society for Microbiology, Washington, D.C.
11. **Feeley, J. C., and W. E. DeWitt.** 1976. Immune response to *Vibrio cholerae*, p. 289–295. *In* N. R. Rose and H. Friedman (ed.), Manual of clinical immunology. American Society for Microbiology, Washington, D.C.
12. **Furniss, A. L., J. V. Lee, and T. J. Donovan.** 1978. The *Vibrios*. PHLS monograph series no. 11. Maidstone Public Health Laboratory. H. M. Stationery Office, London, England.
13. **Hickman, F. W., J. J. Farmer III, D. G. Hollis, G. R. Fanning, A. G. Steigerwalt, R. E. Weaver, and D. J. Brenner.** 1982. Identification of *Vibrio hollisae* sp. nov. from patients with diarrhea. J. Clin. Microbiol. **15:**395–401.
14. **Hollis, D. G., R. E. Weaver, C. N. Baker, and C. Thornsberry.** 1976. Halophilic *Vibrio* species isolated from blood cultures. J. Clin. Microbiol. **3:**425–431.
15. **Hughes, J. M., D. G. Hollis, E. J. Gangarosa, and R. E. Weaver.** 1978. Non-cholera vibrio infections in the United

States. Ann. Intern. Med. **88:**602–606.

16. **Huq, M. I., A. K. M. J. Alam, D. J. Brenner, and G. K. Morris.** 1980. Isolation of *Vibrio*-like group EF-6 from patients with diarrhea. J. Clin. Microbiol. **11:**621–624.
17. **Jean-Jacques, W., K. A. Bajashekaraiah, J. J. Farmer III, F. W. Hickman, J. G. Morris, and C. A. Kallick.** 1981. *Vibrio metschnikovii* bacteremia in a patient with cholecystitis. J. Clin. Microbiol. **14:**711–712.
18. **Joseph, S. W., J. B. Kaper, and R. R. Colwell.** 1982. *Vibrio parahaemolyticus* and related halophilic vibrios. Crit. Rev. Microbiol. **10:**77–124.
19. **Kelly, M. T.** 1986. Cholera: a worldwide perspective. Pediatr. Infect. Dis. **5:**S101–S105.
20. **Kelly, M. T., J. W. Peterson, W. E. Sarles, M. Romanko, D. Martin, and B. Hafkin.** 1982. Cholera on the Texas gulf coast. J. Am. Med. Assoc. **247:**1598–1599.
21. **Kelly, M. T., and E. M. D. Stroh.** 1988. Temporal relationship of *Vibrio parahaemolyticus* in patients and the environment. J. Clin. Microbiol. **26:**1754–1756.
22. **Kelly, M. T., and E. M. D. Stroh.** 1989. Urease-positive, Kanagawa-negative *Vibrio parahaemolyticus* from patients and the environment in the Pacific Northwest. J. Clin. Microbiol. **27:**2820–2822.
23. **Lee, J. V., P. Shread, L. Furniss, and T. N. Bryant.** 1981. Taxonomy and description of *Vibrio fluvialis* sp. nov. (synonym group F vibrios, group EF6). J. Appl. Bacteriol. **50:** 73–94.
24. **Morris, J. G., H. G. Miller, R. Wilson, C. O. Tacket, D. G. Hollis, F. W. Hickman, R. E. Weaver, and P. A. Blake.** 1982. Illness caused by *Vibrio damsela* and *Vibrio hollisae*. Lancet **i:**1294–1297.
25. **Morris, J. G., J. H. Tenney, and G. L. Drusano.** 1985. In vitro susceptibility of pathogenic *Vibrio* species to norfloxacin and six other antimicrobial agents. Antimicrob. Agents Chemother. **28:**442–445.
26. **Morris, J. G., R. Wilson, B. R. Davis, I. K. Wachsmuth, C. F. Riddle, H. G. Wathen, R. A. Pollard, and P. A. Blake.** 1981. Non-O group 1 *Vibrio cholerae* gastroenteritis in the United States: clinical, epidemiologic, and laboratory characteristics of sporadic cases. Ann. Intern. Med. **94:** 656–658.
27. **Pavia, A. T., J. A. Bryan, K. L. Maher, T. R. Hester, Jr., and J. J. Farmer.** 1989. *Vibrio carchariae* infection after a shark bite. Ann. Intern. Med. **111:**85–86.
28. **Sakazaki, R., and A. Balows.** 1981. The genera *Vibrio, Plesiomonas* and *Aeromonas,* p. 1272–1301. *In* M. P. Starr, H. Stolp, H. G. Trüper, A. Balows, and H. G. Schlegel (ed.), The prokaryotes. Springer-Verlag KG, Berlin.
29. **Sakazaki, R., K. Tamura, T. Kato, Y. Obara, S. Yamai, and K. Hobo.** 1968. Studies on the enteropathogenic, facultatively halophilic bacteria, *Vibrio parahaemolyticus* III: enteropathogenicity. Jpn. J. Med. Sci. Biol. **21:**325–331.
30. **Shandera, W. X., J. M. Johnston, B. R. Davis, and P. A. Blake.** 1983. Disease from infection with *Vibrio mimicus,* a newly recognized *Vibrio* species. Ann. Intern. Med. **99:** 169–171.
31. **Tacket, C. O., F. Hickman, G. V. Pierce, and L. F. Mendoza.** 1982. Diarrhea associated with *Vibrio fluvialis* in the United States. J. Clin. Microbiol. **16:**991–992.
32. **World Health Organization Scientific Working Group.** 1980. Cholera and other vibrio-associated diarrhoeas. Bull. W.H.O. **58:**353–374.

Chapter 38

Aeromonas and *Plesiomonas*

ALEXANDER VON GRAEVENITZ AND MARTIN ALTWEGG

Bergey's Manual of Systematic Bacteriology lists the genera *Aeromonas* and *Plesiomonas* as belonging to the family *Vibrionaceae* by virtue of their morphology (asporogenous, gram-negative rods with predominantly polar flagellation), facultative anaerobiosis (respiratory and fermentative metabolism), and guanine-plus-cytosine ratio (41, 45). Recently, addition of a new family, *Aeromonadaceae*, and removal of *Plesiomonas* to the genus *Proteus* have been recommended on the basis of molecular genetic evidence (30).

DESCRIPTION OF THE GENERA

Aeromonas

Members of the genus *Aeromonas* (41) measure 1.1 to 4.4 by 0.4 to 1.0 μm. Most possess polar, usually monotrichous flagella of 1.7-μm wavelength; exceptions are the nonmotile species *A. salmonicida* and *A. media* as well as a few mesophilic strains of the other species. Some strains produce short lateral flagella, and a few produce lophotrichous flagella. Aeromonads produce oxidase and catalase and ferment glucose and other carbohydrates to acid or to acid and gas. Nitrates are reduced to nitrites. Many exoenzymes, i.e., amylase, DNase, esterases, peptidases, arylamidases, and other hydrolytic enzymes, are produced (12, 51). Growth may occur at 0 to 45°C; human (mesophilic) strains grow at 10 to 40°C, and *A. salmonicida* grows only below 37°C. Some strains are biochemically more active at 22 than at 37°C (6, 28). In brain heart infusion medium at 28°C, the growth range is between pH 4.5 and 9.0 and between NaCl concentrations of 0 to 4% (39). Aeromonads are not susceptible to 2,4-diamino-6,7-diisopropylpteridine (O/129); i.e., on Mueller-Hinton agar, there is no zone around disks containing 10 or 150 μg of O/129 phosphate (Oxoid Ltd., Basingstoke, United Kingdom). The guanine-plus-cytosine content of the DNA is 57 to 63 mol%. The main cellular fatty acids are hexadecanoic, hexadecenoic, and octadecenoic acids; also present are 3-hydroxymyristic and occasionally 3-hydroxypentadecanoic acids (11, 29).

Plesiomonas

P. shigelloides (formerly C27 or *A. shigelloides*), the only species of the genus (45), measures 2 to 3 μm by 0.1 to 1.0 μm and generally has two to five lophotrichous polar flagella with a wavelength of 3.5 to 4.0 μm. Young cultures may show lateral flagella with a shorter wavelength. Monotrichous and nonmotile strains occur. *P. shigelloides* is heterotrophic, produces oxidase and catalase, and ferments glucose and a few other carbohydrates to acid without gas. Nitrates are reduced to nitrites. In Trypticase soy broth (BBL Microbiology Systems, Cockeysville, Md.), NaCl tolerance ranges from 0 to 5% and pH tolerance ranges from 4.0 to 9.0; growth occurs at 8 to 45°C (32). Most strains are susceptible to O/129. A few strains share a common antigen with *Shigella sonnei* phase 1; cross-agglutination with *Shigella* spp. A and C antisera has also been reported (40). The species contains the common enterobacterial antigen. The guanine-plus-cytosine content of the DNA is 51 mol%. The main cellular fatty acids resemble those of *Aeromonas* spp. except that 3-hydroxylauric acid is present instead of 3-hydroxypentadecanoic acid (29).

TAXONOMY

Bergey's Manual of Systematic Bacteriology (41) recognizes four phenotypically separable *Aeromonas* species, *A. hydrophila*, *A. caviae*, *A. sobria*, and *A. salmonicida*, the latter with the three subspecies *salmonicida*, *masoucida*, and *achromogenes*. Since 1984, four new species with characteristic phenotypes, i.e., *A. media* (2), *A. veronii* (18), *A. eucrenophila* (46), and *A. schubertii* (17), as well as one new subspecies, *A. salmonicida* subsp. *smithia* (7), have been described. Still, these species do not reflect the genetic heterogeneity of the genus as determined by DNA-DNA hybridization studies (Table 1). Some of the DNA hybridization groups do not occur in clinical specimens and therefore will be disregarded (Table 1). Lack of phenotypic markers does not allow reliable identification of strains to the level of genospecies (e.g., DNA hybridization groups). Identification of phenotypic species, however, is recommended for the diagnostic laboratory because there are differences in epidemiology, antibiotic susceptibility, and possibly clinical significance between species (see below). Identification of genetic species cannot be recommended as yet.

NATURAL HABITAT AND CLINICAL SIGNIFICANCE

Aeromonas

Aeromonas spp. are widely distributed in stagnant and flowing fresh waters, in salt waters interfacing with fresh waters, in fish tanks, in water supplies (even chlorinated ones), and in sewage, with densities ranging from <1 to >1,000 cells per ml (50). These limits to growth apply to natural sources as well. Aeromonads have also been isolated from soil and foodstuffs (green vegetables, raw milk, ice cream, meat, and seafood) (37).

Natural diseases due to *Aeromonas* spp. and carriers are observed in amphibians, reptiles, and fish. These animals as well as guinea pigs and white mice can be

TABLE 1. Phenotypic and genetic species in the genus *Aeromonas* and their occurrence in clinical specimens

Phenotypic species (reference)	Hybridization group[a,b]	Found in clinical specimens	Genetic species
A. hydrophila (41)	1	+	*A. hydrophila*
	2	+	Unnamed
	3	+	*A. salmonicida*[a]
A. caviae (41)	4	+	*A. caviae*
	5A	+	*A. media*
	5B	+	*A. media*
A. media (2)	5B	−	*A. media*
A. eucrenophila (46)	6	−	*A. eucrenophila*
A. sobria (41)	7	−	*A. sobria*
	8[c]	+	*A. veronii*
	9	+	Unnamed
A. veronii (18)	10[c]	+	*A. veronii*
A. veronii-like[b]	11	+	Unnamed
A. schubertii (17)	12	+	*A. schubertii*
A. salmonicida (41)			
subsp. *salmonicida*	3	−	*A. salmonicida*
subsp. *achromogenes*	3	−	*A. salmonicida*
subsp. *masoucida*	3	−	*A. salmonicida*
subsp. *smithia* (7)	3	−	*A. salmonicida*

[a] As defined by the Centers for Disease Control (28).
[b] D. J. Brenner, personal communication.
[c] DNA hybridization groups 8 and 10 have subsequently been shown to be identical (28).

infected experimentally by parenteral routes (41). Fecal carrier strains in livestock are infrequent (49).

Human infections with *Aeromonas* spp. occur predominantly during warm weather. The strains probably originate from water, soil, food, or the human gastrointestinal tract. Each species has been isolated in each disease category (23). Nosocomial and community-acquired strains have been observed in either pure or mixed culture. So far, only one instance of a hospital outbreak (without gastrointestinal involvement) has been reported (31).

Four disease categories are known (22, 51): (i) wound infection or cellulitis, related to exposure to water or soil; (ii) septicemia, mostly in association with hepatic, biliary, or pancreatic disease or with malignancy, particularly acute leukemia and aplastic anemia (some patients, however, show no such predisposing conditions); (iii) other extraintestinal infections, e.g., of the eye and the urinary tract, meningitis, peritonitis, otitis, endocarditis, and osteomyelitis; and (iv) diarrheal disease. Most epidemiological studies have shown *Aeromonas* spp. in stools to be significantly more often associated with diarrhea than with the carrier state (43). Association with the consumption of untreated water was also conspicuous (19). Acute self-limited diarrhea is more frequent in young children; in older patients, chronic enterocolitis with or without predisposing conditions (see item ii above) may also be observed (15). Fever, vomiting, and fecal leukocytes or erythrocytes (colitis) may or may not be present (15, 19). Unusual for a bacterial diarrhea, however, is the lack of secondary spread (no epidemics), the inability to elicit symptoms in volunteers after feeding, and the lack of association with putative virulence factors (19, 34, 43). Among these factors are a heat-"stable" (56°C, 10 min) cytotonic toxin, a heat-labile cytotoxin (beta-hemolysin, aerolysin, Asao toxin), surface adhesins, and invasiveness for Hep-2 cells (19, 22, 40, 53). These factors are produced mainly by *A. hydrophila* and *A. sobria* and are therefore associated with certain biochemical test results (e.g., Voges-Proskauer reaction and lysine decarboxylase positivity). Depending on the geographical location, however, either *A. hydrophila* and *A. sobria* (Australia, Thailand, and Bangladesh) or *A. caviae* (Europe and United States) is more often found in such diarrheal patients (22). Also unusual is the wide variation of carrier rates between continents (0.2 to 27%) (40), a fact not explained by the use of different media. These carrier strains may also exhibit virulence factors. It is not known whether the development of some kind of immunity adds to this phenomenon.

Plesiomonas

The aquatic distribution of *P. shigelloides* is limited by its minimum growth temperature of 8°C and lack of halophilism. It may be found in fresh and estuarine water, particularly in tropical climates. Its animal host range is wider than that of *Aeromonas* (freshwater fish, shellfish, oysters, toads, snakes, monkeys, dogs, cats, goats, pigs, poultry, and cattle) (10). Most human *P. shigelloides* strains have been isolated from stools of diarrheic patients in subtropical and tropical areas (Africa, South Asia, Tahiti, and Cuba), in Japan, and in Australia. They are rare in Europe and in the United States (10). Several epidemiological studies have suggested *P. shigelloides* as a possible agent of human diarrhea (low carrier rate; association with shellfish, oyster, or untreated water consumption; outbreaks with predominant serotypes and identification of no other pathogens) (20, 43). Symptoms are mainly those of colitis (20, 25). Human carriers are very rare except in endemic areas (2 to 24% in Thailand) (40) or in association with epidemics. Invasiveness for HeLa cells as well as production of a heat-labile and a heat-stable enterotoxin have been reported (9). *P. shigelloides* DNA shows no homology to the enterotoxin gene of *Vibrio cholerae* (20). Feeding experiments in humans did not result in diarrhea (16).

Extraintestinal infections with *P. shigelloides* (meningitis and septicemia) are very rare (10).

COLLECTION, TRANSPORT, AND STORAGE OF SPECIMENS

A. hydrophila has been found to survive in glycerol-buffered saline for up to 5 days after inoculation (35). At this point, it must be assumed that collection, transport, and storage for specimens containing *Aeromonas* and *Plesiomonas* spp. do not differ from those outlined in chapter 3.

CULTURE AND ISOLATION

Since *Aeromonas* and *Plesiomonas* grow on routinely used common media (e.g., blood agar and most enteric differential agars) (14), their isolation from clinical specimens other than feces does not pose any problems.

Aeromonas

A wide variety of differential or selective media have been designed for the isolation of *Aeromonas* spp. from environmental and fecal specimens (24). No single medium has received general acceptance. However, blood agar containing ampicillin (10 mg/liter) (26) and cefsulodin-irgasan-novobiocin agar incubated at 25 to 30°C (3) are most widely used at this time. The former allows direct oxidase testing but is not very selective. In addition, some strains are ampicillin susceptible (27). Cefsulodin-irgasan-novobiocin medium (4 mg of cefsulodin per liter, not 15 mg/liter) allows simultaneous isolation of *Yersinia* and *Aeromonas* spp. from feces (3), but direct oxidase testing is not recommended because mannitol fermentation results in a low pH and a possibly false-negative oxidase reaction (21). Thiosulfate-citrate-bile salts-sucrose agar is inhibitory for *Aeromonas* spp. and therefore should not be used (26). Isolation frequencies of *Aeromonas* spp. can be increased by using alkaline peptone water, gram-negative broth, or phosphate-buffered saline (the latter at 4°C for 14 days) as an enrichment medium (33).

Plesiomonas

The low incidence of the genus *Plesiomonas* in the United States and in Europe may preclude the use of a separate medium. If present in large numbers, *Plesiomonas* strains may be isolated on regular enteric media (45, 51). Inositol-bile salts-brilliant green agar is selective for both *Aeromonas* and *Plesiomonas* spp. (52), but direct oxidase testing should be avoided because inositol is fermented by the latter (see above). Ampicillin-containing media should not be used for *Plesiomonas* isolation because in some series, a considerable number of strains were ampicillin susceptible (27, 42). Use of alkaline peptone water as enrichment is controversial.

IDENTIFICATION

Aeromonas

Most strains of *A. hydrophila* and *A. sobria* show large zones of beta-hemolysis around colonies on blood agar, whereas *A. caviae* strains are usually nonhemolytic (Table 2). On enteric differential agars, many strains show no signs of lactose fermentation, but a minority of strains yield lactose-fermenting colonies. Slants of triple sugar iron agar may be acid or alkaline.

In the routine diagnostic laboratory, the most important characteristics that should lead to a presumptive diagnosis of *Aeromonas* spp. are a positive oxidase reaction, growth on MacConkey agar, and fermentation of carbohydrates. These tests separate *Aeromonas* spp. (and *P. shigelloides*) from members of the family *Enterobacteriaceae* and from nonfermentative and fastidious fermentative gram-negative rods. Separation from other members of the family *Vibrionaceae* may be more difficult in light of the multitude of new *Vibrio* species (see chapter 37). Key differential features are resistance to the vibriostatic compound O/129, no growth in 6% NaCl, and absence of ornithine decarboxylase (except in *A. veronii*). Some of the commercial identification kits have been reported to be reliable for identification of members of the *Vibrionaceae* (38). However, two main problems should be mentioned. (i) *A. caviae* may be misidentified as *V. fluvialis*. The two organisms can easily be differentiated by testing the ability to grow in nutrient broth without added NaCl or with 6% NaCl. (ii) To date, most data bases contain only "*A. hydrophila*," which includes *A. hydrophila* sensu stricto, *A. caviae*, and *A. sobria*. It can also be anticipated that strains of the new species *A. veronii* and *A. schubertii* would be misidentified unless additional tests are performed.

Identification to the level of phenotypic species is based on few biochemical tests and usually accomplished without problems (Table 2). However, some tests may be medium or temperature dependent. In our hands, lysine decarboxylase was most reliable at 29°C, using the medium of Fay and Barry (6). Identification by enzymatic tests (peptidases, esterases, and "osidases") has been successful on a limited number of strains (12). As yet, there are no simple biochemical tests that would allow identification of DNA hybridization groups (genetic species).

Plesiomonas

P. shigelloides is not beta-hemolytic on blood agar and generally does not ferment lactose on enteric agars. Triple sugar iron agar slants are most often alkaline. Key tests for a presumptive diagnosis are those listed for *Aeromonas* spp. For separation from *Aeromonas* spp., see above and Table 2. *Vibrio* spp. are either arginine dihydrolase or ornithine decarboxylase negative, DNase positive, and usually mannitol positive and inositol negative (see chapter 37).

TYPING

Typing methods successfully used for the characterization of *Aeromonas* strains include serotyping, protein gel electrophoresis, isoenzyme analysis, bacteriophage typing, restriction fragment length polymorphism, and analysis of rRNA gene restriction patterns (4, 44, 48). There is no obvious correlation with taxonomic grouping except in isoenzyme analysis, which has allowed identification of genospecies on the basis of only four enzymes (M. Altwegg, M. W. Reeves, R. Altwegg-Bissig, and D. J. Brenner, J. Clin. Microbiol., submitted for publication). All of these methods have shown that clinical *Aeromonas* isolates are very diverse, indicating that

TABLE 2. Phenotypic characterization of *P. shigelloides* and *Aeromonas* species known to occur in clinical specimens[a]

Characteristic[b]	Species					
	A. hydrophila	*A. caviae*	*A. sobria*	*A. veronii*	*A. schubertii*	*P. shigelloides*
Oxidase	+	+	+	+	+	+
Catalase	+	+	+	+	+	+
Motility	+	+	+	+	+	+
DNase	+	+	+	+	+	−
Indole	+	+	+	+	−	+
H_2S on triple sugar iron agar	−	−	−	−	−	−
Voges-Proskauer	+	−	+	+	v[c]	−
Urea hydrolysis	−	−	−	−	−	−
Lysine decarboxylase	+	−	+	+	+	+
Ornithine decarboxylase	−	−	−	+	−	+
Arginine dihydrolase	+	+	+	−	+	+
Growth in KCN medium	+	+	v	v	−	−
Esculin hydrolysis	+	+	−	+	−	−
Beta-hemolysis on sheep blood agar	+	−	+	+	v	−
Sensitivity to O/129	−	−	−	−	−	+
Growth in 6.5% NaCl	−	−	−	−	−	−
Gelatin hydrolysis 22°C	+	+	+	+[d]	+[d]	+[d]
Gas from glucose	+	−	+	+	−	−
Acid from:						
Glucose	+	+	+	+	+	+
Arbutin	+	+	−	?	?	?
Lactose	v	v	−	−	−	v
Cellobiose	v	+	v	v	−	−
Sucrose	+	+	+	+	−	−
Maltose	+	+	+	+	+	+
L-Arabinose	+	+	v	−	−	−
Raffinose	−	−	−	−	−	−
myo-Inositol	−	−	−	−	−	+
Dulcitol	−	−	−	−	−	−
D-Sorbitol	v	−	−	−	−	−
Salicin	v	+	−	+	−	v
Mannitol	+	+	+	+	−	−

[a] Data are from references 5, 17, 18, 23, 28, 41, and 51 (see these references for additional data).
[b] Incubation at 29 or 37°C for 2 days. +, ≥80% positive; −, ≤20% positive; v, 20 to 80% positive; ?, data not available.
[c] Depending on method used (17).
[d] After 7 days at 22°C.

not a single clone with increased virulence potential is responsible for the majority of infections.

Typing of *P. shigelloides* is based exclusively on serology. Two antigenic schemes have been published (1, 47), which separate strains according to somatic and flagellar antigens.

SEROLOGICAL INVESTIGATIONS

Very few authors have checked antibody production in systemic *Aeromonas* and *Plesiomonas* infections and found elevated titers (10, 13). In patients with *Aeromonas*- or *Plesiomonas*-associated diarrhea, serum agglutinins were rarely elevated (19, 20).

ANTIBIOTIC SUSCEPTIBILITY

Aeromonas

Most *Aeromonas* strains are resistant to penicillin, ampicillin, carbenicillin, and ticarcillin but susceptible to azlocillin, piperacillin, and the second- and third-generation cephalosporins (36, 42). Development of resistance to these drugs, however, has been observed. There are at least four β-lactamases in this species. Two of them are susceptible to clavulanic acid, which, however, does not reduce the MIC of ampicillin to the susceptible range (8). *A. hydrophila* and *A. caviae* are more often resistant to cephalothin and to cefamandole than *A. sobria*, whereas *A. caviae* is more often susceptible to mezlocillin than are the other two species (36). Most aeromonads are susceptible to the aminoglycosides, chloramphenicol, tetracycline, trimethoprim-sulfamethoxazole, and the quinolones (36, 42).

Plesiomonas

P. shigelloides shows susceptibility patterns similar to those of *A. sobria*, although susceptibility to ampicillin has, in some series, been found more frequently than in *Aeromonas* spp. (27, 42).

LITERATURE CITED

1. **Aldova, E.** 1987. Serotyping of *Plesiomonas shigelloides* strains with our own antigen scheme. An attempted epidemiological study. Zentralbl. Bakteriol. Parasitenkd. Infektionskr. Hyg. Abt. 1 Reihe A **265:**253–262.
2. **Allen, D. A., B. Austin, and R. R. Colwell.** 1983. *Aeromonas media*, a new species isolated from river water. Int. J. Syst. Bacteriol. **33:**599–604.
3. **Altorfer, R., M. Altwegg, J. Zollinger-Iten, and A. von Graevenitz.** 1985. Growth of *Aeromonas* spp. on cefsulo-

din-irgasan-novobiocin agar selective for *Yersinia enterocolitica.* J. Clin. Microbiol. **22:**478–480.

4. **Altwegg, M., R. Altwegg-Bissig, A. Demarta, R. Peduzzi, M. W. Reeves, and B. Swaminathan.** 1989. Comparison of four typing methods for *Aeromonas* species. J. Diarrh. Dis. Res. **6:**88–94.
5. **Altwegg, M., A. G. Steigerwalt, R. Altwegg-Bissig, J. Lüthy-Hottenstein, and D. J. Brenner.** 1990. Biochemical identification of *Aeromonas* genospecies isolated from humans. J. Clin. Microbiol. **28:**258–264.
6. **Altwegg, M., A. von Graevenitz, and J. Zollinger-Iten.** 1987. Medium and temperature dependence of decarboxylase reactions in *Aeromonas* spp. Curr. Microbiol. **14:** 1–4.
7. **Austin, D. A., D. McIntosh, and B. Austin.** 1989. Taxonomy of fish associated *Aeromonas* spp., with the description of *Aeromonas salmonicida* subsp. *smithia* subsp. nov. Syst. Appl. Microbiol. **11:**277–290.
8. **Bakken, J. S., C. C. Sanders, R. B. Clark, and M. Hori.** 1988. Beta-lactam resistance in *Aeromonas* spp. caused by inducible beta-lactamases active against penicillins, cephalosporins, and carbapenems. Antimicrob. Agents Chemother. **32:**1314–1319.
9. **Binns, M. M., S. Vaughan, S. C. Sanyal, and K. N. Timmis.** 1984. Invasive ability of *Plesiomonas shigelloides.* Zentralbl. Bakteriol. Parasitenkd. Infektionskr. Hyg. Abt. 1 Reihe A **257:**343–347.
10. **Brenden, R. A., M. A. Miller, and J. M. Janda.** 1988. Clinical disease spectrum and pathogenic factors associated with *Plesiomonas shigelloides* infections in humans. Rev. Infect. Dis. **10:**303–316.
11. **Canonica, F. P., and M. A. Pisano.** 1988. Gas-liquid chromatographic analysis of fatty acid methyl esters of *Aeromonas hydrophila, Aeromonas sobria,* and *Aeromonas caviae.* J. Clin. Microbiol. **26:**681–685.
12. **Carnahan, A. M., M. O'Brien, S. W. Joseph, and R. R. Colwell.** 1988. Enzymatic characterization of three *Aeromonas* species using API peptidase, API "osidase", and API esterase test kits. Diagn. Microbiol. Infect. Dis. **10:** 195–203.
13. **Caselitz, F.-H., V. Freitag, and G. Jannasch.** 1975. Spezifischer Antikörpernachweis bei Aeromonasinfektionen. Zentralbl. Bakteriol. Parasitenkd. Infektionskr. Hyg. Abt. 1 Reihe A **233:**347–354.
14. **Desmond, E., and J. M. Janda.** 1986. Growth of *Aeromonas* species on enteric agars. J. Clin. Microbiol. **23:** 1065–1067.
15. **George, W. L., M. M. Nakata, J. Thompson, and M. L. White.** 1985. *Aeromonas*-related diarrhea in adults. Arch. Intern. Med. **145:**2207–2211.
16. **Herrington, D. A., S. Tzipori, R. M. Robins-Browne, B. D. Tall, and M. M. Levine.** 1987. In vitro and in vivo pathogenicity of *Plesiomonas shigelloides.* Infect. Immun. **55:**979–985.
17. **Hickman-Brenner, F. W., G. Fanning, M. J. Arduino, D. J. Brenner, and J. J. Farmer III.** 1988. *Aeromonas schubertii,* a new mannitol-negative species found in human clinical specimens. J. Clin. Microbiol. **26:**1561–1564.
18. **Hickman-Brenner, F. W., K. L. MacDonald, A. G. Steigerwalt, G. R. Fanning, D. J. Brenner, and J. J. Farmer III.** 1987. *Aeromonas veronii,* a new ornithine decarboxylase-positive species that may cause diarrhea. J. Clin. Microbiol. **25:**900–906.
19. **Holmberg, S. D., W. L. Schell, G. R. Fanning, I. K. Wachsmuth, F. W. Hickman-Brenner, P. A. Blake, D. J. Brenner, and J. J. Farmer III.** 1986. *Aeromonas* intestinal infections in the United States. Ann. Intern. Med. **105:**683–689.
20. **Holmberg, S. D., I. K. Wachsmuth, F. W. Hickman-Brenner, D. A. Blake, and J. J. Farmer III.** 1986. *Plesiomonas* enteric infections in the United States. Ann. Intern. Med. **105:**690–694.
21. **Hunt, L. K., T. L. Overman, and R. B. Otero.** 1981. Role of pH in oxidase variability of *Aeromonas hydrophila.* J. Clin. Microbiol. **13:**1054–1059.
22. **Janda, J. M., and P. S. Duffey.** 1988. Mesophilic aeromonads in human disease: current taxonomy, laboratory identification, and infectious disease spectrum. Rev. Infect. Dis. **10:**980–997.
23. **Janda, J. M., M. Reitano, and E. J. Bottone.** 1984. Biotyping of *Aeromonas* isolates as a correlate to delineating a species-associated disease spectrum. J. Clin. Microbiol. **19:**44–47.
24. **Joseph, S. W., M. Janda, and A. Carnahan.** 1988. Isolation, enumeration and identification of *Aeromonas* sp. J. Food Safety **9:**23–35.
25. **Kain, K. C., and M. T. Kelly.** 1989. Clinical features, epidemiology, and treatment of *Plesiomonas shigelloides* diarrhea. J. Clin. Microbiol. **27:**998–1001.
26. **Kay, B. A., C. E. Guerrero, and R. B. Sack.** 1985. Media for the isolation of *Aeromonas hydrophila.* J. Clin. Microbiol. **22:**888–890.
27. **Kilpatrick, M. E., J. Escarmilla, A. L. Bourgeois, H. J. Adkins, and R. C. Rockhill.** 1987. Overview of four U.S. Navy overseas research studies on *Aeromonas.* Experientia **43:**365–366.
28. **Kuijper, E. J., A. G. Steigerwalt, B. S. C. I. M. Schoenmakers, M. F. Peeters, H. C. Zanen, and D. J. Brenner.** 1989. Phenotypic characterization and DNA relatedness in human fecal isolates of *Aeromonas* spp. J. Clin. Microbiol. **27:**132–138.
29. **Lambert, M. A., F. W. Hickman-Brenner, J. J. Farmer III, and C. W. Moss.** 1983. Differentiation of *Vibrionaceae* species by their cellular fatty acid composition. Int. J. Syst. Bacteriol. **33:**777–792.
30. **MacDonell, M. T., and R. R. Colwell.** 1985. Phylogeny of the *Vibrionaceae,* and recommendation for two new genera, *Listonella* and *Shewanella.* Syst. Appl. Microbiol. **6:** 171–182.
31. **Mellersh, A. R., P. Norman, and G. H. Smith.** 1984. *Aeromonas hydrophila:* an outbreak of hospital infection. J. Hosp. Infect. **5:**425–430.
32. **Miller, M. L., and J. A. Koburger.** 1986. Tolerance of *Plesiomonas shigelloides* to pH, sodium chloride and temperature. J. Food Prot. **49:**877–879.
33. **Millership, S. E., and B. Chattopadhyay.** 1984. Methods for the isolation of *Aeromonas hydrophila* and *Plesiomonas shigelloides* from faeces. J. Hyg. **92:**145–152.
34. **Morgan, D. R., P. C. Johnson, H. L. Dupont, T. K. Satterwhite, and L. V. Wood.** 1985. Lack of correlation between known virulence properties of *Aeromonas hydrophila* and enteropathogenicity for humans. Infect. Immun. **50:**62–65.
35. **Morgan, D. R., P. C. Johnson, A. H. West, L. V. Wood, C. D. Ericsson, and H. L. DuPont.** 1984. Isolation of enteric pathogens from patients with travelers' diarrhea using fecal transport media. FEMS Microbiol. Lett. **23:**59–63.
36. **Motyl, M. R., G. McKinley, and J. M. Janda.** 1985. In vitro susceptibilities of *Aeromonas hydrophila, Aeromonas sobria,* and *Aeromonas caviae* to 22 antimicrobial agents. Antimicrob. Agents Chemother. **28:**151–153.
37. **Nishikawa, Y., and T. Kishi.** 1988. Isolation and characterization of motile *Aeromonas* from human food and environmental specimens. Epidemiol. Infect. **101:**213–223.
38. **Overman, T. L., J. F. Kessler, and J. P. Seabolt.** 1985. Comparison of API 20E, API Rapid E and API Rapid NFT for identification of members of the family *Vibrionaceae.* J. Clin. Microbiol. **22:**778–781.
39. **Palumbo, S. A., D. R. Morgan, and R. L. Buchanan.** 1985. Influence of temperature, NaCl, and pH on the growth of *Aeromonas hydrophila.* J. Food Sci. **50:**1417–1421.
40. **Pitarangsi, C., P. Echeverria, R. Whitmire, C. Tirapat, S. Formal, G. J. Dammin, and M. Tingtalapong.** 1982. Enteropathogenicity of *Aeromonas hydrophila* and *Plesiomonas shigelloides:* prevalence among individuals with and without diarrhea in Thailand. Infect. Immun. **35:**666–

673.
41. **Popoff, M.** 1984. Genus III. *Aeromonas* Kluyver and van Niel 1936, 398, p. 545–548. *In* N. R. Krieg and J. G. Holt (ed.), Bergey's manual of systematic bacteriology, vol. 1. The Williams & Wilkins Co., Baltimore.
42. **Reinhardt, J. F., and W. L. George.** 1985. Comparative in vitro activities of selected antimicrobial agents against *Aeromonas* species and *Plesiomonas shigelloides*. Antimicrob. Agents Chemother. **27:**643–645.
43. **Sack, D. A., K. A. Chowdhury, A. Hug, B. A. Kay, and S. Sayeed.** 1988. Epidemiology of *Aeromonas* and *Plesiomonas* diarrhea. J. Diarrh. Dis. Res. **6:**107–112.
44. **Sakazaki, R., and T. Shimada.** 1984. O-serogrouping scheme for mesophilic *Aeromonas* strains. Jpn. J. Med. Sci. Biol. **37:**247–255.
45. **Schubert, R. H. W.** 1984. Genus IV. *Plesiomonas* Habs and Schubert 1962, 324, p. 548–550. *In* N. R. Krieg and J. G. Holt (ed.), Bergey's manual of systematic bacteriology, vol. 1. The Williams & Wilkins Co., Baltimore.
46. **Schubert, R. H. W., and M. Hegazi.** 1988. *Aeromonas eucrenophila* species nova, *Aeromonas caviae* a later and illegitimate synonym of *Aeromonas punctata*. Zentralbl. Bakteriol. Parasitenkd. Infektionskr. Hyg. Abt. 1 Reihe A **268:**34–39.
47. **Shimada, T., and R. Sakazaki.** 1985. New O and H antigens and additional serovars of *Plesiomonas shigelloides*. Jap. J. Med. Sci. Biol. **38:**73–76.
48. **Stephenson, J. R., S. E. Millership, and S. Tabaqchali.** 1987. Typing of *Aeromonas* species by polyacrylamide-gel electrophoresis of radiolabelled cell proteins. J. Med. Microbiol. **24:**113–118.
49. **Stern, N. J., E. S. Drazek, and S. W. Joseph.** 1987. Low incidence of *Aeromonas* sp. in livestock feces. J. Food Prot. **50:**66–69.
50. **van der Kooij, D.** 1988. Properties of aeromonads and their occurrence and hygienic significance in drinking water. Zentralbl. Bakteriol. Parasitenkd. Infektionskr. Hyg. Abt. 1 Reihe B **187:**1–17.
51. **von Graevenitz, A.** 1985. *Aeromonas* and *Plesiomonas*, p. 278–281. *In* E. H. Lennette, A. Balows, W. J. Hausler, Jr., and H. J. Shadomy (ed.), Manual of clinical microbiology, 4th ed. American Society for Microbiology, Washington, D.C.
52. **von Graevenitz, A., and C. Bucher.** 1983. Evaluation of differential and selective media for isolation of *Aeromonas* and *Plesiomonas* spp. from human feces. J. Clin. Microbiol. **17:**16–21.
53. **Wadström, T., and A. Ljungh.** 1988. Correlation between toxin formation and diarrhoea in *Aeromonas*. J. Diarrh. Dis. Res. **6:**113–119.

Chapter 39

Campylobacter, Helicobacter, and Related Spiral Bacteria

JOHN L. PENNER

GENUS *CAMPYLOBACTER*

The genus *Campylobacter* was proposed in 1963 when it was recognized that bacteria then known as *Vibrio fetus* were not true *Vibrionaceae.* A decade later, Véron and Chatelain (34) described a system of classifying campylobacteria that forms the basis of the current classification system. They recognized four species, with *Campylobacter fetus* as the type species of the genus. In 1977, Skirrow confirmed that one species, *Campylobacter jejuni,* was a major etiological agent of human enteritis (25). This constituted the stimulus for an intense new interest in spiral-shaped bacteria, and the outcome was an expanded genus that included 15 species. The inclusion of so many species led to great diversity in the genus, and questions concerning the validity of including some species have been the subject of much discussion. The organisms are asaccharolytic, thus obviating the applicability of well-known fermentation tests for characterizing and differentiating the species. The few phenotypic traits that can be used are insufficient or unreliable for systematic classification. It was not surprising, therefore, that results emerging from genetic analysis and phylogenetic studies did not support the housing of all 15 species in the same genus, and two species have been placed in the newly created genus *Helicobacter.*

The species currently in the genera *Campylobacter* and *Helicobacter* are listed in Table 1. They are arranged into groups that have been defined on the basis of homologies of 16S rRNA sequences by Thompson et al. (32). DNA hybridization tests and phylogenic studies reported by other groups are generally in agreement with this grouping (21).

Group I consists of true campylobacteria; in subgroup IA are included the thermophilic enteropathogenic species, *C. jejuni, C. coli, C. laridis* and *"C. upsaliensis."* Criteria that unify these four species are their ability to grow at 42°C and to cause enteritis in humans. Subgroup IB includes the type species of the genus, *C. fetus,* and four other species, *C. hyointestinalis, C. sputorum, C. mucosalis,* and *C. concisus.* This group comprises commensals or animal pathogens that rarely cause human infections. Phenotypic diversity is greater among the species of this subgroup, and unifying phenotypic characteristics are not readily identifiable. The cryophilic species, *C. cryaerophila* and *C. nitrofigilis,* considered not to be true campylobacteria, compose group II. These organisms grow at low temperatures and optimally at temperatures lower than 37°C.

GENERAL CHARACTERISTICS OF THE BACTERIA

The genus name *Campylobacter* (curved rod) was proposed for this group of gram-negative bacteria that are curved, spiral, or S shaped (34). Coccoid forms occur in older cultures of some species. The cells have a single polar unsheathed flagellum at one or both ends, and motility is characteristically rapid in a darting corkscrew fashion. The organisms generally are microaerophilic, but those in group II can grow aerobically in subculture after isolation. Some species can grow anaerobically in media supplemented with fumarate or with formate and fumarate. They have a respiratory-type metabolism, use amino acids and intermediates of the tricarboxylic acid cycle, and do not ferment or oxidize carbohydrate substrates that are used in tests for differentiation in the clinical laboratory. Growth temperatures vary widely with respect to optimum and range, but all species grow at 37°C. All organisms are oxidase positive. The tests for catalase and H_2S production, nitrate reduction, hippurate hydrolysis, and susceptibility to nalidixic acid and cephalothin are useful tests for identification. The G+C content is low, ranging from 28 to 38 mol%.

GROUP I. THE TRUE CAMPYLOBACTERIA

Subgroup IA. The Thermophilic Enteropathogenic Species

Subgroup IA includes *C. jejuni,* which consists of two subspecies, *C. jejuni* subsp. *jejuni,* a major cause of human gastroenteritis, and *C. jejuni* subsp. *doylei* (29). *C. coli* also causes human enteritis but not as frequently as does *C. jejuni. C. laridis* organisms, formally known as nalidixic acid-resistant thermophilic campylobacters, were originally isolated from gulls and subsequently from humans with diarrhea. Recently a group of unusual isolates, referred to as urease-positive thermophilic campylobacters, have been shown to be variants of this species (19). The group of catalase-negative or catalase-weak strains identified as *"C. upsaliensis"* are attracting attention as a fourth species of thermophilic enteropathogenic campylobacteria (24) that should be isolated in the clinical laboratory.

Habitats

Strains of thermophilic bacteria are widely distributed in nature. They are present in the intestines of numerous

TABLE 1. *Campylobacter, Helicobacter,* and related spiral bacteria

Genus *Campylobacter*
I. True campylobacteria
IA. Thermophilic enteropathogenic species
C. jejuni subsp. *jejuni*
subsp. *doylei*
C. coli
C. laridis, urease-negative variants
urease-positive variants
"*C. upsaliensis*"
IB. Other true campylobacteria
C. fetus subsp. *fetus*
subsp. *venerealis*
C. hyointestinalis
C. sputorum biovar sputorum
biovar bubulus
biovar fecalis
C. mucosalis
C. concisus
II. Psychrophilic species
C. nitrofigilis
C. cryaerophila
Genus *Helicobacter* and related campylobacteria
H. pylori (*C. pylori*)
H. mustelae (*C. mustelae*)
C. cinaedi
C. fennelliae

mammalian and avian species and in environmental waters contaminated with their feces. There is evidently some host preference, because *C. jejuni* subsp. *jejuni* is the predominating species in poultry (particularly chickens) and cattle, whereas *C. coli* appears to show a preference for the hog as its host. *C. jejuni* subsp. *doylei* has been isolated only from adult human gastric biopsy specimens and from feces of children with diarrhea. *C. laridis* was originally isolated from sea gulls, but its habitat is not restricted to this one species. The urease-positive variants have been isolated from river water and seawater, from mussels and cockles, and from feces of patients with diarrhea (19). "*C. upsaliensis*" was isolated initially from dogs, but it too has a broader habitat (24). Intestinal carriage of *C. jejuni* subsp. *jejuni* by humans is rare in nations with high levels of sanitary conditions but not infrequent by individuals in developing countries.

Clinical significance

Infections in humans cause diarrhea, abdominal pain, fever, and sometimes vomiting. Blood may be present in the stool, particularly in specimens from pediatric patients. The organisms may be isolated in blood cultures, but extraintestinal infections are more likely to occur in patients with predisposing conditions.

Infections can be acquired through consumption of contaminated water or food products such as poorly cooked meat and unpasteurized milk (5). Waterborne outbreaks have occurred as a result of breakdown in the purification and chlorination of municipal water systems. Handling of animals, including household pets, has also been implicated as a source of human infection. Although infections with campylobacteria are essentially zoonoses, case-to-case transmission among family members and institutionalized patients has been reported.

C. jejuni subsp. *jejuni* causes abortion in sheep and enteritis in cattle. Pathogenicity of the other three species in animals has not been established unequivocally.

Isolation

Four selective plating media are currently in use for isolating campylobacteria (1, 4, 10, 25). These have been modified slightly since their first descriptions and are available from commercial sources. The media contain blood to remove toxic forms of oxygen and antibiotics to prevent overgrowth by other enteric species. The plates are incubated at 42 to 43°C in anaerobic jars for 48 to 72 h, and microaerophilic conditions with oxygen concentrations reduced to 3 to 5% are essential for efficient isolation. Such conditions are readily produced with commercially available gas packs or by replacing the air in the jar with 10% carbon dioxide and 90% nitrogen. The presence of hydrogen in these gas mixtures may enhance the growth of some *Campylobacter* species. Colonies that are nonhemolytic, flat, gray or colorless, less than 1 mm in diameter, or large and spreading appear usually after 48 h.

Use of these isolation methods has been immensely successful in isolating the vast majority of *C. jejuni* subsp. *jejuni, C. coli,* and *C. laridis* from fecal specimens. However, the requirement for sterile blood may be a disadvantage in developing countries because of lack of availability. The finding that charcoal can effectively replace the blood (2) marked an advance in medium development (2, 13). (*Campylobacter* blood-free selective medium is now also commercially available.) Despite these improvements, it is clear that no single medium or procedure is totally effective for recovering campylobacteria from feces (3). Some campylobacteria escape detection presumably because they either fail to grow at 42 to 43°C, are susceptible to the antibiotics in the media, or are present only in small numbers. Proposed measures to improve isolation rates include the simultaneous use of different media or duplicate plates at 42 and 37°C. It has also been suggested that the membrane filtration technique (28) be used in conjunction with a plate isolation procedure (3). The species most likely to be missed in routine diagnosis is "*C. upsaliensis*" because of the wide strain variation in susceptibility to the antibiotics in the isolation media.

Identification

Presumptive identification of thermophilic enteropathogenic campylobacteria can be made based on a positive oxidase reaction and characteristic darting motility in a wet mount. For further differentiation into species and biotypes, tests are performed for catalase, urease, and hydrogen sulfide production, nitrate reduction, hippurate, indoxyl acetate, and DNA hydrolysis, and susceptibility to cephalothin and nalidixic acid (Table 2). Since *C. fetus* subsp. *fetus, C. hyointestinalis, C. cinaedi, C. fennelliae,* and *C. cryaerophila* may be recovered on rare occasions from human fecal samples by the isolation procedures described above, their reactions are also included in Table 2.

Serodiagnosis

Patients with *C. jejuni* subsp. *jejuni* infections have antibody levels measurable by enzyme-linked immunosorbent assay (ELISA) and an acid-glycine-extracted

TABLE 2. Laboratory tests for differentiating *Campylobacter* species after isolation from human feces

Species	Test[a]								
	Catalase	Hippuricase	Nitrate reduction	Urease	H_2S[b]	Susceptibility to:		Growth at[c]:	
						Nalidixic acid	Cephalothin	25°C	42°C
C. jejuni subsp. *jejuni*	+	+	+	−	−	S	R	−	+
C. jejuni subsp. *doylei*	d	+	−	−	−	S	S	−	(+)
C. coli	+	−	+	−	−	S	R	−	+
C. laridis[d]	+	−	+	−	−	R	R	−	+
"*C. upsaliensis*"	(−)	−	+	−	−	S	S	−	+
C. fetus subsp. *fetus*	+	−	+	−	−	R	S	+	(−)
C. hyointestinalis	+	−	+	−	+	R	S	+	+
C. cinaedi	+	−	+	−	−	S	I	−	−
C. fennelliae	+	−	−	−	−	S	S	−	−
C. cryaerophila	+	−	+	−	−	d	R	+	−

[a] +, More than 90% positive; −, more than 90% negative; (+), most strains positive but a low percentage negative; (−), most strains negative but a low percentage positive or weakly positive; d, 10 to 90% positive; S, susceptible; R, resistant; I, intermediate zones of inhibition.
[b] On triple sugar iron.
[c] All species grow at 35 to 37°C.
[d] The urease-positive thermophilic campylobacter variants of *C. laridis* are urease positive and susceptible to nalidixic acid.

antigen from one strain or from several strains as the test antigen. A standardized preparation is not available, and various strains have been used for preparation of the antigenic extract.

Epidemiological typing

Serotyping of *C. jejuni* and *C. coli* can be performed on the basis of thermolabile antigens by the slide agglutination technique and thermostable lipopolysaccharide antigens by passive hemagglutination. Epidemiological studies have also made use of plasmid profiles and restriction endonuclease DNA digest analysis to differentiate strains.

Subgroup IB. Other Species of True Campylobacteria

In subgroup IB of true campylobacteria there are five species genetically related by interspecies 16S rRNA sequence homology values at ≥88% (32). *C. fetus* is the type species of the genus and has received the most attention because of its importance in veterinary medicine. The other four species are *C. hyointestinalis, C. sputorum, C. mucosalis,* and *C. concisus.* Phenotypically, however, the group is diverse. The species differ in their habitats, atmospheric conditions for isolation, and pathogenicity. Only occasional strains of *C. fetus* grow at 42°C, whereas strains of the other four species generally grow at this temperature; only strains of *C. fetus* subsp. *venerealis* do not grow in 1.0% glycine. Only *C. concisus* is resistant to cephalothin, and all but *C. sputorum* (biovar sputorum) are resistant to nalidixic acid. Thus, unifying phenotypic traits unique to this group of species that would confirm the close relatedness seen in genetics studies need to be discovered.

C. fetus

C. fetus is divided into two subspecies, *C. fetus* subsp. *fetus* (formerly subspecies *intestinalis*) and *C. fetus* subsp. *venerealis* (formerly subspecies *fetus*). Some confusion occurred before the adoption of this classification (27) and in the early literature, when *Vibrio fetus* only was used. The two subspecies are genetically so closely related that the validity of the subspecies ranking is questionable, but the recognition of this classification has continued for practical reasons and convenience (22). Although distinguishable by habitat and pathogenesis, identification to the subspecies level on the basis of phenotypic characteristics is difficult in the laboratory. Both subspecies are important pathogens, but only *C. fetus* subsp. *fetus* is recognized as an infectious agent for humans. The most useful laboratory test to differentiate the two subspecies is that *C. fetus* subsp. *fetus* grows in 1% glycine and *C. fetus* subsp. *venerealis* does not. However, it should be noted that authors differ on the reliability of this test. The ability of both subspecies to grow at 25°C and their different antibiotic susceptibilities permit them to be differentiated from the group of thermophilic enteropathogenic campylobacteria.

C. fetus subsp. *fetus*

Organisms of *C. fetus* subsp. *fetus* occur in the intestinal tract of cattle and sheep and are an important cause of sporadic abortion in these animals. In humans, this species is well recognized as a rare cause of extraintestinal infections in patients usually with predisposing conditions and has been involved in cases of septicemia, meningitis, salpingitis, fetal infections, abortions, and other systemic infections. However, the generally held assumption that *C. fetus* subsp. *fetus* does not cause enteritis in humans is being challenged by increasing numbers of reports of its isolation from the intestinal tracts of patients with diarrhea. Some of these isolates multiply at 42°C; however, most do not. This fact raises the possibility that many are missed by incubation of the isolation media at 42°C and that the subspecies may therefore occur more frequently in the human intestine. Isolation of *C. fetus* subsp. *fetus* should be done on media without cephalothin, to which the organisms are generally susceptible, and under microaerophilic conditions at 37°C. In addition, filtration of feces through a 0.6-μm-pore-size membrane filter before inoculation of media has been reported to be a reliable method for isolating these organisms. The use of both methods in the clinical laboratory would enhance the recovery rate, permit a more accurate determination of the frequency of these organisms in the human intestine, and yield data on their importance as causes of human enteritis.

C. fetus subsp. *venerealis*

In contrast to *C. fetus* subsp. *fetus*, *C. fetus* subsp. *venerealis* does not inhabit the intestinal tract of humans or animals. The principal habitat is the preputial cavity of the asymptomatic bull. In cows and heifers, infections occur in the vagina, cervix, uterus, and oviducts, leading to abortions and infertility. Human infections are rare; only two cases have been reported in patients with underlying conditions. Isolation of the bacteria from preputial washings, semen, or vaginal mucus is as described for *C. fetus* subsp. *fetus*.

C. hyointestinalis

A new species, *C. hyointestinalis*, was proposed in 1985 for campylobacteria that were isolated from the intestinal contents of pigs (7). The bacteria have the general characteristics of true campylobacteria but tend to produce filamentous forms rather than coccoid forms in older cultures. Although they grow at 42°C, some strains produce more abundant growth at 37°C. Colonies are yellow, smooth, and nonswarming. They are catalase positive and produce hydrogen sulfide on triple sugar iron medium; DNA relatedness tests confirmed that this group constitutes a new species (7). 16S rRNA sequence data indicate that this species is most closely related to *C. fetus* (32).

Because of the high frequency of isolation of *C. hyointestinalis* from pigs with proliferative ileitis, it was suspected that the bacteria were involved in the disease. However, it has been isolated from feces of healthy and diarrheic cattle, from a hamster with enteritis, and from humans with gastrointestinal disease. All human isolates were from patients with watery diarrhea except one, from a patient who had proctitis. In each case, the condition resolved with elimination of the organism. As for *C. fetus* subspecies *fetus*, isolation of this species should be at 37°C on medium not containing cephalothin.

C. sputorum

As a result of a comprehensive DNA relatedness study (23), classification of this group of bacteria has undergone considerable taxonomic revision. *C. sputorum* subsp. *sputorum*, *C. sputorum* subsp. *bubulus*, and "*C. fecalis*" were found to be so closely related that classification by subspecies was unnecessary; they were therefore separated only at the rank of biovar (biogroup or biotype). The biovars have quite distinct nonoverlapping habitats, but the number of laboratory tests by which they can be differentiated is limited.

C. sputorum biovar sputorum is considered a commensal of the human oral cavity, but by the filtration technique it has been isolated from 2% of stool specimens from healthy humans (14). Moreover, this biovar has also been recovered from a human leg abscess and from the feces of an infant with diarrhea, but the clinical significance of these isolations is unknown. *C. sputorum* biovar bubulus is a bovine commensal with habitats in the preputial cavity in the male and in the genital tract of the female. The bacteria have not been associated with disease in either cattle or humans. *C. sputorum* biovar fecalis has been isolated from sheep feces, bovine semen, and the bovine vagina, but a pathogenic role for this biovar in animals or humans has yet to be demonstrated.

The biovars all grow at 37 and 42°C but not at 25°C. *C. sputorum* biovar fecalis is the only one that is catalase positive; biovar sputorum, in contrast to the other biovars, does not grow in 3.5% NaCl.

Strains of *C. sputorum* are isolated by incubation for 3 to 4 days at 37°C on blood agar with antibiotics in an atmosphere of 3 to 5% oxygen, 2 to 5% carbon dioxide, and the remainder nitrogen. As a result of the development of isolation media by different investigators, the compositions of these media vary with biovars. Formulations for each have been detailed by Smibert (26).

C. mucosalis

C. mucosalis group (formerly classified as *C. sputorum* subsp. *mucosalis*) was elevated from the rank of subspecies to species in 1985 on the basis of DNA relatedness. The bacteria have the general characteristics of true campylobacteria and resemble most closely *C. concisus* in that they are catalase negative and require hydrogen. Either hydrogen or formate is required for microaerophilic growth, and either hydrogen and fumarate or formate and fumarate are required for anaerobic growth. *C. mucosalis* differs from *C. concisus* by its susceptibility to cephalothin, by the ability to grow at 25°C, and by the production of dirty yellow colonies (23).

C. mucosalis is of interest to veterinarians because of a suspected but unproven role in the development of intestinal lesions in pigs. The organisms have been isolated from the mucosa of pigs with intestinal adenomatosis, necrotic ileitis, regional ileitis, and proliferative hemorrhagic enteropathy, but inoculation of healthy pigs with *C. mucosalis* does not produce these symptoms. The organisms have also been isolated from intestinal contents and oral cavities of healthy pigs but not from humans.

Isolation of *C. mucosalis* consists of diluting homogenized specimens of mucosa scraped from the intestine, the chyme, or feces in broth or phosphate-buffered saline and spreading 0.1 ml on solid blood agar. The isolation medium contains 5% lysed horse blood, novobiocin, trimethoprim, and noninhibitory concentrations of brilliant green. Oral swabs are washed in saline, which is then filtered before plating on isolation medium. Incubation in an atmosphere containing hydrogen is essential; satisfactory mixtures consist of hydrogen (77%), nitrogen (10%), oxygen (3%), and carbon dioxide (10%).

C. concisus

A group of bacterial isolates from humans with periodontal disease was found in 1981 to constitute a new *Campylobacter* species to which the name *C. concisus* was given (30). The bacteria are similar in their general characteristics to those described for the genus. They differ, however, from other *Campylobacter* species except *C. mucosalis* in their requirements for hydrogen or formate for microaerophilic growth and formate and fumarate for anaerobic growth. They do not produce catalase, are resistant to both cephalothin and nalidixic acid, and grow at 37 and 42°C but not at 25°C. The organisms are taken from the oral cavity under anaerobic conditions by using an oxygen-free gas-flushed syringe and are isolated on Trypticase soy agar (BBL Microbiology Systems, Cockeysville, Md.) plates supplemented with sheep blood (5%) in an anaerobic atmosphere containing 80% nitrogen, 10% carbon dioxide, and 10% hydrogen (31). Stock cultures of *C. concisus* can be maintained in semisolid brucella medium supplemented with 0.3% fumaric acid. For weekly transfer, the bacteria should be incubated at 37°C in an atmosphere of oxygen (6%), carbon dioxide (5%), hydrogen (15%), and nitrogen (74%) (23).

The species resembles *C. mucosalis* more closely than other campylobacteria and can be differentiated from that species by its inability to grow at 25°C and its resistance to cephalothin. At this time, *C. concisus* has not been isolated from anyone other than patients with periodontitis, but the significance of the organism in this condition has not been determined.

GROUP II. THE PSYCHROPHILIC SPECIES

Two groups of bacteria, named *C. nitrofigilis* (16) and *C. cryaerophila* (20), were assigned to the genus *Campylobacter*. Phenotypically they are quite distinct, and there are few traits that reveal the close relatedness indicated by the genetic analyses. Both species are oxidase, catalase, and nitrate positive and have cell morphology, flagellation, and motility as expected of species in the genus *Campylobacter*. A unique characteristic that does suggest relatedness is the ability of both species to grow at low temperatures and to grow optimally at temperatures below 37°C. Apart from this trait, there is little in common to the two species, and this fact has been a major drawback for proposing a new genus.

C. nitrofigilis

C. nitrofigilis, as its name implies, is capable of fixing nitrogen and is found in the roots of salt marsh grasses. Characteristics that distinguish this species from others in the genus are the production of a brown, water-soluble pigment from tryptophan and a requirement for sodium chloride. Additional details on the characteristics of *C. nitrofigilis* and methods for isolation are found in the report of McClung et al. (16). There is no evidence that *C. nitrofigilis* causes infections in humans or animals.

C. cryaerophila

C. cryaerophila resembles the true campylobacteria in morphology, motility, positive reactions for oxidase and catalase, and moles percent G+C content but differs in its ability to grow at low temperatures and in the presence of air after isolation. Most strains reduce nitrate and nitrite and are resistant to carbenicillin (64 μg/ml) (20).

The species has been isolated from the genital tracts and aborted fetuses of cows, pigs, sheep, and horses, from animal feces, and from milk from a cow with mastitis (20). Six human isolates of *C. cryaerophila* have been reported, but the methods for isolation were not stated and the identification was not subjected to confirmation by DNA hybridization tests. However, a fecal isolate confirmed by DNA hybridization tests to be *C. cryaerophila* has been recovered from a homosexual patient who complained of diarrhea and abdominal pain. The veterinary and medical significance of this species has not been determined.

Isolation and culture

A simplified procedure consisting of two steps has been developed for isolating *C. cryaerophila*. In the first step, leptospira medium (with 5-fluorouracil and 1% rabbit serum) is inoculated and incubated aerobically at 30°C. Growth of the organisms as a distinct zone below the surface of the medium may occur as soon as 24 to 48 h or after up to 4 to 5 weeks. In the second stage, the bacterial growth from the semisolid isolation medium is subcultured on blood agar supplemented with 7% lysed horse blood and carbenicillin (125 μg/ml). Plates are cultured at 30°C under microaerophilic conditions, and small colonies (1 mm in diameter) appear within 48 to 72 h. The microaerophilic atmosphere for this second step has been stressed as important for optimum rates of recovery.

It was generally believed that *C. cryaerophila* would not be isolated in the clinical laboratory because the isolation procedures described above are not routinely used, but a strain has been reported to have been isolated by using blood agar containing 6% lysed horse blood, vancomycin (10 mg/ml), polymyxin B (1,250 IU/ml), and trimethoprim (10 mg/ml). Colonies appeared on agar after 3 days of incubation under microaerophilic conditions at 37°C but not at 42°C. This finding indicates that the occurrence of *C. cryaerophila* in human stools is possible and that this possibility should be taken into consideration in the clinical laboratory.

GENUS *HELICOBACTER* AND RELATED CAMPYLOBACTERIA

The discovery in 1983 (15) that spiral-shaped organisms resembling campylobacteria could be isolated from the human stomach stimulated a renewed interest in the etiology of human type B gastritis and the role of these organisms in this disease. The organisms, now included in *Helicobacter pylori*, were given the name *C. pyloridis*, but this was later changed to *C. pylori* (of the pylorus). The primary criteria for assigning this group of bacteria to the genus *Campylobacter* were their spiral-shaped cells and their G+C content (36 to 37 mol%). A second group of spiral organisms, *Helicobacter mustelae*, isolated from the gastric mucosa of ferrets, was also included in the genus *Campylobacter*, first as a subspecies of *C. pylori* and later as a separate species with the name *C. mustelae* (6). Phylogenetic studies have yielded convincing data that these two species are not true campylobacteria but are more closely related to *Wolinella succinogenes* (21, 22); however, a formal proposal for emending the description of the genus *Wolinella* to include them has yet to be published. On the other hand, Goodwin et al. (8), citing major differences between *Wolinella* species and these two species, proposed that they be placed in a separate new genus, *Helicobacter*. The final solution to this taxonomic problem will be determined by usage.

H. pylori (*C. pylori*)

Much discussion has centered on the role of *H. pylori* in human gastroduodenitis (15), and there is now convincing evidence that it is the etiological agent of antral (type B) gastritis. The organisms are found on the gastric mucosa and in the gastric crypts throughout the stomach and are protected by the mucous layer from gastric acid, to which they are susceptible. They may also occur in the duodenum, but in this site they are associated with metaplastic gastric mucosa. *H. pylori* organisms are not invasive and have not been isolated from the bloodstream, but since they do not grow in commercial blood culture systems their role in bacteremias is inconclusive. Although there is strong circumstantial evidence that *H. pylori* may have a role in the etiology of the gastric and duodenal ulcer and nonulcer dyspepsia, unequivocal evidence has not been forthcoming.

Phenotypic characteristics that separate *H. pylori* from *Campylobacter* species include a smooth cell surface (in contrast to the rugose surface of *C. jejuni*), possession of polar tufts of four to six sheathed flagella, production of urease, and unique fatty acid profiles. The habitat of the organisms appears to be the human stomach; nonhuman sources have not been identified. The frequency of presence in the human population increases with age and varies among groups of different ethnic origins. There are higher incidences among family members and institutions for handicapped patients, suggesting person-to-person spread of the organism.

Isolation and identification of *H. pylori*

Specimens of gastric biopsies, brushings, or aspirate have been used for the detection of *H. pylori*. Of these, the biopsy produces the most reliable results. The organisms may be detected in stained smears, by phase-contrast microscopy, by the production of urease (a presumptive test), and by isolation through culture. The most widely used stains for examining biopsy material are Giemsa, hematoxylin and eosin, and the Warthin-Starry silver stain, but a number of other staining procedures have also been tried and are under evaluation. The three stains produce satisfactory results; however, the Warthin-Starry stain is complex, and silver precipitates may be confused with the bacteria. The Giemsa stain with minor modification (S. F. Gray, J. I. Wyatt, and B. J. Rathbone, Letter, J. Clin. Pathol. **39:**1279, 1986) is simpler and has been recommended for routine examination of biopsy specimens.

H. pylori organisms are prolific producers of urease, and this property is made use of in indirect tests by placing the macerated biopsy specimen into urea broth or Christensen urea agar. A change in color of the medium to alkalinity is a positive test for urease. This is a rapid presumptive test only, and isolation of the bacteria is necessary for confirmation.

The biopsy material is minced or homogenized in 0.9% saline inoculated on the surface of isolation media and incubated microaerophilically at 37°C for up to 7 days (most isolates are seen in 3 to 4 days). There are notable differences in media recipes for isolating and culturing *H. pylori*, and it is clear that the ideal medium remains to be developed. Skirrow campylobacter medium, chocolate agar, and Marshall brain heart infusion medium with horse blood have been used. The antibiotics for isolation of *C. jejuni* are not suitable for isolation of *H. pylori*. Goodwin et al. (9) found that Marshall medium with vancomycin (6 mg/liter), nalidixic acid (20 mg/liter), and amphotericin (2 mg/liter) was more satisfactory than media with the concentrations cited in the original formulation. Fresh media and high humidity are essential for effective recovery of *H. pylori*. Sodium metabisulfite in the FBP supplement (ferrous sulfate, sodium metabisulfite, and sodium pyruvate) added to media for isolation of *C. jejuni* was found to be inhibitory to *H. pylori* (9). As is the case with media, there are marked differences in the compositions of the microaerophilic atmospheres used for culturing *H. pylori*. Concentrations ranging from 7 to 12% carbon dioxide, 0 to 85% hydrogen, and 0 to 85% nitrogen have been reported. Generally, the atmosphere is produced in anaerobic jars with commercial gas-generating envelopes or by evacuating the air and replacing it with a mixture of gases that leads to a final concentration of 5 to 6% for oxygen.

After an incubation period of 3 to 4 days or up to 7 days, the translucent colonies of *H. pylori*, 1 to 2 mm in diameter, are observed. They are identified as oxidase and catalase positive gram-negative spiral bacteria with a characteristic rapid urease. The organisms also produce alkaline phosphatase, γ-glutamylaminopeptidase, and leucine aminopeptidase.

For a noninvasive test for the presence of *H. pylori* in the stomach, patients are administered [^{14}C]urea or [^{13}C]urea, and the production of labeled carbon dioxide in breath samples is analyzed by liquid scintillation or mass spectrometry (11). This urea breath test is recommended for diagnosis, for follow-up of patients after treatment, and for examination of populations in epidemiological studies.

ELISA is the most commonly used technique for serodiagnosis of *H. pylori*. Either an acid-glycine-extracted antigenic preparation from one or more strains or a crude preparation of urease protein is used as the test antigen. A serotyping scheme to differentiate strains for epidemiological investigations has not yet been developed. Currently, bacterial chromosomal DNA restriction endonuclease digest analysis is the technique most frequently used for differentiation.

H. pylori is susceptible to a wide range of antibiotics including erythromycin, tetracycline, penicillin, gentamicin, cephalothin, clindamycin, ciprofloxacin, nitrofurantoin, and rifampin, but is resistant to cefsulodin, nalidixic acid, sulfonamides, trimethoprim, sulfamethoxazole, and vancomycin. Of the agents used for treatment of ulcer disease, it is susceptible to bismuth subcitrate and resistant to cimetidine, ranitidine, and sucralfate at the levels used (17). Many antibiotics with in vitro activity against *H. pylori* are ineffective in vivo, and the most appropriate antibiotic therapy for *H. pylori* remains to be determined by controlled clinical trials.

H. mustelae (*C. mustelae*)

Bacteria resembling *H. pylori* but isolated only from normal and inflamed mucosa of ferrets (*Mustela putorius furo*) were isolated in 1986 and recognized as a new species in 1989 (6). The bacteria resemble *H. pylori* but differ in their ability to reduce nitrate, susceptibility to nalidixic acid, resistance to cephalothin, and the possession of both lateral and polar sheathed flagella. Gastric biopsy specimens taken by endoscopy, at surgery, or at necropsy are examined for mucus-associated bacteria by the modified Giemsa stain (Gray et al., J. Clin. Pathol., 1986). For isolation, homogenized biopsy specimens are inoculated on selective blood agar media and incubated at 37°C for 5 days in microaerophilic atmospheres containing hydrogen. The isolated bacteria are curved or spiral-shaped gram-negative rods with positive reactions for catalase and oxidase and rapid urease production. It has been postulated that since gastritis and ulcers commonly occur in the ferret, this animal may represent an ideal model for investigating the development of these gastric disorders and their therapeutic management.

CAMPYLOBACTERIA RELATED TO THE GENUS *HELICOBACTER*

C. cinaedi and *C. fennelliae*

C. cinaedi and *C. fennelliae* were discovered during investigations of the etiology of enteritis, proctitis, and proctocolitis in homosexual men (33). Since then the species have been obtained from the blood of bacteremic patients, and *C. cinaedi* has been found as normal intestinal flora of the Syrian hamster. The organisms were assigned to the genus *Campylobacter* on the basis of their phenotype, cell morphology, and moles percent G+C content (33). However, it has been demonstrated that *C. cinaedi* and *C. fennelliae* are more closely related to *H. pylori* and to *W. succinogenes* than to other species in the genus *Campylobacter* (32). Moreover, like the species in the genus *Helicobacter*, they possess sheathed flagella (12); a proposal to transfer the two species to the genus *Helicobacter* is likely to be forthcoming in the near future.

By using DNA probes, it was shown that *C. cinaedi* consists of two groups, originally designated CLO-1A (strains isolated from both symptomatic and asymptomatic individuals) and CLO-1B (strains isolated from symptomatic patients). The two groups can be differentiated by phenotypic tests. *C. fennelliae* organisms (formerly CLO-2 strains) were isolated only from symptomatic patients.

Methods for isolating thermophilic campylobacteria are inappropriate for isolating *C. cinaedi* and *C. fennelliae*. A preferred selective isolation medium is *Brucella* agar base with sheep blood (10%), vancomycin (10 mg/liter), polymyxin (2,500 IU/liter), trimethoprim (5 mg/liter), and amphotericin (2 mg/liter). Incubation is at 37°C for 7 days under a microaerophilic atmosphere containing hydrogen obtained with a gas-generating envelope without catalyst (33).

C. cinaedi and *C. fennelliae* are gram-negative, urease-negative, catalase- and oxidase-positive slender, curved, spiral-shaped, or occasionally straight rods. Coccoid forms may occur in older cultures. The bacteria are rapidly motile, grow at 25 or 42°C, and are susceptible to nalidixic acid. *C. fennelliae* is susceptible to cephalothin, whereas *C. cinaedi* shows intermediate zones of inhibition. *C. cinaedi* reduces nitrate, whereas *C. fennelliae* does not, and has colonies with an odor of hypochlorite (33).

OTHER SPIRAL-SHAPED BACTERIA

W. succinogenes

W. succinogenes (formerly *Vibrio succinogenes*) is of interest from a taxonomic standpoint. *H. pylori* is genetically more closely related to *W. succinogenes* than it is to the true *Campylobacter* species (21, 32). It is however, readily differentiated from *H. pylori* on the basis of phenotypic characteristics. The cells are helical, curved, or straight, display rapid, darting motility by means of single polar unsheathed flagella (30), and are oxidase, catalase, and urease negative. The G+C content of the DNA is 46 to 49 mol%. *W. succinogenes* occurs in the bovine rumen; there are no reports of its isolation from humans.

"Gastrospirillum hominis"

The name *"Gastrospirillum hominis"* was proposed by McNulty et al. (18) for unculturable helix-shaped bacteria possessing bipolar lophotrichous sheathed flagella. The bacteria were detected by microscopic examination of stained biopsy specimens in six patients with chronic active gastritis in the absence of *H. pylori*. One biopsy was positive in the rapid urease test, and antibodies against urease were detected in other patients. The clinical significance of this species and other gastric spiral bacteria not fitting existing systems of classification will no doubt be the subject of further studies.

ADDENDUM IN PROOF

A recent proposed revision in nomenclature recommends that *Campylobacter laridis* be revised to *Campylobacter lari* (A. von Graevenitz, Int. J. Syst. Bacteriol. **40:**211, 1990).

LITERATURE CITED

1. **Blaser, M. J., I. D. Berkowitz, F. M. La Force, J. Cravens, L. B. Reller, and W.-L. L. Wang.** 1979. *Campylobacter* enteritis: clinical and epidemiological features. Ann. Intern. Med. **91:**179–185.
2. **Bolton, F. J., D. N. Hutchinson, and D. Coates.** 1984. Blood-free selective medium for isolation of *Campylobacter jejuni* from feces. J. Clin. Microbiol. **19:**169–171.
3. **Bolton, F. J., D. N. Hutchinson, and G. Parker.** 1988. Reassessment of selective agars and filtration techniques for isolation of *Campylobacter* species from faeces. Eur. J. Clin. Microbiol. Infect. Dis. **7:**155–160.
4. **Bolton, F. J., and L. Robertson.** 1982. A selective medium for isolating *Campylobacter jejuni/coli*. J. Clin. Pathol. **35:** 462–467.
5. **Cover, T. L., and M. J. Blaser.** 1989. The pathobiology of *Campylobacter* infections in humans. Annu. Rev. Med. **40:** 269–285.
6. **Fox, J. G., T. Chilvers, C. S. Goodwin, N. S. Taylor, P. Edmonds, L. I. Sly, and D. J. Brenner.** 1989. *Campylobacter mustelae*, a new species resulting from the elevation of *Campylobacter pylori* subsp. *mustelae* to species status. Int. J. Syst. Bacteriol. **39:**301–303.
7. **Gebhart, C. J., P. Edmonds, G. E. Ward, H. J. Kurtz, and D. J. Brenner.** 1985. *"Campylobacter hyointestinalis"* sp. nov.: a new species of *Campylobacter* found in the intestines of pigs and other animals. J. Clin. Microbiol. **21:** 715–720.
8. **Goodwin, C. S., J. A. Armstrong, T. Chilvers, M. Peters, M. D. Collins, L. Sly, W. McConnell, and W. E. S. Harper.** 1989. Transfer of *Campylobacter pylori* and *Campylobacter mustelae* to *Helicobacter* gen. nov. as *Helicobacter pylori* comb. nov. and *Helicobacter mustelae* comb. nov., respectively. Int. J. Syst. Bacteriol. **39:**397–405.
9. **Goodwin, C. S., E. Blincow, J. R. Warren, T. E. Waters, C. R. Sanderson, and L. Easton.** 1985. Evaluation of cultural techniques for isolating *Campylobacter pyloridis* from

endoscopic biopsies or gastric mucosa. J. Clin. Pathol. **38:** 1127–1131.

10. **Goossens, H., M. De Boeck, and J. P. Butzler.** 1983. A new selective medium for the isolation of *Campylobacter jejuni* from human feces. Eur. J. Clin. Microbiol. **2:**389–394.
11. **Graham, D. Y., P. D. Klein, D. J. Evans, L. C. Alpert, A. R. Opekun, and T. W. Boutton.** 1987. *Campylobacter pylori* detected non invasively by the ^{13}C-urea breath test. Lancet **i:**1174–1177.
12. **Han, Y.-H., R. M. Smibert, and N. R. Krieg.** 1989. Occurrence of sheathed flagella in *Campylobacter cinaedi* and *Campylobacter fennelliae.* Int. J. Syst. Bacteriol. **39:** 488–490.
13. **Karmali, M. A., A. E. Simor, M. Roscoe, P. C. Fleming, S. S. Smith, and J. Lane.** 1986. Evaluation of a blood-free, charcoal-based, selective medium for the isolation of *Campylobacter* organisms from feces. J. Clin. Microbiol. **23:**456–459.
14. **Karmali, M. A., and M. B. Skirrow.** 1984. Taxonomy of the genus *Campylobacter,* p. 1–20. *In* J.-P. Butzler (ed.), *Campylobacter* infection in man and animals. CRC Press, Inc., Boca Raton, Fla.
15. **Marshall, B.** 1983. Growth of S-shaped bacteria from gastric antrum. Lancet **i:**1273–1275.
16. **McClung, C. R., D. G. Patriquin, and R. E. Davis.** 1983. *Campylobacter nitrofigilis* sp. nov., a nitrogen-fixing bacterium associated with roots of *Spartina alterniflora* Loisel. Int. J. Syst. Bacteriol. **33:**605–612.
17. **McNulty, C. A. M.** 1989. Bacteriological and pharmacological basis for the treatment of *Campylobacter pylori* infection. Gastroenterol. Clin. Biol. **13:**96B–100B.
18. **McNulty, C. A. M., J. Dent, A. Curry, J. S. Uff, G. A. Ford, M. G. L. Gear, and S. P. Wilkinson.** 1989. New spiral bacterium in gastric mucosa. J. Clin. Pathol. **42:**585–591.
19. **Megraud, F., D. Chevrier, N. Desplaces, A. Sedallian, and J. L. Guesdon.** 1988. Urease-positive thermophilic campylobacter (*Campylobacter laridis* variant) isolated from an appendix and from human feces. J. Clin. Microbiol. **26:**1050–1051.
20. **Neill, S. D., J. N. Campbell, J. J. O'Brien, S. T. C. Weatherup, and W. A. Ellis.** 1985. Taxonomic position of *Campylobacter cryaerophila* sp. nov. Int. J. Syst. Bacteriol. **35:** 342–356.
21. **Romaniuk, P. J., B. Zoltowska, T. J. Trust, D. J. Lane, G. J. Olsen, N. R. Pace, and D. A. Stahl.** 1987. *Campylobacter pylori,* the spiral bacterium associated with human gastritis, is not a true *Campylobacter* sp. J. Bacteriol. **169:** 2137–2141.
22. **Roop, R. M., II, R. M. Smibert, J. L. Johnson, and N. R. Krieg.** 1984. Differential characteristics of catalase-positive campylobacters correlated with DNA homology groups. Can. J. Microbiol. **30:**938–951.
23. **Roop, R. M., II, R. M. Smibert, J. L. Johnson, and N. R. Krieg.** 1985. DNA homology studies of the catalase-negative campylobacters and *"Campylobacter fecalis,"* an emended description of *Campylobacter sputorum,* and proposal of the neotype strain of *Campylobacter sputorum.* Can. J. Microbiol. **31:**823–831.
24. **Sandstedt, K., J. Ursing, and M. Walder.** 1983. Thermotolerant *Campylobacter.* with no or weak catalase activity isolated from dogs. Curr. Microbiol. **8:**209–213.
25. **Skirrow, M. B.** 1977. Campylobacter enteritis: a "new" disease. Br. Med. J. **2:**9–11.
26. **Smibert, R. M.** 1981. The genus *Campylobacter,* p. 609–617. *In* M. P. Starr (ed.), The prokaryotes. A handbook on habitats, isolation and identification of bacteria. Springer-Verlag, New York.
27. **Smibert, R. M.** 1984. Genus *Campylobacter,* p. 111–118. *In* N. R. Krieg and J. G. Holt (ed.), Bergey's manual of systematic bacteriology, vol. 1. The Williams & Wilkins Co., Baltimore.
28. **Steele, T. W., and S. N. McDermott.** 1984. Technical note: the use of membrane filters applied directly to the surface of agar plates for the isolation of *Campylobacter jejuni* from feces. Pathology **16:**263–265.
29. **Steele, T. W., and R. J. Owen.** 1988. *Campylobacter jejuni* subsp. *doylei* subsp. nov., a subspecies of nitrate-negative campylobacters isolated from human clinical specimens. Int. J. Syst. Bacteriol. **38:**316–318.
30. **Tanner, A. C. R., S. Badger, C.-H. Lai, M. A. Listgarten, R. A. Visconti, and S. S. Socransky.** 1981. *Wolinella* gen. nov., *Wolinella succinogenes* (*Vibrio succinogenes* Wolin et al.) comb. nov. and description of *Bacteroides gracilis* sp. nov., *Wolinella recta* sp. nov., *Campylobacter concisus* sp. nov., and *Eikenella corrodens* from humans with periodontal disease. Int. J. Syst. Bacteriol. **31:**432–445.
31. **Tanner, A. C. R., C. Haffer, G. T. Bratthall, R. A. Visconti, and S. S. Socransky.** 1979. A study of the bacteria associated with advancing periodontitis in man. J. Clin. Periodontol. **6:**278–307.
32. **Thompson, L. M., III, R. M. Smibert, J. L. Johnson, and N. R. Krieg.** 1988. Phylogenetic study of the genus *Campylobacter.* Int. J. Syst. Bacteriol. **38:**190–200.
33. **Totten, P. A., C. L. Fennell, F. C. Tenover, J. M. Wezenberg, P. L. Perine, W. E. Stamm, and K. K. Holmes.** 1985. *Campylobacter cinaedi* (sp. nov.) and *Campylobacter fennelliae* (sp. nov.): two new *Campylobacter* species associated with enteric disease in homosexual men. J. Infect. Dis. **151:**131–139.
34. **Véron, M., and R. Chatelain.** 1973. Taxonomic study of the genus *Campylobacter* Sebald and Véron and designation of the neotype strain for the type species, *Campylobacter fetus* (Smith and Taylor) Sebald and Véron. Int. J. Syst. Bacteriol. **23:**122–134.

Chapter 40

Miscellaneous Gram-Negative Bacteria

M. JOHN PICKETT, DANNIE G. HOLLIS, AND EDWARD J. BOTTONE

Gram-negative aerobic bacilli recovered from clinical specimens can be divided into four groups: (i) nonfastidious, fermentative, facultatively anaerobic, oxidase-negative bacilli (members of the family *Enterobacteriaceae*, or enteric bacilli); (ii) nonfastidious, obligately aerobic, nonfermentative bacilli (NFB) (Table 1); (iii) fastidious haemophilic bacilli of *Haemophilus* species; and (iv) unusual bacilli (UB) (Table 2).

These groups are somewhat artificial but are meaningful in terms of methods used for processing their members. Of all aerobic gram-negative rods isolated from clinical specimens, 68 to 78% are enteric bacilli, 12 to 16% are NFB, 8 to 15% are haemophilic bacilli, and fewer than 1% are UB.

Being obligate aerobes and frequently strongly proteolytic, the NFB cannot be processed with the battery of media used for enteric bacilli. However, given appropriate media and methods, most NFB can readily be identified. NFB grow well on the slant but do not acidify the butt of Kligler iron agar (KIA) and triple sugar iron agar (TSIA) media. In contrast, nearly all species within the other three groups either fail to grow on KIA or, if they grow, acidify the butt of the tubed medium. Excepting an occasional nonpigmented strain of *Pseudomonas aeruginosa*, ready identification of NFB is particularly true for strains of the three most commonly encountered species, *P. aeruginosa*, *Acinetobacter baumannii* (*"A. anitratus"*), and *Xanthomonas* (*Pseudomonas*) *maltophilia*. These three species represent nearly 70% of all NFB recovered from clinical specimens (Table 3).

The term UB is used loosely to denote gram-negative rods other than enteric bacilli, *Haemophilus* species, and the NFB. Most isolates of UB, but not some *Aeromonas* species, *Pasteurella* species, and *Vibrio* species, are in fact rarely encountered in clinical specimens. Some UB (*Aeromonas* species, *Plesiomonas* species, and *Vibrio* species), like enteric bacilli, are fermentative and nonfastidious but, differing from enteric bacilli, are oxidase positive. Some (*Campylobacter* species and *Eikenella* species), like some NFB (*Moraxella* species and some pseudomonads), fail to acidify glucose but, unlike most NFB, are fastidious. Several (*Capnocytophaga* species, *Cardiobacterium* species, and some *Brucella* species), differing from both enteric bacilli and NFB, present little or no growth on aerobically incubated, 48-h blood agar (BA) plates. All share one feature: they are encountered infrequently in clinical specimens and may also easily escape detection.

NONFERMENTERS

Materials and methods

The protocols of E. O. King and her successors at the Special Bacteriology Laboratory, Centers for Disease Control (CDC), Atlanta, Ga., are commonly used for identification of NFB. Selection of primary media for isolation depends on the specimen; they should include an aerobically incubated broth (for blood, cerebrospinal fluid, and aspirates) and, for other specimens, aerobically incubated blood and MacConkey agar plates. Initial incubation should be at 35 to 37°C, since most bacteria associated with humans grow better at this temperature than at either 30°C or room temperature (22 ± 2°C). However, an occasional NFB, particularly from an environmental specimen, may grow poorly at 35°C. Hence, a BA plate showing poor growth after 1 or 2 days at 35°C should be held an additional two days at room temperature. Any isolate showing better growth at room temperature than at 35°C should thereafter be processed at 30°C or room temperature.

Either of two approaches or a combination thereof may be used for identification of an NFB. Both approaches assume that an isolate under study is known to be an NFB; that is, it grew on the slant but did not acidify the butt of KIA (or TSIA) medium. The first approach, modified from that of Weaver and Hollis (see Clark et al. [10]), uses the oxidase reaction and growth on MacConkey agar but not acidification of glucose. This omission is admissible since more than 90% of oxidase-positive strains will be glucose positive. Results from screening tests determine which batteries of media (Table 4) should be used to complete an identification. The OF (oxidation-fermentation) basal medium for carbohydrates should be that with phenol red indicator; OF media with bromothymol blue indicator are inhibitory for some nonfermenters (43). The Moeller arginine, lysine, and ornithine media (1 ml per tube) must be heavily inoculated (0.5 to 1.0 mm^3 of cells). The 0.4% agar in enteric motility media is usually not admissible for NFB; either OF basal medium or motility nitrate medium (both contain 0.3% agar) may be used. Inclusion of 0.1% potassium nitrate in the latter medium promotes growth of many NFB and also detects denitrifying strains. Neither of these two soft agar media is as sensitive as a hanging-drop preparation for detecting motility.

The second approach for processing NFB uses the oxidase reaction, acidification of glucose, and motility as screening tests. Generous inocula from a KIA slant are used for a motility nitrate stab and an aerobic low-peptone (ALP) glucose slant (44). Both motility and acidification of glucose are commonly evident within 2 h; however, as screening tests both media are incubated 6 h at 35°C. The ALP basal medium for carbohydrates is more sensitive than an OF basal medium and can be used for fastidious bacteria as well as for nonfermenters. The slant of fluorescence-lactose-denitrification medium is acidified within 48 h, and usually within 24 h, by all lactose-positive acinetobacters (and

TABLE 1. Nonfermentative gram-negative bacilli[a]

Genus, species, and group	Synonyms[b]	% of stains positive		
		Oxidase	Growth on MacConkey agar	Glucose, acidified
Acinetobacter spp.				
Glucose-positive (501)[c]	*A. anitratus, A. calcoaceticus, A. haemolyticus, Herellea* (Table 6)	0	100	100
Glucose negative (253)	*A. lwoffi, A. calcoaceticus* subsp. *lwoffi, A. alcaligenes, Mima polymorpha*	0	97	0
Agrobacterium radiobacter (38)	*A. tumefaciens*, Vd-3[d] (Table 7)	100	100	100
Alcaligenes faecalis[e]	*A. odorans* (49)[c] (Table 10)	100	100	0
—[e]	*Alcaligenes faecalis* (69)	100	100	0
A. piechaudii[f]	*A. faecalis* type I	100	100	0
A. xylosoxidans subsp. *denitrificans*	*A. denitrificans* (34)	100	100	0
A. xylosoxidans subsp. *xylosoxidans*	*Achromobacter xylosoxidans*, IIIa and IIIb (135) (Table 7)	100	100	78
EF-4b (34)		100	71	96
EO-2 (93)		100	74	100
EO-3 (5)		100	100	100
Flavobacterium breve (3)	*Bacillus brevis, Bacterium canale, Pseudobacterium brevis* (Table 8)	100	100	100
F. indologenes	*Flavobacterium balustinum, F. gleum*, IIb (155)	96	63	98
F. meningosepticum (148)	IIa	99	92	99
F. multivorum (22)	*Sphingobacterium multivorum*, IIk-2	100	100	100
F. odoratum (74)	M-4f	99	96	0
F. spiritivorum (11)	*Sphingobacterium spiritivorum*, IIk-3	100	55	100
F. thalpophilum[g]	*Sphingobacterium thalpophilum*, IIk-2	100	100	100
F. yabuuchiae[h]	IIk-2	100	100	100
Moraxella atlantae (23)	M-3 (Table 9)	100	100	0
M. lacunata (25)	*Moraxella liquefaciens*	100	4	0
M. nonliquefaciens (243)		100	10	0
M. osloensis (163)	*Moraxella duplex, Mima polymorpha*	100	70	0
M. phenylpyruvica (50)	*Mima polymorpha*, M-2	100	86	0
M-5 (59)	*Moraxella*-like, *Neisseria parelongata*	100	62	0
M-6 (40)	*Moraxella*-like, *Neisseria elongata*	100	50	0
Ochrobactrum anthropi	*Achromobacter*, Vd (71) (Table 7)	100	100	99
Oligella ureolytica	IVe (37) (Table 10)	100	89	0
O. urethralis	*Moraxella urethralis* (22) (Table 9)	100	96	0
Psychrobacter immobilis[i]	*Micrococcus cryophilus* (Table 7)	100	92	85
Sphingobacterium mizutae[j]	*Flavobacterium mizutaii* (Table 8)	100	0	100
Weeksella virosa	*Flavobacterium* IIf (87) (Table 8)	100	10	0
W. zoohelcum	*Flavobacterium* IIj (41)	100	2	0
IIe (18)	*Flavobacterium* IIe	88	7	100
IIh (21)	*Flavobacterium* IIh	100	0	100
IIi (23)	*Flavobacterium* IIi	100	0	100
IVc-2		100	100	0

[a] Exclusive of the genera *Alteromonas, Chryseomonas, Flavimonas, Methylobacterium, Pseudomonas* (chapter 41), and *Bordetella* (chapter 46).
[b] For additional synonyms, see Gilardi (18).
[c] Numbers in parentheses are the number of strains examined at the CDC (10).
[d] Group designation of the CDC.
[e] The CDC's *Alcaligenes odorans* is now *Alcaligenes faecalis* (31); the CDC's *Alcaligenes faecalis* is not recognized by *Bergey's Manual.*
[f] Data for seven strains are from Kiredjian et al. (33).
[g] Data for seven strains are from Holmes et al. (24).
[h] Data for two strains are from Holmes et al. (28).
[i] Data for 13 strains are from Moss et al. (36).
[j] Data for five strains are from Yabuuchi et al. (66).

also by *Pseudomonas cepacia*). Other NFB rarely acidify this medium. The medium contains nitrite as well as nitrate and hence will show gas production with most strains of *Alcaligenes faecalis* (formerly *A. odorans*), *Flavobacterium odoratum*, and *Oligella* (*Moraxella*) *urethralis*. MBM acetate is the mineral base medium of Gilardi (19) modified by addition of 0.001% bromothymol blue and 0.1% sodium acetate trihydrate (43). This medium is alkalinized by *Moraxella osloensis* and *Oligella urethralis* but not by other moraxellae. Any strongly oxidase-positive, nonmotile NFB is a potential indole-positive flavobacterium. When cell paste for a spot indole test is taken from a 2-day BA plate, a positive test is always reliable and a negative test is usually reliable. However, a tube test (either tryptone broth or buffered tryptophan) for indole should be made when the spot test is negative. Quality control for the spot test is important; the cell paste must be taken from a medium containing adequate tryptophan. After the screening tests listed in Table 4 have been determined, initial grouping of an NFB can be made by using the key in Table 5 as a guide. As noted in Table 4, several

TABLE 2. Unusual gram-negative bacilli[a]

Organism	No. of strains	Capnophilic	% of strains positive				See Table:
			Catalase	Oxidase	TSIA, acid		
					Slant	Butt	
Actinobacillus actinomycetemcomitans	120	+	99	19[b]	100	100	15
A. equuli	19	−	73	100	100	100	13
A. lignieresii	30	−	89	100	100	100	13
A. suis	33	−	85	100	100	100	13
A. (Pasteurella) ureae	97	−	63	99	100	99	13
Capnocytophaga spp.							
DF-1	155	+	7[c]	7	73	55	15
DF-2	27	+	100	96	17	15	15
Cardiobacterium hominis (IId)	65	+	1	100	93	84	15
Chromobacterium violaceum	37	−	97	67	8	94	16
DF-3	21	+	0	0	95	100	15
EF-4a	97	−	100	100	3	73	16
Eikenella corrodens	506	+	8	100	0	0	15
HB-5	44	+	2	54	100	98	15
Kingella denitrificans	60	−	10	100	2	0	16
K. indologenes	6	−	0	100	100	100	16
K. kingae	33	−	0	100	32	12	16
Pasteurella aerogenes	16	−	100	100	94	100	13
P. gallinarum	10	−	100	90	100	100	13
P. haemolytica	67	−	86	95	100	100	13
P. multocida	306[d]	−	98	97	99	99	13
Pasteurella "n. sp. 1" (*P. dagmatis*)	91	−	96	98	100	100	13
P. pneumotropica	107	−	100	99	100	97	13

[a] Exclusive of the genera *Aeromonas, Plesiomonas* (chapter 38), *Brucella* (chapter 44), *Bordetella* (chapter 46), *Francisella* (chapter 43), *Campylobacter* (chapter 39), *Gardnerella* (chapter 48), *Haemophilus* (chapter 45), *Vibrio* (chapter 37), and *Bartonellaceae.* Data from Clark et al. (10). See also Mutters et al. (37), Schlater et al. (50), and Table 14 for newly described species of pasteurellae. Not all strains were tested for some features.

[b] 95% of the strains were either oxidase negative or only weakly positive.

[c] 98% of the strains were either catalase negative or only weakly positive.

[d] *P. multocida* of the CDC charts (10) may contain more than one species (37).

of the commercial kits for nonfermenters give reliable results with oxidase- and glucose-positive NFB. However, these kits usually do not perform well with glucose-negative NFB. Finally, not only commercial kits (40) but also gas-liquid chromatography of cellular fatty acids (59, 63), though not described in this chapter, are increasingly being used for identification of clinical isolates.

Acinetobacter

Acinetobacters are nonmotile rods, 1 to 1.5 μm in diameter and 1.5 to 2.5 μm in length, becoming spherical in the stationary phase of growth. Recent isolates from clinical specimens are usually coccobacillary in smears prepared from 1-day BA plates. However, when they are grown in the presence of penicillin or repeatedly subcultured, rods will be evident in stained preparations. All strains grow well at 30°C, and most also grow at 35°C. All are oxidase negative and catalase positive. Most strains are nutritionally independent (grow well on MBM acetate).

Acinetobacters are widely distributed in nature and as normal flora of human skin. They are opportunistic pathogens and have been recovered from a variety of clinical specimens (2, 54, 55). They are resistant to many antimicrobial agents (16, 49, 55, 60). Most strains grow well on MacConkey agar. Colonies on 1-day BA plates are 1 to 3 mm in diameter. Other features are presented in Table 6.

Only one species of *Acinetobacter, A. calcoaceticus,* is described in *Bergey's Manual* (29). However, past common practice in clinical laboratories was to assign isolates to one of four biovars, "*A. anitratus*" (glucose positive), "*A. haemolyticus*" (hemolytic "*A. anitratus*"), "*A. lwoffi*" (glucose negative), and "*A. alcaligenes*" (hemolytic and gelatin-positive "*A. lwoffi*") (17).

Recent DNA hybridization studies (4, 6) have identified 17 hybridization groups (genospecies) within this genus: *A. baumannii, A. calcoaceticus, A. haemolyticus, A. johnsonii, A. junii, A. lwoffii,* and 11 unnamed genospecies. Former biovar "*A. anitratus*" encompasses three of the genospecies, *A. calcoaceticus* (no growth at 41°C), *A. baumannii* (growth at 44°C), and unnamed genospecies 3 (growth at 41°C but not at 44°C). Most strains formerly assigned to biovar "*A. lwoffi*" are those of genospecies 8 and 9, now named *A. lwoffii.* Finally, most hemolytic strains of *Acinetobacter* species, whether glucose negative or glucose positive, belong to genospecies 4, now *A. haemolyticus,* but a minority of hemolytic strains belong to unnamed genospecies 6. In summary, in clinical laboratories most glucose-positive and nonhemolytic acinetobacters are *A. baumannii,* but a few are *A. calcoaceticus;* most nonhemolytic and glucose-negative acinetobacters are *A. lwoffii,* and most hemolytic acinetobacters are *A. haemolyticus.* Other genospecies are less frequently encountered in clinical specimens. For *A. baumannii,* 17 biotypes, based on utilization of six substrates and useful for epidemiological studies, have been established (5).

"Achromobacter" (*Ochrobactrum*), *Agrobacterium*, and saccharolytic *Alcaligenes*

All are oxidase positive, saccharolytic, and peritrichously flagellated. All are widely distributed in the environment and are opportunistic pathogens.

TABLE 3. Incidence of nonfermenters in clinical bacteriology[a]

Organism	No. of strains	% for each species	Cumulative %
Pseudomonas aeruginosa	2,949	45.9	45.9
Pyocyanogenic	2,876 (45%)		
Apyocyanogenic	73 (1%)		
Acinetobacter spp., glucose positive	1,099	17.1	62.9
Xanthomonas (Pseudomonas) maltophilia	417	6.5	69.4
Acinetobacter spp., glucose negative	209	3.2	72.6
Pseudomonas putida	207	3.2	75.9
Flavobacterium IIb	163	2.5	78.4
Pseudomonas fluorescens	159	2.5	90.9
P. cepacia	154	2.4	83.3
P. stutzeri	127	2.0	85.3
Moraxella spp. and *Oligella urethralis*	95	1.5	86.8
Pseudomonas paucimobilis	79	1.2	88.0
P. acidovorans	76	1.2	89.2
Alcaligenes faecalis	73	1.1	90.3
A. xylosoxidans subsp. *xylosoxidans*	52	0.8	91.1
Flavimonas oryzihabitans (Ve-2)	51	0.8	91.9
P. pseudoalcaligenes	47	0.7	92.6
P. alcaligenes	46	0.7	93.3
"*Alcaligenes faecalis* types I and II"[b]	45	0.7	94.0
Shewanella putrefaciens	44	0.7	94.7
Alcaligenes xylosoxidans subsp. *denitrificans*	38	0.6	95.3
Pseudomonas pickettii	37	0.6	95.9
P. diminuta	35	0.5	96.4
P. vesicularis	28	0.4	96.9
Flavobacterium multivorum	27	0.4	97.3
Weeksella virosa	24	0.4	97.7
Flavobacterium meningosepticum	20	0.3	98.0
Chryseomonas luteola (Ve-1)	16	0.2	98.2
Bordetella bronchiseptica	15	0.2	98.5
Agrobacterium	15	0.2	98.7
Flavobacterium odoratum	15	0.2	98.9
CDC group IVc-2	10	0.2	99.1
Oligella ureolytica	10	0.2	99.2
Pseudomonas testosteroni	9	0.1	99.4
Ochrobactrum anthropi (*Achromobacter* Vd-1)	9	0.1	99.5
Weeksella zoohelcum	8	0.1	99.6
Pseudomonas pseudomallei	7	0.1	99.8
Pseudomonas mendocina	6	0.1	99.8
Ochrobactrum anthropi (*Achromobacter* Vd-2)	4	0.1	99.9
Methylobacterium extorquens[c]	3	<0.1	100.0
Flavobacterium breve	3	<0.1	100.0

[a] Adapted from G. L. Gilardi, personal communication, 1980.
[b] See Table 10.
[c] The several synonyms include *Pseudomonas mesophilica* and *Protomonas extorquens* (18).

Achromobacter is not presently a recognized genus (31). *Achromobacter xylosoxidans* has been transferred to genus *Alcaligenes* as *A. xylosoxidans* subsp. *xylosoxidans* (31, 33), and "*Achromobacter*" sp. group Vd has been named *Ochrobactrum anthropi* (25). An individual cell of *O. anthropi* may bear polar, subpolar, or lateral flagella. Early tabulations from the CDC recognized two biotypes within the Vd group, Vd-1 (mannitol and sucrose negative) and Vd-2 (mannitol and sucrose positive). Lactose is never acidified. Nonpigmented *P. aeruginosa* can be confused with *O. anthropi;* however, the latter is acetamide and gelatin negative, whereas these

TABLE 4. Media for identification of nonfermenters[a]

Screening tests	Additional media or tests	Nonfermenter kit
Oxidase reaction and growth on MacConkey agar		
Oxidase negative, MacConkey positive	OF glucose, OF lactose, OF sucrose, motility, nitrate broth	
Oxidase positive, MacConkey positive	OF glucose, OF lactose, OF maltose, OF mannitol, OF sucrose, OF xylose, motility, nitrate broth, tryptone broth, urea	
Oxidase positive, MacConkey negative	OF glucose, OF lactose, OF mannitol, OF sucrose, motility, tryptone broth, urea	
Oxidase, motility, ALP glucose		
Oxidase negative	FLN slant, motility nitrate stab	Not needed
Oxidase positive, glucose positive	ALP lactose, ALP maltose, ALP mannitol, ALP sucrose, ALP xylose, esculin, nitrate broth, ALP urea, indole	Reliable
Oxidase positive, glucose negative, nonmotile	FLN slant, MBM acetate, gelatin broth, ALP citrate, ALP urea, nitrate broth, indole, catalase	Not reliable
Oxidase positive, glucose negative, motile	FLN, ALP acetamide, ALP allantoin, ALP histidine, ALP malonate, ALP saccharate, ALP urea	Not reliable

[a] Nonfermenters (NFB) are aerobic gram-negative rods that do not acidify the butt but do grow well on the slant of KIA and TSIA media. The oxidase-negative NFB include *Acinetobacter* spp., *Chryseomonas* (Ve-1), *Flavimonas* (Ve-2), and *Xanthomonas* (*Pseudomonas*) *maltophilia* (see chapter 41). Additional tests for acinetobacters are shown in Table 6. Tests for acidification of maltose and decarboxylation of lysine should be included if *X. maltophilia* is suspected. Most strains of Ve present yellow, "warty," and pitting colonies. OF, Oxidation-fermentation basal medium with phenol red; FLN, fluorescence-lactose-denitrification medium; ALP, aerobic low-peptone basal medium; MBM, mineral basal medium; MacConkey positive, growth on MacConkey agar medium.

TABLE 5. Key to identification of NFB (gram-negative rods that do not acidify the butt but grow well on the slant of KIA and TSIA media)[a]

Feature	Organisms
Ox+	
Mac+	
Glu+	
Motility+	*Agrobacterium* spp., *Alcaligenes xylosoxidans* subsp. *xylosoxidans*, *Ochrobactrum* (1% Glu−)
Motility−	EF-4b (4% Glu−), EO-2, EO-3, *Flavobacterium breve*, *Flavobacterium* group IIb (4% Ox−, 2% Glu−), *F. meningosepticum* (1% Ox− and Glu−, 8% Mac−), *F. multivorum*, *F. spiritivorum*, *F. thalpophilum*, *F. yabuuchiae*, *Psychrobacter* sp. (8% Mac−)
Glu−	
Motility+	*Alcaligenes faecalis*, "*A. faecalis* type II" (possible *Bordetella avium*), *A. piechaudii*, *A. xylosoxidans* subsp. *denitrificans* and subsp. *xylosoxidans*, *Oligella ureolytica*, IVc-2
Motility−	*Flavobacterium odoratum* (1% Ox−, 4% Mac−), *Moraxella atlantae*, *M. osloensis*, *M. phenylpyruvica*, *Oligella urethralis* (4% Mac−), *Psychrobacter* sp. (8% Mac−), M-5, M-6
Mac−	
Glu+	
Motility−	EF-4b, EO-2, *Flavobacterium* group IIb (4% Ox−, 2% Glu−), *F. mizutaii*, *F. spiritivorum*, IIe (7% Mac+), IIh, IIi
Glu−	
Motility+	*Oligella ureolytica*
Motility−	*Moraxella lacunata* (4% Mac+), *M. nonliquefaciens* (10% Mac+), *M. osloensis*, *M. phenylpyruvica*, *Weeksella virosa* (10% Mac+), *W. zoohelcum* (2% Mac+), M-5, M-6
Ox−	
Mac+	
Motility−	
Glu+	*Acinetobacter* spp.
Glu−	*Acinetobacter* spp. (3% Mac−)
Mac−, Motility−, Glu+	IIe (7% Mac+)

[a] See chapter 46 for *Bordetella* spp. and chapter 41 for *Chryseomonas*, *Flavimonas*, *Pseudomonas*, and *Xanthomonas* spp. Ox, Oxidase; Mac, growth on MacConkey agar medium; Glu, glucose; +, positive; −, negative.

two tests are usually positive with the former. Colonies of *O. anthropi* are usually less than 1 mm in diameter on 1-day BA plates and enlarge to ca. 2 mm on 2-day plates. *O. anthropi* is resistant to many antimicrobial agents but may be susceptible to amikacin, norfloxacin, tetracycline, and trimethoprim-sulfamethoxazole (49, 56, 61). For other features, see Table 7.

Agrobacterium (from agros, a field) species are primarily associated with tumors of plants (32). The species status of *Agrobacterium tumefaciens* and *A. radiobacter* is controversial. Oncogenic strains carry a tumor-inducing plasmid and are usually addressed as *A. tumefaciens.* Such strains, upon loss of the plasmid, are no longer pathogenic for plants and are frequently addressed as *A. radiobacter.* Most agrobacteria recovered from clinical specimens (CDC group Vd-3) belong to *A. radiobacter* biovar 1 (9, 32, 47). They have been associated with endocarditis, peritonitis, and septicemia. Most strains are susceptible to gentamicin, polymyxin B, and trimethoprim-sulfamethoxazole but may be resistant to other antimicrobial agents (9, 47, 61). All strains of biovar 1 grow at 35°C, and some also grow at 42°C; all produce 3-ketolactonate from lactose (10), and most reduce nitrate. Biovar 2 does not produce 3-ketolactonate and does not grow at 35°C. Most strains grow on MBM acetate (19). This taxon is exceptional in that it acidifies the entire battery of six sugars routinely used at the CDC (10). Stained preparations present cells 0.6 to 1 μm in diameter and 1.5 to 3 μm long, occurring singly or in pairs. Colonies on 1-day BA plates are ca 0.5 mm in diameter and enlarge to ca. 2 mm on 2-day plates.

Alcaligenes species appear in stained preparations as coccobacilli and rods, 0.5 to 1 μm in diameter and 0.5 to 2.6 μm long. Colonies are nonpigmented and similar in size to those of agrobacteria. At present, three species are recognized (31, 33): *A. faecalis* (equivalent to *A. odorans* on the CDC charts), *A. piechaudii* (*A. faecalis* on the CDC charts), and *A. xylosoxidans* (containing two subspecies, *denitrificans* and *xylosoxidans*). *A. faecalis*, *A. piechaudii*, and *A. xylosoxidans* subsp. *denitrificans* are nonsaccharolytic (see Table 10). *A. xylosoxidans* subsp. *xylosoxidans*, a saccharolytic taxon, has been recovered from both clinical and environmental specimens. It has been associated with septicemia, peritonitis, meningitis, and other focal infections. Most strains are resistant to aminoglycosides, chloramphenicol, and tetracycline but susceptible to trimethoprim-sulfamethoxazole and some of the newer penicillins (11, 49, 61). They can be confused with nonpigmented strains of *P. aeruginosa*, but the former are always mannitol and gelatin negative and are usually arginine dihydrolase negative, whereas the latter are always arginine dihydrolase positive and are usually mannitol and gelatin positive (10). Other features are presented in Table 7.

Groups EF-4b, EO-2, and EO-3 and *Psychrobacter*

All are nonmotile. The EF-4b group contains oxidase-, catalase-, and glucose-positive nonfermenters (Table 7). They do not appear to fit well into any named genus. They resemble pasteurellae in being coccobacillary or short rods, nonmotile, glucose positive, and associated with animal bites, but pasteurellae are fermentative and usually acidify sucrose. The microscopic morphology is also suggestive of acinetobacters, but the latter are always oxidase negative, whereas EF-4b is strongly oxidase positive. Their cellular fatty acid profile is suggestive of *Neisseria* species. Strains of EO-2 (EO for eugonic oxidizer) are also coccobacillary or short rods. They have been recovered from numerous body sites, particularly urine, eye, blood, and wounds (10). Recently, 28 of the CDC strains assigned to this group were identified as *Psychrobacter immobilis*, EO-2, and EO-3 by distinctive cellular fatty acid profiles and other phenotypic features (36). Only EO-3 was mannitol pos-

TABLE 6. Features for identification of *Acinetobacter* species[a]

Feature	% Positive strains of given genospecies[b]										
	1 (8)[c]	2 (121)	3 (15)	4 (23)	5 (17)	6 (3)	7 (23)	8/9 (34)	10 (4)	11 (4)	12 (3)
Gelatin, hydrolyzed	0	0	0	96	0	100	0	0	0	0	0
Glucose, acidified	100	95	100	52	0	66	0	6	100	0	33
Growth											
37°C	100	100	100	100	100	100	0	100	100	100	100
41°C	0	100	100	0	90	0	0	0	0	0	0
44°C	0	100	0	0	0	0	0	0	0	0	0
Hemolysis	0	0	0	100	0	100	0	0	0	0	0
Utilized											
trans-Aconitate	100	99	100	52	0	0	0	0	0	0	0
β-Alanine	100	95	94	0	0	0	0	0	100	100	0
DL-4-Aminobutyrate	100	100	100	100	88	0	35	40	100	100	100
Arginine	100	98	100	96	95	100	35	0	0	0	100
Azelate	100	90	100	0	0	0	0	100	50	25	100
Citrate	100	100	100	91	82	100	100	0	100	100	0
Glutarate	100	100	100	0	0	0	0	0	100	100	100
Histidine	100	98	94	96	100	100	0	0	100	100	0
DL-Lactate	100	100	100	0	100	0	100	100	100	100	100
D-Malate	0	98	100	96	100	66	22	76	100	100	0
Malonate	100	98	87	0	0	0	13	0	0	0	100

[a] Data from Bouvet and Grimont (4). Except where noted, all incubations were at 30°C.

[b] The numbered genospecies are based on DNA-DNA hybridizations. 1, *A. calcoaceticus;* 2, *A. baumannii;* 3, unnamed; 4, *A. haemolyticus;* 5, *A. junii;* 6, unnamed; 7, *A. johnsonii;* 8 and 9, *A. lwoffii;* 10, 11, and 12, unnamed. Approximate synonyms are *A. anitratus* for glucose-positive strains (*A. haemolyticus* if hemolytic) and *A. lwoffii* for glucose-negative strains (*A. alcaligenes* if hemolytic).

[c] Number in parentheses is number of strains examined.

itive and formed a yellow pigment. EO-2, but not *P. immobilis,* always formed O-shaped cells and always grew at 35°C.

Flavobacteria, *Weeksella,* and groups IIe, IIh, and IIi

All are nonmotile, oxidase-positive rods, but polar and lateral flagella have been seen on some strains of both *Flavobacterium meningosepticum* and *F. multivorum.* All are in the hospital environment and may be implicated in opportunistic infections. The indole-positive flavobacteria are saccharolytic, and the three named taxa (*F. breve, F. indologenes,* and *F. meningosepticum*) are usually strongly proteolytic; they display diffuse beta-hemolysis (proteolysis) on BA plates and rapidly hydrolyze gelatin. In contrast, the three indole-positive and unnamed taxa, IIe, IIh, and IIi, are usually gelatin negative. The indole-negative, sucrose-positive flavobacteria also differ from other flavobacteria in their cellular fatty acids, and this feature has led to the proposal that they be placed in a new genus, *Sphingobacterium* (66).

Strains of heterogeneous *Flavobacterium* species group IIb are more common in clinical specimens than all other flavobacteria combined (Table 3). Nearly all strains of IIb are strongly pigmented (yellow to orange) and indole positive (spot test) on 2-day BA plates (44). Other flavobacteria are not strongly pigmented on such plates. Colonies are smooth, 0.5 to 1.0 mm in diameter, and usually distinctly pigmented on 1-day BA plates. Colonies on 2-day plates are 1 to 2 mm in diameter. Indole-positive proteolytic strains and indole-negative nonproteolytic strains of flavobacteria are commonly resistant to many antimicrobial agents, including aminoglycosides; indole-positive nonproteolytic strains are less commonly resistant. Importantly, results from disk and MIC tests for sensitivity may differ (61). Other features are presented in Table 8. *F. indologenes* has been proposed as the binomial for some of the IIb group (66). However, present evidence suggests that both this and other binomials (*F. balustinum* and *F. gleum*) represent taxa within and not synonyms for IIb. Colonies of *F. meningosepticum* are smooth and 1 to 2 mm in diameter on 1-day BA plates. Colonies on 2-day plates are 2 to 3 mm in diameter, surrounded by zones of proteolysis, and may be weakly pigmented (yellow). Colonies of *F. odoratum* are spreading, pigmented (yellowish or tan), slightly rough, and 1 to 3 mm in diameter on 1-day BA plates; they enlarge to 2 to 5 mm on 2-day plates. Cultures of *F. odoratum* usually produce a fruity odor. Colonies of the IIk-2 and IIk-3 groups (*F. mizutaii, F. multivorum, F. spiritivorum, F. thalpophilum,* and *F. yabuuchiae*) are similar to those of *F. meningosepticum* on both 1- and 2-day BA plates. *F. spiritivorum* and *F. yabuuchiae* can be distinguished by DNA hybridization, but their biochemical profiles are similar (Table 8). However, the former but not the latter hydrolyzes 2-naphthyl phosphate (28).

The genus *Weeksella* was recently proposed to encompass two *Flavobacterium*-like taxa, groups IIf and IIj (26, 27), and additional *Weeksella*-like strains have been described (3). *Weeksella* species contain rods 0.7 µm in diameter and 2 to 3 µm long. They usually grow at both 35 and 42°C. They are obligatively aerobic, oxidase, catalase, and indole positive, and nonsaccharolytic. Colonies of *Weeksella virosa* (IIf) are 0.2 to 0.8 mm in diameter on 1-day BA plates and 2 to 3 mm on 2-day plates. Always on 2-day and usually also on 1-day plates, the growth as seen by reflected light is unique; it is softly butyrous to mucoid (virosa, slimy) and pale yellow-green. Most strains have been recovered, presumably as commensals and primarily from the uro-

TABLE 7. Features of miscellaneous oxidase-positive, saccharolytic, indole-negative nonfermenters[a]

Feature	% of strains positive[b]						
	Agrobacterium radiobacter (38)[c]	*Alcaligenes xylosoxidans* subsp. *xylosoxidans* (135)	EF-4b (34)	EO-2 (93)	EO-3 (5)	*Ochrobactrum anthropi* (Vd) (71)	*Psychrobacter immobilis* (13)
Acidified (special OF medium [10])							
Glucose	100	78	96	100	100	99	85
Lactose	100	0	0	97	100	0	85
Maltose	100	0	0	21	20	57	17w
Mannitol	100	0	0	20	100w	80	0
Sucrose	100	0	0	0	0	53	0
Xylose	100	99	0	100	100	100	85
Arginine dihydrolase	3	13	0	0	ND	68	5
Catalase	100	98	100	98	100	100	100
Cetrimide agar, growth	0	96	ND	0	ND	3w	ND
Citrate (Simmons)	100	95	20	25	ND	67	18
Esculin, hydrolyzed	100	0	0	0	0	49	0
Gelatin, hydrolyzed	3	0	9	0	0	0	0
Indole	0	0	0	0	0	0	0
MacConkey agar, growth	100	100	71	74	100	100	92
Nitrate reduced	87	100	97	85	0	100	77
Nitrate → gas	5	60	0	2	0	99	0
Urea (Christensen)	100	0	0	77	100	100	15
42°C, growth	34	84	69	35	20	56	0

[a] Most data from Clark et al. (10) and Moss et al. (36). Not all strains were tested for some features.
[b] w, Weak; ND, no data.
[c] Number in parentheses is number of strains examined.

genital tracts of females (10, 26). This species will grow on Thayer-Martin selective medium. Colonies of *Weeksella zoohelcum* (IIj) are similar in size to those of *W. virosa* but are usually sticky and not mucoid. *W. zoohelcum*, unlike *W. virosa*, is urease positive (Table 8). The organism has been recovered from sputum, cerebrospinal fluid, abscesses, and wounds, frequently those associated with animal contacts, particularly dog bites (10, 27).

Moraxella, Oligella urethralis, M-5, and M-6

These nonfermenters are nonmotile, strongly oxidase positive, nonsaccharolytic, usually susceptible to penicillin, and usually coccobacillary upon Gram stain. They may colonize the respiratory tract, urinary tract, and eyes but only rarely cause disease (septicemia, endocarditis, or meningitis). Some strains, particularly those of *Moraxella lacunata* and *M. phenylpyruvica*, may grow poorly in OF basal medium. Biochemical tests on such strains can be made by using generous inocula (from BA or chocolate agar plates) on ALP media. According to Gilardi (19), growth on his mineral base medium plus acetate definitively distinguishes between *M. osloensis* and *Oligella urethralis* (always positive) and the four other named species of *Moraxella* (always negative). *M. osloensis* and *O. urethralis* can easily be distinguished (Table 9). When the data of Table 9 fail to effect identification of other moraxellae or to distinguish between these and glucose-negative psychrobacters (Table 7), the cellular fatty acid profiles can be helpful in differentiation (36).

Colonies of *Moraxella nonliquefaciens*, the most frequently encountered species, are smooth, transparent, and 0.1 to 0.6 mm in diameter on 1-day BA plates; they are translucent and ca. 1 mm in diameter on 2-day plates. All strains are phenylalanine dihydrolase negative (19); none grow on MBM acetate; nearly all strains reduce nitrate to nitrite; and most strains fail to grow on MacConkey agar. Other features are summarized in Table 9. Colonies of *M. osloensis* are similar to those of *M. nonliquefaciens*. *M. osloensis*, differing from *M. nonliquefaciens*, acidifies ethanol and grows on MBM acetate. Colonies of *M. lacunata* are smaller than those of *M. osloensis* and may remain less than 0.5 mm in diameter after several days of incubation. All strains of *M. lacunata* digest Loeffler slants. Most strains hydrolyze gelatin and fail to grow on MacConkey agar. Two cellular fatty acid groups have been reported for strains of *M. lacunata*, thus indicating heterogeneity of this species (36). Colonies of *M. atlantae*, like those of *M. lacunata*, are smaller than those of *M. osloensis*, and some strains present spreading and pitting colonies. All strains grow on MacConkey agar and all are phenylalanine dihydrolase negative. Colonies of *O. urethralis* are smooth, transparent, and 0.1 to 0.5 mm in diameter on 1-day BA plates; they are opaque and 1 to 2 mm on 2-day plates. *O. urethralis*, differing from all moraxellae, alkalinizes ALP citrate, produces gas from nitrite, and is a relatively small coccoid bacterium (43). Most clinical isolates of M-5 are associated with wounds incurred by animal bites. Like most moraxellae, all strains are susceptible to penicillin; none reduce nitrate but most reduce nitrite, and many strains produce a water-soluble yellow-tan pigment. Most strains of M-6 differ from most moraxellae by being catalase negative. Most strains are susceptible to penicillin, and all reduce both nitrate and nitrite. *Neisseria parelongata* has been listed as a synonym for M-5, and *N. elongata* as been given as a synonym for M-6 (18). M-6 has been recovered from numerous body sites (10) and has been implicated in endocarditis and osteomyelitis (10, 14, 42).

TABLE 8. Features of *Flavobacterium* spp., *Weeksella* spp., and groups IIe, IIh, and IIi[a]

Feature	% of strains positive													
	F. breve (7)[b]	*Flavobacterium* group IIb[c] (155)	*F. meningosepticum* (148)	*F. mizutaii* (5)	*F. multivorum* (22)	*F. odoratum* (74)	*F. spiritivorum* (11)	*F. thalpophilum* (7)	*F. yabuuchiae* (2)	IIe (18)	IIh (21)	IIi (23)	*W. virosa* (IIf) (87)	*W. zoohelcum* (IIj) (41)
Acidified														
Ethanol	0	16	57	0	0	0	100	0	100	ND[d]	ND	ND	0	0
Glucose	86	98	99	100	100	0	100	100	100	100	100	100	0	0
Lactose	0	0	57	100	100	0	100	100	100	0	0	100	0	0
Maltose	86	98	100	100	100	0	100	100	100	100	95	100	0	0
Mannitol	0	10	99	0	0	0	100	0	100	0	0	0	0	0
Sucrose	0	14	0	100	100	0	100	100	100	0	0	100	0	0
Xylose	0	31	3	100	100	0	100	100	100	0	5	100	0	0
Catalase	100	99	100	100	100	100	100	100	100	88	100	100	98	100
Citrate (Simmons)	0	3	12	0	0	0	0	0	0	0	0	0	0	0
DNase	100	4	100	0	61	100	100	86	100	0	100	0	0	0
Esculin, hydrolyzed	0	70	99	100	100	0	100	100	100	0	100	96	0	0
Gelatin, hydrolyzed	100	78	91	0	0	96	11	86	100	0	7	0	100	98
Indole	100	98	100	0	0	0	0	0	0	100	100	100	100	98
MacConkey agar, growth	100	63	92	0	100	96	55	100	ND	7	0	0	10	2
Nitrate reduced	0	22	0	0	0	0	0	100	0	0	0	0	0	0
Nitrite reduced	0	20	37	60	0	83	0	0	0	0	ND	ND	0	0
Oxidase	100	96	99	100	100	99	100	100	100	88	100	100	100	100
Urease	0	42	8	20	95	100	91	100	100	0	0	32	0	100
42°C, growth	0	42	45	0	0	31	11	100	0	0	5	36	70	10

[a] Data from Clark et al. (10), Gilardi (17, 19), Holmes et al. (24, 26–28), and Yabuuchi et al. (66). Not all strains were tested for some features.
[b] Number in parentheses is number of strains examined.
[c] See text for proposed binomials.
[d] ND, No data.

TABLE 9. Features of *Moraxella* spp., *Oligella urethralis*, M-5, and M-6[a]

Feature	% of strains positive							
	M. atlantae (23)[b]	*M. lacunata* (25)	*M. nonliquefaciens* (243)	*M. osloensis* (163)	*M. phenylpyruvica* (50)	*O. urethralis* (22)	M-5 (59)	M-6 (40)
Morphology	cb, r	cb, r	cb, f	cb, r	cb, f	cb, r	r	r
Catalase	91	100	95	95	90	100	100	8
Citrate (Simmons)	0	0	0	0	0	46[c]	0	0
Gelatin, hydrolyzed	0	74	0	0	0	0	0	0
Indole	0	0	0	0	0	0	0	0
Loeffler slant, digested	0	100	0	0	0	0	0	0
MBM acetate[d]	42	7	0	100	43	60[c]	25	83
Nitrate reduced	5	100	95	24	68	0	0	100
Nitrite reduced	20	0	0	0	0	100	84	100
Phenylalanine deaminase	0	31	0	14	97	100	73	0
Urea (Christensen)	0	0	0	0	100	0	0	0

[a] Data from Clark et al. (10) and Gilardi (19). Not all strains were tested for some features. cb, Coccobacilli; r, rods (usually in pairs); f, filaments.
[b] Number in parentheses is number of strains.
[c] Some strains of *Oligella* (*Moraxella*) *urethralis* may not grow on Simmons basal medium containing acetate or citrate (43).
[d] MBM acetate is Simmons basal medium plus acetate; positive result indicates growth and alkalinization.

Motile glucose-negative nonfermenters

All seven taxa described in Table 10 are peritrichously flagellated. All except *O. ureolytica* grow well on MacConkey agar and ALP basal media, are probably present in the hospital environment, and may be opportunistic pathogens. Most strains of *A. faecalis* and *Bordetella bronchiseptica* are susceptible to aminoglycosides and some cephalosporins; most strains of IVc-2 are resistant to aminoglycosides but susceptible to some cephalosporins; most strains of *O. ureolytica* are susceptible to aminoglycosides but may be resistant to other antimicrobial agents (19). Most strains of *O. ureolytica*, like some moraxellae, grow poorly on ALP media. Again, however, when generous inocula are used, ALP media are applicable to this species. The normal habitat of *O. ureolytica* is not known. Most of the 20 strains processed at the University of California, Los Angeles, were recovered from urine samples of neurologically compromised adult males.

All taxa of *Alcaligenes* present colonies of workable size (0.5 to 3 mm in diameter) on 1-day BA plates. Colonies of *A. faecalis* are usually smooth but sometimes rough. Growth on 2-day plates is alpha-hemolytic and dirty in appearance. Cultures often exhibit a fruity odor. Nitrate is not reduced, but nitrite is reduced to gas. "*A. faecalis* type I" of the CDC (Table 10) appears to be synonymous with *A. piechaudii* (33), recently associated with chronic ear infection (41). "*A. faecalis* type II" usually presents flat, spreading growth on 2-day plates.

TABLE 10. Features of oxidase-positive, motile, glucose-negative nonfermenters[a]

Feature	% of strains positive						
	Alcaligenes faecalis (22)[b]	*A. piechaudii* (7)	"*A. faecalis* type II" (3)	*A. xylosoxidans* subsp. *denitrificans* (8)	*Bordetella bronchiseptica* (12)	*Oligella ureolytica* (20)	IVc-2 (6)
Acidified							
Ethanol	100	100	100	100	0	76	0
Fructose[c]	0	0	0	0	0	0	0
Alkalinized							
Acetamide	100	100	0	100	0	0	0
Allantoin	0	0	0	0	100	100	100
Histidine	100	100	0	100	0	0	100
Itaconate	0	100	0	100	100	100	100
Malonate	100	100	0	100	100	0	100
Saccharate	0	100	0	100	100	0	100
Urea	0	0	0	0	100	100	100
Catalase	100	100	100	100	100	100	100
Gelatin, hydrolyzed	22	0	0	0	0	0	0
Indole	0	0	0	0	0	0	0
MacConkey agar, growth	100	100	100	100	100	89	100
Nitrate reduced	0	100	0	100	92	75	17
Nitrite → gas	100	0	0	100	0	90	0

[a] Most data, including number of strains examined, are from Pickett and Greenwood (45). Data for hydrolysis of gelatin and growth on MacConkey agar are from Clark et al. (10). Synonyms: *A. faecalis* (31), formerly *A. odorans* (10); *A. piechaudii* (33), formerly *A. faecalis* type I (45); *A. xylosoxidans* subsp. *denitrificans* (33), formerly *A. denitrificans* (10); *O ureolytica*, formerly IVe (43).
[b] Number in parentheses is number of strains examined.
[c] *Pseudomonas acidovorans* and *P. pseudoalcaligenes*, also motile and glucose-negative nonfermenters (see chapter 41), acidify fructose.

It is relatively inert in biochemical tests; its features are similar to those of *Bordetella avium* (chapter 46). Two taxa of Table 10, *B. bronchiseptica* and *O. ureolytica*, are exceptional in their rapid alkalinization of urea media, and alkalinization is also relatively rapid with IVc-2. Members of these three taxa also differ from *Alcaligenes* species in their restricted growth. Colonies of *B. bronchiseptica* are 0.1 to 0.5 mm in diameter on 1-day BA plates and 1 to 1.5 mm on 2-day plates; those of IVc-2 are ca. 0.5 mm on 1-day plates and 1 to 2.5 mm on 2-day plates; those of *O. ureolytica* are less than 0.1 mm on 1-day plates and only 0.3 to 1 mm on 2-day plates.

UB

Materials and methods

The procedures and media of the CDC (10, 65; Table 11) are generally applicable to clinical laboratories. The CDC uses rabbit blood agar plates prepared with heart infusion agar (Difco Laboratories, Detroit, Mich.). Such plates may be more nutritious than commercial plates prepared without infusion. In addition, most commercial plates are prepared with sheep blood and hence may be slightly less sensitive than rabbit blood to bacterial hemolysins. Not only formulation but also age is important for BA plates. The expiration date on commercial plates may not be a reliable guide that the plates are satisfactory for the more fastidious UB; plates more than 2 weeks old may not be optimal. Any isolate that may be capnophilic should be inoculated onto duplicate BA plates for incubation at 35°C, one plate aerobically and the other in a candle jar (3 to 5% carbon dioxide and saturated humidity). Commercial chocolate agar plates may also be less nutritious than those used in the Special Bacteriology Laboratory at the CDC. The latter are prepared with heart infusion agar (Difco) basal medium supplemented with yeast extract and 4% rabbit blood, whereas commercial plates are sometimes prepared with a Mueller-Hinton agar as basal medium.

The oxidase test of Table 11 should be made with the more sensitive tetramethyl, not dimethyl, reagent. The infusion broth and slant media of Table 11 are used when growth fails in infusion-free media. With quite fastidious bacteria, growth may fail in the peptone basal medium (enteric fermentation base) used for sugar fermentation tests. In such instances, each tube should be supplemented with 2 drops of normal rabbit serum. Sera from other animals may contain an enzyme that degrades maltose (22). Alternatively, when growth fails in peptone basal medium, large inocula (0.5 to 1 mm^3 of cell paste) with buffered sugars (such as for neisseriae) or ALP sugars (as for nonfermenters) can be used. No growth is required by these two methods. Similarly, a buffered amino acid broth, large inoculum, and ninhydrin reagent (to test for decarboxylation of lysine and ornithine) obviate the need for growth of the more fastidious bacilli. The motility medium of Table 11 can be that used for pseudomonads, motility nitrate agar used for NFB, or OF basal medium used for NFB (see chapter 121). For indole tests, the CDC incubates the tryptone medium for 2 days and then tests for indole with Ehrlich reagent after extraction with xylene. A more sensitive procedure, at least for flavobacteria (44), is use of a buffered tryptophan broth medium and modified Kovacs reagent. Gram stains are prepared not only from the BA plate but also from an infusion agar slant and infusion broth. Growth on the BA plate is also used for an oxidase test. Infusion agar slants are also used to determine growth at 25, 35, and 42°C, and one of these slants is used for a catalase test (3% hydrogen peroxide).

A key for identification of these bacilli, modified from that of Weaver et al. (65), is given in Table 12. The key should be used only as a guide; variable reactions may be encountered.

TABLE 11. Media and substrates recommended for identification of miscellaneous fermentative and fastidious gram-negative bacilli[a]

Blood agar plate
Oxidase test, Gram stain
Heart infusion agar slants
Heart infusion broth
Triple sugar iron agar slant
Liquid peptone basal medium with:
Glucose
Lactose
Maltose
Mannitol
Sucrose
Xylose
MacConkey agar slant
Simmons citrate agar
Methyl red–Voges-Proskauer medium
Motility medium
Christensen urea agar
Nitrate medium (peptone base)
Nitrate medium (heart infusion base)
2% tryptone medium (for indole test)
Nutrient broth
Nutrient broth with 6% sodium chloride
Gelatin medium
Esculin agar
Lysine and ornithine decarboxylase media

[a] Adapted from Weaver et al. (65).

Actinobacillus

The genera *Actinobacillus* and *Pasteurella* are similar in respect to moles percent G+C of their chromosomal DNA, phenotypic features, and animal reservoirs for human disease. No one phenotypic feature definitively distinguishes these two genera (37), but identification of a recent clinical isolate can usually be effected by reference to features of the species (Table 13).

Actinobacilli were first associated with actinobacillosis of cattle, and they have since been recovered from other animals and humans (10). Several of the human infections were of animal origin, including animal bites. All are susceptible to tetracycline and chloramphenicol (12, 30). The CDC has processed 82 strains, 19 of *Actinobacillus equuli*, 30 of *A. lignieresii*, and 33 of *A. suis*. All are nonmotile, present coccobacilli and small rods upon Gram stain, are oxidase positive, and acidify both slants and butts of TSIA (Table 2). On 1-day BA plates, colonies are translucent and 1 to 2 mm in diameter. Most strains of *A. equuli* and *A. suis*, but none of *A. lignieresii*, ferment melibiose and trehalose. All strains of *A. suis*, but none of *A. equuli* and *A. lignieresii*, hydrolyze esculin. Other features are presented in Table 13. Weaver et al. (65) suggest that the 33 strains tabulated by the CDC as *A. suis* may in fact represent more than one taxon and that some of these strains may be

TABLE 12. Key to identification of miscellaneous gram-negative bacteria[a]

Feature	Organisms
Ox+	
Mac+	
Glu+	
Motility+	*Chromobacterium violaceum*
Motility−	
Ur+	
Ind+	*Pasteurella pneumotropica* (1% Ox−, 4% Ur−, 10%, Ind−)
Ind−	*Actinobacillus equuli, A. hominis, A. lignieresii, A. suis* (6% Mac−), *Pasteurella aerogenes*
Ur−	
Ind+	HB-5
Ind−	EF-4a, *Kingella kingae* (10% Glu−), *Pasteurella gallinarum* (10% Ox−), *P. haemolytica* (5% Ox−)
Mac−	
Glu+	
Motility−	
Ur+	
Ind+	*Pasteurella dagmatis* (2% Ox−, 1% Mac+), *P. pneumotropica* (1% Ox−, 4% Ur−, 10% Ind−)
Ind−	*Actinobacillus equuli, A. lignieresii, A. suis, A. ureae* (1% Ox−)
Ur−	
Ind+	
Cat+	*Pasteurella dagmatis* (2% Ox−, 1% Mac+, 4% Cat−), *P. multocida* (3% Ox−, 1% Ind−, 2% Cat−)
Cat−	*Cardiobacterium hominis* (1% Cat+), HB-5, *Kingella indologenes*
Ind−	
Cat+	*Actinobacillus actinomycetemcomitans* (5% Mac+, 1% Cat−), *Capnocytophaga canimorsus* (3% Ox−, 2% Mac+, 7% Glu−), *C. cynodegmi*, EF-4a, *Pasteurella gallinarum* (10% Ox−), *P. haemolytica* (5% Ox−)
Cat−	*Kingella denitrificans* (8% Glu−, 10% Cat+), *K. kingae* (10% Glu−), *P. haemolytica* (5% Ox−)
Glu−, motility−, Ur−, Ind−, Cat−	*Eikenella corrodens* (8% Cat+)
Ox−	
Mac+	
Glu+	
Motility+	*Chromobacterium violaceum*
Motility−	HB-5
Mac−	
Glu+	
Motility−	
Ur−	
Ind+	
Cat−	DF-3 (4% Ur+), HB-5 (2% Cat+)
Ind−	
Cat+	*Actinobacillus actinomycetemcomitans* (5% Mac+, 1% Cat−)
Cat−	*Capnocytophaga* spp. (DF-1), DF-3 (4% Ur+)

[a] Adapted from Weaver et al. (65). Several genospecies of *Pasteurella* are not included (see Table 14). Ox, Oxidase; Mac+, growth on MacConkey agar; Glu, glucose; Ur, urea; Ind, indole; Cat, catalase; +, positive; −, negative.

"Actinobacillus hominis." "A. hominis," recovered in Copenhagen from patients with chronic lung disease, is not recognized in *Bergey's Manual;* its features are similar to those of *A. suis* (65). In the Special Bacteriology Laboratory at the CDC, the type strain of *"A. hominis"* hydrolyzed esculin and fermented mannitol but did not ferment D-mannose, D-arabinose, or cellobiose.

Recent DNA-DNA hybridization studies indicate that the taxon formerly addressed as *Pasteurella ureae* should be transferred to genus *Actinobacillus* as *A. ureae* (38). It differs from the other three species in being lactose and xylose negative. It has been recovered from the respiratory tract, blood, and cerebrospinal fluid (58).

"Bacterium actinomycetem comitans" (comitans, from accompanying *Actinomyces*) was first recovered from actinomycotic lesions in cattle and humans. This trinomial term was later changed to *Actinobacillus actinomycetemcomitans.* Recent taxonomic studies, including DNA-DNA hybridizations and examination of surface antigens, led to the proposal that this taxon be transferred to the genus *Haemophilus* as *H. actinomycetemcomitans* (46); however, this proposal has not been favorably received (Int. J. Syst. Bacteriol. **37**:474, 1987). This bacterium, probably of endogenous origin, is now particularly associated with periodontitis and endocarditis but has also been associated with other focal infections. Therapy has frequently involved penicillin or ampicillin, but resistance to these agents is common. In vitro, cefazolin, cefotaxime, ceftriaxone, aminoglycosides, and chloramphenicol show good activity (30, 67). These bacteria, like brucellae, *Haemophilus aphrophilus,* and *Francisella tularensis,* appear as small coccobacilli or short rods upon Gram stain. They are relatively fastidious and are obligate capnophiles (a candle jar will satisfy their requirement for elevated carbon dioxide tension). In broth, these bacilli adhere to the wall of the tube, and the medium, except for a slight sediment, remains clear. Colonies on 1-day plates may be less than 0.5 mm in diameter but enlarge to 2 to 3 mm, sometimes with rough surfaces and pitting, after

TABLE 13. Features of *Actinobacillus* spp. and *Pasteurella* spp.[a]

Feature	% of strains positive									
	A. equuli (19)[b]	*A. lignieresii* (30)	*A. suis* (33)	*A. (Pasteurella) ureae* (97)	*P. aerogenes* (16)	*P. dagmatis* (*Pasteurella* "n. sp. 1") (91)	*P. gallinarum* (10)	*P. haemolytica* (67)	*P. multocida* (306)	*P. pneumotropica* (107)
Acidified										
Glucose	100	100	100	100	100	100	100	100	100	100
Lactose	95	78	97	0	57	3	0	42	8	53
Maltose	95	100	100	96	100	100	100	99	2	100
Mannitol	100	100	54	100	6	0	0	39	78	3
Sucrose	100	100	100	100	94	99	100	100	100	100
Xylose	100	100	100	0	81	0	33	69	67	95
Citrate (Simmons)	0	0	0	0	0	0	0	0	0	0
Esculin, hydrolyzed	0	0	100	0	0	0	0	23	0	0
Gelatin, hydrolyzed	47	0	6	0	0	13	0	12	0	0
Glucose, gas	0	0	0	0	100	16	0	0	0	0
Hemolysis	0	4	76	0	0	0	0	72	0	0
Indole	0	0	0	0	0	100	0	0	99	90
Lysine decarboxylase	0	0	0	0	0	2	0	3	0	33
MacConkey agar, growth	89	75	94	0	100	1	30	85	3	53
Nitrate reduced	100	100	100	99	100	100	100	100	99	100
Ornithine decarboxylase	0	0	0	0	88	0	25	10	94	100
Urea (Christensen)	100	100	100	100	100	81	0	0	0	96
VP	12	0	50	21	29	28	50	71	0	13
42°C, growth	31	14	31	5	94	27	67	50	32	8

[a] Adapted from Clark et al. (10). Not all strains were tested for some features. According to present taxonomy (37; Table 14), not all of the 306 strains tabulated here as *P. multocida* are members of this species. See Table 15 for *Actinobacillus actinomycetemcomitans*.
[b] Number in parentheses is number of strains examined.

several days of incubation. Additional features are presented in Tables 2 and 14.

Capnocytophaga

All *Capnocytophaga* strains are capnophilic; this enhanced growth in the presence of carbon dioxide can be effected by incubation in a candle jar. All are gram-negative slender or filamentous rods. All are facultatively anaerobic, and all ferment carbohydrates, though never mannitol and xylose. Most display gliding motility (twitching and translocation), but this may not be evident on some agar media. Gliding can be determined by inoculating cultures onto heart infusion agar containing 5% rabbit serum (8). Growth on BA is usually favored when the basal medium contains heart infusion. As noted above, in tests for acidification of sugars, particularly with strains of the DF-2 group (DF for dysgonic fermenter), positive results may best be obtained when relatively large inocula in small volumes of fluid basal medium or on ALP basal medium are used.

The five species of Table 15 fall into two groups with respect to habitat, pathogenicity, and cultural features: DF-1 (*Capnocytophaga gingivalis*, *C. ochracea*, and *C. sputigena*) and DF-2 (*C. canimorsus* and *C. cynodegmi*). DF-1 is associated with presence in and disease of the oral cavity, particularly periodontitis, and also with septicemia. Most *Capnocytophaga* strains are resistant to aminoglycosides but are susceptible to several other antimicrobial agents, including penicillin (7, 12, 57). Colonies of DF-1 may scarcely be visible on 1-day BA plates but usually enlarge to several millimeters after 2 to 4 days and display flat, spreading, fingerlike edges. DF-1 is oxidase, catalase, and usually arginine dihydrolase negative; in contrast, most strains of the DF-2 group are positive in these three tests. Many strains of DF-2 have been associated with septicemia or meningitis following dog bites.

DNA-DNA hybridizations will distinguish the five species of *Capnocytophaga* (8), but the three species of the DF-1 group cannot always be identified by conventional tests. Indeed, the CDC (10) tabulates these as a group rather than as three separate species. Additional discussion of the capnocytophagas can be found in the fourth edition of this Manual (65).

Cardiobacterium

Cardiobacterium hominis is one of the few capnophilic, nonmotile UB that are oxidase positive but catalase negative. In Gram stains prepared from BA cultures, it appears as a pleomorphic rod-shaped bacillus with bulbous ends, and the cells frequently appear in clusters resembling rosettes. However, when the growth medium is supplemented with yeast extract, it appears as gram-negative rods with little evidence of pleomorphism (64). On 1-day BA plates the colonies are minute, but at 2 days they are 1 mm in diameter, smooth, and butyrous. The colonies of some strains may pit the agar. All strains ferment glucose and maltose but not lactose and xylose; all are indole positive, but positivity is weak with some strains. Other features are presented in Tables 2 and 15. The normal habitat of *C. hominis* is the upper respiratory tract. It is an etiologic agent of endocarditis (65).

Chromobacterium violaceum

The facultatively anaerobic bacillus *Chromobacterium violaceum* is a normal inhabitant of soil and water and is only rarely associated with human disease (15). Most

TABLE 14. Hybridization groups of *Pasteurella* spp.: phenotypic features[a]

Feature	Reaction[b]												
	P. anatis (2)[c]	*P. avium* (3)	*P. canis* (5)	*P. dagmatis* (6)	*P. galli-narum* (3)	*P. lan-gaa* (2)	*P. mul-tocida* subsp. *galli-cida* (6)	*P. mul-tocida* subsp. *mul-tocida* (26)	*P. mul-tocida* subsp. *septica* (9)	*Pasteur-ella* species A (4)	*Pasteur-ella* species B (2)	*P. sto-matis* (6)	*P. volan-tium* (10)
Acidified													
L-Arabinose	−	−	−	−	−	−	d	−	−	+	−	−	−
Dulcitol	−	−	−	−	−	−	+	−	−	−	+	−	−
Maltose	−	−	−	+	+	−	−	−	−	d	+	−	+
Mannitol	+	−	−	−	−	+	+	+	+	d	−	−	+
Sorbitol	−	−	−	−	−	−	+	+	−	−	−	−	d
Trehalose	+	+	d	+	+	−	−	d	+	+	+	+	+
D-Xylose	+	d	d	−	−	−	+	d	+	d	+	−	d
Indole	−	−	d	+	−	−	+	+	+	−	+	+	−
NAD required	−	d	−	−	−	−	−	−	−	+	−	−	+
Ornithine decarboxylase	−	−	+	−	−	−	+	+	+	−	+	−	d
Urea	−	−	−	+	−	−	−	−	−	−	−	−	−

[a] Adapted from Mutters et al. (37).
[b] −, ≧90% of strains negative; +, ≧90% of strains positive; d, different results (11 to 89% of strains positive).
[c] Number in parentheses is number of strains.

TABLE 15. Features of capnophilic bacilli

Feature	% of strains positive									
	Actinobacillus actinomycetemcomitans[a] (120)[d]	*Capnocytophaga canimorsus* (DF-2)[b] (75)	*C. cynodegmi* (DF-2-like)[b] (9)	*C. gingivalis* (DF-1)[c] (25)	*C. ochracea* (DF-1)[c] (27)	*C. sputigena* (DF-1)[c] (6)	*Cardiobacterium hominis*[a] (65)	DF-3[a] (21)	*Eikenella corrodens*[a] (506)	HB-5[a] (44)
Acidified										
Galactose	100	89	67	0	83	0	0	ND[e]	ND	0
Glucose	99	93	100	100	100	100	100	100	0	100
Lactose	0	100	100	8	92	40	0	95	0	0
Maltose	95	95	100	100	100	100	100	100	0	0
Mannitol	82	0	0	0	0	0	95	0	0	0
Raffinose	0	0	89	24	70	17	0	ND	ND	0
Sucrose	0	0	89	100	100	100	98	95	0	0
Xylose	42	0	0	0	0	0	0	100	0	0
Arginine dihydrolase	0	99	100	0	0	0	0	0	0	0
Catalase	99	100	100	0	0	0	1	0	8	2
Citrate (Simmons)	0	0	0	0	0	0	0	0	0	0
Esculin	0	64	100	75	96	83	2	100	0	0
Gelatin, hydrolyzed	0	0	0	17	14	60	0	0	0	0
Indole	0	0	0	0	0	0	100	85	0	100
Lysine decarboxylase	0	0	0	9	5	0	0	9	82	0
MacConkey agar, growth	5	2	0	0	0	0	0	0	0	58
Motility	0	0	0	0	0	0	0	0	0	0
Nitrate reduced	100	0	17	4	8	83	0	0	99	100
Ornithine decarboxylase	0	0	0	0	0	0	0	0	98	0
Oxidase	19	97	100	0	0	0	100	0	100	54
Urease	0	0	0	12	14	0	0	4	0	0

[a] Most data from Clark et al. (10). Not all strains were tested for some features.
[b] Data from Brenner et al. (8). Not all strains were tested for some features.
[c] Data from Socransky et al. (53).
[d] Number in parentheses is number of strains examined.
[e] ND, No data.

cases have occurred in tropical and subtropical climates. In the United States, human infections have been reported from Florida, Louisiana, and South Carolina. *C. violaceum* is susceptible to aminoglycosides, chloramphenicol, and tetracycline (65). Most of the 37 strains processed by the CDC produced a violet pigment (10), violacein, which is soluble in ethanol but insoluble in water and chloroform; this pigment is probably unique to this species. Some strains present both pigmented and nonpigmented colonies on BA plates. Nonpigmented strains resemble *Aeromonas* species but are maltose and mannitol negative (51). *C. violaceum* is susceptible to aminoglycosides and chloramphenicol but resistant to penicillin and cephalosporins (15). Colonies on 1-day BA plates are 0.5 to 1.5 mm in diameter, convex, and smooth. Some strains are hemolytic. Motility is by one polar and one to four lateral flagella. It does not decarboxylate lysine and ornithine or deaminate phenylalanine, but it may be arginine dihydrolase positive. The nonpigmented strains are frequently indole positive. Oxidase-negative strains could be mistaken for enteric bacilli, and oxidase-positive strains could be mistaken for *Vibrio* species or *Aeromonas* species. However, distinction can usually be made on grounds of the features just noted, along with those presented in Tables 2 and 16.

DF-3

DF-3, a small coccobacillus, is described briefly by Clark et al. (10) but is not discussed in the fourth edition of this Manual. It is nutritionally fastidious and facultatively anaerobic. Cultures are described as having a sweet and bitter odor. Its cellular fatty acids present a unique profile that is similar to those of *Capnocytophaga* species (63). It is capnophilic, oxidase negative, and catalase negative (Table 2). It can be distinguished from other UB that share this triad of features by tests for reduction of nitrate and acidification of lactose and xylose (Table 14). It has been recovered from blood, feces, urine, wounds, and other body sites (10, 62).

EF-4a

EF-4a, a nonmotile coccobacillus, resembles pasteurellae in several features, including infections in humans following animal contact, particularly animal bites. Recent studies on RNA and DNA relatedness (48) led to the proposal that the EF-4a, EF-4b, and M-5 groups are members of emended family *Neisseriaceae*. EF-4a differs from pasteurellae in fermenting only glucose, in being arginine dihydrolase positive, and in that some strains are weakly pigmented (yellow to tan). Nitrate is usually reduced to gas, and a few strains reduce both nitrate and nitrite without formation of gas. Other features are shown in Tables 2 and 16.

Eikenella

The genus *Eikenella* contains straight, unbranched rods 1.5 to 4 μm in length. They are nonmotile, but twitching may occur on some media. They are oxidase positive, usually catalase negative, facultatively anaerobic, and nonsaccharolytic. Hemin is usually required for aerobic growth. Strains of *Eikenella* are susceptible to several antimicrobial agents, including the penicillins and tetracycline, but not clindamycin (49). The genus contains only one species, *Eikenella corrodens*.

E. corrodens is part of the normal flora of mucous membranes. It can also be etiologically significant, singly or in mixed infections, in arthritis, empyema, endocarditis, meningitis, pneumonia, postsurgical infection, and abscesses in soft tissue, including the brain (13). It is a capnophilic slender bacillus. On 1-day BA plates colonies may be minute or inapparent, and several days of incubation may be required before colonies of workable size are present. Such colonies have moist, clear centers surrounded by flat, spreading growth. Pitting of the medium is not always apparent. A slight yellow pigmentation may be present in aged cultures. Ornithine and usually also lysine are decarboxylated. The arginine dihydrolase test is negative. All strains appear to be antigenically related. Other features are shown in Tables 2 and 14. *E. corrodens* can be confused with

TABLE 16. *Chromobacterium* sp., *Kingella* spp., and group EF-4a[a]

Feature	% of strains positive				
	C. violaceum (37)[b]	EF-4a (97)	*K. denitrificans* (60)	*K. indologenes* (1)	*K. kingae* (33)
Acidified					
Glucose	100	100	92	100	90
Lactose	0	0	0	0	0
Maltose	3	0	0	100	100
Mannitol	0	0	0	0	0
Sucrose	26	0	0	100	0
Xylose	0	0	0	0	0
Citrate (Simmons)	77	4	0	0	0
Esculin, hydrolyzed	5	0	0	0	0
Gelatin, hydrolyzed	86	60	0	0	0
Hemolysis	48	0	0	0	84
Indole	21	0	0	100	0
MacConkey agar, growth	100	50	0	0	36
Motility	100	0	0	0	0
Nitrate reduced	97	97	93	0	6
Urea (Christensen)	19	0	0	0	0
42°C, growth	85	70	48	0	4

[a] Adapted from Clark et al. (10). Not all strains were tested for some features.
[b] Number in parentheses is number of strains examined.

another pitting or corroding bacterium, obligatively anaerobic *Bacteroides ureolyticus* (formerly *B. corrodens*). However, they differ in that *E. corrodens* is facultatively aerobic, lysine decarboxylase positive, and gelatin negative.

Group HB-5

The capnophilic group HB-5 presents coccobacilli and rods upon Gram stain. On 1-day BA plates, colonies are 0.5 to 1.0 mm in diameter, convex, and smooth. HB-5 is facultatively anaerobic, and all strains are weakly aerogenic. Of the usual battery of six sugars used by the CDC, only glucose is acidified. Other features are summarized in Tables 2 and 14. HB-5 has been recovered from placenta, amniotic fluid, blood, finger lesions, rectal sites, surgical incisions, leg abscesses, and urogenital specimens (1, 65). It is susceptible to many antimicrobial agents.

Kingella

Kingella species are coccobacillary or straight rods 2 to 3 μm in length and commonly appear in pairs or short chains. They are nonmotile but may be piliated and show twitching motility. They are facultatively anaerobic, fermentative, oxidase positive, and usually catalase negative. They are nutritionally fastidious and hence, as noted above for other fastidious bacteria, may require special procedures for fermentation tests. Their normal habitat appears to be the upper respiratory tract of humans.

The taxon *Kingella denitrificans* was first designated TM-1 because of its recovery on Thayer-Martin medium from throat swabs during a survey for carriers of gonococci and meningococci (23). The TM-1 group was later reported to be similar to "saccharolytic *Moraxella* species" (now *Kingella kingae*), and the genus *Kingella* was proposed (52) to encompass these two taxa and *Kingella indologenes*. *K. denitrificans* is rarely if ever pathogenic. Colonies on 1-day BA plates are 0.5 mm or less in diameter and convex; some strains pit the agar. It usually mimics gonococci in its microscopic morphology, its failure to acidify any sugar other than glucose, and its occasional failure to grow on TSIA. It is, however, a rod and also differs from gonococci in reducing nitrate and usually in being catalase negative (Tables 2 and 16).

K. indologenes is only rarely encountered in clinical specimens. Both of the two strains examined by Snell and Lapage (52) and four additional strains processed at the CDC were associated with eye infections. It is susceptible to penicillin. It differs from the other two *Kingella* species in being not only indole positive but also sucrose positive.

The taxon *K. kingae* has been progressively named *Moraxella* new species 1, *Moraxella kingii*, and now *K. kingae* (21). It is an opportunistic pathogen, particularly for young children, and has been recovered from blood, bone, joint fluid, and the nasopharynx. Most strains are susceptible to many antimicrobial agents, including penicillin (35, 65). On 1-day BA plates, colonies are 0.5 mm or less in diameter. The colonies of some strains have a flat periphery and pit the agar. Salient features for identification of this species are hemolysis (usually weak), catalase negativity, and acidification of both glucose and maltose. Other features are presented in Tables 2 and 16.

Pasteurella

In animals, pasteurellae cause fowl cholera, hemorrhagic septicemia, mastitis, septic pleuropneumonia, snuffles, and other focal infections. In humans, they have been recovered from lesions in many parts of the body. Both normal and diseased wild and domestic animals are the reservoirs for most human infections. *Pasteurella* species are coccobacilli or rods 1 to 2 μm in length. They are nonmotile, facultatively anaerobic, and saccharolytic. Most strains recovered from clinical specimens are catalase, indole, oxidase, and sucrose positive; most decarboxylate ornithine; some are capsulated. Most strains are susceptible to penicillin, tetracycline, and chloramphenicol (65). Oxidase tests should be made with cultures grown on BA or chocolate agar medium; negative tests may be obtained with other growth media (20). Tables 2 and 13 present the species (except *Pasteurella ureae*, transferred to the genus *Actinobacillus*) and their features as tabulated by the CDC (10).

As already noted, phenotypic features of *Pasteurella* species are similar to those of *Actinobacillus* species. Indeed, recent DNA hybridization studies (37) disclosed that several taxa previously assigned to the genus *Pasteurella* (*P. aerogenes*, *P. haemolytica*, and *P. pneumotropica*) are more closely related to the genus *Actinobacillus*. These hybridization studies detected 13 taxa in the genus *Pasteurella;* differential phenotypic features of these taxa are shown in Table 14. Two "*P. pneumotropica*-like" taxa of *Pasteurellaceae*, encompassing 11 of 12 strains recovered from hamsters, were neither named nor assigned to a genus within this family (34).

"*P.*" *aerogenes* has been recovered from aborted fetuses of swine and from animal bites, urine, and peritoneal fluid in humans. Colonies on 1-day BA plates are 0.5 to 1 mm in diameter, convex, smooth, translucent, and nonhemolytic. The biochemical profile of this species is distinct from that of other pasteurellae (Tables 13 and 14).

The two strains of *P. anatis* studied were recovered from the intestinal tracts of ducks (37). Important differential tests are for acidification of arabinose, maltose, mannitol, trehalose, and xylose and for decarboxylation of ornithine (Table 14).

Two of the three strains of *P. avium* studied were from chickens, and the third was from a calf. The two from chickens required V factor (NAD) for growth. This species is catalase, oxidase, and sucrose positive and gelatin and lactose negative. Nitrate is reduced to nitrite. Lysine is not decarboxylated. There is no growth on MacConkey and Simmons citrate agars. Other differential tests are for acidification of arabinose, maltose, and mannitol, for production of indole, and for decarboxylation of ornithine (Table 14).

The recently described species *P. caballi* (50) differs from other pasteurellae in being catalase negative. All of the 29 strains recovered from horses were aerogenic, failed to grow on MacConkey agar, acidified neither trehalose nor L-arabinose, and were both urease and indole negative.

Some *Pasteurella* strains assigned to *P. multocida* in

the CDC charts (10) have been reassigned to *P. canis* on grounds of results from hybridization studies (37). Biotype 1 strains of *P. canis*, recovered from dogs (mouth) and dog bites in humans, are indole positive; biotype 2, from cattle, is indole negative. Differential tests are for acidification of dulcitol, maltose, and mannitol and for decarboxylation of ornithine (Table 14).

The name *P. dagmatis* was proposed (37) for a group of pasteurellae addressed by the CDC as *Pasteurella* sp. "n. sp. 1" (*Pasteurella* "gas") (10). It has also been called *Pasteurella pneumotropica* type Henriksen (37). Many of the 91 strains processed at the CDC were recovered from human focal wounds after animal contact, particularly cat and dog bites. On 1-day BA plates, colonies are 1 to 2 mm in diameter and nonhemolytic. Differential tests are for acidification of maltose and xylose, production of indole, decarboxylation of ornithine, and hydrolysis of urea (Tables 13 and 14).

Most strains of *P. gallinarum* were recovered from fowl (10, 37). Important differential tests are for acidification of arabinose, maltose, and mannitol and for production of indole (Tables 13 and 14).

P. haemolytica is relatively common as an agent of septicemia and mastitis in domestic animals but rarely causes disease in humans (65). It is indole and urea negative (Table 13). Freshly isolated strains are hemolytic but may lose this feature upon subculture. The species contains two biotypes. Type A is xylose positive, esculin negative, and usually mannose negative; type T is mannose positive, xylose negative, and usually esculin positive.

P. multocida is probably the least unusual of all "unusual bacilli" encountered in clinical laboratories. The CDC, a reference laboratory, has processed more than 300 strains, as compared with 16 of *P. aerogenes* and 19 of *A. equuli* (10). As noted above, *P. multocida* of the CDC charts (10) may contain more than one species. *P. multocida* is apparently a commensal in the upper respiratory tracts of fowl and mammals and possibly also of humans (65). In humans, it is associated with focal infections following animal bites, with chronic pulmonary disease, and with systemic disease, including meningitis. Colonies on 1-day BA plates are 1 to 2 mm in diameter and nonhemolytic. Like other pasteurellae and actinobacilli, it acidifies both the slant and butt of TSIA. An occasional strain may give a weak or even negative oxidase test; however, tests with the tetramethyl reagent are only rarely negative. Results from tests for indole, ornithine decarboxylase, and acidification of maltose and sucrose provide salient features of this species. Tests for acidification of dulcitol and sorbitol delineate three subspecies (Table 14). Bacteriophage typing as an epidemiological tool has been described (39).

P. pneumotropica was initially associated with pneumonic lesions in laboratory mice, and most of the strains processed at the CDC were recovered from mice and rats (10, 65). It appears to be less common than other species of pasteurellae as an agent of either animal or human disease. On 1-day BA plates, colonies are 0.5 to 1.5 mm in diameter, low convex, and nonhemolytic. Salient features for identification come from tests for ornithine decarboxylase, hydrolysis of urea, and production of gas from glucose (Table 13).

Pasteurella species A and B are provisional taxa in this genus (Table 14).

Strains of *P. stomatis* were recovered from the respiratory tracts of cats and dogs (37). Important differential tests are for acidification of maltose and mannitol, production of indole, and decarboxylation of ornithine (Table 14).

Most strains of *P. volantium* were recovered from fowl, but one strain was from a human tongue (37). All of 10 strains required V factor (NAD) for growth; other features are similar to those of *P. avium* (Table 14).

LITERATURE CITED

1. **Baddour, L. M., M. S. Gelfand, R. E. Weaver, T. C. Woods, M. Altwegg, L. W. Mayer, R. A. Kelley, and D. J. Brenner.** 1989. CDC group HB-5 as a cause of genitourinary infections in adults. J. Clin. Microbiol. **27:**801–805.
2. **Bergogne-Bérézin, E., M. L. Joly-Guillou, and J. F. Vieu.** 1987. Epidemiology of nosocomial infections due to *Acinetobacter calcoaceticus*. J. Hosp. Infect. **10:**105–113.
3. **Botha, W. C., P. J. Jooste, and T. J. Britz.** 1989. The taxonomic relationship of certain environmental flavobacteria to the genus *Weeksella*. J. Appl. Bacteriol. **67:** 551–559.
4. **Bouvet, P. J. M., and P. A. D. Grimont.** 1986. Taxonomy of the genus *Acinetobacter* with the recognition of *Acinetobacter baumannii* sp. nov., *Acinetobacter haemolyticus* sp. nov., *Acinetobacter johnsonii* sp. nov., and *Acinetobacter junii* sp. nov. and emended descriptions of *Acinetobacter calcoaceticus* and *Acinetobacter lwoffii*. Int. J. Syst. Bacteriol. **36:**228–240.
5. **Bouvet, P. J. M., and P. A. D. Grimont.** 1987. Identification and biotyping of clinical isolates of *Acinetobacter*. Ann. Inst. Pasteur Microbiol. **138:**569–578.
6. **Bouvet, P. J. M., and S. Jeanjean.** 1989. Delineation of new proteolytic genomic species in the genus *Acinetobacter*. Res. Microbiol. **140:**291–299.
7. **Bremmelgaard, A., C. Pers, J. E. Kristiansen, B. Korner, O. Heltberg, and W. Frederiksen.** 1989. Susceptibility testing of Danish isolates of *Capnocytophaga* and CDC group DF-2 bacteria. APMIS **97:**43–48.
8. **Brenner, D. J., D. G. Hollis, G. R. Fanning, and R. E. Weaver.** 1989. *Capnocytophaga canimorsus* sp. nov. (formerly CDC group DF-2), a cause of septicemia following dog bite, and *C. cynodegmi* sp. nov., a cause of localized wound infection following dog bite. J. Clin. Microbiol. **27:** 231–235.
9. **Cain, J. R.** 1988. A case of septicaemia caused by *Agrobacterium radiobacter*. J. Infect. **16:**205–206.
10. **Clark, W. A., D. G. Hollis, R. E. Weaver, and P. Riley.** 1984. Identification of unusual pathogenic gram-negative aerobic and facultatively anaerobic bacteria. Centers for Disease Control, Atlanta.
11. **D'Amato, R. F., M. Salemi, A. Mathews, D. J. Cleri, and G. Reddy.** 1988. *Achromobacter xylosoxidans* (*Alcaligenes xylosoxidans* subsp. *xylosoxidans*) meningitis associated with a gunshot wound. J. Clin. Microbiol. **26:**2425–2426.
12. **Finegold, S. M., and E. J. Baron.** 1986. Bailey and Scott's diagnostic microbiology. The C.V. Mosby Co., St. Louis.
13. **Flesher, S. A., and E. J. Bottone.** 1989. *Eikenella corrodens* cellulitis and arthritis of the knee. J. Clin. Microbiol. **27:**2606–2608.
14. **Garner, J., and R. H. Briant.** 1986. Osteomyelitis caused by a bacterium known as M6. J. Infect. **13:**298–300.
15. **Georghiou, P. R., G. M. O'Kane, S. Siu, and R. J. Kemp.** 1989. Near-fatal septicaemia with *Chromobacterium violaceum*. Med. J. Aust. **150:**720–721.
16. **Gerner-Smidt, P.** 1987. The epidemiology of *Acinetobacter calcoaceticus:* biotype and resistance-pattern of 328 strains consecutively isolated from clinical specimens. Acta Pathol. Microbiol. Immunol. Scand. Sect. B **95:**5–11.
17. **Gilardi, G. L.** 1985. Cultural and biochemical aspects for

identification of glucose-nonfermenting gram-negative rods, p. 17–84. *In* G. L. Gilardi (ed.), Nonfermentative gram-negative rods. Laboratory identification and clinical aspects. Marcel Dekker, Inc., New York.

18. **Gilardi, G. L.** 1988. Microbiological terminology update II. Hoffmann-La Roche, Inc., Nutley, N.J.
19. **Gilardi, G. L.** 1989. Identification of glucose-nonfermenting gram-negative rods. North General Hospital, New York.
20. **Grehn, M., and F. Müller.** 1989. The oxidase reaction of *Pasteurella multocida* strains cultured on Mueller-Hinton medium. J. Microbiol. Methods **9:**333–336.
21. **Henriksen, S. D., and K. Bøvre.** 1976. Transfer of *Moraxella kingae* Henriksen and Bøvre to the genus *Kingella* gen. nov. in the family *Neisseriaceae*. Int. J. Syst. Bacteriol. **26:**447–450.
22. **Hollis, D. G., R. E. Weaver, and P. S. Riley.** 1983. Emended description of *Kingella denitrificans* (Snell and Lapage 1976): correction of the maltose reaction. J. Clin. Microbiol. **18:**1174–1176.
23. **Hollis, D. G., G. L. Wiggins, and R. E. Weaver.** 1972. An unclassified gram-negative rod isolated from the pharynx on Thayer-Martin medium (selective agar). Appl. Microbiol. **24:**772–777.
24. **Holmes, B., D. G. Hollis, A. G. Steigerwalt, M. J. Pickett, and D. J. Brenner. 1983.** *Flavobacterium thalpophilum*, a new species recovered from human clinical material. Int. J. Syst. Bacteriol. **33:**677–682.
25. **Holmes, B., M. Popoff, M. Kiredjian, and K. Kersters.** 1988. *Ochrobactrum anthropi* gen. nov., sp. nov. from human clinical specimens and previously known as group Vd. Int. J. Syst. Bacteriol. **38:**406–416.
26. **Holmes, B., A. G. Steigerwalt, R. E. Weaver, and D. J. Brenner.** 1986. *Weeksella virosa* gen. nov., sp. nov. (formerly group IIf), found in human clinical specimens. Syst. Appl. Microbiol. **8:**185–190.
27. **Holmes, B., A. G. Steigerwalt, R. E. Weaver, and D. J. Brenner.** 1986. *Weeksella zoohelcum* sp. nov. (formerly group IIj), from human clinical specimens. Syst. Appl. Microbiol. **8:**191–196.
28. **Holmes, B., R. E. Weaver, A. G. Steigerwalt, and D. J. Brenner.** 1988. A taxonomic study of *Flavobacterium spiritivorum* and *Sphingobacterium mizutae:* proposal of *Flavobacterium yabuuchiae* sp. nov. and *Flavobacterium mizutaii* comb. nov. Int. J. Syst. Bacteriol. **38:**348–353.
29. **Juni, E.** 1984. Genus III. *Acinetobacter* Brisou and Prévot 1954, 727^{AL}, p. 303–307. *In* N. R. Krieg and J. G. Holt (ed.), Bergey's manual of systematic bacteriology, vol. 1. The Williams & Wilkins Co., Baltimore.
30. **Kaplan, A. H., D. J. Weber, E. Z. Oddone, and J. R. Perfect.** 1989. Infection due to *Actinobacillus actinomycetemcomitans:* 15 cases and review. Rev. Infect. Dis. **11:**46–63.
31. **Kersters, K., and J. De Ley.** 1984. Genus *Alcaligenes* Castellani and Chalmers 1919, 936^{AL}, p. 361–373. *In* N. R. Krieg and J. G. Holt (ed.), Bergey's manual of systematic bacteriology, vol. 1. The Williams & Wilkins Co., Baltimore.
32. **Kersters, K., and J. De Ley.** 1984. Genus III. *Agrobacterium* Conn 1942, 359^{AL}, p. 244–254. *In* N. R. Krieg and J. G. Holt (ed.), Bergey's manual of systematic bacteriology, vol. 1. The Williams & Wilkins Co., Baltimore.
33. **Kiredjian, M., B. Holmes, K. Kersters, I. Guilvout, and J. De Ley.** 1986. *Alcaligenes piechaudii*, a new species from human clinical specimens and the environment. Int. J. Syst. Bacteriol. **36:**282–287.
34. **Krause, T., I. Kunstýr, and R. Mutters.** 1989. Characterization of some previously unclassified *Pasteurellaceae* isolated from hamsters. J. Appl. Bacteriol. **67:**171–175.
35. **Morrison, V. A., and K. F. Wagner.** 1989. Clinical manifestations of *Kingella kingae* infections: case report and review. Rev. Infect. Dis. **11:**776–782.
36. **Moss, C. W., P. L. Wallace, D. G. Hollis, and R. E. Weaver.** 1988. Cultural and chemical characterization of CDC groups EO-2, M-5, and M-6, *Moraxella* (*Moraxella*) species, *Oligella urethralis*, *Acinetobacter* species, and *Psychrobacter immobilis*. J. Clin. Microbiol. **26:**484–492.
37. **Mutters, R., P. Ihm, S. Pohl, W. Frederiksen, and W. Mannheim.** 1985. Reclassification of the genus *Pasteurella* Trevisan 1887 on the basis of deoxyribonucleic acid homology, with proposals for the new species *Pasteurella dagmatis*, *Pasteurella canis*, *Pasteurella stomatis*, *Pasteurella anatis*, and *Pasteurella langaa*. Int. J. Syst. Bacteriol. **35:**309–322.
38. **Mutters, R., S. Pohl, and W. Mannheim.** 1986. Transfer of *Pasteurella ureae* Jones 1962 to the genus *Actinobacillus* Brumpt 1910: *Actinobacillus ureae* comb. nov. Int. J. Syst. Bacteriol. **36:**343–344.
39. **Nielsen, J. P., and V. T. Rosdahl.** 1990. Development and epidemiological applications of a bacteriophage typing system for typing *Pasteurella multocida*. J. Clin. Microbiol. **28:**103–107.
40. **Oberhofer, T. R.** 1985. Rapid identification of glucose-nonfermenting gram-negative rods with commercial miniaturized kits, p. 85–116. *In* G. L. Gilardi (ed.), Nonfermentative gram-negative rods. Laboratory identification and clinical aspects. Marcel Dekker, Inc., New York.
41. **Peel, M. M., A. J. Hibberd, B. M. King, and H. G. Williamson.** 1988. *Alcaligenes piechaudii* from chronic ear discharge. J. Clin. Microbiol. **26:**1580–1581.
42. **Perez, R. E.** 1986. Endocarditis with *Moraxella*-like M-6 after cardiac catheterization. J. Clin. Microbiol. **24:**501–502.
43. **Pickett, M. J.** 1988. Moraxellae: identification. Curr. Microbiol. **17:**281–283.
44. **Pickett, M. J.** 1989. Methods for identification of flavobacteria. J. Clin. Microbiol. **27:**2309–2315.
45. **Pickett, M. J., and J. R. Greenwood.** 1986. Identification of oxidase-positive, glucose-negative, motile species of nonfermentative bacilli. J. Clin. Microbiol. **23:**920–923.
46. **Potts, T. V., J. J. Zambon, and R. J. Genco.** 1985. Reassignment of *Actinobacillus actinomycetemcomitans* to the genus *Haemophilus* as *Haemophilus actinomycetemcomitans* comb. nov. Int. J. Syst. Bacteriol. **35:**337–341.
47. **Potvliege, C., L. Vanhuynegem, and W. Hansen.** 1989. Catheter infection caused by an unusual pathogen, *Agrobacterium radiobacter*. J. Clin. Microbiol. **27:**2120–2122.
48. **Rossau, R., G. Vandenbussche, S. Thielemans, P. Segers, H. Grosch, E. Göthe, W. Mannheim, and J. De Ley.** 1989. Ribosomal ribonucleic acid cistron similarities and deoxyribonucleic acid homologies of *Neisseria*, *Kingella*, *Eikenella*, *Simonsiella*, *Alysiella*, and Centers for Disease Control groups EF-4 and M-5 in the emended family *Neisseriaceae*. Int. J. Syst. Bacteriol. **39:**185–198.
49. **Rubin, S. J., P. A. Granato, and B. L. Wasilauskas.** 1985. Glucose-nonfermenting gram-negative bacteria, p. 330–349. *In* E. H. Lennette, A. Balows, W. J. Hausler, Jr., and H. J. Shadomy (ed.), Manual of clinical microbiology, 4th ed. American Society for Microbiology, Washington, D.C.
50. **Schlater, L. K., D. J. Brenner, A. G. Steigerwalt, C. W. Moss, M. A. Lambert, and R. A. Packer.** 1989. *Pasteurella caballi*, a new species from equine clinical specimens. J. Clin. Microbiol. **27:**2169–2174.
51. **Sivendra, R., and S. H. Tan.** 1977. Pathogenicity of nonpigmented cultures of *Chromobacterium violaceum*. J. Clin. Microbiol. **5:**514–516.
52. **Snell, J. J. S., and S. P. Lapage.** 1976. Transfer of some saccharolytic *Moraxella* species to *Kingella* Henriksen and Bøvre 1976, with descriptions of *Kingella indologenes* sp. nov. and *Kingella denitrificans* sp. nov. Int. J. Syst. Bacteriol. **26:**451–458.
53. **Socransky, S. S., S. C. Holt, E. R. Leadbetter, A. C. R. Tanner, E. Savitt, and B. F. Hammond.** 1979. *Capnocytophaga:* new genus of gram-negative gliding bacteria. III. Physiological characterization. Arch. Microbiol. **122:** 29–33.
54. **Traub, W. H.** 1989. *Acinetobacter baumannii* serotyping

for delineation of outbreaks of nosocomial cross-infection. J. Clin. Microbiol. **27:**2713–2716.

55. **Traub, W. H., and M. Spohr.** 1989. Antimicrobial drug susceptibility of clinical isolates of *Acinetobacter* species (*A. baumannii, A. haemolyticus,* genospecies 3, and genospecies 6). Antimicrobial. Agents Chemother. **33:**1617–1619.
56. **Van Horn, K. G., C. A. Gedris, T. Ahmed, and G. P. Wormser.** 1989. Bacteremia and urinary tract infection associated with CDC group Vd biovar 2. J. Clin. Microbiol. **27:**201–202.
57. **Verghese, A., F. Hamati, S. Berk, B. Franzus, S. Berk, and J. K. Smith.** 1988. Susceptibility of dysgonic fermenter 2 to antimicrobial agents in vitro. Antimicrob. Agents Chemother. **32:**78–80.
58. **Verhaegen, J., H. Verbraeken, A. Cabuy, J. Vandeven, and J. Vandepitte.** 1988. *Actinobacillus* (formerly *Pasteurella*) *ureae* meningitis and bacteraemia: report of a case and review of the literature. J. Infect. **17:**249–253.
59. **Veys, A., W. Callewaert, E. Waelkens, and K. Van Den Abbeele.** 1989. Application of gas-liquid chromatography to the routine identification of nonfermenting gram-negative bacteria in clinical specimens. J. Clin. Microbiol. **27:** 1538–1542.
60. **Vila, J., M. Almela, and M. T. Jimenez de Anta.** 1989. Laboratory investigation of a hospital outbreak caused by two different multiresistant *Acinetobacter calcoaceticus* subsp. *anitratus* strains. J. Clin. Microbiol. **27:**1086–1089.
61. **von Graevenitz, A.** 1985. Ecology, clinical significance, and antimicrobial susceptibility of infrequently encountered glucose-nonfermenting gram-negative rods, p. 181–232. *In* G. L. Gilardi (ed.), Nonfermentative gram-negative rods. Laboratory identification and clinical aspects. Marcel Dekker, Inc., New York.
62. **Wagner, D. K., J. J. Wright, A. F. Ansher, and V. J. Gill.** 1988. Dysgonic fermenter 3-associated gastrointestinal disease in a patient with common variable hypogammaglobulinemia. Am. J. Med. **84:**315–318.
63. **Wallace, P. L., D. G. Hollis, R. E. Weaver, and C. W. Moss.** 1989. Characterization of CDC group DF-3 by cellular fatty acid analysis. J. Clin. Microbiol. **27:**735–737.
64. **Weaver, R. E.** 1984. Genus *Cardiobacterium* Slotnick and Dougherty 1964, 271[AL], p. 583–585. *In* N. R. Krieg and J. G. Holt (ed.), Bergey's manual of systematic bacteriology, vol. 1. The Williams & Wilkins Co., Baltimore.
65. **Weaver, R. E., D. G. Hollis, and E. J. Bottone.** 1985. Gram-negative fermentative bacteria and *Francisella tularensis,* p. 309–329. *In* E. H. Lennette, A. Balows, W. J. Hausler, Jr., and H. J. Shadomy (ed.), Manual of clinical microbiology, 4th ed. American Society for Microbiology, Washington, D.C.
66. **Yabuuchi, E., T. Kaneko, I. Yano, C. W. Moss, and N. Miyoshi.** 1983. *Sphingobacterium* gen. nov., *Sphingobacterium spiritivorum* comb. nov., *Sphingobacterium multivorum* comb. nov., *Sphingobacterium mizutae* sp. nov., and *Flavobacterium indologenes* sp. nov.: glucose-nonfermenting gram-negative rods in CDC groups IIK-2 and IIb. Int. J. Syst. Bacteriol. **33:**580–598.
67. **Zambon, J. J.** 1985. *Actinobacillus actinomycetemcomitans* in human periodontal disease. J. Clin. Periodontol. **12:**1–20.

Chapter 41

Pseudomonas and Related Genera

GERALD L. GILARDI

A system is presented for the isolation and progressive identification of pseudomonads and related species and their differentiation from other nonfastidious, glucose-nonfermenting gram-negative rods encountered in clinical specimens. Classification consists of approved and proposed names based on volume 1 of *Bergey's Manual of Systematic Bacteriology* (27), recent Centers for Disease Control (CDC) publications, and issues of the *International Journal of Systematic Bacteriology* and related journals.

METHODS FOR ISOLATION AND IDENTIFICATION OF SPECIES OF *PSEUDOMONAS* AND RELATED GENERA

Isolation media

Nonfastidious, glucose-nonfermenting gram-negative rods (nonfermenters) grow easily on routine primary isolation media used in bacteriology and are readily isolated from clinical specimens and from hospital environments. They are usually isolated on peptone agar media with or without infusion containing 5% sheep or rabbit blood, although media enriched with blood are not essential for their isolation. In addition to blood agar, one of the less inhibitory selective-differential media, e.g., MacConkey or eosin-methylene blue agar, should be used for primary isolation, since the latter may increase the chance of recovering nonfermenters from a source that may contain numerous bacterial species. Media containing cetyltrimethylammonium bromide (cetrimide), 2,4,4-trichloro-2-hydroxydiphenyl ether (irgasan), 9-chloro-9-(4-diethylaminophenyl)-10-phenylacridan (C-390), sodium lauroyl sarcosine, or similar compounds are used for the selective isolation of *P. aeruginosa*. *P. cepacia* medium, containing crystal violet and polymyxin B, OFPBL (oxidation-fermentation base supplemented with agar, lactose, polymyxin B, and bacitracin), or similar media are used for selective isolation of *P. cepacia* from respiratory specimens of cystic fibrosis patients.

Identification methods

The battery of simple routine diagnostic media and tests recommended (Table 1) has been modified over a number of years and may need further revision as additional taxonomic and biochemical information on nonfermenters is obtained.

Screening procedure

A practical screening procedure designed to separate similar genera and to distinguish between species of nonfermenters should collect the following information: odor, pigmentation, and colonial morphology; Gram reaction, somatic shape, and spore formation; motility and flagellar morphology; mode of glucose utilization; production of hydrogen sulfide, arginine dihydrolase, and indophenol oxidase; growth at 42°C; and oxidation of glucose, xylose, lactose, and maltose in oxidative-fermentative (OF) basal medium (Difco Laboratories, no. 1688). Buffered single substrates and oxidative low-peptone medium are more sensitive alternatives to OF basal medium (18).

Somatic morphology

Species of *Pseudomonas* and related genera (*Chryseomonas, Comamonas, Flavimonas, Methylobacterium, Shewanella*, and *Xanthomonas*) are straight or slightly curved asporogenous rods. *Acinetobacter* species are usually very short plump rods often approaching coccoid shape. *Moraxella* species are usually very short plump rods, predominately in pairs and short chains and occasionally pleomorphic. The Gram reaction and spore formation of an isolate suspected of being a nonfermenter should be carefully studied. Troublesome isolates presumptively considered to be nonfermenters may be gram-negative-staining *Bacillus* species or gram-positive coryneforms. Colonies giving questionable Gram reactions can be examined with 3% KOH or L-alanine-4-nitroanilide (LANA test) (4). Growth from colonies of gram-negative rods becomes stringy when emulsified in KOH. The emulsion turns yellow in the LANA test.

Flagellar morphology

Flagellar morphology is readily observed with a light microscope after staining, such as with the method of Gray or Leifson (see chapter 122). Although many nonfermenters can be identified and differentiated without determining their flagellar morphology, this characteristic should be determined for the identification of apyocyanogenic *P. aeruginosa* strains, motile glucose nonoxidizers (e.g., *P. alcaligenes, P. diminuta, Comamonas* spp., *Alcaligenes faecalis*, and *Bordetella bronchiseptica*), and enzymatically aberrant strains.

Most flagellated nonfermenters can be divided into three groups according to attachment of the flagellum or flagella to the bacterial soma. Cells of strains of polar monotrichous species usually have one flagellum per pole or both poles. The number of flagella per pole on cells of strains of species with a tuft of polar flagella varies from zero to six or more. Cells of strains of peritrichous species have one or more flagella arranged on the cell. Cells without flagella often occur in flagellated populations. Some strains may produce subpolar and, under certain growth conditions, lateral flagella.

TABLE 1. Media and tests for isolation and identification of species of *Pseudomonas* and related genera

Purpose	Medium or test
Isolation, presumptive identification, and screening	Blood, infusion, or peptone agar
	MacConkey, Leifson deoxycholate, or eosin-methylene blue agar
	Kligler iron or triple sugar iron agar
	Motility
	OF glucose, lactose, xylose, and maltose media
	Indophenol oxidase
	Arginine dihydrolase (Moeller medium)
	Growth at 42°C
	Odor, colonial morphology, and pigmentation
	Somatic morphology (Gram stain)
	Flagellum stain
	Antibiogram
Further identification	Christensen urea agar
	Phenylalanine deaminase test agar
	Nitrate broth
	Lysine and ornithine decarboxylases
	DNase test medium
	OF fructose and mannitol media
	Esculin hydrolysis agar
	Nutrient gelatin
	Tryptone broth (for indole)
	Acetate assimilation test medium

When species of *Pseudomonas* and related genera are flagellated, the flagellum or flagella are attached at a pole. *Alcaligenes* species, *B. bronchiseptica*, *Agrobacterium* species, and *Ochrobactrum* species are peritrichous when flagellated and produce indophenol oxidase. *Acinetobacter* species are nonmotile rods and do not produce indophenol oxidase, whereas *Moraxella* species are nonmotile rods that produce indophenol oxidase. *Oligella* species are similar to *Moraxella* species except that they produce phenylalanine deaminase, utilize acetate, and may be motile. *Flavobacterium* species are nonmotile rods that produce indophenol oxidase, gelatinase, indole, and an intracellular yellow pigment. *Sphingobacterium* species do not produce indole or gelatinase but otherwise are similar to *Flavobacterium* species. *Weeksella* species are nonoxidizers and usually nonpigmented but otherwise are similar to *Flavobacterium* species.

Additional identification methods

Approximately 15% of all gram-negative isolates from clinical specimens are nonfermenters. Pyocyanogenic *P. aeruginosa* isolates account for about 70% of these isolates. *Acinetobacter* isolates are the second most frequently encountered nonfermenters, followed by *Xanthomonas maltophilia*. Other frequently encountered nonfermenters include *P. fluorescens, P. putida, P. cepacia, P. stutzeri, Flavobacterium indologenes, Alcaligenes* species, and *Moraxella* species, except for the rarely isolated *M. lacunata*. *P. pseudomallei* and *P. mallei* are geographically limited.

Although many nonfermenters can be identified from information collected during the screening procedure, it is necessary to detect additional characteristics (media are listed in Table 1) to identify other isolates. Serological (32, 42), bacteriophage (2), bacteriocin pattern (15), plasmid profile (39), and enzyme profile (38) systems have been used as epidemiological markers or research tools for identification of *P. aeruginosa*, *P. cepacia*, and *X. maltophilia*. Monoclonal antibody (31) and DNA hybridization probe (41) have been applied to the identification of *P. aeruginosa* and *P. fluorescens*. Some diagnostic laboratories find it expedient to use commercial micromethod identification kits or automated or semiautomated systems designed for nonfermenter identification (see chapter 18).

Incubation temperature

Primary isolation media are usually incubated at 35 or 37°C. These media initially incubated at 35°C for 24 to 48 h should be reincubated at 30°C or room temperature (18 to 22°C) to permit the growth of some nonfermenters in clinical specimens that grow slowly at 35°C and may be masked by other bacteria. Media used to detect enzymatic activity of nonfermenters should be incubated at 30°C unless otherwise stated or indicated. Since flagellar proteins are optimally synthesized at low temperature, motility medium and cultures to be stained for flagella should be incubated at room temperature. Some of the methods used in the study of nonfermenters are described in greater detail elsewhere (3, 6, 18, 28, 43, 44).

CHARACTERISTICS OF SPECIES OF *PSEUDOMONAS* AND RELATED GENERA

The common characteristics for identification of most strains of species of *Pseudomonas* and related genera (*Chryseomonas, Comamonas, Flavimonas, Methylobacterium, Shewanella,* and *Xanthomonas*) are presented in Table 2. Useful characteristics for species identification are given in Tables 3 through 18.

rRNA HOMOLOGY GROUP I

On the basis of extensive phylogenetic examinations, the genus *Pseudomonas* eventually may include only the saprophytic phytopathogenic fluorescent pseudo-

TABLE 2. Common characteristics for identification of species of *Pseudomonas* and related genera

Characteristic	Sign
Gram-negative, asporogenous, straight or slightly curved rod	+
Nonfastidious[a]	+
Motility[b]	+
Polar monotrichous or polar tuft of flagella[b]	+
Obligately aerobic[c]	+
Chemoorganotrophic	+
OF glucose medium open, acid (no gas)	+ or −
OF glucose medium sealed, acid	−
Indophenol oxidase	+ or −
Catalase	+
Indole	−
Photosynthetic pigment	−
Fluorescent and nonfluorescent pigments	+ or −

[a] Most grow with acetate as the sole carbon and energy source in a mineral base medium; a few require growth factors. All grow on infusion base agar.
[b] *P. mallei* is nonmotile and without flagella.
[c] Some species utilize nitrogen as a terminal acceptor anaerobically.

monads of the *P. fluorescens* DNA homology group, the nonfluorescent denitrifying species located in the *P. stutzeri* DNA homology group, and the nonpigmented strains with low metabolic activity that constitute the *P. alcaligenes* DNA homology group (10). These three DNA homology groups comprise rRNA homology group I.

P. fluorescens DNA Homology Group (*P. aeruginosa, P. fluorescens,* and *P. putida*)

Most strains of *P. aeruginosa* (24, 43), *P. fluorescens* (22, 43), and *P. putida* (43) (Table 3) produce indophenol oxidase, arginine dihydrolase, and water-soluble, yellow-green, yellow-brown, or colorless fluorescent pigments (pyoverdins). Fluorescent pigments that are not visible with ordinary light can be detected when exposed to UV light (ca. 254 nm). Production of pyoverdin is influenced by nutritional factors, and media that support growth may not promote their synthesis. Most strains are susceptible to polymyxin.

P. aeruginosa

Most *P. aeruginosa* strains are identified on the basis of the characteristic grapelike odor of aminoacetophenone, colonial morphology, growth at 42°C, and production of pyocyanin, a water-soluble blue, nonfluorescent, phenazine pigment. Water-soluble, nonfluorescent red (pyorubin) and brown (pyomelanin) pigments may be synthesized. The combination of yellow pyoverdins and blue pyocyanin give the green color associated with most *P. aeruginosa* strains. Colonies may have a metallic sheen (resembling phage plaques) representing autolysis. Colonial variants (smooth, coliform type, rough, mucoid, gelatinous, dwarf) arising by dissociation of a single strain give the false impression that different bacterial species are present. Mucoid strains frequently are atypical biochemically.

Apyocyanogenic (non-pyocyanin-producing) strains can be recognized as variants of *P. aeruginosa* by several uniform characteristics (Table 3): the presence of polar monotrichous flagella, growth at 42°C, oxidation of glucose, and failure to produce acid from disaccharides.

P. aeruginosa is widely distributed in soil, water, sewage, the mammalian gut, and plants and is frequently isolated from infusion fluids, disinfectants, cosmetics, and foodstuffs. The organism causes disease in humans as well as in certain animals, insects, and plants. *P. aeruginosa* is occasionally associated with community-acquired infections but is most frequently restricted to infections of hospitalized patients with predisposing factors. Sources in the hospital environment, including medical equipment and pharmaceuticals, may serve as transitory vectors. Colonized patients are the major reservoir. Person-to-person transfer serves as the most important mode of transmission. *P. aeruginosa* is an agent of meningitis, septicemia, endocarditis, severe epidemic diarrhea of infants, ocular infection, burn wound infection, cystic fibrosis-related lung infection, hot tub- and whirlpool-associated folliculitis, osteomyelitis, malignant external otitis, pneumonia, and urinary tract infection.

P. aeruginosa produces a variety of toxins and enzymes such as slime glycolipoprotein, alginate, hemolysin, fibrinolysin, lipase, esterase, lecithinase, elastase, DNase, phospholipase, endotoxin, enterotoxin, and exotoxin, some of which may contribute to its pathogenesis. The relationship of *P. aeruginosa* and other

TABLE 3. Characteristics useful for identification of *P. aeruginosa, P. fluorescens,* and *P. putida* strains

Characteristic[a]	Sign[b]		
	P. aeruginosa	*P. fluorescens*	*P. putida*
Pyocyanin	+ or −	−	−
Pyoverdin	+ or −	+	+ or −
Indophenol oxidase	+	+	+
Motility	+	+	+
Polar monotrichous flagella	+	−	−
Polar tuft of flagella	−	+	+
Glucose, acid (OFBM)	+	+	+
Arginine dihydrolase (DBM)	+	+	+
Gelatin hydrolysis	− or +	+	−
Growth at 42°C	+	−	−

[a] Abbreviations: OFBM, OF basal medium; DBM, decarboxylase base Moeller medium.
[b] +, 90% or more positive within 2 days; −, no reaction (90% or more); + or −, most strains positive; − or +, most strains negative.

nonfermenters to human disease has been summarized in a number of reviews (3, 6, 13, 33, 47).

P. fluorescens and *P. putida*

Strains of *P. fluorescens* and *P. putida* have a polar tuft of flagella, do not produce pyocyanin, and do not grow at 42°C. *P. fluorescens* is proteolytic, and a few strains reduce nitrate, occasionally with gas. *P. putida* does not reduce nitrate and is nonproteolytic. This separation on gelatinase activity alone is questionable. Failure to produce pyocyanin or to grow at 42°C and possession of a polar tuft of flagella distinguish *P. fluorescens* and *P. putida* from *P. aeruginosa.* It is rarely necessary to identify *P. fluorescens* and *P. putida* biovars (43) in a clinical laboratory. Some of these biovars may deserve independent species status.

A large number of fluorescent pseudomonads are not readily identified as one of the recognized species. Some of these strains may lack arginine dihydrolase or indophenol oxidase. Such strains are mainly psychrophils, food spoilage organisms, phytopathogens, or soil and water isolates not usually isolated from human sources.

P. fluorescens and *P. putida* are isolated from soil, water, plants, animal sources, the hospital environment, and human clinical specimens. *P. fluorescens* is commonly associated with spoilage of foodstuffs such as fish and meat. Both species are usually environmental contaminants and are rarely opportunistic pathogens for humans. *P. fluorescens* has been associated with empyema, urinary tract infection, postoperative infection, pelvic inflammatory disease, and fatal transfusion reactions due to contaminated blood. *P. putida* has been associated with infections of the extremities, bacteriuria, septic arthritis, septicemia following blood transfusion, and bacteremia associated with contaminated intravascular pressure monitor transducers. Both species are newly recognized as pathogens in cancer patients. Adhesive exopolysaccharides and lipopolysaccharide endotoxin possibly contribute to the pathogenesis of *P. fluorescens* and *P. putida.*

P. stutzeri DNA Homology Group (*P. stutzeri,* CDC Group Vb-3, and *P. mendocina*)

P. stutzeri (36, 43), CDC group Vb-3 (6), and *P. mendocina* (36) (Table 4) grow under strictly anaerobic conditions in nitrate-containing media, as do *P. aeruginosa, P. pseudomallei,* and other bacterial species that reduce nitrate to nitrogen gas. Strains are motile with a polar flagellum. Indophenol oxidase is produced. Acid is produced in glucose and certain other carbohydrates but not in lactose. The species are salt tolerant and nonhalophilic but require sodium cation for growth. Strains are uniformly susceptible to the polymyxins.

P. stutzeri

Most freshly isolated strains produce dry, wrinkled, tough, adherent colonies, smooth colonies, and various intermediate types. The colonies are usually buff to light brown because of a high intracellular concentration of cytochrome *c.* Ability to produce nitrogen gas may be lost on repeated subculture. Maltose and usually starch are attacked. Arginine dihydrolase is not produced, but *P. stutzeri*-like CDC group Vb-3 hydrolyzes arginine. *P. stutzeri* may be confused with *P. pseudomallei,* since the two species produce similar colony types. Flagellar morphology, susceptibility to the polymyxins, and reactions for starch, arginine, and lactose are the main distinguishing characteristics.

P. stutzeri has been isolated from soil, water, animal sources, the hospital environment, and human clinical specimens. This organism represents part of the increased flora during myelosuppressive therapy. Biovar Vb-3 strains have been isolated from human clinical materials and from dialysis supply tanks. *P. stutzeri* has been associated with various infections in humans, including pneumonia and septicemia in a patient with multiple myeloma, infant pleuropneumonia, septicemia caused by contaminated intravenous fluids, hip joint lesion in a diabetic patient, postoperative and posttraumatic infections of the extremities, cervical lymphadenopathy, otitis media, conjunctivitis, corneal ulcer, septic arthritis, urinary tract infection, prosthetic valve endocarditis, and puncture wound osteomyelitis.

P. mendocina

Colonies are flat, smooth, butyrous, and nonwrinkled, and they produce a brown-yellow, intracellular carotenoid pigment. Arginine dihydrolase is produced. Enzymes for maltose and starch are not produced. A polar monotrichous flagellum and growth at 42°C distinguish this species from phenotypically similar nitrogen gas-producing biovars of *P. fluorescens.*

TABLE 4. Characteristics useful for identification of *P. stutzeri,* CDC group Vb-3, and *P. mendocina* strains

Characteristic[a]	Sign[b]		
	P. stutzeri	Group Vb-3	*P. mendocina*
Wrinkled and smooth colonies, buff to light brown color	+	+	−
Smooth colonies and brown-yellow, intracellular pigment	−	−	+
Indophenol oxidase	+	+	+
Motility	+	+	+
Polar monotrichous flagella	+	+	+
Glucose, acid (OFBM)	+	+	+
Lactose	−	−	−
Maltose	+	+	−
Nitrate to gas	+	+	+
Arginine dihydrolase (DBM)	−	+	+

[a] See Table 3, footnote *a*.
[b] See Table 3, footnote *b*.

P. mendocina has been isolated from soil, water, and diseased fleece from sheep. Recovery from human clinical sources other than from urine and leg ulcer specimens has not been documented. Association with infections in humans is unknown.

P. alcaligenes DNA Homology Group (*P. alcaligenes* and *P. pseudoalcaligenes*)

Most strains of *P. alcaligenes* (23, 43) and *P. pseudoalcaligenes* (43) (Table 5) are motile with a single polar flagellum; the wavelength of the flagellum is approximately 1.6 μm. The species are biochemically inert. Indophenol oxidase is produced. Nitrate reduction (usually no gas) is strain variable. Alkali usually accumulates in OF glucose medium. Pigments are not produced.

P. pseudoalcaligenes produces a weak acid reaction from fructose in OF basal medium. Fructose is the only substrate used by all strains of *P. pseudoalcaligenes* and no strains of *P. alcaligenes*. Additional substrates (e.g., citrate, ethanol, and *n*-propanol) not used by any of the latter are used by most of the nutritionally more versatile *P. pseudoalcaligenes* strains. Phenotypic characteristics do not easily distinguish the two species.

P. alcaligenes and *P. pseudoalcaligenes* have been isolated from water, food, animal sources, hospital equipment, and human clinical specimens and are occasional opportunists. *P. alcaligenes* has been associated with endocarditis, neonatal septicemia, empyema, eye infection, and intrauterine infection. *P. pseudoalcaligenes* has been identified as the etiological agent of meningitis, septicemia, postoperative knee infection, pneumonitis, and intrauterine infection.

rRNA HOMOLOGY GROUP II

P. solanacearum DNA Homology Group (*P. pseudomallei, P. mallei, P. cepacia, P. gladioli,* and *P. pickettii*)

rRNA homology group II contains a number of species that are enzymatically, phenotypically, and genotypically related (1). With the exception of the opportunistic *P. pickettii* (*P. thomasii*), the species include the animal pathogens *P. mallei* (*Loefflerella mallei*) and *P. pseudomallei* (*Loefflerella pseudomallei*) and the plant pathogens *P. cepacia, P. gladioli* (*P. marginata, P. allicola*), *P. caryophylli,* and *P. solanacearum.* The latter two species have not been recovered from human sources.

The principal feature shared by *P. pseudomallei* (40), *P. mallei* (21, 40), *P. cepacia* (37), *P. gladioli* (5), and *P. pickettii* (26) (Tables 6 and 7) is nutritional versatility in the type and number of organic compounds utilized as sole sources of carbon and energy. A few strains fail to produce indophenol oxidase, and others produce a slow and very weak indophenol oxidase reaction. None of the isolates of these species are susceptible to the polymyxins.

P. pseudomallei

Colonies vary from mucoid and smooth to rough and wrinkled in texture and from bright orange to cream in color. A characteristic initial putrid odor is followed by an earthy odor. Strains are motile with a polar tuft of flagella. Growth accompanied by gas occurs anaerobically in nitrate-containing media. Gelatin and arginine are hydrolyzed, growth occurs at 42°C, and glucose, lactose, and a wide range of other carbohydrates are oxidized. Identification of suspicious isolates should be confirmed by a reference laboratory. Flagellar morphology and arginine, gelatin, lactose, and other reactions distinguish *P. pseudomallei* from *P. stutzeri.*

P. pseudomallei, a free-living organism, has been isolated from soil and water in restricted geographic regions. It causes melioidosis, an endemic glanders-like disease of humans and animals, in Southeast Asia and northern Australia and rarely in the Western Hemisphere. Patients with acquired immunodeficiency syndrome have developed melioidosis. Infection usually occurs in the United States among those who visited endemic regions. Laboratory-acquired infections occur. Toxins include a lethal factor with anticoagulant activity and a skin-necrotizing proteolytic agent.

P. mallei

Colonies are smooth and range from white to cream in color. Growth is slower than that of *P. pseudomallei* or *P. aeruginosa*. *P. mallei* is the only nonmotile species in the genus *Pseudomonas*. *P. mallei* slowly oxidizes glucose and a wide range of other carbohydrates but

TABLE 5. Characteristics useful for identification of *P. alcaligenes* and *P. pseudoalcaligenes* strains

Characteristic[a]	Sign[b]	
	P. alcaligenes	*P. pseudoalcaligenes*
Indophenol oxidase	+	+
Motility	+	+
Polar monotrichous flagella and normal wavelength	+	+
Glucose, acid (OFBM)	−	− or +
Fructose	−	+
Nitrate to gas	−	−

[a] See Table 3, footnote *a*.
[b] See Table 3, footnote *b*.

TABLE 6. Characteristics useful for identification of *P. pseudomallei* and *P. mallei* strains

Characteristic[a]	Sign[b]	
	P. pseudomallei	*P. mallei*[c]
Smooth to rough colonies, bright orange to cream color	+	−
Smooth colonies, white to cream color	−	+
Motility	+	−
Polar tuft of flagella	+	−
Glucose, acid (OFBM)	+	+
Maltose	+	(+)
Nitrate to gas	+	−
Arginine dihydrolase (DBM)	+	+ or (+)
Growth at 42°C	+	−

[a] See Table 3, footnote *a*.
[b] (+), Reactions delayed 2 or more days; for other signs, see Table 3, footnote *b*.
[c] Data from Hugh (21).

TABLE 7. Characteristics useful for identification of *P. cepacia, P. gladioli,* and biovars of *P. pickettii* strains

Characteristic[a]	Sign[b]				
	P. cepacia	*P. gladioli*	*P. pickettii*		
			Biovar 1	Biovar 2	Biovar 3
Green-yellow, water-soluble pigment	+ or −	+	−	−	−
Indophenol oxidase	+ or +(w)	−[c]	+	+	+
Motility	+	+	+	+	+
Polar monotrichous flagella	−	+	+	+	+
Polar tuft of flagella	+	−	−	−	−
Glucose, acid (OFBM)	+	+	(+)	(+)	(+)
Lactose, maltose	+	−	(+)	−	(+)
Mannitol	+	+	−	−	(+)
Nitrate to gas	−	−	(+)	(+)	(+) or −
Lysine decarboxylase (DBM)	+	−	−	−	−

[a] See Table 3, footnote *a*.
[b] (w), Weakly reactive; for other signs, see Tables 3 and 4, footnotes *b*.
[c] Oxidase-positive strains reported (5).

not xylose or sucrose. Arginine dihydrolase is produced. Negative reactions occur for nitrogen gas production, gelatin hydrolysis, and growth at 42°C.

P. mallei is considered to be the only true parasite of animals in the genus *Pseudomonas.* It is the agent of glanders (farcy) of equines, which is transmitted, although quite rarely, from equine hosts to humans by direct contact and from person to person. The disease is limited to Asia, parts of Africa, and the Middle East. *P. mallei* produces the endotoxin mallein.

P. cepacia

Some *P. cepacia* strains produce a green-yellow, water-soluble, nonfluorescent phenazine pigment. Brown, red, or purple pigments may be produced, depending on the carbon sources used for growth. These water-soluble pigments occur in the bacterial cell but may not diffuse into the surrounding agar medium. Many strains of clinical origin are nonpigmented. Colonies on blood agar are opaque, glistening, occasionally mottled, convex in elevation, and butyrous in consistency. A sweet odor similar to that associated with *P. aeruginosa* is produced by some strains.

P. cepacia is motile with a polar tuft of three to eight flagella. Acid is produced from a wide range of carbohydrates, including lactose and maltose. Most strains hydrolyze *o*-nitrophenyl-β-D-galactopyranoside (ONPG), gelatin, and esculin and decarboxylate lysine and ornithine. A number of classifications into biovars on the basis of enzymatic activity and growth temperature, as well as bacteriocin patterns, plasmid profiles, and serotyping systems, permit epidemiological marking of strains.

P. cepacia has been isolated from rotten onions (as a phytopathogen), soil from a variety of geographic regions, animal sources, disinfectants, pharmaceuticals, hospital equipment, and various clinical specimens. *P. cepacia* colonizes patients during myelosuppressive therapy. This primarily opportunistic organism has been associated with various types of human infections of community-acquired and nosocomial origins, including septicemia, meningitis, endocarditis, pneumonia, postoperative wound and urinary tract infections, septic arthritis, chronic granulomatous disease, cystic fibrosis-related lung infection, cervical osteomyelitis, conjunctivitis, corneal ulcer, and endophthalmitis. Potential virulence factors include protease, lipase, lecithinase, and hemolysin. An intrabacterial toxic complex appears to be responsible for pulmonary necrosis associated with pneumonia.

P. gladioli

P. gladioli closely resembles some yellow-pigmented strains of *P. cepacia* but is distinguished from the latter by a number of attributes. *P. gladioli* is motile with a single polar flagellum and hydrolyzes ONPG and urea. Negative test reactions occur for indophenol oxidase (usually), sucrose, and maltose and for decarboxylation of lysine and ornithine (7).

P. gladioli is a phytopathogen isolated from decayed onions. Strains have been isolated from water, blood, and cerebrospinal fluid and from respiratory specimens of patients with cystic fibrosis; otherwise it has rarely been recovered from human clinical specimens. Clinical significance is undetermined.

P. pickettii

In contrast to other species in the *P. solanacearum* DNA group, colonies of *P. pickettii* are nonpigmented. Growth development on blood agar and other media characteristically is slow. Cells are motile by means of a polar flagellum. Indophenol oxidase and urease are produced. Acid development from carbohydrates in OF medium and nitrate reduction to gas characteristically are slow and may require 48 h of incubation to detect. The optimum temperature of incubation for the detection of nitrogen gas is 30°C. Dihydrolase and decarboxylases are not produced. Several biovars are differentiated by acidification of specific carbohydrates, growth at 42°C, nitrate reduction, and gelatinase production.

P. pickettii has been isolated from wet hospital equipment, hospital solutions, cosmetics, paper mill effluent, teething rings, and patient sources. Primarily opportunistic, this organism has been implicated in a case of acute, nonfatal meningitis, infections of the urinary and respiratory tracts, and a number of cases of septicemia, both in diabetic patients and in patients in cardiac units, resulting from the use of contaminated antiseptics, intravenous fluids, and respiratory therapy solutions.

rRNA HOMOLOGY GROUP III

P. acidovorans DNA Homology Group (*C. acidovorans, C. testosteroni,* and *C. terrigena*)

rRNA homology group III contains the *P. acidovorans* and the *P. facilis-delafieldii* DNA homology groups. *P. acidovorans, P. testosteroni,* and *P. terrigena* (*Vibrio terrigenus*), which constitute the *P. acidovorans* DNA group, are not members of the genus *Pseudomonas*. Flagellar morphology, physiology, and electron microscopy indicate a relationship closer to the genus *Spirillum* than to the genus *Pseudomonas*. The genus *Comamonas* was proposed for the *P. acidovorans* group, and the name *C. terrigena* was revived (9). *P. acidovorans* and *P. testosteroni* were later transferred to the genus (46).

Cells of *Comamonas acidovorans, C. testosteroni,* and *C. terrigena* (9, 46) (Table 8) are motile by means of a polar tuft of one to six flagella with a mean wavelength of 3.1 μm, a distinctive characteristic of the comamonads. Indophenol oxidase is produced. Nitrate is reduced (no gas). Acid is not produced from glucose, and most carbohydrates are not oxidized. Although indole is not produced, *C. acidovorans* strains produce anthranilic acid and kynurenine in tryptone broth, which react to form an orange color with Kovacs reagent. Growth is not pigmented.

Oxidation of fructose and mannitol in OF medium and additional phenotypic features distinguish *C. acidovorans* from *C. testosteroni* and *C. terrigena*. *C. terrigena* is differentiated from *C. testosteroni* in requiring growth factors (methionine and nicotinamide) in a mineral base medium and by utilizing β-alanine but not histidine and phenylalanine. *C. testosteroni* is distinguished from *C. terrigena* in having no growth factor requirements and by utilizing histidine and phenylalanine but not β-alanine as sole source of carbon. Acetamide hydrolysis, mediated by an aliphatic amidase, is a practical reaction for distinguishing *C. acidovorans* from other comamonads. This enzyme occurs also in other nonfermenters.

Comamonads have a wide geographic distribution and are common soil and water saprophytes. Comamonads have been isolated from animal sources, foodstuffs, hospital equipment, and human clinical specimens but are rarely clinically significant. *C. acidovorans* was the etiological agent of a corneal ulcer and (along with *Enterobacter cloacae*) septicemia in five patients undergoing cardiovascular monitoring. Incompletely identified comamonads (either *C. testosteroni* or *C. terrigena*) have been associated with septicemia and endocarditis.

P. facilis-delafieldii DNA Homology Group (*P. delafieldii*)

P. delafieldii (11, 35) (Table 9) possesses a single polar flagellum. Indophenol oxidase is produced. Acid develops in glucose, xylose, and mannitol in OF medium but not in lactose, sucrose, or maltose. Positive test reactions occur for nitrate reduction (no gas), arginine dihydrolase, urease, DNase, and gelatinase.

P. delafieldii has been isolated from soil, pus from cement femur, joint aspiration, and trachea. No information concerning its clinical role is available.

rRNA HOMOLOGY GROUP IV

P. diminuta DNA Homology Group (*P. diminuta* and *P. vesicularis*)

P. diminuta and *P. vesicularis* are more closely related to the genus *Gluconobacter* or *Acetobacter* than to the genus *Pseudomonas* because of the production of acid from primary alcohols, the multiple requirements for growth factors, and the production of orange pigment, among other characteristics. The *P. diminuta* homology group is temporarily placed in the genus *Pseudomonas* and deserves a separate generic rank (8).

The distinctive characteristic of the strains of *P. diminuta* (6, 29) and *P. vesicularis* (6, 12) (Table 10) is the very tightly coiled monotrichous flagellum with a wavelength that varies from 0.62 to 0.98 μm. The wavelength of most polar monotrichous pseudomonads is approximately 2 μm. Indophenol oxidase is produced. Additional characteristics include a requirement for specific growth factors, the production of acid from primary alcohols by all strains that can utilize alcohols, and an otherwise restricted range of biochemical activities. Nitrate is rarely reduced.

Colonies of *P. diminuta* are usually chalk white in color. Most carbohydrates in OF basal medium are not oxidized, although a few strains weakly produce acid from glucose. Pellicle forms in broth culture. Esculin is not hydrolyzed. Panthothenate, biotin, cyanocobalamin, and cystine are required as growth factors.

P. vesicularis is distinguished from *P. diminuta* by weak oxidation (strain variable) of glucose, xylose, and maltose, failure to produce a pellicle in broth culture,

TABLE 8. Characteristics useful for identification of *C. acidovorans, C. testosteroni,* and *C. terrigena* strains

Characteristic[a]	Sign[b]		
	C. acidovorans	*C. testosteroni*	*C. terrigena*
Indophenol oxidase	+	+	+
Motility	+	+	+
Polar tuft of flagella and long wavelength	+	+	+
Glucose, acid (OFBM)	−	−	−
Fructose, mannitol	+	−	−
Mineral base medium + acetate	+	+	−

[a] See Table 3, footnote *a*.
[b] See Table 3, footnote *b*.

TABLE 9. Characteristics useful for identification of *P. delafieldii* strains

Characteristic[a]	Sign[b]
Indophenol oxidase	+
Motility	+
Polar monotrichous flagella	+
Glucose, fructose, xylose, mannitol, acid (OFBM)	+
Maltose	−
Arginine dihydrolase	+
Urease	+
DNase	+
Gelatinase	+

[a] See Table 3, footnote *a*.
[b] See Table 3, footnote *b*.

TABLE 11. Characteristics useful for identification of *X. maltophilia* strains

Characteristic[a]	Sign[b]
Lavender-green color on blood agar	+
Indophenol oxidase	−
Motility	+
Polar tuft of flagella	+
Maltose, acid (OFBM)	+
Lysine decarboxylase (DBM)	+
Esculin hydrolysis	+
DNase	+

[a] See Table 3, footnote *a*.
[b] See Table 3, footnote *b*.

production of an orange, intracellular carotenoid pigment (strain variable), and a requirement for pantothenate, biotin, and cyanocobalamin (but not cystine) as growth factors. The hydrolysis of esculin by *P. vesicularis* is a useful method for distinguishing this species from *P. diminuta*. *P. vesicularis* and most *P. diminuta* strains produce acid from ethanol.

P. diminuta and *P. vesicularis* have been isolated from water, hospital equipment, and human clinical specimens. *P. diminuta* was determined to be the etiological agent in one case of septicemia, but the clinical significance of both species is uncertain.

rRNA HOMOLOGY GROUP V

P. maltophilia-Xanthomonas DNA Homology Group (*X. maltophilia*)

The transfer of *P. maltophilia* to the genus *Xanthomonas* as a separate species, *X. maltophilia*, has been proposed (45). This proposal was based partly on the following common reactions: acid reactions from OF glucose, lactose, and maltose; alkaline reactions from rhamnose and mannitol; negative indophenol oxidase reaction; hydrolysis of ONPG and esculin; and a requirement for growth factors.

Colonies of *X. maltophilia* (6, 43) (Table 11) are opaque and flat with rugose surfaces and uneven borders and develop a characteristic lavender-green color on blood agar media. A greenish discoloration of erythrocytes develops around confluent growth. Brown-colored by-products of metabolism may accumulate in certain agar media. A similar reaction is observed with other nonfermenters. Growth on nutrient agar media is usually accompanied by a very faint yellow, intracellular pigment that is water-soluble but does not diffuse into the agar medium. Growth on blood agar is accompanied by a strong odor of ammonia.

Strains of *X. maltophilia* are motile with a polar tuft of one to six or more flagella. Acid accumulates in glucose, maltose, and other carbohydrates. An ONPG reaction is produced by most strains. Lysine decarboxylase, esculin, DNase, and gelatin reactions are produced. Indophenol oxidase reaction is usually negative. Most (biovar 1) but not all (biovar 2) strains require methionine (or cystine plus glycine) for growth.

X. maltophilia is a free-living, ubiquitous organism with a wide geographic distribution; it has been isolated from water, soil, animal sources, plant material, foods, pharmaceuticals, hospital equipment, and human clinical specimens. *X. maltophilia* is usually a commensal or contaminant and is part of the transient flora of hospitalized patients. *X. maltophilia* has been associated with primary pneumonia and nosocomial infections, including endocarditis, septicemia, bronchial, lobar, and aspiration pneumonia, urinary tract infection, cholangitis, meningitis, acute mastoiditis, postoperative and posttraumatic wound infections, conjunctivitis, corneal ulcer, and ecthyma gangrenosum. A high incidence of infections occurs in patients with malignant solid tumors, leukemia, and lymphoma. Enzymes such as elastase, esterase, lipase, mucinase, hyaluronidase, RNase, and hemolysin may be potential virulence factors.

TABLE 10. Characteristics useful for identification of *P. diminuta* and *P. vesicularis* strains

Characteristic[a]	Sign[b]	
	P. diminuta	*P. vesicularis*
Chalk white color	+ or −	−
Orange, intracellular pigment	−	+ or −
Indophenol oxidase	+	+
Motility	+	+
Polar monotrichous flagella and short wavelength	+	+
Glucose, maltose, acid (OFBM)	− or +(w)	+(w) or −
Esculin hydrolysis	−	+

[a] See Table 3, footnote *a*.
[b] See Table 7, footnote *b*.

SPECIES OF UNCERTAIN RNA HOMOLOGY GROUP AFFILIATION

P. paucimobilis

Evidence from DNA hybridization results, rRNA cistron comparisons, and cellular fatty acid profiles indicates that *P. paucimobilis* is not an authentic member of the genus *Pseudomonas* and that a new genus designation may be justified (10, 34).

Colonies of *P. paucimobilis* (6, 19) (Table 12) are circular, convex, entire, smooth, opaque, and butyrous in consistency except for occasional viscous and mucoid strains. An intracellular, nondiffusible carotenoid (nostoxanthin) yellow pigment develops which is distinct from the pigments of other yellow-pigmented species.

TABLE 12. Characteristics useful for identification of *P. paucimobilis* strains

Characteristic[a]	Sign[b]
Yellow, intracellular pigment	+
Indophenol oxidase	+
Motility	+ or −
Polar monotrichous flagella	+ or −
Glucose, maltose, acid (OFBM)	+
Mannitol	−
ONPG reaction	+
Urease	−
Esculin hydrolysis	+
Lysine decarboxylase (DBM)	−

[a] See Table 3, footnote *a*.
[b] See Table 3, footnote *b*.

Cells are motile by means of a single polar flagellum. Occasionally only a few cells in a population are motile (motility may be difficult to demonstrate). Indophenol oxidase is usually produced. Acid is produced in OF basal medium from a wide range of carbohydrates but not from mannitol or other sugar alcohols. ONPG and esculin are hydrolyzed. Reactions for urease, nitrate, dihydrolase, and decarboxylases are negative. Lack of urease distinguishes nonmotile strains of this species (CDC group IIk-1) from phenotypically similar strains of *Sphingobacterium (Flavobacterium) multivorum* (CDC group IIk-2).

P. paucimobilis has been isolated from water sources, plants, air, hospital equipment, pharmaceuticals, and human clinical specimens. This opportunist has been implicated in human infections of community-acquired and nosocomial origins, including meningitis, urinary tract infection, peritonitis during ambulatory peritoneal dialysis, multiple skin granuloma, splenic abscess (along with *Clostridium difficile*), empyema following orthotopic cardiac transplantation, postoperative and posttraumatic wound infections, and septicemia in patients with chronic leg disease and pulmonary embolism. DNase, lipase, esterase, phosphatase, and an endotoxin-like factor may contribute to its virulence.

P. pertucinogena

P. pertucinogena, on the basis of a study of two strains by Kawai and Yabuuchi (25) (Table 13), produces gray colonies on Bordet-Gengou medium that mimic colonies of rough phase IV strains of *Bordetella pertussis*. Colonies on tryptic soy agar are semitranslucent, entire, smooth, and glistening. Water-soluble pigments are not formed. The organism is polar monotrichous and produces indophenol oxidase, phenylalanine deaminase, a weak delayed reaction in OF glucose, and pertussin, a bacteriocin that inhibits the growth of *B. pertussis*. The source of two collection strains is not recorded but was probably the human respiratory tract. Clinical significance is unknown.

Pseudomonas-like group 2

The flagellar morphology of *Pseudomonas*-like group 2 (CDC group IVd; EF group 1) (7) (Table 14) is similar to that of the comamonads. Colonies on blood agar media have a sticky consistency and are difficult to remove. Indophenol oxidase, urea, ONPG, and phenylalanine deaminase reactions are positive. Acid is produced in glucose, xylose, mannitol, and lactose (variable) but not sucrose and maltose. Nitrate, esculin, gelatin, dihydrolase, and decarboxylase reactions are negative.

Isolates have been recovered from the human respiratory tract (and may be associated with acute or chronic respiratory distress), blood, and dialysate.

Pseudomonas sp. CDC group 1

Pseudomonas sp. CDC group 1 (6) (Table 15) is similar to *P. alcaligenes*. The major phenotypic difference is the reduction of both nitrate and nitrite to gas. The organism has been isolated from environmental sources and human clinical specimens. One isolate caused bacteremia and meningitis.

C. luteola

Chryseomonas luteola was proposed (20) for *Pseudomonas luteola*, which is unrelated to the rRNA homology groups of the genus *Pseudomonas*. Strains of *C. luteola* (6, 20) (Table 16) produce smooth colonies, wrinkled, rough, and adherent colonies, or a mixture of colony types with an intracellular, nondiffusible, water-insoluble, yellow pigment. Strains are motile with a polar tuft of one to six or more flagella. Indophenol oxidase is not produced. Acid is produced from a number of carbohydrates and polyhydric alcohols in OF medium. *C. luteola* is distinguished from motile strains of *P. paucimobilis*, since the former strains use polyhydric alcohols, do not produce indophenol oxidase, and may produce wrinkled colonies. *C. luteola* is dis-

TABLE 13. Characteristics useful for identification of *P. pertucinogena* strains[a]

Characteristic[b]	Sign[c]
Water-soluble pigments	−
Indophenol oxidase	+
Motility	+
Polar monotrichous flagella	+
Phenylalanine deaminase	+
Glucose, acid (OFBM)	− or +(w)
Hydrogen sulfide (Kligler iron agar)	−
Nitrate reduction	−
Urease	−

[a] Data from Kawai and Yabuuchi (25).
[b] See Table 3, footnote *a*.
[c] See Table 7, footnote *b*.

TABLE 14. Characteristics useful for identification of *Pseudomonas*-like group 2 strains

Characteristic[a]	Sign[b]
Indophenol oxidase	+
Motility	+
Polar tuft of flagella and long wavelength	+
Glucose, acid (OFBM)	+
Lactose	− or +
Sucrose, maltose	−
ONPG reaction	+
Phenylalanine deaminase	+
Urease	+
Gelatinase	−

[a] See Table 3, footnote *a*.
[b] See Table 3, footnote *b*.

TABLE 15. Characteristics useful for identification of *Pseudomonas* sp. group 1 strains

Characteristic[a]	Sign[b]
Indophenol oxidase	+
Motility	+
Polar monotrichous flagella and normal wavelength	+
Glucose, acid (OFBM)	−
Nitrate and nitrite to gas	+

[a] See Table 3, footnote *a*.
[b] See Table 3, footnote *b*.

tinguished from *Flavimonas oryzihabitans* by flagellar morphology and by positive test reactions by the former for nitrate reduction (no gas) and hydrolysis of ONPG, esculin, and arginine.

C. luteola is not found in the general environment but is primarily recovered as a saprophyte or commensal from human sources. This opportunistic organism has been associated with prosthetic valve endocarditis, subdiaphragmatic abscess, postoperative infant septicemia (along with *F. oryzihabitans*), septicemia in patients with pancreatic abscess and granulomatous hepatitis, and peritonitis in patients undergoing continuous ambulatory peritoneal dialysis.

F. oryzihabitans

F. oryzihabitans was proposed (20) for *Pseudomonas oryzihabitans,* which is unrelated to any of the five major rRNA hybridization groups of the genus *Pseudomonas.* Colonies of *F. oryzihabitans* (5, 17) (Table 16) (like those of *C. luteola*) may be smooth or wrinkled, rough, and adherent with an intracellular, nondiffusible, water-insoluble, yellow pigment. Strains are motile with a single polar flagellum. Indophenol oxidase is not produced. Acid is produced from a number of carbohydrates and polyhydric alcohols. *F. oryzihabitans* is distinguished from phenotypically related *C. luteola* by flagellar morphology and by negative test reactions by the former for nitrate reduction and hydrolysis of ONPG, esculin, and arginine.

F. oryzihabitans is found in the general environment, including rice paddies and rice flour, in the hospital environment, and as a saprophyte of humans and other warm-blooded animals. The opportunist has been associated with postoperative infant septicemia (along with *C. luteola*), postneurosurgical septicemia, septicemia in patients with severe digestive hemorrhage and metastatic adenocarcinoma of the stomach, and peritonitis in patients on continuous ambulatory peritoneal dialysis.

TABLE 16. Characteristics useful for identification of *C. luteola* and *F. oryzihabitans* strains

Characteristic[a]	Sign[b]	
	C. luteola	*F. oryzihabitans*
Smooth and/or wrinkled colonies	+	+
Yellow, intracellular pigment	+	+
Indophenol oxidase	−	−
Motility	+	+
Polar monotrichous flagella	−	+
Polar tuft of flagella	+	−
Glucose, mannitol, acid (OFBM)	+	+
Esculin hydrolysis	+	−

[a] See Table 3, footnote *a*.
[b] See Table 3, footnote *b*.

Methylobacterium spp.

Red-pigmented facultative methanol oxidizers, e.g., *Pseudomonas mesophilica,* are not pseudomonads and have been placed in the emended genus *Methylobacterium,* family *Methylococcaceae* (16). The nondiffusible pink- to red-pigmented colonies of *Methylobacterium* spp. (13, 14) (Table 17) grow poorly on media used for isolation of other nonfermenters. Growth occurs best, for example, on Sabouraud agar, buffered charcoal-yeast extract agar, or Middlebrook and Cohn 7H11 agar. No growth occurs on MacConkey agar. Growth may occur better at 30 than at 35°C. The slow-growing organisms after 4 or 5 days develop into small, round, raised, shiny, and entire colonies about 1 mm in diameter. Cells are straight to slightly curved, diphtheroid-like rods containing large volutin granules. A tendency to resist Gram decolorization is noted. Most strains are motile (weakly and not readily detectable) with a single polar flagellum. Indophenol oxidase, urease, and amylase are produced. Oxidase reaction may be weak. *Methylobacterium* spp. are facultative methanol oxidizers. Weak acid is produced (strain variable) from a few carbohydrates in OF medium. Acetate is utilized as the sole source of carbon and energy in a mineral base medium without growth factors.

Eight species (*M. extorquens, M. fujisawaense, M. mesophilicum, M. organophilum, M. radiotolerans, M. rhodinum, M. rhodesianum,* and *M. zatmanii*) and additional unassigned biovars are recognized on the basis of substrates utilized as sole carbon source (16, 17).

Methylobacterium spp. are isolated from a wide range of habitats, such as soil, water, air, rice grain, sewage, rumen of cows, and the hospital environment, but primarily from leaf surfaces and leaf nodules of plants (perennial ryegrass, tobacco, soybean, etc.). The species

TABLE 17. Characteristics useful for identification of *Methylobacterium* spp. and unnamed pink-pigmented rod strains

Characteristic[a]	Sign[b]	
	Methylobacterium spp.	Unnamed pink-pigmented rod
Pink, intracellular pigment	+	+
Vacuolated rods	+	−
Indophenol oxidase	+ or +(w)	+ or +(w)
Motility	+	+ or −
Polar monotrichous flagella	+	+ or −
Methanol, acid (OFBM)	+ or −	−
Urease	+	+
Starch hydrolysis	+	+
Mineral base medium + acetate	+	−
Growth at 42°C	−	+ or −

[a] See Table 3, footnote *a*.
[b] See Table 7, footnote *b*.

are occasionally isolated from human clinical specimens. Rarely clinically significant, *Methylobacterium* spp. have been implicated in an outbreak of nosocomial infections in a bone marrow transplant unit, bacteremia in a patient with metastatic adenocarcinoma of the lung, catheter-induced bacteremia, peritonitis in a patient undergoing continuous ambulatory peritoneal dialysis, and probably chronic skin ulcer infection.

Unnamed pink-pigmented rods

Unnamed pink-pigmented rods (14) are phenotypically similar to *Methylobacterium* spp. but probably are not genotypically related. The unnamed pigmented rods (14) (Table 17) grow on Sabouraud agar, and some strains also grow on blood agar media. After 2 to 3 days, the organisms develop into either small, round, raised, shiny, and entire colonies about 1 mm in diameter or larger mucoid colonies about 2 mm in diameter. Cells are short, plump rods in pairs without vacoules. Indophenol oxidase, urease, and amylase are produced. Methanol is not utilized, and growth does not occur with acetate as the sole carbon source in mineral base medium. Weak acid is produced from fructose and occasionally other carbohydrates in OF medium. Motility and growth on MacConkey agar and at 42°C are strain variable.

These bacteria have been isolated from environmental sources and human clinical specimens. The opportunist has been associated with septicemia in patients with acute myelogenous leukemia and pancreatic abscess.

S. putrefaciens

Pseudomonas putrefaciens (*P. rubescens*) does not belong in the genus *Pseudomonas*. Although the name *Alteromonas putrefaciens* for this organism is validly published, the proposed new genus *Shewanella* for the alteromonads within the family *Vibrionaceae* has been supported by analyses of polar lipids, fatty acids, and isoprenoid quinones (30).

Colonies of *Shewanella putrefaciens* (6, 30) (Table 18) are dome shaped, circular, smooth, slightly viscous or mucoid, and usually red-brown or salmon pink in color. Hemodigestion appears in the zone of heavy growth on blood agar. Cells are motile by means of a single polar flagellum. Indophenol oxidase is produced. Abundant hydrogen sulfide is produced in Kligler iron agar. An occasional strain may produce very little or no hydrogen sulfide. Nitrate is reduced (no gas). Gelatinase, ornithine decarboxylase, and DNase tests are positive. Biovars are distinguished on the basis of oxidation of sucrose and maltose, ability to grow in a high (6.5%) salt concentration, and additional properties.

Biovar 1 (CDC group Ib-1) is found primarily in dairy, fishery, and other environmental sources and causes spoilage of protein foods stored at refrigerator temperatures, such as butter, fish, meat, and poultry. Biovar 1 occasionally is isolated from human clinical specimens but rarely is clinically significant. It has been implicated in an intra-abdominal abscess in a patient with colonic carcinoma and was isolated from the bile of a patient with biliary tract disease. The remaining biovars (including CDC group Ib-2) are primarily isolated from human clinical specimens and occasionally from environmental sources. Biovar 2, an occasional opportunist, has been associated with a case of meningitis following head injury, otitis media, and septicemia in patients with chronic leg ulcers.

TABLE 18. Characteristics useful for identification of *S. putrefaciens* biovar strains

Characteristic[a]	Sign[b]		
	Biovar 1	Biovar 2	Biovar 3
Red-brown or pink color	+	+	+
Indophenol oxidase	+	+	+
Motility	+	+	+
Polar monotrichous flagella	+	+	+
Sucrose, maltose, acid (OFBM)	+	−	−
Hydrogen sulfide (Kligler iron agar)	+	+	+
Ornithine decarboxylase (DBM)	+	+	+
DNase	+	+	+
Growth on salmonella-shigella agar	−	+	−
Growth on 6.5% NaCl agar	−	+	−

[a] See Table 3, footnote *a*.
[b] See Table 3, footnote *b*.

ANTIMICROBIAL SUSCEPTIBILITY

Strains of *P. aeruginosa* are generally susceptible to the anti-*Pseudomonas* penicillins (carbenicillin, ticarcillin, piperacillin, mezlocillin, and azlocillin), a large number of third-generation cephalosporins (cefoperazone, cefotaxime, and ceftazidime), and the aminoglycosides (gentamicin, tobramycin, and amikacin) as well as to the newer fluorinated carboxyquinolone compounds (ciprofloxacin), monobactams (aztreonam), and thienamycins (imipenem). Synergy is shown between the anti-*Pseudomonas* penicillins and aminoglycosides. Strains are usually resistant to the antistaphylococcal penicillins, ampicillin, the macrolides, the lincosamides, first- and second-generation cephalosporins, the tetracyclines, chloramphenicol, and trimethoprim-sulfamethoxazole.

P. pseudomallei and related species (e.g., *P. cepacia*) are resistant to the polymyxins and aminoglycosides. Most *P. pseudomallei* strains are susceptible to tetracycline, chloramphenicol, kanamycin, gentamicin, tobramycin, and ceftazidime. *P. cepacia* is susceptible to piperacillin, mezlocillin, minocycline, chloramphenicol, trimethoprim-sulfamethoxazole, and imipenem.

Most *X. maltophilia* strains show multiple resistance. Susceptibility is demonstrated to moxalactam, doxycycline, chloramphenicol, ciprofloxacin, and trimethoprim-sulfamethoxazole; other antimicrobial agents are either constantly ineffective or rarely effective. Antibiograms have been described in detail elsewhere (3, 40, 47). Because of the unpredictable resistance to antimicrobial agents, determination of the specific antibiogram for each clinical isolate is necessary.

LITERATURE CITED

1. **Ballard, R. W., N. J. Palleroni, M. Doudoroff, R. Y. Stanier, and M. Mandel.** 1970. Taxonomy of the aerobic

pseudomonads: *Pseudomonas cepacia, P. marginata, P. alliicola,* and *P. caryophylli.* J. Gen. Microbiol. **60:**199–214.

2. **Bergan, T.** 1978. Phage typing of *Pseudomonas aeruginosa,* p. 169–199. *In* T. Bergan and J. R. Norris (ed.), Methods in microbiology, vol. 10. Academic Press, Inc. (London), Ltd., London.
3. **Bergan, T.** 1981. Human- and animal-pathogenic members of the genus *Pseudomonas,* p. 666–700. *In* M. P. Starr, H. Stolp, H. G. Trüper, A. Balows, H. G. Schlegel (ed.), The prokaryotes. A handbook on habitats, isolation and identification of bacteria. Springer-Verlag, New York.
4. **Carlone, G. M., M. J. Valadez, and M. J. Pickett.** 1983. Methods for distinguishing gram-positive from gram-negative bacteria. J. Clin. Microbiol. **16:**1157–1159.
5. **Christenson, J. C., D. F. Welch, G. Mukwaya, M. J. Muszynski, R. E. Weaver, and D. J. Brenner.** 1989. Recovery of *Pseudomonas gladioli* from respiratory tract specimens of patients with cystic fibrosis. J. Clin. Microbiol. **27:**270–273.
6. **Clark, W. A., D. G. Hollis, R. E. Weaver, and P. Riley.** 1985. Identification of unusual pathogenic gram-negative aerobic and facultatively anaerobic bacteria. Centers for Disease Control, Atlanta.
7. **Dees, S. B., D. G. Hollis, R. E. Weaver, and C. W. Moss.** 1983. Cellular fatty acid composition of *Pseudomonas marginata* and closely associated bacteria. J. Clin. Microbiol. **18:**1073–1078.
8. **De Vos, P., and J. De Ley.** 1983. Intra- and intergeneric similarities of *Pseudomonas* and *Xanthomonas* ribosomal ribonucleic acid cistrons. Int. J. Syst. Bacteriol. **33:**487–509.
9. **De Vos, P., K. Kersters, E. Falsen, B. Pot, M. Gillis, P. Segers, and J. De Ley.** 1985. *Comamonas* Davis and Park 1962 gen. nov., nom. rev. emend., and *Comamonas terrigena* Hugh 1962 sp. nov., nom. rev. Int. J. Syst. Bacteriol. **35:**443–453.
10. **De Vos, P., A. van Landschoot, P. Segers, R. Tytgat, M. Gillis, M. Bauwens, R. Rossau, M. Goor, B. Pot, K. Kersters, P. Lizzaraga, and J. De Ley.** 1989. Genotypic relationships and taxonomic localization of unclassified *Pseudomonas* and *Pseudomonas*-like strains by deoxyribonucleic acid: ribosomal ribonucleic acid hybridizations. Int. J. Syst. Bacteriol. **39:**35–49.
11. **Falsen, E.** 1988. Catalogue of strains: Culture Collection, University of Göteborg, 5th ed. University of Göteborg, Göteborg, Sweden.
12. **Galarneault, T. P., and E. Leifson.** 1964. *Pseudomonas vesiculare* (Büsing et al.) comb. nov. Int. Bull. Bacteriol. Nomencl. Taxon. **14:**165–168.
13. **Gilardi, G. L.** 1976. *Pseudomonas* species in clinical microbiology. Mt. Sinai J. Med. **43:**710–726.
14. **Gilardi, G. L., and Y. C. Faur.** 1984. *Pseudomonas mesophilica* and an unnamed taxon, clinical isolates of pink-pigmented oxidative bacteria. J. Clin. Microbiol. **20:**626–629.
15. **Govan, J. R. W., and G. Harris.** 1985. Typing of *Pseudomonas cepacia* by bacteriocin susceptibility and production. J. Clin. Microbiol. **22:**490–494.
16. **Green, P. N., and I. J. Bousfield.** 1983. Emendation of *Methylobacterium* Patt, Cole, and Hanson 1976; *Methylobacterium rhodinum* (Heumann 1962) comb. nov. corrig.; *Methylobacterium radiotolerans* (Ito and Iizuka 1971) comb. nov. corrig.; and *Methylobacterium mesophilicum* (Austin and Goodfellow 1979) comb. nov. Int. J. Syst. Bacteriol. **33:**875–877.
17. **Green, P. N., I. J. Bousfield, and D. Hood.** 1988. Three new *Methylobacterium* species: *M. rhodesianum* sp. nov., *M. zatmanii* sp. nov., and *M. fujisawaense* sp. nov. Int. J. Syst. Bacteriol. **38:**124–127.
18. **Greenwood, J. R.** 1985. Methods of isolation and identification of glucose-nonfermenting gram-negative rods, p. 1–16. *In* G. L. Gilardi (ed.), Nonfermentative gram-negative rods. Laboratory identification and clinical aspects. Marcel Dekker, Inc., New York.
19. **Holmes, B., R. J. Owen, A. Evans, H. Malnick, and W. R. Willcox.** 1977. *Pseudomonas paucimobilis,* a new species isolated from human clinical specimens, the hospital environment, and other sources. Int. J. Syst. Bacteriol. **27:**133–146.
20. **Holmes, B., A. G. Steigerwalt, R. E. Weaver, and D. J. Brenner.** 1987. *Chryseomonas luteola* comb. nov. and *Flavimonas oryzihabitans* gen. nov., comb. nov., *Pseudomonas*-like species from human clinical specimens and formerly known, respectively, as groups Ve-1 and Ve-2. Int. J. Syst. Bacteriol. **37:**245–250.
21. **Hugh, R.** 1970. *Pseudomonas* and *Aeromonas,* p. 175–190. *In* J. E. Blair, E. H. Lennette, and J. P. Truant (ed.), Manual of clinical microbiology. American Society for Microbiology, Washington, D.C.
22. **Hugh, R., L. Guarraia, and H. Hatt.** 1964. The proposed neotype strains of *Pseudomonas fluorescens* (Trevisan) Migula 1895. Int. Bull. Bacteriol. Nomencl. Taxon. **14:**145–155.
23. **Hugh, R., and P. Ikari.** 1964. The proposed neotype strain of *Pseudomonas alcaligenes* Monias 1928. Int. Bull. Bacteriol. Nomencl. Taxon. **14:**103–107.
24. **Hugh, R., and E. Leifson.** 1964. The proposed neotype strains of *Pseudomonas aeruginosa* (Schroeter 1872) Migula 1900. Int. Bull. Bacteriol. Nomencl. Taxon. **14:**69–84.
25. **Kawai, Y., and E. Yabuuchi.** 1975. *Pseudomonas pertucinogena* sp. nov., an organism previously misidentified as *Bordetella pertussis.* Int. J. Syst. Bacteriol. **25:**317–323.
26. **King, A., B. Holmes, I. Phillips, and S. P. Lapage.** 1979. A taxonomic study of clinical isolates of *Pseudomonas pickettii, "P. thomasii,"* and "group IVd" bacteria. J. Gen. Microbiol. **114:**137–147.
27. **Krieg, N. R., and J. G. Holt (ed.).** 1984. Bergey's manual of systematic bacteriology, vol. 1, 9th ed., p. 141–406. The Williams & Wilkins Co., Baltimore.
28. **Lányi, B.** 1987. Classical and rapid identification methods for medically important bacteria, p. 1–67. *In* R. R. Colwell and R. Grigorova (ed.), Methods in microbiology, vol. 19. Academic Press, Inc. (London), Ltd., London.
29. **Leifson, R., and R. Hugh.** 1954. A new type of polar monotrichous flagellation. J. Gen. Microbiol. **10:**68–70.
30. **Moule, A. L., and S. G. Wilkinson.** 1987. Polar lipids, fatty acids, and isoprenoid quinones of *Alteromonas putrefaciens* (*Shewanella putrefaciens*). Syst. Appl. Microbiol. **9:**192–198.
31. **Mutharia, L. M., and R. E. W. Hancock.** 1985. Monoclonal antibody for an outer membrane lipoprotein of the *Pseudomonas fluorescens* group of the family *Pseudomonadaceae.* Int. J. Syst. Bacteriol. **35:**530–532.
32. **Nakamura, Y., S. Hyodo, E. Chonan, S. Shigeta, and E. Yabuuchi.** 1986. Serological classification of *Pseudomonas cepacia* by somatic antigen. J. Clin. Microbiol. **24:**152–154.
33. **Neu, H. C.** 1985. Ecology, clinical significance, and antimicrobial susceptibility of *Pseudomonas aeruginosa,* p. 117–158. *In* G. L. Gilardi (ed.), Nonfermentative gram-negative rods. Laboratory identification and clinical aspects. Marcel Dekker, Inc., New York.
34. **Owen, R. J., and P. J. H. Jackman.** 1982. The similarities between *Pseudomonas paucimobilis* and allied bacteria derived from analysis of deoxyribonucleic acids and electrophoretic protein patterns. J. Gen. Microbiol. **128:**2945–2954.
35. **Palleroni, N. J.** 1984. Genus I. *Pseudomonas* Migula 1894, 237[AL], p. 141–199. *In* N. R. Kreig and J. G. Holt (ed.), Bergey's manual of systematic bacteriology, vol. 1, 9th ed. The Williams & Wilkins Co., Baltimore.
36. **Palleroni, N. J., M. Doudoroff, and R. Y. Stanier.** 1970. Taxonomy of the aerobic pseudomonads: the properties of the *Pseudomonas stutzeri* group. J. Gen. Microbiol. **60:** 215–231.

37. **Palleroni, N. J., and B. Holmes.** 1981. *Pseudomonas cepacia* sp. nov., nom. rev. Int. J. Syst. Bacteriol. **31:**479–481.
38. **Poh, C. L., and G. K. Loh.** 1988. Enzymatic characterization of *Pseudomonas cepacia* by API ZYM profile. J. Clin. Microbiol. **26:**607–608.
39. **Poh, C. L., E. H. Yap, L. Tay, and T. Bergan.** 1988. Plasmid profiles compared with serotyping and pyocin typing for epidemiological surveillance of *Pseudomonas aeruginosa.* J. Med. Microbiol. **25:**109–114.
40. **Redfearn, M. S., N. J. Palleroni, and R. Y. Stanier.** 1966. A comparative study of *Pseudomonas pseudomallei* and *Bacillus mallei.* J. Gen. Microbiol. **43:**293–313.
41. **Samadpour, M., S. L. Mosely, and S. Lory.** 1988. Biotinylated DNA probes for exotoxin A and pilin genes in the differentiation of *Pseudomonas aeruginosa* strains. J. Clin. Microbiol. **26:**2319–2323.
42. **Schable, B., D. L. Rhoden, R. Hugh, R. E. Weaver, N. Khardori, P. B. Smith, G. P. Bodey, and R. L. Anderson.** 1989. Serological classification of *Xanthomonas maltophilia (Pseudomonas maltophilia)* based on heat-stable O antigens. J. Clin. Microbiol. **27:**1011–1014.
43. **Stanier, R. Y., N. J. Palleroni, and M. Doudoroff.** 1966. The aerobic pseudomonads: a taxonomic study. J. Gen. Microbiol. **43:**159–271.
44. **Stolp, H., and D. Gadkari.** 1981. Nonpathogenic members of the genus *Pseudomonas,* p. 719–741. *In* M. P. Starr, H. Stolp, H. G. Trüper, A. Balows, H. G. Schlegel (ed.), The prokaryotes. A handbook on habitats, isolation, and identification of bacteria. Springer-Verlag, New York.
45. **Swings, J., P. De Vos, M. Van den Mooter, and J. De Ley.** 1983. Transfer of *Pseudomonas maltophilia* Hugh 1981 to the genus *Xanthomonas* as *Xanthomonas maltophilia* (Hugh 1981) comb. nov. Int. J. Syst. Bacteriol. **33:** 409–413.
46. **Tamaoka, J., D.-M. Ha, and K. Komagata.** 1987. Reclassification of *Pseudomonas acidovorans* den Dooren de Jong 1926 and *Pseudomonas testosteroni* Marcus and Talahay 1956 as *Comamonas acidovorans* comb. nov. and *Comamonas testosteroni* comb. nov., with an emended description of the genus *Comamonas.* Int. J. Syst. Bacteriol. **37:** 52–59.
47. **von Graevenitz, A.** 1985. Ecology, clinical significance, and antimicrobial susceptibility of infrequently encountered glucose-nonfermenting gram-negative rods, p. 181–232. *In* G. L. Gilardi (ed.), Nonfermentative gram-negative rods. Laboratory identification and clinical aspects. Marcel Dekker, Inc., New York.

Chapter 42

Legionella

FRANK G. RODGERS AND A. WILLIAM PASCULLE

CHARACTERIZATION

The genus *Legionella* and the family *Legionellaceae* were proposed in 1979 (6) to contain the newly recognized human pneumonic pathogen *Legionella pneumophila*. Since then, the discovery of additional new species, not all of which have been isolated from clinical infections, has resulted in a much expanded genus which at present comprises 29 named species, three subspecies, 21 serogroups, and five tentatively named species (Table 1). Furthermore, six unnamed species have been identified and proposed (49), and others have been partially described. On the basis of colonial autofluorescence and DNA homology, it was suggested that the group be subdivided into three genera, *Legionella, Tatlockia,* and *Fluoribacter* (18). However, this has not received universal acceptance. Of the various species, *L. pneumophila* is the major pathogen and is the most commonly encountered member of the group in the clinical microbiology laboratory. The organism was first isolated from the lung tissues of patients who had died from a form of lobar pneumonia called Legionnaires disease contracted during an American Legion convention in Philadelphia in 1976, and it is for this outbreak that both the organism and the major clinical presentation were named.

The organisms are nutritionally fastidious, nonsporeforming, aerobic, gram-negative, slender rods. From autopsied lung, the bacteria appear as coccobacilli or short rods with nonparallel sides tapering to rounded ends. Each bacterial cell measures approximately 0.5 by 1 to 2 μm; however, after cultivation on bacteriological media a wide variation in size has been reported, with organisms measuring 0.3 to 0.7 μm in width by 2 to 3 μm in length and with long forms in excess of 20 μm relatively common (36). The bacteria replicate by pinching binary fission. Depending upon conditions of culture, *L. micdadei* possesses a densely staining region in the periplasm and an extra layer superjacent to the outer membrane. The significance of these and their role in the variable acid-fast and Gram stain reactions of this organism are unclear. Legionellae show little structural evidence for a peptidoglycan layer. However, *L. pneumophila* has been shown to possess diaminopimelic acid and 2-keto-3-deoxyoctonate, key components of peptidoglycan and lipopolysaccharide, respectively. In addition, sudanophilic poly-β-hydroxybutyrate granules are found in the cytoplasm, and high levels of both branched-chain fatty acids and ubiquinones with 10 or more isoprene units in the side chain occur in the cell wall. Legionellae produce a number of potent cytotoxic exoproteases, and these may influence the expression of pulmonary disease by suppressing phagocytosis, interrupting host-cell oxidative metabolism, and inducing cytolysis. With the exception of *L. oakridgensis*, "*L. nautarum*," and "*L. londiniensis*," all legionellae are motile by means of polar or subpolar flagella, and these flagella appear to share a broad common antigenicity (37). Flagella, which occur singly or occasionally in pairs, are unsheathed and 14 to 20 nm in diameter and possess a structure typical of other gram-negative bacteria. Pili are also present (36).

Phenotypic characteristics are not of major use in designating species of *Legionella*. However, many may be helpful for identifying isolates to the genus level and into broad subgroups. These tests together with a variety of serological assays can be used to distinguish species. The legionellae have a genome size of approximately 2.5×10^9 daltons and a guanine-plus-cytosine content in their DNA of 38 to 52 mol%. DNA-hybridization assay remains the recognized method for species identification. Plasmid content and peptide composition, multilocus enzyme analysis, the use of monoclonal antibodies, and restriction enzyme analysis are powerful tools in epidemiological investigations and may serve to delineate those strains more commonly associated with epidemics.

All species of the genus show a weak catalase and peroxidase activity (exception: "*L. worsleiensis*" is catalase negative but peroxidase positive) and liquefy gelatin (exceptions: *L. micdadei, L. feeleii,* and "*L. nautarum*"), and most produce a soluble brown pigment from tyrosine (Table 1). Hippurate hydrolysis (23) offers a relatively simple method for the differentiation of *L. pneumophila* from other *Legionella* species, while the bromocresol-purple spot test (18) is useful for distinguishing *L. micdadei*. In general, legionellae do not utilize carbohydrates, and early reports confirmed that sugars were neither oxidized nor fermented. However, the Entner-Doudoroff and pentose phosphate pathways are involved in the catabolism of glucose, while the gluconeogenic anabolic enzymes of the Embden-Meyerhof pathway are responsible for sugar synthesis and the Krebs cycle for carbon assimilation. Nitrates are not reduced and urea is not hydrolyzed. Amino acids such as arginine, threonine, methionine, serine, isoleucine, valine, and cystine form the major sources of energy for the organism, which, with the exception of passaged strains of *L. oakridgensis*, shows an absolute nutritional requirement for L-cysteine. Indeed, the legionellae will not grow on ordinary laboratory media which have not been supplemented with iron and L-cysteine. This property may be useful in the clinical microbiology laboratory in that an isolate which is gram negative and catalase positive and grows on buffered charcoal yeast extract (BCYE) agar enriched with L-cysteine, iron, and α-ketoglutarate (BCYEα), but not on BCYEα without L-cysteine or on blood agar, may be tentatively identified as a member of the genus *Legionella*. Additional tests are required to confirm and elaborate the identification.

TABLE 1. Classification and phenotypic properties of the legionellae[a]

Species	No. of serogroups	Isolated from:		Characteristics							
		Humans	Environment	Catalase	β-Lactamase	Oxidase	Hippurate	Gelatin liquefaction	Brown pigment	Autofluorescence	Motility
L. pneumophila[b]	14	+	+[c]	+	+	V	+	+	+	−	+
L. micdadei[d]	1	+	+	+	−	+	−	−	−	−	+
L. dumoffii[e]	1	+	+	+	+	−	−	+	V	BW	+
L. gormanii[e]	1	−	+	+	+	−	−	+	+	BW	+
L. bozemanii[e]	2	+	+[f]	+	V	V	−	+	+	BW	+
L. longbeachae	2	+	−	+	V	+	−	+	+	−	+
L. jordanis	1	+	+	+	+	+	−	+	+	−	+
L. oakridgensis	1	+	+	+	+[g]	−	−	+	+	−	−
L. wadsworthii	1	+	−	+	+	−	−	+	−	−	+
L. feeleii	2	+	+[h]	+	−	−	V	−	+[g]	−	+
L. sainthelensi	1	−	+	+	+	+	−	+	+	−	+
L. anisa	1	−	+	+	+	+	−	+	+	BW(V)	+
L. maceachernii	1	+	+	+	−	+	−	+	+	−	+
L. jamestowniensis	1	−	+	+	+	−	−	+	+	−	+
L. rubrilucens	1	−	+	+	+	−	−	+	+	R	+
L. erythra	1	−	+	+	+	+	−	+	+	R	+
L. hackeliae	2	+	−	+[g]	+	+	−	+	+	−	+
L. spiritensis	1	−	+	+	+	+	+[g]	+	+	−	+
L. parisiensis	1	−	+	+	+	+	−	+	+	BW	+
L. cherrii	1	−	+	+	+	+	−	+	+	BW	+
L. steigerwaltii	1	−	+	+	+	−	−	+	+	BW	+
L. santicrusis	1	−	+	+	+	+	+	+	+	−	+
L. israelensis	1	−	+	+	+	−	−	+[g]	+	−	+
L. birminghamensis	1	+	−	+	+	V	−	+	ND	YG	+
L. cincinnatiensis	1	+	−	+	−	+	−	+	ND	−	+
L. moravica	1	−	+	+	+	+[g]	−	+	ND	−	+
L. brunensis	1	−	+	+	+	−	−	+	ND	−	+
L. quinlivanii	1	−	+	+	−	−	−	+	ND	−	+
L. tuconensis	1	+	−	+	+	−	−	+	ND	BW	+
"*L. londiniensis*"[i]	1	−	+	+[g]	+	−	−/+[g]	+	+	−	−
"*L. geestiae*"[i]	1	−	+	+	−	−	+[g]	+	+[g]	−	+
"*L. quarteiraensis*"[i]	1	−	+	+	+	−	−	+	+	−	+
"*L. nautarum*"[i]	1	−	+	+	+	+	−	−	−	−	−
"*L. worsleiensis*"[i]	1	−	+	+[j]	+	−	−	+	+	−	+

[a] All strains fail to reduce nitrate and do not grow on unsupplemented blood agar, and only laboratory-adapted strains of *L. oakridgensis* grow on BCYEα agar without L-cysteine. V, Variable; YG, yellow-green fluorescence; BW, blue-white fluorescence; R, red fluorescence; ND, no data available.

[b] *L. pneumophila* contains three subspecies, *L. pneumophila* subsp. *pneumophila* (the type species of the group), subsp. *pascullei*, and subsp. *fraseri*.

[c] *L. pneumophila* serogroups 8 and 11 to 14 have not yet been isolated from environmental sources.

[d] *Tatlockia* has been proposed as an alternative genus name for this species.

[e] *Fluoribacter* has been proposed as an alternative genus name for these species.

[f] *L. bozemanii* serogroup 2 has not been isolated from environmental sources.

[g] Some strains are weakly positive only.

[h] *L. feeleii* serogroup 2 has not been isolated from environmental sources.

[i] Proposed new species (P. J. L. Dennis et al., manuscript in preparation). Six additional unnamed species have been proposed (49).

[j] Peroxidase is positive.

Although legionellae do not appear to require iron in greater amounts than do other organisms, the presence of soluble iron stimulates growth. Furthermore, the addition of trace metals such as calcium, cobalt, copper, magnesium, manganese, nickel, vanadium, and zinc enhances growth. Some strains produce more profuse growth on bacteriological media in a humid atmosphere with added CO_2. The charcoal and α-ketoglutarate in BCYEα agar may serve to scavenge toxic oxygen radicals or to remove oleic acid released from the yeast extract in the medium during autoclaving.

CLINICAL SIGNIFICANCE

Legionnaires disease, caused by organisms belonging to the genus *Legionella,* is an acute lobar pneumonia presenting with multisystem manifestations. Although apparent asymptomatic seroconversions have been reported, the disease typically occurs as spectacular outbreaks, sporadic cases, and nosocomial infections. The condition was characterized following the severe outbreak at an American Legion convention in Philadelphia in July 1976. Infection usually begins with acute fever, headache, rigors, weakness, and myalgia in the absence of a productive cough. Upper respiratory tract symptoms may only occur later in the disease, when sputum production may be bloody or purulent. Fatigue, dyspnea, bradycardia, rales, and respiratory difficulties increase as the disease progresses. Extrapulmonary abnormalities are common, with symptoms of confusion, disorientation, agitation, nausea, vomiting, and diarrhea frequent findings. Pulmonary X-ray usually shows a patchy infiltrate with pleural effusions. Progression to dense consolidation is common. Typically, radiological changes, which on average follow the onset of symptoms by 3 days, may be bilateral and slow to resolve. Other nonspecific changes reported for this condition include elevations in creatinine and the erythrocyte sedimentation rates, abnormal liver function tests usually in the absence of jaundice, hyponatremia, hypophosphoremia, proteinuria, hematuria, and renal insufficiency (1).

The disease has its highest incidence in the summer months. Reported factors predisposing to infection with this opportunistic pathogen include a compromised immune system such as one undergoing immunosuppressive therapy or T-cell dysfunction, underlying disease, recent surgery, increased age, and heavy smoking. Exposure to aerosols generated from water sources subsequently shown to contain the organism is a necessary prequisite to disease. The disease is more common in men than in women, and infections in children are rare. Retrospective studies have shown that the disease, although unrecognized, has occurred in epidemics since the 1940s.

In addition to Legionnaires disease, *L. pneumophila* also causes a nonpneumonic, influenzalike illness known as Pontiac fever (19). Pontiac fever is a self-limiting, febrile illness usually affecting healthy individuals. The attack rate, incubation period, symptomatology, and fatality ratio for Legionnaires disease and Pontiac fever, collectively referred to as legionellosis, are outlined in Table 2. That *L. pneumophila* infection manifests as two disparate conditions is perplexing. It is clear that the state of the host at the time of infection is crucial; however, the degree of exposure to the organism, strain-specific virulence traits as yet undefined, or a combination of these may be important factors in disease expression.

In cases of Legionnaires disease, biopsy or autopsy lung specimens usually show a fibrinopurulent disease with focal or lobar consolidation, congestion, edema, and red or, more commonly, grey hepatization. Pleural exudates, vasculitis, and coagulative necrosis are common, and in the majority of cases there is a multilobar diffuse involvement. Hemorrhage, necrosis, and abscess formation may also occur (3). The inflammatory reaction, which consists of fibrin-rich debris and edema fluid with a mixed infiltrate of macrophages and polymorphonuclear leukocytes, occurs in the alveoli and small bronchioles. Leukocytoclasis or lysis of the inflammatory exudate is characteristic. Organisms, which are not detected by hematoxylin-eosin staining, may be visualized by silver impregnation procedures, specific immunofluorescence, or electron microscopy (1). By these techniques, legionellae can be found within alveolar macrophages and polymorphonuclear leukocytes as well as in association with lytic foci.

PATHOGENESIS AND IMMUNITY

Legionellae are facultative intracellular pathogens. The establishment of disease is a multifactorial phenomenon, and critical considerations include the occurrence of bacterial virulence factors, the status of the host, and the dose of infecting bacteria. A crucial step in intracellular multiplication is the binding of the or-

TABLE 2. Clinical presentation of legionellosis

Condition	Named for:	Attack rate (%)	Incubation period (days)	Symptoms[a]	Other organs affected	Case/ fatality ratio (%)
Legionnaires disease[b]	Philadelphia outbreak	1–5	2–10	Pneumonia (dyspnea, hemoptysis, upper respiratory tract infection symptoms, sputum production, abdominal pain)	Central nervous system, kidneys, gastrointestinal tract	0–20 (variable)
Pontiac fever	Pontiac outbreak	95	1–2	Nonpneumonic (pleuritic pain)	None	0

[a] Symptoms common to both conditions include cough, myalgia, headache, confusion, chest pains, nausea or vomiting, diarrhea, and fever.
[b] Reported incidence of Legionnaires disease varies but ranges from <1 to 30% of all pneumonias.

ganism to host cell receptors by means of bacterial "adhesins," followed by breaching of the host cell membranes by "bacteriopexis" or endocytosis (33, 35). This process forms a necessary prelude to the initiation of disease. In human infection the organism proliferates in the cytoplasm of susceptible cells in the respiratory network. However, a number of nonphagocytic cells support the intracellular growth of legionellae in laboratory cultures (2). Bacterial replication occurs rapidly within vacuoles lined with host cell ribosomes and in association with vesicles, cytoplasmic filaments, and mitochondria (33). Host cell destruction leading to tissue damage is probably due to a combination of physical trauma due to bacterial replication along with the production of nuclease, lipase, phosphatase, and potent proteolytic enzymes. Release of organisms from infected host cells is by cell lysis. Both virulent-to-avirulent and avirulent-to-virulent changes have been noted in populations of legionellae.

In human lung the organism replicates preferentially in alveolar macrophages. Although the process of phagocytosis by macrophages is independent of opsonizing antibody and complement, it is enhanced if these are present. On the other hand, phagocytosis by polymorphonuclear leukocytes requires both these serum factors, and the process is not bactericidal (26). Upon ingestion of legionellae, macrophages exhibit an oxidative burst, but acidification of the phagosome and phagosome-lysosome fusion do not occur (25). In this manner, legionellae resist the bactericidal action of superoxide, hydrogen peroxide, and hydroxyl radicals produced by the acetaldehyde-xanthine oxidase system of phagocytes.

Although a number of animal species including guinea pigs, rats, chicken embryos, rabbits, and various primates are susceptible to *Legionella* infection, guinea pigs have proved most useful for the study of pathogenesis and immunity. Humoral antibody may be passively transferred, but may not completely protect against challenge with virulent bacteria. As with other intracellular pathogens, cell-mediated rather than humoral immunity appears to be important in overall host defense mechanisms. Indeed, the participation of sensitized T-cells elaborating lymphokines which in turn mediate macrophages is critical to immunity. Such activated macrophages appear to be nonspecifically armed against legionellae (50). Understanding the role of preexisting immunity resulting from past exposure is crucial to developing viable vaccination strategies in disease prevention.

Plasmids have been found in legionellae, but their occurrence shows no correlation with virulence. However, the presence of plasmids has proved useful in epidemiological studies of epidemics of Legionnaires disease. Deletion of genes encoding for bacterial outer membrane proteins has been shown to reduce virulence of *L. pneumophila*. However, the role of outer membrane proteins and surface components in the interaction of the organism both with host cells in the initiation of infection and with the immune system in resistance to disease is unknown. Despite extensive studies with virulent and avirulent strains, the precise nature of the bacterial virulence factors remains unknown. Although restricted pieces of *L. pneumophila* DNA have been transformed into *Escherichia coli* and their products have been investigated, data are required on the nature of these genes and the part they play in the pathogenic process and genetic regulation of virulence.

These bacteria, although effective pathogens, are not predominantly human parasites, in that humans are inopportune hosts, offering no ecological advantage to the microorganism. Human-to-human spread of the disease has not been observed, but rather infection results from the delivery of an adequate dose of organisms in aerosolized form to the lungs from environmental or aquatic sources.

Environmental implications

The *Legionellaceae* are ubiquitous in natural freshwater habitats (Table 1). Although they constitute only a small proportion of the total bacterial count in the aquatic environment, *L. pneumophila* and other members of *Legionella* have been isolated from lakes, rivers, streams, natural thermal lagoons, mud samples, ground water, and ponds associated with volcanic activity (1, 17). From these sources they gain entry to and colonize man-made water supplies. As a consequence, the organism has been isolated from the water systems of many large buildings and hospitals. Although not thermophiles, these aquatic bacteria are frequently associated with and survive in water at temperatures often in excess of 60°C. Legionellae have been found in potable-, hot-, and cooling-water supplies, whirlpool spas, and the thermally polluted effluent from cooling towers, air conditioners, and evaporative condensers. Aerosols generated from these aquatic environments serve as the major source for disease. Organisms present in water droplets of 5 to 15 μm can readily enter the respiratory tract and colonize the alveolar airspaces of the lung, infect the alveolar macrophages, and induce disease.

Although the legionellae are slow-growing and have relatively complex nutritional requirements in the laboratory, they persist in the environment and are not normally displaced by other aquatic saprophytes. This has led to the suggestion that they are not free-living organisms. Indeed, it has been reported that the growth of *L. pneumophila* may be enhanced in the presence of naturally occurring protozoa, blue-green algae, or other microorganisms (45; B. S. Fields, T. A. Nerad, and T. K. Sawyer, *ATCC Q. Newsl.* **10:**1, 6, 1990). Freshwater amoebae and ciliates of the genera *Acanthamoeba, Echinamoeba, Hartmanella, Naegleria, Tetrahymena,* and *Cyclidium* support the intracellular growth of legionellae and therefore constitute a mechanism for the amplification of bacterial numbers in aquatic habitats (Fields et al., *ATCC Q. Newsl.* **10:**1, 6, 1990). Current evidence suggests that these agents may act as reservoirs for the pathogen by presenting it to the host in suitably sized droplets and in sufficient numbers protected intracellularly in protozoa. Furthermore, cyanobacteria, flavobacteria, and algal material present in the natural environment may either stabilize the bacteria in aerosols or stimulate their growth. Other factors influencing the long-term colonization of man-made water supplies are the nature of the plumbing system, the construction materials used, and the degree of stagnation and sedimentation, as well as the holding temperature and amount of chlorination. Despite these, the number of legionellae in water supplies does not always correlate with disease. However, these associations may be particularly important for the potential exposure of high-risk patients and in the acquisition of nosocomial infections.

Direct observation for legionellae in centrifuged water samples, using a fluorescent-antibody technique, has not proved useful, and culture on selective media preceded by a decontamination step remains the method of choice. In the absence of disease, it is debatable whether screening water samples for legionellae is productive. However, should this be required, multiple samples should be taken at regular intervals, and all *Legionella* isolates should be fully identified.

COLLECTION, TRANSPORT, HANDLING, AND STORAGE OF SPECIMENS

Nature of specimen

Legionellae are most frequently isolated from specimens originating in the respiratory tract. They are also, on rare occasions, isolated from other extrapulmonary sites including pericardial and peritoneal fluids as well as wounds and abscesses, both in the presence and absence of obvious pulmonary infection. In addition, blood cultures are sometimes positive, but the diagnostic value of performing blood culture for *Legionella* has not been established. At autopsy, specimens of liver, spleen, and kidney may be culturally positive.

The legionellae can be recovered from sputum and subsequently identified, provided special selective techniques and media are employed (12, 47). Patients with Legionnaires disease frequently produce scanty amounts of sputum which may be contaminated significantly with oral secretions. Since the legionellae are not known to colonize humans and therefore are not commensals of the respiratory tract, such specimens may prove acceptable for the recovery of legionellae even if they are not suitable for routine culture. Respiratory secretions from those patients who are unable to provide adequate sputum specimens may be collected by transtracheal aspiration or bronchoalveolar lavage. Bronchoalveolar lavage specimens tend to be diluted during collection, and these should be centrifuged prior to examination for legionellae. On occasion it may be necessary to collect lung tissue samples to establish the diagnosis of Legionnaires disease. In these instances open-lung biopsy rather than transtracheal biopsy is preferred, as the former has a much higher diagnostic yield. Pleural effusions may be present in cases of legionellosis, but legionellae are not frequently recovered from pleural fluid.

Specimen collection

Sputum should be collected and transported in sterile containers with tightly fitting lids to prevent spillage and specimen drying during transport. The use of saline in specimen collection fluids should be avoided as sodium ions may be inhibitory for the organism. Bronchoscopists should use minimal amounts of local anesthetic agents, such as lidocaine, as these too are inhibitory for legionellae as indeed they are for other bacteria. Specimens from bronchoalveolar lavage should be centrifuged as quickly as possible and the sediment should be suspended in sterile, nonbacteriostatic water.

Specimen transport

While the legionellae are relatively hardy, care should be taken in handling samples of respiratory secretions since these may contain only small numbers of viable organisms. Special media are not required for transport of specimens as long as they are protected from drying and rapid temperature changes. Specimens can be held at 4°C or transported on wet ice provided they are examined within 48 h of collection. Those which are to be held for longer periods should be stored frozen, preferably at −70°C, and also transported in the frozen state on dry ice. Repeated freezing and thawing should be avoided as each freeze/thaw cycle causes a drop in viability. Quality control materials and other specimens which may be tested repeatedly should be stored frozen in small aliquots.

Tissue samples are handled in a similar fashion. Tissue may be stored and transported at 4°C or frozen, but fresh or frozen tissue is preferable to Formalin-fixed material. Material which has been fixed in Formalin and/or embedded in paraffin wax is satisfactory for direct immunofluorescent-antibody (DFA) testing only and should be employed when no other material is available. With the exception of fixed tissues, the submission of specimens for DFA testing only should be strongly discouraged, as this technique is significantly less sensitive than culture.

Specimen processing

Dilution of sputum and lung tissues is recommended as these samples contain substances which are inhibitory to legionellae. Specimens should be diluted even if albumin is incorporated into the medium. A bacteriologic broth such as Trypticase soy or, alternatively, sterile water is satisfactory for this purpose, and specimens should be diluted 10-fold prior to inoculation of media. Lung or other tissues should be prepared as 10% (wt/vol) suspensions in similar diluents, and these should be further diluted 10-fold after homogenization. Dilute specimens, particularly pleural and pericardial fluids and bronchoalveolar lavage fluids, should be centrifuged before inoculation of culture media. Transtracheal aspirates and bronchial washings may be inoculated onto media directly, and purulent parts of sputum specimens may be inoculated after a 1 to 10 dilution. Smears of tissues, sputum, and fluids should be made for immunofluorescence.

Respiratory specimens are likely to be contaminated with a variety of non-*Legionella* organisms. Decontamination of such specimens results in about a 10% higher yield of positive cultures even when semiselective media are employed (7). These specimens should be diluted 10-fold in KCl-HCl buffer (pH 2.2) and incubated for no more than 4 min at room temperature prior to inoculation onto both semiselective and nonselective media (4). Similar results can be obtained by heating specimens in a water bath at 60°C for 1 to 2 min or at 50°C for 30 min. Prolonged decontamination treatment should be avoided because the legionellae are also slowly inactivated by these treatments. Some laboratories have found it useful on a routine basis to inoculate all potentially contaminated specimens in duplicate using three plates (two semiselective and one nonselective; see chapter 121 for media) without pretreatment and a similar three plates with decontaminated specimen (12). Alternatively, when resources are limited, specimens can be inoculated without decontamination and the remainder of the specimen may be stored at 4°C. If these inoculated media contain heavy growth of contaminating non-*Legionella* bacteria after 48 h of incubation, the specimen may be removed from storage, decontaminated, and recultured (34).

Inoculated plates are typically incubated at 35°C in a humid atmosphere either in ambient air or with 5% CO_2. Proper humidification is crucial to prevent the media from drying out and becoming inhibitory during prolonged incubation. Inoculated plates should be incubated for at least 7 days, but some laboratories prefer to incubate cultures for up to 14 days.

Laboratory safety

Only one case of laboratory-acquired Legionnaires disease has ever been reported, and this was apparently caused by exposure to aerosols during inoculation of experimental animals. Legionellae may be handled safely in any biosafety level 2 (P2) facility, which includes most clinical microbiology laboratories practicing universal infection control precautions. Centrifugation of specimens or suspensions suspected of containing legionellae should be done under sealed conditions. Homogenization of tissues must be performed in a biological safety cabinet to prevent exposure to aerosols (9). Other than these, no extraordinary precautions need be taken when handling most specimens or cultures of the organism.

When handling plates of *Legionella* media it should be borne in mind that other potentially hazardous organisms, such as *Francisella tularensis* (46) or *Coccidioides immitis,* may grow on these media. This is especially so in areas where tularemia and coccidioidomycosis are known to occur. Laboratory personnel handling BCYEα plates should exercise caution when unrecognized bacterial colonies or atypical gram-negative bacilli are found, as microorganisms other than legionellae may not be harmless "contaminants."

LABORATORY DIAGNOSIS

L. pneumophila serogroup 1 (50%) and serogroup 6 (10%), other *L. pneumophila* serogroups (20%), and *L. micdadei* (5%) among them account for the vast majority of clinical disease. Although most infections are of a single etiology, dual infections involving different species of *Legionella* as well as other agents have been reported (10). The diagnosis of infections due to these pathogens may be achieved by the clinical microbiologist using a variety of tests each possessing different degrees of sensitivity and specificity (Table 3). Antigen detection systems for *L. pneumophila* include DFA, radioimmunoassay, enzyme-linked immunosorbent assay (ELISA), nucleic acid probes, and agglutination tests. These have the potential for high specificity (>99%), with sensitivities ranging from 60 to 90%. Demonstration of a serological response to the organism in serum using indirect immunofluorescence (IFA), although retrospective, has proven extremely useful. However, culture affords the mainstay of diagnosis and has a specificity of 100% and a sensitivity of approximately 75% (Table 3).

DIRECT EXAMINATION

Stains

Detection of legionellae directly in clinical specimens offers the most rapid procedure for the diagnosis of Legionnaires disease. However, great care is required in interpretation to ensure against false-positive results due to nonspecificity or cross-reactions which may arise from contaminating organisms or antigens. Organisms may be visualized directly in clinical specimens with variable success using nonspecific staining techniques such as Gram (using carbol-fuchsin as counterstain), modified Gram-Weigert, Giemsa, Gimenez, and Dieterle silver stains (Fig. 1, top left). These staining techniques may prove useful for normally sterile specimens such as lung biopsies or pleural fluids. However, due to their nonspecificity, such staining procedures are generally unhelpful for sputum or other specimens contaminated with normal respiratory tract organisms. Strains of *L. micdadei* stain weakly acid fast. With the exception of silver impregnation, in which the organisms stain dark brown to black, those stains routinely used in histology fail to demonstrate the organism in Formalin-fixed tissue sections.

TABLE 3. Sensitivity and specificity of diagnosis tests for *L. pneumophila*

Test	Commerically available reagents or kits	Specificity (%)	Sensitivity (%)
Direct Gram, Gimenez, silver staining	Yes	No specificity	Variable
DFA[a]	Yes	>99	Up to 75
Immunoassays (radioimmunoassay, ELISA, hemagglutination, latex agglutination)	No	>99	Up to 90
Nucleic acid probes[b]	Yes	>99	75
Serological diagnosis[c]			
IFA	Yes	>99	75
Rapid microagglutination	Yes	95	80
Culture and isolation[d]	Yes	100	75

[a] A monoclonal antibody detecting a 25 to 29-kilodalton protein is also available from Genetic Systems, Seattle, Wash.

[b] Available from Geneprobe Inc., San Diego, Calif.

[c] Some reagents are available commercially or from Centers for Disease Control, Atlanta, Ga., or Division of Microbiological Reagents and Quality Control, London, England.

[d] Bacteriological media may be made or commercially purchased from BBL, Cockeysville, Md.; Difco Laboratories, Detroit, Mich.; or Oxoid Ltd., Basingstoke, England. No particular commercial medium is recommended. Variations in batches occur and control samples should be regularly tested. Formulations for bacteriological media are given in chapter 121.

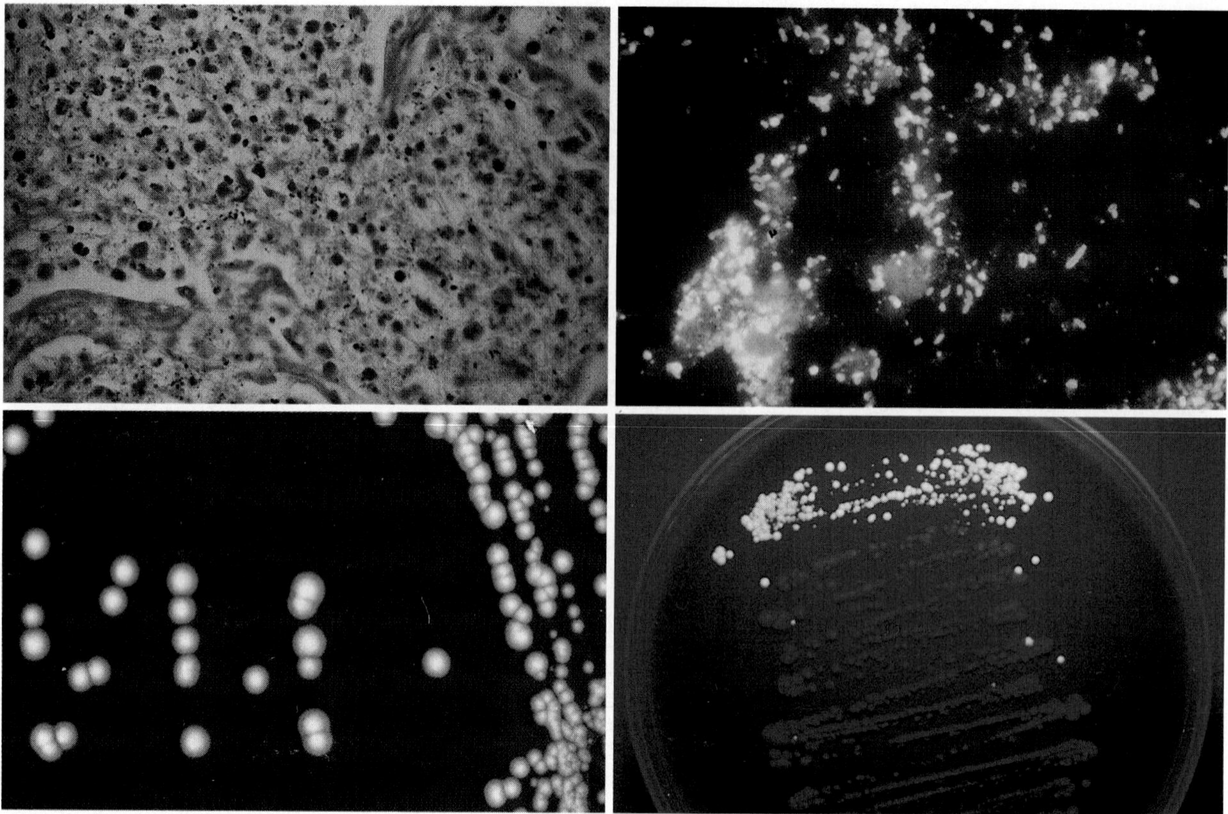

FIG. 1. (Top left) *Legionella* pneumonia. Histological section nonspecifically stained by the Dieterle silver impregnation method. Darkly staining *Legionella* organisms are present in association with pale-staining lung cells. (Such a positive result, while nonspecific, would suggest a potential diagnosis of Legionnaires disease, especially if no pneumonic pathogen was isolated on routine laboratory media and a tissue Gram stain was negative. DFA and culture for *Legionella* should be attempted.) (Top right) *Legionella* pneumonia. Lung suspension smear specifically stained with FITC-conjugated anti-*Legionella* serum. Brightly fluorescing *Legionella* organisms are evident. (Bottom left) Colonies of *L. pneumophila* serogroup 1 (Nottingham N7 strain), growing on BCYEα agar after 4 days of incubation. (Bottom right) Colonies of *L. pneumophila* N7 and *L. bozemanii* serogroup 1 on BCYEα agar illuminated only with long-wave UV light at 366 nm. Note intense blue-white autofluorescence of *L. bozemanii*. *L. pneumophila* does not autofluoresce (Table 1).

DFA

DFA tests have been developed to detect *Legionella* spp. (8, 27) in lung tissue, in transtracheal aspirates and biopsies, in lavage fluids, and in sputum (Fig. 1, top right). When controlled and carefully performed, the DFA test has a specificity close to 100%. The technique is rapid but handicapped by low sensitivity due to the relatively large number of organisms required for microscopic visualization (10^4 to 10^5 organisms per ml). Although the majority of disease is caused by *L. pneumophila* serogroup 1, the multiplicity of species and serogroups and the lack of genus-specific reagents limit the usefulness of the technique. Hence, DFA negative results using available sera do not necessarily exclude disease. Cross-reactions with *Pseudomonas* and *Bacteroides* spp. have been reported, as has nonspecific fluorescence with some strains of streptococci, pneumococci, or staphylococci; however, these are less problematic in laboratories with extensive experience of the technique. The use of monoclonal antibodies has been shown to reduce false-positive reactions while still permitting reaction with a wide range of serotypes of *L. pneumophila*. Indeed, a fluorescein isothiocyanate (FITC)-conjugated monoclonal antibody which recognizes a major outer membrane protein present on all serotypes of *L. pneumophila* has been described (20). Although it cannot be used on Formalin-fixed specimens and the fluorescence of organisms is not intense, this antibody is now commercially available. For these reasons, it is strongly advised that DFA testing be coupled with culture methods despite the extended time required by the latter.

Caution should be used when performing DFA tests to ensure that positive control smears are tested separately from clinical specimens and so avoid carryover of organisms in the wash fluids. In addition, all reagents for DFA should be filter sterilized and slides should be alcohol washed to avoid false-positive reactions arising from environmental legionellae which may be present in the water supply. Many of the polyvalent, serospecific, and individual species-specific antisera used in the test are commercially available. Touch smears from fresh lung biopsies, scrapings from Formalin-fixed tissues, purulent areas of sputum or transtracheal washings, or deposits from centrifuged pleural fluids ($3{,}000 \times g$ for 20 min) are spread thinly on clean glass slides and allowed to air dry. The smears should then be heat fixed to the slides, fixed in 10% neutral buffered Formalin, rinsed in distilled water, dried, and stained with FITC-conjugated antisera used initially as a *Legionella* polyvalent pool. In the event of a positive result, subsequent tests may use a more specific serum to refine detection to the species or serogroup level. After incubation in a humid atmosphere at 37°C for 20 min, slides should be rinsed twice for 5 min each in phosphate-buffered saline, followed by a distilled-water wash. Slides should be air dried, mounted in buffered glycerol (pH 9.0), and examined for bright green, peripherally fluorescent coccobacillary or rod-shaped bacteria in a UV, preferably epifluorescent, microscope equipped with excitation filters appropriate for FITC.

The fluorescent organisms may be found in smears either free or located within phagocytes. Indeed, many such DFA smears may show large amounts of fluorescing, apparently amorphous material derived from lysed macrophages which had been infected with legionellae. This finding is more common in specimens from patients who had received antibiotic therapy. This presumably *Legionella*-specific antigenic material may make finding discrete bacteria difficult and therefore confuse diagnosis. The morphology of the organisms as well as the quantity and degree of fluorescence should be noted. Although unusually shaped legionellae may be found in specimens from patients who had received chemotherapy prior to specimen collection, caution should be exercised in interpreting morphologically atypical fluorescing organisms as *Legionella* due to possible cross-reactions with other bacteria. Positive control samples containing the appropriate serogroup of *Legionella* should be prepared separately and read at the same time. In addition, samples of the clinical specimen under investigation should be treated with FITC-conjugated normal rabbit serum, and this should test negative.

Immunoassays

Rapid detection methods for *Legionella* soluble antigens in urine, respiratory tract secretions, sputum, and serum have been developed using radioimmunoassay, ELISA, and latex agglutination tests (30, 39); however, these are not in routine use, nor have they been fully evaluated, and not all the reagents are commercially available. The sensitivity of these assays was shown to be 80 to 90% and the specificity is almost 100%. Although the sensitivity of the latex test was lower than the others, this test was more rapid and relatively easy to perform. The high degree of serospecificity for these assays makes them somewhat less adaptable for widespread, routine clinical use in screening assays. Excretion of antigen in the urine may commence as early as 3 days after the onset of clinical disease and persist for up to 1 year after infection (30). Although this long excretion period may offer a convenient diagnostic test late in the infection, a positive result may reflect a previous rather than a current infection.

Nucleic acid probes

A commercially available DNA probe appears to be an acceptable substitute for DFA examination in those laboratories which have sufficient test volumes to make this test cost effective (14, 34). The test, which uses a short-half-life ^{125}I-labeled cDNA radioactive probe, is a nucleic acid hybridization assay for a wide range of *Legionella* species rRNA. The product hybridizes strongly with the highly conserved rRNA from *Legionella*. The resultant RNA/DNA duplexes are immobilized by binding to hydroxyapatite, centrifuged, washed to remove cDNA which had not reacted, and evaluated in a gamma counter. Initial problems with low specificity have been resolved by modification of the test reagent, and patient specimens with test/control ratios of ≥5.0 may be considered positive. The DNA probe test shows a specificity similar to DFA and, like DFA, is not sufficiently sensitive to replace culture. Recently, a polymerase chain reaction procedure has been used to enhance the sensitivity of a *Legionella*-DNA probe. However, this technology is not routinely available. Physicians should be discouraged from submitting specimens for direct examination only.

SEROLOGICAL DIAGNOSIS

Serological diagnosis of legionellosis is best achieved by the IFA test using heat- or Formalin-killed *Legionella*-specific antigens and FITC-conjugated anti-human whole immunoglobulin (21, 27, 48). Heat-killed agar-grown organisms suspended in normal chicken yolk sac, or, alternatively, formalinized yolk sac-grown bacteria, are added to wells on glass slides, air dried, and acetone fixed. These slides, which may be stored sealed at −20°C prior to use, are overlaid with dilutions of patients' sera and incubated at 37°C for 30 min. After careful, thorough rinsing in phosphate-buffered saline to remove unbound globulin, slides are similarly incubated in anti-human FITC conjugate, rinsed, and mounted in 10% glycerol. To arrest fluorescence fading, 1% 1,4-diazobicyclo-(2.2.2)-octane (DABCO; Sigma Chemical Co., St. Louis, Mo.) may be added to the mounting medium. Slides are best examined immediately in a fluorescence microscope equipped with an appropriate FITC excitation filter. If only small numbers of sera are to be processed, specimens can be examined at dilutions of 1:32 to 1:1,024. For larger workloads, sera can be initially screened at dilutions of 1:32 or 1:64 and positives can be titrated fully thereafter. The level of fluorescence should be recorded for each serum dilution as 4+ through 1+, to ± (equivocal) and negative. The endpoint is considered as the serum dilution showing organisms which are barely stained yellow-green (1+). Positive control sera should be included. In addition, care should be taken to prevent washover of antibody from highly positive samples during rinsing.

This assay depends on the presence in the patient's serum of immunoglobulin G, M, or A specific to *Legionella* organisms. Acute-phase sera (within 1 week of onset) and convalescent-phase sera (3 to 6 weeks later) from patients suspected of suffering from Legionnaires disease are screened against *Legionella* antigens, and those showing at least a fourfold rise in antibody titer to a level of 1:128 or greater are considered significant. Results from single serum specimens are more difficult to interpret, but an antibody titer of 1:256 or higher to *Legionella* is considered suggestive of infection. As antibody levels in the general population are low (the organism is not carried in the absence of disease) and multiple episodes of Legionnaires disease are rare, such high titers may be useful. However, caution should be used, as high levels of antibody may persist for some years after infection. Furthermore, false-positive reactions have been reported for patients with *Bacteroides*, *Pseudomonas*, *Proteus*, and rickettsial infections, and similar problems of cross-reacting antibodies have been reported in sera from intravenous-drug abusers. The sensitivity of IFA is approximately 75%, and the specificity approaches 100%. As a consequence, the predictive value (the likelihood that positive serological results are not falsely positive) is high. Despite this, the test is more useful in outbreak situations than for sporadic cases.

Other serodiagnostic tests described for legionellosis include ELISA, microagglutination, immune adherence, hemagglutination, immunodiffusion, and counterimmunoelectrophoresis. Many of these are readily adaptable to laboratory automation, and one, the rapid microagglutination test with a sensitivity of 80% and a specificity of 95%, is in routine use in some parts of the world (21). However, these serological procedures have met with varying degrees of success. Indeed, due to its extensive use to date, IFA remains the serological test of choice for Legionnaires disease. Although seroconversion can be detected in some patients as early as 1 week into the infection, the retrospective nature of these serological diagnostic tests limits their usefulness in comparison to culture.

CULTURE AND ISOLATION

Media

Cultivation followed by identification of *Legionella* spp. from human specimens is the definitive method for the diagnosis of Legionnaires disease. Although the sensitivity of culture varies from 50 to 80%, the specificity is 100%. A further major advantage of culture is that, when positive, the isolate is available for further investigation. To date, despite a few apparently immunofluorescence-positive results, legionellae have not been isolated from the normal flora of the upper respiratory tract.

The primary medium for the isolation of legionellae is BCYEα (buffered charcoal yeast extract agar with added α-ketoglutarate). Two semiselective media, both based on BCYEα, are also useful for such specimens as sputum which are often contaminated with other microorganisms. BMPA medium (11) contains cefamandole, polymyxin B, and anisomycin, while modified Wadowski-Yee medium contains glycine (to inhibit other gram-negative bacteria), vancomycin, polymyxin B, and anisomycin. (For *Legionella* medium formulations see chapter 121.) The greatest yield of legionellae occurs when specimens are inoculated onto all three media. Semiselective media should never be used alone, as some species of legionellae, such as *L. micdadei*, are inhibited by the antibiotics present. Furthermore, the growth of small numbers of *L. pneumophila* may also be inhibited on these semiselective media. The incorporation of bromocresol purple and bromothymol blue into these media enhances the recognition of some species. While there is no evidence that the use of these dyes improves the specificity of the media, their addition does not appear to be detrimental either. The addition of 1% (wt/vol) albumin to BCYEα has been shown to increase the detection rate of *L. micdadei* and *L. bozemanii* from tissue specimens and of one isolate of *L. anisa* from the environment, but had no effect on the recovery of a single strain of *L. pneumophila* (32).

The legionellae are nutritionally fastidious and are inhibited by media of poor caliber, so strict attention should be paid to the quality of the ingredients. The pH of the medium, which should be checked when cool, is most critical, and unbuffered media should not be used. Primary growth of the legionellae from clinical specimens does not occur outside the pH range 6.85 to 6.95. Exposure of media to light, particularly when hot, may also result in the accumulation of peroxides which can be inhibitory to the bacteria (24). For this reason, some workers prefer to pour plates in a darkened room and store them in lightproof containers.

Both semiselective and nonselective media for the isolation of *Legionella* are commercially available in powdered form, but their quality may at times be variable (28). Indeed, we have encountered some commercial media which, although they allowed the growth of legionellae, did so only after prolonged incubation. Unfortunately, *Legionella* isolates which have been passaged on BCYEα agar lose their strict growth requirements and do not constitute an adequate quality control challenge for these media. Good quality control specimens preferably require the use of tissues from a human case of Legionnaires disease or experimentally infected guinea pigs, but lacking these, *L. pneumophila* ATCC 33152 has been recommended. Since the production of such materials is normally beyond the capacity of most laboratories, media should be obtained from reputable suppliers, should be quality tested in the user laboratory, and should be stored tightly sealed to prevent drying. Strict attention should also be paid to expiration dates. The quality of media made from dehydrated powders has not been formally compared with that of media made from separate components, but they are most likely equivalent provided the precautions outlined for medium making are exercised.

Isolation

Recognition of the unique colonial morphology of *Legionella* spp. is facilitated by the use of a dissecting microscope. Laboratories which rely only on examination with the naked eye will undoubtedly miss some isolates and delay the identification of others. The legionellae are slow growing, but the characteristic morphology of their colonies is apparent even when these are not macroscopically visible. Colonies are usually microscopically evident after 2 days of incubation on BCYEα medium and visible macroscopically after 3 to 5 days. Growth on semiselective media may be delayed slightly. On rare occasions, colonies may appear as early as 24 h after inoculation, but only from specimens with unusually large numbers of organisms present. On isolation, suspect colonies should be passaged to unsupplemented blood agar or L-cysteine-deficient BCYEα agar to facilitate identification; with few exceptions, the legionellae will not grow on these. Inoculated plates should be examined daily with a dissecting microscope and high oblique illumination. *Legionella* colonies are round with an entire edge, glistening, and low convex to convex and measure 1 to 4 mm in diameter (Fig. 1, bottom left). The edge of the colonies, particularly on the first 2 days of growth, usually displays a pink or blue-green iridescence while the center of the colony is grayish with a characteristic speckled opalescence, the appearance of which resembles cut or ground glass. At this time, the colonies produced by some species of *Legionella* autofluoresce brilliant blue-white when irradiated with long-wave (366-nm) UV light (Fig. 1, bottom right), while others appear bright red (Table 1). *L. pneumophila,* the type species of the group and the most commonly isolated *Legionella,* does not autofluoresce. With continued incubation, the centers of the colonies become creamy white and often lose the ground-glass appearance and much of their iridescence. At this time, large and small colony variants are common. It is a characteristic feature of *Legionella* spp. that the colonies are difficult to pick off the agar with a bacteriological loop; indeed, they appear stringy and do not spread evenly on subculture plates. By about 3 to 4 days of incubation, the colonies may be easily confused with those of other bacteria. Some other organisms growing on BCYEα may at times produce colonies which could be confused with those of legionellae and include *Pseudomonas* spp., *Bacillus* spp., various lactobacilli, and diphtheroids. Usually these are easily differentiated from the legionellae by their larger size and/or Gram stain reaction. Isolates meeting these criteria should be further passaged to regular BCYEα agar to complete the species and serogroup identification.

IDENTIFICATION

The genus *Legionella* presently contains 29 defined species and three subspecies which together account for 47 serovars and a number of others yet to be or tentatively reported. Although useful, traditional phenotypic testing (Table 1) does not permit comprehensive, reliable identification, owing to insufficient phenotypic diversity among the relatively large number of species and serotypes. The identification of the more commonly occurring members of the genus is relatively simple, while many other species and all the subspecies of *L. pneumophila* can be identified only by a few highly specialized laboratories. As the majority of reported human infections are caused by *L. pneumophila* serotypes 1 and 6 together with *L. micdadei,* clinical laboratories should be able to identify most of their isolates by relatively simple, straightforward methods. Since the therapy for all *Legionella* infections is identical, the identification of an isolate beyond the genus level is of value for epidemiological purposes only.

Legionella organisms derived from agar media are pleomorphic gram-negative rods approximately 0.5 by 2 μm in size and with a characteristic tapered shape. Cells from suspect colonies are first examined, preferably as methanol-fixed smears, by Gram stain using either 0.1% basic fuchsin or a prolonged safranin procedure as counterstain. The presumptive assignment of an organism to the genus *Legionella* is achieved by demonstrating that the isolate is a gram-negative rod which requires L-cysteine for growth. The necessity for L-cysteine can be established by subculturing suspicious colonies to either L-cysteine-deficient BCYEα agar or 5% sheep blood agar. Care should be taken not to carry over L-cysteine-containing media in the subculture inoculum. These plates should be incubated at 35°C for 48 h. Organisms growing on these are unlikely to be members of the genus *Legionella.* One exception, *L. oakridgensis,* may only require cysteine for primary isolation. Caution should be exercised when using blood agar alone to establish the demand of an organism for iron and cysteine, particularly when dealing with environmental specimens. Some environmental heterotrophic bacteria exist which will grow on BCYEα without cysteine but not on blood agar, causing possible misidentification of these as legionellae.

Isolates which fail to grow in the absence of cysteine may be presumptively identified as *Legionella.* Several relatively simple tests can further characterize the more common isolates. The simplest method is to serogroup the organism using the DFA test with commercially available FITC-conjugated antisera. Several polyvalent reagents are available which react with the more common species and serotypes. Care must be taken to use bacterial suspensions with relatively small numbers of organisms (10^5 to 10^6 CFU/ml) when preparing smears on glass slides for DFA examination. Many commercial conjugates are of relatively low antibody titer, and fluorescence may be quenched by a prozone effect if the bacterial smear contains too many organisms. Air-dried, Formalin-fixed smears are preferable. A slide agglutination test has also been described for serotyping, but reagents are not commercially available (41). Additionally, a commercially available DNA probe (Gen-Probe, San Diego, Calif.) has been shown to be extremely sensitive and specific for identifying *Legionella* isolates (13). It is important for those working in areas where tularemia is prevalent to recognize that a gram-negative rod growing on BCYEα but not reacting in the DFA test or the *Legionella* DNA probe may be *F. tularensis* (46). The sensitivity and specificity of these tests are shown in Table 3. Phenotypic tests, although of limited diagnostic value, can be useful as a guide. Indeed, the presence in some species of *Legionella* of a pigment which is autofluorescent in long-wave UV light can be helpful. However, serologic, physiologic, or genetic tests are required to complete the identification process.

The identification of species and serogroups for which antibody conjugates are not readily available can be performed only by a small number of specialized laboratories capable of performing more specialized tests. DNA hybridization studies constitute the definitive method for the identification of legionellae. However, in the absence of such sophisticated tests, members of the genus *Legionella* can be identified by serological means including DFA using either polyclonal or monoclonal antibodies directed against serospecific lipopolysaccharide (somatic or O) antigens. These assays are not always easy to interpret, as cross-reacting antigens occasionally occur within the genus. It has been shown by passive hemagglutination that many legionellae share common flagellar or H antigens (37), and this property has been used to identify antibodies in patients' serum. Flagellum-specific antisera are not commercially available but may be prepared by cross-absorbing antisera prepared against whole organisms with the homologous bacteria from which the flagella have been removed by boiling or shearing. In this fashion, previously unrecognized species or uncommon serogroups of legionellae have been confirmed, based on flagellar antigens, by IFA and ELISA.

The cell wall of the legionellae, unlike that of most gram-negative bacteria, is rich in branched-chain fatty acids which can be qualitatively and quantitatively assayed by either gas-liquid chromatography or high-pressure liquid chromatography. Although the fatty acid profiles vary slightly with *Legionella* species, 15-carbon-atom (a-15:0-methyl-12-methyltetradecanoic) and 16-carbon-atom (i-16:0-methyl-14-methylpentadecanoic and 16:1-methylhexadecanoic) fatty acids consistently predominate. Because of the existence of multiple species in the genus, this technique is primarily used for the initial examination of an isolate as it permits the division of the genus into broad taxonomic groups (31). Furthermore, quantitative estimation of ubiquinone content (31), plasmid profiles, and DFA using monoclonal antibodies permit similar differentiation of these organisms into several large groupings.

Definitive identification presently requires genetic analysis, typically by estimation of DNA homology with known *Legionella* species (5). Restriction endonuclease digest analysis of *Legionella* DNA has proved useful for the differentiation of isolates. Another promising tool for the recognition of new species and serogroups as well as for the differentiation of strains is multilocus enzyme electrophoresis. In this procedure, the electrophoretic mobility of a panel of 23 bacterial cytoplasmic enzymes is measured (5, 40). Since small genetically encoded changes in enzyme structure may also alter electrophoretic mobility, these measurements can be used to estimate the genetic relatedness between organisms at the genus, species, or strain level.

ANTIMICROBIAL SUSCEPTIBILITY

Isolates of *Legionella* are susceptible to a wide range of antibiotics in vitro (15, 42). However, this sensitivity is not necessarily reflected clinically. As legionellae are facultative intracellular pathogens, only those antibiotics capable of penetrating the membranes of infected cells to reach intracellular bacteria have an effective role in therapy. From animal and cell culture studies, those antimicrobial agents which inhibit intracellular bacterial growth include erythromycin, rifampin, and the 5-fluoroquinolones (16, 22, 43, 44). Others, such as the aminoglycosides and β-lactam antibiotics, have little or no part to play in chemotherapy, although many possess effective MICs and induce major bacterial damage in vitro (29, 38). Furthermore, with the exception of *L. micdadei, L. feeleii, L. maceachernii, L. cincinnatiensis, L. quinlivanii,* and *"L. geestiae,"* strains of *Legionella* produce a β-lactamase.

When legionellosis is diagnosed early, treatment using appropriate antibiotics is usually successful; however, in untreated patients the prognosis is poor, and respiratory distress, shock, or circulatory collapse may lead to death. The relatively high mortality associated with this disease reflects the nature of those individuals infected: immunocompromised patients and those with underlying conditions such as leukemia, lymphoma, or acquired immunodeficiency syndrome (AIDS). Antibacterial regimes usually include erythromycin, the drug of choice for the treatment of Legionnaires disease, used either alone or with rifampin. Doxycycline, cotrimoxazole, or a number of quinolones may also be clinically effective. However, due to a lack of correlation between in vitro susceptibility and in vivo efficacy as well as the difficulty in standardizing MIC methods, antimicrobial susceptibility testing in the routine laboratory is not appropriate at present. For this reason, some groups have advocated growing legionellae in a variety of cell cultures or animal systems for the evaluation of antibiotics against *Legionella* spp. (16, 22, 43, 44). Although effective, these systems are not readily applicable to the routine clinical laboratory. However, these studies have suggested that combinations of the above drugs may function synergistically and may prove useful in the therapy of Legionnaires disease.

LITERATURE CITED

1. **Bartlett, C. L. R., A. D. Macrae, and J. T. Macfarlane.** 1986. *Legionella* infections. Edward Arnold, London.
2. **Benson, C. E.** 1985. Tissue culture systems, p. 133–141. *In* S. M. Katz (ed.), Legionellosis, vol. 2. CRC Press, Boca Raton, Fla.
3. **Blackmon, J. A., M. D. Hicklin, and F. W. Chandler.** 1978. Special expert pathology panel. Legionnaire's disease; pathological and historic aspects of a "new" disease. Arch. Pathol. Lab. Med. **102:**337–343.
4. **Bopp, C. A., J. W. Sumner, G. K. Morris, and J. G. Wells.** 1981. Isolation of *Legionella* spp. from environmental water samples by low-pH treatment and use of a selective medium. J. Clin. Microbiol. **13:**714–719.
5. **Brenner, D. J., A. G. Steigerwalt, P. Epple, W. F. Bibb, R. M. McKinney, R. W. Starnes, J. M. Colville, R. K. Selander, P. H. Edelstein, and C. W. Moss.** 1988. *Legionella pneumophila* serogroup Lansing 3 isolated from a patient with fatal pneumonia, and descriptions of *L. pneumophila* subsp. *pneumophila* subsp. nov., *L. pneumophila* subsp. *fraseri* subsp. nov., and *L. pneumophila* subsp. *pascullei* subsp. nov. J. Clin. Microbiol. **26:**1695–1703.
6. **Brenner, D. J., A. G. Steigerwalt, and J. E. McDade.** 1979. Classification of Legionnaires' disease bacterium: *Legionella pneumophila,* genus novum, species nova, of the family *Legionellaceae,* family nova. Ann. Intern. Med. **90:**656–658.
7. **Buesching, W. J., R. A. Brust, and L. W. Ayers.** 1983. Enhanced primary isolation of *Legionella pneumophila* from clinical specimens by low-pH treatment. J. Clin. Microbiol. **17:**1153–1155.
8. **Cherry, W. B., B. Pittman, P. P. Harris, G. A. Hebert, B. M. Thomason, L. Thacker, and R. E. Weaver.** 1978. Detection of Legionnaires disease bacteria by direct immunofluorescent staining. J. Clin. Microbiol. **8:**329–338.
9. **Department of Health and Human Services, Centers for Disease Control, and National Institutes of Health.** 1988. Biosafety in microbiology and biomedical laboratories. U.S. Government Printing Office, Washington, D.C.
10. **Dowling, J. N., F. J. Krobroth, M. Karpf, R. B. Yee, and A. W. Pasculle.** 1983. Pneumonia and multiple lung abscesses caused by dual infection with *Legionella micdadei* and *Legionella pneumophila.* Am. Rev. Respir. Dis. **127:**121–125.
11. **Edelstein, P. H.** 1981. Improved semiselective medium for isolation of *Legionella pneumophila* from contaminated clinical and environmental specimens. J. Clin. Microbiol. **14:**298–303.
12. **Edelstein, P. H.** 1984. Legionnaires' disease laboratory manual. National Technical Information Service, Springfield, Va.
13. **Edelstein, P. H.** 1986. Evaluation of the Gen-Probe DNA probe for the detection of *Legionella* in culture. J. Clin. Microbiol. **24:**556–558.
14. **Edelstein, P. H., R. N. Bryan, R. K. Enns, D. E. Kohn, and D. L. Kacian.** 1987. Retrospective evaluation of Gen-Probe rapid diagnostic system for detection of legionellae in frozen clinical respiratory tract specimens. J. Clin. Microbiol. **25:**1022–1026.
15. **Edelstein, P. H., and R. D. Myer.** 1980. Susceptibility of *Legionella pneumophila* to twenty antimicrobial agents. Antimicrob. Agents Chemother. **18:**403–408.
16. **Fitzgeorge, R. B., A. Baskerville, and A. S. R. Feather-**

stone. 1986. Treatment of experimental Legionnaires' disease by aerosol administration of rifampicin, ciprofloxacin and erythromycin. Lancet **i:**502–503.

17. **Fliermans, C. B.** 1985. Ecological niche of *Legionella pneumophila*, p. 75–116. *In* S. M. Katz (ed.), Legionellosis, vol. 2. CRC Press, Boca Raton, Fla.
18. **Garrity, G. M., A. Brown, and R. M. Vickers.** 1980. *Tatlockia* and *Fluoribacter:* two new genera of organisms resembling *Legionella pneumophila*. Int. J. Syst. Bacteriol. **30:**609–614.
19. **Glick, T. H., M. B. Gregg, B. Berman, G. Mallison, W. W. Rhodes, Jr., and I. Kassanoff.** 1978. Pontiac fever. An epidemic of unknown etiology in a health department. I. Clinical and epidemiological aspects. Am. J. Epidemiol. **107:**149–160.
20. **Gosting, L. H., K. Cabrian, J. C. Sturge, and L. C. Goldstein.** 1984. Identification of a species-specific antigen in *Legionella pneumophila* by a monoclonal antibody. J. Clin. Microbiol. **20:**1031–1035.
21. **Harrison, T. G., and A. G. Taylor.** 1982. A rapid microagglutination test for the diagnosis of *Legionella pneumophila* (serogroup 1) infection. J. Clin. Pathol. **40:**77–82.
22. **Havlichek, D., L. Saravolatz, and D. Pohlod.** 1987. Effect of quinolones and other antimicrobial agents on cell-associated *Legionella pneumophila*. Antimicrob. Agents Chemother. **31:**1529–1534.
23. **Hébert, G. A.** 1981. Hippurate hydrolysis by *Legionella pneumophila*. J. Clin. Microbiol. **13:**240–242.
24. **Hoffman, P. S., L. Pine, and S. Bell.** 1983. Production of superoxide and hydrogen peroxide in medium used to culture *Legionella pneumophila:* catalytic decomposition by charcoal. Appl. Environ. Microbiol. **45:**784–791.
25. **Horwitz, M. A.** 1983. The Legionnaires' disease bacterium (*Legionella pneumophila*) inhibits phagosome-lysosome fusion in monocytes. J. Exp. Med. **154:**2108–2126.
26. **Horwitz, M. A., and S. C. Silverstein.** 1981. Interaction of the Legionnaires' disease bacterium (*Legionella pneumophila*) with human phagocytes. 1. *L. pneumophila* resists killing by polymorphonuclear leukocytes, antibody and complement. J. Exp. Med. **153:**386–397.
27. **Jones, G. L., and G. A. Hebert (ed.).** 1979. Legionnaires': the disease, the bacterium and the methodology. Centers for Disease Control, Atlanta, Ga.
28. **Kealthy, J. D., and W. C. Winn, Jr.** 1984. Comparison of media for the recovery of *Legionella pneumophila* clinical isolates, p. 19–20. *In* C. Thornsberry, A. Balows, J. C. Feeley, and W. Jakubowski (ed.), *Legionella:* Proceedings of the 2nd International Symposium. American Society for Microbiology, Washington, D.C.
29. **Kirby, B. D., K. M. Snyder, R. D. Myer, and S. M. Finegold.** 1980. Legionnaires' disease: report of sixty-five nosocomial acquired cases and review of the literature. Medicine **59:**419–422.
30. **Kohler, R. B., W. C. Winn, Jr., and L. J. Wheat.** 1984. Onset and duration of urinary antigen excretion in Legionnaires disease. J. Clin. Microbiol. **20:**605–607.
31. **Lambert, M. A., and C. W. Moss.** 1989. Cellular fatty acid composition and isoprenoid quinone contents of 23 *Legionella* species. J. Clin. Microbiol. **27:**465–473.
32. **Morrill, W. E., J. M. Barbaree, B. S. Fields, G. N. Sanden, and W. T. Martin.** 1990. Increased recovery of *Legionella micdadei* and *Legionella bozemanii* on buffered charcoal yeast extract agar supplemented with albumin. J. Clin. Microbiol. **28:**616–618.
33. **Oldham, L. J., and F. G. Rodgers.** 1985. Adhesion, penetration and intracellular replication of *Legionella pneumophila:* an in vitro model of pathogenesis. J. Gen. Microbiol. **131:**697–706.
34. **Pasculle, A. W., G. E. Veto, S. Krystofiak, K. McKelvey, and K. Vrsalovic.** 1989. Laboratory and clinical evaluation of a commercial DNA probe for the detection of *Legionella* spp. J. Clin. Microbiol. **27:**2350–2358.
35. **Rodgers, F. G.** 1983. The role of structure and invasiveness on the pathogenicity of *Legionella pneumophila*. Zentralbl. Bakteriol. Parasitenkd. Infektionskr. Hyg. **255:**138–144.
36. **Rodgers, F. G.** 1985. Morphology of *Legionella*, p. 39–82. *In* S. M. Katz (ed.), Legionellosis, vol. 1. CRC Press, Boca Raton, Fla.
37. **Rodgers, F. G., and T. Laverick.** 1984. *Legionella pneumophila* serogroup 1 flagellar antigen in a passive hemagglutination test to detect antibodies to other *Legionella* species, p. 42–44. *In* C. Thornsberry, A. Balows, J. C. Feeley, and W. Jakubowski (ed.), *Legionella:* Proceedings of the 2nd International Symposium. American Society for Microbiology, Washington, D.C.
38. **Rodgers, F. G., A. O. Tzianabos, and T. S. J. Elliott.** 1990. The effect of antibiotics that inhibit cell wall, protein, and DNA synthesis on the growth and morphology of *Legionella pneumophila*. J. Med. Microbiol. **31:**37–44.
39. **Sathapatayavongs, B., R. B. Kohler, L. J. Wheat, A. White, and W. C. Winn.** 1983. Rapid diagnosis of Legionnaires' disease by latex agglutination. Am. Rev. Respir. Dis. **127:**559–562.
40. **Selander, R. K., R. M. McKinney, T. S. Whittman, W. F. Bibb, D. J. Brenner, F. S. Nolte, and P. E. Pattison.** 1985. Genetic structure of populations of *Legionella pneumophila*. J. Bacteriol. **163:**1021–1027.
41. **Thacker, W. L., B. B. Plikaytis, and H. W. Wilkinson.** 1985. Identification of 22 *Legionella* species and 33 serotypes with the slide agglutination test. J. Clin. Microbiol. **13:**794–797.
42. **Thornsberry, C., C. N. Baker, and L. A. Kirven.** 1978. In vitro activity of antimicrobial agents on Legionnaires disease bacterium. Antimicrob. Agents Chemother. **13:**78–80.
43. **Tzianabos, A. O., and F. G. Rodgers.** 1989. Pathogenesis and chemotherapy of experimental *Legionella pneumophila* infection in the chick embryo. Zentralbl. Bakteriol. Parasitenkd. Infektionskr. Hyg. A **271:**293–303.
44. **Vildé, J. D., E. Dournon, and P. Rajagopalan.** 1986. Inhibition of *Legionella pneumophila* multiplication within human macrophages by antimicrobial agents. Antimicrob. Agents Chemother. **30:**743–748.
45. **Wadowski, R. M., and R. B. Yee.** 1985. Effect of non-legionellae bacteria on the multiplication of *Legionella pneumophila* in potable water. Appl. Environ. Microbiol. **49:**1206–1210.
46. **Westerman, E. L., and J. MacDonald.** 1983. Tularemia pneumonia mimicing Legionnaires' disease: isolation of the organism on CYE agar and successful treatment with erythromycin. South. Med. J. **76:**1169–1170.
47. **Wilkinson, H. W.** 1987. Hospital laboratory diagnosis of *Legionella* infections. Centers for Disease Control, Atlanta, Ga.
48. **Wilkinson, H. W., A. L. Reingold, B. J. Brake, D. L. McGiboney, G. W. Gorman, and C. V. Broome.** 1983. Reactivity of serum from patients with suspected legionellosis against 29 antigens of *Legionellaceae* and *Legionella*-like organisms by indirect immunofluorescence assay. J. Infect. Dis. **147:**23–31.
49. **Wilkinson, I. J., N. Sangster, R. M. Ratcliff, P. A. Mugg, D. E. Davos, and J. A. Lancer.** 1990. Problems associated with identification of *Legionella* species from the environment and isolation of six possible new species. Appl. Environ. Microbiol. **56:**796–802.
50. **Winn, W. C.** 1988. Legionnaires' disease: a historical perspective. Clin. Microbiol. Rev. **1:**60–81.

Chapter 43

Francisella

SCOTT J. STEWART

CHARACTERIZATION

Francisella tularensis is a small gram-negative coccobacillus (0.2 μm by 0.2 to 0.7 μm). It is nonmotile and nonpiliated, and it possesses a thin capsule composed predominantly of lipid. It is a strict aerobe that usually requires an enriched medium for propagation. The organism is extremely infectious, and it can remain viable for months at low temperatures in such diverse substrates as mud, water, and decaying animal carcasses. Biosafety level 2 is recommended for clinical laboratory work of suspected material, and biosafety level 3 is required for culturing or animal inoculation (24).

ECOLOGY

Tularemia is primarily a disease of wild animals, perpetuated in nature by ectoparasites, contaminated environment, cannibalism, and chronic carriers. Human infection is incidental and is usually the result of interaction with wild animals and their environs.

This organism is extremely widespread (Fig. 1). Literally hundreds of wild and domestic mammals and birds have been found infected with *F. tularensis*, including common house pets. Dozens of biting and blood-sucking insects have been shown to be vectors. Wild rabbits and ticks are the source for most of the human cases in the endemic areas of Arkansas, Missouri, and Oklahoma, which annually report more than 50% of the cases in the United States. Biting flies are the most common vectors in Utah, Nevada, and California, whereas ticks are the most common vectors in the Rocky Mountain states. Beavers and muskrats have been responsible for human outbreaks in areas where they are still commercially trapped for their pelts.

There are two main biovars, type A (*F. tularensis tularensis*) and type B (*F. tularensis palearctica*), with some additional local subgroups currently being proposed. Type A is found only on the North American continent. This biovar produces the more serious disease in humans, with an untreated fatality rate of about 5%. It is usually associated with wild rabbits, ticks, and sheep. Type B is widespread in most parts of the temperate zone in the Northern Hemisphere, including North America. It produces a milder, often subclinical disease. This biovar is usually associated with water, beavers, and muskrats. Only a few poorly documented cases have been reported from the Southern Hemisphere, with no mention of biovars.

TAXONOMY

Tularemia was first described in 1911 as a plaguelike disease in rodents in Tulare County, California (11). The next year the organism was isolated and named *Bacterium tularensis* (12). Edward Francis became involved in 1920 and dedicated his career to describing the clinical manifestations, diagnosis, and histopathology of this disease. His landmark article, published in 1925, is still considered an excellent description of the disease as it occurs in humans today (8). In 1974, the causative organism was renamed *Francisella tularensis* in recognition of his contributions. Early colloquial names such as rabbit fever and deerfly fever in this country, hare fever in Japan, and trapper's ailment in Europe and Asia attest to its long-recognized association with wild animals. Humans are universally susceptible; age, sex, or race pose no barriers to this disease. The annual incidence of tularemia in humans in the United States has decreased from several thousand in the 1930s to a few hundred in the 1980s. The incidence of the disease in humans has declined along with the disappearance of market hunting and trapping. In China, where wild rabbits are still processed for meat, this association continues (17).

CLINICAL SIGNIFICANCE

Tularemia often begins with the sudden onset of flulike symptoms: chills, fever, headache, and generalized aches. Other accompanying symptoms and their respective clinical forms are given below. The usual course of the infection is as follows. The organism penetrates the skin. After an incubation period of 2 to 10 days, an ulcer forms at the site of penetration, which becomes the local focus of infection and may persist for several months. The organism is transported via the lymphatic system to the regional nodes, which enlarge and frequently become necrotic. For a brief period early in the infection, the organism is disseminated through the bloodstream to other organs, including the spleen, liver, lungs, kidneys, intestine, central nervous system, and even skeletal muscles.

The ulceroglandular form of the disease constitutes about 80% of the reported cases. The ulcer is erythemic, indurated, and nonhealing and has a punched-out appearance at 1 to 3 weeks. Ulcers on the upper extremities usually result from exposure to mammalian vectors and occur mostly on rabbit hunters and beaver trappers. Lesions on the lower extremities, head, and back are usually from the bite of a blood-sucking arthropod such as a tick, deerfly, or mosquito.

Oculoglandular tularemia is an unusual variation of the ulceroglandular form. The conjunctivae, usually having been infected by being rubbed with contaminated fingers, are quickly and painfully inflamed with numerous yellowish nodules and pinpoint-size ulcers. Because of the pain and debilitating effect of this form of the infection, the patient usually seeks medical at-

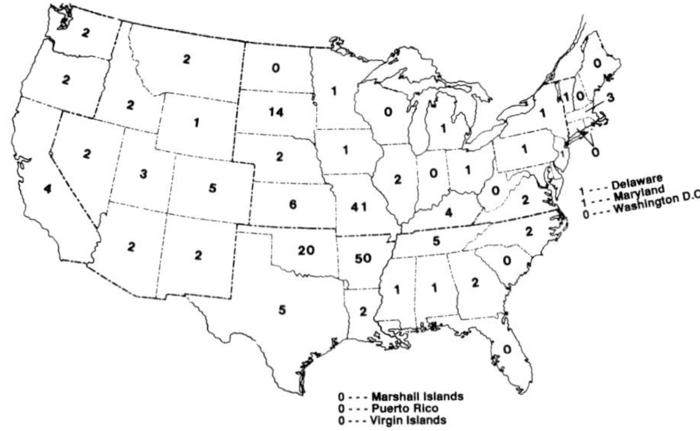

FIG. 1. Average number of tularemia cases per year by state, 1983 to 1988 (5).

tention before regional lymphadenopathy is evident (13). A very painful preauricular adenopathy is unique to tularemia and separates it from cat scratch disease, sporotrichosis, tuberculosis, and syphilis (10).

Oropharyngeal tularemia is described as a sore throat, painful beyond its appearance, that does not respond to penicillin or its analogs (9). The buccal or pharyngeal area is considered the portal of entry because the classic ulcer is frequently found there, and the patient's history usually includes ingestion of contaminated food or water. The tonsils become enlarged and covered with a yellow-white pseudomembrane similar to that described for diphtheria (14).

Glandular tularemia is the term used when an ulcer is not found. On occasion, patients with unexplained regional lymphadenopathy have undergone lymph node biopsy for suspected malignancy (7). Surgical manipulations of otherwise untreated tularemic lymph nodes have initiated severe infections as a result of the release of large numbers of organisms from within the node (19).

Systemic or typhoidal tularemia is the acute form of this infection, with a mortality rate of 30 to 60% (16). If this type of infection is suspected, specific antibiotic therapy must be immediately initiated because the course can be so rapid that death of the patient may precede a diagnostic workup. Systemic tularemia appears as an acute septicemia, lacking the classic external ulcer and lymphadenopathy. Toxemia, severe headache, and continuous high fever are common findings. The patient may be delirious, and prostration and shock may develop.

Pleuropulmonary tularemia can result from either inhalation of an infectious aerosol or dissemination of the organism to and colonization of the pleural cavity (18). Infectious aerosols have been well established as the source of human epidemics.

Gastrointestinal tularemia is almost always traced to the consumption of contaminated food or water (1). This form of the infection is usually associated with abdominal or low-back pain and persistent diarrhea. The course of this type of infection can vary from mild unexplained persistent diarrhea with no other symptoms to a rapidly fulminating fatal disease. When fatal cases have been autopsied, extensive ulceration throughout the bowel has been found, indicating a massive inoculum.

COLLECTION OF SPECIMENS

Collection and manipulation of specimens suspected of containing *F. tularensis* should be done with extreme caution, since tularemia is currently listed as the third most commonly reported laboratory-associated bacterial infection. The operator should be trained for these procedures, should wear protective gloves and a laboratory coat, and should work in an area of limited access. Procedures that have high aerosol potential such as centrifugation or mincing of tissues should be performed in partial containment equipment or a biological safety cabinet. The work area and all wastes should be thoroughly decontaminated upon completion of the procedure (24).

LABORATORY DIAGNOSIS

Conventional microscopy of polychromatic-stained tissue smears or sections show the organism to occur singly and in groups both intra- and extracellularly. A Gram-stained preparation of cultured material shows very small, single, weakly staining, gram-negative coccobacilli. An indirect fluorescent-antibody test can be performed by using commercially available antisera (BBL Microbiology Systems no. 40808; Difco Laboratories no. 2241-47-0).

CULTURE

The fastidious organism usually requires an enriched medium for growth. The historical medium of choice is cystine glucose blood agar (21); however, good growth has been achieved with modified Mueller-Hinton broth, chocolate agar supplemented with IsoVitaleX (BBL), and modified charcoal-yeast agar (2, 6, 25). A heavy inoculum on appropriate medium will yield a growth mass in 18 h, whereas individual colonies may require 2 to 4 days of incubation to reach 2 mm in size. The colonies are blue-gray, round, smooth, and slightly mucoid. On media containing blood, there usually is a small zone of alpha-hemolysis surrounding the colony. Overgrowth by contaminating organisms can be reduced by incorporating 100 to 500 U of penicillin per ml into the medium. A slide agglutination test using commercially available antiserum and positive control antigen (Difco no. 2240-56-9) can be easily performed and is very specific for identification.

During infection, direct isolation is frequently achieved from ulcer scrapings, lymph node biopsies, gastric washings, and sputum. Circulating blood seldom reveals the organism, although this source has become more common through the use of more sensitive blood-culturing systems. Isolations from urine and feces have been extremely rare.

SEROLOGY

Tularemia is most frequently confirmed by serology. Commercially available antigens (BBL no. 4087; Difco no. 2240-56-5) can be used with the standard tube agglutination test. A titer of less than 1:20 is not considered diagnostic because nonspecific cross-reactions are common at this level. A fourfold increase during illness or a single titer of 1:160 or greater is considered diagnostic. Titers into the thousands are common late in the infection and can persist for years at levels of 1:20

to 1:80. A microagglutination test has been described that is about 100-fold more sensitive and should be of great value if the reagents become commercially available (4, 20). Enzyme-linked immunosorbent assay tests have proven useful for detecting both antibodies and antigens (3, 23).

BIOCHEMISTRY

Biochemical reactions are of no particular value and do not justify the additional risk to the diagnostician. *F. tularensis* produces acid but no gas from glucose, maltose, mannose, and fructose. Acid production from glycerol by type A but not type B serves to differentiate the biovars (22).

ANIMAL INOCULATION

Inoculation of common laboratory animals has proven very reliable for isolation of *F. tularensis* because less than 10 organisms can cause infection. With an intraperitoneal injection, type A organisms will kill mice and rabbits in 4 to 8 days, whereas more than 10^6 type B organisms are required to produce a fatal infection in rabbits. These procedures must be performed in biosafety level 3 animal facilities and are therefore no longer used for routine diagnosis.

TREATMENT, PREVENTION, AND CONTROL

Streptomycin is the drug of choice, with defervescence common within 24 h and a relapse rate of less than 5%. Other aminoglycosides have been used with various degrees of success. The organism is also susceptible to tetracycline and chloramphenicol, but relapse rates with these antibiotics can exceed 50% (7). All isolates tested have been found to be resistant to penicillin, cephalosporin, and polypeptide antibiotics (15).

Since there is no effective control of this disease in nature, public awareness of the ubiquitous presence of this organism and potential for human infection should be maintained. In endemic areas, one should avoid handling dead or moribund animals and reduce the possibility of insect bites by wearing protective clothing, using insect repellents, and promptly removing ticks. The chlorination of municipal drinking water has virtually eliminated epidemics from that source, but untreated water should be considered when other routes are not evident.

An investigational live attenuated vaccine is available through the U.S. Army Medical Research and Development Command, Fort Detrick, Frederick, Md. It is recommended for persons working with the agent or with infected animals and for persons working in or entering the laboratory or animal room where cultures or infected animals are maintained (24).

LITERATURE CITED

1. **Amos, H. L., and D. H. Sprunt.** 1936. Tularemia. Review of literature of cases contracted by ingestion of rabbit. J. Am. Med. Assoc. **106:**1078–1080.
2. **Baker, C. N., D. G. Hollis, and C. Thornsberry.** 1985. Antimicrobial susceptibility testing of *Francisella tularensis* with a modified Mueller-Hinton broth. J. Clin. Microbiol. **22:**212–215.
3. **Bavanger, L., J. A. Maeland, and A. I. Naess.** 1988. Agglutinins and antibodies to *Francisella tularensis* outer membrane antigens in the early diagnosis of disease during an outbreak of tularemia. J. Clin. Microbiol. **26:**433–437.
4. **Brown, S. L., F. T. McKinney, G. C. Klein, and W. L. Jones.** 1980. Evaluation of a safranin-O-stained antigen microagglutination test for *Francisella tularensis* antibodies. J. Clin. Microbiol. **11:**146–148.
5. **Centers for Disease Control.** 1983–1988. Summaries—cases of specified notifiable diseases, United States. Morbid. Mortal. Weekly Rep.
6. **Clark, W. A., D. G. Hollis, R. E. Weaver, and P. Riley.** 1984. Identification of unusual pathogenic gram-negative aerobic and facultatively anaerobic bacteria, p. 164. U.S. Department of Health and Human Services publication no. 017-023-00149. U.S. Government Printing Office, Washington, D.C.
7. **Evans, M. E., D. W. Gregory, W. Schaffner, and Z. A. McGee.** 1985. Tularemia: a 30 year experience with 88 cases. Medicine **64:**251–269.
8. **Francis, E.** 1925. Tularemia. J. Am. Med. Assoc. **250:**3216–3224. (Reprint.)
9. **Fulginiti, V. A., and C. Hoyle.** 1966. Oropharyngeal tularemia. Rocky Mount. Med. J. **63:**41–42, 67.
10. **Halperin, S. A., T. Gast, and P. Ferrieri.** 1985. Oculoglandular syndrome caused by *Francisella tularensis.* Clin. Ped. **24:**520–522.
11. **McCoy, G. W.** 1911. A plague-like disease in rodents. Public Health Bull. **43:**53–71.
12. **McCoy, G. W., and C. W. Chapin.** 1912. *Bacterium tularense,* the cause of a plague-like disease of rodents. U.S. Public Health Mar. Hosp. Bull. **53:**17–23.
13. **Nohinek, B., and J. J. Marr.** 1983. Tularemia: two manifestations in modern man. Mo. Med. **80:**687–689, 698.
14. **Ohara, H.** 1934. Oto-rhino-laryngologia. Fukuoka **7:**432–437.
15. **Ohara, S., T. Sato, and M. Homma.** 1978. Geographical differences in susceptibility among naturally occurring strains of *Francisella tularensis.* Jpn. J. Bacteriol. **33:**415–420.
16. **Olsen, P. F.** 1975. Tularemia, p. 191–223. *In* W. T. Hubert, W. F. McCulloch, and P. R. Schnurrenberger (ed.), Diseases transmitted from animals to man. Charles C Thomas, Publisher, Springfield Ill.
17. **Pang, Z. C.** 1987. The investigation of the first outbreak of tularemia in Shandong Peninsula. Chung-Hua Liu Hsing Ping Hsueh Tsa Chih **8:**261–263.
18. **Rubin, S. A.** 1978. Radiographic spectrum of pleuropulmonary tularemia. Am. J. Roentgenol. **131:**277–281.
19. **Saslaw, S., H. T. Eiglesbach, H. E. Wilson, J. A. Prior, and S. Carhart.** 1961. Tularemia vaccine study. Arch. Int. Med. **107:**689–701.
20. **Sato, T., H. Fujita, Y. Ohara, and M. Homma.** 1988. Evaluation of a microagglutination test for early detection of the *Francisella tularensis* antibodies. Ann. Rep. Ohara Hosp. **31:**1–5.
21. **Stewart, S. J.** 1981. Tularemia, p. 705–714. *In* A. Balows and W. J. Hausler, Jr. (ed.), Diagnostic procedures for bacterial, mycotic and parasitic infections, 6th ed. American Public Health Association, Inc., Washington, D.C.
22. **Stewart, S. J.** 1988. Tularemia, p. 519–524. *In* A. Balows, W. J. Hausler, Jr., M. Ohashi, and A. Turano (ed.), Laboratory diagnosis of infectious diseases: principles and practice. Springer-Verlag, New York.
23. **Tarnvik, A., S. Lofgren, L. Ohlund, and G. Sandstrom.** 1987. Detection of antigen in urine of a patient with tularemia. Eur. J. Clin. Microbiol. **6:**318–319.
24. **U.S. Department of Health and Human Services.** 1984. Biosafety in microbiological and biomedical laboratories. U.S. Department of Health and Human Services publication no. 84-8395. U.S. Government Printing Office, Washington, D.C.
25. **Westerman, E. L., and J. McDonald.** 1983. Tularemia pneumonia mimicking legionnaires' disease: isolation of organism on CYE agar and successful treatment with erythromycin. South. Med. J. **76:**1169–1170.

Chapter 44

Brucella

N. P. MOYER, L. A. HOLCOMB, AND W. J. HAUSLER, JR.

DESCRIPTION OF THE GENUS

Habitat

Members of the genus *Brucella* are intracellular parasites that cause epizootic abortions in a variety of animals and septicemic febrile illness or localized infection of bone, tissue, or organ systems in humans. Organisms are isolated from unpasteurized dairy products, infected animals, and clinical specimens such as blood, bone marrow, or tissue. The species infective for humans are *B. suis*, which usually infects swine, *B. abortus*, predominantly a pathogen for cattle, *B. melitensis*, found in goats and sheep, and *B. canis*, a pathogen of dogs. *B. neotomae*, which occurs in the desert wood rat, and *B. ovis*, which is pathogenic for sheep, are not known to cause disease in humans.

Taxonomy

On the basis of DNA-DNA hybridization studies, it has been proposed that the genus *Brucella* consist of a single species, *B. melitensis* (15). The currently recognized species would be designated biovars, with the present numbers conserved. We have retained the existing vernacular names to avoid confusion.

Organism

Brucellae are small, nonmotile, nonsporulating, gram-negative coccobacilli or short rods (0.5 to 0.7 μm by 0.5 to 1.5 μm) arranged singly or in pairs and short chains. Capsules are not produced.

Growth

Growth occurs aerobically, often enhanced by CO_2, but no growth occurs under strict anaerobic conditions. Thiamine, niacin, and biotin are required for growth, and some strains require the addition of serum to the medium for growth. Calcium panthenate and *meso*-erythritol stimulate growth (9). Optimal growth temperature is 37°C, with a temperature range of 10 to 40°C. Optimal pH range is 6.6 to 7.4. Colonies appear on agar surface after 2 to 3 days of incubation and reach 2 to 3 mm after 4 or 5 days. Growth is slower on selective media. Colonies are nonhemolytic and nonpigmented and have a smooth glistening surface. *B. ovis* and *B. canis* occur normally in the rough form, whereas the other four species have been encountered only in the smooth form. Dissociation readily occurs in the laboratory. A cell wall-defective variant of bovine origin has been reported (10).

Physiology

Brucellae are catalase-positive, oxidase-positive (except *B. ovis* and *B. neotomae*), urease-variable organisms that reduce nitrate to nitrite. They are citrate and methyl red negative, do not produce acetylmethylcarbinol or gelatinase, and do not release *o*-nitrophenol from *o*-nitrophenol-β-D-galactoside. Metabolism is mainly oxidative, with little fermentative action on carbohydrates in conventional media. Production of H_2S, resistance to thionin and basic fuchsin, and urea hydrolysis help differentiate the species. Complete biotype or strain identification requires oxidative metabolism studies (19).

Serological identification

Smooth strains of *Brucella* are agglutinated with unabsorbed antisera to smooth *Brucella* (commercially available), with known cross-reactions to *Francisella tularensis*, *Vibrio cholerae*, *Escherichia coli* serotype O157:H7, *Salmonella* serotype O:30, and *Yersinia enterocolitica* serotype O:9 (5). Nonsmooth strains cross-react with some *Pseudomonas* species. Monospecific antisera prepared by differential absorption with *B. melitensis* and *B. abortus* can be used to determine the predominant lipopolysaccharide, M or A. The structure of the A lipopolysaccharide O chain has been determined to be a homopolymer of 1,2-linked 4,6-dideoxy-4-formamido-α-D-mannopyranose, and the M polysaccharide differs from the A lipopolysaccharide O chain by the presence of both 1,2-linked and 1,3-linked 4,6-dideoxy-4-formamido-α-D-mannopyranose subunits. *B. ovis*, *B. canis*, and rough variants of other *Brucella* species cross-react when unabsorbed anti-rough *Brucella* sera are used, but no cross-reactions occur when these organisms are agglutinated with unabsorbed anti-smooth *Brucella* sera.

CLINICAL SIGNIFICANCE

Brucellosis in humans has a variable incubation time, an insidious or abrupt onset, and no pathognomonic symptoms or signs. For these reasons, the majority of laboratory confirmations of brucellosis are based on serological tests rather than isolation of the organism (16). In 10 to 15% of patients with brucellosis, various complications of an articular, osseous, visceral, or neurological nature occur. Osteomyelitis is the most frequent complication in humans (26).

In the United States, brucellosis is largely job related. Most of the 1,654 reported cases during the period 1978 to 1987 occurred in persons with occupational or avocational exposure to animals or laboratory cultures of *Brucella* (7, 24, 26). Only 129 cases were reported in 1987 (7). *B. canis*, a pathogen of dogs, has accounted for more than 30 cases of brucellosis in humans (26). Sporadic episodes of food-associated brucellosis have occurred in recent years. In most instances, the organism responsible was *B. melitensis* and the vehicle was

Mexican or Mediterranean goat cheese (2, 6, 26). Brucellosis has occurred in hunters butchering elk, moose, and bison in the United States and in persons ingesting raw meat, bone marrow, or liver of reindeer, moose, and caribou in Alaska (17). Accidental self-inoculation or corneal contamination with the vaccine strains of *B. abortus* strain 19 and *B. melitensis* strain Rev 1 has been reported (23, 24).

COLLECTION AND TRANSPORT OF SPECIMENS

Multiple blood cultures should be obtained when brucellosis is suspected. Acute-phase serum should be obtained as soon as possible after onset of the disease, followed by a convalescent-phase serum collected 14 to 21 days after onset. Additional sera may be required to establish a diagnosis when blocking antibody is present or when immunoglobulin G studies are indicated. Infected tissues and abscesses should be cultured, as should bone marrow, spleen, and liver biopsies if available. Rarely, cerebrospinal fluid, pleural fluid, peritoneal fluid, urine, and other specimens may be collected for isolation of brucellae. Although brucellae are relatively resistant to adverse environmental conditions, specimens should be cultured as soon as possible. If a delay is expected or specimens are to be sent to a central laboratory for culturing, the specimens should be refrigerated.

CULTURE AND ISOLATION

Infection with *Brucella* spp. is readily acquired by laboratory workers through skin contact, inhalation of aerosols, eye and mouth contact, and accidental inoculation by needle and syringe. Culture work should be done in a biological safety cabinet, and laboratory workers should wear protective clothing (8).

Blood

When blood and other body fluids are cultured, the Castaneda technique is recommended. This technique utilizes a biphasic (solid and liquid) medium in the same bottle. The solid phase is prepared by adding additional agar to Trypticase soy agar (BBL Microbiology Systems, Cockeysville, Md.), tryptose agar, or brucella agar to a final concentration of 2.5%. The liquid phase is prepared from the same basal medium without agar and added aseptically after the agar has solidified. The Castaneda bottle should also have an atmosphere of 5 to 10% CO_2. This procedure using the Castaneda bottle is described by Alton et al. (1). If Castaneda bottles are not available, commercial biphasic or broth blood culture bottles can be used for culturing *Brucella* spp.; however, subcultures must be made from broth blood culture bottles every 4 to 5 days. It is important to use media with added CO_2 and to vent the blood culture bottle. Blood cultures should be incubated at 35 to 37°C and examined for 30 days. The lysis-centrifugation method has been effective for recovery of *Brucella* spp. from blood, bone marrow, and spinal fluid (12).

Abscesses and tissues

Fibrous clots, exudates, and tissue are aseptically ground, and the resulting material is inoculated onto 5% sheep blood agar, brucella agar containing 5% serum, or serum dextrose agar (Oxoid USA Ltd., Columbia, Md.). When significant contamination is likely, a selective medium should be inoculated in addition to the basal medium. Overgrowth of cultures can be controlled by adding 1.4 ml of 0.1% aqueous crystal violet (certified) per liter of medium before sterilization, but this concentration of crystal violet may inhibit small numbers of *B. suis* and *B. melitensis*. The medium developed by Farrell containing bacitracin, polymyxin B, nalidixic acid, vancomycin, cycloheximide, and nystatin (Oxoid) has proven effective (13). Modified Thayer-Martin medium and serum dextrose medium containing vancomycin, colistin, nystatin, and furadantin (BBL) are somewhat less selective than Farrell medium (3, 9). Corner et al. described a biphasic medium for isolation of brucellae from bovine tissue (11).

Incubation

Inoculated plates are incubated at 35 to 37°C in an atmosphere of 5 to 10% CO_2 for 10 days. The high humidity that develops in sealed chambers or jars under these conditions promotes rapid growth of molds, which may contaminate cultures and render them valueless. A layer or tray of dry $CaCl_2$ placed in the bottom of the chamber or jar will help to control humidity.

Examination of cultures

Examine plates for signs of growth. After 4 to 5 days, *Brucella* colonies are 2 to 3 mm in diameter, spheroidal, moist, slightly opalescent, translucent, and bluish white in reflected light. These characteristics may vary somewhat with pH and available moisture. Transfer isolated colonies to several tryptose agar slants or slants of similar media and incubate them under 5 to 10% CO_2 at 37°C for 48 h. If sufficient growth is not obtained, reincubate the specimens for another 24-h period. *Brucella* spp. yield a fine, clear, translucent growth with a slight amber tinge.

IDENTIFICATION

Preliminary identification

Gram stain and examine specimens for gram-negative pleomorphic coccobacilli. Since brucellae take the counterstain poorly, apply counterstain for 1 to 3 min instead of the usual 30 s. Nonhemolytic colonies that are gram-negative coccobacilli, do not ferment lactose or glucose, are obligate aerobes, and are oxidase positive are tested for agglutination in anti-smooth *Brucella* serum (Difco Laboratories).

Suspected *Brucella* colonies are emulsified in 2 separate drops of saline. A drop of anti-smooth *Brucella* serum is added to the first drop, and normal serum is added to the second. The suspensions and sera are mixed and examined for agglutination, which should be rapid and complete unless dissociation has occurred. *B. canis* and *B. ovis* will not agglutinate in anti-smooth *Brucella* serum. Control cultures of known *Brucella* spp. should be used in conjunction with the suspected culture.

A semiquantitative urease spot test can be performed by preparing a dense suspension of the organisms and placing a loopful of the suspension on a slant of Christensen urea agar. *B. suis* and *B. canis* will turn the indicator pink in less than 1 min, whereas *B. abortus* will usually take 5 to 10 min.

The morphological, biochemical, and serological results obtained by these methods are sufficient criteria to place the isolate in the genus *Brucella*. Negative cultures do not rule out brucellosis. Preliminary identification is sufficient laboratory evidence for the physician to initiate therapy.

Definitive identification and biotyping

There are now 6 species and 15 biotypes comprising the genus *Brucella*. There are three recognized biotypes of *B. melitensis*, seven biotypes of *B. abortus*, and five biotypes of *B. suis* (15). Biotyping of *Brucella* strains aids in understanding the epidemiology of brucellosis. The decreasing incidence of this infection, however, does not allow most laboratories to maintain proficiency in identifying species and biotypes. Common criteria for the definitive identification of the species and biotypes of the genus *Brucella* are (i) production of H_2S, (ii) requirement of increased CO_2 for growth, (iii) agglutination in monospecific sera, (iv) urease production, and (v) growth in the presence of basic fuchsin and thionin in solid media (Table 1).

H_2S production. Production of H_2S is detected by suspending a lead acetate paper strip directly over but not touching the inoculated surface of a tryptose agar slant. The strip is examined daily for 4 days and is replaced with a fresh strip each day. Hydrogen sulfide production blackens the strip.

Requirements for additional CO_2. The strain under examination is inoculated on duplicate tryptose agar slants; one slant is incubated in air, and the other is incubated in an atmosphere of 5 to 10% CO_2. Since mutants occur that are no longer dependent on additional CO_2, this test should be carried out immediately after initial isolation of the organism. Good growth in CO_2 and scanty or no growth in air indicates a requirement of CO_2.

Agglutination in monospecific antiserum. A dense suspension of the organism to be tested is prepared in 0.5% phenolized saline and heated at 60°C for 1 h. A drop of the suspension is added to a drop of each monospecific antiserum, and the solution is mixed. Agglutination should occur within 1 min with one of the sera. Control cultures of *B. abortus* biotype 1, *B. melitensis* biotype 1, and *B. ovis* or *B. canis* should be used for this test. These control cultures should agglutinate in their respective homologous sera within 1 min without agglutinating in the other sera.

Tube agglutination test. A culture suspension is prepared by harvesting a fresh slant culture with 0.5% phenolized saline. The harvest is then heated at 60°C for 1 h, diluted, and standardized to 78% light transmission at a wavelength of 650 nm in a spectrophotometer. The monospecific tube test is performed in duplicate, i.e., one set of tubes for each of the monospecific sera. The serum is diluted just beyond its known titer by the double-dilution method, starting at 1:5. An equal amount of the antigen suspension, prepared as described above, is then added to each tube plus the saline control. The tubes are incubated for 24 h at 37°C and read. Usually the strain being studied will be agglutinated by one of the sera to its known titer but not at all by the other antiserum. *B. melitensis* biotype 3 is agglutinated by both monospecific sera at various titers (1).

Growth in the presence of thionin and basic fuchsin. The concentration of basic fuchsin and thionin (Allied Chemical and Dye Co., New York, N.Y.) used in these tests is between 20 and 40 μg of dye per ml of medium. The actual concentration of dye is that which will differentiate among control cultures of *B. melitensis*, *B. abortus*, and *B. suis* biotypes. This concentration will depend on the basal medium used as well as the bacteriostatic action and purity of the dye and must be determined by using control cultures.

The medium is prepared by heating a 0.1% dye solution in a boiling-water bath for 20 min and then adding the required amount to the melted agar base (tryptose agar or Trypticase soy agar). The agar is mixed and poured into petri dishes. The surface of the plates should be dry before inoculation. From each pure culture and control strain to be tested, a suspension is made by suspending a loopful of the organism in 1.0 ml of sterile saline. The suspensions should be of equal density. A sterile cotton swab can be used to inoculate the medium. Six cultures, including reference strains, may be tested on each plate. The plates are incubated under 5 to 10% CO_2 at 37°C for 3 to 4 days and examined for growth. *B. abortus* strain 19 cannot be distinguished from other CO_2-dependent strains of *B. abortus* biotype 1 by the routine identification procedures. Growth inhibition tests utilizing thionin blue (2 μg/ml), erythritol (1 mg/ml), and penicillin (5-U disk), however, will allow differentiation (9, 20).

Results from the routine typing tests mentioned above will identify almost all *Brucella* strains as a particular biotype. Bacteriophage typing and oxidative-metabolic tests are required to identify occasional strains (1).

Phage typing. The phage test is particularly useful in distinguishing *B. abortus* biotypes 3 to 7 from *B. melitensis*. The routine test dilution (RTD) of bacteriophage Tbilisi will completely lyse smooth cultures of *B. abortus*, but *B. suis* and *B. melitensis* cultures are not affected by this phage dilution (1). *B. suis* is partially lysed by a phage concentration of $10^4\times$ RTD, whereas most strains of *B. melitensis* are not lysed by this concentration. Test cultures are grown for 24 h on agar slants and then washed off with enough normal saline solution to produce a suspension containing 10^9 cells per ml. Inoculate a well-dried agar plate with a cotton swab that has been soaked in the bacterial suspension being tested. Using a Pasteur pipette delivering 50 drops/ml, add 1 drop of the RTD of phage on the inoculated areas of the test cultures. Repeat the process for $10^4\times$ RTD on the same agar plate. Allow the plate to dry and incubate it in 5 to 10% CO_2 at 37°C for 48 h. Smooth and smooth-intermediate *B. abortus* cultures are lysed by the RTD and $10^4\times$ RTD; rough and other nonsmooth phases are not lysed. *B. suis* cultures are usually lysed by $10^4\times$ RTD but not the RTD. *B. melitensis* is not lysed by either.

SUSCEPTIBILITY TO ANTIMICROBIAL AGENTS

Since intracellular parasites are relatively inaccessible to antibiotics, prolonged treatment is advised. A combination of one of the tetracyclines with streptomycin is currently regarded as the best treatment for this disease, since the relapse rate for patients receiving antibiotic combinations is significantly lower (26). The recommended regimen for treatment of acute brucel-

TABLE 1. Differential characteristics of the species and biotypes in the genus *Brucella*

Species	Biotype	Characteristic[a]														
		CO_2 required	H_2S production	Urease activity	Growth in the presence of dyes[b]				Growth on:		Agglutination in sera[c]			Lysis by phage Tbilisi		Most common host reservoir
					Basic fuchsin (20 μg)	Thionin 40 μg	Thionin 20 μg	Thionin blue (2 μg/ml)	Erythritol (1 mg/ml)	Penicillin (5 U)	A	M	R	RTD	$10^4 \times$ RTD	
B. melitensis	1	−	−	Var	+	+	+	+	+	+	−	+	−	−	−	Sheep, goats
	2	−	−	Var	+	+	+	+	+	+	+	−	−	−	−	Sheep, goats
	3	−	−	Var	+	+	+	+	+	+	+	+	−	−	−	Sheep, goats
B. abortus	1	(+)	+	1–2 h	+	−	−	+	+	+	+	−	−	+	+	Cattle
	2	(+)	+	1–2 h	−	−	−	−	(−)	−	+	−	−	+	+	Cattle
	3	(+)	+	1–2 h	+	+	+	+	+	+	+	−	−	+	+	Cattle
	4	(+)	+	1–2 h	(+)	−	−	+	+	+	−	+	−	+	+	Cattle
	5	−	−	1–2 h	+	−	+	+	+	+	−	+	−	+	+	Cattle
	6	−	(+)	1–2 h	+	−	+	+	+	+	+	−	−	+	+	Cattle
	7[d]	−	+	1–2 h	+	−	+	+	+	+	−	+	−	+	+	Cattle
Strain 19	1	−	+	1–2 h	+	−	−	−	−	−	+	−	−	+	+	Vaccine
B. suis	1	−	+	0–30 min	(−)	+	+	(−)	+	−	+	−	−	−	+	Pigs
	2	−	−	0–30 min	−	−	+	−	+	−	+	−	−	−	+	Pigs, horses
	3	−	−	0–30 min	+	+	+	+	+	(−)	+	−	−	−	+	Pigs
	4	−	−	0–30 min	(−)	+	+	−	+	−	+	+	−	−	+	Reindeer
	5	−	−	0–30 min	−	+	+		+		−	+	−	−	+	Rodents
B. canis		−	−	0–30 min	−	+	+	(−)	+	−	−	−	+	−	−	Dogs
B. neotomae		−	+	0–30 min	−	−	−	+	+	−	+	−	−	−	+	Wood rat
B. ovis		+	−	−	(−)	+	+	−	−	−	−	−	+	−	−	Sheep (rams)

[a] +, Positive; −, negative; (+), most strains positive; (−), most strains negative; Var, variable.
[b] Species differentiation is obtained on Trypticase soy or tryptose agar with dye concentrations of 20 and 40 μg/ml. Other concentrations may be preferable with other growth media. Interpretation of results should be controlled with the reference strains of each species. Tests should be conducted in CO_2 for strains requiring CO_2.
[c] A, Monospecific *B. abortus* antiserum; M, monospecific *B. melitensis* antiserum; R, anti-rough *Brucella* serum.
[d] Formerly *B. abortus* biovar 9; biovars 7 and 8 were deleted by the International Committee on Bacterial Taxonomy, Subcommittee on Taxonomy of *Brucella*.

losis is tetracycline or doxycycline for 21 days plus streptomycin for 7 to 14 days (27). The combination of cotrimoxazole with rifampin or tetracycline and streptomycin with rifampin is also effective. Most *Brucella* strains are highly resistant to the penicillins and cephalosporins. Kanamycin and gentamicin can replace streptomycin if resistance develops.

Routine susceptibility testing of *Brucella* isolates is not necessary. Relapses that occur in brucellosis and the progression of some acute cases to chronic brucellosis have not been due to the emergence of resistant strains. If resistance to tetracycline or streptomycin is suspected, a standard broth dilution method may be used to determine the susceptibility of the organism (14).

IMMUNOSEROLOGICAL DIAGNOSIS

Since isolation of the organisms from infected patients is difficult, serological tests are relied on for the routine diagnosis of brucellosis in the majority of cases. The agglutination test is the principal test used clinically in the United States (21, 25), although limitations are noted. The standard antigen is prepared from *B. abortus* 1119-3 and is available to state and federal laboratories from the U.S. Department of Agriculture, National Animal Disease Laboratory, Ames, Iowa. The tube agglutination test as described by Meyer (18) is recommended. Laboratories receiving an occasional request for this test should refer the specimen to their state public health laboratory.

The microagglutination test correlates well with the tube agglutination test and is used by public health laboratories as a quantitative screening test for large numbers of sera (4). Serum titers equal to or greater than 1:80 should be retested by the tube agglutination test (21). The 2-mercaptoethanol test for immunoglobulin G is useful in evaluating response to antimicrobial therapy and in diagnosing chronic brucellosis (26). Other tests currently used for serodiagnosis of brucellosis include the Rose Bengal test, complement fixation test, enzyme-linked immunosorbent assay, and gel precipitation tests (22).

If brucellosis is suspected in patients with negative cultures, rising agglutinin titers of ≥1:160 are considered diagnostic. Because of the nature of the brucellosis, acute-phase serum is seldom available. A single-serum agglutinin titer of 1:160 or 1:320 is suggestive of brucellosis when accompanied by a compatible clinical course in a patient with a history of potential exposures. However, these titers lose diagnostic significance in groups repeatedly exposed to brucellae, such as abattoir employees and veterinarians. Serological results must be critically assessed along with clinical findings and occupational and other epidemiological factors before a diagnosis is made.

LITERATURE CITED

1. **Alton, G. G., L. M. Jones, and D. E. Pietz.** 1975. W.H.O. laboratory techniques in brucellosis. W.H.O. Monogr. Ser. 55.
2. **Arnow, P. M., M. Smaron, and V. Ormiste.** 1984. Brucellosis in a group of travelers to Spain. J. Am. Med. Assoc. **251**:505–507.
3. **Brown, G. M., C. R. Ranger, and D. J. Kelley.** 1970. Selective medium for the isolation of *Brucella ovis*. Cornell Vet. **61**:265–280.
4. **Brown, S. L., G. C. Klein, F. T. McKinney, and W. L. Jones.** 1981. Safranin O-stained antigen microagglutination test for detection of *Brucella* antibodies. J. Clin. Microbiol. **13**:398–400.
5. **Bundle, D. R., J. W. Cherwonogrodzky, M. Caroff, and M. B. Perry.** 1987. The lipopolysacchrides of *Brucella abortus* and *B. melitensis*. Ann. Inst. Pasteur Microbiol. **138**:92–98.
6. **Centers for Disease Control.** 1983. Brucellosis—Texas. Morbid. Mortal. Weekly Rep. **32**:548–553.
7. **Centers for Disease Control.** 1988. Summary of notifiable diseases in the United States, 1987. Morbid. Mortal. Weekly Rep. **36**:54.
8. **Centers for Disease Control and National Institutes of Health.** 1988. Biosafety in microbiological and biomedical laboratories, 2nd ed. Document no. 17-40-508-3. U.S. Government Printing Office, Washington, D.C.
9. **Corbel, M. J., and W. J. Brinley-Morgan.** 1984. *Brucella*. *In* N. R. Krieg and J. G. Holt (ed.), Bergey's manual of systematic bacteriology, vol. 1, p. 377–388. The Williams & Wilkins Co., Baltimore.
10. **Corbel, M. J., A. C. Scott, and H. M. Ross.** 1980. Properties of a cell-wall defective variant of *Brucella abortus* of bovine origin. J. Hyg. **85**:103–113.
11. **Corner, L. A., G. G. Alton, and H. Iyer.** 1985. An evaluation of a biphasic medium for the isolation of *Brucella abortus* from bovine tissues. Aust. Vet. J. **62**:187–189.
12. **Etemadi, H., A. Raissadat, M. J. Pickett, Y. Zafari, and P. Vahedifar.** 1984. Isolation of *Brucella* spp. from clinical specimens. J. Clin. Microbiol. **20**:586.
13. **Farrell, I. D.** 1974. The development of a new selective medium for the isolation of *Brucella abortus* from contaminated sources. Res. Vet. Sci. **16**:280–286.
14. **Hall, W. E., and R. E. Manion.** 1970. In vitro susceptibility of *Brucella* to various antibiotics. Appl. Microbiol. **20**:600–604.
15. **International Committee on Systematic Bacteriology, Subcommittee on Taxonomy of *Brucella*.** 1988. Minutes of the meeting, September 5, 1986. Int. J. Syst. Bacteriol. **38**:450–452.
16. **McAllister, T. A.** 1976. Laboratory diagnosis of human brucellosis. Scott. Med. J. **21**:129–131.
17. **Meyer, M. E.** 1974. Advances in research on brucellosis, 1957–1972. Adv. Vet. Sci. Comp. Med. **128**:231–246.
18. **Meyer, M. E.** 1986. Immune response to brucellae, p. 385–387. *In* N. R. Rose, H. Friedman, and J. L. Fahey (ed.), Manual of clinical immunology, 3rd ed. American Society for Microbiology, Washington, D.C.
19. **Meyer, M. E., and H. S. Cameron.** 1961. Metabolic characterization of the genus *Brucella*. II. Oxidative metabolic patterns of the described biotypes. J. Bacteriol. **82**:396–400.
20. **Morgan, W. J. B.** 1961. The use of the thionin blue sensitivity test in the examination of *Brucella*. J. Gen. Microbiol. **25**:135–139.
21. **Moyer, N. P., G. M. Evans, N. E. Pigott, J. D. Hudson, C. E. Farshy, J. C. Feeley, and W. J. Hausler, Jr.** 1987. Comparison of serologic screening tests for brucellosis. J. Clin. Microbiol. **25**:1969–1972.
22. **Moyer, N. P., and L. A. Holcomb.** 1988. Brucellosis, p. 143–154. *In* A. Balows, W. J. Hausler, Jr., M. Ohashi, and A. Turano (ed.), Laboratory diagnosis and infectious diseases: principles and practice, vol. 1. Springer-Verlag, New York.
23. **Nicoletti, P., J. Ring, B. Boysen, and J. Buczek.** 1986. Illness in a veterinary student following accidental inoculation of *Brucella abortus* strain 19. J. Am. Coll. Health **34**:236–237.
24. **Ollé-Goig, J. E., and J. Canela-Soler.** 1987. An outbreak

of *Brucella melitensis* infection by airborne transmission among laboratory workers. Am. J. Public Health **77:**335–338.

25. **Spink, W. W., N. D. McCullough, L. M. Hutchings, and C. K. Mingle.** 1954. A standardized antigen for agglutination technique for human brucellosis. Report no. 3 of the National Research Council, Committee on Public Health Aspects of Brucellosis. Am. J. Pathol. **24:**496–498.
26. **Young, E. J.** 1983. Human brucellosis. Rev. Infect. Dis. **5:**821–842.
27. **Young, E. J.** 1989. Treatment of brucellosis in humans, p. 127–141. *In* E. J. Young and M. J. Corbel (ed.), Brucellosis: clinical and laboratory aspects. CRC Press, Inc., Boca Raton, Fla.

Chapter 45

Haemophilus

MOGENS KILIAN

DESCRIPTION OF THE GENUS

Members of the genus *Haemophilus* are obligate parasites that constitute part of the normal flora of the respiratory tract of humans and many animal species. The type species *Haemophilus influenzae* is responsible for a variety of diseases in humans, ranging from chronic respiratory infection to meningitis. Other species are implicated in venereal disease and conjunctivitis, and some are occasional causes of endocarditis and abscess formation.

In morphology, *Haemophilus* organisms range from coccobacilli to filamentous rods. They are gram negative, non-acid fast, nonmotile, and nonsporeforming. Strains isolated from invasive infections are usually encapsulated.

Members of the genus *Haemophilus* are facultatively anaerobic. In vitro growth requires accessory growth factors: X factor (hemin) and V factor (NAD). *H. influenzae* requires both of these compounds, whereas some of the other species of the genus require only one (Table 1). Growth to sizable colonies on blood agar occurs only around bacteria secreting V factor, e.g., staphylococci. Preferred media are chocolate agar (blood agar base with 10% heated defibrinated horse or bovine blood) or Levinthal agar. *H. ducreyi*, which is notably difficult to cultivate, requires special media (see below). Strains of some of the species grow better in a humid atmosphere with added 5 to 10% CO_2. The optimal temperature is about 33 to 37°C (see below).

With respect to biochemical characteristics, carbohydrates are fermented; end products from the fermentation of glucose are succinic, lactic, and acetic acids. Strains of some species produce gas in fermentation media. Only *H. ducreyi*, which according to recent taxonomic data does not belong in this genus, is negative in traditional fermentation tests. All strains reduce nitrate and produce alkaline phosphatase. The majority of *H. influenzae* strains are oxidase and catalase positive.

CLINICAL SIGNIFICANCE

H. influenzae is one of the three leading causes of bacterial meningitis. There are an estimated 10,000 cases of meningitis caused by this organism in the United States each year, most of which occur in young children. Virtually all of these cases are caused by organisms that possess a serotype b capsule, and about 93% of the strains belong to biotype I (20, 41). The same sero- and biotype is also the major etiological agent of acute epiglottitis (obstructive laryngitis). Occasional cases of meningitis caused by nonencapsulated strains or strains possessing a capsule of one of the other five serotypes usually have a pathogenesis different from that of typical *H. influenzae* meningitis. Such cases are often secondary to trauma or occur in patients with impaired host defenses. Invasion of the bloodstream by encapsulated strains of *H. influenzae* (usually serotype b) may result in suppurative arthritis, osteomyelitis, cellulitis, and pericarditis. Primary *H. influenzae* pneumonia occurs in children as well as in adults but is relatively uncommon.

Although a primary pathogen, *H. influenzae* serotype b may be isolated from upper respiratory tract cultures of healthy individuals. The frequency of pharyngeal *H. influenzae* serotype b colonization is below 1% during the first 6 months of life but averages 3 to 5% throughout the rest of childhood, although it may be considerably higher in selected populations (29, 30, 41).

Haemophilus species constitute approximately 10% of the constant bacterial flora of the healthy upper respiratory tract. The predominant species is *H. parainfluenzae*, which accounts for three-fourths of the *Haemophilus* flora. Nonencapsulated *H. influenzae* strains, usually of multiple biotypes, are present in the pharynx of most healthy children but normally constitute less than 2% of the total bacterial flora. With increasing age of the individual, *H. influenzae* becomes less frequent as a pharyngeal commensal (22). *H. haemolyticus* is rarely encountered in the human respiratory tract.

Nonencapsulated *H. influenzae* of the biotypes found in the healthy respiratory tract (predominantly biotypes II and III) may be isolated from cases of sinusitis, otitis media, chronic or acute exacerbations of lower respiratory tract infections including cystic fibrosis, and chronic conjunctivitis. Cases of *H. influenzae* otitis media are associated with significantly increased proportions (50% of total bacterial flora) of the same biotype in the nasopharynx (27). Although the implication of nonencapsulated *H. influenzae* in such infections may be secondary to viral or trachomatous infection or to obstruction of normal passages, *H. influenzae* is likely to play an important role in the pathogenesis, partly because the bacterium is capable of jeopardizing the normal immune protection of mucous membranes (23). *H. influenzae* and *H. parainfluenzae* are occasionally implicated in nongonococcal urethritis.

An organism closely resembling *H. influenzae* is associated with an acute purulent and contagious form of conjunctivitis that occurs as seasonal endemics, especially in hot climates. This organism, *H. aegyptius* (Koch-Weeks bacillus) (36), is more difficult to cultivate in vitro than is *H. influenzae* but the two species are notably difficult to differentiate in the laboratory (see below). A recently described fulminant pediatric disease, Brazilian purpuric fever, is associated with an apparently unique organism that has been designated *H. influenzae* biogroup aegyptius (6). The disease is manifested by septicemia and vascular collapse, hypotensive

TABLE 1. Principal differential characteristics of *Haemophilus* species

Species	Factor requirement		Hemolysis	Fermentation of:					Presence of catalase	β-Galactosidase ONPG[b] test	CO_2 enhances growth
	X[a]	V		Glucose	Sucrose	Lactose	Mannose	Xylose			
H. influenzae (H. aegyptius)[c]	+	+	−	+	−	−	−	D[d]	+	−	−
H. haemolyticus	+	+	+	+	−	−	−	D	+	−	−
H. ducreyi	+	−	−	−	−	−	−	−	−	−	−
H. parainfluenzae[c]	−	+	−	+	+	−	+	−	D	D	D
H. parahaemolyticus[c]	−	+	+	+	+	−	−	−	+	−	−
H. segnis	−	+	−	w[e]	w	−	−	−	D	D	−
H. paraphrophilus[f]	−	+	−	+	+	+	+	D	−	+	+
H. aphrophilus[f]	−	−	−	+	+	+	+	−	−	+	+

[a] As determined by the porphyrin test.
[b] ONPG, *o*-Nitrophenyl-β-D-galactopyranoside.
[c] For further characteristics, see Table 2.
[d] D, Differences encountered.
[e] w, Weak fermentation reaction.
[f] For further characteristics, see Table 3.

shock, and death, usually within 48 h of onset. It is usually preceded by purulent conjunctivitis that has resolved before the onset of fever. Most cases have occurred in the neighboring São Paulo and Paraná states of Brazil (6). Similar cases have recently been observed in Australia, but these were caused by a different organism.

H. ducreyi is the cause of the venereal disease soft chancre or chancroid. *H. ducreyi* infection is an important cause of genital ulcers in Asia and Africa but less so in North America and most parts of Europe. There is geographical clustering in disease reporting that is primarily attributable to the presence of endemic disease and to large outbreaks. In the United States, since 1981 there have been nine large outbreaks of chancroid, concentrated in a few states. Morbidity figures from the United States show an annual incidence of approximately 1,000 to 5,000 cases. Symptomless cervical carriage of *H. ducreyi* may occur (31, 37). Extragenital chancroid is rare but may occur.

The species *H. parainfluenzae, H. parahaemolyticus, H. aphrophilus, H. paraphrophilus,* and *H. segnis* all form part of the normal oral microflora. The oral *Haemophilus* species, which very rarely encompass *H. influenzae,* amount to a mean number of 4×10^7/ml of saliva (22, 39). Some of these species (*H. aphrophilus, H. paraphrophilus,* and *H. segnis*) are predominantly found in dental plaque. *H. haemolyticus* may be encountered in gingival crevices. Like several other oral bacteria, these species are occasionally implicated in endocarditis and abscesses of internal organs (1). Most cases of meningitis ascribed to *H. parainfluenzae* can probably be explained by misidentification of *H. influenzae* isolates (see below).

There are no reports of human infections caused by the many *Haemophilus* species that occur in animals (21, 22). An exception is a single communication of otitis media caused by *H. haemoglobinophilus,* which is part of the normal mucosal flora of dogs.

COLLECTION OF SPECIMENS

Since most infections caused by *H. influenzae* serotype b are associated with bacteremia, blood samples are important sources for isolation of this organism. This is also true for cases of suspected bacterial endocarditis. Likewise, cerebrospinal fluid (CSF) should be collected for examination whenever the physician suspects or wants to rule out meningitis. Specimens of patient blood and CSF are obtained and processed as described in chapter 3. Prompt transport of these samples to the laboratory is mandatory to ensure the fastest possible diagnosis and survival of microorganisms in the sample. Additional specimens from which *Haemophilus* organisms may be isolated include fluid aspirated from infected joints, pus, nasopharyngeal or throat swabs, and occasionally vaginal swabs. Since *Haemophilus* species are normal inhabitants of the upper respiratory tract, it is important that samples taken from foci in this location remain representative of the infecting flora by avoidance of contamination with the commensal flora as far as possible. Thus, for sampling of the lower respiratory tract, any method that bypasses the upper respiratory tract (bronchial washings, transtracheal aspiration, etc.) is preferred.

Cotton swabs should be moistened in broth before the sample is taken and should be transported to the laboratory in a transport medium. Samples should be kept at room temperature. Viability of *Haemophilus* organisms is readily lost as a result of drying out or chilling; as a rule, these organisms do not survive more than a few days in clinical samples. This is particularly true for the fastidious species which may be isolated from conjunctivae or genital ulcers. Hence, whenever possible, such specimens should be directly inoculated on isolation media.

Specimens for *H. ducreyi* culture should be obtained from the base and undermined margins of the chancroid lesion with a saline- or broth-moistened swab. Ulcers may be precleaned with sterile saline, but this procedure is not required. Cultivation from the ulcer may be supplemented by aspirating pus from infected bubonic lymph nodes, but isolation of *H. ducreyi* from pus is usually less successful than isolation from ulcer material (31).

Isolated *Haemophilus* cultures may be stored for many years after lyophilization in skim milk. An alternative method of storage is freezing of 24-h broth cultures or suspensions of freshly grown cells in 10% glycerol below −60°C. Most strains may also be maintained by weekly transfers on agar media. However, strains of *H. aegyptius* and *H. ducreyi* will rapidly die out.

DIRECT MICROSCOPE EXAMINATION

Direct microscope examination of CSF is particularly important to obtain the fastest possible diagnosis. A film of CSF concentrated by centrifugation or filtration (see chapter 3) is prepared on a microscope slide, allowed to air dry, flame fixed or fixed in absolute methanol for 10 min, and stained by the Gram method. In preparation of the Gram stain, care should be exercised in decolorization, since the coccobacillary form of *H. influenzae* may resemble pneumococci in morphology. However, in CSF the organism generally is relatively pleomorphic, with coccoid, coccobacillary, short-rod, long-rod, and filamentous forms. The bacteria may be few in number but are usually detected by careful examination for 10 to 30 min. The type b capsule, which is present in virtually all strains found in CSF, can be demonstrated by the capsular swelling reaction (see chapter 29). If a sufficient number of organisms is present, a drop of the CSF is mixed on a microscope slide with a drop of an antiserum against the type b capsule. By phase-contrast microscopy, the type b capsule will appear swollen and sharply delineated when compared with a control smear of the organism. Immunofluorescence staining of the capsule with fluorescein-conjugated anti-type b serum provides another excellent means of identifying type b encapsulated strains in clinical samples. Monoclonal antibodies for use in immunofluorescence assays have been developed to detect *H. influenzae* and *H. ducreyi* in smears (16, 31).

Several immunochemical techniques for detecting capsular antigen in the CSF and other body fluids have recently been developed. These include countercurrent immunoelectrophoresis, latex agglutination, staphylococcal coagglutination, enzyme immunoassay, and radioimmunoassay. The reported sensitivities and specificities of these methods have varied, probably because of differences in test reagents, antisera, conditions of testing, and other aspects. However, several of the methods are now available as commercial ready-to-use kits. Comparisons of commercial latex agglutination (Bactigen; Wampole Laboratories, Cranbury, N.J.) and coagglutination (Phadebact Haemophilus Test; Pharmacia Diagnostics, Piscataway, N.J.) diagnostic kits with countercurrent immunoelectrophoresis for detection of type b capsular antigen in CSF found the two agglutination tests to be superior with regard to both sensitivity and specificity (10, 25, 28, 44). Both enzyme immunoassays and radioimmunoassays (13, 25) are highly sensitive but require specialized equipment not generally available in bacteriological laboratories.

Microscope examination of Gram-stained smears from conjunctivae is an important supplement because cultivation is often inadequate for establishing the presence of the implicated microorganism. *H. aegyptius* isolates appear as slender gram-negative rods in smears of conjunctival scrapings.

There is some doubt about the value of direct examination of Gram-stained smears as an aid in the diagnosis of chancroid. Most genital ulcers have a polymicrobial flora, and the arrangements of *H. ducreyi* cells as long chains or "school of fish" previously considered typical appears to be more characteristic of smears prepared from cells grown in vitro (31). Recently developed monoclonal antibodies against *H. ducreyi* may be used in immunofluorescence assays, but further studies are warranted to determine the sensitivity and specificity of this technique.

CULTIVATION

When attempting to isolate infectious microorganisms from sources that may yield *Haemophilus* species, it is important to keep in mind that most conventional agar media do not support growth of this group of microorganisms. Although growth factors X and V are contained in blood cells, only X factor is directly available in ordinary blood agar. To release V factor, the blood cells must be broken up by heating as in chocolate agar or in Levinthal medium. In addition to liberating V factor, this heat treatment is necessary to inactivate V-factor-destroying enzymes present in blood.

Cultivation of samples of spinal fluid or pus, or subcultivation from blood cultures, should be performed on both chocolate agar and blood agar. After inoculation, the blood agar plate is cross-inoculated with a streak of a staphylococcal strain. The staphylococci provide V factor and allow detection of *Haemophilus* organisms growing as satellite colonies.

Swabs from the respiratory tract should be inoculated on blood agar plates which have likewise been cross-inoculated with a staphylococcal strain. If *Haemophilus* organisms are of particular interest, it is advisable to use a selective medium. Even when present in considerable numbers, *Haemophilus* organisms may easily escape detection after incubation because of overgrowth by the remaining flora. Chocolate agar supplemented with bacitracin (300 mg/liter) has been found to give excellent recoveries.

Because of the particularly fastidious nature of *H. aegyptius* and *H. ducreyi*, special media are recommended for their isolation. For *H. aegyptius* (including *H. influenzae* biogroup aegyptius), chocolate agar supplemented with 1% IsoVitaleX (BBL Microbiology Systems, Cockeysville, Md.) provides a good medium for isolation, although primary growth from clinical samples is never luxuriant (42). For the cultivation of conjunctival swabs, it is also recommended that the sample be spread on ordinary blood agar cross-inoculated with a staphylococcal strain. The latter medium facilitates the identification of other pathogens that may be found in this location.

Since chancroid lesions usually contain a mixed flora, it is advisable to use a semiselective medium. Several different media have been tested, but the sensitivity for *H. ducreyi* is never 100% (for a review, see reference 31). GC agar (GIBCO Laboratories, Grand Island, N.Y.) containing 1 to 2% hemoglobin, 5% fetal bovine serum, 10% CVA enrichment (GIBCO), and 3 μg of vancomycin per ml appears to have the highest sensitivity for the isolation of *H. ducreyi* from clinical specimens. However, several investigators have observed that the use of two different media significantly increases the isolation frequency (14, 31).

Agar plates used for isolation of *Haemophilus* organisms should not be allowed to dry before use. A wrinkled surface of the medium indicates a degree of dryness likely to inhibit or delay growth of *Haemophilus* organisms. Cultures should be incubated at 35 to 37°C. An exception is cultures of *H. ducreyi*, which grow significantly better at 33°C. A moist atmosphere supplemented with 5 to 10% CO_2 is preferred by most strains and is mandatory for the isolation of *H. ducreyi*. Given optimal conditions, most *Haemophilus* species grow to at least 1- to 2-mm colonies after incubation for 18 to 24 h. However, *H. aegyptius* requires incubation for 2 to 4 days, and growth of *H. ducreyi* is notoriously slow, often requiring incubation for up to 9 days (21, 31).

With the exception of *H. aphrophilus* and *H. ducreyi*, all *Haemophilus* species that may be isolated from humans require V factor. Therefore, on blood agar these species will grow as satellite colonies around the staphylococcus streak. *H. haemolyticus* and *H. parahaemolyticus* strains show beta-hemolytic zones around colonies, which may resemble those of pyogenic streptococci. The satellite growth of these hemolytic *Haemophilus* strains is often less pronounced because of the release of V factor from lysed blood cells.

H. influenzae colonies on chocolate agar are grayish, semiopaque, smooth, and flat convex, usually with an entire edge. In dense areas of the plate, encapsulated strains tend to grow confluently, in contrast to colonies of nonencapsulated strains, which remain separate. On clear agar media such as Levinthal agar, colonies of encapsulated strains show a bright iridescence when light is obliquely transmitted from behind. The bluish green color of nonencapsulated strains examined in the same way should not be taken as an indication of capsulation. The iridescence of encapsulated strains is most clearly detected in young (10- to 18-h) cultures and will gradually disappear during prolonged incubation. In some strains with capsules of serotypes other than type b, the iridescence is not always clear-cut. Strains from cases of meningitis and epiglottitis virtually always produce indole, which gives the growth on agar media a characteristic pungent smell.

Colonies of *H. parainfluenzae* may be up to 3 mm in diameter after incubation for 24 h and appear smooth or rough and wrinkled. Most colonies are flat, grayish, and semiopaque. *H. aphrophilus* and *H. paraphrophilus* grow as rough, raised colonies which rarely attain a diameter exceeding 1 to 2 mm. When incubated in air without extra CO_2, these species will grow, if at all, in colonies of various sizes, which give the culture a contaminated look. *H. aegyptius, H. segnis*, and *H. ducreyi* grow as small (<1-mm) smooth colonies. The latter species may also grow in colonies of various sizes.

IDENTIFICATION OF CULTURES

The satellite phenomenon, which may be detected in primary agar plate cultures, provides a convenient means for a tentative genus identification of all of the V-factor-requiring species. However, it should be emphasized that other bacteria, such as some streptococci, corynebacteria, occasional strains of *Pasteurella multocida*, and some animal-pathogenic *Actinobacillus* and *Pasteurella* species, may show satellite growth as well.

The prerequisite for detecting the satellite phenomenon is an agar medium which lacks V factor. Since ordinary blood agar contains various amounts of free V factor, depending on the method of preparation and length of storage, it may sometimes be difficult to achieve convincing satellite growth on this medium. The special problem associated with hemolytic strains has already been mentioned. In case of doubtful reactions, far better results are obtained on a blood agar medium to which the blood (5 to 10%) is added before autoclaving. Since NAD is heat labile, this medium is completely devoid of V factor but otherwise satisfies all growth requirements of *Haemophilus* species, including X factor. Instead of being provided by a staphylococcus streak, V factor may be provided by an NAD-containing paper disk placed on the surface of the plate after inoculation.

Once the V-factor requirement has been identified, the most important means for further differentiation is determination of the X-factor requirement. This has often been done by demonstrating growth around an X-factor-containing paper disk placed on an inoculated agar medium or by comparing growth on agar media with and without added blood. The inherent problem of these methods is that probably no complex medium that will otherwise satisfy all growth requirements of *Haemophilus* species is totally free of X factor. Therefore, even when particular care is being exercised to avoid carrying over X factor with inoculum, this method will lead to an erroneous result in about 18% of cases (M. Kilian and K. R. Eriksen, unpublished data). If the identity is not being confirmed by biochemical tests, *H. influenzae* strains may be misidentified as *H. parainfluenzae* and vice versa. This undoubtedly explains some of the reported cases of meningitis ascribed to *H. parainfluenzae*.

The porphyrin test (20) provides a more accurate and rapid means of determining the X-factor requirement. This method is based on the observation (5) that hemin-independent *Haemophilus* strains excrete porphobilinogen and porphyrins, both of which are intermediates in the hemin biosynthetic pathway (Fig. 1), when supplied with δ-aminolevulinic acid. X-factor-requiring strains do not excrete these compounds because of a lack of all the enzymes involved in the biosynthesis of heme. Both porphobilinogen and porphyrins may be visualized by simple methods, which form the basis for the test.

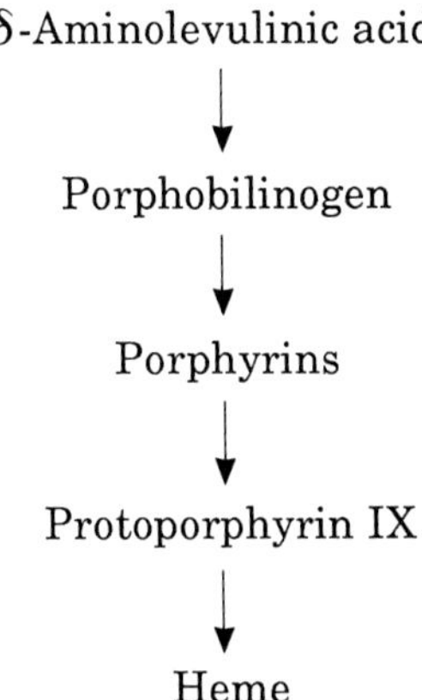

FIG. 1. Principal steps of the heme biosynthetic pathway.

Porphyrin test

Substrate. The substrate consists of 2 mM δ-aminolevulinic acid hydrochloride (Sigma Chemical Co., St. Louis, Mo.) and 0.8 mM $MgSO_4$ in 0.1 M phosphate buffer at pH 6.9. The substrate is distributed in 0.5-ml quantities in small glass tubes and may be stored for several months in a refrigerator.

Inoculation. Suspend a heavy loopful of bacteria from an agar plate culture in the substrate. Incubate for 4 h.

Reading. After incubation, expose to a Wood light (wavelength, approximately 360 nm), preferably in a dark room. A red fluorescence from the bacterial cells or from the fluid indicates porphyrins; i.e., growth of the strain is not dependent on X factor. In cases of doubtful reactions, the tubes may be reincubated for up to 24 h.

Alternative method for reading. After incubation, add 0.5 ml of Kovacs reagent (*p*-dimethylaminobenzaldehyde, 5 g; amyl alcohol, 75 ml; and concentrated HCl, 25 ml), shake the mixture vigorously, and allow the phases to separate. A red color in the lower water phase is indicative of porphobilinogen, which means that growth of the strain is not dependent on X factor. When this method of reading is used, it is advisable to include an inoculated tube without δ-aminolevulinic acid as a negative control. Kovacs reagent gives a red color reaction also with indole. Although an indole reaction will be present in the upper alcohol phase, indole-positive strains of *H. influenzae* may erroneously be identified as X factor independent in the absence of an appropriate control.

Other biochemical tests

Table 1 shows the key tests that are valuable in further differentiating the *Haemophilus* species that may be expected in human samples. Criteria for the identification of species primarily associated with animal diseases may be found elsewhere (21). Fermentation of glucose, sucrose, and lactose are important tests for species identification. Fermentation reactions are performed in 1% solutions of the respective carbohydrates in phenol red broth base (Difco Laboratories, Detroit, Mich.) supplemented with X and V factors (10 mg/liter each) after autoclaving (20). Reactions are usually clear-cut after 24 h of incubation, but some species such as *H. segnis* and *H. aegyptius* show weak reactions. Fermentation tests may also be performed by the use of commercial substrate-containing disks (3). However, studies have not yet been carried out to ensure comparable results, in particular with respect to the lactose fermentation tests, in which differences may be expected as a result of different pH indicators.

H. influenzae and *H. parainfluenzae* can be subdivided into a number of biotypes (7, 11, 15, 20, 34, 40) on the basis of three biochemical reactions: indole production, urease activity, and ornithine decarboxylase activity (Table 2). The biotypes of *H. influenzae* in particular have shown a relationship to source of isolation (2, 20, 22, 34, 40, 43). There is a certain correlation between biotype and capsular serotype of *H. influenzae* strains (20, 43). The vast majority of strains from invasive infections belong to biotype I (20), and biotype IV has been associated with genital infections (43). For epidemiologic purposes, subtyping on the basis of outer membrane proteins, lipopolysaccharides, or isoenzymes is a more sensitive tool than biotyping (4, 18, 26, 32).

The three reactions used for the subdivision of *H. influenzae* and *H. parainfluenzae* into biotypes are performed as rapid tests. In addition to rapidity, the advantage of this type of test is that growth is not required. Hence, the media do not have to include growth factors. All three test media (0.3- to 0.5-ml quantities) are inoculated with a heavy loopful of bacteria from an agar culture, and the results are read after incubation for 4 h. The test for ornithine decarboxylase may in some

TABLE 2. Key to differentiation of the biotypes of *H. influenzae* and *H. parainfluenzae*, *H. aegyptius*, *H. parahaemolyticus*, and *H. segnis*

Species and biotype	Indole	Urease	Ornithine decarboxylase
H. influenzae			
Biotype I	+	+	+
Biotype II	+	+	−
Biotype III[a]	−	+	−
Biotype IV	−	+	+
Biotype V	+	−	+
Biotype VI	−	−	+
Biotype VII	+	−	−
Biotype VIII	−	−	−
H. aegyptius[a]	−	+	−
H. parainfluenzae[b]			
Biotype I	−	−	+
Biotype II	−	+	+
Biotype III	−	+	−
Biotype IV	+	+	+
Biotype VI	+	−	+
Biotype VII	+	+	−
Biotype VIII	+	−	−
H. parahaemolyticus	−	+	−
H. segnis	−	−	−

[a] For tests differentiating *H. aegyptius* and *H. influenzae* biotype III, see text.

[b] V-factor-dependent strains showing negative reactions in all three tests used for biotyping have been referred to as a separate biotype of *H. parainfluenzae*. However, it is yet unclear whether such strains are indeed *H. parainfluenzae* or are strains of *H. segnis* or *H. paraphrophilus*. If they do belong to *H. parainfluenzae*, it would be logical to apply the designation biotype V, which has not yet been used. The reaction pattern used by Sturm (40) to characterize his "biotype V" had previously been published as biotype IV by Bruun et al. (7).

cases require additional incubation for 18 to 20 h. Recommended media are given below.

Indole test. The substrate is 0.1% L-tryptophan in 0.05 M phosphate buffer at pH 6.8. After incubation for 4 h with bacteria, add 1 volume of Kovacs reagent and shake mixture. Red color in the upper alcohol phase indicates the presence of indole.

Urease test. The substrate is 0.1 g of KH_2PO_4, 0.1 g of K_2HPO_4, 0.5 g of NaCl, and 0.5 ml of 1:500 phenol red in 100 ml of distilled water. Adjust the pH to 7.0 with NaOH, autoclave the mixture, and add 10.4 ml of a 20% (wt/vol) filter-sterilized aqueous solution of urea. (For 1:500 phenol red, dissolve 0.2 g of phenol red in NaOH and add distilled water to 100 ml.) Red color developing within 4 h indicates urease activity.

Ornithine decarboxylase test. The substrate is the medium used regularly for other bacteria. However, for *Haemophilus* organisms it is inoculated with a heavy loopful of bacteria. The medium is commercially available from Difco. A purple color developing within 4 to 24 h indicates ornithine decarboxylase activity.

Alternative methods

Several commercial systems that are now available give comparable results when used for biotyping of *H. influenzae* and *H. parainfluenzae:* PathoTec strips (General Diagnostics, Morris Plains, N.J.), API 10S or API 20E strips (Analytab Products, Plainview, N.Y.), and the Minitek system (BBL) (3, 17, 19). However, some of the available kits are less satisfactory for species identification because they do not allow differentiation of the V-factor-requiring species.

If media other than those mentioned above are used for identification and biotyping of *Haemophilus* strains, it is advisable to include strains of known identity as a reference.

Comments on taxonomy

H. aegyptius has the same key biochemical characteristics as *H. influenzae* biotype III (Table 2). Characteristics that may be of use in the separation of the two taxa include poorer in vitro growth of *H. aegyptius,* its more slender and rodlike shape, its ability to agglutinate erythrocytes, its inability to ferment xylose, and its susceptibility to troleandomycin (5 μg) (Roerig-Pfizer Inc., New York, N.Y.) (21, 36). However, none of these characteristics will unequivocally differentiate the two species. The reported distinct outer membrane protein profiles of *H. aegyptius* and *H. influenzae* biotype III may be used as an important adjunct to differentiate the two species (9). Although at present it may seem taxonomically unjustified to maintain the separation, clinical data indicate that the two species are different. The Brazilian purpuric fever isolate (*H. influenzae* biogroup aegyptius) is distinct from other strains of *H. influenzae* and *H. aegyptius* in its unique outer membrane protein profile and isoenzyme pattern and by containing a characteristic 24-megadalton plasmid (6).

The name *H. paraphrohaemolyticus* has been used for weakly hemolytic strains that require extra CO_2 in the incubation atmosphere but are otherwise similar to *H. parainfluenzae.* However, it is questionable whether there is any clinical or taxonomic justification for maintaining these two groups as separate species.

The species *H. aphrophilus* and *H. paraphrophilus* are closely related to *Actinobacillus actinomycetemcomitans* ("*Haemophilus actinomycetemcomitans*"). On primary isolation, *H. aphrophilus* may require X factor. However, this is usually not the case upon subcultivation (20, 24). Biochemical reactions, which are valuable in separating *H. aphrophilus* from related organisms, are provided in Table 3.

SEROLOGICAL IDENTIFICATION

The use of serological methods for species identification of *Haemophilus* strains has not been adequately evaluated. Therefore, serological identification is of value only for encapsulated strains of *H. influenzae.* Such strains can be separated into serotypes a through f on the basis of six serologically distinct capsular polysaccharides (35; M. Pittman, unpublished data). A subdivision of strains on the basis of capsular serotypes is highly relevant, since severe pathogenicity is almost exclusively associated with strains possessing the serotype b capsule. Serotype a, d, e, and f strains are occasionally isolated from infections as well as from the healthy respiratory tract, whereas serotype c strains are rare.

Capsular serotyping may be carried out by slide agglutination, staphylococcal coagglutination, latex agglutination, capsular swelling test, immunofluorescence microscopy, and countercurrent immunoelectrophoresis. The last three methods are of value mainly for direct identification of strains in clinical samples as described above. Once the organism is isolated, the most practical method for serotyping encapsulated strains is slide agglutination.

The cell suspension used for the slide agglutination test must be prepared from a young (6- to 18-h) agar culture, since the capsular structure tends to deteriorate in older cultures. A smooth suspension of bacteria is made in normal saline containing Formalin (0.5%, vol/vol). The cell suspension must be of sufficient density to permit the antigen-antibody reaction to proceed to completion within 1 min. In a strong positive reaction, all bacteria are agglutinated, and the fluid between the clusters is clear.

Antisera for serotyping encapsulated *H. influenzae* are available from Difco, Burroughs Wellcome Co. (Research Triangle Park, N.C.), and some state laboratories. Since such antisera also contain antibodies to some somatic antigens, agglutination may occur as a result of reaction with antigens other than capsules. Therefore, it is important that only strong reactions occurring within 1 min be counted as positive anticapsular reactions.

For screening of nasopharyngeal swab cultures for the presence of encapsulated strains, Levinthal agar containing antiserum is a valuable and sensitive tool (30). However, the method is too slow and expensive for general use for the identification of single strains.

Antigenic similarities to the six capsular polysaccharides of *H. influenzae* have been found in a number of unrelated bacteria. However, these cross-reactions should not create practical problems for laboratory diagnosis. Bacteria possessing antigens cross-reactive with the type b capsule include *Streptococcus pneumoniae* serotypes 6, 15a, 29, and 35a, *Escherichia coli* K100, *Staphylococcus aureus, Staphylococcus epidermidis, Streptococcus pyogenes, Streptococcus faecalis, Bacillus alvei,* and *Bacillus pumilus.*

TABLE 3. Differential tests for *H. aphrophilus*, *H. paraphrophilus*, and some related species

Species	X factor required	V factor required	Indole	Urease	Ornithine decarboxylase	Lysine decarboxylase	Fermentation of: Glucose	Sucrose	Lactose	Mannitol	Nitrate reduction	Presence of catalase
H. aphrophilus	+[a]	−	−	−	−	−	+	+	+	−	+	−
H. paraphrophilus	−	+	−	−	−	−	+	+	+	−	+	−
A. actinomycetemcomitans	−	−	−	−	−	−	+	−	−	D[b]	+	+
Eikenella corrodens	−	−	−	−	+	+	−	−	−	−	+	−
Cardiobacterium hominis	−	−	+	−	−	−	+	+	−	+	−	−
Kingella indologenes	−	−	+	−	−	−	+	+	−	−	−	−
H. haemoglobinophilus	+	−	+	−	−	−	+	+	−	+	+	+

[a] The requirement for hemin is often lost upon subcultivation, and the porphyrin test is positive.
[b] D, Differences encountered.

ANTIBIOTIC SUSCEPTIBILITY

Wild-type strains are susceptible to penicillin and its derivatives and to chloramphenicol, sulfonamides, tetracyclines, and the cephalosporins. However, because of spread of conjugative plasmids, an increasing number of clinical *Haemophilus* isolates are now resistant to the penicillins, in most cases as a result of a TEM-1 type β-lactamase, and to the tetracyclines, and occasional strains (0.6 to 1.4%) are also resistant to chloramphenicol (33). The likelihood that an *H. influenzae* isolate will be resistant to ampicillin is 10 to 30% in most countries but in certain areas may exceed 60%. In a recent collaborative study, the overall rate of β-lactamase production was 15.2% among a total of 3,356 clinical isolates obtained from 22 medical centers distributed throughout the United States. Twenty-one percent of encapsulated type b isolates produced β-lactamase (12, 33). Ampicillin-resistant isolates of *H. influenzae* occur more frequently in children who have received β-lactam therapy within the previous 3 months.

An alarmingly high incidence of antibiotic resistance among *H. influenzae* strains has been recorded in Spain. From 1981 to 1984, 60% of *H. influenzae* strains isolated from patients with meningitis were resistant to ampicillin, 65.7% were resistant to chloramphenicol, and 57% were resistant to both (8). Most strains resistant to chloramphenicol are also resistant to tetracycline (33).

β-Lactamase production has been observed at a frequency of 76% among *H. parainfluenzae* isolates from throat cultures from ambulatory children attending a Canadian hospital (38).

Haemophilus organisms are resistant to bacitracin, which may be used as a selective agent in isolation media.

Methods for susceptibility testing of *Haemophilus* isolates and their many pitfalls have recently been reviewed (33).

LITERATURE CITED

1. **Albritton, W. L.** 1982. Infections due to *Haemophilus* species other than *H. influenzae*. Annu. Rev. Microbiol. **36:** 199–216.
2. **Albritton, W. L., S. Penner, L. Stanley, and J. Brunton.** 1978. Biochemical characteristics of *Haemophilus influenzae* in relationship to source of isolation and antibiotic resistance. J. Clin. Microbiol. **7:**519–523.
3. **Back, A. E., and T. R. Oberhofer.** 1978. Use of the Minitek system for biotyping of *Haemophilus* species. J. Clin. Microbiol. **7:**312–313.
4. **Barenkamp, S. J., R. S. Munson, Jr., and D. M. Granoff.** 1981. Subtyping isolates of *Haemophilus influenzae* type b by outer-membrane protein profiles. J. Infect. Dis. **143:** 668–676.
5. **Biberstein, E. L., P. D. Mini, and M. G. Gills.** 1963. Action of *Haemophilus* cultures on δ-aminolevulinic acid. J. Bacteriol. **86:**814–819.
6. **Brenner, D. J., L. W. Mayer, G. M. Carlone, L. H. Harrison, W. F. Bibb, M. C. C. Brandileone, F. O. Sottnek, K. Irino, M. W. Reeves, J. M. Swenson, K. A. Birkness, R. S. Weyant, S. F. Berkley, T. C. Woods, A. G. Steigerwalt, P. A. D. Grimont, R. M. McKinney, D. W. Fleming, L. L. Gheesling, R. C. Cooksey, R. J. Akko, C. V. Broome, and The Brazilian Purpuric Fever Study Group.** 1988. Biochemical, genetic, and epidemiologic characterization of *Haemophilus influenzae* biogroup aegyptius (*Haemophilus aegyptius*) strains associated with Brazilian purpuric fever. J. Clin. Microbiol. **26:**1524–1534.
7. **Bruun, B., J. J. Christensen, and M. Kilian.** 1984. Bac-

teremia caused by a beta-lactamase producing *Haemophilus parainfluenzae* strain of a new biotype. Acta Pathol. Microbiol. Scand. Sect. B **92:**135–138.

8. **Campos, J., S. Garcia-Tornel, J. M. Gairi, and I. Fabregues.** 1986. Multiply resistant *Haemophilus influenzae* type b causing meningitis: comparative clinical and laboratory study. J. Pediatr. **108:**897–902.
9. **Carlone, G. M., F. O. Sottnek, and B. D. Plikaytis.** 1985. Comparison of outer membrane protein and biochemical profiles of *Haemophilus aegyptius* and *Haemophilus influenzae* biotype III. J. Clin. Microbiol. **22:**708–713.
10. **Collins, J. K., and M. T. Kelly.** 1983. Comparison of Phadebact coagglutination, Bactogen latex agglutination, and counterimmunoelectrophoresis for detection of *Haemophilus influenzae* type b antigens in cerebrospinal fluid. J. Clin. Microbiol. **17:**1005–1008.
11. **Doern, G. V., and K. C. Chapin.** 1987. Determination of biotypes of *Haemophilus influenzae* and *Haemophilus parainfluenzae*. A comparison of methods and a description of a new biotype (VIII) of *H. parainfluenzae*. Diagn. Microbiol. Infect. Dis. **7:**269–272.
12. **Doern, G. V., J. H. Jorgensen, C. Thornsberry, D. A. Preston, and the Haemophilus influenzae Surveillance Group.** 1986. Prevalence of antimicrobial resistance among clinical isolates of *Haemophilus influenzae:* a collaborative study. Diagn. Microbiol. Infect. Dis. **4:**95–107.
13. **Drow, D. L., D. G. Maki, and D. D. Manning.** 1979. Indirect sandwich enzyme-linked immunosorbent assay for rapid detection of *Haemophilus influenzae* type b infection. J. Clin. Microbiol. **10:**442–450.
14. **Dylewski, J., H. Nsanze, G. Maitha, and A. Ronald.** 1986. Laboratory diagnosis of *Haemophilus ducreyi:* sensitivity of culture media. Diagn. Microbiol. Infect. Dis. **4:**241–245.
15. **Gratten, M.** 1983. *Haemophilus influenzae* biotype VII. J. Clin. Microbiol. **18:**1015–1016.
16. **Groeneveld, K., L. van Alphen, N. J. Geelen-van den Broek, P. P. Eijk, H. C. Zanen, and R. J. van Ketel.** 1987. Detection of *Haemophilus influenzae* with monoclonal antibody. Lancet **i:**441–442.
17. **Holländer, R.** 1981. Die biochemische Characterisierung von *Haemophilus*-Stämmen mit Hilfe der API 20E- und API 50E-Testsysteme. Zentralbl. Bakteriol. Parasitenkd. Infektionskr. Hyg. Abt. 1 Orig. Reihe A **250:**322–329.
18. **Inzana, T. J.** 1983. Electrophoretic heterogeneity and interstrain variation of the lipopolysaccharide of *Haemophilus influenzae*. J. Infect. Dis. **148:**492–499.
19. **Juni, B. A., J. M. Rysavy, and D. J. Blazevic.** 1982. Rapid biotyping of *Haemophilus influenzae* and *Haemophilus parainfluenzae* with PathoTec strips and spot biochemical tests. J. Clin. Microbiol. **15:**976–978.
20. **Kilian, M.** 1976. A taxonomic study of the genus *Haemophilus,* with the proposal of a new species. J. Gen. Microbiol. **93:**9–62.
21. **Kilian, M., and E. L. Biberstein.** 1984. *Haemophilus* Winslow, Broadhurst, Buchanan, Krumwiede, Rogers and Smith 1917, 561, p. 558–596. *In* N. R. Krieg and J. G. Holt (ed.), Bergey's manual of systematic bacteriology, vol. 1. The Williams & Wilkins Co., Baltimore.
22. **Kilian, M., W. Frederiksen, and E. L. Biberstein (ed.).** 1981. *Haemophilus, Pasteurella* and *Actinobacillus*. Academic Press, Inc. (London), Ltd., London.
23. **Kilian, M., J. Reinholdt, S. B. Mortensen, and C. H. Sørensen.** 1983. Perturbation of mucosal immune defence mechanisms by bacterial IgA proteases. Clin. Respir. Physiol. **19:**99–104.
24. **King, E. O., and H. W. Tatum.** 1962. *Actinobacillus actinomycetemcomitans* and *Haemophilus aphrophilus*. J. Infect. Dis. **111:**85–94.
25. **Leinonen, M., and H. Käyhty.** 1978. Comparison of counter-current immunoelectrophoresis, latex agglutination, and radioimmunoassay in detection of soluble capsular polysaccharide antigens of *Haemophilus influenzae* type b and *Neisseria meningitidis* of groups A or C. J. Clin. Pathol. **31:**1172–1176.
26. **Loeb, M. R., and D. H. Smith.** 1980. Outer membrane protein composition in disease isolates of *Haemophilus influenzae:* pathogenic and epidemiological implications. Infect. Immun. **30:**709–717.
27. **Long, S. S., F. M. Henretig, M. J. Teter, and K. L. McGowan.** 1983. Nasopharyngeal flora and acute otitis media. Infect. Immun. **41:**987–991.
28. **Marcon, M. J., A. C. Hamoudi, and H. J. Cannon.** 1984. Comparative laboratory evaluation of three antigen detection methods for diagnosis of *Haemophilus influenzae* type b disease. J. Clin. Microbiol. **19:**333–337.
29. **Michaels, R. H., C. S. Poziviak, F. E. Stonebraker, and C. W. Norden.** 1976. Factors affecting pharyngeal *Haemophilus influenzae* type b colonization rates in children. J. Clin. Microbiol. **4:**413–417.
30. **Michaels, R. H., F. E. Stonebraker, and J. B. Robbins.** 1975. Use of antiserum agar for detection of *Haemophilus influenzae* type b in the pharynx. Pediatr. Res. **9:**513–516.
31. **Morse, S. A.** 1989. Chancroid and *Haemophilus ducreyi.* Clin. Microbiol. Rev. **2:**137–157.
32. **Musser, J. M., D. M. Granoff, P. E. Pattison, and R. K. Selander.** 1985. A population genetic framework for the study of invasive diseases caused by serotype b strains of *Haemophilus influenzae*. Proc. Natl. Acad. Sci. USA **82:** 5078–5082.
33. **Needham, C. A.** 1988. *Haemophilus influenzae:* antibiotic susceptibility. Clin. Microbiol. Rev. **1:**218–227.
34. **Oberhofer, T. R., and A. E. Back.** 1979. Biotypes of *Haemophilus* encountered in clinical laboratories. J. Clin. Microbiol. **10:**168–174.
35. **Pittman, M.** 1931. Variation and type specificity of the bacterial species *Haemophilus influenzae*. J. Exp. Med. **53:** 471–492.
36. **Pittman, M., and D. J. Davis.** 1950. Identification of the Koch-Weeks bacillus (*Hemophilus aegyptius*). J. Bacteriol. **59:**413–426.
37. **Plummer, F. A., L. J. D'Costa, H. Nsanze, J. Dylewski, P. Karasira, and A. R. Ronald.** 1983. Epidemiology of *Haemophilus ducreyi* in Nairobi, Kenya. Lancet **ii:**1293–1295.
38. **Scheifele, D. W., and S. J. Fussell.** 1981. Frequency of ampicillin-resistant *Haemophilus parainfluenzae* in children. J. Infect. Dis. **143:**495–498.
39. **Sims, W.** 1970. Oral haemophili. J. Med. Microbiol. **3:**615–625.
40. **Sturm, A. W.** 1986. Isolation of *Haemophilus influenzae* and *Haemophilus parainfluenzae* from genital-tract specimens with a selective medium. J. Med. Microbiol. **21:**349–352.
41. **Turk, D. C., and J. R. May.** 1967. *Haemophilus influenzae*. Its clinical importance. English Universities Press, London.
42. **Vastine, D. W., C. R. Dawson, I. Hoshiwara, C. Yoneda, T. Daghfous, and M. Messadi.** 1974. Comparison of media for the isolation of *Haemophilus* species from cases of seasonal conjunctivitis associated with severe endemic trachoma. Appl. Microbiol. **28:**688–690.
43. **Wallace, R. J., C. J. Baker, F. J. Quinones, D. G. Hollis, R. E. Weaver, and K. Wiss.** 1983. Nontypable *Haemophilus influenzae* (biotype 4) as a neonatal, maternal, and genital pathogen. Rev. Infect. Dis. **5:**123–135.
44. **Welch, D. F., and D. Hensel.** 1982. Evaluation of Bactogen and Phadebact for detection of *Haemophilus influenzae* type b antigen in cerebrospinal fluid. J. Clin. Microbiol. **16:**905–908.

Chapter 46

Bordetella

MARY J. R. GILCHRIST

DESCRIPTION OF THE GENUS

Three *Bordetella* species have been isolated from humans: *Bordetella pertussis, Bordetella parapertussis,* and *Bordetella bronchiseptica.* However, recent molecular genetic studies suggest that these three organisms are insufficiently different to be classified as separate species (35). Moreover, studies show that *B. pertussis, B. parapertussis,* and *B. bronchiseptica* possess all of the genetic information to code for the production of toxins but that only *B. pertussis* elaborates these toxins (41). If the genes coding for the toxins are supplied exogenously to *B. parapertussis,* the organism produces the toxins (33). These studies suggest that the differences between *B. pertussis* and *B. parapertussis,* phenotypic in nature, are a function of the regulation of the toxin genes. In support of such a suggestion, some workers have reported inducing strain interconversion from *B. pertussis* to *B. parapertussis* (26).

If *B. parapertussis* is merely a nontoxigenic strain variant of *B. pertussis,* this fact would explain the enigmatic observations relative to a causal role for *B. parapertussis* in clinical disease. Dual infection with *B. pertussis* and *B. parapertussis* was hypothesized when *B. parapertussis* was isolated from individuals with pertussis who exhibited lymphocytosis (30); lymphocytosis-promoting factor is a toxin produced exclusively by *B. pertussis.* Conversion of *B. pertussis* to *B. parapertussis* was offered as an explanation by another group (14). One can hypothesize that the toxins of *B. pertussis,* subject to coordinate control by the *vir* operon (32, 46) and vulnerable to phenotypic modulation by growth conditions (47), are turned off, and the organism converts to the *B. parapertussis* variant (10). Interconversion among strains would also account for the observation that laboratory strains of *B. pertussis* exhibit growth properties more like those of *B. parapertussis* (10). Although recent data suggest that the bordetellae may not be separate species, at the time of this writing the species designations for the bordetellae have not yet been resolved; therefore, the text that follows will adhere to the taxonomic distinctions now extant (38).

The bordetellae are tiny coccobacillary forms (0.2 to 0.5 by 0.5 to 2.0 μm) that occur singly or in pairs and stain gram negative, often with a bipolar appearance (38). Strict aerobes, these organisms exhibit optimal growth at 35°C. Of the three species, only *B. bronchiseptica* exhibits motility.

NATURAL HABITATS

Whereas humans represent the only known reservoir of *B. pertussis* (29), *B. bronchiseptica* is a well-known pathogen of animals (13), and many cases of human disease with *B. bronchiseptica* can be traced to a history of exposure to animals. Where pertussis is concerned, human-to-human transmission is well established, but the precise epidemiological links are still somewhat obscure. Individuals vaccinated as infants experience waning immunity in young adulthood (4) and are known to acquire pertussis disease that may be somewhat attenuated by their immune status (10). Such atypical infections serve as the source of many known cases of pertussis. In addition, there may be asymptomatic carriers, i.e., individuals who carry strains that are nontoxigenic (47) but convert to toxigenicity upon establishing residence in a new host. Coordinately with conversion to toxin production, the organism undergoes major changes in surface antigens, thus allowing the nontoxigenic strains to elude the antibody surveillance system of the host; such organisms have been termed stealth pathogens. Evolution in our understanding of strain conversion and improvements in our ability to detect these organisms will resolve these issues.

HUMAN DISEASE

In classical pertussis, an incubation period of 7 to 10 days precedes the catarrhal phase, a time period when the patient is often presumed to have a viral respiratory infection. The catarrhal phase evolves into the paroxysmal coughing phase, which is marked by a staccato cough that occurs in paroxysms (one or many per day) and may be accompanied by vomiting or an inspiratory whoop. Lymphocytosis, when present, is often quite pronounced and pathognomonic. The convalescent phase, a persisting cough that may awaken the patient nightly for many weeks, completes the course of disease. In young infants, perhaps with maternal antibody (5), and in adults with waning immunity (7) or AIDS (36), many of the characteristics pathognomonic for clinical pertussis are often absent, and disease is misdiagnosed until another family member develops clinical pertussis. The appellation "whooping cough" was abandoned when it was discovered that not all patients exhibit a "whoop." If interpreted in a similarly strict sense, the species epithet "pertussis," substituted because it alludes to the staccato cough, is now appropriate only to disease in which the cough is a distinctive feature. As a name for the disease, however, the term pertussis is likely to remain, since most milder presentations go largely unrecognized.

B. bronchiseptica is a zoonotic agent that may localize at any body site. There are case reports citing its detection in wounds, sputum, and many body fluids. *B. bronchiseptica* grows readily on routine culture media used in the laboratory. Thus, it is primarily detected in cultures that are not directed *Bordetella* cultures. As such, it must be distinguished from other small, gram-negative, glucose-nonfermenting bacteria; the differentiating characteristics for these purposes are covered in chapter 40.

SPECIMEN COLLECTION AND TRANSPORT

When Bordet-Gengou agar medium for isolation of *B. pertussis* was first devised, there was no suitable collection and transport method for the organism. As a result, the patient was allowed to cough on the surface of the Bordet-Gengou agar medium held several inches in front of the mouth. Some clinicians still refer to a pertussis culture by the archaic term "cough plate." The aspiration of bronchial or nasopharyngeal secretions provides a good alternative specimen (37, 44, 50) but is complicated by difficulty in collection and would not be appropriate in many settings. The pernasal swab is more efficacious than the throat swab (31), presumably because *B. pertussis* adheres to ciliated respiratory cells, and therefore these organisms may preferentially reside in the nasopharynx. Alternatively, since the diversity of flora in the throat exceeds that of the nasopharynx, the isolation of *B. pertussis* from throat swabs may be difficult. Because *B. pertussis* is susceptible to killing by exposure to fatty acids and other deleterious substances in some swabs, careful selection of the swab tip is required. Calcium alginate is superior to Dacron, and both are preferred over rayon or cotton (23, 24). Nasopharyngeal swabs are best collected by passing the swab on a flexible wire handle through the nares until resistance is met by virtue of contact with the nasopharynx. Although a contact time of 30 s is advocated, in practice a few seconds of contact often induces coughing or patient resistance, either of which is adequate incentive to remove the swab. A second swab is collected from the contralateral nostril.

Culture media are directly inoculated at the bedside in some clinical settings where such a procedure is practicable. Although preferred by some (37, 44), direct inoculation is not proven to be superior to some of the transport protocols currently available. A tube of charcoal-blood transport medium (40) is most desirable when transport duration may be prolonged (24). For transport times of less than 24 h, blood-free charcoal transport medium (25), Amies transport medium with charcoal, or Stainer-Scholte broth with cyclodextrin (48) may be used. For very short (<2 h) transport times, a fatty acid-free solution of 1.0% Casamino Acids (Difco Laboratories) may be acceptable (11). To improve collection technique, a collection kit with detailed instructions can be assembled. Sample kit instructions are provided in Appendix 1.

When transport duration is short, the transport device is kept at room temperature. When prolonged transport times are anticipated, there are several possible transport modes; the optimum remains unresolved (17). Some studies of transport conditions have advocated refrigeration (34), whereas others advocate overnight or, preferably, 48-h incubation (16, 23, 24, 27) before shipping. Because of the presence of selective antibiotics, the incubation step takes the form of an enrichment, allowing *B. pertussis* to grow and subsequently outnumber the other components of the nasopharyngeal flora. For such enrichment to effectively take place, the components of the transport or enrichment medium must select for growth of *B. pertussis* at the expense of other bacteria. For some, enrichment proved unsuitable and was therefore abandoned (50). Since studies directed at determining the optimum transport or enrichment conditions have used a variety of different media and other variables, it is not possible to advocate one set of conditions as superior to another.

The selection of appropriate media for the isolation of *B. pertussis* cannot be completely rationalized from data available in the literature, since studies addressing this issue have used media beyond the recommended shelf life or sham cultures rather than field trial conditions. Media containing charcoal (25), charcoal and blood (39), or cyclodextrin resins (2) have been devised to protect *B. pertussis* from the fatty acids and other deleterious substances to which the organism is sensitive. The shelf life of media is extended to several months when blood is absent, but charcoal-blood agar has a 4- to 8-week shelf life, far superior to the 1- to 7-day shelf life of Bordet-Gengou agar (16). Pending further experience with the cyclodextrin medium, charcoal-blood agar medium is a reasonable compromise in efficacy and shelf life (21, 22). Although horse blood was originally recommended, the substitution of sheep blood has been practiced (12, 31) without evident loss of efficacy. However, studies comparing horse, sheep, and human blood show a definite deficit with human blood (20). Although some (1, 27, 37) have advocated the simultaneous use of Bordet-Gengou medium and charcoal-blood agar, available data do not adequately distinguish between enhancement with a second agar type and enhancement with a second swab plated onto a duplicate plate of similar medium.

In a comparison of the efficacy of charcoal-blood agar with that of Bordet-Gengou medium, it was discovered (M. J. R. Gilchrist, unpublished observations) that some commercially prepared plated charcoal-blood agar media do not support the growth of *B. pertussis* from clinical specimens. Although the quality control strain of *B. pertussis* grew well on the commercially prepared medium, only 1 of 12 patient isolates grown on Bordet-Gengou agar was recovered on the charcoal-blood agar medium. This observation emphasizes the importance of using a fresh clinical isolate for the performance of quality control assessments of media. It is not unusual for *B. pertussis* strains to become laboratory adapted and to readily grow on routine blood agar medium. Thus, for adequate quality control challenges, a fresh clinical isolate should be amplified by one passage on laboratory medium and frozen in small portions in sheep blood or glycerol at −70°C. Upon removal from the freezer, the strain should not be passaged more than once before use in the quality control challenge. After adjustment with a turbidity standard and dilution to yield 100 colonies, the organism may be plated on the new and old media. Growth should be scored for colony size and number; these features should be comparable on the new and old media (M. Marcon, personal communication).

The growth of even a few colonies of *Staphylococcus aureus* on an agar medium produces an inhibitory substance that diffuses throughout the plate and may inhibit the growth of *B. pertussis* within a radius of several centimeters (10). Therefore, it is necessary to incorporate into the medium an antibiotic that is selective against *S. aureus*. Cephalexin (42) at 5 to 40 μg/ml is now considered superior to methicillin and penicillin for its stability in solution and for its spectrum of inhibition. Whereas some advocate simultaneous inoculation of a nonselective medium, others have abandoned this practice because of its low yield and large increase in workload (51). A recent study (20) demonstrated no significant enhancement in the growth of *B. pertussis* on nonselective media versus cephalexin medium. It is not uncommon to include an antifungal agent (amphotericin or anisomycin) in media when fungal overgrowth is a problem, perhaps primarily in reference laboratories. Alternatively, the offending fungal colony can be cut out of the agar or a second plate inoculated from the retained transport tube (51). Thus, in many settings a single plate of cephalexin-containing charcoal-blood agar is sufficient for primary isolation of *B. pertussis.*

Primary plates are inoculated and incubated at 35°C in a moist chamber or wrapped with tape to ensure moisture retention. Some authors have cited the use of a candle jar with an unlit candle, since carbon dioxide is contraindicated for the growth of *B. pertussis* (20) and oxygen deprivation may slow the growth of the organism. Depending on the rate of growth on the medium chosen, inoculated plates should generally be incubated for 6 or 7 days before being discarded as negative.

Recognition of growth on agar requires experience. Growth on Bordet-Gengou agar may be detected after 3 to 6 days of incubation. Hemolysis of the agar is difficult to appreciate if there are only a few colonies but is readily detected as a lawn of confluent hemolysis surrounding a cluster of colonies. Growth on charcoal-blood agar medium can be detected within 48 h of incubation, especially if a stereoscopic microscope is used to scan the surface of the agar plates. When examined under the dissecting microscope, young colonies tend to be quite convex, shiny, and silver in color, resembling a drop of mercury. With increasing age, the colonies progress to a whiter color and then resemble a bisected pearl. A new colony blot assay, using monoclonal antibodies for detection, allows for early (within 40 h) localization of *B. pertussis* colonies even in a culture plate containing mixed growth of other organisms (15).

Presumptive identification of colonies on the primary growth plate should be attempted if there is sufficient growth. A Gram stain and oxidase test may be conducted first. Colonies that are oxidase positive are tested for *B. pertussis,* and colonies that are oxidase negative are tested for *B. parapertussis.* Since the oxidase reaction deteriorates with prolonged incubation, it should not be considered reliable with mature colonies on plates incubated for prolonged periods (16). If there is only a small amount of growth on the agar medium, the organisms can be identified presumptively by preparation of a direct fluorescent-antibody (DFA) smear, using specific antisera for the two potential species. Caution in the interpretation of these smears is indicated, however, since false-negative results are known to occur when too heavy a smear preparation is used and false-positive results may occur as a result of cross-reactions with other small gram-negative bacilli. Since some media may support the growth of *Haemophilus* species, it may be prudent to subculture the isolate to a pertussis medium, a chocolate agar medium, and a blood agar medium or subject it to another test for factor requirements. If a large amount of growth is present, a presumptive identification can be made by agglutination of a suspension of these bacteria with specific antisera. In laboratories well acquainted with the bordetellae, a presumptive identification may be sufficient. For those laboratories wishing to confirm the identity of their isolates, the putative species may be derived by performance of the tests listed in Table 1.

DFA TEST

Methods for performing the DFA test for direct detection of *Bordetella* species in human clinical specimens are described in general terms in chapter 11. Since negative control antisera from the homologous animal species are not available with commercial reagents (Difco), it may be helpful to use two patient test wells and stain one each with *B. pertussis* and *B. parapertussis* antiserum. To increase the discriminating powers of the test readers, the magnitude of the reaction of the positive control slide (*B. pertussis*) and the negative control slide (*Haemophilus influenzae* or *B. parapertussis*) should be recorded each time the test is done. When the positive control drops below 3+ or the negative control exceeds 1+, new reagents may be necessary. This exercise will help to detect decay in the performance of the diluted conjugate, a drop in pH of the mounting fluid below 7.2, or performance problems with the fluorescence microscope. Excessive numbers of microorganisms, usually when tested from a culture plate, will damp the fluorescence yield. Thus, the positive control slide should be made to conform to a McFarland turbidity standard and then diluted to yield a reasonable number of fluorescing organisms per microscopic field. Test organisms should not exceed this density.

The sensitivity of the DFA test is limited by the number of organisms present in the secretions and thus visible to the microscopist. Since acutely ill patients who have

TABLE 1. Distinguishing characteristics of the bordetellae

Species	Characteristic					
	Oxidase	Urea	Motility	Browning on Mueller-Hinton agar	Growth on: Sheep blood agar	Growth on: MacConkey agar
B. pertussis	+	−	−	−	−[a]	−
B. parapertussis	−	+	−	+	+	+
B. bronchiseptica	+	+++	+	−	+	+

[a] Laboratory-adapted strains will grow on blood agar.

not been treated with antibiotics shed the largest numbers of organisms, a laboratory serving a practice that sees such patients will tend to have a highly sensitive DFA test compared with culture techniques. Clinical experience suggests that laboratories obtaining a 60 ± 10% sensitivity should consider their performance comparable to that of the most skilled. Those experiencing a higher sensitivity rate might well question the sensitivity of their culture protocol at detecting low numbers of organisms.

The DFA test is prone to produce many false-positive results if not performed in a laboratory where culture results are routinely available for comparison. Depending on the antibiotic-prescribing practices of the area, one can expect a few positive DFA results when organisms have been rendered nonviable for culture. A specificity of less than 90%, however, should lead one to suspect overreading of the DFA test or an insensitive culture protocol. Careful scrutiny of the positive control should assist in reading of the DFA tests. The organisms are tiny, with a dark center surrounded by a rim of bright fluorescence (oval doughnuts). While organisms grown on cephalexin medium may be elongated as a result of antibiotic effects, organisms from human clinical specimens should not be scored as positive unless they conform precisely to the morphology exhibited by an appropriate positive control organism.

Individuals in laboratories equipped with a fluorescence microscope but no medium production capability may be tempted to perform DFA testing in lieu of culture. The maintenance of accurate reading of the DFA test for pertussis, however, is extremely difficult. The best quality assurance for this DFA test is routine monitoring of the specificity and sensitivity as compared with results for culture techniques. Without such monitoring, the accuracy of the reading can deteriorate over time. A laboratory that is monitoring the performance of its DFA test should consider initiating an investigation if the sensitivity falls outside the range 60 ± 10% or if the specificity falls below 90%. Given the capriciousness in reading these results and the low sensitivity, laboratories are generally advised against performing the test without simultaneous culturing (12).

The DFA test should be used to obtain an early presumptive result. A positive result strongly suggests that the patient has pertussis. If the DFA test result is negative, the culture result must be awaited.

RECOMMENDED LABORATORY PROTOCOL

The exact transport and plating protocol for a given laboratory depends on its patient base and experience. The available data supporting one type of protocol in preference to another are insufficiently convincing to compel a laboratory that is currently satisfied with its pertussis protocol to make changes. To avoid elaborate protocols that may not be necessary or cost effective, a hospital laboratory may wish to establish one of the protocols outlined in Appendix 2. If one of the more complex protocols (2 or 3) is adopted, the laboratory should use the data garnered to refine and simplify the protocol. Because of their requirement for prolonged transport, reference laboratory protocols are more complex (27) and should be individualized to the needs of the facility.

ANTIBIOTIC SUSCEPTIBILITY

Erythromycin has for some time been the antibiotic of choice for therapy and prophylaxis of pertussis (10). Where treatment or prophylaxis failures have been reported, compliance has often been a problem, because erythromycin is not without its side effects. Other failures of erythromycin may be due to inadequate drug concentrations in secretions. The estolate form of erythromycin reaches adequate concentrations in secretions and appears efficacious (10). When this form of erythromycin is not advisable, the ethyl succinate and stearate forms have been advocated, using a special twice-per-day dosing regimen (6). With this regimen, patients stopped shedding the organism within 5 days. Surprisingly, their symptoms were ameliorated, even though they had already entered the paroxysmal phase. This new treatment protocol requires confirmation in controlled clinical settings before it is generally adopted.

Surveys of antibiotic susceptibility of *B. pertussis* in Europe (18), Japan (45), and the United States (28) have detected no change in the pattern of susceptibility of *B. pertussis* isolates to erythromycin. The quinolones appear to have good in vitro activity against *B. pertussis* (3, 28), but the clinical utility of the quinolones may be limited by virtue of the proscription against their use in infants and children. Since erythromycin is still universally effective against *B. pertussis,* it is not necessary for laboratories to perform antibiotic susceptibility testing. Such testing is generally limited to surveys because the test must be conducted by special techniques. Agar dilution assays on charcoal agar must be subjected to rigorous quality control assessments, since the charcoal may adsorb or inactivate some of the antibiotics (19).

ALTERNATIVE DIAGNOSTIC TESTS

The culture-DFA test combination is currently the most sensitive and specific method for diagnosis of pertussis. At best, however, one can detect four of five cases of pertussis, and at worst the rate may drop to less than one of two cases. A variety of serological tests (agglutination, complement fixation, hemagglutination, etc.) have long been available to confirm the diagnosis of pertussis. Their utility, however, has been hampered by their requirement for seroconversion in order to distinguish active disease from standing titers due to vaccine (43) or maternal antibodies. Newer methodologies, primarily enzyme-linked immunosorbent assays (ELISA), have been developed that use detection systems for immunoglobulins G, M, and A in serum or secretions. A commercial ELISA test, available in some countries, has not been approved for use in the United States and may not have comparable application, given the background of different vaccination practices. Unfortunately, no significant reduction in time for detection has been achieved because antibody appearance is delayed beyond the time by which diagnosis is required. As scientific tools for epidemiological surveys, these serological assays remain excellent; when applied to the diagnosis of pertussis, these assays should be a part of a comprehensive approach that includes culture and multiple serological parameters.

During the next decade, a variety of newer diagnostic modalities are expected to be introduced. The use of monoclonal antibodies for performance of the DFA test will most likely aid in improving performance of the test. Tests for the detection of adenylate cyclase (49) and pertussis toxin (8) in respiratory secretions show promise as alternatives to culture. Moreover, it is anticipated that tests relying on molecular probes or other specific reporter-probe combinations will improve the reliability of diagnosis of pertussis, particularly if these tests can discriminate between nontoxigenic variants and toxigenic strains. With the introduction of acellular vaccines for pertussis (9), it is possible that new serological tools will become available. For example, in individuals vaccinated with the acellular vaccine, a serological method that detects antibody response to a pertussis antigen that is not in the acellular vaccine would clearly establish that response as due to infection.

APPENDIX 1.

B. PERTUSSIS COLLECTION KIT FOR CULTURE AND IMMUNOFLUORESCENT STAIN

Contents of kit

1. Ziploc bag for transport
2. 1 petri dish of agar medium
3. 1 Calgiswab type 1
4. 1 tube of Casamino Acids transport medium
5. Instructions

Introduction

The enclosed media are optimized for collection of specimens for culture and immunofluorescent stain for *B. pertussis*. The organism is sensitive to drying, heat, cold, cotton, fatty acids, and antibiotics such as erythromycin. Therefore, avoid exposure to these conditions or agents.

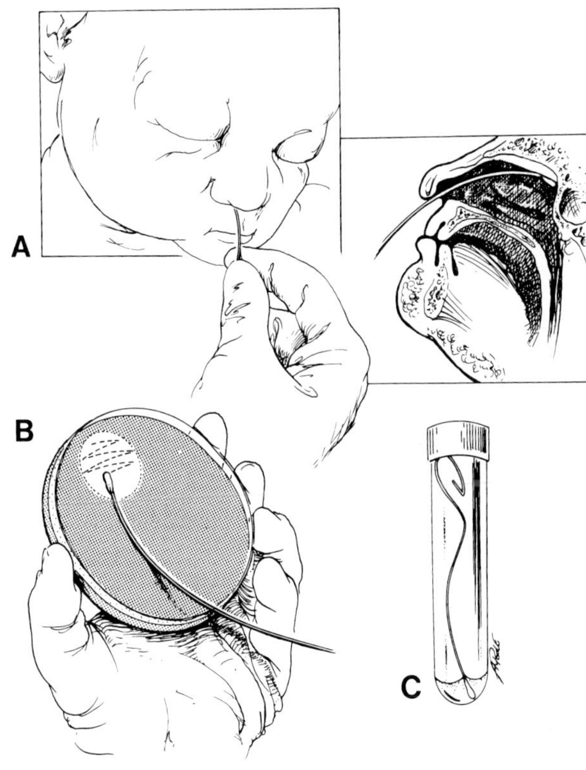

FIG. A1.

Collection

DO NOT USE KIT IF IT IS EXPIRED (SEE LABEL ON OUTSIDE OF BAG). WARM THE CULTURE MEDIA TO ROOM TEMPERATURE FOR AT LEAST 30 MIN. Remove plastic from edge of agar plate and discard. Using a Calgiswab, collect a nasopharyngeal swab specimen by inserting the swab into the posterior nasopharynx (Fig. A1A) and holding it there for 15 to 30 s or until the patient coughs. Alternatively, collect a nasopharyngeal aspirate.

SWAB IMMEDIATELY ONTO THE CULTURE PLATE. Rub secretions into an area the size of a quarter near the edge of the medium (Fig. A1B). Place the swab into transport medium in a tube (Fig. A1C), tighten the lid, place the agar and tube into a Ziploc bag, and transport the specimen to the laboratory immediately.

APPENDIX 2.

SUGGESTED PROTOCOLS FOR LABORATORY TESTING FOR PERTUSSIS

Protocol 1

Using a direct plating collection kit (Appendix 1), inoculate one plate of charcoal-blood agar with cephalexin and prepare one two-well slide from the Casamino Acids solution. (Follow instruction given in the text for quality control assessment of media.) Stain one well each with *B. pertussis* and *B. parapertussis* antiserum. Streak the plate for isolation when it is delivered to the laboratory.

Protocol 2

(Although this protocol and protocol 3 may improve recovery by 10 to 20%, they also double or triple the cost and may not be justifiable in most settings.) Using a direct plating collection kit (Appendix 1) but with two swabs and two agar plates, inoculate two plates of charcoal-blood agar with cephalexin or one plate of charcoal-blood agar with cephalexin and one of Bordet-Gengou agar with cephalexin. (Follow instructions given in the text for quality control assessment of media. There is no compelling reason to add Bordet-Gengou agar medium if quality control assessment of charcoal-blood agar is done well, unless laboratories prefer recognition of *B. pertussis* on Bordet-Gengou agar.) Prepare one two-well slide from the Casamino Acids solution; stain one well each with *B. pertussis* and *B. parapertussis* antiserum. Streak plates for isolation when they are delivered to the laboratory.

Protocol 3

Using the first tube of a two-tube transport collection kit, inoculate one or two plates of media (protocol 2). Use the swab from the second transport tube to prepare slides for DFA stain. Incubate the second tube for 48 h and inoculate a second set of plates.

I am grateful to Teresa Sketch Bretl, Susan Shuptar, Mary Jo Corrigan, Charlotte Rumpke Wiley, Michael Girten, Annamaria Bustamante, Kim Moultney, and Mobeen Rathore for assistance in the investigations that form the basis of this chapter. Furthermore, I acknowledge discussions with Joseph Campos (Children's Hospital National Medical Center, Washington, D.C.), Mohamed Karmali (Hospital for Sick Children, Toronto, Ontario, Canada), Mario Marcon (Children's Hospital, Columbus, Ohio), and David Welch (Children's Hospital, Oklahoma City, Oklahoma) concerning refinement of the procedures outlined in this chapter. Finally, I thank C. C. Linnemann (University of Cincinnati College of Medicine, Cincinnati, Ohio) for critical reading of the manuscript.

LITERATURE CITED

1. **Ahmad, F., and M. A. Calder.** 1984. Isolation of *Bordetella pertussis:* benefits of using both Bordet-Gengou and charcoal media. J. Clin. Pathol. **37:**1071–1072.
2. **Aoyama, T., Y. Murase, T. Iwata, A. Imaizumi, Y. Suzuki, and Y. Sato.** 1986. Comparison of blood-free medium (cyclodextrin solid medium) with Bordet-Gengou medium for clinical isolation of *Bordetella pertussis.* J. Clin. Microbiol. **23:**1046–1048.
3. **Appleman, M. E., T. L. Hadfield, J. K. Gaines, and R. E. Winn.** 1987. Susceptibility of *Bordetella pertussis* to five quinolone antimicrobic drugs. Diagn. Microbiol. Infect. Dis. **8:**131–133.
4. **Bass, J. W., and S. R. Stephenson.** 1987. The return of pertussis. Pediatr. Infect. Dis. J. **6:**141–144.
5. **Bass, J. W., and L. L. Zacher.** 1989. Do newborn infants have passive immunity to pertussis? Pediatr. Infect. Dis. J. **8:**352–353.
6. **Bergquist, S.-O., S. Bernander, H. Dahnsjö, and B. Sundelöf.** 1987. Erythromycin in the treatment of pertussis: a study of bacteriologic and clinical effects. Pediatr. Infect. Dis. J. **6:**458–461.
7. **Cherry, J. D., L. J. Baraff, and E. Hewlett.** 1989. The past, present and future of pertussis. The role of adults in epidemiology and future control. West. J. Med. **150:**319–328.
8. **Friedman, R. L., S. Paulaitis, and J. W. McMillan.** 1989. Development of a rapid diagnostic test for pertussis: direct detection of pertussis toxin in respiratory secretions. J. Clin. Microbiol. **27:**2466–2470.
9. **Fulginiti, V. A.** 1989. The current state of pertussis and pertussis vaccines. Am. J. Dis. Child. **143:**532–533.
10. **Gilchrist, M. J. R., and C. C. Linnemann, Jr.** 1988. Pertussis, p. 403–410. *In* A. Balows, W. J. Hausler, Jr., M. Ohashi, and A. Turano (ed.). Laboratory diagnosis of infectious diseases: principles and practice. Springer-Verlag, New York.
11. **Gilligan, P. H.** 1983. Laboratory diagnosis of *Bordetella pertussis* infection. Clin. Microbiol. Newsl. **5:**115–117.
12. **Gilligan, P. H., and M. C. Fisher.** 1984. Importance of culture in laboratory diagnosis of *Bordetella pertussis* infections. J. Clin. Microbiol. **20:**891–893.
13. **Goodnow, R. A.** 1980. Biology of *Bordetella bronchiseptica.* Microbiol. Rev. **44:**722–738.
14. **Granström, M. M., and P. Askelöf.** 1982. Parapertussis: an abortive pertussis infection? Lancet **i:**1249–1250.
15. **Gustafsson, B., and P. Askelöf.** 1989. Rapid detection of *Bordetella pertussis* by a monoclonal antibody-based colony blot assay. J. Clin. Microbiol. **27:**628–631.
16. **Hoppe, J. E.** 1988. Methods for isolation of *Bordetella pertussis* from patients with whooping cough. Eur. J. Clin. Microbiol. Infect. Dis. **7:**616–620.
17. **Hoppe, J. E.** 1989. Recovery of *Bordetella pertussis* from nasopharyngeal swabs. J. Clin. Microbiol. **27:**595–596.
18. **Hoppe, J. E., and A. Haug.** 1988. Antimicrobial susceptibility of *Bordetella pertussis* (part 1). Infection **16:**126–130.
19. **Hoppe, J. E., A. Haug, and K. Botzenhart.** 1988. Bordetellae and charcoal horse blood agar: inactivation of antibiotics in agar during prolonged incubation for susceptibility testing. Chemotherapy **34:**36–39.
20. **Hoppe, J. E., and M. Schlagenhauf.** 1989. Comparison of three kinds of blood and two incubation atmospheres for cultivation of *Bordetella pertussis* on charcoal agar. J. Clin. Microbiol. **27:**2115–2117.
21. **Hoppe, J. E., and J. Schwaderer.** 1989. Comparison of four charcoal media for the isolation of *Bordetella pertussis.* J. Clin. Microbiol. **27:**1097–1098.
22. **Hoppe, J. E., and R. Vogl.** 1986. Comparison of three media for culture of *Bordetella pertussis.* Eur. J. Clin. Microbiol. **5:**361–363.
23. **Hoppe, J. E., and A. Weib.** 1987. Recovery of *Bordetella pertussis* from four kinds of swabs. Eur. J. Clin. Microbiol. **6:**203–205.
24. **Hoppe, J. E., S. Wörz, and K. Botzenhart.** 1986. Comparison of specimen transport systems for *Bordetella pertussis.* Eur. J. Clin. Microbiol. **5:**671–673.
25. **Jones, G. L., and P. L. Kendrick.** 1969. Study of a blood-free medium for transport and growth of *Bordetella pertussis.* Health Lab. Sci. **6:**40–45.
26. **Kumazawa, N. H., and M. Yoshikawa.** 1978. Conversion of *Bordetella pertussis* and *Bordetella parapertussis.* J. Hyg. **81:**15–23.
27. **Kurzynski, T. A., D. M. Boehm, J. A. Rott-Petri, R. F. Schell, and P. E. Allison.** 1988. Comparison of modified Bordet-Gengou and modified Regan-Lowe media for the isolation of *Bordetella pertussis* and *Bordetella parapertussis.* J. Clin. Microbiol. **26:**2661–2663.
28. **Kurzynski, T. A., D. M. Boehm, J. A. Rott-Petri, R. F. Schell, and P. E. Allison.** 1988. Antimicrobial susceptibilities of *Bordetella* species isolated in a multicenter pertussis surveillance project. Antimicrob. Agents Chemother. **32:**137–140.
29. **Linnemann, C. C., Jr., and J. W. Bass.** 1981. *Bordetella* infections. *In* A. Balows and W. J. Hausler, Jr. (ed.), Diagnostic procedures for bacterial, mycotic and parasitic infections, 6th ed. American Public Health Association, Inc., Washington, D.C.
30. **Linnemann, C. C., Jr., and E. B. Perry.** 1977. *Bordetella parapertussis:* recent experience and a review of the literature. Am. J. Dis. Child. **131:**560–563.
31. **Marcon, M. J., A. C. Hamoudi, H. J. Cannon, and M. M. Hribar.** 1987. Comparison of throat and nasopharyngeal swab specimens for culture diagnosis of *Bordetella pertussis* infection. J. Clin. Microbiol. **25:**1109–1110.
32. **Miller, J. F., J. J. Mekalanos, and S. Falkow.** 1989. Coordinate regulation and sensory transduction in the control of bacterial virulence. Science **243:**916–922.
33. **Monack, D., J. J. Munoz, M. G. Peacock, W. J. Black, and S. Falkow.** 1989. Expression of pertussis toxin correlates with pathogenesis in *Bordetella* species. J. Infect. Dis. **159:**205–210.
34. **Morrill, W. E., J. M. Barbaree, B. S. Fields, G. N. Sanden, and W. T. Martin.** 1988. Effects of transport temperature and medium on recovery of *Bordetella pertussis* from nasopharyngeal swabs. J. Clin. Microbiol. **26:**1814–1817.
35. **Musser, J. M., E. L. Hewlett, M. S. Peppler, and R. K. Selander.** 1986. Genetic diversity and relationships in populations of *Bordetella* species. J. Bacteriol. **166:**230–237.
36. **Ng, V. L., M. York, and W. K. Hadley.** 1989. Unexpected isolation of *Bordetella pertussis* from patients with acquired immunodeficiency syndrome. J. Clin. Microbiol. **27:**337–338.
37. **Parker, C. D., and B. J. Payne.** 1987. *Bordetella* infections, p. 155–166. *In* B. B. Wentworth (ed.), Diagnostic procedures for bacterial infections. American Public Health Association, Inc., Washington, D.C.
38. **Pittman, M.** 1984. Genus *Bordetella* Morena-Lopez 1952, 178, p. 388–393. *In* N. R. Krieg and J. G. Holt (ed.), Bergey's manual of systematic bacteriology, vol. 1. The Williams & Wilkins Co., Baltimore.
39. **Preston, N. W.** 1970. Technical problems in the laboratory diagnosis and prevention of whooping cough. Lab. Pract. **19:**482–486.
40. **Regan, J., and F. Lowe.** 1977. Enrichment medium for the isolation of *Bordetella.* J. Clin. Microbiol. **6:**303–309.
41. **Rozinov, M. N., A. A. Dain, Y. L. Shumakov, I. A. Lapaeva, and T. A. Holzmayer.** 1988. All species of the genus *Bordetella* contain genes for pertussis toxin of *Bordetella pertussis.* Zentralbl. Bakteriol. Parasitenkd. Infektionskr. Hyg. Abt. 1 Orig. Reihe A **269:**205–210.

42. **Stauffer, L. R., D. R. Brown, and R. E. Sandstrom.** 1983. Cephalexin-supplemented Jones-Kendrick charcoal agar for selective isolation of *Bordetella pertussis:* comparison with previously described media. J. Clin. Microbiol. **17:** 60–62.
43. **Thomas, M. G., K. Redhead, and H. P. Lambert.** 1989. Human serum antibody responses to *Bordetella pertussis* infection and pertussis vaccination. J. Infect. Dis. **159:**211–218.
44. **Washington, J. A., II.** 1985. Laboratory procedures in clinical microbiology, 2nd ed., p. 101. Springer-Verlag, New York.
45. **Watanabe, M., Y. Nakase, T. Aoyama, H. Ozawa, Y. Murase, and T. Iwata.** 1986. Serotype and drug susceptibility of *Bordetella pertussis* isolated in Japan from 1975 to 1984. Microbiol. Immunol. **30:**491–494.
46. **Weiss, A. A., and S. Falkow.** 1984. Genetic analysis of phase change in *Bordetella pertussis.* Infect. Immun. **43:** 263–269.
47. **Weiss, A. A., and E. L. Hewlett.** 1986. Virulence factors of *Bordetella pertussis.* Annu. Rev. Microbiol. **40:**661–686.
48. **Wirsing von König, C. H., A. Tacken, and H. Finger.** 1988. Use of supplemented Stainer-Scholte broth for the isolation of *Bordetella pertussis* from clinical material. J. Clin. Microbiol. **26:**2558–2560.
49. **Wirsing von König, C. H., A. Tacken, and E. L. Hewlett.** 1989. Detection of *Bordetella pertussis* by determination of adenylate cyclase activity. Eur. J. Clin. Microbiol. Infect. Dis. **8:**633–636.
50. **Wort, A. J.** 1983. Bacteriological diagnosis of pertussis. Lancet **i:**766.
51. **Young, S. A., G. L. Anderson, and P. D. Mitchell.** 1987 Laboratory observations during an outbreak of pertussis. Clin. Microbiol. Newsl. **9:**176–179.

Chapter 47

Mycoplasmas

GEORGE E. KENNY

CHARACTERIZATION

Mycoplasmas are small (0.2- to 0.3-μm) pleomorphic organisms bounded only by a cell membrane, with no evidence of a cell wall (20); hence, they are not susceptible to β-lactams and do not Gram stain. Individual cells (star-shaped, round, and filamentous forms) from broth cultures can be seen by dark-field and phase-contrast microscopy, but the rich mycoplasmal medium contains many artifacts. On solid media, mycoplasmas form microscopic colonies 10 to 300 μm in diameter; these are visible with magnification, giving a typical "fried egg" appearance (Fig. 1).

GROWTH

Because of their small genome (5×10^8 to 1×10^9 daltons), mycoplasmas are highly fastidious (20) and require enriched media. Unusual growth requirements include cholesterol (from serum supplement), preformed nucleic acid precursors (from yeast extract), and urea for *Ureaplasma urealyticum*. Growth rates vary with generation times in broth from 1 h for some ureaplasmas to 6 h for *Mycoplasma pneumoniae*. The yield of organisms from broth is small (1 to 20 mg of protein per liter), and cultures show at most a faint haze best seen by comparison with uninoculated medium. Colonies on agar are detectable in 2 (*Mycoplasma hominis*) to 20 (*M. pneumoniae*) days. The human species can be categorized into groups by the ability to ferment glucose, utilize arginine, or hydrolyze urea (Table 1).

TAXONOMY AND NOMENCLATURE

The mycoplasmas associated with humans include eight species in the genus *Mycoplasma*, one species in the genus *Ureaplasma*, and *Acholeplasma laidlawii* (Table 1). The *Mycoplasma* species and *U. urealyticum* are classified within the family *Mycoplasmataceae*, order *Mycoplasmatales*, whereas *A. laidlawii* is within the family *Acholeplasmataceae*, order *Acholeplasmatales*. The common names mycoplasmas, ureaplasmas, and acholeplasmas are used for organisms in genus *Mycoplasma*, *U. urealyticum*, and *Acholeplasma* species, respectively. The term "mollicutes" has been proposed as an inclusive common name for all organisms in class *Mollicutes* but has yet to be adopted widely (20). The human *Mycoplasma* species can be distinguished into three groups. (i) *M. pneumoniae* and *M. genitalium* are slow-growing, glycolytic, aerobic species that show serological cross-reactions; (ii) *Mycoplasma fermentans* utilizes both arginine and glucose and grows best under anaerobic conditions, though established strains grow aerobically; (iii) the remaining five human *Mycoplasma* species utilize arginine but not glucose and immunologically cross-react. Ureaplasmas are distinguished by their ability to hydrolyze urea. *A. laidlawii* is glycolytic and makes large colonies; it is distinguished by its growth in media without serum. *Mycoplasma* species are identified by inhibition of growth on agar by disks impregnated with rabbit antiserum (4).

CLINICAL SIGNIFICANCE

M. pneumoniae is a major cause of primary atypical pneumonia and accounts for 10 to 20% of total X-ray-proven pneumonia (6). Four additional species are found in the oral cavity. *Mycoplasma salivarium* is a common inhabitant of the gingival crevice, especially in persons with periodontal disease, and is not observed in edentulous persons. *Mycoplasma orale*, *M. faucium*, and *M. buccale* appear to be normal oral flora. In contrast, *M. pneumoniae* is not a harmless microorganism and persists in the respiratory tract for 1 to several months after infection. Subclinical infections are common, and the disease, called walking pneumonia, is ordinarily mild. Unlike other respiratory diseases, *M. pneumoniae* infections are not seasonal. In large populations, disease is endemic year-round, with periodic increases in incidence, but in smaller populations outbreaks appear as epidemics. Infection spreads slowly in families, and transmission apparently requires close contact.

Carriage of mycoplasmas in the genital tract is common: vaginal carriage of *U. urealyticum* occurs in 60% of normal women, and *M. hominis* is found in 20% (26). Both organisms appear to be effective opportunists and have been recovered from the bloodstream in pure culture from women with mild postpartum fever (17, 26). Ureaplasmas appear to be responsible for a portion of nonspecific urethritis in males.

SPECIAL CONSIDERATIONS FOR CULTURE OF MYCOPLASMAS

Because mycoplasmas grow slowly, forming colonies visible microscopically on agar (Fig. 1), their culture characteristics differ greatly from those of other bacteria. Growth in broth cultures shows only a faint haze and is best judged by the change in pH of the medium through use of an appropriate metabolic marker (Table 1). Since mycoplasmas grow embedded in the agar with only a slight surface growth, transfer of cultures with a wire loop is ineffective. To transfer a colony to broth, the agar around the colony is excised and placed in broth. For transfer to agar, the piece of agar is emulsified in broth and transferred to a plate. Agar plates are observed under a stereoscopic microscope by oblique light at ×20 to ×60 magnification. This procedure provides the best working distance and resolution for observing

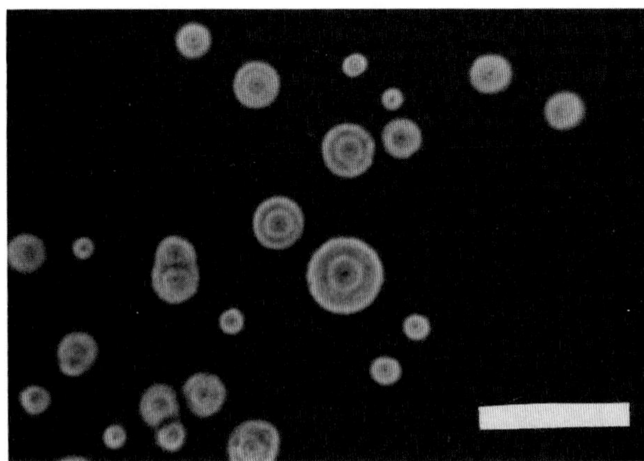

FIG. 1. Colonies of *M. pneumoniae* AP-164 on H agar (10 days of incubation). Bar = 100 μm.

colonies on the agar surface through the bottom without opening the plate and avoids contamination with either bacteria or mycoplasmas during the repeated observations.

Quality control (11) of culture media by using known positive specimens is most important. The critical variable in the media is the lot of peptone and not the serum and fresh yeast extract. Although most lots of soy peptone powder were useful for prototypic strains, only one in three was efficient for isolation of *M. pneumoniae* directly from specimens (15). Dehydrated peptone effective for *M. pneumoniae* appeared to be equally effective for ureaplasmas and *M. hominis*. Therefore, until manufacturers carry out effective quality control, it will be necessary to test individual lots of medium. Clinical specimens known to be positive or first-passage strains from patients are preferable to stock strains. Fortunately, "good" lots of dehydrated powders appear to be stable at room temperature for years; therefore, the initial evaluation of new batches is important. Thereafter, the use of first-passage isolates as controls will detect batches of medium from which a major ingredient such as serum, yeast extract, or urea has been omitted.

Different conditions are required to isolate the various human mycoplasmas. *U. urealyticum* requires a pH of 6.0 for optimum growth and little growth occurs above pH 7.0, whereas most other species grow on media with a pH of 6.5 to 8.0. *M. hominis*, the most pH-tolerant organism, grows well on media with a pH from 5.5 to 8.0, whereas *M. pneumoniae* grows poorly outside the range of 6.0 to 7.5. *M. salivarium*, *M. orale*, *M. faucium*, *M. buccale*, and *M. fermentans* are isolated anaerobically on H agar with little growth aerobically, whereas *M. hominis* and *U. urealyticum* appear indifferent to atmosphere. Both *M. pneumoniae* and *M. genitalium* are obligate aerobes, and growth is enhanced by the presence of CO_2 (Table 1). The requirement for CO_2 is complicated by the pH effects in that the serum supplement contains $NaHCO_3$. The final pH of unbuffered agar medium containing 20% serum may be as much as 0.5 pH unit lower if incubated in 5% CO_2 than in air. Thus, aerobic organisms such as *M. pneumoniae* may appear to grow better in microaerobic environments (95% N_2, 5% CO_2) because of the more favorable neutral pH achieved. Phenol red is included in all media recommended in chapter 121 to aid in monitoring pH.

Only one broth base and one agar base need be prepared, and these differ only in the addition of agarose (chapter 121). Adjustment of the pH to 6.0 with 2-(*N*-morpholino)ethane sulfonic acid (MES) buffer and addition of urea are required for ureaplasmas, and glucose is added to broth medium for glycolytic mycoplasmas. The additives are prepared as sterile stock solutions that store well at room temperature in the dark.

Other media have been recommended (5, 9, 23, 25). Hayflick medium (9) is commonly used but appears to show lot-to-lot variation in the powder. The SP-4 medium of Tully et al. was used to isolate *M. genitalium* (27); however, no strains of this organism have been reported from the genital tract in the time since the initial isolates were recovered.

Artifacts are a major problem in detection of mycoplasmas in clinical specimens. Cells and debris may re-

TABLE 1. Properties of human mycoplasmas and ureaplasmas

Species	Serovar	Metabolic marker			Optimal pH	Growth in atmosphere			Time for colony formation (days)
		Arginine	Urea	Glucose		Air	Anaerobic[a]	Candle jar	
Genital organisms									
U. urealyticum	14	−	+	−	5.5–6.5	++	++	++	1–4
M. hominis	?[b]	+	−	−	5.5–8.0	++	++	++	1–4
M. fermentans	1	+	−	+	~7.0[c]	+	++	ND[d]	3–20
Respiratory organisms									
M. pneumoniae	1	−	−	+	6.5–7.5	++	±	++	3–20
M. salivarium	1	+	−	−	6.0–7.0	+	++	ND	2–5
M. orale[e]	1	+	−	−	~7.0[c]	+	++	ND	3–10
Other[f]									
M. genitalium	?[b]	−	−	+	~7.0[c]	+	±	++	Slow
A. laidlawii	1	−	−	+	6.0–8.0	++	++	++	1–5

[a] Hydrogen plus carbon dioxide with catalyst (GasPak; BBL).
[b] Number of serovars unknown.
[c] Limited data available.
[d] ND, No data available.
[e] Properties of *M. faucium* and *M. buccale* are similar.
[f] Species recovered from both genital and respiratory tracts.

semble the fried-egg colonies; thus, it is imperative that the laboratory demonstrate that the agent is transferable. Certain serum lots induce the formation of pseudocolonies, which are whorls of lipid crystals appearing on the surface of agar plates after extended incubation. These crystals transfer but do not produce metabolic products. Large amounts of cellular material in specimens may show acid production from mammalian enzymes. Excessive moisture on the agar surface can allow the organisms to replicate in the surface fluid and so fail to form colonies. This difficulty, a particular problem with ureaplasmas, can be avoided by pouring plates 24 h before use and holding them at room temperature overnight to lessen surface moisture. Plates can be stored in sealed plastic boxes at 4°C.

Penicillin is the principal selective agent used in mycoplasmal medium. Thallium acetate inhibits gram-negative organisms but should not be used if either *U. urealyticum* or *M. genitalium* is suspected (thallium acetate is toxic, and care should be taken in its use). Amphotericin (1:2,000) is useful for inhibition of yeast cells.

COLLECTION, TRANSPORT, AND STORAGE OF SPECIMENS

Specimens collected on swabs should be placed in 2-ml vials of transport medium. Trypticase soy broth (BBL Microbiology Systems, Cockeysville, Md.) supplemented with 0.5% bovine albumin and with penicillin (200 U/ml) to suppress bacterial overgrowth is satisfactory. Other transport media can be used provided that they contain protein and have been tested. Mycoplasmas are remarkably susceptible to drying; thus, specimens or swabs should be placed in transport medium or cultured promptly. Tissues or sputum specimens are submitted directly to the laboratory. Although specimens may be held at 4°C for up to 48 h, they should not be stored at −20°C. If cultures cannot be inoculated at once, the transport medium should be frozen immediately at −70°C. Mycoplasmas survive freezing and thawing very well provided that the medium contains protein.

ISOLATION OF *M. PNEUMONIAE* FROM THE RESPIRATORY TRACT

Swabs are extracted in 2 ml of transport medium, and portions (0.1 ml) are inoculated both in diphasic H broth and onto H agar. Before inoculation of media, sputum, body fluids, and disrupted tissues should be diluted 1:10 and 1:100 to reduce the amount of inhibitory materials normally present in tissues. Agar plates are incubated aerobically at 37°C in a sealed container and examined regularly (2, 5, 10, 14, and 21 days) for typical colonies. Diphasic cultures should be examined by viewing tubes through the side with a stereoscopic microscope. Growth of *M. pneumoniae* is particularly noteworthy in that small fluid medium colonies or spherules (3) can be seen floating in the medium or attached to bits of agarose. This observation usually precedes the decrease in pH as judged by the phenol red indicator. Diphasic cultures should be transferred to agar on day 21, and these plates should be held for 3 weeks. Specimens are considered presumptively positive if they show typical small colonies on agar and spherule and acid production in fluid medium. Colonies may appear from 4 to 21 days after inoculation. This presumptive diagnosis is confirmed by a test for hemolysis if enough colonies exist. The hemolysis test is done on the isolation plate by overlaying the colonies with a thin layer (1 drop per plate) of 8% guinea pig erythrocytes in saline agar. After incubation overnight at 37°C in a humidified chamber, a zone of hemolysis will be observed around individual colonies. Further identification is carried out by inhibition of growth with specific antiserum (4). Portions (0.1 ml) of 1:1, 1:10, and 1:100 dilutions of the broth culture are spread uniformly over H-agar plates, and filter paper disks (3 to 5 mm) soaked in undiluted mycoplasmal antiserum are added. After incubation for 5 to 7 days, the plates are examined for zones of inhibition of colonial growth. Caution is required, since this test is quite sensitive to excessive numbers of organisms. Unfortunately, this identification procedure does not distinguish *M. genitalium* from *M. pneumoniae*. This was not a problem when *M. genitalium* was thought to be solely a genital organism, but such is no longer the case (1). Other species that may be detected include *M. hominis*, which grows rapidly and forms large colonies. Although the anaerobic oral mycoplasmas such as *M. orale* and *M. salivarium* are abundant in throat swabs, these species are rarely detected aerobically on H agar. Other media may be less selective; 0.002% methylene blue has been used, but this dye also partially inhibits *M. pneumoniae* and is not recommended. Occasionally, *A. laidlawii* is encountered. This organism hemolyzes guinea pig erythrocytes. However, it grows rapidly, forms large colonies, and grows in medium without serum.

Since patients carry the organism for 1 to 2 months after infection, *M. pneumoniae* is relatively easy to isolate, a characteristic that is little hampered by antimicrobial therapy. However, isolation is slow, particularly for specimens that are positive in diphasic culture only (15).

ISOLATION OF GENITAL MYCOPLASMAS

Since both *M. hominis* and *U. urealyticum* are ordinarily sought simultaneously from the genital tract, methods for their isolation are considered together despite the different properties of these organisms. Viability of *U. urealyticum* is difficult to maintain because of the rapid die-off caused by the depletion of urea. In broth cultures, it is necessary to buffer the broth and supply an optimum concentration of urea. *U. urealyticum* will survive for about 12 h in broth after an indicator color change and about 2 days after the appearance of colonies on agar; however, because of local elevation in pH, viability is rapidly lost after staining with the $CaCl_2$-urea stain. MES is an optimum buffer; the molar ratio of MES to urea for broth cultures is 2:1 to 4:1 or 10 to 20 mM MES (pH 5.5) to 5 mM urea. For agar, a ratio of 10:1 or 30 mM MES to 3 mM urea is sufficient to permit maximum colony diameter and limit the increase in pH in the vicinity of the colony. The addition of the reducing agent, 1 mM Na_2SO_3, reduces the lag phase for some but not all isolates. *M. hominis* is the least fastidious of the potential human pathogens and grows well on H agar, in H broth, and in the corresponding U media. *M. hominis* strains show a faint but distinct haze in broth, whereas *U. urealyticum* produces no haze but shows a readily recognizable pH change from the hydrolysis of urea.

For the isolation of genital mycoplasmas, 0.1-ml portions of specimen are inoculated into H and U broths and onto the corresponding agars. Agar plates are incubated aerobically or in 5% CO_2 in air. Broth cultures are incubated aerobically in sealed tubes. Incubation of plates under stringent anaerobiasis gives no advantage for *M. hominis* or *U. urealyticum* but does favor the isolation of *M. fermentans*. *U. urealyticum* is resistant to lincomycin and susceptible to erythromycin, whereas the reverse is true for *M. hominis*. Therefore, addition of lincomycin (25 µg/ml) to U broth and U agar will select for *U. urealyticum*. Because the pH is 7.0 to 7.5, H agar and H broth select against *U. urealyticum* (Table 1); incorporation of erythromycin (25 µg/ml) will further enhance selectivity.

U-agar plates should be observed daily for 4 days and stained on the plate with 1 to 2 drops of $CaCl_2$-urea solution on day 4 for the final reading. Ureaplasmal colonies stain brown within 5 min, whereas *M. hominis* colonies are unaffected. The U broth should be observed twice daily for color changes. When color changes are observed, 1 drop of culture is transferred to 3 ml of U broth, and 0.1 ml of this diluted suspension is inoculated onto a U-agar plate (it is necessary to dilute or streak out the inoculum because confluent lawns of *U. urealyticum* cannot be detected microscopically). Cultures are reported positive for ureaplasmas if the specimen produces a color change from urea and typical colonies that develop a brown color upon reaction with the $CaCl_2$-urea stain.

H-agar plates are observed on days 1, 2, 3, 5, and 10. Colonies of *M. hominis* may appear as early as 1 day but are usually seen in 2 to 5 days. H-broth cultures should be transferred to H agar on days 2 and 4. Nearly all large-colony mycoplasmas are *M. hominis*, but occasionally bacteria that produce colonies resembling *M. hominis* are isolated. These isolates ordinarily grow on bacteriological medium without serum. Large-colony forms can be identified as *M. hominis* if they are transferable, utilize arginine (20 mM L-arginine in H broth), and produce typical large colonies. Their identity can be verified by growth inhibition on agar in a manner similar to that described for *M. pneumoniae*. *M. hominis* colonies will also be seen on U-agar plates and on subcultures from U broth if lincomycin is not included in the medium.

Tissues should be ground in transport medium, diluted 1:10 and 1:100, and inoculated into media. Both species have been recovered from blood (17, 26). Because of the complexity of the blood culture medium used by Lamey et al. (17), it is recommended that a diphasic medium be prepared with 10 ml of U agar overlaid with 50 ml of U broth (both without lincomycin) and that this medium be inoculated with 1 to 5 ml of blood (without anticoagulant). Cultures should be subcultured daily to U agar (without lincomycin) and observed for the presence of mycoplasmal and ureaplasmal colonies.

Because *M. fermentans* and *M. genitalium* are rare isolates, it is not possible to make recommendations for their effective culture. Although *M. fermentans* is well established (20), few isolates exist, suggesting rarity or inadequate media. *M. genitalium* is difficult to cultivate, and only several isolates have been reported from the genital tract. This species has been isolated only in the early 1980s and on SP-4 medium (27). The use of nick-translated whole genomic probes shows a prevalence of about 10% in males (10). The recovery of this organism from respiratory specimens (1) also causes problems for the interpretation of *M. pneumoniae* culture results because of their close cultural similarity.

SIGNIFICANCE OF ISOLATIONS

The isolation of *M. pneumoniae* is always clinically significant because the organism is not a member of the normal flora. For genital organisms, the situation differs because these mycoplasmas colonize the vagina and male urethra of healthy persons. Isolation from internal sources is of importance provided that other organisms are sought as well. When one is sampling the uterus, upper urogenital tract, and other internal sites, care must be taken to avoid contamination from the vagina or the urethra.

ANTIMICROBIAL SUSCEPTIBILITY TESTING

Mycoplasmas have been considered generally susceptible to tetracyclines. However, strains of *M. hominis* and *U. urealyticum* but not *M. pneumoniae* that show high-level tetracycline resistance are now prevalent (21). This resistance is mediated by the transposon *tetM*. Two methods have been used for antimicrobial susceptibility testing: the agar dilution method (14), in which the endpoint is prevention of colony formation on agar, and a broth dilution method (24) that uses a metabolic endpoint (urea hydrolysis, glucose utilization, or arginine hydrolysis). The main concern is to determine whether strains of *U. urealyticum* or *M. hominis* isolated from internal sites are susceptible to tetracycline. Since the resistance due to *tetM* is high level (≥32 µg/ml) and much different from the 0.5 to 2 µg/ml for susceptible strains, such resistance can easily be detected by using either method to test the isolate at a tetracycline concentration of 8 µg/ml. Testing of susceptibility to other antimicrobial agents is less clearly defined because the differences between susceptible and resistant strains are less dramatic.

OTHER CELL-WALL-DEFICIENT BACTERIA

Cell-wall-deficient bacteria or L forms (18) are gram-negative and gram-positive bacteria that have lost their cell walls and can be grown, albeit with difficulty, on medium supplemented with serum and osmotically balanced to prevent lysis of these fragile forms. In vitro, L forms are induced from bacteria by prevention of cell wall synthesis with penicillin or by removal of the cell wall with lysozyme. On agar media, colonies of L forms resemble those of mycoplasmas, and osmotically stable L forms may be encountered occasionally during attempts to isolate mycoplasmas. Colonies are frequently very large, and the organism usually reverts to the parent organism if penicillin is omitted from the medium. Cell-wall-deficient bacteria that depend on osmotic stabilization require a special medium with increased osmotic pressure (wall-defective medium; see chapter 121 and reference 7). The role of L forms in disease has been most difficult to establish (19), they may be involved in urinary tract disease (7). Culture for cell-wall-deficient forms can be attempted with specimen materials from internal sites where evidence of infection exists but no microbes are recovered.

DIRECT EXAMINATION

Considerable attention has been paid to direct detection methods, particularly for *M. pneumoniae* because of its slow growth. The cDNA ribosomal probe (Gen-Probe, San Diego, Calif.) in its current ^{125}I-labeled form has a detection limit of about 2×10^3 CFU from cultures of *M. pneumoniae* (8). Two disadvantages of this assay are that (i) only about half of the throat swab specimens from patients with *M. pneumoniae* pneumonia contain sufficient organisms for detection (15) and (ii) it cannot distinguish between *M. pneumoniae* and *M. genitalium*. The polymerase chain reaction (2) has a lower detection limit (10^2 color-changing units) for *M. pneumoniae* in cultures. The detection limit of a nick-translated whole genomic probe for *U. urealyticum* was 10^3 CFU (22). This detection level might be satisfactory for identification of significant ureaplasmal infections of the genital tract because high concentrations correlate better with disease than does the mere presence of organisms (26).

SERODIAGNOSIS

The complement fixation test with lipid antigen has been a standard method for determining antibodies to *M. pneumoniae* (12, 13, 15). Antibody increases correlate well with the isolation of *M. pneumoniae* from patients with pneumonia (15), but the test can give false-positive reactions in patients with proven bacterial meningitis (16). No general methods are available for detecting antibodies to *M. hominis* or *U. urealyticum*. Serodiagnosis is considered in detail elsewhere (12).

LITERATURE CITED

1. **Baseman, J. B., S. F. Dallo, J. G. Tully, and D. L. Rose.** 1988. Isolation and characterization of *Mycoplasma genitalium* strains from the human respiratory tract. J. Clin. Microbiol. **26:**2266–2269.
2. **Bernet, C., M. Garret, B. DeBarbeyrac, C. Bebear, and J. Bonnet.** 1989. Detection of *Mycoplasma pneumoniae* by using the polymerase chain reaction. J. Clin. Microbiol. **27:**2492–2496.
3. **Boatman, E. S., and G. E. Kenny.** 1971. Morphology and ultrastructure of *Mycoplasma pneumoniae* spherules. J. Bacteriol. **106:**1005–1015.
4. **Clyde, W. A.** 1964. *Mycoplasma* species identification based upon growth inhibition by specific antisera. J. Immunol. **92:**958–965.
5. **Dorman, S. A., D. J. Wilson, and T. F. Smith.** 1983. Comparison of growth of *Mycoplasma pneumoniae* on modified New York City and Hayflick media. Am. J. Clin. Pathol. **79:**235–237.
6. **Foy, H. M.** 1982. *Mycoplasma pneumoniae*, p. 345–366. *In* A. S. Evans and H. A. Feldman (ed.), Bacterial infections of humans: epidemiology and control. Plenum Publishing Corp., New York.
7. **Gutman, L. T., M. Turck, R. G. Petersdorf, and R. J. Wedgwood.** 1965. Significance of bacterial variants in urine of patients with chronic bacteriuria. J. Clin. Invest. **44:**1945–1952.
8. **Harris, R., B. P. Marion, G. Varkanis, T. Kok, B. Lunn, and J. Martin.** 1988. Laboratory diagnosis of *Mycoplasma pneumoniae* infection. 2. Comparison of methods for the direct detection of specific antigen or nucleic acid sequences in respiratory exudates. Epidemiol. Infect. **101:**685–694.
9. **Hayflick, L.** 1965. Tissue cultures and mycoplasmas. Tex. Rep. Biol. Med. **23**(Suppl. 1):285–303.
10. **Hooton, T. M., M. C. Roberts, P. L. Roberts, K. K. Holmes, W. E. Stamm, and G. E. Kenny.** 1988. Prevalence of *Mycoplasma genitalium* as determined by DNA probe in men with urethritis. Lancet **i:**266–268.
11. **Kenny, G. E.** 1985. *Mycoplasma* and *Ureaplasma*, p. 135–143. *In* J. M. Miller and B. B. Wentworth (ed.), Methods for quality control in diagnostic microbiology. American Public Health Association, Inc., Washington, D.C.
12. **Kenny, G. E.** 1986. Serology of mycoplasmal infections, p. 440–445. *In* N. R. Rose, H. Friedman, and J. L. Fahey (ed.), Manual of clinical laboratory immunology. American Society for Microbiology, Washington, D.C.
13. **Kenny, G. E., and J. T. Grayston.** 1965. Eaton pleuropneumonia-like organism (*Mycoplasma pneumoniae*) complement-fixing antigen: extraction with organic solvents. J. Immunol. **95:**19–25.
14. **Kenny, G. E., T. M. Hooton, M. C. Roberts, F. D. Cartwright, and J. Hoyt.** 1989. Susceptibilities of genital mycoplasmas to the newer quinolones as determined by the agar dilution method. Antimicrob. Agents Chemother. **33:**103–107.
15. **Kenny, G. E., G. G. Kaiser, M. K. Cooney, and H. M. Foy.** 1990. Diagnosis of *Mycoplasma pneumoniae* pneumonia: sensitivities and specificities of serology with lipid antigen and isolation of the organism on soy peptone medium for identification of infections. J. Clin. Microbiol. **28:**2087–2093.
16. **Kleemola, M., and H. Kayhty.** 1983. Increase in titers of antibodies in patients with purulent meningitis. J. Infect. Dis. **146:**284–288.
17. **Lamey, J. R., D. A. Eschenbach, S. H. Mitchell, J. M. Blumhagen, H. M. Foy, and G. E. Kenny.** 1982. Isolation of mycoplasmas and bacteria from the blood of postpartum women. Am. J. Obstet. Gynecol. **143:**104–112.
18. **Madoff, S.** 1986. Introduction to the bacterial L-forms, p. 1–20. *In* S. Madoff (ed.), The L-forms of bacteria. Marcel Dekker, Inc., New York.
19. **Pachas, W. N.** 1986. L-forms and bacterial variants in disease, p. 287–318. *In* S. Madoff (ed.), The L-forms of bacteria. Marcel Dekker, Inc., New York.
20. **Razin, S., and E. A. Freundt.** 1984. The mycoplasmas, p. 740–793. *In* N. R. Krieg and J. G. Holt (ed.), Bergey's manual of systematic microbiology, vol. 1. The Williams & Wilkins Co., Baltimore.
21. **Roberts, M. C., S. L. Hillier, J. Hale, K. K. Holmes, and G. E. Kenny.** 1986. Tetracycline resistance and *tetM* in pathogenic urogenital bacteria. Antimicrob. Agents Chemother. **30:**810–812.
22. **Roberts, M. C., M. Hooton, W. Stamm, K. K. Holmes, and G. E. Kenny.** 1987. DNA probes for the detection of mycoplasmas in genital specimens. Isr. J. Med. Sci. **23:**618–620.
23. **Robertson, J. A.** 1978. Bromthymol blue broth: improved medium for detection of *Ureaplasma urealyticum* (T-strain mycoplasma). J. Clin. Microbiol. **7:**127–132.
24. **Senterfit, L.** 1983. Antibiotic sensitivity testing of mycoplasmas, p. 397–404. *In* J. G. Tully and S. Razin (ed.), Methods in mycoplasmology, vol. 2. Academic Press, Inc., New York.
25. **Shepard, M. C.** 1983. Culture media for ureaplasmas, p. 137–146. *In* S. Razin and J. G. Tully (ed.), Methods in mycoplasmology, vol. 1. Academic Press, Inc., New York.
26. **Taylor-Robinson, D., and W. M. McCormack.** 1979. Mycoplasmas in human genito-urinary infections, p. 307–366. *In* J. G. Tully and S. Razin (ed.), The mycoplasmas, vol. 2. Academic Press, Inc., New York.
27. **Tully, J. G., R. M. Cole, D. Taylor-Robinson, and D. L. Rose.** 1981. A newly discovered mycoplasma in the human genital tract. Lancet **i:**1288–1291.

Chapter 48

Gardnerella, Streptobacillus, Spirillum, and *Calymmatobacterium*

PETER PIOT

This chapter deals with some taxonomic orphans and ill-defined bacterial species that have little in common.

GARDNERELLA VAGINALIS

Description

The genus *Gardnerella* contains only one species, *Gardnerella vaginalis*. The type strain is 594 Gardner and Dukes (ATCC 14018; NCTC 10287). On the basis of DNA hybridization and phenotypic taxonomic studies, this genus is not related to any other established taxon (9, 22). Its cell wall is similar to that of a gram-positive bacterium, both morphologically and in chemical composition (12, 29). The cells are nonmotile, pleomorphic, nonencapsulated, gram-negative to gram-variable rods that average 0.5 by 1.5 μm. Fimbriae are present on freshly isolated strains (1). The cellular fatty acids include laurate, myristate, stearate, oleate, and palmitate. The mol% G+C of the DNA is 42 to 44.

G. vaginalis is facultatively anaerobic and fermentative, with acetic acid as the major end product. Catalase and oxidase are not produced. Most strains are fastidious in their growth requirements (4). Colonies on human blood bilayer agar medium are 0.3 to 0.5 mm in diameter after incubation for 48 h at 35 to 37°C in a 5% CO_2 atmosphere. The optimal pH for growth ranges between 6 and 7. A distinct beta-hemolysis is produced on human and rabbit but not on sheep blood agar media. Acid is produced from a wide variety of carbohydrates.

Natural habitat and clinical significance

G. vaginalis is associated with bacterial vaginosis. Bacterial vaginosis is a defined syndrome, the hallmark of which is a malodorous vaginal discharge associated with a significant increase in the number of *G. vaginalis* and various obligate anaerobes, mainly *Bacteroides* spp., *Mobiluncus* spp., and *Peptococcus* spp. (6), and a decrease in the number of vaginal lactobacilli. A minimum diagnostic requirement for bacterial vaginosis is the presence of at least three of the following signs: excessive vaginal discharge, vaginal pH of >4.5, clue cells (vaginal epithelial cells covered by small gram-negative rods), and a fishy, aminelike odor in the KOH test. The succinate/lactate ratio in vaginal secretions is significantly increased (>0.4), and volatile organic acids, including acetic, propionic, and butyric acids, are found in most patients. Although *G. vaginalis* is encountered consistently and in high numbers in women with bacterial vaginosis, the organism can also be isolated from as many as 20 to 40% of healthy women, depending on the sensitivity of the culture technique. The pathogenesis of bacterial vaginosis is unclear.

G. vaginalis is a common blood isolate in postpartum and postabortal fever and has been isolated from amniotic fluid (7). This organism is frequently isolated from the endometrium of women with postpartum endometritis (35). It can cause fatal and nonfatal septicemia and soft tissue infection in neonates. It is a rare cause of urinary tract infection. *G. vaginalis* has also been isolated from vaginal and liver abscesses, bartholinitis, abdominal fluid, and the oropharynx. Though it has been associated with balanoposthitis, its presence in the male urethra or on the glans is usually not associated with clinical manifestations.

Collection, transport, and storage of specimens

Vaginal discharge can be collected with calcium alginate or cotton-tip swabs. One swab is either placed into a transport medium such as Amies or Stuart or, preferably, used to inoculate the isolation medium. A second swab is used to prepare a Gram-stained smear and a wet mount. Isolation media should be inoculated as soon as possible after specimen collection, at most within 24 h when a transport medium is used.

Direct examination

Direct examination of vaginal secretions is more relevant for the diagnosis of bacterial vaginosis than is isolation of *G. vaginalis* from these specimens because *G. vaginalis* can be part of the normal vaginal flora. The presence of clue cells correlates well with a diagnosis of bacterial vaginosis. The classic description of clue cells was based on a wet-mount preparation. However, the observation of clue cells in a Gram-stained smear is preferable (32). This smear allows not only for a better evaluation of the vaginal flora but also for preservation of the preparation for later examination. In typical smears from patients with bacterial vaginosis, clue cells are accompanied by a mixed flora consisting of very large numbers of small gram-negative and gram-variable rods and coccobacilli in the absence of larger gram-positive rods (lactobacilli). Gram-negative curved rods may be found as well. When the clinical examination is normal, *Lactobacillus* spp. morphotypes are found alone or in the presence of small numbers of *G. vaginalis* morphotypes. In general, there is a strong inverse relationship between the numbers of *G. vaginalis* and *Lactobacillus* spp. morphotypes.

Culture and isolation

Semiselective human blood bilayer agar (HBT agar) (34) is inoculated by rolling a swab across a sector of the plate. This inoculum is streaked with a loop to allow a semiquantitative estimate of the growth of the isolate. Plates are incubated in a candle jar or a humid atmosphere containing 5% CO_2. Obligately anaerobic strains of *G. vaginalis* occasionally occur (20), but routine anaerobic incubation is not recommended. After 48 h of incubation, the plates are examined for colonies exhibiting diffuse beta-hemolysis. Alternatively, vaginalis agar (nonselective single-layer human blood agar) (10) may be used. Isolates should be subcultured at least every 72 h, since older cultures are often no longer viable. For isolation of *G. vaginalis* from blood, sodium polyanetholsulfonate SPS should be deleted from the medium, since this ingredient may inhibit the organism.

Identification

A presumptive identification of *G. vaginalis* may be based on the typical cell morphology in the Gram stain, beta-hemolysis with diffuse edges on human blood bilayer agar, and a negative catalase test (10, 23, 33). Laboratory reports should include a quantitative estimate of the growth of *G. vaginalis*.

When a more accurate identification is required, α- and β-glucosidase, hippurate hydrolysis, and starch hydrolysis tests yield a maximum discriminative value (Table 1). Starch hydrolysis can be determined on Mueller-Hinton agar enriched with 5% (vol/vol) sterile horse serum and detected by the addition of Lugol iodine.

Inhibition tests with disks containing 50 μg of metronidazole (zone of inhibition present), 5 μg of trimethoprim (zone of inhibition present), 1 mg of sulfonamide (no zone of inhibition), and 10% bile (zone of inhibition present) are also useful in the differentiation of *G. vaginalis*, vaginal lactobacilli, and unclassified catalase-negative coryneforms. The latter two groups of organisms are resistant to metronidazole, trimethoprim, and bile and are variably susceptible to sulfonamide (23). Traditional identification schemes for *G. vaginalis* were based on sugar fermentation reactions, but these are of little value since other organisms from the vagina frequently give the same reactions as does *G. vaginalis*. Moreover, fermentation tests with *G. vaginalis* are often inconsistent. However, when extragenital isolates must be fully characterized, acid production from the carbohydrates listed in Table 1 is determined. The rapid method of Greenwood et al. is recommended (10). Tests should always be performed with large inocula from cultures not older than 24 h. Gas-liquid chromatography of organic acids may also provide additional information. Most *G. vaginalis* strains produce acetic and lactic acids. However, these acids are also produced by bifidobacteria and some unclassified vaginal coryneforms. *G. vaginalis* can also be diagnosed with the help of the API 20 Strep method.

Isolates can be subdivided into six biovars on the basis of the production of lipase and β-galactosidase and the hydrolysis of hippurate. Antimicrobial susceptibility testing of genital isolates of *G. vaginalis* is not recommended.

TABLE 1. Selected features of *G. vaginalis* (175 strains)[a]

Test	Test result[b]	% Positive
Beta-hemolysis (human blood bilayer agar)	+	99
Hippurate hydrolysis	+	90
Starch hydrolysis	+	100
α-Glucosidase	+	100
β-Glucosidase	−	0
β-Galactosidase	V	45
Lipase	V	64
Growth on MacConkey agar	−	0
Growth on Kligler agar	−	0
Acid from:		
Arabinose	V	38
Glucose	+	100
Maltose	+	100
Mannitol	−	0
Starch	+	100
Sucrose	+	85
Trehalose	V	72
Xylose	V	44
Zone of inhibition with:		
Metronidazole (50 μg)	+	92
Trimethoprim (5 μg)	+	100
Sulfonamide (1 mg)	−	0
Bile (10%)	+	100

[a] From reference 23.
[b] +, Positive; −, negative; V, variability between strains.

Serological investigations

Fluorescent-antibody tests for the identification of *G. vaginalis* have been reported (11). Isolates can be further divided into serovars by using a dot blot technique (14).

STREPTOBACILLUS MONILIFORMIS

Description

There is only one species in the genus *Streptobacillus*, *S. moniliformis* (30). The type strain is ATCC 14647. *S. moniliformis* is a facultatively anaerobic, highly pleomorphic, asporogenous gram-negative rod. The rods are less than 1 μm wide by 1 to 5 μm long, but curved and looping filaments as long as 100 to 150 μm may be formed. The filaments are not branched. Morphology is heavily influenced by cultural conditions and age of culture. In young cultures or in smears from clinical material, cells usually appear to be more uniform, with occasional homogeneous filaments. Irregular coccobacilli are found in older cultures, with granules and bands appearing in the filaments. These may consist of a series of bulbous swellings, giving the appearance of a string of beads, and may contain numerous granules. Oil-like droplets containing various lipids can be found inside and outside the bacterial cells. Older cultures do not stain well in the Gram stain; better results may be obtained with Giemsa or Wayson stain (26). L forms occur easily during cultivation (30). Strains from cases of Haverhill fever can be distinguished from rat bite fever strains on the basis of electrophoretic protein patterns (2). The mol% G+C of the DNA is 24 to 25.

Natural habitat and clinical significance

The nasopharynx of wild and laboratory rats seems to be the natural habitat of *S. moniliformis*. Though most human cases are acquired through rat bites, rare cases have occurred following bites, scratches, or direct contact with other rodents and rodent-ingesting animals. Haverhill fever (erythema arthriticum epidemicum) is acquired by ingesting milk, or rarely other food, contaminated with *S. moniliformis*. In a recent large outbreak of streptobacillary fever, water was the most likely vehicle of transmission (21).

Rat bite fever is characterized mainly by a relapsing fever with sudden onset, chills, headache, vomiting, and a skin rash (27). Diarrhea and weight loss are often found in infants and young children (25). The incubation period is usually less than 10 days. The bite wound usually heals rapidly without severe inflammation. Almost half of the patients develop a migratory polyarthritis, and 75% develop a maculopapular or petechial rash, mostly on the palms and soles. Severe complications include hepatic and splenic congestion, pneumonia, endocarditis, myocarditis, various abscesses, chorioamnionitis, hepatitis, meningitis, and nephritis.

Haverhill fever is also characterized by fever, rash, arthralgia, chills, and vomiting, but gastrointestinal and respiratory symptoms are more common than in rat bite fever (24). It occurs often as small-scale outbreaks, but larger epidemics have been reported (21).

Collection, transport, and storage of specimens

Blood and joint fluid (preferably in substantial quantity) are the major sources for demonstration of *S. moniliformis*. They should be citrated by being mixed with equal volumes of 2.5% sodium citrate (26) to prevent clotting before microscopic examination and culture. No formal studies on the optimal conditions of transport and storage have been published.

Culture and isolation

Media enriched with whole blood, serum, or ascitic fluid are required. A wide variety of broth and agar media have been used for the isolation of *S. moniliformis*, but none has been evaluated in a large clinical trial. Such media include various blood agar bases, chocolate agar, Schaedler agar, thioglycolate broth, meat infusion broth, and tryptose-based media, all enriched with 15% blood, 20% horse or calf serum, or 5% ascitic fluid. Sodium polyanethol sulfonate (SPS) may inhibit *S. moniliformis*, and only blood culture media without SPS are recommended (19). A papain digest of ox liver (Panmede) has been used to supplement brain heart infusion cysteine broth for cultivation of the agent (31). Use of sedimented blood cells to inoculate isolation media has been advocated (26). Some microbiologists recommend the use of a medium that facilitates the isolation of the more fastidious L-phase variants, which can be recovered on heart infusion enriched with horse serum and yeast extract (26).

Specimens should be inoculated into an appropriate broth and on an agar medium. Inoculated media are incubated at 35°C in a humidified 7 to 8% CO_2 atmosphere.

Identification

In broth media, characteristic "puff balls" appear after 2 to 6 days. Colonies on agar are round, grayish, smooth, and glistening, with a diameter of 1 to 2 mm, but L-phase colonies with the typical fried-egg appearance can also appear. It is recommend that the organisms be subcultured as soon as they are detected, since the marked decrease of pH in broth can be lethal to the bacteria.

S. moniliformis is largely an inactive species. The following reactions are negative: indole production, gelatin liquefaction, nitrate reduction, oxidase, catalase, urea hydrolysis, phenylalanine deamination, and casein and serum digestion. Acid without gas is produced from glucose, maltose, fructose, galactose, glycogen, mannose, and starch but not from carbohydrates such as rhamnose, raffinose, mannitol, inositol, sorbitol, and glycerol. Reported reactions with arabinose, xylose, lactose, and sucrose vary (15, 26). Fermentation reactions may be determined in cysteine trypic agar base (19). A typical fatty acid profile can be identified by using gas-liquid chromatography (28). The reader is referred to more extensive reviews for an in-depth discussion (15, 26, 30). Penicillin is the most active drug in vitro and is the drug of choice for treating the infection (5).

Serological investigations

Serum agglutinins against *S. moniliformis* can be demonstrated. A fourfold rise in titer or a titer of 1:80 is considered diagnostic. However, the test has not been standardized, and no large-scale evaluation has been reported.

SPIRILLUM MINUS

Description

According to the 1984 edition of *Bergey's Manual*, *S. minus* does not belong to the genus *Spirillum* and is described under "Species *incertae sedis*" (17). It has not been cultivated in vitro and consists of aerobic motile gram-negative spiral bacteria that are 3 to 5 μm in length and 0.2 to 0.5 μm wide. *S. minus* has two to six very angular windings and pointed ends with one flagellum at each pole (16, 17). The mol% G+C of the DNA is 36 to 38.

Natural habitat and clinical significance

The natural habitat appears to be similar to that of *S. moniliformis*. Spirillary rat bite fever is also known as Sodoku. It is usually acquired via the bite of a rat, mouse, or rodent-ingesting animal and has an incubation period of approximately 2 weeks. In contrast with streptobacillary rat bite fever, inflammation, induration, and occasionally ulceration appear at the inoculation site when the systemic manifestations appear and may be accompanied by lymphangitis and regional lymphadenitis. In addition to the clinical manifestations of *S. moniliformis* infection, approximately half of the patients with Sodoku present with a maculopapular rash that appears initially erythematous to purple and gradually coalesces (27). The case fatality rate is 5 to 10%.

Identification

S. minus can be demonstrated by dark-field microscopy in wet mounts of blood, in exudate of the initial lesion, and in lymph nodes and cutaneous eruptions. Blood specimens should also be stained with Giemsa or Wright stain.

Isolation of *S. minus* from mice and guinea pigs can be attempted by intraperitoneal injection of 1 to 2 ml of blood or of samples of exudate from the initial lesion and lymph nodes. Both peritoneal fluid and blood of the inoculated animals should be examined weekly by dark-field microscopy and stained smears for 4 weeks after inoculation.

CALYMMATOBACTERIUM GRANULOMATIS

Description

C. granulomatis consists of nonmotile gram-negative pleomorphic rods, 0.5 to 1.5 μm wide by 1 to 2 μm in length, with rounded ends. The organisms have a sharply defined capsule and exhibit single or bipolar chromatic condensation (3). Bacterial fimbriae may be seen on electron microscopy (18). In lesions, the bacteria appear in the cytoplasm of histiocytes, polymorphonuclear leukocytes, and plasma cells. Culture in yolk-containing media has been reported in recent years but not confirmed. Strains are apparently not available. The mol% G+C of the DNA is not known.

Natural habitat and clinical significance

C. granulomatis is the cause of donovanosis (granuloma inguinale), a poorly studied disease affecting only humans and occurring mainly in selected areas of the developing world (13). It is probably sexually acquired, though there is some controversy about this (8).

The incubation period is long, probably 8 to 80 days. The disease is characterized by beefy red granulomatous lesions in the anogenital areas. Extragenital locations may also occur. Secondary infection may modify the clinical picture.

Collection of specimens and laboratory diagnosis

The ulcerative lesions should be cleansed with sterile gauze, and tissue debris should be removed. Specimens of tissue are obtained by scraping or punch biopsy at the border of the lesion. A crush preparation from the lesion is obtained by spreading a piece of granulation tissue against a slide. The impression is then air dried and stained with Giemsa or Wright stain.

Donovanosis is characterized by the presence of Donovan bodies, which appear as clusters of blue- or black-staining organisms with a safety-pin appearance in the cytoplasm of mononuclear cells. Formalin-fixed and wax-embedded biopsy specimens are not recommended, since the pathognomonic Donovan bodies are infrequently seen.

Minced specimens can also be inoculated into the yolk sacs of 5-day-old embryonated eggs. The organisms may be detected in the yolk sac fluid after incubation for 72 h. Egg yolk-containing media can be inoculated, but recent experience has not been reported in the literature (3).

LITERATURE CITED

1. **Boustouller, Y. L., A. P. Johnson, and D. Taylor-Robinson.** 1987. Pili on *Gardnerella vaginalis* studied by electron-microscopy. J. Med. Microbiol. **23:**327–329.
2. **Costas, M., and R. J. Owen.** 1987. Numerical analysis of electrophoretic protein patterns of *Streptobacillus moniliformis* strains from human, murine and avian infections. J. Med. Microbiol. **23:**303.
3. **Dienst, R. B., and G. H. Brownell.** 1984. Genus *Calymmatobacterium* Aragao and Vianna 1913, 221[AL], p. 585–587. *In* N. R. Krieg and J. G. Holt (ed.), Bergey's manual of systematic bacteriology, vol. 1. The Williams & Wilkins Co., Baltimore.
4. **Dunkelberg, W. E., and I. McVeigh.** 1969. Growth requirements of *Haemophilus vaginalis.* Antonie van Leeuwenhoek J. Microbiol. Serol. **35:**129–145.
5. **Edwards, R., and R. G. Finch.** 1986. Characterisation and antibiotic susceptibilities of *Streptobacillus moniliformis.* J. Med. Microbiol. **21:**39–42.
6. **Eschenbach, D. A., S. Hillier, C. Critchlow, C. Stevens, T. De Rouen, and K. K. Holmes.** 1988. Diagnosis and clinical manifestations of bacterial vaginosis. Am. J. Obstet. Gynecol. **158:**819–828.
7. **Gibbs, R. S., M. H. Weiner, K. Walmer, and M. J. St. Clair.** 1987. Microbiologic and serologic studies of *Gardnerella vaginalis* in intra-amniotic infection. Obstet. Gynecol. **70:**187–190.
8. **Goldberg, J.** 1964. Studies on granuloma venereum. VII. Some epidemiological considerations of the disease. Br. J. Vener. Dis. **40:**140–147.
9. **Greenwood, J. R., and M. J. Pickett.** 1980. Transfer of *Haemophilus vaginalis* Gardner and Dukes to a new genus, *Gardnerella: G. vaginalis* (Gardner and Dukes) comb. nov. Int. J. Syst. Bacteriol. **30:**170–178.
10. **Greenwood, J. R., M. J. Pickett, W. J. Martin, and E. G. Mack.** 1977. *Haemophilus vaginalis (Corynebacterium vaginale)*: method for isolation and rapid biochemical identification. Health Lab. Sci. **14:**102–106.
11. **Hansen, W., B. Vray, K. Miller, F. Crokaert, and E. Yourassowsky.** 1987. Detection of *Gardnerella vaginalis* in vaginal specimens by direct immunofluorescence. J. Clin. Microbiol. **25:**1934–1937.
12. **Harper, J. J., and G. H. G. Davis.** 1982. Cell wall analysis of *Gardnerella vaginalis (Haemophilus vaginalis).* Int. J. Syst. Bacteriol. **32:**48–50.
13. **Hart, G.** 1975. Chancroid, donovanosis, lymphogranuloma venereum. U.S. Department of Health, Education and Welfare publication no. (CDC) 75-8302. Center for Disease Control, Atlanta.
14. **Ison, C. A., D. G. Harvey, A. Tanna, and C. S. Easmon.** 1987. Development and evaluation of scheme for serotyping *Gardnerella vaginalis.* Genitourin. Med. **63:**196–201.
15. **Josephson, S. L.** 1988. Rat-bite fever, p. 443–447. *In* A. Balows, W. J. Hausler, Jr., M. Ohashi, and A. Turano (ed.), Laboratory diagnosis of infectious disease, vol. 1. Springer-Verlag, New York.
16. **Kowal, J.** 1961. Spirillum fever. Report of a case and review of the literature. N. Engl. J. Med. **264:**123–128.
17. **Krieg, N. R.** 1984. Genus *Aquaspirillum* Hylemon, Wells, Krieg and Jannasch, 1973, 361[AL], p. 72–90. *In* N. R. Krieg and J. G. Holt (ed.), Bergey's manual of systematic bacteriology, vol. 1. The Williams & Wilkins Co., Baltimore.
18. **Kuberski, T., J. M. Papadimitriou, and P. Phillips.** 1980. Ultrastructure of *Calymmatobacterium granulomatis* in lesions of granuloma inguinale. J. Infect. Dis. **142:**744–749.
19. **Lambe, D. W., A. W. McPhedran, J. A. Mertz, and P. Stewart.** 1973. *Streptobacillus moniliformis* isolated from a case of Haverhill fever: biochemical characterization and inhibitory effect of sodium polyanethol sulfonate. Am. J. Clin. Pathol. **60:**854–860.
20. **Malone, B. H., M. Schreiber, N. J. Schneider, and L. V. Holdeman.** 1975. Obligately anaerobic strains of *Corynebacterium vaginale (Haemophilus vaginalis).* J. Clin. Microbiol. **2:**272–275.
21. **McEvoy, M. B., N. D. Noah, and R. Pilsworth.** 1987. Outbreak of fever caused by *Streptobacillus moniliformis.* Lancet **ii:**1361–1363.
22. **Piot, P., E. Van Dyck, M. Goodfellow, and S. Falkow.** 1980. A taxonomic study of *Gardnerella vaginalis (Haemophilus vaginalis)* Gardner and Dukes 1955. J. Gen. Microbiol. **119:**373–396.
23. **Piot, P., E. Van Dyck, P. A. Totten, and K. K. Holmes.** 1982. Identification of *Gardnerella (Haemophilus) vaginalis.* J. Clin. Microbiol. **15:**19–24.

24. **Place, E. H., and L. E. Sutton.** 1934. Erythema arthriticum epidemicum (Haverhill fever). Arch. Intern. Med. **54:**659–684.
25. **Raffin, B. J., and M. Freemark.** 1979. Streptobacillary rat-bite fever: a pediatric problem. Pediatrics **64:**214–217.
26. **Rogosa, M.** 1985. *Streptobacillus moniliformis* and *Spirillum minus*, p. 400–406. *In* E. H. Lennette, A. Balows, W. J. Hausler, Jr., and H. J. Shadomy (ed.), Manual of clinical microbiology, 4th ed. American Society for Microbiology, Washington, D.C.
27. **Roughgarden, J. W.** 1965. Antimicrobial therapy of rat bite fever, a review. Arch. Intern. Med. **116:**39–54.
28. **Rowbotham, T. J.** 1983. Rapid identification of *Streptobacillus moniliformis.* Lancet **ii:**567.
29. **Sadhu, K., P. A. Domingue, A. W. Chow, J. Nelligan, N. Cheng, and J. W. Costerton.** 1989. *Gardnerella vaginalis* has a gram-positive cell-wall ultrastructure and lacks classical cell-wall lipopolysaccharide. J. Med. Microbiol. **29:** 229–235.
30. **Savage, N.** 1984. Genus *Streptobacillus* Levaditi, Nicolau and Poincloux 1925, 1188[AL], p. 598–600. *In* N. R. Krieg and J. G. Holt (ed.), Bergey's manual of systematic bacteriology, vol. 1. The Williams & Wilkins Co., Baltimore.
31. **Shanson, D. C., J. Pratt, and P. Greene.** 1985. Comparison of media with and without "Panmede" for the isolation of *Streptobacillus moniliformis* from blood cultures and observations on the inhibitory effect of sodium polyanethol sulphonate. J. Med. Microbiol. **21:**39–42.
32. **Spiegel, C. A., R. Amsel, and K. K. Holmes.** 1983. Diagnosis of bacterial vaginosis by direct Gram stain of vaginal fluid. J. Clin. Microbiol. **18:**170–177.
33. **Taylor, E., and I. Phillips.** 1983. The identification of *Gardnerella vaginalis.* J. Med. Microbiol. **16:**83–92.
34. **Totten, P. A., R. Amsel, J. Hale, P. Piot, and K. K. Holmes.** 1982. Selective differential human blood bilayer media for isolation of *Gardnerella (Haemophilus) vaginalis.* J. Clin. Microbiol. **15:**141–147.
35. **Watts, D. H., D. A. Eschenbach, and G. E. Kenny.** 1989. Early postpartum endometritis: the role of bacteria, genital mycoplasmas, and *Chlamydia trachomatis.* Obstet. Gynecol. **73:**52–60.

Chapter 49

General Processing of Specimens for Anaerobic Bacteria

PATRICK R. MURRAY AND DIANE M. CITRON

Anaerobic bacteria are the most common organisms colonizing the human body and are a frequent cause of serious infections (22–25, 37, 85). Unless special techniques are used for the collection and transportation of specimens and for the initial laboratory processing, the laboratory will not be able to isolate these bacteria. This problem is particularly significant because most anaerobic infections involve a polymicrobic mixture of both aerobic and anaerobic bacteria. If the specimen is improperly handled or not processed for anaerobes, then the role of these organisms in the infection will not be demonstrated.

At present, clinical laboratories are confronted with the need to provide rapid, clinically relevant information for patient management in a cost-effective fashion. Because some anaerobic bacteria grow slowly and specific identification of isolates is frequently delayed until pure cultures are obtained, the comprehensive workup of specimens for anaerobic bacteria can be time consuming and expensive. Despite the desire to use the many sophisticated tools that are available for isolation and identification of organisms, the clinical microbiologist must provide information that is needed for patient management within a time frame that is medically useful. Thus, the processing of clinical specimens for anaerobic bacteria requires a balance between comprehensive bacteriology in some circumstances and rapid, presumptive reporting in other situations. The decisions influencing these technical choices should be determined by the available financial resources and discussions between the microbiologist and the medical staff.

This chapter presents procedures for the collection, transport, and initial processing of anaerobic specimens as well as for the preliminary characterization of isolates. Descriptions of medically important species of anaerobes and their identification characteristics are discussed in chapters 50, 51, 52, and 56. Antibiotic susceptibility testing with anaerobes is discussed in chapter 113.

GENERAL CHARACTERISTICS

Definition of an anaerobe

Bacteria are categorized as aerobes or anaerobes on the basis of their ability to satisfy their energy requirements for growth in the presence or absence of oxygen. This distinction is, however, an oversimplification. A spectrum of bacteria exists; some organisms require oxygen as a terminal electron acceptor (obligate aerobes), some grow both oxidatively, using oxygen as a terminal electron acceptor, and anaerobically, obtaining energy by fermentative pathways with organic compounds (facultative anaerobes), and some do not use oxygen and are inhibited by it (obligate anaerobes). The group of obligate anaerobes has been further subdivided into strict obligate anaerobes that do not form colonies on agar surfaces exposed to 0.5% or more oxygen and moderate obligate anaerobes that are capable of growth at oxygen levels ranging from 2 to 8% oxygen (49). Whereas strict obligate anaerobes are typically members of the normal flora, most infections are produced by moderate obligate anaerobes (88).

The reasons why anaerobic bacteria are inhibited or killed by oxygen are species specific and incompletely understood. Microorganisms that use oxygen as a terminal electron acceptor generate toxic oxygen reduction products, including hydrogen peroxide, hydroxyl radicals, singlet oxygen, and superoxide anions. These reactive metabolic by-products can cause breaks in DNA and destroy lipid components of cells, as well as inactivate certain enzyme systems crucial to the metabolic activities of the organisms. Many aerobes and facultative anaerobes are protected from these reactive by-products by producing catalase, peroxidase, and superoxide dismutase. It was originally thought that oxygen toxicity in anaerobes depended on the absence of these protective enzymes. However, it is now recognized that most *Bacteroides* species and some other species produce inducible superoxide dismutases after exposure to oxygen (31, 72). The level of superoxide dismutase is generally higher in gram-negative then in gram-positive organisms and correlates with the degree of oxygen tolerance in moderate obligate anaerobes (88). Catalase production has been documented for some species of the genera *Bacteroides*, *Peptostreptococcus*, and *Propionibacterium* but is variable within species and does not correlate with oxygen tolerance (74). Peroxidase activity has not been demonstrated in anaerobes. Thus, enzymes such as superoxide dismutase certainly play an important role in oxygen tolerance and virulence in some anaerobes. However, the reasons why other anaerobes (e.g., *Clostridium perfringens*) are able to survive oxygen exposure for as long as 72 h or more despite the absence of protective enzymes is unknown (73).

Anaerobes as normal flora

Anaerobic bacteria are the predominant bacterial species in and on the human body, outnumbering aerobic organisms by as much as 1,000:1 in the colon and gingival crevices of the mouth (Table 1). Knowledge of the specific anaerobes that colonize the different body sites is important because most anaerobic infections are endogenous; that is, anaerobes spread from their

TABLE 1. Concentrations of anaerobes in different body sites of humans[a]

Site	Total bacteria (per ml or g)	Ratio of anaerobes to aerobes
Mouth		
Nasal washings	10^3–10^4	3-5:1
Saliva	10^8–10^9	1:1
Tooth surface	10^{10}–10^{11}	1:1
Gingival crevice	10^{11}–10^{12}	1,000:1
Gastrointestinal tract		
Stomach	10^2–10^5	1:1
Proximal small bowel	10^2–10^4	1:1
Ileum	10^4–10^7	1:1
Colon	10^{11}–10^{12}	1,000:1
Female genital tract		
Vagina	10^8–10^9	3-5:1
Endocervix	10^8–10^9	3-5:1

[a] From reference 6 with permission.

normal sites of colonization into adjacent, normally sterile tissues where disease is present. Thus, the identity of anaerobes associated with specific infections can frequently be predicted by the involved body site. The *Bacteroides fragilis* group colonizes the large intestine and is most commonly associated with intra-abdominal infections. The *Bacteroides melaninogenicus* group and *Fusobacterium* species are most commonly found in the upper respiratory tract, and these organisms are associated with anaerobic pleuropulmonary infections. (Weakly saccharolytic *Bacteroides* spp. have now been reclassified in the genus *Prevetella* [see chapter 52].) *Actinomyces* species colonize the upper respiratory tract and gastrointestinal tract and are responsible for disease (actinomycosis) of the mouth, chest, and abdominal wall and for infections associated with intrauterine devices. The frequency of the various anaerobes that are found at different human body sites is summarized in Table 2.

Anaerobes as a cause of disease

Typically, anaerobic infections are characterized by polymicrobic mixtures of aerobic and anaerobic organisms that constitute the endogenous microbial flora in humans. Virtually all organ systems may be involved in anaerobic infections (Table 3), although infections of the urinary tract are uncommon unless a preexisting anatomic abnormality exists or invasive manipulation of the urinary tract has occurred (47). Furthermore, anaerobic bacteremias have decreased in frequency in recent years, possibly because of the selective pressures of empiric, broad-spectrum antibiotics, many of which have excellent activity against anaerobes (17, 94). In contrast, anaerobes are involved in most nonsurgical

TABLE 3. Relative incidence of anaerobic bacteria in various infections[a]

Type of infection	Incidence (%)
Bacteremia	5–20
Central nervous system	
Brain abscess	89
Subdural empyema	10
Meningitis	Low[b]
Head and neck	
Ocular	38
Chronic sinusitis	50
Chronic otitis media	30–60
Periodontal abscess	100
Other oral infection	94–100
Pleuropulmonary	
Aspiration pneumonia	85–90
Lung abscess	93
Necrotizing pneumonia	85
Empyema	76
Intra-abdominal	
Peritonitis and abscess	90–95
Liver abscess	>50
Female genital tract	
Salpingitis, pelvic peritonitis	>55
Tubo-ovarian abscess	92
Vulvovaginal abscess	74
Septic abortion	73
Soft tissue	
Gas gangrene (myonecrosis)	100
Crepitant cellulitis	High[b]
Necrotizing faciitis	High[b]
Urinary tract	<1

[a] Adapted from references 22 to 25 and 86.
[b] Percentage data not available.

TABLE 2. Incidence of anaerobes as normal flora of humans[a]

Genus	Incidence[b]					
	Skin	Upper respiratory tract[c]	Intestine	External genitalia	Urethra	Vagina
Gram-negative bacteria						
Bacteroides	0	2	2	1	1	1
Fusobacterium	0	2	1	1	1	±
Veillonella	0	2	1	0	U	1
Gram-positive bacteria						
Peptostreptococcus	1	2	2	1	±	1
Clostridium	±	±	2	±	±	±
Actinomyces	0	1	1	0	0	±
Bifidobacterium	0	1	2	0	0	±
Eubacterium	0	1	2	U	U	1
Lactobacillus	0	1	1	0	±	2
Propionibacterium	2	1	±	U	0	1

[a] Adapted with modification from reference 86.
[b] U, Unknown; 0, not found or rare; ±, irregular; 1, usually present; 2, usually present in large numbers.
[c] Includes nasal passages, nasopharynx, oropharynx, and tonsils.

brain abscesses, chronic pleuropulmonary infections, intra-abdominal infections, and infections of the female genital tract (22–25). Increased numbers of vaginal anaerobes in association with other flora have been shown to increase risk for preterm labor and chorioamnionitis (30, 38, 57).

Exogenous, monomicrobic, anaerobic infections are relatively uncommon, with most exogenous infections associated with sporeforming anaerobes (i.e., clostridia). Examples of these infections include food-borne, wound, or infant botulism mediated by *Clostridium botulinum*, gastroenteritis and enteritis necroticans due to *Clostridium perfringens*, tetanus caused by *Clostridium tetani*, and myonecrosis (gas gangrene) caused by a number of gas-producing clostridia.

Despite the diversity of infections produced by anaerobes, most infections are due to a relatively limited number of bacteria (Table 4; 13, 28). One-third of the anaerobes isolated in clinical laboratories are members of the *B. fragilis* group. Other commonly isolated organisms include peptostreptococci and fusobacteria. Some anaerobes are isolated infrequently but are associated with or responsible for specific diseases: *Clostridium septicum* (associated with colorectal cancer), *Fusobacterium necrophorum* (Vincent's angina), *Propionibacterium acnes* or *Peptostreptococcus magnus* (infections of prosthetic devices), *Mobiluncus* spp. (bacterial vaginosis), and *Bilophila wadsworthia*, a new genus (appendicitis) (5).

Virulence factors are responsible for the enhanced pathogenicity of specific anaerobes. Many of the anaerobes most commonly responsible for disease (e.g., *B. fragilis* and *C. perfringens*) are able to tolerate prolonged exposure to oxygen. Furthermore, the enhanced virulence of *B. fragilis* and some other *Bacteroides* species is associated with the presence of a polysaccharide capsule that is antiphagocytic and promotes abscess formation (11, 69). Production of neurotoxins and cytolytic toxins is very important in the infections caused by many clostridia (e.g., *C. tetani, C. botulinum, C. perfringens, C. difficile*), and the production and release of enzymes such as proteases, lipase, and lecithinase promote the destruction of tissue and spread of anaerobes. This tissue destruction also provides nutrition and an anaerobic environment for the growth of bacteria.

TABLE 4. Incidence of anaerobes in clinical specimens[a]

Organism	No.	% of total
Bacteroides fragilis group	141	34.8
B. fragilis	77	19.0
B. thetaiotaomicron	12	3.0
B. vulgatus	10	2.4
B. distasonis	10	2.4
B. ovatus	6	1.5
B. uniformis	3	0.7
Unidentified	23	5.7
Bacteroides spp.		
Pigmented	26	6.4
Other	45	11.1
Fusobacterium spp.	32	7.9
Peptostreptococcus spp.	117	28.9
Clostridium spp.	9	2.2
Nonsporeforming gram-positive bacilli	20	4.9
Gram-negative cocci	15	3.7

[a] Excluding *Propionibacterium* species. Adapted from reference 28.

Many clinical signs can suggest infection with anaerobes: disease commonly associated with anaerobic infections (periodontal disease, aspiration pneumonia, and intra-abdominal infection), clinical conditions associated with tissue destruction and poor vascular perfusion (trauma and malignancy), infection proximal to mucosal surfaces, human or animal bite, gas in tissue, abscess formation, a foul-smelling discharge, and presence of sulfur granules in discharge from a sinus tract. However, none of the clinical clues are specific for anaerobic infections, and the definitive role of anaerobes in infection must be demonstrated by obtaining the appropriate specimens for specific microbiologic testing.

SPECIMEN COLLECTION AND TRANSPORT

Collection

Because anaerobes may be involved in infections at any body site, all specimens collected in a manner to avoid contamination with the normal endogenous flora should be processed for both aerobic and anaerobic bacteria. Some of the specimens that should not be cultured anaerobically because contamination is unavoidable are as follows:

1. Throat or nasopharyngeal swabs
2. Gingival swabs
3. Expectorated sputum
4. Sputum obtained by nasotracheal or orotracheal suction
5. Bronchoscopy specimens not collected by a protected, double-lumen catheter
6. Gastric and small bowel contents (except in "blind loop" and similar syndromes)
7. Large bowel contents, ileostomy, colostomy, feces (except in suspected disease caused by *C. difficile* or *C. botulinum*)
8. Voided and catheterized urines
9. Vaginal and cervical swabs
10. Surface material from decubitus ulcers, wounds, eschars, and sinus tracts
11. Material adjacent to skin or mucous membranes that has not been adequately decontaminated

When one of these specimens is received for anaerobic culture, the physician or nurse responsible for the patient should be contacted by laboratory personnel to determine whether the appropriate test was requested (e.g., request for anaerobe culture of feces instead of *C. difficile* culture). If the requested test is determined to be inappropriate, the laboratory should not process the specimen because (i) these specimens predictably yield numerous isolates of unknown clinical significance, (ii) the laboratory results may be misleading to the clinician, and (iii) such added work is an unnecessary, costly burden on the resources of the patient and laboratory. The microbiologist must be prepared to suggest appropriate ways to collect the proper specimen. These techniques are summarized in Table 5.

Whereas collection of uncontaminated specimens for anaerobic culture is normally not complicated for specimens from blood, the central nervous system, or abdominal area, the collection of appropriate specimens from other body sites is frequently problematic. Specimens from the lower respiratory tract or paranasal si-

TABLE 5. Recommended procedures for collection of specimens for anaerobic culture[a]

Site	Specimen and method of collection
Central nervous system	Cerebrospinal fluid (especially when turbid)
	Abscess material
	Tissue biopsy
Dental area, ear, nose, throat, and sinuses	Carefully aspirated or biopsy material from abscesses after surface decontamination with povidone-iodine
	Needle aspirates and surgical specimens from sinuses in chronic sinusitis
Pulmonary area	Transtracheal aspiration
	Percutaneous lung puncture
	Thoracotomy specimen
	Bronchoscopic specimen obtained with protective, double-lumen catheter[b]
Abdominal area	Paracentesis fluid
	Needle-and-syringe aspiration of deep abscess under ultrasound or at surgery
	Surgical specimen if not contaminated with intestinal flora
	Bile
Female genital tract	Laparoscopy specimens
	Surgical specimens
	Endometrial cavity specimen obtained with endometrial suction curette[c] after cervical os is decontaminated
Urinary tract	Suprapubic aspirate of urine
Bone and joint	Aspirate of joint (in suppurative arthritis)
	Deep aspirate of drainage material after surgery (e.g., in osteomyelitis)
Soft tissue	Open wounds—deep aspirate of margin or biopsy of the depths of wound only after careful surface decontamination with povidone-iodine
	Sinus tracts—aspiration by syringe and small plastic catheter after careful decontamination of skin orifice
	Deep abscess, anaerobic cellulitis, infected vascular gangrene, clostridial myonecrosis—needle aspirate after surface decontamination
	Surgical specimens, including curettings and biopsy material
	Decubiti and other surface ulcers—thoroughly cleanse area with povidone-iodine by surgical scrub technique; aspirate pus from deep pockets or obtain biopsy from deep tissue at margin

[a] Adapted from reference 20.
[b] Reviewed in reference 3.
[c] Reviewed in reference 55.

nuses are frequently contaminated with organisms colonizing the oropharynx and nasopharynx. Transtracheal aspiration is now rarely performed for the collection of specimens from the lower respiratory tract, and many physicians are reluctant to collect specimens by percutaneous lung aspiration or thoracotomy because of the morbidity associated with these procedures. Bronchoscopy specimens are frequently submitted for anaerobic culture, but these are inappropriate unless a protected, double-lumen catheter (14) is used to circumvent contamination with oral bacteria. The diagnosis of anaerobic infections in the urinary tract must be confirmed by obtaining urine by suprapubic aspiration, a procedure uncommonly performed with adult patients. Although catheterized urine specimens are frequently submitted for anaerobic cultures, these specimens are inappropriate because contamination with anaerobes that colonize the urethra is unavoidable. Soft tissue infections can be reliably diagnosed by microbiologic procedures if (i) the skin surface is properly cleaned and disinfected and (ii) the specimen is collected from the base of the wound, where active multiplication of organisms occurs. Collection of pus from the surface of a deep wound is not recommended because the colonizing organisms rarely reflect the true etiologic agents.

The microbiologic investigation of certain female genital tract infections poses special problems related to anaerobic bacteriology. Puerperal or postpartum endometritis occurs after 1 to 4% of childbirths and, in most instances, involves microorganisms of the normal cervicovaginal microflora (55, 71, 86). Anaerobes, including *B. fragilis*, *B. bivius*, *B. melaninogenicus* and peptostreptococci, can be very significant in these infections. *Clostridium* spp., including *C. perfringens*, may be isolated from the endometrial cavity, but their importance can be interpreted only with a full knowledge of the clinical setting. Most patients do not have myonecrosis of the uterus, but when this condition does occur, it is serious and life threatening. Martens et al. (55) found that by decontaminating the cervix with Betadine and dilating the cervix, samples of endometrium not contaminated with vaginal organisms could be obtained by the use of an endometrial suction curette (Pipelle; Unimar, Wilton, Conn.) or a swab. Both of these techniques were superior to the double-lumen catheter method for obtaining adequate specimens.

Amniotic fluid cultures may be obtained from women in labor or with ruptured amniotic membranes who develop fever, maternal or fetal tachycardia, uterine tenderness, discharge with a foul odor, and leukocytosis (27). Anaerobic cultures of placentas can be performed on swab specimens obtained by carefully peeling apart the amnion and chorion to reveal the uncontaminated extraplacental membrane (38). Amniotic fluid infection and chorioamnionitis have been shown to be associated with preterm labor and premature birth (30, 38). Anaerobic organisms associated with bacterial vaginosis, such as *Mobiluncus*, *Bacteroides*, and *Peptostreptococcus* species, are isolated significantly more frequently from patients with amnionitis than from normal controls.

Whenever possible, specimens for anaerobic culture should be collected by aspiration with a needle and syringe or tissue samples should be submitted. Although many physicians and nurses find collection of specimens with swabs to be more convenient, such specimens are less desirable. A specimen can be easily contaminated with organisms present on a skin or mucosal surface, anaerobes are exposed to ambient oxygen, the specimen is subjected to drying, a relatively small volume of specimen is collected, and swabs are less satisfactory than aspirates for the preparation of smears for direct microscopic examination.

Transport

Successful recovery of anaerobic bacteria requires rapid delivery of the specimen to the clinical laboratory in a transport system that maintains a moist, anaerobic atmosphere. The speed with which the specimen should be delivered to the laboratory depends in part on the quantity of specimen collected. A large volume of pus (2 ml or more) can remain relatively anaerobic for at least a few hours (7). Likewise, if a large tissue sample is collected, anaerobes deep within the tissue will be protected from oxygen toxicity. However, specially designed anaerobic transport systems should be used for small samples of tissues, aspirated fluids, or specimens collected on swabs. Although the transport of specimens in capped syringes has been recommended in the past (86), this practice should now be discouraged because the risk of a needle stick is significant.

A number of systems have been developed for transport of specimens for anaerobic culture. These systems include enclosed tubes or vials with an anaerobic atmosphere and isotonic agar base which maintains a moist environment (e.g., Port-A-Cul system [BBL Microbiology Systems, Cockeysville, Md.], Anaerobic Transport Medium [Anaerobe Systems, San Jose, Calif.], and Anaport and Anatube [Scott Laboratories, Inc., Fiskeville, R.I.]), glass or plastic tubes with catalytic systems for generating an anaerobic atmosphere after swabs are inserted (e.g., Vacutainer anaerobic specimen collector [Becton Dickinson and Co., Cockeysville, Md.], Anaerobic Culturette system [BBL Microbiology Systems, formerly Marion Scientific]), and tubes with an anaerobic atmosphere and reduced transport medium (e.g., PRAS [prereduced anaerobically sterilized] anaerobic transport system [Remel, Lenexa, Kans.] and Anaerobic Transport Medium [Anaerobe Systems]). Each of these systems can be used for transport of anaerobic specimens, although most can only accommodate specimens collected either on swabs or by aspiration. Some systems (e.g., Vacutainer anaerobic specimen collector and Anaerobic Culturette) cannot be used for tissue specimens because the tubes are too narrow to permit insertion or retrieval of the specimen. In addition, recovery of anaerobes in the Vacutainer anaerobic specimen collector was demonstrated to be inferior to that in the Port-A-Cul, particularly when transit times were extended (12). The PRAS anaerobic transport system, based on the systems described by Holdeman et al. (40) and Sutter and associates (86), can be used with swabs, aspirates, or tissues, will maintain the specimen in a moist, anaerobic atmosphere, and is inexpensive in comparison with the alternative systems. Specimens should be maintained at room temperature during transport because refrigeration can decrease the number of viable organisms (33).

DIRECT EXAMINATION OF SPECIMENS

Macroscopic examination

Visual inspection of clinical specimens may provide information about the nature and quality of the material collected. The presence of purulence or necrotic tissue, sulfur granules, or a foul odor should suggest the possibility of anaerobes.

Microscopic examination

Direct microscopic examination of clinical specimens shows the types of host cells present and the number and morphological features of microorganisms. Preliminary clues to an anaerobic infection can frequently be made on the basis of the Gram stain morphology of isolates in the specimen. For example, *Bacteroides* spp. are pale-staining, pleomorphic gram-negative bacilli; *Fusobacterium nucleatum* is a thin, fusiform gram-negative bacillus; *Veillonella* isolates are very small, gram-negative cocci; *Actinomyces* isolates are branching gram-positive bacilli; and *C. perfringens* is a large, rectangular, gram-positive bacillus without spores. Other clostridial species can have quite variable staining properties and appear very pleomorphic, and spores are not always present. This information may help guide the clinician in the selection of therapy until culture and susceptibility test results are available.

The Gram stain is also an important means of quality control. If morphological forms observed by microscopy are not recovered in culture, the procedures may have been defective for one or more of the following reasons: (i) the specimen was improperly transported to the laboratory, (ii) the isolation media were defective, (iii) the anaerobic incubation system was defective, (iv) anaerobic subculture was performed improperly, or (v) growth was inhibited by the presence of other bacteria or antibiotics.

It is important to report the microscopic findings promptly to the attending physician because many anaerobes require 48 h or more before growth can be seen, and additional time is needed to confirm the anaerobic growth requirements of the isolate and to obtain identification and susceptibility test results.

When Gram stains are prepared, methanol is preferable to heat fixation to better preserve the morphology of tissue cells and organisms. Slides should be flooded with absolute methanol for 1 to 2 min and then rinsed with tap water before Gram staining (52). Because many gram-negative anaerobes stain poorly, a 1% aqueous solution of basic fuchsin can be used as a counterstain to enhance detection.

Phase-microscopy and dark-field examination of wet mounts may be useful for the demonstration of spirochetes. A modified Kinyoun acid-fast stain can distinguish non-acid-fast *Actinomyces* species from some *Nocardia* species. Fluorescent-antibody stains have been developed in research and reference laboratories for the rapid identification of many anaerobic species, and commercial fluorescent-antibody reagents have been useful for the preliminary identification of members of the *B. fragilis* group and the *B. melaninogenicus* group (Direct-detect; Organon Teknika, Malvern, Pa.). Because these reagents are relatively expensive and false-positive and false-negative reactions have been reported, they cannot be used to replace culture (65, 95).

Other procedures

The direct analysis of short-chain fatty acids by gas-liquid chromatography can be used for the rapid presumptive identification of anaerobes detected in blood cultures (82, 100) and has also been used for the direct analysis of purulent material (29). Whereas the former application can be quite valuable, the latter lacks sensitivity and specificity and cannot be recommended. A properly performed Gram stain is quicker and more cost effective.

The use of serological tests for the detection of other anaerobes has been limited. One such test, however, is a commercially produced (BBL [formerly Marion Scientific]) latex antigen test for the rapid diagnosis of *C. difficile*-associated diarrhea. The reagent reacts with a cytoplasmic protein antigen present in *C. difficile* as well as some other bacterial species (i.e., *Clostridium sporogenes, Peptostreptococcus anaerobius,* and *Porphyromonas asaccharolyticus* [51, 58]). Use of this test as the sole criterion for the diagnosis of *C. difficile*-associated diarrhea remains controversial (8, 44) since the reagent does not react with either of the toxins. A dot immunobinding assay for the detection of *C. difficile* enterotoxin has been developed (Difco Laboratories, Detroit, Mich.) and evaluated in comparison with other laboratory methods for diagnosis of *C. difficile*-associated diarrhea (99).

INITIAL PROCESSING OF SPECIMENS

Selection of media for primary isolation

Because the majority of anaerobic infections involve a polymicrobic mixture of anaerobic and aerobic organisms, optimum recovery of all significant bacteria requires the use of both nonselective and selective media. The most commonly used media for the recovery of anaerobes from clinical specimens are listed in Table 6. The actual selection of media is determined by the specimen type, amount of specimen received, and financial resources of the laboratory. At a minimum, all specimens received for anaerobic culture should be plated onto a nonselective aerobic and nonselective supplemented anaerobic blood agar plate and on a selective medium for the recovery of organisms in the *B. fragilis* group (48). Freshly prepared media are preferred (36, 64); however, PRAS agar plates are commercially available (Anaerobe Systems). These media are prepared and packaged in an oxygen-free environment, are stored at room temperature, have a prolonged shelf life with minimal adverse effect on the recovery or growth of anaerobes, and have been demonstrated to be superior to other commercially produced media that are prereduced for 24 h before use (53). Storing agar media under anaerobic conditions removes dissolved oxygen but has no effect on oxygen radicals that have formed during aerobic storage. The addition of cysteine or palladium chloride to media stored in air is of questionable value, with palladium chloride demonstrated to be toxic for some organisms (40, 66, 70). Oxyrase (Oxyrase, Inc., Ashland, Ohio) is an oxygen-reducing agent that can be incorporated into anaerobic media (1, 16). However, the effect on growth of a wide selection of anaerobes has not been evaluated.

TABLE 6. Isolation media for the recovery of anaerobes from clinical specimens

Medium	Purpose
Anaerobic blood agar	Supports the growth of strict anaerobic and facultatively anaerobic bacteria.
Bacteroides bile esculin agar	Supports the selective growth of *B. fragilis* group organisms; occasionally other bacteria grow, including *Fusobacterium mortiferum, Klebsiella pneumoniae, Enterococcus* species, and yeasts.
Kanamycin-vancomycin laked blood agar	Supports the selective growth of *Bacteroides* species and enhances pigment production in the *B. melaninogenicus* group. Yeasts and kanamycin-resistant gram-negative bacilli may grow on agar.
Phenylethyl alcohol sheep blood agar	Supports the growth of most gram-positive and gram-negative anaerobes; inhibits facultative anaerobic gram-negative bacilli.
Colistin-nalidixic acid blood agar	Supports the selective growth of anaerobic and facultatively anaerobic gram-positive bacteria; most gram-negative bacteria are inhibited.
Thioglycolate medium (BBL-135C) supplemented with hemin and vitamin K_1	Enrichment broth used as a backup to plated media.
Chopped meat broth	Enrichment broth used as a backup to plated media.

The current National Committee for Clinical Laboratory Standards recommended standards for quality control testing of anaerobic blood agar plates require growth of *B. fragilis* and *C. perfringens* on anaerobic blood agar media after incubation for 2 to 3 days (68). The new standard, to be published in late 1990, will recommend testing of additional, more fastidious strains, including *F. nucleatum, P. anaerobius* and *Bacteroides levii.* Because prolonged storage of anaerobic media decreases their ability to support growth of the more fastidious strains, laboratories may want to test their primary isolation media with a *Fusobacterium* sp. or *P. anaerobius.*

Nonselective media. A number of blood agar bases have been developed for the growth of anaerobes, including brucella, brain heart infusion supplemented with yeast extract, Columbia, CDC, and Schaedler. Each supports the growth of important anaerobes and can be recommended, although anaerobic cocci appear to grow best on CDC agar (79) and anaerobic gram-negative bacilli appear to grow best on brucella agar (79) or Schaedler agar (66). Schaedler agar contains a high concentration of glucose, which supports the rapid growth of saccharolytic organisms but may compromise the viability of organisms exposed to the acids accumulated during bacterial metabolism. Another basal medium is Fastidious Anaerobe Agar (Lab M, Bury, England), which supports the growth of fusobacteria exceptionally well. All nonselective blood agar media should be supplemented with vitamin K_1 and hemin (84).

Selective media. To ensure the isolation of all medically important anaerobes from clinical specimens, selective media should be used. Most anaerobes but not aerobic and facultative anaerobic gram-negative bacilli will grow on phenylethyl alcohol blood agar. Colistin-nalidixic acid blood agar supports the growth of most anaerobes except those that are susceptible to colistin, which includes some strains of *Bacteroides* and *Fusobacterium* spp. Kanamycin-vancomycin laked blood (KVLB) agar inhibits most gram-positive bacteria and facultatively anaerobic gram-negative bacilli while permitting the growth of most *Bacteroides* species and some *Fusobacterium* strains. The laked or lysed blood facilitates rapid pigment production by the pigmented *Bacteroides* species. Vancomycin inhibits most strains of the *Porphyromonas* group, previously called *Bacteroides asaccharolyticus, B. gingivalis,* and *B. endodontalis* (78). Bacteroides bile esculin (BBE) agar contains bile and gentamicin, which inhibit most aerobic bacteria and non-*B. fragilis* group anaerobes (48). *B. fragilis* group organisms grow rapidly in the presence of bile and produce brown to black colonies from esculin hydrolysis. One exception is *Bacteroides vulgatus,* which usually does not hydrolyze esculin and appears as a clear colony. *Bilophila wadsworthia* grows as a small, clear colony with a black center after 3 to 5 days of incubation. *Fusobacterium varium* and *F. mortiferum* can both grow in the presence of bile, although most strains are inhibited by the gentamicin, and *F. mortiferum* can blacken the BBE agar as a result of esculin hydrolysis and H_2S production. Occasional strains of *Enterococcus* spp. can also grow on and blacken BBE agar, but these isolates can be readily identified by their Gram-staining properties.

The routine use of additional selective agar media for specific organisms is not recommended but may be valuable in certain circumstances: supplementation of blood agar media with rifampin for the isolation of *F. mortiferum, F. varium, Clostridium ramosum,* and some *Eubacterium* strains; fusobacterium egg yolk agar for the recovery of *Fusobacterium, Veillonella,* and *Leptotrichia* isolates; cycloserine-cefoxitin-fructose agar (CCFA) for the recovery of *C. difficile;* and mobiluncus agar for the recovery of *Mobiluncus* sp. (26, 63, 80, 86).

Broth media. Clinical specimens can also be inoculated into broth media, with enriched thioglycolate medium (BBL-135C) or chopped meat-glucose medium used most commonly. The major advantage of these media is that if the anaerobic incubation system fails, then the cultured specimen will not be lost. Other applications of broth media include use of enriched thioglycolate medium for the isolation of slow-growing anaerobes such as *Actinomyces* species or chopped meat-glucose medium for the isolation of *Clostridium* species by a heat shock (19) or ethanol spore selection procedure (46). Chopped meat-glucose medium is also an excellent holding medium for isolated anaerobes (19).

Both thioglycolate and chopped meat-glucose media should be supplemented with vitamin K_1 and hemin. Furthermore, non-PRAS broth media should be heated for 10 min in a boiling water bath to drive off oxygen, followed by cooling, before inoculation with clinical specimens. After inoculation, screw caps are tightened and broth media can be incubated aerobically. Alternatively, PRAS broth media should be incubated after gassing of the butyl rubber-stoppered tubes with N_2 or oxygen-free CO_2 as described by Holdeman et al. (40).

Inoculation procedures

Sterile pipettes should be used for the inoculation of primary isolation media. If a large volume of nonpurulent fluid (e.g., thoracentesis fluid) is received, the specimen should be concentrated by centrifugation, and the sediment should be inoculated onto media and used to prepare a Gram stain. Place 1 to 2 drops of purulent fluid or sediment onto each agar plate and, if a broth medium is used, inoculate the specimen near the bottom of the tube. Care should be used to avoid introducing air into the broth medium. Before discarding the pipette, prepare a smear for Gram stain examination.

If the specimen is received on a swab, extract the material in a small volume (0.5 to 1 ml) of thioglycolate broth or other liquid medium and then inoculate the specimen onto the culture media with a pipette. Tissue specimens should be homogenized in approximately 1 ml of thioglycolate or other broth, using a tissue grinder. This should be done as rapidly as possible to minimize exposure to oxygen if an anaerobic chamber is not available for processing the specimen.

Anaerobic holding jar

Anaerobic bacteria vary in tolerance to oxygen (49). Therefore, care must be taken to avoid prolonged oxygen exposure of freshly inoculated media. It is not always practical or economically feasible for a laboratory to incubate plates in an anaerobic atmosphere immediately after they have been inoculated. One alternative is to keep the specimens in the transport medium and set them up in batches, thus incubating several specimens in one anaerobe jar. The use of an anaerobic holding jar is another alternative to immediate incubation (56). One or more anaerobic jars can be used to hold uninoculated media, recently inoculated plates, and plates containing colonies to be subcultured. An alternative to anaerobic jars is a large rectangular Plexiglas holding box, which laboratories must create in-house (3). The anaerobic holding jars or box should be flushed with commercial-grade N_2, but not CO_2, to maintain the media at a neutral pH. When the system is started, a high gas flow should be maintained for 1 to 2 min to purge the air from the system. Then the gas flow should be reduced to a rate at which the anaerobic atmosphere is maintained and the gas is conserved. The gas flow rate can be measured by holding the rubber tubing (0.25-in. [ca. 0.64-cm] diameter), which ordinarily goes into the jar, just under the surface of the water in a small beaker. The gas flow rate should be 1 to 2 bubbles of gas per s.

If a holding jar or box is used for inoculated media or subcultured plates, the anaerobic atmosphere should be tested by inoculating a plate with an oxygen-sensitive organism, such as a *Fusobacterium* sp., and leaving the plate in the system during the holding period. If growth occurs, then the system is performing adequately.

ANAEROBIC INCUBATION SYSTEMS

The primary isolation of obligately anaerobic bacteria from clinical specimens requires the incubation of inoculated media in an anaerobic atmosphere. A variety of systems, including anaerobic jars, disposable bags, chambers, and the Hungate roll tube system have been developed and used successfully (Table 7). The selection of an individual system or combination of systems should be determined by the volume of anaerobic cultures processed in a laboratory, the type of specimens processed, and the financial resources of the laboratory. Any of the systems should be satisfactory for the recovery of anaerobes commonly associated with human disease (75).

TABLE 7. Comparison of culture methods for isolation of anaerobes from clinical specimens[a]

Factor	Anaerobic jar	Disposable anaerobic bags	Anaerobic chamber	Roll tube system
Initial cost	Moderate	Low	High	Moderate
Continuing cost	Moderate	High	Moderate	Moderate
Time	Low	Low	Moderate	Moderate
Space required	Moderate	Small	Moderate–large	Moderate
Recovery of significant anaerobes	Satisfactory and convenient	Satisfactory and convenient	Satisfactory, but technique is time consuming	Satisfactory, but technique is cumbersome
Suitability for tissue grinding, specimen homogenization with blender	Not suitable	Not suitable	Allows processing without exposure to oxygen	Not suitable
Principal advantages	Uncomplicated and convenient; conventional techniques employed	Plates can be inspected at any time without disturbing anaerobic conditions; uncomplicated and convenient; conventional techniques employed	Plates can be inspected at any time under anaerobic conditions; conventional isolation procedures are employed	Tubes can be inspected at any time without disturbing anaerobic conditions
Principal disadvantages	Possibility of prolonged exposure of plates to oxygen during inspection and subculture	Holds only two plates; possibility of prolonged exposure of plates to oxygen during subculture	Space requirement; high initial cost; time consuming	Technique requires more training time; cumbersome to isolate and purify strains; colony morphology frequently not distinctive

[a] Adapted from reference 86.

Anaerobic jar

Anaerobic jars are cylindrical containers made of plastic, glass, or metal. A metal or plastic lid (usually with an O-ring gasket) is clamped to a flange at the top of the jar to create an airtight seal. Several different manufacturers (e.g., BBL, Oxoid Ltd., Difco, and Scott Laboratories, Inc.) produce or distribute anaerobic jars, all of which are satisfactory for use in a clinical laboratory. Some jar lids have vents or valves through which air can be evacuated and an anaerobe gas mixture added. A new, rapid, automated device (Anoxomat; Mart Microbiology Automation, Lichtenvoore, Holland) for automatically setting up jars by the evacuation-replacement method, which also alerts one to leaking, has recently been introduced and evaluated (10). A vented lid is not required if a self-contained H_2-CO_2 generator is used. Gas-generating systems are convenient for laboratories that perform relatively few anaerobic cultures, but they are more expensive than evacuation-replacement gas systems. Trace amounts of oxygen present in the jars will mix with hydrogen and in the presence of a catalyst be reduced to form water.

Failure of a jar to maintain an anaerobic atmosphere is most commonly the result of a cracked O-ring gasket in the lid, cracks around the vents in the lids, or inactive catalyst. The GasPak system (BBL) uses a "cold" catalyst consisting of palladium-coated alumina pellets which is active at room temperature. The catalyst is inactivated by H_2S, by other volatile metabolic products or bacteria, and by excessive moisture. Fresh or rejuvenated catalysts should be used in each anaerobic jar. In most anaerobic jars, the palladium catalysts are stored in removable baskets which are rejuvenated after each use. Palladium catalyst are also included in some gas-generating envelopes (e.g., GasPak Plus disposable generator), thus eliminating the need for reactivation of catalysts. For the other systems, restoration of catalyst activity can be accomplished by heating the catalyst at 160°C in a drying oven for 2 h. If a drying oven is not available, a toaster oven set at 160°C (360°F) may be used.

A redox indicator, such as a methylene blue strip (BBL) or resazurin (Difco or Oxoid), should be included in each jar. The strip should be colorless at the end of the incubation period. If the indicator is colored, then the system has not functioned properly and the plates are invalid for assessing growth of anaerobes. If the specimen was inoculated into broth medium, then the broth should be subcultured onto all primary media and handled as was the original specimen. The defective jar should be carefully examined to determine the reason for its failure, and it should either be repaired or replaced.

At ambient temperature, the O_2 concentration in the GasPak 100 anaerobic system (BBL) was reported to be 0.2 to 0.6% within 60 min after activation of the gas generator (77). At the same time, the CO_2 concentration was 4.6 to 6.2%, and the E_h values of three different media were −30 to −229 mV. These results indicate a rapid lowering of the oxygen concentration and the establishment of reducing conditions in the media, even though the methylene blue redox indicator remained colored for as long as 6 h.

Disposable anaerobic bags

Disposable bags and pouches (BBL GasPak Pouch [Becton Dickinson, formerly Marion Scientific], Bio-Bag, Difco Anaerobic Pouch, and Anaerocult P [E.

Merck AG, Darmstadt, Federal Republic of Germany]) are available as anaerobic incubation systems. One or two agar plates can be placed in these self-contained systems, and they are sealed with either a reusable sealing bar or heat. In the BBL and Becton Dickinson bags, an anaerobic gas generator is activated in the presence of palladium catalyst to achieve anaerobiosis. In the other two systems, an iron powder is activated with water that reduces the molecular oxygen in the atmosphere by generating iron oxide. The establishment of an anaerobic atmosphere can be verified by examining the redox indicator. A recent study demonstrated the superiority of the Difco catalyst-free iron system to the Bio-Bag for recovering anaerobes from clinical specimens (21). Bacterial growth on the agar plates can be detected by examining the plates through the transparent plastic, although the growth may be obscured by condensation on the inner surface of the bags. These systems are convenient, do not require a large incubation space, and permit examination of inoculated plates at any time during incubation. However, they are not cost effective for primary incubation of large numbers of plates.

Anaerobic chambers

An economical approach for handling anaerobic cultures is the use of an anaerobic chamber or glove box. Flexible plastic glove boxes are available in several sizes from Coy Laboratory Products, Ann Arbor, Mich.; a rigid glove box is available from Forma Scientific Inc., Marietta, Ohio; and a rigid glove-free model is available from Anaerobe Systems. The atmosphere inside the chamber consists of 5% H_2, 5 to 10% CO_2, and the balance N_2. The system is kept anaerobic with a palladium catalyst, which is reactivated by heating at 160°C for 2 h several times per week. The atmosphere in the glove boxes is kept relatively dry with silica gel, which can cause desiccation of media and poor growth of anaerobes. The gloveless model has a condensate control system that removes excess condensable moisture while retaining a high humidity, which prevents dehydration of culture media. Specimens and media are passed into the chamber through an entry lock system that automatically exchanges air for the anaerobic gas mixture. The flexible glove box can be maintained at 37°C for incubation of very large numbers of plates, although it is not comfortable for the microbiologist to work with hands in vinyl gloves at this temperature. Alternatively, a separate incubator can be placed inside the chamber. The rigid glove box and the gloveless models have a separate built-in incubator. A microscope adapter can be mounted on the gloveless model, thus allowing the microbiologist the use of a dissecting scope without exposing the plates to oxygen.

Oxygen concentrations should be kept at ≤6 ppm, measured by using an oxygen analyzer (Forma) or resazurin or methylene blue indicators. Leaks or tears that occur can be localized by using a hydrogen leak detector (Anaerobe Systems, Coy, or Forma) and can be repaired by replacing the gloves, patching with electrical tape, or resealing seams with a silicon glue. Performance of the system being used should be routinely monitored by incubating a plate inoculated with one or more fastidious anaerobes, such as fusobacteria or *Porphyromonas* sp.

Roll tube system

The roll tube system using PRAS media was developed by Hungate (41) and then refined by Moore and associates of the Virginia Polytechnic Institute Anaerobe Laboratory (40, 62). In this system, all manipulations are performed under a stream of anaerobic gas. Thus, the specimen and isolated organisms are never exposed to oxygen. This system has been used primarily in research laboratories; it is optimum for the study of extremely oxygen-sensitive anaerobes but is generally not convenient for clinical laboratories or required for the isolation of the moderate obligate anaerobes associated with most human infections.

INCUBATION CONDITIONS

The incubation temperature ordinarily used for primary bacterial isolation is 35°C, although some bacteria, such as *C. perfringens*, will grow more rapidly at higher temperatures (e.g., 42 to 47°C). Inoculated nonselective media (e.g., enriched blood agar) should ordinarily be incubated in an anaerobic atmosphere for at least 48 h before exposure to oxygen, thus protecting cells in logarithmic growth from oxygen toxicity (83). This requirement does not pose a problem for the early detection of growth if incubation is in an anaerobic chamber, roll tube, or anaerobic bag. With each of these systems, the plates or tubes can be examined without removing them from the anaerobic environment. Anaerobic jars and bags should not be opened before 48 h unless the procedure is performed in an anaerobic chamber. Some selective media (e.g., BBE agar for *B. fragilis* group and egg yolk agar for clostridia) can be examined after 24 h of incubation because the selected anaerobes grow rapidly.

No primary plate for isolation of anaerobes should be exposed to air for longer than 15 to 30 min because slow-growing anaerobes may be killed by prolonged oxygen exposure and never detected. Some anaerobic isolates present on subculture plates tend to be more aerotolerant and can survive longer oxygen exposure, whereas others, such as *Fusobacterium* sp., generate hydrogen peroxide and rapidly die. If growth is not present on the primary agar media but the broth culture is turbid, then the broth should be Gram stained and subcultured onto isolation media and reincubated. Nonselective media with no growth observed after 2 days of incubation should be reincubated for a total of at least 5 days, with longer incubation required for fastidious organisms such as *Actinomyces* sp. When selective media (e.g., BBE, KVLB, phenylethyl alcohol, and colistin-nalidixic acid agars) are incubated beyond 72 h, the selective agents start to deteriorate and allow the growth of previously inhibited organisms; however, in some instances it may be desirable to incubate these plates for prolonged periods, such as for the isolation of *Bilophila* sp. on BBE agar or for pigment production of the *B. melaninogenicus* group of organisms on KVLB agar.

INITIAL EXAMINATION OF ANAEROBIC CULTURES

The extent to which anaerobic cultures are worked up depends in large part on the clinical utility of the culture data and the laboratory resources. Because most anaerobic infections are polymicrobic mixtures and involve bacterial species that may be difficult to isolate and identify rapidly, it is important that all laboratories promptly perform and report the Gram stain results and any preliminary culture information (e.g., presence of multiple bacterial species resembling anaerobes). This information alone is frequently adequate for guiding the physician's selection of empiric antibiotic therapy. Every laboratory should also be able to identify *C. perfringens* and members of the *B. fragilis* group, because these virulent organisms are commonly associated with serious infections. Finally, all laboratories should have the capability of isolating all organisms present in the specimen and maintaining them in a viable state. The decision as to whether this is done for all specimens or routinely for only specific ones should be influenced by the specimen type and clinical situation. At a minimum, all laboratories should routinely identify isolates from normally sterile fluids (e.g., blood, cerebrospinal, pleural, and peritoneal fluids) and tissues. Routine identification of all isolates from specimens in which contamination with normal flora can occur (e.g., some wounds and abscesses) is much more difficult to justify, and the need for this procedure should be determined on an individual basis. A group-level identification based on colony morphology, growth on selective media, and Gram stain reaction may be sufficient. The morphological characteristics of anaerobes can guide the identification of isolates present in plated specimens. The following are guidelines for the isolation and identification of anaerobes that might be present in a clinical specimen.

Colonial characteristics

After the appropriate incubation period, the anaerobic media should be examined for evidence of growth. Because many anaerobes grow slowly and colonies may macroscopically appear similar, a dissecting microscope should be used for this examination. Examine isolated colonies as well as areas of heavy growth to detect microorganisms present in small numbers. The characteristics of each colony type, e.g., hemolytic pattern on blood agar (*C. perfringens* typically has a double zone of beta-hemolysis), as well as the colony size, shape, and pigmentation should be recorded. Observe the agar surface for pitting colonies and spreading growth and examine the plate under long-wave UV light (365 nm) to detect fluorescent colonies. The pigmented *Bacteroides* and *Porphyromonas* species often show brick red fluorescence. Weak red fluorescence is seen with most *Veillonella* isolates, but this fades within 5 to 10 min after exposure to air (9). Since colonial morphology can vary on different formulations of anaerobe blood agar, the type of medium and culture age should be recorded.

Microscopic features

The Gram reaction, morphology of vegetative cells, and presence or absence of spores are all key features in the classification and identification of anaerobic bacteria. Gram-stained smears should be examined from both solid and liquid cultures that show good growth. The staining reaction is generally more accurate with young cultures, but spores may be more easily demonstrated with older cultures. Many obligate anaerobes classified as gram positive are gram variable, and certain species (e.g., *C. ramosum* and *C. clostridiiforme*) usually appear as gram negative even though they are classified with gram-positive organisms.

Record the shape and size of the cells, presence of spores, branching, pleomorphism, and the arrangement of cells (singly, pairs, tetrads, chains, clusters, etc.). Spores will appear unstained and will be more refractile than vegetative cells. It is best to examine chopped meat medium or another medium without carbohydrate when searching for spores. It may be necessary to inoculate a chopped meat agar slant (incubated for 5 days at 30°C) and to use a heat shock or alcohol spore selection technique to demonstrate spores (46). Spores of some clostridia (e.g., *C. perfringens*) can seldom be demonstrated in laboratory culture. If spores are seen, note their shape, size, and position in cells (subterminal or terminal) and whether they cause swelling of the cells.

PRESUMPTIVE GROUPING OF ANAEROBES

Each unique morphological type should be picked from the blood agar plate, Gram stained, and subcultured onto another anaerobic blood agar plate and a chocolate agar plate incubated in an air–5% CO_2 atmosphere. The Gram stain will guide the identification tests, and the subculture plates will differentiate between strict anaerobes and facultative anaerobes. A chocolate agar plate should be used for aerobic incubation because *Haemophilus* spp. can grow anaerobically on blood agar plates. Multiple subcultures can be performed onto the chocolate agar plate, but only one subculture should be made onto the anaerobic blood agar plate to ensure that adequate growth will be available for biochemical testing.

Antibiotic disk test (86, 87)

The use of special potency antibiotic disks on the anaerobic blood agar purity plate can aid in the preliminary classification of isolates (Table 8). The plate should be inoculated so that a heavy lawn of growth will be present in the first quadrant, and the other quadrants should be streaked for isolation. Special potency disks should then be placed in the first quadrant: colistin (10 μg), vancomycin (5 μg), and kanamycin (1,000 μg). After good growth is obtained on the plate, a zone size of 10 mm or less is interpreted as indicating resistance. Susceptibility results obtained with these disks cannot be used to predict clinical susceptibility to the antibiotic.

Gram-positive anaerobes are usually susceptible to vancomycin and kanamycin and resistant to colistin. This characteristic can be very helpful because some gram-positive organisms (e.g., *C. clostridiiforme*, *C. ramosum*, and *Peptostreptococcus asaccharolyticus*) consistently stain gram variable or gram negative. Exceptions are some lactobacilli and, rarely, some *Clostridium* strains that are vancomycin resistant. In addition, strains of *Porphyromonas* species (formerly the *B. asaccharolyticus* group) are usually susceptible to vancomycin, which can cause confusion unless a careful Gram stain of the isolated colony is prepared and the presence of pigment is noted. Kanamycin is useful for separating fusobacteria (susceptible) from bacteroides (resistant), although some bacteroides (e.g., *B. ureolyticus* and *B. gracilis*) are susceptible to kanamycin.

TABLE 8. Presumptive grouping of anaerobes with rapid diagnostic tests[a]

Anaerobe	Characteristic														
	Cell morphology	Spores	Double-zone beta-hemolysis	Kanamycin (1 mg)	Colistin (10 μg)	Vancomycin (5 μg)	Growth in 20% bile	Catalase	Alanine peptidase	Indole production	Nitrate reduction	Urease	Lipase	Lecithinase	Motility	Brick red fluorescence
Bacteroides fragilis group	B	–	–	R	R	R	+	V	+	V	–	–	–	–	–	–
Other *Bacteroides* spp.	B	–	–	R	V	R	–	–	+	V	$-^{+}$	–	–	–	–	–
Pigmented *Bacteroides* spp.	CB/B	–	–	R	V	V	–	–	+	V	–	–	V	–	–	+
Bacteroides ureolyticus-like group	B	–	–	S	S	R	–	–	–	–	+	V	–	–	V	
B. ureolyticus	B	–	–	S	S	R	–	–	–	–	+	+	–	–	–	
B. gracilis	B	–	–	S	S	R	–	–	–	–	+	–	–	–	–	
Wolinella	B	–	–	S	S	R	–	–	–	–	+	–	–	–	+	
Fusobacterium	B	–	–	S	S	R	V	–	–	V	–	–	V	–	–	
Veillonella	C	–	–	S	S	R	–	V	–	–	+	–	–	–	–	
Peptostreptococcus	C	–	–	V	R	S	–	V	V	V	$-^{+}$	–	–	–	–	
Clostridium	B	+		V	R	S	V	–	$-^{+}$	V	V	V	V	V	V	
C. perfringens	B	+	+	S	R	S	+	–	–	–	V	–	–	+	–	
C. bifermentans	B	+	–	S	R	S	V	–	–	+	–	–	–	+	+	
C. sordellii	B	+	–	S	R	S	V	–	–	+	–	$+^{-}$	–	+	+	
C. difficile	B	+	–	S	R	S	+	–	–	–	–	–	–	–	+	
Nonsporeforming bacilli	CB/B	–	–	V	R	S	V	–	V	V	V	V	V	–	V	
Propionibacterium acnes	B	–	–	S	R	S	–	+	$+^{-}$	$+^{-}$	+	–	–	–	–	
Eubacterium lentum	CB/B	–	–	S	R	S	–	–	V	–	+	–	–	–	–	

[a] Adapted from reference 86. B, Bacillus; CB, coccobacillus; C, coccus; R, resistant; S, susceptible; –, negative reaction; +, positive reaction for majority of strains (includes weak as well as strong acid production from carbohydrates with saccharolytic organisms); $+^{-}$, most strains positive (helpful if positive); $-^{+}$, most strains negative (some weakly positive); V, variable reaction.

However, their colonies can be readily differentiated because they are smaller and more transparent.

After an isolate is confirmed to be an anaerobe and the preliminary Gram stain classification is determined, additional biochemical tests can be useful for the presumptive identification of the organism (Table 8).

Catalase (35)

Most gram-negative anaerobes are catalase negative, with the exception of many members of the *B. fragilis* group and *Bilophila wadsworthia*. Some strains of gram-positive cocci are catalase positive, as are all strains of *Propionibacterium acnes*. Catalase production is markedly influenced by the selection of growth medium. Hemin supplementation of media enhances catalase production, while the presence of carbohydrates inhibits it (32, 98). To perform the test, colonies should be selected from a blood agar plate (avoid picking up blood, which will give a false-positive reaction) or blood-free medium, such as egg yolk agar, and suspended in 1 drop of 10 to 15% hydrogen peroxide. A positive reaction is indicated by the production of bubbles. The plate does not have to be exposed to air before testing.

Indole production (50)

Production of indole is a useful differential test separating *B. fragilis, B. distasonis*, and *B. vulgatus* (negative reaction) from other members of the *B. fragilis* group (*B. thetaiotaomicron, B. ovatus*, and *B. uniformis;* positive reaction). Growth from a pure culture on a tryptophan-containing medium is rubbed onto a filter paper saturated with 1% *p*-dimethylaminocinnamaldehyde reagent. Alternatively, a sterile blank disk is placed on the heavy-growth area of a pure culture plate for 5 min and then removed to an empty petri dish, after which a drop of reagent is added. Rapid production of a blue color (within 1 min) indicates a positive reaction. Colonies cannot be tested from cultures with mixed growth because indole is diffusible and false-positive reactions may be observed. Different formulations of anaerobic blood agar may contain different amounts of tryptophan, which may affect detection of indole production by some strains. A weakly positive strain should be used for quality control of the medium. Egg yolk agar with Lombard-Dowell base is supplemented with tryptophan and is an excellent medium for detection of indole production.

Nitrate reductase (96)

Most *Veillonella* strains and all strains of *Eubacterium lentum* and the *B. ureolyticus* group are nitrate positive. The test is performed by applying a nitrate disk, which contains potassium nitrate, to an area of the plate with heavy inoculum before incubation. After growth has occurred, nitrate reagents A (sulfanilic acid) and B (1,6-Cleve's acid) (see chapter 122) are added to the disk. A pink or red color indicates the presence of nitrite. Although most positive reactions occur within 1 min, some may take as long as 5 min to develop. If no color change occurs, zinc dust is sprinkled on the disk to determine whether nitrate was reduced beyond nitrite. If a red color develops, nitrate was not reduced; if the disk remains colorless, then nitrate was reduced beyond nitrite (a positive reaction). Nitrate disks are available from several sources, including Anaerobe Systems, Difco, and Remel.

Sodium polyanetholsulfonate (97)

The sodium polyanetholsulfonate test is useful for separating *P. anaerobius* (susceptible) from all other gram-positive cocci (resistant). Some strains of *Peptostreptococcus micros* are susceptible, but they can be distinguished by their cellular morphology. *P. micros* are tiny, gram-positive cocci, whereas *P. anaerobius* are fairly large coccobacilli. The test is performed by placing a sodium polyanetholsulfonate disk (1 mg) onto an inoculated plate. After incubation, a positive reaction is indicated by a >12-mm zone of inhibited growth around the disk. Disks are available from several sources, including Difco, Remel, and Anaerobe Systems.

Growth in bile (93)

The test for growth in bile is useful for preliminary classification of anaerobic gram-negative bacilli. Members of the *B. fragilis* group are resistant to bile, whereas other *Bacteroides* species are inhibited. *F. mortiferum* and *F. varium* (bile resistant) can also be separated from *F. nucleatum* and *F. necrophorum* (inhibited by bile) by this test. *Bilophila wadsworthia* is also bile resistant. A bile disk (15 mg of oxgall) is placed onto an inoculated plate and examined for a zone of inhibition after growth has occurred. A zone of inhibition denotes bile sensitivity. The test can also be performed by inoculating a suspension of organisms into a tube of thioglycolate or PRAS peptone-yeast-glucose broth containing 20% bile (2% commercial oxgall). A control tube without bile should also be inoculated. The tubes are then incubated, and growth is compared. A positive reaction is indicated by either comparable growth in both tubes or stimulated growth in bile. Bile disks are available from several sources, including Remel and Difco.

Alanine peptidase

The alanine peptidase test distinguishes between *Bacteroides* (positive) and *Fusobacterium* (negative) species. *B. ureolyticus* group is also negative but can be distinguished from fusobacteria with the nitrate test (*B. ureolyticus* is nitrate positive). An alanine peptidase disk is placed on a pure culture of gram-negative bacilli, and a drop of cinnamaldehyde reagent is added to the disk. Development of a deep pink to red color indicates a positive reaction, and a yellow color represents a negative reaction. These disks are available from Carr-Scarborough.

Brilliant green disks

The brilliant green test also distinguishes between *Bacteroides* (sensitive) and *Fusobacterium* (resistant) species. The disk is placed on an inoculated blood agar plate, incubated anaerobically for 24 to 48 h, and then read for growth inhibition around the disk. A zone size of ≤10 mm indicates resistance. Disks are available from A. S. Rosco, Taastrup, Denmark.

Urease (59)

B. ureolyticus, C. sordellii, Peptostreptococcus tetradius, Bilophila wadsworthia, and some *Actinomyces* species hydrolyze urea. A heavy suspension of bacteria is removed from an isolation plate and suspended in 0.5 ml of urea broth. The broth is incubated aerobically and observed for as long as 24 h. A positive reaction is the development of a red color, indicative of urea hydrolysis and ammonia production, with a corresponding decrease in pH. The test can also be performed by using urea disks (Difco). A heavy suspension of the organism is prepared in 0.4 ml of sterile water, a urea disk is added, and the test is incubated aerobically. Most positive reactions occur within a few minutes, although a negative test should be incubated for 24 h (59). This test can also be performed with Urease Diagnostic Tablets (Rosco) as follows. Prepare a heavy suspension of the organism in 0.25 ml of saline. Add one tablet and incubate the suspension. A red to purple color indicates a positive reaction. Most positive reactions occur within 4 h; negative tests should be incubated for 24 h.

Lecithinase and lipase

The lecithinase and lipase reactions are helpful for identifying *Clostridium* species and *F. necrophorum.* Most strains of *B. intermedius* also produce lipase. Reactivity is determined by streaking the isolate onto egg yolk agar. A positive lecithinase reaction appears as a milky white precipitate around and below the colonies. A positive lipase reaction appears as a mother-of-pearl sheen on the surface of the agar around the colonies.

Other rapid enzymatic tests

Chromogenic glycosidase tests are included in the rapid identification kits currently being used for identification of anaerobes. Individual tests are available as tablets from Rosco. The test is performed by preparing a heavy suspension of the organism in 0.25 ml of saline and adding one tablet of the substrate. The tube is incubated aerobically for 4 to 24 h. A yellow color denotes a positive reaction. The following substrates are available: β-*N*-acetylglucosaminidase, α-fucosidase, α-galactosidase, β-galactosidase, α-glucosidase, β-glucosidase, β-glucoronidase, α-mannosidase, and β-xylosidase.

DEFINITIVE IDENTIFICATION OF ANAEROBES

The definitive identification of all anaerobes that can be recovered in human infections is frequently time consuming, labor intensive, and relatively costly. No single system can be used exclusively; rather, the "gold standard" for identification consists of a combination of methods, including metabolic end product analysis by gas-liquid chromatography, the use of PRAS biochemicals, and use of a variety of rapid biochemical identification systems. Fortunately, most clinical isolates can be identified by the careful selection of a limited number of simple tests. The precise selection of tests for definitive identification is discussed in subsequent chapters. This discussion will focus on an overview of the available test procedures. For the most part, the more complicated procedures should be used for identification of unusual isolates or for studies of normal flora, in which a greater variety of organisms exists.

Gas-liquid chromatography (40, 62)

Analysis of the end products of bacterial metabolism by gas-liquid chromatography is performed on a broth culture of the organism. Caution should be used when choosing the basal medium because the peptone and carbohydrate content will affect the end products detected (75, 76). Peptone-yeast, peptone-yeast-glucose, and chopped meat with carbohydrates are the broths most commonly used. Typical chromatograms for many anaerobes are depicted in the Virginia Polytechnic Institute *Anaerobe Laboratory Manual* (40, 62).

The broth is acidified with 2 to 3 drops of 50% H_2SO_4 and centrifuged. The supernatant may be injected directly for detection of the volatile acids if a flame ionization detector is used. If a thermal conductivity detector is used, then the sample must first be extracted as follows. Pipette 1 ml of the supernatant into a glass tube. Add 0.2 ml of 50% H_2SO_4, 0.4 g of NaCl, and 1 ml of methyl-*t*-butyl ether. Stopper the tube and mix the contents well by inverting the tube about 20 times. Centrifuge the tube briefly or allow it to stand for about 30 min to separate the water and ether layers. Remove the top ether layer and transfer it to another tube. Add a pinch of 4-20-mesh $CaCl_2$ to remove all traces of water. The sample is now ready for injection. The quantity to be injected will usually be between 5 and 15 μl but will vary with the operating conditions and should be determined by experimenting with an extract of the standard (see below).

For determination of nonvolatile acids, methyl derivatives must be prepared as follows. Pipette 1 ml of the supernatant of the broth culture to be analyzed into a glass tube. Add 2 ml of methanol and 0.4 ml of 50% H_2SO_4. Stopper the tube and shake it vigorously. Heat the tube at 60°C for 30 min or allow it to stand at room temperature overnight. Add 1 ml of H_2O and 0.5 ml of chloroform, replace the stopper, and mix the contents well. If the sample was heated, cool it to room temperature before adding the chloroform. Allow the tube to stand or centrifuge it briefly to separate the chloroform and water layers. Draw the bottom chloroform layer into the syringe, wipe the needle, and inject the chloroform into the column. The amount of sample will vary with the operating conditions. One should use the standard, extracted in the identical manner, to determine the optimum amount.

The standards used in these procedures consist of a mixture of defined quantities of the same short-chain fatty acids as the end products of anaerobic metabolism. One can compare the chromatogram of the isolate with that of the standard, match the locations and relative sizes of the peaks, and define which end products and in what quantities the isolate produces. Premixed standards for the volatile and nonvolatile fatty acids are available from Supelco, Bellefonte Park, Pa.

Because the same fatty acids are sometimes present in uninoculated media, the media should be extracted in the same manner and any peaks detected should be subtracted from the chromatogram of the test organism. Semiquantitation of the fatty acids is usually sufficient for identification of clinical isolates.

Gas-liquid chromatography equipment is available from several sources, including Varian and Hewlett-Packard Co., both in Palo Alto, Calif. A small model equipped with a thermal conductivity detector is available from Dodeca (formerly Capco), Freemont, Calif. Columns are available from Supelco.

PRAS biochemical tests

PRAS media, for determining the biochemical characteristics of anaerobes, have usually been used for taxonomic classification of anaerobes and for reference identification. In this approach, tubes containing medium for carbohydrate fermentation, proteolytic activity, and other tests are inoculated with a special gassing device (40) or with a needle and syringe. After incubation and growth of the organism, saccharolytic activity is determined by measuring the pH of the medium. Other reactions are read according to instructions provided in the Virginia Polytechnic Institute *Anaerobe Laboratory Manual* (40). PRAS biochemicals are available from Carr-Scarborough and Scott Laboratories.

Presumpto plates

The Presumpto plate system, developed by Dowell and associates at the Centers for Disease Control (18, 19), consists of differential tests in quadrant plates. The Presumpto I plate contains media for determination of growth in 20% bile, lecithinase and lipase production, esculin hydrolysis, H_2S production, and indole production. Presumpto II and III plates contain tests for carbohydrate fermentation, starch, casein and gelatin hydrolysis, and DNase activity. Identification tables for use with the Presumpto system have been published elsewhere (18, 19).

Rapid identification systems

In the early 1970s, several micromethods were developed for testing biochemical reactions. The API 20A (Analytab Products, Plainview, N.Y.) is a strip consisting of 16 cupules containing carbohydrate substrates plus 4 cupules for detection of indole production, urease, gelatinase, and esculin hydrolysis. A catalase test is performed by adding 2 drops of H_2O_2 to the mannitol cupule. The test organism is suspended in the inoculum broth and added to the cupules. After a 24- to 48-h incubation, the reactions are manually read and scored. A seven-digit number is generated and matched in a code book for identification. Although some organisms can be identified with this method, it is not useful for most asaccharolytic strains and some fastidious strains that fail to grow in the system (34, 60). In addition, some saccharolytic organisms reduce the bromcresol purple indicator or produce color reactions that are difficult to interpret.

The Minitek system (BBL) consists of disks impregnated with carbohydrate substrates, nitrate, indole, esculin, and urea. These ingredients are dispensed into microdilution plates in a specific configuration, and a broth suspension of the organism is added. The indicator is phenol red. After 48 h of incubation, the results are read and scored. The number obtained is matched in a code book for species identification. The comments made about the API 20A system are applicable to this system (34, 42).

In the 1980s, several companies devised 2- to 4-h rapid systems that are based on the detection of preformed enzymes present in the bacteria in high concentrations (RapID-ANA [Innovative Diagnostic Systems, Inc., Atlanta, Ga.], AN-Ident and API-ZYM [Analytab], ATB 32A [API Systems, Montalieu Vercieu, France], ANI Card [Vitek Systems, Hazelwood, Mo.], ABL system [Austin Biological Systems, Austin, Tex.], and Anaerobe Panel [American MicroScan, Sacramento, Calif.]). These systems contain chromogenic substrates that test for both glycosidases and peptidases and other enzymes and thus are potentially capable of identifying a wider range of organisms. Because preformed enzymes are measured, incubation of these systems in an anaerobic atmosphere is unnecessary, although fresh viable cultures are essential. As more organisms are tested and the data bases are expanded, this approach will most likely replace the older conventional methods for measuring biochemical activity. These systems have been evaluated by a number of investigators (4, 15, 39, 43, 45, 67, 76, 89, 92), with their accuracy for species-level identification varying in each study from 65 to 90%. At the present time, these systems should be supplemented with other rapid methods to avoid misidentification. Accurate genus- and group-level identification is preferable to inaccurate species-level identification.

The procedures for using these systems are similar. The organisms are suspended into inoculating fluid and then transferred into individual cupules, microwells, or a reservoir (which is then used to transfer the inoculum into the test wells). After approximately 4 h of aerobic incubation (2 h with the ABL system), reagents are added and the reactions are interpreted. This information is converted into a numerical code whose numbers are matched in a code book for species identification. The Vitek and MicroScan systems provide computer-assisted identification.

The API-ZYM system has 19 substrates that include peptidases and glycosidases plus other biochemical reactions, but no data base for identification of clinical isolates has been developed. This system has been successfully used for the identification of a variety of anaerobic strains (39, 54).

Alternative systems

A novel method developed for identification of anaerobes is based on analysis of whole-cell long-chain fatty acid methyl ester profiles (Hewlett-Packard Co., Sunnyvale, Calif.). The data base has recently been compiled for anaerobes, and the system is available for use. The organisms are inoculated into 10 ml of peptone-yeast-glucose broth and incubated until good growth is achieved (usually overnight). Specific supplements are required for some organisms. The cells are harvested by centrifugation and saponified in a mixture of methanol and NaOH. The fatty acids are methylated in methanol acidified with 6 N HCl and then extracted into a mixture of hexane and methyl-*t*-butyl ether. After a wash with an NaOH solution, the sample is ready for injection into the chromatograph. The fatty acid methyl esters are identified and quantitated by comparing peak area and retention times with those of a reference standard. The resulting profile is compared with other profiles in the data base, and a computer printout lists the percent probability of a match with several organisms. This system has been used to identify anaerobes and as an adjunct to other methods to define new species (61). The data base and software are available from Microbial ID, Inc., Newark, Del.

USE OF REFERENCE LABORATORIES

Laboratories are encouraged to use the services available in reference laboratories for assistance or confirmation of an identification or for the performance of antimicrobial susceptibility tests when such testing is not performed in the primary laboratory. The primary laboratory should initially evaluate the services available in a reference laboratory to ensure that high-quality services can be provided in a timely fashion. The reference laboratory should be notified in advance that an isolate is to be sent so that unnecessary delays in processing the isolate are avoided. Isolates should be submitted in agar deeps (e.g., motility medium or Thiogel [BBL]), plain cooked meat medium, or a transport medium (e.g., Cary-Blair or an agar-based anaerobic system) that will prevent desiccation and exposure to oxygen. Inoculate the agar deep or cooked meat medium with a capillary pipette and incubate the medium until good growth has occurred before shipment. Inoculate the Cary-Blair or agar-based transport medium with a swab from fresh colonial growth, but do not incubate it before shipment. All tubes should be tightly sealed with a screw cap and should not be exposed to refrigerated temperatures.

LITERATURE CITED

1. **Adler, H. I., and W. D. Crow.** 1981. A novel approach to the growth of anaerobic microorganisms. Biotechnol. Bioeng. Symp. **11:**533–540.
2. **Allen, S. D., and J. A. Siders.** 1982. An approach to the diagnosis of anaerobic pleuropulmonary infections. Clin. Lab. Med. **2:**285–303.
3. **Allen, S. D., J. A. Siders, and L. M. Marler.** 1985. Isolation and examination of anaerobic bacteria, p. 421–422. *In* E. H. Lennette, A. Balows, W. J. Hausler, Jr., and H. J. Shadomy (ed.), Manual of clinical microbiology, 4th ed. American Society for Microbiology, Washington, D.C.
4. **Applebaum, P. C., C. S. Kaufman, and J. W. Depenbusch.** 1985. Accuracy and reproducibility of a four-hour method for anaerobe identification. J. Clin. Microbiol. **21:**894–898.
5. **Baron, E. J., P. Summanen, J. Downes, M. C. Roberts, and S. M. Finegold.** 1989. *Bilophila wadsworthia* gen. nov., sp. nov., a unique gram-negative anaerobic rod recovered from appendicitis specimens and human faeces. J. Gen. Microbiol. **135:**3405–3411.
6. **Bartlett, J. G.** 1990. Anaerobic bacteria: general concepts, p. 1828–1842. *In* G. L. Mandell, R. G. Douglas, and J. E. Bennett (ed.), Principles and practices of infectious diseases, 3rd ed. Churchill Livingstone, New York.
7. **Bartlett, J. G., N. Sullivan-Sigler, T. J. Louie, and S. L. Gorbach.** 1976. Anaerobes survive in clinical specimens despite delayed processing. J. Clin. Microbiol. **3:**133–136.
8. **Bennet, R. G., B. E. Laughton, L. M. Mundy, L. D. Bobo, C. A. Gaydos, W. B. Greenough, and J. G. Bartlett.** 1989. Evaluation of a latex agglutination test for *Clostridium difficile* in two nursing home outbreaks. J. Clin. Microbiol. **27:**889–893.
9. **Brazier, J. S. and T. V. Riley.** 1988. UV red fluorescence of *Veillonella* spp. J. Clin. Microbiol. **26:**383–384.
10. **Brazier, J. S., and S. A. Smith.** 1989. Evaluation of the Anoxomat: a new technique for anaerobic and microaerophilic clinical bacteriology. J. Clin. Pathol. **42:**640–644.
11. **Brook, I.** 1986. Encapsulated anaerobic bacteria in synergistic infections. Microbiol. Rev. **50:**452–457.
12. **Brook, I.** 1987. Comparison of two transport systems for recovery of aerobic and anaerobic bacteria from abscesses. J. Clin. Microbiol. **25:**2020–2022.
13. **Brook, I.** 1988. Recovery of anaerobic bacteria from clinical specimens in 12 years at two military hospitals. J. Clin. Microbiol. **26:**1181–1188.
14. **Broughton, W. A., J. B. Bass, and M. B. Kirkpatrick.** 1987. The technique of protected brush catheter bronchoscopy. J. Crit. Illness **2**(8):63–70.
15. **Burlage, R. S., and P. D. Ellner.** 1985. Comparison of the PRAS II, ANIdent and RapID-ANA systems for identification of anaerobic bacteria. J. Clin. Microbiol. **22:**32–35.
16. **Crow, W. D., R. Machanoff, and H. I. Adler.** 1985. Isolation of anaerobes using an oxygen reducing membrane fraction: experiments with acetone butanol producing organisms. J. Microbiol. Methods **4:**133–139.
17. **Dorsher, C. W., W. R. Wilson, and J. E. Rosenblatt.** 1989. Anaerobic bacteremia and cardiovascular infections, p. 289–310. *In* S. M. Finegold and W. L. George (ed.), Anaerobic infections in humans. Academic Press, Inc., San Diego, Calif.
18. **Dowell, V. R., and T. M. Hawkins.** 1977. Laboratory methods in anaerobic bacteriology. CDC laboratory manual. Department of Health Education and Welfare publication no. (CDC) 78-8272. Center for Disease Control, Atlanta.
19. **Dowell, V. R., G. L. Lombard, F. S. Thompson, and A. Y. Armfield.** 1977. Media for isolation, characterization and identification of obligately anaerobic bacteria. CDC laboratory manual. Center for Disease Control, Atlanta.
20. **Dowell, V. R., Jr., and S. D. Allen.** 1981. Anaerobic bacterial infections, p. 171–214. *In* A. Balows and W. J. Hausler, Jr. (ed.), Diagnostic procedures for bacterial, mycotic, and parasitic infections, 6th ed. American Public Health Association, Washington, D.C.
21. **Downes, J., J. I. Mangels, J. Holden, M. J. Ferraro, and E. J. Baron.** 1990. Evaluation of two single-plate incubation systems and the anaerobic chamber for the cultivation of anaerobic bacteria. J. Clin. Microbiol. **28:**246–248.
22. **Finegold, S. M.** 1977. Anaerobic bacteria in human disease. Academic Press, Inc., New York.
23. **Finegold, S. M., and W. L. George (ed.).** 1989. Anaerobic infections in humans. Academic Press, Inc., San Diego, Calif.
24. **Finegold, S. M., W. L. George, and M. E. Mulligan.** 1985. Anaerobic infections. Disease-a-month, vol. 31, no. 10 and 11. Year Book Medical Publishers, Inc., Chicago.
25. **Finegold, S. M., and H. M. Wexler.** 1988. Therapeutic implications of bacteriologic findings in mixed aerobic-anaerobic infections. Antimicrob. Agents Chemother. **32:**611–616.
26. **George, W. L., V. L. Sutter, D. Citron, and S. M. Finegold.** 1979. Selective and differential medium for isolation of *Clostridium difficile*. J. Clin. Microbiol. **9:**214–219.
27. **Gibbs, R. S., J. D. Blanco, R. J. St. Clair, and Y. S. Castaneda.** 1982. Quantitative bacteriology of amniotic fluid from women with clinical intra-amniotic infection at term. J. Infect. Dis. **145:**1–8.
28. **Goldstein, E. J. C., and D. M. Citron.** 1988. Annual incidence, epidemiology, and comparative in vitro susceptibilities to cefoxitin, cefotetan, cefmetazole, and ceftizoxime of recent community-acquired isolates of the *Bacteroides fragilis* group. J. Clin. Microbiol. **26:**2361–2366.
29. **Gorbach, S. L., J. W. Mayhew, J. G. Bartlett, H. Thadepalli, and A. Onderdonk.** 1976. Rapid diagnosis of anaerobic infections by direct gas-liquid chromatography of clinical specimens. J. Clin. Invest. **57:**478–484.
30. **Gravett, M. G., D. Hummel, D. A. Eschenbach, and K. K. Holmes.** 1986. Preterm labor associated with subclinical amniotic infection and with bacterial vaginosis. Obstet. Gynecol. **67:**229–237.
31. **Gregory, E. M., W. E. C. Moore, and L. V. Holdeman.** 1978. Superoxide dismutase in anaerobes: survey. Appl. Environ. Microbiol. **35:**988–991.
32. **Gregory, E. M., B. J. Veltri, D. L. Wagner, and T. D. Wilkins.** 1977. Carbohydrate repression of catalase synthesis in *Bacteroides fragilis*. J. Bacteriol. **129:**534–535.

33. **Hagen, J. C., W. S. Wood, and T. Hashimoto.** 1977. Effect of temperature on survival of *Bacteroides fragilis* subsp. *fragilis* and *Escherichia coli* in pus. J. Clin. Microbiol. **6**:567–570.
34. **Hansen, S. L., and B. J. Stewart.** 1976. Comparison of API and Minitek to Centers for Disease Control methods for the biochemical characterization of anaerobes. J. Clin. Microbiol. **4**:227–231.
35. **Hansen, S. L., and B. J. Stewart.** 1978. Slide catalase. A reliable test for differentiation and presumptive identification of certain clinically significant anaerobes. Am. J. Clin. Pathol. **69**:36–40.
36. **Hanson, C. W., and W. J. Martin.** 1976. Evaluation of enrichment, storage, and age of blood agar medium in relation to its ability to support growth of anaerobic bacteria. J. Clin. Microbiol. **4**:394–399.
37. **Heseltine, P. N. R., M. D. Appleman, and J. M. Leedom.** 1984. Epidemiology and susceptibility of resistant *Bacteroides fragilis* group organisms to new beta-lactam antibiotics. Rev. Infect. Dis. **6**:S254–S259.
38. **Hillier, S. L., J. Martius, M. Krohn, N. Kiviat, K. K. Holmes, and D. A. Eschenbach.** 1988. A case-control study of chorioamnionic infection and histologic chorioamnionitis in prematurity. N. Engl. J. Med. **319**:972–978.
39. **Hofstad, T.** 1980. Evaluation of the API-ZYM system for identification of *Bacteroides* and *Fusobacterium* species. Med. Microbiol. Immunol. **168**:173–177.
40. **Holdeman, L. V., E. P. Cato, and W. E. C. Moore (ed.).** 1977. Anaerobe laboratory manual, 4th ed. Virginia Polytechnic Institute and State University, Blacksburg.
41. **Hungate, R. E.** 1969. A roll tube method for cultivation of strict anaerobes. Methods Microbiol. **3b**:117–132.
42. **Hussain, Z., R. Lannigan, B. C. Schieven, L. Stoakes, T. Kelly, and D. Groves.** 1987. Comparison of RapID-ANA and Minitek with a conventional method for biochemical identification of anaerobes. Diagn. Microbiol. Infect. Dis. **6**:69–72.
43. **Karachewski, N. O., E. L. Busch, and C. L. Wells.** 1985. Comparison of PRAS II, RapID-ANA and API 20A systems for identification of anaerobic bacteria. J. Clin. Microbiol. **21**:122–126.
44. **Kelly, M. T., S. G. Champagne, S. H. Sherlock, M. A. Nobel, H. J. Freeman, and J. A. Smith.** 1987. Commercial latex agglutination test for detection of *Clostridium difficile*-associated diarrhea. J. Clin. Microbiol. **25**:1244–1247.
45. **Kitch, T. T., and P. C. Applebaum.** 1989. Accuracy and reproducibility of the 4-hour ATB 32A method for anaerobe identification. J. Clin. Microbiol. **27**:2509–2513.
46. **Koransky, J. R., S. D. Allen, and V. R. Dowell, Jr.** 1978. Use of ethanol for selective isolation of sporeforming microorganisms. Appl. Environ. Microbiol. **35**:762–765.
47. **Kunin, C. M.** 1987. Detection, prevention, and management of urinary tract infections, 4th ed., p. 160. Lea & Febiger, Philadelphia.
48. **Livingston, S. J., S. D. Kominos, and R. B. Lee.** 1978. New medium for selection and presumptive identification of the *Bacteroides fragilis* group. J. Clin. Microbiol. **7**:448–453.
49. **Loesche, W. J.** 1969. Oxygen sensitivity of various anaerobic bacteria. Appl. Microbiol. **18**:723–727.
50. **Lombard, G. L., and V. R. Dowell, Jr.** 1983. Comparison of three reagents for detecting indole production by anaerobic bacteria in microtest systems. J. Clin. Microbiol. **18**:609–613.
51. **Lyerly, D. M., D. W. Ball, J. Toth, and T. D. Wilkins.** 1988. Characterization of cross-reactive proteins detected by Culturette brand rapid latex test for *Clostridium difficile*. J. Clin. Microbiol. **26**:397–400.
52. **Mangels, J. I., M. E. Cox, and L. H. Lindberg.** 1984. Methanol fixation: an alternative to heat fixation of smears before staining. Diagn. Microbiol. Infect. Dis. **2**:129–137.
53. **Mangels, J. I., and B. P. Douglas.** 1989. Comparison of four commercial brucella agar media for growth of anaerobic organisms. J. Clin. Microbiol. **27**:2268–2271.
54. **Marler, L., S. Allen, and J. Siders.** 1984. Rapid enzymatic characterization of clinically encountered anaerobic bacteria with the API ZYM system. Eur. J. Clin. Microbiol. **3**:294–300.
55. **Martens, M. G., S. Faro, H. A. Hammill, G. D. Riddle, and D. Smith.** 1989. Transcervical uterine cultures with a new endometrial suction curette: a comparison of three sampling methods in postpartum endometritis. Obstet. Gynecol. **74**:273–276.
56. **Martin, W. J.** 1971. Practical method for isolation of anaerobic bacteria in the clinical laboratory. Appl. Microbiol. **22**:1168–1171.
57. **Martius, J., M. A. Krohn, S. L. Hillier, W. E. Stamm, K. K. Holmes, and D. A. Eschenbach.** 1988. Relationships of vaginal *Lactobacillus* species, cervical *Chlamydia trachomatis,* and bacterial vaginosis to preterm birth. Obstet. Gynecol. **71**:89–95.
58. **Miles, B. L., J. A. Siders, and S. D. Allen.** 1988. Evaluation of a commercial latex test for *Clostridium difficile* for reactivity with *C. difficile* and cross-reactions with other bacteria. J. Clin. Microbiol. **26**:2452–2455.
59. **Mills, C. K., B. Y. Grimes, and R. L. Gherna.** 1987. Three rapid methods compared with a conventional method for detection of urease production in anaerobic bacteria. J. Clin. Microbiol. **25**:2209–2210.
60. **Moore, H. B., V. L. Sutter, and S. M. Finegold.** 1975. Comparison of three procedures for biochemical testing of anaerobic bacteria. J. Clin. Microbiol. **1**:15–24.
61. **Moore, L. H., J. L. Johnson, and W. E. C. Moore.** 1987. *Selenomonas noxia* sp. nov., *Selenomonas flueggeii* sp. nov., *Selenomonas infelix* sp. nov., *Selenomonas dianae* sp. nov., and *Selenomonas artemidis* sp. nov. from the human gingival crevice. Int. J. Syst. Bacterial. **36**:271–280.
62. **Moore, L. V. H., E. P. Cato, and W. E. C. Moore (ed.).** 1987. Anaerobe laboratory manual update. Supplement to the VPI anaerobe laboratory manual, 4th ed., 1977. Virginia Polytechnic Institute and State University, Blacksburg.
63. **Morgenstein, A. A., D. M. Citron, and S. M. Finegold.** 1981. New medium selective for *Fusobacterium* species and differential for *Fusobacterium necrophorum.* J. Clin. Microbiol. **13**:666–669.
64. **Morris, J. G.** 1976. Oxygen and the obligate anaerobe. J. Appl. Bacteriol. **40**:229–244.
65. **Mouton, C., P. Hammond, J. Slots, and R. J. Genco.** 1980. Evaluation of Fluoretec-M for detection of oral strains of *Bacteroides asaccharolyticus* and *Bacteroides melaninogenicus.* J. Clin. Microbiol. **11**:682–686.
66. **Murray, P. R.** 1978. Growth of clinical isolates of anaerobic bacteria on agar media: effects of media composition, storage conditions, and reduction under anaerobic conditions. J. Clin. Microbiol. **8**:708–714.
67. **Murray, P. R., C. J. Weber, and A. C. Niles.** 1985. Comparative evaluation of three identification systems for anaerobes. J. Clin. Microbiol. **22**:52–55.
68. **National Committee for Clinical Laboratory Standards.** 1985. Proposed standard M22-P. Quality assurance for commercially prepared microbiological culture media, vol. 5, p. 543. National Committee for Clinical Laboratory Standards, Villanova, Pa.
69. **Onderdonk, A. B., D. L. Kasper, R. L. Cisneros, and J. G. Bartlett.** 1977. The capsular polysaccharide of *Bacteroides fragilis* as a virulence factor: comparison of pathogenic potential of encapsulated and unencapsulated strains. J. Infect. Dis. **136**:82–89.
70. **Owens, D. W., R. D. Rolfe, and D. J. Hentges.** 1976. Effectiveness of palladium chloride for the isolation of anaerobes. J. Clin. Microbiol. **3**:218–220.
71. **Penn, R. L.** 1983. Gynecological and obstetrical infec-

tions, p. 555–593. *In* R. E. Reese and R. G. Douglas, Jr. (ed.), A practical approach to infectious diseases. Little, Brown & Co., Boston.

72. **Privalle, C. T., and E. M. Gregory.** 1979. Superoxide dismutase and oxygen lethality in *Bacteroides fragilis.* J. Bacteriol. **138:**139–145.
73. **Rolfe, R. D., D. J. Hentges, J. T. Barrett, and B. J. Campbell.** 1977. Oxygen tolerance of human intestinal anaerobes. Am. J. Clin. Nutr. **30:**1762–1769.
74. **Rolfe, R. D., D. J. Hentges, B. J. Campbell, and J. T. Barrett.** 1978. Factors related to the oxygen tolerance of anaerobic bacteria. Appl. Environ. Microbiol. **36:**306–313.
75. **Rosenblatt, J. E., A. Fallow, and S. M. Finegold.** 1973. Comparison of methods for isolation of anaerobic bacteria from clinical specimens. Appl. Microbiol. **25:**77–85.
76. **Schreckenberger, P. C., D. M. Celig, and W. M. Janda.** 1988. Clinical evaluation of the Vitek ANI card for identification of anaerobic bacteria. J. Clin. Microbiol. **26:** 225–230.
77. **Seip, W. F., and G. L. Evans.** 1980. Atmospheric analysis and redox potentials of culture media in the GasPak system. J. Clin. Microbiol. **11:**226–233.
78. **Shah, H. N., and M. D. Collins.** 1988. Proposal for reclassification of *Bacteroides asaccharolyticus, Bacteroides gingivalis,* and *Bacteroides endodontalis* in a new genus, *Porphyromonas.* Int. J. Syst. Bacteriol. **38:**128–131.
79. **Sheppard, A., C. Cammarata, and D. H. Martin.** 1990. Comparison of different medium bases for the semiquantitative isolation of anaerobes from vaginal secretions. J. Clin. Microbiol. **28:**455–457.
80. **Smith, H. J., and H. B. Moore.** 1988. Isolation of *Mobiluncus* species from clinical specimens by using cold enrichment and selective media. J. Clin. Microbiol. **26:** 1134–1137.
81. **Sondag, J. E., M. Ali, and P. R. Murray.** 1979. Relative recovery of anaerobes on different isolation media. J. Clin. Microbiol. **10:**756–757.
82. **Sondag, J. E., M. Ali, and P. R. Murray.** 1980. Rapid presumptive identification of anaerobes in blood cultures by gas-liquid chromatography. J. Clin. Microbiol. **11:**274–277.
83. **Spaulding, E. H., V. Vargo, T. C. Michaelson, M. Korzeniowski, and R. M. Swenson.** 1974. Anaerobic bacteria: culture and identification, p. 87–103. *In* J. E. Prier and H. Friedman (ed.), Opportunistic infections. University Park Press, Baltimore.
84. **Sperry, J. F., M. D. Appleman, and T. D. Wilkins.** 1977. Requirement of heme for growth of *Bacteroides fragilis.* Appl. Environ. Microbiol. **34:**386–390.
85. **Styrt, B., and S. L. Gorbach.** 1989. Recent developments in the understanding of the pathogenesis and treatment of anaerobic infections. N. Engl. J. Med. **321:**240–245.
86. **Sutter, V. L., D. M. Citron, M. A. C. Edelstein, and S. M. Finegold.** 1985. Wadsworth anaerobic bacteriology manual, 4th ed. Star Publishing Co., Belmont, Calif.
87. **Sutter, V. L., and S. M. Finegold.** 1971. Antibiotic disk susceptibility tests for rapid presumptive identification of gram-negative anaerobic bacilli. Appl. Microbiol. **21:** 13–20.
88. **Tally, F. P., B. R. Goldin, N. V. Jacobus, and S. L. Gorbach.** 1977. Superoxide dismutase in anaerobic bacteria of clinical significance. Infect. Immun. **16:**20–25.
89. **Tanner, A. C. R., M. N. Strzempko, C. A. Belsky, and G. A. McKinley.** 1985. API ZYM and API An-Ident reactions of fastidious oral gram-negative species. J. Clin. Microbiol. **22:**333–335.
90. **Turton, L. J., D. B. Drucker, and L. A. Ganguli.** 1983. Effect of glucose concentration in the growth medium upon neutral and acidic fermentation end-products of *Clostridium bifermentans, Clostridium sporogenes* and *Peptostreptococcus anaerobius.* J. Med. Microbiol. **16:**61–67.
91. **Turton, L. J., D. B. Drucker, W. F. Hillier, and L. A. Ganguli.** 1983. Effect of eight growth media upon fermentation profiles of ten anaerobic bacteria. J. Appl. Bacteriol. **54:**295–304.
92. **VanWinkelhoff, A. J., M. Clement, and J. deGraff.** 1988. Rapid characterization of oral and non-oral pigmented Bacteroides species with the ATB Anaerobes ID system. J. Clin. Microbiol. **26:**1063–1065.
93. **Weinberg, L. G., L. L. Smith, and A. H. McTighe.** 1983. Rapid identification of the *Bacteroides fragilis* group by bile disk and catalase tests. Lab. Med. **14:**785–788.
94. **Weinstein, M. P., L. B. Reller, J. R. Murphy, and K. A. Lichtenstein.** 1983. The clinical significance of positive blood cultures: a comprehensive analysis of 500 episodes of bacteremia and fungemia in adults. Laboratory and epidemiologic observations. Rev. Infect. Dis. **5:**35–53.
95. **Weissfeld, A. S., and A. C. Sonnenwirth.** 1981. Rapid detection and identification of *Bacteroides fragilis* and *Bacteroides melaninogenicus* by immunofluorescence. J. Clin. Microbiol. **13:**798–800.
96. **Wideman, P. A., D. M. Citronbaum, and V. L. Sutter.** 1977. Simple disk technique for detection of nitrate reduction by anaerobic bacteria. J. Clin. Microbiol. **5:**315–319.
97. **Wideman, P. A., V. L. Vargo, D. M. Citronbaum, and S. M. Finegold.** 1976. Evaluation of the sodium polyanethol sulfonate disk test for the identification of *Peptostreptococcus anaerobius.* J. Clin. Microbiol. **4:**330–333.
98. **Wilkins, T. D., D. L. Wagner, D. J. Veltri, and E. M. Gregory.** 1978. Factors affecting production of catalase by bacteroides. J. Clin. Microbiol. **8:**553–557.
99. **Woods, G. L., and P. C. Iwen.** 1990. Comparison of a dot blot immunobinding assay, latex agglutination, and cytotoxin assay for the laboratory diagnosis of *Clostridium difficile*-associated diarrhea. J. Clin. Microbiol. **28:**855–857.
100. **Wust, J.** 1977. Presumptive diagnosis of anaerobic bacteremia by gas-liquid chromatography of blood cultures. J. Clin. Microbiol. **6:**586–590.

Chapter 50

Clostridium

STEPHEN D. ALLEN AND ELLEN JO BARON

Sporeforming, catalase-negative, anaerobic bacilli with gram-positive cell wall components belong to the genus *Clostridium*. Detailed descriptions of 85 species are provided in volume 2, section 13, of the 1986 edition of *Bergey's Manual of Systematic Bacteriology* (20). By late 1989 an additional 20 species were characterized and defined, bringing the total to more than 100 validly published species of *Clostridium*. Only limited numbers of these species are commonly encountered in properly collected clinical materials from humans (Table 1). Although botulism, tetanus, and certain other clostridial diseases may arise exogenously, the source of most *Clostridium* species in patients with infectious diseases is the patients' own flora, especially the large bowel flora.

DESCRIPTION OF THE GENUS

The vegetative cells of most species are rod shaped and straight or curved, but cells vary from short coccoid rods to long filamentous forms. Rod-shaped cells may be rounded, tapered, or blunt ended. Cells occur singly, in pairs, or in chains of various lengths. In certain species (e.g., *C. cocleatum* and *C. spiroforme*), many rods may be joined together to form tight coils or spiral-shaped configurations (20). Most species stain gram positive, at least very early in culture, but some, such as *C. ramosum* and *C. clostridiiforme*, almost always appear gram negative after overnight culture. Several species (e.g., *C. tetani*) are usually gram negative by the time their spores are formed. All but a few species are characteristically motile by means of peritrichous flagella. In most instances, the nonmotile species isolated from clinical specimens are *C. perfringens*, *C. ramosum*, and *C. innocuum*. The spores of clostridia are usually ovoid to spherical and distend the vegetative cells. Certain species, e.g., *C. perfringens*, produce spores only under special culture conditions. Although the majority of *Clostridium* species are obligate anaerobes, there is considerable species variation with respect to the ability of isolates to tolerate exposure to oxygen; some (e.g., *C. haemolyticum* and *C. novyi* type B) are strict obligate anaerobes and will not grow when exposed to trace amounts of oxygen, whereas others grow in a gas mixture of 5% O_2, 10% CO_2, and 85% N_2, and a few aerotolerant clostridia show scant growth on plating media incubated in a 5 to 10% CO_2 incubator in air or in a candle jar. Catalase is not produced except in rare instances. If produced, it is only weak or in a small amount. In addition, the clostridia lack a cytochrome system and thus react negatively in the cytochrome oxidase test. They do not have a mechanism for electron transport phosphorylation, and they obtain ATP by substrate-level phosphorylation (17). They are usually fermentative, proteolytic, or both, but some are asaccharolytic and nonproteolytic. Many clostridia produce a range of short-chain fatty acids (e.g., acetate and butyrate) when grown in peptone-yeast extract-glucose or chopped meat carbohydrate medium, and many produce a variety of other kinds of fermentation products (e.g., acetone, butanol, and other alcohols). The metabolisms and energy-yielding mechanisms of clostridia are extremely diverse and interesting (17).

Since some aerotolerant clostridia (e.g., *C. tertium*, *C. histolyticum*, and *C. carnis*) may grow on the surface of a fresh agar medium under aerobic conditions, it is possible to confuse these species with certain facultatively anaerobic *Bacillus* species. However, members of the genus *Clostridium* usually form spores under anaerobic conditions and almost never produce catalase. Also, aerotolerant clostridia show much better growth (i.e., they form larger colonies) under anaerobic conditions than in air, whereas *Bacillus* species often form larger colonies on aerobically incubated media than on media incubated anaerobically.

NATURAL HABITATS AND CLINICAL SIGNIFICANCE

The clostridia are distributed widely in soil and in freshwater and marine sediments throughout the world. Some are psychrophilic and some are thermophilic, but most are mesophilic. *Desulfotomaculum* is an additional genus of sporeforming anaerobic bacilli that is encountered in nature, but *Clostridium* is the only genus of sporeforming anaerobes found in humans, either in nonpathogenic habitats or in infected sites. Several *Clostridium* species inhabit the lower intestinal tract of humans and other animals as part of the normal flora (34). Most species are harmless saprophytes.

Exogenous and endogenous diseases

Exogenous infections, including botulism, *C. perfringens* food-borne illness, gas gangrene associated with traumatic wounds, and tetanus, are well-known historically and are clinically important. Although usually acquired from the patient's own gastrointestinal tract, *C. difficile* may be spread exogenously from person to person during outbreaks of hospital-acquired diarrhea or colitis (53, 71). Endogenous infections involving clostridia of the indigenous flora are much more common, however. As for other endogenous infections involving anaerobes (endocarditis, brain abscess, aspiration pneumonia, intra-abdominal abscess, etc.), special circumstances are required for the development of endogenous infections with the clostridia. Common predisposing factors include trauma, operative procedures, vascular stasis, obstruction, treatment with immuno-

TABLE 1. *Clostridium* species most frequently encountered in clinical specimens at the Indiana University Medical Center Anaerobe Laboratory, 1979 through 1988[a]

Species	No. of isolates	% of total isolates
C. perfringens	472	26
C. ramosum	257	14
C. innocuum	235	13
C. clostridiiforme	200	11
C. difficile	130	7
C. butyricum	90	5
C. cadaveris	83	5
C. bifermentans	64	4
C. sporogenes	63	3
C. septicum	61	3
C. tertium	50	3
C. paraputrificum	42	2
C. glycolicum	25	1
C. subterminale	20	1
Other recognized species[b]	50	3

[a] Based on the data of J. A. Siders and S. D. Allen. The total of 1,842 isolates does not include 252 isolates (12% of 2,094 isolates) that did not belong to a recognized species. All of the isolates were from properly collected specimens. No isolates were from feces, intestinal materials, or other contaminated sources.

[b] Includes 1 to 10 isolates of each of the following: *C. sordellii, C. barati, C. malenominatum, C. sphenoides, C. putrificum, C. symbiosum, C. indolis, C. celatum, C. tetani, C. carnis, C. leptum,* and *C. hastiforme.*

suppressive agents, chemotherapeutic agents used in the treatment of malignancy, prior treatment with antimicrobial agents (as in pseudomembranous colitis), and underlying illness such as leukemia, carcinoma, or diabetes mellitus. Under the right conditions, clostridia can invade and multiply in essentially any area of the body.

C. perfringens, other histotoxic clostridia, and clostridial myonecrosis (or gas gangrene)

C. perfringens, the *Clostridium* species most commonly isolated from human materials, is encountered in a wide variety of clinical settings, ranging from simple contamination of a wound to traumatic or nontraumatic myonecrosis, clostridial cellulitis, intra-abdominal sepsis, gangrenous cholecystitis, postabortion infection with devastating septicemia, intravascular hemolysis, bacteremia in various clinical settings, aspiration pneumonia, necrotizing pneumonia, thoracic empyema, subdural empyema, and brain abscess (12, 30, 31, 90). The organism is ubiquitous, occurring in soil, water, sewage, and the intestinal tracts of animals and many humans. *C. perfringens*, also called *C. welchii* (primarily by British workers), produces a variety of toxins (biologically active proteins) which play an important role in pathogenicity (reviewed by Smith [88] and more recently by Hatheway [43]). Accordingly, five mouse-lethal toxin types of *C. perfringens*, designated A through E, are recognized by the detection and specific neutralization of four toxins, which have been designated alpha, beta, epsilon, and iota, from culture fluids (43, 94; Table 2). In reference laboratories such as those of the Centers for Disease Control (CDC), lethal toxins are detected by using toxicity and toxin-antiserum neutralization tests in mice (26). Most infections of humans involving *C. perfringens* are caused by type A strains. *C. perfringens* type C is the only other toxin type encountered in human illness (90). Type C is associated with a disease called enteritis necroticans (discussed below). All five lethal toxin types of clostridia produce alpha toxin, which is primarily responsible for the mouse lethality. Also referred to as phospholipase C, the alpha toxin has several additional properties. It is the lecithinase that produces the opaque zone of lecithin hydrolysis breakdown products that surrounds colonies of *C. perfringens* growing on egg yolk agar plates. Alpha toxin is also a hemolysin active against erythrocyte cell membranes, giving rise to the outer zone of partial hemolysis that surrounds colonies on sheep blood agar plates. The alpha toxin is also active against the membranes of muscle cells, leukocytes, and platelets, and it has necrotizing activity that leads to the death of a variety of host cells and tissues. In addition to producing alpha toxin, type B strains of *C. perfringens* produce beta and epsilon lethal toxins, type D strains produce epsilon lethal toxin, and type E is the only type that produces iota toxin as well as alpha toxin (Table 2). Beta toxin is a major lethal factor produced by type C strains of *C. perfringens*. This toxin is important in the pathogenesis of pig-bel (i.e., necrotic enteritis or enteritis necroticans), Darmbrand, and certain other forms of necrotizing enteropathy (43).

A variety of other toxins, known as minor toxins, which may or may not serve as virulence factors, are produced by *C. perfringens* (43, 88, 94). These include lambda toxin (a protease), kappa toxin (a collagenase), mu toxin (a hyaluronidase), a neuraminidase, additional hemolysins including theta toxin, which is a heat-labile, oxygen-labile hemolysin that is responsible for the inner zone of complete hemolysis surrounding *C. perfringens* colonies on sheep blood agar media, and a DNase (90, 109).

C. perfringens is commonly considered to be one of a group of organisms referred to as the histotoxic clostridia. The histotoxic clostridia most commonly involved in gas gangrene (myonecrosis) are *C. perfringens* (80%), *C. novyi* (40%), and *C. septicum* (20%), followed by *C. histolyticum* and *C. bifermentans*. Other species such as *C. sordellii, C. fallax, C. sporogenes*, and *C. tertium* have been encountered in myonecrosis, but their pathogenic significance is not certain.

Clostridial myonecrosis (gas gangrene) is not the predisposing bacteriologic infectious process but rather a toxin-mediated breakdown of muscle tissue associated with growth of the organism. It is a rapidly progressive, life-threatening, invasive, clinicopathological condition with liquefactive necrosis of muscle, gas formation, and associated clinical signs of toxemia. Blood cultures are positive in about 15% of patients (39). Many excellent descriptions of the clinical and pathological features of gas gangrene have been published elsewhere (3, 12, 34, 39, 98, 100, 109).

Crepitant cellulitis

The presence of gas in an infected site does not always signal clostridial myonecrosis. Various gas-producing bacteria may form gas in tissue; the most frequent to do so, particularly after laceration-type wounds involving soft tissue other than muscle, are the clostridia, especially *C. perfringens* (2, 99, 109). Crepitant cellulitis caused by clostridia, also called anaerobic cellulitis, characteristically involves subcutaneous tissues or ret-

TABLE 2. Distribution of major toxins among the types of *C. perfringens*[a]

Type	Occurrence (country where originally found)	Major toxin: Alpha — Presence or absence	Alpha — Characteristics	Beta — Presence or absence	Beta — Characteristics	Epsilon — Presence or absence	Epsilon — Characteristics	Iota — Presence or absence	Iota — Characteristics
A	Gas gangrene of humans and animals Intestinal flora of humans and animals Putrefactive processes in soil, etc. (United States) Food poisoning (United Kingdom)	+	Lethal Lecithinase Hemolytic Necrotizing Also called phospholipase C	–	Lethal Necrotizing	–	Lethal Permease	–	Lethal Dermonecrotic ADP ribosylating
B	Lamb dysentery Enterotoxemia of foals (United Kingdom) Enterotoxemia of sheep and goats (Iran)	+		+		+		–	
C	Enterotoxemia of sheep (struck) (United Kingdom) Enterotoxemia of calves and lambs (United States) Enterotoxemia of piglets (United Kingdom) Enteritis necroticans of humans (Darmbrand) (Germany) Enteritis necroticans of humans (pig-bel) (Papua New Guinea)	+		+		–		–	
D	Enterotoxemia of sheep, lambs, goats, and cattle, possibly humans (Australia)	+		–		+		–	
E	Sheep and cattle, pathogenicity doubted (United Kingdom)	+		–		–		+	

[a] Adapted from Sterne and Warrack (94) and Hatheway (43).

roperitoneal tissues (2, 3). In contrast to clostridial myonecrosis, the muscle is usually not invaded extensively and remains viable in crepitant cellulitis. Although both kinds of infections are serious, the outlook for patients who have clostridial infections confined to subcutaneous tissue is usually not so ominous as for those with myonecrosis, provided the correct diagnosis and treatment are initiated early in the course of illness. Pertinent findings in crepitant cellulitis include abundant gas in the tissue, often more than in myonecrosis, tissue swelling without much discoloration of the overlying skin, minimal pain, and a thin, sweet-smelling or sometimes foul-smelling exudate that may contain numerous polymorphonuclear leukocytes and bacteria (2, 12). On occasion, however, polymorphonuclear leukocytes may be absent because of the activity of the leukolytic toxins of the clostridia. The presence of boxcar-shaped gram-variable rods and no leukocytes in a Gram stain of infected tissue should lead one to suspect clostridial infection. These infections may involve clostridia only but are frequently polymicrobial, also containing *Escherichia coli*, *Peptostreptococcus* spp., *Bacteroides* spp., or other bacteria (2, 75). In some patients whose initial presentation is that of clostridial crepitant cellulitis focally, there may be a devastatingly fulminant clinical course, with rapid spread of bacteria, gas, and cellulitis through fascial planes, signs of toxemia, septicemia, shock, and intravascular hemolysis, progressing to renal failure and death.

Acute nonclostridial crepitant cellulitis is another kind of potentially severe clinical entity which spares muscle and is characterized by a rapidly spreading infectious process involving subcutaneous connective tissue and skin, along with extensive gas formation. Numerous polymorphonuclear leukocytes and bacteria other than clostridia, including *Peptostreptococcus* spp., *Streptococcus* spp., *Staphylococcus aureus*, *E. coli*, *Klebsiella* spp., *Proteus* spp., the pigmented *Bacteroides* and *Porphyromonas* groups, and *Bacteroides fragilis* group, are among the organisms most commonly encountered in this condition (2, 75).

The gas present in the clostridial and the nonclostridial gas-producing infections is largely insoluble hydrogen and nitrogen, believed to be derived mostly from anaerobic pathways of fermentation, deamination, and denitrification (75, 100). Because of its high solubility in water or in tissue fluid, carbon dioxide produced as an end product of aerobic metabolism is unlikely to accumulate significantly as free gas in tissue.

Clostridial bacteremia

From year to year at Indiana University Hospitals, approximately 10 to 12% of all blood cultures contain clinically significant bacteria, and about 0.5 to 2% of these bacteria are *Clostridium* species. The species encountered most frequently in positive blood cultures is *C. perfringens*, which accounts for more than 20% to over half of the clostridial isolates (S. D. Allen, unpublished data). Other *Clostridium* species found less frequently in positive blood cultures include *C. septicum*, *C. ramosum*, *C. bifermentans*, *C. sordellii*, *C. difficile*, *C. tertium*, *C. cadaveris*, *C. innocuum*, *C. sporogenes*, *C. sphenoides*, *C. butyricum*, and others (Allen, unpublished data; 1, 18, 40). Underlying conditions commonly associated with clostridial bacteremia have included chronic alcoholism, sepsis following intra-abdominal surgery, necrosis of the small intestine and large bowel, genitourinary tract disorders (including septic abortions), cardiovascular disease, pulmonary diseases, underlying malignancy, diabetes, and decubitus ulcers (18, 40). In many instances of bacteremia involving *C. perfringens* and certain other clostridia, isolates are of doubtful significance and may represent contaminants. Isolates deposited transiently in the perianal area could be spread to a venipuncture site, or isolates could reflect transient bacteremia of no clinical significance. One large retrospective study found that half of all clostridia isolated from blood represented contaminants (106).

C. septicum bacteremia

C. septicum is associated with malignancies, especially leukemia/lymphoma or carcinoma of the large bowel, in as many as 70 to 85% of patients whose blood cultures are positive for this organism (58, 59). Another clinically important association has been observed between *C. septicum* bacteremia, neutropenia, and enterocolitis involving the terminal ileum or cecum (14, 54, 79, 114). The neutropenia has been related not only to chemotherapy for leukemia or other neoplastic disease but also to cyclic neutropenia and drug-induced agranulocytosis. Although the isolation of *Pseudomonas* spp., *E. coli*, *Klebsiella* spp., and other organisms has been described in some older reports of patients with leukemia and necrotizing enterocolitis, increasing numbers of reports of *C. septicum* bacteremia and neutropenic enterocolitis are suggesting that *C. septicum* could be a major etiologic agent of this condition (54, 79, 114).

Not all patients with *C. septicum* bacteremia have malignancy or neutropenic enterocolitis. Diabetes mellitus, severe atherosclerotic cardiovascular disease, and gas gangrene, which may arise spontaneously in the absence of a traumatic wound or an external portal of entry, may antedate the onset of *C. septicum* bacteremia. *C. septicum* is isolated only rarely from the feces of healthy individuals, and it is not recovered often from blood cultures. The portal of entry for *C. septicum* into the bloodstream is believed to be the ileocecal region of the bowel. Whether or not *C. septicum* is part of the indigenous microflora of this site has not been established. *C. septicum* has been found in the lumens of 10 to 68% of normal appendixes and in none of 30 nonlumen appendiceal tissue samples from gangrenous or perforated appendices (13, 34). The clinical importance of recognizing *C. septicum* bacteremia and starting appropriate treatment without delay cannot be overemphasized. Patients with this syndrome are usually acutely and gravely ill, frequently have high temperatures, and often show metastatic spread of myonecrosis to distant anatomic sites. Mortality is very high, yet appropriate antibiotic therapy, especially penicillin G, with aggressive surgical intervention early in the course of the illness, may aid in avoiding a devastating outcome (58, 59).

Intra-abdominal infections

Clostridium species are commonly encountered in a variety of polymicrobial infections involving the abdomen, including peritonitis, intra-abdominal abscesses, and septicemia in patients who have obstructive or perforating lesions of the terminal ileum or large bowel (40). *C. perfringens* and *C. septicum* have been documented in patients with overwhelming sepsis and gangrenous necrosis of the small intestine or large bowel. Prior abdominal surgery with some manipulation of the bowel, penetrating wounds involving the small intestine or large bowel, and carcinoma of the colon, leukemia, or other malignancy, frequently with mucosal ulceration of the distal small intestine or cecum, have been observed in these patients (Allen, unpublished data; 31). Although it is clear that clostridia play a major pathogenic role in some life-threatening necrotizing infections of the intestinal tract, such as enteritis necroticans, clostridial necrotizing enteropathy in adults (discussed below), or *C. septicum* disease (see above), the role of clostridia in intra-abdominal infections, especially posttrauma mixed infections, must be assessed on an individual patient basis in the context of the clinical setting.

Uterine infections

C. perfringens has been isolated from the vaginas and cervixes of approximately 1 to 9% of healthy pregnant and nonpregnant women (22). Gas gangrene of the uterus, which is now rare in the United States, has occurred most frequently as a consequence of illegal or self-induced abortions. It has also followed spontaneous abortion or vaginal delivery in which the postabortal or puerperal uterus contained blood clots and fragments of necrotic placenta or fetal tissue, along with a minimum number of clostridia which could proliferate within the endometrium and subsequently invade the uterine wall. Clostridial myonecrosis of the uterus is associated with fulminant and overwhelming septicemia, marked intravascular hemolysis with a sudden drop in the hemoglobin, and hemolysis, profound anemia, jaundice, hemoglobinuria, and excretion of urine that is burgundy wine in color. Patients become hypotensive, then not uncommonly develop cardiovascular collapse, cardiac failure, pulmonary edema, renal failure, and coma, and may die within hours after the onset of the infection (109). A dirty red-brown, foul-smelling vaginal discharge containing gas bubbles and a Gram-stained smear showing numerous gram-positive bacilli should suggest clostridial myonecrosis of the uterus.

Assessing the clinical significance of *Clostridium* species isolated from miscellaneous specimens

The isolation of *Clostridium* species from a specimen is without meaning unless it is considered in relation to the clinical condition of the patient. Because clostridia are ubiquitous, they are likely to be found in any area that is directly or indirectly contaminated with feces, soil, or dust. Even the toxigenic species are only opportunistic pathogens, and conditions suitable for progressive infection occur only rarely. Therefore, close liaison between the attending physician and the clinical microbiologist is essential for an assessment of the clinical significance of clostridial isolates and the establishment of the correct diagnosis.

This situation is particularly the case with *C. perfringens*. Although this species may cause a host of pathological conditions, many isolates will have doubtful or no clinical significance. *C. septicum*, on the other hand, is rarely isolated except from serious, often fatal clinical conditions. *C. novyi* is seldom isolated in civilian hospital laboratories. During wartime, it has been responsible for gas gangrene as the result of wounds that were contaminated with soil when inflicted (90). Most *C. novyi* strains encountered in wounds belong to type A; only a few belong to type B. The isolation of either type from a wound should be regarded with concern.

The isolation of a pathogenic strain of *C. sordellii* from a human infection is rare; the great majority of isolates appear to lack toxigenicity (90). However, *C. sordellii*, in addition to being demonstrated as an infrequent cause of myonecrosis and involvement in mixed infections, was implicated recently as the cause of fatal spontaneous endometritis (49) and a rapidly lethal toxic shock-like syndrome in postpartum women (68).

The isolation of *C. botulinum*, particularly type A, from a wound suggests the possibility of wound botulism. Nevertheless, toxigenic strains of *C. botulinum* have been isolated from wounds in the absence of clinical evidence of botulism. Wound isolates identified biochemically as *C. sporogenes* should be tested for botulinal toxin production if warranted by clinical circumstances; *C. sporogenes* and the proteolytic group I strains of *C. botulinum* are indistinguishable except by toxin assays (Table 3). In addition to the culturing of wound samples, testing of the patient's serum for toxin is particularly important when wound botulism is suspected (89). Demonstration of toxin in serum is also important for diagnosis of tetanus. Since most people have been immunized with tetanus toxoid, the isolation of *C. tetani* from a wound may not be clinically significant. Even in unimmunized persons, it is not uncommon to find this organism in wounds without the patient showing symptoms and signs of tetanus (90).

C. histolyticum is encountered in far fewer than 1% of civilian wounds. Its presence is without clear significance unless a progressive anaerobic infection of muscle is in progress, and then the prognosis is poor (90).

C. perfringens food-borne illness

C. perfringens generally ranks behind *Salmonella* spp. and *S. aureus* as the third most common cause of food poisoning in the United States (5). Almost all U.S. outbreaks and cases of *C. perfringens* food-borne gastroenteritis appear to be due to type A strains (84). In *C. perfringens* type A food-borne disease, the food vehicle is almost always an improperly cooked meat (e.g., beef, turkey, chicken, or pork) or a meat product, such as gravy, that has cooled slowly after cooking or may have been reheated to a moderate temperature (5). Spores survive the initial cooking; the spores then germinate, and vegetative cells proliferate during slow cooling or reheating. *C. perfringens* type A food-borne illness should be suspected when there is an outbreak of diarrhea with crampy abdominal pain within about 7 to 15 h after the consumption of a suspected food (84). However, the incubation period has ranged up to 30 h. Most patients are afebrile; nausea and vomiting occur in less than a third of patients, and the stools are frequently foamy and foul smelling. Illness results from the ingestion of food with about 10^8 viable vegetative cells which, in the alkaline environment of the intestine, undergo sporulation, producing an enterotoxin in the process (84). The enterotoxin, a 34,000-molecular-weight protein (a structural component of *C. perfringens* spores), induces fluid and electrolyte secretion in the ileum of

TABLE 3. Differential characteristics of commonly encountered clostridia[a]

Species	Spores	Egg yolk agar		Growth on aerobic blood agar	Gelatin hydrolysis	Milk digestion	Indole production	Carbohydrate fermentation						Principal metabolic products PYG or CMC	Other
		LEC	LIP					Glucose	Maltose	Lactose	Sucrose	Salicin	Mannitol		
C. bifermentans	OS	+	−	−	+	+	+	+	w/−	−	−	−	−	A, (p), (ib), (b), (iv), (ic)	Urease negative
C. botulinum[b]															
Group I[c]	OS	−	+	−	+	+	−	+	−/w	−	−	−	−	A, (p), ib, B, IV, (v), (ic)	
Group II[c]	OS	−/+	+	−	+	+	−/+	+	V	−	−	−	−	A, P, B, (v)	
Group III[c]	OS	−	+	−	+	−	−	+	+/w	−	+/w	−	−	A, B	
C. butyricum	OS	−	−	−	−	−	−	+	+	+	+	+	−/+	A, B	
C. cadaveris	OT	−	−	−	+	+	+	+	−	−	−	−	−	A, (p), B (from PY = A, p, ib, b, iv)	
C. chauvoei[d]	OS	−	−	−	+	−	−	+	+/w	+/w	+/w	−	−	A, B	
C. clostridiiforme	OS	−	−	−	−	−	−/+	+	+/w	+/−	+	+/−	−	A	Spores seldom observed; usually gram negative
C. difficile	OS	−	−	−	+	−	−	+	−	−	−	−/w	+/−	A, (p), ib, B, iv, (v), ic	
C. histolyticum	OS	−	−	V	+	+	−	−	−	−	−	−	−	A	Aerotolerant
C. innocuum[e]	OT	−	−	−	−	−	−	+	−	−	+	+	+	A, B	
C. limosum	OS	+	−	−	+	+	−	−	−	−	−	−	−	A	
C. novyi A[c]	OS	+	+	−	+	−	−	+	V	−	−	−/+	−	A, P, B	
C. novyi B[c]	OS	+	−	−	+	+	+/−	+	V	−	−	−	−	A, P, B	
C. paraputrificum	OT	−	−	−	−	−	−	+	+	+	+	+	−	A, B	
C. perfringens[e]	OS	+	−	−	+	+	−	+	+	+	+	−	−	A, (p), B	Spores seldom observed; double zone of hemolysis
C. ramosum[e]	R/OT	−	−	−	−	−	−	+	+	+	+	+	+/−	A	Spores seldom observed; frequently gram negative
C. septicum	OS	−	−	−	+	+	−	+	+	+	−	V	−	A, (p), B	Spreading colony
C. sordellii	OS	+	−	−	+	+	+	+	w/+	−	−	−	−	A, (p), (ib), (iv), (ic)	Usually urease positive
C. sphenoides	RS/T	−	−	−	−	−	+	+	+	w/+	w/−	w/+	w/+	A	Usually gram negative
C. sporogenes	OS	−	+	−	+	+	−	+	−/w	−	−	−	−	A, (p), ib, B, iv, (v), (ic)	
C. subterminale	OS	−/+	−	−	+	+	−	−	−	−	−	−	−	A, (p), ib, B, IV, (ic)	
C. tertium	OT	−	−	+	−	−	−	+	+	+	+	+	+/w	A, B	Aerotolerant
C. tetani	RT	−	−	−	+	+/−	V	−	−	−	−	−	−	A, p, B	

[a] Based on the use of PRAS media as described by Holdeman et al. (50). Key: +, positive reaction; −, negative reaction; V, variable reaction; /, either/or; O, oval; R, round; S, subterminal; T, terminal; LEC, lecithinase production; LIP, lipase production. Fermentation products: A, acetic; B, butyric; F, formic; IB, isobutyric; IC, isocaproic; IV, isovaleric; P, propionic; V, valeric. ( ), May or may not be present. Capital letters indicate major peaks; lowercase letters indicate minor peaks.

[b] Group I contains proteolytic strains (A, B, and F), group II contains types C and D, and group III contains saccharolytic strains (B, E, and F).

[c] Toxin neutralization test required for identification.

[d] Pathogenic for herbivores.

[e] *C. innocuum*, *C. perfringens*, and *C. ramosum* are nonmotile.

mice and other animal models (113). Usually the illness is mild, and most patients recover within 2 to 3 days after onset. The diagnosis is confirmed by the culture of at least 10^5 organisms per g from epidemiologically implicated food and by the demonstration, by a quantitative spore selection technique, of median spore counts of at least 10^6 *C. perfringens* spores per g of feces collected within 24 h of the onset of illness (5, 84). Latex reagents for detecting type A enterotoxin are under development and evaluation (69) but not available in clinical laboratories. Laboratory testing for *C. perfringens* food-borne illness is a public health laboratory function that should be done concomitantly with epidemiologic support. Ideally, isolates of the same serotype should be cultured from epidemiologically incriminated food and ill persons but not from controls. Unfortunately, the experience with serotyping of *C. perfringens* at the CDC has not been highly successful (84).

C. perfringens in enteritis necroticans

C. perfringens produces a much more severe necrotizing disease of the small bowel known as enteritis necroticans, which can occur sporadically or in an epidemic form. The syndrome has been called Darmbrand in Germany and pig-bel in Papua, New Guinea (12, 73, 90, 109).

In this condition, seen mostly in children, there is evidence that *C. perfringens* type C, which is either part of the normal intestinal flora or ingested with contaminated pork or other meat during a feast, proliferates in the small intestine and produces beta toxin. This toxin production probably leads to focal paralysis, inflammation, hemorrhage, and segmental gangrenous necrosis of the intestine, particularly the jejunum. Among the factors likely to be involved in the pathogenesis of enteritis necroticans are (i) overeating, which might distend the bowel and cause partial obstruction; (ii) poor nutrition, which leads to low levels of production of the pancreatic proteases (particularly trypsin, which ordinarily destroys beta toxins); and (iii) a diet that is rich in trypsin inhibitors (such as the semicooked sweet potatoes that are often eaten at pig feasts) (104). The incidence of this condition in the United States is unknown, probably because the disease is rather obscure and would be easy to overlook clinically.

Although the etiology of neonatal necrotizing enterocolitis is unknown, epidemiologic data support a direct role for microorganisms and their toxins in the pathogenesis of this disease. Of the implicated organisms, clostridia, particularly *C. perfringens*, are among the organisms most likely to be involved (55).

C. difficile gastrointestinal illness

C. difficile is a major cause of antibiotic-associated diarrhea and pseudomembranous colitis (61). It is now one of the most commonly detected enteric pathogens and an important cause of nosocomial infections in hospitals and nursing homes (38, 53, 71). The organism has been isolated from diverse natural habitats, including soil, hay, sand, dung from various large mammals (cows, donkeys, and horses), and from dog, cat, rodent, and human feces (33). *C. difficile* is carried asymptomatically in the gastrointestinal flora of as many as half of all healthy neonates, dropping to the adult carrier rate of less than 4% in children older than 2 years (21, 102). Among adults who have received antibiotic therapy, carriage rates as high as 46% have been reported (35). Hospitalized patients frequently become colonized with this organism (35, 101, 102). Antimicrobial agents of all classes and several anticancer chemotherapeutic agents have been implicated in the development of *C. difficile*-associated diarrhea or pseudomembranous colitis (61). The most commonly reported agents are ampicillin, clindamycin, and cephalosporins (33). Patients with bowel stasis, status post-bowel surgery, and those without known risk factors can also contract *C. difficile*-induced gastrointestinal disease, although this form of the disease is rare. Clinical symptoms range from mild diarrhea to toxic megacolon (37). The most severe complications, perforated bowel and death, are unlikely to occur in appropriately treated patients.

Organisms other than *C. difficile* have rarely been shown to be important agents of antibiotic-associated diarrhea. It has been proposed that enterotoxin-producing *C. perfringens* may also cause antibiotic-associated diarrhea (15, 16). This syndrome awaits confirmation by others. Because appropriate antitoxins are not available commercially, clinical laboratories are currently unable to differentiate enterotoxin-producing strains from the normal fecal strains of *C. perfringens*. Although the infection is extremely rare at this time, *S. aureus* has been shown to cause enterocolitis (66).

C. difficile produces at least three potential virulence factors: an enterotoxin (toxin A) that induces a positive fluid response in the rabbit ligated ileal loop model, a cytotoxin (toxin B) that induces cytopathic effects (CPE) in numerous tissue culture cell lines (62, 96), and a substance that inhibits bowel motility (51). Toxin A also produces CPE in cell culture but is 1,000 times less potent than toxin B in the cell lines that have been tested (96). All strains tested for toxin in vitro produce either both toxins or no detectable toxin (61); it is thought that toxins A and B are important in the pathogenesis of *C. difficile*-associated disease, with toxin A being more important. Toxin A seems to interfere with the cytoskeleton of intestinal epithelial cells, thereby rendering the cells nonfunctional. Complete pathogenic mechanisms of *C. difficile*-associated disease have yet to be defined despite active research in the area (23).

No single laboratory test yields definitive diagnosis at this time. Visualization by colonoscopy of the characteristic pseudomembranous plaques remains the method of choice to document pseudomembranous colitis, although microscopic lesions may not be grossly visible in less severe or early cases (37). Pseudomembranous lesions are also produced in the colon in ischemic enterocolitis, shigellosis, amoebiasis, and other conditions that could be mistaken morphologically for *C. difficile*-associated pseudomembranous colitis, and colonoscopy subjects patients to unnecessary trauma and cost. Detection of the organism in culture of feces, detection of a *C. difficile*-associated protein in fecal supernatants by a latex agglutination assay (52, 63, 70, 77), and detection of the cytotoxin by a cell culture assay (11, 105) have all been used to diagnose *C. difficile*-associated disease. Counterimmunoelectrophoresis is not specific enough for routine diagnostic testing (81, 107, 111). Clinically evaluated disease, verified by successful treatment with vancomycin or metronidazole, seems to be associated most strongly with detection of the cytotoxin in cell culture (11, 33, 78), although toxin-negative, culture-positive cases have been reported (60). Enzyme-linked immunosorbent assays (ELISAs) for both toxins have been developed, but they have not yet enjoyed routine use in clinical laboratories (105). One commercial membrane-bound solid-phase ELISA for toxin has been evaluated (110). Gram stain of fecal smears (85) and ELISAs for antibody to *C. difficile* toxins (103) have not proved useful for diagnosis of gastrointestinal disease.

Botulism

Botulism, a neuroparalytic disease produced by the neurotoxins of *C. botulinum*, is currently classified into four categories: (i) classical food-borne botulism, an intoxication caused by the ingestion of preformed botulinal toxin in contaminated food; (ii) wound botulism, the rarest form of botulism (40 cases have been reported), which results from the elaboration of botulinal toxin in vivo after growth of *C. botulinum* in an infected wound; (iii) infant botulism, in which botulinal toxin is elaborated in vivo in the intestinal tract of an infant who has been colonized with *C. botulinum;* and (iv) an undetermined classification of botulism for those cases involving individuals older than 12 months in which no food or wound source is implicated (4, 43). There are seven toxigenic types of *C. botulinum* (A through G) based on antigenically distinct toxins produced by different strains of the organism. Type C can be subdivided into two toxin types, C_1 and C_2; C_1 is a neurotoxin, and C_2 is not a neurotoxin but causes increased vascular permeability. Types A, B, E, and F are the principal causes of botulism in humans; types C and D have been associated with botulism in birds and mammals (43). Type G organisms, now called *Clostridium argentinense* (95), have been isolated from soil in Argentina and from autopsy materials from five individuals who died suddenly, but the type G organisms have not been clearly implicated in cases of botulism (91). The potent neurotoxins of *C. botulinum* are protoplasmic proteins that are synthesized during growth of the organisms and released during lysis (25). The mechanisms of action of the botulinal neurotoxins are not completely known, but a three-step process has been hypothesized: (i) the toxin binds irreversibly to a receptor site at the neuromuscular junction and other peripheral autonomic synaptic sites, but the receptor sites have yet to be identified; (ii) a portion of the toxin molecule probably penetrates the plasma membrane, possibly by receptor-mediated endocytosis, and thus is internalized into the nerve cell; and (iii) the neurotoxin molecule acts within the nerve terminal to prevent release of acetylcholine (43, 86). The characteristic clinical hallmark of botulism is an acute flaccid paralysis, which begins with bilateral cranial nerve impairment involving muscles of the face, head, and pharynx and then descends symmetrically to involve muscles of the thorax and extremities. Death may result from respiratory failure caused by a paralysis of the tongue or muscles of the pharynx that occludes the upper airway or from paralysis of the diaphragm and intercostal muscles. Patients diagnosed with food-borne or wound botulism should immediately receive trivalent (type ABE) antitoxin and promptly receive intensive respiratory care. For further information on botulism in general, see Hatheway (42, 43), Smith and Sugiyama (89), the CDC handbook (4), and Dowell (25).

Infant botulism is the most frequently encountered form of botulism; 760 cases were reported in the United States between 1976 and 1988 (5, 6). Infant botulism has been reported from North and South America, Europe, Asia, and Australia (7). In the United States in general, the geographical distribution of toxin types in infant botulism cases has paralleled the distribution of *C. botulinum* toxin types in soil sampled from across the United States (87). Type A has been the most frequent botulinal toxin type in cases of infant botulism in states west of the Mississippi River, whereas type B cases have predominated east of the Mississippi (7). Interestingly, one infant from Hawaii had two different strains of *C. botulinum;* one strain was type A, and the other was type B (42). Two other cases were caused by a strain(s) of *C. botulinum* which produced toxins that required both type B antitoxin and type F antitoxin for neutralization (42). In another interesting case, type F infant botulism was caused by an organism that most closely resembled *C. barati* in its cultural and biochemical characteristics (41). Type E botulism, caused by toxigenic strains of *C. butyricum,* was confirmed in two infants from Italy (42). Infants have ranged from 6 days to 11.7 months old (92). The ingestion of spores by the infant during the first weeks of life is probably a prerequisite for the development of the disease. Preformed toxin has not been detected in any food or liquid ingested by the babies. To date, the only clearly defined risk factors have been breast feeding and exposure to honey, the latter of which is a potential source of spores. The CDC has recommended that honey not be fed to infants less than 1 year old (92). Another concern is that spores have also been found in a limited number of samples of corn syrup. Corn syrup is often given to infants for treatment of decreased frequency of bowel movements (92). However, *C. botulinum* spores in the corn syrup actually consumed by an infant with botulism are yet to be demonstrated. Whatever the sources of the spores, the ingested spores of *C. botulinum* germinate within the intestinal tract, and the vegetative cells multiply and produce the neurotoxin, which is then absorbed into the bloodstream. Decreased frequency of bowel movements, which may also be a sign of decreased intestinal motility, is an additional risk factor for infant botulism (92). The decreased motility could lead to spread of *C. botulinum* or its toxin from the colon to the small intestine, where the toxin is probably absorbed (92). The first sign of illness is invariably constipation, although this decreased frequency of bowel movements is often overlooked. Patients who are ultimately hospitalized usually develop lethargy and mild weakness with feeding difficulties, pooled oral secretions, and an altered cry. The baby eventually becomes floppy, loses head control, and may go on to develop ophthalmoplegia, ptosis, flaccid facial expression, dysphagia, other signs of cranial nerve deficits, and generalized muscular weakness. Respiratory insufficiency necessitating respiratory therapy also may occur, as in other forms of botulism (7, 8). There is a spectrum of clinical features in infant botulism, ranging from mild illness not requiring hospitalization to sudden death, and this syndrome accounts for a small percentage of cases of sudden infant death syndrome (7, 9). The differential diagnosis of infant botulism has included sepsis, myasthenia gravis, failure to thrive, benign congenital hypotonia, and a variety of other conditions.

Tetanus

Tetanus is an extremely dramatic illness produced by the action of a potent neurotoxin, tetanospasmin, which is elaborated by *C. tetani*. Tetanospasmin is a heat-labile protoplasmic protein that is released after the autolysis of *C. tetani*. The toxin becomes bound to gangliosides in the central nervous system and blocks inhibitory impulses to the motor neurons, thus producing prolonged muscle spasms of both flexor and extensor muscles. Like the botulinal toxins, tetanospasmin acts at myoneural junctions to inhibit the release of acetylcholine. The binding sites for tetanospasmin and botulinal toxins differ; spasticity is characteristic of tetanus, and flaccid paralysis is characteristic of botulism (25). Tetanus is still largely a disease of the unimmunized in the United States and is reported most frequently from areas of the rural South. It would be unusual for the clinical laboratory to be requested to isolate *C. tetani* from a wound, since tetanus usually presents little diagnostic problems for the clinician. For more details on tetanus, see Furste et al. (32), Smith and Williams (90), Willis (109), and the excellent review by Dowell (25).

COLLECTION AND TRANSPORT OF CLINICAL SPECIMENS

As with other anaerobic bacteria, the proper selection, collection, and transport of clinical specimens are extremely important for the laboratory diagnosis of clostridial infections. For recommended collection and transport procedures in general, refer to chapters 3 and 49. Several tissue specimens should be taken from the active site of infection when gas gangrene is suspected, because the clostridia are often not distributed uniformly in pathological lesions.

Specimens for confirmation of *C. perfringens* food-borne illness

For a laboratory confirmation of *C. perfringens* food-borne illness, most clinical laboratories will need to use the services of a reference laboratory (e.g., local or state public health laboratory). For the shipment of food and fecal specimens to a reference laboratory, the samples should be collected in sterile, leakproof containers and transported at 4°C. Rectal swabs should be placed in an anaerobic transport container (chapter 49) and shipped at 4°C (84).

Specimens for *C. difficile* culture and toxin assay

A single, freshly passed fecal specimen (ideally 10 to 20 ml of watery stool; minimum of 5.0 ml or 5 g) is the preferred specimen for *C. difficile* culture and toxin assay. To lessen the chance of obtaining positive culture results from patients merely colonized with the organism, we recommend that only liquid or unformed stool specimens be processed. Results of testing solid, formed stools are not likely to contribute to the diagnosis of *C. difficile*-associated disease. An exception could be made for epidemiologic surveys in which the objective is to determine the degree of *C. difficile* carriage in a population. Swab specimens are inadequate for the toxin assay because the volume of sample obtained is too small, although swabs have been used successfully to detect carriers during epidemiologic investigations (67). Other appropriate specimens include lumen contents and surgical or autopsy samples of the large bowel. Specimens should be transported in tightly sealed, leakproof plastic or glass containers. To yield optimal recovery, stool specimens should be cultured within 2 h of collection; although spores will survive in refrigerated stool for several days, there will probably be a large decrease in the number of viable vegetative cells of *C. difficile* in refrigerated specimens. Stools may be placed in an anaerobic environment (anaerobic transport vial or swab) if culture must be performed after storage. Adequate recovery of *C. difficile* may be expected from stools stored at 5°C for up to 2 days. Specimens for toxin assay may be stored at 5°C for up to 3 days and should be frozen at −70°C if a longer delay is anticipated before the assay is performed. Freezing at −20°C results in a dramatic loss of cytotoxin activity. Specimens to be tested by the CDT latex agglutination assay can be refrigerated for up to 3 days, as recommended by the manufacturer (Culturette Brand CDT *C. difficile* test; Becton Dickinson Microbiology Systems, Cockeysville, Md.). Freezing of stool specimens may result in a loss of sensitivity for the antigen detected by the latex test and is not recommended.

Suspected neutropenic enterocolitis involving *C. septicum*

The specimens of choice for suspected neutropenic enterocolitis involving *C. septicum* are three blood cultures collected from three different venipuncture sites, stool (at least 25 g or 25 ml, if liquid), and lumen contents or tissue from the involved ileocecal area collected at surgery or autopsy and transported in tightly sealed leakproof containers. In addition, a biopsy sample of muscle (or an aspirate of fluid from the involved area, taken by needle and syringe) should be collected if the patient is also suspected of having myonecrosis.

Specimens for *C. botulinum* culture and toxin assay

The clinical diagnosis of food-borne botulism can be confirmed by the demonstration of botulinal toxin in serum, feces, gastric contents, or vomitus or by the recovery of *C. botulinum* from the feces of the patient. The organism has been isolated only rarely from individuals who were not victims of the illness or who had eaten food contaminated with *C. botulinum* that had caused botulism in others during an outbreak (4, 42). The demonstration of botulinal toxin and *C. botulinum* in suspect foods aids in determining the food item responsible for an outbreak, but it provides only indirect evidence to support a clinical diagnosis of botulism. Ideally, 15 to 20 ml of serum (not whole blood), 25 to 50 g of stool, and the suspect food(s) should be collected. Specimens to collect from patients with suspected wound botulism include serum, feces, tissue, exudate, or swab samples from the wound. When infant botulism is suspected, collect serum (2 ml) and as much passed stool as possible. In most instances, the diagnosis of infant botulism has been confirmed by the detection of the toxin or *C. botulinum* or both in feces. Toxin has been detected in serum only infrequently in infants with this diagnosis.

Most hospital laboratories are not properly equipped to process specimens from patients suspected of having botulism. The CDC, Atlanta, Ga., provides epidemiologic aid and emergency laboratory services 24 h a day, every day of the week. The attending physician or state epidemiologist should notify the CDC immediately when there is a suspected case of botulism so that appropriate action can be taken to establish the diagnosis, initiate treatment, and investigate the potential outbreak. The appropriate CDC telephone number (available 24 h/day) for enteric disease epidemiologic aid is (404) 639-3753.

DIRECT EXAMINATION

The direct microscopic examination of clinical materials can provide extremely useful information for the physician in the diagnosis and treatment of clostridial infections. Gas gangrene is an extremely urgent situation, requiring a rapid clinical diagnosis. The direct examination of a Gram-stained smear of the wound may be of special aid to the clinician in establishing the diagnosis. Characteristic findings are the absence of inflammatory cells and other cellular outlines and the presence of clostridia in smears prepared from the central areas of the lesion. It is important to distinguish clostridial myonecrosis, which requires radical surgical excision or amputation of a limb, from anaerobic cellulitis, nonclostridial anaerobic cellulitis, or spreading fasciitis (12, 31). The muscle is usually not necrotic in the last three conditions and should not need to be removed. Nonclostridial anaerobic cellulitis may involve anaerobic cocci, facultatively anaerobic cocci, *Bacteriodes* spp., *Fusobacterium* spp., and other microorganisms. Cell outlines of striated muscle cells and granulocytes remain intact in the latter condition.

The usual Gram stain is satisfactory for the direct examination of a specimen. Special note should be taken of gram-positive rods with or without spores because sporulation in tissue is not common with the two species most frequently encountered in wound and abscess materials, *C. perfringens* and *C. ramosum*. *C. perfringens* usually appears as large, relatively short, fat, gram-positive rods in tissue smears; the cells of *C. ramosum* are more slender, longer, and often curved (56). *C. perfringens* may or may not be encapsulated in smears from wounds; capsules usually are present in smears of endometrial specimens from postabortion *C. perfringens* infections. Special spore stains offer no advantage over Gram stains for the demonstration of spores. Examination with a phase microscope is helpful if the spores are mature or nearly so. If spores are present, note their shape (spherical or oval) and position (terminal or subterminal to central) in the cells. The best single medium for the demonstration of spores is chopped meat medium made up as an agar slant. Incubate the culture anaerobically at 5 to 7°C below the optimum temperature for growth of the clostridia. For most species, 30°C is satisfactory, but 37°C is better for inducing sporulation of *C. perfringens*. If spores are not visible, their presence may be deduced by subjecting a suspension of the isolate to heat (80°C) or ethanol treatment (described below).

CULTURE AND ISOLATION

The general procedures described in chapter 49 for the collection and transport of specimens and for the isolation and examination of cultures apply to the clostridia. Clostridia usually produce good growth on commercially available CDC anaerobe blood agar and phenylethyl alcohol blood agar (PEA) after 1 to 2 days of incubation. Brucella 5% sheep blood agar, Columbia or brain heart infusion agar supplemented with yeast extract, vitamin K_1, and hemin may also be used as the nonselective blood agar medium; colonial characteristics vary on these different media. A few species, such as *C. perfringens*, form colonies after overnight incubation. When clostridia are suspected in wound or abscess specimens (e.g., from gas gangrene), it is recommended that egg yolk agar (modified McClung-Toabe formula; 26) or neomycin egg yolk (NEY) agar be inoculated in addition to blood agar and PEA. To prepare NEY medium, neomycin is added to achieve a final concentration of 100 μg/ml. Neomycin is heat stable and can be added before the medium is autoclaved. Neomycin can also be added to anaerobe blood agar in the same concentration. The purpose of neomycin is to inhibit some of the facultatively anaerobic gram-negative bacilli; thus, NEY medium is moderately selective.

After incubation, examine the blood agar and PEA cultures with a dissecting microscope, noting particularly the hemolysis pattern, colony structure, and any evidence of swarming or of motile colonies. Examine the egg yolk agar or NEY culture for evidence of lecithinase (phospholipase C) or lipase production. Lecithinase activity is indicated in either medium by the development of an insoluble, opaque, whitish precipitate within the agar. An iridescent sheen or oil-on-water appearance (pearly layer) on the surface growth indicates lipase activity. Proteolysis, the third reaction that can be seen on egg yolk agar or NEY medium, is indicated by a zone of translucent clearing in the medium around the colonies. In addition to the modified McClung-Toabe egg yolk agar formulation (26), these same reactions can be determined on the hemin-supplemented egg yolk agar formulation recommended by Sutter et al. (97) or on Lombard-Dowell egg yolk agar (Presumpto plate; 27, 56).

If swarming growth has covered the surface of the agar medium, inoculate another blood agar plate and incubate it anaerobically only overnight. Subculture from the colonies as soon as the plates are taken from the anaerobe jar. If swarming is again observed, subculture the isolate to a PEA blood agar plate to inhibit swarming. Alternatively, anaerobic blood agar made up with 4% (or higher concentration) agar may be useful. This mixture is known as stiff blood agar (26). When isolated colonies can be picked, subculture them to chopped meat medium, incubate the culture overnight, and use it for the inoculation of differential media. In addition, inoculate chopped meat-carbohydrate broth (50) for gas-liquid chromatography.

Spore selection techniques

Most clinical specimens other than blood in which clostridia may be sought (feces, material from wounds and abscesses, muscle and other soft tissue, surgical removal specimens, necropsy materials, etc.) yield a mixture of nonsporeforming bacteria. The possibilities include virtually any nonsporeforming bacteria that grow aerobically or anaerobically. A spore selection technique, with heat or alcohol treatment, is a useful selective means of isolating sporeformers while inhibiting nonsporeformers. Spores of clostridia (or of *Ba-*

cillus spp.) resist the heat or alcohol treatment, whereas vegetative cells are killed. After these treatments, spores will germinate and produce growth under appropriate conditions. Heat treatment alone should not be relied upon, because the spores of various *Clostridium* spp. and strains of species vary in their degree of resistance to heat. Treatment of specimens with at least 50% ethanol (final concentration) for 1 h aids in the selective isolation of clostridia from mixed infections and circumvents the problem of different spore tolerances to heat (57). The major problem to avoid with alcohol treatment is the presence of solid specimen particles that are not adequately penetrated by the alcohol. When the specimen is not sufficiently homogenized, the vegetative cells of nonsporeformers may not be inhibited.

Alcohol treatment. To a 1-ml sample of a fecal suspension, a homogenate of a wound or exudate, etc., in a sterile screw-cap tube, add an equal volume of absolute (or 95%) ethyl alcohol (57). Mix the specimen gently at room temperature (22 to 25°C) for 1 h. An Ames Aliquot Mixer (Miles Laboratories, Inc., Elkhart, Ind.) is a convenient way to provide continuous mixing. Subculture the treated material, and inoculate chopped meat-glucose (or chopped meat-glucose-starch) medium, anaerobe blood agar, or egg yolk agar. Incubate the culture and inspect it for growth as described above (and in chapter 49). For stool specimens, it is often advantageous to alcohol treat separate 1-ml samples from a series of 1:10 dilutions. This treatment helps the alcohol penetrate solid particles.

Heat treatment. For heat treatment (26), preheat a tube of chopped meat-glucose-starch medium in an 80°C water bath for 5 min and then add 1 ml of sample suspension. Heat the culture for 10 min, remove the tube, and cool it in cold water. Subculture the treated sample suspension into an unheated tube of chopped meat-glucose-starch medium and onto an anaerobe blood agar and egg yolk agar plate. Incubate the culture anaerobically and examine it for growth as described above.

Laboratory investigation of *C. perfringens* food-borne illness

Methods for the enumeration of *C. perfringens* in foods and *C. perfringens* spores in feces with egg yolk-free tryptose-sulfite-cycloserine agar are described in detail by Hauschild and colleagues (44–46). Although methods for the detection of *C. perfringens* enterotoxin in feces have been described previously and are of considerable interest, these assays are still considered experimental and are generally not available in clinical laboratories (64, 84).

Primary isolation of *C. difficile* from feces

Stool or fecal swab material should be inoculated to cycloserine-cefoxitin-egg yolk-fructose agar (CCFA; 36), which is commercially available. Plates should be incubated anaerobically for 48 h before observation. Colonies of *C. difficile* are approximately 5 to 8 mm in diameter, yellowish, circular to irregular, and flat, with a rhizoid or erose edge and a ground-glass appearance. The colonies have a distinctive odor like *p*-cresol (or horse manure), and they fluoresce yellow-green under long-wavelength UV light.

In addition to the use of CCFA medium, *C. difficile* from fecal samples can be isolated by using an alcohol or heat shock spore selection technique, as described above. Studies by one of us demonstrated greater recovery of *C. difficile* from stool specimens with the heat shock procedure than with CCFA (i.e., 54 of 362 stools were positive by heat shock, versus 43 of 362 stools positive with use of CCFA); however, the differences were not statistically significant (Allen, unpublished data). If a spore selection technique is used, inoculate the alcohol- or heat-treated sample onto anaerobe blood agar and an egg yolk agar plate after treatment. It is important to realize that *C. difficile* does not produce spores on CCFA medium, so colonies from this medium should not be tested in a spore selection assay. After 48 h of incubation, colonies on anaerobic blood-containing agars are nonhemolytic, 2 to 4 mm in diameter, slightly raised, and flat, with a rhizoid or erose edge. They are gray to translucent and show a crystalline, iridescent internal speckling when viewed under a dissecting microscope. The odor remains distinctive. Gram stain of *C. difficile* reveals gram-positive to gram-variable rods that are thin, even sided, 0.5 μm wide by 3 to 5 μm long, and with subterminal spores (unless the stain was prepared from colonies on CCFA).

Presumptive identification of *C. difficile* from CCFA can be made by demonstrating typical colony morphology, Gram stain morphology, fluorescence, and characteristic odor. Definitive identification depends on demonstration of the unique pattern of short-chain fatty acid metabolic products by using gas-liquid chromatography (Table 3) and by biochemical characterization of isolates. Both API 20A (Analytab Products, Plainview, N.Y.) and API ZYM systems yield acceptable results (47).

Although they are adjuncts to the cytotoxin neutralization test, the isolation and identification of the organism alone or the presumptive demonstration of its presence by latex agglutination assay does not prove that a patient has *C. difficile*-mediated gastrointestinal illness, since the organism can be isolated from the feces of healthy newborns and hospitalized patients who have no evidence of gastrointestinal disease. Also, the latex test has a potential for cross-reactions with other bacteria (although significant numbers of these organisms are not found routinely in normal stool), including *C. sporogenes*, *C. botulinum*, and *Peptostreptococcus anaerobius* (63, 70). When warranted clinically, positive latex agglutination test results should be corroborated by another method, e.g., cytotoxin assay or culture. Diagnosis rests on correlation of laboratory and clinical data.

C. difficile cytotoxin assay

A commercial cytotoxin assay system containing human foreskin fibroblast monolayers in a 96-well microdilution plate format, diluent, toxin control, and neutralizing antiserum (Bartels Immunodiagnostic Supplies, Inc., Bellevue, Wash.) has been found to yield results comparable to those obtained by conventional cytotoxin assays (74, 112). This system uses a 1:40 dilution of the original sample.

Depending on the cells used and the dilution of feces tested, conventional systems have shown different levels of sensitivity (24). Laboratories wishing to develop an in-house cytotoxin assay should determine optimal parameters to correlate with the clinical assessment of disease favored by their clinicians. Neutralization of cytotoxic effects by specific anti-*C. difficile* antiserum or cross-reactive *C. sordellii* antiserum (65) is an essential step for accurate performance of the test. When performed concurrently with cytoxicity testing, neutralization allows reporting of a final result usually within 48 h. Testing stool filtrates diluted from 1:40 to 1:100 should yield reasonable results when HeLa, HEp-2, or WI-38 cell monolayers are used (11, 77). Cells may be purchased, or cell culture lines can be maintained from stock cultures by trypsinizing and passing the cells into fresh flasks with growth medium weekly and by substituting maintenance medium for growth medium after 24 h of incubation. Maintenance medium should be exchanged for fresh medium every 48 h. The media used for tissue culture assays are the same as those used for viral tissue cultures. The following conventional procedure is one variation (29).

1. Prepare a fresh tissue culture monolayer by aseptically pipetting all of the fluid medium from above the cell monolayer in a 25-cm^2 tissue culture flask, washing the cells with two changes of 5 ml of Hanks balanced salt solution (HBSS), and trypsinizing the cells by adding 5.0 ml of 10% trypsin in HBSS. Swirl the flask gently and allow it to sit at room temperature for 5 to 10 min or until most of the cell layer has detached (the cells will be floating in the medium). Add 10 ml of growth medium to dilute out the effects of the trypsin and adjust the cells to 50,000/ml in growth medium, using a hemacytometer. Distribute the well-mixed cell suspensions into flat-bottom tissue culture wells in a 96-well microdilution plate, 180 μl per well. Cover the wells and incubate the plate for 24 h in 5% CO_2 or until a confluent monolayer is established.
2. Dilute stool 1:1 in HBSS or phosphate-buffered saline. Centrifuge diluted stool samples (5 to 10 ml) at 2,500 × *g* for 20 min to produce a clear supernatant. Discard the pellet. Pass the supernatant through a 0.45-μm-pore-size membrane filter; dilute 0.1 ml of the filtrate with 0.1 ml of HBSS or phosphate-buffered saline for the toxin test well and dilute another 0.1 ml with 0.1 ml of antitoxin (*C. difficile* antitoxin, available from T. D. Wilkins, Virginia Polytechnic Institute and State University, Blacksburg, or *C. sordellii* antitoxin, available from the Bureau of Biologics, Food and Drug Administration, Bethesda, Md.) for the neutralization well. Fecal material will be at a 1:4 dilution.
3. Place 20 μl of each diluted filtrate into the growth medium in the fresh (24-h) tissue culture wells showing confluent monolayers, for a final 1:40 dilution of feces.
4. Inoculate control wells with known toxin, toxin plus antitoxin, growth medium alone, and antitoxin alone.
5. Cover the wells and incubate the plate in 5% CO_2 for up to 72 h, observing for CPE (rounding up and detaching of cells) after each 24-h incubation.
6. Positive results will show CPE in the toxin control well and in the well containing patient filtrate with growth medium but not in the well with growth medium alone, the antitoxin alone, or the patient filtrate plus antitoxin. If CPE occurs with both the neutralized and diluted patient filtrates, nonspecific toxicity is present and the test cannot be interpreted. By diluting the patient stool filtrate and repeating the test with several dilutions (up to 1:1,000), the nonspecific toxicity may be eliminated.

DISTINGUISHING FEATURES OF COMMONLY ISOLATED SPECIES

As stated in the beginning of the chapter, isolates that are sporeforming, catalase-negative, anaerobic or aerotolerant bacilli are, by definition, species of the genus *Clostridium*. To avoid misidentification of gram-variable or gram-negative clostridia (e.g., *C. ramosum* and *C. clostridiiforme*) as *Bacteroides* or *Fusobacterium* species, inhibition by vancomycin (5-μg disk; described in chapter 49) should be verified; virtually all *Clostridium* species are inhibited by vancomycin (97).

Some especially useful characteristics for differentiation of the *Clostridium* species are relation to oxygen, spore location in the cell, motility, lecithinase production, lipase production, hydrolysis of gelatin, action on milk, urease activity, indole production, and the fermentation of key carbohydrates (Table 3). Other useful characteristics include short-chain acid metabolic products analyzed by gas-liquid chromatography (described in chapter 49). Certain clinically important clostridia can be differentiated to the species level (e.g., *C. botulinum*) only by the inclusion of toxin neutralization tests.

As reviewed elsewhere (56), several commercial packaged kits have been marketed and evaluated for the rapid identification of anaerobes in general. Three evaluations of the An-Ident system (Analytab Products), which examined clostridia in general, showed that 59 to 81% (overall mean of 64%) of 120 clostridia tested were identified without the use of additional tests (19, 72, 93). The system performed best with *C. perfringens*. In another study, An-Ident was found to identify only 77.9% of the *C. difficile* isolates tested (47). RapID-ANA II (Innovative Diagnostic Systems, Inc., Decatur, Ga.) is a revised and recently marketed system that tests for 18 preformed enzymes and has an expanded code compendium. At this writing, no evaluations of this modified system have been published. Preliminary data indicate that RapID-ANA II permits correct identifications of *C. perfringens* and some of the other commonly encountered clostridia but that it is not able to differentiate all of the *Clostridium* spp. encountered in clinical materials (J. A. Siders and S. D. Allen, unpublished data). The Vitek ANI system (Vitek Systems, Inc., Hazelwood, Mo.) was found to identify 63.7% of 44 clostridia tested to the species level (82). Although it identified 8 of 8 *C. perfringens* correctly, it identified only 7 of 11 (64%) strains of *C. difficile*. Thus, without the use of supplemental tests, no one of these three micromethod systems should be relied on for the identification of clostridia. The biochemical and morphologic characteristics listed in the preceding paragraph (also see Table 3) are within the capabilities of most clinical laboratories, and with the exception of toxicity testing, most of them should be determined for all isolates of clostridia from blood, properly selected and collected deep wound and abscess specimens, and usually sterile body fluids (other than urine). If packaged kit results are generated, these results should be compared against the results obtained from the practical and supplemental tests mentioned above to avoid errors with the kit identification results.

Presumptive identification of a few species can be accomplished fairly rapidly without the need of packaged micromethod kits. Fluorescent-antibody reagents for *C. septicum*, *C. novyi*, *C. chauvoei* (found only in infections of herbivores), and *C. sordellii* (Wellcome Research Laboratories, Beckenham, England) permit the rapid presumptive identification of these species.

C. perfringens is signaled by colonies on blood agar plates that are surrounded by narrow inner zones of complete hemolysis and wider outer zones of discoloration and incomplete hemolysis. Gram-stained smears of 48- to 72-h colonies characteristically show short to intermediate gram-positive or gram-variable rods without spores. Subculture such a colony to an egg yolk agar plate, one-half of which has been spread with *C. perfringens* antitoxin (Cooper Animal Health, Inc., Kansas City, Mo.) and incubate the culture anaerobically overnight. *C. perfringens* will produce a zone of precipitation around colonies on the control side of the plate and little or no precipitation on the side spread with antitoxin (this response is known as the Nagler reaction). Similar reactions will be given by *C. bifermentans*, *C. sordellii*, and *C. barati* (formerly *C. paraperfringens*), but these species should not cause difficulty. *C. bifermentans* does not form a double zone of hemolysis, sporulates readily, is motile, is more proteolytic than *C. perfringens*, produces indole (e.g., with use of the spot indole test described in chapter 49), and varies from *C. perfringens* in other cultural characteristics. *C. sordellii* resembles *C. bifermentans*, but *C. sordellii* is urease positive. None of the other clostridia listed in Table 3 are urease positive. *C. barati* is so seldom encountered in clinical material (Table 1) that it is not likely to be an appreciable source of error. *C. perfringens* liquefies gelatin, but *C. barati* does not.

A recently marketed rapid glutamic acid decarboxylase microdilution test (Carr-Scarborough Microbiologicals, Inc., Stone Mountain, Ga.) was found to aid in the differentiation of commonly isolated clostridia (10). In this test, a semisolid medium contained in a microdilution tube is inoculated heavily with a pure culture of a *Clostridium* isolate; the tube is incubated aerobically at 35°C for up to 4 h and then observed for a change from green to dark blue. Banks et al. showed that organisms producing a positive glutamic acid decarboxylase reaction were *C. perfringens* (30 of 31 strains), *C. sordellii* (10 of 10 strains), *C. barati* (15 of 15 strains), and *C. difficile* (3 of 12 strains); each of the other clostridia tested gave negative reactions (10).

C. difficile is relatively easy to recognize and identify. As indicated above, it has a distinctive odor in culture and produces characteristic colonies on anaerobe blood agar, PEA, and CCFA (36, 56, 97). It produces subterminal spores that are readily seen on Gram stains of colonies on 2- to 3-day-old blood agar plates. *C. difficile* is motile, which can be shown by the preparation of a wet mount from a fresh colony or a broth culture. Metabolic product analysis typically shows acetic, propionic, isobutyric, butyric, isovaleric, valeric, and isocaproic acids. A large peak of isocaproic acid is a key characteristic. Other commonly encountered *Clostridium* species with subterminal spores that may produce isocaproic acid include *C. sporogenes*, *C. bifermentans*, *C. sordellii*, and sometimes *C. subterminale*. *C. sporogenes* produces Medusa-head colonies on anaerobe blood agar that are distinct from those of *C. difficile*. *C. bifermentans* and *C. sordellii* are both indole positive, but *C. difficile* is indole negative. *C. subterminale* differs in several biochemical characteristics (Table 3). The Presumpto plate system, originally developed by Dowell and Lombard (27), permits the rapid differentiation of clostridia in general and is a practical way to separate *C. difficile* from other clostridia (56). In this system, *C. difficile* hydrolyzes esculin and gelatin but is negative for indole and nitrate (analyses are done by rapid disk tests). *C. difficile* is saccharolytic and is one of the few clostridia that ferments mannitol. A useful test which aids in the rapid identification of *C. difficile* is the performance of gas-liquid chromatography on a norleucine-tyrosine broth culture (76). All 120 strains of *C. difficile* tested produced caproic acid and *p*-cresol in the norleucine-tyrosine medium; none of the other clostridia or other bacteria examined produced both products.

It is often difficult to isolate *C. tetani* from a suspected lesion. When this organism is being sought, a freshly poured blood agar plate should be inoculated lightly. Incubate the culture for 1 day and examine it carefully for swarming, which may be in the form of a very thin layer. Transfer cells from the edge of the swarming area to a tube of broth and streak a plate of medium containing 5% agar; incubate the culture and pick an isolated colony. Animal inoculation (a reference laboratory procedure) may be required for demonstration of *C. tetani* in a specimen. A small amount of material from the lesion is emulsified in sterile broth, and 0.1 ml of this material is injected into each of four mice, beside the base of the tail. Two of the mice are injected additionally with 0.1 ml of tetanus antitoxin. Death or symptoms of tetanus in the unprotected mice indicate the presence of *C. tetani* in the specimen. Different approaches to presumptive identification are described in detail elsewhere (56, 97).

IDENTIFICATION

To identify clostridia, inoculate the prereduced anaerobically sterilized (PRAS) tubed media (available commercially) and other media indicated in Table 3, prepared as described by Holdeman et al. (50) (see chapter 49). Although the CHO-based media of Dowell and Hawkins (26) provide an excellent system for characterizing clostridia and can be used, Table 3 is based on results obtained with PRAS media, and a few of the reactions differ. Thus, if CHO-based media are used, other tables should be consulted (26). Incubate the cultures for 24 to 72 h at 35 to 37°C; overnight incubation is often sufficient for many clostridia in PRAS media if growth is prompt and adequate. Examine Gram stains of the chopped meat culture to determine the presence, position, and shape of the spores. If spores are not found, inoculate a tube of chopped meat medium, heat the culture at 70°C for 10 min, and incubate the tube. Growth in this heated tube usually indicates the presence of spores, although none may be apparent microscopically. Alternatively, an alcohol spore selection technique may be helpful for those clostridia with heat-sensitive spores (57).

Determine carbohydrate fermentation by measuring pH (50). Determine the metabolic products from chopped meat-carbohydrate broth culture by gas chromatography (chapter 49). Results will not be identical if peptone-yeast extract-glucose is the culture medium (26, 50). The identification of *Clostridium* species can be made without gas chromatography, but such identification usually involves more time. The information listed in Table 3 will serve to identify most of the clostridia commonly isolated from clinical specimens. Information on additional tests and descriptions of differential characteristics of additional species can be found elsewhere (20, 26, 50, 56, 90, 97).

Toxin tests are necessary for the identification of a few species. *C. sporogenes* cannot be differentiated with certainty from the proteolytic group I strains of *C. botulinum* unless toxin tests are used. A few strains of group III *C. botulinum* produce lecithinase as well as lipase and are difficult to distinguish from *C. novyi* type A except by toxin tests or by the use of a *C. novyi* fluorescent-antibody conjugate (90). To test for toxin, inoculate two tubes of chopped meat-glucose medium; incubate one tube at 37°C overnight and incubate the other tube at 37°C for 3 days. Test the overnight culture first; if no toxin is found, test the 3-day culture. Centrifuge the culture and place 1.2-ml amounts of the supernatant in several tubes. Add 0.3 ml of appropriate antiserum per tube for the various species suspected. Let the well-mixed suspensions stand for 30 min at room temperature or at 37°C and then inject 0.5-ml portions of control supernatant (without antiserum) and antiserum mixtures intraperitoneally into each of two mice. Observe the mice for 3 days and record the deaths that occur. Only specific sera for laboratory testing should be used for toxin identification; therapeutic sera are often unsatisfactory because they may contain antibodies to toxins of species other than those listed on the label. Diagnostic clostridial antisera are available from Wellcome Reagents Ltd., Wellcome Research Laboratories, Beckenham, England BR3 3BS.

If it is necessary to determine the toxin type of an isolate of *C. perfringens* or *C. botulinum,* it is best to send the isolate to a reference laboratory. However, veterinary clinical microbiology laboratories should be familiar with the technique for determining the toxin type of *C. perfringens* isolates.

SUSCEPTIBILITY TO ANTIMICROBIAL AGENTS

Penicillin G shows excellent activity against most but not all strains of *C. perfringens* and has traditionally been considered the antibiotic of choice for the clostridia in general (80, 83). However, resistance is slowly increasing in *C. perfringens,* to the extent that alternative antimicrobial agents will need to be considered (12). β-Lactamase has not been demonstrated in *C. perfringens.* As referred to by Hecht et al., resistance to penicillin in *C. perfringens* has been shown to involve a decreased affinity of penicillin-binding protein 1 for penicillin (48). Resistance to penicillin is especially common in *C. ramosum, C. clostridiiforme,* and *C. butyricum* (28, 80); these species produce β-lactamases that are induced by β-lactam antibiotics (48).

Although clindamycin is still highly active against most species of commonly encountered anaerobic bacteria in the United States, a number of clostridia are frequently resistant to it. These clostridia include strains of the following species: *C. ramosum, C. difficile, C. tertium, C. subterminale, C. innocuum, C. sporogenes,* and some strains of *C. perfringens* (108).

Chloramphenicol, piperacillin, metronidazole, imipenem, and combinations of β-lactam drugs with β-lactam inhibitors (e.g., ampicillin-sulbactam) are active against nearly all of the clostridia, with only a few exceptions (12, 28, 80). The clostridia have shown variable resistance to the cephalosporins and tetracyclines, and they are usually resistant to the aminoglycosides. The quinolones, of which ciprofloxacin is the most active, have not shown remarkable activity against the clostridia (80). Many clostridia other than *C. perfringens* are resistant to cefoxitin, cefotaxime, ceftazidime, ceftizoxime, moxalactam, cefoperazone, and other third-generation β-lactam drugs (28, 80).

Severe *C. difficile*-associated intestinal disease is usually treated with oral vancomycin or metronidazole, although most strains of *C. difficile* are susceptible to a number of antimicrobial agents in vitro (including penicillins, tetracycline, and quinolones). For patients unable to tolerate oral antibiotics whose conditions require therapy, parenteral vancomycin or metronidazole is recommended (33). Antibiotic therapy often results in relapse of disease, so discontinuation of the offending agent or change to an agent less likely to cause diarrhea should be considered the primary intervention of choice (33).

LITERATURE CITED

1. **Alpern, R. J., and V. R. Dowell, Jr.** 1971. Nonhistotoxic clostridial bacteremia. Am. J. Clin. Pathol. **55:**717–722.
2. **Altemeier, W. A., and W. R. Culbertson.** 1948. Acute nonclostridial crepitant cellulitis. Surg. Gynecol. Obstet. **87:**206–212.
3. **Altemeier, W. A., and W. L. Furste.** 1947. Gas gangrene. Surg. Gynecol. Obstet. **84:**507–523.
4. **Anonymous.** 1979. Botulism in the United States, 1899–1977. Handbook for epidemiologists, clinicians and laboratory workers. Center for Disease Control, Atlanta.
5. **Anonymous.** 1983. Foodborne disease outbreaks annual summary 1981. Centers for Disease Control, Atlanta.
6. **Anonymous.** 1989. Summary of notifiable diseases, United States 1988. Morbid. Mortality Weekly Rep. **33:** 165–166.
7. **Arnon, S. S.** 1989. Infant botulism, p. 601–609. *In* S. M. Finegold and W. L. George (ed.), Anaerobic infections in humans. Academic Press, Inc., New York.
8. **Arnon, S. S., and J. Chin.** 1979. The clinical spectrum of infant botulism. Rev. Infect. Dis. **1:**614–624.
9. **Arnon, S. S., K. Damus, and J. Chin.** 1981. Infant botulism: epidemiology and relation to sudden infant death syndrome. Epidemiol. Rev. **3:**45–66.
10. **Banks, E. R., S. D. Allen, J. A. Siders, and N. A. O'Bryan.** 1989. Characterization of anaerobic bacteria by using a commercially available rapid tube test for glutamic acid decarboxylase. J. Clin. Microbiol. **27:**361–363.
11. **Bartlett, J. G.** 1981. Laboratory diagnosis of antibiotic-associated colitis. Lab. Med. **12:**347–351.
12. **Bartlett, J. G.** 1990. Gas gangrene (other *Clostridium*-associated diseases), p. 1850–1860. *In* G. L. Mandell, R. G. Douglas, Jr., and J. E. Bennett (ed.), Principles and practice of infectious diseases, 3rd ed. Churchill Livingstone, Inc., New York.
13. **Bennion, R. S., E. J. Baron, J. E. Thompson, Jr., J. Downes, P. Summanen, D. A. Talan, and S. M. Finegold.** 1990. The bacteriology of gangrenous and perforated appendicitis—revisited. Ann. Surg. **211:**165–171.
14. **Bignold, L. P., and H. P. B. Harvey.** 1979. Necrotizing enterocolitis associated with invasion by *Clostridium septicum* complicating cyclic neutropaenia. Aust. N.Z. J. Med. **9:**426–429.
15. **Borriello, S. P., F. E. Barclay, A. R. Welch, M. F. Stringer, G. N. Watson, R. K. T. Williams, D. V. Seal, and K. Sullens.** 1985. Epidemiology of diarrhoea caused by enterotoxigenic *Clostridium perfringens.* J. Med. Mi-

crobiol. **20:**363–372.

16. **Borriello, S. P., H. E. Larson, A. R. Welch, F. Barclay, M. F. Stringer, and B. A. Bartholomew.** 1984. Enterotoxigenic *Clostridium perfringens:* a possible cause of antibiotic-associated diarrhea. Lancet **i:**305–307.
17. **Brock, T. D., and M. T. Madigan.** 1988. Biology of microorganisms, 5th ed. Prentice-Hall, Inc., Englewood Cliffs, N.J.
18. **Brook, I.** 1989. Anaerobic bacterial bacteremia: 12-year experience in two military hospitals. J. Infect. Dis. **160:**1071–1075.
19. **Burlage, R. S., and P. D. Ellner.** 1985. Comparison of PRAS II, AN-Ident, and RapID-ANA systems for identification of anaerobic bacteria. J. Clin. Microbiol. **22:**32–35.
20. **Cato, E. P., W. L. George, and S. M. Finegold.** 1986. Genus *Clostridium* Prazmowski, p. 1141–1200. *In* P. H. A. Sneath, N. S. Mair, M. E. Sharpe, and J. G. Holt (ed.), Bergey's manual of systematic bacteriology, vol. 2. The Williams & Wilkins Co., Baltimore.
21. **Cooperstock, M.** 1988. *Clostridium difficile* in infants and children, p. 45–64. *In* R. D. Rolfe and S. M. Finegold (ed.), *Clostridium difficile:* its role in intestinal disease. Academic Press, Inc., New York.
22. **Decker, W. H., and W. Hall.** 1966. Treatment of abortions infected with *Clostridium welchii.* Am. J. Obstet. Gynecol. **95:**394–399.
23. **Donta, S. T.** 1988. Mechanism of action of *Clostridium difficile* toxins, p. 169–181. *In* R. D. Rolfe and S. M. Finegold (ed.), *Clostridium difficile:* its role in intestinal disease. Academic Press, Inc., New York.
24. **Donta, S. T., N. Sullivan, and T. D. Wilkins.** 1982. Differential effects of *Clostridium difficile* toxins on tissue-cultured cells. J. Clin. Microbiol. **15:**1157–1158.
25. **Dowell, V. R., Jr.** 1984. Botulism and tetanus: selected epidemiologic and microbiologic aspects. Rev. Infect. Dis. **6**(Suppl. 1):S202–S207.
26. **Dowell, V. R., Jr., and T. M. Hawkins.** 1977. Laboratory methods in anaerobic bacteriology, CDC laboratory manual. Department of Health, Education, and Welfare publication no. (CDC) 78-8272. Center for Disease Control, Atlanta.
27. **Dowell, V. R., Jr., and G. L. Lombard.** 1982. Differential agar media for identification of anaerobic bacteria, p. 258–262. *In* R. C. Tilton (ed.), Rapid methods and automation in microbiology. American Society for Microbiology, Washington, D.C.
28. **Finegold, S. M.** 1989. Therapy of anaerobic infections, p. 793–818. *In* S. M. Finegold and W. L. George (ed.), Anaerobic infections in humans. Academic Press, Inc., New York.
29. **Finegold, S. M., and E. J. Baron.** 1986. Microorganisms encountered in the gastrointestinal tract, p. 260–278. *In* Bailey & Scott's diagnostic microbiology, 7th ed. The C. V. Mosby Co., St. Louis.
30. **Finegold, S. M., and W. L. George (ed.).** 1989. Anaerobic infections in humans. Academic Press, Inc., New York.
31. **Finegold, S. M., W. L. George, and M. E. Mulligan.** 1986. Anaerobic infections. Year Book Medical Publishers, Inc., Chicago.
32. **Furste, W., A. Aquirre, and D. J. Knoepfler.** 1989. Tetanus, p. 611–627. *In* S. M. Finegold and W. L. George (ed.), Anaerobic infections in humans. Academic Press, Inc., New York.
33. **George, W. L.** 1989. Antimicrobial agent-associated diarrhea and colitis, p. 661–678. *In* S. M. Finegold and W. L. George (ed.), Anaerobic infections in humans. Academic Press, Inc., New York.
34. **George, W. L., and S. M. Finegold.** 1985. Clostridia in the human gastrointestinal flora, p. 1–37. *In* S. P. Borriello (ed.), Clostridia in gastrointestinal disease. CRC Press, Inc., Boca Raton, Fla.
35. **George, W. L., R. D. Rolfe, G. M. Harding, R. Klein, C. W. Putman, and S. M. Finegold.** 1982. *Clostridium difficile* and cytotoxin in feces of patients with antimicrobial agent-associated pseudomembranous colitis. Infection **10:**205–207.
36. **George, W. L., V. L. Sutter, D. Citron, and S. M. Finegold.** 1979. Selective and differential medium for isolation of *Clostridium difficile.* J. Clin. Microbiol. **9:**214–219.
37. **Gerding, D. N., R. L. Gebhard, H. W. Sumner, and L. R. Peterson.** 1988. Pathology and diagnosis of *Clostridium difficile* disease, p. 259–286. *In* R. D. Rolfe and S. M. Finegold (ed.), *Clostridium difficile:* its role in intestinal disease. Academic Press, Inc., New York.
38. **Gilligan, P. H., L. R. McCarthy, and V. M. Genta.** 1981. Relative frequency of *Clostridium difficile* in patients with diarrheal disease. J. Clin. Microbiol. **14:**26–31.
39. **Gorbach, S. L.** 1979. Other *Clostridium* species (including gas gangrene), p. 1876–1885. *In* G. L. Mandell, R. G. Douglas, Jr., and J. E. Bennett (ed.), Principles and practice of infectious diseases. John Wiley & Sons, Inc., New York.
40. **Gorbach, S. L., and H. Thadepalli.** 1975. Isolation of *Clostridium* in human infections: evaluation of 114 cases. J. Infect. Dis. **131:**S81–S85.
41. **Hall, J. D., L. M. McCroskey, B. J. Pincomb, and C. L. Hatheway.** 1985. Isolation of an organism resembling *Clostridium barati* which produces type F botulinal toxin from an infant with botulism. J. Clin. Microbiol. **21:**654–655.
42. **Hatheway, C. L.** 1988. Botulism, p. 111–133. *In* A. Balows, W. J. Hausler, Jr., M. Ohashi, and A. Turano (ed.), Laboratory diagnosis of infectious diseases: principles and practice, vol. 1. Springer-Verlag, New York.
43. **Hatheway, C. L.** 1990. Toxigenic clostridia. Clin. Microbiol. Rev. **3:**66–98.
44. **Hauschild, A. H. W.** 1975. Criteria and procedures for implicating *Clostridium perfringens* in food-borne outbreaks. Can. J. Public Health **66:**388–392.
45. **Hauschild, A. H. W., and R. Hilsheimer.** 1974. Enumeration of food-borne *Clostridium perfringens* in egg yolk-free tryptose-sulfite-cycloserine agar. Appl. Microbiol. **27:**521–526.
46. **Hauschild, A. H. W., R. Hilsheimer, and D. W. Griffith.** 1974. Enumeration of fecal *Clostridium perfringens* spores in egg yolk-free tryptose-sulfite-cycloserine agar. Appl. Microbiol. **27:**527–530.
47. **Head, C. B., and S. Ratnam.** 1988. Comparison of API ZYM system with API AN-Ident, API 20A, Minitek Anaerobe II, and RapID-ANA systems for identification of *Clostridium difficile.* J. Clin. Microbiol. **26:**144–146.
48. **Hecht, D. W., M. H. Malany, and F. P. Tally.** 1989. Mechanisms of resistance and resistance transfer in anaerobic bacteria, p. 755–769. *In* S. M. Finegold and W. L. George (ed.), Anaerobic infections in humans. Academic Press, Inc., New York.
49. **Hogan, S. F., and K. Ireland.** 1989. Fatal acute spontaneous endometritis resulting from *Clostridium sordellii.* Am. J. Clin. Pathol. **91:**104–106.
50. **Holdeman, L. V., E. P. Cato, and W. E. C. Moore (ed.).** 1977. Anaerobe laboratory manual, 4th ed. Virginia Polytechnic Institute and State University, Blacksburg, Va.
51. **Justus, P. G., J. L. Martin, D. A. Goldberg, N. S. Taylor, J. G. Bartlett, R. W. Alexander, and J. R. Mathias.** 1982. Myoelectric effects of *Clostridium difficile:* motility-altering factors distinct from its cytotoxin and enterotoxin in rabbits. Gastroenterology **83:**836–843.
52. **Kelly, M. T., S. G. Champagne, C. H. Sherlock, M. A. Noble, H. J. Freeman, and J. A. Smith.** 1987. Commercial latex agglutination test for detection of *Clostridium difficile*-associated diarrhea. J. Clin. Microbiol. **25:**1244–1247.
53. **Kim, K.-H., R. Fekety, D. H. Batts, D. Brown, M. Cudmore, J. Silva, Jr., and D. Waters.** 1981. Isolation of *Clostridium difficile* from the environment and contacts

of patients with antibiotic-associated colitis. J. Infect. Dis. **143:**42–44.
54. **King, A., A. Rampling, D. G. D. Wright, and R. E. Warren.** 1984. Neutropenic enterocolitis due to *Clostridium septicum* infection. J. Clin. Pathol. **37:**335–343.
55. **Kliegman, R. M., and A. A. Fanaroff.** 1984. Necrotizing enterocolitis. N. Engl. J. Med. **310:**1093–1103.
56. **Koneman, E. W., S. D. Allen, V. R. Dowell, Jr., W. M. Janda, H. M. Sommers, and W. C. Winn, Jr.** 1988. Color atlas and textbook of diagnostic microbiology, 3rd ed. J. B. Lippincott Co., Philadelphia.
57. **Koransky, J. R., S. D. Allen, and V. R. Dowell, Jr.** 1978. Use of ethanol for selective isolation of sporeforming microorganisms. Appl. Environ. Microbiol. **35:**762–765.
58. **Koransky, J. R., M. D. Stargel, and V. R. Dowell, Jr.** 1979. *Clostridium septicum* bacteremia: its clinical significance. Am. J. Med. **66:**63–66.
59. **Kornbluth, A. A., J. B. Danzig, and L. H. Bernstein.** 1989. *Clostridium septicum* infection and associated malignancy. Medicine **68:**30–37.
60. **Lashner, B. A., J. Todorczuk, D. F. Sahm, and S. B. Hanauer.** 1986. *Clostridium difficile* culture-positive toxin-negative diarrhea. Am. J. Gastroenterol. **81:**940–943.
61. **Lyerly, D. M., H. C. Krivan, and T. D. Wilkins.** 1988. *Clostridium difficile:* its disease and toxins. Clin. Microbiol. Rev. **1:**1–18.
62. **Lyerly, D. M., D. E. Lockwood, S. H. Richardson, and T. D. Wilkins.** 1982. Biological activities of toxins A and B of *Clostridium difficile*. Infect. Immun. **35:**1147–1150.
63. **Lyerly, D. M., and T. D. Wilkins.** 1986. Commercial latex test for *Clostridium difficile* toxin A does not detect toxin A. J. Clin. Microbiol. **23:**622–623.
64. **Mahony, D. E., E. Gilliatt, S. V. Dawson, E. Stockdale, and S. H. S. Lee.** 1989. Vero cell assay for rapid detection of *Clostridium perfringens* enterotoxin. Appl. Environ. Microbiol. **55:**2141–2143.
65. **Martinez, R. D., and T. D. Wilkins.** 1988. Purification and characterization of *Clostridium sordellii* hemorrhagic toxin and cross-reactivity with *Clostridium difficile* toxin A (enterotoxin). Infect. Immun. **56:**1215–1221.
66. **McDonald, M., P. Ward, and K. Harvey.** 1982. Antibiotic-associated diarrhoea and methicillin-resistant *Staphylococcus aureus*. Med. J. Aust. **1:**462–464.
67. **McFarland, L. V., M. B. Coyle, W. H. Kremer, and W. E. Stamm.** 1987. Rectal swab cultures for *Clostridium difficile* surveillance studies. J. Clin. Microbiol. **25:**2241–2242.
68. **McGregor, J. A., D. E. Soper, G. Lovell, and J. K. Todd.** 1989. Maternal deaths associated with *Clostridium sordellii* infection. Am. J. Obstet. Gynecol. **161:**987–995.
69. **Mclane, B. A., and J. T. Snyder.** 1987. Development and preliminary evaluation of a slide latex agglutination assay for detection of *Clostridium perfringens* type A enterotoxin. J. Immunol. Methods **100:**131–136.
70. **Miles, B. L., J. A. Siders, and S. D. Allen.** 1988. Evaluation of a commercial latex test for *Clostridium difficile* and cross-reactions with other bacteria. J. Clin. Microbiol. **26:**2452–2455.
71. **Mulligan, M. E., L. R. Peterson, R. Y. Y. Kwok, C. R. Clabots, and D. N. Gerding.** 1988. Immunoblots and plasmid fingerprints compared with serotyping and polyacrylamide gel electrophoresis for typing *Clostridium difficile*. J. Clin. Microbiol. **26:**41–46.
72. **Murray, P. R., C. J. Weber, and A. C. Niles.** 1985. Comparative evaluation of three identification systems for anaerobes. J. Clin. Microbiol. **22:**52–55.
73. **Murrell, T. G. C.** 1989. Enteritis necroticans, p. 639–659. *In* S. M. Finegold and W. L. George (ed.), Anaerobic infections in humans. Academic Press, Inc., New York.
74. **Nachamkin, I., L. Lotz-Nolan, and D. Skalina.** 1986. Evaluation of a commercial cytotoxicity assay for detection of *Clostridium difficile* toxin. J. Clin. Microbiol. **23:**954–955.
75. **Nichols, R. L., and J. W. Smith.** 1975. Gas in the wound; what does it mean? Surg. Clin. N. Am. **55:**1289–1296.
76. **Nunez-Montiel, O. L., F. S. Thompson, and V. R. Dowell, Jr.** 1983. Norleucine-tyrosine broth for rapid identification of *Clostridium difficile* by gas-liquid chromatography. J. Clin. Microbiol. **17:**382–385.
77. **Peterson, L. R., J. J. Holter, C. J. Shanholtzer, C. R. Garrett, and D. N. Gerding.** 1986. Detection of *Clostridium difficile* toxins A (enterotoxin) and B (cytotoxin) in clinical specimens; evaluation of a latex test. Am. J. Clin. Pathol. **86:**208–211.
78. **Peterson, L. R., M. M. Olson, C. J. Shanholtzer, and D. N. Gerding.** 1988. Results of a prospective, 18-month clinical evaluation of culture, cytotoxin testing, and Culturette brand (CDT) latex testing in the diagnosis of *Clostridium difficile*-associated diarrhea. Diagn. Microbiol. Infect. Dis. **10:**85–91.
79. **Rifkin, G. D.** 1980. Neutropenic enterocolitis and *Clostridium septicum* infection in patients with agranulocytosis. Arch. Intern. Med. **140:**834–835.
80. **Rosenblatt, J. E.** 1989. Antimicrobial susceptibility of anaerobic bacteria, p. 731–753. *In* S. M. Finegold and W. L. George (ed.), Anaerobic infections in humans. Academic Press, Inc., New York.
81. **Ryan, R. W., I. Kwasnik, and R. C. Tilton.** 1980. Rapid detection of *Clostridium difficile* toxin in human feces. J. Clin. Microbiol. **12:**776–779.
82. **Schreckenberger, P. C., D. M. Celig, and W. M. Janda.** 1988. Clinical evaluation of the Vitek ANI card for identification of anaerobic bacteria. J. Clin. Microbiol. **26:**225–230.
83. **Schwartzman, J. D., L. B. Reller, and W.-L. L. Wang.** 1977. Susceptibility of *Clostridium perfringens* isolated from human infection to twenty antibiotics. Antimicrob. Agents Chemother. **11:**695–697.
84. **Shandera, W. X., C. O. Tacket, and P. A. Blake.** 1983. Food poisoning due to *Clostridium perfringens* in the United States. J. Infect. Dis. **147:**163–170.
85. **Shanholtzer, C. J., L. R. Peterson, M. N. Olson, and D. N. Gerding.** 1983. Prospective study of gram-stained stool smears in diagnosis of *Clostridium difficile* colitis. J. Clin. Microbiol. **17:**906–908.
86. **Simpson, L. L.** 1989. Peripheral actions of the botulinum toxins, p. 153–178. *In* L. L. Simpson (ed.), Botulinum neurotoxin and tetanus toxin. Academic Press, Inc., New York.
87. **Smith, L. D.** 1978. The occurrence of *Clostridium botulinum* and *Clostridium tetani* in the soil of the United States. Health Lab. Sci. **15:**74–80.
88. **Smith, L. D.** 1979. Virulence factors of *Clostridium perfringens*. Rev. Infect. Dis. **1:**254–260.
89. **Smith, L. D., and H. Sugiyama.** 1988. Botulism: the organism, its toxins, the disease, 2nd ed. Charles C Thomas, Publisher, Springfield, Ill.
90. **Smith, L. D., and B. L. Williams.** 1984. The pathogenic anaerobic bacteria, 3rd ed. Charles C Thomas, Publisher, Springfield, Ill.
91. **Sonnabend, O., W. Sonnabend, R. Heinzle, T. Sigrist, R. Dirnhofer, and U. Krech.** 1981. Isolation of *Clostridium botulinum* type G and identification of type G botulinal toxin in humans: report of five sudden unexpected deaths. J. Infect. Dis. **143:**22–27.
92. **Spika, J. S., N. Shaffer, N. Hargrett-Bean, S. Collin, K. L. MacDonald, and P. A. Blake.** 1989. Risk factors for infant botulism in the United States. Am. J. Dis. Child. **143:**828–832.
93. **Stenson, M. J., D. T. Lee, J. E. Rosenblatt, and J. M. Contezac.** 1986. Evaluation of the AnIdent system for the identification of anaerobic bacteria. Diagn. Microbiol. Infect. Dis. **5:**9–15.
94. **Sterne, M., and G. H. Warrack.** 1964. The types of *Clostridium perfringens*. J. Pathol. Bacteriol. **88:**279–283.

95. **Suen, J. C., C. L. Hatheway, A. G. Steigerwalt, and D. J. Brenner.** 1988. *Clostridium argentinense*, sp. nov.: a genetically homogeneous group composed of all strains of *Clostridium botulinum* toxin type G and some nontoxigenic strains previously identified as *Clostridium subterminale* or *Clostridium hastiforme*. Int. J. Syst. Bacteriol. **38:**375–381.
96. **Sullivan, N. M., S. Pellett, and T. D. Wilkins.** 1982. Purification and characterization of toxins A and B of *Clostridium difficile*. Infect. Immun. **35:**1032–1040.
97. **Sutter, V. L., D. M. Citron, M. A. C. Edelstein, and S. M. Finegold.** 1985. Wadsworth anaerobic bacteriology manual, 4th ed. Star Publishing Co., Belmont, Calif.
98. **Swartz, M. N.** 1990. Myositis, p. 812–818. *In* G. L. Mandell, R. G. Douglas, Jr., and J. E. Bennett (ed.), Principles and practice of infectious diseases, 3rd ed. Churchill Livingstone, Inc., New York.
99. **Swartz, M. N.** 1990. Subcutaneous tissue infections and abscesses, p. 808–812. *In* G. L. Mandell, R. G. Douglas, Jr., and J. E. Bennett (ed.), Principles and practice of infectious diseases, 3rd ed. Churchill Livingstone, Inc., New York.
100. **VanBeek, A., E. Zook, P. Yaw, R. Gardner, R. Smith, and J. L. Glover.** 1974. Nonclostridial gas-forming infections. Arch. Surg. **108:**552–557.
101. **Varki, N. M., and T. I. Aquino.** 1982. Isolation of *Clostridium difficile* from hospitalized patients without antibiotic-associated diarrhea or colitis. J. Clin. Microbiol. **16:**659–662.
102. **Viscidi, R., S. Willey, and J. G. Bartlett.** 1981. Isolation rates and toxigenic potential of *Clostridium difficile* isolates from various patient populations. Gastroenterology **81:**5–9.
103. **Viscidi, R. P., R. H. Yolken, B. E. Laughon, and J. G. Bartlett.** 1983. Enzyme immunoassay for detection of antibody to toxins A and B of *Clostridium difficile*. J. Clin. Microbiol. **18:**242–247.
104. **Walker, P. D., T. G. C. Murrell, and L. K. Nagy.** 1980. Scanning electron microscopy of the jejunum in enteritis necroticans. J. Med. Microbiol. **13:**445–450.
105. **Walker, R. C., P. J. Ruane, J. E. Rosenblatt, D. M. Lyerly, C. A. Gleaves, T. F. Smith, P. F. Pierce, Jr., and T. D. Wilkins.** 1986. Comparison of culture, cytoxicity assays, and enzyme-linked immunosorbent assay for toxin A and toxin B in the diagnosis of *Clostridium difficile*-related enteric disease. Diagn. Microbiol. Infect. Dis. **5:** 61–69.
106. **Weinstein, M. P., L. B. Reller, J. R. Murphy, and K. A. Lichtenstein.** 1983. The clinical significance of positive blood cultures: a comprehensive analysis of 500 episodes of bacteremia and fungemia in adults. I. Laboratory and epidemiologic observations. Rev. Infect. Dis. **5:**35–53.
107. **West, S., and T. D. Wilkins.** 1982. Problems associated with counterimmunoelectrophoresis assays for detecting *Clostridium difficile* toxin. J. Clin. Microbiol. **15:**347–349.
108. **Wilkins, T. B., and T. Thiel.** 1973. Resistance of some species of *Clostridium* to clindamycin. Antimicrob. Agents Chemother. **3:**136–137.
109. **Willis, A. T.** 1969. Clostridia of wound infection. Butterworths, London.
110. **Woods, G. L., and P. C. Iwen.** 1990. Comparison of a dot blot immunobinding assay, latex agglutination, and cytotoxin assay for the laboratory diagnosis of *Clostridium difficile*-associated diarrhea. J. Clin. Microbiol. **28:**855–857.
111. **Wu, T. C., and J. C. Fung.** 1983. Evaluation of the usefulness of counterimmunoelectrophoresis for diagnosis of *Clostridium difficile*-associated colitis in clinical specimens. J. Clin. Microbiol. **17:**610–613.
112. **Wu, T. C., and S. M. Gersch.** 1986. Evaluation of a commercial kit for the routine detection of *Clostridium difficile* cytotoxin by tissue culture. J. Clin. Microbiol. **23:**792–793.
113. **Yamamoto, K., I. Ohishi, and G. Sakaguchi.** 1979. Fluid accumulation in mouse ligated intestine inoculated with *Clostridium perfringens* enterotoxin. Appl. Environ. Microbiol. **37:**181–186.
114. **Yeong, M. L., and G. I. Nicholson.** 1988. *Clostridium septicum* infection in neutropenic enterocolitis. Pathology **20:**194–197.

Chapter 51

Anaerobic Gram-Positive Nonsporeforming Bacilli and Cocci

SHARON HILLIER AND BERNARD J. MONCLA

The anaerobic gram-positive cocci and nonsporeforming rods comprise a diverse group of bacteria from 11 genera. They are, for the most part, opportunistic pathogens that are part of the normal mucosal flora of humans. Because they are ubiquitous on mucosal surfaces, they are commonly recovered from clinical specimens from urogenital and oral sites (Table 1). As a group, these organisms are seldom recovered in pure culture. Rather, abscess and wound specimens often yield two or three representatives of this group, usually along with anaerobic gram-negative rods or facultative organisms.

Common features of this group of bacteria are their fastidious growth requirements and slow growth on laboratory media. The obligately anaerobic strains are very sensitive to oxygen during transport, with some species having marked loss of viability in 4 h, even when placed in anaerobic transport media (Fig. 1). Compared with *Bacteroides fragilis* or *Clostridium perfringens*, the anaerobic gram-positive cocci and nonsporeforming rods are very slow growing. A 48-h anaerobic incubation, which is suitable for some *Bacteroides* species, is inadequate for this group of organisms. Many specimens such as neck abscess aspirates or amniotic fluid specimens were reported as "no growth" when the plates or broths were held for 2 days or less. There is no alternative to incubating the media for at least 5 days or, in the case of actinomycosis, for up to 2 weeks.

The added cost of the extended incubation is minimal compared with the cost of repeat computerized axial tomography scans, biopsies, and infectious disease consultations resulting from a culture-negative abscess specimen. While it is certainly difficult to identify many of the members of this group, the most common mistake made with anaerobic rods and cocci is that the organisms are never recovered at all.

ANAEROBIC GRAM-POSITIVE RODS

Characterization

The taxonomy of the gram-positive nonsporeforming anaerobic rods is not well understood. Technical developments and rapid methods that have so dramatically enhanced other areas of clinical microbiology are not yet available for gram-positive nonsporeforming anaerobic rods. Therefore, it is likely that many of these organisms have been misidentified in the past. Furthermore, many of the organisms of this group are fastidious and very slow growing, at least on primary culture. Once obtained in pure culture, the biggest obstacle to identification is placement into the correct genus. Once the genus is determined, it is relatively easy to identify isolates to the species level.

It is helpful to obtain reference strains of the different species for comparison; most species are extremely variable in their colony and cellular morphologies. If these organisms are observed on a direct Gram smear of clinical materials, cultures may require incubation for up to 2 weeks for the organisms to grow.

The genera discussed in this section are *Actinomyces, Bifidobacterium, Lactobacillus, Mobiluncus, Propionibacterium*, and *Rothia*. All except *Mobiluncus* share many phenotypic traits. In cellular morphology, members of these genera are usually pleomorphic gram-positive to gram-variable rods. They are considered anaerobes, but only the genera *Bifidobacterium, Eubacterium*, and *Mobiluncus* are strictly anaerobic; other genera contain species that are facultatively anaerobic, microaerophilic, or capnophilic. Most are slow growing, requiring 3 or more days in culture before colonies are visible on solid media. Some organisms, such as *Actinomyces israelii*, may take up to 2 or more weeks to become visible in primary culture. Members of these genera are inhabitants of the skin and mucosal surfaces such as the oral cavity, intestines, and urogenital tracts of both human beings and lower animals. In the past, many species have been considered part of the normal flora; however, recent studies suggest that some *Eubacterium* species are found only in diseased periodontal pockets (42). Nevertheless, many of the species are considered to be opportunistic pathogens that can cause significant and life-threatening infections at many sites in the body.

Taxonomy

The genera of bacteria discussed in this chapter are taxonomically quite diverse while sharing many phenotypic characteristics. In the past, bacterial taxonomy has relied heavily on descriptive aspects of these organisms, which has resulted in the grouping of genera into families that were probably not appropriate taxonomically.

The gram-positive anaerobic bacteria may be separated into two major subdivisions on the basis of high or low moles percent G+C. The two groups appear to represent separate phylogenetic lines. The low-G+C subdivision represents a more ancient line and includes the genera *Lactobacillus, Clostridium, Eubacterium, Peptostreptococcus*, and *Peptococcus*. The high-G+C subdivision includes the genera *Bifidiobacterium, Actinomyces, Propionibacterium, Rothia, Bacterionema*, and *Mobiluncus* (18, 40, 47, 64). These genera form the so-called *Actinomycetales* branch (18).

TABLE 1. Recovery of anaerobic gram-positive rods and cocci from various specimen types

Site	Reference	No. of patients	Isolates recovered for given genus (%):				
			Peptostrepto-coccus	*Actinomyces*	*Eubacterium*	*Lacto-bacillus*[a]	*Propioni-bacterium*
Kidney abscess	6	6	83	0	17	0	17
Bladder abscess	6	2	100	0	50	0	0
Periurethral abscess	6	7	71	0	0	0	0
Bartholin gland abscess	6	26	42	0	8	4	0
Penile abscess	6	7	86	0	0	0	0
Scrotal/testicular abscess	6	21	48	5	5	0	0
Periapical abscess	10, 63	22	68	14	9	23	0
Orofacial infection	27	55	33	0	13	33	0
Penile wound	6	6	66	0	0	0	0
Periodontal pockets	—[b]	85	60	75	43	NA	15
Breast abscess	7	41	51	0	2	0	27
Peritonsillar abscess	34	42	36	0	0	2	10
Blood	9	587	11	0	2	0.2	36
Nostril (normal)	8	25	16	0	0	0	75
Vagina	—[c]	230	87	7	3	14	22

[a] Obligately anaerobic strains only. NA, No attempts were made to recover *Lactobacillus* isolates in this study.
[b] Moncla, unpublished data.
[c] Hillier, unpublished data.

The eighth edition of *Bergey's Manual of Determinative Bacteriology* discussed the diphtheroid organisms as "*Actinomycetes* and related organisms" and included a rather diverse group of organisms, from *Corynebacterium* to *Actinomyces* to *Mycobacterium* (12). Consistent with the philosophies of the times, considerable effort was expended in attempting to describe the higher taxonomic order. For example, the order *Actinomycetales* was divided into eight families, of which *Actinomycetaceae* was one. Five genera of this family were listed: *Actinomyces, Arachnia, Bifidobacterium, Bacterionema,* and *Rothia*. With the most recent edition of *Bergey's Manual* (53), this type of emphasis has been largely abandoned. Traditionally, inclusion in this group of microorganisms was based primarily on morphologic and biochemical criteria. Although considerable progress has been made in understanding the taxonomy of these bacteria, reliable and accessible tests for identification of many of these species are still not available. As a result, identification in the clinical laboratory is difficult. The genera fall into discrete units based on amino acid content or cell wall, major end products of glucose fermentation, and moles percent G+C content (47, 49, 53). *Actinomyces* cell walls contain lysine, aspartic acid, and ornithine, similar to the cell walls of some *Bifidobacterium* species. *Bacterionema* cell walls have DL-diaminopimelic acid (DL-DAP), whereas *Arachnia* cell walls have LL-DAP. *Rothia* cell walls contain lysine. *Propionibacterium* cell walls may contain *meso*-DAP, LL-DAP, or lysine in place of DAP. There is some overlap in the moles percent G+C content of all of these organisms (Table 2).

The genus *Arachnia* as described in the most recent edition of *Bergey's Manual* (53) contains only one described species, *A. propionica*. However, recent studies have demonstrated that *A. propionica* is more closely related to *Propionibacterium* species. Accordingly, this organism has been reclassified into this genus as *Propionibacterium propionicus* (16). Because it is phenotypically more similar to *Actinomyces* than *Propionibacterium* species, *P. propionicus* is discussed separately from the other propionibacteria. The other monotypic genera, *Rothia* and *Bacterionema,* may represent other, as yet undescribed species; however, additional studies will be required to define further divisions.

Mobiluncus isolates (motile anaerobic curved rods) were first recovered from the uterine discharge of a woman with postpartum endometritis in 1913. Although other workers reported the recovery of similar anaerobic rods from the vaginal specimens, this group of microorganisms was not recognized and given the name *Mobiluncus* until 1984 (55). The genus *Mobiluncus* consists of obligately anaerobic, gram-variable or gram-negative, curved, nonsporeforming rods with tapered ends. The rods occur singly or in pairs and may have a gullwing appearance. They are motile by multiple subpolar flagella. Even though the single organism stains gram negative to gram variable, members of the genus possess a multilayered gram-positive type of cell wall lacking lipopolysaccharide, 2-keto-3-deoxyoctulosonic acid, and hydroxylated fatty acids typically found in the cell walls of gram-negative organisms (14). These organisms are susceptible to vancomycin and resistant to colistin, consistent with the susceptibility patterns of other gram-positive organisms. The genus *Mobiluncus* does not conform to other families of anaerobic bacteria. Because the family *Bacteroidaceae* includes other genera of curved, anaerobic, rod-shaped bacteria that produce succinic acid, the genus *Mobiluncus* was tentatively placed into the family *Bacteroidaceae* in 1984. Recently, partial reverse transcriptase sequencing of the 16S RNA has demonstrated that *Mobiluncus* is more closely related to the genus *Actinomyces* than to members of the family *Bacteroidaceae* (40).

Natural habitat and clinical significance

Information on the occurrence of anaerobes in infectious materials is difficult to obtain, since many data on anaerobic infections are not reliable (23). Both methodologic and taxonomic parameters contribute to our inability to obtain such data. However, data from individual laboratories specializing in anaerobes indicate that the prevalence of anaerobes in various infec-

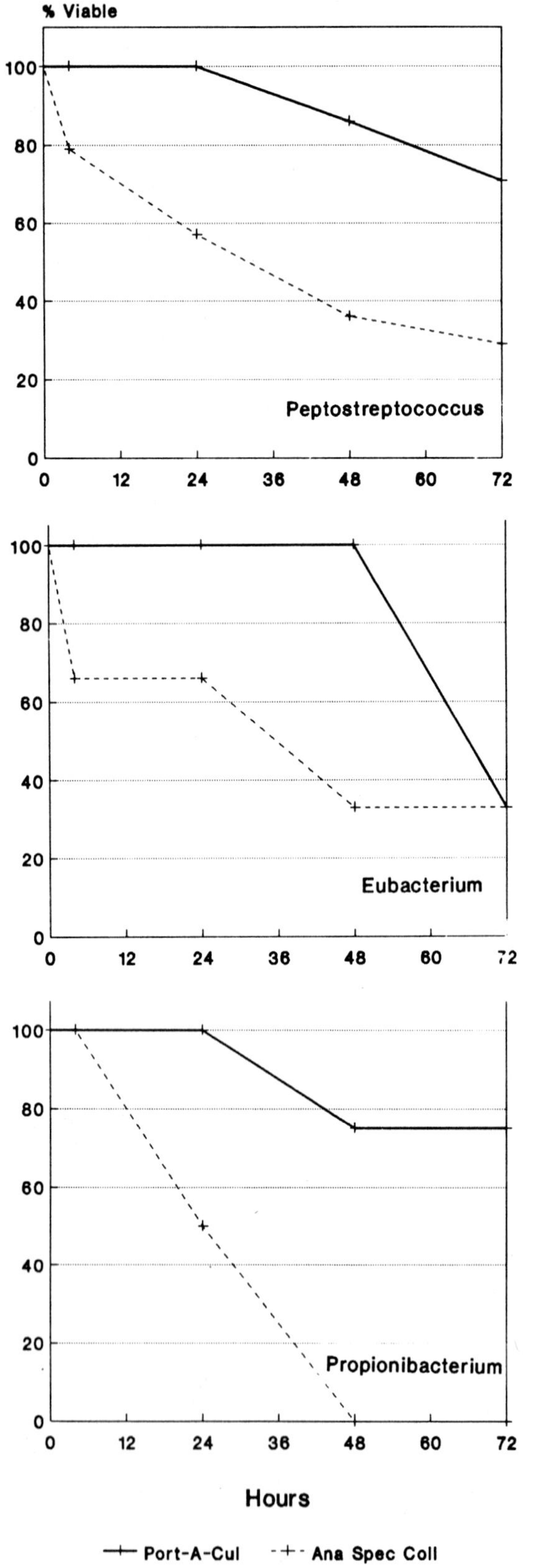

FIG. 1. Survival of anaerobic gram-positive cocci and rods in Port-A-Cul (BBL Microbiology Systems, Cockeyville, Md.) and Anaerobic Specimen Collector (Becton Dickinson Vacutainer Systems, Rutherford, N.J.). (Adapted from data presented in reference 5.)

tions is much greater than is realized by many clinical laboratories. For example, Finegold determined that *Actinomyces* spp. were isolated from 14% of the infections involving anaerobes, while other workers reported a much lower incidence (23). Recovery of anaerobic gram-positive rods from clinical specimens is summarized in Table 1.

There are currently 13 recognized species of *Actinomyces: A. bovis, A. denticolens, A. howellii, A. hordeovulneris, A. humiferus, A. israelii, A. meyeri, A. naeslundii, A. odontolyticus, A. pyogenes, A. slackii, A. suis,* and *A. viscosus.*

With the exception of *A. humiferus,* which is found exclusively in soil, the normal habitat of *Actinomyces* spp. appears to be the oral cavities and mucous membranes of humans and lower animals. *A. bovis, A. denticolens, A. howellii, A. hordeovulneris, A. slackii,* and *A. suis* have not been isolated from humans. *A. bovis* is the etiologic agent of bovine actinomycosis (lumpy jaw) and is capable of producing experimental infections in other animals.

A. israelii, A. naeslundii, A. viscosus, A. odontolyticus, A. pyogenes, and *A. meyeri* are causative agents of disease in humans. These organisms are important constituents of the normal flora of mucous membranes and therefore must be considered opportunistic pathogens. They have on occasion been isolated from stools but are most likely transient colonizers of the gut. All except *A. pyogenes* and *A. meyeri* are found in very high numbers in saliva and subgingival plaque. *A. viscosus* and *A. naeslundii* have been studied extensively and are known to play significant roles in dental caries and periodontal disease (47).

Actinomycosis is the most frequently encountered disease entity. The incidence of actinomycosis in the United States is difficult to determine, since it is not a reportable disease. While there are a few recent reports on this subject, Slack and Gerencser concluded, "Actinomycosis occurs throughout the world and is neither a rare nor a common disease" (52). Actinomycosis is observed twice as frequently in men as in women, and the anatomical distribution is about 60% cervicofacial, 15% thoracic, 20% abdominal, and 5% other types.

Actinomycosis is characterized as a chronic granulomatous lesion that becomes suppurative and forms abscesses and draining sinuses (35, 45). A purulent actinomycotic discharge may be present, usually containing macroscopic sulfur granules (Fig. 2) that appear as whitish, yellow, or brown granular bodies. *A. israelii* is the most common cause of actinomycosis in humans, but the other species of *Actinomyces,* as well as *P. propionicus,* may also be etiologic agents. These infections are usually polymicrobic in nature. Frequently *Fusobacterium* species, *Eikenella corrodens, Capnocytophaga* species, *Actinobacillus actinomycetemcomitans,* black-pigmented *Bacteroides* species, *Porphyromonas asaccharolytica, Porphyromonas gingivalis,* and streptococci in various combinations are isolated along with *Actinomyces* species or *P. propionicus. Actinomyces* species are almost never recovered in pure cultures. It is believed that these associated microorganisms contribute to the pathogenesis of actinomycosis. *Actinomyces* species may also be involved in pelvic inflammatory disease associated with intrauterine devices (65).

Among animals, the incidence of actinomycosis is greatest in cattle, although infections have also been

TABLE 2. Differentiation of gram-positive anaerobic rods

Characteristic	Reaction[a]							
	Actinomyces	*P. propionicus*	*Bifidobacterium*	*Lactobacillus*	*Rothia*	*Propionibacterium*	*Eubacterium*	*Mobiluncus*
Strictly anaerobic	v	−	+	v	−	v	+	+
Motility	−	−	−	−	−	−	v	+
Catalase production	±[b]	−	−	−	+	v	−	−
Metabolic products[c]	S, L, a	A, P, s[d]	A, L[e]	L, (a), (s)	A, L, (s), (py)	A, P, iv, s, l	A, B[f]	S, L, A
Indole production	−	v	−	−	−	−	−	−
Nitrate reduction	v	+	−	−	+	v	v	v
Mol% G+C of DNA	58–68	63–75	57–64	35–53	65–69	59–66	30–40	49–52

[a] Data compiled from references 18, 25, 43, 46–49, and 53. Abbreviations and symbols: v, variable results occur for different species of the same genus; A, acetic acid; S, succinic acid; B, butyric acid; L, lactic acid; P, propionic acid; IV, isovaleric acid; PY, pyruvic acid; ( ), variable or, if produced, usually present only in trace amounts; lowercase letters, products usually produced in small amounts; +, most strains positive; −, most strains negative.

[b] *A. viscosus* is the only member of the genus that produces catalase.

[c] Determined on peptone-yeast extract-glucose broth cultures.

[d] Under anaerobic conditions, *P. propionicus* ferments glucose to CO_2, acetic acid, propionic acid, and small amounts of lactic and succinic acids. In air, glucose is converted to CO_2 and acetic acid.

[e] Acetic and lactic acid are produced in a molar ratio of 3:2.

[f] Metabolic products formed by *Eubacterium* species vary. See Table 4.

reported in swine, dogs, sheep, goats, horses, cats, deer, moose, and antelope (52). Bovine actinomycosis (lumpy jaw) occurs when *A. bovis* gains entrance into the mandibular tissue following traumatic injury after ingestion of rough plant material such as straw or silage or by a broken tooth. As the infection develops, there is a simultaneous destruction of existing bone and stimulation of bone growth, resulting in a proliferative osteitis. The infection can eventually spread to the contiguous tissue, resulting in impairment of mastication or breathing. The yellow discharge from the sinus tracts frequently contains sulfur granules.

A. hordeovulneris is of veterinary importance because it is an agent of actinomycosis (thoracic or abdominal) of dogs (11). Infections are often associated with an irritation of the dog's skin by members of the grass genus *Hordeum* (foxtail). The awns of *Hordeum* have sharp tips with barbed flaring hairs which cause them to become trapped in the coat of the animal. When the dog licks himself, the sharp structures of the foxtail are contaminated by the saliva and penetrate the skin to form a wound. These structures ultimately migrate into the tissues, leaving sites of inflammation and necrosis. The awns may also be inhaled or swallowed. In many cases, *A. viscosus* is isolated with *A. hordeovulneris,* suggesting that the natural habitat of the organism is the canine oral cavity. *A. suis* is believed to be involved in swine mammary gland actinomycosis. The pathogenicity of *A. denticolens, A. howellii,* and *A. slackii* is unknown.

P. propionicus is a recognized agent of lacrimal canaliculitis and actinomycosis, and it produces abscesses in animals when injected. *P. propionicus* was originally described as *Actinomyces propionicus* because of its similarity to *Actinomyces* species (16).

Rothia is a monotypic genus that is considered an opportunistic pathogen. It has been isolated from abdominal infections, infectious endocarditis, and other infections. Its habitat appears to be human supragingival plaque.

Eubacterium species are not frequently encountered in clinical specimens, probably because of the difficulty in recognizing such species. *E. lentum* is the species most frequently observed. *Eubacterium* species are usually isolated in mixed culture from abscesses and wounds and very seldom from blood cultures. Several recently described species have been associated with periodontal disease: *E. nodatum, E. timidum,* and *E. brachy* (31). A recent study by Hill et al. (28) suggests that these species have been involved in numerous infections at other sites, such as head and neck, thorax, bones, skin, and pelvis. *Eubacterium* species are found in the oral cavities of humans and lower animals, soils, and animal and plant products. At least 34 species are currently recognized and at least 19 other distinct groups of unnamed species are known, but only a few are encountered in the clinical laboratory (Table 1).

Bifidobacterium species are seldom encountered in clinical materials. *B. dentium,* formerly *Actinomyces eriksonii* and later *B. eriksonii,* appears to be the only *Bifidobacterium* species with pathogenic potential. It has been isolated from human dental caries, feces of humans, human vaginas, and various clinical materials such as lower respiratory tract specimens. *B. longum* and *B. breve* are found only occasionally in human clinical materials.

Most *Lactobacillus* species recovered from clinical

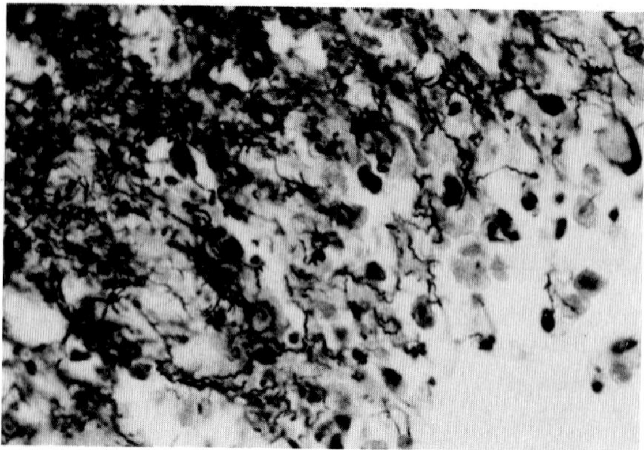

FIG. 2. Microscopic morphology of *Actinomyces* species in a sulfur granule taken from an oral soft tissue section stained with the Brown-Brenn modification of the Gram stain. Note the characteristic appearance of the clubbed-shaped filaments and the numerous polymorphonuclear leukocytes. Magnification, ×100. (Courtesy of Dolphine Oda, Department of Oral Biology, University of Washington, Seattle.)

specimens are microaerophilic, but occasionally an obligately anaerobic isolate can be recovered. They are found as part of the normal flora of the mouth, intestinal tract, and vagina of humans and may therefore be recovered from specimens contaminated by normal flora. They are rarely pathogenic. However, lactobacilli have been reported to cause endocarditis (19, 57), neonatal meningitis, chorioamnionitis (41), amnionitis (17), pleuropulmonary infections, and bacteremia (3) (Table 1). Identification of anaerobic lactobacilli to the species level is extremely difficult and, given the low pathogenicity of the organism, is rarely indicated.

The natural habitats of *Mobiluncus* species are the reproductive tracts and rectums of humans and other primates. *Mobiluncus* species have been reported in 50 to 65% of the vaginal specimens from women with bacterial vaginosis (*Gardnerella vaginalis* vaginitis or nonspecific vaginitis) (33). In our experience, *Mobiluncus* species are recovered from fewer than 10% of specimens from women with normal, *Lactobacillus*-predominant flora. *Mobiluncus* species have also been recovered from the rectums of women with bacterial vaginosis and from the rectal and urethral specimens from the male sex partners of women with bacterial vaginosis (33). In our laboratory, we have also recovered *Mobiluncus* species and the other bacteria associated with bacterial vaginosis from the vaginas of children with no history of sexual abuse. Vaginal specimens from rhesus macaque monkeys have also yielded *Mobiluncus* species (20).

The pathogenic potential of *Mobiluncus* species is not well understood. However, it is unclear whether the rare isolation from clinical specimens is due to the lack of ability of many laboratories to isolate and identify this fastidious microorganism or whether the organism is unlikely to cause invasive disease. While *Mobiluncus* species are present in the vaginal specimens of many women with bacterial vaginosis, the role of the organisms in the etiology of the syndrome is not known. However, studies using fluorescent monoclonal antibodies have demonstrated that *Mobiluncus* species can attach to vaginal epithelial cells with *G. vaginalis* to form the clue cells typically seen in the vaginal fluid of women with bacterial vaginosis (24). Curved rods resembling *Mobiluncus* species can easily be identified in Gram-stained vaginal smears from women with bacterial vaginosis (Fig. 3).

The pathogenic potential of *Mobiluncus* species has been supported by its isolation from breast abscesses, umbilical discharge, breast wounds, and blood cultures (26, 56). The organism can also be recovered from the endometrial aspirates of women with pelvic inflammatory disease and from the chorioamnion of the placenta from preterm deliveries (29). Although *Mobiluncus* species have been recovered in pure cultures from some sterile-site specimens, the organisms are most often recovered with other anaerobic bacteria, including *Bacteroides* and *Peptostreptococcus* species.

Direct microscopic examination of clinical material

Direct microscopic examination of clinical materials is an excellent presumptive method for detection of anaerobic gram-positive rods and should be used whenever possible. In oral pathology laboratories, specimens are sectioned, stained with a Brown-Brenn stain, and examined for sulfur granules, which are considered diagnostic for actinomycosis (Fig. 2). In general, samples

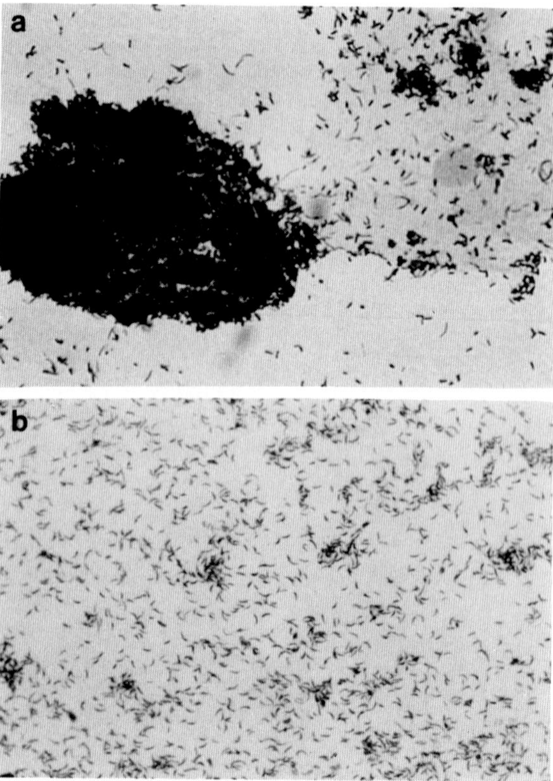

FIG. 3. (a) Gram-stained vaginal smear from a woman with bacterial vaginosis. Note the clue cell (left) and clear squamous epithelial cell (right). Smear contains numerous small gram-negative to gram-variable rods (*Gardnerella* sp.) and curved rods (*Mobiluncus* sp.). (b) Microscopic morphology of a 72-h subculture of *Mobiluncus curtisii*.

should be sent for microbial analysis, and such materials should be stained to guide the workup of the specimen.

A variety of materials are suitable for examination for the presence of sulfur granules: surgically removed tissues, autopsy tissues, bronchial washes, body fluids, purulent exudates, intrauterine devices, Papanicolaou smears, or gauze from draining wounds. Sulfur granules are irregular in shape and size (ranging from 0.1 to 5 mm), hard, and usually yellowish. The sulfur granules may be large enough to see with the unaided eye; granules from oral actinomycosis may sometimes resemble popcorn husks. If sulfur granules are observed, one should be removed with an inoculating needle, loop, or sterile forceps, placed in a drop of water on a microscope slide, and then gently crushed with a second slide. A wet mount should be examined under low power (×100). The granules should have distinctly irregular edges. Upon reduction of the light intensity, the periphery of the granules should give the appearance of a club-shaped mass of filaments, which is usually difficult to distinguish. The clubs should become very distinct at higher magnification (×1,000). The clubs should be refractile, and their appearance has been described as hyaline. Having made these initial observations, one must confirm the presence of filaments. Remove the cover slip and dry, heat fix, and Gram stain the specimen. The presence of gram-positive branched and unbranched filaments should be easily discerned.

It is usually necessary to fix, section, and stain tissue specimens to demonstrate sulfur granules. If stained with hematoxylin-eosin, the eosinophilic clubs should be visible at the periphery of the granules. Diphtheroidal cells and filaments should be apparent at the base of the clubs. Visualization of the filaments in the granules is easier with a modified Gram stain such as MacCallum-Goodpasteur or Brown-Brenn (21). Fixed and sectioned tissues can also be stained with fluorescent-antibody reagents. Other species that may produce granules with clubs are *Nocardia*, *Streptomyces*, and *Staphylococcus* species.

The presence of *Staphylococcus* species can be ruled out by morphology and Gram reaction. To distinguish *Actinomyces* from *Nocardia* isolates, granules should be stained for acid fastness by the method of Kinyoun or Ziehl-Neelsen, since other stains may yield unreliable results (52).

Culture and isolation

A number of agar plate media are available for isolation and cultivation of nonsporeforming anaerobic gram-positive rods. Blood agars (5% sheep blood or rabbit blood) supplemented with hemin and vitamin K are most often recommended; these media include Centers for Disease Control anaerobe blood agar, brain heart infusion, brucella agar, modified Schaedler agar, phenylethyl alcohol blood agar, and heart infusion agar. Media containing vancomycin should not be used. Anaerobic blood culture media, enriched thioglycolate medium, and chopped meat-glucose medium will support growth of these microorganisms.

The usual procedures for anaerobes (see chapter 49) should be used. We have found that fresh medium (less than 7 to 9 days old) works best for primary isolation of these anaerobes. Other authors state that plates should be wrapped in a plastic wrap to prevent desiccation and may be stored for 4 to 6 weeks. In our laboratory, blood agar plates are stored inside a dark plastic garbage bag-lined box at 5°C. This practice prevents desiccation and protects the medium from the generation of oxidizing components by light. Plate media are reduced overnight, in either an anaerobic glove box or an anaerobic jar, before use. This routine has eliminated the need to use anaerobically sterilized medium. Laboratories unable to prepare their own media may wish to consider the use of commercially prepared prereduced anaerobically sterilized (PRAS) blood agar such as is available from Anaerobe Systems (San Jose, Calif.). These media have an extended shelf life of up to 6 months and yield results comparable to those obtained with fresh media.

Primary isolation

Physicians must indicate clearly those specimens to be cultured for the presence of nonsporeforming anaerobic gram-positive rods, since several additional steps are required for proper setup, incubation, and holding times.

Sulfur granules, if present, should be placed in a sterile petri dish and rinsed with thioglycolate broth. They should then be transferred with a sterile Pasteur pipette to a sterile tube or preferably a Ten Broeck grinder (available from various sources) with approximately 0.5 ml of thioglycolate broth. The granules should be crushed with the tip of a sterile glass rod and immediately inoculated to one plate each of anaerobic blood agar and phenylethyl alcohol blood agar (1 drop of inoculum each). Plates should be streaked to achieve well-isolated colonies. Thioglycolate broth medium should be inoculated with 2 drops of inoculum near the bottom of the tube; the screw caps should be left loose to allow the exchange of gases and exposure to anaerobic atmospheres. Media should be incubated in an anaerobic jar or anaerobic chamber at 35 to 37°C. Cultures should be examined after 48 h for growth and then reincubated for 5 to 7 days. It may be necessary to hold plates for as long as 2 to 4 weeks. Incubation of plate media in anaerobic glove boxes may lead to serious desiccation; we therefore prefer to incubate primary cultures in anaerobic jars. However, when anaerobic glove boxes are used, plates may be placed in plastic containers such as Tupperware to prevent drying. A paper towel should be placed on top of the plates in the containers to absorb the moisture that collects from condensation. Additional media appropriate for other anaerobes, capnophilics, and aerobes may also be required (see chapter 49). Specimens without observable granules should be processed as described above and in chapter 49.

Isolation of *Actinomyces* species from specimens rich in microflora may be particularly troublesome. Fluorescent antibodies to *Actinomyces*, *Bifidobacterium*, and *Propionibacterium* species are available from the Centers for Disease Control and may be used on tissue sections and clinical materials.

Selective media and methods have been described for isolation of *Actinomyces* species (1, 39). Cervical swabs or intrauterine devices may present a considerable problem, since the number of organisms may be quite high and many different species are present. Traynor et al. (58) described a method in which swabs are soaked in 5 ml of thioglycolate broth and the samples are diluted 10-fold in the same medium (10^{-1} to 10^{-4} dilutions). Dilutions are plated on Columbia blood agar with and without 2.5 mg of metronidazole per liter. Although this method would not inhibit many organisms such as streptococci and lactobacilli, it appears to give results comparable to those obtained by using fluorescent antibody in a direct microscopic examination.

The importance of *Actinomyces* species in periodontal diseases and caries has spurred workers in the dental research field to develop selective media for recovery of these species from dental plaque (39). However, their usefulness with clinical materials has yet to be tested, and it would probably not be cost effective to maintain a supply of such media in the clinical laboratory.

Identification and distinguishing characteristics

Colony and cell morphologies are perhaps the best means of presumptively separating anaerobic gram-positive rods into genera; however, these characteristics can be both variable and diverse. For example, *Actinomyces* species yield numerous colony types on blood agar, which range from "smooth" to "molar tooth." The microcolony morphologies of *Actinomyces, Propionibacterium, Rothia,* and *Bacterionema* species have been used by some laboratories and are very helpful, but the use of these methods does not lend itself to general clinical microbiology. The colony and cellular morphologies of these genera are quite variable, depending on culture medium used (liquid or solid) and the age and conditions of culture.

The key for the presumptive genus identification of anaerobic gram-positive rods is shown in Table 2; keys for identification of species are presented in Tables 3 to 6. A flow chart for identification of *Eubacterium* species is presented in Table 7. Genera that may have coryneform morphology include *Actinomyces, Eubacterium, Bifidobacterium, Lactobacillus, Propionibacterium, Bacillus, Clostridium, Streptococcus, Nocardia, Corynebacterium, Erysipelothrix,* and *Listeria.* Many may be eliminated from consideration by some relatively simple means. The presence of bacterial endospores would indicate *Bacillus* or *Clostridium* species. Several filamentous clostridia (e.g., *C. clostridiiforme, C. perfringens,* and *C. ramosum*) fail to produce endospores on laboratory media. Growth on egg yolk agar with phospholipase C (lecithinase) production would indicate *C. perfringens.* For identification of *C. clostridiiforme* and *C. ramosum,* see chapter 50. Some organisms appear more rodlike or diphtheroidal on solid medium than in broth culture (*Streptococcus mutans, S. intermedius,* and *Gemella morbillorum*), and some form short coccoid forms on solid media more readily than in broth (*Propionibacterium, Eubacterium, Bifidobacterium,* and *Lactobacillus* species). *Nocardia, Corynebacterium, Erysipelothrix,* and *Listeria* species may be eliminated from the anaerobic gram-positive nonsporeforming bacilli by testing oxygen tolerance. The observation of rods with clubs or bifurcated ends should suggest a species of *Bifidobacterium,* but this morphology may also be observed in other genera. Non-acid-fast branched filaments are good indicators for *Actinomyces* species.

***Actinomyces* spp.** The *Actinomyces* species are facultatively anaerobic except for *A. bovis, A. israelii,* and *A. meyeri,* which are strict anaerobes. All species grow best in primary cultures under anaerobic conditions. It may be difficult to obtain isolates in pure culture; therefore, several subcultures are recommended to ensure purity before biochemical tests are carried out.

The macroscopic appearance of *Actinomyces* colonies on blood agar and cellular morphology are the features most frequently observed, but it should be remembered that these characteristics are extremely variable. Excellent photographs and drawings may be found in references 32, 52, and 53. Differential characteristics for species of *Actinomyces* are presented in Table 3.

Differentiation of several species may be difficult. *A. naeslundii* (Fig. 4c) and *A. viscosus* are very similar but differ in catalase production, *A. viscosus* being positive. *A. israelii* (Fig. 4a) and *P. propionicus* are differentiated by the production of propionic acid by *P. propionicus.* Morphologically, *A. israelii* and other *Actinomyces* species are very similar to *E. nodatum* (28, 32) (Fig. 5a), but the production of butyric acid by some *Eubacterium* species is a differential characteristic. It may be quite

TABLE 3. Differential characteristics of the members of the genus *Actinomyces* and *Propionibacterium propionicus*[a]

Characteristic	Reaction of given species[b]						
	Av	Apy	Am	Ai	An	Ao	Ppr
Catalase production	+	−	−	−	−	−	−
Nitrate reduction	d	−	−	d	+	+	+
Gelatin hydrolysis	−	+	−	−		−	d
H_2S production on triple sugar iron	+	−	−	+	+	+	d
Esculin hydrolysis	d	−	−	+	+	d	−
Pink pigment on blood agar	−	−	−	−	−	+	−
Urease	d	−	d	−	+	−	−
Acid from:							
m-Inositol	d	d	−	+	+	−	d
Glycerol	d	−	d	−	d	d	d[c]
Xylose	−	d	+	+	d	d	−
Raffinose	+	−	−	+	+	−	+
Mol% G+C of DNA	59–69	56–58	64–67	57–65	63–68	62	63–65

[a] Adapted from references 18, 25, 47, 49, 52, and 53.
[b] Abbreviations and symbols: Av, *A. viscosus;* Apy, *A. pyogenes;* Am, *A. meyeri;* Ai, *A. israelii;* An, *A. naeslundii;* Ao, *A. odontolyticus;* Ppr, *P. propionicus;* +, positive reactions for 90 to 100% of strains tested; −, negative reactions for 90 to 100% of strains tested; d, variable reactions.
[c] *P. propionicus* serovar 1, variable reactions; serovar 2, usually negative.

TABLE 4. Characteristics of nonsaccharoclastic species of *Eubacterium*[a]

Species	Morphologic properties		Metabolic products[b]	Utilization of pyruvate	Nitrate reduced	Gelatin hydrolyzed	Esculin hydrolyzed	Hydrogen produced
	Cellular[c]	Colonial						
E. nodatum	Branched, filamentous, or club shaped cells, nonmotile. Cells in PY are 0.5–0.9 by 2.0–12 μm.	Molar tooth, heaped, or raspberry. 0.5–1.0 μm in diameter.	a, B (f, l, s)	+	−	−	−	−
D-6 group[d]	Regular, variable length, occasional chaining, beading, or diphtheroidal.	Circular, entire convex.	a, B, paa (f, l, s)	−	−	−	−	+
E. brachy	Short or coccoidal chaining. Cells in PY are 0.4–0.8 by 0.1–3.0 μm.	Circular, entire low convex, occasionally rough.	ib, iv, ic (a, f, l, s, hc)	−, (+)	−	−	−	+
E. timidum	Short, regular to diphtheroidal, occasional clumps. Cells in PY are 0.8–1.6 by 1.6–3.1 μm.	Circular, entire low convex.	paa (a, f, l, s)	−	−	−	−	−
E. lentum	Short or coccoidal, occasional chains. Cells in PY are 0.2–0.4 by 0.2–2.0 μm.	Circular, entire low convex.	(a, f, l, s)	−	+	−	−	−
E. dolichum	Thin rods in long chains, slightly tapered. Cells in PYG are 0.4–0.6 by 1.6–6.0 μm.	Fails to grow on blood agar plates.	b (l, a)	−	−	w	−	−
E. combesii	Singles, pairs, short chains, and palisade arrangements. Cells are motile. Cells in PYG are 0.6–0.8 by 3.0–10 μm.	Circular, entire to irregular convex, semiopaque, whitish yellow, shiny, smooth.	A, B, iv, l, ib (p, f)	+	−	+	d	+

[a] Data compiled from references 28, 32, and 43.

[b] ic, Isocaproate; iv, isovalerate; ib, isobutyrate; a, acetate; b, butyrate; l, lactate; s, succinate; f, formate; p, propionate; v, valerate; paa, phenylacetate; hc, hydrocinnamate. Capital letters represent an amount of product equal to or greater than 1 meq/100 ml of culture; lowercase letters represent an amount of product less than 1 meq/100 ml of culture; products in parentheses are not produced uniformly. +, Most strains positive; −, most strains negative; (+), usually positive but some strains give negative reaction; w, reaction weak; d, reaction variable.

[c] PY, Peptone-yeast extract; PYG, peptone-yeast extract-glucose.

[d] An undescribed *Eubacterium* species that appears to be of clinical significance.

TABLE 5. Selected characteristics of *Bifidobacterium* species encountered in human normal flora and clinical materials[a]

Species	Fermentation of:					Occurrence in human material[b]			
	Arabinose	Cellobiose	Glycogen	Melezitose	Sucrose	Clinical	Mouth	Intestines-feces	Cervix-vagina
B. dentium	+	+	+	$+^{-}$	+	+	+	+	+
B. bifidum	−	−	−	−	−	+		+	+
B. infantis	−	$-^{+}$	−	−	+			+	+
B. globosum	+	v	+	−	+			+	
B. breve	−	+	$+^{-}$	v	+	+		+	+
B. longum	+	$-^{+}$	−	$+^{w}$	+	+		+	
B. catenulatum	v	+	v	−	+			+	+
B. adolescentis	v	+	+	−	+			+	

[a] Taken from reference 1. Fermentation patterns of *Bifidobacterium* species overlap considerably; polyacrylamide gel electrophoresis or DNA-DNA homology data or both are required for the definitive identification of some species. All *Bifidobacterium* species produce acid from glucose. +, pH below 5.5, or positive; w, pH 5.5 to 5.9, or weak; −, pH above 5.9, or negative; v, variable; superscript, reaction of some strains of a species.

[b] The only documented pathogenic species listed is *B. dentium* (formerly *B. eriksonii*). Few other species have been isolated from clinical specimens; none are commonly encountered.

difficult to distinguish *A. israelii* from *P. propionicus* by the standard bench biochemical tests; however, although both organisms produce acetic and succinic acids as end products of carbohydrate metabolism, *P. propionicus* produces propionic acid whereas *A. israelii* produces lactic acid. Some actinomycetes actually require CO_2 in order to produce succinate.

***Eubacterium* spp.** *Eubacterium* spp. are easily confused with other anaerobic gram-positive rods; however, gas-liquid chromatographic analysis of metabolic end products is very useful in differentiation. Organisms may be either uniform or pleomorphic (Fig. 5) and are obligately anaerobic. They are chemoorganotrophs and may or may not be saccharoclastic. The moles percent G+C for the species range from 30 to 55%, demonstrating that the genus is a heterogeneous group. This conclusion is supported by the fact that there are three groups on the basis of metabolic end products: (i) butyric acid plus other short-chain fatty acids and alcohols; (ii) a combination of lactic, acetic, and formic acids with H_2; or (iii) little or no detectable acids.

***Rothia* sp.** Morphologically, *Rothia* sp. closely resembles *Actinomyces* spp. and to some extent *Nocardia* spp.; differentiation cannot be made by colonial and cellular morphologies. Biochemically, *Rothia* sp. is fermentative, whereas *Nocardia* spp. are not; fermentation of glucose by *Rothia* sp. does not produce succinic acid, whereas fermentation by *Actinomyces* spp. does. When grown aerobically, *Rothia* sp. forms 1-mm colonies in 18 to 24 h that are smooth or granular in appearance. After 4 to 7 days, the colonies may be smooth or convex, with highly convoluted surfaces. When grown anaerobically, the colonies are smaller and highly filamentous, resembling the "spider" colonies of *Actinomyces* spp. By contrast, *Actinomyces* spp. are preferentially anaerobic, requiring CO_2 for maximal growth.

TABLE 6. Identifying characteristics of *Mobiluncus* species

Characteristic	Species	
	M. mulieris	*M. curtisii*
Length (μm)	2.9	1.7
Gram reaction	Negative	Variable
Hippurate hydrolyzed	−	+ (85%)
α-D-Galactosidase	−	+
Arginine dihydrolase	−	+
Proline aminopeptidase	+	+
α-D-Glucosidase	+	+
β-D-Glucosidase	−	−

TABLE 7. Flow chart for identification of selected *Eubacterium* species[a]

I. Butyric acid produced
  A. Caproic acid produced
    E. alactolyticum
  B. Caproic acid not produced, acid from glucose
    1. Indole produced
      E. saburreum
    2. Indole not produced
      a. Nitrate reduced
        i. Esculin hydrolyzed
          E. multiforme
        ii. Esculin not hydrolyzed
          E. monoforme
      b. Nitrate not reduced
        i. Major lactic acid from glucose
          E. rectale
        ii. No major lactic acid from glucose
          aa. Esculin hydrolyzed
            E. limosum
          bb. Esculin hydrolyzed
            No acid from glucose and maltose
            E. combesii

            Weak acid from glucose and maltose
            E. nodatum

II. Butyric acid not produced
  A. Acid from glucose
    1. Indole produced
      E. tenue
    2. Indole not produced
      a. Major lactic acid from glucose
        E. aerofaciens
      b. No lactic acid from glucose
        E. contortum
  B. No acid from glucose
    E. lentum
    E. brachy
    E. timidum

[a] Modified from reference 43.

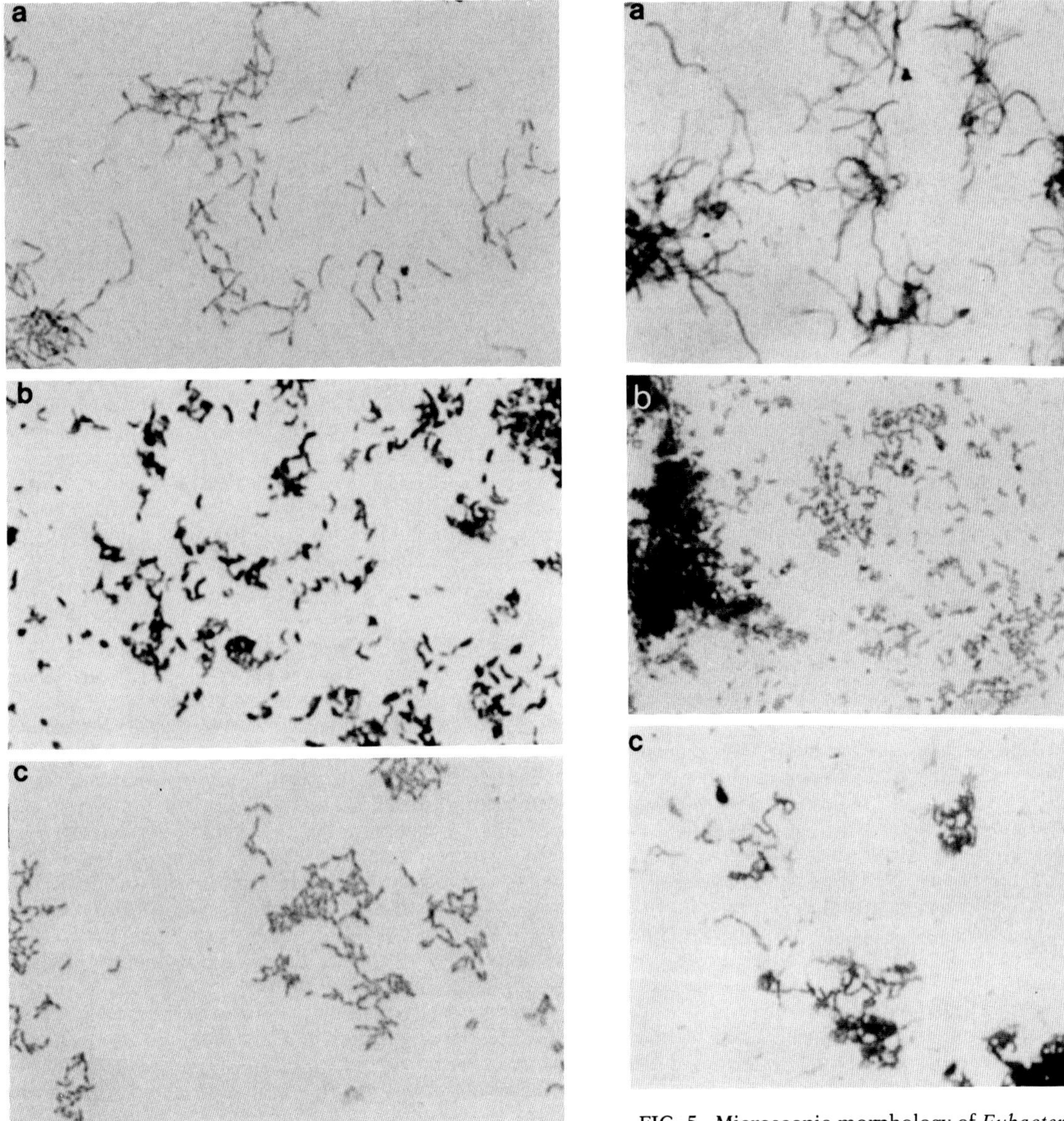

FIG. 4. Microscopic morphology of *Actinomyces israelii* ATCC 12102 (a), *A. meyeri* ATCC 35568 (b), and *A. naeslundii* ATCC 12104 (c). Gram stains prepared from 48-h anaerobic sheep blood agar subculture. Magnification, ×1,000.

FIG. 5. Microscopic morphology of *Eubacterium nodatum* ATCC 33099 (a), *E. timidum* ATCC 33092 (b), and *E. brachy* ATCC 33089 (c). Gram stains prepared from 48-h anaerobic sheep blood agar subculture. Magnification, ×1,000.

***Bifidobacterium* spp.** The key characteristic of *Bifidobacterium* spp. is the production of acetate and lactate at a molar ratio of 3:2, which distinguishes these organisms from other lactic acid- and acetic acid-producing gram-positive anaerobic rods.

***Lactobacillus* spp.** *Lactobacillus* spp. can usually be identified on the basis of Gram stain, a negative catalase test, and gas chromatography showing a major lactic acid peak from glucose.

***Mobiluncus* spp.** There are currently two recognized species of *Mobiluncus: M. curtisii* and *M. mulieris*. They are oxidase, catalase, and indole negative, are weakly saccharolytic, and produce succinic and acetic acids during fermentation, with or without lactic acid. Growth is not stimulated by formate-fumarate. Strains are motile by multiple subterminal flagella. H_2S is not produced. Colonies are colorless, translucent, smooth, and convex and may have a watery appearance, especially on very moist or fresh media. Colonies have a maximum diameter of 2 to 3 mm after 5 days of uninterrupted anaerobic incubation. Colonies may be less than 1 mm in diameter after 2 days of incubation.

M. curtisii can be differentiated from *M. mulieris* most easily by its length and gram-variable, rather than gram-negative, staining. *M. curtisii* is shorter (mean length, 1.7 μm) than *M. mulieris* (mean length, 2.9 μm) (Table 6). *M. curtisii* is reported to hydrolyze hippurate, but up to 15% of *M. curtisii* isolates identified by DNA homology lack the ability to hydrolyze hippurate (S. Hillier, unpublished observation). Gas chromatographic analysis of peptone-yeast extract broth supplemented with starch and 2% serum is of some usefulness in distinguishing

TABLE 8. Identification of anaerobic gram-positive rods and cocci by rapid methods

Species	% Correctly identified to genus and species (no. of isolates tested)[a] by:				
	API 20A	Vitek ANI	PRAS II	RapID ANA	AN-Ident
Actinomyces spp.	14 (7)	50 (6)	NT	58 (26)	86 (7)
Propionibacterium spp.	90 (10)	89 (18)	66 (6)	93 (29)	63 (16)
Eubacterium lentum	100 (4)	33 (6)	100 (2)	100 (10)	100 (6)
Lactobacillus spp.	0 (1)	25 (4)	100 (1)	100 (2)	100 (2)
Bifidobacterium spp.	0 (1)	75 (4)	NT	33 (3)	0 (1)
Peptostreptococcus spp.	60 (25)	76 (58)	92 (24)	92 (51)	100 (13)

[a] Data compiled from references 2, 13, 36, 44, and 50. NT, Not tested.

the two species. *M. curtisii* produces a major succinate and minor acetate peak, whereas *M. mulieris* generally produces major succinate and acetate peaks, with or without a minor lactate peak. Both species of *Mobiluncus* are positive for proline aminopetidase and α-D-glucosidase and negative for phosphatases and β-D-glucosidase. *M. curtisii* is also positive for α-D-galactosidase and arginine dihydrolase, whereas *M. mulieris* is negative for these two enzymes in the RapID ANA system (Innovative Diagnostic Systems, Atlanta, Ga.) (N. E. Hodinka, Abstr. Annu. Meet. Am. Soc. Microbiol. 1988, p. 368, C217).

Rapid identification methods

Commercially available identification systems give excellent identification in some cases and perform unacceptably with other organisms (Table 8). For instance, the Vitek ANI card correctly identified only 66% of 38 nonsporeforming gram-positive rods to the genus and species level in one study (50). This system correctly identified 19 of 21 *Actinomyces* and *Propionibacterium* species but only 3 of 10 *Eubacterium* and *Lactobacillus* species. Published studies have suggested that systems such as the API 20A, AN-Ident (Analytab Products, Plainview, N.Y.), or RapID ANA (Innovative Diagnostic Systems) can reliably identify anaerobic gram-positive rods to the genus but not always the species level (36, 44). No matter how good the identification system (or how strong the claims made by their manufacturers), attempts at identification without gas chromatography can be disastrous. In one study, an isolate identified as a *Propionibacterium* sp. by gas chromatography was identified as an *Actinomyces* sp. by AN-Ident and as *E. lentum* by PRAS II (13). It is essential that any identification made with the assistance of these methods be balanced against the Gram reaction and morphology of the isolate, the specimen source, and the clinical picture.

Antibiotic susceptibility

The anaerobic gram-positive rods, unlike other anaerobes, are not generally susceptible to metronidazole. Metronidazole MICs against *Actinomyces* spp. and *P. propionicus* range from 25 to >125 μg/ml; although 92% of *Eubacterium* spp. are susceptible, there are some strains for which MICs are >128 μg/ml. *M. curtisii* and *M. mulieris* are also resistant to metronidazole (MIC for 90% of strains tested [MIC_{90}] = 256 μg/ml) and its hydroxy metabolite. Most isolates are susceptible to chloramphenicol, piperacillin, mezlocillin, carbenicillin, ticarcillin, cefoxitin, and imipenem (Table 9). Quinolones do not generally have good activity against this group of anaerobic bacteria. The MIC_{50} for ciprofloxacin was at or above the breakpoint for resistance for *Eubacterium* spp., *Lactobacillus* spp., and *Bifidobacterium* spp. (60).

M. curtisii and *M. mulieris* are susceptible to ampicillin, cephalosporins, clindamycin, erythromycin, and

TABLE 9. Susceptibility of anaerobic gram-positive cocci and nonsporeforming rods[a]

Organism	No. of strains	Antimicrobial agent	Breakpoint (μg/ml)	MIC_{90}	Range
Peptostreptococcus spp.	25	Cefoperazone	32	4	0.12–8
	25	Cefoxitin	32	4	0.06–16
	25	Penicillin G	16	8	0.06–8
	25	Imipenem	8	0.12	0.06–2
	25	Clindamycin	4	16	0.06–128
	25	Metronidazole	16	>256	0.25–>256
	25	Chloramphenicol	16	8	0.5–32
	139	Ciprofloxacin	4	4	0.06–32
Anaerobic rods	32	Cefoperazone	32	4	0.125–8
	32	Cefoxitin	32	4	0.06–16
	32	Penicillin G	16	8	0.06–8
	32	Imipenem	8	0.12	0.06–1
	32	Clindamycin	4	256	0.06–>256
	32	Metronidazole	16	256	0.125–>256
	32	Chloramphenicol	16	8	1–64
	147	Ciprofloxacin	4	16	0.06–>64

[a] Data compiled from references 59 and 60.

vancomycin. *M. mulieris* is generally more susceptible to tetracycline (MIC_{90} = 8 μg/ml) than is *M. curtisii* (MIC_{90} = 16 μg/ml) (54).

ANAEROBIC GRAM-POSITIVE COCCI

Characterization

The anaerobic gram-positive cocci include the genera *Peptostreptococcus* and *Peptococcus* as well as some species of *Streptococcus* and *Staphylococcus*. Major revisions in the taxonomy of gram-positive cocci occurred in 1982. The genus *Peptostreptococcus* now includes *P. anaerobius, P. asaccharolyticus, P. indolicus, P. magnus, P. micros, P. prevotii, P. productus,* and *P. tetradius* (22). The genus *Peptococcus* now contains a single species, *Peptococcus niger* (62). The organisms formerly called Gaffkya anaerobia are included in the species *P. tetradius*. These taxonomic changes have been recognized only partially by clinical laboratories and physicians, resulting in the continued reporting of nonexistent species of *Peptococcus* in recent medical literature.

Anaerobic cocci are considered to belong in the genus *Streptococcus* when lactic acid is the major product of glucose fermentation. *S. intermedius* and *S. constellatus*, which were previously included among the anaerobic streptococci, are now considered to be aerotolerant members of the "*S. milleri*" group. Thus, the species of *Streptococcus* currently included as anaerobic streptococci in the most recent edition of *Bergey's Manual* (53) include three strictly anaerobic species (*S. hansenii, S. pleomorphus,* and *S. parvulus*) (15); there is also an aerotolerant species, *Gemella morbillorum* (formerly *S. morbillorum*) (38). The true taxonomic status of these organisms remains unclear, since most numerical taxonomic studies have not included those organisms.

Staphylococcus saccharolyticus (formerly *Peptococcus saccharolyticus*) is the only species of genus *Staphylococcus* that grows well under anaerobic conditions but poorly or not at all under aerobic conditions (37). *S. saccharolyticus* is catalase positive on hemin-supplemented media, but catalase production is weak or absent on media lacking added hemin. Glucose fermentation produces CO_2, ethanol, acetic acid, and small amounts of formic and lactic acids. *S. saccharolyticus* is coagulase negative and susceptible to novobiocin and is thought to be most closely related to *S. epidermidis*.

Other genera of anaerobic gram-positive cocci include *Ruminococcus, Coprococcus,* and *Sarcina*. These organisms can be isolated from the rumen of animals and the stomach and bowel of humans. However, their isolation from clinical specimens is exceedingly rare, and they will not be discussed further. For further information on their isolation and identification, volume 2 of *Bergey's Manual* (53) should be consulted.

The anaerobic gram-positive cocci are widely distributed as normal flora in humans and other animals. They can be recovered routinely from the skin, upper respiratory tract, intestinal tract, and urogenital tract. Anaerobic gram-positive cocci can be recovered from the vaginas of over 80% of premenopausal women (Hillier, unpublished data). Likewise, these organisms can be recovered from 60% of periodontal pocket specimens (B. J. Moncla, unpublished data) but are relatively uncommon in the saliva. Many anaerobic gram-positive cocci recovered from oral and genital tract specimens cannot be identified to the species level (or sometimes even the genus level) by current taxonomic schemes. This fact suggests that there are several species, and perhaps genera, of anaerobic gram-positive cocci that are yet to be described.

Clinical significance

The role of "anaerobic streptococci" in human infections has been recognized since the early 1900s. Schwarz and Dieckman published a report in 1926 on postpartum endometritis in 165 women (51). They recovered *Peptostreptococcus anaerobius* from 28% of the blood and endometrial cultures and other "anaerobic streptococci" from 13%. The importance of anaerobic gram-positive cocci in the etiology of postpartum endometritis has since been confirmed in many studies. In one recent report, a wide variety of species have been reported from the endometria of women with postpartum fever, including *P. anaerobius* (19%), *P. asaccharolyticus* (20%), *P. magnus* (41%), *P. prevotii* (15%), and *P. tetradius* (26%). *Peptococcus niger*, a less frequent isolate, was recovered from only 4% of the endometrial specimens (30). These organisms are also frequently recovered from tubo-ovarian abscess, the fallopian tubes, or endometria of women with pelvic inflammatory disease, septic abortion, amnionitis, and infection of the placental membranes (chorioamnionitis) (29) (Table 1). In pelvic infections, these organisms are often isolated along with *Bacteroides* species (usually not *B. fragilis* group) and facultative bacteria such as *Escherichia coli* or streptococci.

Anaerobic gram-positive cocci are isolated from a wide variety of head and neck infections, including periodontitis, chronic otitis media, chronic sinusitis, and brain abscess. The source of anaerobic cocci in brain abscess is probably related to the presence of these bacteria in otitis and sinusitis and their subsequent spread into the central nervous system. Anaerobic gram-positive cocci present in the gingiva can be spread hematogenously after dental manipulations or extractions to cause brain abscess. The organisms can also spread by aspiration from the oral cavity to cause pulmonary disease, including pneumonitis, lung abscess, empyema, or necrotizing pneumonia. As with obstetric or gynecologic infections, these types of infections typically include other anaerobes, facultative streptococci, and *E. coli*.

Spillage of fecal contents into the peritoneum following appendicitis, diverticulitis, surgery, penetrating trauma, or cancer can lead to intra-abdominal infections involving anaerobic gram-positive cocci, *Bacteroides* and clostridial species, and facultative bacteria. Intestinal perforation or malignancy may also lead to liver abscess, which involves obligate anaerobes in at least half of all cases (4).

Bacteremia due to anaerobic gram-positive cocci most commonly follows obstetric or gynecologic infections, including postpartum endometritis or amnionitis. The most commonly occurring isolates include *P. magnus, P. asaccharolyticus,* and *P. anaerobius* (6). Infection of bone, joints, and grafts may also occur, with *P. magnus* being of principal importance in these sites.

TABLE 10. Flow chart for identification of anaerobic gram-positive cocci

I. Black pigment (may be olive green to mustard), catalase positive
   Peptococcus niger

II. No black pigment
   A. Sensitive to sodium polyanetholsulfonate (61)
      Peptostreptococcus anaerobius
   B. Not sensitive to sodium polyanetholsulfonate
      1. Indole positive
         a. Nitrate positive, coagulase positive
            Peptostreptococcus indolicus
         b. Nitrate negative, coagulase negative
            Peptostreptococcus asaccharolyticus
      2. Indole negative
         a. Urease positive
            i. Nitrate positive
               Staphylococcus saccharolyticus
            ii. Nitrate negative
               Peptostreptococcus tetradius
         b. Urease negative
            i. Esculin positive
               Peptostreptococcus productus
            ii. Esculin negative
               Peptostreptococcus prevotii
               Peptostreptococcus magnus
               Peptostreptococcus micros

Isolation

The anaerobic cocci grow well on most nonselective plating media suitable for anaerobic isolation. Blood, brucella, Centers for Disease Control, and Schaedler agar base supplemented with 5% sheep blood, vitamin K, and hemin, generally yield good growth in 48 to 72 h. Acceptable broth media include peptone-yeast extract-glucose, chopped meat-glucose, and thioglycolate supplemented with hemin, vitamin K, and rabbit serum (5%). Supplementation with Tween 80 (final concentration, 0.02%) may stimulate growth in broth media.

Identification and distinguishing characteristics

Although it seems evident that anaerobic gram-positive cocci should stain as gram-positive cocci, this is not always true. For instance, *P. productus* and *P. anaerobius* may be elongated and resemble gram-positive coccobacilli. Any of the gram-positive cocci may lose gram positivity with age. To add to the confusion, anaerobic gram-negative cocci, including *Veillonella* and *Megasphaera* species, may at times appear to be gram positive. Preparation of Gram stains from a variety of media, both broth and solid, and examination of subcultures at different ages will often help to assess the correct cellular morphology and Gram stain reaction. Gram-positive cocci that resemble rods while on agar medium will assume a more coccoid appearance when grown in broth. Vancomycin susceptibility is useful for establishing that a microorganism is gram-positive in those instances in which gram-variable or gram-negative staining is observed.

Assignment of anaerobic gram-positive cocci to a specific genus can also be somewhat difficult, especially if a gas chromatograph is not available. Any identification of anaerobic gram-positive cocci that is made without the aid of gas chromatographic analysis of growth by-products must be considered presumptive. Even though the rapid identification strips can readily identify many species of anaerobic gram-positive cocci (Table 8), the accuracy of the identification is directly related to the knowledge and experience of the individual reading the test. The flow diagram (Table 10) and Table 11 can be used to further distinguish the genera and species.

***Peptostreptococcus* spp.** The three species of *Peptostreptococcus* most commonly seen in clinical specimens are *P. magnus, P. anaerobius*, and *P. asaccharolyticus*. Colonies of *P. magnus* are minute to 0.5 mm and nonhemolytic. Cells are 0.7 to 1.2 μm in diameter and appear in a tightly packed arrangement. The colonies of *P. anaerobius* are usually somewhat larger (1 mm) and nonhemolytic, and the individual cells are smaller (0.5 to 0.6 μm in diameter) than those of *P. magnus*. Very young cultures of *P. anaerobius* may have elongated cells in chains. The colonies of *P. anaerobius* may have a pungently sweet odor. *P. asaccharolyticus* colonies are minute to 2 mm in diameter and may have a slightly yellow pigment on blood agar. The individual cells are 0.5 to 1.5 μm in diameter and are arranged in pairs, tetrads, or irregular clumps. *P. magnus* can be distinguished from *P. micros* by its larger cell size. Col-

TABLE 11. Identifying characteristics of anaerobic cocci[a]

Organism	Coagulase	Indole	Nitrate	Esculin	Gelatin	Urease	Fermentation of:					GLC analysis[b]
							Cellobiose	Glucose	Lactose	Maltose	Sucrose	
Peptococcus niger	−	−	−	−	−	−	−	−	−	−	−	B, C, iv, a
Peptostreptococcus												
P. anaerobius	−	−	−	−	−	−	−	+ (w)	−	−	−	A, IC, ib, b, iv
P. magnus	−	−	−	−	v	−	−	−	−	−	−	A, (l), (s)
P. micros	−	−	−	−	−	−	−	−	−	−	−	A, (l), (s)
P. indolicus	+	+	+	−	−	−	−	−	−	−	−	A, B, p, (l), (s)
P. asaccharolyticus	−	+	−	−	−	−	−	−	−	−	−	A, B, (l), (p), (s)
P. prevotii	−	−	±	−	−	−	−	−	−	−	−	B, C, iv, a
P. tetradius	−	−	−	−	−	+	−	+	−	+	+	B, L, (a), (p)
P. productus	−	−	−	+	−	−	+	+	+	+	+	A, (l), (s)

[a] Symbols: +, 90% or more positive; −, 90% or more negative; ±, usually negative, some strains positive; v, variable reaction; (w) weak reaction.
[b] Gas-liquid chromatographic (GLC) analysis of fatty acid products in peptone-yeast broth with glucose. Capital letters indicate major metabolic products; lowercase letters indicate minor products; parentheses indicate a variable reaction. A, Acetic acid; P, propionic acid; IB, isobutyric acid; B, butyric acid; IV, isovaleric acid; V, valeric acid; IC, isocaproic acid; C, caproic acid; L, lactic acid; S, succinic acid.

TABLE 12. Biochemical characteristics of the anaerobic streptococci and *Gemella* sp.[a]

Characteristic	Reaction[b]			
	G. morbillorum	*S. hansenii*	*S. pleomorphus*	*S. parvulus*
Aerotolerance	+	−	−	−
Acid from:				
Cellobiose	−	−	−	+
Fructose	−	−	+	+
Galactose	−	+	−	+
Inulin	−	−	NT	+
Lactose	−	+	−	+
Maltose	w	+	−	+
Mannose	w	−	d	+
Salicin	−	−	−	+
Sucrose	w	−	−	+
Raffinose	−	+	NT	−
Production of H_2S	−	+	w	−
Esculin hydrolysis	−	d	NT	+

[a] All species produce lactic acid from fermentation and fail to ferment mannitol, sorbitol, and starch. Adapted from reference 53.
[b] +, Positive; −, negative; w, weak; d, differs among strains; NT, not tested.

onies of *P. micros* are nonhemolytic, minute to 1 mm in diameter, and opaque.

***Peptococcus* sp.** *Peptococcus niger* is rarely recovered from clinical specimens, although it is commonly isolated in low quantities from the vagina (Hillier, unpublished data). In all likelihood, this isolate has gone unnoticed within mixed anaerobic cultures from clinical specimens. On initial isolation, the colonies are black to olive green. The pigment may not be visible to the naked eye but is evident under a dissecting microscope. The black pigment fades quickly upon exposure to oxygen. After subculture, or after the culture is 1 week old, the colony can take on a mustard yellow pigment. The colonies are convex and circular, with a shiny, smooth appearance. They are weakly catalase positive and are indole, urease, and coagulase negative; nitrate is not reduced; esculin and starch are not hydrolyzed. Hydrogen sulfide (in sulfide-indole motility medium) and ammonia are produced. The only definitive means to differentiate *Peptococcus* from *Peptostreptococcus* species is by analyzing G+C content (53). Unfortunately, this analysis is not practical, and peptococci must be presumptively identified on the basis of pigment production and the catalase reaction. The biochemical characteristics of the anaerobic streptococci are given in Table 12.

Other anaerobic cocci. *Streptococcus parvulus* (formerly *Peptostreptococcus parvulus*), *S. hansenii*, and *S. pleomorphus* are obligately anaerobic cocci that differ from *Peptostreptococcus* species in having lactic acid fermentation. *S. parvulus* cells are small (0.3 to 0.6 mm in diameter), occurring in short chains or pairs. The colonies are nonhemolytic and minute to 1.0 mm in diameter after 48 h of incubation in anaerobic blood agar. Growth in broth is stimulated by addition of 0.02% Tween 80. Cells of *S. hansenii* are larger (1.6 to 2.3 mm in diameter) and may have tapered ends. Colonies of anaerobic blood agar are 2 mm in diameter and nonhemolytic. *S. pleomorphus,* as implied by its name, is pleomorphic in size and shape, depending on the growth conditions. Cells stain gram positive initially but may stain gram negative in as little as 24 h. Colonies are 2 to 3 mm in diameter and may be weakly hemolytic. The differential characteristics of these species are summarized in Table 12.

Antibiotic susceptibility (Table 9)

Most *Peptostreptococcus* isolates (96%) are susceptible to β-lactams and most cephalosporin-type antibiotics, although ticarcillin and cefotaxime MICs as high as 64 μg/ml have been reported. Clindamycin and metronidazole are slightly less active (84 and 88%, respectively) (59, 60). Although some published reports have suggested that metronidazole resistance occurs only in microaerophilic strains, we have observed metronidazole resistance in several obligately anaerobic isolates of peptostreptococci.

LITERATURE CITED

1. **Allen, S. D.** 1985. Gram-positive, nonsporeforming anaerobic bacilli, p. 461–472. *In* E. H. Lennette, A. Balows, W. J. Hausler, Jr., and H. J. Shadomy (ed.), Manual of Clinical Microbiology, 4th ed. American Society for Microbiology, Washington, D.C.
2. **Appelbaum, P. C., C. S. Kaufmann, and J. W. Depenbusch.** 1985. Accuracy and reproducibility of a four-hour method for anaerobe identification. J. Clin. Microbiol. **21:** 894–898.
3. **Bayer, A. S., A. W. Chow, D. Betts, and L. B. Guze.** 1978. Lactobacillemia—report of nine cases. Important clinical and therapeutic considerations. Am. J. Med. **64:**808–813.
4. **Bjornson, H. S.** 1989. Biliary tract and hepatic infections, p. 333–347. *In* S. M. Finegold and W. L. George (ed.), Anaerobic infections in humans. Academic Press, Inc., San Diego.
5. **Brook, I.** 1987. Comparison of two transport systems for recovery of aerobic and anaerobic bacteria from abscesses. J. Clin. Microbiol. **25:**2020–2022.
6. **Brook, I.** 1988. Anaerobic bacteria in suppurative genitourinary infections. J. Urol. **141:**889–893.
7. **Brook, I.** 1988. Microbiology of non-puerperal breast abscesses. J. Infect. Dis. **157:**377–379.
8. **Brook, I.** 1988. Aerobic and anaerobic bacteriology of purulent nasopharyngitis in children. J. Clin. Microbiol. **26:** 592–594.
9. **Brook, I.** 1988. Recovery of anaerobic bacteria from clinical specimens in 12 years at two military hospitals. J. Clin. Microbiol. **26:**1181–1188.
10. **Brook, I., S. Grimm, and R. B. Kielich.** 1981. Bacteriology of acute periapical abscess in children. J. Endodont. **7:** 378–380.
11. **Buchanan, A. M., J. L. Scott, M. A. Gerencser, B. L. Beaman, S. Jang, and L. Biberstein.** 1984. *Actinomyces hor-*

deovulneris sp. nov., an agent of canine actinomycosis. Int. J. Syst. Bacteriol. **34:**439–443.

12. **Buchanan, R. E., and N. E. Gibbons (ed.).** 1974. Bergey's manual of determinative bacteriology, 8th ed. The Williams & Wilkins Co., Baltimore.
13. **Burlage, R. S., and P. D. Ellner.** 1985. Comparison of the PRAS II, AN-Ident, and RapID ANA systems for identification of anaerobic bacteria. J. Clin. Microbiol. **22:**32–35.
14. **Carlone, G. M., M. L. Thomas, R. J. Arko, G. O. Guerrant, C. W. Moss, J. M. Swenson, and S. A. Morse.** 1986. Cell wall characteristics of *Mobiluncus* species. Int. J. Sys. Bacteriol. **36:**288–296.
15. **Cato, E. P.** 1983. Transfer of *Peptostreptococcus parvulus* (Weinberg, Nativelle, and Prevot 1937), Smith 1957 to the genus *Streptococcus: Streptococcus parvulus* (Weinberg, Nativelle, and Prevot 1937) comb. nov., nom. rev., emend. Int. J. Syst. Bacteriol. **33:**82–84.
16. **Charfreitag, O., M. D. Collins, and E. Stackebrandt.** 1988. Reclassification of *Arachnia propionica* as *Propionibacterium propionicus* comb. nov. Int. J. Syst. Bacteriol. **38:**354–357.
17. **Cox, S. M., L. E. Phillips, L. J. Mercer, C. E. Stager, S. Waller, and S. Faro.** 1986. Lactobacillemia of amniotic fluid origin. Obstet. Gynecol. **68:**134–135.
18. **Cummins, C. S., and J. S. Johnson.** 1986. Genus I. *Propionibacterium* Orla-Jensen 1909, 337[AL], p. 1346–1353. *In* P. H. A. Sneath, N. S. Mair, M. E. Sharpe, and J. G. Holt (ed.), Bergey's manual of systematic bacteriology, vol. 2. The Williams & Wilkins Co., Baltimore.
19. **Davis, A. J., P. A. James, and P. M. Hawkey.** 1986. *Lactobacillus* endocarditis. J. Infect. **12:**169–174.
20. **Doyle, L., C. L. Young, S. S. Jang, and S. L. Hillier.** 1990. Normal vaginal aerobic and anaerobic bacterial flora of the Rhesus macaque. J. Primatol. **19.**
21. **Emmons, C. W., C. H. Binford, and J. P. Utz.** 1970. Medical mycology, 2nd ed. Lea & Febiger, Philadelphia.
22. **Ezaki, T., N. Yamamoto, K. Ninomiya, S. Suzuki, and E. Yabuuchi.** 1983. Transfer of *Peptococcus indolicus, Peptococcus asaccharolyticus, Peptococcus prevotii,* and *Peptococcus magnus* to the genus *Peptostreptococcus* and proposal of *Peptostreptococcus tetradius* sp. nov. Int. J. Syst. Bacteriol. **33:**683–698.
23. **Finegold, S. M.** 1989. General aspects of anaerobic infection, p. 137–153. *In* S. M. Finegold and W. L. George (ed.), Anaerobic infections in humans. Academic Press, Inc., San Diego.
24. **Fohn, M. J., S. A. Lukehart, and S. L. Hillier.** 1988. Production and characterization of monoclonal antibodies to *Mobiluncus* species. J. Clin. Microbiol. **26:**2598–2603.
25. **Gerencser, M. A., and G. H. Bowden.** 1986. Genus *Rothia.* Georg and Brown 1967, 68[AL], p. 1342–1346. *In* P. H. A. Sneath, N. S. Mair, M. E. Sharpe, and J. G. Holt (ed.), Bergey's manual of systematic bacteriology, vol. 2. The Williams & Wilkins Co., Baltimore.
26. **Glupczynski, Y., M. Labbe, F. Crockaert, F. Pepersack, P. Van Der Auwera, and E. Yourassowsky.** 1984. Isolation of *Mobiluncus* in four cases of extragenital infections in adult women. Eur. J. Clin. Microbiol. **3:**433–435.
27. **Heimdahl, A., L. V. Konow, T. Satoh, and C. E. Nord.** 1985. Clinical appearance of orofacial infections of odontogenic origin in relation to microbiologic findings. J. Clin. Microbiol. **22:**299–302.
28. **Hill, G. B., O. M. Ayers, and A. P. Kohan.** 1987. Characterization and sites of infection of *Eubacterium nodatum, Eubacterium timidum, Eubacterium brachy,* and other asaccharolytic *Eubacteria.* J. Clin. Microbiol. **25:**1540–1545.
29. **Hillier, S. L., J. Martius, M. Krohn, N. Kiviat, K. K. Holmes, and D. A. Eschenbach.** 1988. A case-control study of chorioamnionic infection and histologic chorioamnionitis in prematurity. N. Engl. J. Med. **319:**972–978.
30. **Hillier, S. L., D. H. Watts, M. F. Lee, and D. A. Eschenbach.** 1990. Etiology and treatment of post cesarean section endometritis following cephalosporin prophylaxis. J. Reprod. Med. **35**(Suppl.)**:**322–328.
31. **Holdeman, L. V., E. P. Cato, J. A. Burmeister, and W. E. C. Moore.** 1980. Descriptions of *Eubacterium timidum* sp. nov., *Eubacterium brachy* sp. nov., and *Eubacterium nodatum* sp. nov. isolated from human periodontitis. Int. J. Syst. Bacteriol. **30:**163–169.
32. **Holdeman, L. V., E. P. Cato, and W. E. C. Moore (ed.).** 1977. Anaerobe laboratory manual, 4th ed. Virginia Polytechnic Institute and State University, Blacksburg.
33. **Holst, E., B. Wathne, B. Hovelius, and P.-A. Mårdh.** 1987. Bacterial vaginosis: microbiological and clinical findings. Eur. J. Clin. Microbiol. **6:**536–541.
34. **Jokipii, A. M., L. Jokipii, P. Sipila, and K. Jokinen.** 1988. Semiquantitative culture results and pathogenic significance of obligate anaerobes in peritonsillar abscesses. J. Clin. Microbiol. **26:**957–961.
35. **Juhl, G., and W. A. Brezezkinski.** 1984. Disseminated actinomycosis associated with infection by *Capnocytophaga* species. J. Infect. Dis. **149:**654.
36. **Karachowski, N. O., E. L. Busch, and C. L. Wells.** 1985. Comparison of PRAS II, RapID ANA, and API 20A systems for identification of anaerobic bacteria. J. Clin. Microbiol. **21:**122–126.
37. **Kilpper-Balz, R., and K. H. Schleifer.** 1981. Transfer of *Peptococcus saccharolyticus* Foubert and Douglas to the genus *Staphylococcus: Staphylococcus saccharolyticus* (Foubert and Douglas) comb. no. Zentralbl. Bakteriol. Parasitenkd. Infektionskr. Hyg. Abt. 1 Orig. Reihe C **2:**324–331.
38. **Kilpper-Bälz, R., and K. H. Schleifer.** 1988. Transfer of *Streptococcus morbillorum* to the genus *Gemella* as *Gemella morbillorum* comb. nov. Int. J. Syst. Bacteriol. **38:** 442–443.
39. **Kornman, K. S., and W. J. Loesche.** 1978. New medium for isolation of *Actinomyces viscosus* and *Actinomyces naeslundii* from dental plaque. J. Clin. Microbiol. **7:**514–518.
40. **Lassnig, C., M. Dorsch, J. Wolters, E. Schaber, G. Stöffler, and E. Stackebrant.** 1989. Phylogenetic evidence for the relationship between the genera *Mobiluncus* and *Actinomyces.* FEMS Microbiol. Lett. **65:**17–22.
41. **Lorenz, R. P., P. C. Appelbaum, R. M. Ward, and J. J. Botti.** 1982. Chorioamnionitis and possible neonatal infection associated with *Lactobacillus* species. J. Clin. Microbiol. **16:**558–561.
42. **Moore, L. V. H., W. E. C. Moore, E. P. Cato, R. M. Smibert, J. A. Burmeister, and A. M. Best.** 1987. Bacteriology of human gingivitis. J. Dent. Res. **66:** 989–995.
43. **Moore, W. E. C., and L. V. H. Moore.** 1986. Genus *Eubacterium* Prevot 1938, 294[AL], p. 1353–1373. *In* P. H. A. Sneath, N. S. Mair, M. E. Sharpe, and J. G. Holt (ed.), Bergey's manual of systematic bacteriology, vol. 2. The Williams & Wilkins Co., Baltimore.
44. **Murray, P. R., C. J. Weber, and A. C. Niles.** 1985. Comparative evaluation of three identification systems for anaerobes. J. Clin. Microbiol. **22:**52–55.
45. **Reiner, S. L., J. M. Harrelson, S. E. Miller, G. B. Hill, and H. A. Gallis.** 1987. Primary actinomycosis of an extremity: a case report and review. Rev. Infect. Dis. **9:**581–589.
46. **Schaal, K. P.** 1986. Genus *Actinomyces* Harz 1877, 133[AL], p. 1383–1418. *In* P. H. A. Sneath, N. S. Mair, M. E. Sharpe, and J. G. Holt (ed.), Bergey's manual of systematic bacteriology, vol. 2. The Williams & Wilkins Co., Baltimore.
47. **Schaal, K. P., G. M. Schofield, and G. Pulverer.** 1980. Taxonomy and clinical significance of *Actinomycetaceae* and *Propionibacteriaceae.* Infection **8**(Suppl. 2)**:**S122–S130.
48. **Schofield, G. M., and K. P. Schaal.** 1980. Carbohydrate fermentation patterns of facultatively anaerobic actinomycetes using micromethods. FEMS Microbiol. Lett. **8:** 67–69.

49. **Schofield, G. M., and K. P. Schaal.** 1981. A numerical taxonomic study of members of the *Actinomycetaceae* and related taxa. J. Gen. Microbiol. **127:**237–259.
50. **Schreckenberger, P. C., D. M. Celig, and W. M. Janda.** 1988. Clinical evaluation of the Vitek ANI card for identification of anaerobic bacteria. J. Clin. Microbiol. **26:**225–232.
51. **Schwarz, D., and W. J. Dieckman.** 1926. Anaerobic streptococci: their role in puerperal infection. South. Med. J. **19:**470–479.
52. **Slack, J. M., and M. A. Gerencser.** 1975. *Actinomyces*, filamentous bacteria: biology and pathogenicity. Burgess Publishing Co., Minneapolis.
53. **Sneath, P. H. A., N. S. Mair, M. E. Sharpe, and J. G. Holt (ed.).** 1986. Bergey's manual of systematic bacteriology, vol. 2. The Williams & Wilkins Co., Baltimore.
54. **Spiegel, C. A.** 1987. Susceptibility of *Mobiluncus* species to 23 antimicrobial agents and 15 other compounds. Antimicrob. Agents Chemother. **31:**249–252.
55. **Spiegel, C. A., and M. Roberts.** 1984. *Mobiluncus* gen. nov., *Mobiluncus curtisii* subsp. *curtisii* sp. nov., *Mobiluncus curtisii* subsp. *holmesii* subsp. nov., and *Mobiluncus mulieris* sp. nov., curved rods from the human vagina. Int. J. Syst. Bacteriol. **34:**177–184.
56. **Sturm, A. W.** 1989. *Mobiluncus* species and other anaerobic bacteria in nonpuerperal breast abscess. Eur. J. Clin. Microbiol. **8:**789–792.
57. **Sussman, J., E. J. Baron, S. Goldman, R. Pizzarello, and M. Kaplan.** 1988. Clinical manifestations and therapy of *Lactobacillus* endocarditis. Rev. Infect. Dis. **8:**771–776.
58. **Traynor, R. M., D. Pavatt, H. L. D. Duguid, and I. D. Duncan.** 1981. Isolation of actinomycetes from cervical specimens. J. Clin. Pathol. **34:**914–916.
59. **Wexler, H. M., and S. M. Finegold.** 1988. In vitro activity of cefoperazone plus sulbactam compared with that of other antimicrobial agents against anaerobic bacteria. Antimicrob. Agents Chemother. **32:**403–406.
60. **Whiting, J. L., N. Cheng, and A. W. Chow.** 1987. Interactions of ciprofloxacin with clindamycin, metronidazole, cefoxitin, cefotaxime, and mezlocillin against gram-positive and gram-negative anaerobic bacteria. Antimicrob. Agents Chemother. **31:**1379–1382.
61. **Wideman, P. A., V. L. Vargo, D. Citronbaum, and S. M. Finegold.** 1976. Evaluation of the sodium polyanethol sulfonate disk test for the identification of *Peptostreptococcus anaerobius*. J. Clin. Microbiol. **4:**330–333.
62. **Wilkins, T. D., W. E. C. Moore, S. E. H. West, and L. V. Holdeman.** 1975. *Peptococcus niger* (Hall) Kluyver and van Niel 1936: emendation of description and designation of neotype strain. Int. J. Syst. Bacteriol. **25:**47–49.
63. **Williams, B. L., G. F. McCann, and F. D. Schoenknecht.** 1983. Bacteriology of dental abscesses of endodontic origin. J. Clin. Microbiol. **18:**770–774.
64. **Woese, C. R.** 1987. Bacterial evolution. Microbiol. Rev. **51:**221–271.
65. **Yoonessi, M., K. Crickard, I. S. Cellino, S. K. Satchidanand, and W. Fett.** 1985. Association of *Actinomyces* and intrauterine contraceptive devices. J. Reprod. Med. **30:**48–52.

Chapter 52

Anaerobic Gram-Negative Bacilli and Cocci

HANNELE R. JOUSIMIES-SOMER AND SYDNEY M. FINEGOLD

This chapter deals with members of the genera *Anaerobiospirillum, Anaerorhabdus, Anaerovibrio, Bacteroides, Bilophila, Butyrivibrio, (Campylobacter), Centipeda, Desulfomonas, Desulfovibrio, Fibrobacter, Fusobacterium, Leptotrichia, Megamonas, Mitsuokella, Porphyromonas, Prevotella, Rikenella, Ruminobacter, Sebaldella, Selenomonas, Succinimonas, Succinivibrio, Tissierella* and *Wolinella*. These organisms are part of the normal flora of humans or lower animals in the mouth, upper respiratory tract, intestinal tract, or urogenital tract. Anaerobic spirochetes are covered in chapter 56; anaerobic *Campylobacter* spp. are discussed in chapter 39. The initial differentiation of these genera is based on motility, flagellar arrangement, cellular morphology, and an analysis of metabolic end products by gas-liquid chromatography (GLC) (Table 1) (5, 10, 18, 28, 38, 39). Species definition is based on biochemical characteristics, nucleic acid base composition, and homology (50). In the majority of clinical specimens, only the genera *Bacteroides, Prevotella, Porphyromonas,* and *Fusobacterium,* among bacilli, need to be considered. *Acidaminococcus, Megasphaera,* and *Veillonella* constitute the genera of anaerobic, gram-negative cocci (Table 1). Of these, *Veillonella* is the genus most often encountered in clinical specimens (36, 44).

CHARACTERIZATION OF ANAEROBIC BACILLI

This section will focus on *Bacteroides* spp., *Porphyromonas* spp., *Prevotella* spp., and *Fusobacterium* spp. These species are identified presumptively on the basis of a few observations such as colonial and cellular morphology, pigment production, fluorescence under long-wave UV light, susceptibility to special-potency antibiotic disks, and certain rapidly determined biochemical characteristics. A definite identification requires the determination of multiple characteristics with a battery of biochemical tests. Definitive identification is not feasible for all anaerobic isolates because of financial constraints and is not ordinarily important for clinical purposes. Such detailed bacteriology should be available in certain teaching centers or reference laboratories for special circumstances such as unusual clinical cases, organisms not previously encountered, and publication and teaching purposes. For clinical purposes, it is generally sufficient to know the broad groupings of isolates and their usual patterns of susceptibility to antimicrobial agents. The taxonomy of anaerobic gram-negative bacilli has been in a state of great change in recent years, and this trend will continue. It has been proposed that only the present *Bacteroides fragilis* group (including *B. eggerthii*) should be included in the genus *Bacteroides* and that other species that have not yet been reclassified should be (38). Shah and Collins have proposed a new genus, *Prevotella*, to include the moderately saccharolytic organisms presently in the genus *Bacteroides*. This genus would include the former *B. oris, B. buccae, B. buccalis,* the *B. oralis* group, *B. melaninogenicus, B. denticola, B. loescheii, B. intermedius, B. corporis, B. bivius, B. disiens, B. heparinolyticus, B. oulorum, B. ruminicola,* and *B. zoogleoformans* (39). For recent taxonomic changes, see Table 2.

CHARACTERIZATION OF ANAEROBIC, GRAM-NEGATIVE COCCI

The anaerobic, gram-negative cocci are identified presumptively on the basis of colonial and cellular morphology, fluorescence under long-wave UV light, susceptibility to special-potency antibiotic disks, and some rapidly determined biochemical characteristics. A definite identification relies on carbohydrate fermentation test results and fatty acid profiles of metabolic end products determined by GLC.

OCCURRENCE IN CLINICAL MATERIAL AND SIGNIFICANCE

Gram-negative anaerobic bacilli are the most commonly encountered anaerobes in clinical infections; they are found in more than half of the specimens yielding anaerobes (7, 13). The *B. fragilis* group, which is bile resistant (see Table 4), is the most commonly recovered anaerobe of all types found in clinical specimens and is more resistant to antimicrobial agents than are most other anaerobes. *B. fragilis* and *B. thetaiotaomicron* are the species in the group of greatest clinical significance. They are recovered from most intra-abdominal infections and may be seen in infections at other sites. The *B. fragilis* group constitutes the dominant portion of the normal colonic flora. These organisms may also be found in smaller numbers in the female genital tract but not commonly in the mouth or upper respiratory tract.

The pigmenting anaerobic gram-negative bacilli are composed of saccharolytic and asaccharolytic species of the genera *Prevotella* and *Porphyromonas* (37, 38), respectively. Eight species of these genera (formerly *Bacteroides* spp.) are found in human clinical material (see Table 6). *Prevotella corporis, P. denticola, P. intermedia, P. loescheii, P. melaninogenica, Porphyromonas endodontalis,* and *Porphyromonas gingivalis* are found in the human oral cavity. Some are important pathogens in oral, dental, and bite infections and may produce infections of the head, neck, and lower respiratory tract. Some of the above-mentioned pigmenting organisms

TABLE 1. Differentiation of the genera of gram-negative anaerobic bacteria

Group	Characteristic	Genus
Rod-shaped cells or coccobacilli	I. Nonmotile or peritrichous flagella	
	A. Produce butyric acid (without isobutyric and isovaleric acids)	*Fusobacterium*
	B. Produce major lactic acid	*Leptotrichia*
	C. Produce acetic acid and hydrogen sulfide; reduce sulfate	*Desulfomonas*
	D. Not as above (A, B, or C)	*Anaerorhabdus*
		Bacteroides
		Bilophila
		Fibrobacter
		Megamonas
		Mitsuokella
		Porphyromonas
		Prevotella
		Rikenella
		Ruminobacter
		Sebaldella
		Tissierella
	II. Polar flagella	
	A. Fermentative	
	1. Produce butyric acid	*Butyrivibrio*
	2. Produce succinic acid	
	a. Spiral-shaped cells	*Succinivibrio*
	b. Ovoid cells	*Succinimonas*
	3. Produce propionic and acetic acids	*Anaerovibrio*
	B. Nonfermentative; produce succinic acid from fumarate	*Wolinella/Campylobacter concisus*
	III. Tufts of flagella on concave side of curved cells; fermentative	*Selenomonas*
	IV. Flagella in a spiral arrangement along cell body; fermentative	*Centipeda*
	V. Bipolar tufts of flagella	*Anaerobiospirillum*
Spherical or kidney bean-shaped cells	I. Produce propionic and acetic acids	*Veillonella*
	II. Produce butyric and acetic acids	*Acidaminococcus*
	III. Produce isobutyric, butyric, isovaleric, valeric, and caproic acids	*Megasphaera*

plus *Porphyromonas asaccharolytica* are also prevalent in the urogenital and intestinal tracts and are important in various infections. Three other pigmenting species, *Bacteroides levii, B. macacae,* and *B. salivosus,* are of animal origin and are possibly related to *Porphyromonas* spp. and *Prevotella* spp. (37). These organisms may be encountered in humans with animal bite infections.

The bile-sensitive, saccharolytic gram-negative bacilli (see Table 5) are encountered in the same setting as are the pigmenting gram-negative rods (23). *Prevotella bivia* and *P. disiens* are found particularly in female genital tract infections and less frequently in oral infections. Their recognition is important, since these strains are often resistant to the β-lactam antibiotics, including penicillin, aminopenicillins, and cephalosporins. *Prevotella oris* and *P. buccae* are found in a variety of oral (15) and other infections. The *Prevotella oralis* group is now represented by *P. oralis, P. veroralis, P. buccalis,* and *P. oulora* (29, 39, 40, 49).

Strains that produce a viscous material in broth are represented by *Prevotella zoogleoformans* (indole negative) and *P. heparinolytica* (indole positive) (3, 35); these organisms are found in the oral cavity and oral-associated infections. *Mitsuokella dentalis* (a new genus, formerly *Bacteroides,* and a new species) has been isolated from infected root canals (16).

The bile-sensitive asaccharolytic species *Bacteroides capillosus, B. putredinis,* and *Tissierella preacuta* (formerly *Bacteroides praecutus*) (9) inhabit the intestinal tract and have occasionally been recovered from miscellaneous infections (23). *Bacteroides forsythus* (a new species) (46), a fusiform gram-negative rod, has been recovered from subgingival sites in periodontitis.

The asaccharolytic, formate- and fumarate-requiring, nitrate- or nitrite-reducing gram-negative rods include *Bacteroides ureolyticus, B. gracilis, Wolinella curva, W. recta,* and *W. succinogenes* (Table 1). *B. ureolyticus* has been recovered from a variety of infections, including pulmonary, head and neck, intra-abdominal, urogenital, bone, and soft tissue infections. *B. gracilis* has been recognized relatively recently as an important pathogen in serious visceral or head and neck infections. This organism is relatively often resistant to antimicrobial agents, including penicillins and cephalosporins (20), despite not producing β-lactamase. *Wolinella* spp. are primarily oral isolates found in periodontitis and periodontosis (45). *Bilophila wadsworthia* (a new genus and species) (5) resembles *B. ureolyticus* and *Desulfomonas* spp. but is stimulated by bile, is strongly catalase positive, and does not reduce sulfate. It has been recovered from inflamed and noninflamed appendices and related abscesses as well as from human fecal specimens.

Fusobacterium nucleatum is commonly encountered in clinical infections. There are probably several different species presently included in this one species (14). This organism is found in the mouth and in the genital, gastrointestinal, and upper respiratory tracts. It is often involved in the same types of infection as are the pig-

TABLE 2. Recent taxonomic changes

New nomenclature	Previous nomenclature
Anaerorhabdus furcosus	*Bacteroides furcosus*
Bacteroides caccae	*Bacteroides* sp. "3452A"
B. forsythus	New species
B. galacturonicus	New species
B. merdae	New species
B. pectinophilus	New species
B. salivosus	New species
B. stercoris	New species
B. tectum	New species
Bilophila wadsworthia	New genus and species
Centipeda periodontii	New genus and species
Fibrobacter succinogenes	*Bacteroides succinogenes*
F. intestinalis	New species
Fusobacterium alocis	New species
F. sulci	New species
F. ulcerans	New species
Megamonas hypermegas	*B. hypermegas*
Mitsuokella multiacida	*B. multiacidus*
M. dentalis	New species
Selenomonas artemidis	New species
S. dianae	New species
S. flueggei	New species
S. infelix	New species
S. noxia	New species
Porphyromonas asaccharolytica	*B. asaccharolyticus*
P. endodontalis	*B. endodontalis*
P. gingivalis	*B. gingivalis*
Prevotella bivia	*B. bivius*
P. buccae	*B. buccae*
P. buccalis	*B. buccalis*
P. corporis	*B. corporis*
P. denticola	*B. denticola*
P. disiens	*B. disiens*
P. heparinolytica	*B. heparinolyticus*
P. intermedia	*B. intermedius*
P. loescheii	*B. loescheii*
P. melaninogenica	*B. melaninogenicus*
P. oralis	*B. oralis*
P. oris	*B. oris*
P. oulora	*B. oulorum*
P. ruminicola	*B. ruminicola*
P. veroralis	*B. veroralis*
P. zoogleoformans	*B. zoogleoformans*
Rikenella microfusus	*B. microfusus*
Ruminobacter amylophilus	*B. amylophilus*
Sebaldella termitidis	*B. termitidis*
Tissierella praeacuta	*B. praeacutus*
Wolinella curva	New species

mented *Prevotella* spp. and *Porphyromonas* spp. *Fusobacterium alocis, F. sulci* (both new species) (8), and *F. periodonticum* are primarily isolated from subgingival sites in gingivitis and periodontitis. *Fusobacterium necrophorum* is a very virulent anaerobe that may cause severe infection, usually in children or young adults, originating from pharyngotonsillitis. Local complications include peritonsillar abscess, periapical abscess, and jugular vein septic thrombophlebitis. There may also be multiple metastatic abscesses (most frequently in the lungs, pleural space, liver, and large joints) related to bacteremia (postanginal sepsis syndrome or Lemierre's disease) (31). *F. necrophorum* is encountered much less often now than in the era before antimicrobial agents. *Fusobacterium ulcerans* (a new species) is found in tropical ulcer (1).

Leptotrichia buccalis is a common mouth organism and may be found in the vagina and intestinal tract. It has been involved in cases of septicemia in immunocompromised patients with oral mucosal infections (4).

Selenomonas sputigena and the new species *S. artemidis, S. dianae, S. flueggei, S. infelix,* and *S. noxia* (30) are all oral organisms, as is *Centipeda periodontii* (a new genus and species) (29), which is found in subgingival sites in patients with periodontitis.

Desulfomonas pigra, Desulfovibrio spp., *Succinimonas amylolytica, Succinivibrio dextrinosolvens,* and *Butyrivibrio fibrisolvens* are all found as normal colonic flora but may occasionally be encountered in clinical infections as well (19). The sites of normal carriage of *Anaerobiospirillum succiniciproducens* in humans is unknown at present, but *Anaerobiospirillum* species are common in the fecal flora of cats and dogs (26). Strains of *Anaerobiospirillum* spp. have been isolated from blood cultures in compromised patients (19, 27) and from fecal specimens of patients with diarrhea (26). In the latter case, a zoonotic role for *Anaerobiospirillum* spp. has been proposed (26).

Acidaminococcus fermentans, Megasphaera elsdenii, and *Veillonella parvula* (see Table 8) are part of the normal human fecal flora, and *V. parvula,* as well as *V. atypica* and *V. dispar,* are part of the normal oral flora (36, 42). Anaerobic gram-negative cocci are rare pathogens. *Veillonella* spp. are isolated more frequently from clinical specimens than is *Megasphaera* sp., and *Acidaminococcus* sp. and *Veillonella* spp. have been encountered in oral, bite wound, head and neck, and miscellaneous soft tissue infections (44).

COLLECTION AND TRANSPORT OF SPECIMENS

The collection and transport of specimens are discussed in chapters 3 and 49. The importance of properly collected specimens cannot be overemphasized. An improperly collected or transported specimen, contaminated with normal flora, causes additional work for the laboratory and yields meaningless or misleading results for clinicians.

DIRECT EXAMINATION

Direct examination is of great importance, since it provides immediate semiquantitative information about the types of organisms and host cells present in a specimen; culture results will not be available until at least several days later. Thus, the initial therapy of a sick patient must be undertaken with knowledge of the usual infecting flora in particular types of infections and information provided by direct examination. The following methods of direct examination may be useful for the detection of gram-negative, nonsporeforming anaerobic bacteria: Gram stain, acridine orange stain, dark-field or phase-contrast microscopy, fluorescent-antibody procedures, and GLC.

Nucleic acid probes, used in the direct demonstration of some oral and nonoral gram-negative bacilli, are not yet standardized and produced for commercial distribution. Of the conventional methods, the Gram stain is by far the simplest and the most likely to yield significant information. A Gram stain reveals the type and relative numbers of most organisms, anaerobic and other, that are clinically significant. For the microbiologist, the findings from the Gram-stained smear may suggest the need for special selective media; this method also provides quality control regarding efficiency of isolation. For example, pale, pleomorphic, irregularly staining gram-negative rods are frequently obligate anaerobes. Coccobacillary forms are suggestive of the pigmenting *Prevotella* spp., *Porphyromonas* spp. (Fig. 1), or *Haemophilus* spp. Pale, pleomorphic, or uniform gram-negative rods with irregular or bipolar staining from an intra-abdominal infection are suggestive of *B. fragilis* group organisms (Fig. 2). *F. nucleatum* is a thin gram-negative rod with pointed ends; these organisms are often found in pairs end to end (Fig. 3). This needle-shaped morphology is shared with the microaerophilic *Capnocytophaga* spp. A much larger fusiform rod may suggest the presence of *L. buccalis*. *Fusobacterium mortiferum* is an extremely pleomorphic rod with deformed filaments containing swollen areas along with large, round bodies and exhibiting irregular staining (Fig. 4). *F. necrophorum* may have similar morphology but usually with fewer round bodies. *Bilophila wadsworthia* shows a mild degree of pleomorphism, and intracellular vacuoles are common (Fig. 5). Some clostridia usually stain as gram negative; an example is *Clostridium clostridioforme*. In thick films from exudates and bloody fluids, recognition of organisms may be facilitated by staining with acridine orange (24). Dark-field and phase-contrast microscopy may be helpful in the detection of small, poorly staining organisms (*Bacteroides pneumosintes*), the direct observation of motility (*Wolinella* spp.), the noting of spores (*Clostridium* spp.), and the recognition of morphotypes not cultivable on ordinary media (spirochetes).

Direct immunofluorescence staining of specimens has been used to rapidly detect members of the *B. fragilis* group and some members of the pigmented gram-negative species. Reagents are commercially available (Organon Teknika, Durham, N.C.). Certain cross-reactions

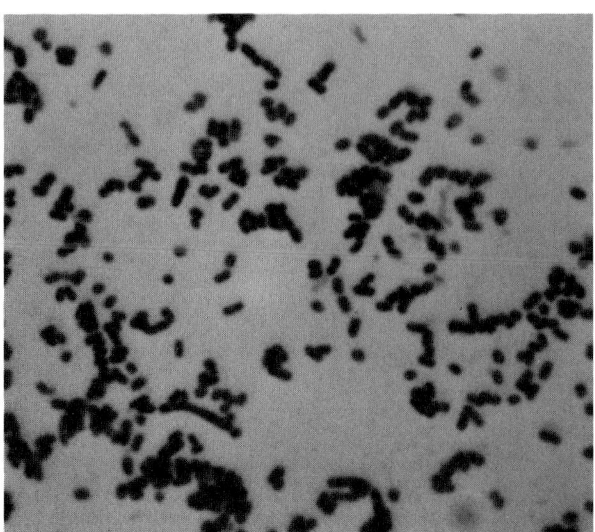

FIG. 1. Coccobacillary cells of *Porphyromonas asaccharolytica*.

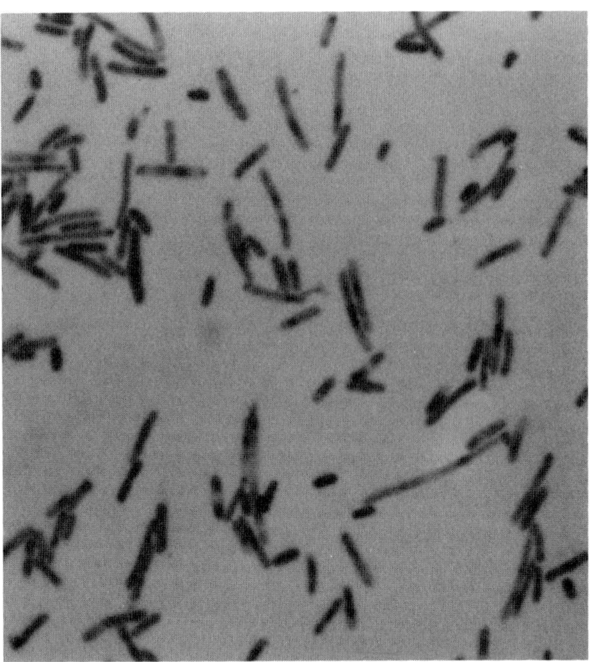

FIG. 2. Pleomorphic, irregularly staining cells of *Bacteroides fragilis*.

(with *P. bivia* and *P. disiens*) may occur, and the possibility of failure to detect *P. gingivalis* and some members (*B. ovatus*, *B. vulgatus*, and *B. distasonis*) of the *B. fragilis* group by individual test kits must be borne in mind (34, 52).

CULTURE AND ISOLATION

The selection and use of primary isolation media are discussed in chapter 49. The following procedures are used in the Wadsworth Clinical Anaerobic Bacteriology Research Laboratory (44) and the Anaerobe Reference Unit of the National Public Health Institute, Helsinki, Finland. Specimens are processed with a minimum of delay after submission. The minimum medium set that we inoculate includes (i) a nonselective, enriched, bru-

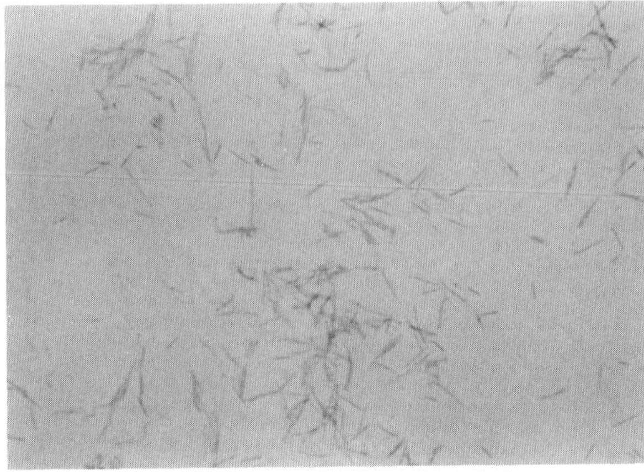

FIG. 3. Cells of *Fusobacterium nucleatum*. Note the slender shape with pointed ends.

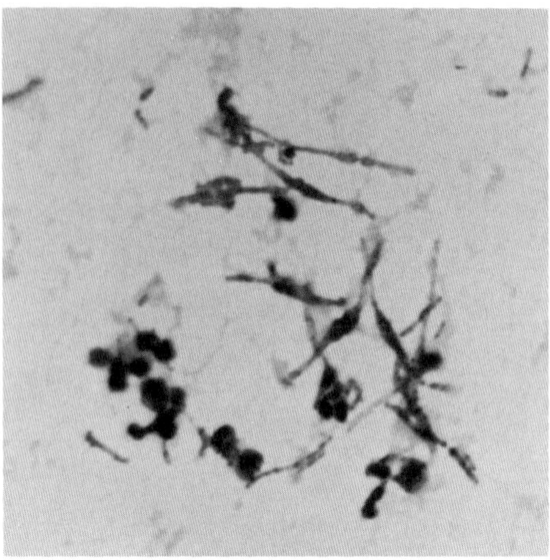

FIG. 4. Microscopic morphology of *Fusobacterium mortiferum*. There is marked pleomorphism and irregularity of staining. Note the filaments with swellings along their course.

cella-base sheep blood agar plate supplemented with vitamin K_1 and hemin (BAP); (ii) a kanamycin-vancomycin laked sheep blood agar for the selection of *Bacteroides* and *Prevotella* spp. (44) (it should be noted, however, that the 7.5-μg/ml concentration of vancomycin in the original formulation of this medium is inhibitory for asaccharolytic *Porphyromonas* spp. [47, 48]; at the National Public Health Institute, we have reduced the amount of vancomycin to 2.0 μg/ml); (iii) a *Bacteroides* bile-esculin agar plate (BBE) for the selection and presumptive identification of the *B. fragilis* group (25) and *Bilophila* sp. (5); and (iv) a phenylethyl alcohol-sheep blood agar plate to prevent overgrowth by aerobic gram-negative rods. Not all clinical laboratories will find it possible to use all four of these plate media. When fusobacteria are clinically suspected as the cause of infection, special selective media may be used (32). Fastidious anaerobe agar (see chapter 49) produces luxuriant growth of fusobacteria and can be used as a base medium with or without selective agents.

The inoculated anaerobic plates are immediately placed in an anaerobic environment, i.e., an anaerobic jar or chamber or an anaerobic pouch (Anaerobe Pouch, Difco Laboratories, Detroit, Mich.; Anaerocult P, Diagnostica Merck, Darmstadt, Federal Republic of Germany). Although not optimal, the holding jar method (chapter 49) may be used until enough plates accumulate to set up a jar. A new rapid, automated device (Anoxomat, Mart Microbiology Automation, Lichtenvoore, The Netherlands), for automatically setting up jars by the evacuation-replacement method and that alerts one to leaking jars, has been introduced commercially (6).

After incubation for 48 h at 35 to 36°C, the plates are examined, and the amount of growth of each colony type is estimated. In the case of a seriously ill patient, the plates may be examined and processed earlier in an anaerobic chamber or viewed through a plastic bag set up as a single or double culture.

To avoid undue exposure of cultures to oxygen, the use of small jars that are opened one at a time is advisable. The colonies are described, preferably with the aid of an 8× hand lens or a stereoscopic dissecting microscope, and they are Gram stained as described in chapter 49. Ideally, different colony types are subcultured to a brucella BAP to which special-potency antibiotic disks (colistin, 10 μg; kanamycin, 1,000 μg; and vancomycin, 5 μg), a nitrate disk, and a blank disk for indole detection are added (Fig. 6); to a chocolate agar plate which is incubated in 5 to 10% CO_2 and to blood agar which is incubated in air (for aerotolerance testing); to a rabbit laked blood agar plate for the rapid demonstration of pigment production; and to an egg yolk agar plate for the demonstration of lipase activity as well as for catalase testing. The primary plates are

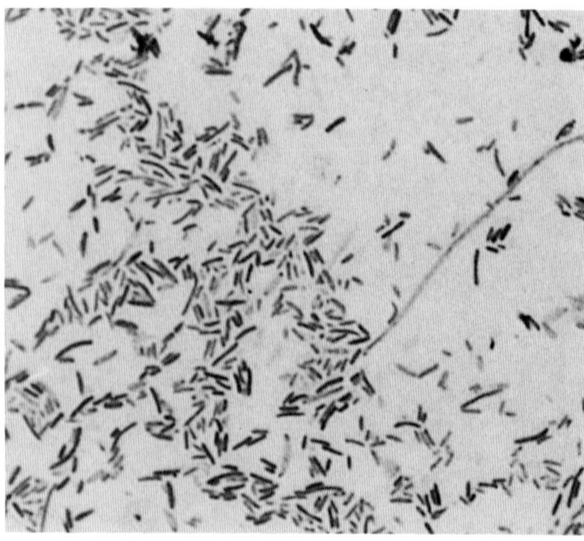

FIG. 5. Microscopic morphology, *Bilophila wadsworthia*.

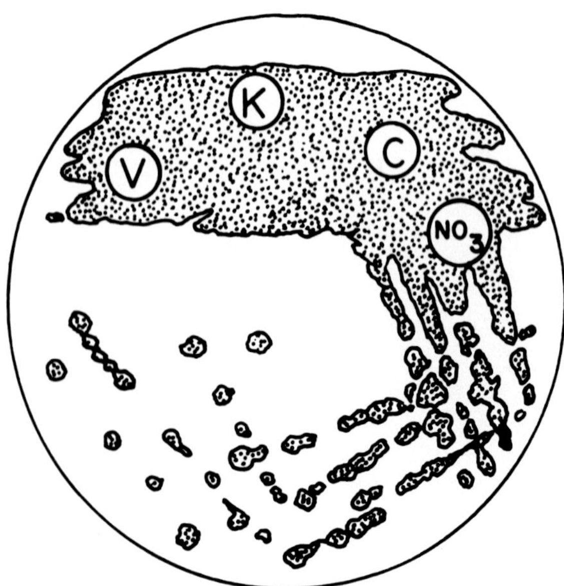

FIG. 6. Placement of special-potency antibiotic and nitrate disks. A blank disk for indole testing may be added (usually after growth has occurred).

reincubated along with the purity and test plates. In routine clinical microbiology, an incubation period of at least 5 to 7 days for primary plates is recommended. With shorter incubation times, several anaerobic species may not be detected.

The following characteristics are noted, and tests are made from the BAP: detailed colony morphology, pigment, fluorescence (long-wave UV light) (the last two are also recorded from the rabbit laked blood agar plate), hemolysis, greening, pitting, spot indole reaction (*p*-dimethylaminocinnamaldehyde reagent), nitrate and nitrite reduction, special-potency antibiotic disk susceptibility, catalase (15% H_2O_2, preferably from egg yolk agar), and motility from broth culture or plate (hanging drop). Motile isolates are studied further as indicated in Table 1; most often these isolates will be *Wolinella* spp. Another approach is the use of a Lombard-Dowell Presumpto 1 plate (see chapter 49), which may give additional important information for the presumptive identification of the anaerobic gram-negative rods (12). Good growth is necessary for the proper interpretation of test results on this medium. The primary plates are reinspected after 4 or more days to detect slow growers, new morphotypes, or late pigmenters. In oral microbiology, two rapid in situ tests have been used. One is used for the rapid differentiation of lactose-fermenting from lactose-nonfermenting species by spraying the colonies with the 4-methylumbelliferyl-D-galactoside reagent (Sigma Chemical Co., St. Louis, Mo, catalog no. M-1633; or Difco or Carr-Scarborough) and screening for fluorescent (lactose-positive) colonies under long-wave UV light (2). The other test is to demonstrate trypsinlike activity of suspected colonies of *P. gingivalis* by spraying the colonies with the carboxy-L-arginine-7-amino-4-methylcoumarin amide hydrochloride reagent (Hoechst AG, distributor; Calbiochem-Behring, La Jolla, Calif., catalog no. 21400) and screening for fluorescent colonies under long-wave UV light (41).

IDENTIFICATION OF SPECIES

Presumptive identification

Most of the clinically significant gram-negative rods can be placed into broad groups with relatively few tests, and some can be presumptively identified with ease (Table 3). The special-potency antibiotic disk pattern can be used to separate the gram-negative rods into several groups. A zone size equal to or greater than 10 mm is considered susceptible. Most of the *Bacteroides* spp. and *Prevotella* spp. are resistant to vancomycin and kanamycin and variable in susceptibility to colistin, whereas *Fusobacterium* strains, the *B. ureolyticus*-like group, and *Bilophila* sp. are resistant to vancomycin but susceptible to both colistin and kanamycin. As noted before, exceptions to this generalization include *Porphyromonas* spp. (*P. asaccharolytica, P. endodontalis,* and *P. gingivalis*), which are usually susceptible to vancomycin and resistant to colistin. *B. ureolyticus, B. gracilis, Wolinella* spp., and *Bilophila* sp. colonies are usually much smaller and more translucent than those of fusobacteria. An anaerobic gram-negative, catalase-negative rod that requires formate and fumarate for growth in broth culture or that pits agar may be presumptively identified as a *B. ureolyticus*-like organism. To document a formate-fumarate requirement, inoculate two tubes of peptone-yeast extract (or thioglycolate) broth medium, one containing the additive and the other without (serving as a control). Compare intensity of growth (see Table 3, footnote *b*). A strongly catalase-positive rod, stimulated by bile and pyruvate, can be presumptively identified as *Bilophila* sp. Organisms that fluoresce brick red under long-wave UV light or produce black colonies are placed in the pigmenting *Prevotella* spp.-*Porphyromonas* spp. group (Fig. 7). The *B. fragilis* group can be presumptively identified by their special-potency antibiotic disk pattern (resistant to all three antibiotics) and growth in 20% bile determined by a tube test, by a bile disk test (51), or on a BBE agar plate (Fig. 8). Most organisms not fitting these groupings are *Bacteroides* spp. or *Prevotella* spp. but occasionally are representatives of the other new genera listed in Table 1.

Gram-negative cocci are susceptible to colistin and usually to kanamycin but resistant to vancomycin. Small, gram-negative cocci reducing nitrate or nitrite and growing as small grayish white, translucent colonies, which fluoresce red under UV light, can be presumptively identified as *Veillonella* sp.

Rapid identification

The anaerobic gram-negative rods that can be rapidly identified are shown in Table 3. *F. nucleatum* is a thin rod with tapering ends and is indole positive. It fluoresces chartreuse under UV light and often produces greening of the agar after exposure to air. At least three different colony morphotypes of *F. nucleatum* exist: speckled (ground glass texture), bread crumb, and smooth. The size of the colonies varies according to type; for the bread crumb variant, it is usually <0.5 to 1 mm (Fig. 9). The new *Fusobacterium* species, *F. alocis* and *F. sulci* (mainly encountered in periodontal microbiology), are distinguished from *F. nucleatum* by their negative indole reaction, but further testing is necessary to separate them from other indole-negative *Fusobacterium* species. *F. necrophorum* is a bile-sensitive, lipase-positive fusobacterium. It is a pleomorphic long rod with round ends and often bizarre forms that produces indole, fluoresces chartreuse, greens the agar, and often produces beta-hemolysis around the dull, umbonate colonies (Fig. 10). Lipase-negative strains require further biochemical testing. A bile-resistant fusobacterium may be presumptively identified as belonging to the *F. mortiferum-F. varium* group; however, other fusobacteria (e.g., *F. necrophorum* and *F. ulcerans*) may grow in 20% bile; therefore, further testing is required to confirm the presumptive identification.

B. ureolyticus, B. gracilis, and *Wolinella* spp. are thin gram-negative rods with rounded ends and possess the *Fusobacterium* disk pattern. The colonies are small and translucent or transparent and may produce greening of the agar. Three colony morphotypes exist: smooth and convex, pitting (Fig. 11), and spreading. All colony types can occur in the same culture. These organisms are asaccharolytic, catalase-negative, and nitrate or nitrite reducing, and they require supplementation of broth media with formate and fumarate for growth (Table 3, footnote *b*). The *Wolinella* spp. are motile and difficult to differentiate from *Campylobacter concisus* (see chapter 39); however, *Wolinella* spp. are oxidase negative or weakly positive, whereas *C. concisus* is strongly oxidase positive. *B. ureolyticus* is urease posi-

TABLE 3. Grouping of anaerobic gram-negative rods

Group and species	Characteristic[a]														
	Kanamycin (1,000 μg)	Vancomycin (5 μg)	Colistin (10 μg)	Growth in 20% bile	Catalase	Indole	Lipase	Slender cells with pointed ends	Growth stimulated by formate-fumarate[b]	Nitrate reduction[c]	Urease[d]	Motility[e]	Pitting of agar	Pigment	Brick red fluorescence
Bacteroides fragilis group	R	R	R	$+^{-}$	V	V	−								−
Other *Bacteroides* spp.	R	R	V	−	−	V	−			$-^{+}$					
Pigmenting species	R	V	V	−	$-^{+}$	V	V							+	$+^{-}$
Prevotella intermedia	R	R	S	−	−	+	$+^{-}$								
P. loescheii	R	R	V	−	−	−	V								
B. ureolyticus-like group[f]	S	R	S	−	−	−	−		+	+	V	V	V		
B. ureolyticus	S	R	S	−	−	−			+	+	+	−	V		
B. gracilis	S	R	S	−	−	−			+	+	−	−	V		
Wolinella spp.	S	R	S	−	−	−			+	+	−	+	V		
Campylobacter concisus[g]	S	R	S	−	−	−			+	+	−	+	−		
Bilophila sp.[h]	S	R	S	+	+	−	−		−	+	$+^{-}$	−	V		
Fusobacterium spp.	S	R	S	V	−	V	V	V							−
F. nucleatum	S	R	S	−		+	−	+							
F. necrophorum	S	R	S	$-^{+}$		+	$+^{-}$	−							
F. varium-mortiferum	S	R	S	+		V	−	−							

[a] R, Resistant; S, susceptible; V, variable; +, positive reaction for majority of strains; −, negative reaction; $+^{-}$, most strains positive, some strains negative; $-^{+}$, most strains negative, some strains positive.

[b] Compare the growth of the organism in an unsupplemented thioglycolate broth with growth in a broth supplemented with formate and fumarate (additive: dissolve 3 g of sodium formate, 3 g of fumaric acid, and 20 pellets of sodium hydroxide in 50 ml of distilled water. Adjust pH to 7. Filter sterilize the sample. Add 0.5 ml of additive to 10 ml of culture broth [17, 44]).

[c] Use the spot nitrate disk test (chapter 49).

[d] Make a heavy suspension of the organism in 0.5 ml of sterile urea broth (Difco) or in sterile saline and insert a urea tablet (Rosco, Taastrup, Denmark). Incubate the tubes aerobically for up to 24 h. A bright pink or red is positive; this color usually appears within 15 to 30 min. If the indicator becomes reduced, add Nessler reagent (chapter 122) to determine the ammonia production (ammonia indicates a positive reaction).

[e] Use the hanging-drop method with colonies from the isolation BAP. If result is negative, check motility with a young broth culture supplemented with formate and fumarate.

[f] Formate and fumarate should be added to test media for this group of organisms.

[g] *C. concisus* is strongly oxidase positive; *Wolinella* spp. are oxidase negative or weakly positive.

[h] Growth stimulated by 1% pyruvate (final concentration).

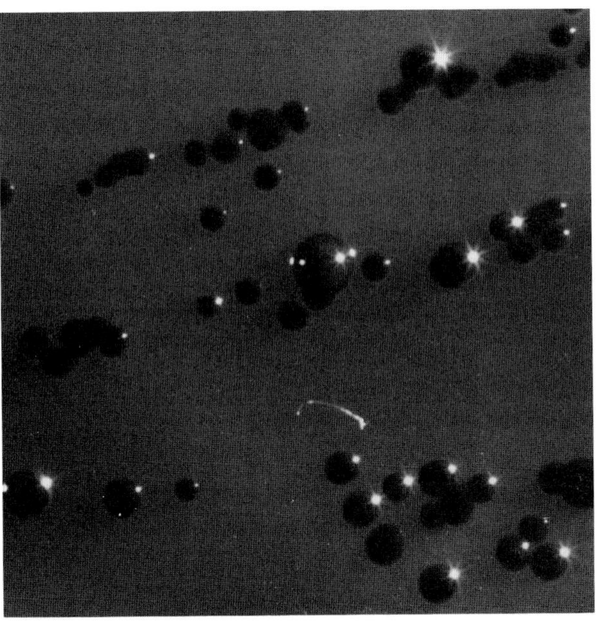

FIG. 7. Black-pigmenting colonies of *Porphyromonas asaccharolytica*.

tive, and *B. gracilis* is nonmotile and urease negative (Table 3, footnotes *d* to *f*). *Bilophila* sp., which phenotypically resembles *B. ureolyticus*, is distinguished from the former three species by its stimulation by bile and strong catalase reaction. An indole- and lipase-positive coccobacillus that forms black-pigmented colonies or fluoresces brick red may be identified as *P. intermedia*. Any lipase-negative strains must be identified further by other biochemical tests. A lipase-positive, indole-negative pigmenting gram-negative rod may be identified as *P. loescheii*, but occasional strains of *P. melaninogenica* may also be lipase-positive (29).

Small, gram-negative cocci, fluorescing red under UV light and reducing nitrate or nitrite, are probably *Veillonella* spp. *Megasphaera* cells are large (>1.5 μm). *Megasphaera* and *Acidaminococcus* colonies do not fluoresce.

Definitive identification

The definite identification of most species requires certain additional biochemical tests and metabolic end product analysis by GLC. Curved rods that are not *Wolinella* spp. should be checked for motility and identified according to Table 1. Organisms with small, translucent, spreading colonies that are not *B. ureolyticus*-like should also be checked for motility. Very large fusiform rods isolated from the mouth or urogenital tract are suggestive of *Leptotrichia* spp. The characteristic GLC pattern should be confirmed. Tables 4 to 7 are based on reactions in prereduced, anaerobically sterilized (PRAS) liquid media (chapter 49) (17, 29, 44). Thioglycolate-based media with a bromthymol blue indicator give similar results (11) (for the use of these media, see chapters 49 and 121). **Do not interpret the results from other systems with these tables.** Gas chromatographic

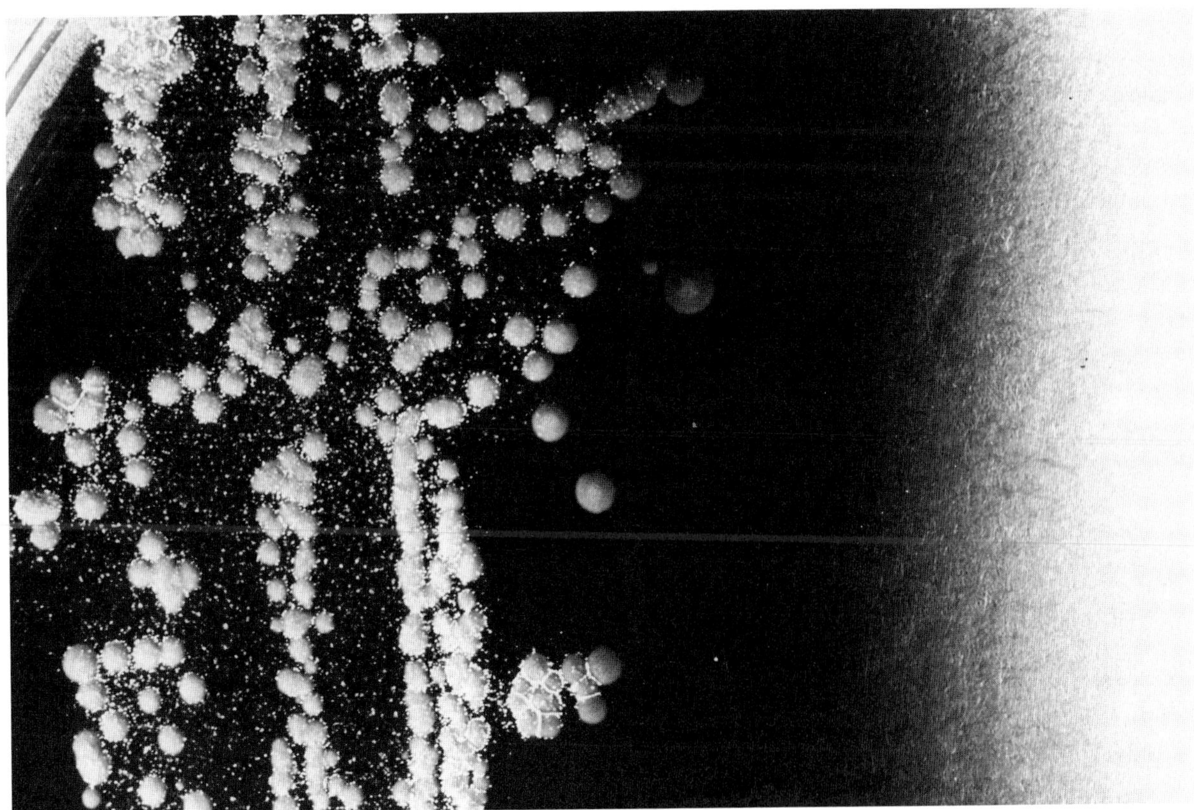

FIG. 8. Colonies of *Bacteroides fragilis* on BBE agar. Note the blackening of the agar and colonies due to esculin hydrolysis and bile precipitation.

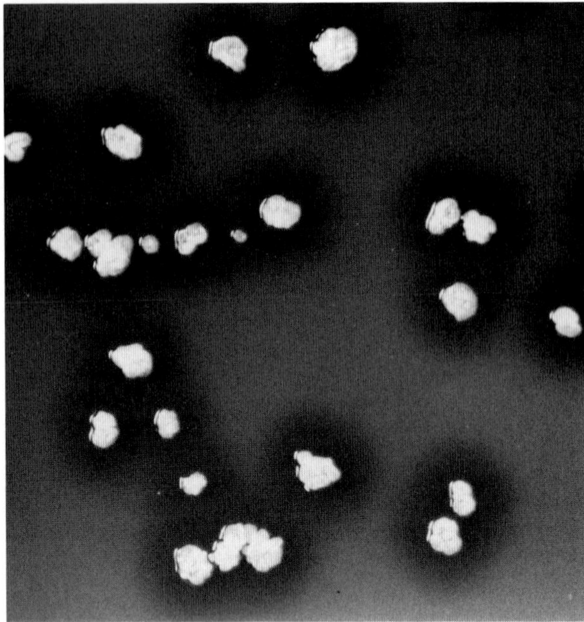

FIG. 9. Bread crumb-shaped colonies of *Fusobacterium nucleatum.*

analysis may be performed on broth that shows good growth of the organism (see chapter 49 for procedures). Each lot of uninoculated broth must be assayed in parallel with samples to determine the background amounts of acetic and succinic acids; if chopped meat broth is used, an uninoculated broth is assayed for lactic acid. Fermentation end products vary depending on the substrate available to the organism, which may lead to misinterpretation of the GLC pattern and misidentification of the organism. For instance, saccharolytic organisms will produce greater amounts of isoacids in the absence of a fermentable carbohydrate, and a fermentable carbohydrate is required for the detection of lactic acid.

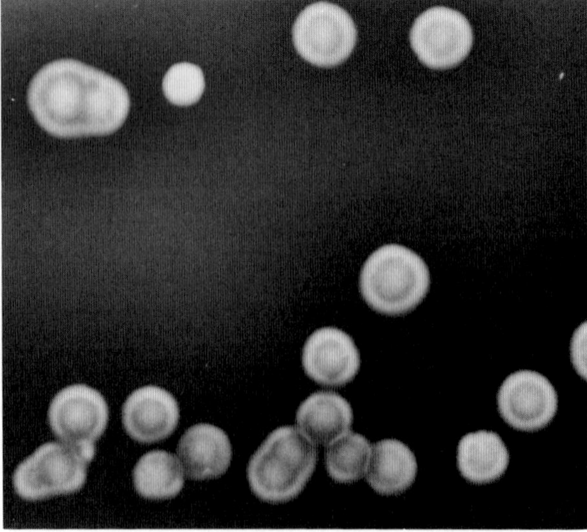

FIG. 10. Umbonate colonies of *Fusobacterium necrophorum.*

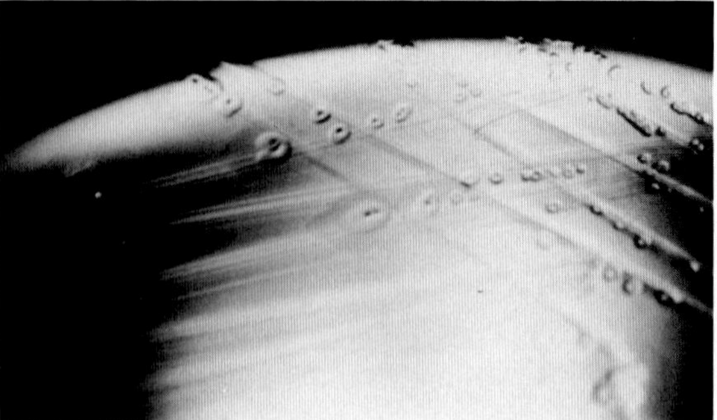

FIG. 11. Pitting colonies of *Bacteroides ureolyticus.*

Colonies of the *B. fragilis* group on brucella BAP are 2 to 3 mm in diameter, circular, entire, convex, and gray to white. Supplementation of media with hemin enhances growth. The cells may be uniform or pleomorphic (some with vacuoles); this difference is medium and age dependent. Good growth in or stimulation by 20% bile (2% oxgall) is characteristic of the *B. fragilis* group; the exception to this rule is the poor growth of *B. uniformis* in bile. Some non-*B. fragilis* group organisms are bile resistant; however, *B. splanchnicus* and *B. eggerthii* are sucrose negative, and *Bilophila* sp. forms much smaller colonies on BBE agar and is asaccharolytic. Most of the *B. fragilis* group organisms blacken the BBE agar (esculin hydrolyzed) except for *B. vulgatus,* which may not hydrolyze esculin. Table 4 is a key for the differentiation of the bile-resistant *B. fragilis* group and related *Bacteroides* spp. *B. thetaiotaomicron* and *B. ovatus* may be difficult to differentiate; xylan and salicin are useful in separating these two species; the former is xylan and salicin positive, and the latter is usually negative for both. More ovoid-shaped cells on Gram stain are suggestive of *B. ovatus.* Differentiation of *B. ovatus* and *B. stercoris* is made by trehalose utilization; *B. ovatus* ferments trehalose, whereas *B. stercoris* does not (21). *B. caccae* and *B. merdae* closely resemble *B. distasonis.* Arabinose is fermented by *B. caccae* but not usually by *B. distasonis* or *B. merdae. B. caccae* and most *B. merdae* strains are catalase negative, and *B. distasonis* is usually positive.

The bile-sensitive, nonpigmenting anaerobic gram-negative bacilli form three major subgroups: (i) saccharolytic, (ii) saccharolytic and proteolytic, and (iii) asaccharolytic. The first two subgroups have been proposed as part of a new genus, *Prevotella,* as mentioned before. Table 5 lists the more commonly encountered or clinically important species in this group.

The saccharolytic organisms fall into two categories, pentose fermenters and nonfermenters (arabinose and xylose are usually tested). *P. oris* and *P. buccae* are pentose fermenters. They are phenotypically very similar, but they can be differentiated by the α-fucosidase and *N*-acetyl-β-glucosaminidase tests (see Table 5, footnote *b*) (15, 22); the former is positive and the latter negative in both tests. *P. buccae* is susceptible to the special-potency colistin disk, whereas *P. oris* is not (22). *P. zoogleoformans,* which is only rarely isolated from clinical specimens, may ferment pentoses. Recently, indole-positive oral strains of this bacterium from both humans and lower animals (cats, dogs, and horses) have been reidentified as *P. heparinolytica* (3, 35). Both produce

TABLE 4. Characteristics of bile-resistant (*B. fragilis* group and related) *Bacteroides* spp.

Group and species	Characteristic[a]												
	Growth in 20% bile	Indole	Catalase	Esculin hydrolyzed	Fermentation of:								Fatty acids from PYG[b]
					Glucose	Sucrose	Maltose	Rhamnose	Salicin	Trehalose	Arabinose	Xylan	
B. fragilis group													
B. distasonis	+	–	$+^-$	+	+	+	+	V	+	+	$-^+$		A, p, S (pa, ib, iv, l)
B. caccae	+	–	–	+	+	+	+	$+^-$	$-^+$	+	+		A, p, S (iv)
B. fragilis	+	–	+	+	+	+	+	–	–	–	–		A, p, S, pa (ib, iv, l)
B. merdae	+	–	$-^+$	+	+	+	+	+	+	+	$-^+$		A, p, S (ib, iv)
B. vulgatus	+	–	$-^+$	$-^+$	+	+	+	+	–	–	+		A, p, S
B. ovatus	+	+	$-^+$	+	+	+	+	+	+	+	+	+	A, p, S, pa (ib, iv, l)
B. stercoris	+	+	–	$+^-$	+	+	+	+	$-^+$	–	$-^+$		A, p, S, f (ib, iv)
B. thetaiotaomicron	+	+	$+^-$	+	+	+	+	+	$-^+$	+	+	–	A, p, S, pa (ib, iv, l)
B. uniformis	W^+	+	$-^+$	+	+	+	+	$-^+$	$+^-$	–	+		a, p, l, S (ib, iv)
B. eggerthii	+	+	–	+	+	–	+	$+^-$	–	–	+		A, p, S (ib, iv, l)
Other													
B. splanchnicus	W^+	+	–	+	+	–	–	–	–	–	+		A, P, ib, b, iv, S (l)

[a] +, Positive reaction for the majority of strains (includes weak as well as strong acid production from carbohydrates); –, negative reaction; W, weak reaction; $+^-$, most strains positive, some strains negative; $-^+$, most strains negative, some strains positive. Sugars: +, pH < 5.5; W, pH 5.5 to 5.7; –, pH > 5.7.

[b] Capital letters indicate major metabolic products from peptone-yeast extract-glucose (PYG), lowercase letters indicate minor products, and parentheses indicate a variable reaction for the following fatty acids: A, acetic; P, propionic; F, formic; IB, isobutyric; B, butyric; IV, isovaleric; V, valeric; L, lactic; S, succinic; PA, phenylacetic. Note that isoacids are primarily from carbohydrate-free media (e.g., peptone-yeast extract) in the case of saccharolytic organisms.

viscous material in broth cultures. The indole reaction differentiates these two species.

Salicin, cellobiose, and xylan are the key sugars in the differentiation of *P. oralis, P. buccalis, P. veroralis,* and *P. oulora* (40). Furthermore, *P. oulora* produces catalase and is lipase-positive (29). Certain strains of the saccharolytic pigmenting *Prevotella* spp. require more than 21 days to develop pigment, and these strains, especially *P. loescheii,* closely resemble the *P. oralis* group organisms. Darker, more opaque colonies and salicin, xylan, and gelatin reactions may aid in differentiating the strains.

P. bivia and *P. disiens* are both saccharolytic and strongly proteolytic. Gelatin and milk are usually digested within 2 to 3 days (milk may take longer). Differentiation is based on lactose fermentation; *P. bivia* is lactose positive, and *P. disiens* is lactose negative. Under long-wave UV light, *P. bivia* colonies may fluoresce a light orange to pink (coral) that should not be confused with the brick red fluorescence of the pigmenting *P. melaninogenica-P. intermedia* group and *Porphyromonas* spp. Tests for the production of indole and the fermentation of mannose, sucrose, and lactose and observation for pigment production on a rabbit laked blood agar plate are useful. Asaccharolytic, nonpigmented, bile-sensitive *Bacteroides* spp. and *Tissierella* spp. are infrequently isolated from clinical specimens. *B. capillosus* may ferment glucose weakly, is esculin positive, coagulates milk, and may grow better with Tween 80-supplemented media. *B. pneumosintes* (not shown in Table 5) is a tiny rod and forms minute colonies. *T. praeacuta* and *B. putredinis* are asaccharolytic and proteolytic; an indole test will differentiate them.

The pigmented *Prevotella* spp. and *Porphyromonas* spp. vary greatly in degree and rapidity of pigmenting, depending primarily on the type of blood used in the agar; laked rabbit blood is most reliable and produces most rapid pigmentation. A period of 2 to 21 days may be required to detect pigmentation, which ranges from buff to tan to black. The identity of strains not showing pigmentation within 21 days must be established by other biochemical tests. *Actinomyces odontolyticus,* a gram-positive, nonsporeforming rod, may be confused initially with these organisms since it may produce a red pigment. A Gram stain will readily differentiate them. The pigmented *Prevotella* spp. and *Porphyromonas* spp. fluoresce pink, orange, chartreuse, or brick red under UV light. Brick red is the only reliable color for presumptive identification, since some nonpigmenting *Prevotella* spp. fluoresce coral or pink. Fluorescence is masked by pigment production in older cultures.

Table 6 is a key for the differentiation of the pigmenting *Prevotella* spp. and *Porphyromonas* spp. *Porphyromonas asaccharolytica, P. endodontalis,* and *P. gingivalis* are all asaccharolytic and phenotypically very similar. Pigment may not be detectable in *P. endodontalis* cultures until 7 days (48). Phenylacetic acid production, trypsinlike activity, and *N*-acetyl-β-glucosaminidase activity of *P. gingivalis* will differentiate it from the other two species (see Table 6, footnote *b*). The α-fucosidase activity of *P. asaccharolytica* in turn separates it from *P. endodontalis.*

The unusual special-potency antibiotic disk pattern (susceptible to vancomycin) in addition to asaccharo-

TABLE 5. Characteristics of nonpigmented, bile-sensitive *Bacteroides* and *Prevotella* spp. and *Tissierella* sp.

Subgroup and species	Characteristic[a]													
	Glucose	Sucrose	Lactose	Arabinose	Xylose	Salicin	Cellobiose	Xylan	Esculin hydrolyzed	α-Fucosidase[b]	*N*-Acetyl-β-glucosaminidase[b]	Indole	Gelatin	Fatty acids from PYG[c]
Saccharolytic pentose fermenters														
Prevotella oris	+	+	+	+⁻	+	+	+		+	+	+	−		A, S (p, ib, iv)
P. buccae	+	+	+	+	+	+	+		+	−	−	−		A, S (p, ib, b, iv, l)
P. heparinolytica[d]	+	+	+	+	+	+	+		+	+	+	+		a, S (p, iv)
P. zoogleoformans[d]	+	+	+	V	V	V	+		+			−		A, P, S (ib, iv)
Saccharolytic pentose nonfermenters														
P. oralis	+	+	+	−	−	+	+	−	+			−		A, f, S (l)
P. buccalis	+	+	+	−	−	−	+	−	+			−		a, iv, S
P. veroralis	+	+	+	−	−	−	+	+	+			−		a, S
P. oulora	+	−	+	−	−	−	−	−	−			−		A, S
Saccharolytic and proteolytic														
P. bivia	+	−	+	−	−	−	−		−			−	+	A, iv, S (f, ib)
P. disiens	+	−	−	−	−	−	−		−			−	+	A, S (f, p, ib, iv)
Weakly or nonsaccharolytic														
Bacteroides capillosus	W⁻	−	−	−	−	−	−		+			−	−	a, s (f, p, l)
Tissierella praeacuta	−	−	−	−	−	−	−		−			−	+	A, p, ib, B, IV, s (f, l)
B. putredinis	−	−	−	−	−	−	−		−			+	+	a, P, ib, b, IV, S (l)

[a] See Table 4, footnote *a*. W⁻, Most strains give weak reaction, some give negative reaction.
[b] Make a heavy suspension (>McFarland no. 2) of the organism in 0.25 ml of sterile saline. Insert a tablet of substrate (Rosco). Incubate the sample for 4 h (or overnight). Yellow color positive; colorless negative.
[c] See Table 4, footnote *b*.
[d] Unique in producing viscous sediment in broth.

TABLE 6. Characteristics of pigmented *Prevotella* spp. and *Porphyromonas* spp.

Species	Characteristic[a]											
	Indole	Lipase	Catalase	Fermentation of:				Esculin hydro-lyzed	α-Fuco-sidase[b]	*N*-Acetyl-β-glucos-aminidase[b]	Tryp-sin	Phenylacetic acid production	Fatty acids from PYG[c]
				Glucose	Maltose	Lactose	Cellobiose						
Asaccharolytic (*Porphyromonas*)													
P. asaccharolytica	+	–	–	–	–	–	–		+	–	–	–	A, p, ib, B, IV, S
P. endodontalis	+	–	–	–	–	–	–		–	–	–	–	A, p, ib, B, IV, S
P. gingivalis	+	–	–	–	–	–	–		–	+	+	+	a, p, ib, B, IV, s, pa
Saccharolytic (*Prevotella*)													
P. intermedia	+	$+^{-}$	–	+	+	–	–						A, iv, S (f, p, ib)
P. corporis	–	–	–	+	+	–	–						A, ib, iv, S, (b)
P. melaninogenica	–	$-^{+}$	–	+	+	+	–	–					A, S (f, ib, iv, l)
P. denticola	–	–	–	+	+	+	–	+					A, S (f, ib, iv, l)
P. loescheii	–	V	–	+	+	+	+	V					a, S (f, l)

[a] See Table 4, footnote *a*.
[b] See Table 5, footnote *b*.
[c] See Table 4, footnote *b*.

TABLE 7. Characteristics of *Fusobacterium* spp.

Species	Characteristic[a]											
	Distinctive cellular morphology	Indole	Growth in 20% bile	Lipase	Gas in glucose agar	Fermentation of:			Esculin hydrolyzed	Lactate converted to propionate	Threonine converted to propionate	Fatty acids from PYG[b]
						Glucose	Fructose	Mannose				
F. nucleatum	Slender, pointed ends	+	$-^{c}$	–	$-^{2}$	$-^{w}$	$-^{w}$	–	–	–	+	a, p, B (F, L, s)
F. gonidiaformans	Gonidia form	+	–	–	4^{2}	–	–	–	–	–	+	A, p, B (f, l, s)
F. necrophorum		+	$-^{+}$	$+^{-}$	4^{2}	$-^{w}$	$-^{w}$	–	–	+	+	a, p, B (l, s)
F. naviforme	Boat shape	+	–	–	$-^{2}$	w^{-}	–	–	–	–	–	a, B, L (f, p, s)
F. varium		$+^{-}$	+	–	4	w^{+}	w^{+}	$+^{w}$	–	–	+	a, p, B, L (s)
F. mortiferum	Bizarre; round bodies	–	+	–	4	$+^{w}$	$+^{w}$	$+^{w}$	+	–	+	a, p, B (f, v, l, s)
F. ulcerans	Pointed ends, some with central round swellings	–	+	–	2	+	–	$+^{-}$	–	–	+	a, p, B, l (s)
F. russii		–	–	–	2^{-}	–	–	–	–	–	–	a, B, L (f)

[a] See Table 4, footnote *a;* $+^{w}$, most positive, some strains weakly positive; $-^{w}$, most strains negative, some strains weakly positive; w^{-}, most strains weakly positive, some strains negative; w^{+}, most strains weakly positive, some strains positive. Gas in peptone-yeast extract-glucose (PYG) agar deep: –, no gas detected; 2, splits agar horizontally; 4, agar displaced to the top of the tube. Sugars: +, pH < 5.5; W, pH 5.5 to 5.7; –, pH > 5.7.
[b] See Table 4, footnote *b*.
[c] Extremely rarely, strains may be positive.

TABLE 8. Characteristics of gram-negative cocci

Organism	Characteristic[a]			
	Nitrate reduction	Catalase	Glucose	Fatty acids from PYG[b]
Veillonella spp.	+	V	−	A, p
Acidaminococcus fermentans	−	−	−	A, B
Megasphaera elsdenii	−	−	+	a, ib, b, iv, v, C

[a] See Table 4, footnote *a*. V, Variable reaction.
[b] See Table 4, footnote *b*.

lytic properties separate the *Porphyromonas* spp. from the other pigmenters. As noted before, *Prevotella melaninogenica*, *P. loescheii*, and *P. denticola* may require a full 21 days to develop pigment and may therefore be confused with the *P. oralis* group organisms. As noted before, salicin and cellobiose are useful tests in differentiating the two groups of organisms. *B. macacae*, *B. levii*, and *B. salivosus* are pigmenting *Bacteroides* species of animal origin and are rarely isolated from human clinical specimens. These species are separated from the human strains by the positive catalase reaction of most of the animal strains.

With the special-potency antibiotic disks, *Fusobacterium* spp. are resistant to vancomycin and sensitive to kanamycin and colistin; they produce butyric acid without isobutyric or isovaleric acid. The fusobacteria are weakly saccharolytic or nonfermentative. Most are nonproteolytic (gelatin negative). Colonial morphology varies greatly. In addition, some strains fluoresce chartreuse under UV light, and other strains cause greening of the agar. The most common clinical isolates, *F. nucleatum* and *F. necrophorum*, are indole positive. These two organisms have been discussed above in the section on rapid identification.

Table 7 characterizes the more commonly isolated fusobacteria. The conversion of threonine and lactate to propionic acid is important in the differentiation of these species. Bizarre pleomorphic rods with very large round bodies are suggestive of *F. mortiferum* (Fig. 4). This organism may grow on BBE agar and turn the agar black. A new species, *F. ulcerans*, isolated from tropical ulcer closely resembles *F. mortiferum* but is esculin negative (1). *F. periodonticum*, an oral isolate, is indole positive and bile sensitive, ferments glucose, fructose, and galactose, and converts threonine but not lactate to propionate. The two recently described, bile-sensitive asaccharolytic fusobacteria, *F. alocis* and *F. sulci*, from the gingival sulci, are indole negative and thus may be distinguished from *F. nucleatum* (8).

Veillonella spp. are nonfermentative and produce acetic and propionic acids (Table 8). *Acidaminococcus fermentans* produces acetic and butyric acids. *Megasphaera elsdenii* is glucose fermenting and produces multiple fatty acids, including caproic acid.

Other approaches to identification

Several microsystems are currently available for the identification of anaerobes. These include the API 20A and AN-Ident (Analytab Products, Inc., Plainview, N.Y.), Minitek (BBL Microbiology Systems, Cockeysville, Md.), IDS RapID ANA II panel (Innovative Diagnostic Systems, Decatur, Ga.), and ATB 32 A panel (API Systems, Montalieu, Vercieu, France). The API 20A and the Minitek systems produce results in 24 to 48 h and have computerized data bases. Both systems are best suited for the identification of fast-growing, saccharolytic organisms. With asaccharolytic and slow-growing strains, problems in interpretation occur; therefore, one should

TABLE 9. Activities of various drugs against *Bacteroides* spp., *Porphyromonas* spp., and *Prevotella* spp. (Wadsworth agar dilution procedure)

Drug	Breakpoint	% Susceptible at breakpoint			
		B. fragilis species	*B. fragilis* group[a]	*B. gracilis*	Other
Chloramphenicol	16	100	100	100	100
Imipenem	8	100	100	100	100
Ticarcillin-clavulanate[b]	128	100	99	60[c]	100
Metronidazole	16	100	100	93	99
Clindamycin	4	93	81	61	100
Cefoxitin	32	92	75	78	99
Ticarcillin[d]	128	78	83	20[c]	100
Penicillin G	16	5	6	67	70
Cefotaxime	32	50	50	78	96
Ceftizoxime	32	43	45[e]	89	97
Cefoperazone	32	57	51	67	94
Moxalactam	16	78	55	78	77
Cefotetan	32	85	56	50	80

[a] Includes the species *B. fragilis*.
[b] Other β-lactam–β-lactamase inhibitor combinations have equivalent activity.
[c] Only five strains studied.
[d] Other broad-spectrum penicillins have similar activity.
[e] This drug is much more active (95% susceptible at breakpoint) with microbroth dilution procedure.

not use these systems for such strains. The color reactions are not always clear-cut; shades of brown (API) and yellow-orange (Minitek) obscure interpretation of reactions. The overall accuracy of both systems is increased if these methods are supplemented by the simple tests mentioned before and by GLC. The AN-Ident and RapID ANA II are 4-h test systems based primarily on the detection of preformed enzymes. The panels are incubated in air. The use of heavy inocula and a short incubation period minimizes the risk of contamination. Interpretation of the color reactions of naphthylamine substrates may cause problems, since borderline reactions often occur. A computerized data base, with the inclusion of the recent changes in nomenclature, is available. In our experience in testing 480 bacterial strains with an earlier version of RapID ANA, the overall accuracy of identification to species level was 74% (43). The precision of this system may be increased when supplemented with the simple tests discussed earlier and GLC. These systems are a good initial approach for the identification of organisms that would otherwise need extensive testing in PRAS biochemicals; organisms not identified by the rapid tests will still require the use of PRAS biochemicals if definitive identification is sought. At present, the Vitek system for anaerobes is quite comparable to the RapID ANA II system.

The ATB 32 A has recently entered the European market. The principle in this system also is the detection of preformed enzymes. So far, there are only limited data on the performance of this system. In one study that examined 250 clinical isolates, the overall accuracy of identification of anaerobes to species level was 84% (W. J. Looney, I. Duca, A. Gallusser, and H. Modde, Abstr. 3rd Eur. Congr. Anaerobic Bacteria Infect., 1989, abstr. PE 6, p. 37).

The Microbial Identification System (MIS) technique is based on the determination of extracted cellular fatty acids of anaerobes by GLC, using a capillary column (33). Fatty acid profiles obtained are compared with those in a library compiled in a computer.

Serological procedures are not yet practical for the identification of colonial growth.

Susceptibility testing of anaerobes is discussed in chapter 113. The usual susceptibility patterns of the most commonly encountered gram-negative rods of clinical significance are noted in Tables 9 and 10; the usual susceptibility patterns of *Veillonella* spp. are noted in Table 10.

TABLE 10. Activities of various drugs against other gram-negative anaerobes

Drug	% Susceptible at breakpoint		
	Fusobacterium spp.	*Bilophila* spp.[a]	*Veillonella* spp.
Chloramphenicol	100	100	100
Imipenem	95	71	100
Ticarcillin-clavulanate	97	22	
Metronidazole	100	100	100
Clindamycin	92	94	95–100
Cefoxitin	99	45	100
Ticarcillin	85	29	100
Penicillin G	100	45	70–90
Cefotaxime	100	73	
Ceftizoxime	100	43	
Cefoperazone	88		
Moxalactam	77		
Cefotetan	81	79	

[a] Inoculum density McFarland no. 2 instead of the standard 0.5.

The β-lactamase-producing (nitrocefin test) gram-negative anaerobic rods are as follows:

B. fragilis group
B. gracilis (occasionally)
B. coagulans
B. splanchnicus
F. mortiferum
F. nucleatum
F. varium
Megamonas hypermegas
Mitsuokella multiacida
Pigmented *Prevotella* spp. and *Porphyromonas* spp.
Prevotella buccae
P. oris
P. disiens
P. oralis group

Not all strains within each species or group produce β-lactamase.

LITERATURE CITED

1. **Adriaans, B., and H. Shah.** 1988. *Fusobacterium ulcerans* sp.nov. from tropical ulcers. Int. J. Syst. Bacteriol. **38:**447–448.
2. **Alcoforado, G. A., T. L. McKay, and J. Slots.** 1987. Rapid method for detection of lactose fermenting oral microorganisms. Oral Microbiol. Immunol. **2:**35–38.
3. **Bailey, G. D., L. V. H. Moore, D. N. Love, and J. L. Johnson.** 1988. *Bacteroides heparinolyticus:* deoxyribonucleic acid relatedness of strains from the oral cavity and oral-associated disease conditions of horses, cats, and humans. Int. J. Syst. Bacteriol. **38:**42–44.
4. **Baquero, F., J. Fernández, F. Dionda, A. Erice, J. Pérez de Oteiza, J. A. Reguera, and M. Reig.** 1990. Capnophilic and anaerobic bacteremia in neutropenic patients: an oral source. Rev. Infect. Dis. **12**(Suppl **2**)**:**S157–S160.
5. **Baron, E. J., P. Summanen, J. Downes, M. C. Roberts, H. Wexler, and S. M. Finegold.** 1989. *Bilophila wadsworthia*, gen. nov. and sp. nov., a unique gram-negative anaerobic rod recovered from appendicitis specimens and human faeces. J. Gen. Microbiol. **135:**3405–3411.
6. **Brazier, J. S., and S. A. Smith.** 1989. Evaluation of the Anoxomat: a new technique for anaerobic and microaerophilic clinical bacteriology. J. Clin. Pathol. **42:**640–644.
7. **Brook, I.** 1988. Recovery of anaerobic bacteria from clinical specimens in 12 years at two military hospitals. J. Clin. Microbiol. **26:**1181–1188.
8. **Cato, E. P., L. V. H. Moore, and W. E. C. Moore.** 1985. *Fusobacterium alocis* sp. nov. and *Fusobacterium sulci* sp. nov. from the human gingival sulcus. Int. J. Syst. Bacteriol. **35:**475–477.
9. **Collins, M. D., and H. N. Shah.** 1986. Reclassification of *Bacteroides praeacutus* Tissier (Holdeman and Moore) in a new genus, *Tissierella*, as *Tissierella praeacuta* comb. nov. Int. J. Syst. Bacteriol. **36:**461–463.
10. **Collins, M. D., and H. N. Shah.** 1987. Recent advances in the taxonomy of the genus *Bacteroides*, p. 249–258. *In* S. P. Borriello, J. M. Hardie, B. S. Draser, B. I. Duerden, M. J. Hudson, and R. J. Lysons (ed.), Recent advances in anaerobic bacteriology. Martinus Nijhoff Publishers, Boston.
11. **Dowell, V. R., Jr., and T. M. Hawkins.** 1974. Laboratory methods in anaerobic bacteriology, CDC manual. Department of Health, Education, and Welfare publication (CDC) 74-8272. Center for Disease Control, Atlanta.

12. **Dowell, V. R., Jr., and G. L. Lombard.** 1977. Presumptive identification of anaerobic nonsporeforming gram-negative bacilli. Center for Disease Control, Atlanta.
13. **Finegold, S. M., and W. L. George (ed.).** 1989. Anaerobic infections in humans. Academic Press, Inc., San Diego, Calif.
14. **Gharbia, S. E., and H. N. Shah.** 1988. Characteristics of glutamate dehydrogenase, a new diagnostic marker for the genus *Fusobacterium*. J. Gen. Microbiol. **134:**327–332.
15. **Haapasalo, M.** 1986. *Bacteroides buccae* and related taxa in necrotic root canal infections. J. Clin. Microbiol. **24:** 940–944.
16. **Haapasalo, M., H. Ranta, H. Shah, K. Ranta, K. Lounatmaa, and R. M. Kroppenstedt.** 1986. *Mitsuokella dentalis* sp. nov. from dental root canals. Int. J. Syst. Bacteriol. **36:**566–568.
17. **Holdeman, L. V., E. P. Cato, and W. E. C. Moore (ed.).** 1977. Anaerobic laboratory manual, 4th ed. Virginia Polytechnic Institute and State University, Blacksburg.
18. **Holdeman, L. V., R. W. Kelley, and W. E. C. Moore.** 1984. Anaerobic gram-negative straight, curved and helical rods. Family 1. *Bacteroidaceae* Pribram 1933, 10^{AL}, p. 602–662. *In* N. R. Krieg and J. G. Holt (ed.), Bergey's manual of systematic bacteriology, vol. 1. The Williams & Wilkins Co., Baltimore.
19. **Johnson, C. C., and S. M. Finegold.** 1987. Uncommonly encountered, motile, anaerobic gram-negative bacilli associated with infection. Rev. Infect. Dis. **9:**1150–1162.
20. **Johnson, C. C., J. F. Reinhardt, M. A. C. Edelstein, M. E. Mulligan, W. L. George, and S. M. Finegold.** 1985. *Bacteroides gracilis,* an important anaerobic bacterial pathogen. J. Clin. Microbiol. **22:**799–802.
21. **Johnson, J. L., W. E. C. Moore, and L. V. H. Moore.** 1986. *Bacteroides caccae* sp. nov., *Bacteroides merdae* sp. nov., and *Bacteroides stercoris* sp. nov., isolated from human feces. Int. J. Syst. Bacteriol. **36:**499–501.
22. **Johnston, B. L., M. A. C. Edelstein, E. Y. Holloway, and S. M. Finegold.** 1987. Bacteriologic and clinical study of *Bacteroides oris* and *Bacteroides buccae*. J. Clin. Microbiol. **25:**491–493.
23. **Kirby, B. D., W. L. George, V. L. Sutter, D. M. Citron, and S. M. Finegold.** 1980. Gram-negative anaerobic bacilli: their role in infection and patterns of susceptibility to antimicrobial agents. I. Little-known *Bacteroides* species. Rev. Infect. Dis. **2:**914–951.
24. **Lauer, B. A., L. B. Reller, and S. Mirrett.** 1981. Comparison of acridine orange and gram stains for detection of microorganisms in cerebrospinal fluid and other clinical specimens. J. Clin. Microbiol. **14:**201–205.
25. **Livingstone, S. J., S. D. Kominos, and R. B. Yee.** 1978. New medium for selection and presumptive identification of the *Bacteroides fragilis* group. J. Clin. Microbiol. **7:**448–453.
26. **Malnick, H., A. Jones, and J. C. Vickers.** 1989. *Anaerobiospirillum:* cause of a "new" zoonosis? Lancet **i:**1145–1146.
27. **McNeil, M. M., W. J. Martone, and V. R. Dowell, Jr.** 1987. Bacteremia with *Anaerobiospirillum succiniciproducens*. Rev. Infect. Dis. **9:**737–742.
28. **Montgomery, L., B. Flesher, and D. Stahl.** 1988. Transfer of *Bacteroides succinogenes* (Hungate) to *Fibrobacter* gen. nov. as *Fibrobacter succinogenes* comb. nov. and description of *Fibrobacter intestinalis* sp. nov. Int. J. Syst. Bacteriol. **38:**430–435.
29. **Moore, L. V. H., E. P. Cato, and W. E. C. Moore.** 1987. Anaerobe laboratory manual update. Published as a supplement to the *Anaerobe Laboratory Manual,* 4th ed., 1977. Virginia Polytechnic Institute and State University, Blacksburg.
30. **Moore, L. V. H., J. L. Johnson, and W. E. C. Moore.** 1987. *Selenomonas noxia* sp. nov., *Selenomonas flueggei* sp. nov., *Selenomonas infelix* sp. nov., *Selenomonas dianae* sp. nov., and *Selenomonas artemidis* sp. nov., from the human gingival crevice. Int. J. Syst. Bacteriol. **36:**271–280.
31. **Moreno, S., J. G. Altozano, B. Pinilla, J. C. Lopez, B. de Quiros, A. Ortega, and E. Bouza.** 1989. Lemierre's disease: postanginal bacteremia and pulmonary involvement caused by *Fusobacterium necrophorum*. Rev. Infect. Dis. **11:**319–324.
32. **Morgenstein, A. A., D. M. Citron, and S. M. Finegold.** 1981. New medium selective for *Fusobacterium* species and differential for *Fusobacterium necrophorum*. J. Clin. Microbiol. **13:**666–669.
33. **Moss, C. W., and O. I. Nunez-Montiel.** 1982. Analysis of short-chain acids from bacteria by gas-liquid chromatography with fused-silica capillary column. J. Clin. Microbiol. **15:**308–311.
34. **Mouton, C., P. Hammond, J. Slots, and R. J. Genco.** 1980. Evaluation of Fluoretec-M for detection of oral strains of *Bacteroides asaccharolyticus* and *Bacteroides melaninogenicus*. J. Clin. Microbiol. **11:**682–686.
35. **Okuda, K., T. Kato, J. Shiozu, I. Takazoe, and T. Nakamura.** 1985. *Bacteroides heparinolyticus* sp. nov. isolated from humans with periodontitis. Int. J. Syst. Bacteriol. **35:** 438–442.
36. **Rogosa, M.** 1984. Anaerobic gram negative cocci. Family I. *Veillonellaceae* Rogosa 1971, 232^{AL}, p. 680–685. *In* N. R. Krieg and J. G. Holt (ed.), Bergey's manual of systematic bacteriology, vol. 1. The Williams & Wilkins Co., Baltimore.
37. **Shah, H. N., and M. D. Collins.** 1988. Proposal for reclassification of *Bacteroides asaccharolyticus, Bacteroides gingivalis,* and *Bacteroides endodontalis* in a new genus, *Porphyromonas*. Int. J. Syst. Bacteriol. **38:**128–131.
38. **Shah, H. N., and M. D. Collins.** 1989. Proposal to restrict the genus *Bacteroides* (Castellani and Chalmers) to *Bacteroides fragilis* and closely related species. Int. J. Syst. Bacteriol. **39:**85–87.
39. **Shah, H. N., and M. D. Collins.** 1990. *Prevotella,* a new genus to include *Bacteroides melaninogenicus* and related species formerly classified in the genus *Bacteroides.* Int. J. Syst. Bacteriol. **40:**205–208.
40. **Shah, H. N., M. D. Collins, J. Watabe, and T. Mitsuoka.** 1985. *Bacteroides oulorum* sp. nov., a nonpigmented saccharolytic species from the oral cavity. Int. J. Syst. Bacteriol. **35:**193–197.
41. **Slots, J.** 1987. Detection of colonies of *Bacteroides gingivalis* by a rapid fluorescence assay for trypsin-like activity. Oral Microbiol. Immunol. **2:**139–141.
42. **Sugihara, P. T., V. L. Sutter, H. R. Attebery, K. S. Bricknell, and S. M. Finegold.** 1974. Isolation of *Acidaminococcus fermentans* and *Megasphaera elsdenii* from normal human feces. Appl. Microbiol. **27:**274–275.
43. **Summanen, P., and H. Jousimies-Somer.** 1988. Comparative evaluation of Rap ID ANA and API 20A for identification of anaerobic bacteria. Eur. J. Clin. Microbiol. Infect. Dis. **7:**771–775.
44. **Sutter, V. L., D. M. Citron, M. A. C. Edelstein, and S. M. Finegold.** 1985. Wadsworth anaerobic bacteriology manual, 4th ed. Star Publishing Co., Belmont, Calif.
45. **Tanner, A. C. R., S. Badger, C.-H. Lai, M. A. Listgarten, R. A. Visconti, and S. S. Socransky.** 1981. *Wolinella* gen. nov., *Wolinella succinogenes* (*Vibrio succinogenes* Wolin *et al.*) comb. nov., and description of *Bacteroides gracilis* sp. nov., *Wolinella recta* sp. nov., *Campylobacter concisus* sp. nov., and *Eikenella corrodens* from humans with periodontal disease. Int. J. Syst. Bacteriol. **31:**432–445.
46. **Tanner, A. C. R., M. A. Listgarten, J. L. Ebersole, and M. N. Strzempko.** 1986. *Bacteroides forsythus* sp. nov., a slow-growing, fusiform *Bacteroides* sp. from the human oral cavity. Int. J. Syst. Bacteriol. **36:**213–221.
47. **van Winkelhoff, A. J., and J. de Graaff.** 1983. Vancomycin as a selective agent for isolation of *Bacteroides* species. J. Clin. Microbiol. **18:**1282–1284.

48. **van Winkelhoff, A. J., T. J. M. van Steenbergen, N. Kippuw, and J. de Graaff.** 1985. Further characterization of *Bacteroides endodontalis,* an asaccharolytic black-pigmented *Bacteroides* species from the oral cavity. J. Clin. Microbiol. **22:**75–79.

49. **Watabe, J., Y. Benno, and T. Mitsuoka.** 1983. Taxonomic study of *Bacteroides oralis* and related organisms and proposal of *Bacteroides veroralis* sp. nov. Int. J. Syst. Bacteriol. **33:**57–64.

50. **Wayne, L. G., D. J. Brenner, R. R. Colwell, P. A. D. Grimont, O. Kandler, M. I. Krichevsky, L. H. Moore, W. E. C. Moore, R. G. E. Murray, E. Stackebrandt, M. P. Starr, and H. G. Trüper.** 1987. Report of the ad hoc committee on reconciliation of approaches to bacterial systematics. Int. J. Syst. Bacteriol. **37:**463–464.

51. **Weinberg, L. G., L. L. Smith, and A. H. McTighe.** 1983. Rapid identification of the *Bacteroides fragilis* group by bile disk and catalase tests. Lab. Med. **14:**785–788.

52. **Weissfeld, A. S., and A. C. Sonnenwirth.** 1981. Rapid detection and identification of *Bacteroides fragilis* and *Bacteroides melaninogenicus* by immunofluorescence. J. Clin. Microbiol. **13:**798–800.

Chapter 53

Leptospira

AARON D. ALEXANDER

CHARACTERIZATION

Members of the genus *Leptospira* constitute a genetically diverse group of pathogenic and nonparasitic organisms, as disclosed by DNA base ratio analysis and DNA homology studies (5, 33). Two species are recognized: *L. interrogans*, for the parasitic members, and *L. biflexa*, for the so-called saprophytic leptospires (10). Strains of *L. biflexa* are omnipresent in fresh surface waters, are frequently found in ordinary and deionized tap water, and are occasionally found in salt water. *L. interrogans* leptospires are distributed throughout the world in approximately 160 different mammalian species, including domestic animals, as well as a large variety of rodents and other feral mammals. The pathogenic leptospires cause acute, febrile, systemic disease of humans and other mammals. Both species comprise a large number of serovars based on agglutinogenic characteristics. Members of the two species are indistinguishable morphologically and are primarily differentiated on the basis of infectivity for laboratory animals. *L. biflexa* strains also differ from those of *L. interrogans* by their ability to grow at 13°C and their greater resistance to growth-inhibiting concentrations in media containing 225 μg of 8-azaguanine per ml (11).

Leptospires are helicoidal, flexible organisms, usually 6 to 20 μm long and approximately 0.1 μm in diameter, with semicircular hooked ends (occasionally, one or both ends are straight) (Fig. 1). They are motile. Electron microscopy reveals a cylindrical body helicoidally wound about two periplasmic flagella that are inserted subterminally at opposite ends of the helicoidal body, with their free ends extending toward the middle of the cell (Fig. 2). A common external sheath covers both structures. Leptospires appear to be faintly colored in preparations stained by Wright or Giemsa stain and are not readily observed in Gram-stained smears. They are invisible by bright-field microscopy but readily seen by dark-field or phase-contrast microscopy. Leptospires can pass through filters that normally retain bacteria. This attribute frequently results in contamination of tissue culture and other filter-sterilized media with *L. biflexa* strains which are omnipresent in water.

Leptospires are aerobic. With few exceptions, strains can be readily cultivated in artificial media containing 10% rabbit serum or 1% bovine serum albumin plus long-chain fatty acids at pH 6.8 to 7.4. The optimum temperature is 30°C, and the incubation time for optimum growth ranges from a few days to 4 weeks or longer (usually 6 to 14 days).

Leptospires within species are not distinguishable on the basis of biochemical characteristics. Classification is based on their agglutinogenic characteristics. The basic taxon is serovar. Serovars are identified by microscopic agglutination and agglutinin-adsorption tests with serovar-specific rabbit antiserum (10). More than 200 serovars of *L. interrograns* have been identified. The serovars have been assembled into 23 serogroups on the basis of shared major agglutinogens. The serogroup has no taxonomic status but is used as an expedient for selecting antisera or antigens to identify isolates or to test sera for antibodies (15).

Pathogenic leptospires produce lethal to subclinical infections in hamsters, guinea pig, gerbils, and weanling rabbits after intraperitoneal inoculation.

NATURAL HABITAT AND CLINICAL SIGNIFICANCE

Many serovars occur predominantly in select mammalian hosts, but the distribution of a specific serovar in a select host is not exclusive. The same animal species may be a primary reservoir for several different serovars and may also carry types occurring primarily in other mammals.

The nesting site for leptospires in the natural host is the lumen of nephritic tubules, whence the organisms are shed into the urine. The persistence and intensity of leptospiruria may vary with the host and with the serovar causing the infection. For example, Norway rats infected with serovar icterohaemorrhagiae shed profuse numbers of leptospires for the remainder of their natural life, whereas strains of serovar canicola apparently persist less efficiently in the kidneys of the rats. Shedding by infected dogs, cattle, and swine may be heavy for only a few months after infection and is usually sparse or absent after 6 months (29).

Infections are incurred directly by contact with the urine of carriers or indirectly by contact with streams, ponds, swamps, or wet soils contaminated with the urine of carriers. Pathogenic leptospires can survive for 3 months or longer in neutral or slightly alkaline waters, but they do not persist in brackish or acid waters. Organisms enter their hosts through abrasions of the skin, through mucosal surfaces of the nasopharynx or esophagus, or through the eye.

Leptospirosis in humans is primarily associated with occupational exposure. Work with animals or in rat-infested surroundings poses infection hazards (e.g., for veterinarians, dairymen, swineherds, abattoir workers, miners, and fish and poultry processors). In various parts of the world, leptospirosis occurs sporadically or in epidemic proportions in agricultural workers engaged in the raising of rice, cane, flax, and vegetables, in rubber planation workers, and in soldiers exposed to natural environments contaminated by animal carriers. The potential infection hazards of bathing or swimming in ponds or streams around which livestock are pastured have been demonstrated repeatedly (4, 13).

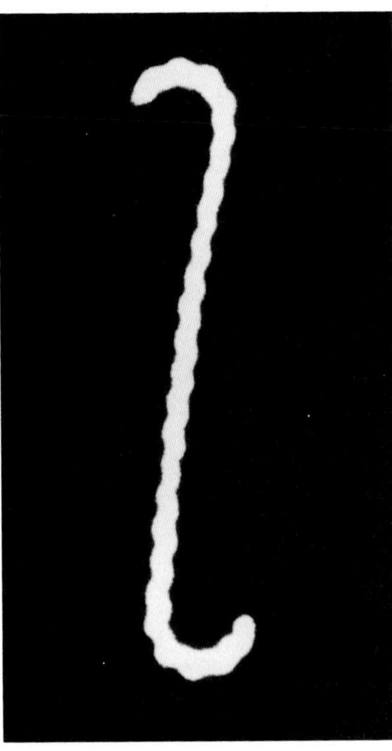

FIG. 1. *Leptospira* sp. Dark-field illumination. ×1,250. (Courtesy of C. D. Cox, Department of Microbiology, University of Massachusetts, Amherst.)

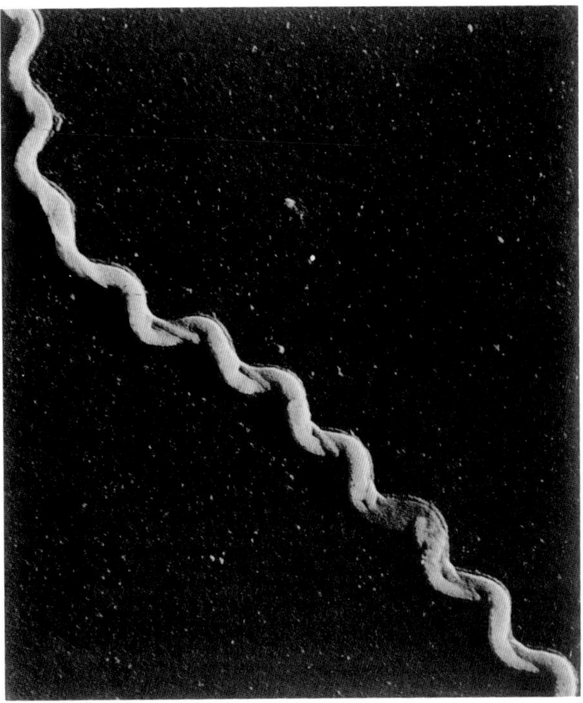

FIG. 2. Electron micrograph of a portion of a leptospire. (Courtesy of the Armed Forces Institute of Pathology, Washington, D.C.)

The clinical manifestations of leptospirosis in humans and animals are variable, ranging from a mild, catarrh-like illness to icteric disease with severe kidney and liver involvement. Diagnosis can be established in the laboratory only by demonstration of the organisms or by serological tests. A variety of procedures are available for laboratory diagnosis. The selection and use of appropriate tests are contingent on an understanding of the course of leptospiral infections.

The incubation period ranges from 3 to 30 days but is usually 10 to 12 days. Leptospiremia occurs at the time of disease onset and persists for approximately 1 week. During this acute phase, leptospires may also be present in cerebrospinal fluid and in the milk of lactating animals. Antibodies become detectable by days 6 to 10 of the disease and reach maximal levels at week 3 or 4. Thereafter, antibody levels gradually recede but may remain detectable for years (4, 31).

In humans and domestic animals, leptospires may be found in the urine after week 1 of disease. Urinary shedding may persist for 2 to 3 months in a large proportion of cases. In some cases, intermittent shedding may occur for longer periods of time. Infection in pregnant livestock during the latter half of gestation may result in abortion several weeks later, at which time the dam may have detectable antibodies and may be a urinary shedder.

DIRECT EXAMINATION

The concentration of leptospires in the blood and cerebrospinal fluid of patients with naturally occurring infections is low, and the organisms are difficult to demonstrate by direct microscopy. The chances of demonstrating leptospires are increased by the centrifugation of blood treated with sodium oxalate or heparin at low speed to remove cellular elements and then at high speed to concentrate the remaining elements, which are examined microscopically (31). Although this method may be valuable in the establishment of a rapid diagnosis, it frequently results in misdiagnosis by the mistaken identification of fibrils or extrusions from cells as spirochetes. Therefore, direct dark-field examination of blood is not recommended as a single diagnostic procedure.

Direct dark-field examination may be of value for the examination of specimens in which there is a high concentration of leptospires, e.g., blood, peritoneal fluid, or liver suspension from hamsters or guinea pigs infected with clinical material or, frequently, urine or kidney suspensions from wildlife, swine, dogs, and other domestic animals, and aborted livestock fetuses.

The examination of blood or other fluids and tissue suspensions is conducted with a minute drop of fluid distributed in a thin layer between a glass slide and a cover slip. It is important to disperse cellular particles; otherwise, too much light may be reflected, and these reflections can interfere with the detection of leptospires. The typical morphology and motility of leptospires should be evident before a presumptive diagnosis is made. The failure to detect leptospires does not rule out their presence. Diagnosis by microscope examination should be confirmed by cultural or serological tests.

Fluorescent-antibody techniques provide a more sensitive method than dark-field microscopic examination for detecting organisms in specimens and are being used by an increasing number of laboratories. The use of serovar-specific as well as more broadly reactive pooled multiple serovar conjugates has been reported (20). Conventional techniques are used to conjugate hyperimmune (usually rabbit) serum and to examine specimens. The National Veterinary Service Laboratory (Animal and Plant Health Inspection Service [APHIS]) of the U.S. Department of Agriculture, Ames, Iowa, has multivalent leptospiral fluorescent-antibody conjugates for diagnostic use for the veterinary profession. Requests for service or reagents should be channeled through local APHIS representatives or state veterinary representatives. Silver deposition techniques are used in some laboratories to demonstrate organisms in tissue sections (9). Enzymatic radioimmunoassay (6) and immunoperoxidase (24) staining procedures have been described but are not used routinely. All of these microscopic detection procedures have limitations in that their successful use depends on the presence of relatively large numbers of organisms. When positive, they can provide a rapid presumptive diagnosis. More sensitive techniques by the use of DNA probes are being used in several reference laboratories and may eventually become more readily applicable in diagnostic laboratories (16, 27, 34).

CULTURAL EXAMINATION

During week 1 of disease, the most reliable way to detect leptospires is by the direct culturing of blood on appropriate media (see chapter 121). Media containing rabbit serum (i.e., Fletcher semisolid and Khorthof liquid media) or bovine serum albumin and long-chain fatty acids (i.e., bovine albumin-Tween 80 liquid or semisolid medium [BA-Tw 80]) will grow most strains of leptospires (9, 31). The BA-Tw 80 media are particularly useful for isolation of the some of the more fastidious serovars (e.g., hardjo). For this purpose, the BA-Tw 80 media may be enriched by the addition of rabbit serum (0.4 to 1.0%) (8). It is advisable to use at least four tubes of medium from two different types or lots of medium for each sample. Media are dispensed in approximately 5-ml amounts to test tubes (16 by 125 mm, preferably screw capped). Prepared media can be stored for months at room temperature. Repeated daily blood cultures with the use of 1 to 2 drops of blood per 5 ml of medium during week 1 of disease are recommended. The use of minimal inocula, particularly after day 4 of disease, serves to minimize the effect of growth-inhibiting substances that may be present in the blood. If media are not available at the time blood is collected, the blood can be defibrinated or mixed with anticoagulants (heparin or sodium oxalate; citrate solutions may be inhibitory) and subsequently cultured. Alternatively, clotted blood can be triturated and cultured. Spinal fluid obtained during the acute phase of the disease can also be cultured.

After week 1 of disease, blood cultures are rarely successful. However, at this time and for several months thereafter, the urine may contain leptospires, which may be isolated by culturing or animal inoculation. In infected humans, the concentration of leptospires in the urine is low; shedding may be intermittent. Therefore, repeated isolation attempts should be made. Isolation attempts should be made as soon as possible after collection of the specimen. Leptospires may not survive in acid urine for more than a few hours. Urine obtained aseptically, e.g., by perforation of the bladder (a technique used for infected dogs) can be cultured directly (23). Because the undiluted urine may contain growth-inhibiting substances, both undiluted urine and a 10-fold dilution of urine are recommended for culture, with the use of 1 to 2 drops of inoculum. Direct culture isolation is also possible with midstream urine samples carefully collected from cleansed genitalia. Urine samples as well as other specimens (e.g., aborted bovine and swine fetuses and abattoir-derived kidney) which are not obtained aseptically can be successfully cultured in media containing 5-fluorouracil (100 μg/ml) (used singly or in combination with fosfomycin [400 μg/ml]) and nalidixic acid (20 μg/ml) (8, 12, 21), which inhibit the growth of contaminating bacteria.

In fatal cases, leptospires may be present in various tissues as well as in the blood. Liver and kidney are the tissues of choice for the recovery of organisms. Tissues are triturated by glass grinders or by the use of sand with a mortar and pestle and are suspended in 9 parts of physiological salt solution or medium. The 10% suspension, and 1:10 and 1:100 dilutions thereof, are cultured as in the method for urine. The higher dilutions of tissue suspensions are cultured to limit the effects of growth-inhibiting substances that may be present. Alternatively, especially under field conditions (for example, in culturing the kidneys of trapped small animals), 0.5 to 1.0 g of kidney can be expressed through the barrel of a 2- or 5-ml syringe (without a needle) directly onto medium, which can then be diluted further and subcultured. For culturing the kidneys of large domestic animals, a representative sample can be obtained by scraping the cortex with sterile metal bottle caps with grated surfaces. The grated surface is prepared by punching holes in the cap with a nail. The ground tissue is collected on the undersurface of the bottle cap. If tissues cannot be processed immediately, they can be collected aseptically in sterile bottles, rapidly frozen, and stored at dry-ice temperatures. The addition of a cryoprotective agent such as glycerol (1 part to 20 parts of tissue) before freezing of the specimen may minimize the deleterious effects of freezing on leptospires.

Cultures are incubated in the dark at 30°C or at room temperature. Most pathogenic strains are detected in culture after 6 to 14 days of incubation. In some cases, leptospires may be seen as early as day 3 or as late as 2 to 4 months after incubation. A few strains, e.g., serovar hardjo from cattle, are difficult to isolate, and recovery may require prolonged incubation for 4 or more months, with periodic topping of cultures with fresh medium or subculturing (8). At the time of optimal growth, the concentration of leptospires may be 1×10^8 to 4×10^8 organisms per ml. Cultures should be examined at 5- to 7-day intervals and discarded if they are negative after 2 to 4 months of incubation.

Growth in tubes of semisolid medium occurs in the form of a linear disk 1 to 3 cm below the surface. The absence of a disk does not necessarily rule out the presence of leptospires. Fluid media inoculated with leptospires become faintly turbid. For the examination of cultures for growth, a minute drop is obtained from a few centimeters below the surface of fluid cultures or from the ringed area of growth in semisolid media. The drop is placed on a slide, covered with a cover slip, and examined by dark-field microscopy, first at low (×150) and then at high dry (×450) magnification. Leptospires are recognized by their characteristic motility as well as by their morphology. In a fluid medium, leptospires appear to rotate along their longitudinal axis, alternately moving backward and forward. The motility is characteristic because of the spinning hooked ends. In a semisolid medium or in a more viscous milieu, serpentine as well as boring and flexing movements occur.

Positive cultures should be transferred to fresh medium. The inoculum should make up 5 to 10% of the volume of the subculture. Stock cultures are best maintained in semisolid medium, such as Fletcher or BA-Tw 80 medium. After ringed growth occurs at 30°C, cultures can be stored at room temperature. Transfers are usually made at 6- to 8-week intervals. Cultures maintained in fluid medium should be transferred more frequently, at 3- to 6-week intervals. For long-term preservation, cultures of leptospires can be stored by liquid nitrogen refrigeration, with use of glycerol or dimethyl sulfoxide as a cryoprotective agent (3).

Contaminated cultures can be purified by passage in media containing 5-fluorouracil or antibiotics with the use of small inocula. If cultures are heavily contaminated, it may be advisable to use three or more serial 10-fold dilutions for the inoculation of subcultures. Cultures can also be purified by filtration through bacteriological filters with average pore sizes ranging from approximately 0.22 to 0.45 μm or by animal inoculation methods. Weanling hamsters or young guinea pigs are inoculated intraperitoneally with 0.5 to 1.0 ml of the contaminated culture. After 10 to 15 min, blood is obtained from the heart and cultured. It may be possible to purify some cultures by subculturing on solid plating medium (30) containing 1% agar, but not all strains readily form colonies in plating medium. Leptospires form subsurface colonies and can be picked for transfer with a sterile capillary pipette.

ANIMAL INOCULATION

Animal inoculation methods are particularly useful for the isolation of strains from tissues or body fluids containing contaminating microorganisms. For material that can be obtained aseptically, animal inoculation techniques provide no greater chances of isolation than do direct cultural methods except for rare instances in which strains are not cultivated easily but can be demonstrated in animals.

The choice laboratory animals for leptospirosis are weanling hamsters and young guinea pigs. *Meriones* species and weanling rabbits have also been used. The laboratory animals selected should be known to be free from natural infections. The course of disease in laboratory animals varies with different serovars or even with different strains of the same serovar and may be inapparent to lethal. Material is inoculated intraperitoneally, preferably in at least three animals. Heart blood for culture and microscope examination is obtained whenever signs of disease are present; otherwise, samples are taken on days 4 and 6 and then at 3- to 4-day intervals up to day 20 after inoculation. Kidney cultures should also be done if animals are alive at the time of the last bleeding.

SEROLOGICAL EXAMINATION

Detection of antibodies

The microscopic agglutination test is the procedure most often used for the detection of antibodies. It is highly sensitive and specific, and it can be used to test both animal and human sera for diagnostic as well as epidemiological purposes. It is highly serovar specific. To ensure the detection of antibodies that may be produced by any of the large number of different serovars, it is necessary to use a battery of different antigens encompassing cross-reactions with most of the known serovars that may be present. In the continental United States, approximately 23 serovars have been demonstrated in nonhuman animal hosts. However, relatively few serovars have been associated with the infections in humans and domestic animals. At this time, the use of the following eight serovars as antigens would serve to detect all but rare cases of leptospirosis: copenhageni, grippotyphosa, canicola, wolffi, pomona, djatzi, autumnalis, and patoc. Serovar patoc, a biflexa-type leptospire, is used because of the frequent occurrence of cross-reactions with this antigen in sera from human leptospirosis patents. The proposed list of antigens may be modified according to local experience and needs. The substitution of local isolates of the same or a related type could provide a more sensitive test.

Antigens used in microscopic agglutination tests consist of 4- to 7-day-old cultures in fluid media. The recommended density of cultures is 2×10^8 organisms per ml (32). These organisms may be used live, or they may be treated with Formalin. A detailed description of the conduct of the microscopic agglutination test is given in reference 1. Generally, test sera are serially diluted two- to fourfold with physiological salt solution to provide serum dilutions from 1:50 to 1:3,200. Amounts of 0.2 ml of each dilution are distributed in a series of agglutination tubes, to each of which is added an equal volume of antigen. The reaction mixtures are shaken, incubated at 30°C for 2 to 3 h, shaken again, and examined microscopically for agglutination by dark-field illumination. The test has been adapted for use with microtitration techniques (23). Titers of 1:100 are considered significant, and they may range as high as 1:25,000 or greater.

The laboriousness of the microscopic agglutination test limits its usefulness for small diagnostic laboratories. A variety of other serological procedures have been proposed (1, 9). Procedures that have been widely used in lieu of microscopic agglutination tests are the macroscopic (slide or plate) agglutination test with a battery of single or pooled Formalin-fixed antigens (23) and three genus-specific tests in which *L. biflexa* antigens (e.g., strain Patoc) are used in macroscopic agglutination (9, 19), indirect hemagglutination or erythrocyte lysis, and complement fixation tests (9). A genus-specific macroscopic agglutination test using a synthetic polymer sensitized with pooled sonicated serovars is also being used (22).

Macroscopic agglutination tests with either single or pooled Formalin-fixed antigens are commercially available from Lee Laboratories, Grayson, Ga., or Fort Dodge Laboratories, Fort Dodge, Iowa. In the genus-specific macroscopic agglutination test (TR/Patoc test), a heat-treated (100°C), concentrated antigen is used. The two types of macroscopic agglutination tests can be used for the serodiagnosis of recent or current infections in humans and animals but have limitations for the detection of antibodies for retrospective studies, e.g., in serological surveys. The hemolytic test entails the use of a 50% ethyl alcohol-soluble–95% ethyl alcohol-insoluble extract of specific *L. biflexa* strains. This test has been used advantageously in areas of multiple-serovar leptospirosis for the diagnosis of human infections (7). The test has been simplified by the use of sensitized sheep or human type O erythrocytes preserved with glutaraldehyde or pyruvic aldehyde in an indirect hemagglutination procedure (23). A complement fixation test in which a fixed *L. biflexa* antigen is used for the diagnosis of human infections is used in some European countries (9).

Enzyme-linked immunosorbent assay procedures have been increasingly used in leptospira diagnostic laboratories to detect leptospiral antibodies in humans and animals (9, 26, 28). However, they have not replaced the microscopic agglutination test, which still serves as the reference procedure in these laboratories. The technique allows a ready assessment of the relative occurrence of specific immunoglobulins M and G, thereby affording insight on the recency of infection. The procedure of Terpstra et al. (26) entails the use of genus-specific, heat-extracted, serovar icterohaemorrhagiae antigen and appears to have good sensitivity in the detection of leptospiral antibodies, irrespective of the infecting serovar.

Culture typing

Microscopic agglutination techniques are used for culture typing. An isolate used as antigen is first screened with a select group of 12 or more serovar antisera to determine its serogroup relationship. Isolates are then tested with different serovars of one or more selected serogroups to determine further antigenic relationships. On the basis of observed cross-reactions, representative strains of serovars are chosen for reciprocal agglutinin adsorption tests. "Two strains are considered to belong to different serovars if, after cross-absorption with adequate amounts of heterologous antigen, 10% or more of the homologous titer regularly remains in at least one of the two antisera in repeated tests" (32). Procedures for the conduct of definitive culture typing are described in detail elsewhere (2, 9). Antigenic factor analysis has been used for the classification of strains (14), but single-factor sera for such tests are not generally available.

The definitive typing of strains is usually done in leptospirosis reference laboratories. In the United States, such tests are done at the World Health Organization Collaborating Center for the Epidemiology for Leptospirosis, Bacterial Zoonoses Activity, Centers for Disease Control, Atlanta, Ga., and at the APHIS laboratory in Ames, Iowa. The APHIS laboratory provides service to the veterinary profession. Presumptive serogroup or serovar identification can usually be made in diagnostic laboratories by cross-agglutination tests with antisera of strains used for serological diagnosis. Antisera are prepared in rabbits by the injection of successive doses of 0.5, 1.0, 2.0, and 4.0 ml of live cultures into the marginal ear vein at 5- to 7-day intervals; 5- to 7-day-old cultures in rabbit serum medium are commonly used as a source of inoculum. A blood sample is obtained 7 days after the last injection, and the serum therefrom is tested with homologous antigen. If the titer is 1:6,400 or greater, blood is removed by cardiopuncture. The separated serum is distributed into vials and stored at −20 to −30°C. Alternatively, it can be stored in the freeze-dried state or preserved by the addition of an equal volume of glycerol or by the addition of Merthiolate (concentration, 1:10,000).

Alternative methods for the classification of leptospires by use of restriction endonuclease DNA analysis and monoclonal antibodies are being applied in several leptospira reference laboratories (17, 18, 25, 27). Findings for the most part are consistent with agglutination procedures, but differences do occur.

DISCUSSION

An unequivocal laboratory diagnosis of current cases of leptospirosis can be established by the isolation of the organism from blood or cerebrospinal fluid or by the demonstration of significant rises in antibody titer in two or more properly timed serum samples.

Direct cultural procedures are relative simple and within the capabilities of the ordinary diagnostic laboratory. Repeated blood culture attempts during week 1 of disease usually are successful. Preferably, blood cultures should be obtained before antibiotic therapy is started. The use of replicate culture tubes is particularly important. The isolation of leptospires from only one of four or more tubes inoculated is not unusual. The recognition of isolated organisms as leptospires is based on their morphology, motility, and cultural characteristics. The cultural isolation of strains also allows their identification by culture typing tests, which may have epidemiological or forensic importance, as in occupational diseases.

The definitive identification of isolates can be established only by recovery and subsequent typing tests and is usually carried out in reference laboratories. The microscopic agglutination test, which is highly serogroup and serovar specific, may provide clues to the identity of the infecting serovar. However, the determination of serovars on the basis of the serological response of the patient has the following limitations: the agglutinins may be cross-reacting antibodies initiated by a type not included among the test antigens, higher titers may occur against serologically heterologous but antigenically related strains as well as against unrelated serologically heterologous strains (paradoxical reactions), and complex serological responses may occur in repeated or simultaneous infections.

From the viewpoint of the clinician, the management and treatment of leptospirosis does not depend on the infecting serovar; thus, a laboratory diagnosis of leptospirosis per se serves as confirmation of the clinical diagnosis. In this respect, the macroscopic agglutination and genus-specific test may suffice. Unfortunately, the current serological tests and isolation procedures rarely provide a rapid laboratory confirmation of infection before the end of week 1 of disease.

Methods for direct detection of leptospires in specimens, when positive, provide a rapid diagnosis, but negative findings do not rule out the presence of leptospires. Current developments in leptospiral DNA detection afford promise for a sensitive, rapid diagnostic procedure.

LITERATURE CITED

1. **Alexander, A. D.** 1986. Serological diagnosis of leptospirosis, p. 435–439. *In* N. R. Rose, H. Friedman, and J. L. Fahey (ed.), Manual of clinical laboratory immunology,

3rd ed. American Society for Microbiology, Washington, D.C.

2. **Alexander, A. D., L. B. Evans, A. J. Toussaint, R. Marchwicki, and F. R. McCrumb.** 1957. Leptospirosis in Malaya. II. Antigenic analysis of 110 leptospiral isolates and other serologic studies. Am. J. Trop. Med. Hyg. **6:**871–889.
3. **Alexander, A. D., E. F. Lessel, L. B. Evans, E. Franck, and S. S. Green.** 1972. Preservation of leptospires by liquid-nitrogen refrigeration. Int. J. Syst. Bacteriol. **22:**166–169.
4. **Alston, J. M., and J. C. Broom.** 1958. Leptospirosis in man and animals. E. and S. Livingstone, Edinburgh.
5. **Brendle, J. J., M. Rogul, and A. D. Alexander.** 1974. Deoxyribonucleic acid hybridization among selected leptospiral serotypes. Int. J. Syst. Bacteriol. **24:**205–214.
6. **Chappel, R. J., B. Adler, S. A. Ballard, S. Faine, R. T. Jones, B. D. Miller, and J. A. Swainga.** 1985. Enzymatic radioimmunoassay for detecting *Leptospira interrogans* serovar pomona in the urine of experimentally-infected pigs. Vet. Microbiol. **10:**179–186.
7. **Cox, C. D., A. D. Alexander, and L. C. Murphy.** 1957. Evaluation of the hemolytic test in the serodiagnosis of human leptospirosis. J. Infect. Dis. **101:**210–218.
8. **Ellis, W. A.** 1986. The diagnosis of leptospirosis in farm animals, p. 13–31. *In* W. A. Ellis and T. W. A. Little (ed.), The present state of leptospirosis and control. Martinus Nijhoff, Dordrecht, The Netherlands.
9. **Faine, S. (ed.).** 1982. Guidelines for the control of leptospirosis. W.H.O. offset publication no. 67. World Health Organization, Geneva.
10. **Johnson, R. C., and S. Faine.** 1984. Family II. *Leptospiraceae* Hovind-Hougen 1979, 245[AL], p. 62–67. *In* N. R. Krieg and J. G. Holt (ed.), Bergey's manual of systematic bacteriology, vol. 1. The Williams & Wilkins Co., Baltimore.
11. **Johnson, R. C., and V. G. Harris.** 1967. Differentiation of pathogenic and saprophytic leptospires. 1. Growth at low temperatures. J. Bacteriol. **94:**27–31.
12. **Johnson, R. C., and P. Rogers.** 1964. 5-Fluorouracil as a selective agent for growth of leptospirae. J. Bacteriol. **87:** 422–426.
13. **Kaufmann, A. F.** 1976. Epidemiological trends of leptospirosis in the United States, 1965–1974, p. 177–189. *In* R. C. Johnson (ed.), The biology of parasitic spirochetes. Academic Press, Inc., New York.
14. **Kmety, E.** 1967. Factorenanalyse von Leptospiren der Icterohaemorrhagiae und einiger verwandter Serogruppen. Edition of Scientific Committees for General and Special Biology of the Slovak Academy of Science, vol. 13, no. 3. Slovak Academy of Sciences, Bratislava, Czechoslovakia.
15. **Kmety, E., and H. Dikken.** 1988. Revised list of *Leptospira* serovars accepted by the Subcommitte on the Taxonomy of Leptospira at the Manchester meeting, 6/7 September 1986. University Press, Groningen, The Netherlands.
16. **LeFebvre, R.** 1987. DNA probe for detection of the *Leptospira interrogans* serovar hardjo genotype hardjo-bovis. J. Clin. Microbiol. **25:**2236–2238.
17. **LeFebvre, R. B., J. W. Foley, and A. B. Thiermann.** 1985. Rapid and simplified protocol for isolation and characterization of leptospiral chromosomal DNA for taxonomy and diagnosis. J. Clin. Microbiol. **22:**606–608.
18. **Marshall, R. B., B. E. Wilton, and A. J. Robinson.** 1981. Identification of leptospiral serovars by restriction endonuclease analysis. J. Med. Microbiol. **14:**163–166.
19. **Mazzonelli, J., G. Dorta de Mazzonelli, and M. Mailloux.** 1974. Possibilité de diagnostic serologique macroscopique des leptospiroses à l'aide d'un antigene unique. Med. Mal. Infect. **4:**253–254.
20. **Miller, D. A., M. A. Wilson, and C. A. Kirkbride.** 1989. Evaluation of multivalent leptospira fluorescent antibody conjugates for general diagnostic use. J. Vet. Diagn. Invest. **1:**146–149.
21. **Oie, S., A. Koshiro, H. Konishi, and Z. Yoshii.** 1986. In vitro evaluation of combined usage of fosfomycin and 5-fluorouracil for selective isolation of *Leptospira* species. J. Clin. Microbiol. **23:**1084–1087.
22. **Seki, M., T. Sato, Y. Arimitsu, T. Matuhasi, and S. Kobayashi.** 1987. One point method for serological diagnosis of leptospirosis: a microcapsule agglutination test. Epidemiol. Infect. **99:**399–405.
23. **Sulzer, C. R., and W. L. Jones.** 1976. Leptospirosis. Methods in laboratory diagnosis (revised edition). Publication no. (CDC) 74-8275. U.S. Department of Health, Education, and Welfare, Washington, D.C.
24. **Terpstra, W. J., J. Jubboury-Postema, and H. Korver.** 1983. Immunoperoxidase staining of leptospires in blood and urine. Zentralbl. Bakteriol. Mikrobiol. Hyg. A **254:**534–539.
25. **Terpstra, W. J., H. Korver, J. van Leeuwen, P. R. Klatser, and Arend H. J. Kolk.** 1985. The classification of sejroe group serovars of *Leptospira interrogans* with monoclonal antibodies. Zentralbl. Bakteriol. Mikrobiol. Hyg. A **259:** 498–506.
26. **Terpstra, E. J., G. S. Ligthart, and G. J. Schoone.** 1980. Serodiagnosis of human leptospirosis by enzyme-linked-immunosorbent assay (ELISA). Zentralbl. Bakteriol. Mikrobiol. Hyg. A **247:**400–405.
27. **Terpstra, W. J., G. J. Schoone, G. S. Ligthart, and J. Ter Schegget.** 1987. Detection of *Leptospira interrogans* in clinical specimens by in situ hybridization using biotin-labelled DNA probes. J. Gen. Microbiol. **133:**911–914.
28. **Thiermann, A. B., and L. A. Garrett.** 1983. Enzyme-linked-immunosorbent assay for the detection of antibodies to *Leptospira interrogans* serovars *hardjo* and *pomona* in cattle. Am. J. Vet. Res. **44:**884–888.
29. **Van der Hoeden, J.** 1958. Epizootiology of leptospirosis. Adv. Vet. Sci. **4:**277–339.
30. **Wannen, J. S.** 1958. Isolation of leptospiras from contaminated cultures by plating. Aust. J. Sci. **20:**239.
31. **Wolff, J. W.** 1954. The laboratory diagnosis of leptospirosis. Charles C Thomas, Publisher, Springfield, Ill.
32. **World Health Organization.** 1967. Current problems in leptospirosis. Report of a World Health Organization Expert Group. W.H.O. technical report series no. 380. World Health Organization, Geneva.
33. **Yasuda, P. H., A. G. Steigerwalt, K. R. Sulzer, A. F. Kaufmann, F. Rogers, and D. J. Brenner.** 1987. Deoxyribonucleic acid relatedness between serogroups and serovars in the family *Leptospiraceae* with proposals for seven new *Leptospira* species. Int. J. Syst. Bacteriol. **37:** 407–415.
34. **Zuerner, R. L., and C. A. Bolin.** 1988. Repetitive sequence element cloned from *Leptospira interrogans* serovar hardjo type hardjo-bovis provides a sensitive diagnostic probe for bovine leptospirosis. J. Clin. Microbiol. **26:**2495–2500.

Chapter 54

Borrelia

WILLY BURGDORFER AND TOM G. SCHWAN

CHARACTERIZATION

According to *Bergey's Manual of Systematic Bacteriology* (36), spirochetes of the genus *Borrelia* belong to the family *Spirochaetaceae* in the bacterial order *Spirochaetales*. Morphologically, they are helical organisms with 4 to 30 coils and are 5 to 25 μm long and 0.2 to 0.5 μm wide. An outer envelope or membrane encloses the coiled protoplasmic cylinder. The protoplasmic cylinder consists of the peptidoglycan layer and the cytoplasmic membrane enclosing the protoplasmic contents of the cell. Beneath the outer envelope and attached subterminally to opposite ends of the protoplasmic cylinder are the periplasmic flagella (axial filaments). The free ends of the periplasmic flagella extend toward the middle of the cell, where they overlap. Thus, in cross sections, 15 to 22 periplasmic flagella are seen at the terminal portions of the cell, and 30 to 44 periplasmic flagella are present at the middle areas of the cell. Borreliae are highly motile. Multiplication is by binary fission.

Borreliae have an affinity for acid dyes, and they stain with nearly all aniline dyes. They can be demonstrated in tissue sections by silver impregnation techniques. Dark-field microscopy is used for the rapid examination and detection of spirochetes in peripheral blood or in vector tissues.

Borreliae are microaerophilic and require long-chain fatty acids for growth. Glucose is metabolized by the glycolytic pathway, resulting in the accumulation of lactic acid.

The moles percent G+C of the DNA for certain borreliae (*B. hermsii, B. turicatae*, and *B. parkeri*) ranges from 28.0 to 30.5. Within the same range are isolates of the recently discovered Lyme disease spirochete now known as *Borrelia burgdorferi* (34).

ECOLOGY OF BORRELIAE

All borreliae are arthropod borne; some are pathogenic for humans, rodents, domestic animals, and birds. Those causing relapsing fever in humans are transmitted either by the body louse, *Pediculus humanus humanus*, or by a large variety of soft-shelled ticks of the genus *Ornithodoros*. The etiologic agent of avian borreliosis is transmitted by various species of *Argas* ticks, whereas that of tick spirochetosis in cattle, horses, and sheep is transmitted by ixodid ticks of the genus *Rhipicephalus* and probably by ticks of other genera.

B. burgdorferi, the causative agent of Lyme disease and related disorders, is transmitted by ixodid ticks of the *Ixodes ricinus* complex, namely, *I. dammini* in the northeastern and midwestern United States, *I. pacificus* in the western United States, *I. ricinus* in Europe, and *I. persulcatus* in Asian countries (3). Other hematophagous arthropods such as tabanids and mosquitoes may also be involved in the transmission of this agent.

B. recurrentis is the etiologic agent of louse-borne relapsing fever, a disease whose prevalence depends on ecological and sociological conditions favoring heavy infestations by body lice. Humans are the only reservoir of this agent. Infection in lice is limited primarily to the hemolymph. Thus, transmission does not occur by bite via saliva but by contamination of the bite wound with the infectious hemolymph of lice that have been smashed or otherwise traumatized by scratching. Borreliae may penetrate normal, unbroken skin.

Borreliae that cause tick-borne relapsing fevers are widely distributed throughout the Eastern and Western Hemispheres. Accordingly, spirochetes causing African, Asiatic, and American relapsing fevers are distinguished from one another (Table 1). There are numerous tick-spirochete associations whose significance in relation to human disease is not known. Vector specificity for *Borrelia* spp. has been reported from several geographic areas. In North America, for instance, *B. hermsii, B. turicatae*, and *B. parkeri* are said to be vector specific; i.e., they are maintained and transmitted only by their specific tick vectors, *Ornithodoros hermsi, O. turicata*, and *O. parkeri*, respectively (20). In other areas, such as Iran and Egypt, even local or regional specificity is common. Thus, *O. tholozani* from one area in Iran failed to transmit *B. persica* from other parts of that country (4). The mechanism of this vector-spirochete specificity is still conjectural.

The development of relapsing fever borreliae in ticks differs from that in the body louse; after entering the hemocele, spirochetes invade all tissues, including those of the salivary glands and, in many instances, also those of the ovary. The passage of spirochetes via eggs to progeny (transovarial infection) occurs in *O. moubata, O. erraticus* (both varieties), *O. tholozani, O. tartakowskyi, O. verrucosus, O. turicata, O. hermsi, Argas persicus*, and *A. arboreus* but not in *O. parkeri, O. talaje, O. rudis, A. streptopelia*, and *A. hermanni*.

Transmission of tick-borne spirochetes to a vertebrate host takes place via either infected saliva or infectious body fluids (coxal fluid). Most known *Ornithodoros* and *Argas* vectors are intermittent, mainly nocturnal, fast feeders that live in the soil of rodent burrows (e.g., *O. turicata* and *O. parkeri*), in the crevices of old tree stumps or between the logs of rodent-infested cabins (e.g., *O. hermsi*), and in the dirt floors of native huts (e.g., *O. moubata*) and animal shelters (e.g., *O. tholozani*).

The Lyme disease spirochete, *B. burgdorferi*, in most of its tick vectors shows a distribution limited to the midgut. However, during tick engorgement, spirochetes penetrate the gut epithelium to invade via hemolymph the salivary glands, from where they are said to be

TABLE 1. Characteristics and distribution of arthropod-borne borreliae

Borrelia sp.	Arthropod vector	Animal reservoir	Distribution	Disease
B. recurrentis (syn. *B. obermeyeri*, *B. novyi*)	*P. humanus humanus*	Humans	Worldwide	Louse-borne, epidemic relapsing fever
B. duttonii	*O. moubata*	Humans	Central, eastern, and southern Africa	East African tick-borne, endemic relapsing fever
B. hispanica	*O. erraticus* (large variety)	Rodents	Spain, Portugal, Morocco, Algeria, Tunisia	Hispano-African tick-borne relapsing fever
B. crocidurae, *B. merionesi*, *B. microti*, *B. dipodilli*	*O. erraticus* (small variety)	Rodents	Morocco, Libya, Egypt, Iran, Turkey, Senegal, Kenya	North African tick-borne relapsing fever
B. persica	*O. tholozani* (syn. *O. papillipes*, *O. crossi*?)	Rodents	From west China and Kashmir to Iraq and Egypt, USSR, India	Asiatic-African tick-borne relapsing fever
B. caucasica	*O. verrucosus*	Rodents	Caucasus to Iraq	Caucasian tick-borne relapsing fever
B. latyschewii	*O. tartakowskyi*	Rodents	Iran, Central Asia	Caucasian tick-borne relapsing fever
B. hermsii	*O. hermsi*	Rodents, chipmunks, tree squirrels	Western United States	American tick-borne relapsing fever
B. turicatae	*O. turicata*	Rodents	Southwestern United States	American tick-borne relapsing fever
B. parkeri	*O. parkeri*	Rodents	Western United States	American tick-borne relapsing fever
B. mazzottii	*O. talaje* (*O. dugesi*?)	Rodents	Southern United States, Mexico, Central and South America	American tick-borne relapsing fever
B. venezuelensis	*O. rudis* (syn. *O. venezuelensis*)	Rodents	Central and South America	American tick-borne relapsing fever
B. burgdorferi	*I. dammini*	Rodents	Eastern and midwestern United States	Lyme disease
	I. pacificus	Rodents	Western United States	Lyme disease
	I. ricinus	Rodents	Europe	Lyme disease
	I. persulcatus	Rodents	Asian countries	Lyme disease
	?	?	Australia	Lyme disease
B. theileri	*Rhipicephalus* spp., probably other ixodid ticks	Cattle, horses, sheep	South Africa, Australia, North America, Europe	Tick spirochetosis
B. coriaceae	*O. coriaceus*	Deer (?) Cattle (?)	Western United States	Epizootic bovine abortion (?)
B. anserina	*Argas* spp. (mites?)	Fowl	Worldwide	Avian borreliosis
B. brasiliensis	*O. brasiliensis*	?	South America (Brazil)	?[a]
B. graingeri	*O. graingeri*	?	East Africa (Kenya)	One laboratory case[a]
B. tillae	*O. zumpti*	Rodents	South Africa	?[a]
B. queenslandica	*O. gurneyi*	Rodents	Australia	?[a]
B. armenica	*O. alactagalis*	Rodents	Armenia	?[a]

[a] Spirochete-tick associations of unknown or little health significance.

transmitted via saliva secreted during late stages of tick engorgement (62). Regurgitation of spirochetes in gut fluids is also considered a potential mode of transmission (14).

The main sources for spirochetal infections of arthropods are rodents (rats, mice, and squirrels) and lagomorphs. Exceptions include (i) humans, who appear to be the sole reservoir of *B. recurrentis* and *B. duttonii*, the respective etiologic agents of louse-borne (epidemic) and tick-borne (endemic) relapsing fevers; (ii) birds, the sources of *B. anserina;* and (iii) domestic animals, the reservoirs of *B. theileri*. Because of the large variety of animals that serve as hosts for the immature and adult stages of the *I. ricinus* complex, isolations of *B. burgdorferi* have been made from various species of small, medium, and large animals, including rodents, lagomorphs, deer, domestic animals (dogs, horses, and cows), and even one bird. So far, small rodents and rabbits are recognized as important sources for infecting ticks with this spirochete (3, 15).

CLINICAL SIGNIFICANCE

Relapsing fever in humans

Relapsing fever in humans is a febrile, septicemic disease with sudden onset after an incubation period of 2 to 15 days. Fever persists for 3 to 7 days and is followed by an afebrile interval of several days to several weeks. Thereafter, as many as 10 relapses may occur, especially in untreated patients, as a result of antigenic variations in the causative borreliae. Detailed clinical descriptions of relapsing fever in humans have been presented by Bryceson et al. (11).

According to medical history, more than 50 million persons contracted louse-borne relapsing fever during the first half of this century. Large epidemics have occurred throughout Europe, Africa, Asia, and South America. During World War II, 1 million reported and more than 9 million unreported cases, with a fatality rate of 5%, are said to have occurred.

Since 1967, louse-borne relapsing fever has been reported primarily from African countries, especially Ethiopia (2,278 to 8,700 cases annually) and Sudan, although recent outbreaks have occurred also in South America (World Health Organization Weekly Epidemiological Record, 1967–1978). Information on its prevalence in the USSR and the People's Republic of China is not available.

Because of the sporadic occurrence of tick-borne relapsing fevers, extremely little is known about their incidence worldwide. In Jordan, where tick-borne relapsing fever is caused by *B. persica* transmitted by *O. tholozani*, 723 cases, 4 ending in death, were recorded from 1959 to 1969 (23). In Rwanda, where *O. moubata* transmits *B. duttonii*, sporadic cases have occurred since 1959. In 1974, however, 103 cases, 2 of them fatal, came to the attention of health authorities and suggested an increase in the incidence in that country (22). Lastly, the microscopic examination of blood during a malarial survey in Iran revealed spirochetes in 13 persons. Most likely, the spirochetes had been transmitted by *O. erraticus* (small form), a vector commonly found in the burrows of gerbils in that area (29).

In the United States, during the period 1964 to 1987, a total of 431 cases of tick-borne relapsing fever were recognized (Table 2). Most occurred within the distributional area of *O. hermsi*, and a few occurred also within that of *O. turicata*. Outbreaks usually are sporadic and rarely involve more than two persons. Even so, one outbreak involved 11 Boy Scouts camping near Spokane, Wash. (61), and another outbreak involved 62 employees and tourists at the North Rim of the Grand Canyon in Arizona (10). Tick-borne relapsing fever is underreported in the United States because it is seldom recognized. Most patients are unaware of a tick bite, and unless a history of wilderness exposure, camping, or spending nights in old, rodent-infested cabins is given, the disease is rarely suspected during the initial period of fever (25).

Lyme disease in humans

Lyme disease is an endemic inflammatory disorder that usually begins in summer with the distinctive skin lesion erythema chronicum migrans, accompanied by headache, stiff neck, myalgias, arthralgias, malaise, fatigue, or swelling of the lymph nodes. Weeks to months later, some patients may develop meningoencephalitis, myocarditis, or migrating musculoskeletal pain. Still later, patients may develop intermittent attacks of oligoarticular arthritis or chronic arthritis in the large joints, particularly the knees. First described after an outbreak among children in Lyme, Conn., in 1975 (58), the disease appears to be more severe than erythema chronicum migrans, a tick-borne associated syndrome observed as early as 1908 in Europe (2) and for the first time in the United States in 1969 (54). The etiologic agent, *B. burgdorferi*, remained obscure until 1981, when it was discovered in *I. dammini* from New York (16). It is closely related, if not identical, to isolates of spirochetes from the European tick vector, *I. ricinus* (17). Other clinical syndromes in Europe that appear to be related to the same agent include lymphocytoma (lymphadenosis benigna cutis), acrodermatitis chronica atrophicans, tick-borne meningoradiculitis (Garin-Bujadoux-Bannwarth syndrome), and myositis (46).

In the United States from 1975 through 1979, about 500 cases of Lyme disease, the majority from the Northeast, were reported. Since 1982, the year the discovery of the causative agent of Lyme disease and related disorders was reported, 13,825 cases, 4,600 in 1988 alone, came to the attention of the Centers for Disease Control (19). Increased incidence is thought to be due to improved awareness and recognition of the disease as well as to actual geographic spread. The number of states with Lyme disease has also increased from 14 in 1979 to 34 in 1987 and to 43 in 1988.

Borrelioses in animals

Borrelioses in rodents and lagomorphs may be similar to the diseases observed in humans. There may be one or more relapses accompanied by spirochetemias in various degrees. Not all animals are equally susceptible

TABLE 2. Cases of tick-borne relapsing fever in the United States, 1964 to 1989[a]

Borrelia sp. and state	No. of cases				
	1964–68	1969–73	1974–78	1979–83	1984–89
B. hermsii					
California	13	17	53	58	32
Arizona	0	62	3	4	5
Oregon	14	5	20	20	14
Washington	12	0	4	5	6
Colorado	0	0	4	20	12
New Mexico	0	0	1	3	9
Idaho	0	0	1	3	9
B. turicatae					
Texas	2	1	3	15	4
Kansas	1	0	1	0	0
Oklahoma	0	0	2	0	0

[a] According to reports from the state health departments.

to the various *Borrelia* species, and even differences in susceptibility to various isolates of a single species of spirochete may be seen. Young animals are generally more susceptible and occasionally die as the result of infection.

Avian borreliosis, caused by *B. anserina*, affects geese, ducks, turkeys, and chickens in Europe, Siberia, India, Africa, Australia, Indonesia, and South, Central, and North America. In certain countries the disease is of great economic importance because it causes severe losses to the poultry industry. Clinically, the disease begins with a high fever after an incubation period of about 4 days. The birds become cyanotic and have yellowish-green diarrhea. During the early stages of the febrile reaction, spirochetes can be readily detected in the blood. Surviving birds recover after about 2 weeks and have long-lasting immunity.

Tick spirochetosis caused by *B. theileri* in cattle, horses, and sheep in South Africa, and recently also in Australia, is a benign disease characterized by one to two attacks of fever, inappetence, weight loss, weakness, and anemia.

The Lyme disease spirochete, *B. burgdorferi*, does not adversely affect wild animals. However, in dogs, cows, and horses, it has been reported to cause arthritic manifestations with lameness, stiffness, and swollen joints (18, 43, 44). Infected white-footed mice (*Peromyscus leucopus*) develop long-lasting (up to 8 months) spirochetemias characterized by alternating low and high concentrations of spirochetes, as suggested by the cyclic pattern of infected ticks feeding upon them (15, 24, 41). New Zealand White rabbits, hamsters, and certain genetic lines of rats have also been shown to be susceptible to *B. burgdorferi* and appear useful for studies related to the pathogenicity of this agent (9, 13, 27, 32).

A borrelialike spirochete has recently been detected in *Ornithodoros coriaceus*, the soft tick implicated in the epizootiology of epizootic bovine abortion, which is a major disease of rangeland cattle in the western United States (39). Genetic and phenotypic characteristics revealed that this spirochete is a new species of *Borrelia*, and the name *B. coriaceae* was proposed (30). As yet, there is only circumstantial evidence that this organism is causally related to epizootic abortion.

DIAGNOSIS OF BORRELIAL INFECTION

Direct examination

Diagnosis of most borrelioses is based primarily on the detection of spirochetes in the peripheral blood of febrile persons and animals or in the hemolymph and tissues of arthropod vectors (12). Unlike the tick-borne relapsing fever borreliae, the Lyme disease spirochete cannot readily be detected in blood preparations by either dark-field or conventional microscopy. However, successful isolation in BSK II medium (see below) injected with blood from a patient or from a tick host suggests the occurrence of spirochetemias of unknown duration and concentrations. Direct diagnosis, however, is possible through the demonstration of silver-stained organisms in sections of biopsied skin lesions.

Detection of spirochetes in the blood

During the febrile period, most spirochetes circulate in the blood and can be detected by light or dark-field microscopy of wet preparations made from a drop of blood mixed with a small drop of sodium citrate and covered with a cover slip. Leishman, Giemsa, May-Grünwald, Wright, and other combinations of Romanowsky stains are used to stain thin- and thick-drop films for examination by conventional light microscopy (Fig. 1). For the initial diagnosis, thick films should always be examined, because spirochetemias may be mild and always tend to become milder with each succeeding relapse. A proper thick film is made by placing a drop of blood on a slide and stirring the drop with a toothpick, an applicator stick, or the corner of a microscope slide in a circular motion until it is evenly spread over an area about 1 cm in diameter. This preparation is then air dried for 30 min. During staining, dehemoglobinization renders the smear transparent, a process necessary for the ready detection of blue-stained spirochetes. A microhematocrit concentration technique previously described (26) detects spirochetes more readily in the blood of mildly infected persons. The most dependable methods for detecting spirochetes in ticks are dark-field examination of tissues removed by dissection and inoculation of susceptible animals with tissue suspensions.

Detection of spirochetes in arthropod vectors

Spirochetes in the body louse are limited to the hemolymph, which can be readily obtained for microscopic examination by the amputation of the distal portion of one or more legs. The hemolymph test is also useful for the detection of borreliae in large tick vectors, e.g., *O. moubata*, *O. parkeri*, *O. turicata*, *O. erraticus* (large form), and *Argas* spp. The test is not infallible, however, because borreliae are not always abundant in body fluid, particularly in ticks that have been without a blood meal for a long period. The feeding of infected ticks on experimental animals does not always lead to the transmission of spirochetes. Thus, testing of ticks by this method is not recommended unless feeding experiments can be carried out repeatedly. Dependable ways to detect spirochetes in ticks are (i) direct immunofluorescence with species-specific fluorescein isothiocyanate-labeled antibodies, (ii) careful dark-field examination of tissues removed by dissection, and (iii) inoculation of susceptible animals with tick triturates. Recently, the polymerase chain reaction has been developed for the identification of DNA specific for *B.*

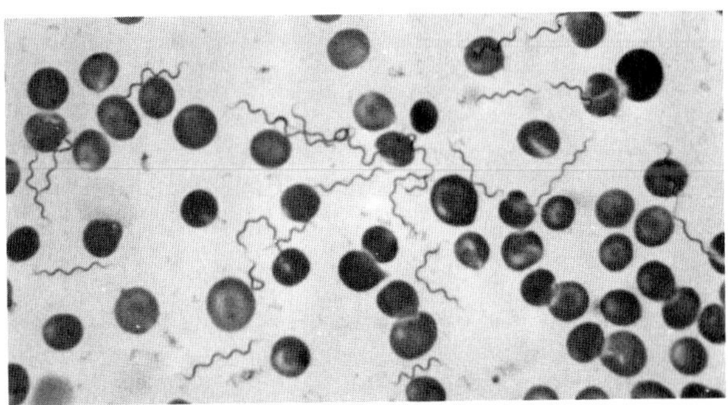

FIG. 1. *B. hermsii* in a thin smear of rodent blood. Giemsa stain; ×740.

burgdorferi, which may allow for the detection of only one to five spirochetes in infected ticks and vertebrate tissues (47).

ANIMAL INOCULATION

During late relapses of relapsing fever, spirochetes in the blood of the infected person or animal may be extremely scarce. Thus, a failure to detect organisms microscopically should never be considered conclusive but should call for the inoculation of susceptible laboratory animals with whole blood or suspensions of triturated blood clots. Suckling Swiss mice and suckling rats are the animals of choice for both louse-borne *B. recurrentis* and tick-borne borreliae. Monkeys, rabbits, and guinea pigs are also useful, depending on the *Borrelia* species involved. The chicken is the animal of choice for *B. anserina*.

Usually, 0.05 to 0.2 ml of a 1:1 dilution of blood in sodium citrate is injected intramuscularly or intraperitoneally into test animals. Any spirochetes in the inoculum may be detected in blood preparations as early as 3 days after inoculation. Blood films should be examined daily for at least 14 days before an animal is considered negative. Laboratory-reared white-footed mice (*P. leucopus*) are used for the isolation of *B. burgdorferi* from ticks and from blood specimens and tissue biopsies from patients. Although microscopically not readily detectable in blood smears, this spirochete can be recovered in BSK II medium (see below) from tissues of mice sacrificed 7 to 10 days after inoculation; urinary bladder, spleen, and skin appear to be most productive (52, 55).

CULTIVATION

Borreliae can be cultivated readily in their arthropod vectors or in a large variety of vertebrate hosts, particularly small rodents. Cultivation has been successful also in embryonated chicken eggs. A growth medium (Kelly medium) has been developed, and so far *B. hermsii, B. parkeri, B. turicatae, B. hispanica,* and *B. recurrentis* have been cultivated in vitro (35).

Modified versions of Kelly medium have also been successfully used for the cultivation of *B. burgdorferi* from ticks as well as from the blood, skin, and cerebrospinal fluid of Lyme disease patients (7, 57). Increased concentrations of agarose have been used to grow *B. burgdorferi* on a solidified medium, allowing production of colonies from single organisms (38). Attempts to cocultivate *B. burgdorferi* with tick and mammalian cells have also been made in an effort to produce a better medium and to address questions concerning spirochete-host cell interactions (37, 60). Although the Lyme disease spirochete can be successfully grown in both liquid and solid media, continuous serial passage may affect many biological changes in the population of cultured spirochetes. Such changes include the loss of infectivity in hamsters (33) and white-footed mice (50, 51), changes in protein profiles, the migration of lipopolysaccharidelike material in acrylamide gels, and the reduction in number of detectable plasmids (5, 28). Thus, it appears that spirochetes cultured for even relatively short periods of time may be quite different from their naturally occurring ancestral strains.

SEROLOGICAL DIAGNOSIS

The ability of relapsing fever spirochetes to spontaneously change their antigenic composition makes the serodiagnosis of these diseases difficult and explains the inefficiency and failure of many serological procedures, including agglutination, adhesion, opsonic activity, immobilization, and borreliolysin, in the detection of antibodies. Nevertheless, promising results have been obtained with the indirect immunofluorescence test with cultured spirochetes as antigens. This test may also be used for the characterization of antigenic types of borreliae and for the detection of mixed populations and serotypes of spirochetes (59). Lyme disease can be identified serologically either by indirect immunofluorescent staining or by the more sensitive and specific enzyme-linked immunosorbent assay (48). However, because these tests and their reagents are not yet standardized, variations in results and in interpretations thereof are common (6, 45, 56). False-negative results may be obtained during the first few weeks of infection, whereas false-positive findings may be recorded for patients with other spirochetal diseases such as syphilis and relapsing fever. Immunoblotting is being used to help identify false-positive reactions. Research is under way to improve the sensitivity and specificity of serological procedures, using as test antigens species-specific proteins of *B. burgdorferi* (42).

ANTIBIOTIC SUSCEPTIBILITY

Although borreliae are susceptible to many antibiotics, tetracyclines are the drugs of choice. They reduce the relapse rate and rid the central nervous system of spirochetes. However, the rapid destruction of organisms may provoke a severe Jarisch-Herxheimer reaction. There is no general agreement about the dosage of the antibiotic and its route of administration. Good results have been obtained with 0.5 g of tetracycline given orally every 6 h for 4 to 5 days or with a single oral dose of 100 mg of doxycycline. To avoid the Jarisch-Herxheimer reaction, a combined penicillin-tetracycline therapy is recommended. This treatment consists of 400,000 U of procaine penicillin administered intramuscularly, to be followed the next day by 500 mg of tetracycline given orally every 6 h for 7 days (49).

Avian borreliosis has been treated successfully with 100,000 U of procaine penicillin given intramuscularly or with oxytetracycline at 2 mg/kg of body weight.

Although all stages of Lyme disease may respond to antibiotic therapy, treatment regimens depend on the nature and severity of clinical manifestations (1, 56). Antibiotics given early in disease shorten the duration of the rash and prevent later illness, although some patients with severe early disease have developed manifestations later despite recommended courses of antibiotics.

Men, nonpregnant women, and children with early disease, mild neurological symptoms, or minor cardiac involvement have been treated orally with doxycycline, 100 mg twice a day, or with tetracycline HCl, 250 to 500 mg three times a day for 10 to 30 days. Amoxicillin, 250 to 500 mg three times a day (20 to 40 mg/kg per day for children) for 10 to 30 days, is also effective and is preferred for children under 8 years of age and for pregnant and lactating women. For patients who cannot take tetracycline and are allergic to penicillin, erythromycin is recommended in a dosage of 250 mg four times a day (or 30 mg/kg per day for children).

Patients with late neurological (focal central nervous system involvement) complications, severe Lyme arthritis, or severe cardiac involvement require intravenous application of penicillin G or ceftriaxone. For details on dosages and length of treatment, the reader is referred to the references cited above.

IDENTIFICATION

Although DNA base (G+C) content and DNA homology studies provide information about the relationship of certain borreliae to other spirochetes of the same genus, these studies are of no value in distinguishing the many relapsing fever spirochetes from one another (31). Similarly, the phenomenon of antigenic phase variations makes a precise serological identification difficult if not impossible. Therefore, the taxonomic identification of borreliae must take into account the geographic distribution and the natural arthropod vectors.

In certain areas, such as the Western Hemisphere, a specific relationship appears to exist between certain *Borrelia* species and their natural tick vectors. Each species of vector tick maintains and transmits its own spirochete, whose physiological behavior is quite distinct from that of other *Borrelia* species (see above). This phenomenon of specificity has permitted the identification by xenodiagnosis of spirochetes isolated from relapsing fever patients (21). This specificity, however, does not hold true for other areas of the world, and exceptions to it have occurred even in the Western Hemisphere. Thus, for most cases of tick-borne relapsing fevers, taxonomic identification of the etiologic agent is presumptive and is based on a history of exposure to a particular vector.

Several molecular procedures are available to identify the Lyme disease spirochete, *B. burgdorferi*, and to differentiate it from other pathogenic spirochetes. Polyacrylamide gel electrophoresis of whole-cell lysates demonstrates two major surface proteins, OspA and OspB, which are unique to *B. burgdorferi*. The presence of these proteins, or that of OspA only, provides a presumptive identification which then can be confirmed by the reactivity to a monoclonal antibody that recognizes an epitope unique to this protein (8). DNA-hybridization probes are also available for the identification of this spirochete (53), and the polymerase chain reaction may also be used (47). Plasmid profiles (5) and restriction endonuclease patterns of total DNA (40) in agar gels are also useful in differentiating isolates of these microorganisms.

LITERATURE CITED

1. **Abramowicz, M.** 1989. The medical letter. Med. Lett. **31:** 57–59.
2. **Afzelius, A.** 1921. Erythema chronicum migrans. Acta Dermato-Venereol. **2:**120–125.
3. **Anderson, J. F.** 1989. Epizootiology of *Borrelia* in lxodes tick vectors and reservoir hosts. Rev. Infect. Dis. **11:**1451–1459.
4. **Baltazard, M., R. Pournaki, and G. Chabaud.** 1954. Sur les fièvres récurrentes à Ornithodores. Bull. Soc. Pathol. Exot. **47:**589–596.
5. **Barbour, A. G.** 1988. Plasmid analysis of *Borrelia burgdorferi*, the Lyme borreliosis agent. J. Clin. Microbiol. **26:** 475–478.
6. **Barbour, A. G.** 1989. The diagnosis of Lyme disease: rewards and perils. Ann. Intern. Med. **110:**501–502.
7. **Barbour, A. G., W. Burgdorfer, S. F. Hayes, O. Péter, and A. Aeschlimann.** 1983. Isolation of a cultivable spirochete from *Ixodes ricinus* ticks of Switzerland. Curr. Microbiol. **8:**123–126.
8. **Barbour, A. G., S. L. Tessier, and W. J. Todd.** 1983. Lyme disease spirochete and ixodid tick spirochetes share a common surface antigenic determinant defined by a monoclonal antibody. Infect. Immun. **41:**795–804.
9. **Barthold, S. W., K. D. Moody, G. A. Terwilliger, R. O. Jacoby, and A. S. Steere.** 1988. An animal model for Lyme arthritis. Ann. N.Y. Acad. Sci. **539:**264–273.
10. **Boyer, K. M., R. S. Munford, G. O. Maupin, C. P. Pattison, M. D. Fox, A. M. Barnes, W. L. Jones, and J. E. Maynard.** 1977. Tick-borne relapsing fever: an interstate outbreak originating at Grand Canyon National Park. Am. J. Epidemiol. **105:**469–479.
11. **Bryceson, A. D. E., E. H. O. Parry, P. L. Perine, D. A. Warrell, D. Vukotich, and C. S. Leithead.** 1970. Louse-borne relapsing fever. A clinical and laboratory study of 62 cases in Ethiopia and a reconsideration of the literature. J. Med. **39:**129–170.
12. **Burgdorfer, W.** 1976. The diagnosis of the relapsing fevers, p. 225–234. In R. C. Johnson (ed.), Biology of parasitic spirochetes. Academic Press, Inc., New York.
13. **Burgdorfer, W.** 1984. The New Zealand White rabbit: an experimental host for infecting ticks with Lyme disease spirochetes. Yale J. Biol. Med. **57:**609–612.
14. **Burgdorfer, W.** 1984. Discovery of the Lyme disease spirochete and its relation to tick vectors. Yale J. Biol. Med. **57:**515–520.
15. **Burgdorfer, W.** 1989. Vector/host relationships of the Lyme disease spirochete, *Borrelia burgdorferi*. Rheum. Dis. Clin. N. Am. **15:**775–787.
16. **Burgdorfer, W., A. G. Barbour, S. F. Hayes, J. L. Benach, E. Grunwaldt, and J. P. Davis.** 1982. Lyme disease—a tick-borne spirochetosis? Science **216:**1317–1319.
17. **Burgdorfer, W., A. G. Barbour, S. F. Hayes, O. Péter, and A. Aeschlimann.** 1983. Erythema chronicum migrans—a tick borne spirochetosis. Acta Trop. **40:**79–83.
18. **Burgess, E. C.** 1988. *Borrelia burgdorferi* infection in Wisconsin horses and cows. Ann. N.Y. Acad. Sci. **539:**235–243.
19. **Centers for Disease Control.** 1989. Lyme disease—United States, 1987 and 1988. Morbid. Mortal. Weekly Rep. **38:** 668–672.
20. **Davis, G. E.** 1942. Species unity or plurality of the relapsing fever spirochetes, p. 41–47. *In* F. R. Moulton (ed.), A symposium on relapsing fever in the Americas. Science Press Printing Co., Lancaster, Pa.
21. **Davis, G. E.** 1956. The identification of spirochetes from human cases of relapsing fever by xenodiagnosis with comments on local specificity of tick vectors. Exp. Parasitol. **5:**271–275.
22. **deClercq, A. G., A. Z. Meheus, E. de Pierpont, and C. Nyirashema.** 1975. Single-dose doxycycline treatment of tick-borne relapsing fever. East Afr. Med. J. **8:**428–429.
23. **deZulueta, J., S. Nasrallah, J. S. Karam, A. R. Anani, G. K. Sweatman, and D. A. Muir.** 1971. Finding of tick-borne relapsing fever in Jordan by the malaria eradication service. Ann. Trop. Med. Parasitol. **65:**491–495.
24. **Donahue, J. G., J. Piesman, and A. Spielman.** 1987. Reservoir competence of white-footed mice for Lyme disease spirochetes. Am. J. Trop. Med. Hyg. **36:**92–96.
25. **Fihn, S., and E. B. Larson.** 1980. Tick-borne relapsing fever in the Pacific Northwest: an underdiagnosed illness? West. J. Med. **133:**203–209.
26. **Goldschmid, J. M., and K. Mahomed.** 1972. The use of the microhematocrit technic for the recovery of *Borrelia duttonii* from the blood. Am. J. Clin. Pathol. **58:**165–169.
27. **Heijka, A., J. L. Schmitz, D. M. England, S. M. Callister,**

and R. F. Schell. 1989. Histopathology of Lyme arthritis in LSH hamsters. Am. J. Pathol. **134:**1113–1123.

28. **Hyde, F. W., and R. C. Johnson.** 1986. Genetic analysis of *Borrelia.* Zentralbl. Bakteriol. Parasitenkd. Infektionskr. Hyg. Abt. 1 Orig. Reihe A **263:**119–122.
29. **Janbakhsh, B., and A. Ardelan.** 1977. The nature of sporadic cases of relapsing fever in Kazeroun area, southern Iran. Bull. Soc. Pathol. Exot. **70:**587–589.
30. **Johnson, R. C., W. Burgdorfer, R. S. Lane, A. G. Barbour, S. F. Hayes, and F. W. Hyde.** 1987. *Borrelia coriaceae* sp. nov.: putative agent of epizootic bovine abortion. Int. J. Syst. Bacteriol. **37:**72–74.
31. **Johnson, R. C., F. W. Hyde, and C. M. Rumpel.** 1984. Taxonomy of the Lyme disease spirochete. Yale J. Biol. Med. **57:**529–537.
32. **Johnson, R. C., C. Kodner, M. Russell, and P. H. Duray.** 1988. Experimental infection of the hamster with *Borrelia burgdorferi.* Ann. N.Y. Acad. Sci. **539:**258–262.
33. **Johnson, R. C., N. Marek, and C. Kodner.** 1984. Infection of Syrian hamsters with Lyme disease spirochetes. J. Clin. Microbiol. **18:**1099–1101.
34. **Johnson, R. C., G. P. Schmid, F. W. Hyde, A. G. Steigerwalt, and D. J. Brenner.** 1984. *Borrelia burgdorferi* sp. nov.: etiologic agent of Lyme disease. Int. J. Syst. Bacteriol. **34:**496–497.
35. **Kelly, R. T.** 1978. Cultivation and physiology of relapsing fever borreliae, p. 87–94. *In* R. C. Johnson (ed.), Biology of parasitic spirochetes. Academic Press, Inc., New York.
36. **Kelly, R. T.** 1984. Genus IV. *Borrelia* Swellengrebel 1907, 582, p. 57–62. *In* N. R. Krieg and J. C. Holt (ed.), Bergey's manual of systematic bacteriology, vol. 1. The Williams & Wilkins Co., Baltimore.
37. **Kurtti, T. J., U. G. Munderloh, G. G. Ahlstrand, and R. C. Johnson.** 1988. *Borrelia burgdorferi* in tick cell culture: growth and cellular adherence. J. Med. Entomol. **25:** 256–261.
38. **Kurtti, T. J., U. G. Munderloh, R. C. Johnson, and G. G. Ahlstrand.** 1987. Colony formation and morphology in *Borrelia burgdorferi.* J. Clin. Microbiol. **25:**2054–2058.
39. **Lane, R. S., W. Burgdorfer, S. F. Hayes, and A. G. Barbour.** 1985. Isolation of a spirochete from the soft tick, *Ornithodoros coriaceus:* a possible agent of epizootic bovine abortion. Science **230:**85–87.
40. **LeFebvre, R. B., G. C. Perny, and R. C. Johnson.** 1989. Characterization of *Borrelia burgdorferi* isolates by restriction endonuclease analysis and DNA hybridization. J. Clin. Microbiol. **27:**636–639.
41. **Levine, J. F., M. L. Wilson, and A. Spielman.** 1985. Mice as reservoirs of the Lyme disease spirochete. Am. J. Trop. Med. Hyg. **34:**355–360.
42. **Magnarelli, L. A., J. F. Anderson, and A. G. Barbour.** 1989. Enzyme-linked immunosorbent assays for Lyme disease: reactivity of subunits of *Borrelia burgdorferi.* J. Infect. Dis. **159:**43–49.
43. **Magnarelli, L. A., J. F. Anderson, A. B. Schreier, and C. M. Ficke.** 1987. Clinical and serologic studies of canine borreliosis. J. Am. Vet. Med. Assoc. **191:**1089–1094.
44. **Magnarelli, L. A., J. F. Anderson, E. Shaw, J. E. Post, and P. C. Palka.** 1988. Borreliosis in equids in northeastern United States. Am. J. Vet. Res. **49:**359–362.
45. **Magnarelli, L. A., J. M. Meegan, J. F. Anderson, and W. A. Chappell.** 1984. Comparison of an indirect fluorescent-antibody test with an enzyme-linked immunosorbent assay for serological studies of Lyme disease. J. Clin. Microbiol. **20:**181–184.
46. **Reimers, C. D., D. E. Pongratz, U. Neubert, A. Pilz, G. Hubner, M. Naegele, B. Wilske, P. H. Duray, and J. de Koning.** 1989. Myositis caused by *Borrelia burgdorferi:* report of four cases. J. Neurol. Sci. **91:**215–226.
47. **Rosa, P. A., and T. G. Schwan.** 1989. A specific and sensitive assay for the Lyme disease spirochete, *Borrelia burgdorferi,* using the polymerase chain reaction. J. Infect. Dis. **160:**1018–1029.
48. **Russell, H., J. S. Sampson, G. P. Smith, H. W. Wilkinson, and B. Plikaytis.** 1984. Enzyme-linked immunosorbent assay and indirect immunofluorescence assay for Lyme disease. J. Infect. Dis. **149:**465–470.
49. **Salih, S. Y., and D. Mustafa.** 1977. Louse-borne relapsing fever. II. Combined penicillin and tetracycline therapy in 160 Sudanese patients. Trans. R. Soc. Trop. Med. Soc. **71:** 49–51.
50. **Schwan, T. G., and W. Burgdorfer.** 1987. Antigenic changes of *Borrelia burgdorferi* as a result of *in vitro* cultivation. J. Infect. Dis. **156:**852–853.
51. **Schwan, T. G., W. Burgdorfer, and C. F. Garon.** 1988. Changes in infectivity and plasmid profile of the Lyme disease spirochete, *Borrelia burgdorferi,* as a result of in vitro cultivation. Infect. Immun. **56:**1831–1836.
52. **Schwan, T. G., W. Burgdorfer, M. E. Schrumpf, and R. H. Karstens.** 1988. The urinary bladder, a consistent source of *Borrelia burgdorferi* in experimentally infected white-footed mice (*Peromyscus leucopus*). J. Clin. Microbiol. **26:**893–895.
53. **Schwan, T. G., W. J. Simpson, M. E. Schrumpf, and R. H. Karstens.** 1989. Identification of *Borrelia burgdorferi* and *B. hermsii* using DNA hybridization probes. J. Clin. Microbiol. **27:**1734–1738.
54. **Scrimenti, R. J.** 1970. Erythema chronicum migrans. Arch. Dermatol. **102:**104–105.
55. **Sinsky, R. J., and J. Piesman.** 1989. Ear punch biopsy method for detection and isolation of *Borrelia burgdorferi* from rodents. J. Clin. Microbiol. **27:**1723–1727.
56. **Steere, A. C.** 1989. Lyme disease. N. Engl. J. Med. **321:** 586–596.
57. **Steere, A. C., R. L. Grodzicki, A. N. Kornblatt, J. E. Craft, A. G. Barbour, W. Burgdorfer, G. P. Schmid, E. Johnson, and S. E. Malawista.** 1983. The spirochetal etiology of Lyme disease. N. Engl. J. Med. **308:**733–740.
58. **Steere, A. C., S. E. Malawista, J. A. Hardin, S. Ruddy, P. W. Askenase, and W. A. Andiman.** 1977. Erythema chronicum migrans and Lyme arthritis. The enlarging clinical spectrum. Ann. Intern. Med. **86:**685–698.
59. **Stoenner, H. G., T. Dodd, and C. Larsen.** 1982. Antigenic variation of *Borrelia hermsii.* J. Exp. Med. **156:**1297–1311.
60. **Thomas, D. D., and L. E. Comstock.** 1989. Interaction of Lyme disease spirochetes with cultured eucaryotic cells. Infect. Immun. **57:**1324–1326.
61. **Thompson, R. S., W. Burgdorfer, R. Russell, and B. J. Francis.** 1969. Outbreak of tick-borne relapsing fever in Spokane County, Washington. J. Am. Med. Assoc. **210:** 1045–1050.
62. **Zung, J. L., S. Lewengrub, M. A. Rudzinska, A. Spielman, S. R. Telford, and J. Piesman.** 1989. Fine structural evidence for the penetration of the Lyme disease spirochete *Borrelia burgdorferi* through the gut and salivary tissues of *Ixodes dammini.* Can. J. Zool. **67:**1737–1748.

Chapter 55

Treponema

THOMAS J. FITZGERALD

CHARACTERIZATION

The genus *Treponema* (order *Spirochaetales*, family *Spirochaetaceae*) contains four human pathogens and at least six human nonpathogens. The most recent edition of *Bergey's Manual of Systematic Bacteriology* (18) has changed the nomenclature for this genus. The pathogens are termed nonculturable treponemes, and the nonpathogens are termed culturable treponemes. The four pathogens are closely similar and can be differentiated only by epidemiology (endemic geographic location), clinical manifestations, and mode of transmission. DNA homology has been compared for the agents that cause syphilis, yaws, and endemic syphilis (12). On the basis of these findings, these three agents have been combined into one species and three subspecies. *T. pallidum* (syphilis) is now *T. pallidum* subsp. *pallidum*, *T. pertenue* (yaws) is now *T. pallidum* subsp. *pertenue*, and *T. endemicum* is now *T. pallidum* subsp. *endemicum*; *T. carateum* (pinta) retains its original name. The diseases caused by these four human pathogens are collectively termed treponematoses.

At least six nonpathogens have been identified as part of the normal flora; they are especially prominent in the oral cavity. Some have also been found in the genital and intestinal tracts. Recent evidence suggests that some of these nonpathogenic treponemes are associated with gingivitis and periodontal disease (14). For an extensive review of these nonpathogens, see reference 17.

Syphilis is found worldwide, yaws is endemic in the tropics, pinta is prevalent in tropical areas of Central and South America, and endemic syphilis is restricted to desert regions. These treponemal infections are very complex in that each exhibits distinct stages of symptomatic manifestations followed by asymptomatic periods. Without antibiotic therapy, these diseases are chronic and may last for 30 to 40 years.

The treponemes are gram-negative bacteria that at one time were considered to be strict anaerobes; incubation in air rapidly killed them. It has been shown that *T. pallidum* subsp. *pallidum* takes up oxygen and possesses an electron transport system (3). *T. pallidum* subspp. *pallidum* and *pertenue* survive better in very low concentrations of oxygen (5), and it is more appropriate to characterize them as microaerophilic. The four pathogens are morphologically identical. They are 6 to 20 μm long and 0.1 to 0.2 μm wide (Fig. 1). They exhibit characteristic motility, with rapid rotation about their longitudinal axis and flexing, bending, and snapping about their full length. The ends are pointed. Division is by transverse fission. Elongation of organisms and eventual splitting apart account for the variation in length.

Hovind-Hougen (8) determined the ultrastructures of pathogenic treponemes by using transmission electron microscopy. Treponemes are coated with an amorphous layer of glycosaminoglycans that are either host derived or synthesized as a capsular material (6). There is an outer membrane (outer envelope) which covers the periplasmic flagella (axial filaments) that wind around the surface of the organisms. Three periplasmic flagella, which impart motility, arise at each end of the cell and extend halfway down the organism, usually overlapping at midpoint. A cell wall and a cytoplasmic membrane enclose the cytoplasmic contents. Six to eight cytoplasmic tubules are located next to the inner surface of the cytoplasmic membrane. These tubules are attached at each end of the cell and wind around the organism, with the free ends extending toward the midpoint of the cell. The cytoplasm contains ribosomes, mesosomes, and a nuclear region. The susceptibility to penicillin indicates the presence of a peptidoglycan layer.

The nonpathogenic treponemes differ morphologically in being slightly wider (0.20 to 0.25 μm) and shorter (3 to 15 μm). They have blunter ends and one to eight periplasmic flagella.

Antigenically, the four pathogens are identical. An individual subspecies-specific antigen has not yet been identified, although promising results should emerge from use of recently developed molecular biology techniques. Serological reactions demonstrate immunological relatedness. Both Wassermann and anti-*T. pallidum* subsp. *pallidum* antibodies develop in response to each treponemal disease. Protective immunogens are also related, as shown by cross-resistance (20). In areas where yaws is endemic, the incidence of syphilis is low. After effective campaigns to eradicate yaws, the incidence of syphilis then increases dramatically. Similar epidemiologic observations have been made in areas where endemic syphilis is eliminated.

Where necessary, the individual treponematosis can be distinguished by infecting different laboratory animals. This, however, is a difficult, time-consuming process not readily available to clinical laboratories. Therefore, the geographic location together with the clinical manifestations of the patient are the key to diagnosis. In general, each of the treponematoses can be divided into an early stage (the first 2 years) and a late stage (beyond 2 years). Syphilis is further subdivided into primary, secondary, and tertiary stages. The diagnosis of treponemal disease can be complicated by frequent overlap of the clinical manifestations of early and late stages and also by the widespread occurrence of uncharacteristic lesion appearance. The clinical manifestations of each treponematosis are quite diverse and highly variable. For detailed descriptions of syphilis, yaws, pinta, and endemic syphilis, see references 4, 10,

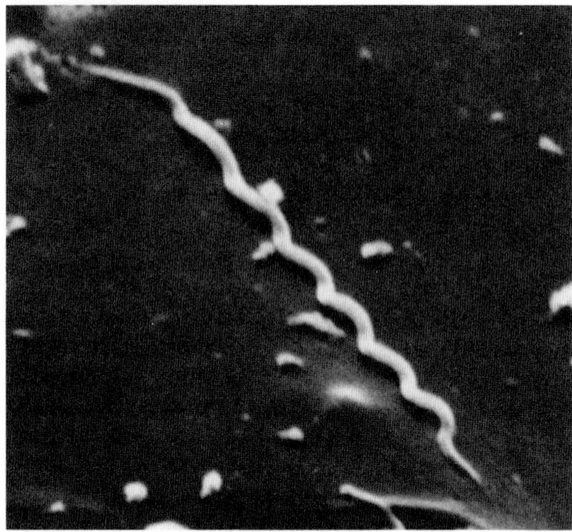

FIG. 1. Scanning electron micrograph of *T. pallidum* (Nichols strain).

and 22. Comparative generalizations for the treponemal diseases are shown in Table 1, as adapted from Vegas (22).

COLLECTION, TRANSPORT, AND STORAGE

Relative to other bacteria, treponemes are very susceptible to environmental influences (20, 23). They are rapidly killed by heat, cold, desiccation, most disinfectants, and osmotic changes. *T. pallidum* subsp. *pallidum* exhibits optimal ranges of pH (7.2 to 7.4), temperature (20 to 35°C), and oxygen concentration (1 to 4%). Because of this delicate nature, it is important to examine lesion material immediately; storage at room or refrigerator temperature even for a few hours is not recommended. Occasionally, tissue samples (from stillborn congenital syphilis-infected babies and tertiary syphilis patients) are required for autopsy. These samples should be cut into small fragments (1 mm^3) and stored at −70°C or in liquid nitrogen. Dimethyl sulfoxide (10%) or glycerol (15%) should be used as a cryoprotectant. The freezing and thawing of specimens should be done very rapidly. Repeated freeze-thaw cycles are to be avoided.

Serum or plasma samples for serological testing are stored at 4°C or at −20°C. A new procedure is especially useful for field surveys which may require prolonged transport to the laboratory (15). A few drops of blood from a finger prick are dropped onto fiber glass disks (the old method used filter paper disks). These disks are dried at room temperature and eluted at the laboratory with phosphate-buffered saline for 2 h. The eluate is then tested for serological activity. Specimens have been kept for as long as 200 days without significant decreases in antibody titers.

Finally, a brief comment should be made about blood obtained from syphilitic donors. The older study of Turner and Diseker (19) had demonstrated that treponemes within blood lost their viability within 2 to 4 days of storage at 4°C. In industrialized countries, donated blood should be screened with a Venereal Disease Research Laboratory (VDRL) or rapid plasma region (RPR) test, and positive results should be confirmed with a fluorescent treponemal antibody absorption (FTA-ABS) or hemagglutination reaction. Two reports (11, 16) discuss potential problems with transfusion-induced syphilis.

DIRECT EXAMINATION

The detection of treponemes within lesion material is an important diagnostic tool. Although these organisms can be stained, their thinness makes them almost impossible to visualize with light microscopy. Dark-field microscopy is recommended. Phase-contrast microscopy may also be used, but the organisms are not as readily apparent. Exudates from the lesions of each treponematosis should contain treponemes. Depending on the development of the lesion, the numbers may vary from 1 organism per 20 fields to 50 organisms per field. Clinical samples should be obtained before antibiotic therapy.

TABLE 1. Characteristics of the treponematoses

Disease	Characteristic[a]					
	Epidemiologic					
	Agent	Other name(s)	Area(s)	Predominant age group(s)	Spread	Congenital infection
Syphilis	*T. pallidum*	Venereal syphilis	Worldwide	Adults	Venereal contact	Yes
Yaws	*T. pertenue*	Frambesia, pian	Tropics	Children	Skin contact	No
Pinta	*T. carateum*	Carate, cute	Tropics, Central and South America	Children, adolescents	Skin contact	No
Endemic syphilis	*T. pallidum* (variant)	Bjel, dichuchwa	Deserts	Children, adults	Mucous membrane contact	Rarely

[a] Common features: highly contagious, generalized infections, regional and general adenopathy, treponemes in exudate of early lesions, chronic and prolonged, some spontaneous healing, latent stage (except pinta), relatively painless, and nonfatal except in some cases of tertiary and congenital syphilis.

Motile organisms rotate around their longitudinal axis and also bend, snap, and flex along their length. Because of their highly characteristic motility, viable treponemes are easy to distinguish. Nonmotile organisms, however, can be easily confused with bits of tissue debris. With specimens from well-developed syphilitic lesions, the exudate may contain large amounts of mucoid material. Besides rotating, the organisms in these specimens may exhibit a smooth, translational, backward-and-forward movement. This directed motility is also occasionally observed in specimens from yaws lesions.

Samples for dark-field microscopy are obtained in different ways, one of which is as follows (4). If multiple lesions are present, choose the smallest wet lesion available. The chances of visualizing treponemes decrease as lesions increase the size of their ulceration. Clean the surface of the lesion with saline and blot it dry. Gently remove any crusts that are present. Superficially abrade the lesion until very slight bleeding occurs and isolate the clear serum exudate from the lesion subsurface by applying gentle pressure at the base of the lesion; wipe away the first few drops of blood. Touch a glass slide to the clear exudate, place a cover slip on the specimen, and immediately examine the slide by dark-field microscopy. The exudate may also be removed with a capillary pipette and then transferred to a glass slide. If no fluid exudes, a small drop of saline may be added to the lesion. Alternatively, lesion material may be aspirated with a 26-gauge needle inserted at the base rather than the center of the lesion. After aspiration, a drop of saline is drawn into the needle, and the material is expressed onto a glass slide for dark-field examination. Whatever method is chosen, examine material immediately, since treponemes rapidly die when placed on a slide and motile organisms are much easier to visualize.

Accidental infection from laboratory exposure is rarely reported. Nevertheless, the high rates of incidence of the treponematoses indicate their contagious nature. Specimens for dark-field and serological examination present potential hazards. If the skin of the examiner is exposed, immediate washing with disinfectant is sufficient to prevent infection, and penicillin prophylaxis is not recommended. If the eyes are exposed, immediate, thorough washing with saline followed by penicillin prophylaxis is recommended. Procain penicillin G, clemizole penicillin, procaine penicillin G with 2% aluminum monostearate, or benzathine penicillin G may be used. In cases of penicillin allergy, tetracycline or erythromycin is effective.

Treponemal lesions frequently exude material that is infectious. For this reason, the examiner should always wear gloves. Slides containing dark-field samples, as well as materials used for obtaining these samples, should be placed directly into disinfectant. Disinfectants rapidly kill treponemes; 70% ethanol is very effective. Freshly isolated serological specimens may contain infectious organisms. Although these organisms are rapidly inactivated in air, good laboratory procedure dictates sterilization of discarded materials, preferably by autoclaving. After clinical or serological specimens are handled, the hands should be washed with soap or disinfectant, and the table top should be swabbed with disinfectant.

CULTURE AND ISOLATION

Since the four pathogenic treponemes cannot be grown in vitro, little is known about their cultural characteristics, biochemical reactions, metabolic activities, and chemical composition. The organisms can be maintained in vitro for 1 to 6 days after extraction from infected tissues. Maintenance media such as Nelson medium contain rabbit serum, reducing agents (cysteine, thioglycolate, and glutathione), vitamins, cofactors, amino acids, and salts. A variety of cell culture media such as Eagle or McCoy medium supplemented with fetal bovine serum and reducing agents may be substituted for Nelson medium.

Animal inoculation is not routinely performed for patient diagnosis. When necessary, the rabbit is the animal of choice for *T. pallidum* subsp. *pallidum*. Primary and secondary infections are quite similar to human infections. The rabbit or the hamster is recommended for *T. pallidum* subspp. *pertenue* and *endemicum*. It is difficult to infect animals with *T. carateum;* minimal

TABLE 1—*Continued*

	Characteristic[a]							
	Disease related							
	Incubation period	Invasiveness	Tissues infected	Predominant cellular infiltrate	Destructive lesions	Granulomas	Gummas	Condyloma lata
Syphilis	10–90 days	High	All	Lymphocytes, plasma cells	Yes	Yes	Yes	Yes
Yaws	14–28 days	Intermediate	Skin, bones, soft tissues	Mostly plasma cells	Yes	Yes	Yes	Yes
Pinta	2–6 mo	Low	Skin	Mostly lymphocytes	No	No	No	No
Endemic syphilis	?	Intermediate	Mucous membranes; skin, muscles, bones	Lymphocytes, plasma cells	Yes	Yes	Yes	Yes

success has been achieved with chimpanzees. In places where either syphilis and yaws or syphilis and endemic syphilis are prevalent, specific differentiation can be extremely difficult because of the overlap in clinical manifestations. In this situation, various laboratory animals are inoculated. Comparisons of lesion development then can be used to identify the specific treponemal disease.

Suspected treponemal material for animal inoculation may be contaminated with other microorganisms. To bypass this obstacle, the material is injected intratesticularly. The treponemes rapidly spread to the draining popliteal lymph nodes. Days or weeks later, the nodes can be removed and injected intratesticularly into other animals to produce uncontaminated treponemal preparations. The temperature of animal quarters is important for lesion development (20). Optimal infection occurs at 16 to 18°C. Higher temperatures decrease the intensity of the infection; temperatures below 16°C adversely affect the animals (rabbits develop higher rates of respiratory infections, and hamsters tend to hibernate).

IDENTIFICATION

Definitive diagnosis of the treponematoses can be difficult. The four pathogenic treponemes are identical morphologically and closely related immunologically. A species-specific antigen has not been isolated, and serological reactions for each disease are quite similar. In addition, there are no differential biochemical reactions. The four criteria used for diagnosis are geographic area, clinical manifestations, dark-field specimens, and serological reactions.

The geographic distributions of the four treponematoses are listed in Table 1. The location of a patient within areas in which the disease is endemic is a key initial observation.

Characteristic clinical manifestations of the treponematoses vary greatly. Distinct overlap occurs: late syphilis mimics late yaws; gummas of syphilis, yaws, and endemic syphilis are indistinguishable; condyloma lata of syphilis, yaws, and endemic syphilis are identical; and skin lesions of syphilis, yaws, and endemic syphilis are similar. Despite these potential problems, clinical manifestations usually differ sufficiently to prevent confusion. To the clinician, differential diagnosis is not always necessary, since penicillin is the drug of choice for each treponematosis.

The importance of the demonstration of treponemes in lesion material has been stressed. Treponemes are readily observed in lesion exudates in each of the treponemal diseases. It is difficult, however, to observe treponemes in specimens from dry lesions not exuding material.

Serology is a critical aspect in the diagnosis of treponemal disease. Two different types of tests are used. Nontreponemal tests detect Wassermann or reaginic antibodies; these are totally different from the reaginic antibodies associated with immunoglobulin E (IgE) in allergy. A few examples of the nontreponemal tests include the VDRL, RPR, automated reagin, Kahn, plasmacrit, Hinton, and Kline tests. In contrast to these tests, treponemal tests detect antibodies specific for treponemal antigens; they include the FTA-ABS, *T. pallidum* immobilization, and hemagglutination tests. Because the pathogenic treponemes are antigenically similar and elicit both nontreponemal and treponemal antibodies, it is not possible to distinguish these diseases serologically.

Depending on the stage of the disease, quantitative and qualitative serological results vary. Nontreponemal tests usually parallel the infection. Titers are high during clinical infection and then decrease either during subclinical infection (latency) or after effective antibiotic therapy. In contrast, the treponemal tests may not become positive until well after the initial clinical manifestations; titers may remain high in latency and after treatment. Therefore, it is recommended that nontreponemal tests be used for diagnosis in the early stages, treponemal tests be used for the diagnosis of latency, and nontreponemal tests be used for the evaluation of cure after antibiotic therapy (6 to 12 months beyond treatment). For an in-depth discussion of serological testing, see references 13 and 21.

Two terms relevant to serological testing are sensitivity and specificity. The perfect test, not yet developed, would detect 100% of the treponemal infections and would be nonreactive in all other diseases. Sensitivity refers to negative serology in patients with clinical treponemal disease. Biological false-negative results may occur early in the infection before antibodies have time to develop. Specificity refers to positive serology in the absence of treponemal disease. Biological false-positive results may be found for patients with chronic diseases such as leprosy, malaria, collagen disorders, and autoimmune problems.

The most recent recommendation by the World Health Organization (1) is to screen sera with a VDRL, RPR, or automated reagin test and to confirm positive sera with the FTA-ABS test. A *T. pallidum* immobilization test will definitively determine equivocal reactions. This immobilization test, however, is not recommended except in extreme cases, since it requires a viable source of freshly harvested treponemes and the maintenance of a large colony of rabbits.

The FTA-ABS test (9) requires a fluorescence microscope with a dark-field condenser. Suspected serum is added to a commercial preparation of treponemal organisms that have been dried and fixed on a slide. Fluorescein-conjugated antibody to human IgG is added. Dark-field microscopy is used to locate the treponemes. Fluorescence microscopy is then used to determine whether the treponemes specifically fluoresce. Problems occur with negative or weakly reactive serum. The switches between dark-field and fluorescence microscopy cause delays during quantitative measurements. A new refinement incorporates the incident illumination of Ploem and a double FTA-ABS reaction. All treponemes are nonspecifically stained with rhodamine-labeled anti-*T. pallidum* subsp. *pallidum* globulin. The fluorescein-labeled antibody to human IgG is then added. Selective emission filters differentiate between rhodamine- and fluorescein-stained organisms.

Recently, microhemagglutination tests have been developed that are equivalent to the FTA-ABS test in terms of sensitivity and specificity. Two similar commercial preparations are available. The kit from Fujirebro Laboratories contains sensitized sheep erythrocytes, and the kit from Difco Laboratories contains sensitized turkey erythrocytes. These hemagglutination reactions are advantageous in that they do not require a fluorescence microscope and positive results are a bit easier to read.

Quality control is crucial to serological testing. Controls that include both positive sera of known titers and negative sera that do not react should be routinely used. In addition, the FTA-ABS test requires subjective evaluations of fluorescence, which are especially troublesome with borderline sera. Occasionally, reagents are defective, improperly reconstituted, or old. The appropriate controls will uncover these problems.

Two final comments are pertinent to treponemal antibody detection. Cerebrospinal fluid should be tested to diagnose symptomatic neurosyphilis or to differentiate between asymptomatic neurosyphilis and latency. This is especially relevant to AIDS patients that have concurrent syphilis. See reference 7 for a recent overview. In addition, the incidence of congenital syphilis is increasing dramatically. This disease is difficult to diagnose serologically. Maternal IgG passes the placenta and enters the fetal circulation. At birth, the baby will be seropositive for at least 3 to 6 months as a result of residual maternal antibodies. Quantitative VDRL or RPR tests should be performed over a period of 6 months. If the titer either increases or stabilizes and does not decrease, congenital syphilis is indicated. Some attempts have been made to detect IgM against *T. pallidum*. For an updated review of problems in diagnosing congenital syphilis, see reference 2. A positive reaction at the time of birth would then indicate infection. These tests, however, are still suboptimal and not routinely used.

Serological tests for syphilis are covered in greater detail in a recent World Health Organization review (21).

LITERATURE CITED

1. **Antal, G. M.** 1979. Present status of therapy and serodiagnosis of syphilis (some selected aspects). W.H.O. document W.H.O./V.D.T./Res. **70**:359.
2. **Baughn, R. E.** 1989. Congenital syphilis: immunologic challenge. Pathol. Immunopathol. Res. **8**:161–178.
3. **Cox, C. D., and M. K. Barber.** 1974. Oxygen uptake by *Treponema pallidum*. Infect. Immun. **10**:123–127.
4. **Crissey, J. T., and D. D. Denenholz.** 1984. Syphilis. Clin. Dermatol. **2**:1–166.
5. **Fieldsteel, A. H., J. G. Stout, and F. A. Becker.** 1979. Comparative behavior of virulent strains of *Treponema pallidum* and *Treponema pertenue* in gradient cultures of various mammalian cells. Infect. Immun. **24**:337–345.
6. **Fitzgerald, T. J., and R. C. Johnson.** 1979. Surface mucopolysaccharides of *Treponema pallidum*. Infect. Immun. **24**:244–251.
7. **Hook, E. W.** 1989. Syphilis and HIV infection. J. Infect. Dis. **160**:530–534.
8. **Hovind-Hougen, K.** 1976. Determination by means of electron microscopy of morphological criteria of value for classification of some spirochetes, in particular treponemes. Acta Pathol. Microbiol. Scand. Suppl. **255**:1–41.
9. **Hunter, E. G., R. M. McKinney, S. E. Maddison, and D. D. Cruce.** 1979. Double-staining procedure of the fluorescent treponemal antibody absorption (FTA-ABS) test. Br. J. Vener. Dis. **55**:105–108.
10. **Lomholt, G.** 1972. Textbook of dermatology, vol. 1, p. 634–679. Blackwell Scientific Publications, Ltd., Oxford.
11. **Meheus, A., and A. De Schryver.** 1989. Syphilis and safe blood. W.H.O. document W.H.O./V.D.T./Res. **89**:444.
12. **Miao, R. M., and A. H. Fieldsteel.** 1980. Genetic relationship between *Treponema pallidum* and *Treponema pertenue*, two noncultivable human pathogens. J. Bacteriol. **141**:427–429.
13. **Miller, J. N.** 1975. Value and limitations of nontreponemal and treponemal tests in the laboratory diagnosis of syphilis. Clin. Obstet. Gynecol. **19**:191–203.
14. **Moore, W. E. C., L. V. Holdeman, R. M. Smibert, D. E. Hash, J. A. Burmeister, and R. R. Ranney.** 1982. Bacteriology of severe periodontitis in young adult humans. Infect. Immun. **38**:1137–1148.
15. **Paris-Hamelin, A., G. Causse, A. Vaisman, S. Fuster-Ibarboure, and N. Tordjman.** 1979. Utilization of fiberglass discs to collect specimens for the serodiagnosis of syphilis by the fluorescent antibody and passive haemagglutination tests. W.H.O. document W.H.O./V.D.T./Res. **79**:360.
16. **Risseeuw-Appel, I. M., and F. C. Kothe.** 1983. Transfusion syphilis; a case report. Sex. Transm. Dis. **10**:200–201.
17. **Smibert, R. M.** 1977. CRC handbook of microbiology, 2nd ed., vol. 1., p. 195–228. CRC Press, Inc., Cleveland.
18. **Smibert, R. M.** 1984. Genus III. *Treponema* Schaudinn 1905, 1728[AL], p. 49–57. *In* N. R. Krieg and J. R. Holt (ed.), Bergey's manual of systematic bacteriology, vol. 1. The Williams & Wilkins Co., Baltimore.
19. **Turner, T. B., and T. M. Diseker.** 1941. Duration of infectivity of *Treponema pallidum* in citrated blood stored under conditions obtaining in blood banks. Bull. J. Hopkins Hosp. **68**:269–279.
20. **Turner, T. B., and D. H. Hollander.** 1957. Biology of the treponematoses. W.H.O. Monogr. Ser. **35**:1–277.
21. **Van Dyck, E., P. Piot, and A. Meheus.** 1989. Benchlevel W.H.O./V.D.T./Res. **89**:443.
22. **Vegas, F. K.** 1975. Clinical, tropical dermatology, p. 79–105. Blackwell Scientific Publications, Ltd., Oxford.
23. **Willcox, R. R., and T. Guthe.** 1966. *Treponema pallidum*. A bibliographical review of the morphology, culture and survival of *T. pallidum* and associated organisms. W.H.O. Suppl. **35**:1–169.

Chapter 56

Anaerobic Spirochetes

ROBERT M. SMIBERT

The genus *Treponema* now consists of two groups of organisms. The first is made up of the treponemes that cause the classical treponematosis in humans. These organisms are usually propagated in laboratory animals. The second group consists of the treponemes that can be grown in artificial media and usually are found as part of the normal flora of the oral cavity, intestines, rumen, and genitals of humans and lower animals. This group of cultivable anaerobic treponemes will be discussed in this chapter, along with isolation methods and identification procedures.

DESCRIPTION OF THE GENUS

The host-associated treponemes are helically coiled organisms that have one or more periplasmic flagella. The protoplasmic cylinder is covered by an outer membrane similar to the outer membrane of other gram-negative organisms. Periplasmic flagella are anchored at each end of the cell and wind around the periplasmic cylinder inside the outer membrane. The periplasmic flagella are thus located in the periplasmic space. Treponemes are motile, with the ability both to stay in place and rotate and to move from place to place. The treponemes range from species that are tightly coiled to ones that are loosely coiled. They range in width from 0.15 to >0.4 μm. Some species are short, and others are long (3 to 4 μm to >30 μm). The G+C ratio of treponemal DNA ranges from 25 to 54 mol% (28, 31). These organisms usually have one or more antigens in common with *Treponema pallidum*.

Growth of most of these organisms requires good anaerobic techniques and the addition of proper nutritional supplements to culture media. Some treponemes require the medium to be supplemented with 10% heat-inactivated animal serum. Organisms needing serum are *T. denticola*, *T. vincentii*, *T. phagedenis*, *T. refringens*, *T. minutum*, *T. scolodontum*, *T. hyodysenteriae*, *T. innocens*, and a large treponeme recently isolated from AIDS patients.

Some oral species (*T. denticola*, *T. vincentii*, and *T. scoliodontum*) require thiamine pyrophosphate (TPP) in addition to serum (5, 38). *T. phagedenis* also needs, in addition to serum, a fermentable energy source such as glucose for growth.

The second group of treponemes requires short-chain volatile fatty acids and a fermentable carbohydrate source as medium supplements. The volatile fatty acids can be found in rumen fluid along with heme and vitamin K. Rumen fluid is added to a medium at a final concentration of 20 to 30%. The medium can be autoclaved. Another source of volatile fatty acids is a mixture of fatty acids (10) used to supplement the medium. The organisms needing short-chain fatty acids are *T. socranskii* (31), *T. pectinovorum* (30), *T. bryantii* (34), *T. succinifaciens* (8), and *T. saccharophilum* (22).

All species except *T. pectinovorum* can use glucose as an energy source. *T. pectinovorum* can ferment only pectin. However, either glucuronic acid or galacturonic acid, both of which are breakdown products of pectin, can replace pectin.

The best method for cultivating treponemes anaerobically is use of prereduced media with either the Virginia Polytechnic Institute (VPI) roll tube method or an anaerobic chamber. An anaerobic jar, such as a GasPak jar (BBL Microbiology Systems), can also be used with prereduced media. The exceptions to the phrase "good anaerobic techniques" are *T. hyodysenteriae*, *T. innocens*, and the large treponeme recently isolated from AIDS patients (12). For their growth aerobically prepared blood agar plates are streaked and incubated in anaerobic jars under anaerobic conditions. Prereduced broth cultures are injected with air to yield 1% oxygen (35). Thus, these organisms appear to be microaerophils.

NATURAL HABITAT AND CLINICAL SIGNIFICANCE

The host-associated cultivable treponemes are part of the normal flora found on the genitals of humans and animals, as part of the flora of the rumen of ruminants, and as part of the intestinal and oral flora of animals and humans. Those found in the genital flora are *T. phagedenis*, *T. refringens*, and *T. minutum*. The treponemes found in the rumen are *T. bryantii* and *T. saccharophilum*. Those found in the intestinal flora are *T. hyodysenteriae* (found in pigs with swine dysentery), *T. innocens* (found in pigs), *T. succinofaciens* (also from pigs), *Brachyspira aalborgii* (from humans), and the recently isolated large treponeme from AIDS patients with diarrhea. Treponemes that are part of the oral flora are *T. denticola*, *T. vincentii*, *T. socranskii*, *T. pectinovorum*, and *T. skoliodontum*. *T. socranskii* and *T. denticola* are the most prominent members of the treponemal flora in humans.

T. hyodysenteriae is the cause of swine dysentery and is found in the mucosa of lesions in the intestine of pigs. The organism produces a hemolysin. *B. aalborgii* was isolated from rectal biopsies from humans with an intestinal disorder (11). There are reports in the literature of treponemes in the intestines of dogs with intestinal problems (23). Recently, a large treponeme was reportedly isolated mainly from AIDS patients with diarrhea (7, 12, 25, 36, 37). This organism is similar to *T. hyodysenteriae* in its growth requirements and in many other characteristics. In the oral cavity, treponemes are hard to find in people with a healthy gingiva and no periodontal disease. In human gingivitis, the incidence and numbers of treponemes in the gingival flora increase. This increase becomes greater as the gingivitis becomes more severe (4, 16, 19). In human periodontal disease, the incidence of treponemes in subgingival samples increased to between 88 and 97%, with an increase in the number of treponemes in the flora (4, 17–20). The species most often predominating in subgingival samples is *T. socranskii*, but *T. denticola* and *T. pectinovorum* are also frequently found in these samples. *T. denticola* has been reported to be linked to the severity of periodontal disease (27). Extracts of *T. denticola* have been found to supress fibroblast proliferation (6) and the human lymphocyte response (26). *T. denticola* has been reported to adhere to epithelial cells (21, 24) and to induce morphologic changes and detachment of the tissue culture cells. It has been reported that oral treponemes may be involved in multiple sclerosis (9). Thus, although *T. hyodysenteriae* is the only cultured treponeme that is known to cause disease, there is some indication that other treponemes might have some pathogenic potential.

COLLECTION, TRANSPORT, AND STORAGE OF SPECIMENS

Collection

Supragingival and subgingival periodontal samples can be taken with a sterile dental scaler with a detachable tip or with paper points. Subgingival samples from periodontal pockets should be taken with great care to prevent contamination with supragingival material. The supragingival plaque should first be cleaned from the tooth surface, and then the subgingival sample is taken with a scaler or paper points. The sample is placed into a tube with anaerobic dilution broth and small glass beads and is dispersed by a few seconds of vortexing (19). Sonic oscillation should not be used to disperse the samples because treponemes are quickly destroyed by brief sonication. The samples are diluted 10-fold, and each dilution is cultured.

Intestinal and rumen samples are diluted in anaerobic dilution broth, and the samples are dispersed by either brief vortexing or shaking. Tenfold dilutions of the sample can be made, if desired, and each dilution can be examined by dark-field microscopy for treponemes and cultured.

Samples from pigs with swine dysentery are usually taken from the large colon of pigs at necropsy. Intestinal material is gently removed from the intestinal lesion, and the surface of the lesion is washed with sterile saline. The lesion is scraped with a sterile instrument, and the resulting colonic mucosal sample is placed in anaerobic dilution broth or streaked directly onto blood agar plates. The plates are incubated in anaerobic jars. Upon dark-field microscopic examination of the samples, a large fat treponeme can be seen.

Stool samples or stool swabs from AIDS patients with diarrhea are examined by dark-field microscopy for a large fat treponeme. Samples positive for treponemes are streaked onto selective blood agar plates, and the plates are incubated in anaerobe jars for 5 to 7 days.

Genital samples can be collected by swabbing the genital region with sterile, moistened swabs. The swabs are placed into anaerobic dilution broth or placed directly into selective isolation medium.

Transport

Samples in prereduced dilution medium or selective broth should be transported at ambient temperature to the laboratory and inoculated onto culture media within 5 to 12 h after collection. Fecal, intestinal, and rumen samples may be placed in a container and transported to the laboratory. They should be cultured within 5 h after collection. Collection and transport of swabs as well as other kinds of samples should be done by using anaerobic systems.

Storage

Intestinal, rumen, fecal, and oral samples may be preserved in liquid nitrogen or in a mechanical freezer at −80°C. Recovery of treponemes from frozen specimens will not be as good as recovery from freshly collected ones. Specimens with only a few treponemes in them may yield no isolation after freezing. Whole sections of intestines from pigs with swine dysentery may be cut into small pieces and frozen for future use in isolation of the treponeme or as a source of infectious material for pigs. Isolated cultures of treponemes are preserved best by growing the organism in broth to the late log phase of growth, adding dimethyl sulfoxide (1 to 2 drops to 1 ml of culture), and freezing the cultures in 1-ml portions in liquid nitrogen or in a −80°C freezer. Freeze-dried cultures have not proven adequate for preservation of treponemes.

DIRECT EXAMINATION

The best method of direct examination of samples is by dark-field microscopy. A phase-contrast microscope can also be used; however, a dark-field microscope is preferred because small treponemes may not be seen or may be very difficult to see by phase-contrast microscopy.

CULTURE AND ISOLATION

Two general methods can be used for the isolation of treponemes. The preferred method uses selective media, while a second method uses a membrane filter with or without antibiotics to make a medium selective. The membrane filter method uses the small cell diameter of some treponemes and their motility to achieve a separation of treponemes from other larger bacteria. Selective media for the obligately anaerobic treponemes in the oral cavity, intestines, and rumen and on the genitals use rifampin (14, 33) or rifampin and polymyxin (19, 31). Selective media for the isolation of microaerophilic-like treponemes use spectinomycin (32) or spectinomycin and polymyxin (12). In addition to these methods, three other, less frequently used techniques will be presented.

Anaerobic treponemes

Selective media. Dilutions of samples are inoculated into rifampin (2 μg/ml) (14) or rifampin-polymyxin (2 μg/ml–800 U/ml) (19, 31) broth or semisolid medium. The cultures are incubated at 37°C for 1 to 2 weeks. Cultures should be examined by dark-field microscopy for treponemes after 1 week of incubation. Supplements in the basic medium will determine which kinds of treponemes are isolated. If only serum (10%) or serum (10%) and TPP (0.0075%) are added, then only serum-requiring organisms will be isolated. If only rumen fluid (20 to 30%), glucose, and pectin are in the medium, then only treponemes needing short-chain fatty acids will be isolated. A general-purpose isolation and culture medium that supports the growth of most described treponemes should contain rumen fluid (or short-chain fatty acid mixture), serum, TPP, glucose, and pectin.

Cultures containing treponemes are transferred to rifampin-polymyxin broth or semisolid medium. If a culture is contaminated with another kind of bacteria, the treponeme can be separated from the contaminant either by streaking the isolate onto selective agar plates or by using a parabiotic chamber (Bellco Glass, Inc.). The Bellco chamber (no. 1945) with rubber stoppers is put together with a membrane filter (25-mm diameter with a pore size of either 0.2 or 0.3 μm [5, 19, 28]) between the two sections of the chamber. The contaminated culture is placed into one of the chambers, and sterile prereduced medium (with or without antibiotics) is placed in the other chamber. The chambers should be gassed with oxygen-free nitrogen during inoculation to ensure that the medium remains anaerobic. After 12 to 18 h of incubation, the motile treponemes migrate through the filter and grow in the medium on the other side of the membrane filter. The purified culture is inoculated into fresh medium. The culture will be free of nontreponemes but will be a mixture of different kinds of treponemes. Pure cultures can be made by streaking agar plates.

Membrane filter method. Membrane filters (45-mm diameter) with a pore size of 0.2 or 0.3 μm are placed onto the surface of agar isolation medium. The isolation medium can contain antibiotics such as rifampin and polymyxin. A sterile O ring is placed on top of the filter and sealed to the filter with sterile 3% molten agar in water. A portion from the various dilutions is placed on the membrane filter, and the plate is quickly placed into an anaerobic jar. The culture is incubated at 37°C for 1 to 2 weeks. After incubation, the filter is removed, a plug of agar from the white hazy growth in the agar under the filter is placed onto a slide, a cover slip is added, and the slide is examined by dark-field microscopy. A plug of the hazy growth is removed with a Pasteur pipette and transferred to broth or semisolid medium.

Single-colony isolation of treponemes is necessary for identification to the species level or for characterization of an unnamed isolate. Colonies can be obtained by quickly streaking prereduced agar plates with a 2- to 3-day-old culture. The plates are incubated in anaerobic jars for 1 to 2 weeks. Two jars are used. One jar contains the prereduced agar medium, and the other is used to receive streaked plates. While both jars are opened, they are gassed with a stream of carbon dioxide. The jar with the streaked plates should be made anaerobic as quickly as possible with a hydrogen-carbon dioxide gas mixture or a GasPak envelope (BBL). The quickest way to obtain anaerobic conditions is to use a jar with a vent and evacuate the jar, fill it with a gas mixture, and clamp the vent. The procedure of evacuating and filling the jar is repeated several times. When a GasPak envelope is used, the envelope is placed in the jar, the jar is evacuated once, and the vent is clamped. This method reduces the amount of oxygen in the jar and helps to establish anaerobic conditions within a few minutes. After incubation for 1 to 2 weeks, the hazy white colonies growing in the agar are plugged with a Pasteur pipette and subcultured in broth or semisolid medium.

The growth of treponemes into an agar medium in plates requires a soft agar medium. A medium with 0.75 to 0.80% Oxoid purified agar (Oxoid USA Ltd., Columbia, Md.) is recommended. This concentration of agar is equivalent to 1.2% Bacto-Agar (Difco Laboratories). The soft agar medium is needed because treponemes grow into rather than on the surface of the agar.

Cultures of treponemes can be transferred weekly and can be preserved by freezing in liquid nitrogen or in a −80°C freezer. Two- to three-day broth cultures are transferred to small sterile plastic freezer tubes (0.5 to 1 ml) under a stream of nitrogen, a drop of dimethyl sulfoxide is added, and the tube is placed in a freezer.

Miscellaneous isolation methods. An older method is the well-plate technique. Agar medium is poured into a petri dish to make a thick plate 12 to 14 mm deep. Thicker plates can be made by using deeper dishes. The agar medium can also contain antibiotics and be selective for treponemes. A well 3 to 5 mm deep is made with a Pasteur pipette. Any fluid in the well should be carefully removed. The inoculum is carefully placed in the well to avoid contamination of the upper edge of the well. The plates are incubated in an anaerobic jar for 1 to 2 weeks. The plates are examined for a circle of white hazy growth in the agar around the well. An agar plug of the growth is removed and inoculated into broth medium (28).

In another method, 10-fold dilutions of a sample are inoculated into molten agar deeps (34). The anaerobic medium should contain 0.7% agar. Selective media can also be used. After incubation, treponeme colonies appear as fluffy white balls in the medium. The soft agar column is removed from the culture tube, and treponeme colonies are picked and subcultured.

Microaerophilic-like treponemes

To isolate *T. hyodysenteriae*, *T. innocens*, and the large treponeme from AIDS patients, the sample is streaked onto blood agar plates containing spectinomycin (400 μg/ml) or spectinomycin (400 μg/ml) and polymyxin (5 μg/ml) (12, 32). The blood agar plated should not be prereduced and can be made and handled the same way as are aerobic media. The plates are incubated in anaerobe jars under anaerobic conditions for 2 to 6 days. The selective plates are examined for areas of hemolysis that show little or no surface growth in the hemolytic zone. Small colonies can usually be seen by indirect lighting. A hemolytic zone is scraped with a loop and either streaked onto a fresh blood agar plate or inoculated into a broth medium such as Trypticase soy broth (BBL) with 10% serum or bovine calf serum. The plates and tubes are incubated in an anaerobic jar for 3 to 5 days. The best way to grow these organisms in broth or semisolid medium is to use prereduced medium like heart infusion broth with 10% inactivated animal serum. It is necessary to aerate the medium. These organisms are microaerophilic-like and will grow best in a medium with 1% oxygen (35). No growth occurs in strict anaerobic conditions. No growth occurs if there is more than 5% oxygen in the culture. If the VPI anaerobic system is used, the gas flow is turned off while the culture is being inoculated. If a sealed tube (16 or 18 mm by 150 to 200 mm) of prereduced serum-broth is used, 1 ml of air is injected into the culture tube. Heavy growth of these organisms occurs in tubes or flasks of broth that have about 1% oxygen and are stirred by magnetic stir bars or are shaken on shakers. A weekly transfer of stock cultures is needed to maintain cultures. Cultures of these organisms can be preserved in broth with dimethyl sulfoxide in liquid nitrogen or in a −80°C freezer.

Special equipment

The culture and identification of treponemes require good anaerobic methods for most organisms. These anaerobic requirements can be met using the VPI anaerobic system (Bellco) or an anaerobic chamber. Anaerobic jars are also needed for some isolations and for colonization of treponemes. For the identification of these organisms, a gas chromatograph or high-pressure liquid chromatograph is helpful in determining their end products of metabolism.

IDENTIFICATION

Examination of a pure culture of treponemes by dark-field microscopy

Estimate the cell diameter and length, whether the cells are tightly or loosely coiled, and whether the ends are hooked or straight. Tables 1, 2, and 3 show the key characteristics of named treponeme species. Start on Table 1 and then go to Table 2 for final identification of the nonfermenting treponemes. Table 3 contains the information on the end products of metabolism.

Additional information on treponemes can be found in *Bergey's Manual of Systematic Bacteriology* (29) and other references (11, 30, 31).

Serological investigations

T. socranskii subsp. *socranskii* can be differentiated from *T. socranskii* subsp. *buccalis* only by a serological test. A slide agglutination test will separate the two subspecies. They form two separate subgroups by DNA homology (31). There are seven serotypes of *T. hyodysenteriae* (15). The serotyping of *T. hyodysenteriae* is based on using the lipopolysaccharide of the organism (hot phenol-water method) as the antigen in an agarose immunodiffusion test.

The moles percent G+C contents of the DNA of treponemes are as follows: *T. phagedenis*, 39; *T. refringens*, 39 to 43; *T. denticola*, 38; *T. pectinovorum*, 39; *T. succinifaciens*, 36; *T. bryantii*, 36; *T. minutum*, 37; *T. vincentii*, 44; *T. socranskii*, 50 to 52; *T. saccharophilum*, 54; *T. pallidum*, 53; *T. hyodysenteriae*, 25 to 26; and *T. innocens*, 25 to 26.

ANTIBIOTIC SUSCEPTIBILITY

With a broth tube dilution method, *T. phagedenis*, *T. refringens*, *T. denticola*, and *T. vincentii* are inhibited by penicillin (0.1 to 1 U/ml) and by (micrograms per milliliter) ampicillin (0.1 to 1), oxacillin (0.1 to 10), cloxacillin (0.1 to 1), cephalothin (0.1 to 10), vancomycin (0.1 to 10), bacitracin (0.1 to 1), erythromycin (0.1 to 1), novobiocin (1 to 500), tetracycline (1), oxytetracycline (1 to 10), chloramphenicol (100 to 500), kanamycin (100 to 1,000), gentamicin (1 to 500), and viomycin (10 to 1,000). All are resistant to (micrograms per milliliter) cycloserine (500 to 1,000), polymyxin B (500 to 1,000), nalidixic acid (500 to 1,000), and methenamine mandelate (500 to 1,000). *T. socranskii* is inhibited by penicillin (10 to 100 U/ml) and by (micrograms per milliliter) ampicillin (10 to 100), oxacillin (100 to 500), cephalothin (0.1 to 1), erythromycin (0.01), vancomycin (1 to 10), tetracycline (1 to 10), chloramphenicol (100), and viomycin (100 to >1,000) (1). Bactericidal concentrations of antimicrobial agents are usually 10 to 100 times higher than the inhibitory concentrations (2). Oral and rumen treponemes are resistant to rifampin (1 to 50 μg/ml) (14, 33). A broth-disk method for determining antimicrobial susceptibility of treponemes has been reported (3). MICs (micrograms per milliliter) for *T. hyodysenteriae* have been reported: carbadox (0.00625), olaquindox (0.025 to 0.1), tiamulin (0.025 to 0.05), monensin (0.05 to 0.1), metronidazole (0.05 to 0.2), furazolidone (0.025), ampicillin (0.39 to 0.78), ceftizoxime (0.1 to 1.56), chloramphenicol (1.56), oxytetracycline (1.56 to 6.25), gentamicin (1.56 to 6.25), virginiamycin (0.39 to 1.56), lincomycin (3.13 to 25), thiopeptin (12.5 to 25), and tylosin (100 to >100) (13).

MEDIA

Oral treponeme isolation medium

This is a general isolation medium that will support the growth of both serum- and short-chain fatty acid-requiring treponemes. See references 19, 30, and 31.

Polypeptone (BBL), 5 g; heart infusion broth (BBL), 5 g; yeast extract, 5 g; glucose, 0.8 g; pectin, 0.8 g; fructose, 0.8 g; soluble starch, 0.8 g; sucrose, 0.8 g; maltose, 0.8 g; ribose, 0.8 g; xylose, 0.8 g; sodium pyruvate, 0.8 g; K_2HPO_4, 2.0 g; NaCl, 5.0 g; $MgSO_4$, 0.1 g; cysteine hydrochloride, 0.68 g; clarified rumen fluid, 500 ml; distilled water, 500 ml. The pH is 7.0. The base medium is made prereduced. Filter-sterilized inactivated rabbit or calf serum (10%) and TPP (0.0075%) are added to the sterile medium. A filter-sterilized fresh yeast autolysate (5%) can also be added.

For a semisolid medium, add Bacto-Agar (0.16%). For a solid medium, add Oxoid Special Agar (0.75 to 0.8%). The rumen fluid can be replaced by a short-chain fatty acid mixture (19). To the medium described above add hemin, 5 mg; vitamin K_1, 1 mg; and 3 ml of the fatty acid mixture. The volatile fatty acid mixture consists of acetic acid, 17 ml; propionic acid, 6 ml; *n*-butyric acid, 4 ml; isobutyric acid, 1 ml; DL-2-methylbutyric acid, 1 ml; isovaleric acid, 1 ml; and *n*-valeric acid, 1 ml.

Rifampin-polymyxin selective medium

See references 19 and 31. Oral treponeme isolation medium or any other medium listed supplemented with rifampin (2 μg/ml) and polymyxin B (800 U/ml).

Medium for serum-requiring treponemes

See reference 19.

TABLE 1. Key characteristics of treponemes

Species	Characteristic[a]														
	Cell size	Rumen fluid or serum	Fermentation of:											Indole production	Esculin hydrolysis
			Glucose	Fructose	Lactose	Mannitol	Sucrose	Arabinose	Rhamnose	Maltose	Raffinose	Xylose	Pectin		
T. phagedenis bv. *reiteri*	M	S	A	A	A	A	–	–	–	–	–	–	–	+	–
T. phagedenis bv. *kazan*	M	S	A	A	A	A	–	–	–	–	–	–	–	+	+
T. socranskii subsp. *socranskii*	S	R	A	A	–	–	A	A	A	A	V	A	V	–	–
T. socranskii subsp. *buccalis*	S	R	A	A	–	–	A	A	A	V	V	A	V	–	–
T. socranskii subsp. *paredis*	S	R	A	A	–	–	A	–	–	A	V	V	V	–	–
T. pectinovorum	M	R	–	–	–	–	–	–	–	–	–	–	A	–	–
T. succinifaciens	M	R	A	–	A		–	A	–	A	–	A			
T. bryantii	M	R	A	–	A		A	A	–	–	–	A	–		
T. saccharophilum	L	R	A	A	A	–	A	A	–	A	A	–	A		
T. hyodysenteriae	L	S	A	A	A	–	A	–	–	A	A	–	A	+	+
T. innocens	L	S	A	A	A	–	A	A	–	A	A	A	A	–	+
T. denticola bv. *denticola*	M	S	–	–	–	–	–	–	–	–	–	–	–	+	+
T. denticola bv. *comandonii*	M	S	–	–	–	–	–	–	–	–	–	–	–	–	+
T. vincentii	M	S	–	–	–	–	–	–	–	–	–	–	–	+	V
T. refringens bv. *refringens*	M	S	–	–	–	–	–	–	–	–	–	–	–	+	+
T. refringens bv. *calligyrum*	M	S	–	–	–	–	–	–	–	–	–	–	–	+	+
T. minutum	S	S	–	–	–	–	–	–	–	–	–	–	–	+	+
T. skoliodontum	S	S	–	–	–	–	–	–	–	–	–	–	–	–	–

[a] S, Small (0.15 to 0.24 μm in diameter); M, medium (0.25 to 0.32 μm); L, large (>0.35 μm); S, needs rumen serum; R, needs rumen fluid or volatile fatty acid mixture; A, acid production with a pH of 6.0 and below in 95% of strains; –, no acid production or negative test result; +, positive test result; V, variable result or test result negative in less than 90% of strains. *T. hyodysenteriae* produces a strong beta-hemolysis on blood agar plates; *T. innocens* produces a weak hemolysis on blood agar plates. Data for *T. hyodysenteriae* and *T. innocens* are from tests done in broth medium aerated to contain 1% oxygen, with the tubes shaken.

T. socranskii subsp. *socranskii* and *T. socranskii* subsp. *buccalis* cannot yet be differentiated by a biochemical test. They can be differentiated by DNA homology and by a serological (slide agglutination) test.

TABLE 2. Some key characteristics of nonfermenting treponemes

Species	Characteristic[a]						
	Phosphatase	H_2S	Makes indole	Grows on 1% glycine	Makes formate	Makes acetate and butyrate	Converts fumarate to succinate
T. denticola bv. *denticola*	+	+	+	−	−	−	−
T. denticola bv. *comandonii*	+	+	−	V	−	−	−
T. vincentii	−	+	+	−	−	+	−
T. refringens bv. *refringens*	−	+	+	−	−	−	+
T. refringens bv. *calligyrum*	−	+	+	+	−	−	+
T. minutum	−	+	+	+	+	−	−

[a] +, Positive test or growth in 90% or more of strains; −, negative test or no growth; V, variable results in less than 90% of strains. Fatty acids determined by gas-liquid chromatography or high-pressure liquid chromatography.

Trypticase (BBL), 20 g; heart infusion broth (BBL), 5 g; yeast extract, 10 g; K_2HPO_4, 2 g; cysteine hydrochloride 0.68 g; distilled water, 900 ml. The pH is 7.0. Add 100 ml of filter-sterilized heat-inactivated serum and TPP (0.0075%). The medium is made prereduced. Solid medium should contain Oxoid Special Agar (0.75 to 0.8%). The selective agents rifampin and polymyxin B can be added.

NOS medium

See reference 14.

Heart infusion broth, 1.24 g; Trypticase (BBL), 1.0 g; yeast extract, 0.25 g; sodium thioglycolate, 0.05 g; cysteine hydrochloride, 0.1 g; L-asparagine, 0.025 g; glucose, 0.2 g; distilled water, 100 ml; Noble agar (Difco), 0.7 g. The base medium is supplemented with 0.2% TPP, 0.3 ml; volatile fatty acid solution, 0.2 ml; 10% sodium bicarbonate, 2.0 ml; and inactivated rabbit serum, 2.0 ml. All supplements are filter sterilized and added to the prereduced base medium. The volatile fatty acid solution consists of isobutyric acid, 0.5 ml; DL-2-methylbutyric acid, 0.5 ml; isovaleric acid, 0.5 ml; and *n*-valeric acid, 0.5 ml dissolved in 100 ml of 0.1 N KOH. Rifampin and polymyxin B can also be added.

Media for the characterization of treponemes

The media described in the *Anaerobe Laboratory Manual* (10) are used for identification of treponemes. These media are supplemented with serum, TPP, and rumen fluid. The rumen fluid can be replaced with the volatile fatty acid mixture as in the medium for serum-requiring treponemes. The manual also explains how to make prereduced media.

Selective medium for *T. hyodysenteriae*, *T. innocens*, and the large treponeme from AIDS patients

See references 12, 32, 36, and 37.

Trypticase soy agar (BBL); citrated bovine blood, 10%; spectinomycin (The Upjohn Co.), 400 μg/ml. Polymyxin B (5 μg/ml) can also be added (12). The blood agar plates are made aerobically.

Selective medium for *B. aalborgii*

See reference 11.

Trypticase soy agar (BBL); calf blood, 10%; spectinomycin, 400 μg/ml; polymyxin B, 5 μg/ml.

For additional information on media, see references 8, 10, 14, 22, 28, 29, 31, and 34.

TABLE 3. Metabolic products of treponemes

Species	Product[a]									
	Ethanol	Propanol	Butanol	Acetic acid	Formic acid	Propionic acid	*n*-Butyric acid	Lactic acid	Succinic acid	H_2 gas
T. phagedenis	+	+	+	+	+	tr	+	−	−	−
T. socranskii	−	−	−	+	−	−	−	+	+	−
T. pectinovorum	−	−	−	+	+	−	−	tr	−	−
T. succinifaciens	−	−	−	+	+	−	−	+	+	−
T. bryantii	−	−	−	+	+	−	−	−	+	−
T. saccharophilum	+	−	−	+	+	−	−	−	−	−
T. hyodysenteriae	−	−	−	+	tr	−	+	−	−	+
T. innocens	−	−	−	+	tr	−	+	−	−	+
T. denticola	−	−	−	+	−	tr	tr	−	−	−
T. vincentii	−	−	−	+	−	−	+	−	−	−
T. refringens	−	−	−	+	−	−	−	−	−	−
T. minutum	−	−	−	+	+	−	−	−	−	−
T. skoliodontum	−	−	−	+	−	−	−	−	−	−

[a] +, Major product; −, not present; tr, trace or small amount present or only occasionally. Determined by gas-liquid chromatography or high-pressure liquid chromatography.

This work was supported in part by Public Health Service grants DE-05054 and DE-05139 from the National Institute of Dental Research and by the Commonwealth of Virginia.

LITERATURE CITED

1. **Abramson, I. J., and R. M. Smibert.** 1972. Inhibition of growth of treponemes by antimicrobial agents. Br. J. Vener. Dis. **47:**407–412.
2. **Abramson, I. J., and R. M. Smibert.** 1972. Bactericidal activity of antimicrobial agents for treponemes. Br. J. Vener. Dis. **47:**413–418.
3. **Abramson, I. J., and R. M. Smibert.** 1972. Method of testing antibiotic sensitivity of spirochaetes, using antibiotic disks. Br. J. Vener. Dis. **48:**269–273.
4. **Addy, M., H. Newman, M. Langeroudi, and J. G. L. Gho.** 1983. Dark-field microscopy of the microflora of plaque. Br. Dent. J. **155:**269–273.
5. **Austin, F. E., and R. M. Smibert.** 1982. Thiamine pyrophosphate, a growth factor for *Treponema vincentii* and *Treponema denticola*. Curr. Microbiol. **7:**147–152.
6. **Boehringer, H., N. S. Taichan, and B. J. Shenker.** 1984. Suppression of fibroblast proliferation by oral spirochetes. Infect. Immun. **45:**155–159.
7. **Coene, M., A. M. Agliano, A. T. Paques, P. Cattani, G. Dettori, A. Sanna, and C. Cocito.** 1989. Comparative analysis of the genomes of intestinal spirochetes of human and animal origin. Infect. Immun. **57:**138–145.
8. **Cwyk, W. M., and E. Canale-Parola.** 1979. *Treponema succinifaciens* sp. nov., an anaerobic spirochete from swine intestine. Arch. Microbiol. **122:**231–239.
9. **Gay, D., and G. Dick.** 1986. Is multiple sclerosis caused by an oral spirochete? Lancet **ii:**75–77.
10. **Holdeman, L. V., E. P. Cato, and W. E. C. Moore (ed.).** 1977. Anaerobe laboratory manual, 4th ed. Virginia Polytechnic Institute and State University, Blacksburg.
11. **Hovind-Hougen, K., A. Birch-Anderson, R. Henrik-Nielsen, M. Orholm, J. O. Pedersen, P. S. Teglbjaerg, and E. H. Thaysen.** 1982. Intestinal spirochetosis: morphological characterization and cultivation of the spirochete *Brachyspira aalborgii* gen. nov., sp. nov. J. Clin. Microbiol. **16:**1127–1136.
12. **Jones, M. J., J. N. Miller, and W. L. George.** 1986. Microbiological and biochemical characterization of spirochetes isolated from the feces of homosexual males. J. Clin. Microbiol. **24:**1071–1074.
13. **Kitai, K., M. Kashiwazaki, Y. Adachi, K. Kunugita, and A. Arakawa.** 1987. In vitro antimicrobial activity against reference strains and field isolates of *Treponema hyodysenteriae*. Antimicrob Agents Chemother. **31:**1935–1938.
14. **Leshine, S. B., and E. Canale-Parola.** 1980. Rifampin as a selective agent for isolation of oral spirochetes. J. Clin. Microbiol. **12:**792–795.
15. **Mapother, M. E., and L. A. Joens.** 1985. New serotypes of *Treponema hyodysenteriae*. J. Clin. Microbiol. **22:**161–164.
16. **Moore, L. V. H., W. E. C. Moore, E. P. Cato, R. M. Smibert, J. A. Burmeister, A. M. Best, and R. R. Ranney.** 1987. Bacteriology of human gingivitis. J. Dent. Res. **66:** 989–995.
17. **Moore, W. E. C., L. V. Holdeman, E. P. Cato, R. M. Smibert, J. A. Burmeister, K. G. Palcanis, and R. R. Ranney.** 1985. Comparative bacteriology of juvenile periodontitis. Infect. Immun. **48:**507–519.
18. **Moore, W. E. C., L. V. Holdeman, E. P. Cato, R. M. Smibert, J. A. Burmeister, and R. R. Ranney.** 1983. Bacteriology of moderate (chronic) periodontitis in mature adult humans. Infect. Immun. **42:**510–515.
19. **Moore, W. E. C., L. V. Holdeman, R. M. Smibert, I. J. Good, J. A. Burmeister, K. G. Palcanis, and R. R. Ranney.** 1982. Bacteriology of experimental gingivitis in young adult humans. Infect. Immun. **38:**651–657.
20. **Moore, W. E. C., L. V. Holdeman, R. M. Smibert, D. E. Hash, J. A. Burmeister, and R. R. Ranney.** 1982. Bacteriology of severe periodontitis in young adult humans. Infect. Immun. **38:**1137–1148.
21. **Olsen, I.** 1984. Attachment of *Treponema denticola* to cultured human epithelial cells. Scand. J. Dent. Res. **92:**55–63.
22. **Paster, B. J., and E. Canale-Parola.** 1985. *Treponema saccharophilum* sp. nov., a large pectinolytic spirochete from the bovine rumen. Appl. Environ. Microbiol. **50:**212–219.
23. **Pindak, F. F., W. E. Claper, and J. H. Sherrod.** 1965. Incidence and distribution of spirochetes in the digestive tract of dogs. Am. J. Vet. Res. **26:**1391–1402.
24. **Reijntjens, F. J., F. H. M. Mikx, J. M. L. Wolters-Lutgerhost, and J. C. Maltha.** 1986. Adherence of oral treponemes and their effect on morphological damage and detachment of epithelial cells in vitro. Infect. Immun. **51:** 642–647.
25. **Ruane, P. J., M. M. Nakata, J. F. Reinhardt, and W. L. George.** 1989. Spirochete-like organisms in the human gastrointestinal tract. Rev. Infect. Dis. **2:**184–196.
26. **Shenker, B. J., M. A. Listgarten, and N. S. Taichman.** 1984. Suppression of human lymphocyte responses by oral spirochetes: a monocyte-dependent phenomenon. J. Immun. **132:**2039–2045.
27. **Simonson, L. G., C. H. Goodman, J. J. Bial, and H. E. Morton.** 1988. Quantitative relationship of *Treponema denticola* to severity of periodontal disease. Infect. Immun. **56:**726–728.
28. **Smibert, R. M.** 1981. The genus *Treponema*, p. 564–577. *In* M. P. Starr, H. Stolp, H. G. Trüper, A. Balows, and H. G. Schlegel (ed.), The prokaryotes. A handbook on habitats, isolation, and identification of bacteria. Springer-Verlag, New York.
29. **Smibert, R. M.** 1984. Genus III. *Treponema* Schaudin 1905, 1728[AL], p. 49–57. *In* N. R. Krieg and J. G. Holt (ed.), Bergey's manual of systematic bacteriology, vol. 1. The Williams & Wilkins Co., Baltimore.
30. **Smibert, R. M., and J. A. Burmeister.** 1983. *Treponema pectinovorum* sp. nov. isolated from humans with periodontitis. Int. J. Syst. Bacteriol. **33:**852–856.
31. **Smibert, R. M., J. L. Johnson, and R. R. Ranney.** 1984. *Treponema socranskii* sp. nov., *Treponema socranskii* subsp. *socranskii* subsp. nov., *Treponema socranskii* subsp. *buccale* subsp. nov., and *Treponema socranskii* subsp. *paredis* subsp. nov. isolated from the human periodontia. Int. J. Syst. Bacteriol. **34:**457–462.
32. **Songer, J. G., J. M. Kinyon, and D. L. Harris.** 1976. Selective medium for isolation of *Treponema hyodysenteriae*. J. Clin. Microbiol. **4:**57–60.
33. **Stanton, T. B., and E. Canale-Parola.** 1979. Enumeration and selective isolation of rumen spirochetes. Appl. Environ. Microbiol. **38:**965–973.
34. **Stanton, T. B., and E. Canale-Parola.** 1980. *Treponema bryantii* sp. nov., a rumen spirochete that interacts with cellulolytic bacteria. Arch. Microbiol. **127:**145–158.
35. **Stanton, T. B., and E. Canale-Parola.** 1988. *Treponema hyodysenteriae* growth conditions under various culture conditions. Vet. Microbiol. **18:**177–190.
36. **Tomkins, D. S., S. A. Foulkes, P. G. R. Godwin, and A. P. West.** 1986. Isolation and characterization of intestinal spirochaetes. J. Clin. Pathol. **39:**535–541.
37. **Tomkins, D. S., M. A. Waugh, and E. M. Cooke.** 1981. Isolation of intestinal spirochetes from homosexuals. J. Clin. Pathol. **34:**1385–1387.
38. **Van Horn, K. G., and R. M. Smibert.** 1983. Albumin requirement of *Treponema denticola* and *Treponema vincentii*. Can. J. Microbiol. **29:**1141–1148.

Chapter 57

Morphology, Taxonomy, and Classification of the Fungi*

DENNIS M. DIXON AND ROBERT A. FROMTLING

Mycology is a well-recognized, valuable component of the daily responsibilities of the clinical microbiology laboratory. The list of opportunistic fungal pathogens is increasing at an impressive rate that is related to the expanding size of the immunocompromised patient population. As a result, clinical laboratory technologists must be able to recognize an increasingly large group of potential fungal pathogens. Moreover, there is the need to recognize that even though a given isolate may not be a documented fungal pathogen, its isolation from a normally sterile site and ability to grow at 37°C should require that it be considered a possible pathogen. With few exceptions, all of the fungi that infect humans have the ability to grow at 37°C. Beyond this, it is difficult to identify traits or factors associated with virulence in the pathogenic fungi.

Mycological identification can be frustrating because of the importance placed on morphology and the need to become familiar with certain structures and terms. However, the investment of a small amount of time to learn a few basic structures and principles of classification can result in the ability to recognize and properly identify many medically important fungi.

DESCRIPTION OF FUNGI

Fungi were among the first microorganisms recognized because some of the fruiting structures, such as the mushrooms, are large enough to be seen without a microscope. The word mycology, in fact, is derived from *mykes*, the Greek word for mushroom. Fungi initially were classified with the plants, and much of the botanical influence is seen today, even though the organisms have been transferred to a separate, fifth kingdom on the basis of cell structure (Table 1). The nomenclature of the fungi is governed by the International Code of Botanical Nomenclature (adopted by the 14th International Botanical Congress, Berlin, August 1987). Morphology retains an important role in the identification of most fungi, which places demands on the observer to become familiar with identification of the organisms through experience. Morphology is more important for identification of moulds than yeasts, but even with the latter, morphology on media such as cornmeal agar is a key first step in the identification process. (For a discussion of the use of "mould" versus "mold," see reference 6.)

Fungi are extremely successful organisms, as evidenced by their ubiquity in nature. They are an important component in the energy cycle, where they function as decomposers. Thus, fungi are valuable as saprophytes in nature. Of the estimated 250,000 species, fewer than 100 are known to be primary pathogens of humans. The infection of humans seems to be an accident of nature, since it represents a "dead end" for the fungus; i.e., most fungal infections are not contagious but are acquired through exposure to a point source in nature where the organism exists as a saprophyte. This fact has practical implications in the laboratory and is why moulds in particular should be manipulated in a biological safety cabinet (see section on laboratory safety, below).

Fungi are eucaryotic, chemoheterotrophic organisms with cell walls containing chitin, cellulose, or both. They may be unicellular or multicellular; there is a tendency to be multinucleate. The body of a fungus is termed the thallus. Fungi can be grouped simply on the basis of morphology as either yeasts or moulds. A yeast can be defined morphologically as a cell that reproduces by budding, a process whereby a progenitor cell pinches off a portion of self to produce a progeny cell. In this connotation, yeasts are generally unicellular and produce circular, restricted, pasty or mucoid colonies, in contrast to moulds, which are multicellular, filamentous forms of fungi consisting of threadlike filaments called hyphae which interweave to form mycelium. The resulting colonies are "fuzzy." Since many medically important fungi, such as *Blastomyces dermatitidis*, can exist in each of these two morphologies, they are called dimorphic. When additional forms are present, the term "polymorphic" (pleomorphic) is applied (Fig. 1).

Fungi reproduce by the formation of spores. These may be either asexual (involving mitosis only) or sexual (involving meiosis; preceded by fusion of protoplasm and fusion of nuclei of two cells). One fungus can produce both sexual and asexual spores. Specialized structures (fruiting bodies or fructifications) may be associated with either sexual or asexual spores (Table 2). Recognition of a particular fruiting structure can be a useful step in the identification process. It is important to determine the type of spore contained in order to establish both the type of fruiting structure and the ultimate identification.

Asexual spores are of two general types: sporangiospores and conidia (Fig. 2). Sporangiospores are asexual spores produced within a containing structure (sporangium); they are characteristic of the lower fungi classified as Zygomycetes such as *Rhizopus* and *Mucor* species. Typically, these fungi have broad, sparingly septate hyphae. In the Oomycetes, classified in kingdom Protista

* The authors are indebted to and dedicate this chapter to the late Billy H. Cooper, author of this chapter in the preceding edition of this Manual.

TABLE 1. Simplified taxonomic scheme illustrating the major groups of Kingdom Fungi (Myceteae) in which medically important fungi are classified[a]

Taxonomic designation	Representative genera	Human disease
Division: Amastigomycota		
Subdivision: Zygomycotina		
Class: Zygomycetes		
Order: Mucorales	*Rhizopus, Mucor, Rhizomucor, Absidia, Cunninghamella, Saksenaea*	Zygomycosis; opportunistic in patients with diabetes, leukemia, severe burns, or malnutrition; rhinocerebral infections
Order: Entomophthorales	*Basidiobolus, Conidiobolus*	Zygomycosis; subcutaneous infections
Subdivision: Ascomycotina		
Class: Ascomycetes		
Subclass: Hemiascomycetidae		
Order: Endomycetales	*Saccharomyces, Pichia* (teleomorphs of some *Candida* spp.)	Numerous mycoses
Subclass: Plectomycetidae		
Order: Onygenales	*Arthroderma* (teleomorphs of *Trichophyton* and *Microsporum* spp.)	Dermatophytoses
	Ajellomyces (teleomorphs of *Histoplasma* and *Blastomyces* spp.)	Systemic mycoses
Order: Eurotiales	Teleomorphs of some *Aspergillus* and *Penicillium* spp.	Aspergillosis; hyalohyphomycosis
Subdivision: Basidiomycotina		
Class: Basidiomycetes		
Subclass: Holobasidiomycetidae		
Order: Agaricales	*Amanita, Agaricus*	Mushroom poisoning from consumption of poisonous species (e.g., of *Amanita*)
Subclass: Teliomycetidae		
Order: Ustilagenales	*Filobasidiella* (teleomorph of *Cryptococcus neoformans*)	Cryptococcosis
Subdivision[b]: Deuteromycotina		
Class: Deuteromycetes		
Subclass: Blastomycetidae (Blastomycetes[c])		
Order: Cryptococcales	Imperfect yeasts: *Candida, Cryptococcus, Trichosporon, Pityrosporum*	Numerous mycoses
Subclass: Hyphomycetidae (Hyphomycetes[c])		
Order: Moniliales		
Family: Moniliaceae	*Epidermophyton, Coccidioides, Paracoccidioides, Sporothrix, Aspergillus*	Numerous mycoses
Family: Dematiaceae	*Phialophora, Fonsecaea, Exophiala, Wangiella, Xylohypha, Bipolaris, Exserohilum, Alternaria*	Chromoblastomycosis, mycetoma, and phaeohyphomycosis
Subclass: Coelomycetidae (Coelomycetes[c])		
Order: Sphaeropsidales	*Phoma*	Phaeohyphomycosis
Division: Mastigomycota		
Subdivision: Diplomastigomycotina		
Class: Oomycetes[d]	*Pythium*	Pythiosis

[a] Modified from references 1 and 2.
[b] This subdivision and all of its taxa are form taxa.
[c] Some taxonomists delete Deuteromycetes as a rank and replace this class with the Blastomycetes, Hyphomycetes, and Coelomycetes rather than using these names as subclass designations.
[d] Some taxonomists place these organisms in Kingdom Protista (Protoctista).

by some taxonomists, the sporangiospores (zoospores) are often motile. Conidia are asexual spores that are borne naked and are nonmotile, as evidenced in *Aspergillus* and *Penicillium* spp. and the dermatophytes. The conidial fungi are classified together as the Deuteromycetes (Fungi Imperfecti).

Sexual spores are the result of meiosis (Fig. 3). The meiotic nuclei are packaged into cells which function as spores. These spores and their mode of production serve as the basis for taxonomic grouping. The Oomycetes undergo a mating process characterized by the production of specialized structures (antheridia and

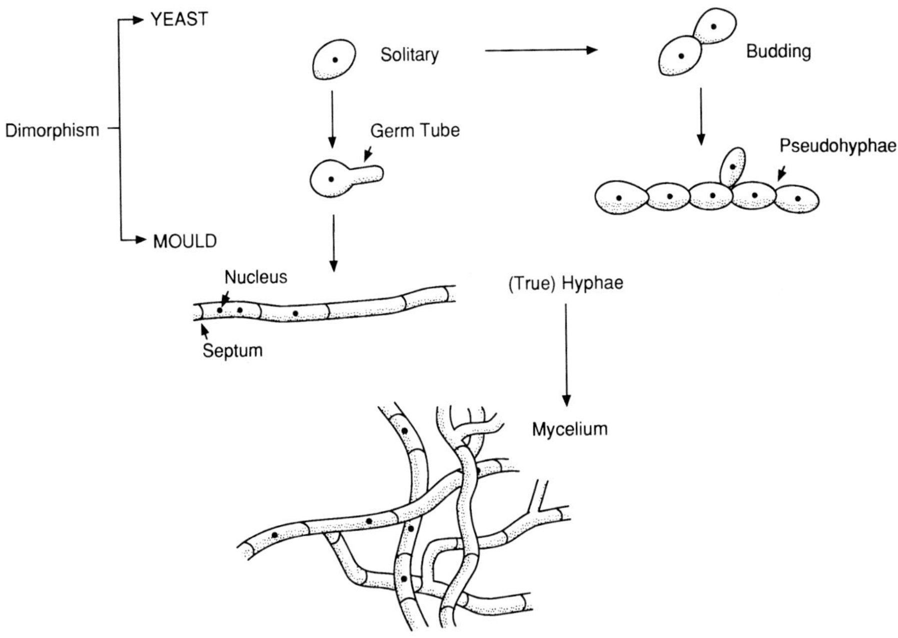

FIG. 1. Simplified representations of the fungal thallus.

oogonia; Fig. 3), resulting in oospores contained in an oogonium. The only medically important fungus in this group thus far is *Pythium* species. The Zygomycetes produce zygospores that are typically large, ornamented cells easily recognized, such as those of *Rhizopus* species. However, zygospores rarely are seen in the clinical laboratory since most of the medically important species are heterothallic; that is, two different strains of compatible mating types are required for the production of sexual spores.

The higher fungi are represented by the Ascomycetes, the Basidiomycetes, and the Deuteromycetes. The sexual spore of the Ascomycetes is the ascospore, characterized by its production within a containing sac (ascus). The sexual spore of the Basidiomycetes is the basidiospore, characterized by extrusion from a club-shaped structure (basidium). The Deuteromycetes produce no known sexual spores. They are included with the higher fungi since they are presumed to represent the conidial stages of Ascomycetes and, more rarely, Basidiomycetes that have lost the ability to produce sexual spores. It also is possible that certain Deuteromycetes never had the ability to produce sexual spores. Since sexual spores hold taxonomic precedence, the Deuteromycetes represent a provisional taxonomic group.

Recognition of a given spore as sexual or asexual is dependent largely on knowledge of the life cycle of the fungus (to determine whether the spore is the result of meiosis or mitosis) and the recognition of the characteristic morphology of the spore. Of particular importance with the conidial fungi is the complication imposed by the subsequent finding of the sexual stage of a fungus that has been named on the basis of its conidial

TABLE 2. Fruiting structures helpful in classification of some medically important fungi

Fruiting structure	Characteristics	Taxonomic group	Representative genera
Sexual (ascomata)			
Perithecium	Spherical or flask-shaped ascoma with opening	Ascomycotina	*Chaetomium, Leptosphaeria*
Cleistothecium	Spherical ascoma; no opening	Ascomycotina	*Pseudallescheria, Eurotium, Ajellomyces,*[a] *Arthroderma*[a]
Asexual (conidiomata)			
Pycnidium	Spherical or flask-shaped conidioma, usually with opening	Deuteromycotina[b]	*Hendersonula, Phoma, Pyrenochaeta*
Synnema	Ropelike tangle of conidiophores, usually with apical fertile region	Deuteromycotina	*Graphium*
Sporodochium	Clump of conidiophores	Deuteromycotina	*Fusarium, Epicoccum*

[a] The term gymnothecium occasionally is used to refer to the characteristic, loosely woven cleistothecium produced by these genera.
[b] Specifically, the Coelomycetes.

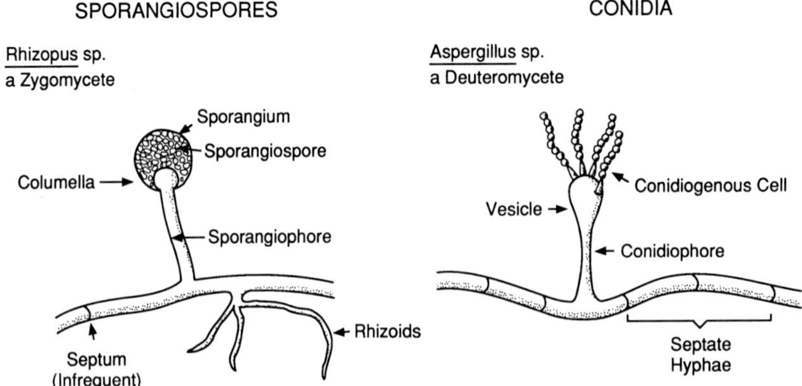

FIG. 2. Stylized representation of two kinds of asexual fungal spores.

(asexual) form. For example, *B. dermatitidis* was named in 1898 on the basis of its asexual characteristics: a fungus (*myces*) that reproduced by budding (*Blasto*) recovered from a case of dermatitis (*dermatitidis*). The fungus grows as a yeast in tissue (37°C) and as a mould in culture (25°C). It produces lateral solitary spores meeting the definition of conidia. In 1968, the fungus was found to complete a life cycle by mating with an opposite mating type to yield a diploid zygote that underwent meiosis to yield ascospores. Since *B. dermatitidis* was the name chosen to describe the entity known only in the asexual form, a new name, *Ajellomyces dermatitidis,* was chosen for the ascomycetous form. The form isolated in clinical microbiology laboratories is *B. dermatitidis,* and this name is retained for that description. However, we now know that *B. dermatitidis* represents the conidial form of an ascomycete; the asexual form of conidial fungi is known as the anamorph, and the sexual form is called the teleomorph. The entire fungus is collectively termed the holomorph. The name of the teleomorph also serves as the name for the holomorph.

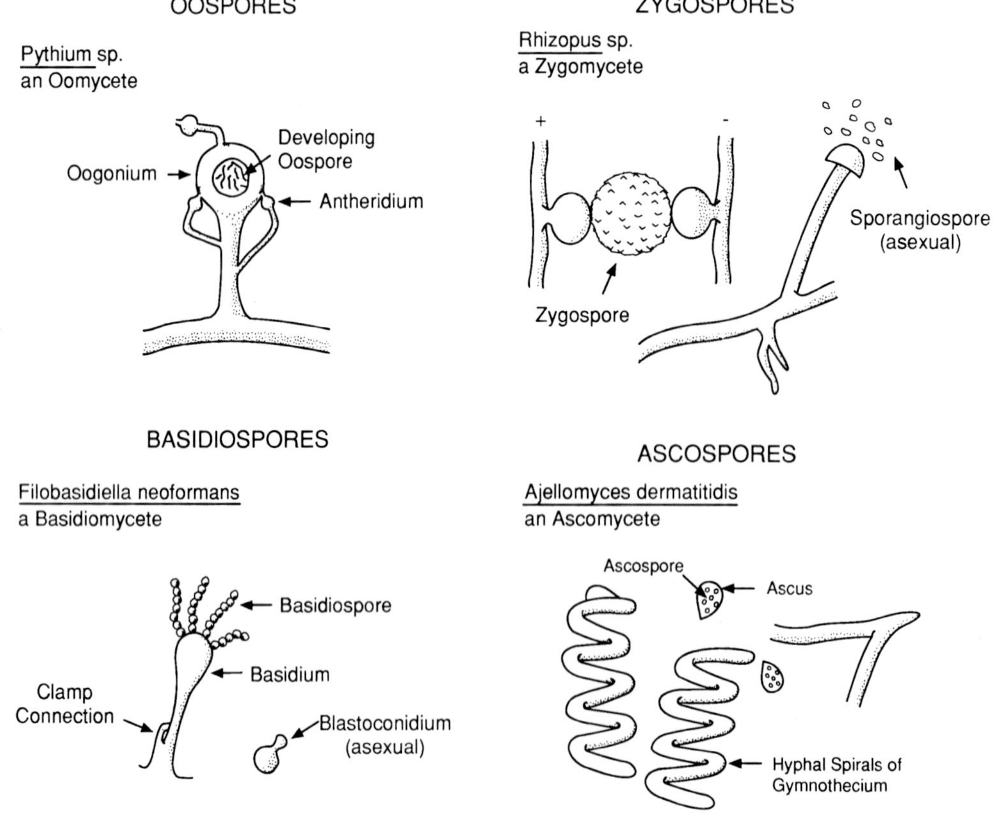

FIG. 3. Stylized representation of four kinds of sexual fungal spores, using medically important examples.

The Deuteromycetes can be segregated into the Blastomycetes, Coelomycetes, and Hyphomycetes. The Blastomycetes contain anamorphs that reproduce by budding; the Coelomycetes contain moulds that produce conidia within a cavity of fungal tissue (pycnidium; Table 2); the Hyphomycetes contain moulds that produce conidia without fruiting structures or with synnemata (Table 2) or produce only sterile hyphae. The Hyphomycetes often are further described as being either dematiaceous (darkly pigmented) or hyaline, although these terms may be used to describe any fungus. Useful separations within the Deuteromycetes are made on the basis of morphology and ontogeny of the conidia and conidiogenous cells (cells that produce conidia). Conidia may develop by either a blastic process (budding) or a thallic process (fragmentation). Some different types of conidiogenesis are summarized in Table 3. Since different fungi can produce conidia that look similar, it often is helpful to study a variety of microscopic fields in order to evaluate the mode of development of the conidium from the conidiogenous cell.

There can be confusion in the use of the term "yeast." Some mycologists restrict this term to a specific group of Ascomycetes that produce ascospores in a free ascus, are primarily unicellular, and reproduce asexually by either budding (e.g., *Saccharomyces* spp.) or fission

TABLE 3. Groupings of conidia on the basis of ontogeny

Conidial group	Characteristic	Representative genera
Thallic development	The hyphal tip ceases to elongate; there is a depolarization of wall growth. An entire segment begins to differentiate, and cell wall growth occurs by a thickening process.	
Arthroconidia	Thallic production whereby hyphal segments fragment into individual cells that have been delimited by the prior development of a septum. All other modes of ontogeny listed below are a modification of blastic production.	*Coccidioides, Geotrichum*
Blastic development	Essentially a budding process whereby localization (polarization) of growth occurs at region of the mother cell which "blows out" to give rise to a conidium.	
Blastoconidia	Conidium originates as a blown-out portion of the mother cell. The developing cell is recognizable before being delimited by a septum. The daughter cell may separate completely or remain attached to form chains.	*Candida, Cryptococcus,* and most other yeasts; *Cladosporium, Xylohypha*
Phialoconidia	Blastic production from a tubular, often flask-shaped conidiogenous cell (phialide) which does not increase in length or width.	*Aspergillus, Fusarium, Lecythophora, Malassezia, Penicillium, Phialophora*
Annelloconidia	Blastic production from a flask-shaped conidiogenous cell (annellide) which extends via percurrent growth (inner layers grow through the outer layers) and often tapers.	*Exophiala, Phaeoannellomyces, Scedosporium, Scopulariopsis*
Poroconidia	Blastic production through a channel in the cell wall of the conidiogenous cell.	*Alternaria, Bipolaris, Curvularia, Drechslera, Exserohilum*
Sympoduloconidia	Successive blastic conidial production characterized by continued growth of the conidiogenous cell to one side of the base of the conidium. This typically results in a zig-zag or distorted ampulliform appearance to the conidiogenous cell. The poroconidia of *Curvularia, Drechslera, Bipolaris,* and *Exserohilum* spp. are produced on sympodial conidiophores.	*Sporothrix, Dactylaria*
Aleurioconidia	Older but useful term describing conidia that typically have a broad base of attachment to a conidiogenous cell and separate by lysis of the conidiogenous hyphal walls, leaving a remnant attached to the conidium as an annular frill. *Epidermophyton, Microsporum,* and *Trichophyton* spp. now are recognized to produce conidia by a thallic process, and their conidia now are termed holothallic conidia. *Blastomyces, Chrysosporium,* and *Histoplasma* spp. produce holoblastic conidia.	*Blastomyces, Chrysosporium, Histoplasma, Epidermophyton, Trichophyton, Microsporum*

(e.g., *Schizosaccharomyces* spp.). In this context, other fungi with budding morphology but without the characteristically borne ascospores are referred to as yeastlike. Thus, although *B. dermatitidis* reproduces by budding and has a teleomorph that produces ascospores, the ascus is contained in a fruiting body (and therefore is not free). Because of this, the budding morphology would be termed "yeastlike" by those holding a strict taxonomic usage and "yeast" by those using a morphological definition. In short, there is confusion because "yeast" is not a formal taxon.

LABORATORY PROCEDURES

Basic bacteriological techniques are applicable to the fungi. However, since fungi have longer generation times than most bacteria, cultures need to be kept longer, and provisions need to be made to prevent media from excessive drying. This can be done by pouring plates with more media than would be used for bacteriological plates, by sealing them with paraffin tape, by incubating them in moist chambers, or by using tubed media where possible.

Yeasts are manipulated in much the same way as bacteria. Moulds, however, require some specialized procedures. Inflexible, straight needles rather than loops generally are preferred, and colonies are transferred by cutting a small portion of growth to be used as a point inoculum. It is possible to streak moulds for isolation if there is sufficient spore production. This can be done with a standard bacteriological loop after using a straight needle to place a portion of inoculum on the plate to be streaked; this procedure is useful in separating mixed cultures. To separate fungi mixed with bacteria, cultures can be streaked on media containing antibacterial antibiotics. If this fails, 1 drop of a broth or saline suspension of the mixed culture can be used to inoculate each of four tubes of Sabouraud broth, to which is added in series either 1, 2, 3, or 4 drops of 1 N HCl (10).

Microscopy is very important in fungal identification. Bright-field optics and a magnification factor of about 500 are sufficient to resolve the features of medically important fungi when the specimens are mounted in lactophenol (for pigmented fungi) or lactophenol cotton blue (Poirrier blue; for unpigmented fungi). Phenol is listed as a hazardous chemical. Solutions containing phenol should be prepared, stored, and used in an approved chemical safety cabinet. Often, however, critical evaluation of conidial ontogeny requires greater magnification (×1,000). Some structures, such as annellations present on annellides or collarettes present on phialides, are clearer with phase-contrast optics. Fluorescent brighteners (calcofluor white) used in conjunction with a UV light source and the proper filter combination are useful not only in detecting fungi in clinical material but also in elucidating fungal structure. One study described the use of a 330- to 380-μm excitation filter, 420-μm barrier filter, and 515W eyepiece side absorption filter (22).

Specimen mounts for microscopic examination of moulds include teased, mashed, and slide culture preparations. The simplest method is use of the teased preparation. Sterile, straight dissecting needles are used to remove a portion of growth, which is teased apart in 95% ethanol; a drop of either lactophenol or lactophenol cotton blue is added, and the mount is sealed with a cover slip. A modification of the teased preparation involves cutting a small section of growth and the uppermost surface of adherent medium from the plate and mashing this in a drop of mounting medium, using a cover slip. In more critical studies to determine conidial ontogeny, it may be necessary to set up a slide culture. This procedure requires sterile glass slides and cover slips and a sterile moist chamber. It is convenient to autoclave a supply of glass petri dishes containing U-shaped bent glass rods. Slides can be labeled, dipped in 95% ethanol, flame sterilized, and placed on the bent rods in the petri dishes. Sporulation agar (potato dextrose, cornmeal, or cereal) is then cut out of plates into squares approximately one-half the size of the cover slip and placed on the slides within the petri dish. These manipulations can be performed by using flame-sterilized spatulas or scalpels. The edges of the agar then are inoculated, and a flame-sterilized cover slip is placed on top of the agar. The result is a glass incubation chamber which is kept moist by the addition of water; the fungus should grow on both glass surfaces in contact with the agar. Thus, it is possible to remove the cover slip to mount in lactophenol on a fresh slide and, after removal of the agar block, place a drop of lactophenol cotton blue and a cover slip on the original slide.

Any of the preparations described above can be kept as reference slides. Nail polish can be added to the corners of the cover slip to fix it to the slide; after excessive mounting medium evaporates or is blotted dry, the edges of the cover slip can be completely sealed to the slide to make a semipermanent mount.

The taxonomy of the medically important yeasts is based not only on morphology but also on extensive physiological characterization as used in clinical bacteriology. Commercial products now are available to assist in compartmentalizing the key physiological reactions necessary to identify these organisms.

Although not as important as in the taxonomy of the yeasts, certain physiological reactions and special tests can be helpful in the identification of the moulds. Examples of selected tests for this purpose are shown in Table 4.

LABORATORY SAFETY

Following established safety procedures when working with any potential human pathogen should be mandatory for clinical laboratory personnel. The two most common means of acquiring infections by fungi in the laboratory are inhalation of conidia that are aerosolized and accidental inoculation with sharps (e.g., needles, scalpel blades, and broken glass) that are associated with clinical specimens.

Biosafety levels, including laboratory practices and techniques, safety equipment, and appropriate laboratory facilities, have been defined to guide those working with infectious agents (18). Biosafety level 1 requires basic laboratory facilities and the use of standard microbiological practices. This level applies to the use of characterized microorganisms not known to cause disease in healthy human adults. Biosafety level 2 requires level 1 practices plus laboratory coats, decontamination of all infectious wastes, limited access to the laboratory, protective gloves, and the posting of biohazard warning signs. This level is used when handling moderate-risk

TABLE 4. Special tests to aid in the identification of selected moulds

Test or procedure	Application	Examples	Reference(s)
Aspergillus flavus differential medium	Differentiates *A. flavus* group from most other aspergilli by production of yellow-orange colony reverse.	*A. flavus* + *A. fumigatus* −	21
Christensen urea agar	Differentiation of dermatophytes.	*Trichophyton mentagrophytes* + *T. rubrum* −	Chapter 59
Exoantigen test	Specific identification of various fungi by immunodiffusion.	*Histoplasma capsulatum* *Blastomyces dermatitidis* *Coccidioides immitis*	9
Mycosel agar	Differentiates certain pathogens from morphologically similar saprophytes. In general, the cycloheximide in Mycosel agar inhibits the saprophytic fungi to a greater degree than the pathogens, but there are notable exceptions, such as the one listed here and *Cryptococcus neoformans*, the pathogenic aspergilli, and the Zygomycetes.	*Dactylaria constricta* var. *gallopava* − var. *constricta* +	20
Nitrate assimilation	Differentiates *Wangiella* spp. from most other dematiaceous pathogens.	*Wangiella dermatitidis* − *Exophiala jeanselmei* +	17; I. F. Salkin, M. E. Kenma, and M. G. Rinaldi, Abstr. X Congr. Int. Soc. Hum. Anim. Mycol., abstr. p-52, 1988
Proteolysis (e.g., 12% gelatin in broth)	May differentiate some pathogenic dematiaceous fungi from saprophytes, but this is medium, fungus, test, and laboratory dependent.	*Fonsecaea* spp. − *Cladosporium* spp. +	4
Sodium chloride tolerance	Differentiation of selected dermatophytic and dematiaceous fungi.	*Exophiala werneckii*, growth in presence of ≥15% NaCl *E. jeanselmei*, no growth	8
Thermotolerance	Differentiation of various fungi. Growth maxima (°C):		
	55	*Rhizomucor* spp.	12
	50–52	*Rhizopus rhizopodiformis*	5, 23
	45	*Aspergillus fumigatus*	19
	45	*D. constricta* var. *gallopava*	20
	42	*Xylohypha bantiana*	3
	40	*Wangiella dermatitidis*	16
	40	*Exserohilum mcginnisii*	15
	40	*Bipolaris spicifera*	15
	37	*Exophiala jeanselmei*	16
	37	*Cladosporium carrionii*	7
Trichophyton agars	Nutritional differentiation of dermatophytes.	*Trichophyton tonsurans*, greater growth on T_4 than on T_1	Chapter 59
Wickerham assimilation and fermentations	Differentiation of selected Zygomycetes.	Selected Zygomycetes	23

microorganisms that are associated with human disease. Biosafety level 3 requires level 2 facilities and practices supplemented by controlled access to the laboratory and use of special laboratory clothing and partial containment equipment, e.g., a biological safety cabinet. This level is used when the potential of infection from aerosols, autoinoculation, or ingestion exists and when personnel are handling microorganisms that may cause severe or lethal infections.

Clinical specimens that may contain fungi pathogenic

for humans should be handled by using biosafety level 2 practices, containment equipment, and facilities as outlined in reference 18. Standard precautions include the use of a biological safety cabinet or biohazard hood when working with any clinical material suspected of containing fungi. These cabinets are the most commonly used primary containment devices in laboratories working with infectious agents. Personnel must be properly trained in the use of the cabinets. An additional advantage of using biological safety cabinets is that they protect the clinical specimens from extraneous, airborne contamination.

Biosafety level 2 procedures are specifically recommended for personnel working with clinical specimens that may contain *B. dermatitidis, Coccidioides immitis, Histoplasma capsulatum, Cryptococcus neoformans, Sporothrix schenckii,* and pathogenic members of the genera *Microsporum, Epidermophyton,* and *Trichophyton.* If *B. dermatitidis, C. immitis,* or *H. capsulatum* is growing in the mould form, biosafety level 3 procedures and containment should be followed (18), since the conidia of these fungi have great potential for causing infection if inhaled.

Additional information on the safe handling and processing of clinical specimens that may contain these and other fungi are outlined in chapters 58 through 65. The reader also may consult reference 13 for valuable information on laboratory safety.

STOCK CULTURES

Stock cultures of fungi are an essential source of material for quality control organisms, for reference cultures to be used in comparative identification, for production of known metabolites, and for teaching collections. Numerous methods of preserving fungal cultures are available (14); these methods vary according to the organisms represented, the size of the collection, and considerations of cost, practicality, and personal preference. Two of the simplest methods involve either freezing actively growing agar slant cultures at −10°C (caution: *Epidermophyton* isolates and many Zygomycetes may not survive freezing) or preparing sterile water suspensions of cultures. In the latter instance, cultures are grown on potato-dextrose agar until mature (several days to 2 weeks), and mycelium, spores, or yeast cells are scraped or washed from the surface of slants by using sterile distilled water and a pipette (11). The resulting fungal suspensions can be sealed in sterile vials to prevent evaporation and stored at room temperature. A time-tested but less commonly used technique is to cover an agar slant culture of a fungus with sterile mineral oil.

For long-term preservation, preparation of lyophilized cultures and storage of cultures at −70°C or in liquid nitrogen are well-established procedures, but they require expensive equipment such as lyophilizers or liquid nitrogen freezers. However, cultures stored by these techniques may be kept for many years without losing viability or biochemical or morphological characteristics.

CONCLUSION

The descriptions, procedures, and guidelines outlined in chapters 58 through 65 present the current knowledge of specialized areas of medical mycology that are relevant to clinical microbiology personnel. The reader also is referred to chapter 96 in the 4th edition of this Manual, which addresses the serology of fungal detection, and chapter 18 of the present edition for information on automated and commercial methods of identifying fungi.

In addition to the cited literature, a list of selected references appears at the end of this chapter for those interested in learning more about basic and medical mycology and related applications. The American Society for Microbiology, the Centers for Disease Control, and several universities frequently conduct workshops and training programs in medical mycology, including specialty courses in clinical mycology. Information on these programs may be found in *ASM News* and in the newsletters of the Medical Mycological Society of the Americas, Mycological Society of America, and International Society for Human and Animal Mycology.

LITERATURE CITED

1. **Alexopoulos, C. J., and C. W. Mims.** 1979. Introductory mycology, 3rd ed. John Wiley & Sons, Inc., New York.
2. **Cooper, B. H.** 1985. Taxonomy, classification, and nomenclature of fungi, p. 495–499. *In* E. H. Lennette, A. Balows, W. J. Hausler, Jr., and H. J. Shadomy (ed.), Manual of clinical microbiology, vol. 4. American Society for Microbiology, Washington, D.C.
3. **Dixon, D. M., T. J. Walsh, W. G. Merz, and M. R. McGinnis.** 1989. Infections due to *Xylohypha bantiana* (*Cladosporium trichoides*). Rev. Infect. Dis. **11:**515–525.
4. **Espinel-Ingroff, A., P. R. Goldson, M. R. McGinnis, and T. M. Kerkering.** 1988. Evaluation of proteolytic activity to differentiate some dematiaceous fungi. J. Clin. Microbiol. **26:**301–307.
5. **Gartenberg, G., E. J. Bottone, G. T. Keusch, and I. Weitzman.** 1978. Hospital-acquired mucormycosis (*Rhizopus rhizopodiformis*) of skin and subcutaneous tissue. Epidemiology, mycology and treatment. N. Engl. J. Med. **299:**1115–1118.
6. **Illman, W. I.** 1970. On the use of mould versus mold for a mycelial fungus. Mycologia **62:**1214.
7. **Iwatsu, T.** A new species of *Cladosporium* from Japan. Mycotaxon **20:**521–533.
8. **Kane, J., and R. C. Summerbell.** 1987. Sodium chloride as an aid in identification of *Phaeoannellomyces werneckii* and other medically important dematiaceous fungi. J. Clin. Microbiol. **25:**944–946.
9. **Kaufman, L., and P. G. Standard.** 1987. Specific and rapid identification of medically important fungi by exoantigen detection. Annu. Rev. Microbiol. **41:**209–225.
10. **McGinnis, M. R.** 1980. Laboratory handbook of medical mycology. Academic Press, Inc., New York.
11. **McGinnis, M. R., A. A. Padhye, and L. Ajello.** 1974. Storage of stock cultures of filamentous fungi, yeasts, and some aerobic actinomycetes in sterile distilled water. Appl. Microbiol. **28:**218–222.
12. **McGinnis, M. R., and I. F. Salkin.** 1986. Identification of molds commonly used in proficiency tests. Lab. Med. **17:** 138–142.
13. **Miller, B. M. (ed.).** 1986. Laboratory safety: principles and practices. American Society for Microbiology, Washington, D.C.
14. **Monaghan, R. L., and S. Currie.** 1985. Preservation of antibiotic production by representative bacteria and fungi. Dev. Indust. Microbiol. **26:**787–792.
15. **Padhye, A. A., L. Ajello, M. A. Wieden, and K. K. Steinbronn.** 1986. Phaeohyphomycosis of the nasal sinuses caused by a new species of *Exserohilum*. J. Clin. Microbiol. **24:**245–249.

16. **Padhye, A. A., M. R. McGinnis, and L. Ajello.** 1978. Thermotolerance of *Wangiella dermatitidis*. J. Clin. Microbiol. **8:**424–426.
17. **Pincus, D. H., I. F. Salkin, N. J. Hurd, I. L. Levy, and M. E. Kemna.** 1988. Modification of potassium nitrate assimilation test for identification of clinically important yeasts. J. Clin. Microbiol. **26:**366–368.
18. **Richardson, J. H., and W. E. Barkley (ed.).** 1988. Biosafety in microbiological and biomedical laboratories, 2nd ed. HHS publication no. (NIH) 88-8395. U.S. Government Printing Office, Washington, D.C.
19. **Rippon, J. W.** 1988. Medical mycology. The pathogenic fungi and the pathogenic actinomycetes, 3rd ed. The W. B. Saunders Co., Philadelphia.
20. **Salkin, I. F., and D. M. Dixon.** 1987. *Dactylaria constricta:* description of two varieties. Mycotaxon **29:**377–381.
21. **Salkin, I. F., and M. A. Gordon.** 1975. Evaluation of *Aspergillus* differential medium. J. Clin. Microbiol. **2:**74–75.
22. **Salkin, I. F., M. R. McGinnis, M. J. Dykstra, and M. G. Rinaldi.** 1988. *Scedosporium inflatum,* an emerging pathogen. J. Clin. Microbiol. **26:**498–503.
23. **Scholer, H. J., E. Mueller, and M. A. A. Schipper.** 1983. Mucorales, p. 9–59. *In* D. H. Howard (ed.), Fungi pathogenic for humans and animals. Marcel Dekker, Inc., New York.

SELECTED REFERENCES FOR FURTHER STUDY

1. **Ainsworth, G. C., F. K. Sparrow, and A. S. Sussmann.** 1973. The fungi. An advanced treatise, vol. 4A and 4B. Academic Press, Inc., New York.
2. **Cole, G. T.** 1986. Models of cell differentiation in conidial fungi. Microbiol. Rev. **50:**95–132.
3. **Cole, G. T., and R. A. Samson.** 1979. Pattern of development in conidial fungi. Fearon Pitman Publishers, Inc., Belmont, Calif.
4. **Dolan, C. T., J. W. Funkhoser, E. W. Koneman, N. Y. Miller, and G. D. Roberts.** 1976. Atlases of medical mycology, vol. 1–6. American Society for Clinical Pathology, Chicago. (Kodachrome slides and explanatory manual.)
5. **Emmons, C. W., C. H. Binford, J. P. Utz, and K. J. Kwon-Chung.** 1977. Medical mycology, 3rd ed. Lea & Febiger, Philadelphia.
6. **Haley, L. D., J. Trandel, and M. B. Coyle.** 1980. Cumitech 11, Practical methods for culture and identification of fungi in the clinical microbiology laboratory. Coordinating ed., J. C. Sherris. American Society for Microbiology, Washington, D.C.
7. **Hawksworth, D. L.** 1974. Mycologist's handbook. Commonwealth Mycological Institute, Kew, Surrey, England.
8. **Hawksworth, D. L., B. C. Sutton, and G. C. Ainsworth.** 1983. Ainsworth & Bisby's dictionary of the fungi, 7th ed. Commonwealth Mycological Institute, Kew, Surrey, England.
9. **Kendrick, B.** 1985. The fifth kingdom. Mycologue Publications, Waterloo, Ontario, Canada.
10. **Koneman, E. W., G. D. Roberts, and S. F. Wright.** 1978. Practical laboratory mycology, 2nd ed. The Williams & Wilkins Co., Baltimore.
11. **Larone, D. H.** 1987. Medically important fungi. A guide to identification. Elsevier, New York.
12. **Phillips, G. D. (ed.).** Review of medical and veterinary mycology. Commonwealth Mycological Institute, Kew, Surrey, England.
13. **Salkin, I. F., and B. E. Robinson.** 1988. Section 1: mycology, p. 1–411. *In* B. B. Wentworth (ed.), Diagnostic procedures for mycotic and parasitic infections. American Public Health Association, Inc., Washington, D.C.

Chapter 58

Detection and Recovery of Fungi from Clinical Specimens

WILLIAM G. MERZ AND GLENN D. ROBERTS

The laboratory diagnosis of fungal infections requires awareness by clinicians, collection of proper specimens, and appropriate mycologic laboratory procedures. This chapter presents guidelines for (i) collection and transport of specimens, (ii) preparation and interpretation of direct microscopic examination of specimens, and (iii) culturing and incubation of mycologic cultures. Since chapter 47 in the fourth edition of this manual was excellent, we have chosen to build on that chapter rather than to create a chapter de novo. To those authors, thank you for your excellent foundation.

SPECIMEN COLLECTION, TRANSPORT, AND STORAGE

Specimen collection, transport, and storage are extremely important for providing rapid, accurate results for the diagnosis and management of mycoses. Specimens must be collected under aseptic conditions or after appropriate hygienic preparation to optimize the significance of the mycologic results. Communication between physicians and the laboratory is essential. Specimens must be accompanied by important information, including the proper patient identifiers, the time of collection, and presumptive diagnosis, which might help the laboratory.

With the increased awareness of safety and concern for health care providers at all levels, all specimens for mycologic studies should be handled as potentially hazardous. Although blood and other body fluids or specimens contaminated with blood require special care, it is suggested that all specimens be treated with the same care; specimens should be sent in double leakproof containers, sealed at the bedside. For example, cerebrospinal fluid (CSF) should be placed in a sterile tube with a leakproof lid, and the tube should be placed in a second container, sealed carry container, or sealed bag. The second container will prevent hazardous contact should the tube leak in transit. Specimens that leak in transit should be judged individually. If the specimen can be recollected, this is the best option. If the specimen is not repeatable (e.g., it is one requiring an invasive procedure), judgment should be exercised, and a comment should be added to the results if the specimen is processed.

Specimens for fungal cultures are best sent in a sterile container. Although there is not an extensive literature, pathogenic fungi can be recovered from specimens sent in most anaerobic bacterial transport media or other transport media. Direct examination should not be attempted from these transport systems.

Transportation to the laboratory should be rapid and safe (in double containers). Fortunately, delayed processing of specimens for fungal culture is not as detrimental as with virologic, parasitologic, or certain bacteriologic specimens. In general, if specimen processing is delayed, storage at 4°C is usually appropriate. There are rare exceptions which are noted below for specific types of specimens. Specimens submitted on Culturette swabs should not be stored before culturing, since *Histoplasma capsulatum*, *Blastomyces dermatitidis*, and *Cryptococcus neoformans* may be inhibited.

Hair, skin, and nails

Specimens for the diagnosis of tinea capitis should include representative abnormal hairs removed with forceps and scalp scales collected by scraping. Skin specimens for both dermatophytosis and primary cutaneous candidiasis should be obtained by scraping the active borders of the lesions with a scalpel or glass microscope slide after wiping the affected area with an alcohol swab.

Nail specimens should be obtained by clipping a generous portion of the affected area of the nail and obtaining scrapings of the excess keratin produced beneath the nail.

All hair, skin, and nail specimens may be placed in an envelope or sterile culture dish for transport to the laboratory. Should storage be required, storage at room temperature is optimum. Storage at 4°C is usually acceptable; however, an occasional dermatophyte might not tolerate refrigeration. The use of swabs for the collection and transport of these specimens should be discouraged. Direct exams cannot be performed, and cultures may not be optimal. If a specimen is received on a swab and a new specimen cannot be obtained, the swab should be used for culture only. The cotton portion should be streaked onto the surface of the agar and left in contact with the agar surface if an agar slant is used.

External eye

Specimens from patients with presumed mycotic keratitis should be obtained with care by an ophthalmologist, usually in an operating room. (For clinical laboratory samples, do not prefix with KOH.) After the surface of the cornea is scraped several times, the Kimura scalpel should be streaked on X's or C's designated on the bottom of appropriate fungal media in petri dishes (6). Another portion of the scraping should be fixed on glass microscope slides for examination by the clinical or pathology laboratory. Inoculated plates should be kept at room temperature if transit time to the laboratory may be delayed.

Sterile body fluids (CSF, pericardial, peritoneal, synovial, and vitreous humor)

All fluids should be obtained under aseptic conditions with the use of a sterile syringe. The fluid can be transferred to a sterile tube for safe transport to the laboratory. Specimens should be stored at 4°C.

Urine samples

All urine specimens should be collected in sterile containers and sent immediately to the laboratory. Specimens may be stored at 4°C for up to 12 h. Twenty-four-hour urine specimens and specimens collected from catheter bags are not acceptable for mycologic studies.

Vaginal secretions

Diagnosis of vaginal candidiasis is better established by clinical characteristics and a positive direct examination of the secretions. Cultures may be misleading, since yeasts are part of the normal vaginal flora of up to 20% of healthy women. However, cultures may be helpful in monitoring therapy, in the management of individuals with chronic recurring disease, or when tests for all other etiologies of infectious vaginitis have been unrewarding. Appropriate specimens are two swabs or one swab and one smear (transported in a closed container) in order to both culture and perform a direct examination. Specimens may be stored at 4°C if needed.

Stool

Diagnosis of many fungal infections of the gastrointestinal tract are better established by biopsy of pathologic tissue than by culture of stool specimens. Positive cultures may be misleading, since up to 40% of healthy individuals and up to 75% of compromised patients are colonized with yeasts. Stool cultures should be submitted in a sterile container or on two rectal swabs. Storage at 4°C is appropriate.

Respiratory secretions

Since most respiratory specimens are collected through the upper respiratory tract, proper specimen collection procedures are extremely important to permit the recovery of fungal pathogens in the presence of normal bacterial and fungal flora. Proper oral hygiene of brushing teeth and rinsing should be performed before specimen collection. Some patients may require induction of sputum performed by experienced personnel. First morning specimens usually are preferred. Twenty-four-hour collections are inappropriate; they should be rejected, and new specimens should be requested. All specimens should be collected in wide-mouth containers with leakproof lids. Specimens may be stored at 4°C if necessary. A total of 5 to 10 ml is more than adequate; specimens grossly contaminated by saliva as evidenced by numerous squamous epithelial cells need not be rejected (7); however, plating of specimens or parts of specimens containing large numbers of macrophages or polymorphonuclear cells may enhance the recovery of pathogenic fungi. Transit times for mycologic cultures are not as critical as those for bacteriologic cultures; fungi have been recovered with delays of up to 2 weeks (5).

Upper respiratory tract

Since fungi may be normal flora of the upper respiratory tract or contaminants from environmental aeroflora, cultures may be misleading. Therefore, direct examination of the specimen is extremely important. Material obtained by curretting is optimal; however, swabs are acceptable, although two are necessary so that direct examination may be performed. Specimens may be stored at 4°C.

Tissues

Tissue specimens should be collected by experienced personnel using strict aseptic procedures. Specimens may be divided by the physician or by the laboratory. They should be placed in a small sterile container and sent to the laboratory immediately. If transport is to be delayed, the specimen may be covered with a minimal amount of sterile saline without preservative. Exceptions are tissue specimens so minute that they are better cultured by the physician, such as a corneal specimen.

Blood

Blood specimens should be collected by experienced personnel using strict aseptic procedures. For a recent update on fungal blood cultures, see Telenti and Roberts (13). If blood culture bottles (radiometric or nonradiometric) are used, they should be inoculated at the bedside. With the lysis-centrifugation method, 10-ml tubes should be used (1). Inoculated blood bottles or lysis tubes may be kept at room temperature but need to be taken immediately to the laboratory. Delayed detection will occur with blood bottles, and recovery will be affected in lysis tubes (11) if specimens are not processed within 8 to 9 h of collection. Collection times are critical.

SPECIMEN HANDLING

The laboratory staff must take the time to verify that all pertinent information about a specimen has been provided, the specimen has not leaked in transit, it was delivered by an appropriate method, and the time between collection and initial mycologic processing is acceptable. Addressing potential problems at this time is far superior to attempting to correct a problem after a culture has become positive.

Safe handling of specimens both for protection of the laboratory staff and for minimization of contamination is important. All blood or body fluid specimens or specimens contaminated by blood or body fluids must be processed by personnel wearing gloves and laboratory coat or gown. For optimal safety, it is essential that all clinical specimens be processed in a biologic safety cabinet by trained personnel wearing laboratory coats and gloves. (Refer to chapter 57.)

DIRECT EXAMINATION

Rapid, non-culture-dependent methods for accurate detection of fungal antigens for diagnosis of mycoses are needed. Cryptococcal antigen testing, however, is the only acceptable method currently available. Experimental methods for *Candida, Aspergillus, Coccidioides,* and *Histoplasma* antigens show promise for the future. The development of nucleic acid probes, nucleic acid amplification, and rapid, simple hybridization formats may provide rapid mycotic diagnosis, but these techniques are not yet available. At present, only the direct examination of clinical specimens to detect fungal elements is used for the rapid diagnosis of mycotic infections. Prompt identification of fungal elements is important, since the sooner a serious fungal infection is diagnosed, the earlier specific antifungal therapy can be initiated, thus increasing the chance for a favorable outcome. Accurate detection and recognition of specific elements can save days to weeks for recovery and identification of the pathogenic fungi. Specifically, a definitive diagnosis of many mycotic infections can be made by trained personnel when fungal elements specific for certain fungi and pathognomic of infection are detected. Some examples include the detection of *H. capsulatum* in blood or bone marrow, *B. dermatitidis*, and *Coccidioides immitis* by direct examination.

Detection of specific fungal elements which are part of our normal flora or our environment may be crucial in making a decision as to whether a specific fungus recovered is a contaminant or an opportunistic pathogen. Detection of wide, wavy hyphae morphologically compatible with the agent of zygomycosis is necessary for specific diagnosis of the acute fulminant infection in patients with diabetes mellitus in acidosis. A culture positive for *Rhizopus* sp. may be a contaminant or a pathogen, and the delay in time of initiation of aggressive antifungal therapy and surgical procedures can be crucial. Similarly important examples include agents of aspergillosis or agents of hyalohyphomycosis and phaeohyphomycosis, cases in which detection of hyphae in a clinical specimen is strongly associated with the presence of disease.

In addition, the detection of specific fungal elements allows the laboratory to add specialized media or increased incubation time for optimal recovery of fungi. An example is the addition of mycobacterium media for better recovery of a *Nocardia* sp. when the typical thin, branching filaments are seen in a direct examination of a specimen. Flagging cultures with a positive direct examination for *B. dermatitidis* or *Coccidioides immitis* has permitted recovery of these pathogens by extending the incubation period beyond the laboratory's normal incubation time.

There are, however, limitations and potential problems with direct examinations. First, a negative direct examination never rules out a fungal infection. The sensitivity varies according to anatomical site, amount of specimen examined, number of organisms, site of pathology, type of patient, and quality of the examiner. Second, false-positive findings unfortunately do occur. Lysed lymphocytes in an India ink preparation of a CSF sample have been mistaken for *C. neoformans*, collagen fibers have been mistaken for *Nocardia* filaments, fat droplets have been confused with budding yeast cells, etc. Equivocal findings always should be reviewed by more than one reader, or a second procedure should be performed to aid in resolving this type of problem. A false-positive direct examination usually is more harmful than a false-negative direct examination.

Since direct examinations are less sensitive than cultures, cultures should be performed on specimens, and direct examinations should be performed only if sufficient volume is provided. Like all policies, exceptions exist; a positive direct examination of a mouth lesion suspected to be candidiasis may be more important than a positive culture.

A number of stains or procedures can be used to detect fungal elements in direct examination of clinical specimens (Table 1). Each method has its advantages and disadvantages. The wet preparation, KOH, Calcofluor white, Gram stain, Wright stain, and Giemsa stain are usually performed in clinical laboratories.

The Papanicolaou stain usually is performed in a cytopathology laboratory, and the periodic acid-Schiff and methenamine silver stains usually are performed by pathology laboratories. Since laboratory personnel occasionally are requested to aid in interpretation, familiarity with these stains may be helpful.

As a group, fungi exhibit great diversity and polymorphism, as exemplified by the various morphologies and structures seen in pathologic tissue. However, recognition of these diverse structures in clinical specimens can provide specific identification of many fungal pathogens or at least a definable list of possible pathogens for others. The characteristic fungal elements seen in clinical specimens are presented in Table 2. Most fungi appear the same in tissue as in other clinical specimens. Figures 1 to 26 illustrate these fungal elements as seen in clinical specimens.

CULTURE GUIDELINES

This section discusses principles and provides laboratory approaches for recovery of pathogenic fungi.

Optimum recovery of medically important fungi from clinical specimens is related to multiple factors. The first is the specimen itself. It must be freshly collected and appropriate for the mycotic infection being considered. Table 3 lists guidelines for the selection of clinical specimens for the major mycoses that may be submitted for mycologic cultures.

The quality of the specimen to be cultured also is important. In general, there are fewer fungal cells at the site of an infection than bacterial cells in a bacterial infection. Therefore, a sufficient volume of specimen must be cultured to ensure optimal recovery. Although pretreatment of specimens may not be done routinely, Table 4 presents guidelines for use in the recovery of fungi. As a general rule, at least 1 to 2 ml of a fluid specimen or enough tissue to properly inoculate three to four media with ~0.5 ml is sufficient. Concentration of fluids, e.g., peritoneal fluid, pericardial fluid, and even CSF at volumes of >1 to 2 ml, should be performed by centrifugation and culturing of the pellet. Alternatively, the specimen may be filtered with a membrane filter (0.45-μm pore size) and then cultured. Most fungi will not survive 2% NaOH treatment as used for recovery of mycobacteria (8).

The value of quantitating by colony counts or semiquantitating by light, moderate, or heavy growth of yeasts is equivocal. Even with urine cultures, there is no clear answer. It has been suggested that a count of $>10^4$ colonies per ml is associated with pyelonephritis and less is associated with contamination (3). Others suggest that any colony count is abnormal (2). Caution: Both false-positive and false-negative results occur, and the physician needs to make a clinical decision on the significance of a positive urine culture for *Candida* sp. on an individual basis.

TABLE 1. Methods for direct microscopic detection of fungal elements in clinical specimens

Method (reference)	Use	Time required	Advantages	Disadvantages
Alcian blue	Detection of *C. neoformans* in CSF	2 min	When positive in CSF, is diagnostic.	Not commonly used; like India ink, does not detect all cases.
Acid-fast	Detection of mycobacteria and *Nocardia* spp.	12 min	Detects *Nocardia* spp. and *B. dermatitidis*.	Tissue specimens are difficult to interpret because of strong background staining.
Calcofluor white (4)	Detection of fungi	1 min	Can be mixed with KOH; detects fungi rapidly as a result of bright fluorescence.	Requires fluorescence microscope; background fluorescence prominent, but fungi exhibit more intense fluorescence. Vaginal secretions are difficult to interpret.
Giemsa	Examination of bone marrow and peripheral blood smear	15 min	Detects intracellular *H. capsulatum*.	Detection is usually limited to *H. capsulatum*.
Gram	Detection of bacteria	3 min	Is commonly performed on most clinical specimens submitted for bacteriology and will detect most fungi, if present.	Some fungi stain well; others, e.g., *Cryptococcus* spp., stain weakly in some instances and exhibit only stippling. Some *Nocardia* isolates fail to stain or stain weakly. Common Gram stain artifacts appear as yeast cells.
India ink	Detection of *C. neoformans* in CSF	1 min	When positive in CSF, is diagnostic of meningitis.	Negative in many cases of meningitis; not reliable.
Potassium hydroxide (KOH)	Clearing of specimen to make fungi more readily visible	5 min; if clearing is not complete, an additional 5–10 min is necessary	Rapid detection of fungal elements.	Experience required, since background artifacts are often confusing. Clearing of some specimens may require an extended time.
Methylene blue	Detection of fungi in skin scrapings	2 min	Usually added to KOH; provides contrast for detection of elements.	Background staining of cells makes reading difficult.
Methenamine silver	Detection of fungi in histologic section	1 h	Best stain to detect fungal elements.	Requires a specialized staining method that is not usually readily available to microbiology laboratories.
Papanicolaou	Examination of secretions for presence of malignant cells	30 min	Cytotechnologist can detect fungal elements.	Required specialized staining and reader familiar with this stain.
Periodic acid-Schiff (PAS)	Detection of fungi	20 min; 5 min additional if counterstain is used	Stains fungal elements well; hyphae and yeasts can be readily distinguished.	*Nocardia* spp. do not stain well; *B. dermatitidis* appears pleomorphic. PAS-positive artifacts can appear as yeast cells.
Wright	Examination of bone marrow or peripheral blood smears	7 min	Detects intracellular *H. capsulatum*.	Detection is usually limited to *H. capsulatum*.

The next important factor is the use of various types of media, since no one fungal medium is best for all medically important fungi. It has been suggested that at least one medium be used that does not contain any antifungal or antibacterial agents, although generally this is not helpful; brain heart infusion agar, inhibitory mold agar, and SABHI agar are examples. To ensure maximum recovery of fastidious dimorphic fungi, one medium (brain heart infusion) containing blood (5 to 10% sheep blood) should be used. Media containing

TABLE 2. Characteristic fungal elements seen in direct examination of clinical specimens

Morphologic fungal elements found	Organism(s)	Size range (diam; μm)	Characteristic features
Yeast	*Histoplasma capsulatum*	2–5	Small; oval to round budding cells; often found clustered within histocytes; difficult to detect when present in small numbers; often intracellular. See Fig. 1 and 2.
	Sporothrix schenckii	2–6	Small; oval to round to cigar shaped; single or multiple buds present; uncommonly seen in clinical specimens. See Fig. 3.
	Cryptococcus neoformans	2–15	Cells varying in size; usually spherical but may be football shaped; buds usually single and "pinched off"; capsule may or may not be evident; rarely pseudohyphal forms with or without a capsule may be seen. See Fig. 4–7.
	Blastomyces dermatitidis	8–15	Cells usually large and spherical, double refractile; buds usually single, but several may remain attached to parent cells; buds connected by a broad base. See Fig. 8 and 9.
	Paracoccidioides brasiliensis	5–60	Cells are usually large and surrounded by smaller buds around the periphery (mariner's wheel appearance); smaller (2–5 μm) cells may be present and resemble *H. capsulatum;* buds have "pinched off" appearance. See Fig. 10 and 11.
Spherules	*Coccidioides immitis*	10–200	Spherules vary in size; some contain endospores, others are empty. Adjacent spherules may resemble *B. dermatitidis;* endospores may resemble *H. capsulatum* but show no evidence of budding. Spherules may produce multiple germ tubes if a direct preparation is kept in a moist chamber for ≥24 h; hyphae may be found in cavitary lesions. See Fig. 12 and 13.
"Sporangium"	*Rhinosporidium seeberi*	6–300	Large, thick-walled sporangia containing sporangiospores; mature sporangia are larger than spherules of *C. immitis.*
Yeast and pseudohyphae or true hyphae	*Candida* spp.	3–4 (yeast) 5–10 (pseudohyphae)	Cells usually exhibit single budding; pseudohyphae, when present, are constricted at the ends and remain attached like links of sausage; true hyphae, when present, have parallel walls and are septate. See Fig. 14 and 15.
Yeast and hyphae	*Malassezia furfur*	3–8 (yeast) 2.5–4 (hyphae)	Short curved hyphal elements usually are present along with round yeast cells that retain their spherical shape in compacted clusters. See Fig. 16.
Wide nonseptate hyphae	Zygomycetes: *Mucor, Rhizopus,* and other genera	10–30	Hyphae are large, ribbonlike, often fractured or twisted; occasionally septa may be present, branching usually at right angles. Smaller hyphae overlap with those of *Aspergillus* spp., particularly *A. flavis.* See Fig. 17–19.
Hyaline septate hyphae	Dermatophytes: skin and nails	3–15	Hyaline septate hyphae are commonly seen. Chains of arthroconidia may be present. See Fig. 20.
	Hair	3–15	Arthroconidia on periphery of hair shaft producing a sheath are indicative of ectothrix infection. Arthroconidia formed by fragmentation of hyphae within the hair shaft are indicative of endothrix infection.
	Hair	3–15	Long hyphal filaments or channels within the hair shaft are indicative of favus hair infection.
	Aspergillus spp.	3–12	Hyphae are septate and exhibit dichotomous, 45°-angle branching; larger hyphae, often disturbed, may resemble those of Zygomycetes. See Fig. 21–23.
	Geotrichum spp.	4–12	Hyphae and rectangular arthroconidia are present and sometimes are rounded. Irregular forms may be present. See Fig. 24.
	Trichosporon spp.	2–4 by 8	Hyphae and rectangular arthroconidia are present and sometimes are rounded. Blastoconidia may be difficult to observe.
	Pseudallescheria boydii (cases other than mycetoma)		Hyphae are septate and are impossible to distinguish from those of other hyaline moulds, e.g., *Aspergillus* spp.

(*Continued on next page*)

TABLE 2—*Continued*

Morphologic fungal elements found	Organism(s)	Size range (diam; μm)	Characteristic features
	Fusarium spp.		Hyphae are septate and are impossible to distinguish from those of other hyaline moulds, e.g., *Aspergillus* spp.
Dematiaceous septate hyphae	*Bipolaris* spp. *Curvularia* spp. *Exserohilum* spp. *Exophiala* spp. *Phialophora* spp. *Wangiella dermatitidis* *Xylohypha bantiana*	2–6	Dematiaceous polymorphous hyphae are seen; budding cells with single septa and chains of swollen rounded cells may be present. Occasionally aggregates may be present in infection caused by *Phialophora* and *Exophiala* spp.
	Phaeoannellomyces werneckii	1.5–5	Usually large numbers of frequently branched hyphae are present along with budding cells.
Sclerotic bodies	*Cladosporium carrionii* *Fonsecaea compacta* *Fonsecaea pedrosoi* *Phialophora verrucosa* *Rhinocladiella aquaspersa*	5–20	Brown, round to pleomorphic, thick-walled cells with transverse septa. Commonly, cells contain two fission plates that form a tetrad of cells. Occasionally, branched septate hyphae may be found in addition to sclerotic bodies. See Fig. 25.
Granules (see Fig. 26)	*Acremonium* *A. falciforme* *A. kiliense* *A. recifei*	200–300	White, soft granules without a cementlike matrix.
	Curvularia *C. geniculata* *C. lunata*	500–1,000	Black, hard grains with a cementlike matrix at periphery.
	Aspergillus nidulans	65–160	White, soft granules without a cementlike matrix.
	Exophiala jeanselmei	200–300	Black, soft granules, vacuolated, without a cementlike matrix, made of dark hyphae and swollen cells.
	Fusarium		White, soft granules without a cementlike matrix.
	F. moniliforme	200–500	
	F. solani	300–600	
	Leptospaeria		
	L. senegalensis	400–600	Black, hard granules; cementlike matrix present.
	L. tompkinsii	500–1,000	Periphery composed of polygonal swollen cells and center of a hyphal network.
	Madurella *M. grisea*	350–500	Black, soft granules without a cementlike matrix, periphery composed of polygonal swollen cells and center of hyphal network.
	M. mycetomatis	200–900	Black to brown, hard granules of two types: (i) rust brown, compact, and filled with cementlike matrix (ii) deep brown, filled with numerous vesicles, 6–14 μm in diameter, cementlike matrix in periphery, and central area of light-colored hyphae.
	Neotestudina rosatti	300–600	White, soft granules with cementlike matrix present at periphery.
	Pseudallescheria boydii	200–300	White, soft granules composed of hyphae and swollen cells at periphery in a cementlike matrix.
	Pyrenochaeta romeri	300–600	Black, soft granules composed of polygonal swollen cells at periphery; center is network of hyphae; no cementlike matrix present.

antibacterial agents should be used with any specimen that might contain normal bacterial flora. Inhibitory mold agar, SABHI, or brain heart infusion plus gentamicin (5 or 50 to 100 μg/ml), chloramphenicol (16 μg/ml), and penicillin (20 μg/ml)-streptomycin (40 μg/ml) commonly have been used. Incorporation of norfloxacin (5 μg/ml) or ciprofloxacin (5 μg/ml) also has proven effective. The eucaryotic protein synthesis inhibitor cycloheximide (0.5 μg/ml), alone or together with antibacterial agents, should be used in one medium. In addition, specialized media for the recovery of specific fungi may be employed: media containing substrates (L-dopa, caffeic acid, etc.) for detection of *C. neoformans* by its phenol oxidase activity; yeast extract-phosphate agar with addition of NH_4OH (10) for inhibition of bacteria and recovery of dimorphic fungi from specimens; media containing or overlaid with a source of long-chain fatty acids, e.g., olive oil, for the recovery of *Malassezia furfur;* DTM media (12) specifically formulated for culture of dermatophytes; or mycobacterial medium (Lowenstein-Jensen) or Middlebrook medium for the recovery of *Nocardia* spp. Sabouraud dextrose (2%) agar containing cycloheximide and chloramphenicol is best used for recovery of dermatophytes.

TABLE 3. Selection of clinical specimens for fungal culture[a]

Specimen	Suspected infection												
	Blasto-mycosis	Coccidioido-mycosis	Histo-plasmosis	Paracoccidi-oidomycosis	Candi-diasis	Crypto-coccosis	Asper-gillosis	Zygo-mycosis	Fusariosis	Dermato-phytosis	Chromoblas-tomycosis	Sporo-trichosis	Mycetoma
Lower respiratory tract	1	1	1	2	X	1	1	1	3			3	
Blood		6	2		1	2			2			X	
Bone	4	X		X		X	X	X	X			X	
Bone marrow		X	3	X	X	X			X				
Brain	X	X		X	X	X	X	3	X		X		
CSF	X	X	X		X	5						X	
Eye			X		X		X	X	5				
Nose/nasal sinus	X	X		X	X		2	2	4			4	
Prostate	X	X			X								
Mucous membrane	3	2	5	3	4	X	X	X	X			X	
Subcutaneous tissue		X			X			X			2	2	1
Joints	X	X			X		X		X				
Urine	5	5	4		2	3	X						
Skin	2	3	X	1	X	X	X	4	1	1	1	1	2
Hair and nails					X		X		6	2			
Multiple systemic sites during disseminated infection	6	4	6	4	3	4	3	5	X			X	

[a] Predominant sites for recovery are ranked in order of importance (based on most common clinical presentations). X indicates other sites from which organisms have been recovered.

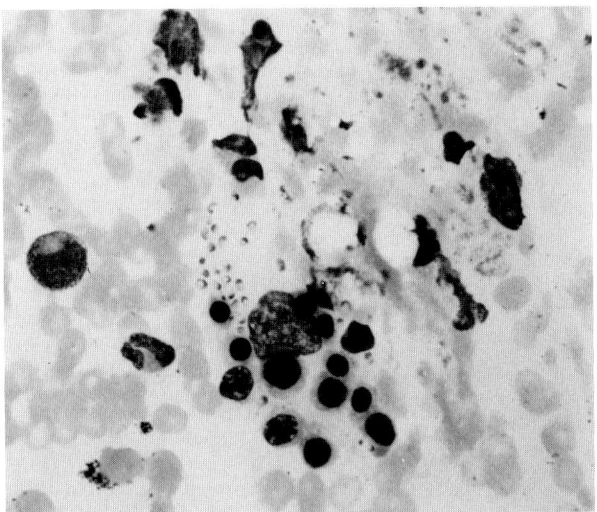

FIG. 1. *Histoplasma capsulatum* in bone marrow. Small intracellular yeast cells are apparent in this Wright-Giemsa preparation. ×2,360.

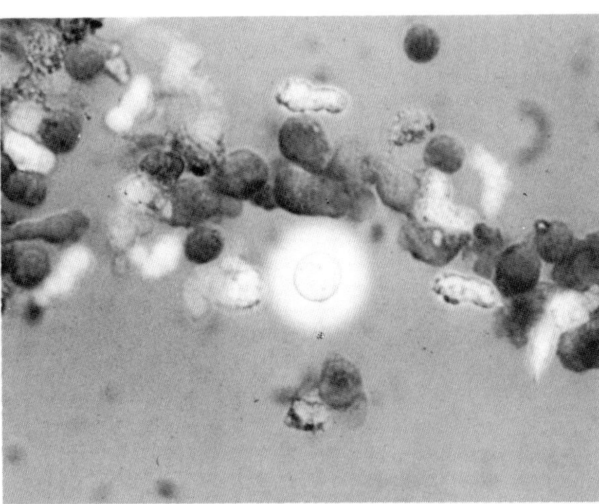

FIG. 4. India ink preparation of cerebrospinal fluid, showing a single encapsulated spherical yeast cell of *Cryptococcus neoformans*. ×2,385.

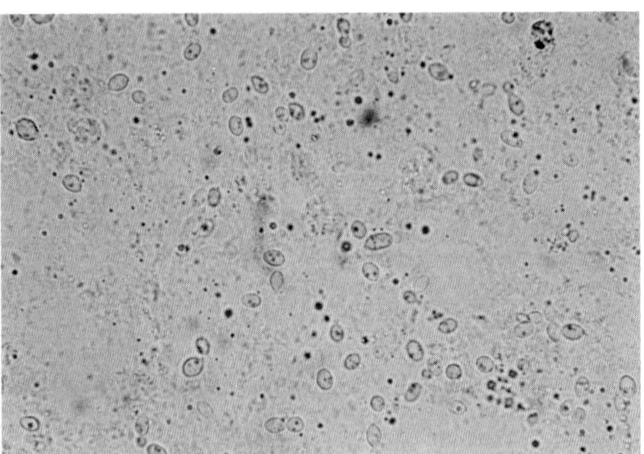

FIG. 2. Numerous small budding yeast cells of *Histoplasma capsulatum* present in sputum as seen by bright-field microscopy. ×1,852.

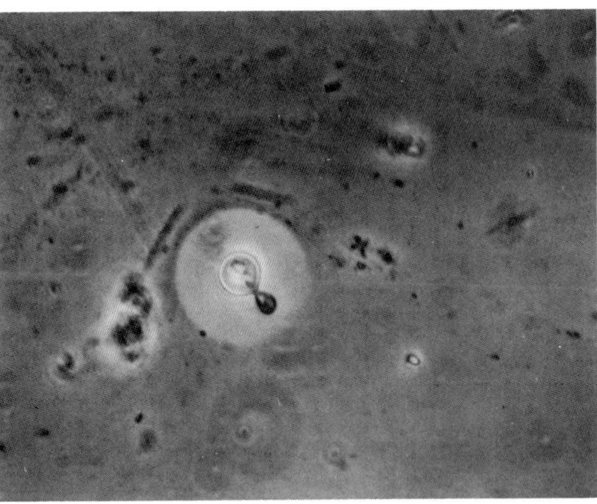

FIG. 5. Phase-contrast photomicrograph of *Cryptococcus neoformans* present in sputum. Note the spherical yeast cell with a "narrow-necked" bud attached. ×2,385.

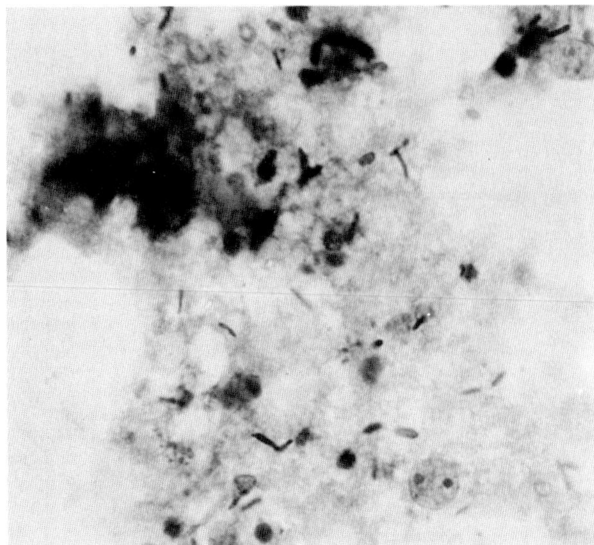

FIG. 3. Periodic acid-Schiff stain of exudate from a cutaneous ulcer, showing numerous elongated yeast cells (cigar bodies) of *Sporothrix schenckii*. ×1,915.

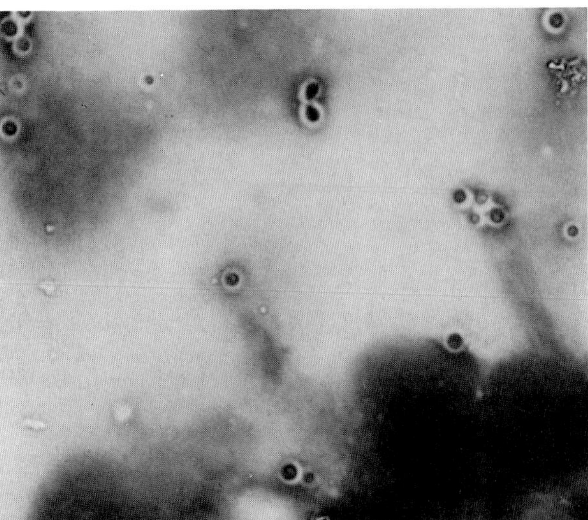

FIG. 6. Periodic acid-Schiff stain of sputum, showing spherical yeast cells of *Cryptococcus neoformans*. Note the presence of a capsule and the variation in size of cells. ×1,590.

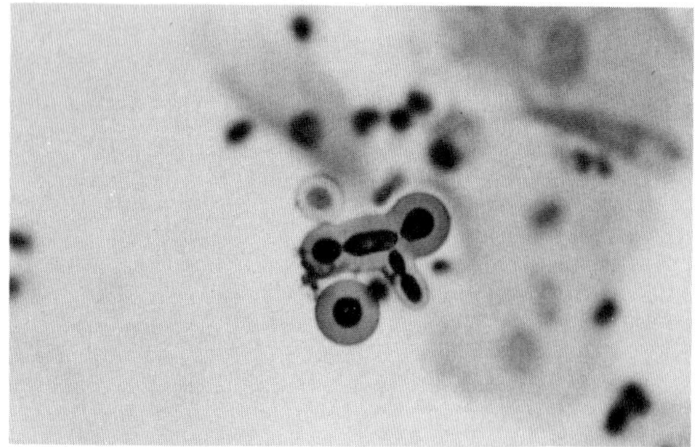

FIG. 7. Papanicolaou stain of sputum showing the rare pseudohyphal form of *Cryptococcus neoformans*. Note the presence of a capsule surrounding all cells. ×2,210.

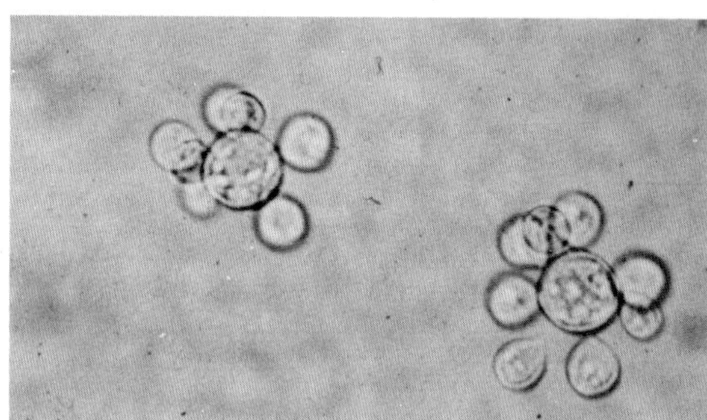

FIG. 10. Bright-field photomicrograph of *Paracoccidioides brasiliensis,* showing multiple budding yeast cells resembling mariner's wheels. ×1,590.

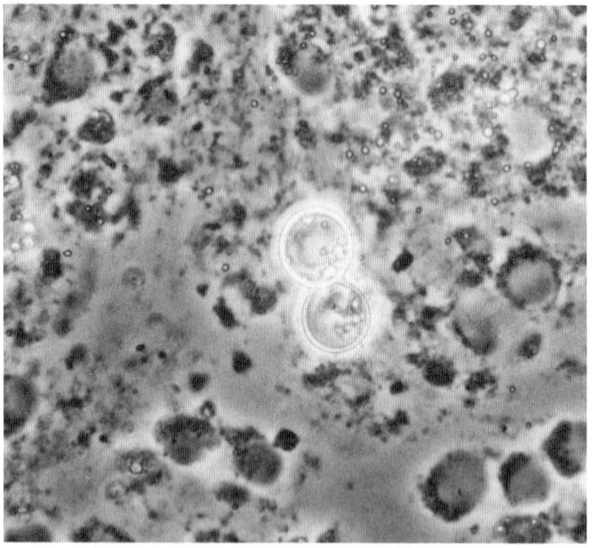

FIG. 8. Phase-contrast photomicrograph of *Blastomyces dermatitidis* in sputum. The presence of a large broad-based budding yeast cell with a "double contoured" wall is characteristic. ×3,040.

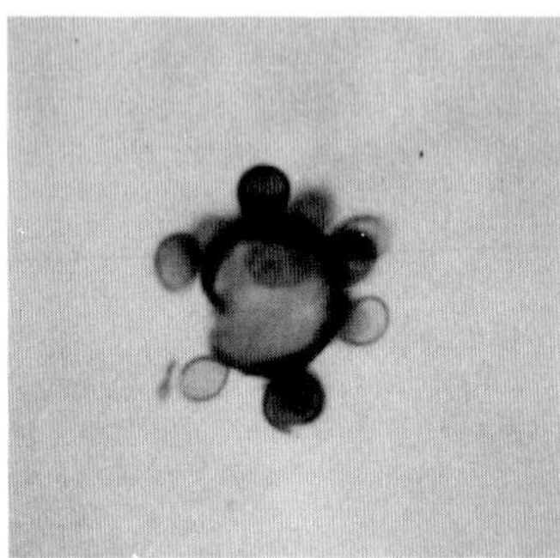

FIG. 11. Methenamine silver stain of *Paracoccidioides brasiliensis* yeast form. ×980.

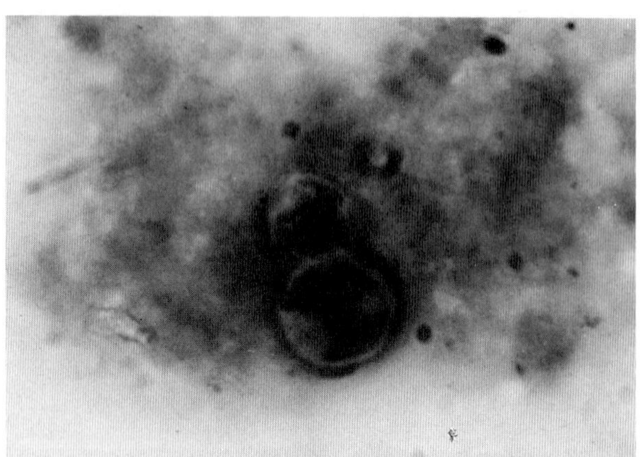

FIG. 9. Gram stain of *Blastomyces dermatitidis* yeast form in sputum. ×1,852.

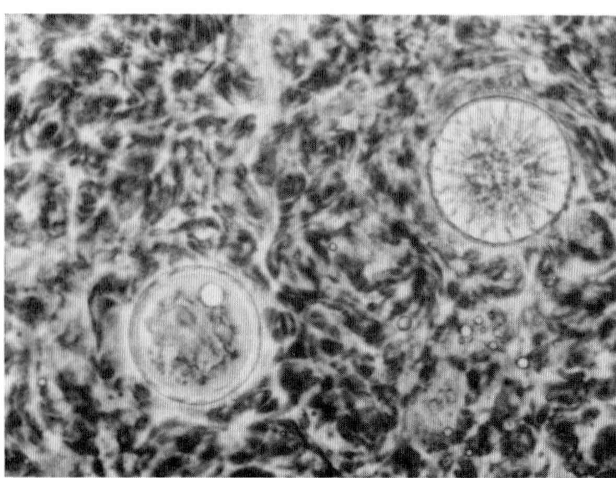

FIG. 12. Phase-contrast photomicrograph of *Coccidioides immitis* spherules in sputum. Note the absence of endospores and the presence of cleavage furrows on one spherule. ×2,400.

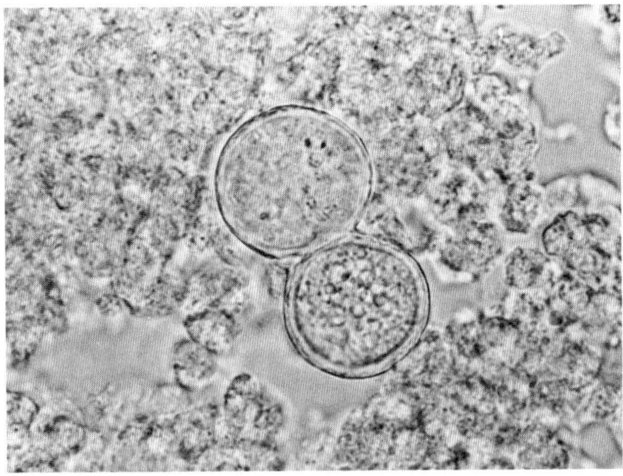

FIG. 13. Bright-field photomicrograph of two adjacent spherules of *Coccidioides immitis* that morphologically resemble *Blastomyces dermatitidis*. Note the presence of endospores in one spherule. ×1,228.

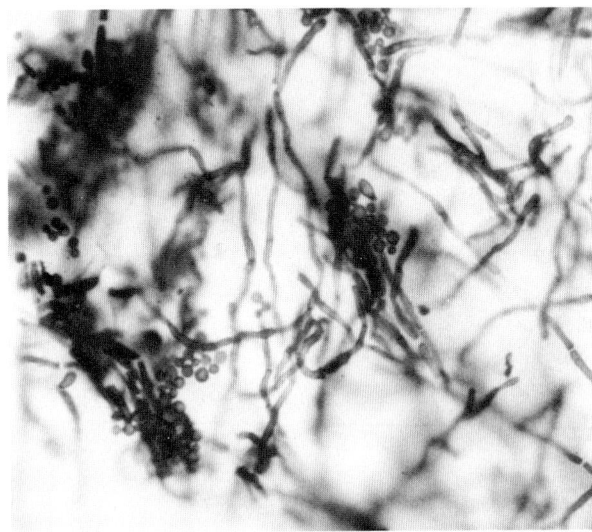

FIG. 16. Periodic acid-Schiff stain of skin, showing hyphal and yeast elements characteristic of *Malassezia furfur*. ×1,590.

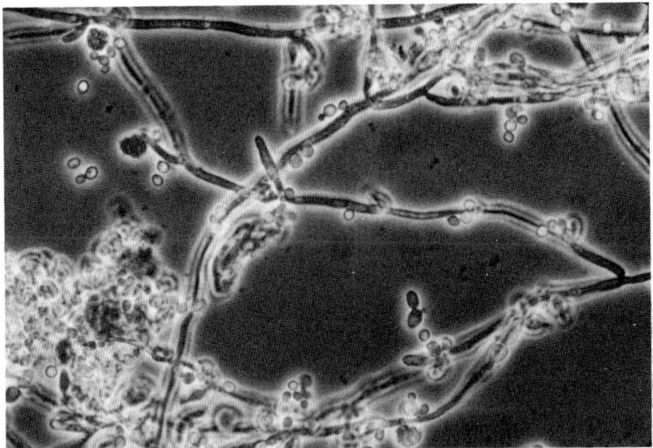

FIG. 14. Phase-contrast photomicrograph of *Candida* sp. in peritoneal fluid. Note the presence of blastoconidia and pseudohyphae characteristic of the genus. ×1,493.

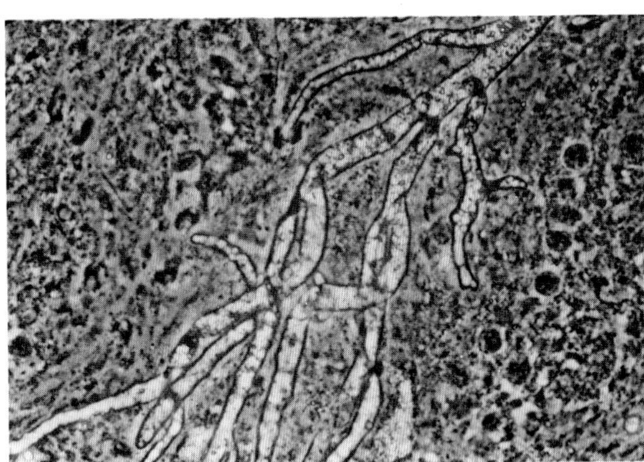

FIG. 17. Phase-contrast photomicrograph of wound exudate, showing large, aseptate, twisted hyphae characteristic of a zygomycete. ×1,496.

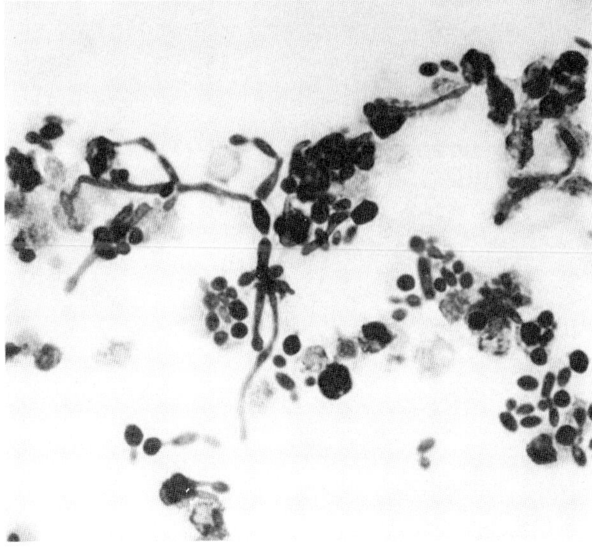

FIG. 15. Periodic acid-Schiff stain of *Candida* sp. ×1,390.

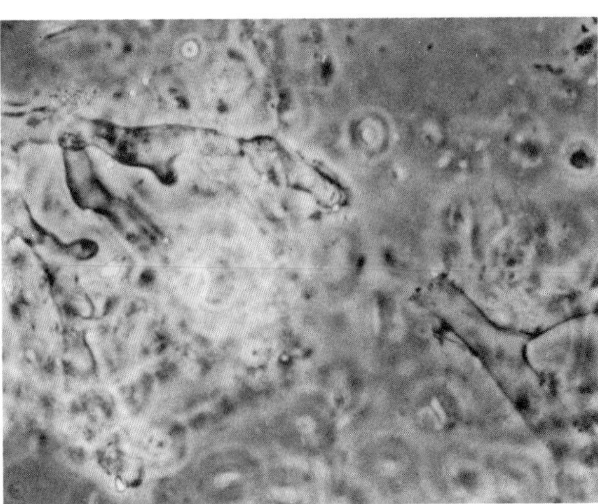

FIG. 18. Phase-contrast photomicrograph showing fractured pieces of large aseptate hyphae characteristic of a zygomycete. ×1,990.

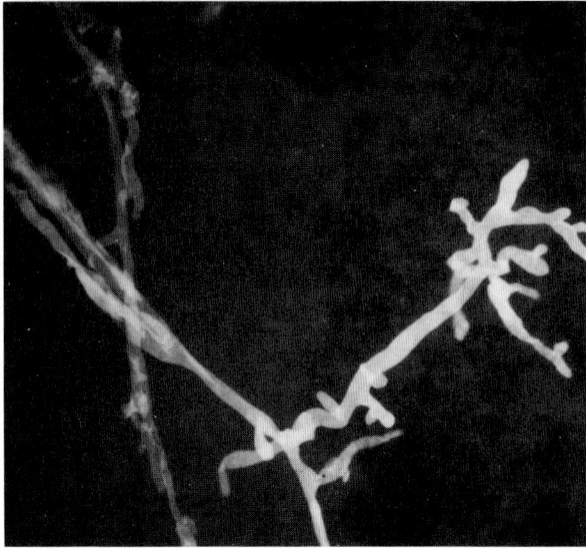

FIG. 19. Calcofluor white-stained sputum showing characteristic hyphae of a zygomycete. ×807.

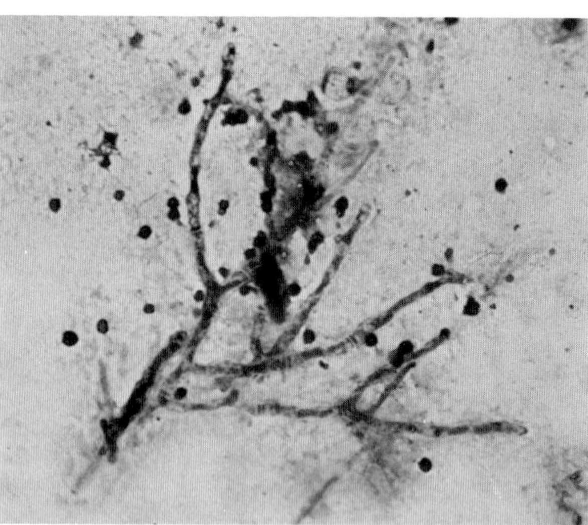

FIG. 22. Gram stain of sputum, showing dichotomously branching septate hyphae consistent with those of *Aspergillus* sp. ×1,860.

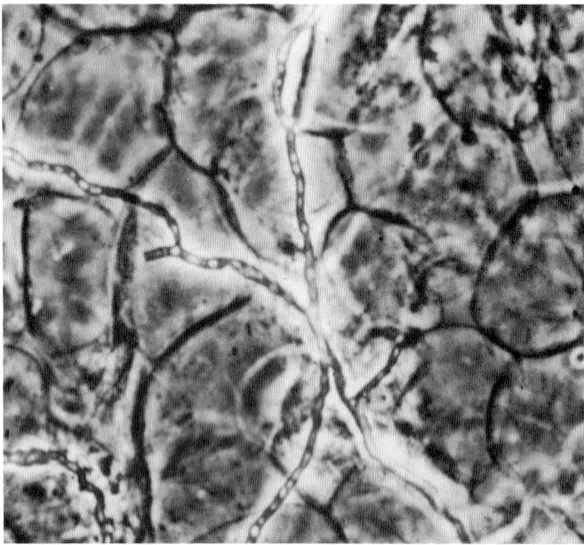

FIG. 20. Phase-contrast photomicrograph of hyphae of a dermatophyte intertwined among squamous cells. ×1,535.

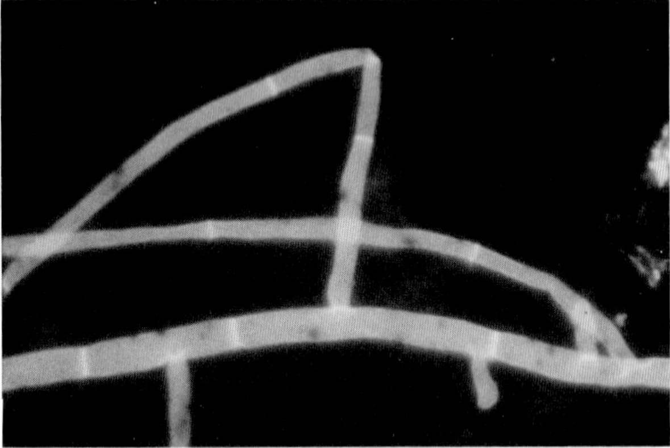

FIG. 23. Calcofluor white stain of hyphae characteristic of *Aspergillus* sp. ×1,597.

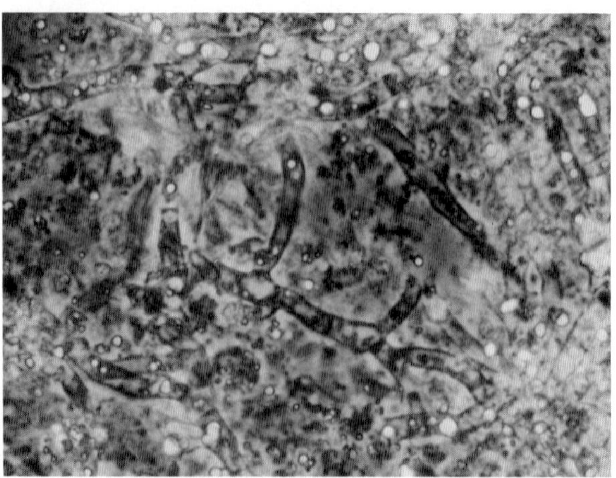

FIG. 21. Phase-contrast photomicrograph of exudate from lung tissue, showing septate hyphae. *Aspergillus* sp. was recovered in culture. ×2,675.

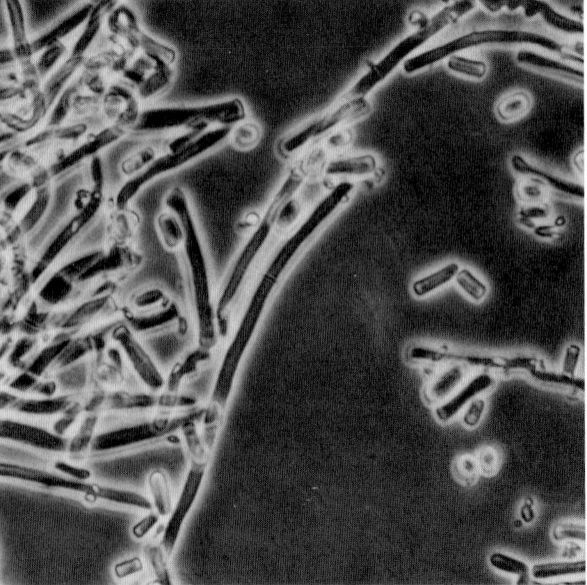

FIG. 24. Phase-contrast photomicrograph showing hyphae and arthroconidia present in sputum. *Geotrichum* sp. was recovered in culture. ×1,549.

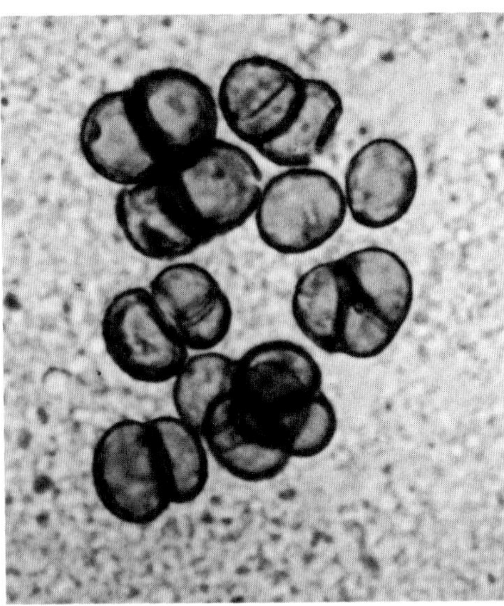

FIG. 25. KOH preparation of sclerotic cells in tissue characteristic of the tissue form of the etiologic agents of chromoblastomycosis. ×1,535.

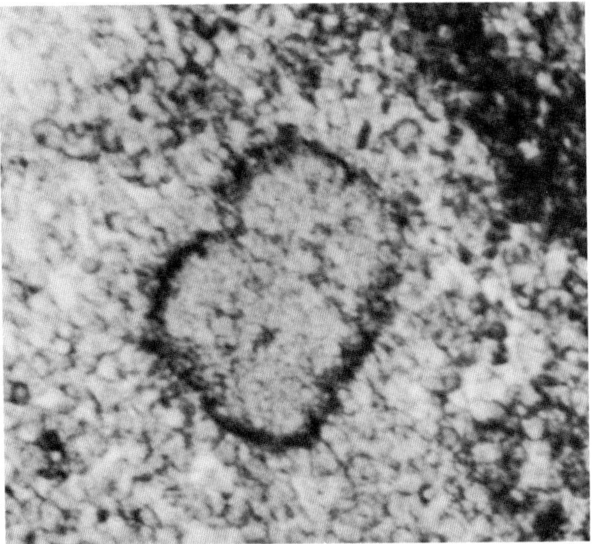

FIG. 26. KOH preparation of a granule in wound exudate characteristically seen in mycetoma. ×500.

Proper incubation temperature, containers, and duration also are important in optimizing recovery of fungi from clinical specimens. It is generally recommended that cultures be incubated at 30°C, since this is near the optimal temperature for growth for many fungi, although culturing at room temperature also is acceptable. Use of culture dishes is best, since they provide a large surface area for the specimens to be spread; however, dehydration may occur. Therefore, use of 40 ml of medium per dish may help prevent surface dehydration. Test tubes (especially larger-diameter tubes) can be used; these usually do not present the problem of dehydration. Large tubes are preferred, and they should be incubated horizontally in racks throughout the incubation period or for at least 24 h to ensure spread of inoculum over a large surface area. Caution: All screw caps must be left loosened for proper aeration; otherwise growth is either inhibited or abnormal, leading to delayed identification.

All specimens should be incubated for at least 4 weeks. Incubation for 6 weeks may be required for maximum recovery of fastidious fungi, e.g., *H. capsulatum* and *B. dermatitidis*. If a single medium (plate or tube) becomes positive for an equivocal pathogen, the remaining media can be incubated and the analysis not completed until the end of the incubation period. Some laboratories may perform surveillance cultures on highly compromised patient populations (9). Multiple skin sites, stool or rectal swabs, urine (with or without centrifugation), throat, nares, and nasopharynx have been used. These specimens need to be inoculated on media containing antibacterial agents and incubated for 5 to 10 days, and all yeasts and filamentous fungi should be identified. Results may help predict what organism is causing an infection.

All cultures should be examined regularly for growth. Any specimens overgrown by a bacterium or a fungus suspected to be a laboratory contaminant should be discarded, and a new specimen should be requested as rapidly as possible. All filamentous fungi (and all fungi, if possible) should be handled in a certified laminar-flow biologic safety cabinet (see chapter 57).

TABLE 4. Pretreatment of clinical specimens prior to plating

Specimen	Pretreatment	Comments
Respiratory secretions	Lysis with mucolytic agents	Optional; may improve yield but also may increase other organisms, i.e., yeasts and bacteria
Body fluids	Centrifugation or filtration	Necessary for optimal recovery; all specimens >1–2 ml
Urine	Centrifugation	Necessary for optimal recovery, especially of agents of deep mycoses
Nails	Macerated in a mortar or broken into very thin sections	Necessary for optimal recovery of dermatophytic and nondermatophytic agents
Tissue	Macerated in a mortar or cut into small pieces	Necessary for optimal recovery of all agents

LITERATURE CITED

1. **Bille, J., L. Stockman, G. D. Roberts, C. D. Horstmeier, and D. M. Ilstrup.** 1983. Evaluation of a lysis-centrifugation system for recovery of yeast and filamentous fungi from blood. J. Clin. Microbiol. **18:**469–471.
2. **Fisher, J. F., W. H. Chew, S. Shadomy, R. J. Duma, C. G. Mayhall, and W. C. House.** 1982. Urinary tract infections due to *Candida albicans*. Rev. Infect. Dis. **4:**1107–1118.
3. **Goldberg, P. K., P. J. Kozinn, G. J. Wise, N. Nouri, and R. B. Brooks.** 1979. Incidence and significance of candiduria. J. Am. Med. Assoc. **241:**582–584.
4. **Hageage, G. J., and B. J. Harrington.** 1984. Use of calcofluor white in clinical mycology. Lab. Med. **15:**109–112.
5. **Hariri, A. R., H. O. Hempel, C. L. Kimberlin, and N. L. Goodman.** 1982. Effects of time lapse between sputum collection and culturing on isolation of clinically significant fungi. J. Clin. Microbiol. **15:**425–428.
6. **Jones, D. B., T. J. Liesegang, and N. M. Robinson.** 1981. Cumitech 13, Laboratory diagnosis of ocular infections. Coordinating ed., J. A. Washington II. American Society for Microbiology, Washington, D.C.
7. **Murray, P. R., R. E. VanScoy, and G. D. Roberts.** 1977. Should yeasts in respiratory secretions be identified? Mayo Clin. Proc. **52:**42–45.
8. **Roberts, G. D., A. G. Karison, and D. R. DeYoung.** 1976. Recovery of pathogenic fungi from clinical specimens submitted for mycobacteriological culture. J. Clin. Microbiol. **3:**47–48.
9. **Sandford, G. R., W. G. Merz, J. R. Wingard, P. Charache, and R. Saral.** 1980. The value of fungal surveillance cultures as predictors of systemic fungal infections. J. Infect. Dis. **142:**503–509.
10. **Smith, C. D., and N. L. Goodman.** 1975. Improved culture method for the isolation of *Histoplasma capsulatum* and *Blastomyces dermatitidis* from contaminated specimens. Am. J. Clin. Pathol. **68:**276–280.
11. **Stockman, L., G. D. Roberts, and D. M. Ilstrup.** 1984. Effect of storage of the Dupont lysis-centrifugation system on recovery of bacteria and fungi in a prospective clinical trial. J. Clin. Microbiol. **19:**283–285.
12. **Taplin, D.** 1965. The use of gentamicin in mycology. J. Invest. Dermatol. **45:**549–550.
13. **Telenti, A., and G. D. Roberts.** 1989. Fungal blood cultures. Eur. J. Clin. Microbiol. Infect. Dis. **8:**825–831.

Chapter 59

Dermatophytes and Agents of Superficial Mycoses

IRENE WEITZMAN AND JULIUS KANE

DERMATOPHYTOSES

The dermatophytoses (tinea or ringworm) are fungal infections of the keratinized tissues (hair, nails, skin, etc.) of humans and lower animals by a group of closely related keratinophilic fungi collectively referred to as dermatophytes, whose anamorphs (asexual form) belong to the genera *Epidermophyton*, *Microsporum*, and *Trichophyton*. Cutaneous infections resembling dermatophytosis may be caused by yeasts or other unrelated filamentous fungi that are normally saprophytes or plant pathogens; these infections are often referred to as opportunistic dermatomycoses (58).

Tissue invasion is essentially cutaneous because of the inability of these fungi to penetrate deeper tissues or organs as a result of nonspecific inhibitory factors in serum (30) and inhibition of fungal keratinases (14). Infection may range from mild to severe as a consequence of the reaction of the host to the metabolic products of the fungus, the virulence of the infecting strain, anatomical location of the infection, and local environment factors. Occasionally, subcutaneous tissue may be invaded, e.g., in Majocchi's granuloma, kerion, mycetomalike processes (8, 60) or, more rarely, a generalized systemic infection (6).

Characterization

Physiologically, the dermatophytes have in common the ability to digest keratin (an insoluble scleroprotein), a tolerance for cycloheximide, and the ability to produce a rise in pH to the alkaline range as a consequence of growth in media containing glucose and peptone.

The three genera of the dermatophytes originally were classified in the phylum Deuteromycota (Fungi Imperfecti). Within recent years, many of the *Microsporum* and *Trichophyton* species were found to reproduce sexually and produce asci and ascospores (56). These species then were classified in the family Gymnoascaceae, phylum Ascomycota, teleomorphic genera *Nannizzia* and *Arthroderma*, respectively. A careful evaluation of the descriptions defining these two genera concluded that the characteristics represent a continuum. Consequently, these two taxa may be considered congeneric, and on the basis of priority, the correct generic name is therefore *Arthroderma* (56). Current taxonomic controversy centers on the classification of the order and family for the placement of the genus *Arthroderma;* some consider the Arthrodermataceae of the Onygenales to be more representative than the Gymnoascaceae of the Eurotiales (12).

Dermatophytes usually are grouped into three categories based on host preference and natural habitat (3). Anthropophilic species almost exclusively infect humans; animals are rarely infected. Geophilic species are soil-inhabiting organisms, and soil serves as a source of infection for both humans and lower animals. Zoophilic species are essentially pathogens of lower animals, although animal-to-human transmission is not uncommon. This grouping (Table 1) may be helpful in determining the source of infection; e.g., human infections caused by *Microsporum canis* are often the result of contact of susceptible children with stray kittens (32).

Geographically, the dermatophytes may vary in distribution (40); some, e.g., *Trichophyton rubrum*, have a global distribution, whereas others, e.g., *Trichophyton concentricum*, are geographically limited to the Pacific Islands and regions in Central and South America.

Clinical Manifestations

Anatomic location

Traditionally, infections caused by dermatophytes have been named according to the anatomical location involved, e.g., tinea barbae (beard and moustache), tinea capitis (scalp, eyebrows, and eyelashes), tinea corporis (face and trunk), tinea cruris (groin, perineal, and perianal areas), tinea pedis (feet), and tinea unguium (nails). Different dermatophyte species may produce clinically identical lesions; conversely, a single species may infect many anatomical sites.

Tinea barbae, usually caused by zoophilic fungi, e.g., *Trichophyton verrucosum* and *T. mentagrophytes* var. *mentagrophytes*, typically are highly inflammatory and may present as acute pustular folliculitis that may progress to suppurative boggy lesions (kerion). A less severe form appearing as dry, erythematous, scaly lesions also may occur. Tinea capitis may vary in its presentation from slightly erythematous, patchy, scaly areas with dull gray hair stumps to highly inflammatory with folliculitis, kerion formation, alopecia, and scarring. *Trichophyton tonsurans* and *M. canis* are the most common agents (40).

Favus (tinea favosa), most commonly caused by *Trichophyton schoenleinii*, is a chronic infection of the scalp and glabrous skin characterized by the formation of cup-shaped crusts resembling honeycombs (scutula). Tinea corporis, which can be caused by any dermatophyte, classically is manifested as circular, erythematous lesions with scaling and a raised active, often vesicular border. Chronic lesions on the trunk and extremities usually are caused by *T. rubrum*. Tinea cruris ("jock itch"), usually caused by *T. rubrum* or *Epidermophyton floccosum*, typically appears as scaly, erythematous to tawny brown, bilateral and asymmetric lesions extending down to the inner thigh and exhibiting a sharply marginated border frequently studded with small vesicles. Tinea pedis varies in appearance; the most com-

TABLE 1. Grouping of the dermatophytes on the basis of host preference and natural habitat

Anthropophilic	Geophilic	Zoophilic
Epidermophyton floccosum	*M. fulvum*	*M. canis* var. *canis*
Microsporum	*M. gypseum*	*M. canis* var. *distortum*
audouinii	*M. nanum*[a]	*M. equinum*
ferruginium	*M. persicolor*[a]	*M. gallinae*
Trichophyton	*M. praecox*	*T. equinum*
concentricum	*M. racemosum*	*T. mentagrophytes* var. *erinacei*, var. *mentagrophytes*, var. *quinckeanum*
gourvilli	*M. vanbreuseghemii*	*T. simii*
megninii		
mentagrophytes var. *interdigitale*		
raubitschekii		*T. verrucosum*
rubrum		
schoenleinii		
soudanense		
tonsurans		
violaceum		
yaoundei		

[a] Some consider *M. nanum* and *M. persicolor* to be zoophilic.

mon manifestation is maceration, peeling, itching, and painful fissuring between the fourth and fifth toes. An acute inflammatory condition with vesicles, pustules, or a hyperkeratotic chronic type ("moccasin foot") are other manifestations. *T. mentagrophytes* var. *mentagrophytes* (granular) frequently causes the more inflammatory type of infection, whereas *T. rubrum* or *T. mentagrophytes* var. *interdigitale* (velvety) cause the more chronic type. Tinea unguium, most often caused by *T. rubrum*, usually appears as thickened, deformed, friable, discolored nails with accumulated subungual debris.

Transmission and contagion

Anthropophilic fungi usually are transmitted by close human contact or indirectly by sharing clothes, combs, brushes, towels, bedsheets, etc. Tinea capitis is highly contagious and may spread rapidly within a family, institution, or school. Transmission of tinea cruris is associated with shared clothing, towels, and sanitary facilities. The transmission of tinea pedis and tinea unguium is controversial (44, 58). Geophilic infections involving transmission from a soil source to humans or lower animals are rare, but outbreaks originating from infected soil with secondary human transmission have been reported (5). Infections involving zoophilic species result from animal to human contact (cats, dogs, cattle, laboratory animals, etc.) or by indirect transmission involving fomites.

Detection

Patients with suspected tinea capitis should be examined in a darkened room with a Wood's lamp (filtered UV light peak of 3,650 Å) for the presence of bright green fluorescent hairs. Such hairs, considered Wood's light positive, typically occur in the small-spored ectothrix type of hair invasion caused by *Microsporum audouinii*, *M. canis*, and *M. ferrugineum*. Hairs infected with *T. schoenleinii* may show a dull green color (42).

A Wood's lamp also may be used to differentiate between infections of the skin that may be similar clinically, e.g., erythrasma (caused by a bacterium, *Corynebacterium minutissimum*) from dermatophytosis. In the former the skin fluoresces orange to coral red, whereas the latter infection is not fluorescent.

The direct microscopic examination of skin, hair, and nails is the most rapid method of determining fungal etiology. This may be accomplished readily by examination of the clinical material in 10% potassium hydroxide (KOH), in 25% sodium hydroxide (NaOH) with 5% glycerin, or in Calcofluor white (43).

Laboratory Methods

Collection and transport of specimens

Aseptic technique should be used whenever feasible to minimize contamination. Sufficient clinical material should be collected for direct microscopic examination and for culture. The following equipment should be available for collection and transport of specimens: sterile nail clippers, scissors, forceps for epilating hairs, scalpels, sterile gauze squares, 70% alcohol for disinfection, sterile water for cleaning painful areas, surface-sterilized clean glass slides, clean pill packets or clean paper envelopes to contain and transport the clinical specimens, and appropriate culture media when feasible. Black photographic paper may be useful to collect and better visualize scrapings. Closed tubes are not recommended for specimens since they retain moisture, which may result in an overgrowth of contaminants. Disposable brushes have been recommended for collection of specimens from the scalp or fur of animals (33).

Hairs from the scalp should be epilated with the sterile forceps. If the specimen is Wood's light positive, epilate only fluorescent hairs. In favus, the scutulum at the mouth of the hair follicle is suitable for culture and microscopic examination. Hairs invaded by endothrix fungi may need to be dug out with the tip of a sterile scalpel blade because the hairs often break off flush at scalp level, making it difficult to grasp them with forceps. Rubbing with a sterile moistened swab was reported to be successful for pediatric patients (19). Active borders of skin lesions should be scraped with a scalpel (after disinfection with alcohol or cleansing with sterile water) to collect epidermal scales. In vesicular tinea pedis, the tops of the vesicles can be removed with sterile scissors for direct examination and culture. Nails should be disinfected with alcohol gauze squares. The most desirable material for culture is the waxy subungual debris which contains the viable fungal elements. The crumbly debris directly underneath the nail near the tip should be removed with a scalpel before collection of material for culture in order to remove contaminating saprophytic fungi and bacteria. Similarly, if the dorsal nail plate is diseased, the outer surface is to be scraped and discarded before the nail is cultured.

Direct microscopic examination

Skin scrapings or hairs are placed in 1 or 2 drops of a KOH or NaOH aqueous solution on a clean glass slide. A cover slip is placed on top, and the preparation is heated gently (short of boiling) by being passed rapidly over a Bunsen burner three or four times and then allowed to sit at room temperature for a few minutes for clearing. Nails may require a stronger alkali solution, up to 25% KOH or NaOH, and a longer clearing time. Demonstration of fungi also may be accomplished by use of Calcofluor white (43). All preparations should be examined under low power and confirmed under high power.

Infected skin and nails may reveal hyaline hyphal fragments, septate, often branched hyphae, and chains of arthroconidia (Fig. 1).

The appearance of infected hairs depends on the invading dermatophyte species. Three main types, ectothrix, endothrix, and favic, are observed by the direct microscopic examination. The terms "ectothrix" and "endothrix" refer to the location of the arthroconidia in relation to the hair shaft. Arthroconidia are formed by the fragmentation of the invading hyphae. The appearance, size, and location of the arthroconidia may suggest the infecting genera or species. The appearances described below are based on the descriptions of Rippon (42).

Ectothrix hairs. Arthroconidia appear as a mosaic sheath around the hair or as chains on the surface of the hair shaft (Fig. 2).

Arthroconidia 1 to 3 μm in diameter appearing as a mosaic sheath around the hair are suggestive of *M. audouinii, M. canis,* or *M. ferrugineum.* Infected hairs are Wood's lamp positive.

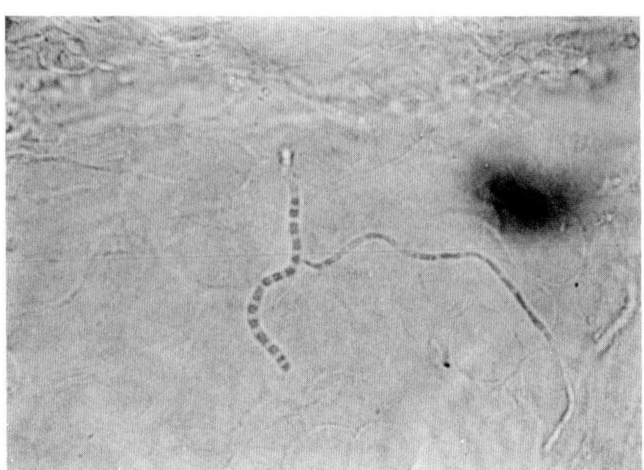

FIG. 1. Dermatophyte hyphae in skin scraping. NaOH mount. ×400.

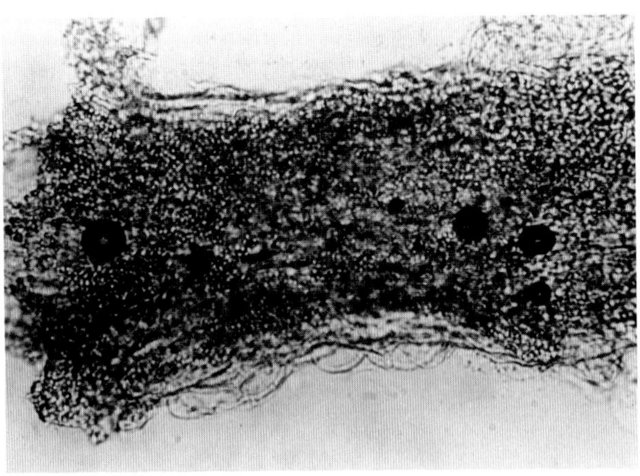

FIG. 2. *M. audouinii,* ectothrix type of hair invasion. ×400.

Arthroconidia 3 to 4 μm in diameter, few in number and scattered around the outside of the hair are suggestive of *Microsporum gypseum* and *M. fulvum.* Hairs are Wood's lamp negative.

Arthroconidia 3 to 4 μm in diameter in chains on the hair surface are suggestive of the *T. mentagrophytes* complex. Hairs are Wood's lamp negative.

Large arthroconidia, 8 to 12 μm in diameter, in large dense chains around the hair are characteristic of *T. verrucosum.* Hairs are Wood's lamp negative.

Endothrix hairs. Endothrix hair invasion produced by *T. tonsurans, T. violaceum,* and *T. gourvilli* are observed as chains of arthroconidia, 3 to 4 μm in diameter, filling the inside of shortened hair stubs (Fig. 3). Hairs are Wood's lamp negative. *T. rubrum,* which rarely infects hair, has been described as both ectothrix and endothrix infections (42).

Favic hairs. Hyphal filaments, air bubbles, or tunnels and fat droplets are observed intrapilar (Fig. 4). These hairs are reported to show a dull green appearance under the Wood's lamp. In general, all infected hairs show hyphae within the hair shaft at some time during the course of infection, usually during the early stages.

Isolation media

In the United States, the most common media used for the isolation of dermatophytes are Sabouraud dex-

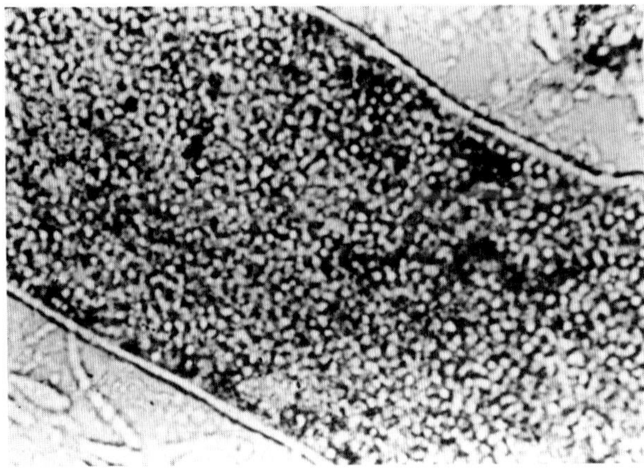

FIG. 3. *T. tonsurans,* endothrix type of hair invasion. ×1,000.

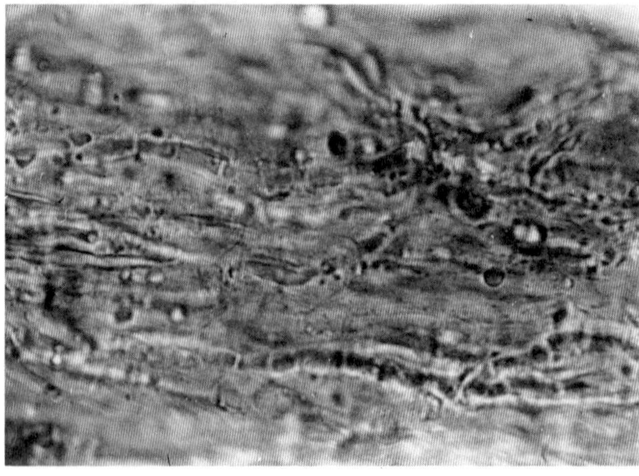

FIG. 4. Hair infected by *T. schoenleinii* from a case of favus. ×1,000.

trose agar (SDA) (pH 5.6) and Emmon's modification, with less dextrose (2% instead of 4%) and a pH of between 6.8 and 7.0, paired with SDA containing chloramphenicol and cycloheximide to inhibit bacterial and saprophytic fungal contamination (available commercially as Mycobiotic agar [Difco Laboratories, Detroit, Mich.] or Mycosel [BBL Microbiology Systems, Cockeysville, Md.]). SDA with chloramphenicol is recommended for the isolation from contaminated specimens of opportunistic fungi that cause clinical infections resembling dermatophytosis but are sensitive to cycloheximide (43). The addition of gentamicin is recommended for specimens heavily contaminated by bacteria (51). SDA with cycloheximide, chloramphenicol, and gentamicin (CCG) is routinely used as an isolation medium in the laboratory of J. Kane, in addition to Casamino Acids (Difco)-erythritol-albumin agar medium plus CCG for positive skin and nail specimens. This medium discourages the growth of *Candida albicans* and encourages the more slowly growing dermatophytes (15). In addition, Littman oxgall agar supplied commercially by Difco and by Remel Laboratories (Lenexa, Kans.) is used routinely for nail scrapings for the isolation of yeasts and moulds sensitive to cycloheximide. Specimens from cattle ranges and farms also should be inoculated onto bromocresol purple (BCP)-milk solids agar plus CCG and 0.5% yeast extract to enhance growth and reveal the characteristic casein hydrolysis of *T. verrucosum* (29).

Some laboratories use dermatophyte test medium (available commercially from Difco and Remel). This selective medium screens for the presence of dermatophytes from heavily contaminated material (feet, nails, etc.). The growth of dermatophytes causes a rise in pH, thus changing the phenol red indicator from yellow to red. The antibiotics gentamicin and chlortetracycline inhibit bacteria, whereas the cycloheximide inhibits saprophytic fungi (52). This medium should be considered only for screening purposes, since fungi other than dermatophytes can grow and turn the medium red (35, 46).

Cultures are routinely incubated at 25 to 30°C and examined weekly for up to 4 weeks. Cultures of specimens suspected for *T. verrucosum* also should be incubated at 37°C, since this temperature enhances growth of this species.

Identification

Identification of the dermatophyte species often is based on colony characteristics in pure culture on SDA and on microscopic morphology. However, these criteria alone may be insufficient, since colonial appearance may vary or be similar for different species; characteristic pigmentation may fail to appear, and some isolates may not sporulate. This situation is especially pertinent for the genus *Trichophyton*. Special media may be required to stimulate pigment production; sporulation and physiological tests also may be necessary in conjunction with morphology to identify the species correctly.

Colony characteristics

The following sets of characteristics are important in observing gross colony morphology: color of the surface and on the reverse of the colony; texture of the surface (powdery, granular, woolly, cottony, velvety, or glabrous; topography (refers to the elevation, type of folding, margins, etc.); and rate of growth.

Microscopic morphology

Microscopic morphology, especially the appearance and arrangement of the conidia (macroconidia or microconidia) and other structures, may be determined by teased mounts or slide culture preparations mounted in lactophenol cotton blue (Poirrer's blue) (phenol is listed as a hazardous chemical; solutions containing phenol should be prepared, stored, and used in an approved chemical safety cabinet) or in more permanent mounting fluids (55). Sometimes special media, such as cornmeal or cornmeal-dextrose agar, potato-dextrose agar, SDA plus 3 to 5% NaCl (24, 28), or lactritmel agar (9, 22), may be required to stimulate sporulation.

Physiological tests

In vitro hair perforation test. The in vitro hair perforation test devised by Ajello and Georg to distinguish between atypical isolates of *T. mentagrophytes* and *T. rubrum* (4) also may be used to distinguish *M. canis* from *M. equinum* (39). Hairs exposed to *T. mentagrophytes* and *M. canis* show wedge-shaped perforations perpendicular to the hair shaft (a positive test result), whereas *T. rubrum* and *M. equinum* do not form these perforating structures. This test also may be useful as an aid in identifying other species (39).

Place short strands of human hair in petri dishes and autoclave the dishes at 120°C for 10 min; add 25 ml of sterile distilled water and 2 to 3 drops of 10% sterilized yeast extract. Inoculate these plates with several fragments of the test fungus that has been grown on SDA; incubate the plates at 25°C and examine them at regular intervals over a period of 21 days. Hairs may be examined microscopically for perforations by removing a few segments and placing them in a drop of lactophenol cotton blue mounting fluid. Gentle heating of the lactophenol cotton blue mounts aids in the detection.

Special nutritional requirements. The nutritional tests originally were described by Georg and Camp as an aid in the routine identification of *Trichophyton* species that seldom produce conidia or resemble each other morphologically (17). Certain species have distinctive nutritional requirements, whereas others do not. The method employs a casein basal medium that is vitamin free (T#1) to which various vitamins are added: #2 inositol, #3 thiamine and inositol, #4 thiamine, #5 nicotine acid, and an ammonium nitrate basal medium #6 to which histidine is added #7. These media are available commercially as trichophyton agars 1 to 7, in dehydrated form from Difco and prepared from Remel. A small fragment (about the size of the head of a pin) is taken from the culture to be tested and placed on the surface of the basal media (controls) and media containing the vitamin and amino acid additives. Care must be taken to avoid transferring agar from the fungus inoculum to the nutritional media. Incubation is carried out at room temperature (or 37°C if *T. verrucosum* is suspected) and read after 7 and 14 days. The amount of growth is graded from 0, ±, to 4+. Charts indicating the nutritional requirements are available as package inserts from the manufacturer, from the original paper (17), and from various texts (42, 58).

Urea hydrolysis. The ability to hydrolyze urea provides additional data to aid in the differentiation of *T. rubrum* (urease negative) from *T. mentagrophytes* (typically urease positive), *T. rubrum* from *T. raubitschekii* (urease positive) (27, 50), and *T. rubrum* from *T. megninii* (urease positive) (45). Both Christensen urea agar and broth may be used; however, some consider the broth to be more sensitive for this purpose (25). After the urea medium is inoculated, it is incubated at 25 to 30°C for 7 days. The tubes should be examined every 2 to 3 days for the color change from orange or pale pink to a purple-red color indicating the presence of urease, a positive test result. Negative and positive controls always should be included and read first.

Growth on BCP-milk solids-glucose medium. Type of growth (profuse versus restricted) and a change in the pH indicator (bromocresol purple) indicating alkalinity are especially useful for differentiating *T. rubrum* from *T. mentagrophytes* and *T. mentagrophytes* from *Microsporum persicolor* (28, 50). *T. rubrum* shows restricted growth and produces no alkaline reaction on this medium, whereas *T. mentagrophytes* typically shows profuse growth and an alkaline reaction. Although *M. persicolor* shows profuse growth, it does not result in an alkaline reaction. Other tests for differentiating *T. mentagrophytes* from *M. persicolor* have been described (36).

Cultures to be tested are inoculated onto slants of BCP-milk solids-glucose medium and examined for a pH change and growth characteristics at the end of a 7-day incubation period at 25°C. A color change from pale blue to violet purple indicates an alkaline reaction.

Growth on polished rice grains. *M. audouinii*, unlike most dermatophytes, grows poorly on rice grains and produces a brownish discoloration (11). *Microsporum equinum* recently was reported to have a growth pattern resembling that of *M. audouinii* (1). This is a useful test for differentiating these species from *M. canis* and from other dermatophytes that typically grow and sporulate on the rice grains.

The medium is prepared in 125-ml flasks by mixing 1 part of raw unfortified rice grains to 3 parts of water (11) or 8.0 g of rice grains to 25 ml of distilled water. Autoclave at 15 lb/in^2 for 15 min. Inoculate the surface of the rice and incubate the sample for 2 weeks at 25 to 30°C.

Temperature tolerance and temperature enhancement. Tests for temperature tolerance and enhancement are useful for differentiating *T. mentagrophytes* from *T. terrestre* (37), *T. mentagrophytes* from *M. persicolor* (28), *T. verrucosum* from *T. schoenleinii* (42), and *T. soudanense* from *M. ferrugineum* (57). At 37°C *T. mentagrophytes* shows good growth, whereas *T. terrestre* does not grow and *M. persicolor* grows poorly or not at all; growth of *T. verrucosum* and *T. soudanense*, but not *T. schoenleinii* or *M. ferrugineum*, is enhanced.

Inoculate two slants of SDA with an equivalent fragment of the culture. Incubate the slants at 25 to 30°C and at 37°C. Compare the growth at both temperatures when mature colonies appear at 25°C. Appropriate controls are recommended and should be compared first.

Description of the Etiologic Agents

For practical purposes, identification of the dermatophytes in the routine clinical laboratory is based on the anamorph, i.e., conidia in culture, rather than on the sexual form (teleomorph).

Two types of hyaline conidia may be produced by the dermatophytes: large multicellular, smooth or rough, thin- or thick-walled macroconidia and smaller unicellular, smooth-walled microconidia. The three genera are grouped according to the presence or absence of these two types of conidia and the appearance of the surface of the macroconidia, i.e., rough versus smooth. Identification of the species is based on the microscopic appearance and arrangement of the conidia, colonial morphology on SDA (Fig. 5–20), and physiological tests (Table 2).

Epidermophyton species

Microconidia are lacking; only smooth-walled, broadly clavate macroconidia are produced with one to nine septa, 20 to 60 μm in length by 4 to 13 μm in width, and borne singly or in clusters of two to three. *E. floccosum* is the only pathogen (genus has only two species); it invades skin and nails but not hair.

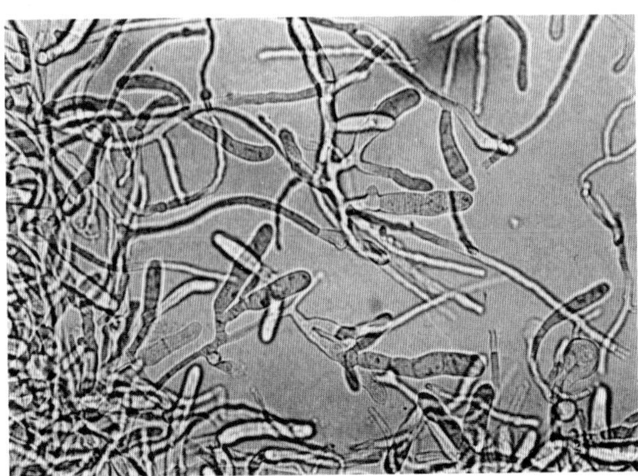

FIG. 5. Macroconidia of *E. floccosum* on SDA. Note the absence of microconidia. ×400.

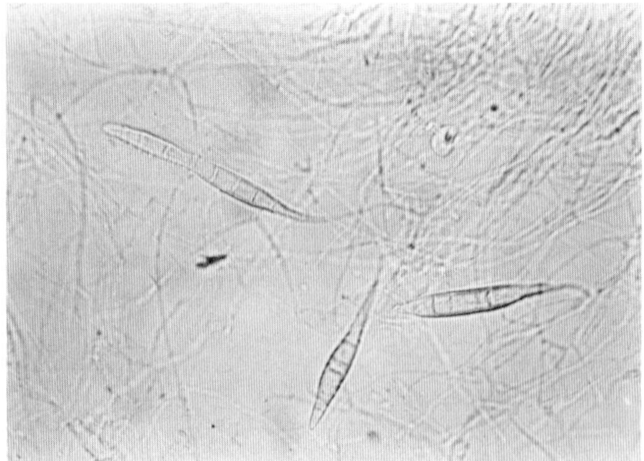

FIG. 6. Macroconidia of *M. audouinii* on SDA plus 3% NaCl. ×400.

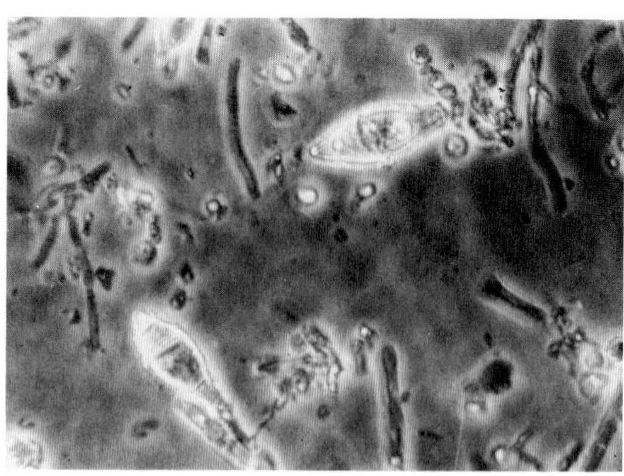

FIG. 9. Fusiform two- to three-septate macroconidia of *M. equinum*. Phase contrast; ×400.

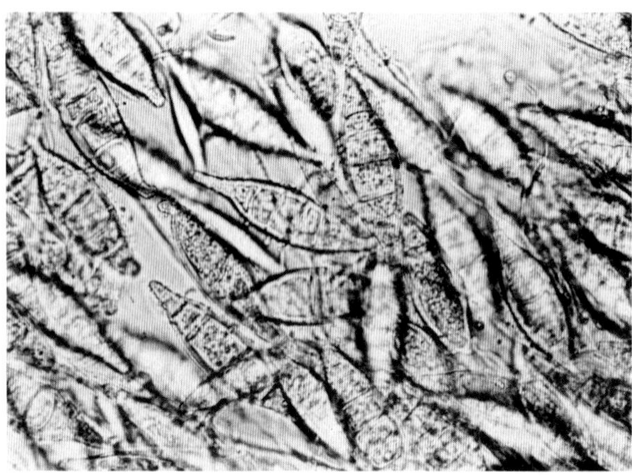

FIG. 7. Macroconidia of *M. canis* with rough thick walls. ×400.

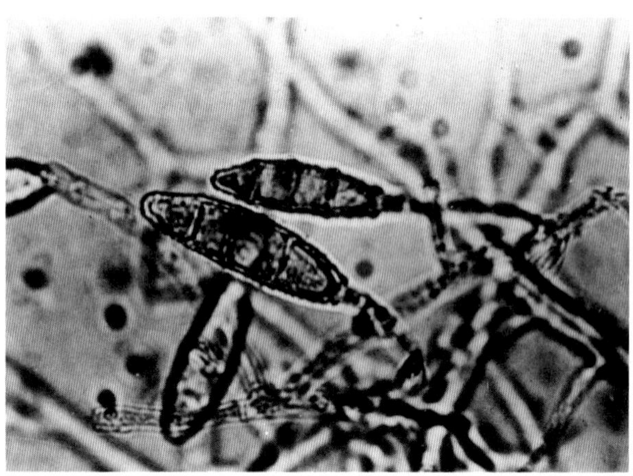

FIG. 10. Macroconidia of *M. gypseum*. ×400.

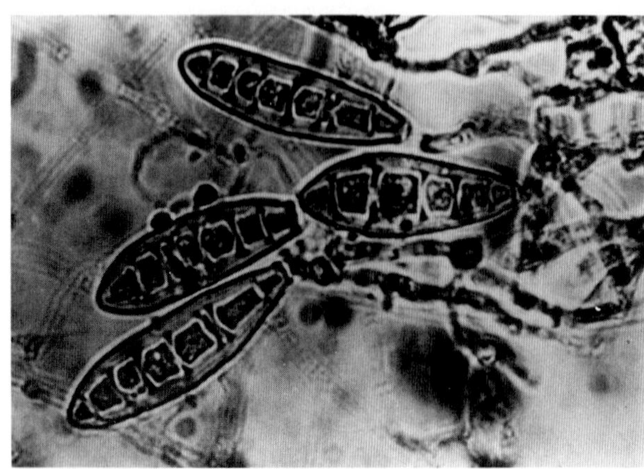

FIG. 8. Macroconidia of *M. cookei* with thick walls and pseudosepta. ×400.

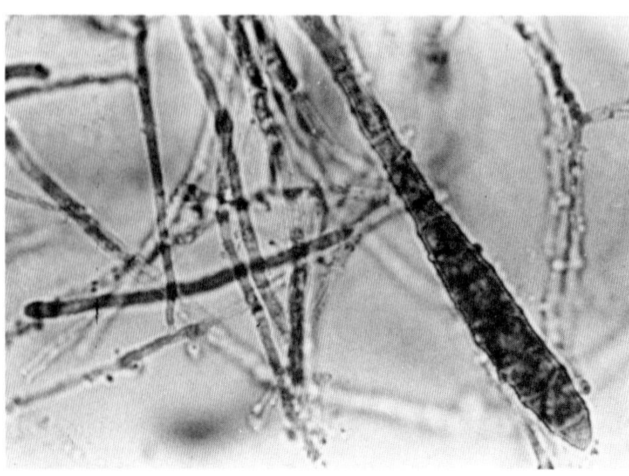

FIG. 11. Rough-walled macroconidium of *M. persicolor* on SDA plus 3% NaCl. ×1,000.

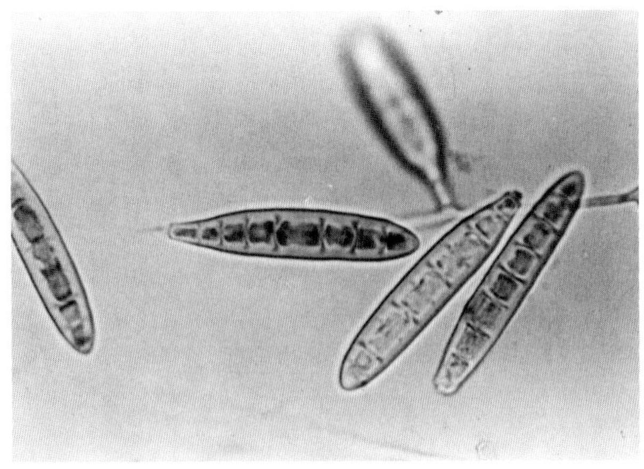

FIG. 12. Smooth-walled macroconidia of *T. ajelloi.* ×400.

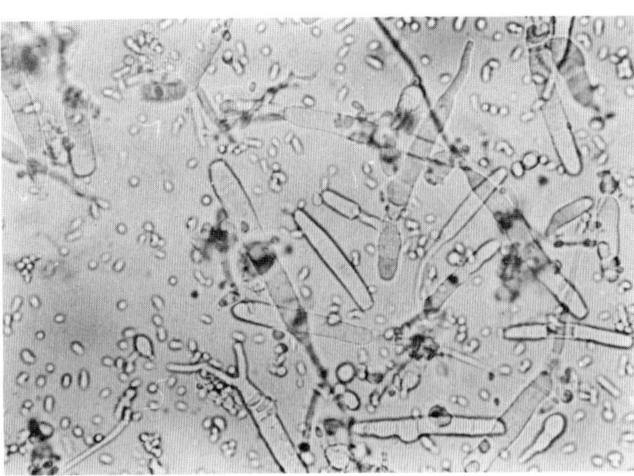

FIG. 15. Smooth-walled macroconidia of *T. raubitschekii* from primary isolate on SDA. ×400.

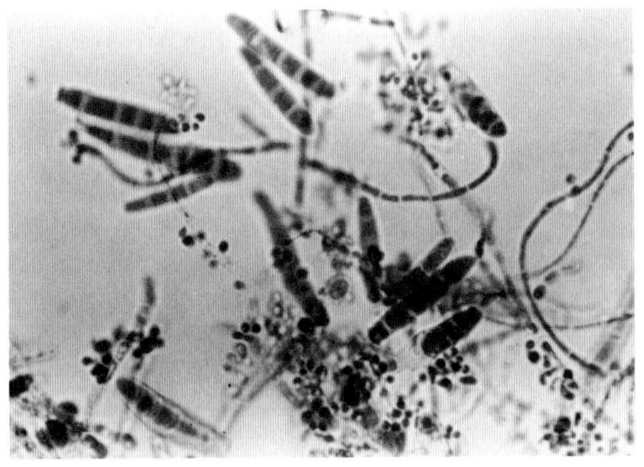

FIG. 13. Macro- and microconidia of *T. mentagrophytes* on SDA, plus 5% NaCl. ×400.

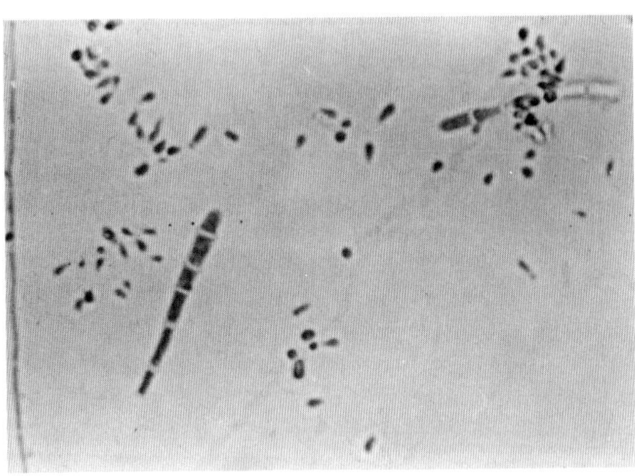

FIG. 16. Long, narrow macroconidium and clavate to pyriform microconidia of *T. rubrum.* ×400.

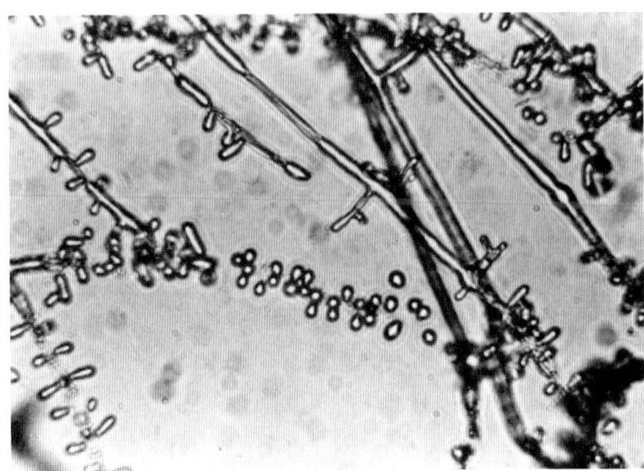

FIG. 14. Clavate and subspherical microconidia of *T. raubitschekii.* ×400.

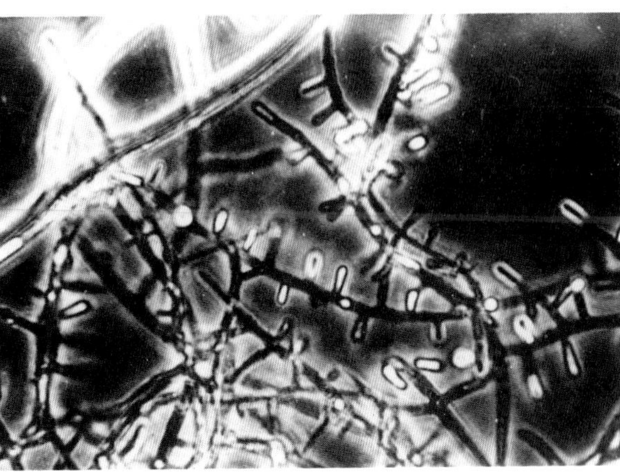

FIG. 17. Clavate macroconidium, microconidia, and intermediate conidia of *T. terrestre.* Phase contrast; ×400.

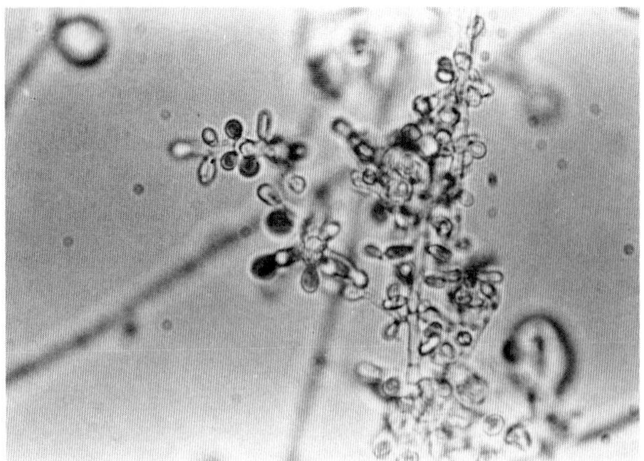

FIG. 18. Microconidia with typical condensed cytoplasm of *T. tonsurans*. ×400.

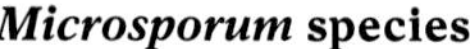

Microsporum species

Microsporum species produce macroconidia and microconidia that may be rare or numerous, depending on the species and substrate. The distinguishing characteristic is the macroconidium, which is rough walled (varying from minutely roughed, echinulate to verrucose). Macroconidia also vary in shape (obovate, fusiform to cylindrofusiform), number of septa (1 to 15), size (6 to 160 by 6 to 25 μm), and width of the cell wall. Microconidia are pyriform or clavate and usually are arranged singly along the sides of the hyphae. *Microsporum* species invade skin and hair, rarely nails.

Trichophyton species

Macroconidia have smooth, thin to thick walls, are variable in shape (clavate, fusiform to cylindrical), range in number of septa (1 to 12) and size (8 to 86 by 4 to 14 μm), and are borne singly or in clusters. Microconidia, which are usually more numerous than macroconidia, may be globose, pyriform, or clavate and are borne singly or in grapelike clusters. Although the production of microconidia is most characteristic of this genus, two species lacking microconidia have been described: *T. (Keratinomyces) longifuscum* (2, 16) and *T. kanei* (49).

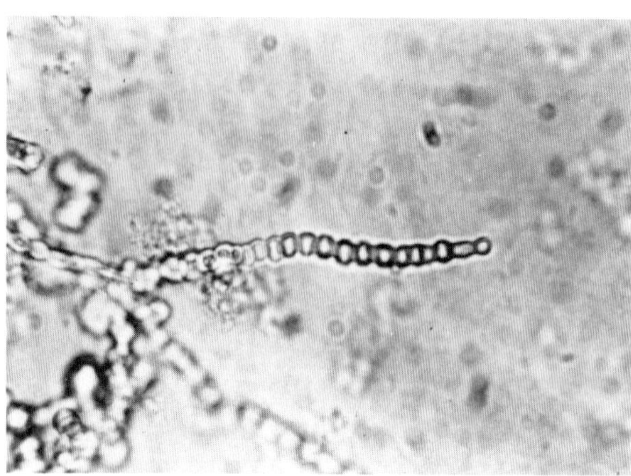

FIG. 19. Characteristic chlamydospores produced by *T. verrucosum* on BCP-casein-yeast extract agar. ×400.

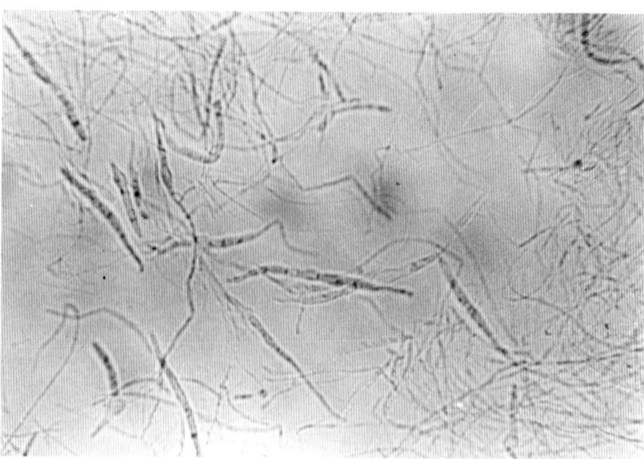

FIG. 20. Rat-tailed macroconidia of *T. verrucosum* on BCP-casein-yeast extract agar. ×400.

Characteristic features of the pathogenic dermatophytes are presented in Tables 3 and 4. These tables also include some similar but rarely pathogenic geophilic *Microsporum* and *Trichophyton* species and *T. fischeri*, which must be differentiated from *T. rubrum*.

SUPERFICIAL MYCOSES

Superficial mycoses include diseases in which the causative fungi colonize the cornified layers of the epidermis or the suprafollicular portion of the hair. There is little tissue damage, and cellular response from the

TABLE 2. Sequence of procedures for the identification of dermatophytes in pure culture[a]

1. Examine the colony for color of the surface and reverse, topography, texture, and rate of growth. Proceed to step 2.
2. Prepare teased mounts and search for identifying microscopic morphology, especially presence, appearance, and arrangement of macroconidia and microconidia (consult Fig. 5–20 and Tables 3 and 4). If results are inconclusive, proceed to step 3.
3. Prepare and examine slide cultures for characteristic morphology as indicated above if teased mounts do not provide sufficient information. Consider special media if sporulation is absent (potato-dextrose agar, SDA + 3–5% NaCl, lactrimel). If results are inconclusive, proceed to step 4.
4. Perform as many of the physiological tests listed below as necessary for identification:
   a. Urease.
   b. Nutritional requirements if a *Trichophyton* sp. is suspected.
   c. Growth on rice grains if a *Microsporum* sp. is suspected.
   d. In vitro hair perforation test.
   e. Temperature tolerance and/or optimum temperature of growth.
   f. Special media to differentiate *T. mentagrophytes* from *M. persicolor* (28), *T. rubrum* from *T. mentagrophytes* (50), and *T. soudanense* from *M. ferrugineum* (57).
   g. Mating studies to be performed in reference laboratories (38).

[a] It may be necessary to incubate cultures on brain heart infusion agar or similar medium to determine absence of bacterial contamination before proceeding to step 4. Procedures are adapted from Weitzman et al. (58).

TABLE 3. Important characteristics of pathogenic *Epidermophyton* and *Microsporum* species[a]

Species	Colony on SDA	Microscopic morphology	Comments
Epidermophyton			
E. floccosum	Yellowish green to khaki; flat to radially folded; powdery to velvety; yellow-brown reverse; white tufts common on surface of older cultures; slow growth.	Abundant, widely clavate, smooth-walled macroconidia, 20–40 by 6–8 μm, single or in clusters, 0–4 septa (Fig. 5); chlamydospores common in older cultures.	Invades skin and nails, not hair. No microconidia.
Microsporum			
M. audouinii	Grayish white, cream to tan, flat, spreading, velvety; light salmon pink to light reddish brown reverse; moderate growth.	Usually no conidia; apiculate, terminal chlamydospores are the only characteristic features; pectinate hyphae may be present.	Prepubertal tinea capitis and tinea corporis; poor growth and brownish discoloration on rice grains; sporulating strains have irregular fusiform and elongated macroconidia with few septa at irregular intervals (Fig. 6); microconidia rare to moderate; does not perforate hair in vitro (39).
M. canis			
var. *canis*	White to pale buff, woolly; yellow-orange to orange-brown, rarely nonpigmented reverse; rapid growth.	Numerous fusiform macroconidia with thick walls, up to 15 septa; 18–125 by 5–25 μm, with asymmetric knobbed apex (Fig. 7), few microconidia.	Good growth and sporulation on rice grains; perforates hair in vitro (39).
var. *distortum*	White to pale buff; usually with radial grooves, colorless to yellowish on reverse; rapid growth.	Macroconidia are distorted, bizarre in shape, 20–60 by 7–27 μm; microconidia abundant.	
M. cookei	Yellowish to reddish tan; flat; powdery, granular or downy; reverse dark purple-red; rapid growth.	Macroconidia numerous, some resembling *M. gypseum* but most have thicker walls (1–5 μm) (Fig. 8); microconidia abundant.	Geophilic species; rarely pathogenic.
M. equinum	White, pale buff to pale salmon; folding; velvety to finely powdery; buff to salmon on reverse.	Macroconidia infrequent on SDA, are elliptical to fusiform, 18–60 by 5–15 μm, 2 to 4 celled; thick walls, may resemble *M. canis* (Fig. 9).	Macroconidia stimulated by Niger seed medium 8 agar (26); does not perforate hair in vitro (39); growth on rice grains resemble that of *M. audouinii* (1).
M. ferrugineum	Yellowish to rust colored; folded; waxy; white, velvety variants found in Balkans (42); very slow grower.	Usually no conidia; numerous chlamydospores, irregular hyphae, and long, straight, coarse hyphae with prominent septa ("bamboo hyphae").	Geographically restricted to parts of Africa, Asia, eastern Europe; light yellow colonies on Lowenstein-Jensen medium differentiates it from dark, reddish brown colonies of *T. soudanense* (53, 58).
M. gallinae	White, tinged with pink, slightly folded, downy; raspberry red, diffusing pigment on reverse; rapid to moderate growth rate.	Macroconidia fairly abundant, blunt tipped, 6–8 by 15–50 μm, 2 to 10 celled; cell walls usually smooth, sometimes echinulate; pyriform microconidia.	Conidia stimulated by growth on media containing yeast extract or thiamine.
M. gypseum complex (*M. gypseum* and *M. fulvum*)	Pale buff, rosy buff to light cinnamon, white border; flat, powdery, granular to floccose; buff to reddish brown on reverse; rapid growth.	Abundant macroconidia, 25–60 by 7.5–15 μm; ellipsoidal to fusiform, up to 6 septa, thin walled (Fig. 10); microconidia moderately abundant.	Definitive identification of species is obtained by inducing the teleomorph by mating tester strains on appropriate media (38, 59).
M. nanum	Cream to buff; powdery reddish brown on reverse; moderate growth.	Abundant obovate to clavate macroconidia, 10.5–30 by 6.5–13 μm, usually 2 celled; microconidia few to moderate.	Grows more slowly than members of *M. gypseum* complex; must be differentiated from *Trichothecium roseum*.

(*Continued on next page*)

TABLE 3—*Continued*

Species	Colony on SDA	Microscopic morphology	Comments
M. persicolor	Yellowish buff becoming peach to pink; flat; powdery to downy; reddish brown on reverse; rapid growth.	Abundant microconidia, spherical to pyriform (few clavate), stalked, borne mostly in grapelike clusters but also singly along the slides of hyphae; thin-walled macroconidia (Fig. 11) often smooth; spiral hyphae common.	Resembles *T. mentagrophytes;* can be differentiated on BCP-milk solids-glucose medium (28); rough-walled macroconidia on SDA + 3% NaCl (28); peach to rose colonies on cereal agar (36). Absence of good growth at 37°C (28).
M. praecox	Cream to yellowish tan; folded, powdery; pale yellow to orange on reverse; moderate growth rate.	Numerous long fusiform macroconidia, some with apical appendages, 40–90 by 7–17 μm, 2–8 septa, thin walled; microconidia absent.	
M. racemosum	White, cream or buff; flat; finely granular; reverse dark purple-red; rapid growth.	Macroconidia abundant, fusiform to ellipsoidal, 41–77 by 9 μm, 3–8 septa, moderately thick walls; numerous microconidia mostly stalked and produced in grapelike clusters.	Macronidia resemble *M. gypseum.*
M. vanbreuseghemii	Pink to deep rose, light buff or yellowish; flat; coarsely granular to downy; reverse cream to pale yellow; rapid growth.	Abundant cylindrofusiform macroconidia, 43.8–87.5 μm, thick walled, up to 12 septa; numerous pyriform to obovate microconidia borne singly along sides of hyphae.	

[a] Adapted from Weitzman et al. (58).

host generally is lacking. The disease is essentially cosmetic, involving changes in the pigmentation of the skin (pityriasis versicolor or tinea nigra) or formation of nodules along the hair shaft distal from the follicle (black piedra and white piedra).

In contrast to the dermatophytoses, the etiologic agents are diverse and unrelated.

Pityriasis Versicolor (Tinea Versicolor)

Pityriasis versicolor is an infection of the stratum corneum caused by the lipophilic yeast *Malassezia furfur* (synonyms: *Pityrosporum furfur, P. orbiculare,* and *P. ovale*). Lesions appear as scaly, discrete or concrescent, hypopigmented or hyperpigmented (fawn, yellow brown, brown, or red) patches chiefly on the neck, torso, and limbs. The infection is largely cosmetic, becoming apparent when the skin fails to tan normally. The disease has a worldwide distribution; it is common in temperate zones and very prevalent in the tropics. *M. furfur* is found on the normal skin and elicits disease only under conditions, local or systemic, that favor the overgrowth of the organism.

M. furfur has been associated with folliculitis (7), obstructive dacryocystitis, systemic infections in patients receiving intralipid therapy (13), and seborrheic dermatitis, especially in patients with acquired immunodeficiency syndrome (AIDS) (18).

Direct examination

The fungus is observed readily when scrapings are mounted in 10% KOH plus ink (10), 25% NaOH plus 5% glycerin, or Kane's formulation (glycerol, 10 ml; Tween 80, 10 ml; phenol, 2.5 g; methylene blue, 1.0 g; distilled water, 480 ml). The presence of short, septate, occasionally branching filaments 2.5 to 4 μm in diameter and of variable length along with clusters of small, unicellular, oval or round budding yeast cells (budding is phialidic) averaging 4 μm (up to 8 μm) in size is diagnostic (Fig. 21).

Isolation and culture

Culture is not essential for identification unless the findings of direct microscopic examination are atypical. If culture is desired, olive oil added to the medium is essential. Scrapings may be inoculated on SDA plus cycloheximide and chloramphenicol (Mycosel [BBL] or Mycobiotic agar [Difco]) or Littman oxgall agar (Difco or Remel) and overlaid with sterile oil (we recommend Gallo or Pompeian) and incubated at 37°C. Growth is slow; colonies are cream colored, glossy, and raised (Fig. 22), later becoming dull, dry, and tan to brownish. Only budding yeast cells appear in culture (Fig. 23); hyphae are not found in routine isolation media, although short germ tubes may be produced.

Tinea Nigra

Tinea nigra is characterized by the appearance, primarily on the palms of the hands and less commonly on the dorsa of the feet, of flat, sharply marginated, brownish black nonscaly macules.

The disease is most common in the tropical areas of Central and South America, Africa, and Asia (41) and has been reported to be prevalent in North Carolina and along coastal areas of southeastern United States (54). Cases diagnosed outside of the endemic areas have resulted from travel to the American tropics or the Caribbean islands (41).

The etiologic agents are *Phaeoannellomyces* (*Exo-*

TABLE 4. Important characteristics of pathogenic *Trichophyton* species[a]

Species	Colony on SDA	Microscopic morphology	Comments[b]
T. ajelloi	Cream or orange-tan, flat, powdery; reverse blackish purple, sometimes nonpigmented; rapid growth.	Microconidia rare, macroconidia numerous, fusiform to cylindrical, thick walled, multiseptate, 5–12 celled (Fig. 12).	Geophilic species, rarely pathogenic.
T. concentricum	Beige, brown, or reddish; elevated and convoluted glabrous to velvety; no undersurface color; slow growing.	Micro- and macroconidia usually absent; chlamydospores may be present.	Geographically restricted; 50% of isolates are stimulated by thiamine, others are autotrophic.
T. equinum	Cream colored; flat; fluffy; reverse yellow becoming reddish brown.	Pyriform or spherical microconidia; macroconidia rare, similar to those of *T. mentagrophytes*.	Requires nicotinic acid; an autotrophic variety has been described (47).
T. fischeri	White, velvety to cottony; reverse brownish red to wine red; closely resembles *T. rubrum*	Pyriform and subglobose micronidia abundant along unbranched hyphae, macroconidia long and sinuous, cylindrical to clavate; thin closterosporelike hypha projections often produced.	Geophilic species not pathogenic, growth at 37°C; urease test negative; in vitro hair perforation test negative; growth restricted on BCPCDA, no pH change within 7 days; no red undersurface pigment on CEAA (23); must be differentiated from *T. rubrum* and *T. raubitschekii* (27).
T. gourvilii	Pink to red; heaped up; convoluted; glabrous; becoming velvety.	Typical *Trichophyton*-type macroconidia and microconidia usually found.	No special nutritional requirements.
T. kanei	White velvety to granular; reverse brownish red to wine red.	Macroconidia predominant, cylindrical to clavate, often with T-shaped bases; microconidia absent; arthroconidia small, mostly cylindrical, pyriform when formed terminally.	Urease test weakly positive; in vitro hair test negative; growth restricted on BCPCDA, no pH change within 7 days.
T. megninii	Pink to rose; radially folded; suedelike; reverse wine red.	Pyriform to clavate microconidia; macroconidia rare, similar to those of *T. rubrum*.	Requires L-histidine; urease positive.
T. mentagrophytes	Cream, tan, or pink; flat; powdery to granular or fluffy; reverse light tan, yellow, red, or reddish brown; sometimes producing a diffusible melanoid pigment.	Round to pyriform microconidia in clusters or singly along the hyphae; clavate macroconidia present in some strains (Fig. 13); coiled hyphae (spirals) are usually seen.	Urease positive; perforates hair in vitro; grows at 37°C; growth profuse on BCPCDA, with alkalinity within 7 days.
T. raubitschekii	Buff; raised center with radial grooves; velvety to granular; reverse blood red.	Microconidia clavate, globose or subspherical, sessile, or on short stalks along unbranched hyphae; macroconidia abundant on primary isolation; thin, elongate with blunt ends, 5–9 celled (Fig. 14 and 15).	Urease positive; in vitro hair perforation test negative; brown pigmentation on CMD agar (27); growth restricted on BCPCDA, no pH change within 7 days.

(*Continued on next page*)

TABLE 4—*Continued*

Species	Colony on SDA	Microscopic morphology	Comments[b]
T. rubrum	White; velvety, seldom powdery; reverse wine red, sometimes yellow, orange, or a diffusible melanoid pigment; growth and color variants have been described (61).	Pyriform microconidia usually along unbranched hyphae; macroconidia absent to rare, thin, cylindrical to clavate in granular cultures (Fig. 16).	Urease test negative; in vitro hair perforation test negative; red undersurface pigment on CMD and CEAA agars except in yellow or hyaline variants (15); growth restricted on BCPCDA, no pH change within 7 days; must be differentiated from *T. raubitschekii* (27) and *T. fischeri* (23).
T. schoenleinii	White to tan; heaped and convoluted; glabrous or waxy, becoming velvety on subculture; reverse lacking pigment; slow growth.	Micro- and macroconidia rarely seen; chlamydospores often numerous; hyphal tips often show "nailhead" morphology and branch to form antlerlike structures (favic chandeliers).	Autotrophic for vitamins, which differentiates it from *T. verrucosum*.
T. simii	White to pale buff; flat or slightly convoluted; powdery; reverse straw to salmon.	Numerous macroconidia, some fragment or develop swellings resembling chlamydospores; pyriform microconidia and spirals may be found.	
T. soudanense	Yellow-orange (like dried apricots); flat with convolutions; suedelike texture; fringed (eyelash) periphery; reverse yellow to orange-yellow; slow growing.	Pyriform microconidia rare; macroconidia very rare; reflex branching characteristic.	Growth stimulated at 37°C (57).
T. terrestre	White, pale yellow, or red; flat; granular to downy; reverse pale yellow, yellowish brown or red; rapid growth.	Microconidia clavate to pyriform, single or clustered, short, intermediate, or fully extended to attain the size of macroconidia; clavate to cylindrical, thin walled, 2–6 celled (Fig. 17).	Geophilic, rarely pathogenic; usually no growth at 37°C; must be differentiated from *T. mentagrophytes*.
T. tonsurans	Color varies with isolate (yellow, cream, white, pink, brown, gray, etc.); convoluted; raised or flat; velvety to powdery; reverse dark brown to mahogany red; slow growing.	Clavate to elongate microconidia, some swollen into balloon forms and attached to branched conidiophore by a short stalk (Fig. 18); macroconidia rare.	Stimulated by thiamine.
T. verrucosum	Cream to tan; flat; discoid; velvety (var. *discoides*); white, heaped, and folded, glabrous to downy (var. *album*); yellow-ochre; convoluted; glabrous (var. *ochraceum*); slow growing.	Usually no micro- or macroconidia; chlamydospores usually numerous and in chains (Fig. 19).	All strains require thiamine; most require inositol as well; growth stimulated at 37°C; growth and hydrolysis within 6 days on BCPCYA medium (29); rat-tailed macroconidia also stimulated (Fig. 20), characteristics differentiating it from *T. schoenleinii*.
T. violaceum	Violet or lavender; heaped and convoluted; glabrous or velvety; purple undersurface; slow growing.	Micro- and macroconidia usually lacking; chlamydospores may be found.	Growth and sporulation stimulated by thiamine.
T. yaoundei	Initially buff, turning to chocolate brown; diffusible; slow growing.	Pyriform microconidia rare; macroconidia not found; chlamydospores seen.	Geographically limited to Africa.

[a] Adapted from Weitzman et al. (58).
[b] CEAA, Casamino Acids-erythritol-albumin agar; CMA, cornmeal agar; BCPCDA, bromocresol purple-casein-dextrose agar; BCPCYA, bromocresol purple-casein-yeast extract agar.

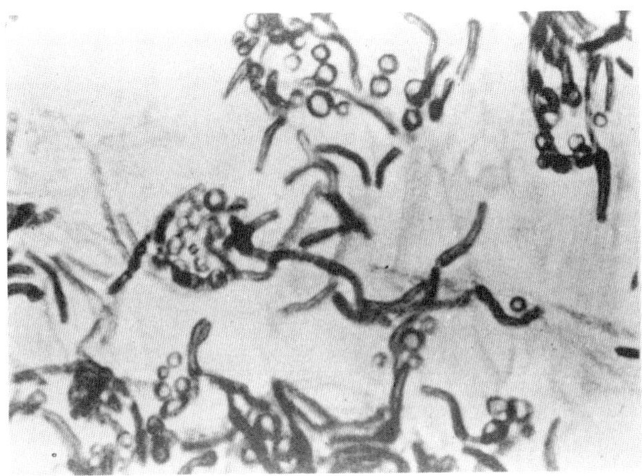

FIG. 21. *Malassezia furfur* in skin scrapings from a lesion of pityriasis versicolor (Kane's stain). ×1,000.

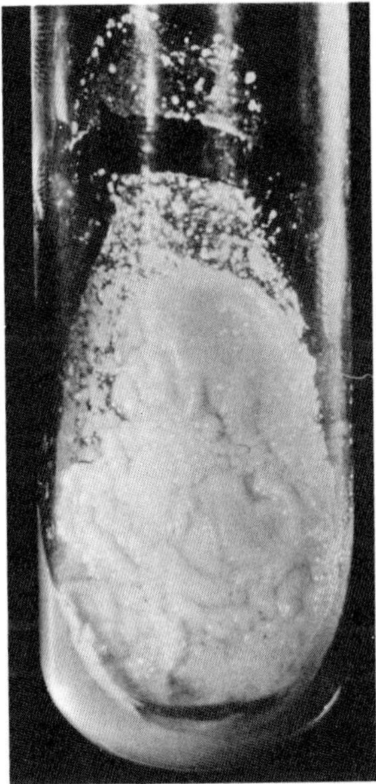

FIG. 22. Culture of *Malassezia furfur* on Littman oxgall agar overlaid with olive oil (Gallo).

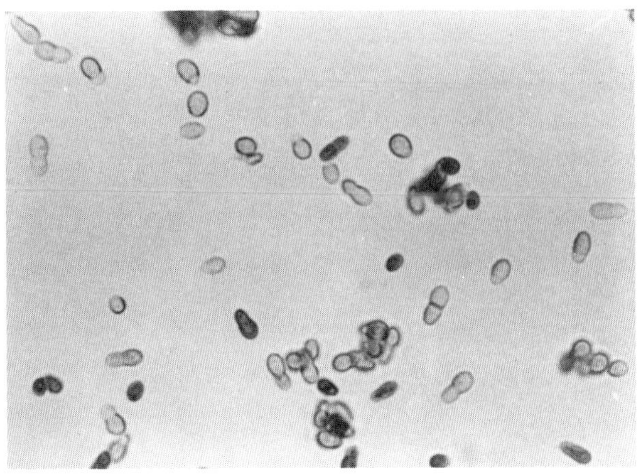

FIG. 23. *Malassezia furfur*, microscopic appearance of yeast cells on Littman oxgall overlaid with olive oil. ×400.

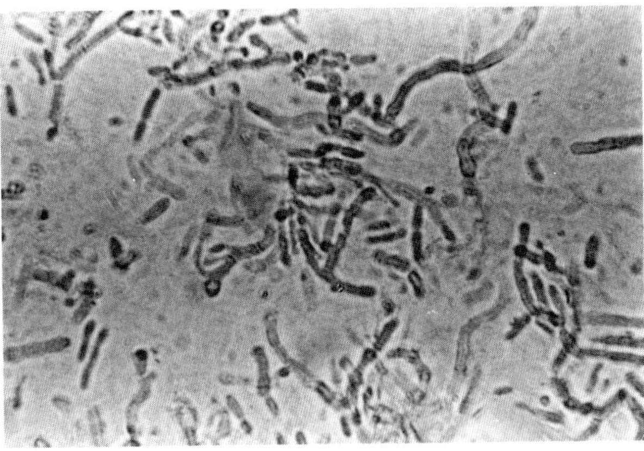

FIG. 24. *P. werneckii* in NaOH mount of skin from lesion of *T. nigra*. ×400.

phiala or *Cladosporium*) *werneckii* (34) and *Stenella araguata*. *S. araguata* is very rare and will not be described here.

Direct microscopic examination

Microscopic examination of skin scrapings with KOH or NaOH reveals numerous light brown, frequently branching septate filaments 1.5 to 5 μm in diameter, short sinuous septate fragments (Fig. 24), and budding cells, some septate.

Isolation, culture, and identification

On SDA with or without antibiotics, *P. werneckii* grows slowly and usually appears within 2 to 3 weeks as moist, shiny, olive to greenish black yeastlike colonies, occasionally only mycelial (34). Microscopic observation of the yeastlike colonies reveals one- to two-celled pale brown to deeply pigmented cylindrical to spindle-shaped cells with some budding. The cells are rounded at one end and tapered toward the other (Fig. 25), with annellations (rings) at the tapered end (34). With prolonged incubation, the colonies develop velvety, greenish gray to grayish black aerial mycelium over portions of the yeastlike growth. As the colonies become more mycelial, microscopic observation will reveal olivaceous, thin or broad, often thick-walled hy-

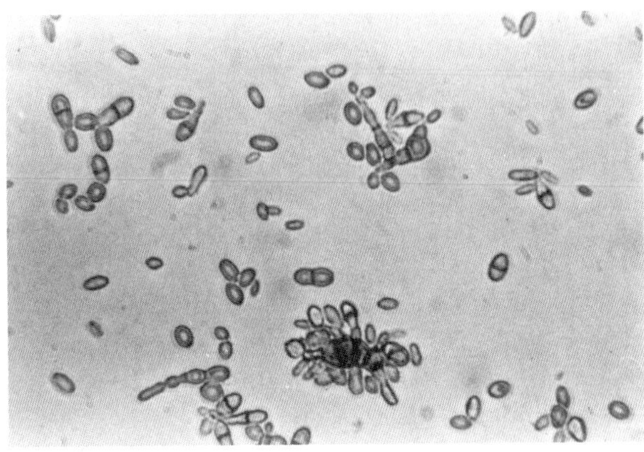

FIG. 25. *P. werneckii* after 2 weeks on SDA. Note dematiaceous unicellular and bicellular annelloconidia. ×400.

phae septate at frequent intervals. Along these hyphae, one- to two-celled hyaline to olivaceous annelloconidia arise from intercalary annellides or from annellides integrated within the hyphae. These annelloconidia tend to accumulate in balls, eventually sliding down along the sides of the hyphae. Seceded conidia may produce new conidia by budding.

Black Piedra

Black piedra is a fungal infection of the scalp hair, less commonly the beard or moustache, and rarely axillary or pubic hairs. The disease is characterized by the presence of discrete, hard, and gritty dark brown to black nodules adhering firmly to the hair shaft (Fig. 26). It is found mostly in tropical regions in Africa, Asia, and Central and South America. Humans as well as primates are infected.

The etiologic agent in humans is *Piedraia hortae,* an ascomycete whose nodules serve as ascostromata containing locules which harbor the asci and ascospores.

Direct microscopic examination

Hair fragments containing the nodules are mounted in 25% NaOH or KOH, heated gently, and carefully squashed without breaking the cover slip (the nodules are very hard). The squashed preparation of a mature nodule should reveal compact masses of dark, septate hyphae around the surface of the hair and round to oval asci containing hyaline, curved, fusiform, aseptate ascospores that bear one or more appendages.

Isolation, culture, and identification

SDA with chloramphenicol and SDA with chloramphenicol and cycloheximide should be used for isolation. Some reports have indicated that cycloheximide may be inhibitory; howèver, others have used this antibiotic successfully.

Colonies are very slow growing, dark brown to black, and heaped in the center with a flat periphery. A greenish brown, short aerial mycelium eventually covers the young glabrous colony. Microscopic examination reveals only dark hyphae; conidia and ascospores are not found on routine mycological media.

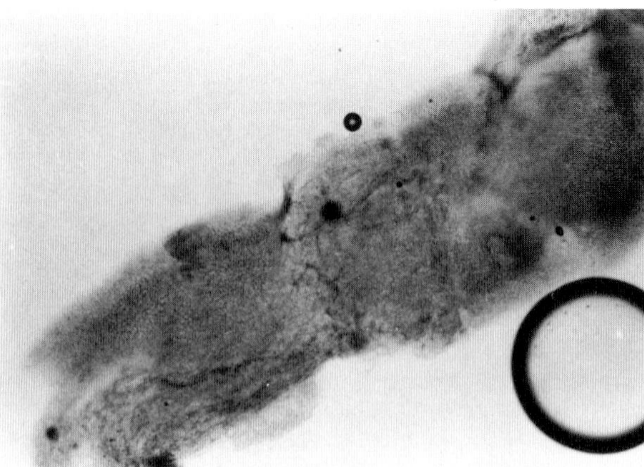

FIG. 27. White piedra nodule on hair from the groin. ×1,000.

White Piedra

White piedra is a fungus infection of the hair shaft characterized by the presence of soft white, yellowish, beige, or greenish nodules found chiefly on facial, axillary, or genital hairs (Fig. 27) and less commonly on scalp, eyebrows, and eyelashes. Nodules may be discrete or more often coalescent, forming an irregular transparent sheath.

The infection occurs sporadically in North America and Europe and more commonly is found in South America and the Orient (41). Although white piedra is an uncommon infection, genital white piedra is more frequent in certain populations (21, 48).

The etiologic agent, *Trichosporon beigelii* (*cutaneum*), is found in the normal flora of the skin and in the environment. Humans as well as domestic animals, especially horses, may be infected (41). *T. beigelii* also has been reported to cause disseminated infections in immunosuppressed patients (20).

Direct microscopic examination

Microscopic examination of hairs containing the adherent nodules mounted in 10% KOH or 25% NaOH plus 5% glycerin and squashed under a cover slip will

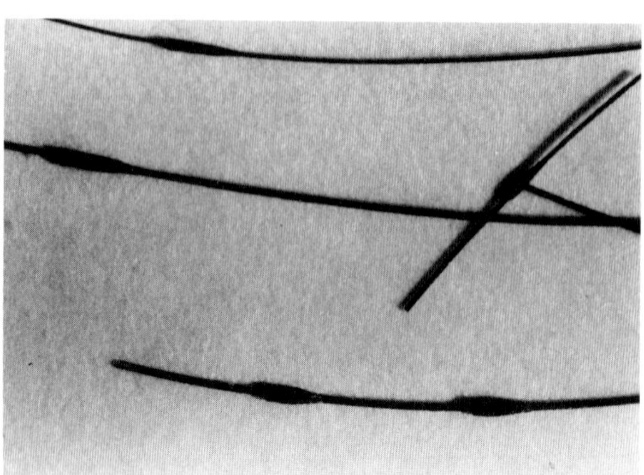

FIG. 26. Black piedra nodules on scalp hair. NaOH mount; ×100.

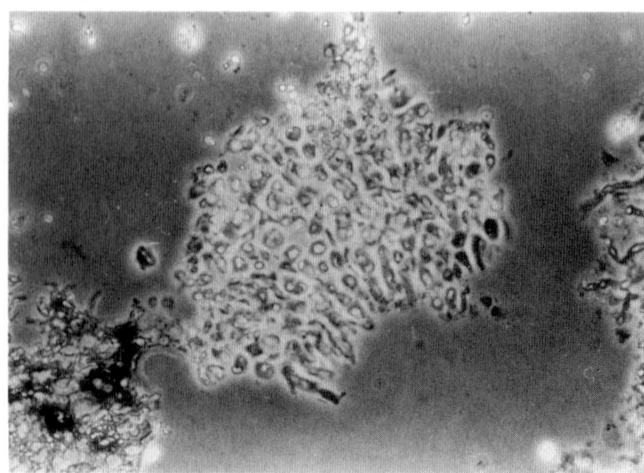

FIG. 28. *T. beigelii* arthroconidia from a crushed nodule of white piedra. ×1,000.

reveal intertwined hyaline septate hyphae, hyphae breaking up into oval or rectangular arthroconidia 2 to 4 μm in diameter (Fig. 28), occasional blastoconidia, and bacteria which may surround the nodule as a zoo-glea.

Isolation, culture, and identification

T. beigelii may be isolated readily on SDA with chloramphenicol or other isolation media containing antibacterial antibiotics. The isolation medium should not contain cycloheximide, since it is inhibitory. Growth on routine culture media is rapid, resulting in cream-colored, soft colonies when young, becoming membranous, wrinkled with radial furrows and irregular folding with age. Microscopically, the presence of hyaline hyphae, arthroconidia, and blastoconidia is characteristic of the genus. Physiological studies are necessary for species identification. *T. beigelii* (*cutaneum*) does not ferment carbohydrates; it assimilates dextrose, lactose, D-xylose, and inositol. The following commonly used carbon compounds are assimilated by some isolates and not by others: galactose, sucrose, maltose, cellobiose, trehalose, raffinose, L-arabinose, and erythritol. This organism does not assimilate potassium nitrate, is urease positive, and gives a positive reaction with diazonium blue B salt (31).

LITERATURE CITED

1. **Aho, R.** 1987. Mycological studies on *Microsporum equinum* isolated in Finland, Sweden and Norway. J. Med. Vet. Mycol. **25:**255–260.
2. **Ajello, L.** 1968. A taxonomic review of the dermatophytes and related species. Sabouraudia **6:**147–159.
3. **Ajello, L.** 1960. Geographic distribution and prevalence of the dermatophytes. Ann. N.Y. Acad. Sci. **89:**30–38.
4. **Ajello, L., and L. K. Georg.** 1957. In vitro cultures for differentiating between atypical isolates of *Trichophyton mentagrophytes* and *Trichophyton rubrum*. Mycopathol. Mycol. Appl. **8:**3–7.
5. **Alsop, J., and A. P. Prior.** 1961. Ringworm infection in a cucumber greenhouse. Br. Med. J. **1:**1081–1083.
6. **Araviysky, A. N., R. A. Araviysky, and G. A. Eschkov.** 1975. Deep generalized trichophytosis. Mycopathologia **56:** 47–65.
7. **Back, O., J. Faergemann, and R. Hornquist.** 1985. Pityrosporum folliculitis: a common disease of the young and middle-aged. J. Am. Acad. Dermatol. **12:**56–61.
8. **Barson, W. J.** 1985. Granuloma and pseudogranuloma of the skin due to *Microsporum canis*. Arch. Dermatol. **121:** 895–897.
9. **Borelli, D.** 1962. Medios caseros para micologıa. Arch. Venez. Med. Trop. Parasitol. Med. **4:**301–310.
10. **Cohen, M. M.** 1954. A simple procedure for staining tinea versicolor (*M. furfur*) with fountain pen ink. J. Invest. Dermatol. **22:**9–10.
11. **Conant, N. F.** 1936. Studies on the genus *Microsporum*. I. Cultural studies. Arch. Dermatol. **33:**665–683.
12. **Currah, R. S.** 1985. Taxonomy of the Onygenales: Arthrodermataceae, Gymnoascaceae, Myxotrichaceae and Onygenaceae. Mycotaxon **24:**1–216.
13. **Danker, W. M., S. A. Spector, J. Fierer, and C. E. Davis.** 1987. *Malassezia* fungemia in neonates and adults: complication of hyperalimentation. Rev. Infect. Dis. **9:**743–753.
14. **Dei Cas, E., and A. Vernes.** 1986. Parasitic adaptation of pathogenic fungi to mammalian hosts. Crit. Rev. Microbiol. **13:**173–218.
15. **Fischer, J. B., and J. Kane.** 1974. The laboratory diagnosis of dermatophytosis complicated with *Candida albicans*. Can. J. Microbiol. **20:**167–182.
16. **Flórián, E., and J. Galgóczy.** 1964. *Keratinomyces longifusus* sp. nov. from Hungary. Mycopathol. Mycol. Appl. **24:**73–80.
17. **Georg, L. K., and L. B. Camp.** 1957. Routine nutritional tests for the identification of dermatophytes. J. Bacteriol. **74:**113–121.
18. **Groisser, D., E. J. Bottone, and M. Lebwohl.** 1989. Association of *Pityrosporum orbiculare* (*Malassezia furfur*) with seborrheic dermatitis in patients with acquired immunodeficiency syndrome (AIDS). J. Am. Acad. Dermatol. **20:**770–773.
19. **Head, E. S., J. C. Henry, and E. M. MacDonald.** 1984. The cotton swab: technic for the culture of dermatophyte infections: its efficacy and merit. J. Am. Acad. Dermatol. **11:**797–801.
20. **Hoy, J., K.-C. Hsu, K. Rolston, R. L. Hopfer, M. Luna, and G. P. Bodey.** 1986. *Trichosporon beigelii* infection: a review. Rev. Infect. Dis. **8:**959–967.
21. **Kalter, D. C., J. A. Tschen, P. L. Cernoch, M. E. McBride, J. Sperber, S. Bruce, and J. E. Wolf, Jr.** 1986. Genital white piedra: epidemiology, microbiology, and therapy. J. Am. Acad. Dermatol. **14:**982–993.
22. **Kaminski, G. W.** 1985. The routine use of modified Borelli's lactritmel (MBLA). Mycopathologia **91:**57–59.
23. **Kane, J.** 1977. *Trichophyton fischeri* sp. nov.: a saprophyte resembling *Trichophyton rubrum*. Sabouraudia **15:**231–241.
24. **Kane, J., and J. B. Fischer.** 1975. The effect of sodium chloride on the growth and morphology of dermatophytes and some other keratolytic fungi. Can. J. Microbiol. **21:** 742–749.
25. **Kane, J., and J. B. Fischer.** 1976. The differentiation of *Trichophyton rubrum* from *T. mentagrophytes* by use of Christensen's urea broth. Can. J. Microbiol. **17:**911–913.
26. **Kane, J., A. A. Padhye, and L. Ajello.** 1982. *Microsporum equinum* in North America. J. Clin. Microbiol. **16:**943–947.
27. **Kane, J., I. F. Salkin, I. Weitzman, and C. Smitka.** 1981. *Trichophyton raubitschekii*, sp. nov. Mycotaxon **13:**259–266.
28. **Kane, J., L. Sigler, and R. C. Summerbell.** 1987. Improved procedures for differentiating *Microsporum persicolor* from *Trichophyton mentagrophytes*. J. Clin. Microbiol. **25:**2449–2452.
29. **Kane, J., and C. Smitka.** 1978. Early detection and identification of *Trichophyton verrucosum*. J. Clin. Microbiol. **8:**740–747.
30. **King, R. D., H. A. Khan, J. C. Foye, J. H. Greenberg, and H. E. Jones.** 1975. Transferrin, iron and dermatophytes. 1. Serum dermatophyte inhibitory component definitively identified as unsaturated transferrin. J. Lab. Clin. Med. **86:**204–212.
31. **Kreger-Van Rij, N. J. W.** 1984. *Trichosporon* Behrend. *In* N. J. W. Kreger-Van Rij (ed.), The yeasts, a taxonomic study, 3rd ed., p. 933–962. Elsevier, Amsterdam.
32. **Lawson, G. T. N., and W. J. McLeod.** 1957. *Microsporum canis*—an intensive outbreak. Br. Med. J. **2:**1159–1160.
33. **Mackenzie, D. W. R.** 1963. "Hairbrush diagnosis" in detection and eradication of nonfluorescent scalp ringworm. Br. Med. J. **2:**363–365.
34. **McGinnis, M. R., W. A. Schell, and J. Carson.** *Phaeoannellomyces* and the Phaeococcomycetaceae, new dematiaceous blastomycete taxa. Sabouraudia **23:**179–188.
35. **Merz, W. G., C. L. Berger, and M. Silva-Hutner.** 1970. Media with pH indicators for the isolation of dermatophytes. Arch. Dermatol. **102:**545–547.
36. **Padhye, A. A., F. Blank, P. J. Koblenzer, S. Spatz, and L. Ajello.** 1973. *Microsporum persicolor* infection in the United States. Arch. Dermatol. **108:**561–562.
37. **Padhye, A. A., and J. W. Carmichael.** 1971. The genus *Arthroderma* Berkeley. Can. J. Bot. **49:**1525–1540.
38. **Padhye, A. A., A. S. Sekohn, and J. W. Carmichael.** 1973. Ascocarp production by *Arthroderma* and *Nannizzia* species

on keratinous and non-keratinous media. Sabouraudia **11:** 109–114.

39. **Padhye, A. A., C. N. Young, and L. Ajello.** 1980. Hair perforation as a diagnostic criterion in the identification of *Epidermophyton, Microsporum* and *Trichophyton* species, p. 115–120. *In* Superficial cutaneous and subcutaneous infections. Scientific publication no. 396. Pan American Health Organization, Washington, D.C.
40. **Rippon, J. W.** 1985. The changing epidemiology and emerging patterns of dermatophyte species, p. 209–234. *In* M. R. McGinnis (ed.), Current topics in medical mycology. Springer-Verlag, New York.
41. **Rippon, J. W.** 1988. Medical mycology: the pathogenic fungi and the pathogenic actinomycetes, 3rd ed., p. 154–168. The W. B. Saunders Co., Philadelphia.
42. **Rippon, J. W.** 1988. Medical mycology: the pathogenic fungi and the pathogenic actinomycetes, 3rd ed., p. 169–275. The W. B. Saunders Co., Philadelphia.
43. **Robinson, B. E., and A. A. Padhye.** 1988. Collection, transport and processing of clinical specimens, p. 11–32. *In* B. B. Wentworth (ed.), Diagnostic procedures for mycotic and parasitic infections, 7th ed. American Public Health Association, Inc., Washington, D.C.
44. **Rosenthal, S. A.** 1974. The epidemiology of tinea pedis, p. 515–526. *In* H. M. Robinson, Jr. (ed.), The diagnosis and treatment of fungal infections. Charles C Thomas, Publisher, Springfield, Ill.
45. **Rosenthal, S. A., and H. Sokolsky.** 1965. Enzymatic studies with pathogenic fungi. Dermatol. Int. **4:**72–79.
46. **Salkin, I. F.** 1973. Dermatophyte test medium: evaluation with nondermatophytic pathogens. Appl. Microbiol. **26:** 134–137.
47. **Smith, J. M. B., R. D. Jolly, L. K. Georg, and M. D. Connole.** 1968. *Trichophyton equinum* var. *autrophicum:* its characteristics and geographic distribution. Sabouraudia **6:**296–304.
48. **Stenderup, A., H. Schonheyder, P. Ebbesen, and M. Melbye.** 1986. White piedra and *Trichosporon beigelii* carriage in homosexual men. J. Med. Vet. Mycol. **24:**401–406.
49. **Summerbell, R. C.** 1987. *Trichophyton kanei,* sp. nov. a new anthropophilic dermatophyte. Mycotaxon **28:**509–523.
50. **Summerbell, R. C., S. A. Rosenthal, and J. Kane.** 1988. Rapid method for differentiation of *Trichophyton rubrum, Trichophyton mentagrophytes,* and related dermatophyte species. J. Clin. Microbiol. **26:**2279–2282.
51. **Taplin, D.** 1965. The use of gentamicin in mycology. J. Invest. Dermatol. **45:**549–550.
52. **Taplin, D., N. Zaias, G. Rebell, and H. Blank.** 1969. Isolation and recognition of dermatophytes on a new medium (DTM). Arch. Dermatol. **99:**203–209.
53. **Vanbreuseghem, R., and R. Zaman.** 1963. Contribution à l'identification du *Trichophyton* (*Langeronia*) *soudanense* et du *Trichophyton ferrugineum.* Ann. Soc. Belge Med. Trop. **3:**259–270.
54. **Van Velsor, H., and H. Singletary.** 1964. Tinea nigra palmaris. Arch. Dermatol. **90:**59–61.
55. **Weeks, R. J., and A. A. Padhye.** 1982. A mounting medium for permanent preparations of micro-fungi. Mykosen **25:** 702–704.
56. **Weitzman, I., M. R. McGinnis, A. A. Padhye, and L. Ajello.** 1986. The genus *Arthroderma* and its later synonym *Nannizzia.* Mycotaxon **25:**505–518.
57. **Weitzman, I., and S. A. Rosenthal.** 1983/1984. Studies in the differentiation between *Microsporum ferrugineum* Ota and *Trichophyton soudanense* Joyeux. Mycopathologia **84:**95–101.
58. **Weitzman, I., S. A. Rosenthal, and M. Silva-Hutner.** 1988. Superficial and cutaneous infections caused by molds: dermatomycoses, p. 33–97. *In* B. B. Wentworth (ed.), Diagnostic procedures for mycotic and parasitic infections, 7th ed. American Public Health Association, Inc., Washington, D.C.
59. **Weitzman, I., and M. Silva-Hutner.** 1967. Non-keratinous agar media as substrates for the ascigerous state in certain members of the gynmoascaceae pathogenic for man and animals. Sabouraudia **5:**335–339.
60. **West, B. C., and K. J. Kwon-Chung.** 1980. Mycetoma caused by *Microsporum audouinii.* Am. J. Clin. Pathol. **73:** 447–454.
61. **Young, C. N.** 1972. Range of variation among isolates of *Trichophyton rubrum.* Sabouraudia **10:**164–170.

Chapter 60

Yeasts of Medical Importance

NANCY G. WARREN AND H. JEAN SHADOMY

NATURAL HABITAT AND CLINICAL SIGNIFICANCE

Yeasts are ubiquitous in our environment, being found on fruits, vegetables, and other plant materials (exogenous). Some live as normal inhabitants in and on our bodies (endogenous). Therefore, they may be found in specimens without having any clinical significance. Yeasts are considered opportunistic pathogens and as such may be cultured from specimens of patients debilitated in some fashion, e.g., by hormone imbalance or by the administration of immunosuppressive agents such as corticosteroids, anticancer drugs, the newer anti-AIDS drugs, or the overuse of broad-spectrum antibiotics. Patients who undergo transplant surgery with the concomitant administration of immunosuppressive drugs often may acquire yeast infections. Diseases such as AIDS and others that cause a diminution or depletion of the immunological system also are predisposing factors for yeast infections. Endocarditis caused by yeasts has been associated with the use of nonsterile equipment by drug addicts. Fungemia may occur when indwelling catheters are not changed or removed at frequent intervals; it also has been reported in infants supported by lipid-supplemented hyperalimentation (12).

Yeasts are by far the most common fungi isolated from human patients. The decision as to the significance of their presence in a specimen ultimately rests with the physician, but accurate, complete information from the laboratory is essential for a reasonable conclusion to be made. Taking careful note of such information as type of specimen (e.g., closed, normally sterile sites rather than sputum or urine), number of specimens positive with the same organism from the same patient, and number of colonies formed is essential if a correct conclusion is to be made.

CHARACTERISTICS OF YEASTS

Yeasts are unicellular, eucaryotic, budding cells, generally round to oval or, less often, elongate or irregular in shape. They multiply principally by the production of blastoconidia (buds). When blastoconidia are produced one from the other in a linear fashion without separating, a structure termed a pseudohypha is formed. Under certain circumstances, some yeasts may produce true septate hyphae. Such circumstances are associated with the diminution of oxygen, e.g., submerged colonies in agar medium, at the bottom of broth media in a test tube, or in the presence of 5 to 10% CO_2. This phenomenon also may occur in host tissues as a result of reduced oxygen tension.

Cultures of yeasts are moist, creamy, or glabrous to membranous in texture. Several produce a capsule which may make the colony mucoid. With rare exceptions, aerial hyphae are not produced. Colonies may be hyaline or brightly colored, or they may be darkly pigmented as a result of the presence of melanins. This latter group, found in the Dematiaceae, is discussed in chapter 62. Dimorphic fungal pathogens possessing a yeast phase in tissue are discussed in the context of each individual organism.

Although there are many genera and hundreds of species termed yeasts, only a relative few produce disease in humans and animals. They generally are identified (classified) by observing the macroscopic and microscopic features mentioned above. Usually, biochemical tests also are required for definitive identification to the species level. Most of the pathogenic yeasts are found in the Deuteromycetes, or Fungi Imperfecti, that is, fungi which do not exhibit the sexual or teleomorphic state in culture.

Yeasts also may be classified by their method of sexual reproduction into the Ascomycetes and Heterobasidiomycetes. A few genera may produce the sexual state on standard mycological media over time. In some instances, it may be necessary to identify the teleomorphic state of a yeast culture. This is best accomplished by submitting it to a reference laboratory for further study.

DIRECT EXAMINATION

The appropriate examination of a clinical specimen is essential prior to proper processing of the material. Additionally, it often will aid the laboratorian and the physician in a preliminary identification, either ruling in or out certain pathogenic yeasts. Certain methods are universal to the preliminary observation of fungi in a specimen, e.g., Gram stain, Calcofluor, and 20% KOH. However, others such as the India ink preparation for the demonstration of a capsule, are used for the yeasts and yeastlike fungi only. This preparation is used with cultures and on specimens of urine, cerebrospinal fluid, etc., that have been centrifuged. It generally is not useful on primary specimens such as sputum or other material that do not allow even distribution of the ink. It must be remembered that if 20% KOH is used on a preparation, neither the India ink nor Gram stain subsequently may be added.

In performing the microscopic examination of a specimen for yeasts, features may be observed that can aid in identification: (i) size and shape of the organism, (ii) mode of attachment of bud(s), (iii) presence or absence of a capsule, (iv) thickness of cell wall, (v) presence of pseudohyphae, and (vi) presence of arthroconidia. Other unusual structures also should be noted.

IDENTIFICATION

A scheme for yeast identification is presented in Fig. 1. As a general guideline, it offers a basic approach to yeast identification but also allows flexibility for adaptation to individual laboratory situations. Morphologic and physiologic properties of the most commonly encountered yeasts in clinical specimens are found in Table 1. Particularly salient characteristics of individual yeasts will be reemphasized in the sections dealing with specific yeast genera. A sound, systematic approach to yeast identification cannot be stressed enough. With the numerous yeast identification systems available today, most yeast species can be identified easily; however, repeat testing sometimes is necessary, and morphologic characteristics on cornmeal or similar agars should be mandatory.

Macroscopic characteristics of yeasts

Most yeasts grow well (*Malassezia furfur* being an exception) on common mycological and bacteriological media. Growth is usually detected in 48 to 72 h, and subcultures or laboratory-adapted strains may grow more rapidly. Colonies have a smooth to wrinkled, creamy appearance; some pigment may be observed initially or intensify with age. Heavily encapsulated yeasts have a very moist, mucoid appearance.

The ability of yeasts to grow at 37°C is a very important characteristic. Most pathogenic species grow readily at 25 and 37°C, whereas saprophytes usually fail to grow at the higher temperature. In addition, some yeast species, e.g., *Candida albicans*, grow in the presence of cycloheximide (Acti-Dione) found in Mycosel (BBL Microbiology Systems, Cockeysville, Md.), Mycobiotic (Difco Laboratories, Detroit, Mich.), and similar agars, whereas most other yeasts, including *Cryptococcus neoformans*, are inhibited.

Pellicle growth on the surface of liquid media such as Sabouraud dextrose broth or malt extract broth has been used in the past to assist with yeast identification. More recent evidence suggests that this characteristic can be variable; however, as an ancillary test, it may be helpful with identifying *Candida tropicalis*, *Candida krusei*, and *Trichosporon* spp.

Microscopic characteristics of yeasts

Upon isolation of a suspected yeast from clinical specimens, the first examination made should be a wet preparation of a colony. A small amount of growth is

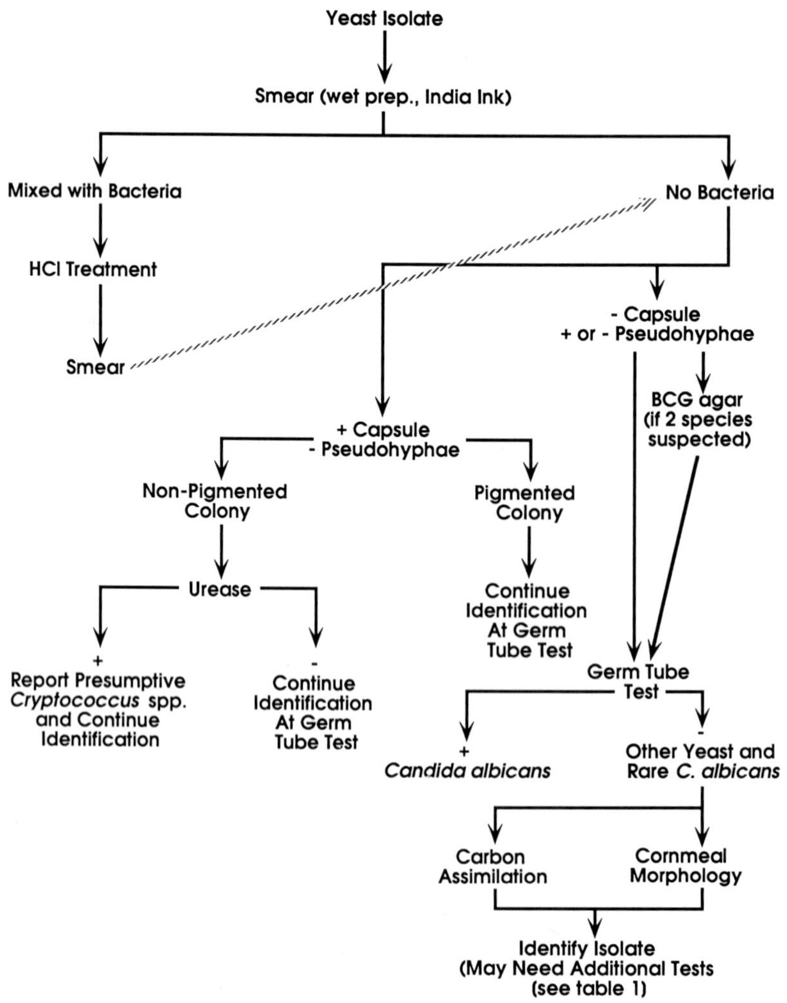

FIG. 1. Scheme for identification of yeasts from clinical specimens.

TABLE 1. Cultural and biochemical characteristics of yeasts frequently isolated from clinical specimens[a]

Species	Growth at 37°C	Pellicle in broth	Pseudo/true hyphae	Chlamydospores	Germ tubes	Capsule, India ink	Assimilation[b]:												Fermentation of:						Urease	KNO_3 utilization	Phenol oxidase	Ascospores
							Dextrose	Maltose	Sucrose	Lactose	Galactose	Melibiose	Cellobiose	Inositol	Xylose	Raffinose	Trehalose	Dulcitol	Dextrose	Maltose	Sucrose	Lactose	Galactose	Trehalose				
Candida albicans	+	−	+	+	+	−	+	+	+*	−	+	−	−	−	+	−	+	−	F	F	−	−	F	F	−	−	−	−
C. catenulata	+*	−	+	−	−	−	+	+	−	−	+	−	−	−	+	−	−	−	F*	−	−	−	−	−	−	−	−	−
C. guilliermondii	+	−	+	−	−	−	+	+	+	−	+	+	+	−	+	+	+	+	F	−	F	−	F*	F	−	−	−	−*
C. kefyr	+	−	+	−	−	−	+	−	+	+	+	−	+*	−	+*	+	−*	−	F	−	F	F*	F	−	−	−	−	−
C. krusei	+	+	+	−	−	−	+	−	−	−	−	−	−	−	−	−	−	−	F	−	−	−	−	−	+*	−	−	−*
C. lambica	+*	+	+	−	−	−	+	−	−	−	−	−	−	−	+	−	−	−	F	−	−	−	−	−	−	−	−	−*
C. lipolytica[c]	+	+	+	−	−	−	+	−	−	−	−	−	−	−	−	−	−	−	−	−	−	−	−	−	+	−	−	−*
C. lusitaniae[d]	+	−	+	−	−	−	+	+	+	−	+	−	+	−	+	−	+	−	F	−	F	−	F	F	−	−	−	−*
C. parapsilosis[e]	+	−	+	−	−	−	+	+	+	−	+	−	−	−	+	−	+	−	F	−	−	−	−	−	−	−	−	−
C. rugosa	+	−	+	−	−	−	+	−	−	−	+	−	−	−	+*	−	−	−	−	−	−	−	−	−	−	−	−	−
C. tropicalis[f]	+	+	+	−	−	−	+	+	+	−	+	−	+	−	+	−	+	−	F	F	F	−	F	F	−	−	−	−
C. zeylanoides	−	−*	+	−	−	−	+	−	−	−	−*	−	−*	−	−	−	+	−	−	−	−	−	−	−	−	−	−	−
Torulopsis glabrata	+	−	−	−	−	−	+	−	−	−	−	−	−	−	−	−	+	−	F	−	−	−	−	F	−	−	−	−
T. candida	+	−	−	−	−	−	+	+	+	+*	+	+	+	−	+	+	+	+*	W	−	W	−	−	W	−	−	−	−*
T. pintolopesii[g]	+	−	−	−	−	−	+	−	−	−	−	−	−	−	−	−	−	−	F	−	−	−	−	−	−	−	−	−
Cryptococcus neoformans	+	−	R	−	−	+	+	+	+	−	+	−	+	+	+	+*	+	+	−	−	−	−	−	−	+	−	+	−
C. albidus	−*	−	−	−	−	+	+	+	+	+*	+*	+	+	+	+	+	+	+*	−	−	−	−	−	−	+	+	−	−
C. laurentii	+*	−	−	−	−	+	+	+	+	+	+	+*	+	+	+	+*	+	+	−	−	−	−	−	−	+	−	−	−
C. luteolus	−	−	−	−	−	−	+	+	+	−	+	+	+	+	+	+	+	+	−	−	−	−	−	−	+	−	−	−
C. terreus	−*	−	−	−	−	+	+	+*	−	+*	+*	−	+	+	+	−	+	−*	−	−	−	−	−	−	+	+	−	−
C. uniguttulatus	−	−	−	−	−	+	+	+	+	−	−*	−	−*	+	+	+*	−*	−	−	−	−	−	−	−	+	−	−	−
Rhodotorula glutinis	+	−	−	−	−	−*	+	+	+	−	+*	−	+	−	+	+	+	−	−	−	−	−	−	−	+	+	−	−
R. rubra	+	−	−	−	−	−*	+	+	+	−	+	−	+*	−	+	+	+	−	−	−	−	−	−	−	+	−	−	−
Saccharomyces cerevisiae	+	−	−*	−	−	−	+	+	+	−	+	−	−	−	−	+	+*	−	F	F	F	−	F	F*	−	−	−	+
Hansenula anomala	+*	−	−	−	−	−	+	+	+	−	+	−	+	−	+	−	+	−	F	F*	F	−	F	−	−	+	−	+
Trichosporon beigelii	+*	+	+	−	−	−	+	+	+	+	+*	+*	+*	+	+	+*	+*	+*	−	−	−	−	−	−	+*	−	−	−
T. pullulans	+*	+	+	−	−	−	+	+	+	+*	+	+*	+	+*	+*	+*	+	−	−	−	−	−	−	−	+	+	−	−
Geotrichum candidum[h]	−*	+	+	−	−	−	+	−	−	−	+	−	−	−	+	−	−	−	−	−	−	−	−	−	−	−	−	−
Blastoschizomyces capitatus	+	+	+	−	−	−	+	−	−	−	+	−	−	−	−	−	−	−	−	−	−	−	−	−	−	−	−	−
Prototheca wickerhamii[h]	+	−	−	−	−	−	+	−	−	−	+	−	−	−	−	−	+	−	−	−	−	−	−	−	−	−	−	−

[a] *, Strain variation; R, rare; F, the sugar is fermented (i.e., gas is produced); W, weak fermentation. Based on data from Barnett et al. (3) and Kreger-van Rij (26).
[b] +, Growth greater than that of the negative control.
[c] *C. lipolytica* assimilates erythritol; *C. krusei* does not. Maximum growth temperature: *C. krusei*, 43 to 45°C; *C. lipolytica*, 33 to 37°C.
[d] *C. lusitaniae* assimilates rhamnose; *C. tropicalis* does not.
[e] *C. parapsilosis* assimilates L-arabinose; *C. tropicalis* usually does not.
[f] Rare strains of *C. tropicalis* produce teardrop-shaped chlamydospores.
[g] *T. pintolopesii* is a thermophilic yeast capable of growth at 40 to 42°C.
[h] Are not yeasts, but may be confused with several yeast genera.

emulsified in a drop of sterile distilled water and examined microscopically with a reduced light source. Observations should include size and shape of the yeast, method of bud attachment, and presence or absence of pseudohyphae, true hyphae, or arthroconidia. Any round or slightly oval budding yeast with rare or no pseudohyphae should be examined further for the presence of a capsule.

The same wet preparation used for the initial microscopic examination can be used for an India ink examination. A small drop of India ink is added close to the edge of the cover slip and allowed to diffuse underneath. The preparation then can be examined for the presence of encapsulated yeasts (Fig. 2). The outline of the yeast cell, surrounded by a clear area that is the mucopolysaccharide capsule, will be obvious against a dark India ink background. False-positive preparations usually are the result of contaminated ink or artifacts, which can exhibit ragged edges. Capsular size cannot be used for identification purposes, since this characteristic may be influenced by culture age, medium composition, and strain variation. The presence of a capsule does not automatically ensure that the yeast is *Cryptococcus neoformans*, since other cryptococci, *Rhodotorula* spp., and rare *Torulopsis* spp. will produce capsules. In practice, any nonpigmented, round, encapsulated yeast recovered from cerebrospinal fluid should be considered as *C. neoformans* until proven otherwise.

Purity of cultures

Before any additional physiologic tests are performed, it is essential to ensure that one has a pure culture. A Gram stain of the culture can verify purity, but often bacterial contamination can be detected during the wet preparation examination. If the culture is mixed with bacteria, the isolate should be inoculated to a blood agar plate, and individual colonies should be picked or, alternatively, treated with hydrochloric acid (Fig. 1). The HCl procedure is performed by inoculating a colony into three tubes of Sabouraud dextrose broth. A capillary pipette is used to add 4 drops of 1 N HCl to the first tube, 2 drops to the second tube, and 1 drop to the third tube. After incubation at 25°C for 24 to 48 h, 0.1 ml of each broth is subcultured onto fresh Sabouraud dextrose agar plates.

It is possible that more than one yeast species will be recovered from a clinical specimen, especially if the specimen is from a normally nonsterile site (59). Careful attention to colonial morphology and microscopic characteristics can offer clues to a mixed population. Subculturing individual isolates to additional media can be helpful, and the use of *Candida* bromcresol green agar or Pagano-Levin agar (Difco; 19, 59) may delineate the presence of more than one yeast species.

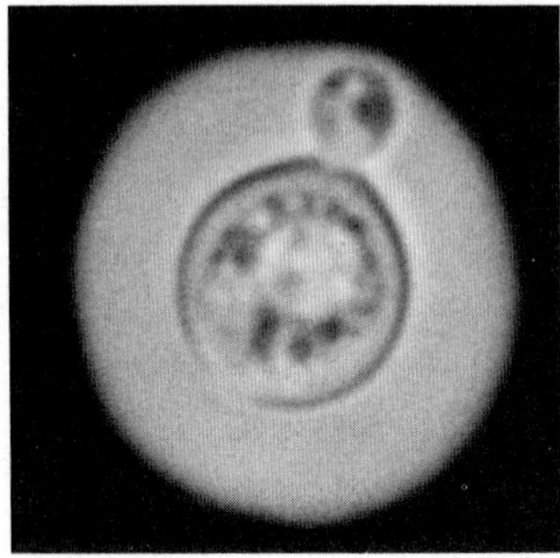

FIG. 2. India ink preparation of *Cryptococcus neoformans*. Magnification, ×400.

Morphology studies

While examination of a wet preparation gives a primary indication of the yeast involved, more extensive study of morphology on cornmeal agar, Wolin-Bevis agar, or rice extract agar will offer the opportunity to correlate morphologic characteristics with results of biochemical testing. These morphology agar plates are inoculated by cutting a small portion of a yeast colony into the agar, making a gridlike pattern. By making three or four parallel scratches in the agar surface, followed by three or four additional perpendicular cuts, dilution of the inoculum is accomplished. A cover slip is added, and the plate is incubated at room temperature for 18 to 48 h. Microscopic examination should reveal thick-walled chlamydospores of *Candida albicans* or other structures of the other yeasts (Table 2). Special attention also should be given to the size and shape of the pseudohyphae and the arrangement of blastoconidia along the pseudohyphae. Figure 3 illustrates several of the morphologic characteristics. Using known control organisms can ensure quality of the medium and offer the opportunity to compare morphologies of the known standard organisms with that of the test culture in question. Experience is needed to detect some of the more subtle characteristics, and these findings should be considered preliminary, i.e., one of the first steps in complete yeast identification.

Germ tube test

One of the most valuable and simplest tests for the rapid presumptive identification of *C. albicans* is the germ tube test (Fig. 4a). Using a capillary pipette, a portion of a yeast colony is emulsified in 0.5 ml of fetal (or newborn) bovine serum. It is not necessary to replace the cap on the test tube, and the pipette can be left in the tube during incubation. The preparation is incubated at 37°C for 2 to 4 h. After incubation, a drop of the serum is examined microscopically for the presence of germ tubes. The short hyphal initials that are produced by *C. albicans* are not constricted at the junction of the blastoconidium and germ tube. Frequently, so many *C. albicans* blastoconidia produce germ tubes that the germ tubes become entwined with each other, producing clumps of cells. *C. tropicalis* also can produce hyphal initials, but the blastoconidia are larger than those of *C. albicans*, and there is a definite constricture where the hyphal initial joins a blastoconidium (Fig. 4b). In addition to using a known culture of *C. albicans* as a positive test control, negative controls using *C. tropicalis* and *Torulopsis glabrata* also should be included. The preparation should not be incubated longer than 4 h, since other hypha-producing yeasts will begin to germinate after this time.

Several preparations for use in the germ tube test are available commercially, as well as egg albumin (6), bovine serum albumin, rabbit coagulase plasma-Trypticase soy broth (5), and sheep serum (13). In the past, pooled human serum was found to be a good substrate (35).

TABLE 2. Microscopic appearance of several yeasts and yeastlike fungi

Organism	Pseudo-hyphae	True hyphae	Blasto-conidia	Arthro-conidia	Annello-conidia	Chlamydo-spores	Asco-spores
Blastoschizomyces capitatus	X	X	X		X		
Candia albicans	X	X	X			X	
Other *Candida* spp.	X[a]	X[a]	X				X[a]
Cryptococcus spp.			X				
Geotrichum spp.		X		X			
Hansenula spp.	X[a]		X				X
Rhodotorula spp.			X				
Saccharomyces spp.	X[a]		X				X
Torulopsis spp.			X				
Trichosporon spp.	X	X	X	X			

[a] Strain variation.

More recently, a medium that combines the germ tube test, colony morphology studies, and phenol oxidase test has been developed (15). In our experience, fetal bovine serum consistently has performed the best and alleviates problems with the potential presence of *C. albicans* antibody, hepatitis, or human immunodeficiency virus.

Ascospore formation

Several yeasts recovered from clinical specimens may be present in their teleomorphic (sexual) state. To enhance production of ascospores, cultures should be inoculated onto media such as Fowell acetate agar, incubated at room temperature for 2 to 5 days, and examined by wet preparation for the presence of ascospores within asci. Some mycologists prefer to perform special stains to detect ascospores. The Ziehl-Nielsen stain routinely employed in mycobacteriology can be used if needed; however, most ascospores can be detected easily in a drop of sterile distilled water. Ascospore production in *Saccharomyces cerevisiae* is evidenced by the presence of one to four globose spores (Fig. 5c); *Hansenula anomala* produces one to four hat-shaped spores (Fig. 5a).

Phenol oxidase test

The phenol oxidase test detects the ability of *Cryptococcus neoformans* to produce phenol oxidase on substrates containing caffeic acid. The most frequently used medium is birdseed agar (containing niger or thistle seeds), and a number of formulations showing varying degrees of success have been described by several investigators. Apparently, test performance is related to the dextrose content of the medium; the more dextrose in the medium, the less likely a valid test will be obtained. When *C. neoformans* is subcultured on the medium, colonies turn a dark brown in 2 to 5 days. The test can be incubated at room temperature, but results are obtained more rapidly at 37°C. Because of the wide variation in medium formulations, the test must be subjected constantly to quality control measures. *C. neoformans* is used for the positive control, and *Cryptococcus albidus* is used for the negative control. This latter yeast may give a tan color on the substrate, whereas *C. neoformans* will turn a chocolate brown. Rapid methods, including a disk procedure, have been developed (9).

Urease

The urease test detects the ability of a yeast to produce the enzyme urease. In the presence of suitable substrates, urease splits urea, producing ammonia, which raises the pH and causes a color shift in the phenol red indicator from amber to pinkish red. The test is performed by inoculating a small portion of a yeast colony to a Christensen urea agar slant, which then is incubated at 25 to 30°C for up to 4 days. A 15-min test also has been described (60). The urease test aids in the identification of *Cryptococcus* spp. and *Rhodotorula* spp., which are all urease positive. Most strains of *Trichosporon* spp. are positive, whereas *Geotrichum* spp. and *Blastoschizomyces capitatus* are negative. Nearly all *Candida* spp. encountered in clinical specimens are urease negative, exceptions being *C. lipolytica, C. humicola,* and some strains of *C. krusei.*

Carbohydrate assimilation tests

The mainstay of yeast identification to the species level is the carbohydrate assimilation test, which measures the ability of a yeast to utilize a specific carbohydrate as the sole source of carbon in the presence of oxygen. The classical Wickerham and Burton method (11) employs tubes containing a yeast nitrogen base broth to which individual carbon sources are added (Table 1). Each of 12 tubes is inoculated with a very dilute suspension of yeast cells and incubated at room temperature for up to 21 days. Assimilation is detected by the presence of growth (turbidity) in each tube. Disadvantages of this method include extended incubation periods and the need to prepare media and inoculum. The major advantage is flexibility; many more carbon sources than the standard 12 listed can be tested if an uncommon yeast is found.

The auxanographic method of Beijerinck frequently has been used in clinical laboratories, and many modifications exist: (i) inoculating the test yeast on the agar surface instead of seeding the agar; (ii) using filter paper disks impregnated with each carbon source rather than adding small amounts of dry carbohydrate; (iii) adding drops of carbohydrate in liquid form to agar plates; and (iv) placing liquid carbohydrate into wells that have been cut in the agar (11).

One of the common forms of auxanography used today is the Minitek system (BBL Microbiology Systems, Cockeysville, Md.). A 20-ml tube of yeast nitrogen base is melted in a boiling water bath. While the medium is cooling to 48°C, a 24- to 72-h yeast culture is suspended in 4 ml of sterile distilled water to equal the turbidity

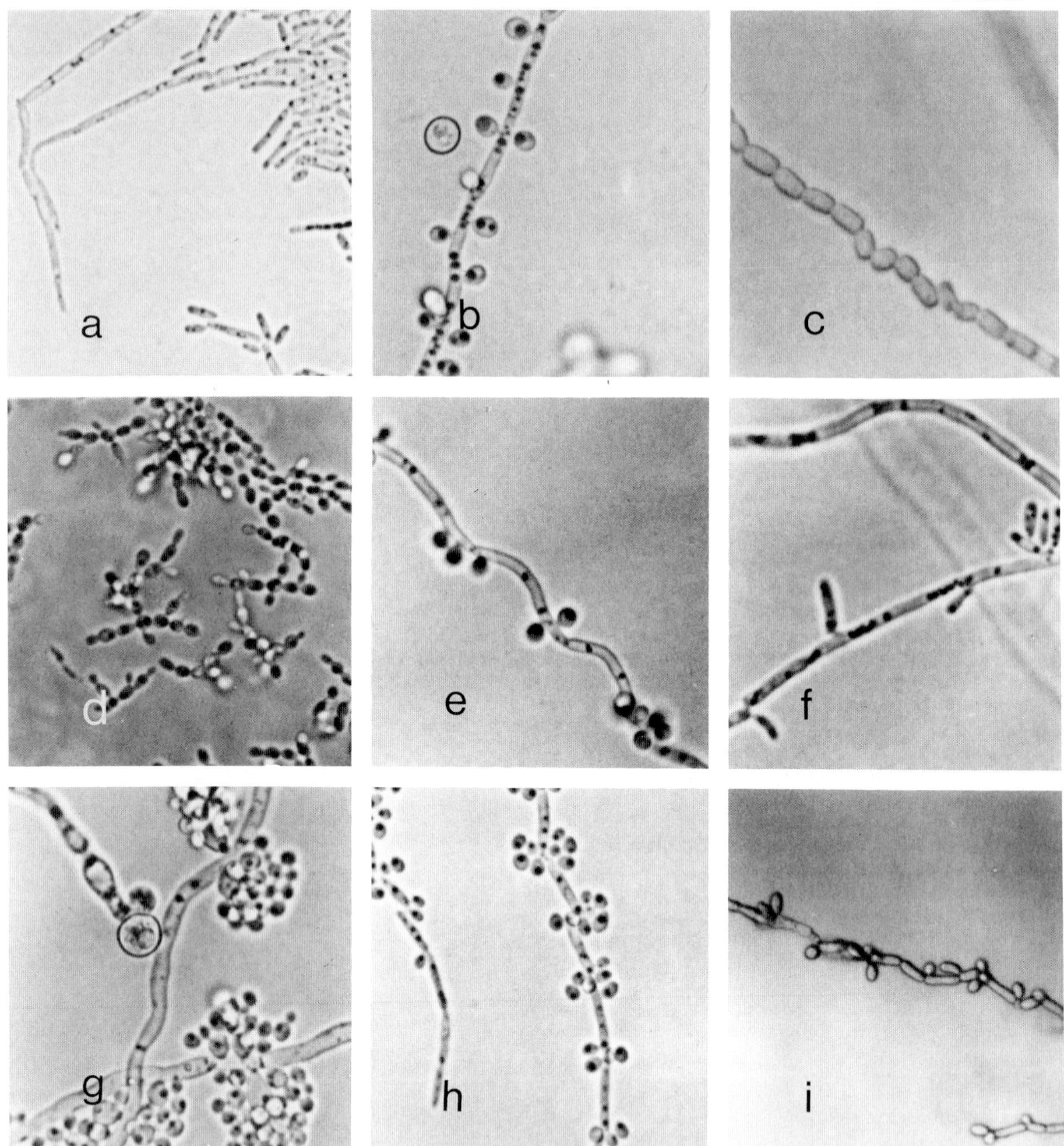

FIG. 3. Morphologic features of some yeast and yeastlike organisms on cornmeal agar at 24 to 48 h, ambient temperature. (a) *Candida krusei:* extremely elongated, rarely branched pseudohyphae; few blastoconidia. (b) *Candida tropicalis:* blastoconidia formed at septa and between septa. (c) *Geotrichum candidum:* arthroconidia. (d) *Candida guilliermondii:* chains of blastoconidia forming sparse pseudohyphae in a young culture. (e) *Candida lusitaniae:* short distinctly curved pseudohyphae with blastoconidia formed at, and occasionally between, septa. (f) *Blastoschizomyces capitatus:* true hyphae, annelloconidia resembling arthroconidia. (g) *Candida albicans:* blastoconidia, chlamydospores, true hyphae, and pseudohyphae. (h) *Candida parapsilosis:* elongated, delicately curved pseudohyphae with blastoconidia at septae. (i) *Trichosporon beigelii:* blastoconidia formed at the corners of arthroconidia. Magnification, ×370. (Courtesy of B. A. Davis.)

of a McFarland No. 4 nephelometer standard. The entire yeast suspension is poured into the tempered medium, and the mixture is added to a sterile plastic petri dish (15 by 150 mm). After the agar-yeast mixture has hardened, 12 carbohydrate disks (listed in Table 1) are added to the surface of the plate, using a disk dispenser or forceps. The plate is incubated at 25 to 30°C for 10 to 24 h and examined for the presence or absence of yeast growth around each disk. The test is best read by removing the top of the petri dish and tilting the bottom of the dish against an indirect light. Growth around a carbon source indicates assimilation of that particular compound. The size of the zone or density of yeast growth around a disk is not important; presence or ab-

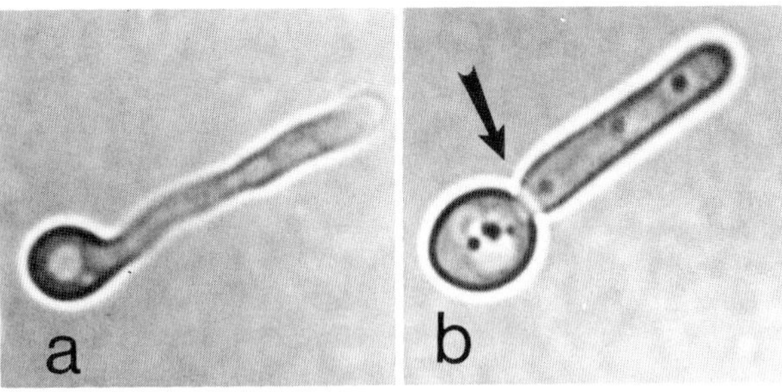

FIG. 4. Germ tube test. (a) Germ tube formation of *Candida albicans*. (b) Blastoconidial germination with constriction (arrow) of *Candida tropicalis* not seen with true germ tubes of *C. albicans*. Magnification, ×400. (Courtesy of B. A. Davis.)

sence of growth is. Some carbohydrate disks contain phenol red, which may diffuse into the medium, giving a yellow color. This color does not indicate the presence of growth. If growth is difficult to detect, the plate may be reincubated for an additional 24 h, although this is rarely necessary.

Probably the most frequently used yeast identification system is the API 20C (Analytab Products, Plainview, N.Y.). This system is similar to the API 20E used for the identification of *Enterobacteriaceae* and consists of a strip with 19 microcupules containing dehydrated carbon substrates and 1 microcupule without carbohydrate, which is a growth control. The basal medium is melted in a boiling water bath and tempered to 50°C. A sterile applicator stick is used to remove a small por-

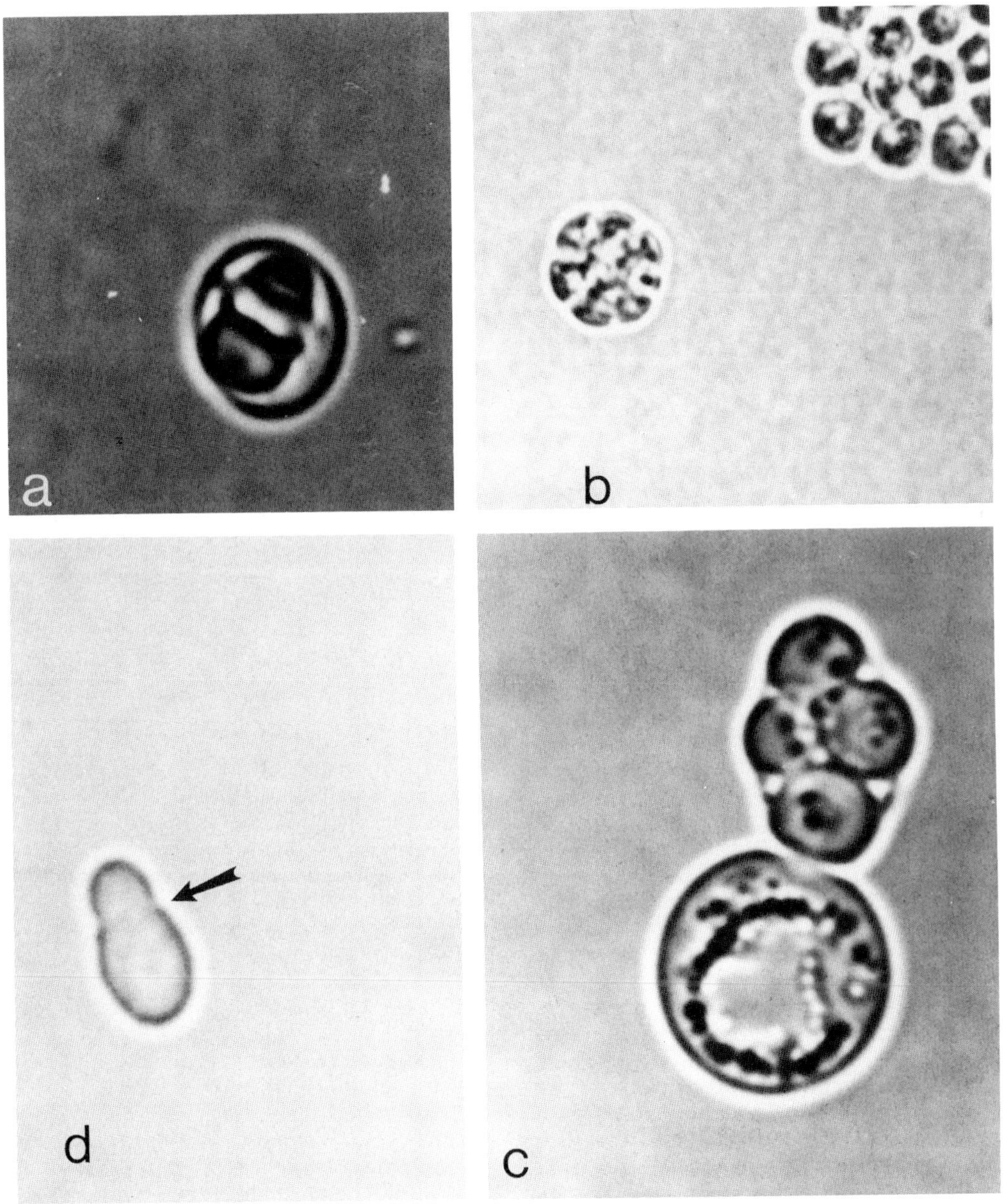

FIG. 5. Diagnostic features of selected yeasts. (a) Ascus of *Hansenula anomala* containing hat-shaped ascospores. (b) Sporangium of *Prototheca wickerhamii* containing sporangiospores. (c) *Saccharomyces cerevisiae* with vegetative cell and ascus containing four globose ascospores. (d) Bottle-shaped, budding yeast demonstrating phialoconidium and collarette (arrow) of *Malassezia furfur*. Magnification, ×1,000. (Courtesy of B. A. Davis.)

tion of a 48- to 72-h yeast culture. The growth is emulsified in the cooled basal medium to achieve a density of <1+ as compared with the Wickerham card provided with the test kit. Each microcupule is filled with the yeast-medium mixture, and the strip is incubated in a moist chamber for up to 72 h at 30°C. Care needs to be taken in the inoculation step to fill each cupule with the same amount of inoculum and to avoid introducing bubbles, which may interfere with reading the reactions. Readings are made daily, and a positive reaction is recorded when turbidity in a carbohydrate cupule is considered heavier than that observed in the growth control cupule. The results are converted to a seven-digit code number and compared with a profile register supplied by the manufacturer. There is excellent correlation of this system with conventional yeast identification methods, and the manufacturer maintains a large data bank for assistance. This method and the Minitek system are the two with which we are the most familiar. Both have yielded highly reproducible, accurate results in our laboratories.

A third method used for yeast identification is the Uni-Yeast-Tek System (Remel Laboratories, Lenexa, Kans.). This system consists of a multicompartment plate containing controls, urea, nitrate, six carbon sources, soluble starch, and cornmeal morphology wells. It offers the advantage of combining several yeast identification test procedures in one contained unit; however, the number of carbohydrate substrates is limited, and the incubation time may need to be extended. When compared with conventional methods, this system identified 92% of commonly encountered yeasts, and accuracy could be increased when the incubation period was extended to 7 days (10).

Several automated or semiautomated systems are available for yeast identification: AMS-YCB (Vitek Systems, Hazelwood, Mo.), Quantum II (Abbott Laboratories, Dallas, Tex.), and more recently MicroScan (Baxter Healthcare Corp., West Sacramento, Calif.). These systems offer the advantages of rapid results and objective interpretation via computer-based instrumentation. In addition, the instruments are versatile in that they can be used for bacterial identification, bacterial sensitivity testing, and in some cases antigen detection. There are numerous comparison studies in the literature which should help mycologists decide whether any of these systems are appropriate for their particular laboratories (33, 41, 52). Accuracy appears to be a potential problem; commonly encountered yeasts are more easily identified correctly than are rare species, and all systems should be improved by an expansion of their data bases.

Nitrate assimilation test

The rationale behind the nitrate assimilation test procedure is similar to that of the carbon assimilation test: it tests the ability of a yeast to utilize nitrate as a sole nitrogen source. Yeast inoculum is prepared as for the auxanographic carbohydrate assimilation test. Yeast carbon base (Difco) is used as the basal medium. After the medium-yeast mixture has been added to the petri dish and allowed to solidify, the nitrate sources are added. Approximately 1 ml of potassium nitrate (KNO_3) and 1 ml of peptone solutions are added to opposite sides of the agar surface. Alternately, 1 mg of each chemical can be added in solid form if care is taken not to contaminate the potassium nitrate with the powdered peptone. The plate is incubated at 25 to 30°C for 48 to 96 h. The test is read by examining the plate for growth around the peptone. Because all yeasts can utilize peptone as a source of nitrogen, this serves as a growth control and validates the test reactions. Then the plate is examined for the presence or absence of growth around the KNO_3.

Several modifications of this test have been suggested. A rapid (15-min) nitrate assimilation test that has been in use for several years utilizes a swab that has been pretreated with reaction chemicals (21). The swab is swept over several yeast colonies, inserted in a test tube, and pressed against the side of the tube to increase contact between reaction chemicals and yeast. The test tube is incubated for 10 min at 45°C (or for 2 h at 37°C). After incubation, the swab is added to another tube containing 3 drops of 0.5% α-naphthylamine and 3 drops of 0.8% sulfanilic acid. Development of a pink to red color, as compared with known positive and negative yeast controls, is considered positive. This method appears to correlate well with expected reactions of most clinical yeasts; however, rarely encountered yeasts and some strains of *Rhodotorula* spp. may give false results.

Another modification of the KNO_3 test recently has been published and provides results in 24 h (43). Modified KNO_3 agar is prepared by dissolving individually 1.4 g of KNO_3, 1.6 g of yeast carbon base, 0.12 g of bromthymol blue, and 16.0 g of Noble agar in 1.0 liter of distilled water. After the pH is adjusted to 5.9 to 6.0, the medium is dispensed in 6-ml portions into screw-cap tubes (16 by 125 mm), autoclaved for 15 min, and allowed to solidify as slants. A portion of a yeast colony is inoculated over the agar surface and incubated at 25 to 30°C. The test is considered positive if the medium color changes from greenish yellow to blue-green or blue.

Although it is not necessary to perform nitrate assimilation studies on every yeast isolate, this information can be helpful with certain groups of yeasts. The test is most beneficial when one is trying to identify *Cryptococcus, Rhodotorula, Trichosporon,* and *Hansenula* spp.

Carbohydrate fermentation tests

Fermentative yeasts recovered from clinical specimens produce carbon dioxide and alcohol. Production of gas and not a pH shift is indicative of fermentation. Therefore, it is essential to perform all tests in tubes containing Durham tube inserts (small inverted glass tubes that trap the CO_2). All carbohydrates that are fermented also will be assimilated; however, not all assimilated carbon sources necessarily will be fermented.

The standard fermentation procedure is that suggested by Wickerham (11). An aqueous suspension of yeast, not to exceed a density of a McFarland No. 1 nephelometer standard, is prepared, and 0.1 ml is added to each of the fermentation broth tubes containing Durham tube inserts and specific carbon sources. Six different carbohydrates are used routinely: glucose, maltose, sucrose, galactose, lactose, and trehalose. Cellobiose can be used also if an additional test is needed to confirm the identity of *Candida lusitaniae.* Caps are tightened on the tubes, which then are incubated at 30°C for 10 to 14 days. The tubes should be agitated daily, taking care not to introduce air bubbles in the

Durham tubes. Positive fermentation is evidenced by gas bubbles being trapped in the Durham tubes.

Rarely are fermentation studies needed to identify most of the commonly isolated yeasts if the mycologist is familiar with typical morphology on cornmeal agar. The test is most helpful in differentiating the various species of *Candida; Cryptococcus* and *Rhodotorula* spp. are nonfermentative.

Maintenance of yeast cultures

Well-characterized yeast isolates should be retained for use as quality control organisms to ascertain the performance of media and to provide examples of known positive and negative biochemical and morphological reactions. Yeasts can be maintained easily in a culture collection by heavily inoculating a tube of sterile distilled water with a 48- to 72-h yeast culture grown on Sabouraud dextrose agar. The yeast suspension should remain viable for at least 2 years if the cap is tightened securely on the tube and the tube is stored at room temperature. To retrieve the culture, 1 to 2 drops of the suspension is removed aseptically from the tube with a sterile capillary pipette, and the suspension is inoculated onto Sabouraud dextrose agar.

Serology

Several serological methods are available for aid in diagnosing yeast infections. Fluorescent-antibody techniques using specific conjugates are extremely useful in instances when yeasts were observed in tissue sections or body fluids but isolation of the etiologic agent was not possible. The number of laboratories equipped to perform these examinations is limited; the Centers for Disease Control is the major resource for this valuable service. Serodiagnostic methods for the detection of cryptococcal antigen and antibody, *Candida* antigen, antibody, and metabolites, and other yeasts are easily performed in the clinical laboratory. It is beyond the scope of this chapter to discuss the performance and interpretation of these procedures; however, the reader is referred to previous editions of this Manual for discussions of these essential components of fungal diagnosis.

ORGANISMS RESEMBLING YEASTS

Occasionally, organisms such as moulds, algae, etc., may grow on mycologic media and produce colonies resembling those produced by yeasts. However, careful attention to morphologic characteristics will differentiate them from each other. The following are several examples of such organisms that are recovered from clinical specimens and superficially can be confused with yeasts.

Genus *Geotrichum*

Members of the genus *Geotrichum* may be confused with yeasts because they produce a white to cream-colored, mealy, subsurface colony on fungal media. Aerial mycelium occasionally may be produced, giving a colony that superficially resembles *Coccidioides immitis*. Microscopic examination reveals septate, hyaline hyphae that break into arthroconidia upon maturation (Fig. 3c). No other structures are observed. *Geotrichum candidum* may be separated from *Trichosporon beigelii* by carbohydrate assimilations and the lack of urease and blastoconidia production. *Geotrichum* spp. occasionally may be isolated from patient specimens but rarely are considered pathogenic except in extremely debilitated individuals.

Genus *Ustilago*

The genus *Ustilago* represents a heterobasidiomycetous fungus that is parasitic on seeds and flowers of many cereals and grasses. It may be inhaled and therefore isolated from sputum specimens. The colonies are slow growing and, when young, are moist, compact, and white. With age, short hyphae are produced, and the colonies become velvety or powdery. Microscopically, the cells are irregular and yeastlike or elongate and spindle-shaped and may resemble arthroconidia. With the production of short hyphae, clamp connections are formed. Physiologically, most isolates are nitrate positive and have a carbohydrate assimilation pattern similar to that of *Cryptococcus albidus*.

Black yeasts

Occasional isolates of *Sporothrix schenckii*, *Aureobasidium pullulans*, and agents of phaeohyphomycosis initially produce white to tan yeastlike colonies on primary isolation media. Identification methods for these organisms are quite different from yeast identification methods and are discussed in chapter 62.

Genus *Prototheca*

Prototheca species are ubiquitous achlorophyllous algae that rarely may produce disease in humans and animals (23). Human infection usually involves the skin and underlying tissues or olecranon bursa. *Prototheca wickerhamii* is recovered most often from human specimens, whereas *P. zopfii* usually is associated with animal infections. Colonies are white to cream colored, yeastlike, and dull or moist to mucoid in appearance. The optimal growth temperature is 30°C, and growth is inhibited by media containing cycloheximide. Microscopically, the cells are variable in size and shape and do not bud (Fig. 5b). Asexual reproduction is by release of sporangiospores from sporangia. Generally, sporangia of *P. zopfii* (14 to 16 μm) are larger than those of *P. wickerhamii* (7 to 13 μm), but this characteristic can be influenced by environmental conditions. Cells of *P. wickerhamii* are round, whereas most strains of *P. zopfii* exhibit cells that are oval to cylindrical in shape. Carbon assimilation studies can be used for identification purposes. Both species assimilate glucose and galactose; in addition, *P. wickerhamii* assimilates trehalose. *Prototheca* is a nonfermentative genus (44).

CHARACTERISTICS OF MEDICALLY IMPORTANT YEAST GENERA

Genus *Blastoschizomyces*

Blastoschizomyces capitatus, a newly proposed combination for *Blastoschizomyces pseudotrichosporon* and *Trichosporon capitatum*, is a rare pathogen of humans (49). It is widely distributed in nature and occasionally has been recovered as normal skin flora. Disseminated disease usually is associated with immunosuppressive conditions (2). Macroscopically, colonies are glabrous with radiating edges, white to cream colored and shiny. Microscopically, isolates produce true hyphae, pseudohyphae, and annelloconidia resembling arthroconidia (Fig. 5f). On the basis of morphologic features alone, *B. capitatus* can be difficult to separate from *Trichosporon* spp., and physiologic tests are needed. *B. capitatus* is nonfermentative and can be separated from *T. beigelii* by growth on Sabouraud dextrose agar at 45°C and on cycloheximide-containing agar at room temperature and by failure to hydrolyze urea.

Genus *Candida*

The heterogeneous genus *Candida* belongs to the family Cryptococcaceae, within the Fungi Imperfecti (Deuteromycetes). *Candida* spp. are ubiquitous yeasts, being found on many plants and as normal flora of the alimentary tract and mucocutaneous membranes of humans. Because *Candida* spp. can be present in clinical specimens as a result of environmental contamination, colonization, or actual disease processes, proper handling of clinical material is essential in achieving an accurate diagnosis. For example, a few *Candida albicans* cells will multiply rapidly in sputum left at room temperature, giving the inaccurate impression that large numbers of yeasts are present. Yeasts that are normal flora can invade tissue and produce life-threatening disease in patients whose immune defenses have been altered by disease or iatrogenic intervention. *C. albicans*, the most common species isolated from clinical specimens, causes mild to severe infections of the skin, nails, and mucous membranes in individuals with normal immune defenses and serious deep-seated infections in debilitated hosts. Oropharyngeal candidiasis is an expected finding sometime during the course of human immunodeficiency virus infection and constitutes one of the opportunistic infections used to define a case of AIDS (8). In addition to *C. albicans*, *C. parapsilosis*, *C. tropicalis*, and *C. guilliermondii* continue to play a major role in the etiology of urinary tract infections, meningitis, pyelonephritis, and fungemia (40). Other *Candida* spp. are emerging as opportunistic pathogens. *C. lipolytica* (57) and *C. krusei* (38) have been associated with fungemia, and *C. lusitaniae* recently has been recognized as an important pathogen because of its general resistance to amphotericin B (18). An extensive review of the genus and diseases produced by *Candida* spp. has been presented by Odds (40).

Blastoconidia of *Candida* spp. vary in shape, from round to oval to elongate. Asexual reproduction is by multilateral budding, and true mycelia may be present. If sexual reproduction occurs, the yeasts are classified by their teleomorphic state. For example, the teleomorph of *C. kefyr* is *Kluyveromyces marxianus*, that of *C. krusei* is *Issatchenkia orientalis*, that of *C. lusitaniae* is *Clavispora lusitaniae*, and that of *C. guilliermondii* is in the genus *Pichia*. Production of pseudohyphae is one of the major differentiating factors separating *Candida* spp. from *Torulopsis* spp. Taxonomists are in disagreement as to whether this is a suitable criterion for keeping the two genera distinct. As in the previous edition of this Manual, we prefer to maintain the separateness of the two genera until additional studies offer further insight into this question.

Appearance of pseudohyphae and attachment of blastoconidia are important characteristics to observe when identifying *Candida* spp. Figure 5 illustrates these morphologic features. Observation of germ tubes and chlamydospores is also helpful in identifying *C. albicans*. Growth on fungal media can be detected as early as 24 h; however, colonies usually are visible in 48 to 72 h as white to cream colored or tan. They are creamy in texture and may become more membranous and convoluted with age. Most *Candida* spp. grow well aerobically at 25 to 30°C, and many will grow at 37°C or above. Carbon assimilation and occasionally fermentation studies are needed to differentiate the species (Table 1). Of the *Candida* spp. usually recovered from clinical specimens, *C. guilliermondii* is the only one to assimilate dulcitol, and *C. kefyr* (*C. pseudotropicalis*) assimilates lactose. The assimilation of rhamnose can be helpful in separating *C. lusitaniae* from the biochemically similar but rhamnose-negative variants of *C. tropicalis*. Certain rare strains of *C. tropicalis* may assimilate cellobiose weakly and exhibit an assimilation pattern similar to that of *C. parapsilosis*. The inclusion of arabinose is helpful, since *C. parapsilosis* readily assimilates this carbohydrate whereas most strains of *C. tropicalis* do not. Urease generally is not produced nor is KNO_3 utilized by the *Candida* spp. listed in Table 1.

Genus *Cryptococcus*

The genus *Cryptococcus* contains many species, six of which are noted in Table 1. Of these, *Cryptococcus neoformans* is considered the only human pathogen, although *C. albidus* (27) and a few others rarely have been implicated in disease in severely debilitated individuals. *Cryptococcus* species are round to oval yeastlike fungi ranging greatly in size, from 3.5 to 8 μm or more in diameter, with single budding and a narrow neck between parent and daughter cell (Fig. 2). Occasionally, several buds may be seen; pseudohyphae are rarely observed. The cell wall is quite fragile, and it is not unusual to find collapsed or crescent-shaped cells, especially in stained tissue sections. Cells are characterized by the presence of a mucopolysaccharide capsule varying from a wide halo to a nearly undetectable, lighter zone around the cells, depending on the strain and the medium used. Use of India ink with wet preparations, or the mucicarmine stain for mucopolysaccharide with fixed preparations, may be helpful in elucidating the capsule. Colonies typically are mucoid as a result of the presence of capsular material, become dry and duller with age, and exhibit a wide range of color (cream, tan, pink, or yellow). The color may darken with age. Strains possessing only a slight capsule may appear similar to colonies of *Candida* isolates. All members of the genus produce urease, utilize various carbohydrates, and are nonfermentative.

C. neoformans was the first serious fungal pathogen of humans to be identified as a heterobasidiomycetous yeast. Mating studies (29) have demonstrated two separate mating pairs, depending on serotype. At least four serotypes of *C. neoformans* have been identified: A, B, C, and D. Serotypes A and D were found to produce the teleomorphic state *Filobasidiella neoformans*, and serotypes B and C produce the teleomorph originally named *Filobasidella bacillispora* (31). The latter species was found to be identical to *C. neoformans* var. *gattii* (55). Although there are certain differences besides serotype, e.g., utilization of creatinine and certain dicarboxylic acids, temperature tolerance, and virulence for mice, all serotypes now are considered variants of *F.*

neoformans. Standard laboratory tests do not differentiate between the serotypes. However, media have been recommended for separating serotypes A and D from serotypes B and C, but these media are not available commercially (32, 50).

Serotype A is by far the most common serotype isolated in human disease and is found worldwide. In the past, serotype B has been seen almost exclusively on the West Coast of the United States. Recently, however, serotype B has been recovered from patients with AIDS throughout the United States. Serotype C thus far has been most prevalent in tropical areas, whereas serotype D is found in Europe and other temperate regions. Serotypes B and C never have been recovered from nature (4, 30).

Other than in cases of AIDS, cryptococcosis, particularly cryptococcal meningitis, is seen primarily in individuals with debilitating conditions such as lupus erythematosis, sarcoidosis, leukemia, lymphomas, and Cushing's syndrome. However, individuals not known to have underlying disease also occasionally are seen.

All *Cryptococcus* species are nonfermentative aerobes. Separation of species is based on assimilation of various carbohydrates and KNO_3 (Table 1). *C. neoformans* may be distinguished from other *Cryptococcus* species by these biochemical studies as well as by growth at 37°C, which also may be seen with *C. albidus* and *C. laurentii*. *C. neoformans* may be differentiated from other yeasts and from other *Cryptococcus* species by its production of brown colonies on birdseed agar, although with occasional isolates (particularly serotype C) the production of phenol oxidase may have to be induced. Differentiation from the genus *Rhodotorula*, which also forms a capsule, produces urease, and is nonfermentative, usually is accomplished by noting utilization of inositol (Table 1) and absence of carotenoid pigments characteristically present in *Rhodotorula* species.

Genus *Hansenula*

Two species in the genus *Hansenula* have been reported to cause disease in humans. *Hansenula anomala* has been associated with catheter-related infections (24), and *H. polymorpha* has been recovered from mediastinal lymph nodes of a child with chronic granulomatous disease (37). Variations in colony morphology may cause confusion with *Cryptococcus* and *Candida* spp. Texture may be smooth to wrinkled, and color may be white, cream, or tan. Microscopically, multilateral budding cells are observed. Pseudohyphae and true hyphae have been reported as characteristics of the genus; however, they have not been observed with the two species discussed here. Individual species are either homothallic or heterothallic. Although *H. anomala* is heterothallic, the diploid form is the one usually recovered from clinical specimens. The asci contain one to four hat-shaped spores (Fig. 5a). All members of the genus are nitrate positive. Carbohydrate assimilation and fermentation studies are needed to identify the individual species (28).

Genus *Malassezia*

The genus *Malassezia* consists of lipophilic yeasts that reproduce by unipolar bud fission. Previously named species *Pityrosporum ovale* and *P. orbiculare* have been combined and renamed *Malassezia furfur* (48). No teleomorphic state has been described; however, cell wall structure and a positive diazonium blue B staining reaction suggest that this form-genus may be closely related to the Basidiomycetes (54). *M. furfur* is the etiologic agent of tinea versicolor and has been associated with seborrheic dermatitis (53; see also chapter 59). Although this fungus was once thought to be solely an agent of superficial fungal infections, reports of recovery of the organism from folliculitis (25), peritonitis (56), and the upper respiratory tract (39) suggested the potential for a more pathogenic role. *M. furfur* now has been established as a causal agent of severe fungemia and bronchopneumonia associated with intralipid therapy in neonates and adults (12, 46). The second species in this genus, *M. pachydermatis*, has been isolated from dogs and other animals but rarely from humans (51). Several isolates of *M. pachydermatis* have been recovered from tissue fluids and blood, but the role of this organism in disease awaits further clarification (17).

Although it is not absolutely necessary to culture routine skin scrapings in order to arrive at a diagnosis of tinea versicolor, the mycologist should be prepared to isolate this organism when fungemia or other serious infections are suspected. *M. furfur* has an absolute requirement for long-chain fatty acids (C_{12} to C_{24}), whereas *M. pachydermatis* will grow on such media as Sabouraud dextrose agar without the extra lipid additive. Many mycologists overlay the medium with several drops of sterile olive oil when attempting to isolate *M. furfur*. An alternate medium, Sabouraud dextrose agar with olive oil and Tween 80 incorporated into the agar, works well and offers the opportunity for colony quantitation.

After incubation at 35 to 37°C under normal atmospheric conditions, growth usually appears as creamy colonies in 2 to 4 days. Microscopically, *Malassezia* spp. appear, in culture, as small (1 to 2 by 2 to 4 μm) bottle-shaped, budding yeasts; hyphal forms also may be observed in tissue. Careful observation will reveal that the junction between the bud and the mother cell (a phialide with a collarette) is rather broad and not as constricted in appearance as seen in *Torulopsis* or *Candida* spp. (Fig. 5d). Routine biochemical testing for the identification of *Malassezia* spp. usually is not attempted. Identification to the genus level is accomplished by demonstrating typical microscopic and macroscopic morphology and good growth at 37°C but no or poor growth at 25°C. Growth on Sabouraud dextrose agar with and without lipid additives will separate *M. furfur* from *M. pachydermatis*. *Malassezia* spp. are nonfermentative and urease positive.

Genus *Pichia*

The teleomorphic genus *Pichia* encompasses several species of *Candida* (for example, *C. lambica* and *C. guilliermondii*). Generally, the anamorphic (asexual) state is the one recovered from clinical specimens, since mating studies usually are needed to produce the teleomorphic (sexual) form. The biochemical and physiologic reactions of the teleomorph should be identical to those of the anamorph as listed in Table 1.

Genus *Rhodotorula*

Rhodotorula spp. are normal inhabitants of moist skin and can be recovered from such environmental sources as shower curtains, bathtub grout, and toothbrushes (11). In rare instances, *Rhodotorula* spp. have been reported to cause septicemia (42), meningitis (45), and systemic infection (47).

Rhodotorula spp. are similar in many physiologic and morphologic properties to *Cryptococcus* spp. Both are round to oval-shaped, multilateral budding yeasts with capsules, produce urease, and fail to ferment carbohydrates. *Rhodotorula* spp. differ from cryptococci by their inability to assimilate inositol and their obvious carotenoid pigment.

Genus *Saccharomyces*

Saccharomyces cerevisiae is the most common species of the genus recovered in the clinical laboratory. Usually thought to be nonpathogenic, it has been reported occasionally to cause thrush, vulvovaginitis (11), and fungemia (14).

Multilateral budding yeast cells are round to oval, and short rudimentary (occasionally well-developed) pseudohyphae may be formed. Ascospore production can be enhanced easily by growing the yeast on Fowell acetate agar for 2 to 5 days at room temperature. Asci contain one to four round, smooth ascospores (Fig. 5c). Other physiologic properties are listed in Table 1. Assimilation of raffinose by *S. cerevisiae* is noteworthy. Very few yeasts encountered in the clinical laboratory utilize this carbon source; when this characteristic is observed, *S. cerevisiae* should be considered.

Genus *Torulopsis*

Torulopsis glabrata is regarded as a symbiont of humans and can be isolated routinely from the oral cavity and from the genitourinary, alimentary, and respiratory tracts of most individuals. As an agent of serious infection, it has been associated with endocarditis (7), meningitis (1), and multifocal, disseminated disease (20). It is recovered often from urine specimens and has been estimated to account for as many as 21% of urinary yeast isolates (16).

T. glabrata consists of oval, multilateral budding yeasts, 2 to 4 μm in size, which do not form pseudohyphae. *T. glabrata* typically assimilates glucose and trehalose only. Lack of pseudohyphae, growth at 37°C, and fermentation of glucose separate it from *C. zeylanoides*.

Genus *Trichosporon*

Trichosporon spp. belong to the family Cryptococcaceae. *T. beigelii* is the usual species seen in the clinical laboratory; *T. capitatum* has been renamed *Blastoschizomyces capitatus* (49). *T. beigelii*, previously known as *T. cutaneum*, is the etiologic agent of white piedra, which is a superficial infection on the distal portion of the scalp, beard, and axillary and pubic hair. The true nature of the invasive capability of *T. beigelii* was not recognized until 1970 (58). Since then, occasional reports of disseminated disease have appeared (34, 36). The largest series of cases was presented by Hoy et al. (22), in which the majority of patients were neutropenic and pneumonia usually preceded dissemination of the disease.

Trichosporon spp. produce blastoconidia of various shapes, well-developed hyphae, pseudohyphae, and arthroconidia. If a *Trichosporon* isolate produces only few blastoconidia, differentiation from *Geotrichum* spp. may be difficult. Inoculation of malt extract broth at room temperature will encourage blastoconidia production in *Trichosporon* spp., usually within 48 to 72 h. Growth usually is observed within 1 week on solid media, and young colonies are cream colored, smooth, and shiny, later becoming dry, membranous, and cerebriform. *T. beigelii* and *T. pullulans* are urease positive; *T. pullulans* is also nitrate positive. Most *Trichosporon* spp. are nonfermentative.

LITERATURE CITED

1. **Anhalt, E., J. Alvarez, and R. Bert.** 1986. *Torulopsis glabrata* meningitis. South Med. J. **79:**916.
2. **Baird, D. R., M. Harris, R. Menon, and R. Stoddart.** 1985. Systemic infection with *Trichosporon capitatum* in two patients with leukemia. Eur. J. Clin. Microbiol. **4:**62–64.
3. **Barnett, J. A., R. W. Payne, and D. Yarrow.** 1983. Yeasts: characteristics and identification. Cambridge University Press, New York.
4. **Bennett, J. E., K. J. Kwon-Chung, and D. H. Howard.** 1977. Epidemiological differences among serotypes of *Cryptococcus neoformans*. Am. J. Epidemiol. **105:**582–586.
5. **Berardinelli, C., and D. J. Opheim.** 1985. New germ tube induction medium for the identification of *Candida albicans*. J. Clin. Microbiol. **22:**861–862.
6. **Buckley, H. R., and N. van Uden.** 1963. The identification of *Candida albicans* within two hours by the use of an egg white preparation. Sabouraudia **2:**205–208.
7. **Carmody, T. J., and K. K. Kane.** 1986. *Torulopsis (Candida) glabrata* endocarditis involving a bovine pericardial xenograft heart valve. Heart Lung **15:**40–42.
8. **Centers for Disease Control.** 1987. Revision of the CDC surveillance case definition for acquired immunodeficiency syndrome. Morbid. Mortal. Weekly Rep. **36**(Suppl.)**:** 3S–15S.
9. **Cooper, B. H.** 1980. Clinical laboratory evaluation of a screening medium (CN Screen) for *Cryptococcus neoformans*. J. Clin. Microbiol. **11:**672–674.
10. **Cooper, B. H., J. B. Johnson, and E. S. Thaxton.** 1978. Clinical evaluation of the Uni-Yeast-Tek system for rapid presumptive identification of medically important yeasts. J. Clin. Microbiol. **7:**349–355.
11. **Cooper, B. H., and M. Silva-Hutner.** 1985. Yeasts of medical importance, p. 526–541. *In* E. H. Lennette, A. Balows, W. J. Hausler, Jr., and H. J. Shadomy (ed.), Manual of clinical microbiology, 4th ed. American Society for Microbiology, Washington, D.C.
12. **Danker, W. M., S. A. Spector, J. Fierer, and C. E. Davis.** 1987. *Malassezia* fungemia in neonates and adults: complication of hyperalimentation. Rev. Infect. Dis. **9:**743–753.
13. **Dolan, C. T., and D. M. Ihrke.** 1970. Further studies of the germ tube test for *Candida albicans* identification. Am. J. Clin. Pathol. **55:**733–734.
14. **Eschete, M. L., and B. C. West.** 1980. *Saccharomyces cerevisiae* septicemia. Arch. Intern. Med. **140:**1539.
15. **Fleming, W. H., III, K. L. Knezek, and G. L. Doern.** 1987. Evaluation of SOC for the presumptive identification of *Candida albicans* and *Cryptococcus neoformans*. Mycopathologia **97:**25–31.
16. **Frye, K. R., J. M. Donovan, and G. W. Drach.** 1988. *Torulopsis glabrata* urinary infections: a review. J. Urol. **139:** 1245–1249.
17. **Gueho, E., R. B. Simmons, W. R. Pruitt, S. A. Meyer, and D. G. Ahearn.** 1987. Association of *Malassezia pachydermatis* with systemic infections of humans. J. Clin. Microbiol. **25:**1789–1790.
18. **Hadfield, T. L., M. B. Smith, R. E. Winn, M. G. Rinaldi, and C. Guerra.** 1987. Mycoses caused by *Candida lusitaniae*. Rev. Infect. Dis. **9:**1006–1012.
19. **Haley, L. D., and C. S. Callaway.** 1978. Laboratory meth-

ods in medical mycology, p. 112–113. DHEW Publication no. (CDC) 78-8361. Centers for Disease Control, Atlanta, Ga.

20. **Hickey, W. F., L. H. Sommerville, and F. J. Schoen.** 1983. Disseminated *Candida glabrata:* report of a uniquely severe infection and a literature review. Am. J. Clin. Pathol. **80:**724–727.
21. **Hopkins, J. M., and G. A. Land.** 1977. Rapid method for determining nitrate utilization by yeasts. J. Clin. Microbiol. **5:**497–500.
22. **Hoy, J., K.-C. Hsu, K. Rolston, R. L. Hopfer, M. Luna, and G. P. Bodey.** 1986. *Trichosporon beigelii* infection: a review. Rev. Infect. Dis. **8:**959–967.
23. **Kaplan, W.** 1978. Protothecosis and infections caused by morphologically similar green algae, p. 218–232. *In* The black and white yeasts. Pan American Health Organization publication 356. Proceedings of the IV International Conference on Mycoses. Pan American Health Organization, Washington, D.C.
24. **Klein, A. S., G. T. Tortora, R. Malowitz, and W. H. Greene.** 1988. *Hansenula anomala:* a new fungal pathogen. Arch. Intern. Med. **148:**1210–1213.
25. **Klotz, S. A., D. J. Drutz, M. Huppert, and J. E. Johnson.** 1982. *Pityrosporum* folliculitis, its potential for confusion with skin lesions of systemic candidiasis. Arch. Intern. Med. **142:**2126–2129.
26. **Kreger-Van Rij, N. J. W. (ed.).** 1984. The yeasts, a taxonomic study, 3rd ed. Elsevier Science Publishers, B.V., Amsterdam.
27. **Krumholz, R. A.** 1972. Pulmonary cryptococcosis. A case due to *Cryptococcus albidus.* Am. Rev. Respir. Dis. **105:** 421–424.
28. **Kurtzman, C. P.** 1984. Genus 11. *Hansenula* H. et P. Sydow, p. 165–213. *In* N. J. W. Kreger-van Rij (ed.), The yeasts, a taxonomic study, 3rd ed. Elsevier Science Publishers, B.V., Amsterdam.
29. **Kwon-Chung, K. J.** 1975. A new genus, *Filobasidiella,* the perfect state of *Cryptococcus neoformans.* Mycologia **67:** 1197–1200.
30. **Kwon-Chung, K. J., and J. E. Bennett.** 1984. High prevalence of *Cryptococcus neoformans* var. *gattii* in tropical and subtropical regions. Zentralbl. Bakteriol. Mikrobiol. Hyg. **257:**213–218.
31. **Kwon-Chung, K. J., J. E. Bennett, and T. S. Theodore.** 1978. *Cryptococcus bacillisporus* sp. nov. serotype B-C of *Cryptococcus neoformans.* Int. J. Syst. Bacteriol. **28:**616–620.
32. **Kwon-Chung, K. J., I. Polacheck, and J. E. Bennett.** 1982. Improved diagnostic medium for separation of *Cryptococcus neoformans* var. *neoformans* (serotypes A and D) and *Cryptococcus neoformans* var. *gattii* (serotypes B and C). J. Clin. Microbiol. **15:**535–537.
33. **Land, G., R. Stotler, K. Land, and J. Staneck.** 1984. Update and evaluation of the AutoMicrobic yeast identification system. J. Clin. Microbiol. **20:**644–652.
34. **Leblond, V., O. Saint-Jean, A. Datry, G. Lecso, C. Frances, S. Bellefigh, M. Gentilini, and J. L. Binet.** 1986. Systemic infections with *Trichosporon beigelii* (*cutaneum*). Cancer **58:**2399–2405.
35. **Mackenzie, D. W. R.** 1962. Serum tube identification of *Candida albicans.* J. Clin. Pathol. **15:**563–565.
36. **Manzella, J. P., I. J. Berman, and M. D. Kubrika.** 1982. *Trichosporon beigelii* fungemia and cutaneous dissemination. Arch. Dermatol. **118:**343–345.
37. **McGinnis, M. R., D. H. Walker, and J. D. Folds.** 1980. *Hansenula polymorpha* infection in a child with chronic granulomatous disease. Arch. Pathol. Lab. Med. **104:**290–292.
38. **Merz, W. G., J. E. Karp, D. Schron, and R. Saral.** 1986. Increased incidence of fungemia caused by *Candida krusei.* J. Clin. Microbiol. **24:**581–584.
39. **Oberle, A. D., M. Fowler, and W. D. Grafton.** 1981. *Pityrosporum* isolate from the upper respiratory tract. Am. J. Clin. Pathol. **76:**112–116.
40. **Odds, F. C.** 1988. *Candida* and candidosis, 2nd ed. The W. B. Saunders Co., Philadelphia.
41. **Pfaller, M. A., T. Prestion, M. Bale, F. P. Koontz, and B. A. Body.** 1988. Comparison of the Quantum II, API Yeast Indent, and AutoMicrobic systems for identification of clinical yeast isolates. J. Clin. Microbiol. **26:**2054–2058.
42. **Pien, F. D., R. L. Thompson, D. Deye, and G. D. Roberts.** 1980. *Rhodotorula* septicemia: two cases and a review of the literature. Mayo Clin. Proc. **55:**258–260.
43. **Pincus, D. H., I. F. Salkin, N. J. Hurd, I. L. Levy, and M. A. Kemna.** 1988. Modification of potassium nitrate assimilation test for identification of clinically important yeasts. J. Clin. Microbiol. **26:**366–368.
44. **Pore, R. S.** 1985. *Prototheca* taxonomy. Mycopathologia **90:**129–139.
45. **Pore, R. S., and J. Chen.** 1976. Meningitis caused by *Rhodotorula.* Sabouraudia **14:**331–335.
46. **Richet, H. M., M. M. McNeil, M. C. Edwards, and W. R. Jarvis.** 1989. Cluster of *Malassezia furfur* pulmonary infections in infants in a neonatal intensive-care unit. J. Clin. Microbiol. **27:**1197–1200.
47. **Rusthoven, J. J., R. Feld, and P. J. Tuffnell.** 1984. Systemic infection by *Rhodotorula* spp. in the immunocompromised host. J. Infect. **8:**244–246.
48. **Salkin, I. F., and M. A. Gordon.** 1977. Polymorphism of *Malassezia furfur.* Can. J. Microbiol. **23:**471–475.
49. **Salkin, I. F., M. A. Gordon, W. M. Samsonoff, and C. L. Rieder.** 1985. *Blastoschizomyces capitatus,* a new combination. Mycotaxon **22:**373–380.
50. **Salkin, I. F., and N. J. Hurd.** 1982. New medium for differentiation of *Cryptococcus neoformans* serotype pairs. J. Clin. Microbiol. **15:**169–171.
51. **Sanguinetti, V., M. P. Tampieri, and L. Morganti.** 1984. A survey of 120 isolates of *Malassezia* (*Pityrosporum*) *pachydermatis.* Mycopathologia **85:**93–95.
52. **Sekhon, A. S., A. A. Padhye, A. K. Gorg, and W. R. Pruitt.** 1986. Evaluation of the Abbott Quantum II yeast identification system. Mykosen **30:**408–411.
53. **Shuster, S.** 1984. The aetiology of dandruff and the mode of action of therapeutic agents. Br. J. Dermatol. **111:**235–242.
54. **Simmons, R. B., and D. G. Ahearn.** 1987. Cell wall ultrastructure and DBB reaction of *Sporopachydermia quercuum, Bullera tsugae* and *Malassezia* spp. Mycologia **79:** 38–43.
55. **Vanbreuseghem, R., and M. Takashio.** 1970. An atypical strain of *Cryptococcus neoformans* (San Felice) Vuillemin 1894. II. *C. neoformans* var. *gattii* var. nov. Ann. Soc. Belg. Med. Trop. **50:**695–702.
56. **Wallace, M., H. Bagnall, D. Glen, and S. Averill.** 1979. Isolation of lipophilic yeasts in "sterile" peritonitis. Lancet **ii:**956.
57. **Walsh, T. J., I. F. Salkin, D. M. Dixon, and N. J. Hurd.** 1989. Clinical, microbiological and experimental animal studies of *Candida lipolytica.* J. Clin. Microbiol. **27:**927–931.
58. **Watson, K. C., and S. Kallichurum.** 1970. Brain abscess due to *Trichosporon cutaneum.* J. Med. Microbiol. **3:**191–193.
59. **Yamane, N., and Y. Saitoh.** 1985. Isolation and detection of multiple yeasts from a single clinical sample by use of Pagano-Levin agar medium. J. Clin. Microbiol. **21:**276–277.
60. **Zimmer, B. L., and G. D. Roberts.** 1979. Rapid selective urease test for presumptive identification of *Cryptococcus neoformans.* J. Clin. Microbiol. **10:**380–381.

Chapter 61

Dimorphic Fungi Causing Systemic Mycoses

THOMAS J. WALSH AND THOMAS G. MITCHELL

Fungal dimorphism may be defined as growth of a mould form in the natural environment or in the laboratory at 25 to 30°C and as growth in the yeast or spherule form in tissues or when incubated on enriched media at 37°C (55, 62, 68). The dimorphic fungi that cause endemic systemic mycoses are *Histoplasma capsulatum* var. *capsulatum, Histoplasma capsulatum* var. *duboisii, Blastomyces dermatitidis, Coccidioides immitis,* and *Paracoccidioides brasiliensis.* These fungi also have been termed primary or systemic fungal pathogens. In the environment, they all produce a filamentous or mycelial form with hyaline, branching, septate hyphae. The conidia or hyphae of *B. dermatitidis, P. brasiliensis* and both varieties of *H. capsulatum* convert to budding yeast cells in tissue or on enriched media at 37°C in the laboratory. *C. immitis* produces spherules in tissue or in vitro under the appropriate conditions. Temperature is a critical variable in inducing dimorphism in these fungi. The mycelial form at 25 to 30°C undergoes morphological conversion to the yeast or spherule form at 37°C. *B. dermatitidis* and *P. brasiliensis* may convert to their yeast forms in response to temperature alone (42). *H. capsulatum* requires elevated temperature and the presence of reducing conditions, such as free thiol groups from cysteine (38). The conversion of *C. immitis* from arthroconidia to spherules requires changes in temperature, CO_2 content, and nutrients (6). The mechanisms that regulate dimorphism are the subject of active investigations.

Although *Sporothrix schenckii* is classically regarded as a dimorphic fungus, this fungus will be discussed elsewhere (chapter 62). *Penicillium marneffei,* which also undergoes a hyphal-to-yeastlike transformation from environment to host tissue, is discussed in chapter 63. The term "dimorphism" may be more broadly defined to encompass morphological transformations of other fungi, such as *Candida albicans, Wangiella dermatitidis,* and *Phialophora verrucosa* (as well as other fungi causing chromoblastomycosis) (68).

The purpose of this chapter is to provide a guide to the laboratory identification of the dimorphic fungi that cause systemic mycoses (Table 1). Discussions of taxonomy, mycology, ecology, and clinical manifestations are provided to facilitate understanding of the dimorphic fungi and their diseases as they pertain to the clinical microbiology laboratory.

TAXONOMY AND MYCOLOGY

Dimorphic fungi causing systemic mycoses are assigned to the form-class Deuteromycetes. The names *H. capsulatum* var. *capsulatum, H. capsulatum* var. *duboisii, B. dermatitidis, C. immitis,* and *P. brasiliensis* designate the anamorphs (asexual stage) of these fungi. The teleomorphs (sexual stage) of *H. capsulatum* and *B. dermatitidis* are classified in the subdivision Ascomycotina and family Gymnoascaceae (34, 35, 39, 40). The teleomorphs of *C. immitis* and *P. brasiliensis* are not known.

On routine fungal culture at 25 to 30°C in the laboratory, the five species usually grow as moulds and produce colonies that may be indistinguishable from each other, as well as many saprophytic species. Colonies usually develop within days to a week, although some specimens do not become positive for many weeks. After colony formation, conidia usually appear in 1 to 2 weeks. The geographic distribution, morphologic features, and teleomorphs are summarized in Table 2.

Histoplasma capsulatum Darling 1906

The name *H. capsulatum* was suggested by the appearance of the yeast cells within macrophages of a patient who had died of an infection thought to be due to a protozoan (9). Despite its name, which was based on early descriptions of the histopathological lesions, *H. capsulatum* is neither protozoan nor encapsulated. The fungus was first cultured from the blood of an infected child (12). The sexual stage or teleomorph of *H. capsulatum* was demonstrated by Kwon-Chung and named *Emmonsiella capsulata* (34). The new term, *Ajellomyces capsulatus,* was proposed by McGinnis and Katz on taxonomic grounds (41).

H. capsulatum grows at 25 to 30°C on Sabouraud glucose agar (SGA) as a white to buff colony. The mycelium is characterized by hyphae with slender conidiophores and spherical or pyriform tuberculate and nontuberculate macroconidia measuring 8 to 16 µm in diameter. Finely roughened microconidia of 2 to 5 µm in diameter may be abundant in fresh clinical isolates.

When the mould phase of *H. capsulatum* is incubated at 37°C on enriched medium, such as brain heart infusion (BHI) agar with blood and cysteine, conidia will germinate and convert to yeast cells. After subculture, blastoconidia develop that are ovoid to spherical and measure 2 to 4 µm in diameter. This same yeast morphology is present in tissue. Although *H. capsulatum* now should be technically termed *Histoplasma capsulatum* var. *capsulatum,* the former term will be retained throughout this chapter for simplicity.

Histoplasma capsulatum var. *duboisii* Drouhet 1957

Originally designated *Histoplasma duboisii* by Vanbreuseghem, this organism was later recognized by Drouhet as a variant of *H. capsulatum* and is thus designated *Histoplasma capsulatum* var. *duboisii* (56). Mating studies have confirmed that *H. capsulatum* and *H. capsulatum* var. *duboisii* are variants of the same species (36). The in vitro morphological features of the mycelial

TABLE 1. General epidemiological features of the primary systemic mycoses

Feature	Mycosis			
	Histoplasmosis	Blastomycosis	Coccidioidomycosis	Paracoccidioidomycosis
Saprobic form (<35°C) with hyaline septate hyphae	Yes	Yes	Yes	Yes
Tissue form	Yeasts	Yeasts	Spherules	Yeasts
High infection rate in endemic areas	Yes	?	Yes	Yes
≥90% of infections are initiated via respiratory tract	Yes	Yes	Yes	Yes
≥90% of infections are asymptomatic	Yes	?	Yes	Yes
≥90% of infections are self-limiting	Yes	?	Yes	Yes
≥90% of infections involve immunocompetent hosts	Yes	Yes	Yes	Yes
Approx % of males among patients with disease	80–90	50–90	75–90	95

and yeast phases of *H. capsulatum* var. *duboisii* are virtually identical to those of *H. capsulatum* (51). In vivo, however, *H. capsulatum* var. *duboisii* develops larger, thick-walled oval yeast cells, 10 to 15 μm in diameter. This organism will hereafter be referred to as *H. capsulatum* var. *duboisii.*

Blastomyces dermatitidis Gilchrist et Stokes 1898

B. dermatitidis was originally isolated from a cutaneous lesion (16). The teleomorph of *B. dermatitidis* was identified as *Ajellomyces dermatitidis* (39, 40). At 25 to 30°C, *B. dermatitidis* grows as a mould with conidia and septate hyphae. The mould form of *B. dermatitidis* produces abundant conidia from aerial hyphae and lateral conidiophores. These conidia are spherical, ovoid, or pyriform in shape and 3 to 5 μm in diameter, resembling the microconidia of *H. capsulatum*. However, unlike the microconidia of *H. capsulatum*, the conidia of *B. dermatitidis* are smooth. Thick-walled chlamydospores 7 to 18 μm in diameter also may be observed in *B. dermatitidis*. Isolates may vary in rate of growth, colony appearance, and degree and type of conidiation. Colonies usually require 2 or more weeks for full development.

TABLE 2. Characteristics of systemic dimorphic fungi

Anamorph (teleomorph)	Ecology	Mycelial form	Tissue form
Histoplasma capsulatum (Ajellomyces capsulatus)	Alkaline soil, bird and bat guano; Ohio, Missouri, and Mississippi River valleys	Hyphae, globose microconidia, 3–5 μm in diameter; tuberculate and nontuberculate macroconidia (8–16 μm)	Small oval yeasts; 2–4 μm in diameter
Histoplasma capsulatum var. *duboisii (Ajellomyces capsulatus)*	Central Africa	Hyphae, microconidia, tuberculate and nontuberculate macroconidia identical to those of *H. capsulatum*	Thick-walled yeasts; narrow-based budding; 10–15 μm in diameter
Blastomyces dermatitidis (Ajellomyces dermatitidis)	River banks? Ohio and Mississippi River valleys	Hyphae and oval, pyriform, to globose terminal and lateral conidia, 2–10 μm	Thick-walled yeasts; wide-based single budding; 8–15 μm in diameter
Coccidioides immitis	Soil; semiarid regions of southwestern United States; Mexico, Central America, and South America	Hyphae and arthroconidia, 3–6 μm	Spherules, 20–60 μm in diameter, containing endospores, 2–4 μm
Paracoccidioides brasiliensis	Soil?; Central and South America	Hyphae; rare oval to globose terminal and lateral microconidia; intercalary chlamydospores	Thick-walled multiply budding yeasts; 15–30 μm in diameter

On enriched media at 37°C, *B. dermatitidis* grows as a yeast with colonies that are folded, pasty, and moist. The yeast cells of *B. dermatitidis* in vitro or in tissue are thick walled and spherical; they produce single buds with a characteristically broad base of attachment between the bud and parent cell.

Coccidioides immitis Rixford et Gilchrist 1896

The life cycle of *C. immitis* involves development of hyphae, arthroconidia, and spherules. In native soil or on routine laboratory culture, *C. immitis* produces branching, septate hyphae and arthroconidia that usually, but not invariably, develop in alternate hyphal cells. As the arthroconidia mature, the hyphal cells between them disintegrate, and the arthroconidia are released as unicellular structures. The arthroconidia are characteristically barrel shaped, measuring approximately 3 by 6 µm, and often bear remnants of cell wall material from the disrupted adjacent hyphal cells.

In tissue or on special media, the arthroconidia become spherical, enlarge, and develop into spherules that may contain endospores. Spherules range in size up to 80 µm. At maturity, the spherules rupture to release the endospores, which may themselves develop into spherules.

Paracoccidioides brasiliensis (Splendore) Almeida 1930

P. brasiliensis at 25 to 30°C initially produces a nonspecific mycelial colony that may later bear a variety of conidia (e.g., chlamydospores, arthroconidia, and single conidia) (53). In tissue or on enriched media at 37°C, the characteristic yeast form develops. The budding yeast cells are globose to pyriform; they may become quite large (10 to 30 µm in diameter), produce numerous small buds (2 to 10 µm), and resemble a "mariner's wheel" or "pilot wheel."

SYSTEMIC MYCOSES DUE TO DIMORPHIC FUNGI

Systemic fungal infections have become increasingly important problems with the advent of new and expanding populations of immunocompromised patients (4, 5, 28, 31, 43, 66, 70, 72, 74). Patients with the acquired immunodeficiency syndrome (AIDS) represent the newest and most rapidly expanding group at risk for systemic mycoses (4, 43, 72). Improved transportation and mobility of contemporary society no longer restrict the presentation of histoplasmosis, blastomycosis, coccidioidomycosis, and paracoccidioidomycosis to their respective endemic areas. Newer advances in antifungal therapy have expanded therapeutic options and reduced the toxicity of treating these mycoses (71). The successful diagnosis of a systemic mycosis requires coordination of the expertise of the clinical microbiology laboratory and the physicians caring for the patients. Clear communication of a patient's medical condition and of the laboratory data are essential for an accurate and efficient mycological diagnosis. A basic understanding of the pathogenesis, epidemiology, and clinical manifestations of the systemic mycoses caused by the dimorphic fungi will permit a better approach to laboratory identification and clinical diagnosis.

Pathogenesis

In most cases, human systemic mycoses due to the dimorphic fungi are initiated when aerosolized conidia are inhaled. The conidia are sufficiently small to reach the lower respiratory tract, including the alveolar air spaces. Upon entry of the conidia into the lower respiratory tract, the interaction of host defenses and various fungal factors determines the outcome of infection (28). For *H. capsulatum* and *P. brasiliensis*, the conidia are initially contained by alveolar macrophages, which are modulated by T lymphocytes, resulting in localized granulomatous inflammation (10, 46, 58, 60). By comparison, a combined acute (pyogenic) and chronic (mononuclear or macrophage) inflammatory response often is observed with *C. immitis* and *B. dermatitidis* (11, 19). More than 95% of cases of histoplasmosis, coccidioidomycosis, and paracoccidioidomycosis are estimated to be self-limiting and produce minimal symptoms. In most cases, the only evidence of infection is the development of an immune response, which is manifested by conversion to a positive delayed-type skin reaction and the production of specific precipitins and complement-fixing antibodies (13, 44, 59). The small percentage of these episodes that advance to progressive pulmonary infection or clinically overt disseminated infection often is associated with predisposing risk factors, particularly underlying defects in cell-mediated immunity.

Epidemiology and clinical manifestations

Histoplasmosis. *H. capsulatum* has been isolated from soil with high nitrogen concentrations, especially related to droppings of starlings, chickens, and bats (17). Outbreaks of pulmonary histoplasmosis have been associated with exposure to these reservoirs (18, 56, 58, 73). *H. capsulatum* is found principally along the Ohio, Mississippi, and St. Lawrence rivers but is found in other areas of the United States and throughout the world. Histoplasmosis has been discussed in depth in several recent reviews (10, 24, 43, 45, 72, 73).

The clinical manifestations of histoplasmosis may be classified according to site (pulmonary, extrapulmonary, or disseminated infection), by duration of infection (acute, subacute, and chronic), and by pattern of infection (primary versus reactivation). Primary acute pulmonary histoplasmosis may develop in a normal, immunocompetent host who is exposed to a heavy inoculum (18, 73). Yeast cells of *H. capsulatum* may be observed on direct examination of sputum.

Histoplasmosis may reactivate years later in isolated tissues, particularly the brain, adrenal glands, mucocutaneous surfaces, and other sites. This pattern of histoplasmosis, which often occurs in elderly and immunocompromised patients, must be differentiated from other mycoses, tuberculosis, or neoplastic disease (25, 72). Tissue from any of these sites may be submitted for culture and histopathological studies.

Disseminated histoplasmosis may develop in immunocompromised patients with cellular immunodeficiencies (20, 43, 72, 74). However, disseminated histoplasmosis of infancy may develop in otherwise apparently healthy infants less than 2 years of age. Specimens for culture include blood, urine, bone marrow, and sputum. Patients with AIDS and disseminated histoplasmosis also may have cutaneous lesions. Biopsy and culture of these cutaneous lesions may reveal *H. capsulatum*.

African histoplasmosis. African histoplasmosis is caused by *H. capsulatum* var. *duboisii* and is limited to equatorial Africa between 20° N and 10° S. African histoplasmosis is distinguished from histoplasmosis due to *H. capsulatum* var. *capsulatum* by (i) larger, thick-walled yeast cells (10 to 15 µm in diameter) in tissue biopsies; (ii) diminished pulmonary involvement; (iii) greater frequency of skin and bone lesions; and (iv) pronounced giant cell formation (14, 32, 56). Isolated lesions may develop in the cutaneous and subcutaneous tissues or bone (14, 32). Another presentation is multiple, disseminated lesions that may involve the skin, subcutaneous tissues, bone, lymph nodes, or abdominal organs.

Blastomycosis. Human and canine cases of blastomycosis occur principally in the Ohio and Mississippi River valleys but are not limited to these regions (15, 45). *B. dermatitidis* has been isolated from river bank soil and beaver dams associated with outbreaks of blastomycosis (29, 30, 45).

B. dermatitidis may cause self-limited or localized pulmonary lesions. Chronically progressive blastomycosis may involve one or more organs, most commonly the lungs, followed by skin, genitourinary tract, bone, or central nervous system in nonimmunocompromised patients (3, 11, 45, 63). Sputum samples, bronchial lavage fluid, or lung biopsies may be submitted for microscopy and culture. Sputum cytology collected to identify malignant cells in patients with chronic pulmonary infiltrates may reveal unsuspected yeast cells of *B. dermatitidis*. Lung biopsy may reveal a pyogranulomatous reaction with marked fibrosis. Cutaneous lesions may be ulcerative or verrucous and resemble a variety of chronic infections or skin cancer. Biopsy demonstrates pseudoepitheliomatous hyperplasia, acanthosis, and intraepidermal and dermal abscesses containing blastoconidia of *B. dermatitidis*. Osteomyelitis develops in up to one-third of patients with blastomycosis. The genitourinary tract, especially the prostate and epididymis, is another target of blastomycosis. Urine collected for culture after prostatic massage may also reveal *B. dermatitidis*. Meningitis due to blastomycosis is uncommon and difficult to diagnose by culture of lumbar cerebrospinal fluid; recovery of *B. dermatitidis* may be improved with ventricular or cisternal fluid (33).

Coccidioidomycosis. *C. immitis* is distributed in regions of the southwestern United States and northwestern Mexico, Argentina, and other areas of Central and South America (48). Clinical manifestations of coccidioidomycosis have been classified in three general groups: (i) initial pulmonary infection, which is usually self-limiting; (ii) pulmonary complications; and (iii) extrapulmonary disease (5, 23, 31). Primary infections in normal hosts usually resolve spontaneously without antifungal therapy. However, primary pulmonary infection, particularly in immunocompromised patients, may evolve into one of several complications: pulmonary nodules, thin-walled cavities, progressive pneumonia, pyopneumothorax, and bronchopleural fistula. Certain patient populations with defective cellular immunity are apparently more susceptible to progressive pneumonia, complicated pneumonia, and dissemination.

Dissemination to extrapulmonary sites may result in cutaneous and soft tissue infection, osteomyelitis, arthritis, and meningitis. Cerebrospinal fluid, other body fluids, and biopsies of tissues infected by *C. immitis* may be submitted to the clinical microbiology laboratory for microscopic examination and culture. More detailed discussion of the clinical manifestations of coccidioidomycosis may be found in several informative reviews (5, 23, 31, 48, 65).

Paracoccidioidomycosis. *P. brasiliensis* is restricted to Central and South America, but within this vast area, the endemicity varies considerably (52). More than 95% of patients who progress to symptomatic paracoccidioidomycosis are males, possibly because of estrogen-mediated inhibition of mycelial-to-yeast transformation (54, 64). Paracoccidioidomycosis may be considered to have three patterns of infection: acute pneumonia, chronic pneumonia, and disseminated infection (66). These infections may be further classified as primary infection or reactivation. Fever, cough, sputum production, chest pain, dyspnea, hemoptysis, malaise, and weight loss may occur with pneumonia and disseminated infection. Extrapulmonary lesions often develop on the face and oral mucosa. Other sites include lymph nodes, spleen, liver, gastrointestinal tract, and adrenal glands. The epidemiology and clinical manifestations of paracoccidioidomycosis are discussed in greater detail elsewhere (56, 66).

COLLECTION, TRANSPORT, AND STORAGE OF SPECIMENS

Methods of collection, transport, and storage of specimens are detailed in chapter 58. Since the respiratory tract is the most common portal of entry of the dimorphic fungi, most specimens from patients with suspected endemic mycoses are sputum, bronchoalveolar lavage, transtracheal aspirates, or lung biopsy. From extrapulmonary sites that also may be infected, tissue specimens (e.g., skin, liver, and bone) as well as body fluids (e.g., blood, urine, and synovial fluid) may be submitted.

Several aspects of collection and transport of specimens are particularly relevant to the dimorphic fungi. Sputum often is contaminated by bacteria, saprophytic yeasts endogenous to the oral cavity, and airborne conidia of saprophytic moulds. Care must be taken to transport, process, and properly culture such contaminated specimens promptly to avoid overgrowth by more rapidly growing bacteria or saprophytic fungi.

Blastomycosis and coccidioidomycosis may cause suppurative cutaneous and visceral lesions. For example, the prostate may be the site of an abscess due to *B. dermatitidis*. Specimens consisting of pus or exudate should be submitted, whenever possible, in syringes. Swabs should be avoided but, when they are used to collect specimens, should be transported directly to the laboratory, preferably in commercial transport systems to prevent drying.

Normally sterile fluids and tissues also should be transported promptly to the laboratory, especially if their collection required an invasive procedure. Extreme care should be given to such specimens because the repetition of an invasive procedure to replace a lost or damaged specimen subjects the patient to further discomfort and risk of complications. Tissue should be divided and submitted for histopathological and mycological examination. Where available and appropriate, special tissue stains should be requested, such as the Grocott-Gomori methenamine silver (GMS), periodic acid-Schiff (PAS), and Giemsa stains. Direct fluorescent-antibody methods may identify fungal cells that are sparsely present or atypical in morphology.

BIOSAFETY

The conidia of the mycelial form of dimorphic fungi are highly infectious and easily transmissible by aerosolization. The arthroconidia of *C. immitis* have a propensity for airborne transmission. The yeast forms of dimorphic fungi in tissue are also infectious if aerosolized (e.g., during specimen processing) and inhaled or accidentally injected by direct percutaneous inoculation. Laboratory-acquired infections due to the systemic dimorphic fungi have been well documented (70); overall, laboratory-acquired fungal infections are more common than bacterial, parasitic, and chlamydial infections and second only to viral infections (50). Coccidioidomycosis and histoplasmosis constituted 46% of these fungal infections.

All plating of specimens and study of cultures should be performed within a biosafety cabinet (chapters 57 and 58). Plates with a suspicious hyaline mould should be opened only in a biosafety cabinet. Slants are preferable to plates for isolation of dimorphic fungi. Slants are safer, require less space, and are more resistant to desiccation during protracted incubation. However, plates are appropriate for initial recovery of dimorphic fungi from lysis-centrifugation blood cultures. If colonies of dimorphic fungi, such as *C. immitis*, are identified on plates, they should be sealed with tape in the biosafety cabinet, properly decontaminated, and disposed of.

LABORATORY DIAGNOSIS

General guidelines

The dimorphic fungi that cause systemic mycoses are identified by direct microscopic examination of specimens, by isolation and characterization of the fungus in cultures, or by demonstration of specific exoantigens produced in culture (Table 3).

TABLE 3. Summary of methods for microbiological identification of dimorphic fungi that cause systemic mycoses

Direct microscopic examination
- Wet preparations of fresh clinical specimens[a]
  - Calcofluor white or KOH
  - Combination of Calcofluor white and KOH
- Preparations of fixed specimens
  - Wright or Giemsa stain (especially of bone marrow aspirates or buffy coat smears to detect *H. capsulatum* within monocytes or macophages)
  - Cytopathology (*B. dermatitidis* or *H. capsulatum* or the spherules of *C. immitis*) by Papanicolaou staining methods
  - Indirect fluorescent-antibody staining
  - Staining of a paraffin-embedded clot section of bone marrow aspirate (by H&E, PAS, GMS, Giemsa, and Wright stains), especially for *H. capsulatum*
  - Histopathological examination of paraffin-embedded tissue specimens (by H&E, PAS, GMS, Giemsa, and Wright stains)

Culture
- Nonsterile specimens
  - Primary isolation on media[b] containing antibacterial antibiotics (e.g., chloramphenicol, gentamicin, streptomycin, or penicillin) with and without cycloheximide to inhibit saprophytic fungi
  - Yeast extract agar with concentrated ammonium hydroxide (inhibits the growth of *Candida* spp. but not the systemic dimorphic fungi)
  - Cultures incubated at 30°C under aerobic conditions
  - Tubes or plates to be held for 4–8 weeks or longer[c,d]
- Sterile specimens[e]
  - Primary isolation on media[b]
  - Cultures incubated at 30°C under aerobic conditions
  - Subculture suspicious mycelial colonies to promote sporulation[c]
  - Tubes or plates to be held for 4–8 weeks or longer[d,f]
- Conversion of mycelial form to yeast form

Exoantigen identification
- Detection of cell-free antigens produced by the mycelial-form cultures

[a] Touch preparations of freshly resected tissues also may be stained with Calcofluor white.
[b] Such as blood agar, BHI agar, inhibitory mould agar, SGA, enriched broth, and BHI broth.
[c] Potato-dextrose agar or SGA.
[d] Subculture suspicious colonies.
[e] Tissues should be minced or homogenized before plating. Mincing is preferable to homogenization.
[f] Laboratories in the endemic regions also may consider incubating cultures directly at 37°C.

The systemic dimorphic fungi produce hyaline, septate hyphae at 25 to 30°C in the laboratory. The conidia or hyphae of most isolates of *B. dermatitidis*, *P. brasiliensis*, and both varieties of *H. capsulatum* will convert to budding yeast cells in tissue or on enriched media at 37°C in the laboratory. Mycelial-to-yeast conversion appears to be more reliable at 37 than at 35°C. Conversion from the mycelial to yeast form usually requires 7 to 14 days or longer. During the early phases of conversion, a mixture of mycelial and yeast forms is found. *C. immitis* produces spherules in vitro under the appropriate conditions; however, this conversion is not a routine procedure in most clinical microbiology laboratories.

On routine culture at 25 to 30°C in the laboratory, the five species of dimorphic fungi discussed in this chapter grow as moulds and produce colonies that may be indistinguishable from each other, as well as many saprophytic species. Their colonies do not exhibit reliably consistent characteristics with regard to texture, pigmentation, or growth rate. Colonies may develop within days to a week, although some species, such as *H. capsulatum*, may not grow until after 4 to 6 weeks of incubation or longer. Detection of circulating antibodies and fungal antigens in serum and other sterile body fluids of infected patients is useful in establishing a clinical diagnosis of certain endemic mycoses, particularly coccidioidomycosis and histoplasmosis.

Direct examination. Careful direct microscopic examination of specimens may provide rapid presumptive diagnosis of a systemic mycosis, which is advantageous since these dimorphic fungi tend to grow slowly. Fresh, wet preparations of sputum, centrifuged cerebrospinal fluid or urine, pus, skin scrapings, tissue impression smears, and similar specimens should be examined directly with Calcofluor white, KOH, or both. Calcofluor white binds nonspecifically to fungal cell wall polysaccharides such that the walls fluoresce brightly under UV illumination (21). Calcofluor white is a sensitive staining procedure that offers excellent visualization of the morphology of pathogenic fungi. This method is further described in chapter 57.

Additional procedures for examining sputum for fungi are provided in chapter 58. Sputum may be concentrated and stained directly with Wright or Giemsa stain to detect *H. capsulatum* within monocytes or macrophages. Patients with pulmonary mycoses due to dimorphic fungi have chronic pulmonary infiltrates often resembling lung cancer. Papanicolaou staining methods used by cytopathologists are valuable for detection of the spherules of *C. immitis* and the yeast cells of *B. dermatitidis* and *H. capsulatum* (57). Indeed, routine Papanicolaou staining of sputum from patients with suspected endemic pulmonary mycoses may be an effective method of rapid diagnosis. Indirect fluorescent-antibody staining is another rapid, sensitive, and specific method of diagnosis by direct examination.

Bone marrow aspirates, buffy coat smears, and peripheral blood smears are valuable for the early detection of *H. capsulatum* in disseminated histoplasmosis (20, 43). Giemsa or Wright stain reveals the yeast cells within circulating monocytes or tissue macrophages. Staining of a paraffin-embedded clot section of bone marrow aspirate by PAS, GMS, Giemsa, and Wright stains is another method that allows detection of *H. capsulatum* in granulomas (69).

Touch preparations of bone marrow biopsies, lymph nodes, and other tissues are an efficient means of detecting fungi in these tissues. The same group of special stains, as well as Calcofluor white, may be applied to slides to which the freshly cut surface of a tissue specimen has been pressed, dried, and fixed with heat or ethanol. Histopathological examinations of specimens are usually completed within 24 h and may provide definitive diagnostic information.

Culture. Several considerations pertain to the systemic dimorphic fungi. As indicated previously, nonsterile specimens, such as sputum or skin, often are contaminated with bacteria and saprophytic fungi that can overgrow the slower growing dimorphic fungi. Therefore, primary isolation media should contain antibacterial antibiotics (e.g., chloramphenicol, gentamicin, streptomycin, or penicillin) with cycloheximide to inhibit saprophytic fungi. Media without cycloheximide also should be included because this compound inhibits many opportunistic pathogens, such as *Cryptococcus neoformans*, *Candida* spp., *Aspergillus* spp., and Zygomycetes. Alternatively, such specimens can be plated on yeast extract agar to which a drop of concentrated ammonium hydroxide is allowed to diffuse from the edge of the plate; this inhibits the growth of *Candida* species but not the systemic dimorphic fungi (61).

Normally sterile specimens may be inoculated directly onto blood agar, BHI agar, inhibitory mould agar, SGA, and enriched broth such as BHI broth. Tissues should be minced or homogenized before plating. All cultures for systemic dimorphic fungi should be incubated at 25 to 30°C under aerobic conditions. Since tubes or plates are to be held for 4 to 8 weeks or longer, the incubator should be well humidified to prevent desiccation of the agar. Culture tubes are preferable; however, if plates are used, 25 ml of agar should be used per plate. Laboratories in the endemic regions also may consider incubating cultures simultaneously at 37°C.

Exoantigen identification. The mycelial forms of *H. capsulatum*, *B. dermatitidis*, *C. immitis*, and *P. brasiliensis* are often indistinguishable microscopically. The exoantigen technique is a simple diagnostic method that detects the presence of cell-free antigens, known as exoantigens, which are produced by the mycelial-form cultures. A specific exoantigen detected in the aqueous extract of a mycelial culture may identify any of the systemic dimorphic fungi (Table 4). This procedure is relatively rapid and applicable to nonsporulating cultures. Exoantigens are demonstrated by immunodiffusion of specific antigens in either a concentrated aqueous extract of the colony on solid medium or the supernatant fluid of a broth culture of the isolate. Reference antisera identify specific antigens in the isolate and the control antigen.

Methods to detect exoantigens have been developed by Kaufman and Standard (26, 27). To test a culture on solid medium, the mature slant culture is overlaid with Merthiolate (1:5,000) at room temperature. After overnight incubation, the fluid is aspirated and a 5-ml sample is concentrated 50-fold (Minicon B-15; Amicon Corp.) or tested unconcentrated for *C. immitis*. The concentrate is placed on a microimmunodiffusion well opposite reference antigens and antisera. Note that antiserum is placed in the center well 1 h before the control antigens and concentrate are added to adjacent wells. The microimmunodiffusion plate is incubated for 24 h at room temperature, the template is removed, the surface of the agarose plate is washed and covered with distilled water, and the plate is read over indirect light for lines of identity. Any line of identity with control antigen-antibody is significant.

Some isolates produce more readily detectable antigen when grown in liquid medium at 25°C for 3 or more days. For this procedure, one or more 30-ml BHI cultures are established in 125-ml flasks, which are incubated on a gyratory shaker at 150 rpm. After 3 days, all or a portion of the culture is removed and 1% Merthiolate is added to give a final concentration of 1:5,000. The Merthiolate-treated sample is shaken for another day and centrifuged. Five-milliliter samples of the supernatant fluid are concentrated 10- and 25-fold as described above and tested for the presence of specific exoantigen. Note that *C. immitis* does not require concentration. If 3-day cultures are unproductive, concentrated culture supernatants from older cultures may be tested.

TABLE 4. Species-specific exoantigens for the identification of systemic dimorphic fungal pathogens

Fungus	Exoantigen(s)[a]
Histoplasma capsulatum	h, m
Blastomyces dermatitidis	A
Coccidioides immitis	HS, F, HL
Paracoccidioides brasiliensis	1, 2, 3

[a] Exoantigens are detected by precipitin lines of identity in immunodiffusion tests of concentrated culture supernatant fluids versus reference antigens and antisera (27).

Laboratory identification of specific dimorphic fungi

Histoplasma capsulatum. Direct examination of specimens for *H. capsulatum* is best accomplished with special stains. The budding yeast cells of *H. capsulatum* (2 to 4 μm) on a Calcofluor white or KOH preparation of sputum may be too small for reliable detection or may be confused with *Torulopsis glabrata,* which is similar in size and shape and often colonizes the human oropharynx (Fig. 1 and 2). The small yeast cells of *H. capsulatum* are observed frequently within the cytoplasm of macrophages. In contrast, the yeast cells of *T. glabrata* are seldom found within macrophages. Nevertheless, the only reliable methods to distinguish between these two species are culture and indirect fluorescent-antibody staining. Giemsa and hematoxylin and eosin (H&E) stains reveal the intracellular yeasts of *H. capsulatum* more readily, especially in sputum, blood smears, bone aspirates, and biopsy specimens. The GMS stain delineates the yeast cells but not the cellular detail of the host inflammatory cells.

Histopathological examination of paraffin-embedded specimens by H&E and PAS stains reveals that *H. capsulatum* elicits a granulomatous inflammatory response. Different patterns of inflammation may be evident, depending on the duration and severity of infection. Large numbers of the tiny yeasts pack the cytoplasm of macrophages in acute pulmonary or disseminated histoplasmosis (Fig. 3). The yeast cells of *H. capsulatum* must be distinguished from cells of the intracellular parasites *Leishmania donovani* and *Toxoplasma gondii. L. donovani* contains a kinetoplast, which is not present in the yeast cells of *H. capsulatum.* The tachyzoites of *T. gondii* are not stained by GMS. Chronic lesions of histoplasmosis are characterized by epithelioid granulomas and fewer numbers of budding yeast cells within the macrophages. As lesions become fibrotic and calcified, the number of yeasts continues to diminish. The GMS stain is preferable for detection of the small numbers of yeasts. Budding may not be observed in the chronic lesions of histoplasmosis.

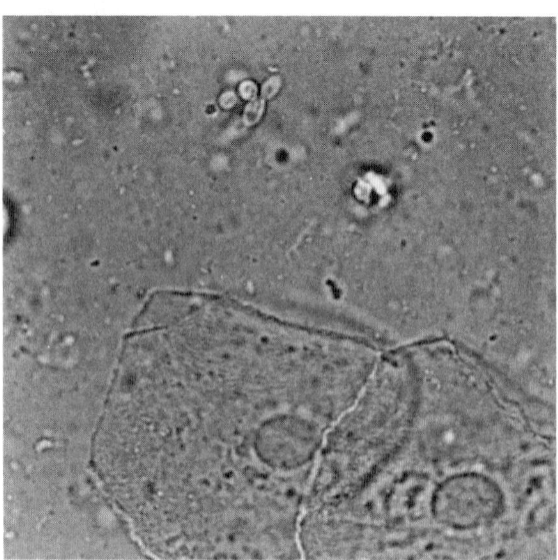

FIG. 1. KOH wet mount of sputum showing blastoconidia of *Histoplasma capsulatum* adjacent to epithelial cells. Original magnification, ×400.

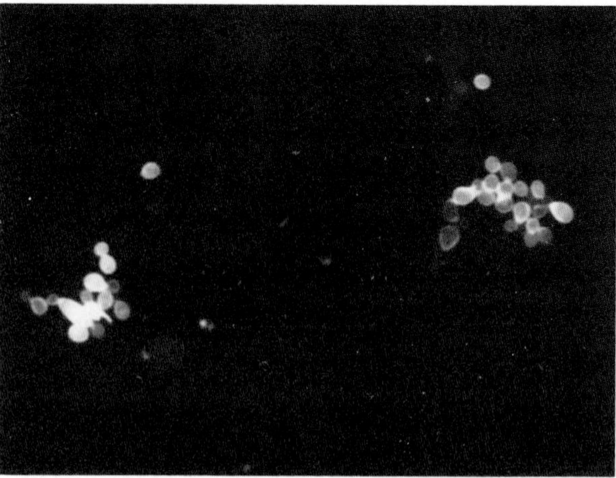

FIG. 2. Calcofluor white wet mount of sputum showing blastoconidia of *Histoplasma capsulatum.* Original magnification, ×400.

H. capsulatum also should be distinguished histologically from the small form of *B. dermatitidis,* endospores or young spherules of *C. immitis,* and yeast cells of *Cryptococcus neoformans.* Yeast cells of *B. dermatitidis* have a broader base of attachment between the bud and parent cell than do those of *H. capsulatum.* The presence of spherules of various sizes distinguishes *C. immitis* in tissue. Alcian blue or Mayer mucicarmine stain will stain the polysaccharide capsule of *Cryptococcus neoformans* but will not stain *H. capsulatum,* which lacks a capsule.

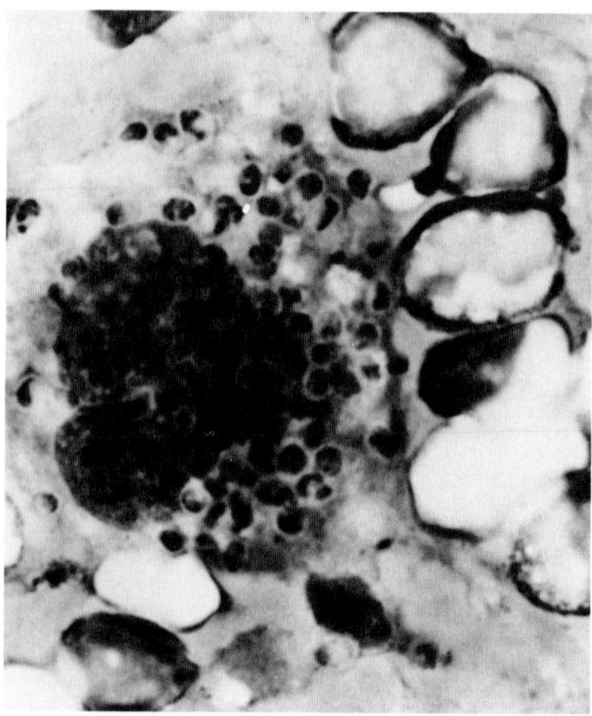

FIG. 3. Bone marrow aspirate with macrophage containing numerous blastoconidia of *Histoplasma capsulatum.* Giemsa stain; original magnification, ×1,250.

Culture of specimens infected with *H. capsulatum* at 25 to 30°C reveals a fluffy, slowly growing colony with aerial mycelium that varies in color from white to buff to brown (1). During early growth of the mycelial culture, spherical to oval to pyriform microconidia (2 to 5 μm in diameter) are present. These microconidia may be sessile on the sides of hyphae or attached to short lateral conidiophores. With continued growth, the mould develops slender conidiophores and characteristic globose or pyriform, tuberculate or nontuberculate macroconidia measuring 8 to 16 μm in diameter (Fig. 4). Since these macroconidia may resemble those of the saprophytic genus *Sepedonium*, a suspicious isolate must be converted to the yeast form or be shown to produce the h or m exoantigen to identify it as *H. capsulatum*. Furthermore, *H. capsulatum* grows on media with cycloheximide, but the monomorphic *Sepedonium* spp. are inhibited. *Chrysosporium* spp. develop conidia that resemble the microconidia of *H. capsulatum;* however, *Chrysosporium* spp. do not develop macroconidia and are not dimorphic. The *Chrysosporium* state of *Renispora flavissima* also may resemble the mycelium of *H. capsulatum.*

Conversion of the mycelial form of *H. capsulatum* to the yeast form is performed by incubating the mycelial culture at 37°C on enriched medium, such as BHI agar with cysteine. This conversion may be difficult but can be performed best at 37 instead of 35°C. When the mycelium is incubated at 37°C, spherical to oval budding yeast cells (2 to 5 μm in diameter) develop. Hyphal cells may form buds directly or develop enlarged, transitional cells that subsequently begin to bud (Fig. 5). The microconidia also may convert to budding yeast cells. Complete conversion rarely is achieved, but the presence of a mixture of typical yeast cells with hyphal elements is sufficient to confirm the identification. Yeast cells of *H. capsulatum*, in vitro or in vivo, are small and ellipsoidal, approximately 1 to 3 by 3 to 5 μm. This conversion usually requires at least 7 to 10 days. Such yeast cells also may be isolated directly on blood agar plates or other enriched media incubated at 37°C. Buds often are formed at the smaller end of ellipsoidal yeast cells and attached by a narrow connection.

The lysis-centrifugation technique (Isolator; E. I. du Pont de Nemours & Co., Inc., Wilmington, Del.) is the optimal method to most effectively recover *H. capsulatum* and other dimorphic fungi from blood specimens (2, 47, 49). The tube in which the blood is collected for culture contains a mixture (saponin, propylene glycol, sodium polyanetholesulfonate, and EDTA) that lyses leukocytes, prevents coagulation, and inhibits comple-

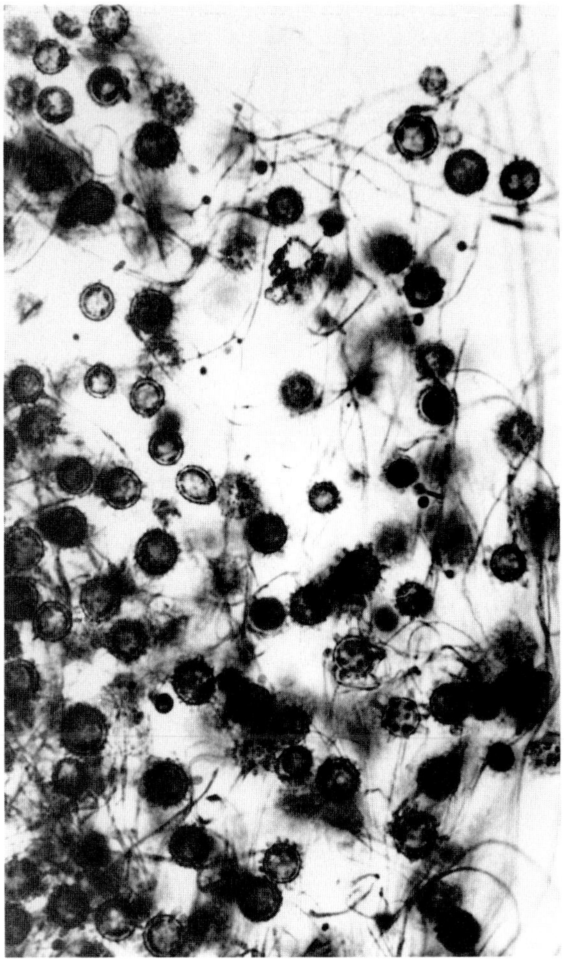

FIG. 4. Mycelial phase of *Histoplasma capsulatum* demonstrating tuberculate and nontuberculate macroconidia, grown on potato-dextrose agar at 25°C. Original magnification, ×400.

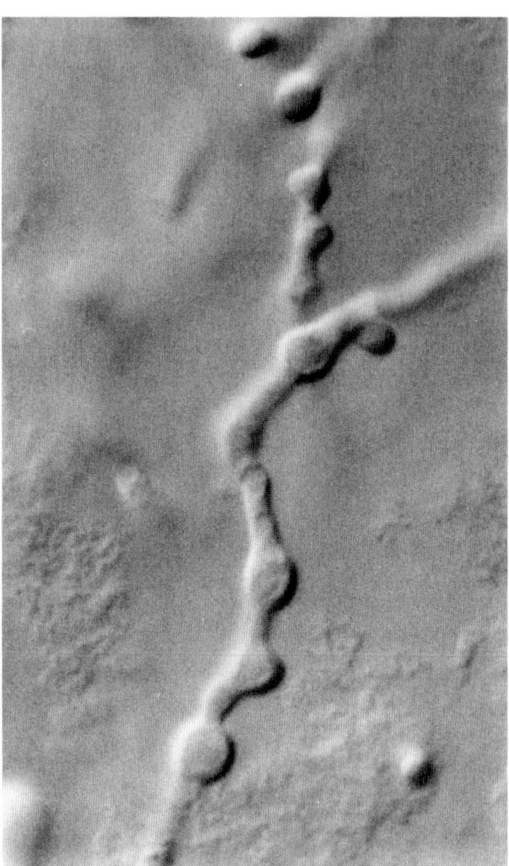

FIG. 5. Transitional phase of *Histoplasma capsulatum* during conversion from mycelial to yeast phase on chocolate agar at 36°C. Original magnification, ×400.

ment. After the tube is centrifuged at 3,000 × *g* for 30 min, the supernatant is withdrawn from the tube and the concentrate is transferred via pipette from the bottom of the tube to culture media. A variety of media may be used, including inhibitory mould agar, SGA, BHI, or chocolate agar plates. *H. capsulatum* may be isolated as a mixture of yeast cells and hyphae directly from lysis-centrifugation blood cultures, which are routinely incubated at 35°C. The application of lysis-centrifugation and biphasic media to blood cultures, especially in patients with AIDS, has increased the recovery of *H. capsulatum* from blood (49).

***Histoplasma capsulatum* var. *duboisii*.** *H. capsulatum* var. *duboisii* differs reliably from *H. capsulatum* var. *capsulatum* only in its tissue form. Direct examination of purulent material or tissue biopsy specimens (usually skin, bone, or lymph nodes) treated with Calcofluor white or KOH reveals large, thick-walled, budding yeasts of *H. capsulatum* var. *duboisii* that measure 10 to 15 µm in diameter. The spherical to ellipsoidal yeast cells in infected tissue are found within the abundant multinucleate giant cells in a fibrogranulomatous inflammatory reaction (Fig. 6). Retraction of the cytoplasm of the phagocytes from the yeasts produces an artifactual "capsule" on H&E stain. With GMS stain, the narrow attachment between the buds and yeasts creates a "figure-eight" or "double-cell" budding configuration. The yeast cells occasionally may be connected in short chains. *B. dermatitidis* also may infect skin and bone. However, *H. capsulatum* var. *duboisii* is distinguishable from *B. dermatitidis* in tissue by the presence of narrow-based budding in the former and broad-based budding in the latter yeasts. Moreover, the abundance of many intracellular thick-walled yeasts in numerous multinucleate giant cells is more typical of *H. capsulatum* var. *duboisii* than of *B. dermatitidis*.

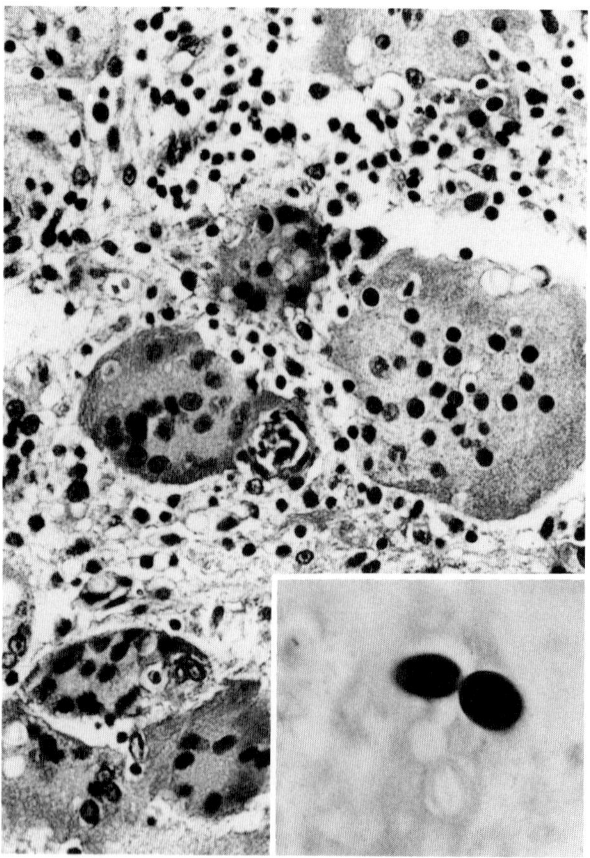

FIG. 6. Bone biopsy showing multinucleate giant cells and intracytoplasmic blastoconidia of *Histoplasma capsulatum* var. *duboisii*. PAS stain; magnification, ×250. (Specimen kindly provided by Andrew Smith.) (Insert) Bone biopsy revealing budding yeasts of *Histoplasma capsulatum* var. *duboisii*. GMS stain; original magnification, ×1,250.

The colonial morphology and microscopic appearance of the mould form of *H. capsulatum* var. *duboisii* grown at 25 to 30°C are the same as for *H. capsulatum*, including the typical microconidia and macroconidia. Distinction between the in vitro yeast phases of *H. capsulatum* var. *duboisii* and *H. capsulatum* var. *capsulatum* may be difficult. When the mould is incubated at 37°C, the fungus converts to yeast cells that are similar in size and shape to those of *H. capsulatum* var. *capsulatum*, especially in early cultures. Some cells of *H. capsulatum* var. *duboisii* may be larger and more thick walled; however, these cells are not the same as the characteristic larger and thick-walled yeast forms present in tissue of cases of African histoplasmosis (51). Thus, histopathological documentation of the characteristic tissue forms of *H. capsulatum* var. *duboisii* is a critical step for establishing the laboratory diagnosis of this organism.

***Blastomyces dermatitidis*.** Direct Calcofluor white or KOH mounts of sputum, exudates, and tissues can demonstrate the yeast cells of *B. dermatitidis*, which are large, spherical, and thick walled and measure approximately 8 to 15 µm in diameter (Fig. 7 and 8). The yeast cells bud singly and have a wide base of attachment between the bud and parent yeast cell. This characteristic can be used to distinguish the yeast cells of *B. dermatitidis* from those of *H. capsulatum* var. *duboisii*, the latter of which have a narrow base of attachment and usually are found in multinucleate giant cells. The bud of *B. dermatitidis* often attains the same size as the parent yeast before becoming detached. Infected tissues stained with GMS will reveal these characteristic yeast forms (Fig. 9). These yeast cells also have been recognized on cytological specimens of sputum (often submitted to rule out primary lung cancer) treated with Papanicolaou stain. Communication with the patient's physician concerning travel history greatly facilitates the distinction between *B. dermatitidis* and *H. capsulatum* var. *duboisii*.

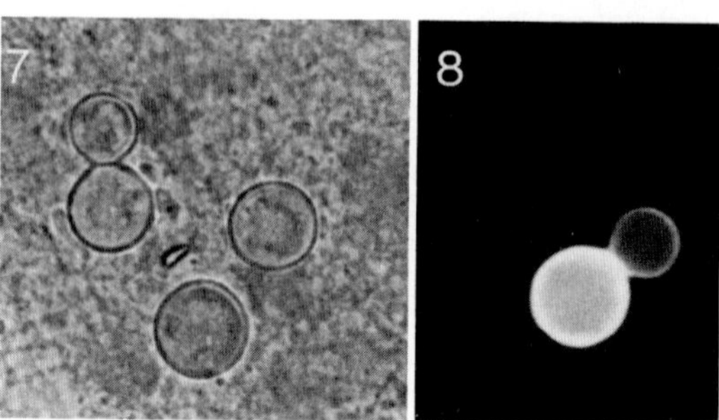

FIG. 7. KOH wet mount of sputum showing budding yeast of *Blastomyces dermatitidis*. Magnification, ×400.

FIG. 8. Calcofluor white wet mount of sputum showing budding yeast of *Blastomyces dermatitidis*. Original magnification, ×400.

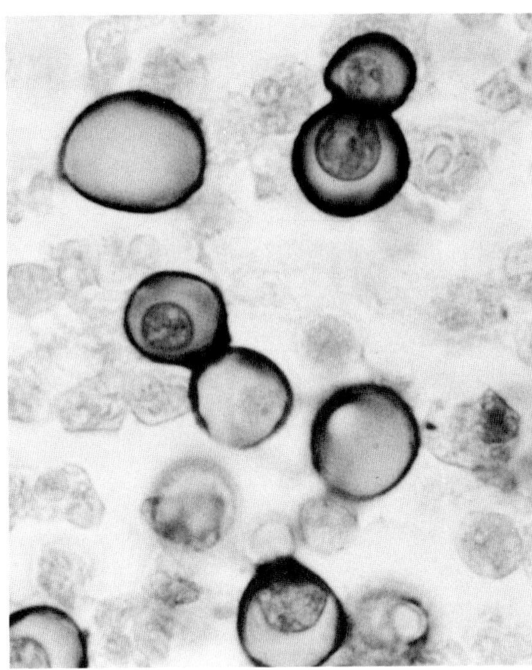

FIG. 9. Lung biopsy demonstrating blastoconidia of *Blastomyces dermatitidis*. GMS stain; original magnification, ×1,250.

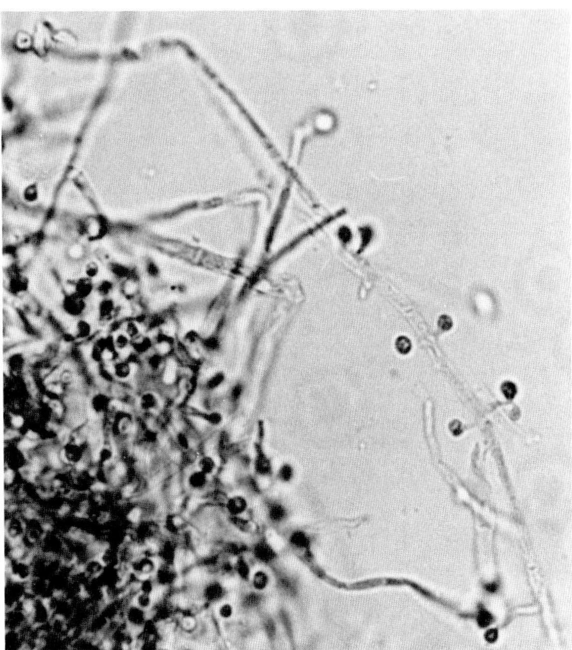

FIG. 10. Mycelial phase of *Blastomyces dermatitidis* demonstrating pyriform and globose terminal and lateral conidia, grown on potato-dextrose agar at 25°C. Original magnification, ×400.

When specimens are cultured at 25 to 30°C, *B. dermatitidis* initially produces a fluffy, white colony on routine mycological media. Some strains develop tan, glabrous colonies without conidia, and others may produce light brown colonies with concentric rings. The mould form of *B. dermatitidis* produces conidia measuring 2 to 10 µm in diameter that are located on short terminal or lateral hyphal branches (Fig. 10). These conidia are typically spherical, ovoid, or pyriform in shape and 3 to 5 µm in diameter. Thick-walled chlamydospores 7 to 18 µm in diameter also may be observed. The colony and conidia resemble those of *Chrysosporium* spp. and may not be distinguishable from an early culture of *H. capsulatum* having only hyphae, conidiophores, and microconidia. The identification is confirmed by conversion to the yeast form by growth at 37°C or detection of exoantigen A (27). However, conversion or exoantigen is probably not necessary if a tissue diagnosis of blastomycosis also is established.

At 37°C, the yeast form grows as a white to light brown, wrinkled colony. In vitro or in tissue, the yeast cells of *B. dermatitidis* are thick walled and spherical; they produce single buds with a characteristically wide base of attachment between the bud and parent cell. The microscopic morphology of *B. dermatitidis* isolates may vary. A small form produces yeast cells in tissue resembling *H. capsulatum* (56). Although most of these small forms of *B. dermatitidis* possess the characteristic features of broadly attached buds, cells with narrow attachments may be observed. Rarely, hyphae also are seen in tissue along with yeast cells of *B. dermatitidis* (22).

Coccidioides immitis. Because of the risks to laboratory personnel when working with the mould form of *C. immitis*, direct examinations of sputum, exudates, and tissue are highly recommended. Mature spherules are thick walled, usually 20 to 60 µm in diameter, and easily recognized on wet mounts using KOH or Calcofluor white (Fig. 11 to 14). Larger spherules may measure up to 80 µm in diameter. Endospores (2 to 4 µm) can be observed in intact or recently disrupted spherules. During maturation, spherules undergo progressive cleavages that lead to the formation of the uninucleate endospores. Immature or smaller spherules (10 to 20 µm in diameter) lacking endospores may resemble phagocytic cells, artifacts, or other fungi. Mature

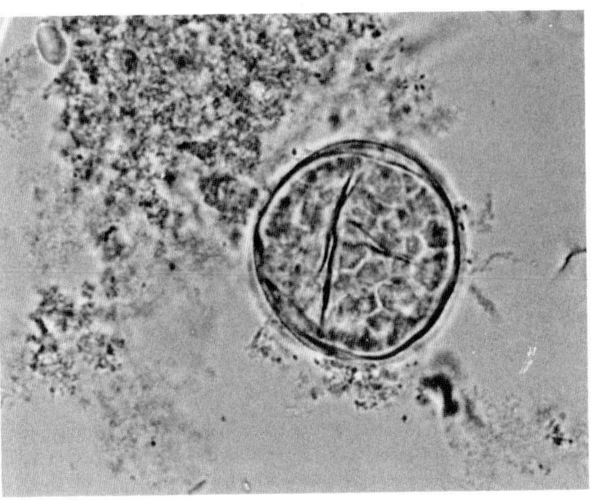

FIG. 11. KOH wet mount of sputum showing spherule with endospores of *Coccidioides immitis*. Original magnification, ×400.

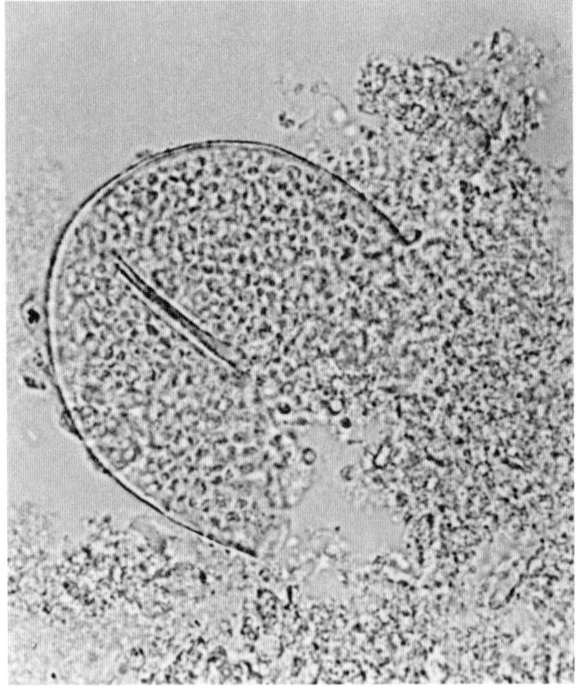

FIG. 12. KOH wet mount of sputum showing disrupted spherule and endospores of *Coccidioides immitis*. Original magnification, ×400.

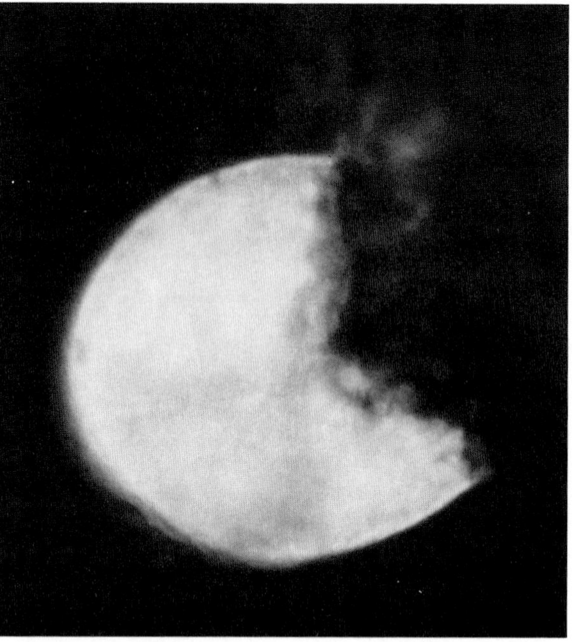

FIG. 14. Calcofluor white wet mount of sputum showing disrupted spherule and faintly visible endospores of *Coccidioides immitis*. Original magnification, ×400.

spherules rupture to release the endospores. Hyphae may develop in chronic cavitary and granulomatous lesions of pulmonary coccidioidomycosis.

Histopathology of coccidioidomycosis presents a variable inflammatory response ranging from an acute pyogenic to a chronic granulomatous reaction. This variability may be due to an acute inflammatory reaction to endospores after rupture of spherules. A granulomatous response is observed in association with intact spherules. Foci of calcification and fibrosis may be present in resolving granulomatous lesions. Spherules are sparse in tissue from patients with resolving infection, but they are numerous during progressive disease. Spherules of *C. immitis* are identified easily in tissue by routine H&E, GMS, and PAS stains, particularly the latter (Fig. 15). Endospores within the spherules of infected tissue may be observed histologically by H&E and PAS stains.

Endospores and small spherules may be confused with atypical forms of *B. dermatitidis* and nonbudding yeasts of *H. capsulatum*, *P. brasiliensis*, *T. glabrata*, and

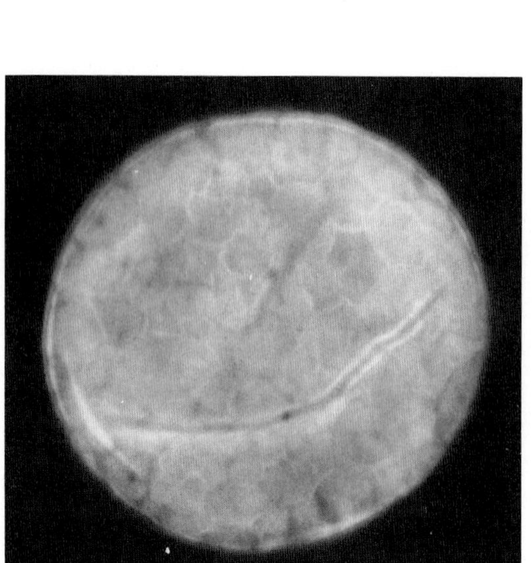

FIG. 13. Calcofluor white wet mount of sputum showing spherule of *Coccidioides immitis*. Original magnification, ×400.

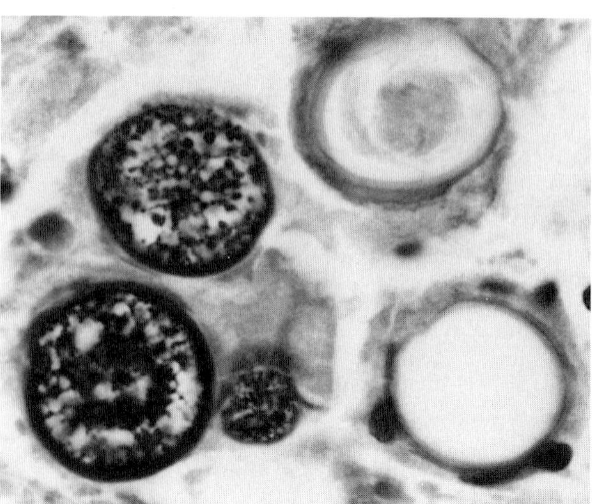

FIG. 15. Lung biopsy demonstrating empty spherules and spherules filled with endospores of *Coccidioides immitis*. PAS stain; original magnification, ×763.

Cryptococcus neoformans. Prototheca wickerhamii may resemble small spherules, and *Rhinosporidium seeberi* may simulate larger spherules of *C. immitis*. Some pollen grains found in sputum also look like spherules.

When spherules of *C. immitis* cannot be identified on wet mounts, specimens should be cultured on slants instead of plates. *C. immitis* grows readily on conventional media at 25 to 30°C usually within 1 week as a floccose colony composed of hyaline, septate hyphae with arthroconidia (Fig. 16). The pigmentation and texture of colonies are highly variable. Colors range from buff to yellow to tan; the texture may be floccose to powdery, depending on the degree of fragmentation of the hyphae into arthroconidia.

The arthroconidia of *C. immitis* develop initially in the lateral hyphal branches and are thick-walled, barrel-shaped cells, 2 to 4 by 3 to 6 μm, that alternate with empty, thin-walled disjunctor cells. As the walls of these disjunctor cells deteriorate, the arthroconidia become detached and dispersed. The mycelium of *C. immitis* must be distinguished from those of other genera that produce hyphae and arthroconidia, including *Malbranchea, Uncinocarpus, Arthroderma, Auxarthron, Geotrichum*, and *Oidiodendron*.

Conversion of the mould form of *C. immitis* to the tissue form is not routinely performed in clinical microbiology laboratories, although a synthetic broth can be used to generate viable endospores (7, 8). An agar medium for cultivation of spherules also may be used for rapid in vitro conversion and identification of *C. immitis* (67). Alternatively, spherules may be produced by intraperitoneal injection of hyphae and arthroconidia into laboratory animals in approved facilities. However, demonstration of exoantigen HS production is the safest and fastest method of confirmation (27).

Paracoccidioides brasiliensis. *P. brasiliensis* may be identified by direct examination of sputum, bronchoalveolar lavage, pus from draining lymph nodes, scrapings from ulcer, or tissue biopsies. A wet mount of such material may reveal the characteristic thick-walled pilot wheel or mariner's wheel configuration of the yeast form of *P. brasiliensis* (Fig. 17 and 18). The parent yeast cell measures 15 to 30 μm in diameter, whereas the buds are 2 to 10 μm and have a narrow base of attachment. Some yeast cells may measure as much as 60 μm in diameter. The presence of multiple budding distinguishes this yeast from *Cryptococcus neoformans* and *B. dermatitidis.*

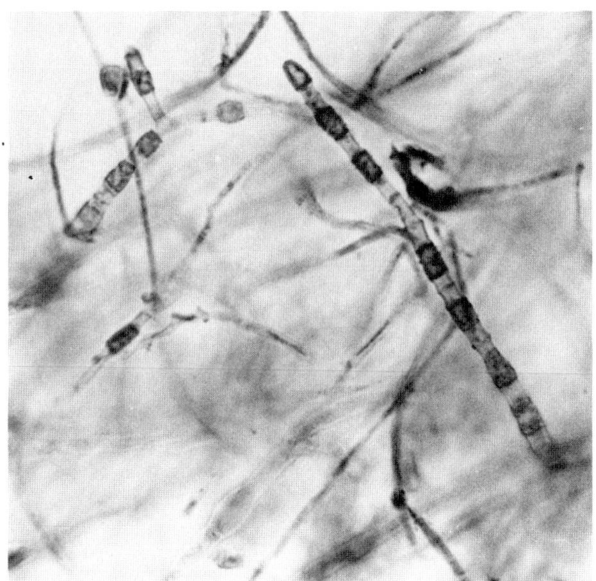

FIG. 16. Mycelial phase of *Coccidioides immitis* demonstrating hyphae with thick-walled arthroconidia alternating with thin-walled empty (disjunctor) cells, grown on potato-dextrose agar at 25°C. Original magnification, ×400.

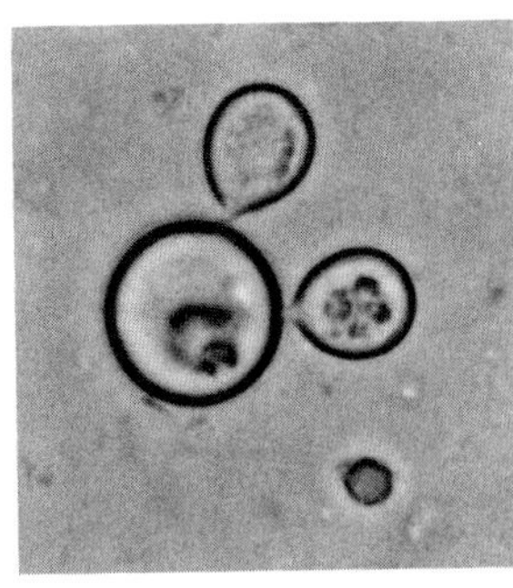

FIG. 17. KOH wet mount of sputum showing blastoconidia of *Paracoccidioides brasiliensis*. Original magnification, ×400.

Histopathological examination using H&E, GMS, and PAS stains of tissue infected with *P. brasiliensis* reveals a pyogranulomatous process with infiltrating polymorphonuclear leukocytes, mononuclear cells, macrophages, and multinucleate giant cells. Single budding forms occasionally are observed that resemble *B. dermatitidis;* however, the multiply budding forms seen elsewhere in the specimen distinguish *P. brasiliensis* from *B. dermatitidis.*

At 25 to 30°C, isolates of *P. brasiliensis* grow slowly and produce colonies that vary in gross morphology, ranging from glabrous, brown colonies to wrinkled, floccose, beige or white colonies. Primary isolation is improved on yeast extract agar (53). The mould form of *P. brasiliensis* may require growth for several weeks before conidia develop. These conidia may be absent to infrequent. When present, the microconidia appear laterally along the hyphae and may resemble those of *B. dermatitidis.* Chlamydoconidia may predominate in the mycelium. Rectangular arthroconidia and interca-

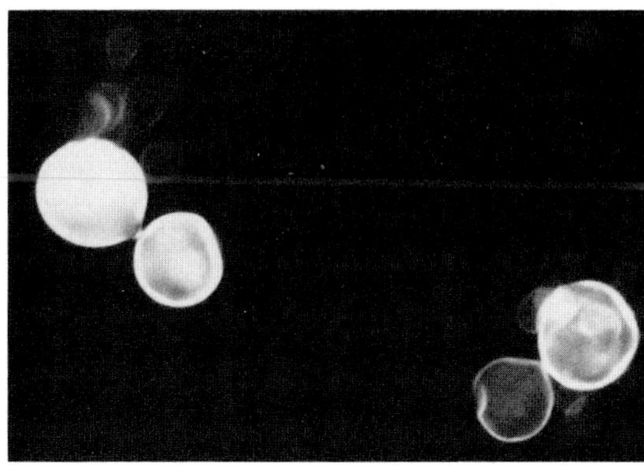

FIG. 18. Calcofluor white wet mount of sputum showing blastoconidia of *Paracoccidioides brasiliensis*. Original magnification, ×400.

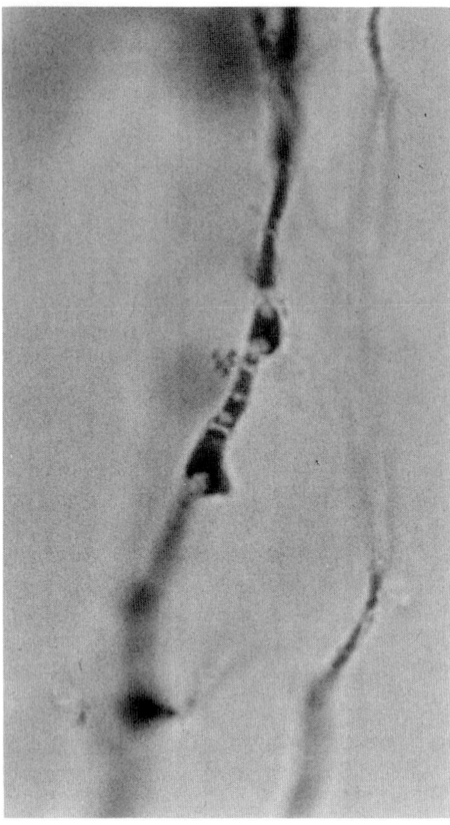

FIG. 19. Mycelial phase of *Paracoccidioides brasiliensis* showing early formation of intercalary chlamydospores, grown on potato-dextrose agar at 25°C. Original magnification, ×400.

lary chlamydospores also may be produced (Fig. 19). Since the microscopic features of the mycelial form of *P. brasiliensis* are not specific, conversion to the yeast form or detection of specific antigen is necessary for definitive identification.

When the hyphae are incubated at 35 to 37°C on BHI or Kelly medium, the yeast form develops slowly. The yeast colony is folded, friable, and white to gray and consists of singly and multiply budding cells. The multiply budding yeast cells demonstrate the characteristic mariner's wheel configuration, similar to that seen in tissue. The parent yeast cell measures 10 to 25 µm in diameter and the progeny buds, which are narrowly attached, are up to 10 µm in diameter.

LITERATURE CITED

1. **Berliner, M.** 1968. Primary subcultures of *Histoplasma capsulatum*. 1. Macro- and micromorphology of the mycelial phase. Sabouraudia **6:**111–118.
2. **Bille, J. L., L. Stockman, G. D. Roberts, C. D. Horstmeier, and D. M. Ilstrup.** 1983. Evaluation of a lysis-centrifugation system for recovery of yeasts and filamentous fungi from blood. J. Clin. Microbiol. **18:**469–471.
3. **Bradsher, R. W.** 1988. Systemic fungal infections: diagnosis and treatment. I. Blastomycosis. Infect. Dis. Clin. North Am. **2:**877–898.
4. **Bronnimann, D. A., R. D. Adam, J. N. Galgiani, M. P. Habib, E. A. Petersen, B. Porter, and J. W. Bloom.** 1987. Coccidioidomycosis in the acquired immunodeficiency syndrome. Ann. Intern. Med. **106:**372–379.
5. **Bronnimann, D. A., and J. N. Galgiani.** 1989. Coccidioidomycosis. Eur. J. Clin. Microbiol. Infect. Dis. **8:**466–473.
6. **Cole, G. T., and S. H. Sun.** 1985. Arthroconidium-spherule-endospore transformation in *Coccidioides immitis*, p. 281–333. *In* P. J. Szaniszlo (ed.), Fungal dimorphism with emphasis on fungi pathogenic for humans. Plenum Publishing Corp., New York.
7. **Converse, J. L.** 1955. Growth of spherules of *Coccidioides immitis* in a chemically defined liquid medium. Proc. Soc. Exp. Biol. Med. **90:**709–711.
8. **Converse, J. L.** 1956. Effect of physico-chemical environment on spherulation of *Coccidioides immitis* in a chemically defined medium. J. Bacteriol. **72:**784–792.
9. **Darling, S. T. A.** 1906. A protozoan general infection producing pseudotubercles in the lungs and focal necrosis in the liver, spleen, and lymph nodes. J. Am. Med. Assoc. **46:** 1283–1285.
10. **Davies, S. F.** 1988. Diagnosis of pulmonary fungal infections. Semin. Respir. Infect. **3:**162–171.
11. **Davies, S. F., and G. A. Sarosi.** 1989. Blastomycosis. Eur. J. Clin. Microbiol. Infect. Dis. **8:**474–479.
12. **de Monbreun, W. A.** 1934. The cultivation and cultural characteristics of Darling's *Histoplasma capsulatum*. Am. J. Trop. Med. Hyg. **14:**93–135.
13. **de Repentigny, L.** 1989. Serological techniques for diagnosis of fungal infection. Eur. J. Clin. Microbiol. Infect. Dis. **8:**362–375.
14. **Drouhet, E.** 1989. African histoplasmosis, p. 221–247. *In* R. J. Hay (ed.), Tropical fungal infections. Bailliere's clinical tropical medicine and communicable diseases. International practice and research, vol. 4. Bailliere Tindall, Philadelphia.
15. **Furcolow, M. L., J. F. Busey, R. W. Menges, et al.** 1970. Prevalence and incidence studies of human and canine blastomycosis. II. Yearly incidence studies in three states, 1960–1967. Am. J. Epidemiol. **92:**121–131.
16. **Gilchrist, T. C., and W. R. Stokes.** 1898. A case of pseudo-lupus vulgaris caused by a Blastomyces. J. Exp. Med. **3:** 53–78.
17. **Goodman, N. L., and H. W. Larsh.** 1967. Environmental factors and growth of *Histoplasma capsulatum* in soil. Mycopathol. Mycol. Appl. **33:**145–156.
18. **Goodwin, R. A., J. E. Loyd, and R. M. Des Prez.** 1981. Histoplasmosis in normal hosts. Medicine **60:**231.
19. **Graham, A. R., R. E. Sobonya, D. A. Bronnimann, and J. N. Galgiani.** 1988. Quantitative pathology of coccidioidomycosis in acquired immunodeficiency syndrome. Hum. Pathol. **19:**800–806.
20. **Graybill, J. R.** 1988. Histoplasmosis and AIDS. J. Infect. Dis. **158:**623–626.
21. **Hageage, G. J., and B. J. Harrington.** 1984. Use of calcofluor white in clinical mycology. Lab. Med. **15:**109–112.
22. **Hardin, H. F., and D. I. Scott.** 1974. Blastomycosis. Occurrence of filamentous forms in vivo. Am. J. Clin. Pathol. **62:**104–106.
23. **Hobbs, E. R.** 1989. Coccidioidomycosis. Dermatol. Clin. **7:**227–239.
24. **Johnson, P. C., and G. A. Sarosi.** 1989. Community-acquired fungal pneumonias. Semin. Respir. Infect. **4:**56–63.
25. **Kauffman, C. A., and M. S. Terpenning.** 1988. Deep fungal infections in the elderly. J. Am. Geriatr. Soc. **36:**548–557.
26. **Kaufman, L., and P. G. Standard.** 1978. Improved version of the exoantigen test for identification of *Coccidioides immitis* and *Histoplasma capsulatum* cultures. J. Clin. Microbiol. **8:**42–45.
27. **Kaufman, L., and P. G. Standard.** 1987. Specific and rapid identification of medically important fungi by exoantigen detection. Annu. Rev. Microbiol. **41:**209–225.
28. **Khardori, N.** 1989. Host-parasite interaction in fungal infections. Eur. J. Clin. Microbiol. Infect. Dis. **8:**331–351.
29. **Klein, B. S., J. M. Vergeront, A. F. DiSalvo, L. Kaufman, and J. P. Davis.** 1987. Two outbreaks of blastomycosis along rivers in Wisconsin. Isolation of *Blastomyces der-*

matitidis from riverbank soil and evidence of its transmission along waterways. Am. Rev. Respir. Dis. **136:**1333–1338.

30. **Klein, B. S., J. M. Vergeront, R. J. Weeks, U. N. Kumar, G. Mathai, B. Varkey, L. Kaufman, R. W. Bradsher, J. F. Stoebig, and J. P. Davis.** 1986. Isolation of *Blastomyces dermatitidis* in soil associated with a large outbreak of blastomycosis in Wisconsin. N. Engl. J. Med. **314:**529–534.
31. **Knoper, S. R., and J. N. Galgiani.** 1988. Systemic fungal infections: diagnosis and treatment. I. Coccidioidomycosis. Infect. Dis. Clin. North Am. **2:**861–875.
32. **Kotloff, K. L., P. A. Vial, J. W. R. Young, and A. G. Smith.** 1987. *Histoplasma duboisii* infection in a Liberian girl. Pediatr. Infect. Dis. J. **6:**202–205.
33. **Kravitz, G. R., S. F. Davies, M. R. Eckman, et al.** 1981. Chronic blastomycotic meningitis. Am. J. Med. **71:**501–505.
34. **Kwon-Chung, K. J.** 1972. Sexual stage of *Histoplasma capsulatum.* Science **175:**326.
35. **Kwon-Chung, K. J.** 1973. Studies on *Emmonsiella capsulata.* I. Heterothallism and development of the ascocarp. Mycologia **65:**109–121.
36. **Kwon-Chung, K. J.** 1975. Perfect state (*Emmonsiella capsulata*) of the fungus using large-form African histoplasmosis. Mycologia **67:**980.
37. **Kwon-Chung, K. J., R. J. Weeks, and H. W. Larsh.** 1974. Studies on *Emmonsiella capsulata* (*Histoplasma capsulatum*). II. Distribution of the two mating types in 13 endemic states of the United States. Am. J. Epidemiol. **99:**44–49.
38. **Maresca, B., and G. S. Kobayashi.** 1989. Dimorphism in *Histoplasma capsulatum:* a model for the study of cell differentiation in pathogenic fungi. Microbiol. Rev. **53:**186–209.
39. **McDonough, E. S., and A. L. Lewis.** 1967. *Blastomyces dermatitidis:* production of the sexual stage. Science **156:** 528–529.
40. **McDonough, E. S., and A. L. Lewis.** 1968. The ascigerous stage of *Blastomyces dermatitidis.* Mycologia **60:**76–83.
41. **McGinnis, M. R., and B. Katz.** 1979. *Ajellomyces* and its synonym *Emmonsiella.* Mycotaxon **8:**157–164.
42. **Medoff, G., A. Painter, and G. S. Kobayashi.** 1987. Mycelial- to yeast-phase transitions of the dimorphic fungi *Blastomyces dermatitidis* and *Paracoccidioides brasiliensis.* J. Bacteriol. **169:**4055–4060.
43. **Minamoto, G., and D. Armstrong.** 1988. Fungal infections in AIDS. Histoplasmosis and coccidioidomycosis. Infect. Dis. Clin. North Am. **2:**447–456.
44. **Mitchell, T. G.** 1988. Serodiagnosis of mycotic infections, p. 303–323. *In* B. B. Wentworth (ed.), Diagnostic procedures for mycotic and parasitic infections, 7th ed. American Public Health Association, Inc., Washington, D.C.
45. **Mitchell, T. G.** 1988. Blastomycosis, p. 1927–1938. *In* R. D. Feigin and J. D. Cherry (ed.), Textbook of pediatric infectious diseases, 2nd ed. The W. B. Saunders Co., Philadelphia.
46. **Moscardi-Bacchi, M., A. Soares, R. Mendes, S. Marques, and M. Franco.** 1989. In situ localization of T lymphocyte subsets in human paracoccidioidomycosis. J. Med. Vet. Mycol. **27:**149–158.
47. **Musial, C. E., W. R. Wilson, I. R. Sinkeldam, and G. D. Roberts.** 1987. Recovery of *Blastomyces dermatitidis* from blood of a patient with disseminated blastomycosis. J. Clin. Microbiol. **25:**1421–1423.
48. **Pappagianis, D.** 1988. Epidemiology of coccidioidomycosis. Curr. Top. Med. Mycol. **2:**199–238.
49. **Paya, C. V., G. D. Roberts, and F. R. Cockerill III.** 1987. Laboratory methods for the diagnosis of disseminated histoplasmosis: clinical importance of the lysis-centrifugation blood culture technique. Mayo Clin. Proc. **62:**480–485.
50. **Pike, R. M.** 1979. Laboratory-associated infections: incidence, fatalities, cases, and prevention. Annu. Rev. Microbiol. **33:**41–66.
51. **Pine, L., E. Drouhet, and G. Reynolds.** 1964. A comparative morphological study of the yeast phases of *Histoplasma capsulatum* and *Histoplasma duboisii.* Sabouraudia **3:**211–224.
52. **Restrepo, A.** 1985. The ecology of *Paracoccidioides brasiliensis:* a puzzle still unresolved. Sabouraudia **23:**323–334.
53. **Restrepo, A., and I. Correa.** 1973. Comparison of two culture media for primary isolation of *Paracoccidioides brasiliensis* from sputum. Sabouraudia **10:**260–265.
54. **Restrepo, A., M. E. Salazar, L. E. Cano, E. P. Stover, D. Feldman, and D. A. Stevens.** 1984. Estrogens inhibit mycelium-to-yeast transformation in the fungus *Paracoccidioides brasiliensis:* implications for resistance of females to paracoccidioidomycosis. Infect. Immun. **46:**346–353.
55. **Rippon, J. W.** 1980. Dimorphism in pathogenic fungi. Crit. Rev. Microbiol. **8:**49–97.
56. **Rippon, J. W.** 1988. Medical mycology. The pathogenic fungi and the pathogenic actinomycetes, 3rd ed., p. 1–797. The W. B. Saunders Co., Philadelphia.
57. **Sanders, J. S., G. A. Sarosi, D. J. Nollett, and J. L. Thompson.** 1977. Exfoliative cytology in the rapid diagnosis of pulmonary blastomycosis. Chest **72:**193–196.
58. **Schwarz, J.** 1981. Histoplasmosis. Plenum Publishing Corp., New York.
59. **Segal, G. P.** 1987. Serodiagnostic procedures in the systemic mycoses. Semin. Respir. Med. **9:**136–144.
60. **Singer-Vermes, L. M., E. Burger, M. F. Franco, M. M. Di-Bacchi, M. J. Mendes-Giannini, and V. L. Calich.** 1989. Evaluation of the pathogenicity and immunogenicity of seven *Paracoccidioides brasiliensis* isolates in susceptible inbred mice. J. Med. Vet. Mycol. **27:**71–82.
61. **Smith, C. D., and N. L. Goodman.** 1975. Improved culture method for the isolation of *Histoplasma capsulatum* and *Blastomyces dermatitidis* from contaminated specimens. Am. J. Clin. Pathol. **62:**276–280.
62. **Soll, D. R.** 1985. *Candida albicans,* p. 167–195. *In* P. J. Szaniszlo (ed.), Fungal dimorphism with emphasis on fungi pathogenic for humans. Plenum Publishing Corp., New York.
63. **Steck, W. D.** 1989. Blastomycosis. Dermatol. Clin. **7:**241–250.
64. **Stevens, D. A.** 1989. The interface of mycology and endocrinology. J. Med. Vet. Mycol. **27:**133–140.
65. **Stevens, D. A. (ed.).** 1980. Coccidioidomycosis: a text. Plenum Publishing Corp., New York.
66. **Sugar, A. M.** 1988. Paracoccidioidomycosis. Infect. Dis. Clin. North Am. **2:**913–924.
67. **Sun, S. H., M. Huppert, and K. R. Vukovich.** 1976. Rapid *in vitro* conversion and identification of *Coccidioides immitis.* J. Clin. Microbiol. **3:**186–190.
68. **Szaniszlo, P. J., and J. L. Harris (ed.).** 1985. Fungal dimorphism—with emphasis on fungi pathogenic for humans. Plenum Publishing Corp., New York.
69. **Walsh, T. J., R. Catchatourian, and H. Cohen.** 1983. Disseminated histoplasmosis complicating bone marrow transplantation. Am. J. Clin. Pathol. **79:**509–511.
70. **Walsh, T. J., and P. A. Pizzo.** 1988. Nosocomial fungal infections: a classification for hospital-acquired fungal infections and mycoses arising from endogenous flora or reactivation. Ann. Rev. Microbiol. **42:**517–545.
71. **Walsh, T. J., and P. A. Pizzo.** 1988. Treatment of systemic fungal infections: recent progress and current problems. Eur. J. Clin. Microbiol. Infect. Dis. **7:**460–475.
72. **Wheat, L. J.** 1988. Systemic fungal infections: diagnosis and treatment. I. Histoplasmosis. Infect. Dis. Clin. North Am. **2:**841–859.
73. **Wheat, L. J.** 1989. Diagnosis and management of histoplasmosis. Eur. J. Clin. Microbiol. Infect. Dis. **8:**480–490.
74. **Wheat, L. J., T. G. Slama, J. A. Horton, et al.** 1982. Risk factors for disseminated or fatal histoplasmosis. Analysis of a large urban outbreak. Ann. Intern. Med. **96:**159–163.

Chapter 62

Dematiaceous Fungi

MICHAEL R. McGINNIS, IRA F. SALKIN, WILEY A. SCHELL, AND LESTER PASARELL

CHARACTERIZATION

Dematiaceous fungi are characterized by the development of a brown to olive to black color in the cell walls of their vegetative cells, conidia, or both, which results in colonies that are olive to black. The dark pigmentation of the majority of medically important fungi is caused by the deposition of dihydroxynaphthalene melanin (44) formed via pentaketide metabolism. This substance differs from the dihydroxyphenylalanine melanin associated with *Cryptococcus neoformans* formed by the oxidation of *ortho-* and *para*-diphenols. These ubiquitous and cosmopolitan opportunistic pathogens normally are associated with soil and plants, but occasionally they may cause infections in humans and lower animals (17, 26, 39). In medical mycology, dematiaceous fungi often are thought of as being exclusively Hyphomycetes. This idea is in error because some Ascomycetes, Basidiomycetes, Coelomycetes, and Zygomycetes may be dematiaceous.

Mycotic infections caused by dematiaceous fungi include chromoblastomycosis, mycetoma, phaeohyphomycosis, and sporotrichosis. In this chapter, only the agents of chromoblastomycosis, phaeohyphomycosis, and sporotrichosis will be considered. Sporotrichosis is treated here because the etiologic agent is dematiaceous in culture, even though the yeast form in tissue appears hyaline. However, use of the Masson-Fontana stain has revealed that a low concentration of melanin exists in the walls of the yeastlike cells.

Deciding whether a particular dematiaceous fungus is involved in the disease process can be difficult at times because these fungi occasionally are recovered from clinical specimens as contaminants. Documentation of a dematiaceous fungus as the etiologic agent of a mycotic infection necessitates sound evidence that the infection is compatible with a mycosis, that the suspected etiologic agent is seen in clinical specimens, that the morphology of the fungus in the clinical specimens is compatible with the suspected etiologic agent, and that the recovered fungus is identified properly. The repeated recovery of a suspected etiologic agent, especially from more than one type of clinical specimen and on more than one isolation medium, is highly significant. Isolation of a dematiaceous fungus from body sites that normally are sterile is suspicious and should not be quickly dismissed as contamination. The ability of the suspected etiologic agent to grow on media at 37°C may serve as corroborative evidence of its potential to cause an infection.

COLLECTION, TRANSPORT, AND STORAGE OF SPECIMENS

Clinical specimens must be collected aseptically and then promptly transported to the clinical laboratory in a properly labeled sterile container. Swabs are an inferior means of specimen collection, and their use should be avoided. Transport media should not be used if specimens cannot be completely and easily retrieved. An adequate quantity of clinical material is necessary if the information obtained in the laboratory is to be meaningful. Refer to chapter 58 for further information.

The specimens most frequently submitted for the recovery of dematiaceous fungi include aspirates, biopsy material, scrapings, and surgical tissue specimens. Specimens other than skin scrapings must be protected from dehydration by addition of a few drops of sterile distilled water to the specimens at the time of collection. Biopsy and tissue specimens can be kept moist by placing them between two pieces of sterile gauze moistened with sterile distilled water. Clinical specimens never should be placed on cotton pads, since cotton fibers can be confused with hyphae in the direct microscopic examination. In addition, it is often impossible to recover all of the clinical specimen from among the cotton fibers. Direct microscopic examination of the specimens and subsequent plating must be done promptly.

PROCESSING AND DIRECT EXAMINATION OF SPECIMENS

Clinical specimens obtained for the recovery of dematiaceous fungi usually do not require extensive processing. If aspirated specimens contain a substantial amount of purulent material, this material can be dissolved with *N*-acetyl-L-cysteine without sodium hydroxide. Highly suspicious areas consisting of necrotic, purulent, or caseous material are selectively examined microscopically, and portions are inoculated onto isolation media. Tissue specimens and biopsy material should be minced with scalpels into 0.5- to 1.0-mm pieces and inoculated directly to culture media. Tissue homogenizers should not be used because a zygomycete may be present. Zygomycetes do not have compartmentalized hyphae (regularly septate when in tissue) and can be damaged easily by homogenization.

Traditionally, specimens have been examined microscopically in 10% KOH. The clearing process can be accelerated by gently heating the KOH preparation. Specimens can be examined microscopically, using a fluorescent compound such as Calcofluor white in 10% KOH. Because penetration of Calcofluor white into tissue is limited, material for microscopic examination should be minced to a pulp, spread thinly on a microscope slide, and then mixed thoroughly with the Calcofluor white. When fungal cells are found, they must be examined by bright-field illumination for the presence of melanin. This is accomplished without moving the slide, by blocking off the UV lamp, rotating the filter out of the light path, and then turning on the incandescent lamp. It must be noted that heavily melanized fungal cells like muriform cells and granules may not be reliably detected by Calcofluor white staining. When either chromoblastomycosis or mycetoma is suspected, examination of clinical specimens by bright-field microscopy is required. In some instances, the dark color of dematiaceous fungi can be seen in tissue sections stained with hematoxylin and eosin. If not, however, and if a dematiaceous fungus is suspected, an unstained tissue section should be examined microscopically by bright-field microscopy. A drop of immersion oil can be placed directly onto a paraffin section mounted on a microscope slide, and then the section is examined microscopically. To determine whether fungal cells are dematiaceous, it is imperative that the microscope's illumination be correctly adjusted according to the Koehler technique.

The etiologic agents of chromoblastomycosis may be filamentous at the surface of the skin. In the deeper subcutaneous tissues, they occur as muriform cells (sclerotic bodies) (Fig. 1). Muriform cells are typically chestnut brown, subglobose, and 5 to 13 μm in size and possess thick cross walls. By definition, mature muriform cells have intersecting cross walls. Many of the cells found represent younger stages of development and have one or no septa. The cells result from vegetative growth without the elongation seen in hyphae; they divide by fission along the septa. The presence of muriform cells in clinical specimens is diagnostic of chromoblastomycosis. However, since the appearance of the muriform cells formed by chromoblastomycotic agents is similar, the identity of the fungus in a given case cannot be determined on the basis of tissue morphology.

Phaeohyphomycosis (1, 17, 26) is characterized by the presence in tissue of dematiaceous yeastlike cells, hyphae, or both. The hyphae may be regular and uniform in diameter or irregular in shape with many swollen cells, and they can be either short or very long (Fig. 2). The name phaeohyphomycosis is not meant to be restricted to Hyphomycetes; it encompasses all fungi having dark hyphae associated with disease in tissue, regardless of the taxonomic classification of the etiologic agent. As with chromoblastomycosis, the etiologic agents of phaeohyphomycosis cannot be identified from clinical specimens. These fungi must be grown on laboratory culture media before they can be identified.

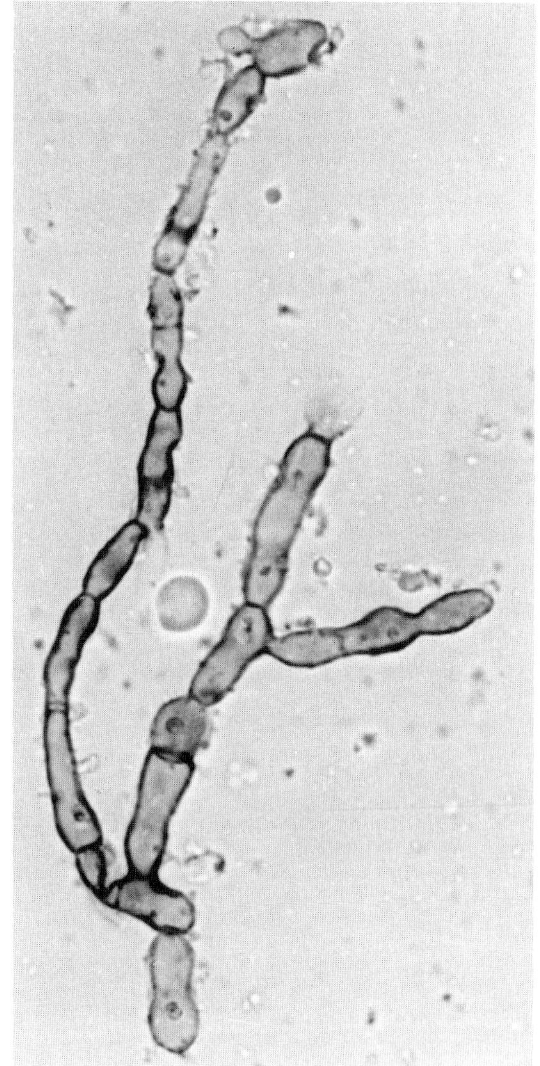

FIG. 2. Dematiaceous hyphae in a subcutaneous aspirate of a cyst mounted in potassium hydroxide.

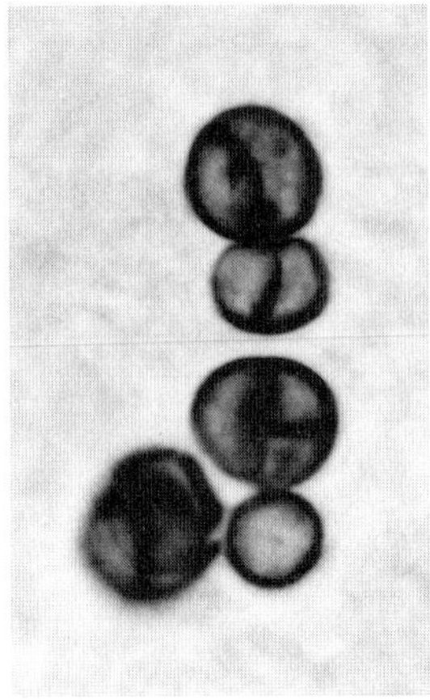

FIG. 1. Muriform cells in cutaneous tissue mounted in potassium hydroxide.

Most mycologists consider it fruitless to examine clinical specimens for the yeast form of *Sporothrix schenckii*. The number of yeast cells in the specimen typically is very limited, and their small size and shape are not distinctive. The yeast form of *S. schenckii* is not seen easily in sections of tissue stained with hematoxylin and eosin. The fungus usually can be seen in tissue sections when the sections first are treated with diastase and then stained by the Gomori or periodic acid-Schiff technique. Fluorescent-antibody-specific conjugates are ideal, although they are available only at some reference laboratories.

CULTURE AND ISOLATION

Dematiaceous fungi are isolated easily on most routine media. Some of them are sensitive to the 0.5-mg/ml concentration of cycloheximide (36) used in some isolation media; for that reason, a medium such as Sabouraud dextrose agar (2% dextrose) or mould-inhibitory agar, with and without antibacterial agents, should be used in conjunction with a medium containing cycloheximide. Most dematiaceous fungi grow well at 30°C; some species grow poorly or not at all at 37°C. Most of the pathogenic dematiaceous fungi usually are visible on isolation media within a week. However, cultures should not be discarded as negative until 4 weeks after inoculation. Once a dematiaceous fungus is isolated, it must be determined whether the isolate is in pure culture. If the culture is not pure, then the fungus must be purified by the isolation of hyphal tips or individual germinating conidia or by streaking the organism onto 100-mm petri plates containing a fungal culture medium with antibacterial agents and isolating individual colonies for subculture to a similar medium (25). This purification is extremely important because many of the opportunistic dematiaceous pathogens are polymorphic; that is, they can produce several different kinds of conidia in the same culture. For an accurate identification, it must be known whether the various types of conidia present in a culture were formed by one fungus or by several fungi. The colony characteristics and microscopic morphology used for the identification of dematiaceous fungi are based on cultures that have been grown for approximately 2 weeks at 25 to 30°C on a medium such as potato-dextrose agar or cornmeal-dextrose agar. These media usually stimulate the formation of conidia. If a suspected pathogen does not produce conidia under such conditions, exposure to a naked incandescent light bulb for several days in a 12-h light/12-h dark cycle while the pathogen is growing on a medium such as 2% water agar, V-8 juice agar, potato-dextrose agar, cornmeal-dextrose agar, moistened sterile wooden sticks, or filter paper may stimulate it to form conidia. The culture also can be exposed to UV light (310 to 410 nm), grown at both high and low temperatures, and grown on hay infusion agar, soil extract agar, and cereal agar, lyophilized, and then regrown, any of which may stimulate the development of conidia and other kinds of structures. Isolates believed to be *S. schenckii* should be subcultured in an enriched medium such as brain heart infusion broth containing 0.1% agar and grown under 5% CO_2 at 35 to 37°C to assess their ability to convert to the yeast phase. When temperature studies are conducted, it is important concurrently to incubate at 25°C an additional tube of medium inoculated with the fungus to demonstrate viability of the inoculum. For an isolate to be considered dimorphic, only a few cells of its typical tissue form need to develop; the entire colony does not have to be converted to its corresponding tissue form.

IDENTIFICATION

The identification of dematiaceous fungi (3, 4, 6, 14, 15, 25) ultimately rests on their microscopic morphology (Table 1) and, to a lesser extent, on their gross colony morphology. The importance of conidium development in defining the numerous genera of dematiaceous fungi makes it essential to determine how a particular fungus forms its conidia. For this reason, slide culture preparations (25) using potato-dextrose agar or cornmeal-dextrose agar are ideal for identification purposes.

Our understanding of conidium development (7, 20, 25) has resulted in the redefinition of many genera of medically important fungi. Terms such as spore and conidium (plural, conidia) no longer should be used interchangeably. Many mycologists consider spores to be propagules that arise either from meiosis (ascospores, basidiospores, oospores, or zygospores) or by mitosis within a sporangium (sporangiospores). All other asexual, nonmotile propagules are considered conidia. Conidia usually occur on specialized hyphae or hyphal branches called conidiophores. The actual cells that give rise to the conidia are referred to as conidiogenous cells. The distinction between the various kinds of conidiogenous cells is important for the identification of dematiaceous fungi. A phialide is a conidiogenous cell that forms a succession of conidia from a locus inside its apex. The apex increases in neither length nor width during conidial production. Phialides usually are flask shaped to cylindrical. A cup-shaped structure called a collarette may be present at the apex of the phialide (Fig. 3). In contrast to a phialide, an annellide (Fig. 4) is a conidiogenous cell characterized by an annellated apex that becomes longer and usually narrower as it forms a succession of conidia. The apex lengthens, and each annellation results when the newest conidium detaches and leaves a scar on top of the scar formed by the previous conidium.

Some fungi produce conidia by a blowing-out process. Such conidia are called blastoconidia. They may occur individually or in chains. The term acropetal is used when new conidia are formed at the apex of the chain. The term basipetal denotes the condition in which new conidia are formed at the base of the chain. A number of the medically important dematiaceous fungi produce conidiophores that are sympodial. In this type of development, a conidium is formed at the apex of the conidiophore. The conidiophore then increases in length by the formation of a new growing point just below and to one side of the conidium. At the apex of this new growth, a second conidium develops. The entire process is repeated, which often results in a conidiophore that has the appearance of a series of bent knees, which is said to be geniculate (Fig. 5).

The term anamorph is used to characterize an asexual reproductive structure or form produced by a fungus. Occasionally, some fungi seen in the clinical laboratory produce more than one asexual form, or anamorph. An example of this polymorphic nature is *Fonsecaea pedrosoi*, which may form a sympodial anamorph (*Rhinocladiella* form), a phialide anamorph (*Phialophora* form), and an anamorph consisting of branched chains of blastoconidia (*Cladosporium* form). When a single fungus produces more than one anamorph, the term synanamorph can be used to designate any of these concurrently existing forms. The *Rhinocladiella*, *Phialophora*, and *Cladosporium* forms are synanamorphs of *F. pedrosoi*.

A small number of medically important fungi have the ability to produce sexual forms. The sexual form of a fungus is referred to as a teleomorph. *Pseudallescheria boydii* is characterized by the formation of cleistothecia; hence, it is a teleomorph. *P. boydii* also may produce two anamorphs, namely, *Scedosporium* and *Graphium*.

TABLE 1. Diagnostic features for some medically important dematiaceous fungi

Genus	Diagnostic characteristics	Comments	Selected references
Alternaria	Conidiophores dark, septate, simple, or branched. Conidia muriform, obclavate, with a beak, darkly pigmented, in simple or branched acropetal chains.	Recognized by the distinctive muriform, obclavate conidia with a beak (tapering apex).	14, 15, 25
Aureobasidium	Conidiogenous cells phialides, undifferentiated from hyphae. Conidia borne laterally, hyaline, one celled, often producing secondary blastoconidia. Large, dark, one- or two-celled, thick-walled arthroconidia commonly present.	Differentiated from *Hormonema* spp. by the production of conidia in a synchronous manner. Differentiated from *Phaeococcomyces* spp. by the lack of dematiaceous yeast cells.	10, 14, 15, 25
Bipolaris	Conidiophores dark, erect, geniculate as a result of sympodial development. Conidia multiseptate, cylindrical to oblong, dark, septal walls thickened with slightly protruding hila.	Differentiated from *Curvularia* spp. by possessing conidia that are oblong to cylindrical with thickened septal walls.	2, 29, 34
Cladosporium	Conidiophores dark, erect, often septate. Conidia one to several celled in some species, with dark hila, occurring in fragile, branched acropetal chains. Conidia at branch points of chains usually shield shaped.	*C. carrionii* grows up to 37°C and forms branching chains of conidia from distinct conidiophores, with conidia ca. 5 μm long.	25
Curvularia	Conidiophores dark, erect, geniculate as a result of sympodial development. Conidia multiseptate, usually curved, with central cell larger and darker than end cells, thickness of septal and outer cell wall approximately the same.	Differentiated from *Bipolaris* spp. by possessing (i) curved conidia that have an enlarged and darker central cell and (ii) narrow septa.	14, 15, 25
Dactylaria	Condiophores hyaline and erect but occasionally may be geniculate as a result of sympodial development. Conidia two celled, cylindrical to oblong, dark. One-celled, globose phialoconidia may be present in young colonies.	*D. constricta* var. *gallopava* grows at 45°C, is inhibited on Mycosel, is late gelatin positive, and is pathogenic to fowl and humans. *D. constricta* var. *constricta* does not grow at 45°C, grows on Mycosel, is rapidly gelatin positive, and is not known to be pathogenic. Both form a diffusible red pigment on Sabouraud glucose medium.	11, 35
Exophiala	Conidiophores hyaline to subhyaline, hyphalike or distinct. Conidiogenous cells annellides that are cylindrical to lageniform. Conidia are one to several celled (one species), hyaline to pale brown, accumulating in balls at the apices of the annellides. *Phaeoannellomyces* synanamorph usually present.	*E. jeanselmei* has cylindrical to lageniform annellides produced from conidiophores, with some annellides intercalary. Growth up to ca. 37°C. *E. jeanselmei* is differentiated from *W. dermatitidis* by lack of the ability to grow at 40°C, by the development of annellides instead of phialides, and by the ability to assimilate KNO_3.	10, 16, 22–25, 31
Exserohilum	Conidiophores dark, erect, geniculate as a result of sympodial development. Conidia multiseptate, cylindrical to oblong, dark, with strongly protruding hila.	Differentiated from *Bipolaris* spp. by having strongly protruding, truncate hila.	2, 29, 34
Fonsecaea	Conidiophores pale brown, usually erect, swollen apically as a result of sympodial development. Conidia one celled, pale brown; primary conidia function as sympodial conidiogenous cells to produce secondary conidia. Tertiary conidia may be formed in the same manner. *Rhinocladiella*, *Cladosporium*, or *Phialophora* synanamorphs often are present.	*F. pedrosoi* is differentiated from *F. compacta* by having conidia that are more elongate and in loose conidial heads.	25

(*Continued on next page*)

TABLE 1—*Continued*

Genus	Diagnostic characteristics	Comments	Selected references
Phaeoannellomyces	Conidiophores and hyphae absent. Yeast cells one or two celled, pale to brown to black, annellides; pseudohyphae may be formed. Often occurs as a synanamorph associated with *Exophiala* spp.	*P. werneckii* produces one- to two-celled yeast cells that are annellides, the latter predominant; cells tapering toward one or both ends, bearing annellations.	24, 30
Phaeococcomyces	Conidiophores and hyphae absent. Yeast cells one celled, pale brown to black; pseudohyphae may be formed; conidia, blastoconidia, annelloconidia absent. May occur as a synanamorph associated with species of *Wangiella* and other genera.	Often will produce synanamorphs when grown on either cornmeal agar or potato-dextrose agar.	8, 10, 25
Phialophora	Conidiophores absent or present, pale brown. Conidiogenous cells phialides with distinct collarettes. Conidia one celled, hyaline to pale brown, accumulating as balls at the apices of the phialides.	*P. verrucosa* produces flask-shaped phialides with cup-shaped, dark, often deep collarettes. *P. parasitica* produces phialides of variable length, some isolates forming extremely long phialides swollen near the base, with prominent encrustations on the cell wall. Conidia elliptical to cylindrical, often curved. *P. repens* produces intercalary phialides without basal septa or phialides cylindrical to slightly lageniform with a delicate collarette. *P. richardsiae* produces phialides of variable size and shape, some phialides long with flaring, flattened collarettes. Conidia of two shapes: globose conidia from phialides with flattened collarettes and cylindrical, often curved conidia from other phialides.	14, 15, 18, 25
Rhinocladiella	Conidiophores pale brown, erect, usually with distinct scars, and sympodial in development. Conidia one celled, fusiform to obovate, pale brown, with a dark basal scar.	Conidia occur along the conidiophore.	15, 16, 25, 40
Scedosporium	Conidiophores hyaline, short or long. Predominant conidiogenous cells annellides with slight swelling just below the apex, with or without swollen bases. Conidia one celled, obovate, truncate, subhyaline to light black, single or in balls.	*S. apiospermum* grows at 37°C but lacks a swelling at base of its conidiogenous cell. *S. inflatum* grows at 37°C, conidiogenous cells have swollen bases, and most isolates do not grow on media containing cycloheximide. Several species of ascomycetes besides *Pseudallescheria boydii* may produce an *S. apiospermum* anamorph.	13, 21, 25, 28, 38
Scytalidium	Hyphae produce one- to two-celled arthroconidia, pale brown to brown, subglobose to ellipsoidal.	May occur as synanamorphs with *Aureobasidium* spp. and *Nattrassia mangiferae*.	9, 25, 43
Wangiella	Conidiophores hyphalike, subhyaline to pale brown. Conidiogenous cells phialides without distinct collarettes, intercalary or lateral from hyphae. Phialides cylindrical with rounded apices. Conidia one celled, subglobose, pale brown, occurring as balls that slip down the conidiogenous cells. Annellidic and apical sympodial developing synanamorphs often present.	*W. dermatitidis* is differentiated from *E. jeanselmei* and similar fungi by the production of phialides and the ability to grow at 40°C. Nitrate assimilation negative.	16, 22, 32
Xylohypha	Conidiophores hyphalike, pale brown. Blastoconidia one celled, without evident darkly pigmented hila, occurring as long, sparsely branching chains.	*X. bantiana* is differentiated from *Cladosporium carrionii* by growing faster, having longer conidia (2–2.5 by 4–7 μm), being neurotropic, and growing at 42–43°C.	27, 33

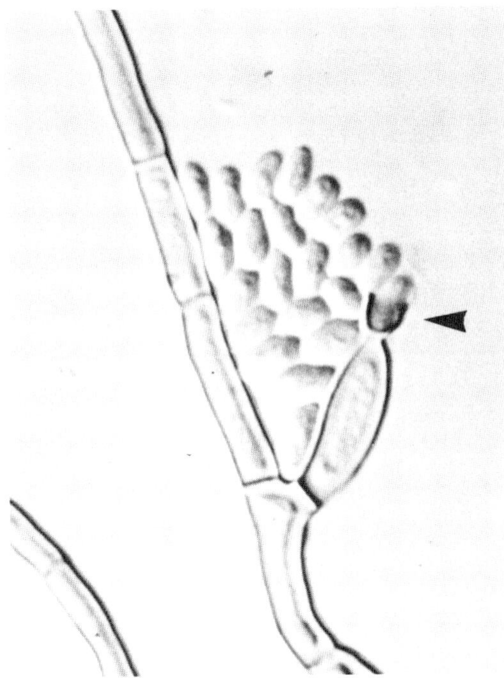

FIG. 3. *Phialophora verrucosa*. Note presence of collarette (arrowhead) at apex of the phialide.

The term holomorph is used to encompass the whole fungus. In this example, the whole fungus consists of the *Pseudallescheria*, *Scedosporium*, and *Graphium* forms. Because fungi must be classified by sexual structures when possible, the name used for the teleomorph also is used for the whole fungus (holomorph). Problems occasionally arise with anamorph-teleomorph connections because a teleomorph may have more than one anamorph and a single anamorph may be produced by several different teleomorphs. For example, *Scedosporium apiospermum* is one anamorph that is produced by several species of *Pseudallescheria* and *Petriella*.

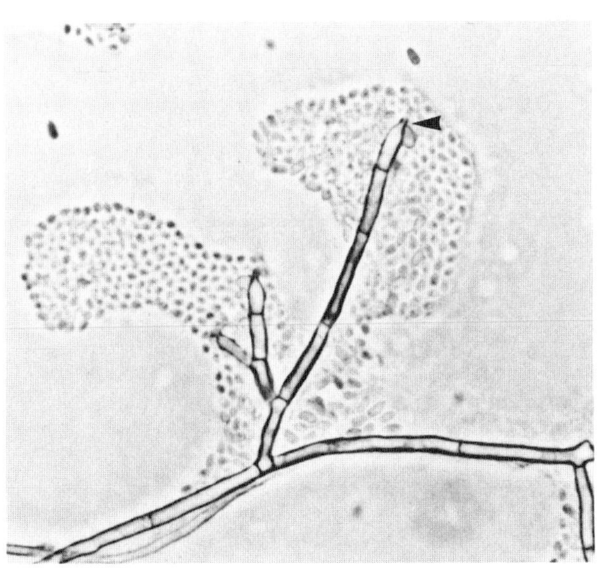

FIG. 4. *Exophiala spinifera*. The apex of an annellide (arrowhead) becomes longer and narrower as it grows.

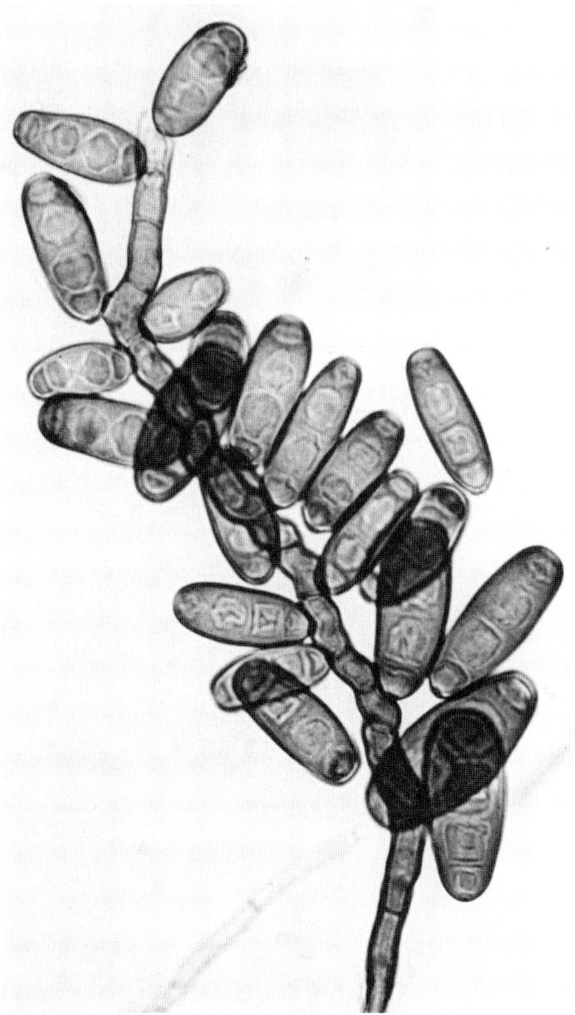

FIG. 5. *Bipolaris spicifera*. The geniculate appearance of the conidiophore results from sympodial development.

The black yeasts are at times extremely difficult and frustrating to identify. Black yeasts typically represent one growth form or anamorph of polymorphic fungi. The genera *Phaeococcomyces* and *Phaeoannellomyces* were established (8, 10, 30) to accommodate isolates that consisted of black, budding yeasts and occasional short elements of pseudohyphae, or toruloid hyphae. The assumption that a black yeast, regardless of whether the colony is initially dematiaceous or not, should be identified as *Aureobasidium pullulans* is incorrect. One of the most frequently isolated black yeasts in the clinical laboratory is the *Phaeoannellomyces* synanamorph of *Exophiala jeanselmei*. When fresh isolates of this fungus are transferred from Sabouraud dextrose agar to potato-dextrose agar or cornmeal agar, the typical conidiogenous cells and conidia of *E. jeanselmei* rapidly become evident.

Sterile isolates represent a second group of medically important fungi that are especially difficult to identify. They commonly are referred to as members of the form-order Mycelia Sterilia. These fungi have been shown to cause phaeohyphomycosis and mycetoma. When sterile dematiaceous fungi are isolated, one should attempt the induction of conidia or fruiting bodies as previously discussed. The cultures should be kept for several weeks before they are discarded. With time, some of these fungi may develop structures that produce spores or conidia, such as ascocarps, pycnidia, or synnemata, either in the agar or at the colony surface.

Alternaria spp.

Members of the genus *Alternaria* occasionally are implicated as agents of phaeohyphomycosis. These fungi have been associated with infections involving bone, cutaneous tissue, ears, eyes, paranasal sinuses, and the urinary tract. An *Alternaria* sp. and *Alternaria alternata* (synonym, *A. tenuis*) (19) are the only well-documented human pathogens in this genus. The *Alternaria* anamorph of *Pleospora infectoria* has been reported to be a pathogen of humans but has not been documented convincingly. In clinical specimens, the hyphae are mostly or entirely hyaline.

Alternaria colonies are rapidly growing, cottony, and gray to black. The erect conidiophores are dematiaceous, simple or branched, and usually solitary, but they occasionally occur in small groups. The conidia of *Alternaria* spp. develop at the apex of the conidiophore in acropetal, branching chains (Fig. 6). The conidia are dematiaceous, muriform, smooth or rough, tapering toward the distal end, and typically with a short cylindrical beak at their apices.

Alternaria isolates are difficult to identify beyond the generic level. If an isolate is recovered that must be identified to species, it should be sent to a specialist.

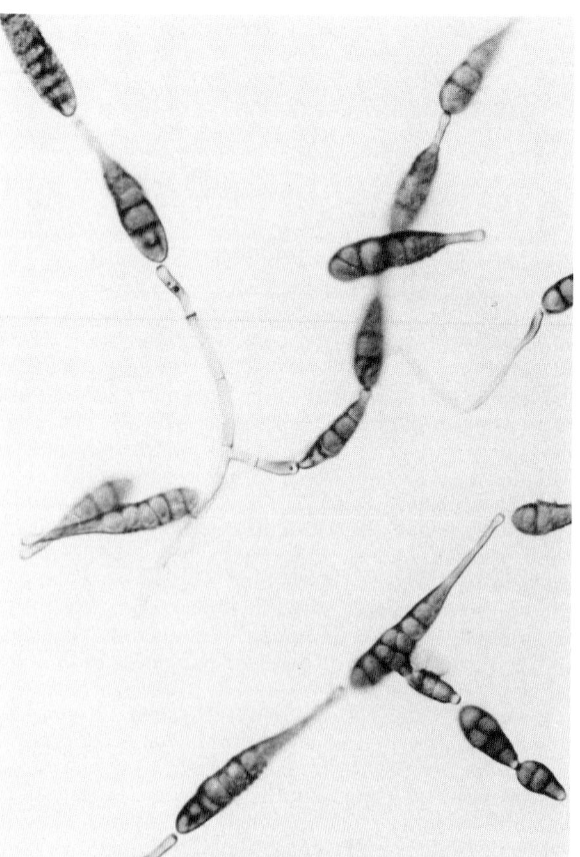

FIG. 6. *Alternaria* sp. Muriform conidia having beaks arise in branching chains from the conidiophore.

Aureobasidium spp.

Aureobasidium pullulans has been implicated as an agent of phaeohyphomycosis in humans and other animals (37). This hyphomycete is capable of causing opportunistic infections and has been reported from skin, nail, subcutaneous, and deeper tissues.

Colonies of *A. pullulans* are smooth, moist, and yellow, white, cream, light pink, or light brown, finally becoming black as a result of the development of arthroconidia. The conidiogenous cells are undifferentiated from the vegetative hyphae and may be intercalary, terminal, or arising as short lateral branches from the hyphae. The conidia are hyaline, one celled, smooth, ellipsoidal, and variable in shape and size. The conidia develop in a synchronous manner from the conidiogenous cells (Fig. 7). Blastoconidia commonly are produced from the conidia that arise from the undifferentiated hyphal cells. A *Scytalidium* synanamorph consisting of dematiaceous arthroconidia typically is present. *Hormonema* spp. often are confused with *Aureobasidium* spp. In the genus *Hormonema*, the conidia arise in a basipetal succession from either hyaline or dematiaceous, hyphalike conidiogenous cells. In contrast, *A. pullulans* produces its conidia in a synchronous manner (10). Because of the confusion that has surrounded these two genera, some of the reported cases of infection ascribed to *A. pullulans* may have been caused by misidentified isolates of *Hormonema* spp. This speculation is based on the fact that several authors have illustrated *Hormonema* spp. under the name *Aureobasidium*.

Bipolaris spp.

Several *Bipolaris* species, including *Bipolaris australiensis*, *B. hawaiiensis*, and *B. spicifera*, have caused

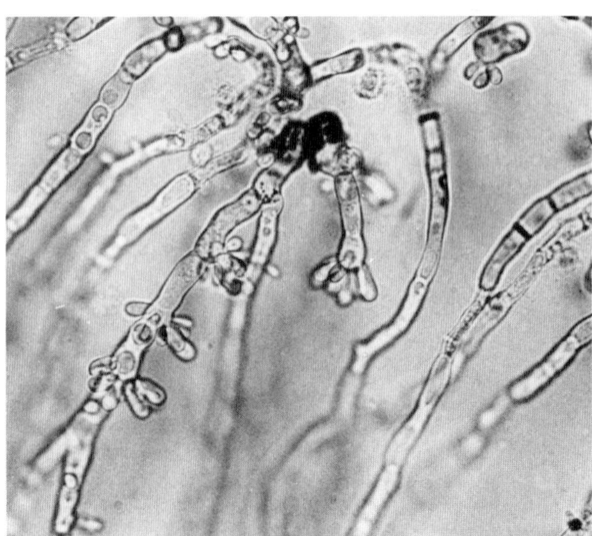

FIG. 7. *Aureobasidium pullulans*. Conidia develop in a synchronous manner.

a spectrum of infections in humans, including meningitis, paranasal sinusitis, cutaneous, eye, and pulmonary infections (29). In clinical specimens, the hyphae are frequently hyaline. In the past, some medical microbiologists have confused species of *Drechslera, Exserohilum,* and *Helminthosporium* with *Bipolaris* species. Recent taxonomic studies (2, 29) have established useful criteria for the recognization of *Bipolaris* spp. and their separation from species classified in similar genera.

Bipolaris, Drechslera, Exserohilum, and *Helminthosporium* spp. all form rapidly growing, woolly, gray to black colonies. Their conidiophores are dematiaceous, solitary or in groups, simple or branched, and septate. The conidiophores of *Bipolaris, Drechslera,* and *Exserohilum* spp. are sympodial and geniculate, whereas those of *Helminthosporium* spp. are straight and stop lengthening when the terminal conidium is formed. The conidia produced by these fungi are dematiaceous, oblong to cylindrical, and multicelled.

Bipolaris spp. (Fig. 5) are characterized by having a hilum (basal scar) that slightly protrudes below the contour of the basal cell of the conidium and a germ tube that arises adjacent to the hilum and grows along the conidial axis, with the first conidial septum being median. *Drechslera* spp. have hila that are continuous with the conidial walls and germ tubes that arise perpendicular to the conidial axis from the basal conidial cell, and the first conidial septum delineates the basal portion; that is, it is not median. The diagnostic features for the genus *Exserohilum* are discussed in the section on that genus.

Cladosporium spp.

Occasionally, isolates of *Cladosporium* spp. are reported from cutaneous, eye, and nail infections. *Cladosporium* isolates are rapidly growing, velvety or cottony, and usually some shade of olive gray to olive brown or black. Erect, tall, branching, dematiaceous conidiophores arise from the hyphae. One- to several-celled, smooth or rough, dematiaceous blastoconidia form in acropetal branching chains at the apex of the conidiophore (Fig. 8). The conidia have a dark hilum at each end. The conidia at the branch points of the chains tend to have a shieldlike shape and are commonly referred to as shield cells.

Curvularia spp.

Curvularia geniculata, C. lunata, C. pallescens, C. senegalensis, and *C. verruculosa* have been implicated in a number of opportunistic infections (25), including paranasal sinusitis, endocarditis, eye infections, mycetoma, and pulmonary phaeohyphomycosis. In clinical specimens, the hyphae may be hyaline.

Curvularia colonies are rapidly growing, woolly, and gray to grayish black or brown. Their conidiophores are dematiaceous, solitary or in groups, simple or branched, septate, sympodial, and geniculate. The conidia are two to several celled, usually curved, dark with pale ends, solitary, and typically with a dark hilum (Fig. 9). The works by Ellis (14, 15) should be consulted if a *Curvularia* isolate must be identified to species.

Dactylaria spp.

Dactylaria constricta recently was proposed by Dixon and Salkin (11) as a new combination for two previously

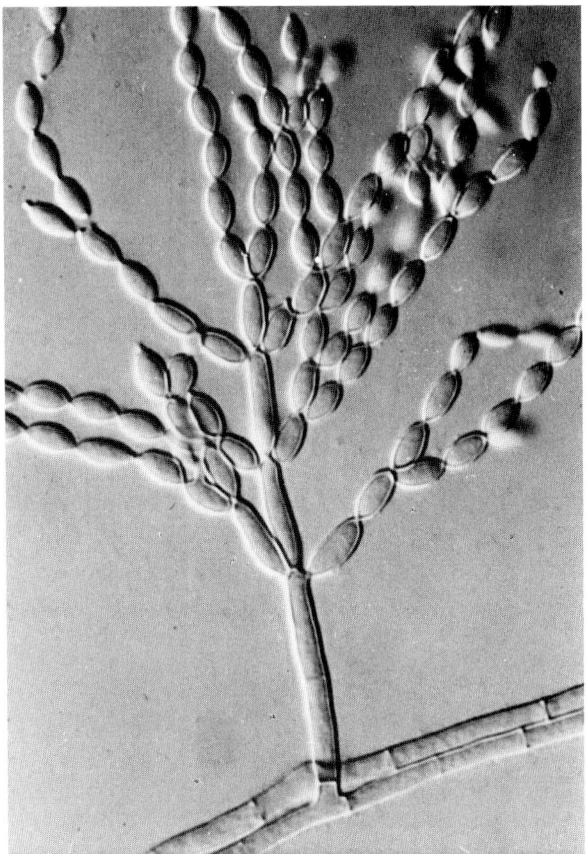

FIG. 8. *Cladosporium carrionii.* Branching chains of blastoconidia have developed from an erect conidiophore.

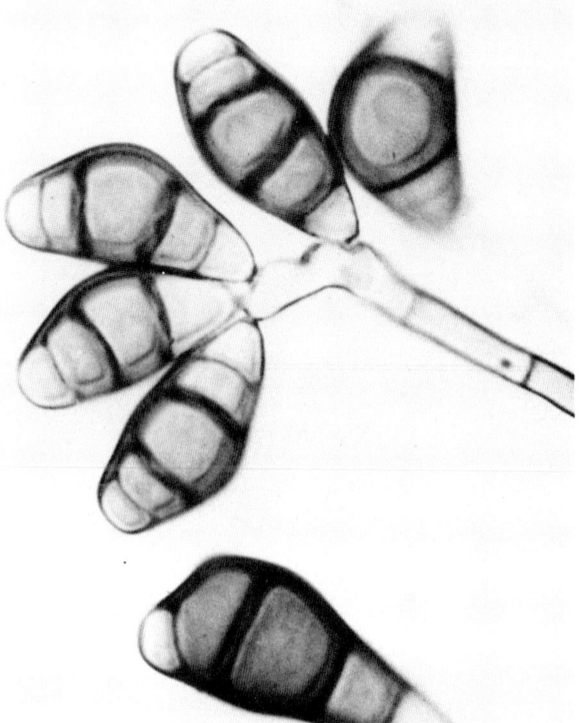

FIG. 9. *Curvularia* sp. Curved conidia developing from a geniculate conidiophore.

described dematiaceous Hyphomycetes, *D. gallopava* and *Scolecobasidium constrictum*. The fungus has been reported as the cause of epizootic encephalitis in flocks of turkeys and chickens as well as of disseminated infections in immunocompromised human hosts.

D. constricta colonies are flat and olive gray and usually form a bordeaux red diffusible pigment when grown on Sabouraud dextrose agar. Two-celled, holoblastic conidia with rhexolytic dehiscence are formed on solitary conidiophores, which is the predominant and most characteristic anamorphic structure (Fig. 10). However, one may find that holoblastic conidia are formed occasionally on sympodially proliferating conidiophores. Globose, single-celled phialoconidia developing from phialides with fine collarettes have been observed in young colonies (11, 35).

D. constricta may be differentiated into two varieties on the basis of physiologic characteristics and pathogenicity, as assessed in an experimental mouse model (35). In contrast to *D. constricta* var. *constricta*, *D. constricta* var. *gallopava* grows on Sabouraud glucose agar at 37 and 45°C, is inhibited on Mycosel agar, gives a delayed (≧21 days) positive gelatin reaction, and is pathogenic in Swiss albino mice when inoculated intravenously. This variety has been associated with infections in fowl and humans.

Exophiala **spp.**

Exophiala jeanselmei is a common etiologic agent of mycotic subcutaneous abscesses. This dematiaceous hyphomycete may cause either mycetoma or phaeohyphomycosis. *E. moniliae* and *E. spinifera* also have been reported as agents of phaeohyphomycosis (22). *E. werneckii* recently has been renamed *Phaeoannellomyces werneckii* (30) and is discussed in the section on the genus *Phaeoannellomyces*.

The colonial morphology of *Exophiala* spp. is varied. Colonies are slow to rapidly growing, moist and yeastlike at first, becoming woolly with age, and gray to black. Some isolates, which are predominantly the *Phaeoannellomyces* synanamorph of *E. jeanselmei*, may remain black and yeastlike. Conidiophores are dematiaceous, simple, or hyphalike. The conidiogenous cells are annellides. In *E. jeanselmei*, the annellides are lageniform to cylindrical, tapering to a narrow apex; in *E. moniliae*, they are inflated to elliptical, tapering to a very long, narrow apex; in *E. spinifera*, they are lageniform to cylindrical, tapering to a narrow apex, and arise from distinct spinelike conidiophores. *E. jeanselmei* assimilates potassium nitrate.

The conidia are one celled in most species and accumulate in balls at the apices of the annellides. With careful study using the oil immersion objective, annellations (rings) usually can be seen at the apices of the annellides. *E. jeanselmei* was believed incorrectly by some to belong to the genus *Phialophora* (23). The fungus later was transferred to the genus *Exophiala* when it was discovered that the conidiogenous cells of *E. jeanselmei* were annellides and not phialides. An identical situation occurred when it was discovered that the conidiogenous cells of *E. spinifera* (Fig. 4) were annellides.

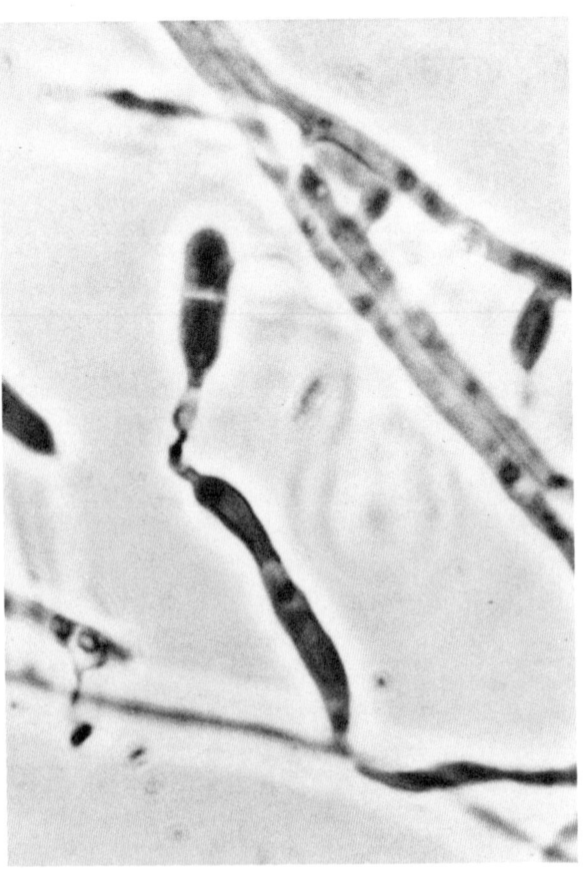

FIG. 10. *Dactylaria constricta*. Two-celled conidium is attached by a narrow denticle to the conidiophore.

Exserohilum **spp.**

The genus *Exserohilum* contains three recognized pathogens, *Exserohilum longirostratum*, *E. mcginnisii*, and *E. rostratum*. Like *Bipolaris* spp., members of the genus *Exserohilum* have been confused with *Drechslera* and *Helminthosporium* spp. The confusion has been resolved as a result of recent taxonomic studies (1, 29).

Exserohilum spp. produce ellipsoidal to fusoid conidia that have a strongly protruding truncate hilum (Fig. 11). When a germ tube originates from the basal conidial cell, it arises adjacent to the hilum and grows along the conidial axis. Like *Bipolaris* spp., *Exserohilum* spp. form the first conidial septum nearly median. The large, multicelled (profusely produced) conidia arise from sympodial conidiophores.

Fonsecaea **spp.**

The genus *Fonsecaea* contains two species, *Fonsecaea compacta* (incorrectly spelled *compactum*) and *F. pedrosoi*. Both are agents of chromoblastomycosis. *Fonsecaea* colonies are slowly growing, velvety to woolly, and olive to black. *Fonsecaea* isolates are extremely polymorphic. They are characterized by the development of one-celled primary conidia that form on erect, dark, sympodial conidiophores. The primary conidia in turn become conidiogenous cells and form secondary one-celled conidia. This process usually results in only three levels of conidia (Fig. 12). Another form of development (incorrectly called *Acrotheca*-like) may occur that is similar to the form seen in the genus *Rhinocladiella*. Yet another anamorph may be seen in which the conidia occur as branching chains of blastoconidia,

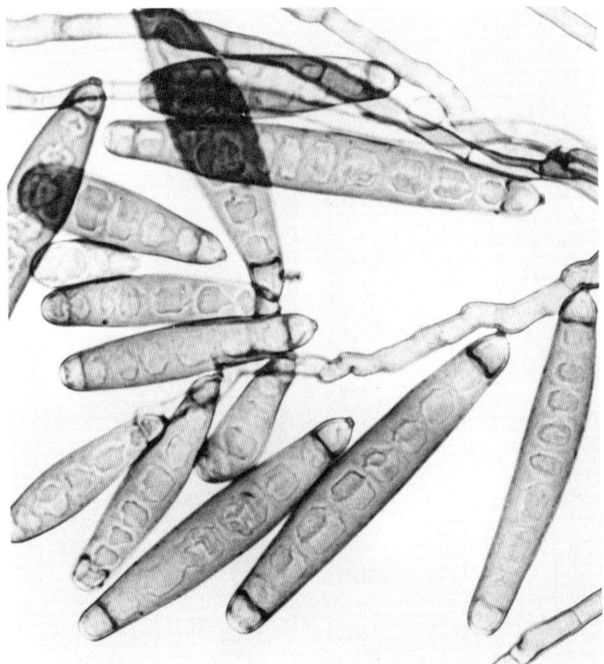

FIG. 11. *Exserohilum rostratum.* Ellipsoidal conidia having protruding hila are developing from a sympodial conidiophore.

similar to those found in the genus *Cladosporium. Fonsecaea* spp. also may produce phialides with collarettes bearing balls of one-celled conidia that are typical of the genus *Phialophora.*

F. pedrosoi and *F. compacta* are morphologically distinct (25). *F. pedrosoi* is differentiated from *F. compacta* by its elongate conidia that occur in loose heads, in contrast to the rounded conidia in compact heads produced by *F. compacta.* As a result of their polymorphic nature, *F. pedrosoi* and *F. compacta* have been placed inappropriately in the genera *Phialophora* and *Rhinocladiella.*

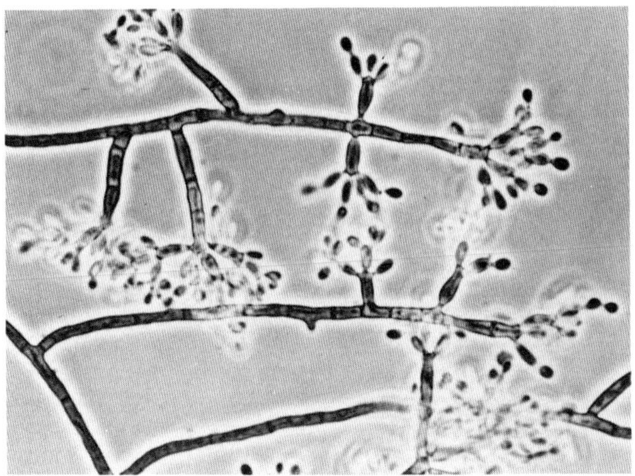

FIG. 12. *Fonsecaea pedrosoi.* Series of conidia arise from each other at the apices of sympodial conidiophores.

Phaeoannellomyces spp.

Phaeoannellomyces is a genus of the black yeasts that is characterized by the development of yeast cells that function as annellides (30). *Phaeoannellomyces werneckii* (syn. *Cladosporium werneckii, Exophiala werneckii*) and *P. elegans* are known opportunistic pathogens.

P. werneckii, which is a cause of superficial phaeohyphomycosis (1, 17, 26), produces two-celled yeast cells that produce annelloconidia from their distal ends (Fig. 13). Hyphae giving rise to terminal and intercalary annellides like those produced by *Exophiala* spp. may develop. *P. werneckii* is classified in the blastomycete genus *Phaeoannellomyces* because the yeast anamorph is stable, distinct, predominant, and unique. *P. elegans,* which is a synanamorph associated with *E. jeanselmei,* is distinguished from *P. werneckii* by having one-celled yeast cells.

P. elegans forms slimy, mucoid, slow-growing, smooth colonies that are grayish black. Budding yeast cells, which are at first subhyaline, are abundant. With age, some of the cells become larger and darker and may have thickened cell walls. Some pseudohyphae usually are present. Hyphal development may become dominant in some isolates of this species with subsequent subculture.

Phaeococcomyces spp.

Phaeococcomyces is a genus containing black yeasts that often are synanamorphs associated with several of the medically important polymorphic dematiaceous Hyphomycetes such as *Wangiella dermatitidis. Phaeococcomyces,* which was originally named *Phaeococcus* (8, 10), contains species that are distinguished from each

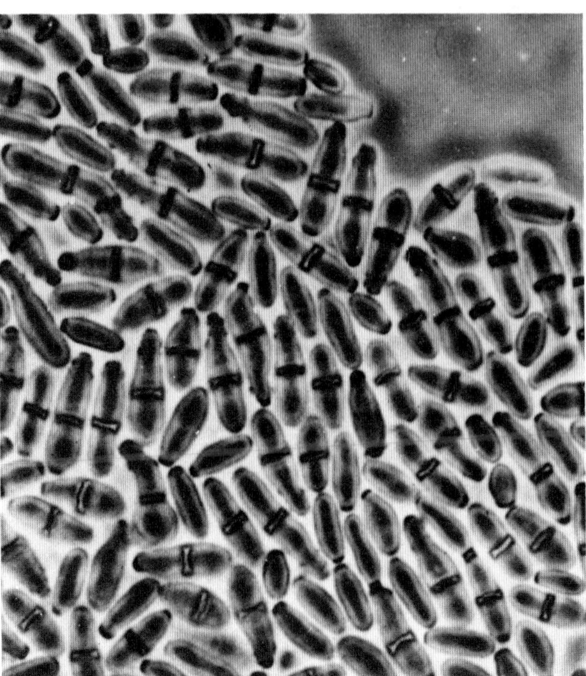

FIG. 13. *Phaeoannellomyces werneckii.* The yeastlike cells are annellides.

other primarily on morphological criteria. The genus is characterized by the development of holoblastic, multilateral blastoconidia, in contrast to the annelloconidia produced by *Phaeoannellomyces* spp. (30).

Black yeasts occasionally are isolated in the clinical laboratory. They are recognized by their black, usually mucoid, yeastlike colonies. When grown on cornmeal agar or potato-dextrose agar, many black yeasts rapidly produce hyphae and conidiogenous cells typical of genera such as *Exophiala*. Because of the diverse modes of conidiogenesis in this heterogenous group of fungi, additional genera probably will be needed in the future to fully accommodate the black yeasts.

Phialophora spp.

Members of the genus *Phialophora* are well-recognized etiologic agents of phaeohyphomycosis and chromoblastomycosis. In addition to causing cutaneous and subcutaneous tissue invasion, some species have caused endocarditis and mycotic keratitis. The pathogenic *Phialophora* species include *Phialophora bubakii, P. parasitica, P. repens, P. richardsiae*, and *P. verrucosa*.

Phialophora colonies are rapidly growing, cottony to velvety, and usually some shade of olive gray. When conidiophores are present, they usually are short. The conidiogenous cells are hyaline to dematiaceous phialides that are cylindrical to flask shaped. At the apices of the phialides, distinct collarettes are present (Fig. 3). The conidia are one celled and usually hyaline, and they occur in balls that occasionally may slip down along the phialides in some species. Some species commonly produce intercalary phialides; a yeast form may occur in some isolates.

P. mutabilis and *P. hoffmannii* traditionally have been considered species of *Phialophora*. Gams and McGinnis (18) have reclassified these species in the genus *Lecythophora*. This reclassification was necessary because these fungi produce intercalary phialides with short, lateral, conically tapering tips exceeding 1.2 μm with periclinal wall thickenings and have conidia accumulating in balls at the apices of the phialides. Collarettes are present at the tips of the phialides.

Rhinocladiella spp.

Rhinocladiella aquaspersa, previously known as *Acrotheca aquaspersa*, is a rare etiologic agent of chromoblastomycosis (40), human cases having been reported in Brazil and Mexico.

Colonies of *R. aquaspersa* are rapidly growing, velvety, slightly elevated, and olive black. The conidiophores are sympodial, unbranched, erect, and usually darker than the vegetative hyphae. Conidia are one celled, rarely two celled, fusiform, elliptical or obovate, smooth, light brown, and with a dark basal scar (Fig. 14). Annellides like those of *Exophiala* spp. and phialides like those of *Wangiella* spp. may be present.

Scedosporium spp.

Scedosporium apiospermum, previously known as *Monosporium apiospermum*, is an anamorph of *Pseudallescheria boydii*, a fungus once classified as *Petriellidium boydii* and *Allescheria boydii* (28). The fungus may cause mycetoma as well as infections involving the lungs and brain, in which the fungus grows in the form of hyphae that look like those produced by *Aspergillus* spp.

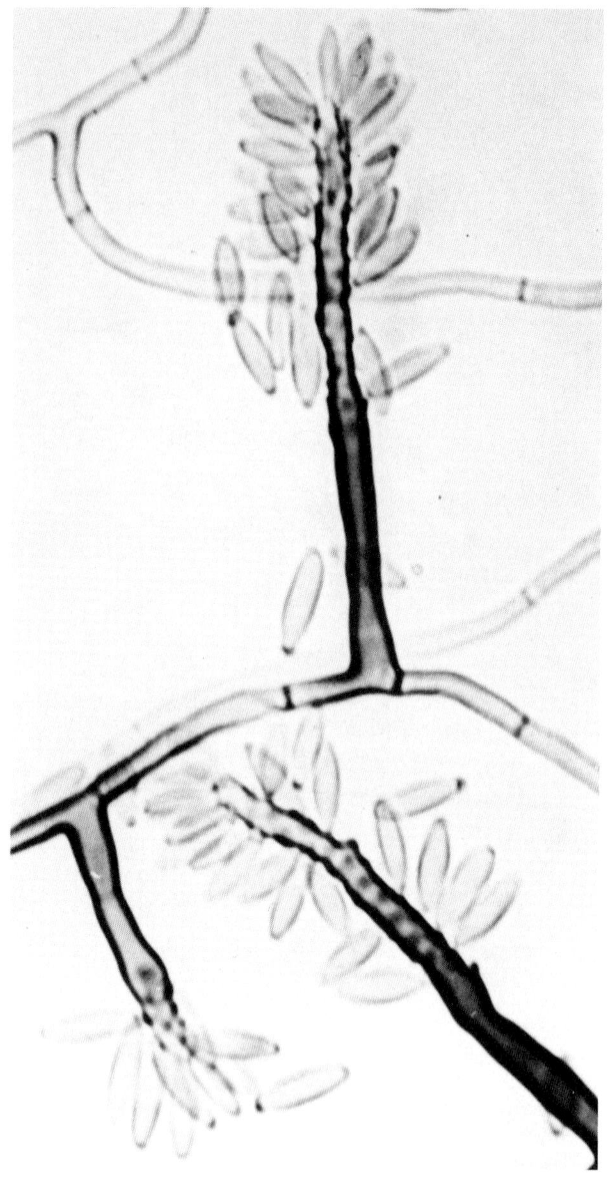

FIG. 14. *Rhinocladiella aquaspersa*. One-celled conidia arise from erect conidiophores.

S. apiospermum rapidly produces colonies that are cottony and smoky gray to dark brown. One-celled conidia may occur singly along the hyphae or in clusters at the apices of annellides (Fig. 15). The annellides often are characterized by noticeably swollen rings (annellations). The conidia are obovate, truncate, and subhyaline to light black.

S. apiospermum occasionally has a *Graphium* synanamorph present. Several members of the genera *Pseudallescheria* and *Petriella* may produce a *S. apiospermum* anamorph. Therefore, without having the teleomorph present, it is not possible to determine whether an isolate of *S. apiospermum* was produced by *Pseudallescheria boydii*.

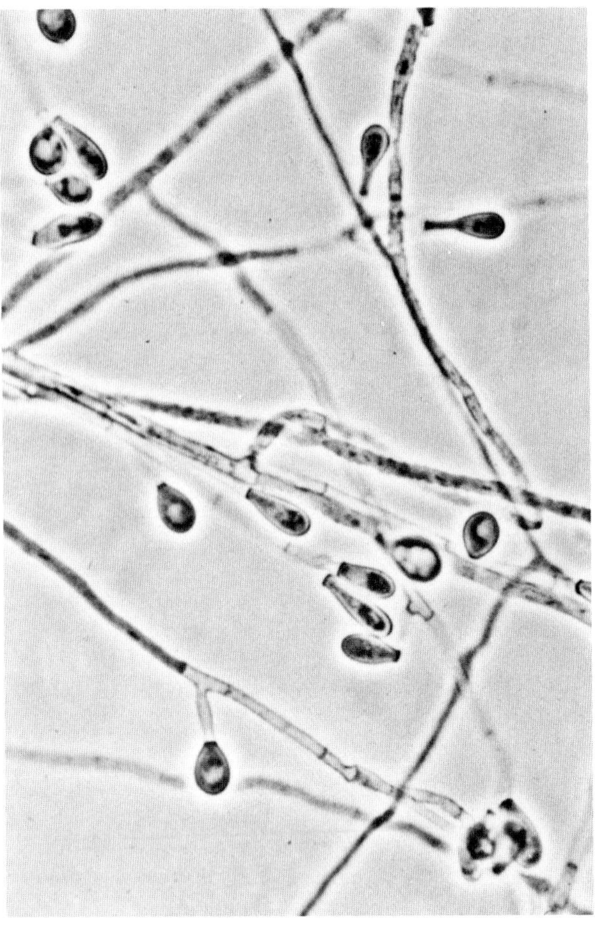

FIG. 15. *Scedosporium apiospermum*. One-celled conidia with truncate bases occur in groups at the apices of annellides.

S. inflatum has been described recently as a new *Scedosporium* species that was isolated from a bone biopsy specimen (21). *S. inflatum* differs from *S. apiospermum* by having a more rapid growth rate on standard nutrient media, brown to black, flat, nearly mucoid colonies when young, the formation of one-celled annelloconidia from annellides with swollen bases, and cycloheximide sensitivity. Although the conidiogenous cells of *S. inflatum* occasionally may appear in light microscopy to proliferate sympodially, this is an artifact (13).

Scytalidium spp.

Members of the genus *Scytalidium* (25) have been well documented as opportunistic fungal pathogens of nail, skin, and subcutaneous tissue. *Scytalidium dimidiatum*, a synanamorph associated with the pycnidial fungus *Nattrassia mangiferae* (syn. *Hendersonula toruloidea*), and *S. hyalinum* have caused disease. *S. hyalinum*, because of its hyaline nature, would be classified best in a genus other than *Scytalidium*. *Scytalidium* spp. produce rapidly growing colonies that are at first white, becoming dark gray with age. *S. dimidatum* (Fig. 16) forms arthroconidia that are brown, cylindrical at first, becoming rounded, barrel shaped or subglobose, and one or two celled.

In 1989, Sutton and Dyko (43) reclassified the pycnidial fungus *H. toruloidea* into the new genus *Nattrassia*

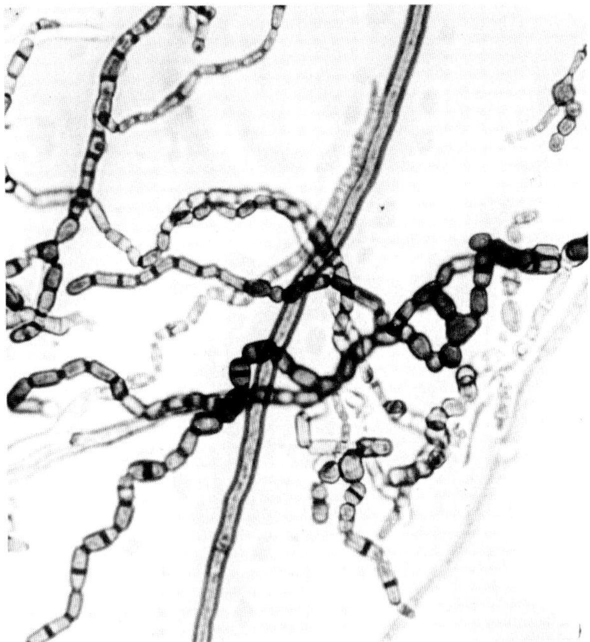

FIG. 16. *Scytalidium dimidiatum*. Chains consisting of one- or two-celled arthroconidia are present.

as a synonym of *N. mangiferae*. These authors proposed the new combination *S. dimidiatum*, which nicely accommodates the anamorph commonly referred to as the *Scytalidium* synanamorph of *H. toruloidea*. *S. dimidiatum* is the form isolated in the clinical laboratory, and an additional medium like banana chips is required for the *N. mangiferae* anamorph to be formed. The monograph on *Malbranchea* spp. by Sigler and Carmichael (41) and the study of *Hendersonula* by Sutton and Dyko (43) should be consulted for the identification of *Scytalidium* spp.

Sporothrix spp.

Sporothrix schenckii, a dimorphic fungus, is considered the only pathogenic member of the genus *Sporothrix*. Recently, a new species, *S. cyanescens*, was added to the genus (9). Some of the isolates upon which the species description was based were recovered from patients with mycosis involving the skin. Recent experiments in an animal model clearly demonstrate that this species is not pathogenic (42). Colonies of *S. schenckii* are rapidly growing and at first moist, flat, and yeastlike, later developing aerial hyphae. They are initially white, becoming brown to black with age. The conidia are of two kinds in most fresh isolates. Hyaline, one-celled conidia develop solitarily upon denticles along the hyphae; laterally from sympodial, slender, tapering, erect conidiophores; and terminally in clusters at the apices of swollen conidiophores (Fig. 17). The second type of conidia are one celled, thick walled, and black. These conidia develop along the hyphae. At 37°C on enriched media, the mould form of *S. schenckii* converts to a yeast form.

Isolates recovered from environmental sources, e.g., sphagnum moss, form colonies that are neither flat nor moist and usually do not become black with age, which

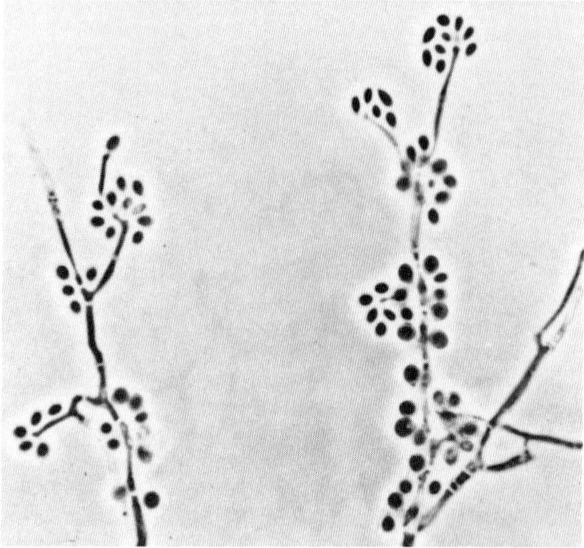

FIG. 17. *Sporothrix schenckii.* Solitary conidia on threadlike denticles arise from sympodial conidiophores.

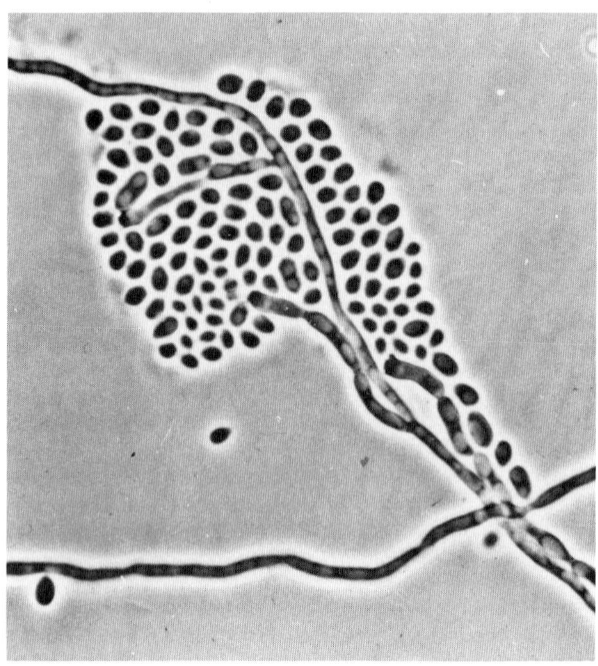

FIG. 18. *Wangiella dermatitidis.* One-celled conidia are produced from phialides.

is due to the absence of the thick-walled conidia. While the hyaline conidia in natural isolates develop in a manner similar to those found in isolates recovered from human infections, they are clavate in shape, as opposed to the oval shape of conidia in pathogenic isolates. Both environmental and clinical isolates will form a yeast phase when grown on appropriate media at 37°C. Although the ascomycete *Ceratocystis stenoceras* has been associated as the teleomorph of environmental isolates of *S. schenckii,* no teleomorph has been found for isolates recovered from human infections.

The etiologic agent of sporotrichosis originally was described as *S. schenckii.* Later, the fungus erroneously was transferred to the genus *Sporotrichum.* Members of the genus *Sporotrichum* are Basidiomycetes, characterized by the formation of large hyphae with clamp connections and large, one-celled, thick-walled, golden conidia (25). They are neither dimorphic nor pathogenic for humans and other animals.

Wangiella spp.

Wangiella dermatitidis is an agent of phaeohyphomycosis that typically causes infections involving cutaneous and subcutaneous tissue. The infection most frequently has been seen in patients living in Japan. Insignificant isolates are occasionally isolated from sputum specimens.

The colonies of *W. dermatitidis* are moist and yeastlike at first, developing some aerial hyphae with age. They are olive to black. Distinct conidiophores are absent. The conidiogenous cells are phialides that do not have collarettes (Fig. 18). Some conidiogenous cells appear to possess a group of slightly raised, truncate denticles at their apices that occur as a result of polyphialidic development. Rare annellides may be produced by isolates of this fungus. The one-celled, light to dark, smooth phialoconidia form in balls at the apices of the phialides and then slide down their sides. The phialides develop from conidiophores that are indistinguishable from the hyphae. Most isolates produce an abundant yeast form (*Phaeococcomyces* anamorph) and large amounts of toruloid hyphae. Potassium nitrate is not assimilated (16).

The genus *Wangiella* was established to accommodate the fungus known as *Hormiscium dermatitidis* and *Phialophora dermatitidis* (22). The genus *Wangiella* was necessary because the phialides without collarettes that are typical of *W. dermatitidis* could not be accommodated in any existing genus. *W. dermatitidis* can be recognized by its ability to grow at 40°C, whereas similar dematiaceous Hyphomycetes do not grow at that temperature (32).

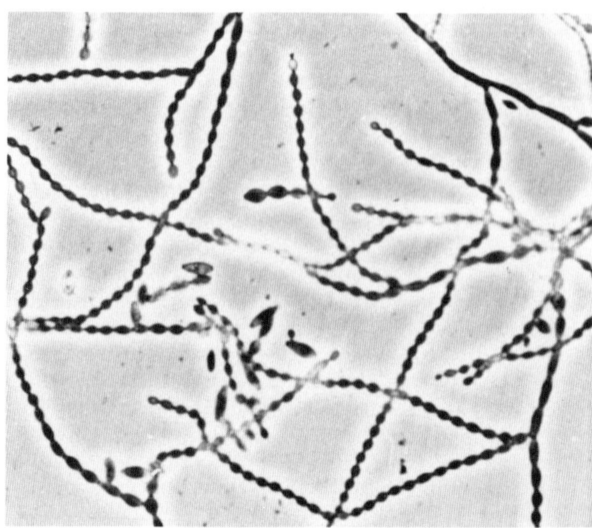

FIG. 19. *Xylohypha bantiana.* Long, sparsely branching chains of blastoconidia arise from nondifferentiated hyphae.

Xylohypha spp.

The genus *Xylohypha* contains at least two medically important species, *Xylohypha bantiana* and *X. emmonsii*. *Xylohypha bantiana*, which previously was known as *Cladosporium trichoides* and *C. bantianum* (5, 27), is the major pathogen in the genus (12). The fungus was transferred to the genus *Xylohypha* because it produces conidiophores that are indistinguishable from the vegetative hyphae, as well as one-celled blastoconidia, without evident darkly pigmented hila, that are borne in long, sparsely branching chains. Colonies of *X. bantiana* are olive gray and floccose. *X. bantiana* (Fig. 19) isolates should be handled with extreme care within a biological safety cabinet.

X. bantiana and *Cladosporium carrionii* (Fig. 8) are similar morphologically. *C. carrionii* has a slower growth rate and shorter conidia (2 to 3 by 4 to 5 μm versus 2 to 2.5 by 4 to 7 μm, with some being 3 by 15 to 20 μm), is dermatotropic rather than neurotropic, and has a maximum growth temperature of 35 to 36°C, in comparison with 42 to 43°C for *X. bantiana*.

LITERATURE CITED

1. **Ajello, L.** 1975. Phaeohyphomycosis: definition and etiology. Pan Am. Health Org. Sci. Publ. **304:**126–133.
2. **Alcorn, J. L.** 1983. Generic concepts in *Drechslera*, *Bipolaris* and *Exserohilum*. Mycotaxon **17:**1–86.
3. **Barnett, H. L., and B. B. Hunter.** 1972. Illustrated genera of imperfect fungi, 3rd ed. Burgess Publishing Co., Minneapolis.
4. **Barron, G. L.** 1968. The genera of Hyphomycetes from soil. The Williams & Wilkins Co., Baltimore.
5. **Borelli, D.** 1960. *Torula bantiana*, agente di un granuloma cerebrale. Riv. Anat. Patol. Oncol. **17:**615–622.
6. **Carmichael, J. W., B. Kendrick, I. L. Conners, and L. Sigler.** 1980. Genera of Hyphomycetes. University of Alberta Press, Edmonton, Alberta, Canada.
7. **Cole, G. T., and R. A. Samson.** 1979. Patterns of development in conidial fungi. Pitman Press, London.
8. **de Hoog, G. S.** 1979. Nomenclatural notes on some black yeast-like hyphomycetes. Taxon **28:**347–348.
9. **de Hoog, G. S., and G. A. deVries.** 1973. Two new species of *Sporothrix* and their relations to *Blastobotrys nivea*. Antonie van Leeuwenhoek J. Microbiol. Serol. **39:**515–520.
10. **de Hoog, G. S., and E. J. Hermanides-Nijhof.** 1977. The black yeasts and allied Hyphomycetes. Studies in mycology no. 15. Centraalbureau voor Schimmelcultures, Baarn, The Netherlands.
11. **Dixon, D. M., and I. F. Salkin.** 1986. Morphologic and physiologic studies of three dematiaceous pathogens. J. Clin. Microbiol. **24:**12–15.
12. **Dixon, D. M., T. J. Walsh, W. G. Merz, and M. R. McGinnis.** 1989. Infections due to *Xylohypha bantiana* (*Cladosporium trichoides*). Rev. Infect. Dis. **11:**515–525.
13. **Dykstra, M. J., I. F. Salkin, and M. R. McGinnis.** 1990. An ultrastructural comparison of conidiogenesis in *Scedosporium apiospermum*, *Scedosporium inflatum*, and *Scopulariopsis brumptii*. Mycologia **81:**896–904.
14. **Ellis, M. B.** 1971. Dematiaceous Hyphomycetes. Commonwealth Mycological Institute, Kew, England.
15. **Ellis, M. B.** 1976. More dematiaceous Hyphomycetes. Commonwealth Mycological Institute, Kew, England.
16. **Espinel-Ingroff, A., P. R. Goldson, M. R. McGinnis, and T. M. Kerkering.** 1988. Evaluation of proteolytic activity to differentiate some dematiaceous fungi. J. Clin. Microbiol. **26:**301–307.
17. **Fader, R. C. and M. R. McGinnis.** 1988. Infections caused by dematiaceous fungi: chromoblastomycosis and phaeohyphomycosis. Infect. Dis. Clin. N. Am. **2:**925–938.
18. **Gams, W., and M. R. McGinnis.** 1983. *Phialemonium*, a new anamorph genus intermediate between *Phialophora* and *Acremonium*. Mycologia **75:**977–987.
19. **Goodpasture, H. C., T. Carlson, B. Ellis, and G. Randall.** 1983. *Alternaria* osteomyelitis. Evidence of specific immunologic tolerance. Arch. Pathol. Lab. Med. **107:**528–530.
20. **Kendrick, W. B. (ed.).** 1971. Taxonomy of Fungi Imperfecti. University of Toronto Press, Toronto.
21. **Malloch, D., and I. F. Salkin.** 1984. A new species of *Scedosporium* associated with osteomyelitis in humans. Mycotaxon **21:**247–255.
22. **McGinnis, M. R.** 1978. Human pathogenic species of *Exophiala*, *Phialophora*, and *Wangiella*. Pan Am. Health Org. Sci. Publ. **356:**35–59.
23. **McGinnis, M. R.** 1979. Taxonomy of *Exophiala jeanselmei* (Langeron) McGinnis and Padhye. Mycopathologia **65:**79–87.
24. **McGinnis, M. R.** 1979. Taxonomy of *Exophiala werneckii* and its relationship to *Microsporum mansonii*. Sabouraudia **17:**145–154.
25. **McGinnis, M. R.** 1980. Laboratory handbook of medical mycology. Academic Press, Inc., New York.
26. **McGinnis, M. R.** 1983. Chromoblastomycosis and phaeohyphomycosis: new concepts, diagnosis, and mycology. J. Am. Acad. Dermatol. **8:**1–16.
27. **McGinnis, M. R., D. Borelli, A. A. Padhye, and L. Ajello.** 1986. Reclassification of *Cladosporium bantianum* in the genus *Xylohypha*. J. Clin. Microbiol. **23:**1148–1151.
28. **McGinnis, M. R., A. A. Padhye, and L. Ajello.** 1982. *Pseudallescheria* Negroni et Fischer, 1943, and its later synonym *Petriellidium* Malloch, 1970. Mycotaxon **14:**94–102.
29. **McGinnis, M. R., M. G. Rinaldi, and R. E. Winn.** 1986. Emerging agents of phaeohyphomycosis: pathogenic species of *Bipolaris* and *Exserohilum*. J. Clin. Microbiol. **24:**250–259.
30. **McGinnis, M. R., W. A. Schell, and J. Carson.** 1985. *Phaeoannellomyces* and the Phaeococcomycetaceae, new dematiaceous blastomycete taxa. Sabouraudia **23:**179–188.
31. **Padhye, A. A.** 1978. Comparative study of *Phialophora jeanselmei* and *P. gougerotii* by morphological, biochemical, and immunological methods. Pan Am. Health Org. Sci. Publ. **356:**60–65.
32. **Padhye, A. A., M. R. McGinnis, and L. Ajello.** 1978. Thermotolerance of *Wangiella dermatitidis*. J. Clin. Microbiol. **8:**424–426.
33. **Padhye, A. A., M. R. McGinnis, L. Ajello, and F. W. Chandler.** 1988. *Xylohypha emmonsii* sp. nov., a new agent of phaeohyphomycosis. J. Clin. Microbiol. **26:**702–708.
34. **Pasarell, L., M. R. McGinnis, and P. G. Standard.** 1990. Differentiation of medically important isolates of *Bipolaris* and *Exserohilum* with exoantigens. J. Clin. Microbiol. **28:**1655–1657.
35. **Salkin, I. F., and D. M. Dixon.** 1987. *Dactylaria constricta:* description of two varieties. Mycotaxon **29:**377–381.
36. **Salkin, I. F., and N. Hurd.** 1972. Quantitative evaluation of the antifungal properties of cycloheximide. Antimicrob. Agents Chemother. **1:**177–184.
37. **Salkin, I. F., J. A. Martinez, and M. E. Kemna.** 1986. Opportunistic infection of the spleen caused by *Aureobasidium pullulans*. J. Clin. Microbiol. **23:**828–831.
38. **Salkin, I. F., M. R. McGinnis, M. J. Dykstra, and M. G. Rinaldi.** 1988. *Scedosporium inflatum*, an emerging pathogen. J. Clin. Microbiol. **26:**498–503.
39. **Schell, W. A., and M. R. McGinnis.** 1988. Molds involved in subcutaneous infections, p. 99–171. *In* B. B. Wentworth (ed.), Diagnostic procedures for mycotic and parasitic infections, 7th ed. American Public Health Association, Inc., Washington, D.C.
40. **Schell, W. A., M. R. McGinnis, and D. Borelli.** 1983. *Rhinocladiella aquaspersa*, a new combination for *Acrotheca aquaspersa*. Mycotaxon **17:**341–348.
41. **Sigler, L., and J. W. Carmichael.** 1976. Taxonomy of *Mal-*

branchea and some other Hyphomycetes with arthroconidia. Mycotaxon **4:**349–488.

42. **Sigler, L., J. L. Harris, D. M. Dixon, A. L. Flis, I. F. Salkin, M. Kemna, and R. A. Duncan.** 1990. Microbiology and potential virulence of *Sporothrix cyanescens,* a fungus rarely isolated from blood and skin. J. Clin. Microbiol. **28:** 1009–1015.
43. **Sutton, B. C., and B. J. Dyko.** 1989. Revision of *Hendersonula.* Mycol. Res. **93:**466–488.
44. **Wheeler, M. H., and A. A. Bell.** 1987. Melanins and their importance in pathogenic fungi. Curr. Top. Med. Mycol. **2:**338–387.

Chapter 63

Opportunistic Hyaline Hyphomycetes

ALVIN L. ROGERS AND MICHAEL J. KENNEDY

Historically, clinical microbiologists have given little attention to the isolation and identification of most fungi that exist as ubiquitous saprophytes of soil and decomposing organic matter, dismissing the growth of such organisms on laboratory media as "contaminants." Today, with the increased use of antimicrobial agents and immunosuppressive and cytotoxic drugs, the introduction into clinical medicine of highly technical methods for advanced life support, and the recognition of newer diseases and physiologic problems, the overall incidence of infections caused by fungi once considered contaminants has increased to the point that the microbiologist now must consider isolates of such fungi with suspicion. Indeed, the list of saprophytic and plant parasitic moulds that have latent pathogenic capabilities and have been found to cause opportunistic infections in humans and animals has grown so long that it is now necessary to categorize them into accessible groups (71).

For the sake of convenience, and to discourage the coining and proliferation of unnecessary new disease names based on the genera of the etiologic agents, two major disease groups have been proposed for those fungi that exist ubiquitously in nature and are not generally considered pathogens but have been found to cause disease: phaeohyphomycosis and hyalohyphomycosis (2, 3, 53, 54). The division is based on the presence or absence of pale brown to black pigmented fungal elements in tissue. Phaeohyphomycosis broadly defined is a heterogeneous group of infections characterized by the presence of dark pigmented fungal elements in tissue (see chapter 62). Phaeohyphomycosis is differentiated from other mycoses (e.g., chromoblastomycosis and mycetoma) involving dematiaceous fungi that present as specific clinical entities having a characteristic pathology (see chapter 65) (53). The term "hyalohyphomycosis" was proposed as a complement to phaeohyphomycosis, in which the fungi involved have a basic tissue form consisting of hyaline, septate mycelial elements that may be branched and are occasionally toruloid (63). The term "hyalohyphomycosis" was not intended to replace such well-established disease names as aspergillosis, but it allows hyaline Hyphomycetes which cause opportunistic infections to be categorized until such time as it is recognized that a particular organism causes infections with regularity or that there is some other aspect that is particularly distinctive to warrant assignment of a specific disease name. In this chapter, some of the well-established and infrequent hyaline Hyphomycetes most likely to be encountered in clinical specimens will be discussed, together with a listing of unique or very rare agents of hyalohyphomycosis.

ETIOLOGIC AGENTS OF HYALOHYPHOMYCOSIS

There are thousands of Hyphomycetes that are ubiquitous in nature and are distributed worldwide in the soil on decaying vegetation and other organic matter, fouling numerous man-made surfaces, as well as existing as airborne conidia. Some of these organisms may be involved in clinical disease as either primary or secondary opportunists, particularly in the compromised host (71). The majority of Hyphomycetes, however, are not considered pathogenic and appear unlikely to be able to adapt to or take advantage of most situations that have been shown to predispose to opportunistic infections. Therefore, when such fungi are suspected as etiologic agents, repeated isolation of a particular fungus from the same or multiple specimens and the direct demonstration of fungal elements within tissue or body fluids are needed for the establishment of the etiology of disease. It should be stressed, however, that no fungal isolate should be discarded as a contaminant without thorough examination of the clinical specimens and careful consideration of the diagnosis. The use of biopsies thus may be necessary in some instances, and close communication between laboratory personnel and physicians is essential. Careful quality control to ensure that isolation media are not contaminated and careful inspection of the location on a slant or plate where growth of a fungus occurs in relation to where a specimen was placed are also important factors in the determination of whether an isolate is involved in disease.

The opportunistic hyaline Hyphomycetes that have been proven to cause infections in humans and animals are listed in Table 1. To date, 74 species of fungi belonging to 20 genera that meet the requirements mentioned above and qualify as true etiologic agents of aspergillosis or hyalohyphomycosis have been described in the literature under various disease names (Table 1). Reports that appear to be invalid or are at least questionable as to the involvement of other hyaline Hyphomycetes in various infections are discussed elsewhere (2, 3, 71).

Nomenclature, classification, and taxonomy

The 74 species of proven etiologic agents of aspergillosis and hyalohyphomycosis listed in Table 1 are distributed throughout the Kingdom Fungi and belong to genera of the Ascomycota, Basidiomycota, and Deuteromycota. The majority of these fungi have no known sexual cycle (teleomorph) and reproduce asexually (anamorph) by budding or conidiation. These are referred to as Fungi Imperfecti and are accommodated in the phylum or division Deuteromycota, which is fur-

TABLE 1. Currently known agents of aspergillosis and hyalohyphomycosis[a]

Acremonium	*Beauveria*	*Penicillium*
A. alabamensis	*B. alba*	*P. casei*
A. falciforme	*B. bassiana*	*P. chrysogenum*
A. kiliense		*P. citrinum*
A. potroni	*Chrysosporium*	*P. commune*
A. recifei	*Chrysosporium* sp.	*P. expansum*
A. roseo-griseum		*P. glaucum*
A. strictum	*Coprinus*	*P. marneffei* (as a schizo-yeast and mycelium in tissue)
	C. cinereus	*P. spinulosum*
Anxiopsis	*C. delicatulus*	
A. fulvescens		*Scedosporium*
A. sterocari	*Cylindrocarpon*	*S. apiospermum*
	C. lichenicola	*S. inflatum*
Arthrographis	*C. tonkinense*	
A. kalrae	*C. vaginae*	*Schizophyllum*
		S. commune
Aspergillus	*Fusarium*	
A. amstelodami	*F. chlamydosporum*	*Scopulariopsis*
A. candidus	*F. dimerum*	*S. acremonium*
A. carneus	*F. moniliforme*	*S. brevicaulis*
A. clavatus	*F. nivale*	
A. conicus	*F. simifectum*	*Scytalidium*
A. deflectus	*F. oxysporum*	*S. hyalinum*
A. fischeri	*F. proliferatum*	
A. flavipes	*F. roseum*	*Trichoderma*
A. flavus	*F. solani*	*T. viride*
A. fumigatus	*F. verticillioides*	
A. nidulans		*Tritiarchium*
A. niger	*Microascus*	*T. oryzae*
A. niveus	*M. cinerereus*	
A. ochraceus		*Volutella*
A. oryzae	*Myriodontium*	*V. cinerscens*
A. parasiticus	*M. keratinophylum*	
A. repens		
A. restrictus	*Paecilomyces*	
A. ruber	*P. fumoso-roseus*	
A. sydowi	*P. javanicus*	
A. terreus	*P. lilacinus*	
A. ustus	*P. marquandii*	
A. versicolor	*P. variotii*	

[a] Data from references 49, 63, 69, 71, and 86.

ther separated into three form-classes: Blastomycetes, Hyphomycetes, and Coelomycetes. The perfect forms of some of the fungi listed in Table 1 are included here because they occasionally are isolated in culture, although the anamorphic forms of these fungi induce disease and are the forms that usually are observed in tissues and cultures in the clinical laboratory. Members of the form-class Hyphomycetes are separated into various groups on the basis of the following morphologic similarities: (i) the presence or absence of dark pigment in hyphal structures, (ii) types of conidia, and (iii) mode of conidiogenesis (13). Refer to chapter 57 for additional information on nomenclature, classification, and taxonomy.

Clinical manifestations

The spectrum of disease caused by hyaline Hyphomycetes is diverse. The disease state is largely determined by the local and general immunologic and physiologic state of the host and may be symptomatic or asymptomatic. In most instances, the portal of entry for a fungus is either through a break in the epidermis or by way of the lungs. Noted exceptions include introduction into the body by means of contaminated surgical instruments, intraocular lenses, prosthetic devices, or other contaminated materials or solutions associated with surgery, routine health care, or both.

Although hyaline Hyphomycetes can grow in most body tissues and fluids, colonization or invasion is commonly, but not solely, associated with subcutaneous soft tissue and mucous membranes. Individuals whose resistance is lowered as a result of a severe debilitating disease or immunosuppressive therapy, for instance, typically suffer from invasive pulmonary or paranasal sinus infections (71). Noninvasive forms of aspergillosis and hyalohyphomycosis also have been noted in debilitated individuals as well as in individuals with apparently normal defense mechanisms. In such cases, the fungus colonizes a preexisting cavity in the lungs such as an ectatic bronchus, a tuberculous cavity, or a lung cyst (11). In addition to the various pulmonic forms of hyalohyphomycosis, clinical syndromes involving other organs or tissues also are recognized. Infections of the ear canal, nail, cutaneous and subcutaneous tissues, cornea, and other sites manifesting as cellulitis, bursitis, nephritis, endocarditis, peritonitis, fungemia, and rarely involvement of the central nervous system all have been documented.

Collection, transport, storage, and processing of specimens

Specimens from patients with suspected fungal infections are to be collected with prudence and transported to the laboratory and processed as soon as possible, using standard procedures described elsewhere in this volume (see chapter 58). Because of the diverse manifestations of aspergillosis and hyalohyphoycosis, various sites may need to be examined for fungal elements. Biopsy material, transtracheal aspirates, and sputum samples collected in the early morning all may be useful specimens for the isolation and detection of hyaline Hyphomycetes, as are infected nails.

Swabs taken from mucous membranes and skin lesions and blood cultures (86) are generally of little help in diagnosing infections caused by hyaline Hyphomycetes and are not recommended unless multiple specimens are obtained.

Media containing antibacterial agents such as chloramphenicol, gentamicin, or penicillin plus streptomycin should be useful because the growth of indigenous bacteria will be inhibited. Media that contain cycloheximide, such as Mycobiotic agar (Difco Laboratories) or Mycosel agar (Becton Dickinson and Co.), should not be used because most hyaline Hyphomycetes are sensitive to this compound. If possible, the specimen should be inoculated onto several types of media and incubated at 25 and 37°C.

ASPERGILLUS SPECIES

Aspergillosis now is considered the second most common fungal infection requiring hospitalization in the United States (24, 70). The pathologic responses caused by members of the genus *Aspergillus* vary in severity and clinical course and may occur as both primary and secondary infections. These responses include (i) toxicity due to ingestion of foods contaminated with mycotoxins or other metabolites produced by aspergilli; (ii) allergy and sequelae to the presence of conidia or transient growth of the organism in body orifices; (iii) colonization without extension in preformed cavities and debilitated tissues within the respiratory tract, often called aspergilloma or fungus ball; (iv) superficial infection of the skin, paranasal sinuses, external ear canal, and, more rarely, burn eschar, nail, and other sites; (v) invasive, inflammatory, granulomatous, necrotizing infection of the lungs; and (vi) systemic and fatal disseminated disease (10, 11, 70, 71). The clinical manifestations of aspergillosis are determined largely by the local or general immunologic and physiologic state of the host, but it should be noted that various forms of the disease may integrate and overlap (70). The differentiation of species of aspergilli causing human disease is considered below.

Nomenclature, morphology, and identification

Of the hundreds of recognized species of aspergilli, only about 20 have been verified to cause infections in humans, and only about 4 of these consistently and regularly are encountered as causes of disease (69, 71). In the clinical laboratory, aspergilli are readily isolated on most mycological media and tend to reproduce in the asexual (anamorphic) form. Periodically, some species also may develop a teleomorph, which may aid in identification, but it is the anamorphs that induce disease and are seen in tissue and culture. Thus, isolates of the genus *Aspergillus* usually are distinguished and identified on the basis of anamorphic characteristics (Table 2). It should be noted that although many species of aspergilli produce morphologic characteristics required for identification, some species require transfer to special media for observation of their diagnostic features. Subculture of an isolate to Czapek-Dox agar and 2% malt extract agar with incubation at 25°C allows identification of most aspergilli, using standard monographs and taxonomic keys (65, 66).

The anamorphic appearance typically observed in culture consists of septate, hyaline, branching hyphae, which may or may not give rise to asexual reproductive structures called conidiophores (Fig. 1). The conidiophore is an erect, hyaline to brown, stalklike hypha that varies greatly in length among different species. It is usually nonseptate and may have a smooth or textured surface (65, 71). Conidiophores arise directly from the vegetative hyphae, or more typically from a specialized hyphal cell called the foot cell, and terminate in a bulbous head, the vesicle. The vesicle may appear as a globose, hemispherical, flask-shaped, or clavate structure and may be covered, either entirely or partially, by a row of flask-shaped conidiogenous cells called phialides. Phialides may arise either directly from the vesicle (uniseriate), from metulae on the vesicle (biseriate), or from a combination of the two, as is observed in some species such as *Aspergillus flavus* (Fig. 2). Phialides form long chains of phialoconidia at their tips as they mature. These are formed simultaneously by a budding or blowing-out process, with the youngest conidium at the base and the most mature at the tip. The conidia are typically globose to subglobose and vary in size, color, wall texture, and thickness, depending upon the species.

Some species of aspergilli also may develop other morphological structures that may be helpful in the identification of an isolate. For example, cleistothecia, which consist of spherical structures whose outer walls are composed of interwoven hyphae and whose interiors are filled with asci and ascospores (sexual structures), are produced by species assigned to both the Glaucus and Nidulans groups (Table 2). Similarly, thick-walled single cells called Hülle cells may be present in clusters; these cells most often are associated with cleistothecia of the *Aspergillus nidulans* group but occasionally are found in colonies of some other groups (Table 2).

Because the large numbers of species within the genus *Aspergillus* makes identification to the species level difficult for even the experienced microbiologist, the aspergilli have been placed into distinct, accessible groups. Listed in Table 2 are the distinctive groups that have been established to aid in the identification of aspergilli; the basic common morphologic and physiologic characteristics also are indicated. The morphologic characteristics are based on fungal structures present in culture when the organisms are grown at 25°C on Czapek-Dox agar or 2% malt agar. Each group except the Glaucus group is named after a representative species within it. There is no species "*Aspergillus glaucus*" because original descriptions for such a species were presented in such vague terms that subsequently the name was used for a number of different species of aspergilli (52). It should be noted that some species may be placed in more than one group. The excellent monograph by Raper and Fennell (65) will help to further identify isolates when an exact species name is required.

Occasionally, nonconidiating isolates of aspergilli are encountered in the laboratory. In such cases, exoantigen tests have proved useful for the rapid identification to the genus level and, in the case of *Aspergillus fumigatus*, to the species level (39, 79).

Histopathologic examination

Assessment of the pathological importance of any species of *Aspergillus* isolated from clinical specimens can be as difficult as the identification of an isolate to the species level, because aspergilli are routinely isolated from respiratory secretions, skin scrapings, and other specimens. Stimlam et al. (85), for instance, reported that when isolated, aspergilli are significant in only 10% of the cases. Thus, it is imperative that the organism be (i) demonstrated by direct microscopic examination in fresh clinical material and (ii) repeatedly isolated from the same specimen or multiple body sites to demonstrate clinical significance.

In tissue sections, aspergilli typically are seen as hyaline, closely septate (without constrictions) hyphae that are 3 to 6 μm in diameter, branch dichotomously at acute (45°) angles, and have smooth parallel walls (Fig. 3). Most hyphae proliferate throughout the tissue, often in parallel or radial arrays. The hyphae may be stained with hematoxylin and eosin if the tissue is properly fixed, is not understained with hematoxylin, and is not necrotic. Viable hyphae are often basophilic to amphophilic, whereas hyphae in macerated or necrotic tissue tend to be eosinophilic (10). However, fungal elements and the details of hyphal morphology of aspergilli are best demonstrated with the special fungal stains, particularly Gomori methenamine silver stain. When hyphal elements typical of aspergilli are present in histologic sections, a presumptive diagnosis can be made. But because it is not always possible to distinguish the hyphae of aspergilli from the hyphae of other oppor-

TABLE 2. Characteristics of a representative species of some *Aspergillus* groups grown on Czapek-Dox agar[a]

Group and organism	Colony color	Conidiophore	Vesicle	Seriation: Uni	Seriation: Bi	Conidial head	Conidia	Cleisto-thecia	Hülle cells	Comment
Fumigatus group *A. fumigatus*	White to green to gray-green; slate gray with age; reverse side variable in color	Length, up to 300 µm (rarely to 500 µm); width, 5–8 µm; smooth walled; greenish, especially in upper portion	Dome shaped; conidiophore gradually enlarges, merging into vesicle; 20–30 µm in diameter; phialides on upper half only, with axes parallel to that of the conidiophore	+		Strongly columnar, compact	Globose to subglobose, elliptical in some isolates; echinulate to rarely smooth; most are 2.5–3.0 µm in diameter			Grows well at 45°C; one of the most commonly occurring moulds in nature; most common human pathogen
Flavus group *A. flavus*	Yellow to yellowish green to green with age	Length, 400–850 µm (rarely to 2.5 mm); uncolored; thick walled; coarsely roughened	Elongate, becoming subglobose to globose; 10–65 (commonly 25–45) µm in diameter	+	+	Radiate, splitting into columns with age	Globose; smooth to echinulate; 3–6 (most are 3.5–4.5) µm in diameter			Some strains produce toxins; growth usually enhanced at 37°C; small uniseriate vesicles; often produces dark-brown to black sclerotia; common human pathogen
Niger group *A. niger*	White, becoming black; reverse side occasionally pale yellow	Length, 1.5–3.0 mm; width, 15–20 µm; smooth walls; colorless with brownish shade on upper half	Globose; most are 45–75 µm in diameter		+	Globose, then radiate, splitting into columns with age	Globose; thick walls; brown; irregularly roughened; most are 4–5 µm in diameter			Frequent cause of otomycosis; sometimes associated with colonization of cavities
Terreus group *A. terreus*	Cinnamon buff to brown, rarely orange-brown	Length, 100–250 µm; width, 4.5–6 µm; flexous; smooth walled; colorless	Hemispherical or domelike, merging into conidiophore; 10–16 µm in diameter		+	Long, columnar; uniform in diameter throughout length	Globose to slightly elliptical; smooth; 1.8–2.4 µm in diameter			May form single globose conidia on submerged hyphae (aleurioconidia, 6–7 µm)
Versicolor group *A. versicolor*	Variable, white to yellow, orange-yellow, tan to yellowish green	Length, up to 500–700 µm; width, 5 µm, merging into funnel shape at vesicle; smooth walled; uncolored or yellowish	Hemispherical or semielliptical; 12–16 µm in diameter		+	Radiate	Globose; strongly to delicately echinulate; most are 2–3 µm in diameter		+	Hülle cells, when present, resemble *A. nidulans* type; *A. versicolor* and *A. sydowi* most common pathogens in this group

(*Continued on next page*)

TABLE 2—*Continued*

Groups and organism	Colony color	Conidiophore	Vesicle	Seriation		Conidial head	Conidia	Cleistothecia	Hülle cells	Comment
				Uni	Bi					
Glaucus group *A. repens*	Green to yellow-green to gray-green; orange-yellow areas of cleistothecia with age	Length, 0.5–1.0 mm; smooth walled; uncolored; broadens toward the vesicle	Domelike, hemispherical, 25–40 µm in diameter		+	Radiate to loosely columnar	Ovate to globose; spinulose; most are 5–6.5 µm in diameter	+		Abundant yellow cleistothecia; most of the Glaucus group grow poorly at 37°C; *A. repens*, *A. ruber*, and *A. amstelodami* are most common pathogens in this group
Clavatus group *A. clavatus*	Blue-green	Length, 1.5–3.0 mm; width, 20–30 µm; smooth walled; uncolored; merging into vesicle	Clavate; fertile over area up to 250 µm long; 40–60 µm in diameter	+		Clavate; splits into 2–3 compact columns with age	Elliptical; thick walled; smooth; 3–4.5 by 2.5–3.5 µm; occasionally larger in some strains			May be involved in allergic conditions
Nidulans group *A. nidulans*	Dark green in conidial forms; buff to yellow in primarily cleistothecial forms; reverse side purplish red	Length, 60–130 (most are 75–100) µm; width, 2.5–3 µm, increasing to 3.5–5 µm near vesicle; smooth walls; brown	Hemispherical; 8–10 µm in diameter		+	Short; columnar	Globose; rugulose; 3–3.5 µm in diameter	+	+	Cleistothecia small, usually abundant; completely enveloped by or associated with Hülle cells
Flavipes group *A. flavipes*	White to buff to darker; color due to off-white conidial mass and brownish conidiophores	Length, 500–800 µm (2–3 mm at margin in old colonies); thick walled; yellow to brown; smooth to faintly granular (occasionally disklike concretions on surface)	Subglobose to vertically elongated; up to 18 by 25 µm		+	Loosely columnar to radiate	Globose to subglobose; smooth; 2–3 µm in diameter		+	Hülle cells irregularly swollen, twisted, or branched; *A. niveus* and *A. carneus* included in group

[a] Modified from reference 86.

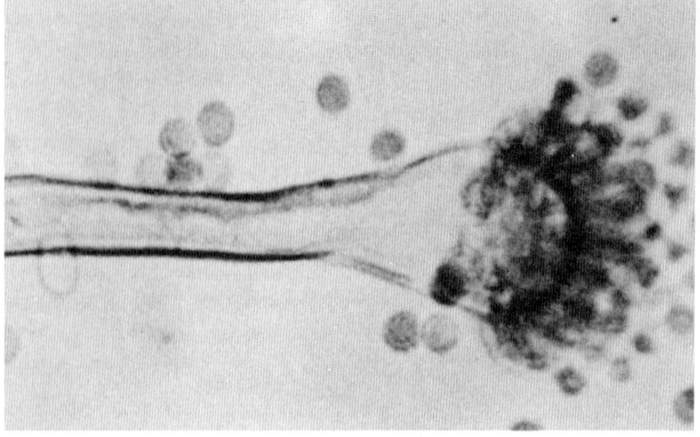

FIG. 1. *Aspergillus* species. Conidiophore. (Reprinted with permission from reference 5a.)

tunistic hyaline Hyphomycetes such as *Fusarium* species and *Scedosporium apiospermum*, a presumptive histologic diagnosis always must be confirmed by culture or immunologic techniques. Occasionally, however, typical conidial heads may be present in tissue sections, which will aid in the diagnosis. These usually are seen when the fungus colonizes preexisting cavities in the lungs. It should be noted that in such specimens conidia may become detached and lie free in tissue or tissue cavities, resembling small yeast cells when stained with Gomori methenamine silver stain.

In some instances, hyphal elements also may exhibit atypical morphologic features and may be seen as short globose and distorted hyphae that measure up to 12 μm in diameter and lack conspicuous septa. These may be mistaken for the hyphae of Zygomycetes, which generally are broader (up to 15 μm) and infrequently septate, with nonparallel walls that often appear collapsed and acutely twisted. The branching pattern of the Zygomycetes, however, is not as acute as that of the aspergilli, and the hyphal elements of the Zygomycetes in tissue generally are not oriented in the same direction. In addition, the Zygomycetes generally do not take the special fungus stains as uniformly or as intensely as do the aspergilli (11). Nevertheless, problems in differential diagnosis under atypical or typical conditions when aspergilli are suspect usually can be resolved by direct immunofluorescence.

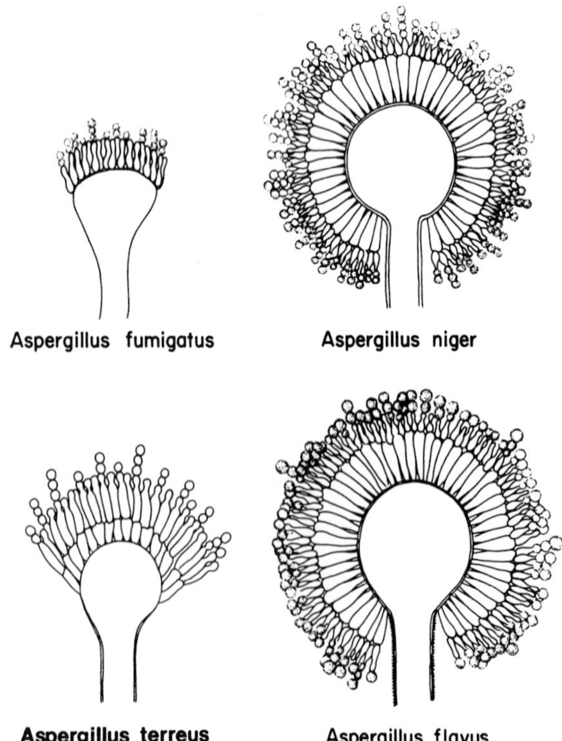

FIG. 2. Conidiophores of uniseriate (*A. fumigatus*) and biseriate (*A. niger*, *A. terreus*, and *A. flavus*) aspergilli. (Reprinted with permission from reference 71; courtesy of J. W. Rippon.)

Serologic diagnosis

Serologic tests for the detection of circulating *Aspergillus* antigens or antibodies to aspergilli have proven useful in the diagnosis of aspergillosis in patients yielding negative cultures and in distinguishing between various clinical forms of the disease. For instance, serologic tests may be useful in defining the etiology of pulmonary infections in the absence of cultures, since a number of fungi such as *Pseudallescheria boydii* may form fungus balls in the lungs resembling those caused by aspergilli (71). Moreover, tests for *Aspergillus* antibodies or antigens may be extremely useful for rapid diagnosis of aspergillosis in patients with invasive infections, for whom early treatment may be required to resolve this potentially fatal form of the disease.

A number of serologic tests have been used in a variety of patients with aspergillosis. The techniques that appear to be the most reliable are the immunodiffusion and counterimmunoelectrophoresis tests for detecting circulating antibody and the radioimmunoassays and enzyme-linked immunosorbent assays (ELISAs) for detecting circulating antigens (86). Other tests such as complement fixation tests also have been described, but their diagnostic role remains uncertain (70). Summarized in Table 3 are the serologic responses in different types of aspergillosis with various assays. As can be noted from the table, a significant number of patient sera respond positively to most tests. However, antibodies to aspergilli have been unpredictable in patients with invasive or disseminated infections, in part because of the underlying immunosuppression or therapy and the acute and fulminant course of these infections (94). False-positive results also have been noted in individuals with pulmonary infections caused by other fungi or tuberculosis (27). Thus, although immunologic tests have proven useful for the diagnosis of aspergillosis, improvements in sensitivity and practicality still are needed.

PENICILLIUM SPECIES

Members of the genus *Penicillium* are the common blue-green moulds that exist ubiquitously in nature and seem to be ever present in the hospital environment. Moulds belonging to this genus grow at a wide range of incubation temperatures (4 to 45°C), are among the most common of all laboratory contaminants, and can be isolated easily from sputum, bronchial secretions, and other secretions and body surfaces. Therefore, even repeated isolation of a *Penicillium* species from patient specimens does not necessarily indicate an etiologic

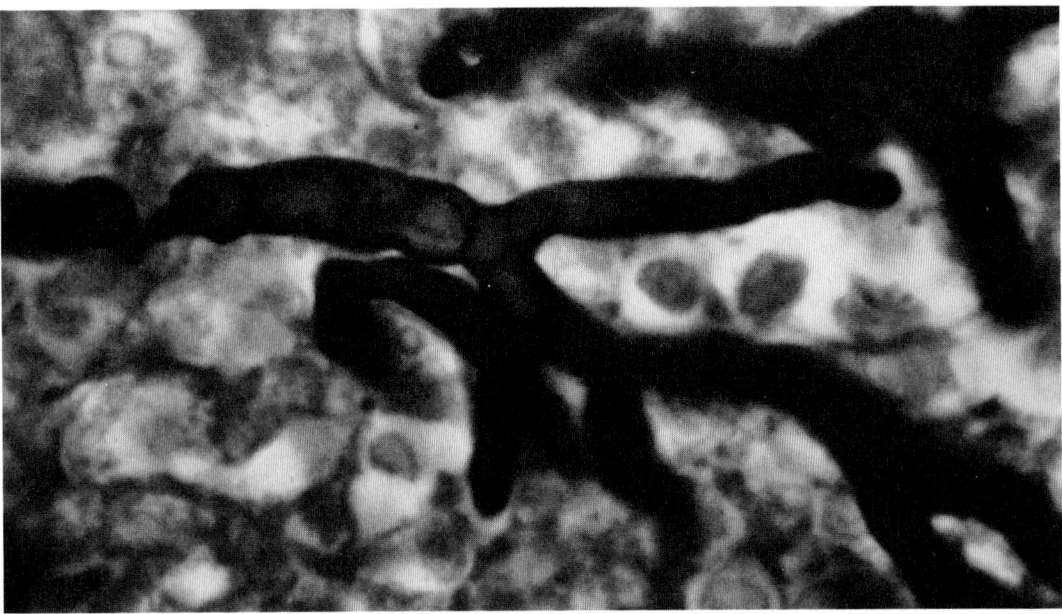

FIG. 3. Invasive aspergillosis. Dichotomous branching and septation of hyphae. Sometimes there is an indentation of the hyphal wall at the point of septal formation. Gomori methenamine silver stain. (Reprinted with permission from reference 71; micrograph courtesy of J. W. Rippon.)

role. A diagnosis of a species of *Penicillium* as the etiologic agent, therefore, can be made only by demonstrating typical fungal elements in tissue specimens or smears of lesional exudate and by isolating and identifying the fungus in culture.

Because members of the genus *Penicillium* are among the most ubiquitous of all fungi and have been isolated from a variety of anatomical sites in humans, a long list of diseases has developed over the years in which these organisms have been the purported etiologic agents (71). As noted by Rippon (71), however, in the vast majority of these cases the mould isolated was a contaminant and not associated with the pathology. Nevertheless, the literature does contain several authenticated cases of human infections caused by *Penicillium* species. Gillium and Vest (28), for instance, reported a urinary tract infection caused by *Penicillium citrinum*. The patient had sporadic attacks of fever and right flank pain,

TABLE 3. Serological responses in different types of aspergillosis[a]

Assay	Response (no. positive/total [%])			
	Colonization	Aspergilloma	Allergic	Invasive or disseminated
Immunodiffusion		36/44 (82)	20/31 (66)	4/7 (57)
		28/30 (93)	7/14 (50)	14/16 (88)
	46/60 (77)	19/19 (100)	2/3 (67)	1/3 (33)
		7/8 (88)	2/5 (40)	
		21/22 (95)	39/51 (77)	
		17/17 (100)	14/18 (78)	6/8 (75)
		12/13 (92)	29/29 (100)	
		17/17 (100)	5/5 (100)	1/1 (100)
	11/121 (9)	23/23 (100)	14/17 (82)	
		13/13 (100)	5/6 (83)	1/8 (12)
		22/23 (90)	13/14 (93)	
	202/224 (90)	6/7 (86)	1/1 (100)	
Complement fixation		23/29 (79)	7/14 (50)	1/5 (20)
	49/60 (82)	19/19 (100)	3/3 (100)	3/3 (100)
Radioimmunoassay		39/41 (95)	27/28 (96)	2/3 (67)
ELISA				
IgE			11/15 (73)	
IgG			13/15 (87)	
IgG		20/22 (91)	343/51 (67)	
	9/9 (100)	6/9 (67)	8/9 (89)	
		17/17 (100)	18/18 (100)	3/8 (38)
Indirect fluorescent antibody	17/17 (100)	4/5 (80)	1/1 (100)	

[a] Adapted from reference 94.

and several boli of mycelial mats were voided in the urine. Huang and Harris (36) reported on and verified a case of systemic infection caused by *Penicillium commune* in a leukemic patient who had disseminated cerebral and pulmonary infection. At autopsy, vascular invasion, thrombosis, and infarction were noted, and masses of septate, hyaline mycelia were demonstrated in the thrombi. Similarly, *Penicillium chrysogenum* and other penicilli also have been shown to cause endocarditis after mitral or aortic valve replacement (16, 33, 42, 88), mycotic keratitis (22, 31), external ear infections (71), hypersensitivity pneumonitis (83), and colonization of necrotic pulmonary tissue (48).

Infections caused by *Penicillium marneffei* manifesting as either granulomatous pulmonary lesions or skin abscesses also have been reported in about 20 patients (10, 71). Some of these patients acquired the infection naturally, whereas others had underlying disabilities or were immunocompromised, but all resided or had traveled in Southeast or Far East Asia, where this mycosis appears to be endemic (10). The potential pathogenicity of *P. marneffei* also was revealed in a laboratory accident when an investigator infected his right index finger with a syringe while inoculating laboratory rodents with this fungus (11). A small nodule developed at the puncture site 9 days after the incident, and *P. marneffei* was isolated from the digital nodule 12 days after the inoculation.

In tissue sections, most species of *Penicillium* are seen as hyaline, septate, branching (45° angle) mycelial elements (15 to 20 μm) (9, 75, 76). An exception is the tissue form of *P. marneffei*, which is found as small ovoid yeastlike cells measuring 2.5 to 5 μm in diameter and resembling the yeast cells of *Histoplasma capsulatum* var. *capsulatum*. These yeastlike cells can be distinguished easily from the yeast cells of *H. capsulatum* var. *capsulatum* because they reproduce by planate division and by their failure to stain with specific fluorescent-antibody conjugates of *H. capsulatum* (19, 26, 40). Occasionally, elongated sausagelike forms of *P. marneffei* with one or more septa also may be formed in necrotic and cavitary lesions (10). In addition, hyaline, septate hyphae such as those already described also may be seen (9, 75, 75).

On Sabouraud dextrose agar, Czapek agar, and other standard mycological media at 25°C, all *Penicillium* species grow rapidly at first as downy, white colonies that change color with maturation. The most commonly isolated species are blue-green or yellow-green, but because colony color is characteristic for each species, other shades of color can develop (64). *P. marneffei* produces a diffusible red pigment and red-stained hyphae that may aid in identification. An exoantigen test also has been described and is a rapid and specific method to identify isolates of *P. marneffei* (78).

Microscopically, *Penicillium* species are characterized by 1.5- to 5-μm-wide hyaline, septate mycelia that produce branched or unbranched, smooth to rough, hyaline to colored conidiophores (100 to 250 μm). The conidiogenous cells are groups of flask-shaped phialides that are produced directly on a central branch of a single conidiophore or on a secondary branch of the conidiophore called the metula (Fig. 4). This branched part of the conidiophore forms the characteristic brushlike structure referred to as the penicillius and is the major characteristic upon which species of *Penicillium* are identified and categorized into groups or series. Branching patterns among the penicilli include simple (not branched; the Monoverticillata), one or two staged and symmetrical (the Biverticillata-symmetrica), one or two staged and asymmetrical (the Asymmetrica), and three or more staged (the Polyverticillata) (64). The phialoconidia of *Penicillium* species are usually round with a smooth to finely roughened surface, may be hyaline, dark green, or blue green in color, measure 2 to 5 μm in diameter, and are formed in basipetal chains 50 to 75 μm in length. Sclerotia and sexual fruiting bodies also may be present in culture. It should be noted that the genus *Penicillium* contains the anamorphs of several Ascomycetes. The most common teleomorph states include *Eupenicillium*, *Penicilliopsis*, and *Talaromyces* (71).

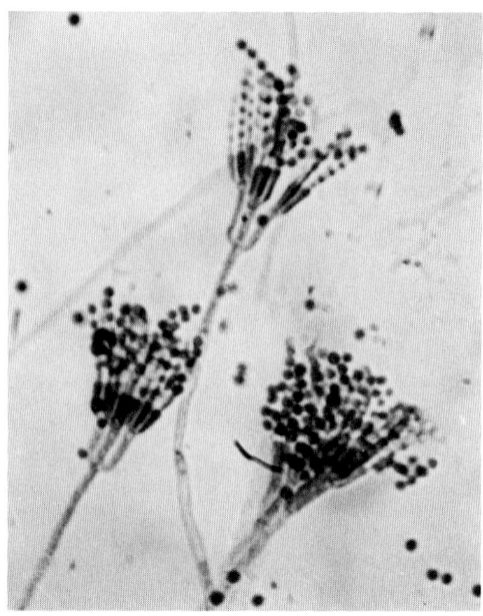

FIG. 4. *Penicillium* species. Brushlike penicillius and conidiophores showing primary branches and metulae and ending in phialides that bear chains of conidia (basocatenulate).

FUSARIUM SPECIES

Fusarium species are ubiquitous soil saprophytes and plant pathogens. Several species have caused a variety of superficial and invasive human infections. *Fusarium moniliforme*, *F. oxysporum*, and *F. solani* are the most common species isolated from clinical specimens and usually are confined to cases of keratitis, onychomycosis, and colonization of burned skin. Cutaneous infections other than colonization of burn wounds also have been reported and include a spectrum of skin lesions manifesting as erythematous or necrotic nodules that enlarge and ulcerate and may be painful (92). Infections of the deeper tissues causing endophthalmitis, leg ulcers, facial granuloma, osteomyelitis, infection of the central nervous system, and several other types of systemic infections also have been reported (60, 68). Most of these infections are associated with trauma or the use of corticosteroids and immunosuppression, and they typically occur in patients with neoplastic or other debilitating disease (92).

In histologic sections, *Fusarium* species present as septate branching hyaline hyphae that are 3 to 8 µm in width. These hyphae are haphazardly dispersed throughout the lesion and are indistinguishable from the hyphae of aspergilli or other hyaline Hyphomycetes. Dichotomous branching of the hyphae is frequent, with branches generally formed at an angle of approximately 45°; the branches often are constricted at their sites of origin from parent hyphae (11). Chandler and Watts (10) also have noted that hyphal varicosities and terminal or intercalated chlamydospores sometimes are found in the lesions of invasive or disseminated infections involving *Fusarium* species. Immunofluorescence and immunosorbent assays may help distinguish between infections caused by some hyaline Hyphomycetes, but definitive diagnosis requires isolation and identification of the fungus.

In culture, *Fusarium* species grow rapidly and produce white, downy colonies that become grayish to purple with age. All species grow well on most mycological media, but the medium used can have a profound influence on conidiogenesis and the texture and surface character of the colonies. For this reason, potato-dextrose agar typically is used for examining macroscopic and microscopic characteristics of *Fusarium* species. On this medium, *Fusarium* species produce a white and cottony colony that quickly develops a pink or violet center with a lighter periphery. Some species remain white or become tan, and the reverse side of the colony is generally light in color. *F. moniliforme* produces a purple to violet pigment that diffuses into the agar and has a gray-white surface. *F. oxysporum* varies in color from brown-white to violet-brown, whereas the colony of *F. solani* is dull brown or "dirty" tan with a hint of pale green.

Microscopically, *Fusarium* species are characterized by the production of both macro- and microphialoconidia. The macrophialoconidia are hyaline, two-celled to multicelled, fusiform or sickle-shaped conidia (3 to 8 by 11 to 80 µm) and typically occur in bananalike clusters (Fig. 5). The microphialoconidia are ovoid to cylindrical, one- or two-celled hyaline conidia (2 to 3 by 4 to 8 µm) that generally are borne as mucous balls or occasionally as short chains. In rare instances, some isolates lack the curved macrophialoconidia typical of the genus *Fusarium* and may be considered to be a species of *Acremonium*. The conidiophores bearing microphialoconidia of *Fusarium* species generally are shorter than those of *Acremonium* species. If an isolate is suspected to be a *Fusarium* species but lacks typical macrophialoconidia, subculture to another medium may stimulate macrophialocondia production. Microscopic and colonial features of the most commonly isolated *Fusarium* species are shown in Fig. 5 and summarized in Table 4.

PAECILOMYCES SPECIES

Species of *Paecilomyces* occur worldwide as saprophytes and exist as airborne contaminants that are resistant to most sterilizing techniques (71). Of the 31 recognized species (74), only a few species have been documented to cause infections in humans (63). Most of the cases reported have been mycotic keratitis, endocarditis following valve replacement, and endophthalmitis following lens implantation (1, 4, 32, 37, 38,

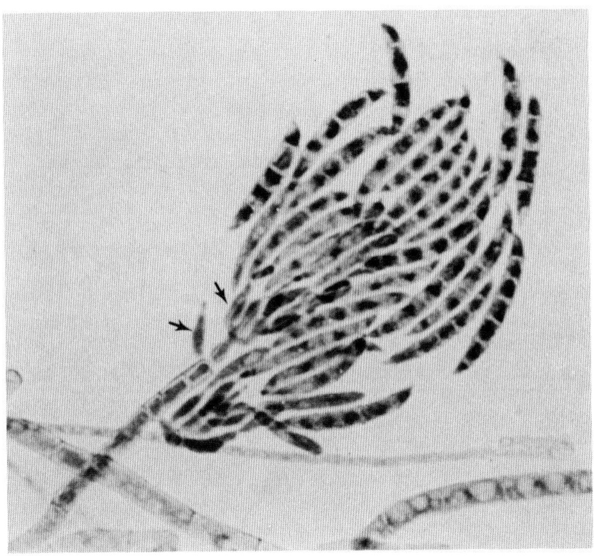

FIG. 5. *Fusarium* species. Phialides (arrows) give rise to macroconidia. Microconidia, when present, also are produced from phialides. (Reprinted with permission from reference 71; micrograph courtesy of J. W. Rippon.)

50, 82, 87). Several cases of cutaneous infections (38), pulmonary infection (29, 35), pyelonephritis (81), corneal ulcers (30), chronic maxillary sinusitis (72), orbital cellulitis (5), pulmonary infusion (15, 23) and pneumonia (18), sinusitis (62), and a deep cutaneous cellulitis of the leg of a renal transplant patient (34) have been reported. In most instances in which *Paecilomyces* species have been proven to cause infection, especially in immunocompromised patients, the patient history noted contact and usually trauma, either surgically or accidentally, of the infected tissue. In several cases of nosocomial infections, for example, the organism was found contaminating unopened packages containing intraocular lenses or the disinfectant used for surgical instruments (55, 59, 61).

Histological examination of tissues infected with *Paecilomyces lilacinus* and *P. variotii* have revealed hyaline, septate mycelial elements about 2 to 4 µm wide that are strongly Gomori methenamine silver stain positive (89). In some instances, mycelia had projected into lumina of necrotic tissue, and conidiophores bearing flask-shaped phialides were seen (11). Chains of smooth, spherical conidia also were noted either free or attached to the tapered ends of the phialides. Hyphal and rounded, budding cellular forms also have been noted in tissue sections from which *Paecilomyces marquandii* was grown (34). Examination of tissue from chameleons infected with *Paecilomyces viridis* also has shown spherical to oval budding yeast cells that were 2 to 7 µm in diameter (77).

All *Paecilomyces* species grow well on Sabouraud dextrose agar, giving rise to white floccose colonies that may change color with time. *P. lilacinus* grows rapidly on Sabouraud dextrose agar and most other media and produces a low and spreading colony that turns lilac colored or vinaceous. *P. variotii* colonies also are fast growing but are velvety and tan to gray in color, depending on the age of the culture. Microscopically, *Paecilomyces* species resemble *Penicillium* species in

TABLE 4. Morphologic features of three commonly isolated *Fusarium* species[a]

Characteristic	*F. moniliforme*	*F. oxysporum*	*F. solani*
Growth (cm) on potato-dextrose agar (7–10 days)	4–5	4–5	3–3.5
Colonies	Peach, salmon, vinaceous, purple to violet	Grayish white to gray to purple to violet	Dull brown
Microconidia	Fusoid to clavate, 5–12 by 1.5–2.5 μm, produced in chains from lateral phialides	Oval, ellipsoid, cylindric, or slightly curved, 5–12 by 2–3.5 μm from simple lateral phialides	Cylindric to oval, 8–16 by 2–4 μm, from laterally branched conidiophores bearing phialides
Macroconidia	Not produced in some strains; when present, equilaterally fusoid, 3–7 septate, 25–60 by 2.5–4 μm	3–5 septate, 27–60 by 3–4 μm	Inequilaterally fusoid, with widest point above center, length variable, 1–5 septate (32–55 by 4–6 μm), 5–9 septate (35–100 by 4.3–8 μm)
Chlamydospores	Generally absent	Globose, smooth, borne singly or in pairs, intercalary or on short lateral branches	Globose, smooth, borne singly or in pairs or short lateral branches or intercalary

[a] Adapted from reference 63.

some characteristics (Fig. 6). The most commonly isolated species, *P. lilacinus,* was once classified as *Penicillium lilacinum* by Raper and Thom (66). The primary microscopic characteristics of *Paecilomyces* species are hyaline mycelia that are 2 to 4 μm wide and septate. Long conidiophores, 400 to 600 μm, are produced with verticillate branches that bear whorls of several phialides. The phialides are flask shaped with a tapered neck and bear chains of phialoconidia 50 to 75 μm in length. The phialoconidia are ellipsoidal to fusiform, with a smooth to finely roughened surface, and measure 1 to 2 by 2 to 3 μm.

SCOPULARIOPSIS SPECIES

Members of the genus *Scopulariopsis* are common soil fungi, and isolates of *Scopulariopsis* frequently are recovered in the clinical laboratory. Human infections with *Scopulariopsis* species, however, are caused essentially by one species, *Scopulariopsis brevicaulis.* Although *Scopulariopsis koningii* also has been reported to cause infections on several occasions, it was concluded that all of the isolates were actually *S. brevicaulis* (58).

Infections with *S. brevicaulis* usually are confined to the nails. Direct examination in KOH of scrapings or

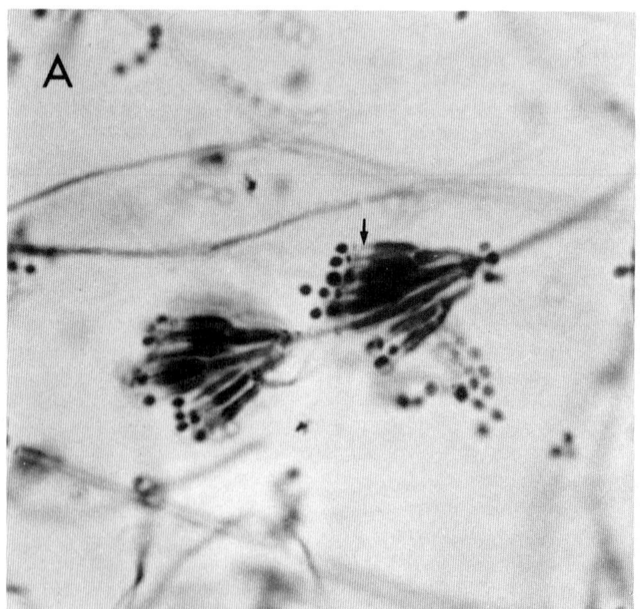

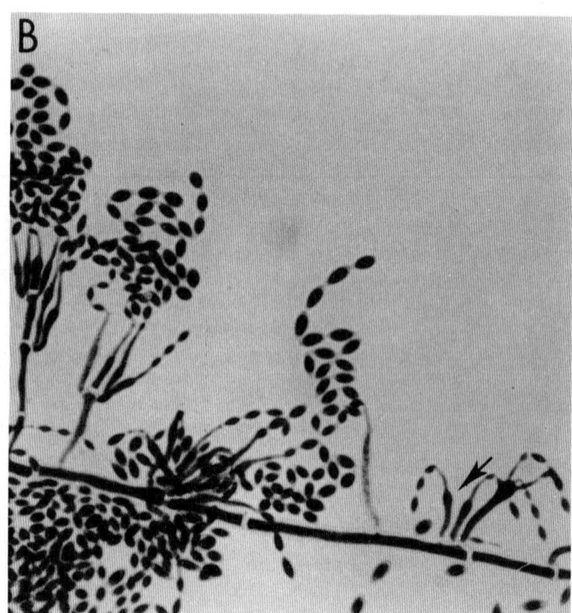

FIG. 6. (A) Slide culture of *Paecilomyces lilacinus* showing compactly arranged phialides with a long narrow neck (arrow), with a small young conidium at the tip of the phialide, which is attached to a chain of older conidia. Note the resemblance to *Penicillium* species. (B) *Paecilomyces* species. Note well-developed conidiophores (left) with phialides, which are the long, tapering tubes developing on the terminus of the conidiophore. They also arise directly from the main hypha (arrow). (Reprinted with permission from reference 71; micrographs courtesy of J. W. Rippon.)

clippings of infected nails shows chains of conidia typical of the genus, unlike the hyphal elements observed with dermatophytes. Occasionally, invasion of deep tissue has been reported. Sekhon et al. (80) reported the isolation of *S. brevicaulis* from a deep lesion in soft ankle tissue after the swollen ankle had been drained for a primary bacterial infection. *S. brevicaulis* also has been isolated from a fungus ball in a preformed pulmonary cavity (47), causing pneumonia in a patient with acute myeloblastic leukemia (95), and was observed growing and producing annelloconidia on necrotic tissue behind an eye in a patient with diabetes (52).

Scopulariopsis species grow moderately to rapidly at room temperature on all laboratory media. Colonies are white and glabrous at first, becoming gray to light brown and powdery as conidia develop. The reverse side of the colony is generally tan with a brownish center. Microscopically, *Scopulariopsis* species superficially resemble some species of *Paecilomyces* and *Penicillium* because their conidiogenous cells (annellides) may be produced singly or grouped into penicillate structures on a conidiophore (Fig. 7). Annellides proliferate percurrently during the production of conidia and so become annellated (ringed). Annelloconidia are produced in chains, with the youngest conidium at the base (basocatenulate). Mature conidia usually are flattened at the basal edge where they are released from the annellide and are thick-walled, round to lemon shaped, rough and spiny, and hyaline to brown in color.

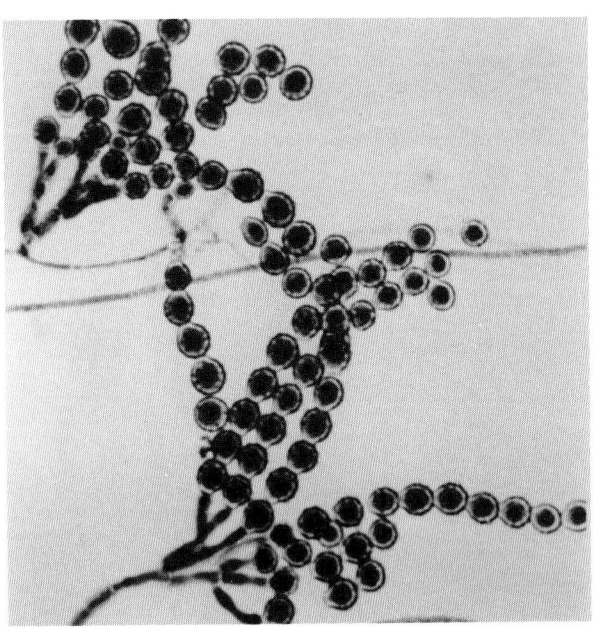

FIG. 7. *Scopulariopsis* species. Annellophores variously arranged, with conidia arising from the top of the annelide; the youngest conidium is at the bottom of the chain (basocatenulate). (Reprinted with permission from reference 71; micrograph courtesy of J. W. Rippon.)

ACREMONIUM SPECIES

Species of the genus *Acremonium*, which now includes the organism formerly called *Cephalosporium*, are abundant in soil, sewage, and other environmental sources and represent the anamorphs of several teleomorph fungi (71). Teleomorphs include, among others, *Emericellopsis*, *Nectria*, *Wallrothiella*, *Mycocitrus*, *Ceratocystis*, and *Hypocrea* (other anamorph states also may be present in the same colony). *Acremonium* spp. have been isolated from many cases of mycetoma, onychomycosis, and mycotic keratitis and as colonizers of soft contact lenses (71). More rarely, these fungi have been associated with other types of human infection. *Acremonium strictum* was found in invasive pulmonary disease in a boy with chronic granulomatous disease (7). Biopsy material from another case involving a midline granuloma with eroding destruction of the hard palate and involvement of the maxilla and mandible revealed the presence of hyaline hyphae in tissue sections, and *Acremonium* sp. was repeatedly isolated on several occasions (14). Meningitis developed in a 33-year-old woman receiving steroids during her second pregnancy after administration of a spinal anesthetic given for a cesarean section of her first pregnancy. Biopsy revealed hyphal units in tissue section, and *Acremonium* sp. was cultured (20). A fatal infection in a patient undergoing dialysis (46) and cerebritis in an intravenous drug abuser have been reported (93). Other cases also have documented species of *Acremonium* in endocarditis in a prosthetic valve (45), infection in arthritis (91) and osteomyelitis of the calvarium following trauma (8), and infection of subcutaneous tissue following renal transplant (90).

Acremonium species grow well on Sabouraud dextrose agar and also will grow on dermatophyte agar and other mycological media. White, low spreading colonies that are moist in appearance, becoming velvety to cottony and white, gray, or rose at maturity, rapidly grow. The colony reverse is generally colorless but may vary from pale yellow to pinkish in some species. Microscopically, *Acremonium* species are characterized by the presence of solitary, erect, hyaline, unbranched, tapering phialides that arise from vegetative hyphae or fascicles. At the apex of each phialide, an extremely delicate ball of one-celled and occasionally two-celled, globose to cylindrical, hyaline phialoconidia (2 to 3 by 4 to 8 μm) is formed. The conidia are disrupted easily and often form clusters at the tips of the phialides; occasionally, short chains of phialoconidia can be seen. The characteristic structures of the genus are shown in Fig. 8.

BEAUVERIA SPECIES

Members of the genus *Beauveria* are common soil saprophytes that are not generally noted as a serious cause of infections in humans but rather as insect pathogens and the organisms responsible for the disease known as muscardine of silkworms (71). *Beauveria* species, however, occasionally are recovered in the clinical laboratory and have been proven to cause infections in humans. Freour and Lahourcade (25), for instance, reported on an infection of the lung in a 22-year-old female who had ulcerative cervical lymphadenopathy and was diagnosed as having tuberculosis. A chest X-ray examination revealed a thick-walled pulmonary cavity plus other small pulmonary lesions from which *Beauveria bassiana* later was isolated. Hyphae were visible in tissue sections as well as in bronchial aspirates. *B. bassiana* and *B. alba* also have been isolated from mycotic keratitis (51, 73).

The genus *Beauveria* is characterized by dense clus-

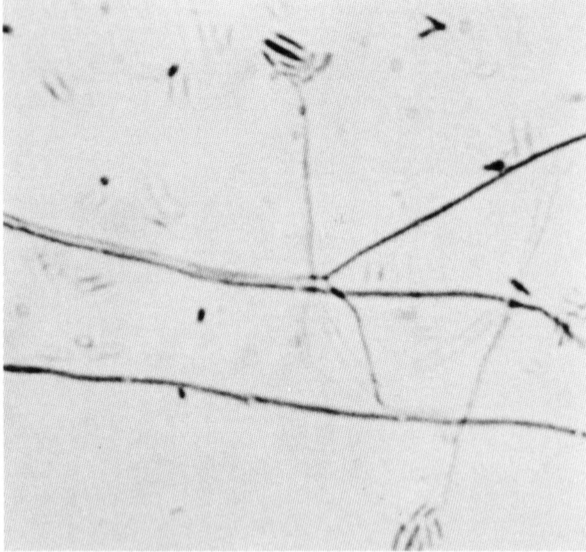

FIG. 8. *Acremonium* species. Tapered conidiogenous cell (phialide) giving rise to single-cell conidia. These accumulate as balls or heads (cephalosporia) and also may occur as chains. (Reprinted with permission from reference 5a.)

ters of hyaline, flask-shaped conidiogenous cells that are inflated at the base and proliferate sympodially in a zigzag (rachiform or geniculate) fashion (Fig. 9). The conidiogenous cells often are aggregated into sporodochia or synnemata, making it difficult at times to observe the characteristic structures, and produce small one-celled, hyaline, globose to ovoid, blastic conidia (2.5 to 4.5 μm in diameter) along the rachis at each bend point. Colonies of *Beauveria* species are moderately fast growing, appearing white to tan at first but becoming powdery in time to resemble the colonies of *Histoplasma* species or some species of dermatophytes.

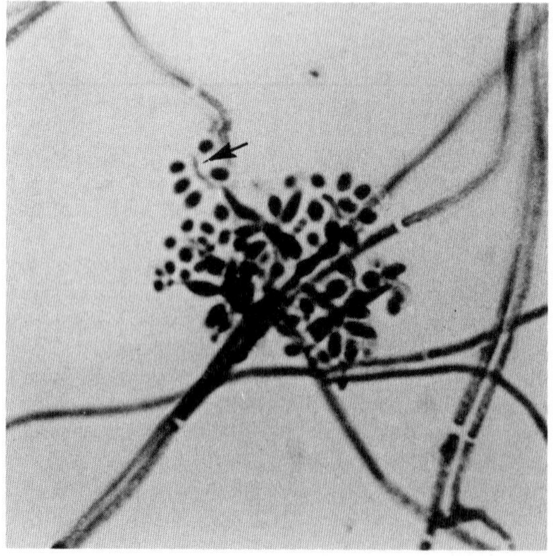

FIG. 9. *Beauveria* species. Group of conidiogenous cells that produce zigzagging rachis (arrow) growth that is sympodial in development. A conidium is produced first on one side and then on the other. (Reprinted with permission from reference 71; micrograph courtesy of J. W. Rippon.)

SCEDOSPORIUM SPECIES

Scedosporium species are soil- and water-inhabiting fungi that can cause opportunistic infections in humans who are compromised as a result of debilitating disease or drugs or who undergo trauma with introduction of the organism into the dermal or subcutaneous tissue (71). A number of case reports have documented infections involving the eye, ear, sinuses, central nervous system, internal organs, and lungs (6, 71, 96). Involvement of the lungs includes both colonizing and invasive pulmonary infections that can be difficult to distinguish from pulmonary aspergillosis (10).

In tissue sections, the hyphae of *Scedosporium* species resemble those of aspergilli and other agents of hyalohyphomycosis in that they are hyaline, septate, branched, and hematoxylinophilic. There are subtle differences between the hyphae of *Scedosporium* species and aspergilli and other hyaline Hyphomycetes in histopathologic sections, but hyphae of the former can be reliably distinguished from these fungi only by direct immunofluorescence. The hyphae of *Scedosporium* species are somewhat narrower (2 to 5 μm) than those of aspergilli and exhibit a branching pattern that is not progressive and is generally more haphazard than that of most hyaline Hyphomycetes (10). Nevertheless, culture and serologic analysis are necessary to establish the diagnosis, especially since both aspergilli and *Scedosporium* species or its teleomorphs (e.g., *P. boydii*) have been found to coexist in the same infection (71). Serologic procedures and exoantigen tests may aid in prognostic evaluation (44, 57).

Scedosporium species can be isolated on almost all mycological media that do not contain cycloheximide and occasionally can be observed growing as a teleomorph (*P. boydii*). The taxonomy of both the teleomorph and anamorph stages of this fungus is complicated and has been summarized by Rippon (71). The fungus grows readily and rapidly at first as a white colony that turns brown with age as abundant aerial mycelia produce conidia. The colony reverse typically shows areas of gray to black pigmentation. Rare strains also may produce colonies that are ivory colored and membranous, tan or cinnamon brown, and annular in growth (71).

The genus *Scedosporium* is characterized by hyaline, septate hyphae that are 1 to 3 μm in diameter and one-celled, light- to dark-brown annelloconidia that are 4 to 9 by 6 to 10 μm in size (Fig. 10). The conidia are smooth, subglobose, and ovoid to elongate (pear shaped) and are borne singly or in small groups upon short, denticlelike lateral hyphal outgrowths from elongate, simple, or branched conidiophores, or they may occur sessile or laterally on the hyphae. When detached from the conidiophore, the conidia appear to be cut off at the base (i.e., truncate). Two species have been documented to cause infections in humans: *Scedosporium apiospermum* and *S. inflatum*. The chief characteristic separating the two species is that *S. inflatum* has an inflated conidiophore. The conidiophores are extremely variable in length, are produced singly or in clusters, and are distinctly flask shaped and swollen at the base. Occasionally, *Scedosporium* may be associated with the genus *Graphium*, which produces tufts of conidiophores (synnemata) in culture. It is characterized by long, erect, narrow conidiophores that appear cemented together, diverge at the apex, and bear clusters of oval, truncate conidia (2 to 3 by 5 to 7 μm). Each

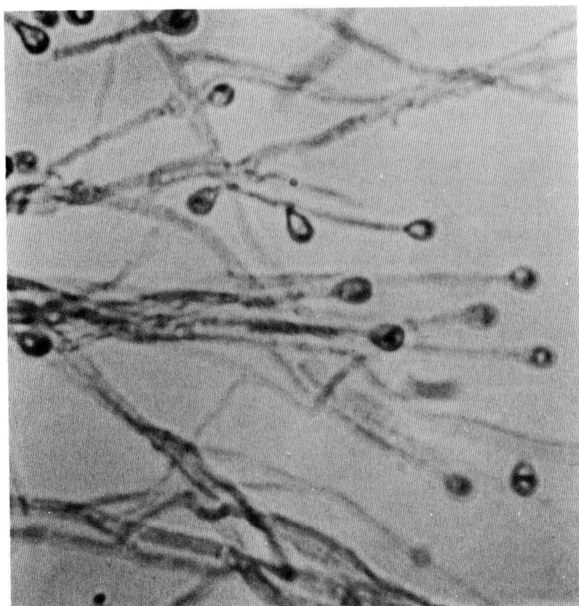

FIG. 10. *Scedosporium apiospermum* anamorph of *Pseudallescheria boydii.* Single-celled conidia being produced on short hyphae and on elongate conidiophores.

conidiophore bears one conidium. Therefore, because more than one member of the Microascaceae may form a *Scedosporium* anamorph that is identical to the one formed by *P. boydii,* the mycologist must not assign an isolate of *S. apiospermum* with the name *P. boydii* without the presence of typical cleistothecia.

RARE OPPORTUNISTIC HYALINE HYPHOMYCETES

Allergic reactions due to inhalation of fungal spores and toxicosis due to the ingestion of mushrooms have been reported frequently, but the incidence of human infections by Basidiomycetes is very rare. Several reports have described the isolation of Basidiomycetes from various anatomical sites. Speller and MacIves (84) reported on the isolation of the mushroom *Coprinus cinereus* (later identified by De Vries et al. [17] as *C. delicatulus*) from acute inflammatory endocarditis after surgical implantation of a mitral valve prosthesis, where heavily branched septate hyphae were observed in the aortic valve and within myocardial tissue. Emmons (21) also reported on the observation of mycelial strands on direct examination and the repeated isolation of *Coprinus micaceus* from the sputa of one patient. Similarly, *Schizophyllum commune* also has been isolated and mycelial elements observed in sputa from a patient with chronic lung disease (12). *S. commune* also has been isolated from infected fingernails (43), the cerebrospinal fluid of a patient with meningitis, from several patients with maxillary sinusitis (41, 71), and from an ulcerative lesion perforating the hard palate of a 4-year-old girl who had no underlying disease (67). In the latter instance, biopsies from the submucosal tissue revealed irregular hyphae with clamp connections (Fig. 11). Meningitis was attributed to an *Ustilago* sp. by Moore and Russel (56), who observed structures that resembled the sprout mycelium and echinulate spores of *Ustilago zeae.*

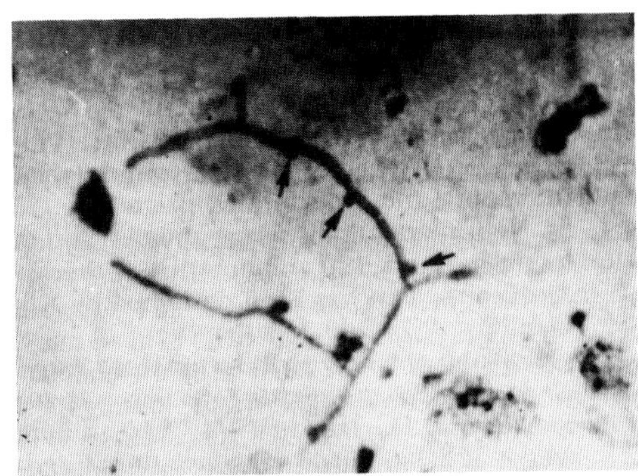

FIG. 11. *Schizophyllum commune.* Hyphae and clamp connections (arrow) are evident in a KOH mount of scrapings from the roof of a mouth.

LITERATURE CITED

1. **Agarwal, P. K., B. Lal, S. Waheb, O. P. Srivastava, and S. C. Misra.** 1979. Orbital paecilomycosis due to *Paecilomyces lilacinus* (Thom) Samson. Sabouraudia **17:**363–370.
2. **Ajello, L.** 1982. Hyalohyphomycosis: a disease entity whose time has come. Newsl. Med. Mycol. Soc. N.Y. **10:**3–5.
3. **Ajello, L.** 1986. Hyalohyphomycosis and phaeohyphomycosis: two global diseases entities of public health importance. Eur. J. Epidemiol. **2:**243–251.
4. **Allevato, P. A., J. M. Ohorodnik, E. Mezger, and J. F. Eisses.** 1984. *Paecilomyces javanicus* endocarditis of native and prosthetic aortic valve. Am. J. Clin. Pathol. **82:** 247–252.
5. **Austwick, P. K. C.** 1984. *Fusarium* infections in man and animals, p. 129–140. *In* M. Moss and J. E. Smith (ed.), The applied mycology of *Fusarium.* Cambridge University Press, London.

5a. **Beneke, E. S., and A. L. Rogers.** 1980. Medical mycology manual with the human mycoses monograph, 4th ed. Macmillan Publishing Co., New York.

6. **Bloom, S. M., R. R. Warner, and I. Weitzman.** 1982. Maxillary sinusitis: isolation of *Scedosporium* (*Monosporium*) *apiospermum* anamorph of *Petrillidium* (*Allescheria*) *boydii.* Mt. Sinai J. Med. **49:**492–494.
7. **Boltansky, H., K. J. Kwon-Chung, A. Macher, and J. I. Gillin.** 1984. *Acremonium strictum*-related pulmonary infection in a patient with chronic granulomatous disease. J. Infect. Dis. **149:**653.
8. **Brabender, W., and J. Ketcherside.** 1985. *Acremonium kiliense* osteomyelitis of the calvarium. Neurosurgery **16:** 554–556.
9. **Capponi, M., and P. Sureau.** 1956. Penicillose de *Rhizomys sinensis.* Bull. Soc. Pathol. Exot. **49:**418.
10. **Chandler, F. W., and J. C. Watts.** 1987. Pathologic diagnosis of fungal infections. American Society of Clinical Pathologists, Inc., Chicago.
11. **Chandler, F. W., W. Kaplan, and L. Ajello.** 1980. Color atlas and text of the histopathology of mycotic diseases. Year Book Medical Publishers, Inc., Chicago.
12. **Ciferri, R., and A. Chavez Batista.** 1956. Isolation of *Schizophyllum commune* from sputum. Atti Ist. Bot. Lab. Crittogam. Pavia **14:**118–120.
13. **Cole, G. T.** 1986. Models of cell differentiation in conidial fungi. Microbiol. Rev. **50:**95–132.
14. **Cowen, D. E., and D. E. Dines.** 1965. *Cephalosporium* midline granuloma. Ann. Intern. Med. **62:**791–795.

15. **Dekhkan-Khodzhaeva, N. A., and S. Shamsiev.** 1982. Role of *Paecilomyces* in the etiology of protracted recurrent bronchopulmonary disease in children. Pediatriya **9:** 12–14.
16. **DelRossi, A. J., D. Morse, P. M. Spagna, and G. M. Lemole.** 1980. Successful management of *Penicillium* endocarditis. J. Thorac. Cardiovasc. Surg. **80:**945–947.
17. **De Vries, G. A., R. F. O. Kemp, and D. C. E. Speller.** 1971. Endocarditis caused by *Coprinus delicatulus*, p. 185–186. Proceedings of the Fifth Congress of the International Society for Human and Animal Mycology. Comptes Rendus Communications, Paris.
18. **Dharmasena, F. M., G. S. R. Davies, and D. Catovsky.** 1985. *Paecilomyces variotii* pneumonia complicating hairy cell leukemia. Br. Med. J. **290:**967–968.
19. **DiSalvo, A. F., A. Fickling, and L. Ajello.** 1972. Infection caused by *Penicillium marneffei*. Am. J. Clin. Pathol. **59:** 259–263.
20. **Drouhet, E., and L. Martin.** 1965. Mycose meningocerebrale a *Cephalosporium*. Presse Med. **31:**1809–1814.
21. **Emmons, C. W.** 1954. Isolation of *Myxotrichum* and *Gymnoascus* from lungs of animals. Mycologia **46:**334–338.
22. **Eschete, M. L., J. W. King, C. West, and A. Aberle.** 1981. *Penicillium chrysogenum* endophthalmitis. Mycopathologia **74:**125–127.
23. **Fench, F. F., and C. P. Mallia.** 1972. Pleural effusion caused by *Paecilomyces lilacinus*. Br. J. Dis. Chest **66:**284–290.
24. **Fraser, D. W., J. I. Ward, L. Ajello, and B. D. Plikaytis.** 1979. Aspergillosis and other systemic mycoses. J. Am. Med. Assoc. **242:**1631–1635.
25. **Freour, P., and M. Lahourcade.** 1965. Une mycose nouvelle. Etude clinique et mycologique d'une localisation pulmonaire de *"Beauveria."* Bull. Soc. Med. Hop. Paris **117:**197–206.
26. **Garrison, R. G., and K. S. Boyd.** 1973. Dimorphism of *Penicillium marneffei* as observed by electron microscopy. Can. J. Microbiol. **19:**1305–1309.
27. **Gerber, J. D., and R. D. Jones.** 1973. Immunologic significance of aspergillin antigens of six species of *Aspergillus* in the serodiagnosis of aspergillosis. Am. Rev. Respir. Dis. **108:**1124–1129.
28. **Gillium, J., and S. A. Vest.** 1951. *Penicillium* infection of the urinary tract. J. Urol. **65:**485–489.
29. **Gordon, M. A.** 1984. *Paecilomyces lilacinus* (Thom) Sampson, from systemic infection in an armadillo (*Dasypus novemcinectus*). Sabouraudia **22:**109–116.
30. **Gordon, M. A., and S. A. Norton.** 1985. Corneal transplant infection by *Paecilomyces lilacinus*. Sabouraudia **23:**295–301.
31. **Gugnani, H. C., S. Gupta, and R. S. Talwar.** 1978. Role of opportunistic fungi in ocular infections in Nigeria. Mycopathologia **65:**155–166.
32. **Haldane, E. V., and J. L. MacDonald.** 1974. Prosthetic valvular endocarditis due to the fungus *Paecilomyces*. Can. Med. Assoc. J. **111:**963–965.
33. **Hall, W. J.** 1974. *Penicillium* endocarditis following open heart surgery and prosthetic valve insertion. Am. Heart J. **87:**501–506.
34. **Harris, L. F., B. M. Dan, and A. W. Lefkowitz.** 1979. *Paecilomyces* cellulitis in a renal transplant patient; successful treatment with intravenous miconazole. South. Med. J. **72:**897–898.
35. **Heard, D. J., G. H. Cantor, E. R. Jacobson, B. Purich, L. Ajello, and A. A. Padhye.** 1986. Hyalohyphomycosis caused by *Paecilomyces lilacinus* in an Aldabra tortoise. J. Am. Vet. Med. Assoc. **189:**1143–1145.
36. **Huang, S. N., and L. S. Harris.** 1963. Acute disseminated penicillosis. Am. J. Clin. Pathol. **39:**167–174.
37. **Jade, K. B., M. F. Lyons, and J. W. Gnan.** 1986. *Paecilomyces lilacinus* in an immunocompromised patient. Arch. Dermatol. **122:**1169–1170.
38. **Kalish, S. B., and R. Goldschmidt.** 1982. Infective endocarditis carditis caused by *Paecilomyces varioti*. J. Clin. Pathol. **78:**249–252.
39. **Kaufman, L.** 1981. Current methods for serodiagnosing systemic fungus infections and identifying their etiologic agents. Estr. Ig. Mod. **76:**422–442.
40. **Kaufman, L., and W. Kaplan.** 1961. Preparation of a fluorescent antibody specific for the yeast phase of *Histoplasma capsulatum*. J. Bacteriol. **82:**729–735.
41. **Kern, M. E., and F. A. Uecker.** 1986. Maxillary sinus infection caused by the homobasidiomycetous fungus *Schizophyllum commune*. J. Clin. Microbiol. **23:**1001–1005.
42. **Kinare, S. G., and A. P. Chaukar.** 1978. Fungal endocarditis after cardiac valve surgery. J. Postgrad. Med. **24:**164–170.
43. **Klingman, A. M.** 1950. A basidiomycete probably causing onychomycosis. J. Invest. Dermatol. **14:**67–70.
44. **Kohler, U.** 1982. Entzundlicher Tranen-Nasenwegsuerschluss dirch *Monosporium apiospermum*. Klin. Monatsbl. Augenheilk. **181:**480–482.
45. **Lacaz, C. da S., and M. E. Porto.** 1981. Endocardite em protese de dura-mater provocada pelo *Acremonium kiliense*. Rev. Inst. Med. Trop. Sao Paulo **23:**274–275.
46. **Landay, M. E., J. H. Greenwald, A. Sterner, and D. L. Ashbach.** 1982. *Cephalosporium* (*Acremonium*) in dialysis-connected peritonitis. J. Indiana State Med. Assoc. **75:**391.
47. **Larsh, H. W.** 1977. Opportunistic fungi in chronic disease other than cancer and related problems, p. 221–229. *In* K. Iwata (ed.), Recent advances in medical and veterinary mycology. Proceedings of the Sixth Congress of the International Society for Human and Animal Mycology. University Park Press, Baltimore.
48. **Liebler, G. A., G. J. Magovern, P. Sadighi, S. B. Park, and W. J. Cushing.** 1977. *Penicillium* granuloma of the lung presenting as a solitary pulmonary nodule. J. Am. Med. Assoc. **234:**671.
49. **Matsumoto, T., and T. Matsuda.** 1988. Critical review of hyalohyphomycosis caused by *Fusarium* species, p. 292–296. *In* J. M. Torres-Rodriguez (ed.), Proceedings of the Tenth Congress of the International Society for Human and Animal Mycology-ISHAM. J. R. Prous S. A., Barcelona.
50. **McClellen, J. R., J. D. Hamilton, J. A. Alexander, W. G. Wolfe, and J. B. Reed.** 1976. *Paecilomyces varioti* endocarditis on a prosthetic aortic valve. J. Thorac. Cardiovasc. Surg. **71:**472–475.
51. **McDonnell, P. J., T. P. Werblin, L. Sigler, and W. R. Green.** 1985. Mycotic keratitis due to *Beauveria albi*. Cornea **3:**213–216.
52. **McGinnis, M. R.** 1980. Laboratory handbook of medical mycology. Academic Press, Inc., New York.
53. **McGinnis, M. R.** 1983. Chromoblastomycosis and phaeohyphomycosis: new concepts, diagnosis, and mycology. J. Am. Acad. Dermatol. **8:**1–16.
54. **McGinnis, M. R., L. Ajello, and W. A. Schell.** 1985. Mycotic diseases: a proposed nomenclature. Int. J. Dermatol. **24:**9–15.
55. **Miller, G. P., and G. Rebell.** 1978. Intravitreal antimycotic therapy and the cure of mycotic endophthalmitis caused by a *Paecilomyces lilacinus* contaminated pseudophakos. Ophthalmic Surg. **9:**54–63.
56. **Moore, M., and W. O. Russel.** 1946. Chronic leptomeningitis and ependymitis caused by *Ustilago*, probably *U. zeae:* ustilagomycosis, the second reported instance of human infection. Am. J. Pathol. **22:**761–773.
57. **Morace, G., and P. L. Polonelli.** 1981. Exoantigen test for identification of *Petriellidium boydii*. J. Clin. Microbiol. **14:** 237–240.
58. **Morton, F. J., and G. Smith.** 1963. The genera *Scopulariopsis* Bainier, *Microascus* Zukal, and *Doratomyces* Corda. Mycology paper 86. Commonwealth Mycologial Institute, Kew, Surrey, England.
59. **Mosier, N. A., and B. Lusk.** 1977. Fungal endophthalmitis following intraocular lens implantation. Am. J. Ophthalmol. **240:**378–380.

60. **Nadler, J. P.** 1990. Disseminated fusarial infection. Rev. Infect. Dis. **12:**162.

61. **O'Day, D. M.** 1977. Fungal endophthalmitis caused by *Paecilomyces lilacinus* after intraocular lens implantation. Am. J. Ophthalmol. **83:**130–131.

62. **Otcenasek, M., Z. Jirousek, Z. Nozicka, and K. Mencl.** 1984. Paecilomycosis of the maxillary sinus. Mykosen **27:** 242–248.

63. **Padhye, A. A.** 1988. Hyalohyphomycosis, p. 654–662. *In* A. Balows, W. J. Hausler, Jr., M. Ohashi, and A. Turano (ed.), Laboratory diagnosis of infectious diseases: principles and practice, vol. I. Bacterial, mycotic and parasitic diseases. Springer-Verlag, New York.

64. **Ramirez, C.** 1982. Manual and atlas of the Penicillia. Elsevier Biomedical Press, New York.

65. **Raper, K. B., and D. I. Fennell.** 1965. The genus *Aspergillus.* The Williams & Wilkins Co., Baltimore.

66. **Raper, K. B., and C. Thom.** 1949. A manual of the penicillia. The Williams & Wilkins Co., Baltimore.

67. **Restrepo, A., D. L. Greer, M. Robledo, O. Osorio, and H. Mondragon.** 1973. Ulceration of the palate caused by a basidiomycete *Schizophyllum commune.* Sabouraudia **9:** 201–204.

68. **Richardson, S. E., R. M. Bannatyne, R. C. Summerbell, J. Milliken, R. Gold, and S. S. Weitzman.** Disseminated fusarial infection in the immunocompromised host. Rev. Infect. Dis. **10:**1171–1181.

69. **Rinaldi, M. G.** 1983. Invasive aspergillosis. Rev. Infect. Dis. **5:**1061–1066.

70. **Rinaldi, M. G.** 1988. Aspergillosis, p. 559–572. *In* A. Balows, W. J. Hausler, Jr., M. Ohashi, and A. Turano (ed.), Laboratory diagnosis of infectious diseases: principles and practice, vol. I. Bacterial, mycotic and parasitic diseases. Springer-Verlag, New York.

71. **Rippon, J. W.** 1988. Medical mycology: the pathogenic fungi and the pathogenic actinomycetes, 3rd ed. The W. B. Saunders Co., Philadelphia.

72. **Rockhill, R. C., and M. D. Klein.** 1980. *Paecilomyces lilacinus* as the cause of chronic maxillary sinusitis. J. Clin. Microbiol. **11:**737–739.

73. **Sachs, S. W., J. Baum, and C. Mies.** 1985. *Beauveria bassiana* keratitis. Br. J. Ophthalmol. **69:**548–550.

74. **Samson, R. A.** 1974. *Paecilomyces* and some allied hyphomycetes. Studies in mycology no. 6. Centraalbureau voor Schimmelcultures, Baarn, The Netherlands.

75. **Segretain, G.** 1959. *Penicillium marneffei* n. sp. agent d'une mycose du systeme reticuloendothelial. Mycopathologia **11:**327–353.

76. **Segretain, G.** 1962. Some new or infrequent fungous pathogens, p. 33–49. *In* G. Dalldorf (ed.), Fungi and fungous diseases. Charles C Thomas, Publisher, Springfield, Ill.

77. **Segretain, G., H. Fromentin, P. Destombes, E. R. Brygoo, and A. Dodin.** 1964. *Paecilomyces virdis* n. sp. champignon dimorphique, agent d'une mycose generalisee de *Chameleo lateralis* Gray. C. R. Acad. Sci. **259:**258–261.

78. **Sekhon, A. S., J. S. K. Li, and A. K. Garg.** 1982. Penicilliosis marneffei: serological and exoantigen studies. Mycopathologia **77:**51–57.

79. **Sekhon, A. S., P. G. Standard, L. Kauffman, A. K. Garg, and P. Cifuentes.** 1986. Grouping of *Aspergillius* species with exoantigens. Diagn. Immunol. **4:**112–116.

80. **Sekhon, A. S., D. J. Williams, and J. H. Harvey.** 1974. Deep scopulariopsis: a case report and sensitivity studies. J. Clin. Pathol. **27:**837–843.

81. **Sherwood, J. A., and A. S. Dansky.** 1983. *Paecilomyces* pyelonephritis complicating nephrolithiasis and a review of *Paecilomyces* infections. J. Urol. **130:**526–528.

82. **Silver, M. D., P. G. Tuffinell, and W. G. Bigelow.** 1971. Endocarditis caused by *Paecilomyces varioti* affecting an aortic valve allograft. J. Thorac. Cardiovasc. Surg. **61:**278–281.

83. **Solley, G. O., and R. E. Hyatt.** 1980. Hypersensitivity pneumonitis induced by *Penicillium* species. J. Allergy Clin. Immunol. **65:**65–70.

84. **Speller, D. C. E., and A. C. MacIves.** 1971. Endocarditis caused by a *Coprinus* species. A fungus of the toadstool group. J. Med. Microbiol. **4:**370–374.

85. **Stimlam, C. V., D. E. Dines, R. F. Rodgers-Sullivan, G. D. Roberts, and W. C. Sheehan.** 1980. Respiratory tract *Aspergillus*—clinical significance. Minn. Med. **63:**25–30.

86. **Swatek, F., C. Halde, M. J. Rinaldi, and H. J. Shadomy.** 1985. *Aspergillus* and other opportunistic saprophytic hyaline hyphomycetes, p. 584–594. *In* E. H. Lennette, A. Balows, W. J. Hausler, Jr., and H. J. Shadomy (ed.), Manual of clinical microbiology, 4th ed. American Society for Microbiology, Washington, D.C.

87. **Takayasu, S., M. Akagi, and Y. Shimizu.** 1977. Cutaneous mycosis caused by *Paecilomyces lilacinus.* Arch. Dermatol. **113:**1687–1690.

88. **Upshaw, C. B.** 1974. *Penicillium* endocarditis of aortic valve prosthesis. J. Thorac. Cardiovasc. Surg. **68:**428–431.

89. **Uys, C. J., and P. A. Don.** 1963. Endocarditis following cardiac surgery due to the fungus *Paecilomyces.* South Afr. Med. J. **37:**1276–1280.

90. **Van Etta, L. L., L. R. Peterson, and D. N. Gerding.** 1983. Mycetoma in a renal transplant patient. Arch. Dermatol. **119:**707–708.

91. **Ward, H. P., W. J. Martin, J. C. Ivins, and L. A. Weed.** 1961. *Cephalosporium* arthritis. Proc. Staff Meet. Mayo Clin. **36:**337–343.

92. **Weitzman, I.** 1988. Saprophytic molds as agents of cutaneous and subcutaneous infection in the immunocompromised host. Arch. Dermatol. **122:**1161–1168.

93. **Wetli, C. V., S. D. Weiss, T. J. Cleary, and E. Gyori.** 1984. Fungal cerebritis from intravenous drug abuse. J. Forensic Sci. **29:**260–268.

94. **Wheat, L. J.** 1986. The role of the serologic diagnostic laboratory and the diagnosis of fungal disease, p. 43–68. *In* G. A. Sarosi and S. F. Davies (ed.), Fungal diseases of the lung. Grune and Stratton, Inc., New York.

95. **Wheat, L. J., M. Bartlett, M. Ciccarelli, and J. W. Smith.** 1984. Opportunistic *Scopulariopsis* pneumonia in an immunocompromised host. South. Med. J. **77:**1608–1609.

96. **Zapater, R. C., and E. J. Albesi.** 1979. Corneal monosporiosis. Ophthalmologica **178:**142–147.

Chapter 64

Agents of Zygomycosis

NORMAN L. GOODMAN AND MICHAEL G. RINALDI

Zygomycosis is an umbrella term for an array of diseases caused by fungi placed in the taxonomic class Zygomycetes. The archaic, obsolete term phycomycosis should be discarded altogether. Human pathogens in this class are further classified in two orders, Mucorales and Entomophthorales. Some investigators prefer to call mycoses incited by members of the Mucorales mucormycosis and those caused by species classified in the Entomophthorales as entomophthoromycosis. More recently, a species classified in the class Oomycetes of the Kingdom Protoctista has been demonstrated as an agent of human disease. This organism previously was considered to be a fungus and is considered here for that reason. Zygomycetous species are etiologic agents of a broad range of mycoses in both normal and immunocompromised hosts, although infections most often occur in the latter. Table 1 summarizes one system of classification of the pathogenic Zygomycetes and Oomycetes (25, 26, 44).

BIOLOGY OF THE ZYGOMYCETES

The agents of zygomycosis are distributed universally and frequently are associated with plant debris and soil. Some of the moulds found in this group are major plant pathogens, food spoilage organisms, and sources of food in the Orient. Many species commonly are observed as saprobes or contaminants. Zygomycetes are not particularly fastidious or difficult to grow and generally require no special media or enhancements for cultivation. Zygomycetous fungi are generally rapid growers, with the exception of some entomophthoraceous species. Whereas they proliferate well in the laboratory environment, some species (e.g., strains of *Conidiobolus*, *Basidiobolus*, and *Saksenaea* species) do not readily produce the characteristic fruiting structures upon which specific identification depends. With such isolates, the special techniques discussed below may be used to obtain characteristic morphology necessary for identification.

Most mucoraceous species easily fill a petri dish within 3 to 5 days and demonstrate a grayish white aerial mycelium with a woolly texture. Care must be taken, since such colonies are tenacious and often get stuck on a teasing needle when the microbiologist attempts to remove a portion of the colony in preparation for microscopic examination. As with most medically significant moulds, colonial morphology serves as an adjunct to identification; moulds must be examined microscopically for proper identification. Entomophthoraceous Zygomycetes exhibit a distinctly different colonial appearance in contrast to mucoraceous genera. These fungi grow in 3 to 5 days as flat, waxy-appearing colonies that often may develop radial grooves and are gray to pale yellow in color. They also are difficult to remove from the agar surface. Some mucoraceous Zygomycetes, when grown in liquid media at 35 to 37°C with increased carbon dioxide tension, demonstrate the ability to transform to a yeastlike form. This observation is uncommon in most clinical laboratories because the necessary growth conditions are not used. This interesting phenomenon of dimorphism may be valuable for identifying some species of *Mucor* and *Cokeromyces recurvatus* (45). Zygomycetes pathogenic for humans grow at both 25 and 37°C, but as noted below, a single temperature of 30°C is acceptable and adequate.

The hyphae of Zygomycetes, both in culture and in tissue, most often are broad (5 to 15 μm in diameter) and irregular and lack septa (cross walls) except near fruiting structures or in old cultures. A lack of septate hyphae properly is termed coenocytic and reflects that most Zygomycetes consist of one long, complex piece of hypha with cytoplasm essentially continuous throughout the fungus. To provide an accurate genus and species designation, Zygomycetes must be identified microscopically. Characteristic and distinctive fruiting structures serve to distinguish between genera and species within genera. There are presently no identification kits, nucleic acid probes, or commercially available immunological or serological means to identify Zygomycetes, and so the eye and brain, a good reference text with keys, and a fair amount of patience and persistence are necessary for proper identification. As noted above, colonial morphology may serve as a useful aid in identification; e.g., colonies of *Rhizopus* species often produce voluminous numbers of sporangial fruiting heads which appear as black dots nestled in whitish gray aerial mycelium, whereas entomophthoraceous fungi may exhibit short, white, velvety collections or blooms of asexual propagules. In all cases, microscopic examination is essential.

The one oomycetous protist discussed here, *Pythium insidiosum*, previously was considered a fungus classified in the division Mastigomycota. Most contemporary investigators now believe that species of the genus *Pythium* are not fungi, and they appropriately are classified in the Kingdom Protoctista (Table 1). This species incites disease primarily in animals (equines in particular) but recently has been documented as a devastating human pathogen (16, 73; M. G. Rinaldi, S. M. Seidenfeld, A. W. Fothergill, and D. A. McGough, Abstr. Annu. Meet. Am. Soc. Microbiol. 1989, F11, p. 460). Because it previously has been considered a fungus and long has been studied under the purview of medical mycology, it is included here and will be discussed further below.

TABLE 1. One system of classification of Zygomycetes and Oomycetes pathogenic for humans[a]

Superkingdom: Eukaryota—Cells containing genetic material that is surrounded or enclosed by a true membrane system.
Kingdom: Fungi—Absorptive nutrition; zygotic meiosis; unicellular or filamentous; cell walls chitinous.
Division: Zygomycotina—Motile spores not produced; mycelium, when present, aseptate (coenocytic). Teleomorph (sexual form) characterized by production of zygospores.
Class: Zygomycetes—Saprobic, parasitic, or predaceous. Mycelium emersed in host tissue when parasitic or predaceous.
Order 1: Mucorales
Family 1: Mucoraceae
Genera: *Absidia, Apophysomyces, Mucor, Rhizomucor, Rhizopus*
Pathogenic species: 1. *Absidia corymbifera*
2. *Apophysomyces elegans*
3. *Mucor circinelloides* form *circinelloides*
4. *Mucor hiemalis*
5. *Mucor racemosus*
6. *Mucor ramosissimus*
7. *Mucor rouxianus*
8. *Rhizomucor miehei*
9. *Rhizomucor pusillus*
10. *Rhizopus arrhizus*
11. *Rhizopus microsporus* variety *microsporus*
12. *Rhizopus microsporus* variety *oligosporus*
13. *Rhizopus microsporus* variety *rhizopodiformis*
Family 2: Cunninghamellaceae
Genus: *Cunninghamella*
Pathogenic species: *Cunninghamella bertholletiae*
Family 3: Mortierellaceae
Genus: *Mortierella*
Pathogenic species: *Mortierella wolfii*
Family 4: Saksenaeaceae
Genus: *Saksenaea*
Pathogenic species: *Saksenaea vasiformis*
Family 5: Syncephalastraceae
Genus: *Syncephalastrum*
Pathogenic species: Etiologic agents classified in this genus have not been identified to species level.
Family 6: Thamnidiaceae
Genus: *Cokeromyces*
Pathogenic species: *Cokeromyces recurvatus*
Order 2: Entomophthorales
Family 1: Ancylistaceae
Genus: *Conidiobolus*
Subgenus: *Conidiobolus*
Pathogenic species: 1. *Conidiobolus coronatus*
2. *Conidiobolus incongruus*
Family 2: Basidiobolaceae
Genus: *Basidiobolus*
Pathogenic species: *Basidiobolus ranarum*
Kingdom: Protoctista—Ingestive, absorptive, or photosynthetic nutrition; mitotic reproduction; unicellular or multicellular; flagella or cilia with microtubules in 9 + 2 arrangement.
Class: Oomycetes—Biflagellate zoospores; anterior tinsel-type flagellum; posterior whiplash-type flagellum.
Order: Peronosporales
Family: Pythiaceae
Genus: *Pythium*
Pathogenic species: *Pythium insidiosum*

[a] This system does not necessarily reflect the opinion of every taxonomic authority but serves as a guide to those zygomycetous fungi and oomycetous protists that have been documented as agents of human disease and may be observed in clinical microbiology laboratories.

ZYGOMYCOTIC DISEASES

As noted previously, zygomycosis encompasses a spectrum of diseases. Because of changes in taxonomy and the expanded range of etiologic agents, the designation zygomycosis is preferred over the older and still frequently used term mucormycosis. To reiterate, the term phycomycosis should be eliminated from the nomenclature of medical mycology (65). In general, fungi in the order Mucorales cause the more severe forms of disease while those in the order Entomophthorales cause disease of the nasal mucosa and subcutaneous tissue (65). The diseases occur predominantly in individuals who are compromised physically, physiologically, or immunologically. The diseases may be acquired by many routes, but the most common are inhalation of spores, traumatic implantation of fungal elements in tissue, and invasion of fungal elements across compromised membrane barriers.

When normal protective barriers have been breached, the fungal elements invade adjacent tissue and spread via blood vessels to adjacent organ systems, in time becoming widely disseminated. A hallmark of zygomycosis, in all forms except those due to entomophthoraceous species, is blood vessel invasion with subsequent thrombosis, ischemia, and necrosis.

Predisposing conditions to zygomycosis are numerous, but the most common are diabetic acidosis, diseases and disorders leading to severe leukopenia and phagocytic dysfunction, immunosuppression, AIDS, malnutrition, severe burns, alcoholism, intravenous drug abuse, and dialysis (12, 55, 60, 65, 66). Recent information indicates an association between zygomycosis and the use of deferoxamine in patients on dialysis (70).

Zygomycetous infections have been reported from virtually all anatomic sites but are usually placed in five categories: rhinocerebral, pulmonary, gastrointestinal, cutaneous, and widely disseminated. Other, miscellaneous forms of infection also have been reported (65).

Rhinocerebral zygomycosis

The rhinocerebral form of zygomycosis is the most common form of the disease. It has been reported in very young to elderly patients, a vast majority of whom suffered from poorly controlled diabetes (12, 24, 37, 51, 62, 67, 70). Other underlying diseases of note are leukemia, chronic alcoholism, and profound immunosuppression, as in organ and bone marrow transplant patients (12, 42, 55, 60, 65, 66). Several species of Zygomycetes have been reported as the etiologic agents of this disease, but the majority of cases are caused by *Rhizopus arrhizus* (12, 55, 60, 65).

Rhinocerebral zygomycosis is usually an acute, rapidly progressive, fulminant disease, although it may be chronic and subclinical (12, 55, 60, 65). Infection is acquired by inhaling sporangiospores, which subsequently grow in the nose and extend to adjacent tissue or deposit in the paranasal sinuses, where they germinate and grow.

Symptoms of rhinocerebral zygomycosis usually develop rapidly and are unilateral. They usually start as progressive headaches, retro-orbital pain, and fever. Periorbital edema and bloody nasal discharge are symptoms of advanced disease. Ophthalmoplegia, with ptosis and proptosis, is common. Decreased visual acuity is common, and facial paralysis may occur (6, 12, 37, 38, 48, 55, 60, 65). Abnormal mental status often signals brain involvement. These symptoms may develop in a few hours or over many days, depending on the site infected, status of the host, and degree of pathology. Concurrent with the varying degree of symptoms, the fungus at first causes local tissue necrosis, simulating sinusitis, and then invades the arterial walls and reaches the periorbital tissue and cranial vault. Alternatively, the fungus may invade the soft palate, forming a white to black plaquelike lesion or fistula (12, 55, 60, 65, 66).

Pulmonary zygomycosis

The clinical picture of pulmonary zygomycosis is extremely variable. Infection of the lung primarily is caused by inhalation of aerosolized sporangiospores of zygomycetous fungi, although the lung also may be involved in disseminated zygomycosis, with evidence of spread from other sites. The population most commonly acquiring pulmonary zygomycosis includes patients with leukemia, lymphoma, profound immunosuppression (e.g., those with bone marrow transplants), and uremia. Pulmonary disease is not frequent in diabetic patients (12, 55, 60, 65, 66).

The acute form of pulmonary zygomycosis is severe. Symptoms include fever, pleuritic chest pain, and leukocytosis. Radiologically, the disease may present as extensive infiltrate, consolidation, or miliary pattern or as nodules, ill-defined infiltrates, or small wedge-shaped peripheral lesions. Cavitation may occur, and "fungus balls" have been reported (6, 39, 61, 68, 81).

Subacute zygomycosis, an increasingly frequent finding, is largely limited to the airways, with no or minimal parenchymal involvement. When parenchyma is involved, the chest X-ray examination shows small peripheral densities or ill-defined infiltrates. Bronchial plugging may occur, with fungal elements growing in mucus within a bronchus, without invasion (6, 65).

Pulmonary zygomycosis is similar in pathology to other forms of the disease. The fungus invades adjacent tissue through blood vessels, resulting in thrombosis, infarction, and necrosis. Because of the rapidity of invasion and destruction of tissue in the acute form of the disease, most patients do not survive (65, 66).

Gastrointestinal zygomycosis

Intestinal zygomycosis is a rare infection in humans, usually acquired by ingestion of fungi or spread from the abdomen after surgery, from dirty trauma to the abdomen, or from a contaminated ileostomy. Intestinal zygomycosis in children is associated with severe undernourishment, amebic colitis, typhoid, pellagra and kwashiorkor (12, 20, 42, 55, 60, 65).

Gastrointestinal infections may be caused by species of Mucorales or by Entomophthorales. In cases in which isolations and identifications were made, *Absidia corymbifera* was the most frequent agent of the Mucorales, with *Basidiobolus* and *Conidiobolus* species being etiologic agents of the Entomophthorales.

Symptoms of gastrointestinal zygomycosis vary considerably, depending on the site and extent of involvement. Nonspecific abdominal pain, diarrhea, "coffee ground" hematemesis, and bloody stools have been reported (42, 65, 66).

As with other forms of zygomycosis, the fungus invades blood vessels, with thrombosis and subsequent necrosis in the gastrointestinal tract or adjacently infected organs. Traumatized tissue infected with Zygomycetes often appears as large plaquelike areas of gray and blackened eschar on the surface (20, 42, 65, 66).

Cutaneous zygomycosis

Clinical manifestations of cutaneous zygomycosis are as variable as the other forms of this disease (12, 55, 60, 65). Primary cutaneous zygomycosis may be caused by injection of the organism into the cutaneous or subcutaneous tissue or by implantation through agents such as elastoplastic bandages (17, 36, 56, 83), by major trauma of automobile accidents, or by machinery (71, 78, 80). Cutaneous and subcutaneous zygomycosis also may occur as a result of hematogenous spread or direct invasion from other organs to cutaneous and subcutaneous tissue. As in other forms of zygomycosis, cutaneous disease occurs predominantly in patients compromised by the same diseases, including burns. Furthermore, it should be noted that patients with this form of disease range from neonates to adults of all ages (12, 22, 36, 56, 65, 66, 71, 78, 80).

Many species of several genera of the class Zygomycetes have been reported to cause cutaneous and subcutaneous disease. Of those causes for which a specific identification has been made, *Rhizopus microsporus* variety *rhizopodiformis* and *R. arrhizus* are most common (65, 66); however, other species have been isolated. *Cunninghamella bertholletiae* recently has been shown to cause a cutaneoarticular infection in a patient with AIDS (49). *Apophysomyces elegans* and a species of *Syncephalastrum* also recently have been shown to cause cutaneous disease (32, 82). The list of etiologic agents will undoubtedly become longer as the number of compromised patients increases and as the fungal isolates are more specifically identified (R. J. Fetchick, M. G. Rinaldi, and S. H. Sun, Abstr. Annu. Meet. Am. Soc. Microbiol. 1986, F35, p. 403).

The lesion of cutaneous zygomycosis is nonspecific and appears initially as a small erythematous nodule or plaque that rapidly progresses, within hours or days, to an indurated cellulitis, often with a central black eschar or central necrotic ulcer. Gangrenous changes may occur, and hemorrhagic bullae appear. Vascular invasion often occurs, with rapid spread of the fungus to adjacent organs. Histopathological findings may include hyperkeratosis of the epidermis, accumulation of neutrophils, proteinaceous fluids, and cellular debris. There is often a mixed suppurative and necrotizing inflammatory reaction in the dermis, subcutaneous tissue, and skeletal muscle. Foci of suppurative necrosis and hemorrhages usually are found in association with necrotizing vasculitis of blood vessels. Broad, nonseptate hyphae usually are present in the newly invaded tissue and blood vessels (65, 66).

Disseminated zygomycosis

The prevalence of disseminated zygomycosis has increased with the increasing number of compromised patients, and the extent of dissemination probably is more evident because clinicians and laboratorians are more aware of these diseases; therefore, they perform more extensive laboratory tests.

The primary site of disseminated zygomycosis is the lung, with spread to the central nervous system, where abscesses and infarcts are found (65, 66), or to the vascular system with seeding to the heart and subsequently via emboli to other organs of the body (9, 29, 31, 69, 79). There also is indication that spread may occur from the sinuses to the brain and other organs. Recent literature and personal experience illustrate that no organ of the body is spared in disseminated disease of the profoundly compromised patient.

The previously mentioned predisposing factors are associated with disseminated disease. Profound leukopenia is a major factor associated with many cases of disseminated zygomycosis (65, 66). Recent reports of the association between deferoxamine use and disseminated zygomycosis, particularly in dialysis patients, have added another factor to the list (8, 70, 84).

Clinical manifestations of disseminated zygomycosis are as variable as the organs involved. Since most cases occur in compromised patients, the symptoms of the primary disease or condition may mask the symptoms of the fungal disease.

As expected, disseminated disease has been reported to be caused by all of the Zygomycetes associated with the more restricted forms of the disease (40, 50, 55, 60, 63, 65, 66, 72). Specimens such as blood, pus, urine, spinal fluid, and other fluids usually do not yield the infecting zygomycete in culture, so tissue biopsy often is necessary to obtain a definitive diagnosis. As a consequence, premortem diagnosis of disseminated zygomycosis is infrequent.

Because the mortality rate of disseminated zygomycosis is very high and diagnosis is difficult, clinicians and laboratorians should make special efforts to obtain good specimens and examine them thoroughly for the presence of fungi. The presence of nonseptate hyphae in the specimen or growth of a zygomycete from any clinical specimen should initiate an aggressive workup of the patient.

Other forms

Other miscellaneous types of zygomycosis include endocarditis, resembling other forms of fungal endocarditis, with large vegetations and emboli spreading to major vessels. Burn wound infections and traumatic wound infections are not infrequent (9, 12, 31, 55, 60, 65). Brain abscesses are a growing problem in drug addicts (34, 40, 52, 55, 85) and AIDS patients (15, 77). These infections appear to be primary to introduction of the fungi in the injection material. Osteomyelitis, unassociated with contiguous spread of rhinocerebral disease, has been seen in a patient with neutropenia and anemia who had been receiving glucosteroids (18). Another patient required amputation after injury to the tibia led to *Saksenaea vasiformis* infection (58).

Infections caused by entomophthoraceous fungi

Zygomycosis due to entomophthoraceous fungi is caused by members of two genera, *Conidiobolus* and *Basidiobolus* (Table 1). The former are involved primarily in disease of the head and face, sometimes referred to as chronic rhinofacial zygomycosis, and the latter are associated with disease of the trunk and arms. There are, however, reports of disseminated disease by *Conidiobolus* species (65, 66), so these anatomic designations probably are not appropriate.

Most cases of this form of zygomycosis have been reported from Africa, India, and other parts of Asia (43, 66), but recent cases have been reported in the United States, the Caribbean, and South America (7, 65, 66). Rhinofacial disease probably is caused by the inhalation or inoculation of the fungus and is characterized by swelling of the perinasal tissue, nose, and mouth. Symptoms are nasal stuffiness, drainage, and sinus pain. Infection begins as swelling of the inferior nasal turbinates, with extension into adjacent structures. Nodular subcutaneous masses can be palpated through the skin. As the disease progresses, generalized facial swelling occurs. Systemic signs and symptoms are usually absent (43, 65, 66).

Subcutaneous entomophthoraceous zygomycosis begins as nodular subcutaneous lesions that are firm and not painful. The trunk, arms, legs, and buttocks most often are affected (7, 43, 65, 66). Invasion of muscle and gastrointestinal involvement also has been reported (1, 7, 33). Most cases of this disease will progress slowly unless therapy is administered.

Disseminated mycoses also may occur. One case presented with cough, low-grade fever, weight loss, and a breast mass (11). The patient died of massive pulmonary hemorrhage. Autopsy findings showed fungal involvement throughout the body.

Histological findings are the same for all forms of the disease. Acute and chronic inflammatory reactions are found around the hyphae. Hyphae may be surrounded by eosinophilic material either in a stellate formation or as a simple sheath (Splendore-Hoeppli phenomenon). In contrast to disease caused by the Mucorales, the Entomophthorales do not invade blood vessels; thus, tissue infarction and necrosis are not found (66).

Pythiosis

Dating back to 1884, a disease was recognized in horses that subsequently has been called by several names, such as swamp cancer and bursatti. The disease has been observed most often in tropical areas and is chronic and progressive, with substantial morbidity. The causative agent was of uncertain taxonomic affinity but at the time was felt to most closely resemble a "lower" zygomycete. Later, the organism was considered to be a species of *Mortierella*. Investigations by Austwick and Copeland showed that the organism produced biflagellate zoospores at 25°C when incubated under special conditions, and they concluded the entity was a species of *Pythium* (2). Further detailed taxonomic studies revealed the organism to be a new species of *Pythium*, *P. insidiosum* (16). As noted previously, *Pythium* species presently are classified in the Kingdom Protoctista and therefore are not fungi. The disease is properly termed pythiosis and has remained associated with medical mycology even though it properly belongs in medical protistology.

Pythiosis recently has been documented as an authentic infectious disease of humans, and in some cases has been devastating (16, 73; Rinaldi et al., Abstr. Annu. Meet. Am. Soc. Microbiol. 1989). It is difficult to induce characteristic morphological features in laboratory isolates; special cultural conditions must be used. For this reason, it is, as always, beneficial for the clinician to give the microbiologist information regarding the patient's disease and appearance. If pythiosis is included in the differential diagnosis, the laboratorian can take steps to maximize the proper identification of *P. insidiosum*.

LABORATORY METHODS

The laboratory methods for collecting, processing, and culturing specimens are covered in chapter 58. There are, however, a few important points relative to zygomycosis that should be emphasized.

Specimen collection

As discussed throughout this chapter, most lesions of zygomycosis are abscesses and necrotic tissue. Within the abscesses, the fungus is exposed to the lytic activities of phagocytic cells and the enzymes of lysed cells. It is unlikely that these hyphal elements are viable, and one should collect the specimen for culture by curettage or other surgical procedure. Swabs should not be used for collecting specimens to detect fungi. The ideal specimen for detecting zygomycotic infection is surgically excised.

Direct microscopic examination of clinical specimens

Because zygomycosis is a serious and often rapidly fatal disease, a timely diagnosis is important for early detection and management. An early, tentative diagnosis often can be made by observing fungal elements in a well-collected clinical specimen. Scrapings of lesions in the upper turbinates, aspirated material from the sinuses, and sputum or bronchial brushings from the lungs, when examined in a 10 to 20% KOH preparation, will contain broad (10 to 15 μm), pleomorphic, nonseptate, ribbonlike hyphae (Fig. 1). Demonstrating hyphae in a clinical specimen is more indicative of disease than detecting them in a culture because of the ubiquitous nature of the Zygomycetes. There are numerous methods for staining fungal elements in clinical specimens. The Calcofluor white stain commonly is used in wet preparations and requires no more time or effort than the KOH preparation. The Calcofluor stains the fungal elements bright yellow-green when the appropriate filters are used. Other stains such as periodic acid-Schiff, Giemsa, and Wright stains may be used, but they require more time for preparation. More information about these stains may be found in chapters 120 and 122. A word of caution: the Gram stain is not a good stain for demonstrating fungi in clinical specimens, especially if heat fixation is used.

Culture

A listing of media for isolating fungi can be found in chapter 121. Most of the etiologic agents of zygomycosis grow in 24 to 48 h on most enriched laboratory media when incubated at 30°C. Many of these fungi do not grow on media containing cycloheximide; therefore, at least 1 U of enriched medium not containing cycloheximide should be used in a routine battery of mycological media. It also should be noted that most of these fungi grow on nonselective bacteriological media. Thus, these fungi may be isolated in the bacteriology laboratory as well as the mycology laboratory. Often it is not appreciated that grinding or macerating of tissue to be cultured for zygomycetous fungi results in their destruction. Hence, specimens submitted for recovery of this group of moulds never should be ground or mashed before plating; rather, intact blocks of material should be aseptically cut away from the main specimen and

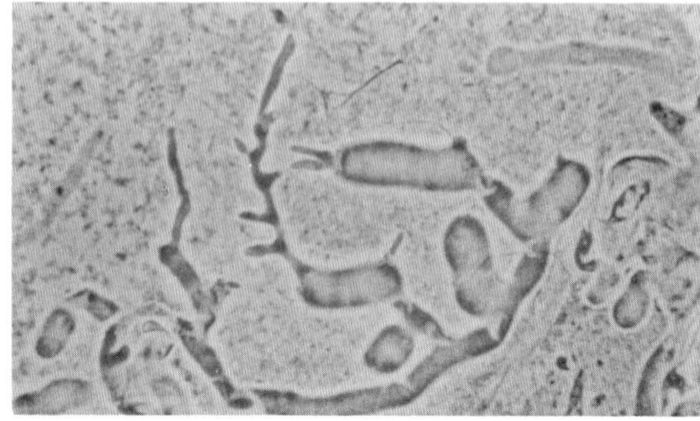

FIG. 1. Wet preparation of scrapings from an oral lesion of a patient with rhinocerebral zygomycosis. Note broad, ribbonlike pleomorphic hyphae. Phase microscopy, ×400.

plated in toto. Another helpful aid in the isolation of Zygomycetes from clinical materials is the use of "bread baiting." One simply scatters small pieces of fresh bread over the surface of the plate and inoculates the intact blocks of specimen thereon.

Histopathology

The main histopathologic feature of zygomycosis is necrosis with acute and chronic infiltrates. Blood vessels at the infected site may be surrounded by hyphae, with walls invaded and the vessel occluded. The organism appears as ribbonlike, filamentous, nonseptate hyphae, 10 to 25 μm in diameter (Fig. 2). Branching is irregular, and branches usually arise at right angles. Staining reactions by the various tissue stains are variable. The hyphae sometimes do not stain well by the Gomori methenamine silver stain but generally stain better by this method than by the hematoxylin-and-eosin or the periodic acid-Schiff stain.

The histologic pattern of entomophthoromycosis is one of a chronic inflammatory process and many small abscesses surrounded by epithelioid and giant cells. Fungal elements often are surrounded by an eosinophilic sleeve or halo (Splendore-Hoeppli phenomenon) (13, 65, 66).

Serology

Serological tests are being developed for zygomycosis, but commercial serological reagents currently are not available for these diseases. Some research centers, e.g., the Division of Bacterial and Mycotic Diseases, Center for Infectious Diseases, Centers for Disease Control, Atlanta, Ga., have accomplished promising work in the serological diagnosis of zygomycosis and in identification of some of its agents (30, 35, 35a, 40).

CULTURAL AND MICROSCOPIC CHARACTERISTICS

For identification of pathogenic genera and species (11, 16, 19, 21, 23, 25, 26, 28, 53, 59, 64, 66, 74–76), all descriptions provided below are based on growth on media and conditions designated in the aforementioned references (mainly malt extract agar in standard petri dishes). If more than one species is described in a genus, generic characteristics are noted as well.

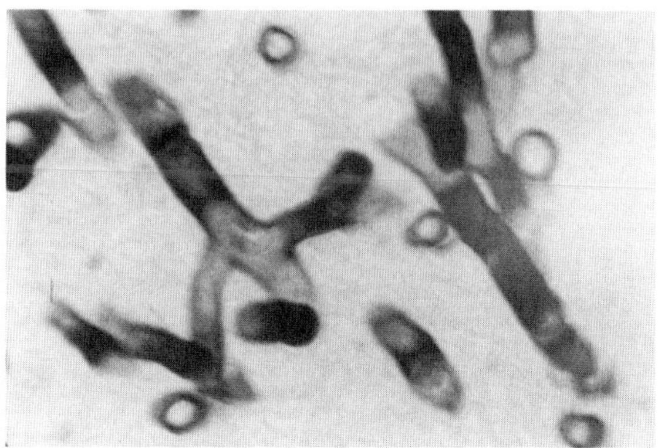

FIG. 2. Lung tissue from a case of disseminated zygomycosis. Note broad, nonseptate hyphae with branches at right angles. Gomori methenamine silver stain, ×400.

Absidia corymbifera (Cohn) Saccardo et Trotter (incorrect, older name *Absidia ramosa*)

A. corymbifera is a very rapidly growing zygomycete that may cover the surface of a petri dish in 24 h at 37°C. Colonies are initially white and then become pale gray. Microscopically, *A. corymbifera* produces internodal (i.e., produced between rhizoids, as contrasted to nodal, or produced directly across from rhizoids), light gray, abundantly branching long sporangiophores that are up to 450 μm in length and 4 to 8 μm in diameter; they often are arranged in whorls. Rhizoids (rootlike hyphae extending into the substrate) are sparingly produced, 12 μm in diameter and up to 370 μm in length, and hyaline. Numerous smaller and irregularly shaped sporangiophores also may be produced. The sporangiophores branch repeatedly to form corymbs (arranged in clusters; hence the species epithet name). Sporangia (usually round or pear-shaped saclike fruiting structures in which are produced asexual sporangiospores) are small, 20 to 35 μm in diameter, hyaline to gray, and pyriform (pear shaped) with almost conical columellae (a columella is the swollen tip of a sporangiophore projecting into the sporangium), 16 to 27 μm in diameter and also pyriform, possessing distinctive apophyses (an apophysis is a swelling at the end of a sporangiophore below the sporangium) that are not bell or funnel shaped and often have a short projection at the top. Sporangiophores are never thickened or darkened at the apex. Sporangiospores (asexual propagules produced within sporangia) are ellipsoid and are 2 to 3.5 by 3 to 4.5 μm in size. This species is thermophilic and can grow at 45°C; some strains can grow at 50°C (53, 59).

Apophysomyces elegans Misra, Srivastava et Lata

Apophysomyces elegans resembles *Absidia corymbifera* in producing pyriform, apophysate sporangia borne at the tips of sporangiophores that arise from stolons not always opposite rhizoids. It also has much more pronounced funnel- or bell-shaped apophyses. The sporangiophores are always darkened and thickened at the apex. Colonies are rapid growing at first and remain low and near the agar surface. As they mature, they form flocculent aerial mycelium filling the petri dish within 7 days. Colonies initially are white, becoming brownish gray with the reverse pale yellow. Aerial hyphae are branched, hyaline, smooth, generally aseptate and 3.4 to 8.0 μm in diameter. Sporangiophores are formed slowly, generally arise singly, and develop at right angles from aerial hyphal branches. A segment of the hyphal branch at the place of origin of sporangiophore generally becomes delimited by two septa, and the segment then becomes slightly thick walled and light grayish brown. After forming a lateral sporangiophore, the hyphal branch proceeds to form a second sporangiophore and terminates the branch after some further growth. Sporangiophores are straight or curved, slightly tapered toward the apex, unbranched, light grayish brown, often darker near the base, up to 532 μm long, and 3.4 to 5.7 μm wide near the base, gradually tapering to a width of 2.3 to 3.4 μm just below the apophyses. The wall is thick, smooth, and occasionally slightly darker and thicker toward the inside at a point about 4 to 18 μm below the apophyses. Sporangia are produced terminally and singly on the sporangiophores and are pyriform, multispored, distinctly apophysate, columellate, white at first, light yellowish brown by reflected light when mature, and 20 to 58 μm in diameter. The sporangial wall is transparent, thin, smooth, and deliquescent, leaving a small collar at the base of the columella. Apophyses are conspicuous, funnel shaped or bell shaped, 10 to 46 μm high and 11 to 40 μm in diameter at the widest part. The wall of the apophyses is smooth, light grayish brown, and slightly thicker than the columella walls. Columellae are hemispherical, thin walled, subhyaline to light grayish brown, and 18 to 28 μm in diameter. Sporangiospores are mostly oblong, occasionally subglobose, very light brown in mass, subhyaline individually, thin walled, smooth, and 5.4 to 8.0 by 4.0 to 5.7 μm in size (Fig. 3). Zygospores are not seen.

The manner of development of the *Apophysomyces* sporangiophores is reminiscent of that described below for *Saksenaea vasiformis*. The sporangium-forming hypha from its end produces a rhizoidal complex, some of which is submerged in agar; an erect sporangiophore develops in the opposite direction. However, the similarity stops there, as the sporangial morphology is entirely different for the two species.

This zygomycete does not sporulate well under routine laboratory conditions. The same holds true for the zygomycete *S. vasiformis* (see below). Fortunately, a simple technique has been developed that induces consistent sporulation in both species (54; Table 2). The method consists of growing isolates on Sabouraud dextrose agar, aseptically cutting out blocks of agar permeated with mycelia, transferring the blocks to a petri plate containing 2.0 ml of sterile, distilled water supplemented with 0.2 ml of 10% filter-sterilized yeast extract medium, and incubating the blocks at 37°C. In addition, exoantigen tests have been developed for the rapid and specific identification of *A. elegans* and *S. vasiformis* (41).

Mucor species

Typically, *Mucor* species grow rapidly, forming sphere-shaped columellae, which, unlike *Absidia* columellae, are borne entirely within the sporangial wall and which collapse irregularly if at all. Sporangiophores are solitary, simple or branched, and globose. Sporangia that deliquesce at maturity are characteristic. In contrast to *Rhizopus* species, rhizoids and stolons are absent. The spores of *Mucor* species are mucus bound. *Mucor* species are the least common etiologic agents of human zygomycosis.

***Mucor circinelloides* form *circinelloides* van Tieghem (Schipper).** We accept the taxonomic treatment of Schipper (74) in which several forms (i.e., shapes) of the species *M. circinelloides* are described. The only instance of human disease incited by this species is the case noted previously caused by *M. circinelloides* form *circinelloides*. Colonies often spread across the entire petri dish, but growth is relatively low and sparse, appearing pale gray or yellowish. Coloration appears more brown at 37°C than at 25°C. Sporangiophores are borne from aerial hyphae and often are branched and formed sympodially (in a zigzag pattern). Sporangia are spherical, 25 to 30 μm in diameter, and sometimes up to 80 μm in size. Columellae are roughly spherical and are

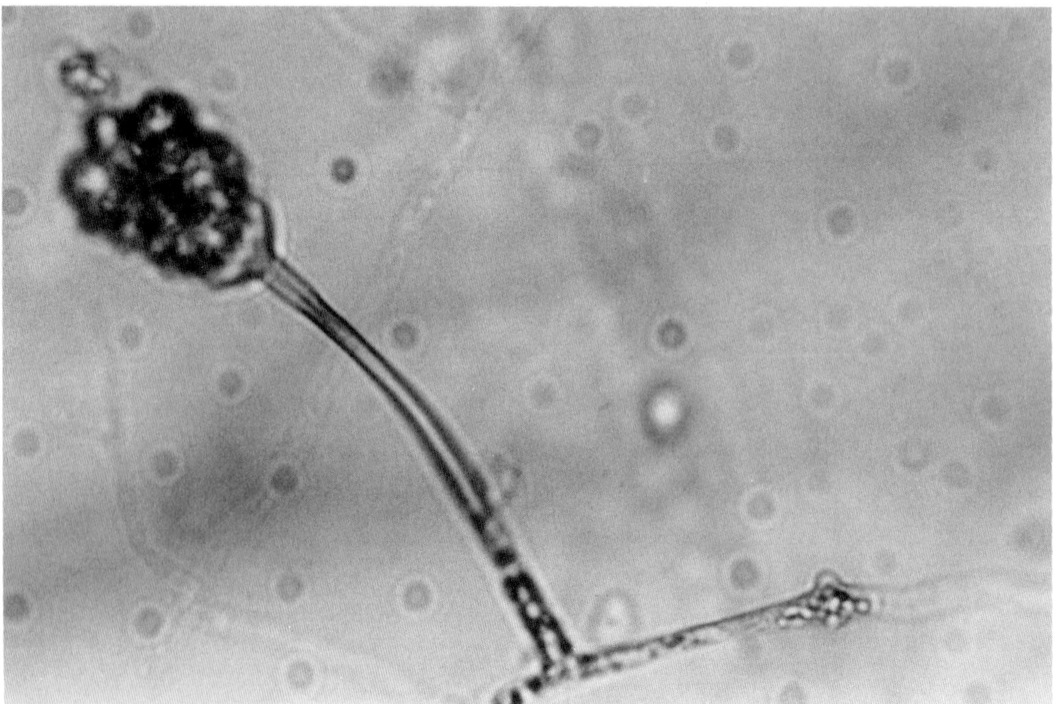

FIG. 3. *Apophysomyces elegans*: 12 days, 10% yeast extract in water, 37°C. Note sporangiophore, apophysate sporangium, and subglobose sporangiospores. Water mount, ×400.

TABLE 2. Method of inducing sporulation by *Apophysomyces elegans* and *Saksenaea vasiformis*[a]

Sporulation medium:	1. 20 ml of sterile, distilled water 2. 10% yeast extract solution (filter sterilized and stored at 4°C before use)
Procedure:	1. Inoculate isolate onto Sabouraud dextrose agar; incubate the specimen at 37°C for 4–5 days. 2. Using aseptic technique, cut out 1-cm² agar blocks permeated with hyphal growth. 3. Transfer two blocks to a petri dish containing 20 ml of sterile, distilled water. 4. Add 3 drops (0.2 ml) of the filter-sterilized 10% yeast extract solution to the dish. 5. Incubate the dish at 37°C in the dark. 6. Examine the dish daily, commencing at 5 days (fungal growth will be a thin film over the surface of the water) and for up to 13 days. 7. Optimal or characteristic sporulation likely will be observed after 10–12 days of incubation.

[a] From references 68 and 71.

up to 50 μm in diameter. Sporangiospores are hyaline, ellipsoidal, 4.5 to 7 μm in length, and smooth walled. Formation of chlamydoconidia is not common, but when seen they are spherical, cylindrical or irregular, and up to 15 μm in diameter. Zygospores are not formed in pure culture (Fig. 4).

***Mucor hiemalis* Wehmer.** Colonies often fill an entire petri dish; growth is relatively sparse and grayish with a pale reverse. Sporangiophores generally are unbranched and are less commonly sympodially branched; sporangia are up to 60 μm in diameter; columellae are ellipsoidal, 15 to 30 μm in diameter; sporangiospores are hyaline, narrowly to broadly ellipsoidal or reniform (kidney shaped), 5 to 11 μm long, and smooth walled. Chlamydoconidia are uncommon, spherical to cylindrical or irregular, and up to 15 μm in diameter. Zygospores are not formed in pure culture.

M. hiemalis is similar to *M. circinelloides* but produces larger sporangiospores, which are sometimes reniform, and usually has unbranched sporangiophores. Of most note, however, is the inability of *M. hiemalis* to grow at 37°C, which raises doubt as to its validity as a human pathogen, at least as an invader of deep tissue. Its pathogenic role may be limited to cutaneous infections.

***Mucor racemosus* Fresenius.** Colonies spread across the petri dish and are low to moderately raised. Mycelium is colorless, with overall color light to mid-brown due to sporangia and chlamydoconidia. Sporangiophores are borne from surface or aerial mycelium and are branched sympodially or irregularly. Sporangia are up to 80 μm in diameter and light brown, with encrusted walls. Columellae are ellipsoidal to pyriform and are up to 40 μm long. Sporangiospores are hyaline to pale brown, broadly ellipsoidal to subspheroidal, commonly 5 to 8 μm in diameter, and smooth walled. Chlamydoconidia and arthroconidia are formed abundantly and are 5 to 20 μm in diameter or have a long axis. Zygospores are not formed in pure culture. The maximum growth temperature for this species appears to be 35°C; poor growth is obtained at 37°C, which again raises the question of authenticity of this species as a pathogen in deep, invasive zygomycosis.

***Mucor ramosissimus* Samutsevitsch.** The colony is rapid growing and cinnamon buff to olive gray in color; the reverse is grayish and slightly yellow at the point of inoculation. Sporangiophores are up to 17 μm in diameter, always arise from substrate mycelium, and become progressively smaller in diameter upwards, sometimes ending in a sterile filament. They are colorless to faintly colored, with septa. Sporangiospores typically are roughened and erect and branch regularly in a sympodial fashion, with as many as 11 fertile branches; first branches bear the larger sporangia, which are 15 to 33 μm in length and are somewhat constricted below the sporangia. Each successive branch is shorter and smaller in diameter, with swollen and racket-shaped regions located especially toward the top of sporangiophores and often successively above one another. Sporangia are 15 to 70 μm in diameter and few to many spored; smaller sporangia lack columellae. Sporangia at first appear white in transmitted light and then olive gray; they are globose to dorsiventrally flattened, especially in larger sporangia. Some larger sporangial walls are deliquescent, but the great majority have extremely persistent walls that remain in one or two pieces when crushed; they are roughened, encrusted, and transparent. Columellae are 20 to 37 μm in diameter and 17 to 30 μm in length, applanate (flattened) to almost globose, smooth, hyaline, and empty, with collars. Sporangiospores are 3.3 to 5.5 by 3.5 to 8 μm, irregularly ovoid to globose, somewhat variable in size, smooth, thin walled, singly hyaline, and brownish in mass, with contents uniform. Chlamydoconidia are not seen, but specialized cells called oidia often are formed; they are 6.5 to 13 μm in diameter, terminal in chains or intercalary, hyaline with dense cytoplasm, thick walled, and compressed to globose to elongate, arising at the ends of hyphae or arising along the side of substrate hyphae. Zygospores are not seen. Colonial spread is restricted, and the species grows well at 37°C.

Characteristics of *M. ramosissimus* that aid in species-level identification are extremely low colonies on all media; tough, persistent sporangial walls; many sporangia devoid of columellae and thus resembling the condition in sporangia of *Mortierella* species; short sporangiophores that repeatedly branch sympodially as many as 12 times; and the occurrence of racket-shaped enlargements in the sporangiophores (23).

***Mucor rouxianus* (Calmette) Wehmer.** Colonial turf is low, at most 4 mm high, white, yellow or gray, delicate, and loose. Large, thick-walled, irregular cells may be formed in submerged mycelium. Sporangiophores are weakly sympodially branched. Sporangia are bright yellow or golden brown, usually 50 (20 to 100) μm in diameter, with columellae up to 40 μm high, globose or flattened, and often with a colored membrane. Sporangiospores are oval and 4 to 5 μm long. Chlamydoconidia are black, numerous, located on aerial hyphae, variably sized, and up to 100 μm in diameter. On submerged hyphae, budding yeastlike cells may appear. Zygospores are not present. Abundant fat globules may develop in the mycelium when the organism is grown on starchy substrates. The globules are deep yellow in color. Optimum growth temperature is approximately 37°C, with a temperature range of 9 to 45°C.

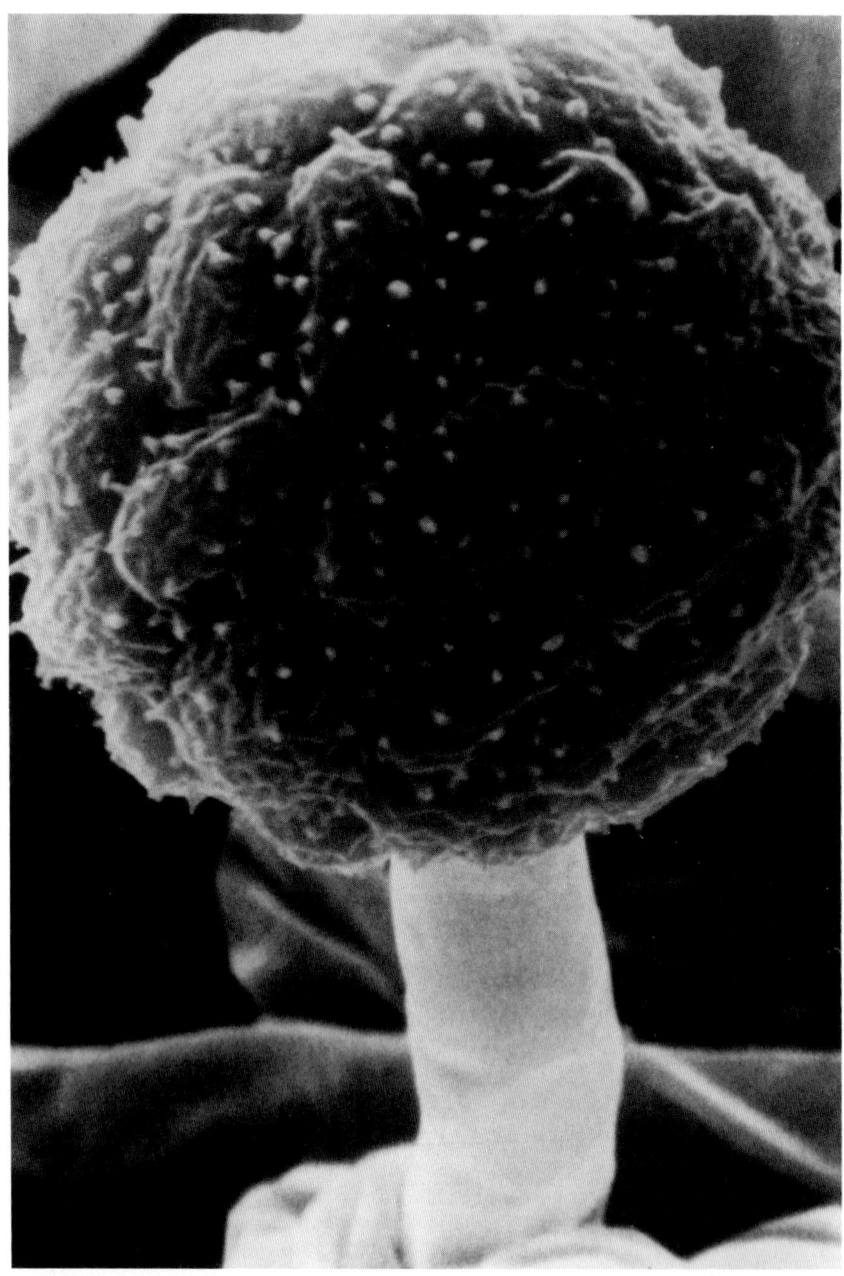

FIG. 4. *Mucor circinelloides* form *circinelloides*: 5 days on potato flakes agar, 30°C. Electron micrograph of sporangiophore. Note intact sporangium exhibiting small, knobby protuberances and containing sporangiospores. ×950.

Rhizomucor species

Rhizomucor species formerly were considered species of *Mucor* but currently are distinguished by the production of stolons and their thermophilic nature.

***Rhizomucor miehei* (Cooney et Emerson) Schipper.** *R. miehei* is similar in most respects to *R. pusillus* (see below), but spiny-walled sporangia, up to 50 to 60 μm in diameter, with columellae rarely larger than 30 μm in diameter serve to render it a separate species.

***Rhizomucor pusillus* (Lindt) Schipper.** Colonies are up to 25 to 35 mm in diameter and colorless to white, with floccose mycelium surmounted by brown sporangia. At 37°C, colonies are more dense and are brown to dark gray. This species of *Rhizomucor* is a true thermophile with the ability to grow at temperatures as high as 60°C. Sporangiophores are borne from surface hyphae and sometimes are unbranched, but they usually are extensively and irregularly branched. Poorly formed rhizoids may be present but not adjacent to the sporangiophore base (note the distinction with *Rhizopus* species; see below). Sporangia are spherical, brown or gray, and 40 to 60 (or to 80) μm in diameter. Columellae are spherical, ellipsoidal, or pyriform, and 20 to 45 μm in diameter, sometimes collapsing irregularly (note similarity to *Mucor* species); sporangiospores are hyaline, spherical to broadly ellipsoidal, 3 to 4 μm in diameter, and smooth walled. Zygospores occasionally may be produced by some isolates. They are black, broadly ellipsoidal, and 60 to 70 μm in diameter.

Rhizopus species

Rhizopus species are among the most well known fungi in biology. Coarse, rampant growth and rapidly maturing spores are characteristic of *Rhizopus* species. *Rhizopus* is distinguished from other genera in the order Mucorales by the formation of rhizoids which are conspicuous at the base of the sporangiophores, by columellae which often collapse into umbrella shapes with age, and by dry sporangiospores with striate walls (Fig. 5).

***Rhizopus arrhizus* Fisher (synonym *R. oryzae*;** *R. oryzae* is considered by many investigators as a separate species and by still others as the correct name of the fungus, with *R. arrhizus* being the synonym [75]). Colonies spread across the entire petri dish but are rather low and sparse, with fine, gray mycelium, small black-gray sporangia, and a pale reverse. Sporangiophores are borne in clusters of one to three across from rhizoids and are usually unbranched, with spherical sporangia up to 150 μm in diameter, white at first and then becoming grayish black at maturity. Columellae usually are spherical, are up to 100 μm in diameter and pale brown, and in age collapse downward to form umbrella shapes. Sporangiospores are brown, variably shaped, ellipsoidal to broadly fusiform or irregularly angular, and commonly 5 to 8 μm long, with striate (striped) walls. This species is the most common agent of human zygomycosis.

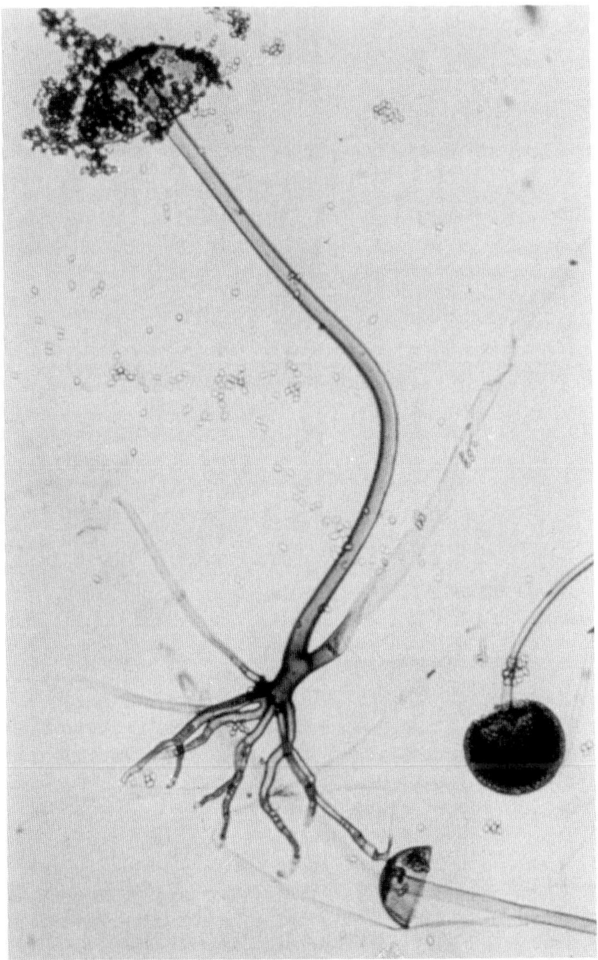

FIG. 5. *Rhizopus* species: 4 days on potato flakes agar, 30°C. Note rhizoids, sporangiophores, dark sporangia, sporangiospores, and collapsed columellae. ×304.

***Rhizopus microsporus* van Tieghem variety *microsporus* (Schipper et Stalpers) (synonym *R. microsporus*).** We accept the taxonomic treatment of Schipper and Stalpers (75). Colonies are pale brownish gray. Rhizoids are simple. Sporangiophores are produced on stolons up to 400 μm long and 10 μm wide but mostly are smaller, brownish, and often in pairs. Sporangia are grayish black, appear powdery, and are up to 80 μm in diameter. Columellae are subglobose to globose to conical and mouse gray in color, with indefinite apophyses. Sporangiospores are angular to broadly ellipsoidal to lemon shaped, up to 6.5 to 7.5 μm in length, homogeneous, and distinctly striate. Good growth occurs at 46°C, with no growth at 50°C.

***Rhizopus microsporus* van Tieghem variety *oligosporus* (Saito) Schipper et Stalpers (synonym *R. oligosporus*).** Colonies are pale yellowish brown to gray. Rhizoids are simple and subhyaline. Sporangiophores are produced on stolons and are up to 300 μm in length, 15 μm wide, brownish, and in groups of one to three. Sporangia are black and up to 80 to 100 μm but are predominantly 50 to 60 μm in diameter. Columellae are subglobose to globose to subglobose-conical and are mouse gray in color. Sporangiospores are subglobose to globose, up to 9 μm in diameter, and heterogeneous; larger spores are irregular. Zygospores are unknown. Restricted growth occurs at 45°C; good growth and sporulation occur at 40°C.

***Rhizopus microsporus* van Tieghem variety *rhizopodiformis* (Cohn) Schipper et Stalpers (synonyms *R. cohnii, R. rhizopodiformis*).** Colonies are dark grayish brown; rhizoids are simple. Sporangiophores are produced on stolons up to 500 μm in length and are 8 μm in width and brownish, with one to four produced together. Sporangia are bluish to grayish black, powdery in appearance, and up to 100 μm in diameter. Larger columellae are pyriform and mouse gray in color (columella/sporangia ratio, 4/5). Sporangiospores are subglobose to globose, up to 5 to 6 μm in diameter, homogeneous, and minutely spinulose (spiny) (Fig. 6).

Cunninghamella bertholletiae Stadel

Colonies are extremely floccose and whitish, becoming gray as spores develop; the reverse is off-white. Hyphae are broad, sparsely septate with rhizoids, with conspicuous, abundant oil globules. They are erect, usually branched (dichotomous, verticillate, or bizarre). Sporangiophores are up to 16 μm in diameter and terminate in fertile, typically globose vesicles that are up to 40.5 μm in diameter. The vesicles bear unispored pedicillate (stalked) sporangiola (small sporangia without columellae, generally having a small number of spores) that are mostly smooth, spherical, and 6 to 13 μm in diameter. They also may be subglobose, broadly ellipsoidal and ellipsoidal, and 6.5 to 15.5 by 7.8 to 20 μm in size; they are felt by some investigators to rep-

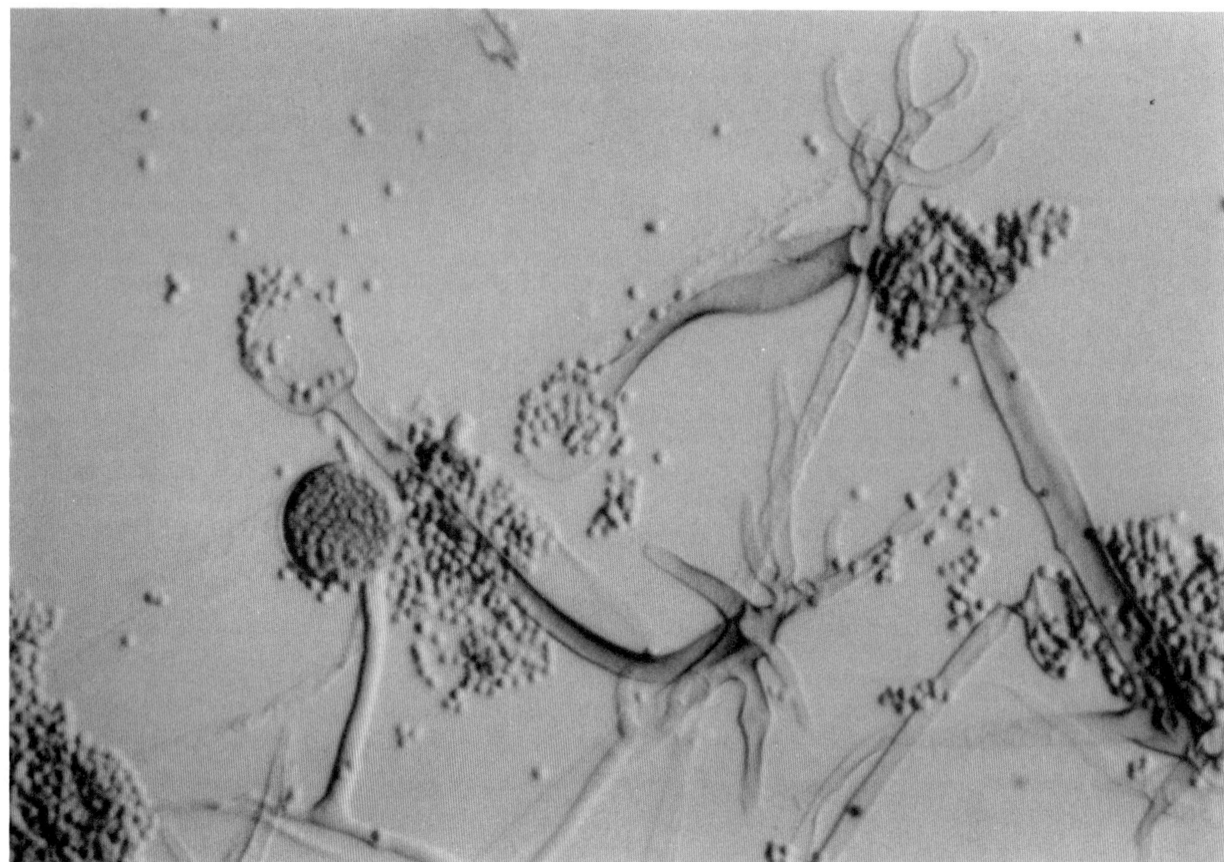

FIG. 6. *Rhizopus microsporus* var. *rhizopodiformis*: 4 days on potato flakes agar, 30°C. Note rhizoids, stolons, sporangiophores, columellae, sporangia, and globose sporangiospores. Nomarski differential interference microscopy, ×400.

resent conidia. Zygospores may be formed when compatible mating types are crossed. The appearance of whorled branches, originating on the primary sporangiophore, at a variable distance from the terminal vesicle and terminating in smaller vesicles bearing sporangiola, is typical of *Cunninghamella* species, including *C. bertholletiae* (Fig. 7).

Mortierella wolfii Mehrotra et Baijal

Although it is an authentic pathogen of animals involved particularly in bovine abortion, the role of *M. wolfii* as a human pathogen is less certain. Colonial growth is white, fine, and cottony; often there is an associated garliclike odor. Colonies frequently demonstrate the appearance of rosettes of overlapping lobes. Hyphae are distinctively uneven, with production of numerous chlamydoconidia. Sporangiophores arise from rhizoids on substrate hyphae and taper from 10 to 20 μm at the base to 3 to 5 μm at the tip. Sporangiophores are delicate and may be simple or branched. Sporangia are globose, lack columellae, are 15 to 48 μm in diameter, and rapidly deliquesce, leaving a large collarette. Sporangiospores are small, 2 by 2 to 4 μm, and cylindrical to kidney shaped with a double wall. Small, one-celled conidia called stylospores also may develop. This zygomycetous species grows well at 40°C. Often it is difficult to induce sporulation in *M. wolfii* in vitro. Seviour et al. have described a medium, silage extract agar, that facilitates characteristic sporulation of numerous authentic and suspected isolates of *M.*

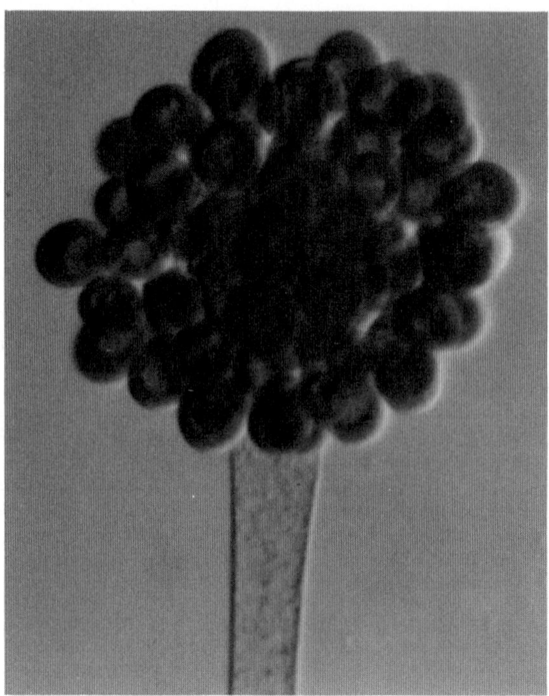

FIG. 7. *Cunninghamella bertholletiae*: 4 days on potato flakes agar, 30°C. Note sporangiophore, globose vesicle, and pedicillate sporangiola. ×400.

wolfii recovered from bovine abortion and pneumonia cases (76). The key ingredient is filtered silage, resulting in an extract solidified with 2% (wt/vol) agar at pH 4.5 to 4.7. For *M. wolfii*, as with many fungi, conditions that are optimal for vegetative growth are not good for sporulation induction and vice versa.

Saksenaea vasiformis Saksena

The genus *Saksenaea* is monotypic (contains only one species, *S. vasiformis*), and unless the sporulation induction method outlined in Table 2 is used, this rapidly growing zygomycete will produce only broad, aseptate to sparsely septate, branched, hyaline hyphae. When induced by the 10% yeast extract method, however (54), very characteristic sporangia are produced. Rhizoids are dichotomously branched, are 3.2 to 4.8 μm in size, and are broad and stalked; sporangiophores are 6.4 to 9.6 by 24 to 64 μm long. Sporangia are flask shaped with a spherical venter (the swollen, hollow portion at the midpoint of the flask-shaped sporangium) and are 16 to 43.2 by 22.4 to 51.2 μm in size, with distinct dome-shaped columellae. The venter is surmounted by a long neck, 6.4 to 11.2 by 54.4 to 200 μm, with the apex of the neck slightly broader, 8 to 14.4 μm in diameter, and is closed by a mucilaginous plug. Sporangiospores are oblong to rectangular, 1.4 to 2.1 by 2.8 to 4.2 μm, and one celled and are released through an opening in the sporangial apex. Zygospores are unknown. Maximum growth temperature is 44°C.

Syncephalastrum racemosum Cohn ex Schröter

Syncephalastrum is another monotypic genus. *S. racemosum* produces colonies that are rapidly growing and cover the entire petri dish with sparse to moderately dense, sometimes very dense, mid- to deep-gray mycelium, with the reverse pale or yellowish brown. Sporangiophores are borne from aerial hyphae and are long and branched or produced as short side branches from fertile hyphae. Sporangial heads are 30 to 80 μm in diameter, with sporangiospores formed linearly within cylindrical sacs called merosporangia borne on spicules around the columella. The columellae are spherical or nearly so, 10 to 50 μm in diameter, and brown, with smooth walls except at the points of attachment of merosporangia; they usually collapse irregularly. Sporangiospores adhere in chains of up to 10 and become brown, irregular in size and shape, spherical to cylindrical, 3 to 5 (up to 10) μm in diameter, or long and smooth walled. The fingerlike tubular merosporangia each contain a single row of sporangiospores that are characteristic for this species. Septa often are formed in sporangiophores as merosporangia mature. The maximum growth temperature is 40°C. *S. racemosum* appears to be a rare agent of human disease (Fig. 8).

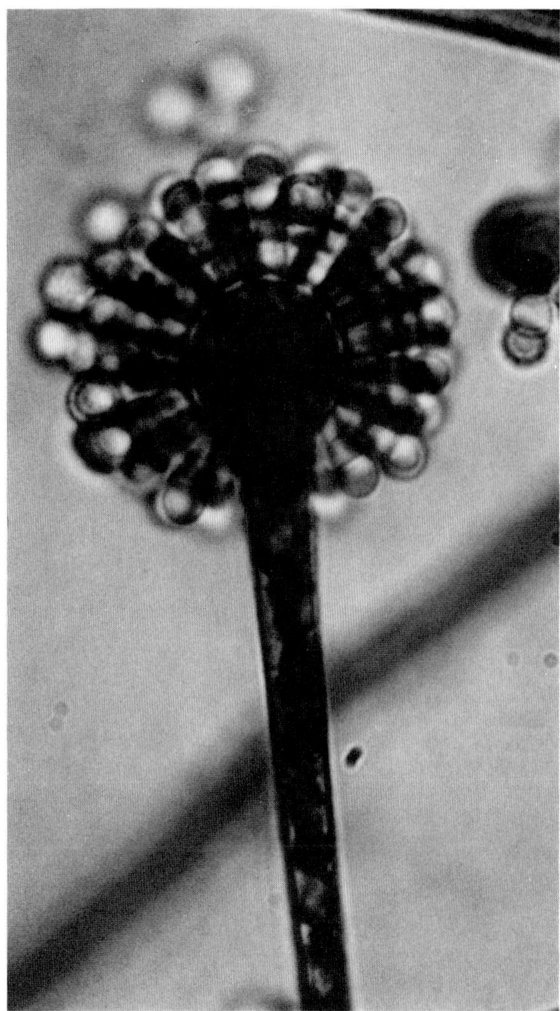

FIG. 8. *Syncephalastrum racemosum*: 4 days on potato flakes agar, 30°C. Note coenocytic hyphae, sporangiophore, columella, and merosporangia with linear chains of sporangiospores. ×400.

Cokeromyces recurvatus Poitras

Although the pathogenicity of *C. recurvatus* remains to be resolved, its implication in two cases of human genitourinary mycotic disease merits notice (3, 45). This organism (as well as some isolates of *Mucor* species; 4, 5) displays dimorphism in that it can grow under certain environmental conditions in a yeastlike form. Others have noted colonization of the genitourinary tract by dimorphic zygomycetous fungi (G. D. Roberts, personal communication to K. J. Kwon-Chung, cited in reference 3; 14, 66). *C. recurvatus* also has a distinctive appearance of its mould-form asexual fruiting structures, and it readily produces zygospores in culture; it is homothallic (i.e., requires only one thallus for production of sexual spores).

In host tissue and in culture at 35°C on enriched medium, such as brain heart infusion agar with 5% sheep erythrocytes incubated in 5 to 7% carbon dioxide, *C. recurvatus* grows after 2 days as a tan, flat, slightly wrinkled, tenacious colony, 3 to 5 mm in diameter. Microscopically, in culture and in clinical specimens, the organism appears as thin-walled yeast cells, some of which may demonstrate multipolar budding, resembling the parasitic form of *Paracoccidioides brasiliensis*. In culture at 25°C on potato flakes agar (64), colonies attain diameters of 15 to 20 mm after 5 days of incubation, are tan, and are radially wrinkled with gray central areas due to sporangiospore production. Mature colonies turn brown with production of zygospores in 10 days. Hyphae are sparsely septate, 5 to 15 μm in diameter. Sporangiophores arise from vegetative hyphae and are 100 to 500 µm in length and 9 µm wide. Terminal vesicles are formed at apices of sporangiophores and are 12.6 to 31.5 µm in diameter. Sporangiole stalks recurve and twist when mature; walls are thicker and darker than that of the vesicles and are 60 to 120 µm long by 2.2 µm wide. Sporangiola are globose, are 8.4 to 12.6 µm in diameter, and contain 12 to 20 sporangiospores when mature. Sporangiospores are smooth walled, variably sized, and 2.5 by 4.5 µm in diameter; they lack striations and are usually ovoid to ellipsoidal but may be variably shaped (Fig. 9). Zygospores produced in abundance between copulating branches arise from superficial hyphae, outgrowths from sporangiophores, or suspensors of mature zygospores. Zygospores are 33.5 to 54.5 µm in diameter. When mature, they are brown, globose and rough walled as a result of sharply pointed projections; they are homothallic (Fig. 10).

Conidiobolus species

The only mycologically authenticated human pathogens, *Conidiobolus coronatus* and *C. incongruus*, recently have undergone taxonomic change and now are classified in the family Ancylistaceae (25, 26). Mycelium is inconspicuous when young and sparse to luxuriant when mature. It is often infrequently septate, with aerial mycelium nonexistent to abundant. Vegetative growth always occurs as walled cells, often forming variably shaped hyphal bodies by pinching off or dissociation of intercalary cells devoid of cytoplasm. It grows readily on nutritionally simple media but cannot utilize nitrate or nitrite. Conidiophores are simple or (rarely) branched dichotomously and are positively phototrophic. Conidiogenous cells usually are undistinguished in diameter or appearance from vegetative hyphae (but occasionally clavate or distinctly thicker than vegetative hyphae) and have a basal septum that produces apical conidia. Primary conidia are unitunicate (i.e., the outer wall layer does not separate from the conidial surface) and pyriform to obovoid or globose; papillae are rounded to apiculate and are forcibly discharged toward a light source by papillar eversion against the conidiogenous cell. Secondary conidia usually have the shape of primary conidia but are smaller. They are formed singly on short secondary conidiophores and are forcibly discharged toward a light source by papillar eversion. Secondary conidia also may be ovoid to cylindrical capilloconidia that are dispersed passively from apices of capillary secondary conidiophores. These may be produced singly from a primary conidium or as three or more small, forcibly discharged microconidia on spikelike projections (villae). Species capable of forming capilloconidia or microconidia also produce single, forcibly discharged secondary conidia. Capilloconidia or microconidia never are formed by the same species. Rhizoids usually are absent. If rhizoids are present, they are thicker than conidiophores, occur singly, and terminate in a platelike holdfast. Resting spores are globose, with two thickened wall layers; they are colorless to cream, yellowish, or amber in mass. Zygospores are produced inside a layer of two (sometimes inconspicuous) conjugating cells and remain in the axis of these cells or only slightly displaced laterally at maturity (but not budded laterally through a narrow isthmus). They germinate to produce a germ conidiophore and germ conidium or limited germ mycelium with several germ conidiophores. Germ conidia resemble primary conidia and are forcibly discharged by papillar eversion. Other resting spore types include chlamydoconidia (usually irregular in shape, with a single thickened wall layer) or villose conidia (produced by decoration of the primary conidial wall with numerous short to long, hairlike appendages).

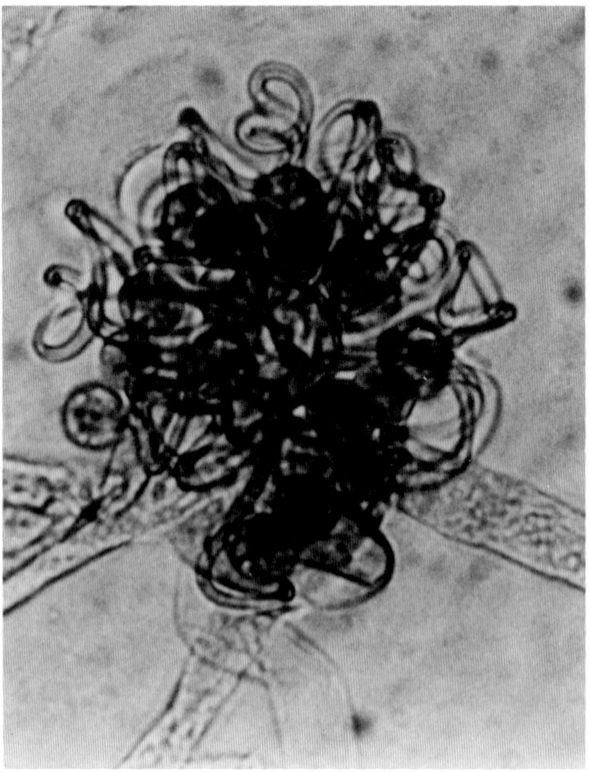

FIG. 9. *Cokeromyces recurvatus*: 4 days on potato flakes agar, 30°C. Note hyphae, sporangiophore with terminal vesicle presenting with twisting and recurving sporangiolar stalks, and sporangiola containing globose, smooth-walled sporangiospores. ×400.

Conidiobolus coronatus **(Constantin) Batko (synonym *Entomophthora coronata*).** Colonies grow rapidly, are glabrous and adherent initially, and then develop furrowing and folding, particularly at 37°C. With time, colonies become covered with short, white aerial mycelium and conidiophores. Conidia are forcibly discharged from the conidiophores and may adhere to the lid of the culture dish or tube. Colony color becomes tannish to light brown with age. Short, erect unbranched conidiophores produce single-celled, large conidia, 25 to 45 µm in diameter. The conidia are ejected and travel distances up to 30 mm. These conidia may germinate to produce one or more hyphal germ tubes. The conidia have prominent papillae on the walls that give rise to secondary conidia. Several papillae and conidia may be produced, giving the original conidium a corona of secondary conidia (hence the species epithet name). A conidium also may produce multiple, short, hairlike appendages called villae that characterize this particular species of *Conidiobolus*. Conidia falling on glass or plastic will produce a short conidiophore and

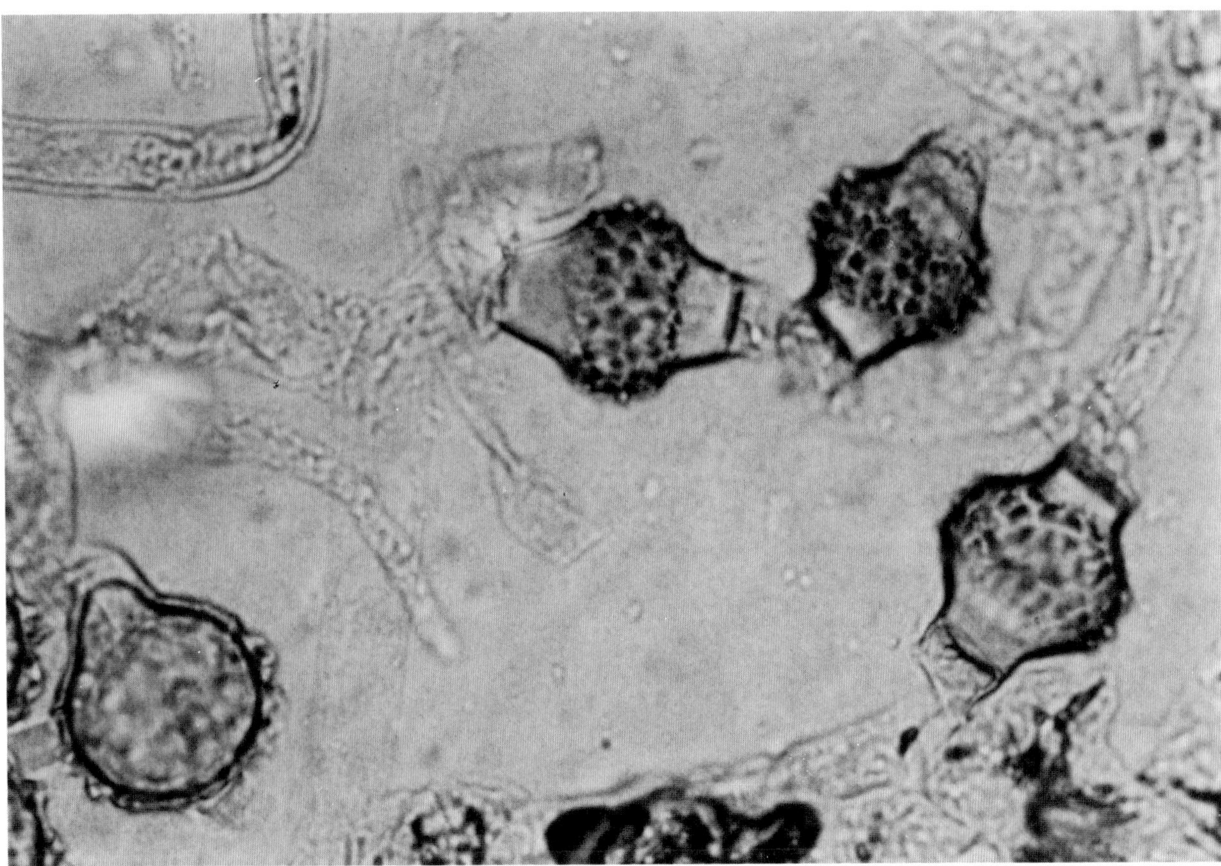

FIG. 10. *Cokeromyces recurvatus*: 12 days on potato flakes agar, 30°C. Note rough-walled, brown zygospores and suspensors. ×400.

eject another conidium. This conidium will, in turn, germinate to produce another conidium, and this process repeats itself until stored nutrients are exhausted. Chlamydoconidia may be formed abundantly and submerged in the growth medium. Zygospores are rare.

Conidiobolus incongruus **Drechsler.** *C. incongruus* is very similar to *C. coronatus* and also produces multiplicative conidia with papillae, but the villose corona characteristic of *C. coronatus* is not produced.

Basidiobolus ranarum Eidam (synonyms *B. haptosporus, B. meristosporus, B. heterosporus*)

Rapid growth occurs at 30°C, with variable growth at 37°C. Colonies are yellow-gray, flat, folded, furrowed, and waxy, and they adhere to the agar. Large vegetative hyphae, 8 to 20 μm, become increasingly septate as maturation occurs. After 7 to 10 days, the colony becomes overgrown with mycelia as masses of zygospores, chlamydoconidia, and conidia are formed. Zygospores are 20 to 50 μm in diameter and have smooth to undulated thick walls; most human isolates produce smooth-walled zygospores. Zygospores produce prominent single "beaks" attached to one side, representing remnants of copulatory tubes. Conidiophores produce unicellular conidia at their apices. The apical portion of the conidiophore initially enlarges and then becomes a vesicle immediately beneath the conidium. The conidium is blown out of the top of the swelling, carrying with it the top of the vesicle as a residual attachment. The subconidial swelling or vesicle then emits a stream of fluid that propels the conidium, a characteristic of the genus *Basidiobolus* (Fig. 11; 28). Secondary or replicative spores can be produced from discharged primary conidia.

It should be noted that students of the entomophthoraceous fungi refer to the asexual reproductive propagules as conidia rather than sporangiospores. Both terms are used in the literature, sometimes in the same discussion (21).

Pythium insidiosum De Cock, Mendoza, Padhye, Ajello et Kaufman (synonyms *P. gracile, P. destruens*)

As noted previously, the oomycetous protoctistan *P. insidiosum* organism currently is not classified in the Kingdom Fungi. However, because it has been discussed and retained in the field of medical mycology, it is described here (16). Colonies are submerged or have very short aerial mycelium with a vague or distinct, finely radiate pattern. They are colorless to white or yellowish white, and an undulating radiate pattern is observed on Sabouraud dextrose agar (Fig. 12). Main hyphae mostly measure 4 to 6 (up to 10) μm in diameter, do not taper and have rounded tips (Fig. 13). The lateral branches are often perpendicular to and as wide as the main hyphae; they sometimes are thinner than the main

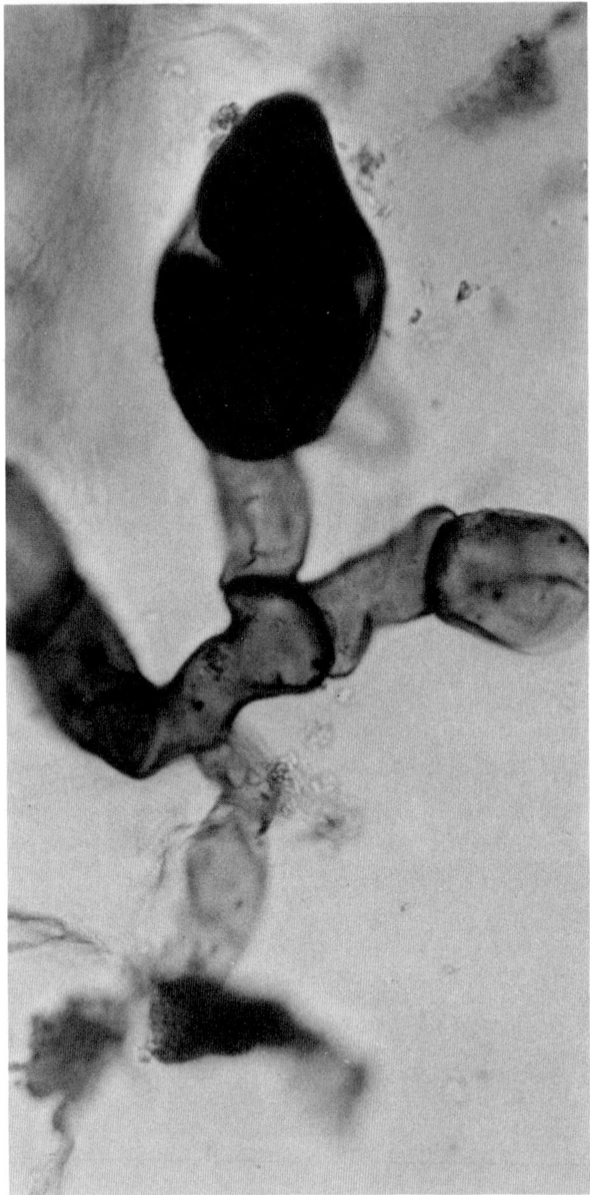

FIG. 11. *Basidiobolus ranarum*: 14 days on potato flakes agar, 30°C. Note septate conidiophore giving rise to dark unicellular conidium that will be forcibly discharged. ×400.

hyphae and measure 2.5 μm or more in diameter. Septa are present in viable plasma-filled hyphae, particularly the main hyphae, but are generally sparse in young hyphae; however, the presence or absence of septa depends heavily on the type of medium used for growth. The septa apparently double when hyphae disarticulate into segments with blunt ends, especially in "squash" preparations. In squash preparations, hyphal segments of various lengths with one or more side branches measuring 12 to 50 by 300 μm more generally are observed. Club-shaped appressoria (intercalary, globose hyphal swellings measuring 12 to 28 μm in diameter, which presumably represent undeveloped oogonia) also are observed.

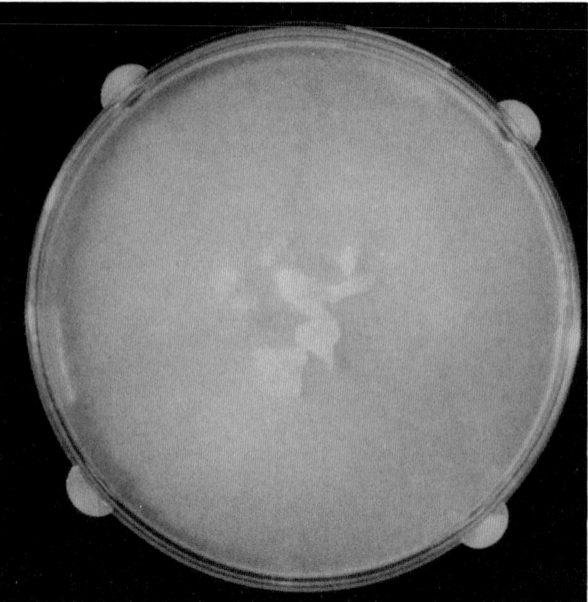

FIG. 12. *Pythium insidiosum*: hyaline colony on potato flakes agar, 10 days, 30°C. Radiate, short aerial mycelia are characteristic for this oomycete.

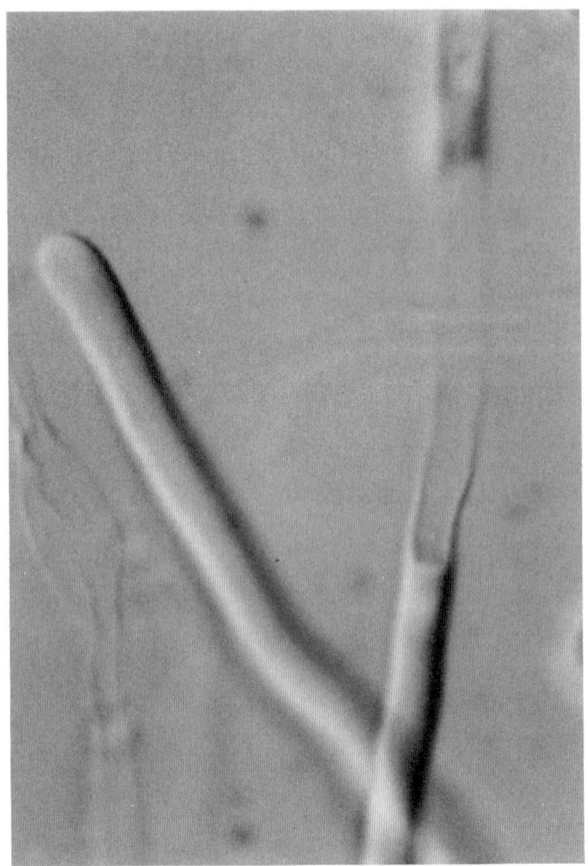

FIG. 13. *Pythium insidiosum*: 10 days on potato flakes agar, 30°C. Hyaline hyphae, 5 μm in diameter, with rounded tips. Nomarski differential interference microscopy, ×400.

Zoosporangia are produced only in water cultures; they are filamentous and not differentiated from vegetative hyphae. Either a terminal part of a sparsely septate hypha or a complete segment of a hypha may function as a sporangium. Discharge tubes develop at the tip of a hypha or laterally on a segment, are thin walled and irregular in outline, are 45 to 700 µm or more in length and 3 to 4 µm in diameter, and widen at the tip to measure 5 to 8 µm. The transition from a thin hypha into a discharge tube is not always distinct. At maturity, sporangial protoplasm flows through an apical opening in the discharge tube and forms a vesicle. The vesicles are globose to subglobose and hyaline and measure 20 to 60 µm in diameter. Through progressive cleavage, biflagellate zoospores are formed inside the vesicle, while the vesicle wall continues to extend during this process. Zoospores have two laterally inserted flagella and measure 12 to 14 by 6 to 8 µm; they are released through a break in the vesicle wall. Zoospores are attracted by nonsterile human and canine hair. The encysted zoospores are globose, measure 8 to 12 µm in diameter, and germinate by means of germ tubes.

Oogonia may develop on cornmeal agar at 24 and 30°C and often are in clusters around the solid parts in the agar. They are intercalary and occasionally subterminal in position and are colorless, smooth, and subglobose, including a small part of the subtending hypha at both ends. They often appear deformed because of the rigid fertilization tube that measures 19 to 36 (usually 23 to 30) µm in diameter. One, two, or rarely three antheridia (male sexual apparatuses) per oogonium (female sexual apparatus) may be observed. Antheridia are diclinous (located on different hyphae than the oogonia), terminal, and inflated clavate to tubular in shape and measure 11 to 37 by 6 to 10 µm. The antheridia are attached to the oogonium over its entire length. The tips of antheridia produce fertilization tubes which indent the oogonial walls. These fertilization tubes present a persistent but slightly shriveled appearance after fertilization. The fertilization tube is relatively thick walled

TABLE 3. Differential characteristics of some clinically significant zygomycete genera

Genus	Colonial morphology	Microscopic morphology
Rhizopus	Rapid growth, cottony, white, becoming gray to brown	Long, unbranched sporangiophores, solitary or in clusters arising from rhizoids; sporangia dark, globose, containing mostly angulated, striated sporangiospores; columellae hemispheric
Mucor	Rapid growth, cottony, white, becoming gray to brown	Rhizoids absent; branched or simple sporangiophores arise from hyphae; sporangia globose; sporangiospores globose to cylindrical; columellae variable
Absidia	Rapid growth, cottony, gray to olive	Finely branched sporangiophores arise from stolons between rhizoids; pear-shaped sporangia contain globose sporangiospores; conspicuous apophysis merges with round columellae; septum usually present in sporangiophore below apophysis
Rhizomucor	Rapid growth, white, becoming gray-brown, low aerial mycelium	Sporangiophores arise from branched aerial hyphae or stolons; rhizoids poorly developed; globose sporangia contain small, round sporangiospores; thermotolerant (growth up to 55°C)
Cunninghamella	Rapid growth, white, becoming dark gray	Erect sporangiophores terminate in globose vesicles; additional smaller, whorled branches of sporangiophores occur beneath primary vesicle; vesicles bear one-spored sporangiola on short stalks (denticles)
Syncephalastrum	Rapid growth, white, becoming gray to black	Branched sporangiophores terminate in globose vesicles; tubular sporangia (merosporangia) contain single row of globose sporangiospores; rhizoids usually present
Saksenaea	Rapid growth, white, woolly	Sporulation induced on nutritionally deficient media; flask-shaped sporangia on short sporangiophores; rhizoids at base of sporangiophore
Apophysomyces	Rapid growth, white, cottony	Sporulation induced on nutritionally deficient media; sporangiophores arise from hyphae, with supporting "foot cells"; pear-shaped sporangia, pronounced dark apophysis; sporangiospores oblong
Mortierella	Rapid growth, white, cottony, garliclike odor; colonies appear as overlapping "rosettes"	Short tapering sporangiophores arise from rhizoids; small, multispored sporangia rapidly deliquesce; sporangiospores kidney shaped with double wall
Cokeromyces	Moderate growth, tan, flat, tenacious, becoming brown-gray	Dimorphic yeast at 37°C; sporangiole stalks arise from vesicle and recurve backward, terminating in multispored sporangiola; zygospores abundant

and measures 4 to 6 µm in diameter. Oospores are aplerotic (not filling the oogonium) and occasionally almost pleurotic (filling the oogonium) and are pressed to one side of the oogonium by the rigid fertilization tube. Oospores measure 17 to 20 by 25 to 27 µm in diameter, with walls 1 by 3 to 4 µm thick. The oospore contents often appear yellowish and finely granular and show a distinct ooplast. Optimal growth temperature is 34 to 36°C, with maximum growth occurring between 40 and 45°C. *P. insidiosum* differs from all known *Pythium* species by the septation of the main hyphae and by the formation of conspicuous, thick-walled fertilization tubes. Although it possesses filamentous, noninflated sporangia like other *Pythium* species, it is unique because of its large antheridia and the high optimum growth temperature.

This organism may be encountered in the clinical laboratory, albeit rarely. To identify *P. insidiosum*, special conditions must be used to induce sporulation; e.g., for studies of sporangium development, water cultures should be used (colonized grass leaves or small pieces of agar cultures in distilled water or soil extract are recommended). Soil extract is prepared by shaking 400 g of sandy soil in 1 liter of distilled water, followed by filtering and autoclaving of the extract. Water cultures should be kept in the dark in a room at 25 to 30°C or in an incubator at 33°C (16). Recent investigations have shown that *P. insidiosum* has been the species responsible for all cases of human and animal disease, as judged by morphology and serology studies (16, 46). In addition, methods for obtaining rapid zoosporogenesis (47) and immunohistochemical and immunodiffusion diagnostic techniques have been reported (10, 27).

Most clinical microbiologists, with sustained study and careful observation, can effectively deal with the genus and species identification of most Zygomycetes. When difficulties are encountered, reference laboratories may offer access to some of the special techniques discussed above, as well as provide definitive species identification. Outlined in Table 3 are some salient identification characteristics of selected, clinically significant genera of Zygomycetes.

LITERATURE CITED

1. **Aguiar de, E., W. C. Moraes, and A. T. Londero.** 1980. Gastrointestinal entomophthoramycosis caused by *Basidiobolus haptosporus*. Mycopathologia **72:**101–105.
2. **Austwick, P. K. C., and J. W. Copeland.** 1974. Swamp cancer. Nature (London) **250:**84.
3. **Axelrod, P., K. J. Kwon-Chung, P. Frawley, and H. Rubin.** 1987. Chronic cystitis due to *Cokeromyces recurvatus*: a case report. J. Infect. Dis. **155:**1062–1064.
4. **Bartnicki-Garcia, S.** 1972. The dimorphic gradient of *Mucor rouxianus*: a laboratory exercise. ASM News **38:** 456–458.
5. **Bartnicki-Garcia, S., and W. J. Nickerson.** 1962. Induction of yeast-like development in *Mucor* by carbon dioxide. J. Bacteriol. **84:**829–840.
6. **Bigby, T. D., M. L. Serota, L. M. Tierney, and M. A. Matthay.** 1986. Clinical spectrum of pulmonary mucormycosis. Chest **89:**435–439.
7. **Bittencourt, A. L., A. T. Londero, M. D. Araujo, N. Mendonca, and J. L. A. Bastos.** 1979. Occurrence of subcutaneous zygomycosis caused by *Basidiobolus haptosporus* in Brazil. Mycopathologia **68:**101–104.
8. **Boelaert, J. R., G. F. van Roost, P. L. Vergauwe, J. J. Verbanck, C. de Vroey, and M. F. Segaert.** 1988. The role of desferrioxamine in dialysis-associated mucormycosis: report of three cases and review of the literature. Clin. Nephrol. **29:**261–266.
9. **Bosken, C. H., A. H. Szporn, and J. Kleinerman.** 1987. Superior vena cava syndrome due to mucormycosis in a patient with lymphoma. Mt. Sinai J. Med. **54:**508–511.
10. **Brown, C. C., J. J. McClure, P. Triche, and C. Crowder.** 1988. Use of immunohistochemical methods for diagnosis of equine pythiosis. Am. J. Vet. Res. **11:**1866–1868.
11. **Busapakum, R., U. Youngchaiyud, S. Sriumpai, G. Segretain, and H. Fromentin.** 1983. Disseminated infection with *Conidiobolus incongruus*. Sabouraudia **21:**323–330.
12. **Carbone, K. M., L. R. Pennington, L. R. Gimenez, C. R. Burrow, and A. J. Watson.** 1985. Mucormycosis in renal transplant patients: a report of two cases and review of the literature. Q. J. Med. **57:**825–831.
13. **Chandler, F. W., W. Kaplan, and L. Ajello.** 1980. A colour atlas and textbook of the histopathology of mycotic diseases. Wolfe Medical Publications, London.
14. **Cooper, B. H.** 1987. A case of pseudoparacoccidioidomycosis: detection of the yeast phase of *Mucor circinelloides* in a clinical specimen. Mycopathologia **97:**189–193.
15. **Cuadrado, L. M., A. Guerrero, J. A. Garcia Asenjo, F. Martin, E. Palau, and D. Garcia Urra.** 1988. Cerebral mucormycosis in two cases of acquired immunodeficiency syndrome. Arch. Neurol. **45:**109–111.
16. **De Cock, A. W. A. M., L. Mendoza, A. A. Padhye, L. Ajello, and L. Kaufman.** 1987. *Pythium insidiosum* sp. nov., the etiologic agent of pythiosis. J. Clin. Microbiol. **25:**344–349.
17. **Dennis, J. E., K. H. Rhodes, D. R. Cooney, and G. D. Roberts.** 1980. Nosocomial *Rhizopus* infection (zygomycosis) in children. J. Pediatr. **96:**924–928.
18. **Echols, R. M., D. G. Selinger, C. Hallowell, J. S. Goodwin, M. H. Duncan, and A. H. Cushing.** 1979. *Rhizopus* osteomyelitis: a case report and a review. Am. J. Med. **66:**141–145.
19. **Ellis, J. J., and L. Ajello.** 1982. An unusual source of *Apophysomyces elegans* and a method for stimulating sporulation of *Saksenaea vasiformis*. Mycologia **74:**144–145.
20. **Gordon, G., M. Indeck, J. Bross, D. A. Kapoor, and S. Brotman.** 1988. Injury from silage wagon accident complicated by mucormycosis. J. Trauma **28:**866–867.
21. **Greer, D. L., and A. L. Rogers.** 1985. Agents of zygomycosis (phycomycosis), p. 575–583. *In* E. H. Lennette, A. Balows, W. J. Hausler, Jr., and H. J. Shadomy (ed.), Manual of clinical microbiology, 4th ed. American Society for Microbiology, Washington, D.C.
22. **Hall, J. C., J. H. Brewer, W. A. Reed, D. M. Steinhaus, and K. R. Watson.** 1988. Cutaneous mucormycosis in a heart transplant patient. Cutis **42:**183–186.
23. **Hesseltine, C. W., and J. J. Ellis.** 1964. An interesting species of *Mucor, M. ramosissimus*. Sabouraudia **3:**151–154.
24. **Huddle, K. R. L., M. J. Hale, C. A. Joseph, and K. L. Chang.** 1987. Rhinocerebral mucormycosis in diabetic keto-acidosis. South Afr. Med. J. **72:**713–714.
25. **Humber, R. A.** 1989. Synopsis of a new classification of the Entomophthorales (Zygomycotina). Mycotaxon **37:** 441–460.
26. **Humber, R. A., C. C. Brown, and R. W. Kornegay.** 1989. Equine zygomycosis caused by *Conidiobolus lamprauges*. J. Clin. Microbiol. **27:**573–576.
27. **Imwidthaya, P., and S. Srimuang.** 1989. Immunodiffusion test for diagnosing human pythiosis. Mycopathologia **106:** 109–112.
28. **Ingold, C. T.** 1934. The spore discharge mechanism in *Basidiobolus ranarum*. New Phytol. **33:**273–277.
29. **Iqbal, S. M., and R. L. Scheer.** 1986. Myocardial mucormycosis with emboli in a hemodialysis patient. Am. J. Kidney Dis. **8:**455–458.
30. **Jones, K. D., and L. Kaufman.** 1978. Development and evaluation of an immunodiffusion test for diagnosis of sys-

temic zygomycosis (mucormycosis): preliminary report. J. Clin. Microbiol. **7:**97–103.

31. **Kalayjian, R. C., R. H. Herzig, A. M. Cohen, and M. C. Hutton.** 1988. Thrombosis of the aorta caused by mucormycosis. South. Med. J. **81:**1180–1182.
32. **Kamalam, A., and A. S. Thambiah.** 1980. Cutaneous infection by *Syncephalastrum.* Sabouraudia **18:**19–20.
33. **Kamalam, A., and A. S. Thambiah.** 1984. Muscle invasion by *Basidiobolus haptosporus.* Sabouraudia J. Med. Vet. Mycol. **22:**273–277.
34. **Kasantikul, V., S. Shuangshoti, and C. Taecholarn.** 1987. Primary phycomycosis of the brain in heroin addicts. Surg. Neurol. **28:**468–472.
35. **Kaufman, L., L. F. Turner, and D. W. McLaughlin.** 1989. Indirect enzyme-linked immunosorbent assay for zygomycosis. J. Clin. Microbiol. **27:**1979–1982.

35a. **Kaufman, L., L. Mendoza, and P. G. Standard.** 1990. Immunodiffusion test for serodiagnosing subcutaneous zygomycosis. J. Clin. Microbiol. **28:**1887–1890.

36. **Kerr, P. G., H. Turner, A. Davidson, C. Bennett, and M. Maslen.** 1988. Zygomycosis requiring amputation of the hand: an isolated case in a patient receiving haemodialysis. Med. J. Aust. **148:**258–259.
37. **Kline, M. W.** 1985. Mucormycosis in children: review of the literature and report of cases. Pediatr. Infect. Dis. **4:** 672–675.
38. **Kotzamanoglou, K., G. Tzanakakis, E. Michalopoulos, and M. Stathopoulou.** 1988. Orbital cellulitis due to mucormycosis. Graefe's Arch. Clin. Exp. Ophthalmol. **226:** 539–541.
39. **Lake, F. R., R. McAleer, and A. E. Tribe.** 1988. Pulmonary mucormycosis without underlying systemic disease. Med. J. Aust. **149:**323–325.
40. **Lawrence, R. M., W. T. Snodgrass, G. W. Reichel, A. A. Padhye, L. Ajello, and F. W. Chandler.** 1986. Systemic zygomycosis caused by *Apophysomyces elegans.* J. Med. Vet. Mycol. **24:**57–65.
41. **Lombardi, G., A. A. Padhye, P. G. Standard, L. Kaufman, and L. Ajello.** 1989. Exoantigen tests for the rapid and specific identification of *Apophysomyces elegans* and *Saksenaea vasiformis.* J. Med. Vet. Mycol. **27:**113–120.
42. **Lyon, D. T., T. T. Schubert, A. G. Mantia, and M. H. Kaplan.** 1979. Phycomycosis of the gastrointestinal tract. Am. J. Gastroenterol. **72:**379–394.
43. **Martinson, F. D.** 1972. Clinical, epidemiological and therapeutic aspects of entomophthoromycosis. Ann. Soc. Belg. Med. Trop. **52:**329–342.
44. **McGinnis, M. R., and W. A. Shell.** 1985. Classifying the medically-important fungi. Diagn. Med. **8:**30–36.
45. **McGough, D. A., A. W. Fothergill, and M. G. Rinaldi.** 1990. *Cokeromyces recurvatus* Poitras, a distinctive zygomycete and potential pathogen: criteria for identification. Clin. Microbiol. Newsl. **12:**113–117.
46. **Mendoza, L., L. Kaufman, and P. Standard.** 1987. Antigenic relationship between the animal and human pathogen *Pythium insidiosum* sp. nov., the etiologic agent of pythiosis. J. Clin. Microbiol. **25:**344–349.
47. **Mendoza, L., and J. Prendas.** 1988. A method to obtain rapid zoosporogenesis of *Pythium insidiosum.* Mycopathologia **104:**59–62.
48. **Morduchowicz, G., D. Shmueli, Z. Shapira, S. L. Cohen, A. Yussim, C. S. Block, J. B. Rosenfeld, and S. D. Pitlik.** 1986. Rhinocerebral mucormycosis in renal transplant recipients: report of three cases and review of the literature. Rev. Infect. Dis. **8:**441–446.
49. **Mostaza, J. M., F. J. Barbado, J. Fernandez-Martin, J. Pena-Yanez, and J. J. Vasquez-Rodriguez.** 1989. Cutaneoarticular mucormycosis due to *Cunninghamella bertholletiae* in a patient with AIDS. Rev. Infect. Dis. **11:**316–318.
50. **Nimmo, G. R., R. F. Whiting, and R. W. Strong.** 1988. Disseminated mucormycosis due to *Cunninghamella bertholletiae* in a liver transplant recipient. Postgrad. Med. J. **64:**82–84.
51. **Oakley, L. A., J. F. Fisher, and J. H. Dennison.** 1986. Bread mold infection in diabetes. Postgrad. Med. **80:**93–102.
52. **Oliveri, S., E. Cammarata, G. Augello, P. Mancuso, R. Tropea, L. Ajello, and A. A. Padhye.** 1988. *Rhizopus arrhizus* in Italy as the causative agent of primary cerebral zygomycosis in a drug addict. Eur. J. Epidemiol. **4:**284–288.
53. **Onions, A. H. S., D. Allsopp, and H. O. W. Eggins.** 1981. Zygomycetes, p. 27–49. *In* Smith's introduction to industrial mycology, 7th ed. Edward Arnold, London.
54. **Padhye, A. A., and L. Ajello.** 1988. Simple method of inducing sporulation by *Apophysomyces elegans* and *Saksenaea vasiformis.* J. Clin. Microbiol. **26:**1861–1863.
55. **Parfrey, N. A.** 1986. Improved diagnosis and prognosis of mucormycosis. Medicine **65:**113–123.
56. **Patterson, J. E., G. E. Barden, and F. J. Bia.** 1986. Hospital-acquired gangrenous mucormycosis. Yale J. Biol. Med. **59:**453–459.
57. **Pierce, P. F., S. I. Soloman, L. Kaufman, V. F. Garagusi, R. H. Parker, and L. Ajello.** 1982. Zygomycetes brain abscesses in narcotic addicts with serological diagnosis. J. Am. Med. Assoc. **248:**2881–2882.
58. **Pierce, P. F., M. B. Wood, G. D. Roberts, R. H. Fitzgerald, C. Robertson, and R. S. Edson.** 1987. *Saksenaea vasiformis* osteomyelitis. J. Clin. Microbiol. **25:**933–935.
59. **Pitt, J. I., and A. D. Hocking.** 1985. Zygomycetes, p. 143–167. *In* Fungi and food spoilage. Academic Press, Sydney.
60. **Rangel-Guerra, R., H. R. Martinez, and C. Saenz.** 1985. Mucormycosis, report of 11 cases. Arch. Neurol. **42:**578–581.
61. **Reed, A. E., B. A. Body, M. B. Austin, and H. F. Frierson.** 1988. *Cunninghamella bertholletiae* and *Pneumocystis carinii* pneumonia as a fatal complication of chronic lymphocytic leukemia. Hum. Pathol. **19:**1470–1472.
62. **Reich, H., W. Behr, and J. Barnert.** 1985. Rhinocerebral mucormycosis in a diabetic ketoacidotic patient. J. Neurol. **232:**115–117.
63. **Rex, J. H., A. M. Ginsberg, L. F. Fries, H. I. Pass, and K. J. Kwon-Chung.** 1988. *Cunninghamella bertholletiae* infection associated with deferoxamine therapy. Rev. Infect. Dis. **10:**1187–1195.
64. **Rinaldi, M. G.** 1982. The use of potato flakes agar in clinical mycology. J. Clin. Microbiol. **15:**1159–1160.
65. **Rinaldi, M. G.** 1989. Zygomycosis. Infect. Dis. Clin. North Am. **3:**19–41.
66. **Rippon, J. W.** 1988. Medical mycology. The pathogenic fungi and the pathogenic Actinomycetes, 3rd ed. The W. B. Saunders Co., Philadelphia.
67. **Rippon, J. W., and C. T. Dolan.** 1979. Colonization of the vagina by fungi of the genus *Mucor.* Clin. Microbiol. Newsl. **11:**4–5.
68. **Rothstein, R. D., and G. L. Simon.** 1986. Subacute pulmonary mucormycosis. J. Med. Vet. Mycol. **24:**391–394.
69. **Rozich, J., H. P. Holley, F. Henderson, J. Gardner, and F. Nelson.** 1988. Cauda equina syndrome secondary to disseminated zygomycosis. J. Am. Med. Assoc. **260:**3638–3640.
70. **Ryan-Poirier, K., R. M. Eiseman, J. H. Beaty, P. G. Hunt, G. A. Burghen, and R. J. Leggiadro.** 1988. Post-traumatic cutaneous mucormycosis in diabetes mellitus. Clin. Pediatr. **27:**609–612.
71. **Sands, J. M., A. M. Macher, T. J. Ley, and A. W. Nienhuis.** 1985. Disseminated infection caused by *Cunninghamella bertholletiae* in a patient with beta-thalassemia. Ann. Intern. Med. **102:**59–63.
72. **Sane, A., S. Manzi, J. Perfect, A. J. Herzberg, and J. O. Moore.** 1989. Deferoxamine treatment as a risk factor for zygomycete infection. J. Infect. Dis. **159:**151–152.
73. **Sathapatayavongs, B., P. Leelachaikul, R. Prachaktam, V. Atichartakarn, S. Sriphojanart, P. Trairatvorakul, S.**

Jirasiritham, S. Nontasut, C. Eurvilaichit, and T. Flegel. 1989. Human pythiosis associated with thalassemia hemoglobinopathy syndrome. J. Infect. Dis. **159:**274–280.

74. **Schipper, M. A. A.** 1976. On *Mucor circinelloides, Mucor racemosus,* and related species. Stud. Mycol. **12:**1–40.
75. **Schipper, M. A. A., and J. A. Stalpers.** 1984. A revision of the genus *Rhizopus.* II. The *Rhizopus microsporus* group. Stud. Mycol. **25:**20–34.
76. **Seviour, R. J., A. L. Cooper, and N. W. Skilbeck.** 1987. Identification of *Mortierella wolfii,* a causative agent of mycotic abortion in cattle. J. Med. Vet. Mycol. **25:**115–123.
77. **Smith, A. G., C. I. Bustamante, and G. D. Gilmore.** 1989. Zygomycosis (absidiomycosis) in an AIDS patient. Mycopathologia **105:**7–10.
78. **Tintelnot, K., and B. Nitsche.** 1988. *Rhizopus oligosporus* as a cause of mucormycosis in man. Mycoses **32:**115–118.
79. **Tuder, R. M.** 1985. Myocardial infarct in disseminated mucormycosis: case report with special emphasis on the pathogenic mechanisms. Mycopathologia **89:**81–88.
80. **Venezio, F. R., D. J. Sexton, R. Forsythe, M. Williams, and B. Reisberg.** 1985. Mucormycosis after open fracture injury. South. Med. J. **78:**1516–1517.
81. **Ventura, G. J., H. M. Kantarjian, E. Anaissie, R. L. Hopfer, and V. Fainstein.** 1986. Pneumonia with *Cunninghamella* species in patients with hematologic malignancies. Cancer **58:**1534–1536.
82. **Wieden, M. A., K. K. Steinbronn, A. A. Padhye, L. Ajello, and F. W. Chandler.** 1985. Zygomycosis caused by *Apophysomyces elegans.* J. Clin. Microbiol. **22:**522–526.
83. **White, C. B., P. J. Barcia, and J. W. Bass.** 1986. Neonatal zygomycotic necrotizing cellulitis. Pediatrics **78:** 100–102.
84. **Windus, D. W., T. J. Stokes, B. A. Julian, and A. Z. Fenves.** 1987. Fatal *Rhizopus* infections in hemodialysis patients receiving deferoxamine. Ann. Intern. Med. **107:** 678–680.
85. **Woods, K. R., and B. J. Hanna.** 1986. Brain stem mucormycosis in a narcotic addict with eventual recovery. Am. J. Med. **80:**126–128.

Chapter 65

Fungi Causing Eumycotic Mycetomas

ARVIND A. PADHYE AND LIBERO AJELLO

DEFINITION OF THE DISEASE

A mycetoma is a localized, chronic, granulomatous infection involving cutaneous and subcutaneous tissues and eventually, in some cases, the bones. Mycetomas generally are confined to the feet or hands, but occasionally other parts of the body such as the back, shoulders, and buttocks may be involved. The lesions contain granulomas and abscesses that suppurate and drain through sinus tracts. The pus contains granules (grains) that vary from microscopic in size to 2 mm in diameter. Size, color, shape, and texture of the granules vary with the species and sometimes suggest the specific etiology. Both filamentous fungi and Actinomycetes are known to cause mycetomas. Mycetomas caused by Actinomycetes are called actinomycotic mycetomas, and those incited by species of filamentous fungi are referred to as eumycotic mycetomas. The disease is distributed worldwide and is more commonly seen in humans than in lower animals. Only a few authentic veterinary cases of mycetoma involving such animals as dogs, horses, and goats have been described in the literature (2, 10, 27).

OCCURRENCE OF THE CAUSAL AGENTS IN NATURE

The causal agents of eumycotic mycetomas are saprophytes that live on organic debris in soil. The various causal agents have been isolated from either soil or plant material (1, 4, 18, 24). Segretain (42) and Segretain and Mariat (45), using specific media and techniques, showed that *Leptosphaeria senegalensis* and *Leptosphaeria tompkinsii* were found on about 50% of the dry thorns of the *Acacia* trees that were examined, particularly those that had been stained by mud during the rainy season. *Neotestudina rosatii* was isolated from sandy ground (28), and *Madurella mycetomatis* was recovered from soil and anthills (41, 49). *Acremonium* spp., *Curvularia* spp., *Aspergillus nidulans*, and *Pseudallescheria boydii* frequently have been isolated from soil. Borelli (6) isolated *Madurella grisea* from soil in Venezuela.

MODE OF INFECTION AND SYMPTOMS

A mycetoma develops after a traumatic injury by contaminated thorns, splinters from plants, fish scales or fins, snake bites, insect bites, farm implements, knives, etc. In recent years, development of mycetoma after surgery (38) and in renal transplant recipients (19) also has been reported. The initial lesions are characterized by a feeling of discomfort and pain at the point of inoculation. Weeks or months later, the subcutaneous tissue at the site of inoculation becomes indurated, abscesses develop, and sinuses may drain to the surface. The lesions are characterized by swelling, suppurating abscesses, granulomas, and sinuses from which serosanguinous fluid containing granules oozes out. The mycetoma develops slowly beneath thick fibrosclerous tissue. The subsequent phase of proliferation involves the invasion of muscles and intramuscular layers. The granulomatous lesions can extend as deep as bony tissue, causing severe destruction of bone. Regardless of the etiologic agent involved, the causal organisms develop in the form of soft or hard, compact mycelial masses, known as granules or grains, within the infected tissue. The hallmark of a mycetoma is the granule composed of nonconidiating mycelium that may or may not be embedded in a cementlike matrix.

Mycetomas develop mainly among people, such as field workers, farmers, sugarcane workers, and fishermen, who are in contact with contaminated materials. Even though, because of increased exposure, the prevalence of mycetomas is much higher in males than in females, women and children who walk barefoot also are vulnerable to infection.

Fungus balls, caused by *Aspergillus* species, *Coccidioides immitis*, or *P. boydii* in preformed lung cavities, sometimes mistakenly are called mycetomas (20). In the absence of well-organized granules, they should be referred to appropriately as fungus balls, aspergillomas, or coccidioidomas (29). Similarly, mycelial aggregates formed by dermatophytes in deep tissues differ in many respects from the granules of the mycetomas. Such infections caused by dermatophytes are best referred to as pseudomycetomas rather than mycetomas (3).

GEOGRAPHIC DISTRIBUTION OF EUMYCOTIC MYCETOMAS

Eumycotic mycetomas occur primarily in the tropical and hot temperate zones of the world. They frequently are reported from countries near the Tropic of Cancer, but they also occur beyond this area. Numerous cases have been described from Africa, Asia, and South and Central America. Mycetomas are not seen as commonly in the United States as in tropical countries. A survey of the literature from 1979 to 1988 revealed that not more than 10 cases of eumycotic mycetoma had been reported in the United States.

CLIMATIC CONDITIONS

Climate has a definite influence on the prevalence and distribution of mycetomas. Rivers that flood each year during the wet season in many countries of Africa and Asia influence the distribution of the causal agents. Rainfall also favors the spread of the etiologic agents on organic matter (14).

COLLECTION AND EXAMINATION OF THE GRANULES

Since all of the agents of eumycotic mycetomas are soil saprophytes and some are encountered as contaminants of clinical specimens, their etiologic role in mycetomas must be established carefully. A definitive diagnosis must be based on the demonstration of granules in tissue and repeated isolation of the causal fungus from granules aspirated from preferably unopened sinuses.

Pus, exudate, or biopsy material should be examined for the presence of granules, which vary in size from 0.2 to 2 mm or more and are usually detectable with the naked eye. Their color, texture, size, and shape give a fair indication of the identity of the etiologic agent. Actinomycotic and eumycotic mycetomas are differentiated by the examination of crushed granules in Gram-stained preparations. Actinomycotic granules are composed of gram-positive, interwoven, thin filaments, 0.5 to 1.0 μm in diameter, as well as coccoid and bacillary forms. Granules of the eumycotic agents, on the other hand, are composed of broad, interwoven, septate hyphae, 2 to 5 μm in diameter, with many bizarre-shaped, swollen cells up to 15 μm in diameter, especially at the periphery of the granules. In many species, the granules also contain a cementlike material.

To maximize the chances of obtaining pure cultures of the etiologic agents, granules from the eumycotic mycetomas should be washed several times with saline containing antibacterial antibiotics such as penicillin and streptomycin. The granules thus freed from the surface bacteria are cultured in several petri dishes of Sabouraud dextrose agar (SDA; Difco Laboratories, Detroit, Mich.) containing chloramphenicol (50 mg/liter) and Sabouraud agar containing chloramphenicol and cycloheximide (500 mg/liter). Several of these plates should be incubated at 25°C, and the others should be incubated at 37°C. All should be observed at 48-h intervals. Since many of the fungi that cause eumycotic mycetomas grow slowly, culture plates should be incubated for 6 weeks before being discarded as negative. Identification of the isolated fungus, when possible, is based on gross colony morphology and pigmentation, the morphology of its conidiophores and conidia, and the mechanism of conidiogenesis. Since certain species (*M. grisea, M. mycetomatis, N. rosatii, Pyrenochaeta mackinnonii,* and *Pyrenochaeta romeroi*) do not sporulate readily, sporulation media and physiologic tests, such as those for carbohydrate and nitrate utilization, must be used for identification.

ETIOLOGIC AGENTS AND THEIR CLASSIFICATION

The 22 species known to cause eumycotic mycetomas are listed below. Of these species, 5 belong to the division Ascomycota and 17 are classified under the division Deuteromycota (Fungi Imperfecti).

Ascomycota
- *Emericella nidulans* (*Aspergillus nidulans*) (26)
- *Leptosphaeria senegalensis* (28)
- *Leptosphaeria tompkinsii* (16)
- *Neotestudina rosatii* (43)
- *Pseudallescheria boydii* (32)

Deuteromycota
- *Acremonium falciforme* (21, 33)
- *Acremonium kiliense* (21)
- *Acremonium recifei* (21, 27)
- *Curvularia geniculata* (10)
- *Curvularia lunata* (26, 27)
- *Corynespora cassicola* (10)
- *Exophiala jeanselmei* (31, 37)
- *Fusarium moniliforme* (27, 28)
- *Fusarium solani* (7, 28, 48)
- *Madurella grisea* (6, 23, 25, 26)
- *Madurella mycetomatis* (6, 23, 28)
- *Phialophora cyanescens* (15)
- *Plenodomus avramii* (8)
- *Polycytella hominis* (12)
- *Pseudochaetosphaeronema larense* (9, 39)
- *Pyrenochaeta mackinnonii* (7, 39)
- *Pyrenochaeta romeroi* (5, 39, 44)

CHARACTERISTICS OF THE GRANULES IN TISSUE

The granules of eumycotic mycetomas are composed of septate mycelial filaments that are at least 2 to 4 μm in diameter. The mycelium may be distorted and bizarre in form and size. Chlamydospores are frequently present, especially at the periphery of the granule. The mycelium of the granules may or may not be embedded in a cementlike substance, depending on the species involved. Often the granules elicit an immunological response, the so-called Splendore-Hoeppli reaction (13). This reaction is seen histologically in the form of a deposit of an eosinophilic material around the granule.

Depending on the etiologic agent involved, the granules are white to yellow-brown to black and range from 200 μm to 5 mm in diameter. The color gives some clue to the species involved. Most textbooks on medical mycology mention a definitive relationship between the color of the granules and the causal species.

The causal agents that produce hyaline mycelium and conidia generally produce white granules in tissue, whereas those that are pigmented or dematiaceous produce dark granules in tissue. There are several exceptions to this rule. For example, hyaline fungi such as *A. kiliense* and *F. solani* have been described in the literature as producers of black granules (21, 48). In a reverse manner, dematiaceous etiologic agents such as *P. boydii* and *Phialophora cyanescens* (15) have been described as producers of white granules in tissue. Although the gross and microscopic characteristics of the granules provide insight into the identity of the etiologic agent or of a particular group in which it belongs, definitive identification should be based on repeated isolation of the same fungus from several granules, and identification of the etiologic agent should be based on its colonial features, microscopic characteristics of conidia, and conidiophores, and mechanism of conidiogenesis. The gross characteristics of the granules formed by each of the 22 species cited are summarized in Table 1.

DESCRIPTION OF THE MORE PREVALENT ETIOLOGIC AGENTS

The 11 etiologic agents described below represent the species that have been isolated most commonly from

TABLE 1. Gross characteristics of the granules of the eumycotic mycetoma agents

Kind of granule and species	Texture	Size range (mm)	Cementlike matrix
White grain in tissue			
Acremonium falciforme	Soft	0.2–0.5	Absent
Acremonium kiliense	Soft	0.2–0.5	Absent
Acremonium recifei	Soft	0.2–0.5	Absent
Aspergillus nidulans	Soft	1–2	Absent
Fusarium moniliforme	Soft	0.2–0.5	Absent
Fusarium solani	Soft	0.2–0.6	Absent
Neotestudina rosatii	Soft	0.5–1	Present, peripheral
Phialophora cyanescens	Soft	?	Absent
Polycytella hominis	Soft	0.5–1	Absent
Pseudallescheria boydii	Soft	0.5–1	Absent
Black grain in tissue			
Corynespora cassicola	Hard	0.2–0.5	Absent
Curvularia geniculata	Hard	0.5–1	Present, peripheral
Curvularia lunata	Hard	0.5–1	Present, peripheral
Exophiala jeanselmei	Soft	0.2–0.3	Absent
Leptosphaeria senegalensis	Hard	0.5–2	Present, peripheral
Leptosphaeria tompkinsii	Hard	0.5–2	Present, peripheral
Madurella grisea	Soft	0.3–0.6	Present, peripheral
Madurella mycetomatis	Hard	0.5–5	Present, homogeneous
Plenodomus avramii	Soft	0.5–0.8	Absent
Pseudochaetosphaeronema larense	Soft	0.2–0.5	Absent
Pyrenochaeta mackinnonii	Soft	0.2–0.5	Absent
Pyrenochaeta romeroi	Soft	0.2–0.6	Absent

human or lower animal mycetomas. The physiologic characteristics of the five species that are isolated most commonly from eumycotic mycetomas are summarized in Table 2. In the United States, cases of eumycotic mycetoma are not common. Among the cases studied, the following species, in diminishing order of frequency, were isolated: *P. boydii, A. falciforme, M. mycetomatis, M. grisea,* and *E. jeanselmei.*

Acremonium falciforme (Carrion) Gams 1971

Three *Acremonium* species (*A. falciforme, A. kiliense,* and *A. recifei*) are known to cause mycetomas. *Acremonium falciforme* is the second most common cause of mycetoma in the United States. It was found to be an agent of eumycotic mycetomas in the San Francisco Bay area of California (21). It also was reported as causing mycetoma in a renal transplant recipient (19) and as an etiologic agent of mycetoma in a patient from New York (33).

The granules of *A. falciforme* are white to pale yellow, soft, and 0.2 to 0.5 mm in diameter. They are composed of slender, polymorphic, septate hyphae 1.5 to 2.0 μm in diameter with irregular bulbous swellings and peripheral cementing material (Fig. 1). In tissue sections, the granules resemble those produced by *P. boydii.* The diagnosis, therefore, should rest not on the structure of granules in tissues alone but also on the isolation and identification of the causal fungus.

Colonies of *A. falciforme* on SDA agar are slow growing, reaching 60 to 65 mm in diameter in 2 weeks. They are downy and gray-brown, becoming gray-violet. The reverse of the colony develops a violet-purple pigment. The hyphae are hyaline, septate, smooth, branched, and 1.5 to 2.5 μm in diameter. They bear erect, undifferentiated, unbranched, repeatedly septate conidiophores. The conida are borne at the tip of the phialidic conidiogenous cells in mucoid clusters. The conidia are sausage shaped, slightly curved, and nonseptate to monoseptate. In size they measure 7 to 8.5 by 2.7 to 3.2 μm (Fig. 2). The intercalary or, rarely, terminal chlamydospores are smooth, thick walled, and 5 to 8 μm in diameter.

The other two species, *A. kiliense* and *A. recifei,* are not known to cause mycetomas as frequently as does

TABLE 2. Physiologic characteristics of some causal agents of eumycotic mycetomas

Etiologic agent	Utilization of:					Starch hydrolysis	Utilization of:			Protease activity	Optimum growth temp (°C)
	Galactose	Glucose	Lactose	Maltose	Sucrose		Asparagine	KNO_3	$(NH_4)_2SO_4$		
Acremonium falciforme	+	+	−	+	+	−	+	+	+	±	30
Exophiala jeanselmei	+	+	−	+	+	+	+	±	±	−	30
Madurella grisea	+	+	−	+	+	+	+	+	+	±	25
Madurella mycetomatis	+	+	+	+	−	+	+	+	+	±	37
Pseudallescheria boydii	±	+	−	−	±	−	+	+	+	+	30

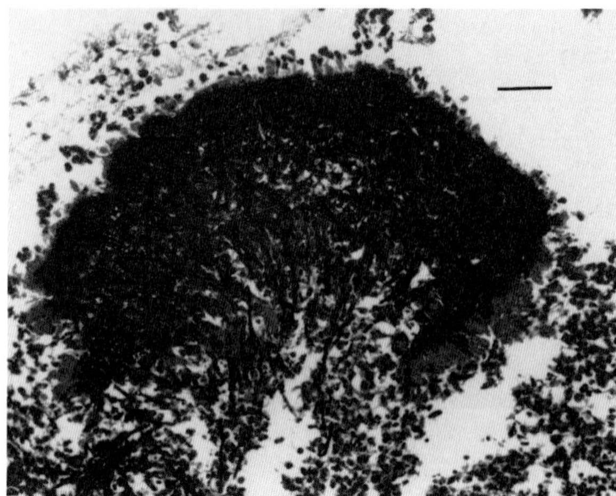

FIG. 1. White, soft granule of *Acremonium falciforme* composed of septate hyphae and peripheral cementing material, Gomori methenamine silver plus hematoxylin and eosin stain. Bar = 10 μm.

A. falciforme. Their granules are similar in morphology to those of *A. falciforme*. They cannot be differentiated from each other or from those produced by *P. boydii*. When isolated, *A. kiliense* develops pinkish orange, glabrous colonies with coremia. Conidia are broadly elliptical to cylindrical and nonseptate, occurring in gleoid masses at the tips of lateral, long, tapering phialides with vestigial collarettes. Chlamydospores are present. Colonies of *A. recifei* are white to pinkish buff and moist to glabrous. Their conidiophores are branched, bearing long, tapering phialides. Conidia are claviform and nonseptate to monoseptate.

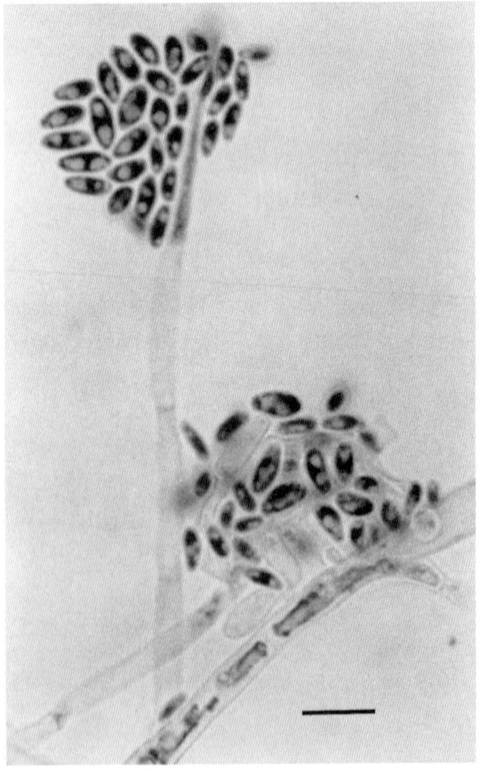

FIG. 2. *Acremonium falciforme*. Slide culture on SDA showing erect, septate conidiophore, phialidic conidiogenous cell, and slightly curved conidia. Bar = 10 μm.

Curvularia geniculata (Tracy and Earl) Boedijin, 1933

C. geniculata has been found to be the etiologic agent of mycetomas in dogs in the United States (10). Its granules are black to dark brown, firm, and 0.5 to 1.0 mm or more in size. In tissue sections, the granule is spherical, ovoid, or irregularly shaped and often surrounded by a zone of epithelioid cells. The periphery of the granule is composed of a dense, interwoven mass of dematiaceous mycelium and thick-walled, chlamydosporelike cells embedded in a cementlike substance. The interior of the granules is vacuolar and consists of a loose network of septate, hyphal filaments.

In culture, *C. geniculata* develops a cottony to downy, olive gray to black colony. Microscopically, the dematiaceous, septate hyphae bear solitary, geniculate conidiogenous cells. The conidia are without protruding hila. They are smooth walled, predominantly five celled, and curved, with the median cell pale to dark brown.

Curvularia lunata (Wakker) Boedijin

C. lunata has been described as an etiologic agent of mycetomas among humans in Senegal and Sudan (26). Its granules resemble those of *C. geniculata* in their morphologic characteristics. In culture, *C. lunata* produces geniculate conidiophores producing terminal, sympodial conidiogenous cells. Conidia are without protruding hila. They are smooth and predominantly four celled, with the penultimate cell pale to dark brown.

Exophiala jeanselmei (Langeron) McGinnis and Padhye 1977

E. jeanselmei is known as an agent of eumycotic mycetomas in India (46, 47), Malaya, Thailand (40), Argentina (36), and the United States (37). *E. jeanselmei* produces dark granules in host tissue. They are brown to black, irregular in shape, and fragile. Detached portions or fragments of the granules often are found within giant cells. When extruded through open sinuses, the granules often look like worm cases because of their elongated shape and irregular surface. In tissue sections, they appear as hollow spheres or as sinuous bands that are worm shaped in appearance. The external surface is composed of brown, thick-walled hyphae and thick-walled chlamydosporelike cells. The granules are cement free. Within the hollow granules, smaller, degenerated hyphal fragments with leukocytes and giant cells may be seen.

Initially, the colonies of *E. jeanselmei* may be yeastlike and black, gradually spreading, raised or dome shaped, and 20 to 25 mm in diameter. After 2 weeks on SDA, the colonies are covered with short aerial hyphae. At this stage, the colony is mousey gray to olive gray with an olive black reverse. The septate mycelium is sometimes toruloid, branched, and pale brown. The conidiophores are partially differentiated from the vegetative hyphae, solitary, branched or unbranched, smooth walled, and pale brown. The conidiogenous cells produce conidia from one or more areas of their cells. The tips of the conidiogenous cells are closely annellated, cylindrical, obclavate, smooth walled, pale brown to black, and elongate as a result of successive conidial formation. The conidia, which aggregate in masses at the tips of the conidiophores, tend to slide down the conidiophore or along hyphae. The smooth conidia are exogenous, nonseptate, subglobose, and ellipsoidal to cylindrical, measuring 1.5 to 2.8 μm.

Leptosphaeria senegalensis Baylet, Camain et Segretain 1959, and *Leptosphaeria tompkinsii* El Ani, 1966

L. senegalensis and *L. tompkinsii* are known to cause mycetomas in the northern tropical zone of West Africa, especially in Senegal and Mauritania, and in India. The granules of the two species are indistinguishable from each other. They are black, 0.5 to 2 mm in size, and firm to hard in texture. In tissue sections, the granules are round to polylobulated, with large vesicles. At the periphery, the mycelium is embedded in a black, cementlike substance. The central portion of the granules consists of a loose network of hyphae.

In culture, *L. senegalensis* and *L. tompkinsii* grow rapidly and produce gray-brown colonies. On cornmeal agar, both species produce perithecia that are nonostiolate, scattered, immersed or superficial, globose to subglobose, black, and covered with brown, flexuous hyphae. The asci are numerous, eight spored, clavate to cylindrical, and double walled. The major differences between the two species are found in the ascospores, which differ in size, shape, and septation as well as in the nature of the gelatinous sheath that surrounds them (16, 17).

Madurella grisea Mackinnon, Ferrada and Montemayer, 1949

M. grisea occurs as an etiologic agent of black grain mycetomas in South America, India, Africa, and North and Central America (25). In the United States, five cases caused by *M. grisea* have been described (11, 34).

The granules are black, 0.3 to 0.6 mm, and soft to firm. In tissue sections, the granules are oval, lobulated or kidney shaped (reniform), and sometimes vermiform. They are composed of a dense network of hyphae, weakly pigmented in the center and brown to blackish brown in the peripheral region as the result of the presence of a brown, cementlike interstitial material.

In culture, *M. grisea* forms slow-growing velvety colonies that are cerebriform, radially furrowed or smooth, and dark gray to olive brown to black. The reverse of the colonies is black. In old cultures, a red-brown diffusible pigment is produced by many isolates. Microscopically, the hyphae are septate, dematiaceous, 1 to 3 μm in diameter, and nonsporulating. Chlamydospores rarely are observed. Large, moniliform hyphae 3 to 5 μm in diameter often are seen. Some isolates of *M. grisea* have been described as producing abortive or fertile pycnidia (30). Such isolates are indistinguishable from *Pyrenochaeta romeroi* (44).

Madurella mycetomatis (Laveran) Brumpt, 1905

The granules produced by *M. mycetomatis* are reddish brown to black. They may reach 5 mm or more in diameter and are firm to hard. In tissue sections, the granules are compact, variable in size and shape, and frequently multilobulated. They are composed of hyphae 1 to 5 μm in diameter that terminate in enlarged hyphal cells at the periphery of the granule and measure 12 to 15 μm in diameter. The cell wall pigment is minimal, but the hyphal cells contain brown particles. The hyphae are embedded in a conspicuous brown matrix that is characteristic of *M. mycetomatis*. Some granules are vesicular and more regular in size and shape. The vesicles are prominently visible in the peripheral zone in a dense, brown, cementlike matrix (Fig. 3).

In culture, *M. mycetomatis* shows wide variation. Colonies are slow growing and white at first, becoming olivaceous, yellow, or brown, flat or dome shaped, and velvety to glabrous, with a characteristic brown diffusible pigment. On nutritionally deficient media, sclerotia 750 μm in diameter develop. These are black and made of undifferentiated polygonal cells. On SDA, the mycelium is sterile. On nutritionally poor media, such as soil extract or hay infusion agar, about 50% of the isolates produce round to pyriform conidia 3 to 4 μm in diameter from the tips of phialides. The phialides are long and tapering, often with a collarette. They range from 3 to 15 μm in length. Occasionally, two or three phialides may arise from a lateral branch (Fig. 4).

M. mycetomatis grows better at 37 than at 30°C, whereas *M. grisea* grows better at 30 than at 37°C. The ability of *M. mycetomatis* isolates to grow at temperatures as high as 40°C serves as a useful diagnostic criterion to distinguish them from *M. grisea*. *M. mycetomatis* is slowly proteolytic and utilizes glucose, maltose, and galactose but not sucrose. It utilizes potassium nitrate, ammonium sulfate, asparagine, and urea, and it hydrolyzes starch. *M. grisea*, on the other hand, is weakly proteolytic and assimilates glucose, maltose, and sucrose but not lactose (Table 2).

Neotestudina rosatii Segretain and Destombes, 1961

The granules of *N. rosatii* are white to brownish white, 0.5 to 1.0 mm in size, and soft. In tissue sections, they

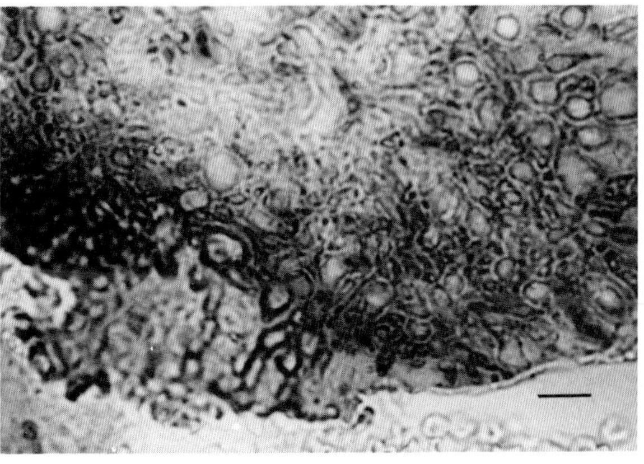

FIG. 3. Black, vesicular granule of *Madurella mycetomatis* showing conspicuous cementlike matrix. Hematoxylin and eosin stain. Bar = 10 μm.

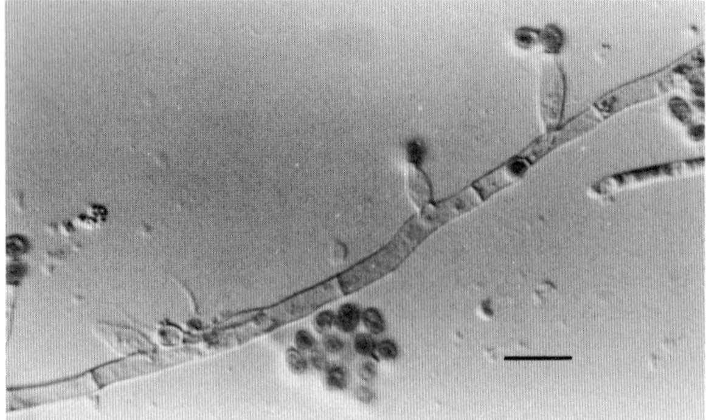

FIG. 4. *Madurella mycetomatis.* Slide culture on soil extract agar showing phialides and phialoconidia. Bar = 10 μm.

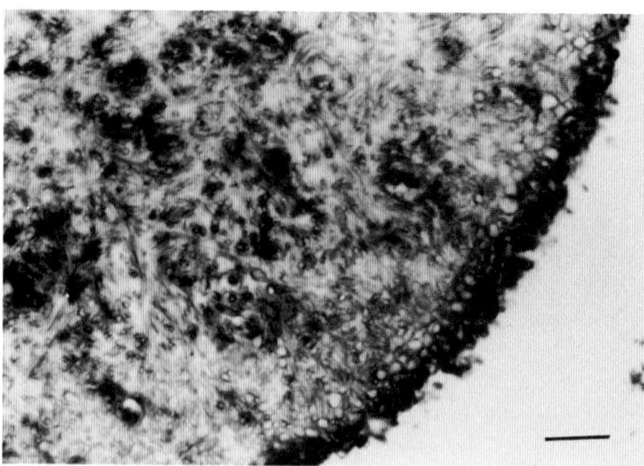

FIG. 5. White, soft granule of *Pseudallescheria boydii* showing central area of the granule consisting of loosely interwoven, hyaline, septate hyphae and lack of cementing material at the periphery. Gomori methenamine silver stain. Bar = 10 μm.

appear to be polyhedral to subregular. The hyphae are embedded in a peripheral cementing material with an eosinophilic border. The central portion of the granules consists of more or less disintegrated mycelium and chlamydospores. Mycetomas caused by *N. rosatii* have been described in Australia, Cameroon, Guinea, Senegal, and Somalia (28, 43).

In culture, colonies of *N. rosatii* are slow growing, attaining 25 to 28 mm in diameter in 2 weeks, with aerial mycelium that is grayish black to brownish black. On potato-carrot or cornmeal agar incubated at 30°C, most of the cleistothecia are submerged. The cleistothecial walls are smooth and surrounded by a weft of brown to hyaline hyphae. The eight-spored asci, 12 to 35 by 10 to 25 μm, are scattered in the central part of the cleistothecium and are globose to subglobose, thick walled, and bitunicate, becoming evanescent as ascospores mature. Ascospores vary in size (9 to 12.5 by 4.5 to 8.0 μm) and shape, ranging from ellipsoidal to bicampanulate, asymmetrical, or slightly curved, and are constricted at the median transverse septum, with brown, smooth walls.

Pseudallescheria boydii (Shear) McGinnis, Padhye, and Ajello, 1982
Anamorph: *Scedosporium apiospermum* Sacc. ex Castellani and Chalmers, 1919

The granules produced by *P. boydii* are white to yellowish white and soft to firm; they vary from spherical to subspherical to lobulated and measure from 0.2 to 2.0 mm in diameter. In tissue sections, the granules are composed of hyaline hyphae 1.5 to 5.0 mm in diameter, which radiate from the center into terminal and thick-walled cells 15 to 20 μm in diameter at the periphery of the granules. The granules of *P. boydii* lack a cementlike matrix. The central portion of the granules consists of loosely interwoven hyaline mycelium (Fig. 5).

Colonies grow rapidly and are floccose and white at first, becoming gray as conidia are produced. With age, the colonies become dark brown. The anamorphic state, *S. apiospermum*, produces conidia that are egg shaped to clavate, truncate at the tapered end, and subhyaline, becoming pale gray to pale brown in mass. Conidia are produced singly. They remain attached at the tips of conidiogenous cells or multiply from annellides (Fig. 6). Annellations can be detected at the tip of the conidiogenous cell as swollen rings. Occasionally, some isolates also produce a *Graphium* synanamorph, which is characterized by ropelike bundles of hyphae with annellidic conidiogenesis. The hyphae are fused into long stalks known as synnemata. The conidia produced are hyaline, cylindric to clavate, and truncate at the base (Fig. 7).

The ascocarps of the teleomorphic state may be produced when isolates are grown on cornmeal agar. The cleistothecia develop submerged in the agar and appear as black dots. They are spherical, nonostiolate, 140 to 200 μm in diameter, and often covered with brown, thick-walled, septate hyphae, 2 to 3 μm wide, with a wall 4 to 6 μm thick composed of two to three layers of interwoven, flattened, dark brown cells 2 to 6 μm wide. The cleistothecia open at maturity by an irregular rupture of the wall. The eight-spored asci are ellipsoidal to

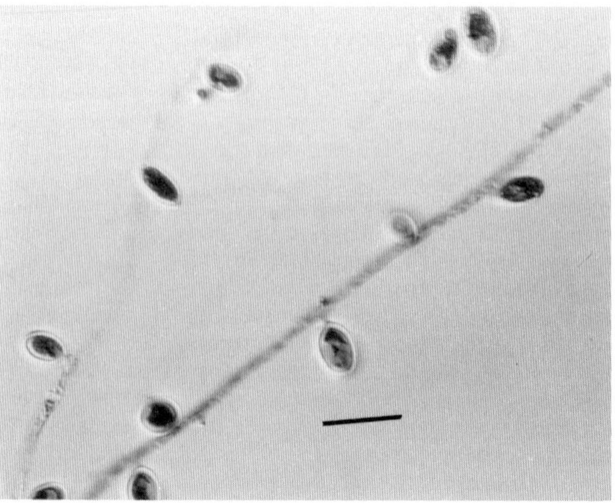

FIG. 6. *Scedosporium apiospermum* anamorph of *P. boydii.* Slide culture on cornmeal agar showing clavate, truncate conidia. Bar = 10 μm.

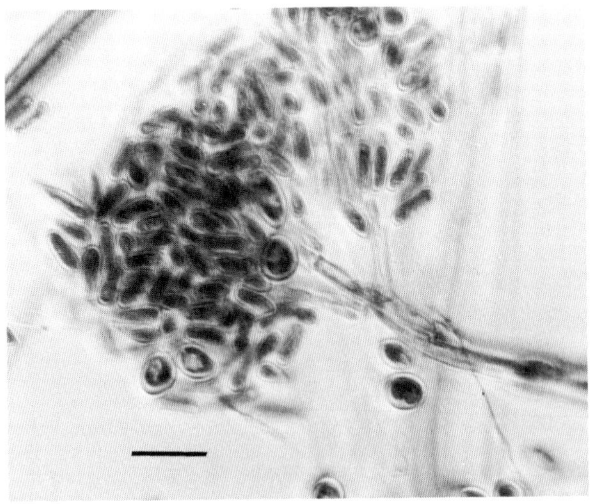

FIG. 7. *Graphium* anamorph of *Scedosporium apiospermum*. Slide culture showing bundles of hyphae (synnemata) and cylindric to clavate conidia. Bar = 10 μm.

nearly spherical. They measure 12 to 18 by 9 to 13 μm. The ascospores are ellipsoidal to oblate (football shaped), symmetrical or slightly flattened, and straw colored. They have two germ pores and measure 6 to 7 by 3.5 to 4 μm.

Even though *P. boydii* is homothallic, many clinical and soil isolates do not form ascocarps. Their identification, then, is based on the morphology of the conidial state alone. *P. boydii* is the commonest agent of mycetoma in humans as well as lower animals in the United States. It has been isolated frequently from manure, soil, and water. It is often encountered as a contaminant of respiratory specimens from patients with chronic lung disease. It is also isolated frequently from open, dirty wounds. Its isolation from such specimens does not always implicate *P. boydii* as an etiologic agent. On the other hand, *P. boydii* is known to cause necrotizing pneumonia and disseminated infections in immunocompromised patients. The significance of its isolation always should be determined after communication with the attending physician and pathologist.

Pyrenochaeta romeroi Borelli, 1959

Mycetomas caused by *P. romeroi* have been reported from Somalia, India, and South America (22, 28). *P. romeroi* produces soft to firm, black granules that are oval, lobulated, and sometimes vermiform. They resemble those of *M. grisea* (44).

In culture, colonies of *P. romeroi* are fast growing and floccose to velvety, with a gray surface and whitish margin. The reverse of the colony is black, with no diffusible pigment. The hyphae are hyaline to brown, septate, and branched. On nutritionally poor media, *P. romeroi* produces ostiolate, isolated or aggregated pycnidia, 50 to 160 by 40 to 100 μm, bearing subhyaline, elliptical pycnidiospores, 0.8 to 1.0 by 1.5 to 1.0 μm.

The close resemblance of the granules produced by *P. romeroi* to those produced by *M. grisea* and the morphological similarity of the pycnidia formed by some isolates of *M. grisea* and by *P. romeroi* suggest that these two species may be closely related. However, according to Murray and Buckley (35), the two species show serological differences that allow differentiation between them.

LITERATURE CITED

1. **Ajello, L.** 1962. Epidemiology of human fungus infections, p. 69–83. *In* G. Dalldorf (ed.), Fungi and fungous diseases. Charles C Thomas, Publisher, Springfield, Ill.
2. **Ajello, L.** 1978. Animal mycetomas—a review, p. 270–275. *In* Proceedings, Primer Simposio Internacional de Micetomas. Universidad Centro Occidental, Barquisimeto, Venezuela.
3. **Ajello, L., W. Kaplan, and F. W. Chandler.** 1980. Dermatophyte mycetomas: fact or fiction?, p. 135–140. *In* Superficial, cutaneous and subcutaneous infections. Scientific publication no. 396. Pan American Health Organization, Washington, D.C.
4. **Baylet, R., R. Camain, and M. Rey.** 1961. Champignons de mycétomes isolés des épineux au Sénégal. Bull. Soc. Med. Afr. Noire Lang. Fr. **6:**317–319.
5. **Borelli, D.** 1959. *Pyrenochaeta romeroi* n. sp. Rev. Dermatol. Venez. **1:**325–327.
6. **Borelli, D.** 1962. *Madurella mycetomi* y *Madurella grisea*. Arch. Venez. Med. Trop. Parasitol. Med. **4:**195–211.
7. **Borelli, D.** 1976. *Pyrenochaeta mackinnonii* nova species agente de micetoma. Castellania **4:**227–234.
8. **Borelli, D.** 1978. *Plenodomus avramii* nova species agente de micetoma, p. 116–126. *In* Proceedings, Primer Simposio Internacional de Micetomas. Universidad Centro Occidental, Barquisimeto, Venezuela.
9. **Borelli, D., R. Zamora, and G. Senabre.** 1976. *Chaetosphaeronema larense* nova specie agente de micetoma. Gac. Med. Caracas **84:**307–318.
10. **Brodey, R. S., H. S. Schryver, M. J. Deubler, W. Kaplan, and L. Ajello.** 1967. Mycetoma in a dog. J. Am. Vet. Med. Assoc. **151:**442–451.
11. **Butz, W. C., and L. Ajello.** 1971. Black grain mycetoma. Arch. Dermatol. **104:**197–201.
12. **Campbell, C. K.** 1987. *Polycytella hominis* gen. et sp. nov., a cause of human pale grain mycetoma. J. Med. Vet. Mycol. **25:**301–305.
13. **Chandler, F. W., W. Kaplan, and L. Ajello.** 1980. A colour atlas and textbook of the histopathology of mycotic diseases. Wolfe Medical Publications Ltd., London, England.
14. **Destombes, P., A. Poirier, and O. Nazimoff.** 1970. Mycoses profundes reconnues en 9 ans de pratique histopathologique à l'Institut Pasteur du Cameroun. Bull. Soc. Pathol. Exot. **63:**310–315.
15. **De Vries, G. A., G. S. De Hoog, and H. P. De Bruyn.** 1984. *Phialophora cyanescens* sp. nov., with *Phaeosclera*-like synanamorph, causing white-grain mycetoma in man. Antonie van Leeuwenhoek J. Microbiol. Serol. **50:**149–153.
16. **El-Ani, A. S.** 1966. A new species of *Leptosphaeria*, an etiologic agent of mycetoma. Mycologia **58:**406–411.
17. **El-Ani, A. S., and M. A. Gordon.** 1965. The ascospore sheath and taxonomy of *Leptosphaeria senegalensis*. Mycologia **57:**275–278.
18. **Emmons, C. W.** 1962. Soil reservoirs of pathogenic fungi. J. Wash. Acad. Sci. **52:**3–9.
19. **Etta, L. L. Van, L. R. Peterson, and D. Gerding.** 1983. *Acremonium falciforme* (*Cephalosporium falciforme*) mycetoma in a renal transplant patient. Arch. Dermatol. **119:** 707–708.
20. **Fahey, P. J., M. J. Utell, and R. W. Hyde.** 1981. Spontaneous lysis of mycetomas after acute cavitating lung disease. Am. Rev. Respir. Dis. **123:**336–339.
21. **Halde, C., A. A. Padhye, L. D. Haley, M. G. Rinaldi, D. Kay, and R. Leeper.** 1976. *Acremonium falciforme* as a cause of mycetoma in California. Sabouraudia **14:**319–326.
22. **Klokke, A. H., G. Swamidasan, R. Anguli, and A. Verghese.** 1968. The causal agents of mycetoma in South India. Trans. R. Soc. Trop. Med. Hyg. **62:**509–516.

23. **Mackinnon, J. E.** 1954. A contribution to the study of the causal organisms of maduromycosis. Trans. R. Soc. Trop. Med. Hyg. **48:**470–480.
24. **Mackinnon, J. E., I. A. Conti-Diaz, E. Gezuele, and E. Civila.** 1971. Datos sobre ecologia de *Allescheria boydii,* Shear. Rev. Urug. Pathol. Clin. Microbiol. **9:**37–43.
25. **Mackinnon, J. E., L. V. Ferrada, and L. Montemayor.** 1949. *Madurella grisea* n. sp., a new species of fungus producing the black variety of maduromycosis in South America. Mycopathol. Mycol. Appl. **4:**385–392.
26. **Mahgoub, E. S.** 1973. Mycetomas caused by *Curvularia lunata, Madurella grisea, Aspergillus nidulans,* and *Nocardia brasiliensis* in Sudan. Sabouraudia **11:**179–182.
27. **Mahgoub, E. S., and I. Murray.** 1973. Mycetoma. William Heinemann Medical Books Ltd., London, England.
28. **Mariat, F., P. Destombes, and G. Segretain.** 1977. The mycetomas: clinical features, pathology, etiology and epidemiology. Contrib. Microbiol. Immunol. **4:**1–39.
29. **Matsumoto, T., and L. Ajello.** 1986. No granules, no mycetomas. Chest **90:**151–152.
30. **Mayorga, R., and J. E. Close De Leon.** 1966. Sur une souche de *Madurella grisea* sporifere isolée d'un mycétome Guatemaltèque a grains noirs. Sabouraudia **4:**210–214.
31. **McGinnis, M. R., and A. A. Padhye.** 1977. *Exophiala jeanselmei,* a new combination for *Phialophora jeanselmei.* Mycotaxon **5:**341–352.
32. **McGinnis, M. R., A. A. Padhye, and L. Ajello.** 1982. *Pseudallescheria* Negroni et Fischer, 1943, and its later synonym *Petriellidium* Malloch, 1970. Mycotaxon **14:**94–102.
33. **Milburn, P. B., D. M. Papayanopulos, and B. M. Pomerantz.** 1988. Mycetoma due to *Acremonium falciforme.* Int. J. Dermatol. **27:**408–410.
34. **Montes, L. F., R. G. Freeman, and W. McClarin.** 1969. Maduromycosis due to *Madurella grisea.* Arch. Dermatol. **99:**74–79.
35. **Murray, I. G., and H. R. Buckley.** 1969. Serological differences between *Pyrenochaeta romeroi* and *Madurella grisea.* Sabouraudia **7:**62–63.
36. **Negroni, R.** 1970. Estudio micologico del primer caso de micetoma por *Phialophora jeanselmei* observado en la Argentina. Med. Cutanea **5:**625–630.
37. **Neilson, H. S., N. F. Conant, T. Weinberg, and J. F. Reback.** 1968. Report of a mycetoma due to *Phialophora jeanselmei* and undescribed characteristics of the fungus. Sabouraudia **6:**330–333.
38. **Pankovich, A. M., B. J. Auerbach, W. I. Metzer, and T. Barreta.** 1981. Development of maduromycosis (*Madurella mycetomi*) after nailing of a closed tibial fracture. A case report. Clin. Orthoped. Relat. Res. **154:**220–222.
39. **Punithalingam, E.** 1979. Sphaeropsidales in culture from humans. Nova Hedwigia **37:**119–158.
40. **Pupaibul, K., W. Sindhuphak, and A. Chindamporn.** 1982. Mycetoma of the hand caused by *Phialophora jeanselmei.* Mykosen **25:**321–330.
41. **Segretain, G.** 1964. Recherches sur l'écologie de *Madurella mycetomi* au Sénégal. Bull. Soc. Fr. Mycol. Med. **3:** 121–124.
42. **Segretain, G.** 1972. Epidémiologie des mycétomes. Ann. Soc. Belge Med. Trop. **52:**277–286.
43. **Segretain, G., and P. Destombes.** 1961. Description d'un nouvel agent de maduromycose, *Neotestudina rosatii,* n. gen., n. sp. isolé en Afrique. C.R. Acad. Sci. **253:**2577–2579.
44. **Segretain, G., and P. Destombes.** 1969. Recherches sur les mycétomes à *Madurella grisea* et *Pyrenochaeta romeroi.* Sabouraudia **7:**51–61.
45. **Segretain, G., and F. Mariat.** 1968. Recherches sur la présence d'agents de mycetomes dans le sol et sur les epineux du Senegal et de la Mauritanie. Bull. Soc. Pathol. Exot. **61:**194–202.
46. **Talwar, P., and S. C. Sehgal.** 1979. Mycetomas of North India. Sabouraudia **17:**287–291.
47. **Thammayya, A., and M. Sanyal.** 1980. *Exophiala jeanselmei* causing mycetoma pedis in India. Sabouraudia **18:** 91–95.
48. **Thianprasit, M., and A. Sivayathorn.** 1984. Black dot mycetoma. Mykosen **27:**219–226.
49. **Thirumalachar, M. J., and A. A. Padhye.** 1968. Isolation of *Madurella mycetomi* from soil in India. Hind. Antibiot. Bull. **10:**314–318.

Chapter 66

Diagnostic Parasitology: Introduction and Methods

JAMES W. SMITH AND MARILYN S. BARTLETT

Parasitic diseases continue to cause significant morbidity and mortality in the world, particularly in less-developed tropical and subtropical countries. In the United States, indigenous malaria was eradicated long ago, and indigenous nematode infections such as ascariasis, trichuriasis, and hookworm infection have markedly decreased in both incidence and severity. Some other infections are increasing. Giardiasis is a frequent public health problem, with outbreaks related to water supplies and day care centers for children. *Pneumocystis carinii*, *Cryptosporidium* species, *Strongyloides stercoralis*, *Enterocytozoon bienusi*, and *Toxoplasma gondii* are increasingly important causes of serious infections in immunocompromised hosts, especially those with AIDS (acquired immune deficiency syndrome).

The incidence of fecal parasites in specimens submitted to United States public health laboratories in 1978 (14) is summarized in Table 1. These figures do not represent prevalence in the United States population but show incidence in the fecal specimens submitted for parasite examination. Prevalence for most parasites is probably much lower than these figures indicate.

In addition to infections which are indigenous to the United States, a wide variety of infections may be seen in U.S. citizens who have traveled or worked in foreign countries, or in foreign nationals who are visiting or now residing in the United States. Many of these people, such as persons infected with malaria, may be asymptomatic for months or years before disease develops or relapses occur. Some people are recognized as having malaria only when a recipient of their blood develops transfusion-induced malaria or when a baby develops congenital malaria. Other diseases such as echinococcosis may require years before becoming clinically evident.

Efforts to eradicate parasite infections have had variable success. Sanitary fecal disposal, improved water supplies, and improved hygiene in food production and preparation have aided in the control of intestinal parasites. However, much of the earlier enthusiasm for the eradication of malaria has been tempered by the realization that malaria eradication is going to be difficult because parasites are becoming resistant to chemotherapeutic agents, mosquito vectors are becoming resistant to common insecticides, and the use of some insecticides may harm the environment. Human modifications of the environment, such as the building of dams and irrigation systems, have provided an appropriate environment for vectors such as snails and thus allowed diseases such as schistosomiasis to flourish in areas where these diseases had been uncommon. In addition, immunization programs for parasite infections have developed more slowly than was anticipated.

HOST-PARASITE RELATIONS

A knowledge of parasite life cycles is crucial in the understanding of the ways infection is acquired and spread, the pathogenesis of disease, and the ways in which disease might be controlled. Some parasites which infect only humans, such as *Enterobius vermicularis* (pinworm), have a narrow host specificity, whereas others such as *Trichinella spiralis* infect numerous species. When other animals harbor the same parasite stage as humans, these animal species may serve as reservoir hosts. Humans infected with a parasite stage usually seen in other animal species are referred to as accidental hosts.

In the simplest life cycle, a parasite stage from humans is immediately infective for other humans, as in pinworm infection or giardiasis. In other infections such as ascariasis or trichuriasis, a maturation period outside the body is required before the parasite is infective. However, for many parasite infections, a second or even a third host is required for completion of the life cycle. Hosts are defined as intermediate hosts if they do not contain the sexual stage and as definitive hosts if they do contain the sexual stage. Some protozoa, such as the amebae, flagellates, and hemoflagellates, do not have a recognized sexual stage. In the intermediate host, there may be massive proliferation of organisms, as occurs in humans harboring malaria parasites or snails harboring schistosome intermediate stages, or there may be no proliferation, as in mosquitoes which harbor microfilariae undergoing maturation. There may be proliferation in definitive hosts, as in mosquitoes harboring the sexual stage of malaria in which thousands of sporozoites are produced. There may be no proliferation, as in helminth infections in which one adult is developed from each infective larva; however, the adult helminths do produce numerous eggs or larvae.

In some helminth infections, a migration through various body tissues is essential for maturation, as in ascariasis or schistosomiasis, whereas in other infections the larva leaves the egg and simply matures in the intestinal tract, as in trichuriasis and enterobiasis. Host tissues involved vary depending upon the parasite. In severely immunocompromised patients, sites may be involved that are not involved in normal hosts.

Parasites of humans proliferate tremendously at certain stages, with thousands or even millions of forms being produced for every one that survives to perpetuate the parasite. Parasites may be quite hardy. For example, certain stages, particularly eggs and cysts, may survive for weeks or months in the environment.

Parasites often have developed unique ways of protection from the defense mechanisms of the host. These mechanisms include the ability to change antigenic characteristics so that although the host forms antibody,

TABLE 1. Incidence of intestinal parasites in 322,735 fecal specimens examined by state health department laboratories, 1978[a]

Parasite	No. of examinations	% of positive specimens
Protozoa		
Giardia lamblia	12,947	4.0
Entamoeba histolytica	2,409	0.8
Dientamoeba fragilis	1,880	0.6
Balantidium coli	7	
Isospora spp.	1	
Nonpathogenic	21,120	6.5
Nematodes		
Trichuris trichuria	5,481	1.7
Ascaris lumbricoides	4,630	1.4
Enterobius vermicularis	4,344	1.4
Hookworm	2,035	0.6
Strongyloides stercoralis	602	0.2
Trichostrongylus spp.	14	
Trematodes		
Clonorchis-Opisthorchis	205	0.06
Schistosoma mansoni	48	
Fasciola hepatica	1	
Paragonimus westermani	1	
Cestodes		
Hymenolepis nana	1,068	0.3
Taenia spp.	251	0.08
Diphyllobothrium latum	20	
Hymenolepis diminuta	12	
Dipylidium caninum	7	

[a] Adapted from *Centers for Disease Control: Intestinal Parasite Surveillance. Annual Summary, 1978* (issued August 1979). The survey does not include laboratories in Guam, Puerto Rico, or the Virgin Islands. One or more parasites were found in 14.7% of specimens. Percentages are not calculated for parasites identified less than 100 times.

the antibody does not react with the modified parasite; or the parasite may be coated with host antigens, as in schistosomiasis, so that the host does not recognize the parasite as foreign. Macrophages and both cell-mediated and humoral immunities appear to be important in the host responses to parasitic infections. Eosinophils are particularly important in the defense against tissue-invading helminths.

DIAGNOSIS OF PARASITIC INFECTIONS

The diagnosis of most parasitic infections is dependent upon the laboratory. For intestinal and blood parasites, morphologic demonstration of diagnostic stage(s) is the principal means of diagnosis, whereas for tissue infections, immunodiagnostic techniques are generally more important. During the early stages before diagnostic forms are produced (prepatent period), patients may be symptomatic. For example, patients may have pulmonary symptoms and eosinophilia due to ascaris larval migration at a time when there are no adults in the intestine and thus there are no eggs in feces. In such patients the physician may suspect parasite infection, but the actual diagnosis must be based on a clinical impression or immunodiagnostic tests, or diagnosis must await the production of diagnostic stages.

In establishing a diagnosis, the clinician places a great deal of trust in the laboratory. This trust can be misplaced if laboratory personnel are not competent to identify or exclude parasites. The literature clearly documents instances in which outbreaks have been overlooked due to incompetent laboratory diagnosis or in which inflammatory cells or other objects have been identified as parasites and outbreaks have been diagnosed when none existed (31). The results of proficiency-testing programs (43, 47) also suggest that laboratories have difficulty with the identification of some parasites, especially intestinal protozoa (Table 2).

Identification may be by gross examination for adult helminths or, more commonly, by microscopic examination for protozoa, helminth eggs, and larvae. The diagnostic forms of some parasites, such as the eggs of *Ascaris* spp., are present on a regular basis. Other forms, such as malaria parasites, *Taenia* eggs, or *Giardia* cysts, vary from day to day.

Most immunodiagnostic tests used today for parasitic infections detect antibody. In recent years, the sensitivity and specificity of many such tests have improved. A number of antigen detection tests and nucleic acid probes have recently been described and show promise. These are more thoroughly discussed in chapter 67 on nonmorphologic diagnostic methods. For those wishing to know more about clinical disease caused by parasites there are a number of excellent books (5, 10, 26, 33, 54, 56). Morphology of parasites in histologic sections is summarized in a recent book by Gutierrez (27).

LABORATORY PROCEDURES

Many methods for diagnostic parasitology have been described. There are advantages and disadvantages to each method. Some are particularly valuable for epidemiologic studies or for evaluations of new therapeutic agents, whereas other methods are used primarily for laboratory diagnosis. In this chapter we have selected from the numerous methods those which are widely used in this country and which are sensitive and relatively easy to perform. These methods should prove adequate for most laboratories. For additional procedures, laboratory manuals (3, 23, 41) or parasitology books (10, 36) should be consulted. When alternative methods

TABLE 2. Participant performance in College of American Pathologists parasitology survey program, 1973 through 1977[a]

Parasite	No. of specimens	Avg correct identification (%)
Formalin-fixed fecal specimens		
Ascaris lumbricoides eggs	6	90
Hookworm	6	92
Strongyloides stercoralis larvae	4	88
Trichuris trichuria eggs	6	93
Diphyllobothrium latum eggs	6	81
Hymenolepis diminuta eggs	5	91
Taenia sp. eggs	6	87
Paragonimus westermani eggs	5	83
Giardia lamblia cysts	8	65
Entamoeba coli cysts	9	88
No parasite seen	6	92
PVA-fixed specimens		
Entamoeba histolytica	5	73
Entamoeba coli	4	52
Endolimax nana	4	51
Negative for parasites	3	77

[a] See reference 47.

or methods for specific parasites are indicated, references will be given, but the methods will not be described.

PROCEDURES FOR INTESTINAL AND BILIARY PARASITES

Intestinal and biliary parasites are generally diagnosed by finding diagnostic stages in feces or other intestinal material such as duodenal or sigmoidoscopic aspirates. Studies have shown that the eggs of most parasites are uniformly distributed in the fecal mass due to the mixing action of the colon (38), although some, such as schistosome eggs, which originate in the distal colon, may be more numerous on the surface of formed fecal specimens. The distribution of protozoan forms is more variable. There may be fewer protozoan trophozoites in the first part of an evacuation than in the last because they have deteriorated while in the lower colon.

Collection and Handling of Fecal Specimens

The numbers and times of collection for fecal specimens depend somewhat on the diagnosis suspected. As a routine, because some organisms are shed in a variable pattern, it is advisable to examine multiple specimens before excluding parasites. The general recommendation is to collect a specimen every second or third day, for a total of three specimens. From a hospitalized patient, one specimen each day for 3 days may be more cost effective.

A number of substances may interfere with stool examination. Particulate materials such as barium, antacids, kaolin, and bismuth compounds interfere with morphologic examination, and oily materials such as mineral oil create small, refractile droplets that make examination difficult. Antimicrobial agents, particularly broad-spectrum antimicrobial agents, may suppress amebae. If any of these substances have been used, specimens should not be submitted until the substances have been cleared (generally 5 to 10 days). A fecal specimen may appear satisfactory by gross examination when there is still barium, etc., which can interfere with microscopic examination.

Fecal specimens are best collected into wide-mouthed, watertight containers with tight-fitting lids such as waxed, pint-sized ice cream cartons or plastic containers. Usually patients can defecate directly into such containers. Urine should not be allowed to contaminate specimens, as it is harmful to some parasites. If specimens are to be collected in a bed pan, the patient should urinate into a separate container before the specimen is collected. Toilet paper should not be included with the specimen. Stool should not be retrieved from toilet bowl water, as various free-living protozoa or nematodes in water might be confused with the parasites. In addition, water is harmful to some parasites such as schistosome eggs and amebic trophozoites. If the patient is producing formed specimens, stool may be collected by having the patient squat over waxed paper to defecate.

Purgation with sodium sulfate or buffered phospho-soda may be helpful for establishing the diagnosis of amebiasis (2, 60), giardiasis, or strongyloidiasis (21) in some patients. Purgation (requiring the order of a physician) is usually done after a series of fecal specimens have been negative. Prior arrangements must be made with the laboratory, and specimens must be collected during regular laboratory hours. The patient is given the appropriate salt solution orally. In approximately 1 to 1.5 h, the patient will begin to pass stool specimens, and each specimen should be promptly transported to the laboratory for examination.

Clinical information such as the suspected diagnosis, travel history of the patient, and clinical findings should be included on the requisition for all specimens submitted. In addition, the time the specimen was passed and the time it was placed in fixative should be noted. If the specimen is in fixative, the consistency of the original specimen should be stated, or a portion of unfixed specimen should be included with the fixed specimen.

A laboratory may have specimens placed in fixatives in the home or patient care area immediately after passage, may place portions of specimen in fixatives at the time they are received in the laboratory, or may examine the specimen unfixed. Many laboratories use a combination of these methods depending on the location of the patient, consistency of the specimen, time of day, and laboratory work load. Prompt examination or fixation is particularly important for soft, loose, or watery specimens, which are most likely to contain protozoan trophozoites (35). A number of kits for fecal collection, fixation, and/or laboratory processing are available from commercial sources and are widely used.

Formed specimens, which are likely to contain protozoan cysts or helminth eggs or larvae, can remain satisfactory for a number of hours at room temperature or overnight in a refrigerator. Soft and liquid specimens should be examined or placed in fixatives promptly (within 1 h). Specimens which cannot be examined or fixed promptly should be either refrigerated or left at room temperature. They should not be incubated, as incubation speeds the deterioration of the organisms. Feces for parasite examination must not be frozen and thawed.

The fixative system generally used is a two-vial technique with one vial containing 5 to 10% buffered Formalin and the other vial containing polyvinyl alcohol (PVA) fixative. A portion of the specimen is added to the fixative in a ratio of approximately 3 parts fixative to 1 part specimen and thoroughly mixed to ensure adequate fixation. If unfixed specimens are processed in the laboratory, fecal films may be prepared and immediately fixed in Schaudinn fixative. An alternative to Formalin is Merthiolate-iodine-Formalin (MIF), which fixes and stains at the same time (46); however, there are some reservations about this method (3). Sodium acetate-Formalin (59) is used by many laboratories. It is satisfactory for concentration and wet mount examination and for permanent staining. It has the advantages that it does not contain mercury which may present disposal problems, that only one vial is required, and that it is not as poisonous as mercury-containing fixatives; however, the permanent stains are not as good as those with Schaudinn's or PVA fixative. Most laboratories in the United States use the two-vial Formalin-PVA fixative combination.

Gross Examination of Feces

Specimens should be examined grossly to determine the consistency (hard, formed, loose, or watery), color, and presence of gross abnormalities such as worms, mucus, pus, or blood. It may be profitable to examine flecks of mucus, pus, or blood for parasites. If adult worms or portions of tapeworms are sought, the feces may be carefully washed through a wire screen. (Small worms may be difficult to see if gauze is used.) The identification characteristics of adult worms are not discussed in this chapter, so parasitology books should be consulted (10, 36).

Procedures for Microscopic Examination

The three principal microscopic examinations performed on stool specimens are direct wet mount, wet mount after concentration, and permanent stain. Although each examination can contribute to diagnosis, the yield of some methods is small with certain kinds of specimens. Procedures to be performed on various types of specimens are outlined in Table 3. As a minimum, formed specimens should be examined by a concentration procedure. Soft specimens should be examined by concentration and permanent stain and, if submitted fresh, by direct wet mount. Loose and watery specimens should be examined by wet mount and permanent stain. If specimens are received in fixative and the consistency is not known, concentration and permanent stain should be performed. Other examinations may be helpful (Table 3). Special procedures which may assist in the diagnosis of specific parasites are noted below in discussions of the parasites.

Calibration and use of an ocular micrometer

Size is important in the differentiation of parasites and is most accurately determined with a calibrated ocular micrometer; thus, each laboratory performing diagnostic parasitology must have such a micrometer.

An ocular micrometer is a disk on which is etched a scale in units from 1 to 50 or 100. To determine the micrometer value of each unit in a particular eyepiece and at a specific magnification, the unit must be calibrated with a stage micrometer. A stage micrometer has a scale 2 mm long ruled in five intervals of 0.01 mm (10 µm).

Calibration of the ocular micrometer

1. Insert the micrometer in the eyepiece so that the micrometer rests on the diaphragm, with the etched scale facing the eye. In many new microscopes, the micrometer can be dropped in and secured with a ring retainer. (It is helpful to have an extra ocular in which the micrometer may be retained.)
2. Place the stage micrometer on the microscope stage.
3. Focus on the etched scale. Since the micrometer must be calibrated for each objective, begin with the lowest magnification (e.g., ×10).
4. Align the two scales so that the zero points are superimposed (Fig. 1).

TABLE 3. Laboratory examination for various types of fecal specimens

Type of specimen	Method[a]		
	Direct wet mount	Concentration	Permanent stain
Unpreserved			
Formed	+	++	±
Soft	++	++	++
Loose and watery	++	±[b]	++
Preserved			
Formalin			
Formed or soft	+	++	−
Loose or liquid	++	±[b]	−
PVA fixative			
Formed	−	−	±
Soft, loose, or liquid	−	−	++

[a] ++, Essential for basic examination; +, recommended for basic examination; ±, optional for basic examination; −, not recommended for basic examination.

[b] Concentration is recommended if *Cryptosporidium* sp. is suspected.

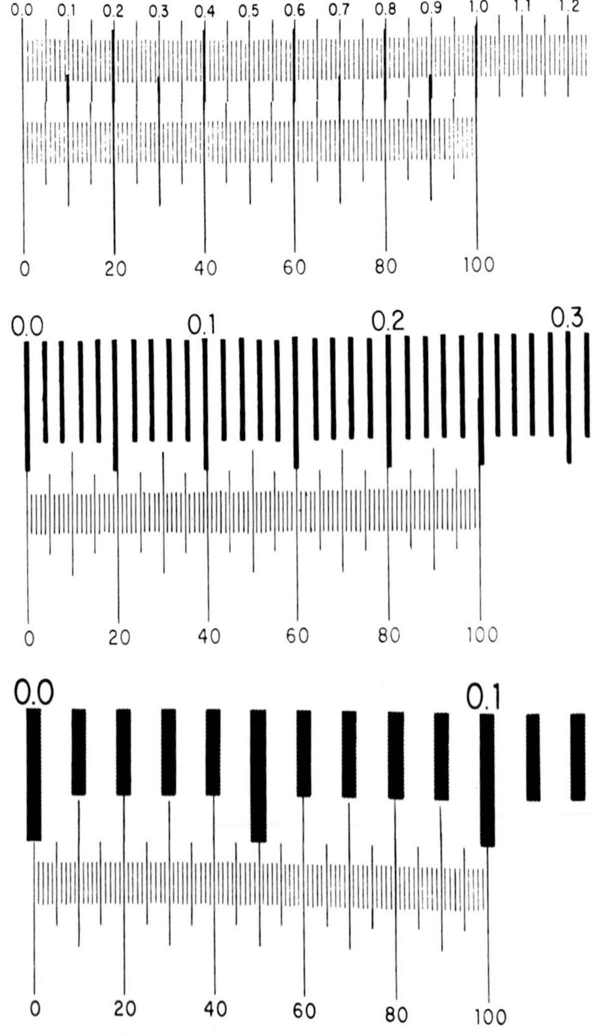

FIG. 1. Calibration of ocular micrometer. The ocular micrometer (lower scale) and stage micrometer (upper scale) appear like this under low (top), high dry (middle), and oil immersion (bottom) magnifications. In these examples, the values of one ocular unit are: low, 10 µm; high dry, 2.5 µm; and oil immersion, 1.0 µm.

5. Find a point far down the scales at which a line of the stage micrometer coincides with a line of the ocular micrometer. Count the number of ocular units and the number of stage units from zero to these coinciding lines.

6. Multiply the number of stage micrometer units by 1,000 to convert millimeters to micrometers.

7. Divide the product of step 6 by the number of ocular units to determine the value of an ocular unit.

Repeat the calibration for each objective. Keep a record of the unit value for each objective for each microscope used. Calibration must be done separately for each microscope and must be repeated if an ocular or objective is changed.

Use of the micrometer. Insert the eyepiece containing the calibrated ocular micrometer in the microscope. Count the number of ocular units which equal the structure to be measured. Multiply the number by the micrometer value of the ocular unit for the objective being used. If an ocular micrometer is properly used, parasites which are similar in appearance but different in size can be readily differentiated.

Direct wet mount

The direct wet mount made from unconcentrated fresh feces is most useful for the detection of the motile trophozites of intestinal protozoa and the motile larvae of *Strongyloides* spp. It is also useful for the detection of protozoan cysts and helminth eggs. For fixed feces, the direct wet mount may allow the detection of parasites which do not concentrate well. This method is also useful for the examination of specific portions of feces, such as flecks of blood or mucus.

Direct wet mounts are prepared by placing a small drop of 0.85% saline toward one end of a glass slide (2 by 3 in. [ca. 5 by 7.5 cm]) and a small drop of appropriate iodine solution (see below) toward the other end. With an applicator stick, a small portion of specimen (1 to 2 mg) is thoroughly mixed in each diluent, and a no. 1 cover slip (22 mm) is added. The density of fecal material should be such that newspaper print can be read with difficulty through the smear. The material should not overflow the edges of the cover slip. Grit or debris may prevent the cover slip from seating and may be removed with a corner of the cover slip or an applicator stick. Mounts may be sealed with Vaspar (50% petroleum jelly, 50% paraffin) which is melted on a hot plate (not over an open flame). A cotton applicator or small brush is used to apply small drops of Vaspar to opposite corners to attach the cover slip and then to seal it with even strokes. The amount of Vaspar on top of the cover slip should be minimal. Sealing slows drying and allows oil-immersion magnification to be used. Alternatively, drying can be slowed by placing wet gauze or paper toweling in a petri dish, laying portions of applicator sticks or glass rods on the moist material, laying the slide on the sticks or rods, and replacing the lid of the dish.

The iodine solution should be that of Dobell and O'Connor (1%) or a 1:5 dilution of Lugol iodine. Iodine solution, if too weak, will not stain organisms properly and, if too strong, will cause clumping of fecal material. Stock iodine solution should be stored in a tightly stoppered brown bottle away from sunlight. Keep the iodine and saline solutions in small dropper bottles, and replace (don't replenish) the solutions weekly. Iodine solution keeps longer if it is refrigerated. Iodine stain solution can be quality controlled by the observation of appropriate staining of positive clinical specimens or Formalin-fixed specimens kept for that purpose.

For the examination of wet mounts, the light of the microscope must be properly adjusted. To achieve optimal resolution, the condenser should be centered and focused for Kohler illumination (racked up). To achieve contrast of the objects in the field, light intensity is diminished with the iris diaphragm of the condenser rather than by lowering the condenser.

The entire saline wet mount cover slip should be systematically scanned at ×100 to ×200 magnification. Suspicious objects are confirmed at higher magnification. In addition, the preparation should be scanned at higher power (×400 to ×500) for several passes across the cover slip to look for protozoan cysts which might be missed with lower power. Screening a slide should take an experienced microscopist about 10 min. If debris is covering a suspicious object, the debris may be moved by pressing or tapping on the cover slip with an applicator stick. This pressure may also help in reorienting an egg, as when one is looking for an operculum or spine. The saline wet mount is best for the detection of helminth eggs and larvae, and it is especially good for protozoan cysts, which appear refractile. The principal usefulness of the iodine mount is to study the morphology of protozoan cysts, as this stain shows nuclear detail and glycogen masses (but does not stain chromatoid material). If suspicious objects are seen, they can be examined under oil immersion (×1,000). If definite or possible protozoan cysts or trophozoites are detected which cannot be identified in wet mounts, permanent stains are required.

A solution of buffered methylene blue (pH 3.6) may be used as a vital stain for the examination of fresh specimens for protozoa (42). The wet mount is prepared as described above, with buffered methylene blue substituted as diluent and 5 to 10 min allowed for the dye to become incorporated by the organisms before examination. Organisms become overstained in 20 to 30 min.

Concentration procedures

Concentration procedures are used to separate parasites from fecal detritus. These procedures are based on differences in the specific gravity of parasite forms and fecal material. In sedimentation, the parasite forms are heavier than the solution and are found in the sediment, whereas in flotation, solutions of high specific gravity are used, and parasite forms float to the surface. An initial washing step removes some of the soluble or finely particulate material, and straining removes larger portions of debris. A wide variety of sedimentation and flotation methods have been described. The Formalin-ethyl acetate modification of the Formalin-ether sedimentation technique and a zinc sulfate flotation technique are widely used and are the only methods described in this chapter. Both methods require that centrifugation be performed in centrifuges with free-swinging carriers. Squeeze bottles for Formalin, saline, or water simplify the processing of large numbers of specimens.

Formalin-ethyl acetate centrifugal sedimentation. The original procedure from which the Formalin-ethyl acetate centrifugal sedimentation technique was adapted was the Formalin-ether concentration method of Ritchie (44). The Formalin-ethyl acetate procedure (61) avoids problems with the flammability and storage of ether. This procedure can be performed on specimens which have been fixed in Formalin for a time or on specimens with Formalin added during the processing. The procedure can also be performed on material fixed in MIF fixative or sodium acetate-Formalin fixative.

The procedure with Formalin-preserved specimens is as follows.

1. Thoroughly mix the formalinized specimens.

2. Depending on the density of the specimen, strain a sufficient quantity through two layers of wet gauze into a 15-ml conical centrifuge tube to give the desired amount of sediment. (Wet gauze in a 4-oz [ca. 120-ml] conical paper cup with the tip cut off can be used for straining.)

3. Add tap water or saline, mix the solution thoroughly, and centrifuge it at 650 × *g* for 1 min. The amount of the resulting sediment should be about 1 ml. The amount of sediment may be adjusted by the addition of more feces and centrifugation again or by the addition of water, suspension again, the removal of an appropriate amount of material, and then recentrifugation.

4. Decant the supernatant and wash it again with tap water, if desired.

5. To the sediment, add 10% Formalin to the 9-ml mark, and mix the solution thoroughly.

6. Add 4 ml of ethyl acetate, stopper the tube, and shake the tube vigorously in an inverted position for 30 s. Remove the stopper with care.

7. Centrifuge the solution at 450 to 500 × *g* for 1 min. Four layers should result: ethyl acetate, plug of debris, Formalin, and sediment.

8. Free the plug of debris from the sides of the tube by ringing the tube with an applicator stick, and carefully pour the top three layers into a discard container. With the tube still tipped, use a swab to remove debris from the sides of the tube. This step is very important, for lipid droplets which reach the sediment make examination difficult.

9. Mix the remaining sediment with the small amount of fluid that drains back down from the sides of the tube (or add a drop of saline or Formalin). If mounts are to be prepared later, a small amount of Formalin may be added to the sediment and the tube may be stoppered.

10. Prepare wet mounts as described above, and examine them.

The procedure for Formalin-ethyl acetate concentration of fresh specimens is as follows.

1. Comminute a portion of stool about 1.5 cm in diameter in about 10 ml of saline or water.

2. Strain about 10 ml of the fecal suspension into a 15-ml conical centrifuge tube.

3. Centrifuge the suspension at 650 × *g* for 2 min. This step should provide about 1 ml of sediment. If not, adjust the amount of sediment as described above.

4. Wash the sediment again if desired.

5. To the sediment, add 10% buffered Formalin to the 9-ml mark, mix thoroughly, and allow the mixture to stand for 5 min or longer.

6. Proceed as for step 6 of the procedure for fixed specimens.

(Note that either saline or water can be used. Tap water will lyse *Blastocystis hominis*. If schistosomiasis is suspected, the specimen should be preserved in Formalin before concentration to prevent hatching.)

Zinc sulfate centrifugal flotation. The zinc sulfate concentration method originally described by Faust et al. (20) may be performed on unfixed or Formalin-fixed specimens, although the specific gravity of the zinc sulfate solution required differs. The disadvantages of the zinc sulfate concentration are: (i) dense schistosome eggs do not concentrate well; (ii) opercula often pop, and thus operculate eggs may be missed; and (iii) larvae and cysts may collapse. The modified procedure with Formalin-fixed feces (6) slows the collapse of larvae and cysts and largely prevents the popping of opercula. The advantages are that it leaves a rather clean background, has less grit than the sedimentation procedure, and is better for the concentration of some parasites, such as *Giardia* cysts.

The procedure for Formalin-preserved specimens (6) is as follows. The specific gravity of the zinc sulfate must be 1.20. Centrifugation must be performed in round-bottomed tubes such as 16-by-100-mm disposable tubes.

1. The Formalin-preserved fecal material is mixed, strained through one layer of cheesecloth into a conical paper cup, poured into the tube to a level about 1 cm from the top, and then centrifuged.

2. The tubes are centrifuged for 3 min at about 650 × *g*. There should be 1 to 1.5 cm of sediment.

3. Decant the supernatant from each tube, and drain the last drop against a clean section of paper towel.

4. To the packed sediment of each tube, add zinc sulfate to within 1 cm of the rim.

5. Insert two applicator sticks, and thoroughly mix the packed sediment.

6. Immediately centrifuge the suspension at 500 × *g* for 1.5 min and allow the centrifuge to stop without vibrations.

7. Very carefully transfer the tubes to a rack of the proper size, so that the tubes remain vertical. Do not disturb the surface films, which now contain the parasites. Allow the tubes to stand for 1 min to compensate for any movement. The countertop must be vibration free.

8. With a loop which is bent at a right angle, transfer to a slide (2 by 3 in. [ca. 5 by 7.5 cm]) 2 loops of surface material beside 1 drop of saline and 2 loops beside 1 drop of iodine. With the heel of the loop, mix first the saline and then the iodine with surface material. Cover each mixture with a 22-mm no. 1 cover slip. The slide should be made within 20 min.

9. To retard drying, place each prepared slide on a bent glass rod or portions of applicator sticks in a petri dish containing a damp paper towel. Petri dishes may be placed in the refrigerator if examination will be delayed. Alternatively, cover slips may be sealed with Vaspar.

The procedure with fresh specimens is as follows:

1. Comminute a fecal specimen about 1 cm in diameter in a tube (16 by 100 mm) half filled with tap water. Add additional water to within 1 to 2 cm of the top.

2. Centrifuge the tube at 650 × *g* for 1 min.

3. Discard the supernatant, and add a zinc sulfate solution of specific gravity 1.18 to within 1 cm of the rim.

4. Proceed as from step 5 above.

Sheather sugar flotation. Sheather sugar flotation is recommended for the concentration of *Cryptosporidium* cysts (15). Although these oocysts will concentrate when the Formalin-ethyl acetate or zinc sulfate technique is used, they are more readily detected with the Sheather sugar flotation, for they stand out sharply from the background in this solution of high specific gravity. This procedure may be performed on unfixed or Formalin-fixed feces. The procedure for Sheather sugar flotation is outlined below.

1. (a) Formed stool. Place approximately 0.5 g of stool in a tube (16 by 100 mm) about half full of Sheather sugar solution. Mix the solution thoroughly, and then add more sugar solution to within 1 cm of the top.

(b) Watery stool. Centrifuge the fecal specimen and mix 0.5 to 1 ml of sediment with Sheather solution as described above.

2. Centrifuge the solution at 400 × *g* for 5 to 10 min.

3. Remove the top portion of the sample with a wire loop bent at a right angle. Place several loopfuls on a glass slide (2 by 3 in.). Cover the specimen with a 22-mm cover slip, and examine the slide with a ×40 objective. Oocysts are found just beneath the cover slip and are refractile. Saline or iodine is not used in the preparation of these mounts.

Baermann concentration. The Baermann concentration technique (57) has greater sensitivity for the detection of *Strongyloides* larvae than do the standard concentration techniques described above. This technique is useful clinically for the diagnosis and monitoring of therapy of *Strongyloides* infections, and it is useful epidemiologically for the examination of soil for the larvae of nematode parasites.

A funnel with a clamped rubber tube on the stem is placed in a ring stand. A circular mesh screen is placed across the funnel approximately one-third from the top, a portion of coarse fabric such as muslin is placed on the screen, and feces is added. Tap water at 37°C is added so that the water just touches the feces. Let the specimen stand 1 h, remove 2 ml of fluid from the stem, and centrifuge the sample at 300 × *g* for 3 min. Prepare a wet mount of sediment, and examine it for larvae.

Hatching technique for detection of viable schistosome eggs. Place a large amount of feces (5 to 10 g) in a large flask (1 to 2 liters), and add water while mixing to break up the feces to a fine suspension. Bring the water level to 2 to 5 cm from the top of the flask. Cover the sides of the flask with foil or other material to shield all but the top of the liquid from light. Allow the flask to stand at room temperature for several hours. With a hand lens, examine the material at the top of the flask neck for swimming miracidia. Remove the miracidia with a Pasteur pipette for examination with a 10× objective. It is not possible to determine the species of schistosome from the miracidia.

Other concentration procedures. Concentration procedures have been described for feces preserved in MIF (11), sodium acetate-Formalin (59), or PVA fixative (23). MIF- or sodium acetate-Formalin-fixed feces may be used in place of Formalin-fixed feces in the Formalin-ethyl acetate concentration procedure. Some workers feel that organisms do not concentrate as well from material fixed in PVA fixative (13) or from material which has been in MIF for extended periods (3, 10).

If large amounts of specimen are to be concentrated, as when specimens of eggs are prepared for teaching, gravity sedimentation is usually used. The feces is thoroughly mixed in liquid (water, saline, or 10% Formalin) and allowed to settle in a sedimentation jar or funnel for several hours or overnight. Supernatant fluid is discarded, and the sediment is again suspended and allowed to settle. This procedure can be continued if desired until the supernatant is clear.

Permanent stains

Permanent stains of fecal smears are most needed for the detection and identification of protozoan trophozoites, but they are also used for the identification of cysts (22, 34, 55). Wet mounts of fresh feces, even with stains such as methylene blue, are not as sensitive for trophozoites and therefore do not substitute for permanent stains (24). It is sometimes difficult to identify cysts which are detected in wet mounts; thus, for each specimen, regardless of consistency, it may be worthwhile to fix a portion in PVA fixative or to prepare two fecal films fixed in Schaudinn fixative so that permanent stains can be performed if needed. Permanent stains also provide a permanent record and are easily referred to consultants if there are questions on identification.

A number of staining procedures have been described. Some stains, such as chlorazol black (25), require fresh specimens and are not widely used. A variety of stains for fecal smears preserved by Schaudinn or PVA fixative have been described, including various hematoxylin stains (3, 41).

The stain most widely used in the United States is the Wheatley trichrome stain (58), which is the only permanent stain described in this chapter. The trichrome staining procedure uses reagents with a relatively long shelf life and is easy to perform. The procedure is outlined below and in Table 4. Note that there are differ-

TABLE 4. Trichrome stain procedure

Step	Reagent	Staining time		Purpose
		PVA fixative	Schaudinn fixative	
1	70% alcohol plus iodine	10 min	1 min	Removal of mercuric chloride, hydration
2	70% alcohol	5 min	1 min	Removal of iodine, hydration
3	70% alcohol	5 min	1 min	Wash, hydration
4	Trichrome stain	6–8 min	2–8 min	Stain
5	90% alcohol acidified	5–10 s	Brief dip	Destain
6	95% alcohol	Rinse	Rinse	Stop destaining
7	95% alcohol	5 min	Rinse	Dehydration
8	Carbol-xylene	10 min	1 min	Clearing and dehydration
9	Xylene	10 min	1–3 min	Clearing

ences in staining times depending on whether the specimen is fixed in Schaudinn or PVA fixative, as penetration is slower in the latter.

Preparation of smears. (i) Unpreserved specimens with Schaudinn fixative

1. To prepare thin, uniform smears, place a drop of saline on a glass slide (1 by 3 in. [ca. 2.5 by 7.5 cm]). With an applicator stick, transfer a small, representative portion of the specimen to the drop of saline, and mix the two. Spread the solution into a film by rolling the applicator stick along the surface. Remove any lumps.

Before watery specimens are smeared, apply an adhesive such as serum or albumin to the slide. Liquid specimens may be centrifuged, and the sediment may be used for smear preparation.

2. Place fresh smears immediately into Schaudinn fixative. Do not allow the smears to dry at any time before they are stained. Smears should fix for at least 1 h at room temperature or for 5 min at 50°C; however, they can be left in fixative for several days. After fixation, slides may be kept in 70% alcohol indefinitely before they are stained.

(ii) Unpreserved specimens with PVA fixative

1. On a slide (1 by 3 in.), thoroughly mix 1 drop of unfixed specimen with 1 drop of PVA fixative.
2. Spread the specimen as described below.
3. Allow the smear to dry, preferably overnight, before it is stained.

(iii) PVA fixative-preserved specimens

1. Preserve 1 part specimen in 3 parts PVA fixative. Mix thoroughly. Fix for at least 1 h. Specimens keep indefinitely.
2. Add 1 drop of PVA-fixed specimen to a slide.
   (a) If there is little sediment, remove a portion of the sediment with a Pasteur pipette.
   (b) If there is abundant sediment, mix the specimen thoroughly, and add 1 drop of specimen to a slide with applicator sticks or a Pasteur pipette.
3. Spread the material over the center third of the slide by rolling the specimen with an applicator stick. Remove any lumps. The film should extend to both the top and bottom edges of the slide, as this helps prevent peeling.
4. Allow the slide to dry overnight at room temperature or 35°C. In an urgent situation the slide can be dried for 4 h at 35°C and then stained.

Trichrome staining procedure. Table 4 outlines the steps in the trichrome staining procedure.

Permanently stained slides may be mounted with a cover slip or may be air dried and examined after oil is added. Slides should be examined at a magnification of ×400 to ×500 or greater after they are scanned under lower power to find optimal areas. A 50× oil-immersion objective is particularly helpful, as it allows the easy use of a 100× oil-immersion objective for the detailed examination of organisms while allowing more rapid screening with a 50× objective. Oculars of 5× or 6× can provide the same result. A 20× dry objective may also assist in screening.

Permanently stained slides should be kept for 2 years.

Stain reactions. In an ideal stain, the cytoplasm of cysts and trophozoites is blue-green tinged with purple. *Entamoeba coli* cyst cytoplasm is often more purple than that of other species. Nuclear chromatin, chromatoid bodies, erythrocytes, and bacteria stain red or purplish red. Other ingested particles such as yeasts often stain green. Parasite eggs and larvae usually stain red. Inflammatory cells and tissue cells stain in a fashion similar to that of protozoa. Color reactions may vary from the above.

Incompletely fixed cysts may stain predominantly red, and organisms which have degenerated before fixation often stain pale green. Poor fixation due to an inadequate mixing of the specimen in fixative may result in both of these appearances. In some specimens, degeneration has occurred before the specimen is placed in fixative, either in the patient before the specimen was evacuated or because of delay in fixing the specimen.

Troubleshooting the trichrome stain. Except for problems with delayed or inadequate fixation as noted above, problems with the trichrome stain are usually related to reagents other than the stain. If crystalline material is apparent after the specimen is stained, the crystals are probably mercuric chloride in the fixative which was not adequately removed because the iodine in the alcohol-iodine solution was too weak or because the slide was in this solution too short a time. If crystals are present after treatment with proper-strength iodine-alcohol, they are present in the specimen, which is thus unsatisfactory, and another specimen should be requested.

If the stain appears washed out, it is likely that the slide was destained too much. This washed-out appearance can be either because the specimen was left too long in the acid-alcohol destain or because the alcohol wash after the acid-alcohol destain had become acidic as a result of transfer by previous slides.

The trichrome may become diluted by carry-over alcohol if more than 10 slides per day are stained in one Coplin jar. To restore the stain, the lid may be left off for several hours to allow alcohol to evaporate, and then the volume is replaced with new stain.

Control slides should be used to monitor the staining. Specimens containing protozoa are best for controls; however, feces containing inflammatory cells or added buffy-coat leukocytes also are satisfactory.

Restaining. Should the stain be unsatisfactory, the slide can be destained by placing it in xylene to remove the cover slip or immersion oil and then placing it in 50% alcohol for 10 min to hydrate the slide. Destain the slide in 10% acetic acid in water for several hours, and then wash it thoroughly first in water and then in 50 and 70% alcohols. Place the slide in stain for 8 min, and then complete the stain procedures. It is helpful to eliminate or shorten the destain step.

Acid-fast stain for *Cryptosporidium* sp. Acid-fast staining for *Cryptosporidium* sp. has recently become important because this parasite is now recognized as a cause of severe diarrhea in immunodeficient patients such as those with AIDS, and it can cause transient diarrhea in immunocompetent individuals. A variety of acid-fast and fluorochrome staining procedures have been described for *Cryptosporidium* spp. (12), and all the procedures appear to work. The modified acid-fast stain described is that used to stain *Nocardia* spp. in that it uses milder acid decolorization.

The following procedure (28) may be used on fresh or Formalin-fixed material or on material from concentration procedures. If the specimen is liquid, centrifuge it, and use the sediment to prepare a smear. Albumin may be required on slides to assist in adherence of fixed or concentrated material.

1. Pick a portion of material with an applicator stick, mix the material in a drop of saline, spread it on a glass slide (1 by 3 in.), and allow to dry.
2. Fix the dried film in absolute methanol for 1 min, and air dry the slide.
3. Flood the slide with Kinyoun carbol-fuchsin, and stain for 5 min.
4. Wash the slide with 50% ethyl alcohol in water, and immediately rinse it with water.
5. Destain the smear with 1% sulfuric acid for 2 min or until no color runs from the slide.
6. Wash the slide with water.
7. Counterstain the smear with Loeffler methylene blue for 1 min.
8. Rinse the slide with water, dry it, and examine the smear with oil immersion.

The results are that *Cryptosporidium* oocysts stain bright red and background materials stain blue or pale red.

Egg counts

Egg-counting methods are used in clinical studies to assess the intensity of infections (especially infections by intestinal nematodes) and the efficacy of therapeutic agents, and these methods are commonly used for epidemiologic studies. Methods used for scientific studies, such as Kato thick smear (30) or Stoll egg counting (53), require greater accuracy than methods used for patient care. The simplest, most practical method is to use a standard fecal suspension which contains approximately 2 mg of feces mixed in a drop of saline and covered with a cover slip. The entire cover slip is examined at a magnification of ×100, field by field, and the number of eggs is counted. For research work, the density of the smear can be standardized with a light meter (9), but this standardization is not essential for patient care. The number of eggs per cover slip provides a rough index of the severity of the infection.

Duodenal material

The examination of duodenal fluid or duodenal biopsy material may be useful for the diagnosis of giardiasis, strongyloidiasis, or other upper intestinal parasite infections in patients in whom parasites cannot be detected in the feces. In addition, duodenal fluid occasionally can be useful in showing whether helminth eggs are originating in the biliary tract or the intestinal tract. Duodenal material may be obtained by passing a tube through the nose and stomach into the upper small intestine and then aspirating enteric fluid. As an alternative, a string test (Enterotest, Hedeco Corp., Mountain View, Calif.) may be used (8). A weighted gelatin capsule attached to a string is swallowed, and the proximal end of the string is taped to the face of the patient. Over a period of several hours, helped with small sips of water, the string reaches the upper small intestine. After 4 to 5 h, the string is retrieved, and the material on the bile-stained portion is stripped from the string and examined for parasites with direct wet mounts or with permanent stains when wet-mount findings are questionable. Aspirated duodenal fluid is examined in a similar fashion. The material for permanent stains can be fixed in Schaudinn or PVA fixative, although the latter may adhere better to the slide. If questionable organisms are seen in the direct wet mount, the cover slip can be removed, the material can be mixed with a drop of PVA fixative, and a film can be made for later permanent staining.

A duodenal biopsy can be used to demonstrate *Giardia* organisms. A biopsy is usually obtained by a swallowed biopsy capsule. In searching for *Giardia* spp., it is generally preferable to make both impression smears and sections of biopsy tissue. *Giardia* spp. are usually present in mucus or attached to epithelium rather than in tissue. Biopsies occasionally can confirm a diagnosis of strongyloidiasis or cryptosporidiosis.

Sigmoidoscopic material

Materials obtained by sigmoidoscopy may be helpful in the diagnosis or monitoring of amebiasis, schistosomiasis, or cryptosporidiosis. Patients suspected of having amebiasis may have ulcerations of the colon which can be visualized by sigmoidoscopy or colonoscopy. Scrapings or aspirates of material from ulcers can be examined by direct wet mounts and permanent stains as described above. The finding of typical, erythrophagocytic, motile trophozoites in direct wet mounts or in permanently stained preparations allows a diagnosis of amebiasis. Material is best aspirated with a pipette or scraped with an instrument. Swabs should not be used, as the parasites may be killed or trapped by swab material.

Biopsy material for amebiasis should be processed for surgical pathology and then examined for ulcers containing amebae. The periodic acid-Schiff stain counterstained with hematoxylin is particularly helpful because amebae stain more intensely with periodic acid-Schiff stain than do inflammatory cells, and amebae show typical amebic nuclei. Of course, there are no amebic cysts in tissue.

Biopsy material for schistosomiasis is better examined in teased preparations than in sections, as the entire thickness can be examined at once, and the viability of eggs can be determined by observation of movement of the larvae within the eggs (32).

In cryptosporidiosis, biopsy material shows organisms at the luminal surface of the epithelial cells, but the organisms are small, and the study of structural detail requires electron microscopy.

Abscess material

Abscesses suspected of being caused by *Entamoeba histolytica* may be aspirated, and the material may be submitted to the laboratory. The last material aspirated is most likely to contain amebae. Material may be examined microscopically in wet mounts and permanent stains, and in addition, it can be cultured for amebae if bacteria are also added to the culture as described below. Abscess material is often thick and difficult to examine. It may be treated with streptokinase and streptodonase enzymes to liquefy the specimen.

1. Reconstitute streptokinase and streptodornase (Varidase; Lederle Laboratories, Pearl River, N.Y.) per the instructions of the manufacturer.
2. Add 1 part enzyme solution to 5 parts aspirated material.
3. Incubate the mixture at 35 to 37°C for 1 h. Shake the mixture at intervals.
4. Centrifuge the mixture at 300 to 400 × *g* for 5 min.
5. The sediment may be used for microscopic ex-

aminations for amebae (wet mounts and permanent stains) and for the culture of amebae.

Cellophane tape

Cellophane tape is used for finding the eggs of *Enterobius vermicularis* or *Taenia* species from the perianal area. The tape used must be clear cellophane and not slightly cloudy or opaque. The procedure for obtaining specimens is outlined in Fig. 2. Alternatively, a Vaspar swab may be used (37, 41). Specimens from more than 1 day may be required to diagnose light infections (45).

Examination of cellophane tape

1. If the specimen is difficult to examine, raise the tape from the front of the glass slide, add a drop of toluene to the slide, and replace the tape smoothly with an applicator stick. (Remember, *Enterobius vermicularis* and *Taenia solium* eggs are infective!)
2. Examine the entire tape, including the edges, with ×100 magnification (10× objective).
3. Confirm suspicious objects with high-dry objectives (40× to 50×).

Culture for amebae

Cultures for amebae have improved detection in some studies (19, 39), but they are not widely used. Although *Giardia* spp. have been cultured in research laboratories, cultures are not useful for diagnosis.

A variety of culture media for amebae have been described, and some may be purchased from commercial medium manufacturers. The method described here

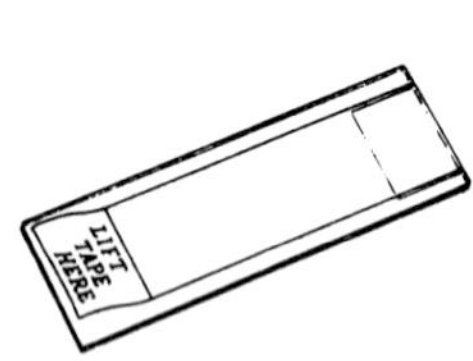

a. Cellulose-tape slide preparation

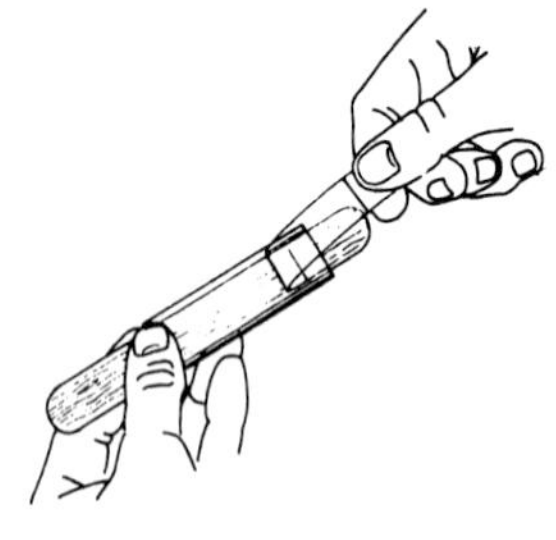

b. Hold slide against tongue depressor one inch from end and lift long portion of tape from slide

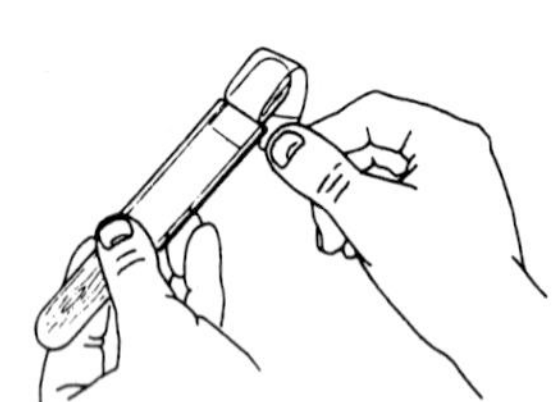

c. Loop tape over end of depressor to expose gummed surface

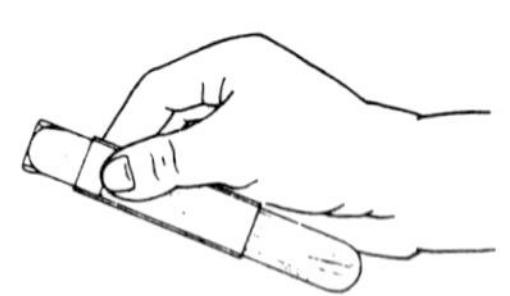

d. Hold tape and slide against tongue depressor

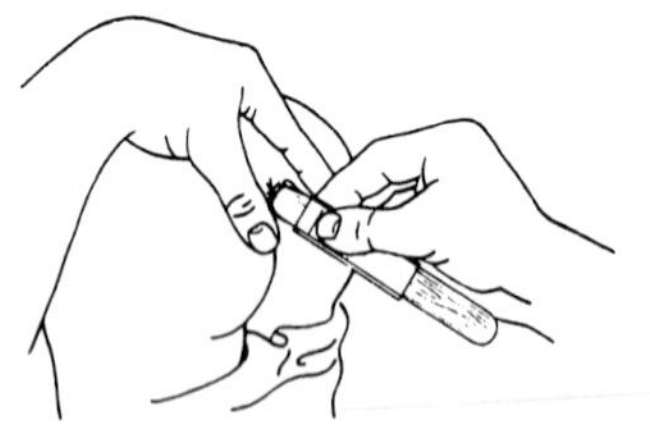

e. Press gummed surfaces against several areas of perianal region

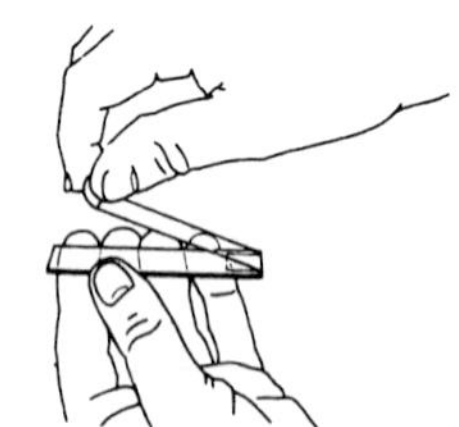

f. Replace tape on slide

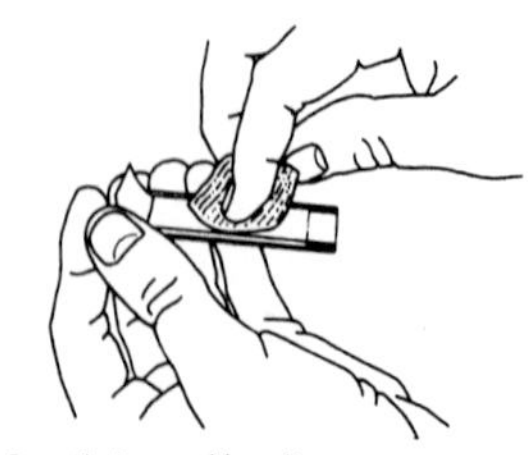

g. Smooth tape with cotton or gauze

Note: Specimens are best obtained a few hours after the person has retired, perhaps at 10 or 11 P.M., or the first thing in the morning before a bowel movement or bath.

FIG. 2. Use of cellulose tape preparation for the diagnosis of pinworm infections. From Melvin and Brooke (41).

uses the modified charcoal agar slant diphasic medium described by McQuay (39).

1. Place 3 ml of sterile 0.5% phosphate-buffered saline on a charcoal agar slant.
2. Add approximately 30 mg of sterile rice starch to the tube.
3. Warm the medium to 35°C before it is inoculated.
4. (a) Inoculate the medium with fecal specimen (approximately 0.5 ml of liquid specimen or a 0.5-cm sphere of formed specimen) which is mixed with the saline overlay.

   (b) If abscess material is cultured, bacteria must be inoculated into the culture in addition to the inoculation with 0.5 ml of specimen. A heavy inoculum with *Clostridium perfringens* or *Escherichia coli* is satisfactory.
5. Incubate the culture at 35°C.
6. At 24 and 48 h, remove 1 drop of liquid from the lowest point of the overlay, and prepare a wet mount.
7. Examine the wet mount for amebae.
8. Permanent stains can be prepared by the fixation of sediment in PVA fixative, with the subsequent preparation of smears and staining.

Larval maturation

Larval maturation studies, sometimes referred to as cultures, can be performed on fecal specimens applied to wet filter paper. Nematode larvae such as *Strongyloides* spp. or hookworm mature to the filariform stages in the culture container and migrate from feces into water, where they are detected microscopically. The procedure can be performed in a petri dish with a square of filter paper or in a large test tube with a strip of filter paper (3, 10, 41).

1. Smear approximately 0.5 g of feces on the filter paper.
2. (a) For the tube method, insert the filter paper strip into the tube so that the bottom of the strip is in 3 ml of water. The feces-smeared portion of the strip need not be immersed in the water.

   (b) For the petri dish method, place feces on one half of a piece of filter paper. Lay the feces-bearing end of the filter paper on a glass rod or a portion of an applicator stick in the petri dish. Add approximately 3 ml or sufficient water so that the feces-free end of the filter paper is in the liquid.
3. Leave the tube or dish at room temperature in the dark. Add water as needed to ensure that the filter paper is in contact with the water.
4. Examine the liquid for larvae either by direct microscopic examination with an inverted microscope or by examination of a wet mount of sediment from the liquid. With the petri dish method, the surface of the feces also may be examined with a dissecting microscope.
5. Examine the specimen on days 2, 3, 5, and 7. *Strongyloides* filariform larvae are likely to be found on days 2 and 3, and hookworm larvae may be found on days 5 through 7. Larvae are identified by their morphological characteristics.

Adult worms

Adult worms, or objects suspected to be adult worms, may be submitted to the laboratory. The laboratory must determine if these are helminths and, if so, if they are parasites. Identification characteristics are described in standard references (10). Tapeworm proglottids, particularly those of the *Taenia* species, are difficult to differentiate grossly unless they are cleared so that the internal structure can be seen and the number of lateral uterine branches can be counted. One procedure for clearing the proglottids is outlined below.

Clearing *Taenia* proglottids and other helminths. Proglottids are first relaxed by placing them in warm saline (56°C) for 1 h and then cleared by immersion in carbol-xylene while they are kept flat. One way is to press a proglottid between two glass slides held together with membrane clips or string. Frosted slides are easier to use. Clearing takes from several hours to overnight.

The proglottid is examined under a dissecting microscope or with a hand lens, and the uterine branching is observed. Glycerine and beechwood creosote can also be used with good results. Cleared proglottids may be mounted or stained if desired.

Small nematodes may also be cleared in carbol-xylene or beechwood creosote and mounted in Permount or balsam. This method is particularly good for hookworm adults.

BLOOD AND TISSUE PARASITES

Blood and tissue parasites whose diagnostic forms circulate in the peripheral blood are generally diagnosed by the demonstration of parasites in Giemsa-stained thick or thin films of blood. Special concentration techniques may be helpful for the diagnosis of some diseases such as filarial or trypanosomal infections. Other tissue parasites which do not circulate in the blood may be diagnosed by the detection of parasites in skin snips, lesion scrapings, body fluids, or biopsy material or by the detection of antibody or antigen in serum or other body fluids.

Collection and Handling of Specimens

Blood

The timing of the collection of blood specimens depends on the parasite disease suspected. For example, for certain filarial infections, specimens are best obtained between 10:00 p.m. and midnight, whereas for other infections, specimens are best obtained during the day. In malaria, the numbers and stages of parasites in the peripheral blood vary with different parts of the cycle.

Blood films are best made from blood which is not anticoagulated, such as that obtained from finger stick or ear lobe puncture. Anticoagulants may interfere with parasite morphology and staining. Care should be taken that the alcohol disinfectant is allowed to dry before the area is punctured, or there may be fixation of erythrocytes, which will interfere with the preparation and staining of thick films. Both thick and thin films can be prepared from blood obtained by venipuncture, although it is best if the blood remaining in the needle of the venipuncture device is used, because it is anticoagulant free. Thick and thin films can be prepared from blood that is anticoagulated, but the staining characteristics are not as good. EDTA-anticoagulated blood is better for staining than citrate- or heparin-anticoagulated blood.

Both thick and thin blood films are useful. Thick films are more sensitive because the same amount of blood can be examined in a thick film in 5 min as can be examined in a thin film in 30 min. However, thin films allow the study of the effects of parasites on erythrocytes and provide better parasite morphology.

Thick and thin films may be prepared on separate slides or on the same slide, with the thick film at one end and the thin film at the other end.

The thick film is prepared by spreading 1 drop or puddling several small drops of blood into an area approximately 1.5 cm in diameter. A properly prepared thick film should be thin enough so that newspaper print can barely be read through it. If the film is too thick, it will fragment and peel, and if the film is too thin, the increased sensitivity will be lost. Thick films should be allowed to dry overnight and should be stained within 3 days. They must not be heated, and they should be protected from dust. If the erythrocytes are fixed, they will not dehemoglobinize. If prompt examination is required, prepare a slightly thinner thick film, dry it for 1 h, and stain it.

The thin film is prepared in the same manner as a film for a differential leukocyte count. A small drop of blood is placed on one end of a microscope slide. A second slide held at an acute angle of 30 to 45° is backed into the drop of blood, which spreads along the junction of the slides. The spreader slide is then pushed along the slide, and it pulls the drop of blood along behind the angled edge of glass. A properly prepared thin film should have a significant area near the end which is only one erythrocyte thick and in which the erythrocytes show good morphology. The angle and speed of the spreader slide and size of the drop of blood will influence the thickness and size of the film.

Slides with only a thin film can be fixed by being immersed in absolute methyl or ethyl alcohol for 1 min and allowed to air dry. If the thick film is on one end of the slide and the thin film is on the other end, the thin film is fixed by a brief flooding or by immersion in alcohol and allowed to air dry, while the thick film is protected from alcohol or alcohol fumes. In a well-ventilated area, the slide may be dried vertically with the thick film up or horizontally after the thick film is covered with a dry paper towel.

Thick and thin films are best stained with Giemsa stain, as it provides the most detailed and intense staining of parasites. Wright stain or various rapid Giemsa stains can be used for thin films but not for thick films. Wright stain contains alcohol, which will fix the erythrocytes. Wright stain and rapid Giemsa stains do not stain parasites as well as Giemsa stain. The staining procedure is outlined below.

Tissue

Biopsy or necropsy tissue may be examined by histology sections or impression smears.

To prepare impression smears (49), tissue should be blotted to remove as much blood or other fluid as possible and then pressed against glass slides (1 by 3 in.) to make a series of impressions. Tissue should be dry enough so that it sticks to the slide and leaves an irregular film on the slide. Similar impressions may be made on multiple slides from the same portion of tissue. Portions of biopsy tissue with different gross appearances can be used with the impressions from each portion placed in a longitudinal row. Impressions must be close together, preferably with slight overlapping to make slide scanning easier. Impressions from small fragments may be placed in a small area (1 cm in diameter). After being dried, the area with impressions may be circled with a diamond marker to facilitate the location and scanning of the material. Fixatives and stains appropriate for the parasites suspected are used. If amebiasis is suspected, impression smears must be fixed promptly in Schaudinn fixative and not allowed to air dry. For most other parasites, the slides are allowed to dry before fixation in methyl alcohol. Giemsa is the usual stain, but other stains such as methenamine silver or hematoxylin may be used depending on the parasite suspected.

Aspirates of bone marrow or spleen

Aspirates of bone marrow or spleen may be useful in the diagnosis of infections such as leishmaniasis, trypanosomiasis, and occasionally malaria. In such instances, Giemsa stains of alcohol-fixed bone marrow films are most useful. Splenic aspiration is rarely performed in the United States because it is dangerous.

Fluids

Fluids such as tissue aspirates, cyst fluid, bronchial washings, cerebrospinal fluid, pleural fluid, and peritoneal fluid can be examined directly, or they can be centrifuged and the sediment can be examined by wet mounts or stains (or both), depending on the parasite suspected, as described above for abscesses or tissue.

Skin snips

Skin snips may be useful in the diagnosis of microfilarial infections such as onchocerciasis in which the parasites circulate in the skin and not the blood. A small (2-mm) skin snip is taken with a needle and a knife. The needle point is stuck into the skin, and the skin is raised. With a sharp knife or razor blade, the skin is excised just below the needle. Alternatively, a scleral punch may be used. The skin snip is then placed in a small volume (0.2 ml) of saline in a tube or a microtiter well, teased, and allowed to stand for 30 min or more. The microfilariae migrate from the tissue into the saline, which is then examined microscopically to demonstrate the wiggling microfilariae.

Concentration Procedures for Blood

A number of procedures have been described for the concentration of blood specimens. Most of these procedures have been developed to diagnose filarial infections.

The three most widely used methods are membrane filter (17, 18), saponin lysis (40), and Knotts concentration (29). Procedures for the first two methods will be given here, as these methods are the most sensitive. Membrane filter techniques use 5- or 3-μm filters produced by Millipore Corp., Bedford, Mass., or Nuclepore Corp., Pleasanton, Calif. Both filters give satisfactory results, but the procedures with the Nuclepore filters do not require the lysis of erythrocytes (1). Parasites on filters are often not as suitable for morphologic study as those in thick films.

Membrane filter concentration for filariae

1. Collect approximately 7 ml of blood in EDTA.
2. With a syringe and firm pressure, pass 5 to 7 ml of blood through a 5-µm Nuclepore filter held in a Swinney adapter.
3. Wash the membrane several times with a small amount of distilled water or physiologic saline.
4. The moist filter may be examined directly or fixed and stained in the usual fashion for a thin blood film.

Saponin lysis concentration for filariae

The saponin lysis method (40) can be performed on either EDTA- or citrate-anticoagulated blood. Saponin solution to lyse erythrocytes is available in most laboratories for use with automated hematology instruments.

1. Centrifuge up to 10 ml of blood at 150 × *g* for 10 min.
2. Remove and discard the plasma.
3. Mix the packed erythrocytes with 50 ml of 0.5% saponin solution in 0.85% saline.
4. Mix the solution at intervals for 15 min.
5. Centrifuge the solution at 650 × *g* for 10 min.
6. Decant and discard the supernatant (there should be about 1 ml of sediment).
7. Spread several drops of sediment on a glass slide (1 by 3 in.), and examine two such uncovered wet mounts for motile microfilariae. Allow the wet mounts to dry before they are fixed and stained.
8. Prepare four or five similar wet mounts and examine them as described above. To each slide, immediately add 2 drops of 1% acetic acid solution and mix it well (microfilariae will be killed and straightened). Allow the slide to air dry.
9. Dip the dried slides in buffered methylene blue-phosphate solution.
10. Rinse the slides in distilled water, and let them air dry.
11. Stain the mounts for 10 min in a 1:20 dilution of Giemsa stain in buffered water.
12. Examine the slides microscopically.

Staining Procedures

Giemsa stain procedure

The procedures for staining thick and thin films differ. Staining is usually done in a Coplin jar. The stain must be made fresh each day.

Stain slides with only a thin film as follows.

1. Fix and dry the blood film as described above.
2. Prepare a 1:40 dilution of stock Giemsa stain in neutral buffered water (pH 7.0 to 7.2) (generally, 2 ml of Giemsa stock plus 38 ml of buffered water with 0.01% Triton X-100).
3. Stain the film for approximately 60 min (the time, which will vary slightly with different lots of stock Giemsa stain, can be determined by the staining of leukocytes and erythrocytes).
4. Wash the slide briefly by dipping it in buffered water.
5. Air dry the slide in a vertical position.

Note that, alternatively, a 1:20 dilution for 20 to 30 min may be used.

Stain slides with only a thick film as follows.

1. Do not fix the slide.
2. Prepare a 1:50 dilution of stock Giemsa stain in neutral buffered water (pH 7.0 to 7.2).
3. Stain the film for approximately 50 min (the optimal time may vary with different lots of stain).
4. Wash the slide by placing it in buffered water for 3 to 4 min.
5. Air dry the slide in a vertical position.

For combination thick and thin films, the procedure is as follows.

1. Fix the thin film but not the thick film as described above.
2. Stain the film in a 1:50 dilution of Giemsa stain in neutral buffered water (pH 7.0 to 7.2) for approximately 50 min.
3. Rinse the thin film briefly by dipping it in buffered water. Wash the thick film by immersing it in buffered water for 3 to 5 min.
4. Dry the slide in a vertical position with the thick film down.

For staining cysts of *Pneumocystis carinii*, rapid methenamine silver stain or toluidine blue O stain are recommended (see chapter 122, Reagents and Stains).

Culture Procedures for Blood and Tissue Parasites

Culture procedures have been developed for a number of blood and tissue parasites, but these procedures are used primarily in research. The culturing of *Leishmania* spp. and *Trypanosoma cruzi* may be helpful for diagnosis, and the procedures are easy to use (3).

Biopsy or blood specimens may be cultured for *Leishmania* spp. or *T. cruzi* with Novy-MacNeal-Nicolle medium. Biopsy specimens are ground in a small amount of saline. Biopsies from skin lesions or other tissues which may contain bacteria may have penicillin (0.1 ml of 1,000 U/ml) added to the medium with the inoculum. The inoculum is 1 drop of ground tissue or blood. Incubate the culture at room temperature (22°C), and at days 3 and 7, examine a direct mount of liquid from the bottom of the slant at ×400 magnification. These cultured organisms are potentially infective for humans.

URINE

Urine specimens usually are examined for the eggs of *Schistosoma haematobium* or the trophozoites of *Trichomonas vaginalis*, although occasionally the larvae of *Strongyloides stercoralis* may be found in urine of patients with hyperinfection syndrome. Urine is the usual specimen for the diagnosis of *Trichomonas* infection in males. See below (Vaginal Material) for culture method. Urine is centrifuged, and the sediment is examined microscopically.

SPUTUM

Sputum may be examined to diagnose *Paragonimus* infection or hyperinfection due to *Strongyloides stercoralis*. Occasionally an amebic abscess or hydatid cyst may rupture, and amebic trophozoites or hydatid sand, respectively, may be found in sputum. *Entamoeba histolytica* must be differentiated from *Entamoeba gingivalis*, which may be found in the oral cavity of over 30% of people (16). Occasionally, the migrating larvae of ascarids, strongyloides, or hookworm can be found.

Sputum may be examined directly by wet mount or treated with a mucolytic agent such as *N*-acetyl-cysteine and then concentrated by simple centrifugation, with subsequent examination of the sediment.

Specially induced sputum can be useful for diagnosis of *Pneumocystis* infection in patients with AIDS but requires collection of specimens by specially trained personnel and experienced laboratory personnel to process and evaluate the material. Bronchoalveolar lavage is the preferred specimen if the above conditions are not fulfilled.

VAGINAL MATERIAL

Trichomonas vaginalis frequently infects the vagina, and *Enterobius vermicularis* adults or eggs occasionally may be found. Direct wet mounts of vaginal material for typical, tumbling *Trichomonas vaginalis* organisms are widely used and generally allow the diagnosis of symptomatic infection, but wet mounts are not as sensitive as culture methods.

Vaginal material is best submitted as liquid in a tube, although swabs submitted in a small amount of saline may be used. A drop of the material is covered with a cover slip and examined with reduced light. To culture, 1 or 2 drops of urine sediment or vaginal exudate are inoculated into tubes of warmed, modified Diamond medium. If vaginal swabs are submitted, the swab is immersed in the medium and pressed against the side of the tube to express material. Tubes are incubated at 35°C, and drops of culture are examined by wet mount at 48 and 72 h for motile trophozoites.

TABLE 5. Handling of specimens for referral

Specimen	Handling
Feces, for:	
Helminths	Fix in 10% Formalin.
Protozoa	Fix a portion in 10% buffered Formalin and either fix a portion in PVA fixative or prepare three Schaudinn-fixed fecal films.
Cryptosporidium spp.	Fix a portion in 10% buffered Formalin.
Material from suspected amebic abscess	Place the last material aspirated in a sterile tube and send it on ice for culture (do not freeze). Prepare Schaudinn-fixed films, or fix a portion in PVA fixative. Obtain serum for serology.
Duodenal aspirate	Centrifuge, and remove the supernatant. Prepare two films from sediment. Fix in Schaudinn or PVA fixative. Preserve the remainder of sediment in 10% Formalin.
Urine, for:	
Trichomoniasis	Centrifuge. Cover the sediment with sterile saline and send it on ice (not frozen) for direct mounts and culture.
Schistosomiasis	Centrifuge entire midday urine. Add an equal volume of 10% buffered Formalin to the sediment.
Sputum, for:	
Nematode larvae or *Paragonimus* eggs	Break up mechanically or digest 1 part sputum plus 5 parts 3% NaOH for 1 h. Centrifuge, and preserve the sediment in an equal volume of 10% buffered Formalin.
Amebae	Prepare films fixed in Schaudinn fixative, or fix a portion in PVA fixative.
Blood	
Malaria and babesiosis	Send unstained and, if available, Giemsa-stained thick and thin films. Fix thin film (but not thick) in alcohol before it is sent.
Filariasis	Send 5 ml of citrate- or EDTA-anticoagulated blood on ice (not frozen). Unfixed thick films may be sent in addition. Send serum for serologic tests.
Trypanosomiasis	Send 5 ml of anticoagulated blood as for filariasis (above). Send fixed thin films.
Cerebrospinal fluid	
Trypanosomes, *Toxoplasma, Leishmania,* trichinella	Send on ice (not frozen).
Free-living amebae	Send in a sterile container without refrigeration.
Sigmoidoscopic material	Fix films in Schaudinn fixative or mix material with PVA fixative and prepare film.
Tissue	For impression smears when *Entamoeba histolytica* is suspected, fix in Schaudinn or PVA fixative. When *Toxoplasma, Leishmania, Pneumocystis,* or *Trypanosoma* is suspected, prepare multiple impression smears and fix in 100% methyl alcohol. For surgical pathology, fix the tissue in buffered Formalin.
Whole worms or proglottids	Wash debris from the specimen and send it in saline. If there are multiple worms or proglottids, some may be fixed in Formalin.

REFERRAL OF MATERIALS

Few laboratories perform complete parasitological examination, whereas many perform limited studies and some perform none. Referral laboratories may provide services not available in the individual laboratory and can provide consultation on specimens with questionable laboratory findings. Referral laboratories with a special interest and competence in parasitology may be found in major cities, university medical centers, and state public health laboratories. The major national resource is the Centers for Disease Control in Atlanta, Ga. Specimens for the Centers must be sent via a state public health laboratory, and appropriate clinical information must be provided. Guidelines for handling specimens to be sent to a referral laboratory are outlined in Table 5. Of course, the recommendations of the specific referral laboratory should supersede these guidelines.

SAFETY

The parasitology laboratory has infection hazards for personnel. Blood, feces, and other body materials as well as parasite cultures may be infective for a variety of microbial agents. Eggs of *Ascaris* spp. can survive and embryonate even in Formalin, and *Cryptosporidium* oocysts are hardy. In fresh fecal specimens, the cysts of *Entamoeba histolytica* and *Giardia* spp., the oocysts of *Cryptosporidium* spp., the eggs of *Enterobius vermicularis, Taenia solium,* and *Hymenolepis nana,* and the larvae of *Strongyloides stercoralis* may be infective. In addition, feces may contain other infectious agents such as hepatitis A virus, rotavirus, *Salmonella* spp., *Shigella* spp., and *Campylobacter* spp. Blood and tissue specimens can be infectious for trypanosomes, *Leishmania* spp., malaria, and *Babesia* spp., as well as for hepatitis B, hepatitis C, and AIDS.

Reagents such as mercury-containing fixatives (Schaudinn and PVA fixatives) may be toxic, and solvents such as ether may be flammable. These materials must be handled and discarded properly.

QUALITY ASSURANCE

The parasitology laboratory must have an up-to-date procedure manual and appropriate reference materials, which might include color atlases (4, 52) or 35-mm slide collections (48, 50, 51), permanently stained glass slides, wet fecal material containing parasites, and one or more standard reference books on laboratory methods (3, 23, 41) or general medical parasitology (5, 10, 36). It must have an ongoing quality control program for equipment, reagents, and procedures (7). The persons performing parasitic examinations must be competent in the identification of parasites which might be found in patients from whom they receive specimens. Methods should allow the ready use of outside consultants, if there is a question of diagnosis. Personnel may maintain proficiency through participation in formal courses or workshops, review of self-study sets, and periodic review of known positive materials. Participation in external survey programs is particularly valuable, as the performance of the laboratory in the identification of unknown specimens can be compared with the performance of other laboratories (47).

If a laboratory is unable to do accurate parasitology because of either the types of procedures offered or the quality of personnel available, it should arrange to have specimens appropriately prepared and submitted to a reference laboratory.

LITERATURE CITED

1. **Abaru, D. E., and D. A. Denham.** 1976. A comparison of the efficacy of the Nucleopore and Millipore filtration systems for detecting microfilariae. Southeast Asian J. Trop. Med. Public Health **7:**367–369.
2. **Andrews, J.** 1934. The diagnosis of intestinal protozoa from purges and normally passed stools. J. Parasitol. **20:**253–254.
3. **Ash, L. R., and T. C. Orihel.** 1987. Parasites: a guide to laboratory procedures and identification. ASCP Press, American Society of Clinical Pathologists, Chicago.
4. **Ash, L. R., and T. C. Orihel.** 1990. Atlas of human parasitology, 3rd ed. American Society of Clinical Pathologists Press, Chicago.
5. **Balows, A., W. J. Hausler, Jr., M. Ohashi, and A. Turano (ed.).** 1988. Laboratory diagnosis of infectious diseases. Principles and practice, vol. 1. Bacterial, mycotic, and parasitic diseases. Springer Verlag, New York.
6. **Bartlett, M. S., K. Harper, N. Smith, P. Verbanac, and J. W. Smith.** 1978. Comparative evaluation of a modified zinc sulfate flotation technique. J. Clin. Microbiol. **7:**524–528.
7. **Bartlett, M. S., and K. L. Harper.** 1985. Parasitology, p. 145–166. *In* J. M. Miller and B. B. Wentworth (ed.), Methods for quality control in diagnostic microbiology. American Public Health Association, Washington, D.C.
8. **Beal, C. B., P. Viens, R. G. L. Grant, and J. M. Hughes.** 1970. A new technique for sampling duodenal contents. Am. J. Trop. Med. Hyg. **19:**349–352.
9. **Beaver, P. C.** 1950. The standardization of fecal smears for estimating egg production and worm burden. J. Parasitol. **36:**451–455.
10. **Beaver, P. C., R. C. Jung, and E. W. Cupp.** 1984. Clinical parasitology, 9th ed. Lea & Febiger, Philadelphia.
11. **Blagg, W., E. L. Schlaegel, N. S. Mansour, and G. I. Khalaf.** 1955. A new concentration technic for the demonstration of protozoa and helminth eggs in feces. Am. J. Trop. Med. Hyg. **4:**23–28.
12. **Brondson, M. A.** 1984. Rapid dimethyl sulfoxide-modified acid-fast stain of *Cryptosporidium* oocysts in stool specimens. J. Clin. Microbiol. **19:**952–953.
13. **Carroll, M. J., J. Cook, and J. A. Turner.** 1983. Comparison of polyvinyl alcohol- and Formalin-preserved fecal specimens in the Formalin-ether sedimentation technique for parasitological examination. J. Clin. Microbiol. **18:**1070–1072.
14. **Center for Disease Control.** 1979. Intestinal parasite surveillance, annual summary, 1978. Center for Disease Control, Atlanta, Ga.
15. **Current, W. L., N. C. Reese, J. V. Ernst, W. S. Bailey, M. B. Heyman, and W. M. Weinstein.** 1983. Human cryptosporidiosis in immunocompetent and immunodeficient persons. N. Engl. J. Med. **308:**1252–1257.
16. **Dao, A. H., D. P. Robinson, and S. W. Wong.** 1983. Frequency of *Entamoeba gingivalis* in human gingival scrapings. Am. J. Clin. Pathol. **80:**380–383.
17. **Dennis, D. T., E. McConnell, and G. B. White.** 1976. Bancroftian filariasis and membrane filters: are night surveys necessary? Am. J. Trop. Med. Hyg. **25:**257–262.
18. **Desowitz, R. S., and J. C. Hitchcock.** 1974. Hyperendemic bancroftian filariasis in the Kingdom of Tonga: the application of the membrane filter technique to an age-stratified blood survey. Am. J. Trop. Med. Hyg. **23:**877–879.
19. **Edelman, M. H., and C. L. Spingarn.** 1977. Cultivation of *Entamoeba histolytica* as a diagnostic procedure: a brief review. Mt. Sinai J. Med. **43:**27–32.
20. **Faust, E. C., J. S. D'Antoni, V. Odom, M. J. Miller, C. Peres, W. Sawitz, L. F. Thomen, J. E. Tobie, and J. H.**

Walker. 1938. A critical study of clinical laboratory technics for the diagnosis of protozoan cysts and helminth eggs in feces. Am. J. Trop. Med. Hyg. **18:**169–183.

21. **Finkelman, D., C. Hines, Jr., and W. D. Davis.** 1981. Value of purgation in examining stool for parasites. South. Med. J. **74:**679–680.
22. **Garcia, L. S., T. C. Brewer, and D. A. Bruckner.** 1979. A comparison of the formalin-ether concentration and trichrome stained smear methods for the recovery and identification of intestinal protozoa. Am. J. Med. Technol. **45:** 932–935.
23. **Garcia, L. S., and D. A. Bruckner.** 1988. Diagnostic medical parasitology. Elsevier, New York.
24. **Gardner, B. B., D. J. Del Junco, J. Fenn, and J. H. Hengesbaugh.** 1980. Comparison of direct wet mount and trichrome staining techniques for detecting *Entamoeba* species trophozoites in stools. J. Clin. Microbiol. **12:**656–658.
25. **Gleason, N. N., and G. R. Healy.** 1965. Modification and evaluation of Kohn's one-step staining technic for intestinal protozoa in feces or tissue. Am. J. Clin. Pathol. **43:**494–496.
26. **Goldsmith, R., and D. Heyneman (ed.).** 1989. Tropical medicine and parasitology. Appleton and Lange, Norwalk, Conn.
27. **Gutierrez, Y.** 1989. Diagnostic pathology of parasitic infections, with clinical correlations. Lea & Febiger, Philadelphia.
28. **Haley, L. D., and P. G. Standard.** 1973. Laboratory methods in medical mycology, 3rd ed. Center for Disease Control, Atlanta, Ga.
29. **Knott, J. I.** 1939. A method for making microfilarial surveys on day blood. Trans. R. Soc. Trop. Med. Hyg. **33:**191–196.
30. **Komiya, Y., and A. Kobayashi.** 1966. Evaluation of Kato's thick smear technic with a cellophane cover for helminth eggs in feces. Jpn. J. Parasitol. **19:**59–64.
31. **Krogstad, D. J., H. C. Spencer, Jr., G. R. Healy, N. N. Gleason, D. J. Sexton, and C. A. Herron.** 1978. Amebiasis: epidemiologic studies in the United States, 1971–1974. Ann. Intern. Med. **88:**89–97.
32. **Lichtenberg, F., and C. Valladares.** 1955. Compression examination of fresh tissue for ova of *Schistosoma mansoni*. Am. J. Clin. Pathol. **25:**1099–1102.
33. **Manson-Bahr, P. E. C., and D. R. Bell (ed.).** 1987. Manson's tropical diseases, 19th edition. The W. B. Saunders Co., Philadelphia.
34. **Markell, E. K., L. R. Ash, D. M. Melvin, D. V. Moore, F. Songandares-Bernal, and M. Voge.** 1977. Procedures suggested for use in examination of clinical specimens for parasitic infection. A statement by the Subcommittee on Laboratory Standards, Committee on Education, American Society of Parasitology. J. Parasitol. **63:**959–960.
35. **Markell, E. K., and P. M. Quinn.** 1977. Comparison of immediate polyvinyl alcohol (PVA) fixation with delayed Schaudinn's fixation for the demonstration of protozoa in stool specimens. Am. J. Trop. Med. Hyg. **26:**1139–1142.
36. **Markell, E. K., M. Voge, and D. T. John.** 1986. Medical parasitology, 6th ed. The W. B. Saunders Co., Philadelphia.
37. **Markey, R. L.** 1950. A vaseline swab for the diagnosis of *Enterobius* eggs. Am. J. Clin. Pathol. **20:**493.
38. **Martin, L. K.** 1965. Randomness of particle distribution in human feces and the resulting influence on helminth egg counting. Am. J. Trop. Med. Hyg. **14:**747–759.
39. **McQuay, R. M.** 1956. Charcoal medium for growth and maintenance of large and small races of *Entamoeba histolytica*. Am. J. Clin. Pathol. **26:**1137–1141.
40. **McQuay, R. M.** 1970. Citrate-saponin-acid method for the recovery of microfilariae from blood. Am. J. Clin. Pathol. **54:**743–746.
41. **Melvin, D. M., and M. M. Brooke.** 1982. Laboratory procedures for the diagnosis of intestinal parasites, 3rd ed. U.S. Department of Health, Education and Welfare publication no. (CDC) 82-8282. Centers for Disease Control, Atlanta, Ga.
42. **Nair, C. P.** 1953. Rapid staining of intestinal amoebae on wet mounts. Nature (London) **172:**1051.
43. **National Research Council, Office of International Affairs, Board on Sciences and Technology for International Development, and the Institute of Medicine, National Academy of Sciences.** 1987. The US capacity to address tropical infectious disease problems, p. 93–96. National Academy Press, Washington, D.C.
44. **Ritchie, L. S.** 1948. An ether sedimentation technique for routine stool examinations. Bull. U.S. Army Med. Dept. **8:** 326.
45. **Sadun, E. H., and D. M. Melvin.** 1956. The probability of detecting infections with *Enterobius vermicularis* by successive examinations. J. Pediatr. **48:**431–438.
46. **Sapero, J. J., and D. K. Lawless.** 1953. The "MIF" stain preservation technique for the identification of intestinal protozoa. Am. J. Trop. Med. Hyg. **2:**613–619.
47. **Smith, J. W.** 1979. Identification of fecal parasites in the special parasitology survey of the College of American Pathologists. Am. J. Clin. Pathol. **72**(Suppl.):371–373.
48. **Smith, J. W., L. R. Ash, J. H. Thompson, R. M. McQuay, D. M. Melvin, and T. C. Orihel.** 1976. Diagnostic parasitology—intestinal helminths. American Society of Clinical Pathologists, Chicago.
49. **Smith, J. W., and M. S. Bartlett.** 1982. Laboratory diagnosis of *Pneumocystis carinii* infection, p. 393–406. *In* W. C. Winn (ed.), Clinics in laboratory medicine. The W. B. Saunders Co., Philadelphia.
50. **Smith, J. W., R. M. McQuay, L. R. Ash, D. M. Melvin, T. C. Orihel, and J. H. Thompson.** 1976. Diagnostic parasitology—intestinal protozoa. American Society of Clinical Pathologists, Chicago.
51. **Smith, J. W., D. M. Melvin, T. C. Orihel, L. R. Ash, R. M. McQuay, and J. H. Thompson.** 1976. Diagnostic parasitology—blood and tissue parasites. American Society of Clinical Pathologists, Chicago.
52. **Spencer, F. M., and L. S. Monroe.** 1982. The color atlas of intestinal parasites, 2nd ed. Charles C Thomas, Publisher, Springfield, Ill.
53. **Stoll, N. R.** 1923. Investigations on the control of hookworm disease. XV. An effective method of counting hookworm eggs in feces. Am. J. Hyg. **3:**59–70.
54. **Strickland, G. T. (ed.).** 1984. Tropical medicine, 6th ed. The W. B. Saunders Co., Philadelphia.
55. **Thornton, S. A., B. S. Hanna-West, H. L. Dupont, and L. K. Pickering.** 1983. Comparison of methods for identification of *Giardia lamblia*. Am. J. Clin. Pathol. **80:**858–860.
56. **Warren, K. S., and A. A. F. Mahmoud (ed.).** 1984. Tropical and geographic medicine. McGraw-Hill Book Co., New York.
57. **Watson, J. M., and R. Al-Hafidh.** 1957. A modification of the Baermann funnel technique and its use in establishing the infection potential of human hookworm carriers. Ann. Trop. Med. Parasitol. **51:**15–16.
58. **Wheatley, W. B.** 1951. A rapid staining procedure for intestinal amoebae and flagellates. Am. J. Clin. Pathol. **21:** 990–991.
59. **Yang, J., and T. Scholten.** 1977. A fixative for intestinal parasites permitting the use of concentration and permanent staining procedures. Am. J. Clin. Pathol. **67:**300–304.
60. **Yarinsky, A., and S. D. Sternberg.** 1963. A study of paired purged stool specimens for the recovery of *Entamoeba histolytica*. Am. J. Clin. Pathol. **40:**598–600.
61. **Young, K. H., S. L. Bullock, D. M. Melvin, and C. L. Spruill.** 1979. Ethyl acetate as a substitute for diethyl ether in the Formalin-ether sedimentation technique. J. Clin. Microbiol. **10:**852–853.

Chapter 67

Nonmorphologic Diagnosis of Parasitic Infections

MARIANNA WILSON AND PETER SCHANTZ

Many papers have been published on serologic tests for parasitic diseases. The types of tests, discussed in previous editions of this Manual (53, 93), have evolved through the years from simple gel diffusion to sophisticated immunoblots as technology has advanced. Major improvements have been made in test parameters as a result of more sensitive techniques and development of more specific antigens. Specificity has always been a problem in the serodiagnosis of helminthic infections; recent use of purified antigens such as the glycoprotein antigens of *Taenia solium* (91) have greatly improved these assays.

Diagnosis of parasitic infections is definitively made by observation of parasites in host tissue or excreta. This is rarely possible in infections such as toxoplasmosis or toxocariasis, when parasites are located in deep tissue sites, or in infections such as cysticercosis or echinococcosis, when invasive techniques are necessary to obtain material at some risk to the patient. Detection of antibodies can be valuable in indicating whether a nonimmune individual with no previous exposure to the parasite may have acquired an infection while traveling in a disease-endemic area. However, detection of parasite-specific antibodies in an individual native to a parasite-endemic area may reflect only a past infection unrelated to the patient's current status. In general, detecting antibodies to parasitic diseases can indicate only that infection occurred at some time in the past and does not necessarily reflect acute or current infection. Antibodies may slowly decline after the patient is cured of infection but will generally last from at least 1 year to many years and so are not usually a reliable indication of successful cure. The detection of parasitic-specific immunoglobulin M (IgM) antibodies can be of value in determining the time of initial *Toxoplasma* infection, but detection of IgM or IgA antibodies for any other parasitic disease is not currently recommended because of insensitivity or lack of ability to interpret the results.

The past decade has seen several changes in the availability of parasitic serologic tests (Table 1). Several private laboratories now offer tests that were previously available only at the Centers for Disease Control (CDC). Because commercial kits for parasitic diseases (other than toxoplasmosis and amebiasis) are not available in the United States, each laboratory has obtained its own reagents and set up its own tests. Duplication of a published procedure does not necessarily mean that the results of the laboratory attempting to duplicate it are identical to those found by the laboratory that developed the procedure without exchange of reagents and sera. Therefore, the interpretation derived from the original results should not be applied to a duplicated test procedure without in-house evaluation to establish test sensitivity, specificity, and interpretation for the new test. The user should insist on interpretation criteria for the specific test performed.

Toxoplasma antibody detection tests are now performed by a large number of state health department, hospital, and private laboratories because of the availability of commercial kits. It is virtually impossible to compare results obtained with kits from different companies, other than as just positive or negative, because of the lack of standardization in expressing results (99). To obtain Food and Drug Administration (FDA) approval for a commercial kit, the manufacturer or potential distributor must present data to the FDA showing that the kit is substantially equivalent to one that has received FDA approval. If each subsequent kit is not quite as good as the FDA-approved one with which it is compared, then results obtained with additional kits may reflect cumulative drift from the originally approved kit. A good proficiency testing program could perhaps mitigate some of these problems, but unfortunately no organization in the United States has offered a proficiency testing program for any serologic test for parasitic diseases since 1986.

The diagnosis of human intestinal protozoan infections depends on the microscopic detection of the various parasite stages in feces, duodenal fluid, or biopsied material from the small intestine. Since fecal examination is very labor-intensive and requires a skilled microscopist, both antibody tests and antigen detection tests have been investigated as alternatives. Antibody tests have been shown to be of limited value except for invasive amebiasis. Detection of parasite antigens should be more indicative of current infection and could be quickly performed by laboratory personnel other than an experienced morphologist. Much work has been accomplished during the last 10 years on the development of antigen detection systems, resulting in commercially available reagents for *Giardia*, *Cryptosporidium*, *Pneumocystis*, and *Trichomonas* species.

Molecular biology shows promise for improving diagnosis of a variety of parasitic infections. Nucleic acid probes may allow detection of parasite nucleic acid in material from patients with various infections, including malaria (49, 50) and leishmaniasis (100). In addition, probes may allow improved strain recognition and taxonomy, which will clarify epidemiology. Molecular biology may also allow development of improved antigens for serologic tests that will show less cross-reactivity with antibody to other parasites, as has recently been described for Chagas' disease (13, 22). There are as yet no commercially available probes for diagnosis of parasitic infections, but a number are likely to become available in the next decade. Even though these probes

TABLE 1. Antibody and antigen tests for parasitic diseases[a]

Disease	Antibody tests performed at CDC	Test(s) performed at commercial or other labs	Antigen detection kits available commercially
Amebiasis	IHA	Yes	
Babesiasis	IIF		
Chagas' disease (*Trypanosoma cruzi*)	IIF, CF	Yes	
Cryptosporidiosis			IIF
Cysticercosis	IB	Yes	
Fascioliasis		Yes	
Filariasis		Yes	
Echinococcosis	IHA, IB	Yes	
Giardiasis		Yes	EIA, IIF
Leishmaniasis	IIF, CF	Yes	
Malaria	IIF	Yes	
Paragonimiasis	IB	Yes	
Pneumocystosis			IIF
Schistosomiasis	EIA, IB	Yes	
Strongyloidiasis	EIA	Yes	
Toxocariasis	EIA	Yes	
Toxoplasmosis	IIF, EIA-IgM	Yes	
Trichinellosis	BF	Yes	
Trichomoniasis			EIA, DIF

[a] BF, Bentonite flocculation; CF, complement fixation; DIF, direct immunofluorescence; EIA, enzyme immunoassay; IB, immunoblot; IHA, indirect hemagglutination; IIF, indirect immunofluorescence.

may show improved accuracy and may be less labor-intensive, they are likely to be much too expensive for routine use in underdeveloped countries.

PROTOZOAL DISEASES

Amebiasis

Amebiasis is one of the more prevalent parasitic diseases in the United States. It may be found in individuals from rural areas, those confined to institutions for mental or physical disabilities, homosexual men, and individuals who have traveled or lived in Third World countries. Several clinical syndromes are recognized: asymptomatic infections, involving only luminal colonization of the gut, account for the vast majority of human infections; symptomatic infections may be limited to the gastrointestinal tract (amebic colitis) or may be extraintestinal (amebic liver abscess). Serologic testing is most useful in patients with extraintestinal disease in which organisms are not generally found on stool examination.

The indirect hemagglutination (IHA) test has been in use at CDC for more than 20 years. The IHA test detects antibody specific for *Entamoeba histolytica* at titers of ≥1:256 in approximately 95% of patients with extraintestinal amebiasis, in 70% of patients with active intestinal infection, and in 10% of asymptomatic individuals who are passing cysts of *E. histolytica*. Positive titers may persist for months or years even after successful treatment, so the presence of a titer does not necessarily indicate acute or current infection. Specificity is excellent: false-positive reactions rarely occur at titers of ≥1:256 (53, 94).

Several commercial procedures, including IHA, immunodiffusion, and enzyme immunoassay (EIA), are available in the United States. Although the immunodiffusion test is specific, it is slightly less sensitive than the IHA test and requires a minimum of 24 h to obtain an answer, in contrast to the 2 h required for the IHA test. However, the simplicity of the procedure makes it ideal for the laboratory that has only an occasional specimen to test. The IHA and EIA tests are more suitable for laboratories that have frequent requests for amebiasis serology. EIA tests have been found to be as sensitive and specific as the IHA test (57). Although the detection of IgM antibodies specific for *E. histolytica* has been reported, sensitivity is only about 60% in patients with current invasive disease.

Immunologic detection of specific amebic antigens in fecal specimens from patients with intestinal disease might prove to be more cost-effective than the labor-intensive microscopic examination of stools by skilled technicians. There have been several reports of successful detection of *E. histolytica* antigens in fecal specimens by EIA (2). However, these procedures are not quite as sensitive and specific as visual examination (42), and no commercial kits are currently available.

Babesiosis

Natural transmission of *Babesia microti* occurs in the coastal areas of the northeastern United States and rarely in Minnesota and Wisconsin. Because the tick vector also transmits the causative agent of Lyme disease, dual infections have been reported in New York. Diagnosis of *Babesia* infection should be made by observation of parasites in patient blood films. However, serology has been shown to be useful in detecting infected individuals with very low levels of parasitemia, such as asymptomatic blood donors, for posttherapy diagnosis after parasitemia is no longer detectable, and for discrimination between *Plasmodium falciparum* and *Babesia* infection in patients whose blood film examination is inconclusive and whose travel histories cannot exclude either parasite (36).

The indirect immunofluorescence (IIF) test is quite sensitive for *B. microti* infection (10). Patient titers generally rise to ≥1:1,024 during the first weeks of illness and fall gradually over 6 months to 1:16 to 1:256, remaining at that level for up to 13 months or longer.

Specificity is 100% in patients with other tick-borne diseases or individuals not exposed to the parasite. However, cross-reactions may occur in serum specimens from patients with malaria infections, but generally titers are highest with the homologous antigen (11).

Chagas' disease

Infections with *Trypanosoma cruzi* are common in Central and South America. During the acute stage of illness, blood film examination generally reveals the presence of trypomastigotes. During the chronic stage of infection, the parasites are rare or absent from the circulation, and immunodiagnosis may be the only means of disease detection other than xenodiagnosis.

Currently, the IIF and complement fixation (CF) tests are used at CDC. Although the IIF test is very sensitive, cross-reactivity occurs with antibodies to *Leishmania* organisms, which occur in the same geographic areas as *T. cruzi*. The CF test is less sensitive but more specific than the IIF test (53). Although differentiating between acute and chronic infection is very important in determining therapy, serology cannot be used to do so. A positive titer in all tests is indicative only of infection at some unknown time, not of acute infection.

Sensitivity and specificity of EIA tests for antibody detection using crude antigens are similar to those of the IIF test. Research during the past decade has indicated that increased specificity may be obtained with the use of purified antigens of 90, 72, and 25 kilodaltons (kDa) (55) or use of antigens produced by molecular biologic techniques (13), but reagents are not yet available. Antigen detection in both serum and urine has been reported but is still not an established procedure (23).

Cryptosporidiosis

Cryptosporidium parvum is an important intestinal protozoan pathogen in humans. Like *Giardia lamblia*, the organisms cause diarrhea; the organisms are transmitted by person-to-person contact or may be waterborne. The disease can be very severe in immunocompromised patients. One commercial company offers a monoclonal antibody to *Cryptosporidium* oocyst cell wall with a fluorescein isothiocyanate (FITC)-labeled anti-immunoglobulin for the detection of oocysts in stools by IIF (27). No kits are currently available for detection of soluble antigen. Antibody tests are not recommended because of lack of ability to discriminate between acute and old infection.

Giardiasis

G. lamblia, the most common human intestinal protozoan pathogen in the United States, is an important cause of diarrhea in children and adults. Outbreaks of disease are common within day-care centers through person-to-person contact; they may also occur from drinking water contaminated by infected human or animal feces. Infected individuals often excrete cysts intermittently, so multiple stools collected over at least several days must sometimes be examined to detect the parasite.

Commercial reagents are available for the detection of soluble *Giardia* antigens and whole parasites in stools. One EIA detects *Giardia*-specific antigen 65 cyst antigen in eluates of fresh or fixed stools with a sensitivity of 96% and specificity of 100%, compared with stool examination, which has 74% sensitivity and 100% specificity (80). This fecal antigen assay does not detect trophozoite antigens and so will not detect individuals who are passing trophozoites only at the time the stool is obtained. Another EIA kit requires a fresh stool specimen but detects multiple cyst and trophozoite antigens. The manufacturer's evaluation found kit sensitivity to be 91% and specificity to be 96%. A third EIA kit also detects multiple cyst and trophozoite antigens but can be used to test fresh, frozen, or fixed specimens. The manufacturer's stated test sensitivity is 96%; stated test specificity is 97%. A monoclonal antibody to *Giardia* cyst wall is available from one company in a kit that includes FITC-labeled anti-monoclonal immunoglobulin for use in an IIF procedure to detect *Giardia* cysts in stools. Antibody detection tests are insensitive and so are not recommended for individual patient diagnosis.

Leishmaniasis

Of the three clinical forms of leishmaniasis, cutaneous, mucocutaneous, and visceral, the last is the most difficult to diagnose. Biopsy of liver, spleen, or bone marrow is necessary to demonstrate the parasite in tissue. Antibody detection is a useful adjunct for diagnosing visceral leishmaniasis but is less useful for cutaneous leishmaniasis.

The IIF and CF tests are used at CDC for detection of antibodies (77). These procedures can differentiate leishmaniasis from other clinically similar conditions but cannot determine the species of *Leishmania*, which is necessary for selecting the appropriate therapy. Cross-reactions occur in patients with antibodies to *T. cruzi* (Chagas' disease), which is endemic in some of the same areas as leishmaniasis in Central and South America. Only the IIF test is performed in cases of suspected cutaneous leishmaniasis. Sensitivity of all antibody tests for cutaneous leishmaniasis is poor, since many patients do not have a detectable circulating antibody response to the parasite.

The immunology and classification of *Leishmania* species have been very active areas of research. Biochemical, immunologic, and molecular biology techniques have been used extensively, resulting in more specific antigens and probes for detection and identification of parasites (4, 6, 44).

Malaria

The serodiagnosis of malaria is not recommended except for screening blood donors involved in cases of transfusion-induced malaria when the donor's parasitemia may be below the detectable level of blood film examination (89). IIF tests with the human species of *Plasmodium* used for antibody detection are very sensitive and specific, but the presence of antibodies indicates only that infection occurred at some time in the past and does not indicate the individual's immune status (see also chapter 68).

Pneumocystosis

Pneumocystis carinii pneumonia is the primary cause of death among persons with acquired immunodeficiency syndrome (AIDS) and a cause of morbidity among other immunocompromised individuals. The parasites are usually limited to the alveoli of the lung, and in the past, invasive procedures have been necessary to obtain material for definitive diagnosis. Rapid antibody tests that detect current active infections would be invaluable tools for diagnosis. Unfortunately, none of the tests now available can be recommended for individual patient diagnosis. Antibody detection with IIF or EIA has been evaluated, but these tests are of little clinical value (66). Tests for circulating soluble antigens have also been shown to be of little value in determining the current status of individuals because of the high incidence of detectable antigen in asymptomatic people.

The current preferred method of diagnosing *P. carinii* pneumonia in patients with AIDS is examining pulmonary specimens (bronchoalveolar lavage or induced sputum) for the presence of parasites (69). Immunofluorescence has been found to be the most sensitive stain, detecting organisms in 10 to 15% more specimens than Diff-Quik or toluidine blue O stains. Four U.S. companies offer kits for an IIF procedure to detect parasites, employing monoclonal antibodies to human *P. carinii*.

Toxoplasmosis

Because of the incidence of *Toxoplasma* infection (24) and the availability of commercial kits, antibody detection of *Toxoplasma* infection constitutes the largest number of serologic test requests for parasitic diseases in the United States. Comparisons of kits indicated that most perform comparably in detecting *Toxoplasma*-specific IgG antibodies (99) but vary markedly in detecting *Toxoplasma*-specific IgM antibodies (98).

The IIF and EIA tests for IgG and IgM antibodies are most commonly used today. Individuals should be initially tested for the presence of *Toxoplasma*-specific IgG antibodies to determine their immune status. A positive IgG titer indicates infection with the organism; a high IgG titer (i.e., IIF titer of >1:1,024) may indicate infection within the past several years. If more precise knowledge of the time of infection is necessary, then an IgG-positive individual should have an IgM test performed by a procedure with minimal nonspecific reactions, such as IgM-capture EIA (21, 72). Newborn infants suspected of congenital toxoplasmosis should always be tested by an IgM-capture EIA; the IIF-IgM test has been shown to be much less sensitive (25 versus 75%) than the EIA in detecting infant IgM antibodies (70). *Toxoplasma*-specific IgM antibodies may be detected by EIA for as long as 18 months after acute acquired infection (71, 98), but high levels may indicate infection within the past 3 to 4 months. Table 2 summarizes the interpretation of serology results obtained at CDC (see also chapter 68).

Serologic determination of active central nervous system toxoplasmosis in immunocompromised patients is not possible at this time (61). *Toxoplasma*-specific IgG antibody levels in AIDS patients often are only low to moderate, but occasionally no specific IgG antibodies can be detected. Test results for IgM antibodies are generally negative. Detection of circulating antigen in AIDS patients has been evaluated, but the procedures lack sensitivity.

Trichomoniasis

Trichomoniasis, an infection caused by *Trichomonas vaginalis*, is a common sexually transmitted disease. Diagnosis is usually made by the detection of trophozoites in vaginal secretions or urethral specimens by wet-mount microscopic examination or after culture. A kit that uses FITC- or enzyme-labeled monoclonal antibodies for use in a direct immunofluorescence or EIA procedure is available for the detection of whole parasites in fluids. Sensitivity appears to be equal to that of wet-mount examination, but the results obtained by using the kits have not been compared with those obtained by using cultured specimens, a technique known to be more sensitive than direct examination.

TABLE 2. Interpretation of *Toxoplasma* serological test results

Titer		Interpretation
IIF-IgG	EIA-IgM[a]	
<1:16	Negative	No evidence of exposure
>1:16	Negative	Infection probably acquired more than 1 year ago
≥1:1,024	1:4–1:256	Infection probably acquired within past 18 months
≥1:1,024	≥1:1,024	Recent infection probably acquired within past 4 months

[a] Presence of any IgM titer suggests infection within the last 18 months. A titer of ≥1:1,024 suggests infection acquired within 4 months; however, many persons with infection within 4 months will have titers lower than 1:1,024 but generally ≥1:64. Thus, for some patients, IgM titers may be difficult to interpret as to time when infection occurred.

HELMINTHIC DISEASES

Cysticercosis (larval *Taenia solium*)

Computerized tomographic and magnetic resonance imaging techniques have greatly increased the ability of clinicians to detect and define the nature of space-occupying lesions in the central nervous system. The appearance of cysticerci by these techniques is variable, however, and not entirely specific. Serodiagnostic tests may be helpful in confirming the diagnosis.

Many currently available serologic tests for cysticercosis use crude or purified extracts of cysticerci as antigens in EIA to detect antibodies in serum or cerebrospinal fluid (CSF) (20, 82); the sensitivity of these assays has varied from 75 to 100%, both in serum and in CSF. The predominant immunoglobulin class of *Cysticercus*-specific antibody detected was IgG; IgM, IgA, and IgE antibodies cannot be correlated with the patient's clinical status or prognosis and so are of little value. A major problem in serodiagnosis of *T. solium* cysticercosis has been nonspecificity related to cross-reacting components in crude antigens derived from cysticerci. These components bind antibodies produced by other helminth infections, especially hydatidosis and filariasis (85). Most partially purified fractions evaluated in EIA appear to have lower sensitivity than crude antigens and do not necessarily achieve higher specificity.

Development at CDC of the immunoblot assay using purified glycoprotein antigens (91) has eliminated the nonspecific problems observed in all other tests while increasing test sensitivity. At least one of seven glycoprotein antigens, ranging from 13 to 50 kDa, was recognized by serum specimens from 97% of 108 parasitologically confirmed cases of cysticercosis. No serum of 376 patients with heterologous infections reacted with any of the *Cysticercus*-specific antigens.

The CDC immunoblot assay is both more specific (100%) and more sensitive than the EIA systems with which it has been compared. The most important factors identified as determining positive immunoblot reactions are the number of cysticerci and stage of development demonstrable by imaging. Continuing prospective evaluation of the immunoblot assay has demonstrated sensitivity greater than 93% in serum of patients with clinically diagnosed active cysticercosis. Sensitivity in CSF of the same patients is somewhat less (80%). Seropositivity in patients with single, enhancing parenchymal cysts has been <50% in serum. These figures are reduced further in patients with a single calcified cyst. Seropositivity in serum and CSF of patients with multiple but only calcified cysts has been 82 and 77%, respectively. Serologic tests for cysticercosis do not distinguish between active and inactive infection and thus have not been useful in evaluating the outcome and prognosis of medically treated patients.

Fascioliasis

The acute manifestations of human fascioliasis may precede the appearance of eggs in the stool by several weeks; therefore, serologic methods are of greatest interest to the clinician in the early stages of disease. Serodiagnosis is also useful for the confirmation of chronic fascioliasis when egg production is low or sporadic and for ruling out "pseudo-fascioliasis" associated with ingested parasite eggs in sheep or calf liver.

Fasciola hepatica infection causes the induction of multiple antibodies of varying degrees of specificity detectable within 2 to 4 weeks after infection. One approach to immunodiagnosis is the use of crude *Fasciola* antigens in an enzyme-linked immunosorbent assay (ELISA) (8, 46). For serum specimens of patients from areas where *Schistosoma mansoni* is endemic, a circumoval precipitin (COP) test must also be done to determine reactivity to *Schistosoma* antigens. A positive *Fasciola* ELISA reaction with a negative COP test strongly suggests fascioliasis. The COP test does not cross-react with *Fasciola* infected serum (47). Crude or purified excretory-secretory (ES) antigens appear to provide the most sensitive and early diagnosis; however, some cross-reactivity is apparent with serum samples of patients with schistosomiasis (45). Recently, a 17-kDa ES antigen revealed by immunoblot was reported to be present in serum samples of all patients with fascioliasis and was not recognized by patients with schistosomiasis or other parasitic infections, whose sera sometimes react with *Fasciola* antigens in quantitative assays (48). Antibody levels decrease shortly after chemotherapeutic cure and can be used to predict the success of therapy.

Filariasis

Lymphatic: *Wuchereria bancrofti* and *Brugia* spp. Because filaria and microfilaria can be present in small numbers or sequestered in inaccessible sites, and because the means to detect them parasitologically are relatively insensitive, immunologic techniques have often been used for diagnosis. Immunodiagnostic tests traditionally used for diagnosis of human filariasis have been serologic or skin test measures of antibodies. The antigens used have been crude or fractionated extracts from filarial worms of other mammals, especially *Dirofilaria immitis* of dogs (54). Such antigens are usually reactive with serum samples of patients with various forms of filariasis but are completely lacking in specificity. ES or surface antigens of homologous (*Wuchereria* or *Brugia*) parasites are more specific antigen preparations than whole-worm somatic extracts (67), but supplies of such material have been limited because of the lack of animal models and difficulties of in vitro cultivation. EIAs that measure only IgG4 or IgE antibodies to *Brugia* antigens greatly reduce nonspecificity because humans do not produce IgG4 antibodies to phosphocholine, an immunodominant molecule present on a wide range of organisms, including filariae (59).

Important shortcomings of antibody detection methods are their inability to distinguish past exposure from current infection and their lack of correlation with worm burden. Detection of parasite material (antigen or other products) in blood or urine offers potential advantages for assessing the state of individual infections. Although circulating antigens can be detected in patients with bancroftian filariasis, positive results have been confined almost exclusively to serum specimens from individuals with microfilaremia (3, 95, 96). Another problem is the binding of antigen into immune complexes, which interferes with their detection by some antigen detection methods (62). Many of the lymphatic filarial syndromes are not associated with microfilaremia, and what is sorely needed for diagnosis of such conditions is a tool for sensitively detecting the presence of parasite material (e.g., antigen) in the body fluids of an infected individual (63). Until these assays become available, diagnosis of these amicrofilaremic syndromes must be made clinically (76).

At present, positive serum antibody tests or skin tests are of little diagnostic value except in patients not native to the endemic areas. This is because most residents of regions in which filariasis is endemic have been sensitized to filarial antigens through years of exposure to infected mosquitoes and because of the fact that filarial antigens may be cross-reactive with those of other nematode parasites also found in these areas. Thus, a positive immunodiagnostic test is a necessary but not sufficient prerequisite for the diagnosis of brugian or bancroftian filariasis (76). Conversely, a negative test result in an American or European whose symptoms suggest lymphatic filariasis after travel in an area where filariasis is endemic is highly predictive of the absence of infection.

Onchocerciasis. Current diagnostic methods are limited to the detection of parasites in the skin or the eye or the presence of suggestive clinical changes. These are crude, invasive, and often laborious and insensitive techniques. Accurate serodiagnostic tests are needed to identify individuals requiring treatment, to evaluate the success of treatment, and for epidemiologic surveys.

Host antibodies of the IgG and IgE isotypes that react with onchocercal antigens are readily detected in the sera of infected individuals; however, they are not specific for the presence or extent of the infection, nor do they allow discrimination between onchocerciasis and other filarial infections. Tests based on IgE detection are more specific than those based on IgG (97). EIA restricted to the IgG4 class and using purified, surface-derived onchocercal antigens of low molecular mass was highly sensitive and specific, although tests still cross-reacted with serum specimens of some patients with *W. bancrofti* infection (7). Antigen detection methods are feasible, but these and antibody assays require refinement of the reagents to control specificity (17).

Echinococcosis

Cystic hydatid disease (*Echinococcus granulosus*). Since hydatid cysts are located in deep-seated organs, and since closed biopsy is usually contraindicated because of the danger of inducing anaphylaxis or dissemination, accurate serodiagnostic tests can be very helpful in confirming or ruling out a presumptive diagnosis.

IHA, IIF, and EIA are highly sensitive tests for detecting antibodies in serum of patients with cystic hydatid disease (CHD); diagnostic sensitivity varies from approximately 60 to 90%, depending on the characteristics of the cases (83). Tests using whole *E. granulosus* antigens are not specific, however, and false-positive reactions occur commonly in sera of patients with other helminth infections, liver cirrhosis, and cancer. Serodiagnostic tests based on the detection of antibody to the *Echinococcus* antigen 5 or the 8-kDa antigen have the highest degree of specificity. Demonstration of the arc-5 in patient serum may be considered diagnostic for hydatid disease with an important exception: serum specimens from 5 to 10% of patients with *Taenia solium* cysticercosis give false-positive arc-5 reactions. The immunoblot assay, based on recognition of the 8-kDa antigen which does not react with cysticercal antibodies, appears absolutely specific (65). At CDC, the immunoblot assay was more sensitive (80%) than the arc-5 double-diffusion assay (54%) in serum samples of 70 patients with CHD. At CDC, all serum specimens are now screened in the IHA test, and all IHA-reactive specimens (titers ≥ 1:64) are tested in the immunoblot assay.

Correct interpretation of echinococcal serodiagnostic tests requires an understanding of the factors that can influence the results (83). Negative test results do not rule out echinococcosis because some cyst carriers do not have detectable antibody. Detectable immune responses have been associated with the location, the integrity, and the vitality of the larval cyst. Cysts in the liver are more likely to elicit antibody response than are cysts in the lungs, and regardless of localization, tests are least sensitive for diagnosing intact hyaline cysts. Such healthy metacestodes produce a low level of antigenic stimulation, and nearly 50% of carriers of this kind of cyst in the lungs may have negative serologic results. Cysts in the brain and in the spleen, like pulmonary cysts, are associated with lowered serodiagnostic reactivity, whereas those in bone appear to more regularly stimulate detectable antibody. Fissuration or rupture of a cyst is followed by an abrupt stimulation of antibodies. Senescent, calcified, or dead cysts apparently cease to stimulate the host, who may be seronegative.

Another cause of false-negative test results is antibody binding with antigen in circulating immune complexes. Circulating antigen was detectable in up to 50% of such serum specimens (14). Although tests for circulating antigen may provide a useful adjunct to antibody tests for diagnosis (37), such tests are not available in the United States.

Alveolar hydatid disease (*Echinococcus multilocularis*). Problems of sensitivity appear less important in serodiagnosis of *E. multilocularis* infections than of *E. granulosus* infections. Most infected persons have a detectable immune response, and most patients with alveolar hydatid disease (AHD) are positive in serologic tests using heterologous *E. granulosus* antigens. With crude *Echinococcus* antigens, nonspecific reactions create the same difficulties as described above for diagnosis of CHD; however, purified *E. multilocularis* antigens (Em2) used in EIA give positive serologic reactions in more than 95% of AHD cases (38). Comparing serologic reactivity to Em2 antigen with that to antigens containing components of both *E. multilocularis* and *E. granulosus* permits discrimination of patients with AHD from those with CHD (39, 60).

Paragonimiasis

The passage of eggs in sputum or feces of patients with pulmonary paragonimiasis is usually sporadic and sometimes absent; therefore, serodiagnosis is often necessary. Other indications for serodiagnostic tests are to confirm or rule out cases of presumed extrapulmonary paragonimiasis (cerebral or cutaneous) and for monitoring the results of individual chemotherapy. In the United States, serodiagnostic tests have been useful to physicians for differentiating paragonimiasis from tuberculosis in Indochinese immigrants (52).

The CF test has been the standard test for paragonimiasis; it is highly sensitive for diagnosis and assessing cure after therapy (52, 102). An EIA procedure was compared with the CF test at CDC and agreed favorably in terms of sensitivity and specificity (D. Moore and D. Allain, unpublished data). EIA was positive in 88 of 98 Indochinese patients (90%) with paragonimiasis. Cross-reactions were common with serum specimens of patients with clonorchiasis or schistosomiasis but were not a problem in serum specimens of patients with high titers to cestode and nematode infections. The problem of nonspecificity has been resolved at CDC by development of an immunoblot assay using a comparatively crude antigen extract (86). Positive reactions, based on demonstration of an 8-kDa antigen-antibody band, were obtained with the serum samples of 96% of patients with parasitologically confirmed *Paragonimus westermani* infection. Specificity was ≥99%; of 210 serum specimens from patients with other parasitic and nonparasitic infections, only 1 serum specimen from a patient with *Schistosoma haematobium* reacted positively.

Most published literature deals with pulmonary paragonimiasis due to *P. westermani*, although in some geographic areas other *Paragonimus* species cause similar or distinct clinical manifestations in human infections. Serologic test development has been reported for infections due to *Paragonimus miyazakii* (58, 101) and *P. africanus* and *P. uterobilateralis* (56). The extent of cross-reactivity of the *P. westermani* antigen used in the CDC immunoblot assay with antibodies from patients infected with other *Paragonimus* spp. is unknown.

Schistosomiasis

Detection of antibodies to schistosomes can be useful to indicate infections when eggs cannot be easily demonstrated in fecal or urine specimens. At CDC, all serum specimens are initially tested by EIA using *S. mansoni* adult worm antigen (43). A positive reaction (greater than 10 U/μl of serum) indicates infection with *Schistosoma* spp. Specificity of this assay in detecting schistosome infection is 99%. Sensitivity is 99% for *S. mansoni* infection, ≥90% for *S. haematobium* infection, and ≥50% for *S. japonicum* infection. Because the EIA using *S. mansoni* adult worm antigen is not as sensitive for detection of the other species as for detection of *S. mansoni*, immunoblots of all three species are used (based on the patient's travel history) to ensure detection of *S. haematobium* and *S. japonicum* infections. Species-specific diagnosis is achieved by using adult worm antigens on immunoblots (92). The presence of antibody is indicative only of schistosome infection at some time and cannot be correlated with worm burden, egg production, clinical status, or prognosis. Test sensitivity and specificity vary widely among the many tests currently available for the serologic diagnosis of schistosomiasis and are dependent on the type of antigen preparations used (crude, purified, adult worm, egg, or cercarial) (12, 64).

Strongyloidiasis

Early diagnosis and treatment of strongyloidiasis in the chronic intestinal phase are critical for preventing dissemination of the infection, which may prove lethal in immunosuppressed patients. Serodiagnostic tests for strongyloidiasis are indicated when the infection is suspected and the organism cannot be demonstrated by repeated stool examinations or duodenal aspiration or by enterotests. Currently recommended serologic tests use antigens derived from *Strongyloides stercoralis* filariform larvae (74). With use of such antigens, EIA was more sensitive (84 to 92%) than IIF or IHA when the tests were compared in the same groups of patients (9, 15, 25, 41, 74, 81, 90). Immunocompromised persons with disseminated strongyloidiasis usually have detectable IgG antibodies despite their immunodepression (28). Cross-reactions with patients with filariasis and some other nematode infections are common (40, 73). Other important limitations are the fact that 8 to 16% of *Strongyloides* carriers are seronegative in currently available tests and that antibody test results cannot be used to differentiate between past and current infections. Despite these shortcomings, serum samples of patients scheduled for potentially immunocompromising therapies should be screened for *Strongyloides* antibody. A positive test warrants continuing efforts to establish a parasitologic diagnosis, followed by appropriate anthelminthic treatment.

Serologic monitoring may be of use in the follow-up of immunocompetent treated patients. In a limited number of patients, antibody titers decreased markedly, and in some cases disappeared, after successful thiabendazole therapy (29, 78). However, until more data become available, serodiagnosis should not replace stool examinations for demonstration of cure.

Toxocariasis (larva migrans)

Serodiagnostic tests are usually the only way the pediatrician or ophthalmologist can confirm a presumptive clinical diagnosis of toxocaral visceral larva migrans (VLM) or ocular larva migrans (OLM), the two most common clinical syndromes associated with *Toxocara* infections. The currently recommended serologic test for toxocariasis is EIA with larval-stage antigens. Such antigens can be extracted from embryonated eggs or released in vitro by cultured infective larvae (16). The latter, *Toxocara* excretory-secretory (TES) antigens, are preferable to larval extracts because they are convenient to produce and because an absorption-purification step is not required to obtain maximum specificity (31). When testing serum specimens from patients with high titers of antibody to other helminth antigens, we rarely found reactions positive for TES antigens (35); the few samples that did react with TES antigens showed patterns of banding by immunoblot identical to those of patients with toxocaral larva migrans, thus suggesting concurrent infection (P. Schantz and B. Gottstein, unpublished data). We did not obtain cross-reactions with anti-A and anti-B blood group antibodies (33) or C-reactive protein, although such cross-reactivity with *Toxocara* antigens has been reported by others (87, 88).

Evaluation of the true sensitivity and specificity of serologic tests for toxocariasis in human populations is not possible because of the lack of parasitologic methods to diagnose the disease definitively and to exclude infection in controls. These inherent problems result in underestimations of sensitivity and specificity. Evaluation of the *Toxocara* EIA in groups of patients with presumptive diagnoses of VLM indicated sensitivity and specificity at a titer of ≥1:32 of 78 and 92%, respectively (34). At a given cutoff titer, the sensitivity of EIA for the diagnosis of OLM is less than that for VLM (79, 84); in our experience, sensitivity and specificity were 73 and 95%, respectively. When the cutoff titer was lowered to 1:8, the sensitivity was 90% (79). In some clinical situations, the lower cutoff titer would make the test more efficient for ruling out toxocariasis. The reduced sensitivity of serologic tests for OLM is probably related to the low larval burden or to the longer period between onset of infection and serodiagnostic testing. Further confirmation of the specificity of the serologic diagnosis of OLM can be obtained by examining aqueous or vitreous humor samples (5, 30).

When interpreting the serologic findings for patients, clinicians must be aware that a measurable titer is not positive proof of a causative relationship between *Toxocara canis* infection and the current illness. In most human populations, a small number of those tested have positive EIA titers that apparently reflect the prevalence of asymptomatic toxocariasis. In the United States, this was reported as 2.8% (cutoff titer, 1:32) of nearly 9,000 persons tested but varied significantly according to age, race, and socioeconomic status (32).

Work in progress promises new techniques that may yield much more clinically useful information than the positive or negative result provided by current antibody assays. Such studies include the detection of circulating TES antigens (1); with further evaluation, such tests may be suitable for clinical use. Monoclonal antibody-based tests reportedly distinguished between *T. canis* and *T. cati* and distinguished recent from chronic infections (68).

Trichinellosis

Human patients rarely develop detectable antibody before 3 to 5 weeks postinfection, well after the onset of acute-stage illness. Therefore, it is advisable to take multiple serum specimens spaced several weeks apart in order to demonstrate seroconversion in patients whose initial specimen was negative. Since serologic tests tend to remain positive for several months to a year, serodiagnostic test results by themselves do not provide data on the time course of infection.

Currently used tests include bentonite flocculation (75), IIF, and EIA. Antigens are prepared from muscle larva and may be crude antigens prepared from homogenates of whole larvae, or partially purified stichocyte antigens obtained by cell fractionation and immunoaffinity chromatography (18), or ES products produced by cultured larvae (26). Positive reactions are detectable in serum samples of 80 to 100% of patients with clinically symptomatic trichinellosis. Antibody levels are often below cutoff levels in the first month postinfection, peak in the second or third month postinfection, and then decline slowly. IgG, IgM, and IgE antibodies are all detectable in many patients; however, tests based on IgG antibodies are most sensitive (19). In our experience at CDC, no statistical difference in sensitivity has been observed between the bentonite flocculation and EIA tests with either crude or ES antigens (F. O. Richards et al., unpublished data); therefore, the bentonite flocculation test is used for routine serodiagnosis. Recent studies have demonstrated circulating antigens in patients with trichinellosis; however, tests for antibodies were more sensitive diagnostic indicators (51).

LITERATURE CITED

1. **Aguilar, C., C. Cuellar, S. Fenou, and J. L. Guillen.** 1987. Comparative study of assays detecting circulating immune complexes and specific antibodies in patients infected with *Toxocara canis*. J. Helminthol. **61:**196–202.
2. **Arvind, A. S., N. Shetty, and M. J. G. Farthing.** 1988. Serodiagnosis of amoebiasis. Serodiagn. Immunother. Infect. Dis. **2:**79–84.
3. **Au, A. C. S., D. A. Denham, M. W. Steward, C. C. Draper, M. D. Ismail, C. K. Rao, and J. W. Mak.** 1981. Detection of circulating antigens and immune complexes in feline and human lymphatic filariasis. Southeast Asian J. Trop. Med. Public Health **12:**492–498.
4. **Barker, D. C.** 1987. DNA diagnosis of human leishmaniasis. Parasitol. Today **3:**177–184.
5. **Biglan, A. W., L. T. Glickman, and L. A. Lobes.** 1979. Serum and vitreous *Toxocara* antibody in nematode endophthalmitis. Am. J. Ophthalmol. **88:**898–901.
6. **Blaxter, M. L., M. A. Miles, and J. M. Kelly.** 1988. Specific serodiagnosis of visceral leishmaniasis using a *Leishmania donovani* antigen identified by expression cloning. Mol. Biochem. Parasitol. **30:**259–270.
7. **Cabrera, Z., R. M. E. Parkhouse, K. Forsyth, A. Gomez Priego, R. Pabon, and L. Yarzabol.** 1989. Specific detection of human antibodies to *Onchocerca volvulus*. Trop. Med. Parasitol. **40:**454–459.
8. **Carlier, Y., D. Bout, and A. Capron.** 1979. Application de l'ELISA (enzyme linked immunosorbent assay) en parasitologie et mycologie. Rev. Inst. Pasteur Lyon **12:** 25–33.
9. **Carrol, S. M., K. T. Karthigasu, and D. I. Grove.** 1981. Serodiagnosis of human strongyloidiasis by an enzyme-linked immunosorbent assay. Trans. R. Soc. Trop. Med. Hyg. **75:**706–709.
10. **Chisholm, E. S., T. K. Ruebush II, A. J. Sulzer, and G. R. Healy.** 1978. *Babesia microti* infection in man: evaluation of an indirect immunofluorescent antibody test. Am. J. Trop. Med. Hyg. **27:**14–19.
11. **Chisholm, E. S., A. J. Sulzer, and T. K. Ruebush II.** 1986. Indirect immunofluorescence test for human *Babesia microti* infection: antigenic specificity. Am. J. Trop. Med. Hyg. **35:**921–925.
12. **Correa-Oliveira, R., L. M. S. Dusse, I. R. C. Viana, D. G. Colley, O. S. Carvalho, and G. Gazzinelli.** 1988. Human antibody responses against schistosomal antigens. I. Antibodies from patients with *Ancylostoma, Ascaris lumbricoides* or *Schistosoma mansoni* infections react with schistosome antigens. Am. J. Trop. Med. Hyg. **38:** 348–355.
13. **Cotrim, P. C., G. S. Paranhos, R. A. Mortara, J. Wanderley, A. Rassi, M. E. Camargo, and J. F. DaSilveira.** 1990. Expression in *Escherichia coli* of a dominant immunogen of *Trypanosoma cruzi* recognized by human chagasic sera. J. Clin. Microbiol. **28:**519–524.
14. **Craig, P. S., E. Zeyhle, and T. Romig.** 1986. Hydatid disease: research and control in Turkana. II. The role of immunological techniques for the diagnosis of hydatid disease. Trans. R. Soc. Trop. Med. Hyg. **80:**183–192.
15. **Dafalla, A. A.** 1972. The indirect fluorescent antibody test for serodiagnosis of strongyloidiasis. J. Trop. Med. Hyg. **75:**109–111.
16. **de Savigny, D. H.** 1975. *In vitro* maintenance of *Toxocara canis* larvae and a simple method for the production of *Toxocara* ES antigen for use in serodiagnostic tests for visceral larva migrans. J. Parasitol. **61:**781–782.
17. **des Moutis, I., A. Ouaissi, J. M. Grzych, L. Yarzabal, A. Haque, and A. Capron.** 1983. *Onchocerca volvulus:* detection of circulating antigen by monoclonal antibodies in human onchocerciasis. Am. J. Trop. Med. Hyg. **32:** 533–542.
18. **Despommier, D. D., andA. Laccetti.** 1981. *Trichinella spiralis:* partial characterization of antigens isolated by immuno-affinity chromatography from the large particle fraction of the muscle larva. J. Parasitol. **67:**322–339.
19. **Feldmeier, H., H. Fischer, and G. Blaumeiser.** 1987. Kinetics of humoral response during the acute and the convalescent phase of human trichinosis. Zentralbl. Bakteriol. Parasitenkd. Infektonskr. Hyg. Abt. 1 Reihe A **264:** 221–234.
20. **Flisser, A., and C. Larralde.** 1986. Cysticercosis, p. 109–161. *In* K. W. Walls and P. M. Schantz (ed.), Immunodiagnosis of parasitic diseases, vol. 1. Academic Press, Inc., New York.
21. **Franco, E. L., K. W. Walls, and A. J. Sulzer.** 1981. Reverse enzyme immunoassay for detection of specific anti-*Toxoplasma* immunoglobulin M antibodies. J. Clin. Microbiol. **13:**859–864.
22. **Frasch, A. C. C., and M. B. Reyes.** 1990. Diagnosis of Chagas disease using recombinant DNA technology. Parasitol. Today **6:**137–139.
23. **Freilij, H. L., R. S. Corral, A. M. Katzin, and S. Grinstein.** 1987. Antigenuria in infants with acute and congenital Chagas' disease. J. Clin. Microbiol. **25:**133–137.
24. **Frenkel, J. K.** 1990. Toxoplasmosis in human beings. J. Am. Vet. Med. Assoc. **196:**240–248.
25. **Gam, A. A., F. A. Neva, and W. A. Krotoski.** 1987. Comparative sensitivity and specificity of ELISA and IHA for serodiagnosis of strongyloidiasis with larval antigens. Am. J. Trop. Med. Hyg. **37:**157–161.
26. **Gamble, H. R., and C. E. Graham.** 1984. Monoclonal antibody-purified antigen for the immunodiagnosis of trichinosis. Am. J. Med. Vet. Res. **45:**67–73.
27. **Garcia, L. S., T. C. Brewer, and D. A. Bruckner.** 1987. Fluorescence detection of *Cryptosporidium* oocysts in human fecal specimens by using monoclonal antibodies. J. Clin. Microbiol. **25:**119–121.
28. **Genta, R. M., R. W. Douce, and P. D. Walzer.** 1986. Diagnostic implications of parasite-specific immune responses in immunocompromised patients with strongyloidiasis. J. Clin. Microbiol. **23:**1099–1103.
29. **Genta, R. M., and G. H. Weil.** 1982. Antibodies to *Stron-*

gyloides stercoralis larval surface antigen in chronic strongyloidiasis. Lab. Invest. **47:**87–90.

30. **Glickman, L. T., R. Cypess, D. Hiles, and T. Gessner.** 1979. *Toxocara* specific antibody in the serum and aqueous humor of a patient with presumed ocular and visceral toxocariasis. Am. J. Trop. Med. Hyg. **28:**29–35.
31. **Glickman, L. T., R. B. Grieve, S. S. Lauria, and D. L. Jones.** 1985. Serodiagnosis of ocular toxocariasis: a comparison of two antigens. J. Clin. Pathol. **38:**103–107.
32. **Glickman, L. T., and P. M. Schantz.** 1981. Epidemiology and pathogenesis of zoonotic toxocariasis. Epidemiol. Rev. **3:**230–250.
33. **Glickman, L. T., and P. M. Schantz.** 1985. Do *Toxocara canis* larva antigens used in enzyme-linked immunosorbent assay for visceral larva migrans cross-react with AB iso-hemagglutinins and give false positive results? Parasitenkunde **71:**394–400.
34. **Glickman, L. T., P. M. Schantz, R. Dombroske, and R. Cypess.** 1978. Evaluation of serodiagnostic tests for visceral larva migrans. Am. J. Trop. Med. Hyg. **27:**492–498.
35. **Glickman, L. T., P. M. Schantz, and R. B. Grieve.** 1986. Toxocariasis, p. 201–231. *In* K. W. Walls and P. M. Schantz (ed.), Immunodiagnosis of parasitic diseases, vol. 1. Academic Press, Inc., New York.
36. **Golightly, L. M., L. R. Hirschhorn, and P. E. Weller.** 1989. Fever and headache in a splenectomized woman. Rev. Infect. Dis. **11:**629–637.
37. **Gottstein, B.** 1984. An immunoassay for the detection of circulating antigens in human echinococcosis. Am. J. Trop. Med. Hyg. **33:**1185–1191.
38. **Gottstein, B.** 1985. Purification and characterization of a specific antigen from *Echinococcus multilocularis*. Parasite Immunol. **7:**202–212.
39. **Gottstein, B., P. M. Schantz, T. Todorov, A. G. Saimot, and P. Jacquier.** 1986. An international study on the serological differential diagnosis of human cystic and alveolar echinococcosis. Bull. WHO **64:**101–105.
40. **Grove, D. I.** 1980. Strongyloidasis in allied ex-prisoners of war-Asia. Br. Med. J. **1:**598–601.
41. **Grove, D. I., and A. J. Blair.** 1981. Diagnosis of human strongyloidiasis by immunofluorescence, using *Strongyloides ratti* and *S. stercoralis* larvae. Am. J. Trop. Med. Hyg. **30:**344–349.
42. **Grundy, M. S., A. Voller, and D. Warhurst.** 1987. An enzyme-linked immunosorbent assay for the detection of *Entamoeba histolytica* antigens in faecal material. Trans. R. Soc. Trop. Med. Hyg. **81:**627–632.
43. **Hancock, K., and V. C. W. Tsang.** 1986. Development and optimization of the FAST-ELISA for detecting antibodies to *Schistosoma mansoni*. J. Immunol. Methods **92:**167–176.
44. **Handman, E., G. F. Mitchell, and J. W. Goding.** 1987. *Leishmania major:* a very sensitive dot-blot ELISA for detection of parasites in cutaneous lesions. Mol. Biol. Med. **4:**377–383.
45. **Hillyer, G. V.** 1986. Fascioliasis, paragonimiasis, clonorchiasis and opisthorchiasis, p. 39–68. *In* K. W. Walls and P. M. Schantz (ed.), Immunodiagnosis of parasitic diseases, vol. 1. Academic Press, Inc., New York.
46. **Hillyer, G. V., R. H. Bermudez, and G. Ramirez de Arellano.** 1984. Use of immunologic techniques to predict success of therapy in human fascoliasis: a case report. Bol. Asoc. Med. P.R. **76:**116–119.
47. **Hillyer, G. V., and L. Sagramoso de Ateca.** 1980. Antibody responses in murine schistosomiasis and fascioliasis. Am. J. Trop. Med. Hyg. **29:**598–601.
48. **Hillyer, G. V., and M. Sole de Galanes.** 1988. Identification of a 17-kilodalton *Fasciola hepatica* immunodiagnostic antigen by the enzyme-linked immunoelectrotransfer blot technique. J. Clin. Microbiol. **26:**2048–2053.
49. **Holmberg, M., A. B. Vaidya, F. C. Shenton, R. W. Snow, B. M. Greenwood, H. Wigzell, and U. Pettersson.** 1990. A comparison of two DNA probes, one specific for *Plasmodium falciparum* and one with wider reactivity, in the diagnosis of malaria. Trans. R. Soc. Trop. Med. Hyg. **84:**202–205.
50. **Ihler, G. M., and A. C. Rice-Ficht.** 1989. Detection of hemotropic parasites by DNA hybridization, p. 233–247. *In* F. C. Tenover (ed.), DNA probes for infectious diseases. CRC Press, Inc., Boca Raton, Fla.
51. **Ivanoska, D., K. Cuperlovic, H. R. Gamble, and K. D. Murrell.** 1989. Comparative efficacy of antigen and antibody-detection tests for human trichinellosis. J. Parasitol. **75:**38–41.
52. **Johnson, R. J., and J. R. Johnson.** 1983. Paragonimiasis in Indochinese refugees: roentgenographic findings with clinical correlations. Am. Rev. Respir. Dis. **128:**534–538.
53. **Kagan, I. G.** 1980. Serodiagnosis of parasitic diseases, p. 724–750. *In* E. H. Lennette, A. Balows, W. J. Hausler, Jr., and J. P. Truant (ed.), Manual of clinical microbiology, 3rd ed. American Society for Microbiology, Washington, D.C.
54. **Kagan, I. G., L. Norman, and D. S. Allain.** 1963. An evaluation of the bentonite flocculation and indirect hemagglutination tests for diagnosis of filariasis. Am. J. Trop. Med. Hyg. **12:**548–555.
55. **Kirchhoff, L. V., A. A. Gam, R. d'A. Gusmao, R. S. Goldsmith, J. M. Rezende, and A. Rassi.** 1987. Increased specificity of serodiagnosis of Chagas' disease by detection of antibody to the 72- and 90-kilodalton glycoproteins of *Trypanosoma cruzi*. J. Infect. Dis. **155:**561–564.
56. **Knobloch, J., and R. Lederer.** 1983. Immunodiagnosis of human paragonimiasis by an enzyme immunoassay. Tropenmed. Parasitol. **34:**21–23.
57. **Knobloch, J., and E. Mannweiler.** 1983. Development and persistence of antibodies to *Entamoeba histolytica* in patients with amebic liver abscess. Am. J. Trop. Med. Hyg. **32:**727–732.
58. **Kobayashi, A., S. Suzuki, K. Horiuchi, M. Yokogawa, and K. Araki.** 1975. Four human cases of paragonimiasis miyazakii. Jikeikai Med. J. **22:**127–135.
59. **Lal, R. B., and E. A. Ottesen.** 1988. Enhanced diagnostic specificity in human filariasis by IgG_4 antibody assessment. J. Infect. Dis. **158:**1034–1037.
60. **Lanier, A. P., D. E. Trujillo, P. M. Schantz, J. F. Wilson, and B. Gottstein.** 1987. Comparison of serologic tests for diagnosis and followup of alveolar hydatid disease. Am. J. Trop. Med. Hyg. **37:**609–615.
61. **Luft, B. J., and J. S. Remington.** 1987. Toxoplasmic encephalitis. J. Infect. Dis. **157:**1–6.
62. **Lunde, M. N., R. Paranjape, T. J. Lawley, and E. A. Ottesen.** 1988. Filarial antigen in circulating immune complexes from patients with *Wuchereria bancrofti* filariasis. Am. J. Trop. Med. Hyg. **38:**366–371.
63. **Lutsch, M. N., J. Y. Cesbron, D. Henry, J. P. Dessaint, K. Wandji, M. Ismail, and A. Capron.** 1988. Lymphatic filariasis: detection of circulating and urinary antigen and differences in antibody isotypes complexed with circulating antigen between symptomatic and asymptomatic subjects. Clin. Exp. Immunol. **71:**253–260.
64. **Maddison, S. E.** 1987. The present status of serodiagnosis and seroepidemiology of schistosomiasis. Diagn. Microbiol. Infect. Dis. **7:**93–105.
65. **Maddison, S. E., S. B. Slemenda, P. M. Schantz, J. A. Fried, M. Wilson, and V. C. W. Tsang.** 1989. A specific diagnostic antigen of *Echinococcus granulosus* with an apparent molecular weight of 8 kDa. Am. J. Trop. Med. Hyg. **40:**377–383.
66. **Maddison, S. E., K. W. Walls, H. W. Haverkos, and D. D. Juranek.** 1984. Evaluation of serologic tests for *Pneumocystis carinii* antibody and antigenemia in patients with acquired immunodeficiency syndrome. Diagn. Microbiol. Infect. Dis. **2:**69–73.
67. **Maizels, R. M., M. Philipp, and B. M. Ogilivie.** 1982. Molecules on the surface of parasitic nematodes as probes

of the immune response in infection. Immunol. Rev. **61:** 109–136.

68. **Maizels, R. M., and B. D. Robertson.** 1989. *Toxocara canis:* secreted glycoconjugate antigens in immunobiology and immunodiagnosis, p. 1–9. *In* M. W. Kennedy (ed.), Parasitic nematodes—antigens, membranes and genes. Taylor and Francis Ltd., New York.
69. **Masur, H., H. C. Lane, J. A. Kovacs, C. J. Allegra, and J. C. Edman.** 1989. Pneumocystis pneumonia: from bench to clinic. Ann. Intern. Med. **111:**813–826.
70. **Naot, Y., G. Desmonts, and J. S. Remington.** 1981. IgM enzyme-linked immunosorbent assay test for the diagnosis of congenital *Toxoplasma* infection. J. Pediatr. **98:** 32–36.
71. **Naot, Y., D. R. Guptill, and J. S. Remington.** 1982. Duration of IgM antibodies to *Toxoplasma gondii* after acute acquired toxoplasmosis. J. Infect. Dis. **145:**770.
72. **Naot, Y., and J. S. Remington.** 1980. An enzyme-linked immunosorbent assay for detection of IgM antibodies to *Toxoplasma gondii:* use for diagnosis of acute acquired toxoplasmosis. J. Infect. Dis. **142:**757–766.
73. **Neva, F. A.** 1986. Biology and immunology of human strongyloidiasis. J. Infect. Dis. **153:**397–406.
74. **Neva, F. A., A. A. Gam, and J. Burke.** 1981. Comparison of larval and enzyme-linked immunosorbent assay for strongyloidiasis in humans. J. Infect. Dis. **144:**427–432.
75. **Norman, L., and I. Kagan.** 1975. An evaluation of crude and fractionated trichina antigens in the diagnosis of trichinosis. Bol. Chil. Parasitol. **30:**58–64.
76. **Ottesen, E. A.** 1984. Filariasis and tropical eosinophilia, p. 390–411. *In* K. S. Warren and A. F. Mahmoud (ed.), Tropical and geographical medicine. McGraw-Hill Book Co., New York.
77. **Pappas, M. G., P. B. McGreevy, R. Hajkowski, L. D. Hendricks, C. N. Oster, and W. T. Hockmeyer.** 1983. Evaluation of promastigote and amastigote antigens in the indirect fluorescent antibody test for American cutaneous leishmaniasis. Am. J. Trop. Med. Hyg. **32:**1260–1267.
78. **Pelletier, L. L., C. B. Baker, A. A. Gam, T. B. Nutman, and F. A. Neva.** 1988. Diagnosis and evaluation of treatment of chronic strongyloidiasis in ex-prisoners of war. J. Infect. Dis. **157:**573–576.
79. **Pollard, Z. F., W. H. Jarrett, W. S. Hagler, D. S. Allain, and P. M. Schantz.** 1979. ELISA for diagnosis of ocular toxocariasis. Ophthalmology **86:**750–752.
80. **Rosoff, J. D., C. A. Sanders, S. S. Sonnad, P. R. de Lay, W. K. Hadley, F. F. Vincenzi, D. M. Yajko, and P. D. O'Hanley.** 1989. Stool diagnosis of giardiasis using a commercially available enzyme immunoassay to detect *Giardia*-specific antigen 65 (GSA 65). J. Clin. Microbiol. **27:**1997–2002.
81. **Sato, Y., M. Takara, and M. Otsuru.** 1985. Detection of antibodies in strongyloidiasis by enzyme-linked immunosorbent assay (ELISA). Trans. R. Soc. Trop. Med. Hyg. **79:**51–55.
82. **Schantz, P. M.** 1987. Improvements in the serodiagnosis of helminthic zoonoses. Vet. Parasitol. **25:**95–120.
83. **Schantz, P. M., and B. Gottstein.** 1986. Echinococcus (hydatidosis), p. 69–107. *In* K. W. Walls and P. M. Schantz (ed.), Immunodiagnosis of parasitic diseases, vol. 1. Academic Press, New York.
84. **Schantz, P. M., D. Myer, and L. T. Glickman.** 1979. Clinical, serologic, and epidemiologic characteristics of ocular toxocariasis. Am. J. Trop. Med. Hyg. **28:**24–28.
85. **Schantz, P. M., D. Shanks, and M. Wilson.** 1980. Serologic cross-reactions with sera from patients with echinococcosis and cysticercosis. Am. J. Trop. Med. Hyg. **21:**609–612.
86. **Slemenda, S. B., S. E. Maddison, E. C. Jong, and D. D. Moore.** 1988. Diagnosis of paragonimiasis by immunoblot. Am. J. Trop. Med. Hyg. **39:**469–471.
87. **Smith, H. V., H. R. Hinson, and R. W. A. Girdwood.** 1985. Serodiagnosis of human toxocariasis. Trans. R. Soc. Trop. Med. Hyg. **81:**516.
88. **Smith, H. V., J. R. Kusel, and R. W. A. Girdwood.** 1985. The production of human A and B blood group like substances by *in vitro* maintained second stage *Toxocara canis* larvae: their presence on the outer larval surfaces and in their excretions/secretions. Clin. Exp. Immunol. **54:**625–633.
89. **Sulzer, A. J., and M. Wilson.** 1971. The indirect fluorescent antibody test for the detection of occult malaria in blood donors. Bull. WHO **45:**375–379.
90. **Tribouley-Duret, J., J. Tribouley, M. Apprious, and R. N. Mergroud.** 1978. Application du test ELISA au diagnostic de la strongyloidose. Ann. Parasitol. Hum. Comp. **53:**641–8.
91. **Tsang, V. C. W., J. A. Brand, and A. E. Boyer.** 1989. An enzyme-linked immunoelectrotransfer blot assay and glycoprotein antigens for diagnosing human cysticercosis (*Taenia solium*). J. Infect. Dis. **159:**50–59.
92. **Tsang, V. C. W., K. Hancock, S. E. Maddison, A. L. Beatty, and D. M. Moss.** 1984. Demonstration of species-specific and cross-reactive components of the adult microsomal antigens from *Schistosoma mansoni* and *S. japonicum* (MAMA and JAMA). J. Immunol. **132:**2607–2613.
93. **Walls, K. W.** 1985. Serodiagnostic tests for parasitic diseases, p. 945–948. *In* E. H. Lennette, A. Balows, W. J. Hausler, Jr., and H. J. Shadomy (ed.), Manual of clinical microbiology, 4th ed. American Society for Microbiology, Washington, D.C.
94. **Walls, K. W., and M. Wilson.** 1984. The use of the solid phase indirect immunofluorescent assay (FIAX) in the serodiagnosis of amebiasis. Ann. N.Y. Acad. Sci. **420:**422–430.
95. **Weil, G. J., D. C. Jain, S. Santhanam, A. Malhotra, H. Kumar, K. V. P. Sethumadhavan, F. Liftis, and T. K. Ghosh.** 1987. A monoclonal antibody-based enzyme immunoassay for detecting parasite antigenemia in Bancroftian filariasis. J. Infect. Dis. **156:**350–355.
96. **Weil, G. J., K. V. P. Sethomadhavan, S. Santhanam, D. C. Jain, and T. K. Gosh.** 1988. Persistence of parasite antigenemia following diethylcarbamazine therapy of Bancroftian filariasis. Am. J. Trop. Med. Hyg. **38:**589–595.
97. **Weiss, N., R. Hussain, and E. A. Ottesen.** 1982. IgE antibodies are more species-specific than IgG antibodies in human onchocerciasis and lymphatic filariasis. Immunology **45:**129–137.
98. **Wilson, M., D. A. Ware, and D. D. Juranek.** 1990. Serologic aspects of toxoplasmosis. J. Am. Vet. Med. Assoc. **196:**277–281.
99. **Wilson, M., D. A. Ware, and K. W. Walls.** 1987. Evaluation of commercial serodiagnostic kits for toxoplasmosis. J. Clin. Microbiol. **25:**2262–2265.
100. **Wirth, D. F., W. D. Rogers, H. Dourado, and B. Albuquerque.** 1989. Leishmaniasis: DNA probes for diagnosis, p. 249–258. *In* T. C. Tenover (ed.), DNA probes for infectious diseases. CRC Press, Inc., Boca Raton, Fla.
101. **Yokogawa, M., K. Arki, K. Saito, T. Momose, M. Kimura, S. Suzuki, and N. Chiba.** 1974. *Paragonimus miyazakii* infections in man first found in Kanto district, Japan.—Especially, the methods of immunosero-diagnosis. Jpn. J. Parasitol. **23:**167–179.
102. **Yokogawa, M., M. Tsuji, and T. Okura.** 1962. Studies on the complement fixation test for paragonimiasis as the method of criterion of cure. Jpn. J. Parasitol. **11:**117–122.

Chapter 68

Blood and Tissue Protozoa

DONALD J. KROGSTAD, GOVINDA S. VISVESVARA, KENNETH W. WALLS, AND JAMES W. SMITH

Pathogenic protozoa may infect the gastrointestinal or genitourinary tracts (chapter 69) or invade the blood or deep tissues. Protozoan infections are usually diagnosed morphologically if the parasites are present in the blood (malaria and babesiosis) or in areas readily accessible to biopsy (cutaneous leishmaniasis). In contrast, protozoan infections at sites difficult to biopsy (e.g., systemic toxoplasmosis) are typically diagnosed serologically or by other, less direct methods.

MALARIA

Malaria is of overwhelming importance in the developing world. Each year, there are 200 million to 300 million cases of malaria and 2 million to 3 million deaths from the disease. Although malaria is distinctly less common in developed countries such as the United States and Canada, 700 to 1,000 cases are diagnosed in the United States and reported to the Centers for Disease Control (CDC) each year (10). Despite their smaller numbers, these cases are of concern because (i) they occur primarily among nonimmune travelers, who are at increased risk for severe and complicated malaria (11), and (ii) they are often misdiagnosed initially by physicians unfamiliar with the signs and symptoms of malaria.

Life cycle

Malaria is transmitted to humans by sporozoites from the salivary glands of female anopheline mosquitoes. After their inoculation by the mosquito, sporozoites travel via the bloodstream to the liver, where they infect hepatocytes. After 8 to 25 days (depending on the species), sporozoites mature to infectious tissue schizonts and release 2,000 to 30,000 merozoites, which reenter the bloodstream and infect erythrocytes (Fig. 1). The asexual replication cycle then recurs in erythrocytes in the bloodstream at regular intervals (48 h for *Plasmodium falciparum, P. vivax,* or *P. ovale;* 72 h for *P. malariae*) until treatment, acquisition of immunity, or death supervenes. In the relapsing malarias (*P. vivax* and *P. ovale*), some sporozoites become dormant hypnozoites after entering hepatocytes. These hypnozoites can develop to mature tissue schizonts (and release merozoites) 6 to 24 months later. Thus, they provide a morphologic explanation for the phenomenon of relapsing malaria (44, 45). Primaquine, which is used to prevent relapse, eradicates hypnozoites and gametocytes, whereas chloroquine is not effective against either. Although gametocytes do not produce disease in humans, they are essential to complete the parasite life cycle. In the anopheline mosquito, macro- and microgametocytes (derived from infected erythrocytes) fuse to form an ookinete, which undergoes reduction division to produce infectious sporozoites (Fig. 1).

Epidemiology

For practical purposes, malaria is endemic only in tropical areas of the developing world. However, the anopheline mosquito vector necessary for malaria transmission is also present in the developed countries such as the United States. As a result, malaria transmission can and does occur in the United States after the introduction of large numbers of infected persons (e.g., following the Korean and Vietnam wars and the more recent influx of refugees from Southeast Asia) (10). Malaria may also be transmitted by the transfusion of infected blood or blood products, by the sharing of syringes among drug addicts, or by disruption of the normal placental barrier at birth (congenital malaria) (43). Because the most common presenting symptoms of malaria (fever, chills, and myalgia) are nonspecific and may not develop until after the infected person returns to a nonmalarious area, rapid laboratory diagnosis is typically the most important factor in determining the clinical outcome in a nonimmune traveler.

Differences among plasmodial species

Infections caused by *P. falciparum* are more fulminant than those caused by other plasmodia and may produce coma and cerebral malaria within 2 to 3 days in nonimmune persons (11). In addition, *P. falciparum* infections are often resistant to chloroquine (31, 42). The other plasmodia that infect humans are all chloroquine susceptible (*P. vivax, P. ovale,* and *P. malariae*). The laboratory must diagnose the infecting species correctly and rapidly for the clinician to choose appropriate antimalarial agents (42) and to anticipate the likely complications (11). For reasons noted above, it is particularly important to differentiate *P. falciparium* from the other species.

P. vivax and *P. ovale* infections are very similar clinically and morphologically. Both parasites produce limited parasitemias and milder illnesses than *P. falciparum* because they preferentially invade young erythrocytes (52); both produce late relapses from persistent infection of hepatocytes (hypnozoites), and both produce enlargement of and Schuffner stippling in their host erythrocytes. Fortunately, this potential for confusion rarely has adverse clinical consequences because both *P. vivax* and *P. ovale* infections are treated with the same antimalarial agents (42).

Because *P. malariae* rarely causes acute illness, the differential diagnosis of malaria in the acutely ill patient is usually between *P. falciparum* and *P. vivax* (or *P. ovale*).

Diagnosis of malaria

Morphology. Examination of stained blood smears is the only readily available way to diagnose malaria

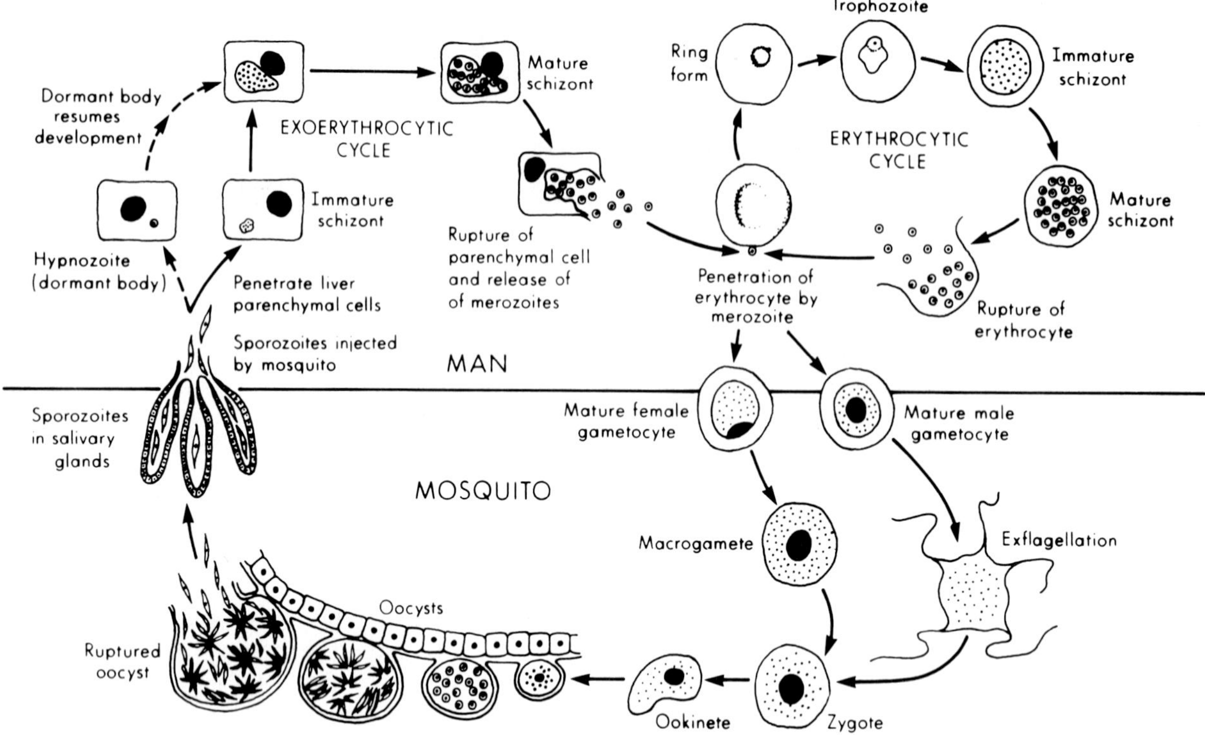

FIG. 1. Life cycle of the malaria parasite. (Reproduced with permission from reference 42.)

within the clinically relevant time frame (1 to 3 h). Thick and thin blood smears should be prepared and stained with Giemsa stain as described in chapter 66. Although parasites may also be seen with other stains, Wright stain cannot be used with thick films. Giemsa stain is preferred by most investigators and should be used if malaria is suspected.

Thick blood smears are more sensitive than thin smears because they permit one to examine 10-fold-greater volumes of blood per unit area (or time) on the microscope slide. The sensitivity of the thick smear is greater because the erythrocytes are dehemoglobinized by exposure to the hypotonic Giemsa stain without prior fixation in methanol (as in the thin smear). The result is that only parasites and leukocytes remain after staining. Most experienced malariologists prefer thick smears because of their greater sensitivity. However, thick smears are more difficult to read than thin smears because the erythrocytes are no longer evident. As a result, one cannot determine the effect of the parasite on the size of its host erythrocyte (Table 1), the presence of Schuffner stippling, or the position of the parasite within the erythrocyte (Table 2). For these reasons, thin smears may be necessary to identify the infecting species (Fig. 2 to 7) and are often preferable to thick smears (Fig. 8 to 10) for laboratories that have only occasional experience with positive specimens.

Potential pitfalls in Giemsa staining. The most common problem in Giemsa staining is failure to control the pH of the phosphate buffer, which should be between 7.0 and 7.2. Because the detection of Schuffner stippling in erythrocytes infected by *P. vivax* or *P. ovale* is particularly pH dependent, incorrectly buffered stain may cause *P. vivax* or *P. ovale* infection to be mistaken for *P. falciparum* infection.

Pitfalls in microscopy. In examining the stained blood film, inexperienced observers commonly make two mistakes.

1. Inadequate magnification. Ring-stage malaria parasites are characteristically ≤2 μm in diameter. For this reason, oil immersion magnification (≥ ×1,000) is essential. Standard high-power magnification (×440) is inadequate to distinguish malaria parasites from platelets, precipitated stain, or nonspecific debris.
2. Confusion of parasites with platelets. Platelets are similar in size to malaria parasites and are often mistaken for plasmodia when they are on top of an erythrocyte in the blood film. This problem can usually be resolved by identifying other platelets

TABLE 1. Simplified identification of plasmodia[a]

Characteristic	*P. vivax* (and *P. ovale*)	*P. falciparum*	*P. malariae*
Enlarged infected cells	+	0	0
Schuffner stippling	+	0	0
Multiple erythrocytic stages on smear	+	0	+
Multiply infected erythrocytes	±	+	0

[a] The most reliable criteria are erythrocyte enlargement and Schuffner stippling. Other criteria (in the bottom two lines of the table) are relative and should not be taken as absolute (see the text for details).

TABLE 2. Morphology of *Plasmodium* species infecting humans[a]

Species	Appearance of erythrocyte		Appearance of parasite			Stages found in circulating blood
	Size	Schuffner stippling	Cytoplasm	Pigment	No. of merozoites	
P. vivax	Enlarged; maximum size (attained with mature trophozoites and schizonts) may be 1.5 to 2 times normal erythrocyte diameter	Present with all stages except early ring forms	Irregular, ameboid in trophozoites; has "spread-out" appearance	Golden brown, inconspicuous	12–24; avg, 16	All stages; wide range of stages may be seen on given film
P. malariae	Normal	Absent (Ziemann's dots rarely seen)	Rounded, compact trophozoites with dense cytoplasm; band-form trophozoites occasionally seen	Dark brown, coarse, conspicuous	6–12; avg, 8; "rosette" schizonts occasionally seen	All stages; wide variety of stages usually not seen; relatively few rings or gametocytes generally present
P. ovale	Enlarged; maximum size may be 1.25 to 1.5 times normal erythrocyte diameter; ~20% or more of infected erythrocytes are oval or fimbriated or both (border has irregular projections)	Present with all stages except early ring forms	Rounded, compact trophozoites; occasionally slightly ameboid; growing trophozoites have large chromatin mass	Dark brown, conspicuous	6–14; avg, 8	All stages
P. falciparum	Normal; multiply infected erythrocytes are common	Absent (Maurer's dots occasionally seen)	Young rings are small, delicate, often with double chromatin dots; gametocytes are crescent or elongate	Black; coarse and conspicuous in gametocytes	6–32; avg, 20–24	Rings or gametocytes or both; other stages develop in blood vessels of internal organs but are not seen in peripheral blood except in severe infections

[a] See reference 72.

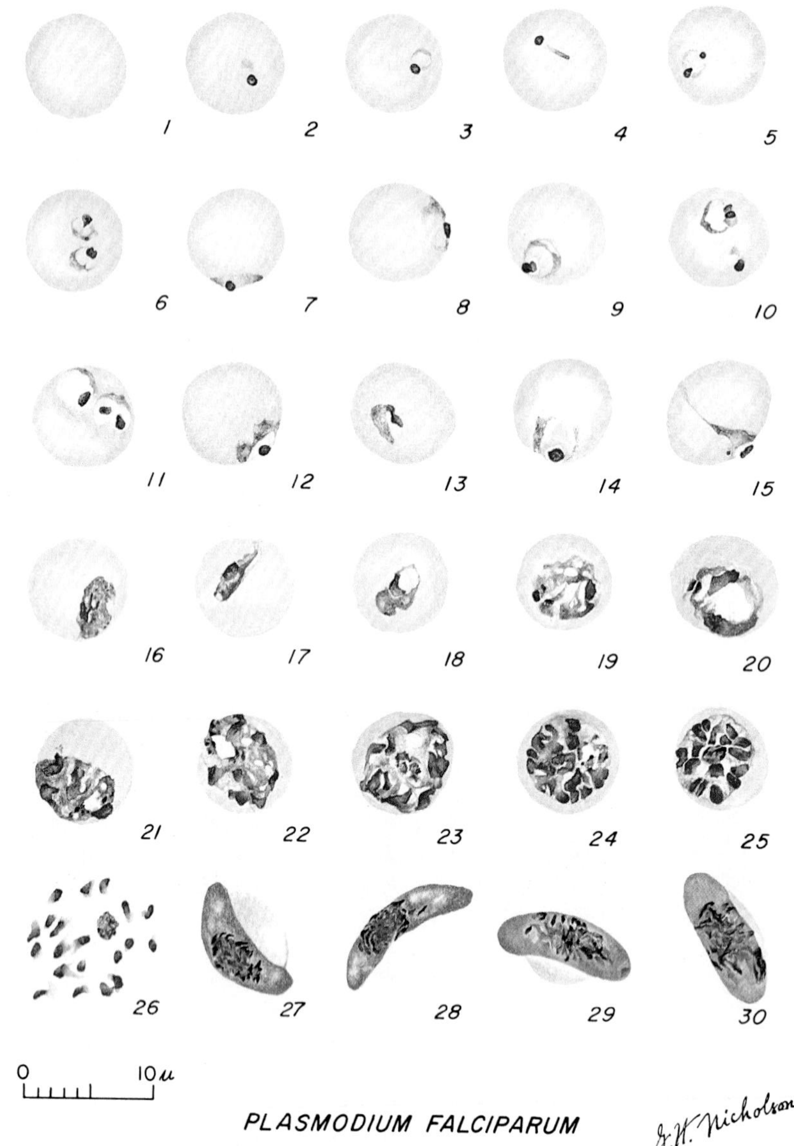

FIG. 2. *Plasmodium falciparum* growth stages: successive developmental stages as they appear in stained blood films. Rings and gametocytes will be found in peripheral blood films; other stages occur in erythrocytes but are sequestered in the capillaries of internal organs and hence are rarely found in peripheral blood films. Drawings: 1, normal erythrocyte; 2 to 11, young trophozoites; 12 to 15, growing trophozoites; 16 to 18, mature trophozoites; 19 to 22, immature schizonts; 23 to 26, nearly mature and mature schizonts; 27 and 28, mature macrogametocytes; 29 and 30, mature microgametocytes. (Reproduced with permission from reference 12.)

that are not near erythrocytes by their morphology on thin smears and by determining that no pigment, chromatin dots, or signet rings are present.

Alternative methods. In malaria-endemic areas, there is a need to examine relatively large numbers of specimens within short periods of time. To address this need, a rapid detection system based on fluorescence microscopy has recently been developed (73). In this test, acridine orange is used to stain and visualize the parasite. The parasite is identified by its morphology and by its characteristic position at the top of the erythrocyte layer after centrifugation in a microhematocrit tube. Preliminary studies with this technique suggest that it has a sensitivity approximately eightfold greater than that of the thick smear and that a specimen can be examined in 30 to 40 s (versus the several hours necessary to dry, stain, and examine a thick smear).

Serologic tests (antibody detection) are not useful for the diagnosis of acute malaria because most patients

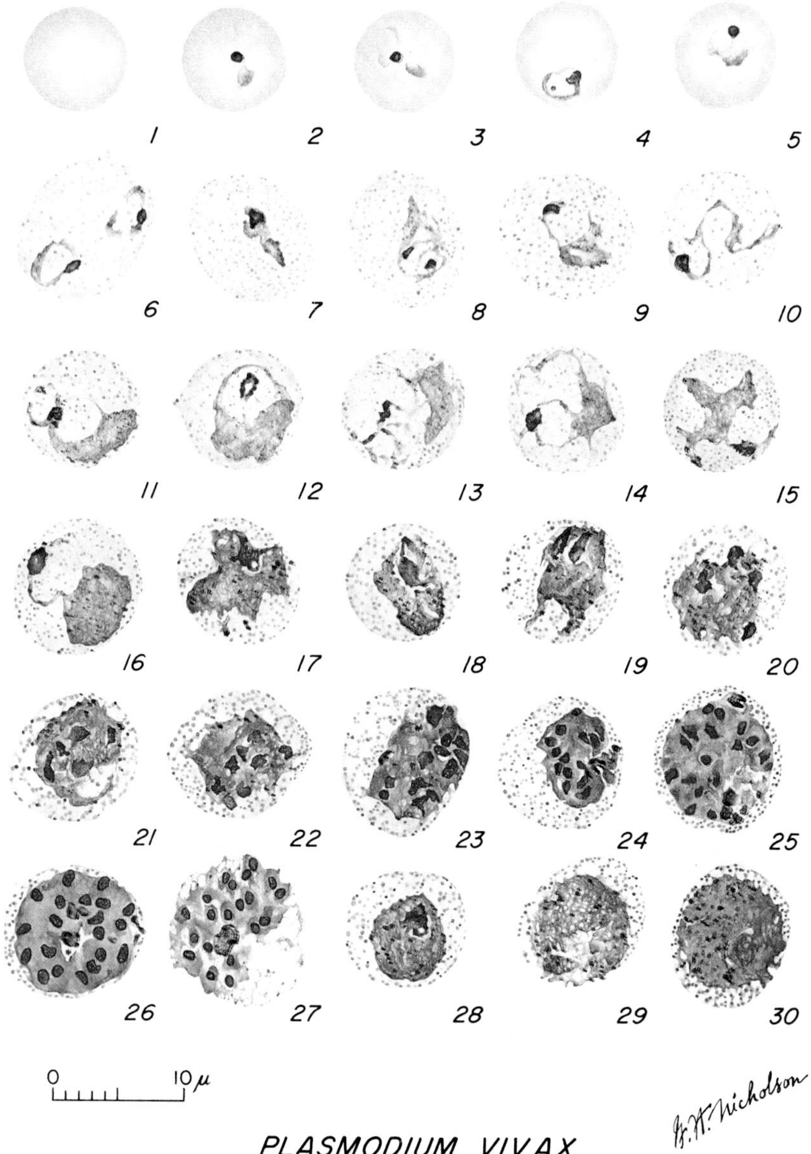

FIG. 3. *Plasmodium vivax* growth stages: successive developmental stages as they appear in stained blood films. Drawings: 1, normal erythrocyte; 2 to 5, young trophozoites; 6 to 16, growing trophozoites; 17 and 18, mature trophozoites; 19 to 21, young (early) immature schizonts; 22 and 23, older immature schizonts; 24 to 27, nearly mature and mature schizonts; 28 and 29, nearly mature and mature macrogametocytes; 30, mature microgametocyte. (Reproduced with permission from reference 12.)

require 3 or more weeks to produce a diagnostic rise in antibody titer.

Diagnosis of the infecting species

Morphology. In acutely ill patients, the infecting species is typically either *P. falciparum* or *P. vivax* and can usually be identified morphologically by using simple criteria such as the size of the parasitized erythrocyte, Schuffner stippling, and the variety of parasite stages present (Tables 1 and 2). However, if most parasites are early (ring) stages and Schuffner stippling is not seen, it may be difficult or impossible to distinguish between *P. falciparum* and *P. vivax* or *P. ovale*. In such situations and in patients with mixed infections (5 to 7% of patients with malaria have mixed infections), more subtle morphologic criteria must be used, such as the number of parasites per erythrocyte or the central versus peripheral location of the parasite within the erythrocyte (Table 2). Unfortunately, these criteria are less reliable and may be misleading. For example, *P. vivax* infections may have more than one parasite per erythrocyte, may have double chromatin dots, and may have parasites at the

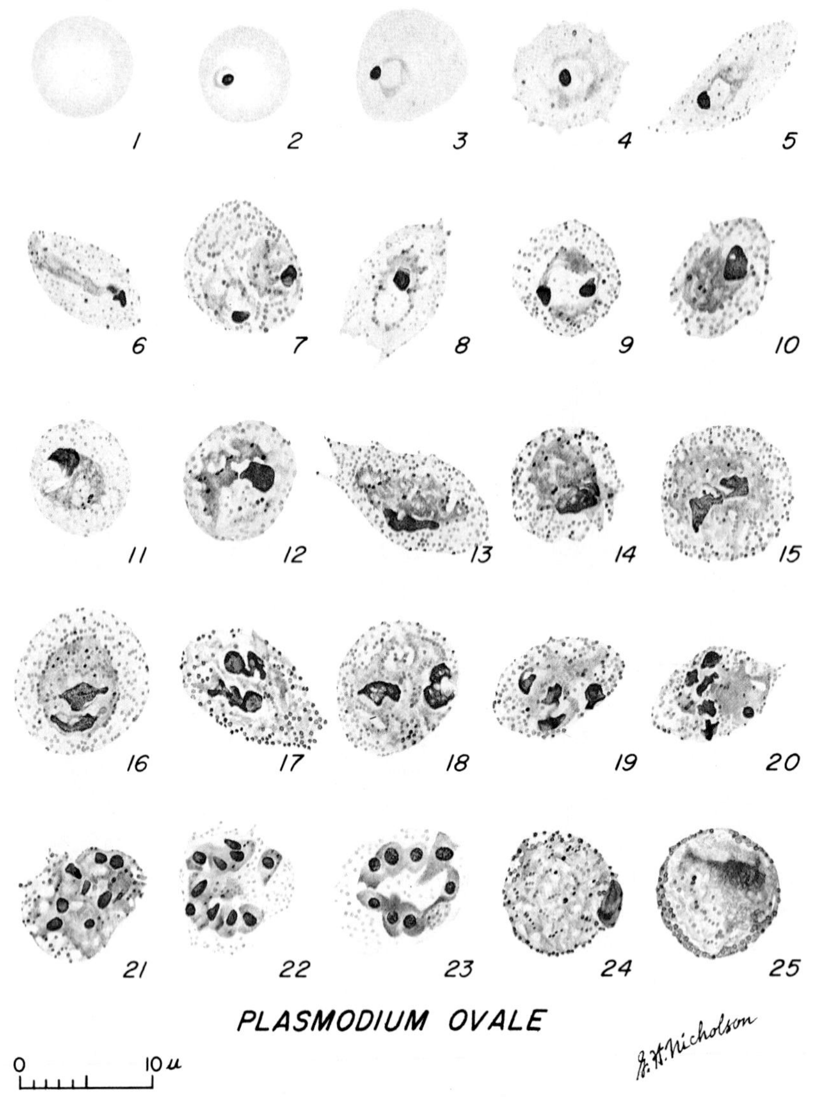

FIG. 4. *Plasmodium ovale* growth stages: successive development stages as they appear in stained blood films. Drawings: 1, normal erythrocyte; 2 to 5, young trophozoites; 6 to 12, growing trophozoites; 13 to 15, mature trophozoites; 16 to 22, immature schizonts; 23, mature schizont; 24, mature macrogametocyte; 25, mature microgametocyte. (Reproduced with permission from reference 12.)

periphery (rather than the center) of the erythrocyte (72). Other potentially useful criteria include the intensity of the parasitemia (*P. falciparum* produces the highest parasitemias because it can invade erythrocytes of all ages) (Table 3) (52), the number of merozoites in a mature schizont, and the variety of asexual forms present on the peripheral smear (the only asexual forms present in *P. falciparum* infections are ring forms). These criteria are summarized in Table 3.

Although banana-shaped gametocytes are diagnostic of *P. falciparum* infection, their absence does not exclude that diagnosis. Because *P. falciparum* gametocytes take longer to mature than the asexual forms of the parasite (8 to 10 days versus 2 days), nonimmune travelers often become severely ill before sufficient time has elapsed to permit the maturation of diagnostic ga-

TABLE 3. Plasmodial infection and erythrocyte age[a]

Plasmodium species	Erythrocyte age	Maximal parasitemia (per μl)
P. malariae	Old	10,000
P. vivax (and *P. ovale*)	Young	25,000
P. falciparum	Any age	≥1,000,000

[a] Adapted from Neva (52).

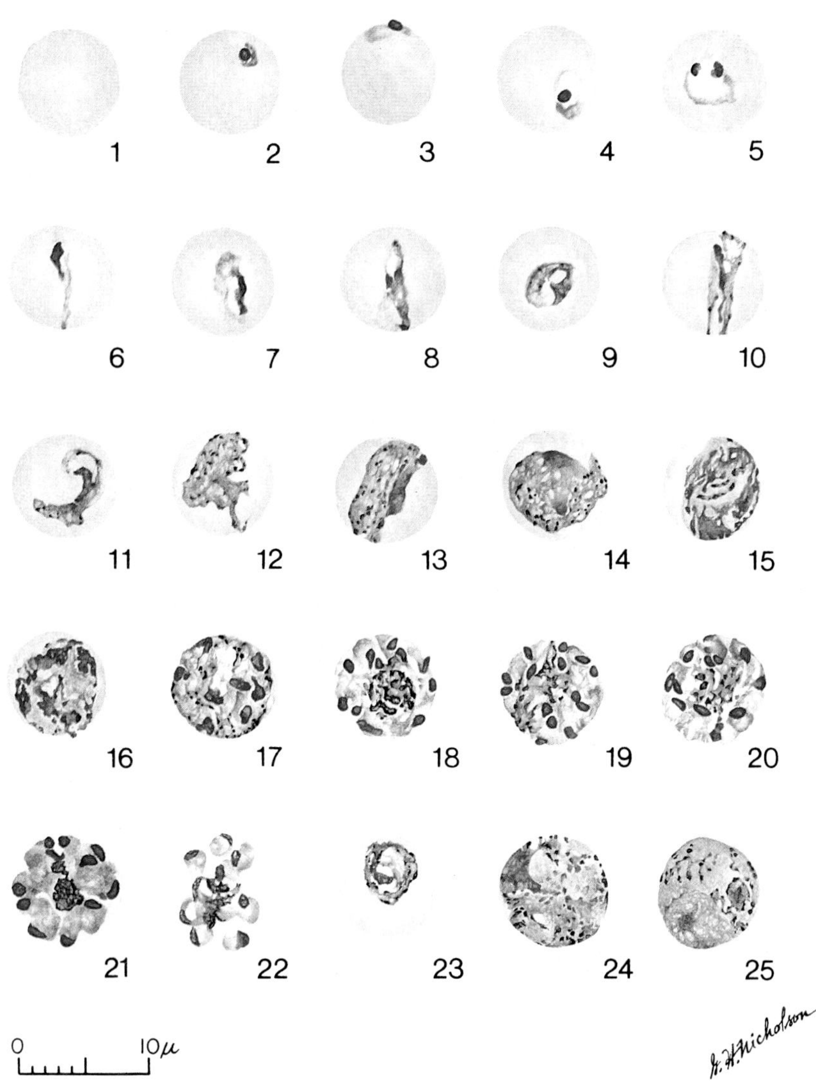

FIG. 5. *Plasmodium malariae* growth stages: successive developmental stages as they appear in stained blood films. Drawings; 1, normal erythrocyte; 2 to 5, young trophozoites; 6 to 11, growing trophozoites; 12 and 13, nearly mature and mature trophozoites; 14 to 20, immature schizonts; 21 and 22, mature schizonts; 23, developing gametocyte; 24, mature macrogametocyte; 25, mature microgametocyte. (Reproduced with permission from reference 12.)

metocytes in vivo. Thus, despite their prominence in textbooks, gametocytes are rarely present in blood smears obtained from acutely ill nonimmune persons. In contrast, gametocytes alone are frequently observed in smears from semi-immune residents of malaria-endemic areas.

Alternative methods. Several laboratories are studying DNA probes for the specific diagnosis of malaria. The most interesting probes are directed at multiply repeated regions of the genome in *P. falciparum* to diagnose infections with that species (1, 19). The current sensitivity of this method is similar to that of the thick smear, but the technique requires the use of radioisotopes. Although the sensitivity of the method has been enhanced by use of the polymerase chain reaction (68), the polymerase chain reaction may also produce false-positive test results. Both the false-positive test results and the need for a nonradioactive detection system must be addressed before this method can be applied in the developing world where malaria is endemic. Fluorescence microscopy of acridine orange-stained blood specimens (73) will need to be studied in greater detail to define its accuracy in diagnosing the infecting parasite species.

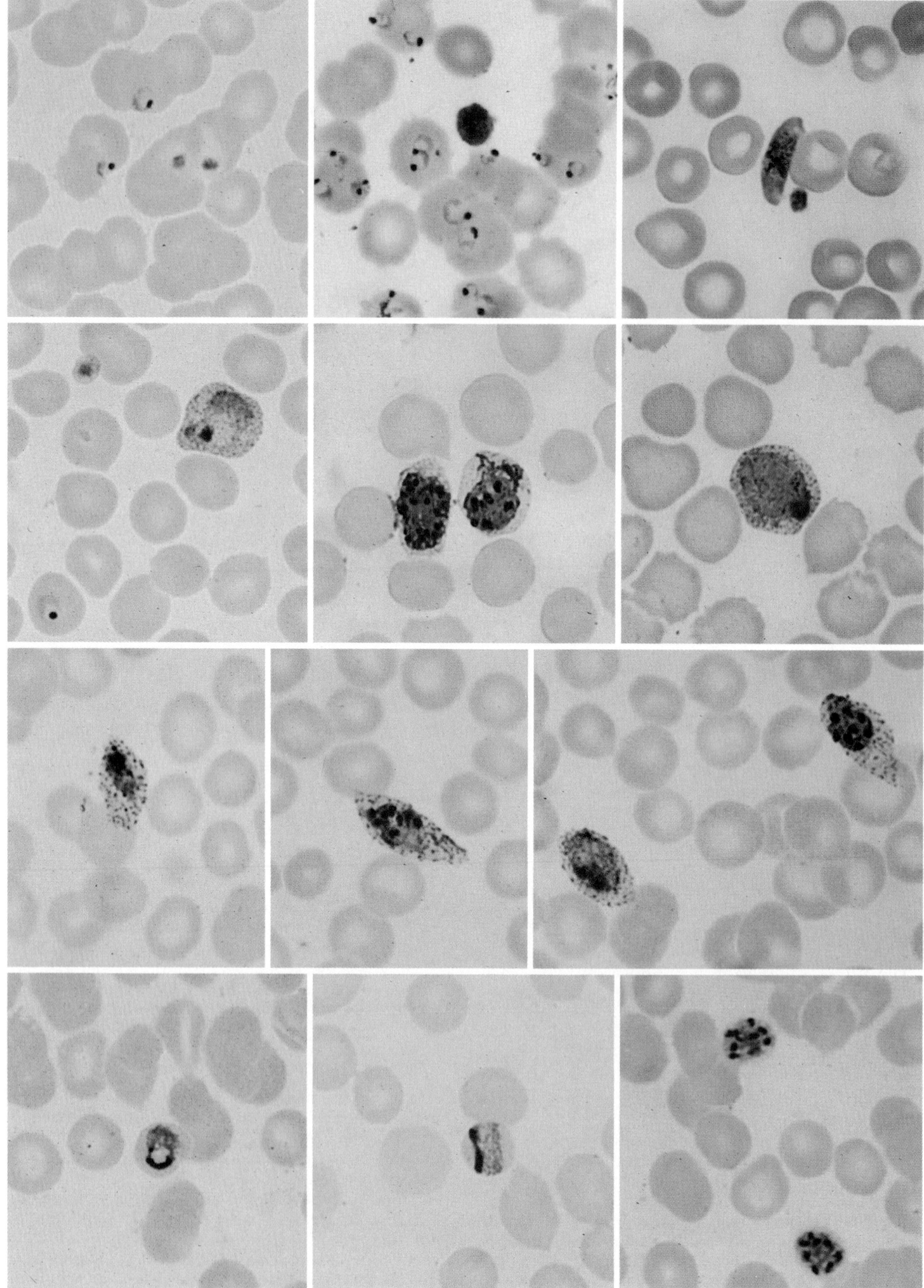

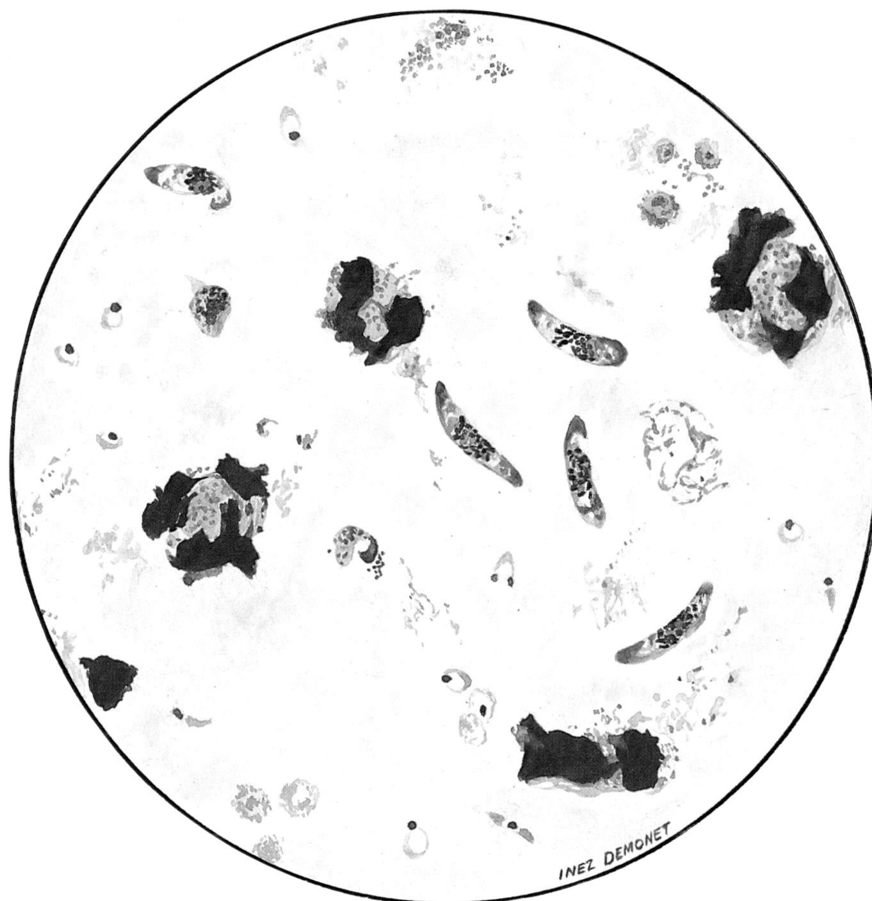

FIG. 7. Morphology of *Plasmodium falciparum* in thick blood film. There are multiple small (ring-form) trophozoites and sausage-shaped gametocytes. In addition, there are two gametocytes toward 10 o'clock which have other shapes. (Reproduced from reference 89.)

Effects of treatment

Morphology. Treatment with antimalarial agents may change the morphology of parasites in the bloodstream within hours. Typical changes observed with chloroquine and quinine include vacuolation of the parasite cytoplasm resulting from enlargement of the parasite's food vacuole (lysosome) and its other acid vesicles. Although patients may improve clinically within hours after treatment (in part from the antipyretic effects of many antimalarial agents), short-term changes in the magnitude of the parasitemia are determined in large measure by the synchronous nature of most malaria infections. Thus, the parasitemia may remain relatively constant for 24 to 30 h even when treatment is effective. Conversely, the parasitemia may fall on alternate days in *P. falciparum* infection even with ineffective treatment as a result of the peripheral sequestration of trophozoite- and schizont-containing erythrocytes. For these reasons, apparent changes in the morphology and number of circulating parasites in the first 1 to 2 days after treatment should be interpreted with caution. Effective treatment should either eliminate or dramatically reduce the number of circulating parasites within 3 to 6 days after treatment (92). Gametocytes are not killed by chloroquine and thus may be found in blood films after successful therapy.

Alternative methods. Both DNA probes and fluorescence microscopy have been used to monitor the response of malaria to treatment. Although both methods offer promise, the amount of experience with each is insufficient to recommend them for general use at this time.

FIG. 6. Photomicrographs of *Plasmodium* species in thin blood films; Giemsa stain, ×1,000. (First row) *Plasmodium falciparum*. Left: Two erythrocytes contain ring-form trophozoites. In addition, two platelets are present. Center: Numerous rings in erythrocytes of a patient with severe *P. falciparum* malaria. Right: Sausage-shaped microgametocyte. (Second row) *Plasmodium vivax*. Left: Growing trophozoite in enlarged erythrocyte with Schuffner stippling. A ring-form trophozoite is present in another erythrocyte. Center: Immature and mature schizonts. Right: Macrogametocyte. (Third row) *Plasmodium ovale*. Left: Growing trophozoite which is compact in an enlarged, elongated erythrocyte with fimbriae and Schuffner stippling. Center: Mature schizont. Right: Schizont and macrogametocyte. (Fourth row) *Plasmodium malariae*. Left: Normal-size erythrocyte containing growing trophozoite. Center: Band-shaped trophozoite. Right: Two mature schizonts. (Photomicrographs from Lawrence Ash, used with permission.)

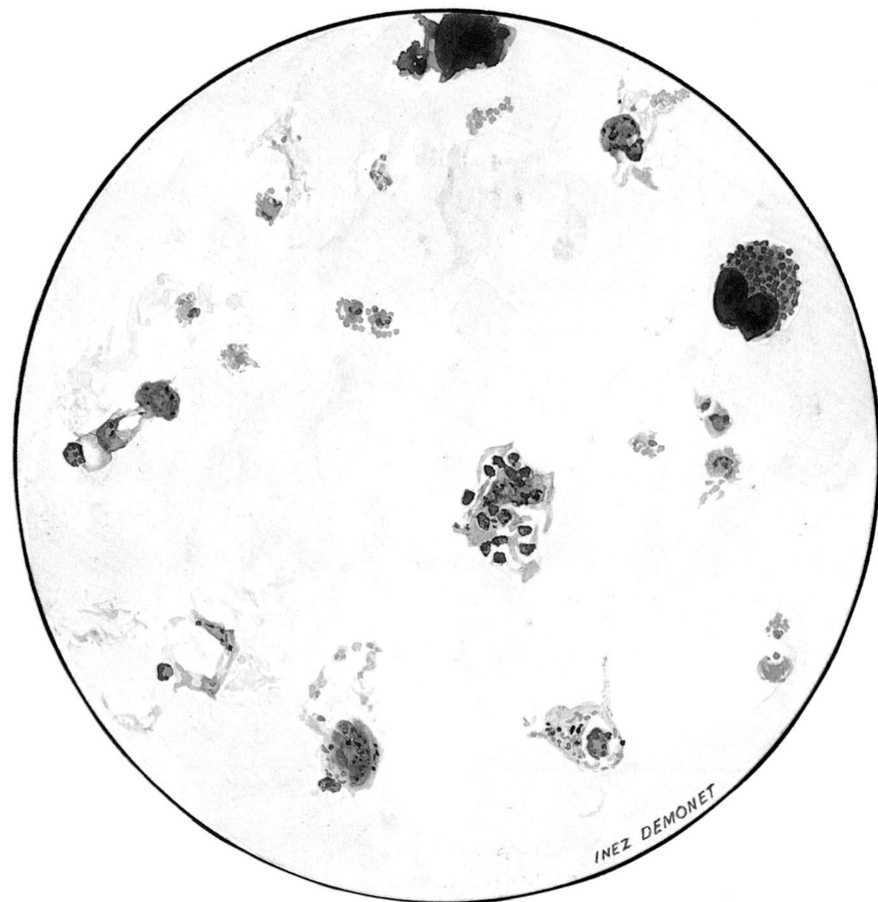

FIG. 8. Morphology of *Plasmodium vivax* in thick blood film. There are ameboid trophozoites at 2, 8, and 9 o'clock, an immature schizont with two chromatic masses at 7 o'clock, a macrogametocyte at 5 o'clock, and a mature schizont near the center. (Reproduced from reference 89).

Serologic diagnosis

Serologic testing for antibodies is not useful for the diagnosis of malaria in acutely ill patients because the time delays involved are greater than the time frame for clinical decision making. The decision as to whether (or how) to treat an acutely ill patient must be made in 1 to 3 h, whereas 3 or more weeks are required to produce a diagnostic rise in antibody titer and another several weeks are needed to send the specimens to CDC or another reference laboratory for testing.

However, if the morphologic diagnosis is not clear because smears were obtained only after treatment, because the patient was treated empirically, or because of a low parasitemia with only ring forms, retrospective serologic testing may be helpful. For example, a 14-day course of primaquine should be given to persons with indirect fluorescence (IIF) test results suggestive of recent *P. vivax* infection to prevent late relapse due to persistent hypnozoites in the liver even if the original illness responded to treatment with chloroquine alone. Chloroquine is active against the asexual erythrocytic forms that produce clinical symptoms but not against the hypnozoites that produce relapse.

Serologic testing is also helpful in the identification of infected blood donors associated with transfusion malaria and has been used in epidemiologic studies of transmission in malaria-endemic areas. Serologic testing is not particularly useful for the study of individual patients in malaria-endemic areas because of cross-reactivity among species and because titers may remain elevated for years after infection.

Specific-antibody testing is currently performed at CDC for antibodies to *P. falciparum*, *P. vivax*, and *P. malariae*. No commercial reagents or kits are available. In persons with a single defined exposure (e.g., tourists), titers of <1:64 suggest no exposure, titers of 1:64 suggest recent exposure, and titers of >1:64 indicate recent exposure and clinical illness.

BABESIOSIS

Babesia species that may infect humans include *B. microti*, a rodent parasite, and *B. bovis*, a parasite of cattle which has been associated with disease in splenectomized patients. In the United States, babesiosis is generally caused by *B. microti*. Like plasmodia, babesia live in erythrocytes and (in severe infections) may produce massive hemolysis. In contrast to plasmodia, ba-

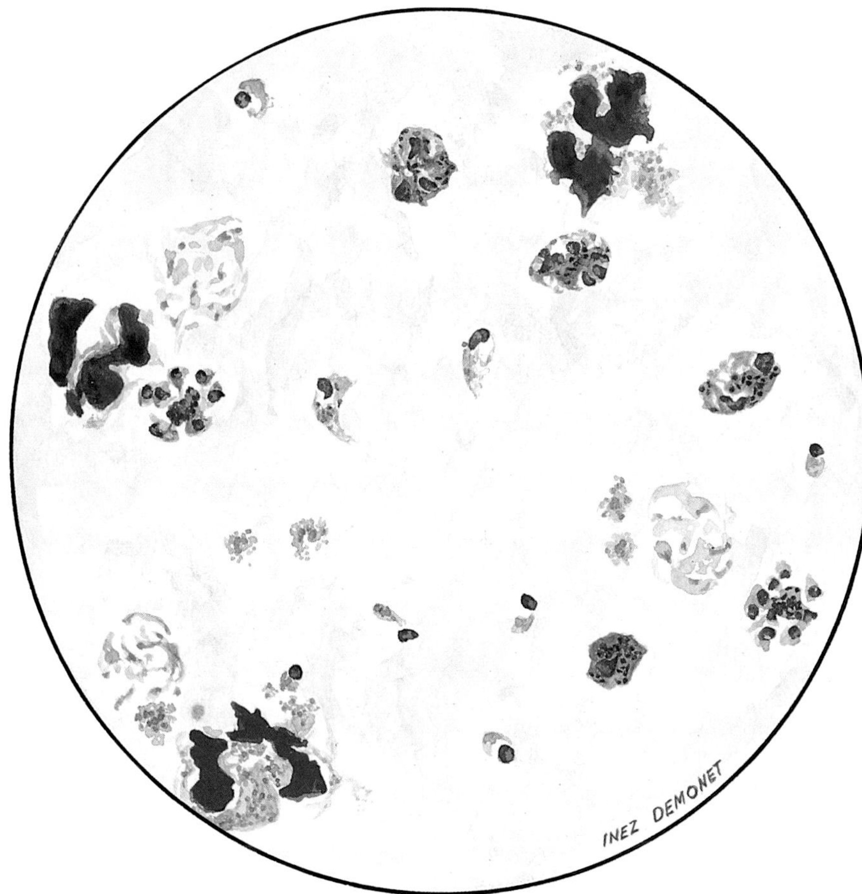

FIG. 9. Morphology of *Plasmodium malariae* in thick blood film. There are small trophozoites toward 6 o'clock, growing trophozoites slightly above the center, mature trophozoites at 5 o'clock, immature schizonts at 12, 1, and 3 o'clock, and mature schizonts at 4 and 9 o'clock. (Reproduced from reference 89.)

besia have no known exoerythrocytic stages. Babesiosis was first described in humans as a fatal infection of splenectomized patients and other immunosuppressed hosts. Subsequent serologic studies have shown that undiagnosed babesia infections are common in endemic areas such as Martha's Vineyard and that most patients recover uneventfully (61).

Life cycle and epidemiology

Babesiosis is a zoonosis that involves humans only accidentally. Its reservoirs are wild mammals, such as deer and mice, and the tick vector, which can perpetuate the infection by transovarian transmission. The distributions of infected wildlife and of the tick vector are consistent with the prevalence of babesiosis on the East Coast of the United States, including Martha's Vineyard, Nantucket Island, and Shelter Island. Additional foci of transmission have now been identified in Wisconsin and Indiana.

Diagnosis

Because most persons with babesiosis have subacute or chronic illnesses, serologic studies (antibody titers) are often diagnostic because the 3 to 4 weeks necessary to produce a diagnostic rise in antibody titer may transpire months before the patient consults a physician. In contrast, the speed of morphologic diagnosis is essential for critically ill patients, who must be diagnosed and treated rapidly.

Morphology. Babesiosis is usually diagnosed by the examination of Giemsa-stained thin blood smears. In contrast to plasmodia, babesia parasites have no pigment even in multiply infected erythrocytes. Babesia parasites are typically smaller than plasmodia but are often mistaken for plasmodia or platelets (30). Thus, if only ring forms are observed and if neither pigment nor gametocytes are present, it may be virtually impossible to differentiate babesia from plasmodia on a single smear. This distinction is important clinically because chloroquine is ineffective for babesiosis (50), which should be treated with the combination of quinine plus clindamycin (91).

Except in splenectomized patients, babesia parasitemias are typically low. The most diagnostic stage is the tetrad, which has four pyriform organisms grouped together without pigment (Fig. 10). Trophozoites may occasionally be seen free (outside erythrocytes) on peripheral smears (30).

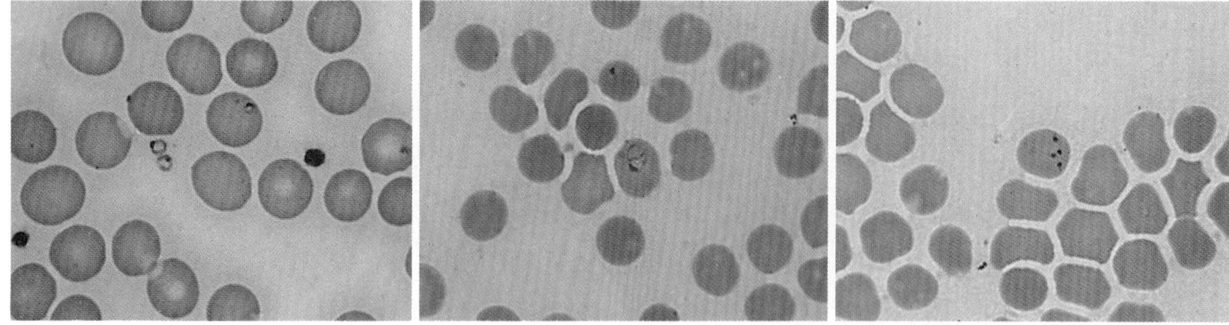

FIG. 10. Morphology of *Babesia microti* in thin blood films; Giemsa stain. (Left) Erythrocyte containing ring form plus two extraerythrocytic babesia organisms. (Middle) Erythrocyte containing a small ring and erythrocyte containing more mature trophozoites without pigment. (Right) Erythrocyte containing a tetrad. (Courtesy of George Healy, CDC.)

Serology. Antibody testing is used most frequently for epidemiologic studies. It is also useful for the evaluation of individual patients with subacute or chronic illnesses who have negative blood smears. These persons often have parasitemias of ≤0.1%, which are difficult or impossible to diagnose by morphology alone. Unfortunately, the value of serologic testing is compromised by cross-reactivity with malaria. Because both morphologic and serologic testing may produce false-positive results with malaria-infected persons, a careful history of overseas travel and exposure is essential before a positive (morphologic or serologic) result is interpreted as diagnostic of babesiosis. The IIF for babesiosis is performed at CDC (see chapter 66).

Alternative methods. Chronically infected patients with low parasitemias may be impossible to diagnose by morphology. In these patients, serology and the inoculation of susceptible animal hosts (5) may be the only way to make the diagnosis. Animal inoculation is available only in research laboratories.

KINETOPLASTIDA

Leishmania spp. and *Trypanosoma* spp., commonly referred to as the hemoflagellates, are kinetoplastida which are characterized by the presence of a kinetoplast. They are spread by arthropod hosts and have animal reservoirs such as dogs, rodents, and cattle, depending on the species. There are four stages of organisms in the kinetoplastida. The amastigote, which measures 2 to 5 μm, has a nucleus, kinetoplast, and axoneme but no flagellum and lives intracellularly. The promastigote is slender and elongated with a central nucleus and anterior kinetoplast, axoneme, and flagellum. The epimastigote is similar to the promastigote, but the kinetoplast is closer to the nucleus and there is a small undulating membrane with axoneme, then the anterior flagellum. The trypomastigote has the kinetoplast at the posterior end and an undulating membrane with axoneme extending the length of the organism, emerging as an anterior flagellum. Amastigotes and trypomastigotes are the most common forms in humans, with the other forms being found primarily in arthropod vectors. In leishmaniasis, amastigotes are found in humans and promastigotes are found in arthropod vectors.

Leishmaniasis

Leishmaniasis is caused by *Leishmania* spp. which parasitize monocytes and macrophages and in humans live as obligate intracellular parasites. Some are able to proliferate at a temperature of 37°C and cause visceral leishmaniasis; others prefer lower temperatures and cause cutaneous or mucocutaneous leishmaniasis. The infection is spread by sandflies of the genera *Phlebotomus* in the Old World and *Lutzomia* in the New World, which host the promastigote stage. The epidemiology, clinical manifestations, and species of *Leishmania* differ (22, 93). As with many infections, host factors are important and immunocompromised persons such as those with acquired immunodeficiency syndrome (AIDS) may develop more severe disease.

Cutaneous leishmaniasis in the Old World (Mediterranian, Middle East, and Central Africa) is caused by *Leishmania major*, *L. tropica*, or *L. aethiopica*. Mucocutaneous lesions (affecting mucous membranes such as those of the nose, lips, and cheeks) may be caused by *L. aethiopica*. Cutaneous leishmaniasis in the New World (Central and South America) is caused by *Leishmania* organisms of various species which may be placed into the *Leishmania braziliensis* group, the *L. mexicana* group, or *L. peruviana*. The most aggressive infections are caused by the *L. braziliensis* group, which may cause mucocutaneous lesions. The clinical syndromes may differ in various geographic areas.

Visceral leishmaniasis in the Old World is found in the Mediterranean area, Afghanistan, Pakistan, India, China, and Africa and is caused by *Leishmania donovani* of various subspecies. In the New World, visceral leishmaniasis is found in South and Central America and is caused by *L. donovani* of the subspecies *chagasi*. The amastigotes proliferate in cells of the reticuloendothelial system, causing particularly noticeable manifestations in the liver, spleen, lymph nodes, and bone marrow. Many patients have mild or asymptomatic infections, but some have severe disease which may prove fatal if untreated.

Diagnosis

Morphologic diagnosis is the most accepted method for the identification of these intracellular parasites,

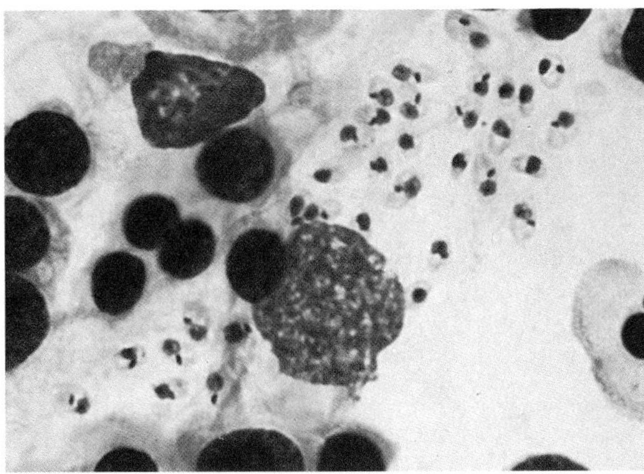

FIG. 11. Macrophages containing an intracellular amastigote of *Leishmania donovani*. (Reproduced with permission from reference 72.)

which are typically found in mononuclear cells or macrophages. In tissue sections or impression smears stained with Giemsa, the amastigote form of the parasite (Fig. 11) is identified by the presence of both the darkly staining kinetoplast and a lighter-staining nucleus (26). The kinetoplast aids in differentiating amastigotes from *Histoplasma*, *Toxoplasma*, or *Sarcocystis* species. Of these, only *Histoplasma* organisms stain with methenamine silver nitrate. *L. donovani* is usually diagnosed in specimens from liver, spleen, bone marrow, or lymph nodes. When scrapings or biopsies of cutaneous or mucocutaneous lesions are obtained for other leishmania, care must be taken to sample the active margin of the lesion and to avoid confusing gram-positive cocci (which are normal skin flora) with leishmania. Gram-positive cocci typically resemble the kinetoplast alone, without a nucleus or a surrounding mononuclear phagocytic cell.

Culture of promastigotes from the blood (or buffy coat) in systemic forms or of aspirates or skin scrapings in the cutaneous forms of the disease is definitive (chapter 66). However, such culture may provide false-negative results if antibiotics are not added to the cultures to suppress bacterial growth or if the biopsy or scrapings are inadequate.

According to one study (88), the sensitivity of histologic sections stained with hematoxylin and eosin is 14%, that of imprints is 19%, that of cultures is 58%, and that of all methods combined is 67%.

Serologic tests may be of value in visceral leishmaniasis but are of more limited usefulness in the cutaneous form of the disease. Positive serologic results are especially helpful in residents of the developed world who have had defined exposures (see chapter 67).

Trypanosomiasis

In trypanosomiasis, trypomastigotes may be found in the blood at some times during the disease process.

Neither American trypanosomiasis (Chagas' disease) nor African trypanosomiasis (sleeping sickness) is a major health problem in the United States or other developed countries. Although almost all human cases of these diseases in the United States are imported, occasional endogenous human cases of Chagas' disease may occur in the south, southeast, and southwest United States (66).

Trypanosomes known to cause disease in humans include *Trypanosoma cruzi* (the cause of Chagas' disease) and *T. brucei gambiense* and *T. brucei rhodesiense* (which cause sleeping sickness). A third species, *T. rangeli*, has been described in humans but has not been associated with clinical illness.

Chagas' disease

The life cycle of *T. cruzi* requires both an animal reservoir (usually rodents) and an insect vector. Both the reduviid (triatomid) vector and an animal reservoir exist in an area extending from Georgia to California and presumably account for the few reported cases of Chagas' disease in lifelong residents of the United States (97). Infectious parasite forms are present in feces of the vector and are rubbed into the bite wound, causing a local lesion (the chagoma). Proliferation of the amastigote stage occurs in organs such as the heart. Trypomastigotes may be present in peripheral blood early in the disease, but they do not proliferate. Acute disease usually resolves without treatment but can prove fatal in children. More chronic sequelae of the disease such as myocardial conduction defects, myocardial scarring, megacolon, and megaesophagus develop years after the initial infection and frequently lead to death.

African trypanosomiasis

The transmission of African trypanosomiasis to humans requires tsetse flies. These insects are not present in the United States, which helps to limit this disease to Africa. The reservoir of African trypanosomiasis is primarily in humans in West Africa (*T. brucei gambiense*) and in animals such as cattle, bushbuck, and impala in East Africa (*T. brucei rhodesiense*) (94).

Infection with *T. brucei rhodesiense* classically produces septicemic disease with generalized lymphadenopathy and may also cause fatal encephalitis within a few months. In contrast, *T. brucei gambiense* causes a more indolent disease which rarely produces encephalitis (sleeping sickness) in less than 2 to 3 years.

Diagnosis

In Chagas' disease, trypomastigote forms of the parasite may be found in the peripheral blood early in the disease (within the first several months). Later, the organisms can be seen in the amastigote form on histopathologic examination of involved organs such as the heart (Fig. 12), although the organisms are often difficult to find. Culture of peripheral blood on NNN medium when positive is also diagnostic. Trypomastigotes of *T. cruzi* are typically less sinuous than those of the African trypanosomes and have a larger kinetoplast (Fig. 12). However, the diagnosis is usually established by serologic testing (see chapter 67).

In contrast to *T. cruzi*, the organisms of African trypanosomiasis remain extracellular as trypomastigotes and proliferate in that stage. They are more sinuous and have a kinetoplast smaller than that of *T. cruzi* (Fig. 13). They circulate in the peripheral blood acutely and may be seen in biopsies or aspirates of involved lymph nodes as well as in bone marrow. Late in the disease, trypanosomes may be found in cerebrospinal fluid by Giemsa stain of smears of the cell pellet after centrif-

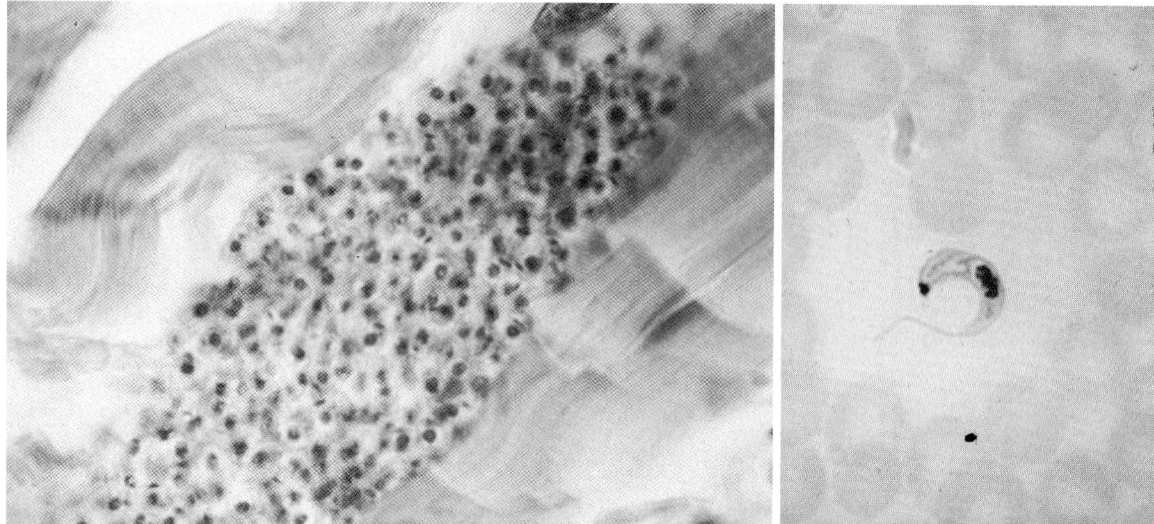

FIG. 12. *Trypanosoma cruzi* amastigotes in skeletal muscle (hematoxylin and eosin stain) and trypomastigote in peripheral blood (Giemsa stain). (Reproduced with permission from reference 72.)

ugation. Increased levels of immunoglobulin M (IgM) in spinal fluid are characteristic although not diagnostic.

Because single exposures tend to produce titers that remain positive, serologic testing is most valuable for the study of tourists who have had only a single defined exposure (see chapter 67).

TOXOPLASMOSIS

Toxoplasmosis is recognized to have a worldwide distribution, with prevalence rates as high as 80 to 90% in some areas and less than 1% in others. Since the majority of infections are asymptomatic and persist for the life of the patient, both tachyzoites (trophozoites) and bradyzoites (cystizoites) can be found in apparently normal individuals (Fig. 14). Similarly, IgG antibody levels persist for life but usually at relatively low levels. These features of the infection create major problems in the pathologic and serologic diagnosis of toxoplasmosis.

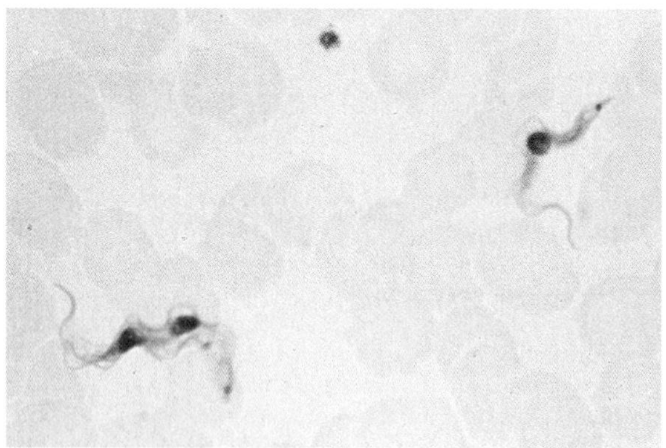

FIG. 13. Trypomastigotes of *Trypanosoma brucei rhodesiense* in mouse; thin film, Giemsa stain. One trypomastigote is in the process of cell division. (Reproduced with permission from reference 72.)

Toxoplasma gondii, the causative agent, is an obligate intracellular parasite found in most warm-blooded animals. Only members of the family *Felidae* serve as the definitive host, in which the parasite transforms into male and female gametes which unite and form oocysts, which are passed in the feces (20). The oocytes mature to the infective stage in the environment and are then infective for a variety of animals, including humans. This major mode of transmission in part explains the high prevalence rates in some populations. Severe illness has rarely resulted from exposure to cat feces. Most infections are asymptomatic or cause mild nonspecific symptoms such as sore throat or fever.

Beef, pork, lamb, and chicken have all been shown to harbor the encysted form of the parasite and therefore serve as a source of infection through the ingestion of undercooked meat. Epidemiologic studies of outbreaks have indicated that undercooked meat serves as a common mode of transmission. Acquired in this way, the disease frequently is mildly symptomatic but rarely of major consequence.

Much less frequent but perhaps of greater clinical importance is the person-to-person transmission by blood products and tissue transplantation. Since many patients receiving transfusions or tissue are immunosuppressed for therapeutic reasons, the introduction of material containing viable *T. gondii* into these immunocompromised patients has led to severe and fatal infections.

Of the acquired infections, perhaps the most devastating consequences result from transplacental transfer of infection to the fetus when the mother acquires her primary infection during pregnancy. Consequences vary according to the stage of pregnancy in which the infection occurs. Fetal death or major abnormalities may occur when infection is acquired during the first trimester, whereas apparently normal deliveries are common when infection is acquired in the third trimester. However, this latter group, left untreated, may develop major symptoms months or years later. With rare

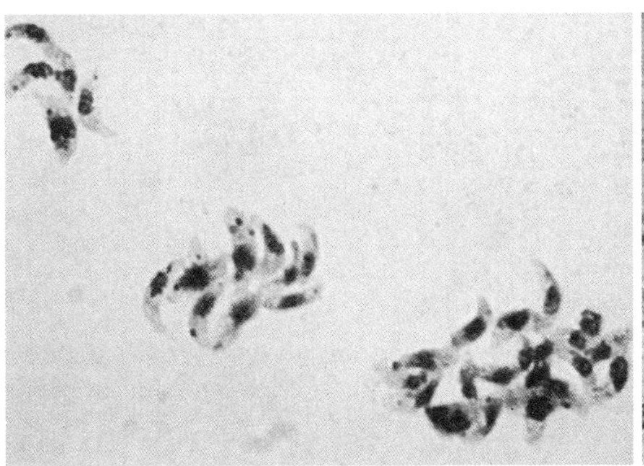
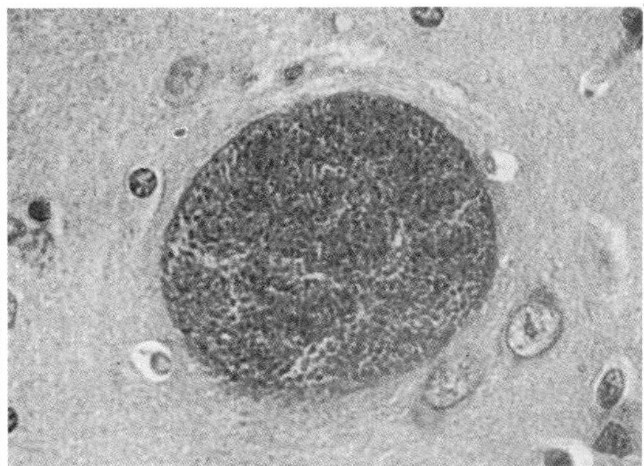

FIG. 14. *Toxoplasma gondii.* (Left) Tachyzoites (trophozoites). (Right) Tissue cyst in brain containing numerous bradyzoites. (Reproduced with permission from reference 72.)

exceptions, women with preexisting antibody will not transmit the infection to the fetus.

Reactivation of subclinical infection acquired in utero or occasionally in childhood or later is considered to be responsible for severe adult disease. Ocular toxoplasmosis is one of the leading causes of adult retinochoroiditis and frequently leads to blindness in the affected eye. Although this condition is seen in congenital disease as well, it is most commonly seen in adults. Acquired cases have been reported, but frequently multiple healed lesions are present, suggesting that long-lasting infection has preceded the clinical problem.

Toxoplasmosis affecting the central nervous system (CNS) is now one of the leading causes of death among AIDS patients. Characteristic manifestations of the disease in AIDS include encephalitis, pneumonitis, and myocarditis (41, 62). With over 200 reports in only the last 3 years, toxoplasmosis is now the most frequent cause of CNS complications in patients with AIDS. It is assumed that the CNS involvement is usually the result of reactivation of a preexisting toxoplasmosis infection as a result of immunosuppression by human immunodeficiency virus but occasionally may be acquired by needle sharing or other exposure after development of AIDS.

Clinical, histologic, or pathologic diagnosis of each of these conditions is difficult and complicated by the presence of viable organisms in otherwise normal individuals and the lack of pathognomonic features. Acquired and congenital infections frequently mimic infectious mononucleosis, rubella, cytomegalovirus disease, or other virus infections. CNS lesions are somewhat typical, but not diagnostic, in computer-assisted tomography. They usually are not readily available for pathologic study. Ocular lesions are the exception to this dilemma since the lesions, although not absolutely diagnostic, are quite typical and easily recognized by the experienced ophthalmologist. Isolation of the parasite or demonstration of cysts in tissue is not absolutely diagnostic since it has been shown that viable cysts are present in chronic subclinical cases. The demonstration of tachyzoites or antigen in the tissue by immunohistologic stains, however, is considered diagnostic of active infection.

Fortunately, infection is accompanied by good antibody response; unfortunately, the chronic nature of the disease results in the persistence, perhaps for life, of the antibodies. Many serologic procedures have been shown to be effective, but only five have been routinely accepted. The Sabin-Feldman dye test (63), once the standard against which all other tests were compared, is still an excellent procedure but is complex and performed by only a few laboratories. IIF is sensitive and accurate and is used widely throughout the world. Indirect hemagglutination, used primarily for screening, is losing favor and is less common. Enzyme-linked immunosorbent assay (ELISA) is increasingly popular because it is useful for both screening and quantitation of IgG and IgM antibodies. Latex agglutination tests are used primarily for screening and are readily adaptable to use in small laboratories or clinics.

Perhaps as much as in any other disease, the measurement of IgM antibodies is critical to the serologic diagnosis of toxoplasmosis. The differentiation of acute versus chronic infection can often be determined by the presence of IgM, or passively transferred antibody from mother to fetus can be ruled out by the presence of IgM antibody. Some indication of recency of acquisition of infection can be made by the level of IgM antibody present.

The detection and measurement of IgM antibodies are fraught with problems. Initially, IIF was the only acceptable test, but it was recognized as having limitations. False-positive reactions, caused by rheumatoid factor (8), could be removed only by absorption, and false-negative reactions were not uncommon (59), especially in newborns. These false-negative reactions were caused by anti-*Toxoplasma* IgG, which blocked the detection of anti-*Toxoplasma* IgM (58) and could be removed only with the use of column fractionation or ultracentrifugation to separate the IgG from IgM. Now, tests such as the reverse (or capture) ELISA (16, 67) and IgM immunosorbent agglutination assay (14) and the use of immunocolumns have all been shown to be highly effective in the accurate detection of IgM antibody. Each, however, has its shortcomings, and serologic interpretations should be made cautiously. The most popular of these are the ELISA systems that use a capture method. IgM antibody is captured by anti-μ antibody on the solid phase, and conventional ELISA techniques are then used to complete the test. By this method, IgM is separated from IgG and both rheumatoid factor reactions and blocking by IgG can be eliminated. Although the sensitivity of this test is greater than that of the IIF tests, false-negative results may occur, especially in newborns. Both the capture system and immunocolumns in conjunction with ELISA are available in kit form for the detection of IgM antibody.

A separate interpretation of serologic test results is required for each of the clinical forms of the disease: asymptomatic infection, congenital infection, maternal infection acquired during pregnancy, ocular infection, adult disseminated infection, and infections manifested in AIDS patients. The serodiagnosis of congenital infection depends on the accurate measurement of specific IgM antibodies. IgG antibodies are efficiently transported from maternal to fetal circulation and in some cases may be slightly higher (twofold) in the fetus. IgM antibodies, on the other hand, are not shared by mother and fetus except when placental damage and leakage occur. This situation occurs in only a small percentage of cases. IgM antibody in the newborn circulation is generally considered of fetal origin and is diagnostic of congenital infection. The diagnosis of toxoplasmosis in a newborn requires a positive toxoplasma IgM test and an IgG titer equivalent to the maternal IgG titer. Infant sera must always be tested in parallel with maternal samples.

Most tests on obstetric patients are performed as qualitative screening tests rather than as quantitative tests for diagnosis. The presence of antibody before conception indicates immunity, although a few exceptions have been documented. In general, serologic procedures for screening are used merely to test for the presence of antibody, and the absolute titers are less important. Infections acquired during pregnancy are associated with a risk of transmission to the fetus. To determine whether a positive titer in a pregnant woman represents acute infection, a prepregnancy or very early pregnancy sample is extremely valuable. Unfortunately, in most cases these samples are not available, and clinical decisions must be based on more limited serologic information. Since approximately one-third of pregnant women in the United States have IgG antibody without evidence of active disease, IgG levels must be unusually high to be of significance. IgM antibodies, on the other hand, do not persist, and their presence indicates a relatively recent infection. For the serodiagnosis of acute infection, titers of 1:64 are usually accepted as minimal for IgM, and titers of 1:1,024 are minimal for IgG in adults. Interpretations based on these serologic guidelines are, of course, influenced by the clinical presentation. Significant levels of IgM antibody are assumed to indicate that the infection was acquired within the past 6 months, although newer tests can measure IgM in some patients for up to 1 year. The absence of IgM antibody, particularly by newer procedures, militates strongly against recent infection.

Ocular toxoplasmosis is usually diagnosed clinically, and serology serves only for confirmation. These cases are often confusing because the antibody level may be very low when the major, or only, clinical manifestation is ocular. These patients commonly have titers as low as 1:8, which is far below those accepted as diagnostic in other adult infections. Although the importance of these low levels is questionable, an absence of IgG antibody would indicate that the likelihood of ocular toxoplasmosis is nil. Since virtually all ocular cases are considered a reactivation of an old infection, IgM antibody testing rarely plays a role in serodiagnosis of the ocular disease.

Adult disseminated cerebral toxoplasmosis is a clinical entity that was extremely rare until the appearance of AIDS. As high as 40% of AIDS patients develop CNS toxoplasmosis (46), yet serologic diagnosis is still a dilemma. The presence of relatively low IgG titers and the apparent absence of IgM antibodies in many of these cases suggests that they represent the reactivation of chronic toxoplasmosis rather than recent infection (29). The newer tests (reverse ELISA, IgM immunosorbent agglutination assay, and agglutination assay) show great promise but still detect only 75 to 80% of proven cases (77). It has been shown that these tests can be used to demonstrate intrathecal production of antibody (57), which would indicate a progressive CNS involvement from reactivated cases, and to detect seroconversion from negative to positive even in immunosuppressed patients (71). The obvious shortcomings of each of these tests further emphasize that the interpretation of serologic results is still uncertain and serology can serve only as an adjunct to clinical and pathologic diagnosis.

A variety of serologic procedures are available both commercially and at specialty laboratories. In general, these procedures can be divided into three types: screening tests, quantitative tests, and tests for measuring specific class antibodies (IgM and IgG subclasses). Qualitative screening tests include latex agglutination, direct agglutination, indirect hemagglutination, and ELISA. These tests have all been evaluated and shown to be reliable. For diagnosis, screening tests should not be used alone. Rather, positive results and questionable negative results should be confirmed by quantitative testing.

Quantitative procedures include IIF (37), Sabin-Feldman methylene blue dye (63), and ELISA (85) tests. ELISA has now been accepted as one of the tests of choice but requires more training and experience than IIF. Numerous reports have shown the comparability of the IIF and dye tests (86). Because of its ease of performance and the availability of reagents, IIF is the test of choice of the clinical laboratory. It is both specific and sensitive and, with limitations, can be used for IgM testing.

A variety of reagents and kits are available commercially. All have been evaluated and found adequate, although quality control problems continue to plague the industry. Latex, direct agglutination, indirect hemagglutination, ELISA, and IIF kits are available. Consumers should restrict products precisely to their intended use. Screening tests or semiquantitative procedures should not be used for clinical diagnosis.

PNEUMOCYSTOSIS

Pneumocystosis is caused by *Pneumocystis carinii*, a protist of unsettled taxonomy. Although it has generally been considered a protozoan, recent evaluation of RNA (17) suggests that it is more closely related to fungi. However, the issue is not settled (21, 34), and for this edition of the Manual it will be included with the parasites.

Pneumocystosis usually presents as diffuse bilateral interstitial pneumonitis in patients who have AIDS or are immunosuppressed by therapy for malignancies or transplantation (87, 96). In the United States, *Pneumocystis* pneumonia occurs in up to 80% of AIDS patients, frequently recurs after therapy, and is a leading cause of death in these patients. With the recent widespread use of prophylactic aerosol pentamidine (39), *Pneumocystis* infections of other organs are becoming more common (78). Infection is acquired by the airborne route, and most persons in the United States appear to have had asymptomatic infection as children. The infection remains quiescent in the lungs; however, if the person becomes immunosuppressed, the infection may become active and lead to pneumonia. Infections may be acquired from exogenous sources and outbreaks have been described (27, 64).

Diagnosis of *Pneumocystis* pneumonia is established by morphologically demonstrating *Pneumocystis* organisms in material from the lungs or occasionally other organs. Although antigen detection in serum has been described (56), it is not useful clinically (33). Antibody detection is not very useful because most normal persons have had subclinical infections and many immunosuppressed persons do not develop an immune response (55).

Specimen collection and handling

For diagnosis of *Pneumocystis* pneumonia, the laboratory will examine material from the lung. A variety of specimens can be used, but some are better than others. The most widely used specimen is bronchoalveolar lavage fluid (47). In bronchoalveolar lavage, the bronchoscope is wedged into a bronchus, and fluid is forced into the lung and then reaspirated. This allows materials to be washed from the alveoli, where the *Pneumocystis* exudates with organisms are found. Bronchoalveolar lavage fluid is much better for diagnosis than bronchial washings which are obtained by placing fluid in the tracheobronchial tree but without wedging the bronchoscope and forcing fluid into the alveoli. Bronchial washing fluid is frequently negative in patients with *Pneumocystis* pneumonia. Transbronchial biopsies have proven quite useful, sometimes allowing diagnosis when bronchoalveolar lavage fluid is negative. Bronchial brushes have not been useful in our experience but have produced good results at some institutions (28). Open lung biopsy may be performed in some patients when it is crucial to determine the etiology of the pulmonary problem. Impression smears of the cut surface of the lung or histopathologic sections can be examined.

Properly induced sputum has been useful for diagnosis of *Pneumocystis* pneumonia in AIDS patients at some institutions (3, 40). Highly motivated employees must spend the 30 min to 1 h required to induce good specimens by using hypertonic saline, and laboratory personnel must be experienced in examining for *Pneumocystis* organisms. It is important to obtain deep-cough-induced specimens that contain alveolar material. Random sputum specimens and specimens obtained after minimal induction effort are unlikely to prove useful, and the laboratory should not examine such specimens. If an induced specimen is to be examined, the physician must be ready to progress to bronchoalveolar lavage or transbronchial biopsy if the induced sputum proves to be negative. AIDS patients not on prophylaxis with aerosol pentamidine usually have infections with numerous *Pneumocystis* organisms, often in clumps, whereas organisms may be less numerous in *Pneumocystis* infections of AIDS patients on aerosol pentamidine prophylaxis or other immunocompromised patients. There are no good data on the usefulness of induced sputum to diagnose *Pneumocystis* pneumonia in non-AIDS patients.

Three types of stains may be used for *P. carinii:* organism stains, cyst stains, and immunologic stains. There are advantages and disadvantages of each. The principal organism stain is Giemsa or various rapid modifications that stain *Pneumocystis* organisms. Both free trophozoites and intracystic organisms are stained, but cyst walls do not stain and are seen as halos around the intracystic organisms (Fig. 15). Nuclei stain red to violet, and the cytoplasm stains pale blue. The Giemsa stain gives a more delicate stain than do the rapid methods.

In bronchoalveolar lavage fluid or induced sputum, the *Pneumocystis* organisms are usually in large clumps (Fig. 15) and can easily be overlooked. In the Giemsa technique, staining of host cells on the slide provides an internal control for each slide, and special control slides are not needed.

Cyst stains stain walls of *Pneumocystis* cysts. The most widely used cyst stains are methenamine silver nitrate and toluidine blue O, although others, such as cresyl echt violet, Gram-Weigert, and Cellufluor, are used by some laboratories. A laboratory should select one cyst stain that is found to be convenient and reliable. Positive control slides for cyst stains, preferably containing *Pneumocystis* organisms, should be included each time slides are stained. Various rapid methenamine silver stains are satisfactory (6, 32) and are preferred to the classic stain because they take much less time. Toluidine blue O is a useful stain, and a recent modification that does not require ether reduces the hazard (24). Disposal of the concentrated acids may present a problem to some laboratories. Cellufluor (also called Calcofluor white) staining has been used as a nonimmunologic fluorescent stain (2). With both toluidine blue O and Cellufluor, the specific lot of stain should be checked for appropriate staining before being put in service (90).

All of the cyst wall stains stain the walls of the cysts and do not stain intracystic organisms or free trophozoites. There is a thickened area of the wall that may appear as a dark dot or as a parenthesis (Fig. 15). Cysts are often collapsed or folded and may be cup shaped. Some of these may be cysts that have already ruptured and released their intracystic organisms.

Immunofluorescent stains based on monoclonal antibodies to *Pneumocystis* organisms have been described (23, 40). These research reagents have shown good sensitivity and specificity when compared with other methods. The usefulness of commercially available immunofluorescence staining reagents should be determined from published evaluations rather than from the results obtained with the research reagents. A method using immunoperoxidase has also been described (4). Both cysts and trophozoites are stained with immunologic reagents, and the appropriate organism morphology must be demonstrated before a slide is considered positive.

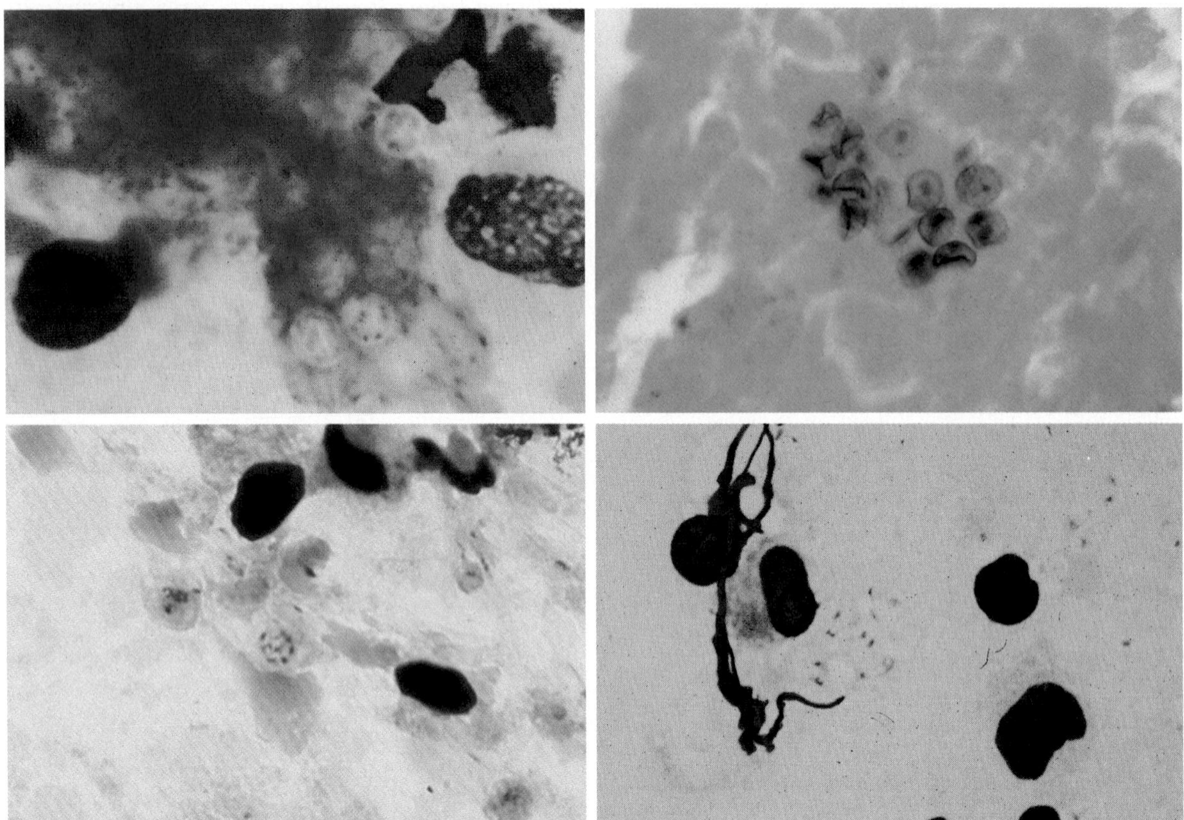

FIG. 15. *Pneumocystis carinii* organisms. (Top, left) Clump of *P. carinii* in bronchoalveolar lavage specimen; Giemsa stain. Both cysts and trophozoites are present, but only some are in the plane of focus. (Top, right) Cysts in tissue section; methenamine silver stain. (Bottom, left) Cyst in impression smear showing intracystic bodies; Giemsa stain. (Bottom, right) Trophozoites in impression smear; Giemsa stain.

Each laboratory must select the stains most appropriate for its situation. We routinely use Giemsa and rapid methenamine silver since they are useful for detecting not only *Pneumocystis* organisms but also other infectious agents. For example, *Histoplasma capsulatum*, *Cryptococcus neoformans*, or *Aspergillus* species can be detected by silver stain and Giemsa stain, and nocardiae, legionellae, pneumococci, and other bacteria as well as toxoplasmas and cytomegalovirus may be detected by Giesma stain. All of these organisms may infect immunocompromised patients and sometimes cause clinical disease resembling *Pneumocystis* pneumonia.

The types of specimens that will be obtained, the laboratory that will perform the examination (microbiology, cytopathology, or surgical pathology), and the procedures used in examining the specimen will vary among institutions and will depend on the skills and availability of personnel and the available resources. Thus, each institution will need to apply the information presented above to its specific situation.

FREE-LIVING PATHOGENIC AMEBAE

Description

Small free-living amebae belonging to the genera *Naegleria*, *Hartmannella*, and *Acanthamoeba* are commonly found in soil, fresh water, and even sewage and sludge (25, 48, 60, 70). Several species of *Acanthamoeba* have also been isolated from brackish water and seawater (65). Organisms of the genera *Naegleria* and *Acanthamoeba* have been known to cause fatal infections of the CNS in humans (9, 25, 35, 48, 60). The concept that these small free-living amebae could become human pathogens was proposed by Culbertson and colleagues, who isolated *Acanthamoeba* sp. strain A-1 (now designated *A. culbertsoni*) from tissue culture medium thought to contain an unknown virus (13). They also demonstrated amebae in the brain lesions of mice and monkeys that died within 1 week after intracerebral inoculation with these amebae. Culbertson hypothesized that similar infection might exist in nature in humans. Fowler and Carter in 1965 (18) were the first to describe a fatal infection due to free-living amebae, which they presumed to be *Acanthamoeba* species, in the brain of an Australian patient (9). The infection is now believed to have been due to *Naegleria* species (25). In 1966, Butt described the first case of free-living ameba infection in the United States and coined the term primary amebic meningoencephalitis (PAM) (7). *Naegleria* amebae cause an acute and fulminating PAM, generally leading to death 5 to 7 days after the onset of symptoms (9, 25, 35, 48). Since all but a few isolations from human cerebrospinal fluid and brain tissue have yielded only *Naegleria* organisms and the clinical picture from the onset of illness to death closely resembles that described for *Naegleria* species, it is now generally believed that most human infections have been due to *Naegleria* amebae. The portal of entry of these amebae is the nasal passage. When people swim in lakes and other bodies of water that harbor these amebae, the organisms may enter the nostrils and make their way into the olfactory lobes via the cribriform plate. More than 140 cases of PAM have been reported worldwide; only a few patients have survived. As of 1 September 1989, 63 cases of PAM had occurred in the United States. *Naegleria* amebae are not generally known to produce cysts in the brain tissue. However, on the basis of the presence and morphology of the cysts in the affected tissues in some cases, immunofluorescence staining of the amebae in the tissues (25, 48, 80, 81), and the epidemiologic and clinical pictures, it is known that *Acanthamoeba,* as well as some other free-living amebae, also causes a usually fatal granulomatous amebic encephalitis (GAE). GAE is usually chronic, and it may last for more than a week and sometimes even for months. Since most of the patients with GAE had no history of contact with fresh water, it is believed that the route of invasion and penetration into the CNS is hematogenous, probably from a primary focus in the lower respiratory tract or the skin (48). In some patients with GAE, chronic ulceration of the skin containing trophozoites and cysts has been reported. Since *Acanthamoeba* cysts have been isolated from dust in the air (25, 48), it is quite likely that some persons, especially those who are immunologically compromised, inhale cyst forms of these amebae when passing through areas where soil has been freshly turned. The amebae subsequently may undergo excystation into trophozoites and invade the nasal mucosa. More than 40 cases of GAE have been recorded worldwide, and 27 of these cases had occurred in the United States as of 1 September 1989. Because of the confusion that existed in the earlier literature with regard to the nomenclature of *Acanthamoeba* and *Hartmannella,* some workers in the field referred to these amebas as belonging to the *Hartmannella-Acanthamoeba* group. Since no true *Hartmannella* species has as yet been found to be pathogenic to humans, all references to *Hartmannella* in human tissues should be corrected to read as *Acanthamoeba* or some other, yet unknown ameba. Only one species of *Naegleria, N. fowleri,* is known to cause human disease, although several species of *Acanthamoeba* (*A. culbertsoni, A. castellanii, A. polyphaga,* and *A. astronyxis*) are considered pathogenic to humans (25, 48).

In addition to causing GAE, *Acanthamoeba* causes a painful vision-threatening disease of the human cornea, *Acanthamoeba* keratitis. If the infection is not treated promptly, it may lead to ulceration of the cornea, loss of visual acuity, and eventually blindness and enucleation (15, 36, 74, 75, 79, 95). As of 1 September 1989, more than 250 cases of *Acanthamoeba* keratitis had been reported to CDC. The first case of *Acanthamoeba* keratitis in the United States was reported in 1973 in a south Texas rancher with a history of trauma to his right eye (36). Both trophozoites and cyst stages of *A. polyphaga* not only were demonstrated in corneal sections but also were repeatedly cultured from the corneal scrapings and biopsy specimens. Between 1973 and July 1988, 208 cases were diagnosed and reported to CDC (75). The number of cases gradually increased between 1973 and 1984, with a dramatic increase beginning in 1985. On the basis of an in-depth epidemiologic and case control study (74, 75), it was found that a major risk factor was the use of contact lenses, predominantly daily-wear or extended-wear soft lenses, and that patients with *Acanthamoeba* keratitis were significantly more likely than controls to use homemade saline instead of commercially prepared saline (78 versus 30%), disinfect their lenses less frequently than recommended by the lens manufacturers (72 versus 32%), and wear their lenses while swimming (63 versus 30%). *Acanthamoeba* organisms have also been isolated from ear discharge, pulmonary secretions, nasopharyngeal swabs, maxillary sinuses, mandibular autografts, and stool samples (25, 48, 81, 85). *Acanthamoeba* spp. also may harbor legionellae and mycobacteria and contribute to their persistence in the environment. Excellent reviews (9, 25, 35, 81) and several books (48, 60, 70) have been published on the biology, disease potential, pathogenicity, and epidemiology of these amebae and the diseases they cause.

Morphology

N. fowleri in its trophic form is a small limaxlike ameba measuring 10 to 35 μm; it exhibits an eruptive locomotion by producing smooth hemispherical bulges. The posterior end, called the uroid, appears to be sticky and often has several trailing filaments. During its life cycle, it produces a transient pear-shaped biflagellate stage because of altered environmental conditions and smooth-walled cysts (25, 35, 70, 81) (Fig. 16a to d). The flagellates do not have a cytosome. Cysts are usually spherical and measure 7 to 15 μm. According to recent work (6), the cyst wall may have one or more pores plugged with a mucoid material.

Acanthamoeba organisms are slightly larger (15 to 45 μm) and produce from the surface of the body fine, tapering, hyaline projections called acanthopodia (Fig. 16e and f). The ameba has no flagellate stage but produces a double-walled cyst (10 to 25 μm) with a wrinkled outer wall (ectocyst) and a stellate, polygonal, or even round inner wall (endocyst) (25, 48, 54, 70, 81).

Both *Naegleria* and *Acanthamoeba* organisms are uninucleate, and the nucleus is characterized by a large, dense, centrally located nucleolus. The *Naegleria* amebae exhibit the promitotic pattern of cell division, wherein the nucleolus and the nuclear membrane persist during nuclear division. *Acanthamoeba* organisms, however, divide by conventional mitosis whereby the nucleolus and the nuclear membrane disappear during cell division.

Collection, handling, and storage of specimens

For isolating the etiologic agent, cerebrospinal fluid, small pieces of tissue (brain, lungs, corneal biopsy material, etc.), or corneal scrapings from the affected area must be obtained aseptically. The specimens should be kept at room temperature (24 to 28°C) and should never be frozen. The specimens may be kept at 4°C for short periods of time but never for more than 24 h. Personnel handling the specimens must take appropriate precautions, such as wearing surgical masks and gloves and working in a biological safety cabinet. Remaining tissues must be preserved in 10% neutral buffered Formalin so that they can be examined histologically for amebae.

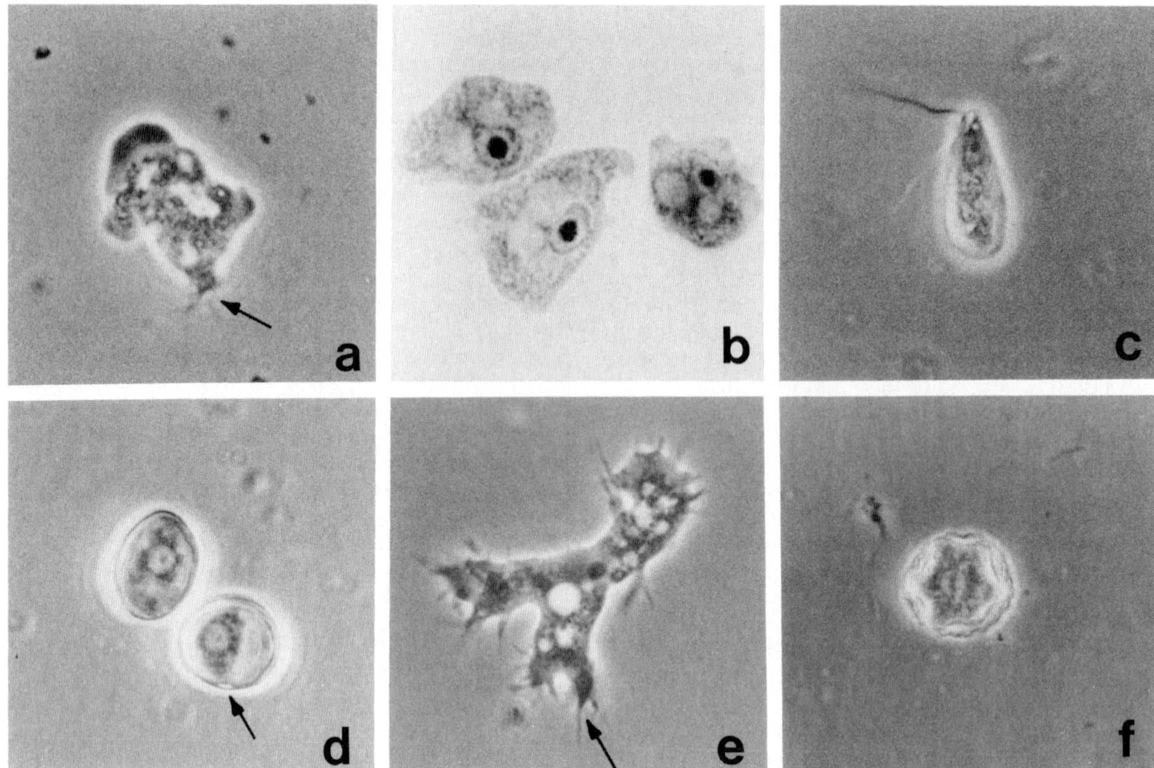

FIG. 16. Free-living pathogenic amebae. (a to d) *Naegleria fowleri:* (a) trophozoites, phase contrast (note the uroid and filaments at arrow); (b) trophozoites, trichrome stain; (c) biflagellate, phase contrast; (d) smooth-walled cyst, phase contrast (note the pore at arrow). (e and f) *Acanthamoeba castellanii:* (e) trophozoite, phase contrast (note the acanthopodia at arrow); (f) double-walled cyst, phase contrast. All magnifications are ×1,100.

Methods of examination

Direct examination. Direct examination of the sample as a wet-mount preparation is of paramount importance in the diagnosis of PAM and other diseases caused by these amebae. Since the amebae tend to attach to the surface of the container, the container should be shaken gently; then a small drop of fluid is placed on a clean microscope slide and covered with a no. 1 cover slip. The cerebrospinal fluid may have to be centrifuged at 150 × *g* for 5 min to concentrate the amebae. After the specimen has been centrifuged, most of the supernatant is carefully aspirated, and the sediment is gently suspended in the remaining fluid. A drop of this suspension is prepared as described above for microscopic observation.

The slide preparation should be examined under a compound microscope with 10× and 40× objectives. Phase-contrast optics are preferable. If regular bright-field illumination is used, the slide should be examined under diminished light. A step in which the slide is warmed to 35°C is optional. Amebae, if present, can easily be detected by their active directional movement.

Permanently stained preparations. A small drop of the sedimented cerebrospinal fluid or other sample is placed in the middle of a slide and allowed to stand in a moist chamber for 5 to 10 min at 37°C. This will allow any amebae to attach to the surface of the slide. Several drops of warm (37°C) Schaudinn fixative are placed directly on the sample and allowed to stand for 1 min. The slide is then transferred to a Coplin jar containing the fixative and fixed for 1 h. It may be stained in Wheatley trichrome or Heidenhain iron hematoxylin stain (see chapter 122) for various staining procedures). Corneal scrapings smeared on microscope slides may be fixed with methanol and stained with Hemacolor stain (Harleco, a division of EM Industries, Inc.) (79).

Isolation

The recommended procedure for isolating free-living pathogenic amebae from biological specimens is as follows.

Materials

Page ameba saline (53) (see chapter 121 for preparation)
Nonnutrient agar plates with ameba saline (see chapter 121 for preparation)
Culture of *Escherichia coli* or *Enterobacter aerogenes*, 18 to 24 h old
Sterile distilled water
Bacteriologic loop
Fine spatula made of nichrome wire
Sterile Pasteur pipettes, rubber bulbs
Sterile 1-ml serologic pipettes
Sterile screw-cap test tubes, 100 by 13 mm or 125 by 16 mm
Moist chamber
Vaspar (1:1 petrolatum-paraffin), melted

Microscope slides, 3 by 1 or 3 by 2 in. (7.6 by 2.5 or 7.6 by 5 cm)

Cover slips, 22 mm square, no. 1 thickness

Preparation of agar plates

1. Remove plates from refrigerator and place them in a 37°C incubator for 30 min.

2. Add 0.5 ml of ameba saline to a slant culture of *E. coli* or *E. aerogenes*. Gently scrape the surface of the slant with a sterile bacteriologic loop (do not break the agar surface). Using a sterile Pasteur pipette, gently and uniformly suspend the bacteria. Add 2 to 3 drops of this suspension to the middle of a warmed (37°C) agar plate and spread the bacteria over the surface of the agar with a bacteriologic loop.

Inoculation of plates with specimens

1. For cerebrospinal fluid samples, centrifuge the cerebrospinal fluid at 1,000 rpm for 5 to 8 min. With a sterile serologic pipette, carefully transfer all but 0.5 ml of the supernatant to a sterile tube and store the sample at 4°C for possible future use. Mix sediment with remaining fluid; with a sterile Pasteur pipette, place 2 to 3 drops in the center of the agar plate precoated with bacteria and incubate the plate at 37°C.

2. For tissue samples, triturate a small piece of the tissue in a small quantity of ameba saline. With a sterile Pasteur pipette, place 2 to 3 drops in the center of the agar plate. Incubate the plate at 37°C.

3. Water and soil samples are handled in the same manner as cerebrospinal fluid and tissue specimens, respectively.

Examination of plates

1. Using the low-power (10×) objective of a microscope, observe the plates daily for 7 days for amebae.

2. If you see amebae, circle that area with a wax pencil. With the fine spatula, cut a small piece of agar from the circled area and place it face down on the surface of a fresh agar plate precoated with bacteria; incubate the plate as described above. Both *Naegleria* and *Acanthamoeba* organisms can easily be cultivated in this way and, with periodic transfers, maintained indefinitely. When the plate is examined under a microscope, the amebae will look like small blotches; if they are observed carefully, their movement can be discerned. After 2 to 3 days of incubation, the amebae will start to undergo encystation. If a plate is examined after 4 to 5 days of incubation, both trophozoites and cysts will be visible.

Identification and culture

Identification of living specimens to the genus level is based on characteristic patterns of locomotion, morphologic features of the trophic and cyst forms, and the enflagellation experiments. Immunofluorescence or immunoperoxidase tests using monoclonal antibodies are helpful in identifying the species, especially those of *Acanthamoeba*, in fixed tissue.

Enflagellation experiment

1. Mix a drop of the sedimented cerebrospinal fluid containing amebae with about 1 ml of sterile distilled water in a sterile tube or, with a bacteriologic loop, scrape the surface of a plate that is positive for amebae. Transfer a loopful of scraping to a sterile tube containing approximately 1 ml of distilled water.

2. Gently shake the tube and transfer a drop of this suspension to the center of a cover slip, the edges of which have been coated thinly with petroleum jelly. Place a microscope slide over the cover slip and invert the slide. Seal the edges of the cover slip with Vaspar (a warmed half-and-half mixture of petroleum jelly and paraffin). Place the slide in a moist chamber and incubate it as described above for 2 to 3 h. In addition, incubate the tube as described above.

3. Periodically examine the tube and the slide preparation microscopically for free-swimming flagellates. *Naegleria* spp. have a flagellated stage; *Acanthamoeba* spp. do not. If the sample contains *N. fowleri*, about 30 to 50% of the amebae will have undergone transformation into pear-shaped biflagellated organisms.

Other culture methods. (i) Axenic culture. *Acanthamoeba* spp. can easily be cultivated, without the addition of serum or host tissue, axenically in many different types of nutrient media, e.g., Proteose Peptone-yeast extract-glucose medium (82) (see chapter 121 for preparation), Trypticase soy broth medium (25, 48), or chemically defined medium (25). *N. fowleri*, however, requires fetal calf serum or brain extract in the medium, e.g., Nelson medium (70, 83) (see chapter 121 for preparation). A chemically defined medium for *N. fowleri* has been developed only recently (51).

Axenic cultures are prepared as follows. Actively growing amebae, 24 to 36 h old, are scraped from the surface of the plate, suspended in 50 ml of ameba saline, and centrifuged at 800 rpm for 5 min. The supernatant is aspirated, and the sediment is inoculated into Proteose Peptone-yeast extract-glucose medium or Nelson medium, depending on the ameba isolate, and incubated at 37°C. Penicillin and streptomycin to final concentrations of 400 U/ml and 400 g/ml, respectively, are added aseptically to the medium before the amebae are inoculated. Three subcultures into the antibiotic-containing medium at weekly intervals are usually sufficient to eliminate the associated bacteria (*E. coli* or *E. aerogenes*).

(ii) Cell culture. Pathogenic *Acanthamoeba* and *Naegleria* amebae can also be inoculated onto many types of mammalian cell cultures as well as onto chicken fibroblasts. The amebae grow vigorously in these cell cultures and produce cytopathic effects. These amebae were mistaken for transformed cell types presumed to contain viruses which were erroneously termed lipovirus and Ryan virus (25, 82).

Animal inoculation. Two-week-old Swiss-Webster mice, weighing 12 to 15 g, can be infected with these amebae. Mice are anesthetized with ether, and a drop of ameba suspension is instilled into their nostrils. The mice die within 5 to 7 days after developing characteristic signs such as ruffled fur, aimless wandering, partial paralysis, and finally coma and death. Amebae can be demonstrated in the mouse brain either by culture or by histologic examination.

Antigenic characteristics

Pathogenic *N. fowleri* is morphologically indistinguishable from the nonpathogenic *N. gruberi* at the trophic stage. Differences between these amebae, however, have been demonstrated antigenically by the gel diffusion, immunoelectrophoresis, and IIF techniques (25, 81). Antigenic differences have also been shown between various species of *Acanthamoeba* (25, 60, 70, 79, 82). Some recent studies indicate that *N. fowleri* can be distinguished from other *Naegleria* species on the basis of their isoenzyme electrophoretic patterns (60) as well as the restriction fragment length polymorphisms of the genomic DNA (49).

Serology

Not much information is available on the antibody response to these amebae in humans. Serologic tests are not useful for diagnosis and are available only in research laboratories.

Complement fixation antibody to *Acanthamoeba* organisms has been demonstrated in serum samples of patients suffering from upper respiratory tract distress and those with optic neuritis and macular disease (25, 82). Kenney (38) demonstrated increasing complement fixation antibody titers to *Acanthamoeba* organisms in three successive serum samples from each of two patients. The first sample of one of the patients, a 57-year-old man with an old brain infarct, had a 1:8 titer against *A. culbertsoni.* A second serum sample taken 1 month later showed an increase in titer to 1:16. A third serum sample, taken 1 month after the second, showed a further increase in the titer to 1:64. The patient later died of cerebral hemorrhage, and amebae were demonstrated in the brain. Three successive serum samples taken 1 month apart from a 39-year-old man hospitalized with acute gastritis also showed an increase from 2 to 16 in the complement fixation titers to *A. culbertsoni* antigens. Amebae were seen in the stool samples of this patient but were identified as *Iodamoeba bütschlii.* He was treated with dehydroemetine and chloroquine, and the complement fixation titer decreased to 1:2 in a serum sample obtained 2 months later. Precipitin antibody was also demonstrated in the serum of a patient suffering from *A. polyphaga* keratitis (48, 79, 80). An increase in the ameba immobilization antibody titer over a 16-month period was recently demonstrated in the serum of a Nigerian patient, who made a partial recovery from an *Acanthamoeba rhysodes*-induced CNS disease (80).

An antibody response to *N. fowleri,* however, has not yet been defined. Most of the patients with *Naegleria* PAM have died within a very short time (5 to 10 days), before they have had sufficient time to produce detectable levels of antibody. In one case, however, in which the patient survived PAM due to *Naegleria,* an IIF titer of 1:4,096 against *N. fowleri* was detected in the serum after 42 days of hospitalization (69).

Treatment

Pathogenic *N. fowleri* is exquisitely sensitive to amphotericin B (9, 35, 48). At least three PAM patients were reported to have recovered after receiving intrathecal and intravenous injections of this drug alone or in combination with miconazole (9, 35, 48, 69). Culbertson found sulfadiazine to be active against experimental *Acanthamoeba* infections in mice (see references 25 and 48). Jones et al. (36) found that paromomycin, clotrimazole, and hydroxystilbamidine isethionate were active against *A. polyphaga* in vitro. In one study, propamidine isethionate 0.1% eye drops (Brolene) and 0.15% dibromopropamidine ointment together with topical neomycin sulfate were found to be successful in the management of *Acanthamoeba* keratitis (15). In another recent study, 1% clotrimazole when used in combination with Brolene and neosporin on four patients gave excellent results (95).

LITERATURE CITED

1. **Barker, R. H., Jr., L. Suebsaeng, W. Roeney, G. C. Aleerim, H. V. Dourado, and D. F. Wirth.** 1986. Specific DNA probe for the diagnosis of *Plasmodium falciparum* malaria. Science **231:**1434–1436.
2. **Baselski, V. S., M. K. Robison, L. W. Pifer, and D. R. Woods.** 1990. Rapid detection of *Pneumocystis carinii* in bronchoalveolar lavage samples by using Cellufluor staining. J. Clin. Microbiol. **28:**393–394.
3. **Bigby, T. D., D. Margolskee, J. L. Curtis, P. F. Michael, D. Sheppard, W. K. Hadley, and P. C. Hopewell.** 1986. The usefulness of induced sputum in the diagnosis of *Pneumocystis carinii* pneumonia in patients with the acquired immunodeficiency syndrome. Am. Rev. Respir. Dis. **133:**515–518.
4. **Blumenfield, W., and J. A. Kovacs.** 1988. Use of a monoclonal antibody to detect *Pneumocystis carinii* in induced sputum and bronchoalveolar lavage fluid by immunoperoxidase staining. Arch. Pathol. Lab. Med. **112:**1233–1236.
5. **Brandt, F., G. R. Healy, and M. Welch.** 1977. Human babesiosis: the isolation of *Babesia microti* in golden hamsters. J. Parasitol. **63:**934–937.
6. **Brinn, N. T.** 1883. Rapid metallic histological staining using the microwave oven. J. Histotechnol. **6:**125–129.
7. **Butt, C. G.** 1966. Primary amebic meningoencephalitis. N. Engl. J. Med. **274:**1473–1476.
8. **Camargo, M. G., P. G. Leser, and A. Rocca.** 1972. Rheumatoid factors as a cause for false-positive IgM antitoxoplasma fluorescent tests: a technique for specific results. Rev. Inst. Med. Trop. Sao Paulo **14:**310–313.
9. **Carter, R. F.** 1972. Primary amoebic meningo-encephalitis: an appraisal of present knowledge. Trans. R. Soc. Trop. Med. Hyg. **66:**193–208.
10. **Centers for Disease Control.** 1987. Malaria surveillance report. U.S. Public Health Service, Atlanta.
11. **Chongsuphajaisiddhi, T., C. H. M. Gilles, D. J. Krogstad, L. A. Salako, D. A. Warrell, N. J. White, P. F. Beales, J. A. Najera, U. K. Sheth, H. C. Spencer, and W. H. Wernsdorfer.** 1986. Severe and complicated malaria. Trans. R. Soc. Trop. Med. Hyg. **80**(Suppl):1–50.
12. **Coatney, G. R., W. E. Colling, M. Warren, and P. G. Contacos.** 1971. The primate malarias. U.S. Department of Health, Education and Welfare, Washington, D.C.
13. **Culbertson, C. G., J. W. Smith, and J. R. Minner.** 1958. *Acanthamoeba:* observations on animal pathogenicity. Science **127:**1506.
14. **Desmonts, G., Y. Naot, and J. S. Remington.** 1981. Immunoglobulin M-immunosorbent agglutination assay for diagnosis of infectious diseases: diagnosis of acute congenital and acquired *Toxoplasma* infections. J. Clin. Microbiol. **14:**486–491.
15. **Driebe, W. T., G. A. Stern, R. J. Epstein, G. S. Visvesvara, M. Adi, and T. Komadina.** 1988. Potential role for topical clotrimazole in combination chemotherapy. Arch. Ophthalmol. **106:**1196–1201.
16. **Duermeyer, W., F. Wielaard, and J. Van der Veen.** 1979. A new principle for the detection of specific IgM antibodies applied in an ELISA for hepatitis. Am. J. Med. Virol. **4:**25–32.
17. **Edman, J. C., J. A. Kovacs, H. Masur, D. V. Santi, H. J. Elwood, and M. L. Sogin.** 1988. Ribosomal RNA sequence shows *Pneumocystis carinii* to be a member of the fungi. Nature (London) **334:**519–522.
18. **Fowler, M., and R. F. Carter.** 1965. Acute pyogenic meningitis probably due to *Acanthamoeba* sp.: a preliminary report. Br. Med. J. **2:**740–742.
19. **Franzen, L., G. Westin, R. Shabo, L. Aslund, H. Perlmann, T. Persson, H. Wigzell, and U. Petterson.** 1984. Analysis of clinical specimens by hybridisation with probe containing repetitive DNA from *Plasmodium falciparum.* Lancet **i:**525–528.
20. **Frenkel, J. K., J. P. Dubey, and N. L. Miller.** 1970. *Toxo-*

plasma gondii in cats: fecal stages identified as coccidian oocysts. Science **167**:893–896.

21. **Frenkel, J. K., M. S. Bartlett, and J. W. Smith.** 1990. RNA homology and the reclassification of *Pneumocystis*. Diagn. Microbiol. Infect. Dis. **13**:1–2.
22. **Giannini, A. H., M. Schittini, J. S. Keithly, P. W. Warburton, C. R. Cantor, and L. H. T. Van der Ploeg.** 1986. Karyotype analysis of *Leishmania* species and its use in classification and clinical diagnosis. Science **232**:762–765.
23. **Gill, V., G. Evans, F. Stock, J. Parrillo, H. Masur, and J. Kovacs.** 1987. Detection of *Pneumocystis carinii* by fluorescent-antibody stain using a combination of three monoclonal antibodies. J. Clin. Microbiol. **25**:1837–1840.
24. **Gosey, L. L., R. M. Howard, F. G. Witebsky, F. P. Ognibene, T. C. Wu, V. J. Gill, and J. D. MacLowry.** 1985. Advantages of modified toluidine blue O stain and bronchoalveolar lavage for diagnosis of *Pneumocystis carinii* pneumonia. J. Clin. Microbiol. **22**:803–807.
25. **Griffin, J. L.** 1978. Pathogenic free-living amebae, p. 507–549. *In* J. P. Kreier (ed.), Parasitic protozoa, vol. 5. Academic Press, Inc., New York.
26. **Gutierrez, Y.** 1990. Diagnostic pathology of parasitic infections with clinical correlations. Lea & Febiger, Philadelphia.
27. **Haron, E., G. P. Bodey, M. A. Luna, R. Dekmezian, and L. Elting.** 1988. Has the incidence of *Pneumocystis carinii* pneumonia in cancer patients increased with the AIDS epidemic? Lancet **ii**:904–905.
28. **Hartmann, B., M. Koss, A. Hui, W. Baumann, L. Athos, and T. Boylen.** 1985. *Pneumocystis carinii* pneumonia in the acquired immunodeficiency syndrome (AIDS). Diagnosis with bronchial brushings, biopsy and bronchoalveolar lavage. Chest **87**:603–607.
29. **Hauser, W. E., B. J. Loft, F. K. Conley, and J. S. Remington.** 1982. Central nervous system toxoplasmosis in homosexual and heterosexual adults. N. Engl. J. Med. **307**: 498–499.
30. **Healy, G. R., and T. K. Ruebush II.** 1980. Morphology of *Babesia microti* in human blood smears. Am. J. Clin. Pathol. **73**:107–109.
31. **Herwaldt, B. L., D. J. Krogstad, and P. H. Schlesinger.** 1988. Antimalarial agents: specific chemoprophylaxis regimens. Antimicrob. Agents Chemother. **32**:953–956.
32. **Hinds, I.** 1988. A rapid and reliable silver impregnation method for *Pneumocystis carinii* and fungi. J. Histotechnol. **11**:27–29.
33. **Hughes, W. T.** 1985. Serodiagnosis of *Pneumocystis carinii* [letter]. Chest **87**:700.
34. **Hughes, W. T.** 1989. *Pneumocystis carinii:* taxing taxonomy. Eur. J. Epidemiol. **5**:265–269.
35. **John, D. T.** 1982. Primary amoebic meningoencephalitis and the biology of *Naegleria fowleri*. Annu. Rev. Microbiol. **36**:101–123.
36. **Jones, D. B., G. S. Visvesvara, and N. M. Robinson.** 1975. *Acanthamoeba polyphaga* keratitis and *Acanthamoeba* uveitis associated with fatal meningoencephalitis. Trans. Ophthalmol. Soc. U.K. **95**:221–232.
37. **Kelen, A. E., L. Ayllon-Leindl, and N. A. Labzoffsky.** 1962. Indirect fluorescent antibody method in serodiagnosis of toxoplasmosis. Can. J. Microbiol. **8**:545–554.
38. **Kenney, M.** 1971. The micro-Kolmer complement fixation test in routine screening for soil ameba infection. Health Lab. Sci. **8**:5–10.
39. **Kovacs, J. A., and H. Masur.** 1989. Prophylaxis of *Pneumocystis carinii* pneumonia: an update. J. Infect. Dis. **160**: 882–886.
40. **Kovacs, J. A., V. L. Ng, H. Masur, G. Leoung, W. K. Hadley, G. Evens, H. C. Lane, F. P. Ognibene, J. Shelhamer, J. E. Parrillo, and V. J. Gill.** 1988. Diagnosis of *Pneumocystis carinii* pneumonia: improved detection in sputum with use of monoclonal antibodies. N. Engl. J. Med. **318**:589–593.
41. **Krick, J. A., and J. S. Remington.** 1978. Toxoplasmosis in the adult—an overview. N. Engl. J. Med. Hyg. **32**:703–715.
42. **Krogstad, D. J., B. L. Herwaldt, and P. H. Schlesinger.** 1988. Antimalarial agents: specific treatment regimens. Antimicrob. Agents Chemother. **32**:957–961.
43. **Krogstad, D. J., and M. A. Pfaller.** 1983. Prophylaxis and treatment of malaria. Curr. Clin. Top. Infect. Dis. **3**:56–73.
44. **Krotoski, W. A., W. E. Collins, R. S. Bray, P. C. C. Garnham, F. B. Cogswell, R. W. Gwadz, R. Killick-Kendrick, R. Wolf, R. Sinden, L. C. Koontz, and P. S. Stanfill.** 1982. Demonstration of hypnozoites in sporozoite-transmitted *Plasmodium vivax* infection. Am. J. Trop. Med. Hyg. **31**: 1291–1293.
45. **Krotoski, W. A., D. M. Krotoski, P. C. C. Garnham, R. S. Bray, R. Killick-Kendrick, C. C. Draper, G. A. T. Targett, and M. W. Guy.** 1980. Relapses in primate malaria: discovery of two populations of exoerythrocytic stages—preliminary note. Br. Med. J. **1**:153–154.
46. **Luft, B. J., and J. S. Remington.** 1985. Toxoplasmosis of the central nervous system, p. 315–358. *In* J. S. Remington and M. N. Swartz (ed.), Current clinical topics in infectious diseases, vol. 6. McGraw-Hill Book Co., New York.
47. **Martin, W. J., II, T. F. Smith, D. R. Sanderson, W. M. Brutinel, F. R. Cockerill III, and W. W. Douglas.** 1987. Role of bronchoalveolar lavage in the assessment of opportunistic pulmonary infections: utility and complications. Mayo Clin. Proc. **62**:549–557.
48. **Martinez, A. J.** 1985. Free-living amebas: natural history, prevention diagnosis, pathology, and treatment of the disease. CRC Press, Inc., Boca Raton, Fla.
49. **McLaughlin, G. L., F. H. Brandt, and G. S. Visvesvara.** 1988. Restriction fragment length polymorphisms of the DNA of selected *Naegleria* and *Acanthamoeba* amoebae. J. Clin. Microbiol. **26**:1655–1658.
50. **Miller, L. H., F. A. Neva, and F. Gill.** 1978. Failure of chloroquine in human babesiosis (*Babesia microti*): case report and chemotherapeutic trials in hamsters. Ann. Intern. Med. **88**:200–202.
51. **Nerad, T. A., G. S. Visvesvara, and P. M. Daggett.** 1983. Chemically defined media for the cultivation of *Naegleria:* pathogenic and high temperature tolerant species. J. Protozool. **30**:383–387.
52. **Neva, F. A.** 1977. Looking back for a view of the future: observations on immunity to induced malaria. Am. J. Trop. Med. Hyg. **26**(Suppl.):211–215.
53. **Page, F. C.** 1967. Taxonomic criteria for limax amoebae, with descriptions of 3 new species of *Hartmanella* and 3 *Vahlkampfia*. J. Protozool. **14**:499–521.
54. **Page, F. C.** 1967. Redefinition of the genus *Açanthamoeba* with descriptions of three species. J. Protozool. **14**:709–724.
55. **Peglow, S. L., A. G. Smulian, M. J. Linke, C. L. Pogue, S. Nurre, J. Crisler, J. Phair, J. W. M. Gold, D. Armstrong, and P. D. Walzer.** 1990. Serologic responses to *Pneumocystis carinii* antigens in health and disease. J. Infect. Dis. **161**:296–306.
56. **Pifer, L. L.** 1985. Serodiagnosis of *Pneumocystis carinii* [letter]. Chest **87**:698–700.
57. **Potasman, I., L. Resnick, B. J. Luft, and J. S. Remington.** 1988. Intrathecal production of antibodies against *Toxoplasma gondii* in patients with toxoplasmic encephalitis and the acquired immunodeficiency syndrome (AIDS). Ann. Intern. Med. **108**:49–51.
58. **Pyndiah, J., U. Krech, P. Price, and J. Wilhelm.** 1979. Simplified chromatographic separation of immunoglobulin M from G and its application to toxoplasma indirect immunofluorescence. J. Clin. Microbiol. **9**:170–174.
59. **Remington, J. S., and G. Desmonts.** 1973. Congenital toxoplasmosis: variability in the IgM fluorescent antibody response and some pitfalls in diagnosis. J. Pediatr. **83**:27–30.
60. **Rondanelli, E. G. (ed.).** 1987. Amphizoic amoebae human pathology. Piccin Nuova Libraria, Padua, Italy.

61. **Ruebush, T. K., II, D. D. Juranek, E. S. Chisholm, P. C. Snow, G. R. Healy, and A. J. Sulzer.** 1977. Human babesiosis on Nantucket Island: evidence for self-limited and subclinical infections. N. Engl. J. Med. **297:**825–827.
62. **Ruskin, J., and J. S. Remington.** 1976. Toxoplasmosis in the compromised host. Ann. Intern. Med. **84:**193–199.
63. **Sabin, A. B., and H. A. Feldman.** 1948. Dyes as microchemical indicators of a new immunity phenomenon affecting a protozoan parasite (toxoplasma). Science **108:** 660–663.
64. **Santiago-Delpin, E. A., E. Mora, Z. A. Gonzalez, L. A. Morales-Otero, and R. Bermudez.** 1988. Factors in an outbreak of *Pneumocystis carinii* in a transplant unit. Transplant. Proc. **20:**462–465.
65. **Sawyer, T. K., G. S. Visvesvara, and B. A. Harke.** 1976. Pathogenic amoebas from brackish and ocean sediments, with description of *Acanthamoeba hatchetti*, n. sp. Science **196:**1324–1325.
66. **Schiffler, R. J., G. P. Mansur, T. R. Navin, and K. Limpakarnjanarat.** 1984. Indigenous Chagas' disease (American trypanosomiasis) in California. J. Am. Med. Assoc. **251:**2983–2984.
67. **Schmitz, H., V. von Diemling, and B. Flehmig.** 1980. Detection of IgM antibodies to cytomegalovirus (CMV) using enzyme-labelled antigen. J. Gen. Virol. **50:**59–68.
68. **Schochetman, G., C. Y. Ou, and W. K. Jones.** 1988. Polymerase chain reaction. J. Infect. Dis. **158:**1154–1157.
69. **Seidel, J. S., P. Harmatz, G. S. Visvesvara, A. Cohen, J. Edwards, and J. Turner.** 1982. Successful treatment of primary amebic meningoencephalitis. N. Engl. J. Med. **306:** 346–348.
70. **Singh, B. N.** 1975. Pathogenic and non-pathogenic amebae. Halsted Press, Division of John Wiley & Sons, Inc., New York.
71. **Sluiters, J. F., A. H. M. M. Balk, C. E. Essed, B. Mochtar, W. Weimar, M. L. Simoons, and E. P. F. Ijzerman.** 1989. Indirect enzyme-linked immunosorbent assay for immunoglobulin G and four immunoassays for immunoglobulin M to *Toxoplasma gondii* in a series of heart transplant recipients. J. Clin. Microbiol. **27:**529–535.
72. **Smith, J. W., D. M. Melvin, T. C. Orihel, L. R. Ash, R. M. McQuay, and J. H. Thompson, Jr.** 1976. Atlas of diagnostic medical parasitology: blood and issue parasites. American Society of Clinical Pathologists, Chicago.
73. **Spielman, A., J. B. Perrone, A. Teklehaimanot, F. Blacha, S. C. Wardlaw, and R. A. Levine.** 1988. Malaria diagnosis by direct observation of centrifuged samples of blood. Am. J. Trop. Med. Hyg. **39:**337–342.
74. **Stehr-Green, J. K., T. M. Bailey, F. H. Brandt, J. H. Carr, W. W. Bond, and G. S. Visvesvara.** 1987. *Acanthamoeba* keratitis in soft contact lens wearers: a case-control study. J. Am. Med. Assoc. **258:**57–60.
75. **Stehr-Green, J. K., T. M. Bailey, and G. S. Visvesvara.** 1989. The epidemiology of *Acanthamoeba* keratitis in the United States. Am. J. Ophthalmol. **107:**331–336.
76. **Sulzer, A. J., and M. Wilson.** 1971. The fluorescent antibody test for malaria. Crit. Rev. Clin. Lab. Sci. **2:**601–609.
77. **Suzuki, Y., D. M. Israelski, B. R. Danneman, P. Stepick-Biek, P. Thulliez, and J. S. Remington.** 1988. Diagnosis of toxoplasmic encephalitis in patients with acquired immunodeficiency syndrome by using a new serologic method. J. Clin. Microbiol. **26:**2541–2543.
78. **Telzak, E. E., R. J. Cote, J. W. M. Gold, S. W. Campbell, and D. Armstrong.** 1990. Extrapulmonary *Pneumocystis carinii* infections. Rev. Infect. Dis. **12:**380–386.
79. **Theodore, F. H., F. A. Jakobiec, K. B. Juechter, P. Ma, R. C. Troutman, P. M. Pang, and T. Iwamoto.** 1985. The diagnostic value of a ring infiltrate in acanthamoebic keratitis. Ophthalmologica **92:**1471–1479.
80. **Visvesvara, G. S.** 1987. Laboratory diagnosis, p. 193–215. *In* E. G. Rondanelli (ed.), Amphizoic amoebae human pathology. Piccin Nuova Libraria, Padua, Italy.
81. **Visvesvara, G. S.** 1988. Acanthamoebiasis and naegleriosis, p. 723–730. *In* A. Balows, W. J. Hausler, Jr., M. Ohashi, and A. Turano (ed.), Laboratory diagnosis of infectious diseases: principles and practice, vol. 1. Springer-Verlag, New York.
82. **Visvesvara, G. S., and W. Balamuth.** 1975. Comparative studies on related free-living and pathogenic amebae with special reference to *Acanthamoeba*. J. Protozool. **22:**245–256.
83. **Visvesvara, G. S., and G. R. Healy.** 1975. Comparative antigenic analysis of pathogenic and free-living *Naegleria* species by the gel diffusion and immunoelectrophoresis techniques. Infect. Immunol. **11:**95–108.
84. **Visvesvara, G. S., S. S. Mirra, F. H. Brandt, D. M. Moss, H. M. Mathews, and A. J. Martinez.** 1983. Isolation of two strains of *Acanthamoeba castellanii* from human tissue and their pathogenicity and isoenzyme profiles. J. Clin. Microbiol. **18:**1405–1412.
85. **Walls, K. W., S. L. Bullock, and D. K. English.** 1977. Use of the enzyme-linked immunosorbent assay (ELISA) and its microadaptation for the serodiagnosis of toxoplasmosis. J. Clin. Microbiol. **5:**273–277.
86. **Walton, B. C., B. M. Benchoff, and W. H. Brooks.** 1966. Comparison of the indirect fluorescent antibody test and the methylene blue dye test for the detection of antibodies to *Toxoplasma gondii*. Am. J. Trop. Med. Hyg. **15:**147–152.
87. **Walzer, P. D., C. K. Kim, and M. T. Cushion.** 1989. *Pneumocystis carinii*, p. 83–178. *In* P. D. Walzer and R. M. Gertor (ed.), Parasitic infections in the compromised host. Marcel Dekker, Inc., New York.
88. **Weigle, K. A., M. Daralos, P. Heredia, R. Molineros, N. G. Saravia, and A. D. Alessandro.** 1987. Diagnosis of cutaneous and mucocutaneous leishmaniasis in Colombia: a comparison of seven methods. Am. J. Trop. Med. Hyg. **36:**489–496.
89. **Wilcox, A.** 1960. Manual for the microscopical diagnosis of malaria in man. U.S. Department of Health, Education and Welfare, Washington, D.C.
90. **Witebsky, F. G., J. W. B. Andrews, V. J. Gill, and J. D. MacLowry.** 1988. Modified toluidine blue O stain for *Pneumocystis carinii:* further evaluation of some technical factors. J. Clin. Microbiol. **26:**774–775.
91. **Wittner, M., K. S. Rowin, H. B. Tanowitz, J. F. Hobbs, S. Saltzman, B. Wenz, R. Hirsch, E. Chisholm, and G. R. Healy.** 1982. Successful chemotherapy of transfusion babesiosis. Ann. Intern. Med. **96:**601–604.
92. **World Health Organization.** 1973. Chemotherapy of malaria and resistance to antimalarials: report of a WHO Scientific Group. Tech. Rep. Ser. no. 529. World Health Organization, Geneva.
93. **World Health Organization.** 1984. The leishmaniases. Tech. Rep. Ser. no. 701. World Health Organization, Geneva.
94. **World Health Organization.** 1986. Epidemiology and control of African trypanosomiasis. Tech. Rep. Ser. no. 739. World Health Organization, Geneva.
95. **Wright, P., D. Warhurst, and B. R. Jones.** 1985. Acanthamoeba keratitis successfully treated medically. Br. J. Ophthalmol. **69:**778–782.
96. **Young, L. S.** 1984. *Pneumocystis carinii* pneumonia: pathogenesis, diagnosis, treatment. *In* C. Enfant (ed.), Lung biology in health and disease, vol. 22. Marcel Dekker, Inc., New York.
97. **Zeledon, R.** 1974. Epidemiology, modes of transmission and reservoir hosts of Chagas' disease, p. 51–85. *In* K. Elliott, M. O'Connor, and G. E. W. Wolstenholme (ed.), Trypanosomiasis and leishmaniasis: a Ciba Foundation symposium. Elsevier/North-Holland Publishing Co., Amsterdam.

Chapter 69

Intestinal and Urogenital Protozoa

GEORGE R. HEALY AND JAMES W. SMITH

The protozoa that parasitize the intestinal and urogenital systems of humans belong to five groups: amebae, flagellates, ciliates, coccidia, and microsporidia (Table 1). With the exception of *Trichomonas vaginalis* and microsporidia of the genera *Pleistophora, Nosema,* and *Encephalitozoon,* all of the organisms live in the intestinal tract.

The species of intestinal protozoa vary in prevalence and in pathogenicity (Table 1). Some species are rarely encountered in patients in the United States but may be found in Americans who travel to areas in which the organisms are endemic and in persons from those areas who visit or emigrate to the United States. Therefore, clinicians and laboratory personnel should be aware of both common and uncommon parasite species that might be found in their patients.

In addition to the protozoan species generally considered human parasites, some species parasitic in animals may also infect humans. For example, *Cryptosporidium* species, long recognized as pathogens in calves, lambs, turkeys, and other animals, have recently been found in humans and have caused severe infections in patients with acquired immunodeficiency syndrome (AIDS).

Most of the intestinal protozoa (except *Sarcocystis hominis* and *S. suihominis,* which are acquired by ingestion of the infective stages in raw or improperly cooked beef and pork, respectively) are transmitted through fecally contaminated food, water, or other materials. Prevalence of intestinal protozoa is correlated with socioeconomic conditions, and higher rates of infection occur in people who have poor personal hygiene or who live in areas with poor sanitation. Contaminated water supplies are a particular problem because cysts are not killed by usual levels of chlorination. Filtration is required. Endemic and epidemic disease has been traced to water supplies which use surface water that either is not filtered or has improperly functioning filters. Several species of microsporidia have caused disease in patients with AIDS or individuals with suppressed immune function (35) (Table 1).

Some of the intestinal protozoa are commensals or nonpathogenic organisms that produce no evidence of disease; however, microscopists must be able to distinguish pathogenic from nonpathogenic species. In addition, the presence of nonpathogenic species indicates that the person has been exposed to fecal contamination. Several species are capable of causing mild to severe gastrointestinal symptoms. *Entamoeba histolytica* may produce extraintestinal lesions in various areas of the body, and microsporidia have been diagnosed in tissues other than the intestine, such as muscle, liver, brain, kidney, and cornea. However, pathogenic or potentially pathogenic protozoa do not always produce symptoms in infected people or may remain after symptoms have resolved. Such asymptomatic persons may serve as reservoirs for the infection. In addition, detection of a potentially pathogenic protozoan does not necessarily prove that the organism is causing the illness. Patients may have diarrhea caused by other organisms such as *Salmonella* spp. *Shigella* spp., *Escherichia coli,* or rotavirus. The pathogenicity of some species (*Blastocystis* spp., for example) has been questioned. *T. vaginalis,* a urogenital protozoan, is also considered pathogenic and may cause mild to severe vaginitis and other urogenital problems.

This chapter covers information on the morphologic identification of organisms (presented in tabular form and diagrams), recommended procedures for laboratory diagnosis, and clinical aspects of important pathogens. Serology and antigen detection are discussed in chapter 67.

In the descriptions of diseases, the clinical manifestations noted refer to findings in patients with symptomatic disease and do not necessarily refer to findings in every person infected with the parasite species.

LABORATORY DIAGNOSIS

Because the symptoms produced by pathogenic intestinal protozoa are usually nonspecific, diagnosis requires laboratory detection of the parasite by the microscopic examination of feces or other body material. Immunodiagnostic methods are useful for the diagnosis of extraintestinal amebiasis, but they are of limited usefulness for intestinal diseases.

Although not all intestinal protozoa are pathogenic, microscopists must be capable of identifying both pathogenic and nonpathogenic species, with the possible exception of species that are rarely found in patients in the United States. Morphology, especially that of amebae, varies, and species characteristics often overlap such that individual nonpathogenic organisms may have characteristics resembling those of pathogens and vice versa. Thus, for reliable identification, microscopists must be able to differentiate all species regardless of their potential for causing disease. Special attention will be given to the recognition and identification of the clinically significant pathogens, especially *E. histolytica, Giardia lamblia,* and *Cryptosporidium* spp.

The identification of protozoan species is based on the morphology of the diagnostic stages. The particular features or characteristics used for identification vary with the group of organisms (for example, amebae or flagellates), the species, and the stage(s) of parasite present. The diagnostic stages are trophozoites or cysts for the amebae, flagellates, and ciliates; oocysts or spo-

TABLE 1. Intestinal and urogenital protozoa that may be found in specimens from patients in the United States

Type and species	Relative prevalence[a]	Pathogenicity
Amebae		
Entamoeba histolytica	+	+
Entamoeba hartmanni	+	−
Entamoeba coli	++	−
Entamoeba polecki	R	−
Endolimax nana	++	−
Iodamoeba bütschlii	+	−
Ciliate		
Balantidium coli	R	+
Flagellates		
Dientamoeba fragilis	+	+
Giardia lamblia	++	+
Trichomonas vaginalis	++	+
Trichomonas hominis	+	−
Chilomastix mesnili	+	−
Enteromonas hominis	R	−
Retortamonas intestinalis	R	−
Coccidia		
Isospora belli	R	+
Sarcocystis spp.	R	?
Cryptosporidium sp.	+	++
Blastocystis hominis	+	±
Microsporidia		
Pleistophora	R	+
Encephalitozoon	R	+
Enterocytozoon	R	+
Nosema	R	+

[a] R, Rare.

rocysts for the coccidia; vacuolated forms for *Blastocystis hominis;* and spores for the microsporidia.

The type of material to be examined depends on the parasite and its location in the body. For the intestinal protozoa, feces are commonly submitted for examination, although other materials such as duodenal or sigmoidoscopic aspirates or biopsies are occasionally obtained.

Four types of procedures are used to recover and demonstrate intestinal protozoa: direct wet-mount examinations, concentration techniques, permanently stained preparations, and cultivation (27) (procedures are discussed in detail in chapter 66). All of these methods may not be needed in every case. The selection of appropriate techniques depends on the species of parasite suspected and the stage(s) of parasite likely to be found in the specimen. For example, trophozoite stages of amebae and flagellates are more likely to be present in soft or diarrheic stools, and cysts are more likely in formed feces. Thus, the techniques used to examine diarrheic fecal specimens may differ from those used for formed specimens.

For accurate and reliable identification, specimens must be properly collected and handled before examination. Protozoa, especially trophozoites, may develop atypical morphology in old or poorly collected specimens (24). Ideally, fecal specimens should be placed in fixative immediately after being evacuated or should reach the laboratory within 1 to 2 h after passage; other materials such as urine, aspirate, or biopsy from duodenum or colonic lesions should be sent to the laboratory immediately after collection. If transportation is delayed, specimens should be appropriately preserved to maintain the diagnostic characteristics of organisms that might be present.

AMEBAE

Six species of intestinal amebae may live in the cecum and colon of humans: *Entamoeba histolytica, Entamoeba hartmanni, Entamoeba polecki, Entamoeba coli, Endolimax nana,* and *Iodamoeba bütschlii.* Infection is acquired by the ingestion of cysts, which excyst in the intestine. The cysts are quite hardy and can survive for days or weeks in water or soil. Infection is usually diagnosed by the identification of organisms in feces, although other materials may be examined in symptomatic cases. Immunodiagnostic tests are useful for the diagnosis of extraintestinal amebiasis and may assist in diagnosis of invasive intestinal disease (see chapter 67).

Entamoeba histolytica

E. histolytica causes amebiasis and is the only ameba pathogenic for humans (30). Infections with *E. histolytica* are classified as amebiasis irrespective of whether the person exhibits symptoms. A number of outbreaks have occurred in the United States (23), usually from contaminated food or water. A recent outbreak was caused by inadequate disinfection of a colonic irrigation apparatus (20). Strains isolated from patients with clinical disease have been shown by isoenzyme analysis to differ from commensal strains (33), which suggests that only strains with certain isoenzyme patterns are capable of causing invasive disease. The incubation period is variable, from as short as a few days to weeks or even months (12). Clinical amebiasis, i.e., infection with symptoms produced, presumably by an amebic invasion of colonic tissue, may present with various manifestations, including dysentery, colitis, and ameboma. Amebic dysentery is an acute diarrhea with ulcerations of the colonic mucosa. Symptoms include crampy, lower abdominal pain, with bloody mucoid diarrhea in severe cases, and occasionally may be complicated by intestinal perforation. In some people, an increased frequency of bowel movements with or without blood and mucus may occur. A chronic form, amebic colitis, produces symptoms similar to those of ulcerative colitis or other forms of inflammatory bowel disease, with diarrhea, sometimes bloody, occurring over a long period, sometimes alternating with periods of constipation or normal bowel function. Some patients with amebiasis have been misdiagnosed as having ulcerative colitis (20). Another, less common form of intestinal disease, ameboma, is produced by the growth of granulomatous tissue in response to the infecting amebae, resulting in a large local lesion of the bowel which radiologically resembles a carcinoma.

Infections with *E. histolytica,* with or without a history of antecedent, gastrointestinal symptoms, may result in hematogenous spread of the organisms to the liver via the portal system, resulting in amebic abscess or abscesses of the liver. This occurs in up to 5% of patients with symptomatic intestinal amebiasis. Approximately 40% of patients with amebic liver abscess do not have a history of prior bowel symptoms, and in some patients *E. histolytica* may not be present in stool at the time liver disease becomes manifest. Amebic abscesses occasionally occur in the lung, brain, or other organs.

Intestinal infection is usually diagnosed by the microscopic identification of organisms in feces or in sigmoidoscopic material from ulcerations. Only trophozoites are found in tissue lesions, but both trophozoites and cysts may be found in the intestinal lumen. Some patients with invasive disease may have only trophozoites in fecal specimens, and direct wet mount of fresh material or the more sensitive permanent stain may be required to establish the diagnosis. Trophozoites are difficult to recognize in wet mounts of fixed material or concentration material. Depending on the type of fecal specimen, morphologic examination by direct wet mount, concentration, and permanent stain may be useful. Purged stool specimens occasionally show parasites when they are not detected in normally passed stools. Cultures for amebae may be helpful and are essential if isoenzyme patterns are to be examined but are not routinely used in most laboratories (11, 27) (see chapter 66). Suspected amebic abscesses are generally diagnosed by positive serologic tests (see chapter 67), although organisms may sometimes be identified microscopically in abscess aspirates or liver tissue biopsy. The last material aspirated is more likely to contain amebae. Cultivation of liver abscess fluid is not routinely attempted. Aspirates of abscesses or intestinal lesions may show amebic trophozoites, sometimes containing ingested erythrocytes in direct wet mounts or with permanent stains such as trichrome. In sections of liver or intestinal lesions, periodic acid-Schiff (PAS) stain counterstained with hematoxylin is particularly helpful. Amebic trophozoite cytoplasm is more PAS positive than most tissue and inflammatory cells, and identification is confirmed by demonstrating the typical *Entamoeba* nucleus (17).

Other species of intestinal amebae are not pathogenic but must be differentiated from *E. histolytica* (see below). *E. polecki* is seen occasionally in refugees from Southeast Asia and may be confused with *E. histolytica* (16).

Entamoeba gingivalis is a common inhabitant of the oral cavity, particularly in patients with poor oral hygiene (10). It resembles *E. histolytica* but does not have a cyst stage. As a result, trophozoites of *E. gingivalis* may cause confusion in diagnosing amebic lung abscess by morphologic examination of pulmonary material.

Morphologic identification of amebae in fecal specimens

Both trophozoites and cysts are diagnostic stages of the amebae, and either or both stages can be detected in feces. Microscopists must be familiar with the morphologic characteristics used for the differentiation of species and must be able to distinguish trophozoites from epithelial cells, polymorphonuclear leukocytes, and macrophages, as well as from pus cells, yeasts, pollen, molds, and other objects that may be present in feces.

Characteristics used to distinguish species of amebae are as follows.

- Trophozoites
  - Motility (progressive or nonprogressive; most evident in saline wet mounts of fresh feces)
  - Cytoplasm
    - Appearance (finely granular or coarse)
    - Inclusions (erythrocytes, yeast cells, molds, or bacteria)
  - Nucleus
    - Peripheral chromatin (present or absent; if present, the arrangement and size and uniformity of peripheral chromatic granules)
    - Karyosome (size and position)
- Cysts
  - Nucleus
    - Number
    - Peripheral chromatin (present or absent, distribution)
    - Karyosome (size and position)
  - Cytoplasmic inclusions (chromatoid bodies or glycogen; these are more often seen in young cysts)

Size is not a reliable feature for species differentiation of either trophozoites or cysts except in separating *E. histolytica* and *E. hartmanni*.

Not all of the characteristics listed can be seen in a single type of preparation; stained and unstained wet mounts and permanent stained smears are necessary to demonstrate all of the features (Table 2). Unstained wet mounts may reveal trophozoites and cysts. The motility of trophozoites in physiological saline mounts of fresh material and the presence of cytoplasmic inclusions such as erythrocytes in trophozoites and chromatoid bodies in cysts can be observed. However, stained preparations are usually needed for reliable species identification. Buffered methylene blue solution (Nair stain) can be used for temporary stains of trophozoites in fresh specimens and will permit the microscopist to distinguish host cells from amebae and trophozoites of *Entamoeba* spp. from those of other genera. Iodine solutions are used for temporary cyst stains of fresh or fixed specimens. Characteristics of cysts are less variable than those of trophozoites, and species of cysts can frequently be identified in iodine-stained wet mounts, especially if the organisms are examined with oil immersion magnification.

Regardless of the types of materials examined or the methods used to demonstrate organisms, species identifications are based on microscopic observations of morphologic characteristics. The typical characteristics of trophozoites and cysts of the ameba species are listed in Tables 3 and 4; diagrams of amebic cysts and trophozoites are presented in Fig. 1. Diagrams of nuclei are shown in Fig. 2; photomicrographs are presented in Fig. 3 through 5. Although *Dientamoeba fragilis* is a flagellate, it is included in these tables and figures because it resembles and must be differentiated from the amebae.

Morphologic characteristics of species overlap, and some organisms may be atypical, thus making identification difficult. For example, distinguishing trophozoites of *E. histolytica* from those of *E. coli* is often difficult because of morphologic variations. Rarely can species of trophozoites be identified from a single feature, such as karyosome location, or from a single organism. The microscopist must observe both the cytoplasmic and nuclear characteristics of several organisms before making a species identification. Although cysts are more easily identified than trophozoites, several cysts (particularly if they are immature) should be observed to ensure that the identification is reliable. If two species are identified, there should be distinct populations of each.

Sometimes, although amebic organisms are recognized, species cannot be identified. In these instances,

TABLE 2. Characteristics of intestinal amebae visible in different types of fecal preparations[a]

Characteristic	Unstained		Temporary stain		Permanent stain
	Saline	Formalin	Iodine (cysts)	Buffered methylene blue (trophozoites)[b]	
Trophozoite					
Motility	+	−		−	−
Cytoplasm					
Appearance	+	+		+	+
Inclusions (erythrocytes, bacteria)	+	+		+	+
Nucleus	−	+[c]		+	+
Cyst					
Nucleus	−	+	+		+
Chromatoid bodies	+	+	+[d]		+
Glycogen	−	−	+		− (vacuole present)

[a] From Brooke and Melvin (4).
[b] Quensel stain may be substituted for buffered methylene blue.
[c] Nuclei of trophozoites are visible in Formalin-fixed material but are usually not sufficiently distinctive for species identification.
[d] Chromatoid bodies are more easily seen in unstained wet mounts than in iodine preparations.

the laboratory should report "unidentified ameba trophozoites (or cysts)"; if the genus can be determined but the species cannot, "unidentified *Entamoeba* trophozoites or cysts" should be reported, and another specimen should be requested.

FLAGELLATES

The flagellates inhabit the intestinal and atrial areas. Intestinal infections by flagellates that have cyst stages are acquired by the ingestion of cysts. Infections are usually diagnosed by morphologic examinations of feces or other body materials. For *G. lamblia*, immunodiagnostic tests have been reported for the detection of antibody in serum specimens and parasite antigens in stool specimens (see chapter 67). Species identifications are generally based on microscopic identification of morphologic features of trophozoites or cysts. Two species, *G. lamblia* and *D. fragilis*, cause clinically significant intestinal disease, and *T. vaginalis* is a frequent cause of vaginitis.

Giardia lamblia

Giardiasis is acquired by the ingestion of the hardy cysts of *G. lamblia*. Outbreaks related to contaminated water are common in the United States, and infections are frequent in day-care centers (44) and among campers and male homosexuals (39, 46). Trophozoites infect the upper small intestine but do not invade the tissues to produce ulcers. Infection may elicit a variety of symptoms (46) or may be asymptomatic. The incubation period is variable, ranging from a few days to several weeks, with an average of about 9 days (21). In acute giardiasis, symptoms include nausea, upper intestinal cramping or pain, and malaise. There is often explosive, watery diarrhea, characterized by foul-smelling stools. These symptoms are accompanied by flatulence and abdominal distention. The acute stage of clinical giardiasis may be followed by a chronic stage, or the chronic type of infection may be the first indication of infection. In such infections, there are flatulence, mushy, foul-smelling stools, upper intestinal cramping, and abdominal distention. A number of patients also exhibit belching, nausea, anorexia, vomiting, and symptoms of heartburn. Fever and chills may be present, but to a lesser degree. Symptoms may mimic peptic ulcer or gallbladder disease. In some patients the cysts may be excreted in stools in a variable pattern, although the reasons for this are not clear (9). This variable presence of cysts may occur even when there are classic symptoms of disease and numerous trophozoites in the upper small intestine.

Diagnosis is usually established by the demonstration of cysts or, occasionally, trophozoites in feces or of trophozoites in duodenal contents obtained by string test (1), aspiration, or biopsy (Fig. 5 to 7). Because of the variable shedding of organisms, several stool specimens should be examined before the infection is ruled out. It is best to examine a total of three specimens collected 2 to 3 days apart, although daily specimens for a total of three can be used. If viable trophozoites are present, they can be readily identified by the characteristic falling-leaf or tumbling motion in saline mounts of fresh feces. The large, ventral sucking disk can be seen as the organism turns. In a lateral view, the trophozoite appears spoon shaped. Permanent stains may be needed if organisms cannot be identified in wet mounts or by concentration (43). Immunofluorescent and antigen detection methods are discussed in chapter 67. Small plant cells can resemble *Giardia* cysts, so organisms should be carefully examined for the fibrils and nuclei characteristic of *Giardia* species. Permanent stains may help.

When *Giardia* organisms are not found in stool specimens, duodenal aspirates, string test mucus, or biopsied mucosal tissue can be examined. The string test (1) is used to collect mucus from the duodenal area and may be less traumatic for the patient than other methods. Materials obtained by drainage, aspiration, or the string test can be examined by simple, direct wet mounts. Biopsy tissue may be processed and stained by the usual histopathologic methods; however, before preservation, a fresh imprint smear of the mucosal surface on a slide can be made and stained with trichrome or Giemsa stain.

TABLE 3. Differential morphology of ameba trophozoites found in human stool specimens[a]

Species	Size (diam or length)	Motility	Nucleus			Cytoplasm	
			No. and characteristics	Peripheral chromatin	Karyosomal chromatin	Appearance	Inclusions
Entamoeba histolytica	10–60 μm; usual range, 15–20 μm, commensal form[b]; >20-μm invasive form[c]	Progressive, with hyaline, fingerlike pseudopods	1, not visible in unstained preparations	Fine granules; usually evenly distributed and uniform in size	Small, discrete; usually centrally located but occasionally eccentric	Finely granular	Erythrocytes occasionally; noninvasive organisms may contain bacteria
Entamoeba hartmanni	5–12 μm; usual range, 8–10 μm	Usually nonprogressive, but may be progressive occasionally	1, not visible in unstained preparations	Similar to *E. histolytica*	Small, discrete, often eccentric	Finely granular	Bacteria
Entamoeba coli	15–50 μm; usual range, 20–25 μm	Sluggish, nonprogressive, with blunt pseudopods	1, often visible in unstained preparations	Coarse granules, irregular in size and distribution	Large, discrete, usually eccentric	Coarse, often vacuolated	Bacteria, yeast cells, or other material
Entamoeba polecki	10–25 μm; usual range, 15–20 μm	Usually sluggish, similar to *E. coli;* occasionally in diarrheic specimens, motility may be progressive	1, may be slightly visible in unstained preparations; occasionally distorted by pressure from vacuoles in cytoplasm	Usually fine granules evenly distributed; occasionally granules may be irregularly arranged; chromatin sometimes in plaques or crescents	Small, discrete, eccentric; occasionally large, diffuse, or irregular	Coarsely granular, may resemble *E. coli;* contains numerous vacuoles	Bacteria, yeast cells
Endolimax nana	6–12 μm; usual range, 8–10 μm	Sluggish, usually nonprogressive with blunt pseudopods	1, visible occasionally in unstained preparations	None	Large, irregularly shaped, blotlike	Granular, vacuolated	Bacteria
Iodamoeba bütschlii	8–20 μm; usual range, 12–15 μm	Sluggish, usually nonprogressive	1, not usually visible in unstained preparations	None	Large, usually central; surrounded by refractile, achromatic granules often not distinct even in stained slides	Coarsely granular, vacuolated	Bacteria, yeast cells, or other material
Dientamoeba fragilis[d]	5–15 μm; usual range, 9–12 μm	Pseudopods are angular, serrated, or broad lobed; hyaline, almost transparent	2 (in ca. 20% of organisms, only 1 nucleus is present), nuclei invisible in unstained preparations	None	Large cluster of 4–8 granules	Finely granular	Bacteria; occasionally erythrocytes

[a] From Brooke and Melvin (4).
[b] Commensal form usually found in asymptomatic or chronic cases; may contain bacteria.
[c] Invasive form usually found in acute cases; often contains erythrocytes.
[d] Flagellate included with amebae for diagnostic purposes.

TABLE 4. Differential morphology of ameba cysts found in human stool specimens[a]

Species	Size	Shape	Nucleus: No. and characteristics	Nucleus: Peripheral chromatin	Nucleus: Karyosomal chromatin	Cytoplasm: Chromatoid bodies	Cytoplasm: Glycogen
Entamoeba histolytica	10–20 μm; usual range, 12–15 μm	Usually spherical	4 in mature cyst; immature cysts with 1 or 2 occasionally seen	Present; fine, uniform granules, evenly distributed	Small, discrete, usually centrally located	Present; elongated bars with bluntly rounded ends	Usually diffuse; concentrated mass often present in young cysts; stains reddish brown with iodine
Entamoeba hartmanni	5–10 μm; usual range, 6–8 μm	Usually spherical	4 in mature cyst; immature cysts with 1 or 2 often seen	Similar to *E. histolytica*	Similar to *E. histolytica*	Present; elongated bars with bluntly rounded ends	Similar to *E. histolytica*
Entamoeba coli	10–35 μm; usual range, 15–25 μm	Usually spherical occasionally oval, triangular, or other shapes	8 in mature cyst; supernucleated cysts with 16 or more occasionally seen; immature cysts with 2 or more occasionally seen	Present; coarse granules irregular in size and distribution but often more uniform than in trophozoites	Large, discrete, usually eccentric but occasionally centrally located	Present but less frequently seen than in *E. histolytica;* usually splinterlike with pointed ends	Usually diffuse, but occasionally a well-defined mass in immature cysts; stains reddish brown with iodine
Entamoeba polecki	9–18 μm; usual range, 11–15 μm	Spherical or oval	1, rarely 2; occasionally visible in unstained preparations	Usually fine granules evenly distributed	Usually small and eccentric	Present; many small bodies with angular or pointed ends or few large bodies; may be oval, rodlike, or irregular	Usually small, diffuse masses; stains reddish brown with iodine; dark area called inclusion mass (possibly concentrated cytoplasm) often also present; mass does not stain with iodine
Endolimax nana	5–10 μm; usual range, 6–8 μm	Spherical, ovoidal, or ellipsoidal	4 in mature cysts; immature cysts with less than 4 rarely seen	None	Large (blotlike), usually central	Occasionally granules or small oval masses, but bodies as seen in *Entamoeba* spp. are not present	Usually diffuse; concentrated mass seen occasionally in young cysts; stains reddish brown with iodine
Iodamoeba bütschlii	5–20 μm; usual range, 10–12 μm	Ovoidal, ellipsoidal, triangular, or other shapes	1 in mature cyst	None	Large, usually eccentric; refractile, achromatic granules on one side of karyosome; indistinct in iodine preparations	Occasionally granules present, but chromatoid bodies as seen in *Entamoeba* spp. are not present	Compact, well-defined mass; stains dark brown with iodine

[a] From Brooke and Melvin (4).

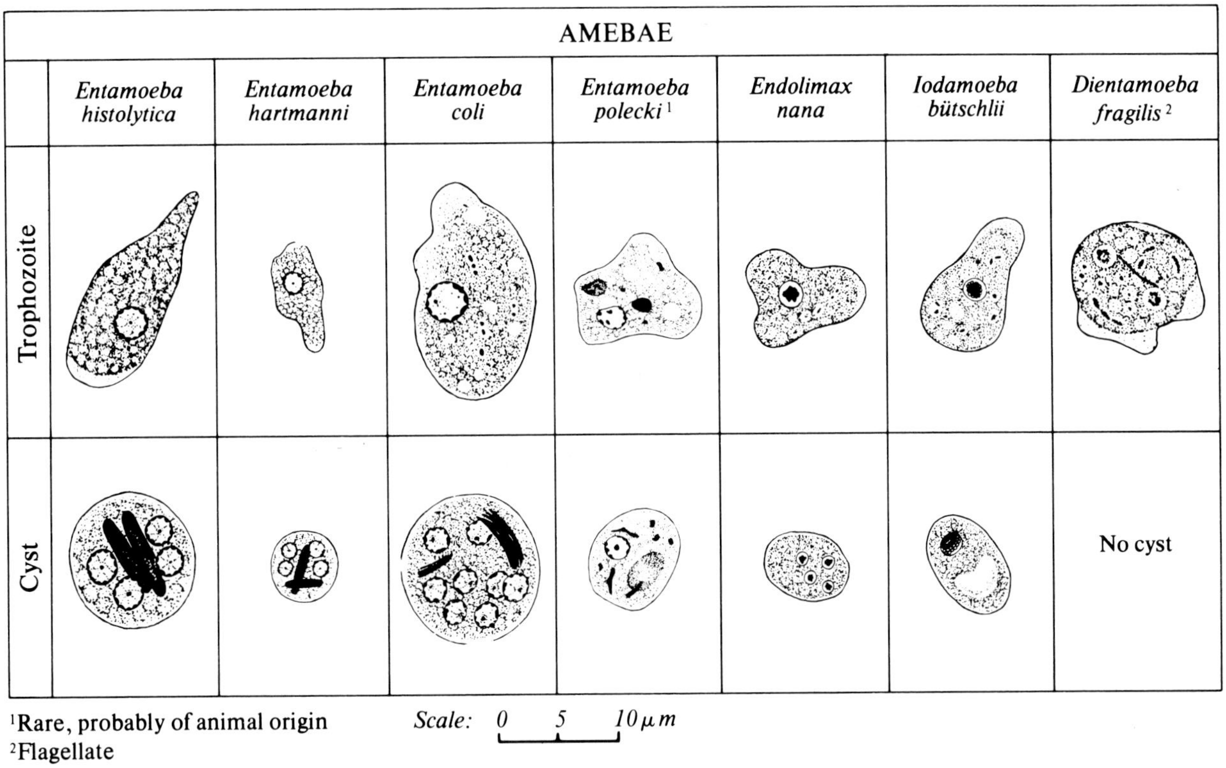

AMEBAE
Entamoeba histolytica
Entamoeba hartmanni
Entamoeba coli
Entamoeba polecki[1]
Endolimax nana
Iodamoeba bütschlii
Dientamoeba fragilis[2]
Trophozoite
Cyst
No cyst
[1]Rare, probably of animal origin
[2]Flagellate
Scale: 0 5 10 μm

FIG. 1. Amebae found in human stool specimens. (From Brooke et al. [4].)

Entamoeba histolytica
Entamoeba hartmanni
Entamoeba coli
Endolimax nana
Dientamoeba fragilis*
Iodamoeba bütschlii**

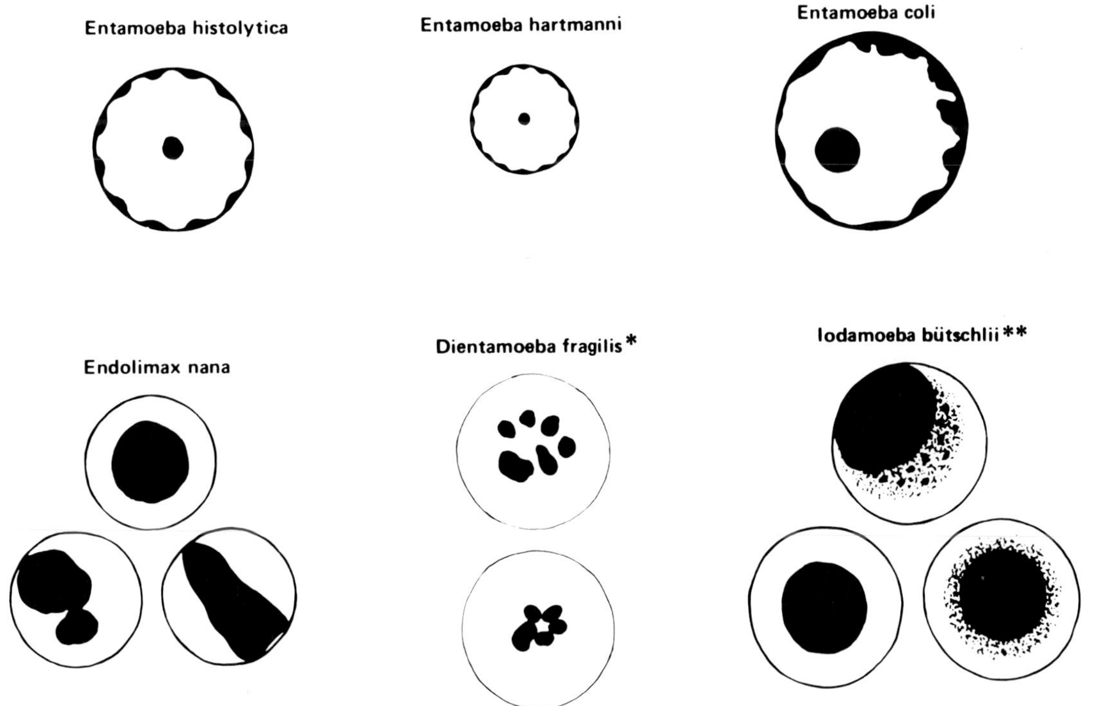

FIG. 2. Nuclei of amebae. *Flagellate. ***Iodamoeba* cysts often have eccentric karyosomes against the nuclear membrane, as in the upper *Iodamoeba* nucleus, whereas the trophozoite nuclei are usually not against the nuclear membrane. Achromatic granules are not always visible (lower left) in *Iodamoeba* nuclei. (From Smith et al. [38].)

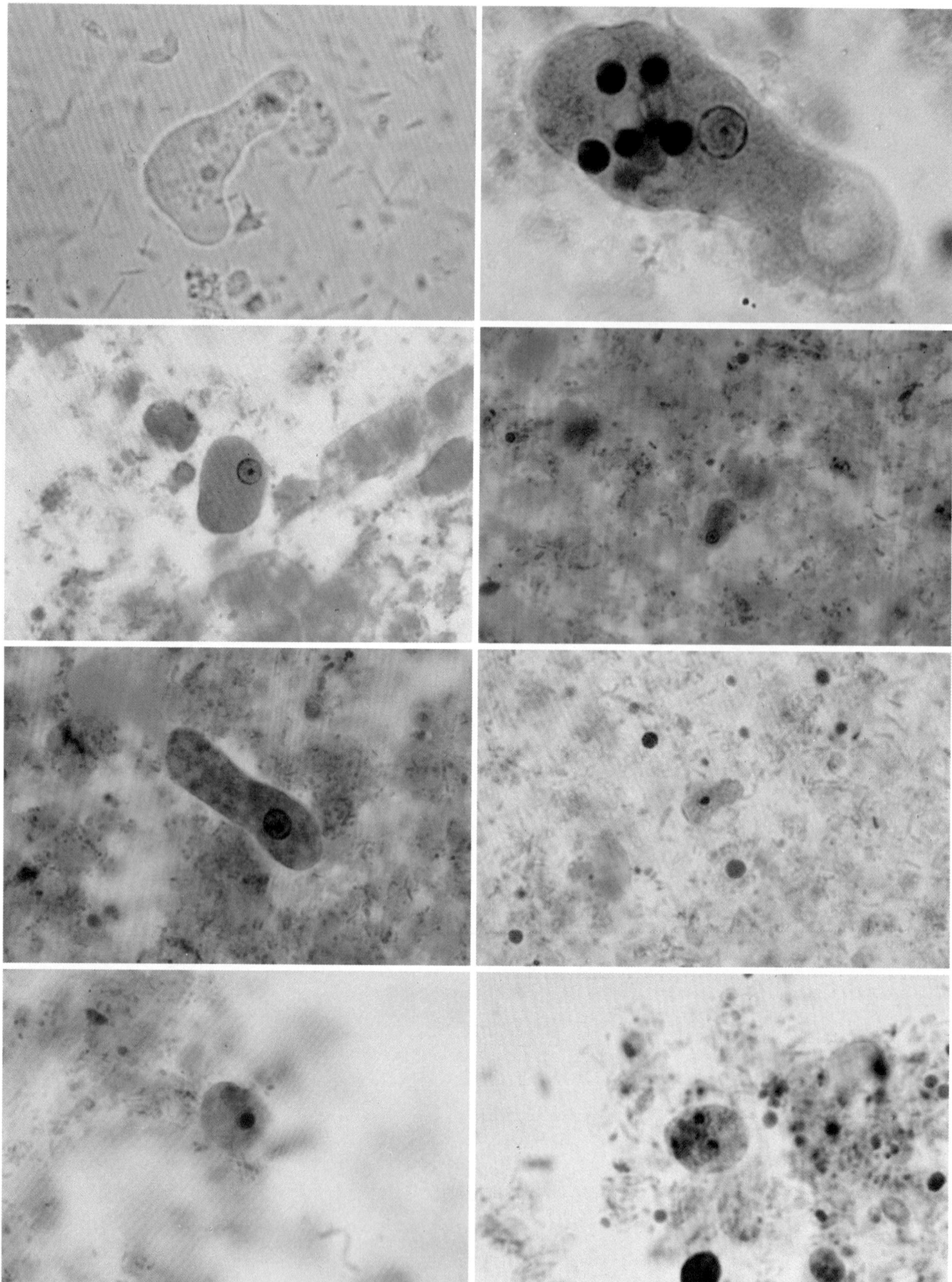

FIG. 3. Ameba trophozoites (trichrome stain, except upper left; oil immersion magnification). Row 1: (left) *E. histolytica*, unstained. The clear pseudopod is evident at the bottom of the organism. Several ingested erythrocytes are present in the cytoplasm. The nucleus is not visible. (Right) *E. histolytica*. This large trophozoite contains numerous ingested erythrocytes to the left of the nucleus. The nucleus has a small, dotlike central karyosome and peripheral chromatin which although granular

Chilomastix mesnili

C. mesnili is a nonpathogenic flagellate that inhabits the cecum and colon. The diagnostic stages, trophozoites and cysts, are passed in feces. The trophozoites have a characteristic rotating, wobbling motion that is readily recognized in saline mounts of fresh material. The spiral groove, which extends along the body, is sometimes visible as the organism turns. In permanent stained preparations, trophozoites are usually lightly stained and sometimes distorted, and they may be overlooked. The most prominent feature is the long cytostome which extends about one-third to one-half the length of the body. The nucleus also may have a collection of chromatin along one side, giving it a lopsided look (Fig. 6 and 7).

The presence of the cytostome and spiral groove, the location of the nucleus at one end with tapering of the opposite end, and nuclear characteristics aid in the differentiation of *C. mesnili* from other intestinal protozoa.

C. mesnili cysts are often identified by their usual lemon shape, single large nucleus, and fibrils (Fig. 6). Cysts are not always lemon shaped; they may be rounded or, if viewed on end, may appear round.

Dientamoeba fragilis

D. fragilis is a flagellate with no external flagellum; thus, the disease dientamebiasis is discussed in the flagellate section, but the organism is included in Fig. 1 to 3 and Tables 2 and 3, which concern amebae, because it must be differentiated from the amebae. The organism does not have a cyst stage, and the exact means of spread is not clear. *D. fragilis* infection is commonly associated with enterobiasis, and it has been suggested that *D. fragilis* may infect *Enterobius* eggs and thus bypass gastric acidity (5). Although clinical infections with *D. fragilis* occur, they are infrequently reported, probably because of the self-limited nature of the infection such that stool examination is not requested and because of the difficulty in detecting and identifying the trophozoites in stool specimens from individuals with suggestive symptoms. The incubation period for clinical dientamebiasis is not known with certainty. Symptoms have been reported more frequently in children than in adults and are predominately diarrhea and abdominal distention (41). Outbreaks in day-care centers have been described (44). Nausea, vomiting, and weight loss have been recorded in from one-third to one-fifth of the cases reported in the literature.

Permanent stains are usually required to diagnose this infection, and multiple specimens may be required, since shedding varies from day to day (47). The delicately staining trophozoites are usually (60 to 80%) binucleate, though the nuclei may be in different planes of focus. They must be differentiated from the trophozoites of *E. nana*, *I. bütschlii*, and *E. hartmanni*. Nuclear characteristics, the presence of binucleate forms, and the absence of cysts aid in identification of this organism.

Trichomonas hominis

T. hominis, a nonpathogenic protozoan that inhabits the colon, has only a trophozoite stage. The motile trophozoites in saline wet mounts display a nervous, jerky motion. They possess an undulating membrane which extends most of their length (Fig. 6 and 7) and often can be seen in wet mounts, especially if the organisms have slowed down or are trapped in fecal debris. Iodine stains are of little value for the identification of *T. hominis* because the organisms tend to become distorted. Permanent stains are also of limited value; although organisms can be seen, they are often distorted and difficult to recognize.

Trichomonas vaginalis

T. vaginalis inhabits the urogenital systems of both males and females and is considered a pathogen. The trophozoites (the only stage) are found in the urine of both sexes, in material from the vagina, and in prostatic secretions. It is estimated that approximately 5 million women in the United States have trichomoniasis and that roughly 1 million men harbor the parasite. Infection is usually, but not always, acquired by sexual contact. The infection in males is generally asymptomatic, but 25 to 50% of infected women exhibit symptoms (45), which include dysuria, vaginal itching and burning, and in severe infections a foamy, yellowish-green discharge with a foul odor. In many women the infection becomes symptomatic and chronic, with periods of relief in response to therapy. Recurrences of infection and disease may be caused by reinfection from an asymptomatic sexual partner, in the true sense of a sexually transmitted disease, or by failure of the drug metronidazole to completely eliminate the parasite. Symptomatic infections in males are rarely reported but include prostatitis, urethritis, epididymitis, and urethral stricture. Rarely, *T. vaginalis* infections occur in ectopic sites, and parasites may be recovered from areas of the body other than the urogenital system (26).

Infections with *T. vaginalis* are usually detected by finding the motile trophozoites in wet mounts of vaginal

is distributed in fairly uniform fashion. This large erythrophagocytic trophozoite is from a patient with amebic dysentery. Row 2: (left) *E. histolytica*. The trophozoite is typical of the commensal form of *E. histolytica*. It is smaller than the invasive form seen in row 1, right, and does not contain ingested erythrocytes. The nucleus is typical, with a dotlike central karyosome and evenly distributed peripheral chromatin. (Right) *E. hartmanni*. This organism has characteristics similar to those of *E. histolytica* but is smaller. The nucleus is at the lower portion of the trophozoite. Row 3: (left) *E. coli*. This elongated trophozoite of *E. coli* has a nucleus with a large eccentric karyosome. There is some unevenness in distribution of peripheral chromatin. Cytoplasm contains numerous vacuoles. (Right) *E. nana*. This trophozoite has a nucleus with a large karyosome and no peripheral chromatin on the nuclear membrane. A clear halo surrounds the karyosome and extends to the nuclear membrane. It is most evident beneath the karyosome. Cytoplasm is delicate and vacuolated. Row 4: (left) *I. bütschlii*. This organism has a large karyosome and no chromatin on the nuclear membrane. Distinct achromatic granules are not evident in the nucleus, but the karyolymph is "muddy" in contrast to the clearer karyolymph noted above for *E. nana*. The cytoplasm of this organism is rather homogeneous, although the cytoplasm of *I. bütschlii* trophozoites often contains numerous ingested bacteria. (Right) *D. fragilis* trophozoites. This flagellate is included here because it must be differentiated from the amebae. There are two nuclei, one above the other. The granular karyosome of the lower nucleus is evident. There is no chromatin on the nuclear membrane. Cytoplasm is vacuolated.

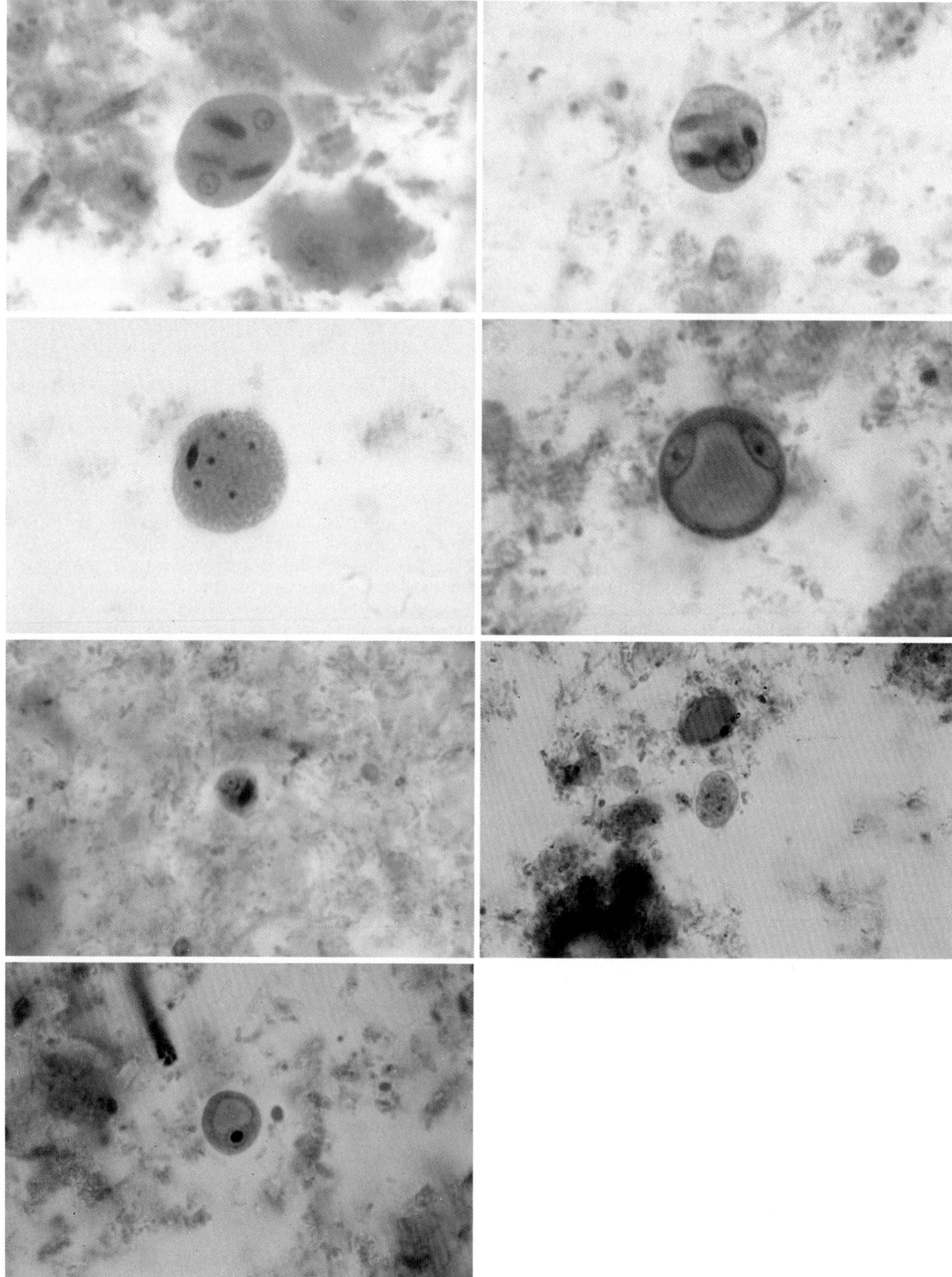

FIG. 4. Ameba cysts (trichrome stain; oil immersion magnification). Row 1: (left) *E. histolytica*. Two of the four nuclei are seen in this plane of focus. Three chromatoid bodies are evident which stain dark blue and have rounded contours. (Right) *E. histolytica*. This uninucleate cyst has numerous rounded chromatoid bodies which in this organism stain red. The pale-staining areas represent glycogen masses. Row 2: (left) *E. coli*. Five nuclei are evident in this plane of focus, and there is a red chromatoid

fluid, prostatic fluid, or sediments of freshly passed urine. In wet mounts, the trophozoites move with a nervous, jerky motion and possess an undulating membrane, which extends only half the length of the organism. In old urine specimens, the organisms may be dead or badly distorted and thus cannot be identified or may be confused with host cells. In addition, old urine specimens may be contaminated with airborne, free-living flagellates, especially if the urine collection vessel is open to the air and not sterile.

Vaginal materials commonly used for the diagnosis of *T. vaginalis* infections are vaginal fluid, scrapings, or washings. These samples may be examined morphologically in a saline wet mount or as a stained smear, or the material can be cultured. Although some workers feel that wet mount examinations are as efficient as cultures in revealing infections, current evidence suggests that cultivation methods are superior (15, 34). Immunofluorescent and enzyme-linked immunoassay (ELISA) methods have recently been described (see chapter 67).

Morphologic identification of flagellates

The characteristics of trophozoites and cysts which aid in identification are outlined below. The flagellates are a more diverse group than the amebae.

Trophozoites
- Motility (in saline mounts, the type of trophozoite movement is characteristic and species specific)
- Shape
- Number of nuclei (the character of the nucleus is not generally used for species identification)
- Other features (undulating membrane, sucking disk, prominent cytostome, spiral groove)
- Flagella (number and location; since flagella are difficult to see and count, they are not practical diagnostic features for species identification, but their presence distinguishes the organism as a flagellate trophozoite)

Cysts
- Shape
- Size
- Number of nuclei
- Fibrils (arrangement or pattern within the cyst; their presence distinguishes the cyst as a flagellate rather than an ameba cyst)

Not all of the features listed can be seen in a single type of preparation (Table 5). In many cases, species can be determined by the examination of either direct or concentrated wet mounts, without resorting to permanent stains. If viable trophozoites are present, identification can readily be made by the type of motility in direct saline mounts; no further observations are necessary. Species of cysts can usually be identified in iodine-stained mounts. However, permanent stains are necessary if organisms are atypical, are degenerate, or cannot be positively identified in wet mounts. The diagnostic features of flagellate trophozoites and cysts are described in Tables 6 and 7, respectively; diagrams are shown in Fig. 6, and photomicrographs are presented in Fig. 5 and 7.

CILIATE

Balantidium coli, a pathogenic ciliate inhabiting the colon, is the only ciliate and the largest protozoan parasitizing humans. Both trophozoites and cysts may be found in the feces.

Balantidiasis in humans is rarely reported in the United States. The disease is more prevalent where there is a close association of humans with pigs, the natural hosts from which humans contract the infection. The organism also infects nonhuman primates, especially the great apes. The symptoms of infection with *B. coli* are referable to the large bowel and similar to those of amebiasis: lower abdominal pain, nausea, vomiting, and tenesmus. Chronic infections may present with cramps, frequent episodes of watery, mucoid diarrhea, and rarely with bloody diarrhea. Chronic infections have been known to last for several months. In tropical areas in which the parasite is endemic, the infection often is severe in patients who may also have other parasitic, bacterial, or viral infections or are undernourished. *B. coli* causes colonic ulcers similar to those caused by *E. histolytica*, but it does not spread to other organs.

In human feces, trophozoites are readily recognized by their large size, shape, and rapid, rotating motion. Cysts are less easily identified, but they usually cause few diagnostic problems. The morphology of trophozoites and cysts is described in Table 8; diagrams are shown in Fig. 8. Characteristics that are visible in different types of preparations are listed in Table 5.

The examination of direct saline mounts is the most practical method of detecting infections. Cysts can be recovered by concentration, but in human infections trophozoites are usually more numerous than cysts. Iodine-stained mounts and permanent stains are of little value because the organisms tend to overstain.

COCCIDIA

The intestinal coccidia that parasitize humans belong to the subphylum Sporozoa and are obligatory tissue parasites that inhabit the mucosa of the small intestine. Species of three genera, *Isospora*, *Sarcocystis*, and *Cryptosporidium*, parasitize humans. The intestinal phase of toxoplasmosis which occurs in cats is similar to the intestinal infections of *Isospora* and *Sarcocystis* species in humans. The growth stages resemble those of malaria (also a sporozoan) and involve asexual and sexual generations. Therefore, the diagnostic stages, which are passed in feces, are unlike those of other intestinal protozoa. For both *Isospora* and *Cryptosporid-*

---

body to the left. Nuclear karyosomes are large and central. Although karyosomes are typically eccentric, they may be centered as in nuclei of this cyst. Cytoplasm is granular. (Right) *E. coli*. This binucleate cyst of *E. coli* contains a large glycogen vacuole. Immature cysts such as this are typical of *E. coli*. Row 3: (left) *E. hartmanni*. This small cyst has one nucleus in this plane of focus. A large chromatoid body is present on the right. (Right) *E. nana*. All four dotlike nuclei are evident at this focal plane. Halos are evident around some of them. Row 4: *I. bütschlii*. This cyst has a large glycogen vacuole, with the nucleus below it. Achromatic granules are not evident, and the karyosome is large and rounded.

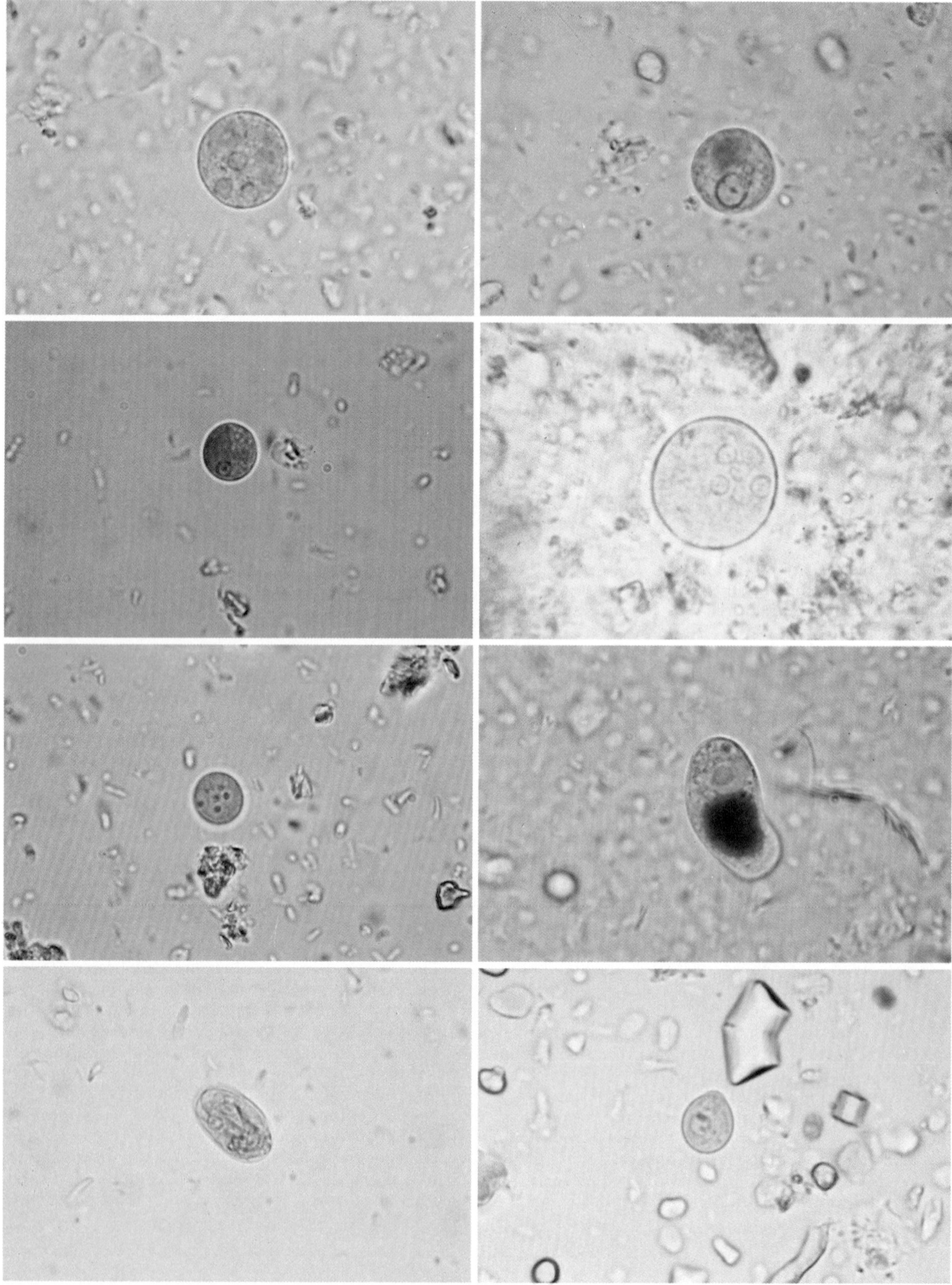

FIG. 5. Ameba and flagellate cysts (iodine-stained wet mounts; oil immersion magnification). Row 1: (left) *E. histolytica*. Three nuclei are evident in this focal plane. (Right) *E. histolytica*. This immature uninucleate cyst has a reddish-staining glycogen mass above the nucleus. Row 2: (left) *E. hartmanni*. There is one nucleus in this focal plane. An irregular reddish glycogen mass is evident above the nucleus. (Right) *E. coli*. In this focal plane, a cluster of six nuclei may be recognized toward the right of the

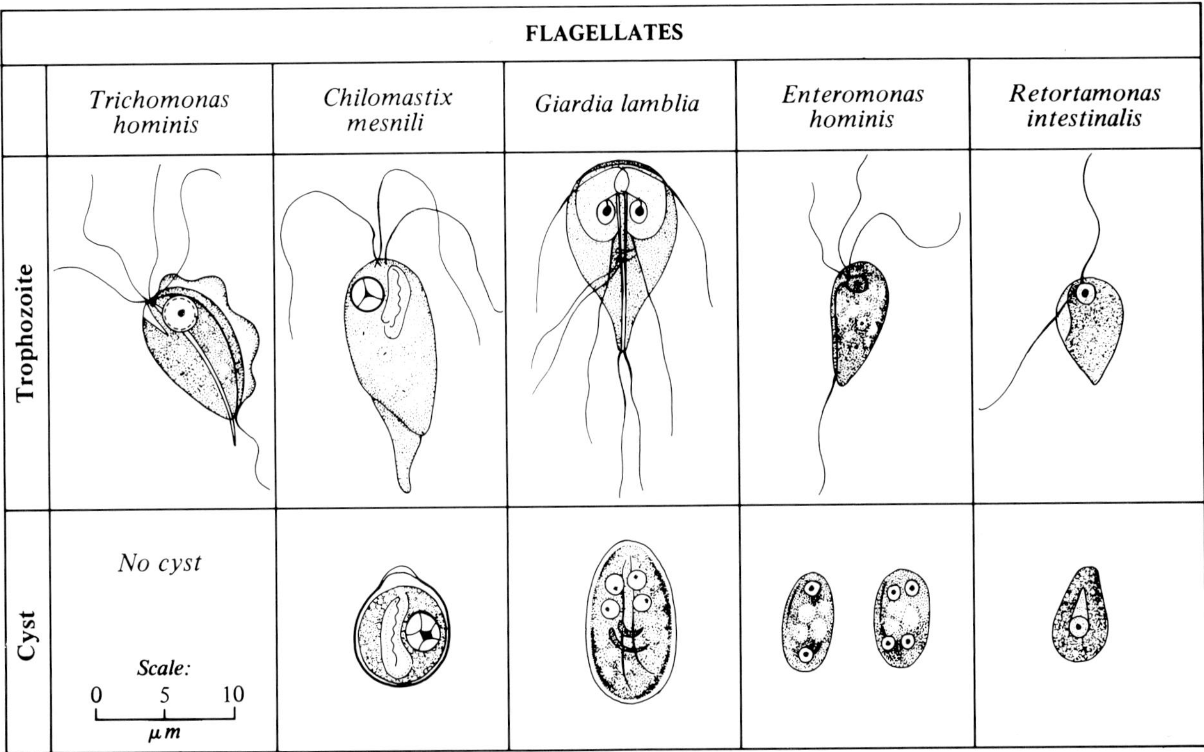

FIG. 6. Flagellates found in human stool specimens. (From Brooke and Melvin [4].)

ium species, oocysts, either unsporulated (immature) as in *Isospora belli* or sporulated (mature) as the cryptosporidia, are diagnostic stages. The diagnostic stages for *Sarcocystis* species are free sporocysts and mature oocysts. Oocysts and sporocysts are transparent and are difficult to see in unstained preparations unless the microscope light is reduced and carefully regulated. Descriptions of the diagnostic stages are presented in Table 8; diagrams are shown in Fig. 8; photomicrographs are presented in Fig. 9. Characteristics that are visible in different types of mounts are listed in Table 5.

Isospora and *Sarcocystis* species

Isosporiasis is caused by *I. belli* and, although infrequently recognized, can produce severe intestinal disease (3). The disease has been found to occur in AIDS patients (40). Deaths from overwhelming infections have been reported in immunocompromised patients. Organisms infect the overall intestine, and symptoms, apparently caused by the schizogony of the developing forms in the epithelial cells and perhaps by the toxins produced, include diarrhea, nausea, fever, steatorrhea, headache, and weight loss. The disease may persist for months or years.

Sarcocystis infection occurs in a variety of hosts, including humans. The sexual stage of *Sarcocystis* species, similar to that of *Isospora* species, occurs in the intestine of the carnivorous definitive host (19), and the asexual stage occurs in the muscles of an intermediate host animal that ingests infective sporozoites from the feces of the carnivore. Humans are infected with the sexual stages of *S. hominis* (formerly called *Isospora hominis*), acquired from ingestion of improperly cooked or raw beef, and *S. suihominis*, acquired from ingestion of pork. Infected humans excrete sporulated oocysts that possess a thin oocyst wall (32). Humans are occasionally infected with a number of other species of *Sarcocystis*, in which the asexual stages parasitize skeletal and cardiac muscles (2).

Isospora and *Sarcocystis* intestinal infections are diagnosed by the identification of the organisms in direct or concentrated wet mounts of feces. Iodine stains the oocysts and sporocysts and makes them more readily visible. The oocysts usually stain acid fast. Trichrome stains, however, are of little or no value for demonstration of the organisms. In addition to being difficult to detect microscopically, oocysts of *I. belli* are sometimes not passed in feces until the symptoms of the infection have subsided. The duration of oocyst passage varies considerably, from a few days to a few weeks; therefore, in attempting to establish the diagnosis, several stool specimens should be collected and examined. This pattern of passage of diagnostic stages of coccidia in feces may also be true of *Sarcocystis* species (13). The diagnostic stage of *I. belli* is an unsporulated or immature

---

cyst. Row 3: (left) *E. nana*. Four nuclei are evident, though the one in the center is out of focus. (Right) *I. bütschlii*. The large, reddish glycogen mass is prominent. Above it is the nucleus, which has a large pale karyosome surrounded by a muddy irregular karyolymph space. Row 4: (left) *G. lamblia*. Two nuclei are evident toward the upper left, and multiple fibrils are present. (Right) *C. mesnili*. This small, lemon-shaped cyst has the nucleus on the left and faint fibrils on the right.

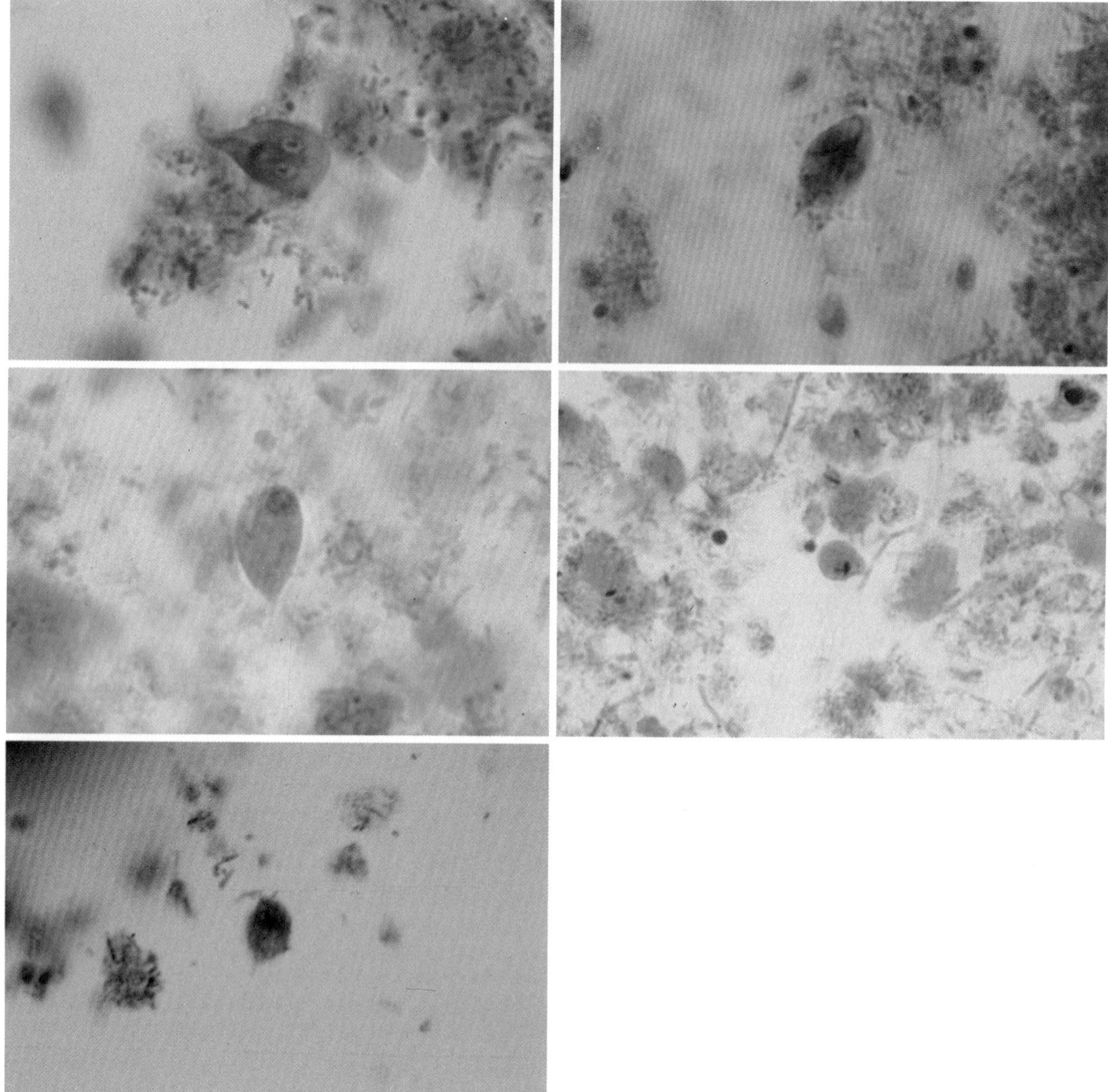

FIG. 7. Flagellates (trichrome stain; oil immersion magnification). Row 1: (left) *G. lamblia* trophozoite. Two nuclei and prominent median body are evident in this pyriform organism. (Right) *G. lamblia* cyst. There are two nuclei toward the bottom in this plane of focus. Fibrils are evident in the cytoplasm. Row 2: (left) *C. mesnili* trophozoite. The nucleus is at the upper end. The pale cytosome is evident to the left of the nucleus. The posterior end is tapered. (Right) *C. mesnili* cyst. The lemon-shaped cyst is in the center of this field. The nucleus is in the lower portion of the cyst. Fibrils are faintly visible. Row 3: (left) *T. hominis* trophozoite. The nucleus is toward the top of the organism. A portion of the undulating membrane is evident to the right of the nucleus. The axostyle is evident at the bottom of the organism.

oocyst that will mature in several days at room temperature to an oocyst containing two sporocysts, which in turn contain four sporozoites each. *Sarcocystis* species already have mature sporocysts, sometimes surrounded by a thin-walled oocyst.

Cryptosporidium species (*Cryptosporidium parvum* in mammals) (8)

Cryptosporidium species infect the brush border of columnar epithelial cells and cause crytosporidiosis (14). Human infections are caused by *C. parvum*. They may occasionally infect the cells of other organs in immunocompromised hosts. Clinically apparent infections with *Cryptosporidium* species can be separated into two groups. Patients with intact immune function develop a profuse, watery diarrhea accompanied by mild epigastric cramping pain, nausea, and anorexia which is generally self-limited, lasting for 10 to 15 days (22). Immunocompromised patients, such as those having AIDS or receiving immunosuppressive therapy, develop a more severe, long-lasting infection. Symptoms are as

TABLE 5. Characteristics of intestinal flagellates, a ciliate, and coccidia visible in different types of fecal preparations[a]

Group characteristics	Unstained		Temporary stain		Permanent stain
	Saline	Formalin	Iodine (cysts)	Neutral red[b] (trophozoites)	
Flagellates					
Trophozoites					
Motility	+	−		+	−
Shape	+	+		+	+ (may be distorted)
Nucleus	−	+		+	+
Flagella	±	−		+	±
Other features[c]	+	+		+	+
Cyst					
Shape	+	+	+		+
Nucleus	−	+	+		+
Fibrils	±	+	+		+
Ciliate (*Balantidium coli*)					
Trophozoites					
Motility	+	−		+	−
Macronucleus	+	+		+	+
Cilia	+	+		+	+
Cyst					
Macronucleus	+	+	±		+
Coccidia					
Oocyst and sporocyst	+	+	+		+[d]

[a] Adapted from Brooke and Melvin (4).
[b] Neutral red dye in Methocel solutions.
[c] The undulating membrane of *Trichomonas* and the spiral groove of *Chilomastix* may not be visible in all cases.
[d] *Cryptosporidium* oocysts can be demonstrated in acid-fast stains.

noted above, but the disease is prolonged, with profuse, watery diarrhea persisting from several weeks to months or years. There is no effective specific therapy for cryptosporidiosis. Outbreaks have been reported in day-care centers and associated with contaminated municipal water supplies (18).

Specimens from patients suspected of having cryptosporidiosis should be preserved in Formalin before being sent to the laboratory or immediately upon receipt. *Cryptosporidium* oocysts are very small (4 to 5 µm) and can easily be overlooked in fecal preparations or confused with yeast cells. The infection has likely

TABLE 6. Differential morphology of flagellate trophozoites found in human stool specimens[a]

Species	Length	Shape	Motility	No. and characteristics of nuclei	No. and location of flagella[b]	Other features
Trichomonas hominis	8–20 µm; usual range, 11–12 µm	Pear shaped	Nervous, jerky	1, not visible in unstained mounts	3–5 anterior 1 posterior	Undulating membrane extending length of body
Chilomastix mesnili	6–24 µm; usual range, 10–15 µm	Pear shaped	Stiff, rotary	1, not visible in unstained mounts	3 anterior 1 in cytostome	Prominent cytostome extending 1/3–1/2 length of body; spiral groove across ventral surface
Giardia lamblia	10–20 µm; usual range, 12–15 µm	Pear shaped	Falling leaf	2, not visible in unstained mounts	4 lateral 2 ventral 2 caudal	Sucking disk occupying 1/2–3/4 of ventral surface; median bodies lying horizontally or obliquely in lower part of body
Enteromonas hominis	4–10 µm; usual range, 8–9 µm	Oval	Jerky	1, not visible in unstained mounts	3 anterior 1 posterior	One side of body flattened: posterior flagellum extends free posteriorly or laterally
Retortamonas intestinalis	4–9 µm; usual range, 6–7 µm	Pear shaped or oval	Jerky	1, not visible in unstained mounts	1 anterior 1 posterior	Prominent cytostome extending ca. 1/2 length of body

[a] From Brooke and Melvin (4).
[b] Not a practical feature for the identification of species in routine fecal examinations.

TABLE 7. Differential morphology of flagellate cysts found in human stool specimens[a]

Species	Size	Shape	No. and characteristics of nuclei	Other features
Trichomonas hominis	No cyst			
Chilomastix mesnili	6–10 μm; usual range, 8–9 μm	Lemon shaped with anterior hyaline knob	1, not visible in unstained preparations	Cytostome with supporting fibrils; usually visible in stained preparations
Giardia lamblia	8–19 μm; usual range, 11–12 μm	Oval or ellipsoidal	Usually 4, not distinct in unstained preparations; usually located at one end	Fibrils or flagella longitudinally in unstained cysts; deep-staining fibers or fibrils lying laterally or obliquely across fibrils in lower part of cyst; cytoplasm often retracts from a portion of cell wall
Enteromonas hominis	4–10 μm; usual range, 6–8 μm	Elongated or oval	1–4, usually 2 lying at opposite ends of cyst; not visible in unstained mounts	Resembles *E. nana* cyst; fibrils or flagella usually not seen
Retortamonas intestinalis	4–9 μm; usual range, 4–7 μm	Pear shaped or slightly lemon shaped	1, not visible in unstained mounts	Resembles *Chilomastix* cyst; shadow outline of cytostome with supporting fibrils extending above nucleus

[a] From Brooke and Melvin (4).

been common in humans but was undiagnosed because the organisms were not recognized by the usual diagnostic methods. Both immature and mature oocysts may be present, although usually those present are mature and contain four naked sporozoites; sporocysts are not present (Table 8, Fig. 8, and Fig. 9). Identification is often difficult. Direct wet mounts can be used to examine feces, but oocysts are difficult to differentiate from yeasts, and in light infections, organisms may not be detected. Specimens can also be concentrated by

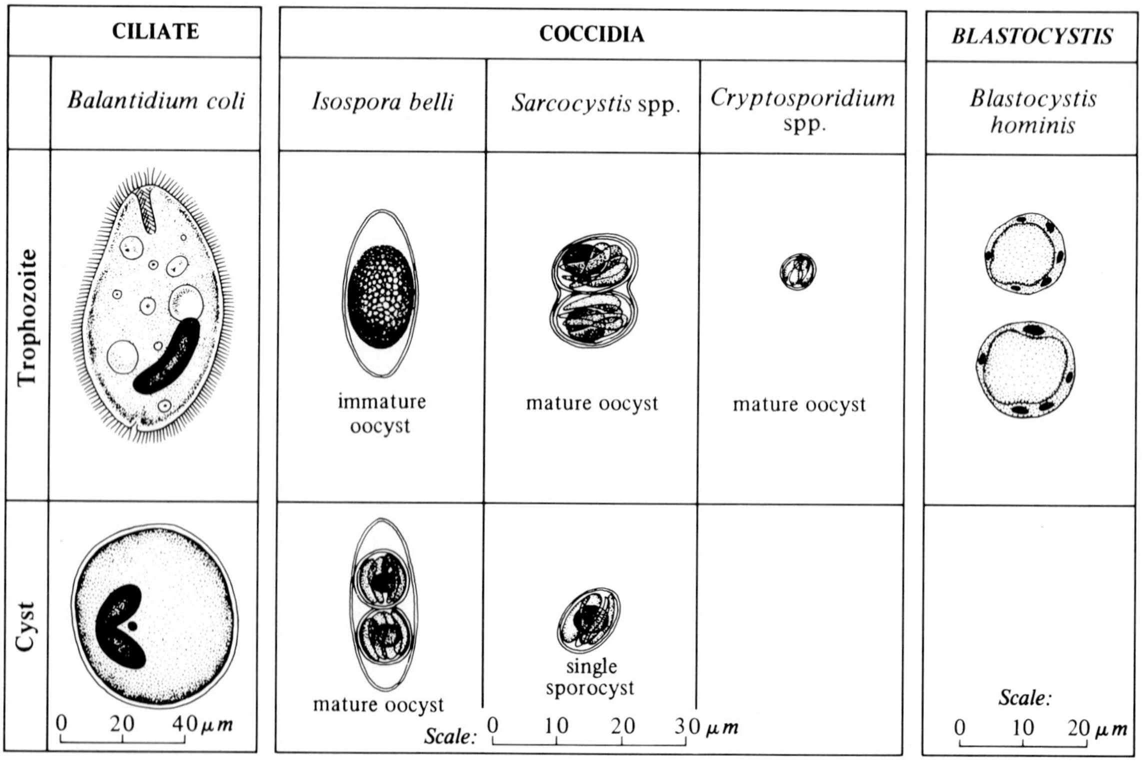

FIG. 8. Ciliate, coccidia, and *B. hominis* found in human stool specimens. (From Brooke and Melvin [4].)

TABLE 8. Differential morphology of ciliate, coccidia, and *Blastocystis* species found in human stool specimens[a]

Type, species, and form	Size (length)	Shape	Motility	No. and characteristics of nuclei	Other features
Ciliate					
Balantidium coli					
Trophozoite	40–70 µm or more; usual range, 40–50 µm	Ovoid with tapering anterior end	Rotary, boring	1 large, kidney-shaped macronucleus; 1 small, subspherical micronucleus immediately adjacent to macronucleus; macronucleus occasionally visible in unstained preparations as hyaline mass	Body surface covered by spiral, longitudinal rows of cilia; contractile vacuoles present
Cyst	45–65 µm; usual range, 50–55 µm	Spherical or oval		1 large macronucleus visible in unstained preparations as hyaline mass	Macronucleus and contractile vacuole are visible in young cysts; in older cysts, internal structure appears granular
Coccidia					
Isospora belli	Oocyst: 25–30 µm; usual range, 28–30 µm	Ellipsoidal	Nonmotile		Usual diagnostic stage is immature oocyst with single granular mass (zygote) within; mature oocyst contains 2 sporocysts with 4 sporozoites each
Sarcocystis spp.	Sporocyst[b]	Oval	Nonmotile		Mature oocysts with thin wall collapsed around 2 sporocysts or free, fully mature sporocysts with 4 sporozoites inside are usually seen in feces
S. hominis	13–17 µm; usual range, 14–16 µm				
S. suihominis	11–15 µm; usual range, 12–13 µm				
Cryptosporidium spp.	Oocyst: 3–6 µm; usual range, 4–5 µm	Spherical or oval	Nonmotile	Mature oocyst contains 4 naked sporozoites; no sporocysts	
Blastocystis					
Blastocystis hominis[c]					
Vacuolated form	5–30 µm; usual range, 8–10 µm	Spherical, oval, or ellipsoidal	Nonmotile	1, usually, but 2–4 may be present; located in rim of cytoplasm; in binucleated organism, nuclei may be at opposite poles; in quadrinucleated forms, nuclei are evenly spaced around the periphery of the cell	Cell contains large central body, or vacuole, with a thin band, or rim, of cytoplasm around the periphery; occasionally a ring of granules may be seen in cytoplasm, and the cell appears to have a beaded rim

[a] Adapted from Brooke and Melvin (4).
[b] Sizes are based on information from Rommel and Heydorn (32) and Heydorn et al. (19).
[c] Description based on information from Zierdt (48) and McClure et al. (25).

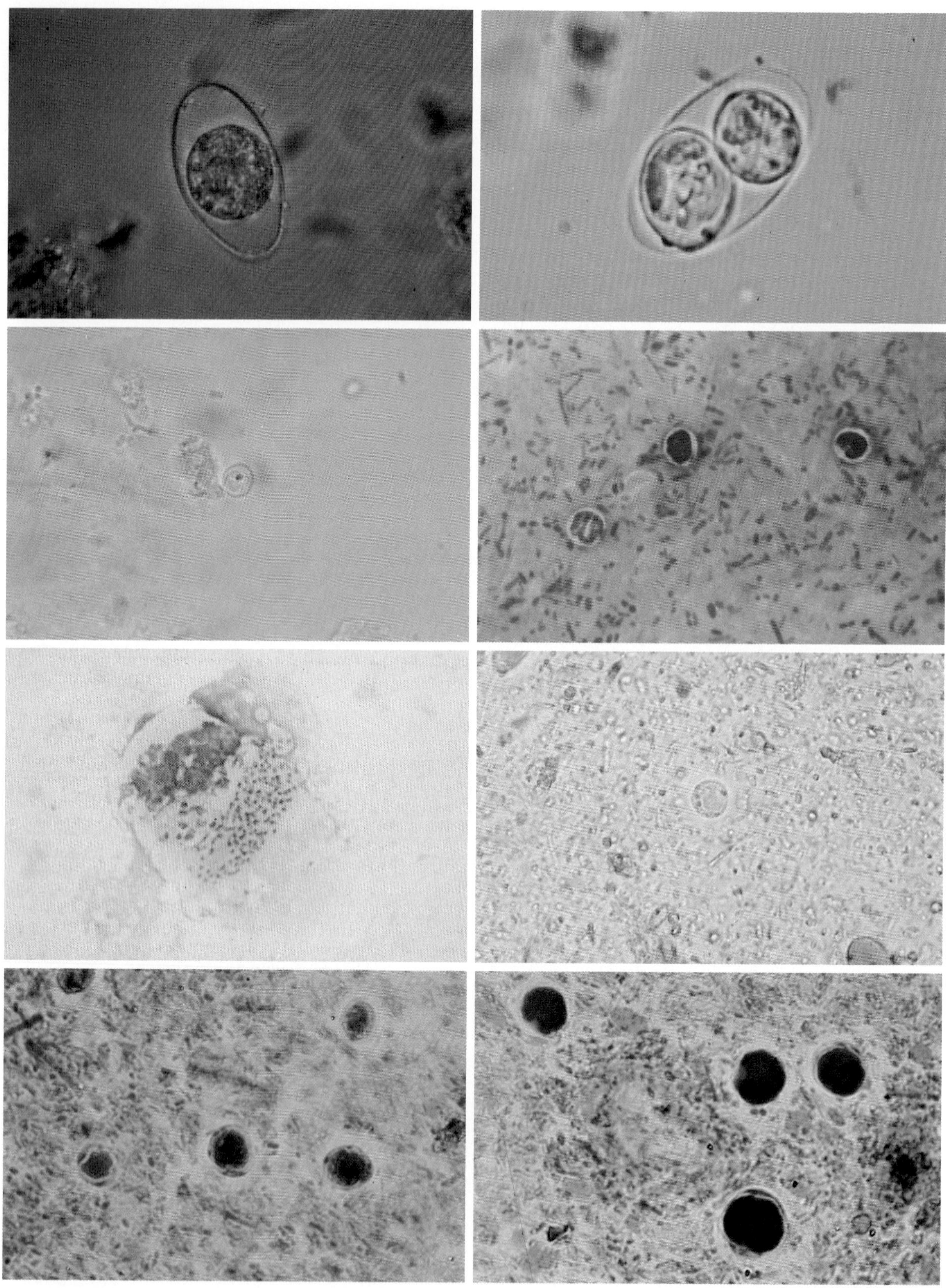

FIG. 9. Coccidia, stained and unstained. Magnification, ×1,000 except row 3, left (×2,000). Row 1: (left) *I. belli,* immature oocyst, unstained; (right) *I. belli* mature oocyst, unstained. Row 2: (left) *Cryptosporidium* oocyst, unstained; (right) *Cryptosporidium* oocysts with acid-fast stain. Row 3: (left) *Enterocytozoon* spores in intestinal cell, Giemsa stain (courtesy of Elizabeth Canning, used with permission); (right) *B. hominis,* vacuolated forms, iodine stain. Row 4: (left) *B. hominis,* vacuolated forms, trichrome stain; (right) *B. hominis,* vacuolated forms, trichrome stain.

the Sheather sugar flotation method or the Formalin-ethyl acetate method. Both unstained and iodine-stained mounts as well as slides for acid-fast staining should be prepared. In unstained mounts containing mature oocysts, the refractile residual body can be detected but the sporozoites may not be distinct. Oocysts do not stain with iodine (unless they are exposed to it for long periods), but yeast cells do stain, thus helping to distinguish oocysts from yeast cells. Various acid-fast stains are more sensitive than wet mounts and are the usual methods used to detect oocysts in feces or concentrates or to confirm the identification of organisms seen in other preparations. Oocysts stain intensely acid fast, whereas yeast cells and fecal material do not. There is usually some irregularity in staining of organisms, which aids in differentiating them from homogeneously staining particles sometimes seen in feces. In many mature oocysts, sporozoites can be seen. Both fluorochrome and carbol-fuchsin acid-fast stains are useful. An immunofluorescent stain has recently been reported and is commercially available (42).

MICROSPORIDIA

The microsporidian organisms that parasitize humans belong to the phylum Microspora, order Microsporida. The microsporidia are obligate, intracellular parasites of invertebrate and vertebrate animals. Although the four genera that have been implicated in human infections are acquired by the ingestion of the small (1 to 2 μm) spores containing a coiled polar tubule, only *Enterocytozoon* remains as a parasite of the intestine. The other three genera (*Nosema*, *Encephalitozoon*, and *Pleistophora*) are found in a variety of tissues (6, 36). Microsporidial keratoconjunctivitis has recently been recognized in patients with AIDS (7).

The parasites have been diagnosed primarily in AIDS patients or other immunocompromised individuals. Diagnosis of biopsied tissues has been usually made from electron microscopic studies. Since the spores are small (1 to 2 μm), efforts to find them in stool specimens by light microscopy have been unrewarding. Recently, spores have been identified in Giemsa-stained intestinal biopsies (31) (Fig. 9) by using oil immersion light microscopy. Less costly and less cumbersome diagnostic methods are needed.

BLASTOCYSTIS HOMINIS

B. hominis inhabits the large intestine, and organisms are passed in feces. Three morphologic forms have been described: amebic, granular, and vacuolated (48, 49). The vacuolated form is most commonly seen in fecal specimens (25).

Although *B. hominis* may be found in up to 25% of stool specimens examined, only occasional patients have clinical symptoms, and there is much controversy about whether *B. hominis* is sometimes or never a pathogen (28, 29, 37). Blastocystosis may be suspected when the complete battery of parasitologic, bacterial, and viral tests on stools has failed to disclose any agent other than *B. hominis* and *Blastocystis* organisms are numerous in the specimen. The predominant and virtually only symptom has been persistent, mild diarrhea.

Infection is diagnosed by finding the familiar spherical or ovoid form with a large vacuole or area in the center and granules arranged around the periphery. The organism is described in Table 8 and shown in Fig. 8 and 9. *Blastocystis* organisms can be demonstrated by any of the methods usually used for the diagnosis of intestinal parasite infections, although exposing unfixed feces to water in the performance of concentration procedures causes lysis of *Blastocystis* organisms.

LITERATURE CITED

1. **Beal, C. B., P. Viens, R. G. L. Grant, and J. M. Hughes.** 1970. A new technique for sampling duodenal contents. Am. J. Trop. Med. Hyg. **19:**349–352.
2. **Beaver, P. C., R. K. Gadgil, and P. Morera.** 1979. Sarcocystosis in man: a review and report of five cases. Am. J. Trop. Med. Hyg. **28:**819–844.
3. **Brandborg, L. L., S. B. Goldberg, and W. C. Breidenbach.** 1970. Human coccidiosis—a possible cause of malabsorption. N. Engl. J. Med. **283:**1306–1313.
4. **Brooke, M. M., and D. M. Melvin.** 1984. Morphology of diagnostic stages of intestinal parasites of humans, 2nd ed. U.S. Department of Health and Human Services publication no. (CDC) 84-8116. Centers for Disease Control, Atlanta.
5. **Burrows, R. B., and M. A. Swerdlow.** 1956. *Enterobius* vermicularis as a probable vector of *Dientamoeba fragilis.* Am. J. Trop. Med. Hyg. **5:**258–265.
6. **Canning, E. U., and W. S. Hollister.** 1987. Microsporidia of mammals—widespread pathogens or opportunistic curiosities. Parasitol. Today **3:**267–273.
7. **Centers for Disease Control.** 1990. Microsporidian keratoconjunctivitis in patients with AIDS. Morbid. Mortal. Weekly Rep. **39:**188–189.
8. **Current, W. L.** 1988. The biology of *Cryptosporidium.* ASM News **54:**605–611.
9. **Danciger, M., and M. Lopez.** 1975. Numbers of *Giardia* in the feces of infected children. Am. J. Trop. Med. Hyg. **24:**237–242.
10. **Dao, A. H., D. P. Robinson, and S. W. Wong.** 1983. Frequency of *Entamoeba gingivalis* scrapings. Am. J. Clin. Pathol. **80:**380–383.
11. **Diamond, L. S.** 1988. Cultivation of *Entamoeba histolytica* in vitro, p. 27–40. *In* J. I. Ravdin (ed.), Amebiasis: human infection by *Entamoeba histolytica.* John Wiley & Sons, Inc., New York.
12. **Elsdon-Dew, R.** 1968. The epidemiology of amoebiasis. Adv. Parasitol. **6:**1–62.
13. **Fayer, R.** 1982. Other protozoa: *Eimeria, Isospora, Cystosospora, Besnoitia, Hammondia, Frenkelia, Sarcocystis, Encephalitozoon,* and *Nosema,* p. 187–196. *In* L. Jacobs (ed.), Handbook series in zoonoses, section C. Parasitic zoonoses, vol. 1. CRC Press, Inc., Boca Raton, Fla.
14. **Fayer, R., and B. Ungar.** 1986. *Cryptosporidium* spp. and cryptosporidiosis. Microbiol. Rev. **50:**458–483.
15. **Fouts, A. C., and S. J. Kraus.** 1980. *Trichomonas vaginalis:* reevaluation of its clinical presentation and laboratory diagnosis. J. Infect. Dis. **141:**137–143.
16. **Gay, J. D., T. L. Abell, J. H. Thompson, Jr., and V. Loth.** 1985. *Entamoeba polecki* infection in southeast Asian refugees: multiple cases of a rarely reported parasite. Mayo Clin. Proc. **60:**523–530.
17. **Gutierrez, Y.** 1990. Diagnostic pathology of parasitic infections with clinical correlations. Lea & Febiger, Philadelphia.
18. **Hayes, E. B., T. D. Matte, T. R. O'Brien, T. W. McKinley, G. S. Logsdon, J. B. Rose, B. P. Ungar, D. M. Word, P. F. Pinsky, M. L. Cummings, M. A. Wilson, E. G. Long, E. S. Hurwitz, and D. D. Juranek.** 1989. Large community outbreak of cryptosporidiosis due to contamination of a filtered public water supply. N. Engl. J. Med. **320:**1372–1376.
19. **Heydorn, A. O., R. Gestrich, M. Melhorn, and M. Rom-**

mel. 1975. Proposal for a new nomenclature of the *Sarcosporidia*. Z. Parasitenkd. **48:**73–82.

20. **Istre, G. R., K. Kreiss, R. S. Hopkins, G. R. Healy, M. Benziger, T. M. Canfield, P. Dickinson, T. R. Englert, R. C. Compton, H. M. Mathews, and R. A. Smith.** 1982. An outbreak of amebiasis spread by colonic irrigation at a chiropractic clinic. N. Engl. J. Med. **307:**339–342.
21. **Jokipii, A. M. M., M. Hemilia, and L. Jokipii.** 1985. Prospective study of acquisition of *Cryptosporidium, Giardia lamblia*, and gastrointestinal illness. Lancet **ii:**487–489.
22. **Jokipii, L., and A. M. M. Jokipii.** 1986. Timing of symptoms and oocyst excretion in human cryptosporidiosis. N. Engl. J. Med. **315:**1643–1648.
23. **Krogstad, D. J., H. C. Spencer, G. R. Healy, N. N. Gleason, D. J. Sexton, and C. A. Herron.** 1978. Amebiasis: epidemiologic studies in the United States, 1971–1974. Ann. Intern. Med. **88:**89–97.
24. **Markell, E. K., and P. M. Quinn.** 1977. Comparison of immediate polyvinyl alcohol (PVA) fixation with delayed Schaudinn's fixation for the demonstration of protozoa in stool specimens. Am. J. Trop. Med. Hyg. **26:**1139–1142.
25. **McClure, H. M., E. A. Strobert, and G. R. Healy.** 1980. *Blastocystis hominis* in a pig-tailed macaque: a potential enteric pathogen for nonhuman primates. Lab. Anim. Sci. **30:**890–894.
26. **McLaren, L., L. Davis, G. Healy, and G. James.** 1983. Isolation of *Trichomonas vaginalis* from the respiratory tract of infants with respiratory diseases. Pediatrics **71:** 888–890.
27. **Melvin, D. A., and M. M. Brooke.** 1982. Laboratory procedures for the diagnosis of intestinal parasites, 3rd ed. U.S. Department of Health and Human Services publication no. (CDC) 82-8282. Centers for Disease Control, Atlanta.
28. **Miller, R. A., and B. H. Minshew.** 1988. *Blastocystis hominis:* an organism in search of a disease. Rev. Infect. Dis. **10:**930–938.
29. **Quadri, S. M. H., G. A. Al-Okaili, and F. Al-Dayel.** 1989. Clinical significance of *Blastocystis hominis*. J. Clin. Microbiol. **27:**2407–2409.
30. **Ravdin, J. I.** 1988. Amebiasis. Human infection by *Entamoeba histolytica*. John Wiley & Sons, Inc., New York.
31. **Rijpstra, A. C., E. U. Canning, R. J. VanKetel, J. K. J. Eeftinck-Schattenkerk, and J. J. Laarman.** 1988. Use of light microscopy to diagnose small-intestinal microsporidiosis in patients with AIDS. J. Infect. Dis. **157:**1827–1831.
32. **Rommel, M., and A. O. Heydorn.** 1972. Beitrage rum Lebenszykles der Sarkosporidien. III. *Isospora hominis* (Raillet und Lucet, 1891) Wenyon, 1923, eine Dauerform der Sarkosporidien des Rindes und des Schweins. Berl. Muench. Tiertaerztl. Wochenschr. **85:**143–145.
33. **Sargeaunt, P. G., and J. E. Williams.** 1980. A comparative study of *Entamoeba histolytica* (NIH: 200, HK9, etc.), "*E. histolytica*-like" and other morphologically identical amoebae using isoenzyme electrophoresis. Trans. R. Soc. Trop. Med. Hyg. **74:**469–474.
34. **Schmidt, G. P., L. C. Matheny, A. A. Zaidi, and S. J. Kraus.** 1989. Evaluation of six media for the growth of *Trichomonas vaginalis* from vaginal secretions. J. Clin. Microbiol. **27:**1230–1233.
35. **Shadduck, J. A.** 1989. Human microsporidiosis and AIDS. Rev. Infect. Dis. **11:**203–207.
36. **Shadduck, J. A., and E. Greeley.** 1989. Microsporidia and human infections. Clin. Microbiol. Rev. **2:**158–165.
37. **Sheehan, D. J., B. G. Raucher, and J. C. McKitrick.** 1986. Association of *Blastocystis hominis* with signs and symptoms of human disease. J. Clin. Microbiol. **24:**548–550.
38. **Smith, J. W., R. M. McQuay, L. R. Ash, D. M. Melvin, T. C. Orihel, and J. H. Thompson, Jr.** 1976. Atlas of diagnostic parasitology. II. Intestinal protozoa. American Society for Clinical Pathology, Chicago.
39. **Smith, J. W., and M. W. Wolfe.** 1980. Giardiasis. Annu. Rev. Med. **31:**373–383.
40. **Soave, R., and W. D. Johnson.** 1988. AIDS commentary. *Cryptosporidium* and *Isospora belli* infection. J. Infect. Dis. **157:**225–229.
41. **Spencer, M. J., L. S. Garcia, and M. R. Chapin.** 1979. *Dientamoeba fragilis:* an intestinal pathogen in children. Am. J. Dis. Child. **133:**329–393.
42. **Sterling, C. R., and M. J. Arrowood.** 1986. Detection of *Cryptosporidium* spp. infections using a direct immunofluorescent assay. Pediatr. Infect. Dis. **5:**S139–S142.
43. **Thornton, S. A., A. H. West, H. L. DuPont, and L. K. Pickering.** 1983. Comparison of methods for identification of *Giardia lamblia*. Am. J. Clin. Pathol. **80:**858–860.
44. **Turner, J. A.** 1985. Giardiasis and infections with *Dientamoeba fragilis*. Pediatr. Clin. North Am. **32:**865–880.
45. **Walsh, J.** 1982. Human helminthic and protozoan infections in the north, p. 45–62. *In* K. W. Warren and J. Z. Bowers (ed.), Parasitology, a global perspective. Springer-Verlag, New York.
46. **Wolfe, M. S.** 1984. Symptomatology, diagnosis, and treatment, p. 147–161. *In* S. L. Erlandsen and E. A. Meyer (ed.), *Giardia* and giardiasis. Plenum Publishing Corp., New York.
47. **Yang, J., and T. H. Scholten.** 1977. *Dientamoeba fragilis*. A review with notes on its epidemiology, pathogenicity, mode of transmission and diagnosis. Am. J. Trop. Med. Hyg. **26:**16–22.
48. **Zierdt, C. H.** 1973. Studies of *Blastocystis hominis*. J. Protozool. **20:**114–121.
49. **Zierdt, C. H., C. D. Donnally, J. Muller, and G. Constantopoulos.** 1988. Biochemical and ultrastructural study of *Blastocystis hominis*. J. Clin. Microbiol. **26:**965–997.

Chapter 70

Tissue Helminths

THOMAS C. ORIHEL AND LAWRENCE R. ASH

There are a large number of helminth parasite species, including nematodes, flukes, and tapeworms, which, as adults or larvae, live in the tissues of humans. The nematodes include the filariae, *Trichinella*, and *Capillaria hepatica*, as well as zoonotic species of ascarids, metastrongyles, and hookworms. The cestodes are represented by larval tapeworms which produce cysticercosis, coenurosis, sparganosis, and hydatid disease. Schistosomes (blood flukes) inhabit blood vessels of the abdomen but are discussed in the chapter on intestinal helminths (chapter 71) because their eggs are passed in feces and urine.

NEMATODES

Filariae

The filarial worms are arthropod-transmitted parasites of the lymphatic, subcutaneous, and cutaneous tissues of humans. All share a unique characteristic: the adult female worm produces a primitive larva called a microfilaria, which is found in the peripheral blood or in the skin. Certain species of microfilariae circulate in the blood with a well-defined circadian rhythm or "periodicity" which may be nocturnal or diurnal; other species lack periodicity and circulate in the blood at all hours of the day and night. When absent from the peripheral blood, microfilariae are to be found in the deeper visceral capillaries. Because adult worms are typically sequestered in the tissues, diagnosis of filarial infections depends on finding microfilariae in the blood or skin. The microfilaria is simple in its structure. It is vermiform in shape and, in stained preparations, appears to be composed of a column of nuclei which is interrupted along its length by spaces or special cells which are the precursors of the body organs. Some species of microfilariae are enveloped in a sheath, whereas in others the sheath is absent.

All filariae are transmitted by species of bloodsucking arthropods such as mosquitoes, midges, blackflies, and tabanid flies, in which the microfilaria develops to the infective stage. Development of the infective larva to the gravid, adult stage in the vertebrate host requires several months, in some cases as long as a year or more. Although these parasites are not endemic in humans in the United States, they are often seen in immigrants or in individuals who have resided or traveled in endemic areas. There are several species of filariae which infect humans.

Wuchereria bancrofti, causing an infection often referred to as bancroftian filariasis, is the most common and widespread species of filaria infecting humans. It has cosmopolitan distribution throughout tropical and subtropical areas of the world. Adult worms live in the host's lymphatic system and produce lymphangitis, lymphadenitis, and obstructive fibrosis which restricts the flow of lymph, with a resultant lymphedema. Long-term chronic infection may result in elephantiasis of the extremities and genitalia. The microfilaria circulates in the peripheral blood with a nocturnal periodicity in most regions of the world; however, in the South Pacific region, the microfilaria is essentially without any periodicity. The microfilaria is sheathed, lies in smooth curves, and measures about 298 μm in length by 7.5 to 10 μm in diameter. Column nuclei are dispersed; there is a short head space, and the pointed tail is devoid of nuclei (Fig. 1A). In Giemsa stain, the sheath stains faintly or not at all. The microfilaria must be distinguished from other sheathed microfilariae. This is done most easily on the basis of the arrangement of nuclei, particularly in the tail (Fig. 2). Since microfilariae may be present in the blood only in small numbers, sensitive procedures such as thick blood films, Saponin lysis, Knott concentration, or membrane filter concentration are used routinely to detect infections.

Brugia malayi is another mosquito-borne filaria which inhabits the lymphatic system of humans. It is restricted in its geographical distribution to Asia and the Indian subcontinent. In some regions it is coendemic with *W. bancrofti*. Lymphatic pathology similar to that produced in bancroftian filariasis is seen in chronic infections with this parasite. The microfilaria, which circulates in the blood, may be periodic or subperiodic. It is similar in its structure to that of *W. bancrofti*, being sheathed but somewhat smaller in size (270 μm by 5 to 6 μm). It can be differentiated from the *W. bancrofti* microfilaria by the presence of subterminal and terminal nuclei in the tail (Fig. 1B and 2b). With Giemsa stain, the sheath stains a bright pink color, whereas that of *W. bancrofti* does not.

Another species of *Brugia*, *B. timori*, infects humans in the Lesser Sunda Islands in the Indonesian archipelago. It too is a lymphatic dweller and produces a microfilaria very similar to that of *B. malayi*. The two can be most easily differentiated on the basis of size. *B. timori* is larger, measuring more than 300 μm in length; also, its sheath tends not to stain with Giemsa stain.

Loa loa, a common filarial parasite of humans, is endemic only in West and Central Africa. It is often called the eye worm because the adult worms, which live in the subcutaneous tissues, often migrate into the conjunctiva and the cornea. The adult worms move freely through the tissues, often producing transient inflammatory reactions referred to as "Calabar" swellings. The microfilariae circulate in the blood, often in large numbers, with a diurnal periodicity. They are sheathed and measure up to 300 μm in length. In contrast to the other sheathed microfilariae, nuclei extend to the end of the

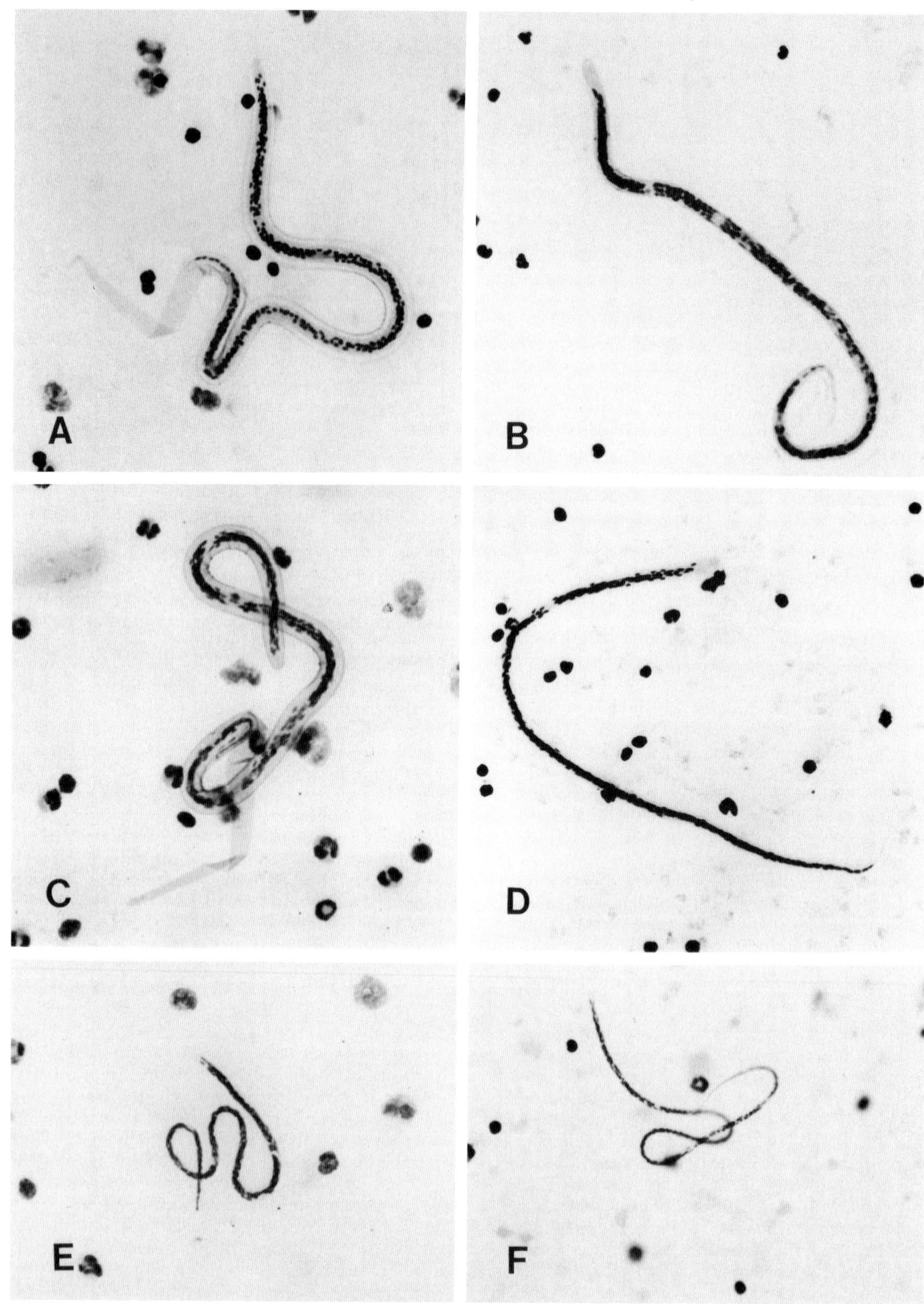

FIG. 1. Common microfilariae found in humans. Hematoxylin stain, ×400. (A) *Wuchereria bancrofti*, (B) *Brugia malayi*, (C) *Loa loa*, (D) *Onchocerca volvulus*, (E) *Mansonella perstans*, and (F) *Mansonella ozzardi*.

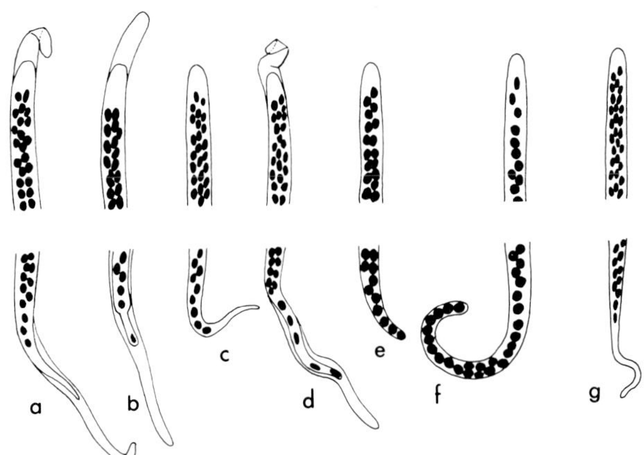

FIG. 2. Diagrammatic representation of the anterior and posterior extremities of the common microfilariae found in humans. (a) *Wuchereria bancrofti*, (b) *Brugia malayi*, (c) *Onchocerca volvulus*, (d) *Loa loa*, (e) *Mansonella perstans*, (f) *Mansonella streptocerca*, and (g) *Mansonella ozzardi*.

tapered tail; however, they are somewhat irregularly arranged along the length of the tail (Fig. 1C and 2d). It should be noted that the sheath of the microfilaria does not stain with Giemsa stain. When adult worms enter the conjunctiva, they can be surgically extracted. Diagnosis of infection depends on identification of the microfilaria in diurnal blood films or removal of adult worms from the conjunctivae.

Onchocerca volvulus is an important human parasite in both hemispheres. It occurs in people across Central Africa, in a small area in the Middle East (Yemen), in Mexico, in portions of Central America, and in several countries in the northern part of South America. Adult worms are found embedded in fibrous nodules in the subcutaneous tissues and sometimes in deeper tissues. These nodules or "onchocercomata" may be found on the head, trunk, and extremities; their anatomical location frequently correlates with the geographical strain of the parasite. The microfilaria is found in the skin. It lacks a sheath and measures approximately 309 μm in length by 5 to 9 μm in diameter. The tail is tapered, usually bent or flexed, and without nuclei (Fig. 1D and 2c). The microfilaria is rarely found in the blood but may appear there as well as in the urine, particularly after treatment with diethylcarbamazine. Diagnosis is made by finding the typical microfilaria in skin snips teased in water or saline, in the fluid expressed from scarified skin, or in aspirates from nodules. Also, adult worms may be demonstrated in excised nodules which have been sectioned and stained. Adult worms may be freed from the fibrous tissues of the nodule by using digestive enzymes such as collagenase (10). Microfilariae may also be seen in the cornea and in the anterior chamber of the eye viewed with the aid of a slit lamp.

Skin snips are best obtained using a biopsy punch. Samples should be taken from the region of the scapula or the iliac crest, although other sites (near nodules) are acceptable. Teasing the skin snip tends to liberate the microfilariae from the tissues.

Mansonella streptocerca is another skin-dwelling filaria found in humans in the rainforest belt of Africa. This filaria has been known by a variety of generic names including *Acanthocheilonema, Dipetalonema,* and *Tetrapetalonema*, but has recently been placed in *Mansonella* (8). The adult worms are found in the dermal layers of the skin, as are the microfilariae. The microfilaria has no sheath, is long and slender, and measures approximately 210 μm by 5 to 6 μm. Its most characteristic feature is its "crooked" tail (Fig. 2f); in addition, the column of nuclei extends to the end of the tail. In areas where this species overlaps in its distribution with *O. volvulus*, great care must be given to proper identification of the microfilariae found in skin snips.

Two other species of *Mansonella* are parasites of humans. One of these, *Mansonella ozzardi*, is restricted in its geographical distribution to the Western Hemisphere. It is endemic in portions of Mexico, Panama, and northern South America, especially in the Amazon Basin and as far south as northern Argentina. It is also found in several Caribbean islands including Hispaniola. The adult worms inhabit the subcutaneous tissues, and the microfilariae circulate in the blood. The microfilaria is small, measuring about 224 μm by 4 to 5 μm, and has a long attenuated tail devoid of nuclei (Fig. 1F and 2g). It circulates in the blood at all hours of the day and night. It has been observed in experimental animals that an infection requires approximately 5 months to reach the patent (microfilaremic) state. This filaria, like *L. loa*, readily infects visitors to endemic areas and is frequently found in missionaries and others residing temporarily in endemic areas.

Mansonella perstans (formerly *Dipetalonema perstans*), a filaria with wide geographical distribution in tropical Africa but less widely seen in South America, also is seen frequently in individuals who have lived temporarily in endemic areas. The location of the adults of this filaria is not certain, but it is believed that they inhabit the peritoneal cavity and mesenteries of humans. The microfilaria has no sheath, is small (measuring approximately 203 μm by 4 to 5 μm), and circulates in the peripheral blood without any periodicity. Its most characteristic feature is its blunt tail filled with nuclei (Fig. 1E and 2e). In the Western Hemisphere, *M. perstans* often is found in association with *M. ozzardi*. In areas where the two species coexist, special care must be taken to make accurate identifications.

Laboratory diagnosis of filariasis. Microfilariae may be detected in samples of blood by a variety of techniques. In thick, wet blood films prepared during either the day or night, microfilariae may be quickly recognized by their size and rapid movement in the blood. However, individual species are not likely to be identified in this manner, so that stained blood films are generally required. Thin blood films usually are not adequate because of the small volume of blood used. In contrast, thick blood films of approximately 20 μl, dehemoglobinized and stained with Giemsa or hematoxylin stains, bring out the diagnostic morphological features of each species.

Often the numbers of microfilariae in the blood may be too scanty to find even in thick blood films so that it is necessary to examine a larger volume. Procedures for this are given in chapter 66. Microfilariae are readily identified on the basis of their size, the presence or absence of a sheath and its staining characteristics with Giemsa, and the structure of the tail.

Skin snips must be examined when searching for mi-

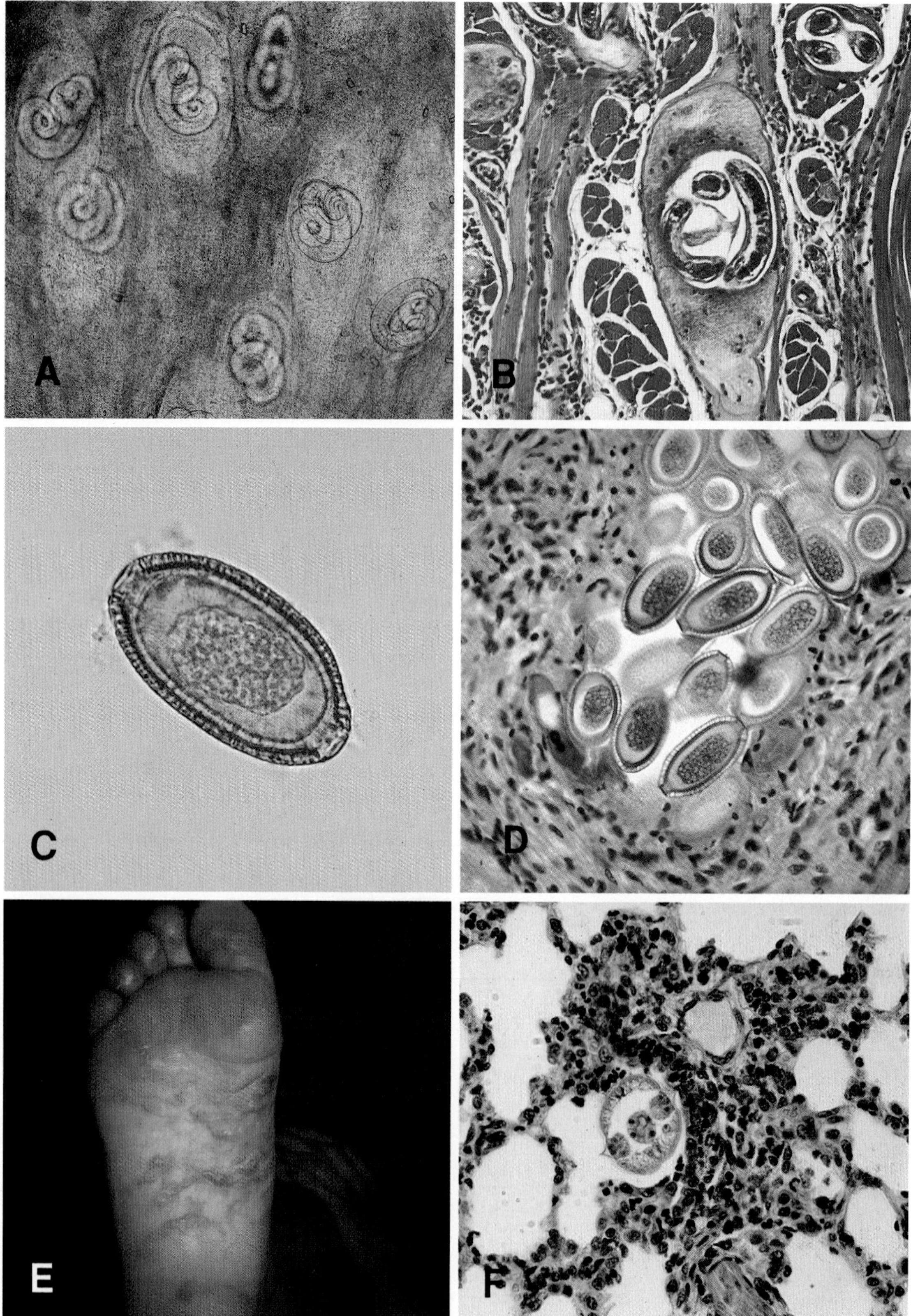

FIG. 3. Nematode parasites in tissues. (A) *Trichinella spiralis* infective-stage larvae. In this press preparation of diaphragm muscle, one can see the encapsulated, infective larvae (×100). (B) *Trichinella spiralis* infective-stage larva in section of rat tongue; hematoxylin-eosin stain (×200). (C) *Capillaria hepatica* egg. Note that this unembryonated egg resembles that of *Trichuris* spp. However, the plugs at either end are less prominent, and the shell has a striated appearance (×750). (D) *Capillaria hepatica* eggs in liver; hematoxylin-eosin stain. Unembryonated eggs are expelled by the female into the burrows produced by the adult.

crofilariae of *O. volvulus* and *M. streptocerca*. Care should be taken to obtain "bloodless" snips so as not to contaminate the sample with other species of microfilariae that may be present in the blood. Techniques have been described in which one simply abrades a small area of skin and collects the exuded tissue juices on a slide, which be either examined immediately for living microfilariae or allowed to dry and then stained and examined. Serological tests have poor sensitivity and specificity and generally are not useful for diagnosis. The patient's history of travel and residencies is particularly helpful when considering a diagnosis of filariasis.

Trichinosis

Trichinella spiralis, the agent of human trichinosis, is a parasite of carnivores with very little evidence of host specificity. Infection in humans results from the ingestion of insufficiently cooked or raw pork and pork products containing the encysted larvae. Bear meat is also a frequent source of human infection. Adult worms live in the mucosa of the small intestine. The female produces and discharges larvae which enter the bloodstream and invade the skeletal musculature, where they undergo further development and encapsulation. These larvae remain viable for many years. Initially there may be a nonspecific gastroenteritis, fever, eosinophilia, myositis, and circumorbital edema. The adult worms survive in the intestine for up to 6 to 8 weeks and then are expelled from the host.

The definitive diagnosis is made by demonstration of encapsulated larvae in biopsy specimens from skeletal muscle, particularly deltoid and gastrocnemius muscles (Fig. 3A and B). The digestion of muscle tissue in artificial gastric juice followed by examination of the sediment for larvae is more sensitive. Serological tests are widely used with good results. A highly antigenic parasite, *Trichinella* stimulates a very strong antibody response that can be measured by a variety of procedures. For many years the bentonite flocculation procedure has been the test of choice (6). Although somewhat difficult to perform, this test is highly specific and a reliable indicator of infection. There is some correlation between infective dose and level of antibody activity, and in some cases very light infections are serologically negative. Measurable antibody does not appear until 3 to 4 weeks postinfection, so that sera negative during the acute attack should be confirmed by testing a second specimen 2 to 4 weeks later. Although the specificity is excellent, titers persist for years, not becoming negative for 2 to 3 years.

Capillariasis

Though normally a parasite of rodents, *Capillaria hepatica* can produce infection in humans. Human and animal infections are acquired by ingestion of infective eggs in soil; adult worms mature and deposit eggs directly into the liver parenchyma, where they remain in an undeveloped state until the liver is eaten and the eggs are digested free to pass in the feces of the predator animal. If, as in the human host, the liver is not eaten, the eggs are never liberated into the external environment. Diagnosis is established by liver biopsy or necropsy. In genuine human cases, eggs are not passed in feces (2). When humans are found passing eggs of *C. hepatica* it is indicative of spurious infection and represents an instance where the livers of infected animals have been eaten (e.g., squirrel pie). Eggs will be passed for several days and will then disappear from the stool.

The eggs of *C. hepatica* must be distinguished from the eggs of *Trichuris* or other species of human *Capillaria*. Eggs are 51 to 67 μm long by 30 to 35 μm wide and have thick, striated walls and inconspicuous "plugs" at both ends (Fig. 3C). These eggs are unembryonated when seen in feces. Eggs in liver biopsy specimens can be readily recognized on the basis of their characteristic morphological features (Fig. 3D).

Other nematode infections

Larva migrans. Several species of nematode parasites which are natural parasites of lower animals may gain entry into the human host and undergo partial development. The severity of subsequent disease manifestations may vary from asymptomatic to serious in the form of skin rash, pneumonitis, and involvement of the central nervous system.

(i) Cutaneous larva migrans. Cutaneous larva migrans, also known as creeping eruption or ground itch, refers to the production of serpiginous, inflamed trails in the skin (Fig. 3E) resulting in intense pruritus, and may be caused by various species of *Strongyloides*, *Ancylostoma*, or other animal hookworm species. It occurs as a result of skin contact with sandy-loam types of soil that contain filariform larvae of hookworms and *Strongyloides* spp. discharged in the feces of dogs, cats, and other animals. In the southeastern part of the United States this may be an occupational hazard of electricians, plumbers, and construction workers who inadvertently come in contact with infected soil when working under or near houses where animals have defecated. In addition, species of *Strongyloides* occurring in wild animals such as nutria and raccoons have been incriminated in causing dermatitis in oil field workers and trappers in Louisiana. *Ancylostoma braziliense*, a hookworm of dogs and cats, has been the species usually identified with classical creeping eruption acquired along sandy beaches, but other species of the genus may be involved too. Invasion of human skin by the dog hookworm, *Ancylostoma caninum*, can produce creeping eruption; these larvae may also invade other tissues and organs of the body, including the eye, where they produce granulomatous, visceral larva migrans-like lesions.

Diagnosis of cutaneous larva migrans is based almost entirely on clinical findings and the demonstration of the classical serpiginous trails (Fig. 3E).

(ii) Visceral larva migrans. Visceral larva migrans is a syndrome originally associated with the larval migration in humans, especially children, of dog and cat

Characteristic features of eggs are seen even in tissue sections (×290). (E) Hookworm, cutaneous larva migrans. Infective-stage larvae of dog or cat hookworms wander through the layers of skin, producing serpiginous trails; this condition is often referred to as creeping eruption. (F) *Ascaris* larva in section of lung; hematoxylin-eosin stain (×675).

ascarids of the genus *Toxocara*. Although many other helminths of animals may infect humans and migrate through organs and deeper tissues of the body, *Toxocara canis* is still the classical example of this kind of infection.

Toxocara canis, the dog ascarid, is more important as a human parasite than is *T. cati*, the species occurring in felines. Toxocariasis results from the ingestion of infective eggs from soil and is characterized by hypereosinophilia, hepatomegaly, fever, pneumonitis, and sometimes death. The visceral larva migrans syndrome may persist for many years and may result in severe complications involving the eye and central nervous system. Ocular larva migrans may mimic retinoblastoma, a malignant tumor of the eye. Other nematode larvae producing the syndrome include *A. caninum* (the dog hookworm), *Gnathostoma spinigerum* (a spirurid parasite of dogs and cats in Southeast Asia), and some trematode and cestode larval parasites of wild animals that also invade human tissues.

Diagnosis of visceral larva migrans is difficult and is generally based on clinical findings and immunodiagnostic procedures. These procedures are described elsewhere (chapter 67).

Occasionally, diagnosis is established by finding focal inflammatory lesions containing larvae in tissue specimens such as the liver and brain as well as other organs. Sections of nematode larvae can sometimes be identified in human tissues after biopsy or necropsy, and these can be identified by specialists expert in helminth microanatomy (Fig. 3F).

Anisakiasis. The growing popularity of eating raw fish dishes—sushi, sashimi, ceviche, "Tahitian salad," and others—has led to increased human infection with various larval ascaridoid nematodes. A number of genera, including *Anisakis* and *Pseudoterranova*, are parasites, as adults, of marine mammals, utilizing shrimplike crustaceans as first intermediate hosts and fish and squid as second intermediate hosts in their life cycle. Larval stages in the mesenteries or flesh of fish have the ability to pass from one fish to another when they are ingested without maturing to adult worms. When humans accidentally ingest the larval stages of these nematodes, the larvae may partially penetrate the wall of the stomach or the intestine and produce an eosinophilic granuloma. Many human infections present with acute abdomen or other signs suggestive of intestinal obstruction. In some instances the long, whitish worms, up to several centimeters long, may be coughed up by the patient or be removed from the throat.

Diagnosis of the nematodes producing anisakiasis can be accomplished by study of the distinctive morphological features of the whole worms or by examination of the microanatomy of the parasites in histologic section (Fig. 4F).

Eustrongylidiasis. Nematode larvae of the genus *Eustrongylides*, parasites belonging to the family Dioctophymatoidea, have in recent years been responsible for a number of cases of human infection. These parasites normally occur as adult worms in the alimentary tracts of fish-eating birds and utilize fish, amphibians, and reptiles as intermediate hosts. Although five of the cases have occurred in individuals who have eaten live minnows while fishing, one of the cases occurred as a result of eating home-prepared sushi (11). In most instances, these large, bright red larvae have invaded the abdominal cavity of patients, from which they have been surgically removed. These parasites, along with the anisakine nematodes, further illustrate the potential for acquisition of parasitic infections by eating raw, infected fish.

***Angiostrongylus cantonensis* and *A. costaricensis*.** Metastrongylid nematodes of the genus *Angiostrongylus* have been found to be important human parasites (2). *A. cantonensis*, a lungworm that lives in the pulmonary artery of rats (*Rattus* spp.), is a cause of human eosinophilic meningitis or eosinophilic meningoencephalitis in many Pacific islands including Hawaii, in Thailand, Indonesia, and other parts of Southeast Asia, and in Cuba. Though human cases have not been reported, the parasite has been found in rats in Puerto Rico and in New Orleans. In the life cycle, rats excrete first-stage larvae in the feces, and these penetrate directly into, or are ingested by, many species of terrestrial snails or slugs. Larvae reach the infective, third stage in the molluscs, and when the molluscs are eaten by rats, the larvae make a prolonged month-long migration through the brain before they become adults in the pulmonary artery. Here the worms mate and the females lay eggs which will develop and hatch in the lung tissue; larvae will be found in feces 7 weeks after rats ingest infected molluscs.

Infective larvae in terrestrial molluscs may be eaten by a wide range of vertebrate and invertebrate animals including planarians, shrimp, crabs, fish, amphibians, and reptiles. In these hosts the larvae remain in various tissues in the infective stage. Human infections are rarely derived from eating ordinary terrestrial molluscs; instead, infection is acquired by eating raw or poorly cooked infected shrimp, crabs, or large edible snails such as *Pila*. Accidental infection also may result from eating infected planarians or small slugs on improperly washed vegetables, such as lettuce, or fruits, such as strawberries.

In the human host, larvae migrate to the brain, spinal cord, or eye, where they become immature adults. Rarely can the worms complete the migration to the pulmonary artery; instead, they usually die in the meninges or the parenchyma of the brain, giving rise to meningeal symptoms. Diagnosis is usually based on a history of being in an area where the parasite occurs, combined with the development of appropriate clinical symptoms such as severe and prolonged headaches, nerve involvement, and the presence of eosinophils in cerebrospinal fluid. Occasionally, immature worms may be found in aspirated cerebrospinal fluid. Serological diagnosis has not been reliable.

A closely related parasite, *A. costaricensis*, causes human abdominal angiostrongyliasis in most countries of Central and South America. This parasite normally lives in small arteries and arterioles of the ileocecal region of various rodents. Eggs are produced and develop in the intestinal wall, and first-stage larvae then migrate into the intestinal lumen to pass in feces. Various terrestrial slugs serve as intermediate hosts; most likely, as is the case for *A. cantonensis*, most terrestrial snails and slugs will support development of the parasite to the infective third stage. Infection is acquired by accidental ingestion of slugs or other hosts. Transport hosts probably play an important role in human infection. Most human infections occur in children, but all age groups may be infected. The distal small intestine is the

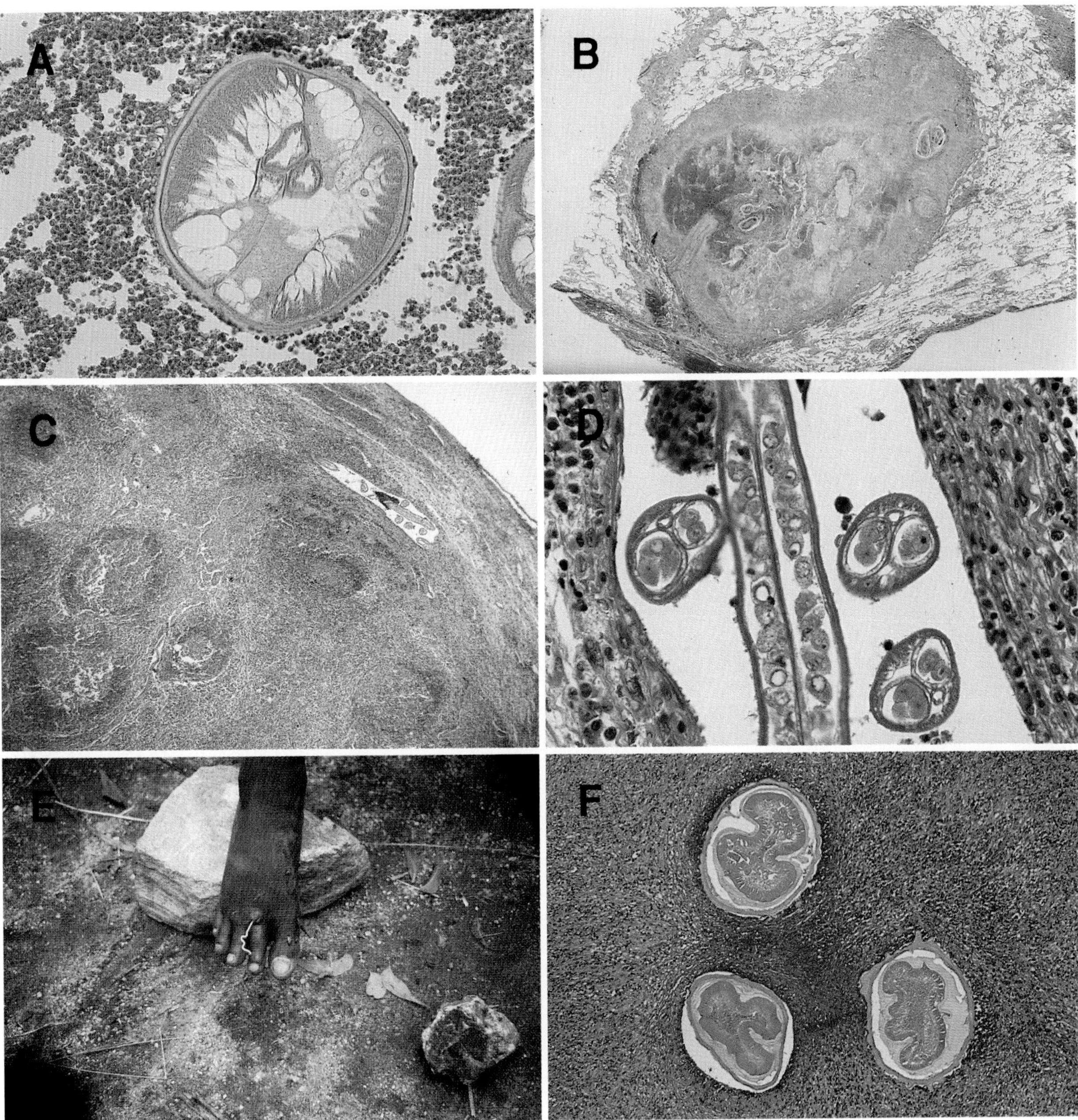

FIG. 4. Helminth parasites in tissues. (A) *Dirofilaria tenuis* in the cheek of a man from Florida; hematoxylin-eosin stain. Although this female worm is dead, most of the normal architecture of body wall remains, i.e., cuticle, hypodermis, and musculature, allowing identification of the filaria (×125). (B) *Dirofilaria immitis* in granulomatous nodule in human lung; hematoxylin-eosin stain. The immature worm is trapped in a small pulmonary artery (×7). (C) *Brugia* species, immature worm in a subcapsular vessel of lymph node from a human in Ohio; hematoxylin-eosin stain (×23). (D) High-power view of the parasite in panel C to illustrate morphology of the filaria (×300). (E) *Dracunculus medinensis,* adult worm partially extruded from a lesion at the base of the toe of an individual in Cameroon, West Africa. (F) Anisakid worm in peritesticular tissue of a man; hematoxylin-eosin stain. Although the worm is dead, morphological features, e.g., hypodermal cords, help identify the parasite (×350). Panels A and B courtesy of Paul Beaver, Tulane University, New Orleans, La.; panels C and D courtesy of Y. Gutierrez, Case-Western Reserve University, Cleveland, Ohio; panel E courtesy of Mark Eberhard, Centers for Disease Control, Atlanta, Ga.

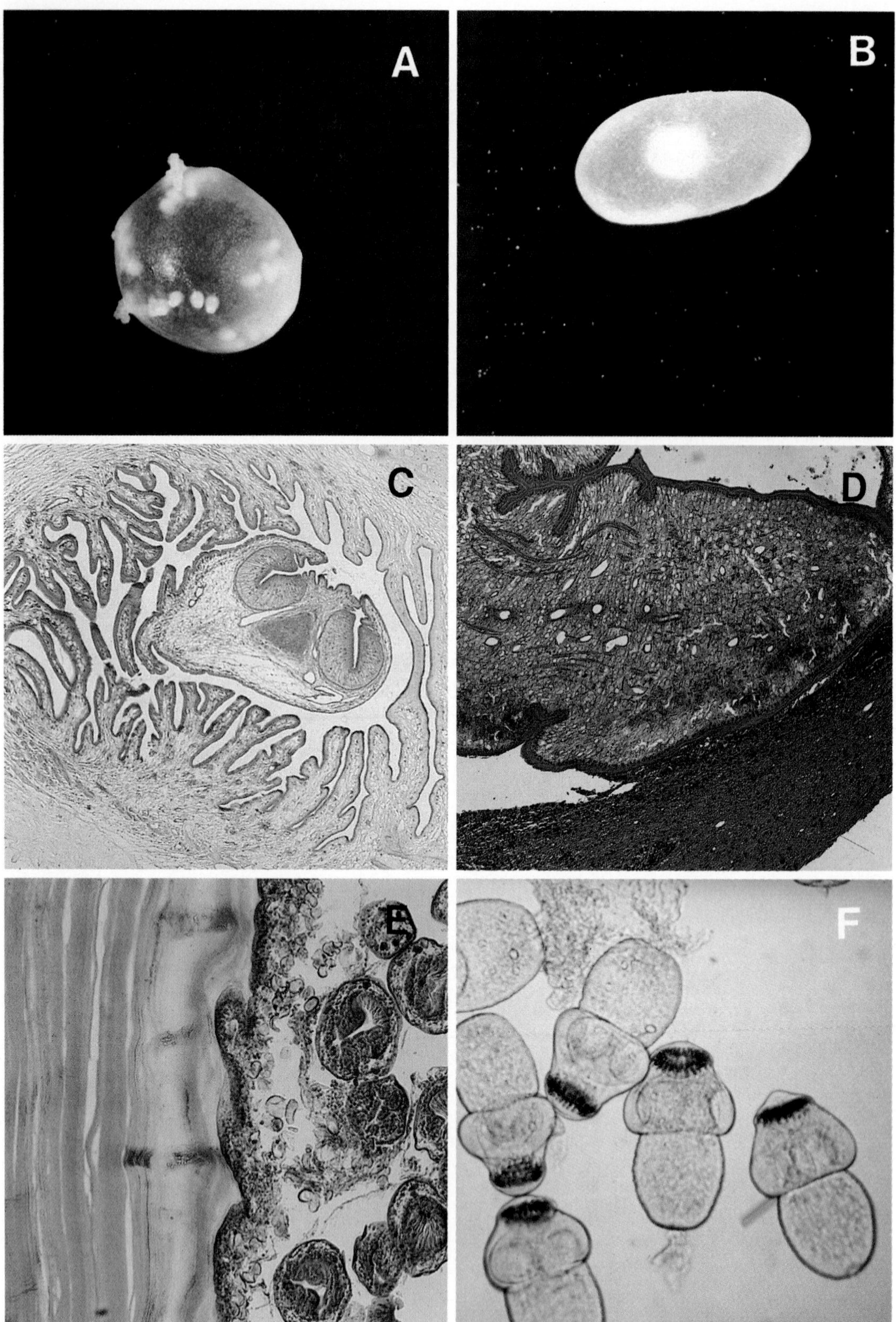

FIG. 5. Helminth parasites in tissues. (A) Coenurus of *Taenia multiceps* from the eye of a man (×6). (B) Cysticercus of *Taenia solium*, also called *Cysticercus cellulosae* (×10). (C) Cysticercus of *Taenia solium* in human brain; hematoxylin-eosin stain. Note that two of the suckers and rostellar elements are seen but hooks are not present in this section (×10). (D) Section of sparganum in human brain; hematoxylin-eosin stain. Note bluish-staining calcareous corpuscles in parasite tissue which help identify its cestode nature (×10). (E) *Echinococcus granulosus*, hydatid cyst in liver; hematoxylin-eosin stain. Note laminated membrane, germinal layer, and individual scoleces (×65). (F) *Echinococcus granulosus*, hydatid sand. Here the scoleces are everted and the hooks are clearly evident (×150). (Panel F from reference 1, used by permission.)

usual site, where eggs stimulate a granulomatous inflammation which leads to symptoms of acute abdomen. Surgery is often performed and the affected tissues may be resected; infection is subsequently diagnosed by finding eggs in tissue. Larvae have not been found in human feces. Though serological tests have been described, their reliability is still in question.

Zoonotic filariae. In recent years, a wide variety of filarial worms which are natural parasites of wild mammals have been recovered from the tissues of people in many parts of the world. Infections have been recorded with greatest frequency in the United States and the Mediterranean region. These filariae are transmitted by bloodsucking arthropods that, in some cases, feed on both animals and humans. Their feeding behavior, together with the overlapping environments of certain (infected) animals and humans, makes it possible for the infective stages of these filariae to accidentally infect humans.

Species of *Dirofilaria*, among them *D. tenuis*, *D. repens*, and *D. ursi*, which have been found in the subcutaneous tissues of their animal hosts and are transmitted by mosquitoes, are the filariae most frequently encountered in human infections (2). These infections are characteristically cryptic, i.e., there is no microfilaremia; female worms may be sexually mature but are usually infertile. The worms have a propensity for migration to the face, orbit, and conjunctivae but may be found, dead or alive, in subcutaneous nodules on any part of the body. Diagnosis is based on recovery of the intact worm from the tissues or by the identification of the filaria in histological sections of the affected tissues (Fig. 4A). Usually, only a single worm is recovered from human tissues although two or more have been found on rare occasions.

Dirofilaria immitis, the heartworm of dogs and other canidae, has been reported from humans wherever the filaria is found in dogs. Typically, immature stages of the parasite lodge in and obstruct small pulmonary arteries, producing an infarct and eventually a granulomatous nodule (Fig. 4B) which appears as a "coin lesion" in the lung on X rays (2, 9). At present, diagnosis depends on microscopic examination of the excised lesion; there are no serologic or immunologic tests that will differentiate the parasitic lesion from neoplastic tumors. On rare occasions, adult worms have been found in the right side of the heart or in the great vessels.

Lymphatic-dwelling *Brugia* species are natural parasites of animals in many parts of the world. Human infections of zoonotic origin have been reported most frequently from the northeastern United States and northern South America (7). The worms are invariably located in lymph nodes or lymphoid tissues (Fig. 4C and D). As stated for the dirofilarias, patent infections are extremely rare; most often the female worms recovered are immature and infertile. The animal reservoirs of infection in the natural environment have not been precisely established but raccoons, rabbits, and wild felines and possibly others may be involved.

Dracontiasis. The parasite *Dracunculus medinensis* is frequently referred to as "guinea worm." It is still widely distributed in Africa, the Middle East, and parts of India and Pakistan. The adult worms live in the subcutaneous tissues, and infection becomes evident when the female migrates to the body surfaces, usually on the feet or ankles, and produces a blister on the skin. On contact with water, the blister ruptures and the female worm discharges swarms of motile larvae into the water. Only a small portion of the female is extruded from the lesion (Fig. 4E). However, it can be removed from the body by gentle traction. If the female fails to reach the surface of the body, it dies in the tissues and may calcify. Male worms, which are very small, are rarely seen and also die in the tissues. Secondary bacterial infections of the lesions are common and may be temporarily disabling.

The life cycle involves transmission of the parasite by a biologic vector, a copepod, which ingests first-stage larvae liberated by the female worm. After development of the larvae to infectivity, ingestion of infected copepods by humans in their drinking water can result in transmission of infection. Diagnosis depends on the appearance of the female worm on the surface of the skin (Fig. 4E). The administration of various drugs, e.g., metronidazole, thiabendazole, and antihistamines or corticosteroids help relieve symptoms and may facilitate removal of worms from the tissues by traction. Guinea worm infection can be controlled easily by provision of piped water or covered wells for drinking purposes.

CESTODES

There are a number of tapeworm species that, as adults, live in the intestine of humans or animals and whose larval stages often are found in human tissues. They can be recognized in most cases on the basis of their morphological features. These are described below.

Sparganosis

Human sparganosis is caused by larval cestodes of the genus *Spirometra*, which are parasites of cats, dogs, and various wild canids and felids. These parasites are closely related to *Diphyllobothrium* and have similar life cycles involving copepods as first intermediate hosts and fish as second intermediate hosts. *Spirometra mansoni* is found in many parts of Asia, in particular in China, Japan, Korea, Vietnam, and other areas, and *Spirometra mansonoides* is the common species in the United States. Characteristically, in sparganosis, the plerocercoid larva (also called a sparganum) migrates in the tissues of the human host after ingestion of these larvae in poorly cooked fish, ingestion of infected copepods containing procercoid larvae, or the use of infected hosts such as frogs and snakes as poultices, a practice followed in many Asian countries. In the United States, typical cases of sparganosis present as subcutaneous swellings which may be migratory and sometimes tender; usually there is little or no peripheral eosinophilia. Diagnosis is usually made after surgical removal of the mass and histopathological study (Fig. 5D).

Coenurosis

Coenurosis is produced by the larval stage of the tapeworm *Taenia multiceps*, which in the adult stage is a common intestinal parasite of canid and felid species, e.g., dogs, foxes, and cats. The adult worms live in the small intestine of their host. They produce eggs indistinguishable from those of other species of *Taenia*. Herbivores and omnivores, as well as some rodents, are the usual intermediate hosts. The hexacanth embryo that hatches from the egg migrates to extraintestinal sites such as the brain, subcutaneous tissues, or musculature and develops to the coenurus stage. Typically, the coenurus, which may vary from a few millimeters to several centimeters in diameter, has multiple scoleces which develop from the germinal layer lining the bladderlike larva (Fig. 5A). Humans usually acquire the infection by ingesting the eggs from dog feces. Diagnosis is usually made from material surgically removed from the human host.

Cysticercosis

Human cysticercosis is produced by the ingestion of the eggs of the pork tapeworm, *Taenia solium*. It can be found throughout the world, although it has its greatest prevalence in Mexico, other areas of Latin America, India, China, Africa, and Europe. Acquisition of cysticercosis in the United States is uncommon, but immigrants from endemic areas are frequently diagnosed with the infection, and reports of cysticercosis in the U.S. are increasing (5).

The cysticercus or bladder worm is round to oval and translucent and measures about 5 mm or more in diameter (Fig. 5B). It has an invaginated scolex bearing four suckers and a circle of hooks. This cysticercus will develop in any organ or tissue of the body; they are most serious when they occur in the central nervous system and the eye (4). Diagnosis of the infection may be difficult. It may be established by the recovery of whole cysticerci or the histologic demonstration of cysticerci in surgically removed tissues (Fig. 5C). Diagnosis may also be accomplished by detection of calcifying cysticerci by X ray and the use of computerized tomography.

Hydatid disease

Various forms of hydatid disease are caused by a number of species of the tapeworm *Echinococcus*. *E. granulosus* is a minute tapeworm, measuring 3 to 6 mm in length, found in domestic and wild canids. It occurs extensively in sheep- and cattle-raising areas of the world. Unilocular hydatid infection results from humans ingesting the taeniidlike eggs of this parasite. The normal life cycle of the parasite involves canids as definitive hosts, who pass eggs in feces which are ingested by sheep, cattle, and other animals. In these animals, the embryo released from the egg migrates to various organs, principally the liver and lungs, where it develops into a hydatid cyst. Within this cyst scoleces develop and proliferate from a germinal membrane (Fig. 5E), so that ultimately the cysts may become very large and contain many hundreds, and even thousands, of scoleces, usually referred to as "hydatid sand" (Fig. 5F); each of these is a potentially infective organism should the cyst rupture. When canids ingest cysts in the tissues of sheep, each of the scoleces ingested will mature in the intestine to produce an adult tapeworm. Thus, infected dogs may harbor heavy worm burdens.

Only the larval stage, the hydatid cyst, develops in humans as a result of accidental ingestion of *E. granulosus* eggs, and this may take many years. Hydatid cysts may grow in almost all organs and tissues of the body, as they do in normal intermediate hosts, but they are most common in the liver and lungs. Involvement of the central nervous system and bone is not uncommon. These cysts continue to grow, and their presence frequently goes undetected until they reach sufficient size to cause clinical symptoms. Infections of the central nervous system usually become apparent much earlier than those of other organs.

Diagnosis of hydatid infection may be difficult but can be accomplished by several means. X rays, ultrasonic scanning, and computerized tomography can detect cysts in tissues. When combined with an appropriate residential or travel history, or an occupation such as sheep raising in endemic areas, observation of tissue cysts provides reasonable grounds for suspicion of infection. Many immunodiagnostic tests have been utilized, but there is wide variability in their sensitivity and specificity (2). Aspiration of material from a hydatid cyst in situ is dangerous and not a recommended procedure, since accidental spillage of cyst material in the body may result in further dissemination of infection, an anaphylactic reaction, or both.

Multilocular hydatid (alveolar hydatid) infection

A second form of hydatidosis occurring in humans is alveolar hydatid disease, caused by the larval stage of *Echinococcus multilocularis*. The life cycle of this parasite involves foxes, wolves, and dogs as definitive hosts for the small tapeworms, and small rodents and voles as intermediate hosts. Human ingestion of the typical taeniid eggs may result in the development of this invasive cyst in the liver. These cysts usually lack scoleces in the human host, and they may ramify throughout the tissue. The geographical distribution of this infection is usually the northern parts of Europe, Japan, and North America, but the infection is also present in Australia, New Zealand, and South America. Diagnosis is difficult and frequently is accomplished only by histological examination of tissues removed surgically. Serological tests are of some value, although their sensitivity and specificity, as mentioned, are a problem.

Polycystic hydatid infection

A third type of hydatid disease, caused by *Echinococcus vogeli* in Latin America, has been reported (3). The normal life cycle of this parasite involves bush dogs and large rodents, or pacas. A polycystic hydatid develops primarily in the liver where, in humans, it is an invasive type of cyst. Diagnosis has been by examination of pathological specimens removed by surgery.

LITERATURE CITED

1. **Ash, L. R., and T. C. Orihel.** 1990. Atlas of human parasitology, 3rd ed. American Society of Clinical Pathologists, Chicago.
2. **Beaver, P. C., R. C. Jung, and E. W. Cupp.** 1984. Clinical parasitology, 9th ed. Lea & Febiger, Philadelphia.
3. **D'Alessandro, A., R. L. Rausch, C. Cuello, and N. Aristizabal.** 1979. *Echinococcus vogeli* in man with a review on polycystic hydatid disease in Colombia and neighboring countries. Am. J. Trop. Med. Hyg. **28:**303–317.
4. **Del Britto, O. H., and J. Sotelo.** 1988. Neurocysticercosis: an update. Rev. Infect. Dis. **10:**1075–1087.
5. **Flisser, A., K. Willms, J. P. Laclette, C. Larralde, C. Ridaura, and F. Beltran (ed.).** 1982. Cysticercosis: present state of knowledge and perspectives. Academic Press, Inc., New York.
6. **Norman, L., and I. G. Kagan.** 1963. Bentonite, latex and

cholesterol flocculation tests for the diagnosis of trichinosis. Public Health Rep. **78:**227–232.

7. **Orihel, T. C., and P. C. Beaver.** 1989. Zoonotic *Brugia* infections in North and South America. Am. J. Trop. Med. Hyg. **40:**638–647.
8. **Orihel, T. C., and M. L. Eberhard.** 1982. *Mansonella ozzardi:* a redescription with comments on its taxonomic relationships. Am. J. Trop. Med. Hyg. **31:**1142–1147.
9. **Ro, J. Y., P. J. Tsakalabis, V. A. White, M. A. Luna, E. G. Chang-Tung, L. Green, L. Cribbett, and A. C. Ayala.** 1989. Pulmonary dirofilariasis: the great imitator of primary metastatic lung tumor. A clinicopathologic analysis of seven cases and a review. Hum. Pathol. **20:**69–76.
10. **Schulz-Key, H.** 1988. The collagenase technique: how to isolate and examine adult *Onchocerca volvulus* for evaluation of drug effects. Trop. Med. Parasitol. **39:**423–440.
11. **Wittner, M., J. W. Turner, G. Jacquette, L. R. Ash, M. P. Salgo, and H. B. Tanowitz.** 1989. Eustrongyloidiasis—a parasitic infection acquired by eating sushi. New Engl. J. Med. **320:**1124–1126.

Chapter 71

Intestinal Helminths

LAWRENCE R. ASH AND THOMAS C. ORIHEL

Intestinal helminths are usually diagnosed by detection of eggs or larvae in fecal specimens. Characteristics used in identifying eggs (Fig. 1) include size, shape, thickness of shell, special structures of the shell (mammillated covering, operculum, knob, spine), and development stage of egg contents (undeveloped, developing, embryonated).

Objects that might be confused with helminth eggs include pollen grains, mushroom spores, portions of vegetable material, and mite eggs. Plant hairs may be confused with nematode larvae. Confusing objects usually do not show the proper structure and content and may not be the correct size.

In the period after infection is acquired but before helminths have matured to produce eggs (prepatent period), infections are difficult to diagnose. Larvae occasionally may be found in sputum as a result their migration through the lungs, but in most instances diagnosis during the prepatent periods can be established only on the basis of clinical symptomatology, if at all.

NEMATODES

The nematodes, or roundworms, are small to large, elongate, cylindrical parasites living primarily as adult worms in the intestinal tract. Nematodes mainly have life cycles that are direct and require no intermediate hosts, but some utilize one or more intermediate hosts. All of the nematodes of humans, with the exception of *Strongyloides* spp., are dioecious (have two sexes) and characteristically have four larval stages and a fifth, adult stage. The stage of infectivity for the human host varies from the first- to the third-stage larva, depending on the species of parasite involved. The infective stages of nematodes are usually within eggs, but in a few species (hookworms, *Strongyloides* spp.) the larvae hatch from the eggs and become infective in the soil. Diagnosis of most of the human intestinal nematode parasites depends on finding characteristic eggs in feces. An important exception to this is *Strongyloides stercoralis* infection, in which first-stage larvae are excreted in fresh feces.

The parasites that commonly infect humans are described below.

Enterobius vermicularis

Infection with *Enterobius vermicularis,* the human pinworm parasite, is worldwide in its distribution, and its true prevalence is probably considerably underestimated. The organism is primarily a parasite of young children; the rapid development of its eggs to the infective stage and their ability to persist for extended periods on fomites lead to rapid dissemination of the infection from child to child and to adults.

Pinworm adults are small, with females being 8 to 13 mm long and barely visible to the naked eye as white, motile worms on the surface of stool specimens or on the perianal skin. Males are only 2 to 3 mm long and usually are not seen. The adult female has a characteristic long and pointed tail, whereas in males the posterior end is blunt. Adult worms typically live in the cecum, colon, appendix, and rectum. Usually, adult females migrate out of the anal orifice at night and lay their eggs in the perianal area, where they adhere to the skin, hair, or bed clothing and bed linen that come in contact with these eggs. Because they live so low in the intestinal tract, females often lay their eggs on top of the fecal mass, where they are not well mixed into the fecal stream and often are not detected in routine stool examinations.

Enterobius eggs are elongate and flattened on one side, with a thick, colorless shell. They are 50 to 60 μm long by 20 to 40 μm wide and are partially embryonated when laid. The eggs develop rapidly and become infective within 4 to 6 h, at which time the egg contains a tadpolelike larva (Fig. 2A). Adherence of these eggs to fingers and fomites results in their ready transfer to the mouth and further infection.

The infection is especially troublesome in young children; large worm burdens may cause extreme pruritus, loss of sleep, and irritability. Adult females occasionally may enter the vagina and subsequently the uterus or fallopian tubes, where they die. Disintegration of the dead worms and liberation of the eggs contained in utero result in an inflammatory response and granuloma formation about the eggs in these sites.

Infection is best diagnosed by the use of a cellophane tape procedure (see chapter 66). Examinations on multiple days may be required to diagnose infection. The proportion of specimens positive correlates with severity of infection (7).

Other methods have been used to demonstrate this infection, in particular the use of Vaspar anal swabs; however, the cellophane tape method is the most widely used.

Ascaris lumbricoides

The largest and probably the most prevalent of the human intestinal roundworms, *Ascaris lumbricoides* has a worldwide distribution. The flesh-colored adult worms are large; adult females usually range from 20 to 35 cm long by 3 to 6 mm wide, and males range from 15 to 31 cm by 2 to 4 mm. Males, with their ventrally curved tails, can be readily distinguished from females, which have straight tails. Females produce large numbers of eggs, perhaps up to 200,000 per female worm per day.

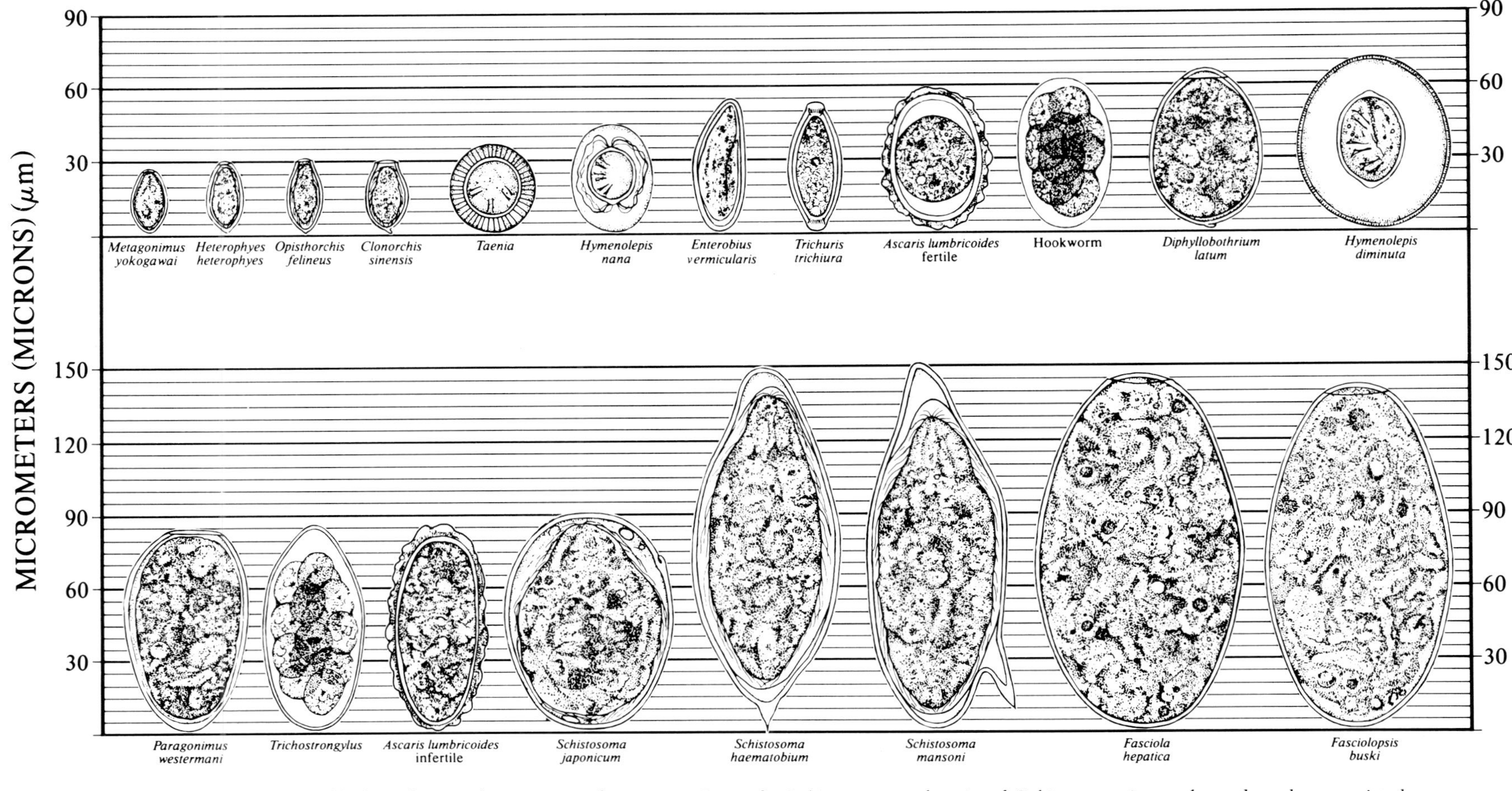

FIG. 1. Relative sizes of helminth eggs (from Centers for Disease Control). *Schistosoma mekongi* and *Schistosoma intercalatum* have been omitted.

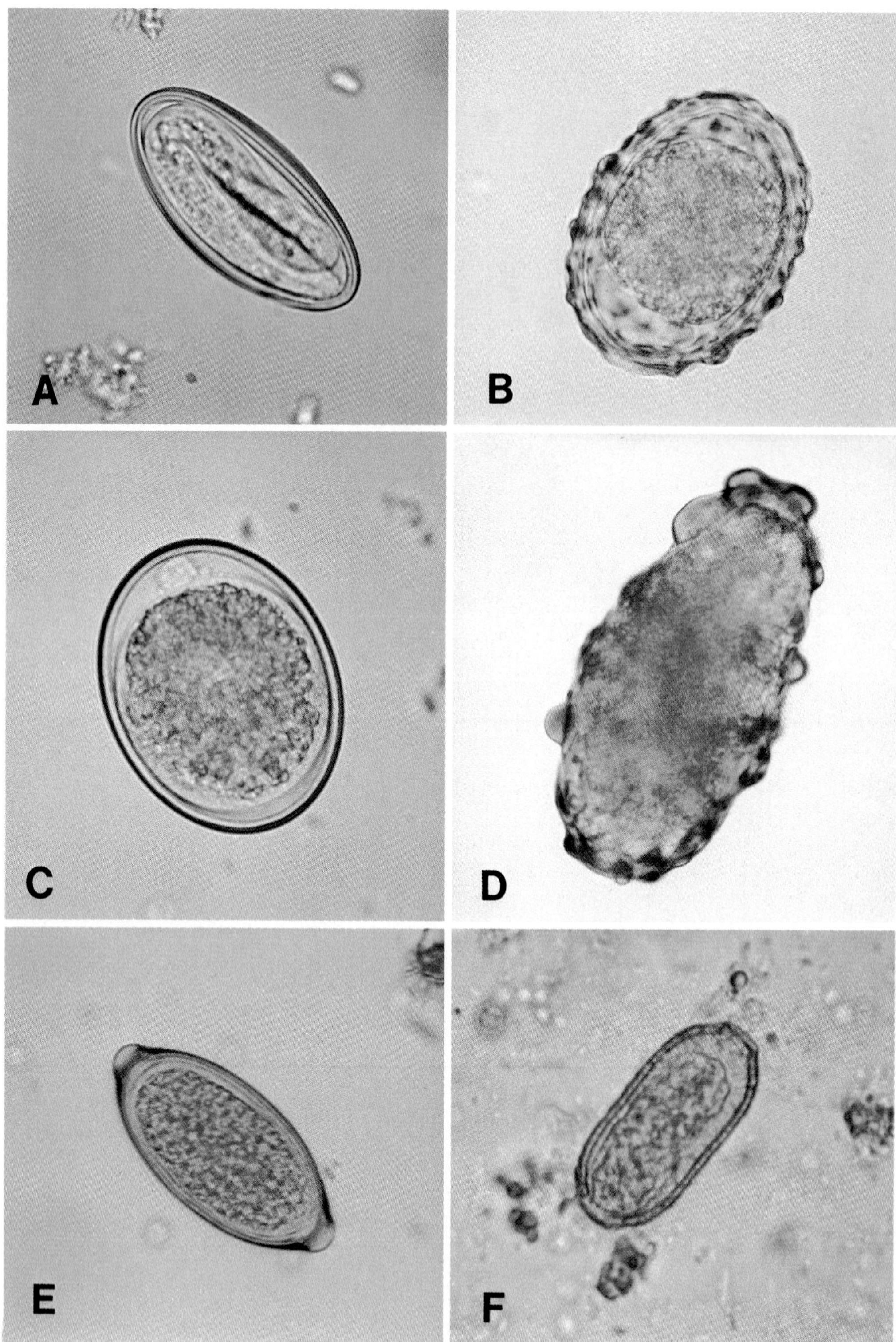

FIG. 2. Eggs of intestinal nematode parasites (×850). (A) Embryonated, infective egg of *Enterobius vermicularis.* (B) Fertile egg of *Ascaris lumbricoides.* (C) Decorticated, fertile egg of *A. lumbricoides.* (D) Infertile egg of *A. lumbricoides.* (E) *Trichuris trichiura.* (F) *Capillaria philippinensis.* (Panels A, C, and D from reference 2, used with permission.)

These eggs must undergo a developmental period in soil of approximately 2 to 3 weeks before they are infective.

In the human host, infective eggs hatch in the intestine, and the second-stage larvae undergo an obligatory migration through the liver to the lungs, where they grow and develop for 8 to 9 days to a length of approximately 1 mm before returning to the small intestine to complete maturity. The prepatent period is approximately 2 months.

Pathology in humans can be caused by both larval and adult *A. lumbricoides*. The larval migration phase in infections with large numbers of eggs, and in particular with repeated infections, may result in *Ascaris* pneumonitis (Loeffler's syndrome) consisting of dyspnea, cough, rales, eosinophilia, and transient, shifting lung infiltrates as seen by X-ray examination. Adult worms may cause intestinal blockage when present in large numbers. However, the presence of small numbers or even one adult worm is potentially dangerous because of their tendency to migrate to ectopic sites, particularly the liver, when febrile illness occurs. The normal life span for adult worms is approximately 1 year, although female worms may persist for 16 to 20 months.

Infection is usually diagnosed by demonstration of typical fertile eggs in feces. Fertile eggs are ovoid, contain a single-celled ovum, and measure 55 to 75 μm long by 35 to 50 μm wide. Eggs are yellow-brown and have a thick, transparent shell that is covered by a mammillated albuminoid outer layer (Fig. 2B). Occasionally, the outer mammillated layer is absent; these eggs are called decorticated eggs (Fig. 2C). Female worms that have never been fertilized or have exhausted their supply of sperm will produce infertile eggs. These are elongate, 85 to 90 μm by 43 to 47 μm, and have a thin shell that may lack mammillations entirely or may have grossly irregular mammillations scattered unevenly over the surface of the shell. These eggs contain a mass of disorganized, highly refractive granules and fat globules of various sizes (Fig. 2D). Because of the large numbers of eggs produced by the female worms, the eggs can usually be found in direct fecal smears and are readily detected by either flotation or sedimentation concentration procedures. Infertile eggs do not float in the standard zinc sulfate solution (specific gravity, 1.18), and they may be missed if only this flotation concentration is used. Adult worms may be spontaneously passed in feces or emerge from the anus, mouth, or nares; young developing worms, especially in heavy infections, may be found in feces. The characteristic, prominent three lips at the anterior end of the worm aid in the diagnosis of these immature or adult parasites.

Trichuris trichiura

Infection with *Trichuris trichiura*, known as whipworm infection, is worldwide in geographic distribution and is found in the warmer, moist regions of the world. Adult worms live attached to the wall of the cecum and, less commonly, to the wall of the large intestine, appendix, and lower part of the ileum. Males and females are of similar size, ranging from 30 to 50 mm long, and have a long attenuated anterior portion and a thicker, short posterior end. The long, slender anterior end is threaded into the mucosal epithelium, and the posterior portion hangs free in the lumen. Adult worms are long-lived, commonly up to 10 years and often longer. Though frequently found in association with *A. lumbricoides* infection, because soil requirements for the development of infective eggs are similar, *Trichuris* infections are more frequently seen in older children because of the longer life span of the adult parasites. Egg production by *Trichuris* females probably does not exceed several thousand eggs per day.

Eggs are barrel shaped and yellow-brown, have thick shells, and usually measure 50 to 55 μm long by 22 to 24 μm wide. At both ends of the egg are prominent, clear, mucoid "plugs" (Fig. 2E). The eggs contain an unsegmented ovum when passed in feces, and once the eggs are in the soil it takes 2 to 3 weeks for the infective, first-stage larva to develop. When infected eggs are ingested, the prepatent period in humans is approximately 3 months.

Light infections with *T. trichiura* usually are not troublesome, but when large numbers of parasites are present there may be diarrhea or even dysentery with abdominal cramping, and occasionally rectal prolapse may occur. Heavy infections may result in dehydration, weight loss, and anemia.

Diagnosis, in particular with heavy infections, is readily made by finding the characteristic eggs in direct wet mounts of feces. In light infections, when eggs are few in number, the use of concentration procedures is required to find the eggs. In some instances, larger than normal eggs (65 to 83 μm by 27 to 36 μm wide) are produced by female worms for reasons not well understood (10). In addition, the dog whipworm (*Trichuris vulpis*) can reach maturity in humans; the eggs of this parasite are normally larger than those in typical *T. trichiura* infections, being 72 to 90 μm long by 32 to 40 μm wide. The eggs of *T. vulpis*, though similar in length to the large eggs occasionally seen in *T. trichiura* infections, are usually wider and more barrel shaped.

Capillaria philippinensis

Capillaria philippinensis has been recognized since the mid-1960s as causing human infection. Although its geographic distribution was thought to be restricted to the Philippines and Thailand, occasional cases in recent years from Japan, Egypt, and Iran suggest that the parasite may be found in other parts of Southeast Asia, the Middle East, and possibly other areas. *C. philippinensis* is normally a parasite of fish-eating birds, and various fish serve as obligatory intermediate hosts. In endemic areas, human infection is acquired by the ingestion of raw or poorly cooked fish harboring infective larvae in their tissues. Patent infections develop in approximately 1 month. Female worms may contain thick-shelled, unembryonated eggs, thin-shelled, embryonated eggs, or first-stage larvae in their uteri (4). Internal autoinfection from the larvae is a normal feature of the life cycle in mammalian hosts, resulting in large worm burdens that cause diarrhea, wasting, dehydration, and, if untreated, death of the host.

Diagnosis of the infection depends on finding the characteristic thick-shelled, unembryonated eggs in feces. The eggs are 36 to 45 μm long by 21 μm wide, have a moderately thick, striated shell, and possess inconspicuous mucoid "plugs" at both ends of the egg (Fig. 2F). It is not uncommon in individuals with chronic diarrhea for eggs, larvae, and even adult worms to be passed simultaneously in feces.

Hookworm infection

The two principal human hookworm parasites are *Necator americanus* and *Ancylostoma duodenale*, but other species of the genus *Ancylostoma* may also produce infections in humans in various parts of the world. *N. americanus* is found in the United States as well as other parts of the world, but *A. duodenale* is not present in the United States, although its geographic distribution elsewhere frequently overlaps that of *N. americanus*. Hookworm infection is widely distributed in the tropics and subtropics and also extends into moist, temperate climates.

Adult hookworms are characterized by an anterior end modified into a buccal capsule that contains either teeth or cutting plates with which they can anchor themselves to the wall of the small intestine. Male hookworms are further characterized by having posterior ends modified to form an umbrellalike structure referred to as a bursa; this structure does not occur in female worms, which have straight, pointed tails. *Necator* adults are 7 to 11 mm long by 0.3 mm wide, and they have a buccal capsule provided with cutting plates. *A. duodenale* adults are somewhat larger, 8 to 13 mm long by 0.4 mm wide, and they have a buccal capsule containing two pairs of teeth.

The thin-shelled eggs of *N. americanus* and *A. duodenale* are unembryonated when passed in feces, and they are essentially indistinguishable from each other (Fig. 3A): their size ranges from 55 to 75 µm long by 36 to 40 µm wide. In the soil, the eggs embryonate and hatch within 1 to 2 days as first-stage, rhabditoid larvae measuring 250 to 350 µm long by 17 µm wide.

In the hookworm life cycle, the first-stage larvae that hatch in the soil develop into infective, third-stage, filariform larvae in approximately 1 week, and these larvae initiate human infection by direct penetration of the skin. *A. duodenale* infective larvae can also infect via the mouth, but *N. americanus* cannot; in addition, *N. americanus* requires an obligatory lung migration, whereas if *A. duodenale* infection is acquired orally, there is direct maturation in the intestine to the adult stage. Patent infections develop in 5 to 6 weeks, and the life span of the adults of both species is usually only 1 to 2 years but may be as long as 10 years or more.

The pathogenesis of hookworm infections is directly related to the worm burden. Light infections are well tolerated and exhibit few symptoms. Acute, heavy infections may result in fatigue, weakness, abdominal pain, and diarrhea with blood loss; the latter is more severe in *A. duodenale* infections. Chronic hookworm infection results in an iron-deficient anemia, listlessness, pallor, and general retardation of development in afflicted children.

Diagnosis is accomplished by demonstration of characteristic eggs in feces (Fig. 3A). Counts of fewer than five eggs per cover slip in wet mounts indicate light infections unlikely to cause anemia. Counts of over 25 eggs per cover slip suggest heavy infection. If there has been prolonged delay in examination of the feces (usually more than a day), larvae may develop and hatch, and it is then necessary to differentiate hookworm first-stage larvae from those of *S. stercoralis*, the stage typically passed in the feces in human strongyloidiasis. Hookworm rhabditoid larvae have a long, narrow buccal chamber (Fig. 3E) and an inconspicuous genital primordium which is an elongate cluster of cells located midway along the intestine, between it and the ventral body wall.

Accurate identification of the hookworm species causing infection depends on recovering and examining adult worms or on culturing larval stages from eggs to the infective, filariform stage, with subsequent morphological study of these larvae to distinguish between *Necator* and *Ancylostoma* species (1).

Trichostrongylus species

Human infection with species of the genus *Trichostrongylus* are found throughout the world, in particular in rural areas where herbivorous animals are raised. Although these infections are rarely troublesome in terms of human disease, they do cause some diagnostic difficulties, since trichostrongyle eggs resemble hookworm eggs in shape, although they tend to be much larger in size.

Adult worms are rarely seen in feces. They are small, slender worms, usually measuring less than 1 cm in length, and males have a large prominent bursa. Many different *Trichostrongylus* species may infect humans, depending on the area of the world in which the infections are acquired.

Trichostrongyle eggs are larger than hookworm eggs, 75 to 95 µm long by 40 to 50 µm wide. They have a colorless, thin shell, and the egg is tapered slightly at one end. The inner vitelline membrane is frequently wrinkled at the tapered end of the egg, and the germinal mass does not fill the shell (Fig. 3B).

Strongyloides stercoralis

Strongyloidiasis is widely distributed in the tropics and subtropics and also extends into moist, temperate regions. Even in endemic areas its distribution is extremely focal because the existence of the parasite is dependent on a high groundwater table. Adult parasitic females are parthenogenetic, and parasitic males do not occur. These minute females, only 2 to 3 mm long, live within the mucosal epithelium of the small intestine, where they produce thin-shelled eggs which embryonate and hatch in the mucosa of the intestine. The first-stage larvae migrate into the intestinal lumen and are the usual stage passed in feces (Fig. 3C).

In the soil, first-stage larvae may follow a direct or indirect course of development. In the direct cycle, the larvae develop into filariform, third-stage infective larvae that can initiate human infection by direct penetration of the skin. Alternatively, the first-stage larvae may have an indirect cycle in the external environment in which the larvae develop into a free-living generation of adult male and female worms. When these free-living adults mate, the female lays eggs which embryonate and hatch in the soil as first-stage larvae; the eggs then develop into filariform larvae, which may initiate infection by skin penetration. Although multiple free-living generations have been suggested to occur, it appears that this is not common.

Infection may persist for decades as a result of autoinfection either in the colon or in the perianal area (6). Such infection may be asymptomatic or produce minimal symptoms; however, former prisoners of war in the Far East continue to experience recurrent bouts of serpiginous urticarial rashes due to larval migration on the trunk, buttocks, and groin (3). Individuals with latent infections who develop malnutrition, frequently in association with alcoholism, and patients who are immunocompromised or receive immunosuppressive therapy are at great risk for developing hyperinfection

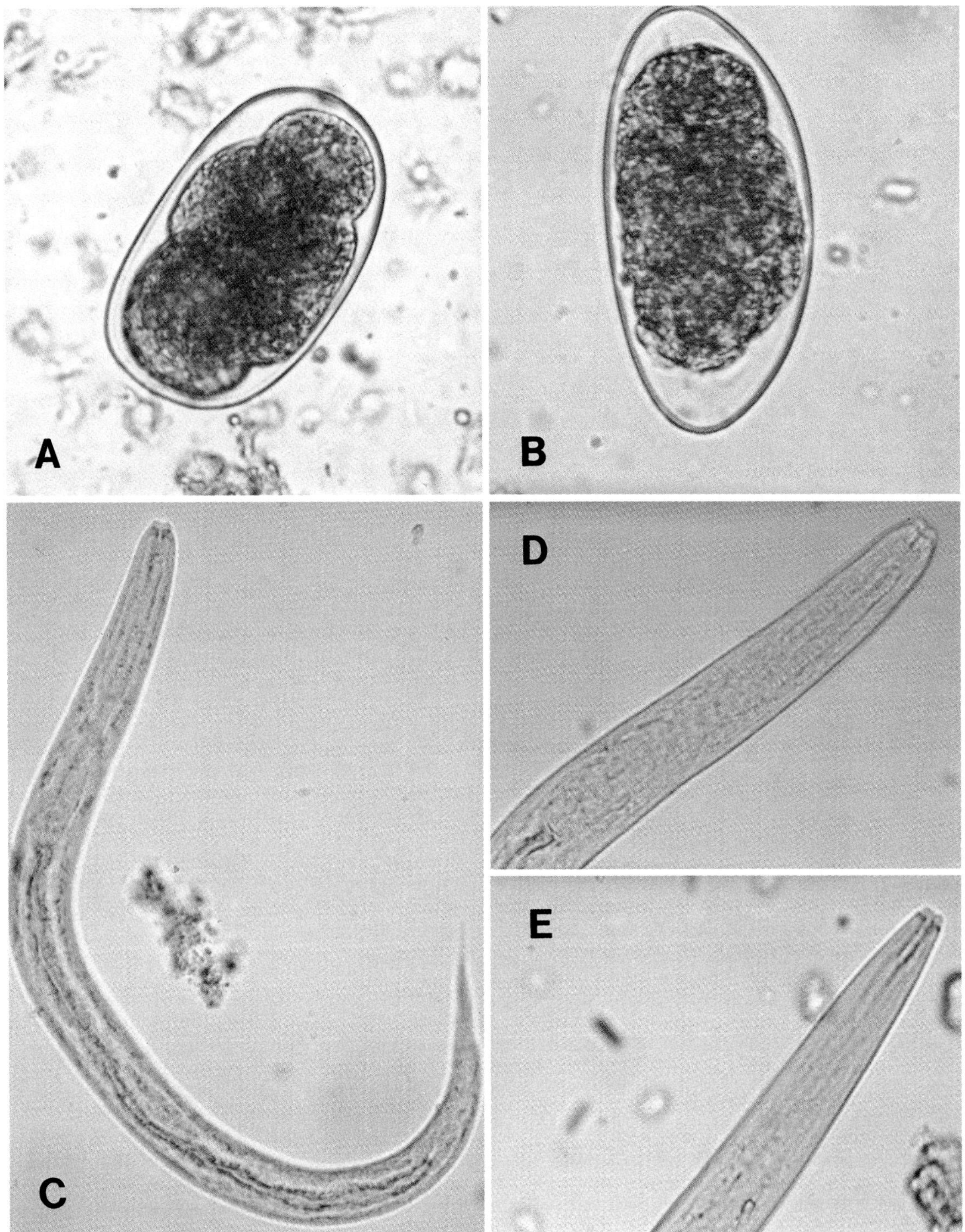

FIG. 3. Eggs and larvae of intestinal nematode parasites (×850). (A) Hookworm egg. (B) *Trichostrongylus* sp. (C) First-stage larva of *Strongyloides stercoralis*. (D) Anterior end of first-stage larva of *S. stercoralis* to show short buccal cavity. (E) Anterior end of first-stage hookworm larva to show long buccal cavity. (Panels A, C, and E from reference 2, used with permission.)

with the parasite (5, 8). Hyperinfection results in rapid multiplication of these parasites within the intestinal tract and subsequent reinvasion of the bowel wall or perianal skin, with migration of third-stage larvae through the viscera and back to the intestine to develop into adult females. This greatly accelerated life cycle can result in overwhelming infection, with massive numbers of adult parasites in the intestinal epithelium and migrating larvae invading all organs and tissues of the body. Unless detected rapidly, these fulminating infections may result in death. Interestingly, although latent strongyloidiasis may be a serious complication in individuals who are immunocompromised or immunosuppressed, this hyperinfection syndrome does not appear to be an important complication in individuals with the acquired immunodeficiency syndrome (AIDS).

Diagnosis may be difficult, in particular in individuals with longstanding chronic infections. In patients with no symptoms and in whom few parasites are present, direct wet mount and standard concentration procedures may fail to reveal the first-stage larvae. Individuals who are candidates for immunosuppressive therapy, and who are from known geographic areas where strongyloidiasis is endemic (e.g., many parts of Latin America and Southeast Asia), must be carefully screened for the possible presence of this infection. In latent infections it is common for only small numbers of larvae to be passed in feces, and in many instances the larvae will be passed on an irregular basis. Thus, multiple stool examinations, several days apart, should be performed. In addition to normal concentration procedures, it is recommended that whole fecal specimens be examined by the Baermann procedure (see chapter 66). Multiple examinations performed in this manner are likely to detect light infections, if present. Duodenal aspiration techniques, including the Enterotest, have also resulted in improved diagnosis of this infection.

First-stage *Strongyloides* larvae are the diagnostic stage found in feces; they measure 180 to 380 μm in length by 14 to 20 μm in width. They have a short buccal chamber and a prominent cluster of cells, the genital primordium, located midway along the intestine between it and the ventral body wall (Fig. 3C and D). If stool specimens have been allowed to sit at warm room temperatures for more than 24 h before examination, it may be necessary to distinguish between *Strongyloides* first-stage larvae and the first-stage larvae of hookworm that may have embryonated and hatched from eggs present in the feces. Hookworm first-stage larvae are of the same size as *Strongyloides* larvae, but they have a long buccal chamber (Fig. 3E) and the genital primordium is inconspicuous and usually cannot be seen.

Occasionally, third-stage larvae of *Strongyloides* may be seen in feces, particularly in cases of hyperinfection. These larvae are approximately 500 μm long; they have a ratio of esophagus length to intestine length of 1:1, and the tail of the larva is notched.

TREMATODES

Adult trematode parasites of humans live in the intestine, liver, lung, or blood vessels. The flukes, as they are frequently called, all have complex life cycles that involve snails as first intermediate hosts, and many must utilize a second intermediate host, most frequently fish, in which the infective stage for humans will develop. In the life cycles of the various flukes, specific freshwater molluscs are used as first intermediate hosts by each species of trematode. The molluscs are infected by a ciliated larva, the miracidium, which emerges from the trematode eggs. Within the snail tissues a complex developmental process involving several different parasite stages results finally in the production of a tailed larva called a cercaria. Cercariae are released into water, and some (as in the schistosomes) may infect humans directly, although in most species the cercariae invade the tissues of a second intermediate aquatic host within which the cercaria develops into the infective, metacercaria stage. Some metacercariae occur on various types of aquatic vegetation rather than in the flesh of second intermediate hosts. Human infection with trematodes is usually acquired by ingestion of infective stages, although schistosomiasis is produced by direct skin invasion by cercariae. Trematode infections usually are diagnosed by identification of eggs in feces or, more rarely, in sputum or urine. The eggs of all human trematodes except the schistosomes have an operculum through which the miracidium escapes. Small trematode eggs usually contain a fully developed miracidium when passed in feces, as do the schistosome eggs; larger trematode eggs are undeveloped when passed and must undergo a period of development in water for several weeks before the miracidium is produced.

Intestinal flukes

Fasciolopsis buski. *F. buski* is the largest and most pathogenic of the human intestinal flukes. It occurs in many parts of Asia, including China, India, Indonesia, Taiwan, Thailand, and Vietnam. Pigs and humans are the primary hosts for this parasite, and infection is acquired by ingestion of various types of aquatic vegetation upon which the metacercarial stage is encysted. Such plants as water chestnuts and the water caltrop are important sources of infection. It takes approximately 3 months from ingestion of metacercariae until eggs are found in feces. The eggs are large, 130 to 140 μm by 80 to 85 μm, ovoid, and unembryonated when passed in feces. The operculum is not conspicuous, and at the abopercular end the relatively thin shell often appears to be blemished (Fig. 4A). *Fasciolopsis* eggs are essentially indistinguishable from those of *Fasciola hepatica*, the sheep, cattle, and human liver fluke. Since *F. buski* is restricted to the Orient, whereas *Fasciola hepatica* is of worldwide distribution, it is important to establish the geographic history of the patient with the infection as well as any clinical symptomatology to establish the correct diagnosis.

Heterophyid infections. There are a large number of genera and species of minute intestinal flukes that parasitize humans in many parts of the world. Though of little medical significance, heterophyid eggs resemble those of the liver flukes *Clonorchis* and *Opisthorchis*, which may pose diagnostic problems in the laboratory. The most important species are *Heterophyes heterophyes* and *Metagonimus yokogawai*, both of which occur principally in Asia, although the former also is found in Egypt and Turkey and the latter extends into the Balkan states. All of the heterophyids show little host specificity, and dogs, cats, and various wild animals are the usual definitive hosts in nature. Adult flukes live in the crypts of the small intestine and are only a few millimeters long. Patent infections develop within 2 to 3 weeks of ingestion of infected, poorly cooked fish harboring metacercariae under their scales. When large numbers of worms are present there may be a mild diarrhea and abdominal cramping, but ordinarily there is little or no symptomatology associated with the infections.

All heterophyid eggs are small, 20 to 30 μm long by 13 to 17 μm wide, are ovoid, and have an inconspicuous operculum. The eggs contain a miracidium when laid (Fig. 4B). Though somewhat similar in morphology to the *Clonorchis* eggs, heterophyid eggs lack the seated

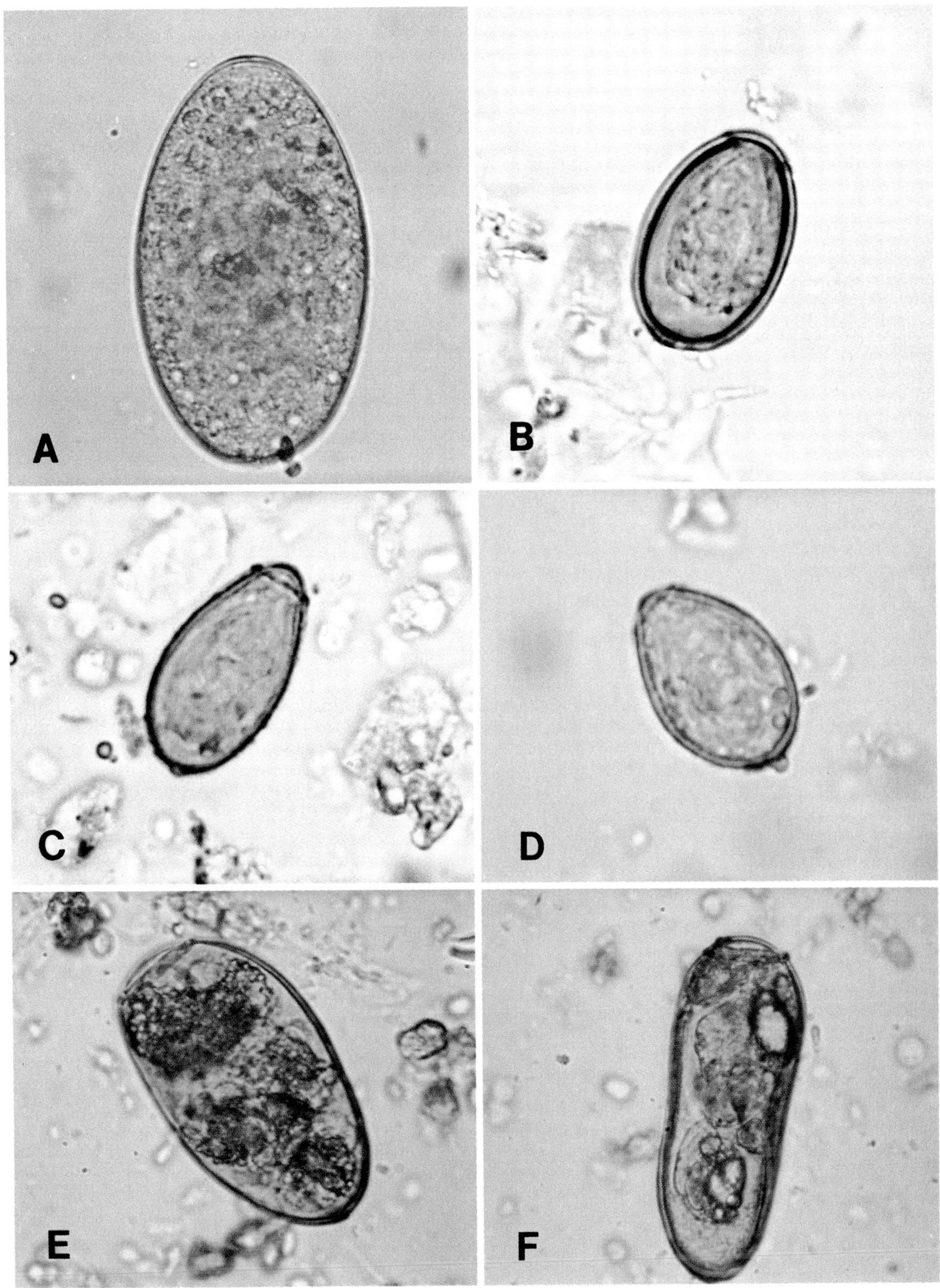

FIG. 4. Eggs of trematode parasites. (A) Egg of *Fasciolopsis buski* (×500). (B) Egg of *Heterophyes heterophyes* (×1,500). (C) Egg of *Clonorchis sinensis* (×1,500). (D) Egg of *Opisthorchis viverrini* (×1,500). (E) Egg of *Paragonimus westermani* (×600). (F) Somewhat atypical egg of *P. westermani* (×600). (Panels B through F from reference 2, used with permission.)

operculum characteristic of *Clonorchis* and *Opisthorchis* eggs. These eggs are usually passed in small numbers, and the infections are self-limiting, rarely lasting for more than several months.

Liver flukes

Fasciola hepatica. *F. hepatica* has a worldwide distribution in sheep- and cattle-raising areas of the world, where it causes occasional human infections. Infection is acquired by ingestion of aquatic vegetation, such as watercress in salads, on which metacercariae have encysted. Metacercariae migrate from the intestine to the bile ducts of the liver by passing through the intestinal wall into the abdominal cavity and entering the liver through its outer surface. As a consequence of this migration, migrating worms may end up in ectopic locations such as the body wall and cutaneous tissues. The prepatent period is approximately 3 months. Adult worms are large, fleshy flukes that may cause severe liver damage, particularly when present in large numbers.

Eggs are large, 130 to 150 µm long by 63 to 90 µm wide, are ovoid, and have a yellow-brown shell. There is an inconspicuous operculum, and the eggs are unembryonated when laid. These eggs are morphologically similar to *Fasciolopsis buski* eggs. Geographic history and symptomatology aid in diagnosis. Since the ingestion of eggs in infected cattle or sheep liver will result in the passage of these eggs in feces, it is necessary to rule out spurious infection by examination of feces several days after individuals have stopped eating liver.

Clonorchis sinensis. The so-called Oriental liver fluke is commonly seen in the United States, particularly in immigrants from Southeast Asia. *C. sinensis* and the closely related species *Opisthorchis viverrini* live as adults in the bile ducts of humans and reservoir host animals, including cats and dogs, throughout the Orient. Infections are acquired by ingestion of metacercariae encysted under the scales of fish that have been insufficiently cooked. Infections may persist for 20 years or longer. Pickled fish imported from the Orient have been occasional sources of human infection in the United States.

Diagnosis of infection depends on finding the characteristic eggs in feces. Embryonated *Clonorchis* eggs measure 27 to 35 µm long by 12 to 19 µm wide, are ovoid, and have a yellow-brown, moderately thick shell with a seated operculum (Fig. 4C). At the end opposite the operculum, there is usually a small knob or short, commalike extension of the shell. *Clonorchis* and *Opisthorchis* eggs (Fig. 4D) are similar in size and appearance to heterophyid eggs except that the latter lack the knob at the abopercular end and do not have a seated operculum.

Lung flukes

Paragonimus westermani. Human lung fluke infections are caused by a number of species of *Paragonimus* in various parts of the world. *P. westermani,* found in the Orient, is the most important species, but other species in Central and South America, Africa, and other parts of Asia are also responsible for human disease. Dogs, cats, and wild animals serve as reservoirs of infection. Adult flukes usually live in pairs in fibrous capsules in the lung parenchyma of their hosts. Eggs that are produced pass up the bronchial tree and may be found in sputum or in feces after they have been swallowed. Crabs and crayfish are second intermediate hosts, and human infections derive from eating raw or poorly cooked infected crustaceans.

In the human host, metacercariae migrate from the intestine into the body cavity through the diaphragm and invade the lungs, where the worms mature and lay eggs after 5 to 6 weeks. These infections may be long-lived, frequently 10 to 20 years. In the course of larval migration, the flukes may take aberrant migratory routes and end up in ectopic locations such as the body wall, the rib cage, and the brain. In the brain, the infection is frequently fatal.

Diagnosis depends on finding eggs in feces or, less frequently, in sputum. The broadly ovoid eggs are thick shelled, yellow-brown, and unembryonated and have a distinct operculum. They measure 80 to 120 µm long by 45 to 70 µm wide. At the abopercular end the shell is distinctly thickened but does not have a knob (Fig. 4E). Though the eggs of the other species of *Paragonimus* may differ somewhat in size, shape, and morphology, they are usually sufficiently similar that the diagnosis of paragonimiasis can be made (Fig. 4E and F).

Blood flukes (schistosomes)

Schistosomiasis (bilharziasis) afflicts more than 250 million people in the world and as such is, along with malaria, one of the most important of all human parasitic diseases. The etiologic agents are the blood flukes, which are markedly different from the other human trematodes. The schistosomes have separate sexes and live in blood vessels of the abdominal cavity. The three most important human schistosomes are *Schistosoma mansoni, S. japonicum,* and *S. haematobium;* there are a number of other species of lesser importance which infect humans in Africa and Asia. Though each of the schistosomes utilizes specific and different snail intermediate hosts, their life cycles are similar. Each produces thin-shelled eggs that lack an operculum and contain a miracidium when excreted in feces or urine. Infected snails produce fork-tailed cercariae which directly penetrate the skin and establish infection in human and animal hosts. In the mamalian host, the larval blood flukes migrate through the lungs and become established in venous blood vessels of the mesenteries or the bladder, where they mature and females deposit eggs. Through a mechanism not well understood, the eggs make their way through the wall of the intestine or bladder and pass in feces or urine. Pathology due to schistosome infection is primarily attributed to egg deposition in tissue at the site of adult worms or the areas of venous drainage (liver or lung).

S. mansoni. *S. mansoni* has the widest geographic distribution of the schistosomes, including Africa, the Arabian peninsula, Brazil, Surinam, Venezuela, Puerto Rico, and a number of Caribbean islands. Adult worms live in the portal system of the liver and the small venules of the lower ileum and colon. Eggs are laid in the blood vessels, make their way through the wall of the intestine, and are passed in feces. *S. mansoni* eggs measure 114 to 175 µm long by 45 to 70 µm wide; they contain a miracidium, and the shell has a prominent

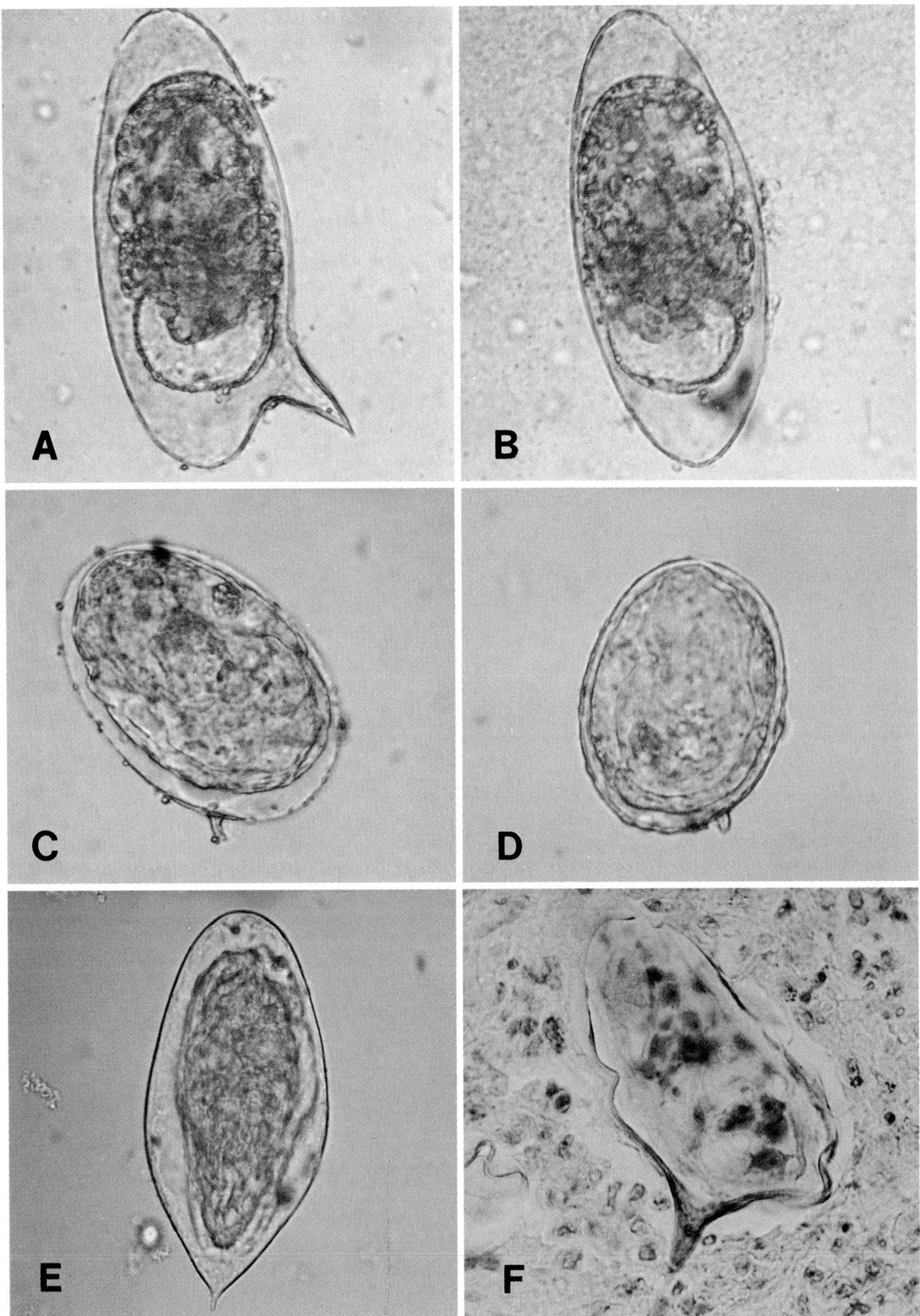

FIG. 5. Eggs of schistosome species (×600). (A) Egg of *Schistosoma mansoni.* (B) *S. mansoni* egg with typical lateral spine not in view. (C) *S. japonicum.* (D) *S. mekongi.* (E) *S. haematobium.* (F) *S. mansoni* egg showing lateral spine in tissue section. (Panels C through E from reference 2, used with permission.)

lateral spine (Fig. 5A and B). In acute schistosomiasis, blood and mucus appear in feces along with the lateral-spined eggs. The prepatent period for the infection is approximately 6 weeks. In chronic schistosomiasis, eggs will accumulate in the walls of the intestine and rectum and also the liver (Fig. 5F); correspondingly, fewer eggs will be found in feces, and concentration procedures will be required to diagnose infection reliably. Rectal biopsies may also be useful in diagnosis (see chapter 66).

S. japonicum. *S. japonicum* is found in China, the Philippines, and other countries of Southeast Asia. A zoophilic strain of the parasite infects animals but not humans in Taiwan, and the infection has been virtually eliminated from Japan, where occasional infections may be found in cattle. Animal reservoirs of infection are important and include water buffaloes, pigs, dogs, cats, and wild rodents. Adult worms live in mesenteric veins, and the prepatent period is 5 to 6 weeks. The embryonated eggs found in feces are round to ovoid, lack an operculum, and measure 70 to 100 μm long by 55 to 65 μm wide. The thin shell has a small, inconspicuous spine which frequently is not seen (Fig. 5C). In addition, the surface of the egg frequently has fecal debris adhering to it, which can make the eggs difficult to see or recognize. Rectal biopsy may be an important diagnostic tool when fecal examinations are negative.

S. mekongi. Closely related to *S. japonicum* but described as a separate species, *S. mekongi* is a parasite of humans and dogs in countries bordering on the Mekong River, specifically Laos and Kampuchea. The egg is similar in morphology to that of *S. japonicum* but smaller (9), ranging from 51 to 78 μm long by 39 to 66 μm wide. Eggs from dogs are usually smaller than those from human cases. There is a small, knoblike spine on the shell that may be difficult to see (Fig. 5D).

S. haematobium. *S. haematobium* occurs in Africa, Lebanon, Syria, Iran, the Arabian peninsula, and Malagasy, where it causes urinary schistosomiasis. Adult worms reside in the venous plexuses of the bladder, and eggs that are laid move through the wall of the bladder and pass in urine. In chronic infections, accumulation of eggs in the bladder wall can lead to bladder and ureter pathology. The thin-shelled eggs of the parasite measure 112 to 170 μm long by 40 to 70 μm wide, are embryonated, and have a terminal spine (Fig. 5E). Hematuria is frequently present with this infection, and diagnosis is made by finding eggs in urine sediment. Eggs can sometimes be found in feces and in the wall of the rectum as well as in the bladder.

S. intercalatum. *S. intercalatum* is a human schistosome that occurs in Zaire, Gabon, Cameroon, and the Central Africa Republic. The eggs of this species are found in feces and have a terminal spine and thus must be differentiated from *S. haematobium* eggs. Eggs are usually larger than those of *S. haematobium*, measuring 140 to 240 μm long by 50 to 85 μm wide.

CESTODES

The four most common adult tapeworm parasites of the human small intestine are *Diphyllobothrium latum, Taenia saginata, Taenia solium*, and *Hymenolepis nana*. Two other tapeworms, primarily animal parasites, reach maturity in humans and may cause infrequent infections; they are *Hymenolepis diminuta* and *Dipylidium caninum*. In addition to the adult tapeworms, a number of larval cestodes can produce serious human disease, including cysticercosis (*Taenia solium*), hydatid disease (*Echinococcus* spp.), and coenurosis (*Taenia multiceps*). The large adult tapeworms, *D. latum, T. saginata*, and *T. solium*, usually occur singly in the intestine and may live up to 20 years or longer. Diagnosis of tapeworm infections is achieved by finding characteristic eggs, proglottids, or both in feces, depending on the species involved. All of the adult tapeworms in humans require an intermediate host with the exception of *H. nana*, which may or may not utilize an intermediate host. Morphologically, adult tapeworms consist of the anterior head end or scolex; a short, undifferentiated neck region that gives rise to the proglottids; and the main body (strobila) of the tapeworm, consisting of immature, mature, and gravid proglottids. As tapeworms increase in age and size, the most posterior gravid proglottids may break off or disintegrate and pass in feces. Some tapeworms (*D. latum, H. nana*, and *H. diminuta*) lay eggs which pass in feces; others (*T. saginata* and *T. solium*) typically have proglottids which break off and pass in feces or actively migrate out of the anus. Sometimes *Taenia* proglottids rupture in the intestine, and eggs will then appear in feces. The eggs of all species of *Taenia* and the related genus *Echinococcus* are morphologically identical and cannot be distinguished from one another. The eggs of *T. solium, T. multiceps*, and *Echinococcus* spp. can infect humans directly and cause disease; the eggs of *T. saginata* are not directly infective to humans.

Diphyllobothrium latum

Known as the fish tapeworm, *D. latum* differs from other adult tapeworms infecting humans in its morphology, biology, and epidemiology. Its geographic distribution includes areas with cold, clear lakes as in Scandinavia, other areas of northern Europe, the USSR, northern Japan, and North America, principally the upper Midwest, Canada, and Alaska. The adult parasite can attain a length of 10 to 15 m, is ivory in color, and has a scolex that is provided with shallow grooves (bothria) on its dorsal and ventral aspects.

In its life cycle, unembryonated, operculate eggs, resembling those of trematodes, are passed in feces and must undergo embryonation in water for several weeks. Ciliated, six-hooked embryos (coracidia) hatch from these eggs and must be ingested by appropriate species of freshwater copepods. Within the copepod a solid-bodied larval stage, the procercoid, develops and becomes infective to the second intermediate host, fish. In fish, the procercoids migrate into the flesh and develop into the plerocercoid (sparganum) stage, which is then infective to the human or animal hosts. After ingestion of the sparganum stage, it takes 3 to 5 weeks for the adult tapeworm to attain maturity and begin to lay eggs. The parasite may produce no clinical symptoms in some people, but when it reaches a large size it may cause mechanical obstruction of the bowel, may cause diarrhea and abdominal pain, and in some individuals, particularly in northern European countries, may be responsible for a vitamin B_{12} deficiency resulting in pernicious anemia.

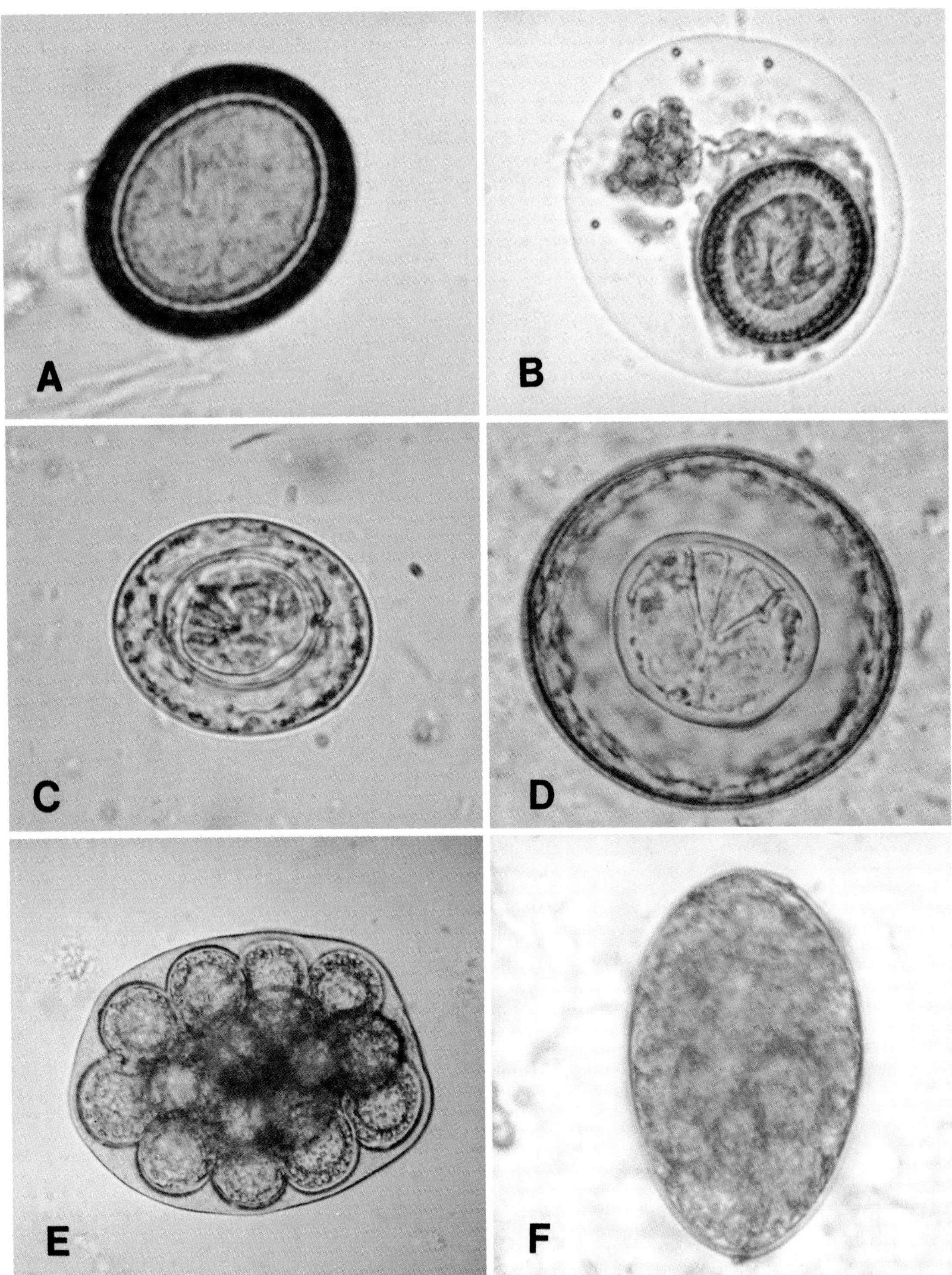

FIG. 6. Eggs of cestodes. (A) Egg of *Taenia* spp. Eggs of all species of *Taenia* and *Echinococcus* are identical (×1,000). (B) *Taenia* egg surrounded by the primary membrane frequently seen around eggs directly liberated from gravid proglottids (×800). (C) *Hymenolepis nana* (×900). (D) *Hymenolepis diminuta* (×900). (E) Egg packet of *Dipylidium caninum*. (F) *Diphyllobothrium latum* (×800). (Panels B through F from reference 2, used with permission.)

Diagnosis is made by finding the characteristic operculated eggs in feces. They measure 58 to 75 μm in length by 40 to 50 μm in width. At the abopercular end there is frequently a small knoblike protrusion (Fig. 6F). Individuals with longstanding infection are likely to have large numbers of eggs in feces. As infections grow older, one or a small chain of proglottids may break off and be passed in feces. These proglottids are wider than long (3 by 1 mm), and the genital pore is situated on the midventral surface rather than laterally as in the other human tapeworms. In freshly passed proglottids, the coiled uterus has a yellow-brown color in the center of the proglottid.

Taenia saginata

T. saginata, the beef tapeworm, has a worldwide distribution but is particularly prevalent in Mexico, South America, eastern and western Africa, and many countries of Europe. Cattle serve as the intermediate host, and ingestion of eggs on contaminated pastureland by grazing cattle results in the development in their tissues of the infective cysticercus stage (*Cysticercus bovis*).

The cysticercus is 0.5 to 2.0 mm in diameter and has a pearl-like appearance in tissues, where the unarmed scolex is invaginated into a fluid-filled bladder. After ingestion of the cysticercus in raw or poorly cooked beef, it takes approximately 2 to 3 months for the infection to become patent in the human host. Adult tapeworms attain lengths of 4 to 8 m and have a scolex with four suckers and an unarmed rostellum; gravid proglottids are longer than they are wide (18 to 20 mm by 5 to 7 mm). Each proglottid has a genital pore at the midlateral margin. In mature proglottids, the ovary has only two lobes and a vaginal sphincter muscle is present. Gravid proglottids, which are highly muscular and active, will break off from the strobila and can actively migrate out of the anus. Although patients may exhibit no symptomatology with this infection, the mature worm may cause abdominal discomfort, diarrhea, and occasionally intestinal obstruction as a result of its large size.

Diagnosis of species usually is made by identification of gravid proglottids that have been passed in feces or have actively migrated out of the anus. Identification of the proglottids is based on morphology of the uterus which has been either injected via the genital pore with India ink or stained with carmine or hematoxylin stains or on morphology after the specimen has been cleared (see chapter 66). In *T. saginata* there are 15 to 20 lateral branches on each side of the central uterine stem. If the proglottids rupture in the intestine, the typical *Taenia* eggs can be seen in feces, although specific identification on the basis of these eggs is impossible. Taeniid eggs are spherical and have a thick, yellow-brown, prismatic shell (Fig. 6A). Within the egg is a six-hooked embryo, the oncosphere. Occasionally, especially when eggs are liberated directly from proglottids, there is a thin outer membrane around the eggs (Fig. 6B). Eggs measure 31 to 43 μm in diameter.

It is generally accepted that the eggs of *T. saginata* are not directly infective to humans, but caution should be exercised in the handling of all proglottids and taeniid eggs since the eggs of *T. solium*, *T. multiceps*, and *Echinococcus* spp. are directly infective and can cause cysticercosis, coenurosis, and hydatidosis, respectively.

In Taiwan, the Philippines, and perhaps other parts of Southeast Asia there is a human tapeworm morphologically identical as an adult worm to *T. saginata*. With this species, however, the cysticercus stage is limited to the liver of pigs and less frequently cattle, and the scolex has hooklets. The adult stage of the tapeworm is not distinguishable from the typical *T. saginata*, including lack of hooks on the scolex. Studies are ongoing to determine the exact status of this parasite.

Taenia solium

Known as the pork tapeworm, *T. solium* has an extensive geographic distribution throughout Europe, Mexico, Central and South America, China, and India. It is no longer commonly found in the United States. Human infection is acquired by ingestion of infective cysticerci (*Cysticercus cellulosae*) in poorly cooked pork or pork products. The adult worms may reach lengths of 2 to 7 m; they have a scolex with four suckers and a rostellum armed with two rows of hooklets. In mature proglottids, the ovary has two lobes and an accessory lobe, and a vaginal sphincter muscle is lacking. Gravid proglottids have 7 to 13 lateral uterine branches off the central uterine stem. Since the eggs of *T. solium* are infective to humans and can cause cysticercosis, extreme caution in the handling of these proglottids is recommended (see chapter 70).

Hymenolepis nana

H. nana is the smallest of the adult tapeworms infecting humans, attaining lengths of 2.5 to 4.0 mm, and is the most common tapeworm infection of humans in the United States. Though it is normally a parasite of mice, in which the life cycle characteristically involves various beetles as intermediate hosts, transmission to humans, by direct ingestion of eggs containing six-hooked embryos, is common. When eggs are ingested by humans, a solid-bodied larva, the cysticercoid, first develops in the wall of the small intestine and subsequently migrates back into the intestinal lumen, where it reaches maturity as an adult tapeworm in 2 to 3 weeks. In beetles that ingest eggs of *H. nana*, the cysticercoids develop in the body cavity and have a thick protective wall about them. Although humans may acquire infection by accidental ingestion of infected beetles, direct infection is far more common and is the primary reason why *H. nana* usually occurs in institutional and familial settings where hygiene is substandard. A feature of human *H. nana* infection is the opportunity for internal hyperinfection, which may result in the presence of large numbers of adult tapeworms.

Diagnosis of *H. nana* infection rests on finding the spherical to subspherical, embryonated eggs in feces. The eggs are 30 to 47 μm in diameter and thin shelled, and they contain an oncosphere (Fig. 6C). There are two thickenings at opposite poles of the membrane around the embryo, and from these arise four to six polar filaments which extend into the space between the embryo and the outer shell.

Hymenolepis diminuta

An occasional human parasite, *H. diminuta* is primarily a parasite of rats. Beetles and other arthropods serve as obligatory intermediate hosts, with humans generally acquiring infection accidentally by ingestion of infected meal beetles present in various grains and cereals. Cysticercoids, the infective stage, develop in the hemocoel of beetles after ingestion of eggs. As an adult, *H. diminuta* may be 20 to 60 cm long, and numerous tapeworms may be present in the same host. In humans, hyperinfection or direct infection by ingestion of eggs, as occurs with *H. nana*, does not occur.

Diagnosis of *H. diminuta* infection is by demonstration of eggs in feces. The eggs are spherical and large, 70 to 85 μm by 60 to 80 μm, and have a yellow-brown, moderately thick shell (Fig. 6D). The six-hooked embryo in the egg is considerably separated from the outer membrane. Since there are no polar filaments, the combination of size and lack of these filaments allows for ready differentiation of these eggs from those of *H. nana*.

Dipylidium caninum

D. caninum is the most common and widespread adult tapeworm of dogs and cats. Human infection has been reported in many parts of the world. Children are more frequently infected as a result of more intimate contact with dogs and their fleas, which serve as obligatory intermediate hosts. Because the infection is not a troublesome one and is self-limiting, there are probably many more cases of it than are reported in the literature.

Adult tapeworms may be present in considerable numbers and may vary in length from 10 to 70 cm. The scolex is conical in shape, with four prominent suckers and a small retractile rostellum that bears multiple rows of small spines. Gravid proglottids are elongate (23 by 8 mm), have a genital pore on each lateral margin (hence the name double-pored tapeworm), and are divided into small compartments, each of which contains 8 to 15 six-hooked oncospheres that are enclosed in a thin, embryonic membrane. In dogs, proglottids are frequently passed in small chains; when they undergo dehydration on carpets and floors, they resemble grains of rice. In the life cycle, larval fleas ingest the eggs and cysticercoids develop in the hemocoel; the cysticercoids remain viable when larval fleas undergo metamorphosis to the adult flea, and human and animal infections usually are acquired by ingestion of the adult fleas. The tapeworms reach maturity in the small intestine in approximately 1 month.

Diagnosis of infection is usually made by finding the typical, double-pored, compartmented proglottids in feces or by finding packets of oncospheres liberated by disintegration of the proglottids (Fig. 6E).

LITERATURE CITED

1. **Ash, L. R., and T. C. Orihel.** 1987. Parasites: a guide to laboratory procedures and identification. ASCP Press, Chicago.
2. **Ash, L. R., and T. C. Orihel.** 1990. Atlas of human parasitology, 3rd ed. ASCP Press, Chicago.
3. **Cook, G. C.** 1987. *Strongyloides stercoralis* hyperinfection syndrome: how often is it missed? Q. J. Med. **64:**625–629.
4. **Cross, J. H., and V. Basaca-Sevilla.** 1989. Intestinal capillariasis. Prog. Clin. Parasitol. **1:**105–119.
5. **Genta, R. M.** 1989. Global prevalence of strongyloidiasis: critical review with epidemiologic insights into the prevention of disseminated disease. Rev. Infect. Dis. **5:**755–767.
6. **Pelletier, L. L.** 1984. Chronic strongyloidiasis in World War II Far East ex-prisoners of war. Am. J. Trop. Med. Hyg. **33:**55–61.
7. **Sadun, E. H., and D. M. Melvin.** 1956. The probability of detecting infections with *Enterobius vermicularis* by successive examination. J. Pediatr. **48:**438–441.
8. **Scowden, E. B., W. Schaffner, and W. J. Stone.** 1978. Overwhelming strongyloidiasis: an unappreciated opportunistic infection. Medicine **57:**527–544.
9. **Voge, M., D. Bruckner, and J. I. Bruce.** 1978. *Schistosoma mekongi* sp. n. from man and animals, compared with four strains of *Schistosoma japonicum*. J. Parasitol. **64:**577–584.
10. **Yoshikawa, H., M. Yamada, Y. Matsumoto, and Y. Yoshida.** 1989. Variations in egg size of *Trichuris trichiura*. Parasitol. Res. **75:**649–654.

Chapter 72

Arthropods of Medical Importance

HARRY D. PRATT AND JAMES W. SMITH

Arthropods may affect human health in several ways. Arthropods may transmit disease-causing pathogens mechanically, as when flies carry bacteria causing diarrhea and dysentery from filth to human food. Other arthropods are biological vectors in the transmission of viruses, bacteria, protozoa, and metazoa that cause human disease. For example, mosquitoes may transmit malaria parasites, or fleas may transmit bacteria causing plague (3, 16, 25).

Arthropods such as lice, scabies mites, and tissue-invading maggots also may be parasites on a patient. Others may attack a patient: mosquitoes, certain flies, fleas, bedbugs, some spiders, ticks, and mites, which bite with their mouthparts, or bees, wasps, and scorpions, which sting with an apparatus at their posterior end. Such bites or stings usually cause only temporary local swelling and itching which are treated with calamine or other soothing lotions, although secondary infection may occur. A few persons become sensitized to protein in the insect bite or sting, and if they are bitten or stung at a later date, these people develop larger, more severe welts around each lesion. For example, a person repeatedly infested with scabies mites may develop a generalized rash and intense itching over much of the body, not just in the areas of scabies mite infestation. A few people who are sensitized to the stings of bees, wasps, or hornets may, if stung again, have a severe anaphylactic reaction and may die. Such reactions usually occur within 1 h after the sting.

Arthropods are very widespread in the environment, and excrement and fragments of arthropods are present in soil and dust. Persons may become hypersensitive to these materials and develop allergic manifestations such as asthma and hay fever (6, 15, 16).

Parasitism by arthropod parasites that are attached to the skin or temporarily invade superficial tissues is generally called infestation. In contrast, parasitism of body tissues, intestine, or atria by protozoan or helminth parasites is generally called infection.

The arthropods are the largest of the animal phyla, with over a million species. It is beyond the scope of this chapter to deal with all of the arthropods of medical importance or the therapy and control of arthropod infestations. The most common ectoparasites submitted to laboratories for identification in the United States are discussed, and pictorial keys showing the principles of identification are presented. Microbiologists can recognized the major groups of arthropods sent to laboratories and in some cases, as with head or crab lice, can identify a specimen to the genus and species levels with reasonable confidence. Arthropods may be brought to the laboratory because a person wishes to know whether they are of concern and what might be done to control them. Some, such as cockroaches, clothes moths, termites, and stored-food insects, are widespread and require special literature on household pest control (4, 8, 28). More detailed information on arthropods of medical importance and their identification, treatment, and control is available in various references (4, 16, 25, 28, 36, 39).

PHYLUM ARTHROPODA

The phylum Arthropoda comprises invertebrate animals with a segmented body, several pairs of jointed appendages, and a rigid chitinous exoskeleton which is molted periodically and renewed as the animal grows. Two classes are of importance to the clinical microbiologist.

Arthropods develop from egg to adult through a developmental process known as metamorphosis, literally a change in form (4). Insects with gradual metamorphosis pass through three stages during their lives: egg, nymphs, and adult. Examples are sucking lice, bedbugs, and cockroaches. Nymphs are smaller but resemble adults. They change (metamorphose) gradually through a succession of molts until they become adults. In some with gradual metamorphosis, such as cockroaches and kissing bugs, the nymphs have wing pads while adults have wings. Nymphs are always sexually immature, while adults are sexually mature, ready to mate and reproduce. Nymphs have the same type of mouthparts as adults and live in the same environment, for example, head lice nymphs and adults on the scalp.

Insects with complete metamorphosis pass through four stages during their lives: egg, larva, pupa, and adult. Examples are flies, fleas, mosquitoes, and bees. Insects with this type of metamorphosis differ greatly in the immature and adult stages. Typical larvae are wigglers of mosquitoes, maggots of flies, and caterpillars of moths and butterflies. The pupa is a nonfeeding stage during which the larva undergoes profound external and internal changes to become the adult. Typically larvae have different mouthparts and live in a different environment than the adults.

Ticks and mites have a still different type of metamorphosis, typically with four stages: egg, larva, nymph (or several nymphal stages), and adults. Tick and mite larvae have three pairs of legs, while nymphs and adults have four.

Class Insecta

Representatives. Lice, bugs, fleas, flies, cockroaches, and others.

Characterization. As adults with three body regions (head, thorax, and abdomen), one pair of antennae, three pairs of legs, and wings in many species.

Medical importance. May be venomous or parasitic or acts as vectors of disease.

Class Insecta includes the following important species:

- Order Dictyoptera, family Blattellidae (cockroaches)
- Order Dictyoptera, family Blattidae (cockroaches)
- Order Hemiptera, family Cimicidae (bedbugs)
- Order Anoplura, family Pediculidae (human lice)
- Order Anoplura, family Pthiridae (crab lice)
- Order Siphonaptera, family Pulicidae (fleas)
- Order Diptera (flies, maggots)

Class Arachnida

Representatives. Ticks, mites, spiders, and scorpions.

Characterization. As adults with one or two body regions (cephalothorax and abdomen, or one body region in ticks and mites), no antennae, four pairs of legs, and no wings. Larvae of ticks and mites have only three pairs of legs.

Medical importance. May be venomous or parasitic or act as vectors of disease.

Class Arachnida includes the following important species:

- Order Araneida, family Theridiidae (black widow spider)
- Order Araneida, family Loxoscelidae (brown recluse spider)
- Order Acarina, family Ixodidae (hard ticks)
- Order Acarina, family Argasidae (soft ticks)
- Order Acarina, family Sarcoptidae (scabies mites)
- Order Acarina, family Demodecidae (follicle mites)
- Order Acarina, family Trombiculidae (chiggers)
- Order Acarina, family Dermanyssidae (rodent and bird mites)
- Order Acarina, family Pyroglyphidae (house dust mites)

SPECIMEN HANDLING AND EXAMINATION

Clinical microbiologists are often asked to identify arthropods or arthropod larvae. Specimens of ectoparasites should be preserved and shipped for identification in 70% ethyl alcohol (Formalin is irritating to the eyes of the identifier). Fly larvae should be washed in water to remove debris, particularly those collected from fecal samples or wounds, and then killed in hot (not boiling) water (about 80°C) for a few minutes so that they do not become dark when placed in 70% alcohol.

Most ectoparasites can be identified with a dissecting microscope with magnifications of ×25 to ×75 power. However, some may have to be mounted on microscope slides and examined with a compound microscope. Some fleas, fly larvae, lice, and mites may have to be treated overnight with cold 10% potassium or sodium hydroxide to remove the internal flesh and permit better visibility of key characters. Such specimens can then be washed in water, dehydrated serially in 70% ethyl alcohol, Cellosolve, and clove oil, and then mounted in Canada balsam as permanent slides. Quick nonpermanent mounts can be made with commercially available clearing and mounting medium, such as Hoyer mounting medium, or by mounting the specimen directly in 85% lactic acid in water (39).

Assistance in identifying arthropods may be obtained from entomologists in public health laboratories, educational institutions, natural history museums, or agriculture extension agencies.

COCKROACHES, ORDER DICTYOPTERA

(4, 7, 8, 12, 16, 25, 28, 34, 36)

Over 3,500 species of cockroaches have been described for the entire world, but less than 1% are domiciliary, and only about 8 are commonly found in buildings in the United States (Fig. 1). Cockroaches are often more important pests in hospitals and laboratories than are flies, fleas, or lice.

Cockroaches are usually classified in the order Orthoptera, but many modern authorities place them in the order Dictyoptera, suborder Blattaria (34). Cockroaches are flattened dorsoventrally like a pancake, with long, filiform antennae, and legs adapted for running. They vary in size from immatures 1 to 2 mm long to giant tropical species 75 mm or more in length. Cockroaches develop by gradual metamorphosis with three stages in the life cycle: eggs in a capsule, nymphs without wings which are sexually immature, and adults, usually with wings, which are sexually mature. They have chewing mouthparts and feed on many types of organic matter, including fecal material loaded with pathogens.

Five species of cockroaches are commonly found in buildings in the United States and throughout the world. They can be divided into two groups: the small species less than 15 mm long in the family Blattellidae include the German and brown-banded cockroaches; and the large species more than 15 mm long in the family Blattidae include the Oriental, American, and smoky brown cockroaches (Fig. 1).

The German cockroach (*Blattella germanica*) is easily recognized by its small size (adults are 10 to 13 mm long) and the two black longitudinal bars on the pronotum of both nymphs and adults. The National Pest Control Association considers this the number one pest in buildings in this country, especially prevalent in kitchens and bathrooms.

The brown-banded cockroach (*Supella longipalpa*, formerly *Supella supellectilium*) receives its name from the brown bands across the wings of the adult or the thorax and abdomen of the nymph. The adult averages 10 to 13 mm long and has a single broad, dark, longitudinal strip in the middle of the pronotum. It is found in many parts of the buildings besides the kitchen and bathroom and often chews the bindings of books in laboratories and offices.

The Oriental cockroach (*Blatta orientalis*) is a large, entirely dark insect; adults are 18 to 24 mm long. The male has short, truncate wings extending two-thirds to three-fourths the length of the abdomen, and the female has short, triangular wing pads. The Oriental cockroach is more abundant in the cooler parts of the United States and is found particularly in kitchens, basements, and sewers.

The American cockroach (*Periplaneta americana*) is the largest cockroach commonly found in buildings; adults are 27 to 35 mm long. This chestnut brown species has indistinct yellowish markings on the pronotum, wings of the adult extending beyond the tip of the abdomen, and cerci tapering, the last segment twice as long as wide. It is found throughout buildings, but it prefers warm, damp basements, steam tunnels, and sewers.

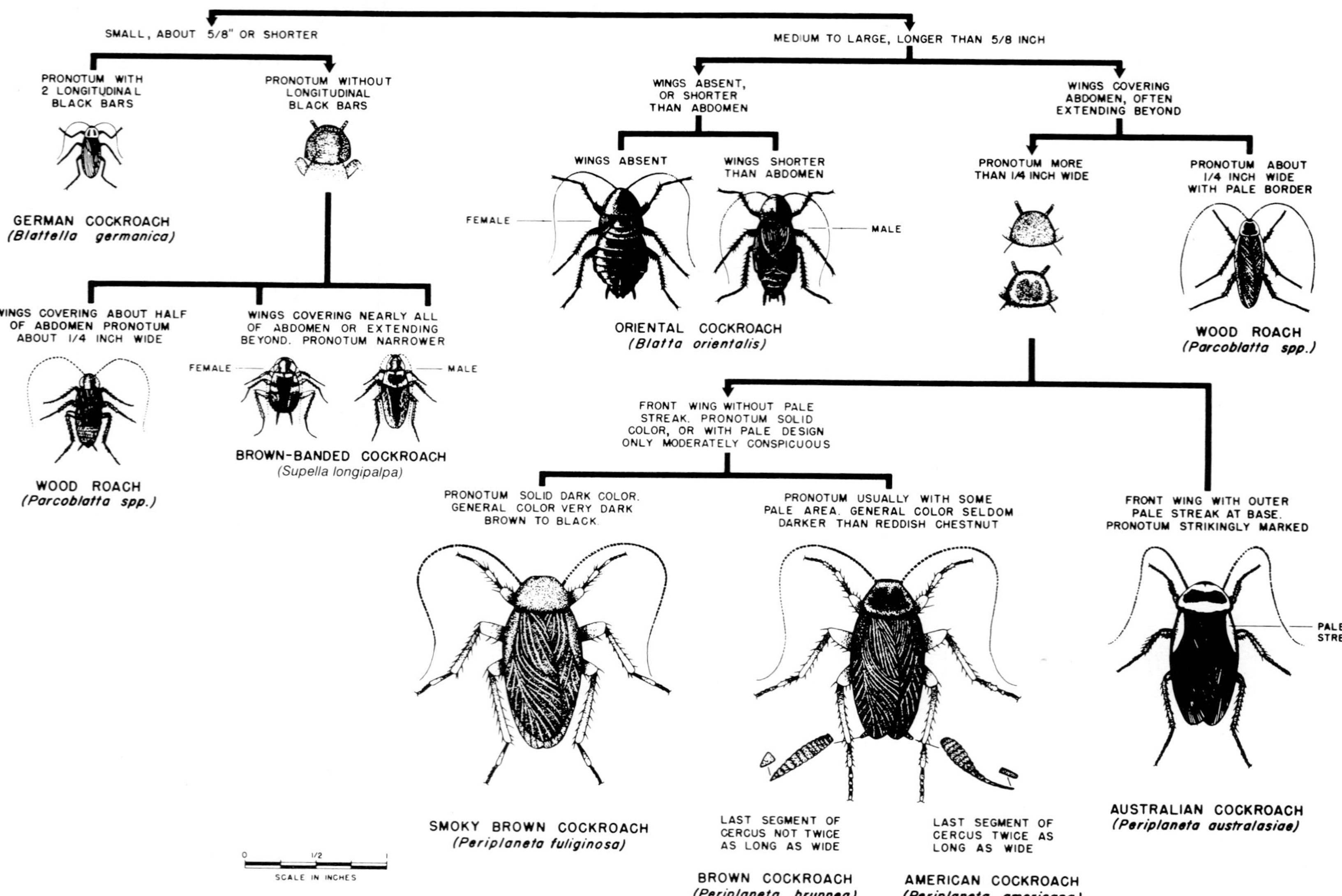

FIG. 1. Pictorial key to some common species of cockroaches (8).

The smoky brown cockroach (*Periplaneta fuliginosa*) is a large, entirely dark species with wings extending beyond the tip of the abdomen. It is an outdoor species found in the southern United States that invades buildings in warm weather, particularly in suburban areas with considerable vegetation near the buildings.

Cockroaches are repulsive pests which taint an area with a repugnant odor and foul with excrement all surfaces with which they come in contact. They may be carriers of salmonellae, a cause of food poisoning. Although a variety of aerosols, dusts, and residual sprays are available for private individuals and professional pest control technicians, there are many places with computers, television sets, and delicate electronic equipment where the use of small, plastic bait boxes containing hydramethylnon or other pesticides or sticky cockroach traps should be used.

BEDBUG, ORDER HEMIPTERA

(4, 5, 16, 25, 28, 36)

The bedbug (*Cimex lectularius*) is a reddish brown insect 4 to 5 mm long, with a pair of four-segmented antennae and a three-segmented, blood-sucking proboscis which lies in a groove on the underside of the head and thorax (Fig. 2). It has short wing pads but cannot fly. The pronotum is broad and concave on the anterior margin. The abdomen is flattened and somewhat heart shaped.

Normally, bedbugs feed at night and hide during the day in cracks and crevices in bedsteads, in seams or tufts of mattresses, or under loose wallpaper in bedrooms. However, infestations also occur in overstuffed chairs, sofas, and furniture in theaters and clubs. Sometimes the first signs of these insects are tiny spots of blood on bedding or the dead insects themselves, killed as people crushed them rolling in their sleep. Some people are very sensitive to bedbug bites and have reddish wheals as big as a quarter or half dollar, while other people are hardly aware of them. In addition to causing local lesions, bedbugs can cause nervous disorders and sleeplessness in children and adults. Although bedbugs feed repeatedly on humans, they have not been incriminated in the transmission of any disease.

HUMAN LICE, ORDER ANOPLURA

(4, 5, 16, 20, 25, 26, 28, 32, 35, 36)

The sucking lice are small, wingless, dorsoventrally flattened insects belonging to the order Anoplura. They differ from other ectoparasites by their specialized legs, each ending in a single (usually curved) claw. This claw and the opposing thumblike process enable lice to cling to hair or fibers of clothing or bedding. Three types of sucking lice are specific parasites of humans, usually but not always confined to a certain part of the body. They are named according to the region of the body that they infest or their general appearance: head louse, body louse, and pubic or crab louse (Fig. 3).

The head louse (*Pediculus humanus capitis*) is 1 to 2 mm long, with three pairs of legs of approximately equal size and an elongate abdomen with slightly darkened margins but without lateral hair tufts. The adults and immatures, called nymphs, are found on the head and neck, particularly behind the ears and on the back of the neck. The eggs, called nits, are glued to the hairs.

The body louse (*Pediculus humanus humanus*) is usually 2 to 4 mm long, with three pairs of legs of approximately equal size and an elongate abdomen with pale margins but without lateral hairy tufts. The adults and immatures are found on the hairy parts of the body below the neck and frequently rest on clothing when they are not feeding. Typically the eggs are laid on clothing, particularly along the seams.

The pubic or crab louse (*Pthirus pubis*) is 0.8 to 1.8 mm long, with the first pair of legs much smaller and more slender than the second and third pairs of legs, and having a short crablike abdomen with lateral hairy tufts. The adults and immatures are typically found on the pubic (hence the species name "pubic louse") and anal areas of the body or on other parts of the body with widely spaced hairs, such as the chest, armpits, mustaches, beard, eyebrows, or eyelashes. The eggs are glued to hairs.

These three species can be identified by referring to Fig. 3.

Body lice are the vectors of pathogens that cause epidemic typhus, epidemic relapsing fever, and trench fever. Fortunately, none of these diseases occurs in the United States today. Infestations with body lice are not common in this country, possibly as a result of the widespread use of automatic washing machines and hot-air dryers to launder clothing regularly. However, infestations of crab lice are reported frequently, possibly as a result of a more permissive society in recent years. Crab lice usually are transmitted from person to person during sexual intercourse; rarely are they acquired from infested toilet seats.

Epidemics of head lice are reported frequently in the United States and in many other parts of the world, particularly among schoolchildren who wear infested garments such as caps, scarves, and other clothing left in crowded cloakrooms, use infested combs or brushes, or lie on infested carpet, beds, or other upholstered furniture. In examining a person for head lice, check especially the area behind the ears and on the back of the neck, looking for adults and nymphs on the scalp and nits on the head hair. Head lice attach their eggs to hairs very close to the scalp, normally within 0.25 in. (ca. 0.6 cm) of the scalp surface. Hatched eggs will be 0.5 in. (ca. 1.3 cm) or more from the scalp—the so-called half-inch rule for determining whether nits are live. The best method for determining whether the eggs have hatched is to examine them with a hand lens or under a dissecting microscope. Live eggs have an embryo inside and a cap (or operculum); hatched eggs have no cap. It is important to differentiate nits from hair casts and globs of hair spray (32) (Fig. 3).

FLEAS, ORDER SIPHONAPTERA

(4, 5, 7, 8, 13, 16, 17, 25, 28)

Fleas are small, wingless insects with bodies compressed from side to side and long legs adapted for jumping. The name of the flea order, Siphonaptera, refers to their blood-sucking or "siphoning" mouthparts and to their lack of wings. They vary from 1 to 8.5 mm in length, averaging about 2 to 4 mm. Fleas develop through complete metamorphosis, with four stages in the life cycle: egg, larva, pupa, and adult. Fleas often cause loss of blood, irritation, and extreme discomfort. Public health workers are concerned with fleas as vec-

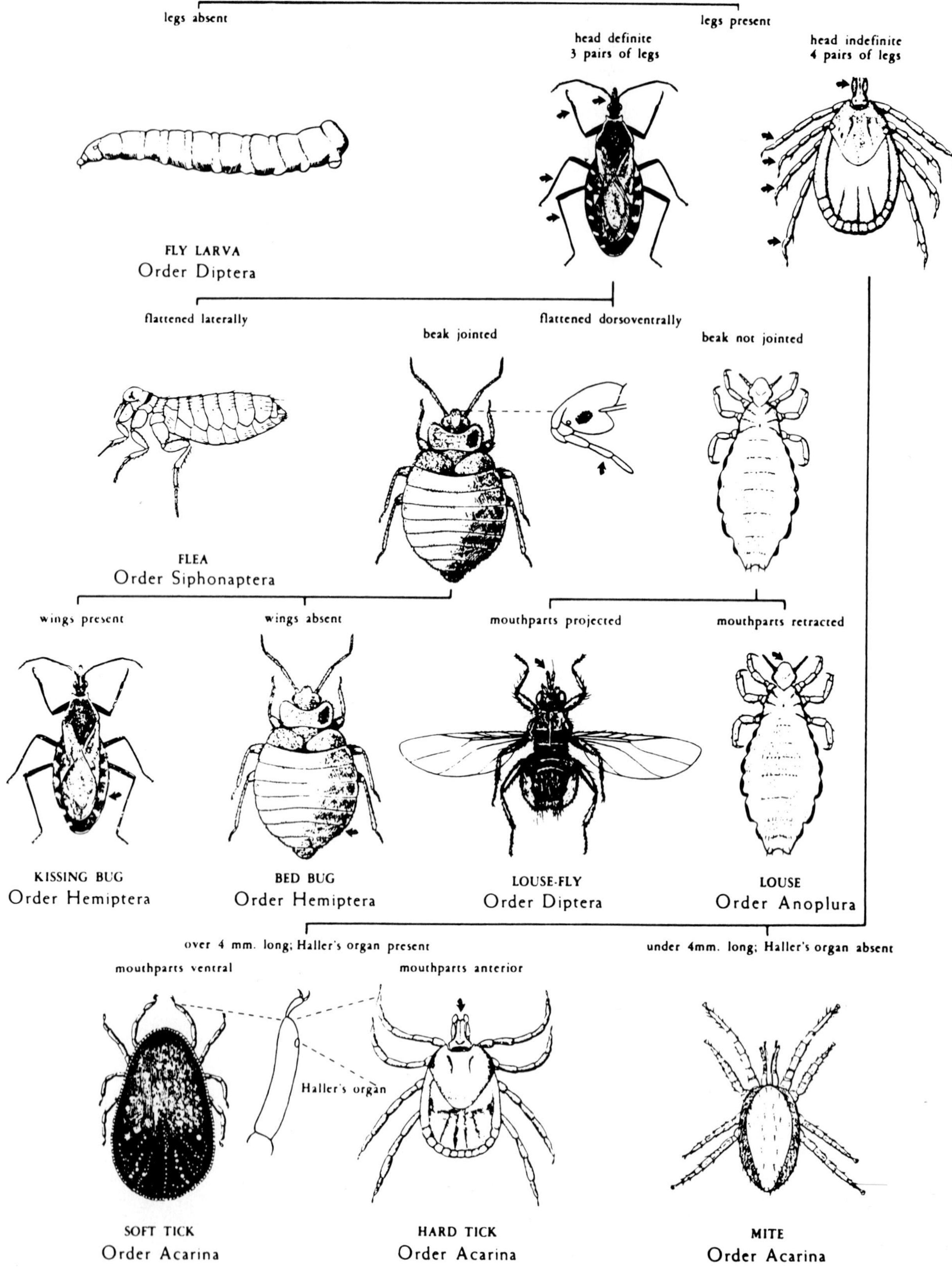

FIG. 2. Pictorial key to common groups of human ectoparasites (C. J. Stojanovich and H. G. Scott, Centers for Disease Control, Atlanta, Ga.).

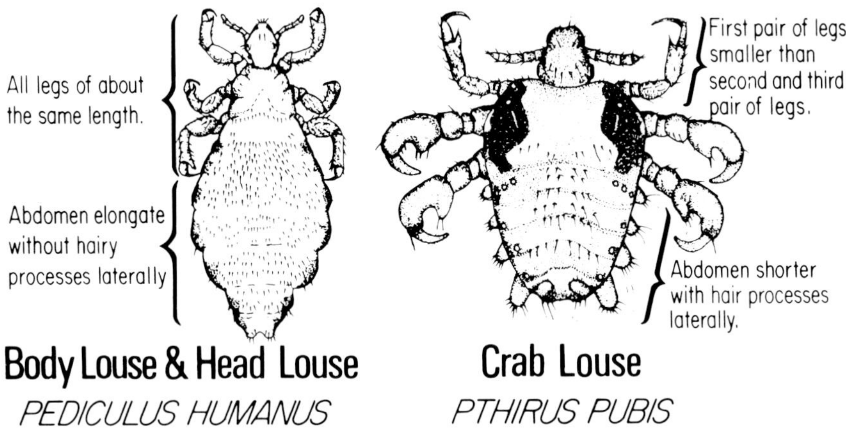

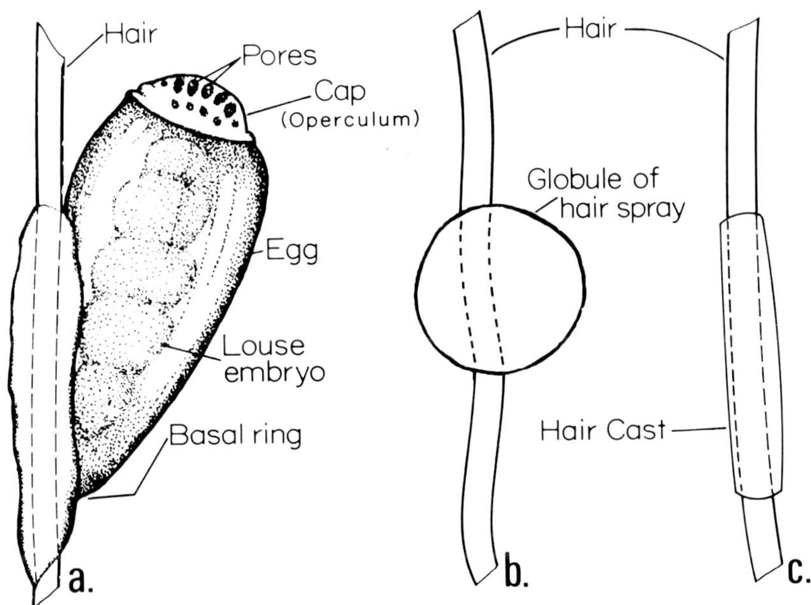

FIG. 3. Identification characteristics of lice and nits commonly found on humans. The upper figures show the important identifying characteristics of adult lice. In the lower figure are shown (a) an egg (nit) and (b) a globule of hair spray and (c) a hair cast, which must be differentiated from the nit (H. D. Pratt and K. S. Littig, Centers for Disease Control, Atlanta, Ga.).

tors of plague and flea-borne or murine typhus from rats to humans and as vectors of rural or sylvatic plague among wild rodents and occasionally to humans. In addition, fleas are intermediate hosts for the double-pored dog tapeworm (*Dipylidium caninum*) and two rodent tapeworms (*Hymenolepis diminuta* and *Hymenolepis nana*) that occasionally infect humans (16, 25). In the United States, most problems with fleas occur when persons are bitten by dog or cat fleas. This is more frequent when the preferred host (dog or cat) is no longer available, as when the animal dies or leaves home.

Causative organisms

The important structures used in identifying fleas are shown in Fig. 4. The presence or absence of the genal or pronotal combs, the shape of the head and spermatheca in the female, the length of the labial palpi, and the number and position of bristles on the head, abdomen, and tarsi offer important characters of identification.

The Oriental rat flea (*Xenopsylla cheopis*) is the chief vector of the rickettsiae causing flea-borne or murine typhus from rats to humans. It was the most important species transmitting urban plague in the United States during the period 1900 to 1925. The Oriental rat flea normally parasitizes Norway and roof rats, but it bites humans readily. It has neither genal nor pronotal combs, the front margin of the head is rounded and the thorax is of normal length, the mesopleuron is divided by a vertical thickening, the ocular bristle is inserted in front of the eye, and the female has a large, dark, C-shaped spermatheca (Fig. 4).

The cat flea (*Ctenocephalides felis*) and the dog flea (*Ctenocephalides canis*) both have genal and pronotal

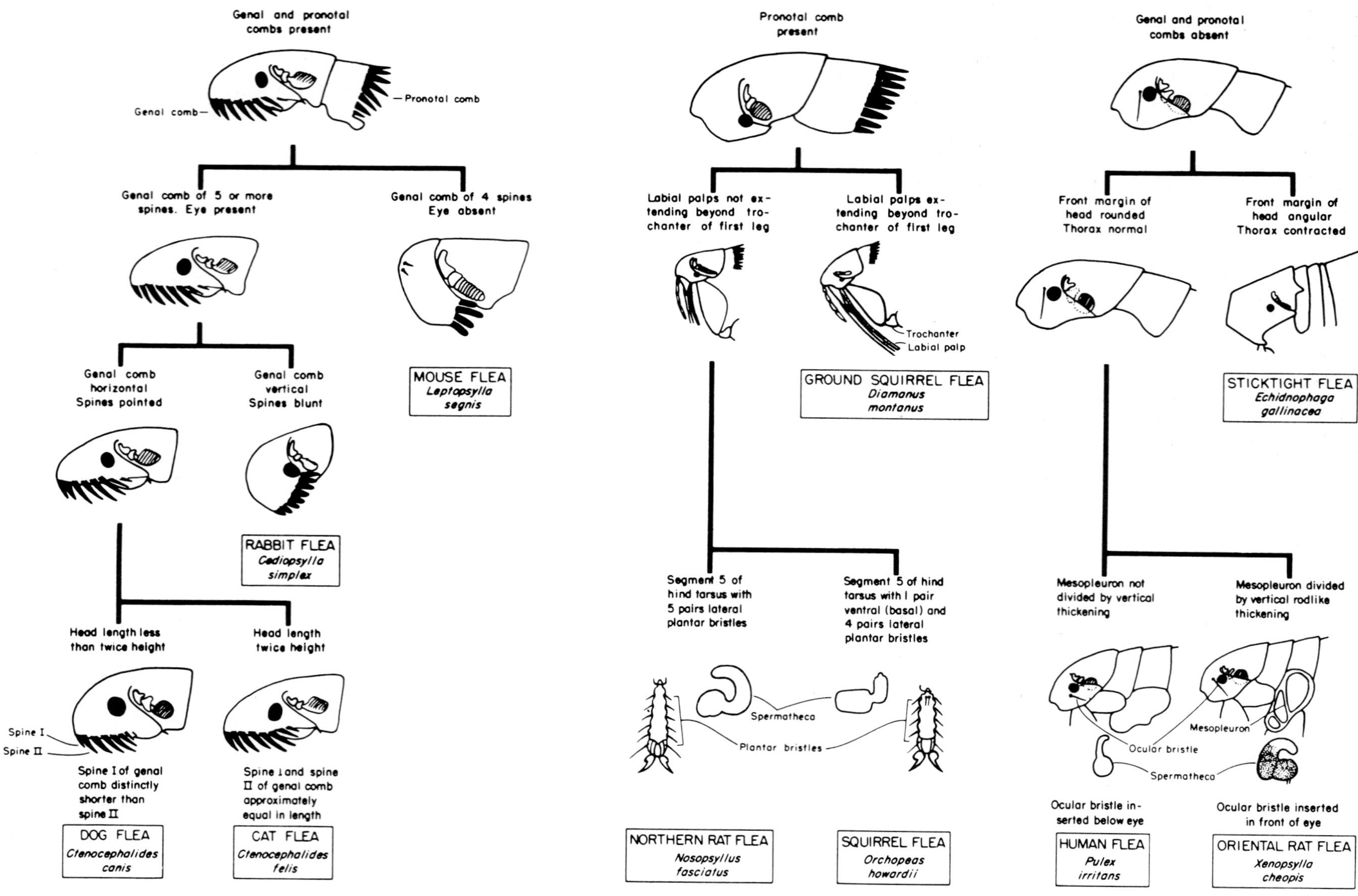

FIG. 4. Pictorial key to some common fleas in the United States (H. D. Pratt, Centers for Disease Control, Atlanta, Ga.).

combs, each with seven or eight pointed black teeth on each side of the body (Fig. 4). The head of the cat flea is about twice as long as it is high and the first two spines of the genal comb are almost the same length, whereas the head of the dog flea is less than twice as long as it is high and the first spine of the genal comb is definitely shorter than the second. It is usually not necessary to distinguish between these two species because they have similar habits and both species attack cats, dogs, rats, and humans.

FLY MAGGOTS, ORDER DIPTERA
(2, 4, 6, 8, 19, 25, 36)

Flies belong to the insect order Diptera, or two-winged insects. Flies develop by complete metamorphosis, with four stages in the life cycle: egg, larva, pupa, and adult. Fly larvae are often called maggots. Clinical microbiologists may receive specimens of fly larvae submitted from wounds or sinuses, the umbilical area of newborn babies, or stool or urine samples.

A typical muscoid fly larva is legless and somewhat cone shaped, with a narrow anterior end bearing the mouthparts and anterior spiracles and a broader posterior end with two prominent posterior spiracles (Fig. 5). The structure of the mouthparts and the anterior and posterior spiracles provide characters used in identification. Most muscoid fly larvae are rather similar and are identified by characters shown in Fig. 6. Two types easily recognized with the naked eye are the lesser house fly and latrine fly (*Fannia* spp.), which have prominent lateral processes, and the rat-tailed maggot (*Eristalis tenax*), which has a long, telescopic respiratory tube.

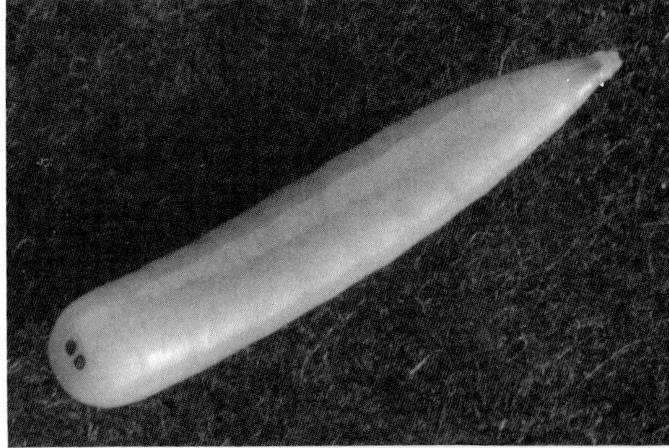

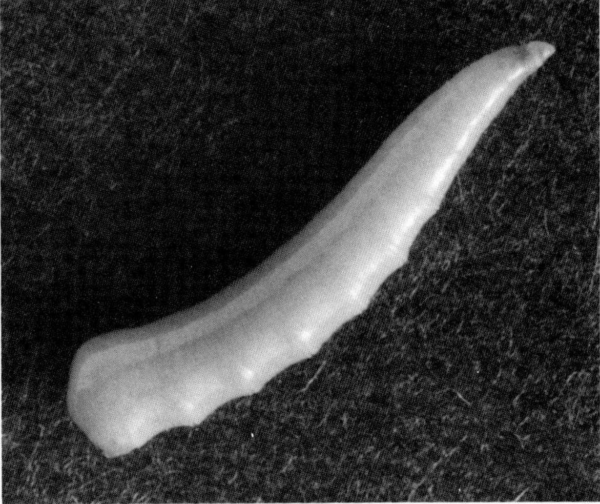

FIG. 5. Larva of house fly, *Musca domestica*. Dorsal view (above) and lateral view (below) with dark spiracles evident at posterior end (left) and mouthparts at anterior end (right).

Clinical manifestations and epidemiology

Infestation with fly maggots causes a condition known as myiasis, in which the fly larvae feed on living or dead tissues of humans or on food in the human intestinal tract. A number of terms have been used to describe the various types of myiasis, depending on the location of the fly larvae: enteric or gastrointestinal (digestive tract); dermal, subdermal, or cutaneous (skin); auricular (ear); ocular (eye); nasopharyngeal (nose); and urinary or urogenital (urogenital tract) (19).

Fly larvae in the alimentary canal cause nausea, pain in the abdomen, diarrhea, dysentery (with actual discharge of blood as a result of injury to the intestinal mucosa), and nervousness. Fifty species of fly larvae have been reported, either positively or questionably, from cases of enteric myiasis in humans (19). Many of these cases involved flies which lay their eggs or larvae on fish, cold meat, cheese, ripe fruit, and other foods. Normally such eggs or larvae are destroyed by the digestive juices in the human alimentary tract. However, there are apparently reliable records of living larvae found in the stool or vomit or both. These cases include children who drank "dirty water" from a ditch or container containing rat-tailed maggots (*Eristalis*) and people who ate meat or fish containing larvae (*Sarcophaga*).

Laboratory workers should be very careful in reporting enteric myiasis. Stool samples can easily be contaminated in the laboratory, particularly by flesh flies (*Sarcophaga* spp.), which are strongly attracted by the smell of feces. Flesh flies lay larvae rather than eggs, and the first two larval stages are often completed in a day, so that it is possible to find third-stage larvae in stool samples only 1 day old. In cases of "questionable enteric myiasis," a second stool sample should be passed in a fly-free room and the material should be examined at once.

Although myiasis due to maggots feeding on dead tissue may be found in wounds when dressings or casts are removed, invasive disease with maggots invading living tissue is uncommon in the United States. On the other hand, in the tropics of Central and South America, Africa, and Asia, humans may develop skin infestations with fly larvae causing painful, festering "boils." The spiracles of the fly larvae are usually evident, since the larvae depend on outside air for respiration. In these days of rapid airplane transportation, we have seen larvae of the human bot fly (*Dermatobia hominis*) pressed from "boils" on people who were infected earlier in Central or South America when bitten by a mosquito, fly, or tick carrying the human bot fly egg. People who have flown back from Africa to the United States have been shocked to press from a "boil" a larva of the tumbu fly (*Cordylobia anthropophaga*). In these cases, in confirming the identification of the fly larva, it has been most helpful to the laboratory worker to ask the patient, "Where have you been recently?," since these flies do not occur in the United States. Good identification keys,

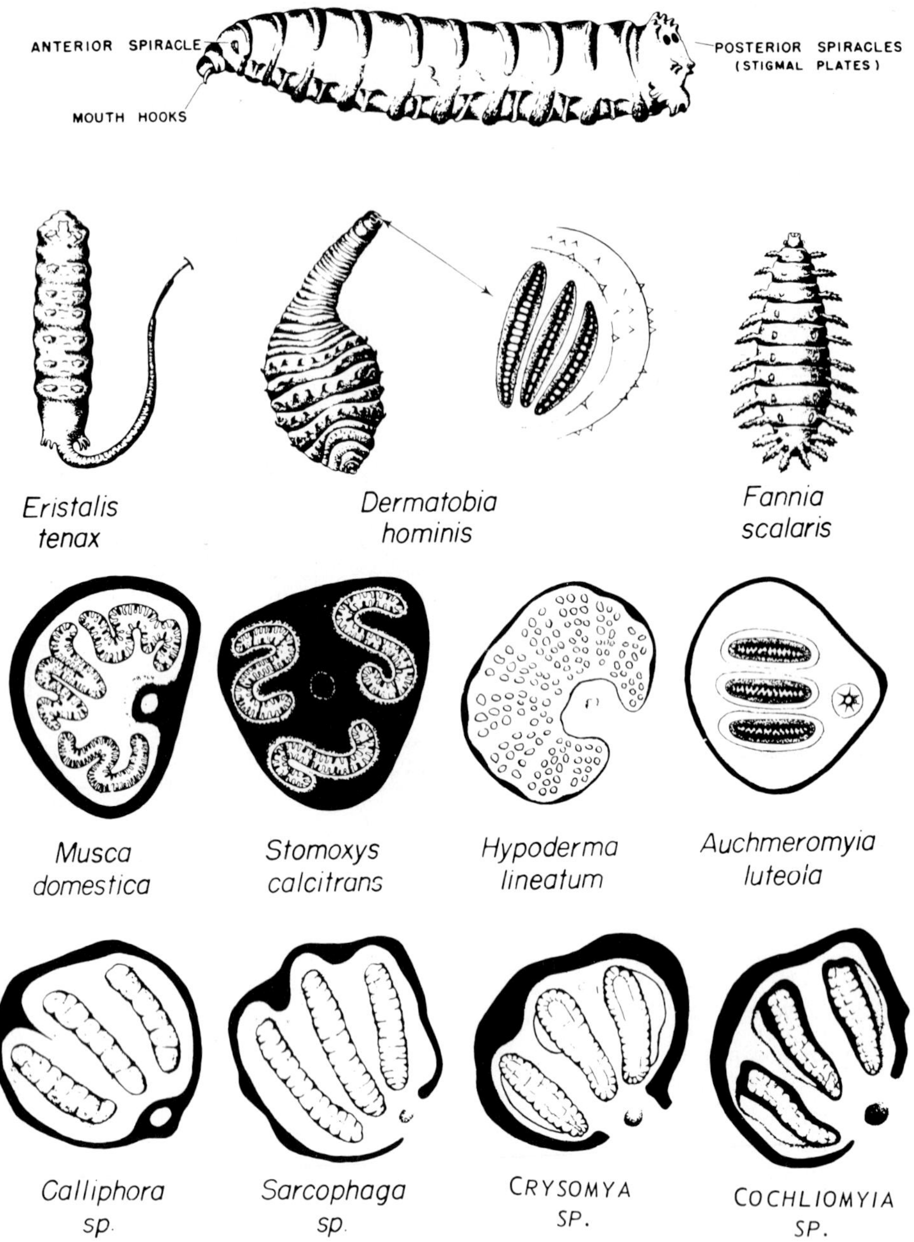

FIG. 6. Key characters of myiasis-producing fly larvae (Centers for Disease Control, Atlanta, Ga.). Top, Mature larva of a muscoid fly (from R. Hegner et al., © 1938 by D. Appleton-Century Co., Inc., New York).

illustrations, and accounts of the biology of these flies are found in James (19), Harwood and James (16), and Smith (36).

SPIDERS, ORDER ARANEIDA

(5, 8, 13, 16, 22, 36)

Spiders are readily identified by a number of characters: eight legs, no antennae, body divided into two regions (cephalothorax and abdomen) joined by a narrow pedicel, and unsegmented abdomen with spinnerets at the tip. All spiders kill their prey by biting and injecting venom. Therefore, it is not surprising that there are reports of some 50 species of spiders biting humans, usually in self-defense (13). In most cases the bite is no worse than the sting of a bee or wasp, with some redness, swelling, and pain for a few hours, but it can occasionally be more severe. However, the bite of two spiders, the black widow spider and the brown recluse spider (and their relatives), can cause serious illness or death, as discussed below.

The black widow spider (*Latrodectus mactans*) is easily recognized in all stages by the orange or reddish hourglass marking on the ventral side of the abdomen (Fig. 7). Females vary from 5 to 13.5 mm in body length, with a globose, shiny black abdomen with one or more reddish dots on the dorsal side and all-black legs. Males and immatures are smaller than the females and have additional reddish or pale spots on the abdomen and

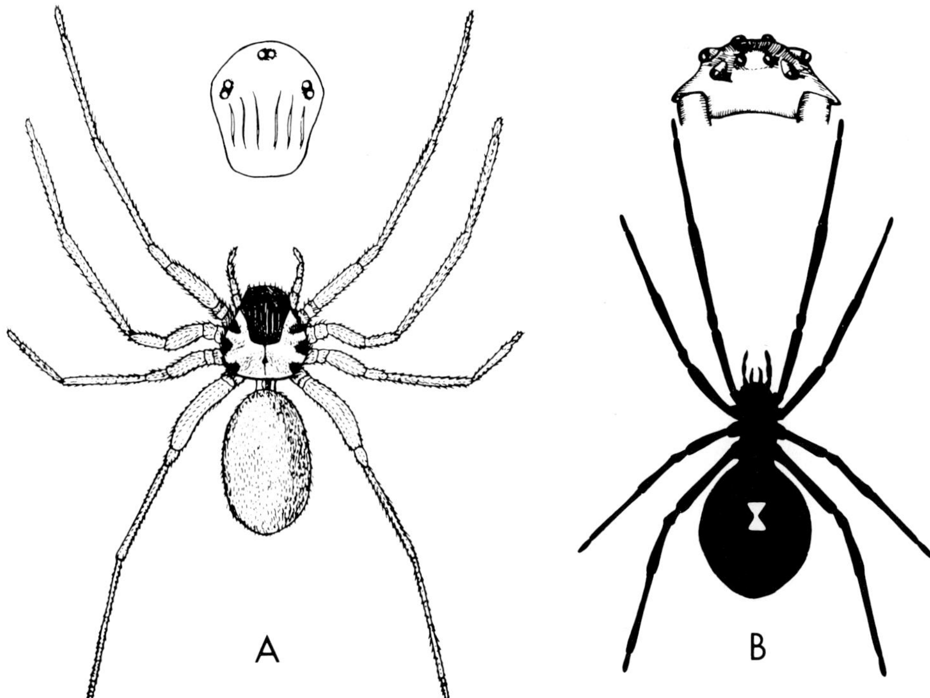

FIG. 7. Key characters of *Loxosceles reclusa* (brown recluse spider) and *Latrodectus mactans* (black widow spider). The brown recluse (A) has a fiddle-shaped marking on the cephalothorax and has six eyes in three pairs. The black widow (B) has a red hourglass on the underside of the abdomen and has eight eyes (Centers for Disease Control, Atlanta, Ga.).

banded legs. The venom injected by the female is a neurotoxin and can cause severe pain within an hour, a "boardlike abdomen," severe illness for a day or more, or even death. In the United States, the venom of four other species of *Latrodectus*, *L. bishopi*, *L. geometricus*, *L. hesperus*, and *L. variolus*, also can cause illness.

The brown recluse or violin spider (*Loxosceles reclusa*) is a brownish species with two characteristics in combination: a dark fiddle or violin marking on the tan or brownish cephalothorax, and six eyes arranged in three pairs forming a semicircle (Fig. 7). The body is 8 to 9 mm long. The venom injected by the female or male is a necrotoxin which causes necrotic lesions with deep tissue damage that extend for several days after the initial bite, heal very slowly (often 6 to 8 weeks or longer), and leave disfiguring scars. In the United States, the venom of three other species of *Loxosceles*, *L. arizonica*, *L. deserta*, and *L. laeta*, can also cause serious illness and leave ugly scars.

TICKS, ORDER ACARINA (4, 5, 8–11, 14, 16, 18, 23, 24, 28, 36, 37, 38, 40–42)

Ticks are blood-sucking arachnids that are ectoparasites of many vertebrates such as reptiles, birds, mammals, and humans. Ticks have a four-stage life cycle: egg; six-legged larva; eight-legged, sexually immature nymph; and eight-legged, sexually mature adult. Usually a blood meal is necessary for the larva to molt to become a nymph, and another blood meal is needed for the nymph to molt before becoming an adult. Hard ticks have only one nymphal stage, whereas soft ticks may have more than one.

There are two families of ticks (Fig. 8): hard ticks in the family Ixodidae and soft ticks in the family Argasidae. Hard ticks have a hard dorsal plate or scutum, and the mouthparts are clearly visible from above. Soft ticks have a leathery body but no hard plate on the dorsal part of the body, and the mouthparts are located ventrally and are not visible from above. Both hard and soft ticks can bite humans and can cause painful, itching lesions.

Causative organisms

Four important species of hard ticks in the United States are the American dog tick (*Dermacentor variabilis*), the Rocky Mountain wood tick (*Dermacentor andersoni*), the lone star tick (*Amblyomma americanum*), and the brown dog tick (*Rhipicephalus sanguineus*). In addition, several species of the genus *Ixodes* are important as vectors of Lyme disease. Ticks in the genera *Dermacentor* and *Amblyomma* are often called "ornate" ticks because they have whitish markings on the scutum easily seen with the naked eye, hand lens, or stereoscopic microscope. The ticks in the other genera of North American hard ticks do not have these whitish markings and are called "inornate" ticks.

The American dog tick (*D. variabilis*) is found in most of the eastern United States and in limited areas on the Pacific Coast, in northern Idaho, and in eastern Washington. Small males of these brownish ticks may be only

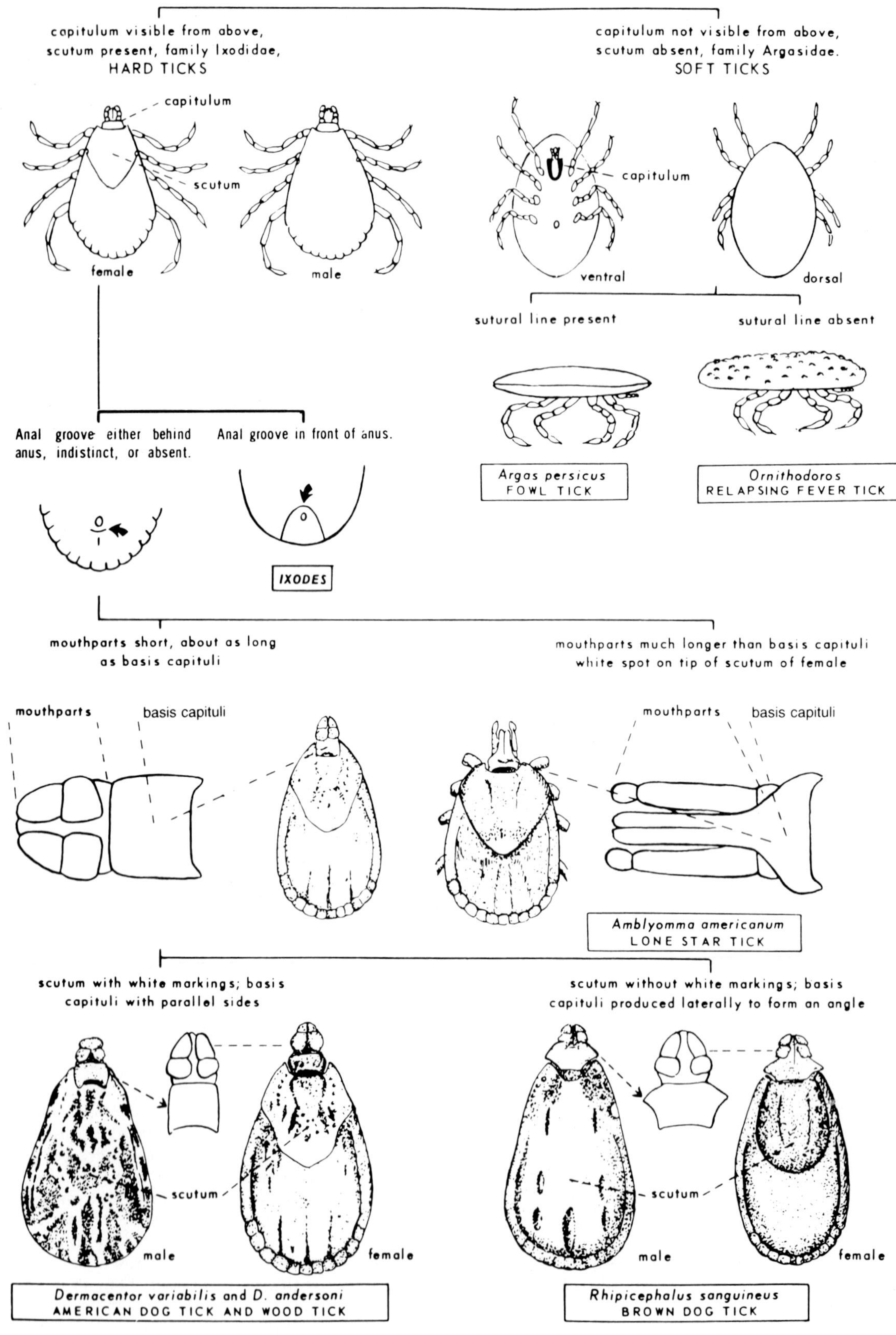

FIG. 8. Pictorial key to some common ticks.

3 mm long, whereas engorged females may grow from 5 to 13 mm or more in length. As shown in the pictorial key (Fig. 8), the mouthparts (palpi and hypostome) are about as long as the basis capituli, and the sides of the basis capituli are parallel. The scutum has diffuse whitish markings that may be faint or well defined. The fine punctuation, called goblets, on the spiracular plates on the underside of the abdomen, behind and lateral to the fourth pair of coxae, is finer in *D. variabilis* than in *D. andersoni*. The American dog tick is the important vector of Rocky Mountain spotted fever in the eastern United States. It may also transmit pathogens causing tularemia and Q fever.

The American dog tick, Rocky Mountain wood tick, and lone star tick all have been reported to cause tick paralysis. After these ticks feed for several days, they inject a toxin which causes an ascending flaccid paralysis that can progress to death. The paralysis can be reversed by removal of the tick. Use forceps to remove the tick by a slow steady pull that will not break off the mouthparts and leave them in the wound. Sometimes a drop of chloroform, ether, alcohol, Vaseline, or fingernail polish will help make the tick detach its mouthparts. After removal of the tick, the wound should be disinfected.

The Rocky Mountain wood tick (*D. andersoni*) is similar to the American dog tick. However, the whitish markings on the scutum are generally more evident, and the goblets on the spiracular plate are larger and less numerous than in the American dog tick. *D. andersoni* is the major vector of Rocky Mountain spotted fever and Colorado tick fever in the Rocky Mountain region. It may transmit tularemia, Q fever, and Powassan encephalitis and may cause tick paralysis.

The lone star tick (*A. americanum*) has mouthparts much longer than the basis capituli. The female has a conspicuous whitish marking on the scutum, from which is derived the name "lone star tick," for the Lone Star State of Texas. This tick may serve as a vector for Rocky Mountain spotted fever and tularemia and may cause tick paralysis. Unlike the American dog and Rocky Mountain wood ticks, whose larvae and nymphs do not normally feed on humans, the larvae, nymphs, and adults of the lone star tick all feed on persons. There are many reports of people who were bitten by lone star tick larvae and nymphs and developed severe itching and redness comparable to attacks of chiggers.

The brown dog tick (*R. sanguineus*) rarely bites humans in North America. However, it is commonly found on dogs and in buildings where both dogs and humans live. It is an inornate brown species which varies from 3 mm long when unengorged to 13 mm or more in engorged females. The sides of the basis capituli are angled. It is not uncommon to find larvae, nymphs, and adults of the brown dog tick in homes, kennels, veterinary hospitals, or laboratory animal houses, because all stages obtain their blood meals from dogs. The brown dog tick is probably the vector from dog to dog, but not from dog to humans, of *Ehrlichia canis*, which causes human ehrlichiosis (14, 25).

The deer tick (*Ixodes dammini*) often bites humans in the United States from March to December. It transmits protozoan parasites (*Babesia microti*) that cause human babesiosis and spirochetes (*Borrelia burgdorferi*) that cause Lyme disease. The black-legged tick (*Ixodes scapularis*) may be the vector of Lyme disease in the southern United States, and *Ixodes pacificus* is the vector in the west. Other species of *Ixodes* are the vectors in Europe, Asia, and Australia. Lyme disease is now the most commonly reported tick-borne disease in the United States, with about 5,000 cases in 1988, and the most prevalent tick-borne illness in the world (4, 37, 38).

Several other species of *Ixodes* are of considerable interest because of their role in the transmission of Powassan encephalitis and other diseases. *Ixodes* ticks are easily recognized because they have the anal groove curved in a U shape in front of the anus, whereas other genera of hard ticks have the anal groove behind the anus or absent. Species identification of ticks in the genus *Ixodes* is difficult, and the services of a specialist may be required (11, 23, 24).

Soft ticks in the genus *Ornithodoros*, family Argasidae, transmit relapsing fever spirochetes (*Borrelia* spp.) in limited areas in 13 western states. These ticks are dull-colored, leathery species with the mouthparts on the underside of the body, not visible from above. In the United States, at least four species of *Ornithodoros* (*O. hermsi*, *O. parkeri*, *O. talaje*, and *O. turicata*) are proven vectors of *Borrelia* spp., which cause tick-borne relapsing fever. Their identification requires specialized literature (10). Many of these cases of relapsing fever were contracted in rural cabins inhabited by small rodents, such as chipmunks. As they slept, people were bitten by infected relapsing fever ticks which came from rodent nests in the cabins (41).

MITES, ORDER ACARINA
(1, 2, 5, 8, 16, 21, 25, 27, 31, 33)

Mites are tiny arthropods with eight legs in the adult stage, a saclike body, and no antennae. Clinical laboratories may be requested to identify mites which parasitize humans. Because of their small size, mites are generally difficult for the nonspecialist to identify. However, well-mounted specimens of the more common and important parasitic mites may be identified by reference to pictorial keys (Fig. 9) or to illustrations in specialized literature (1, 8, 27). Some of the most important mites are discussed below.

The scabies, itch, or mange mite (*Sarcoptes scabiei*) causes an infectious skin disease called scabies, mange, or "the itch." Diagnosis is made by locating the mite, usually a female with an egg, in a papule or vesicle in the epidermis or in a tiny burrow in the superficial skin. In young children, the mites may be found on any part of the body. In adults, up to 80% of the mites occur on some part of the hands or arms, particularly the webbing between the fingers or the folds of the wrists, on the external genitalia of males, and on the breasts of women. Mellanby (29) recommends teasing the mite from its burrow or papule with a needle (or cutting a tiny bit of skin with a razor blade), mounting the specimen on a slide with a cover glass, and then examining it under a compound microscope. Muller et al. (30) prefer scraping the skin with a sharp scalpel with a drop of mineral oil and then examining this liquid with a microscope having a magnification of at least 50 diameters. The mites average 0.3 to 0.4 mm in length, with an oval saclike body in which the first and second pairs of legs are widely separated from the third and fourth pairs (Fig. 9). The mouthparts at the anterior end have che-

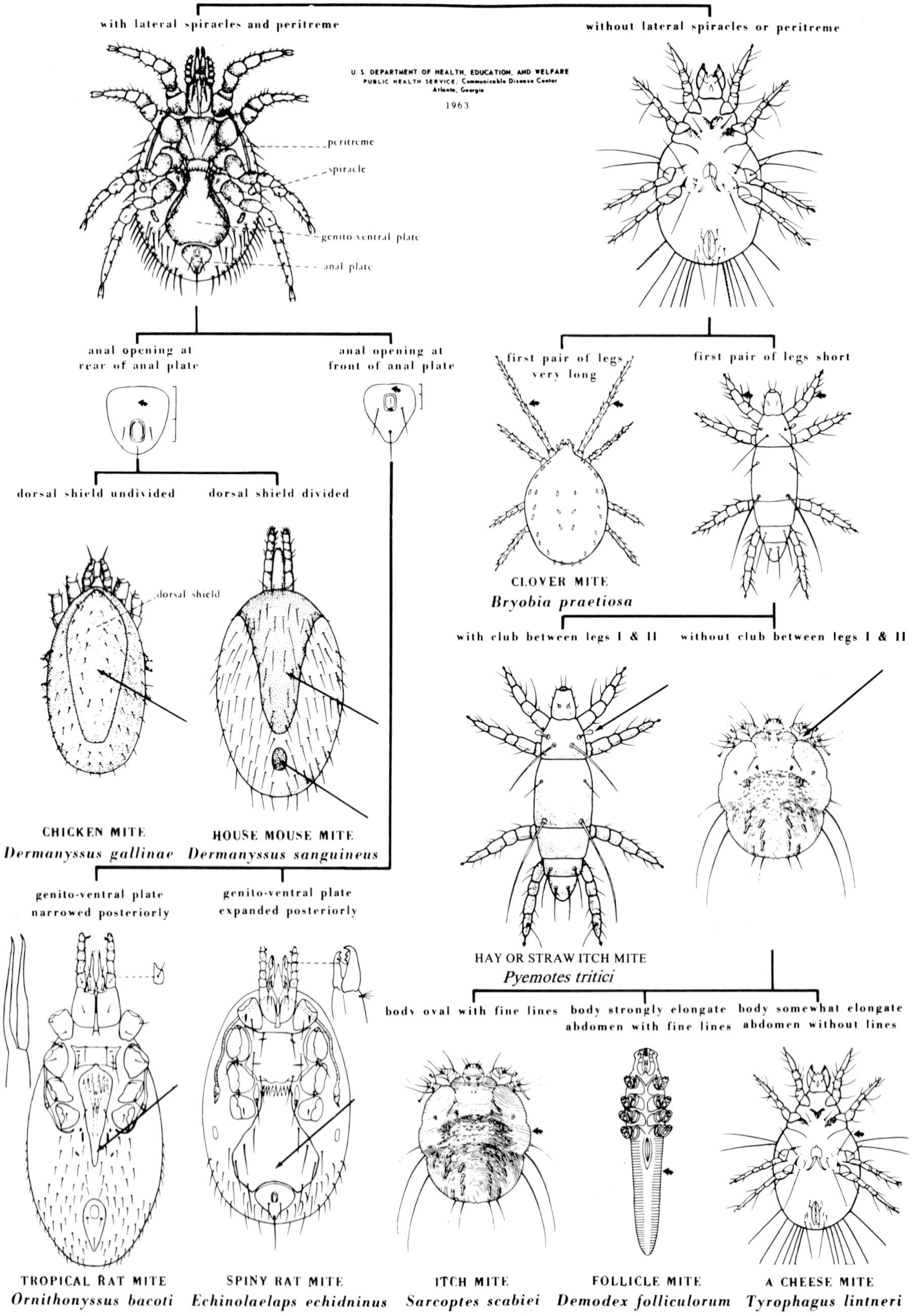

FIG. 9. Pictorial key to some mites of public health importance (H. G. Scott and C. J. Stojanovich, Centers for Disease Control, Atlanta, Ga.).

licerae and palpi, and the anus is at the posterior end. The skin has fine wrinkles on the dorsal side, with a number of prominent blunt spines and many backward-projecting triangular points.

The scabies mites cause intense itching and rash, particularly at night. In a previously unexposed individual, a month or more may elapse between initial infestation and onset of symptoms; in reinfested persons, rash and itching may develop quickly after penetration of even a single mite, suggesting that both the itching and rash are due to hypersensitivity to the mite. Although the majority of the papules or burrows with mites are found on the hands or arms, the "scabies rash" has a characteristic distribution in the armpits, waist, buttocks, inner thigh, and ankles, areas that do not correspond with the location of the mites.

Scabies is often considered to be a "family disease," with mites transferred from husband to wife, or from one child to another, by simple contact such as touching or shaking hands. The disease is also acquired through sexual contact. Outbreaks may occur in hospitals or institutions. If one member of a family or group of persons has scabies, it is advisable to treat all close contacts (29, 31, 33).

The hair follicle mite (*Demodex folliculorum*) and the sebaceous gland mite (*Demodex brevis*) are microscopic, cigar-shaped creatures with eight stumpy legs and annulate abdomens. They are found in hair follicles and sebaceous glands, particularly on the nose and face. They probably infest over half of middle-aged adults. The infestation is usually asymptomatic but may be associated with blackheads. The mites may be squeezed out of hair follicles, often by pressing with a slide against the nose, or they may be incidental findings in histological sections of facial skin (33).

Chiggers are larvae of mites in the family Trombiculidae. In Asia, these mites are vectors of scrub typhus. In other parts of the world, trombiculid mites infest grass and bushes, and their six-legged larvae, i.e., chiggers (red bugs, harvest mites), may attack humans. Mite larvae appear as tiny reddish dots attached to skin, usually in areas where clothing is tight, such as the ankles at the tops of socks, or skin touched by belts or elastic bands. Sensitive individuals react to the secretions of the larvae with swollen itching areas at the sites of attachment which persist for days. Scratching may lead to secondary infections. The six-legged larvae have characteristic branched, featherlike hairs. The eight-legged nymphs and adults are nonparasitic vegetarians.

The straw or hay itch mite (*Pyemotes tritici*) normally is a parasite of insect larvae which infest straw, hay, grains, wood, and other plant products. These mites may attack people who handle these products, such as people sleeping on hay or crawling under houses infested with wood borers, and may cause severe itching and rash. Adult mites have a characteristic club-shaped hair between the first and second pairs of legs. In gravid females, the abdomen becomes enormously enlarged, resembling a small pearl (33).

Mites of the family Dermanyssidae are normally parasites of rodents or birds but may attack people, causing dermatitis. People raising domestic fowl may suffer from attacks of the chicken mite (*Dermanyssus gallinae*), northern fowl mite (*Ornithonyssus sylviarum*), or tropical bird mite (*Ornithonyssus bursa*). These same species are often parasites of birds nesting in buildings, such as pigeons, starlings, or sparrows, and may leave the bird nest and attack people.

The tropical rat mite (*Ornithonyssus bacoti*) is a common parasite of rats, particularly in the southern United States. There are many reports of this species attacking humans when rats are killed in buildings. The mites leave the dead animal and seek a blood meal from the nearest warm-blooded animals, people.

The house mouse mite (*Liponyssoides sanguineus*), often reported as belonging to the genera *Allodermanyssus* or *Dermanyssus*, is a parasite of house mice. It is sometimes abundant in buildings in the northeastern United States and may transmit the rickettsiae causing rickettsial pox from mice to people (36).

Grain and cheese mites are frequently found in tremendous numbers in flour, grain, cheese, and dried fruits, particularly when humidity and temperatures are high. Some of these mites may cause dermatitis among persons who handle these infested foods.

In recent years, there have been many reports of allergic reactions to mites (entire or in fragments) and their excreta that produce conditions similar to asthma in some persons. The chief offenders seem to be the house dust mites (*Dermatophagoides farinae* and *Dermatophagoides pteronyssoides*), which occur in great numbers in dust from mattresses and bedroom floors and in smaller numbers in other parts of houses (4, 27).

LITERATURE CITED

1. **Baker, E. W., T. M. Evans, D. J. Gould, W. B. Hull, and H. L. Keegan.** 1956. A manual of parasitic mites of medical or economic importance. National Pest Control Association, Inc., New York.
2. **Beaver, P. C., R. C. Jung, and E. W. Cupp.** 1984. Clinical parasitology, 9th ed. Lea & Febiger, Philadelphia.
3. **Benenson, A. S.** 1985. Control of communicable diseases in man, 14th ed. American Public Health Association, Inc., Washington, D.C.
4. **Bennett, G. W., J. M. Owens, and R. M. Corrigan.** 1988. Truman's scientific guide to pest control operations. Edgell Communications, Duluth, Minn.
5. **Borror, D. J., N. F. Johnson, and C. A. Triplehorn.** 1989. An introduction to the study of insects, 6th ed. Saunders College Publishing Co., Philadelphia.
6. **Brown, H. W., and F. A. Neva.** 1983. Basic clinical parasitology, 5th ed. Appleton-Century-Crofts, Norwalk, Conn.
7. **Busvine, J. R.** 1980. Insects and hygiene. Chapman & Hall, Ltd., London.
8. **Communicable Disease Center.** 1967. Pictorial keys: arthropods, reptiles, birds, and mammals of public health significance. Communicable Disease Center, Atlanta, Ga.
9. **Cooley, R. A.** 1938. The genera *Dermacentor* and *Otocentor* (Ixodidae) in the United States with studies in variation. Natl. Inst. Health Bull. no. 171.
10. **Cooley, R. A., and G. M. Kohls.** 1944. The Argasidae of North America, Central America, and Cuba. Am. Midl. Nat. Monogr. 1.
11. **Cooley, R. A., and G. M. Kohls.** 1945. The genus *Ixodes* in North America. Natl. Inst. Health Bull. no. 184.
12. **Cornwell, P. B.** 1968. The cockroach, a laboratory insect and an industrial pest. Rentokil Library, Hutchinson, London.
13. **Ebeling, W.** 1975. Urban entomology. Division of Agriculture Sciences, University of California, Richmond.
14. **Fishbein, D. B., L. A. Sawyer, C. J. Holland, E. D. Hayes, W. Okoroanyanwu, D. Williams, K. Sikes, M. Ristic, and J. E. McDade.** 1987. Unexplained febrile illnesses after exposure to ticks: infection with an *Ehrlichia*. J. Am. Med. Assoc. **257**:3100–3104.
15. **Frazier, C. A., and P. K. Brown.** 1980. Insects and allergy

and what to do about them. University of Oklahoma Press, Norman.

16. **Harwood, R. F., and M. T. James.** 1979. Entomology in human and animal health, 7th ed. Macmillan Publishing Co., New York.
17. **Holland, G. P.** 1949. The Siphonaptera of Canada. Canadian Department of Agriculture Tech. Bull. no. 70.
18. **Hoogstraal, H.** 1981. Changing patterns of tickborne diseases in modern society. Annu. Rev. Entomol. **26:**75–99.
19. **James, M. T.** 1948. The flies that cause myiasis. USDA miscellaneous publication no. 631.
20. **Juranek, D. D.** 1984. *Pediculus capitis* in school children: epidemiologic trends, risk factors, and recommendations for control, p. 199–211. *In* M. Orkin and N. L. Maibach (ed.), Cutaneous infestations and insects bites. Marcel Dekker, Inc., New York.
21. **Juranek, D. D., R. W. Currier, and L. E. Millikan.** 1984. Scabies control in institutions, p. 139–158. *In* M. Orkin and N. L. Maibach (ed.), Cutaneous infestations and insect bites. Marcel Dekker, Inc., New York.
22. **Kaston, B. J.** 1978. How to know the spiders, 3rd ed. W. C. Brown Co., Dubuque, Iowa.
23. **Keirans, J. E., and C. M. Clifford.** 1978. The genus *Ixodes* in the United States: a scanning electron microscope study and key to the adults. J. Med. Entomol. 1978, Suppl. 2.
24. **Keirans, J. E., and T. R. Litwak.** 1989. Pictoral key of the adults of hard ticks, family Ixodidae (Ixodida: Ixodoidea) east of the Mississippi river. J. Med. Entomol. **26:** 435–448.
25. **Kettle, D. S.** 1982. Medical and veterinary entomology. John Wiley & Sons, Inc., New York.
26. **Kim, K. C., H. D. Pratt, and C. J. Stojanovich.** 1986. The sucking lice of North America. Pennsylvania State University Press, University Park.
27. **Kratz, G. W.** 1978. A manual of acarology, 2nd ed. Oregon State University Book Store, Corvallis.
28. **Mallis, A. (ed.).** 1982. Handbook of pest control. Franzak and Foster, Cleveland.
29. **Mellanby, K.** 1972. Scabies. E. W. Classey, Ltd., Hampton, Middlesex, England.
30. **Muller, G., P. H. Jacobs, and N. E. Moore.** 1973. Scraping for human scabies. Arch. Dermatol. **107:**70.
31. **Orkin, M., and H. I. Maibach.** 1985. Cutaneous infestations and insect bites. Marcel Dekker, Inc., New York.
32. **Osgood, S. B., W. B. Jellison, and G. M. Kohls.** 1961. An epidemic of pseudopediculosis. J. Parasitol. **47:**985–986.
33. **Parish, L. C., W. B. Nutting, and R. M. Schwartzman.** 1983. Cutaneous infestation of man and animal. Praeger, New York.
34. **Pratt, H. D.** 1988. Annotated checklist of the cockroaches (Dictyoptera) of North America. Ann. Entomol. Soc. Am. **81:**882–885.
35. **Pratt, H. D., and K. S. Littig.** 1973. Lice of public health importance and their control. Center for Disease Control, Atlanta, Ga.
36. **Smith, K. G. V. (ed.).** 1973. Insects and other arthropods of medical importance. British Museum (Natural History), London.
37. **Spielman, A.** 1988. Lyme disease and human babesiosis: evidence incriminating vector and reservoir hosts, p. 147–165. *In* P. T. Englund and A. Sher (ed.), The biology of parasitism. Alan R. Liss, Inc., New York.
38. **Steere, A. C.** 1989. Lyme disease. N. Engl. J. Med. **321:** 585–596.
39. **Steyskal, G. C., W. L. Murphy, and E. M. Hoover.** 1987. Insects and mites: techniques for collection and preservation. USDA miscellaneous publication no. 1443.
40. **Strickland, G. T. (ed.).** 1984. Hunter's tropical medicine, 6th ed. The W. B. Saunders Co., Philadelphia.
41. **Thompson, R. S., W. Burgdorfer, R. Russell, and B. J. Francis.** 1969. Outbreak of tick-borne relapsing fever in Spokane, Washington. J. Am. Med. Assoc. **210:**1045–1050.
42. **Yunker, C. E., J. E. Keirans, C. M. Clifford, and E. H. Easton.** 1986. *Dermacentor* ticks (Acari, Ixodoidea: Ixodidae) of the New World; a scanning electron microscope atlas. Proc. Entomol. Soc. Wash. **88:**609–627.

Chapter 73

Taxonomy of Viruses

JOSEPH L. MELNICK

Viruses are separated into families on the basis of the type and form of the nucleic acid genome and the size, shape, substructure, and mode of replication of the virus particle. Within each family, classifications of genera and species are based on antigenicity in addition to other properties.

Significant developments in classification and nomenclature of viruses are documented in the reports of the International Committee on Taxonomy of Viruses, formerly the International Committee on Nomenclature of Viruses. These reports, published in 1971 (8), 1976 (3), 1979 (5), and 1982 (6), have dealt with viruses of humans, lower animals, insects, plants, bacteria, and fungi and have included summaries of the properties of those groups of viruses as related to their taxonomic placement. Recent decisions of the committee were summarized in an interim report published in 1989 (2).

It seems probable that most of the major groups of viruses have been recognized, particularly with regard to those infecting humans and the vertebrate animals of direct importance to humans. Many of them now have been officially placed in families, genera, and species; within some families, subfamilies or subgenera or both also have been established. Although the focus of this chapter is on these families, progress also has been made with respect to the taxonomy of the viruses of other host groups. For more detailed discussion of virus taxonomy, references 1 through 8 are recommended to the reader.

In Table 1, properties of the major families of RNA-containing viruses of humans and other vertebrate animals are summarized; in Table 2, vertebrate viruses with a DNA genome are similarly treated. In Table 3, these families are listed along with the genera and the individual members that may be of special concern for the viral diagnostic laboratory. Subfamilies are also included if they represent agents having direct or indirect bearing on human diseases. Since most of these virus agents are dealt with more fully in the other chapters of this section, the text that follows is confined to explanation and commentary on some examples from the tables, together with some notes about recent developments.

PICORNAVIRIDAE

Picornaviridae, the smallest of the vertebrate viruses with RNA genomes, have been classed in four genera and several hundred species.

More than 70 members of the genus *Enterovirus* are known to infect humans; these include polioviruses, coxsackieviruses of the A and B groups, echoviruses, and enterovirus serotypes that have been assigned sequential numbers rather than being placed in the echovirus or coxsackievirus subgroups (since the distinctions among these groups have been found to be less sharp than was recognized when these subdivisions were initially established).

More than 100 viruses infecting humans belong to the genus *Rhinovirus*. A third genus in the family is *Cardiovirus*, typified by encephalomyocarditis virus of mice, which may also (rarely) infect humans. A fourth genus, *Aphthovirus*, includes the economically important foot-and-mouth disease viruses of cattle.

The picornavirus genome is one piece of linear, single-stranded positive-sense RNA of low molecular weight (about 2.5×10^6). The RNA is infectious and serves as its own messenger for protein translation. The virion is about 27 nm in diameter; it contains 60 copies of each of the four major polypeptides (molecular weights of 33,000, 27,000, 23,000, and 60,000). The enteroviruses and cardioviruses are acid stable and have a buoyant density in CsCl of about 1.34 g/cm^3; in contrast, the rhinoviruses and aphthoviruses are acid labile and have a higher buoyant density, about 1.4 g/cm^3. The base sequences of representative viral genomes have been determined, and the three-dimensional structure of the virion has been established.

After decades of investigation, hepatitis A virus has been classified as a picornavirus. Although it resembles enteroviruses in many respects, it differs in amino acid sequences and also in its greater resistance to thermal inactivation. It belongs in a separate genus (*Heparnavirus*).

The diseases caused by picornaviruses range from paralytic poliomyelitis to aseptic meningitis, hepatitis, pleurodynia, myocarditis, skin rashes, and common colds; inapparent infection is very common. Different viruses may produce the same syndrome; on the other hand, a single picornavirus may cause several different syndromes. Strain differentiation among the polioviruses is of direct concern in public health and medical virology. In the years since 1951 (when the existence of three poliovirus serotypes became known), genomic differences within serotypes have been demonstrated, but the old established strains used in the vaccines continue to confer excellent immunity against current wild strains.

REOVIRIDAE

For all of the virus families listed in Table 1, the RNA genome is single stranded except in the case of the family *Reoviridae*, whose RNA is double stranded. The genus *Reovirus* differs somewhat from the other genera in its possession of an outer protein shell and the larger molecular weight of its genome (15×10^6 versus 12×10^6). There are three serotypes within the genus *Reovirus* that infect humans, monkeys, dogs, and cattle; in

TABLE 1. Current classification of RNA-containing viruses of vertebrates

Characteristic	Classification											
Nucleic acid core	RNA											
Capsid symmetry	Icosahedral					Helical						Icosahedral
Virion: naked or enveloped	Naked			Enveloped		Enveloped						Enveloped
Site of capsid assembly	Cytoplasm			Cytoplasm		Cytoplasm						Cytoplasm
Site of nucleocapsid envelopment				Surface membrane	Intracytoplasmic membranes	Surface membrane				Intracytoplasmic membranes		Surface membrane
Reaction to ether treatment	Resistant			Sensitive	Sensitive	Sensitive				Sensitive		Sensitive
No. of capsomeres	32	32	32	?	?							
Ribonucleoprotein helix diam (nm)						9–15	18		18	11–13	10–12	
Virion diam (nm)	24–30	35–39	60–80	70	40–50	80–120	150–300	50–300	60 × 180	80–130	80–110	About 100
Mol wt of nucleic acid in virion (10^6)	2.3–2.8	2.6	12–15	3–4	4	4–5	5–8	3–5	3.5–4.6	5–6	6–7	6–7
Family	*Picornaviridae*	*Caliciviridae*	*Reoviridae*	*Togaviridae*	*Flaviviridae*	*Orthomyxoviridae*	*Paramyxoviridae*	*Arenaviridae*	*Rhabdoviridae*	*Coronaviridae*	*Bunyaviridae*	*Retroviridae*

TABLE 2. Current classification of DNA-containing viruses of vertebrates

Characteristic	Classification						
Nucleic acid core	DNA	DNA	DNA	DNA	DNA	DNA	DNA
Capsid symmetry	Icosahedral	Icosahedral	Icosahedral	Icosahedral	Icosahedral	Icosahedral	Complex
Virion: naked or enveloped	Naked	Naked	Naked	Enveloped	Enveloped	Enveloped	Complex coats
Site of capsid assembly	Nucleus	Nucleus	Nucleus	Nucleus	Nucleus	Cytoplasm	Cytoplasm
Site of nucleocapsid envelopment				Cytoplasm	Nuclear membrane	Cytoplasmic membrane	
Reaction to ether or other lipid solvents	Resistant	Resistant	Resistant	Resistant	Sensitive	Sensitive	Resistant
No. of capsomeres	32	72	252		162	1,500	
Virion diam (nm)	18–26	45–55	70–90	40–50	100	130–300	230 × 300
Mol wt of nucleic acid (10^6)	1.5–2.0	3.0–5.0	20–30	2.1	80–150	100–250	160
Family	*Parvoviridae*	*Papovaviridae*	*Adenoviridae*	*Hepadnaviridae*	*Herpesviridae*	*Iridoviridae*	*Poxviridae*

addition, at least five avian reoviruses are known. In the genus *Orbivirus*, important human pathogens include Colorado tick fever virus and the Kemerovo viruses; other important orbiviruses are the bluetongue viruses of sheep and the viruses of African horse sickness. The most recently established genus is *Rotavirus*, which includes several viruses that infect humans as well as viruses of many other mammalian species, typified by simian virus SA-11 and Nebraska calf diarrhea virus. The human rotaviruses are increasingly being recognized as the cause of a large share of the serious episodes of nonbacterial infantile diarrhea. Rotavirus gastroenteritis is one of the most common childhood illnesses throughout the world and is a leading cause of infant deaths in developing countries. These viruses also infect adults, particularly those in close contact with infants and children, but infected adults usually experience no symptoms or may have only minor illness.

CALICIVIRIDAE

Other recent additions to the taxonomic roll of RNA-containing viruses are the members of the families *Caliciviridae* and the *Bunyaviridae*. The *Caliciviridae* include a number of viruses of pigs, cats, and sea lions and may include agents that infect humans. Calicivirus-like particles have been observed in human feces in association with gastroenteric disease; preliminary results have failed to show relationship to the feline calicivirus. The possible relationship of these agents to the virus of Norwalk gastroenteritis also remains to be resolved. Norwalk virus, a widespread human agent causing acute epidemic gastroenteritis, has a virion protein structure similar to that of the caliciviruses; it also resembles caliciviruses in several other characteristics. Because these agents have not yet been successfully adapted to tissue culture, it has been difficult to study their properties.

BUNYAVIRIDAE

Members of the *Bunyaviridae* form a family of more than 220 viruses, at least 145 of them belonging to the Bunyamwera supergroup of serologically interrelated arboviruses. With the taxonomic placement of this large group, the vast majority of the viruses of the classical arbovirus groupings, initially based on ecological properties and subdivided by serological interrelationships, have been assigned to families on the basis of biophysical and biochemical characteristics. Human illness caused by Hantaan virus has been recognized in the Far East as Korean hemorrhagic fever, and a variant is known in Scandinavian and eastern European countries as epidemic nephropathy. The illness has been variously named "hemorrhagic fever with renal syndrome" or "muroid virus nephropathy." These agents are now established as a genus, *Hantavirus*. The virus has a labile membrane and a tripartite single-stranded RNA genome. The most common natural hosts are mice (in Korea) and voles (in Europe). There have been several instances of infection of staff members handling laboratory rats infected with the virus, both in the Far East and more recently in Europe.

RETROVIRIDAE

The family *Retroviridae* includes not only the RNA tumor viruses (oncornaviruses and leukoviruses) that are now assigned to a subfamily, *Oncovirinae*, but also the slow viruses of the maedi-visna group (now subfamily *Lentivirinae*) and the foamy virus group of agents that form syncytia in cell cultures (now assigned to the subfamily *Spumavirinae*). The human immunodefi-

TABLE 3. Members of virus families, with emphasis on viruses that infect humans

Family[a]	Genus	Common species	No. of members
Picornaviridae	*Enterovirus*	Polioviruses	3
		Coxsackieviruses, group A	23
		Coxsackieviruses, group B	6
		Echoviruses	31
		Enteroviruses 68 through 71	4
		Viruses of other vertebrates	>34
	Heparnavirus	Hepatitis A virus	1
		Hepatitis A virus of monkeys	>2
	Cardiovirus	Encephalomyocarditis virus and mengovirus; mouse encephalomyelitis virus	3
	Rhinovirus	Virus types infecting humans	>115
		Viruses of cattle	2
	Aphthovirus	Foot-and-mouth disease viruses of cattle and other cloven-hoofed animals	7
Caliciviridae	*Calicivirus*	Vesicular exanthema of swine virus	13
		Viruses of cats and sea lions (possible member: Norwalk gastroenteritis virus of humans)	Many >5
Reoviridae	*Reovirus*	Viruses of humans, monkeys, and lower vertebrates	3
		Viruses of birds	>5
	Orbivirus	17 subgroups, including Colorado tick fever and Kemerovo viruses of humans; also bluetongue virus of sheep and African horse sickness virus	>90
	Rotavirus	Human rotaviruses	>6
		Rotaviruses of many mammals, including SA-11 virus of monkeys and Nebraska calf diarrhea virus	Many
Birnaviridae	*Birnavirus*	Infectious pancreatic necrosis virus of fish; infectious bursal disease virus of chickens	2
Togaviridae	*Alphavirus*	Sindbis virus and many other mosquito-borne viruses, including the viruses of eastern equine, Venezuelan, and western equine encephalitis and Semliki Forest virus	23
	Rubivirus	Rubella virus	1
	Pestivirus	Viruses of cattle and pigs	>3
Flaviviridae	*Flavivirus*	Yellow fever virus and other mosquito-borne viruses, including the viruses of dengue, of Japanese, Murray Valley, and St. Louis encephalitis, and of West Nile fever	26
		Tick-borne viruses, including the viruses of Kyasanur Forest disease, Omsk hemorrhagic fever, European and Far Eastern tick-borne encephalitis of humans, and louping ill of sheep	11
		Viruses whose vectors are unknown	17
Orthomyxoviridae	*Influenzavirus*	Influenza virus type A	Many
		Influenza virus type B	Several
		Influenza virus type C	1
Paramyxoviridae	*Paramyxovirus*	Human parainfluenza viruses, including Sendai virus	4
		Mumps virus	1
		Newcastle disease virus of fowl; viruses of other diseases of birds and mammals	>6
	Morbillivirus	Measles virus	1
		Rinderpest virus of cattle	1
		Distemper virus of dogs	1
		Peste-des-petits-ruminants virus of sheep and goats	1
	Pneumovirus	Human respiratory syncytial virus	1
		Respiratory disease viruses of cattle and mice	?
Rhaboviridae	*Vesiculovirus*	Vesicular stomatitis virus of horses, cattle, and pigs	Several
	Lyssavirus	Rabies virus	1
		Lagos bat virus and others	>5
Filoviridae	*Filovirus*	Marburg virus	1
		Ebola virus	2
Coronaviridae	*Coronavirus*	Human coronavirus	2
		Mouse hepatitis virus, infectious bronchitis virus of fowl, and other agents infecting pigs and other vertebrates	>4
Bunyaviridae	*Bunyavirus*	Bunyamwera virus	>145
		California encephalitis viruses	
		LaCrosse virus, other serologically cross-related groups, and several ungrouped viruses	
	Phlebovirus	Sandfly fever viruses	>30
		Other viruses of humans and lower animals, including Rift Valley fever virus of sheep and other ruminants, which may cause human disease	

(*Continued on next page*)

TABLE 3—*Continued*

Family[a]	Genus	Common species	No. of members
	Nairovirus	Crimean-Congo hemorrhagic fever virus	>27
		Viruses of 5 other serogroups, including the virus of Nairobi sheep disease	
	Uukuvirus	Uukuniemi virus and six other agents, all belonging to the same serogroup (infect rodents and ticks)	7
	Hantavirus	Hantaan virus of hemorrhagic fever with renal syndrome	Many
Retroviridae			
Oncovirinae	Type C oncovirus group	Sarcoma and leukemia viruses of mice, cats, cattle, birds, snakes, and primates	>15
		Human T-cell leukemia-associated virus types I and II	>2
	Type B oncovirus group	Mammary tumor virus of mice (and humans?)	?
	Type D oncovirus group	Monkey (mammary tumor?) virus (Mason-Pfizer monkey virus)	?
Spumavirinae	*Spumavirus*	Syncytial and foamy viruses of humans, monkeys, cattle, and cats	>4
Lentivirinae	*Lentivirus*	Human immunodeficiency virus	2
		Visna, maedi, and progressive pneumonia viruses of sheep	?
Arenaviridae	*Arenavirus*	Lymphocytic choriomeningitis virus of mice	1
		Lassa fever virus	1
		Viruses of the Tacaribe complex, including Junin and Machupo viruses of South American hemorrhagic fevers	>8
Parvoviridae	*Parvovirus*	Human parvoviruses B19 and RA-1	>2
		Aleutian mink disease virus; viruses of rodents, pigs, cattle, cats, and dogs	Many
	Dependovirus	Adeno-associated virus (adeno-satellite virus): human (types 1–5); monkey (type 4); also of cattle, dogs, and birds	>8
Papovaviridae	*Papillomavirus*	Human papilloma viruses (warts)	Many
		Rabbit (Shope) papillomavirus	1
		Papillomaviruses of other mammals	Many
	Polyomavirus	Polyomavirus of mice	1
		JC and BK viruses of humans	2
		Simian virus 40 of rhesus monkeys	1
		Lymphotropic virus of African green monkeys	1
		Viruses of mice, rabbits, and baboons	>5
Adenoviridae	*Mastadenovirus*	Human adenoviruses	>36
		Viruses of other mammals	>45
	Aviadenovirus	Viruses of birds	>13
Hepadnaviridae	*Hepadnavirus*	Human hepatitis B virus	1
		Hepatitis B viruses of woodchucks, ground squirrels, and ducks	>3
Herpesviridae			
Alphaherpesvirinae	*Simplexvirus*	Human herpes simplex virus types 1 and 2	2
		Bovine mammillitis virus	1
		Herpes B virus of monkeys	1
	Varicellovirus	Varicella-zoster virus	1
		Pseudorabies virus	1
		Equine rhinopneumonitis virus	1
Betaherpesvirinae	*Cytomegalovirus*	Human cytomegalovirus	1
	Muromegalovirus	Mouse cytomegalovirus	1
Gammaherpesvirinae	*Lymphocryptovirus*	Epstein-Barr virus	1
	Thetalymphocryptovirus	Marek's disease herpesvirus of fowl	1
	Rhadinovirus	Herpesvirus saimiri and others	>2
Iridoviridae	*Iridovirus*	Iridescent insect viruses	Several
		African swine fever virus (?)	1
	Ranavirus	Frog viruses	>30
	Piscinivirus	Fish viruses	Several
Poxviridae			
Chordopoxvirinae (poxviruses of vertebrates)	*Orthopoxvirus*	Vaccinia virus	1
		Smallpox virus (variola)	1
		Poxviruses of lower animals	>6
	Parapoxvirus	Orf virus and other viruses of ungulates	?
		Virus of milker's nodule	1
	Avipoxvirus	Fowlpox virus and other viruses of birds	8
	Capripoxvirus	Viruses of sheep and goats	3
	Leporipoxvirus	Myxoma virus of hares	4
		Fibroma viruses of rabbits and squirrels	
	Suipoxvirus	Swinepox virus	1
	Yatapoxvirus	Yabapox and tanapox viruses	2
	Molluscipoxvirus	Molluscum contagiosum virus	1
Entomopoxvirinae		Poxviruses of insects	>24

[a] Where subfamilies have been designated, they are listed in this column, indented below the family name.

ciency viruses (HIV) associated with AIDS are members of *Lentivirinae*.

Retroviruses characteristically have a reverse transcriptase (RNA-dependent DNA polymerase) within the virion. The genome is an inverted dimer of linear, single-stranded positive RNA that dissociates readily into two or three pieces. Replication of the viral RNA involves a DNA provirus that is integrated into host cellular DNA.

Endogenous members of the *Oncovirinae* may be part of the germ line of vertebrate hosts, being inherited as Mendelian genes. The oncovirus genes may not be expressed, but they can be activated by physical and chemical agents, by superinfection with other oncoviruses, and even by herpesviruses. It was through studies of oncoviruses that the cellular oncogenes became recognized.

With some exceptions, oncoviruses fall into host-species-specific groups of agents, including either leukemias or sarcomas, that is, leukemia-sarcoma complexes of avian, murine, feline, and hamster oncoviruses. Other groups are murine mammary tumor virus and primate oncoviruses.

The subfamily *Oncovirinae* has been divided into types according to morphological, antigenic, and enzymatic differences. The type B oncovirus group includes the mouse mammary tumor virus and probably similar viruses from guinea pig and perhaps other species. The type C oncovirus group includes mammalian, avian, and reptilian subgenus groupings as well as a number of ungrouped species. Two members of *Oncovirinae* type C that infect humans, human T-cell leukemia-associated virus types I and II, have been recognized; they are associated with human T-cell leukemias. Type D includes viruses of monkeys.

Members of the subfamily *Spumavirinae*, foamy viruses, do not induce tumors or cellular transformation but cause persistent asymptomatic infections in natural and experimental host animals. Foamy or syncytial viruses are known for a number of mammalian species, including humans.

The slow viruses of the maedi-visna group, which have been placed in the subfamily *Lentivirinae*, are morphologically and chemically like other members of the family *Retroviridae* but do not induce tumors. Natural infections are known only in sheep. Visna virus causes panleukoencephalitis. Serologically related viruses (variously designated in different countries as maedi or progressive pneumonia viruses) cause interstitial pneumonitis.

Two types of the human lentivirus, HIV, have been recognized; type 1 is more widespread and more virulent. HIV is a completely exogenous virus, in contrast to the transforming retroviruses. However, after an individual is exposed to and infected by HIV, proviral DNA is integrated into the cellular DNA of infected cells. The many different isolates of HIV exhibit considerable divergence, particularly in the gene that codes for viral envelope proteins. Visna virus, the prototype of the genus *Lentivirus*, is also known to undergo progressive antigenic variation in reaction to the host's immune response during persistent infection.

PARVOVIRIDAE

All of the virus families shown in Table 2 have their DNA genomes in double-stranded form except the *Parvoviridae*, whose DNA is single stranded within the virion. Members of the family *Parvoviridae* are very small viruses (Table 2). The molecular weight of the nucleic acid in the virion is relatively very low, 1.5×10^6 to 2.0×10^6 (as compared, for example, with 160×10^6 for the DNA of poxviruses). Some members display resistance to high temperatures (60°C, 30 min).

The family *Parvoviridae* encompasses viruses of numerous species of vertebrates, including humans. Two members of the genus *Parvovirus*, the members of which are able to replicate independently, have been found to be associated with disease problems of human beings. Parvovirus B19 has been shown to cause a transient shutdown of erythrocyte production by killing the late erythroid progenitor cells. This shutdown presents particular problems for individuals already suffering from hemolytic anemias such as sickle cell anemia, causing aplastic crises. A virus named RA-1, which is associated with rheumatoid arthritis, is another newly identified member of the genus.

A host range mutant of feline panleukopenia parvovirus, known as canine parvovirus, induces acute enteritis with leukopenia in young and adult dogs as well as myocarditis in puppies. Infections with this virus have reached enzootic proportions around the world.

Several serotypes of adeno-associated viruses, belonging to the genus *Dependovirus*, are known to infect humans, but they have not been shown to be associated with any human disease. Members of this genus cannot multiply in the absence of a replicating adenovirus which serves as a helper virus. The single-stranded DNA is present within the virion as either plus or minus complementary strands in separate particles. Upon extraction, the plus and minus DNA strands unite to form a double-stranded helix.

HEPADNAVIRIDAE

Ample evidence has accumulated for the formation of a new virus family. The name *Hepadnaviridae* reflects the DNA-containing genomes of its members and their replication within hepatocytes. These viruses have a circular DNA genome that is double stranded except for a region of variable length that is single stranded. In the presence of appropriate substrates, DNA polymerase within the virion can complete the single-stranded region to its full length of 3,200 nucleotides.

Hepatitis B virus of humans and three similar viruses found in woodchucks, Beechey ground squirrels, and Pekin ducks share many basic features. All members of the family share antigens as well as similar morphology and behavior in the infected host. Large amounts of excess viral coat protein are produced in the form of small 22-nm spherical and tubular particles (in the human virus, the antigen is known as hepatitis B surface antigen). The viruses replicate in the liver and are associated with acute and chronic hepatitis. More than 300 million persons are persistent carriers of the human virus and are at very high risk of developing liver cancer. The woodchuck hepatitis B virus also causes liver cancer in its natural host. Fragments of viral DNA may be found in the liver cancer cells of both species.

LITERATURE CITED

1. **Andrewes, C. H., H. G. Pereira, and P. Wildy.** 1978. Viruses of vertebrates, 4th ed. Macmillan Publishing Co., New York.

2. **Brown, F.** 1989. The classification and nomenclature of viruses: summary of the results of meetings of the International Committee on Taxonomy of Viruses, Edmonton, Canada, 1987. Intervirology **30:**181–186.
3. **Fenner, F.** 1976. Classification and nomenclature of viruses: second report of the International Committee on Taxonomy of Viruses. Intervirology **7:**1–16.
4. **Fields, B. N., D. M. Knipe, R. M. Chanock, J. L. Melnick, B. Roizman, and T. P. Monath (ed.).** 1990. Virology, 2nd ed. Raven Press, New York.
5. **Matthews, R. E. F.** 1979. Classification and nomenclature of viruses: third report of the International Committee on Taxonomy of Viruses. Intervirology **12:**129–296.
6. **Matthews, R. E. F.** 1982. Classification and nomenclature of viruses: fourth report of the International Committee on Taxonomy of Viruses. Intervirology **17:**1–199.
7. **Melnick, J. L.** 1966. Summaries on viral taxonomy (published annually). Prog. Med. Virol.
8. **Wildy, P.** 1971. Classification and nomenclature of viruses: first report of the International Committee on Nomenclature of Viruses. Monogr. Virol. **5:**1–81.

Chapter 74

Preparation of Specimens for Virological Examination

DAVID A. LENNETTE

GENERAL CONSIDERATIONS

The objective of specimen processing is to optimize the recovery or detection of any viruses that may be present in samples as they arrive at the processing laboratory. Since only a few factors are known to affect this goal, processing of virologic specimens is not especially complicated. However, relatively few papers deal with studies of specimen processing methods, and it is possible that previously overlooked approaches will prove to be both fruitful and needed.

Storage temperature

Virus isolation in cell cultures, from appropriately selected specimens, is capable of recovering many different agents and is the approach chosen when many viruses are plausible etiologic agents. Proper storage of specimens is important, since periods of up to several days may elapse before some specimens are finally inoculated into isolation systems. Most virus-containing specimens can be held at 4 to 8°C for several days before there is an excessive loss of infectivity. Freezing specimens to −70°C or below will preserve residual viral infectivity of most specimens almost indefinitely, although a significant loss of infectivity may occur with each freeze-thaw cycle. Many viruses lose infectivity rapidly if stored at −15 to −20°C, the temperature range found in most standard combination refrigerator-freezers; the temperature cycling associated with frost-free freezers may cause even more rapid loss of infectivity.

Samples for virus isolation attempts should be kept at 4 to 6°C, but not frozen, until just before they are inoculated into the appropriate host systems. If residual specimen material is to be kept for possible retrieval at a later date, it is usually best to freeze it to −70°C (or below). If lability to freezing of a virus suspected to be present is a concern, the sample may be mixed with an equal volume of 2SP (0.2 M sucrose in 0.02 M sodium phosphate buffer at pH 7.2). Many laboratories have found that this commonly used chlamydia transport medium (or even a 2× concentration, 4SP) is effective in preserving infectivity of viruses that are labile to freezing, especially members of the herpesvirus group; the use of older cryopreservatives, such as sorbitol syrup or glycerin, has been largely abandoned.

Specimen inspection

All specimens received should be inspected to determine that they are properly labeled, with adequate patient identification by name or code number. The specimen site should be given on the label, and submitters who do not provide this information should be requested to do so. Any discrepancies between specimen label information and the accompanying submission form should be noted on the form, and appropriate follow-up actions should be taken. Unlabeled specimens are not acceptable and should be rejected. Leaking specimen containers should be identified as soon as possible; they should be decontaminated with a general laboratory disinfectant or kept isolated in a closed ziplock plastic bag. Submitters of leaking specimens should be advised of the event and instructed on how to avoid the problem in the future. If the received specimen volume is less than the minimum that is normally processed, usually 1 to 2 ml for fluid samples, this fact should be noted and reported to the submitter. Initial specimen processing is completed when the laboratory accession number is affixed to the specimen container and the specimen is recorded, either on paper or in a data processing system.

STERILE AND NONSTERILE SPECIMENS FOR VIRAL CULTURE

The following sections describe processing of different types of specimens, which fall into two broad categories: specimens that are normally sterile and those that are microbially contaminated. Normally sterile specimens may be inoculated for isolation as soon as the indicated processing steps are completed. Contaminated specimens are processed to obtain a fluid volume of 2 to 3 ml, which is then treated with a mixture of antibiotics. The latter mixture is chosen to substantially reduce overgrowth of microorganisms in the host cell cultures during the time in which virus isolation attempts are in progress. Antibiotics are also added to the maintenance medium of the cell cultures used for isolation attempts. Although it may seem redundant to use antimicrobial agents to treat both the specimen extracts and the cell cultures to which they are added, no studies have been published to show the relative efficacy of omitting either step. No consensus has developed for the preference of a particular antibiotic mixture, although one study has indicated that better results could be obtained with the combination of vancomycin with gentamicin and amphotericin B than with the combination of penicillin with gentamicin and amphotericin B (3); a number of antibiotics are commercially available, usually packaged at 100 times the intended final concentration. Some commonly used reagents are penicillin-streptomycin-neomycin (5 mg of penicillin G, 5 mg of streptomycin sulfate, and 10 mg of neomycin sulfate per ml), nystatin (10,000 U/ml), Fungizone (0.25 mg of amphotericin B and 0.25 mg of sodium deoxycholate per ml), and gentamicin reagent solution (10 mg of gentamicin sulfate per ml).

Swabs

Swabs are frequently submitted to the laboratory and are taken from various sources: conjunctiva, oral cavity, oropharynx, nares, skin lesions, rectum, and various genital sites. The swabs may already be in a suitable fluid viral transport and storage medium; if not, they should be transferred to a vial containing 2 to 3 ml of such a medium. Dry swabs are not acceptable; most commonly isolated viruses lose infectivity rapidly on a dry swab. Swabs should be regarded as microbially contaminated unless obtained from a normally sterile site, e.g., an internal organ during a surgical procedure.

Washes

Washes collected from different sections of the respiratory tract—nasal, pharyngeal, bronchial, and bronchoalveolar washes—may all be submitted to the virology laboratory for virus isolation. All such specimens contain some cells and variable amounts of microbial contaminants. It is recommended that washes be centrifuged to pellet the cells and microbes and that the centrifuged wash fluid be used as inoculum; microbially contaminated cell cultures will be less frequent, and the recovery of viruses is not lower than with inoculation of uncentrifuged specimens. Centrifugation for 10 to 15 min at 3,000 × *g* is usually sufficient for this purpose. Heavily contaminated fluids may need to be filtered through a 200-nm-pore-size membrane filter. The cell-containing pellet may be used to prepare smears for direct antigen detection techniques, e.g., immunofluorescent staining.

Normally sterile body fluids

Normally sterile body fluids include cerebrospinal fluid, pleural fluid, amniocentesis fluid, synovial fluid, and culdocentesis fluid. These specimens should not be diluted in any transport medium, preservative, etc. These fluids contain variable amounts of cells, but centrifugation of the specimens is not needed, since microbial contamination is rarely encountered during isolation attempts with specimens of this type.

Blood

Blood represents a special case of a normally sterile body fluid and is best regarded as a tissue. Viruses are normally recovered from the cellular components of blood, and plasma (or serum) is seldom used for the isolation of viruses (except enteroviruses in the newborn). The high density of cells, particularly erythrocytes, will interfere in the examination of inoculated cell cultures; therefore, the specimens must be fractionated before inoculation. This is usually done by processing a sample of at least 5 ml of anticoagulated whole blood with a commercially available separatory medium. Blood collected with citrate as an anticoagulant gives the fewest problems; that obtained with heparin was found to give the same rate of cytomegalovirus (CMV) detection as that collected with EDTA (8).

A widely used procedure combines the use of Ficoll-Hypaque (Pharmacia, Inc.) centrifugation with Macrodex (Pharmacia, Inc.) sedimentation to recover both mononuclear (MN) cells and polymorphonuclear leukocytes (PMNs) (5). All procedures are carried out at room temperature.

1. Equal (5-ml) volumes of whole blood and sterile phosphate-buffered saline (PBS) are mixed together and then gently layered over 3 ml of Ficoll-Hypaque in a 15-ml conical centrifuge tube.
2. The tube is centrifuged at 400 × *g* for 30 min. The diluted plasma is removed and discarded, and the band of cells visible above the Ficoll-Hypaque interface is removed and saved.
3. This mononuclear cell-containing band is washed with 10 ml of cell culture medium twice, using 800 × *g* centrifugation for 15 min to collect the cells from each wash cycle. The fractionated MN cell sample is ready for direct inoculation of cell cultures.
4. PMNs are recovered from the erythrocyte-rich pellet at the bottom of the tube. The pellet is pipetted into a tube containing 2.5 ml of Macrodex solution; wash the remaining cells out of the original centrifuge tube with an equal volume of PBS and transfer the cells to the Macrodex tube.
5. The tube with the suspension is allowed to stand for 2 h, after which the supernatant PMN-enriched fraction is collected and the sedimented erythrocytes are discarded. The Macrodex-PMN fraction is washed in the same manner as the MN cell fraction and may be combined with the MN cell fraction for inoculation of cell cultures.

Recently, a colloidal silica preparation (Sepracell-MN; Sepratech Corp.) has been introduced for the recovery of MN cells; it offers a more convenient alternative to the use of Hypaque-Ficoll, since MN cells and PMNs can be recovered in a single step (8). Several separation procedures are provided by the manufacturer of this reagent. The procedure for separating whole blood by using colloidal silica as described in reference 8 is as follows.

1. Gently mix 5 ml of blood and 6.7 ml of Sepracell-MN in a tightly capped conical centrifuge tube and then centrifuge the tube at 1,500 × *g* for 20 min at room temperature in a swinging-bucket rotor.
2. Collect two layers of cells from the continuous gradient; collect the MN cell layer just below the meniscus and transfer it to a centrifuge tube containing 5 ml of PBS; then collect the layer of PMNs found just above the packed erythrocytes and transfer them to the tube with the PBS-MN cell mixture.
3. The collected cells are washed once by centrifugation at 700 × *g* for 10 min and then resuspended to a 2.5-fold concentration relative to the original blood volume; e.g., a 5-ml blood specimen should give a 2-ml cell sample. The fractionated cell sample is ready for direct inoculation of cell cultures.

A similar procedure using Percoll (Pharmacia, Inc.) is possible.

Semen

Semen may be submitted to the virology laboratory for isolation of CMV but is highly toxic to cell cultures. Recovery of other viruses from semen is possible but uncommon. Special processing is required to reduce cytotoxicity and enhance CMV recovery (4). The best results have been obtained with the following method.

1. Transfer semen to a 1.5-ml microcentrifuge tube

(Eppendorf style) and centrifuge the tube for 5 min at high speed in a compatible microcentrifuge system.

2. Remove and discard the supernatant fraction; suspend the pellet in 1 ml of maintenance medium and disperse the contents thoroughly by vortexing.

3. Inoculate the sample in 0.2-ml amounts into shell vial cultures or conventional tube cultures. Do NOT centrifuge the shell vials. Incubate the sample for 2 h at 33 to 35°C to allow the virus absorption to take place.

4. Remove the inoculum and replace it with 2 ml of maintenance medium.

5. Examine the cultures as usual for evidence of CMV infection.

Tissue samples

Most soft tissue samples are received as small fragments in a small volume of viral transport medium; they can be dispersed using a sonication bath. Larger samples (and harder tissues) should be triturated by using a sterile mortar-pestle set. Grinding in a mortar should be done in very small volumes, with little added fluid; addition of a pinch of sterile sand or alumina may speed the processing of hard or tough tissue samples. The ground-up sample material is then extracted into enough Hanks balanced salt solution to form an approximately 10% (wt/vol) suspension, which is then centrifuged as for a wash specimen. If viable cells for explantation or cocultivation are to be obtained, the sample should be finely minced (to fragments smaller than 0.5 mm) in a petri dish with a scalpel or a set of dissecting scissors; using a minimum volume of fluid may make this procedure easier.

Bone marrow

Bone marrow aspirates, if properly collected with an anticoagulant, may be diluted in a small volume of Hanks balanced salt solution and then processed in the same manner as a blood specimen. If the volume is small, it is practical to simply inoculate the diluted specimen and then remove the inoculum from the cell culture tubes after an absorption period of 1 h or more in the cell culture incubator.

Urine

Urine specimens are commonly cytotoxic and often acidic; unprocessed samples frequently adversely affect inoculated cell cultures, necessitating passages to new cell cultures within a few days. To alleviate these problems, dilute a portion of a urine sample with an equal volume of chlamydia transport medium (2SP) containing 0.1% (added) sodium bicarbonate. Most specimens need not be diluted further. With experience, one can adjust inoculum volumes to give the best results.

The virus most often recovered from urine specimens is CMV, for which the added 2SP serves as a fairly effective cryoprotective agent.

Stools

Because stool consistency varies from watery to well formed, dilution of specimens to obtain an extract for processing requires some adjustment of the volume of added fluid. Add enough Hanks balanced salt solution to dilute liquid stool at least 1:2, but do not dilute a formed stool more than about 1:10. Use only enough specimen to obtain a volume that is easily processed; usually 3 to 5 ml is ample. An extract of the diluted stool is obtained by centrifugation; a small, high-speed angle centrifuge that can run 12- by 75-mm tubes to at least $3,000 \times g$ is ideal for this purpose. Centrifugation for 10 min at $\geq 3,000 \times g$ usually results in a well-clarified supernatant fluid extract; mucoid stools may require pretreatment with a mucolytic agent such as 1.0% *n*-acetylcysteine or dithiothreitol to obtain satisfactory results. Because of their consistency and very high microbial content, stool specimens result in cell culture contamination more often than do other specimens; addition of antibiotics does not alleviate this problem, although it can be dealt with, if necessary, by filtering specimen extracts through 200-nm-pore-size membrane filters.

ENHANCEMENT OF VIRAL INFECTIVITY

Postinoculation centrifugation

Although the mechanisms are not yet understood, enhancement of viral infectivity by low-speed centrifugation of inoculated cell cultures has been recognized for more than 20 years (7). Centrifuged shell vial cultures, analogous to those used for *Chlamydia* isolation, are widely used for the recovery of herpes simplex viruses (HSV) and CMV. There is some indication that the effect may extend to varicella-zoster virus (VSV) (10). Centrifugation leads to a much greater infectivity enhancement for CMV than it does for HSV (6). Laboratories that have previously optimized their recovery of HSV in freshly grown cell cultures may find no advantage in using the centrifugation method for recovery of HSV; this is subject to determination by each laboratory, of course.

Sterile shell vials containing monolayer cell cultures grown on 12-mm circular cover slips are inoculated with specimens for the isolation of HSV, CMV, or VZV. The inoculated vials are then plugged and centrifuged in a swinging-bucket rotor for 1 h at approximately $1,000 \times g$, at ambient temperature (up to 35°C, in an uncooled centrifuge). The inoculum is then removed from the vials and replaced with 1 to 2 ml of maintenance medium. The centrifugation technique is used in conjunction with examination by immunofluorescence after 2 or 3 days of incubation.

Biochemical enhancement of infectivity

Reoviruses and rotaviruses, which are tedious or difficult to isolate in cell culture from clinical specimens, may have their infectivity greatly enhanced by treatment with proteolytic enzymes, notably trypsin (1, 9). Laboratories that wish to isolate these agents should adopt two simple procedures:

1. Add trypsin (0.01 mg/ml) to processed stool extracts and other specimens of interest.

2. Substitute serum-free cell culture maintenance medium containing 0.5% bovine serum albumin and 0.005 mg of trypsin per ml for use with cell cultures inoculated with the trypsin-treated specimens.

It is reported that pretreatment of human diploid fibroblast cells with 10 μM dexamethasone will significantly increase the sensitivity of the cells to infection with CMV (11). At the time this is written, the method has not yet been widely evaluated, and one study has failed to confirm these results (2). This subject needs additional study before any recommendations can be offered.

PROCESSING SPECIMENS FOR IMMUNOFLUORESCENT STAINING

Many common viruses may be readily detected by immunofluorescent or immunoperoxidase staining of appropriately prepared smears or tissue sections. All specimens for such procedures are prepared as cells deposited on microscope slides; plain, precleaned 1-mm-thick glass slides are suitable for use with any specimen. For work with cell suspensions, some laboratories prefer slides that have a printed overlay having wells for cell spots.

Samples for immunofluorescent staining may be prepared from tissue obtained at biopsy or autopsy. Thin frozen sections (<7 μm thick) are excellent for almost any tissue. If cut sections are unavailable, impression smears may be adequate, although they do not allow the examination of as many cells; touch preparations can be made with a freshly cut piece of tissue. Partially dry the wet surface by gently blotting it against the dry surface of a petri dish. The cut surface is then pressed firmly, with a sliding motion, against a microscope slide.

Cells recovered from the processing of wash specimens (see above) can be used to prepare immunofluorescence smears. Any pellet available from the wash centrifugation is dispersed in the smallest possible volume, 0.01 to 0.05 ml, of PBS containing 0.1% bovine serum albumin and spotted onto slides as required.

All slides should be air dried as rapidly as possible (the intake grid of a laminar-flow biological safety cabinet is excellent for this purpose) and then fixed briefly. The standard fixation for most purposes is 5 min in acetone at room temperature (cold acetone absorbs water from the air and soon loses efficacy). Staining for some agents may be improved by methanol fixation. Tissues that have been fixed in Formalin are generally unsuitable for immunofluorescent staining because of denaturation of viral antigens. Some success has been obtained by careful digestion with trypsin in order to reexpose viral antigen epitopes, but this procedure is not routine for most virology laboratories.

LITERATURE CITED

1. **Clark, S. M., J. R. Roth, M. L. Clark, B. B. Barnett, and R. S. Spendlove.** 1981. Trypsin enhancement of rotavirus infectivity: mechanism of enhancement. J. Virol. **39:**816–822.
2. **Espy, M. J., A. D. Wold, D. M. Ilstrup, and T. F. Smith.** 1988. Effect of treatment of shell vial cultures with dimethyl sulfoxide and dexamethasone for detection of cytomegalovirus. J. Clin. Microbiol. **26:**1091–1093.
3. **Forrer, C. B., O. M. Blahy, A. L. Maiatico, J. M. Campos, and H. M. Friedman.** 1982. Comparison of vancomycin and penicillin for viral isolation. J. Clin. Microbiol. **16:** 295–298.
4. **Howell, C. L., M. J. Miller, and D. A. Bruckner.** 1986. Elimination of toxicity and enhanced cytomegalovirus detection in cell cultures inoculated with semen from patients with acquired immunodeficiency syndrome. J. Clin. Microbiol. **24:**657–660.
5. **Howell, C. L., M. J. Miller, and W. J. Martin.** 1979. Comparisons of rates of virus isolation from leukocyte populations separated from blood by conventional and Ficoll-Paque/Macrodex methods. J. Clin. Microbiol. **10:**533–537.
6. **Hudson, J. B., V. Misra, and T. R. Mosmann.** 1976. Cytomegalovirus infectivity: analysis of the phenomenon of centrifugal enhancement of infectivity. Virology **72:**235–243.
7. **Osborn, J. E., and D. L. Walker.** 1968. Enhancement of infectivity of murine cytomegalovirus in vitro by centrifugal inoculation. J. Virol. **2:**853–858.
8. **Paya, C. V., A. D. Wold, and T. F. Smith.** 1988. Detection of cytomegalovirus from blood leukocytes separated by Sepracell-MN and Ficoll-Paque/Macrodex methods. J. Clin. Microbiol. **26:**2031–2033.
9. **Spendlove, R. S., M. E. McClain, and E. H. Lennette.** 1970. Enhancement of reovirus infectivity by extracellular removal or alteration of the virus capsid by proteolytic enzymes. J. Gen. Virol. **8:**83–94.
10. **West, P. G., B. Aldrich, R. Hartwig, and G. J. Haller.** 1988. Increased detection rate for varicella-zoster virus with combination of two techniques. J. Clin. Microbiol. **26:**2680–2681.
11. **West, P. G., B. Aldrich, R. Hartwig, and G. J. Haller.** 1988. Enhanced detection of cytomegalovirus in confluent MRC-5 cells treated with dexamethasone and dimethyl sulfoxide. J. Clin. Microbiol. **26:**2510–2514.

Chapter 75

Herpes Simplex Viruses

ANN M. ARVIN AND CHARLES G. PROBER

CLINICAL BACKGROUND

The common clinical manifestations of herpes simplex virus (HSV) infection have been recognized for centuries. With the development of methods for the laboratory isolation and characterization of HSV, two biologically distinct serotypes, HSV-1 and HSV-2, were identified. Furthermore, with the development and refinement of a variety of serological techniques able to identify HSV infections, a better understanding of the epidemiology and pathogenesis of these infections in the human host has been achieved (42, 56). The prevalence of HSV-1 infections increases gradually beginning in childhood, reaching 70 to 80% in later adult years, whereas HSV-2 infection is typically acquired as a sexually transmitted disease, so that its incidence increases from adolescence (8). The prevalence rates for HSV-2 infection range from about 15% to more than 50% in adults, depending on a variety of demographic variables (26, 53). As with the other members of the herpesvirus group (varicella-zoster virus, Epstein-Barr virus, and cytomegalovirus), initial infection with HSV results in the establishment of viral latency, with the potential for subsequent viral reactivation. The initial mucocutaneous infection caused by HSV-1 or HSV-2 is followed by latent infection of neuronal cells in the dorsal root ganglia (5, 23, 52). Subsequent viral reactivation is accompanied by viral excretion from the original mucocutaneous sites of infection, with or without the concomitant appearance of clinical signs and symptoms. HSV transmission can result from direct contact with infected secretions from a symptomatic or an asymptomatic host (10). Although previous infection with HSV-1 does not prevent infection upon exposure to HSV-2, preexisting HSV-1 immunity may modify the severity of HSV-2 infection, rendering it clinically mild or asymptomatic.

The classic presentation of primary HSV-1 infection is herpes gingivostomatitis, an infection of the oral mucosa resulting in extensive, painful vesicular lesions associated with a high temperature and marked submandibular lymphadenopathy. Recurrences of orolabial infections are referred to as fever blisters or cold sores. Other clinical manifestations of HSV-1 infection are conjunctivitis, keratitis, and herpetic whitlow. The most serious infection caused by HSV-1 is sporadic encephalitis, which occurs in older children and adults (58). This infection has an untreated mortality rate of approximately 70%.

The classic presentation of a primary HSV-2 infection is herpes genitalis, an infection characterized by the appearance of extensive, bilaterally distributed lesions in the genital area accompanied by fever, inguinal lymphadenopathy, and dysuria. Symptomatic primary genital HSV is caused by HSV-2 in approximately 85% of cases, with the remaining cases caused by HSV-1. Because genital HSV-1 infection is much less likely to produce recurrences, 99% of recurrent genital herpes is due to HSV-2 (21). The most serious consequence of genital HSV infection is neonatal herpes. This infection usually results from exposure of neonates to virus being excreted by mothers at the time of vaginal delivery (11). Unfortunately, the majority (70%) of mothers who infect their neonates are experiencing asymptomatic genital infections at delivery (62). If the neonate is exposed to a mother having a recurrent infection at delivery, the attack rate is quite low, probably less than 5% (40). However, if the mother is experiencing a primary infection at delivery, the attack rate is probably greater than 50% (59). Neonates may present with infection localized to the skin, eyes, and mucosa or the central nervous system, or the infant may present with a disseminated infection. The untreated mortality rate for infants who develop disseminated infection exceeds 70% (62).

Many individuals with primary HSV-1 or HSV-2 infection do not manifest characteristic clinical disease. In fact, primary infections are often entirely asymptomatic. Similarly, despite the apparently universal establishment of latency, most individuals with past HSV infections do not experience symptomatic recurrences. Nevertheless, individuals who have had HSV-1 or HSV-2 infection are subject to asymptomatic reactivations associated with the isolation of infectious virus from oral or genital sites. Therefore, prevention of the transmission of HSV-1 and HSV-2 in the population is very difficult.

Because of the high prevalence of past HSV infections in the general population, many patients who develop malignancy, an immunodeficiency such as AIDS, or other diseases that require immunosuppressive therapy may contract HSV-1 or HSV-2 infection. These infections, which may be primary or may arise from reactivation of a past infection, can be severe (48). They can be locally invasive, causing considerable mucocutaneous necrosis, or they can spread to contiguous organs, causing infections such as esophagitis or proctitis. Herpes infections in these immunocompromised hosts can also produce viremia with dissemination to multiple organs, causing meningoencephalitis, pneumonitis, hepatitis, and coagulopathy. In addition to the susceptibility of classically immunosuppressed patients, some individuals with chronic skin diseases, particularly eczema, can experience severe primary HSV-1 infection, referred to as Kaposi's varicelliform eruption.

While a presumptive diagnosis of HSV infection can often be made on the basis of clinical findings, a definitive diagnosis is important in many circumstances. Appropriate laboratory testing allows the proper evaluation of mucocutaneous lesions in high-risk patients who are likely to benefit from specific antiviral therapy if the lesion is herpetic (51). The laboratory documentation of

HSV infection also provides critical information for managing patients with disseminated disease or encephalitis. In addition, laboratory diagnosis is valuable for many patients with HSV infections that are not life threatening. For example, proving that a genital infection is herpes facilitates counseling regarding the advisability of acyclovir therapy, the risk of recurrences, and the measures to reduce HSV transmission to contacts.

DESCRIPTION OF AGENT

HSV-1 and HSV-2, along with varicella-zoster virus, are the human herpesviruses that are classified in the alphaherpesvirus subfamily of herpesviruses (45). Important characteristics of this subfamily include a short replication cycle, producing lytic infection in tissue culture, and the establishment of latency in neural ganglia. Like other herpesviruses, HSV-1 and HSV-2 have an icosahedral capsid, consisting of 162 capsomeres, surrounding a core that contains the viral DNA. The phospholipid-rich viral envelope is acquired when the virion buds through regions of the nuclear membrane that have been modified by insertion of viral proteins. The complete virion has a diameter of between 110 and 120 nm. Tegument proteins have been identified between the capsid and the viral envelope. HSV DNA is linear, double stranded, and relatively G+C rich, with a molecular weight of 96×10^6. The viral genome consists of a long unique and a short unique region, each of which is flanked by inverted-repeat regions. Extensive sequence homologies, involving about 40% of the genome, can be demonstrated between HSV-1 and HSV-2 DNAs, to which the antigenic cross-reactivity of the two serotypes and other biological similarities are attributable. The overall pattern of nucleotide sequences composing HSV DNA is conserved; however, restriction endonuclease analysis demonstrates sufficient variability of cleavage sites among clinically unrelated isolates to permit the investigation of HSV transmission by using molecular epidemiologic methods.

The HSV genome codes for more than 50 polypeptides, including at least nine glycoproteins, designated glycoprotein A (gA) through gI, at least six capsid proteins, viral protein kinase, DNA polymerase, other enzymes, and DNA-binding proteins that are involved in viral replication (11, 45). The immediate-early proteins of the virus, such as ICP0 and ICP4, constitute products of the alpha genes of HSV that are involved in initiating the cascade by which the expression of HSV genes is regulated. With respect to the glycoproteins, gB and gD carry major epitopes to which neutralizing antibodies bind and appear to be involved in viral attachment to the target cell. gC has been shown to bind to the cell surface complement receptor, C3b; gE and gI are involved in constituting the receptor for immunoglobulin that appears on infected-cell membranes. gB, gD, and gH apparently affect the movement of adsorbed virus from the surface into the cytoplasm of the cell. Although these and other functions of some HSV proteins have been defined or suggested, the understanding of specific effects on virus entry and virus-induced changes in mammalian cells remains quite limited. Because the host-cell-derived viral envelope is phospholipid rich, the virus is readily inactivated by lipid solvents; exposure to a pH of <4 and temperatures of $\geq 56°C$, maintained for ≥ 0.5 h, also eliminates infectivity.

COLLECTION AND STORAGE OF SPECIMENS

HSV-1 and HSV-2 can be recovered from clinical specimens obtained by swabbing mucocutaneous lesions or previously involved mucocutaneous sites in patients with asymptomatic infection. Fresh vesicles, which contain a high concentration of virus, should be aspirated with a small-gauge (e.g., 25-gauge) needle attached to a tuberculin syringe. After aspiration, the surface of the vesicle should be removed, and a premoistened swab should be used to absorb any remaining fluid. Cotton swabs are preferred for taking specimens for HSV culture because calcium alginate swabs can reduce viral recovery (13). The base of the lesion should then be swabbed vigorously to recover infected epithelial cells. Ideally, specimens should be directly inoculated, at the bedside, into tubes of cell culture. If direct inoculation is not feasible, the swab specimens should be placed directly into 1 to 2 ml of viral transport medium consisting of veal infusion broth, Trypticase soy broth (BBL Microbiology Systems, Cockeysville, Md.), or commercial transport medium with antibiotics added to suppress bacterial growth. Clinical specimens that might contain HSV can be shipped effectively to reference laboratories at ambient temperatures in Virocult transport tubes (Medical Wire and Equipment Co., Cleveland, Ohio). HSV can survive in these tubes for about 2.75 days at 22°C, and the tubes are compact, enclosed, and resistant to breakage (25).

HSV can be isolated directly from cerebrospinal fluid obtained from patients with meningitis or from peripheral blood leukocytes in those with disseminated infection. HSV can also be isolated from homogenized sterile tissue specimens, such as brain tissue from patients with encephalitis. When such specimens are homogenized, a 10% tissue suspension in sterile broth should be prepared. Trypsinizing the tissue may enhance the efficiency of virus isolation from such samples (4). Heparin, which may be present in buffy coat preparations of peripheral blood leukocytes, can interfere with viral isolation and therefore should be avoided. HSV-2 can sometimes be isolated from urine samples obtained from patients with genital herpes complicated by urethritis or cystitis. Rectal swab specimens rarely yield HSV.

Highest isolation rates of HSV are likely if specimens are inoculated on the day they are taken. If a delay in inoculation is unavoidable, careful attention must be given to conditions of transport and storage, which can affect the recovery of HSV. In particular, specimens should not be frozen at −20°C before processing. Specimens may be maintained at 4°C during transport and for periods of up to 48 h (6, 65). See chapter 74 for additional information.

ISOLATION OF VIRUS

Viral culture is the most sensitive method for the laboratory diagnosis of HSV, and it also allows for typing of the viral isolate. HSV-1 and HSV-2 cause typical cytopathic effects (CPE) in a wide variety of cell culture systems (17). Primary human embryonic cells and human diploid cell lines, such as MRC-5, are commonly used because they are commercially available and because other viruses can be isolated in these cell types. Primary rabbit kidney and mink lung are particularly sensitive cell lines specifically for HSV isolation. Continuous human or primate cell lines, such as HEp-2 and Vero, are somewhat less sensitive. The inoculation of two different cell lines in parallel can minimize the periodic variations in sensitivity of different cell lines that are often difficult to avoid (7). The percentage difference in the rate of recovery of HSV in either of two acceptable cell lines is less than 5% and is apparent, for the most part, in clinical specimens that contain low concentrations of virus. If primary cells are used, the recovery of HSV is optimal when the cells are used at low passage. Most procedures for HSV culture incorporate a 1-h adsorption at 36 to 37°C before incubation with a standard tissue culture medium such as Eagle minimal essential medium supplemented with 2% fetal calf serum and antibiotics.

The presence of HSV is detected by observing foci of enlarged, refractile cells in the monolayer; some clinical isolates also induce the formation of syncytia with multinucleated giant cells. Although the CPE induced by HSV-1 tends to be more diffuse throughout the monolayer than that induced by HSV-2, this observation is not sufficiently specific to be of differentiating value. The incubation time required to observe CPE depends on the concentration of virus in the sample and the condition of the tissue culture cells. With careful maintenance of tissue culture cells, samples with high concentrations of virus produce CPE within 18 to 24 h, and samples containing low concentrations of virus should be identifiable as positive within 4 to 5 days. Cultures from oral or genital lesions can be expected to be positive within 3 days (7). In one study, CPE was observed within 4 days in more than 99% of genital tract specimens from women with asymptomatic HSV-2 reactivation (64). Adding dexamethasone to the culture medium may hasten the appearance of viral CPE in standard tube cultures (63) or may increase the number of infected cell foci that are visible (57).

The interval to virus identification can be shortened somewhat by preparing the tissue culture cells on removable glass cover slips and inoculating multiple cultures with each specimen. At prescribed intervals after inoculation, the cover slip is removed and the monolayer is stained by using HSV antibodies labeled with fluorescein, biotin-avidin complexes, staphylococcal protein A, or immunoperoxidase reagents (41, 47). Immunologic staining can reveal foci of virus-infected cells before typical CPE is apparent. This immunologic approach has also been applied to regular tissue culture systems and to shell vial systems incorporating centrifugation of the specimen onto the monolayer (21). The yield for earlier viral diagnosis with these techniques depends on the specific tissue culture cell line used, the quality of the HSV-specific antibody reagents, and the viral inoculum in the clinical specimen (16, 24, 35, 38, 66). Typically, results with early immunologic staining at 24 h are not as sensitive as those for standard tube cell cultures that are maintained for 5 to 7 days (46, 63). In an alternative approach, the cells from one of the replicate cultures are lysed with detergent at periodic intervals after inoculation and the supernatant is tested by an enzyme immunoassay method for HSV antigen detection. Earlier detection of HSV has also been accomplished by using HSV-specific DNA probes to demonstrate the presence of virus. The cumulative experience with early detection methods used at 48 h, when compared with standard tube cultures, indicates that the sensitivity with which HSV is identified in clinical specimens is maintained but not enhanced. For clinical purposes, shortening the interval to virus isolation by 24 to 48 h is usually not critical. However, the fact that some of these procedures lend themselves to the semiautomated processing of specimens may be useful for large diagnostic laboratories.

In the case of mucocutaneous HSV infection, the success with which the laboratory can isolate the etiologic agent from clinical specimens depends substantially on the type of lesion being evaluated. For example, in one study HSV was recovered from 94% of genital herpes lesions cultured during the vesicular stage, from 87% cultured during the pustular phase, and from 70% cultured during the ulcer stage but from only 27% cultured during the crusted stage (33). Whether the virus is recovered is also influenced by the specific nature of the infection. Examples include the observation that HSV-1 is rarely isolated from the cerebrospinal fluid of patients with herpes encephalitis and the observation that HSV-2 is more likely to be recovered from the usual site of lesion recurrences than from the cervix in women with asymptomatic reactivation of genital HSV-2 infection (2).

IDENTIFICATION OF VIRUS

Confirmation that CPE is due to HSV and not to varicella-zoster virus, to cytomegalovirus, or to nonspecific toxic changes is the optimal approach to processing HSV cultures. Although in the past HSV serotypes have been differentiated by biochemical and biological differences, the availability of HSV-specific monoclonal antibody reagents has facilitated a simplified immunologic means of verifying and typing HSV isolates recovered in tissue culture (4, 22, 31). Identification of viral isolates with monoclonal antibodies has replaced inoculation of chicken embryo chorioallantoic membrane and guinea pig cells as well as neutralization endpoint and other immunologic procedures for differentiating HSV-1 and HSV-2 isolates. Although in theory a specific monoclonal antibody might not react with epitopes of the relevant viral protein as produced by all HSV strains, in practice it has been possible to develop reagents that are not significantly affected by this potential for antigenic variation. HSV typing with monoclonal antibody reagents is significantly more accurate than typing with polyclonal type-specific rabbit antisera. Three pairs of commercially available monoclonal antibodies (Electro-Nucleonics, Inc., Syva, Inc., and Kallestad Laboratories, Inc.) tested in parallel performed very satisfactorily (30). The Syva and Kallestad Laboratories detection systems were somewhat less time consuming than the Electro-Nucleonics system for the identification of HSV isolates, but the latter system was slightly more sensitive and specific (30). The specificity of the results corresponds closely with typing of isolates by restriction enzyme analysis, which defines the HSV type at the molecular level (4). Use of both HSV-1 and HSV-2 monoclonal antibody reagents makes strain differentiation a component of the confirmation procedure.

Another approach for virus identification involves DNA-DNA hybridization in a dot blot system, using cloned or synthetic DNA probes that are specific for unique nucleotide sequences of HSV-1 and HSV-2 (16,

37). Such methods are comparable to restriction endonuclease analysis in specificity with which HSV types are distinguished and may be more widely used when better nonradioactive labeled probes are developed. The fact that HSV-1 is inhibited by antiviral agents such as bromovinyldeoxyuridine, to which HSV-2 strains are resistant, has also been exploited to differentiate HSV types.

DIRECT EXAMINATION

When mucocutaneous lesions are present, direct detection methods can provide a rapid diagnosis of HSV infection. The most common method used for the direct detection of HSV in clinical specimens is direct immunofluorescence or immunoperoxidase staining of cells taken from mucocutaneous lesions (4, 11). These samples are best obtained by exposing the base of the lesion, removing cells with the blunt end of a cotton applicator stick, and immediately streaking the sample onto a glass slide. Since a negative result is reliable only if intact cells are transferred to the slide, the laboratory should confirm the adequacy of the specimen before processing it. With use of fluorescein-conjugated monoclonal antibodies to HSV to stain cytologic preparations of lesion scrapings, sensitivities compared with that of tissue culture isolation are as high as 78 to 88%, with relatively few false-positive reactions (22, 39, 49, 54). However, a sample for viral culture should be obtained when the lesion scraping is made to allow confirmation of the direct detection result, since both false-positive and false-negative results can occur with the immunofluorescence and immunoperoxidase staining methods. The Papanicolaou (Pap) stain or Tzanck test can be used to demonstrate cytologic changes in specimens obtained from suspected HSV lesions. The cytologic changes being sought include syncytial giant cells, "ballooning" cytoplasm, and Cowdry type A intranuclear inclusions. These pathologic examinations can be useful inexpensive methods for evaluating patients with non-life-threatening illness. However, these methods are not specific for HSV and are much less sensitive than direct detection using immunologic reagents (11). Therefore, a negative Tzanck or Pap smear cannot be relied on for the diagnosis of HSV in critical situations such as infections in newborns, pregnant women at term, patients with encephalitis, or immunosuppressed patients.

Direct detection of infected cells with immunologic reagents has been established as reliable for identifying virus-infected cells in brain tissue from patients with HSV encephalitis, but its sensitivity in this setting results from the fact that many cells harbor HSV. This method should not be extended to the analysis of other samples, such as testing cells from cerebrospinal fluid of patients with encephalitis, attempting to detect HSV-infected cells in genital tract specimens from asymptomatic pregnant women, or examining cells in tracheal aspirate or bronchoalveolar lavage samples from immunocompromised patients with pneumonia.

Monoclonal antibodies capable of binding HSV proteins have also been used to enhance the detection of HSV antigens in clinical specimens by using enzyme-linked immunosorbent assays, (ELISAs), immunoperoxidase assays, immunohemagglutination assays, or avidin-biotin enzyme conjugate assays (1, 32, 36, 43, 49, 50). Most of these methods are applied to the detection of viral antigen in samples collected as described for viral culture. Antigen detection may be enhanced by concentrating the sample by membrane filtration or by collecting the original sample in a special transport system (14, 44). The sensitivities of these methods compared with that of viral isolation range from 70 to 95%, with specificities of 65 to 90%. However, none of the antigen detection techniques has been proved to be sensitive enough to detect the asymptomatic shedding of HSV (36).

Whereas methods that identify HSV proteins in the clinical sample are not likely to be improved sufficiently to permit the detection of asymptomatic HSV infection, the sensitivity of the polymerase chain reaction method appears to be adequate for this purpose (D. A. Hardy, A. M. Arvin, L. L. Yasukara, D. M. Lewinsohn, P. A. Hensleigh, and C. G. Prober, J. Infect. Dis., in press). Viral culture methods effectively amplify HSV by allowing viral replication. Similarly, the polymerase chain reaction method can amplify the "signal" of HSV DNA up to 10^6-fold and should be much more sensitive than methods to detect viral proteins.

Direct viral detection by DNA hybridization using radiolabeled or biotinylated probes has also been evaluated for identifying HSV in pathologic specimens (18, 19, 28). These methods, as well as the use of electron microscopy, are sensitive for demonstrating infected cells in tissue sections but are not widely used in clinical laboratories.

SEROLOGICAL DIAGNOSIS

Assessing HSV immune status to document whether an individual has had past infection with HSV can be done with many serological methods, including complement fixation, indirect immunofluorescence, enzyme immunoassays, solid-phase radioimmunoassay, indirect hemagglutination, latex agglutination, and neutralization. These methods are generally quite sensitive for detecting HSV immunoglobulin G (IgG) antibodies in individuals with past HSV infection regardless of whether the patient has had any recent signs of HSV disease. For most laboratories, HSV serological testing is accomplished most efficiently by using commercial kits based on ELISA or latex agglutination procedures (15, 20). However, the extensive cross-reactivity between HSV-1 and HSV-2 makes it impossible to differentiate past HSV-1 from past HSV-2 infection with any of these methods, including the cumbersome neutralization procedure (53). Since physicians are not often aware of this problem, serological reports that list HSV-1 and HSV-2 antibody titers separately are likely to be misleading.

Recurrent HSV infections are not always accompanied by a significant rise in antibody titer. Therefore, serological tests should not be used to diagnose recurrent HSV infections. In contrast, primary HSV infection can be documented by seroconversion in paired sera by using any of the standard methods, assuming that the patient has no detectable HSV antibodies in the acute-phase serum. However, just as cross-reactivity prevents the distinction of past HSV-1 from past HSV-2 infection, the serotype of HSV responsible for the seroconversion cannot be determined with commercially available serological tests.

Testing for IgM antibodies does not improve the specificity of the serological diagnosis in patients with clinical signs of HSV infection. HSV IgM assays cannot be used to distinguish primary from recurrent infections because the host response to reactivation can also include IgM antibody production. In addition, the maintenance of quality control for HSV IgM antibody assays is very difficult and is complicated particularly by false-positive results, even when efforts are made to fractionate serum IgG and IgM before testing.

Testing for local production of HSV IgG in cerebrospinal fluid samples can be used to document HSV encephalitis in some patients, but a 2- to 4-week interval is required before positive results can be demonstrated (34). Therefore, serological testing is not helpful in providing an early diagnosis to guide the use of antiviral therapy. There is no known diagnostic value in testing cerebrospinal fluid for HSV IgM antibodies.

Recently, serological methods have been developed that circumvent the problem of cross-reactivity between HSV-1 and HSV-2 antibodies. Testing serum samples against HSV-1 and HSV-2 antigens by Western blot (immunoblot) can be used to demonstrate reactivity with type-specific viral proteins (2). The fact that the gG of HSV-1 differs significantly from the HSV-2 homolog has also permitted the development of type-specific serological assays (3, 9, 29, 53). Monoclonal antibody to HSV-2 gG is used either to capture the protein from an HSV-infected cell sonic extract in a solid-phase ELISA or to prepare immunoaffinity-purified HSV-2 gG for use as antigen in a dot blot assay. With use of the capture ELISA method, antibodies to HSV-2 gG were detected in 96 to 98% of persons with previous episodes of culture-proved HSV-2 infections, with very few false-positive results (53). Western blot analysis or assays detecting antibodies to HSV-2 gG can also be used to document primary HSV-2 infections even in patients who have had previous infections caused by HSV-1 (3). At present, none of these HSV type-specific serological tests are commercially available.

EVALUATION, INTERPRETATION, AND REPORTING OF RESULTS

Rapid diagnostic test

Encephalitis caused by HSV and HSV infections in neonates have untreated mortality rates approximating 70% (58, 62). In recent years, effective antiviral therapy has been developed for these life-threatening infections, resulting in the potential to reduce their mortality rates by at least 50% (58, 61). In addition, the course of severe mucocutaneous and disseminated HSV infections in immunosuppressed hosts can be favorably altered by antiviral chemotherapy (51). Furthermore, genital HSV infections, which are the cause of substantial morbidity, can now be effectively managed with acyclovir therapy; the course of clinical attacks can be abrogated, and the frequency of recurrences can be significantly reduced (52). Thus, optimal patient management demands the availability of accurate diagnostic tests for HSV.

For non-life-threatening HSV infections, the availability of a diagnostic laboratory able to perform viral cultures is adequate. Since these infections can usually be recognized clinically, it generally is sufficient for a clinician to obtain virologic confirmation within several days of specimen submission. This can be accomplished readily with viral cultures. However, for life-threatening infections which mandate prompt antiviral therapy, an accurate and rapid diagnostic test for HSV must be available. The best currently available test is immunofluorescence staining. It has been shown that patients with HSV encephalitis are more likely to have a favorable outcome if their antiviral therapy is administered early in the infection (58). Since HSV encephalitis is a difficult infection to diagnose clinically, brain biopsies are recommended for these patients (58). Although antiviral therapy can be started before a definitive diagnosis is made, a positive rapid diagnostic test assures the clinician that optimal therapy has been initiated. A rapid diagnostic test for HSV also must be available to physicians involved with the treatment of newborn infants because prompt therapy of newborns presenting with skin lesions as the only sign of an HSV infection will usually result in an excellent outcome. However, if the diagnosis and treatment of this infection are delayed, dissemination beyond the skin will soon follow and the outcome will be significantly worse (60).

It is important to recognize that rapid diagnostic tests for HSV have not been rigorously evaluated in the assessment of asymptomatic HSV infections, and their clinical use in these circumstances should be discouraged (55).

Isolate typing

Although the serotype of HSV responsible for the clinical infection is important epidemiologically, there are only a few situations in which a clinician needs this information. However, it would be prudent to save the HSV isolate, at least until the clinician has been contacted, to be sure that typing is not desired. One situation in which it is mandatory to type HSV isolates is when the isolate is from the genital tract of a young child. A type 2 isolate recovered from the genital tract of a child should raise concern about the possibility of sexual abuse, whereas a type 1 isolate might be explained on the basis of autoinoculation from the oropharynx.

The type of HSV responsible for the infection also can have prognostic implications. For example, genital infections caused by HSV-1 are less likely to recur than genital infections caused by HSV-2 (27), and HSV encephalitis occurring in newborn infants is likely to be less severe if caused by HSV-1 (12). Although these observations are interesting, they do not demand the immediate availability of viral typing.

Serology

Currently available serological tests for HSV cannot reliably differentiate type 1 and type 2 antibodies. This fact underscores the futility of attempting to differentiate past infections with either of these viruses serologically, using commercially available tests. Since most adults have had HSV-1 infection, often without any primary or recurrent symptoms, this observation means that the serological diagnosis of acute or past HSV-2 infection is not possible with available methods. Serological tests can be used to diagnose a true primary HSV infection only if there is no HSV antibody in the acute-phase serum. In this circumstance, if antibody to HSV is present in the convalescent serum sample, a seroconversion can be diagnosed. However, because of the cross-reactivity between HSV-1 and HSV-2, the specific serotype of HSV responsible for the acute infection cannot be established. It is important to recognize that recurrent infections with HSV cannot be diagnosed serologically. Although a rise in antibody titer might be evident, such rises can also be nonspecific, occurring, for example, in response to recent infections with other herpesviruses (e.g., varicella-zoster virus).

Considering these limitations, laboratories using commercially available serological kits should not attempt to report any type-specific HSV antibody titers. Laboratories should report only that serological evidence of a prior or recent HSV infection is evident. In addition, because the assays detect cross-reacting antibodies, the practice of testing serum samples against both HSV-1 and HSV-2 antigens is not cost effective for the laboratory.

LITERATURE CITED

1. **Adler-Storthz, K., C. Kendall, R. C. Kennedy, R. D. Henkel, and G. R. Dreesman.** 1983. Biotin-avidin amplified enzyme immunoassay for detection of herpes simplex virus antigen in clinical specimens. J. Clin. Microbiol. **18:** 1329–1334.
2. **Arvin, A. M., P. A. Hensleigh, C. G. Prober, D. S. Au, L. L. Yasukawa, A. E. Wittek, P. E. Palumbo, S. G. Paryani, and A. S. Yeager.** 1986. Failure of antepartum maternal cultures to predict the infant's risk of exposure to herpes simplex virus at delivery. N. Engl. J. Med. **315:**796–800.
3. **Ashley, R. L., J. Militoni, F. Lee, A. Nahmias, and L. Corey.** 1988. Comparison of Western blot (immunoblot) and glycoprotein G-specific immunodot enzyme assay for detecting antibodies to herpes simplex virus types 1 and 2 in human sera. J. Clin. Microbiol. **26:**662–667.
4. **Balachandran, N., B. Franme, M. Chernesky, E. Kraiselburd, Y. Kouri, D. Garcia, C. Lavery, and W. E. Rawls.** 1982. Identification of typing of herpes simplex viruses with monoclonal antibodies. J. Clin. Microbiol. **16:** 205–208.
5. **Baringer, J. R., and P. Swoveland.** 1973. Recovery of herpes simplex virus from trigeminal ganglions. N. Engl. J. Med. **288:**648–650.
6. **Bernard, D. L., K. Farnes, D. F. Richards, G. F. Croft, and F. B. Johnson.** 1986. Suitability of new chlamydia transport medium for transport of herpes simplex virus. J. Clin. Microbiol. **24:**692–695.
7. **Callihan, D. R., and M. Menegus.** 1984. Rapid detection of herpes simplex virus in clinical specimens with human embryonic lung fibroblast and primary rabbit kidney cell cultures. J. Clin. Microbiol. **19:**563–565.
8. **Coleman, R. M., L. Pereira, P. D. Bailey, D. Dondero, C. Wickliffe, and A. J. Nahmias.** 1983. Determination of herpes simplex virus type-specific antibodies by enzyme-linked immunosorbent assay. J. Clin. Microbiol. **18:**287–291.
9. **Corey, L., H. G. Adams, Z. A. Brown, and K. K. Holmes.** 1983. Genital herpes simplex virus infections: clinical manifestations, course, and complications. Ann. Intern. Med. **98:**958–972.
10. **Corey, L., and K. K. Holmes.** 1983. Genital herpes simplex virus infections: current concepts in diagnosis, therapy, and prevention. Ann. Intern. Med. **98:**973–983.
11. **Corey, L., and P. G. Spear.** 1986. Infections with herpes simplex viruses. N. Engl. J. Med. **314:**686–691, 749–757.
12. **Corey, L., E. F. Stone, R. J. Whitley, and K. Mohan.** 1988. Difference between herpes simplex virus type 1 and type 2 neonatal encephalitis in neurological outcome. Lancet **i:**1–4.
13. **Crane, L. R., P. A. Gutterman, T. Chapel, and A. M. Lerner.** 1980. Incubation of swab materials with herpes simplex virus. J. Infect. Dis. **141:**531.
14. **Dascal, A., J. Chan-Thim, M. Morahan, J. Portnoy, and J. Mendelson.** 1989. Diagnosis of herpes simplex virus infection in a clinical setting by a direct antigen detection enzyme immunoassay kit. J. Clin. Microbiol. **27:**700–704.
15. **DeGirolami, P. C., J. Dakos, K. Eichelberger, and S. Biano.** 1988. Evaluation of a new latex agglutination method for detection of antibody to herpes simplex virus. J. Clin. Microbiol. **26:**1024–1025.
16. **Espy, M. J., and T. F. Smith.** 1988. Detection of herpes simplex virus in conventional tube cell cultures and in shell vials with a DNA probe kit and monoclonal antibodies. J. Clin. Microbiol. **26:**22–24.
17. **Fayram, L., S. L. Aarnaes, E. M. Peterson, and L. M. de la Maza.** 1986. Evaluation of five cell types for the isolation of herpes simplex virus. Diagn. Microbiol. Infect. Dis. **5:** 127–133.
18. **Forghani, B., K. W. Dupuis, and N. J. Schmidt.** 1985. Rapid detection of herpes simplex virus DNA in human brain tissue by in situ hybridization. J. Clin. Microbiol. **22:** 656–658.
19. **Fung, J. C., J. Shanley, and R. C. Tilton.** 1985. Comparison of the detection of herpes simplex virus in direct clinical specimens with herpes simplex virus-specific DNA probes and monoclonal antibodies. J. Clin. Microbiol. **22:** 748–753.
20. **Gleaves, C. A., and J. D. Meyers.** 1988. Determination of patient herpes simplex virus immune status by latex agglutination. J. Clin. Microbiol. **26:**1402–1403.
21. **Gleaves, C. A., D. J. Wilson, A. D. Wold, and T. F. Smith.** 1985. Detection and serotyping of herpes simplex virus in MRC-5 cells by use of centrifugation and monoclonal antibodies 16 h postinoculation. J. Clin. Microbiol. **21:**29–32.
22. **Goldstein, L. C., L. Corey, J. K. McDougall, E. Tolentiono, and R. C. Nowinski.** 1983. Monoclonal antibodies to herpes simplex viruses: use in antigenic typing and rapid diagnosis. J. Infect. Dis. **147:**829–837.
23. **Hill, T. J.** 1985. Herpes simplex virus latency, p. 201–206. *In* B. Roizman (ed.), The herpesviruses, vol. 3. Plenum Publishing Corp., New York.
24. **Hughes, J. H., D. R. Mann, and V. V. Hamparian.** 1986. Viral isolation versus immune staining of infected cell cultures for the laboratory diagnosis of herpes simplex virus infections. J. Clin. Microbiol. **24:**487–489.
25. **Johnson, F. B., R. W. Levitt, and D. F. Richards.** 1984. Evaluation of the Virocult transport tube for isolation of herpes simplex virus from clinical specimens. J. Clin. Microbiol. **20:**120–122.
26. **Johnson, R. E., A. J. Nahmias, L. S. Magder, F. K. Lee, C. A. Brooks, and C. B. Snowden.** 1989. A seroepidemiologic survey of the prevalence of herpes simplex virus type 2 infection in the United States. N. Engl. J. Med. **321:** 7–12.
27. **Lafferty, W. E., R. W. Coombs, J. Benedetti, C. Critchlow, and L. Corey.** 1987. Recurrences after oral and genital herpes simplex virus infection. Influence of site of infection and viral type. N. Engl. J. Med. **316:**1444–1449.
28. **Langenberg, A., R. Zbanysek, J. Dragavon, R. Ashley, and L. Corey.** 1988. Detection of herpes simplex virus DNA from genital lesions by in situ hybridization. J. Clin. Microbiol. **26:**933–937.
29. **Lee, F. K., R. M. Coleman, L. Pereira, P. D. Bailey, M. Tatsumo, and A. J. Nahmias.** 1985. Detection of herpes simplex virus type 2-specific antibody with glycoprotein G. J. Clin. Microbiol. **22:**641–644.
30. **Lipson, S. M., T. E. Schutzbank, and K. Szabo.** 1987. Evaluation of three immunofluorescence assays for culture confirmation and typing of herpes simplex virus. J. Clin. Microbiol. **25:**391–394.
31. **Miller, M. J., and C. L. Howell.** 1983. Rapid detection and identification of herpes simplex virus in cell culture by a

direct immunoperoxidase staining procedure. J. Clin. Microbiol. **18:**550–553.
32. **Miranda, Q. R., G. D. Bailey, A. S. Fraser, and H. J. Tenoso.** 1977. Solid-phase enzyme immunoassay for herpes simplex virus. J. Infect. Dis. **136**(Suppl.):S304–S310.
33. **Moseley, R. C., L. Corey, D. Benjamin, C. Winter, and M. L. Remington.** 1981. Comparison of viral isolation, direct immunofluorescence, and indirect immunoperoxidase techniques for detection of genital herpes simplex virus infection. J. Clin. Microbiol. **13:**913–918.
34. **Nahmias, A. J., R. J. Whitley, A. N. Visintine, Y. Takei, C. A. Alford, and the Collaborative Antiviral Study Group.** 1982. Herpes simplex virus encephalitis: laboratory evaluations and their diagnostic significance. J. Infect. Dis. **145:**829–836.
35. **Nerurkar, L. S., A. J. Jacob, D. L. Madden, and J. L. Sever.** 1983. Detection of genital herpes simplex infections by a tissue culture–fluorescent-antibody technique with biotin-avidin. J. Clin. Microbiol. **17:**149–154.
36. **Nerurkar, L. S., M. Namba, G. Brashears, A. J. Jacob, Y. S. Lee, and J. L. Sever.** 1984. Rapid detection of herpes simplex virus in clinical specimens using a capture biotin-streptavidin enzyme-linked immunosorbent assay. J. Clin. Microbiol. **20:**109–114.
37. **Peterson, E. M., S. L. Aarnaes, R. N. Bryan, J. L. Ruth, and L. M. de la Maza.** 1986. Typing of herpes simplex virus with synthetic DNA probes. J. Infect. Dis. **153:**757–762.
38. **Peterson, E. M., B. L. Hughes, S. L. Aarnaes, and L. M. de la Maza.** 1988. Comparison of primary rabbit kidney and MRC-5 cells and two stain procedures for herpes simplex virus detection by a shell vial centrifugation method. J. Clin. Microbiol. **26:**222–224.
39. **Pouletty, P., J. J. Chomel, D. Thouvenot, F. Catalan, V. Rabillon, and J. Kadouche.** 1987. Detection of herpes simplex virus in direct specimens by immunofluorescence assay using a monoclonal antibody. J. Clin. Microbiol. **25:** 958–959.
40. **Prober, C. G., W. M. Sullender, L. L. Yasukawa, D. S. Au, A. S. Yeager, and A. M. Arvin.** 1987. Low risk of herpes simplex virus infections in neonates exposed to the virus at the time of vaginal delivery to mothers with recurrent herpes simplex virus infections. N. Engl. J. Med. **316:**240–244.
41. **Pruneda, R. C., and I. Almanza.** 1987. Centrifugation-shell vial technique for rapid detection of herpes simplex virus cytopathic effect in vero cells. J. Clin. Microbiol. **25:** 423–424.
42. **Rawls, W. E.** 1985. Herpes simplex virus, p. 527–561. *In* B. Fields (ed.), Virology. Raven Press, New York.
43. **Redfield, D. C., D. D. Richman, S. Albanil, M. N. Oxman, and G. M. Wahl.** 1983. Detection of herpes simplex virus in clinical specimens by DNA hybridization. Diagn. Microbiol. Infect. Dis. **1:**117–128.
44. **Richman, D. D., P. H. Cleveland, D. C. Redfield, M. N. Oxman, and G. M. Wahl.** 1984. Rapid viral diagnosis. J. Infect. Dis. **149:**298–310.
45. **Roizman, B., and W. Batterson.** 1985. Herpes viruses and their replication, p. 497–517. *In* B. Fields (ed.), Virology. Raven Press, New York.
46. **Rubin, S. J., and S. Rogers.** 1984. Comparison of culture set and primary rabbit kidney cell culture for the detection of herpes simplex virus. J. Clin. Microbiol. **19:**920–922.
47. **Salmon, V. C., R. B. Turner, M. J. Speranza, and J. C. Overall.** 1986. Rapid detection of herpes simplex virus in clinical specimens by centrifugation and immunoperoxidase staining. J. Clin. Microbiol. **23:**683–686.
48. **Saral, R.** 1988. Management of mucocutaneous herpes simplex virus infections in immunocompromised patients. Am. J. Med. **85**(2A):57–60.
49. **Schmidt, N. J., J. Dennis, V. Devlin, D. Gallo, and J. Mills.** 1983. Comparison of direct immunofluorescence and direct immunoperoxidase procedures for detection of herpes simplex virus antigen in lesion specimens. J. Clin. Microbiol. **18:**445–448.
50. **Sewell, D. L. L., and S. A. Horn.** 1985. Evaluation of a commercial enzyme-linked immunosorbent assay for the detection of herpes simplex virus. J. Clin. Microbiol. **21:** 457–458.
51. **Shepp, D. H., B. A. Newton, P. S. Dandliker, N. Flournoy, and J. D. Meyers.** 1985. Oral acyclovir therapy for mucocutaneous herpes simplex virus infections in immunocompromised marrow transplant recipients. Ann. Intern. Med. **102:**783–785.
52. **Straus, S. E., J. F. Rooney, J. L. Sever, M. Seidlin, S. Nusinoff-Lehrman, and K. Cremer.** 1985. Herpes simplex virus infection: biology, treatment, and prevention. Ann. Intern. Med. **103:**404–419.
53. **Sullender, W. M., L. L. Yasukawa, M. Schwartz, L. Periera, P. A. Hensleigh, C. G. Prober, and A. M. Arvin.** 1988. Type-specific antibodies to herpes simplex virus type 2 (HSV-2) glycoprotein G in pregnant women, infants exposed to maternal HSV-2 infections at delivery, and infants with neonatal herpes. J. Infect. Dis. **157:**164–171.
54. **Volpi, A., A. D. Lakeman, L. Pereira, and S. Stagno.** 1983. Monoclonal antibodies for rapid diagnosis and typing of genital herpes infections during pregnancy. Am. J. Obstet. Gynecol. **146:**813–815.
55. **Warford, A. L., R. A. Levy, K. A. Rekrut, and E. Steinberg.** 1986. Herpes simplex virus testing of an obstetric population with an antigen enzyme-linked immunosorbent assay. Am. J. Obstet. Gynecol. **154:**21–28.
56. **Wentworth, B. B., and E. R. Alexander.** 1971. Seroepidemiology of infections due to members of the herpesvirus group. Am. J. Epidemiol. **94:**496–507.
57. **West, P. C., B. Aldrich, R. Hartwig, and G. J. Haller.** 1989. Increased detection of herpes simplex virus in MRC-5 cells treated with dimethyl sulfoxide and dexamethasone. J. Clin. Microbiol. **27:**770–772.
58. **Whitley, R. J.** 1988. Herpes simplex virus infections of the central nervous system. A review. Am. J. Med. **85**(2A):61–67.
59. **Whitley, R. J.** 1990. Herpes simplex, p. 282–305. *In* J. O. Klein and J. S. Remington (ed.), Infectious diseases of the fetus and newborn infants, 3rd ed. The W. B. Saunders Co., Philadelphia.
60. **Whitley, R. J., L. Corey, A. Arvin, F. D. Lakeman, C. V. Sumaya, P. F. Wright, L. M. Dunkle, R. W. Steele, S.-J. Soong, A. J. Nahmias, C. A. Alford, D. A. Powell, V. S. San Joaquin, and the NIAID Collaborative Antiviral Study Group.** 1988. Changing presentation of herpes simplex virus infection in neonates. J. Infect. Dis. **158:**109–116.
61. **Whitley, R. J., A. J. Nahmias, S.-J. Soong, G. G. Galassco, C. L. Fleming, and C. A. Alford.** 1980. Vidarabine therapy of neonatal herpes simplex virus infections. Pediatrics **66:** 495–501.
62. **Whitley, R. J., A. J. Nahmias, A. M. Visintine, C. L. Fleming, and C. A. Alford.** 1980. The natural history of herpes simplex virus infection of mother and newborn. Pediatrics **66:**489–494.
63. **Woods, G. L., and R. D. Mills.** 1988. Effect of dexamethasone on detection of herpes simplex virus in clinical specimens by conventional cell culture and rapid 24-well plate centrifugation. J. Clin. Microbiol. **26:**1233–1235.
64. **Yeager, A. S., A. M. Arvin, and P. A. Hensleigh.** 1982. The validity of reporting results for herpes simplex virus after four days. J. Reprod. Med. **27:**447–448.
65. **Yeager, A. S., J. E. Morris, and C. G. Prober.** 1979. Storage and transport of cultures for herpes simplex virus, type 2. Am. J. Clin. Pathol. **72:**977–979.
66. **Zhao, L., M. L. Landry, E. S. Balkovic, and G. D. Hsiung.** 1987. Impact of cell culture sensitivity and virus concentration on rapid detection of herpes simplex virus by cytopathic effects and immunoperoxidase staining. J. Clin. Microbiol. **25:**1401–1405.

Chapter 76

Human Cytomegalovirus

RICHARD L. HODINKA AND HARVEY M. FRIEDMAN

CLINICAL BACKGROUND

Cytomegalovirus (CMV) infections are common and usually asymptomatic; however, the incidence and spectrum of disease in newborns and in immunocompromised hosts establish this virus as an important human pathogen. CMV infections can be classified as those acquired before birth (congenital), at the time of delivery (perinatal), or later in life (postnatal).

CMV infection has been detected in 0.5 to 2.5% of newborn infants and is the most common identified cause of congenital infection. Fewer than 5% of congenitally infected infants develop symptoms during the newborn period; possible manifestations range from severe disease with jaundice, hepatosplenomegaly, petechiae, and central nervous system abnormalities to more limited involvement. Symptomatic infants may die of complications within the first months of life; more commonly, they survive but are neurologically damaged. It is now recognized that even those congenitally infected infants who are asymptomatic early in life may develop hearing defects.

Newborns can also acquire infection at the time of delivery by contact with virus in the birth canal. Such infants begin to excrete virus at 3 to 12 weeks of age but usually remain asymptomatic. Thus far, it appears that such perinatally infected infants do not develop late neurological sequelae of infection.

Most postnatal infections are acquired by close contact with individuals who are shedding virus. Since CMV has been detected in several body fluids, including saliva, urine, breast milk, cervical secretions, blood, and semen, transmission can occur in a variety of ways. Prolonged shedding of virus after congenital or acquired CMV infection contributes to the ease of virus spread. In addition, CMV can be transmitted by blood transfusion and organ transplantation.

The vast majority of children and adults who acquire CMV infection postnatally remain asymptomatic. In high-risk premature newborns infected as a result of blood transfusions, hepatosplenomegaly and thrombocytopenia have been described. In children attending daycare centers, 20 to 70% of those who enter as toddlers acquire CMV infection over a 1- to 2-year period. Infection is usually asymptomatic, but the children may transmit CMV to their parents, posing a risk to an unborn fetus if the mother is pregnant at the time. In adults, sexual transmission of CMV may occur. Symptoms in young adults include fever, lethargy, and atypical lymphocytosis that can mimic symptoms caused by Epstein-Barr virus.

CMV infections are frequent and occasionally severe in children or adults with congenital or acquired defects of cellular immunity, such as patients with the acquired immunodeficiency syndrome (AIDS), cancer patients (particularly those with leukemia and lymphoma), and recipients of organ transplants. Infections in these patients may be due to reactivation of latent virus or infection with exogenous virus, which may be introduced by blood transfusions or by the grafted organ. Symptoms tend to be most severe after primary infection; however, reactivation infection in a severely immunocompromised host may also cause serious illness. Symptoms in organ transplant patients include fever, leukopenia, thrombocytopenia, pneumonitis, hepatitis, retinitis, and encephalitis. Death may occur as a result of various complications, including bacterial and fungal superinfections. CMV infection, particularly when associated with pneumonitis, is an important cause of morbidity and mortality after bone marrow transplantation. In patients infected with human immunodeficiency virus, CMV is an important cause of fever, sight-threatening retinitis, ulcerative enteritis, and bilateral pneumonia.

DESCRIPTION OF THE AGENT

CMV is a member of the family *Herpesviridae*, which includes Epstein-Barr virus, herpes simplex virus types 1 and 2, varicella-zoster virus, and human herpesvirus 6. Complete CMV particles consist of a core containing double-stranded DNA, an icosahedral capsid, and a surrounding envelope. Electron microscopic features of CMV include virions morphologically indistinguishable from those of other herpesviruses, a high ratio of defective viral particles, and the presence of spherical particles called dense bodies.

Molecular virological techniques have been used to study variation among CMV strains. By DNA-DNA reassociation kinetics analysis, various CMV strains have been found to share considerable homology with AD-169, a standard laboratory strain; by restriction endonuclease analysis, DNAs from various strains have been shown to have similar but distinctive fragment migration patterns (22). These studies suggest that CMV strains are closely related, more so than are herpes simplex virus types 1 and 2. Antigenic heterogeneity among CMV strains has been detected in cross-neutralization and other serological assays, but evidence for distinct serotypes is limited (52).

CMV is inactivated by a number of physical and chemical treatments, including heat (56°C for 30 min), low pH, ether, and cycles of freezing and thawing.

COLLECTION AND STORAGE OF SPECIMENS

Specimens for virus isolation

CMV can be isolated from a variety of body fluids; however, urine, throat washings, and blood (buffy coats) are most common for diagnostic purposes. Urine specimens should be clean-voided specimens. Because excretion of CMV in urine is intermittent, increased recovery of the virus is possible by processing more than one specimen. In the evaluation of immunocompromised patients, buffy coat cultures are particularly useful. Detection of CMV in leukocytes is often a better indicator of symptomatic CMV infection than is shedding of virus in urine or throat. Bronchial washings, biopsies, and autopsy specimens, particularly of lung, kidney, spleen, liver, brain, and retina, can also be processed for virus isolation. The details of specimen collection and processing are given in chapter 74. Since CMV loses infectivity when subjected to freezing and thawing, specimens should be kept at 4°C in an ice water bath or in a refrigerator until they can be used to inoculate cultures, preferably within a few hours after collection. When prolonged transport times are unavoidable, infectivity is reasonably well preserved for at least 48 h at 4°C. If storage in the frozen state is necessary, an equal volume of 0.4 M sucrose-phosphate added to the specimen helps to preserve viral infectivity (19).

Specimens for serology

Single-serum specimens are useful to screen for evidence of past infection with CMV and to identify those individuals at risk for CMV infection. This approach is especially helpful when testing sera from organ transplant donors and from donors of blood products that are to be administered to premature infants or bone marrow transplant patients. For the diagnosis of recent CMV infection, paired sera should be obtained at least 2 weeks apart. If congenital infection is suspected, both maternal and infant sera should be submitted.

DIRECT EXAMINATION OF SPECIMENS

Histopathology

Characteristic large cells with intranuclear and, on occasion, cytoplasmic inclusions can be seen in routine sections of biopsy or autopsy material. Wright-Giemsa-stained touch imprints of lung or other biopsy specimens may demonstrate such cells (43). Although the presence of characteristic cytological changes suggests CMV infection, virological or serological confirmation is suggested. Since CMV can infect tissues without producing morphological changes, failure to find typical cytomegalic cells does not exclude the possibility of CMV infection.

Exfoliative cytology

With exfoliative cytological techniques, a presumptive diagnosis of CMV can be made in 25 to 50% of cases of symptomatic congenital infection. Specimens from older infected individuals are rarely positive. Several fresh urine specimens should be submitted, since exfoliated cells disintegrate rapidly and may be shed only intermittently. Characteristic large cells (cytomegalic) with prominent inclusions are seen in positive preparations. Exfoliative cytology is most useful when virus isolation techniques are not available. This technique can be applied to other specimens, such as bronchoalveolar lavage and cervical secretions.

Immunofluorescence

Monoclonal antibodies to CMV can be used for the direct detection of CMV antigens by immunofluorescence tests on tissues obtained by biopsy or autopsy (16, 51). Cytospin preparations of bronchoalveolar lavage specimens (31), blood leukocytes (50), and urine sediments (28) have also been examined in this manner. The sensitivity of the assay is improved when mixtures of monoclonal antibodies are used (51). An advantage of immunofluorescence staining is its rapidity; results are available within several hours after tissue is obtained. This method is less sensitive than the shell vial culture technique described below, which has largely replaced tissue immunofluorescence as a rapid test for CMV diagnosis.

Electron microscopy

The pseudoreplica method of electron microscopy can be used to detect CMV in urine and oral specimens of congenitally infected infants (29). Positive results can be obtained with almost all specimens that have infectivity titers of $\geq 10^4$ PFU/ml. An advantage of electron microscopy is its rapidity; also, stored or contaminated specimens, unsuitable for isolation attempts, can be examined. The main disadvantages of the technique are its relative insensitivity and the need for experienced personnel and expensive equipment.

Hybridization

Molecular dot blot hybridization techniques have been described for detection of the CMV genome in urine (3, 4, 45) and peripheral blood leukocytes (30, 45). Recently, in situ hybridization has been used for the direct detection of CMV in Formalin-fixed lung (35), Kaposi's sarcoma tissue (17), and cytospin preparations of bronchoalveolar lavage and peripheral blood leukocytes (14, 49). Biotinylated or horseradish peroxidase-labeled CMV-specific DNA probe kits are commercially available. In situ hybridization has the advantage of being rapid and easy to read by light microscopy. However, current methods lack the sensitivity needed for routine use in clinical laboratories.

PCR DNA amplification

The polymerase chain reaction (PCR) is a newly introduced, highly sensitive method for amplifying and detecting small quantities of specific nucleic acid in clinical specimens. The sensitivity and specificity of PCR for diagnosis of active CMV infection have been evaluated (8, 21, 36, 42). In several studies, gene fragments from immediate-early and late CMV genes were amplified to increase the sensitivity of the assay. Use of both gene fragments enabled detection of a variety of clinical isolates, indicating that strain variability is not a limiting factor for PCR diagnosis of CMV. PCR has been used successfully to identify CMV DNA in peripheral blood mononuclear cells and in urine specimens of newborns, transplant patients, and those coinfected with human immunodeficiency virus and CMV.

An unresolved issue with PCR for CMV diagnosis is whether the test can distinguish between active and latent infection. A study by Stanier et al. (48) detected CMV in peripheral blood mononuclear cells of seropositive healthy blood donors, suggesting that a positive

PCR result may correlate better with seropositivity than with active infection. Perhaps amplification of specific CMV transcripts (RNA) that are expressed only during active infection can be used to distinguish active from latent infection. At present, our limited knowledge of CMV transcription during latency precludes performance of such assays.

DETECTION OF CMV IN CELL CULTURE

Processing of specimens

Adjustment of urine specimens to pH 7.0 with 0.1 N NaOH or 0.1 N HCl is recommended to reduce toxicity to cell cultures. Centrifuging urine specimens to obtain sediment-enriched samples has been advocated but is usually unnecessary. Sediment-enriched urines of renal transplant recipients may produce toxicity more frequently than do uncentrifuged urines (27).

A number of procedures have been described for obtaining buffy coat cells. We have found density gradient centrifugation using either Ficoll-Hypaque (11, 20) or Sepracell-MN (39) to be most suitable for a clinical laboratory. Fresh blood collected in the presence of heparin, sodium citrate, or EDTA may be used. Both mononuclear cells and granulocytes are efficiently separated from erythrocytes in a single step. The procedure is rapid and easy to perform, and the reagents are commercially available. When compared with traditional sedimentation methods, the technique results in a greater number of virus isolates and an increased yield of infectious foci or plaques (20).

Throat, biopsy, autopsy, and other specimens are processed as described in chapter 74. All specimens are treated with antibiotics before inoculation of cell cultures. Portions of specimens not used to inoculate cell cultures should be mixed with equal volumes of 0.4 M sucrose-phosphate and frozen at −70°C; some infectivity may be preserved if further isolation attempts are necessary.

Cell cultures

Human fibroblast cells best support the growth of CMV and therefore are used for diagnostic purposes. CMV will not replicate in standard laboratory cell cultures such as HeLa, HEp-2, or monkey kidney cells. Acceptable fibroblast cultures include those prepared from human embryonic tissues or foreskins and serially passaged diploid human fetal lung strains such as WI-38, MRC-5, or IMR-90. Several of these fibroblast cell cultures are commercially available.

Isolation of virus

Specimens to be tested are added in a volume of 0.2 ml to duplicate tubes of confluent fibroblasts maintained on Eagle minimal essential medium with 2% fetal bovine serum. Alternatively, the tubes are drained of medium, the inocula are allowed to absorb for 1 h, and then fresh medium is added. After inoculation, the tubes can be rolled or kept stationary at 36°C. Twenty-four hours later, the medium is changed for tubes inoculated with urine or buffy coat specimens. Thereafter, and for other types of specimens, medium is changed once a week, or more frequently if toxicity appears. When toxicity necessitates passage of the culture, cells rather than culture medium should be passaged, since CMV remains cell associated. Cells are removed by addition of 0.25% trypsin–0.1% EDTA to the monolayers and incubation at 36°C for 5 or 10 min. When the cells detach, minimal essential medium with 2% fetal bovine serum is added, and the cells are used to inoculate fresh tubes. Tubes are examined for cytopathic effect (CPE) daily for the first 5 days and then twice a week for at least 4 weeks for most specimens and for 6 weeks for buffy coat specimens. Control, uninoculated cultures are handled in the same manner as those inoculated with clinical specimens.

The time of appearance and the extent of CPE depend on the amounts of virus present in specimens. In cultures inoculated with urine from a congenitally infected newborn, CPE may develop by 24 h and progress rapidly to involve most of the monolayer if the virus titer of the urine is extremely high. More commonly, foci of CPE, consisting of enlarged, rounded, refractile cells, appear during the first week, and progression of CPE to surrounding cells proceeds slowly (Fig. 1). In cultures inoculated with urine or throat specimens from older individuals, CPE usually appears within 2 weeks. Buffy coat cultures may not become positive until after 3 to 6 weeks. The usual slow progression of CPE in cultures inoculated with clinical specimens is due, at least in part, to limited release of virus into extracellular fluid. With strains of CMV that have been serially passaged, including laboratory-adapted strains, greater amounts of extracellular virus are released, and CPE progresses more rapidly.

For storage of fresh isolates, monolayers exhibiting CPE are treated with trypsin-EDTA, and the cells obtained are suspended in Eagle minimal essential medium with 10% fetal bovine serum and 10% dimethyl sulfoxide and then frozen at −70°C. Infectivity can be better maintained for long periods of time by storage in liquid nitrogen.

Identification of isolates

In many laboratories, CMV isolates are identified solely on the basis of characteristic cytopathology and host cell range. However, viruses such as adenovirus and varicella-zoster may occasionally produce cytopathicity indistinguishable from that of CMV. Suspected CMV isolates can be confirmed by indirect immunofluorescence (IFA), using commercially available monoclonal or polyclonal antibodies. The appearance of typical nuclear fluorescence of infected cells indicates the presence of CMV.

Spin amplification shell vial assay

The spin amplification shell vial assay as described by Gleaves et al. (15) has gained wide acceptance as a rapid method for the detection of CMV from clinical specimens. The technique is based on the amplification of virus in cell cultures after low-speed centrifugation and detects viral antigens produced early in the replication of CMV before the development of CPE. Even low titers of virus present in specimens are easily amplified and rapidly detected within 24 h. Monoclonal antibodies are commercially available and have been used for detection of CMV early antigens. In situ hybridization using commercially available DNA probes to CMV has also been employed (13, 33, 44).

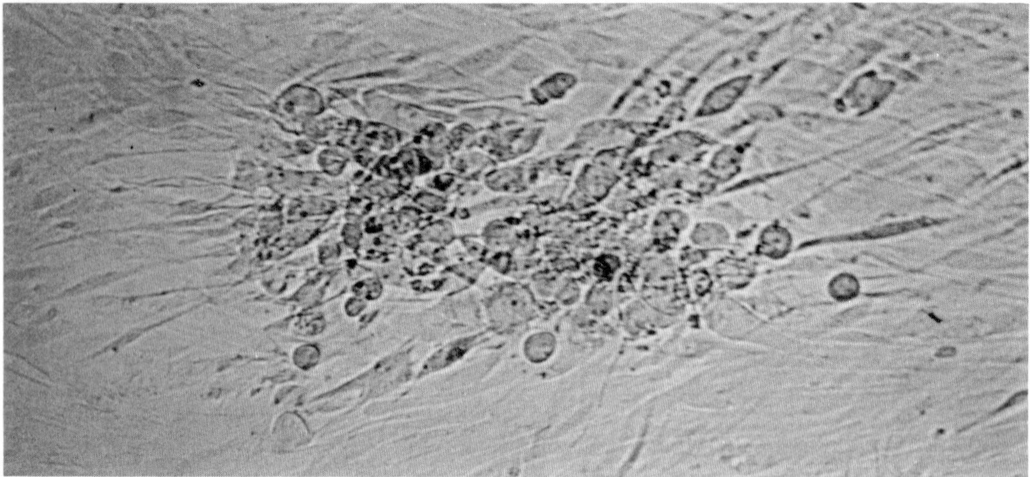

FIG. 1. CPE produced by a CMV isolate in human skin fibroblasts 10 days postinoculation. Unstained preparation; ×100. (Courtesy of Sergio Stagno.)

MRC-5 cells are grown to confluency on 12-mm round cover slips in 1-dram shell vials and inoculated with 0.2 ml of specimen. Shell vials of MRC-5 cells can be obtained commercially or prepared in the laboratory. Monolayers should be inoculated within 1 week after preparation, since older monolayers demonstrate decreased sensitivity to CMV and increased toxicity (10). Two vials should be inoculated for urine, tissue, and bronchoalveolar lavage specimens, and three should be inoculated for blood specimens (38). After inoculation, vials are centrifuged at 700 × *g* for 40 min at 25°C, and then 2.0 ml of Eagle minimum essential medium containing 2% fetal bovine serum and antibiotics is added. The cultures are incubated at 37°C for 16 to 24 h, fixed with acetone, and stained. A longer incubation time may be used but should be determined by each laboratory on the basis of individual experience, reagents and staining technique employed, and whether monolayers are purchased or prepared in the laboratory. Uninfected and CMV-infected monolayers are included as negative and positive controls, respectively. Our laboratory utilizes an IFA to detect the immediate-early antigen of CMV, using the E-13 mouse anti-CMV monoclonal antibody as the primary antiserum followed by a biotin-labeled goat anti-mouse antibody and avidin conjugated with fluorescein isothiocyanate. The monolayers are counterstained with Evans blue. Cover slips are scanned at ×200 to ×250 magnification, and specific staining is confirmed at ×400 to ×630. Positive cells contain apple green fluorescent nuclei against a red background. Staining of immediate-early antigen appears as an even matte green fluorescence with specks of brighter green (Fig. 2A). Viral inclusions (owl's eyes) may be visible in the nuclei (Fig. 2B).

The spin amplification shell vial assay is a valuable adjunct to conventional virus isolation. It has the important features of being rapid, sensitive, and specific. However, skilled technical personnel and attention to

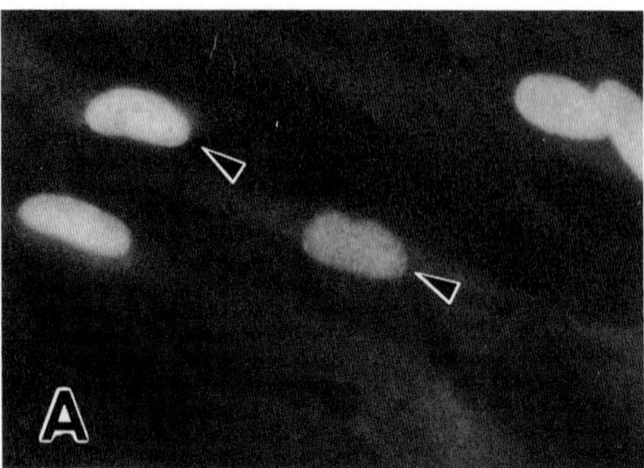

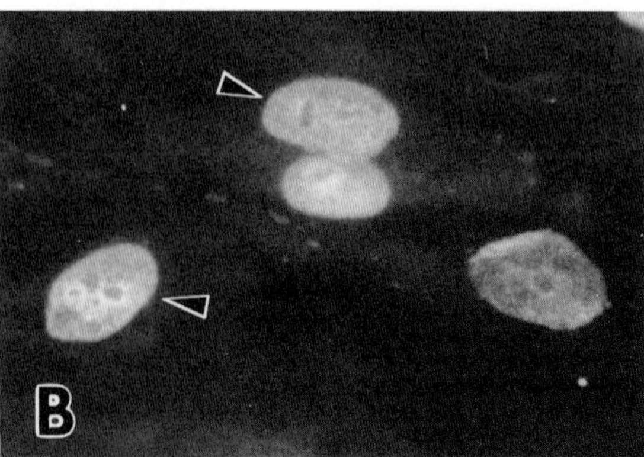

FIG. 2. Demonstration of CMV early antigens in the nuclei of infected MRC-5 cells after shell vial culture and indirect immunofluorescence staining; ×400.

the quality of specimens, monolayers, and reagents are required for optimum performance.

SEROLOGICAL DIAGNOSIS

A variety of tests are available for serodiagnosis of CMV infection. In deciding which test to perform, such factors as cost, turnaround time, equipment needs, and ease of performance should be considered. Which method is chosen will depend on which best meets the needs of individual laboratories.

EIA

Over the last several years, enzyme immunoassays (EIA) have largely replaced other traditional methods for detecting antibodies to CMV. The EIA has the main advantages of being rapid, sensitive, and specific (32, 34, 40). In addition, multiple specimens can be handled daily. The EIA can be used effectively to determine the immune status of a patient (2, 9) and to detect significant rises in antibody titers (32). Kits that detect CMV immunoglobulin G (IgG) are available from a number of commercial sources. The kits are easy to use, and the manufacturers provide detailed instructions. All of the materials necessary to perform the assay are included, and the reagents are stable with time. Some companies also provide a spectrophotometer and automated plate washer, which otherwise must be purchased separately at considerable expense.

The tests are performed as follows. Microdilution wells are precoated with CMV antigen. A small volume (for example, 10 μl) of patient serum is added to a diluent, which is then incubated with CMV antigen in microdilution wells. Unbound antibody is removed by washing, and the conjugate (such as alkaline phosphatase-conjugated anti-human IgG) is added. After incubation, unbound conjugate is removed by washing, and enzyme substrate is added. The reaction is stopped by addition of tribasic sodium phosphate, and the intensity of the color reaction is quantified in a spectrophotometer. Known positive and negative serum controls and calibrated standards are included in each run. Absorbance values of the calibrated standards are used to perform a best-fit linear regression analysis, and the EIA values of the patient specimens are calculated. Results are available within 2 h.

Passive latex agglutination assay

The passive latex agglutination assay provides a simple and rapid means for the detection of antibodies to CMV in human sera and plasma. The method is highly sensitive and specific (1, 23, 32, 34), and it may serve to determine the immune status of patient or blood donor populations (1, 23) or be used to satisfactorily detect significant antibody rises in paired sera (32, 34). Commercial kits are available.

In the passive latex agglutination assay, latex particles are coated with CMV antigens and agglutinate if CMV antibody is present. Agglutination is detected by visual inspection, and positive and negative controls are provided for comparison. The procedure detects both IgG and IgM antibodies. When one is quantifying antibody titer, reactivity is reported as the highest serum dilution showing agglutination. The assay can be completed in 10 to 15 min and does not require extensive washes, long incubation times, or expensive equipment. The main disadvantages are that agglutination patterns can be difficult to discern and readings are subjective.

CF test

The complement fixation (CF) test has been used for many years in clinical laboratories and is suitable for detecting rises in antibody titers. However, the method is technically demanding, requires rigid standardization, and has a slow turnaround time. The CF test is also less sensitive than other methods described for detecting low levels of antibody. Therefore, it may be more desirable to adopt an alternative system, such as the previously described EIA or latex agglutination assay, for routine diagnostic testing.

Reagents for the CF test are commercially available. Generally, the broadly reactive AD-169 antigen is used. It can be prepared by glycine extraction (26) or by freeze-thawing (18). The CF test with glycine-extracted antigen is more sensitive for distinguishing seropositive from seronegative specimens (26), whereas the freeze-thawed antigen is slightly better for detection of fourfold or greater rises in titer (6). Choice of antigen preparation should in part depend on the purpose of the serological test.

Titrations of antigen, hemolysin, and complement are made so that 2 U of each reagent can be used in the assay (see reference 37 for details of the CF test). For performance of the test, patient serum is diluted 1:8 and is heat inactivated for 30 min at 56°C. Each serum is tested at dilutions of 1:8 to 1:1,024 against CMV antigen, at dilutions of 1:8 and 1:16 against control antigen (prepared from uninfected cells), and against buffer alone (to detect anticomplementary activity in the serum). Two units of complement are used, and complement controls contain 2.0, 1.5, 1.0, and 0.5 U of complement that has reacted with 2 U of CMV antigen or 2 U of control antigen. After overnight incubation at 4°C, a 1.4% suspension of hemolysin-sensitized sheep erythrocytes is added to each well, and plates are incubated at 37°C until the 2.0-, 1.5-, and 1.0-U complement control wells clear (15 to 30 min). Results of the antibody testing can then be read immediately, but generally endpoints are easier to interpret if the plates are incubated at 4°C for 1 to 2 h. A 3+ or greater cell button (on a scale of 0 to 4) is considered a positive reaction.

The antibody titer is the highest dilution of serum that gives a 3+ or greater reaction against CMV antigen while giving no reaction against control antigen or against buffer alone. For sera that react against control antigen or buffer, an endpoint can still be determined if the reaction against CMV is at least 2 dilutions higher than the reaction in the control wells.

It is unnecessary to carry out hemolysin and complement titrations each time the CF test is performed. Hemolysin is very stable at 4°C and can be titrated every 3 to 6 months. Complement, once titrated, can be dispensed into volumes appropriate for a single day's tests and frozen at −70°C. As controls, reference sera of known negative and positive titers can be included in each run.

ACIF test

The anticomplement immunofluorescence (ACIF) test is an immunofluorescence assay that detects CMV antibody (25, 41). An important advantage of this assay compared with the CF test is its rapidity, since results can be available within 2 to 3 h. In addition, sera that are anticomplementary by the CF procedure can be tested by the ACIF test. Also, nonspecific cytoplasmic staining caused by binding of antibody to Fc receptors is avoided. Disadvantages of the ACIF test are that fewer specimens can be handled daily, the test requires cell culture facilities and an immunofluorescence microscope, and examination of slides requires considerable time and experience.

For performance of the ACIF test, human embryonic lung fibroblasts are infected with CMV (generally the AD-169 strain) and are harvested with trypsin-EDTA treatment when the fibroblasts show advanced CPE. The cells are sedimented at $300 \times g$ for 5 min and are suspended to approximately 5×10^6 cells per ml. One drop is placed in each well of an eight-well Teflon-coated slide. One 75-cm^2 flask provides enough cells for 16 slides. The slides are air dried, fixed in cold acetone for 10 min, and stored at −20 or −70°C for subsequent use. Cells can be stored for several months without loss of CMV antigens. Heat-inactivated (56°C for 30 min) serum is added to each well in dilutions of 1:8 to 1:1,024. The slides are incubated for 30 min at 37°C in a moist chamber, washed, and then reacted for 45 min at 37°C with an optimal dilution of cold guinea pig complement. Slides are again washed and reacted with an optimal dilution of anti-guinea pig C3 fluorescent conjugate (commercially available) for 30 min at 37°C.

As controls for the test, known positive and negative samples are included in each run. In addition, a single dilution of serum (1:8) is allowed to react with uninfected cells to detect antinuclear antibodies, which can produce false-positive results. The antibody titer is the highest dilution of serum producing 3+ or greater (on a scale of 0 to 4) nuclear fluorescence against CMV-infected fibroblasts while giving no reaction against uninfected control cells.

IFA

As an alternative to the ACIF test, the IFA can be performed (41). This test is slightly faster than the ACIF test but has the disadvantage that the assay should be performed on monolayers of infected cells; these are more difficult to prepare than the cell suspensions used for the ACIF test. In addition, specific nuclear fluorescence, which indicates a positive result, is sometimes difficult to distinguish from nonspecific cytoplasmic fluorescence. The latter occurs because CMV infection of fibroblasts induces a cytoplasmic Fc receptor that binds viral and nonviral IgG antibody (24).

For performance of the test, fibroblasts are grown in cell culture chamber slides and infected with CMV (generally the AD-169 strain). When CPE is 3 to 4+ (approximately 3 days after inoculation), cells are fixed in cold acetone and stored (−20 or −70°C) or are used directly for antibody determination. Human sera are serially diluted from 1:8 to 1:1,024 and allowed to react with infected fibroblasts. As a control for antinuclear antibodies, serum diluted 1:8 is allowed to react with uninfected cells. Slides are incubated at 37°C for 30 min in a moist chamber, washed, and stained with an optimal dilution of fluorescein-conjugated anti-human IgG. After a 30-min incubation at 37°C, slides are washed and mounted for microscopic reading. The antibody titer is the highest serum dilution producing 3+ or greater (on a scale of 0 to 4) nuclear fluorescence when allowed to react with CMV-infected fibroblasts while giving no nuclear staining of uninfected control cells.

Several immunofluorescence assay systems for CMV antibody detection are commercially available. These include a solid-phase fluorescence immunoassay (trademarked as FIAX) in which CMV antigen and control antigen are absorbed onto solid surfaces. A single dilution of patient serum is applied to the solid surfaces, an anti-human IgG fluorescein conjugate is added, and the intensity of fluorescence is measured in a fluorometer (12). CMV-infected culture cells on glass slides are also available commercially for measuring CMV antibodies.

CMV IgM antibodies

Methods for measuring CMV IgM antibodies include IFA, EIA, and radioimmunoassays. The procedures are essentially the same as those employed for detecting IgG antibodies except that anti-human IgM antibodies labeled with suitable markers are used. A recognized pitfall of CMV IgM assays is the occurrence of false-positive and false-negative reactions. False-positive reactions occur when sera contain unusually high levels of rheumatoid factor in the presence of specific CMV IgG (7). Rheumatoid factor is an immunoglobulin, usually of the IgM class, that reacts with IgG. It is produced in some rheumatological, vasculitic, and viral diseases, including CMV infection (46). IgM rheumatoid factor forms a complex with IgG that may contain CMV-specific IgG. The CMV IgG binds to CMV antigen, carrying nonviral IgM with it. A test designed to detect IgM will produce a false-positive result. Therefore, testing for rheumatoid factor and removing it if present is important when one is measuring IgM antibodies. False-negative reactions occur if high levels of specific IgG antibodies competitively block the binding of IgM to CMV antigen. Separation of IgG and IgM fractions before testing decreases the incidence of false-negative results.

Rapid and simple methods for the removal of interfering rheumatoid factor and IgG molecules from serum have been developed. These include gel filtration, affinity chromatography, selective absorption of IgM to a solid phase, and removal of IgG by using hyperimmune anti-human IgG, staphylococcal protein A, or recombinant protein G from group G streptococci. Serum pretreatment methods are now incorporated within the procedures of commercially available immunofluorescence and EIA kits, which has resulted in more reliable IgM tests. Recently, reverse capture solid-phase IgM assays have been used as an alternative approach to avoiding false-positive or -negative results. This method uses a solid phase coated with an anti-human IgM antibody to capture the IgM from a serum specimen, after which competing IgG antibody and immune complexes are removed by washing. The bound IgM antibody is then exposed to specific CMV antigen, followed by the addition of an enzyme-conjugated second antibody and substrate.

Although the detection of CMV-specific IgM may be useful in the determination of recent or active infection, results should be interpreted with caution. IgM antibody can appear in both primary and reactivated CMV infections and can persist for extended periods after a primary infection. Also, patients with Epstein-Barr virus-induced infectious mononucleosis may produce heterotypic IgM responses causing false-positive IgM results.

Other serological tests

Immune adherence hemagglutination, indirect hemagglutination, and the neutralization test are other serological tests that are used to measure CMV antibody.

INTERPRETATION OF RESULTS

Recovery of CMV from urine, throat, or other body fluids within the first week of life is the preferred method for diagnosis of congenital infection. Serological tests are less useful because of transplacental passage of maternal antibody and because of technical problems with detection of CMV-specific IgM. Most symptomatic congenitally infected infants have relatively high initial CF antibody titers, which persist at stable levels for many months (47). Congenital infection should therefore be suspected in infants with typical symptoms whose CMV titers remain high 2 to 3 months after birth. Infants not previously tested and found to be excreting virus after 1 week of age may have either congenital or acquired infection. Standard serological tests do not differentiate between these possibilities.

Interpretation of serological tests performed on sera of patients 6 months of age or older is facilitated by the absence of passively acquired maternal antibody. If the initial serum is negative for CMV antibodies and the second serum is positive, a diagnosis of primary infection can be made. If a serum sample from early in an illness contains CMV antibodies and a second sample taken several weeks later demonstrates a fourfold or greater rise in titer, a diagnosis of recent infection, due to reactivation or reinfection, can be made. Fourfold falls in titer are seldom observed early enough to be useful for laboratory diagnosis, since antibody levels tend to decline slowly over several months after infection. If acute- and convalescent-phase sera are both positive for CMV antibody but the antibody titer is unchanged, the result is interpreted as CMV infection at some time in the past. If the titers of the positive sera are high and the first specimen was obtained late in the illness, the results may indicate active infection, and appropriate specimens for viral isolation should be obtained. Whenever possible, serological diagnoses of CMV infection should be confirmed by virus isolation, particularly since fourfold fluctuations in CMV antibody titers have been noted in some apparently healthy seropositive individuals (53).

Virological or serological detection of CMV indicates active infection but does not establish whether such infection is responsible for symptomatic illness. To implicate CMV as a cause of an illness, laboratory confirmation of active infection in an appropriate clinical setting is required. When CMV is isolated from buffy coat cells, the likelihood that the infection is symptomatic increases, but asymptomatic viremia has also been described (5) and is common in patients with AIDS. Isolation of CMV from liver and particularly lung biopsy specimens must be interpreted with caution, since other pathogens (*Chlamydia trachomatis, Pneumocystis carinii*, bacteria, or fungi) may also be present; when dual infection is documented, the relative importance of each pathogen in producing clinical illness may be difficult to determine.

LITERATURE CITED

1. **Beckwith, D. G., D. C. Halstead, K. Alpaugh, A. Schweder, D. A. Blount-Fronefield, and K. Toth.** 1985. Comparison of a latex agglutination test with five other methods for determining the presence of antibody against cytomegalovirus. J. Clin. Microbiol. **21:**328–331.
2. **Booth, J. C., G. Hannington, T. M. F. Bakir, H. Stern, H. Kangro, P. D. Griffiths, and R. B. Heath.** 1982. Comparison of enzyme-linked immunosorbent assay, radioimmunoassay, complement fixation, anticomplement immunofluorescence and passive haemagglutination techniques for detecting cytomegalovirus IgG antibody. J. Clin. Pathol. **35:**1345–1348.
3. **Buffone, G. J., G. J. Demmler, C. M. Schimbor, and M. D. Yow.** 1988. DNA hybridization assay for congenital cytomegalovirus infection. J. Clin. Microbiol. **26:**2184–2186.
4. **Chou, S., and T. C. Merigan.** 1983. Rapid detection and quantitation of human cytomegalovirus in urine through DNA hybridization. N. Engl. J. Med. **308:**921–925.
5. **Cox, F., and W. T. Hughes.** 1975. Cytomegaloviremia in children with acute lymphatic leukemia. J. Pediatr. **87:** 190–194.
6. **Cremer, N. E., M. Hoffman, and E. H. Lennette.** 1978. Analysis of antibody assay methods and classes of viral antibodies in serodiagnosis of cytomegalovirus infection. J. Clin. Microbiol. **8:**152–159.
7. **Cremer, N. E., M. Hoffman, and E. H. Lennette.** 1978. Role of rheumatoid factor in complement fixation and indirect hemagglutination tests for immunoglobulin M antibody to cytomegalovirus. J. Clin. Microbiol. **8:**160–165.
8. **Demmler, G. J., G. J. Buffone, C. M. Schimbor, and R. A. May.** 1988. Detection of cytomegalovirus in urine from newborns by using polymerase chain reaction DNA amplification. J. Infect. Dis. **158:**1177–1184.
9. **Dylewski, J. S., L. Rasmussen, J. Mills, and T. C. Merigan.** 1984. Large-scale serological screening for cytomegalovirus antibodies in homosexual males by enzyme-linked immunosorbent assay. J. Clin. Microbiol. **19:**200–203.
10. **Fedorko, D. P., D. M. Ilstrup, and T. F. Smith.** 1989. Effect of age of shell vial monolayers on detection of cytomegalovirus from urine specimens. J. Clin. Microbiol. **27:**2107–2109.
11. **Ferrante, A., and Y. H. Thong.** 1980. Optimal conditions for simultaneous purification of mononuclear and polymorphonuclear leukocytes from human peripheral blood by the Hypaque-Ficoll method. J. Immunol. Methods **36:** 109–117.
12. **Friedman, H. M., N. B. Tustin, M. M. Hitchings, and S. A. Plotkin.** 1981. Comparison of complement fixation and fluorescent immunoassay (FIAX) for measuring antibodies to cytomegalovirus and herpes simplex virus. Am. J. Clin. Pathol. **76:**305–307.
13. **Gleaves, C. A., D. A. Hursh, D. H. Rice, and J. D. Meyers.** 1989. Detection of cytomegalovirus from clinical specimens in centrifugation culture by in situ DNA hybridization and monoclonal antibody staining. J. Clin. Microbiol. **27:** 21–23.
14. **Gleaves, C. A., D. Myerson, R. A. Bowden, R. C. Hackman, and J. D. Meyers.** 1989. Direct detection of cytomegalovirus from bronchoalveolar lavage samples by using

a rapid in situ DNA hybridization assay. J. Clin. Microbiol. **27:**2429–2432.

15. **Gleaves, C. A., T. F. Smith, E. A. Shuster, and G. R. Pearson.** 1984. Rapid detection of cytomegalovirus in MRC-5 cells inoculated with urine specimens by using low-speed centrifugation and monoclonal antibody to an early antigen. J. Clin. Microbiol. **19:**917–919.
16. **Goldstein, L. C., J. McDougall, R. Hackman, J. D. Meyers, E. D. Thomas, and R. C. Nowinski.** 1982. Monoclonal antibodies to cytomegalovirus: rapid identification of clinical isolates and preliminary use in diagnosis of cytomegalovirus pneumonia. Infect. Immun. **38:**273–281.
17. **Grody, W. W., K. J. Lewin, and F. Naeim.** 1988. Detection of cytomegalovirus DNA in classic and epidemic Kaposi's sarcoma by in situ hybridization. Human Pathol. **19:**524–528.
18. **Hanshaw, J. B.** 1966. Cytomegalovirus complement fixing antibody in microencephaly. N. Engl. J. Med. **275:**476–479.
19. **Howell, C. L., and M. J. Miller.** 1983. Effect of sucrose phosphate and sorbitol on infectivity of enveloped viruses during storage. J. Clin. Microbiol. **18:**658–662.
20. **Howell, C. L., M. J. Miller, and W. J. Martin.** 1979. Comparison of rates of virus isolation from leukocyte populations separated from blood by conventional and Ficoll-Paque/Macrodex methods. J. Clin. Microbiol. **10:**533–537.
21. **Hsia, K., D. H. Spector, J. Lawrie, and S. A. Spector.** 1989. Enzymatic amplification of human cytomegalovirus sequences by polymerase chain reaction. J. Clin. Microbiol. **27:**1802–1809.
22. **Huang, E.-S., H. A. Kilpatrick, Y.-T. Huang, and J. S. Pagano.** 1976. Detection of human cytomegalovirus and analysis of strain variation. Yale J. Biol. Med. **49:**29–43.
23. **Hursh, D. A., A. D. Abbot, R. Sun, J. P. Iltis, D. H. Rice, and C. A. Gleaves.** 1989. Evaluation of a latex particle agglutination assay for the detection of cytomegalovirus antibody in patient serum. J. Clin. Microbiol. **27:**2878–2879.
24. **Keller, R., R. Peitchel, J. N. Goldman, and M. Goldman.** 1976. An IgG-Fc receptor induced in cytomegalovirus-infected human fibroblasts. J. Immunol. **116:**772–777.
25. **Kettering, J. D., N. J. Schmidt, D. Gallo, and E. H. Lennette.** 1977. Anti-complement immunofluorescence test for antibodies to human cytomegalovirus. J. Clin. Microbiol. **6:**627–632.
26. **Kettering, J. D., N. J. Schmidt, and E. H. Lennette.** 1977. Improved glycine-extracted complement-fixing antigen for human cytomegalovirus. J. Clin. Microbiol. **6:**647–649.
27. **Lee, S. L., and H. H. Balfour.** 1977. Optimal method for recovery of cytomegalovirus from urine of renal transplant patients. Transplantation **24:**228–230.
28. **Lucas, G., J. M. Seigneurin, J. Tamalet, S. Michelson, M. Baccard, J. F. Delagneau, and P. Deletoille.** 1989. Rapid diagnosis of cytomegalovirus by indirect immunofluorescence assay with monoclonal antibody F6b in a commercially available kit. J. Clin. Microbiol. **27:**367–369.
29. **Macris, M. P., A. J. Nahmias, P. D. Bailey, F. K. Lee, A. M. Visintine, and A. W. Braun.** 1981. Electron microscopy in the routine screening of newborns with congenital cytomegalovirus infection. J. Virol. Methods **2:**315–320.
30. **Martin, D. C., D. A. Katzenstein, G. S. M. Yu, and M. C. Jordan.** 1984. Cytomegalovirus viremia detected by molecular hybridization and electron microscopy. Ann. Intern. Med. **100:**222–225.
31. **Martin, W. J., II, and T. F. Smith.** 1986. Rapid detection of cytomegalovirus in bronchoalveolar lavage specimens by a monoclonal antibody method. J. Clin. Microbiol. **23:** 1006–1008.
32. **Mayo, D. R., T. Brennan, S. P. Sirpenski, and C. Seymour.** 1985. Cytomegalovirus antibody detection by three commercially available assays and complement fixation. Diagn. Microbiol. Infect. Dis. **3:**455–459.
33. **McClintock, J. T., S. R. Thaker, M. Mosher, D. Jones, M. Forman, P. Charache, K. Wright, J. Keiser, and F. E. Taub.** 1989. Comparison of in situ hybridization and monoclonal antibodies for early detection of cytomegalovirus in cell culture. J. Clin. Microbiol. **27:**1554–1559.
34. **McHugh, T. M., C. H. Casavant, J. C. Wilber, and D. P. Stites.** 1985. Comparison of six methods for the detection of antibody to cytomegalovirus. J. Clin. Microbiol. **22:** 1014–1019.
35. **Myerson, D., R. C. Hackman, and J. D. Meyers.** 1984. Diagnosis of cytomegaloviral pneumonia by in situ hybridization. J. Infect. Dis. **150:**272–277.
36. **Olive, D. M., M. Simsek, and S. Al-Mufti.** 1989. Polymerase chain reaction assay for detection of human cytomegalovirus. J. Clin. Microbiol. **27:**1238–1242.
37. **Palmer, D. F., L. Kaufman, W. Kaplan, and J. J. Cavallaro.** 1977. Serodiagnosis of mycotic diseases. Charles C Thomas, Publisher, Springfield, Ill.
38. **Paya, C. V., A. D. Wold, D. M. Ilstrup, and T. F. Smith.** 1988. Evaluation of number of shell vial cell cultures per clinical specimen for rapid diagnosis of cytomegalovirus infection. J. Clin. Microbiol. **26:**198–200.
39. **Paya, C. V., A. D. Wold, and T. F. Smith.** 1988. Detection of cytomegalovirus from blood leukocytes separated by Sepracell-MN and Ficoll-Paque/Macrodex methods. J. Clin. Microbiol. **26:**2031–2033.
40. **Phipps, P. H., L. Gregoire, E. Rossier, and E. Perry.** 1983. Comparison of five methods of cytomegalovirus antibody screening of blood donors. J. Clin. Microbiol. **18:** 1296–1300.
41. **Rao, N., D. T. Waruszewski, J. A. Armstrong, R. W. Atchison, and M. Ho.** 1977. Evaluation of anti-complementary immunofluorescence test in cytomegalovirus infection. J. Clin. Microbiol. **6:**633–638.
42. **Shibata, D., W. J. Martin, M. D. Appelman, D. M. Causey, J. M. Leedom, and N. Arnheim.** 1988. Detection of cytomegalovirus DNA in peripheral blood of patients with human immunodeficiency virus. J. Infect. Dis. **158:**1185–1192.
43. **Shulman, H. M., R. C. Hackman, G. E. Sale, and J. D. Meyers.** 1982. Rapid cytological diagnosis of cytomegalovirus interstitial pneumonia on touch imprints from open-lung biopsy. Am. J. Clin. Pathol. **77:**90–94.
44. **Sorbello, A. F., S. L. Elmendorf, J. J. McSharry, R. A. Venezia, and R. M. Echols.** 1988. Rapid detection of cytomegalovirus by fluorescent monoclonal antibody staining and in situ DNA hybridization in a dram vial cell culture system. J. Clin. Microbiol. **26:**1111–1114.
45. **Spector, S. A., J. A. Rua, D. H. Spector, and R. McMillan.** 1984. Detection of human cytomegalovirus in clinical specimens by DNA-DNA hybridization. J. Infect. Dis. **150:** 121–126.
46. **Stagno, S., R. F. Pass, D. W. Reynolds, M. A. Moore, A. J. Nahmias, and C. A. Alford.** 1980. Comparative study of diagnostic procedures for congenital cytomegalovirus infection. Pediatrics **65:**251–257.
47. **Stagno, S., D. W. Reynolds, A. Tsiantos, D. A. Fuccillo, W. Long, and C. A. Alford.** 1975. Comparative serial virologic and serologic studies of symptomatic and subclinical congenitally and natally acquired cytomegalovirus infections. J. Infect. Dis. **132:**568–577.
48. **Stanier, P., D. L. Taylor, A. D. Kitchen, N. Wales, Y. Tryhorn, and A. S. Tyms.** 1989. Persistence of cytomegalovirus in mononuclear cells in peripheral blood from blood donors. Br. Med. J. **299:**897–898.
49. **Stockl, E., T. Popow-Kraupp, F. X. Heinz, F. Muhlbacher, P. Balcke, and C. Kunz.** 1988. Potential of in situ hybridization for early diagnosis of productive cytomegalovirus infection. J. Clin. Microbiol. **26:**2536–2540.
50. **van der Bij, W., R. Torensma, W. J. van Son, J. Anema, J. Schirm, A. M. Tegzess, and T. H. The.** 1988. Rapid immunodiagnosis of active cytomegalovirus infection by

monoclonal antibody staining of blood leukocytes. J. Med. Virol. **25:**179–188.

51. **Volpi, A., R. J. Whitley, R. Ceballos, S. Stagno, and L. Pereira.** 1983. Rapid diagnosis of pneumonia due to cytomegalovirus with specific monoclonal antibodies. J. Infect. Dis. **147:**1119–1120.
52. **Waner, J. L., and T. H. Weller.** 1978. Analysis of antigenic diversity among human cytomegaloviruses by kinetic neutralization tests with high-titered rabbit antisera. Infect. Immun. **21:**151–157.
53. **Waner, J. L., T. H. Weller, and S. V. Kevy.** 1973. Patterns of cytomegaloviral complement-fixing antibody activity: a longitudinal study of blood donors. J. Infect. Dis. **127:**538–543.

Chapter 77

Varicella-Zoster Virus

ANNE A. GERSHON, SHARON P. STEINBERG, AND NATHALIE J. SCHMIDT*

CLINICAL BACKGROUND

Varicella (chickenpox) and zoster represent different clinical manifestations of infection with the same virus. Varicella occurs most frequently in children and is characterized by fever and a generalized vesicular exanthem. Zoster (shingles) generally occurs in adults and consists of a painful, circumscribed eruption of vesicular lesions with accompanying inflammation of associated dorsal root or cranial nerve sensory ganglia. Varicella constitutes the primary infection, whereas zoster is a secondary infection due to reactivation of latent varicella-zoster virus (VZV) in sensory ganglia. It is now widely accepted that zoster results from reactivation of latent virus rather than reintroduction of virus into the host. This is supported by the fact that zoster does not exhibit the seasonal prevalence seen with varicella (late winter and spring), nor does zoster occur frequently in parents of young children, who are often exposed to chickenpox via their own children. Moreover, molecular studies of VZV isolates from patients with zoster occurring only a short time after either natural chickenpox or varicella vaccination have revealed that the viruses causing the primary infection and zoster are the same (36, 39). Although there may be no apparent inciting factors preceding an episode of zoster in all patients, zoster frequently appears in immunocompromised persons (including those with AIDS) and the elderly. Results of certain serological studies after natural varicella or immunization also indicate that reinfection and reactivation of VZV may occur in the absence of clinical symptoms (1, 17–20).

There are several situations in which providing a specific laboratory diagnosis of VZV infection is crucial. VZV infection may cause severe or fatal disease in individuals who are on immunosuppressive therapy or who have genetic defects in their immune responses. Progressive, generalized varicella occurs in as many as 30% of children who acquire chickenpox while receiving chemotherapy and radiotherapy for cancer, and mortality in these cases has ranged from 7 to 28% (7, 8). In older immunodeficient patients, there is an increased risk of disseminated zoster, and mortality rates are similar to those for varicella (23, 26). Providing a specific diagnosis of VZV infection in immunosuppressed patients or their contacts may guide in the administration of antiviral agents or passive immunization with varicella-zoster immunoglobulin. Determining the immunity status (presence or absence of antibody) in high-risk immunocompromised individuals and adults (who are also at some risk to develop severe varicella) exposed to VZV infection also guides in the management of these individuals. Live attenuated varicella vaccine is expected to be licensed soon, and determination of immunity status will also be useful, particularly for adults with no history of varicella, since only about 20% of such individuals are actually susceptible to chickenpox. It is important to provide a specific diagnosis of some of the less common manifestations of VZV infection, such as varicella pneumonia and encephalitic complications, particularly since antiviral agents are now available. It is sometimes necessary to differentiate VZV infection from the vesicular eruptions caused by certain enteroviruses, bacterial agents, or hypersensitivity reactions, and also from generalized vesicular eruptions caused by herpes simplex virus (HSV).

DESCRIPTION OF THE AGENT

VZV has the typical morphology of members of the family *Herpesviridae*. It has a DNA genome with a molecular mass of 80 to 87 megadaltons, consisting of approximately 125,000 base pairs. The DNA is a linear double-stranded molecule that exists in multiple configurations (14, 20). The DNA exists in at least two isomeric forms that differ by inversion of one short terminal genome segment. There is a 5.8×10^6-dalton long unique DNA segment, U_L, flanked by terminal and internal repeats, and a 3.4×10^6-dalton short unique sequence, U_S, flanked by internal and terminal repeats. The virion has a diameter of 150 to 200 nm and consists of an inner icosahedral capsid composed of 162 capsomeres and surrounded by an envelope composed of two or more membranes. The envelope contains essential lipid, and thus infectivity of the virus is inactivated by lipid solvents (37). The virus produces approximately 30 structural and nonstructural proteins, including at least 5 glycoproteins, designated I through V. To date, antigenic variation of VZV isolates has not been demonstrated, although strain differences can be demonstrated by restriction enzyme analysis of the viral genome (35). Restriction enzyme profiles of VZV isolates reveal the following: (i) there are no detectable differences between varicella and zoster isolates, (ii) the agent is remarkably stable after passage in vitro and in vivo, and (iii) nonepidemiologically related strains may be differentiated with only one or two restriction enzymes. Multiple VZV strains are believed to be able to coexist in latent form in the same host. VZV DNA shares partial homology with HSV, Epstein-Barr virus (EBV), equine herpesviruses, and pseudorabies viruses (14). VZV shares major antigens with herpesviruses that produce varicellalike disease in various simian species (9), and it appears to share minor antigens with HSV (26, 34).

* Deceased.

COLLECTION, SHIPMENT, AND STORAGE OF SPECIMENS

Specimens usually examined for VZV are smears of vesicular lesions, vesicular fluid and scrapings, and tissues obtained at autopsy. Virus has been demonstrated in buffy coat or cerebrospinal fluid of immunosuppressed patients (2, 21). Lung is the autopsy tissue from which VZV is most frequently recovered. Smears of cellular material from vesicular lesions should be collected for immunofluorescence (IF) staining wherever feasible, since this technique is more sensitive than isolation in cell culture for virus detection (6, 33). An acute-phase blood specimen should be taken as soon as possible after the onset of symptoms, to be tested in parallel with a convalescent-phase specimen, collected at least 14 days later, in an effort to demonstrate a diagnostically significant increase in VZV antibody titer or the presence of specific immunoglobulin M (IgM). VZV immunity status is determined by testing a single blood specimen collected before, or as soon as possible after, exposure to VZV infection.

Smears of cellular material from lesions

Smears of cellular material from the base of fresh lesions are used for direct examination by IF or histological staining. This is the best method to distinguish between VZV and HSV. Since differentiation of VZV and HSV by IF staining is accomplished by testing against conjugates to each of these viruses and demonstrating staining with only a single conjugate, it is essential to prepare at least two smears of cellular material for IF examination. If insufficient material is available for IF examination, what is available should be submitted for virus isolation only. Cellular material should be placed in holding medium (see chapter 74) to be used for virus isolation. VZV is a very labile agent, however, so the time that the specimen is kept in holding medium prior to culture should be as brief as possible. Care should also be taken to avoid dilution of the specimen as much as possible.

Vesicular fluids

Vesicular fluids collected into capillary pipettes or syringes can be used for virus isolation attempts and electron microscopy, but fluids are unsatisfactory for IF staining. Fluids collected onto swabs and placed in holding medium (see chapter 74) may also be used for virus isolation. Lesions more than 4 days old rarely yield infectious virus, but the fluids may give positive results by electron microscopy, countercurrent immunoelectrophoresis (12), dot blot molecular hybridization (32), or enzyme immunofiltration (4, 43).

Crusts from lesions

Crusts do not yield infectious virus and are not suitable for IF staining or other specific antigen detection methods, but if nothing else is available they may be used for electron microscopy.

Lung, liver, or skin tissue

Smears of autopsy tissue for IF staining are prepared by excising three or four pieces of autopsy tissue about 10 to 15 mm in size, holding the tissue with forceps, and gently pressing the cut surface to the clean area of a slide. A series of impressions is made over an area 30 to 40 mm in length. Three or four slides should be prepared from each specimen. The slides are allowed to dry at room temperature for 15 to 20 min and then are fixed in acetone for 10 min at room temperature and stained as described below. Suspensions of tissue are prepared for virus isolation as described in chapter 74.

Storage and transport of specimens

Specimens for virus isolation attempts should be inoculated into suitable cell cultures as soon as possible after collection. If inoculation must be delayed (realistically for no longer than 12 h), specimens may be transported or held on wet ice or in a refrigerator. For longer periods of holding, dry-ice temperatures are required. Refrigeration is not necessary for smears or fluids to be examined for viral antigen or intranuclear inclusions. It should be remembered that fluid from vesicular lesions may be infectious, and suitable precautions should be taken in packing and storage to protect postal and laboratory personnel.

DIRECT EXAMINATION OF LESION MATERIAL

Examination of vesicular material for virus or viral antigen provides the most accurate and rapid diagnosis of VZV infection. The Tzanck test is less specific than tests for virus antigen (6, 27).

Cytological examination of smears from vesicular lesions

Smears of cellular material collected from the base of vesicular lesions are prepared as described in chapter 74. They are fixed with methanol and stained with buffered Giemsa stain at pH 7.0 to 7.2. Microscopic examination reveals the presence of multinucleated, giant epithelial cells with altered chromatin patterns (Fig. 1); these are characteristic of infection with either VZV or HSV.

Electron microscopy

Vesicular fluids may be examined by electron microscopy. Crusts from lesions may be ground in 1 or 2 drops of distilled water. When transportation of specimens to the laboratory presents a problem, heavy smears of fluids and crusts may be prepared on glass microscope slides and air dried; material from these smears is reconstituted in a drop of water for examination by electron microscopy.

A drop of the specimen is placed on a grid and blotted with filter paper. A drop of 3% phosphotungstic acid (prepared in distilled water buffered to neutrality with 1 N KOH) is then added and blotted. The specimen should be examined in an electron microscope as soon as possible. The demonstration of virus with morphology typical of herpesviruses (Fig. 2) identifies the etiological agent as a member of this group and distinguishes it from the orthopoxviruses, but it does not provide a specific diagnosis of VZV infection.

IF staining

Smears properly collected from the base of fresh vesicular lesions may be used for IF staining for the spe-

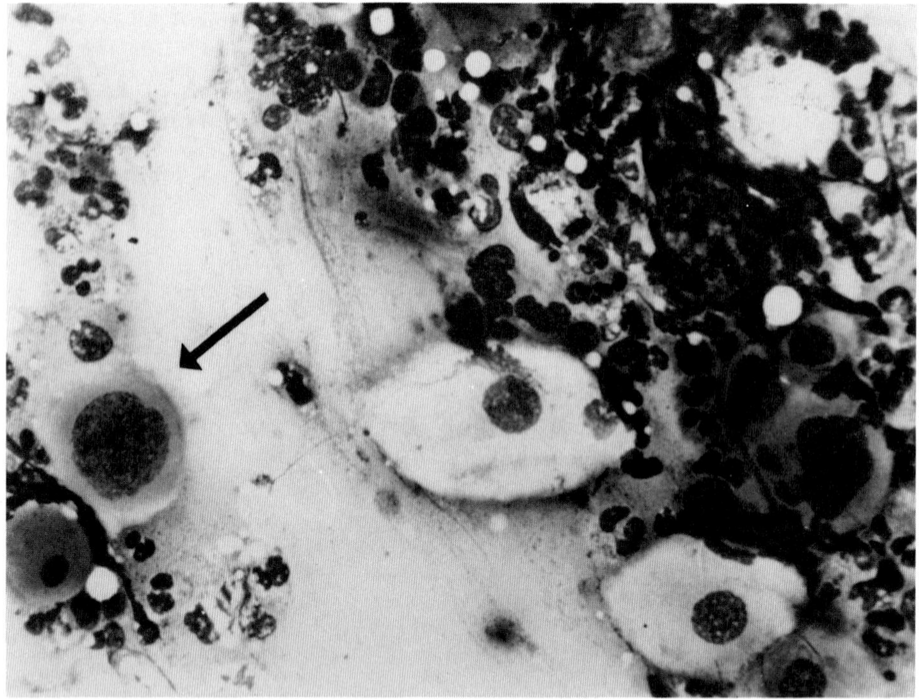

FIG. 1. Giemsa-stained preparation of material from the base of a vesicular lesion. Magnification, ×250. Arrow shows a giant cell with folded nucleus characteristic of VZV or HSV infection.

cific demonstration of VZV antigen in the infected epithelial cells. It is essential that the smears contain a large number of infected cells, and at least two smears should be made to permit staining with conjugates to VZV and HSV (and in very special situations vaccinia virus). The direct method of staining, with the use of fluorescein-conjugated mouse monoclonal antibodies to VZV or HSV glycoproteins available from commercial sources, is the most specific procedure. Direct IF staining is described below. IF staining on frozen sections of punch biopsies from prevesicular skin lesions has also been reported for the rapid and early diagnosis of VZV infections (24).

ISOLATION AND IDENTIFICATION OF VZV

Host systems

Diploid human cell lines or primary human cell cultures are the most sensitive host system for isolation of

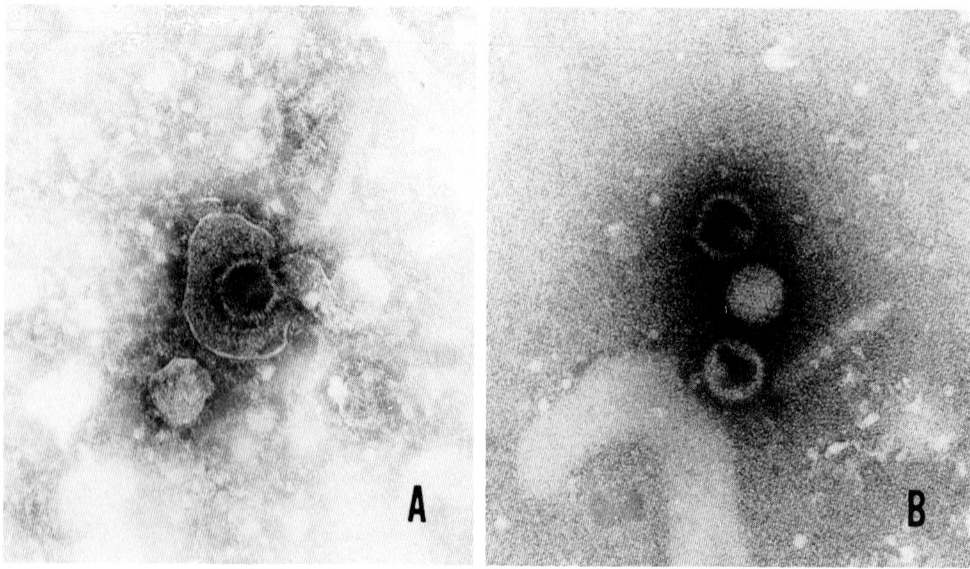

FIG. 2. Electron micrograph of VZV in a preparation from a lesion swab. Magnification, ×80,000. (A) Enveloped virus. (B) Naked nucleocapsids.

VZV from clinical materials. Human fetal diploid kidney (HFDK) or human fetal diploid lung (HFDL) cells have been found to be highly satisfactory for primary isolation of VZV; these cells are available from commercial sources. Some laboratories have used human foreskin fibroblasts for isolation of VZV; sensitivity as compared with that of human fetal diploid cells is uncertain. Cell cultures are initiated with Eagle minimum essential medium (MEM) prepared in a Hanks or Earle balanced salt solution base and supplemented with 10% heat-inactivated (56°C for 30 min) fetal bovine serum. Inoculated cell cultures are maintained in Eagle MEM prepared in Earle balanced salt solution supplemented with 2% fetal bovine serum. Although this medium will maintain the cultures for 14 days without a fluid change, a period usually sufficient for the development of a specific viral cytopathic effect (CPE), we prefer to change the medium at least once a week. Primary monkey kidney cells are less sensitive than human fetal diploid cells for virus isolation, but isolates are sometimes recovered in these cells.

Studies have shown virus isolation, even in optimal cell culture systems, to be less sensitive than IF staining on lesion materials for diagnosis of VZV infection (2, 12). The lability of viral infectivity in vesicular fluid and the strongly cell-associated nature of VZV probably both contribute to the difficulty of virus isolation.

VZV cannot be isolated in mouse or embryonated egg host cell systems.

Evidence of infection in cell cultures

Figure 3 shows the characteristic CPE of VZV in HFDK cells. Initially, the CPE consists of small, discrete foci of rounded and swollen refractile cells; in HFDK and HFDL cells, these may appear from 2 to 14 days after inoculation of the cultures with clinical materials, but in most instances CPE is first apparent at 3 to 7 days. The foci of infected cells enlarge and may slowly involve much of the monolayer. The spread of infection can be accelerated by dispersing cells in the infected culture with trypsin (see below) and replanting them in growth medium in the same culture vessel.

Subpassage and storage of virus

Infectious VZV remains in close association with the host cell, and therefore it is necessary to use virus-infected cells, rather than culture fluids, as an inoculum for serial propagation of the virus. Trypsin-dispersed infected cells are most suitable for subpassage of VZV. The medium is removed from cell cultures in which CPE involves approximately 50% of the cell sheet, and 1 ml of 0.25% trypsin solution is added to each tube culture. After 60 s at room temperature, most of the trypsin is removed, and the small amount of residual trypsin is flooded over the monolayer; as soon as the cells detach from the glass surface, they are dispersed in the original volume of growth medium and inoculated into fresh cell cultures.

Virus in infected cells can be stored in the frozen state if the viability of the cells is maintained through the use of a cryoprotective agent such as dimethyl sulfoxide in the freezing medium. Infected cells are dispersed with trypsin as described above and then suspended in Eagle MEM supplemented with 10% fetal bovine serum and 10% dimethyl sulfoxide. Infectious virus can be recovered after 18 months or more of storage at −70°C, but infectivity is preserved more effectively by storage of the infected cells in liquid nitrogen.

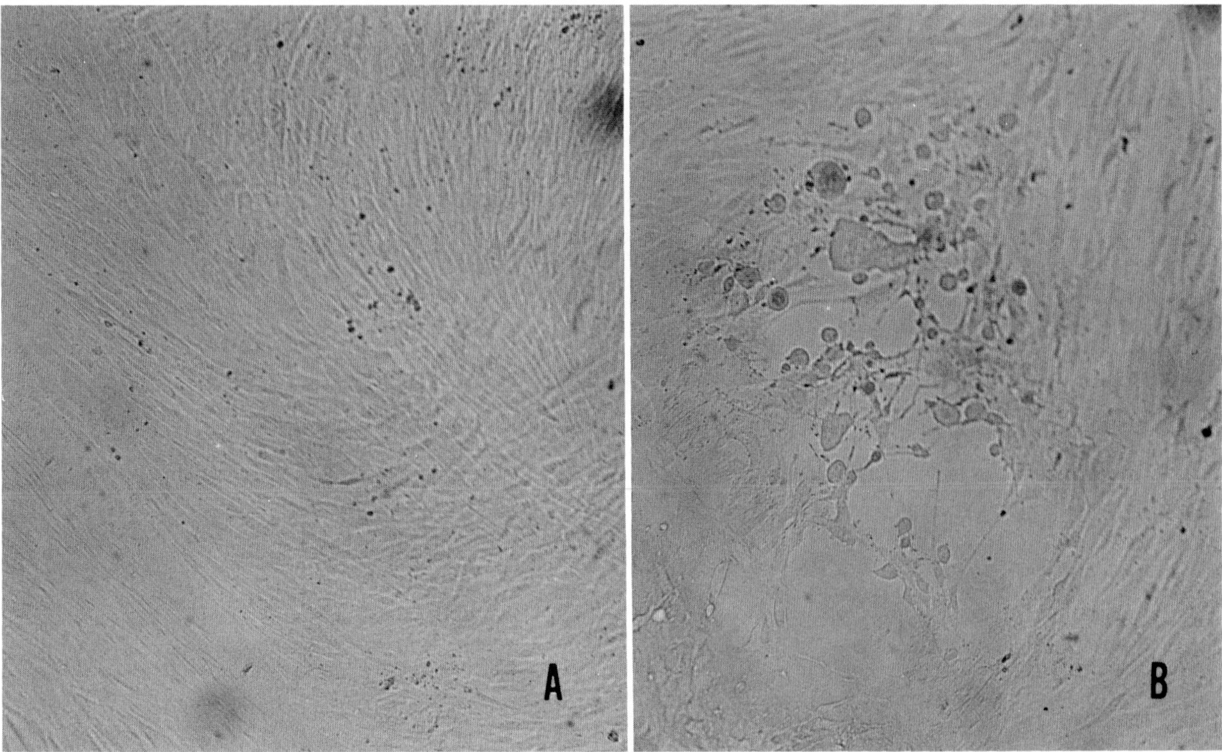

FIG. 3. CPE of VZV in HFDK cells. Magnification, ×100. (A) Uninfected cells. (B) Virus-infected cells.

High-titered cell-free virus prepared by sonic treatment of infected cells is stable at −70°C in MEM with 10% sorbitol and 10% fetal bovine serum for at least 5 years (31). In our experience, cell-free virus is stable for as long as 1 year when similarly frozen in Hanks solution alone.

Identification of VZV isolates

Presumptive identification. Presumptive identification of VZV may be made on the basis of a typical CPE, which is more focal in nature and progresses more slowly than that of HSV. VZV may also be differentiated from HSV by its failure to produce a CPE in rabbit or hamster kidney cell cultures, whereas HSV rapidly produces a CPE. The source of the specimen and the clinical manifestations of the illness should usually prevent confusion between VZV and human cytomegalovirus (CMV). However, if isolations are made from tissue specimens, there may be a need to distinguish between these herpesviruses. VZV grows well in epithelial cells, whereas CMV generally produces a CPE only in human fibroblast cells. Production of CPE by CMV generally is slower and more focal in nature than that produced by VZV. Furthermore, human CMV strains fail to produce CPE in primary monkey kidney cells, but after initial isolation VZV strains will generally do so.

Specific identification. Specific identification of VZV isolates is made by demonstrating their ability to react with a known positive antiserum. Monoclonal antibodies to VZV are available commercially, and these have overcome problems previously encountered with immune VZV serum produced in animals. In the absence of monoclonal antibodies to VZV, acute- and convalescent-phase sera from a known case of varicella may be used. Identification is based on the demonstration of a greater degree of IF reactivity of the isolate with the convalescent-phase serum than with the acute-phase serum. However, the use of human sera of uncertain antibody content for identification of viral isolates is not as reliable as the use of monoclonal antibodies. Human sera used for identification of VZV should be free from antibodies to other human herpesviruses from which it is important to distinguish VZV, namely, HSV and CMV.

Specific identification of VZV isolates is accomplished most readily by IF staining using the direct method. An alternative method is indirect IF staining (38).

Antisera to VZV

Problems encountered in production of VZV antisera have been related in large part to the strongly cell-associated nature of the virus, and various approaches have been used to produce adequately potent VZV antisera free from unwanted antibodies to host proteins, such as immunization of monkeys with virus grown in monkey kidney cell cultures. Other approaches have included use of density gradient-purified virus for immunization of rabbits, guinea pigs, mice, or rats and immunization of rabbits made tolerant to human IgG with antigen immunoprecipitated with human immunoglobulin. Hybridoma technology has been used to produce monoclonal antibodies of high potency and specificity (11, 38). Methods for preparation of antisera to VZV are given in the original publications (see references 11, 37, and 41). However, most clinical virology laboratories will depend on commercially available immune reagents for virus detection and identification. The commercial reagents, monoclonal antibodies for the most part, may be obtained as fluorescein-labeled immunoglobulins for use in direct IF staining or unlabeled for use in indirect IF staining.

IF STAINING FOR VZV

Preparation of VZV slides for IF staining

Smears of VZV-infected cells are required for standardization of IF reagents and as positive controls when IF staining is used for virus detection in clinical materials.

The stock virus is subpassaged two to three times to increase infectivity by inoculating trypsinized infected cells from one culture into two cultures of uninfected cells. When cultures show a 3+ CPE at 24 h after inoculation, they are used for slide preparation. In some laboratories, the following technique has been used to control for nonspecific IF staining. The infected cells are dispersed with trypsin and mixed with trypsin-dispersed cells from two uninfected cultures. The inclusion of uninfected cells in the infected cell smears controls for specificity of IF staining, since only roughly one-third of the cells in the smear should exhibit positive staining. In addition, uninfected cell controls are prepared from trypsinized uninfected cells of the same lot as those infected with VZV. The dispersed cells are suspended in 0.01 M phosphate-buffered saline (PBS) and sedimented by centrifugation by 1,000 × *g* for 5 min. The supernatant fluids are removed, and the packed cells are resuspended in PBS, using a volume of 0.01 ml per tube culture or 0.4 ml per 32-oz (ca 0.95-liter) flask culture. Smears approximately 5 mm in diameter are made from this cell suspension by placing small drops (approximately 0.005 ml) on microscope slides or by using a cytospin apparatus. The smears are dried at room temperature, fixed with acetone at room temperature for 10 min, and then dried at room temperature. Smears can be stored at −70°C until they are used. Before staining, the smears are ringed with a liquid embroidery pen, wax pencil, or diamond pen to retain the conjugate.

Standardization of immune reagents

Fluorescein-conjugated VZV immune conjugates (preferably monoclonal antibodies to VZV) should be titrated against smears of VZV-infected cells to determine the appropriate working dilution for use in virus identification. Ideally, this should be determined in each laboratory, although commercially available labeled monoclonal antibodies are packaged in convenient plastic dropper bottles at working dilutions. If unlabeled VZV antibodies are to be used in indirect IF staining, optimal working dilutions of both the viral immune reagent and the conjugated antispecies immune reagent must be determined by preliminary block titrations.

IF staining is done by either the direct or indirect method (see below), using dilutions of the reagent against smears of VZV-infected and uninfected cells, and the degree of specific immunofluorescence is graded as ±, 1+, 2+, 3+, and 4+. A reading of 4+ indicates glaring yellow-green fluorescence; 3+ indicates bright green but not glaring fluorescence; 2+ is dull green fluorescence; and 1+ and ± designate faint and questionable fluorescence, respectively. The working dilution of the reagent is the highest dilution giving specific staining of 4+ and showing no reactivity with uninfected control cells.

Direct IF staining for VZV detection and identification

Direct IF staining of vesicular lesions or tissue specimens should be done whenever suitable specimens are available, since this technique has been found to be more sensitive than isolation in cell culture for detection of VZV (6, 33).

Smears of epithelial cells from the base of vesicular lesions or impression smears of autopsy or biopsy tissue are prepared as described above; the cytospin method is preferable. It is essential to make enough smears to permit staining with VZV and HSV (and in certain instances CMV) immune reagents.

Working dilutions of the immune conjugates are prepared in PBS. Each of the conjugates is added to the specimen smear in a volume sufficient to cover the ringed area (about 0.005 ml). Positive control slides for VZV and HSV are also stained with each conjugate in every run as a control on the specificity and reactivity of the conjugates. After addition of the conjugates, tests are incubated in a humidified atmosphere at 35 to 37°C for 30 min, and the slides are then rinsed twice in PBS (10 min for each rinsing), followed by a rinse in distilled water. They are allowed to dry and are then mounted in buffered glycerol solution (9 parts glycerol and 1 part PBS).

In specimens that are diagnostic of VZV, examination with a fluorescence microscope should reveal specific staining of 3+ to 4+ intensity, associated with both the cytoplasm and nucleus of the epithelial cells stained with the VZV conjugate, and little or no staining in cells treated with the HSV conjugate. Vesicular lesion specimens containing too few epithelial cells for definitive examination are reported as unsatisfactory rather than negative.

Identification of VZV isolated in cell cultures is performed by direct IF staining when the inoculated cultures show a 2+ viral CPE. Trypsin-dispersed cells from an infected tube culture (or infected cells mixed with those from two uninfected cultures of the same lot as described above) are suspended in PBS, and cells are sedimented by centrifugation. Smears for IF staining are prepared on microscope slides from these cells as described above. Four smears of each suspension are made to permit staining with both VZV and HSV conjugates (and/or CMV conjugate if appropriate). Smears from uninfected cultures are prepared similarly. The smears are fixed and stained as described above. Positive VZV and HSV control slides are included in each run. Again, positive results are based on staining of 3+ to 4+ intensity with the VZV conjugate, little or no staining with HSV or CMV conjugate, and no staining with the uninfected control cells.

Indirect IF staining for VZV detection and identification

Unconjugated monoclonal antibodies can be used for indirect detection of VZV in clinical specimens or for identification of virus isolated in cell culture (38), although direct detection as described above is simpler and preferable. It is essential when using the indirect method to use a conjugate against mouse immunoglobulins which is free from nonspecific reactivity with host tissues and host serum components in clinical specimens. This is determined by testing dilutions of the conjugate against infected and uninfected cell smears in the absence of intermediate mouse antibodies. The appropriate working dilutions of the VZV reagent and the anti-mouse globulin conjugate are determined by preliminary block titration. The working dilution of the VZV immune reagent is applied to the specimen smear, and the specimen is also stained with HSV antibodies as a control. Slides are incubated at 35 to 37°C in a humidified atmosphere for 30 min and then are washed twice in PBS. The working dilution of the conjugate is then added, and tests are incubated at 35 to 37°C for 30 min. The slides are washed twice in PBS and mounted in buffered glycerol. Positive results are based on 3+ to 4+ staining of the specimen with the VZV reagent and little or no staining with the HSV reagent.

Identification of VZV isolates by using shell vials

Identification by use of shell vials is a combination technique involving virus isolation and early specific identification of virus with monoclonal antibody before development of obvious CPE. It is a very convenient means for identification of VZV in clinical specimens. It has been found to be more sensitive than either virus isolation or the Tzanck test for diagnosis of VZV infection, and it compares favorably with the direct IF test on smears of specimens (27). Commercially available shell vials containing cover slips on which HFDL cells are growing in a monolayer are used. Vesicular fluid (1 to 2 drops) is inoculated directly (or swabs are rinsed in approximately 1 ml of medium and 0.2 ml is inoculated) into each of four shell vials from which medium has been removed and centrifuged for 40 min at 700 × *g* at room temperature. After centrifugation, 2 ml of maintenance medium is added to each vial. Two uninfected vials are used as controls. Three vials are incubated at 35 to 37°C for 24 h, and three are incubated similarly for 72 h. At the appointed time, the vials are rinsed twice with 1 ml of PBS, with aspiration of PBS between washings. Monolayers are fixed by removing the medium, washing the sample gently with PBS two times, and adding 2 ml of cold acetone for 10 min. The cover slips are either stored at −70°C, or washed by addition of 1 ml of PBS for immediate use. For staining, one vial is incubated with 1 to 2 drops of commercial fluorescein-conjugated monoclonal antibody to VZV (already diluted to a working dilution as sold in the bottle), and the other vial is incubated with 1 drop of fluorescein-conjugated monoclonal antibody to HSV for 30 min at room temperature or 37°C. The vials are again washed with PBS twice and rinsed with distilled water once; the cover slips are removed from the vials, air dried, and placed cell side down on microscope slides in mounting medium (buffered glycerol). The cover slips are sealed with nail polish, and the slides are examined as above by fluorescence microscopy. Positive results are based on staining of 3+ to 4+ intensity with the VZV conjugate, little or no staining with the HSV conjugate, and no staining with the uninfected control cells. If all vials are negative after 24 h of incubation, the vials incubated for 72 h should be examined. Suggested controls to be included in each run are an uninfected culture with conjugate and a known infected culture with conjugate.

SEROLOGICAL METHODS

Serological procedures are used for laboratory diagnosis of varicella or zoster infections and also for determining immunity status (presence or absence of VZV antibody). Testing for immunity status is particularly useful for healthy adults who have no prior history of varicella, since about 75% of those raised in the continental United States will have detectable VZV antibody and thus have already experienced an episode of varicella (usually without symptoms).

Serodiagnosis

The value of serological procedures for diagnosis of VZV infection is limited to some extent by the fact that heterotypic antibody titer rises to VZV may occur in certain patients with HSV infection who have experienced a prior infection with VZV. This would appear to be a heterotypic antibody response to common antigens in the two viruses (28, 34).

In the past, the complement fixation (CF) test had been the most widely used procedure for serodiagnosis of VZV infections. However, as viral diagnostic laboratories are increasingly adopting enzyme immunoassays (EIAs) as their principal serological tool for viral diagnosis, the CF test has largely been displaced by EIA.

VZV antigens for EIA are available from commercial sources, or they can be prepared from infected HFDL or HFDK cultures. Cultures are inoculated with a high concentration of trypsin-dispersed infected cells and harvested several days later, when the cultures show advanced CPE. Glycine-buffered saline (0.043 M glycine, 0.15 M NaCl, pH 9) is used to rinse infected monolayers, which are then scraped off the glass or plastic with a rubber policeman into approximately 1/20 of the original culture volume of fresh glycine-buffered saline and disrupted by sonication for 30 to 60 s at 2.2 to 2.6 A; the antigen is then clarified by centrifugation at 1,000 × *g* for 5 min at room temperature. Uninfected control antigen is prepared in the same manner. Antigens may be stored at −70°C.

For serodiagnosis of infection, acute- and convalescent-phase sera must be tested in the same run. A fourfold or greater increase in antibody titer between acute- and convalescent-phase sera is considered diagnostically significant. In varicella, antibodies are usually demonstrable within several days after onset of rash, and they reach a peak 2 to 3 weeks later. The antibody increase is usually more rapid in zoster, and it is common for antibodies to be detectable at the time of onset of zoster.

The technique for the EIA test is described in detail in references 10, 15, and 33; a description of one EIA test for VZV antibody follows (10). Tests are performed in microtiter plates marketed specifically for EIA procedures. Wells are coated with an optimal dilution of VZV antigen or control antigen in 0.06 M bicarbonate buffer (pH 9.5) in a volume of 0.2 ml. After overnight incubation at 4°C, the unadsorbed antigen is removed by vacuum suction, the wells are washed with PBS containing 0.05% Tween 20, and protein adsorption sites are saturated by addition of 0.35 ml of a 5% bovine albumin solution in PBS and incubation for 4 h at room temperature. The fluids are then aspirated, and the wells are washed with PBS. Serial twofold dilutions of serum are prepared with 0.05-ml microdilutions in wells coated with VZV antigen and with control antigen. PBS in a volume of 0.05 ml is added to each well, and tests are incubated overnight at room temperature. (Alternatively, a shorter incubation period of 1 to 5 h may be tried.) Controls include (i) known positive and negative sera and (ii) wells incubated with diluent instead of serum. After the incubation with serum, the contents of the wells are aspirated, and the wells are washed three times with PBS. An optimal dilution of alkaline phosphatase-labeled antibodies to human IgG, prepared in PBS with 5% bovine serum albumin, is added in a volume of 0.1 ml, and tests are incubated for 2 h at room temperature. The conjugate is then aspirated from the wells, which are then washed three times with PBS. The enzyme substrate, *p*-nitrophenylphosphate (1 mg/ml) in diethanolamine (10%) buffer (pH 9.8) with 10^{-3} M $MgCl_2$, is added in a volume of 0.1 ml; after incubation at room temperature for 30 min, the reaction is stopped by the addition of 0.05 ml of 3 N NaOH per well. Results can be read by visual inspection against a white background or preferably with an EIA reader. It is preferable to test a known battery of VZV antibody-negative and -positive sera when standardizing this assay and introducing it into a laboratory for the first time for purposes of quality control.

A number of commercially marketed tests for measurement of VZV antibody by EIA are available and have been evaluated (3, 5, 22). In general, these tests are fairly specific; however, since they may lack sensitivity, some adults with immunity to varicella may be misidentified as susceptible to chickenpox when tested by these methods. These methods may also fail to identify individuals who have been immunized with live attenuated varicella vaccine (3).

Alternative methods that are applicable to the routine serodiagnosis of VZV infections are the immune adherence hemagglutination test (10) and anticomplement immunofluorescence (ACIF) staining (13, 25). Neutralizing antibody to VZV can be assayed by plaque reduction techniques with cell-free virus obtained by sonic treatment of infected human diploid cells (28); however, this is primarily a research rather than a diagnostic tool.

Determination of immunity status

A rapid and sensitive serological method is required for determining past infection and presumed immunity to varicella. The CF test is not adequately sensitive for detection of antibody elicited by past infection, giving positive results in only 50% or fewer of individuals with VZV antibody demonstrable by more sensitive methods. EIA assays are more sensitive than CF, and demonstration of VZV antibody by this method is good evidence of prior infection with VZV (varicella). In approximately 10 to 15% of sera in which VZV antibody cannot be detected by EIA, however, antibody is detectable by fluorescent-antibody staining of membrane antigen in VZV-infected cells (FAMA) (40). FAMA has been used as a method for determining immunity status, and results have correlated well with resistance or susceptibility to infection in clinical settings. The FAMA method is somewhat cumbersome, requiring use of live unfixed VZV-infected cells; however, its sensitivity and specificity make it ideal for determining immunity status. In immunocompromised children such as those with leukemia, it is preferable to consider a history of previous varicella as the best indication of immunity rather than the results of a serological test which may, for example, be falsely positive in a child who has recently received blood products.

The FAMA test is performed as follows. Doubling dilutions of serum are made in PBS beginning at 1:2 in a 96-well round bottom microtiter plate. Heat inactivation of serum is not required for this assay and should not be done, since it may lead to nonspecific results. Cells infected with VZV are harvested when they exhibit 90% CPE. Cells are scraped into PBS, centrifuged at 700 × *g* for 2 min, taken up in PBS, and dispersed in 0.025-ml samples into microtiter plates containing dilutions of serum. Cells are then incubated for 30 min at room temperature in a moist chamber. PBS is then added to fill the wells, and the plate is centrifuged at 1,000 × *g* at 4°C for 10 min, after which the PBS is removed by rapidly flipping the plate upside down (this can be done successfully with practice). The washing steps are repeated two more times. A working dilution of fluorescein-labeled anti-human globulin (0.025 ml) is added to each well, and incubation for 30 min at room temperature is again carried out. (This assay may also be used to measure specific VZV IgM antibody [16], in which case a fluorescein-labeled anti-human IgM conjugate is used.) After two washes, a drop of buffered glycerol is added to each well, and the cells are removed with an aspirator and placed on microscope slides. The cells are covered with a glass cover slip, which is sealed with nail polish. The slides are then examined by fluorescence microscopy. The sensitivity of this assay is believed to derive from the fact that live cells are used, which preserves the conformational structure of VZV glycoprotein antigens on the surface of infected cells. This structure is probably altered by fixation, which leads to decreased sensitivity for detection of antibody. A modified FAMA assay in which cells are briefly fixed in dilute glutaraldehyde (0.075% for 60 s at 0°C) and stored at −70°C has, however, been described (42).

A method that yields results comparable to those obtained with FAMA and may be more convenient to perform is the ACIF test (13, 25). This method avoids nonspecific reactivity which may be encountered in indirect IF staining and permits examination of serum at dilutions as low as 1:2 and 1:4 (as does FAMA). Smears of VZV-infected and uninfected cells are prepared as described above for IF staining. Optimal dilutions of complement and conjugate are determined by box titrations of various dilutions of each reagent (diluted in Veronal-buffered saline, pH 7.2) against VZV-infected cells treated with appropriate dilutions of known positive and negative sera. Smears of VZV-infected and uninfected cells are treated with dilutions of inactivated (56°C, 30 min) test serum prepared in PBS for 30 min at 37°C in a humidified chamber. After a 5-min rinse in PBS, an optimal dilution of fluorescein-conjugated anti-guinea pig complement is added, and incubation is conducted for 30 min at 37°C in a moist chamber. After a 5-min rinse, the slides are air dried, mounted in 50% glycerol in PBS, and examined under UV illumination.

EVALUATION AND INTERPRETATION OF RESULTS

Demonstration of viral antigen in or virus isolation from lesion material or autopsy tissue is diagnostic of a current VZV infection. With the increasing availability of VZV-specific immune reagents from commercial sources, specific identification of isolates readily can be made by IF staining or other methods for antigen detection. Pitfalls in the use of human sera for specific identification have been indicated. Isolation of VZV is a relatively slow method and is less sensitive than electron microscopy and IF staining, since infectious virus persists for a shorter length of time in vesicles and is more labile than the viral particles and antigens which can be detected by electron microscopy and IF. The combination of virus isolation and early IF staining before obvious CPE in shell vials is a practical alternative and provides significant information within 24 to 48 h. Other means for presumptive identification of isolates as VZV include failure of VZV to multiply on rabbit or hamster kidney cells (in contrast to HSV) and ability of VZV to propagate in primary monkey kidney cells and human epithelial cells (such as thyroid), which distinguishes it from human CMV.

A fourfold or greater increase in antibody titer to VZV antigen in the absence of a similar rise to HSV antigen is diagnostic of a current VZV infection. However, a high proportion (up to one-third) of individuals with primary HSV infections who have experienced a prior VZV infection show a heterotypic antibody response to VZV antigen, making a differential diagnosis between VZV and HSV infection difficult in the absence of clear-cut clinical findings. Frequently, a differential diagnosis can be made on the basis of the fact that antibody to the infecting virus type is absent or at very low titer in the acute-phase specimen, whereas antibody to the viral heterotype is already present. Demonstration of the presence of VZV IgM in serum is indicative of acute VZV infection, but it will not distinguish between varicella and zoster (16).

Although negative results by FAMA, ACIF, and EIA are reliable indicators of susceptibility to varicella, the occurrence of clinical varicella in a few individuals with low titers of VZV antibody demonstrated by FAMA and ACIF indicates that low levels of antibody demonstrable by these sensitive methods are not always a reliable indication of protection against clinical illness. However, the detection of serum antibody to VZV by FAMA has correlated with protection in up to 96% of individuals in one study (17).

LITERATURE CITED

1. **Arvin, A. M., C. M. Koropchak, and A. C. Wittek.** 1983. Immunologic evidence of reinfection with varicella-zoster virus. J. Infect. Dis. **148:**200–205.
2. **Asano, Y., N. Itakura, Y. Hiroishi, S. Hirose, T. Ozaki, K. Kuno, T. Nagai, T. Yazaki, K. Yamanishi, and M. Takahashi.** 1985. Viral replication and immunologic responses in children naturally infected with varicella-zoster virus and in varicella vaccine recipients. J. Infect. Dis. **152:**863–868.
3. **Balfour, H. H., C. K. Edelman, C. L. Dirksen, D. R. Palermo, C. S. Suarez, J. T. Kentala, and D. D. Crane.** 1988. Laboratory studies of acute varicella and varicella immune status. Diagn. Microbiol. Infect. Dis. **10:**149–158.
4. **Cleveland, P. H., and D. D. Richman.** 1987. Enzyme im-

munofiltration staining assay for immediate diagnosis of herpes simplex virus and varicella-zoster virus directly from clinical specimens. J. Clin. Microbiol. **25:**416–420.

5. **Demmler, G., S. P. Steinberg, G. Blum, and A. A. Gershon.** 1988. Rapid enzyme-linked immunosorbent assay for detecting antibody to varicella-zoster virus. J. Infect. Dis. **157:**211–212.
6. **Drew, W. L., and L. Mintz.** 1980. Rapid diagnosis of varicella-zoster virus infection by direct immunofluorescence. Am. J. Clin. Pathol. **73:**699–701.
7. **Feldman, S., W. C. Hughes, and C. Daniel.** 1975. Varicella in children with cancer: 77 cases. Pediatrics **56:**388–397.
8. **Feldman, S., and L. Lott.** 1987. Varicella in children with cancer: impact of antiviral therapy and prophylaxis. Pediatrics **80:**465–472.
9. **Felsenfeld, A. M., and N. J. Schmidt.** 1977. Antigenic relationships among several simian varicella-like viruses and varicella-zoster virus. Infect. Immun. **15:**807–812.
10. **Forghani, B., N. J. Schmidt, and J. Dennis.** 1978. Antibody assays for varicella-zoster virus: comparison of enzyme immunoassay with neutralization, immune adherence hemagglutination, and complement fixation. J. Clin. Microbiol. **8:**545–552.
11. **Forghani, B., N. J. Schmidt, C. K. Myoraku, and D. Gallo.** 1982. Serological reactivity of some monoclonal antibodies to varicella-zoster virus. Arch. Virol. **73:**311–317.
12. **Frey, H., S. P. Steinberg, and A. A. Gershon.** 1981. Varicella-zoster infections: rapid diagnosis by countercurrent immunoelectrophoresis. J. Infect. Dis. **143:**274–280.
13. **Gallo, D., and N. J. Schmidt.** 1981. Comparison of anticomplement immunofluorescence and fluorescent antibody-to-membrane antigen test for determination of immunity status to varicella-zoster virus and for serodifferentiation of varicella-zoster and herpes simplex virus infections. J. Clin. Microbiol. **14:**539–543.
14. **Gelb, L.** 1990. Varicella-zoster virus, p. 2011–2053. *In* B. N. Fields (ed.), Virology. Raven Press, New York.
15. **Gershon, A., H. M. Frey, S. P. Steinberg, and M. D. Seeman.** 1981. Enzyme-linked immunosorbent assay for measurement of antibody to varicella-zoster virus. Arch. Virol. **70:**169–172.
16. **Gershon, A. A., S. P. Steinberg, W. Borkowsky, D. Lennette, and E. Lennette.** 1982. IgM to varicella-zoster virus: demonstration in patients with and without clinical zoster. Pediatr. Infect. Dis. **1:**164–167.
17. **Gershon, A. A., S. P. Steinberg, and L. Gelb.** 1984. Clinical reinfection with varicella-zoster virus. J. Infect. Dis. **149:** 137–142.
18. **Gershon, A., S. P. Steinberg, P. LaRussa, A. Ferrara, M. Hammerschlag, L. Gelb, and the NIAID Varicella Vaccine Collaborative Study Group.** 1988. Immunization of healthy adults with live attenuated varicella vaccine. J. Infect. Dis. **157:**132–137.
19. **Gershon, A., S. P. Steinberg, and the NIAID Varicella Vaccine Collaborative Study Group.** 1989. Persistence of immunity to varicella in leukemic children immunized with live varicella vaccine. N. Engl. J. Med. **320:**892–898.
20. **Grose, C., and R. Giller.** 1988. Varicella-zoster virus infection and immunization in the healthy and the immunocompromised host. Crit. Rev. Hematol. Oncol. **8:**27–64.
21. **Jemsek, J., S. B. Greenberg, L. Taber, D. Harvey, A. A. Gershon, and R. Couch.** 1983. Herpes zoster-associated encephalitis: clinopathologic report of 12 cases and review of the literature. Medicine **62:**81–97.
22. **LaRussa, P., S. P. Steinberg, E. Waithe, B. Hanna, and R. Holzman.** 1987. Comparison of five assays for antibody to varicella-zoster virus to the fluorescent antibody to membrane antigen assay. J. Clin. Microbiol. **25:**2059–2062.
23. **Locksley, R. M., N. Fluornoy, K. M. Sullivan, and J. D. Meyers.** 1985. Infection with varicella-zoster virus after marrow transplantation. J. Infect. Dis. **152:**1172–1181.
24. **Olding-Stenkvist, E., and M. Grandien.** 1978. Early diagnosis of virus-caused vesicular rashes by immunofluorescence on skin biopsies. I. Varicella, zoster, and herpes simplex. Scand. J. Infect. Dis. **8:**27–35.
25. **Preissner, C. M., S. P. Steinberg, A. A. Gershon, and T. Smith.** 1982. Evaluation of the anticomplement immunofluorescence test for detection of antibody to varicella-zoster virus. J. Clin. Microbiol. **16:**373–376.
26. **Schepp, D. H., P. S. Dandliker, and J. D. Meyers.** 1986. Treatment of varicella-zoster virus infection in severely immunocompromised patients: a randomized comparison of acyclovir and vidarabine. N. Engl. J. Med. **314:**208–212.
27. **Schirm, J., J. J. Meulenberg, G. W. Pastoor, P. C. van Voorst-Vader, and F. P. Schroder.** 1989. Rapid detection of varicella-zoster virus in clinical specimens using monoclonal antibodies on shell vials and smears. J. Med. Virol. **28:**1–6.
28. **Schmidt, N. J.** 1982. Further evidence for common antigens in herpes simplex and varicella-zoster viruses. J. Med. Virol. **9:**27–36.
29. **Schmidt, N. J., D. Gallo, V. Devlin, J. D. Woodie, and R. W. Eammons.** 1980. Direct immunofluorescence staining for detection of herpes simplex and varicella-zoster virus antigens in vesicular lesions and certain tissue specimens. J. Clin. Microbiol. **12:**651–655.
30. **Schmidt, N. J., and E. H. Lennette.** 1975. Neutralizing antibody responses to varicella-zoster virus. Infect. Immun. **12:**606–613.
31. **Schmidt, N. J., and E. H. Lennette.** 1976. Improved yields of cell-free varicella-zoster virus. Infect. Immun. **14:**709–715.
32. **Seidlin, M., H. E. Takiff, H. A. Smith, J. Hay, and S. E. Straus.** 1984. Detection of varicella-zoster virus by dot-blot hybridization using a molecularly cloned viral probe. J. Med. Virol. **13:**53–61.
33. **Shehab, Z., and P. A. Brunell.** 1983. Enzyme-linked immunosorbent assay for susceptibility to varicella. J. Infect. Dis. **148:**472–476.
34. **Shiraki, K., T. Okuno, K. Yamanishi, and M. Takahashi.** 1982. Polypeptides of varicella-zoster virus (VZV) and immunological relationship of VZV and herpes simplex virus (HSV). J. Gen. Virol. **61:**255–269.
35. **Straus, S. E., J. Hay, H. Smith, and J. Owens.** 1983. Genome differences among varicella-zoster virus isolates. J. Gen. Virol. **64:**1031–1041.
36. **Straus, S. E., W. Reinhold, H. A. Smith, W. Ruyechan, D. Henderson, R. M. Blaese, and J. Hay.** 1984. Endonuclease analysis of viral DNA from varicella and subsequent zoster infections in the same patient. N. Engl. J. Med. **311:**1362–1364.
37. **Takahashi, M.** 1983. Chickenpox virus. Adv. Virus Res. **28:**285–356.
38. **Weigle, K. A., and C. Grose.** 1983. Common expression of varicella-zoster viral glycoprotein antigens in vitro and in chickenpox and zoster vesicles. J. Infect. Dis. **148:**630–638.
39. **Williams, D., A. A. Gershon, L. Gelb, T. Kim, C. Alvarado, M. Spraker, S. P. Steinberg, and A. Ragab.** 1985. Herpes zoster following varicella vaccine in a child with acute lymphocytic leukemia. J. Pediatr. **106:**259–261.
40. **Williams, V., A. A. Gershon, and P. A. Brunell.** 1974. Serological response to varicella-zoster membrane antigens measured by immunofluorescence. J. Infect. Dis. **130:** 669–672.
41. **Wroblewska, Z., M. Devlin, R. Reilly, H. van Trieste, M. Wellish, and D. H. Gilden.** 1982. The production of varicella-zoster virus antiserum in laboratory animals. Arch. Virol. **74:**233–238.
42. **Zaia, J. A., and M. Oxman.** 1977. Antibody to varicella-zoster virus-induced membrane antigen: immunofluorescence assay using monodisperse glutaraldehyde-fixed target cells. J. Infect. Dis. **136:**519–530.
43. **Zeigler, T.** 1984. Detection of varicella-zoster viral antigens in clinical specimens by solid-phase enzyme immunoassay. J. Infect. Dis. **150:**149–154.

Chapter 78

Epstein-Barr Virus

EVELYNE T. LENNETTE

CLINICAL BACKGROUND

Epstein-Barr virus (EBV), the etiologic agent of infectious mononucleosis (IM), has a worldwide distribution, 80 to 90% of all adults having been infected. Primary infections occur during the first decade of life in areas with crowded living conditions and poor hygiene. Childhood infections are mostly asymptomatic but infrequently are associated with classical IM. In contrast, 50 to 75% of young adults experience primary EBV infections, with illness ranging from mild to severe (10).

In most cases of IM, clinical diagnosis can be made from the characteristic triad of fever, pharyngitis, and cervical lymphadenopathy lasting for 1 to 4 weeks. Normally a self-limiting illness, IM may be complicated by splenomegaly, hepatitis, pericarditis, or central nervous system involvement. Rare fatal primary infections occur in patients with histiocytic hemophagocytic syndrome or with a genetic X-linked lymphoproliferative syndrome (8, 33). Hematologic features of IM include lymphocytosis with prominent atypical lymphocytes. In 85 to 90% of IM patients, Paul-Bunnell heterophile tests are positive; false-positive results may occur in 2 to 3% of patients and can be excluded only by EBV-specific serology. Specific laboratory diagnosis is also needed to differentiate the 10 to 15% of heterophile-negative EBV infections from mononucleoses induced by other agents, such as cytomegalovirus, adenovirus, and *Toxoplasma gondii*. In primary infections of adults with clinically atypical diseases and of children with negative heterophile response, EBV-specific laboratory diagnosis may also be helpful.

Transmission of EBV requires salivary contact; airborne or bloodborne transmissions are not important routes of infection (15). As with other herpesviruses, EBV causes a persistent, latent infection with intermittent reactivations. Infectious virus can be recovered from the oropharynx of the majority of seropositive, asymptomatic individuals as well as from IM patients. The degree of shedding varies from individual to individual but remains constant within the same individual (34). Salivary EBV shedding in healthy individuals constitutes the primary reservoir for person-to-person transmission. With immunosuppression, infectious virus can be recovered from patients at greater frequency and at higher titers (35). Because of the ubiquitousness of the virus in seropositive individuals, it has been difficult to ascertain the degree of morbidity attributable to EBV reactivations. Although most of the reactivations are asymptomatic (14), there is evidence that they can be associated with severe, chronic diseases in rare instances (32).

EBV is unique among the herpesviruses in its ability to transform and to immortalize human B lymphocytes. In vitro, EBV induces polyclonal immunoglobulin production (31) and leads to establishment of permanent lymphoblastoid lines. In vivo, EBV-infected lymphoid cells are associated with a number of lymphoproliferative conditions, varying from hyperplasia to neoplasia (9).

EBV has long been suspected of having a contributory role in the etiology of Burkitt's lymphoma (BL) and nasopharyngeal carcinoma (NPC) (12). BL is primarily a tumor of children in Africa and New Guinea. Elsewhere in the world, EBV-associated BL has been reported mostly in adults and among severely immunosuppressed male homosexuals (36). EBV has also been consistently associated with undifferentiated squamous cell carcinoma of the nasopharynx, with a particularly high incidence among southern Chinese. In both tumors, viral antigens and genomes can be detected in malignant tissues (21, 23, 26, 38). Unusually high titers of antibodies to several antigens can be correlated with the patient's tumor burden. Serology can be helpful in the management of patients with malignancies and in monitoring the effectiveness of their therapies (12, 13, 19).

With the advent of aggressive and immunosuppressive therapies during organ transplantations, EBV lymphoproliferative disorders are seen at an increasing frequency. They may range from benign, polyclonal hyperplasias with no cytogenetic abnormalities to oligoclonal as well as monoclonal malignant lymphomas. As in BL and NPC, both viral antigens and genomes can be readily demonstrated in the tumors (9).

DESCRIPTION OF THE AGENT

As a member of the family *Herpesviridae*, EBV has the characteristic herpetic 120-nm enveloped morphology, with 162 capsomeres in an icosohedral arrangement. Its double-stranded 172-kilobase-pair DNA exists both as a linear form in the mature virion and as a circular episomal form in latently infected cells. Its linear structure consists of a series of unique sequences alternating with internal repeat sequences, all sandwiched between two terminal repeat elements that are joined during circularization (2, 29).

In vivo, the virus infects both lymphoid and epithelial cell-derived tissues of the nasopharynx. In vitro, EBV has been propagated only in B lymphocytes from human and subhuman primates. Although it shares common antigenic determinants with other EBV-like subhuman primate viruses, EBV is antigenically distinct from other human herpesviruses.

Infection of lymphocytes by EBV leads to their transformation into lymphoblastoid cell lines, capable of continuous growth in culture. Infected cells rarely produce infectious virus in vitro. In most transformed cell lines, the viral genome is maintained latently at a constant copy number per cell, with genome expression restricted to a small number of nuclear and latent membrane proteins (2, 4).

COLLECTION AND STORAGE OF SPECIMENS

Generally, only a single acute-phase serum sample (1 to 5 ml) is needed for diagnosis by serological testing. Convalescent serum collected 1 to 2 months after onset is occasionally needed for confirmation and interpretations. If collected aseptically, serum can be stored at 5°C for several months. For longer-term storage, freezing at −20°C is recommended.

For isolation of excreted virus, 5 to 10 ml of throat gargle collected in serum-free tissue culture medium or Hanks balanced salts solution is satisfactory. Fetal bovine serum (2 to 5%) can then be added as a stabilizer, and antibiotics can be added to suppress microbial growth. With added serum, specimens can be held for 2 to 3 days with prompt refrigeration or frozen at −70°C for long-term storage.

Tissues to be examined for viral antigens are collected aseptically and refrigerated in tissue culture medium. Suitable for this purpose are lymph nodes, spleen, and biopsies of tumors. Thin (5-μm) cryosections, but not Formalin-fixed tissues, are also suitable. Fresh biopsies may be examined for the presence of virus either by selection of EBV-transformed cells or by direct examination of EBV antigens by specific immunostaining.

Cerebrospinal fluid has not been found to be useful for documentation of EBV-associated central nervous system disease. Neither infectious virus nor the corresponding antibodies have been detected in cerebrospinal fluid, suggesting an immunologic rather than virologic etiology of the central nervous system disease.

For cultivation of EBV-infected peripheral blood lymphocytes, 10 ml of heparinized (5 to 10 U/ml) blood from IM patients is sufficient. Blood specimens should be processed as soon as possible, although refrigeration for up to 24 h is adequate.

DIRECT EXAMINATION

Direct detection of Epstein-Barr virions in lymphoid tissues is generally not practical, since infected cells are usually in a latent phase. Mature viral particles are rarely seen in infected lymphocytes, even during IM. Infection of the tongue epithelium, however, is fully permissive. A high concentration of mature virions can be readily demonstrated by electron microscopy in tongue lesion biopsies from patients with hairy oral leukoplakia (7).

In most instances, the presence of EBV can be demonstrated by the detection of induced proteins or of viral genome. The presence of the EBV-induced nuclear antigen complex (EBNA) can be readily shown in touch preparations or cryosections of affected tissues, using the anticomplement indirect immunofluorescence staining technique (30). With a larger quantity of available tissue, EBNA can also be detected by Western immunoblotting (4).

Alternatively, nucleic acid hybridization techniques such as the Southern slot blot method and cytohybridization can be used to demonstrate the presence of EBV genomes in the tissues (1, 27).

ISOLATION

Cord B lymphocytes are favored as indicator cells for EBV isolation because of their good susceptibility to infection. Lymphoid tissues and leukocytes from seronegative adults are, for practical purposes, not useful for the cultivation of EBV because of suppressive interference from T cells usually found in partially fractionated lymphocyte preparations.

Indicator cells

For optimal recovery of lymphocytes, 10 ml of human umbilical cord blood collected aseptically with 5 to 10 U of preservative-free heparin per ml should be fractionated through polysaccharide density gradients (Hypaque-Ficoll, Histopaque, etc.) as recommended by the supplier. During centrifugation, aggregated erythrocytes and granulocytes sediment to the bottom. Lymphocytes can be recovered at the plasma-gradient interphase, washed once with saline, and suspended to a density of 5×10^6 cells per ml in RPMI 1640 medium supplemented with 10% fetal bovine serum. After overnight incubation at 37°C in 5% CO_2 to check for sterility, the lymphocytes are ready for inoculation and should be used as soon as possible. In our laboratory, uninfected lymphocytes thus prepared can be frozen at liquid N_2 temperature in 10% dimethyl sulfoxide. After thawing and a brief washing to remove the preservative, they are usable for EBV isolation, though not without some loss in viability and sensitivity.

Inoculation

Throat garglings must be centrifuged at $1,500 \times g$ for 10 min. The supernatant fluid is filtered through a 0.45-μm-pore-size filter to remove remaining cell debris and microorganisms. Prompt inoculation is recommended, although the specimen can be frozen at −70°C at this stage for future inoculations. Just before inoculation, 1 ml of the fractionated leukocyte suspension is centrifuged and suspended in 0.5 ml of growth medium. A 0.5-ml sample of the filtered throat specimen is added to the leukocyte suspension. After an adsorption period of 1 to 2 h at 37°C, 5 ml of culture medium with 10% fetal bovine serum is added. An uninfected cell control and EBV-infected control should be included in parallel, since rare cord lymphocyte preparations have shown spontaneous transformation. All cultures are incubated for 4 weeks, with weekly replacements of growth medium. Necrosis of uninfected cultures is usually observable after 2 weeks, whereas virus-positive cultures should show clusters of large proliferating lymphoblastoid cells. The transforming agent can then be identified by using the ACIF procedure to detect EBNA in these cells.

IDENTIFICATION

Virus expression in transformed cell lines varies widely, from almost silent with only a few detectable viral antigens to a fully productive cycle with late proteins, such as viral capsid antigen (VCA) and infectious particles. Depending on the exact "block" on viral genome expression, various spectra of EBV antigens are detectable in the transformed cells. The only antigen complex present in all EBV-infected cells, however, is EBNA. It can be reliably used as an EBV marker, assayable by anticomplement indirect immunofluorescence assay (30). Since no commercial hyperimmune animal anti-EBNA sera are available as yet, human sera provide the only source of reagents suitable for EBNA detection. For typing reagents, sera from EBV-infected and -susceptible individuals should be used in parallel. Care should be taken in the selection of negative sera to exclude those with nonspecific antinuclear antibodies.

To detect EBNA in transformed cells in culture, the centrifuged cell pellet is suspended in saline containing 0.5% bovine serum albumin. The cell density is adjusted to 5×10^6 cells per ml, and the suspension is dropped on glass slides. The air-dried slides are fixed for 1 min with an acetone-methanol (1:1) mixture. Fixed smears can be held at −20°C until tested. Several slides should be prepared in this manner to allow for necessary controls.

Identification of individual viral isolates is now possible with the discovery that the sizes of many of the EBNA proteins (EBNA 1 to 6) induced are virus dependent. Each isolate induces proteins with distinctive patterns in Western blotting, thus allowing the fingerprinting or "Ebnotyping" of each virus (6).

SEROLOGICAL DIAGNOSIS

EBV isolation is diagnostically not useful because of the narrow host range of EBV in vitro, the long period needed for isolation of cell-free virus, and the ubiquity of EBV in healthy individuals. Serological testing is the method of choice for the diagnosis of primary infections (17). In patients with symptoms compatible with IM, a positive Paul-Bunnell heterophile antibody result is diagnostic, and no further testing is necessary. Rapid qualitative agglutination or enzyme-linked immunoassay test kits for Paul-Bunnell heterophile antibodies are widely available and are effective for 80 to 85% of IM patients. Quantitative testing procedures include several variations on the Paul-Bunnell differential test (3, 28), the ox cell hemolysis assay (25), and the immune adherence hemagglutination assays (22). Moderate to high levels of heterophile antibodies are seen during the first month of illness and decrease rapidly after week 4. The false-positive rate for the Paul-Bunnell antibodies is approximately 3%, mostly from individuals who maintain a low but persistent level of these antibodies long after their primary illness (18). The false-negative rate is 10 to 15% and is more frequent among children than adults. For these patients, EBV-specific serological testing is needed.

Humoral responses to primary EBV infections appear to be quite rapid. Eighty percent of patients usually have peak titers by the time they consult their physicians (17). Hence, in most cases testing of paired sera is not useful in demonstrating significant antibody changes. On the other hand, effective laboratory diagnosis can be made on a single acute-phase serum by testing antibodies to several EBV-associated antigens measured simultaneously. The level and spectrum of antibodies are sufficiently distinct in most cases to allow determination of whether the patient (i) is still susceptible, (ii) has a current primary infection, (iii) has had a recent (within 2 to 3 months) primary infection, (iv) had a past infection, or (v) may be having reactivated EBV infection (Table 1).

Antibodies to four antigen complexes may be measured: VCA, early antigen-diffuse component (EA/D), early antigen-restricted component (EA/R), and EBNA. In addition, differentiation of immunoglobulin G (IgG), IgM, and IgA subclasses to VCA can often be helpful for confirmatory purposes.

Anti-VCA

During the acute phase, both IgG-VCA and IgM-VCA are detectable. Whereas IgM-VCA disappears after about 4 weeks, IgG-VCA declines to a lower level but persists for life. Neutralizing antibodies can also be detected early after onset and persist for life. In practice, the complex neutralizing assays are rarely used to test immunity. Since all patients with IgG-VCA also have neutralizing antibodies, anti-VCA titers are an accurate indicator of immunity. In patients with BL and NPC, IgG-VCA titers are maintained at very high levels, usually 8 to 10 times the geometric mean titers of healthy adults. NPC patients have an additional high IgA-VCA titer, an outstanding serological feature of EBV.

Anti-EA/D and EA/R

In most patients, antibodies to EA/D show a transient rise in the acute phase. They are generally undetectable 3 to 6 months after onset. Anti-EA/R antibodies follow the disappearance of anti-EA/D and can be transiently detectable up to 2 years after onset (20). Antibodies to either or both EA components at moderate titers can reappear during EBV reactivation. With BL patients, anti-EA/R titers are present at moderate to high levels, whereas with NPC patients, high anti-EA/D titers are common. In the latter patients, both IgG and IGA subclasses of anti-EA/D are present in high titers.

TABLE 1. Serological profiles of EBV-associated syndromes

Antibody-antigen	Profile[a]						
	Nonimmune	Current primary	Recent primary	Past	Reactive	BL	NPC
IgM-VCA	−	+	−	−	−	−	−
IgG-VCA	−	+	+	+	+	++	++
IgA-VCA	−	+/−	−	−	+/−	−	++
IgG-EA/D	−	+	+	−	+/−	−	++
IgA-EA/D	−	−	−	−	*	−	++
IgG-EA/R	−	+/−	+/−	−	+/−	++	−
Anti-EBNA	−	−	+/−	+	+	+	+

[a] −, Negative (<1:10); +, positive (>1:10); +/−, either positive or negative; *, not known.

Anti-EBNA

Antibodies to the EBNA complex, as measured by the standard anticomplement indirect immunofluorescence assay using Raji cells, are rarely present in acute-phase serum. A gradual increase in EBNA antibodies occurs during convalescence, and near-peak titers are maintained for life. With severe immunosuppression, the anti-EBNA titers may gradually decrease but rarely disappear.

Anti-EBNA 1 to 6

By using transfected cell cultures, it is now possible to measure antibody responses to individual EBNA components in human sera (4). After IM infection in healthy individuals, anti-EBNA 2 antibodies increase in titer within the first 3 months of onset. As anti-EBNA 2 titers wane and even disappear, anti-EBNA 1 emerges to reach a peak titer between 6 and 12 months. In contrast, many patients with chronic, poorly defined illnesses or complicated courses of EBV primary infections have abnormal EBNA 1-to-EBNA 2 titer ratios of ≤1, primarily as a result of the persistence of EBNA 2. Unfortunately, no clear associations can be made between the anti-EBNA 1/2 ratio with the duration or nature of illness (16). The significance of antibodies to other EBNA components is still under investigation.

The levels of each of the mentioned antibodies are usually lower in young patients. However, the profile does not differ with age. The exact titers to each antigen and the time needed to develop a full spectrum of antibodies vary widely among individuals. Also, many individuals may maintain EBV antibodies at high levels with or without reactivations (34). For these reasons, diagnosis based on "screening" titers is not feasible.

The optimal combination for EBV serology consists of titration to three markers: IgG-VCA, IgG-EA, and EBNA. The inclusion of EBNA extends the time during which primary infections can be reliably diagnosed to 2 to 3 months. Diagnosis of primary infection should not rely on the detection of IgM-VCA alone. Both false-positive and false-negative results occur in IgM-VCA testing. The former are due to the presence of rheumatoid factor (11), and the latter result from late collection of serum samples.

FLUORESCENT-ANTIBODY TESTS

Listed below are the cell lines most commonly used for measuring antibodies to VCA, EA/D, EA/R, and EBNA (18). All cell lines grow well in RPMI 1640 supplemented with 10% fetal bovine serum.

(i) P3-HR1 is a virus-producing cell line. From 10 to 15% of the cells in the culture express VCA at any given time. This degree of viral expression can be maintained indefinitely. To prepare smears, centrifuged cells from a 1-week-old culture are suspended to a final density of 5×10^6 to 10^7 cells per ml in phosphate-buffered saline containing 0.5% bovine serum albumin. The cell suspension (5 to 10 μl) is dropped on glass slides with a Pasteur pipette. Air-dried slides are fixed for 1 min in acetone. Fixed slides can be stored at −20°C indefinitely.

(ii) The Raji line, in contrast, is positive only for the EBNA complex. VCA is not produced, and EA antigens are rarely detectable if this cell line is grown under normal culture conditions. Hence, Raji cells are suitable for the detection of anti-EBNA. Air-dried smears from 3- to 5-day-old cultures are prepared as described for P3-HR1 cells. Fixation, however, is with a mixture of equal volumes of acetone and methanol for 1 to 2 min.

(iii) EA-positive cells can be prepared several ways. The conventional method involves superinfection of Raji cells with infectious virus concentrated from a P3-HR1 culture, with centrifugation of the culture fluid for 1 h at 10,000 × *g*. EA smears of consistent quality can be prepared with a pretitered virus stock frozen at −70°C. The advantage of this method lies in the ability to control the number of EA-positive cells. The alternative method involves EA induction of Raji cells by treatment with various chemicals, including tumor-promoting agents (37), iododeoxyuridine, and sodium butyrate (5, 24). By controlling the concentration and duration of the treatment with the various chemicals, various degrees of EA expression can be achieved.

(iv) An EBV-negative cell line is necessary as a negative control to exclude nonspecific antinuclear antibodies in some sera. The most appropriate cell line is BJAB, a B-lymphocyte EBV-negative line, although MOLT-4, a T-lymphoid line, is sometime used as an alternative.

For the indirect immunofluorescent-antibody assay, fourfold dilutions of patient serum are incubated with the fixed cells, followed by fluorescein isothiocyanate (FITC)-conjugated antiserum to the appropriate anti-human immunoglobulin subclasses. The samples are incubated for 30 min at 37°C in moist chambers. Acetone-fixed P3-HR1 cells can be used for measurements of IgG, IgM, and IgA antibodies to VCA. IgM-VCA testing is sometime prolonged to 3 h in the first incubation; this may be necessary to enhance the intensity of the staining.

Acetone-fixed EA smears are suitable for indirect immunofluorescent-antibody assays of antibodies to both EA/D and EA/R, since both antigens are present in the EA-producing cells. The corresponding antigens can be differentiated by their characteristic staining morphologies. EA/D-positive cells appear as cells with diffusely distributed speckled staining in the cytoplasm. These cells frequently have a halo of fine granular staining where the antigens have leaked out during fixation. EA/R, in contrast, is restricted to the cytoplasmic regions within the cells. Methanol fixation of the EA smears preferentially removes EA/R only and thus can be used to prepare smears for differentiation of the two antigens.

The concentration of EBNA in EBV-transformed cells is usually low, and the more sensitive anticomplement indirect immunofluorescence assay must be used to detect anti-EBNA. Raji smears are incubated with patient serum, followed by successive 30-min incubations with EBV-negative complement (either pretested human or guinea pig) and appropriately FITC-conjugated anti-C3 antiserum. If human complement is used, FITC-conjugated anti-β_1C/β_1A is preferable. The staining pattern is nuclear and should be present in all of the cells.

Commercial smears are now available for all of the antigens discussed above. Enzyme-linked immunoassays are still under development and have not been fully evaluated in the clinical setting.

INTERPRETATIONS

From the titers and profiles of antibodies to VCA, EA, and EBNA in the acute-phase serum, the patient can be classified as (i) susceptible if anti-VCA is absent (<1:10), (ii) with primary EBV infection if anti-VCA is present and anti-EBNA is absent, or (iii) immune with past infection if both anti-VCA and EBNA are present. Eighty percent of patients with active EBV infections produce anti-EA/D titers. These antibodies can be very useful as indicators of current or reactivated infections. In the absence of anti-EBNA, an anti-EA titer confirms a primary infection. In the presence of anti-EBNA, an anti-EA titer suggests a reactivated infection.

IgM-VCA titers are present in approximately 85 to 90% of sera from IM patients submitted to our laboratory for EBV testing. Most of the 10 to 15% IgM-VCA-negative sera had low or undetectable levels of anti-EBNA, indicative of a primary infection within the past 6 to 8 weeks. A second serum tested 4 to 6 weeks later would show significant rises in anti-EBNA titers in all patients with primary disease. Hence, reliance on anti-EBNA instead of IgM-VCA effectively "extends" the acute phase of the illness. IgM-VCA titers found in the presence of elevated anti-EBNA titers (e.g., >1:20) are almost without exception false results due to rheumatoid factors which can be completely removed by absorption (11).

As with all serological testing, significant changes in EBV antibodies can be demonstrated only with parallel assays. In general, the antibody titers to the various antigens are remarkably stable throughout an individual's lifetime. Significant changes in titers are seldom seen except during the early acute phase of the infection. Antibody level changes seen in EBV-associated tumors occur slowly and are seldom detectable at intervals shorter than 3 to 4 months. In patients with chronic conditions other than malignancies, profiles of EBV antibodies compatible with a reactivated pattern are already established by the time most patients seek clinical diagnosis. Their EBV profiles do not undergo observable changes. Serial EBV serology on these patients is not needed.

LITERATURE CITED

1. **Andiman, W., L. Gradoville, L. Heston, R. Neydorff, M. E. Savage, G. Kitchingman, D. Shedd, and G. Miller.** 1983. Use of cloned probes to detect Epstein-Barr viral DNA in tissues of patients with neoplastic and lymphoproliferative diseases. J. Infect. Dis. **148:**967–977.
2. **Dambaugh, T., K. Hennessy, S. Fennewald, and E. Kieff.** 1986. The virus genome and its expression in latent infection, p. 13–45. *In* M. A. Epstein and B. G. Achong (ed.), The Epstein-Barr virus: recent advances. W. Heinemann Medical Books, London.
3. **Davidsohn, I., and C. L. Lee.** 1969. The clinical serology of infectious mononucleosis, p. 177–200. *In* R. L. Carter and H. G. Penman (ed.), Infectious mononucleosis. Blackwell Scientific Publications, Ltd., Oxford.
4. **Dillner, J., and B. Kallin.** 1988. The Epstein-Barr virus proteins. Adv. Cancer Res. **50:**95–158.
5. **Gerber, P., and S. Lucas.** 1972. Epstein-Barr virus associated antigens activated in human cells by 5-bromodeoxyuridine. Proc. Soc. Exp. Biol. Med. **141:**431–435.
6. **Gratama, J. W., M. A. P. Oosterveer, F. E. Zwaan, G. Klein, and I. Ernberg.** 1988. Eradication of Epstein-Barr virus by allogeneic bone marrow transplantation: implications for sites of viral latency. Proc. Natl. Acad. Sci. USA **85:**8693–8696.
7. **Greenspan, J. S., D. Greenspan, E. T. Lennette, D. I. Abrams, M. A. Conant, V. Petersen, and U. K. Freese.** 1985. Replication of Epstein-Barr virus within the epithelial cells of oral "hairy" leukoplakia, an AIDS-associated lesion. N. Engl. J. Med. **313:**1564–1571.
8. **Grierson, H., and D. T. Purtillo.** 1987. Epstein-Barr virus infections in males with the X-linked lymphoproliferative syndrome. Ann. Intern. Med. **106:**538–545.
9. **Hanto, D. W., and J. S. Najarian.** 1985. Advances in the diagnosis and treatment of EBV-associated lymphoproliferative disease in immunocompromised hosts. J. Surg. Oncol. **30:**215–220.
10. **Henle, G., and W. Henle.** 1979. The virus as the etiologic agent of infectious mononucleosis, p. 197–307. *In* M. A. Epstein and B. G. Achong (ed.), The Epstein-Barr virus. Springer-Verlag KG, Berlin.
11. **Henle, G., E. T. Lennette, M. A. Alspaugh, and W. Henle.** 1979. Rheumatoid factor as a cause of positive reactions in tests for Epstein-Barr virus specific IgM antibodies. Clin. Exp. Immunol. **36:**415–422.
12. **Henle, W., and G. Henle.** 1974. Epstein-Barr virus and human malignancies. Cancer **34:**1368–1374.
13. **Henle, W., and G. Henle.** 1979. Seroepidemiology of the virus, p. 61–102. *In* M. A. Epstein and B. G. Achong (ed.), The Epstein-Barr virus. Springer-Verlag KG, Berlin.
14. **Henle, W., and G. Henle.** 1980. Consequences of persistent Epstein-Barr virus infections, p. 3–9. *In* M. Essex, G. Todaro, and H. zur Hausen (ed.), Viruses in naturally occurring cancers. Cold Spring Harbor Conferences on Cell Proliferation, vol. 7. Cold Spring Harbor Laboratory, Cold Spring Harbor, N.Y.
15. **Henle, W., and G. Henle.** 1985. Infection, immunity, and blood transfusion, p. 201–209. Alan R. Liss, Inc., New York.
16. **Henle, W., G. Henle, J. Andersson, I. Ernberg, G. Klein, C. A. Horwitz, G. Marklund, L. Rymo, C. Wellinder, and S. E. Straus.** 1987. Antibody responses to Epstein-Barr virus-determined nuclear antigen (EBNA)-1 and EBNA-2 in acute and chronic Epstein-Barr virus infection. Proc. Natl. Acad. Sci. USA **84:**570–574.
17. **Henle, W., G. Henle, and C. A. Horwitz.** 1974. Epstein-Barr virus specific diagnostic tests in infectious mononucleosis. Hum. Pathol. **5:**551–564.
18. **Henle, W., G. Henle, and C. A. Horwitz.** 1979. Infectious mononucleosis and Epstein-Barr virus associated malignancies, p. 441–470. *In* E. H. Lennette and N. J. Schmidt (ed.), Diagnostic procedures for viral, rickettsial and chlamydial infections, 5th ed. American Public Health Association, Inc., Washington, D.C.
19. **Henle, W., J. H. C. Ho, G. Henle, J. C. W. Chan, and H. C. Kwan.** 1977. Nasopharyngeal carcinoma: significance of changes in Epstein-Barr virus related antibody patterns following therapy. Int. J. Can. **20:**663–672.
20. **Horwitz, C. A., W. Henle, G. Henle, H. Rudnick, and E. Latts.** 1985. Long term serological follow-up of patients for Epstein-Barr virus after recovery from infectious mononucleosis. J. Infect. Dis. **151:**1150–1153.
21. **Huang, D. P., J. H. C. Ho, W. Henle, and G. Henle.** 1974. Demonstration of Epstein-Barr virus-associated nuclear antigen in nasopharyngeal carcinoma cells from fresh biopsies. Int. J. Cancer **14:**580–588.
22. **Lennette, E. T., G. Henle, W. Henle, and C. A. Horwitz.** 1978. Heterophil antigen in bovine sera detectable by immune adherence hemagglutination with infectious mononucleosis sera. Infect. Immun. **19:**923–927.
23. **Lindahl, T., G. Klein, B. Johansson, and S. Singh.** 1974. Relationship between Epstein-Barr virus (EBV) DNA and the determined nuclear antigen (EBNA) in Burkitt lymphoma biopsies and other lymphoproliferative diseases. Int. J. Cancer **13:**764–772.
24. **Luka, J., B. Kallin, and G. Klein.** 1979. Induction of the Epstein-Barr virus (EBV) cycle in latently infected cells by N-butyrate. Virology **94:**228–231.
25. **Mikkelsen, W., C. J. Tupper, and J. Murray.** 1958. The ox cell hemolysin test as a diagnostic procedure in infectious mononucleosis. J. Lab. Clin. Med. **52:**648–652.

26. **Nonoyama, M., C. H. Huang, J. S. Pagano, G. Klein, and S. Singh.** 1973. DNA of Epstein-Barr virus detected in tissue of Burkitt's lymphoma and nasopharyngeal carcinoma. Proc. Natl. Acad. Sci. USA **70:**3265–3268.
27. **Pagano, J. S., and E. S. Huang.** 1974. Application of RNA-DNA cytohybridization in viral diagnostics, p. 279–299. *In* E. Kurstak and R. Morissett (ed.), Viral immunodiagnosis. Academic Press, Inc., New York.
28. **Paul, J. R., and W. W. Bunnell.** 1932. The presence of heterophile antibodies in infectious mononucleosis. Am. J. Med. Sci. **183:**80–104.
29. **Pritchett, R. F., S. D. Hayward, and E. D. Kieff.** 1975. DNA of Epstein-Barr virus. I. Comparative studies of the DNA of EBV from HR-1 and B95-8 cells. Size, structure and relatedness. J. Virol. **15:**556–569.
30. **Reedman, B. M., and G. Klein.** 1973. Cellular localization of an Epstein-Barr virus (EBV)-associated complement fixing antigen in producer and nonproducer lymphoblastoid cell lines. Int. J. Cancer **11:**499–520.
31. **Rosen, A., P. Gergely, M. Jondal, G. Klein, and S. Britton.** 1977. Polyclonal Ig production after Epstein-Barr virus infection of human lymphocytes in vitro. Nature (London) **267:**52–56.
32. **Schooley, R. T., R. W. Carey, G. Miller, W. Henle, R. Eastman, E. J. Mark, K. Kenyon, E. O. Wheeler, and R. Rubin.** 1986. Chronic Epstein-Barr virus infection associated with fever and interstitial pneumonitis. Clinical and serological features and response to antiviral chemotherapy. Ann. Intern. Med. **104:**636–643.
33. **Wilson, E. R., A. Malluh, S. Stagno, and W. M. Crist.** 1981. Fatal Epstein-Barr virus-associated hemophagocytic syndrome. J. Pediatr. **98:**260–262.
34. **Yao, Q. Y., A. B. Rickinson, and M. A. Epstein.** 1985. A reexamination of the Epstein-Barr virus carrier state in healthy seropositive individuals. Int. J. Cancer **35:**35–42.
35. **Yao, Q. Y., A. B. Rickinson, J. S. H. Gaston, and M. A. Epstein.** 1985. In vitro analysis of the Epstein-Barr virus-host balance in long term renal allograft recipients. Int. J. Cancer **35:**43–49.
36. **Ziegler, J. L., R. C. Miner, E. Rosenbaum, E. T. Lennette, E. Shillitoe, C. Casavant, W. L. Drew, L. Mintz, J. Gershow, J. Greenspan, J. Beckstead, and K. Yamamoto.** 1982. Outbreak of Burkitt's lymphoma in homosexual men. Lancet **ii:**631–636.
37. **zur Hausen, H., F. J. O'Neill, and U. K. Freese.** 1978. Persisting oncogenic herpesvirus induced by the tumor promoter TPA. Nature (London) **272:**373–375.
38. **zur Hauzen, H., H. Schulte-Holthausen, G. Klein, W. Henle, G. Henle, P. Clifford, and L. Santesson.** 1970. EBV DNA in biopsies of Burkitt's tumours and anaplastic carcinomas of the nasopharynx. Nature (London) **228:** 1056–1058.

Chapter 79

Other Herpesviruses

JOHN A. STEWART

HHV-6

Clinical background

HHV-6 and roseola. Roseola (exanthem subitum) is a common human herpesvirus 6 (HHV-6)-associated infectious disease of infancy, most commonly occurring in infants 6 months to 3 years of age. The illness is characterized by an abrupt rise in temperature to as high as 40°C, followed in 2 to 4 days by a rapid drop in temperature that coincides with the appearance of an erythematous maculopapular rash that persists for 1 to 2 days. The other major symptoms are listlessness, irritability, and drowsiness, though convulsions may occur during the febrile episode. Encephalitis may occur as a rare complication. Despite the fever, the child often continues to eat and play normally and does not seem nearly as sick as the high temperature might indicate. Other physical findings that may occur before the rash appears are palpebral edema and suboccipital, postauricular, and cervical lymphadenopathy. The skin lesions are pale pink, vary from 1 to 5 mm in diameter, and are surrounded by a clear area that separates them from other lesions. The lesions are macular and sometimes papular but never vesicular. They appear first on the neck, behind the ears, and on the back and may spread quickly to involve the scalp, chest, abdomen, and thighs. The face and distal extremities are usually spared. The total illness may last from 2 to 7 days.

It has long been believed that roseola is caused by a virus because of leukopenia in patients, the failure to isolate bacteria, the lack of clinical response to antimicrobial agents, a relatively long incubation period of about 10 days (4), and evidence from experimental infection studies in humans (12, 16). Yamanishi et al. (34) were the first to isolate HHV-6 (as evidenced by electron microscopy) from peripheral blood lymphocytes of four children with roseola. In addition, all four acute- and convalescent-phase serum pairs had a significant rise in anticomplement immunofluorescence (ACIF) HHV-6 antibody. All acute-phase titers were less than 10, and convalescent-phase HHV-6 titers ranged from 20 to as high as 320 against antigens from both a Japanese isolate and CDC strain Z29. Convalescent-phase serum samples from seven other roseola patients, collected at least 14 days after onset of illness, were all positive when tested against HHV-6 (Z29). Other investigators reported similar findings from small series of cases (28, 30).

The most extensive study of the role of HHV-6 in roseola was reported by Asano et al. (2). HHV-6 was isolated from mononuclear cell samples collected between days 0 and 7 of disease from 38 of 43 children with roseola. HHV-6 was also isolated from 10 of 36 plasma samples. No virus was isolated from 37 samples on day 8 or later. Neutralizing antibody to HHV-6 was first detected on day 3 of disease (2 of 11 samples) and was positive in all 37 samples collected more than 7 days after onset. Thus, clearance of the virus from the blood was associated with the induction of specific neutralizing antibody.

These studies clearly indicate that HHV-6 is the causative agent of roseola. In concordance with seroepidemiologic studies of several populations, they also indicate that HHV-6 infection is very common and usually occurs early in life. Infants younger than 6 months of age appear to be protected by maternal antibodies, and infection is most commonly acquired between 6 and 18 months of age. The route of infection in infants is unknown, but oral and respiratory secretions of asymptomatic family members are a likely source of infection. In most cases, symptomatic infants have been exposed only to well family members, and secondary cases are quite infrequent.

HHV-6 infection and adult disease. A number of studies have reported a higher prevalence of immunofluorescence assay (IFA) antibody to HHV-6 in patients with connective tissue diseases (e.g., sarcoidosis), lymphomas, lymphoid hyperplasia, and immune suppression or deficiency (1, 18). It now appears that many of the IFAs were insensitive, and the actual seropositive rate in the normal population may exceed 80 to 90% (25). Thus, the studies showing an increased seroprevalence rate in patients with certain diseases may simply indicate that higher mean antibody titers to HHV-6 are present in these patients than in controls. However, higher mean antibody titers to a number of viruses are present in patients with connective tissue diseases, leukemia, lymphoid hyperplasia, human immunodeficiency virus infection, and even chronic fatigue syndrome. This finding may reflect a polyclonal B-cell stimulation or increased reactivation of latent viruses in patients with these diseases.

One of the most convincing reports of HHV-6-associated adult disease described three patients with serological evidence of HHV-6 infection (21). These patients had a mild, afebrile illness of 1 to 3 weeks in duration characterized by dull headache, slight fatigue, and enlarged, bilateral, nontender, cervical lymph nodes that persisted for up to 3 months. No hepatosplenomegaly was noted, but two patients had transiently raised serum liver enzyme levels. Leukopenia was noted with increased mononuclear cells (37 to 56%), of which 3 to 14% were atypical lymphocytes. Immunoglobulin G (IgG) antibody to HHV-6 was elevated at titers of 160 to 2,560, but no rises in titer were found. Specific HHV-6 IgM antibody was found at a low titer of 10 during early illness in two patients. None of the patients had antibodies for cytomegalovirus (CMV) or toxoplasma, and only one patient was positive for Epstein-Barr virus (EBV) with stable titers. One previously EBV-seronegative patient was noted to have classic infectious mononucleosis with typical hematological and serological (EBV seroconversion and positive heterophile) responses 15 months after his HHV-6-associated illness. At this time, the HHV-6 IgM titer sharply increased to 160 and the IgG titer remained elevated at 2,560. It was believed that this dual rise in antibody titer was due to polyclonal B-cell activation or reactivation of latent HHV-6 infection with the primary EBV infection. Another well-documented case of HHV-6 infection with clinical illness was noted in a 21-year-old HHV-6-seronegative patient after liver transplantation from an HHV-6-seropositive donor (32). Primary infection with HHV-6 should be a rare event in adults in most population groups because of the high rate of infection in childhood, but when it occurs, it may have some of the features of a mild "mono-like" illness.

Description of the agent

HHV-6 is a newly recognized member of the family *Herpesviridae* that was initially named human B-lymphotropic virus (24). However, since the virus was shown in several laboratories to have a major tropism for T cells (20, 27) as well as the ability to grow in several other cell types, it was subsequently called human herpesvirus 6, a designation independent of its cell type. HHV-6 is serologically (24) and genetically (13, 14, 19) distinct from the other human herpesviruses and from many animal herpesviruses (1) as well. The virus envelope encloses an icosahedral capsid of 162 capsomeres with a core containing a double-stranded DNA genome of approximately 170 kilobases (14, 19). HHV-6 is readily inactivated by ether and lipid solvents. Cell-free virus does not survive cycles of freezing and thawing unless stored in a protein-rich environment such as skim milk medium. More than 20 polypeptides ranging in size from 30 to 220 kilodaltons are found in solubilized purified virions (M. Yamamoto, personal communication). One of these, a 100-kilodalton polypeptide, is strongly reactive on Western immunoblot analysis with both HHV-6-positive human sera and a murine monoclonal antibody and may prove valuable in diagnostic testing.

HHV-6 DNA is clearly distinct from the DNAs of the other human herpesviruses, herpes simplex virus type 1 (HSV-1), herpes simplex virus type 2 (HSV-2), varicella-zoster virus (VZV), CMV, and EBV, by both restriction endonuclease digestion and nucleic acid hybridization (19). The DNA from strain HHV-6(Z29) hybridizes under stringent conditions with DNA from the NIH strain HHV-6(GS) (13, 19). DNA restriction enzyme patterns of the two strains are very similar (13, 19).

Other HHV-6 isolates from AIDS patients in Africa (9, 29) have been shown to hybridize under stringent conditions with the DNA of HHV-6(GS). HHV-6 isolates from infants with roseola in Japan showed strong antigenic similarity to HHV-6(Z29) (34). In addition, DNA studies by P. Pellett (personal communication) show strong homology among eight Japanese isolates, an African isolate (Z29), and a U.S. isolate. Restriction enzyme comparisons of these isolates show so little variation in fragment size and number that several isolates cannot be distinguished from one another. This variation is less than that seen among HSV-1 isolates. Careful analysis will be required to distinguish true differences between strains.

Collection and storage of specimens

HHV-6 has been isolated only from peripheral blood samples, without confirmed reports of virus isolation from other bodily secretions such as saliva or urine. Heparinized blood samples should be collected, and the mononuclear cells should be purified on Ficoll gradients. The cells are usually cocultivated with phytohemagglutinin-stimulated cord blood cells, but primary culture in RPMI 1640 media may be attempted. For best results, cultures should be set up within 24 h of blood collection. Freezing mononuclear cells for later isolation is not recommended because the virus is highly labile and survives freeze-thaw cycles poorly.

Direct examination

The polymerase chain reaction has been used to recognize HHV-6-specific sequences in the peripheral blood of AIDS patients and patients with lymphoproliferative disorders (5). As yet, no base-line studies in normal individuals in the general population have been reported to help evaluate the positive results. Positive polymerase chain reaction findings could result from the presence of only a few copies of HHV-6 DNA in a single nonmalignant or circulating cell.

Virus isolation

HHV-6 has been isolated from the peripheral blood by primary culture of mononuclear cells and by cocultivation of these cells with either stimulated cord blood or adult lymphocytes. The best results are usually obtained with cord blood cells. For cocultivation studies, mononuclear cells are purified from fresh human cord blood on Ficoll gradients and stimulated to blast formation by culturing for 1 to 3 days with 0.002% phytohemagglutinin and 5% interleukin-2 in growth medium (RPMI 1640 with 10% fetal calf serum, 0.01 mg of hydrocortisone per ml, and antibiotics). The cord cells are cocultivated with an equal volume of mononuclear cells from patients and checked for the appearance of HHV-6 antigen by ACIF after 7 to 10 days.

Identification of HHV-6

Large balloonlike cells may appear after cocultivation with cord blood lymphocytes, suggesting that infection is present; however, such cells may also occur in the absence of infection, and therefore immunological tests are needed to confirm infection. The IFA, using well-characterized human sera, has been used for the confirmation of HHV-6, but the ACIF assay is more sensitive and specific. A few laboratories have reported the development of monoclonal antibodies to HHV-6, but these are not readily available for identification purposes. Monoclonal and well-characterized high-titered human polyclonal antibodies to the other human herpesviruses should not react with HHV-6-infected cells.

Serological diagnosis

The serological diagnosis of recent HHV-6 infection is based on finding a fourfold or greater increase in IFA or ACIF titer or a significant increase in enzyme immunoassay (EIA) values between acute- and convalescent-phase sera. Seroconversion in paired serum specimens may provide evidence of a primary infection with HHV-6. However, with insensitive methods, seroconversion may be difficult to distinguish from a rising titer in a person with reactivated infection. The serological diagnosis of recent infection has been most clearly established in children with roseola (exanthem subitum), as reviewed previously (2, 30, 34).

IFA. One of the most widely used serological procedures for HHV-6 is the IFA. The initial IFA procedure described by Salahuddin et al. (24), in which infected cord blood lymphocytes were used as antigen, detected antibody at a serum dilution of 1:40 in all six patients from whom the virus was isolated. In contrast, only 4 of 220 serum specimens from normal donors were positive at that dilution.

As IFA tests have become more sensitive, the estimation of antibody prevalence in the general population has risen dramatically. A more sensitive test, using infected J Jhan cells as the IFA substrate, was reported by Tedder et al. (29). Using a conservative endpoint, the authors showed that 12 (18%) of 66 patients from the United Kingdom were clearly positive, with another 16 (24%) minimally positive. With the discovery that HHV-6(GS) would grow well in several T-cell lines such as HSB-2 (1), the IFA became easier to perform and possibly more reproducible. The seroprevalence rate in normal blood donors in the United States and Canada found by Ablashi et al. (1) was still only 26%, whereas a 52% prevalence rate was found in serum specimens collected from persons in West Africa. Some of the problems encountered in interpretation of the IFA are pointed out by the report of Krueger et al. (18), who noted an antibody prevalence to HHV-6 of 26% in a normal population if a strict criterion (a titer of at least 40) for positivity was applied. However, if a titer of at least 10 was considered positive, antibody was noted in 63% of the population. Another highly sensitive IFA was developed by Knowles and Gardner (17) with the use of a strict criterion for specificity (diffuse fluorescence only in the enlarged infected cells when a 1:10 dilution of serum was used). They found an almost universal prevalence of antibody, with over 90% of children positive at age 5 and 98% positive at age 17.

ACIF. To avoid problems with strong nonspecific fluorescent staining of cord blood lymphocytes frequently observed with the IFA, an ACIF assay was adopted that greatly reduced nonspecific fluorescence and gave a stronger signal with positive cells (19). The ACIF has been effectively used by Yamanishi et al. (34) in detecting the antibody response of roseola patients and in seroprevalence studies (22). The specificity of the ACIF for HHV-6 has been shown in the following ways. (i) The percentage of infected cells found by ACIF correlates with the proportion of infected cells found by electron microscopy. (ii) No cross-reactivity is found with the other human herpesviruses when high-titered, well-characterized patient serum samples are used. (iii) Cross-adsorption of dually reactive serum specimens is done with CMV-, HSV-, or VZV-infected cells, respectively, before tests for residual antibody. Antibody to the homologous virus is effectively adsorbed, whereas no change in response to HHV-6 is noted. (iv) Seroconversion to either CMV or EBV usually fails to boost HHV-6 reactivity.

The ACIF test is performed by adding heat-inactivated serum specimens to the wells on slides containing acetone-fixed HHV-6 (strain GS or Z29)-infected cord blood cells. After incubation and wash steps, a human serum containing complement is added. After further incubation and wash steps, complement fixation is detected by addition of fluorescein-labeled goat anti-human C3 reagent. Characteristically, cytoplasmic fluorescence is somewhat granular, whereas nuclear fluorescence is solid and bright.

Other serological procedures. The other tests that have been used to detect HHV-6 antibodies include Western immunoblots, immunoprecipitation, neutralization, and the EIA. The Western blot and immunoprecipitation assays (3, 26, 35) are key procedures in the detailed analysis of the individual polypeptides and proteins involved in the immune response to HHV-6. To date, the neutralization test has been evaluated in only one study (2).

To perform an EIA for antibody to HHV-6, virions were harvested from infected HSB-2 cell cultures, disrupted in a Tris–Triton X-100 buffer, and used to coat microdilution plates (25). Bound antibody was detected by alkaline phosphatase reagents. The specificity of the reaction was determined by preincubation of sera with soluble HHV-6, HSB-2 control, CMV, EBV, HSV, and VZV antigens. The other herpesvirus antigens showed no competitive cross-reactivity with IgG antibodies to HHV-6 antigens, whereas the HHV-6-adsorbing antigens reduced binding to HHV-6 by more than 90%. The EIA serum results were normally distributed over a broad range of values, with no evidence of bimodality. This result precluded the designation of a cutoff level between negative and positive sera. Samples showing HHV-6-specific absorption of at least 50% were regarded as positive.

Interpretation of results

The recovery of virus from peripheral blood lymphocytes is the best indicator of active HHV-6 infection but does not distinguish primary infection from reactivation. The results of serological tests are more difficult to interpret. Demonstration of a fourfold rise in IFA or ACIF antibody titer in a young child with a febrile rash illness confirms the diagnosis of HHV-6 infection with roseola. However, in older children and adults, a concurrent rise in antibody to CMV or EBV has been reported quite frequently in connection with a rise in HHV-6 antibody. When serological evidence of dual infection is obtained, the relative importance of each pathogen in producing illness may be difficult to ascertain. Confirmation by virus isolation would help to resolve such problems. Some caution is also needed in interpreting seroprevalence studies. A positive result in adequately controlled tests indicates infection at some undetermined time in the past, but a negative result can be obtained with insensitive procedures and may not indicate absence of infection.

B VIRUS

Clinical background

B virus, or *Herpesvirus simiae*, is a member of the herpes group of viruses that is indigenous to Old World monkeys such as rhesus (*Macaca mulatta*), cynomolgus

(*Macaca fascicularis*), and other Asiatic monkeys of the genus *Macaca*. As the simian counterpart of herpes simplex virus, B virus causes subclinical infections as well as dermal, oral, eye, or genital lesions in monkeys. The importance of the virus to humans is its ability to cause life-threatening central nervous system infections. The virus can be transmitted by monkey bites, by direct or indirect contact with saliva, or even by contact with monkey cell cultures that are widely used in the virus laboratory (33).

After an incubation period of a few days to a month or more, an infected person may show localized redness and vesicles and may have pain at the site of virus inoculation. Vesicles on the mucous membranes, pneumonia, diarrhea, abdominal pain, pharyngitis, and lymphocytic pleocytosis have been reported. In almost all untreated symptomatic cases, an ascending myelitis and encephalopathy occurs that is frequently fatal; most who survive are left with severe brain damage (23). Although the risk of disease with B virus appears to be low (on the basis of the small number of known cases compared with the thousands of macaque contacts yearly), human infection is a potential hazard of working with Old World monkeys, and precautionary measures to protect workers from infection are of critical importance. The identification of four human cases in Florida in 1987 (6) and two cases in Michigan in 1989 (8), after a 13-year period with no reported cases, emphasizes this need.

Description of the agent

B virus is similar to HSV in morphology and size and is inhibited by antiviral agents that suppress DNA synthesis. An enveloped herpesvirus, it is sensitive to lipid solvents, acid pH, and detergent solutions. There is an antigenic relationship between HSV and B virus such that antisera to B virus will neutralize both viruses equally well, whereas antisera to HSV will neutralize homologous virus at much higher titers than B virus (10, 31). The extent of the cross-reaction is enhanced by complement. B virus appears hardier than HSV; it may survive for 7 days at 37°C and for weeks at 4°C and is very stable when stored at −70°C. The virus can be isolated in a number of cell and animal systems that also support the growth of HSV. Rhesus monkey kidney cells readily support the growth of B virus, whereas HSV isolates grow poorly in these cells. The cytopathic effect produced by B virus in many cell lines is quite similar to that produced by HSV, and specific serological or molecular procedures are needed to identify B virus.

Safety

Because of the potential hazards of B-virus infections, guidelines for preventing infection in monkey handlers have been established (7), and caution should be exercised by laboratory workers in processing specimens suspected of containing B virus. Laboratory assistance in investigating such specimens can be obtained from the Southwest Foundation for Biomedical Research, San Antonio, Tex., phone (512) 674-1410, or from the Virus Reference Laboratory Inc., San Antonio, Tex., phone (512) 696-5510.

Collection and storage of specimens

Vesicular fluid of lesions, swabs from the oropharynx, conjunctiva, and skin lesions, or skin biopsy specimens from affected areas can be used for the diagnosis of B-virus infection. The cotton tips of the applicators used to swab the lesions should be broken off into screw-cap vials containing 2 ml of tryptose phosphate broth with 0.5% gelatin or another viral transport medium that contains protein (skim milk or veal infusion broth). Specimens for virus isolation should be kept cold (4 to 8°C) at all times (but not frozen), properly packaged, and promptly shipped to the appropriate laboratory. Inquiries can also be directed to the Division of Viral and Rickettsial Diseases of the Centers for Disease Control, phone (404) 639-1338.

Virus isolation and serological procedures

Since B-virus propagation should be handled under biosafety level 4 conditions, laboratory investigation of specimens from patients or monkeys suspected of B-virus infection is best referred to experienced laboratories equipped to handle B-virus cultures. The serological diagnosis of recent B-virus infection requires the demonstration of at least a fourfold rise in specific antibody titer against B virus in paired serum specimens. Specific antibody assays such as the immunoblot (11) or an EIA for specific antibodies using adsorption procedures (15) are currently available in only a few reference laboratories equipped to handle B virus. In B-virus-infected patients, a rise in titer against HSV may be seen along with an increase in titer to B virus. An increase in antibody is usually observed 10 to 14 days after the onset of illness but may be greatly delayed if the patient is treated with an antiviral medication such as acyclovir.

LITERATURE CITED

1. **Ablashi, D. V., S. F. Josephs, A. Buchbinder, K. Hellman, S. Nakamura, T. Llana, P. Lusso, M. Kaplan, J. Dahlberg, S. Memon, F. Imam, K. L. Ablashi, P. D. Markham, B. Kramarsky, G. R. F. Krueger, P. Biberfeld, F. Wong-Staal, S. Z. Salahuddin, and R. C. Gallo.** 1988. Human B-lymphotropic virus (human herpesvirus-6). J. Virol. Methods **21:**29–48.
2. **Asano, Y., T. Yoshikawa, S. Suga, T. Yazaki, T. Hata, T. Nagai, Y. Kajita, T. Ozaki, and S. Yoshida.** 1989. Viremia and neutralizing antibody response in infants with exanthem subitum. J. Pediatr. **114:**535–539.
3. **Balachandran, N., R. E. Amelse, W. W. Zhou, and C. K. Chang.** 1989. Identification of proteins specific for human herpesvirus 6-infected human T cells. J. Virol. **63:**2835–2840.
4. **Breese, B.** 1941. Roseola infantum (exanthema subitum). N.Y. State J. Med. **41:**1854.
5. **Buchbinder, A., S. F. Josephs, D. Ablashi, S. Z. Salahuddin, M. E. Klotman, M. Manak, G. R. F. Krueger, F. Wong-Staal, and R. Gallo.** 1988. Polymerase chain reaction amplification and in situ hybridization for the detection of human B-lymphotropic virus. J. Virol. Methods **21:**191–197.
6. **Centers for Disease Control.** 1987. B virus infection in humans—Pensacola, Florida. Morbid. Mortal. Weekly Rep. **36:**289–290, 295–296.
7. **Centers for Disease Control.** 1987. Guidelines for prevention of *Herpesvirus simiae* (B virus) infection in monkey handlers. Morbid. Mortal. Weekly Rep. **36:**680–682, 687–689.

8. **Centers for Disease Control.** 1989. B virus infections in humans—Michigan. Morbid. Mortal. Weekly Rep. **38:**453–454.
9. **Downing, R. G., N. Sewankambo, D. Serwadda, R. Honess, D. Crawford, R. Jarrett, and B. E. Griffin.** 1987. Isolation of human lymphotropic herpesviruses from Uganda. Lancet **ii:**390.
10. **Gary, G. W., Jr., and E. L. Palmer.** 1977. Comparative complement fixation and serum neutralization antibody titers to herpes simplex virus type 1 and *Herpesvirus simiae* in *Macaca mulatta* and humans. J. Clin. Microbiol. **5:**465–470.
11. **Heberling, R. L., and S. S. Kalter.** 1987. A dot-immunobinding assay on nitrocellulose with psoralen inactivated *Herpesvirus simiae* (B virus). Lab. Anim. Sci. **37:**304–308.
12. **Hellstrom, B., and B. Vahlquist.** 1951. Experimental inoculation of roseola infantum. Acta Paediatr. Scand. **40:** 189–197.
13. **Josephs, S. F., D. V. Ablashi, S. Z. Salahuddin, B. Kramarsky, R. B. Franza, P. Pellett, A. Buchbinder, S. Memon, F. Wong-Staal, and R. C. Gallo.** 1988. Molecular studies of HHV-6. J. Virol. Methods **21:**179–190.
14. **Josephs, S. F., S. Z. Salahuddin, D. V. Ablashi, F. Schachter, F. Wong-Staal, and R. C. Gallo.** 1986. Genomic analysis of the human B-lymphotropic virus (HBLV). Science **234:**601–603.
15. **Katz, D., J. K. Hilliard, R. Eberle, and S. L. Liper.** 1986. ELISA for detection of group-common and virus-specific antibodies in human and simian viruses. J. Virol. Methods **14:**99–109.
16. **Kempe, C. H., E. B. Shaw, J. R. Lackson, and H. K. Silver.** 1950. Studies on the etiology of exanthem subitum (roseola infantum). J. Pediatr. **37:**561–568.
17. **Knowles, W. A., and S. D. Gardner.** 1988. High prevalence of antibody to human herpesvirus-6 and seroconversion associated with rash in two infants. Lancet **ii:**912–913.
18. **Krueger, G. R. F., B. Koch, A. Ramon, D. V. Ablashi, S. Z. Salahuddin, S. F. Josephs, H. Z. Streicher, R. C. Gallo, and U. Habermann.** 1988. Antibody prevalence to HBLV (human herpesvirus-6, HHV-6) and suggestive pathogenicity in the general population and in patients with immune deficiency syndromes. J. Virol. Methods **21:** 125–131.
19. **Lopez, C., P. Pellett, J. Stewart, C. Goldsmith, K. Sanderlin, J. Black, D. Warfield, and P. Feorino.** 1988. Characteristics of human herpesvirus-6. J. Infect. Dis. **157:** 1271–1273.
20. **Lusso, P., S. Z. Salahuddin, D. V. Ablashi, R. C. Gallo, F. M. Veronese, and P. D. Markham.** 1987. Diverse tropism of human B-lymphotropic virus (human herpesvirus 6). Lancet **ii:**743–744.
21. **Niedermann, J. C., C.-R. Liu, M. H. Kaplan, and N. A. Brown.** 1989. Clinical and serological features of human herpesvirus 6 infection in three adults. Lancet **ii:**817–819.
22. **Okuno, T., K. Takahashi, K. Balachandra, K. Shiraki, K. Yamanishi, M. Takahashi, and K. Baba.** 1989. Seroepidemiology of human herpesvirus 6 infection in normal children and adults. J. Clin. Microbiol. **27:**651–653.
23. **Palmer, A. E.** 1987. B virus, *Herpesvirus simiae:* historical perspectives. J. Med. Primatol. **16:**99–130.
24. **Salahuddin, S. Z., D. V. Ablashi, P. D. Markham, S. F. Josephs, S. Sturzenegger, M. Kaplan, G. Halligan, P. Biberfeld, F. Wong-Staal, B. Kramarsky, and R. C. Gallo.** 1986. Isolation of a new virus, HBLV, in patients with lymphoproliferative disorders. Science **234:**596–601.
25. **Saxinger, C., H. Polesky, N. Eby, S. Grufferman, R. Murphy, G. Tegtmeier, V. Parekh, S. Memon, and C. Hung.** 1988. Antibody reactivity with HBLV (HHV-6) in U.S. populations. J. Virol. Methods **21:**199–208.
26. **Shiraki, K., T. Okuno, K. Yamanishi, and M. Takahashi.** 1989. Virion and nonstructural polypeptides of human herpesvirus-6. Virus Res. **13:**173–178.
27. **Takahashi, K., S. Sonoda, K. Higashi, T. Kondo, H. Takahashi, M. Takahashi, and K. Yamanishi.** 1989. Predominant CD4 T-lymphocyte tropism of human herpesvirus 6-related virus. J. Virol. **63:**3161–3163.
28. **Takahashi, K., S. Sonoda, K. Kawakami, K. Miyata, T. Oki, and T. Nagata.** 1988. Human herpesvirus 6 and exanthem subitum. Lancet **i:**1463.
29. **Tedder, R. S., M. Briggs, C. H. Cameron, R. Honess, D. Robertson, and H. Whittle.** 1987. A novel lymphotropic herpesvirus. Lancet **ii:**390–392.
30. **Ueda, K., K. Kusuhara, M. Hirose, K. Okada, C. Miyazaki, K. Tokugawa, M. Nakayama, and K. Yamanishi.** 1989. Exanthem subitum and antibody to human herpesvirus-6. J. Infect. Dis. **158:**750–752.
31. **Veda, Y., I. Tagaya, and K. Shiroki.** 1968. Immunological relationship between herpes simplex virus and B virus. Arch. Gesamte Virusforsch. **24:**231–244.
32. **Ward, K. N., J. J. Gray, and S. Efstathiou.** 1989. Brief report: primary human herpesvirus 6 infection in a patient following liver transplantation from a seropositive donor. J. Med. Virol. **28:**69–72.
33. **Wells, D. L., S. L. Lipper, J. K. Hilliard, J. A. Stewart, G. P. Holmes, K. L. Herrmann, M. P. Kiley, and L. B. Schonberger.** 1989. *Herpesvirus simiae* contamination of primary rhesus monkey cell cultures: CDC recommendations to minimize risks to laboratory personnel. Diagn. Microbiol. Infect. Dis. **12:**333–336.
34. **Yamanishi, K., T. Okuno, K. Shiraki, M. Takahashi, T. Kondo, Y. Asano, and T. Kurata.** 1988. Identification of human herpesvirus 6 as a causal agent for exanthem subitum. Lancet **i:**1065–1067.
35. **Yoshida, T., H. Yoshiyama, E. Suzuki, S. Harada, K. Yanagi, and N. Yamamoto.** 1989. Immune response of patients with exanthema subitum to human herpesvirus type 6 (HHV-6) polypeptides. J. Infect. Dis. **160:**901–902.

Chapter 80

Poxvirus Infections in Humans*

JOSEPH J. ESPOSITO AND JAMES H. NAKANO

CLINICAL EPIDEMIOLOGICAL BACKGROUND

Molluscum contagiosum virus, the sole member of the proposed genus Molluscipoxvirus, is transmitted strictly between humans. All other poxviruses known to infect humans by natural transmission are zoonoses, including members of the genus *Orthopoxvirus* (monkeypox, buffalopox, and cowpox viruses), the genus *Parapoxvirus* (orf, milker's nodule, and papulosa stomatitis viruses), and the proposed genus Yatapoxvirus (tanapox virus). Three recent comprehensive sources of information describe orthopoxviruses in detail (10, 12, 15). Variola (smallpox) viruses are orthopoxviruses that are no longer naturally occurring; the so-called whitepox viruses, which had been implicated as naturally occurring strains of variola virus that emanated as mutants of monkeypox virus, have been determined to have arisen inadvertently by cross-contamination in the laboratory (9, 10). The only remaining sources of variola virus today are specimens retained by the World Health Organization (WHO) Collaborating Centers for Smallpox and Other Poxvirus Infections at the Centers for Disease Control (CDC), Atlanta, Ga., and the Research Institute of Viral Preparations, Moscow, USSR. Vaccinia virus, the virus in smallpox vaccine, is a laboratory virus and one used for vaccinating military personnel in certain countries and civilians working with orthopoxviruses that infect humans. Vaccinia virus has not generally been regarded as naturally occurring, but DNA data (10) suggest that certain recent isolates of buffalopox virus that infect humans, cattle, and milking buffaloes in India are actually vaccinia virus subspecies that derive from the smallpox vaccination era. Also, there are bioengineered recombinants of vaccinia virus currently in or proposed for human or animal vaccine trials in clinical or field trial settings (5). For example, vaccinia-human immunodeficiency (*env* gene) recombinant vaccines for acquired immunodeficiency syndrome are now being evaluated in Africa and in the United States. Although other members of the families *Entomopoxvirinae* and *Chordopoxvirinae*, including mammalian poxviruses in the genera *Suipoxvirus*, *Avipoxvirus*, *Capripoxvirus*, and *Leporipoxvirus*, are not known to naturally infect humans, anecdotal reports indicate that some of these viruses can do so.

Variola (smallpox)

The last reported case of naturally occurring smallpox was in Somalia in 1977, and two laboratory-associated cases occurred in England in 1982, before variola virus was restricted to WHO Collaborating Centers. Certification of smallpox eradication was made by a Global Commission on 9 December 1979 and accepted by the World Health Assembly in May 1980 (10).

Smallpox was caused by variola virus, which was transmitted naturally among humans by aerosol and by contact, apparently without establishing an animal reservoir (9, 10). Classically, the disease is differentiated epidemiologically as variola major with severe prodrome, fever, prostration, and rash, with case fatality rates of up to 40%, and variola minor (synonyms: alastrim, amass, and Kaffir pox) with less severe systemic reactions and case fatality rates of less than 1%. Smallpox rarely developed without rash, but it was sometimes confused with severe acute leukemia, meningococcemia, or idiopathic thrombocytopenic purpura. The smallpox rash progresses from an enanthem (oropharyngeal lesions) to an exanthem (centrifugal distribution with more lesions on the face and extremities than on the trunk). A severe chickenpox rash, caused by varicella-zoster virus, may be confused with and misdiagnosed as smallpox.

Four clinical manifestations of smallpox are defined: (i) the ordinary form (90% of all cases), summarized above; (ii) the modified form (5% of all cases), which produced mild prodrome with few skin lesions and occurred in previously vaccinated persons; (iii) the flat type (5% of all cases), which produced slowly developing focal lesions with generalized infection and had a 50% fatality rate; and (iv) the hemorrhagic form (<1% of all cases), which led to bleeding into the skin and mucous membranes and was invariably fatal within 1 week after onset (10).

Monkeypox

Monkeypox is currently the most severe naturally occurring poxvirus disease of humans. The clinical appearance of human monkeypox is much like that of smallpox, with a centrifugally distributed vesiculopustular rash predominating, but lymphadenopathy is more prominent and the epidemiology is different (15). The disease is a zoonosis, with virus transmission between humans occurring rarely. Final differentiation between human monkeypox and smallpox generally depends on the isolation and identification of monkeypox virus. Because all orthopoxviruses are antigenically so closely related, serodifferentiation of the diseases is quite difficult.

Like variola virus, monkeypox virus enters the system mainly through the mucosa of the upper respiratory tract or through skin abrasions and migrates to regional lymph nodes. The virus is carried to internal organs during a primary viremia and is then disseminated throughout the body during a secondary viremia. During

* This chapter is dedicated to James Hiroto Nakano, a leader in the smallpox eradication effort at the Centers for Disease Control, who died on 9 February 1990.

the onset period (prodrome), lymphadenopathy, fever, and generalized headache are common symptoms. The rash usually appears first on the face, followed by eruptions on the rest of the body. The lesions develop through stages of macules, papules, vesicles, and pustules. Sequelae involve scarring and pitting at the site of the lesions.

Monkeypox was first recognized in 1958 as an exanthem of primates; hence, the virus was designated monkeypox virus. The disease was subsequently reported in other captured animals and was first recognized in humans in Zaire (Congo), Africa, in 1970. With the ebbing of smallpox, and now in posteradication times, human monkeypox has gained recognition clinically as a rare sporadic zoonosis. Serosurveys and virological investigations of wild animals have suggested that primates are also sporadically infected. The role of wild primates in sustaining virus transmission or as a source of human infection has been difficult to define. Serosurvey data and one report of virus isolation have implicated African arboreal squirrels (*Funisciurus* and *Heliosciurus* spp.) as a reservoir maintaining monkeypox. From 1970 to date, human monkeypox has been observed mostly in Zaire but has also been reported in Liberia, Ivory Coast, Sierra Leone, Nigeria, Benin, Cameroon, and recently in Gabon, where two patients showed hemorrhagic manifestations. Human monkeypox is rare, and its occurrence depends on direct contact with infected animals. The virus presents little risk of being introduced widely in the human populace; in Zaire, for example, 209 cases in a population of about 8 million were observed during the postsmallpox, postvaccination years from 1980 to 1984. The fatality rate for human monkeypox is about 15%. Severe cases are often associated with unvaccinated children. Malaria and other immunodeficiency cofactors may also influence prognoses.

Vaccinia

Except for military personnel in a few countries and persons at risk of contracting laboratory infection with human orthopoxviruses, routine smallpox vaccination has been discontinued worldwide. However, insertion of foreign genes into vaccinia virus has led to genetically engineered human and animal vaccine candidates that have advanced into clinical and field trials (5). The Immunization Practices Advisory Committee for the United States recommends as a safeguard that clinical and research personnel who work directly with human orthopoxviruses or who are otherwise at high risk of virus contact should be vaccinated within 3 years before such contact. In the United States, CDC currently provides smallpox vaccine for human use and vaccinia virus immunoglobulin for treatment of rarely occurring smallpox vaccination side effects.

Serious complications seldom occur after smallpox vaccination with vaccinia virus strains currently recommended by the WHO and authorized in the country of use (e.g., the New York Board of Health strain in the United States). Such complications include postvaccinal encephalitis and encephalopathy, severe skin reactions (e.g., eczema vaccinatum), progressive vaccinia (e.g., vaccinia necrosum), and generalized vaccinia (5, 10). Also, on rare occasions, vaccinia virus lesions may develop in family members and other close contacts of persons recently vaccinated. Vaccinia infections can be life threatening in persons with compromised immune systems.

In India, Egypt, Bangladesh, Pakistan, Indonesia, and the USSR, sporadic outbreaks of so-called buffalopox virus infections have been reported that involve virus transmission between milking buffaloes, cattle, and humans. Lesions have been observed on the animals' teats and the milkers' hands. Biological data and limited DNA analyses have indicated that buffalopox virus isolates from Maharashtra State in India in 1985, after cessation of routine smallpox vaccination, were subspecies of vaccinia virus that may have derived from transmissions between humans and livestock during the smallpox vaccination era. The natural history of buffalopox viruses is not fully determined, and it is not known whether buffalopox viruses are rodent borne like cowpox virus.

Cowpox

Classically, cowpox has been viewed as a rare occupational infection in humans that results from contact with infected cows (12). Infected rodents, felines, and various zoo and circus animals (e.g., elephants) have also been a source of disease transmission. Rodents and felines appear to be the reservoir species maintaining the virus in nature. Cowpox virus has been isolated from such animals in the United Kingdom, Holland, Germany, Denmark, and the USSR. The lesions in humans, usually found on the fingers with reddening and swelling, are likened to those of a primary smallpox vaccination. The site becomes papular, and in 4 to 5 days a vesicle develops; healing takes about 3 weeks (11).

Tanapox

Tanapox virus, Yaba-like disease virus (YLDV), and Yaba monkey tumor virus (YMTV) are serologically related viruses of the proposed genus Yatapoxvirus (11, 16). DNA maps of tanapox virus and YLDV are similar to each other and different from YMTV DNA maps, but all three viral DNAs cross-hybridize extensively (16). The agent of tanapox, an endemic zoonosis across equatorial Africa thought to be transmitted to humans by blood-sucking insects during the rainy season, was first isolated from human skin biopsy specimens taken during outbreaks in 1957 and 1962 that occurred in the Tana River Valley, Kenya (1). During surveillance for human monkeypox in the early 1980s in Zaire, six tanapox virus isolates from different years and locales showed DNA profiles identical to those of Kenya tanapox virus (16). YLDV was first recognized during epizootics in 1965 and 1966 in primate centers in California, Oregon, and Texas; the origin of the epizootics was subsequently traced to a primate-importing company. During these outbreaks, animal handlers had contracted YLDV infections that appeared clinically identical to tanapox virus infections. There have been no recent reports of YLDV infections. Tanapox and Yaba-like disease viruses produce a brief fever that is followed by development of firm, elevated, round, necrotic maculopapular nodules that are discernible from the vesiculopustular lesions produced by infection with the orthopoxviruses. Lesions are primarily on the skin of the upper arm, face, neck, or trunk (11); they umbilicate without pustulation and usually heal in 2 to 4 weeks.

YMTV, isolated in 1958 during an outbreak in a colony of rhesus monkeys in Yaba, near Lagos, Nigeria, produces epidermal histiocytomas, i.e., tumorlike masses of polygonal mononuclear cell infiltrates that advance to suppurative inflammatory reactions in monkeys. Animal handlers have been accidentally infected with YMTV, but there have been no reports of YMTV infection in at least a decade. The natural history of yatapoxviruses is not known.

Parapox

Three different parapoxviruses cause infections in humans, usually presenting clinically as the following occupational diseases: milker's nodule, known as pseudocowpox in dairy cattle; orf, known as contagious ecthyma, contagious pustular dermatitis, contagious pustular stomatitis, or sore-mouth in sheep and goats; and papulosa stomatitis, known as bovine papular stomatitis in calves and beef cattle (11). Infection is transmitted by direct contact with the etiologic agent through abraded skin on hands and fingers that have been in direct contact with infected animal skin or by livestock vaccination. Milker's nodule is a reddened hemispheric papule that matures to a purplish, smooth, firm nodule that varies in size up to 2 cm; lesions usually are not painful and last for up to 6 weeks. Orf infection in humans is usually found on the fingers, hands, and arms but may also be found on the face and neck; there may be fever and swelling of draining lymph nodes, and lesions ulcerate and are painful. Wildlife (e.g., skinning animals such as deer and reindeer) can be sources of orf virus infections in humans.

Molluscum contagiosum

Molluscum contagiosum is present worldwide, occurring in two clinical forms in humans. Molluscum that occurs in children in lesions on the face, trunk, and limbs (except palms and soles) is generally transmitted by direct or indirect skin contact (e.g., among wrestlers or in public baths and swimming pools). Molluscum in young adults, with lesions mostly in the lower abdominal wall, pubis, inner thighs, and genitalia, is a sexually transmitted disease. Lesions of both forms are pearly, flesh-colored, raised, firm, umbilicated nodules about 4 cm in diameter (11). Two virus types have been differentiated by DNA restriction assay. Type I is the most common cause of both clinical forms of the disease (21).

DESCRIPTION OF AGENTS

All poxviruses described in this chapter belong to the family *Poxviridae*, subfamily *Chordopoxvirinae*. Intracellular naked virions (INVs) are large, brick shaped with rounded corners or ovoid, and 220 to 450 by 140 to 260 nm, with an outer membrane, composed of lipid and a matrix of surface tubular protein, enclosing two lateral bodies lying in the concavities of a core membrane, which encases the genome. Virus particles contain about 100 structural proteins, including uncoating enzyme and enzymes associated with transcription of viral genes. Depending on cell type and virus strain, up to 20% of virions may be released in cell culture via the Golgi by exocytosis or release via microvilli. Virions released via cell membranes obtain a single- or double-layer envelope composed of cell membrane interspersed with viral proteins, so-called extracellular enveloped virions (EEVs), which are infectious and have distinct antigenic properties. INVs are released by natural cytolysis or by physical disruption of infected cells; these are also infectious. The genomes of poxviruses consist of a linear molecule of double-stranded DNA of 130 to 375 kilobase pairs. The DNA ends, called hairpin ends or telomeres, are covalently closed; near the left and right ends are sets of repeated sequences called inverted terminal repeats (11, 12).

Histopathology, electron microscopy, determination of virus growth features, antigenic testing, and DNA analyses can be used to characterize poxviruses in clinical samples. Poxvirus growth in the cytoplasm produces perinuclear B-type inclusions that represent the site of viral replication, called virus factories or Guarnieri bodies. Certain species, such as cowpox virus, also produce acidophilic, A-type inclusions, which are proteinaceous deposits detectable histopathologically or by thin-section electron microscopy. A-type inclusions may or may not contain virions, depending on the virus strain. When one visualizes samples by negative-stain electron microscopy, the human orthopoxviruses mentioned above cannot be distinguished morphologically from each other, but tanapox and molluscum contagiosum viruses often can be distinguished by microscopists experienced in examining poxviruses, especially when good clinical histories accompany specimens (11). Parapoxviruses are indistinguishable from each other morphologically, but their distinctive ovoid shape differentiates them from orthopoxviruses and from tanapox and molluscum contagiosum viruses. Members of poxvirus genera are antigenically readily distinguishable, although there is a common poxvirus nucleoprotein antigen, which is prepared by acid extraction and can be resolved by immunofluorescence microscopy and complement fixation (CF) tests. Orthopoxviruses are so closely related that routine serological tests cannot be used to differentiate species. Orthopoxviruses are different from viruses of humans of other poxvirus genera in that they produce a hemagglutinin which is separable from virions and distinctive pocks on embryonated chicken egg chorioallantoic membranes (CAMs). Parapoxviruses and tanapox and molluscum contagiosum viruses usually do not show such features. Restriction endonuclease assay of virion DNA gives genome structural data which are extremely powerful for determining differences between genera, species, strains, and variants (3, 4, 8, 11, 12).

COLLECTION, HANDLING, AND STORAGE OF SPECIMENS

In the United States and its territories, a suspected case of smallpox is immediately reportable by telephone to the state or territorial health department. If smallpox is still suspected after review by the health department, the case should be immediately reported to CDC. The poxvirus laboratories at CDC and at the Research Institute of Viral Preparations (Moscow) serve internationally as WHO Collaborating Centers for Smallpox and Other Poxvirus Infections. The CDC laboratory includes high-containment facilities for working with variola, monkeypox, and exotic poxviruses. In the United States and its territories, other poxvirus specimens should be handled locally through private or governmental health laboratories and not sent directly to CDC.

The basic procedures for collecting clinical specimens can be found in chapter 74. It is important to collect an amount of specimen sufficient to permit effective testing; use of an inadequate amount of specimen decreases the dependability of laboratory tests for diagnosing poxvirus diseases. Suitable specimens for virological tests of most suspected poxvirus infections are biopsies, scabs, and vesicular fluids, including the cells at the base of the vesicles. Vesicular fluid should be collected in two capillary tubes (the preferred method) or on glass microscope slides (four separate slides) as a thick droplet and allowed to air dry without spreading the smear. Alternatively, one can collect sufficient fluid on at least four swabs or about four scabs or lesion biopsies (send air-dried material; do not use transport media or glycerol). Suitable autopsy specimens include sections of skin, liver, spleen, lung, or kidney. After contacting the appropriate laboratory, send the specimens in a Parafilm-sealed container (e.g., screw-cap glass or plastic vial or bottle; slides in a small holder) in a plastic bag. Specimens collected from poxvirus infections can be stored at 4°C for a short time, but temperatures of −20 to −70°C should be used for long-term storage. Take precautions to prevent changes in the pH of specimens such as may occur when dry ice vapors enter containers. A metal, plastic, or paperboard outer container should be used for sending specimens. International, U.S., and local packing and shipping regulations must be followed.

LABORATORY DIAGNOSTIC METHODS

Methods used for diagnosis of smallpox and other orthopoxvirus diseases are listed in Table 1. The CDC Poxvirus Laboratory uses a combination of electron microscopy and virus growth in cell culture and on the CAM of 12-day-old chicken embryos to obtain initial results; comments on these techniques are presented below. These assays are accurate, dependable, and relatively rapid; protocols have been detailed in the previous edition of this Manual (18) and elsewhere (11, 17, 19). The other methods (immunofluorescence microscopy, immunodiffusion in agar, histopathology of stained sections, and CF) do not provide additional advantages to the efficacy of laboratory virus diagnosis; protocols for these procedures have also been described previously (11, 17–19). The most powerful definitive poxvirus identification methods involve electrophoresis of viral DNA digested with restriction endonucleases and DNA hybridizations. These methods generally require special expertise, including background in molecular biological and radioisotope techniques. Because poxvirus DNA assays are not generally performed in clinical diagnostic laboratories, they are beyond the scope of this chapter; however, these methods are described in references 3, 4, 8, 12, and 18. The reader is encouraged to consult these references, which may be useful for clinical laboratories using poxvirus DNA assays.

TABLE 1. Virological methods for the laboratory diagnosis of smallpox, human monkeypox, vaccinia, and cowpox virus infections

Method	Purpose
Primary	
Electron microscopy	Direct visualization of virus
CAM virus culture	Growth of smallpox, human monkeypox, vaccinia, cowpox, whitepox, and herpes simplex viruses with definitive pock characteristics
Tissue culture	Growth of smallpox, human monkeypox, vaccinia, whitepox, and herpes simplex viruses with definitive CPE characteristics
Other	
Immunodiffusion in agar	Antigenic identification
Stained smear	Visualization of elementary bodies
Fluorescent antibody	Visualization of virus-antibody complex; antigenic identification
CF	Visualization of reaction dependent on virus-antibody complex; antigenic identification

Electron microscopy

Negative-stain electron microscopy is well established in advanced clinical laboratories and is very useful for rapidly identifying poxviruses in specimens (11, 13, 18). At the CDC laboratories, the reliability of this method for detecting viruses in specimens collected from smallpox and human monkeypox cases has been more than 98%, and an even higher percentage of positive specimens could have been detected if the quantity of vesicular, pustular, or scab materials had been adequate. Compared with the reliability of electron microscopy for positive diagnosis of smallpox and human monkeypox, the reliability for detecting vaccinia virus in specimens has been only 67%. This low percentage can be partially explained by the inadequate amounts of specimens that were sent for assay or, more likely, by the fact that specimens were obtained when the numbers of virus particles in the lesion were less than needed for visualization. Newer methods of sample preparation that use sample concentration or immunoelectron microscopy should improve the virus identification rate. In examining a prepared grid, one must note that a dense grid showing no transparency indicates that too much material has been applied, and a grid not dense enough and showing too much transparency indicates that too little material has been used. Either condition greatly diminishes the reliability of the test; therefore, it is useful to examine twofold sample dilutions in filtered sterile distilled water.

Electron microscopy is an effective method for distinguishing poxviruses from herpesviruses, especially varicella-zoster virus (chickenpox), which, especially in developing countries, is clinically confused with smallpox and human monkeypox because of the rash (11, 18). Simple negative-stain electron microscopy is not useful for differentiating orthopoxviruses. Although there are no data on the degree of reliability for detecting viruses of milker's nodule, orf, tanapox, and molluscum contagiosum, we have found this procedure most useful (18). Parapoxviruses are smaller, and their morphological characteristics are distinctly different from those of orthopoxviruses and of tanapox and molluscum contagiosum viruses. Parapoxviruses are elongated (ovoid), with tubules on the viral surface arranged in parallel, thereby forming a parallel criss-cross surface pattern. The orthopoxviruses and tanapox and molluscum contagiosum viruses are brick shaped, with surface tubules in a studded, nonparallel arrangement. Tanapox virus morphology is similar to that of orthopoxviruses, but in about 80% of specimens examined tanapox virions have shown a double-layered lipid envelope surrounding the virus outer membrane that contains the tubules. Vaccinia, variola, and monkeypox viruses in clinical lesion specimens usually have no such envelope. Molluscum contagiosum virus has not yet been propagated successfully in cell culture; therefore, its precise morphogenesis is not fully resolved. In clinical lesions, virions resemble orthopoxviruses, but the molluscum surface tubules are more pronounced on virion M forms (i.e., particles into which the negative stain has not fully permeated). Because of the distinctive appearance of molluscum contagiosum lesions, visualization of poxviruses is usually adequate for confirming the diagnosis.

Virus growth on CAM

A detailed technique for preparing chicken embryos so that the air sac can be displaced to the side of the egg to permit inoculation of the CAM has been described by Westwood et al. (23). Fertile chicken eggs must be rotated slowly in a standard egg incubator at 38°C for 12 days to be useful for isolating and identifying orthopoxviruses. Lower embryo growth incubation temperatures render the CAM less susceptible or totally unsusceptible to virus growth. Eggs with infected CAMs are then incubated at 35°C to produce characteristic pocks instead of at higher temperatures, which could give atypical pock morphology. Eggs are opened for examination at 72 h postinfection. Sometimes one or two viral blind passages are required to adapt virus or increase titer to visualize pocks from virus in clinical materials.

The following suggestions may be helpful for differentiating viruses grown on the CAM of 12-day-old chicken embryos.

First, reliable sources of good-quality embryonated eggs, good laboratory technique, and experience are important in the diagnostic culture of viruses on the CAM. CAMs have sometimes not supported the growth of viruses, possibly for one or more of the following reasons: (i) eggs were from unhealthy or malnourished flocks of hens, (ii) unusual antibiotics were used to treat the flock, (iii) there was an infection in the flock, (iv) eggs were improperly incubated, resulting in physiologically less developed embryos, (v) there was insufficient humidity during incubation, (vi) improper solutions were used to dilute specimens, and (vii) inoculated eggs were incubated at an improper temperature. When the eggs are candled, examine the pointed end of the egg to determine whether the CAM is adequately developed. Eggs with underdeveloped CAMs should not be used because they are less sensitive to poxviruses. Eggs showing albumin sac encroachment into the area of the CAM for virus cultivation will yield about 10-fold less vaccinia virus pocks than will a normal area in which blood supply to the CAM is unhampered.

Second, variola, monkeypox, vaccinia, cowpox, and herpes simplex virus types 1 and 2 at 72 h postinfection can be differentiated by pock morphology (11) on less than confluently infected (about 30 pocks) CAMs. Herpes simplex virus is included here because it is isolated at times during examination of suspected poxvirus clinical materials. Varicella-zoster virus does not grow on the chicken CAM.

Variola virus pocks are raised, round, convex (dome-shaped) pocks about 1 mm in diameter with a regular border and smooth surface; they are nonhemorrhagic, with a white, opaque appearance. All pocks appear uniformly the same, and at ×10 magnification pocks resemble fried eggs "sunny side up."

Monkeypox virus pocks are not as raised as variola virus pocks and are 1 mm in diameter with a regular border; many pocks are opaque but with considerable hemorrhage and show a pinpoint-size hole in the center. All pocks on the CAM are uniformly the same except for an occasional nonhemorrhagic (white) variant in some specimens incubated at 34 to 35°C.

Vaccinia virus pocks are white, flattened, and 3 to 4 mm in diameter with a central necrosis and ulceration. Different strains produce more or less hemorrhagic pocks, and hemorrhagic strains produce occasional white variants.

Cowpox virus pocks are 2 to 4 mm in diameter, flattened, and fairly round, with a bright red hemorrhagic central area. Under ×10 magnification, with cowpox the erythrocytes are in the pock, whereas with monkeypox and vaccinia viruses erythrocytes appear to be on the pock.

Herpes simplex virus type 1 produces irregular-shaped, flat, pinpoint-size, nonopaque pocks that have a latticelike appearance on confluently infected CAMs. Herpes simples virus type 2 produces 1-mm-diameter, white, flat, and irregular-shaped pocks of variable size; pocks are large and mucoid when initially grown from clinical specimens.

Tanapox, milker's nodule, orf, and molluscum contagiosum viruses do not grow on CAM.

During the smallpox eradication era, the reliability of the CAM culture method at CDC for detecting variola and monkeypox viruses from adequate specimens of clinically diagnosed cases had been estimated at 91%. Usually specimens were in transit to CDC from Africa for 2 to 4 weeks; if they had been at CDC within 1 or 2 days, the value likely would have been near 100%.

When examining pocks on an infected CAM, one must be careful not to mistake nonspecific lesions or bits of egg shell for true pocks. Of the several causes for the appearance of nonspecific lesions, the most common is mechanical trauma; improper buffers used for diluting virus can induce a high incidence of nonspecific lesions. To avoid this problem, use a phosphate-buffered saline (PBS; 150 mM NaCl, 10 mM sodium phosphate [pH 7.4]).

A large dose of inactivated (heated or UV light irradiated) virus or of nonviable virus can cause a general thickening of the CAM and obscure the effect of a small amount of viable virus which may be present. A similar effect is observed when CAMs are inoculated with diagnostic specimens containing very high amounts of virus. Viral blind passages of serially diluted CAMs inoculated with large doses of such material sometimes is useful.

Tissue cultures

Cell culture systems must be used routinely for virus isolation in the diagnostic laboratory because occasional batches of chicken embryos are refractory to growth of orthopoxviruses on the CAM. Orthopoxviruses generally can be isolated from diagnostic specimens by using human and nonhuman primate cell cultures (e.g., embryonic human diploid, primary monkey kidney, or other cell lines, including BSC, $LLCMK_2$, Vero, and CV-1).

Variola virus in clinical specimens may produce a cytopathic effect (CPE) within 1 to 3 days, usually with a rounding up of the cells and the presence of hyperplastic foci, followed by the formation of small plaques (1 to 3 mm). The CPE spreads rapidly when a high-titered inoculum is used, and the cells eventually slough off. Monkeypox, vaccinia, and cowpox viruses may also cause CPE in 1 to 3 days, characterized usually by fused cells and the formation of rounded-cell foci, followed by the formation of distinct 2- to 6-mm-diameter plaques in 2 to 3 days. Plaques of these virus species under liquid overlay usually show cytoplasmic bridging, and with a high-titered inoculum the entire cell sheet becomes involved and soon sloughs off. When one is producing viral plaques for morphological characterization, several dilutions of the virus or specimen should be inoculated so that plaques are well separated. Plaque morphology at 60 to 72 h postinfection should be documented to avoid including satellite plaques, especially with poxviruses that produce diagnostic "comet"-shaped plaques (12), which are indicative of high levels of EEVs. Because certain tissue specimens may be toxic to cell culture but not to CAMs (or, conversely, toxic to CAMs but not to cell cultures), the use of both systems is recommended for routine diagnostic laboratories.

In some instances, orf virus can be isolated by primary rhesus monkey kidney cells or embryonic human fibroblasts; in other instances, ovine cells may be required for initial isolation (11). After initial virus isolation, orf virus may grow in embryonic human fibroblast cells or nonhuman primate cells. Diagnostic testing of milker's nodule virus is more demanding and usually requires bovine cells for initial isolation, but once isolated, the virus can also be propagated in embryonic human fibroblasts or primate cells.

Tanapox virus in monkey kidney cell lines usually produces distinctive CPE (11, 16) which includes nuclear vacuolation at about 5 days postinoculation at 34°C with established cultures. With fresh clinical lesion material, our experience has been that many specimens are grossly contaminated, perhaps because of secondary infections. Cultivation with high levels of antimycotic and antibacterial agents has required about two blind passages with 6 to 8 days of incubation in Vero or CV-1 cells for successful virus isolation.

Molluscum contagiosum virus has been reported to produce CPE in various cells, including primary human amnion, primary rhesus monkey kidney, BSC-1, WI-38, MRC, FL, and human foreskin cells, but the virus has never been successfully passaged continuously in culture (11).

SEROLOGICAL DIAGNOSIS

For rapid and accurate diagnosis of poxvirus infections, virological studies are preferred over serum antibody assays. However, since appropriate specimens for virological studies may at times be unavailable, for example, because the patient was seen too late in the course of infection, antibody assessment may be the only course for diagnosing the disease. Serum specimens are important in epidemiologic surveillance of the poxvirus-immune status of a population. It is important to note that no one serological test can be equated to a person's level of protection against human poxviruses. Protection is genetically defined and requires a concert of cell-mediated and humoral immune factors. Subsequent infection with members of the same poxvirus genus and species can occur. This section gives some practical comments that may be useful with respect to various serological tests for poxvirus antibodies.

Serological methods used routinely at CDC to assay antibodies evoked by variola, monkeypox, vaccinia, and cowpox viruses during the latter days of smallpox eradication, and now on occasion in posteradication times, include hemagglutination inhibition (HI), neutralization (NT), indirect fluorescent-antibody (IFA), immunodiffusion in agar, enzyme-linked immunosorbent assay (ELISA), radioimmunoassay (RIA), and radioimmunoassay adsorption (RIAA) tests. The techniques for HI and NT (17), IFA (19, 20), immunodiffusion in agar (2), ELISA (22), RIA (24), and RIAA (14, 15) tests have previously been described. In each serological test, a fourfold rise in titer between serum drawn at the acute and convalescent phases is considered diagnostic. Often only a single serum specimen taken at one phase or the other is available. In such situations, it is often very difficult to properly interpret test results.

Because orthopoxviruses are very closely related, the HI, NT, IFA, immunodiffusion in agar, ELISA, and RIA tests are not useful for direct serological differentiation of infection by variola, monkeypox, vaccinia, or cowpox viruses. The RIAA and other serum cross-absorption tests such as those utilizing IFA or immunodiffusion methods have been used with variable success with patient and animal sera, but more research is needed to further optimize such tests, especially antigen standardization and cross-absorption protocols to ensure reproducibility. Cross-absorption of hyperimmune animal sera has been successful in virological tests, but generally sera from patients do not have the antibody levels and specificities of sera from hyperimmunized laboratory animals.

HI test

Not all chicken erythrocytes work in the HI test. It is important to pretest erythrocyte preparations with a standardized hemagglutinin preparation, generally from vaccinia virus. The appendix describes the CDC method of preparing chicken erythrocytes and vaccinia hemagglutinin for the orthopoxvirus serum HI test. The HI test appears to detect one of the earliest rising antibodies after an infection by variola, monkeypox, vaccinia, or cowpox virus. The HI antibody titers in patients with recent smallpox or human monkeypox are generally greater than 1:80 and at times greater than 1:1,000. Sera with extremely high HI titers should be suspected of containing nonspecific HI substances, especially if serum specimens are old and have been improperly stored or if they were collected during autopsy. The appendix describes periodate treatment of serum specimens, which has been very useful and at times used routinely for eliminating nonspecific substances. HI antibodies have variable half-lives after infection, but they may persist for years. For example, we found HI titers of 1:10 to 1:20 at 3 to 4 years after onset in confirmed cases of human monkeypox.

NT test

The antigen for routine poxvirus NT antibody assay can be lysates of infected-cell cultures clarified by low-speed centrifugation or a variety of purified or partially purified virus preparations that may contain INVs, EEVs, or both forms. Purified virus preparations are more defined and, depending on the particle-to-PFU ratio, may be more suitable than lysates which can bind neutralizing antibodies via virions as well as via other intracellular viral antigens. The appendix describes a commonly used method for preparing INVs from poxvirus-infected cell cultures; in different poxvirus laboratories, the procedure has been adapted to purify poxviruses in homogenates from various sources (nodules, CAMs, etc.). Neutralizing antibody for variola, monkeypox, cowpox, and vaccinia viruses may be detectable as early as 6 days postinfection (postvaccination). NT antibodies have variable half-lives, but they have been detected more than 20 years after smallpox vaccination. When only one serum specimen is taken from an infected patient sometime after the onset of rash and it shows only a moderate titer (less than 1:50), the diagnosis is difficult, especially if the patient had been vaccinated previously. A vaccination scar (most countries have not vaccinated civilians for about 10 years) and perhaps a titer of greater than 1:100 is presumptive evidence for the diagnosis of a superinfection by a second orthopoxvirus.

IFA

The general methods for IFA can be found elsewhere in this Manual and in reference 20. The predominant antigen used for the orthopoxvirus IFA diagnostic test at CDC has been monkeypox virus-infected cells that are not fixed but are simply air dried overnight onto microscope slides. A titer of ≥1:32 for a patient without previous vaccination indicates recent orthopoxvirus infection. IFA titers generally begin to decrease about 6 months after the onset of illness, and for this reason the test must be used judiciously in epidemiologic studies.

ELISA

In original versions of the ELISA method utilizing 96-well microdilution plates (22) adapted at CDC for assay of orthopoxvirus antibodies, a crude concentrate of orthopoxvirus-infected cell culture lysate was used as an antigen for testing sera from various sources. Experience indicated that crude-lysate antigens gave more variable titers with different antigen batches, and the need for antigen standardization has become apparent. The antigen now being evaluated at CDC for use in ELISA tests for orthopoxvirus antibodies consists of purified INVs prepared by sucrose gradient centrifugation (see Appendix). Some of the reasons for investigating the use of INVs are that (i) antibodies against virion structural proteins on INVs may be longer lasting than those against other viral antigens, (ii) fewer antigens are present on INVs as compared with infected-cell lysates that contain multiple (e.g., poxviruses produce more than 200 proteins) viral antigens whose quality and quantity could be affected by culture conditions, and (iii) INVs can be quantified spectrophotometrically, which would be an asset to antigen standardization.

RIA

Although no direct comparisons of all poxvirus serological tests have been made, the RIA test for orthopoxvirus antibodies in humans appears to be the most sensitive and most useful assay for detecting long-existing antibodies (24). Because the RIA test requires radioisotopes and specialized, expensive equipment, it has been used to only a limited extent for routine diagnostics. Titers found in humans with recent infection by monkeypox virus ranged from 1:3,000 to 1:20,000 or more. The specificity of this test becomes questionable with titers of <1:50. Antigen standardization is also a problem; no comparative data have been developed on use of more defined antigens.

RIAA

RIAA is a sensitive method by which specific antibodies to monkeypox, vaccinia, and variola viruses can be differentiated. The RIAA using infected CAM homogenates of different orthopoxvirus species as antigen and cross-adsorbing antigen and ^{125}I-staphylococcal protein A immune complex indicator (14) has been used to differentiate specific antibodies to monkeypox virus in a serosurvey of African wildlife to search for animals maintaining transmission of this zoonotic agent. Further evaluation is needed to define which viral antigen is the key component rendering specificity to the test. Studies on cross-adsorbing hyperimmune rabbit sera with soluble antigen preparations of various orthopoxviruses for use in immunodiffusion in agarose indicate that a 78-kilodalton viral protein contains the species-specific determinants (6, 7). It seems that establishing an ELISA version of the RIAA test would be most useful, especially if species-specific antigens become better defined.

Tests for milker's nodule, orf, and tanapox

The serological methods of choice for diagnosing milker's nodule and orf virus infections have been the ELISA (using infected-cell culture concentrated antigen) and IFA tests. For tanapox virus infections, the ELISA (with infected-cell culture concentrate antigen), IFA, and standard NT tests have been used with moderate effectiveness. As in orthopoxvirus serology, there is hope that improvements in serological diagnosis of these infections may be aided by development of more defined antigens. Perhaps because of the relatively less extensive nature of the infections found in these diseases (usually only one to a few lesions on the skin), the serum should be collected at 3 to 5 weeks after onset. Any positive results have been considered useful for diagnosis, since the immunology of these infections is poorly understood and prior vaccinia vaccination does not obfuscate data interpretation.

Molluscum contagiosum

There are no practical serodiagnostic tests for routine or large-scale studies of molluscum contagiosum because the virus cannot be propagated readily.

Other methods

Immunodiffusion and CF tests (17, 18) are less sensitive than the tests mentioned above. With immunodiffusion (2, 6, 19), precipitating antibodies are not seen in many clinically proven cases of variola, monkeypox, or vaccinia virus infection, but the test has been useful with hyperimmune animal sera. It is rarely positive in persons recently vaccinated or revaccinated against smallpox. In the CF test, antibodies in smallpox patients often do not appear until the second week after clinical diagnosis. A significant proportion of sera from unvaccinated smallpox patients tested for CF antibodies, even after day 8 of onset, have been negative. After primary vaccination or revaccination for smallpox, CF antibodies may not be detected. For orf virus and milker's nodule infections, antibodies are also not always detected. For these diseases, negative results are not useful. Experience suggests that the CF test may be of limited value for diagnosis of poxvirus.

VIROLOGICAL DIAGNOSTIC METHODS

Our experience has been that orthopoxvirus infections, especially smallpox and human monkeypox, can be confidently diagnosed in the laboratory by a combination of three tests: electron microscopy, CAM culture, and cell culture. It must be emphasized, however, that appropriate viral specimens in adequate amounts are needed, since frequently the problem is making a negative diagnosis with confidence. The diagnostic confidence for orf, milker's nodule, and tanapox has been relatively less than that for orthopoxvirus infections because the viruses of these diseases have been more difficult to propagate than orthopoxviruses upon primary cultivation of specimens. Furthermore, although visualization of virus particles by electron microscopy in suspected tanapox specimens has generally been successful, it has been more difficult to correctly confirm clinical diagnoses of orf and milker's nodule because the chances of receiving unsuitable specimens are greater.

APPENDIX

Diagnostic reagents and antigen preparations for poxvirus diagnostic tests are not generally available commercially. The previous edition of this Manual (18) contains detailed methods for preparing poxvirus-infected CAM homogenates for use in a variety of tests (low-speed centrifugation was an added step used in preparing RIA and RIAA antigens [14, 24]). Because the hemagglutination and HI tests for orthopoxviruses are useful for screening in epidemiological surveys and recently as a selection system for recombinant vaccinia viruses expressing foreign genes, the following methods for preparing chicken erythrocytes, hemagglutinin antigen, removal of nonspecific HI test inhibitors from sera, and preparation of vaccinia hyperimmune antisera have been carried over from the previous edition (18). These methods could be used to form the essence of a poxvirus diagnostic laboratory. Also presented is a protocol for purification of orthopoxvirus INVs for those laboratories desiring to perform poxvirus ELISA, RIA, or RIAA tests or poxvirus DNA studies.

Chicken erythrocytes for hemagglutination

Our experience has been that about 50% of chickens tested have erythrocytes that can be agglutinated by vaccinia hemagglutinin; thus, samples of erythrocytes from several chickens must be pretested to select those that do hemagglutinate.

Selection of chicken

1. Obtain 5 ml of blood from several 7- to 14-month-old chickens.
2. Wash the erythrocytes from each of the chickens three times with PBS (pH 7.2) by centrifugation (500 × *g* for 10 min).
3. Prepare in PBS a 0.5% erythrocyte suspension from each chicken.
4. Set up the standard hemagglutinin titration for each erythrocyte suspension by using a known positive vaccinia hemagglutinin antigen.
5. Use only the chickens whose erythrocytes are agglutinated by the HA antigen at a dilution equal to or greater than 1:64.

Preparation of erythrocytes for the HI test

1. Collect 50 ml of blood from a pretested chicken and mix the blood in a bottle at a ratio of 1 part of blood to 4 parts of Alsever solution. (Blood-Alsever mixture can be stored at 4°C up to 2 weeks.)
2. Wash erythrocytes three times with PBS (pH 7.2) by centrifugation in 15-ml graduated conical centrifuge tubes.
3. Remove and discard the supernatant and cell buffy coat at each wash.
4. After the third wash, resuspend the packed cells in an equal volume of PBS; the 50% cell suspension is used only on the day of the test.
5. Dilute the suspension to prepare a 0.5% erythrocyte suspension for the HI test.

Preparation of vaccinia antigen for the HI test

1. Inoculate eight BHK-21 cell cultures (150-cm^2 monolayers) with 2 ml of vaccinia virus (titer of ca. 10^7 PFU/ml).
2. Absorb the inoculum for 1 h at 35°C; add 50 ml of prewarmed Dulbecco high-glucose or other minimal essential medium (MEM) containing 0.4% bovine albumin.
3. Harvest infected cells at 80 to 100% CPE (about 2 days).
4. Centrifuge the cells at 500 × *g* for 15 min.
5. Wash the cells three times with 30 ml of reticulocyte swelling buffer (RSB)–0.01 M Tris–0.01 M NaCl–0.0015 M $MgCl_2$ (pH 7.8).
6. After the third washing, suspend the cells in 8 ml of RSB and incubate the suspension overnight at 4°C.
7. Rupture the cells by 20 to 30 strokes with a Dounce homogenizer.
8. Centrifuge the cells at 100 × *g* for 15 min to pellet the nuclei and cell debris.
9. Save the supernatant fluid.
10. Recycle the pellet as in steps 6 and 7 if intact cells are seen microscopically.
11. Centrifuge the cells as in step 8.
12. Pool the supernatant fluids of steps 8 and 11.
13. Centrifuge the supernatant fluid at 75,000 × *g* for 45 min in a Beckman SW28 rotor.
14. Resuspend the pellet in 20 ml of RSB; add Merthiolate to 0.0001%.
15. Evaluate antigen by hemagglutination and HI tests.

Preparation of rabbit antiserum to vaccinia virus

1. Inoculate 2 ml of vaccinia virus (titer of ca. 10^7 PFU/ml) into one confluent cell monolayer (150 cm^2) of primary rabbit kidney cells that have been grown with MEM containing 10% inactivated normal rabbit serum.
2. Absorb virus at 35°C for 1 h; add 50 ml of prewarmed MEM with 2% inactivated normal rabbit serum.
3. Incubate the preparation at 36°C until 100% CPE is observed (2 to 3 days).
4. Harvest infected cells into 10 ml of McIlvaine buffer (pH 7.4).
5. Freeze and thaw cells through three cycles. Titer the virus on CAMs or by plaque titration on cell cultures (chick fibroblasts, monkey kidney cells, etc.); 10^7 to 10^8 PFU/ml is acceptable.
6. Mix the suspension with an equal volume of acceptable adjuvant.

7. Inoculate each prebled rabbit (older than 6 months) in both front footpads with 0.3 ml of the mixture in each footpad.

8. Inoculate 1 ml of the mixture subcutaneously in the right hindquarter.

9. Twenty days later, inoculate a 1-ml booster intramuscularly in the hindquarter.

10. Exsanguinate the rabbit 2 to 4 weeks after the booster.

11. Prepare serum from the blood; store serum in small portions at −20°C.

Periodate treatment of serum to remove nonspecific hemagglutinating and hemagglutination-inhibiting substances

1. Prepare a fresh 0.011 M solution of KIO_4 (do not substitute $NaIO_4$) by dissolving 0.256 g of KIO_4 in 100 ml of PBS. Stir the solution constantly with a magnetic stirrer (do not use heat).

2. Prepare 3% glycerol in PBS.

3. To 0.1 ml of serum in a test tube, add 0.3 ml of the 0.011 M KIO_4 solution and incubate the mixture at room temperature for exactly 15 min.

4. Add 0.1 ml of the 3% glycerol–PBS solution and incubate the solution at room temperature for at least 15 min to stop oxidation; this removes hemagglutination-inhibiting substances.

5. Add 0.05 ml of the 50% chicken erythrocytes and incubate the preparation at 4°C for 1 h for removal of nonspecific hemagglutinating substances present in some sera.

6. Centrifuge the treated serum at 600 × *g* for 10 min and then transfer the supernatant fluid to a fresh tube. The treated serum is considered to be a 1:5 dilution when one is calculating the HI endpoint.

7. Inactivate the treated serum at 56°C for 30 min; then proceed with further dilution of the serum and test for HI antibodies.

Purification of orthopoxvirus INVs from infected-cell monolayers

1. Inoculate each of 30 cell culture monolayers (150 cm^2, FL human amnion, RK-13, etc.) with 2 ml of vaccinia virus (titer, ca. 10^7 PFU/ml); absorb the inoculum for 1 h at 35°C in a CO_2 incubator and then add 50 ml of prewarmed Dulbecco high-glucose or other reinforced MEM containing 2% fetal calf serum.

2. Harvest infected cells at 100% CPE (about 2 to 3 days) by scraping cells into the medium; cooling cultures to 4°C also dislodges cells.

3. Centrifuge the cells at 600 × *g* for 10 min (Beckman JA-10 rotor).

4. Combine and suspend pellets in 300 ml of cold hypotonic RSB–10 mM Tris–10 mM NaCl–1.5 mM $MgCl_2$ (pH 7.8).

5. Pellet the cells as in step 4, resuspend the cells in 40 ml of RSB, and incubate the suspension for 2 h to overnight at 4°C to swell the cells.

6. Rupture the cells by 20 to 30 strokes with a Dounce homogenizer; observe the release of nuclei microscopically.

7. Centrifuge the cells at 100 × *g* for 15 min to pellet the nuclei; save the supernatant fluid.

8. Recycle the pellet as in steps 5 to 7 if intact cells are seen microscopically.

9. Pool the supernatant fluids of steps 7 and 8. (Sonication or Potter-Elvejhem homogenization of supernatant fluid may give better recovery because virions are more dispersed for the next step.)

10. In a Beckman SW28 rotor tube, layer the supernatant fluid onto a 15- to 20-ml cushion of 40% (wt/wt) sucrose (40 g of sucrose in 60 ml of 10 mM Tris buffer [pH 8 to 9]. With a plastic 1-ml pipette, lay a 0.1-ml pad of 100% glycerol beneath the sucrose cushion (to prevent formation of hard pellets of virus particles). Centrifuge the preparation at 50,000 × *g* for 90 min at 4°C.

11. Aspirate the supernatant fluid and most of the sucrose. Resuspend the virus soft pellet, including the glycerol pad and the bottom 1 ml of sucrose.

12. Dilute the pellet about 1:3 with 10 mM Tris buffer (pH 8 to 9) to reduce density so that the virion suspension can be layered gently onto a prechilled sucrose gradient (20 to 40% [wt/wt] sucrose in 10 mM Tris buffer [pH 8 to 9]) cast at room temperature in SW28 rotor tubes (load gradients with less than 5 ml of sample). Before loading gradients, sonicate or Potter-Elvejhem homogenize the pellet to disperse virions.

13. Centrifugation of the gradient at 20,000 × *g* and 4°C will sediment virions to the middle of the gradient (the speed may be increased or decreased for optimized banding of specific poxviruses; poxviruses have a sedimentation coefficient of about 5,000 Svedberg units). Aspirate sucrose above the viral band. Harvest the viral band and dispense it in 0.5-ml samples; store the samples frozen at −20 to −70°C. A small sample of the preparation is diluted (1:20 to 1:30) to determine the optical density at 260 nm (use disposable UV cuvettes). One unit of optical density at 260 nm equals 1.2×10^{10} particles (vaccinia) per ml. Titrate the preparation on monkey kidney cells (CV-1, Vero, BSC-40, etc.) to obtain the particle-to-PFU ratio.

14. Antigen for ELISA is prepared by diluting virus to 10^8 particles per ml in carbonate-bicarbonate ELISA buffer to coat 96-well microdilution plates (or plastic rods used in the rapid ELISA). Concentrated stock antigen for the NT test is made by storing a portion of the samples at −20°C after dilution with an equal volume of sterile 100% glycerol.

15. DNA can be prepared from purified virions essentially as described in references 3, 4, 8, and 19.

LITERATURE CITED

1. **Downie, A. W., C. H. Taylor-Robinson, A. E. Caunt, G. S. Nelson, P. E. C. Manson-Bahr, and T. C. H. Matthews.** 1971. Tanapox: a new disease caused by a poxvirus. Br. Med. J. **1:**363–368.
2. **Dumbell, K. R., and M. Nizamuddin.** 1959. An agar gel precipitation test for the laboratory diagnosis of smallpox. Lancet **i:**916–917.
3. **Esposito, J. J., R. Condit, and J. F. Obijeski.** 1981. The preparation of orthopoxvirus DNA. J. Virol. Methods **2:** 175–179.
4. **Esposito, J. J., and J. C. Knight.** 1985. Orthopoxvirus DNA: a comparison of restriction profiles and maps. Virology **143:**230–251.
5. **Esposito, J. J., and F. A. Murphy.** 1989. Infectious recombinant vectored virus vaccines. Adv. Vet. Sci. Comp. Med. **33:**195–247.
6. **Esposito, J. J., J. F. Obijeski, and J. H. Nakano.** 1977. Serological relatedness of monkeypox, variola, and vaccinia viruses. J. Med. Virol. **1:**35–47.
7. **Esposito, J. J., J. F. Obijeski, and J. H. Nakano.** 1977. The virion and soluble antigen proteins of variola, monkeypox, and vaccinia viruses. J. Med. Virol. **1:**95–110.
8. **Esposito, J. J., J. F. Obijeski, and J. H. Nakano.** 1978. Orthopoxvirus DNA: strain differentiation by electrophoresis of restriction endonuclease fragmented virion DNA. Virology **89:**53–66.
9. **Esposito, J. J., J. F. Obijeski, and J. H. Nakano.** 1985. Can variola viruses be derived from monkeypox virus? An investigation based on DNA mapping. Bull. W.H.O. **63:** 695–703.
10. **Fenner, F., D. A. Henderson, I. Arita, Z. Jezek, and I. Ladnyi.** 1988. Smallpox and its eradication. World Health Organization, Geneva.
11. **Fenner, F., and J. H. Nakano.** 1988. Poxviridae: the poxviruses, p. 177–207. *In* E. H. Lennette, P. Halonen, and F. A. Murphy (ed.), Laboratory diagnosis of infectious diseases, vol. 2. Viral, rickettsial, and chlamydial diseases. Springer-Verlag, New York.
12. **Fenner, F., R. Wittek, and K. R. Dumbell.** 1989. The orthopoxviruses. Academic Press, Inc., New York.

13. **Harris, W. J., and J. C. W. Westwood.** 1964. Phosphotungstate staining of vaccinia virus. J. Gen. Microbiol. **34:** 491–495.
14. **Hutchinson, H. D., D. W. Ziegler, D. E. Wells, and J. H. Nakano.** 1977. Differentiation of variola, monkeypox, and vaccinia antisera by radioimmunoassay. Bull. W.H.O. **55:** 613–623.
15. **Jezek, Z., and F. Fenner.** 1988. Human monkeypox. Monogr. Virol. **17:**1–140.
16. **Knight, J. C., F. J. Novembre, D. R. Brown, C. S. Goldsmith, and J. J. Esposito.** 1989. Studies on tanapox virus. Virology **172:**116–124.
17. **Nakano, J. H.** 1979. Poxviruses, p. 257–308. *In* E. H. Lennette and N. J. Schmidt (ed.), Diagnostic procedures for viral, rickettsial, and chlamydial infections, 5th ed. American Public Health Association, Inc., Washington, D.C.
18. **Nakano, J. H.** 1985. Poxviruses, p. 733–741. *In* E. H. Lennette, A. Balows, W. J. Hausler, Jr., and H. J. Shadomy (ed.), Manual of clinical microbiology, 4th ed. American Society for Microbiology, Washington, D.C.
19. **Nakano, J. H., and J. J. Esposito.** 1989. Poxviruses, p. 224–265. *In* N. J. Schmidt and R. W. Emmons (ed.), Diagnostic procedures for viral, rickettsial, and chlamydial infections, 6th ed. American Public Health Association, Inc., Washington, D.C.
20. **Riggs, J. L.** 1989. Immunofluorescent staining, p. 123–134. *In* N. J. Schmidt and R. W. Emmons (ed.), Diagnostic procedures for viral, rickettsial, and chlamydial infections, 6th ed. American Public Health Association, Inc., Washington, D.C.
21. **Scholz, J., A. Rosen-Wolff, J. Bugert, H. Reisner, M. I. White, G. Darai, and R. Postlethwaite.** 1988. Epidemiology of molluscum contagiosum using genetic analysis of the viral DNA. J. Med. Virol. **27:**87–90.
22. **Voller, A., D. Bidwell, and A. Bartlett.** 1980. Enzyme-linked immunosorbent assay, p. 359–371. *In* N. R. Rose and H. Friedman (ed.), Manual of clinical immunology, 2nd ed. American Society for Microbiology, Washington, D.C.
23. **Westwood, J. C. N., P. H. Phipps, and E. A. Boulter.** 1957. The titration of vaccinia virus on the chorioallantoic membrane of the developing chick embryo. J. Hyg. **52:** 123–139.
24. **Ziegler, D. W., H. D. Hutchinson, J. P. Koplan, and J. H. Nakano.** 1975. Detection by radioimmunoassay of antibody in human smallpox patients and vaccines. J. Clin. Microbiol. **1:**311–317.

Chapter 81

Influenza Viruses

MAURICE W. HARMON AND ALAN P. KENDAL

CLINICAL BACKGROUND

Influenza is an acute respiratory disease that characteristically occurs in epidemic form. Virus is spread from person to person by the aerosol route, and there is an incubation period of 1 to 4 days. Infection with influenza virus can result in a spectrum of clinical responses ranging from asymptomatic infection to primary viral pneumonia that rapidly progresses to a fatal outcome. The typical clinical disease begins abruptly with chills, followed by fatigue, headache, and myalgia. Fever occurs early and persists for 2 to 4 days. Constitutional symptoms are more striking with influenza than with other respiratory diseases. A nonproductive cough is usually present after the first several days of illness, but coryza and pharyngitis are less common. Clinical manifestations of influenza in children can be similar to those in adults, but there are some distinct differences as well. Children may have higher fever, and the incidence of gastrointestinal symptoms, otitis media, croup, and myositis is more frequent in children. Recovery from uncomplicated influenza begins 3 to 4 days after onset, although weakness, fatigue, and cough may persist for a week or longer. Lower respiratory tract complications of influenza, which can be fatal, include primary viral pneumonia, combined viral-bacterial pneumonia, and secondary bacterial pneumonia. Elderly persons and persons with underlying health problems, such as pulmonary or cardiovascular disease, are at increased risk for complications of influenza infection. Reye's syndrome, characterized by noninflammatory encephalopathy and fatty infiltration of the liver, can occur in children after influenza infection. A risk factor for Reye's syndrome is the use of salicylate-containing medications in infections with influenza or varicella virus.

Like several other viral respiratory infections, influenza is a seasonal disease which occurs in the Northern Hemisphere usually between November and April and in the Southern Hemisphere between May and October. In tropical regions influenza may be endemic, with periods of increased activity occurring more than once a year.

Epidemics are often preceded by sporadic cases and isolated outbreaks until community-wide activity causes a rapid increase in visits to clinics, physician offices, or emergency rooms for a period of about 1 month in a given locality. Epidemics of type A influenza occur in about 2 of every 3 years. Outbreaks of type B generally occur every 2 to 3 years. In recent years, cocirculation of influenza A and B viruses, or cocirculation of influenza A virus of two subtypes (H1N1 and H3N2), has been common. Influenza type C is associated with subclinical or mild common cold-like illness and does not cause recognizable epidemics.

Influenza cases do not always follow the classic clinical course, nor do they always occur in epidemic patterns. Sporadic cases, particularly among children, may be difficult to recognize clinically when observed against a background of other febrile respiratory diseases. Laboratory diagnosis of cases early in the season provides advance warning that influenza virus is spreading in the community before it causes an epidemic. Diagnosis is important to support continuing vaccination activities as well as to permit rational use of antiviral agents such as amantadine and rimantadine. Laboratory diagnosis of late-season isolates is also significant. In the United States, strains that appear late in the season and are the minority type or subtype often reappear in epidemic form the next season. Therefore, laboratory diagnosis of influenza by isolation and identification outside as well as inside epidemic periods contributes to the national surveillance effort and improves the prospect of incorporating the correct strains of virus into the vaccine.

A number of chapters and books are available for more detailed information on influenza (10, 17, 25).

DESCRIPTION OF AGENT

The structures of influenza virus types A and B are similar when examined by electron microscopy. Negatively stained preparations of viruses that have had multiple passages in eggs or tissue culture reveal irregularly shaped spherical particles approximately 120 nm in diameter. In contrast, influenza isolates examined after a single passage in culture may show a greater variation in shape and size, including greatly elongated forms. Influenza type C viruses are generally similar but may reveal a reticular structure on their envelope. Influenza viruses contain a single-stranded, segmented genome that is enclosed within a virus-modified host cell membrane. The genome RNA is complementary to the mRNA and is therefore negative sense. The eight segments of influenza types A and B both code for 10 proteins known to be expressed in infected cells. Seven or eight are structural proteins of the virion, the others being nonstructural proteins found only in infected cells.

The three largest RNA segments (segments 1, 2, and 3) code for the three polymerase proteins. The polymerase proteins are named PB1, PB2, and PA on the basis of their electrophoretic mobility and whether they are acidic (PA) or basic (PB) upon isoelectric focusing. PB1 and PB2 are believed to be involved in mRNA synthesis, whereas PA may have a role in virion RNA replication.

The three intermediate-size RNA segments code for the hemagglutinin, the neuraminidase, and the nucleoprotein. The hemagglutinin derives its name from its role in the agglutination of erythrocytes. It is also responsible for attachment to cells at the initiation of infection and has a role in the subsequent penetration of the virus genome into the cell cytoplasm. Virions brought inside the cell in vesicles release ribonucleoprotein after a membrane fusion event mediated by the hemagglutinin. The hemagglutinin polypeptide is synthesized as a single chain that trimerizes and undergoes posttranslational modification whereby each chain is cleaved to give two polypeptide chains (HA1 and HA2) which remain linked by a single disulfide bond. Cleavage of the hemagglutinin polypeptide is necessary for the membrane fusion activity to occur. The three-dimensional structure of the hemagglutinin is known from X-ray crystallography and consists of a stalk with the membrane-anchoring site near the C-terminal end of HA2 and a globular head formed by HA1 at the distal end (35). The receptor-binding site is located in the globular head. Four or five antigenic sites have been identified in the HA1 polypeptide from amino acid sequence changes in antigenic variants. Antibodies to the hemagglutinin neutralize viral infectivity, and it is variation in this molecule that is mainly responsible for the recurring outbreaks of influenza and the difficulty in controlling influenza through immunization.

The second surface glycoprotein, the neuraminidase, is a tetramer held together by disulfide bonds. It is mushroom shaped, with a head that contains the enzymatic and antigenic sites and a stalk which contains a hydrophobic region that anchors the molecule in the membrane (3). The enzymatic action of the molecule cleaves sialic acid from the hemagglutinin and from the infected-cell surface, which is thought to prevent self-aggregation and to promote release of virus from the infected cell. Antibody to the neuraminidase does not neutralize infectivity effectively but does restrict multiple cycles of replication and may attenuate illness.

The nucleoprotein is the major protein of the helical internal ribonucleoprotein complex associated with the RNA segments and the three polymerase proteins. It contains type-specific antigenic determinants that permit influenza A, B, and C viruses to be distinguished. The nucleoprotein molecule is probably phosphorylated at one serine residue per molecule, but the function of the phosphate is not known.

RNA segment 7 of influenza A virus codes for two proteins. The M1 (matrix) protein is a highly conserved, type-specific protein with considerable hydrophobicity. It is located just beneath the viral envelope and is thought to serve a structural function. This protein may also be involved in control of virion RNA polymerase activity and may participate in virus assembly. The coding region of the M1 protein involves only 75% of segment 7 RNA. A second open reading frame exists, and the mRNA for this second protein uses the same code for the first nine amino acids as the M1 protein, but then nearly 600 nucleotides are spliced out and the reading frame is changed (+1). The resultant spliced mRNA codes for a 97-amino-acid polypeptide, designated M2. This is a membrane-spanning protein found in large amounts in infected cells and in reduced amounts in virions (18). The function of this protein is unknown, but single amino acid changes in certain positions in the membrane-spanning region render influenza A viruses resistant to inhibition by amantadine and rimantadine (15). Although a second coding region in RNA segment 7 has been identified in influenza B virus, no protein analogous to M2 has been detected. However, an analogous protein (NB) is expressed by the neuraminidase gene (segment 6), which has a second open reading frame.

Two nonstructural proteins (NS1 and NS2) are coded by RNA segment 8 and are translated from separate mRNAs, of which one is generated by a splicing mechanism similar to that described for M2. Thus, polypeptides NS1 and NS2 also have in common the nine amino acids at their N termini, but the rest of each protein is distinct due to a shift in the mRNA reading frame. The functions of NS1 and NS2 have not been established. NS1 is made in large amounts early in infection and accumulates in the nucleus, whereas NS2 is made late in infection and is found predominantly in the cytoplasm.

In many respects, influenza C virus resembles influenza A and B viruses, but some important differences do exist. The most important is that influenza C virus has only seven RNA segments and no neuraminidase activity. The receptor-binding and receptor-destroying enzyme functions of influenza C virus are distinct from those of influenza A and B viruses. The epidemiology of influenza C virus is one of a mild pediatric respiratory pathogen that only occasionally affects adults.

Influenza virus infectivity may be destroyed by heating to 56°C or treatment with lipid solvents, acid, formaldehyde, β-propiolactone, UV light, or gamma radiation. Infectivity is lost with repeated freezing and thawing or over time by storage in standard −20°C freezers. Infectious virus may be preserved for the long term by lyophilization (with 0.5% gelatin) or by freezing liquid suspensions to −60°C or below in the presence of at least 1% protein as a stabilizer.

Influenza viruses are divided into types A, B, and C on the basis of the antigenic differences of their nucleoprotein antigens. Influenza A viruses are further subdivided into subtypes on the basis of antigenic differences in the hemagglutinin and neuraminidase. The nomenclature system recommended by the World Health Organization includes the virus type, geographic origin, strain number, and year of isolation (36). The antigenic description of the hemagglutinin and neuraminidase is given in parentheses, e.g., A/Shanghai/11/87 (H3N2). The host of origin is also given for animal influenza virus isolates, e.g., A/equine/Prague/1/56 (H7N7). A total of 13 hemagglutinin subtypes and 9 neuraminidase subtypes are recognized, including those isolated from horses, pigs, and birds, but only 3 hemagglutinin and 2 neuraminidase subtypes have been found in human epidemic strains. Prototypes for the three hemagglutinin/neuraminidase combinations that have ever been proven to circulate in humans are A/Puerto Rico/8/34 (H1N1), A/Japan/305/57 (H2N2), and A/Hong Kong/1/68 (H3N2). Each hemagglutinin and neuraminidase subtype may encompass strains exhibiting a considerable degree of antigenic heterogeneity (most evident in human strains) which may be differentiated by hemagglutination inhibition (HI) and neuraminidase inhibition tests (Table 1).

Antigenic variation of influenza viruses occurs primarily in the surface glycoproteins and is mediated by multiple determinants in the hemagglutinin and neuraminidase antigens. Abrupt change in the antigenic

TABLE 1. HI reactions of influenza A (H1N1) viruses isolated from 1977 to 1986

Virus antigen	Reaction with ferret antisera[a]				
	A/USSR/ 90/77	A/Brazil/ 11/78	A/England/ 333/80	A/Chile/ 1/83	A/Taiwan/ 1/86
A/USSR/90/77	*320*	320	160	80	—[b]
A/Brazil/11/78	40	*640*	160	160	—
A/England/333/80	80	320	*640*	320	—
A/Chile/1/83	20	80	40	*160*	—
A/Taiwan/1/86	10	20	20	40	*2,560*

[a] Italicized numbers represent homologous reactions.
[b] —, Less than 10.

composition of influenza A viruses is called antigenic shift and, in the case of the hemagglutinin, may be associated with worldwide epidemics such as those occurring in 1957 with the Asian (H2) virus and in 1968 with the Hong Kong (H3) virus. The appearance in 1977 of the "Russian" influenza virus (H1N1) constituted an antigenic shift, although the virus was antigenically indistinguishable from strains previously isolated in 1950. The ensuing worldwide epidemic was limited, affecting primarily persons born after about 1955. Persons born earlier have been largely protected by virtue of previous infection with strains of the H1N1 subtype which circulated from at least 1918 to 1957.

More gradual changes in the antigens within a subtype are described as antigenic drift, which may or may not be associated with epidemics. Examples of antigenic drift variants and their characterization by postinfection ferret sera are shown in Table 1. Influenza virus types A, B, and C all undergo antigenic drift.

COLLECTION AND STORAGE OF SPECIMENS

Specimens for virus isolation should be taken within the first 3 days of illness, as they are then most likely to yield an isolate. The most practical procedure is a swab culture of the throat and nasal passage of acutely ill patients. To collect a throat swab, vigorously rub the tonsils, soft palate, and back wall of the lower pharynx with a dry cotton applicator. The cotton tip of the applicator is then broken off into screw-cap vials containing 2 to 5 ml of transport medium. For nasal swabs, a wire nasopharyngeal swab is passed into the nostril parallel with the palate, gently rotated, and withdrawn. The secretions on the swab are eluted into the same vial of transport medium used for the throat swab.

Higher isolation rates can be achieved with nasal washes, nasal aspirates, or bronchioalveolar lavage specimens. Collection of such specimens should be attempted with hospitalized patients when success and speed of diagnosis are critical for proper patient management. Nasal washes are collected by instilling 3 ml of transport medium alternately in each nostril while the patient sits with head tipped back and closes the airway by beginning to say "car." Fluid is then collected in a cup by having the patient tip the head forward and blow through the nose. A suitable transport medium is veal infusion broth or tryptose broth containing 0.1% gelatin or 0.5% bovine serum albumin.

Nasal aspirates containing large numbers of epithelial cells may be collected from the nasopharynx by passing a fine plastic catheter (infant feeding tube) through the nose. The catheter is connected to a mucus trap and a suction machine. Suction can also be applied by using a syringe if a suction machine is not available.

Specimens should be transported to the laboratory on wet ice and maintained at 4°C before inoculation. The isolation rate is essentially the same when specimens are held at 4°C for up to 4 days (1). If inoculation is not possible within that time, specimens should be frozen to −70°C immediately after collection and maintained in a mechanical freezer or on dry ice. If dry ice is used, vials should be tightly sealed to prevent entry of CO_2, which will inactivate viral infectivity by lowering the pH. A 10× solution of antibiotics should be added to a portion of the specimen used for virus isolation to yield a final concentration of 800 U of penicillin and 400 μg of streptomycin or 50 μg of gentamicin per ml. Specimens should be gently agitated and then centrifuged for 15 min to remove particulate debris and bacteria.

A diagnosis can be made by direct detection using fluorescence microscopy on specimens with adequate numbers of epithelial cells. The cells contained in aspirates or in nasal washes are sedimented by centrifugation and suspended in phosphate-buffered saline (PBS) by gentle pipetting. This procedure is repeated until mucus cannot be seen, and the cells are spotted onto glass slides. After being allowed to dry, the cells are fixed with acetone for 10 min and stained with immunofluorescent reagents.

Specimens for immunoassay procedures are collected as described above for immunofluorescent examination, but the cells, which often contain large amounts of antigen, are not separated. The entire specimen is diluted in PBS containing a blocking protein (such as 20% fetal calf serum) and a detergent (such as 2% Tween 20). The specimen can then be sonicated, diluted further (fivefold final) in the same buffer, and tested by enzyme immunoassay (EIA) or by time-resolved fluorescence immunoassay.

Blood specimens for serological diagnosis are drawn by venipuncture during the acute stage of the disease, usually at the time a throat swab is collected, and again 2 to 3 weeks later during the convalescent stage. Sera collected aseptically from the blood clots need not be refrigerated during transport to the laboratory but should be stored at 4 or −20°C.

DIRECT DETECTION OF VIRAL ANTIGEN

Direct detection of viral antigen in clinical specimens can be accomplished in a matter of hours and is the most rapid method for establishing a diagnosis of influenza virus infection. Rapid diagnosis has many benefits, particularly in the treatment of hospitalized patients.

Amantadine and rimantadine are effective for antiviral therapy of influenza type A infections but not for influenza type B disease. Rapid diagnosis may also help in the management of immunocompromised patients with influenza as well as help control nosocomial spread. Prompt diagnostic information is important in educating physicians and informing patients. Inappropriate therapy can be eliminated, as can the expense of unnecessary diagnostic tests. On a larger scale, rapid diagnosis of outbreaks can alert public health officials to the possible onset of an epidemic and assist them in the appropriate use of specific control measures, such as vaccination and antiviral prophylaxis of high-risk persons.

As early as 1956, rapid diagnosis by fluorescent-antibody (FA) staining of influenza-infected nasal epithelial cells was demonstrated by Lui (19). Since then, numerous investigators have confirmed the initial findings and have shown the technique to be applicable to a number of other respiratory viruses (7). These early studies established the importance of high-quality clinical specimens, in particular the need for an adequate number of nasal epithelial cells to be present. A summary of more recent trials shows that direct detection by FA can detect 46 to 86% of cases diagnosed by culture (Table 2). In recent studies using high-quality monoclonal antibody reagents, 69 to 100% of cases diagnosed by culture were also detected by FA (Table 2). These results were obtained with the indirect method, in which attention to nonspecific binding of the conjugate is also required. Directly labeled monoclonal antibody reagents are now commercially available and can eliminate or minimize this concern.

The FA technique differs from other immunoassays for antigen detection (see below) in the role of the laboratory worker performing the test. Thus, a negative result with a clinical sample in which only a few nasal epithelial cells are present can be attributed to a poor sample. With immunoassay procedures, this measure of quality control (i.e., identifying poor samples) is not available. Sensitivity comparisons of test methods need to take this factor into account. Some disadvantages of the FA method are that it probably requires greater expertise in test performance and interpretation, lacks an objective endpoint, and is unlikely to be automated to a significant degree. The time-consuming nature of the test may limit its application to surveillance programs, but for urgent hospital laboratories it remains the most rapid diagnostic test.

Immunoassay systems for direct antigen detection overcome some of the drawbacks of the FA technique. A number of assay configurations have been proposed, but the most common utilize a capture antibody bound to a solid phase, usually a microdilution well or plastic bead. Incubation with a clinical specimen results in the binding of viral antigen to the antibody and thus to the solid phase. The bound antigen is then detected by addition of labeled specific antibody (direct method) or by addition of unlabeled specific antibody followed by labeled, anti-species-specific immunoglobulin G (indirect method). The amount of bound antigen is quantitated by the development of color when the appropriate substrate is added if an enzyme-labeled detection system is used or by an alternative detection method if an isotope- or fluorescence-labeled detection system is used. For example, a time-resolved fluorescence immunoassay has been developed and evaluated (34). Such immunoassays can be performed with automated machinery, and the results can be read objectively in spectrophotometers or fluorometers. The data can be promptly manipulated and analyzed by computer.

TABLE 2. Sensitivity of rapid diagnosis of influenza A virus by direct detection of antigen in clinical specimens by immunofluorescence

Antiserum	No. isolation positive	% Immunofluorescence positive	Reference
Polyclonal	15	73	4
	28	86	22
	13	46–77	31
Monoclonal	13	69–77	31
	25	100	20
	10	80	26

In several studies, EIA was found to be as sensitive as the FA technique for detecting viral antigen in nasal aspirate specimens (Table 3) but not as sensitive as virus isolation.

Although EIA kits for influenza virus are not yet commercially available, they are available for other respiratory viruses such as respiratory syncytial virus, herpesvirus, and adenovirus. Hopefully, they will be developed for influenza.

ISOLATION OF VIRUS

Cell culture

Influenza A and B viruses may be isolated in primary rhesus monkey kidney or cynomolgus monkey kidney cells. However, periodic foamy-virus contamination of these cells can pose problems. Influenza A and B viruses can also be easily isolated in Madin-Darby canine kidney (MDCK) cells if trypsin (2 μg/ml) is included in the medium. The trypsin should be treated with 1-tosylamide-2-phenylethyl chloromethyl ketone (i.e., TPCK trypsin), which is available from a number of sources.

The use of the continuous MDCK cell line particularly facilitates rapid culture confirmation that should in many circumstances be the method of choice. The concept of rapid culture confirmation, i.e., the isolation and identification of influenza virus within 1 to 3 days of specimen receipt, is the most practiced advance in influenza diagnosis for many laboratories. It offers speed and simplicity compared with traditional methods of cell culture that may take up to 2 weeks. The diagnosis is based on positive FA or EIA tests performed on cell cultures inoculated 24 to 72 h earlier. Monoclonal antibodies for this purpose are commercially available. About 75 to 85% of cultures are positive 18 to 40 h after inoculation (21, 32, 33). Screening for influenza virus in MDCK cells is more cost effective, since large numbers of specimens can be handled by FA or EIA each day. Reports are possible in 24 h after specimen receipt. This approach is also a good backup for rapid diagnosis by antigen detection, which is likely to replace isolation of respiratory viruses as reagents and tests improve. Influenza isolates are still needed, however, for subtype and strain determinations and eventually for screening for antiviral resistance. Overall, rapid culture confirmation represents good laboratory management in that

TABLE 3. Comparison of immunoassay with other methods for direct detection of influenza antigen in clinical samples

Specimen	Antisera	Method[a]	Reference method	% Positive	Reference
Nasopharyngeal aspirate	Polyclonal	EIA	FA	100	28
Throat swab	Polyclonal	EIA	Isolation	53	11
Nasal wash	Polyclonal	EIA[b]	Isolation	75–87[c]	14
Nasopharyngeal aspirate	Monoclonal	TR-FIA	Serology	85	34
	Poly-monoclonal	EIA	Isolation	64	5
	Poly-monoclonal	ELFA[b]	Isolation	68	5
Nasal wash	Polyclonal	ELFA[b]	Isolation	50–66[d]	2
	Polyclonal	USERIA[e]	Isolation	67–91[d]	2

[a] TR-FIA, Time-resolved fluorescence immunoassay; ELFA, enzyme-linked fluorescence assay; USERIA, ultrasensitive enzyme radioimmunoassay.
[b] EIA used a fluorogenic substrate.
[c] Specimens collected within 24 h of onset of illness.
[d] Samples in the first 4 days of illness. Samples taken on days 5 to 8 showed equivalent or greater sensitivity compared with isolation.
[e] EIA used a tritiated substrate.

diagnosis is rapid and provides an isolate for further study, yet it requires a minimum of time and personnel. Pilot testing of rapid culture confirmation with specimens mailed to a central laboratory by sentinel physicians resulted in about 40% being positive after 3 days in culture during the peak of an epidemic (27).

The traditional method for virus isolation is inoculation of cell cultures maintained in screw-cap test tubes. Rapid culture confirmation has also used cell cultures on cover slips in shell vials or 24-well plates or cell cultures in chamber slides. Before inoculation of specimens, cell cultures should be washed with serum-free medium to remove nonspecific inhibitors that may neutralize virus. After inoculation of 0.3 ml of specimen per tissue culture tube or well (two or three tubes or wells per specimen), cultures are incubated at 34°C for at least 2 h. Two uninoculated tubes or wells of cells are maintained in parallel as controls. After 2 h (but not more than 24 h), medium is removed and cultures are refed with 1.5 ml of serum-free minimal essential medium. For tissue culture other than primary cells, all media should be supplemented with 2 μg of TPCK trypsin per ml. Cultures should be incubated at 34°C (roller drum for tubes) and observed daily for development of viral cytopathic effect, and they should be tested every other day to detect hemadsorption (or tested by FA or EIA for rapid culture confirmation). In the absence of serum, frequent adding or changing of medium is required to maintain cell cultures.

Cultures should be harvested as soon as cytopathic effect is evident. Fluid is transferred to screw-cap vials, and a drop of 10% gelatin is added as a protein stabilizer for freezing. Tissue culture tubes not showing cytopathic effect should be tested by hemadsorption for the presence of virus. Fluid is decanted from each tube into a 2-ml screw-cap vial and kept on ice. Tissue cultures are washed three times with 1.0 ml of guinea pig erythrocytes (0.4%). The last milliliter is left on the cell sheet and incubated for 20 to 30 min at 4°C in a slanted position, with the guinea pig erythrocytes covering the tissue culture cells. The cell sheet is examined microscopically, and a positive tube can be recognized by hemadsorption of guinea pig erythrocytes to the tissue culture cells. Uninfected control tubes should be tested to rule out nonspecific adsorption or the presence of simian viruses (such as types 5 and 40).

If a culture is positive, a portion of the harvest should be frozen at −70°C after addition of gelatin as described above. If the tube is negative, it should be washed, refed with minimal essential medium, and reincubated. If the tube is negative at day 10, the harvest from that tube should be repassaged into fresh tissue culture. In addition to freezing for future reference, titers of positive harvests should be determined by hemagglutination with 0.4% guinea pig erythrocytes at 4°C. If the hemagglutinin titer is negative or less than 8, the harvested material should be repassaged. When viruses produce low hemagglutinin titers in cell culture, passage into eggs may speed up the process of amplifying the titer to a level adequate for identification.

Embryonated eggs

Influenza A and B viruses may be isolated in embryonated hen eggs as well as cell culture. Influenza A viruses grow nearly as well in embryonated eggs as in cell culture, whereas cell culture systems are clearly superior for isolation of influenza B viruses. Some human influenza A and B viruses only grow in the amniotic cavity of the eggs on first inoculation and subsequently adapt to grow in the allantoic cavity of the chicken embryo. Influenza C virus will grow only in the amniotic cavity of eggs and cannot be adapted to grow in the allantoic cavity. Influenza viruses are still cultivated in eggs for vaccine production and for production of large quantities of virus used in laboratory studies.

Adaptation of influenza virus to growth in eggs or MDCK cells exclusively can lead to the selection of host range variants that are distinguishable in HI tests. Molecular studies indicate that this variability arises as a consequence of amino acid changes in the hemagglutinin that affect receptor binding to different host cells (29). This variation does not appear to pose problems in virus identification procedures but is an active area of research interest.

Clinical specimens should be prepared as described above. Viruses that have been already isolated may be diluted before reinoculation, depending on their titers. When high-titer stock viruses are being repeatedly grown in eggs for reagent production, they may be diluted to contain about 10^4 50% egg infectious doses per ml to limit production of defective interfering virus particles.

Ten- to eleven-day-old embryonated eggs are swabbed with 70% alcohol directly over the air sac, and a small hole is punched in the shell in the center of the area. The egg is placed on a candler, with the air sac up, and rotated to locate the embryo. A 23-gauge, 3.8-cm needle attached to a 1-ml syringe is inserted into the amniotic sac with a jabbing motion. The needle is in the correct position when the embryo can be moved. An inoculum of 0.2 ml is injected into the amniotic cavity. The needle is withdrawn slightly, and an additional 0.2 ml is injected into the allantoic cavity. The hole is sealed with wax or glue. Two or three eggs are inoculated per specimen. Eggs are incubated at 33°C for 2 to 3 days. Eggs as young as 7 days may be used to permit longer periods of virus growth while allowing amniotic fluid to be recovered in reasonable yields, such as for poorly growing influenza C viruses. Incubator temperatures should not exceed 35°C because many influenza viruses have an inherent temperature sensitivity.

To minimize bleeding at the time of harvest, after incubation the eggs are left overnight at 4°C. The area over the air sac is swabbed with 70% alcohol, and the shell is broken away to the level of the allantoic membrane. Sterile forceps are used to clear away the membrane so that the allantoic fluid can be collected with a pipette. Amniotic fluid is harvested with a short 20- to 22-gauge needle and a 1-ml syringe. If volumes of amniotic fluid are small, the amnions can be flushed with 1 ml of allantoic fluid to obtain a reasonable working volume. Pools of amniotic fluid are prepared from all eggs inoculated with the same specimen, but allantoic fluids are maintained separately. Fluids are clarified by centrifugation at $800 \times g$ for 15 min.

Undiluted samples of both types of fluids are tested in microdilution plates (50-µl volumes) for the presence of virus by adding an equal volume of guinea pig, chicken, or human O erythrocytes. Erythrocytes should be collected at a ratio of 1 volume of whole blood to 4 volumes of Alsever solution. Suspensions in Alsever solution may be held for as long as 1 week at 4°C. Just before use, the erythrocytes are washed three times with PBS and resuspended to a concentration of 0.4% for guinea pig or human O cells and 0.5% for chicken cells. For the hemagglutination test, the virus-erythrocyte mixtures are incubated at room temperature for 30 to 60 min or at 4°C for several hours until control cells have settled. Some viruses, particularly influenza C, may rapidly elute from erythrocytes at ambient temperature, and influenza C virus does not agglutinate guinea pig erythrocytes. Guinea pig or human O cells may be more sensitive for detecting some strains of influenza A virus in early passage. Titration with chicken erythrocytes at ambient temperature is the most rapid test for detecting virus hemagglutinin in egg fluids.

Two or three blind passages, via both allantoic and amniotic routes, should be performed before a specimen is considered negative. Once influenza A and B viruses have been adapted to grow in the allantoic cavity, amniotic inoculation can be discontinued. Influenza C virus, however, will grow only in the amnion.

Caution should be exercised to avoid cross-contamination when working with egg harvests of influenza viruses because of the high titers that can be achieved and the large number of manipulations involved. Precautions that can be taken include designation of separate work areas for diagnostic specimens and reference or research work and use of disposable material such as pipettes and test tubes whenever possible.

IDENTIFICATION OF VIRUS

HI test

Identification by HI is still a useful method for laboratories that can obtain or prepare up-to-date antisera. Simple typing as to A or B is possible for any laboratory by FA or EIA methods by using monoclonal antibodies to the nucleoprotein antigen. However, that method does not give the virus subtype. Each year, the Centers for Disease Control makes available to state health laboratories and World Health Organization National Influenza Centers such monoclonal and HI antisera to current strains.

For those wishing to prepare their own reagents, HI sera can be prepared in chickens by intravenous inoculation of 5 ml of allantoic fluid containing a minimum hemagglutinin titer of 160. Birds are exsanguinated 10 days after inoculation. For current influenza B strains, two doses of antigen 14 to 21 days apart are needed, and birds are exsanguinated 10 days after the second inoculation.

For more definitive characterization of antigenic relationships, strain-specific antiserum produced in ferrets is recommended. Ferrets are infected by intranasal instillation of 1 ml of allantoic or amniotic fluid containing at least 10^4 infectious particles. Animals are bled 14 days after infection. Ferrets are highly susceptible to infection with influenza virus; therefore, preinfection serum should be tested to rule out prior natural infection. Infected animals should also be kept in isolators to prevent cross-contamination when antisera to more than one virus strain is being prepared. Precautions must be taken to prevent introduction of influenza into the ferret colony. Both of the above procedures for producing antisera have the advantage that antibodies will not be produced to host (i.e., allantoic or amniotic fluid) components or to host membrane antigens, as may occur if hyperimmune antisera are produced in heterologous animal species.

Sera with HI titers of 160 or greater to the homologous antigen are required to be useful in diagnostic tests, and sera should not react with strains outside the type or subtype of the immunizing virus. Occasionally, heterotypic cross-reactivity is observed which cannot be explained on the basis of known antigenic properties of viruses, such as the observation that chickens immunized with A/Texas/1/77 (H3N2) usually produce antibodies that react with A/PR/8/34 (H1N1).

Hemagglutinin titration. The following procedure is described for microtitration techniques with 96-well microdilution plates and multichannel pipettes. (Titration may be done in test tubes by using 10-fold-greater volumes of all reagents. The ratio of all reagents is similar regardless of the total test volume so that expression of titer is independent of the test volumes.) Beginning with undiluted virus, prepare twofold serial dilutions of the virus in 0.1 M PBS (pH 7.2) in 50-µl volumes. Add 50 µl of chicken, guinea pig, or human type O erythrocytes to each well in the series, using erythrocytes that give the highest titer with prevalent strains. Include one well for the erythrocyte suspension as a cell control (diluent plus erythrocytes). Mix and incubate at room temperature until the cells settle (about 30 min with chicken erythrocytes at room temperature and up to several hours with guinea pig or human O cells at 4°C). The results are read by viewing the bottom of the plates. Complete agglutination of the cells produces a uniform film which covers the bottom of the well; in wells without agglutination, the cells settle into a button which flows when the plate is tilted. The highest dilution of the antigen giving complete agglutination is considered to contain 1 hemagglutinating unit (HAU).

Preparation of test antigen. The HI test is performed with the most sensitive erythrocyte system and a test antigen preparation containing 4 HAU in 25 µl. To determine the antigen dilution factor, divide its hemagglutinin titer by 8. For example, if the hemagglutinin titer is 160, then a 1:20 dilution would contain 8 HAU in 50 µl (or 4 HAU in 25 µl used in HI tests).

After an appropriate volume of the antigen is diluted for use in the test, its unitage is checked by a back-titration. Place 50 µl of PBS in wells 1 through 5 in each row and in the cell control wells. Add 50 µl of the test antigen in the first well and prepare serial twofold dilutions through the fifth well. Add 50 µl of the appropriate erythrocyte suspension to all wells and mix; allow the contents to settle. Include a cell control containing diluent and erythrocytes. If the test antigen was prepared correctly (i.e., 8 HAU/50 µl), then the first three dilutions (containing 4, 2, and 1 HAU, respectively) should show complete hemagglutination, while the fourth and fifth dilutions should have partial or no hemagglutination. The cell control should settle to a compact button. Adjust the virus concentration of the working dilution, if necessary, by adding PBS or virus as appropriate. If adjustment of the working antigen dilution is required, confirm the hemagglutinin titer of the final sample by retitration as described above before performing the HI test proper.

Serum treatment. Many influenza isolates are sensitive to serum factors that nonspecifically inhibit agglutination. The inhibitors are mucoproteins and contain carbohydrate side chains that resemble the receptors of erythrocytes. They inhibit hemagglutination by combining with the virus and blocking its attachment to the erythrocytes. Such inhibitors in human, chicken, and most rabbit sera can often be successfully removed by treatment with the receptor-destroying enzyme (RDE) of *Vibrio cholerae* (16). A number of different inhibitors exist, however, and sensitivity varies with the virus to be tested. Successful removal of different inhibitors at times may require treatment with potassium periodate (sometimes in conjunction with trypsin) or kaolin (16). RDE treatment is performed as follows. Add 4 volumes of RDE (100 U/ml) to each volume of serum. Incubate the mixture overnight in a water bath at 37°C. Add 5 volumes of 1.5% sodium citrate and incubate the mixture at 56°C for 30 min. This results in a 1:10 dilution of the serum.

Occasionally, serum contains nonspecific agglutinins that are detected when serum controls are tested. To remove these agglutinins, adsorb the RDE-treated serum at a rate of 0.1 ml of 50% erythrocytes to 1 ml of the 1: 10 serum dilution. Allow adsorption to proceed for 1 h at 4°C and remove the erythrocytes by centrifugation.

HI tests. Prepare twofold dilutions of treated reference antiserum from 1:10 to 1:2,560 in 25-µl volumes in 96-well microdilution plates. Add 25 µl of the test virus suspension containing 4 HAU to each well. To test for erythrocyte agglutinins in the serum, add diluent instead of antigen to a well containing the lowest dilution of serum. Also prepare cell controls (PBS only) and antigen controls (PBS and antigen) for each test. Shake the preparations and incubate them at room temperature for 30 min.

Add 50 µl of erythrocytes to each well; shake the contents and incubate them at room temperature (4°C for influenza C) until the cell control shows the button of normal settling. The HI titer is defined as the reciprocal of the highest serum that completely inhibits agglutination. Complete inhibition is determined by tilting the plates and observing the tear-shaped streaming of cells which flow at the same rate as the cell controls.

FA technique

Influenza virus isolates growing in cell culture may easily be identified by the FA procedure. This procedure may also be used with cells recovered from allantoic or amniotic fluid. Cells are scraped from tissue culture tubes (or centrifuged from egg fluid), and multiple samples are spotted onto glass slides, air dried, and fixed with acetone. Cell monolayers grown on cover slips and maintained in shell vials or 24-well plates have also been used. Infected cells are then stained with FA preparations by direct or indirect procedures. Generally, influenza-typing sera used for this purpose are reactive with the nucleoprotein, M1 protein, or both, so that the test is type specific. Monoclonal antibodies for this purpose are now commercially available. The greatest value of the test is that rapid discrimination between commonly encountered respiratory viruses may be obtained by staining samples from a single tube of cells with an appropriate battery of typing sera. Use of sera specific for the hemagglutinin can enable the test to distinguish between subtypes (30); however, such sera are generally not commercially available. If it is important to distinguish between strains within one subtype, virus antigen will require testing by the HI test with appropriate antisera.

EIA

Just as immunoassays are equivalent to FA procedures for direct detection of antigen in clinical samples, they may also be used to type influenza isolates. Cell culture fluids of virus isolates can be directly adsorbed to microdilution wells and detected with unlabeled monoclonal antibody and enzyme-labeled goat anti-mouse IgG (34). This procedure is more sensitive than detection by hemagglutination and appears to be the way of the future.

SEROLOGICAL DIAGNOSIS

Serological diagnosis of influenza is based on demonstration of a fourfold or greater increase in antibody titer between acute-phase (up to 7 days after onset) and convalescent-phase (14 to 60 days after onset) sera. Thus, it requires collection of a pair of serum samples, which is often not feasible or desirable. Although serological diagnosis is retrospective and therefore of limited usefulness in many clinical situations, it is more economical than virus isolation attempts and can establish the diagnosis when isolation attempts fail. Its main practical value is for epidemiologic investigations or other research studies. Overall, however, every effort should be made to emphasize rapid virus isolation over serological diagnosis as the way to provide an up-to-date, clinically useful virus diagnostic service.

The conventional methods for serological diagnosis are HI, complement fixation (CF), and neutralization. The HI test is simple, inexpensive, and relatively sensitive for most influenza type A viruses. The assay measures antibody to the hemagglutinin and therefore provides information about immune status. Since the test is strain specific, antigens for the HI test for serological diagnosis must be carefully selected to represent strains similar to currently prevalent strains. The HI test is not very sensitive in detecting antibody to influenza type B strains. Although it is possible to increase the sensitivity of the HI test by disrupting virus with ether (23), some loss of specificity may result.

The CF test as usually performed measures antibody to the conserved nucleoprotein antigen and is therefore useful for type-specific diagnosis when variants with new surface antigens emerge. An advantage of the test is that fewer test antigens are required. However, this advantage is offset by the large number of biological reagents to standardize, the occurrence of anticomplementary sera, and the relative insensitivity of the test. For these reasons, the CF test will undoubtedly be replaced by EIA tests in the near future (see below).

The neutralization test for serological diagnosis measures antibody to the hemagglutinin for the most part and generally correlates well with HI results. However, the conventional tube neutralization test and plaque reduction assays are too cumbersome, time consuming, and expensive for use with large numbers of samples. Modifications of the test to a microneutralization assay have largely solved those problems. The use of continuous cell lines and detection of virus by hemagglutination has made the test practical in processing large numbers of sera and in lowering the cost (6). Detection of virus growth by use of a monoclonal antibody to the nucleoprotein and an EIA format has enabled large numbers of serum specimens to be processed in approximately 24 h (13).

The most recent additions to methods for serological diagnosis of influenza are EIA tests, which are more sensitive than CF tests and at least as sensitive as HI tests. More important, however, they offer greater flexibility in measuring antibody to the various proteins of influenza virus. The tests can be designed to measure the antibody response to the hemagglutinin by coating the plates with hemagglutinin protein that has been purified (24), or it can measure antibody to the type-specific nucleoprotein by coating with nucleoprotein that has been purified or expressed from recombinant DNA (9). If EIA plates are coated with whole virus, both type- and strain-specific antigens will be present. The EIA test is the only test that can conveniently measure the specific antibody response in various antibody classes or isotypes. Well-characterized monoclonal antibodies to various human immunoglobulin isotypes have been shown to work well for this purpose (12). Isotype-specific assays may become more important for studying influenza virus, and respiratory viruses in general, because of the high frequency and magnitude of the immunoglobulin A antibody response in serum and nasal secretions after infection.

EVALUATION, INTERPRETATION, AND REPORTING OF RESULTS

The laboratory diagnosis of influenza is based on the isolation and identification of the virus or on the demonstration of a fourfold or greater increase in antibody titer (Fig. 1). Identification of the virus isolate should be reported only as type A, B, or C, unless tests with hemagglutinin- or neuraminidase-specific antisera have been performed to fully characterize the surface antigens. If the virus was identified with hemagglutinin-specific antisera, the corresponding subtype of the neuraminidase is usually inferred, because thus far epidemic isolates of human influenza A have rarely been found to have exchanged hemagglutinin and neuraminidase antigens, even when two subtypes (H1N1 and H3N2) cocirculate.

Serological results should also be interpreted with caution in the absence of virus isolation. A fourfold or greater increase in antibody titer measured by the CF or EIA test with nucleoprotein antigen is indicative only of infection or vaccination with type A (or type B) virus and does not provide information about the virus subtype causing the infection.

Results of HI or neutralization testing of patient sera are also subject to interpretation errors. The specific antigen used in HI or neutralization tests does not necessarily identify the infecting strain because of anamnestic responses that occur frequently as a result of the patient's previous immunologic experience with other influenza strains. Thus, an antibody response may actually be highest to an earlier circulating virus than to the strain causing the current infection.

Interpretation of serological data from immunoassays as they are introduced into general practice needs precise information regarding the nature of the antigen added to the solid phase. In most cases, antigen will probably include the nucleoprotein or M1 protein, and results will be reported as a type-specific antibody response. Only if purified hemagglutinin antigen is used can the virus subtype responsible for infection be determined. Since immunoassays are generally quite sensitive, one should also be aware of the possibility of detecting antibody directed toward a "contaminating" protein, such as neuraminidase in a "pure" hemagglutinin preparation. For this reason, the purity of antigen preparations added to the solid phase should be documented to ensure accurate interpretation of the resulting data.

When an outbreak of influenza is suspected, a rapid presumptive diagnosis can often be made by examining single serum specimens from a group of selected individuals (8). Serum specimens are collected from 10 or more patients who are in the acute stage of the disease and from the same number of age-matched controls who experienced the same symptoms 10 or more days earlier and are now in the convalescent phase of disease. All sera are tested simultaneously for antibody titers by HI, CF, neutralization, or EIA tests. If the outbreak was due to influenza virus, then the geometric mean antibody titer for influenza virus should be significantly higher in the sera from the convalescent group than in the sera drawn from the group in the acute phase of illness. A diagnosis made on this basis should be confirmed, if possible, by conventional methods of virus isolation and by serological diagnosis using paired sera.

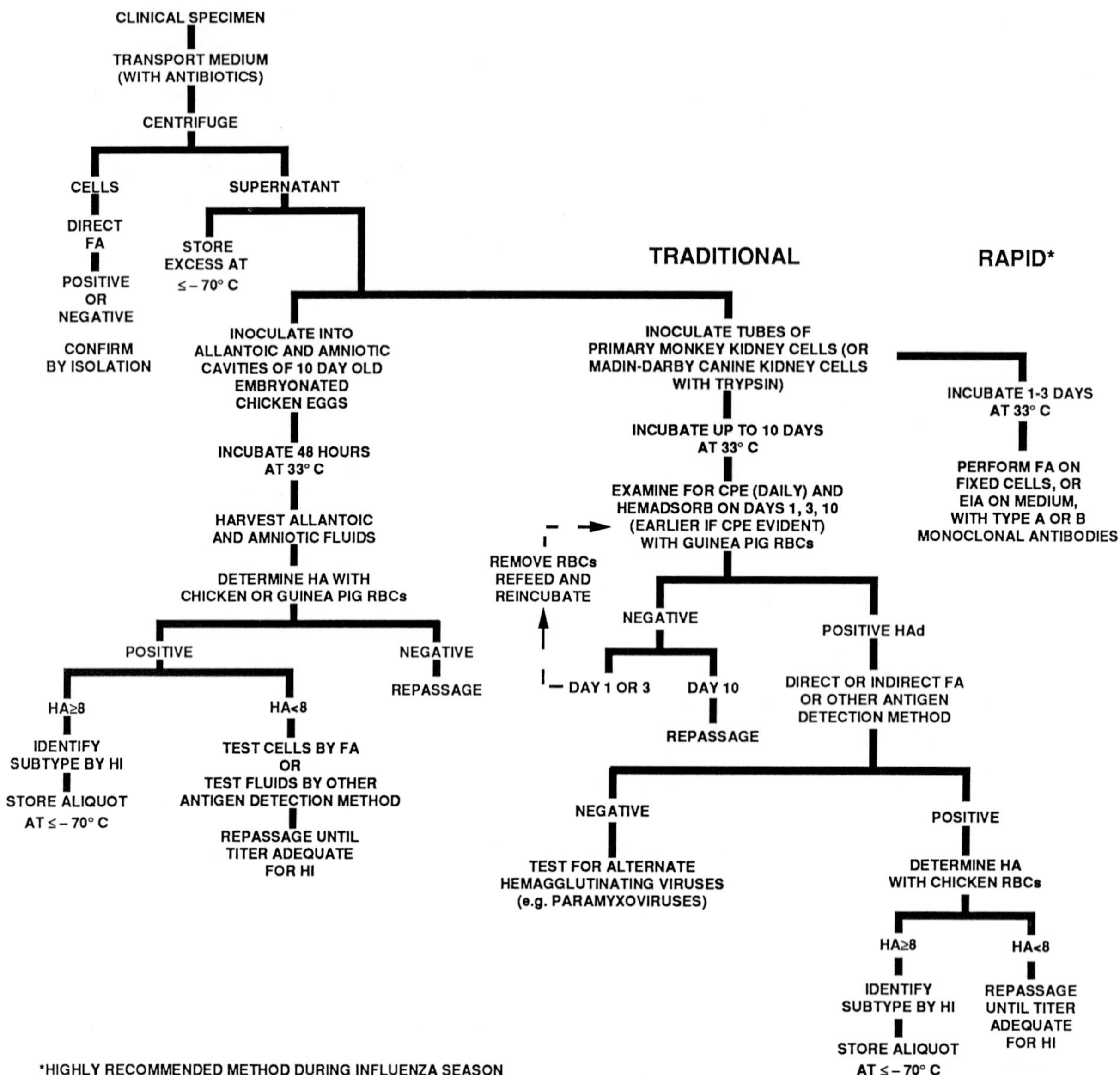

FIG. 1. Schematic for influenza virus isolation. FA, Fluorescent antibody; HA, hemagglutination; HI, hemagglutination inhibition; RBC, erythrocytes; CPE, cytopathic effect; HAd, hemadsorption.

It should be stressed that the comparison must be made between antibody titers of sera from two groups of age-matched ill individuals, one acute and the other convalescent, rather than by comparing antibody titers of sera from a group of convalescent individuals with sera from a group without any recent influenzalike illness. The reason for this is that a group without recent illness may contain a large proportion of persons who have sufficiently high antibody titers to have prevented infection or who have had an asymptomatic infection.

LITERATURE CITED

1. **Baxter, B. D., R. B. Couch, S. B. Greenberg, and J. A. Kasel.** 1977. Maintenance of viability and comparison of identification methods for influenza and other respiratory viruses of humans. J. Clin. Microbiol. **6:**19–22.
2. **Berg, R. A., R. H. Yolken, S. I. Rennard, R. Dolin, B. R. Murphy, and S. E. Straus.** 1980. New enzyme immunoassays for measurement of influenza A/Victoria/3/75 virus in nasal washes. Lancet **ii:**851–853.
3. **Coleman, P. M., J. N. Varghese, and W. G. Laver.** 1983. Structure of the catalytic and antigenic sites in influenza virus neuraminidase. Nature (London) **303:**41–44.
4. **Daisy, J. A., F. S. Lief, and H. M. Friedman.** 1979. Rapid diagnosis of influenza A infection by direct immunofluorescence of nasopharyngeal aspirates in adults. J. Clin. Microbiol. **9:**688–692.
5. **Evans, A. S., and B. Olson.** 1982. Rapid diagnostic methods for influenza virus in clinical specimens: a comparative study. Yale J. Biol. Med. **55:**391–403.
6. **Frank, A. L., J. Puck, B. J. Hughes, and T. R. Cate.** 1980. Microneutralization test for influenza A and B and parainfluenza 1 and 2 viruses that uses continuous cell lines and fresh serum enhancement. J. Clin. Microbiol. **12:**426–432.
7. **Fulton, R. E., and P. J. Middleton.** 1974. Comparison of immunofluorescence and isolation techniques in the diagnosis of respiratory viral infections of children. Infect.

Immun. **10:**92–101.
8. **Grist, N. R., J. Kerr, and A. Isaacs.** 1961. Rapid serological diagnosis of an outbreak of influenza. Br. Med. J. **2:**431.
9. **Harmon, M. W., I. Jones, M. Shaw, W. Keitel, C. B. Reimer, P. Halonen, and A. P. Kendal.** 1989. Immunoassay for serologic diagnosis of influenza type A using recombinant DNA produced nucleoprotein antigen and monoclonal antibody to human IgG. J. Med. Virol. **27:**25–30.
10. **Harmon, M. W., and A. P. Kendal.** 1989. Influenza viruses, p. 631–668. *In* N. J. Schmidt and R. W. Emmons (ed.), Diagnostic procedures for viral, rickettsial and chlamydial infections, 6th ed. American Public Health Association, Inc., Washington, D.C.
11. **Harmon, M. W., and K. M. Pawlik.** 1982. Enzyme immunoassay for direct detection of influenza type A and adenovirus antigens in clinical specimens. J. Clin. Microbiol. **15:**5–11.
12. **Harmon, M. W., D. J. Phillips, C. B. Reimer, and A. P. Kendal.** 1986. Isotype-specific enzyme immunoassay for influenza antibody with monoclonal antibodies to human immunoglobulins. J. Clin. Microbiol. **24:**913–916.
13. **Harmon, M. W., P. A. Rota, H. H. Walls, and A. P. Kendal.** 1988. Antibody response in humans to influenza virus type B host-cell-derived variants after vaccination with standard (egg-derived) vaccine or natural infection. J. Clin. Microbiol. **26:**333–337.
14. **Harmon, M. W., L. L. Russo, and S. Z. Wilson.** 1983. Sensitive enzyme immunoassay with β-D-galactosidase–Fab conjugate for detection of type A influenza virus antigen in clinical specimens. J. Clin. Microbiol. **17:**305–311.
15. **Hay, A. J., A. J. Wolstenholme, J. J. Skehel, and M. H. Smith.** 1985. The molecular basis of the specific anti-influenza action of amantadine. EMBO J. **4:**3021–3024.
16. **Kendal, A. P., J. J. Skehel, and M. S. Pereira.** 1982. Concepts and procedures for laboratory-based influenza surveillance. Centers for Disease Control, Atlanta, Ga.
17. **Kilbourne, E. D.** 1987. Influenza. Plenum Publishing Corp., New York.
18. **Lamb, R. A., C.-J. Lai, and P. W. Choppin.** 1981. Sequences of mRNAs derived from genome RNA segment 7 of influenza virus: colinear and interrupted mRNAs code for overlapping proteins. Proc. Natl. Acad. Sci. USA **78:** 4170–4174.
19. **Liu, C.** 1956. Rapid diagnosis of human influenza infection from nasal smears by means of fluorescein-labeled antibody. Proc. Soc. Exp. Biol. Med. **92:**883–887.
20. **McQuillin, J., C. R. Madeley, and A. P. Kendal.** 1985. Monoclonal antibodies for the rapid diagnosis of influenza A and B virus infections by immunofluorescence. Lancet **ii:**911–914.
21. **Mills, R. D., K. J. Cain, and G. L. Woods.** 1989. Detection of influenza virus by centrifugal inoculation of MDCK cells and staining with monoclonal antibodies. J. Clin. Microbiol. **27:**2505–2508.
22. **Minnich, L., and C. G. Ray.** 1980. Comparison of direct immunofluorescent staining of clinical specimens for respiratory virus antigens with conventional isolation techniques. J. Clin. Microbiol. **12:**391–394.
23. **Monto, A. S., and H. F. Maassab.** 1981. Ether treatment of type B influenza virus antigen for the hemagglutination inhibition test. J. Clin. Microbiol. **13:**54–57.
24. **Murphy, B. R., M. A. Phelan, D. L. Nelson, R. Yarchoan, D. Tierney, W. Alling, and R. M. Chanock.** 1981. Hemagglutinin-specific enzyme-linked immunosorbent assay for antibodies to influenza A and B viruses. J. Clin. Microbiol. **13:**554–560.
25. **Murphy, R. R., and R. G. Webster.** 1989. Orthomyxovirus, p. 1091–1152. *In* B. N. Fields and D. M. Knipe (ed.), Virology. Raven Press, New York.
26. **Ray, C. G., and L. L. Minnich.** 1987. Efficiency of immunofluorescence for rapid detection of common respiratory viruses. J. Clin. Microbiol. **25:**355–357.
27. **Reichelderfer, P. S., K. D. Kappus, and A. P. Kendal.** 1987. Economical laboratory support system for influenza virus surveillance. J. Clin. Microbiol. **25:**947–948.
28. **Sarkkinen, H. K., P. E. Halonen, and A. A. Salmi.** 1981. Detection of influenza A virus by radioimmunoassay and enzyme-immunoassay from nasopharyngeal specimens. J. Med. Virol. **7:**213–220.
29. **Schild, G. C., J. S. Oxford, J. C. de Jong, and R. G. Webster.** 1983. Evidence for host-cell selection of influenza virus antigenic variants. Nature (London) **303:**706–709.
30. **Schmidt, N. J., M. Ota, D. Gallo, and V. L. Fox.** 1982. Monoclonal antibodies for rapid, strain-specific identification of influenza virus isolates. J. Clin. Microbiol. **16:** 763–765.
31. **Shalit, I., P. A. McKee, H. Beauchamp, and J. L. Waner.** 1985. Comparison of polyclonal antiserum versus monoclonal antibodies for the rapid diagnosis of influenza A virus infections by immunofluorescence in clinical specimens. J. Clin. Microbiol. **22:**877–879.
32. **Stokes, C. E., J. M. Bernstein, S. A. Kyger, and F. G. Hayden.** 1988. Rapid diagnosis of influenza A and B by 24-h fluorescent focus assays. J. Clin. Microbiol. **26:**1263–1266.
33. **Swenson, P. D., and M. H. Kaplan.** 1987. Rapid detection of influenza virus in cell culture by indirect immunoperoxidase staining with type-specific monoclonal antibodies. Diagn. Microbiol. Infect. Dis. **7:**265–268.
34. **Walls, H. H., K. H. Johansson, M. W. Harmon, P. E. Halonen, and A. P. Kendal.** 1986. Time-resolved fluoroimmunoassay with monoclonal antibodies for rapid diagnosis of influenza infections. J. Clin. Microbiol. **24:**907–912.
35. **Wilson, I. A., J. J. Skehel, and D. C. Wiley.** 1981. Structure of the hemagglutinin membrane glycoprotein of influenza virus at 3 A resolution. Nature (London) **289:**366–373.
36. **World Health Organization.** 1980. A revision of the system of nomenclature for influenza viruses: a WHO memorandum. Bull. W.H.O. **58:**585–591.

Chapter 82

Parainfluenza Viruses

JOSEPH L. WANER

CLINICAL BACKGROUND

The four parainfluenza viruses (PIVs) of humans cause upper respiratory disease in children and adults. PIV types 1 and 2 (PIV-1 and -2) are the principle causes of laryngotracheobronchitis (croup), although PIV-3 and other infectious agents may also cause croup. PIV-3 is second only to respiratory syncytial virus in importance as a cause of bronchiolitis and pneumonia in infants (3, 4, 8, 16, 17). Type 4 causes mild upper respiratory disease but is rarely encountered in the laboratory because of difficulties in identifying the virus in cell cultures (6). Types 1 and 2 behave similarly, although type 2 generally produces milder illness. The most severe illness caused by PIV-1 and -2 occurs in children between 2 and 4 years of age; type 3 infection produces the most severe illness in infants less than 1 year old. Reinfections with PIVs are common but are generally less severe clinically than primary infections (1, 9). PIV infections in older children and adults are more likely to be asymptomatic or to result in mild disease resembling the common cold syndrome (23). PIV-3 was isolated for prolonged periods from adults without acute symptoms (12).

PIV-1 and -2 occur in alternate-year patterns, tending to produce epidemics in the autumn and early winter (3, 10). Type 3 is predominantly endemic and shows little or no seasonality. PIVs are transmitted via infected respiratory secretions through close person-to-person contact and aerosols. The viruses are labile outside of the host and are readily inactivated by heat and detergents. Laboratory-associated infections should not occur if careful laboratory practices are followed.

DESCRIPTION OF THE VIRUS

PIVs belong to the family *Paramyxoviridae*, genus *Paramyxovirus*. The viruses have helical symmetry and single-stranded, nonsegmented RNA genomes with negative polarity. Virions have envelopes obtained by budding from the host cell cytoplasmic membrane. PIVs have six structural proteins, although coding strategies and the total number of gene products may differ among the paramyxoviruses (2, 19, 20). The HN (hemagglutinin-neuraminidase) and F (fusion) proteins are found in the envelope and are glycosylated. The HN protein is larger than the F protein and is necessary for adsorption to the host cell. After adsorption, the F protein mediates virion entry into the cell. The F protein is also responsible for cell-to-cell spread, manifested morphologically in cell cultures as syncytium. The remaining structural proteins are the large nucleocapsid protein, the nucleoprotein, the phosphoprotein, and the matrix protein.

There are common antigens shared by the four PIVs, mumps virus, Newcastle disease virus, Sendai virus (PIV-1 of mice), bovine PIV-3, and simian virus 5. Isolates of human PIVs can be distinguished individually with the use of specific antisera, particularly monoclonal antibodies (MAbs) (22). Cross-reacting antibodies in patient sera make serological diagnosis of serotypes unreliable.

COLLECTION AND STORAGE OF SPECIMENS

The object of specimen collection is to obtain secretions from the respiratory tract. Efforts should also be made to obtain cellular material, particularly if direct procedures for viral identification are to be attempted. The greatest quantity of virus is excreted early in the course of illness, making the prompt collection of specimens critical for efficient isolation of virus.

Collection of specimens is most commonly accomplished with a wash of the nasopharynx. However, respiratory secretions may be aspirated by a suction device without the addition of a wash. A convenient and effective adaptation of the method described by Hall and Douglas (13) is recommended. The nasopharynx is vigorously swabbed with a Dacron swab on a flexible aluminum or plastic shaft to loosen mucous and cellular material. Approximately 2 ml of sterile saline is then introduced into the nasopharynx through small tubing attached to a 5-ml syringe; a convenient source of tubing is a Butterfly-21 infusion set. The wash is placed in 1.5 ml of transport medium and carried to the laboratory on wet ice. The swab should be placed in the transport medium with the wash.

Adults and older children may resist nasopharyngeal washes. Throat or nasopharyngeal swabs may be used but are generally not as effective as nasopharyngeal washes. The swab should be placed in the transport medium, and the specimen should be taken promptly on wet ice to the laboratory.

Specimens should not be frozen before processing but should be stored at 4°C. A sample (approximately 0.3 ml) should be stored at −70°C for possible use in reevaluating the specimen or for future reference.

Transport medium should consist of a buffered salt solution, pH 7.0, containing a protein-stabilizing agent and antibiotics. In this laboratory, a medium consisting of tryptic soy broth with 0.5% gelatin, gentamicin (50 μg/ml), chloramphenicol (5.0 μg/ml), and amphotericin B (2.0 μg/ml) is used.

ISOLATION IN CELL CULTURE

Primary human embryonic kidney and primary monkey kidney are the most sensitive cell cultures for the isolation of PIVs. PIV isolates may be adapted to grow in continuous cell lines (Vero, HEp-2, LLC-MK2, and HeLa), but these cell lines are not recommended for isolation of virus from clinical specimens. Other viruses that may be present as pathogens in the respiratory tract replicate in primary monkey kidney cultures, which should be an essential component of the laboratory's isolation protocol; primary rhesus monkey kidney (PRMK) cells are recommended. Tubes of uninfected PRMK cultures are maintained on Eagle minimal essential medium (MEME) with 5% newborn calf serum and held at 35°C. Cultures are refed every 4 to 5 days until used but should not be used after 10 days of receipt.

Before inoculation of cell cultures, specimen material is vigorously mixed, the collection swab is pressed against the side of the container to express fluid, and the swab is discarded. The maintenance medium is removed from two PRMK cultures, and the cultures are washed twice with Hanks balanced salt solution (HBSS). Each tube is inoculated with 0.2 ml of the specimen and the cultures are absorbed at 37°C. The inoculum is removed after 1 h, and the cultures are washed once with serum-free medium containing trypsin (SFM) and refed with SFM. Cultures are incubated in a roller drum at 35°C; stationary incubation is also satisfactory. SFM is used because the spread of PIVs and influenza virus in the cell culture is susceptible to serum inhibitors. In our experience, serum may delay hemadsorption (HAd) of PIVs by 1 to 3 days and also diminish the degree of HAd seen. A suitable SFM consists of 50 ml of medium 199, 46 ml of MEME, 3 ml of 100× vitamins for MEME, 0.5 ml of glucose (50% solution), 1 ml of glutamine (200 mM), 0.1 ml of trypsin (0.025%), 50 μg of gentamicin per ml, and 2 μg of amphotericin B per ml; the medium 199 and MEME should be buffered with HEPES (*N*-2-hydroxyethylpiperazine-*N'*-2-ethanesulfonic acid). Cultures that are refed every 4 days may be maintained on SFM for 10 to 14 days.

Cultures are observed daily for cytopathic effect (CPE) to detect not only PIVs but other viruses that may have been in the specimen and replicate in PRMK. In our experience, approximately 50% of the PIV isolates show CPE between 4 and 5 days after inoculation. CPE of the PIVs may range from unrecognizable to destructive, depending on the PIV type and the isolate. Typically, PIV-1 is identified by HAd before CPE appears. CPE consists of small rounded cells that are often difficult to discern as CPE (Fig. 1b). CPE of PIV-2 is often syncytial (Fig. 1c); PIV-3 may show "bridging" of the infected monolayer (Fig. 1d). Degeneration of the entire monolayer often characterizes the CPE of PIV-4, the PIV least commonly encountered in the laboratory.

The detection of a PIV in cell culture after the appearance of CPE is confirmed by HAd. However, HAd may be detected before identifiable CPE and may be used as an inexpensive rapid method for the detection of hemadsorbing viruses, including the PIVs. More than 50% of the PIV-1 and PIV-3 isolates hemadsorb by 48 h after inoculation (15). A convenient strategy is to examine cultures for HAd 24 h after inoculation and at 48-h intervals thereafter; cultures should also be examined for HAd at the earliest sighting of CPE. Guinea pig erythrocytes (RBCs) are washed four times with HBSS and prepared as a 4% solution that may be stored at 4°C for 3 to 4 days. The medium from the cultures to be tested is removed and held at 4°C for possible future analysis. Then 1 ml of cold HBSS is added to each tube, followed by 0.2 ml of a 0.4% solution of RBCs prepared in cold HBSS from the stock solution. The tubes are incubated first at 4°C for 30 min, viewed, and reincubated at room temperature for 30 min; influenza should hemadsorb at 4°C and room temperature, whereas the PIVs hemadsorb only at 4°C. This is not an absolute phenomenon, but it is helpful. The temperature differences seen are associated with degrees of HAd and are not absolute reactions. Uninfected culture tubes of the same lot number as those inoculated should be hemadsorbed at the same time to control for the presence of hemadsorbing monkey viruses in the cell cultures. Human PIVs are more likely to hemadsorb in a diffuse pattern; monkey viruses often do so in batches. Virus proteins may adhere to the glass, particularly on the edge of monolayers, resulting in RBCs adsorbing to glass in the absence of visible cellular material.

Alternatively, cells may be scraped from an inoculated tube 48 h or later after inoculation and prepared for immunofluorescence (IF) as described below. The cells are stained with a pool of MAbs to PIV-1, -2, and -3 or with MAbs to each type (21). The remaining inoculated tube(s) should be held in case the IF procedure is false-negative or to identify a possible dual infection.

DETECTION OF ANTIGEN

IF

The most commonly used method of detecting PIV antigens directly in patient specimens or in infected cell cultures is direct or indirect IF (Fig. 2). MAbs to PIV-1, -2, and -3 are available commercially as individual reagents or in a PIV pool and are the reagents of choice for IF procedures (7, 22, 24).

For direct examination of cells obtained from nasopharyngeal washes, specimens should be obtained as described above; the nasopharynx should be swabbed before washing to obtain increased numbers of nasopharyngeal cells. Cells in the specimen are washed with phosphate-buffered saline, pH 7.0 (PBS), until mucus is virtually removed, which usually requires one to three washes. The cells are resuspended in 0.25 ml of PBS, and 10 to 20 μl of the cell suspension is applied to 8-mm wells circumscribed on eight-well enamel-coated glass slides (Cell-Line Associates, Newfield, N.J.). Wells are examined at ×100 magnification to assess the number and morphology of the cells present. Specimens yielding less than an average of 20 columnar epithelial cells per well should be rejected; squamous epithelial cells are unsatisfactory. The slides are air dried, fixed in cold acetone for 10 min, rinsed in distilled H_2O, and air dried before staining. Slides may be stored with a desiccating agent for several months at −70°C.

Cells sufficient to prepare 20 or more wells are usually obtained. The specimen can be comprehensively examined by staining three or four wells each with antibodies to the common respiratory viruses of the season, i.e., respiratory syncytial virus, influenza virus types A and B, adenovirus, and PIVs. MAbs to these viruses are the immune reagents of choice and are commercially available. A pool of MAbs to PIV-1, -2, and -3 may be applied to the specimen; application of the antibodies to four to six wells provides a good expectation of sensitive and specific results. The diagnosis of a PIV without knowing the type is sufficient for clinical purposes and may be made rapidly with less expense by using the pool; if desired, specific typing can be done later.

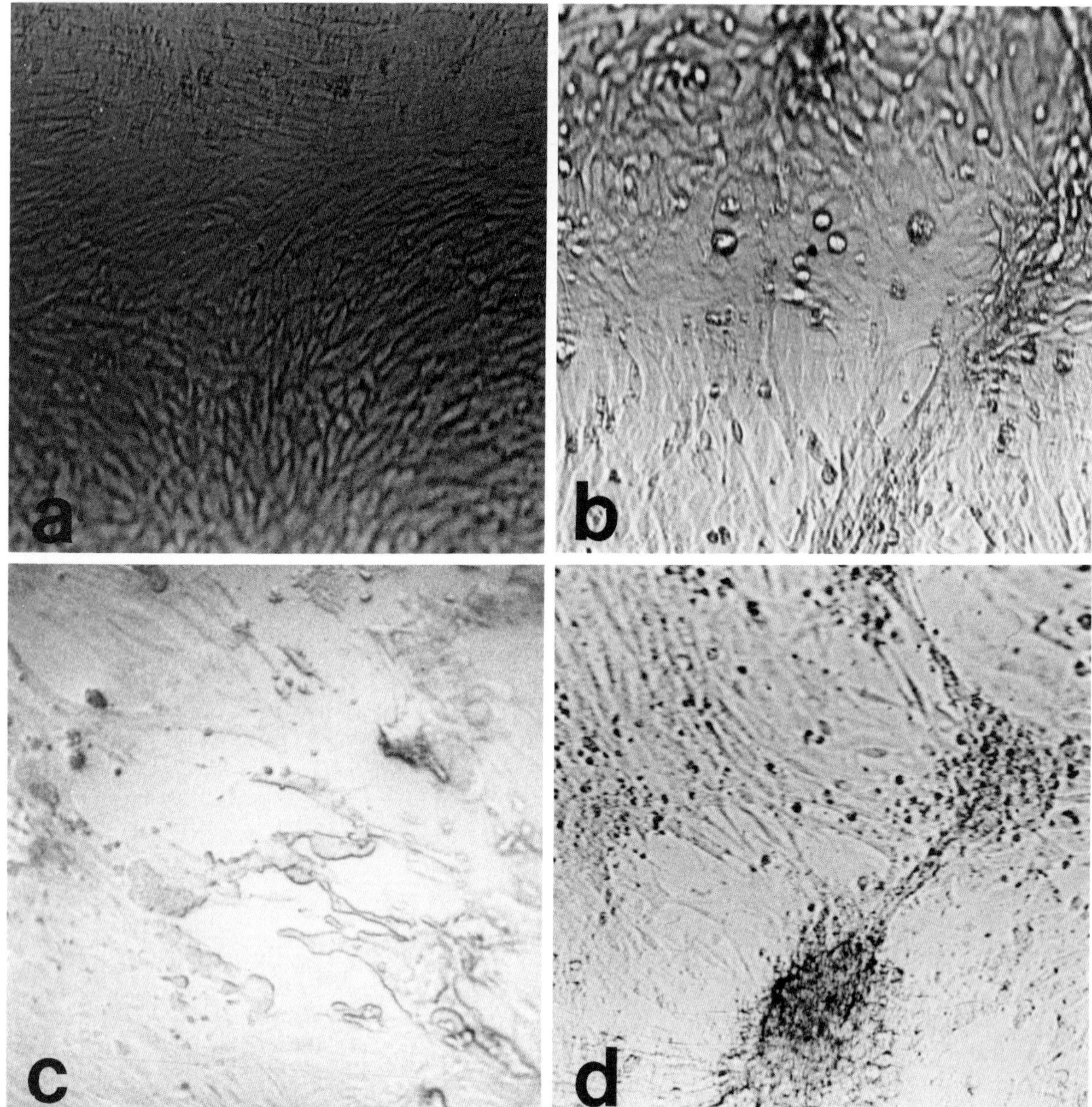

FIG. 1. CPE effect of PIVs in PRMK cell cultures. (a) Uninfected; (b to d) infected with PIV-1 (b), PIV-2 (c), and PIV-3 (d).

EIA

PIV antigens can be identified in infected cell cultures or clinical specimens by enzyme immunoassay (EIA) (18), comparable in sensitivity and specificity to IF (11). Time-resolved fluoroimmunoassay may be more sensitive than EIA or IF (14). Commercial test kits are not available. However, EIA tests can be constructed from reagents prepared locally or purchased as single components. Chapter 12 should be referred to for preparation of EIA tests.

SEROLOGY

Antibody to the PIVs can be detected by complement fixation, hemagglutination inhibition (HI), neutralization, and EIA tests. However, serology is retrospective and rarely provides a helpful diagnosis during acute illness. Some antigens are shared among the PIVs and between the PIVs and other paramyxoviruses, notably mumps virus. Cross-reactions are therefore likely to occur in serological tests. In addition, heterotypic responses may occur in patients and, with the possibility of cross-reactions, make a specific serological diagnosis of a PIV difficult. Antibody determinations are used primarily to make a retrospective diagnosis or to obtain seroepidemiological data on PIV in a community.

Blood samples are collected and allowed to clot; serum is collected after centrifugation at low speed. Paired sera taken during the acute phase of illness and at least 2 weeks later should be tested simultaneously. An increase of fourfold or greater in the antibody titer of the convalescent serum over that of the acute serum

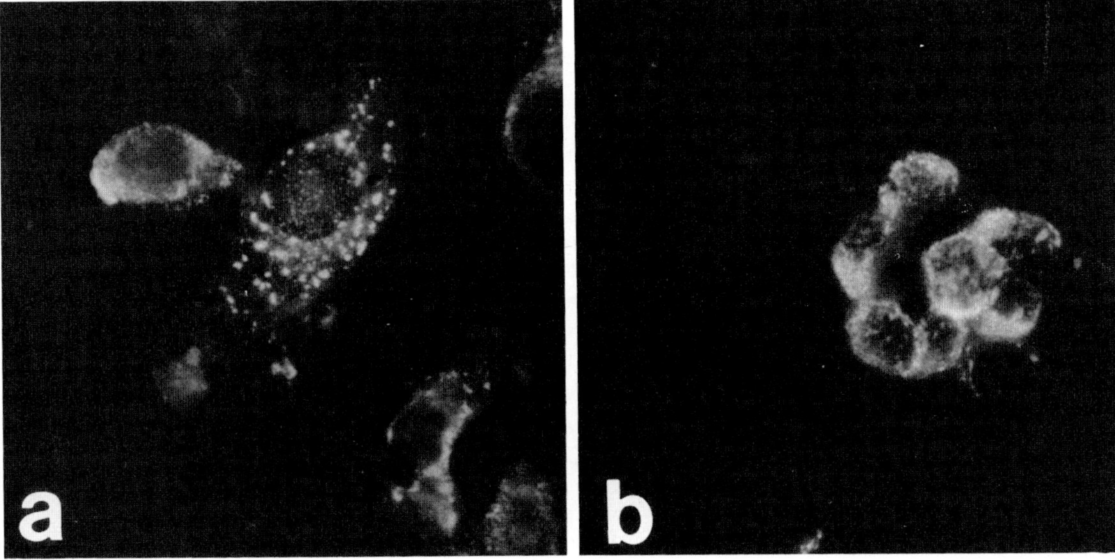

FIG. 2. Indirect IF reactions obtained by using a pool of MAbs to PIV-1, -2, and -3. (a) Infected cell culture; (b) antigen-positive cells from a nasopharyngeal wash.

is diagnostic of recent infection. A fourfold diminution of antibody titer or the presence of antibody in a single serum does not have diagnostic significance. The possible presence of maternal antibody and the immature status of the immune system in infants less than 6 months old make serological diagnosis in this age group unreliable.

PIV antigens for use in complement fixation and HI tests may be purchased. These antigens may also be used in EIA tests; commercial EIA kits are not available. The HI test is recommended, although EIA may function well as a rapid screening test. The neutralization test is relatively specific but is cumbersome to perform and not amenable to routine use in most laboratories (5).

HI antigens (hemagglutinin)

Antigens for the HI test may be prepared from infected cell cultures. Primary monkey kidney cultures are recommended, although continuous cell lines may be used if the PIV is adapted to replicate. Culture fluids may be taken at the time of maximum HAd. Alternatively, culture fluids can be tested for hemagglutination (HA) daily beginning at 3 days after inoculation; the fluids are taken for HI antigen at the time of maximum HA titer, usually within 4 to 6 days after inoculation. The fluids should be treated with Tween 80 and diethyl ether to increase the titer of antigen. Dissolve 0.125 ml of Tween 80 in 2 ml of SFM and add 0.1 ml of the solution per 5 ml of culture fluid. Shake the mixture for 5 min at room temperature and then add diethyl ether to make a final concentration of 33%. Shake the mixture for 15 min at 4°C and then centrifuge it at 2,000 rpm for 30 min. The aqueous layer should be removed, and nitrogen should be bubbled through it to remove the ether; alternatively, the antigen can be placed in an open container to allow the ether to evaporate. Glycerol or albumin at a final concentration of 0.5% should be added as a stabilizer, and the pH should be adjusted to 7.0. Aliquots of the antigen are frozen at −70°C; culture fluids may be stored at −70°C until treated. A control antigen preparation should be prepared in the same manner from uninfected cell cultures of the same type and passage level as that used for the PIV antigen.

Titration of HI antigen

Serial twofold dilutions of antigen are made in PBS and distributed in 0.05-ml volumes to duplicate wells of microdilution plates. An equal volume of 0.4% guinea pig RBCs (prepared as described above) is added to each well. Control wells consist of PBS in place of antigen. The control antigen preparation may be titrated in parallel to test for nonspecific agglutination associated with the cell cultures in which the PIV antigen was prepared. The contents of the wells are mixed by gently tapping the plate. Hold the plate at room temperature until RBC "buttons" appear in the control wells, usually about 30 min. An HA reaction appears as a thin layer of RBCs on the bottom of the well; a partial HA reaction shows a button of various sizes. The highest dilution of antigen that shows partial agglutination of the RBCs is the endpoint. The endpoint dilution is divided by 8 to arrive at the dilution of antigen required to provide 4 U of hemagglutinin in 0.025 ml for subsequent use in HI tests.

HI test

Sera must be treated before testing to remove nonspecific inhibitors and agglutinins. Equal volumes of receptor-destroyer enzyme and serum (0.1 ml is recommended) are incubated together overnight at 37°C. After inactivation at 56°C for 30 min, the serum is incubated with 0.2 ml of 15% guinea pig RBCs for 1 h at 4°C; the RBCs are removed by centrifugation. The serum dilution at this point is 1:4.

Serial twofold dilutions of the treated serum (0.025 ml) are made in microdilution wells, using PBS as a diluent. Four units of antigen (0.025 ml) is added to each well, and the reactants are mixed. Antigen, antibody, RBCs, and serum controls must be included.

In each test, twofold dilutions of the antigen should be made such that 4, 2, 1, 0.5, and 0.25 U of antigen are evaluated for HA activity. A reference serum of known antibody titer is tested to control for specificity and sensitivity; an erythrocyte control consists of RBCs incubated only with PBS; serum controls consisting of 1:8 dilutions of each serum tested are incubated only with PBS.

The reaction mixtures are incubated for 1 h at room temperature, followed by the addition of 0.4% guinea pig RBCs (0.05 ml) to each well. Incubate the test mixture at room temperature until RBC buttons are distinct in the RBC and serum control wells. Hemolysis or agglutination indicates nonspecific reactions associated with the RBCs or the serum. The 4- and 2-U antigen control wells should show complete agglutination, the 1-U well should show partial agglutination, and the 0.5- and 0.25-U wells should not show agglutination. The endpoint is the highest dilution of a serum that completely inhibits agglutination, as evidenced by a complete RBC button in the well.

EVALUATION OF TEST RESULTS

The isolation of virus or the identification of viral antigen in a clinical specimen is the most valuable information to be conveyed to a clinician. PIVs are rarely present in healthy individuals, and their presence in the context of disease is diagnostic. A policy of reporting isolation or positive antigen detection immediately by telephone is recommended. The length of time required to identify replication of PIV in cell cultures usually compromises the usefulness of isolation in patient care. Efforts should therefore be made to use rapid techniques to identify PIV antigen directly in clinical specimens or in infected cell cultures. The identification of a PIV without designation of type is sufficient, since specific therapies are not available.

The time required for paired sera to be obtained to evaluate antibody rises negates the usefulness of serology as a diagnostic tool in acute disease. In addition, antibody rises may not be detectable in infants or in patients with reinfections. Heterologous antibody responses in patients make serological typing of PIVs unreliable. Therefore, serology is primarily retrospective and useful for some epidemiological purposes.

LITERATURE CITED

1. **Chanock, R. M., J. A. Bell, and R. H. Parrott.** 1961. Natural history of parainfluenza virus infection, p. 126–137. *In* M. Pollard (ed.), Perspectives in virology, vol. 2. Burgess Publishing Co., Minneapolis.
2. **Chanock, R. M., and K. McIntosh.** 1985. Parainfluenza viruses, p. 1241–1253. *In* B. N. Fields (ed.), Virology. Raven Press, New York.
3. **Chanock, R. M., and R. H. Parrott.** 1965. Acute respiratory disease in infancy and childhood: present understanding and prospects for prevention. Pediatrics **36:**21–39.
4. **Chanock, R. M., A. Vargosko, A. Luckey, M. K. Cook, A. Z. Kapikian, T. Reichelderfer, and R. H. Parrott.** 1959. Association of hemadsorption viruses with respiratory illness in childhood. J. Am. Med. Assoc. **169:**548–553.
5. **Frank, A. L., J. Puck, B. J. Hughes, and T. R. Cate.** 1980. Microneutralization test for influenza A and B and parainfluenza 1 and 2 viruses that uses continuous cell lines and fresh serum enhancement. J. Clin. Microbiol. **12:**426–432.
6. **Gardner, S. D.** 1969. The isolation of parainfluenza 4 subtypes A and B in England and serological studies of their prevalence. J. Hyg. **67:**545–550.
7. **Gardner, P. S., and J. McQuillen.** 1974. Paramyxoviruses, p. 142. *In* P. S. Gardner and J. McQuillin (ed.), Rapid virus diagnosis: application of immunofluorescence. Butterworths, London.
8. **Glezen, W. P., and F. W. Denny.** 1973. Epidemiology of acute lower respiratory disease in children. N. Engl. J. Med. **288:**498–505.
9. **Glezen, W. P., A. L. Frank, L. H. Taber, and J. A. Kasel.** 1984. Parainfluenza virus type 3: seasonality and risk of infection and reinfection in young children. J. Infect. Dis. **150:**851–857.
10. **Glezen, W. P., F. A. Loda, and F. W. Denny.** 1982. Parainfluenza viruses, p. 441–454. *In* A. S. Evans (ed.), Viral infections of humans. Epidemiology and control. Plenum Publishing Corp., New York.
11. **Grandien, M., C.-A. Petterson, P. S. Gardner, A. Linde, and A. Stanton.** 1985. Rapid viral diagnosis of acute respiratory infections: comparison of enzyme-linked immunosorbent assay and the immunofluorescence technique for detection of viral antigens in nasopharyngeal secretions. J. Clin. Microbiol. **22:**757–760.
12. **Gross, P. A., R. H. Green, and M. G. M. Curnen.** 1973. Persistent infection with parainfluenza type 3 virus in man. Am. Rev. Respir. Dis. **108:**894–898.
13. **Hall, C. B., and R. G. Douglas, Jr.** 1975. Clinically useful method for the isolation of respiratory syncytial virus. J. Infect. Dis. **131:**1–5.
14. **Hierholzer, J. C., P. G. Bingham, R. A. Coombs, K. H. Johansson, L. J. Anderson, and P. E. Halonen.** 1989. Comparison of monoclonal antibody time-resolved fluoroimmunoassay with monoclonal antibody capture-biotinylated detector enzyme immunoassay for respiratory syncytial virus and parainfluenza virus antigen detection. J. Clin. Microbiol. **27:**1243–1249.
15. **Minnich, L. L., and C. G. Ray.** 1987. Early testing of cell cultures for detection of hemadsorbing viruses. J. Clin. Microbiol. **25:**421–422.
16. **Parrott, R. H., A. J. Vargosko, H. W. Kim, J. A. Bell, and R. M. Chanock.** 1962. III. Myxoviruses: parainfluenza. Am. J. Public Health **52:**907–917.
17. **Parrott, R. H., A. Vargosko, A. Luckey, H. W. Kim, C. Cumming, and R. Chanock.** 1959. Clinical features of infection with hemadsorption viruses. N. Engl. J. Med. **260:**731–738.
18. **Sarkkinen, H. K., P. E. Halonen, and A. A. Salmi.** 1981. Type-specific detection of parainfluenza viruses by enzyme immunoassay and radioimmunoassay in nasopharyngeal specimens of patients with acute respiratory disease. J. Gen. Virol. **56:**49–58.
19. **Spriggs, M. K., and P. L. Collins.** 1986. Human parainfluenza virus type 3: messenger RNAs, polypeptide coding assignments, intergenic sequences, and genetic map. J. Virol. **59:**646–654.
20. **Storey, D. G., K. Dimock, and C. Y. Kang.** 1984. Structural characterization of virion proteins and genomic RNA of human parainfluenza virus 3. J. Virol. **52:**761–766.
21. **Stout, C., M. D. Murphy, S. Laurence, and S. Julian.** 1989. Evaluation of a monoclonal antibody pool for rapid diagnosis of respiratory viral infections. J. Clin. Microbiol. **27:**448–452.
22. **Waner, J. L., N. J. Whitehurst, T. Downs, and D. G. Graves.** 1985. Production of monoclonal antibodies against parainfluenza 3 virus and their use in diagnosis by immunofluorescence. J. Clin. Microbiol. **22:**535–538.
23. **Wenzel, R. P., D. P. McCormick, and W. E. Beam, Jr.** 1972. Parainfluenza pneumonia in adults. J. Am. Med. Assoc. **221:**294–295.
24. **Wong, D. T., R. C. Welliver, K. R. Riddlesberger, M. S. Sun, and P. L. Ogra.** 1982. Rapid diagnosis of parainfluenza virus infection in children. J. Clin. Microbiol. **16:**164–167.

Chapter 83

Respiratory Syncytial Virus

ANDREA TALIS AND KENNETH McINTOSH

CLINICAL BACKGROUND (21)

Respiratory syncytial virus (RSV) is the most important cause of pneumonia and bronchiolitis in infants and small children (6, 7). Like the other respiratory viruses, RSV causes a range of respiratory illness, the most common being a cold with profuse rhinorrhea. Of infants infected for the first time, 25 to 40% develop some lower respiratory tract disease. Between 1 and 2% of infected infants require hospitalization, the most severe disease occurring in the first year of life and in those with underlying cardiopulmonary disease. RSV infections appear in large outbreaks every winter.

RSV is very contagious, and most children have experienced infection with RSV by 2 years of age. Immunity to RSV is not complete, and reinfections occur throughout life. Reinfections tend to be less severe than primary infections. RSV is also an unusual cause of significant respiratory illness in normal and elderly adults.

In normal infants and children, the virus is shed for 2 to 3 weeks overall or 1 to 2 weeks after the children appear in the hospital (15). Because of its high infectivity and because hospital staff as well as patients are susceptible, RSV has emerged as the most frequent cause of nosocomial infections on pediatric wards. Atypically long virus shedding as well as off-season isolation of RSV has been noted in our pediatric human immunodeficiency virus-infected and immunosuppressed populations (20).

The studies of Hall and Taber and their colleagues established that RSV bronchiolitis and pneumonia could be successfully treated by administration of ribavirin aerosol (16, 27). This finding has made accurate, rapid identification of cases through laboratory methods an important part of the care of children in hospitals.

DESCRIPTION OF THE AGENT (21)

RSV belongs to the family *Paramyxoviridae* and the genus *Pneumovirus*. It is morphologically similar to other paramyxoviruses with the exception that the diameter of its helical nucleocapsid is smaller, 13 to 14 nm rather than 18 nm. Biochemically, it is also distinct: there is no neuraminidase, and to date hemagglutinating activity has not been described. The single-stranded, negative-sense RNA genome contains 10 separate genes, with several unique features which also differentiate it from other paramyxoviruses.

RSV is an antigenically heterogeneous species, with strain differences which are due primarily to differences in one of the two antigenically active surface components (17). These differences between strains are probably of little or no practical importance from a diagnostic point of view, since available reagents, including monoclonal antibodies, react equally with all clinical isolates (9).

The infectivity of RSV is very sensitive to freezing and thawing. This characteristic is of great importance in the handling of clinical specimens, since recovery of RSV from specimens that have been frozen is uncommon.

RSV grows best in continuous cell lines of human origin, particularly HEp-2 cells and some strains of HeLa cells (Bristol HeLa), but can also be recovered in human diploid cell strains (2) and primary monkey kidney cells. Laboratory strains have a somewhat broader host range. Several simian and small animal species can be infected by the respiratory route. The virus has not been adapted to growth in embryonated eggs.

COLLECTION AND STORAGE OF SPECIMENS

RSV is recovered almost exclusively from the respiratory tract. The specimens containing the most abundant virus are secretions obtained early in the course of the illness. Secretions are ideally obtained as such, either by aspiration through a catheter (11, 22) or by suction into a soft rubber bulb (14). Swabs, either nasopharyngeal or throat, may also be used (3) but are somewhat inferior to aspirated secretions (1). Swabs must be immediately mixed with a suitable volume of holding medium at 4°C. In all instances, specimens should be inoculated onto tissue cultures as soon as possible (4).

In infants and small children, we obtain secretions as follows. A no. 8 French soft plastic feeding tube is attached through a valve-containing trap to an electric suction apparatus. The sterile catheter tip is introduced through the nares to the back of the nose, and suction is intermittently applied by means of the thumb valve while the catheter is slowly withdrawn. This process may in most infants be repeated once so that 0.2 to 0.8 ml of secretion is obtained in the trap. Given the clinical course of RSV, secretions are usually plentiful. However, if use of this procedure yields no secretions, 0.5 to 1 ml of sterile saline can be injected into the posterior nares via the catheter and resuctioned into the trap. The trap must be placed immediately on wet ice and transported to the laboratory, where processing for isolation and rapid antigen detection procedures are performed.

For lower respiratory tract infections, tracheal secretions or bronchoalveolar lavage specimens will contain the virus and should be handled in the same manner.

Swabs are more convenient in adults or older children and are adequate but inferior to secretions. Throat and nasopharyngeal swabs may both be used and combined in a single vial of viral transport medium, which consists of a buffered saline solution containing a pH indicator and a carrier protein (usually bovine serum albumin or gelatin) to stabilize the virus. We also add antibiotics consistent with our tissue culture medium formulation to minimize contamination problems in the virus cultures.

Rapid transport to the laboratory is desirable. Specimens to be cultured should be inoculated as soon as possible, although a delay of minutes to a few hours probably has little effect on the success of virus recovery as long as specimens are kept cold (4). In any case, materials should be held at 4°C in wet ice and not frozen unless the delay before cell culture inoculation is longer than 72 h. If freezing is necessary, it should be accomplished rapidly in a bath of dry ice and acetone or alcohol. Slow freezing (for example, by placing the vial on the shelf of a −20°C freezer) virtually always destroys the infectivity of RSV in clinical specimens.

DIRECT EXAMINATION

Direct examination of secretions is the preferred method for the diagnosis of RSV for several reasons. It is rapid, and the information obtained is therefore more clinically useful with respect to both treatment and the prevention of nosocomial spread. Problems of virus lability are not an issue, since detection and identification of the virus are not dependent on infectivity. Finally, given the current availability of good serological reagents, the methods are widely applicable.

A number of methods have now been described: immunofluorescence (IF) staining (3, 9, 11, 23), enzyme-linked immunosorbent assay (ELISA) (5, 8, 13, 19, 22, 25, 26), immunoperoxidase staining (18), and nucleic acid probe technologies (28). There are good kits available from several commercial suppliers for IF and ELISA tests. The choice of method depends on consideration of a number of factors related to each particular clinical setting.

The two most widely used rapid methods are IF and ELISA. The methods are both considered sensitive and specific enough to be useful in the clinical setting, although it is difficult to set exact figures on their practical sensitivity and specificity because published studies inevitably fail to reflect precisely the events in a working diagnostic laboratory. We prefer IF because it is probably slightly more sensitive than ELISA (1, 13, 22), and it also allows for screening for other respiratory pathogens for which reagents are available.

The technique for rapid IF is described in detail by Gardner and McQuillin (11). Four elements are essential to success in this venture: (i) meticulous attention to collection and preparation of specimens, (ii) high-quality antisera and conjugates, (iii) a good fluorescence microscope, and (iv) practice. Despite these requirements, an increasing number of laboratories are using the method and finding it helpful.

The best specimens for IF tests, as for ELISA or culture (1, 11, 22), are obtained by aspiration of secretions. About 0.2 to 0.4 ml of straight secretion is mixed with 2 ml of cold phosphate-buffered saline (PBS) by using a Pasteur pipette and gently suctioning the specimen and blowing it out with a rubber bulb. This material is then made up to about 10 ml with PBS from a squeeze bottle and centrifuged at 800 to 1,000 rpm for 10 min in a clinical centrifuge. The supernatant wash fluid is pipetted off with a Pasteur pipette, leaving the loosely packed cell button at the bottom. The process is repeated until the cells are free from mucus. Thorough washing of cells minimizes nonspecific fluorescence.

The cells are then suspended in several drops of PBS (experience dictates the volume of PBS to be used at this stage), and about 20 µl is placed in each of six to nine spots on two or three Teflon-coated slides. We use slides with three 14-mm spots on each and find that they are clean enough for use when taken directly from the box. Alternatively, 10-mm squares can be etched on plain slides with a glass-marking pencil.

The drops of suspended cells are spread to cover each spot, allowed to dry, and then fixed for 10 min in acetone at 4°C. At this point they are either stained or stored in airtight boxes at 4°C for up to 1 week and −20°C for longer.

Staining procedures vary but are simple: usually 30 min in a humidified 37°C atmosphere using the antiviral monoclone, followed by three 10-min washes in PBS at room temperature and 30 min of incubation at 37°C for the conjugate, followed by three 10-min washes in PBS. Finally, the slides are rinsed in distilled water and air dried. We prefer the indirect IF method over faster direct procedures for enhanced fluorescein isothiocyanate staining of low positives, using the two-step indirect procedure. In addition, we find the use of two fluorescein isothiocyanate conjugates, each containing a different counterstain (amido black or Evans blue), useful in differentiating specific from nonspecific IF.

Fluorescence microscopes of high quality are widely available, albeit expensive. Epi-illumination is preferred. An oil or glycerol immersion 40× objective is essential for examination of specimens. Filter systems must be individualized for instruments from each manufacturer.

Experience is gained through the examination of specimens that have been also inoculated into tissue culture. This point must be emphasized: each laboratory must develop confidence in IF technique and reading ability. This can be done only by comparing readings with virus recovery. IF does not become a substitute for cell culture until such confidence has been achieved through extensive practice.

The ELISA methods that are currently available are all similar to that described by Chao et al. (8) and use a capture antibody attached to a plastic surface with which the respiratory specimen is incubated. The detector antibody may be directly enzyme conjugated or unconjugated, with a requirement for subsequent incubation with a suitable antispecies reagent. One of the antiviral antibodies is usually monoclonal. In some kits the secretion is treated with a mild detergent or mucolytic agent before being added to the test.

CULTIVATION OF THE AGENT

Different strains of HEp-2 or HeLa cells, as well as different passages of the same strain, vary greatly in sensitivity to RSV. Most diagnostic laboratories use certain precautionary measures to ensure that sensitivity is optimal. HEp-2 cells may be removed from a frozen source at intervals. Alternatively, a known source of RSV may be periodically titrated in the cells in use. HEp-2 cells will, at certain passages, permit growth of virus but cease to demonstrate a syncytial cytopathic effect (CPE). At other passages, sensitivity may be markedly reduced. It is important to be aware of such pitfalls. Variation in the sensitivity of diploid strains and primary cultures is not so evident.

HEp-2 cells should be seeded lightly (5×10^4 to 6×10^4 cells per tube) and inoculated preconfluent when cells are still actively growing. Maintenance medium is Eagle minimal essential medium or its equivalent, supplemented with glutamine, 2% fetal calf serum, and antibiotics. Bovine sera may contain antibody to RSV and should be avoided except in the form of precolostral fetal calf serum. Cultures should be incubated at 33 to 36°C in a stationary rack.

Virus growth is detected by the characteristic syncytium formation in HEp-2 cells. Adjacent cells fuse into irregular, refractile "blobs" or into large sheets of cellular material with indistinct borders and multiple nuclei. Fibroblast strains show areas of destruction that follow the lines of cell growth and occasional syncytia. Primary monkey kidney cells show clusters of enlarged cells.

A change of medium at 5 to 7 days is often very helpful in accelerating CPE of RSV. Cell cultures that are read as negative at 1 week may develop typical changes soon after the medium is changed.

In addition to standard inoculation of tissue culture tube monolayers for the isolation of virus, techniques involving centrifugation to enhance virus infectivity have been used for respiratory virus detection in some laboratories. Adapted from spin-enhanced inoculation procedures developed for cytomegalovirus (12), the methods use cover slips covered by monolayers permissive for respiratory virus growth and detection by IF after brief incubation. In our hands, the spin-enhanced inoculation procedures for respiratory viruses, although more rapid than traditional tube cultures, have suffered from variable and unpredictable sensitivity. They have therefore not replaced IF for rapid detection or routine tissue culture for isolation of RSV.

IDENTIFICATION OF ISOLATES

The usual syncytial CPE in HEp-2 cells is sufficiently characteristic to permit presumptive identification of RSV. Many laboratories end their identification efforts at this point. With the possible exceptions of parainfluenza virus type 3 and mumps virus, no other virus from the human respiratory tract produces a similar CPE in human heteroploid cells. Cell culture-adapted strains of measles virus (including vaccine strains) also do so but are unlikely to present problems. However, we believe that passage of isolates and production of a characteristic CPE a second time is an important identifying feature. Moreover, specific identification is always desirable. We primarily use IF for identification. Complement fixation (CF) may also be used, but achieving an adequate titer of antigen is sometimes difficult. Neutralization is problematic because of the unpredictability of infectivity titers in sample frozen for storage.

SEROLOGICAL METHODS

In general, it is more satisfactory to make a specific diagnosis of RSV infection by recovery of the virus (or identification by rapid methods) from a properly obtained and handled secretion specimen than by serological methods. This is true for several reasons. First, virus rarely is excreted by asymptomatic children, and therefore recovery during illness is fairly convincing evidence of the etiological involvement of the virus in the illness. Second, rises in serum antibody often fail to occur in very young children with RSV infections. Finally, it is frequently not possible to obtain 2- to 3-week convalescent sera, particularly from young infants, in a clinical setting. Therefore, serological methods are often of secondary importance, although in large studies they may give valuable information, and in individual instances in which cultures were not obtained they may be well worth performing. If, however, a virus has been recovered, the presence or absence of a homologous serum antibody titer rise adds little clinically useful information.

As with infection by other viruses, a fourfold antibody rise is considered evidence of infection. Neither a single high titer nor a fourfold fall in titer can be interpreted with any confidence as evidence of recent infection.

A number of tests for serum antibody to RSV have been developed: CF, tube neutralization, plaque reduction, and ELISA. At present, either ELISA (24) or the CF test is the most practical. A plaque reduction neutralization test (10), which includes fresh guinea pig serum in the reaction mixture as a source of complement, is a very sensitive test for serum antibody and offers some advantage in the detection of antibody rises during infection. Likewise, the ELISA offers precision and sensitivity not found in most other serological tests, and significant changes in titer may be found when they are not detectable by more traditional methods (24).

The CF test is performed by standard methods. The antigen is available commercially or may be made from infected HEp-2 cells harvested by freezing when the CPE has been 4+ for several days. When paired sera from infants are being tested, there is some advantage to using the antigen at two to four times normal concentrations (8 to 16 U). Even with this modification, however, the CF test remains insensitive for infants under 6 months of age undergoing what is assumed to be primary infection.

EVALUATION AND REPORTING

Often, the piece of information most valuable to the clinician is a report of whether a particular clinical specimen contains a virus rather than identification of the precise viral species. For this reason, a preliminary report (often by telephone) should be made as soon as a tentative recognition of CPE is made. Often the label "Tentative RSV" can be attached at this point, with more definitive information to follow.

Since RSV is rarely present in normal healthy individuals, it is likely that recovery of the virus during an appropriate respiratory illness means both the presence of an infection and the etiological association of the virus with the disease in question. A negative report, on the other hand, does not prove the absence of infection. There are many possible reasons for a false-negative result, the most likely of which is faulty specimen collection and transport. In highly suspicious clinical circumstances, a repeat specimen should be obtained.

LITERATURE CITED

1. **Ahluwalia, G., J. Embree, P. McNicol, B. Law, and G. W. Hammond.** 1987. Comparison of nasopharyngeal

aspirate and nasopharyngeal swab specimens for respiratory syncytial virus diagnosis by cell culture, indirect immunofluorescence assay, and enzyme-linked immunosorbent assay. J. Clin. Microbiol. **25:**763–767.

2. **Anderson, J. M., and M. O. Beem.** 1966. Use of human diploid cell cultures for primary isolation of respiratory syncytial virus. Proc. Soc. Exp. Biol. Med. **121:**205–209.
3. **Bell, D. M., E. E. Walsh, J. F. Hruska, K. C. Schnabel, and C. B. Hall.** 1983. Rapid detection of respiratory syncytial virus with a monoclonal antibody. J. Clin. Microbiol. **17:**1099–1101.
4. **Bromberg, K., D. Bennett, L. Clarke, and M. F. Sierra.** 1984. Comparison of immediate and delayed inoculation of HEp-2 cells for isolation of respiratory syncytial virus. J. Clin. Microbiol. **20:**123–124.
5. **Bromberg, K., G. Tannis, B. Daidone, L. Clarke, and M. F. Sierra.** 1985. Comparison of Ortho respiratory syncytial virus enzyme-linked immunosorbent assay and HEp-2 cell culture. J. Clin. Microbiol. **22:**1071–1072.
6. **Chanock, R. M., and L. Finberg.** 1957. Recovery from infants with respiratory illness of a virus related to chimpanzee coryza agent (CCA). II. Epidemiologic aspects of infection in infants and young children. Am. J. Hyg. **66:** 291–300.
7. **Chanock, R. M., H. W. Kim, A. J. Vargosko, A. Deleva, K. M. Johnson, C. Cumming, and R. H. Parrott.** 1961. Respiratory syncytial virus. I. Virus recovery and other observations during 1960 outbreak of bronchiolitis, pneumonia, and minor respiratory diseases in children. J. Am. Med. Assoc. **176:**647–653.
8. **Chao, R. K., M. Fishaut, J. D. Schwartzman, and K. McIntosh.** 1979. An enzyme-linked immunosorbent assay (ELISA) for detection of respiratory syncytial virus in human nasal secretions. J. Infect. Dis. **2:**483–486.
9. **Cheesman, S. H., L. T. Pierik, D. Leombruno, K. E. Spinos, and K. McIntosh.** 1986. Evaluation of a commercially available direct immunofluorescent staining reagent for the detection of respiratory syncytial virus in respiratory secretions. J. Clin. Microbiol. **24:**155–156.
10. **Coates, H. V., D. W. Alling, and R. M. Chanock.** 1966. An antigenic analysis of respiratory syncytial virus isolates by a plaque reduction neutralization test. Am. J. Epidemiol. **89:**299–313.
11. **Gardner, P. S., and J. McQuillin.** 1980. Rapid viral diagnosis: application of immunofluorescence, 2nd ed. Butterworth & Co. Ltd., London.
12. **Gleaves, C. A., T. F. Smith, E. A. Shuster, and G. R. Pearson.** 1984. Rapid detection of cytomegalovirus in MRC-5 cells inoculated with virus specimens by using low-speed centrifugation and monoclonal antibody to an early antigen. J. Clin. Microbiol. **19:**917–919.
13. **Grandien, M., C. A. Petterson, P. S. Gardner, A. Linde, and A. Stanton.** 1985. Rapid viral diagnosis of acute respiratory infections: comparison of enzyme-linked immunosorbent assay and the immunofluorescence technique for detection of viral antigens in nasopharyngeal secretions. J. Clin. Microbiol. **22:**757–760.
14. **Hall, C. B., and R. Douglas.** 1975. Clinically useful method for the isolation of respiratory syncytial virus. J. Infect. Dis. **131:**1–4.
15. **Hall, C. B., R. G. Douglas, and J. M. Geiman.** 1976. Respiratory syncytial virus infections in infants: quantitation and duration of shedding. J. Pediatr. **89:**1–15.
16. **Hall, C. B., J. T. McBride, E. E. Walsh, D. M. Bell, C. L. Gala, S. Hildreth, L. G. TenEyck, and W. J. Hall.** 1983. Aerosolized ribavirin treatment of infants with respiratory syncytial virus infection. N. Engl. J. Med. **308:**1443–1447.
17. **Hendry, R. M., A. L. Talis, E. Godfrey, L. J. Anderson, B. F. Fernie, and K. McIntosh.** 1986. Concurrent circulation of antigenically distinct strains of respiratory syncytial virus during community outbreaks. J. Infect. Dis. **153:**291–297.
18. **Jalowayski, A. A., B. L. England, C. J. Temm, T. J. Nunemacher, J. F. Bastian, G. A. MacPherson, W. M. Dankner, R. C. Straube, and J. D. Connor.** 1987. Peroxidase-antiperoxidase assay for rapid detection of respiratory syncytial virus in nasal epithelial specimens from infants and children. J. Clin. Microbiol. **25:**722–725.
19. **Lauer, B. A., H. A. Masters, C. G. Wren, and M. J. Levin.** 1985. Rapid detection of respiratory syncytial virus in nasopharyngeal secretions by enzyme-linked immunosorbent assay. J. Clin. Microbiol. **22:**782–785.
20. **McIntosh, K.** Respiratory viral infections. *In* P. A. Pizzo and C. M. Wilfert (ed.), Pediatric AIDS: the challenge of HIV infection in infants, children and adolescents, in press. The Williams & Wilkins Co., Baltimore.
21. **McIntosh, K., and R. M. Chanock.** 1990. Respiratory syncytial virus, p. 1045–1072. *In* B. N. Fields and D. M. Knipe (ed.), Virology. Raven Press.
22. **McIntosh, K., R. M. Hendry, M. L. Fahnestock, and L. T. Pierik.** 1982. Enzyme-linked immunosorbent assay for detection of respiratory syncytial virus infection: application to clinical samples. J. Clin. Microbiol. **16:**329–333.
23. **Minnich, L., and C. G. Ray.** 1980. Comparison of direct immunofluorescence staining of clinical specimens for respiratory virus antigens with conventional isolation techniques. J. Clin. Microbiol. **12:**391–394.
24. **Richardson, L. S., R. H. Yolken, R. B. Belshe, L. E. Camargo, H. W. Kim, and R. M. Chanock.** 1978. Enzyme-linked immunosorbent assay for measurement of serological response to respiratory syncytial virus infection. Infect. Immun. **23:**660–664.
25. **Sarkkinen, H. K., P. E. Halonen, P. P. Arstila, and A. Q. Salmi.** 1981. Detection of respiratory syncytial, parainfluenza type 2, and adenovirus antigens by radioimmunoassay and enzyme immunoassay on nasopharyngeal specimens from children with acute respiratory disease. J. Clin. Microbiol. **13:**258–265.
26. **Swenson, P. D., and M. H. Kaplan.** 1986. Rapid detection of respiratory syncytial virus in nasopharyngeal aspirates by a commercial enzyme immunoassay. J. Clin. Microbiol. **23:**485–488.
27. **Taber, L. H., V. Knight, B. E. Gilbert, H. W. McClung, S. Z. Wilson, H. J. Norton, J. M. Thurson, W. H. Gordon, R. L. Atmar, and W. R. Schlaudt.** 1983. Ribavirin aerosol treatment of bronchiolitis associated with respiratory syncytial virus infection in infants. Pediatrics **72:**613–618.
28. **Van Dyke, R. B., and M. Murphy-Corb.** 1989. Detection of respiratory syncytial virus in nasopharyngeal secretions by DNA-RNA hybridization. J. Clin. Microbiol. **27:**1739–1743.

Chapter 84

Rhinoviruses

MARIE L. LANDRY

CLINICAL BACKGROUND

The rhinovirus group derives its name from the predominant site of its replication and symptomatology, the nose. Rhinoviruses constitute the major virus group associated with the acute respiratory illness known as the common cold. The average person suffers two to five colds per year, one-third to one-half of which are due to rhinoviruses (11). Although the common cold is a trivial illness, it is acutely disabling. The annual cost of the common cold in days lost from work, cold remedies, and analgesics is in the billions of dollars.

In 1930, it was first recognized that the common cold was caused by a "filterable agent" (15a). With the development of tissue culture techniques in the 1950s, rhinovirus was isolated, first in organ culture (3) and then in monkey kidney cells (33, 34). With the development of the more sensitive human embryonic lung cell culture and the use of growth conditions that mimicked those of the nose, a number of different serological types were isolated in the 1960s. In 1967, types 1A to 55 were designated; in 1971 and 1987, types 56 to 89 and 90 to 100, respectively, were designated (26).

In temperate climates, rhinovirus infections peak in early fall, with a second peak in the spring, yet they continue to cause colds throughout the summer. Multiple types appear to circulate in a given area at any time (23). Serotypes with lower numbers have been gradually replaced by those with higher numbers or strains that cannot be typed. The reason for the changing serotypes is not known, but this phenomenon could represent recirculation of a large number of antigenically stable types or antigenic drift (23, 36).

Studies in volunteers have shown that inoculation of virus into the nose or conjunctiva is the most efficient way to initiate infection. Several investigators have found little evidence for aerosol transmission in the spread of rhinoviruses (12). Instead, they found that virus is present in highest titers in the nose and that hands of infected persons are commonly contaminated. The virus can be transmitted to others via hand-to-hand contact (24), followed by self-inoculation of virus into the nose or conjunctivae (27). A recent study, however, has demonstrated the potential for aerosol transmission as well (15).

From studies in volunteers, the incubation period of rhinoviruses after inoculation has been found to be 2 to 3 days (16). The peak of virus shedding coincides with the acute rhinitis. Virus may become undetectable by 4 to 5 days or be present in low titers for up to 2 weeks. Nasal epithelial cells are infected and are shed into nasal mucus. However, the symptoms of rhinovirus infection are produced in part by chemical mediators of inflammation such as bradykinin and lysylbradykinin (23). Symptoms persist for 7 days on average and include profuse watery discharge, nasal congestion, sneezing, headache, mild sore throat, and cough, with little or no fever. Infection of the lower respiratory tract may also occur (13). Rhinovirus infections have been shown to exacerbate chronic bronchitis and asthma (29, 32), especially in children, and have also been associated with otitis media and sinusitis (20). Immunity is type specific and correlates best with local production of immunoglobulin A (IgA) antibody (4).

DESCRIPTION OF AGENT

Rhinoviruses are members of the family *Picornaviridae*, which includes the enteroviruses. The rhinovirus virion consists of a nonenveloped icosahedral nucleocapsid, 28 to 34 nm in diameter, with capsomeres composed of four structural polypeptides, VP1, VP2, VP3, and VP4. These structural polypeptides are obtained by posttranslational cleavage of a large polypeptide precursor (2, 30). The virion nucleic acid is single-stranded, positive-sense RNA that is more than 7,000 nucleotides long and has a molecular weight of 2.6×10^6. Rhinovirus genomes have been sequenced and found to share 45 to 62% homology with poliovirus (7). Replication occurs in the cytoplasm of infected cells, producing infectious virions that sediment at a buoyant density of 1.38 g/ml in cesium chloride. Empty capsids and particles lacking one or more structural polypeptides are also produced. Infectious and noninfectious particles are immunologically distinct and are referred to as D (dense or native virions), which are fully infectious, and C (coreless virion antigens), which lack VP4 (30).

Because they have no lipid-containing envelope, rhinoviruses are resistant to inactivation by organic solvents such as ether, chloroform, ethanol, and 5% phenol. They are susceptible to heat inactivation at 50 to 56°C within minutes to hours but can be stabilized by addition of $MgCl_2$. Rhinoviruses are differentiated from enteroviruses by their loss of infectivity upon exposure to pH 3 for 3 h at room temperature. After both heat and acid inactivation, rhinoviruses lack VP4, which is important for attachment of virions to cell receptors (30).

At present, 100 rhinovirus serotypes have been numbered on the basis of neutralization tests. There is no group antigen, but by using high-titered hyperimmune rabbit and guinea pig antisera, cross-reactions between antigenic types have been detected and 16 rhinovirus subgroups have been defined (10). The native D antigenicity of rhinoviruses can be changed to C antigenicity by treatment with low pH, heat, or 2 M urea, producing virus particles that react with heterologous antisera (31).

X-ray crystallography studies have suggested that the large depressions or "canyons" found on each icosahedral face are sites for cell receptor binding (35). It has also been recently shown that rhinoviruses can be placed into two groups on the basis of binding to cell receptors (1).

COLLECTION AND STORAGE OF SPECIMENS

In natural infections, rhinovirus can be isolated from 1 day before to 6 days after onset of cold symptoms but is shed in highest concentration during the first 2 days of illness. Since the virus is excreted in highest titers from the nose, nasal rather than throat specimens should be obtained for isolation. Sputum is also a low-yielding specimen for the isolation of rhinovirus. A comparison of nasal wash, nose swab, throat gargle, and throat swab specimens for isolation from clinical specimens revealed nasal wash to be the best (8). Nasal wash specimens are obtained as follows. Tilt the patient's head backward and place 1 ml of sterile phosphate-buffered saline into one of the nostrils. Then ask the patient to lean forward and allow the washing to drip into a sterile petri dish or other collection container. Repeat with the other nostril until each has been washed with 5 ml of phosphate-buffered saline. The washings are then transferred into a sterile container with an equal volume of viral transport medium (VTM) containing antibiotics. Inclusion of phenol red in the VTM allows the detection of acid pH, which would adversely affect the isolation of rhinovirus.

Nasopharyngeal swabs are obtained by inserting a cotton-tip applicator into the nasopharynx. The swab is then immersed in a vial containing 2 ml of VTM.

Specimens should be transported promptly to the laboratory. Best results are obtained with rapid inoculation of cell cultures; however, specimens can be held for up to 24 h at 4°C in VTM with neutral pH. If longer delays are necessary, specimens should be frozen at −70°C and thawed just before inoculation.

DIRECT EXAMINATION

Because of the great number of rhinovirus serotypes and the lack of a group antigen, it has been difficult to develop tests for direct detection of viral antigen in clinical specimens. Studies in the 1970s using immunofluorescence to detect rhinovirus antigens in nasopharyngeal specimens revealed a poor correlation between immunofluorescence and virus isolation (19).

Recently, enzyme-linked immunosorbent assays (ELISAs) using antisera to human rhinovirus EL (an untyped virus) and human rhinovirus type 2 antigens have been developed for detection of rhinovirus directly in clinical specimens and after overnight amplification in cell culture (14). Each ELISA detected between 56 and 69% of rhinovirus types investigated and when used in combination detected over 80%. In addition, nucleic acid hybridization using cDNA and oligonucleotide probes from the 5′ noncoding region of the genome has shown positive hybridization signals from over 90% of rhinoviruses tested (6). The limit of detection appeared to be about 10^3 50% tissue culture infective doses ($TCID_{50}$)/ml under optimal conditions. Because of genome homology with enteroviruses, however, cross-reactions may occur. Polymerase chain reaction has also been applied to rhinovirus detection in clinical material with some success (21). These techniques remain research tools at present.

ISOLATION OF VIRUS

Cell culture

Rhinoviruses are best isolated in sensitive cell culture systems and grow only in cells of human or monkey origin. Although rhinoviruses were originally isolated in primary monkey kidney cells, these cells have not been consistent in yielding a broad range of isolates. The use of sensitive human diploid fibroblasts (HDF) has provided superior results. Rhinoviruses were originally separated into M and H strains on the basis of their ability to replicate in monkey and human cells (M strains replicate in both monkey and human cells, whereas H strains replicate only in human cells). However, this distinction is no longer used, since H strains can be adapted to grow in monkey cells.

The most commonly used cells in clinical laboratories are HDF cells such as human embryonic lung strains WI-38, WI-26, and MRC-5. Human embryonic kidney cells can also support rhinovirus replication. A sensitive strain of HeLa cells, HeLa M cells, supports rhinovirus replication to high titers and has been used to prepare rhinovirus antigens (9). Some isolates have been obtained only in HeLa M cells; however, passage may be necessary before cytopathic effect (CPE) is apparent. Recently, a human fetal tonsil cell line was found to be more sensitive than MRC-5 and HeLa M cells for primary isolation (22). Unfortunately, different lots of normally sensitive cell lines have been found to vary over 100-fold in sensitivity to rhinovirus (5); the reasons for this variation are not known. Therefore, for optimal results, simultaneous use of several sensitive systems is recommended.

After inoculation, cultures are incubated in standard tissue culture medium such as Eagle minimum essential medium with 2% fetal calf serum and antibiotics at a neutral pH. It is important that culture conditions mimic those of the nose; cultures should be incubated at 33°C with continuous rotation in a roller drum to provide aeration of the monolayer. CPE can be observed as early as 24 to 48 h after inoculation and is usually seen by day 4. In fibroblasts, cellular changes are easier to read and therefore often detected earlier than in epithelial cell lines. Both large and small rounded, refractile cells with pyknotic nuclei are observed in foci that also contain cellular debris (Fig. 1). Rhinovirus CPE is often similar to enterovirus CPE but may sometimes be confused with nonspecific changes. The CPE progresses over a 2- to 3-day period, with the degree of cellular change depending on the serotype and the inoculum dose. It should be noted that rhinovirus CPE can regress or virus may inactivate if left too long. Therefore, cultures should be promptly passaged when CPE is clearly apparent. Passage is also necessary to increase viral titers before identification tests are performed.

HDF cell cultures should be observed for 14 days. HeLa cell cultures can be observed for only up to 8 days, when passage becomes necessary because of cell degeneration and rounding.

Organ culture

Organ cultures of human fetal nasal epithelium or trachea have been used to isolate rhinoviruses not detected in standard cell cultures. However, studies com-

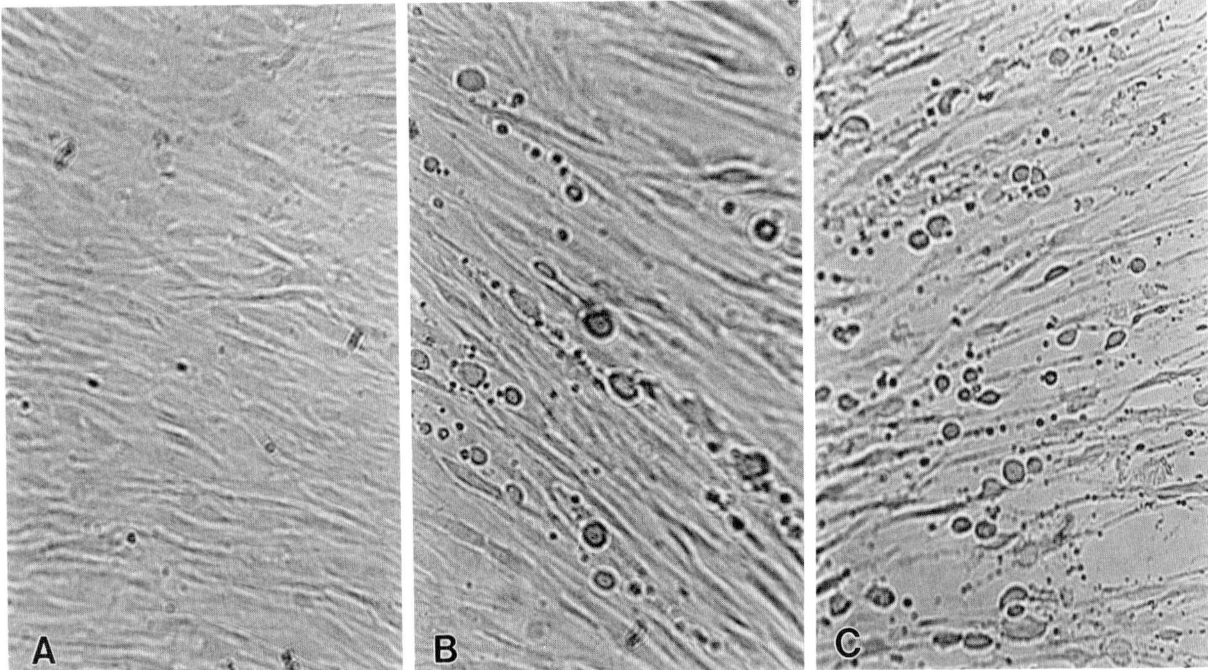

FIG. 1. Rhinovirus CPE in human fibroblast monolayers. (A) Uninfected cells; (B) early focus of rhinovirus CPE; (C) more advanced rhinovirus CPE. Magnification, ×98.

paring organ cultures with standard cell cultures have shown that a combination of both systems is necessary for optimal recovery (28). Because of the limited supply of fetal material, this approach is not widely used. Details of the procedure have been reviewed elsewhere (2, 24, 30). In brief, pieces of nasal epithelium or trachea are incubated in culture tubes at 33°C in a roller drum, examined daily for ciliary activity, and monitored for pH changes. If rhinovirus is replicating, ciliary activity ceases within 5 to 7 days. Virus can be harvested from the supernatant fluids and passaged to fresh organ cultures or cell culture.

IDENTIFICATION OF VIRUS

A presumptive diagnosis of a rhinovirus isolate is made by the appearance and progression of characteristic CPE in the appropriate clinical setting. Further identification requires the confirmation of properties such as sensitivity to temperature and acid pH and resistance to lipid solvents. For routine viral diagnostic laboratories, these tests are sufficient (Fig. 2). Since 100 rhinovirus serotypes have been identified and no group antigen has been found, specific serotype identification by neutralization is time consuming and costly. Only for isolates from unusual clinical situations or in research settings is further serotype identification by neutralization warranted. Before these tests are performed, isolates must be passaged to obtain a minimum titer of 10^3 $TCID_{50}$/ml.

Acid pH stability

Rhinoviruses are sensitive to low pH, whereas enteroviruses are stable. Thus, a reduction in virus titer by 2 to 3 $\log_{10}$ $TCID_{50}$ can be expected upon exposure of rhinovirus to low pH. First, prepare two solutions of a buffer such as *N*-2-hydroxyethylpiperazine-*N'*-2-ethanesulfonic acid (HEPES), one at pH 3.0 and one at pH 7.0. Add 0.2 ml of unknown virus suspension to 1.8 ml of pH 3.0 HEPES and 0.2 ml of virus to 1.8 ml of pH 7.0 HEPES. Keep the mixtures at room temperature for 3 h, adjust the pH to 7.0, make serial dilutions of the mixtures, and inoculate the dilutions into cell cultures. If the unknown virus is a rhinovirus, a minimum 2 $\log_{10}$ reduction in viral titer should be evident in the acid-treated sample. A known rhinovirus and a known enterovirus should be included as control cultures and treated similarly.

Resistance to lipid solvents

Since rhinoviruses lack a lipid envelope, they are resistant to treatment with lipid solvents such as chloroform or ether, and infectivity titers should not be affected. Add 0.1 ml of chloroform to 1 ml of isolate, shake the mixture vigorously for 10 min at room temperature, and then centrifuge it at 1,000 × *g* for 5 to 10 min. Remove the upper aqueous phase and use it to determine the infectivity titer in cell cultures.

Alternatively, add 0.2 ml of diethyl ether to 0.8 ml of isolate in a stoppered tube, shake the tube vigorously, and let it stand at room temperature for 1 to 2 h, with intermittent shaking. Then transfer the mixture into an open glass petri dish in a fume hood and allow the ether to evaporate. Prepare serial dilutions and inoculate them into cell cultures.

An equal volume of unknown virus should be handled in a similar manner but not treated with chloroform or ether. A known picornavirus and a lipid-sensitive virus, such as herpes simplex virus, should also be included as controls. The picornavirus should be unaffected, and

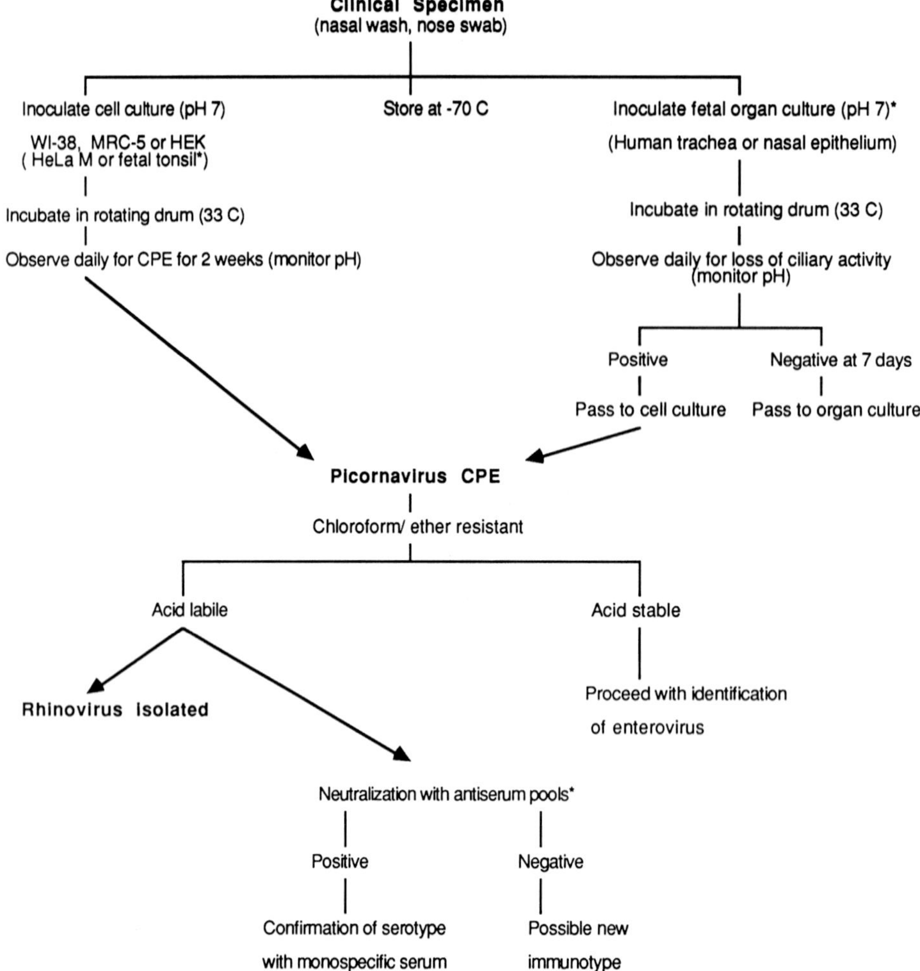

FIG. 2. Flow scheme for the isolation and identification of rhinovirus. Techniques reserved for the research laboratory are marked by an asterisk. HEK, Human embryonic kidney cells.

the herpes simplex virus should be completely inactivated.

Temperature sensitivity

Since rhinoviruses grow best at 33°C, they can be distinguished from enteroviruses by inoculation of serial dilutions of the unknown virus and incubation of one set of cultures at 33°C and a replicate set at 37°C. The onset of CPE should be more rapid and the infectivity titer of virus should be higher at the lower temperature.

Neutralization tests

Specific identification of rhinoviruses by serotyping is an expensive and labor-intensive procedure performed only by specialized laboratories. Hyperimmune antisera for types 1A to 89 are available from the American Type Culture Collection. Intersecting serum pools similar to those used for enterovirus identification have been prepared, and isolates are usually tested in a microneutralization procedure to conserve reagents. Serotype confirmation is then performed by using monospecific antiserum. Neutralization generally involves the neutralization of 30 to 100 $TCID_{50}$ of virus-induced CPE by 20 U of antiserum. Nontypeable isolates are occasionally found. Detailed procedures are described elsewhere (2, 25, 30).

Other tests

Recently, ELISAs that can detect rhinovirus antigens in cell culture have been developed (14). Nucleic acid hybridization techniques and polymerase chain reaction can also be used to identify rhinovirus isolates in cell culture (6, 21). These methods are currently used for research, but as antiviral agents become available for rhinovirus infections (18), rapid, accurate diagnostic methods will assume greater importance.

SEROLOGICAL DIAGNOSIS

Although demonstration of an antibody rise to rhinovirus in natural infections may identify many infections not detected by virus isolation (23), the large number of serotypes makes blind serological testing impractical. However, if a virus has been recovered, patient serum can be tested against that isolate.

The standard serological assay to measure antibody in serum or nasal wash specimens is the neutralization test (17). For maximum sensitivity, a low challenge dose

(3 to 30 $TCID_{50}$) should be used. Plaque reduction neutralization has also been described. Complement fixation detects heterotypic antibody responses to rhinoviruses and enteroviruses, and the findings do not parallel neutralization results. Hemagglutination inhibition has also been used; however, this test is not as sensitive as neutralization, and not all rhinoviruses hemagglutinate.

Recently, ELISAs using human rhinovirus type EL and 2 antigens have been used to detect serum and nasal IgG and IgA in volunteers inoculated with these two viruses (4). ELISA was 100 to 10,000 times more sensitive than neutralization. The problem of detecting antibodies to multiple serotypes in natural infection was not addressed.

EVALUATION, INTERPRETATION, AND REPORTING OF RESULTS

The laboratory diagnosis of rhinovirus infection is based on isolation of virus with characteristic CPE in cell systems sensitive for isolation, such as human fibroblasts, human embryonic kidney cells, and HeLa cells. Both incubation at 33°C and rotation of cultures are essential for virus replication. Differentiation of rhinoviruses from enteroviruses, with which their CPE can be confused, is based primarily on acid stability testing of isolates. Rhinoviruses are inactivated by pH 3 to 5, whereas enteroviruses are unaffected. Sensitivity to 37°C temperature and to organic solvents are additional features of rhinovirus isolates.

Because of the large number of rhinovirus serotypes, identification by neutralization tests is reserved for specialized laboratories. Serotype identification is primarily useful in epidemiologic or research studies. In clinical laboratories, rhinoviruses are rarely specifically sought. Since there is no treatment, cultures are rarely taken from outpatients with the common cold. Instead, isolates are usually found when the clinical diagnosis is influenza or respiratory syncytial virus. However, if specific therapy becomes available, this situation will change. Serological assays for antibody to rhinovirus are also not performed outside the research setting but can provide useful information in studies of viral pathogenesis and immunity.

Because of the tremendous economic cost of rhinovirus infections, much work is being done to understand the pathogenesis of the agent and to develop treatment. Thus, the development of rapid and accurate diagnostic tests should prove useful to clinical laboratories in the near future.

LITERATURE CITED

1. **Abraham, G., and R. J. Colonno.** 1984. Many rhinovirus serotypes share the same cellular receptor. J. Virol. **51:** 340–345.
2. **Al-Nakib, W., and D. A. U. Tyrrell.** 1988. Picornaviridae: rhinoviruses–common cold viruses, p. 723–742. *In* E. H. Lennette, P. Halonen, and F. A. Murphy (ed.), Laboratory diagnosis of infectious diseases, principles and practice, vol. II. Springer-Verlag, New York.
3. **Andrewes, C. H., D. M. Chaproneiri, A. E. H. Gompels, H. G. Pereira, and A. T. Roden.** 1953. Propagation of common cold virus in tissue cultures. Lancet **i:**546–547.
4. **Barclay, W. S., and W. Al-Nakib.** 1987. An ELISA for the detection of rhinovirus specific antibody in serum and nasal secretion. J. Virol. Methods **15:**53–64.
5. **Brown, P. K., and D. A. J. Tyrrell.** 1964. Experiments on the sensitivity of strains of human fibroblasts to infection with rhinovirus. Br. J. Exp. Pathol. **45:**571–578.
6. **Bruce, C. B., W. Al-Nakib, D. A. Tyrrell, and J. W. Almond.** 1988. Synthetic oligonucleotides as diagnostic probes for rhinoviruses. Lancet **ii:**53.
7. **Callahan, P. L., S. Mizutani, and R. J. Colonno.** 1985. Molecular cloning and complete sequence determination of RNA genome of human rhinovirus type 14. Proc. Natl. Acad. Sci. USA **82:**732–736.
8. **Cate, T. R., R. B. Couch, and K. M. Johnson.** 1964. Studies with rhinovirus in volunteers; production of illness, effect of naturally acquired antibody, and demonstration of a protective effect not associated with serum antibody. J. Clin. Invest. **43:**56–67.
9. **Conant, R. M., N. L. Somerson, and V. V. Hamparian.** 1968. Rhinovirus: basis for a numbering system. 1. HeLa cell for propagation and serologic procedures. J. Immunol. **100:**107–113.
10. **Cooney, M. K., J. P. Fox, and G. E. Kenny.** 1982. Antigenic groupings of 90 rhinovirus serotypes. Infect. Immun. **37:**642–647.
11. **Couch, R. B.** 1990. Rhinoviruses, p. 607–629. *In* B. N. Fields and D. M. Knipe (ed.), Virology, 2nd ed. Raven Press, New York.
12. **Couch, R. B., R. G. Douglas, Jr., K. M. Lindgren, P. J. Gerone, and V. Knight.** 1970. Airborne transmission of respiratory infection with coxsackievirus A type 21. Am. J. Epidemiol. **91:**78–86.
13. **Craighead, J. E., J. Meier, and M. H. Cooley.** 1969. Pulmonary infection due to rhinovirus type 13. N. Engl. J. Med. **281:**1403–1404.
14. **Dearden, C. J., and W. Al-Nakib.** 1987. Direct detection of rhinoviruses by an enzyme-linked immunosorbent assay. J. Med. Virol. **23:**179–189.
15. **Dick, E. C., L. C. Jennings, K. A. Mink, C. D. Wartgow, and S. L. Inhorn.** 1987. Aerosol transmission of rhinovirus colds. J. Infect. Dis. **156:**442–448.

15a. **Dochez, A. R., G. S. Shibley, and K. C. Mills.** 1930. Studies in the common cold. IV. Experimental transmission of the common cold to anthropoid apes and human beings by means of a filtrable agent. J. Exp. Med. **52:**701–716.

16. **Douglas, R. G., Jr.** 1970. Pathogenesis of rhinovirus common colds in human volunteers. Ann. Otol. Rhinol. Laryngol. **79:**563–571.
17. **Douglas, R. G., Jr., W. F. Fleet, T. R. Cate, and R. B. Couch.** 1968. Antibody to rhinovirus in human sera. I. Standardization of a neutralization test. Proc. Soc. Exp. Biol. Med. **127:**497–502.
18. **Douglas, R. M., B. W. Moore, H. B. Miles, L. M. Davis, N. M. H. Graham, P. Ryan, D. A. Warswick, and J. K. Albrecht.** 1986. Prophylactic efficacy of intranasal alpha-2 interferon against rhinovirus infections in the family setting. N. Engl. J. Med. **314:**65–70.
19. **Dreizin, R. S., N. M. Borovkova, T. I. Ponomareva, E. M. Vikhnovich, A. A. Kheinitis, and T. V. Leichinskaya.** 1975. Diagnosis of rhinovirus infections by virological and immunofluorescent methods. Acta Virol. **19:** 413–418.
20. **Evans, E. O., J. B. Sydnor, and W. E. C. Moore.** 1975. Sinusitis of the maxillary antrum. N. Engl. J. Med. **293:** 735–739.
21. **Gama, R. E., R. J. Hughes, C. B. Bruce, and G. Stanway.** 1988. Polymerase chain reaction amplification of rhinovirus nucleic acids from clinical material. Nucleic Acids Res. **16:**9346.
22. **Geist, F. C., and F. G. Hayden.** 1985. Comparative susceptibilities of strain MRC-5 human embryonic lung fibroblast cells and the Cooney strain of human fetal tonsil cells for isolation of rhinoviruses from clinical specimens. J. Clin. Microbiol. **22:**455–456.
23. **Gwaltney, J. M., Jr.** 1989. Rhinoviruses, p. 593–615. *In* A. S. Evans (ed.) Viral infections of humans. Plenum Med-

ical Book Co., New York.

24. **Gwaltney, J. M., Jr., P. B. Moskalski, and J. O. Hendley.** 1978. Hand-to-hand transmission of rhinovirus colds. Ann. Intern. Med. **88:**463–467.

25. **Hamparian, V. V.** 1979. Rhinoviruses, p. 535–575. *In* E. H. Lennette and N. J. Schmidt (ed.), Diagnostic procedures for viral, rickettsial and chlamydial infections. American Public Health Association, Inc., Washington, D.C.

26. **Hamparian, V. V., R. J. Colonno, M. K. Cooney, E. C. Dick, et al.** 1987. A collaborative report: rhinoviruses—extension of the numbering system from 89 to 100. Virology **159:**191–192.

27. **Hendley, J. O., R. P. Wenzel, and J. M. Gwaltney, Jr.** 1973. Transmission of rhinovirus colds by self-inoculation. N. Engl. J. Med. **288:**1361–1364.

28. **Higgins, P. G., E. M. Ellis, and D. A. Woolley.** 1969. A comparative study of standard methods and organ culture for the isolation of respiratory viruses. J. Med. Microsc. **2:** 109.

29. **Horn, M. E. C., and I. Gregg.** 1973. Role of viral infection and host factors in acute episodes of asthma and chronic bronchitis. Chest **64:**44–48.

30. **Levandowski, R. A.** 1985. Rhinoviruses, p. 391–405. *In* R. B. Belshe (ed.), Human virology. PSG Publishing Co. Inc., Littleton, Mass.

31. **Longberg-Holm, K., and F. H. Yin.** 1973. Antigenic determinants of infective and inactivated human rhinovirus type 2. J. Virol. **12:**114–123.

32. **Minor, T. E., E. C. Dick, A. N. DeMeo, J. J. Ouellette, M. Cohen, and C. E. Reed.** 1974. Viruses as precipitants of asthmatic attacks in children. J. Am. Med. Assoc. **227:** 292–298.

33. **Pelon, W., W. J. Mogabgab, I. A. Phillips, and W. E. Pierce.** 1957. A cytopathogenic agent isolated from naval recruits with mild respiratory illness. Proc. Soc. Exp. Biol. Med. **94:**262–267.

34. **Price, W. H.** 1956. The isolation of a new virus associated with respiratory clinical disease in humans. Proc. Natl. Acad. Sci. USA **42:**892–896.

35. **Rossman, M. G., E.. Arnold, J. W. Erickson, E. A. Frankenberger, J. P. Griffith, H. J. Hecht, J. E. Johnson, G. Kramer, M. Luo, A. G. Mosser, R. R. Rueckert, B. Sherry, and G. Vriend.** 1985. Structure of a human common cold virus and functional relationship to other picornaviruses. Nature (London) **317:**145–153.

36. **Stott, E. J., and M. Walker.** 1969. Antigenic variation among strains of rhinovirus type 51. Nature (London) **224:** 1311–1312.

Chapter 85

Coronaviruses

C. GEORGE RAY

CLINICAL BACKGROUND

The first human coronaviruses (HCV) were reported in 1965, when respiratory specimens that had been inoculated into organ cultures of human fetal tracheal or nasal epithelium yielded cytopathic agents (17). The 229E strain was subsequently isolated in cell cultures from medical students with acute upper respiratory tract illnesses (4). Coronaviruslike particles in human feces were described later and have subsequently been associated with diarrheal diseases. These latter agents are discussed in chapter 95.

Respiratory transmission from person to person is apparently common. Serological surveys from different areas of the world have shown antibody prevalences among adults of 86% or more for both HCV OC43 and HCV 229E.

Coronaviruses have been determined to be responsible for about 15% of upper respiratory tract infections in adults (1). Infection and seroconversion rates are highest among young children, declining during the second decade and thereafter (12, 16).

The incubation period for HCV infection ranges from 2 to 5 days, and the usual illness lasts 3 to 18 days (mean, 7 days). In adults, HCV-caused illnesses appear similar to those associated with rhinovirus infections except that symptoms of nasal discharge and malaise seem to be more common in coronavirus infections and cough more frequent in rhinovirus infections (1).

The role of HCV in lower respiratory tract illnesses is less clear. Infections have been associated with pneumonia and pleural reactions in military recruits (19). In children, sore throat, cough, coryza, and fever are common (7), and a few patients have developed pulmonary crackles (8). Acute attacks of wheezing can also occur, particularly among persons known to be asthmatic or disposed to recurrent lower respiratory tract infections (6, 10).

DESCRIPTION OF AGENT

The family *Coronaviridae* consists of enveloped, generally spherical virions with helical nucleocapsids containing a single, plus-stranded RNA genome. Their overall diameters range from 80 to 160 nm, and they are distinguished by distinctly separated petal-shaped spikes (peplomers) attached to the envelope surface (Fig. 1). Infectivity is lost upon exposure to acid, trypsin, ether, or chloroform. The major structural proteins include a matrix glycoprotein (E1) embedded into the lipid bilayer envelope, an E2 glycoprotein located on the peplomer, and a nucleocapsid phosphoprotein.

The E1 glycoprotein determines virion budding from the rough endoplasmic reticulum and Golgi membranes. Antibodies to E1 can neutralize the virus only in the presence of complement. Functions of E2 include binding to host cell receptors and induction of cell fusion; antibodies to E2 directly neutralize viral infectivity and can mediate antibody-dependent cell-mediated cytotoxicity.

The binding site for virion attachment via E2 appears to be a sialic acid-containing receptor similar to that recognized by influenza virus type C (18). Virus replication occurs entirely in the cellular cytoplasm, with release either by cell death or via secretory mechanisms.

The family has been divided into four antigenic groups on the basis of serological comparisons. The two recognized human strains, 229E and OC43, are in groups 1 and 2, respectively, along with other mammalian strains. Groups 3 and 4 include avian strains. Extensive genetic variation within strains is well recognized for agents such as mouse hepatitis virus; such variation also occurs in strains specific to humans, but the extent and significance are not yet well defined. There is no evidence that cross-species transmission occurs in nature.

COLLECTION AND STORAGE OF SPECIMENS

Isolations are usually made from pooled nasal and pharyngeal swabs or from nasal washings. Specimens should be collected within 3 days, and not later than 4 to 5 days, after the onset of symptoms. If possible, the specimen should be inoculated onto cell cultures within 2 to 3 h of collection; during the interval between collection and inoculation, it is best to keep the specimen at approximately 4°C. If storage is necessary, the specimens can be frozen at −70°C; if dry ice is used, the specimen must be stored in a flame-sealed glass ampoule, or other provisions must be made to prevent absorption of CO_2 by the specimen. This is especially important for storage, because coronaviruses are inactivated at low pH. The recommended procedures for collection of nasal washings and nasal and pharyngeal swabs are described in chapter 74.

DIRECT EXAMINATION

Direct examination of clinical material for the presence of HCV or HCV antigen is not currently practical for many laboratories. Because of the distinctive morphology and size of HCV, virus particles have been occasionally recognized by electron microscopic examination of clinical specimens. Antigen detection methods, using immunofluorescence of respiratory cells or enzyme-linked immunosorbent assay (ELISA) of respiratory secretions, have been reported (6, 11). The development of murine monoclonal antibodies will likely enhance the sensitivity, specificity, and convenience of these approaches (2). Nucleic acid hybridiza-

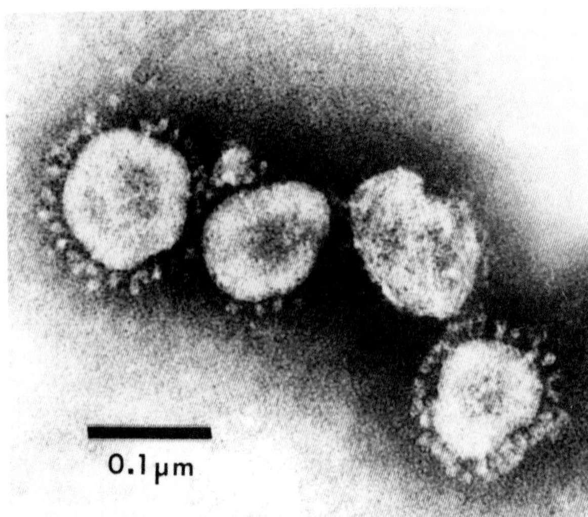

FIG. 1. Electron micrograph of HCV 229E, demonstrating the petal-shaped peplomers projecting from the envelope surfaces. (Courtesy of Claire M. Payne and Charles Bjore.)

tion has also been used experimentally to detect HCV 229E in nasal washings (13).

ISOLATION OF VIRUS

Primary isolation of HCV is difficult. HCV 299E can be cultivated in several human diploid fibroblast cell strains or lines, but organ cultures remain the system of choice for HCV OC43. Details of organ culture methods for HCV isolation have been described (15). Both viruses can be adapted to replicate in a variety of diploid and heteroploid cell lines, and OC43 strains have been adapted in vivo in suckling mouse brains. For the isolation of HCV 229E, the procedure described for rhinovirus isolation in chapter 84 is recommended.

HCV 229E can produce focal degenerative changes upon initial isolation in human diploid cell cultures, but these changes are frequently minimal, and an additional passage may be required before the cytopathic effect is readily visible. Eventually, with additional passage, the cytopathic effect becomes more granular in appearance, the cells detach from the glass surface, and degenerative changes eventually involve the entire cell monolayer.

IDENTIFICATION OF VIRUS

An isolate can be presumptively identified as a coronavirus by determining that it possesses the essential characteristics of the family *Coronaviridae:* ether and acid lability, virus growth in the presence of DNA inhibitors, and typical size and morphology in the electron microscope. Details of these methods have been published (3). Definitive serological identification of HCV 229E is made by the neutralization test in human diploid cells (15).

A group-specific mouse monoclonal antibody to coronaviruses is commercially available, and strain-specific monoclonal antibodies are now emerging (2). These, as well as some polyclonal antibodies, may be shown to be convenient for virus identification by immunofluorescence or ELISA.

SEROLOGICAL DIAGNOSIS

In most instances, the diagnosis of HCV infection has been made by demonstrating a fourfold or greater increase in antibody. The neutralization and complement fixation tests have been used for both virus types. The hemagglutination inhibition test has had broad acceptance for HCV OC43; however, it is important to test and, if necessary, treat the sera for the presence of nonspecific inhibitors (10). More recently, ELISA has been reported to be quite sensitive (9, 16), and indirect immunofluorescence testing can also be applied.

The neutralization test is performed in human diploid cells, using a virus challenge dose of 32 to 100 50% tissue culture infective doses.

Complement-fixing antigens are readily prepared in human diploid cells for HCV 229E and OC43. In addition, infected suckling mouse brain is an excellent source of complement-fixing HCV OC43 antigen. The general procedure for the complement fixation test is as described by Palmer et al. (14).

EVALUATION AND INTERPRETATION OF RESULTS

The fastidious nature of the HCV group has been a serious impediment to developing a better understanding of the natural history of these viruses. Because of these difficulties, diagnoses have usually been made serologically. Hopefully, the wider availability of better immunological reagents for direct virus detection will facilitate more routine and rapid diagnosis in the future.

There is usually an active antibody response to HCV infections that can confer some resistance to reinfection for a year or longer. However, it appears that sufficient antigenic heterogeneity exists among variants of the same strain to allow multiple, symptomatic reinfections to occur.

LITERATURE CITED

1. **Bradburne, A. F., M. L. Bynoe, and D. A. J. Tyrrell.** 1967. Effects of the "new" human respiratory virus in volunteers. Br. Med. J. **3:**767–769.
2. **Fleming, J. O., F. A. K. El Zaatari, W. Gilmore, J. D. Berne, J. S. Burks, S. A. Stohlman, W. W. Tourtellotte, and L. P. Weiner.** 1988. Antigenic assessment of coronaviruses isolated from patients with multiple sclerosis. Arch. Neurol. **45:**629–633.
3. **Hamparian, V. V.** 1979. Rhinoviruses, p. 535–575. *In* E. H. Lennette and N. J. Schmidt (ed.), Diagnostic procedures for viral and rickettsial infections. American Public Health Association, Inc., New York.
4. **Hamre, D., and J. J. Procknow.** 1966. A new virus isolated from the human respiratory tract. Proc. Soc. Exp. Biol. Med. **121:**190–193.
5. **Hovi, T. H., H. Kainulainen, B. Ziola, and A. Salmi.** 1979. OC-43 strain related coronavirus antibodies in different age groups. J. Med. Virol. **3:**313–320.
6. **Isaacs, D., D. Flowers, J. R. Clarke, H. B. Valman, and M. R. MacNaughton.** 1983. Epidemiology of coronavirus respiratory infections. Arch. Dis. Child. **59:**500–503.
7. **Kaye, H. S., and W. R. Dowdle.** 1975. Seroepidemiologic survey of coronavirus (strain 229E) infections in a population of children. Am. J. Epidemiol. **101:**238–244.
8. **Kaye, H. S., H. B. Marsh, and W. R. Dowdle.** 1971. Seroepidemiologic survey of coronavirus (strain OC43) related infection in a children's population. Am. J. Epidemiol. **94:**43–49.
9. **Kraaijeveld, C. A., S. E. Reed, and M. R. MacNaughton.**

1980. Enzyme-linked immunosorbent assay for the detection of antibody in volunteers experimentally infected with human coronavirus strain 229E. J. Clin. Microbiol. **12:**493–497.

10. **McIntosh, K., E. F. Ellis, L. S. Hoffman, T. G. Lybass, J. J. Eller, and V. A. Fulginiti.** 1973. The association of viral and bacterial respiratory infections with exacerbations of wheezing in young asthmatic children. J. Pediatr. **82:**578–593.
11. **McIntosh, K., J. McQuillin, S. E. Reed, and P. S. Gardner.** 1978. Diagnosis of human coronavirus infection by immunofluorescence: method and application to respiratory disease in hospitalized children. J. Med. Virol. **2:** 341–346.
12. **Monto, A. S., and S. K. Lim.** 1974. The Tecumseh study of respiratory illness. VI. Frequency of and relationship between outbreaks of coronavirus infections. J. Infect. Dis. **129:**271–276.
13. **Myint, S., S. Siddell, and D. Tyrrell.** 1989. The use of nucleic acid hybridization to detect human coronaviruses. Arch. Virol. **104:**335–337.
14. **Palmer, D. F., L. Kaufman, W. Kaplan, and J. J. Cavallaro.** 1977. Serodiagnosis of mycotic diseases. Charles C Thomas, Publisher, Springfield, Ill.
15. **Schieble, J. H., and A. Z. Kapikian.** 1979. Coronaviruses, p. 709–723. *In* E. H. Lennette and N. J. Schmidt (ed.), Diagnostic procedures for viral and rickettsial infections. American Public Health Association, Inc., New York.
16. **Schmidt, O. W., I. D. Allan, M. K. Cooney, H. M. Foy, and J. P. Fox.** 1986. Rises in titers of antibody to human coronaviruses OC43 and 229E in Seattle families during 1975–1979. Am. J. Epidemiol. **123:**862–868.
17. **Tyrrell, D. A. J., and M. L. Bynoe.** 1965. Cultivation of a novel type of common-cold virus in organ cultures. Br. Med. J. **1:**1467–1470.
18. **Vlasak, R., W. Luytjes, W. Spaan, and P. Palese.** 1988. Human and bovine coronaviruses recognize sialic acid-containing receptors similar to those of influenza C viruses. Proc. Natl. Acad. Sci. USA **85:**4526–4529.
19. **Wenzel, R. P., J. O. Hendley, J. A. Davies, and J. M. Gwaltney, Jr.** 1974. Coronavirus infections in military recruits. Am. Rev. Respir. Dis. **109:**621–624.

Chapter 86

Adenoviruses

JOHN C. HIERHOLZER

CLINICAL BACKGROUND

Adenoviruses have been recovered from virtually every organ system of humans and have been associated with many clinical syndromes (Table 1). Adenovirus illnesses are endemic throughout the year and occur in all age groups, although they are most common among school-age children, for whom approximately 50% of the infections are asymptomatic. They cause localized outbreaks of respiratory disease in the winter and spring, outbreaks of swimming pool-associated pharyngoconjunctival fever in the summer, and epidemics of keratoconjunctivitis associated with industrial eye trauma or ophthalmologic procedures at any time of the year. Adenoviruses cause 5 to 15% of cases of gastroenteritis in infants and preschool children (3, 25). Epidemics of acute respiratory disease that can occur whenever new military recruits are housed together are now preventable by active immunization with the appropriate serotypes in enteric-coated capsules (24). Of the 47 serotypes so far described, the most common are types 1 to 8, 11, 21, 35, 37, and 40 (1–3, 5, 8, 12, 13, 20, 21, 25, 27–30).

Upper respiratory illness caused by adenoviruses can be in the form of common colds, pharyngitis, or tonsillitis and occurs chiefly in infants and young children. It is associated primarily with types 1 to 7 (5, 20, 21). Findings include coryza, fever, cough, exudate on the pharyngeal walls, a granular appearance of the mucosa, and tender, enlarged cervical nodes. A notable feature of infection with types 1, 2, 5, and 6 is the persistence of virus in a latent state in adenoidal and tonsillar tissues in about 50% of infected children. Another epidemiologically important feature is the excretion of virus in the stool for many months without recurrence of symptoms.

Lower respiratory illness, including bronchitis, bronchiolitis, and pneumonia, often complicates adenovirus infection. Severe pneumonia, sometimes fatal, occurs in infants and children and rarely in adults; it is caused primarily by types 3, 4, 7, and 21 (5, 20–23). Extrapulmonary signs, such as renal involvement, hepatomegaly, and encephalomeningitis, can be seen, especially in infants and immunocompromised patients, and in such patients the generalized disease usually has a fatal outcome. Some children who recover from type 3, 7, or 21 pneumonia have residual lung disease. A cough syndrome similar to whooping cough has been reported in children after type 5 and rarely type 1, 2, and 3 infections (12).

Pharyngoconjunctival fever is characterized by fever, pharyngitis, conjunctivitis, and cervical lymphadenopathy, often with headache, diarrhea, and rash. Typical illness with follicular conjunctivitis is generally evident 5 to 6 days after exposure, with infected individuals shedding virus for about 10 days. Types 1 to 7 are usually incriminated in these infections (20, 21).

Epidemic keratoconjunctivitis (EKC) as sporadic cases is caused by many adenoviruses, but in epidemic form it is caused by type 8, 19, or 37 (17, 30). This severe eye disease becomes apparent after an 8- to 10-day silent incubation period. The initial onset of follicular conjunctivitis with preauricular lymphadenopathy can be accompanied by headache, malaise, and, depending on the serotype, mild upper respiratory illness. After 1 to 2 weeks of these symptoms, subepithelial corneal keratitis develops that may persist for an extended period. Contaminated eye instruments, ophthalmic wash solutions, hands of medical personnel, and towels are the vehicles by which ocular infections are spread to susceptible persons; thus, most cases of EKC in nonindustrial communities are spread iatrogenically. Spread of adenoviruses in eye clinics can be eliminated, however, by triaging patients, cohorting patients and staff, thorough hand washing, using unit-dosage eyedrops, avoiding invasive procedures on patients with EKC, and properly disinfecting equipment and surfaces. In industrial settings with high levels of airborne particulates, EKC outbreaks have resulted from eye-fomite-eye transmission. Trauma to the corneal epithelium is required for initiating virus infection, particularly with type 8. In type 19- or 37-associated EKC, infection can spread to the eye from respiratory or genital sites (11, 12, 27).

Acute hemorrhagic conjunctivitis and acute hemorrhagic cystitis are both sometimes caused by type 11 and rarely by type 21. The virus is readily recovered from eye secretions or urine, as appropriate (4, 12).

Immunocompromised host disease in patients with severe combined immune deficiency, patients with kidney, liver, and marrow transplants or undergoing cancer chemotherapy, and those with AIDS is a major problem because these infections are often fatal. Adenoviruses cause generalized illness in perhaps 10% of such patients; virus has been recovered from brain, throat, leukocytes, lung, urine, stool, cerebrospinal fluid, kidney, liver, and pancreas (4, 12, 13, 28).

Gastroenteritis and related syndromes have been associated with adenovirus infection in infants and children (12, 21). Types 40 and 41 and to a lesser extent 2 and 31 cause acute gastroenteritis (3, 6, 9, 10, 14, 15, 25).

Neurologic disease is sometimes caused by adenoviruses, usually as part of multisystem disease, with type 7 being particularly severe. Reye's syndrome is infrequently associated with the childhood serotypes, especially type 3. Types 1 to 3, 6, 7, 12, and 32 have been isolated from cerebrospinal fluid or brain tissue (12, 21).

TABLE 1. Adenovirus infections and serotypes involved

Syndrome	Signs and symptoms	Serotypes involved	
		Frequently	Infrequently
Upper respiratory illness	Coryza, pharyngitis, fever, tonsillitis, diarrhea	1–3, 5, 7	4, 6, 11, 18, 21, 29, 31
Lower respiratory illness	Bronchitis, pneumonia, fever, coryza, cough	3, 4, 7, 21	1, 2, 5, 35
Pertussis syndrome	Paroxysmal cough, vomiting, fever, upper respiratory illness	5	1–3
Acute respiratory disease	Tracheobronchitis, fever, myalgia, coryza, pneumonia	4, 7	3, 14, 21, 35
Pharyngoconjunctival fever	Pharyngitis, conjunctivitis, fever, coryza, headache, diarrhea, rash, nodes	3, 4, 7	1, 11, 14, 16, 19, 37
Epidemic keratoconjunctivitis	Keratitis, headache, preauricular nodes, coryza, pharyngitis, diarrhea	8, 19, 37	3, 4, 7, 10, 11, 21
Acute hemorrhagic conjunctivitis	Chemosis, follicles, subconjunctival hemorrhage, preauricular nodes, fever	11	2–8, 14, 15, 19, 37
Cystitis	Cystitis (usually hemorrhagic), fever, pharyngitis	11	7, 21, 34, 35
Immunocompromised host disease	Diarrhea, rash, upper respiratory illness, pneumonia; hepatitis, cystitis, otitis media	11, 34, 35	1, 2, 5, 7, 21, 29, 31, 37–39
Gastroenteritis (infant)	Diarrhea, fever, nausea, vomiting, mild upper respiratory illness	31, 40, 41	1, 2, 12–17, 21, 25, 26, 29
Central nervous system disease	Meningitis, encephalitis, Reye's syndrome	7	3, 32
Venereal disease	Ulcerative genital lesions, urethritis, cervicitis	2, 19, 37	1, 5, 7, 11, 18, 31

Serotypes 2, 19, and 37 have been recovered from herpeslike genital lesions, often associated with orchitis, cervicitis, or urethritis. Other syndromes have also been described (11, 12, 21). Finally, adenoviruses are often incriminated in nosocomial transmission. This is not surprising because (i) adenoviruses cause 10% of the pneumonia cases in hospitalized children, (ii) intensive supportive therapy is required for these patients, (iii) adenoviruses are shed for long periods in the stool and are transmissible both by fomites and by aerosolized droplets, and (iv) the viruses can readily infect respiratory and ocular tissues of other patients and of susceptible hospital personnel (3, 5, 8, 20, 21, 23).

DESCRIPTION OF AGENT

Human adenoviruses are nonenveloped, double-stranded DNA viruses of the family *Adenoviridae*, genus *Mastadenovirus*. They are 70 to 90 nm in diameter and icosahedral in shape, comprising 10 structural proteins of molecular weight 5,000 to 120,000. They have a buoyant density in cesium chloride of 1.33 to 1.34 g/cm^3 and a molecular weight by sedimentation coefficient of 170×10^6 to 175×10^6.

Adenoviruses replicate in the cell nucleus and tend to be host species specific. The viruses produce a characteristic cytopathic effect (CPE) that is accompanied by accumulation of multiple antigenic components and organic acids in the host cell culture fluids. Adenoviruses do not hemadsorb erythrocytes (RBC) or replicate in embryonated chicken eggs; all possess genus-specific antigenic determinants on the hexon capsomeres. The capsid proteins of adenoviruses are arranged in an icosahedron having 20 triangular faces and 12 vertices. In each virion are 240 hexons and 12 pentons. The hexons are dispersed on the triangular faces and edges, and the pentons are located in the vertices of the icosahedron. Each penton consists of a base (or vertex capsomere) and a fiber which is a rodlike outward projection of variable length with a terminal knob. Inside the capsid is a single molecule of linear, double-stranded DNA of molecular weight 20×10^6 to 30×10^6. The G+C base composition of the genome for the different human adenoviruses ranges from 47 to 60% (19, 26, 27).

Crude suspensions of most adenoviruses are stable for prolonged periods at −20 to −100°C at pH 6 to 9. Infectious virus is rapidly inactivated at 56°C and by exposure to 0.25% sodium dodecyl sulfate, free chlorine at 0.5 μg/ml, UV irradiation, or 1:400 to 1:4,000 concentrations of Formalin. The agents are not affected by treatment with ether or chloroform, and they can be readily lyophilized without special precautions. The lyophilized viruses appear to retain their infectivity indefinitely at 4°C, −10°C, or below.

A classification scheme based on hemagglutination (HA) properties allows a useful separation of the human adenoviruses into six subgroups (Table 2). The scheme is based primarily on complete agglutination of monkey or rat RBC, partial agglutination of rat RBC, and level (titer) of agglutination and secondarily on complete agglutination of human, chicken, and other RBC. Other viral properties such as antigenic relationships, oncogenicity, fiber length, percent DNA homology within and between subgroups, percent G+C content of the DNA, number of cleavage fragments after digestion with *Sma*I endonuclease, and molecular weight of certain internal proteins tend to coincide with this classification (2, 12, 14, 19, 26, 27).

The replication of adenoviruses is accompanied by the excess formation of antigenic components liberated into the culture fluids as soluble antigens. These proteins are complex structures that carry many antigenic determinants; in particular, the hexons, vertex capsomeres, and fibers possess distinct type- and subgroup-specific antigens. The type-specific determinants on the hexon and fiber are exposed on the surface of the virion and give rise to serum neutralizing (SN) antibodies. In addition, the fiber is a strong hemagglutinin and thus elicits hemagglutination inhibition (HI) antibodies. The genus-specific antigen is the principal determinant on the hexon but resides on the internal part of the capsid and thus is not exposed externally and does not elicit protective antibodies. The vertex capsomere is the toxic factor seen in overinoculated cultures. Additional determinants on these components evoke heterotypic SN and HI antibody responses. These determinants are mostly subgroup specific, although intersubgroup relationships may exist (19, 27).

The complete agglutination of monkey and rat RBC by adenoviruses of subgroups B and D is associated with intact virus particles and three forms of soluble hemagglutinins. The complete soluble forms consist of dodecons (groups of 12 pentons), dimers of pentons, and dimers of fibers. The partial agglutination of rat RBC seen with subgroup C viruses is due to the relative excess of monomeric pentons and fibers in cell culture fluids. These soluble antigens, however, produce complete agglutination of rat RBC in the presence of a heterotypic subgroup C antiserum in the test diluent (19, 21, 27). Thus, the adenovirus components have specific biological properties and serological reactivities, which form the basis of many laboratory tests.

COLLECTION AND STORAGE OF SPECIMENS

Adenoviruses are stable viruses and are readily recovered from obvious sites of infection. Nasopharyngeal swabs or aspirates, nasal swabs or aspirates, swabs of eye exudates, stool or rectal swabs, urine, urethral or cervical swabs, and biopsy or autopsy tissues are all adequate specimens as dictated by the symptoms. Viral detection rates are greatly enhanced by proper collection of specimens early in the disease and by prompt cold or frozen shipment to the laboratory. Details of collection of respiratory, conjunctival, rectal, and other specimens are described in chapter 74.

Paired blood samples are needed to establish or confirm a diagnosis by serological methods. The first specimen should be collected as soon as possible after the onset of symptoms, and the second should be collected 2 to 4 weeks later. After clotting, serum is separated under sterile conditions and stored at −10 to −20°C.

DIRECT EXAMINATION

Many methods have been used for direct detection of adenoviruses in clinical materials, and research in this area is still keen because of the ongoing need to quickly and accurately diagnose a viral infection. Electron microscopy and immunoelectron microscopy have been the principal means of identifying adenoviruses in clinical materials. In one procedure, tissue sections obtained at biopsy or autopsy are fixed, stained, and examined for inclusions or crystalline arrays of mature virions in the cell nucleus. In the other method, specimens of respiratory secretions, urine, or stool (as 10 to 20% extracts) are clarified and observed directly by pseudoreplica negative-stain electron microscopy. Sensitivity is increased by concentrating the specimen (in the case of throat or nasal wash, bronchial aspirate, and urine) by ultracentrifugation or membrane ultrafiltration. Sensitivity is further increased by immunoelectron microscopy, in which the specimen (whether concentrated or not) is incubated with a hyperimmune antiserum or a human convalescent serum before grids are prepared for electron microscopy; aggregates of virus particles then indicate both the viral morphology and a specific reaction with the serum used. The first method has proven useful for diagnosis in tissue samples and for pathological studies. The latter has been highly useful for diagnosis of adenovirus gastroenteritis (6, 15).

For immunofluorescence assay (IFA) examination, cells in unfrozen specimens are washed, suspended in phosphate-buffered saline (PBS), fixed on slides in acetone, and reacted with antihexon serum and antiglobulin conjugate (see chapter 11). Dense nuclear and stippled cytoplasmic staining are positive reactions for adenoviruses. A sensitive extension of IFA is the time-resolved fluoroimmunoassay, in which a purified adenovirus monoclonal antibody (MAb) is used as capture

TABLE 2. Subdivision of the human adenoviruses by HA properties[a]

Subgroup	Serotypes	Oncogenicity	HA subgroup	HA titers with:
A	12, 18, 31	High	3B[b]	Rat (incomplete)
B	3, 7, 11, 16, 34, 35	Weak	1A	Monkey
	14, 21	Weak	1B[c]	Monkey
C	1, 2, 5, 6	Negative	3A	Rat (incomplete)
D	8, 9, 37	Negative	2A	Rat, mouse, human, guinea pig, dog
	10, 19, 26, 27, 36, 38, 39	Negative	2B	Rat, mouse, human
	13, 43	Negative	2C	Rat, mouse, human, monkey
	15, 22, 23, 30, 44, 45, 46, 47	Negative	2D	Rat, mouse, monkey
	17, 24, 32, 33, 42	Negative	2E	Rat, mouse
	20, 25, 28, 29	Negative	2F[c]	Rat (atypical), monkey
E	4	Negative	3A	Rat (incomplete)
F	40, 41	Negative	3A[c]	Rat (atypical)

[a] Adapted from reference 12.
[b] Very low HA titers.
[c] Moderate-range HA titers.

antibody in plastic wells, the specimen is added to the wells, and a europium-labeled adenovirus MAb is used as the detector antibody. The specific fluorescence of the sample is measured by a fluorometer after a time delay to allow the autofluorescence to decay (12, 22).

For antigen detection by enzyme immunoassay (EIA), a polyclonal capture antibody is adsorbed to the plates, and then antigens or specimens, a second polyclonal antibody (detector) from a different animal species, enzyme-conjugated antispecies antibody, and the substrate or color system are added in that order (see chapter 12). Sensitivity is increased by using MAbs at the detector antibody position and further increased by using MAbs in both positions in the assay (12, 15).

Radioimmunoassay is equal in sensitivity and ease of performance to EIA but carries the problem of disposal of the radioactive wastes produced. Radioimmunoassay tests have been used to detect adenoviruses in respiratory secretions and stool specimens (16). Counterelectrophoresis is a convenient test for detecting adenoviruses in toxic and environmental samples but is not as sensitive as EIA. This technique has identified adenovirus antigens in swimming pool water, serum specimens, ophthalmic drops used in eye clinics, and stool specimens (12).

Restriction enzyme (RE) analysis has found limited application in direct detection, being useful only for finding types 40 and 41 in stool specimens (3, 25). The most recent concept for direct detection of adenoviruses is DNA probe technology (see chapter 17). Labeled probes have been most successful with enteric adenoviruses (9, 12, 18).

ISOLATION OF VIRUS

All of the human adenoviruses except types 40 and 41 replicate and produce CPE in continuous human cell lines of epithelial origin such as HeLa, KB, or HEp-2, in primary human embryonic kidney (HEK) cells, and, after adaptation, in human embryonic lung fibroblasts (HELF, WI-38, and MRC-5) and other embryonic fibroblast cells. Types 40 and 41 replicate poorly in the aforementioned cells but do grow to consistent (but low) titers in tertiary cynomolgus monkey kidney cells and in the Graham-293 adenovirus type 5-transformed secondary HEK cell line. For cultivating adenoviruses, Eagle minimal essential medium supplemented with 2% heat-inactivated fetal calf serum and antibiotics is satisfactory as a maintenance medium. Infected cells become enlarged, rounded, and very refractile, and they aggregate into irregular clusters typical of adenovirus CPE (3, 5, 6, 8, 10, 14).

Preparation of the specimen for isolation is important. Respiratory and urine specimens are treated with antibiotics and clarified by low-speed centrifugation for 3 min to remove cells, fibers, and other debris. Stool specimens are brought to 10 to 20% suspensions with PBS or maintenance medium, shaken with glass beads if necessary, and clarified by centrifugation for 30 min. Biopsy or autopsy tissue specimens are minced into small fragments by using sterile surgical scissors and then homogenized in a glass tissue grinder or in a sterile mortar with a sand abrasive and 5 ml of PBS or maintenance medium. A 10 to 20% suspension is made in this manner and then clarified by low-speed centrifugation. Blood monocytes are prepared for culture by applying 3 ml of heparinized blood cells on a Ficoll-Hypaque gradient. The cells are washed and suspended in RPMI medium with 20% fetal calf serum to a final concentration of 1.5×10^6 cells per ml. Portions (0.5 ml) of the cell suspensions are then placed on human embryonic fibroblast feeder monolayers for cocultivation.

Specimens are inoculated onto cell cultures as soon as practical after they are received. Undiluted test material (0.4 to 0.5 ml) is inoculated into one or two cell culture tubes, adsorbed for 1 h at ambient temperature, overlayed with 1 ml of maintenance medium, and incubated at 35 to 36°C either stationary or on a roller drum. Several uninoculated tubes of each cell type used should be incubated and observed for evidence of nonspecific cellular degeneration and for eventual use as negative controls in identity tests. Sometimes, inoculation of a clinical specimen, especially stool, blood, and urine, leads to transient or irreparable toxic effects on cell culture. Such toxicity is apparent within 24 h but can be minimized by washing the cell cultures or at least decanting the inoculum after the 1-h adsorption period. All cultures should be read for CPE twice a week, fed with fresh maintenance medium as required, and subpassaged once after 2 weeks (for HEK and fibroblast cells) or three times at weekly intervals (for continuous epithelial cells), so that all cultures are held and read for at least 28 days. This regimen will yield highest isolation rates. For identification, degeneration should progress until all the cells are affected (4+ CPE) in order to obtain sufficient yields of soluble antigens, hemagglutinins, and infectious virus for identifying the isolate. Soluble antigen yields are highest in HEp-2 and KB cells; infectious virus yields are highest in HEK cells for types 1 to 39 and 42 to 47 and in Graham-293 cells for types 40 and 41.

IDENTIFICATION OF VIRUS

Grouping tests

All of the tests used for direct detection are also used for identifying an isolate as adenovirus. Immunoelectron microscopy, IFA, time-resolved fluoroimmunoassay, and radioimmunoassay are solely genus-specific tests. Counterelectrophoresis, EIA, and DNA hybridization assays are genus specific but can be made type specific if selected antisera, MAbs, or DNA fragments are used, as appropriate. RE analysis is type specific if the electrophoretic pattern matches that of a prototype strain (which is unlikely); no antisera are used. It is apparent, therefore, that the test procedure selected is determined by the level of typing desired. In general, an IFA, EIA, or complement fixation (CF) test is used to classify an isolate as a member of the family *Adenoviridae;* then, agglutination with monkey, human, and rat RBC is used to place the virus into a subgroup; finally, HI and SN tests with selected antisera are used to serotype the virus.

The genus-specific IFA, EIA, and CF tests are based on the reactions of soluble hexons in the supernatant fluids and antihexon serum that is readily made in any animal. Procedures for the IFA and EIA tests are described in chapters 11 and 12); the CF test is described below (see Serological Diagnosis). The choice of test system to use depends on convenience; all will easily identify hexons in cell supernatants.

Typing tests

Adenovirus serotyping is based on type-specific neutralization, although HI is a more practical and convenient test (12, 21, 27). In laboratories unable to procure fresh RBC for HA and HI tests, the only typing method available is SN. In this case, antisera to types 1 to 8, 11, 21, 35, and 37 should be routinely included unless clinical or epidemiological data for the isolate suggest a smaller set of sera (Table 1).

HI test

Microtiter HA and HI tests are performed in either flexible or hard plastic U plates. Serial twofold dilutions (1:2 to 1:4,096) of the isolate in 0.05-ml volumes are prepared in plain PBS diluent, in PBS with 1% type 4 antiserum (for subgroup C strains), and in PBS with 1% type 6 antiserum (for subgroup E). (The type 4 and 6 animal antisera are required for adenoviruses giving incomplete HA patterns. The sera should have titers of at least 1:320, be heat inactivated at 56°C for 30 min, and be absorbed with rat RBC. The absorption is performed by adding 0.1 ml of RBC for every 1.0 ml of a 1:10 dilution of serum, incubating the mixture overnight at 4°C, and pelleting the cells by centrifugation at 1,800 × *g* for 5 min at 4°C.)

RBC are collected and stored in Alsever solution in the usual fashion. Monkey and rat RBC must be handled gently and used within 4 days of collection; immediately before use, the RBC are washed and adjusted to 0.4% in PBS. An equal volume of 0.4% rhesus or vervet RBC is now added to one set of duplicate PBS diluent dilutions, and rat RBC are added to others. The same volume of each RBC suspension is added to two separate wells containing 0.05 ml of each type of diluent to serve as cell controls. The plates are then covered with tape, shaken gently, and incubated in a 37°C water bath for 1 h. After this time, the RBC control wells should exhibit complete sedimentation and a teardrop pattern when the plates are slightly tilted. An HA titer is defined as the reciprocal of the highest dilution of virus that shows complete HA; the dilution endpoint is then considered to contain 1 HA unit per 0.05 ml. The pattern of HA titers with monkey, human, and rat RBC in the PBS diluent, and with rat RBC in the heterotypic serum diluent, thus defines the subgroup to which the isolate belongs (Table 2) (12).

For HI, the typing antisera are heat inactivated and absorbed with the appropriate RBC as described above for type 4 and 6 immune sera. The antisera are diluted serially in 0.025-ml amounts in PBS diluent, and the virus at 4 HA units per 0.025 ml (i.e., the HA titer divided by 8) is added to each well. For a subgroup C or E isolate, antiserum dilutions are prepared in the appropriate heterotypic serum diluent as described above. The mixtures are agitated briefly and incubated at ambient temperature for 1 h before the appropriate RBC suspension is added (at 0.05 ml per well). A back-titration, i.e., serial twofold dilutions of the test antigen dose (0.05 ml in 0.05 ml of PBS or heterotypic serum diluent, as appropriate), and cell controls are included in each test. The plates are incubated in the 37°C water bath for 1 h. After this time, the first four serial dilutions of the back-titration should exhibit a complete HA pattern, thus indicating that the proper antigen dose was used in the test. The isolate is identified by the typing serum which completely inhibits HA to or near the known homologous titer of the antiserum. Cross-reactions may be observed within antisera of the same subgroup; these are discussed below (see Evaluation, Interpretation, and Reporting of Results). Further characterization of the isolate may be obtained with the appropriate antisera in SN tests.

SN tests

SN tests are readable with definitive results and are the closest approximation the laboratory has to the human serum response after infection but are not as convenient to run as HA and HI tests. Three types of SN test can be carried out: the 7-day test in epithelial cell cultures, the 3-day test in monkey kidney cells, and microneutralization tests (5, 8, 12, 14, 21).

Conventional 7-day SN tests may be carried out in HEp-2, KB, HeLa, HEK, or Graham-293 cells. The virus isolate must be titrated for infectivity in the cells to be used in the test by preparing serial 10-fold dilutions of virus in Hanks balanced salt solution and inoculating the tubes in triplicate with 0.1 ml of dilution. After 7 days of incubation at 36°C, the endpoint (or titer) is read by CPE and is considered to be 1 50% tissue culture infective dose ($TCID_{50}$) of virus per 0.1 ml. Since the slow and inconsistent development of CPE at high dilutions of an adenovirus culture tends to obscure the endpoint, a working dilution of virus is used which has a titer of 100 $TCID_{50}$ per 0.1 ml. Type-specific antisera are then selected for the SN test, heat inactivated at 56°C for 30 min, and diluted in Hanks balanced salt solution in a twofold series from 1:10 to 1:1,280 (or slightly beyond the homologous titer of each antiserum). For the SN step, 0.3 ml of virus dilution is mixed with 0.3 ml of each antiserum dilution, incubated at ambient temperature for 1 h, and inoculated onto fresh cell cultures in triplicate at 0.2 ml per tube. Uninoculated cell controls and a back-titration, consisting of a 10-fold dilution series from the working dilution used in the test, are included in the test. The tubes are incubated, fed, and read as usual, with the final reading taken at 7 days. The back-titration should show CPE ending around the second dilution. As in the HI test, the virus type is indicated by inhibition (of CPE) to or near the homologous titer of an antiserum. The antibody endpoint is thus defined as the reciprocal of the highest dilution of serum which completely neutralizes CPE.

The most widely used SN procedure is the 3-day test in primary rhesus monkey kidney cell cultures. This test does not measure inhibition of infectivity but rather measures inhibition of the viral toxicity induced by the vertex capsomere. If primary rhesus monkey kidney cells are not available, the test can be done in established monkey kidney lines such as Vero, LLC-MK2, or BSC-1. To determine the challenge dose of virus to be used in the test, 0.1 ml of each serial twofold dilution (1:1 to 1:128) prepared in maintenance medium is inoculated into three cell cultures that contain 1 ml of maintenance medium. The titration is incubated at 35 to 36°C, and the degree of CPE is read at 3 days. The highest dilution of virus producing 1+ to 2+ CPE (i.e., 25 to 50% of the cell sheet is affected) in the cells at 3 days is considered the endpoint, and the virus dose to be used in the SN test is one dilution back from this endpoint. As described above, the selected antisera are heat inactivated, diluted serially to encompass the known homologous antibody titer of each, mixed with an equal volume (0.3 ml) of the isolate dilution, and incubated at ambient temperature for 1 h. Then 0.2 ml of each virus-serum mixture is inoculated onto fresh cells in triplicate. Uninoculated cell control tubes and three virus control tubes, consisting of 0.1 ml of the working dilution used in the test, are included in the test. The tubes are incubated, fed, and read as usual, with the final reading taken at 3 days. At this time, the virus controls should show 1+ to 2+ CPE; the virus type is indicated by inhibition of CPE to or near the homologous titer of an antiserum.

Microneutralization tests can be done in secondary rhesus monkey kidney cells, Vero cells, and HEp-2 cells. In the Vero test, the virus titration is performed in flat-bottom 96-well plates in replicas of six, with the virus being serially diluted in growth medium by an automatic diluter with flame-sterilized loops, manually with a multichannel pipettor, or automatically with a programmable diluter and disposable tips. Then 0.05 ml of a Vero cell suspension at 175,000 cells per ml is dropped into all wells, including cell control wells. The plate is gently shaken, sealed with sterile tape or lid, incubated at 35 to 36°C for 5 days, and read by staining with a crystal violet-formaldehyde solution. The endpoint is the highest dilution of virus showing 0 to 1+ staining (4+ to 3+ CPE) in 5 days. SN tests then utilize serial dilutions of heat-inactivated antisera made with sterile diluting equipment as described above, 2 U of virus (one dilution back from the endpoint) per well, and the cell suspension. Plates are sealed, incubated, and stained as described above. Cell controls and a virus back-titration should be included. The test is read visually for uninfected (stained) cells, and the antibody endpoint is defined as described above. Types 40 and 41 have peculiar features that separate them from the other adenoviruses with respect to growth and identification in cell cultures; recent reviews concerning the enteric adenoviruses should be consulted for details of these specialized procedures (3, 12, 14, 25, 27).

SEROLOGICAL DIAGNOSIS

Serodiagnosis is accomplished with an acute-phase and convalescent-phase serum pair collected at an interval of 2 to 4 weeks. The timing for collection of the convalescent-phase serum is not critical provided the acute-phase serum was taken early in the illness. Because of the ubiquity of the adenoviruses and the numerous cross-reactions between related serotypes, seroconversion involving a fourfold or greater rise in antibody titer is necessary to document infection. Adenovirus infection can be documented by a genus-reactive test such as CF or EIA, either of which can include the adenovirus antigen as part of a battery of antigens. For illnesses in which adenoviruses play an important role, such as acute respiratory disease, EKC, or pharyngoconjunctival fever, genus-reactive tests can be followed by type-specific tests to pinpoint the serotype involved, or the type-specific test alone can be carried out for the serotypes usually involved (8).

CF test

The CF test is the most widely used serological test for adenovirus infection and is the best standardized. The test antigen is commercially available or is easily made by propagating a common serotype in HEp-2 or KB cells and harvesting by three freeze-thaw cycles 2 or 3 days after 4+ CPE. The supernatant fluid after clarification serves as the CF antigen, which is tested for potency by block titrations against a reference human or animal antiserum. Alternatively, the sensitivity of the CF test can be improved by using a semipurified hexon preparation. The adenovirus CF antigen is stable and group specific, enabling it to detect all 47 human serotypes plus intermediate and atypical strains with equal reliability. Furthermore, it can be part of a battery of a dozen or more viral antigens tested simultaneously, thereby making the test cost effective and efficient in terms of labor and materials. The main disadvantage of the CF test is its low sensitivity; although CF titers are highly reproducible between tests and between laboratories, they detect infection in only 50 to 70% of cases in general and in <50% of cases in young children and in adenovirus-immunized military recruits (12, 16, 22, 24).

EIA

EIA is much more sensitive than CF and is becoming increasingly used in diagnostic laboratories (16). Good reagents and automated EIA readers are now commercially available. The test can be carried out either of two ways. In the first, a common adenovirus (e.g., type 2, 4, or 7) is cultured to produce a high titer of soluble antigens as for the CF antigen. After clarification and dialysis against an alkaline buffer, the supernatant fluid is added to each well of 96-well microdilution plates and incubated overnight at 4°C to prepare the solid-phase antigen. A purified or semipurified hexon preparation is preferable for this step because cellular and medium proteins as well as the type-specific soluble components (fiber, dodecon, etc.) would be removed. After three washes with PBS containing 0.5% gelatin and 0.15% Tween 20, serial dilutions (in PBS-gelatin-Tween 20) of the patient paired sera (1:200 to 1:25,600) are added to parallel rows, and the reaction is incubated at 37°C for 1.5 h. After another three washings, a commercially available anti-human immunoglobulin G (IgG)-peroxidase conjugate at about a 1:1,000 dilution in PBS-gelatin-Tween 20 is added. The plates are placed at 37°C for 1 h, washed, and developed for color (see chapter 12).

In the second procedure, ammonium sulfate-precipitated IgG from an adenovirus antiserum in alkaline buffer is attached to each well of a plate for the solid phase, to serve as the capture antibody. After washing, antigen (either crude or purified as described above) is added and the plates are incubated at 37°C for 1.5 h. The plates are again washed, and serial dilutions of the patient paired sera (the detector antibody) are added. The patient sera must be diluted (1:200 to 1:25,600) in PBS-gelatin-Tween 20 solution containing 1.5% heat-inactivated normal serum of the capture antibody species; this procedure greatly reduces the nonspecific background color. After another incubation at 37°C for 1.5 h and subsequent wash, the anti-human IgG-peroxidase conjugate is added and the plates are incubated at 37°C for 1 h. The plates are then washed and the substrate is added as described above.

Both procedures are highly sensitive and can be made

quite reproducible if adequate care is taken throughout the test. Controls should include negative virus (cell controls), reagent controls, and positive and negative human sera. The background color in a well-devised test should be negligible and, in most EIA readers, is automatically subtracted from the test serum readings.

HI test

HI and SN tests are more sensitive than the CF test and are capable of measuring type-specific antibody rises. Although some reagents are available commercially, most laboratories prepare their own stock cultures of the common adenovirus serotypes for use as HA antigens or infectious virus in HI and SN tests (12, 22, 27). Human serum specimens are treated for HI tests by heat inactivation (56°C, 30 min) and removal of nonspecific agglutinins by absorption with 50% suspensions of rhesus or rat erythrocytes, as appropriate. Sera are then diluted 1:8 to 1:1,024 in the microdilution plate, leaving 0.025 ml in each well. A virus suspension diluted to contain 4 HA units per 0.025 ml is added to each well; the contents are mixed gently and incubated at ambient temperature for 1 h. Then 0.05 ml of erythrocyte suspension is added per well, and the plate is agitated, sealed with tape, and incubated in a 37°C water bath for 1 h. A virus back-titration, serum controls, and cell controls should be included in the test. The endpoint (serum titer) is the highest dilution of serum that completely inhibits the hemagglutination of 4 HA units of virus.

SN tests

SN tests are performed as described above. Acute- and convalescent-phase serum specimens are inactivated at 56°C for 30 min and serially diluted (1:4 to 1: 512) in maintenance medium in sterile tubes, leaving 0.3 ml of each dilution in the tubes. To each tube is added 0.3 ml of the dilution of seed virus. The tubes are shaken and incubated at ambient temperature for 1 h, and 0.2 ml of each virus-serum mixture is then added to each of two cell cultures. A virus control is made with a 1:2 dilution of the working virus dilution used in the test and is inoculated at 0.2 ml per tube; a back-titration is made with four serial 10-fold dilutions of the working virus dilution and is inoculated at 0.1 ml per tube. Uninoculated or sham-inoculated tubes serve as cell controls. Occasionally, known positive and negative sera should be included in the test as a check on the entire system. The cultures are read daily, and the test is concluded when 32 to 320 $TCID_{50}$/0.1 ml is apparent in the virus back-titration. The highest serum dilution in which both tubes show no adenovirus CPE is considered the endpoint.

Alternatively, the 3-day test in MK cells or a micro-SN test such as in Vero cells may be carried out by the same principles. In both tests, cell controls and a virus back-titration should be included. The micro-SN test is ideal for serum surveys because a large number of tests can be carried out in a single run, with little cost in cells, media, and supplies. Also, the test is read visually for uninfected (stained) cells. A fourfold or greater increase in titer between the acute- and convalescent-phase sera is indicative of a type-specific seroconversion (12, 22, 27).

EVALUATION, INTERPRETATION, AND REPORTING OF RESULTS

IFA, CF, and EIA tests for antigen identify all human adenoviruses by the group-specific hexon-antihexon reaction. The three tests perform equally well for this task. HI and SN tests, being type specific, are subject to interpretative problems arising from the multitude of antigenic cross-reactions that occur among the human adenoviruses (7, 12, 14, 17, 19, 21, 22, 27, 29). For instance, all three viruses in subgroup A (Table 2) cross-react in SN tests. Types 12 and 18 exhibit a bilateral cross-reaction between themselves, and type 31 antisera cross-react with types 12 and 18 viruses. Among subgroup B viruses, the most significant reciprocal cross-reactions observed in both HI and SN tests are among types 7, 11, and 14 and between types 3 and 7. Types 34 and 35 are not readily discernible by HI but are by SN. The subgroup C viruses are devoid of any cross-reactions except in occasional antisera.

The major HI and SN cross-reactions in subgroup D do not always coincide, and therefore this subgroup presents the most difficulties in serotyping. Neither types 8 and 9, types 24, 32, and 33, types 10, 19, and 37, nor types 13, 38, and 39 are easily distinguishable by HI, but they are readily typed by SN. Other major HI cross-reactions are type 13 with type 30 and type 22 with type 15. Conversely, types 15, 23, and 29 are clearly identified by HI but are closely related by SN. Other cross-reactions in either test are unilateral and low titered.

A notable reciprocal intergroup cross-reaction, seen only in the SN test, occurs between type 4 (in subgroup E) and type 16 (in subgroup B). Type 4 also cross-reacts with types 40 and 41 of subgroup F. Type 40 is difficult to distinguish from type 41 by HI but can be distinguished by carefully constructed SN tests, EIA with MAbs, DNA hybridization probes, and RE analyses (25). Similarly, isolates with RE patterns different from that of the prototype are the rule rather than the exception, and these "DNA variants" appear to be common for all serotypes (1, 2, 12, 26, 27). Thus, RE patterns with selected enzymes are often part of the laboratory study of clinical isolates and have epidemiological value but can give misleading results when applied to serotyping (7, 10, 13, 28).

For serological tests, a significant rise in antibody titer (fourfold or greater) between the acute- and convalescent-phase sera is required for diagnosis or confirmation of infection. Consequently, the test cannot be performed until late in the convalescent period, when results are of lesser clinical importance than in the acute illness. Nevertheless, the results may be of epidemiological importance or of clinical interest in establishing an association of an unusual illness with adenovirus infection. Since CF and EIA tests detect antibody stimulated by infection with any human adenovirus, they are valuable only as screening tests for adenovirus infection; they will not yield information on the infecting serotype. Also, the CF test is less sensitive than the HI and SN tests, especially in younger children and in superficial infections such as conjunctivitis, and the EIA test is not yet standardized. For both tests, reagent controls (complement, hemolysin, etc. for CF; diluent, enzyme, etc. for EIA), antigen controls and back-titration, and positive and negative human serum controls should be included in the test for proper interpretation of results.

The HI and SN tests are more sensitive provided the infecting serotype is included as an antigen in these tests. Rises in antibody titers to heterotypic adenoviruses may occur with both HI and SN tests in as high as 25% of adult infections, generally between types of the same HA subgroup (12). For these reasons, serology on individual patients cannot be considered to establish the infecting serotype in the absence of virus isolation or epidemiological factors.

Whether an illness is due to adenovirus infection is a more difficult question. Many infections are asymptomatic and persistent. In infants, antibody may not develop until months after the onset of infection. Isolation of an adenovirus, and even serological evidence of infection, may be coincidental to a disease caused by infection with a different agent. On the other hand, isolation of an adenovirus (especially to high titer) from a diseased organ or its secretions, or previous epidemiological association of a syndrome with a particular adenovirus, is considered valid evidence that the adenovirus is the etiological agent of the illness.

LITERATURE CITED

1. **Adrian, T., M. Becker, J. C. Hierholzer, and R. Wigand.** 1989. Molecular epidemiology and restriction site mapping of adenovirus 7 genome types. Arch. Virol. **106:**73–84.
2. **Adrian, T., G. Wadell, J. C. Hierholzer, and R. Wigand.** 1986. DNA restriction analysis of adenovirus prototypes 1 to 41. Arch. Virol. **91:**277–290.
3. **Albert, M. J.** 1986. Enteric adenoviruses. Arch. Virol. **88:** 1–17.
4. **Ambinder, R. F., W. Burns, M. Forman, P. Charache, R. Arthur, W. Beschorner, G. Santos, and R. Saral.** 1986. Hemorrhagic cystitis associated with adenovirus infection in bone marrow transplantation. Arch. Intern. Med. **146:** 1400–1401.
5. **Brandt, C. D., H. W. Kim, A. J. Vargosko, et al.** 1969. Infections in 18,000 infants and children in a controlled study of respiratory tract disease. I. Adenovirus pathogenicity in relation to serologic type and illness syndrome. Am. J. Epidemiol. **90:**484–500.
6. **Brown, M., M. Petric, and P. J. Middleton.** 1984. Diagnosis of fastidious enteric adenoviruses 40 and 41 in stool specimens. J. Clin. Microbiol. **20:**334–338.
7. **de Jong, J. C., R. Wigand, G. Wadell, et al.** 1981. Adenovirus 37: identification and characterization of a medically important new adenovirus type of subgroup D. J. Med. Virol. **7:** 105–118.
8. **Fox, J. P., C. E. Hall, and M. K. Cooney.** 1977. The Seattle virus watch. VII. Observations of adenovirus infections. Am. J. Epidemiol. **105:**362–386.
9. **Hammond, G., C. Hannan, T. Yeh, K. Fischer, G. Mauthe, and S. E. Straus.** 1987. DNA hybridization for diagnosis of enteric adenovirus infection from directly spotted human fecal specimens. J. Clin. Microbiol. **25:** 1881–1885.
10. **Hammond, G. W., G. Mauthe, J. Joshua, and C. K. Hannan.** 1985. Examination of uncommon clinical isolates of human adenoviruses by restriction endonuclease analysis. J. Clin. Microbiol. **21:**611–616.
11. **Harnett, G. B., P. A. Phillips, M. M. Gollow.** 1984. Association of genital adenovirus infection with urethritis in men. Med. J. Aust. **141:**337–338.
12. **Hierholzer, J. C.** 1989. Adenoviruses, p. 219–264. *In* N. J. Schmidt, and R. W. Emmons (ed.), Diagnostic procedures for viral, rickettsial and chlamydial infections, 6th ed. American Public Health Association, Inc., Washington, D.C.
13. **Hierholzer, J. C., R. Wigand, L. J. Anderson, T. Adrian, and J. W. Gold.** 1988. Adenoviruses from patients with AIDS: a plethora of serotypes and a description of 5 new serotypes of subgenus D (types 43–47). J. Infect. Dis. **158:** 804–813.
14. **Hierholzer, J. C., R. Wigand, and J. C. de Jong.** 1988. Evaluation of human adenoviruses 38, 39, 40, and 41 as new serotypes. Intervirology **29:**1–10.
15. **Leite, J. P., H. G. Pereira, R. S. Azeredo, and H. G. Schatzmayr.** 1985. Adenoviruses in faeces of children with acute gastroenteritis in Rio de Janeiro, Brazil. J. Med. Virol. **15:**203–209.
16. **Meurman, O., O. Ruuskanen, and H. Sarkkinen.** 1983. Immunoassay diagnosis of adenovirus infections in children. J. Clin. Microbiol. **18:**1190–1195.
17. **Newland, J. C., and M. K. Cooney.** 1978. Characteristics of an adenovirus type 19 conjunctivitis isolate and evidence for a subgroup associated with epidemic conjunctivitis. Infect. Immun. **21:**303–309.
18. **Niel, C., S. A. Gomes, J. P. Leite, and H. G. Pereira.** 1986. Direct detection and differentiation of fastidious and nonfastidious adenoviruses in stools by using a specific nonradioactive probe. J. Clin. Microbiol. **24:**785–789.
19. **Norrby, E.** 1969. The structural and functional diversity of adenovirus capsid components. J. Gen. Virol. **5:**221–236.
20. **Schmitz, H., R. Wigand, and W. Heinrich.** 1983. Worldwide epidemiology of human adenovirus infections. Am. J. Epidemiol. **117:**455–466.
21. **Sohier, R., Y. Chardonnet, and M. Prunieras.** 1965. Adenoviruses: status of current knowledge. Prog. Med. Virol. **7:**253–325.
22. **Stalder, H., J. C. Hierholzer, and M. N. Oxman.** 1977. New human adenovirus (candidate adenovirus type 35) causing fatal disseminated infection in a renal transplant recipient. J. Clin. Microbiol. **6:**257–265.
23. **Straube, R. C., M. A. Thompson, R. B. van Dyke, et al.** 1983. Adenovirus type-7b in a childrens hospital. J. Infect. Dis. **147:**814–819.
24. **Takafuji, E. T., J. C. Gaydos, R. G. Allen, and F. H. Top.** 1979. Simultaneous administration of live, enteric-coated adenovirus types 4, 7, and 21 vaccines: safety and immunogenicity. J. Infect. Dis. **140:**48–53.
25. **van der Avoort, H. G., A. G. Wermenbol, T. P. Zomerdijk, J. A. Kleijne, J. A. van Asten, P. Jensma, A. D. Osterhaus, A. H. Kidd, and J. C. de Jong.** 1989. Characterization of fastidious adenovirus types 40 and 41 by DNA restriction enzyme analysis and by neutralizing monoclonal antibodies. Virus Res. **12:**139–158.
26. **Wadell, G.** 1984. Molecular epidemiology of human adenoviruses. Curr. Top. Microbiol. Immunol. **110:**191–220.
27. **Wadell, G.** 1988. Adenoviridae: the adenoviruses, p. 284–300. *In* E. H. Lennette, P. Halonen, and F. A. Murphy (ed.), Laboratory diagnosis of infectious diseases: principles and practice, vol II. Viral, rickettsial, and chlamydial diseases. Springer-Verlag, New York.
28. **Webb, D. H., A. F. Shields, and K. H. Fife.** 1987. Genomic variation of adenovirus type 5 isolates recovered from bone marrow transplant recipients. J. Clin. Microbiol. **25:**305–308.
29. **Wigand, R., N. Sehn, J. C. Hierholzer, J. C. de Jong, and T. Adrian.** 1985. Immunological and biochemical characterization of human adenoviruses from subgenus B. I. Antigenic relationships. Arch. Virol. **84:**63–78.
30. **Wishart, P. K., C. James, M. S. Wishart, and S. Darougar.** 1984. Prevalence of acute conjunctivitis caused by chlamydia, adenovirus, and herpes simplex virus in an ophthalmic casualty department. Br. J. Ophthalmol. **68:**653–655.

Chapter 87

Measles Virus

AIMO A. SALMI

CLINICAL BACKGROUND

Measles virus (MV) causes an acute, generalized infection that until recently has been one of the most common viral diseases of childhood worldwide (8, 12). The typical epidemiologic pattern of rapidly spreading outbreaks is most often observed in springtime (2). Epidemic peaks coincide with the school year in developed countries. Measles epidemics at 2- to 5-year intervals were common in densely populated countries before the licensure of measles vaccine. Now the goal of the expanded global program for immunization is to eliminate measles entirely. This goal has not yet been achieved. In developing countries in particular, vaccination programs have been only partially successful. Small epidemics of measles have been observed in vaccinated populations even in developed countries in recent years (10).

Measles is rarely fatal in North America and Europe, but mortality after MV infection can be as high as 20% in developing countries. Poor nutrition and suboptimal hygienic conditions are contributing factors. Measles is traditionally a disease of early childhood, but vaccination programs seem to be changing the epidemiologic pattern. Occasional cases or even small epidemics have recently been observed in schoolchildren and young adults (9).

Measles is spread from an MV-infected to a susceptible person mainly via aerosol. Virus is excreted late during the 9- to 12-day incubation period, and the patient continues to be infectious until early convalescence. The primary site of infection is the mucosal cells of the respiratory tract. The infection spreads to local lymph nodes, and viremia is established. Circulating virus is found in T cells, B cells, and monocytes. Virus spreads to other susceptible organs during the viremic phase. Virus has been found in lung, gut, bile duct, bladder, skin, and lymphoid organs (7).

The prodromal symptoms of measles are similar to those of other upper respiratory tract infections: running nose, sneezing, cough, and fever. Redness of eyes and photophobia are also early symptoms. Koplik's spots on the mouth epithelium, which usually appear after the prodromal symptoms, are the hallmark of the clinical signs of measles. At the time of the viremia, a typical macular or maculopapular exanthem appears. High fever is characteristic at the time of rash onset. Patients are infectious a few days before the onset of rash and continue to excrete virus until the rash has disappeared. If no complicating sequelae appear, the disease disappears in 1 to 2 weeks after the onset of rash. If the infection is severe and generalized, total recovery may take weeks.

Changes in electroencephalograms are seen in about 50% of patients with uncomplicated measles, indicating central nervous system (CNS) involvement. An increased number of immune cells in the cerebrospinal fluid (CSF) is also frequently found in measles patients. Although MV can replicate in brain cells, it is not clear whether it regularly infects brain tissue during uncomplicated measles or whether the changes observed are due to autoimmune reactions.

MV rarely causes an acute encephalitis, but postinfectious encephalomyelitis has been reported to occur in about 0.1% of patients. MV readily causes persistent infection in vitro and may also establish persistence in vivo, especially in the CNS. A rare complication of measles is subacute sclerosing panencephalitis (SSPE), which occurs at a frequency of about 1/1 million. Patients with SSPE, most often boys, usually have a history of an uneventful MV infection early in life. After a latent period of 1 to 10 years, a progressive neurological disease develops which is lethal within a few years. Virologically, a persistent, defective infection progresses in the CNS of these patients.

Persistent MV infection has also been suspected in other chronic autoimmune diseases. Patients with multiple sclerosis as well as those with systemic lupus erythematosus have consistently been found to have elevated levels of antibodies to MV. This finding does not necessarily indicate any role of the virus in the etiology or pathogenesis of these diseases but may reflect polyclonal activation of B cells known to occur during the course of the diseases.

Variants of clinical measles have been observed. Atypical measles may occur in persons previously immunized if the immunity after vaccination was only partial. In such patients, the rash may be hemorrhagic or vesicular and develops first on the extremities. Enlargement of lymph nodes and spleen is frequently seen. Such atypical cases may be difficult to diagnose clinically. Diarrhea may be a prominent sign of measles in developing countries. Measles may be unusually severe in patients in whom T-cell functions are impaired. These patients frequently develop giant-cell pneumonia and severe involvement of other organ systems.

A clinical diagnosis of measles is usually obvious from the clinical symptoms, especially in the Caucasian population. However, recognition of measles rash may be difficult on the background of a dark skin. Laboratory diagnosis by specific virological tests is necessary to confirm the clinical diagnosis in all atypical cases. Even typical measles patients may not be properly diagnosed clinically by physicians who have not previously seen typical measles. Since small measles epidemics are still found even in vaccinated populations in Europe and North America, specific laboratory confirmation is an important addition to the clinical evaluation of patients suspected of having MV infection.

DESCRIPTION OF THE AGENT

MV belongs to the family *Paramyxoviridae* and is a member of the genus *Morbillivirus* (12). Other members of this genus are distemper virus of dogs and rinderpest virus of cattle. The only natural hosts of MV are humans and monkeys, but the virus can be adapted to grow in rodents as well. MV is monotypic, but small biological antigenic variations at the epitope level have been described (19). Such variations have no effect on protective immunity, since measles infection provides a lifelong immunity against reinfection.

The main biochemical and structural features of MV are similar to those of other members of the family *Paramyxoviridae*. MV genetic information is carried by a single-stranded linear RNA that sediments at 50S to 52S and has a molecular weight of about 5×10^6. The enveloped measles virions are pleomorphic and 100 to 250 nm in diameter. The envelope is composed of a cell-derived lipid bilayer from which two types of viral glycoproteins protrude. They are seen by electron microscopy as surface projections of 9 to 15 nm.

MV is composed of six major structural polypeptides, three of which are associated with the envelope. The two protruding glycoproteins, the hemagglutinin (H) and fusion (F) proteins, are the most important from the standpoint of protection. Most of the neutralizing antibodies are against the H protein; the antibodies against the F protein inhibit the spread of MV in tissue. The third virus protein associated with the envelope and lining its inner surface is the hydrophobic matrix (M) protein. The helical nucleocapsid enclosed in the envelope is composed of the RNA genome surrounded by the major internal protein of MV, the nucleoprotein (NP). Two minor proteins associated with the nucleocapsid core are the polymerase (phospho) protein (P) and the large (L) protein, both of which are involved with the RNA polymerase function of the virion.

MV is a labile virus and can be readily inactivated with chemicals affecting the lipid envelope. It is also sensitive to heat inactivation, but its infectivity can be readily maintained by storage at −70°C. Storage at −20°C does not guarantee the maintenance of infectivity for long periods of time. In contrast, MV antigens are relatively stable; hemagglutinating antigens and antigens to be used for enzyme immunoassay (EIA) can be stored at 4°C for months without significant loss of antigenic activity.

COLLECTION AND STORAGE OF SPECIMENS

The success rate for isolation of MV from clinical specimens is low. MV has been isolated from nasopharyngeal and conjunctival specimens during the prodrome and early rash illness and from stool and urine specimens during late illness. Although the CNS is frequently involved in the pathogenetic process of measles, virus isolation from CSF is only rarely successful. Specimens for virus isolation are taken by using standard procedures, refrigerated (but not frozen), and transported to the virus laboratory as soon as possible. Since the infectivity of MV is labile, the transport medium should contain protein to stabilize MV infectivity. Media with bovine serum albumin or fetal calf serum are good for this purpose (see chapter 3).

Direct demonstration of MV antigen in infected cells is successful more often than virus isolation, since large amounts of virus antigens accumulate in infected cells. Therefore, a specimen for antigen detection should have a high number of infected cells. The best specimen for this purpose is nasopharyngeal secretions collected through the nose by a mucus extractor with a mucus trap of the type commonly used in infectious diseases wards. The collected mucus is refrigerated and sent immediately to the laboratory for direct immunofluorescence or antigen detection by immunoassay. Virus antigen may also be detected in circulating peripheral blood cells. Heparinized blood or isolated lymphoid cells are sent refrigerated to the virus laboratory for this examination.

Serological diagnosis is generally based on demonstration of a significant increase in antibody titer in paired serum specimens. The first specimen should be taken as soon as possible after the onset of the disease. The second specimen can be taken as early as 7 days, but preferably 10 to 14 days, after the first specimen. Since antibodies are stable in the presence of other serum proteins, no special precautions are needed for transport of the serum specimen to the virus laboratory. Even ordinary mail service is sufficient if the transport time is not longer than a couple of days. Serum can be stored in the laboratory at 4°C for a few days, but long-term storage should be at −20°C or below.

Testing of paired acute- and convalescent-phase serum specimens is important for the diagnosis of patients who have been immunized against measles but who subsequently become infected. Such patients usually have a record of measles immunization and often have detectable but low titers of immunoglobulin G (IgG) antibodies to MV in their acute-phase serum specimens. The acute-phase sera do not, however, have detectable IgM antibodies to MV. Acute- and convalescent-phase paired sera will show diagnostic rises in IgG MV-specific antibody titers.

A single serum specimen is sufficient for demonstrating MV-specific IgM antibodies provided that it has been taken within 4 to 5 weeks of the onset of measles. Intrathecal MV antibody synthesis is pathognomonic for SSPE. Such synthesis can be demonstrated by titrating antibodies in both serum and CSF. For that purpose, paired serum and CSF specimens are taken during the same day and sent to the virus laboratory. Since the protein concentration is lower in CSF than in serum, immunoglobulins are more labile and require refrigerated transport to the laboratory.

DIRECT EXAMINATION

Typical paramyxoviruslike viruses may be seen under the electron microscope in clinical specimens from measles patients. Since all members of family *Paramyxoviridae* are similar morphologically, no specific diagnosis can be made by such an examination. MV-infected cells are typically multinucleated and formed by fusion of a large number of infected cells. Such cells are pathognomonic for measles, and their presence in throat washings or peripheral blood mononuclear cells can be used as an indication of MV infection. Eosinophilic inclusions are found in the cytoplasm or nuclei of infected cells. The inclusions represent accumulated viral nucleocapsid material and are considered to be diagnostic in SSPE patients.

Although histological examination may aid in the diagnosis of measles, specific diagnosis requires a direct demonstration of virus antigens in the cells. This can be done by immunofluorescence staining of tissue cells obtained from patients (4). The most useful substrate for staining is cells from nasopharyngeal secretions, peripheral blood, and urine sediment. Virus antigen is also found in skin biopsies during the rash. For immunofluorescence, the specimen is spread on a glass slide, air dried, and fixed in ice-cold acetone for 10 min. Fixed slides can be stored frozen, preferably at −70°C, for months.

The fixed cells are stained for MV antigens by hyperimmune measles antiserum and fluoresceinated secondary antibodies specific for the immunoglobulins of the hyperimmune serum. Standard staining conditions commonly used in immunofluorescence staining should be employed (see chapter 11). The stained samples are examined for a specific staining pattern that is typically cytoplasmic; late during the infectious cycle and in chronic measles such as SSPE, it may also be intranuclear. MV-infected cells, especially late during the infectious cycle, contain a large mass of virus antigens. Especially prominent are the NP and P antigens, which can be seen in small spots or large fluorescing bodies in the cytoplasm. For reference purposes, cells infected with a laboratory strain of MV should be included as a positive control.

Direct demonstration of viral antigens by radioimmunoassay or EIA has been used for rapid diagnosis of respiratory virus infections in recent years. Nasopharyngeal specimens without fixation can be directly used in such tests. A few nanograms of MV antigen per milliliter can be detected by EIA (17). There is as yet no information on whether such a test is useful for the laboratory diagnosis of MV infection.

Recently introduced hybridization tests for MV RNA in tissues have been used in research laboratories (3) but have not yet been used in diagnostic laboratories.

ISOLATION OF VIRUS

MV can be isolated from patients during the prodromal state, at the time of the rash, and a few days afterwards. Since the success rate for virus isolation is low (16), this approach cannot be used as the primary means for the laboratory diagnosis of MV infection. Virus isolation is more important for patients with a poor or delayed antibody response, which occurs in many atypical cases of measles.

Although laboratory strains of MV grow readily in a number of continuous cell lines of human or primate origin, the growth of strains from measles patients is poor. The best cells for virus isolation are primary human fetal kidney cells. Since such cells are not generally available, primary monkey kidney cells are the second choice. These cells can be prepared from monkey kidney tissue, if available in the virus laboratory, or may be obtained from commercial sources. Primary human amniotic cells have also been used to isolate MV from patients, but the success rate is lower than in primary kidney cells.

The cytopathic effect (CPE) appears late after the inoculation of an MV-containing sample. The inoculated cultures should be observed for typical CPE for at least 2 weeks. Two types of CPE may be observed in the cultures: (i) spindle-shaped single cells that increase in number when the infection advances and (ii) multinucleated giant cells (syncytia) that increase in size during the culture time. The type of CPE depends on the multiplicity of infection, the virus strain, and the cells used to propagate the virus.

In chronic MV infections (i.e., in SSPE patients), the virus is in a defective, cell-associated form and cannot be isolated by ordinary techniques (6). Instead, cocultivation of patient brain or peripheral blood cells with susceptible monkey cell lines is required. The procedure may take a few weeks and requires many passages of the cell mixture before the CPE appears or antigens can be demonstrated in the coculture. MV isolated by the cocultivation technique may remain cell associated.

IDENTIFICATION OF VIRUS

Methods

A finding that the CPE caused by the isolated virus is syncytial suggests that the virus has a fusion protein. This observation combined with the clinical information justifies an educated guess that the isolated virus may be MV. A preliminary test that can easily be done is hemadsorption with monkey erythrocytes, but this test is not specific for MV. Proper identification of the virus causing the CPE requires use of specific antisera.

A hyperimmune animal antiserum specific for MV, monoclonal antibodies specific for the internal polypeptides (NP, P, and M), or a mixture of different monoclonal antibodies can be used to identify the isolated virus. The most convenient identification test is direct immunofluorescence using specific antisera. Cells with CPE are scraped off, spread on a glass slide, and fixed in ice-cold acetone for 10 min. Staining with MV-specific antibodies and fluoresceinated secondary antibodies is done by standard procedures (see chapter 11). Fluorescence of typical intracellular inclusions stained with the specific antiserum identifies the isolated virus as MV. Staining with a serum specimen taken from a hyperimmunized animal before the immunization should be used, if available, as a negative control.

The isolated virus can also be identified by the neutralization test, but this method is more cumbersome and time-consuming than the fluorescence method. Virus antigen in infected cells can also be identified by a specific EIA test for MV antigens (17).

Preparation of hyperimmune sera

Hyperimmune polyclonal antibodies are available from commercial sources but can also be prepared in different species such as sheep, rabbits, or guinea pigs. The following protocol has been successfully used to prepare a high-titered measles antiserum in rabbits. Concentrated virus purified from supernatants of MV-infected cells as described elsewhere in this chapter is a good immunizing antigen. A total of 0.5 to 1 mg of virus in a 0.2-ml volume of a physiological buffer is mixed with an equal volume of Freund incomplete adjuvant and mixed thoroughly. The antigen is injected intradermally on multiple sites of the shaved back of a rabbit. After 3 weeks, a booster injection of 0.1 to 0.2 mg of MV in an acceptable adjuvant is given subcutaneously. The boosting is repeated after 3 weeks. Two weeks later, a serum sample is taken and tested by immunofluorescence and EIA tests for antibodies binding to noninfected and MV-infected cells. A specific titer of 1/1,000 or higher by immunofluorescence and 1/100,000 or higher by EIA is normally reached in about 2 months of total immunization time. If the titers have reached that level and the binding of antibodies to noninfected cells is less than 1/100 of the specific binding, the antiserum is acceptable and a larger amount of the serum can be collected. If binding of the antiserum to noninfected cells is too high, the antiserum might still be useful after absorption with packed, noninfected cells.

SEROLOGICAL DIAGNOSIS

General principles of serological diagnosis apply to measles. The presence of specific antibodies in a single serum specimen indicates past MV infection or vaccination. Demonstration of a significant increase of specific antibody titers in a serum pair taken at a 7- to 14-day interval is the basis of the diagnosis of an acute infection. Alternatively, demonstration of MV-specific IgM antibodies in only one specimen gives a specific diagnosis. Since the presence of virus-specific IgM can be determined in less than 24 h, its detection can be used as a rapid diagnostic test.

In all serological tests, proper controls should be included in the series. This practice is important because test conditions have a great effect on the level of sensitivity and the degree of nonspecific reactivity in all of these tests. The most important controls are known positive and negative specimens, results of which are the basis for interpretation of the sample results.

Hemagglutination inhibition

The hemagglutination inhibition (HI) test is based on the ability of MV H protein to bind to monkey erythrocytes. If the H protein is in a dimeric form or in a larger particle such as the measles virion, erythrocytes are aggregated and can easily be seen. Specific antibodies inhibit this aggregation, a phenomenon on which the HI antibody test is based.

Preparation of the HI antigen. The antigen for the HI test is available commercially but can also be prepared in a virus laboratory. Continuous cell lines known to give a high yield of MV such as Vero, CV-1, or HeLa should be used. Since MV is considered to be homotypic, any virus strain can be used for hemagglutinin preparation. When the CPE is spread throughout the cell layer, the culture is harvested. Because a large amount of H protein is found both in the cellular membranes and in released virus, whole cultures can be harvested and used for antigen preparation. The material is frozen and thawed five times and centrifuged at 15,000 rpm for 20 min; the supernatant is divided into smaller portions and stored at −20°C. The hemagglutinating ability of the antigen can be increased a minimum of fourfold by treatment with Tween 80 and ether (11).

The hemagglutination is titrated on round-bottom microtiter plates by using erythrocytes from Old World monkeys such as African green or rhesus monkeys. Add 0.05 ml of 0.5% monkey erythrocytes to 0.025-ml volumes of twofold antigen dilutions and incubate the plates for 1 h at 37°C. The pattern of hemagglutination is read, and the last dilution giving a clear agglutination is considered to contain 1 hemagglutinating unit (HAU) of measles antigen. All reagents are diluted in phosphate-buffered saline (PBS). If the erythrocytes aggregate spontaneously, the dilutions are made in PBS supplemented with 0.2 to 1% bovine serum albumin.

HI test. Human sera frequently contain nonspecific inhibitors of hemagglutination, which are removed by addition of an equal volume of 25% kaolin in PBS and incubation for 20 min at room temperature. The mixture is then centrifuged, and the supernatant which represents a 1:2 dilution of the original serum can be stored at −20°C. Some human sera agglutinate monkey erythrocytes, which necessitates absorption of such sera with an equal volume of 50% monkey erythrocytes for at least 4 h at 4°C.

For the HI test, twofold dilutions of serum specimens starting with a 1:2 or 1:4 dilution are made on microtiter plates in a volume of 0.025 ml, and 4 HAU of measles antigen is added in a volume of 0.025 ml. After 1 h of incubation at room temperature, 0.05 ml of 0.5% monkey erythrocytes is added; the plates are then shaken and incubated at 37°C for 1 h. The agglutination pattern is read, and the HI titer is determined as the last dilution inhibiting agglutination. As a control, the hemagglutinating MV antigen is back-titrated to make sure that the amount of hemagglutinin is 4 HAU in the test.

Complement fixation

Antigen for the measles complement fixation (CF) test can be obtained from commercial sources or can be prepared in any virus laboratory capable of tissue culture, using the procedure described above for the HI antigen. The crude antigen containing both the cellular material and culture supernatant can be used as the CF antigen. The Tween 80 and ether treatment of the crude antigen is not required for optimal results, since the main antigen in the CF test is the NP antigen, and the Tween-ether treatment has no significant effect on it.

The CF test for MV antibodies is done by using the standard techniques with microtiter plates and other equipment suitable for that purpose (see chapter 10). For reliable and reproducible results, it is important to determine the optimal concentration of the virus antigen and other components of the system. Positive and negative control specimens are also necessary in every test series.

Although all MV proteins are, in principle, capable of binding antibodies, the bulk of the CF antibodies are against the NP antigen. These antibodies are not protective as such, but their presence reflects the general immune status of the patient. Because the CF test has low sensitivity, it is not well suited for determining immunity. On the other hand, the CF test is as good as the other serological tests for demonstrating a significant titer increase in a serum pair.

Enzyme immunoassay

A recently introduced alternative to the CF test is the EIA antibody test, which is more sensitive than the CF test and has good reproducibility. The most convenient way of setting up the EIA test for MV antibodies is to use microtitration equipment and record the results by using automatic readers with analyzing and printing capability.

EIA test kits for MV antibodies are commercially available, but such tests can also be set up in any virus laboratory. MV antigen is available from commercial sources but can also be prepared by using standard laboratory virus strains and continuous cell lines supporting MV growth, such as the monkey kidney cell line Vero. The cells are maintained in Eagle minimal essential medium without or with 2% or less fetal bovine serum and are infected with a high multiplicity of infectious virus. When the CPE has spread throughout the cell monolayer, the supernatant and infected cells are harvested separately and processed for antigens.

Infected cells contain a large amount of the NP, P, and H proteins and lesser amounts of the M, F, and L proteins. For practical purposes, a crude antigen prepared from infected cells is satisfactory for measuring an increase in the IgG antibodies and determining the immunity status of the patient. If it is important to measure antibodies to all viral structural components or if the antigen is used in the IgM assays, purified virus should be used.

Preparation of EIA antigen. For preparation of the crude cellular antigen, the infected cells are washed three times with cold PBS and resuspended in 10-fold-diluted PBS. The cells are disrupted with powerful ultrasonic equipment or in a tightly fitting Dounce homogenizer. The debris including the nuclei is removed by low-speed centrifugation in an ordinary tabletop refrigerated centrifuge at 500 × *g* for 15 min. The particulate material in the supernatant is pelleted in an ultracentrifuge at 80,000 × *g* for 2 h. The pellet is resuspended in a small volume of PBS. The resuspension might require vigorous homogenization. The amount of protein in the antigen is determined, and the antigen is divided into smaller portions and stored frozen, preferably at −70°C. Storage at −20°C is acceptable, but the antigen tends to aggregate, especially if the storage temperature occasionally rises above −20°C.

Purification of MV. MV for use as EIA antigen is purified from supernatants of infected cells collected at the time when the CPE has spread to 75 to 100% of the cells. After the supernatant has been clarified by centrifugation at 10,000 × *g* for 20 min, it can be stored for a few days at 4°C before further purification. Concentration by 10- to 20-fold is then done in a hollow fiber or membrane concentration apparatus. To the concentrated supernatant, NaCl and α-D-methylmannoside are added to final concentrations of 2 mol/liter and 4%, respectively. These additives reduce the nonspecific binding of cellular debris to the virions. After 30 min on ice, the supernatant is layered onto a step gradient consisting of 10 ml of 18% and 5 ml of 36% potassium tartrate in a buffer consisting of 0.2 M glycine, 0.2 M NaCl, 20 mM Tris, and 2 mM EDTA, pH 7.8 (GNTE buffer). The gradients are centrifuged at 80,000 × *g* for 90 min. The virus material at the 18%–36% interface is collected, diluted with GNTE buffer to a tartrate concentration less than 18%, and layered on a 24-ml linear 18 to 36% potassium tartrate gradient prepared in GNTE buffer. The gradients are centrifuged at 80,000 × *g* for 3 h or overnight. The virus band is collected, diluted in GNTE, and pelleted at 80,000 × *g* for 30 min. The virus is suspended in PBS and stored at −70°C.

EIA for MV antibodies. Flat-bottom microtiter plates are first coated with crude antigen or purified virus material. The plates should be of special EIA type or reliable tissue culture-treated plastic. For coating, the antigen is diluted in PBS or 50 mM carbonate buffer, pH 9.6, to a concentration giving the best binding of specific antibodies. This concentration should be determined experimentally by checkerboard titration, but a concentration of 5 to 50 μg/ml for a crude lysate antigen or 0.5 to 5 μg/ml for purified virions is a good guess for a proper coating concentration. A 0.1-ml volume of the diluted antigen is added to each well in the microtiter plate, and the plate is incubated overnight at room temperature or at 4°C. Blocking of all available protein-binding sites on the plastic plate is done by incubating the wells for 1 to 2 h with 0.1 ml of EIA incubation buffer, consisting of PBS supplemented with 0.5% bovine serum albumin and 0.5% Tween 20.

Serum dilutions are made in two- or fourfold series in EIA incubation buffer, starting from a dilution of 1:50 to 1:200. Dilutions can be made with a multichannel pipette directly on the antigen-coated plates. Incubation with the serum dilutions is for 1 h at 37°C or 2 h at room temperature, after which the plates are washed three times with washing buffer (PBS supplemented with 0.1% Tween 20).

The next step is addition of enzyme-labeled antibodies that recognize human immunoglobulins. The antibodies can be specific for human IgG, which is the major immunoglobulin class of antibodies during measles convalescence and in immune individuals. For demonstration of a titer increase in a specimen pair or the immunity status of an individual, the antibody can also be specific for all human immunoglobulins. The use of heavy-chain (μ-chain)-specific labeled antibodies is necessary only if IgM antibodies are searched for. Incubation with the labeled antibodies is for 1 h at 37°C or 2 h at room temperature, after which the plates are washed as described above. The final step in the assay is incubation of the plates with the substrate solution. The composition of the substrate depends on the enzyme coupled to the anti-human antibodies. For example, a reliable substrate for horseradish peroxidase is hydrogen peroxide (6 mmol/liter) and *o*-phenylenediamine (17 mmol/liter) in phosphate (50 mmol/liter)–citrate (20 mmol/liter) buffer, pH. 5.5.

Titers of the serum specimens can be determined from the absorbance values of the different serum dilutions by criteria established in the laboratory. As in other serological tests, a fourfold increase in antibody titer can be considered proof of an ongoing virus infection. Since there are no standards for EIA tests, the series should always include positive and negative serum specimens.

IgM determinations

The presence of IgM antibodies in a serum specimen indicates an early phase of an immune response. Nearly 100% of serum specimens taken during acute MV infection or in early convalescence are positive for MV-specific IgM antibodies (15, 21). Since an IgM determination can normally be made in less than 24 h in the laboratory, this test can be used for rapid virological diagnosis of an acute MV infection. The main pitfall of the IgM tests is the possibility of nonspecific positive reactions due to rheumatoid factor interference (20, 21).

IgM can be separated from other classes of human

immunoglobulins by physical separation methods such as ultracentrifugation in sucrose gradients and exclusion chromatography in columns. The fraction containing the 19S immunoglobulins (IgM) is then tested for antibody activity by any available method. Physical separation is, however, laborious and time-consuming. It is easier to use specific antibodies that recognize the μ chain of human IgM bound to MV antigen in a test.

IgM determination by fluorescent-antibody techniques requires MV-infected, fixed cells, fluoresceinated antibodies specific to human IgM, and a microscope equipped with a UV light source and proper fluorescence filters. Any laboratory strain of MV can be used to infect a continuous cell line. Cells left uninfected should also be prepared and used as negative controls. Infected and control cultures are washed three times with PBS, fixed in ice-cold acetone for 10 min, and air dried. Fixed cells can be stored for a couple of months at −20°C without a significant loss of antigenicity. Slides taken from cold storage should first be brought to room temperature and rinsed in PBS. The serum specimen to be tested is incubated at 37°C in a moist chamber for 30 min, and the slide is washed three times in PBS. A predetermined dilution of fluorescein-labeled antibodies to human IgM (μ chain specific) is added to the slide and incubated for 30 min at 37°C. After three more washings with PBS, the slides are sealed with cover slips and examined under a fluorescence microscope.

Different immunoassays offer more objective and reliable means of IgM determination. Although radioimmunoassay (1) is still used, EIA has replaced it because of the hazards associated with use of radioactive material. Some enzyme substrates are carcinogenic, but EIA is nevertheless generally less hazardous than radioimmunoassay. Other immunoassays use fluorescent tracers coupled to the antibodies specific for the heavy chain of IgM, but such assays are not yet in a common use.

MV-specific IgM antibodies can be measured by the direct EIA as described for IgG antibodies except that specific antibodies for human μ chain tagged with an enzyme are used for detection of IgM antibodies bound to MV antigen on the solid phase. Testing of only one serum dilution is sufficient for IgM determination. The best dilution depends on the technical requirements of the system used, but a dilution of 1:50 to 1:200 is generally optimal.

The EIA test for MV-specific IgM antibodies is done in the following sequence (for details, see above). (i) Coat microtiter plates with MV antigen; purified virus is preferable, but good-quality lysate antigen is also satisfactory. (ii) Incubate serum dilutions on the coated plates. (iii) Incubate the plates with enzyme-labeled antibodies specific for human μ chain. (iv) Incubate the plates with the substrate. (v) Read the absorbance and interpret the results.

Since many human serum specimens have IgM antibodies capable of binding to cellular proteins, it is necessary to use either antigens prepared from infected and noninfected cells or highly purified virions. Another pitfall in the direct IgM EIA is the nonspecific reaction due to IgM class rheumatoid factor, which binds to IgG. Such binding of the indicator antibodies to IgM class rheumatoid factor that is attached to MV-specific IgG gives a false-positive reaction. Therefore, if the level of rheumatoid factor is elevated in the serum specimen, the IgM test results are not reliable. Such specimens should be absorbed with heat-aggregated human immunoglobulins or latex particles coated with human IgG (21).

The problems with rheumatoid factor can be avoided if the order of reagents in the IgM test is reversed (20). In this system, the first layer coated to the solid phase consists of antibodies to human IgM (commercially available). The second step is incubation of the test specimens on the solid phase, which specifically adsorbs a layer of IgM. The presence of IgM antibodies specific for MV can be detected in two ways. First, specific purified MV is added to the solid phase, and the bound virus is detected by specific antibodies directly bound to an enzyme marker. If the antibodies are used unconjugated, an extra layer of conjugated antibodies specific for the animal species of the MV-specific antiserum is required (20). The second approach is use of purified MV directly labeled with an enzyme (18).

It is easy to recognize negative and strong positive serum specimens. Difficulties arise when the absorbance reading is only slightly elevated. The only way to decide the cutoff level for positivity in such cases is to test a large number of randomly selected serum specimens likely to be IgM negative and determine the mean and standard deviation, which can then be used to determine the 95% probability level of true IgM positivity.

Other serological tests

A number of other tests have been used to determine the presence of MV antibodies in a serum specimen or an increase in the titer of a serum pair. The precipitation-in-gel test is now rarely used as a test for MV antibodies, but indirect immunofluorescence tests for MV IgG and IgM antibodies are still practical alternatives. These tests should be done according to the protocol used for immunofluorescence tests for other viral antibodies. Research laboratories have measured antibodies to different polypeptides of MV by immunoprecipitation of radiolabeled MV proteins and Western immunoblotting (5, 14), but such tests are better suited for qualitative assessment of the immune response against each of the viral polypeptides than for quantitative measurement of the immune response. The neutralization and hemolysis inhibition (HLI) tests can be used for diagnostic tests, since they measure antibodies of direct biological significance. Information about immunity obtained with these tests may be important if epidemics of MV infection appear in a vaccinated population.

Neutralization. The neutralization test is relevant as a marker of immunity, since it measures antibodies capable of inhibiting virus growth. It is more cumbersome than most of the other antibody tests, since it is based on the inhibition of MV growth in tissue culture. The test requires no special equipment beyond the ordinary tissue culture facility. The test can be used as a plaque reduction or CPE inhibition assay variant, the latter of which is briefly described below.

Stock MV is diluted to contain 100 50% tissue culture infective doses per 0.1 ml. Equal amounts of serially diluted serum specimen and the diluted virus are incubated together at 4°C for 60 min. A 0.2-ml volume of this mixture is added to each of three to six tissue culture tubes and incubated at 37°C until CPE appears in half of the control tubes with 1 50% tissue culture infective dose of virus alone. The titer is determined to be the dilution at which the CPE is inhibited in more than half of the tubes.

HLI test. The HLI test measures the presence of antibodies inhibiting hemolysis caused by the F protein of MV. However, since the expression of hemolytic activity requires that virus particles be anchored to erythrocytes via the hemagglutinin, antibodies to the H protein will also interfere with the hemolysis reaction. Because the HLI antibodies are effective in inhibiting virus spread in tissues, their measurement is of relevance, especially if there is a measles outbreak in a vaccinated population (13).

Antigen used in the HLI test should have a large amount of MV F protein, which may vary from one preparation to another. The best cell-virus combination for preparing such an antigen should be experimentally determined. Infected cells in a 10% suspension or 10- to 20-times-concentrated supernatant of MV-infected cells is the starting material for preparing the hemolyzing antigen. The material is disrupted by five cycles of freezing and thawing or by vigorous sonication. The hemolyzing activity of the antigen is determined by adding 0.1 ml of washed 10% green monkey erythrocytes to a twofold dilution series of 0.4 ml of hemolyzing antigen in PBS. After 3 h of incubation at 37°C, the erythrocytes are centrifuged at 1,500 rpm for 10 min and the optical density of the supernatant is measured at 540 nm. An antigen dilution giving an optical density value of about 0.5 is selected as the working dilution.

For the HLI test, add 0.2 ml of the working dilution of the hemolyzing antigen to equal volumes of serial twofold dilutions of the serum specimen. After incubation for 1 h at room temperature, add a 0.1-ml volume of a 10% suspension of monkey erythrocytes. After incubation for 3 h at 37°C, centrifuge the erythrocytes and read the optical density of the supernatant. The HLI titer of the serum is the dilution giving at least 50% reduction of hemolysis, as calculated from the control hemolysis with added PBS but without serum specimen.

EVALUATION AND INTERPRETATION OF RESULTS

Isolation of MV indicates, without exception, active virus replication in the patient and is the basis for a specific virological diagnosis. Negative results for virus isolation do not exclude MV infection, since the efficiency of the isolation method is low. Careful timing of the specimens and testing of more than one specimen are important for successful virus isolation. This is an especially important consideration for patients with abnormal immunity and atypical measles, since the antibody response may be delayed or impaired. Cocultivation of cells from SSPE patients results in virus isolation only in a small percentage of cases. Therefore, negative virus isolation results for these patients do not exclude the diagnosis of SSPE.

HI is one of the best methods for determining the immunity status of an individual, since it is easy to perform and the presence of HI antibodies is known to correlate with protective immunity. HI titers of 1/10 or higher are considered protective against secondary infection, but the lower limit of protection clearly depends on the sensitivity of the test system used. The presence of neutralizing antibodies also correlates well with protective immunity, but the neutralization test is more cumbersome and less often done. EIA measures antibodies to all viral components and can be used as a very sensitive test to determine whether an individual has been in contact with MV. There are rare individuals, however, who are strongly positive in EIA tests but have only low levels of HI or neutralizing antibodies. It is not clear whether such individuals are protected against reinfection by MV.

All of the serological tests described above can be used to demonstrate a significant increase of antibody level in a serum pair. A fourfold or greater increase indicates an ongoing MV infection. If the first serum specimen is taken during the first 2 days of the rash and the second one is taken a minimum of 7 days later, a significant increase in antibody titer can usually be demonstrated. This is true for patients with ordinary measles, but patients with impaired immunity or with atypical measles may synthesize only a low amount of antibodies, and no significant increase may be demonstrated in a pair taken at an interval of a few days. An increase may still be seen if the serum specimens are taken a few weeks apart.

Most SSPE patients have a stable level of antibodies, but significant increases in serum antibody levels can occasionally be demonstrated in some of these patients. This finding probably indicates activation of a latent MV infection. A diagnostic serological test for SSPE patients is the demonstration of intrathecal MV-specific antibody synthesis. This can be done by calculating the CSF/serum titer ratio. The normal ratio is about 1/200 to 1/500, but in SSPE patients it is from 1/5 to 1/50. Such a low ratio indicates intrathecal antibody synthesis provided that ratios of other viral antibodies are normal.

Demonstration of MV-specific IgM antibodies is the best rapid diagnostic test. All patients with ordinary measles have IgM antibodies in specimens taken late during the rash and until 4 to 5 weeks later. Delayed elevation of MV-specific IgM antibodies is not found in patients late after infection, and only low levels of IgM antibodies are seen in some SSPE patients early after the onset of the disease (22). The only pitfall of the measles IgM tests is nonspecific positive results due to rheumatoid factor and occasional binding of IgM to nonviral cellular antigens. If these possibilities are excluded, the assays for MV-specific IgM antibodies can be considered very reliable and rapid diagnostic tests.

LITERATURE CITED

1. **Arstila, P., T. Vuorimaa, K. Kalimo, P. Halonen, M. Viljanen, K. Granfors, and P. Toivanen.** 1977. A solid phase radioimmunoassay for IgG and IgM antibodies against measles virus. J. Gen. Virol. **34:**167–176.
2. **Black, F. L.** 1989. Measles, p. 451–469. *In* A. S. Evans (ed.), Viral infections of humans. Epidemiology and control, 3rd ed. Plenum Publishing Corp., New York.
3. **Fournier, J. G., M. Tardieu, P. Lebon, O. Robain, G. Ponsot, S. Rozenblatt, and M. Bouteille.** 1985. Detection of measles virus RNA in lymphocytes from peripheral blood and brain perivascular infiltrates of patients with subacute sclerosing panencephalitis. N. Engl. J. Med. **313:** 910–915.
4. **Fulton, R. E., and P. J. Middleton.** 1975. Immunofluorescence in diagnosis of measles infections in children. J. Pediatr. **86:**17–22.

5. **Hankins, R. W., and F. L. Black.** 1986. Western blot analysis of measles virus antibody in normal persons and in patients with multiple sclerosis, subacute sclerosing panencephalitis, or atypical measles. J. Clin. Microbiol. **24:** 324–329.
6. **Katz, M., and H. Koprowski.** 1973. The significance of failure to isolate infected viruses in cases of SSPE. Arch. Gesamte Virusforsch. **41:**390–393.
7. **Moench, T. R., D. E. Griffin, C. R. Obriecht, A. J. Vaisberg, and R. T. Johnson.** 1988. Acute measles in patients with and without neurological involvement: distribution of measles virus antigen and RNA. J. Infect. Dis. **158:**433–442.
8. **Morgan, E. M., and F. Rapp.** 1977. Measles virus and its associated diseases. Bacteriol. Rev. **41:**636–666.
9. **Mouallem, M., E. Friedman, R. Pauzner, and Z. Farfel.** 1987. Measles epidemic in young adults: clinical manifestations and laboratory analysis in 40 patients. Arch. Intern. Med. **147:**1111–1113.
10. **Nkowane, B. M., S. W. Bart, W. A. Orenstein, and M. Baltier.** 1987. Measles outbreak in a vaccinated school population: epidemiology, chains of transmission and the role of vaccine failures. Am. J. Public Health **77:**434–438.
11. **Norrby, E.** 1962. Hemagglutination by measles virus. 4. A simple procedure for production of high potency antigen for hemagglutination-inhibition (HI) tests. Proc. Soc. Exp. Biol. Med. **111:**814–818.
12. **Norrby, E.** 1985. Measles, p. 1305–1321. *In* B. N. Fields (ed.), Virology. Raven Press, New York.
13. **Norrby, E., G. Enders-Ruckle, and V. ter Meulen.** 1975. Differences in the appearance of antibodies to structural components of measles virus after immunization with inactivated and live virus. J. Infect. Dis. **132:**262–269.
14. **Norrby, E., C. Örvell, B. Vandvik, and D. J. Cherry.** 1981. Antibodies against measles virus polypeptides in different disease conditions. Infect. Immun. **34:**718–724.
15. **Pedersen, I. R., A. Antonsdottir, T. Evald, and C. H. Mordhorst.** 1982. Detection of measles IgM antibodies by enzyme linked immunosorbent assay (ELISA). Acta Pathol. Microbiol. Scand. **90:**153–160.
16. **Sakaguchi, M., Y. Yoskikawa, K. Yamanouchi, K. Takeda, and T. Sato.** 1986. Characteristics of fresh isolates of wild measles virus. Jpn. J. Exp. Med. **56:**61–67.
17. **Salmi, A., and G. Lund.** 1984. Immunoassays for measles virus nucleocapsid antigen: effect of antigen-antibody complexes. J. Gen. Virol. **65:**1655–1663.
18. **Salonen, J., R. Vainionpää, and P. Halonen.** 1986. Assay of measles virus IgM and IgG class antibodies by use of peroxidase labelled viral antigens. Arch. Virol. **91:**93–106.
19. **Sheshberadaran, H., S.-N. Chen, and E. Norrby.** 1983. Monoclonal antibodies against five structural components of measles virus. I. Characterization of antigenic determinants on nine strains of measles virus. Virology **128:** 341–353.
20. **Tuokko, H.** 1984. Comparison of non-specific reactivity in indirect and reverse immunoassays for measles and mumps immunoglobulin M antibodies. J. Clin. Microbiol. **20:**972–979.
21. **Tuokko, H., and A. Salmi.** 1983. Detection of IgM antibodies to measles virus by enzyme immunoassay. Med. Microbiol. Immunol. **171:**187–198.
22. **Ziola, B., P. Halonen, and G. Enders.** 1986. Synthesis of measles virus-specific IgM antibodies and IgM-class rheumatoid factor in relation to clinical onset of subacute sclerosing panencephalitis. J. Med. Virol. **18:**51–59.

Chapter 88

Mumps Virus

ELLA M. SWIERKOSZ

CLINICAL BACKGROUND

Mumps is an acute, usually self-limited, systemic illness characterized most commonly by bilateral or unilateral parotitis, although approximately one-third of infections may be asymptomatic. Extra-salivary gland manifestations include meningitis, encephalitis, epididymoorchitis, oophoritis, polyarthritis, and pancreatitis. Nephritis, thyroiditis, mastitis, prostatitis, hepatitis, thrombocytopenia, and deafness have been reported as rare manifestations of mumps infection. Humans are the only natural host of mumps virus. Infection confers long-lasting immunity to clinical disease (2). Most cases of mumps occur in children ages 5 to 14 (1). The incubation period of the virus ranges from 2 to 4 weeks, with an average of 16 to 18 days. Transmission is by droplet, with primary viral replication occurring in the upper respiratory mucosal epithelium (12). Virus can be isolated from saliva from 9 days before and up to 8 days after the onset of parotitis (12, 39). Viruria can be detected up to 2 weeks after onset of symptoms (40). Virus can also be recovered from the cerebrospinal fluid (CSF) during meningitis (39). A live, attenuated mumps vaccine is administered to children at 15 months in a trivalent form combined with live, attenuated vaccines to rubella and measles viruses (1). Although vaccine administration has dramatically reduced the incidence of mumps, outbreaks continue to occur in unvaccinated populations (15, 35, 41).

DESCRIPTION OF AGENT

Mumps virus is a member of the genus *Paramyxovirus* in the family *Paramyxoviridae*. The paramyxoviruses include, in addition to mumps, Newcastle disease virus and the parainfluenza viruses. Like other paramyxoviruses, mumps is a pleomorphic, enveloped virus containing a helical nucleocapsid composed of negative-sense, single-stranded RNA and three nucleocapsid-associated proteins, L, NP, and P, the last of which is presumed to be RNA-dependent RNA polymerase (42). Two surface glycoproteins, F (fusion) and HN (hemagglutinin-neuraminidase), project from the lipid envelope and are visualized as spikes by electron microscopy. The HN glycoprotein, which has both hemagglutinating and neuraminidase activities, mediates adsorption of the virus to host cells, whereas the F glycoprotein mediates fusion of lipid membranes, allowing penetration of the nucleocapsid into the cell (42). The HN glycoprotein is also responsible for mediating hemolysis of erythrocytes (RBCs) (7). Antibody against the HN glycoprotein neutralizes viral infectivity (7). A third membrane-associated protein, called the M or matrix protein, is believed to mediate assembly of the virion along the inner surface of the virus-modified host cell membrane (42). Until recently, only one antigenic type of mumps had been detected by hemagglutination inhibition (HI) or neutralization assays. Antigenic differences among mumps strains have now been demonstrated with an HN-specific monoclonal antibody (34). Moreover, strain-dependent differences in cytopathology and neurovirulence have been described (22). More recent studies with monoclonal antibodies have demonstrated that the paramyxo group viruses share common epitopes (29).

Mumps infectivity is destroyed by organic solvents, by detergents, by heating to 56°C, by UV irradiation, and by Formalin treatment (7, 28). Mumps, like other paramyxoviruses, is relatively unstable, losing infectivity when stored for longer than 4 h in protein-free medium (7).

Mumps virus was first cultivated in vitro in chicken embryos (20) and was subsequently successfully cultivated in tissue culture derived from chicken embryos and in mammalian cell cultures (10).

SPECIMEN SELECTION, COLLECTION, AND TRANSPORT

Laboratory diagnosis of mumps is achieved by virus isolation or by serological testing. Virus can be recovered from saliva up to 8 days after onset of symptoms (12, 39), from urine up to 2 weeks after onset (40), from CSF of patients with meningitis (39), and from swabs obtained from the area around Stensen's duct (39). Specimens should be obtained early in the course of illness, when virus titer is highest.

Urine and CSF should be collected in sterile containers and maintained at 4°C until inoculated into cell culture. Swab specimens should be placed in 2 to 3 ml of viral transport medium (VTM). Cotton-, Dacron-, or rayon-tip swabs should be used. A number of transport media are acceptable: Hanks balanced salt solution, veal infusion broth, and tryptose phosphate broth (18). VTM should be supplemented with protein to stabilize virus and with antibiotics to suppress normal bacterial and fungal flora. Bovine serum albumin (0.5%) and gelatin (0.5%) have been used successfully. Antibiotics such as gentamicin (50 μg/ml), penicillin (100 U/ml), and amphotericin B (5 μg/ml) are also added to the VTM to suppress normal bacterial and fungal flora. Specimens in VTM should be held at 4°C until inoculated into cell culture. If inoculation of the specimen into cell culture is to be delayed more than 48 h, the specimen should be frozen at −70°C or below. Repeated freezing and thawing of the specimen decreases the viral titer.

For serological diagnosis, acute- and convalescent-phase blood should be submitted. Acute-phase blood should be collected as soon as possible after onset of symptoms, whereas the convalescent-phase blood is collected 14 or more days after onset. Mumps-specific immunoglobulin M (IgM) can be measured on a single serum specimen. Antibody titers of CSF can also be determined in cases of meningitis (6, 24, 37). A serum specimen should be collected at the same time as the CSF. Serum and CSF specimens for serological studies can be stored at 4°C if tests will be performed within a few days. If longer delays in testing are anticipated, specimens should be stored at −20°C.

DETECTION OF VIRAL ANTIGEN

Development of non-culture-dependent methods of diagnosing mumps have been hampered by the limited commercial availability of mumps-specific antibody and, until the last few years, the decline in the number of cases of mumps. At present, virus isolation and serology are the mainstays of laboratory diagnosis.

VIRUS ISOLATION

Mumps virus can be cultured in a variety of primary and continuous cell lines as well as embryonated hen eggs. In the diagnostic virology laboratory, commercially available primary rhesus monkey kidney (RhMK) and human embryonic kidney cells are commonly used (25). Before inoculation of cell cultures, the culture medium should be discarded and fresh medium should be added. The most commonly used medium is Eagle minimal essential medium supplemented with 2% sterile fetal bovine serum and antibiotics.

Urine should be collected into a sterile container and kept at 4°C until inoculated into cell culture. Before inoculation, the pH of the urine should be adjusted to neutrality, and an antibiotic mixture is added to suppress the growth of bacteria and fungi that may be present in the specimen. The final concentrations of antibiotics are as follows: gentamicin, 50 μg/ml; penicillin, 100 U/ml; and amphotericin B, 5 μg/ml. The urine is centrifuged at 600 × *g* at 4°C, and 0.2 ml of the supernatant is inoculated to each cell culture tube.

Swab specimens are placed in 2.5 ml of VTM and held at 4°C until inoculated into cell culture. Antibiotics are added as described above, and the specimen is vortexed. Unless the specimen is grossly turbid, it can be inoculated into cell culture tubes without centrifugation. Because saliva specimens are often contaminated with normal flora, antibiotics may fail to inhibit their growth. Saliva should be mixed with an equal volume of VTM and filtered through a 0.22-μm-pore-size filter before inoculation into cell cultures. CSF can be inoculated into cell culture tubes without pretreatment.

Cell culture tubes are incubated at 35 to 37°C. Placing the tubes on a roller drum apparatus may hasten the appearance of virus-specific cytopathic effect (CPE) and the production of hemagglutinins. Cell cultures should be examined under low-power microscopy (×40 to ×100) on a daily basis for the first week of incubation and every third or fourth day thereafter for a total of 14 days. The appearance of multinucleated giant cells is suggestive of a paramyxovirus, but CPE may not appear or may be very subtle in appearance. It should be noted that primary monkey kidney cells may contain indigenous viruses that produce CPE. The method of choice for detecting the presence of mumps virus in cell culture is the hemadsorption test (4). At days 5 to 7 and day 14, the medium is removed from the RhMK or human embryonic kidney cell culture tube, and 0.5 ml of a 0.5% suspension of guinea pig RBCs in sterile phosphate-buffered saline (PBS) is added. Guinea pig RBCs should be obtained weekly; a 0.5% suspension prepared in PBS should be stored at 4°C and is good for 3 days after preparation. The tubes are placed on their sides in a stationary rack such that the monolayer is covered and are refrigerated (4°C) for 20 min. The tubes are then examined microscopically for adherence of the RBCs to the cell culture monolayer that is due to the presence of viral hemagglutinin. Uninfected control tubes should be tested in parallel with the inoculated tubes to rule out nonspecific adsorption of RBCs and to detect endogenous simian paramyxoviruses.

Medium from the hemadsorption-positive tubes should be passaged to at least four fresh cell culture tubes to produce enough virus for typing. The passaged tubes should be incubated at 35 to 37°C and checked daily for CPE. When 75 to 100% of the monolayer displays CPE, or at day 7 if no CPE is apparent, hemadsorb one of the tubes. Sufficient antigen for typing the isolate is present when 75 to 100% of the monolayer is hemadsorption positive. Hemadsorption-negative tubes can be washed with PBS, refed with 1.5 ml of maintenance medium, and reincubated. Alternatively, the hemadsorption-negative tubes may be discarded if additional cell culture tubes remain in culture.

IDENTIFICATION OF VIRUS

IF

Because of the decline in the incidence of mumps, few commercial sources produce mumps-specific antiserum, and immunofluorescence (IF) reagents may be difficult to locate. Nevertheless, identification of virus by IF is a rapid and technically simple procedure. Antisera should be titered against parainfluenza viruses to determine the degree of cross-reactivity with these viruses.

Hemadsorption-positive tubes are filled with 2.0 ml of PBS and incubated at 37°C to elute the RBCs from the monolayer. Alternatively, a second passage culture tube showing maximal CPE or hemadsorption can be used. Subsequently, the monolayer is scraped off the wall of the tube and suspended in approximately 1.0 ml of PBS. After low-speed centrifugation of the suspension in a microcentrifuge, the supernatant is removed and the pellet is resuspended in approximately 50 μl of PBS. Portions of the suspension are applied to wells of a Teflon-coated microscope slide and then dried. The slide is fixed in acetone at −20°C for 10 min and air dried. The wells are stained with mumps-specific antiserum conjugated to fluorescein isothiocynate for use in the direct IF test or unconjugated for use in the indirect IF test (31). Cells from an uninfected tube should be stained as a negative control.

CF

Reagents for performance of the complement fixation (CF) test are commercially available (Whittaker Bioproducts, Walkersville, Md.). Antigen is prepared from at least three infected cell culture tubes by three cycles of freezing and thawing, followed by low-speed centrifugation to eliminate cell debris. All but 0.3 ml of medium should be removed from the tubes before freezing. This crude antigen is tested against serial twofold dilutions of immune serum, using the microtiter CF test outlined by Schmidt and Emmons (33). Preimmune serum should be run in parallel with the immune serum to detect nonspecific reactions. Immune serum should also be tested against parainfluenza virus antigens to detect cross-reactivity with these viruses.

HI

Antigen from infected cell culture tubes is prepared as described above. It may be necessary to treat the antigen preparation with Tween 80 and ether to boost the hemagglutinin titer (3). The hemagglutinin titer is determined by a microtiter procedure (16). Crude antigen is diluted in twofold serial dilutions in 0.1 M PBS (pH 7.2) in 0.05-ml volumes in V-bottom plates. To each well is added 0.05 ml of a 0.5% suspension of guinea pig RBCs. An RBC control well containing 0.05 ml of PBS and 0.05 ml of RBCs is also included. The plate is mixed and incubated at room temperature until the RBC control well settles (usually 30 to 60 min). The highest dilution causing agglutination is the endpoint; this dilution contains one hemagglutination unit (HAU) per 0.05 ml. For the HI test, 4 HAU contained in a volume of 0.025 ml is used, which is calculated by dividing the hemagglutinin titer by 8. Thus, if the hemagglutinin titer is 32, a 1:4 dilution of antigen contains 4 HAU.

To ensure that sufficient antigen is used in the HI test, a retitration of the diluted antigen is performed. To a row of six wells is added 0.05 ml of PBS. Add 0.05 ml of the diluted antigen to the first well and make twofold serial dilutions through the fifth well. To the sixth well add 0.05 ml of PBS instead of test antigen. Add 0.05 ml of 0.5% guinea pig RBCs to each well and mix the contents. When the sixth well shows settling of the RBCs, observe the hemagglutination pattern of the other five wells. The first three wells should show hemagglutination, and the last two wells should show compact buttons of settled cells. Adjust the dilution of the working antigen if necessary and retitrate as described above.

The immune serum for the HI test must first be pretreated to remove nonspecific inhibitors of agglutination. Potassium periodate treatment has been successfully used (26). Add 0.3 ml of 0.11 M KIO_4 in PBS to 0.1 ml of heat-inactivated serum. The mixture is incubated at room temperature for 15 min. Subsequently, 0.6 ml of 0.6% glycerol in PBS is added to neutralize the periodate. The final dilution is 1:10. Treatment of serum with receptor-destroying enzyme of *Vibrio cholerae* is an alternate method of removing nonspecific inhibitors of agglutination. Add 0.4 ml of receptor-destroying enzyme (100 U/ml) to 0.1 ml of serum; incubate the mixture overnight in a water bath at 37°C. Add 0.5 ml of 1.5% sodium citrate and incubate the mixture in a water bath at 56°C for 30 min. To remove nonspecific hemagglutinins in the serum, add 0.05 ml of packed guinea pig RBCs to the serum and leave the mixture at 4°C for 1 h. Remove the RBCs by low-speed centrifugation.

Twofold serial dilutions of treated serum in 0.025-ml volumes are prepared in microtiter V-bottom plates. To each well is added 0.025 ml of antigen containing 4 HAU. A serum control well containing undiluted serum (0.025 ml) and 0.025 ml of PBS is included to test for nonspecific serum agglutinins. An RBC control well containing 0.05 ml of PBS is also prepared. The plate is shaken and incubated at room temperature for 30 to 60 min. Add 0.05 ml of the guinea pig RBC suspension to each well, shake the plate, and incubate it at room temperature until the RBC control well shows a button of settled cells. Observe the wells containing diluted immune serum for inhibition of agglutination manifested by buttoning of the RBCs. To facilitate reading of the endpoint, the plate is tilted; nonagglutinated RBCs will form a tear-shaped stream of cells while hemagglutination patterns are undisturbed. Inhibition of agglutination identifies the test antigen as mumps. Immune serum must also be tested against parainfluenza viruses to rule out heterologous reactions.

Hemadsorption inhibition

The hemadsorption inhibition test is less sensitive than the HI test but is technically simpler to perform (16). High-titered mumps antiserum must be used (HI titer of ≥80). Serum is pretreated to remove nonspecific inhibitors of agglutination as described above. Infected cell cultures are first washed twice with PBS, followed by the addition of 0.2 ml of pretreated serum and 0.6 ml of PBS. A hemadsorption-positive control tube containing 0.8 ml of PBS alone is also prepared. Tubes are incubated for 30 min at room temperature on a stationary rack in a horizontal position so that the monolayer is completely covered. To each tube is added 0.2 ml of 0.5% guinea pig RBCs. The tubes are refrigerated for 20 min in a horizontal position and then are examined microscopically for the presence of hemadsorption. The isolate is identified as mumps if the tube with the immune serum fails to hemadsorb but the PBS-treated tube is hemadsorption positive.

Neutralization

The neutralization test (28) requires pretitration of virus. Supernatant from a culture tube exhibiting 75 to 100% hemadsorption is diluted in serial 10-fold dilutions, and 0.2 ml of each dilution is added to duplicate tubes of freshly fed RhMK cells. The tubes are incubated at 35 to 37°C on a rotating drum for 7 days and are examined daily for the development of CPE. At day 7, the tubes are scored either for the presence of CPE or for hemadsorption. The dose of virus that infects 50% of the cultures is calculated (33). For the neutralization assay 30 to 100 50% tissue culture infective doses are required. Heat-inactivated immune serum is mixed with an equal volume of titered virus, and the mixture is incubated for 1 h at 37°C. Subsequently, 0.2 ml of the mixture is inoculated in duplicate into RhMK cell culture tubes. Virus mixed with PBS alone is inoculated as a positive control. Cultures are incubated at 35 to 37°C. Tubes are examined for the presence of CPE or, if no CPE is apparent, are hemadsorbed at 7 days. The absence of hemadsorption in the tubes with antiserum identifies the isolate as mumps.

SEROLOGICAL DIAGNOSIS

The serological diagnosis of mumps, traditionally based on the demonstration of a significant titer rise between acute- and convalescent-phase sera, is limited by the retrospective nature of the diagnosis, the cross-reactions between mumps and parainfluenza viruses, and delays in collection of the acute-phase serum so that titer rises are missed. Newer tests, such as the enzyme-linked immunosorbent assay (ELISA), though more sensitive than the CF and HI tests (23, 30), are hindered by the same disadvantages. Tests for determination of immune status to mumps are now commercially available.

HI

The procedure is identical to that for the HI test described above for the identification of viral isolates. Commercially available antigens and immune sera may be difficult to find. Antigen titers are calculated to determine the dilution containing 4 HAU. Patient serum is pretreated to remove nonspecific inhibitors and nonspecific agglutinins and is diluted serially in twofold dilutions, followed by addition of mumps antigen. Virus-serum mixtures are incubated at 37°C for 1 h. A 0.5% suspension of guinea pig RBCs is added to each well, and the plate is shaken and incubated at room temperature for 30 to 60 min. Wells are observed for the absence or inhibition of agglutination, manifested as a button at the bottom of the well. The highest dilution of serum exhibiting inhibition of hemagglutination is the endpoint. To facilitate reading of the endpoint, the plate is tilted; nonagglutinated RBCs will form a tear-shaped stream of cells while hemagglutination patterns are undisturbed. Positive and negative control sera should be assayed in parallel with the patient sera. Other controls include a well containing test serum and RBCs to test for nonspecific agglutinins, an RBC control well containing cells plus diluent, and an antigen control well containing 4 HAU plus RBCs.

CF

The CF test has been used for several decades for the serological diagnosis of mumps. Mumps S and V antigens, which correspond to the NP and HN virus proteins, respectively, are commercially available (13). The CF test is performed as previously described (33). For maximal detection of seroconversions, both antigens should be tested (5, 11).

Neutralization

Neutralization assays can be performed in either RhMK, human embryo kidney, or primary chicken embryo cell culture tubes as described above or in microtiter plates seeded with Vero cells (17, 28). The microtiter procedure conserves reagents and patient sera and correlates well with the tube test.

IF

The IF procedure allows determination of both IgG and IgM antibodies to mumps. Each infected cell culture tube showing approximately 75% CPE is trypsinized to remove cells from the surface on which they are growing and are centrifuged to remove the trypsin. Pellets are washed in PBS and recentrifuged. The supernatant is discarded, and the remaining pellet is resuspended in 100 µl of PBS. A 10-µl sample is applied to the wells of a Teflon-coated microscope slide, which is air dried. The slide is fixed in acetone at −20°C for 10 min. Serial dilutions of patient serum are applied to fixed wells, and the slide is incubated at 37°C for 30 to 60 min. After washing, fluorescein isothiocyanate-conjugated anti-human IgG or IgM is applied to each well, and the slide is incubated at 37°C for 30 min. The slide is washed in PBS, mounted with buffered glycerol mounting medium, and observed under a fluorescence microscope. The highest dilution of serum showing intracytoplasmic fluorescence is the endpoint. Slides containing uninfected cells should be prepared as a control for nonspecific fluorescence. An IF kit for determination of mumps titers is commercially available (Pharmacia-ENI Diagnostics, Fairfield, N.J.).

ELISA

A number of ELISA protocols that measure IgG and IgM antibodies to mumps virus have been described (9, 21, 23, 25, 27, 30, 32, 36). Antigens used include whole virus, sonicated virus, purified HN (V) and NP (S) antigens, and peroxidase-labeled antigen. Microtiter plates are coated with antigen or, in the case of IgM capture assays, with anti-human IgM. Serum specimens are added to coated wells, and plates are incubated. Plates are washed, anti-human immunoglobulin conjugated to peroxidase or alkaline phosphatase is added, and the plates are reincubated. Plates are washed, and substrate is added to each well. After incubation, the absorbance of each well is read. A threshold value for positive is calculated, i.e., three times the absorbance of the control wells. Controls include wells without serum and conjugate, without serum, and with antibody-positive and -negative sera. A commercially available ELISA, the Mumps STAT Test (Whittaker Bioproducts) is a 1-h test designed to measure IgG antibody in single serum samples for the purpose of identifying mumps-susceptible individuals.

Hemolysis in gel

The hemolysis-in-gel test (8, 28) is based on the principle that mumps antigen-coated RBCs are lysed by specific antibody in the presence of complement. Antigen-coated RBCs are suspended in 1.5% agarose. After solidification in petri plates, 3-mm holes are punched into the gel. The holes are filled with heat-inactivated patient serum, and the plates are incubated for 24 h at 4°C, followed by the addition of guinea pig complement as an overlay. The plates are reincubated at 37°C for 2 h, after which the zone of hemolysis is measured to the nearest 0.1 mm. Plates containing uncoated RBCs are tested in parallel as a control for nonspecific lysis. The diameter of the hemolytic zone is plotted against the serum dilution, and a regression analysis is performed. The diameter of the zone is directly proportional to the antibody titer of the serum.

FIAX

A solid-phase IF assay (FIAX; Whittaker Bioproducts) is available for measurement of IgG to mumps. It is intended for determination of immune status by using single serum samples. Mumps antigen is coated onto one side of a dual-surface "sampler"; the reverse side contains no antigen and serves as a blank. The sampler is immersed in diluted serum and incubated. After a wash step, the sampler is immersed in fluorescein-labeled anti-human IgG antibody. After a final wash, the sampler is inserted into a fluorometer, which measures the amount of bound, labeled antibody and expresses it as fluorescence signal units (FSU). The FSU of the blank side is measured and subtracted from the antigen side FSU. A calibration curve is constructed by plotting the ΔFSU versus titer for each calibrator. Patient titers are then obtained by interpolation of the calibration curve.

CSF antibody

IgG and IgM antibody titers of CSF can be measured in cases of meningitis. CSF titers have been measured by ELISA, HI, CF, hemolysis inhibition, and mixed hemadsorption (6, 24, 37).

EVALUATION AND INTERPRETATION OF RESULTS

The isolation of mumps virus from CSF, respiratory specimens, or urine establishes a diagnosis of mumps. A preliminary report of "hemadsorbing virus" should be made as soon as a positive hemadsorption test is obtained. It is critical to ensure that uninfected cell cultures are hemadsorption negative to rule out the presence of endogenous viruses.

Serological diagnosis of mumps is problematic because of the cross-reactions between mumps and other paramyxoviruses (14, 19, 27). Paired sera exhibiting a fourfold or greater titer rise against mumps should be tested against the parainfluenza viruses. If a titer rise to one or more parainfluenza viruses is observed, it is not possible to make a definitive diagnosis of mumps without a compatible clinical picture.

It has been accepted for many years that serological testing by CF should include measurement of antibody to both V and S antigens of mumps. Moreover, early work describing the CF test demonstrated that antibody to the S antigen arises earlier and more rapidly in developing cases of mumps and that low or absent S antibody in the presence of V antibody indicates long past infection (11). More recent work casts doubt on this interpretation (5). Of 40 mumps cases, V antibody appeared earlier in 14 cases, whereas S antibody appeared earlier in only 2 cases. This study confirms the necessity of testing both V and S antigens for demonstration of seroconversions and extends this recommendation to include HI for detection of the maximum number of mumps cases.

Assays for IgM are more useful, since cross-reactions between mumps and parainfluenza viruses have not been observed for IgM antibody (9, 23, 38). However, false-positive IgM assays due to the presence of rheumatoid factor and false-negative IgM assays due to the presence of high levels of IgG have been observed (32). IgM capture ELISA (9, 21, 32) is highly sensitive and specific and is diagnostic of a current mumps infection. Studies to date have demonstrated that IgM antibody, measured by IgM capture, is present in all patients with mumps by day 5 of illness and that peak IgM titers are reached at 1 week of illness and persist for at least 6 weeks (9, 32).

ELISA is more sensitive than neutralization for determination of immune status (21), although cross-reactions with paramyxoviruses are also observed by ELISA. ELISA is more sensitive than CF and HI for detection of low levels of antibodies (30). For diagnosis of acute mumps infections, significant titer rises may be more difficult to detect than by CF because of the earlier appearance of antibody by ELISA (23).

Two commercially available tests, the Mumps STAT EIA (enzyme immunoassay) and the FIAX Mumps-G, are designed for determination of immune status. However, positive antibody results with these tests may be due to cross-reactions with the parainfluenza viruses.

In cases of mumps meningitis, mumps-specific IgG may be found in CSF. CF and HI methods are less sensitive than ELISA for detection of CSF antibody (6, 24, 37). CSF IgG is present in CSF within a few days after onset of disease and peaks at 7 to 10 days (37).

LITERATURE CITED

1. **ACIP.** 1989. Mumps prevention. Morbid. Mortal. Weekly Rep. **38:**388–392, 397–400.
2. **Baum, S. G., and N. Litman.** 1990. Mumps virus, p. 1260–1265. *In* G. L. Mandell, R. G. Douglas, Jr., and J. E. Bennett (ed.), Principles and practice of infectious diseases, 3rd ed. Churchill Livingstone, New York.
3. **Buynak, E. B., J. E. Whitman, Jr., R. R. Roehm, D. H. Morton, G. P. Lampson, and M. R. Hilleman.** 1967. Comparison of neutralization and hemagglutination-inhibition techniques for measuring mumps antibody. Proc. Soc. Exp. Biol. Med. **125:**1068–1071.
4. **Chanock, R. M., K. M. Johnson, M. K. Cook, D. C. Wong, and A. Vargosko.** 1961. The hemadsorption technique, with special reference to the problem of naturally occurring simian parainfluenza virus. Am. Rev. Respir. Dis. **83:** 125–129.
5. **Freeman, R., and M. H. Hambling.** 1980. Serological studies on 40 cases of mumps virus infection. J. Clin. Pathol. **33:**28–32.
6. **Fryden, A., H. Link, and E. Norrby.** 1978. Cerebrospinal fluid and serum immunoglobulins and antibody titers in mumps meningitis and aseptic meningitis of other etiology. Infect. Immun. **21:**852–861.
7. **Ginsberg, H. S.** 1988. Paramyxoviruses, p. 239–259. *In* R. Dulbecco and H. S. Ginsberg (ed.), Virology, 2nd ed. J. B. Lippincott Co., Philadelphia.
8. **Grillner, L., and J. Blomberg.** 1976. Hemolysis-in-gel and neutralization tests for determination of antibodies to mumps virus. J. Clin. Microbiol. **4:**11–15.
9. **Gut, J. P., C. Spiess, S. Schmitt, and A. Kirn.** 1985. Rapid diagnosis of acute mumps infection by a direct immunoglobulin M antibody capture enzyme immunoassay with labeled antigen. J. Clin. Microbiol. **21:**346–352.
10. **Henle, G., and F. Deinhardt.** 1955. Propagation and primary isolation of mumps virus in tissue culture. Proc. Soc. Exp. Biol. Med. **89:**556–560.
11. **Henle, G., S. Harris, and W. Henle.** 1948. The reactivity of various human sera with mumps complement fixation antigens. J. Exp. Med. **88:**133–147.
12. **Henle, G., W. Henle, K. K. Wendell, and P. Rosenberg.** 1948. Isolation of mumps virus from human beings with induced apparent or inapparent infections. J. Exp. Med. **88:**223–232.
13. **Jensik, S. C., and S. Silver.** 1976. Polypeptides of mumps virus. J. Virol. **17:**363–373.
14. **Julkunen, I.** 1984. Serological diagnosis of parainfluenza virus infections by enzyme immunoassay with special emphasis on purity of viral antigens. J. Med. Virol. **14:**177–187.
15. **Kaplan, K. M., D. C. Marder, S. L. Cochi, and S. R. Preblud.** 1988. Mumps in the workplace. J. Am. Med. Assoc. **260:**1434–1438.
16. **Kendal, A. P., W. R. Dowdle, and G. R. Noble.** 1985.

Influenza viruses, p. 755–762. *In* E. H. Lennette, A. Balows, W. J. Hausler, Jr., and H. J. Shadomy (ed.), Manual of clinical microbiology, 4th ed. American Society for Microbiology, Washington, D.C.

17. **Kenny, M. T., K. L. Albright, and R. P. Sanderson.** 1970. Microneutralization test for the determination of mumps antibody in Vero cells. Appl. Microbiol. **20:**371–373.
18. **Lennette, D. A.** 1985. Collection and preparation of specimens for virological examination, p. 687–693. *In* E. H. Lennette, A. Balows, W. J. Hausler, Jr., and H. J. Shadomy (ed.), Manual of clinical microbiology, 4th ed. American Society for Microbiology, Washington, D.C.
19. **Lennette, E. H., F. W. Jensen, R. W. Guenther, and R. L. Magoffin.** 1963. Serologic responses to para-influenza viruses in patients with mumps virus infection. J. Lab. Clin. Med. **61:**780–788.
20. **Leymaster, G. R., and T. G. Ward.** 1947. Direct isolation of mumps virus in chick embryos. Proc. Soc. Exp. Biol. Med. **65:**346–348.
21. **Linde, G. A., M. Granstrom, and C. Orvell.** 1987. Immunoglobulin class and immunoglobulin G subclass enzyme-linked immunosorbent assays compared with microneutralization assay for serodiagnosis of mumps infection and determination of immunity. J. Clin. Microbiol. **25:**1653–1658.
22. **Merz, D. C., and J. S. Wolinsky.** 1981. Biochemical features of mumps virus neuraminidases and their relationship with pathogenicity. Virology **114:**218–227.
23. **Meurman, O., P. Hanninen, R. V. Krishna, and T. Ziegler.** 1982. Determination of IgG- and IgM-class antibodies to mumps virus by solid-phase enzyme immunoassay. J. Virol. Methods **4:**249–257.
24. **Morishima, T., M. Miyazu, T. Ozaki, S. Isomura, and S. Suzuki.** 1980. Local immunity in mumps meningitis. Am. J. Dis. Child. **134:**1060–1064.
25. **Mufson, M. A.** 1989. Parainfluenza viruses, mumps virus, Newcastle disease virus, p. 669–691. *In* N.J. Schmidt and R. W. Emmons (ed.), Diagnostic procedures for viral, rickettsial, and chlamydial infections, 6th ed. American Public Health Association, Inc., Washington, D.C.
26. **Nakano, J. H.** 1985. Poxviruses, p. 733–741. *In* E. H. Lennette, A. Balows, W. J. Hausler, Jr., and H. J. Shadomy (ed.), Manual of clinical microbiology, 4th ed. American Society for Microbiology, Washington, D.C.
27. **Nicolai-Scholten, M. E., R. Ziegelmaier, F. Behrens, and W. Hopken.** 1980. The enzyme-linked immunosorbent assay (ELISA) for determination of IgG and IgM antibodies after infection with mumps virus. Med. Microbiol. Immunol. **168:**81–90.
28. **Norrby, E.** 1985. Mumps virus, p. 774–778. *In* E. H. Lennette, A. Balows, W. J. Hausler, Jr., and H. J. Shadomy (ed.), Manual of clinical microbiology, 4th ed. American Society for Microbiology, Washington, D.C.
29. **Orvell, C., R. Rydbeck, and A. Love.** 1986. Immunological relationships between mumps virus and parainfluenza viruses studied with monoclonal antibodies. J. Gen. Virol. **67:**1929–1939.
30. **Popow-Kraupp, T.** 1981. Enzyme-linked immunosorbent assay (ELISA) for mumps virus antibodies. J. Med. Virol. **8:**79–88.
31. **Riggs, J. L.** 1989. Immunofluorescence staining, p. 123–133. *In* N. J. Schmidt and R. W. Emmons (ed.), Diagnostic procedures for viral, rickettsial, and chlamydial infections, 6th ed. American Public Health Association, Inc., Washington, D.C.
32. **Sakata, H., M. Tsurudome, M. Hishiyama, Y. Ito, and A. Sugiura.** 1985. Enzyme-linked immunosorbent assay for mumps IgM antibody: comparison of IgM capture and indirect IgM assay. J. Virol. Methods **12:**303–311.
33. **Schmidt, N., and R. W. Emmons.** 1989. General principles of laboratory diagnostic methods for viral, rickettsial and chlamydial infections, p. 21–28. *In* N. J. Schmidt and R. W. Emmons (ed.), Diagnostic procedures for viral, rickettsial, and chlamydial infections, 6th ed. American Public Health Association, Inc., Washington, D.C.
34. **Server, A. C., D. C. Merz, M. N. Waxham, and J. S. Wolinsky.** 1982. Differentiation of mumps virus strains with monoclonal antibody to the HN glycoprotein. Infect. Immun. **35:**179–186.
35. **Sosin, D. M., S. L. Cochi, R. A. Gunn, C. E. Jennings, and S. R. Preblud.** 1989. Changing epidemiology of mumps and its impact on university campuses. Pediatrics **84:**779–784.
36. **Ukkonen, P., M. L. Granstrom, and K. Penttinen.** 1981. Mumps-specific immunoglobulin M and G antibodies in natural mumps infection as measured by enzyme-linked immunosorbent assay. J. Med. Virol. **8:**131–142.
37. **Ukkonen, P., M. L. Granstrom, J. Rasanen, E. M. Salonen, and K. Penttinen.** 1981. Local production of mumps IgG and IgM antibodies in the cerebrospinal fluid of meningitis patients. J. Med. Virol. **8:**257–265.
38. **Ukkonen, P., O. Vaisanen, and K. Penttinen.** 1980. Enzyme-linked immunosorbent assay for mumps and parainfluenza type 1 immunoglobulin G and immunoglobulin M antibodies. J. Clin. Microbiol. **11:**319–323.
39. **Utz, J. P., J. A. Kasel, H. G. Cramblett, C. F. Szwed, and R. H. Parrott.** 1957. Clinical and laboratory studies of mumps. I. Laboratory diagnosis by tissue-culture technics. N. Engl. J. Med. **257:**497–502.
40. **Utz, J. P., C. F. Szwed, and J. A. Kasel.** 1958. Clinical and laboratory studies of mumps. II. Detection and duration of excretion of virus in urine. Proc. Soc. Exp. Biol. Med. **99:**259–261.
41. **Wharton, M., S. L. Cochi, R. H. Hutcheson, J. M. Bistowish, and W. Schaffner.** 1988. A large outbreak of mumps in the postvaccine era. J. Infect. Dis. **158:**1253–1260.
42. **Wolinsky, J. S., and A. C. Server.** 1985. Mumps virus, p. 1255–1284. *In* B. N. Fields, D. M. Knipe, R. M. Chanock, J. L. Melnick, B. Roizman, and R. E. Shope (ed.), Virology. Raven Press, New York.

Chapter 89

Rubella Virus

MAX A. CHERNESKY AND JAMES B. MAHONY

DESCRIPTION OF THE GENUS

Rubella virus is classified as a rubivirus and is a member of the family *Togaviridae,* which also contains the arthropod-borne alpha- and flaviviruses as well as members of the genus *Pestivirus.* Classification is based on morphologic, antigenic, and physicochemical properties. Only one type or species of rubella virus has been recognized so far, and it is immunologically distinct from all other known viruses. The virus possesses three major structural proteins. Two glycoproteins, E1 (58,000 daltons) and E2 (42,000 to 47,000 daltons) are associated with the envelope. A nucleocapsid protein C (33,000 daltons) is found internally. The virus is spherical, with a diameter of 60 to 70 nm, and contains a dense central core surrounded by a lipid bilayer. Replication of viral RNA and protein synthesis occur in the cytoplasm of the cell, which matures by budding into cytoplasmic vesicles or from the marginal plasma membrane. The virus is destroyed by lipid solvents or trypsin but not by freezing and thawing or ultrasonication.

NATURAL HISTORY

Rubella virus is found only in human populations and causes rubella (German measles). Postnatal rubella is transmitted chiefly through direct or droplet contact from nasopharyngeal secretions. The peak incidence of infection is in the late winter and early spring. Subclinical infection is common. The period of maximum communicability appears to be the few days before and 5 to 7 days after onset of the rash. Volunteer studies indicate the presence of rubella virus in nasopharyngeal secretions from 7 days before to 14 days after the onset of the rash. Infants with congenital rubella may continue to shed virus in nasopharyngeal secretions and urine for 1 year or more and may transmit infection to susceptible contacts. Virus can be isolated from the nasopharynx at 6 months of age in approximately 10 to 20% of these patients.

Before the widespread use of rubella vaccine, rubella was an epidemic disease with 6- to 9-year cycles; the majority of cases occurred in children. Currently in North America, the incidence of rubella has declined by more than 99% compared with the incidence in the prevaccine era. Although the risk of acquiring rubella has declined sharply in all age groups, including adolescents and young adults, a greater percentage of the cases are in young, unvaccinated adults in settings in which young adults are grouped together. Recent serological surveys have indicated that 10 to 20% of young adults are susceptible to rubella. This degree of susceptibility in young adults is due predominantly to underutilization of vaccine in this population and not to waning immunity in immunized persons.

The incubation period for postnatal rubella ranges from 10 to 21 days and is usually 16 to 18 days. It is usually a mild disease characterized by an erythematous maculopapular discrete rash, postauricular and suboccipital lymphadenopathy, and slight fever. Some 25 to 50% of infections are asymptomatic. Transient polyarthralgia and polyarthritis occur occasionally in children but are extremely common in older individuals. Encephalitis and thrombocytopenia are rare complications.

The most commonly described anomalies associated with congenital rubella are ophthalmologic (cataracts, microphthalmia, glaucoma, and chorioretinitis), cardiac (patent ductus arteriosus, peripheral pulmonary artery stenosis, and atrial or ventricular septal defects), auditory (sensorineural deafness), and neurologic (microcephaly, meningoencephalitis, and mental retardation). Infants with congenital rubella frequently are growth retarded and have radiolucent bone disease, hepatosplenomegaly, thrombocytopenia, jaundice, and purpuralike skin lesions ("blueberry muffin" appearance).

Antibodies to the virus appear as the rash fades (Fig. 1), and initially both immunoglobulin G (IgG) and IgM antibodies can be detected. Antibodies of the IgM class generally do not persist beyond 4 to 5 weeks after onset of illness, but IgG antibodies usually persist throughout life. Reinfection with the virus can occur, but it is almost always asymptomatic and can be detected by a rise in IgG antibodies. The risk of fetal damage resulting from rubella reinfection during pregnancy is negligible. The attenuated virus vaccines induce the production of IgM and IgG antibodies similar to that observed with natural infections except that the titers are somewhat lower. Reinfection rates with wild virus are greater among vaccinees than among persons previously infected under natural conditions.

COLLECTION AND STORAGE OF SPECIMENS

For details of procedures for the collection and storage of serum, urine, nasopharyngeal, throat, or cerebrospinal specimens, see chapter 74.

LABORATORY INVESTIGATION

Reliable laboratory technology has been developed for (i) determination of immune status to rubella, (ii) diagnosis of postnatal rubella, and (iii) diagnosis of congenital rubella. Because antibody responses are rapid and specific and virus isolation procedures are slow and expensive, serological procedures are usually performed in disease diagnosis (the exception would be virus isolation in a congenitally infected newborn).

A wide variety of cell types are susceptible to infection

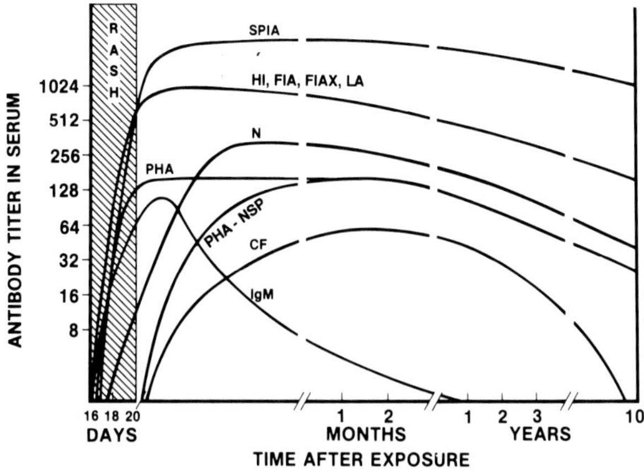

FIG. 1. Antibody response after rubella virus infection. N, Neutralization; CF, complement fixation; HI, hemagglutination inhibition; SPIA, solid-phase immunoassay; PHA, passive hemagglutination (PHAST test); PHA-NSP, passive hemagglutination to nonstructural protein (Rubacell).

by rubella virus. For primary isolation of rubella virus from clinical specimens, however, primary African green monkey kidney (AGMK), Vero, or RK-13 cell cultures are recommended. Isolation of rubella virus in primary cultures of AGMK cells has been considered the standard method (12). Rubella virus is detected in this cell type by interference with the cytopathic effects (CPE) of a challenge virus.

For virus isolation in AGMK, four tubes containing cell monolayers are drained of medium; 0.2 ml of the specimen is inoculated into each tube and allowed to adsorb for 1 h at 35 to 36°C. A 1.5-ml amount of maintenance medium (Eagle basal medium with 2% inactivated fetal bovine serum) is then added to each tube, and the tubes are incubated in stationary racks at 35 to 36°C for 10 days. Uninoculated AGMK cell cultures serve as controls. At the end of the incubation period, the tubes are examined for CPE. If none is found, two inoculated and two control tubes are challenged with 100 to 1,000 50% tissue culture infective doses of a challenge virus. The viruses most commonly used as the challenge agent for rubella isolation in AGMK cells are echovirus type 11 or coxsackievirus A9. Challenged tubes are read 3 to 4 days after challenge. The presence of rubella virus is indicated by complete destruction of the control cells but little or no CPE in the inoculated tubes. Absolute identification of the isolate requires specific neutralization of the interference with rubella antibody.

Specimens with low concentrations of rubella virus may produce little or partial interference in the culture tubes initially inoculated. The culture fluids may have to be passaged to demonstrate the virus. Fluid from the cultures that were not challenged should be inoculated into an additional four tubes of AGMK cells. Control tubes are also included. These tubes should be incubated for an additional 7 to 8 days. Two inoculated tubes and two control tubes are then challenged with echovirus type 11 and observed for CPE. The absence of interference with the echovirus cytopathogenicity on passage of fluid from tubes that did not demonstrate interference initially confirms the absence of an interfering agent. If virus is not found after such a passage, it is rarely found by further passages.

Some laboratories use RK-13 or Vero cells for isolation of rubella virus. In these cell systems, rubella virus produces CPE; however, the CPE is not always clear on primary isolation, and cell culture fluids may need to be passaged several times for full detection of virus. These cell systems, however, do offer the advantage of direct neutralization for identification of an isolate. Furthermore, an indirect immunofluorescence staining method has been shown to be specific and sensitive for identifying rubella virus isolates in these cells (11).

Fresh unfrozen tissue specimens may be of particular value in attempts to isolate virus from fetal tissues and organs. A convenient method is to explant a minced tissue fragment with growth medium and allow sufficient time for the outgrowth of cells. When the cells have formed monolayers, the extracellular fluids can be harvested and tested for the presence of an interfering agent as described above. This is a more sensitive method for rubella virus isolation than the method in which tissue extracts or homogenates of ground tissue are used.

Rubella virus can be specifically neutralized with rubella antiserum prepared in rabbits. Such antisera are available from several commercial sources. Immune rabbit serum is diluted to contain 4 U of neutralizing antibody. A normal preimmune (rubella antibody-free) rabbit serum is diluted similarly for the control titration. The media from the two companion, unchallenged cultures containing the interfering agent are pooled, and serial 10-fold dilutions are made in maintenance medium (undiluted to 10^{-6}); 0.1-ml samples of each dilution are inoculated into three culture tubes. The 10^{-1}, 10^{-2}, and 10^{-3} dilutions are also combined with an equal volume of the prediluted rubella antiserum and of the prediluted normal rabbit serum. After 1 h of incubation at 35°C, 0.2 ml of each of the mixtures is inoculated into three AGMK tubes. The tubes are incubated at 35 to 36°C for 7 to 8 days, challenged with echovirus type 11, and observed for the development of enterovirus CPE. Destruction of the AGMK monolayers inoculated with the isolate dilution containing between 10 and 100 50% tissue culture infective doses plus the immune rabbit serum, but not of those with the normal rabbit serum, indicates that the isolate is rubella virus.

Serological techniques for the detection of antibodies to rubella virus provide the approach of choice for laboratory diagnosis of acute and congenital rubella infections and for the determination of rubella immune status. Methods currently available include hemagglutination inhibition (HI), passive hemagglutination (PHA), hemolysis in gel, latex agglutination, enzyme immunoassay, fluorescence immunoassay, radioimmunoassay, complement fixation (CF), and a variety of rubella-specific IgM antibody assays.

Investigation of the pregnant patient who has been in contact with another person with rubella presents a challenge for a rapid and accurate serological diagnosis. If the patient develops clinical signs, a serum specimen should be collected at that time and paired with a second serum collected 5 or more days later. Both are investigated in parallel (same test, same day). A fourfold or greater rise in hemagglutinating or CF antibodies, together with clinical symptoms, is diagnostic for recent infection. Alternatively, a significant change in optical densities or binding ratios of the sera would be diagnostic in a solid-phase immunoassay (SPIA). A seroconversion in any patient is conclusive for recent rubella virus infection. If SPIA is available for rubella IgM testing, a single serum collected between days 3 and 21 after onset of rash will usually yield a positive diagnosis (3). Patients without clinical symptoms but with rising titers to rubella virus (the first serum containing antibodies) pose a special problem. They may have a primary infection or reinfection with an anamnestic antibody boost. To confirm these cases, a rubella IgM determination may be performed. The absence of late-rising passive hemagglutinating or CF antibodies in the first serum of this type of patient would provide evidence that the infection was primary. Measurement of rubella IgM avidity (6) by enzyme immunoassay may help to determine primary infection or reinfection. A third type of problem case involves patients whose sera are collected several days after the infection, when all serological tests are in plateau (Fig. 1); testing for IgM may be helpful. Serological examination of the suspected contacts may also be helpful in these situations.

Serological investigation of a suspected case of congenital rubella could involve two approaches. One approach is to make serial determinations of rubella HI or SPIA antibodies during the first 6 months of life; a persistence of titer in the infant during this time (Fig. 2) is highly suggestive of congenital rubella. As a second approach, the demonstration of rubella-specific IgM antibody in infant serum during the neonatal period would be diagnostic of congenital rubella.

TEST PROCEDURES

PHA

Two popular PHA tests are available from commercial sources (Rubacell II, Abbott Laboratories, North Chicago, Ill.; PHAST, Calbiochem-Behring, La Jolla, Calif.). Rubacell antibodies parallel CF and neutralization responses after infection, whereas PHAST responses are more closely aligned with HI and SPIA. Both antibodies remain measurable for years after infection or immunization as an index of immunity. Rubacell employs human erythrocytes, stabilized with formaldehyde-pyruvic aldehyde, which have been sensitized with a soluble rubella virus antigen (J. W. Safford, Jr., and R. Whittington, Fed. Proc. **35:**813, 1976). The erythrocytes agglutinate in the presence of specific rubella antibody. To perform the test, 25 µl of phosphate buffer is added to V-bottom microwells. Specimens, as well as positive and negative controls, are added (10 µl) and then mixed before the addition of 25 µl of the sensitized cells. We routinely set up alongside the test sera a row of erythrocytes without soluble rubella antigen as a control, which allows more objective scoring of results. The plates are incubated for 2 h at room temperature. A button of erythrocytes signifies the absence of antibody (susceptibility to rubella), whereas a disperse settling of erythrocytes indicates a positive reaction (immunity to rubella).

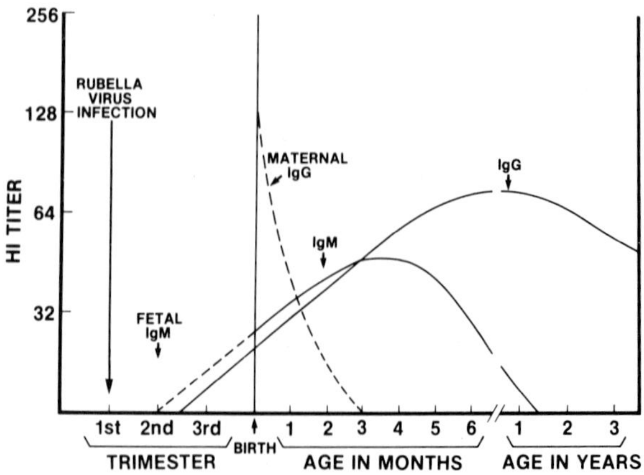

FIG. 2. Antibody responses in an infant congenitally infected with rubella virus.

Radial hemolysis

Radial hemolysis is popular in Europe and can be used to screen large numbers of sera by preparing plates in advance and storing them at 4°C. We have successfully used the method of Russell et al. (9). Freshly drawn sheep erythrocytes are washed with dextrose-gelatin-Veronal buffer, treated with 2.5 mg of trypsin (Difco Laboratories, Detroit, Mich.) per ml in dextrose-gelatin-Veronal for 1 h at room temperature, and sensitized with rubella hemagglutinating antigen (Flow Laboratories, McLean, Va.; 240 hemagglutination units [HAU] per ml) in HEPES (*N*-2-hydroxyethylpiperazine-*N'*-2-ethanesulfonic acid)-saline-albumin-gelatin buffer (HSAG) (pH 6.2) for 1 h at 4°C. Sensitized erythrocytes (0.15 ml of a 50% suspension) are mixed with 0.4 ml of guinea pig complement (Behringwerke, Marburg, Federal Republic of Germany) and then added to 10 ml of 0.8% agarose preheated to 43°C and poured into a square petri dish (100 by 15 mm). Plates can be stored at 4°C and used for up to 14 days. Prepoured radial hemolysis plates are available from Orion Diagnostics, Helsinki, Finland. Sera are inactivated at 56°C for 30 min, pipetted into 3-mm-diameter wells punched in the agarose, and allowed to diffuse overnight at 4°C in a humidified atmosphere. Plates are then incubated for 2 h at 37°C. Plates with incomplete hemolysis are flooded with 4 ml of guinea pig complement (diluted 1:3) and reincubated. All sera are tested in control plates containing unsensitized erythrocytes to monitor nonspecific hemolysis. Zones of hemolysis in control plates may range from 3.5 to 5 mm in diameter. Zone diameters of >5 mm are taken to indicate immunity.

Agglutination

Two very rapid agglutination tests are commercially available and are predominantly used for immunity screening. Rubascan (BBL Microbiology Systems, Cockeysville, Md.) uses antigen-coated latex particles, and the test is performed on a card. Rubaquick (Abbott) is an agglutination test using rubella antigen-coated erythrocytes that are stabilized. The test is performed in a tray. Both kits lend themselves to processing small numbers of specimens.

HI

Procedure. Although different laboratories use modifications of the standard rubella HI test, the following is a description of the test that we have found consistently to give good results. The test is conveniently performed in disposable plastic or vinyl V-bottom microtiter plates. The rubella hemagglutinating antigen is titrated each time the test is performed. Serial twofold dilutions of the antigen are made in 0.025 ml of HSAG (pH 6.2) to which 0.05 ml of a 0.25% washed suspension of pigeon erythrocytes is added. Control cups containing no antigen are included. The plates are sealed and placed at 4°C for 1 h, after which time they are placed at room temperature for 15 min before being read. The highest dilution that produces a pattern of complete hemagglutination is considered 1 HAU; 4 HAU is used in the HI test.

Before the HI test is performed, nonspecific inhibitors of hemagglutination and nonspecific agglutinins must be removed from sera. Test serum (0.1 ml) is added to 0.1 ml of HSAG and 0.6 ml of a 25% suspension of kaolin. The suspension is mixed and allowed to sit at room temperature for 20 min with frequent agitation. The kaolin is pelleted in a clinical centrifuge, and the supernatant fluid is transferred to a clean tube containing 0.05 ml of a 50% suspension of pigeon erythrocytes. After 60 min of incubation at 4°C, the erythrocytes are centrifuged; the supernatant fluid is removed and heated at 56°C for 30 min. This final sample, which represents a dilution of 1:8, is now ready to be incorporated into the test. Alternatively, nonspecific inhibitors may be removed by precipitation with heparin and manganous chloride. The serum sample is diluted 1:4 with 0.15 M NaCl. To each 0.8 ml of diluted serum are added 0.03 ml of sodium heparin (200 U) and 0.04 ml of 1 M manganous chloride. The sample is held at 4°C for 20 min, and the precipitate which forms is pelleted by centrifugation. The supernatant fluid is then adsorbed with pigeon erythrocytes as described above.

Known positive and negative control sera are treated similarly. Further serial twofold dilutions of each serum are made in 0.025-ml amounts of HSAG. An area of the plate is reserved for duplication of the first three dilutions of each serum. These dilutions receive HSAG in place of antigen and serve as serum controls. To each other dilution of serum is added 4 HAU of antigen in a volume of 0.025 ml. The antigen is back-titrated in a separate section of the plate by doubling dilutions in 0.025 ml of HSAG to represent 4, 2, 1, and 0.5 HAU. The plates are incubated for 1 h at room temperature, after which 0.05 ml of a 0.25% suspension of pigeon erythrocytes is added to each well and the plates are mixed on a plate vibrator. The hemagglutination pattern is read after 1 h at 4°C. The highest dilution of serum that completely inhibits hemagglutination is taken as the endpoint or rubella titer.

Since the original description of the HI test for rubella (12), several modifications have been introduced. These include the choice of indicator erythrocytes (4), optimal pH of reagents (5), methods for removal of nonspecific inhibitors from sera (7), methods for preparation of the antigen (10), and duration of incubation of antigen with the sera (8). Commercially available HI tests include Rubindex (Ortho Diagnostics, Inc., Raritan, N.J.) and Rubatech (Abbott).

Reagents. To prepare hemagglutinating antigen, we infect monolayers of BHK-21 cells grown in 32-oz (960-ml) bottles with 5 to 10 ml of rubella stock containing 10^4 or more 50% tissue culture infective doses per ml. After the virus has adsorbed for 2 h at 37°C, the monolayers are covered with Eagle medium containing 2% fetal calf serum that has previously been adsorbed with kaolin. The medium is changed after 24 h and then harvested for hemagglutinating antigen after days 5 and 7 of incubation. High-titered antigen can be extracted from the monolayers by extracting the cell-associated antigen with alkaline buffers. The cell-associated antigen preparations have CF activity and can be used as the antigen source in the CF test. We have found that good-quality CF and hemagglutinating antigens in lyophilized form can be purchased from commercial sources such as Flow Laboratories, M.A. Bioproducts (Walkersville, Md.), Ortho Diagnostics, or Connaught Laboratories (Toronto, Ontario, Canada).

Whole blood is collected by drawing a sample from a pigeon wing vein into modified Alsever solution. The erythrocytes are washed three times in HSAG, and the packed cells are suspended in an equal volume of HSAG to make a 50% suspension; part of this suspension is used to absorb nonspecific agglutinins from the test sera. A 10% working suspension is made in HSAG, from which the 0.25% suspension to be used in the test is prepared.

Acid-washed kaolin powder can be purchased from most scientific supply companies. A 25-g amount of kaolin is washed with Tris buffer until a pH of 7.0 or greater is achieved. The Tris buffer is made by mixing 12.1 g of Trizma base (Sigma Chemical Co., St. Louis, Mo.), 80 ml of 1 N HCl, and 0.85 g of NaCl and bringing the volume to 1 liter. This solution is then further diluted 1:10 in distilled water for washing the kaolin. After the final wash in Tris buffer, the kaolin pellet is suspended in 100 ml of Tris-bovine albumin buffer. This buffer is made by adding to 96.67 ml of Tris buffer the following ingredients: 0.33 ml of a 35% sterile solution of bovine serum albumin (BSA; Nutritional Biochemicals Corp., Cleveland, Ohio), 1 ml of a 0.5% $MgCl_2 \cdot 6H_2O$ solution, 1 ml of an 8% NaN_3 solution, and 1 ml of a 0.5% $CaCl_2$ solution.

HSAG is made from three different stock solutions: (i) 5× HEPES-saline, (ii) 2× BSA, and (iii) 100× gelatin. HEPES-saline is made by adding 29.8 g of HEPES powder, 40.95 g of NaCl, and 0.74 g of $CaCl_2 \cdot 2H_2O$ to 1 liter of water and adjusting the pH to 6.2. BSA is made by adding 20 g of BSA powder to 1 liter of water. Gelatin is made by adding 25.0 mg of gelatin to 2 liters of water. All solutions are filtered. A working solution of HSAG is made by adding 200 ml of HEPES-saline to 500 ml of BSA solution and 100 ml of gelatin stock solution. The volume is made up to 1 liter by adding 200 ml of sterile distilled water. The pH of the working solution should be 6.25. The solution can be stored for 2 months if it remains sterile. HSAG may be purchased from commercial sources such as Flow Laboratories, GIBCO Laboratories (Grand Island, N.Y.), or M.A. Bioproducts.

CF

The CF test is performed by a standard technique (13) (see chapter 10).

SPIA

SPIA kits are now commercially available from a number of North American and European suppliers. Four of the most popular are Rubazyme (Abbott), Rubelisa (M.A. Bioproducts), Cordia R (Cordis Laboratories, Miami, Fla.), and Enzygnost (Calbiochem-Behring). Although SPIA tests have been developed for rubella IgG and IgM, the majority of SPIA tests performed are enzyme immunoassays. Our laboratory uses the Rubazyme test. Although this test does not contain a negative control bead, it has been highly accurate and reproducible and may also be used to determine differences in antibody levels of paired sera by the formation of diagnostic ratios by comparing optical densities. For this test, sera are diluted 1:20 and tested without pretreatment and according to the manufacturer's instructions. One negative control, one positive control, and two immune status controls supplied with the kit are run in each test. Optical densities are determined by using the Quantum spectrophotometer (Abbott). Immune status is determined by comparing the optical density of the test serum with that of the mean immune status controls as instructed by the manufacturer. Automated SPIAs provide high degrees of sensitivity and specificity and facilitate the screening of a large number of sera.

Fluorescence immunoassay

An indirect fluorescent-antibody (IFA) test for rubella antibody using chronically infected LLC-MK_2 cell cultures as the solid-phase antigen was first described in 1964 (2). Other acutely infected cell systems or even purified rubella antigens have since been used for rubella IFA. For the classic IFA test, acutely infected cells are grown either on Leighton tube cover slips or in culture flasks, which are then trypsinized and deposited on slides to form smears. The cytoplasm of cells infected with rubella virus contains rubella antigens. These antigens are used to detect specific antibodies by the indirect method in which an anti-human globulin conjugated with fluorescein isothiocyanate is employed. The technique is rapid and relatively inexpensive and allows quantitation of IgG and IgM antibodies; however, IFA results are read visually with a fluorescence microscope and are open to subjective interpretation.

More recently, a soluble rubella antigen immobilized on an opaque plastic surface has been used in the indirect fluorescence immunoassay test. In this test system, marketed commercially as the FIAX test (Whittaker Bioproducts, Walkersville, Md.), the antigen-sensitized surface is allowed to react in a two-step procedure with the serum and the fluorescein-labeled conjugate, and the resulting fluorescence signal is measured objectively with a fluorometer. The intensity of the fluorescence signal correlates with the titer of rubella antibody. The sensitivity and specificity of this assay method correlate well with those of the HI test.

Other assays for detecting rubella antibody include mixed hemadsorption and time-resolved fluoroimmunoassay. These tests have their own characteristics and have not gained widespread usage.

Specific rubella IgM assays

Detection of rubella-specific IgM antibodies can be achieved by sucrose density gradient fractionation followed by HI or SPIA. Density gradient centrifugation entails diluting the test serum 1:3 in phosphate-buffered saline and adsorbing it with pigeon erythrocytes. After removal of the erythrocytes, the serum is placed on a gradient which is constructed by layering the various sucrose solutions in phosphate-buffered saline in a 5-ml cellulose nitrate tube (37, 33, 28, 24, 18, and 12% [wt/vol], as determined by refractometer readings). Before the test serum is layered, the gradient is allowed to equilibrate by overnight diffusions at 4°C. The specimen is carefully laid on top and then centrifuged for 16 to 18 h at 150,000 × *g*. The bottom of the tube is carefully punctured with a needle-type fraction collector, and 10 to 12 fractions are collected (0.3 ml per fraction; about 20 drops). Fractions 2 to 4 usually contain IgM; fractions 6 to 9 contain IgG, and the top two fractions contain nonspecific inhibitors of hemagglutination. Alternatively, other immunoglobulin separation techniques such as gel filtration, staphylococcal protein A absorption, quaternary aminoethyl-Sephadex chromatography, and 2-mercaptoethanol destruction have been used with variable success. Commercial SPIAs now available for testing whole sera for rubella IgM include Rubazyme M (Abbott), Rubelisa M (M.A. Bioproducts), Rubenz M. (Northumbria Biologicals Ltd., U.K.), and Enzygnost Rubella (Calbiochem-Behring). These SPIAs employ a pretreatment step to eliminate rheumatoid factor false-positive results and possess a high level of sensitivity and specificity (1, 3).

Confirmation of clinical rubella requires the demonstration of a fourfold rise in antibody titers between paired sera or the presence of rubella-specific IgM. There is considerable variability in the antibody titers maintained during life, and a firm diagnosis cannot be made on the basis of the absolute titer of a single serum sample. Because of day-to-day variations in the results of tests, paired sera must be tested in parallel. Differences in titers of paired sera tested on different days may reflect test-to-test variation and not a true change in antibody concentration. This consideration is especially important when paired sera are collected from pregnant women who have not experienced clinical illness. Judgments regarding therapy should be withheld until the sera have been reexamined in parallel. Sera positive for rubella IgM in SPIA should be examined for rheumatoid factor to rule out a false-positive result.

Costs are an important consideration for any laboratory performing rubella serology. As expected, the cost per test for all methods decreases as the number of sera tested in a single run increases. The individual cost of testing small numbers of sera (<10) is highest for radial hemolysis and HI, since these tests are labor intensive and a large proportion of the cost is for the technician's salary. PHA is the least expensive test for testing 10 or fewer sera. As larger numbers of sera are tested, the large difference in the cost per test decreases; the costs are similar for pHA, radial hemolysis, HI, and SPIA, with HI being the least expensive of the four.

INTERPRETATION

The presence of antibody in patient serum indicates that the patient has been previously infected with the virus and is probably immune to rubella. It is still not certain whether minute amounts of antibody, detected by highly sensitive SPIA, are protective. Whenever possible, SPIA responses should be converted to HI antibody equivalence. Patients without detectable antibodies are usually susceptible to infection by rubella virus; however, a small percentage of adults may not have detectable antibodies and yet are immune. Neutralizing antibodies at low dilutions can usually be detected in the sera of these patients. The lack of serological responses to rubella virus vaccine in women who do not have detectable antibodies is often due to low levels of neutralizing antibodies. With the HI test described above, the first dilution in the test is 1:8. A patient serum sample positive only at 1:8 should be retitrated to rule out a possible false-positive reaction.

LITERATURE CITED

1. **Best, J., S. Palmer, P. Morgan-Capner, and J. Hodgson.** 1984. A comparison of Rubazyme-M and MACRIA for the detection of rubella-specific IgM. J. Virol. Methods **8:**99–109.
2. **Brown, G. C., H. F. Maassab, J. A. Veronelli, and T. J. Francis.** 1964. Rubella antibodies in human serum: detection by the indirect fluorescent-antibody technique. Science **145:**943–945.
3. **Chernesky, M. A., L. Wyman, J. B. Mahony, S. Castriciano, J. T. Unger, J. W. Safford, and P. S. Metzel.** 1984. Clinical evaluation of the sensitivity and specificity of a commercially available enzyme immunoassay for detection of rubella virus-specific immunoglobulin M. J. Clin. Microbiol. **20:**400–404.
4. **Gupta, J. D., and J. D. Harley.** 1970. Use of formalinized sheep erythrocytes in the rubella hemagglutination-inhibition test. Appl. Microbiol. **20:**843–844.
5. **Gupta, J. D., and V. J. Peterson.** 1971. Use of a new buffer system with formalinized sheep erythrocytes in the rubella hemagglutination-inhibition test. Appl. Microbiol. **21:**749–750.
6. **Hedman, K., and S. A. Rousseau.** 1989. Measurement of avidity of specific IgG for verification of recent primary rubella. J. Med. Virol. **27:**288–292.
7. **Liebhaber, H.** 1970. Measurement of rubella antibody by hemagglutination inhibition. II. Characteristics of an improved HAI test employing a new method for removal of nonimmunoglobulin HA inhibitors from serum. J. Immunol. **104:**826–834.
8. **Pattison, J. R., D. S. Dane, and J. E. Mace.** 1975. Persistence of specific IgM after natural infection with rubella virus. Lancet **i:**185–187.
9. **Russell, S. M., S. R. Benjamin, M. Briggs, M. Jenkins, P. P. Mortimer, and S. B. Payne.** 1978. Evaluation of the single radial hemolysis (SRH) technique for rubella antibody measurement. J. Clin. Pathol. **31:**521–526.
10. **Schmidt, N. J., and E. H. Lennette.** 1966. Rubella complement fixing antigens derived from the fluid and cellular phases of infected BHK-21 cells: extraction of cell-associated antigen with alkaline buffers. J. Immunol. **97:**815–821.
11. **Schmidt, N. J., E. H. Lennette, J. D. Woodie, and H. H. Ho.** 1966. Identification of rubella virus isolates by immunofluorescent staining, and a comparison of the sensitivity of three cell culture systems for recovery of virus. J. Lab. Clin. Med. **68:**502–509.
12. **Stewart, G. L., P. D. Parkman, H. E. Hopps, R. D. Douglas, J. P. Hamilton, and H. M. Meyer, Jr.** 1967. Rubellavirus hemagglutination-inhibition test. N. Engl. J. Med. **276:**554–557.
13. **U.S. Public Health Service.** 1965. Standardized diagnostic complement fixation method and adaptation to Micro Test. U.S. Public Health Service. Public Health Monogr. 74.

Chapter 90

Human Parvoviruses

J. R. PATTISON

There are three genera in the family *Parvoviridae*. The densoviruses infect members of the order *Insecta* but do not infect humans or other vertebrates. The dependoviruses infect a number of animal species, and serological examination shows that adeno-associated viruses 1 to 4 are common human infections. However, to date they are not associated with any human disease, and there is no requirement to test for them in diagnostic laboratories.

The autonomous parvoviruses are widespread in nature and frequently cause disease in their natural hosts. Some of the animal parvoviruses such as feline panleukopenia virus and canine parvovirus are of particular concern to veterinarians, and immunization against these infections is a routine practice.

With respect to humans, one autonomous parvovirus, designated B19 (39), is of considerable importance, and the remainder of this chapter is concerned with this virus. It is quite possible that some of the small round viruses seen in human feces (29) are also autonomous parvoviruses, but at present there are no data on the exact nature of these viruses or proof of their pathogenicity.

PROPERTIES OF THE VIRUS

B19 virions are relatively uniform, isometric, unenveloped particles ranging in diameter from 20 to 25 nm (mean, 23 nm) (13). The mean buoyant density in $CsCl_2$ has been found to be 1.43 g/ml (range, 1.41 to 1.45 g/ml), with a minor peak at 1.39 g/ml possibly representing empty capsids (10). There are certainly two capsid proteins of approximately 83 and 60 kilodaltons, of which the latter constitutes about 80% of the total protein mass (43). There is also a possible third capsid protein of 48 kilodaltons (10). B19 is resistant to lipid solvents, as would be expected of a parvovirus, but appears to be relatively sensitive to acid and alkali and to heat denaturation. However, in the absence of a cell culture system for the easy replication of the virus, it is not possible to perform definitive studies.

The genome of B19 is a single-stranded DNA 5.5 kilobases in length (40). The virus packages plus and minus DNA strands into separate virions in approximately equal proportions (40). Parvovirus DNA is organized as a linear coding region bounded at each end by terminal palindromic sequences which fold into hairpin duplexes. In B19, these hairpins are relatively long (330 nucleotides versus 100 to 250 nucleotides in animal parvoviruses) and are probably inverted terminal repeats (35). This latter property, like the packaging of both plus and minus strands, is shared by B19 and the dependoviruses. Although all of the evidence available suggests that B19 is an autonomous parvovirus, the similarity in terminal genome structure with the dependoviruses suggests that like these helper-dependent viruses, B19 may be capable of integration into the host genome.

The coding regions of B19 are confined to the plus strand and comprise two open reading frames, coding for nonstructural proteins at the 3′ end and for structural proteins at the 5′ end. Restriction endonuclease analysis of multiple isolates of B19 obtained between 1972 and 1984 indicates that the genome of B19 is relatively stable (24).

There appears to be a single, stable antigenic type of B19. Infection is followed by lifelong immunity, indicating a single neutralizable type. Limited studies using immunodiffusion have revealed antigenically identical viruses from different clinical situations. The occasional minor variation in reactivity with mouse monoclonal antibodies has been noted but has so far not proved to be of epidemiological or diagnostic significance (11).

CLINICAL SIGNIFICANCE

There is a spectrum of disease caused by parvovirus B19 infection, from the wholly asymptomatic to serious, potentially fatal disease in a minority with particular underlying abnormalities.

Nonspecific illness

Parvovirus B19 was first recognized in the sera of asymptomatic blood donors (13). The first report of associated clinical illness involved patients with a mild febrile illness and lymphopenia; volunteer studies indicated that the viremic phase of the infection may be associated with fever, headache, chills, myalgia, and malaise (38). A study in a residential school for boys (17) has defined more closely the occurrence of asymptomatic infection and nonspecific illness caused by B19 infection. Among a group of boys 11 to 15 years old who were seronegative before the outbreak began, 72% seroconverted. Approximately two-thirds of these patients were asymptomatic. One quarter of the infections were associated with an influenzalike illness indistinguishable clinically from the disease caused by influenza A and B viruses, which circulated in the boys at approximately the same time as B19 infection. Only 10% had an erythematous rash that was sufficiently typical (see below) to suggest that laboratory investigations for B19 infection were indicated. Thus, it appears that the majority of infections in childhood are asymptomatic or associated with a nonspecific illness.

Rash illness

The most common illness caused by B19 virus consists of an erythematous maculopapular rash which in its most clinically distinct form is called erythema infectiosum (EI) (1). EI is common in children between 4 and 11 years of age and is sometimes called fifth disease, since it was the fifth of six erythematous rash illnesses of childhood in an old classification. Classically, it starts with an intense erythema of the cheeks (hence another of its names, slapped-cheek disease). The rash then proceeds to involve the trunk and limbs and lasts only 1 or 2 days, although transient recrudescences may occur when the individual is hot (as a result of exercise, bathing, or sunlight). The rash on the limbs tends to have a lacy or reticular appearance. There may be associated lymphadenopathy and joint symptoms (see below).

The association between EI and B19 infection was first described in relation to an outbreak in London (7). Cases in Europe, Scandinavia, North America, Australia, and Japan were later shown to be caused by B19, but it is now clear that the illnesses are not always diagnosed clinically as EI. B19 causes an erythematous rash illness very similar to that caused by rubella virus. Erythema of the cheeks is not always prominent, and the rash often does not have a lacy appearance. It sometimes occurs on the palms and soles. In the absence of laboratory tests, EI is most frequently misdiagnosed as rubella, allergy, or viral illness unless there is an associated outbreak of typical EI with red cheeks in young children. With such epidemiological support, the diagnosis of EI can often be made correctly.

In a few cases of B19 infection, the rash is purpuric (22). In most cases the platelet count is normal, but thrombocytopenia occasionally occurs (26). The purpura is transient in these patients, and there is no evidence that B19 causes idiopathic thrombocytopenic purpura.

Joint disease

Symptoms and signs of joint involvement occur frequently in B19 infection (1, 7). Approximately 80% of adult females report joint symptoms, although the figure is only approximately 10% in childhood cases. The arthropathy of B19 infection is very similar to that seen with rubella. The most common presentation is a symmetrical arthralgia or arthritis in the small joints of the hands, with wrists, knees, and ankles affected in some cases. There is a tendency for the arthropathy to be more severe in children. The symptoms and signs usually resolve within 2 weeks, but in a few cases they persist for months and very occasionally for years (33, 42). Some of these patients may be classified clinically as having early benign rheumatoid arthritis, but they will be found to be rheumatoid factor negative. B19 virus infection does not seem to be related to rheumatoid arthritis in any way; the frequency of B19 antibody is no greater in patients with seropositive rheumatoid arthritis than in controls, and B19 seroconversion occurs in patients who have had rheumatoid arthritis for years (23).

Aplastic crisis

An aplastic crisis is a transient, acute event that complicates chronic hemolytic anemia. There is a fall in hemoglobin from steady-state values, a disappearance of reticulocytes from the peripheral blood, and a virtual absence of erythrocyte precursors in the bone marrow at the beginning of the crisis. The cessation of erythropoiesis lasts 5 to 7 days, and patients present with symptoms of worsening anemia. The situation is serious in most patients and occasionally fatal. Blood transfusion is required in the acute phase, but after a week or so the bone marrow recovers rapidly, there is a reticulocytosis, and the hemoglobin concentration returns to steady-state values.

The association between B19 infection and aplastic crisis was first noted in patients with sickle cell anemia in 1981 (28); even with the insensitive diagnostic criteria of the time, B19 infection was shown to be responsible for 90% of cases (36). It is now clear that B19 is the principal cause of aplastic crises worldwide. There have been B19-associated cases in the West Indies, Europe, and North America, and evidence suggests that B19 has been the principal cause of aplastic crisis in sickle cell anemia for at least the last 20 years (34, 36).

Aplastic crisis occurs in hemolytic states other than sickle cell anemia. Investigation of aplastic crises in patients with hereditary spherocytosis, pyruvate kinase deficiency, transfusion-independent beta-thalassemia intermedia, and the dyserythropoietic anemia called HEMPAS has shown that B19 infection is the cause (15, 18, 32, 41).

B19 infection in immunosuppressed patients

Cases of persistent B19 infection have been described in patients with underlying immunodeficiency states (Nezelof's syndrome-affected, acute lymphatic leukemic, and human immunodeficiency virus-positive individuals) (20, 21). The illness is characterized by either persistent anemia or a remitting and relapsing anemia. Viremia occurs and recurs in periods of anemia, and only a weak humoral immune response can be detected. The bone marrow is typical of that seen in aplastic crisis complicating hemolytic anemia. In one patient with acute lymphocytic leukemia, administration of B19 antibodies resulted in a transient fall in virus titer, a reticulocytosis, and symptoms of EI (fever, rash, and arthralgia).

B19 in pregnancy

The intense viremia that is a consistent feature of B19 infection gives ample opportunity for the virus to reach the placenta and fetus should infection occur during pregnancy, and animal parvoviruses are associated with fetal loss in hamsters, pigs, and cattle.

Early clinical studies showed that there was no increase in birth defects during the year after large outbreaks of EI in the United States and United Kingdom. When B19 diagnostic tests became available, no viral antigen or specific immunoglobulin M (IgM) antibody could be found in sera taken during the first month of life from infants with birth defects (25). However, this diagnostic approach depends on analogy with rubella virus and cytomegalovirus infection. Both of these viruses cause persistent infection of the fetus, and it may be that B19 causes an acute infection that is rapidly cleared. Nevertheless, there is as yet no evidence that B19 causes birth defects.

Early studies indicated that B19 infection does not occur with the expected frequency in pregnant women (6, 25), possibly because B19 infection leads to early fetal loss before pregnancy is confirmed. Moreover, in studies of B19 infection in women known to be pregnant, the spontaneous abortion rate appeared to be high. In early studies the numbers were small, usually less than 10, but the fetal loss rates as a consequence of first-trimester B19 infection were of the order of 35% (16, 25). The largest study is still under way in the United Kingdom, but the results to date suggest that 1 in 10 of the pregnancies complicated by B19 infection ends in spontaneous abortion and that the pregnancy is lost, on average, 4 to 6 weeks after the onset of symptoms of EI in the mother.

Most pregnancies complicated by B19 continue to full-term delivery of normal infants. However, damage sometimes occurs as a consequence of second- or third-trimester infection, and in these cases fetal hydrops appears to be a consistent feature. Maternal B19 infection appears to occur 2 to 12 weeks before the diagnosis of hydrops fetalis (5, 8, 9). B19 infection of the fetus is suggested by cells with eosinophilic intranuclear inclusions, and presence of the virus can be confirmed by in situ or filter hybridization. The percentage of fetal hydrops accounted for by B19 infection is not clear at present. One study reviewed 50 cases of nonimmunological hydrops fetalis that were seen in a single pathology department in the United Kingdom between 1974 and 1983. Cardiovascular anomalies and chromosomal abnormalities were the most common causes, but 13 remained unexplained or had features of unidentified virus infections. Of these 13, 4 had evidence of B19 infection by in situ hybridization (29). Thus, it is clearly worth investigating B19 as a cause of nonimmunological hydrops fetalis either by detecting virus in fetal blood samples, by detecting the B19 genome in extracted tissue, or by specific in situ hybridization. Raised maternal α-fetoprotein levels are also a marker for intrauterine B19 infection.

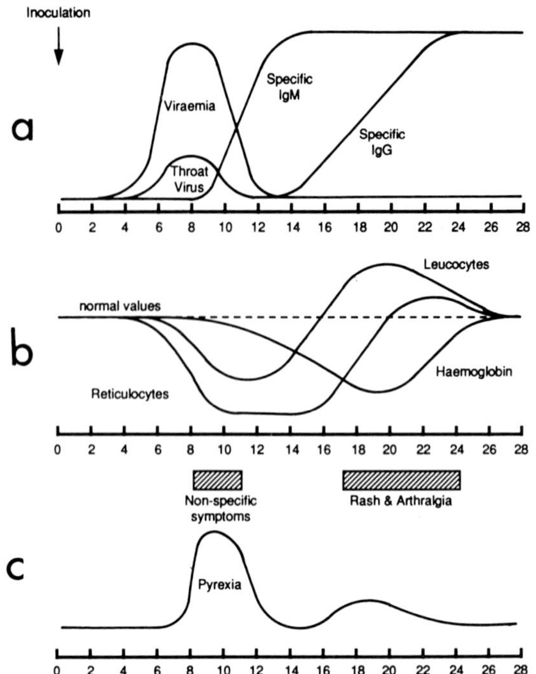

FIG. 1. Events that follow intranasal inoculation of virus. At the time of inoculation, virus was administered as nasal drops to susceptible volunteers. The virological (a), hematological (b), and clinical (c) events occurring during the subsequent 28 days are illustrated schematically. (Reproduced with permission from *Principles and Practice of Clinical Virology*, John Wiley & Sons Ltd., Chichester, England, 1987.)

Pathogenesis of B19 infection

An understanding of the pathogenesis of B19 virus infection provides the key to understanding the diagnostic approaches used in investigating clinical diseases that might be a consequence of infection. Knowledge of the events of pathogenesis has been accumulated from both volunteer studies and cell culture experiments (3, 31, 43). It is assumed that the natural mode of infection is via the respiratory route, since virus is infectious when given as nasal drops and can be found in nasal secretions at the time of the viremia.

Figure 1 illustrates the various events that follow intranasal inoculation of the virus. One week later, an intense viremia (10^{11} particles per ml at peak) develops. In most individuals, this viremia lasts for a matter of days and is followed by a specific antibody response initially of the IgM class but, after a day or so, also of the IgG class.

At the time of the viremia, hematological changes take place. No erythroid precursors are present in the bone marrow of normal individuals 10 days after inoculation, and the expected disappearance of reticulocytes from the peripheral blood and small fall in hemoglobin takes place during week 2 after inoculation. Lymphocytes, neutrophils, and platelets also show a transient drop, but this is not due to lack of precursors in the bone marrow. Studies with cultured bone marrow cells confirm the in vivo observations. B19 selectively inhibits erythroid colony formation but has no effect on the cells of the myeloid series (27). Secondary cultures of erythroid cells are inhibited by virus, indicating a direct effect on committed erythroid cells, and there is morphological and antigenic evidence of intracellular virus.

A second phase of illness occurs in infected volunteers during week 3 after inoculation. The characteristic features are rash and arthralgia. As yet there are no studies of the pathology of either of these features, but since they follow the disappearance of the viremia and occur at a time when there is an easily detectable immune response, the rash and arthralgia may be immune mediated.

The viremia that is characteristic of B19 infection gives ample opportunity for infection of the placenta and fetus if it occurs during pregnancy. In infected fetuses there appears to be a persistent infection, with damage to hematopoietic cells leading to (it is assumed) anemia, heart failure, and hydrops fetalis.

COLLECTION AND STORAGE OF SPECIMENS

Serum is the principal specimen used for the laboratory diagnosis of B19 infection (Fig. 2). This approach is suitable for virus detection in cases of aplastic crisis, persistent infection in immunosuppressed patients, and persistent fetal infection. The detection of specific IgM antibody in serum is the cornerstone of the diagnosis of rash illness and arthropathy. Standard blood specimens are drawn at the time of presentation, and serum is removed aseptically from the blood clots in the usual way. These specimens can be stored at 4°C before test-

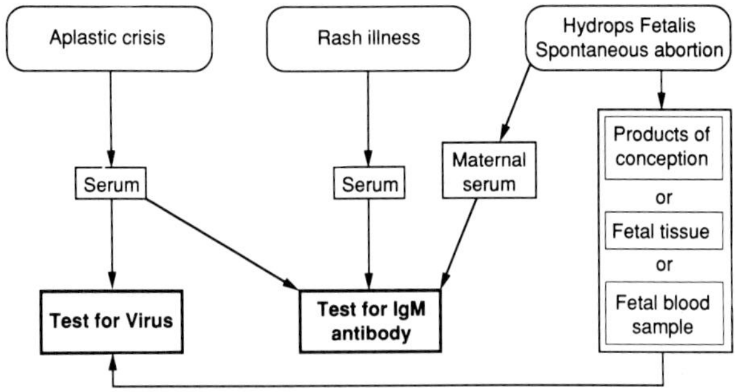

FIG. 2. Schematic diagram of clinical conditions (upper rank), specimens required (middle rank), and tests done (bold type) for the diagnosis of B19 infection.

ing unless there will be a long delay. Subsequent long-term storage is generally at −20°C for antibody-positive specimens, although −70°C is preferred for virus-positive specimens.

Detection of B19 virus by in situ hybridization can be performed on Formalin-fixed, paraffin-embedded tissue so that standard pathology protocols can be observed for fetal tissue.

DETECTION OF VIRUS

A variety of techniques have been described for the detection of B19 virus. Laboratories choose from the list of possible tests on the basis of their overall preferences and whether they are using the techniques in other contexts.

CIE

Counterimmunoelectrophoresis (CIE) is one of the simplest methods. Although insensitive, it can be undertaken by most laboratories and gives results within 1 h (36). Agarose gel (10% in barbitone acetate buffer) is poured to a depth of at least 1 mm on a glass slide or plate resting on a level surface. Two rows of wells (3 mm in diameter and 5 mm from center to center) are punched into the gel. The wells are filled with test or control sera in one row and B19 antibody-positive sera in the other row. The gel is placed so that the wells filled with known antibody-positive sera are on the anode side, and electrophoresis is carried out for 1 h at 120 V (17 mA). The gels are examined for lines of precipitate with indirect back illumination at the end of electrophoresis and after holding the samples at 4°C for 1 h.

EM

Electron microscopy (EM) is a technique in routine use in many laboratories. It is most frequently used for detection of virus in serum by using a negative staining technique but can also be used for examination of thin sections of tissue. For detection of viremia, immunoelectron microscopy is often used. The specimen is mixed with an equal volume of high-titer B19 antibody-positive serum and held at 37°C for 30 min. The sample is diluted 1:10 in phosphate-buffered saline and centrifuged at 40,000 × *g* for 1 h. The pellet is then suspended in a small volume of distilled water, mixed with phosphotungstic acid (pH 6.3) to a final concentration of 3%, and touched onto a Formvar-coated electron microscope grid. A preparation containing an antibody-negative serum should be processed in parallel as a control. The grids should be scanned at a magnification of ×30,000, and suggestive structures should be examined at ×100,000.

Immunoassays

In any laboratory providing B19 diagnostic services, immunoassays should be in routine use for the detection of B19 antibody. Such techniques can be adapted to detect virus. A solid phase is coated with anti-μ-chain antibody and reacted with a serum containing B19-specific IgM antibody. The test material is then reacted with this coated solid phase, and any bound virus is detected by sequential incubation with monoclonal B19 antibody and a labeled anti-mouse immunoglobulin.

The specimen most commonly tested for virus is serum, and a satisfactory working dilution for test serum is 1:10. Other specimens such as nasal or throat washes should be diluted 1:2. A number of variations of the basic test described above are in use, and each requires a different set of detailed steps. The reader is referred to original or recent descriptions for details (2, 11, 12). In general, it must be remembered that appropriate controls must always be included and that if any single reagent or step is changed, the test may need to be reoptimized by making other changes.

Viral genome detection

A variety of techniques have been described for the detection of B19 DNA in serum, body fluids, and tissues. Again, the details of the techniques vary according to whether dot blot hybridization with a radioactive label (4) or a nonradioactive label (14) is being described and whether B19 DNA in tissue is detected after extraction or in situ (5, 30). Most recently, techniques involving amplification of the B19 DNA by using the polymerase chain reaction have been described (34), but such techniques have not been fully validated for routine diagnostic purposes.

A variety of DNA probes are available from laboratories that have described their use, and there are published sequences suitable for use as primers for PCR. Laboratories also require some experience of hybridization and an ability to perform gel electrophoresis and endonuclease restriction to validate the results of hybridization.

Interpretation of results

The relative sensitivities of the methods described above are different. CIE will detect approximately 10^8 to 10^9 particles per ml. Electron microscopy, especially if used after antibody aggregation of virus, will detect 10^5 to 10^6 particles per ml. In the diagnostic setting, this difference in sensitivity does not matter as much as might be expected. The viremia of a primary infection is intense and short-lived, and with acute-phase specimens taken at presentation in aplastic crisis, CIE can be expected to be positive in about 30% of cases. With use of dot blot hybridization, this figure rises to about 60% (4). If an urgent answer is required, CIE and EM should be performed; if the results are negative, radioimmunoassay or DNA-DNA hybridization must be done. The latter is occasionally positive when the former is negative, possibly because of the presence of host antibody coating the virus at the time when the viremia is being cleared. If the only positive result on a specimen is by DNA-DNA hybridization, confirmation must include Southern blotting of the putative B19 DNA to ensure that it is of the correct size. If tissue samples such as placenta are to be tested for B19 DNA, confirmation by Southern blotting with and without endonuclease restriction is mandatory, since weak, false-positive dot blot signals do occur with such samples.

DETECTION OF ANTIBODY

Solid-phase radiolabeled or enzyme-labeled immunoassays are in routine use in virus diagnostic laboratories. These are the preferred methods for the serological diagnosis of B19 infection, although CIE and IEM can be used as relatively insensitive tests of seroconversion.

Specific IgM antibody detection

Procedure. The assay most commonly used is based on the antibody capture principle (12). Polystyrene beads are often used as the solid phase, but microdilution wells in strips or plates are also suitable. The solid phase is coated with anti-IgM, and the test serum is reacted with this preparation. Any specific IgM is then detected by the addition of B19 antigen, followed by a mouse monoclonal anti-B19 antibody and then by either a radiolabeled or enzyme-labeled detector antibody. The antigen most commonly used is native virus from viremic individuals, but a variety of synthetic antigens are being evaluated.

The amount of specific IgM in a serum is quantified by comparing results with those for a set of local standards. The quantification is based on designating a highly reactive serum as containing 100 arbitrary units and including a set of standards in each test (12).

Interpretation of results. Sera found to contain 10 or more arbitrary units of B19 IgM antibody are unequivocally associated with recent infection. Such antibody concentrations usually appear within 3 to 4 days of the onset of symptoms but occasionally (particularly in cases of aplastic crisis) may not appear until 7 to 10 days after onset. A B19 IgM-negative serum taken within 10 days of the onset of illness should also be tested for viral DNA, or a second specimen taken 10 to 14 days later should be requested.

Specific IgM is detectable for 2 to 3 months after acute infection. Interpretation is difficult when equivocal low concentrations of specific IgM are found in sera taken after this time. Testing the sera for IgG may be helpful. Sera containing high concentrations of rubella virus-specific IgM may give low false-positive results when tested for parvovirus-specific IgM, and this fact must be borne in mind when sera taken within 2 weeks of a rubelliform illness are tested (19).

Specific IgG antibody detection

Procedure. Assays for anti-B19 IgG analogous to those for specific antibody of the IgM class but differing in some details have been described. Again, there are radioisotope and enzyme-linked versions of the test, and the choice will depend on local preferences (2, 11). The amount of specific IgG antibody present should be quantitated by comparison of the test serum reading with a standard curve as described for specific IgM.

Interpretation of results. The test can be used on paired sera to detect seroconversion for the diagnosis of B19 infection. Patients have relatively high concentrations (>50 arbitrary units) of specific IgG for a period of 12 months after acute infection, and such values support the diagnosis of infection during that time. However, individual variation in absolute amounts is very large, and the finding of only low values (<20 arbitrary units) does not exclude recent infection.

Past exposure to B19 virus (and therefore immunity in most individuals) is indicated by the detection of >1.0 arbitrary unit of anti-B19 IgG provided that the test serum/negative serum ratio is greater than 2. Because of the relative insensitivity of the test, a negative result is not synonymous with susceptibility. A positive signal depends on a minimum proportion of the IgG having B19 specificity, and thus sera with low concentrations may not bind sufficient antigen to be detected by the indicator antibody.

There is a poor humoral immune response in immunocompromised patients with chronic parvovirus infection, and only low concentrations of anti-B19 IgG (and IgM) can be expected in these patients. None of the detectable antibody neutralizes virus infectivity, and this is taken to be an essential component of the pathogenesis of the chronic infection.

LITERATURE CITED

1. **Ager, E. A., T. D. Y. Chin, and J. P. Poland.** 1966. Epidemic erythema infectiosum. N. Engl. J. Med. **275:**1326–1331.
2. **Anderson, L. J., C. Tsou, R. A. Parker, T. L. Chorba, H. Wulff, P. Tattersall, and P. P. Mortimer.** 1986. Detection of antibodies and antigens of human parvovirus B19 by enzyme-linked immunosorbent assay. J. Clin. Microbiol. **24:**522–526.
3. **Anderson, M. J., P. G. Higgins, L. R. Davis, J. S. Williams, S. E. Jones, I. M. Kidd, J. R. Pattison, and D. A. J. Tyrrell.** 1985. Experimental parvoviral infection in humans. J. Infect. Dis. **152:**257–265.
4. **Anderson, M. J., S. E. Jones, and A. C. Minson.** 1985. Diagnosis of human parvovirus infection by dot-blot hybridisation using cloned viral DNA. J. Med. Virol. **15:**163.
5. **Anderson, M. J., M. N. Khousam, D. J. Maxwell, S. J. Gould, L. C. Happerfield, and W. J. Smith.** 1988. Human parvovirus B19 and hydrops fetalis. Lancet **i:**535.
6. **Anderson, M. J., I. M. Kidd, and P. Morgan-Capner.** 1985. Human parvovirus and rubella-like illness. Lancet **ii:**663.
7. **Anderson, M. J., E. Lewis, I. M. Kidd, S. M. Hall, and B. J. Cohen.** 1984. An outbreak of erythema infectiosum associated with human parvovirus infection. J. Hyg. **92:** 85–93.
8. **Bond, P. R., E. O. Caul, J. Usher, B. J. Cohen, J. P. Clewley, and A. M. Field.** 1986. Intrauterine infection with human parvovirus. Lancet **ii:**448.
9. **Brown, T., A. Anand, L. D. Ritchie, J. P. Clewley, and A. M. Field.** 1986. Intrauterine infection with human parvovirus. Lancet **i:**48.
10. **Clewley, J. P.** 1984. Biochemical characterization of human parvovirus. J. Gen. Virol. **65:**241.
11. **Cohen, B. J.** 1988. Laboratory tests for the diagnosis of infection with B19 virus, p. 69–83. *In* J. R. Pattison (ed.), Parvoviruses and human disease. CRC Press, Inc., Boca Raton, Fla.

12. **Cohen, B. J., P. P. Mortimer, and M. S. Pereira.** 1983. Diagnostic assays with monoclonal antibodies for the serum parvovirus-like virus (SLPV). J. Hyg. **91:**7113.
13. **Cossart, Y. E., B. Cant, A. M. Field, and D. Widdows.** 1975. Parvovirus-like particles in human sera. Lancet **i:** 72.
14. **Cunningham, D., J. R. Pattison, and R. D. Craig.** 1988. Detection of parvovirus DNA in human serum using biotinylated RNA hybridisation probes. J. Virol. Methods **19:** 279–288.
15. **Duncan, J. R., M. D. Capellini, M. J. Anderson, C. G. Potter, J. B. Kurtz, and D. J. Weatherall.** 1983. Aplastic crisis due to parvovirus infection in pyruvate kinase deficiency. Lancet **ii:**14–16.
16. **Gray, E. S., A. Anand, and T. Brown.** 1986. Parvovirus infections in pregnancy. Lancet **i:**208.
17. **Grilli, E. A., M. J. Anderson, and T. W. Hoskins.** 1989. Concurrent outbreaks of influenza and parvovirus B19 in a boys' boarding school. Epidemiol. Infect. **103:**359–370.
18. **Kelleher, J. F., P. P. Mortimer, and T. Kanimura.** 1983. Human serum 'parvovirus,' a specific cause of aplastic crisis in hereditary spherocytosis. J. Pediatr. **102:**720.
19. **Kurtz, J. B., and M. J. Anderson.** 1985. Cross-reactions in rubella and parvovirus specific IgM tests. Lancet **ii:**1356.
20. **Kurtzman, G. J., B. Cohen, P. Meyers, A. Amunullah, and N. S. Young.** 1988. Persistent B19 parvovirus infection as a cause of severe chronic anaemia in children with acute lymphocytic leukaemia. Lancet **i:**1159–1162.
21. **Kurtzman, G. J., K. Ozawa, B. Cohen, G. Hanson, R. Oseas, and N. S. Young.** 1987. Chronic bone marrow failure due to persistent B19 parvovirus infection. N. Engl. J. Med. **317:**287–294.
22. **Lefrere, J.-J., A.-M. Courouce, J.-Y. Muller, M. Clark, and J.-P. Soulier.** 1985. Human parvovirus and purpura. Lancet **ii:**730.
23. **Lefrere, J.-J., O. Meyer, C.-J. Menkes, M.-J. Beaulier, and A.-M. Courouce.** 1985. Human parvovirus and rheumatoid arthritis. Lancet **i:**982.
24. **Morinet, F., J.-D. Tratschin, Y. Perol, and G. Siegl.** 1986. Comparison of 17 isolates of the human parvovirus B19 by restriction enzyme analysis. Bret report. Arch. Virol. **90:**165–172.
25. **Mortimer, P. P., B. J. Cohen, M. M. Buckley, J. E. Cradock-Watson, M. K. S. Ridehalgh, F. Burkhardt, and U. Schilt.** 1985. Human parvovirus and the fetus. Lancet **ii:** 1012.
26. **Mortimer, P. P., B. J. Cohen, M. A. Rossiter, S. M. Fairhead, and A. F. M. S. Rahman.** 1985. Human parvovirus and purpura. Lancet **ii:**730.
27. **Mortimer, P. P., R. K. Humphries, J. G. Moore, R. H. Purcell, and N. S. Young.** 1983. A human parvovirus-like virus inhibits haemopoietic colony formation in vitro. Nature (London) **302:**426–429.
28. **Pattison, J. R., S. E. Jones, J. Hodgson, L. R. Davis, J. M. White, C. E. Stroud, and L. Murtuza.** 1981. Parvovirus infections and hypoplastic crises in sickle cell anemia. Lancet **i:**664.
29. **Paver, W. K., E. O. Caul, C. R. Ashley, and S. K. R. Clarke.** 1973. A small virus in human faeces. Lancet **i:**237.
30. **Porter, H. J., T. Y. Khong, M. F. Evans, V. T.-W. Chan, and K. A. Fleming.** 1988. Parvovirus as a cause of hydrops fetalis: detection by in situ DNA hybridisation. J. Clin. Pathol. **41:**381–383.
31. **Potter, C. G., A. C. Potter, C. S. R. Hatton, H. M. Chapel, M. J. Anderson, J. R. Pattison, D. A. J. Tyrell, P. G. Higgins, J. S. Willman, H. F. Parry, and P. M. Cotes.** 1987. Variation of erythroid and myeloid precursors in the marrow and peripheral blood of volunteer subjects infected with human parvovirus (B19). J. Clin. Invest. **79:**1486.
32. **Rao, K. R. P., A. R. Patel, M. J. Anderson, J. Hodgson, S. E. Jones, and J. R. Pattison.** 1983. Infection with a parvovirus-like virus and aplastic crisis in chronic haemolytic anaemia. Ann. Intern. Med. **98:**930–932.
33. **Reid, D. M., T. M. S. Reid, T. Brown, J. A. N. Rennie, and C. J. Eastmond.** 1985. Human parvovirus-associated arthritis: a clinical and laboratory description. Lancet **ii:** 422.
34. **Saarinen, U. M., T. L. Chorba, P. Tattersall, N. S. Young, L. J. Anderson, and P. F. Coccia.** 1986. Human parvovirus B19 induced epidemic red cell aplasia in patients with hereditary hemolytic anemia. Blood **67:**1411.
35. **Salimans, M. M. M., S. Holsappel, F. M. van de Rijke, N. M. Jiwa, A. K. Raap, and H. T. Weiland.** 1989. Rapid detection of human parvovirus B19 DNA by dot-blot hybridization and the polymerase chain reaction. J. Virol. Methods **23:**19–28.
36. **Sergeant, G. R., J. M. Topley, K. Mason, B. E. Serjeant, J. R. Pattison, S. E. Jones, and R. Mohamed.** 1981. Outbreak of aplastic crisis in sickle cell anaemia associated with parvovirus-like agent. Lancet **ii:**595–597.
37. **Shade, R. O., M. C. Blundell, S. F. Cotmore, P. Tattersall, and C. R. Astell.** 1986. Nucleotide sequence and genome organization of human parvovirus B19 isolated from the serum of a child during aplastic crisis. J. Virol. **58:**921–936.
38. **Shneerson, J. M., P. P. Mortimer, and E. M. Vandervelde.** 1980. Febrile illness due to a parvovirus. Br. Med. J. **2:**1580.
39. **Siegl, G., R. C. Bates, K. I. Berns, B. J. Carter, D. C. Kelly, E. Kurstak, and P. Tattersall.** 1985. Characteristics and taxonomy of Parvoviridae. Intervirology **23:**61.
40. **Summers, J., S. E. Jones, and M. J. Anderson.** 1983. Characterisation of the genome of the agent of erythrocyte aplasia permits its classification as a human parvovirus. J. Gen. Virol. **64:**2567.
41. **West, N. C., R. E. Meigh, M. Mackie, and M. J. Anderson.** 1986. Parvovirus infection associated with aplastic crisis in a patient with HEMPAS. J. Clin. Pathol. **37:**1144.
42. **White, D. G., P. P. Mortimer, D. R. Blake, A. D. Woolf, B. J. Cohen, and P. A. Bacon.** 1985. Human parvovirus arthropathy. Lancet **i:**419.
43. **Young, N., and K. Ozawa.** 1988. Studies of B19 virus in bone marrow cell culture, p. 5–42. *In* J. R. Pattison (ed.), Parvovirus and human disease. CRC Press, Inc., Boca Raton, Fla.

Chapter 91

Arboviruses

ROBERT E. SHOPE

CLINICAL BACKGROUND

The arboviruses are a heterogeneous group of animal viruses, usually biologically transmitted by hematophagous arthropods (mosquitoes, ticks, phlebotomine sand flies, and culicoid midges). One or more of the following syndromes may be associated with human infection: fever, encephalitis, aseptic meningitis, hemorrhagic fever, rash, acute arthritis, hepatitis, and retinitis. Subclinical infection is common. Arboviruses may be recovered from blood and occasionally from cerebrospinal fluid or throat washings. At autopsy, they may be recovered from the central nervous system, liver, and spleen. However, isolation attempts are frequently unsuccessful, and diagnosis must depend largely on serological tests.

Hantaviruses, rodent-associated agents that cause hemorrhagic fever with renal syndrome in Asia and Europe, will also be considered in this chapter.

DESCRIPTION OF AGENTS

Important New World human pathogens include the viruses of eastern, western, Venezuelan, St. Louis, Powassan, and California encephalitis; yellow fever; dengue; and Oropouche, Caraparu, Guaroa, Chagres, and Colorado tick fevers. These viruses contain RNA, are spherical, and except for Colorado tick fever virus have an essential lipid envelope.

The laboratory host of choice is the baby mouse. Other, sometimes less susceptible hosts are wet chicks, hamsters, primary cell cultures of chicken embryo and hamster kidney, and continuous lines such as Vero, BHK-21, and CER. Mosquitoes and insect cell cultures are highly susceptible but often do not respond with cytopathic effect.

Arboviruses pass 0.22-µm- and in many cases 0.1-µm-pore-size membrane filters or the equivalent. They are readily heat inactivated, and most of them agglutinate chick and goose erythrocytes. Most are inactivated by sodium deoxycholate (SDC), diethyl ether, and chloroform.

Serological grouping is done by use of polyvalent sera in enzyme-linked immunosorbent assay (ELISA), immunofluorescence, complement fixation (CF), hemagglutination inhibition (HI), and neutralization tests. Typing is done by use of type-specific sera in these same tests. Arboviruses embrace five families: *Togaviridae* (*Alphavirus*), *Flaviviridae* (*Flavivirus*), *Rhabdoviridae*, *Bunyaviridae*, and *Reoviridae* (*Orbivirus*), defined by physical characteristics that include appearance by electron microscopy, but these groupings are not generally useful to the diagnostic laboratory.

COLLECTION AND STORAGE OF SPECIMENS

Virus isolation is usually successful only if specimens are obtained within the first few days of illness. For virus isolation, collect blood, cerebrospinal fluid, and brain or other organs aseptically; refrigerate the specimens at 4°C. Separate the serum from the clot. Heparinized (0.16 mg/ml) whole blood or homogenized clots are satisfactory for virus isolation and are preferable to serum for some viruses, such as Colorado tick fever virus. If immediate inoculation of the specimen is not possible, store the material at −60°C or colder. Store it in sealed ampoules if dry ice is used. Collect throat washings in 0.75% bovine albumin in Hanks balanced salt solution or phosphate buffers (BAP) prepared from 0.12 M NaCl, 0.02 M sodium phosphate buffer, and bovine albumin (fraction V) powder (final pH, 7.2).

For antibody study, collect acute-phase and 3-week or later convalescent-phase sera and store them at 4°C or colder. Collect acute-phase cerebrospinal fluid from encephalitis patients. Specimens may be shipped without refrigeration.

For long-term virus storage, add 50% normal serum or 7.5% BAP, and store the virus at −60°C or colder. Freeze-drying is excellent for the preservation of both virus and antibody.

ISOLATION OF VIRUS

Preparation of specimens

Mince the tissue with scissors and grind in a mortar or tissue grinder, or use a homogenizer. For safety, work in a vertical laminar-flow containment cabinet. Make a 10% suspension in 0.75% BAP, and centrifuge it at 480 × *g* for 10 min. If bacterial contamination is suspected, centrifuge the suspension for 1 h at 12,000 × *g* in the cold (4°C), or add penicillin (1,200 U/ml) and streptomycin (10 mg/ml). Serum and cerebrospinal fluid are inoculated without preparation or dilution.

Mouse inoculation

Mice are susceptible to most arboviruses. Inoculate 0.015 ml intracerebrally into one or two litters of 1- to 4-day-old Swiss mice from a colony as free as possible from contaminating murine viruses. Observe the animals for 21 days for illness (lethargy, nonfeeding, tremor, loss of equilibrium, alopecia, paralysis, apnea, cyanosis, hyperexcitability, clonus, or circling) or death. Kill such mice by exsanguination (ether and chloroform inactivate arboviruses), and passage a pool of liver and brain intracerebrally until mice uniformly sicken. Test harvested tissues from each passage for bacterial sterility.

Alternative laboratory hosts

If wet chicks are used, inoculate them subcutaneously (4); inoculate baby hamsters intracerebrally. Monolayer cell cultures (chicken embryo, hamster kidney, Vero, BHK-21, HeLa, LLC-MK2, and others) should be inoculated with 0.1 ml and observed for cytopathic effect (18); cell cultures under agar should also be inoculated with 0.1 ml and observed for plaques (11, 12). If dengue virus is suspected, inoculate mosquitoes and test the heads for antigen at 7 days by the fluorescent-antibody test (15); alternatively, inoculate an *Aedes* cell culture (14). If Hantaan-related virus is suspected, inoculate Vero E6 or A549 cells.

Reisolation of the virus is important to rule out laboratory contamination or a murine virus. Alternatively, it is necessary to show an antibody rise in an infected natural host to prove the validity of the isolation.

IDENTIFICATION OF VIRUS

Characterization of the isolate

Pathogenicity for laboratory hosts, incubation periods, infectivity titers by various routes of inoculation, filterability, biochemical tests for RNA, and sensitivity to chemicals may aid in identification. A comprehensive listing of these properties for 504 arboviruses and other zoonotic viruses is available (10).

The World Health Organization Collaborating Centers for Arbovirus Reference and Research at the Division of Vector-Borne Infectious Diseases of the Centers for Disease Control, P.O. Box 2087, Fort Collins, CO 80521, and the Yale Arbovirus Research Unit, Box 3333, New Haven, CT 06510, do special diagnostic tests, accept presumed arboviral isolates for identification, and offer consultation and technical training.

SDC test

Inactivation by SDC is a reliable method of ruling out enteroviruses such as encephalomyocarditis virus, mouse encephalomyelitis virus, and coxsackievirus, but not myxoviruses, poxviruses, rabies virus, lymphocytic choriomeningitis virus, and herpes simplex virus. For the SDC test, prepare a 10% virus (usually brain) suspension in 0.75% BAP and centrifuge the suspension at 12,000 $\times$ *g* for 1 h at 4°C. Mix the supernatant fluid with an equal volume of 1:500 SDC in 0.75% BAP; mix equal volumes of virus and BAP as a control. After incubating both mixtures for 1 h at 37°C, prepare 10-fold dilutions of SDC and control mixtures, and inoculate them intracerebrally into baby mice. A reduction of titer of 1 $\log_{10}$ or more is significant. Include SDC tests of a known arbovirus and an enterovirus as a control. Enteroviruses may give a higher titer in SDC than in the control. Arboviruses of the genus *Orbivirus* (Colorado tick fever) are relatively insensitive to SDC.

Inactivation of arboviruses by ether or chloroform is equally satisfactory in distinguishing them from enteroviruses.

SEROLOGICAL IDENTIFICATION

Principle

Compare the new virus by the neutralization, CF, immunofluorescence, ELISA, and HI tests with viruses known or suspected to be in the geographical region of isolation (3, 10). Initially, test the new virus against polyvalent antibodies, prepared with agents known to exist in the geographical area. Polyvalent antibodies are available from the World Health Organization Collaborating Centers. Once grouping is accomplished, test the virus with type-specific antibodies against viruses in the group. For definitive identification, the new virus and homologous immune antibody must be compared in reciprocal cross-tests with type strain reagents.

Mouse-pathogenic viruses that might be isolated in the United States and for which antibodies should be prepared are listed in Table 1.

Preparation of antibodies

The mouse is the animal of choice for preparation of antibody. Alternatively, guinea pigs, rabbits, monkeys, or horses are used. Mice are preferred because they are susceptible to most arboviruses, they do not usually produce mouse tissue antibody when inoculated with infected mouse brain, and the antibody is useful in CF, HI, immunofluorescence, ELISA, and neutralization tests. Immunize mice with uncentrifuged, infected, 10% mouse brain suspension in saline emulsified with an equal volume of Freund complete adjuvant according to the following schedule: 0.2 ml intraperitoneally on days 0, 7, 14, and 21, with Freund complete adjuvant (1) alone intraperitoneally on day 18. Mice will form ascitic fluid, which can be paracentesed on days 28 and 35 (alternative method: 0.2 ml of infected mouse brain in saline intraperitoneally on days 1, 3, 10, 15, and 20; bleed on day 27). For polyvalent (grouping) antibody, immunize the mice with a mixture of viruses (polyvalent inoculum). For type-specific sera, use a single-virus inoculum. If the virus is lethal intraperitoneally, inactivate the 10% brain suspension by incubation for 1 h at 37°C in 0.1% β-propiolactone in normal saline (12).

Neutralization test

The plaque reduction neutralization test (16) is used to assay antibody and is usually quite sensitive and specific. An established cell line such as Vero is used. Inactivate the test serum at 56°C for 30 min. Mix equal volumes of 1:5 test serum and virus prepared in Eagle minimal essential medium with 5% fetal bovine serum, pretitrated to yield a final count of 100 PFU per well of a six-well plate. A simultaneous titration of virus in normal serum serves to indicate the virus titer. Neutralization of some viruses is enhanced by addition of 10% fresh guinea pig, human, or monkey serum to the serum-virus mixture. Incubate the mixture 16 h at 4°C. Remove the growth medium from the monolayer of cells in six-well plates. Inoculate the mixture onto duplicate wells. Incubate the cells for 1 h at 37°C in 5% CO_2 to permit virus adsorption. Wash the cells with Hanks balanced salt solution and overlay them with equal parts of 1% agarose solution and a nutrient overlay solution containing 10% inactivated (56°C for 30 min) fetal bovine serum. Place the cultures in 5% CO_2 at 37°C for a predetermined incubation period; then add a second over-

TABLE 1. Mouse-pathogenic viruses occurring in the United States (including Puerto Rico and the Virgin Islands)

Family	Virus
Togaviridae	Venezuelan encephalitis (Everglades)
	Eastern encephalitis
	Western encephalitis
	Fort Morgan
	Highlands J
Flaviviridae	Dengue, types 1–4
	Cowbone Ridge
	San Perlita
	Sal Vieja
	Modoc
	St. Louis encephalitis
	Powassan
	Rio Bravo
	Montana *Myotis* leukoencephalitis
	Tyuleniy
	Yellow fever[a]
Bunyaviridae	Tensaw
	Northway
	Cache Valley
	California encephalitis (including LaCrosse virus and several other closely related viruses)
	Buttonwillow
	Mermet
	Pahayokee
	Shark River
	Mahogany Hammock
	Gumbo Limbo
	Lokern
	Main Drain
	Hantaan-related viruses[b]
	Turlock
	Rio Grande
	Sunday Canyon
	Hughes
	Silverwater
	Santa Rosa
	Lone Star
	Virgin River
	Aransas Bay
Rhabdoviridae	Vesicular stomatitis, New Jersey
	Vesicular stomatitis, Indiana
	Flanders
	Hart Park
	New Minto
	Sawgrass
	Connecticut
	Kern Canyon
	Klamath
Reoviridae	Colorado tick fever
	Bluetongue
	Epizootic hemorrhagic disease of deer
	Mono Lake
	Yaquina Head
	Sixgun City
	Llano Seco
Nonarbovirus, SDC sensitive	Tamiami
	Lymphocytic choriomeningitis
	Herpes simplex
	Poxviruses
	Newcastle disease
	Rabies
	Mouse hepatitis

[a] May be recovered from individuals inoculated with live, attenuated virus vaccine.
[b] May not always be mouse pathogenic.

lay with the same composition as the first but containing 10% of a 1:1,000 solution of neutral red. Continue incubation at 37°C until plaques appear, usually in 2 days. A reduction in plaque numbers of 90% is considered significant.

There are numerous modifications that vary the cells, temperature and time of incubation, composition of media, concentration of neutral red, and percentage of plaque reduction considered significant. Some laboratories continue to use the varying virus-constant serum neutralization test in baby mice (18). This test is reliable but expensive.

CF test

See reference 13 for details of the CF test.

Sucrose-acetone-extracted mouse brain (or liver) is the preferred antigen because it is useful in CF, HI, and ELISA tests (5). Alternatively, 10% brain in Veronal buffer can be used as a CF antigen.

Use a vertical laminar-flow cabinet for safety. Prepare brains (20%, wt/vol) in 8.5% sucrose by use of a blender, and express the mixture through an 18-gauge needle into 20 volumes (20 times the volume of the sucrose suspension) of chilled acetone. Shake the mixture thoroughly and then decant the acetone. Immediately add 20 volumes of acetone and shake the mixture again; the sediment should appear as a finely dispersed particulate. Let the mixture stand for 1 h at 4°C without shaking. Carefully decant the acetone and dry the sediment (vacuum pump for 1 h). Rehydrate the powder with normal saline in a volume twice the original brain weight, and centrifuge the specimen at 12,000 × *g* for 30 min. The supernatant fluid is the antigen.

For the identification of isolates, antigen made from the new isolate is used in two dilutions: the optimal dilution, as determined in grid titration with homologous antibody (usually 1:32 to 1:64), and the lowest dilution (most concentrated antigen) that is not significantly anticomplementary (usually 1:4). The antigen is tested with polyvalent antibodies to determine the group and then with type-specific antibodies to determine the type. Definitive identification involves reciprocal cross-CF tests, with the use of antigen and antibody of the new isolate and antigen and antibody of the type virus in a checkerboard scheme.

Fluorescent-antibody test

The indirect fluorescent-antibody test to assay antibody is used for Colorado tick fever virus (6) and has been adapted for other arboviruses. BHK-21 cell cultures are inoculated with virus; after 24 h, cells are removed from the culture vessel with 0.25% trypsin in phosphate-buffered saline (PBS; pH 7.5) and concentrated to give 2.0×10^7 cells per ml. Smears of 0.05 ml of cells are placed on microscope spot slides, air dried, fixed in acetone at room temperature, air dried again, and stored at −65°C.

Test serum and known positive and negative control sera are inactivated at 56°C for 30 min, rinsed briefly in PBS, washed twice for 10 min in PBS (pH 7.3), and rinsed in distilled water. Rabbit anti-species-specific serum conjugated to fluorescein isothiocyanate is added to the slide and incubated for 20 min at 36°C; the slide is washed in PBS and distilled water and then dried and examined for specific staining.

This test has been adapted to rapid, specific typing of dengue virus and other arboviruses grown in C6/36 *Aedes albopictus* mosquito cells by using monoclonal antibodies. The dengue virus antibodies were developed at the Walter Reed Army Institute of Research (7) and are distributed by the World Health Organization Collaborating Centers for Arbovirus Reference and Research at the Centers for Disease Control and Yale University.

Enzyme immunoassay

The ELISA is comparable in sensitivity to the plaque reduction neutralization test, and it is simple and rapid. A commonly used assay for antibody is as follows. Ammonium sulfate precipitate of hyperimmune mouse, mouse monoclonal, or rabbit serum diluted in PBS or carbonate-bicarbonate buffer (pH 9.6) is used to coat wells of polystyrene microplates. This antibody captures antigen from infected mouse tissue or cell culture or from patient tissues. Alternatively, purified antigen may be coated directly. The wells are blocked with 1% horse serum or other protein in PBS, and then positive serum of a species different from that of the coat antibody is detected by antispecies antibody conjugated to peroxidase or other enzyme. A color change is detected when substrate is added; the reaction is assayed in a spectrophotometer. The wells are washed at least three times between each step with PBS containing 0.05% Tween 20. PBS containing 0.05% Tween 20 and 5% horse or fetal bovine serum is used as the diluent in all steps after blocking. Incubation periods and temperatures are best determined for each antigen on a case-by-case basis. The test is adaptable also to antigen detection and is used in some laboratories for surveillance of antigen in naturally infected mosquitoes (8).

The immunoglobulin M (IgM) capture ELISA is applied to the detection of recent infection by using a single serum or cerebrospinal fluid of patients with arbovirus or hantavirus infection. The test has special application to diagnosis of central nervous system infection because most encephalitis patients are positive when admitted to the hospital. IgM in patient material is captured by anti-mu-chain antibody attached to the solid phase. Antigen is added, and the plate is washed; peroxidase-conjugated antiviral antibody and substrate lead to a color change in a positive test (2, 9).

Immunoblot assay using electrophoresed hantavirus-infected cell lysates as antigens has been used to diagnose the subtype of virus causing hemorrhagic fever with renal syndrome. Adsorption of immune sera with homologous and heterologous infected-cell sonic fluids was needed to distinguish between subtypes. The technique is still experimental and is not widely applied (19).

Hemagglutination and HI tests

Antigen preparation. Sucrose-acetone antigen prepared as for the CF test is used. Alternative methods are described in the previous edition of this manual (17).

Chemical reagents. Borate-saline buffer (0.05 M borate, 0.12 M NaCl; pH 9.0) plus 0.4% bovine albumin (Armour fraction V) is used as the diluent of antigens and sera; 0.15 M NaCl–0.2 M Na_2HPO_4 in the proportions shown in Table 2 is used as an adjusting diluent for the addition of cell suspensions. For bunyaviruses (Table 1), 0.4 M NaCl–0.2 M NaH_2PO_4 as an adjusting diluent may give higher antigen titers.

TABLE 2. Composition of adjusting diluents used for the addition of cell suspensions[a]

Final pH[b]	0.15 M NaCl–0.2 M Na_2HPO_4 (%)	0.15 M NaCl–0.2 M NaH_2PO_4 (%)
5.75	3.0	97.0
6.0	12.5	87.5
6.2	22.0	78.0
6.4	32.0	68.0
6.6	45.0	55.0
6.8	55.0	45.0
7.0	64.0	36.0

[a] Adapted from Clarke and Casals (5).
[b] Final pH is that pH realized by mixing equal volumes of the adjusting diluent and borate-saline buffer, pH 9.0.

Treatment of sera. See reference 5. Test sera are adsorbed with kaolin or extracted with acetone for removal of nonspecific inhibitors of viral hemagglutinins. The acetone method is the more reliable and is described here. Dilute the serum 1:10 in PBS; then express the diluted serum through a 23-gauge needle into 12 volumes (with reference to the volume of the diluted serum) of chilled acetone and shake the mixture. After 5 min, centrifuge the mixture lightly (bring the mixture to 270 × *g* on an International PR-2 centrifuge or the equivalent and then turn the machine off). Excessive centrifugation packs the sediment and hinders subsequent extraction. Decant the acetone, replace it immediately with 12 volumes of chilled acetone, and shake the mixture. Centrifuge it for 5 min in the cold at 750 × *g*. Decant the acetone. Spread the sediment over the surface of the tube and dry it for 1 h (vacuum pump). Several sera may be dried simultaneously in a vacuum jar. Rehydrate the mixture to 10 times the original serum volume with borate-saline buffer (pH 9.0) and let the mixture stand overnight at 4°C.

Remove erythrocyte agglutinins (if present) by mixing diluted serum 1:50 with the packed cells (1 part cells, 49 parts 1:10 serum); keep the mixture at 4°C for 20 min with occasional shaking. Centrifuge it at 400 × *g* for 10 min at 4°C. The supernatant serum is used in testing.

Preparation of erythrocytes. See reference 5. Goose or chick erythrocytes are washed and stored for not longer than 2 weeks in a solution of dextrose-gelatin-Veronal (recrystallized Veronal, 0.58 g; gelatin, 0.60 g; sodium Veronal, 0.38 g; $CaCl_2$, 0.02 g; $MgSO_4 \cdot H_2O$, 0.12 g; NaCl, 8.5 g; dextrose, 10.0 g; made up to 1 liter and autoclaved) as an 8% suspension and are diluted 1:24 in an adjusting diluent (Table 2) just before use.

Hemagglutinin titrations. Ninety-six-well plastic microplates are used. Serial twofold antigen dilutions made in tubes are transferred to plates, 25 µl per well. Rows of antigen dilutions are made to correspond to different pH values (for instance, pH 5.75, 6.0, 6.2, 6.4, etc.). For each pH used, 25 µl of diluent (borate-saline buffer with 0.4% bovine albumin) is added to each well, and 50 µl is added to the control well. Cells are suspended in adjusting diluents corresponding to the desired final pH values, and 50 µl of cell suspension is added to each well. The plates are shaken by tapping their corners while holding them on a tabletop, and then the cells are allowed to settle (about 30 min) at room temperature or 37°C. Results are recorded in four grades: complete, nearly complete, partial, and no agglutination.

One unit is contained in the antigen dilution that gives complete or nearly complete agglutination; 4 to 8 U is used in the test. The pH that gives an adequate titer and is on the alkaline side of the optimal pH (to increase the sensitivity of the HI test) is chosen for the HI test.

HI test. Serial twofold dilutions of serum, 25 μl per well, are added to plates, followed by 25 μl of antigen per well. Serum controls (test serum plus diluent) and positive control serum are included in each test. The antigen titration is repeated with each test. The test is incubated for 16 h at 24°C (the HI test is more sensitive with incubation at 24°C than at 2 to 4°C). Erythrocytes in appropriate pH-adjusting diluent are added, 50 μl per well, the cells are allowed to agglutinate and settle, and the test is read as described above. Complete inhibition is considered positive. Serum controls must show no agglutination. For identification of a new isolate, reciprocal cross-HI testing is needed to establish identity with the type virus.

SEROLOGICAL DIAGNOSIS

Neutralization test

Test the patient sera in twofold dilutions in a plaque reduction neutralization test in cell culture. A fourfold rise in antibody titer between the acute- and convalescent-phase sera is of diagnostic significance.

CF test

Use antigen in two dilutions: optimal, as determined in a grid titration with homologous serum, and the most concentrated which at the same time is not significantly anticomplementary (for example, antigen dilutions of 1:64 and 1:4). A fourfold rise in antibody titer between the acute- and convalescent-phase sera is of diagnostic significance.

HI test

For the HI test, 4 to 8 U of antigen is used. Test the sera in twofold dilutions, starting at 1:10. A fourfold rise in antibody titer between the acute- and convalescent-phase sera is of diagnostic significance.

Fluorescent-antibody and ELISA tests

A fourfold rise in antibody titer between acute- and convalescent-phase sera is of diagnostic significance. In the IgM capture ELISA, a positive test indicates recent infection; titers of 1:40 or more probably indicate infection within the prior 6 weeks.

INTERPRETATION OF LABORATORY RESULTS

Definitive diagnosis can be made only with the isolation and identification of virus. A presumptive diagnosis can be made on the basis of a diagnostically significant rise in antibody titer between acute- and convalescent-phase blood specimens; however, antibody may be heterologous (related to a virus of the same group). A high titer of CF (≥1:32) or HI (≥1:320) antibody in a single convalescent-phase specimen or a fall in antibody titer during convalescence is indicative of recent infection, but it must be interpreted cautiously. The detection of IgM usually indicates a recent infection. The detection of specific viral IgM in the cerebrospinal fluid is excellent evidence of viral encephalitis. Isolation of the virus and serological diagnosis indicate association of the virus with clinical illness, but they are not proof of causation.

LITERATURE CITED

1. **Brandt, W. E., E. L. Buescher, and F. M. Hetrick.** 1967. Production and characterization of arbovirus antibody in mouse ascitic fluid. Am. J. Trop. Med. Hyg. **16:**339–347.
2. **Burke, D. S., A. Nisalak, M. A. Ussery, T. Laorakpongse, and S. Chantavibul.** 1985. Kinetics of IgM and IgG responses to Japanese encephalitis virus in human serum and cerebrospinal fluid. J. Infect. Dis. **151:**1093–1099.
3. **Casals, J.** 1961. Procedures for identification of arthropod-borne viruses. Bull. WHO **24:**723–734.
4. **Chamberlain, R. W., R. K. Sikes, and R. E. Kissling.** 1954. Use of chicks in eastern and western encephalitis studies. J. Immunol. **73:**106–144.
5. **Clarke, D. H., and J. Casals.** 1958. Techniques for hemagglutination and hemagglutination-inhibition with arthropod-borne viruses. Am. J. Trop. Med. Hyg. **7:**561–573.
6. **Emmons, R. W., D. V. Dondero, V. Devlin, and E. H. Lennette.** 1969. Serologic diagnosis of Colorado tick fever. A comparison of complement-fixation, immunofluorescence, and plaque-reduction methods. Am. J. Trop. Med. Hyg. **18:**796–802.
7. **Henchal, E. A., J. M. McCown, M. C. Seguin, M. K. Gentry, and W. E. Brandt.** 1983. Rapid identification of dengue virus isolates by using monoclonal antibodies in an indirect immunofluorescence assay. Am. J. Trop. Med. Hyg. **32:** 164–169.
8. **Hildreth, S. W., B. J. Beaty, H. K. Maxfield, R. F. Gilfillan, and B. J. Rosenau.** 1984. Detection of eastern equine encephalomyelitis and Highlands J virus antigens within mosquito pools by enzyme immunoassay (EIA). II. Retrospective field test of the EIA. Am. J. Trop. Med. Hyg. **33:** 973–980.
9. **Jamnback, T. L., B. J. Beaty, S. W. Hildreth, K. L. Brown, and C. B. Gundersen.** 1982. Capture immunoglobulin M system for rapid diagnosis of La Crosse (California encephalitis) virus infections. J. Clin. Microbiol. **16:**577–580.
10. **Karabatsos, N. (ed.).** 1985. International catalogue of arboviruses. American Society of Tropical Medicine and Hygiene, San Antonio, Tex.
11. **Karabatsos, N., and S. M. Buckley.** 1967. Susceptibility of the baby hamster kidney-cell line (BHK-21) to infection with arboviruses. Am. J. Trop. Med. Hyg. **16:**99–105.
12. **Lennette, E. H., M. I. Ota, H. Ho, and N. J. Schmidt.** 1961. Comparative sensitivity of four host systems for the isolation of certain arthropod-borne viruses from mosquitoes. Am. J. Trop. Med. Hyg. **10:**897–904.
13. **Palmer, D. F., L. Kaufman, W. Kaplan, and J. J. Cavallero.** 1977. Serodiagnosis of mycotic diseases. Charles C Thomas, Publisher, Springfield, Ill.
14. **Race, M. W., R. A. J. Fortune, C. Agostini, and M. G. R. Varma.** 1978. Isolation of dengue viruses in mosquito cell cultures under field conditions. Lancet **i:**48–49.
15. **Rosen, L., and D. Gubler.** 1974. The use of mosquitoes to detect and propagate dengue viruses. Am. J. Trop. Med. Hyg. **23:**1153–1160.
16. **Russell, P. K., A. Nisalak, P. Sukhavachana, and S. Vivona.** 1967. A plaque reduction test for dengue virus neutralizing antibody. J. Immunol. **99:**285–290.
17. **Shope, R. E.** 1985. Arboviruses, p. 785–789. *In* E. H. Lennette, A. Balows, W. J. Hausler, Jr., and H. J. Shadomy (ed.), Manual of clinical microbiology, 4th ed. American Society for Microbiology, Washington, D.C.

18. **Webb, P. A., K. M. Johnson, R. B. Mackenzie, and M. L. Kuns.** 1967. Some characteristics of Machupo virus, causative agent of Bolivian hemorrhagic fever. Am. J. Trop. Med. Hyg. **16:**531–538.

19. **Zoller, L., J. Stohwasser, L. B. Giebel, K. K. Sethi, E. K. F. Bautz, and G. Darai.** 1989. Immunoblot analysis of the serological response in hantavirus infections. J. Med. Virol. **27:**231–237.

Chapter 92

Rabies Virus

JEAN S. SMITH

CLINICAL BACKGROUND

Rabies is a fatal, infectious disease of the central nervous system to which humans and all warm-blooded animals are susceptible. The virus is often present in the saliva of rabid animals and consequently transmitted by bite. There then begins a series of events that determines the infectious course. Rabies virus can remain at the site of its entry into the body for days to weeks (4), replicating first extraneurally in myocytes (40). At this point, before the virus enters peripheral nerves, immune intervention will most likely prevent a fatal outcome. Antirabies prophylaxis should include both passive immunity, acquired through instillation of rabies immunoglobulin at the bite site, and induction of active immunity through administration of rabies vaccine, and both should be given in a timely fashion (7). Since humans exposed to rabies ordinarily know when their exposure occurs and can seek treatment promptly, disease prevention is virtually ensured in every case. This treatment is expensive, however, and not without risk to the recipient. Therefore, before treatment is initiated, each biting incident must be evaluated for the probability of rabies transmission. For this reason, the diagnosis of rabies in suspect animals is a critical function of the public health laboratory.

Endemic dog rabies presents the greatest risk to humans, particularly in Africa, Asia, and parts of Latin America, which report 50,000 to 60,000 dog rabies cases each year. Where postexposure prophylaxis is unavailable, human rabies is a common occurrence and probably exceeds the 20,000 cases recorded by the World Health Organization (5, 56, 65).

In Europe and North America, where programs for dog rabies control are present and rabies prophylaxis is readily available, only a few hundred dog rabies cases and less than 10 human rabies deaths are reported each year. These countries are not free of rabies, however, and a diverse and pervasive reservoir of disease in wildlife (more than 30,000 cases per year in a variety of wild carnivore and chiropteran species) requires a continuing program of rabies prevention for humans and domestic animals (8, 66).

DESCRIPTION OF AGENT

The rabies virion contains a single-stranded, negative-sense RNA genome of approximately 12,000 nucleotides encoding five proteins from an equal number of monocistronic mRNAs (11, 29, 59). Electron microscopy has shown that the virus particle has the characteristic structure of the family *Rhabdoviridae;* it is a rigid, bullet-shaped virus, approximately 180 nm in length and 75 nm in diameter (30). The external surface of the virus consists of a lipid bilayer envelope, derived from the host cell plasma membrane, and transmembrane glycoprotein spikelike projections encoded by the virus. It is this surface glycoprotein (or G protein) which may bind specifically to cellular receptors and in turn confer the neurotropism observed in infected animals (36, 37).

On the inner surface of the viral envelope, closely associated with the membrane-bound glycoprotein, is a second membrane or matrix (M) protein thought to play a role in virus budding (13).

The internal, nucleocapsid core of the virus particle is a helix of RNA associated with a phosphorylated nucleoprotein (N), a nucleocapsid-associated phosphoprotein (NS), and a transcriptase protein (L). By analogy with vesicular stomatitis virus, the only rhabdovirus whose biochemistry is known in detail, this RNA-nucleoprotein complex (RNP) is thought to function in the transcription and replication of the virion RNA (14, 67).

Of the five rabies proteins, the N and G proteins serve important roles in diagnosis and treatment. The G protein is responsible for the induction and binding of neutralizing antibodies. Vaccines containing only the G protein, either as purified viral protein or as recombinant DNA-derived protein, confer protective immunity to lethal infection with rabies virus. Detection of antibody to this protein is used to assess vaccine efficacy (12, 17, 63).

The internal proteins of rabies were thought to contribute little or nothing to protection from rabies infection until recent work showed that vaccines containing purified RNP or recombinant DNA-produced N protein would protect animals from a lethal challenge of rabies virus (18; J. W. Sumner, M. Fekadu, J. H. Shaddock, J. J. Esposito, and W. J. Bellini, submitted for publication). Although no neutralizing antibody is induced by these proteins, there is some evidence that they stimulate accessory cells which expedite the production of these antibodies and that they serve a role complementary to that of the G protein in whole-virion vaccines (21).

Accumulations of viral RNP form the intracytoplasmic inclusions diagnostic for rabies infection (50). Observation of these inclusions by histopathologic means (the Negri body) or indirectly by their reaction with fluorescein-labeled antiserum has long been the bulwark of rabies control. Recent advances are the availability of (i) effective diagnostic reagents containing N-protein-specific monoclonal antibodies (24) or immune serum (46a) and (ii) a specific adsorption control material produced from recombinant DNA-derived N protein (46a).

COLLECTION AND STORAGE OF SPECIMENS

Brain material

Direct examination of brain material for rabies-specific inclusions is by far the most common rabies diagnostic procedure the clinical laboratory is asked to perform. There are no reliable methods for the antemortem diagnosis of rabies in animals. Any animal suspected of having rabies should be killed immediately, and brain tissue should be sent to the laboratory for examination. Both wild and stray animals that have bitten a human or domestic animal are always considered possibly rabid and must be killed immediately. A domestic or pet animal that has bitten a human or another animal but otherwise has no signs of illness and has had no contact with rabid animals should be confined and observed for 14 days (64).

Preservation of tissues by fixation in Formalin is not recommended if rabies diagnosis is desired. Although a number of procedures are available for the examination of Formalin-fixed brain tissue (22, 31, 46, 62), they are inadequate replacements for examination of fresh tissue. Immunofluorescent-antibody tests of Formalin-fixed tissue are less sensitive than tests of fresh tissue (46, 62), and artifacts in the enzyme-mediated detection system are difficult to control for and may result in false-positive tests (52). The only advantage of Formalin fixation is that rabies virus in the tissue is inactivated, thereby reducing the risk of exposure to the specimen during handling; however, this is also the major limitation of the test, since questionable results cannot be confirmed by virus isolation.

All material collected for rabies diagnosis should be considered infectious, and appropriate handling and shipping precautions should be taken (9, 60). Preexposure rabies immunization is recommended for veterinarians, animal control personnel, and diagnosticians (7). Those assisting in the removal of the brain from a rabies-suspect animal should wear heavy rubber gloves, a face shield, and protective clothing.

Specimens for antemortem diagnosis in humans

Methods for the antemortem diagnosis of rabies are based on previous studies of rabies pathogenesis (19, 41, 43). These studies showed that after multiplication in the central nervous system, rabies virus may be transmitted centrifugally along nerves to peripheral organs. Peripheral nerves, cornea, salivary glands, and other tissues may be infected; viral antigen is accessible in frozen sections of skin biopsy (58) and touch impressions of corneal epithelium (49), and virus may be isolated from saliva (1). Other satisfactory methods of diagnosis are the demonstration of a significant rise in the titer of antibodies to rabies virus in serum in the absence of passive or active immunization, and especially the appearance of antibody in cerebrospinal fluid (CSF) (1, 2, 28).

Although a positive result on any of the currently used tests is an indication of rabies infection, no single tissue sample has been positive in every case of rabies; therefore, every diagnosis should include tests of a skin biopsy, saliva, and serum. Repeated samples taken later in the clinical course may be necessary if rabies is still suspected despite negative results on initial tests.

Skin biopsy

Biopsy of the skin, 5 to 6 mm in diameter and of the same depth, should be taken from the posterior region of the neck just above the hairline. The biopsy should include a minimum of 10 hair follicles.

Corneal impression

Corneal impressions should be made on cleaned, sterile microscope slides pressed firmly onto the cornea and released (one impression per slide). Two slides should be prepared from each eye.

Saliva

Oral secretions for virus isolation may be collected by using a sterile eyedropper pipette, which is then rinsed into a screw-cap vial containing 1 to 2 ml of a buffered cell culture medium. If the patient does not salivate, a swab of the oral cavity is rotated in the medium, and fluid is then expressed from the swab by rolling it against the side of the tube.

Serum and CSF

Antibody does not usually appear in the serum until days 8 to 10 of clinical illness (which may be several months after the rabies exposure). Specimens collected before day 8 are usually not helpful except as the first of paired samples. Antibody may also appear in the CSF a day to a week (or longer) after antibody is detected in the serum. No significant amount of rabies antibody has been detected in the CSF of rabies-immunized subjects; therefore, rabies antibody in the CSF, regardless of the rabies immunization history, confirms rabies infection.

Postvaccine serum samples

Because seroconversion after immunization with current vaccines is almost 100%, routine postvaccination serological testing is not recommended (7).

DIRECT EXAMINATION

Four methods are currently available to the clinical laboratory for the diagnosis of rabies: direct immunofluorescent antibody (dIFA), virus isolation, detection of Negri bodies (51), and a rapid rabies enzyme-mediated immunodiagnosis (6, 44, 45). The dIFA test for rabies antigen in brain tissue, because of its great sensitivity and specificity, the speed and ease with which it can be performed, and the economy of its reagents, is now the preferred test for rabies diagnosis. Isolation methods, although the most specific of all techniques, lack the speed of direct observation, a critical element in effective rabies prophylaxis. However, techniques for rabies isolation should be available to the laboratory as a confirmatory test of inconclusive dIFA results. Histologic stains for Negri bodies, although fast, inexpensive, and specific, detect only 50 to 80% of dIFA-positive samples. This lack of sensitivity severely limits their usefulness except when dIFA is unavailable. The recently introduced rapid rabies enzyme-mediated immunodiagnosis may be a better, more economic alternative to histologic methods for laboratories without fluorescence microscopes. However, it lacks the specificity gained from direct immunofluorescence observation of rabies intracytoplasmic inclusions, and the relatively high cutoff between negative and positive responses somewhat diminishes its sensitivity. The relative sensitivities of these four techniques are compared in Tables 1 and 2.

dIFA

Although rabies virus may be detected in all parts of the CNS of infected animals, its distribution is frequently uneven (39), and reliable diagnoses can be made only by examining several areas of the brain, which should include the medulla (brain stem), the cerebellum, and the hippocampus. Thin-tissue impressions are made by lightly touching cut sections from each of the three areas of the brain to clean microscope slides. Duplicate impressions are also prepared.

Before staining, impressions are fixed in acetone at −20°C for 1 to 4 h or overnight. Fixation times of less than 1 h result in less brilliant and possibly incomplete staining. In emergency situations, a positive diagnosis can be made by examination of slides fixed for shorter intervals, although a second test of slides fixed for the longer intervals should be used to confirm negative results (33).

After removal from the acetone, the slides are allowed to air dry for 10 to 15 min (acetone-fixed slides should be handled as containing potentially infectious material) (23). Each impression is then reacted with fluorescein-conjugated antirabies antibody for 30 min at 37°C in a humidified chamber. The slides are then rinsed and mounted with a phosphate-buffered glycerol mounting medium (pH 8.5). A standard microscope equipped with a UV light source and appropriate filters is used to observe fluorescing rabies antigen in infected tissues, typically at a magnification of ×400 to ×1,000.

Each test should include slides made from known positive and known negative animals. The rabies-positive control slide serves as a sensitivity control for the antirabies conjugate, and the negative control slide is used to detect nonspecific staining or adherence of aggregates of labeled antibody, which may be mistaken for rabies antigen.

Fluorescein isothiocyanate-labeled antirabies antibody conjugates can be prepared against whole rabies virions (15, 25), against purified RNP (50), or as a mixture of monoclonal antibodies reactive with the N protein (24). No differences in sensitivity or specificity have been observed in over 1,000 tests comparing N-protein-specific monoclonal antibody reagent and hyperimmune serum reagents (J. Smith, unpublished observation). These preparations are available commercially (Centocor Inc., Malvern, Pa.; BBL Microbiology Systems, Cockeysville, Md.; Pasteur Diagnostics, Paris, France).

Antirabies conjugates should be diluted so that antigen in the positive control slide stains with a glaring, apple-green brilliance (+3 to +4 staining intensity) and no background or nonspecific fluorescence is observed on negative tissue. Slides used for conjugate evaluation should contain rabies-specific intracytoplasmic inclusions revealed both as fluorescing dustlike particles of <1 μm and as large, round to oval masses and strings 2 to 10 μm in diameter. Detection of the dustlike particles requires a stronger dilution of conjugate and thus is a more stringent evaluation of the reagent. Positive tests (both the control and test slides) are also graded by the amount of antigen present and its distribution. This distribution may vary from a massive green infiltration of large inclusions and dustlike particles in every area of the tissue impression (+4 antigen distribution) to isolated small inclusions in only a few microscopic fields (+1 antigen distribution).

Although currently available commercial conjugates are both sensitive and specific in their reactions, occasionally inclusions may be observed which are irregular in morphology and distribution or may stain with less than a +3 intensity. A more confident diagnosis may be made on these occasions if the test is repeated with a second antirabies conjugate (preferably prepared with antibody from a different source) and additional specificity controls are included. When these controls are used, two impressions are made on each slide. The specificity of the reaction is ensured by adsorbing the antirabies conjugate with either normal brain tissue (on one impression) or with rabies-infected brain tissue (on the other). When the slide contains rabies antigen, rabies antibody remaining in the conjugate adsorbed with normal brain tissue should react with the antigen on test slides. If the reaction is specific for rabies, tissue stained with the conjugate adsorbed with rabies antigen should not fluoresce. These controls are unnecessary for clear-cut positive or negative tests. However, if the staining intensity is <+3 or the inclusions are sparse and of an unusual morphology, specificity controls may lead to a more confident diagnosis.

Care should be taken to avoid repeated freeze-thaw cycles of the antirabies conjugates and long-term storage at +4°C. These practices promote the formation of antibody aggregates which nonspecifically adhere to tissue. Because of the variable morphology of rabies-specific inclusions and their sometimes sparse distribution, these aggregates are easily mistaken for specific inclu-

TABLE 1. Comparison of dIFA with mouse inoculation (MI) and detection of Negri bodies (NB)[a]

dIFA result	No. of results															
	Predominantly dog rabies area						Predominantly wildlife rabies area, California									
	California				Thailand, MI not done		All samples				Bat samples					
	MI+		MI−				MI+		MI−		MI+		MI−			
	NB+	NB−	NB+	NB−	NB+	NB−	NB+	NB−	NB+	NB−	NB+	NB−	NB+	NB−		
Positive	42	6	0	0	391	13	235	120	4	2	27	26	1	0		
Negative	2	3	0	190	0	220	0	2	0	3,867	0	0	0	369		

[a] Taken from references 35 and 54.

TABLE 2. Comparison of dIFA with rapid rabies enzyme-mediated immunodiagnosis (RREID) and isolation in cell culture (ICC) for diagnosis of rabies in 4,361 samples[a]

dIFA result	No. of results					
	ICC+		ICC−		ICC not done	
	RREID+	RREID−	RREID+	RREID−	RREID+	RREID−
Positive	280	5	7	10	1,079	44
Negative	0	0	3	1,985	16	932

[a] Taken from references 6, 44, and 45.

sions. Aggregates can be removed by centrifugation at 10,000 × *g* for 20 min.

There are also other less often recognized reagents whose quality must be ensured for a reliable diagnosis by dIFA. Acetone must be of high quality and free from contaminants, and the pH of rinse buffers and water should be checked often. An inappropriate mountant can be particularly deleterious when a monoclonal antibody reagent is used (20, 62).

Also important in maintaining high-quality tests is confirmation of dIFA results by virus isolation, which may be done occasionally (e.g., when dIFA results are equivocal) or routinely (e.g., for all dIFA-negative samples involving human exposure or dIFA-negative tissue from large animal brains, for which the larger sample size afforded by isolation techniques may result in a more sensitive test).

dIFA of skin biopsy and corneal epithelium

Serial frozen sections of skin biopsy (3 to 6 mm thick) and corneal impression slides are fixed in cold acetone for 10 min, air dried for 10 min, and stained by dIFA as described above. Rabies-specific intracytoplasmic inclusions may be seen in the cutaneous nerves surrounding the hair shaft. Serial sections should show antigen throughout the nerve fiber. Only rarely is antigen seen in contiguous tissue. Rabies inclusions in infected corneal epithelium are identical to those observed in infected cell cultures; however, only rarely are more than 1% of cells infected. Testing of specimens containing only a few cells is a less sensitive diagnostic method than skin biopsy, and given the difficulty in obtaining adequate samples from clinically ill patients, corneal impression slides are not often used for diagnosis.

ISOLATION OF VIRUS

Mouse

A 20% suspension of approximately 0.3 g of tissue from medulla, cerebellum, and hippocampus is prepared in phosphate-buffered saline containing a protein stabilizer (such as 0.75% bovine albumin fraction V), penicillin (500 U/ml), and streptomycin (2 mg/ml). Five weanling mice or two families of suckling mice are then inoculated intracerebrally with a 1:2 dilution of centrifuged suspension (500 × *g* for 5 min) and observed daily for 30 days for signs of rabies (trembling, humping, paralysis, or prostration). A 7- to 20-day incubation period is expected in mice inoculated with street virus preparations, but incubation periods of 30 days or more are sometimes observed. Virus can be detected by dIFA of the brain of inoculated mice well in advance of the appearance of clinical signs or death. An earlier diagnosis can be made if extra mice are inoculated and their brains are subsequently examined at daily intervals.

If not collected into medium containing antibiotics, saliva samples for virus isolation should be diluted 1:3 into medium with antibiotics, vortexed vigorously, frozen and thawed once, and centrifuged at 2,000 × *g* for 20 min. The supernatant should be inoculated as described above.

Cell culture

Many different cell lines and all conventional methods can be used for rabies virus propagation in cell cultures. Rabies is poorly cytopathic; therefore, evidence of virus growth is by dIFA detection of viral antigen in acetone-fixed cell monolayers. As observed in our laboratory and others (47, 55), murine neuroblastoma (MNA) cell lines are the most sensitive to street rabies virus strains. However, virus strain differences and interlaboratory differences in culture conditions may determine a laboratory's preference for a particular cell line (61).

The procedure used in our laboratory is as follows. An MNA line obtained from the late T. J. Wiktor at the Wistar Institute and maintained at the Centers for Disease Control is used for all isolations. A similar cell line (CCL131) may be obtained from the American Type Cell Collection. These cells prefer an acidic medium, with increased vitamins which may be prepared from commercially available stocks. Eagle minimum essential medium (GIBCO Laboratories, Grand Island, N.Y.) is supplemented with an additional 2× vitamins, 2× glutamine, and 10% fetal bovine serum. Penicillin (100 U/ml), streptomycin (100 μg/ml), and amphotericin B (0.25 μg/ml) are also added. The final concentration of sodium bicarbonate should be 0.7 mg/ml. This medium is optimized for cell growth in closed culture. Open-flask cultures or cell culture slides (e.g., for virus isolation) should be incubated in an atmosphere of 0.5% CO_2 at 37°C and 90% humidity. Higher CO_2 levels require a higher concentration of sodium bicarbonate in the medium.

Brain material for virus isolation is prepared in Eagle minimum essential medium as a 20% suspension of medulla, cerebellum, and hippocampus. After centrifugation at 500 × *g* for 10 min, 0.5 ml of the supernatant is added to a suspension of 4 × 10^6 MNA cells. If not collected into medium containing antibiotics, saliva samples for virus isolation should be diluted 1:3 into medium with antibiotics, vortexed vigorously, frozen and thawed once, and centrifuged at 2,000 × *g* for 20 min. The supernatant should be inoculated as described above. The cells and virus are incubated for 1 h at 37°C. Unless there was obvious evidence of bacterial contamination of the sample, the inoculum may be left on the cells and the suspension may be diluted for incubation as flask or slide cultures.

After 40 to 48 h of culture, the slides (or plates) are fixed in cold (−20°C) acetone for 5 min and examined by dIFA. Most but not all cultures are positive at 20 h, but the inclusions are smaller at 20 h and cultures of low initial infectivity are more difficult to detect. There is little advantage to examination of later cultures other than to increase the number of cells examined, since secondary spread from the original foci of infection is slow and primarily cell to cell. Expansion of a culture of low initial infectivity (i.e., a culture likely to be mistaken as negative on first examination) is best done by trypsinization of the primary culture flask on day 6 or 7 and seeding of a new flask and slide cultures. There is no need to include supernatant from the primary culture. Each infected cell in the primary foci should seed new infectious centers, which are then visualized by dIFA as before. Samples that are negative upon examination of these secondary cultures are considered negative.

Although almost all dIFA-positive samples are also positive on first passage in cell culture, there is a clear advantage to secondary passage of samples for which the dIFA result was inconclusive. In one group of 25 samples in which dIFA revealed a +1 distribution of antigen, 5 were positive in cell culture only at the second passage level (J. Smith and P. Yager, unpublished results).

SEROLOGICAL DIAGNOSIS

Exposure to rabies virus, either as a consequence of infection or as a result of immunization with whole-virion vaccines, induces serum antibody to at least four of the five rabies proteins. The sensitivity and specificity of an assay method for these individual antibody populations vary greatly, and the suitability of a particular method is determined by the purpose for which the results are intended. Assays of vaccine efficacy should measure antibody to the G protein, usually as neutralizing antibody. G-protein-specific ELISAs are also applicable. Diagnostic tests, however, should detect any specific antibody present, regardless of the viral protein that induced it, and enzyme-linked immunosorbent assay (ELISA), using whole-virus immunosorbents, is the most sensitive assay available.

Neutralization test

Although an immune response to G protein is no longer thought to be the only element of protective immunity, antibody to G protein is taken as a reliable indicator for the success of active immunization. Care should be taken in serological assays of vaccine efficacy to avoid detection of antibodies to other viral proteins. The standard test for antibody to G protein measures the ability of a serum to neutralize a challenge inoculum, usually indicated by a reduction in the number of fluorescent-antibody-stained microscopic foci of infected cells. There are several modifications of this procedure (10, 16, 32, 34, 68), but the following (57) is used in our laboratory.

First, an appropriate inoculum of the challenge virus standard strain of rabies virus (ATCC VR959) is determined by serial dilution. Tenfold increments are prepared in eight-well Lab-Tek slides, leaving a final volume of 0.1 ml per well. An equal volume of MNA cells (50,000 to 100,000 cells) in Eagle minimum essential medium (see above) is added. After a 20-h incubation, infected cells are stained by fluorescent-antibody technique. At an ocular magnification of ×160, approximately 50 microscopic fields may be observed in each well of an eight-well slide. One infectious unit of virus is that contained in the virus suspension at which 50% of the observed fields contain one or more infected cells (50% focus-forming dose). In a rabies antibody titration, each serum dilution receives 32 to 100 50% focus-forming doses of virus. The antibody titer is the reciprocal of the serum dilution that reduces the challenge virus to one 50% focus-forming dose (a 97 to 99% virus reduction). The number of international units of rabies antibody in a test serum is determined by comparison with a titration of a rabies reference serum standard included in each test. A minimum post-vaccine titer of 0.5 IU is recommended by the World Health Organization (53).

If large serosurveys are anticipated, it is possible to perform all titrations in microdilution plates and detect changes in virus concentration by enzyme immunoassay (38). This procedure permits automation of all pipetting, spectrophotometric reading of color development, and titer calculation by computer analysis of data.

ELISA

Although not yet in wide use, several ELISAs for determination of antibodies have been developed (3, 27, 42). The rabies antigen may be a commercially prepared rabies vaccine, a whole-virus preparation of purified rabies virus, or isolated glycoproteins. Assays based on whole virus as the immunosorbent also detect antibodies against proteins other than G and consequently may lead to erroneous estimates of protection, a particular problem with nerve tissue-based vaccines (26). Simple methods for the purification of G protein have been published (27), and materials for a G-protein-specific ELISA are available in kit form from Pasteur Diagnostics.

If estimates of vaccine efficacy are required, dilutions of the rabies reference serum standard titrated to contain 0.5 IU of antibody are included, and a positive serum is one which yields an absorbance value equal to that of the reference serum. Although extensive comparative trials have not been conducted, data suggest that ELISA is a reliable and simple alternative to the neutralization test.

In contrast to serological tests of vaccine efficacy, for which specificity is the primary requirement, diagnostic tests should emphasize sensitivity and ideally should detect antibody induced to any of the virion proteins. As could be expected, ELISA, especially when a whole-virion immunosorbent is used, is one of the most sensitive assay methods available. Using such an assay, Savy and Atanasiu (48) were able to detect immunoglobulin M antirabies antibody very early in the clinical course of three human rabies cases and well before neutralizing antibodies could be detected.

LITERATURE CITED

1. **Anderson, L. J., K. G. Nicholson, R. V. Tauxe, and W. G. Winkler.** 1984. Human rabies in the United States, 1960 to 1979: epidemiology, diagnosis, and prevention. Ann. Intern. Med. **100:**728–735.
2. **Arko, R. J., L. G. Schneider, and G. M. Baer.** 1973. Nonfatal canine rabies. Am. J. Vet. Res. **34:**937–938.
3. **Atanasiu, P., P. Perrin, and J. F. Delagneau.** 1980. Use of an enzyme immunoassay with protein A for rabies antigen and antibody determination. Dev. Biol. Stand. **46:** 207–221.
4. **Baer, G. M., and W. F. Cleary.** 1972. A model in mice for the pathogenesis and treatment of rabies. J. Infect. Dis. **125:**520–527.
5. **Blancou, J.** 1988. Epizootiology of rabies: Eurasia and Africa, p. 243–265. *In* J. B. Campbell and K. M. Charlton (ed.), Rabies. Kluwer Academic Publishers, Boston.
6. **Bourhy, H., P. E. Rollin, J. Vincent, and P. Sureau.** 1989. Comparative field evaluation of the fluorescent-antibody test, virus isolation from tissue culture, and enzyme immunodiagnosis for rapid laboratory diagnosis of rabies. J. Clin. Microbiol. **27:**519–523.
7. **Centers for Disease Control.** 1984. Rabies prevention–United States. 1984. Recommendations of the Immunization Practices Advisory Committee (ACIP). Morbid. Mortal. Weekly Rep. **33:**393–402.
8. **Centers for Disease Control.** 1989. Rabies surveillance. United States, 1988. CDC surveillance summaries. Morbid. Mortal. Weekly Rep. **38:**1–21.
9. **Centers for Disease Control and National Institutes of Health.** 1988. Biosafety in microbiological and biomedical laboratories. U.S. Government Printing Office, Washington, D.C.
10. **Cho, H. C., and P. Fenje.** 1975. Rabies neutralizing antibody determination in tissue culture by direct fluorescent antibody technique. J. Biol. Stand. **3:**101–105.
11. **Coslett, G. D., B. P. Holloway, and J. F. Obijeski.** 1980. The structural proteins of rabies virus and evidence for their synthesis from separate monocistronic RNA species. J. Gen. Virol. **49:**161–180.
12. **Cox, J. H., B. Dietzschold, and L. G. Schneider.** 1977. Rabies virus glycoprotein. II. Biological and serological characterization. Infect. Immun. **16:**754–759.
13. **Cox, J. H., F. Weiland, B. Dietzschold, and L. G. Schneider.** 1981. Reevaluation of the structural proteins M1 and M2 of rabies virus, p. 639–645. *In* D. H. L. Bishop and R. W. Compans (ed.), The replication of negative strand viruses. Elsevier North-Holland, Inc., Amsterdam.
14. **De, B. P., and A. K. Banerjee.** 1984. Specific interaction of vesicular stomatitis virus L and NS proteins with heterologous genome ribonucleoprotein template lead to mRNA synthesis in vitro. J. Virol. **51:**628–634.
15. **Dean, D. J., and M. K. Abelseth.** 1973. The fluorescent antibody test, p. 73–84. *In* M. M. Kaplan and H. Koprowski (ed.), Laboratory techniques in rabies. World Health Organization, Geneva.
16. **Debbie, J. G., J. A. Andrulonis, and M. K. Abelseth.** 1972. Rabies antibody determination by immunofluorescence in tissue culture. Infect. Immun. **5:**902–904.
17. **Dietzschold, B., J. H. Cox, L. G. Schneider, T. J. Wiktor, and H. Koprowski.** 1978. Isolation and purification of a polymeric form of the glycoprotein of rabies virus. J. Gen. Virol. **40:**131–139.
18. **Dietzschold, B., H. Wang, C. E. Rupprecht, E. Celis, M. Tollis, H. Ertl, E. Heber-Katz, and H. Koprowski.** 1987. Induction of protective immunity against rabies by immunization with rabies virus ribonucleoprotein. Proc. Natl. Acad. Sci. USA **84:**9165–9169.
19. **DiVestea, A., and G. Zagari.** 1889. La transmission de la rage par voie nerveouse. Ann. Inst. Pasteur (Paris) **3:**237–248.
20. **Durham, T. M., J. S. Smith, F. L. Reid, C. T. Hale-Smith, and M. B. Fears.** 1986. Stability of immunofluorescence reactions produced by polyclonal and monoclonal antibody conjugates for rabies virus. J. Clin. Microbiol. **24:** 301–303.
21. **Ertl, H. C., B. Dietzschold, M. Gore, L. Otvos, J. K. Larson, W. H. Wunner, and H. Koprowski.** 1989. Induction of rabies virus-specific T-helper cell epitopes of the viral ribonucleoprotein. J. Virol. **63:**2885–2892.
22. **Fekadu, M., P. W. Greer, F. W. Chandler, and D. W. Sanderlin.** 1988. Use of the avidin-biotin peroxidase system to detect rabies antigen in formalin-fixed paraffin-embedded tissues. J. Virol. Methods **19:**91–96.
23. **Fischman, H. R., and F. E. Ward.** 1969. Infectivity of fixed impression smears prepared from rabies virus-infected brain. Am. J. Vet. Res. **30:**2205–2208.
24. **Flamand, A., T. J. Wiktor, and H. Koprowski.** 1980. Use of hybridoma monoclonal antibodies in the detection of antigenic differences between rabies and rabies-related virus proteins. I. The nucleocapsid protein. J. Gen. Virol. **48:**97–104.
25. **Goldwasser, R. A., and R. E. Kissling.** 1958. Fluorescent antibody staining of street and fixed rabies virus antigen. Proc. Soc. Exp. Biol. Med. **98:**219–223.
26. **Grandien, M.** 1977. Evaluation of tests for rabies antibody and analysis of serum responses after administration of three different types of rabies vaccines. J. Clin. Microbiol. **5:**263–267.
27. **Grassi, M., A. I. Wandeler, and E. Peterhans.** 1989. Enzyme-linked immunosorbent assay for determination of antibodies to the envelope glycoprotein of rabies virus. J. Clin. Microbiol. **27:**899–902.
28. **Hattwick, M. A. W., T. T. Weiss, C. J. Stechschulte, G. M. Baer, and M. G. Gregg.** 1972. Recovery from rabies. Ann. Intern. Med. **76:**931–942.
29. **Holloway, B. P., and J. F. Obijeski.** 1980. Rabies virus-induced RNA synthesis in BHK-21 cells. J. Gen. Virol. **49:** 181–195.
30. **Hummeler, K., and H. Koprowski.** 1967. Structure and development of rabies virus in tissue culture. J. Virol. **1:** 152–170.
31. **Johnson, K. P., P. T. Swoveland, and R. W. Emmons.** 1980. Diagnosis of rabies by immunofluorescence in trypsin-treated histologic sections. J. Am. Med. Assoc. **244:**41–43.
32. **King, D. A., D. L. Croghan, and E. L. Shaw.** 1965. A rapid quantitative in vitro serum neutralization test for rabies antibody. Can. Vet. J. **6:**187–193.
33. **Kissling, R. E.** 1975. The fluorescent antibody test in rabies, p. 401–416. *In* G. M. Baer (ed.), The natural history of rabies, vol. 1. Academic Press, Inc., New York.
34. **Lennette, E. H., and R. W. Emmons.** 1971. The laboratory diagnosis of rabies: review and perspective, p. 77–90. *In* Y. Nagano and F. Davenport (ed.), Rabies. Proceedings of the Working Conference on Rabies, sponsored by the Japan-United States Cooperative Medical Science Program. University of Tokyo Press, Tokyo.
35. **Lennette, E. H., J. D. Woodie, K. Nakamura, and R. L. Magoffin.** 1965. The diagnosis of rabies by fluorescent antibody method (FRA) employing immune hamster serum. Health Lab. Sci. **2:**24–34.
36. **Lentz, T. L., T. G. Burrage, A. L. Smith, J. Crick, and G. Tignor.** 1982. Is the acetylcholine receptor a rabies virus receptor? Science **215:**182–184.
37. **Lentz, T. L., P. T. Wilson, E. Hawrot, and D. W. Speicher.** 1984. Amino acid sequence similarity between rabies virus glycoprotein and snake venom curare-mimetic neurotoxins. Science **226:**847–848.
38. **Mannen, K., K. Mifune, F. L. Reid-Sanden, J. S. Smith, P. A. Yager, J. W. Sumner, D. B. Fishbein, T. C. Tong, and G. M. Baer.** 1987. Microneutralization test for rabies virus based on an enzyme immunoassay. J. Clin. Microbiol. **25:**2440–2442.
39. **Maserang, D. L., and L. Leffingwell.** 1981. Single-site localization of rabies virus: impact on laboratory reporting

policy. Am. J. Public Health **71**:428–429.

40. **Murphy, F. A., S. P. Bauer, A. K. Harrison, and W. C. Winn.** 1973. Comparative pathogenesis of rabies and rabies-like viruses. Viral infection and transit from inoculation site to the central nervous system. Lab. Invest. **28:** 361–376.
41. **Murphy, F. A., A. K. Harrison, W. C. Winn, and S. P. Bauer.** 1973. Comparative pathogenesis of rabies and rabies-like viruses. Infection of the CNS and centrifugal spread of virus to peripheral tissues. Lab. Invest. **29:**1–16.
42. **Nicholson, K. G., and H. Prestage.** 1982. Enzyme-linked immunosorbent assay: a rapid reproducible test for the measurement of rabies antibody. J. Med. Virol. **9:**43–49.
43. **Perl, D. P.** 1975. The pathology of rabies in the central nervous system, p. 236–242. *In* G. M. Baer (ed.), The natural history of rabies, vol. 1. Academic Press, Inc., New York.
44. **Perrin, P., P. E. Rollin, and P. Sureau.** 1986. A rapid rabies enzyme immuno-diagnosis (RREID): a useful and simple technique for the routine diagnosis of rabies. J. Biol. Stand. **14:**217–222.
45. **Perrin, P., and P. Sureau.** 1987. A collaborative study of an experimental kit for rapid rabies enzyme immuno-diagnosis (RREID). Bull. W.H.O. **65:**489–493.
46. **Reid, F. L., N. H. Hall, J. S. Smith, and G. M. Baer.** 1983. Increased immunofluorescent staining of rabies-infected, formalin-fixed brain tissue after pepsin and trypsin digestion. J. Clin. Microbiol. **18:**968–971.

46a. **Reid-Sanden, F. L., J. W. Sumner, J. S. Smith, M. Fekadu, J. H. Shaddock, and W. J. Bellini.** 1990. Rabies diagnostic reagents prepared from a rabies N gene recombinant expressed in baculovirus. J. Clin. Microbiol. **28:** 858–863.

47. **Rudd, R. J., and C. V. Trimarchi.** 1987. Comparison of sensitivity of BHK-21 and murine neuroblastoma cells in the isolation of a street strain rabies virus. J. Clin. Microbiol. **25:**1456–1458.
48. **Savy, V., and P. Atanasiu.** 1978. Rapid immunoenzymatic technique for titration of rabies antibodies IgG and IgM. Dev. Biol. Stand. **40:**247–250.
49. **Schneider, L. G.** 1969. The cornea test: a new method for the intra-vitam diagnosis of rabies. Zentralbl. Veterinaermed. Reihe B **16:**24–31.
50. **Schneider, L. G., B. Dietzschold, R. E. Dierks, W. Matthaeus, P. J. Enzmann, and K. Strohmaier.** 1973. Rabies group-specific ribonucleoprotein antigen and a test system for grouping and typing of rhabdoviruses. J. Virol. **11:**748–755.
51. **Sellers, T. F.** 1927. A new method for staining Negri bodies of rabies. J. Public Health **17:**1080–1081.
52. **Shi, Z.-R., S. H. Itzkowitz, and Y. S. Kim.** 1988. A comparison of three immunoperoxidase techniques for antigen detection in colorectal carcinoma tissues. J. Histochem. Cytochem. **36:**317–322.
53. **Sinecker, H., P. Atanasiu, H. M. Bahmanyar, M. Selimov, A. I. Wandeler, and K. Boegel.** 1978. Vaccine potency requirements for reduced immunization schedules and pre-exposure treatment. Dev. Biol. Stand. **40:**268–270.
54. **Sitthi-Amorn, C., V. Jiratanavattana, J. Keoyoo, and N. Sonpunya.** 1987. The diagnostic properties of laboratory tests for rabies. Int. J. Epidemiol. **16:**602–605.
55. **Smith, A. L., G. H. Tignor, R. W. Emmons, and J. D. Woodie.** 1978. Isolation of field rabies virus strains in CER and murine neuroblastoma cell cultures. Intervirology **9:** 359–361.
56. **Smith, J. S., and G. M. Baer.** 1988. Epizootiology of rabies: the Americas, p. 267–300. *In* J. B. Campbell and K. M. Charlton (ed.), Rabies. Kluwer Academic Publishers, Boston.
57. **Smith, J. S., P. A. Yager, and G. M. Baer.** 1973. A rapid reproducible test for determining rabies neutralizing antibody. Bull. W.H.O. **48:**535–541.
58. **Smith, W. B., D. C. Blenden, F. Tsu-Huei, and L. Hiler.** 1972. Diagnosis of rabies by immunofluorescent staining of frozen sections of skin. J. Am. Vet. Med. Assoc. **161:** 1495–1501.
59. **Tordo, N., O. Poch, A. Ermine, G. Keith, and F. Rougeon.** 1988. Completion of the rabies virus genome sequence determination: highly conserved domains among the L (polymerase) proteins of unsegmented negative-stranded RNA viruses. Virology **165:**565–576.
60. **Velleca, W. M., and F. T. Forrester.** 1981. Laboratory methods for detecting rabies. U. S. Government Printing Office, Washington, D.C.
61. **Webster, W. A., and G. A. Casey.** 1987. Growth characteristics in cell culture and pathogenicity in mice of two terrestrial rabies strains indigenous to Canada. Can. J. Microbiol. **34:**19–23.
62. **Webster, W. A., and G. A. Casey.** 1988. Diagnosis of rabies infection, p. 201–223. *In* J. B. Campbell and K. M. Charlton (ed.), Rabies. Kluwer Academic Publishers, Boston.
63. **Wiktor, T. J., R. I. Macfarlan, K. J. Reagan, B. Dietzschold, P. J. Curtis, W. H. Wunner, M.-P. Kieny, J.-P. Lecocq, M. Mackett, B. Moss, and H. Koprowski.** 1984. Protection from rabies by a vaccinia virus recombinant containing the rabies virus glycoprotein gene. Proc. Natl. Acad. Sci. USA **81:**7194–7198.
64. **World Health Organization.** 1984. Expert Committee on Rabies, seventh report. World Health Organization, Geneva.
65. **World Health Organization.** 1987. World survey of rabies XXII (for years 1984/85). World Health Organization, Geneva.
66. **World Health Organization and Collaborating Centre for Rabies Surveillance and Research.** 1989. Rabies surveillance report. Rabies Bull. Eur. **12:**1–39.
67. **Wunner, W. H., J. K. Larson, B. Dietzschold, and C. L. Smith.** 1988. The molecular biology of rabies virus. Rev. Infect. Dis. **10:**S771–S784.
68. **Zalan, E., C. Wilson, and D. Pukitis.** 1979. A microtest for the quantitation of rabies virus neutralizing antibodies. J. Biol. Stand. **7:**213–220.

Chapter 93

Enteroviruses

MARILYN A. MENEGUS

CLINICAL BACKGROUND

Enteroviruses commonly infect humans, and the consequences of infection are either asymptomatic virus shedding or a broad spectrum of acute diseases, including undifferentiated febrile illness, aseptic meningitis, encephalitis, paralysis, a sepsislike picture in neonates, myopericarditis, pleurodynia, conjunctivitis, enanthems, exanthems, pharyngitis, and pneumonia. Clinical illness is most frequently seen in infants and young children. In addition, a role has been hypothesized for enteroviruses in the etiology of diabetes, chronic cardiomyopathy, and fetal malformations. An expanded treatment of the clinical aspects of enteroviral disease can be found in several textbooks of virology and infectious disease (3, 4, 17, 23, 24).

In temperate climates, enteroviruses are prevalent in the summer and fall; outbreaks occur each year and are associated with significant morbidity. A more endemic prevalence pattern is seen in tropical and semitropical areas. By 2 years of age, regardless of where they reside, most children have already experienced several asymptomatic or mildly symptomatic enterovirus infections. The viruses are highly transmissible and are spread for the most part via the fecal-oral route. In a family setting and in crowded populations, the rate of infection among nonimmune individuals can reach as high as 80%, with children more likely to be infected than adults. Antibody appears to offer significant protection against disease and also reduces the likelihood of, but does not prevent, infection (14, 17, 24).

The incubation period for most enteroviruses ranges from 1 day to 3 weeks but is generally 3 to 5 days. The viruses enter the alimentary tract via the mouth and begin replicating in the lymphoid tissue of the pharynx and gut. In some cases, viremia then occurs, leading to the involvement of target organs such as the spinal cord, heart, and skin. Virus can be found in the pharynx for 1 to 2 weeks postinfection and may be excreted in feces for even longer periods (2 to 6 weeks). Viremia, on the other hand, is present for only a short time (several days) and is found only early in infection (17, 24, 29).

DESCRIPTION OF THE AGENTS

Viruses belonging to two genera of the family *Picornaviridae*, *Enterovirus* and *Rhinovirus*, commonly infect humans. They share the following composition: a naked, ether-resistant, 20- to 30-nm icosahedral capsid made up of four proteins and a single-stranded, unsegmented, plus-sense RNA genome with a molecular weight of 2.5 $\times 10^6$ to 3.0 $\times 10^6$. The main characteristics that distinguish enteroviruses from rhinoviruses are the stability at acid pH (3.0) and the lower buoyant density in CsCl of the enteroviruses. In addition, enteroviruses, unlike rhinoviruses, replicate better at 36 than 33°C and can be isolated from feces as well as from the respiratory tract (10, 19, 35).

The viruses belonging to the genus *Enterovirus* were initially divided into four groups (poliovirus, echovirus, coxsackievirus A, and coxsackievirus B) on the basis of their pathogenicity for laboratory animals. However, later it was realized that with this system, the lines of demarcation between groups were not sufficiently clear. Therefore, beginning in 1970, new members of the genus were merely called enteroviruses and designated by sequential numbers beginning with 68. There are presently 68 distinct enterovirus serotypes: polioviruses 1 through 3, echoviruses 1 through 34, group A coxsackieviruses 1 through 24, group B coxsackieviruses 1 through 6, and enteroviruses 68 through 72. The numbers are not additive because four of the echovirus serotypes have been reclassified (echovirus 10 as reovirus 1, echovirus 28 as rhinovirus 1A, and echovirus 34 as a prime strain of coxsackievirus A-24; also, echovirus 9 and coxsackievirus A-23 were found to be identical) (10, 14, 19). The latest addition to the genus, hepatitis A virus, was officially designated enterovirus 72 by the International Committee on Taxonomy of Viruses in 1983, but to avoid unnecessary confusion, the committee also recommended retaining the name hepatitis A virus. However, now most feel that hepatitis A virus should be reclassified into a separate genus in the family *Picornaviridae* because of its dissimilarity from other enteroviruses (30).

COLLECTION AND STORAGE OF SPECIMENS

Specimens for enterovirus isolation should be collected as soon after the onset of clinical symptoms as possible. Depending on the clinical picture, one or more of the following specimens may be appropriate: throat swab, feces or rectal swab, cerebrospinal fluid, blood, vesicular fluid, and tissue and conjunctival swab (for selected serogroups only). Methods for specimen collection are described in chapter 74. Occasionally enteroviruses are also isolated from urine, but the significance of such isolates is unknown, and urine is not a recommended specimen. The sampling of multiple sites does result in maximal enterovirus recovery, but before this approach is accepted, some consideration should be given to the clinical usefulness of the information provided relative to the cost. While the greatest sensitivity can be achieved by examining stool specimens, the specificity associated with virus recovery from blood and cerebrospinal fluid renders such findings far more meaningful (6–8).

Enteroviruses are hardier than most other viruses sought in clinical specimens, and they survive well under the conditions recommended in chapters 3 and 74 for specimen shipment and storage. Unlike many other viruses, enteroviruses can be held at 4°C for weeks or frozen at either −20 or −70°C indefinitely without loss of infectivity. A measurable loss of infectivity does occur, however, if specimens are kept at room temperature for many hours or allowed to dry (10, 14, 19).

Paired sera for antibody studies can also be useful in the diagnosis of enterovirus infections. Blood specimens should be collected and processed as described in chapter 74; however, particular emphasis should be placed on the collection of acute-phase blood as soon as possible after the onset of illness. The antibody responses to enteroviruses are often brisk, and titer rises can be missed by even a few days of delay (10, 14, 19, 24).

DIRECT EXAMINATION OF SPECIMENS

Enteroviruses can be demonstrated in clinical specimens by a number of direct diagnostic techniques, including electron microscopy, enzyme-linked immunoassay, and immunofluorescence staining. However, none of these methods is yet in widespread use, and the sensitivity and specificity of each method relative to cell culture are poorly defined (10, 14, 19).

Recent work on the direct detection of enteroviruses by using molecular techniques shows more promise. The presence of highly conserved sequences in both the 3′ and 5′ ends of the enterovirus genome raised the hope that nucleic acid technology could be used to devise a pan-specific probe to detect all enterovirus serotypes (13, 25, 34). Copy DNA and RNA probes as well as synthetic probes have now been developed and successfully used in blot assays to detect almost all human enterovirus serotypes in infected cell culture lysates, but when applied directly to clinical specimens, these probes have been disappointing in terms of sensitivity. In most studies done with cDNA probes, few if any cell culture-positive clinical specimens have been detected by using hybridization assays. The limits of detection in terms of infectious particles have ranged from 10^4 to 10^6 (5, 13, 27, 33, 34). Under experimental conditions, greater sensitivity appears to have been realized by those using cRNA (riboprobes). Nevertheless, sensitivity remained a problem when clinical specimens were examined, with only 50% of culture-positive stool specimens detected in one study (5).

Amplification of viral DNA and RNA (in the form of DNA copies) in clinical specimens by using the polymerase chain reaction (PCR) has resulted in enormous increases in the sensitivity that can be achieved with nucleic acid detection techniques. Recently, PCR was applied to the detection and identification of enteroviruses. A pair of generic enterovirus PCR primers was successfully used to amplify 33 different enterovirus serotypes. In addition, these investigators used a genotype-specific primer pair derived from sequences that code for a capsid protein to demonstrate the usefulness of PCR as an identification tool (2). A significant improvement in our ability to diagnose enteroviral disease by exploiting the power and sensitivity of PCR is a very real possibility in the 1990s.

CULTIVATION OF VIRUSES

Isolation in cell culture

With the exception of most group A coxsackieviruses, isolation in cell culture is the method of choice for the diagnosis of enterovirus infection. For virus recovery from clinical specimens, primary monkey (rhesus, African green, or cynomolgus) kidney (PMK) cells and human diploid fibroblast (e.g., WI-38) are the most efficient and widely used dual culture system (1, 10–12, 14, 19, 36). Because primary kidney cell cultures derived from other species of monkeys and other animals may not be as susceptible as PMK, these alternative cell cultures should not be used as substitutes for PMK cell cultures (12). Unfortunately, no specific fibroblast strain can be recommended, since data are limited regarding the relative sensitivity of fibroblasts for primary enterovirus isolation. The use of two continuous cell lines, RD and BGM, in addition to the PMK and WI-38 cell lines can improve enterovirus isolation in terms of speed, sensitivity, and the spectrum of serotypes detected (1, 6, 9, 21), but many laboratories may find the cost of this approach prohibitive. RD cells also appear to be useful for the propagation and recovery of some of the group A coxsackieviruses (32). In addition to the cell types already mentioned, various other commonly used cells, including HeLa, human embryonic kidney, and HEp-2, also support the growth of a variety of enterovirus serotypes, but their sensitivity for primary isolation is not as well defined as that of PMK and WI-38 cells (10, 14, 19). For the most part, all of the cultures referred to above are now readily available from commercial sources.

Inoculated cultures should be incubated at 37°C on a roller drum. They can also be held in a stationary position, but this may delay the development of viral cytopathic effect (CPE) in some cases. The CPE produced by enteroviruses in cell culture is quite distinctive and can be recognized with greater than 90% accuracy by experienced technologists (11). Enterovirus CPE is often evident quite early; up to 69% of all positive cultures can be detected within 4 days of specimen inoculation (6, 9). Therefore, daily culture readings through day 4 or 5 are recommended to laboratories that place a high priority on providing clinically useful results. Inoculated cultures should be examined for CPE for 10 to 14 days before being discarded as negative. Blind passage of cultures yields only a small number of additional positives.

The growth characteristics of enteroviruses in vitro vary considerably. Polioviruses, both wild and vaccine strains, produce CPE in a wide range of cell types, including PMK, human embryonic kidney and fibroblasts, HeLa, BGM, and RD. The CPE develops quickly and often destroys the monolayer within 3 days. Group B coxsackieviruses, on the other hand, do not replicate well in RD cells or human fibroblasts, but they do replicate well in the other cell systems mentioned. The growth characteristics of echoviruses and group A coxsackieviruses vary from type to type; in general, however, these viruses can be detected with equal frequency in PMK, RD, and human fibroblast cells but seldom in BGM cells. For the most part, the CPE caused by these viruses does not progress as rapidly as that caused by the polioviruses (1, 6, 9–11, 14, 19, 36, 37).

Isolation in suckling mice

Inoculation into suckling mice (24 to 48 h old) is the method of choice for the primary isolation of most of the group A coxsackieviruses; once isolation is accomplished, the viruses can then be adapted to growth in cell culture. Group B coxsackieviruses and some of the newer strains of enterovirus are also pathogenic for suckling mice, but because cell culture is so much simpler, it remains the preferred method for the isolation of these viruses. Only rare strains of echovirus replicate and cause pathology in suckling mice.

Specimens should be inoculated by three routes: 0.02 ml intracerebrally, 0.05 ml intraperitoneally, and 0.03 ml subcutaneously; after inoculation, the mice should be observed for at least 14 days. Signs of illness and then death generally occur in infected animals within 4 to 7 days if virus is present. Group A coxsackievirus infections are characterized by progressive, flaccid paralysis without signs of encephalitis and, histologically, by a generalized myositis, whereas group B coxsackievirus infections cause spastic paralysis, frequently accompanied by encephalitis. Marked panniculitis is also a common feature of group B coxsackievirus infection, but myositis is generally absent or limited and focal (10, 14, 19).

IDENTIFICATION OF THE AGENTS

It is possible to identify an isolate as enterovirus with reasonable certainty on the basis of the clinical history of the patient, the time of year when the specimen was obtained, the type of specimen, the cell culture system(s) that supports its growth, and its CPE. Reporting a presumptive diagnosis of enterovirus infection without waiting for the specific typing of the isolate can be of real value in the clinical management of the patient (6–8).

Specific identification of the serotype is most readily accomplished by virus neutralization, with intersecting pools of hyperimmune serum. Pools may be constructed in many ways, but the most widely used system is that of Lim and Benyesh-Melnick (LBM), which consists of equine antisera combined into eight pools (A through H) (15). With the LBM pools, it is possible to identify 42 of the enteroviruses that grow readily in cell culture. The Research Resources Branch of the National Institute of Allergy and Infectious Diseases once supplied the LBM pools. However, the responsibility for the preparation and distribution of the LBM pools is now in the hands of the World Health Organization, and recently new pools were made from antiserum reserves that had been stored frozen for two decades (20). It is important to conserve these valuable reagents, because the supply is limited. Therefore, if an epidemic due to a single serotype is in progress, the use of a single hyperimmune serum to identify isolates is clearly indicated. It should also be added that it is not always necessary to identify the serotype of each isolate. In most cases, it is probably sufficient for the physician to know simply that a nonpoliovirus enterovirus was isolated. However, it is important to exclude poliovirus as a possibility, because generally such isolates represent clinically irrelevant, long-term shedding of a vaccine strain virus. Poliovirus can be excluded if antisera to the three poliovirus serotypes are pooled and a simple neutralization test is performed.

Mouse neutralization tests are used to identify isolates that do not replicate in cell culture systems. Again, intersecting serum pools (J through P) are available for this purpose (18); these pools are still being distributed by the National Institute of Allergy and Infectious Diseases.

A number of other methods, including hemagglutination inhibition (for strains that hemagglutinate), complement fixation (CF), immunofluorescence, counterimmunoelectrophoresis, and virus agglutination, can be used for virus identification, but none is as specific or widely used as neutralization (10, 14, 19).

If a virus isolate cannot be identified, it may represent a new enterovirus, a mixture of viruses, or some other kind of virus. If there is uncertainly about the identity of an isolate, the determination of size, nucleic acid content, ether stability, and acid lability should show whether or not it is an enterovirus.

SEROLOGICAL PROCEDURES

Traditional methods (serum neutralization and complement fixation)

Detailed descriptions of the standard procedures used for the serodiagnosis of enterovirus infections have been published in previous editions of this Manual and elsewhere (10, 14, 19). Therefore, only the general principles of serological testing and newer developments will be covered below.

A number of factors limit the convenient application of serodiagnostic methods to the diagnosis of enterovirus infections. Foremost, the absence of a group-specific antigen makes it necessary to address each enterovirus serotype individually. Thus, standard serology is impractical for the specific diagnosis of enterovirus infections unless the field of suspected serotypes can be narrowed on clinical or epidemiological grounds or by isolation of the infecting virus from the patient.

The serum neutralization (SN) and CF tests have over the years been our mainstay for the serodiagnosis of enterovirus infections. With both tests, paired acute and convalescent sera taken 2 to 3 weeks apart are required to demonstrate acute infection; traditionally, a fourfold or greater rise in antibody titer is considered significant. However, it is not uncommon for infected individuals, especially those with late disease manifestations, to have already reached the peak of their antibody response by the time the acute-phase serum is drawn. This is particularly true for SN antibody. SN antibodies appear early after infection, are for the most part type specific, persist for years, probably for life, and correlate well with immunity to disease, although they do not invariably protect against reinfection. Individual variation in the peak level of antibody reached as a consequence of infection is considerable, and the rate of SN antibody decline is unpredictable. High (>512) SN antibody titers commonly persist for years; therefore, no conclusions about just when an individual's infection took place should be drawn from "high" SN antibody titers. In contrast, CF antibodies appear a bit later during the course of the clinical illness, are more short-lived (3 to 4 months), and thus appear to be somewhat better suited for the diagnosis of acute infection.

Heterotypic antibody responses further complicate the interpretation of serological studies. They occur frequently during enterovirus infections, and the magnitude of the heterotypic response may equal or even exceed that of the homotypic response. A heterotypic antibody response is seen more frequently with the CF test than with the SN test. Unfortunately, the heterotypic response does not occur with any predictable frequency.

IgM assays

A variety of enterovirus-specific immunoglobulin M (IgM) tests have been developed, but both technical and biological problems associated with IgM detection have restricted their use to research laboratories (10, 16, 22). In the past, gradient separation of IgM followed by virus neutralization tests with the M-rich fractions and precipitin tests were used to detect enterovirus-specific IgM in serum specimens; more recently, enzyme-linked immunosorbent assay tests have been applied to the task. Although IgM can be detected by all of these methods, they do not as yet appear to be sufficiently sensitive or specific for routine diagnostic use (10, 14, 26, 28, 31, 32).

Other methods

A number of other techniques, including immunoprecipitation, indirect fluorescent antibody, passive hemagglutination, and enzyme-linked immunoassay, have been used to detect antibody to enteroviruses (10, 14, 19).

EVALUATION AND INTERPRETATION OF RESULTS

In the individual patient, it is difficult to establish that an enterovirus infection is causally related to disease because these viruses are so prevalent in the general population, particularly during epidemic periods. A causal relationship is most likely if virus is isolated from a normally sterile body site (e.g., blood, cerebrospinal fluid, brain, or liver), but the causal relationship is presumptive if virus is isolated only from pharyngeal or fecal specimens. The latter can be positive in up to 50% of well individuals. A significant rise in antibody titer adds weight to a postulated etiological role for a pharyngeal or fecal isolate, but single high titers are not useful, because neutralizing antibodies can remain elevated for years after an acute infection. Serological tests alone are not useful for the determination of the specific enterovirus serotype causing disease, because heterotypic antibody responses are common and unpredictable in both magnitude and diversity.

LITERATURE CITED

1. **Bell, E. J., and B. P. Cosgrove.** 1980. Routine enterovirus diagnosis in a human rhabdomyosarcoma cell line. Bull. WHO **58:**423–428.
2. **Chapman, N. M., S. Tracy, C. J. Gauntt, and U. Fortmueller.** 1990. Molecular detection and identification of enteroviruses using enzymatic amplification and nucleic acid hybridization. J. Clin. Microbiol. **28:**843–850.
3. **Cherry, J. D.** 1987. Enteroviruses: polioviruses, coxsackieviruses, echoviruses and enteroviruses, p. 1729–1790. *In* R. D. Field and J. D. Cherry (ed.), Textbook of pediatric infectious diseases, 2nd ed. The W. B. Saunders Co., Philadelphia.
4. **Cherry, J. D.** 1990. Enteroviruses, p. 325–366. *In* J. S. Remmington and J. O. Klein (ed.), Infectious diseases of the fetus and newborn infant, 3rd ed. The W. B. Saunders Co., Philadelphia.
5. **Cova, L., H. Kopecka, M. Aymard, and M. Girard.** 1988. Use of cRNA probes for the detection of enteroviruses by molecular hybridization. J. Med. Virol. **24:**11–18.
6. **Dagan, R., J. A. Jenista, and M. A. Menegus.** 1985. Clinical, epidemiological and laboratory aspects of enterovirus infection in young infants, p. 123–151. *In* L. M. de la Maza and E. M. Peterson (ed.), Medical virology IV. Lawrence Erlbaum Associates, Hillsdale, N.J.
7. **Dagan, R., J. A. Jenista, and M. A. Menegus.** 1988. The association of clinical presentation, laboratory findings and virus serotype with the presence of meningitis in hospitalized infants with enterovirus infection. J. Pediatr. **113:**975–978.
8. **Dagan, R., J. A. Jenista, S. L. Prather, K. R. Powell, and M. A. Menegus.** 1985. Viremia in hospitalized children with enterovirus infections. J. Pediatr. **106:**397–401.
9. **Dagan, R., and M. A. Menegus.** 1986. A combination of four cell types for rapid detection of enteroviruses in clinical specimens. J. Med. Virol. **19:**219–228.
10. **Grandian, M., M. Forsgren, and A. Ehrnst.** 1989. Enteroviruses and reoviruses, p. 513–578. *In* N. J. Schmidt and R. W. Emmons (ed.), Diagnostic procedures for viral, rickettsial and chlamydial infections, 6th ed. American Public Health Association, Washington, D.C.
11. **Herrmann, E. C., Jr., D. A. Person, and T. F. Smith.** 1972. Experience in laboratory diagnosis of enterovirus infections in routine medical practice. Mayo Clin. Proc. **47:**577–586.
12. **Hsiung, G. D., and J. L. Melnick.** 1957. Comparative susceptibility of kidney cells from different monkey species to enteric viruses (poliomyelitis, coxsackie, and ECHO groups). J. Immunol. **78:**137–146.
13. **Hyypiä, T., P. Stålhandske, R. Vainionpää, and U. Pettersson.** 1984. Detection of enteroviruses by spot hybridization. J. Clin. Microbiol. **19:**436–438.
14. **Kapsenberg, J. G.** 1988. *Picornaviridae:* the enteroviruses, p. 692–742. *In* E. H. Lennette, P. Halonen, and F. A. Murphy (ed.), Laboratory diagnosis of infectious diseases, vol. 2. Viral, rickettsial, and chlamydial diseases. Springer-Verlag, New York.
15. **Lim, K. A., and M. Benyesh-Melnick.** 1960. Typing of viruses by combinations of antiserum pools. Application to typing of enteroviruses (coxsackie and echo). J. Immunol. **84:**3009–3317.
16. **Magnius, L. O., L. H. Saleh, T. Vikerfors, and H. Norder.** 1988. A solid-phase reverse immunosorbent test for the detection of enterovirus IgM. J. Virol. Methods **20:**73–82.
17. **Melnick, J. L.** 1989. Enteroviruses, p. 191–263. *In* A. S. Evans (ed.), Viral infections of humans, 3rd ed. Plenum Medical Book Co., New York.
18. **Melnick, J. L., N. J. Schmidt, B. Hampil, and H. H. Ho.** 1977. Lyophilized combination pools of enterovirus equine antisera: preparation and test procedures for the identification of field strains of 19 group A coxsackievirus serotypes. Intervirology **8:**172–181.
19. **Melnick, J. L., H. A. Wenner, and C. A. Phillips.** 1980. Enteroviruses, p. 471–534. *In* E. H. Lennette and N. J. Schmidt (ed.), Diagnostic procedures for viral, rickettsial and chlamydial infections, 5th ed. American Public Health Association, Inc., New York.
20. **Melnick, J. L., and I. L. Wimberly.** 1985. Lyophilized combination pools of enterovirus equine antisera: new LBM pools prepared from reserves stored frozen for two decades. Bull. WHO **63:**543–550.
21. **Menegus, M. A., and G. E. Hollick.** 1982. Increased efficiency of group B coxsackievirus isolation from clinical specimens by use of BGM cells. J. Clin. Microbiol. **15:**945–948.
22. **Meurman, O.** 1983. Detection of antiviral IgM antibodies and its problems. A review. Curr. Top. Microbiol. Immunol. **104:**101–131.
23. **Modlin, J. F.** 1990. Coxsackieviruses, echoviruses, and newer enteroviruses, p. 1367–1383. *In* G. L. Mandell, R. G. Douglas, and J. E. Bennett (ed.), Principles and prac-

tice of infectious disease, 3rd ed. Churchill Livingstone Inc., New York.

24. **Moore, M., and D. M. Morens.** 1984. Enteroviruses, including polioviruses, p. 407–483. *In* R. B. Belshe (ed.), Textbook of human virology. PSG Publishing Co., Inc., Littleton, Mass.
25. **Nonoto, A., H. Toyoda, M. Kohara, T. Suganuma, T. Omata, and N. Imura.** 1984. Approaches to the development of new polio virus vaccines based on molecular genetics. Rev. Infect. Dis. **6:**494–498.
26. **Pattison, J. R.** 1983. Tests for coxsackie B virus-specific IgM. J. Hyg. **90:**327–332.
27. **Petitjean, J., M. Quibriac, F. Freymuth, F. Fuchs, N. Laconche, M. Aymard, and H. Kopecka.** 1990. Specific detection of enteroviruses in clinical samples by molecular hybridization using poliovirus subgenomic riboprobes. J. Clin. Microbiol. **28:**307–311.
28. **Pozzetto, B., O. G. Gaudin, M. Aouni, and A. Ros.** 1989. Comparative evaluation of immunoglobulin M neutralizing antibody response in acute-phase sera and virus isolation for the routine diagnosis of enterovirus infection. J. Clin. Microbiol. **27:**705–708.
29. **Prather, S. L., R. Dagan, J. A. Jenista, and M. A. Menegus.** 1984. The isolation of enteroviruses from blood: a comparison of four processing methods. J. Med. Virol. **14:**221–227.
30. **Purcell, R. H., J. H. Hoofnagle, J. Ticehurst, and J. L. Gerin.** 1989. Hepatitis viruses, p. 957–1065. *In* N. J. Schmidt and R. W. Emmons (ed.), Diagnostic procedures for viral, rickettsial and chlamydial infections, 6th ed. American Public Health Association, Inc., Washington D.C.
31. **Reigel, F., F. Burkhardt, and U. Schilt.** 1984. Reaction pattern of immunoglobulin M and G antibodies to echovirus 11 structural proteins. J. Clin. Microbiol. **19:**870–874.
32. **Reigel, F., F. Burkhardt, and U. Schilt.** 1985. Cross-reactions of immunoglobulin M and G antibodies with enterovirus-specific viral structural proteins. J. Hyg. **95:**469–481.
33. **Rotbart, H. A., P. S. Eastman, J. L. Ruth, K. K. Hirata, and M. J. Levin.** 1988. Nonisotopic oligomeric probes for the human enteroviruses. J. Clin. Microbiol. **26:**2269–2271.
34. **Rotbart, H. A., M. J. Levin, and L. P. Villarreal.** 1984. Use of subgenomic poliovirus DNA hybridization probes to detect the major subgroups of enteroviruses. J. Clin. Microbiol. **20:**1105–1108.
35. **Rueckert, R. R.** 1985. Picornaviruses and their replication, p. 705–738. *In* B. N. Fields, D. M. Knipe, R. M. Chanock, J. L. Melnick, B. Rosman, and R. E. Shope (ed.), Virology. Raven Press, New York.
36. **Schmidt, N. J.** 1972. Tissue culture in the laboratory diagnosis of viral infections. Am. J. Clin. Pathol. **57:**820–828.
37. **Schmidt, N. J., H. H. Ho, and E. H. Lennette.** 1975. Propagation and isolation of group A coxsackieviruses in RD cells. J. Clin. Microbiol. **2:**183–185.

Chapter 94

Reoviruses

MARILYN A. MENEGUS

CLINICAL BACKGROUND

Reoviruses infect humans and lower animals and are found worldwide. Through serosurveys, we know that infection of humans is common and occurs at an early age. Although reoviruses have been isolated from individuals with a variety of illnesses, no firm association between infection and human disease has been established. Apparently, most infections are subclinical (2–4).

DESCRIPTION OF THE AGENT

The family *Reoviridae* is composed of three genera: *Reovirus*, *Orbivirus*, and *Rotavirus*. The genus *Reovirus* consists of three virus serotypes, designated 1, 2, and 3. Reoviruses have a naked, double capsid, 70 nm in diameter, with icosahedral symmetry. The capsid contains a genome consisting of 10 segments of double-stranded RNA. Reoviruses are resistant to lipid solvents and are acid stable. Virus synthesis and maturation occur in the cytoplasm of the cell and are associated with the formation of large, eosinophilic, intracytoplasmic inclusions (1).

COLLECTION AND STORAGE OF SPECIMENS

Reoviruses can be recovered from throat swabs, nasal secretions, and feces. Since the viruses are quite stable, specimens can be collected and processed as described in chapter 74.

VIRUS CULTIVATION

Reoviruses replicate and produce cytopathic effect in a wide variety of cell cultures, including primary monkey and human embryonic kidney, HeLa, and human diploid fibroblasts. However, the recognition of reovirus-induced cytopathology can be challenging even for experienced personnel. Infected cells become granular, remain loosely fastened to the glass, and flutter in the medium when agitated. These changes are easily mistaken for nonspecific cell degeneration. The presence of reovirus in cell cultures can be confirmed by the demonstration of cytoplasmic inclusions in stained preparations of the infected cells and hemagglutinating activity (human O erythrocytes) in the cell culture media. The viruses can be definitively identified by a hemagglutination inhibition test with type-specific antisera (2–4). Despite their prevalence, reoviruses are seldom isolated from clinical specimens.

IDENTIFICATION OF THE AGENT

Since all three reovirus serotypes hemagglutinate human erythrocytes, the method of choice for the identification of specific serotypes is the hemagglutination inhibition test. The test is carried out as follows. Typing sera are adsorbed with kaolin by mixing a 1:5 dilution of a serum in 0.85% saline with an equal volume of a 25% suspension of acid-washed kaolin in 0.85% NaCl (25 g of kaolin plus 100 ml of saline solution), and the mixture is allowed to stand for 20 min at room temperature. The mixture is then centrifuged briefly to sediment the kaolin, and the decanted supernatant fluid is considered a 1:10 dilution of serum. A 0.2-ml amount of hemagglutinin diluted in 0.85% NaCl to contain 20 U/ml (4 U/0.2 ml) is added to 0.2-ml amounts of serial twofold dilutions of serum in 0.85% NaCl. Each serum is used from a dilution of 1:10 to, or beyond, its endpoint. Mixtures are shaken briefly and then allowed to stand for 1 h at room temperature before the addition of 0.2 ml of the standard (0.75%) erythrocyte suspension. Erythrocytes are allowed to settle at room temperature, and the titer of the serum is then taken as the dilution that completely inhibits agglutination. The lowest dilution of each serum used is tested for the presence of nonspecific erythrocyte agglutinins by substituting 0.2 ml of saline solution for the antigen. An antigen titration is also included in the test.

An isolate is considered typed if it is inhibited at a titer of at least 1:40 by one of the typing antisera and not at a dilution of 1:10 by the other antisera (2, 3).

SEROLOGICAL METHODS

Practically all naturally occurring and experimental infections with reoviruses are accompanied by a fourfold or greater rise in homologous hemagglutination inhibition antibody. Antibody can be detected for at least 1 year after natural infection and probably persists much longer (2–4). However, tests for reovirus antibody are seldom requested because no clinical situation demands them.

EVALUATION AND INTERPRETATION OF RESULTS

The ubiquity of reoviruses and their lack of association with human disease make it impossible to attach any significance to the isolation of virus from nonsterile body sites. If there is some compelling clinical reason to build a case for a causal relationship with the illness of the patient, additional diagnostic methods (e.g., histopathology and serology) must be employed.

LITERATURE CITED

1. **Joklik, W. K.** 1983. The reovirus particle, p. 9–78. *In* W. K. Joklik (ed.), The reoviridae. Plenum Publishing Corp., New York.
2. **Rosen, L.** 1968. Reoviruses, p. 73–107. *In* H. A. Wenner

and A. M. Behbehani (ed.), Echoviruses and reoviruses. Springer-Verlag, New York.

3. **Rosen, L.** 1979. Reoviruses, p. 577–584. *In* E. H. Lennette and N. J. Schmidt (ed.), Diagnostic procedures for viral, rickettsial, and chlamydial infections, 5th ed. American Public Health Association, Inc., New York.
4. **Stanley, N. F.** 1977. Diagnosis of reovirus infections: comparative aspects, p. 385–421. *In* E. Kurstak and C. Kurstak (ed.), Comparative diagnosis of viral diseases, vol. 1. Human and related viruses. Academic Press, Inc., New York.

Chapter 95

Viruses Causing Gastroenteritis

MARY L. CHRISTENSEN AND CYNTHIA HOWARD

CLINICAL BACKGROUND

Viral gastroenteritis is the second most common clinical disease occurring in developed countries, exceeded only by viral upper respiratory tract illness. A number of viruses have been implicated in gastroenteritis. These include rotaviruses, fastidious fecal (enteric) adenoviruses, caliciviruses, astroviruses, coronaviruses, Norwalk, and Norwalk-like viruses (5). Of these, rotaviruses are the most common known cause of viral gastroenteritis in infants and young children, and they can occasionally cause gastroenteritis in the elderly. The fastidious fecal adenoviruses are probably the second most common cause of gastroenteritis in the pediatric population (5). Calici-, astro-, and coronaviruses are probably responsible for a minority of illness in the young age group (5). In contrast, the Norwalk and Norwalk-like viruses have frequently caused outbreaks of gastroenteritis among older children, adolescents, and adults (17). As a group, all of these viruses are fastidious and cannot be cultivated in routine cell cultures. They were discovered during the 1970s by use of the techniques of electron microscopy (EM) and immunoelectron microscopy EM (IEM), although other, relatively simple detection techniques have been developed for routine use with rotaviruses and fastidious adenoviruses (5).

Rotaviruses

Rotavirus gastroenteritis is ubiquitous, occurring in all parts of the world. It occurs during the cooler months in countries that have temperate climates, although it can occur throughout the year in tropical countries (5).

Rotaviruses are double-stranded RNA (dsRNA) viruses in the family *Reoviridae* (Table 1). Most rotaviruses causing epidemic and endemic pediatric as well as geriatric gastroenteritis share a common group antigen and are classified as group A. Two new groups, B and C, have recently been discovered (5).

Rotavirus infection is by the fecal-oral route. The virus primarily infects the epithelial cells lining the small intestine. After an incubation period of about 1 to 2 days, the onset of rotavirus gastroenteritis is sudden, with vomiting and diarrhea, fever, occasionally abdominal pain, and even respiratory symptoms (5). Loss of fluids and electrolytes in rotavirus gastroenteritis can lead to severe dehydration, hospitalization, and even death. Treatment consists primarily of fluid and electrolyte replacement, either orally or intravenously. Asymptomatic virus shedding in all age groups also occurs with rotavirus. Nosocomial infections are frequent and can account for up to 50% of rotavirus cases occurring in hospitals. Transmission of the virus may be difficult to control, since 10^{10} or more virions per g of stool may be shed by patients, while less than 10 focus-forming units of virus can initiate an infection (5).

Rotavirus infections appear to be repetitive, and reinfection usually involves different serotypes. Antibody that develops after infection may persist for as long as 6 months; antibodies can either protect individuals from reinfection or reduce the severity of reinfection (5).

Various experimental vaccines for rotavirus have been developed and are being evaluated. These are live attenuated vaccines administered by the oral route.

Adenoviruses

Fastidious fecal or enteric adenoviruses are probably the second most common cause of infantile gastroenteritis (5). Like the rotaviruses, they are found throughout the world. Although infection by these adenoviruses is usually endemic with no seasonal variation, more cases tend to occur during the warmer months (5). The fastidious fecal adenoviruses are not readily cultivable in routine cell cultures and primarily comprise the newer serotypes, 40 and 41.

In patients with adenovirus gastroenteritis, diarrhea is usually the predominant symptom. These patients have milder disease, with less vomiting and fever than do rotavirus-infected patients. Symptoms can last from a few days to a few weeks (5). In various reports, fastidious adenoviruses (types 40 and 41) have been associated with respiratory symptoms; however, respiratory adenoviruses (lower-numbered types) have also been associated with gastroenteritis (5). This creates a problem of determining the exact role of these various adenoviruses in either gastroenteritis or viral respiratory disease. Treatment of adenovirus gastroenteritis includes maintaining proper electrolyte balance and fluid levels.

Experimental adenovirus 40 and 41 vaccines have not been pursued, since (i) adenovirus gastroenteritis is apparently not as common or as serious as rotavirus infection and (ii) problems exist with the replication of serotypes 40 and 41 in vitro (5).

Calici-, astro-, and coronaviruses

Calici-, astro-, and coronaviruses account for only a minority of cases of pediatric viral gastroenteritis. Caliciviruses are 30- to 35-nm round RNA viruses in the family *Caliciviridae* (Table 1). Caliciviruses are ubiquitous throughout the world. They cause gastroenteritis in infants and very young children, usually ranging from 1 to 24 months of age. At least one geriatric outbreak has been reported (8). Calicivirus infections can be sporadic or epidemic and occur throughout the year, with peaks in the winter months (7). The infections are as severe as with rotavirus (7). Diarrhea is the predominant

TABLE 1. Classification and characteristics of gastroenteritis viruses

Virus	Family	RNA or DNA	Size (nm)	Envelope	Symmetry and description
Rotavirus	*Reoviridae*	dsRNA	70	No	Icosahedral, double shell
Adenovirus	*Adenoviridae*	dsDNA	70–75	No	Icosahedral
Calicivirus	*Caliciviridae*	RNA	30–35	No	Round, Star of David configuration on surface, cuplike depressions, spiked periphery
Astrovirus	Unclassified	Unknown	28–30	No	Round, 5- or 6-pointed star configuration on surface, smooth periphery
Coronavirus	*Coronaviridae*	RNA, positive stranded	80–150	Yes	Round or pleomorphic, club-shaped surface projections
Norwalk	Unclassified	Unknown	25–30	No	Round

symptom, which can occur without or with vomiting. The duration of the disease averages about 4 days and is usually no longer than 10 days.

Astroviruses are 28- to 30-nm smooth round unclassified viruses with a star configuration on their surfaces. Astroviruses are also ubiquitous, causing both symptomatic and asymptomatic infection in children 0 to 7 years old (5). Exposed adults can develop mild disease, but they develop disease less frequently than do children. There has been at least one astrovirus outbreak among the elderly, caused by the Marin County agent (5). The incubation period is about 24 to 36 h. Symptoms, which last from 0.5 to 4 days, consist of diarrhea with or without vomiting and, to a lesser extent, abdominal pain and fever. The disease appears to be less severe than with rotaviruses, and treatment consists of maintaining fluid and electrolyte balance.

Coronaviruses, in the family *Coronaviridae*, are medium-size enveloped RNA viruses, first recovered from patients with upper respiratory tract illness. Viruslike particles, which by the EM examination of diarrheal stools resemble coronaviruses, may or may not be actual coronaviruses and could be artifactual in some instances (25). These coronaviruses or coronaviruslike particles (CVLP) have been associated with a small percentage of infantile gastroenteritis and necrotizing enterocolitis (5). However, CVLP are associated with a large percentage of pediatric diarrhea cases in Arizona, especially during the cooler, drier months (24). Most patients with CVLP-associated gastroenteritis are under the age of 2 years. Diarrhea is the most common symptom seen in these patients; vomiting and fever occur in about one-half of patients, and occult blood is seen in about one-fifth (24). The disease lasts about 1 week. Treatment is similar to that for the other viral gastroenteritides. Little is known about immunity in coronavirus-associated gastroenteritis.

Norwalk and Norwalk-like viruses

Whereas the viruses discussed above primarily cause disease in infants and small children, Norwalk and Norwalk-like viruses more commonly affect older children and adults in developed countries. By EM, Norwalk virus is a small round virus 27 to 30 nm in diameter. Several other Norwalk-like viruses resemble Norwalk virus in their morphology, the type of clinical disease they cause, and their low concentration in infected stools. However, some of these Norwalk-like viruses vary from Norwalk virus in their antigenic relatedness. These other agents include the Snow Mountain agent, the Hawaii agent, and the Montgomery County agent. Norwalk virus shows at least a one-way serological cross-relatedness with caliciviruses (5).

Norwalk and Norwalk-like viruses have been responsible for outbreaks in schools, colleges, camps, cruise ships, communities, nursing homes, and family groups (17). The sources of infection in these outbreaks included water supplies, swimming areas, ingestion of contaminated food, and person-to-person transmission. Little is known about the role of these viruses in endemic illness, since most infected patients are not hospitalized, and routine diagnostic laboratories do not have the reagents available for detecting these viruses or their viral antibodies.

The clinical features of infections caused by either Norwalk or Norwalk-like agents are similar (17). After an incubation period of 24 to 48 h, the onset is sudden, with severe nausea and vomiting, diarrhea, and low-grade fever. Children are more likely to have vomiting, whereas adults are more likely to have diarrhea. Abdominal pain or cramps, headache, and malaise may also occur. Respiratory symptoms do not appear to be a manifestation, differing from rotavirus and possibly adenovirus infection. The attack rate is high, often with 50% or more of the attendees at a school, camp, or other institution being affected.

Antibody to Norwalk virus is ubiquitous around the world. In American subjects, acquisition of antibody to Norwalk virus is minimal during childhood, rises rapidly throughout adolescence and early adulthood, and then declines in old age. In underdeveloped nations, antibody acquisition develops earlier, during childhood (5).

Immunity to Norwalk and similar viruses appears to last at least 3 months after infection but wanes within 2 to 3 years. Immunity to Norwalk virus appears to be complex; some individuals are susceptible to repeated infections, whereas others appear resistant even to primary Norwalk virus infection (5).

DESCRIPTION OF THE AGENTS

Rotaviruses

Rotaviruses are in the family *Reoviridae*, the members of which possess a double layer of icosahedral shells of approximately 70 nm in diameter, with a core of dsRNA. The dsRNA genome consists of 11 segments, which can be separated by polyacrylamide gel electrophoresis. Different rotavirus isolates frequently exhibit differences in the electrophoretic mobilities of their 11 segments (5).

Three gene segments that code for three major rotaviral antigens are of particular interest (5). Gene segment 4 codes for VP4, originally called VP3. VP4 is an outer capsid protein that can elicit neutralizing antibody. Gene segment 6 codes for VP6, the major inner core structural protein. VP6 is the major subgroup antigen which can specify one of two rotavirus subgroups (subgroups I and II) in group A. Gene segment 8 or 9, depending on the strain of rotavirus, codes for VP7. VP7, the major outer capsid protein which is glycosylated, is responsible for the serotype specificity of the virus, which can be determined by neutralization tests and by enzyme immunoassay (EIA). Four human serotypes, 1 through 4, have been well recognized and characterized. Subgroup I includes human rotavirus strains of serotype 2, and subgroup II includes serotypes 1, 3, and 4. Two new human serotypes, 8 and 9, have more recently been described (23); serotypes 5, 6, and 7 are animal serotypes.

Rotaviruses can be cultivated by using special techniques, described below in the section Detection of Rotaviruses. However, only a minority of virions are infectious to cell cultures.

Adenoviruses

Adenoviruses are 70- to 75-nm nonenveloped icosahedral viruses. There are 41 human adenovirus types. The 41 mammalian adenoviruses share a common group-specific determinant that can be measured by the complement fixation test and by EIA tests. Type specificities can be measured by neutralization or EIA tests (5). Several different tests and criteria have been used to place the 41 adenovirus types into five different subgroups, A through F (5). Types 40 and 41 constitute subgroup F.

Fastidious adenoviruses can be cultivated in Graham 293 cells, in Chang conjunctival cells, or in HEp-2 cells (2, 5).

Calici-, astro-, and coronaviruses

Caliciviruses are 30- to 35-nm round RNA viruses in the family *Caliciviridae*. Caliciviruses derive their name from the 32 cup-shaped depressions on the surface of their virions. This gives their periphery a spiky appearance and causes the formation of a Star of David configuration at certain rotations of the virion. The Star of David configuration is formed by six peripheral hollows surrounding a seventh central hollow (20). Human caliciviruses cannot be cultivated in routine cell cultures (8), although other mammalian caliciviruses can readily be propagated in cells of their species (5).

Astroviruses are unclassified viruses of unknown nucleic acid composition. They are 28- to 30-nm round virus particles with a smooth edge, in contrast to the caliciviruses, which have a rough, spiky edge. The appearance of astroviruses has been described in detail by Madeley (20). Most astrovirus particles have a star-shaped configuration on their surface. This star configuration can have either five or six points, whereas caliciviruses have only six-pointed stars. The points of the astrovirus star radiate out from a central point or knob, and thus there is no hollow center as seen in the calicivirus star. There appear to be at least five distinct serotypes of astroviruses, 1 through 5. Serotype 1 accounts for about 77% of human astroviruses detected (19). Astroviruses can be isolated and propagated in human embryonic kidney cells, to which trypsin-containing medium is added (19). Infected human embryonic kidney cells can be used for immunofluorescence tests or EIAs (18, 19).

Coronaviruses are enveloped medium-size positive-stranded RNA viruses. They are approximately 80 to 150 nm in diameter. They appear as rounded or pleomorphic particles that on their surface have club-shaped projections called peplomers. These projections give the particles the appearance of the corona of the sun.

There are CVLP observed in diarrheal stools by EM that may actually represent a heterogeneous group of particles (5). In some instances, the particles may be true enteric coronaviruses. In other instances, the particles may be similar to the newly described toroviruses, which are medium-size negative-stranded RNA viruses with a peplomer-bearing envelope. In still other instances, the particles may be artifactual, such as R bodies (rod-containing bodies) and C bodies (coccoid or glycocalyceal bodies), which are normal intestinal epithelial cell components (25).

Enteric coronaviruses are apparently difficult to propagate in vitro. Mortensen et al. (24) could not propagate them in a number of routine cell types or in cell lines of human embryonic intestine, human embryonic tonsil, or human rectal tumor. However, Resta et al. (26) reported propagating human enteric coronaviruses in human fetal intestinal organ cultures.

Norwalk and Norwalk-like viruses

Norwalk and Norwalk-like agents (Snow Mountain, Hawaii, and Montgomery County agents) are small round particles 27 to 30 nm in diameter. They have been described as picorna/parvoviruslike, as well as resembling caliciviruses. Originally, their fine morphology was difficult to distinguish because of their small size and because, by IEM, the virions are coated with antibody. However, by direct EM, their particles appear to be more structured than picorna- or parvoviruses and thus more closely resemble the caliciviruses (3). Norwalk and similar viruses resemble caliciviruses in having (i) a single primary structural protein of similar molecular weight and (ii) similar buoyant densities in cesium chloride (5). These agents cannot be cultivated in vitro. Attempts at propagating Norwalk virus in a number of types of cell cultures have failed. There are other small round viruses that were originally thought to be Norwalk-like viruses but are now considered to be candidate parvoviruses; these include the Cockle agent and the Ditchling agent (3).

In addition, various other, unclassified small round virus particles (SRVP) have been observed in diarrheal stools by various investigators. Their various descriptions have included structured SRVP, picornavirus/parvoviruslike, smooth SRVP, and unstructured or featureless SRVP (3). These various particles, in the range of 20 to 30 nm, approach the limits of resolution of the electron microscope. This feature may account for some of the differences in the descriptions of these particles. In addition, some microscopes may have better resolution than others, allowing for the observation and thus reporting of more ultrafine detail.

COLLECTION AND STORAGE OF SPECIMENS

For the direct detection of virus, stool specimens should be collected during the acute phase of the illness. Specimens for Norwalk and similar viruses should be collected within 48 h of onset of illness; specimens for other viruses should be collected within the first week and preferably the first 3 to 5 days of illness. Specimens should be placed directly into plastic or glass screw-cap jars or cups for submission to the laboratory. The specimen container should not contain any preservatives, detergents, metal ions, viral transport media, or tissue culture media which could interfere with EIA, latex agglutination (LA), or other tests. In addition, the specimens should not be added to viral transport media, which (i) can dilute out the specimen beyond the limits of detection of virus particles and (ii) might contain serum albumin or animal sera containing antibodies to rotavirus or other enteric viruses.

Very liquid stool specimens from pediatric patients in diapers can be obtained in several ways. Liquid diarrheal stool can be prevented from being absorbed into a diaper either by placing the disposable diaper, inside out, on the infant or by placing a layer of plastic wrap inside a clean diaper. Also, a clean pediatric urine bag can be placed over the anal area to collect very watery stool. Rectal swabs per se should not be submitted, since sufficient virions may not be present on the swab for detection. Specimens that are transported and processed the same day can be kept at 4°C. If transportation and holding take more than 24 h, specimens should be shipped on dry ice in an airtight container and stored frozen at −70°C.

Detection of virus in stools is the major approach used for diagnosing viral gastroenteritis in the routine diagnostic laboratory. Blood or serum is usually not submitted, since serology for diagnosing viral gastroenteritis is not usually done in most diagnostic laboratories. Serological studies using EIA, radioimmunoassay, and other methods have been carried out primarily in research laboratories for (i) typing or grouping new isolates or (ii) epidemiologic purposes (5). Blood or serum may be submitted to a diagnostic laboratory that does IEM. In this instance, convalescent serum, obtained 2 weeks after the onset of symptoms, can be used to aggregate virus particles occurring in patient stools during the acute phase of illness. An acute-phase serum sample from the same patient should be submitted for control purposes.

DETECTION OF ROTAVIRUSES

Since rotaviruses are difficult to propagate in cell culture, other detection methods have been developed and used. Rotaviruses traditionally have been detected by EM, which is described below. The EM method has several advantages. It is relatively rapid, especially when a small number of samples are evaluated. EM can detect both group A and non-group A rotaviruses as well as other enteric viruses. However, there are several disadvantages as well. The technique requires the use of expensive equipment. It may also be less sensitive than EIA. When a large number of specimens are run at once, EM can be slower and more tedious than other methods now available.

There are two methods that can be easily carried out in diagnostic laboratories and on large numbers of specimens, often without specialized equipment: the LA test and EIA. These two tests are antibody-based tests that utilize antigen-antibody reactions. There are a number of commercial LA and EIA kits available for use (Table 2). LA tests have the advantages of requiring very little equipment and being very rapid, usually completed within 30 min. Most LA tests have a high level of specificity (5, 10, 16, 28), due in part to the incorporation in the test procedure of negative control latex particles coated with nonimmune serum or globulin. However, LA tests are usually not as sensitive as EIAs.

The commercially available EIAs are three-layer double-antibody sandwich assays. They may utilize one of several modifications and vary in several respects. First, either polyclonal or monoclonal antibodies may be used for the capture and detector antibody systems, although some of the assays use polyclonal antibodies for both. Second, one commercial kit incorporates a negative control well that is coated with nonimmune serum or

TABLE 2. General characteristics of commercial rotavirus tests

Test	Kit name (manufacturer)	Monoclonal or polyclonal antibody: capture antibody/ detector antibody (EIA); antibody on latex (LA)	Negative control beads or wells	Form for final reading	Total incubation time (min)
EIA	Pathfinder (Kallestad)	Polyclonal/monoclonal	No	Tube	75
	Rotaclone (Cambridge BioScience)	Monoclonal/monoclonal	No	Microtiter	70
	Rotazyme II (Abbott Laboratories)	Polyclonal/polyclonal	No	Tube	150
	Rotavirus EIA (International Diagnostic Laboratories; Isolab)	Polyclonal/polyclonal	Yes	Microtiter	105
EIA, rapid	TestPack Rotavirus (Abbott Laboratories)	Polyclonal/monoclonal-polyclonal mixture	No	Reaction disk	7
	Rota-Cube (Difco Laboratories)	Unspecified/polyclonal	No	Membrane cube	3
LA	Rota-Stat (International Diagnostic Laboratories; Isolab)	Polyclonal	Yes	Latex beads	13–14
	Meritec-Rotavirus (Meridian Diagnostics)	Polyclonal	Yes	Latex beads	5
	Virogen Rotatest (Wampole Laboratories)	Polyclonal	Yes	Latex beads	17
	Rotavirus Latex (Wellcome Diagnostics)	Polyclonal	Yes	Latex beads	17
	ImmunoScan (Bartels)	Polyclonal	Yes	Latex beads	5
	Rotalex (Medical Technology Corp.)	Polyclonal	Yes	Latex beads	2

globulin, although most of the EIA kits do not include this control. Third, either microtiter wells, larger wells, or test tubes are used for the reaction mixtures. A standard laboratory spectrophotometer can be used for reading the tubes, whereas a microtiter reader is needed for the microtiter wells. One company furnishes a computerized spectrophotometer for reading the tubes. Some manufacturers suggest that visual readings can be carried out; however, with low-level positive or borderline readings, spectrophotometric readings and mathematical calculations of cutoff values based on the manufacturer's directions are recommended.

There are several criteria to take into consideration when choosing an EIA or when choosing between EIA and LA tests. Total incubation times of the standard EIAs can range from 75 min to several hours, which is significantly more time than is needed to report results of LA tests. However, actual hands-on time for EIA is significantly less than the total incubation times. EIAs are usually more sensitive than LA tests (5, 10, 16, 21, 28), although this criterion can vary from manufacturer to manufacturer. Monoclonal antibody-based kits appear to be more sensitive than polyclonal antibody-based kits (5, 10, 16, 21, 28). Kits that contain negative control wells or beads tend to be more specific, since they minimize false-positive reactions. However, neither LA tests nor EIAs detect group B or C rotaviruses, and they may not detect certain group A serotypes (24). Some EIAs give false-positive results on a small percentage of stool specimens from asymptomatic neonates (5, 6, 15).

More recently, simple, easy-to-read 10-min qualitative EIAs have become commercially available (TestPack Rotavirus, Abbott Laboratories; Rota-Cube, Difco Laboratories) (4). In these tests, a stool sample and the necessary reagents are added to either a small reaction disk or cube. Results are easily read visually after several minutes, either as a plus sign or a dot, depending on the commercial test used. If a negative test is carried out correctly, a minus sign or a C will appear, depending on the brand of test. No special equipment or expertise is needed, and these EIAs are sensitive and specific (4). This type of test can be used in small hospital laboratories, as stat tests in large hospital laboratories, or in physician offices.

All of the commercially available EIAs and LA tests are carried out as specified by the manufacturers. Quality control standards specified in the kits should be adhered to. Positive and negative controls are provided in the kits and should be used as instructed by the manufacturers.

Other rotavirus detection methods that are being used primarily as research tools are polyacrylamide gel electrophoresis and dot hybridization with cDNA probes (1, 14). These methods can detect both group A and nongroup A rotaviruses. However, polyacrylamide gel electrophoresis requires special laboratory equipment and expertise. It cannot distinguish among various rotavirus groups and serotypes, and many different electrophoretic patterns may exist within one serotype. A commercial DNA probe test is available that is somewhat labor intensive and has a turnaround time of several hours (1). Radioimmunoassays have been used as research tools (5).

Culture of human rotaviruses is usually not done in diagnostic laboratories, since the virus is found in large quantities in stool specimens and can be rapidly detected by antigen detection tests. However, some research laboratories have cultivated rotaviruses by using various manipulations, including pretreating specimens with trypsin, adding low levels of trypsin to cell culture maintenance medium, and rolling the cell cultures (5). With these methods, the virus can be propagated in primary kidney cells or lines of kidney cells from various species of monkeys. Cytopathic effect (CPE) can usually be observed after several passages and may consist of cell fusion, cell rounding, granularity of cells, cell lysis, and sloughing of cells. Viruses from patient specimens may grow better in primary cells but can then be passaged in the cell lines (5, 29).

DETECTION OF ADENOVIRUSES

Several methods are available to detect adenoviruses in stools. Although the fastidious adenoviruses, types 40 and 41, are responsible for a significant minority of gastroenteritis cases, lower-numbered adenoviruses may also be responsible for some gastroenteritis (5). Direct detection by EM can be used and is described in the next section. EM cannot distinguish between adenovirus types 40 and 41 and lower-numbered adenoviruses excreted in the stool. However, types 40 and 41 tend to be present in the stool in larger numbers than the lower-numbered adenoviruses.

Direct detection by EIA is also available. Adenovirus EIAs are commercially available, are relatively easy and rapid to perform, and can be carried out on a large number of specimens. These advantages are similar to those seen with the rotavirus EIAs. The commercial EIA kits available to detect adenovirus types 40 and 41 directly on stool samples are Adenoclone-Type 40/41 (Cambridge BioScience, Worcester, Mass.) and API Adenovirus 40/41 ELISA (Analytab Products, Plainview, N.Y.). In addition, a group adenovirus EIA that detects all adenovirus serotypes directly from stools can be obtained from either company. Lower-numbered adenoviruses as well as types 40 and 41 may be responsible for some gastroenteritis (5), and this fact should be considered when one is choosing an EIA test to use. Some laboratories first use the group adenovirus EIA test on stool specimens; the group EIA-positive specimens are then tested by EIA for adenovirus types 40 and 41 to distinguish the latter. Other commercial adenovirus type 40 and 41 tests are available in Great Britain and Europe. Positive and negative controls are included in the kits; quality control standards specified by the manufacturers should be followed.

Fastidious adenovirus types 40 and 41 can also be propagated in Graham 293 cells (27), especially when the cells are subconfluent at the time of inoculation (2). Typical adenovirus CPE will develop after several days. Since lower-numbered adenoviruses also grow well in 293 cells (2), CPE in these cells cannot be used to differentiate between the fastidious and nonfastidious types. However, fastidious adenoviruses can be differentiated from lower-numbered adenoviruses by the pattern of fluorescence seen in the fluorescent-antibody test (27). Lower-numbered adenoviruses may also overgrow the fastidious adenoviruses if both are present in a stool sample (2). Approximately 40% of fastidious adenoviruses from stool will also grow in the Chang human conjunctival cell line and HEp-2 cells, with the development of typical adenoviral CPE (5).

EM DETECTION OF VIRUSES

General comments

The gastroenteritis viruses cannot usually be propagated by using routine cell culture types and methods. Thus, EM is frequently used to detect those agents for which no commercial EIA or LA kits are available. These include the non-group A rotaviruses, astro-, calici-, and coronaviruses, Norwalk and Norwalk-like viruses, and other unclassified SRVP. A few research laboratories have developed radioimmunoassays, EIAs, or biotin-avidin EIAs for many of these viruses, often using patient stool specimens for sources of virus and patient convalescent sera for sources of antibody (5). Since the research reagents are not routinely available, EM or IEM is the most feasible way of detection for most diagnostic laboratories.

By EM, one has the advantage of examining a specimen and detecting a number of different viruses. EM methods also take relatively little technical time and preparation. However, access to an electron microscope and a darkroom for developing and printing electron micrographs is needed. EM methods also require a skilled technologist familiar with both (i) instrument operation and routine maintenance and (ii) detecting virus particles and distinguishing them from artifacts. With direct EM, the limit of sensitivity is approximately 10^6 virus particles per ml of specimen. If virus particles are suspected of being excreted in small numbers, IEM can be performed. IEM methods (described below) have the advantage of concentrating virus particles if present. These methods are used particularly if Norwalk or Norwalk-like viruses are suspected.

For direct EM or IEM, it is necessary to negatively stain the virus particles with a heavy metal salt such as phosphotungstic acid (PTA). The metallic salts form an electron-dense matrix around the more electron-transparent virions (12). Thus, the lighter-appearing virus particles can be seen as contrasted against a darker surrounding halo of electron-dense metallic salts. PTA is usually prepared as a 2% aqueous suspension, and the pH is adjusted to 6.5 by addition of 1 N KOH.

If a large number of stool specimens are received from gastroenteritis patients, a laboratory may first choose to screen the specimens by one of the rotavirus EIA or LA assays, since during the winter months up to 40 to 50% of diarrheal stools may be rotavirus positive. EM can then be carried out on the EIA or LA rotavirus-negative samples to detect non-group A rotaviruses and other gastroenteritis viruses. However, with this approach, dual infections with rotavirus and another virus may be missed. A laboratory may also choose to screen specimens by one of the adenovirus EIA tests before performing EM.

Direct EM procedures

A very rapid direct EM procedure has been described by Middleton et al. (22). Basically, a stool suspension is prepared, added to an EM grid, stained with PTA, and viewed by EM. More specifically, an approximate 20% stool suspension is initially prepared, using either distilled water or a 1% aqueous ammonium acetate solution. Some laboratories clarify specimens by low-speed centrifugation to remove debris, but we have found this to be unnecessary. Copper EM grids, 300- or 400-mesh size, are recommended. They should be coated with Formvar, a polyvinyl formol plastic, which forms a stable support film for the specimen and PTA stain (12). An additional thin layer of carbon on the grid over the Formvar provides maximum stability (12).

To prepare the grids, first assemble 75-mm petri dishes lined with filter paper, using one dish per specimen. Use no. 5 tweezers to hold the grid. The tweezers can be held closed by rolling a rubber O-ring gasket over the tweezers toward the tip until the tip is held closed. The tweezers may be laid over the side of the petri dish so that the grid is over the filter paper. Using a fine-bore 9-inch (ca. 23-cm) Pasteur pipette, add a small drop of the 20% stool suspension to the Formvar-carbon-coated surface (dull side) of the grid so that the suspension forms a meniscus. After 10 to 30 s, remove the excess specimen by touching the edge of the grid with the torn edge of a piece of filter paper or lens tissue held perpendicular to the grid. The roughly torn edges enhance capillary action. If the sample on the grid appears particulate or very dense, add a drop of distilled water to the grid, leave it on for 10 to 30 s, and remove it with torn filter paper as before. Alternatively, the dense grid surface can be inverted and touched to 1 or more drops of distilled water placed on Parafilm. While the grid is still damp, immediately add a drop of 2% PTA so that it forms a meniscus, leave it on for 10 to 30 s, and remove it with torn filter paper.

It is recommended that duplicate grids be made, since a grid may have too heavy or too thin a film for viewing, whereas the duplicate grid may be the correct thickness for viewing. Most viruses will be found in areas of moderate density. If a grid is too thick, it will be unviewable. If this is the case, use a more diluted sample or add the distilled water rinse step between adding the specimen and adding the stain. Rinsing steps may also be necessary if ultracentrifugation methods for concentration are used (9, 12). If a grid is too sparse, another grid containing more material needs to be prepared. For this reason, it is usually more convenient to initially prepare grids in duplicate.

Inactivate any viruses on the grid by exposing them to UV light, using 900 $\mu W/cm^2$ at a distance of 15 to 20 cm for at least 10 min (11). The grids are now ready for examination.

In addition to the direct application method given above, virus in stool specimens can be concentrated by one of several methods. One simple, rapid method is ultracentrifugation in a Beckman Airfuge fitted with an EM-90 rotor (12). Up to six samples can be concentrated by this method. First, the stool suspensions are clarified by low-speed centrifugation. A 90-µl sample of each of the clarified supernatant fluids is then centrifuged onto Formvar-carbon-coated grids in the Airfuge at 90,000 rpm for 30 min. The grids are then negatively stained by placing the inverted grids onto individual drops of PTA placed on Parafilm (12), blotting them dry, and applying UV radiation. This Airfuge centrifugation method increases the sensitivity of detection of virus by 1.5 to 3.0 $\log_{10}$.

Virus in clarified stool specimens can also be concentrated by centrifugation in an ultracentrifuge at $100{,}000 \times g$ in a swinging-bucket rotor for 1 h at 40°C (9). After centrifugation, the supernatant fluid should be removed and thoroughly drained. The viral pellet is then suspended in a small volume of distilled water, from which the grids are prepared (9, 12).

Still another method for concentrating virus, as well as removing excessive salts from specimens, is the agar diffusion method (12). In this method, a 1% agar or agarose solution in distilled water is prepared in the wells of a sterile microtiter plate. The plate is sealed and stored at 4°C. For use, one agar-filled well is cut away for each specimen. A drop of stool suspension is applied to the top of the agar well. A grid is then inverted on top of the drop. As the suspension is absorbed into the agar well, virus particles are concentrated on the grid surface. After the grid lies flat onto the agar surface, it is removed and negatively stained.

IEM procedures

If the amount of virus in stools is below the limits of detection by direct EM, several IEM procedures can be carried out to concentrate the virus for detection. One major problem with the IEM procedure is obtaining virus-specific antisera. However, three possible sources of antisera may be used (12). First, patient convalescent sera can be used to clump virus particles in stool samples taken during the acute phase of illness. This method has been frequently used to detect Norwalk and Norwalk-like viruses. However, results are obtained retrospectively. Second, pooled immune serum globulin containing gamma globulin and with a broad population of specific antibodies can be used. This procedure will also increase the trapping efficiency of any virus particles occurring in stool samples. These two methods permit virus in specimens to be assigned to a major group on the basis of morphology (12). A third source of specific antisera is a research laboratory.

There are at least three IEM methods that can be carried out, using convalescent serum, pooled immune globulin, and/or specific immune serum. One of them is direct IEM. By this method, a stool suspension is mixed with an equal volume of antiserum and incubated at 37°C for 1 h. The immune complexes are then sedimented at 10,000 to 15,000 rpm for 30 min. The pellet is suspended in distilled water, added to a grid, and stained with PTA (12).

Another IEM method is solid-phase IEM. In this method, viral antibodies are first adsorbed onto an EM grid. A viral suspension is added, and the antibodies on the grid increase the attraction of viral particles. The grid is then negatively stained and examined. Greater trapping of antibody and therefore virus is achieved by first adding *Staphylococcus aureus* protein A to the grid, to which the gamma globulin then adheres (12).

A third IEM method is the serum-in-agar method (12). It is similar to the agar diffusion method except that antiserum is incorporated into the molten agar at about 45°C, just before it is poured into microtiter wells and hardens. The grid is placed dull side up on top of the agar, and a drop of specimen is placed on top of the grid. The antibody-agar below the grid "pulls" the suspension onto and through the grid, leaving virus particles on the grid.

Examination of grids

As soon as the EM and IEM grids have been stained and UV irradiated, they are ready for examination in the electron microscope. We examine grids at 80 kV; less voltage reduces ease of detection. Initially examine the grid at ×1,000 magnification to assess the general quality of the preparation and select a grid square or set of squares that are neither too dense nor too light. Most viruses will be found in areas of moderate density. If the grid is too thick, it will be unviewable; if it is too sparse, virus particles may not be observed.

Once grid squares of moderate density are found, slowly take the magnification up to ×10,000. Then bring the magnification up to ×40,000 or a higher magnification at which the grids will be examined. One high magnification should be chosen and used consistently. This practice helps in determining the relative size of the various virions that are detected. Most electron microscopes have a circle or bar on the viewing screen that can be used at an appropriate magnification as a guide to determine the approximate diameter size of the virions observed on the screen. Examine grid squares for small round light areas that may represent virus particles surrounded by a dark electron-dense stained fringe area.

The resolving power of the electron microscope enables viruses to be identified on the basis of size and characteristic morphology. The criteria used in classifying and identifying various gastroenteritis viruses are listed in Table 1. Electron photomicrographs of four of the viruses are shown in Fig. 1.

Rotaviruses are approximately 70 nm in diameter with a double icosahedral shell. Depending on the rotation of the virion, some of the capsomeres may appear ringlike, and others may appear to be cylindrical, radiating outwardly.

Adenoviruses are icosahedrons approximately 75 nm in diameter. Their outer edge will appear to be hexagon shaped. The virion surface consists of identical-appearing, closely packed capsomeres. Depending on the rotation of the virion, groups of capsomeres may appear to form one, two, or more triangles on the virion surface.

The caliciviruses are 30- to 35-nm virions. Their capsid surface has a total of 32 cuplike depressions, similar to golf ball depressions, which appear to be filled with PTA stain. In certain orientations, six stain-filled peripheral hollows surrounding a central stain-filled hollow produce a six-pointed Star of David pattern. The peripheral outline of the virions appears to be spiky as a result of the undulation formed by the succession of cuplike depressions on the periphery. Caliciviruses are often seen as single virions.

Astroviruses are slightly smaller than caliciviruses, being approximately 28 to 30 nm in diameter. Most astrovirus particles have a five- or six-pointed star configuration on their surface. The points of the astrovirus star radiate out from a central point or knob, and the virion has no hollow center as does the calicivirus virion. The star shape appears to be formed by stain-filled triangles. The periphery of the virus appears to be smooth, not spiky. Astroviruses are frequently seen in small or large clumps.

Coronaviruses are enveloped virions, being pleomorphic in both size (80 to 150 nm) and shape, although rounded forms are sometimes seen. Coronaviruses have club-shaped projections, called peplomers, on their outer surface. Coronaviruslike particles and artifacts resembling coronaviruses may also be observed in stools.

Norwalk and Norwalk-like viruses are small round viruses approximately 27 to 30 nm in diameter. They

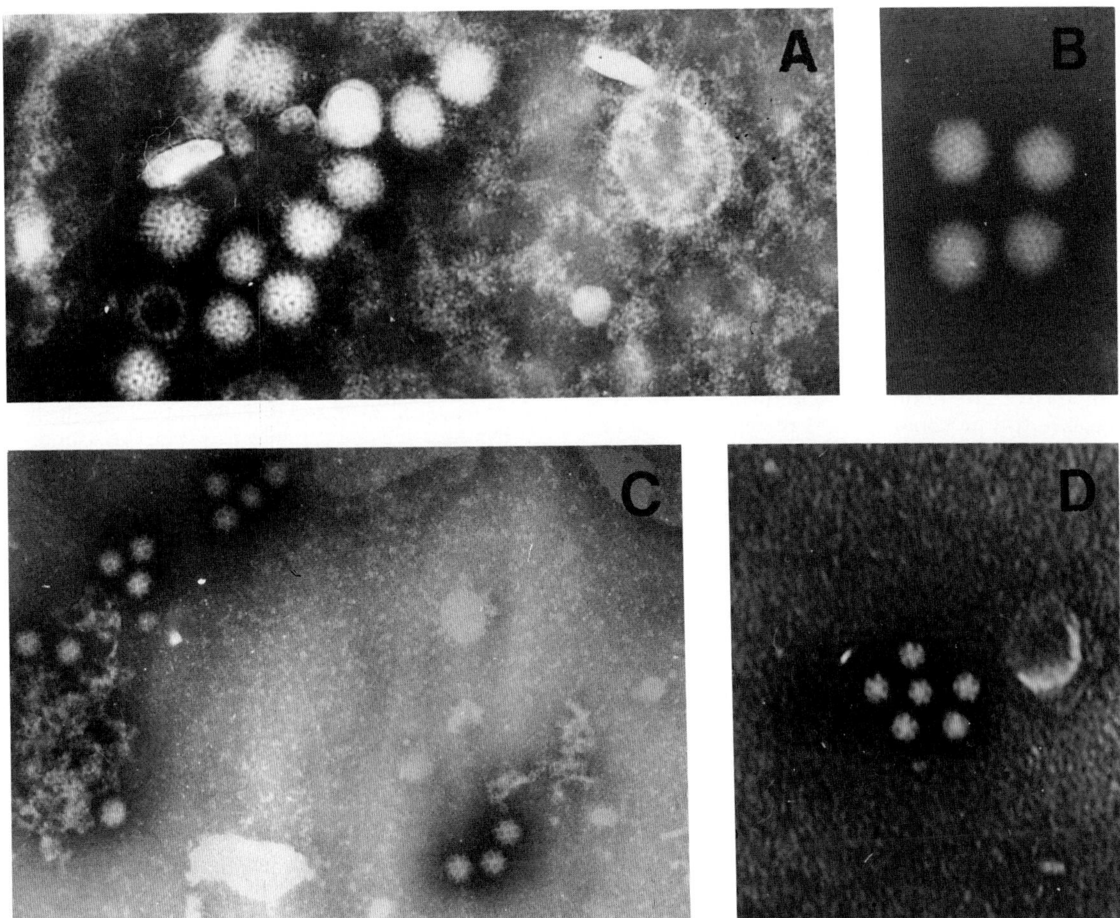

FIG. 1. Common gastroenteritis viruses from stool specimens of pediatric patients with acute gastroenteritis. For each, an approximate 20% stool suspension was prepared in 1% ammonium acetate and negatively stained with 2% PTA. ×140,000. (A) Rotaviruses, complete virions and empty virions; (B) adenoviruses in stool; (C) caliciviruses; (D) astroviruses. (Electron photomicrographs by Cynthia Howard, The Children's Memorial Hospital, Chicago, Ill. From reference 5.)

are usually observed by IEM, using patient convalescent sera. Hence their exact structure is often difficult to distinguish, since by IEM the virions are coated with antibody molecules. However, in a few instances these viruses have been observed by direct EM. They appear to have some observable surface structure and ragged edges, similar to but not identical with those of caliciviruses (3). Norwalk-like viruses have also been described as structured SRVP because of their surface structure and undulating edges (3).

In addition, various other unclassified SRVP have been reported in the literature (3). In some instances, the surface structure of the SRVP cannot be distinguished, either because they are coated with antibody or because of the limits of resolution of the microscope being used. Some SRVP observed by EM have been described as unstructured, or featureless, since they have no observable surface structure and have smooth edges. Unstructured SRVP have also been described as parvoviruslike or picornaviruslike (3). Since these various viruses cannot be grown in routine cell culture, they have not been well studied or classified, and their relationships to one another and to classified viruses are unknown.

Some virion suspensions, especially of rotavirus and enterovirus, may contain both complete and empty virions. The complete virions will appear light, whereas the empty virions will have a light periphery and a dark stain-filled core.

Many artifacts and other constituents can be present in negatively stained preparations of fecal extracts (13): bacterial cell wall components, host cell membranes and subcellular particles, and bacteriophages. The last group contains a variety of morphologic types. Some bacteriophages are hexagonal with a 75-mm diameter, similar to the diameter of adenoviruses. Others, 27 to 30 nm in diameter, are hexagonal and similar to SRVP. These may be confusing to an inexperienced electron microscopist, particularly when the phage tail is missing. A regular lattice array of a bacterial cell wall may resemble the crystalline array sometimes seen with small icosahedral virus particles. Fragments of cell membranes with surface fringe as well as other artifacts may resemble coronaviruses. However, an experienced microscopist is able to discriminate between artifactual constituents and gastroenteritis virus particles (13). Larger virus particles like rotaviruses and adenoviruses, as well as the smaller calici- and astroviruses, are characteristic enough that there is usually no problem in identifying them. However, nondistinctive SRVP may be difficult to distinguish from tail-less bacteriophage and other artifacts.

When one or more virions, or particles suspected of being virions, are found, an electron photomicrograph should be taken to provide a permanent record of the observed virions as well as to show greater detail than can be seen on an EM screen. Especially when small round particles in the range of 25 to 30 nm are observed on the screen, the photomicrograph may more exactly resolve the structure of small particles.

When a laboratory decides to undertake EM for the detection of gastroenteritis viruses, it is suggested that positive control grids containing known viruses with varying sizes and morphologies be reviewed at the beginning of each EM session. This practice will also help the microscopist identify lighting or alignment problems before attempts are made to examine patient grids. The microscopist should also calibrate the electron microscope magnification, using a carbon replica of a diffraction line grating or other standard, which can be obtained from an EM supply company. To accurately measure virus particles, especially those that are unclassified, one should photograph the magnification standard during the same session that one is photographing the virus particles. Methods for measurement and calibration can be obtained from a basic EM methods book.

LITERATURE CITED

1. **Arens, M., and E. M. Swierkosz.** 1989. Detection of rotavirus by hybridization with a nonradioactive synthetic DNA probe and comparison with commercial enzyme immunoassays and silver-stained polyacrylamide gels. J. Clin. Microbiol. **27:**1277–1279.
2. **Brown, M.** 1985. Selection of nonfastidious adenovirus species in 293 cells inoculated with stool specimens containing adenovirus 40. J. Clin. Microbiol. **22:**205–209.
3. **Caul, E. O., and H. Appleton.** 1982. The electron microscopal and physical characteristics of small round human fecal viruses: an interim scheme for classification. J. Med. Virol. **9:**257–265.
4. **Chernesky, M., S. Castriciano, J. Mahony, M. Spiewak, and L. Schaeffer.** 1988. Ability of TESTPACK ROTAVIRUS enzyme immunoassay to diagnose rotavirus gastroenteritis. J. Clin. Microbiol. **26:**2459–2461.
5. **Christensen, M. L.** 1989. Human viral gastroenteritis. Clin. Microbiol. Rev. **2:**51–89.
6. **Cromien, J. L., C. A. Himmelreich, R. I. Glass, and G. A. Storch.** 1987. Evaluation of new commercial enzyme immunoassay for rotavirus detection. J. Clin. Microbiol. **25:**2359–2362.
7. **Cubitt, W. D., and D. A. McSwiggan.** 1981. Calicivirus gastroenteritis in North West London. Lancet **ii:**975–977.
8. **Cubitt, W. D., P. J. Pead, and A. A. Saeed.** 1981. A new serotype of calicivirus associated with an outbreak of gastroenteritis in a residential home for the elderly. J. Clin. Pathol. **34:**924–926.
9. **Davies, H. A.** 1982. Electron-microscopy and immune electron microscopy for detection of gastroenteritis viruses, p. 37–49. *In* D. A. J. Tyrrell and A. Z. Kapikian (ed.), Virus infections of the gastrointestinal tract. Marcel Dekker, Inc., New York.
10. **Dennehy, P. H., D. R. Gauntlett, and W. E. Tente.** 1988. Comparison of nine commercial immunoassays for the detection of rotavirus in fecal specimens. J. Clin. Microbiol. **26:**1630–1634.
11. **Doane, F. W., and N. Anderson.** 1987. Pretreatment of clinical specimens and viral isolates, p. 4–13. *In* Electron microscopy in diagnostic virology. Cambridge University Press, New York.
12. **Doane, F. W., and N. Anderson.** 1987. Methods for preparing specimens for electron microscopy, p. 14–31. *In* Electron microscopy in diagnostic virology. Cambridge University Press, New York.
13. **Doane, F. W., and N. Anderson.** 1987. Bacteriophages, non-viral structures, and artifacts, p. 163–175. *In* Electron microscopy in diagnostic virology. Cambridge University Press, New York.
14. **Eiden, J., S. Sato, and R. Yolken.** 1987. Specificity of dot hybridization assay in the presence of rRNA for detection of rotaviruses in clinical specimens. J. Clin. Microbiol. **25:** 1809–1811.
15. **Giaquinto, C., G. Errico, E. Ruga, I. Naso, and R. D'Elia.** 1986. Evaluation of ELISA test for rotavirus diagnosis in neonates. J. Pediatr. **109:**565–566.
16. **Gilchrist, M. J. R., T. S. Bretl, K. Moultney, D. R. Knowlton, and R. L. Ward.** 1987. Comparison of seven kits for detection of rotavirus in fecal specimens with a sensitive, specific enzyme immunoassay. Diagn. Microbiol. Infect. Dis. **8:**221–228.
17. **Kaplan, J. E., G. W. Gary, R. C. Baron, N. Singh, L. B. Schonberger, R. Feldman, and H. B. Greenberg.** 1982. Epidemiology of Norwalk gastroenteritis and the role of Norwalk virus in outbreaks of acute nonbacterial gastroenteritis. Ann. Intern. Med. **96:**756–761.
18. **Kurtz, J. B., and T. W. Lee.** 1984. Human astrovirus serotypes. Lancet **ii:**1405.
19. **Lee, T. W., and J. B. Kurtz.** 1982. Human astrovirus serotypes. J. Hyg. **89:**539–540.
20. **Madeley, C. R.** 1979. Comparison of the features of astroviruses and caliciviruses seen in samples of feces by electron microscopy. J. Infect. Dis. **139:**519–523.
21. **Mathewson, J. J., D. K. Winsor, Jr., H. L. DuPont, and S. L. Secor.** 1989. Evaluation of assay systems for the detection of rotavirus in stool specimens. Diagn. Microbiol. Infect. Dis. **12:**139–141.
22. **Middleton, P. J., M. T. Szymanski, and M. Petric.** 1977. Viruses associated with acute gastroenteritis in young children. Am. J. Dis. Child. **131:**733–737.
23. **Midthun, K., J. Valdesuso, A. Z. Kapikian, Y. Hoshino, and K. Y. Green.** 1989. Identification of serotype 9 human rotavirus by enzyme-linked immunosorbent assay with monoclonal antibodies. J. Clin. Microbiol. **27:**2112–2114.
24. **Mortensen, M. L., C. G. Ray, C. M. Payne, A. D. Friedman, L. L. Minnich, and C. Rousseau.** 1985. Coronaviruslike particles in human gastrointestinal disease. Am. J. Dis. Child. **139:**928–934.
25. **Payne, C. M., and C. G. Ray.** 1984. Coronavirus? Pediatrics **74:**560–562.
26. **Resta, S., J. P. Luby, C. R. Rosenfeld, and J. D. Siegel.** 1985. Isolation and propagation of a human enteric coronavirus. Science **229:**978–981.
27. **Takiff, H. E., S. E. Straus, and C. F. Garon.** 1981. Propagation and in vitro studies of previously non-cultivable enteral adenoviruses in 293 cells. Lancet **ii:**832–834.
28. **Thomas, E. E., M. L. Puterman, E. Kawano, and M. Curran.** 1988. Evaluation of seven immunoassays for detection of rotavirus in pediatric stool samples. J. Clin. Microbiol. **26:**1189–1193.
29. **Ward, R. L., D. R. Knowlton, and M. J. Pierce.** 1984. Efficiency of human rotavirus propagation in cell culture. J. Clin. Microbiol. **19:**748–753.

Chapter 96

Hepatitis Viruses*

PAUL D. SWENSON

CLINICAL AND EPIDEMIOLOGICAL FEATURES

Viral hepatitis is a systemic disease primarily involving the liver. Most cases of acute viral hepatitis seen in children and adults are caused by one of the following agents (Table 1): hepatitis A virus (HAV), the etiological agent of hepatitis A (infectious hepatitis or short-incubation hepatitis); hepatitis B virus (HBV), which is associated with hepatitis B (serum hepatitis or long-incubation hepatitis); and the recently discovered hepatitis C virus (HCV), the causative agent of hepatitis C. The disease caused by HCV was previously designated parenterally transmitted non-A, non-B hepatitis because it was predominantly blood borne, no specific serological assays were available for its identification, and the hepatitis could not be ascribed to either HAV, HBV, cytomegalovirus, or Epstein-Barr virus. Hepatitis C accounts for most of the transfusion-associated hepatitis cases seen in the United States and a sizable portion of sporadic hepatitis. Hepatitis D virus (HDV), previously called the delta agent, is a defective virus that requires concomitant HBV infection for its own replication and expression. In the United States, most cases of hepatitis D occur in intravenous drug users and hemophiliacs. Hepatitis E virus (HEV) is associated with epidemics and sporadic cases of hepatitis E (enterically transmitted non-A, non-B hepatitis) in parts of Asia, Africa, the Middle East, and Central America. Only rare imported cases of hepatitis E have been recognized in the United States. Other well-characterized viruses that infrequently cause sporadic hepatitis, such as yellow fever virus, cytomegalovirus, Epstein-Barr virus, herpes simplex virus, rubella virus, and the enteroviruses, are discussed in other chapters of this Manual.

The pertinent clinical and epidemiological features of hepatitis A, B, and C are presented in Table 2. All of these agents produce characteristic but generally indistinguishable histopathological lesions in the liver. In individual cases, differentiation among the various types of hepatitis on clinical grounds alone is not feasible. Moreover, clinical expression of disease is extremely variable, ranging from asymptomatic infection to anicteric or icteric hepatitis to fulminant hepatitis and even death. The prodromal or preicteric phase is frequently characterized by low-grade fever (<39.5°C), fatigability, malaise, myalgia, blunting of olfactory and gustatory senses, anorexia, nausea, vomiting, and, especially in patients with HBV infection, maculopapular and urticarial rash, arthralgias, or polyarthritis (seen in 10 to 15% of cases). Symptoms are followed by right upper quadrant discomfort or pain associated with hepatomegaly and the appearance of dark urine and clinical jaundice. Patients with acute viral hepatitis usually recover completely. The frequency of fulminant hepatitis among icteric hepatitis B patients is probably less than 2% now that posttransfusion hepatitis B has been significantly reduced by the screening of donor units for hepatitis B surface antigen (HBsAg). Mortality data for hepatitis A suggest that the frequency of fulminant disease in icteric cases is less than 0.5%. The importance of HDV is its ability to convert an asymptomatic or mild, acute, or chronic HBV infection into fulminant or severe, progressive disease. A striking characteristic of hepatitis E is the 10 to 20% case fatality rate in pregnant women.

Distinguishing between hepatitis A and B assumes practical importance in light of demonstrations that hepatitis A, an infection spread by close contact via the fecal-oral route, can, on rare occasions, be transmitted parenterally, and hepatitis B, which occurs sporadically after parenteral inoculation of virus-contaminated blood or blood products, can also be spread by close intimate contact. The discovery of a unique hepatitis B antigen by Blumberg and his associates (3) and its specific relationship to HBV infection allow serological identification of hepatitis B cases. Now that serological markers for HAV and HCV infections are also available, nearly all cases of acute viral hepatitis can be categorized serologically as hepatitis A, B, or C.

DESCRIPTION OF AGENTS (5, 21, 22, 56, 62)

HAV is a nonenveloped icosahedral 27- to 32-nm particle (Fig. 1) which may appear full or empty under an electron microscope. Its peak buoyant density in cesium chloride is 1.33 to 1.34 g/cm^3, but both heavier and lighter particles exist; the virus has a sedimentation coefficient ($s_{20,w}$) of 160S in a neutral sucrose solution. Studies of its nucleic acid composition indicate that HAV is an RNA virus with a linear, single-stranded genome of approximately 2.3×10^6 daltons. HAV has four major, structural polypeptides similar in molecular weight to those of poliovirus, and it localizes exclusively in the cytoplasm of hepatocytes. Lipid is not an integral component of HAV, which is stable to treatment with 20% ether, acid, and heat (60°C for at least 1 h); its infectivity can be preserved for years at −20°C and for at least 1 month after being dried and stored at 25°C. Viral infectivity is destroyed by autoclaving (121°C for 20 min), by boiling in water for 1 min, by dry heat (180°C for 1 h), by UV irradiation (1 min at 1.1 W), by treatment with Formalin (1:4,000 [wt/vol] for 3 days at 37°C), or by treatment with chlorine (10 to 15 ppm for 30 min) or chlorine-containing compounds (e.g., sodium hypochlorite, 10 mg/liter for 15 min). Only one serotype of HAV has been defined. It does not cross-react with

* This is an update of the chapter by F. Blaine Hollinger and Jules L. Dienstag in the fourth edition of this Manual.

TABLE 1. Terminology of viral hepatitis

Agent	Preferred terminology	Equivalent terminology
Hepatitis A virus	Hepatitis A	Infectious hepatitis Epidemic jaundice Short-incubation hepatitis
Hepatitis B virus	Hepatitis B	Serum or transfusion hepatitis Homologous serum jaundice Long-incubation hepatitis
Hepatitis C virus	Hepatitis C	Parenterally transmitted non-A, non-B hepatitis
Hepatitis D virus	Hepatitis D	Delta hepatitis
Hepatitis E virus	Hepatitis E	Enterically transmitted non-A, non-B hepatitis

HBV, and its host range appears to be limited to humans, marmosets, owl monkeys, Malaysian cynomolgus monkeys, and chimpanzees. Its properties most closely resemble those of the enterovirus subgroup of the family *Picornaviridae*, and it has been classified as enterovirus type 72.

Sera from patients with HBV infections reveal three distinct morphological entities in varying proportions (Fig. 2). The more numerous forms (by a factor of 10^3 to 10^4) are the small pleomorphic spherical particles measuring 17 to 25 nm in diameter (mean of 22 nm). Particle counts of 10^{13} or higher have been detected in some sera. Tubular or filamentous forms of various lengths, but with a diameter similar to that of the smaller particles, are also observed. HBV is a complex, double-shelled particle with a diameter of 42 nm. Originally designated the Dane particle, it consists of a 27-nm core surrounded by a 7- to 8-nm viral protein coat.

The nomenclature used for hepatitis B is shown in Table 3. HBV is the prototype agent for a new family of viruses designated *Hepadnaviridae*. The complex antigen found on the surface of HBV is called HBsAg. Previous designations include Australia or Au antigen and hepatitis-associated antigen. HBsAg on the hepatitis B virion is biochemically identical to that detected on the smaller particles and the filamentous forms and is composed of proteins, carbohydrates, and lipids. HBsAg contains three proteins called the major, the middle, and the large proteins. The major protein is encoded by the S gene and exists as two polypeptides with molecular weights of 24,000 and 27,000, the larger of which is glycosylated. The middle protein is encoded by the pre-S2 region and S gene and is present as two glycosylated polypeptides with molecular weights of 33,000 and 36,000. The large protein is encoded by the pre-S1

TABLE 2. Epidemiology and clinical features of viral hepatitis A, B, and C

Feature	Hepatitis A	Hepatitis B	Hepatitis C
Incubation period	2–7 weeks (avg, 4 ± 1)	4–20 weeks (avg, 11 ± 4)[a]	2–20 weeks (avg, 7 ± 2)
Principal age distribution	Children,[b] young adults	Adults[c]	?
Seasonal incidence	Throughout the year, but tends to peak in autumn	Throughout the year	Throughout the year
Route of infection	Predominantly fecal-oral	Parenteral, sexual contact	Predominantly parenteral
Occurrence of virus			
Blood	2 weeks before to <1 week after jaundice	Months to years	Months to years
Stool	2 weeks before to 2 weeks after jaundice	Absent	Probably absent
Urine	Rare	Absent	Probably absent
Saliva, semen	Rare (saliva)	Frequently present	Unknown
Clinical and laboratory features			
Onset	Usually abrupt	Usually insidious	Insidious
Fever > 38°C	Common early	Less common	Less common
Duration of transaminase elevation	2–6 weeks	2–6+ months	2–6+ months
Immunoglobulins (IgM levels)	Elevated	Normal to slightly elevated	Normal to slightly elevated
Complications	Uncommon, no chronicity	Chronicity in 5 to 10%	Chronicity in 30 to 50%
Mortality rate (icteric cases)	<0.5%	<1–2%	0.5–1%
HBsAg	Absent	Present	Absent
Immunity			
Homologous	Yes	Yes	?
Heterologous	No	No	No
Duration	Probably lifetime	Probably lifetime	?
Gamma globulin (immune globulin USP) prophylaxis	Regularly prevents jaundice	Prevents jaundice only if gamma globulin is of sufficient potency against HBV	?

[a] Longer incubation periods (up to 9 months) have been observed, but the delay has usually been due to the administration of specific antibody (anti-HBs) after infection with HBV.

[b] Nonicteric hepatitis A is common in children.

[c] Among the 15- to 29-year age group, hepatitis B is often associated with drug abuse or promiscuous sexual behavior. Patients with transfusion-associated hepatitis B are generally over age 29.

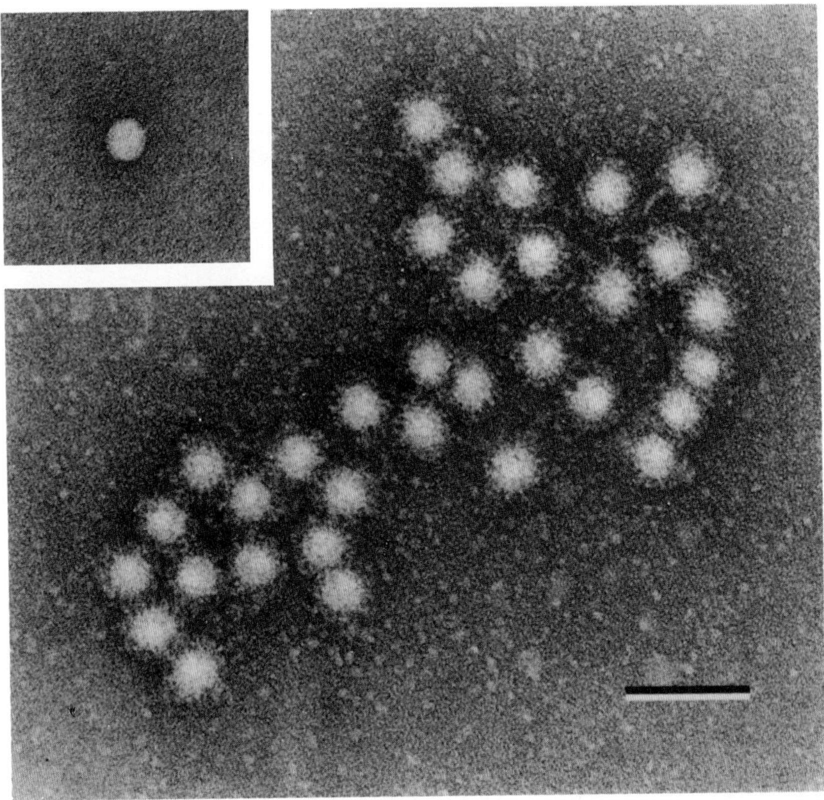

FIG. 1. Electron micrograph of 27-nm HAV particles purified by a combination of isopycnic banding in CsCl, column chromatography, and rate-zonal separation in sucrose. A single isolated HAV particle (upper left) is compared with the same preparation after incubation with convalescent-phase serum from a patient with hepatitis A. ×165,000; bar = 100 nm. (From reference 47.)

region, pre-S2 region, and S gene and consists of two polypeptides with molecular weights of 39,000 and 42,000, the larger being glycosylated. HBsAg on hepatitis B virions and filaments contains up to 20 times more large protein than do 22-nm particles. The 22-nm particles have an average buoyant density of 1.20 g/cm^3 in CsCl and 1.17 g/cm^3 in sucrose, a molecular weight of 3.7×10^6 to 4.6×10^6, and a sedimentation coefficient that ranges from 39 to 54S. Analysis has revealed that one antigenic specificity, designated *a*, is common to all HBsAg preparations. In addition, there are two sets of mutually exclusive determinants, *d* or *y* and *w* or *r*. This results in four principal subtypes of HBsAg: *adw*, *ayw*, *adr*, and *ayr*. Because of antigenic heterogeneity of the *w* determinant, there are 10 major serotypes of HBV. The predominant subtype found in North America is *adw*, followed by *ayw*. HBV subtypes do not change after infection. This fact is useful when one is attempting to trace an infection from one source to another. Complete (DNA-containing) HBV has a buoyant density of 1.28 g/cm^3 in CsCl. The 27-nm internal core of HBV contains the hepatitis B core antigen (HBcAg), a small (3,200 base pairs), circular, partially double-stranded DNA molecule, and specific DNA polymerase activity. The presence of a single-stranded region of variable length in the circular DNA molecules results in genetically heterogeneous particles with buoyant densities in CsCl that range from 1.28 to 1.38 g/cm^3. The core particle contains one major polypeptide with a molecular weight of 22,000. The hepatitis B e antigen (HBeAg) is an integral component of the HBV core particle, presumably existing in a cryptic form. In the serum, HBeAg is a soluble protein with a molecular weight of 15,000 which results from proteolytic cleavage of the core protein.

The stability of HBV does not always coincide with that of HBsAg. Immunogenicity and antigenicity are retained after exposure to ether, acid (pH 2.4 for at least 6 h), heat (98°C for 1 min; 60°C for 10 h), and up to 40 cycles of freeze-thawing. HBV is stable at 37°C for 60 min but not at 60°C for 10 h. However, inactivation may be incomplete under these conditions if the concentration of virus is excessively high. Exposure of HBsAg to 0.25% sodium hypochlorite for 3 min destroys antigenicity (and presumably infectivity). Infectivity in serum is lost after direct boiling for 2 min, autoclaving at 121°C for 20 min, or dry heat at 160°C for 1 h. More recent studies have shown that HBV is inactivated by exposure to sodium hypochlorite (500 mg of free chlorine per liter) for 10 min, 0.1 to 2% aqueous glutaraldehyde, Sporicidin (pH 7.9), 70% isopropyl alcohol, 80% ethyl alcohol at 11°C for 2 min, Wescodyne diluted 1:213, or combined β-propiolactone and UV irradiation (4, 40, 49). HBV has been shown to retain infectivity when stored at 30 to 32°C for at least 6 months and, when frozen at −20°C, for 15 years.

HCV is a 30- to 60-nm enveloped virus which has a single-stranded linear RNA genome, approximately 10 kilodaltons in size, that is positive stranded. These properties suggest that HCV is a togavirus or flavivirus.

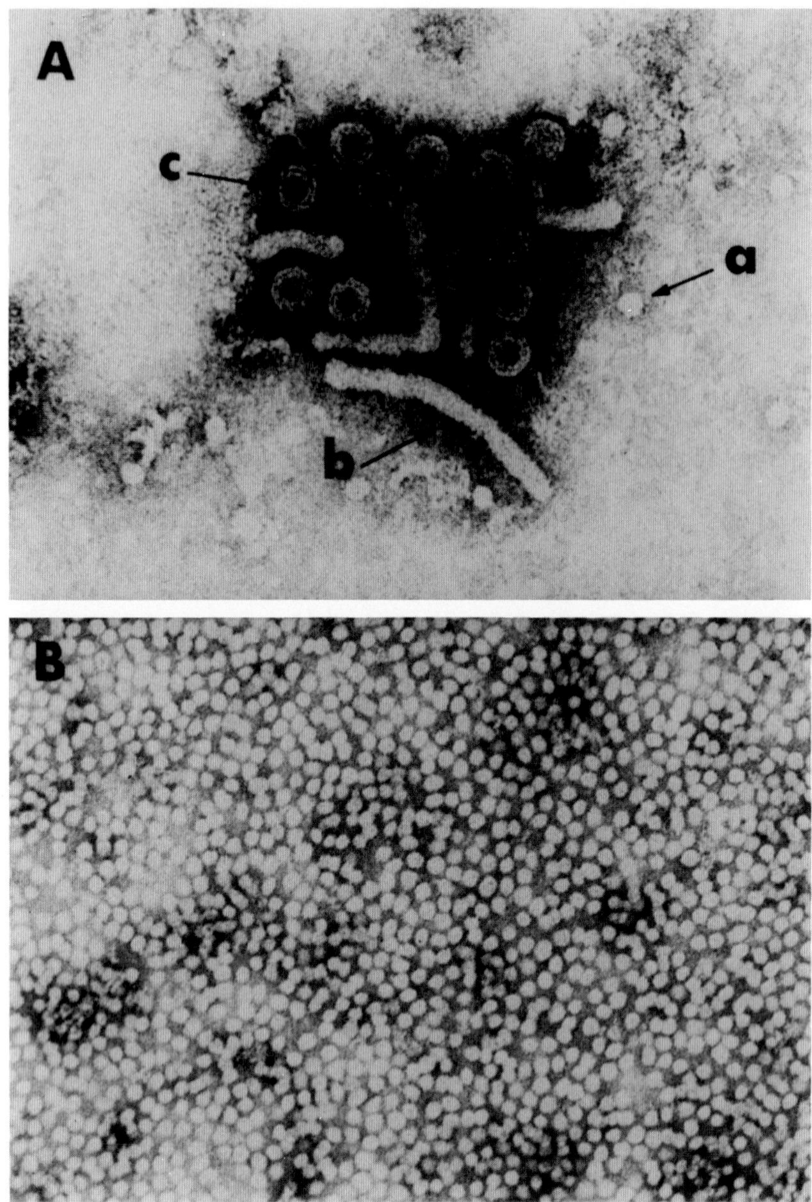

FIG. 2. (A) Electron micrograph of serum showing the presence of three distinct morphological entities: a, 20-nm pleomorphic spherical particles; b, tubular or filamentous forms with a diameter of 20 nm; and c, 42-nm spherical particles now considered to be HBV (Dane particle). ×132,000. (B) Electron micrograph of a purified preparation of 17- to 25-nm pleomorphic spherical particles containing HBsAg. ×77,000. Similar preparations currently are being used in human hepatitis B vaccines.

HDV is a 35- to 37-nm virus composed of an HDV antigen-expressing core encapsidated by HBsAg and requiring the helper function of HBV to support its replication. As anticipated, HDV assumes the HBsAg subtype of the HBV infection present in the host. HDV has a small circular RNA genome (5.5×10^5 daltons) that is nonhomologous with HBV DNA; HDV antigen (HDVAg) is a 68,000-dalton protein. The virus particle has a buoyant density of 1.25 g/cm^3 and a sedimentation coefficient intermediate between those of HBsAg and intact HBV particles. It is inactivated by Formalin under conditions similar to those which inactivate HBV (53).

HEV is a 32- to 34-nm nonenveloped virus with a sedimentation coefficient of 183S and biophysical properties resembling those of some human caliciviruses. Its host range appears to be limited to humans, cynomolgus monkeys, marmosets, and African green monkeys.

PROCESSING OF SPECIMENS AND ENVIRONMENTAL CONTROL

The stability of the various serological markers for HBV and HAV eliminates the need for extraordinary collection and storage procedures if bacterial contamination is minimized. Samples can be stored at 2 to 8°C if testing is to take place within 5 days. Should longer delays be anticipated, specimens must be frozen. The

TABLE 3. Nomenclature for viral hepatitis B

Term	Abbreviation	Description
Hepatitis B virus	HBV	The 42-nm double-shelled particle that consists of a 7-nm outer shell and a 27-nm inner core. The core contains a small, circular, partially double-stranded DNA molecule and DNA polymerase activity. Originally called the Dane particle. This is the prototype for the family *Hepadnaviridae*.
Hepatitis B surface antigen	HBsAg	The complex antigen that is found on the surface of HBV and on the 22-nm particles and tubular forms. Formerly designated Australia antigen or hepatitis-associated antigen.
Hepatitis B core antigen	HBcAg	The antigen associated with the 27-nm core of HBV.
Hepatitis B e antigen	HBeAg	An antigen that is closely associated with the nucleocapsid of HBV. Also found as a soluble protein in serum.
Antibody to HBsAg, HBcAg, and HBeAg	Anti-HBs, anti-HBc, and anti-HBe	Specific antibodies produced in response to their respective antigens.

addition of a bacteriostatic agent to the samples is rarely indicated. Should this become necessary, a final concentration of 0.01% thimerosal, 0.1% sodium azide, or gentamicin sulfate at 25 to 50 µg/ml is preferred. The use of anticoagulants or the presence of severely hemolyzed blood may occasionally cause false-positive immunoassay responses. Serum samples can be shipped at ambient temperatures if delivery is expected to be made within 48 h. Unseparated clotted blood sent in the original collection tube and received in the laboratory within 24 h does not adversely affect assay results. However, safety is best achieved by shipping serum samples frozen in dry ice and in doubly sealed containers, as stipulated by the Interstate Quarantine Regulations (Code of Federal Regulations, Title 42, Part 72.25, Etiologic Agents). Although antibodies to HAV and HBV antigens are stable for years at −20°C and for at least 10 days at 37°C, repetitive freezing and thawing may lead to substantial losses in titer.

Laboratory personnel should regard all specimens collected from hepatitis patients as potentially dangerous, especially stool samples from hepatitis A candidates and blood or body fluids collected from patients with hepatitis B or hepatitis C. In our laboratories, the use of needles is avoided whenever possible; when used, they are placed in puncture-resistant "sharps" containers and incinerated or autoclaved before being discarded. All other materials are placed in discard pans and autoclaved at 121°C for 40 min. Work areas are decontaminated with 0.5% sodium hypochlorite, e.g., a 1:10 dilution of Clorox, that is prepared fresh each month. It is used for physical cleaning of environmental surfaces, for washing hands that have been inadvertently contaminated with virus, and for decontaminating metal instruments or rotors and most labile plastics. Because hypochlorites may be corrosive to many metals, the solutions are not allowed to remain in contact with such materials for more than 10 min. Disposable gloves and gowns are worn when personnel are working with blood products or stool specimens, and handwashing procedures are strictly enforced. Additional safety recommendations can be found in the cited literature (5, 67).

HAV

Direct examination

Immunofluorescence and immunoperoxidase staining techniques as well as thin-section electron microscopic techniques have been applied to the demonstration of HAV in hepatocytes from chimpanzees and marmosets infected with HAV. However, methods for detecting intrahepatic HAV are not applicable to clinically available specimens, for liver biopsy is rarely, if ever, performed on patients with hepatitis A. On the other hand, immunoelectron microscopy (IEM), which was the first method used successfully to visualize HAV (21), remains an important reference technique. By allowing visualization of specific immune aggregates, which are more easily detected than are monodispersed virions, this procedure enhances the sensitivity of conventional electron microscopy approximately 1,000-fold (sensitivity threshold of 10^5 to 10^6 particles per ml for IEM, compared with 10^8 to 10^9 particles per ml for electron microscopy).

For detecting HAV in stools, a 2% fecal extract is prepared from an early-acute-phase stool specimen by mixing 0.2 g of stool in 10 ml of veal infusion broth supplemented with 0.5% bovine serum albumin (BSA). The suspension is homogenized by shaking it vigorously for 5 to 10 min in a securely sealed tube containing glass beads and then is clarified by centrifugation at 4°C for 1 h at 1,000 × *g*. Subsequently, the supernatant fluid is passed through a series of 1.2- and 0.45-µm microfiltration membranes premoistened with 0.5% BSA to minimize virus adsorption. To reduce the hazard of infection in the laboratory, preparation of stool filtrates and of electron microscope grids must be done in an appropriate containment facility. A 0.9-ml volume of stool filtrate is incubated with 0.1 ml of a 1:10 dilution of convalescent-phase serum known to contain antibody to HAV (anti-HAV). Important controls include stool filtrates incubated with diluent alone (phosphate-buffered saline [PBS], pH 7.4) and with preillness serum from a patient with hepatitis A. (Reference chimpanzee preinoculation and convalescent-phase serum samples are available from the Research Resources Branch, National Institute of Allergy and Infectious Diseases, Bethesda, MD 20205.)

After incubation for 1 h at room temperature or, alternatively, overnight at 4°C, the suspension is centrifuged at 47,000 × *g* for 90 min at 4°C to pellet antigen-antibody complexes. The resulting pellet is suspended in 50 μl (1 to 2 drops) of distilled water and then mixed with an equal volume of 2% phosphotungstic acid (pH 7.2). One drop of this preparation is applied to a 400-mesh Formvar carbon-coated copper grid. After 1 min, excess fluid is absorbed with filter paper, and the grid is air dried. Grids are examined by electron microscopy at a magnification of ×40,000 to ×60,000, and antibody-coated aggregates or single antibody-coated particles are counted (Fig. 1). Quantitation is achieved if a reference antiserum is used and the particles in a fixed number of grid squares are enumerated.

Because antibody-coated viruslike particles other than HAV may appear in fecal extracts, a comparison between stool filtrates incubated with preillness serum and convalescent-phase serum is mandatory and preferably is done under code. This technique for visualizing HAV can be applied with minor modifications to detection of HAV in homogenates of liver (from experimental animals) and to HAV purified from liver or stool. IEM can also be modified to quantitate anti-HAV in serum (see below).

Finally, in choosing fecal specimens for visualization of HAV, an attempt should be made to collect the earliest possible sample, for the bulk of fecal HAV shedding precedes the onset of jaundice (Fig. 3). Because such early specimens are rarely available, detection of fecal HAV is usually not a practical clinical diagnostic technique. Instead, clinical diagnosis relies on the demonstration of a serological response.

Biological investigations

Nonhuman primates, primarily chimpanzees (15, 45) and marmosets (specifically genus *Saguinus*) (11, 51), have been experimentally infected with fecal specimens and blood samples and have been found to develop viremia and to excrete the virus in bile and stool. Both naturally and experimentally infected animals can transmit HAV to animal caretakers. Attempts to isolate and propagate HAV in cell or organ cultures were unsuccessful until 1979, when marmoset-adapted HAV was cultivated serially in primary explant cultures of adult *Saguinus labiatus* marmoset livers and in a normal fetal rhesus monkey kidney cell line (FRhK6) (50). A noncytopathic infection occurs with this marmoset-adapted virus.

Recently, HAV has been cultivated in vitro in a large variety of cell lines (African green monkey kidney, additional strains of fetal rhesus monkey kidney, Vero cells, the Alexander human hepatoma cell line, and human diploid lung cells). Although direct inoculation of feces and serum containing HAV has led to successful virus cultivation in vitro, isolation of HAV from clinical

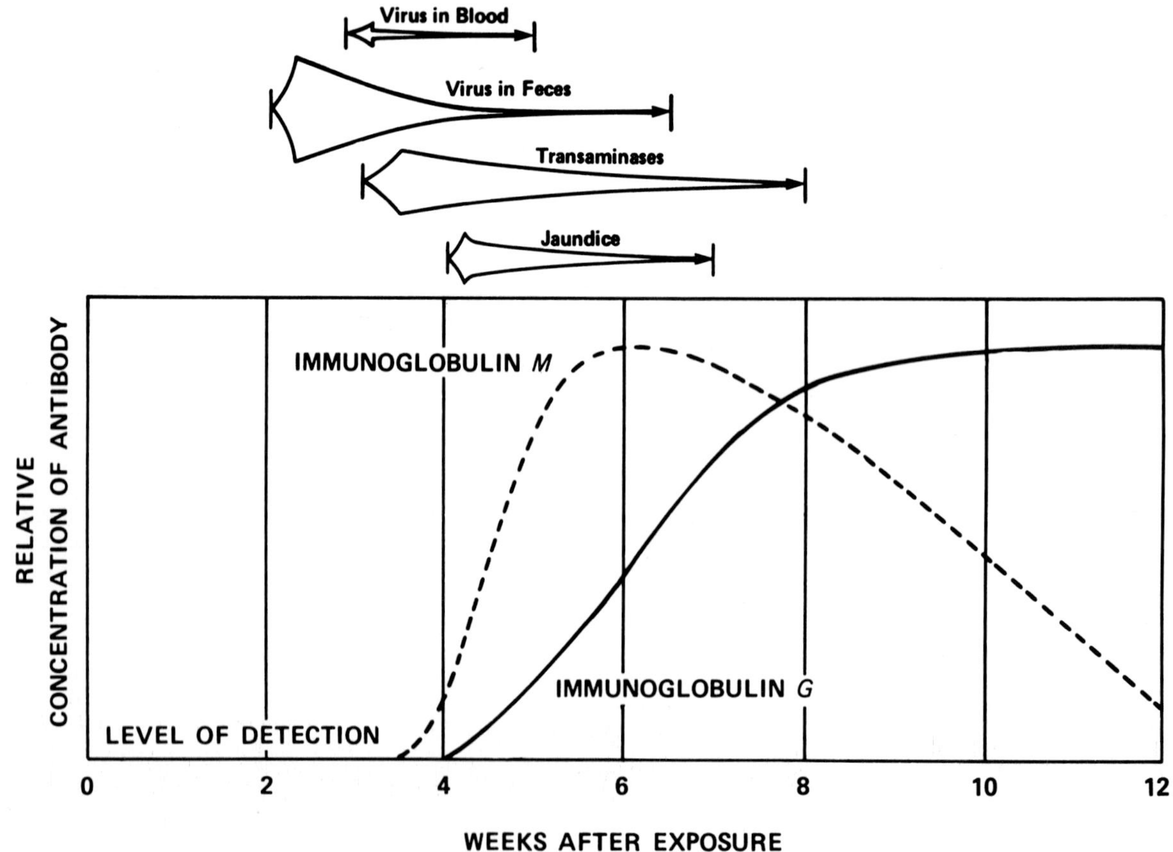

FIG. 3. Immunological and biological events associated with hepatitis A.

specimens is not sufficiently sensitive for routine diagnostic purposes. Moreover, inoculation is usually followed by a long eclipse period, rendering virus isolation attempts impractical for rapid viral diagnosis. Because HAV is not cytopathic in cell culture, detection of virus in vitro requires demonstration of HAV antigen by immunoassay or immunofluorescence microscopy. A byproduct of in vitro cultivation of HAV is a limitless supply of HAV antigen as a diagnostic reagent. In addition, cell culture provides a simple, sensitive method for testing the infectivity of clinical specimens. Still, cultivation of HAV remains limited to a select group of research laboratories. Practical, rapid viral diagnosis is achieved most readily by serological testing.

Serological methods to identify HAV and its antibody

After the visualization of HAV in human stools and marmoset livers, a variety of in vitro assays were developed to detect HAV and its antibody, anti-HAV (Table 4). Of these methods, IEM is valuable as a research and reference tool but impractical for routine diagnostic purposes. Similarly, techniques for localizing HAV in tissue have limited clinical applications. Although complement fixation is a potentially quantitative, rapid assay, its usefulness is limited by its low sensitivity, its nonspecificity, and the high frequency of anticomplementarity in acute-phase hepatitis serum. The immune adherence hemagglutination assay (IAHA) was a popular diagnostic approach to hepatitis A, but, eclipsed by more sensitive, practical assays, this method is rarely used. In contrast, radioimmunoassay (RIA) and enzyme immunoassay (EIA) have been applied widely and will be described in detail below.

Preparation of reagents. The availability of commercial assays for the diagnosis of HAV infection has diminished the need for preparing reagents except in research laboratories. A combination of preparative techniques (including differential centrifugation, isopycnic ultracentrifugation, isopycnic banding in cesium chloride, rate-zonal separation in sucrose, preparative electrophoresis, gel filtration, ion-exchange chromatography, affinity chromatography, and organic solvent extraction) can be used to purify HAV from human or nonhuman primate stool, from homogenized marmoset liver, or from cell culture for use in serological assays. If stool specimens are to be used, they should be collected as early during acute illness as possible, preferably before the onset of jaundice, after which virus excretion declines rapidly (Fig. 3). Thus, most patients presenting with clinically obvious hepatitis A are poor sources of virus-rich stool. Success is much more likely if stool is collected from close contacts of the index case, even in the absence of clinical signs of hepatitis. Although generally impractical, this approach has been rewarding in the setting of large common-source outbreaks (16, 23). Now that HAV has been grown in cell culture, an inexhaustible supply of virus antigen for diagnostic purposes has become available. Details of these purification techniques can be found in the third edition of this Manual.

Little difficulty is encountered in obtaining a source of anti-HAV-positive serum, for the antibody response after natural infection is brisk, reaching peak titers (on the order of 1:100,000) approximately 2 to 3 months after acute illness. Furthermore, relatively high titers of serum anti-HAV are maintained years after infection (59). If necessary, anti-HAV can be raised in animals by immunization with purified HAV (17). Depending on the purity of the HAV preparation used for immunization, antisera raised in animals may have antibodies to normal liver proteins, to stool antigens, or to cell culture components. Therefore, under certain circumstances, appropriate control antigens and antisera must be used, as discussed below.

IEM. IEM can be used to detect either HAV (see Direct Examination of HAV, above) or anti-HAV. The presence of anti-HAV in serum is determined by incubating the serum with a source of HAV containing at least 50 HAV particles per electron microscope grid square. Traditionally, a 2% stool filtrate containing HAV has been used for this purpose, although other sources may be substituted. Paired serum samples (acute phase, or preillness and convalescent phase) are tested under code to allow comparison between them and to avoid observer bias. Serum diluted 1:10 in PBS is incubated with the HAV-positive sample, and IEM is performed as described above. Particles visualized are rated on a scale of 0 to 4+, with 0 signifying no antibody and 4+ representing such heavy antibody coating that the particle surfaces are almost obscured. A rise in antibody rating of 1+, which corresponds roughly to a 10-fold increase in titer by IAHA, is considered a serological response indicative of acute infection. Preillness samples should be anti-HAV negative, acute-phase samples will be negative or barely positive (1 to 2+), and late-convalescent-phase samples, taken several weeks to months after illness, will have high antibody ratings (3 to 4+).

Difficulties in interpretation may arise when serum contains antibodies to other viruslike particles that may be prevalent in stools. Generally, these particles are smaller than the 27-nm HAV particles, and an increase in antibody coating is not observed when paired sera are examined. The presence of these ubiquitous particles emphasizes the importance of testing paired serum samples simultaneously for anti-HAV and of using HAV purified from cell culture. Correspondingly, tests for

TABLE 4. In vitro techniques for detecting HAV and anti-HAV

Technique	HAV	Anti-HAV	Remarks
Immunoelectron microscopy	+	+	
Complement fixation	±	+	Less useful for detecting HAV in unpurified clinical specimens
Immune adherence hemagglutination	±	+	
Radioimmunoassay	+	+	
Immunofluorescence/immunoperoxidase	+	−	Detection of HAV in liver cells
Enzyme immunoassay	+	+	

HAV should include anti-HAV-negative (preinoculation or preillness) control sera.

IAHA. IAHA is a complement-dependent assay 10 to 100 times more sensitive than complement fixation and easily adapted for quantitative determinations on large numbers of samples (46, 47). Although it can be used to detect HAV during virus purification, it is poorly suited to detection of HAV in unpurified liver or stool homogenates. Its widest application, therefore, has been as a serological test to detect anti-HAV. At present, IAHA is used more frequently in areas of the world other than the United States.

IAHA takes advantage of the fact that primate erythrocytes bear surface receptors for the third component of complement (C3). When a finite concentration of partially purified HAV is added to a heat-inactivated serum sample containing anti-HAV, immune complexes form. These immune complexes are incubated with a fresh complement source, followed by exposure to dithiothreitol, which stabilizes the immune complex containing C1, C4, C2, and C3 by protecting it from attack by C3b inactivator. After the addition of human group O erythrocytes, a stable complex forms between C3 and C3 receptors on the erythrocytes, resulting in hemagglutination. Hemagglutination is evaluated on a scale of 0 to 4+. All wells with hemagglutination patterns of 3+ and 4+ are considered positive if hemagglutination is absent in buffer control wells. Details of the assay can be found in the third edition of this Manual.

Because a prozone effect may be encountered, serum samples to be tested are screened at dilutions of 1:10, 1:100, and 1:1,000, and endpoint titers are determined by serial twofold dilutions within or beyond these limits. It is also important to realize that not all erythrocytes are suitable. A large number of donors must be screened; only about 20% of group O donors show marked hemagglutination activity. Once appropriate donors are found, their erythrocytes, stored in Alsever solution, can be used for 2 to 4 weeks. In addition to the difficulties of maintaining a steady source of erythrocytes, IAHA has other limitations. Stool- and liver-derived HAV for IAHA must be purified by one or more biophysical techniques, and only high-titer preparations work satisfactorily. Furthermore, nonionic detergents and CsCl, both used in purification of HAV, interfere with IAHA and must be removed by dialysis. Unlike other techniques for identifying anti-HAV, IAHA reactions cannot be tested for immunological specificity by blocking with purified antigen; instead, specificity must be inferred from a panel of positive and negative control sera. In addition, development of anti-HAV, as measured by IAHA, is delayed from 1 to 4 weeks compared with the earlier detection of antibody possible with other techniques. Finally, nonspecific hemagglutination is encountered when IAHA is used to measure anti-HAV in lots of immune serum globulin; treatment with kaolin has been used to minimize this problem (46).

RIA (Table 5). Commercial RIA kits are available for diagnosing acute HAV infection (HĀVAB-M, Abbott Laboratories, North Chicago, Ill.), for determining the immune status of an individual to HAV after exposure, or for assessing risk in a person traveling to an endemic area or working in a high-risk environment (HĀVAB, Abbott Laboratories). Advantages of RIA over other assay systems include excellent precision, ease of performance, and unexcelled specificity and sensitivity. Limiting factors include the need for a gamma counter and the relatively short shelf life of the radiolabeled reagent.

Because anti-HAV is present in the serum of about 40% of normal urban adults, its detection cannot, by itself, establish a diagnosis of acute disease without further analysis. In some patients, seroconversion or a rise in anti-HAV titer may eventually result in a correct diagnosis. However, the antibody titer is already high in most patients at the time medical attention is sought, thereby limiting the value of this approach. On the other hand, a diagnosis of acute HAV infection can readily be achieved if distinction can be made between anti-HAV of the immunoglobulin M (IgM) class, which appears during acute illness, and IgG antibody, which becomes pronounced during convalescence and remains elevated for years.

The HĀVAB-M assay is a specific and sensitive solid-phase RIA that measures IgM-specific anti-HAV in serum or plasma (10, 57, 65). Conceptually, anti-HAV of the IgM class is removed from the serum by anti-human IgM (μ-chain specific) bound to polystyrene beads. The subsequent addition of HAV results in the attachment of the antigen to IgM anti-HAV that has combined with the solid-phase anti-human IgM. The "sandwich" is completed by adding radiolabeled anti-HAV. Specifically, serum is diluted 1:200 in 0.15 M normal saline, and 10 μl is added to the bottom of a well, followed by the addition of 0.2 ml of specimen diluent (final serum concentration is 1:4,000). A goat anti-human IgM-coated bead is then added to each well, and the trays are covered with an adhesive-backed cardboard and incubated for 2 h at 15 to 30°C. Two negative and three positive control samples are included in every test run. Then the fluid is aspirated from the wells, and the beads are washed two times with distilled or deionized water, followed by the addition of 0.2 ml of formaldehyde-inactivated HAV reagent. The covered trays are incubated for 18 to 22 h at 15 to 30°C, after which the beads are washed again. Next, 0.2 ml of ^{125}I-labeled human anti-HAV is added to each well, the trays are covered, and incubation is continued for 4 h in a 45°C water bath. Finally, the beads are washed, transferred to counting tubes, and counted in a gamma scintillation counter. A cutoff value is calculated based on the positive and negative control samples and on the potency of the HAV and ^{125}I-labeled anti-HAV reagents used. This value is determined by dividing the mean positive control counts per minute by 10 and adding this to the mean negative control counts per minute. Samples with net (minus gamma counter background) counts repeatably greater than or equal to the cutoff are considered positive; those with counts within 10% of the cutoff should be retested to confirm the original results. The validity of the test is verified by checking the ratio of the positive to negative kit control counts, which should be >5.

Other approaches have been developed to detect IgM-specific anti-HAV. These use either concanavalin A to preferentially bind IgM (unpublished data) or staphylococcal protein A to adsorb IgG from serum samples (6). Details of these procedures can be found in the third edition of this Manual.

The HĀVAB test measures total anti-HAV antibody (IgG and IgM). It is based on the principle of competition between anti-HAV in test serum or plasma and ^{125}I-labeled anti-HAV for binding to HAV coated on a polystyrene bead. A 10-µl sample of each specimen is added to the bottom of a well, followed by the addition of 0.2 ml of ^{125}I-labeled human anti-HAV. Three negative and two positive controls are incorporated into every test run. A bead coated with formaldehyde-inactivated HAV (human) is added to each well, and an adhesive cover-sealer is applied to the tray. Trays are incubated for 4 h in a 45°C water bath or for 18 to 24 h at 15 to 30°C. During this time, anti-HAV, if present in the test serum, competes with the labeled antibody for HAV binding sites on the bead. After the incubation period, the fluid contents of the wells are aspirated, and the beads are washed two times with distilled or deionized water and then transferred to counting tubes. Radioactivity bound to the beads is measured in a gamma scintillation counter, and the net (minus gamma counter background) count rate of the test sample is compared with a calculated cutoff value (one-half of the combined negative control mean and the positive control mean). Specimens with counts greater than the cutoff value are negative (no anti-HAV was available to interfere with binding of ^{125}I-labeled anti-HAV to HAV), and specimens with a count rate repeatably lower than the cutoff value are considered positive for anti-HAV. If necessary, an anti-HAV titer can be derived by testing serial serum dilutions from 1:50 to 1:3,200. Dilutions are made in PBS, which is also substituted for negative control serum in this situation. The anti-HAV titer is considered to be that dilution with mean counts most nearly equivalent to, but not greater than, the cutoff value. The validity of these tests is verified by checking the ratio of the negative to positive kit control counts, which should be >5.

For clinical investigators interested in preparing their own RIAs for detecting HAV antigen in stool filtrates or cell culture homogenates or during the various stages of purification, a simple microtiter solid-phase RIA is the most direct method available. Both microtiter solid-phase and competitive-inhibition RIAs have been used for anti-HAV.

The microtiter solid-phase RIA utilizes the sandwich principle, an arrangement created when antibody adsorbed to an inert surface binds an antigen that is subsequently detected by the addition of specific antibody tagged with ^{125}I (65). To test for HAV antigen, 100 to 150 µl of a predetermined optimal concentration of high-titer anti-HAV is added to each well of a polyvinyl microtiter U plate. In most instances, the optimal antibody dilution lies between 1:100 and 1:10,000. The antibody is diluted in 0.05 M glycine buffer (pH 7.2) or in PBS (pH 7.4). An immune globulin preparation may also be used for coating the wells, but purified IgG is usually unnecessary. The plates are incubated overnight at 25°C (or for 2 h at 37°C). Desiccation is minimized by covering the plates with Parafilm "M" (Dixie/Marathon, Greenwich, Conn.) held in place by a close-fitting plastic lid (Falcon no. 3041, Becton Dickinson Labware, Oxnard, Calif.). The plates are washed four times with 0.15 M NaCl containing 0.02% sodium azide and then once with PBS containing 2% fetal bovine serum. The PBS-fetal bovine serum is allowed to remain in contact with the wells at 25°C for at least 30 min to saturate any remaining binding sites. One percent BSA or gelatin works equally well. After the wash procedure, residual fluid is removed to avoid subsequent dilution of samples or reagents if the plates are to be used immediately. Conversely, the plates can be stored at 4°C for at least 6 months without significant loss of reactivity. Duplicate 25- to 75-µl samples of the material suspected of containing HAV are added to the coated wells, and incubation is continued for 2 h at 45°C by floating the Parafilm-covered plates in a water bath. Alternatively, the incubation period may be extended for 1 to 2 days at 4°C.

Appropriate controls should also be evaluated. These include HAV-positive reference material, PBS, and HAV-negative stool or gradient material, e.g., CsCl. After incubation, the wells are aspirated and washed four times with saline or PBS containing 2% fetal bovine serum or 0.05% Tween 20, and the residual fluid is removed before the addition of ^{125}I-labeled IgG containing high-titer anti-HAV. Specific activity of the antibody preparation should range from 15 to 25 µCi/µg, and a total of 200,000 to 300,000 cpm per well is used. In general, the volume of labeled IgG added to each well should not exceed the sample volume used. To reduce background counts significantly without altering the specific binding, the label is diluted in PBS containing 50% fetal bovine serum and 10% normal human serum. Each lot of fetal bovine serum and normal human serum should be evaluated separately before use. After an additional incubation period of 1 h at 45°C (or 4 h at 25°C) and a corresponding wash step, clear adhesive tape (no. 1-220-30, Dynatech Laboratories, Inc., Alexandria, Va.) is applied to the plate, and the wells are numbered. Each well is cut out, and residual radioactivity is measured in a gamma scintillation counter. Mean counts per minute of duplicate samples are compared with mean counts per minute for at least five negative control samples. The test for HAV is considered positive if the ratio of counts in the sample to the mean counts in the negative control wells is ≥2.1 (sample/negative ratio). Specificity is demonstrated by blocking the binding of ^{125}I-labeled anti-HAV (IgG) with convalescent-phase, but not with preinoculation, serum from persons or experimental animals previously infected with HAV, by comparing results with appropriate antigen-negative controls, such as HAV-negative stool filtrates or gradient fractions, or by both methods.

The microtiter solid-phase RIA can also be modified in a number of ways to detect anti-HAV. Perhaps the most sensitive method is an indirect blocking or inhibition assay. Briefly, 0.1 ml of a 1:10 serum dilution is preincubated for 30 min at 25°C with an equal volume of a partially purified standard preparation of HAV. Specimens containing anti-HAV will combine with HAV antigen, thus reducing the amount of HAV available for binding to an antibody-coated microtiter well. Duplicate samples (75 µl) of the reaction mixture are placed in microtiter wells coated with anti-HAV, and incubation is carried out as described above. After the addition of labeled anti-HAV, the wells are counted. A reduction in residual radioactivity of ≥40% as compared with an anti-HAV-negative control sample is indicative of anti-HAV in the test serum.

A second approach substitutes serum dilutions of the sample to be tested for known anti-HAV-positive serum to coat the microtiter wells. If the serum contains anti-HAV, specific binding will result when HAV antigen is added to the microtiter well. Bound antigen will subsequently be detected after the addition of labeled anti-HAV to the wells. The test is considered positive if the sample/negative ratio is ≥2.1. A shortcoming of this procedure, however, is a reduction in sensitivity that occurs at serum dilutions of <1:200 (i.e., at higher protein concentrations).

EIA (Table 5). EIA was first used in hepatitis research to detect HBsAg and anti-HBs, using the sandwich principle employed in the solid-phase RIA procedure. In this technique, an enzyme-labeled antibody is substituted for a radionuclide-labeled preparation, its presence being reflected by hydrolysis of a subsequently added enzyme substrate. The color produced can be quantitated colorimetrically. The development of EIA technology has led to a decline in the popularity of RIA procedures. Major objections to RIA include the expense of a gamma counter and the presence of a radiation hazard. However, in many situations, the large, expensive, general-purpose gamma counters with automatic sample changers are not necessary, and hand-operated gamma counters or ^{125}I spectrometers are similar in price to colorimeters. In addition, the radiation hazard is greatly overstated; 10 μCi of ^{125}I (commercial kits usually contain a total of 15 to 76 μCi of ^{125}I) held at a distance of 10 cm for 1 h yields an exposure rate of only 0.06 mrem (milliroentgen equivalent, man). The exposure rate is inversely proportional to the square root of the distance in centimeters. For comparison, background radiation exposure rates are about 150 mrem per year, a chest X-ray examination provides 10 mrem of exposure, and a gastrointestinal series provides about 8,000 mrem. Nevertheless, EIA has a number of advantages that could recommend it over RIA, particularly in those countries where restrictive laws govern the handling of radioisotopes and the disposal of radioactive wastes. A major factor is the stability of the enzyme-antibody conjugates. These have a shelf life of months to years, compared with radionuclide-labeled antibody conjugates, which must be freshly prepared every 3 to 5 weeks. On the other hand, an additional manipulation is required during EIA in that a specific substrate must be added to detect fixation of the enzyme-antibody conjugate. In addition, some of the enzyme substrates used are potentially carcinogenic; therefore, they should be handled with caution. Both tests are objective, quantitative, reliable, and reproducible.

Simplified, standardized commercial EIA test kits are available to measure IgM-specific anti-HAV and total anti-HAV (HĀVAB-M EIA and HĀVAB EIA, Abbott Laboratories). These commercial tests are analogous to the commercial RIA procedures developed by the same manufacturer (see preceding section).

In the HĀVAB-M EIA for IgM-specific anti-HAV, 10 μl of a serum or plasma sample is added to 2.0 ml of 0.15 M normal saline; 10 μl of the diluted sample is then added to the bottom of a well, followed by the addition of 0.2 ml of specimen diluent (final serum concentration of 1:4,000). Two negative and three positive controls are included in every test run. Polystyrene beads coated with goat antibody to human IgM (μ-chain specific) are added to each well, and the trays are incubated for 1 h in a 40°C water bath, after which the fluid contents of the well are aspirated and the beads are washed three times in distilled or deionized water. Next, 0.2 ml of a solution containing formaldehyde-inactivated HAV (human) is added to each well, and the plates are incubated for 18 to 22 h at 15 to 30°C, after which the wells are aspirated and the beads are washed three more times. Then, 0.2 ml of horseradish peroxidase-conjugated human anti-HAV is added to each well, and the trays are incubated at 40°C for 2 h. After the fluid is aspirated from the wells, the beads are washed and transferred to reaction tubes. Freshly prepared *o*-phenylenediamine solution (0.3 ml) containing H_2O_2 is added to each tube containing a bead as well as to two empty tubes to serve as substrate blanks, and the tubes are covered and incubated for 30 min at 15 to 30°C. The reaction is terminated by adding 1.0 ml of 1 N sulfuric acid to each tube, and A_{492} is determined (within 2 h after the addition of sulfuric acid) in a spectrophotometer. Samples with absorbance levels repeatably equal to or above the cutoff value (the sum of the negative control mean absorbance plus 1/10 of the positive control mean absorbance) are considered positive for IgM-specific anti-HAV, and samples with absorbance values below the cutoff level are considered negative. Because of low confidence in values near the cutoff, samples with absorbances within 10% of the cutoff should be retested to confirm the initial result. Validity of the test requires that the difference in the mean ab-

TABLE 5. Principles of the procedures for various hepatitis assays

Serological assay	Vol required (μl)	Principle of procedure (RIA or EIA)	Type of support system	Adsorbed reagent	Label or conjugate	Positive result (cpm or absorbance value)	
						Low	High
HBsAg	200	Sandwich	Bead, tube, well	Anti-HBs	Anti-HBs		X
Anti-HBc	100	Competitive binding	Bead, well	HBcAg	Anti-HBc	X	
IgM anti-HAV	10	Sandwich[a]	Bead, well	Anti-IgM	Anti-HAV		X
Anti-HAV	10	Competitive binding	Bead, well	HAV antigen	Anti-HAV	X	
Anti-HBs	200	Sandwich	Bead, tube, well	HBsAg	HBsAg		X
HBeAg	200	Sandwich	Bead, well	Anti-HBe	Anti-HBe		X
Anti-HBe	50/100[b]	Competitive binding[c]	Bead, well	Anti-HBe	Anti-HBe	X	
IgM anti-HBc	10	Sandwich[a]	Bead	Anti-IgM	Anti-HBc		X

[a] Modified sandwich: IgM-specific antibody (anti-HAV or anti-HBc) that is immunologically bound to the bead is detected by adding the corresponding antigen (HAV antigen or HBcAg), followed by the appropriate antibody label or conjugate.

[b] RIA requires 100 μl; EIA requires 50 μl.

[c] Anti-HBe in the test sample and adsorbed anti-HBe compete for a standardized amount of HBeAg added to the reaction well before the addition of anti-HBe label or conjugate.

sorbance between the positive and negative control samples be ≥0.400.

In the HĀVAB EIA for total anti-HAV, 10 μl of each serum or plasma specimen is added with 0.2 ml of horseradish peroxidase-conjugated human anti-HAV to a reaction tray well. Three negative and two positive controls are incorporated into every test run. An HAV (human)-coated polystyrene bead is added to each well, and the trays are sealed and incubated for 3 h in a 40°C water bath or for 18 to 24 h at 15 to 30°C. After the incubation period, the fluid contents of the wells are aspirated, and the beads are washed three times with distilled or deionized water and transferred to reaction tubes. Then 0.3 ml of freshly prepared *o*-phenylenediamine substrate solution containing H_2O_2 is added to each tube as well as to two substrate blank tubes. After another 30 min of incubation, shielded from light and at 15 to 30°C, the reaction is stopped by adding 1.0 ml of 1 N sulfuric acid to each tube. A_{492} is determined in a spectrophotometer, and the presence of anti-HAV is determined by comparing the absorbance value of the specimen with a cutoff value (one-half the sum of the negative control mean and the positive control mean absorbance). Specimens with absorbance levels higher than the cutoff value are negative, and those with absorbance values repeatably equal to or below the cutoff are considered positive for anti-HAV. As noted above, samples with absorbance levels within 10% of the cutoff should be retested to confirm the original result. Validity of the test procedure is determined by calculating the difference between the negative and positive control mean absorbances, which should be ≥0.400. If desired, the titer of anti-HAV can be derived by testing serial dilutions of serum from 1:50 to 1:3,200 in PBS. PBS should also be used as the negative control instead of the negative control serum. The titer of anti-HAV is considered to be the sample dilution whose absorbance is most nearly equivalent to, but not greater than, the cutoff value.

Similar microtiter solid-phase EIA test kits are now commercially available to measure IgM-specific anti-HAV and total anti-HAV (Hepanostika Anti-HAV IgM and Anti-HAV Microelisa systems; Organon Teknika, Durham, N.C.).

Commercial EIA tests for HAV antigen are not available. To conduct such an assay (44), 75 μl of a predetermined optimal dilution of anti-HAV (diluted in PBS) is added to wells of polyvinyl microtiter U plates, which are incubated at 4°C for 4 h and then washed three times with PBS containing 0.05% Tween 20. The antibody-coated wells are incubated overnight at 4°C with PBS containing 1% BSA and then are aspirated and washed once before the 25-μl samples being evaluated for HAV antigen are added. The plates are covered and incubated for 15 to 18 h at 4°C; they are then washed once, and 25 μl of PBS-Tween is added and left for 15 min at room temperature. Concurrently, several wells should be incubated with preillness and convalescent-phase sera instead of PBS-Tween; these will serve to demonstrate specificity of the assay. To each well is added 25 μl of anti-HAV conjugated to horseradish peroxidase (type VI, RZ = approximately 3.0; Sigma Chemical Co., St. Louis, Mo.) by the method of Nakane and Kawaoi (48). The enzyme conjugate is diluted in PBS containing 50% BSA. The plates are incubated at room temperature for 2 h and washed three times with PBS-Tween; 100 μl of freshly prepared *o*-phenylenediamine–H_2O_2 substrate is then added. After an additional 30-min incubation period in the dark, 50 μl of 2 M H_2SO_4 is added to each well to stop the reaction, and the optical density is measured at 492 nm in a spectrophotometer. Alternatively, color can be quantitated visually on a scale of 0 to 3+ (43). Before a sample is considered positive for HAV, specificity of the reaction should be checked by demonstrating that binding of enzyme-labeled anti-HAV is blocked with convalescent-phase but not with preillness serum from a patient with previously documented hepatitis A.

Interpretation of test results

Because viremia is limited (28, 30) and because cell culture techniques are cumbersome and insensitive, demonstration of circulating HAV is difficult, impractical, and probably unwarranted for diagnostic purposes. Furthermore, because fecal shedding of virus occurs so early and because liver and bile are not routinely available as diagnostic specimens, a diagnosis of HAV infection can be made most practically by demonstrating a specific antibody response. Classically, this is done by measuring an increase in serum anti-HAV between the acute phase and convalescence; however, the interval required to demonstrate a perceptible change in antibody titer may be as long as 4 to 6 weeks. In many situations appropriately spaced serum specimens are not available; in any event, the ability to make a diagnosis during acute illness, without having to wait for a convalescent-phase sample, is preferable. This can be achieved by demonstrating the presence of anti-HAV of the IgM class, and this approach has become the method of choice for making a diagnosis of acute hepatitis A (Fig. 3).

When one is testing for the presence of HAV in stool or using HAV prepared from stool to detect anti-HAV in serum, it is important to realize that a false-positive test may result from binding of antibodies in serum to non-HAV antigens in stool. Therefore, to ensure specificity of positive results, testing with preinoculation and convalescent-phase reference reagents or appropriate blocking of the specific reaction between HAV antigen and anti-HAV conjugate with convalescent-phase, but not preinoculation, serum is necessary. Many of the difficulties encountered with false-positive results can be eliminated or minimized by using highly purified antigen, by using high-titered hyperimmune animal sera, or by using antigen and antibody reagents derived from heterologous sources. For example, nonspecific binding of antibodies in human serum to human stool components can be eliminated by using antigen derived from marmoset liver or cell culture.

Selection of the best test method in any laboratory depends on the facilities and expertise available. For detection of HAV in stool, IEM, solid-phase RIA, and EIA are of comparable sensitivity, although the EIA may be less specific, especially in competitive binding assays. Although RIA and EIA are the most sensitive tests for anti-HAV, levels of anti-HAV achieved during illness and persisting thereafter are so substantial that any of the available methods is quite satisfactory. Prevalence of anti-HAV in populations determined with all assays is virtually the same.

HBV

Direct examination

Immunofluorescence, immunoperoxidase staining, and electron microscopy have been used extensively to examine pathological specimens and serum samples for the presence of HBV-associated antigens or particles (37, 52). These procedures are not applicable to rapid, large-scale screening of HBV infections by clinical laboratories, but they have been invaluable in elucidating the biosynthetic origin of the various antigens within infected cells and for detecting the presence of immune complexes. Within the liver, HBcAg-containing particles are found predominantly in the nuclei of hepatocytes, whereas HBsAg reactivity is observed exclusively in the cytoplasm. Detection of complete virions is uncommon. The techniques used for immunoperoxidase or immunofluorescence are well known. As a general rule, immunofluorescence staining of cryostat sections is superior to the use of paraffin sections. However, cryostat sections are not always available, and cellular outlines are better resolved in uniformly cut paraffin sections than in frozen sections. Reduction of nonspecific background staining of Formalin-fixed sections can be achieved by treating tissue for 2 to 6 h at 37°C with 0.1% trypsin before staining. Muscle tissue is more resistant to digestion than liver and kidney tissue. In situations in which autologous antibody might bind to cell-associated antigen, cryostat sections can be treated for 5 min with 0.1 M glycine hydrochloride buffer (pH 1.2) before specific antibody (labeled or unlabeled) is added.

Recently, biotin-avidin systems have been introduced for detecting viral antigens in cells or in tissues. This system offers a number of advantages over other immunodiagnostic clinical techniques: (i) the binding of avidin to biotin is extremely rapid and essentially irreversible because of the high affinity constant ($>10^{15}$ M^{-1}) that exists between these two proteins (affinity constants of antibody for most antigens are generally 10^6-fold lower); (ii) sensitivity is enhanced, even when highly diluted primary antibody is used, because the four binding sites on avidin permit amplification of the response; (iii) Formalin-fixed, paraffin-embedded histological sections, smears, and frozen sections can be examined by conventional light microscopy; and (iv) background stain is greatly reduced. Many types of immunoperoxidase staining procedures are available. The ABC (avidin-biotin-labeled horseradish peroxidase complex) procedure developed by Hsu and his associates (35, 36) has been found to be highly sensitive and specific. Briefly, Formalin-fixed tissue sections are deparaffinized and hydrated through xylene and a graded alcohol series. The fixation process should employ a buffered Formalin, not exceeding 4% formaldehyde, sufficient to maintain integrity of the tissue without destroying the antigenic determinants being evaluated. Sections are incubated for 30 min with primary antibody raised against the antigen of interest. The antiserum is diluted in buffer (10 mM PBS, pH 7.6). Slides are washed for 10 min in buffer, after which diluted, biotin-labeled secondary antibody is added and incubation is continued for 30 min. This antibody, directed against the immunoglobulin class of the species used as primary antiserum, introduces biotin-labeled residues into the section at the location of the primary antibody. After washing, an avidin-biotin-labeled horseradish peroxidase complex (Vectastain ABC reagent, Vector Laboratories, Burlingame, Calif.) is added, which binds to the biotin-labeled secondary antibody during a 30- to 60-min incubation period. The slides are rewashed for 10 min in buffer, and tissue antigen is localized by incubating the sections for 5 min in freshly prepared peroxidase substrate solution, i.e., equal volumes of 0.1% diaminobenzidine tetrachloride prepared in 0.1 M Tris buffer (pH 7.2) and 0.02% hydrogen peroxide prepared in distilled water. The hydrogen peroxide should be prepared fresh from a concentrated stock solution. Sections are washed for 5 min in tap water, counterstained with hematoxylin, eosin, or both, and mounted. Sections should not be allowed to dry out during the staining procedure; therefore, a humidified chamber is recommended for incubations. If antigen concentration is low, the peroxidase substrate incubation step may be lengthened to achieve maximal staining. Many mammalian tissues contain endogenous peroxidase. If this problem exists, sections may be incubated for 30 min in 0.3% hydrogen peroxide in methanol either before primary antibody is added or before the ABC reagent step. The latter point is desirable for cases in which the antigenic determinant may be destroyed by hydrogen peroxide. If nonspecific staining occurs, it can be reduced by incubating the sections for 20 min with diluted normal serum prepared from the species in which the secondary antibody is made. Excess serum is blotted from the sections before the primary antibody is added.

Cell cultures and animal models

Despite strong evidence for the growth of HBV in some cell and organ cultures, serial propagation over a prolonged period of time has not been accomplished. Chimpanzees and other high-order primates are highly susceptible to experimental induction of hepatitis B but are not routinely available (2). The pattern of infection is similar to that observed in humans except that the disease is milder; e.g., jaundice is rare. Nevertheless, the chimpanzee system continues to play an essential role in inactivation studies (vaccine safety, disinfection kinetics), infectivity determinations, and immunopathology.

Serological identification of hepatitis B antigens and antibodies

A number of serological techniques with different degrees of sensitivity have been developed for the detection of HBV antigens and their specific antibodies (Table 6). These methods include agarose gel diffusion, counterimmunoelectrophoresis, rheophoresis, complement fixation, latex agglutination, hemagglutination, IEM, EIA, and RIA. Each method offers certain advantages and disadvantages and differs markedly in sensitivity, specificity, simplicity, and expense from the others. A description of these and other methods follows, with emphasis on the RIA and EIA procedures. Readers interested in detailed information concerning the purification of hepatitis B-associated antigens, production of anti-HBV, agarose gel diffusion, discontinuous counterimmunoelectrophoresis, rheophoresis, reverse passive hemagglutination, and hemagglutination are referred to the third edition of this Manual. A complete list of licensed manufacturers for hepatitis B products can be obtained by writing to Professional Inquiries,

TABLE 6. Relative sensitivity of methods used to detect HBV antigens and antibodies

Relative sensitivity (HBsAg)	Assay method	Time to complete test (h)
Least (≥10 μg/ml)	Agarose gel diffusion	24–72
Intermediate (1–5 μg/ml)	Counterimmunoelectrophoresis	1–2
	Rheophoresis	24–72
	Complement fixation	18
Most (0.1–40 ng/ml)	Latex agglutination (third generation)	1
	Hemagglutination	1–3
	Immune adherence	4–24
	Radioimmunoassay	3–24
	Enzyme immunoassay	4–24

HFB-142, Center for Biologics, Evaluation and Research, Food and Drug Administration, 5600 Fishers Lane, Rockville, MD 20857.

Purification of hepatitis B-associated antigens (19, 32). The widespread availability of sensitive and specific commercial kits for the detection of hepatitis B antigens and antibodies has markedly diminished the laboratory's need to prepare highly purified antigens or antibody of high specificity, affinity, and avidity. However, situations may exist (e.g., subtyping) in which reagent preparation may be desirable. For those who are interested, methods for purifying HBsAg or HBcAg are described in the third edition of this Manual. The HBsAg procedure can be completed in 1 week and incorporates a low-pH step to help remove antibody specific for HBsAg and other proteins nonspecifically associated with the particles. The low pH also results in partial disruption of the 42-nm HBV particles and the tubular forms. This may have additional benefits, since 27-nm core particles with their higher densities (1.32 to 1.36 g/cm^3 in CsCl versus 1.24 to 1.28 g/cm^3 for HBV particles) are more easily separated from the lighter 22-nm HBsAg particles, thereby producing a final product that is less likely to be contaminated with HBcAg or to be infectious. Finally, immunogenicity and radioisotopic labeling of these purified HBsAg preparations seem to be superior to those found with other methods of purification that lack a low-pH step (31).

Production of antibodies to hepatitis B (19). Antisera from multiply transfused (or immunized) individuals have provided investigators with a rich source of anti-HBs of moderate titer. The major advantage of human (or chimpanzee) serum is its freedom from anti-normal human serum contaminants. Satisfactory anti-HBs for screening sera for HBsAg also has been prepared in a variety of animals, including horses, goats, guinea pigs, rabbits, mice, rhesus monkeys, baboons, and chimpanzees. However, virtually all of these preparations have detectable levels of antibody to human serum proteins, particularly albumin. These contaminating antibodies can be effectively removed by adsorption with glutaraldehyde cross-linked preparations of normal human serum.

Techniques for immunizing goats, guinea pigs, and rabbits can be found in the third edition of this Manual. Antibody with excellent antigen-precipitating capacity can be prepared in goats. In general, the predominant antibody is directed against the group-specific *a* antigenic determinant unless specimens are obtained early in the course of immunization. Therefore, goat antiserum is better for screening than for subtyping. Antiserum prepared in guinea pigs is an excellent reagent for subtyping and for screening tests. Specificity of antisera produced against subtype *ay* is better than that produced against subtype *ad*, which suggests that the *a* subdeterminant in the *ad* preparation may be more immunogenic, resulting in a more broadly reacting antiserum. Rabbits are also useful for preparing subtyping reagents (especially against the *w* and *r* determinants) and for preparing antiserum to HBcAg. For subtyping, monospecific IgG containing anti-*d* or anti-*y* can be obtained by affinity chromatographic techniques in which the HBV-specific antiserum is passed through a column containing the heterologous HBsAg subtype. Anti-*a* (and presumably anti-*w*) can subsequently be recovered from the column by elution with acid or potassium thiocyanate. More recently, monoclonal antibodies have been produced which have precise, quantifiable specificity and antiserum homogeneity directed against the group *a* determinant and subtypes *ad* and *ay*.

Agarose gel diffusion. Agarose gel diffusion is the least sensitive method available for detecting HBsAg, but it permits direct comparisons to be made between positive specimens regarding their identity, partial relatedness, or nonidentity. Reinforcement of weak precipitin lines is accomplished by placing reference HBsAg-positive specimens in peripheral wells between the unknown specimens. Because HBsAg is a large molecule and diffuses slowly compared with IgG antibody, preincubation of the slides for 2 h at room temperature in a humidified chamber before the addition of anti-HBs in the center well permits precipitin lines to develop more distal to the peripheral well. The slides are observed for the development of precipitin lines at 24, 48, and 72 h.

For subtyping HBsAg, the same reinforcement pattern can be used. Monospecific anti-HBs containing only anti-*d* or anti-*y* antibody can be substituted for the reference antiserum to enhance specificity. Slides are observed for lines of identity or for the formation of a "spur" signifying different antigenic determinants.

Discontinuous counterimmunoelectrophoresis. Discontinuous counterimmunoelectrophoresis or counterelectrophoresis was the method most widely used for detecting HBsAg before the introduction of more sensitive and specific assays such as RIA. It is still used for subtyping. The method is based on the principle that in a relatively alkaline environment, HBsAg, which has an isoelectric pH between 4.4 and 5.2, is negatively charged and migrates in an electrophoretic field toward the anode. Conversely, IgG, being closer to its isoelectric pH, travels by electroendosmosis toward the cathode. This condition is caused by charged groups within the agarose that promote the movement of buffer through the gel toward the cathode, thereby drawing the gamma globulin with it. In this regard, agarose powders with high relative mobility (m_r) are available, making these gels especially suitable for counterimmunoelectrophoresis. A precipitin line forms when optimal concentrations of the antigen and antibody meet. By reducing the ionic strength of the agarose buffer, as compared with that of the buffer used in the electrophoresis chambers, a discontinuous buffer system can be prepared which enhances the movement of acidic proteins toward the anode and globulins toward the cathode. This results in increased sensitivity and speed of reaction and in sharper, more easily read precipitin lines (64). Plates must be examined carefully for weak precipitin lines; a magnifying lens, a darkened room, and a good oblique viewing light are helpful. Artifacts may be encountered in this system, which must not be confused with a true positive reaction. These include a halo of precipitation around the well and movement of lipid over the surface of the agarose adjacent to the sample well. The latter artifact can easily be distinguished from a true precipitin reaction within the gel by wiping the area gently with a cotton swab.

Both specificity and sensitivity depend on the use of potent precipitating antibody rendered free from anti-normal human serum by prior adsorption. False-positive results are uncommon. An imbalance between reactants, either excess HBsAg or anti-HBs, can lead to the establishment of a prozone and a false-negative result. The prozone phenomenon, which occurs in the region of HBsAg excess, can be minimized by diluting the reagent antibody in normal homologous whole serum or its globulin fraction rather than in a buffer (20). Two-dimensional box titrations are essential to determine the optimal concentration of reagent antibody needed in subsequent tests. Specifics of the test can be found in the third edition of this Manual.

Rheophoresis. The bidimensional immunorheophoresis (rheophoresis) method relies on continuous evaporation of water through a central hole placed directly over an antigen or antibody well (38). Protein solutions placed in peripheral wells are transported by hydrodynamic forces to the central area of dehydration through the flow of low-ionic-strength buffer (0.01 M Tris, pH 7.6) placed external to the agarose. Sensitivity is equivalent to that of counterimmunoelectrophoresis.

Reverse passive latex agglutination. The major advantages of the reverse passive latex agglutination method for detecting HBsAg (39) are speed (1 h) and simplicity, coupled with a reagent shelf life of 5 months. These advantages makes the method useful for emergency situations that do not allow ample time to evaluate a sample by standard testing procedures, provided the person performing the assay has experience in reading agglutination reactions. Unfortunately, a relatively high number of false-negative (about 5%) and false-positive (about 20%) reactions occur. The causes of these unwanted reactions include the presence of rheumatoid factor, autoimmune antibodies, heterophile antibodies, lipemic serum, albumin/globulin imbalance, electrolyte abnormalities, pH imbalance, and various drug metabolites. The false-positive rate can be cut in half by heat inactivation and by adsorbing out the rheumatoid factor. All other agglutination reactions should be confirmed by a blocking test. Confirmation of weak positive reactions by another method of equivalent or greater sensitivity and specificity is essential.

Hemagglutination (32, 33). A commercial reverse passive hemagglutination kit is available for detection of HBsAg (AUSCELL, Abbott Laboratories). It is based on the agglutination of human erythrocytes, sensitized with guinea pig anti-HBs, by HBsAg when it is present in the sample being tested. Only about 15% of specimens reactive in this test actually contain HBsAg. Therefore, specimens showing agglutination must be confirmed by specific blocking of the reaction with human anti-HBs.

Detailed methodology for preparing erythrocytes and for conjugating them with IgG or HBsAg can be found in the second edition of this Manual. Erythrocytes (human group O, turkey, or sheep) are coated with purified HBsAg (passive hemagglutination) or with anti-HBs (reversed passive hemagglutination). Anti-HBs antisera are prepared in guinea pigs, sheep, chimpanzees, or horses. Hemagglutination tests have been used extensively for the detection of anti-HBs or HBsAg in human serum or recalcified plasma. Their major advantages are the conservation of sera (less than 10 μl is required), the absence of a requirement for expensive equipment, rapid completion (1 to 3 h), good proficiency, and easy quantification. Disadvantages include a relatively large number of nonspecific reactions and the need for personnel experienced in hemagglutination techniques. False-positive reactions frequently occur at dilutions below 1:8, thereby reducing the sensitivity accordingly. Antibodies against ruminant IgG and Forssman antigen may be removed after heat inactivation by adsorbing the sera with uncoated erythrocytes. However, the use of control erythrocytes coated with normal immunoglobulin from the same species is preferred. False-positive reactions may also occur if the serum or buffer is contaminated with certain microorganisms or if it contains rheumatoid factor. Low dilution of high-titered antibody or HBsAg may result in a false-negative reaction because of the formation of a prozone. The use of a vibration-free surface is also required in the reversed passive hemagglutination test to avoid false-negative results.

RIA (Tables 5 and 7). The RIA technique continues

TABLE 7. Comparison of commercial solid-phase RIAs for the detection of HBsAg

Assay	Source[a]	Support system	Adsorbed antibody	Sample vol (μl)	Incubation: Total time (h)	Incubation: Temp (°C)	Wash solution	Labeled antibody
AusRia II	Abbott	Polystyrene beads	Guinea pig	200	3/18	45	DW[b]	Human
Clinical Assays	ADI	Polystyrene tubes	Guinea pig	200	3/18	45	NaCl	Chimpanzee
NML HBsAg	Centocor	Polystyrene beads	Mouse monoclonal antibody	100/200	4/18	45	DW	Mouse monoclonal antibody
AB-AUK-3	Sorin	Polystyrene beads	Mouse monoclonal antibody	200	3/18	45	DW	Sheep

[a] Abbott, Abbott Laboratories, North Chicago, Ill.; ADI, ADI Diagnostics, Toronto, Ontario, Canada (distributed in the United States by Baxter Healthcare Corp., Dade Division, Cambridge, Mass.); Centocor, Centocor, Inc., Malvern, Pa. (distributed by Organon Teknika Corp., Irving, Tex.); Sorin, Sorin Biomedica, Saluggia, Italy (distributed in the United States by Clinical Sciences, Inc., Whippany, N.J.).

[b] DW, Distilled water.

to be a sensitive and specific method for detecting the various serological markers of hepatitis B (HBsAg, HBeAg, anti-HBs, anti-HBc, anti-HBe, and IgM anti-HBc). The methods most commonly employed utilize the solid-phase sandwich RIA technique. The double-antibody procedure, a research tool that measures the primary interaction between antigen and antibody, can be used for studying the kinetics of this reaction (31, 32). It is highly sensitive, specific, and reproducible. Complete details of this technique, including labeling of purified HBsAg, can be found in the second edition of this Manual.

The solid-phase sandwich method (65) for HBsAg detection is comparable in sensitivity to the double-antibody RIA method, is less cumbersome, and currently is the principal system used by all manufacturers of commercially licensed RIA kits in the United States (Table 7). These assays are capable of detecting HBsAg to a level of 0.1 to 0.5 ng/ml. The concept is identical to that described above for the hepatitis A RIA. Briefly, 200 μl of serum or plasma is added to a solid-phase system to which anti-HBs is adsorbed. The solid-phase support systems currently used in HBsAg assays include polystyrene beads or polystyrene tubes. During incubation (usually 2 h at 45°C or 16 h at room temperature), HBsAg forms an immunological complex with the anti-HBs at the liquid-surface interface. After washing, anti-HBs tagged with ^{125}I is added and incubation is continued (1 h at 45°C). The labeled antibody binds to any HBsAg on the support system, creating an antibody–antigen–^{125}I-antibody sandwich. The washed beads or tubes are counted in a gamma counter. By dividing counts per minute of the test sample (S) by the mean counts per minute of the negative control samples (N), an S/N ratio is calculated. Values of 2.1 and above are generally considered to be reactive (positive). Within limits, there is a direct correlation between the final count rate and the concentration of HBsAg in the specimen. However, size of the HBsAg and surface area of the support system restrict the working range to between 0.1 ng/ml and 1 μg/ml, above which level saturation (a plateau) is reached. Sera from some carriers have HBsAg concentrations above 100 μg/ml. In these situations, further dilutions are required to permit quantitation. Repeatably positive reactions that cannot be confirmed as positive for HBsAg are highly unusual (<0.1%). Nevertheless, the seriousness of the diagnosis, with its attendant personal, social, and economic repercussions, mandates that a confirmatory test be attempted on all repeatably reactive specimens. This can be approached in one of two ways: (i) specimens may be tested with another licensed HBsAg assay, or (ii) a blocking or inhibition assay can be performed to see whether unlabeled anti-HBs will specifically inhibit the reaction. The detection of anti-HBc in the absence of anti-HBs also corroborates a positive HBsAg result.

To avoid an erroneous interpretation, the negative control samples must be comparable to the test specimen. Unfortunately, the kit "negative control" values are usually 10 to 40% higher than values obtained by using fresh normal (nonreactive) sera. Thus, S/N values between 1.5 and 2.1 should be viewed with suspicion whenever the kit negative control is used. Correspondingly, tests for HBsAg in cerebrospinal fluid must use "normal" cerebrospinal fluid as the control. In general, protein-deficient specimens and recalcified plasma result in higher background levels.

In an emergency, the solid-phase RIA may be modified to provide an answer within 1 h. Sensitivity is slightly less than that of the regular assay, but the number of positive specimens likely to be missed should be relatively small. To further reduce the number of false-negative values, at the expense of increasing the number of false-positive reactions, the cutoff value can be reduced to 1.5 times the negative control. Ultimately, verification of a positive reaction by the regular procedure is essential.

Commercial RIA kits are available from several manufacturers for the detection of anti-HBs (Ausab, Abbott Laboratories; Clinical Assays, ADI Diagnostics, Toronto, Ontario, Canada [distributed in the United States by Baxter Healthcare Corp., Dade Division, Cambridge, Mass.]; AB-AUK-3, Sorin Biomedica, Saluggia, Italy [distributed in the United States by Clinical Sciences, Inc., Whippany, N.J.]). Solid-phase RIA for the detection of anti-HBs is similar in principle to HBsAg detection except that the specimen is incubated with polystyrene beads or tubes coated with HBsAg. Radiolabeled HBsAg is used to detect anti-HBs bound to the fixed HBsAg. Specimens with a count rate equal to or greater than 2.1 times the negative control mean counts are reactive. Unfortunately, inter- and intralot variations in commercial anti-HBs kits and diminishing sensitivity as the kits approach the expiration date limit the usefulness of the S/N ratio for comparative purposes. With the advent of the HBsAg vaccine, the need for precision and accuracy in the assay has become more important. To permit results that can be expressed in milli-international units per milliliter, Hollinger et al. (26) have modified the RIA test. Anti-HBs concentrations are based on the First International World Health Organization (WHO) Reference Preparation for HBIG (lot 26.1.77) provided by the International Laboratory for Biological Standards, Central Laboratory of The Netherlands Red Cross Transfusion Services. An arbitrary value of 50 IU of anti-HBs has been assigned to this product. To determine milli-international units per milliliter, an S/R ratio is computed as follows: (sample cpm − negative control mean cpm)/(reference control cpm − negative control mean cpm). The WHO anti-HBs reference standard is diluted to contain 125 mIU/ml. Regression of the S/R ratio on the WHO reference anti-HBs concentration (0.1 to 500 mIU/ml) (Fig. 4) by using the computer nonlinear regression program BMDP3R (18) yielded the following formula: mIU/ml = 130.75 [$e^{0.66765(S/R)}$ − 1][reciprocal of dilution].

The lower limit of detection for anti-HBs with one of the commercially available solid-phase RIAs (Ausab) is 0.7 mIU/ml. Dilutions are usually required when anti-HBs concentrations exceed 200 mIU/ml. To conserve the WHO reference reagent, the laboratory can prepare a large batch of reference anti-HBs and determine its relationship to the WHO reference standard (diluted to 125 mIU/ml) by using the S/R ratio. The exponential in the formula must be adjusted proportionally to agree with the new laboratory standard. For example, if the S/R relationship between the laboratory standard and the WHO reference standard is 0.500, the exponential value in the formula (0.66765) must be reduced by a factor of 0.5. Conversely, an S/R ratio of 1.5 would increase it by a factor of 1.5. Once this adjustment is made, the laboratory reference standard can be substituted

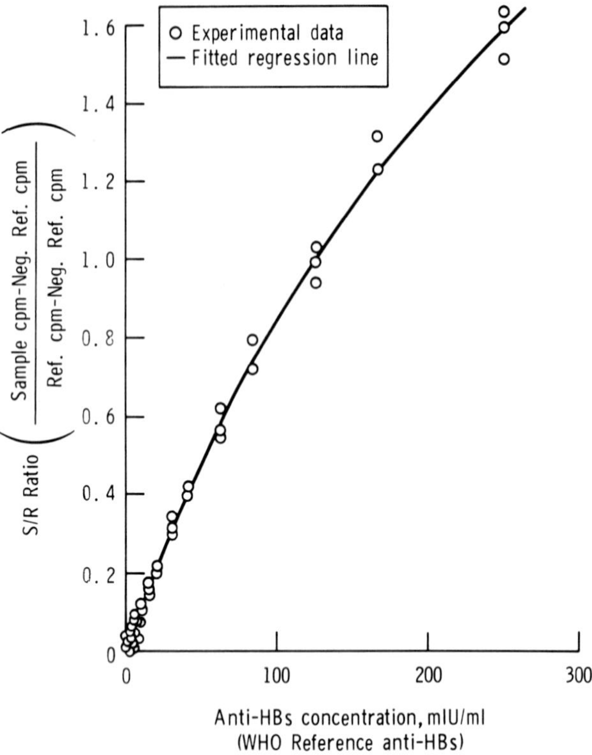

FIG. 4. RIA standard curve for anti-HBs. Regression of the S/R ratio on the anti-HBs concentration (in milli-international units per milliliter). (From reference 26.) For the regression equation, see text.

for the WHO reference standard. Periodic reevaluation against the WHO standard should be performed to verify the accuracy of the laboratory standard, which is stored in small samples at −30°C.

Currently, two RIA kits for anti-HBc are commercially available (Corab, Abbott Laboratories; AB-COREK, Sorin Biomedica). These tests are competitive binding assays in which anti-HBc from the test sample (100 µl) competes with a constant amount of human ^{125}I-tagged anti-HBc for a limited number of binding sites found on beads coated with HBcAg. Within limits, the proportion of radioactive anti-HBc bound to the bead is inversely proportional to the concentration of anti-HBc in the test specimen. Incubation is carried out at room temperature for 20 h. A specimen is considered to be reactive for anti-HBc if the count rate of the unknown is less than the cutoff value (one-half the sum of the negative control mean and the positive control mean).

Other RIA tests available from Abbott Laboratories include those for IgM-specific anti-HBc (Corab-M) and HBeAg and anti-HBe (Abbott HBe). The concept of the Corab-M test is analogous to that for the HĀVAB-M assay for IgM-specific anti-HAV. The tests for HBeAg and anti-HBe are performed with the same commercial kit but use different assay principles. The HBeAg test uses the sandwich principle to measure HBeAg in serum or plasma (200 µl). Polystyrene beads coated with anti-HBe are added to the test samples, and incubation proceeds at 15 to 30°C for 20 h. After the beads are washed, anti-HBe tagged with ^{125}I is added and incubation is continued at 45°C for 3 h. Count rates are increased when HBeAg is present in the serum. A positive reaction is one that is equal to or greater than the cutoff value of 2.1 times the negative control mean count rate. The test for anti-HBe is a modified competitive binding assay in which anti-HBe in the test serum (100 µl) competes with anti-HBe-coated beads for a standardized amount of added HBeAg (100 µl). Trays containing the beads are incubated for 20 h at 15 to 30°C, at the end of which time the beads are washed. If anti-HBe is present in the test sample, less HBeAg would be coupled to the bead and therefore less ^{125}I-labeled anti-HBe would bind to the bead to complete the sandwich. Within limits, the greater the amount of anti-HBe in the specimen, the lower the count rate. The count rate is compared with the cutoff value, which is one-half the sum of the count rates of the negative control mean plus the positive control mean. Specimens with count rates equal to or less than the cutoff are considered reactive for anti-HBe, as for the other competitive binding assays.

EIA (Table 5). The EIA technique is at least as sensitive as RIA and is superior to reversed passive hemagglutination and reverse passive latex agglutination. Improvements in the test have reduced the number of repeatable false-positive reactions, and specificity is now comparable to that observed by RIA. EIA has now replaced RIA as the most popular method for detecting the various serological markers of hepatitis B.

Currently, five EIA procedures are licensed in the United States for the detection of HBsAg in human serum or plasma. These are Auszyme Monoclonal and Auszyme IV (Abbott Laboratories), NML ELISA (Organon Teknika), ELISA Test System 2 (Ortho Diagnostic Systems, Raritan, N.J.), and Anti-HBs ELISA (Pharmacia ENI Diagnostics, Columbia, Md.). Specific details of the assays can be obtained from the package insert accompanying each kit. In the two assays from Abbott Laboratories, HBsAg is detected by incubating 150 to 200 µl of human serum or plasma and 50 µl of horseradish peroxidase-conjugated mouse monoclonal (Auszyme Monoclonal) or goat (Auszyme IV) anti-HBs with a polystyrene bead coated with mouse monoclonal anti-HBs. Trays are sealed with an adhesive cover, and incubation proceeds overnight (usually 16 h) at room temperature. During this incubation period, HBsAg binds to the antibody-coated bead and also combines with the enzyme-labeled antibody to form an antibody-antigen-labeled antibody sandwich. Contents of the wells are aspirated, and the beads are washed. The colorless enzyme substrate solution, containing *o*-phenylenediamine and hydrogen peroxide, is added to the beads, resulting in hydrolysis and the production of a yellow-orange color in tubes containing beads with adsorbed HBsAg and conjugate. After a 30-min incubation period, the enzyme reaction is stopped by adding 1 ml of 1 N sulfuric acid. A_{492} is read in a spectrophotometer. Specimens giving absorbance values equal to or greater than the absorbance value of the negative control mean plus the factor 0.050 are considered positive for HBsAg. Runs are not valid if the difference between the positive and negative controls is less than 0.400 absorbance units. The NML ELISA assay (24, 66) uses microtiter wells coated with guinea pig anti-HBs. The conjugate is chimpanzee anti-HBs labeled with alkaline phosphatase, and the enzyme substrate is *p*-nitrophenyl phosphate. NaOH is used to stop the reaction, which is read colorimetrically at 405 nm. The ELISA Test System 2 and Anti-HBs ELISA assays use polystyrene microtiter wells coated with mouse monoclonal anti-HBs. The conjugate is mouse monoclonal (ELISA Test System 2) or goat (Anti-HBs ELISA) anti-HBs labeled with horseradish peroxidase. Hydrolysis of the substrate (*o*-phenylenediamine–hydrogen peroxide) is stopped with H_2SO_4, and the reaction is read colorimetrically at 492 nm.

In each of these assays, appropriate positive and negative controls are added to ensure specificity of the test. The total incubation times are about 18 h for Auszyme Monoclonal, Auszyme IV, NML ELISA, and Anti-HBs ELISA and 3.5 h for ELISA Test System 2 (although shorter times of 1.5 to 3.5 h can be used). The incubation temperatures are 15 to 30°C for Auszyme Monoclonal and Auszyme IV, room temperature and 45°C for NML ELISA, and 37° and 15 to 30°C for ELISA Test System 2 and Anti-HBs ELISA. Depending on the assay, final readings should be made within 30 min to 2 h after the addition of acid (or base for the NML ELISA test). The blank should be repeated whenever prolonged interruptions occur. Care should be taken to avoid splashing specimens or reagents outside of wells or high up on the rim of the well, since such splashes may not be removed in subsequent washing and could be transferred to tubes, causing test interference. Sodium azide will poison the enzyme substrate, so care should be taken that this reagent is not present in the wash reagent.

Solid-phase EIA for the detection of anti-HBs is similar in principle to HBsAg detection except that the specimen is incubated with polystyrene beads or in microtiter wells coated with HBsAg. Two commercial kits are available (Ausab EIA, Abbott Laboratories; Microplate EIA, ADI Diagnostics [distributed in the United States by Organon Teknika]). Anti-HBs bound to the fixed HBsAg is detected with either a complex consisting of biotin-labeled HBsAg and horseradish peroxidase-conjugated rabbit anti-biotin (Ausab EIA), or horseradish peroxidase-conjugated HBsAg (Microplate EIA).

Three anti-HBc EIA kits that are licensed in the United States (Corzyme, Abbott Laboratories; Hepanostika Anticore, Organon Teknika; AB-COREK EIA, Sorin Biomedica) are competitive binding assays in which anti-HBc from the test sample competes with a constant amount of horseradish peroxidase-conjugated human anti-HBc for a limited number of binding sites found on beads or in wells coated with HBcAg. Within limits, the amount of anti-HBc present in the sample is inversely proportional to the amount of color development. Another commercial EIA kit for anti-HBc (HBc Antibody ELISA, Ortho Diagnostic Systems) is a solid-phase sandwich method in which the specimen is incubated in microtiter wells coated with HBcAg and bound anti-HBc is detected with horseradish peroxidase-conjugated mouse monoclonal anti-human IgG and IgM.

Commercial EIA kits are also available for the detection of IgM-specific anti-HBc (Corzyme-M, Abbott Laboratories) and HBeAg and anti-HBe (Abbott HBe EIA, Abbott Laboratories; Hepanostika HBeAg/anti-HBe, Organon Teknika). The Corzyme-M test uses a modified sandwich technique to measure IgM-specific anti-HBc in serum or plasma. In this assay, 10 µl of an appropriately diluted specimen (10 µl in 0.5 ml of specimen diluent) is added to the bottom of a well, followed by the addition of 0.2 ml of specimen diluent (final serum concentration is 1:1,000). A polystyrene bead coated with antibody specific for human IgM (µ-chain specific) is added to each well. This removes IgM from the patient samples. The wells are sealed with an adhesive cover, and incubation proceeds at 40°C for 1 h. Liquid is then aspirated, and the beads are washed three times with distilled or deionized water. HBcAg and horseradish peroxidase-conjugated human anti-HBc are added to the bead to which IgM-specific anti-HBc may be immunologically bound, and the trays are sealed. After another incubation period at room temperature for 18 to 22 h, the beads are rewashed three times as previously described. The beads are transferred to tubes, and *o*-phenylenediamine solution containing hydrogen peroxide is added. After incubation at 15 to 30°C for 30 min, 1 ml of 1 N sulfuric acid is added to each tube to stop the reaction. A yellow-orange color develops in proportion to the amount of HBcAg–anti-HBc–horseradish peroxidase that bound to the bead during the previous incubation. The intensity of the color is measured with a spectrophotometer at 492 nm. The absorbance is proportional to the quantity of IgM-specific anti-HBc present in the patient serum. A cutoff value of 0.25 times the positive control mean plus the negative control mean is determined. Specimens giving absorbance values equal to or greater than the cutoff are considered positive for IgM antibodies to HBcAg. If rapid results are essential, the second incubation period can be reduced to 3 h at 40°C so that the test can be completed the same day.

The tests for HBeAg and anti-HBe are performed with the same commercial kit but use different assay principles. In the Abbott kit, the HBeAg test uses a sandwich principle to measure HBeAg in serum or plasma. Plastic beads coated with human anti-HBe are added to test samples (200 µl). After the trays are sealed, the samples are incubated at room temperature for 18 to 22 h. The fluid is aspirated, the beads are washed, and anti-HBe (human) conjugated to horseradish peroxidase is then added. After an additional incubation period of 2 h at 40°C, the beads are washed again and transferred to tubes. *o*-Phenylenediamine solution (with hydrogen peroxide) is added, and the reactants are allowed to incubate for another 30 min at 15 to 30°C. The reaction is stopped with 1 N sulfuric acid, and A_{492} values are determined. Specimens giving absorbancy values equal to or greater than the absorbancy value of the negative control mean plus a factor of 0.060 are considered positive for HBeAg. The test for anti-HBe, performed with the same Abbott kit, is a modified competitive binding assay in which anti-HBe in the test serum (50 µl) competes with anti-HBe-coated beads for a standardized amount of added HBeAg. If anti-HBe is present in the test sample, less HBeAg would be coupled to the bead and therefore less horseradish peroxidase-conjugated anti-HBe would bind to the bead to complete the sandwich. The greater the amount of anti-HBe in the specimen, the lower the absorbancy after incubation of the beads in *o*-phenylenediamine solution containing hydrogen peroxide. The Hepanostika tests for HBeAg and anti-HBe are similar in principle to the Abbott assays, but they are carried out in anti-HBe-coated microtiter wells, they use two incubations at 37°C for 2 h, and in the anti-HBe test, the sample is preincubated with HBeAg overnight.

Tests for HBV-associated DNA polymerase (55). Samples are diluted 3- to 30-fold in Tris-saline buffer (pH 7.4; 0.01 M Tris hydrochloride and 0.15 M NaCl) and are clarified at 10,000 × *g* for 10 min; 3.0 ml is then layered over 2.5 ml of 30% (wt/vol) sucrose containing Tris-saline buffer, 0.001 M EDTA, 0.1% 2-mercaptoethanol, and 1 mg of BSA per ml which has been precentrifuged for 10 min at 10,000 × *g* to remove precipitated BSA. After centrifugation for 4 h at 250,000 × *g* (50,000 rpm in an SW65 rotor), the supernatant fluid is removed, residual fluid is adsorbed with paper, and the pellet is resuspended in 50 μl of Tris-saline buffer containing 0.1% Nonidet P-40 and 0.1% 2-mercaptoethanol. For evaluation of a larger number of specimens, a Beckman type 25 rotor that holds 100 1-ml tubes can be used. A 200-μl sample of a precentrifuged undiluted serum is layered over 0.5 ml of 30% (wt/vol) sucrose. The tubes are centrifuged at 24,000 rpm for 15 h at 4°C, and the pellets are recovered as described above. The removal of serum proteins from the pelleted material is essential because their presence will result in high background counts that cannot be washed away. To the resuspended pellet is added 25 μl of the reaction mixture (0.2 M Tris [pH 7.4], 0.08 M $MgCl_2$, 0.24 M NH_4Cl, 1.0 mM dATP, 1.0 mM TTP, 0.025 mM each [^{3}H]dCTP and [^{3}H]dGTP, both at 21 Ci/mmol). The reactants are incubated at 37°C for 3 h, and then 50 μl is placed on a Whatman 3-mm paper disk, washed, and assayed for acid-precipitable ^{3}H. Confirmation that the reactivity is associated with HBV is accomplished by its immunoprecipitation with anti-HBs before Nonidet P-40 detergent treatment and with anti-HBc after the addition of Nonidet P-40.

Hybridization techniques (58). Although hybridization procedures are beyond the scope of most clinical laboratories, an awareness of their availability is desirable. Human serum can be analyzed for HBV DNA sequences by using molecular hybridization techniques. To conduct these studies, 10 to 15 μl of serum is applied to a 0.45-μm nitrocellulose filter sheet, using 5 μl for each application. The paper should be dried between applications. Known positive and negative control samples are included in each assay. The paper is treated with 0.5 N NaOH neutralized with 1 M Tris hydrochloride (pH 7.4) containing 0.5 M NaCl and treated with proteinase K at 200 U/ml for 1 h at 37°C. After this treatment, the paper is washed twice with 0.3 M NaCl containing 0.3 M sodium citrate and then baked in vacuum at 80°C for 2 h, prehybridized, and hybridized for 24 to 36 h in a solution containing Denhardt solution (0.1% BSA, 0.1% Ficoll, 0.1% polyvinylpyrrolidone), 0.6 M NaCl, 0.06 M sodium citrate, 0.1% sodium dodecyl sulfate, 0.025 M sodium phosphate buffer (pH 6.5), 200 μg of denatured calf thymus DNA per ml, and 10^7 cpm of repurified recombinant cloned HBV DNA labeled with ^{32}P (specific activity, 2×10^8 to 4×10^8 cpm/μg of DNA). After hybridization, the nitrocellulose filter is washed, dried, and autoradiographed. This method is capable of detecting visually quantities from 0.2 to 0.5 pg of HBV DNA sequences within 24 h with a 2- to 10-fold increase after 5 days of autoradiography. Similar hybridization studies can be performed by using DNA extracted from small portions of frozen biopsy specimens (58). Recently, the polymerase chain reaction has been used for amplification of HBV DNA in serum, which enables detection of as few as five HBV DNA molecules (63).

A commercial liquid-phase molecular hybridization assay for detection and quantitation of HBV DNA in serum has recently become available for research purposes (Abbott Genostics Hepatitis B Viral DNA, Abbott Laboratories). In this assay, the serum specimen being tested is solubilized and incubated with a ^{125}I-labeled HBV DNA probe overnight at 65°C. The mixture is then loaded onto a column and hybridized HBV DNA is eluted from the column, whereas unhybridized ^{125}I-labeled HBV DNA is retained. The eluate is collected and counted for 10 min in a gamma counter. The assay can detect as little as 1×10^4 to 3×10^4 HBV molecules, or about 0.1 pg of HBV DNA.

Interpretation of test results

Successful detection of HBV serological markers depends not only on the relative sensitivity of the test procedures but also on the availability of experienced personnel who comprehend the procedure used and its idiosyncrasies and are meticulous in performance of the test. Provided that these conditions are met, the final evaluation and interpretation of any positive test result will be determined by the specificity of the reagents used. It is essential for the diagnostic virologist to appreciate the difficulties encountered in preparing from human sources quality reagents that are free from contaminating human proteins. These contaminants result in the production of low concentrations of unwanted antibodies during immunization. The preparation of monospecific antibody, the prior adsorption of antisera with an insoluble immunoadsorbent prepared from normal serum, or the use of monoclonal antibodies has eliminated most of these problems, as has the production of HBV antigens by using recombinant DNA methodology. Specificity testing with a reference antigen or antiserum also provides confirmation of the laboratory result. Additional verification of an HBsAg reaction is generated when anti-HBc is also detected.

The marked increase in sensitivity of the RIA, EIA, or hemagglutination tests as compared with the discontinuous counterimmunoelectrophoresis test should not imply that an equivalent increase in the number of HBsAg-positive persons will be detected. Experience indicates that 70% of the positive carriers in the United States have HBsAg concentrations that are detectable by second-generation assays, leaving 30% undetectable except by the more sensitive procedures. HBsAg levels between 0.1 and 0.5 ng/ml (the lower level of sensitivity for most third-generation tests) are found in less than 5% of the HBV carriers, representing about 0.01% of the donor population. Conversely, 10 to 15% of the HBV carrier population will have HBsAg concentrations above 100 μg/ml.

As shown in Fig. 5 and summarized in Table 8, the presence of HBsAg in a serum is indicative of an active HBV infection, either acute or chronic. In a typical HBV infection, HBsAg will be detected 2 to 4 weeks before the transaminase level becomes abnormal and 3 to 5 weeks before the patient develops symptoms or becomes jaundiced. Anti-HBc, primarily of the IgM immunoglobulin class, usually appears when the transaminase levels begin to increase. The presence of IgM-specific anti-HBc in high titer (>1:1,000) is evidence of an acute infection. These elevated titers decline regardless of whether the disease is resolved or becomes

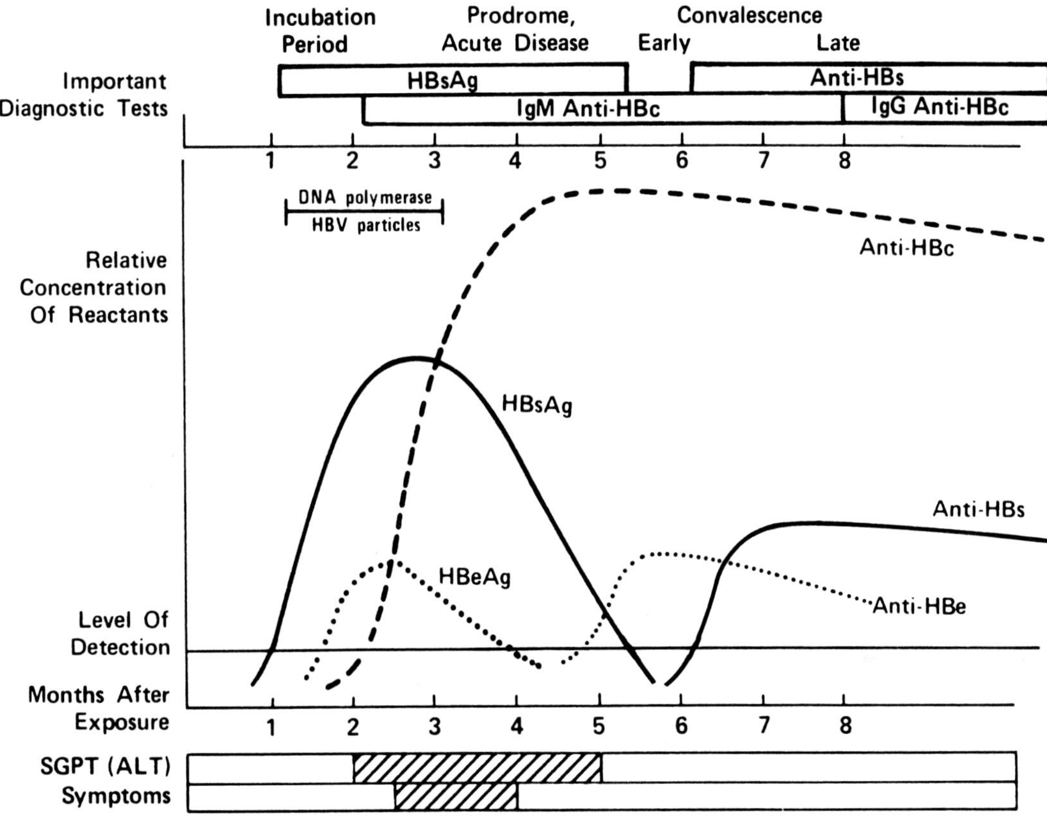

FIG. 5. Serological and clinical patterns observed during acute HBV infection. SGPT, Serum glutamic pyruvic transaminase; ALT, alanine aminotransferase.

chronic. HBsAg that persists for more than 4 to 6 months after the onset of clinical illness specifies those persons who are likely to become carriers of HBV. The HBsAg level rises and falls steadily in acute hepatitis B, whereas the HBsAg concentration is maintained within a very narrow range in untreated chronic carriers. Thus, it is possible to predict the potential for chronicity in patients with acute HBV disease, e.g., those who are positive for IgM-specific anti-HBc, by performing a quantitative RIA or EIA test on paired sera collected 2 to 3

TABLE 8. Interpretation of viral hepatitis screening profile

Assay results			Interpretation
IgM-specific anti-HAV	HBsAg	Anti-HBc	
Positive	Negative	Negative	Recent acute HAV infection.
Negative	Positive	Negative	Early acute HBV infection. Confirmation is required to exclude nonrepeatable or nonspecific reactivity.
Negative	Positive	Positive	HBV infection, either acute or chronic.[a] Symptoms may be unrelated to hepatitis B.
Negative	Negative	Positive	Active HBV infection cannot be excluded. Test for anti-HBs and anti-HBe. A positive anti-HBs test indicates a previous HBV infection and confirms immunity to hepatitis B.[b] A negative anti-HBs and a positive anti-HBe indicate recent HBV infection (<5% of cases). Confirm by demonstrating anti-HBs seroconversion in 2–6 weeks or by examining the sample for high-titer IgM-specific anti-HBc.
Negative	Negative	Negative	Possible hepatitis C, other viral infections, or toxic (drug-induced) liver disease.
Positive	Positive	Positive	Recent acute HAV infection in an HBV carrier.

[a] Differentiate acute from chronic hepatitis by examining the sample for high-titer IgM-specific anti-HBc. Use HBsAg quantitation of paired specimens to predict the potential for chronicity or to verify existing chronic hepatitis B. The presence of HBeAg indicates those specimens which exhibit the potential for enhanced infectivity. HBeAg is found only in the presence of HBsAg. Other HBV serological markers that may be present at the same time include HBV (Dane) particles observable by electron microscopy. By disrupting the virion, HBcAg and viral DNA polymerase can be measured.

[b] Exclude recent transfusions, immune globulin administration, or a maternal antibody source within the previous 6 months.

weeks apart. Most comparisons can be evaluated at a dilution of 1:10,000 (prepared in PBS containing 0.5% BSA), although some samples may require a lower dilution to obtain an S/N ratio that is on the descending slope of the assay dose-response curve. Extreme care must be used in preparing the dilutions. A decline in HBsAg concentration predicts eventual recovery, whereas no change in the concentration indicates that the patient has developed a persistent infection.

Because the anti-HBc test is invariably positive when HBsAg is present in a clinically ill patient (see Fig. 5 and Table 8 for rare exceptions to this statement), its immunodiagnostic value is to validate the HBsAg reaction. Tests with discordant results always should be repeated. However, in perhaps 5 to 10% of the acute cases of hepatitis B (especially those with fulminant disease), and more frequently during early convalescence, serum levels of HBsAg may be undetectable (Fig. 5). Examination of these sera for IgM-specific anti-HBc may help in establishing the correct diagnosis. In the absence of anti-HBc and HBsAg, active hepatitis B disease can be excluded. In contrast, the presence of anti-HBc alone is presumptive evidence for an active HBV infection. However, this relationship is not infallible, as many patients who have recovered from hepatitis B with the development of anti-HBs and anti-HBc eventually lose one or the other.

Specimens that are HBsAg positive may be evaluated for HBeAg, anti-HBe, specific DNA polymerase reactivity, or HBV particles to determine their potential for enhanced infectivity. HBeAg-positive specimens contain high concentrations of HBV particles and are more likely to transmit hepatitis B, in contrast to anti-HBe-positive samples, in which the number of HBV particles is markedly reduced.

Antibody to HBsAg usually becomes detectable 1 to 2 months after the disappearance of HBsAg. It is assumed that anti-HBs production occurs much earlier but is not observed as a result of the formation of immune complexes with excess HBsAg. Antibody to HBsAg, with or without anti-HBc, specifies immunity against reinfection. However, RIA S/N ratios lower than 10 or EIA absorbance values just above the cutoff should be viewed with caution in the absence of anti-HBc. It has been proposed that anti-HBc, not anti-HBs, be used to determine susceptibility or immunity to HBV or to decide whether to recommend vaccination with HBsAg. Conversely, only anti-HBs develops in persons who receive the HBsAg vaccine. Depending on the circumstances, passive transfer of anti-HBs or anti-HBc is often observed in patients receiving these antibodies during blood transfusions, after hepatitis B immune globulin administration, or in neonates of mothers with recent or past hepatitis B. Recognition of these possibilities will avoid an erroneous diagnosis of HBV infection, since passive antibodies gradually disappear over a 2- to 4-month observation period, in contrast to actively produced antibodies, which are remarkably stable over many years.

Subtyping of specimens by the clinical laboratory provides additional information to the clinician or hospital epidemiologist, since the mutually exclusive *d* and *y* subdeterminants are virus specific and not host determined. This fact can be helpful in determining the source of infection or can provide epidemiological evidence for the relatedness among cases.

HDV

Direct examination

Immunofluorescence and immunoperoxidase staining of liver tissue from patients or experimental animals (chimpanzees or woodchucks with woodchuck hepatitis virus) are reliable approaches for the identification of HDV antigen (HDVAg); however, these methodologies are restricted to specialized pathology laboratories and are not practical for adoption as rapid screening tests by clinical laboratories. The methodologies for such immunohistochemical staining are routine for pathology and immunology laboratories. The anti-HDV probe, to which fluorescein or peroxidase is conjugated, is usually derived from serum or plasma that contains a higher titer of anti-HDV and a low level of antibody to HBcAg. Thus, the anti-HBc reactivity can be reduced substantially or eliminated entirely by dilution. However, an anti-HDV-negative, anti-HBc-positive control probe should be used in parallel with the anti-HDV probe to substantiate the anti-HDV specificity of staining. Controls for other sources of nonspecificity, including autoantibodies to nuclear antigens, should be incorporated into procedures for immunohistochemical staining. With these techniques, investigators have shown that the HDVAg localizes primarily to the liver cell nucleus and rarely can be detected in the cytoplasm. Although frozen cryostat sections are preferable, HDVAg is stable to Formalin fixation and paraffin embedding. Therefore, HDVAg can be studied in stored paraffin-embedded tissue after digestion of the section with trypsin or pronase (9).

Serological identification of HDVAg and anti-HDV

Antibodies to HDVAg (anti-HDV) have been identified and quantitated primarily by RIA or EIA (8, 54). The major limitation to wider availability of these diagnostic techniques has been a shortage of HDVAg-containing clinical material for use in immunoassays. As discussed below, however, the ability to perform these tests is increasing among diagnostic laboratories.

Purification of HDVAg and preparation of antibodies. Tests for anti-HDV require a source of HDVAg. Previously, the HDVAg used for these purposes had been obtained from HDVAg-positive human (postmortem) or chimpanzee liver or serum. More recently, a more reliable source, HDVAg-positive woodchuck liver, has become available. HDVAg can be extracted from human liver with strong dissociating agents such as 6 M guanidine hydrochloride or 8 M urea. When liver tissue is obtained from experimentally infected chimpanzees or woodchucks at the peak of intrahepatic HDVAg expression, i.e., before the appearance of anti-HDV, HDVAg can be harvested by simple aqueous extraction. Although HDVAg is rarely detectable in patients with acute HDV infection, occasionally sufficient HDVAg is present in serum to serve as a source of antigen for diagnostic testing.

Serum containing anti-HDV can be obtained from patients or experimental animals with acute or chronic HDV infection. As mentioned above, anti-HBc reactivity, invariably present in anti-HDV-positive serum, is often low in serum samples with a high level of anti-HDV activity. Residual anti-HBc activity can be diluted out, and HBsAg is removed by ultracentrifugation.

RIA. Because the availability of HDVAg remains limited, the only practical approach to routine laboratory immunodiagnosis is commercial immunoassays in which HDVAg is derived from the livers of woodchucks with experimental woodchuck hepatitis virus and HDV infection. A commercial RIA for anti-HDV is available for diagnostic purposes (Abbott Anti-Delta, Abbott Laboratories). The test is a competitive-binding RIA in which anti-HDV in the test serum competes with ^{125}I-labeled human anti-HDV for woodchuck liver-derived HDVAg coating a solid-phase polystyrene bead. In this assay, 100 μl of ^{125}I-labeled anti-HDV and 100 μl of serum or plasma to be tested are delivered to a well and an HDVAg-coated bead is added. Three negative control and two positive control wells are incorporated into each test run. The trays are incubated for 18 to 22 h at room temperature. After incubation, liquid is aspirated from the wells. The beads are washed three times with distilled or deionized water and transferred to counting tubes, and the tubes are assayed in a gamma scintillation counter. The net counts per minute (minus background) for the test sample is compared with a calculated cutoff (0.4 of the mean negative control counts plus 0.6 of the mean positive control counts). Samples with a count rate equal to or below the cutoff are considered reactive for anti-HDV; counts above the cutoff range are considered negative. Validity of the test requires that for each run, the ratio of the mean negative control counts to the mean positive control counts be >4.0.

HDVAg can be detected by solid-phase sandwich RIA as described by Rizzetto et al. (54). The test is based on binding of HDVAg in serum to anti-HDV adherent to a solid phase, followed by incubation with an ^{125}I-labeled purified IgG anti-HDV probe. Because HDVAg always circulates within an HBsAg-encapsidated virion, detection of HDVAg requires detergent (0.5% Tween 80, Nonidet P-40, or deoxycholate) disruption of the virion to expose the internal, otherwise sequestered antigen. Adding to the difficulty of HDVAg detection is the transience of HDV antigenemia, occurring during early infection. This simple solid-phase RIA for HDVAg can be modified for detection of anti-HDV in an RIA blocking assay. A standardized quantity of HDVAg is added to beads to which anti-HDV is adsorbed. Anti-HDV from the test serum or plasma competes with a constant amount of ^{125}I-labeled anti-HDV for the HDVAg immunologically bound to the beads. A reduction in the count rate of ≥50% is evidence for the presence of anti-HDV in the sample. Measurement of anti-HDV titers is achieved by diluting serum and determining the dilution that inhibits 50% of binding as compared with negative control sera (54).

Acute HDV infection (simultaneous with acute HBV infection or acute HDV superinfection of an HBV carrier) is accompanied by an early anti-HDV response predominantly of the IgM class. An antibody class-capture solid-phase RIA for IgM anti-HDV has been described in which antibody to human IgM (μ-chain specific) is bound to a solid phase and test serum is added. If the test serum contains IgM anti-HDV, it will bind to the solid phase. When HDVAg is added subsequently, it binds to the IgM anti-HDV. The sandwich is completed when the labeled probe, ^{125}I-conjugated IgG anti-HDV, binds to the HDVAg (60). The methodology for this technique is analogous to that for the detection of IgM-specific anti-HBc and IgM-specific anti-HAV. Interested readers are referred to the sections above in which details of these assays are provided.

EIA. A commercial EIA for anti-HDV, based on the configuration described above for the commercial RIA, is available for diagnostic purposes (Abbott Anti-Delta EIA, Abbott Laboratories).

Hybridization techniques. Because HDVAg is rarely detectable in serum, even when the serum is known to be infectious, and because anti-HDV is present indefinitely in patients with chronic HDV infection, liver biopsy with immunohistochemical staining for intrahepatic HDVAg is the only reliable way to demonstrate ongoing HDV replication. A noninvasive approach for detecting HDV RNA in serum has been made possible with the recent availability of cloned cDNA probes (61). The cDNA probe for HDV-associated RNA is incubated with serum, and HDV RNA is identified by dot blot hybridization analysis. This technique remains limited to a small number of research laboratories but holds promise as a simple, noninvasive test for the diagnosis of chronic HDV infection.

Interpretation of test results

Infection with HDV can occur in the presence of acute or chronic HBV infection. The duration of HBV infection determines the duration of HDV infection. When acute HDV and HBV infection occur simultaneously, clinical and biochemical features may be indistinguishable from those of HBV infection alone. The presence of HDV infection can be identified by demonstrating intrahepatic HDVAg or, more practically, an anti-HDV seroconversion (a rise in titer of anti-HDV or de novo appearance of IgM-specific anti-HDV, which is briefly if at all detectable). Because IgM-specific anti-HDV is transient and IgG anti-HDV is often undetectable once HBsAg disappears, retrospective serodiagnosis of acute, self-limited, simultaneous HBV and HDV infection is difficult.

In contrast to patients with acute HBV infection, patients with chronic HBV infection can support HDV replication indefinitely. This can happen when acute HDV infection occurs in the presence of a nonresolving acute HBV infection. More commonly, acute HDV infection becomes chronic when it is superimposed on an underlying chronic HBV infection (Fig. 6). In such cases, the HDV superinfection appears as a clinical exacerbation or an episode resembling acute viral hepatitis in someone already chronically infected with HBV. In the past, events resembling acute hepatitis in an HBV carrier or a patient with chronic hepatitis B were attributed to superimposed non-A, non-B hepatitis or to the natural history of the disease. A proportion of such episodes, however, represents acute superinfection with HDV.

When a patient presents with acute hepatitis and has HBsAg and anti-HDV in the serum, determination of the class of anti-HBc is helpful in establishing the relationship between infection with HBV and HDV. Although IgM-specific anti-HBc does not distinguish absolutely between acute and chronic HBV infection, its presence is a reliable indicator of recent infection and its absence is a reliable indicator of infection in the remote past. In simultaneous acute HBV and HDV infections, IgM-specific anti-HBc will be detectable, whereas in acute HDV infection superimposed upon

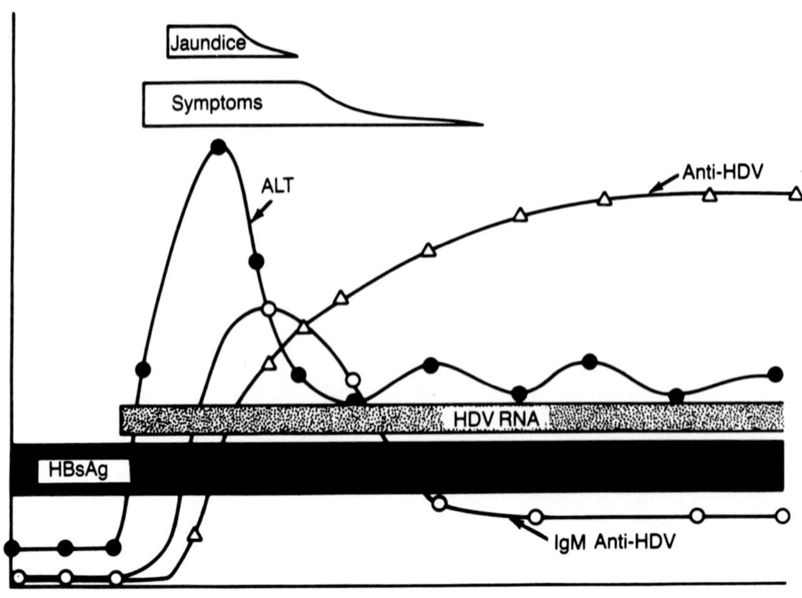

FIG. 6. Typical serological course of acute HDV superinfection in an HBsAg carrier. ALT, Alanine aminotransferase. (From reference 34.)

chronic HBV infection, anti-HBc will primarily be of the IgG class.

As noted above, cDNA tests for the presence of HDV-associated RNA will be useful in the future for determining the presence of ongoing HDV replication and relative infectivity. Currently, probes for this marker are restricted to a limited number of research laboratories.

NON-A, NON-B HEPATITIS (12, 13, 27)

Non-A, non-B hepatitis accounts for approximately 90% of the cases of transfusion-associated hepatitis seen in the United States and may be responsible for up to 20% of endemic and sporadic hepatitis (1, 14). Transmission mechanisms are similar to those for hepatitis B. The incubation period ranges from 5 to 10 weeks, although longer and shorter periods have been observed. Clinical characteristics are similar to those observed after hepatitis B except that chronic liver disease may be more prominent. Experimental transmission of non-A, non-B hepatitis agents has been accomplished in chimpanzees (27, 29). Patients with or without biochemical evidence of liver disease can transmit this disease, although the risk is significantly greater when the donor has alanine aminotransferase abnormalities (25) or detectable levels of anti-HBc. Viremia appears to precede the liver disease by at least 12 days. Evidence for at least two distinct non-A, non-B hepatitis agents has been obtained (27).

Until recently, diagnosis of this entity was by exclusion of HAV, HBV, cytomegalovirus, and Epstein-Barr virus in a patient who presented biochemical evidence of hepatitis. The discovery of HCV and the molecular cloning of its genome and production of a recombinant antigen permitted the recent development of an EIA for detection of antibodies to HCV (7, 42). A commercial EIA for anti-HCV is now available for diagnostic purposes (ORTHO HCV Antibody ELISA Test System, Ortho Diagnostic Systems). In this assay, anti-HCV is detected by incubating 20 μl of serum or plasma to be tested and 200 μl of specimen diluent in a microtiter well coated with recombinant HCV antigen. Plates are covered and incubated at 37°C for 1 h. The fluid contents of the wells are aspirated, and the wells are washed five times with PBS-polysorbate. Then mouse monoclonal anti-human IgG conjugated to horseradish peroxidase is added, and the plates are covered and incubated at 37°C for 1 h. Next, the wells are washed and substrate solution containing *o*-phenylenediamine and hydrogen peroxide is added. After 30 min at room temperature, the enzyme reaction is stopped by adding 50 μl of 4 N sulfuric acid. Specimens giving absorbance values equal to or greater than the absorbance value of the negative control mean plus the factor 0.400 are considered positive for anti-HCV. Antibody to HCV does not become detectable until 3 to 6 months after exposure and thus may be undetectable at the onset of clinical illness (Fig. 7). Anti-HCV persists in patients with chronic HCV infection. Although most cases of parenterally transmitted non-A, non-B hepatitis are apparently due to HCV, it is possible that some cases are caused by at least one other unidentified virus.

The successful propagation of HEV in cynomolgus monkeys has provided a dependable source of virus for laboratory studies. Frozen sections of infected livers from these animals have been recently used in a fluorescent-antibody blocking assay to detect antibody to HEV in serum samples taken during outbreaks of enterically transmitted non-A, non-B hepatitis (41). The

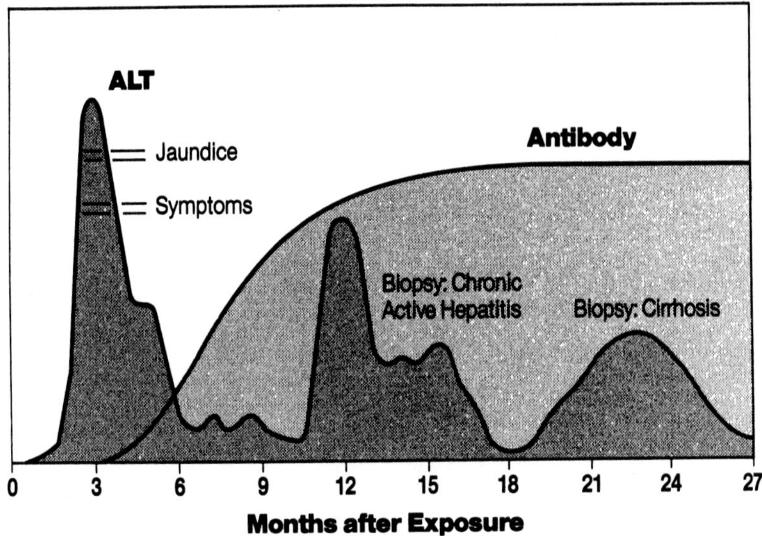

FIG. 7. Serological and clinical course of acute HCV infection, with development of chronic hepatitis and a persistent antibody response to HCV. ALT, Alanine aminotransferase. (Courtesy of Ortho Diagnostic Systems.)

development of these assays for hepatitis C and E represents significant progress toward the eventual control of non-A, non-B hepatitis.

LITERATURE CITED

1. **Aach, R. D., W. Szmuness, J. W. Mosley, F. B. Hollinger, R. A. Kahn, C. E. Stevens, V. M. Edwards, and J. Werch.** 1981. Serum alanine aminotransferase of donors in relation to the risk of non-A, non-B hepatitis in recipients. N. Engl. J. Med. **304:**989–994.
2. **Barker, L. F., J. E. Maynard, R. H. Purcell, J. H. Hoofnagle, K. R. Berquist, and W. T. London.** 1975. Viral hepatitis, type B, in experimental animals. Am. J. Med. Sci. **270:**189–195.
3. **Blumberg, B. S., A. I. Sutnick, W. T. London, and L. Millman.** 1971. The discovery of Australia antigen and its relation to viral hepatitis. Perspect. Virol. **7:**223–240.
4. **Bond, W. W., M. S. Favero, N. J. Petersen, and J. W. Ebert.** 1983. Inactivation of hepatitis B virus by intermediate-to-high-level disinfectant chemicals. J. Clin. Microbiol. **18:**535–538.
5. **Bond, W. W., N. J. Petersen, and M. S. Favero.** 1977. Viral hepatitis B: aspects of environmental control. Health Lab. Sci. **14:**235–252.
6. **Bradley, D. W., H. A. Fields, K. A. McCaustland, J. E. Maynard, R. H. Decker, R. Whittington, and L. R. Overby.** 1979. Serodiagnosis of viral hepatitis A by a modified competitive binding radioimmunoassay for immunoglobulin M anti-hepatitis A virus. J. Clin. Microbiol. **9:** 120–127.
7. **Choo, Q. L., G. Kuo, A. J. Weiner, L. R. Overby, D. W. Bradley, and M. Houghton.** 1989. Isolation of a cDNA clone derived from a blood-borne non-A, non-B viral hepatitis genome. Science **244:**359–361.
8. **Crivelli, O., M. Rizzetto, C. Lavarini, A. Smedile, and J. L. Gerin.** 1981. Enzyme-linked immunosorbent assay for detection of antibody to the hepatitis B surface antigen-associated delta antigen. J. Clin. Microbiol. **14:**173–177.
9. **Crivelli, O., J. W. K. Shih, and M. Rizzetto.** 1983. Methods for detection of the delta antigen and antibody in liver and serum, p. 121–126. *In* G. Verme, F. Bonino, and M. Rizzetto (ed.), Viral hepatitis and delta infection. Alan R. Liss, Inc., New York.
10. **Decker, R. H., S. M. Kosakowski, A. S. Vanderbilt, C.-M. Ling, R. Chairez, and L. R. Overby.** 1981. Diagnosis of acute hepatitis A by HAVAB-M, a direct radioimmunoassay for IgM anti-HAV. Am. J. Clin. Pathol. **76:**140–147.
11. **Deinhardt, F., D. Peterson, G. Cross, L. Wolfe, and A. W. Holmes.** 1975. Hepatitis in marmosets. Am. J. Med. Sci. **270:**73–80.
12. **Dienstag, J. L.** 1983. Non-A, non-B hepatitis. I. Recognition, epidemiology, and clinical features. Gastroenterology **85:**439–462.
13. **Dienstag, J. L.** 1983. Non-A, non-B hepatitis. II. Experimental transmission, putative virus agents and markers, and prevention. Gastroenterology **85:**743–768.
14. **Dienstag, J. L., A. Alaama, J. W. Mosley, A. G. Redeker, and R. H. Purcell.** 1977. Etiology of sporadic hepatitis B surface antigen-negative hepatitis. Ann. Intern. Med. **87:** 1–6.
15. **Dienstag, J. L., S. M. Feinstone, R. H. Purcell, J. H. Hoofnagle, L. F. Barker, W. T. London, H. Popper, J. M. Peterson, and A. Z. Kapikian.** 1975. Experimental infection of chimpanzees with hepatitis A virus. J. Infect. Dis. **132:**532–545.
16. **Dienstag, J. L., J. A. Routenberg, R. H. Purcell, R. R. Hooper, and W. O. Harrison.** 1975. Foodhandler-associated outbreak of hepatitis type A. An immune electron microscopic study. Ann. Intern. Med. **83:**647–650.
17. **Dienstag, J. L., A. N. Schulman, R. J. Gerety, J. H. Hoofnagle, D. E. Lorenz, R. H. Purcell, and L. F. Barker.** 1976. Hepatitis A antigen isolated from liver and stool: immunologic comparison of antisera prepared in guinea pigs. J. Immunol. **117:**876–881.
18. **Dixon, W. J., and M. B. Brown.** 1979. BMDP-79. University of California, Berkeley.
19. **Dreesman, G. R., F. B. Hollinger, R. M. McCombs, and J. L. Melnick.** 1972. Production of potent anti-Australia antigen sera of high specificity and sensitivity in goats. Infect. Immun. **5:**213–221.
20. **Dreesman, G. R., F. B. Hollinger, and J. L. Melnick.** 1972. Detection of hepatitis B antigen by counter-immunoelectrophoresis: enhancing role of homologous serum diluents. Appl. Microbiol. **24:**1001–1002.
21. **Feinstone, S. M., Y. Moritsugu, J. W.-K. Shih, J. L. Gerin, and R. H. Purcell.** 1978. Characterization of HAV, p. 41–48. *In* G. N. Vyas, S. N. Cohen, and R. Schmid (ed.), Viral hepatitis. The Franklin Institute Press, Philadelphia.

22. **Gerin, J. L., and J. W.-K. Shih.** 1978. Structure of HBsAg and HBcAg, p. 147–158. *In* G. N. Vyas, S. N. Cohen, and R. Schmid (ed.), Viral hepatitis. The Franklin Institute Press, Philadelphia.
23. **Gravelle, C. R., C. L. Hornbeck, J. E. Maynard, C. A. Schable, E. H. Cook, and D. W. Bradley.** 1975. Hepatitis A: report of a common source outbreak with recovery of a possible etiologic agent. II. Laboratory studies. J. Infect. Dis. **131**:167–171.
24. **Halbert, S. P., and M. Anken.** 1977. Detection of hepatitis B surface antigen (HBsAg) with use of alkaline phosphatase-labeled antibody to HBsAg. J. Infect. Dis. **136**(Suppl.): 318–323.
25. **Hollinger, F. B.** 1984. Prevention of posttransfusion hepatitis, p. 319–337. *In* G. N. Vyas, J. L. Dienstag, and J. H. Hoofnagle (ed.), Viral hepatitis and liver disease. Grune & Stratton, Inc., Orlando, Fla.
26. **Hollinger, F. B., E. Adam, D. Heiberg, and J. L. Melnick.** 1981. Response to hepatitis B vaccine in a young adult population, p. 451–466. *In* W. Szmuness, H. J. Alter, and J. E. Maynard (ed.), Viral hepatitis, 1981 International Symposium. The Franklin Institute Press, Philadelphia.
27. **Hollinger, F. B., H. J. Alter, P. V. Holland, and R. D. Aach.** 1981. Non-A, non-B posttransfusion hepatitis in the United States, p. 49–70. *In* R. J. Gerety (ed.), Non-A, non-B hepatitis. Academic Press, Inc., New York.
28. **Hollinger, F. B., D. W. Bradley, J. E. Maynard, G. R. Dreesman, and J. L. Melnick.** 1975. Detection of hepatitis A viral antigen by radioimmunoassay. J. Immunol. **115:** 1464–1466.
29. **Hollinger, F. B., G. L. Gitnick, R. D. Aach, W. Szmuness, J. W. Mosley, C. E. Stevens, R. L. Peters, J. M. Weiner, J. B. Werch, and J. J. Lander.** 1978. Non-A, non-B hepatitis transmission in chimpanzees: a project of the transfusion-transmitted viruses study group. Intervirology **10:** 60–68.
30. **Hollinger, F. B., N. C. Khan, P. E. Oefinger, D. H. Yawn, A. C. Schmulen, G. R. Dreesman, and J. L. Melnick.** 1983. Posttransfusion hepatitis type A. J. Am. Med. Assoc. **250**:2313–2317.
31. **Hollinger, F. B., M. Morrison, R. Chairez, and G. R. Dreesman.** 1975. Immunological and biophysical properties of hepatitis B antigen labeled by the chloramine-T and by the lactoperoxidase methods. J. Immunol. Methods **8**:67–84.
32. **Hollinger, F. B., V. Vorndam, and G. R. Dreesman.** 1971. Assay of Australia antigen and antibody employing double-antibody and solid-phase radioimmunoassay techniques and comparison with the passive hemagglutination methods. J. Immunol. **107**:1099–1111.
33. **Hollinger, F. B., C. Wasi, G. R. Dreesman, and J. L. Melnick.** 1973. Subtyping hepatitis B antigen using monospecific antibody-coated cells. J. Infect. Dis. **128**:753–760.
34. **Hoofnagle, J. H.** 1989. Type D (delta) hepatitis. J. Am. Med. Assoc. **261**:1321–1325.
35. **Hsu, S.-M., L. Raine, and H. Fanger.** 1981. A comparative study of the peroxidase-antiperoxidase method and an avidin-biotin complex method for studying polypeptide hormones with radioimmunoassay antibodies. Am. J. Clin. Pathol. **75**:734–738.
36. **Hsu, S.-M., L. Raine, and H. Fanger.** 1981. Use of avidin-biotin-peroxidase complex (ABC) in immunoperoxidase techniques: a comparison between ABC and unlabeled antibody (PAP) procedures. J. Histochem. Cytochem. **29:** 577–580.
37. **Huang, S., H. Minassian, and J. D. More.** 1976. Application of immunofluorescent staining on paraffin sections improved by trypsin digestion. Lab. Invest. **35**:383–390.
38. **Jambazian, A., and J. C. Holper.** 1972. Rheophoresis: a sensitive immunodiffusion method for detection of hepatitis associated antigen. Proc. Soc. Exp. Biol. Med. **140:** 560–564.
39. **Kachani, Z. F., and D. J. Gocke.** 1973. An agglutination-flocculation test for rapid detection of hepatitis B antigen. J. Immunol. **111**:1564–1570.
40. **Kobayashi, H., M. Tsuzuki, K. Koshimizu, H. Toyama, N. Yoshihara, T. Shikata, K. Abe, K. Mizuno, N. Otomo, and T. Oda.** 1984. Susceptibility of hepatitis B virus to disinfectants or heat. J. Clin. Microbiol. **20**:214–216.
41. **Krawczynski, K., and D. W. Bradley.** 1989. Enterically transmitted non-A, non-B hepatitis: identification of virus-associated antigen in experimentally infected cynomolgus macaques. J. Infect. Dis. **159**:1042–1049.
42. **Kuo, G., Q.-L. Choo, H. J. Alter, G. L. Gitnick, A. G. Redeker, R. H. Purcell, T. Miyamura, J. L. Dienstag, M. J. Alter, C. E. Stevens, G. E. Tegtmeier, F. Bonino, M. Colombo, W.-S. Lee, C. Kuo, K. Berger, J. R. Shuster, L. R. Overby, D. W. Bradley, and M. Houghton.** 1989. An assay for circulating antibodies to a major etiologic virus of human non-A, non-B hepatitis. Science **244**:362–364.
43. **Locarnini, S. A., S. M. Garland, N. I. Lehmann, R. C. Pringle, and I. D. Gust.** 1978. Solid-phase enzyme-linked immunosorbent assay for detection of hepatitis A virus. J. Clin. Microbiol. **8**:277–282.
44. **Mathiesen, L. R., S. M. Feinstone, D. C. Wong, P. Skinhøj, and R. H. Purcell.** 1978. Enzyme-linked immunosorbent assay for detection of hepatitis A antigen in stool and antibody to hepatitis A antigen in sera: comparison with solid-phase radioimmunoassay, immune electron microscopy, and immune adherence hemagglutination assay. J. Clin. Microbiol. **7**:184–193.
45. **Maynard, J. E., D. Lorenz, D. W. Bradley, S. M. Feinstone, D. H. Krushak, L. F. Barker, and R. H. Purcell.** 1975. Review of infectivity studies in nonhuman primates with virus-like particles associated with MS-1 hepatitis. Am. J. Med. Sci. **270**:81–85.
46. **Miller, W. J., P. J. Provost, W. J. McAleer, O. L. Ittensohn, V. M. Villarejos, and M. R. Hilleman.** 1975. Specific immune adherence assay for human hepatitis A antibody, application to diagnostic and epidemiologic investigations. Proc. Soc. Exp. Biol. Med. **149**:254–261.
47. **Moritsugu, Y., J. L. Dienstag, J. Valdesuso, D. C. Wong, J. Wagner, J. A. Routenberg, and R. H. Purcell.** 1976. Purification of hepatitis A antigen from feces and detection of antigen and antibody by immune adherence hemagglutination. Infect. Immun. **13**:898–908.
48. **Nakane, P. K., and A. Kawaoi.** 1974. Peroxidase-labeled antibody. A new method of conjugation. J. Histochem. Cytochem. **22**:1084–1091.
49. **Prince, A. M., W. Stephan, and B. Brotman.** 1983. β-Propiolactone/ultraviolet irradiation: a review of its effectiveness for inactivation of virus in blood derivatives. Rev. Infect. Dis. **5**:92–107.
50. **Provost, P. J., and M. R. Hilleman.** 1979. Propagation of human hepatitis A virus in cell culture *in vitro*. Proc. Soc. Exp. Biol. Med. **160**:213–221.
51. **Provost, P. J., W. J. Miller, B. S. Wolanski, O. L. Ittensohn, V. M. Villarejos, W. J. McAleer, and M. R. Hilleman.** 1978. Studies of human HAV strain CR326, p. 49–64. *In* G. N. Vyas, S. N. Cohen, and R. Schmid (ed.), Viral hepatitis. The Franklin Institute Press, Philadelphia.
52. **Ray, M. B.** 1979. Hepatitis B virus antigens in tissue. University Park Press, Baltimore.
53. **Rizzetto, M.** 1983. The delta agent. Hepatology **3**:729–737.
54. **Rizzetto, M., J. W. Shih, and J. L. Gerin.** 1980. The hepatitis B virus-associated δ antigen: isolation from liver, development of solid-phase radioimmunoassays for δ antigen and anti-δ and partial characterization of δ antigen. J. Immunol. **125**:318–324.
55. **Robinson, W. S.** 1975. DNA and DNA polymerase in the core of the Dane particle of hepatitis B. Am. J. Med. Sci. **270**:151–159.
56. **Robinson, W. S.** 1978. Hepatitis B Dane particle DNA structure and the mechanism of the endogenous DNA polymerase reaction, p. 139–145. *In* G. N. Vyas, S. N.

Cohen, and R. Schmid (ed.), Viral hepatitis. The Franklin Institute Press, Philadelphia.

57. **Roggendorf, M., G. G. Frosner, F. Deinhardt, and R. Scheid.** 1980. Comparison of solid phase test systems for demonstrating antibodies against hepatitis A virus (anti-HAV) of the IgM-class. J. Med. Virol. **5:**47–62.
58. **Shafritz, D. A., and S. J. Hadziyannis.** 1984. Hepatitis B virus DNA in liver and serum, viral antigens and antibodies, virus replication, and liver disease activity in patients with persistent hepatitis B virus infection, p. 80–90. *In* F. V. Chisari (ed.), Advances in hepatitis research. Mason Publishing USA, Inc., New York.
59. **Skinhøj, P., F. Mikkelsen, and F. B. Hollinger.** 1977. Hepatitis A in Greenland: importance of specific antibody testing in epidemiologic surveillance. Am. J. Epidemiol. **105:**140–147.
60. **Smedile, A., C. Lavarini, O. Crivelli, G. Raimondo, M. Fassone, and M. Rizzetto.** 1982. Radioimmunoassay detection of IgM antibodies to the HBV-associated delta (δ) antigen: clinical significance in δ infection. J. Med. Virol. **9:**131–138.
61. **Smedile, A., M. Rizzetto, F. Bonino, J. Gerin, and B. Hoyer.** 1984. Serum delta-associated RNA (DAR) in chronic HBV carriers infected with the delta agent, p. 613–614. *In* G. N. Vyas, J. L. Dienstag, and J. H. Hoofnagle (ed.), Viral hepatitis and liver disease. Grune & Stratton, Inc., Orlando, Fla.
62. **Tiollais, P., C. Pourcel, and A. Dejean.** 1985. The hepatitis B virus. Nature (London) **317:**489–495.
63. **Ulrich, P. P., R. A. Bhat, B. Seto, D. Mack, J. Sninsky, and G. N. Vyas.** 1989. Enzymatic amplification of hepatitis B virus DNA in serum compared with infectivity testing in chimpanzees. J. Infect. Dis. **160:**37–43.
64. **Wallis, C., and J. L. Melnick.** 1971. Enhanced detection of Australia antigen in serum hepatitis patients by discontinuous counter-immunoelectrophoresis. Appl. Microbiol. **21:**867–869.
65. **Wide, L.** 1970. Solid phase antigen-antibody systems, p. 199–206. *In* K. E. Kirkham and W. M. Hunter (ed.), Radioimmunoassay methods. E. & S. Livingstone, Edinburgh.
66. **Wolters, G., L. P. C. Kuijpers, J. Kacaki, and A. H. W. M. Shuurs.** 1977. Enzyme-linked immunosorbent assay for hepatitis B surface antigen. J. Infect. Dis. **136**(Suppl.): 311–317.
67. **World Health Organization Scientific Group.** 1973. Viral hepatitis. WHO Tech. Rep. Ser. no. 512.

Chapter 97

Filoviruses and Arenaviruses

PETER B. JAHRLING

CLINICAL BACKGROUND

Viruses from two families, *Arenaviridae* (14) and *Filoviridae* (19), are important human pathogens causing severe, frequently fatal viral hemorrhagic fevers. Although exotic to North America, these viruses are important public health problems in Africa and South America and may be introduced by travelers returning from these areas. The arenavirus and filovirus pathogens have been associated with severe nosocomial outbreaks involving health care workers and laboratory personnel. The similarity of initial isolation, clinical management, and viral diagnostic procedures for patients with suspected arenavirus or filovirus infections is the rationale for grouping these taxonomically distinct viruses together in this chapter. Patients with these infections frequently exhibit similar, nonspecific clinical signs resembling malaria, typhoid, and pharyngitis. A detailed travel history coupled with a high index of suspicion should facilitate rapid viral diagnosis and the timely implementation of appropriate patient isolation and clinical management procedures.

Arenaviruses are maintained in nature by association with specific rodent hosts (Table 1), in which they produce chronic viremia or viruria. Naturally occurring human disease can usually be traced to direct or indirect contact with infected rodents. Aerosol infectivity is also thought to be an important natural route of infection. Attempts to implicate arthropod vectors have been negative, but occasionally ectoparasites taken from viremic mammalian hosts have yielded arenavirus isolates.

Among the 14 recognized members of the family *Arenaviridae* (14), 4 are human pathogens. Lassa virus (LAS) is the etiologic agent of Lassa fever, a West African disease. The original, isolated outbreaks described were hospital associated, occurring first in Nigeria in 1969 and later in Liberia and Sierra Leone. Case fatality rates ranging from 20 to 40% were reported. Subsequently, extensive clinical disease and high seroprevalence were well documented in Nigeria, Sierra Leone, and Liberia. Other countries with serologic evidence of Lassa fever include Guinea, Ivory Coast, Ghana, Senegal, Upper Volta, the Gambia, and Mali. The true incidence of human Lassa fever cases is believed to be thousands to tens of thousands annually. Related viruses, possibly not pathogenic for humans, have been isolated in Mozambique, Zimbabwe, and the Central African Republic (Table 1). Lassa virus is now recognized to persist in endemic foci in Liberia and Sierra Leone. In hospitals located near endemic foci in Sierra Leone, 30% of all medical deaths are attributed to Lassa fever, and mortality among hospitalized Lassa fever cases is still estimated to be 15 to 20%. Overall mortality, including subclinical cases identified serologically, is substantially less, perhaps less than 1%. Deaths occur year-round, with some increases during the dry season.

Junin virus (JUN), causing Argentine hemorrhagic fever (AHF), was first isolated in 1959, although the disease was recognized as early as 1943 in Argentina. JUN infections occur primarily among young male agricultural workers. Annual fluctuations in AHF cases from 1958 to the present have ranged from 100 to 3,500, with several hundred cases occurring most years. Peak seasonal incidence is from March to June, coinciding with the seasons for both corn harvesting and expansion of wild rodent populations, including *Calomys musculinis.* The reported mortality rate for patients with laboratory-confirmed AHF was 14 to 17% before the routine use of immune plasma therapy was implemented.

Machupo virus (MAC), the etiologic agent of Bolivian hemorrhagic fever (BHF), was first isolated in 1963, although reports of sporadic outbreaks began in 1959 and a series of devastating epidemics occurred from 1962 to 1964; these outbreaks involved more than 1,000 patients, with an 18% mortality rate. *Calomys callosus* was implicated as the rodent reservoir, and the incidence of human cases was correlated with the presence of infected rodents in households. Control of *C. callosus* has eliminated epidemic BHF and reduced the annual incidence of cases to less than 10. Another severe outbreak of BHF occurred in Cochabamba, Bolivia, in 1971 and was associated entirely with nosocomial spread from a single index case who had returned from the endemic region. This outbreak, plus the explosive human-to-human chain of lethal transmission for LAS and anecdotal reports of nosocomial spread for JUN highlight the necessity for biocontainment precautions when one is dealing with arenavirus-infected patients and materials.

The relatively limited geographic distributions of LAS, MAC, and JUN probably relate to the limited distributions of the chronically infected rodent hosts. In contrast, lymphocytic choriomeningitis virus (LCM) is associated with the house mouse, *Mus musculus,* and the virus, like its rodent reservoir, is much more widespread (22). The presence of LCM is well documented in the Americas and Europe but not Scandinavia. LCM has also not been isolated from sources in Australia or Africa. Infected mouse colonies have long been associated with transmission to humans; more recently, the role of infected hamster colonies in dissemination, particularly to laboratory workers and pet owners, has become evident, as has the occupational hazard of manipulating certain human tumor cell lines propagated in rodents, including hamsters and nude mice. The absence of LCM from Africa is surprising, and it is plausible that many of the new LAS-like viruses being isolated

TABLE 1. Currently recognized arenaviruses and associated human disease

Virus and date isolated	Natural host	Geographic distribution	Naturally occurring human disease	Human laboratory infections
Old World				
Lymphocytic choriomeningitis, 1933	*Mus musculus* (house mouse)	Americas, Europe	Undifferentiated febrile illness, aseptic meningitis; rarely serious	Common, usually mild, but two fatal
Lassa, 1969	*Mastomys* sp. (multimammate, rat)	West Africa	Lassa fever; mild to severe and fatal disease	Common, often severe
Ippy, 1984	*Arvicanthus* sp.	Central African Republic	Unknown	None
Mopeia, 1977	*Mastomys natalensis*	Mozambique, Zimbabwe	Unknown	None; little experience
Mobala, 1983	*Praomys* sp.	Central African Republic	Unknown	None, little experience
New World				
Junin, 1958	*Calomys musculinus*	Argentina	Argentine hemorrhagic fever	Common, often severe
Machupo, 1963	*Calomys callosus*	Bolivia	Bolivian hemorrhagic fever	Common, often severe
Tacaribe, 1956	Artibeus bats	Trinidad, West Indies	None detected	One suspected; moderately symptomatic
Amapari, 1966	*Oryzomys gaeldi* *Neacomys guianae*	Brazil	None detected	None detected
Parana, 1970	*Oryzomys buccinatus*	Paraguay	None detected	None detected
Tamiami, 1970	*Sigmodon hispidus* (cotton rat)	United States (Florida)	Antibodies detected	None detected
Pichinde, 1971	*Oryzomys albigularis*	Colombia	None detected associated with high concentrations; mild to asymptomatic	Occasional
Latino, 1973	*Calomys callosus*	Bolivia	None detected	None detected
Flexal, 1977	*Oryzomys* spp.	Brazil	None detected; moderately severe	One recognized

from that continent are taxonomically related as closely to LCM as they are to LAS.

Marburg and Ebola hemorrhagic fevers are caused by taxonomically distinct viruses that are prototype members of the new family *Filoviridae* (19). Marburg virus (MBG) was first recognized in 1967 when 25 persons in Germany and Yugoslavia became infected after contact with monkey kidneys or primary tissue cultures derived from monkeys imported from Uganda. Seven of these patients died. In addition, six secondary human cases occurred. Since then, sporadic, virologically confirmed MBG cases have occurred in Zimbabwe, South Africa, and Kenya. Ebola virus (EBO) first emerged in two major disease outbreaks, which occurred almost simultaneously in Zaire and Sudan in 1976. Over 500 cases were reported, with case fatality rates of 88% in Zaire and 53% in Sudan. Despite the simultaneous emergence of EBO strains from Zaire (EBO-Z) and Sudan (EBO-S), these EBO isolates are serologically distinguishable and differ in host range, virulence potential, and biochemical properties. Serologic studies to date suggest that infections with EBO or related viruses have occurred in Zaire, Sudan, the Central African Republic, Gabon, Nigeria, Ivory Coast, Liberia, Cameroon, and Kenya. The geographic range of EBO strains may extend to other African countries, for which adequate serosurveys are lacking. The serologic studies, if valid, suggest that subclinical infections may occur frequently. The natural reservoirs for human infection with MBG and EBO have not been identified. Recently, however, a third filovirus, serologically related to EBO, was isolated from cynomolgus monkeys. These animals originated in the Philippines and were being held in a quarantine facility in Reston, Va., during 1989, when an explosive epizootic occurred; most of the monkeys died, and a filovirus, closely related by serologic criteria to EBO-S, was isolated (15). Early indications are that this virus (tentatively called Ebola-Reston or, alternatively, Reston virus [EBO-R]) is infectious for humans but does not cause serious human disease. The epidemiology and significance of this newly recognized virus strain is a subject for intensive investigation. Additional serologic and molecular data are required to understand the degree of taxonomic relatedness among the three isolates from Zaire, Sudan, and Reston, Va., called Ebola virus.

CLINICAL PRESENTATION

Among the arenavirus pathogens, LCM produces the least severe infection (22). A modest proportion of LCM infections are thought to be subclinical. A "typical" LCM case is usually heralded by fever, myalgia, retro-orbital headache, weakness, and anorexia. Especially during the first week, prominent symptoms include sore throat, chills, vomiting, cough, retrosternal pain, and arthralgias. Rash occurs, but infrequently. In about one-third of the patients, fever recurs, coinciding with the onset of frank neurologic involvement, usually aseptic meningitis or, less frequently, meningoencephalitis. Complete recovery is almost always the rule. Thus, LCM infections are temporarily debilitating but rarely fatal, even when neurologic complications arise.

LAS, JUN, and MAC infections are more severe. For LAS infection, fever and myalgia develop insidiously between 3 and 16 days after exposure and increase in severity during the following week. There are few specific clinical manifestations. Lassa fever patients usually come to the hospital within 5 to 7 days of onset with sore throat, severe lower back pain, and conjunctivitis. These symptoms usually increase in severity during the following week and are accompanied by nausea, vomiting, diarrhea, chest and abdominal pain, headache, cough, dizziness, and tinnitus. Later, pneumonitis and pleural and pericardial effusions with friction rub frequently occur. A maculopapular rash may develop, but frank hemorrhage is seen only in a proportion of the more severe cases. Oozing from puncture sites and mucous membranes and melena are more common. Approximately 15 to 20% of hospitalized patients die. Death relates to sudden cardiovascular collapse resulting from hepatic, pulmonary, and myocardial damage. Few Lassa fever patients develop central nervous system signs, although tinnitus or deafness may develop as recovery begins. Lassa fever is a particularly severe disease among pregnant women, for whom mortality rates are somewhat higher. The disease course for children is similar to that for adults; in infants, a condition described as swollen baby syndrome, characterized by anasarca, abdominal distention, and bleeding, has been described (27). Clinical laboratory studies are not usually helpful for Lassa fever; specific virologic testing is required, especially in a setting in which Lassa fever is less common or mild, atypical cases are occurring.

The clinical pictures for AHF (JUN) and BHF (MAC) are similar to each other and are frequently discussed as a single entity, South American hemorrhagic fevers. Incubation periods range from 7 to 14 days, and very few subclinical cases are thought to occur. Following a gradual onset of fever, anorexia, and malaise over several days, constitutional signs involving gastrointestinal, cardiovascular, and central nervous systems become apparent by the time patients appear at the hospital. On initial examination, AHF and BHF patients are febrile, acutely ill, and mildly hypotensive. They frequently complain of back pain, epigastric pain, headache, retro-orbital pain, photophobia, dizziness, constipation or diarrhea, and coughing. Vascular phenomena, including flushing of the face, neck, and chest, and bleeding from the gums are common. Enanthem is almost invariably present; petechiae or tiny vesicles spread over erythematous palate and fauces. Neurologic involvement, ranging from mild irritability and lethargy to abnormalities in gait, tremors of the upper extremities, and, in severely ill patients, coma, delirium, and convulsions occurs in more than half of the patients. During the second week of illness, clinical improvement may begin or complications may develop. The latter include extensive petechial hemorrhages, oozing from puncture wounds, melena, and hematemesis. These manifestations of capillary damage and thrombocytopenia do not result in life-threatening blood loss. However, hypotension and shock may develop, often in combination with serious neurologic signs among the 15% of patients who die. Survivors begin to show improvement by the third week. Recovery is slow; weakness, fatigue, and mental difficulties may last for weeks, and a significant proportion relapse with a late neurologic syndrome. In contrast with Lassa fever, clinical laboratory studies are frequently useful. Total leukocyte counts usually fall to 1,000 to 2,000 cells per mm^3, although the differential remains normal. Platelet counts fall precipitously, usually to 25,000 to 100,000/mm^3 but occasionally lower. Routine clotting parameters are usually normal or slightly deranged, but in severe cases evidence of disseminated intravascular coagulation is apparent.

MBG and EBO infections are clinically similar, although the frequencies of reported signs and symptoms vary. Following incubation periods of 4 to 16 days, onset is sudden, marked by fever, chills, headache, anorexia, and myalgia. These signs are soon followed by nausea, vomiting, sore throat, abdominal pain, and diarrhea. When first examined, patients are usually overtly ill, dehydrated, apathetic, and disoriented. Pharyngeal and conjunctival injection are usual. Within several days, a characteristic maculopapular rash over the trunk, petechiae, and mucous membrane hemorrhages appear. Gastrointestinal bleeding, accompanied by intense epigastric pain, is common, as are petechiae and bleeding from puncture wounds and mucous membranes. Development of shock occurs soon before death, often 6 to 16 days after onset of illness. Abnormalities in coagulation parameters include fibrin split products and prolonged prothrombin and partial thromboplastin times, suggesting that disseminated intravascular coagulation is a terminal event. Clinical laboratory studies usually reveal profound leukopenia early, followed by a rapid rise in association with secondary bacteremia. Platelet counts decline to 50,000 to 100,000/mm^3 during the hemorrhagic phase.

DESCRIPTION OF THE AGENTS

Arenaviridae

The family *Arenaviridae* comprises 14 named viruses which share unique morphological and physiochemical characteristics. In nature, arenaviruses are associated with unique mammalian hosts, usually rodents (Table 1). Antigenic relationships are established mainly on the basis of broadly reactive antibody binding assays, historically the complement fixation (CF) test, and more recently the indirect fluorescent-antibody (IFA) test and enzyme-linked immunosorbent assay (ELISA). Finer discriminations among virus strains have employed neutralization tests; more recently, monoclonal antibodies have been used for fine discriminations in IFA and ELISA formats. Two taxonomic complexes are generally accepted (4, 38). The LCM, or Old World, complex includes LCM and LAS, including a number of LAS-like strains recently isolated from Mozambique, Zimbabwe, and the Central African Republic. These may be unique viruses or substrains of LAS. All have been isolated from rodents of the family *Muridae*. The Tacaribe, or New World, complex includes Tacaribe, JUN, MAC, Amapari, Parana, Latino, Pichinde, Tamiami, and Flexal viruses. All New World complex viruses have been isolated from rodents of the family *Cricetidae* or, in the case of Tacaribe virus, from bats. Old and New World complex viruses are distantly related, and cross-reactions by CF or IFA with use of crude antigens are obtained only when high-titered antisera are used.

Cross-reactivity with use of synthetic peptides for conserved antigenic epitopes is much broader.

The morphology of arenaviruses is distinctive in thin-section electron microscopy (29) and was the basis for first associating LCM with MAC and ultimately all viruses in the present family. Individual virions are pleomorphic and range in size from 60 to 280 nm (mean, 110 to 130 nm). A unit membrane envelopes the structure and is covered with club-shaped, 10-nm projections. No symmetry has been discerned. The most prominent and distinctive feature of these virions is the presence of varying numbers of electron-dense particles (usually 2 to 10) which may be connected by fine filaments. These particles, 20 to 25 nm in diameter, have been shown to be identical with host cell ribosomes by biochemical and oligonucleotide analysis. Three major virion structural proteins are usually found (36). Two are glycosylated; G1 (50,000 to 72,000 daltons [Da]) and G2 (31,000 to 41,000 Da) constitute the virion envelop and spikes. Both G1 and G2 serve as highly type specific neutralization targets. G2 has not been demonstrated for Tacaribe or Tamiami virus. The N protein (63,000 to 72,000 Da) is clearly associated with the virion RNA and is considered the nucleocapsid protein. The N protein in intact cells or virions is not accessible to antibody but can readily be detected in acetone-fixed cells by immunofluorescence. Nucleocapsids can be isolated by treatment of intact virions with detergent. Liberated nucleocapsids are 10 nm in diameter and range to 450 nm in length. Two size classes of closed or circular nucleocapsid have been identified, 640 and 1,300 nm. Small, 3- to 4-nm beaded strands can also be resolved. Some arenaviruses elaborate a soluble protein antigenically related to the N protein into supernatant fluids of infected-cell cultures. The group-reactive arenavirus antigen measured in both the CF and IFA tests is associated with the nucleocapsid and is probably N protein. No hemagglutinins have been found.

Four RNA species with distinct oligonucleotide fingerprints can be isolated from intact arenavirus virions. The large-RNA (31S) and small-RNA (22S) species are virus specific; the 28S and 18S species, isolated in varying proportions, are ribosomal. The molecular sizes of large and small viral RNAs have been estimated to be 2.6×10^6 and 1.4×10^6 Da, respectively. The coding strategy for arenaviruses is unique and has been termed "ambisense," since the 3′ half of the small RNA codes for N protein in the viral complementary sense and is separated by an intragenic hairpin structure from the 5′ region, which codes for GPC, the precursor of GP1 and GP2, in the viral sense (31). Through this mechanism, GPC and N gene expressions are independently regulated. Viral RNA must be translated before GPC can be expressed, and this regulation may be fundamental to the maintenance of persistent infections in chronically infected hosts and cells in culture.

Arenaviruses mature by budding at the cytoplasmic membrane, and host proteins are incorporated into the virion envelope. Buoyant densities of intact arenavirus particles in cesium chloride range from 1.17 to 1.18 g/ml. All arenaviruses are readily inactivated by ethyl ether, chloroform, sodium deoxycholate, and acid media (pH less than 5). Beta-propiolactone (35) and gamma irradiation (10) are both reported to inactivate arenavirus infectivity while preserving reactivity in standard serologic tests.

Filoviridae

The filoviruses, MBG and EBO, are similar in morphology, density, and polyacrylamide gel electrophoresis profile and have some RNA sequence homology. These viruses were originally classified as members of the *Rhabdoviridae* but now are considered sufficiently distinct by biochemical, ultrastructural, and serologic criteria to warrant separate taxonomic status as members of the *Filoviridae* (19). Detailed characterization of the newly isolated EBO-related filovirus from Reston (tentatively called EBO-R) will eventually determine its correct taxonomic position. MBG and EBO virions mature by the budding of cytoplasmic tubular structures, which contain the nucleocapsids, through the cell membrane. The resulting viral particles are very large, typically 790 to 970 nm in length and consistently 80 nm in diameter. Bizarre structures of widely varying lengths, sometimes exceeding 14,000 nm, as well as branching, circular, or "6" shapes, probably resulting from coenvelopment of multiple nucleocapsids during budding, are frequently found in negatively stained preparations (28) (Fig. 1). When infected tissue culture fluids are purified by rate zonal centrifugation, the infectivity is associated with uniform-size, bacilliform particles 790 nm in length for MBG and 970 nm for EBO, with sedimentation coefficients of 1,400S (20). These infectious particles contain a nucleocapsid with a 20- to 30-nm central axis surrounded by a helical capsid, 40 to 50 nm in diameter, with cross-striations at 3- to 5-nm intervals. The nucleocapsid is surrounded by a host cell-derived envelope bearing 7- to 10-nm projections in a regular array. MBG and EBO virion RNA is monopartite, single stranded, 4.0×10^6 to 4.5×10^6 Da, of negative polarity, and noninfectious (9).

Both viruses have at least seven virus-specific proteins, including a large glycoprotein and two nucleoproteins. Two proteins play a role in viral replication, and two are membrane associated. For EBO, the ribonucleoprotein complex contains L (180 kDa), NP (104 kDa), VP30 (30 kDa), and VP35 (35 kDa) in loose association. GP (125 kDa) is the major spike protein, and VP40 plus VP24 make up the remaining protein content of the multilayered envelope (20). Tryptic peptide maps comparing MBG and EBO structural proteins are entirely dissimilar except for some minimal homology among the NP proteins (9, 20). Serologically, MBG and EBO strains are distinct. EBO-Z, EBO-S, and EBO-R do cross-react in broadly reactive tests such as IFA, but tryptic peptide and oligonucleotide maps show substantial differences among these strains (2). Maps of MBG RNA suggest 40 to 50% homology with EBO-Z. EBO-Z and EBO-S share about 70% homology. Neutralization tests for MBG and EBO have not yet been shown to be sufficiently reliable to enable determination of taxonomic relationships.

Despite their unusual morphologic properties, MBG and EBO resemble the arenaviruses and other lipid-enveloped viruses in being susceptible to lipid solvents, beta-propiolactone (35), formaldehyde, UV light, and gamma radiation (10). These viruses are stable at room temperature for several hours but are inactivated by incubation at 60°C for 1 h.

COLLECTION AND STORAGE OF SPECIMENS

For virus isolation, serum, heparinized plasma, or, less ideally, whole blood should be collected during the

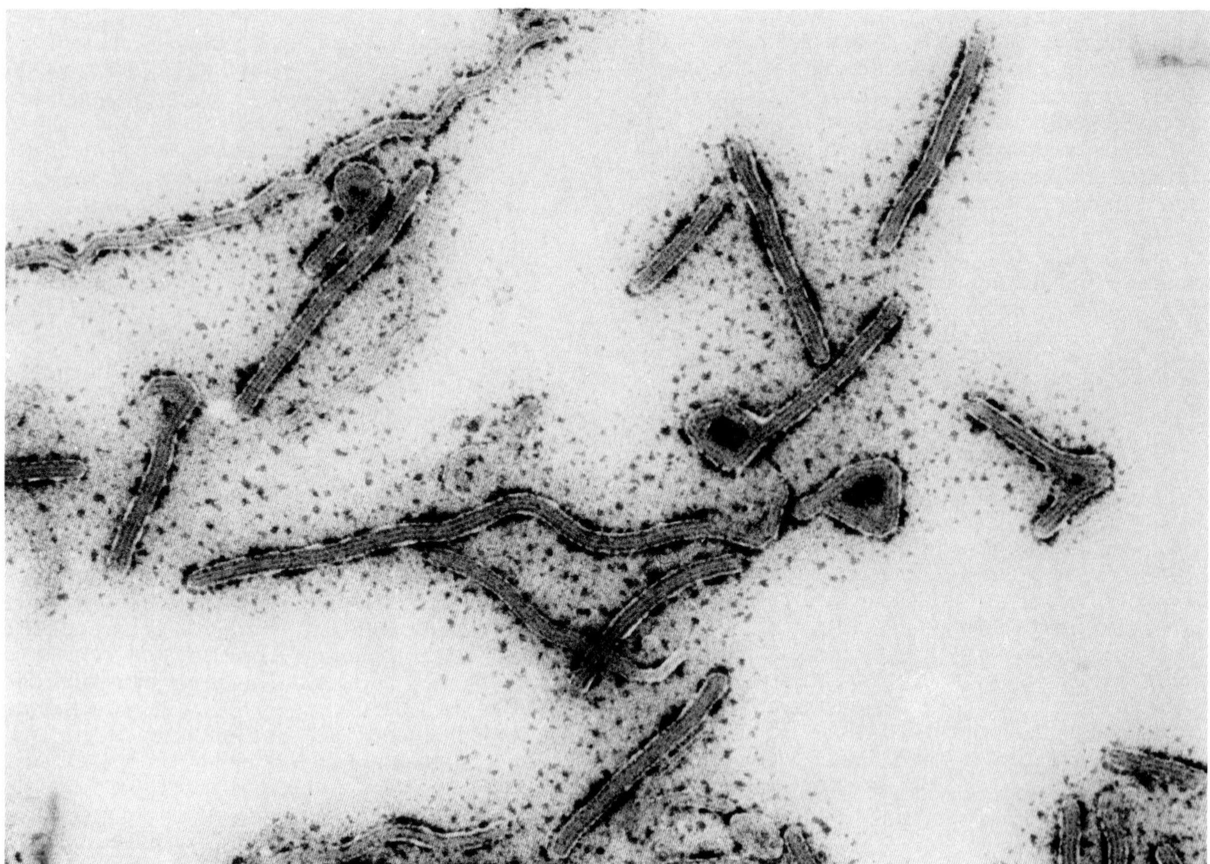

FIG. 1. Electron micrograph of EBO-R. Filamentous particles, 80 nm in diameter with 50-nm cores and various lengths, some >10,000 nm. Negative stain (sodium phosphotungstate) of supernatant fluids from MA-104 cells; magnification, ×32,550. (Courtesy of T. W. Geisbert.)

acute, febrile stages of the illness and frozen on dry ice in liquid nitrogen vapor. Throat wash and urine specimens should also be collected and mixed with an equal volume of buffered diluent containing serum proteins to stabilize viral infectivity prior to freezing. Storage at higher temperatures (over −40°C) may be unavoidable but will lead to rapid losses in infectivity. The success of isolating LAS from most acute-phase sera and throat washings obtained within several weeks of onset is high; LAS is isolated less frequently from urine. JUN is usually recoverable from serum for a period of 3 to 10 days after onset, and often from throat washings for a similar period, but rarely from urine. MAC is recovered from only one in five acute-phase sera and even less frequently from throat washings or urine. LCM may be recovered from acute-phase sera obtained within the first week after onset but rarely, if ever, from throat washings or urine specimens. LCM may also be isolated from the cerebrospinal fluid during the period of meningeal involvement and from the brain at autopsy. MBG and EBO are usually recoverable from acute-phase sera; various specimens, including throat wash, urine, soft tissue effusates, semen, and anterior eye fluid, have yielded these viruses, even when the specimens were obtained late in convalescence. LAS, MAC, JUN, MBG, and EBO are all readily isolated from spleen, lymph nodes, liver, and kidney obtained at autopsy but rarely, if ever, from brain or other central nervous system tissues. Notably, LAS is usually isolated from the placentas of infected pregnant women. Specimens collected for viral isolation are also suitable for testing by antigen capture ELISA; maintenance at −20°C for periods up to several weeks is adequate for antigen preservation. Impression smears of infected tissues, prepared as described in the next section, may be fixed by immersion in cold acetone and stored frozen for viral antigen staining by IFA. Formaldehyde-fixed tissues and paraffin-embedded blocks are also suitable for immunohistochemical identification of viral antigens.

Blood obtained in early convalescence for serodiagnosis may be infectious despite the presence of antibodies and should be handled accordingly (6, 7). Maintenance of samples at −20°C or below is sufficient to preserve antibody titers and antigenicity, but lower temperatures are required to preserve infectivity. Certain anticoagulants should be avoided: citrate interferes with the IFA test, both citrate and oxalate cause nonspecific cytopathic effects in Vero and MA-104 cells used for virus isolation, and EDTA can interfere with some ELISA techniques. Heparinized plasma or serum samples are best.

Manipulation of these specimens and tissues, including sera obtained from convalescent patients, may pose a serious biohazard, and their handling should be minimized outside a maximum containment laboratory. Current recommendations in the United States are that such samples be manipulated only at biosafety level 4 (6). At a minimum, barrier nursing procedures should be implemented, and personnel caring for the patient and handling diagnostic specimens should wear disposable caps, gowns, shoe covers, surgical gloves, and face masks (preferably full-face respirators equipped with high-efficiency particulate air [HEPA] filters). Gloves should be disinfected immediately if they come in direct contact with infected blood or secretions. All disposable and reusable equipment should be placed directly in a suitable disinfectant solution such as sodium hypochlorite, phenolic detergent, or a solution of quaternary ammonium compounds. Reusable equipment can then be sterilized. To minimize the risk of autoinoculation, needle sheaths should not be replaced on used needles; needles should be placed immediately in disinfectant. Glass equipment (e.g., microscope slides, microhematocrit tubes, and syringes) poses a significant hazard also; substitutes should be found for all glass equipment except Vacutainer tubes for blood collection. Use of Vacutainers is considered safer than use of syringes and needles, which must be disassembled before transfer of the contents to another tube. Procedures that generate aerosols (e.g., trituration and centrifugation) should be minimized and done only if additional protective equipment, such as a flexible film plastic isolator capable of maintaining negative pressure and HEPA-filtered exhaust, is available. For specialized procedures, samples may be inactivated by the addition of beta-propiolactone and may then be safely tested by serologic or antigen capture assays in the field. Heating to 60°C for 1 h will render diagnostic specimens noninfectious and is feasible for measurement of heat-stable substances such as electrolytes, blood urea nitrogen, and creatinine.

For all testing of infectious material, samples should be packaged in accordance with current recommendations (5) and forwarded, after consultation, to one of the following laboratories that maintain biosafety level 4 facilities and a diagnostic capability for these agents:

1. Centers for Disease Control
   Special Pathogens Branch
   Division of Viral and Rickettsial Diseases
   Center for Infectious Diseases
   Atlanta, GA 30333
   Telephone: (404)639-1115; Fax: (404)639-3163
2. U.S. Army Medical Research Institute of Infectious Diseases
   Disease Assessment Division
   Fort Detrick
   Frederick, MD 21701
   Telephone: (301)663-7193; Fax: (301)662-2492
3. Center for Applied Microbiology and Research
   Special Pathogens Unit
   Salisbury
   Porton Down
   Wiltshire SP4 OJG
   England
   Telephone: 0980-610391; Fax: 0980-611093
4. National Institute for Virology
   Private Bag X4
   Sandringham, Johannesburg
   South Africa
   Telephone: 27-11-882-9910; Fax: 27-11-882-0596

DIRECT EXAMINATION

MBG and EBO have been successfully visualized directly by electron microscopy of both heparinized blood and urine obtained during the febrile period as well as of tissue culture supernatant fluids. These materials are processed by immediate fixation with 0.5% glutaraldehyde, followed by low-speed centrifugation. Virions are then sedimented at 12,000 $\times$ *g* for 15 min, resuspended in 1/100 original sample volumes, and placed on Formvar-carbon-coated electron microscope grids, which are then negatively stained with 1% phosphotungstic acid for 30 s and examined. The combination of size and shape of the virions is sufficiently characteristic to allow a morphologic diagnosis of filovirus (28) even when the isolate is a new entity such as EBO-R (15). Differentiation of these virions and identification as MBG or EBO are accomplished by immunoelectron microscope techniques (11). Murine monoclonal antibodies and guinea pig polyclonal antisera have been successfully applied to recent filovirus isolates (Fig. 2). Adaptation of these techniques for diagnosis of arenavirus infections is now being developed. Retrospective examination of ultrathin sections of Formalin-fixed tissues obtained from patients at autopsy have occasionally revealed typical MBG, EBO, or arenavirus particles,

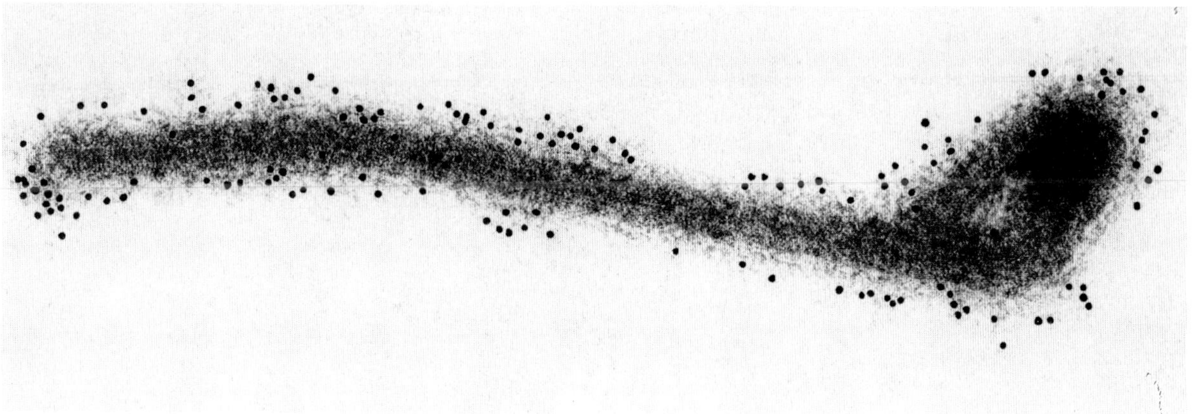

FIG. 2. Immunoelectron microscopic staining of EBO-R after incubation with polyclonal guinea pig anti-EBO serum, followed by anti-guinea pig IgG labeled with gold spheres; magnification ×119,000. (Courtesy of T. W. Geisbert.)

most often in the liver, spleen, or kidney, but only when infectious virus concentrations are very high. EBO-R particles were easily demonstrated by thin-section electron microscopy in tissues of monkeys dying in the 1989 epizootic (15) (Fig. 3).

Direct fluorescent-antibody (DFA) and indirect (IFA) immunofluorescence staining of impression smears or air-dried suspensions from liver, spleen, or kidney have been used successfully to detect cytoplasmic inclusion bodies associated with MBG infection; clumps of MBG antigen have also been observed by DFA examination of infected, dried, citrated blood smears (33). This approach was successfully adapted to the diagnosis of EBO-R in impression smears from blood, tissues, nasal turbinates, and urine. The approach has also been successfully applied to JUN-infected cells in peripheral blood and urinary sediment. Examination of frozen sections of infected tissues by DFA techniques should be feasible but is impractical because of the biohazard associated with this procedure and the difficulty in obtaining fresh, well-preserved tissues. Experience with DFA staining of tissues from monkeys experimentally infected with LAS suggests that antigens for this virus can be detected in diverse tissues when infectious virus concentrations exceed 6 $\log_{10}$ PFU per g. Development of immunohistochemical techniques for detection of filovirus and arenavirus antigens in Formalin-fixed tissues has recently advanced to the point that results are even more satisfactory than for IFA examination of frozen, acetone-fixed sections (21). For filoviruses, paraffin blocks of tissues are sectioned and mounted on silane-coated slides. They are deparaffinized, hydrated, digested with protease, and stained for the presence of viral antigens with cocktails of murine monoclonal antibodies (15). Biotinylated horse anti-mouse antiserum is then reacted, and the product is developed with a streptavidin-alkaline phosphatase system. This technique is expected to prove especially useful for the retrospective diagnosis of viral infections in archived tissues and paraffin blocks. However, extensive collections of field materials have not yet been examined.

Significant progress in development of in situ nucleic acid hybridization techniques has been reported, especially for LCM (34), but application of these methods in the clinical setting has not been reported. Likewise, significant progress has been achieved in the development of primer pairs for polymerase chain reaction techniques to detect viral nucleic acids in clinical materials, especially for EBO and EBO-related viruses. Comparisons with conventional isolation and antigen capture sensitivity and selectivity are under investigation.

ISOLATION OF VIRUS

The best general method currently available for isolation of MBG, EBO, and the pathogenic arenaviruses is the inoculation of appropriate cell cultures, usually Vero cells, followed by IFA or other immunologically specific testing of the inoculated cells for the presence

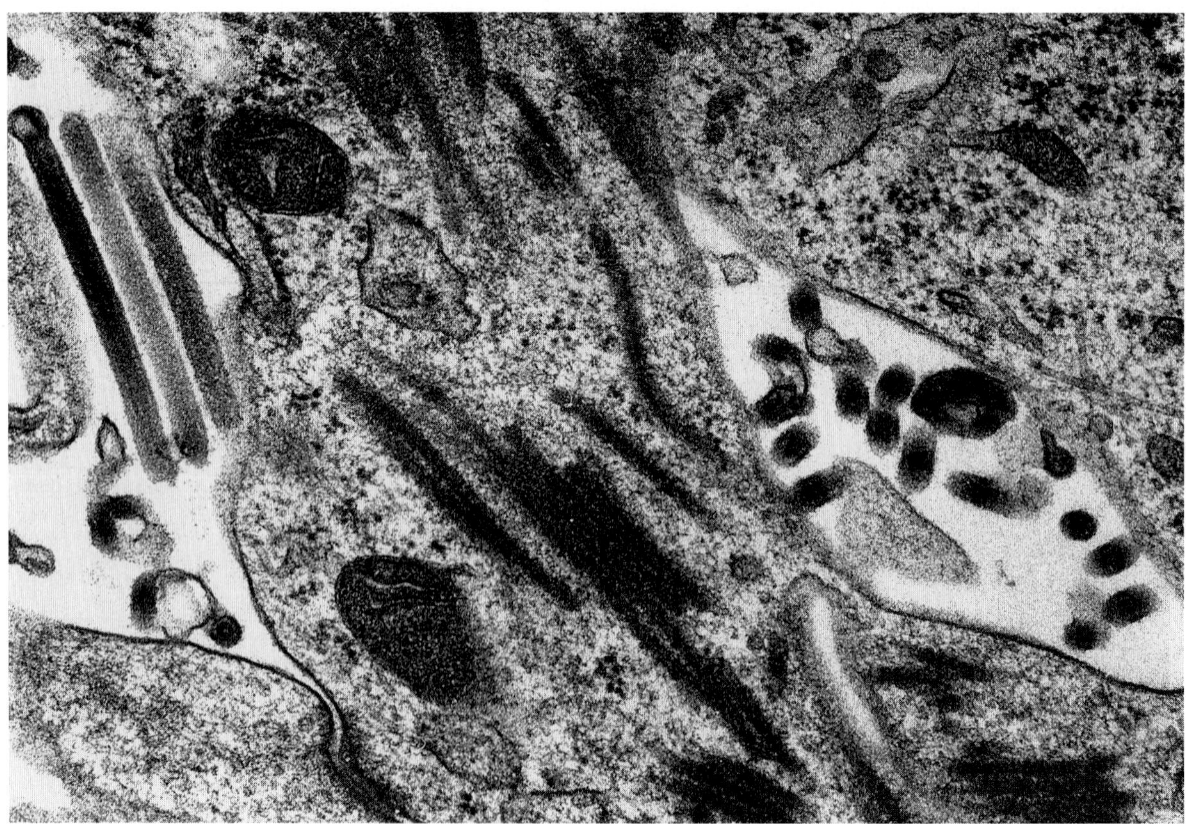

FIG. 3. Thin section of infected MA-104 cells, with EBO virions budding into intracytoplasmic vacuoles in longitudinal and cross section and intracytoplasmic inclusions formed by nucleocapsids; magnification, ×54,000. (Courtesy of T. W. Geisbert.)

of viral antigens. Especially for EBO-R and EBO-S, recent evidence suggests that MA-104 cells (from a fetal rhesus monkey kidney cell line) are more sensitive than Vero cells. Supernatant fluids should be collected for back-titration and confirmatory testing, as detailed below. Primary isolations in cell cultures have been routinely used for years to obtain LAS, MAC, JUN, MGB, and EBO-Z from field-collected materials. Vero cell inoculation should also work for LCM, but intracranial (i.c.) inoculation of weanling mice is still regarded as the most sensitive established indicator of LCM (13). EBO-S has also been isolated by Vero cell inoculation, but less reliably since several blind passages are usually required (26); SW-13 and MA-104 cells are reported to be more sensitive. Other cell lines, including human diploid lung (MRC-5) and BHK-21 cells, also support viral replication. Although historically MAC and JUN were isolated by i.c. inoculation of newborn hamsters and mice, respectively, Vero cells are approximately as sensitive and are far less cumbersome to manage in biosafety level 4 containment. Furthermore, Vero cells permit isolation and identification, usually within 1 to 5 days, a significant advantage over animals, which require 7 to 20 days of incubation for illness to develop.

Clinical specimens and clarified tissue homogenates (usually 10% [wt/vol]) are diluted in a suitable maintenance medium, such as Eagle minimal essential medium with Earle salts and 2% heat-inactivated calf serum, and adsorbed in small volumes to cell monolayers grown in suitable vessels, such as tissue culture T-25 flasks or 60-mm-diameter petri dishes. It is important to test higher dilutions of these specimens as well as more concentrated material, since autointerference (probably from defective interfering particles present in lower dilutions) may totally inhibit viral replication as measured by IFA, ELISA, or plaque formation. After adsorption, sufficient maintenance medium is added to maintain the cells for 7 days. Inoculation of replicate vessels permits destructive testing of cells at frequent intervals. Cells inoculated with high-titered samples contain antigen within 1 to 2 days of inoculation. Cells inoculated with low-titered material may require up to 7 days to accumulate detectable antigen. If no antigen is detected after 7 days, the sample is considered negative, but supernatant fluids should be blind passaged to confirm the absence of virus. When EBO-S is suspected, the requirement for blind passage is anticipated, and supernatant fluids are harvested and passaged at 3- to 5-day intervals. To confirm the presence and identity of the virus, supernatant fluids are tested for evidence of viral replication by plaquing (requires 4 to 8 days) or by ELISA techniques when available (requires several hours). Cocultivation of Ficoll-Hypaque-separated peripheral blood leukocytes with susceptible cells has increased the frequency of isolating JUN (1). Cocultivation of lymphocytes from spleens of experimentally infected animals has yielded LAS late in convalescence, even after neutralizing antibody has appeared. The technique merits systematic development for the remaining arenavirus and filovirus pathogens.

Although adequate cell culture systems exist for the isolation of LCM, most isolations to date have been obtained in mice. Weanling mice, 3 to 4 weeks old, are inoculated i.c. with undiluted samples. Since the "high dose" phenomenon of viral interference is occasionally a problem, a dilution of each sample (perhaps 1:100) is usually also inoculated into a second group of mice. Many LCM isolates produce a characteristic convulsive disease within 5 to 7 days, but some isolates take longer or may not produce death at all. To circumvent the problem of variable responses to different LCM strains, endotoxin (100 μg/0.2 ml), obtained from *Escherichia coli,* is inoculated intraperitoneally into mice 4 to 7 days after virus inoculation. All LCM-infected mice will die with a typical LCM disease within 24 h of endotoxin inoculation, regardless of the virus strain, whereas uninfected mice are unaffected (13). Brains from dead mice may be used to prepare CF or ELISA antigens or may be stained by IFA to obtain presumptive identification. Clarified mouse brain may also be used as an antigen for confirmatory testing by neutralization.

For primary isolation of the other arenaviruses, and for MBG and EBO, animal inoculations are still recommended only when adequate biocontainment facilities exist to maintain animals and when cell cultures are not available. Newborn mice (1 to 3 days old) are highly susceptible to JUN inoculated i.c.; newborn hamsters are believed to be more susceptible to MAC, although newborn mice have been used with success. Newborn hamsters and mice die 7 to 20 days after i.c. inoculation, usually exhibiting a characteristic "tail-spin" reaction. For the South American hemorrhagic fever viruses, particularly JUN, young adult guinea pigs inoculated either i.c. or peripherally have been used; the option to inoculate large volumes of potentially infectious material compensates for lower sensitivity of guinea pigs than of newborn mice and hamsters. Guinea pigs die 7 to 18 days after JUN inoculation. Most LCM strains are lethal for guinea pigs also. For LAS, animals have never been used routinely for virus isolation, although inbred strain 13 guinea pigs are exquisitely sensitive to most LAS strains and uniformly die 12 to 18 days after inoculation; outbred Hartley strain guinea pigs are somewhat less susceptible. The pathogenicity of virulent LAS strains for outbred Swiss albino mice inoculated i.c. seems to vary with different sources; mice should not be seriously considered for LAS isolations. MBG, EBO-Z, and EBO-S produce febrile responses in guinea pigs 4 to 10 days after inoculation; however, none of these viruses kills guinea pigs consistently on primary inoculation, and only EBO-Z has been adapted to uniform lethality by sequential guinea pig passages. EBO-Z is usually pathogenic for newborn mice inoculated i.c., but EBO-S, EBO-R, and MBG are not.

IDENTIFICATION OF VIRUS

Typing antisera

Detection of viral antigens in infected tissue culture cells (usually Vero) merits a presumptive diagnosis, provided the serologic reagents have been tested against all of the prototype arenaviruses and filoviruses expected in a given laboratory, thus permitting an interpretation of viral cross-reactions. Virus isolates in cell culture supernatant fluids or tissue homogenates are presumptively or specifically identified by their reactivities with diagnostic antisera in various serologic tests, described below. Specific polyclonal antisera are prepared in adult guinea pigs, hamsters, rats, or mice inoculated intraperitoneally with infectious virus. Rhesus and cynomolgus monkeys, convalescent from experimental infections, are also reasonable sources for larger quantities of immune sera. To compensate for any expected mortality, additional animals should be inoculated and the virus dose should be adjusted to ensure uniform infection with minimum mortality. Mortality may also be reduced by treatment of the animals with appropriate antiviral drugs, such as ribavirin or specific immune plasma (17). Diagnostic antisera produced in this way are less cross-reactive and usually higher titered than those produced by multiple injections of inactivated antigens. To further reduce the induction of extraneous antibodies, inoculum virus should be derived from tissues or cells homologous to the species being immunized; likewise, the virus suspension should be stabilized with homologous serum or serum proteins. Sera produced for use in the CF, DFA, and IFA tests should be collected 30 to 60 days after inoculation; sera for neutralization tests should be collected later. All sera must be rigorously tested for the presence of live virus before removal from a maximum containment system.

Production and use of specific murine monoclonal antibodies with fine specificities for N and GP epitopes of LCM, JUN, and other arenaviruses have been reported (3), and monoclonal antibodies for LAS, MBG, EBO-Z, and EBO-S with similar potential exist. Such antibodies have proven useful for defining epitopes and taxonomic relationships among these virus strains. One antibody, raised to a conserved sequence in the G2 region of LCM, has been found to react by ELISA and IFA with all arenavirus strains tested. This antibody might find utility as a pan-arenavirus detector in IFA and antigen capture ELISA procedures. Success has also been achieved with use of rats immunized with LCM and cells fused to the rat myeloma line Y3/Ag.1.2.3 (8). Reference reagents for LAS, MAC, MBG, and EBO are not generally available; hyperimmune mouse ascitic fluids for LCM and JUN are available from the Research Resources Branch, National Institutes of Health, Bethesda, Md.

Immunofluorescence procedures

To process infected cells for DFA examination and presumptive identification, inoculated cell monolayers are dispersed by trypsinization (0.05% trypsin with 0.02% EDTA for 10 min at 37°C), diluted in phosphate-buffered saline (PBS) containing 10% calf serum, and centrifuged at 400 × g for 10 min. The cell pellet is washed by resuspension in PBS and then centrifuged and resuspended in PBS to a final concentration of 10^6 cells per ml. Small drops (10 to 20 μl) of cell suspensions are placed onto circular areas of specially prepared epoxy-coated slides, cleaned previously by immersion in ethanol followed by polishing to remove residual oily deposits. These "spot slides" are air dried, fixed in acetone at room temperature for 10 min, and either stained immediately or stored frozen at −70°C. Although acetone fixation greatly reduces infectious intracellular virus, spot slides prepared in this manner should still be considered infectious and handled accordingly. Recently, spot slides have been rendered noninfectious by gamma radiation (10), with no diminution in fluorescent-antigen intensity. Alternatively, infected cells may be biologically inactivated with beta-propiolactone (35). Gamma radiation is recommended if the appropriate equipment is available.

For DFA tests, specific immunoglobulin, prepared by ethanol or ammonium sulfate precipitation of immune sera followed by conjugation with fluorescein, is diluted to a working concentration predetermined by box titration and flooded onto the infected cells, which are incubated at room temperature for 30 min in a moist chamber. After incubation, the slides are washed by immersion in PBS for two 10-min periods, dipped in water to remove salts, dried by evaporation, and mounted under cover slips in PBS-glycerol (pH 7.8). Specific viral fluorescence is characterized as intense, punctate to granular aggregates confined to the cytoplasm of infected cells. Specific MBG and EBO fluorescence may include large, bizarre-shaped aggregates up to 10 μm across. Nonspecific fluorescence is rarely a problem in DFA procedures for these viruses. Detection of MBG, EBO, LAS, and LCM antigens by DFA is usually considered sufficient for a definitive diagnosis, although LAS and LCM cross-react at low levels in this test. Detection of JUN or MAC antigens by DFA constitutes a presumptive diagnosis, since these viruses can be reliably distinguished from each other only by neutralization tests.

CF test

The CF test was routinely used in early investigations for detection and presumptive identification of the arenaviruses and MBG. However, the CF test is rarely used now, since the development of reliable, simplified, and more sensitive immunofluorescence procedures described above. Detailed instructions for performing the CF test for arenaviruses are available (4), and the method can be applied to MBG and EBO as well. In brief, CF antigens are prepared from infected Vero cell culture supernatant fluids or from suckling mouse or suckling hamster brains extracted by sucrose-acetone. For reasons of safety, CF antigens are frequently inactivated by addition of beta-propiolactone, and they may be stored frozen at −70°C indefinitely or preserved by lyophilization.

ELISA

Availability of an ELISA for quantitative detection of arenavirus and filovirus antigens in viremic sera and tissue culture supernatants would facilitate early detection and identification of these agents. An antigen capture ELISA for LAS antigens (30) is now undergoing field testing in West Africa, using IFA and conventional isolation for comparison. The threshold sensitivity for the assay is approximately 2.1 $\log_{10}$ PFU per ml, so it may be sufficiently sensitive to detect antigen in most acute-phase LAS viremias as well as virus concentrations in throat wash and urine samples. Since the test reliably detects LAS antigen in beta-propiolactone-inactivated samples, it can be conducted safely without elaborate containment facilities. The basic approach is that of a triple-antibody (sandwich) capture assay in which antigen is captured by antibody as a solid phase and then detected by an additional two-antibody sandwich. A detection system using alkaline phosphatase and *p*-nitrophenylphosphate (PNPP) is then applied to determine how much of the detection antibody has been retained on the solid phase of the system. For LAS, the successful development of the system depended critically on the use of highly avid, LAS-specific, affinity-purified globulin preparations. Polystyrene microtiter plates (Dynatech no. M29AR) have provided the most uniform results in our system. Briefly, plates are coated with an antibody capable of capturing viral antigen from the test sample. For LAS, affinity-purified monkey anti-LAS immunoglobulin G (IgG) is used at a predetermined dilution (1:200). After overnight incubation at 4°C, plates are washed and test sample dilutions are added. After incubation and washing of the reaction wells, guinea pig anti-LAS immunoglobulin is added as a detector antibody, followed by rabbit anti-guinea pig IgG and then alkaline phosphatase-labeled swine anti-rabbit IgG; finally, PNPP diluted in 1 M diethanolamine buffer is added. Plates are incubated and washed after each reagent except PNPP. The reaction is read spectrophotometrically after 20 min at room temperature. A sample is considered positive if the optical density (OD) is significantly higher than the mean background (average of 30 negative samples plus 2 standard deviations). All samples are tested in duplicate. To detect nonspecific binding (i.e., "sticky" sera), each serum sample is also added to one well treated as described above but with normal (nonimmune) guinea pig immunoglobulin substituted for LAS-immune guinea pig immunoglobulin. At present, sticky sera for which the OD of the control well appears positive cannot be tested reliably. Other detection systems have been successfully used, especially horseradish peroxidase–2,2′-azino-di-(3-ethylbenzthiazoline sulfonate [6]) (ABTS), but the experience with African sera is that lower backgrounds are achieved with the alkaline phosphatase-PNPP system.

For JUN detection, a test similar in principle has been developed, utilizing anti-JUN mouse monoclonal antibody for capture, anti-JUN rabbit serum as the detector, and horseradish peroxidase-conjugated goat anti-rabbit IgG plus ABTS for color development. The test has been compared favorably with virus isolation in mice for sensitivity in detection of viremia in AHF patients in Argentina. Similar techniques for LCM exist but have not been systematically tested in the clinical setting. Substitution of monoclonal antibody of high avidity and appropriate specificities for polyclonal sera generally increases the sensitivities and specificities of these antigen capture ELISAs. However, monoclonal antibodies with broad cross-reactivity (36) are potentially useful for development of a general pan-arenavirus detector system.

Recently, an antigen capture ELISA was also developed for EBO. Although it utilizes murine monoclonal antibodies produced against EBO-Z and EBO-S, it proved extremely sensitive and accurate in detecting EBO-R in tissues from monkeys dying in the 1989 epizootic (15). The principle is similar to that used in the LAS antigen capture ELISA, with some modifications. The assay is a double-sandwich capture ELISA (Fig. 4). Plates are coated overnight with a mixture of monoclonal antibodies and washed, and unknowns are added in fourfold dilutions in SerDil. After incubation and wash steps, polyclonal rabbit anti-EBO serum is added, the specimen is incubated and washed, and anti-rabbit IgG is added. Color development, by the horseradish peroxidase-ABTS system, is proportional to the quantity of EBO antigen captured on the plate. Samples are considered positive if the OD exceeds the mean plus 3 standard deviations for the normal controls. During the EBO-R epizootic, very close concordance was obtained between conventional isolation and the antigen capture ELISA techniques. The suitability of this test for clinical

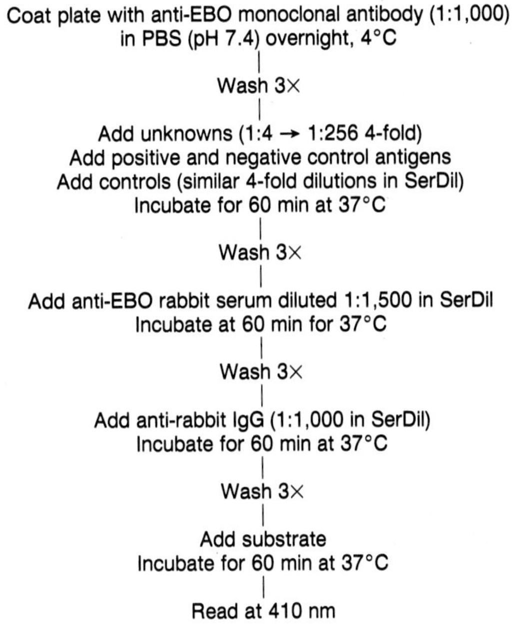

Coat plate with anti-EBO monoclonal antibody (1:1,000)
in PBS (pH 7.4) overnight, 4°C

Wash 3×

Add unknowns (1:4 → 1:256 4-fold)
Add positive and negative control antigens
Add controls (similar 4-fold dilutions in SerDil)
Incubate for 60 min at 37°C

Wash 3×

Add anti-EBO rabbit serum diluted 1:1,500 in SerDil
Incubate at 60 min for 37°C

Wash 3×

Add anti-rabbit IgG (1:1,000 in SerDil)
Incubate for 60 min at 37°C

Wash 3×

Add substrate
Incubate for 60 min at 37°C

Read at 410 nm

FIG. 4. Flow chart for EBO antigen capture ELISA (all volumes = 100 μl).

materials from human patients infected with EBO-Z and EBO-S is predicted to be good but awaits systematic testing of field-collected materials.

Neutralization tests

Neutralization tests for these viruses take many forms; depending on the virus, neutralization tests range from extremely sensitive and reliable (e.g., for JUN and MAC) and moderately insensitive but reliable (for LAS and LCM) to totally unreliable (for MBG and EBO). The common denominator in all neutralization tests is measurement of an inhibition of viral replication by reaction with immune serum. Thus, the form of the test is determined in part by the availability of tools to measure infectious virus or viral antigens (e.g., plaques, DFA, CF, ELISA, or animal infectivity) as well as the kinetics of the virus-antibody interactions. The unreliability of the MBG and EBO neutralization tests may be partially a function of the primitive and cumbersome viral quantitation procedures available as well as low-avidity antibody. For the New World arenaviruses (JUN and MAC), the most generally applied neutralization test is a plaque reduction test using Vero cells and the serum dilution-constant virus format. The serum dilution calculated (by probit analysis) to reduce the control number of plaques by 50% is usually taken as the endpoint, although in some laboratories the highest serum dilution producing 80% reduction (PRN-80) is used. The PRN-80 test is commonly used to distinguish JUN from MAC. For LAS and LCM, neutralizing antibody activity is rapidly lost upon dilution; for this reason, the constant serum dilution-varying virus format is preferred. Neutralization of Old World arenaviruses is also markedly enhanced by addition of complement; thus, 10% fresh guinea pig serum is routinely added to the diluent. Plaque reduction is further enhanced by addition of either anti-immunoglobulin or protein A. Plaque reduction tests in various formats have largely replaced animal protection tests, which were notoriously imprecise for measurement of arenavirus neutralizing antibody.

SEROLOGIC DIAGNOSIS

IFA test

The IFA test is clearly the method of choice for documenting recent infections with MBG, EBO, and the arenaviruses. Preparation of spot slides with use of infected Vero cells is identical to the procedure described above. Uninfected cells are often admixed with the virus-infected cells to aid discrimination between specific and nonspecific fluorescence. Although monovalent spot slides are usually desired and are prepared with cells optimally infected with a single virus, polyvalent spot slides can also be prepared by mixing cells infected with different viruses selected from these or other taxonomic groups which have similar geographic distributions (18). Test sera are diluted serially, usually in twofold increments, starting at 1:4 or 1:10. Prozones may occur in low dilutions. Thus, for screening procedures, sera are commonly tested at both 1:10 and 1:80 dilutions. Infected cells (and uninfected control cells) are incubated with serum dilutions, washed, reincubated with appropriate fluorescein-conjugated antiglobulin (or specific anti-IgM or anti-IgG), washed, mounted, and observed. Endpoint determination is very subjective. Most experienced observers consider the endpoint to be the highest dilution producing typical cytoplasmic fluorescence clearly positive relative to that produced by uninfected cells. Although it is possible to obtain reproducible endpoints within individual laboratories, discrepancies in titers determined by different laboratories are common and probably relate to variations in interpretation, epi-illumination intensity, filtration systems, and fluorescein conjugates. The presence of specific IgM antibodies or a rising IFA titer constitutes a presumptive diagnosis of acute infection. IgM antibodies measured by IFA decline to undetectable titers within several months, whereas IgG antibodies, which are thought to compete with IgM in IFA tests, persist for at least several years (37).

CF test

The CF test was used initially to classify the arenaviruses and to detect seroconversions. However, the CF test is rarely used now because it is inferior to the IFA test for both arenavirus and filovirus infections. CF antibody titers evolve more slowly (3 to 4 weeks after onset) and recede rapidly to undetectable levels (usually within 1 year). The CF test is less specific than the IFA test, and anticomplementary sera are frequently encountered. Since the CF test is often used to screen aseptic meningitis specimens against a battery of antigens, a CF antigen for LCM is often appropriately included in this battery.

Neutralization tests

As described above, reliable protocols for measuring neutralizing antibody to MBG and EBO are not available. For the arenaviruses, plaque reduction tests using Vero cells are generally used. For measuring neutralizing antibody to LAS and LCM, which are both difficult to neutralize and poor inducers of this antibody, test sera are diluted, usually 1:10, in medium containing 10% guinea pig serum as a complement source and mixed with serial dilutions of challenge virus. Titers are expressed as a $\log_{10}$ neutralization index, defined as $\log_{10}$ PFU in control $-$ $\log_{10}$ PFU in test serum. For JUN and MAC, the more conventional serum dilution-constant virus format is usually used, although the constant serum-virus dilution format is equally useful for distinguishing among strains. Neutralizing antibody responses require weeks to months to evolve but persist for years. Performance of these tests is restricted to laboratories equipped to handle the infectious viruses.

ELISA for detection of IgG and IgM antibodies

ELISA procedures for LAS-specific IgG and IgM have been developed (30) and successfully used on field-collected human sera. With these techniques in combination with the LAS antigen capture ELISA described above, virtually all LAS fever patients can be specifically diagnosed within hours of hospital admission. As for the antigen capture ELISA, success is critically dependent on highly avid, purified capture antibodies or globulins. For detection of LAS IgG, guinea pig anti-LAS is diluted (1:200) in coating buffer and incubated in 100-μl volumes in wells of 96-well polystyrene plates. After incubation for 1 h at 37°C, the plates are washed four times, 100 μl of inactivated (gamma-irradiated) LAS antigen is added, and the specimen is incubated for 1 h. After four washes, 100 μl of test serum dilutions (usually starting at 1:1,000) is added. After incubation and washing, 100 μl of alkaline phosphate-labeled anti-human IgG (1:200 dilutions) is added, and the specimen is incubated and washed. Finally, PNPP in diethanolamine buffer is added for color development, and the reaction is read after 20 min at 405 nm. For detection of IgM, an IgM capture ELISA using goat anti-human IgM (μ-chain specific) diluted 1:200 has been most successful. After incubation for 2 h at 37°C and four washes in SerDil, test sera, diluted 1:400 in ELISA buffer, are added (100 μl per well). After 1 h of incubation at 37°C, 100 μl of inactivated LAS antigen is added, and the plates are reincubated for 1 h at 37°C. Four washes are followed by guinea pig anti-LAS immunoglobulin, diluted 1:200 in ELISA buffer (100 μl), and incubation for 1 h at 37°C. After another four washes, goat anti-guinea pig IgG conjugated with alkaline phosphatase (Kirkegaard & Perry Laboratories), diluted 1:400 in ELISA buffer, is added. The plates are incubated again for 1 h at 37°C and washed four times, and 100 μl of PNPP is added. The reaction is read after 15 min at room temperature by use of a spectrophotometer at 405 nm. For detection and control of nonspecific binding, all samples (both IgG and IgM) are run in duplicate wells, on plates with LAS antigens and on plates with uninfected Vero cell culture fluids substituted for LAS antigens. A sample is considered positive when the OD is higher than the mean (plus 2 standard deviations) of the OD of 20 sera known to be negative. A significant advantage of these ELISA procedures is that beta-propiolactone or other methods can be used to inactivate viral infectivity in clinical samples, thus adding an extra measure of safety. For JUN, similar IgG ELISAs have provided promising results with use of paired sera, but detection of IgM antibodies has been less successful. ELISA procedures for specific IgG and IgM responses to EBO and MBG have not been sufficiently developed to merit field testing.

Other serologic tests

Other serologic tests have been applied to diagnosis. Gel diffusion tests have been used for arenaviruses, but those tests detect antibodies directed primarily against nucleocapsid and are less sensitive than the IFA or even the CF test; thus, gel diffusion tests have little role in modern diagnosis. Another test developed for LAS (and antibodies) is a reversed passive hemagglutination (and inhibition) test using LAS antibody-coated erythrocytes that agglutinate in the presence of viral antigen (12). The test has not gained widespread acceptance, perhaps because meticulous care is required to obtain satisfactory antibody-erythrocyte conjugates. For EBO, a radioimmunoassay using ^{125}I-labeled staphylococcal protein A was successfully used on many human and animal sera and discriminated EBO-Z from EBO-S strains (32). Radioimmunoassay and Western immunoblotting procedures have also been used in specialized laboratories to confirm the results of serosurveys based on the IFA test. The places that these specialized procedures will assume in the routine diagnosis of MGB, EBO, and arenavirus infections remains to be determined.

EVALUATION AND INTERPRETATION OF RESULTS

Early diagnosis of arenavirus and filovirus infection is desirable, since specific immune plasma and appropriately selected antiviral drugs are often effective when treatment is initiated soon after onset. Early recognition of these infections should also trigger strict isolation procedures to prevent spread of the disease to patient contacts. In areas where specific viruses are endemic, the index of suspicion is often high, and experienced clinicians may be remarkably accurate in rendering an accurate diagnosis of fully developed cases on clinical grounds alone. Yet even in these areas, specific virologic and serologic tests are required to confirm clinical impressions, since many other diseases, including malaria, typhoid, rickettsiosis, idiopathic thrombocytopenia, and viral hepatitis, may masquerade as an arenavirus or filovirus infection. Although the availability of inactivated-antigen spot slides for IFA in field hospitals has facilitated diagnosis, based on seroconversion by IFA, timely diagnosis requires a means to detect infectious virus or antigen in the field. The ELISA for LAS antigen detection holds promise, since it will detect clinically relevant viremia in beta-propiolactone-inactivated sera. Similar detection systems are urgently required for the other viruses.

Inoculation of tissue cultures for DFA examination and isolation of these viruses should not be conducted outside a maximum containment laboratory, with the exception of LCM, which may be handled at a lower containment level (6). The detection of viral antigens by DFA in Vero cells inoculated with patient specimens constitutes a definitive diagnosis, except for JUN and MAC, which are reliably discriminated from each other only by the neutralization test. Other virus strains that cross-react by DFA, such as LAS with LCM and EBO-Z with EBO-S, can be distinguished in quantitative cross-testing by DFA. For virus isolates originating from areas where the geographic distributions of related viruses overlap, it is essential that quantitative DFA testing be done and desirable that identification be confirmed by neutralization tests when available.

Although interpretation of serologic data is usually facilitated by the generally restricted geographic ranges of these viruses, ranges do overlap and occasionally IFA and CF data are ambiguous. In one documented outbreak, patients with clinical AHF developed CF antibody rises to both JUN and LCM (23). The geographic distributions of JUN and MAC certainly overlap that of LCM in South America. In Africa, the distribution of LAS may overlap those of newly isolated virus strains from rodents in Zimbabwe, Mozambique, and the Central African Republic which cross-react strongly by IFA with LAS and, to a lesser extent, with LCM. Although these strains are not known to be associated with human disease, their presence may confuse interpretation of serologic data from African surveys. The extent to which heterologous arenavirus infection or reinfection broadens antibody specificity has not been systematically evaluated for any of the available serologic tests. For EBO, antibodies reacting in the IFA test have been detected in populations such as Panamanian Indians that have never experienced clinical EBO infections, thus casting doubt on the validity of this test for any population, including those in which EBO infections have been documented virologically. Despite these potential problems, the experience to date has been that in the midst of outbreaks caused by MBG, EBO, or the arenaviruses, identifications of the etiologic agents by using DFA and IFA have been clear and unambiguous, especially when the diagnoses were confirmed by neutralization tests.

Because of the biohazard, virus isolation data for these viruses is usually available only retrospectively. MBG and EBO-Z are usually isolated from acute-phase sera, whereas EBO-S is isolated less often, perhaps because of the need for blind passage. LAS is usually recovered from acute-phase sera of hospitalized patients soon after admission, frequently in the presence of specific IgM antibody. JUN, MAC, and LCM are recovered less frequently, and diagnosis is usually based on seroconversion. The IFA response is the earliest for all of these viruses, detectable 7 to 10 days after onset for LAS and LCM, 10 to 14 days for MBG and EBO, 12 to 17 days for JUN, and 17 to 30 days for MAC. The CF antibodies evolve several days after the IFA response. The presence of specific IgM antibodies detected by the IFA test is indicative of recent infection, since IFA IgM titers persist for less than 3 months. The presence of specific IFA IgM in the cerebrospinal fluid of LCM patients constitutes a definitive diagnosis. For all of the arenavirus and filovirus pathogens, a rising IFA IgM or IgG titer constitutes a strong presumptive diagnosis. Since IFA IgM titers, as well as CF titers, do not persist long, a decreasing titer suggests a recent infection that occurred perhaps several months previously.

For Lassa fever patients, a detectable IFA response does not necessarily signal imminent recovery; viremia frequently persists, and patients die after an IFA response. For JUN, LCM, MBG, and EBO infections, the appearance of antibodies detectable by IFA coincides with disappearance of viremia and with recovery. In MAC infection, IFA titers appear even later, 1 week or more after the crisis has passed. For the arenaviruses, neutralizing antibodies appear much later in convalescence than do IFA or CF antibodies. Reliable neutralizing antibody data for MBG and EBO infections are not available. Neutralizing antibodies against arenaviruses persist for long periods, perhaps for life, and thus provide the most reliable basis for determining the minimum resistance of a population to reinfection. The role of neutralizing antibody in acute recovery is less clear. The protective efficacy of passively administered immune plasma is believed to be a function of neutralizing antibody titers (24), and selection of plasma should be on this basis, especially for Lassa fever, since protective efficacy is predicted by neutralizing antibody titers and not by IFA (16). A serologic test to predict the efficacy of MBG- and EBO-immune plasma is urgently needed.

The highest priority for future development is refinement of the available diagnostic tools to permit definitive virus identifications in the field. A reasonable approach is adaptation of the available LAS and EBO antigen capture ELISAs to the other viruses, using biologically inactivated samples. For broad screening procedures, a highly avid, cross-reactive monoclonal antibody might be used, while a battery of type-specific monoclonal antibodies could be used for definitive identification. This investment in rapid diagnosis will permit more timely intervention with effective treatment regimens and, through implementation of appropriate public health measures, may reduce dissemination of these highly virulent viral pathogens.

LITERATURE CITED

1. **Ambrosio, A. M., D. A. Enria, and J. I. Maiztegui.** 1986. Junin virus isolation from lympho-mononuclear cells of patients with Argentine hemorrhagic fever. Intervirology **25:**97–102.
2. **Buchmeier, M. J., R. U. DeFries, J. B. McCormick, and M. P. Kiley.** 1983. Comparative analysis of the structural polypeptides of Ebola viruses from Sudan and Zaire. J. Infect. Dis. **147:**276–281.
3. **Buchmeier, M. J., H. A. Lewicki, O. Tomori, and M. B. A. Oldstone.** 1981. Monoclonal antibodies to lymphocytic choriomeningitis and Pichinde viruses: generation, characterization, and cross-reactivity with other arenaviruses. Virology **113:**73–85.
4. **Casals, J.** 1977. Serologic reactions with arenaviruses. Medicina (Buenos Aires) **37**(Suppl. 3)**:**59–68.
5. **Centers for Disease Control.** 1980. Interstate shipment of etiologic agents. Fed. Regist. **45:**48626–48629.
6. **Centers for Disease Control.** 1983. Biosafety in microbiology and biomedical laboratories. Centers for Disease Control, Atlanta, Ga.
7. **Centers for Disease Control.** 1988. Management of patients with suspected viral hemorrhagic fever. Morbid. Mortal. Weekly Rep. **37**(Suppl. 3)**:**1–16.
8. **Clark, M., S. Cobbold, G. Hale, and H. Waldmann.** 1983. Advantages of rat monoclonal antibodies. Immunol. Today **4:**100–101.
9. **Cox, N. J., J. B. McCormick, K. M. Johnson, and M. P. Kiley.** 1983. Evidence for two subtypes of Ebola virus based on oligonucleotide mapping of RNA. J. Infect. Dis. **147:** 272–275.
10. **Elliott, L. H., J. B. McCormick, and K. M. Johnson.** 1982. Inactivation of Lassa, Marburg, and Ebola viruses by gamma irradiation. J. Clin. Microbiol. **16:**704–708.
11. **Geisbert, T. W., and P. B. Jahrling.** 1990. Use of immunoelectron microscopy to show Ebola virus during the 1989 United States epizootic. J. Clin. Pathol. **43:**813–816.
12. **Goldwasser, R. A., L. H. Elliott, and K. M. Johnson.** 1980. Preparation and use of erythrocyte-globulin conjugates to Lassa virus in reversed passive hemagglutination and inhibition. J. Clin. Microbiol. **11:**593–599.
13. **Hotchin, J., and E. Sikora.** 1975. Laboratory diagnosis of lymphocytic choriomeningitis. Bull. WHO **52:**555–558.
14. **International Committee on Taxonomy of Viruses.** 1982. Arenaviruses. Intervirology **17:**119–122.
15. **Jahrling, P. B., T. W. Geisbert, D. W. Dalgard, E. D. Johnson, T. G. Ksiazek, W. C. Hall, and C. J. Peters.** 1990. Preliminary report: isolation of Ebola virus from monkeys imported to USA. Lancet **335:**502–505.
16. **Jahrling, P. B., and C. J. Peters.** 1984. Passive antibody therapy of Lassa fever in cynomolgus monkeys. Infect. Immun. **44:**528–533.
17. **Jahrling, P. B., C. J. Peters, and E. L. Stephen.** 1984. Enhanced treatment of Lassa fever by immune plasma combined with ribavirin in cynomolgus monkeys. J. Infect. Dis. **149:**420–427.
18. **Johnson, K. M., L. H. Elliott, and D. L. Heymann.** 1981. Preparation of polyvalent viral immunofluorescent intracellular antigens and use in human serosurveys. J. Clin. Microbiol. **14:**527–529.
19. **Kiley, M. P., E. T. W. Bowen, G. A. Eddy, et al.** 1982. Filoviridae: a taxonomic home for Marburg and Ebola viruses? Intervirology **18:**24–32.
20. **Kiley, M. P., N. J. Cox, L. H. Elliott, et al.** 1988. Physiochemical properties of Marburg virus: evidence for three distinct virus strains and their relationship to Ebola virus. J. Gen. Virol. **69:**1957–1967.
21. **Lascano, E. F., M. I. Berria, and N. A. Candurra.** 1981. Diagnosis of Junin virus in cell cultures by immunoperoxidase staining. Arch. Virol. **70:**79–82.
22. **Lehmann-Grube, F.** 1971. Lymphocytic choriomeningitis virus. Virol. Monogr. **10:**1–173.
23. **Maiztegui, J. I., G. M. Aguirre, M. S. Sabattini, and J. G. B. Oro.** 1971. Activated de dos "arenavirus" en seres humanos y roedores en un mismo lugar de la zona endemica de fiebre hemorragica Argentina. Medicina (Buenos Aires) **31:**509–510.
24. **Maiztegui, J. I., N. J. Fernandez, and A. J. de Damilano.** 1979. Efficacy of immune plasma in treatment of Argentine hemorrhagic fever and association between treatment and a late neurological syndrome. Lancet **ii:**1216–1217.
25. **Martini, G. A.** 1971. Marburg virus disease. Clinical syndrome, p. 1–9. *In* G. A. Martini and R. Siegert (ed.), Marburg virus disease. Springer-Verlag, New York.
26. **McCormick, J. B., S. P. Bauer, L. H. Elliott, P. A. Webb, and K. M. Johnson.** 1983. Biologic differences between strains of Ebola virus for Zaire and Sudan. J. Infect. Dis. **147:**264–267.
27. **Monson, M. H., A. K. Cole, J. D. Frame, J. R. Serwint, S. Alexander, and P. B. Jahrling.** 1987. Pediatric Lassa fever: a review of 33 Liberian cases. Am. J. Trop. Med. Hyg. **36:**408–415.
28. **Murphy, F. A., G. Van der Groen, S. G. Whitfield, and J. V. Lange.** 1978. Ebola and Marburg virus morphology and taxonomy, p. 61–84. *In* S. R. Pattyn (ed.), Ebola virus haemorrhagic fever. Elsevier/North-Holland Biomedical Press, Amsterdam.
29. **Murphy, F. A., and S. G. Whitfield.** 1975. Morphology and morphogenesis of arenaviruses. Bull. WHO **52:**409–419.
30. **Niklasson, B. S., P. B. Jahrling, and C. J. Peters.** 1984. Detection of Lassa virus antigens and Lassa-specific immunoglobulins G and M by enzyme-linked immunosorbent assay. J. Clin. Microbiol. **20:**239–244.
31. **Pedersen, I. R.** 1979. Structural components and replication of arenaviruses. Adv. Virus Res. **24:**277–330.
32. **Richman, D. D., P. H. Cleveland, J. B. McCormick, and K. M. Johnson.** 1983. Antigenic analysis of strains of Ebola virus: identification of two Ebola virus serotypes. J. Infect. Dis. **147:**268–271.
33. **Siegert, R., and W. Slencyka.** 1971. Laboratory diagnosis

and pathogenesis, p. 157–160. *In* G. A. Martini and R. Siegert (ed.), Marburg virus disease. Springer-Verlag, New York.

34. **Southern, P. J., and M. B. A. Oldstone.** 1986. Molecular anatomy of viral infection: study of viral nucleic acid sequences and proteins in whole body sections. *In* M. B. A. Oldstone (ed.), Concepts in viral pathogenesis II. Springer-Verlag, New York.
35. **Van der Groen, G., and L. H. Elliott.** 1982. Use of beta-propiolactone-inactivated Ebola, Marburg, and Lassa intracellular antigens in immunofluorescent antibody assay. Ann. Soc. Belg. Med. Trop. **62:**49–54.
36. **Weber, E. L., and J. J. Buchmeier.** 1988. Fine mapping of a peptide sequence containing an antigenic site conserved among arenaviruses. Virology **164:**30–38.
37. **Wulff, H., and K. M. Johnson.** 1979. Immunoglobulin M and G responses measured by immunofluorescence in patients with Lassa or Marburg virus infections. Bull. WHO **57:**631–635.
38. **Wulff, H., J. V. Lange, and P. A. Webb.** 1978. Interrelationships among arenaviruses measured by indirect immunofluorescence. Intervirology **9:**344–350.

Chapter 98

Papillomaviruses

DENNIS J. McCANCE

The genera *Papillomavirus* and *Polyomavirus* constitute the family *Papovaviridae*. The virions of the two genera are similar physically in that they are icosahedral in structure, but a number of properties, such as genome size, genomic organization, and pathogenesis, suggest that the genera are quite different.

The papillomaviruses (Latin: *papilla,* nipple; Greek: *oma,* tumor) produce in their hosts, whether animal or human, benign epithelial tumors (papillomas or warts) which have been recognized lesions for centuries. Common hand warts and plantar warts are among the most frequent skin lesions in humans, but since they are benign and only a cosmetic nuisance, they have generated little clinical or scientific interest. Since papillomaviruses have been associated with (i) squamous cell carcinomas in patients with the rare autosomal recessive disease epidermodysplasia verruciformis (EV) and (ii) genital cancer in both males and females, interest has grown. However, the inability to propagate the viruses in conventional tissue culture remains a major obstacle to research.

DESCRIPTION OF THE AGENT

The capsid of the papillomaviruses has an icosahedral symmetry containing 72 capsomeres and is 52 to 55 nm in diameter.

The papillomavirus genome is a double-stranded circular, supercoiled DNA molecule of approximately 5.0×10^6 daltons. Viral transcripts appear to be coded for by one strand only, with the other strand containing numerous stop codons. The genome codes for 8 to 10 proteins; the number is uncertain because a function or protein product has not been assigned to each of the open reading frames (ORFs) (Fig. 1) predicted from the DNA sequence. As Fig. 1 shows, the genome arrangement is very similar between different human papillomavirus (HPV) types.

The ORFs designated with an E prefix are produced early in infection; those with an L prefix are produced late in the replicative cycle (3). In fact, this convention does not hold true for all ORFs, since E4 is known to be produced late in infection in warts containing HPV type 1 (HPV-1) and HPV-2 (6).

The major capsid protein, L1, has a molecular size of approximately 55,000 daltons, and the minor capsid, L2, has a size of approximately 76,000 daltons. The capsid proteins of animal and human papillomaviruses are highly conserved, and polyclonal antibodies against a disrupted virus particle, such as bovine papillomavirus type 1 (BPV-1), will cross-react with other disrupted particles of animal and human papillomaviruses. This characteristic provides the basis for the immunocytochemical detection of papillomaviruses in the epithelia of various lesions.

Between the carboxyl terminus of the L1 ORF and the amino terminus of E6 is a noncoding region that contains enhancer and promoter elements and an origin of replication (Fig. 1). The origin of replication was detected in BPV-1 (30), but an equivalent region in HPV has yet to be established.

The activities of some of the early proteins (E) are known and are summarized below.

The E6/E7 region is important for the transformation of primary rodent cells in cooperation with an activated *ras* gene. It appears that E7 has a dominant role in this process (20). For the immortalization of primary human keratinocytes, both E6 and E7 are required (11, 17). Both E6 and E7 ORF products have been detected in cells transformed in vitro and in cells grown from fresh cervical tumor tissue by immunoprecipitation using antibodies raised against bacterial fusion proteins. In addition, E7 has been immunoprecipitated from fresh cervical tumor tissue (23, 26) and has been shown to have transactivation activities similar to those of E1A of adenovirus (20). Recently E7, which has a region of homology with the E1A gene of adenovirus and large T gene of simian virus 40, has been shown to bind to the retinoblastoma gene (RB) product (8). Mutations of both alleles of RB predispose to retinoblastoma and other sarcomas, and consequently this gene has been classified as an antioncogene; i.e., in its absence, tumors arise. The E1A gene of adenovirus and large T gene of simian virus 40 are also transforming genes, and they bind to the RB product. This finding has led to the theory that these viruses may transform cells through a common, as yet unknown pathway.

E1 has been shown, at least for BPV-1, to be involved in replication and maintenance of episomal DNA in rodent cell cultures. The E1 ORF may code for more than one protein. The 3′ half is known to be essential for transient and long-term extrachromosomal replication of BPV-1 DNA in mouse C-127 cells. The 5′ portion encodes a 23-kilodalton protein, called the modulator, which establishes and maintains 100 to 200 copies of BPV-1 DNA per cell in long-term, stable replication assays (28). However, since 5′ mutants are capable of replication in C-127 cells in transient assays, the product encoded by this region is not necessary for the initial phase of BPV-1 replication. Since this region is highly conserved between papillomaviruses, it is likely that the E1 of HPV has the same or similar activities.

E2 is known to be a strong transactivator of the noncoding region of BPV and HPV DNAs (19, 27). The ORF appears to code for at least two proteins, one a full-length product that transactivates and the other a trun-

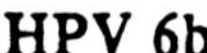

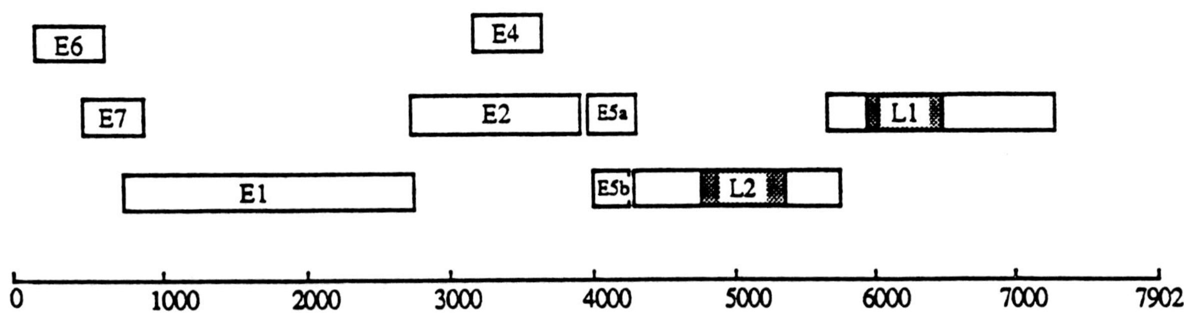

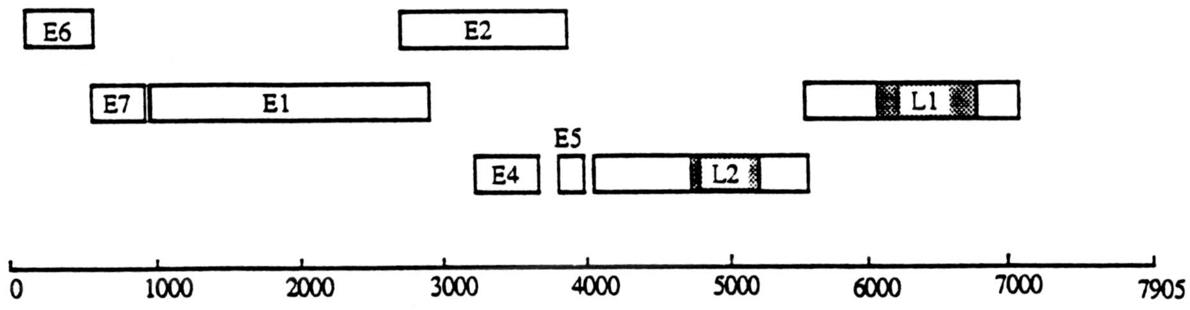

FIG. 1. Organization of the ORFs of HPV-6b and HPV-16.

cated (carboxy-terminal half) product that inhibits transactivation (14). The carboxyl-terminal half is thought to bind DNA, while the amino-terminal part contains the transactivating function.

E5 is the major transforming gene of BPV-1 (5). This region of HPV does not appear to have a similar, or at least as efficient, function. However, all E5 regions of both animal and human viruses so far sequenced are predicted to code for proteins with similar physicochemical properties. Each has three hydrophobic peaks (two in the case of BPV-1) and a hydrophilic carboxy terminus (1). Each hydrophobic region is long enough to transverse the cell membrane, and E5 has been shown by immunoprecipitation studies to be membrane associated. It is therefore conceivable that the functions of the E5 proteins are similar, but perhaps to different degrees in different cell types. For instance, BPV-1 DNA replicates in rodent fibroblasts but HPV cannot. Therefore, there are probably different host-specific cellular factors necessary for viral functions within the genus *Papillomavirus*.

All of the major ORFs are read off one strand and are of comparable size and in similar positions in all papillomaviruses sequenced so far. The sequences are usually highly homologous within ORFs E1, E2, and L1 and diverge most in E4 and E5, in part of L2, and in the noncoding region between the end of L1 and the start of E6.

NATURAL HISTORY OF HPV INFECTIONS

HPVs infect and replicate in squamous epithelium on both keratinized and nonkeratinized (mucosal) surfaces. Most people are infected with the common HPVs, types 1, 2, 3, and 4, which infect cutaneous surfaces usually on the hands and feet and occur commonly in childhood or early adolescence. Some of the HPVs, such as type 7, cause lesions in certain groups of individuals and are found in warts on the skin of people in the meat industry, especially those handling fresh meat carcasses, although this virus has not been related to any animal papilloma. A small group of individuals with EV harbor a number of virus types not found in normal people (4, 13). Two common presentations are (i) multiple warts that may be so numerous as to produce coalescent areas and (ii) dry, scaly, flat lesions that may be red or heavily pigmented. These latter skin lesions, although not having a wartlike appearance, contain many of the unusual types of HPV listed in Table 1. Squamous cell carcinomas develop in nearly a third of patients with EV, usually in areas of skin exposed to the sun (face, neck, and hands being the commonest areas affected); HPV-5 and -8 are commonly found and HPV-14 is rarely found in these lesions. It is not clear whether HPVs induce malignancy since less than 50% of lesions contain HPV genomes, although this low percentage could be due to the fact that there are as yet undetected types.

TABLE 1. HPVs and associated lesions

HPV type	Associated lesions[a]
1	Plantar and common hand warts
2	Common hand warts
3	Flat and juvenile warts
4	Plantar and common hand warts
5	Macular lesions in EV patients
6	Condylomata acuminata, CIN, VIN, laryngeal warts
7	Butchers' warts
8	Macular lesions in EV patients
9	Macular lesions in EV patients
10	Flat warts (rarely condylomata acuminata)
11	Condylomata acuminata, CIN, VIN, laryngeal warts
12	Macular lesions in EV patients
13	Hyperplastic Heck lesions of the oral cavity
14	Flat warts
15	Flat warts
16	CIN, VIN, PIN, bowenoid papulosis, malignant genital carcinomas
17	Macular lesions in EV patients
18	CIN, malignant genital carcinomas
20	Macular lesions in EV patients
21–25	Macular lesions in EV patients
26	Cutaneous warts
27	Flat warts
28	Cutaneous warts
29	Cutaneous warts
30	A laryngeal carcinoma, CIN
31	CIN
32	Hyperplastic Heck lesions of the oral cavity
33	CIN, malignant cervical carcinoma
34	Bowen's disease (cutaneous)
35	CIN, malignant cervical carcinoma
36	Actinic keratosis in EV patients
37	Keratoacanthoma
38	A malignant melanoma
39	CIN, PIN
40	CIN, PIN
41	Cutaneous warts, carcinoma
42	CIN, condylomata acuminata
43	CIN
44	CIN, condylomata acuminata
45	CIN, malignant cervical carcinoma
46	Macules in patients with Hodgkin's disease
47	Wart in EV patient
48	Squamous cell carcinoma in transplant patient
49	Warts in transplant patients
50	Wart in EV patient
51	CIN, malignant cervical carcinoma
52	CIN, malignant genital carcinoma
53	Found in normal genital tissue; no associated lesions
54	Condylomata acuminata
55	Bowenoid papulosis
56	CIN, malignant cervical carcinoma
57	Oral lesions, CIN
58	CIN
59	VIN
60	Epidermoid cyst

[a] EV, Epidermodysplasia verruciformis; CIN, cervical intraepithelial neoplasia; VIN, vulvar intraepithelial neoplasia; PIN, penile intraepithelial neoplasia.

Mucosal surfaces can also be infected with HPVs, and HPV-6 and -11 infect both the genital tract and the mucosa of the larynx. Infection of the larynx is rare but usually requires several episodes of surgery or laser treatment for removal of recurrent lesions. Frequent recurrences may be due to the fact that only the visible lesions are treated although healthy areas of mucosal tissue may harbor HPV genomes. The oral cavity is also infected with other HPVs, and oral warts or hyperkeratoses have been found to contain viral genomes. HPV-13 has been found in an oral carcinoma.

Infection of the genitals and genital mucosa is increasing and involves thousands of new cases each year, usually among sexually active individuals 18 to 35 years old (cf. common hand wart). There is with this infection an increased risk of carcinoma of the cervix and perhaps other areas of the lower genital tract. Benign warts (condylomata acuminata) on the penis, vulva, cervix, and perianal areas commonly contain HPV-6 and -11, but there are other recently recognized lesions of the female genital tract that harbor HPVs; these infections are discussed in the next section.

PATHOGENESIS

Apart from the benign lesions such as common hand warts and verrucas associated with HPV infections, premalignant and malignant lesions, especially of the female genital tract, have been associated with the presence of papillomaviruses.

Oncogenic potential of papillomaviruses

Most of the evidence for an oncogenic potential of HPVs comes from research with animal papillomaviruses. Work in the 1930s showed that the cottontail rabbit papillomavirus produced benign warts in this animal, its natural host, and that these benign tumors in 25% of cases would become malignant after 12 months. Benign tumors produced in domestic rabbits became malignant more frequently and within a shorter time. Also, application of hydrocarbons or tar produced in both animal species a higher and more rapid malignant conversion. The virus DNA was detected in both the benign and malignant lesions. These results suggested that cottontail rabbit papillomavirus produced the benign lesion but that other factors, genetic and environmental, may be necessary for production of malignant disease. More recently, esophageal, intestinal, and bladder papillomas produced by BPV-4 were shown to become malignant when cattle were fed on a diet of bracken (12). In this case, the BPV-4 DNA was detected only in the benign lesion, not after malignant conversion.

In humans, one-third of patients with EV develop squamous cell carcinomas, usually in areas exposed to sunlight. As mentioned previously, approximately 30% of these lesions contain HPV-5 or -8 DNA sequences. This finding suggests that given the right environmental or genetic conditions, benign lesions may develop into a carcinoma with the help of HPVs. Other evidence of a helper function associated with malignant conversion concerns laryngeal papillomas, which may convert from a benign to a malignant state when treated by X irradiation. Studies from Queensland, Australia, where squamous cell carcinoma is common among Caucasians, show papillomaviruslike particles in hyperkeratotic lesions in sun-damaged skin. In Western Australia and Queensland, BPV-like DNA sequences have been found in skin carcinomas of sheep and cattle in sun-exposed areas around the nose and mouth and on the genitals.

The studies with animal papillomaviruses and EV patients show the association of these viruses with malignant conversion and set a precedent for investigating the association of HPVs and genital cancers. Unfortunately, there is no animal model for investigation of carcinomas of the genital tract.

Carcinomas associated with HPV infection

Most of the evidence for a causal association between squamous cell cancers and infection with HPVs comes from work with the genital tract wart viruses (21, 25, 31). The genital HPVs, types 6 and 11, are found in condylomata acuminata, which are predominantly benign lesions; however, a few cases have been reported in which malignant conversion took place in vulvar condylomata and invasion resulted (24). This finding has been documented only in females with vulvar warts who had an underlying immunodeficiency usually associated with lymphomas. Various intraepithelial neoplasias (premalignant lesions in which abnormal cells are confined to the epithelium) of the female lower genital tract and the penis contain HPV DNA in the lesions as detected by DNA-DNA hybridization. HPV-6 and -11 are found in premalignant lesions of the cervix—the so-called cervical intraepithelial neoplasias (CIN), which are graded I to III in increasing order of severity, with CIN III including carcinoma in situ. These lesions are seen only with the colposcope and after addition of 5% acetic acid to the exocervix. They occur between the squamous epithelium of the exocervix and the columnar epithelium of the endocervical canal in the transformation zone, and they are white in appearance (acetowhite epithelium). Neither HPV-6 or HPV-11 has been found in malignant lesions of the cervix or of other areas of the genital tract. On the other hand, HPV-16 and -18 DNA sequences have been found both in CIN and invasive disease of the cervix (7). HPV-16 has been found in 70% of cases of CIN III in Germany (29) and the United Kingdom (15) and has been found in up to 80% of cases of invasive carcinoma of the cervix. In the United States, a survey of pregnant women showed that of those with CIN, HPV-16, -18, or -31 was found in 53% of lesions (10). HPV-16 and -18 have also been detected in a high percentage (58%) of penile carcinomas in Brazil (16), where in one area in the northeast of the country the incidence of penile carcinoma is 10 to 20 times higher than in Europe or North America. There appears to be some geographical differences in HPV types associated with carcinoma of the cervix, since HPV-18, which is not commonly found in Europe or North America, is present in a quarter of invasive lesions of the cervix in African and South American women.

There is a difference in the state of the HPV-16 DNA in premalignant and malignant lesions. In CIN lesions, the HPV-16 DNA sequences are free and not integrated into the chromosome. In malignant disease of the cervix, the HPV-16 DNA appears in most cases to be integrated into the host cell chromosome. Whether this is a significant difference and accounts for malignant change is not clear, but it is known that at least BPV-1 can transform rodent cells in vitro without detectable integrated sequences present.

Other areas of the genital tract are affected by HPV infection, and intraepithelial neoplasias of the vaginal wall (vaginal intraepithelial neoplasia) and vulva (vulvar intraepithelial neoplasia) contain HPV-6, -11, and -16. Again, these lesions are graded on a basis of severity from I to III. Some patients have a multicentric distribution of disease, with intraepithelial lesions appearing on the cervix, vaginal wall, vulva, perineum, and perianal areas and into the rectum. A few of these individuals have some underlying immunodeficiency that necessitates immunosuppressive chemotherapy (e.g., sarcoidosis or idiopathic thrombocytopenic purpura), but others do not appear to be abnormal in this respect.

Infection with genital HPV is also common in males, with condylomata acuminata appearing on the penis and sometimes scrotum and groin. Detection of HPV lesions in males may be difficult without thorough examination because the condylomata may be in the distal end of the urethra and, being small, may remain undetected unless examination is careful and thorough. HPV-6 and to a lesser extent HPV-11 are found in these benign lesions. HPV-16 has been found in intraepithelial neoplasias on the penis in 50% of men who are the regular sexual partners of women with CIN disease.

Malignant disease of the male genitals is rare, although as stated above, it may be high in such countries as Brazil; in these cases, HPV-16 and less frequently HPV-18 are found in these invasive lesions.

Whether the association between HPV and malignant disease is causal or casual remains to be determined. However, if HPVs are involved in inducing malignancy, there are probably other factors that need to be present for malignant change to occur. For example, a genetic background may render some individuals more susceptible than others. Other cofactors, such as smoking, are important. It has been shown that individuals who smoke are at greater risk of carcinoma of the cervix than those who do not if all the other factors (social status, sexual history, etc.) are controlled. More information on the progression of the disease and interaction of HPVs with epithelial cells needs to be gathered before the role of these viruses in malignant disease is unraveled.

Persistence of HPV infections

Circumstantial evidence suggests that HPVs may persist in squamous epithelium without producing recognizable lesions, similar to the persistence of polyomaviruses in the kidney. Up to 42% of allograft recipients develop cutaneous warts within a year after transplant, a high proportion compared with the incidence in age-matched controls. This finding suggests that transplanted patients experience either new infections or reactivation of persistent virus, the latter being supported by the finding of HPV DNA sequences in biopsies of normal areas of the larynx from individuals with recurrent warts. Since the recurrence rate of laryngeal papillomas is high, this finding suggests that the virus is capable of persisting somewhere in the respiratory tract or oral cavity without producing recognizable lesions (an inapparent infection).

In none of the situations described above is there any direct evidence as to which cells harbor the virus. The lower layers of the epithelium are a possibility, although since there is considerable turnover of cells in squamous epithelium, the viral DNA would have to be replicating to remain in such cells and hence persist in the epithelium.

DIAGNOSIS

Apart from the familiar hand wart or verruca, the clinical appearance of wart virus infections varies considerably, from the scaly flat lesions on cutaneous epithelium of individuals with EV to the aceto-white flat lesion on the cervix (CIN lesions).

Since HPVs are associated with benign lesions that spontaneously regress, diagnosis of a particular infecting agent is not necessary. However, since some genital isolates, notably HPV-6 and -11, are found in benign lesions whereas HPV-16 and -18 are found in progressive lesions and malignant lesions, it is thought that a viral diagnosis might help with clinical management. At present there is no easy serological screening test, and the techniques used either are very time-consuming and technically complex for a busy diagnostic laboratory or are not very sensitive. The following sections describe the methods currently used, but most of the work is being carried out in research laboratories rather than routine laboratories.

Culture methods

Although several efforts have been made, no cell type has been found capable of supporting replication, with production of infectious papillomavirus particles.

Immunochemical methods

As stated above, difficulties have been encountered in producing specific antibodies against single papillomavirus types. Currently, antibody directed against common epitopes in the major capsid protein (L1) is used to detect HPV in lesions. This antibody is raised against disrupted BPV extracted from bovine warts, which are generally large and provide a plentiful supply of virions. These antibodies recognize disrupted papillomaviruses from different animal species and can be used for two types of immunochemical staining. In all cases, the principle of the test is the same. The tissue to be investigated can be either Formalin fixed or "snap" frozen in liquid nitrogen. Sections cut from snap-frozen blocks can then be fixed in methanol at −20°C or acetone at room temperature after cryostat sectioning.

The specific antipapillomavirus antibodies are interacted with the sections, which are washed and then stained with antispecies antibodies tagged with a reagent that will visualize the specific antibody interactions. Antispecies antibodies are usually tagged with (i) a fluorescent dye, such as fluorescein isothiocyanate or rhodamine, or (ii) an enzyme, alkaline such as phosphatase or peroxidase. Use of the latter enhances sensitivity and also makes tissue definition much easier, for fluorescent dyes can be seen only against a dark background. The positive cells are in the peripheral layers of the epithelium, and these cells produce structural antigens and mature virus particles. The staining is confined to the nucleus. There are now monoclonal antibodies to HPV-6, -16, and -18 L1 epitopes which can be used on Formalin-fixed sections and differentiate between these three genital isolates (2, 18).

Although the detection rate of HPV antigens by this method in condylomata acuminata and CIN lesions varies from study to study, about 30 to 50% of biopsies exhibit positive staining with antibody directed against the common structural antigen. However, CIN I lesions are more likely to be positive than CIN III lesions, probably because mature particles are seen mainly in the differentiated cells of the epithelium and few or no differentiated cells are seen in the outer cell layers of the epithelium in CIN III lesions.

DNA-DNA hybridization

Southern blot hybridization. Southern blot hybridization is the "gold standard" for detection of HPV DNA. Total DNA, extracted from biopsy tissue or from cervical cells taken by a conventional spatula, is digested by restriction endonucleases, which are bacterial enzymes that digest DNA at specific nucleotide sequences, and then electrophoresed through an agarose horizontal gel. This procedure separates the total DNA into fragments of various sizes, with the smaller ones moving faster than the larger. The DNA is then transferred from the agarose gel to a solid matrix (usually nitrocellulose or nylon filters) by a process called Southern blotting. Before transfer, the DNA is denatured in the gel (i.e., single-stranded DNA is produced) by alkaline treatment. After transfer, the filter can be hybridized with HPV DNA probes labeled with ^{32}P. The labeling of DNA is carried out by a process called nick translation or by random oligonucleotide priming (see chapter 17).

Hybridization is carried out in a plastic bag, with the HPV probe DNA in solution and the tissue DNA attached to the solid matrix. The tissue DNA is already single stranded as a result of denaturation before blotting, and the probe DNA is made single stranded by heating above the melting temperature before addition to the hybridization solution. Hybridization can take place for a couple of hours to 18 to 24 h, depending on the concentration of probe DNA. After hybridization, the filters are washed thoroughly to remove any nonspecific binding of probe to the solid matrix, and then the filter is exposed to X-ray film for various periods of time.

The Southern blot technique is very specific for two reasons: (i) at high stringency, only homologous DNA is detected (e.g., HPV-16 is detected with an HPV-16 probe and not with a HPV-6 probe), and (ii) when the DNA is digested with restriction enzymes, certain band sizes are seen with different HPV types. For example, the enzyme *Pst*I digests HPV-16 six times and gives band sizes ranging from 200 to 2,800 base pairs, whereas HPV-6a gives four bands ranging in size from 960 to 3,800 base pairs. Therefore, there is a double check on the specificity of the hybridization. This method will detect one DNA copy per cell.

Filter in situ hybridization. The filter in situ hybridization method, which detects HPV sequences in cells from a cervical smear, is more rapid than Southern blotting and can be carried out in two ways. First, the cervical cells can be placed directly onto nitrocellulose filters by using suction. The cells are broken open, and the DNA is denatured by alkaline treatment; these filters can then be treated as described above. An alternative method, referred to as dot blot hybridization, is to extract the DNA from the cells, add the DNA to the filter, and then treat the filter as described above.

An advantage of the first method is that it is rapid, and if only very few cells have HPV DNA, this DNA may be detected; in contrast, when the DNA is extracted before it is placed on the filter, these copies are diluted among the total host DNA. However, hybridization with the whole cells on the filter sometimes results in background noise on the X-ray film, which could be taken as a positive result; therefore, there is a higher incidence of false-positives with this technique. The dot blot method is longer because the DNA must be extracted from the biopsy specimen and may be less sensitive when all of the HPV genome copies are in a few cells and so become diluted out in the extraction.

A new hybridization kit on the market uses ^{32}P-labeled HPV RNA as the probe in the dot blot assay. The advantage of using RNA is that hybridization temperatures can be closer to the melting temperature because DNA-RNA binding is more stable than DNA-DNA duplexes and therefore specificity is increased. In addition, after hybridization the filters can be treated with RNase to remove unhybridized probe and reduce background. One major disadvantage is that RNA is more labile than DNA, and thus care must be taken to avoid breakdown of the probe.

Polymerase chain reaction. The recently developed polymerase chain reaction method provides a way to amplify specific target DNA sequences by using primers and a heat-stable polymerase called *Taq* polymerase (9, 22). The sensitivity of the method is 100,000 times that for Southern blotting, so that a single HPV DNA molecule is able to be detected in 100,000 cells. The specificity of the reaction depends on two oligonucleotide primers that flank the HPV DNA segment to be amplified. Denaturation and reannealing of the primers to their complementary sequences, followed by extension using the *Taq* polymerase, are repeated sequentially. Each cycle doubles the amount of target DNA. The problem with such sensitivity is the risk of contamination affecting the results, since contaminants as well as the test DNA can be amplified.

Contamination can come from a number of sources. There may be cross-contamination of biopsy samples if the same instruments are used for different biopsies or in a laboratory where plasmid-cloned HPV DNA is produced in large amounts for use as probes. This DNA could contaminate test samples via aerosols or instruments. Carryover of DNA from one tube to another is a possible source of contamination, and extreme care must be taken to avoid this occurrence. To eliminate false-positives, extreme care must be taken to avoid cross-contamination, a requirement that may make this technique difficult to adapt to a busy diagnostic laboratory.

Because the polymerase chain reaction method is so sensitive and can detect a few copies of HPV DNA, it is difficult to know the significance of a small number of HPV genomes harbored in cervical cells. These few copies convey very little about the infectivity of the virus. This problem, however, is not confined to HPV detection and is one that will have to be addressed with other viruses, especially human immunodeficiency virus.

Future of diagnostic tests for HPV

The value of diagnosing the type of HPV infection, especially of the genital tract, is not clear. It is felt by many that typing would aid in the management of patients, since some types are associated with lesions that progress to malignant disease. However, at present no diagnostic screening is warranted. The new methods of detection such as the polymerase chain reaction may be the way forward, but because of its sensitivity and problems with cross-contamination, this technique is not applicable to diagnostic laboratories at present.

LITERATURE CITED

1. **Budd, F., D. J. McCance, and R. Schlegel.** 1989. DNA sequence of HPV16 E5 ORF and the structural conservation of its encoded protein. Virology **613:**243–246.
2. **Cason, J., D. Patel, J. Naylor, D. Lunny, P. S. Shepherd, J. M. Best, and D. J. McCance.** 1989. Identification of immunogenic regions of the major coat protein of human papillomavirus type 16 that contain type restricted epitopes. J. Gen. Virol. **70:**2973–2987.
3. **Danos, O., M. Katinka, and M. Yaniv.** 1982. Human papillomavirus 1a complete DNA sequence: a novel type of genome organization among *Papovaviridae.* EMBO J. **1:** 231–236.
4. **deVilliers, E. M.** 1989. Heterogeneity of the human papillomavirus group. J. Virol. **63:**4898–4903.
5. **di Maio, D., D. Guralski, and J. T. Schiller.** 1986. Translation of open reading frame E5 of bovine papillomavirus is required for its transforming activity. Proc. Natl. Acad. Sci. USA **83:**1797–1801.
6. **Doorbar, J., D. Campbell, R. J. A. Grand, and P. H. Gallimore.** 1986. Identification of the human papillomavirus-1a E4 gene products. EMBO J. **5:**355–362.
7. **Durst, M., L. Gissmann, H. Ikenberg, and H. zur Hausen.** 1983. Papillomavirus DNA from a cervical carcinoma and its prevalence in cancer biopsy samples from different geographical regions. Proc. Natl. Acad. Sci. USA **80:**3812–3815.
8. **Dyson, N., P. M. Howley, K. Munger, and E. Harlow.** 1989. The human papillomavirus 16 E7 oncoprotein is able to bind to the retinoblastoma gene product. Science **243:** 934–937.
9. **Erlich, H. A., D. H. Gelfand, and R. K. Saiki.** 1988. Product review: specific DNA amplification. Nature (London) **331:**461–462.
10. **Fife, K. H., R. E. Rogers, and B. W. Zwickl.** 1987. Symptomatic and asymptomatic cervical infections with human papillomavirus during pregnancy. J. Infect. Dis. **156:**904–911.
11. **Hudson, J. B., M. A. Bedell, D. J. McCance, and L. A. Laimins.** 1990. Immortalization and alteration of differentiation of human keratinocytes in vitro by the E6 and E7 open reading frames of human papillomavirus type 18. J. Virol. **64:**519–526.
12. **Jarrett, W. F. H., P. E. McNeil, H. M. Laird, B. W. O'Neill, J. Murphy, M. S. Campo, and M. H. Moar.** 1981. Papillomaviruses in benign and malignant tumors of cattle, p. 215–222. *In* M. Essex, G. Todaro, and H. zur Hausen (ed.), Human cancer viruses. Cold Spring Harbor Laboratory, Cold Spring Harbor, N.Y.
13. **Kremsdorf, D., M. Favre, S. Jablonska, S. Obalek, A. L. Rueda, M. A. Lutzner, C. Blanchet-Bardon, P. C. van Vorst Vader, and G. Orth.** 1984. Molecular cloning and characterization of the genomes of nine newly recognized human papillomavirus types associated with epidermodysplasia verruciformis. J. Virol. **52:**1013–1018.
14. **Lambert, P. F., B. A. Spalholz, and P. M. Howley.** 1987. A transcriptional repressor encoded by BPV1 shares a common carboxy-terminal domain with the E2 transactivator. Cell **50:**69–78.
15. **McCance, D. J., M. J. Campion, P. K. Clarkson, P. M. Chesters, D. Jenkins, and A. Singer.** 1985. The prevalence of human papillomavirus type 16 DNA sequences in cervical intraepithelial neoplasia and invasive carcinoma of the cervix. Br. J. Obstet. Gynaecol. **92:**1011–1105.
16. **McCance, D. J., A. Kalache, K. Ashdown, L. Andrache, F. Menezes, P. Smith, and R. Doll.** 1986. Human papillomavirus types 16 and 18 in carcinomas of the penis from Brazil. Int. J. Cancer **37:**55–60.

17. **Munger, K., W. C. Phelps, V. Bubb, P. M. Howley, and R. Schlegel.** 1989. The E6 and E7 genes of human papillomavirus type 16 together are necessary and sufficient for transformation of primary human keratinocytes. J. Virol. **63:**4417–4421.

18. **Patel, D., P. J. Shepherd, J. A. Naylor, and D. J. McCance.** 1989. Reactivities of polyclonal and monoclonal antibodies raised to the major capsid protein of human papillomavirus type 16. J. Gen. Virol. **70:**69–77.

19. **Phelps, W. C., and P. M. Howley.** 1987. Transcriptional transactivation by the human papillomavirus type 16 E2 gene product. J. Virol. **61:**1630–1638.

20. **Phelps, W. C., C. L. Yee, K. Munger, and P. M. Howley.** 1988. The human papillomavirus type 16 E7 gene encodes transactivation and transformation functions similar to those of adenovirus E1A. Cell **53:**539–547.

21. **Reid, R., C. R. Laverty, M. Coppleson, et al.** 1982. Non condylomatous cervical wart virus infection. Obstet. Gynecol. **50:**377–387.

22. **Saiki, R. K., D. H. Gelfand, S. Stoffel, S. J. Scharf, R. Higuchi, G. T. Horn, K. B. Mullis, and H. A. Erlich.** 1988. Primer directed enzymatic amplification of DNA with a thermostable DNA polymerase. Science **239:**487–491.

23. **Seedorf, K., T. Oltersdorf, G. Krammer, and W. Rowekamp.** 1987. Identification of early proteins of the human papillomaviruses type 16 (HPV16) and type 18 (HPV18) in cervical carcinoma cells. EMBO J. **6:**139–144.

24. **Shokri-Tabibzadeh, S., L. G. Koss, J. Mohnar, and S. Rommey.** 1981. Association of human papillomavirus with neoplastic process in the genital tract of four women with impaired immunity. Gynecol. Oncol. **12:**5129–5140.

25. **Singer, A., P. G. Walker, and D. J. McCance.** 1984. Genital wart virus infections: nuisance or potentially lethal. Br. Med. J. **288:**735–737.

26. **Smotkin, D., and F. O. Wettstein.** 1986. Transcription of human papillomavirus type 16 early genes in a cervical cancer and a cancer derived cell line and identification of the E7 protein. Proc. Natl. Acad. Sci. USA **83:**4680–4684.

27. **Spalholz, B. A., P. F. Lambert, C. L. Yee, and P. M. Howley.** 1987. Bovine papillomavirus transcriptional regulation: localization of the E2 response elements of the long control region. J. Virol. **61:**2128–2137.

28. **Thorner, L., N. Bucay, J. Choe, and M. Botchan.** 1988. The product of the bovine papillomavirus type 1 modulator gene (M) is a phosphoprotein. J. Virol. **62:**2474–2482.

29. **Wagner, D., H. Ikenberg, N. Boehm, and L. Gissmann.** 1986. Identification of human papillomavirus in cervical swabs by deoxyribonucleic acid *in situ* hybridization. Obstet. Gynecol. **64:**767–772.

30. **Waldeck, W., F. Rosl, and H. Zentgraf.** 1984. Origin of replication in episomal bovine papillomavirus type 1 DNA isolated from transformed cell. EMBO J. **3:**2173–2178.

31. **zur Hausen, H., L. Gissmann, and J. R. Schlehofer.** 1984. Viruses in the etiology of human genital cancer. Prog. Med. Virol. **30:**170–186.

Chapter 99

Polyomaviruses

RAY R. ARTHUR AND KEERTI V. SHAH

The human polyomaviruses BKV and JCV are ubiquitous, infect a high proportion of the population, and sometimes produce disease with a fatal outcome in specific patient populations. Despite these features, few clinical laboratories have the capability to detect and identify these viruses. Their efforts have been hampered by the fastidious nature of these viruses, the lack of readily available permissive cell lines for virus propagation, and the lack of commercially available immunological reagents. The increasing incidence of progressive multifocal leukoencephalopathy (PML), a fatal degenerative neurological disease caused by JCV, in immunosuppressed populations and recent advances in techniques for the detection of nucleic acids should make diagnostic methods more accessible to clinical laboratories in future years.

CLINICAL BACKGROUND

Human polyomavirus infections occur early in life, and by adulthood nearly 100 and 70% of the population are infected with BKV and JCV, respectively (11, 44, 53). Primary infections with these viruses, although usually symptomless, produce a viremia by which the virus reaches the kidney, where it persists for an indefinite period of time (12, 29). Primary infections occur in seronegative renal allograft recipients who receive kidneys from seropositive donors (2). Reactivation, the result of viral replication in the urinary tract, occurs when there is impairment of cell-mediated immunity. Immunological changes as subtle as those in pregnancy (15), as well as more severe immunosuppression such as that required in organ transplant recipients (8, 13, 24, 30, 36, 43, 59), induce reactivation. With severe immunosuppression, reactivation occurs in about one-half of the seropositive individuals (8).

PML is the most severe clinical manifestation of JCV infection (60). The onset of PML is insidious, with impairment of speech, vision, and mental function. Progressive neurological deterioration, resulting in limb paralysis, cortical blindness, sensory abnormalities, and eventually death, occurs within 6 months of onset. Fever and headache are uncommon during the course of illness, and cerebrospinal fluid is normal. Remission or stabilization of disease may occur in situations where it is possible to ameliorate the immunosuppression by discontinuing immunosuppressive therapy (45).

Pathologically, focal areas of demyelination due to lytic infection of oligodendrocytes are seen most commonly in the cerebrum and less commonly in the cerebellum and brain stem. Affected oligodendrocytes, containing characteristic enlarged basophilic nuclei with occasional basophilic or eosinophilic inclusion bodies (Fig. 1A), are seen in or around early lesions and at the periphery of larger demyelinated lesions. The inflammatory response is minimal; only a few mononuclear cells are observed in infected foci. Bizarre, giant astrocytes with hyperchromatic nuclei are also seen in PML lesions (Fig. 1A).

The immunosuppressive effects of human immunodeficiency virus infection have resulted in a dramatic increase in the incidence of PML in recent years. Presently, PML is estimated to occur in 4% of AIDS patients with neurological symptoms (35). Before the advent of AIDS, PML was a rare disease associated with lymphoproliferative malignancy, most frequently chronic lymphocytic leukemia and Hodgkin's disease (45). Other leukemias, various immunodeficiency syndromes, renal transplantation, lupus erythematosus, pulmonary sarcoidosis, rheumatoid arthritis, and pulmonary tuberculosis were other predisposing conditions. Most of these patients were receiving immunosuppressive chemotherapy including steroids for malignancy, organ transplantation, or other conditions.

The other clinical manifestations of polyomavirus infections occur in the urinary tract and are the result of BKV infection. Hemorrhagic cystitis in recipients of bone marrow transplants is associated with BKV viruria (3, 7). BKV reactivation occurs and is temporally related to hemorrhagic cystitis in as many as 80% of the cases of this frequent complication of bone marrow transplantation (7). The onset of cystitis occurs 2 to 4 weeks after transplantation, continues for approximately 3 weeks, and then resolves spontaneously. For unknown reasons, JCV reactivation occurs infrequently in marrow transplant patients. In renal allograft recipients, BKV infection is associated with ureteral stenosis, an infrequent complication of renal transplantation (14, 24, 59). Several cases of polyomavirus-associated cystitis have been reported in otherwise healthy individuals (28, 41, 46).

DESCRIPTION OF AGENTS

The polyomavirus virion is nonenveloped, has icosahedral symmetry, and is 40 to 45 nm in diameter. A circular, superhelical, double-stranded DNA genome of approximately 3×10^6 daltons (5 kilobases) is enclosed within the viral capsid. BKV and JCV virions form two bands in CsCl isopycnic gradients. A dense band of 1.34 g/cm^3 is composed of complete particles, and a less dense band at 1.29 g/cm^3 consists of empty noninfectious particles. The major capsid protein, VP1, contains internal epitopes that are common to all members of the polyomavirus family (54). Antisera produced by inoculating animals with disrupted virions will react with all polyomaviruses, whereas sera produced by inoculation of intact virions will be virus specific (54). BKV

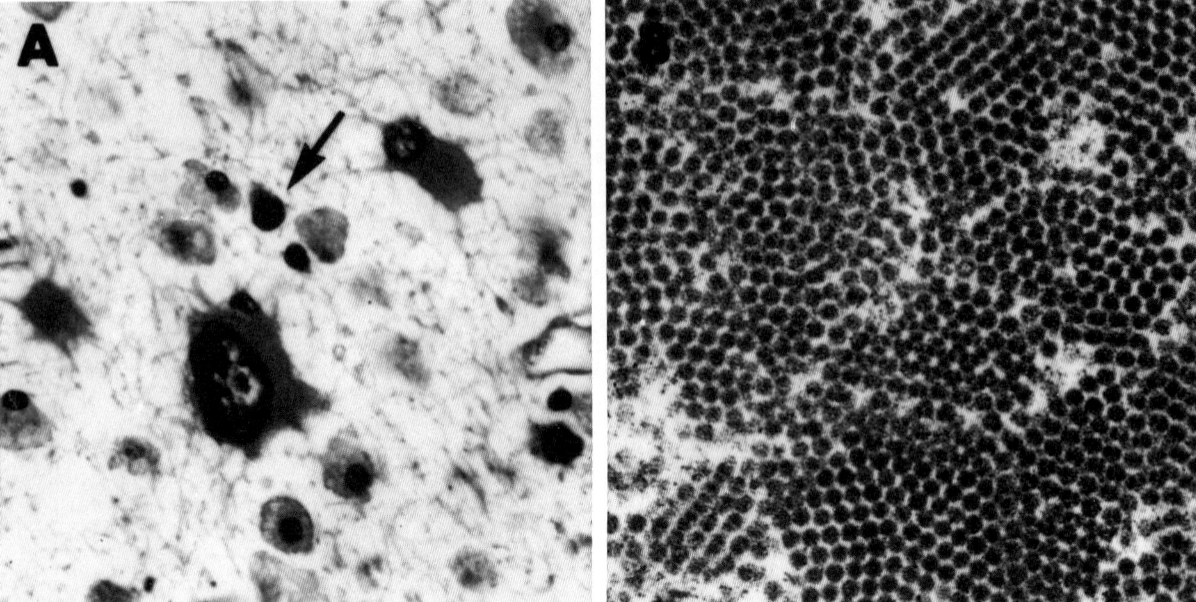

FIG. 1. (A) Characteristic cytopathology of PML: bizarre giant astrocytes and oligodendrocyte with enlarged deeply staining nucleus (arrow). (B) Crystalloid array of JCV particles in an infected oligodendroglial nucleus. (Reproduced with permission from reference 6.)

and JCV hemagglutinate erythrocytes from humans, guinea pigs, and chickens. Polyomaviruses are highly specific for their host species. The viruses are oncogenic for laboratory animals (37, 52, 62) and capable of transforming rodent cells (22, 38). Neither BKV nor JCV appears to have a significant role in human malignancy, although BKV has been associated with tumors of the brain and pancreas in humans (16, 17).

COLLECTION AND STORAGE OF SPECIMENS

Specimens examined for the diagnosis of BKV and JCV infections are usually serum, brain tissue, and urine. The presence of BKV- and JCV-specific antibodies in serum indicates prior infection with the virus. Brain tissue is examined for JCV to confirm the diagnosis of PML. Urine is tested for both BKV and JCV to detect active infections that are usually the result of reactivation of latent virus.

Brain tissue collected by directed biopsy or at autopsy is processed by methods appropriate for the diagnostic technique that will be used for virus detection. Fresh tissue is required for culture. Frozen material is suitable for nucleic acid detection and immunofluorescent staining. Fixed, embedded tissue can be utilized for electron microscopy, immunohistochemical staining, and detection of viral DNA. Urinary sediment produced by low-speed centrifugation (1,500 $\times$ *g*, 15 min) is examined for cytological diagnosis, immunofluorescent staining, culture, and detection of viral DNA. The virus-infected cells display intranuclear inclusions that are filled with virions. Supernatant urine is used for detection of viral antigens by enzyme-linked immunosorbent assay (ELISA). Virus present in urine is pelleted by ultracentrifugation for examination by electron microscopy. For nucleic acid and antigen studies, urine specimens can be held at 4°C for up to 1 week. The pellet and supernatant are stored separately at −70°C until testing.

DIRECT EXAMINATION

Methods for detecting human polyomaviruses by direct examination include electron microscopy, cytological examination, and techniques for detection of viral antigens and DNA. Direct visualization of virus particles by electron microscopy has been used to detect the human polyomaviruses in both urine and brain tissue (23, 56, 64). In urine specimens, 40- to 45-nm particles appear singly or in aggregates bound together by virus-specific antibody that may be present in the urine (48). In specimens in which virions are not coated with antibody, specific identification of BKV and JCV can be made by reacting the virions with specific antisera and examining the virus particles for aggregation or antibody coating (59). Intranuclear crystalline arrays of JCV are seen in infected oligodendrocytes in the brain tissue of PML patients (Fig. 1B). The virions may be somewhat smaller than those seen in urine. Filamentous forms are occasionally observed. A similar pattern of viral arrays is seen in examination of ultrathin sections of exfoliated inclusion-bearing urinary cells (15).

The presence of characteristic inclusions in exfoliated urinary cells is indicative of polyomavirus infection, although viruria is not always associated with excretion of affected cells. A typical polyomavirus-infected urothelial cell is enlarged, with a prominent deeply staining basophilic nucleus containing a single inclusion (34, 59). The intranuclear inclusions in some cells have contracted and separated from the nuclear membrane and have an indistinct halo. Membrane filtration is recommended for the preparation of urines for cytological examination. A highly skilled observer is required to differentiate the cytopathic effect (CPE) of polyomaviruses from that of other viruses such as cytomegalovirus, herpes simplex virus, or adenovirus. Malignant cells may also be mistaken for polyomavirus-infected cells and require careful examination of the nuclear chromatin pattern for diagnosis (34). It is not possible to determine by cytological examination whether the cell is infected with BKV or JCV.

Antigen detection techniques that are commonly performed in many laboratories can be applied to the detection of BKV and JCV. However, polyomavirus-specific antisera are not widely available. Immunofluorescent staining of inclusion-bearing exfoliated urothelial cells (32) and immunohistochemical staining of brain tissue from PML patients (25), with either genus- or virus-specific antiserum, can be used to detect and identify BKV and JCV. Double-antibody antigen capture ELISA can be used to detect virus in supernatant urine and is an efficient technique for examining large numbers of specimens (9).

Various nucleic acid hybridization techniques are being used with increasing frequency for the direct detection of human polyomaviruses. Filter in situ hybridization involves minimal processing of the sample and is an efficient technique for testing large numbers of specimens. Urine sediments are spotted onto nitrocellulose membranes, the cells are lysed, the DNA is denatured with NaOH, and the filter is hybridized with a ^{32}P-labeled molecularly cloned BKV or JCV probe (4). Alternatively, whole urine is boiled and added to the membrane, and the hybridization is performed (26). BKV and JCV have 75% nucleotide sequence homology (21, 51, 63), and genomic probes will cross-hybridize with the heterologous virus (27). The infecting virus can be identified by performing parallel hybridizations with both BKV and JCV probes and comparing the intensities of the autoradiographic signals. Southern hybridization is the "gold standard" for identifying polyomavirus genomic sequences in tissue and urine specimens (6), but it requires extraction of DNA from the sample, digestion with restriction endonucleases, electrophoresis, and transfer of the nucleic acid to a membrane for hybridization (57). Tissue in situ hybridization can be used to detect and localize virus in tissue sections or cytological preparations but is technically demanding (1). The techniques described above require the use of molecularly cloned DNA probes that are not readily available to many laboratories. The use of isotopic labels on the probes similarly reduces the attractiveness of these procedures in the clinical laboratory.

The recent development of the polymerase chain reaction (PCR) overcomes these obstacles (49, 50). The reagents and instrumentation to perform this procedure are commercially available. The nucleotide sequences of BKV and JCV are known (21, 51, 63). The sequences of synthetic oligonucleotide primers used in PCR provide specificity for the amplification of the desired DNA target. Once the desired sequences for the primers are chosen, the oligomers can be purchased. BKV and JCV have been detected in urine and tissue specimens by PCR with use of a single pair of primers, 20 nucleotides in length, that are complementary to the same regions of both viruses (5). The sequences flanked by the primers are unique for each virus. Therefore, the amplified segments can be differentiated on agarose gel after treatment with the restriction endonuclease *Bam*HI (which cuts JCV but not BKV) or by hybridization with virus-specific ^{32}P-labeled oligonucleotide probes complementary to the unique sequences in the amplified segment. The DNA fragments resulting from amplification of BKV and JCV are 176 and 173 base pairs, respectively, in length. Detection of 10 to 100 copies of cloned BKV and JCV DNA is possible by PCR when the reaction products are tested by hybridization. Gel electrophoresis is approximately 100-fold less sensitive than hybridization for detection of viral sequences in the PCR reaction products but is suitable for testing urines from high-risk patient populations with high levels of viruria.

ISOLATION OF VIRUSES

The isolation of human polyomaviruses in cell culture is difficult. Permissive cells are not readily available, the CPE exhibited by these viruses may be subtle, and prolonged periods of cultivation and blind passages may be required for virus isolation. JCV has a highly restricted host cell range, and replication is restricted to a limited number of cells of human origin (61). Primary fetal human glial (PHFG) cells are the preferred cells for the primary isolation of JCV (47). PHFG cell cultures contain a mixed cell population and are not uniform in the susceptibility to JCV replication. Incubation at 39°C is more efficient for isolation of JCV than incubation at 37°C. The CPE produced by JCV in unstained PHFG cells is subtle and is first observed in spongioblasts after 2 to 3 weeks of incubation. These cells are eventually destroyed several weeks after the CPE is first seen. Intranuclear inclusions are seen in stained-cell preparations. Primary human urine-derived epithelial (UDE) cells, although not as sensitive as PHFG cells, can also be used for primary isolation of JCV (10). Neither PHFG nor UDE cells are commercially available. Recently, several continuously culturable transformed cell lines have been used to isolate JCV, but they too are not widely available (39, 40). Virological and serological reagents for JCV can be obtained by propagation of laboratory-adapted virus in human amnion and human embryonic kidney cells (42, 58).

BKV is less restricted in its host cell range than JCV. BKV replicates efficiently in human embryonic kidney cells and can also be isolated by using several primary human cell cultures, including embryonic lung cells, PHFG cells, UDE cells, foreskin cultures, and fetal fibroblasts (31). Monkey kidney cell cultures (e.g., Vero and CV-1) are permissive for BKV. Optimal incubation temperatures range from 37 to 40°C, with the elevated temperatures better for monkey cells. The infected cells show cytoplasmic vacuolation, enlargement of nuclei with inclusions, and cell rounding, followed by detachment from the surface of the culture vessel. Two to four weeks and occasionally longer periods of incubation with blind passages may be required before CPE is evident. Large quantities of reagents for use in serological and other tests may be produced by inoculation of widely available human fibroblast lines (e.g., WI-38 and MRC-5) with laboratory-adapted BKV.

IDENTIFICATION OF VIRUSES

BKV and JCV replication in cell cultures can be detected by electron microscopy, by detection of viral antigens with immunofluorescence microscopy, or by hemagglutination when erythrocytes are mixed with culture supernatants. Virus-specific antisera must be used in immunoelectron microscopy and immunofluorescence assays to identify the virus in infected cells. Similarly, specific antisera are required for viral identification by the hemagglutination inhibition (HI) technique (described below). Most of the virus is cell associated, and several freeze-thaw cycles and neuraminidase treatments are necessary to obtain high concentrations of virions in the culture supernatant (58).

SEROLOGICAL DIAGNOSIS

Serological studies are of limited value in diagnosing active human polyomavirus infections. Primary infections are usually asymptomatic, and most individuals are seropositive, given the high prevalence of BKV and JCV infections in the general population. Serological studies that measure increases of BKV- and JCV-specific antibodies are useful in assessing reactivation in mildly immunosuppressed individuals, such as pregnant women (15) and renal transplant recipients (24, 30), but are of little value for severely compromised patients, such as bone marrow transplant recipients (8) and AIDS patients. Changes in antibody titers in the latter groups of patients do not correlate with viruria. In AIDS patients, for example, serological markers for BKV infections are sometimes lost during the late stages of the disease (18). Serological tests have not contributed to the diagnosis of PML.

The methods most frequently used for measurement of BKV- and JCV-specific antibodies are HI, indirect immunofluorescence assay, virus neutralization, and ELISA. The methods for preparation of infected cells and viral antigens are described above. Of these techniques, HI is relatively simple to perform (53). For the HI test, 4 to 8 hemagglutinating units of antigen in 25-μl volumes is mixed with an equal volume of doubling dilutions of serum, and the mixtures are incubated at 37°C for 1 h. The mixtures are placed on wet ice, and 50 μl of 0.5% human O erythrocytes in cold phosphate-buffered saline is added. The test is read when the cells in the negative control have settled ($\approx$1 h). The HI titer of the serum is the reciprocal of the highest dilution of the serum that completely inhibits hemagglutination. The HI test has several limitations. Human sera contain low levels of nonspecific inhibitors of hemagglutination, and some sera contain nonspecific agglutinins. Inhibitors can be removed by pretreating the sera with acetone (55), and agglutinins, if present, can be removed by adsorption with erythrocytes before testing. HI titers of less than 40 in untreated sera cannot be interpreted with confidence, whereas titers of 20 or greater in acetone-treated sera are indicative of past polyomavirus infection.

ELISA is suitable for testing a large number of sera and is more reliable than HI, since the technique is not affected by the presence of nonspecific hemagglutination inhibitors. Infected cells (33) or culture supernatants (19) as well as purified virus (6) can be used as antigen to coat microdilution plates. Appropriate negative control antigens are required to verify specificity. Negative sera for use as controls can be identified by screening sera from young children. Titers are determined by endpoint dilution (19, 33) or by extrapolation from a standard curve generated by using a high-titered serum standard (6).

The measurement of BKV- and JCV-specific immunoglobulin M (IgM), which is present in serum after primary infections and reactivations, can be measured by either HI or ELISA after separation of the IgM from IgG by sucrose gradient centrifugation, column chromatography, or treatment with protein A. A capture IgM ELISA can be used to measure IgM virus-specific antibody without pretreatment of the serum (20).

EVALUATION, INTERPRETATION, AND REPORTING OF RESULTS

The majority of active polyomavirus infections, either primary infections or reactivations, are not associated with disease. At present, the two clinical conditions most frequently associated with JCV and BKV replication are PML and hemorrhagic cystitis, respectively. Detection of JCV in brain tissue collected at biopsy or autopsy from patients with suspected PML establishes the diagnosis of PML. Concomitant viruria may or may not be present. Prognosis for survival is poor. In bone marrow transplant recipients with BKV-related hemorrhagic cystitis, the viruria and cystitis usually resolve spontaneously in several weeks. Transient viruria undoubtedly occurs in healthy individuals. The use of a sensitive technique such as PCR for the detection of polyomaviruria may detect low-level shedding that has no clinical relevance.

Serological studies are of little diagnostic importance as compared with detection of virus. Infections in severely immunocompromised patients are often not associated with an increase in antibody titers. The tests have utility in seroepidemiologic investigations and in studying reactivation in immunocompetent individuals that escapes virological detection.

LITERATURE CITED

1. **Aksamit, A. J., P. Mourrain, J. L. Sever, and E. O. Major.** 1985. Progressive multifocal leukoencephalopathy: investigation of three cases using in situ hybridization with JC virus biotinylated DNA probe. Ann. Neurol. **18:**490–496.
2. **Andrews, C., K. V. Shah, R. Rubin, and M. Hirsch.** 1982. BK papovavirus infections in renal transplant recipients: contribution of donor kidneys. J. Infect. Dis. **145:**276.
3. **Apperley, J. F., S. J. Rice, J. A. Bishop, Y. C. Chia, T. Krausz, S. D. Gardner, and J. M. Goldman.** 1987. Late-onset hemorrhagic cystitis associated with urinary excretion of polyomaviruses after bone marrow transplantation. Transplantation **43:**108–112.
4. **Arthur, R. R., A. M. Beckmann, C. C. Li, R. Saral, and K. V. Shah.** 1985. Detection of the human papovavirus BK in urine of bone marrow transplant recipients: comparison of DNA hybridization with ELISA. J. Med. Virol. **16:**29–36.
5. **Arthur, R. R., S. Dagostin, and K. V. Shah.** 1989. Detection of BKV and JCV in urine and brain tissue by the polymerase chain reaction. J. Clin. Microbiol. **27:**1174–1179.
6. **Arthur, R. R., and K. V. Shah.** 1988. Papovaviridae: the polyomaviruses, p. 317–332. *In* P. Halonen, E. Lennette, Jr., and F. Murphy (ed.), The laboratory diagnosis of infectious diseases: principles and practice, vol. 2. Springer-Verlag, New York.
7. **Arthur, R. R., K. V. Shah, S. J. Baust, G. W. Santos, and R. Saral.** 1986. Association of BK viruria with hemorrhagic cystitis in recipients of bone marrow transplants. N. Engl. J. Med. **315:**230–234.

8. **Arthur, R. R., K. V. Shah, P. Charache, and R. Saral.** 1988. BK and JC virus infections in recipients of bone marrow transplants. J. Infect. Dis. **158:**563–569.
9. **Arthur, R. R., K. V. Shah, R. H. Yolken, and P. Charache.** 1983. Detection of human papovaviruses BKV and JCV in urines by ELISA. Clin. Biol. Res. **105:**169–176.
10. **Beckmann, A. M., K. V. Shah, and B. L. Padgett.** 1982. Propagation and primary isolation of papovavirus JC in epithelial cells derived from human urine. Infect. Immun. **38:**774–777.
11. **Brown, P., T. Tsai, and D. C. Gajdusek.** 1975. Seroepidemiology of human papovaviruses: discovery of virgin populations and some unusual patterns of antibody prevalence among remote peoples of the world. Am. J. Epidemiol. **102:**331–340.
12. **Chesters, P. M., J. Heritage, and D. J. McCance.** 1983. Persistence of DNA sequences of BK virus and JC virus in normal human tissues and in diseased tissues. J. Infect. Dis. **147:**676–684.
13. **Coleman, D. V., S. D. Gardner, and A. M. Field.** 1973. Human polyomavirus infection in renal allograft recipients. Br. Med. J. **3:**371–375.
14. **Coleman, D. V., E. F. D. Mackenzie, S. D. Gardner, J. M. Poulding, B. Amer, and W. J. I. Russell.** 1978. Human polyomavirus (BK) infection and ureteric stenosis in renal allograft recipients. J. Clin. Pathol. **31:**338–347.
15. **Coleman, D. V., M. R. Wolfendale, R. A. Daniel, N. K. Dhanjal, S. D. Gardner, P. E. Gibson, and A. M. Field.** 1980. A prospective study of human polyomavirus infection in pregnancy. J. Infect. Dis. **142:**1–8.
16. **Corallini, A., M. Pagnani, P. Viadana, E. Silini, M. Mottes, G. Milanesi, G. Gerna, R. Vettor, G. Trapella, V. Silvani, G. Gaist, and G. Barbanti-Brodano.** 1987. Association of BK virus with human brain tumors and tumors of pancreatic islets. Int. J. Cancer **39:**60–67.
17. **Dorries, K., G. Loeber, and J. Meixenberger.** 1987. Association of polyomaviruses JC, SV40 and BK with human brain tumors. Virology **160:**268–270.
18. **Flaegstad, T., H. Permin, A. Husebekk, G. Husby, and T. Traavik.** 1988. BK virus infection in patients with AIDS. Scand. J. Infect. Dis. **20:**145–150.
19. **Flaegstad, T., and T. Traavik.** 1985. Detection of BK virus antibodies measured by enzyme-linked immunosorbent assay (ELISA) and two haemagglutination inhibition methods: a comparative study. J. Med. Virol. **16:**351–356.
20. **Flaegstad, T., and T. Traavik.** 1985. Detection of BK virus IgM antibodies by two enzyme-linked immunosorbent assays (ELISA) and a haemagglutination inhibition method. J. Med. Virol. **17:**195–204.
21. **Frisque, R. J., G. L. Bream, and M. T. Cannella.** 1984. Human polyoma JC virus genome. J. Virol. **51:**459–469.
22. **Frisque, R. J., D. B. Rifkin, and D. L. Walker.** 1980. Transformation of primary hamster brain cells with JC virus and its DNA. J. Virol. **35:**265–269.
23. **Gardner, S. D., A. M. Field, D. V. Coleman, and B. Hulme.** 1971. New human papovavirus (BK) isolated from urine after renal transplantation. Lancet **i:**1253–1257.
24. **Gardner, S. D., E. F. D. MacKenzie, C. Smith, and A. A. Porter.** 1984. Prospective study of the human polyomaviruses BK and JC and cytomegalovirus in renal transplant recipients. J. Clin. Pathol. **37:**578–586.
25. **Gerber, M. A., K. V. Shah, S. N. Thung, and G. ZuRhein.** 1980. Immunohistochemical demonstration of common antigen of polyomaviruses in routine histological tissue sections of animal and man. Am. J. Clin. Pathol. **73:**794–797.
26. **Gibson, P. E., S. D. Gardner, and A. A. Porter.** 1985. Detection of human polyomavirus DNA in urine specimens by hybridot assay. Arch. Virol. **84:**233–240.
27. **Grinell, B. W., B. L. Padgett, and D. L. Walker.** 1983. Distribution of nonintegrated DNA from JC papovavirus in organs of patients with progressive multifocal leukoencephalopathy. J. Infect. Dis. **147:**669–675.
28. **Hashida, Y., P. C. Gaffney, and E. J. Yunis.** 1976. Acute hemorrhagic cystitis of childhood and papovavirus-like particles. J. Pediatr. **89:**85–87.
29. **Heritage, J., P. M. Chesters, and D. J. McCance.** 1981. The persistence of papovavirus BK DNA sequences in normal human renal tissue. J. Med. Virol. **8:**143–150.
30. **Hogan, T. F., E. C. Borden, J. A. McBain, B. L. Padgett, and D. L. Walker.** 1980. Human polyomavirus infections with JC virus and BK virus in renal transplant patients. Ann. Intern. Med. **92:**373–378.
31. **Hogan, T. F., B. L. Padgett, and D. L. Walker.** 1984. Human polyomaviruses, p. 969–995. *In* R. B. Belshe (ed.), Textbook of human virology. PSG Publishing Co., Inc., Littleton, Mass.
32. **Hogan, T. F., B. L. Padgett, D. L. Walker, E. C. Borden, and J. A. McBain.** 1980. Rapid detection and identification of JC virus and BK virus in human urine using immunofluorescence microscopy. J. Clin. Microbiol. **11:**178–183.
33. **Iltis, J. P., C. S. Cleghorn, D. L. Madden, and J. L. Sever.** 1983. Detection of antibody to BK virus by enzyme-linked immunosorbent assay compared to haemagglutination inhibition and immunofluorescent antibody staining. Clin. Biol. Res. **105:**157–168.
34. **Kahan, A., D. Coleman, and L. Koss.** 1980. Activation of human polyomavirus infection-detection by cytologic technics. Am. J. Clin. Pathol. **74:**326–332.
35. **Krupp, L. B., R. B. Lipton, M. L. Swerdlow, N. E. Leeds, and J. Llena.** 1985. Progressive multifocal leukoencephalopathy: clinical and radiographic features. Ann. Neurol. **17:**344–349.
36. **Lecatsas, G., O. W. Prozesky, J. Van Wyk, and H. J. Els.** 1973. Papova virus in urine after renal transplantation. Nature (London) **241:**343–344.
37. **London, W., S. Houff, D. Madden, D. Ficcillo, M. Gravell, W. Wallen, A. Palmer, J. Sever, B. Padgett, D. Walker, G. ZuRhein, and T. Ohashi.** 1978. Brain tumors in owl monkeys inoculated with a human polyomavirus (JC virus). Science **201:**1246–1249.
38. **Major, E. O., and G. di Mayorca.** 1973. Malignant transformation of BHK_{21} clone 13 cells by BK virus—a human papovavirus. Proc. Natl. Acad. Sci. USA **70:**3210–3212.
39. **Major, E. O., A. E. Miller, P. Mourrain, R. G. Traub, E. deWidt, and J. L. Sever.** 1985. Establishment of a line of human fetal glial cells that supports JC virus replication. Proc. Natl. Acad. Sci. USA **82:**1257–1261.
40. **Mandl, C., D. L. Walker, and R. J. Frisque.** 1987. Derivation and characterization of POJ cells, transformed human fetal glial cells that retain their permissivity for JC virus. J. Virol. **61:**755–763.
41. **Mininberg, D. T., C. Watson, and M. Desquitado.** 1982. Viral cystitis with transient secondary vesicoureteral reflux. J. Urol. **127:**983–985.
42. **Miyamura, T., K. Yoshiike, and K. K. Takemoto.** 1980. Characterization of JC papovavirus adapted to grow in human embryonic kidney cells. J. Virol. **35:**498–504.
43. **O'Reilly, R. J., F. K. Lee, E. Grossbard, N. Kapoor, D. Kirkpatrick, R. Dinsmore, C. Stutzer, K. V. Shah, and A. J. Nahmias.** 1981. Papovavirus excretion following marrow transplantation: incidence and association with hepatic dysfunction. Transplant. Proc. **13:**262–266.
44. **Padgett, B. L., and D. L. Walker.** 1973. Prevalence of antibodies in human sera against JC virus, an isolate from a case of progressive multifocal leukoencephalopathy. J. Infect. Dis. **127:**467–470.
45. **Padgett, B. L., and D. L. Walker.** 1983. Virological and serologic studies of progressive multifocal leukoencephalopathy. Clin. Biol. Res. **105:**107–117.
46. **Padgett, B. L., D. L. Walker, M. M. Desquitado, and D. U. Kim.** 1983. BK virus and non-hemorrhagic cystitis in a child. Lancet **i:**770.
47. **Padgett, B. L., D. L. Walker, G. M. ZuRhein, R. J. Eckroade, and B. H. Dessell.** 1971. Cultivation of papova-like virus from human brain with progressive multifocal leu-

koencephalopathy. Lancet **i:**1257–1260.

48. **Reese, J. M., M. Reissig, R. W. Daniel, and K. V. Shah.** 1975. Occurrence of BK virus and BK-specific antibodies in the urine of patients receiving chemotherapy for malignancy. Infect. Immun. **11:**1375–1381.
49. **Saiki, R. K., D. H. Gelfand, S. Stoffel, S. J. Scharf, R. Higuchi, G. T. Horn, K. B. Mullis, and H. A. Erlich.** 1988. Primer-directed enzymatic amplification of DNA with a thermostable DNA polymerase. Science **239:**487–491.
50. **Saiki, R. K., S. Scharf, F. Faloona, K. B. Mullis, G. T. Horn, H. A. Erlich, and N. Arnheim.** 1985. Enzymatic amplification of β-globin genomic sequences and restriction site analysis for diagnosis of sickle cell anemia. Science **230:**1350–1354.
51. **Seif, I., G. Khoury, and R. Dhar.** 1979. The genome of human papovavirus BKV. Cell **18:**963–977. (Erratum, **19:** 567, 1980.)
52. **Shah, K. V., R. W. Daniel, and J. D. Strandberg.** 1975. Sarcoma in a hamster inoculated with BK virus, a human papovavirus. J. Natl. Cancer Inst. **54:**945–950.
53. **Shah, K. V., R. W. Daniel, and R. Warszawski.** 1973. High prevalence of antibodies of BK virus, an SV40 related papovavirus, in residents of Maryland. J. Infect. Dis. **128:** 784–787.
54. **Shah, K. V., H. L. Ozer, H. N. Ghazey, and T. J. Kelly.** 1977. Common structural antigen of papovaviruses of the simian virus 40-polyoma subgroup. J. Virol. **21:**179–186.
55. **Shope, R. E., and G. E. Sather.** 1979. Arboviruses, p. 767–814. *In* E. H. Lennette and N. J. Schmidt (ed.), Diagnostic procedures for viral, rickettsial and chlamydial infections, 5th ed. American Public Health Association, Inc., Washington, D.C.
56. **Silverman, L., and L. J. Rubinstein.** 1965. Electron microscopic examination observations of a case of progressive multifocal leukoencephalopathy. Acta Neuropathol. **5:**215–224.
57. **Southern, E.** 1975. Detection of specific sequences among DNA fragments separated by gel electrophoresis. J. Mol. Biol. **98:**503.
58. **Takemoto, K. K., P. M. Howley, and T. Miyamura.** 1979. JC human papovavirus replication in human amnion cells. J. Virol. **30:**384–389.
59. **Traystman, M. D., P. K. Gupta, K. V. Shah, M. Reissig, L. T. Cowles, W. D. Hillis, and J. K. Frost.** 1980. Identification of viruses in the urine of renal transplant recipients by cytomorphology. Acta Cytol. **24:**501–510.
60. **Walker, D., and B. L. Padgett.** 1983. Progressive multifocal leukoencephalopathy, p. 161–193. *In* H. Fraenkel-Conrat and R. R. Wagner (ed.), Comprehensive virology, vol. 18. Plenum Publishing Corp., New York.
61. **Walker, D. L., and R. J. Frisque.** 1986. The biology and molecular biology of JC virus, p. 327–377. *In* N. P. Salzman (ed.), The papovaviridae: the polyomaviruses, vol. I. Plenum Publishing Corp., New York.
62. **Walker, D. L., B. L. Padgett, G. M. ZuRhein, A. E. Albert, and R. F. Marsh.** 1973. Human papova-virus (JC): induction of brain tumors in hamsters. Science **181:**674–676.
63. **Yang, R. C. A., and R. Wu.** 1979. BK virus DNA: complete nucleotide sequence of human tumor virus. Science **206:** 456–462.
64. **ZuRhein, G. M., and S. M. Chou.** 1965. Particles resembling papova viruses in human cerebral demyelination disease. Science **148:**1477–1479.

Chapter 100

Human Immunodeficiency Viruses

SUSAN W. BARNETT AND JAY A. LEVY

CLINICAL BACKGROUND

In the early 1980s, reports of the unusual occurrence of *Pneumocystis carinii* pneumonia and Kaposi's sarcoma in previously healthy young men in the United States led to the recognition of AIDS as a new disease syndrome (21, 29). Further studies indicated that this disease was also found in Haiti and Africa. Initial epidemiologic evidence strongly suggested that an infectious agent was responsible for the disease and that the agent was transmitted by blood and by sexual contact.

By early 1983, scientists at the Pasteur Institute isolated a novel retrovirus from a young homosexual man with lymphadenopathy (3). This virus, called lymphadenopathy-associated virus, was shown to be distinct from other known human retroviruses, human T-cell leukemia virus type I (HTLV-I), and a more rare virus also isolated from leukocytes, HTLV-II. Soon afterward, biologically and molecularly similar viruses were isolated from AIDS patients in the United States and termed human T-cell lymphotropic virus type III (19) and AIDS-associated retrovirus (39). These AIDS viruses differed from HTLV-I and HTLV-II in that they replicated quickly and to high titers in T-lymphocyte cultures, causing distinct cytopathic effects, they were unable to transform cells, and they demonstrated unique antigenic and molecular properties.

In 1986, a subcommittee of the International Committee on Taxonomy of Viruses recommended that this new subfamily of viruses be named human immunodeficiency virus (HIV) (J. Coffin, A. Haase, J. A. Levy, L. Montaignier, A. Orosczlan, N. Teich, H. Temin, K. Toyoshima, H. Varmus, P. Vogt, and R. Weiss, Letter, Science **232:**697, 1986). It was also suggested that the various strains of the virus be designated by a code with geographically informative letters and sequential numbers placed in brackets or as a subscript (for example, HIV-1_{SF33} for San Francisco isolate 33).

The World Health Organization has estimated that between 500,000 and 800,000 persons in the United States were infected with HIV as of 1988 (54); worldwide, 5 million to 10 million persons are now infected with HIV. It is expected that in the absence of curative therapies, the number of AIDS cases will reach well past 1 million in the 1990s. HIV infection can lead to a variety of disease states, including an acute mononucleosis-like syndrome, prolonged asymptomatic infection, AIDS-related complex, and frank AIDS (29). In a large proportion of cases, adults may experience the acute syndrome at or near the time of seroconversion (12). The distinctive symptoms of acute infection include lymphadenopathy, macular rash, fever, myalgia, arthralgia, headache, fatigue, diarrhea, sore throat, and neurological manifestations. This syndrome may last for a few days up to a couple of weeks, after which the patient generally recovers and remains asymptomatic for months to years. For an extensive discussion of HIV infection and AIDS, see reference 37.

Persistent antibodies to HIV usually develop within 1 week to 3 months of infection, but there have been reports of delayed seroconversion. For example, one recent study of high-risk individuals has revealed that HIV infection may occur up to 3 years before antibodies to the virus appear (28). On occasion, a loss of seropositive status has been observed in infected individuals (16). Thus, in rare situations, some people appear to be persistently infected for as long as a few years and do not mount an antibody response. In some of these cases, HIV can be detected only by a very sensitive assay that detects proviral DNA, the polymerase chain reaction (PCR; see below) (28). The extent and consequences of these silent HIV infections require further study.

Progression from HIV infection to AIDS differs among population groups and has changed over time. From studies of several different cohorts in the United States, it appears that in the absence of treatment, 40 to 50% of infected individuals will progress to develop AIDS 7 to 10 years after infection (49, 75). The majority of HIV-infected individuals remain asymptomatic for at least 2 to 5 years (36). Persistent lymphadenopathy, which often appears during acute infection, was originally believed to predict progression to AIDS in HIV-infected homosexual men but now appears not to be a good predictor (53). The most commonly reported clinical symptoms predictive for progression to AIDS are persistent herpes zoster infections, oral candidiasis (thrush), oral hairy leukoplakia, and constitutional symptoms such as sustained weight loss, fatigue, night sweats, and persistent diarrhea. Some of these symptoms characterize what has been referred to as AIDS-related complex. Herpes zoster is an early sign of progression, thrush and hairy leukoplakia occur later, and the persistent constitutional symptoms appear later and are highly indicative of imminent progression to AIDS (49).

AIDS patients suffer from Kaposi's sarcoma, *P. carinii* pneumonia, chronic diarrhea often caused by cryptosporidia, cryptococcal meningitis, toxoplasmosis, encephalopathies, and dementia, as well as anal or rectal carcinomas and B-lymphocytic lymphomas. In Africa, HIV infection and AIDS are also characterized by chronic diarrhea, a wasting syndrome, resistant tuberculosis, aggressive Kaposi's sarcoma, and persistent herpes zoster (59). Most AIDS patients in the United States have died from *P. carinii* pneumonia, whereas in Africa they frequently succumb to cryptococcal meningitis or chronic dehydration secondary to the severe diarrhea, a condition called slim disease (66). Some HIV-infected individuals also develop autoimmune diseases such as immune thrombocytopenic purpura, neutropenia, and peripheral neuropathy as a result of production of autoantibodies to normal cellular proteins (38). AIDS is therefore a complex of diseases resulting from primary immune disorders induced by the causative agent, HIV.

In 1986, a new subtype of HIV, HIV-2, was isolated from West African AIDS patients and from seropositive, asymptomatic individuals (9). More recently, HIV-2 has been found increasingly in Europe and Brazil (13). Several cases, mostly in immigrant West Africans, have been reported in the United States (2, 6, 7). Although HIV-2 isolates exhibit several biological characteristics in common with HIV-1, they can be serologically and molecularly distinguished from HIV-1. Antigenic cross-reactivity between these subtypes is generally limited to the viral core and polymerase proteins, but most HIV-2-positive sera can be identified by using HIV-1-based serological tests (57). Nevertheless, the spread of HIV-2 and the failure to consistently detect HIV-2-infected specimens by using HIV-1-specific reagents highlight the need to employ HIV-2-specific tests where such an infection is suspected.

DESCRIPTION OF AGENT

HIV subtypes are classified in the family *Retroviridae*, subfamily *Lentivirinae*, by virtue of their physicochemical, molecular, and biological characteristics. The human *Lentivirinae* are distinct from the other subfamilies of human retroviruses, the *Spumavirinae* (human foamy virus) and the *Oncovirinae* (HTLV-I and HTLV-II). In particular, lentivirus genomes are large and contain several viral genes, the viruses frequently induce cytopathic effects in infected cells, and the disease they cause has a long incubation period resulting in immunological and neurological disorders (Table 1). Lentiviruses have been identified in other animals and include visna-maedi virus of sheep, equine infectious anemia virus, caprine encephalitis virus, and bovine, feline, and simian immunodeficiency viruses.

Retrovirus virions are spherical, measure 80 to 130 nm in diameter, and have a unique three-layered structure (Fig. 1). Innermost is the genome-nucleocapsid complex, which is associated with reverse transcriptase (RT) molecules. This complex is enclosed within an icosahedral capsid, which is then surrounded by a host cell membrane-derived envelope from which project viral glycoprotein spikes. The virion genome is a single-stranded positive-sense RNA molecule about 9 kilobases in length. Each virion is diploid, containing two identical copies of its RNA genome.

The HIV-1 and HIV-2 genomes are similar in structure, although subtype-specific genes have been identified (Fig. 2). These genomes contain the three genes common to all retroviruses: the *gag* (group-specific antigen) gene, which encodes the virion core proteins; the *pol* gene, which encodes the RT (or RNA-dependent DNA polymerase), a protease, and the endonuclease (or integrase); and the *env* gene, which encodes the two major envelope glycoproteins, gp120 and gp41 (for a review, see reference 58).

The 53-kilodalton precursor core polypeptide (p53 or p55) encoded by the *gag* gene is cleaved by the HIV protease (p10) into four major components. The most abundant and only phosphorylated of the *gag* proteins is p25, which noncovalently associates with the viral genome to form a nucleoid shell. Other *gag*-encoded core proteins are the p7 and p9 proteins that derive from a p15 precursor which is cleaved from the carboxy

TABLE 1. Characteristics of lentiviruses

Category	Characteristic
Biological	Host species specific
	Exogenous and nononcogenic
	Cytopathic effects in certain infected cells, e.g., $CD4^+$ T helper T cells for HIV (cell fusion and formation of multinucleated giant cells or syncytia)
	Tropic for cells of macrophage lineage; in vivo infection of macrophages usually noncytopathic, with low levels of virus replication
	Accumulation of unintegrated circular and linear forms of proviral DNA in infected cells
	Can cause a persistent low-level productive infection or exist in latent state
	Morphology of virus particle by electron microscopy: cylindrical nucleoid
Molecular	Large provirus size (~9 kilobases)
	Primer binding site for virus replication is $tRNA^{Lys}$.
	Genome contains several regulatory genes that control expression of structural genes during viral replication.
	Truncated *gag* gene; several processed *gag* proteins
	env gene products are highly glycosylated.
	Polymorphism, particularly in *env* region, resulting in high degree of antigenic variation among different viral isolates
Clinical	Persistent infection can lead to a wasting disease after a variable incubation of months to years.
	Involvement of the hematopoietic system
	Involvement of the central nervous system
	Causes clinical conditions that include immune deficiency, autoimmunity, arthritis, and encephalitis

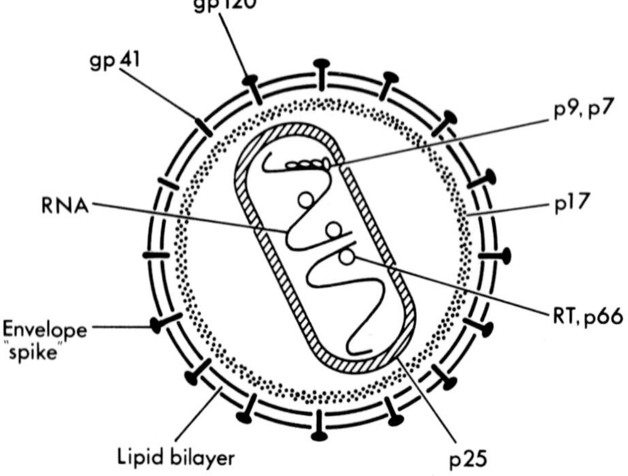

FIG. 1. Basic structure of HIV. Locations of the envelope glycoproteins (gp120 and gp41) and of the major viral core proteins (p25, p17, p9, and p7) are shown. Core protein p17 is found outside the viral nucleoid and forms the matrix of the virion. (Reprinted with permission from reference 38.)

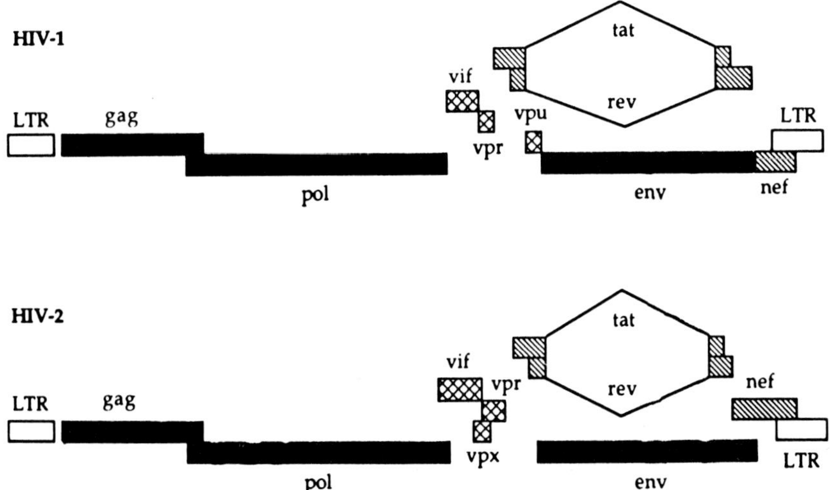

FIG. 2. Genetic structures of HIV-1 and HIV-2. Shown are the genes for the three major structural proteins (*gag, pol,* and *env*) and the regulatory proteins (*tat, rev,* and *nef*) and the genes whose functions are not yet fully characterized (*vif, vpr, vpu* [for HIV-1], and *vpx* [for HIV-2]. *tat* and *rev* are translated from overlapping reading frames and spliced RNA regions that join to coding exons. The major viral regulatory region, the long terminal repeat (LTR), contains sequences that are responsive to viral (e.g., *tat*) and cellular proteins. Further details on the HIV genes can be found in references 58 and 60. (Reprinted with permission from reference 38.)

terminus of p53. p17 comes from the amino terminus of p53 and forms the matrix of the virion (Fig. 1).

The *pol* polyprotein (p160) precursor is cleaved into the self-cleaving viral protease, p10; the RT, which is active in two forms, p66 and p51; and the endonuclease, p32. The RT also possesses an RNase H activity required for viral replication. In the course of viral replication, these enzymes catalyze the synthesis of a double-stranded DNA provirus by using the viral RNA template. Proviral cDNA is integrated into the host cell genome in reactions involving the viral endonuclease. During a productive infection, high levels of viral RNA are transcribed from this proviral template. In a latent or silent infection, very little viral RNA (or protein) is made from the integrated proviral DNA (see reference 60 for details).

The *env* gene encodes a glycosylated precursor polypeptide, gp160, which is processed by host cellular proteases into gp120, the external envelope glycoprotein which forms the spikes on the virion, and the transmembrane protein gp41. During infection, gp120 binds to the CD4 surface receptor before penetration (of cells of the lymphocytic and monocytic lineages). The envelope protein, especially gp120, can differ substantially among HIV-1 and HIV-2 strains. In addition to substantial genetic variability in *env* among these strains, some HIV-2 subtypes possess an external glycoprotein of slightly higher molecular weight, gp140. The gp120 (or gp140) external glycoprotein is attached to the infected cell surface by noncovalent interactions with the viral gp41 protein, whose hydrophobic carboxy terminus serves as a transmembrane anchor.

In addition to these three characteristic retroviral genes, the HIV genomes encode at least four regulatory proteins. Two major genes, *tat* and *rev*, code for proteins (p14 and p19, respectively) that are essential positive regulators of viral replication. *tat* is believed to act at both the transcriptional and posttranscriptional levels to increase viral gene expression. *rev* is required for the transport of full-length mRNA molecules (which encode the viral structural proteins) out of the nucleus (46). The *nef* gene (formerly, *orf-B* or *3'orf*) encodes a 27-kilodalton myristylated protein that down regulates viral replication in some cells and may be important in viral latency (45). *vif* is a 23-kilodalton protein that appears to be important in later stages of virion maturation. Other viral genes include *vpu*, which is HIV-1 specific, *vpx*, which is HIV-2 specific, and *vpr*. Recent studies indicate that the *vpu* gene functions in the release of virus particles from infected cells (70, 71) and that the *vpr* gene plays a role in viral growth kinetics (52). Transcriptional regulation of the viral genome appears to be mediated through indirect and direct viral and cellular protein interactions with DNA sequences within the viral 5' long terminal repeat in proviral DNA. Several binding sites for known *trans*-acting regulatory factors have been mapped in these sequences (for reviews of the molecular biology of HIV, see references 58 and 60).

EPIDEMIOLOGY, PREVENTION, AND CONTROL

HIV is transmitted through intimate sexual contact, contaminated blood and blood products, and passage from mother to child during perinatal events (14). The virus does not appear to be spread by casual contact or by insect vectors. Transmission most likely occurs via virus-infected cells, since high titers of free virus are not usually found in the plasma phase of blood or in other cell-free body fluids (35, 38). Levels of virus when found in cell-free plasma or semen are several orders of magnitude less (11, 25, 38) than the 10^8 to 10^9 particles per ml of cell-free infectious hepatitis B virus particles found in some blood samples of hepatitis B virus-infected individuals. This property of HIV explains the relatively low risk of infection to health care workers from needle sticks (20). The cell-free virus titers in saliva, tears, urine, and milk are at least 10-fold lower than that in plasma (38).

A major route of sexual transmission of HIV is anal intercourse. The anal-receptive partner is more susceptible to infection than is the insertive partner (78). The virus may infect the mucosal epithelial cells of the bowel directly (40, 50) or gain access to other susceptible cells via injured areas in the mucosal lining of the bowel. Transmission of the virus also occurs by vaginal intercourse, with the female showing the highest sensitivity. Sexual transmission of either kind is enhanced in the presence of other sexually transmitted diseases, including syphilis, gonorrhea, and especially ulcerating diseases such as genital herpes and chancroid, as observed in African populations (59).

The major groups infected with HIV in the early stages of its spread in the United States and western Europe were homosexual (and bisexual) men and intravenous drug users. The number of heterosexuals infected by sexual contacts with these groups is increasing, as is the number of babies born to HIV-infected mothers. The other groups at risk for HIV infection have been hemophiliacs and blood transfusion recipients. Fortunately, transmission in the latter groups has been almost eliminated as the result of serological screening of blood donors and heat treatment of clotting factor preparations (41) in countries where these programs have been possible.

At present, there is no vaccine to protect against HIV infection and there are no curative therapies. The best means to prevent the spread of infection is through education. Simply stated, one must avoid contaminated blood and blood products and intimate sexual contact with HIV-infected persons. Condoms should be used during sexual activities involving potentially infected individuals. Intravenous drug users must avoid sharing contaminated needles and syringes. As noted above, blood and blood products should be serologically tested and donors should be screened to eliminate infected individuals, some of whom may yet be seronegative.

On the positive side, there is some hope of controlling the progression from HIV infection to AIDS. Several antiviral approaches are now being developed and tested. The primary molecular target for several of the antiviral drugs is the viral enzyme, RT. The only drug licensed to date by the U.S. Food and Drug Administration for the primary treatment of AIDS is zidovudine (azidothymidine), a nucleoside analog that specifically inhibits the RT enzyme.

In addition to other inhibitors of viral replication (e.g., dideoxyinosine and alpha interferon), antiviral agents are being developed that target the viral protease and the receptor-binding functions of the viral gp120 (e.g., soluble recombinant CD4 and its immunoconjugates). Another promising antiviral approach is identification of agents that specifically kill HIV-infected cells. A potentially good example of this treatment is compound Q (trichosanthin or GLQ223), a substance derived from the root of a Chinese cucumber which has been shown to selectively kill HIV-infected T cells and macrophages in vitro (48).

COLLECTION AND STORAGE OF SPECIMENS; LABORATORY SAFETY

Blood samples, routinely collected by venipuncture, are generally used for viral detection and serological analyses. To isolate virus from peripheral blood mononuclear cells (PBMC), heparinized or EDTA-treated blood samples must be collected. HIV can also be detected and isolated from other body fluids such as plasma, serum, cerebrospinal fluid, saliva, tears, milk, urine, and genital secretions and from biopsy specimens from infected tissues such as the bowel. Even though the amount of virus present in these latter specimens may be low, precautions should be taken during handling of any potentially HIV-infected clinical specimens. Gloves should be worn, and needles should be handled by safe procedures after collection of blood.

Plasma, serum, or other body fluids to be tested serologically should be stored at −20 or −70°C. For later detection of viral antigens, clinical specimens should be stored at −70°C. For best results, virus isolations should be performed immediately after specimen collection (see below). Nevertheless, PBMC and other infected cells may be stored in liquid nitrogen in culture medium plus 10% dimethyl sulfoxide, with reasonable recovery of virus from the PBMC in most cases.

HIV can be inactivated readily under clinical laboratory conditions by several methods (62, 67). Although relatively stable in a dry or lyophilized state (41), the virus is very sensitive to many detergents (for example, Triton X-100 and Nonidet P-40, but not Tween 20), including soap, and can be eliminated rapidly by bleach (0.5% sodium hypochlorite). Greater than 70% alcohol and acetone-alcohol mixtures can also inactivate virus efficiently at room temperature. HIV strains are also sensitive to iodophores such as organic iodine compounds, pH extremes (pH 2, pH 12), UV and X irradiation, and heating in liquid solution at 56°C. For inactivation of virus in serum before serological testing, specimens should be routinely heated at 56°C for 30 min.

DIRECT AND INDIRECT DETECTION OF VIRUS

ELISA for p25 antigen

Enzyme-linked immunosorbent assay (ELISA) (see also chapter 12) is presently the predominant antigen assay for HIV used for clinical investigations. The viral core antigen, p25 (also called p24), which occurs in relatively high abundance in both virions and infected cells, is generally the target of this assay. ELISA in the capture (or sandwich) format (47) has been used by several biotechnology companies in the development of commercial kits for the detection of HIV antigens. In the original assay (47), a high-titered (1:800,000) human antiserum to HIV was used to coat 96-well microdilution plates. The commercial kits use purified animal or human antibodies against a specific HIV antigen, usually the p25 *gag* protein, or against whole virus.

In these kits, plates with antibodies fixed to them are supplied to the user ready for the addition of the test sample, which can be serum, culture supernatant, or other body fluids. The sample volume to be tested is usually 200 µl and is first treated with detergent (0.05% Triton X-100) to disrupt virions. The incubation times vary but are often 2 h for culture supernatants and overnight for serum and other fluids. An antibody specific for HIV antigen(s) is then added and incubated for 2 to 4 h to complete the antigen capture. This antibody may be itself enzyme conjugated or biotin labeled, or it can be detected by a similarly modified secondary antibody. When biotinylated antibodies are used, enzyme-conjugated streptavidin is added in the following step. After washing, the color reaction is initiated with the addition of enzymatic substrate, and the results are measured by spectrophotometry. Results with uninfected controls are used to determine the cutoff value above which the optical density of the sample is considered positive (usually two times the average of the optical density of the uninfected samples). ELISA can also be performed by using a competition format (27). ELISAs have proven to be one of the most sensitive means with which to detect HIV in both laboratory and clinical samples. With this procedure, one is able to detect as little as 30 pg of viral protein per ml or about a few thousand virions per ml (27). ELISAs are also used routinely to detect serum antibodies to HIV (see below).

IFA

The indirect immunofluorescence assay (IFA) also is useful both as a means of detecting the presence of virus in infected cells and as a serological assay with which to detect the presence of antibodies to HIV in serum from infected individuals (see below and chapter 11). In the former application, the presence of virus in PBMC cultures or in other cells can be confirmed by the detection of viral antigens, using HIV-specific antiserum in an IFA (31). For this analysis, cells are washed three times in a neutral-pH, isotonic solution (e.g., phosphate-buffered saline [PBS]) and resuspended at an appropriate concentration before 10 to 20 μl is spotted onto each dot of an IFA slide. After air drying, samples are fixed in acetone (or acetone-alcohol; see below), dried, and reacted with a known anti-HIV antibody containing serum for 30 min at 37°C. Fixed cells can be stored frozen at −20°C for several days and at −70°C for longer periods of time. The sera used to detect viral antigens must be prescreened to ensure that they lack antibodies to normal cell antigens, and uninfected-cell control samples should always be run in parallel with test cells. Monoclonal antibodies to specific HIV antigens can also be used. After incubation with antibody, the cells are washed in PBS, incubated with fluorescent labeled anti-human immunoglobulin G (IgG) for 20 min at 37°C, and then washed again. After washing, the cells are overlaid with 90% glycerol and a glass cover slip for microscopic examination with a fluorescence microscope. The staining pattern for HIV is characteristic (Fig. 3): the distribution of labeled viral antigen may be both diffuse and reticular in the cytoplasm, localized at the periphery of the cell (crescent formation), or found in discrete areas of high intensity (31).

These methods can also be adapted for fluorescence-activated cell sorting analysis. For this method of analysis to measure viral infectivity, monoclonal antibodies are preferable as primary antibodies, and uninfected cells are run separately to measure background fluorescence. IFA is a rapid, sensitive method in which as little as a single HIV-expressing cell can be detected in a population of hundreds or thousands of cells exam-

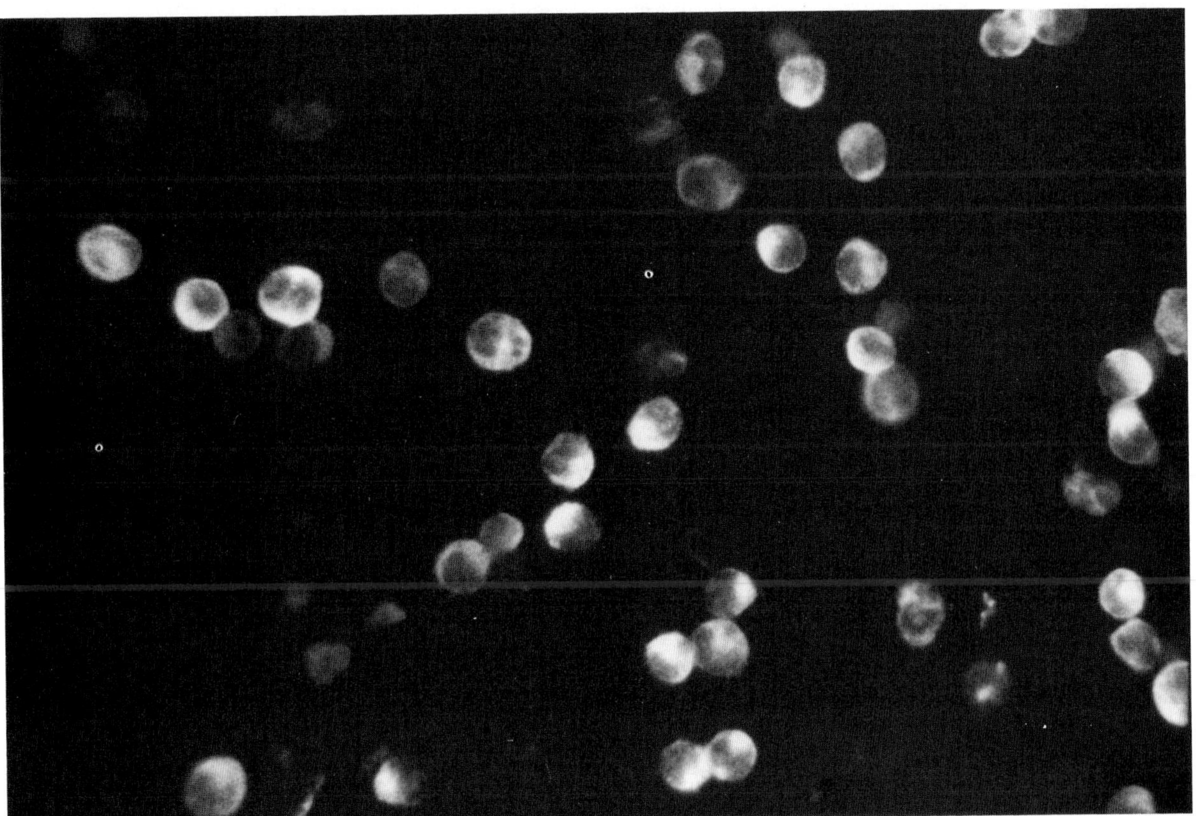

FIG. 3. Photograph of typical IFA-positive cells (magnification, ×225). Note crescent-shaped fluorescence indicative of specific staining of HIV antigens.

ined. However, when microscopy is used to determine HIV reactivity, the success of the assay is dependent on the experience of the reader in interpreting fluorescence patterns.

Immunoperoxidase assay

The immunoperoxidase assay is an enzymatic immunochemical assay by which HIV antigens can be detected in tissue sections or cells (18). Specimens are fixed and mounted on slides, washed with PBS, incubated for 30 min in absolute methanol containing 0.3% hydrogen peroxide to block endogenous peroxidase activity, and washed again in PBS. To reduce nonspecific binding, monoclonal anti-HIV antibodies or antiserum preabsorbed with similar uninfected cells (or tissue) should be used as primary antibodies. After 20 to 30 min of incubation at 37°C with the primary antibody, a species-specific biotinylated IgG fraction is reacted with the sample for 30 min. This procedure is followed by the final color-producing incubation (45 min) with horseradish peroxidase, streptavidin-biotin complex, and substrate (H_2O_2 plus *o*-phenylenediamine). When HIV antigens are present, typical confluent color spots are observed. Secondary antibody complexed with other enzymes such as alkaline phosphatase also can be used. For both this assay and IFA, double-staining experiments are possible to identify infected cell types. Thus, the immunoperoxidase technique is useful in establishing the presence of HIV in particular cell types and tissues. In some cases, this technique can detect HIV in infected cells before the more sensitive p25 antigen ELISA. This observation can be attributed perhaps to the fact that in culture, HIV proteins accumulate inside cells before their release with virions into the culture fluid.

In situ hybridization

In situ hybridization is a histomolecular method to detect the presence of HIV nucleic acids in different cells and tissues. Kits are available commercially which employ enzyme-conjugated HIV detection systems and provide all of the reagents necessary for in situ hybridization. Although these kits are sometimes less sensitive than earlier in situ hybridization protocols (23, 69, 77), their use obviates the need for radioactive materials and autoradiography. A sample protocol is as follows.

To be prepared for hybridization, cells must be washed and concentrated to about 10^7/ml. Then 5 to 10 μl of cells is spotted onto a slide, allowed to air dry, and fixed in 4% paraformaldehyde (freshly made in PBS) for 5 min. Samples are rinsed with PBS and stored in 70% ethanol at 4°C until hybridization is performed. Tissue sections are fixed and treated similarly. Samples are rehydrated in PBS containing 5 mM $MgCl_2$ for 10 min at room temperature and placed in a solution of 70% formamide (deionized) in 2× SSC (1 liter of 20× SSC stock solution contains 175.3 g of NaCl and 88.2 g of sodium citrate) at 70°C for 10 min to denature cellular nucleic acids (prehybridization). After a brief rinse in 5× SSC, excess buffer is removed by careful blotting (avoid touching cells in all steps), and a hybridization solution containing an enzyme (e.g., alkaline phosphatase)-conjugated denatured HIV-specific oligonucleotide probe is added to the cells. Incubation is allowed to proceed at 50°C for 45 min, after which the cells are washed twice in 1× SSC at room temperature and then once at 45°C. Cells that are positive for hybridization are detected after incubation of the sample with the enzyme substrate. Cell nuclei are counterstained with methyl green, and the samples are air dried, mounted by using Permount and a cover slip, and microscopically examined for darkly colored spots over cells indicative of intracellular HIV.

Immunoblot assay

The immunoblot (Western blot) assay (72; see also chapter 13), more commonly used to detect HIV antibodies in serum (see below), also can be used to analyze infected-cell lysates or concentrates of culture supernatants for the presence of HIV proteins. The advantage of this method is that the different HIV gene products can be identified and distinguished by their sizes. For antigen detection, a high-titer control serum with activity against all or most HIV proteins is preferable. When low antigen levels are to be detected, the use of a radiolabeled probe such as ^{125}I-protein A in the final step may be preferred over enzyme conjugates. Reactive bands are revealed by autoradiography or the appropriate enzymatic reactions, and their molecular weights are determined by comparison with molecular weight markers run on the same gel. The immunoblot assay is very useful in distinguishing HIV-1 and HIV-2 isolates after virus culture. In most cases, HIV-1 and HIV-2-specific sera can be used to unambiguously identify which HIV subtype is present. In addition, the sizes of the envelope glycoproteins generally are distinct (gp120 for HIV-1 and gp140 for HIV-2); differences in the core protein may also be observed.

PCR

At present, the most sensitive method of detecting HIV infection is the PCR assay (33, 55). The molecular targets of this procedure are most commonly HIV proviral DNA sequences, but the assay can be modified to permit detection of HIV RNA (24). The PCR assay for HIV DNA can be performed readily with use of only 1 μg of cellular DNA, which is equivalent to only 21 μl of whole blood (33). This DNA amplification procedure uses two oligonucleotide primers that are complementary to the plus and minus strands of target DNA. To ensure detection of many different HIV strains, the sequence of the primers should correspond to regions of the HIV genome that are highly conserved among different HIV isolates. Such regions have been found in *gag*, *env*, and the long terminal repeat. Repeated denaturation, renaturation, and elongation of the primers with a thermostable DNA polymerase are achieved by repeated temperature cycling, which results in an exponential increase in the number of copies of the DNA region flanked by the primers. This DNA is then denatured and hybridized in solution to a radioactively labeled HIV probe that contains sequences complementary to those amplified. When HIV sequences are present, a target-probe complex is formed which can be visualized by autoradiography after polyacrylamide gel electrophoresis. For some studies, the use of multiple primer pairs (and their respective probes) is recommended to further guarantee detection of HIV variants (55). The sensitivity of detection of HIV sequences by using PCR is reported to be as good as one HIV DNA molecule in 100,000 lymphocytes (44). Although low levels of HIV can often be detected after in vitro propagation of infected cells in culture (see below), the PCR method offers the unique advantage that it can detect nonreplicating (latent) viral genomes. Also, PCR procedures can be applied to DNA isolated directly from PBMC of fresh blood, eliminating the need for cell culturing. The disadvantages are that (i) it is technically not yet suitable for routine testing and (ii) because of the extreme sensitivity of the assay, cross-contamination of samples and reagents must be vigilantly avoided (32).

ISOLATION AND CULTIVATION OF VIRUS

Whereas current serological tests (described below) determine whether an individual has been exposed to HIV, a definitive test for an active infection is the recovery of HIV from cells of the infected individual. The initial isolation of HIV was made by cultivating PBMC from a person with lymphadenopathy syndrome (3). In these experiments and others, the mitogen phytohemagglutinin (PHA), which stimulates DNA replication and cellular proliferation of T lymphocytes, is used to amplify the number of infected cells (presumed to be primarily $CD4^+$ helper T lymphocytes) and to increase the release of virus by the cells. Although this procedure was very effective in isolating virus from samples from patients with minimal lymphopenia and mild HIV-associated disease, the recovery rate of virus from some clinical groups (e.g., asymptomatic individuals and patients with severe AIDS) was not more than 50% (42). More efficient viral isolation has been achieved by omitting PHA from the initial sample cultures (5). Instead, PBMC from seronegative donors that have been previously stimulated with PHA are added directly to the PBMC from the person under study. The success of this approach may be due to the avoidance of a PHA induction of suppressor T-lymphocyte ($CD8^+$) cell activity that may reduce viral replication (73). In our laboratory, this cocultivation approach permits the identification of HIV in more than 90% of seropositive individuals with different clinical conditions and allows for the detection of one productively infected $CD4^+$ cell in a population of more than 10^6 PBMC (5). A description of this method follows.

Primary viral isolation from patient material depends on the amplification of HIV being expressed in at most 1/1,000 $CD4^+$ T cells (23, 65). Thus, an adequate amount of heparinized blood is needed (as little as 3 to 5 ml from children and as much as 30 ml from adults). For best results, the blood specimen should be cultured within a few hours after venipuncture. Nevertheless, whole blood can be held for up to 36 h at room temperature without significant reduction of virus recovery. It should not be stored at 4°C for the first 24 h, since it is often difficult to later separate the buffy coat of leukocytes. Any blood sample to be kept for more than 36 h should be stored at room temperature for 24 h and then put at 4°C or should first be subjected to buffy coat separation. In the latter case, leukocytes can then be maintained in serum-containing medium for 7 to 10 days before culture for virus.

For virus isolation, heparinized blood is first spun in a clinical desktop centrifuge at 2,000 rpm for 10 min to separate the buffy coat. The leukocytes are removed from the blood sample, diluted in Hanks balanced salt solution (HBSS; 1:3 [vol/vol]), and overlaid on a Ficoll-Hypaque gradient cushion (HBSS-Ficoll, 3:1 [vol/vol]). This preparation is centrifuged at 2,000 rpm (800 × g) for 15 min without a brake, and the separated PBMC are carefully removed from the Ficoll-HBSS interface and washed at least three times with HBSS. Washed PBMC are suspended at 3×10^6 cells per ml in RPMI 1640 medium supplemented with 10% fetal calf serum, 2% glutamine, 100 IU of penicillin per ml, 100 μg of streptomycin per ml, 5% human interleukin-2 (T-cell growth factor), and 2 μg of Polybrene per ml. The fetal calf serum should be prescreened to avoid possible toxicity to human lymphocytes, and the interleukin-2 should be tested to guarantee that the optimal concentration is used. The latter can be achieved by titrating the interleukin-2 effect on cell viability counts or [^{3}H]thymidine uptake by PBMC.

Usually 3×10^6 to 6×10^6 cells prepared as described above are mixed with an equal number of uninfected PBMC (which were previously stimulated with PHA for 3 days and washed) to initiate the culture. In cases of low numbers of PBMC (e.g., infants), as few as 10^6 cells can be used if the culture vessel is kept small (5). Subsequently, fresh mitogen-stimulated uninfected PBMC are added as needed to maintain viable cell concentrations (at approximately 3×10^6 cells per ml). Cultures are kept at 37°C in a 5% CO_2 atmosphere. They are monitored for the presence of virus, and the medium is replaced every 3 to 4 days. For the detection of virus in the culture fluid, the fluid is first filtered (0.45-μm pore size) or centrifuged at 3,000 rpm (2,000 × g) for 15 min to remove cell debris and then subjected to the RT assay described elsewhere (26) or to the p25 antigen ELISA described above. Culture supernatants possessing substantial levels of p25 antigen or RT activity can also be stored at −70°C for further studies. For most HIV-infected individuals, virus growth will become apparent within the first 2 weeks of culture; by 30 days, more than 90% of those infected will yield a positive viral culture (5). When very low levels of infectious virus are present, these cultures may take longer, sometimes up to 60 days. These methods (minus the PBMC separation steps) can also be adapted to detect and isolate HIV in other body fluids and in biopsy specimens. Recently, good virus recovery has been reported after the addition of fresh patient plasma (200 μl is recommended) to PHA-activated PBMC from normal donors (11, 25). For general information on cell culturing, see chapter 19.

For viral cultivation in vitro, cells (PBMC or established cell lines) are pretreated with Polybrene (2 μg/ml) or DEAE-dextran (25 μg/ml) in culture medium for 30 min at 37°C, centrifuged at low speed to recover cells, and inoculated with a viral stock. Usually the viral stock is simply a viral culture supernatant exhibiting substantial virus titer (measured by p25 ELISA or RT assay). After addition of virus, absorption of the virus onto the cells in a small volume is allowed for at least 30 min at 37°C before the addition of culture medium. The cells are centrifuged and placed in fresh medium every 3 to 4 days, and the supernatant is assayed for RT activity or p25 antigen production to detect viral replication. Some virus isolates can be passaged to several different established human cell lines and maintained as chronically infected cultures (15, 43). Passage of an isolate to an established cell line may require cell-to-cell contact, in which case infected primary leukocytes must be added directly to the cell line for infection of the latter (15). As with primary cultures in PBMC, HIV-infected human cell lines may exhibit cytopathology and cell death, but after a few days a viable subpopulation sometimes emerges that is chronically infected and grows continuously.

DETECTION OF ANTIBODIES TO HIV

ELISA

The indirect ELISA is one of the most sensitive methods for detecting antibodies to HIV and is currently in widespread use as the primary screening method with which to protect blood supplies (76). The assay, which was originally developed to detect antibodies to HTLV-I (64), employs either ruptured purified virus or infected-cell lysates as an antigen. More recently, ELISAs have been developed that use recombinant DNA-derived (4, 8, 51) or synthetic (74) HIV proteins or oligopeptides, most commonly containing conserved regions of gp41. The desired antigen preparation is used to coat the wells of a 96-well plate and serves as the immunosorbent. When purified virus or infected-cell lysates are used, virus is first inactivated by the addition of detergent and heating at 56°C for 30 min. Patient or donor serum or plasma is similarly inactivated, diluted, and allowed to react with the antigen. When whole-cell viral preparations are used as the antigen source, it is necessary to dilute serum (or plasma) samples (approximately 1:50) to avoid nonspecific reactions. Subsequently, an enzyme-conjugated secondary antibody (usually horseradish peroxidase- or alkaline phosphatase-conjugated goat anti-human IgG) is added, and the presence of reactive antibodies in the sample is detected by a color reaction after the addition of enzyme substrate. This color reaction can be quantified by spectrophotometry. There are numerous variations of this assay as well as many commercial kits, most of which provide proprietary conveniences that add to the speed and simplicity of testing. Although the ELISA for HIV antibodies was originally developed to screen donated blood, it is now also routinely used as a diagnostic tool for HIV infection. Unfortunately, this very sensitive assay has a false-positive rate which gives it a poor predictive value in populations with a low prevalence to HIV (61). Therefore, positive ELISA results must always be confirmed by additional testing.

Recently, an ELISA has been described which uses a panel of six recombinant proteins derived from the HIV *gag*, *pol*, and *env* genes (51). It was developed as a supplemental (or confirmatory) test for the presence of antibodies to HIV-1 in sera reactive in the whole-cell-derived virion-screening ELISAs currently licensed for primary blood screening (described above). The advantage of this assay over other supplemental tests (immunoblot and immunofluorescence assays; see below) is that it should prove suitable for large-volume, automated testing.

IFA

The IFA as it applies to the detection of antibodies in patient serum or plasma is performed essentially as described above for viral detection. In this case, cells that have been chronically infected with the virus (such as established T-cell lines) are used as the substrate. It is important that the majority of infected cells be expressing viral proteins (nearly 100% IFA positive) at the time slides are prepared. Infected cells are best mixed 1:1 with uninfected cells of the same type to provide a known background of nonreacting cells as an internal negative control (31). Cells are prepared for staining as described above. It has recently been reported that although acetone is the preferred fixative for good antigen preservation in the IFA, it may not inactivate HIV (17). It has been suggested that acetone-fixed slide preparations be stored at −70°C for at least 40 days to achieve optimal antigen preservation and virus inactivation. We have found that prepared slides can be stored for up to 3 months at this temperature. We sometimes use an alcohol-acetone (1:1) fixative that eliminates infectious virus and preserves antigen. As described above, the staining pattern for HIV is characteristic (Fig. 3) and can therefore be used to determine a true antibody reaction. This assay is rapid and, when necessary, can be performed in less than 1 h. The IFA can be used as a supplemental test for ELISA-positive serum samples and is most useful when a limited number of samples are tested.

Immunoblot assay

The immunoblot assay for the detection of antibodies to HIV in patient samples has been adapted from the original Western blot procedure (72); it is described extensively in other reports (30, 56) and in chapter 13. The assay allows for detection of antibody to specific viral proteins and is therefore clinically useful both as a supplemental test for HIV infection and as a diagnostic tool to monitor disease progression (Fig. 4) (56). For this assay, either purified virus or infected-cell lysates are separated by sodium dodecyl sulfate-polyacrylamide gel electrophoresis and then transferred to nitrocellulose paper by standard blotting procedures. The blot is then cut into narrow strips for blocking and incubation with test sera. Such strips, often prepared with recombinant viral protein preparations, are also available commercially in complete kits containing detector systems. Each strip is incubated separately with a serum specimen (usually diluted 1:50), and after washing, any of several detector systems is used. Detection with ^{125}I-protein A or an alkaline phosphatase-conjugated secondary antibody appears to be most sensitive. If infected-cell lysates are used as the antigen source, one can detect antibody binding to the precursor envelope protein, gp160, as well as to the precursor *gag* protein, p55. These antigens are not detectable when purified viral preparations are used. Because some individuals exhibit antibodies only to gp160 (56), there is an advantage to its presence in this assay.

Variations in the procedures now used to perform immunoblot assays have been described, and several different sets of criteria are used to determine a positive anti-HIV reaction. Many of these procedures and criteria have been reviewed, tested, and critically evaluated by the Consortium for Retrovirus Serology Standardization (10). This publication is worthwhile reading for anyone using this assay to determine HIV infection status. In brief, the Consortium consensus criteria for a positive anti-HIV reaction are the presence of antibodies to either p25 (*gag*) or p31 (endonuclease) and the presence of antibodies to either gp41 (*env*) or gp120/gp160 (*env*). The presence of reactivity to any other HIV proteins in a pattern that does not meet these criteria for positive is considered indeterminate; the absence of

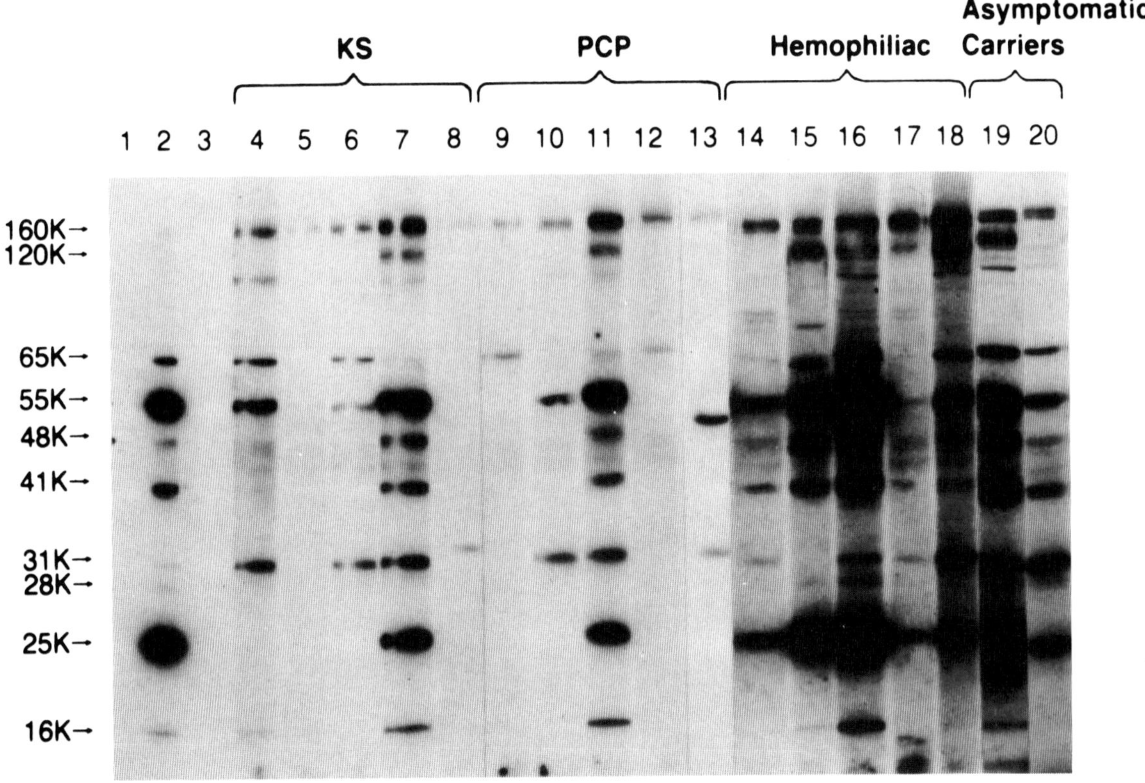

FIG. 4. Immunoblot analysis of sera from patients with Kaposi's sarcoma (KS) and *P. carinii* pneumonia (PCP) and from asymptomatic and hemophiliac men. The viral proteins detected are to the envelope (gp160, gp120, and gp41), the polymerase (p65 and p31), and the core (p55, p48, p25, and p16) proteins. (Reprinted with permission from reference 56.)

reactivity to HIV proteins (no specific bands) is considered negative.

INTERPRETATION OF TEST RESULTS

Since the discovery of the HIV virus as the causative agent of AIDS, the screening of individuals as well as the blood supply for HIV infection has primarily relied on the use of HIV antibody assays (30, 31, 63). Positive antibody status is considered equivalent to HIV infection, and the epidemiologic evidence appears to support this assumption. However, the absence of antibodies to HIV is sometimes an unreliable indicator of the absence of infection, especially in the early stages of infection and in certain populations at high risk for infection. As discussed above, HIV has been identified in individuals known to be at risk who have remained seronegative for up to 3 years after infection (28). Thus, risk status should be considered when evaluating an individual for HIV infection, and tests should be chosen accordingly. In addition, self-deferral of high-risk individuals as blood donors is essential.

A general scheme for the determination of HIV infection is outlined in Fig. 5. Most individuals are initially tested for serum antibodies to HIV by ELISA, but other assays, especially IFA, are also applicable. HIV antibodies can be detected as well in other body fluids from infected individuals. If the patient has been recently infected, antibodies to HIV can develop within 2 to 6 weeks but may take longer. Testing for IgM antibodies (12) or for antibodies to HIV regulatory proteins (e.g., *nef* [1]) may prove useful for the detection of early-stage or latent infections. After initial screening, confirmation of the presence of HIV antibodies is necessary. This is particularly important after ELISA screening because of the occurrence of nonspecific reactions which yield false-positive results. In general, sera giving a positive ELISA are retested by a second ELISA. If this result is also positive, the presence of HIV antibodies in the sample is examined further by IFA or immunoblot, using appropriate control sera and cells.

The nature of the antibody response to HIV analyzed by immunoblots also can be helpful in evaluating the infection status of patients. In most acutely infected individuals, the first antibodies produced are to the *gag* proteins and, in some cases, the *env* proteins. As the disease progresses, antibodies to all of the viral proteins become detectable, particularly the polymerase proteins p65 and p31. Then, when antibodies to the core and the polymerase proteins decrease, a more advanced disease state is usually observed (30, 34, 68). This progression may reflect enhanced virus release into the blood and formation of immune complexes or a decrease in specific antibody production. Neutralizing antibodies and antibodies to gp160 may remain relatively constant until the terminal stages of AIDS (56).

When serological tests for HIV antibodies are inconclusive, viral detection methods may be desirable, especially in high-risk individuals who, for treatment purposes, might benefit from early diagnosis. Although time consuming and technically involved, virus cultivation and PCR assays are the most reliable tests for the de-

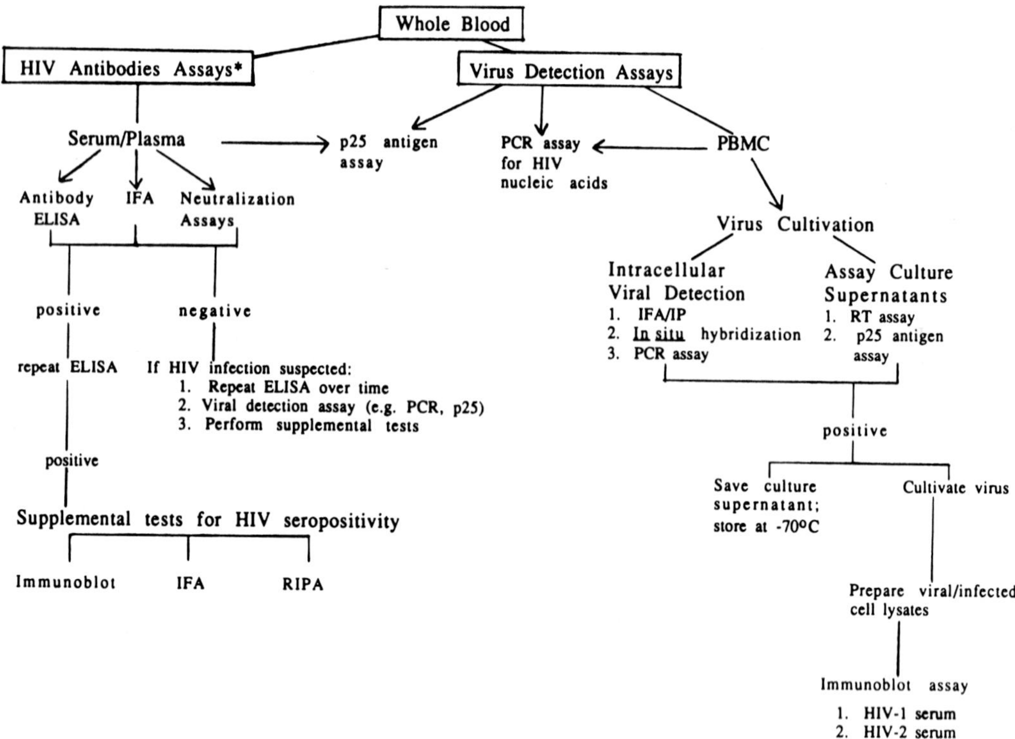

FIG. 5. Scheme for determination of HIV infection.

termination of HIV infection in these individuals. Nevertheless, the predominant HIV assay for clinical investigation is the p25 antigen ELISA. This assay can sometimes detect an initial antigenemic stage (in both blood and cerebrospinal fluid samples) occurring immediately after HIV infection (22). However, this antigenemia is usually transient; a negative antigen status is generally found a few weeks afterward, corresponding to a rise in anti-HIV antibody levels. This finding may reflect the formation of antibody-antigen complexes that mask p25 detection. Thus, although this assay is technically easy and commercially available, its usefulness is limited for diagnostic and screening purposes. In addition, recent findings indicate that p25 antigenemia does not necessarily correlate with plasma viremia as measured by the cultivation (and titration) of infectious virus in patient plasma (11, 25). Plasma infectious virus titers appear to be more reliable indicators of disease progression than p25 antigen levels (11, 25).

If HIV infection is highly suspected and HIV-1-specific test results are inconclusive, serological tests for HIV-2 which employ HIV-2-specific reagents should be used. In addition, viral cultivation may be desirable to further identify possible HIV-2 by immunoblot methods that use viral lysates and HIV subtype-specific sera. This strategy may become more important as the prevalence of HIV-2 increases in countries other than those of West Africa (2, 6, 7).

In conclusion, HIV-1 and HIV-2 are members of the lentivirus subfamily of human retroviruses. These viruses are the causative agents of a complex array of diseases that characterize various clinical states of HIV infection, including AIDS-related complex and frank AIDS. As described above, several serological and viral detection assays are available for use in identifying HIV infection (Fig. 5). While the development of more effective antiviral therapies is awaited, early testing for HIV in potentially infected individuals is recommended to allow prompt medical treatment and surveillance and to prevent the spread of the virus to other individuals. At present, medical treatment is limited to the use of the antiviral drug azidothymidine and treatment of the many opportunistic infections and conditions that afflict HIV-infected individuals. For the moment, continual education on how to prevent HIV transmission must be given major emphasis.

LITERATURE CITED

1. **Ameisen, J.-C., B. Guy, S. Chamaret, et al.** 1989. Antibodies to the *nef* protein and to *nef* peptides in HIV-1-infected seronegative individuals. AIDS Res. Hum. Retroviruses **5:**279–291.
2. **Ayanian, J. Z., J. H. Maguire, R. G. Marlink, M. Essex, and P. J. Kanki.** 1989. HIV-2 infection in the United States. N. Engl. J. Med. **320:**1422–1423.
3. **Barre-Sinoussi, F., M. Nuguyre, C. Dauguet, E. Vilmer, C. Griscelli, F. Brun-Vezinet, C. Rouzioux, J. Gluckman, J. Chermann, and L. Montagnier.** 1983. Isolation of a T-lymphotropic retrovirus from a patient at risk for acquired immunodeficiency syndrome. Science **220:**868–871.
4. **Cabradilla, C. D., J. E. Groopman, J. Lanigan, J. M. Renz, L. A. Lasky, and D. Capon.** 1986. Serodiagnosis of antibodies to the human AIDS retrovirus with a bacterially synthesized *env* polypeptide. Bio/Technology **4:**128–133.

5. **Castro, B. A., C. D. Weiss, L. D. Wiviott, and J. A. Levy.** 1988. Optimal conditions for recovery of the human immunodeficiency virus from peripheral blood mononuclear cells. J. Clin. Microbiol. **26:**2371–2376.
6. **Centers for Disease Control.** 1987. AIDS due to HIV-2 infection—New Jersey. Morbid. Mortal. Weekly Rep. **37:** 969.
7. **Centers for Disease Control.** 1989. Update: HIV-2 infection—United States. Morbid. Mortal. Weekly Rep. **38:**572–580.
8. **Chang, T. W., I. Kato, S. McKinney, P. Chanda, A. D. Barone, F. Wong-Staal, R. C. Gallo, and N. T. Chang.** 1985. Detection of antibodies to human T-cell lymphotropic virus-III (HTLV-III) with an immunoassay employing a recombinant E. coli derived viral antigenic peptide. Bio/Technology **3:**905–909.
9. **Clavel, F., K. Mansinho, S. Chamaret, D. Guetard, V. Favier, J. Nina, M. O. Santos-Ferreira, J. L. Champalimaud, and L. Montaignier.** 1987. Human immunodeficiency virus type 2 infection associated with AIDS in West Africa. N. Engl. J. Med. **316:**1180–1185.
10. **Consortium for Retrovirus Serology Standardization.** 1988. Serological diagnosis of human immunodeficiency virus infection by Western blot testing. J. Am. Med. Assoc. **260:**674–679.
11. **Coombs, R. W., A. C. Collier, J.-P. Allain, B. Nikora, M. Leuther, G. F. Gjerst, and L. Corey.** 1989. Plasma viremia in human immunodeficiency virus infection. N. Engl. J. Med. **321:**1626–1631.
12. **Cooper, D., A. A. Imrie, and R. Penny.** 1987. Antibody response to human immunodeficiency virus after primary infection. J. Infect. Dis. **155:**1113–1118.
13. **Cortes, E., R. Detels, D. Aboulafia, X. Ling Li, T. Moudgil, M. Alam, C. Bonecker, A. Gonzag, L. Oyafuso, M. Tondo, C. Boite, N. Hammershlak, C. Capitani, D. J. Slamon, and D. Ho.** 1989. HIV-1, HIV-2, and HTLV-1 infection in high-risk groups in Brazil. N. Engl. J. Med. **320:**953–958.
14. **Curran, J. W., H. W. Jaffe, A. M. Hardy, W. M. Morgan, R. M. Selik, and T. J. Dondero.** 1988. Epidemiology of HIV infection and AIDS in the United States. Science **239:** 610–616.
15. **Evans, L., T. McHugh, D. Stites, and J. A. Levy.** 1987. Differential ability of human immunodeficiency virus isolates to productively infect human cells. J. Immunol. **138:** 3415–3418.
16. **Farzadegan, H., M. A. Polis, S. M. Wolinsky, C. R. Rinaldo, Jr., J. J. Sninsky, S. Kwok, R. L. Griffith, R. A. Kaslow, J. P. Phair, B. F. Polk, and A. J. Saah.** 1988. Loss of human immunodeficiency type 1 (HIV-1) antibodies with evidence of viral infection in asymptomatic homosexual men. Ann. Intern. Med. **108:**785–790.
17. **Fauvel, M., and G. Ozanne.** 1989. Immunofluorescence assay for human immunodeficiency virus antibody: investigation of cell fixation for virus inactivation and antigen preservation. J. Clin. Microbiol. **27:**1810–1813.
18. **Gabuzda, D. H., D. D. Ho, S. M. de la Monte, M. S. Hirsch, T. R. Rota, and R. A. Sobel.** 1986. Immunohistochemical identification of HTLV-III antigen in brains of patients with AIDS. Ann. Neurol. **20:**289–295.
19. **Gallo, R. C., S. Z. Salahuddin, M. Popovic, G. M. Shearer, M. Kaplan, B. F. Haynes, T. J. Parker, R. Redfield, J. Oleske, B. Safai, G. White, P. Foster, and P. D. Markham.** 1984. Frequent detection and isolation of cytopathic retroviruses (HTLV-III) from patients with AIDS and at risk for AIDS. Science **224:**500–502.
20. **Gerberding, J. L., C. E. Bryant-LeBlanc, K. Nelson, A. R. Moss, D. Osmond, H. F. Chambers, J. R. Carlson, W. L. Drew, J. A. Levy, and M. A. Sande.** 1987. Risk of human immunodeficiency virus, cytomegalovirus, and hepatitis B virus transmission to health care workers exposed to patients with acquired immunodeficiency syndrome (AIDS) and AIDS-related conditions. J. Infect. Dis. **156:**1–8.
21. **Gottlieb, M. S., R. Schroff, H. M. Schanker, et al.** 1981. *Pneumocystis carinii* pneumonia and mucosal candidiasis in previously healthy homosexual men. N. Engl. J. Med. **305:**1425–1430.
22. **Goudsmit, J., D. A. Paul, and J. M. A. Lange.** 1986. Expression of human immunodeficiency virus antigen (HIV-Ag) in serum and cerebrospinal fluid during acute and chronic infection. Lancet **ii:**177–180.
23. **Harper, M. E., L. M. Marselle, R. C. Gallo, and F. Wong-Staal.** 1986. Detection of lymphocytes expressing human T-lymphotropic virus type III in lymph nodes and peripheral blood from infected individuals by *in situ* hybridization. Proc. Natl. Acad. Sci. USA **83:**772–776.
24. **Hart, C., T. Spira, J. Moore, J. Sninsky, G. Schochetman, A. Lifson, J. Galphin, and C.-Y. Ou.** 1988. Direct detection of HIV RNA expression in seropositive subjects. Lancet **ii:** 596–599.
25. **Ho, D. D., T. Moidgil, and M. Alam.** 1989. Quantitation of human immunodeficiency virus type 1 in the blood of infected persons. N. Engl. J. Med. **321:**1621–1625.
26. **Hoffman, A. D., B. Banapour, and J. A. Levy.** 1985. Characterization of the AIDS-associated retrovirus, reverse transcriptase and optimal conditions for its detection in virions. Virology **147:**326–335.
27. **Homsy, J., G. A. Thomson-Honnebier, C. Cheng-Mayer, and J. A. Levy.** 1988. Detection of human immunodeficiency virus (HIV) in serum and body fluids by sequential competition ELISA. J. Virol. Methods **19:**43–56.
28. **Imagawa, D. T., M. H. Lee, S. M. Wolinsky, K. Sano, F. Morales, S. Kwok, J. J. Sninsky, P. G. Nishanian, J. Giorgi, J. L. Fahey, J. Dudley, B. R. Visscher, and R. Detels.** 1989. Human immunodeficiency virus type 1 infection in homosexual men who remain seronegative for prolonged periods. N. Engl. J. Med. **320:**1458–1462.
29. **Jaffe, H., D. Bregman, and R. Selik.** 1983. Acquired immune deficiency syndrome in the United States: the first 1000 cases. J. Infect. Dis. **148:**339–345.
30. **Kalyanaraman, V. S., C. D. Cabradilla, J. P. Getchell, R. Narayanan, E. H. Braff, J.-C. Chermann, F. Barre-Sinoussi, L. Montagnier, T. J. Spira, J. Kaplan, D. Fishbein, H. W. Jaffe, J. W. Curran, and D. P. Francis.** 1984. Antibodies to the core protein of lymphadenopathy-associated virus (LAV) in patients with AIDS. Science **225:**321–323.
31. **Kaminsky, L., T. McHugh, D. P. Stites, P. Volberding, G. Henle, and J. A. Levy.** 1985. High prevalence of antibodies to AIDS-associated retroviruses (ARV) in acquired immune deficiency syndrome and related conditions and not in other disease states. Proc. Natl. Acad. Sci. USA **82:** 5535–5539.
32. **Kwok, S., and R. Higuchi.** 1989. Avoiding false positives with PCR. Product review. Nature (London) **339:**237.
33. **Kwok, S., D. H. Mack, J. J. Sninsky, G. D. Ehrlich, B. J. Poiescz, N. L. Dock, H. J. Alter, D. Mildvan, and M. H. Grieco.** 1988. Diagnosis of human immunodeficiency virus in seropositive individuals: enzymatic amplification of HIV viral sequences in peripheral blood mononuclear cells, p. 243–255. *In* P. A. Luciw and K. S. Steimer (ed.), HIV detection by genetic engineering methods. Marcel Dekker, Inc., New York.
34. **Lange, J. M. A., R. A. Coutinho, W. J. A. Krone, L. F. Verdonck, S. A. Danner, J. Van der Noorda, and J. Goudsmit.** 1986. Distinct IgG recognition pattern during progression of subclinical and clinical infection with lymphadenopathy associated virus/human T lymphotropic virus. Br. Med. J. **292:**228–230.
35. **Levy, J. A.** 1988. The transmission of AIDS: the case of the infected cell. J. Am. Med. Assoc. **259:**3037–3038.
36. **Levy, J. A.** 1988. Retroviridae: human immunodeficiency viruses, p. 677–691. *In* E. H. Lennette, P. Halonen, and F. A. Murphy (ed.), Laboratory diagnosis of infectious diseases, vol. II. Viral, rickettsial and chlamydial diseases. Springer-Verlag, New York.

37. **Levy, J. A. (ed.).** 1989. AIDS: pathogenesis and treatment. Marcel Dekker, Inc., New York.
38. **Levy, J. A.** 1989. Human immunodeficiency virus and the pathogenesis of AIDS. J. Am. Med. Assoc. **261:**2997–3006.
39. **Levy, J. A., A. D. Hoffman, S. Kramer, J. Landis, J. Shimabukuro, and L. Oshiro.** 1984. Isolation of lymphocytopathic retroviruses from San Francisco patients with AIDS. Science **225:**840–842.
40. **Levy, J. A., W. Margaretten, and J. Nelson.** 1989. Detection of HIV in enterochromaffin cells in the rectal mucosa of an AIDS patient. Am. J. Gastroenterol. **84:**787–789.
41. **Levy, J. A., G. A. Mitra, M. F. Wong, and M. Mozen.** 1985. Survival of AIDS-associated retrovirus (ARV) during factor VIII purification from plasma: inactivation by wet and dry heat procedures. Lancet **i:**1456–1457.
42. **Levy, J. A., and J. Shimabukuro.** 1985. Recovery of AIDS-associated retrovirus from patients with AIDS or AIDS-related conditions and from clinically healthy individuals. J. Infect. Dis. **152:**734–738.
43. **Levy, J. A., J. Shimabukuro, T. McHugh, C. Casavant, D. Stites, and L. Oshiro.** 1985. AIDS-associated retroviruses (ARV) can productively infect other cells besides human T helper cells. Virology **147:**441–448.
44. **Loche, M., and B. Mach.** 1988. Identification of HIV-infected seronegative individuals by a direct diagnostic test based on hybridization to amplified viral DNA. Lancet **ii:** 418–421.
45. **Luciw, P. A., C. Cheng-Mayer, and J. A. Levy.** 1987. Mutational analysis of the human immunodeficiency virus; the *orf-B* region down-regulates virus replication. Proc. Natl. Acad. Sci. USA **84:**1434–1438.
46. **Malim, M. H., J. Hauber, S.-Y. Le, J. V. Maizel, and B. R. Cullen.** 1989. The HIV-1 *rev* trans-activator acts through a structured target sequence to activate nuclear export of unspliced viral mRNA. Nature (London) **338:** 254–259.
47. **McDougal, J. S., S. P. Cort, M. S. Kennedy, C. D. Cabradilla, P. M. Feouno, D. P. Francis, D. Hicks, V. S. Kalyanaraman, and L. S. Martin.** 1985. Immunoassay for the detection and quantitation of infectious human retrovirus, lymphadenopathy-associated virus (LAV). J. Immunol. Methods **76:**171–183.
48. **McGrath, M. S., K. M. Hwang, S. E. Caldwell, I. Gaston, K.-C. Luk, P. Wu, V. L. Ng, S. Crowe, J. Daniels, J. Marsh, T. Deinhart, P. V. Lekas, J. C. Vennari, H.-W. Yeung, and J. Lifson.** 1989. GLQ223: an inhibitor of human immunodeficiency virus replication in acutely and chronically infected cells of lymphocyte and mononuclear phagocyte lineage. Proc. Natl. Acad. Sci. USA **86:**2844–2848.
49. **Moss, A. R., and P. Bacchetti.** 1989. Natural history of HIV infection. AIDS **3:**55–61.
50. **Nelson, J. A., C. A. Wiley, C. Reynolds-Kohler, C. E. Reese, W. Margaretten, and J. A. Levy.** 1988. Human immunodeficiency virus detected in bowel epithelium from patients with gastrointestinal symptoms. Lancet **i:** 259–262.
51. **Ng, V. L., C. S. Chiang, C. Debouck, M. S. McGrath, T. H. Grove, and J. Mills.** 1989. Reliable confirmation of antibodies to human immunodeficiency virus type 1 (HIV-1) with an enzyme-linked immunoassay using recombinant antigens derived from the HIV-1 *gag, pol,* and *env* genes. J. Clin. Microbiol. **27:**977–982.
52. **Ogawa, K., R. Shibata, T. Kiyomasu, I. Higuchi, Y. Kishida, A. Ishimoto, and A. Adachi.** 1989. Mutational analysis of the human immunodeficiency virus *vpr* open reading frame. J. Virol. **63:**4110–4114.
53. **Osmond, D., R. E. Chaisson, A. R. Moss, P. Bacchetti, and W. Krampf.** 1987. Lymphadenopathy in asymptomatic patients seropositive for HIV. N. Engl. J. Med. **317:**246.
54. **Osmond, D., and A. R. Moss.** 1989. The prevalence of HIV infection in the United States; a revision of the CDC estimates, p. 1–17. *In* P. Volberding and M. Jacobsen (ed.), AIDS clinical review. Marcel Dekker, Inc., New York.
55. **Ou, C.-Y., S. Kwok, S. W. Mitchell, D. H. Mack, J. J. Sninsky, J. W. Krebs, P. Feorino, D. Warfield, and G. Schochetman.** 1988. DNA amplification for direct detection of HIV-1 in DNA of peripheral blood mononuclear cells. Science **239:**295–297.
56. **Pan, L.-Z., C. Cheng-Mayer, and J. A. Levy.** 1987. Patterns of antibody response in individuals infected with the human immunodeficiency virus. J. Infect. Dis. **155:**626–632.
57. **Peeters, M., E. Delaporte, M.-C. Dazza, and F. Brun-Vezinel.** 1988. Detection of HIV-2 antibodies using five commercial HIV enzyme immunoassays. AIDS **2:**389–390.
58. **Peterlin, B. M., and P. A. Luciw.** 1988. Molecular biology of HIV. AIDS **2**(Suppl. 1):S29–S40.
59. **Quinn, T. C., J. M. Mann, J. W. Curran, and P. Piot.** 1986. AIDS in Africa: an epidemiologic paradigm. Science **234:**955–963.
60. **Rabson, A. B.** 1989. The molecular biology of HIV infection: clues for possible therapy, p. 231–256. *In* J. A. Levy (ed.), AIDS: pathogenesis and treatment. Marcel Dekker, Inc., New York.
61. **Reesnick, H. W., P. N. Lelie, J. G. Huisman, W. Schassbert, M. Gonsalves, C. Aaij, I. N. Winkel, J. A. van der Does, A. C. Hekker, and J. Desmyter.** 1986. Evaluation of six enzyme immunoassays for antibody against human immunodeficiency virus. Lancet **ii:**483–486.
62. **Resnick, L., K. Veren, S. Z. Salahuddin, S. Tondreau, and P. D. Markham.** 1986. Stability and inactivation of HTLV III/LAV under clinical and laboratory environments. J. Am. Med. Assoc. **255:**1887–1891.
63. **Sarngadharan, M. G., M. Popovic, L. Bruch, J. Schubach, and R. C. Gallo.** 1984. Antibodies reactive with human T cell lymphotropic retroviruses (HTLV-III) in the serum of patients with AIDS. Science **224:**506–508.
64. **Saxinger, W. C., and R. C. Gallo.** 1983. Application of the indirect enzyme-linked immunosorbent assay microtest to the detection and surveillance of human T-cell leukemia-lymphoma virus (HTLV). Lab. Invest. **49:**371–377.
65. **Schnittman, S. M., M. C. Psallidopoulos, H. C. Lane, L. Thompson, M. Baseler, F. Massari, C. H. Fox, N. P. Salzman, and A. S. Fauci.** 1989. The reservoir for HIV-1 in human peripheral blood is a T cell that maintains expression of CD4. Science **245:**305–308.
66. **Serwadda, D., R. D. Mugerwa, N. K. Sewankambo, A. Lwegaba, J. W. Carswell, G. B. Kirya, A. C. Bayley, R. G. Downing, R. S. Tedder, S. A. Clayden, R. A. Weiss, and A. G. Dalgleish.** 1985. Slim disease: a new disease in Uganda and its association with HTLV-III infection. Lancet **ii:**849–852.
67. **Spire, B., F. Barre-Sinoussi, and D. Dormont.** 1985. Inactivation of lymphadenopathy-associated virus by heat, gamma rays, and ultraviolet light. Lancet **i:**188–189.
68. **Steimer, K., J. P. Puma, M. D. Power, M. A. Powers, C. George-Nascimento, J. C. Stephens, L. A. Levy, R. Sanchez-Pescador, P. A. Luciw, and P. J. Barr.** 1986. Differential antibody responses of individuals infected with AIDS-associated retroviruses surveyed using the viral core antigen $p25^{gag}$ expressed in bacteria. Virology **150:**283–290.
69. **Stoler, M. H., T. A. Eskin, S. Benn, R. C. Angerer, and L. M. Angerer.** 1986. Human T-cell lymphotropic virus type III infection of the central nervous system: a preliminary *in situ* analysis. J. Am. Med. Assoc. **256:**2360–2364.
70. **Strebel, K., T. Klimkait, F. Maldarelli, and M. A. Martin.** 1989. Molecular and biochemical analyses of human immunodeficiency virus type 1 *vpu* protein. J. Virol. **63:**3784–3791.
71. **Terwilliger, E. F., E. A. Cohen, Y. Lu, J. G. Sodroski, and W. A. Haseltine.** 1989. Functional role of human immunodeficiency virus type 1 *vpu*. Proc. Natl. Acad. Sci. USA **86:**5163–5167.
72. **Towbin, H., T. Staehelin, and J. Gordon.** 1979. Electrophoretic transfer of proteins from polyacrylamide gels to nitrocellulose sheets: procedure and some applications.

Proc. Natl. Acad. Sci. USA **76:**4340–4354.

73. **Walker, C. M., D. J. Moody, D. P. Stites, and J. A. Levy.** 1986. CD8+ lymphocytes can control HIV infection *in vitro* by suppressing virus replication. Science **234:**1563–1566.
74. **Wang, J. J. G., S. Steel, R. Wisniewolski, and C. Y. Wang.** 1986. Detection of antibodies to human T-lymphotrophic virus type III by using a synthetic peptide of 21 amino acid residues corresponding to a highly antigenic segment of gp41 envelope protein. Proc. Natl. Acad. Sci. USA **83:**6159–6163.
75. **Ward, J. W., T. J. Bush, H. A. Perkins, L. E. Lieb, J. R. Allen, D. Goldfinger, S. M. Samson, S. H. Pepkowitz, I. P. Fernando, P. V. Holland, S. H. Kleinman, A. J. Grindon, J. L. Garner, G. W. Rutherford, and S. D. Holmberg.** 1989. The natural history of transfusion-associated infection with human immunodeficiency virus. N. Engl. J. Med. **321:**947–952.
76. **Weiss, S., J. Goedert, M. Sarngadharan, A. Bodner, R. Biggar, J. Clark, R. Dodd, E. Geimann, J. Giron, M. Greene, M. Melbye, M. Popovic, M. Robert-Guroff, C. Saxinger, M. Simberkoff, D. Winn, R. Gallo, and W. Blattner.** 1985. Screening test for HTLV-III (AIDS agent) antibodies. J. Am. Med. Assoc. **253:**221–225.
77. **Wiley, C. A., R. D. Schrier, D. D. Richman, J. A. Nelson, P. W. Lambert, and M. B. A. Oldstone.** 1986. Cellular localization of human immunodeficiency virus infection within the brains of AIDS patients. Proc. Natl. Acad. Sci. USA **83:**7089–7093.
78. **Winkelstein, W., Jr., D. M. Lyman, N. Padian, R. Grant, M. Samual, J. A. Wiley, R. E. Anderson, W. Lang, J. Riggs, and J. A. Levy.** 1987. Sexual practices and risk of infection by the human immunodeficiency virus: the San Francisco Men's Health Study. J. Am. Med. Assoc. **257:** 321–325.

Chapter 101

Other Human Retroviruses

MICHAEL D. LAIRMORE, RIMA F. KHABBAZ, AND THOMAS M. FOLKS

CLINICAL BACKGROUND

Human T-lymphotropic virus type I (HTLV-I) is the first human retrovirus discovered (6). It causes a chronic latent infection and is associated with two diseases, adult T-cell leukemia/lymphoma (ATL) (4) and a progressive myelopathy known as HTLV-I-associated myelopathy-tropical spastic paraparesis (HAM/TSP) (2). Areas of HTLV-I endemicity include southern Japan and the Caribbean basin, where infection rates of 5 to 10% have been reported. High rates of HTLV-I seropositivity have been reported in the United States in intravenous-drug users (7 to 49%), recipients of multiple blood transfusions (2.8%), and female prostitutes (7%). Lower rates have been reported in volunteer blood donors (0.025%). Surveys conducted in areas where HTLV-I is endemic show that HTLV-I seropositivity increases with age and that this age-related increase is sharper for females, resulting in markedly higher rates of infection in women than in men (3). In the Caribbean basin, reported rates are higher in blacks than in other ethnic groups.

HTLV-I can be transmitted by transfusion of HTLV-I-positive cellular blood products, by the sharing of injection equipment contaminated with infectious blood, from infected mother to infant through breast feeding, and by sexual contact. In general, HTLV-I appears to be less efficiently transmitted than human immunodeficiency virus, probably because HTLV-I is highly cell associated.

HTLV-I has been etiologically associated with ATL. ATL is a highly aggressive lymphoma of mature T cells ($T4^+$) first described in Japan in 1978; it is endemic in areas like Japan and the Caribbean where HTLV-I infection is endemic. The latency between infection and disease has been estimated to be between 10 and 40 years, and the lifetime risk of ATL among HTLV-I-infected persons is 2 to 4%. The association of HTLV-I and HAM/TSP is more recent. HAM/TSP is characterized by progressive difficulty in walking, weakness in the lower extremities, sensory disturbances, and urinary incontinence. The latent period for the disease is less than for ATL, and HAM/TSP, unlike ATL, has been caused by blood transfusion.

Human T-lymphotropic virus type II (HTLV-II) is closely related to HTLV-I; the two viruses have a genomic homology of 60%, resulting in extensive serological cross-reactivity. The seroepidemiology and modes of transmission of HTLV-II remain largely ill defined. There is emerging evidence, however, that HTLV-I seropositivity in intravenous-drug users in the United States may be largely due to HTLV-II (5). No specific disease entities have yet been clearly associated with HTLV-II. HTLV-II has been isolated from two patients with a variant of hairy-cell leukemia. However, a serosurvey has shown no serological evidence of HTLV-II infection in 21 patients with this disease.

DESCRIPTION OF AGENTS

Retroviruses are currently grouped into three genera, *Oncovirus, Lentivirus,* and *Spumavirus,* on the basis of genomic organization, biochemical structure, and biological activities. The origin of retroviruses remains an enigma, and their contribution to mammalian gene evolution is only conjectural. Also not known is how retroviral sequences found in the human genome arose. Are these viral sequences just remnants of past retroviral infections, or is their presence the result of a function needed during vertebrate evolution? Because of the findings that retroviral sequences, especially reverse transcriptase, have been located in the human genome, one might presume that such agents provided a critical function in the origin of the species. Some of these eucaryotic dispersed repetitive sequences in vertebrates, known as retrotransposons or retroposons, appear to have a movable element that utilizes an RNA intermediate. Even though particles are not necessarily associated with these RNA intermediates, it is assumed that reverse transcriptase-coding sequences are present within the RNA (9). Such a mechanism of movable genetic material might allow for rapid changes in host genomic structure and facilitate gene displacement or gene reorganization within a species.

Additional links between retroviruses and the human genome can be found in oncogenes. Viral oncogenes have cellular counterparts that maintain extremely high sequence homology to some internal cellular signaling genes, such as *myc, fos,* and *jun* (1). In many cases, retroviruses appear to have incorporated these normal cellular genes into their own genomes and placed them under control of their own regulation.

What do retrotransposons and oncogenes have to do with understanding retroviruses? It seems that the future of new human retroviral discovery will depend on recognizing the mechanism by which movable elements capture and utilize cellular regulatory components. We have begun to identify this mechanism in retroviral *trans*-acting genes. Human immunodeficiency virus and HTLVs are teaching us about RNA transport and stabilization through their *rev* and *rex trans*-acting genes, respectively. How did these viruses acquire such sophistication in such a small genome? Do vertebrates have their own *rev* and *rex* genes? It is logical to suppose that an understanding of these mechanisms will provide insight into new human retroviral isolations.

An exciting question is, where will the next group of human retroviruses be found? One source might be found in patients suffering from autoimmune diseases which for a long time have been the "catch" for possible retroviral etiologies. This is well documented in diseases such as systemic lupus erythematosus, Kawasaki disease, and, recently, in Graves disease. Also, a new human retrovirus (HTLV-V) has been identified in cutaneous T-cell lymphomas and reported to have sequence divergence from HTLV-I or HTLV-II.

Methods for detecting these agents have taken a great leap forward and have contributed significantly to the identification of many infectious agents, including the HTLVs. The recent finding of HTLV-I sequences in patients with multiple sclerosis is an excellent example of how the new technology of polymerase chain reaction (PCR) has expanded our ability to search for new human retroviruses (8). PCR, along with advances in culture techniques using recombinant growth factors, should provide some of the important tools to help determine the potential retroviral etiology of many idiopathic diseases.

It now appears that both of the HTLVs are much more widespread than was previously thought and are gaining in importance as agents that are transmissible not only by blood transfusion but also by sexual contact. This chapter describes the current epidemiological, serological, and molecular aspects of HTLV-I and -II detection necessary to provide insight into the mechanisms of spread and pathogenesis of these two viruses.

LABORATORY DIAGNOSIS

Viruses belonging to the family *Retroviridae* have been described in various animal species for many years; however, the first human retrovirus isolate was not reported until 1980. The delay in the discovery of human retroviruses was due in part to limitations of laboratory techniques for specifically identifying these human pathogens. Techniques that allowed the measurement of a reverse transcriptase (necessary for retrovirus replication) and the ability to culture human lymphocytes for extended periods of time by using soluble growth factors (e.g., interleukin-2) have provided the initial tools for discovering human retroviruses. Recent improvements in both serological (enzyme immunoabsorbent assays [EIA] and immunoblotting [IB] techniques) and virological (PCR) methods of identifying human retroviruses have allowed improvements in the sensitivity and specificity of diagnostic tests for these viruses.

HTLV-I is associated with both lymphoproliferative (ATL) and chronic neurological (HAM/TSP) disorders. Antibodies to HTLV-I are detected in 70 to 90% of patients diagnosed with these diseases, and the virus is found monoclonally integrated with the genome of the lymphoma cells; these observations and epidemiological studies of HTLV-I transmission strengthen the causal linkage of the virus to these disorders. Infected individuals who are producing antibodies against the virus frequently carry the virus in a latent state (integrated viral DNA with no antigen expression). It is only after culturing in appropriate conditions that HTLV-I proteins begin to be detectable from infected cells. Therefore, sensitive and specific methods to detect antibodies directed against HTLV-I or HTLV-II are critical for diagnostic and research investigations of these viruses.

Collection of specimens

The serological diagnosis of HTLV-I and HTLV-II requires serum, plasma, or cerebrospinal fluid. The specimens should be collected and tested or stored frozen in sealed and properly labeled cryovials. Excessive freeze-thaw cycles of specimens may cause false-positive reactions in EIA tests and therefore should be avoided. In addition, samples that contain hemolyzed blood may cause excessive background or false bands in IB and radioimmunoprecipitation assays (RIPA). Lipemic serum may be centrifuged to clear the sample and improve background problems during EIA, IB, or RIPA.

To isolate and identify HTLV, properly collected heparinized blood (approximately 20 to 60 ml) should be collected and transferred as quickly as possible (within 24 h) at room temperature to the laboratory. Mononuclear leukocytes should be separated by Ficoll techniques (see chapter 19), and the resulting leukocytes should be cultured in the presence of mitogen (i.e., phytohemagglutinin P) in RPMI 1640 medium containing serum and interleukin-2. Coculture with either mitogen-stimulated cord blood lymphocytes or leukocytes from normal donors may improve the efficiency of isolation. Concurrent cryopreservation of specimens should be instituted if reculture or alternative diagnostic procedures (i.e., PCR) are considered. Donor samples used for coculture procedures should be prescreened for HTLV.

Serological methods

In November 1988, the U.S. Food and Drug Administration allowed the licensure of EIA screening tests for HTLV-I (see chapter 12). Commercially available EIA tests use detergent to disrupt HTLV-I antigens linked to polystyrene plates or beads. The Food and Drug Administration initially established the sensitivity (97.3 to 100%) and specificity (99.3 to 99.9%) of these tests by using panels of donor sera from various geographic regions. However, the low predictive value of these tests in low-prevalence populations indicates the need for more specific testing of EIA-reactive specimens. In addition, these assays do not distinguish between antibody reactivity of HTLV-I and that of HTLV-II, nor do more specific serological methods such as IB. Additional screening tests available for detection of HTLV antibodies include particle agglutination assay, immunofluorescence, and competitive EIA. Limitations of EIA tests potentially include less than optimal envelope antigen within viral preparations as well as inability to detect antibody reactivity to specific gene products of the virus. As with screening tests for human immunodeficiency virus, most algorithms used to confirm HTLV-I antibody reactivity rely on more specific techniques, including IB and RIPA (see chapter 13). Recent comparisons of these techniques suggest that IB antigen preparations derived from whole lysates of infected cells are superior for full viral gene product representation. Seroreactivities potentially detected by IB and RIPA include *gag* products p19, p24, and precursor p53 and *env* products gp46 and precursor gp61/68. IB is the more sensitive method for detecting *gag* product reactivity, whereas RIPA appears more sensitive for detecting antibodies to HTLV *env*. The quantities and molecular weights of HTLV proteins produced by various cell lines may vary, and specificity of reactive bands should be verified by comparison with molecular weight standards and reactivity to monoclonal antibodies. Specific tests used to verify HTLV reactivity should be able to detect both *gag* (in particular p24) and *env* (gp46 and/or gp61/68). Recently, the U.S. Public Health Service recommended that a serum sample be considered positive only if it demonstrates reactivity both to *gag* p24 and to *env* gp46 and/or gp61/68 (7). Specimens not satisfying these criteria but having immunoreactivity to at least one suspected HTLV gene product (such as p19 only, p19 and p28, or p19 and gp46) are designated "indeterminate," and those without reactivity to a viral gene product should be considered negative. Because of the inherent differences between IB and RIPA in the ability to detect envelope antibodies, both tests may have to be used to classify a reactive serum sample as positive. The immunoreactivities of the polymerase (*pol*) and transactivator (*tax*) proteins have not been adequately defined by the serological methods now available. Because no current serological assay will adequately differentiate between antibodies to HTLV-I and HTLV-II, virus isolation and PCR are required to specifically detect and identify these viruses.

Cell culture and PCR

Virus isolation of HTLV is dependent on activation of T cells, culturing of cells in appropriate conditions for long-term growth of lymphocytes, and selection of adequately primed target cells (6). The viruses are transmitted by cell-to-cell transfer, and successful infections with cell-free virions have been reported only in the presence of high concentrations of the virus. Both HTLV-I and HTLV-II exhibit helper T-cell ($CD4^+$) tropism predominantly, but transformation of $CD8^+$ cells has been reported. In addition, HTLV exhibits broad species in vitro tropism and has been demonstrated to replicate in rat, rabbit, feline, and monkey cells. Initial cultures should be stimulated with mitogen (e.g., phytohemagglutinin) or antibodies against T-cell receptors (anti-CD3) and monitored for the presence of HTLV. Reverse transcriptase is often of limited value for monitoring cultures because of the low levels produced by this cell-associated virus. Recently, antigen capture assays have allowed sensitive (detection of as low as 0.1 ng of core antigen per ml) and specific detection of virus antigen in culture supernatants. In addition, immunofluorescence is useful to monitor cultures for the expression of cell surface or cytoplasmic viral antigens. Recently, PCR (see chapter 17) has allowed the differentiation of HTLV-I from HTLV-II by employing specific amplification of gene regions unique for each virus, using probes specific for each virus or restriction enzyme sites unique for each virus. The success of this method depends on strict adherence to laboratory controls and exacting procedures to prevent contamination of specimens and primer pairs. Appropriate controls should include both negative and positive controls, molecular weight standards, sensitivity controls (serial dilution of positive cell lines), and specificity controls (related but different from amplified target virus, e.g., HTLV-II for HTLV-I amplification). Controls and test samples should be prepared in the same manner to prevent variability in lysing procedures. DNA for PCR can be prepared from cells simply by lysing cells in the presence of detergents (e.g., Nonidet P-40) or using more rigorous methods of phenol extraction. Amplified products are detected after separation in agarose or acrylamide gels, followed by transfer and probing by hybridization with labeled (i.e., ^{32}P) probes (see chapter 17).

All procedures involving DNA extraction should be separated physically from rooms used for amplification of the target DNA to prevent contamination of primer pairs or probes. The development of PCR procedures for HTLV-I and HTLV-II has, for the first time, allowed investigations of the prevalence and potential disease associations of HTLV-II. In addition, the use of PCR to directly diagnose individuals with HTLV infection has in part precluded the need to culture cells from these patients.

LITERATURE CITED

1. **Bishop, J. M.** 1983. Cellular oncogenes and retroviruses. Annu. Rev. Biochem. **52:**301–320.
2. **Gessain, A., F. Barin, J. C. Vernant, O. Gout, L. Maurs, and A. Calender.** 1985. Antibodies to human T-lymphotropic virus type-I in patients with tropical spastic paraparesis. Lancet **ii:**407–410.
3. **Kajiyama, W., S. Kashiwagi, H. Ikematsu, J. Hayashi, H. Nomura, and K. Okahi.** 1986. Intrafamilial transmission of adult T-cell leukemia virus. J. Infect. Dis. **54:**851–857.
4. **Kuefler, P. R., and P. A. Bunn.** 1986. Adult T-cell leukemia/lymphoma. Clin. Haematol. **15:**695–726.
5. **Lee, H., P. Swanson, V. S. Shorty, et al.** 1989. High rate of HTLV-II infection in seropositive IU drug abusers in New Orleans. Science **244:**471–475.
6. **Poiesz, B. J., F. W. Ruscetti, A. F. Gazdar, P. A. Bunn, J. D. Minna, and R. C. Gallo.** 1980. Detection and isolation of type C retrovirus particles from fresh and cultured lymphocytes of a patient with cutaneous T-cell lymphoma. Proc. Natl. Acad. Sci. USA **77:**7415–7419.
7. **Public Health Service Working Group (FDA/CDC/NIH).** 1988. Licensure of screening tests for antibody to human T-lymphotropic virus type 1. Morbid. Mortal. Weekly Rep. **37:**736–747.
8. **Reddy, P., M. Sanberg-Wollheim, R. V. Mehus, P. E. Ray, E. Defreitas, and A. Koprowski.** 1988. Amplification and molecular cloning of HTLV-I sequences from DNA of multiple sclerosis patients. Science **243:**529.
9. **Varmus, H. E.** 1985. Reverse transcriptase rides again. Nature (London) **314:**583.

Chapter 102

Spongiform Encephalopathies

DAVID M. ASHER

The spongiform encephalopathies comprise a group of two or three infectious diseases of humans and at least four of animals (Table 1), with roughly similar clinical courses and histopathological findings (24). All are elicited by similar unique pathogenic agents. They are often called "slow" infections, a term coined by Sigurdsson (69) to describe a pattern of long incubation period, protracted clinical course (months or years) with fatal outcome, pathology restricted to a single organ system, and a limited range of susceptible hosts.

EPIDEMIOLOGY

Kuru was the most common cause of death in women of the Fore language group of Papua New Guinea in the 1950s and early 1960s, also affecting many children of both sexes over the age of 4 years and a few adult males (26). The disease has almost completely disappeared among the Fore and has never affected anyone born after 1960. This peculiar epidemiological pattern suggests that the infection was naturally transmitted only by cannibalism, which ended in the late 1950s, and implies that the incubation period may be as short as 4 years or longer than 30 years (44).

Creutzfeldt-Jakob disease (CJD) (42) is an uncommon cause of dementia, affecting an estimated one per million per year or less in most populations studied, although frequencies in several isolated areas may be more than 30 times higher (52). Males and females are affected in approximately equal numbers. The natural mechanisms of transmission are not yet understood; however, in a growing number of cases, iatrogenic sources of infection have been recognized (24). Contaminated surgical instruments (60, 74), corneal transplants (23) and dural grafts (53, 71) from infected donors, and contaminated human pituitary hormones (10a) were clearly implicated as the origin of CJD in young people. After iatrogenic transmission, incubation periods as short as 14 months and longer than 20 years have been reported.

A single instance of conjugal CJD (37), two cases in neuropathology technicians (57, 70), and one in a neurosurgeon (25) have been described. However, the empirical risk for medical personnel and for other contacts of CJD patients is clearly very small.

Scrapie is an important disease of sheep in Great Britain and on the European continent and has become increasingly common in American sheep in recent years (30). No epidemiological evidence implicates scrapie as a source of human CJD. However, the recent outbreak of bovine spongiform encephalopathy ("mad cow disease") in England, apparently introduced by accidental incorporation into cattle feed of contaminated meat and bone meal prepared from renderings of scrapie-infected sheep (73), has raised fears that the scrapie agent, having crossed one species barrier from sheep into cattle and affecting other ungulates as well (33), may broaden its range of susceptible hosts to include humans (39). This possibility is under intense scrutiny.

Transmissible mink encephalopathy (50) is postulated to have resulted from feeding contaminated beef to mink (49). Nothing is known about the origin and occurrence in the wild of "wasting disease" of American elk and mule deer (75).

CLINICAL PICTURE AND COURSE OF ILLNESS

Kuru is characterized by progressive loss of coordination, cerebellar ataxia of the extremities and trunk, and a variety of signs of brain stem degeneration. There is relatively little clinical evidence of cerebral cortical involvement and no frank dementia. Most patients have the shivering tremors that gave kuru its name in the Fore language. Convulsive seizures and myoclonic jerks have not been observed. Patients become progressively incapacitated and usually die within a year from pneumonia, infected decubitus ulcers with septicemia, or accidental burns (26). The disease has never been recognized outside Papua New Guinea (24).

CJD, first described almost 70 years ago (42), typically affects middle-aged adults, though iatrogenically infected young adults and older adolescents have been described (10a). The disease usually begins insidiously with vague complaints of sensory disturbance, particularly visual, or confusion. Patients become progressively demented, sometimes quite rapidly over only a few weeks. Most patients eventually have repetitive myoclonic jerking movements of the extremities and may have generalized "startle" myoclonus as well. Rigidity and pathological cortical-release reflexes appear as the cerebral gray matter degenerates. A variety of other neurological abnormalities, including convulsions and asymmetrical weakness and spasticity that may suggest a space-occupying lesion, occur less commonly. Most patients die in less than a year after onset, though a few patients survive much longer. Death usually results from pneumonia or one of the other complications to which patients with terminal neurological diseases are subject. Remission of CJD has been claimed but never well documented. In many series of CJD, about 10% of patients have a family history of presenile dementia.

Gerstmann-Sträussler syndrome (GSS) is an extremely rare familial spongiform encephalopathy with progressively severe cerebellar ataxia and relatively later onset of dementia (51). It may be considered a variant of familial CJD.

TABLE 1. Slow infections of the nervous system caused by unconventional agents (spongiform encephalopathies)

Disease	Naturally infected hosts
Creutzfeldt-Jakob disease, Gerstmann-Sträussler syndrome	Humans
Kuru	Humans
Bovine spongiform encephalopathy ("mad cow disease")	Cattle, other captive ungulates, ?cats
Chronic wasting disease	American elk, mule deer
Scrapie	Sheep, goats
Transmissible mink encephalopathy	Mink

Scrapie, transmissible mink encephalopathy, wasting disease of mule deer and elk, and bovine spongiform encephalopathy are degenerative brain diseases that have been recognized in a variety of animals and resemble the human diseases to some degree in clinical picture and course and strikingly in histopathological findings (24).

PATHOLOGY

The spongiform encephalopathies are all characterized by progressive relentless degeneration of the central nervous system (5, 6), most severe in the gray matter, though there may be secondary loss of myelin and white-matter involvement as well. The histopathology consists of neuronal vacuolation and ultimately loss of neurons; vacuolation in humans with CJD and in some animals with CJD and scrapie may be severe enough to cause status spongiosus of the cerebral gray matter, giving the group of diseases its name. Neuronal loss is usually accompanied by proliferation and hypertrophy of fibrous astrocytes. The cerebellum is prominently involved in kuru, with marked loss of Purkinje and granule cells; cerebellar degeneration also occurs in CJD, though it is generally not so severe as in kuru.

There is an accumulation in the brain of an abnormal protein, relatively resistant to protease digestion, that was first recognized morphologically by negative-stain electron microscopy (55) as scrapie-associated fibrils (SAF) and later as a unique band of protein with apparent molecular mass of 27 to 30 kilodaltons on sodium dodecyl sulfate-polyacrylamide gel electrophoresis (9). The protein, designated PrP27-30 (54), was found to be a sialoglycoprotein (10) consisting of some 55 amino acids (58) with attached carbohydrates, a neuraminic acid (10), and an inositol (17). Particularly in disease of long duration, this protein (abbreviated here as SAF/PrP) may form amyloid plaques—staining with Congo red dye and birefringent under polarized light—visible by light microscopy. Plaques are most common and striking in the cerebellum but occur elsewhere in the brain as well. The amyloid plaques of spongiform encephalopathies resemble those of Alzheimer's disease, but antibodies prepared against SAF/PrP do not react with Alzheimer amyloid and vice versa (7, 62). Plaques are found in the brains of some 15% of patients with CJD, 70% of those with kuru, and probably all patients with GSS. Even in brains without plaques, immunostaining reveals extracellular accumulations of SAF/PrP in subependymal and periventricular areas (20) and within neurons in the Golgi apparatus or endoplasmic reticulum (62). Notably lacking in the brain in spongiform encephalopathies is any inflammatory response to infection.

PATHOGENESIS

Most studies investigating the pathogenesis of the spongiform encephalopathies have been conducted with scrapie, both natural and experimental (1, 31). The agent appears to enter the body through the integument; in sheep, the intact intestinal tract may be a portal of entry as well. The agent appears to replicate first in local lymph nodes draining the portal of entry. Later there is replication in spleen and other lymphoid organs throughout the body. There appears to be "viremia" in some animals and possibly in humans as well. In mice with scrapie, the agent may ascend peripheral nerves to the spinal cord (31). In any event, the agents enter the nervous system only relatively late in the course of experimental infections initiated by the subcutaneous route that presumably most closely mimics natural disease. Tissues and body fluids demonstrated to contain the infectious agent in patients dying of CJD are summarized in Table 2 (2).

Scrapie has not been transmitted from affected rodents to offspring in utero, nor have pregnant women with kuru or CJD transmitted disease to their children (24). However, sheep can apparently be infected with scrapie in utero as well as by contact with affected animals after birth.

In none of the spongiform encephalopathies has the presence of antibodies or cell-mediated immune response to the infectious agents been detected, nor have interferons been found.

EFFECT OF HOST GENETICS

In families with CJD, the disease occurs in a pattern suggestive of an autosomal dominant gene (4) and may affect subjects bearing a mutation (29) in the gene coding for the SAF/PrP protein, located on human chromosome 20 (46) and designated the PRIP gene. GSS, generally diagnosed only in families, is even less common than CJD; it has the same apparent pattern of inheritance as familial CJD, and its occurrence correlates with the presence of one of three different mutations in the PRIP gene (19, 21, 22, 29, 34, 61). (Mutations in the PRIP gene have also been detected in patients with "sporadic" CJD [28] as well as in healthy subjects, and their value for predicting disease is under study.) The

TABLE 2. Infectivity of tissues, body fluids, and excretions from patients with CJD

Tissues consistently contain infectious agent (≥50% of attempts)	Tissues sometimes contain infectious agent (4–33% of attempts)	Tissues reported to contain infectious agent (occasionally)
Brain	Kidney	Blood
Spinal cord	Liver	Urine
Eye	Lung	
	Lymph node	
	Spleen	
	CSF	

genes coding for SAF/PrP protein are closely linked or identical to those controlling incubation periods of scrapie in sheep and mice (15, 35, 36, 72); animals with some genotypes have incubation periods so long that they appear resistant to disease (4).

The SAF/PrP proteins of various species are very similar in amino acid sequence and antigenicity but are not identical (8, 45). They are derived from a larger precursor protein of some 250 amino acids, usually designated PrP33-35 (56). PrP33-35 extracted from brain tissue with spongiform encephalopathy is, like SAF/PrP, relatively resistant to protease digestion, while that from normal brains is sensitive; the difference is apparently due to a difference in glycosylation, since the amino acid sequences of the two proteins are identical. PrP33-35 is present in a variety of normal cells, in which it has a relatively rapid rate of turnover (16); its functions are not yet known.

INFECTIOUS AGENTS

The agents of the spongiform encephalopathies are unique in their physical properties. They are all experimentally transmissible to a variety of animals, including monkeys and rodents (24). Although cell cultures have been infected (14, 65), the cells display no cytopathic effects and generally the agents propagate to much lower titers in cultures than in brain tissue. Most studies characterizing the properties of the spongiform encephalopathy agents have used strains of scrapie agent adapted to mice and hamsters, in which incubation periods as short as 60 days and infectivity titers of more than 10^{10} 50% lethal doses per g of brain tissue have been achieved.

The infectious agents display extreme resistance to physical inactivation by heat and by both ionizing and UV radiation, as well as to chemical inactivation by a wide array of substances that destroy most viruses. This behavior, plus the fact that the agents show significant decreases in titers of infectivity after exposure to proteases (18) and other treatments that denature or degrade proteins (63), has convinced some authorities these are most probably replicating proteins devoid of nucleic acid. Prusiner suggested that these novel agents be called "prions" in recognition of their protein content and in anticipation that they would be found to lack nucleic acids (63). Others remain unconvinced that the evidence favors such a structure and suspect that the agent must contain small but unique nucleic acids (38). Those favoring the "all-protein" hypothesis place great emphasis on the aberrant physical behavior of the agents, concluding that they are inconsistent with properties of nucleic acids, and the fact that infectivity has seldom if ever been separated from SAF/PrP protein, which they propose to be the "prion" (64) or "infectious amyloid" (24). However, skeptics have claimed at least partial success in separating infectivity from SAF/PrP, point to discrepancies between the behaviors of infectivity and SAF/PrP, note that all infectious preparations of the scrapie and CJD agents have contained contaminating nucleic acids as well as protein, and finally stress that since SAF/PrP is clearly encoded by a normal host gene and has normal host-encoded primary amino acid sequence, it is unlikely to be able to transmit agent-specific information, as the pathogens of spongiform encephalopathies must (24, 38, 40, 41, 47, 48). Those favoring the hypothesis of all-protein agents have put forth ingenious hypotheses to explain how such proteins might transmit self-replicating information not encoded in their amino acid sequences: these include frameshifting (76), posttranslational differences in glycosylation (64), and association with inorganic molecules that accelerate crystallization of precursor molecules into β-pleated sheets of amyloid protein (12, 24). Despite more than 20 years of controversy, the nature of the spongiform encephalopathy agents remains disputed. Whatever their structure proves to be, the etiological agents of the spongiform encephalopathies are obviously unique, being radically different from any other pathogens known in microbiology.

LABORATORY DIAGNOSIS

The spongiform encephalopathies are generally diagnosed during life by typical constellations of clinical findings. CJD is suspected in a middle-aged patient (or in a younger person with a history suggestive of iatrogenic transmission) having progressive dementia and myoclonic jerks. Later in disease, the electroencephalogram frequently shows periodic high-voltage complexes on a slow and disorganized background (27). Hematological studies and clinical chemistries are unrevealing. Some patients with CJD have abnormal liver function studies suggestive of parenchymal disease (67), the significance of which is not known. The cerebrospinal fluid (CSF) often contains moderately increased amounts of protein, which is not diagnostic; cell content of the CSF is normal.

A research technique involving two-dimensional electrophoresis and isoelectric focusing of CSF in gels has proven useful in diagnosis of CJD; silver staining reveals the presence of two abnormal polypeptides (designated 130 and 131) in CSF of most patients with CJD but not in those with Alzheimer's disease (32). The polypeptides have not yet been identified or fully sequenced. They are apparently not related to SAF/PrP or its precursor or to other known proteins. The presence of the 130 and 131 peptides in CSF is not specific to CJD; they were also found in about half of the CSF specimens from patients with acute herpes encephalitis. In practice, however, the usual diagnostic problem is to differentiate between CJD and Alzheimer's disease, and the presence of the 130 and 131 peptides in CSF strongly militates against the latter. This test is available only in a few research laboratories.

Definitive laboratory diagnosis of spongiform encephalopathies can be made only from brain tissue. Histopathological examination by a skilled and experienced neuropathologist remains the standard by which other tests must be judged. In addition to evaluation of neuronal vacuolation in sections stained with hematoxylin and eosin, stains for astrocytes (gold stains, if available, or immunostaining for glial fibrillary acidic protein) and for amyloid help in diagnosis. Immunostaining of amyloid may be enhanced by pretreating sections with formic acid (43).

Although inoculation of brain tissue suspensions intracerebrally into susceptible animals with induction of typical spongiform encephalopathy is diagnostic, it is extremely time-consuming and expensive; for example, squirrel monkeys, perhaps the most consistently susceptible to experimental CJD agent among commercially available animals, must be observed for at least 3 years before a transmission attempt is considered tentatively negative. Although laboratory rodents are susceptible to some strains of CJD agent, in our experience less than 20% of primary transmission attempts to rodents from well-documented cases have been successful. Attempts at primary transmission to animals have sometimes been confusing because of problems with contamination in laboratories that are studying the agents of spongiform encephalopathies.

The demonstration of SAF/PrP in brains of patients with progressive dementia can be useful in confirming the diagnosis of spongiform encephalopathy (11). Until recently, preparation of the protein required amounts of brain tissue larger than those generally obtained by biopsy; recent reports suggest that modified techniques permitting detection of very small amounts of SAF/PrP either by electron microscopy (59) or by immunostaining on nitrocellulose after guanidine isothiocyanate treatment (68) may be suitable for studying small fragments of biopsy tissue. However, since there is still no effective therapy for the spongiform encephalopathies, biopsy can be recommended only in cases for which other potentially treatable diseases are also under consideration. Limited evidence suggests that demonstration of SAF/PrP in autopsy specimens is more consistently successful when tissue has not been stored frozen for very long periods of time (11). Unfortunately, the techniques for detecting SAF/PrP remain available only by special arrangement with research laboratories.

LABORATORY SAFETY

Although, as discussed above, the risk to laboratory personnel of accidental infection with spongiform encephalopathy agents appears to be very small, because of the uniformly fatal outcome of the diseases, the extreme resistance of the etiological agents to disinfection, and the difficulty of detecting their presence, potentially contaminated tissues should be handled with caution (3). The recent introduction of universal precautions into medical laboratories responsible for testing of human tissues and body fluids may reduce the risk of accidental infection with the spongiform encephalopathy agents while protecting staff against more common exposures to human immunodeficiency virus and hepatitis viruses. Whenever possible, disposable materials should be used and discarded carefully by laboratories handling potentially contaminated specimens, if possible by incineration. Although the spongiform encephalopathy agents may not be completely destroyed by heat, even at very high temperatures (12), titers of infectivity are reduced markedly by heating (66); 2 h in a steam autoclave at 132°C is currently recommended to decontaminate objects that withstand such treatment. The infectivity titers of spongiform encephalopathy agents are also reduced substantially by exposure to 5.25% sodium hypochlorite (undiluted commercial chlorine bleach) and sodium hydroxide (2 M or stronger recommended) (3). Recent evidence suggests that the same formic acid treatment that improves immunostaining of amyloid in tissue sections may inactivate the spongiform encephalopathy agents (13).

LITERATURE CITED

1. **Asher, D. M., C. J. Gibbs, Jr., and D. C. Gajdusek.** 1976. Pathogenesis of spongiform encephalopathies. Ann. Clin. Lab. Sci. **6:**84–103.
2. **Asher, D. M., C. J. Gibbs, Jr., and D. C. Gajdusek.** 1985. Subacute spongiform encephalopathies: slow infections of the nervous system. Clin. Microbiol. Newsl. **7:**129–133.
3. **Asher, D. M., C. J. Gibbs, Jr., and D. C. Gajdusek.** 1986. Slow viral infections: safe handling of the agents of the subacute spongiform encephalopathies, p. 59–71. *In* B. Miller, D. Gröschel, J. Richardson, D. Vesley, J. Songer, R. Housewright, and W. Barkley (ed.), Laboratory safety: principles and practice. American Society for Microbiology, Washington, D.C.
4. **Asher, D. M., C. L. Masters, D. C. Gajdusek, and C. J. Gibbs, Jr.** 1983. Familial spongiform encephalopathies, p. 273–291. *In* S. Kety, L. Rowland, R. Sidman, and S. Matthysse (ed.), Genetics of neurological and psychiatric disorders. Raven Press, New York.
5. **Beck, E., P. M. Daniel, A. J. Davey, D. C. Gajdusek, and C. J. Gibbs, Jr.** 1982. The pathogenesis of spongiform encephalopathies: an ultrastructural study. Brain **104:**755–786.
6. **Beck, E., P. M. Daniel, W. B. Matthews, D. L. Stevens, M. P. Alpers, D. M. Asher, D. C. Gajdusek, and C. J. Gibbs, Jr.** 1969. Creutzfeldt-Jakob disease: the neuropathology of a transmission experiment. Brain **92:**699–716.
7. **Bobin, S. A., J. R. Currie, P. A. Merz, D. L. Miller, J. Styles, W. A. Walker, G. Y. Wen, and H. M. Wisniewski.** 1987. The comparative immunoreactivities of brain amyloids in Alzheimer's disease and scrapie. Acta Neuropathol. (Berlin) **74:**313–323.
8. **Bode, L., M. Pocchiari, H. Gelderblom, and H. Diringer.** 1985. Characterization of antisera against scrapie-associated fibrils (SAF) from affected hamster and cross-reactivity with SAF from scrapie-affected mice and from patients with Creutzfeldt-Jakob disease. J. Gen. Virol. **66:**2471–2478.
9. **Bolton, D. C., M. P. McKinley, and S. B. Prusiner.** 1982. Identification of a protein that purifies with the scrapie prion. Science **218:**1309–1311.
10. **Bolton, D. C., R. K. Meyer, and S. B. Prusiner.** 1985. Scrapie PrP 27-30 is a sialoglycoprotein. J. Virol. **53:**596–606.

10a. **Brown, P.** 1990. Iatrogenic Creutzfeldt-Jakob disease. Aust. N.Z. J. Med. **20:**633–635.

11. **Brown, P., M. Coker-Vann, K. Pomeroy, M. Franko, D. M. Asher, C. J. Gibbs, Jr., and D. C. Gajdusek.** 1986. Diagnosis of Creutzfeldt-Jakob disease by Western blot identification of marker protein in human brain tissue. N. Engl. J. Med. **314:**547–551.
12. **Brown, P., P. P. Liberski, A. Wolff, and D. C. Gajdusek.** 1990. Resistance of scrapie infectivity to steam autoclaving after formaldehyde fixation and limited survival after ashing at 360°C: practical and theoretical implications. J. Infect. Dis. **161:**467–472.
13. **Brown, P., A. Wolff, and D. C. Gajdusek.** 1990. A simple and effective method for inactivating virus infectivity in formalin-fixed tissue samples from patients with Creutzfeldt-Jakob disease. Neurology **40:**887–890.
14. **Butler, D. A., M. R. Scott, J. M. Bockman, D. R. Borchelt, A. Taraboulos, K. K. Hsiao, D. T. Kingsbury, and S. B. Prusiner.** 1988. Scrapie-infected murine neuroblastoma cells produce protease-resistant prion proteins. J. Virol. **62:**1558–1564.
15. **Carlson, G. A., D. T. Kingsbury, P. A. Goodman, S. Coleman, S. T. Marshall, S. DeArmond, D. Westaway, and S. B. Prusiner.** 1986. Linkage of prion protein and scrapie incubation time genes. Cell **46:**503–511.
16. **Caughey, B., R. E. Race, and B. Chesebro.** 1988. Detection of prion protein mRNA in normal and scrapie-infected tissues and cell lines. J. Gen. Virol. **69:**711–716.
17. **Caughey, B., R. E. Race, D. Ernst, M. J. Buchmeier, and B. Chesebro.** 1989. Prion protein biosynthesis in scrapie-infected and uninfected neuroblastoma cells. J. Virol. **63:**175–181.

18. **Cho, H. J.** 1980. Requirement of a protein component for scrapie infectivity. Intervirology **14:**213–216.
19. **Collinge, J., A. E. Harding, F. Owen, M. Poultier, R. Lofthouse, A. M. Boughey, T. Shah, and T. J. Crow.** 1989. Diagnosis of Gerstmann-Sträussler syndrome in familial dementia with prion protein gene analysis. Lancet **ii:**17.
20. **DeArmond, S. J., M. P. McKinley, R. A. Barry, M. B. Braunfeld, J. R. McColloch, and S. B. Prusiner.** 1985. Identification of prion amyloid filaments in scrapie-infected brain. Cell **41:**221–235.
21. **Doh-ura, K., J. Tateishi, T. Kitamoto, H. Sasaki, and Y. Sakaki.** 1990. Creutzfeldt-Jakob disease patients with congophilic kuru plaques have a missense variant prion protein common to Gerstmann-Sträussler syndrome. Ann. Neurol. **27:**121–126.
22. **Doh-ura, K., J. Tateishi, H. Sasaki, T. Kitamoto, and Y. Sakaki.** 1989. Pro → leu change at position 102 of prion protein is the most common but not the sole mutation related to Gerstmann-Straussler syndrome. Biochem. Biophys. Res. Commun. **163:**974–979.
23. **Duffy, P., G. Collins, A. G. DeVoe, B. Streeten, and D. Cohen.** 1974. Possible person-to-person transmission of Creutzfeldt-Jakob disease. N. Engl. J. Med. **290:**693.
24. **Gajdusek, D.** 1990. Subacute spongiform encephalopathies: transmissible cerebral amyloidoses caused by unconventional viruses, p. 2289–2324. *In* B. Fields and D. Knipe (ed.), Virology. Raven Press, New York.
25. **Gajdusek, D. C., C. J. Gibbs, Jr., K. Earle, G. J. Dammin, W. C. Schoene, and H. R. Tyler.** 1974. Transmission of subacute spongiform encephalopathy to the chimpanzee and squirrel monkey from a patient with papulosis maligna of Köhlmeier-Degos. Excerpta Med. Int. Congr. Ser. **319:** 390–392.
26. **Gajdusek, D. C., and V. Zigas.** 1957. Degenerative disease of the central nervous system in New Guinea: epidemic occurrence of "kuru" in the native population. N. Engl. J. Med. **257:**974–978.
27. **Gloor, P., O. Kalabay, and N. Giard.** 1968. The electroencephalogram in diffuse encephalopathies: electroencephalographic correlates of grey and white matter lesions. Brain **91:**779–801.
28. **Goldfarb, L. G., P. Brown, D. Goldgaber, R. Garruto, R. Yanagihara, D. M. Asher, and D. C. Gajdusek.** 1990. Identical mutation in unrelated patients with Creutzfeldt-Jakob disease. Lancet **ii:**174–175.
29. **Goldgaber, D., L. G. Goldfarb, P. Brown, D. M. Asher, W. T. Brown, W. S. Linn, J. W. Teener, S. M. Feinstone, R. Rubenstein, R. J. Kascsak, J. W. Boellard, and D. C. Gajdusek.** 1989. Mutations in familial Creutzfeldt-Jakob disease and Gerstmann-Sträussler-Scheinker's syndrome. Exp. Neurol. **106:**204–206.
30. **Hadlow, W. J.** 1990. An overview of scrapie in the United States. J. Am. Vet. Med. Assoc. **196:**1676–1677.
31. **Hadlow, W. J., R. C. Kennedy, and R. E. Race.** 1982. Natural infection of Suffolk sheep with scrapie virus. J. Infect. Dis. **146:**657–664.
32. **Harrington, M. G., C. R. Merril, D. M. Asher, and D. C. Gajdusek.** 1986. Abnormal proteins in the cerebrospinal fluid of patients with Creutzfeldt-Jakob disease. N. Engl. J. Med. **315:**279–283.
33. **Hourrigan, J. L.** 1990. The scrapie control program in the United States. J. Am. Vet. Med. Assoc. **196:**1679.
34. **Hsiao, K., H. F. Baker, T. J. Crow, M. Poulter, F. Owen, J. D. Terwilliger, D. Westaway, J. Ott, and S. B. Prusiner.** 1989. Linkage of a prion protein missense variant to Gerstmann-Sträussler syndrome. Nature (London) **338:**342–345.
35. **Hunter, N., J. D. Foster, A. G. Dickinson, and J. Hope.** 1989. Linkage of the gene for the scrapie-associated fibril protein (PrP) to the Sip gene in Cheviot sheep. Vet. Rec. **124:**364–366.
36. **Hunter, N., J. Hope, I. McConnell, and A. G. Dickinson.** 1987. Linkage of the scrapie-associated fibril protein (PrP) gene and Sinc using congenic mice and restriction fragment length polymorphism analysis. J. Gen. Virol. **68:** 2711–2716.
37. **Jellinger, K., F. Seitelberger, W. Heiss, and W. Holczabek.** 1972. Konjugale Form der subakuten spongiose Encephalopatie (Jakob-Creutzfeldt Erkrankung). Wien. Klin. Wochenschr. **84:**245–249.
38. **Kimberlin, R. H.** 1986. Scrapie: how much do we really understand? Neuropathol. Appl. Neurobiol. **12:**131–147.
39. **Kimberlin, R. H.** 1990. Detection of bovine spongiform encephalopathy in the United Kingdom. J. Am. Vet. Med. Assoc. **196:**1675–1676.
40. **Kimberlin, R. H., S. Cole, and C. A. Walker.** 1987. Temporary and permanent modifications to a single strain of mouse scrapie on transmission to rats and hamsters. J. Gen. Virol. **68:**1875–1881.
41. **Kimberlin, R. H., C. A. Walker, and H. Fraser.** 1989. The genomic identity of different strains of mouse scrapie is expressed in hamsters and preserved on reisolation in mice. J. Gen. Virol. **70:**2017–2025.
42. **Kirschbaum, W.** 1968. Jakob-Creutzfeldt disease. Elsevier, New York.
43. **Kitamoto, T., K. Ogomori, J. Tateishi, and S. B. Prusiner.** 1987. Formic acid pretreatment enhances immunostaining of cerebral and systemic amyloids. Lab. Invest. **57:**230–236.
44. **Klitzman, R. L., M. P. Alpers, and D. C. Gajdusek.** 1985. The natural incubation period of kuru and the episodes of transmission in three clusters of patients. Neuroepidemiology **3:**3–20.
45. **Kretzschmar, H. A., L. E. Stowring, D. Westaway, W. H. Stubblebine, S. B. Prusiner, and S. J. DeArmond.** 1986. Molecular cloning of a human prion protein cDNA. DNA **5:**315–324.
46. **Liao, Y. C., R. V. Lebo, G. A. Clawson, and E. A. Smuckler.** 1986. Human prion protein cDNA: molecular cloning, chromosomal mapping, and biological implications. Science **233:**364–367.
47. **Manuelidis, L., and E. E. Manuelidis.** 1989. Creutzfeldt-Jakob disease and dementias. Microb. Pathog. **7:**157–164.
48. **Manuelidis, L., T. Sklaviadis, and E. E. Manuelidis.** 1987. Evidence suggesting that PrP is not the infectious agent in Creutzfeldt-Jakob disease. EMBO J. **6:**341–347.
49. **Marsh, R. F.** 1990. Bovine spongiform encephalopathy in the United States. J. Am. Vet. Med. Assoc. **196:**1677.
50. **Marsh, R. F., and R. H. Kimberlin.** 1975. Comparison of scrapie and transmissible mink encephalopathy in hamsters. II. Clinical signs, pathology and pathogenesis. J. Infect. Dis. **131:**104–110.
51. **Masters, C. L., D. C. Gajdusek, and C. J. Gibbs, Jr.** 1981. Creutzfeldt-Jakob disease virus isolation from the Gerstmann-Sträussler syndrome, with an analysis of the various forms of amyloid plaque deposition in the virus-induced spongiform encephalopathies. Brain **104:**559–588.
52. **Masters, C. L., J. O. Harris, D. C. Gajdusek, C. J. Gibbs, Jr., C. Bernoulli, and D. M. Asher.** 1979. Creutzfeldt-Jakob disease: patterns of world-wide occurrence and the significance of familial and sporadic clustering. Ann. Neurol. **5:**177–188.
53. **Masullo, C., M. Pocchiari, G. Macchi, G. Alema, G. Piazza, and M. A. Panzera.** 1989. Transmission of Creutzfeldt-Jakob disease by dural cadaveric graft. J. Neurosurg. **71:**954–955.
54. **McKinley, M. P., D. C. Bolton, and S. B. Prusiner.** 1983. A protease-resistant protein is a structural component of the scrapie prion. Cell **35:**57–62.
55. **Merz, P. A., R. A. Somerville, H. M. Wisniewski, and K. Iqbal.** 1981. Abnormal fibrils from scrapie-infected brain. Acta Neuropathol. (Berlin) **54:**63–74.
56. **Meyer, R. K., M. P. McKinley, K. A. Bowman, R. A. Barry, and S. B. Prusiner.** 1986. Separation and properties of cellular and scrapie prion proteins. Proc. Natl. Acad. Sci. USA **83:**2310–2314.
57. **Miller, D.** 1988. Creutzfeldt-Jakob disease in histopathology

technicians. N. Engl. J. Med. **318:**853–854.

58. **Multhaup, G., H. Diringer, H. Hilmert, H. Prinz, J. Heukeshoven, and K. Beyreuther.** 1985. The protein component of scrapie-associated fibrils is a glycosylated low molecular weight protein. EMBO J. **4:**1495–1501.
59. **Narang, H. K., D. M. Asher, and D. C. Gajdusek.** 1987. Tubulofilaments in negatively stained scrapie-infected brains: relationship to scrapie-associated fibrils. Proc. Natl. Acad. Sci. USA **84:**7730–7734.
60. **Nevin, S., W. H. McMenemy, D. Behrman, and D. P. Jones.** 1960. Subacute spongiform encephalopathy: a subacute form of encephalopathy attributable to vascular dysfunction (spongiform cerebral atrophy). Brain **83:**519–564.
61. **Owen, F., M. Poulter, R. Lofthouse, J. Collinge, T. J. Crow, D. Risby, H. F. Baker, R. M. Ridley, K. Hsiao, and S. B. Prusiner.** 1989. Insertion in prion protein gene in familial Creutzfeldt-Jakob disease [letter]. Lancet **i:**51–52.
62. **Piccardo, P., J. Safar, M. Ceroni, D. C. Gajdusek, and C. J. Gibbs, Jr.** 1990. Immunohistochemical localization of prion protein in spongiform encephalopathies and normal tissue. Neurology **40:**518–522.
63. **Prusiner, S.** 1982. Novel proteinaceous particles cause scrapie. Science **216:**136–144.
64. **Prusiner, S. B.** 1989. Scrapie prions. Annu. Rev. Microbiol. **43:**345–374.
65. **Race, R. E., B. Caughey, K. Graham, D. Ernst, and B. Chesebro.** 1988. Analyses of frequency of infection, specific infectivity, and prion protein biosynthesis in scrapie-infected neuroblastoma cell clones. J. Virol. **62:**2845–2849.
66. **Rohwer, R. G.** 1984. Virus-like sensitivity of scrapie agent to heat inactivation. Science **223:**600–602.
67. **Roos, R., D. C. Gajdusek, and C. J. Gibbs, Jr.** 1973. The clinical characteristics of transmissible Creutzfeldt-Jakob disease. Brain **96:**1–20.
68. **Serban, D., A. Taraboulos, S. J. DeArmond, and S. B. Prusiner.** 1990. Rapid detection of Creutzfeldt-Jakob disease and scrapie prion proteins. Neurology **40:**110–117.
69. **Sigurdsson, B.** 1954. Observations on three slow infections of sheep. Br. Med. J. **110:**255–270, 307–322, 341–354.
70. **Sitwell, L., B. Lach, E. Atack, and D. Atack.** 1988. Creutzfeldt-Jakob disease in histopathology technicians. N. Engl. J. Med. **318:**854.
71. **Thadani, V., P. L. Penar, J. Partington, R. Kalb, R. Janssen, L. B. Schonberger, C. S. Rabkin, and J. W. Prichard.** 1988. Creutzfeldt-Jakob disease probably acquired from a cadaveric dura mater graft. Case report. J. Neurosurg. **69:** 766–769.
72. **Westaway, D., P. A. Goodman, C. A. Mirenda, M. P. McKinley, G. A. Carlson, and S. B. Prusiner.** 1987. Distinct prion proteins in short and long scrapie incubation period mice. Cell **51:**651–662.
73. **Wilesmith, J. W., G. A. Wells, M. P. Cranwell, and J. B. Ryan.** 1988. Bovine spongiform encephalopathy: epidemiological studies. Vet. Rec. **123:**638–644.
74. **Will, R. G., and W. B. Matthews.** 1982. Evidence for case-to-case transmission of Creutzfeldt-Jakob disease. J. Neurol. Neurosurg. Psychiatr. **45:**235–238.
75. **Williams, E. S., and S. Young.** 1982. Spongiform encephalopathy of Rocky Mountain elk. J. Wildl. Dis. **18:** 465–471.
76. **Wills, P. R.** 1989. Induced frameshifting mechanism of replication for an information-carrying scrapie prion. Microb. Pathog. **6:**235–249.

Section VIII. Rickettsiae and Chlamydiae

Chapter 103

Taxonomy

EMILIO WEISS

Section 9 of *Bergey's Manual of Systematic Bacteriology* (6) describes in detail the orders *Rickettsiales* and *Chlamydiales*. The *Rickettsiales*, even though separated from the endosymbionts in this edition of *Bergey's Manual*, represent a complex taxon, which includes the families *Rickettsiaceae*, *Bartonellaceae*, and *Anaplasmataceae*. The *Chlamydiales*, on the other hand, include a single family and a single genus, possibly underclassified. Numerous observations, isolations of new species, and phylogenetic analyses made during the past decade and for the most part after the publication of *Bergey's Manual* suggest that we should take another look at the classification of the family *Rickettsiaceae* and the genus *Chlamydia*.

Table 1 lists the species in the family *Rickettsiaceae* and in the genus *Chlamydia*, including species that have recently been added, and summarizes the information thus far obtained through comparisons of 16S rRNA sequences (20).

Among the changes that have occurred during the past decade, human infection in Europe with the spotted fever group rickettsia *Rickettsia conorii* was found to occur more frequently and to produce a more severe disease than in the past (10, 11). To the large number of rickettsial species in the spotted fever group, some established pathogens and others most likely commensals in the invertebrate host, two have been added, the pathogen *R. japonica* (14) and the commensal *R. helvetica* (8). The commensal *R. bellii* was isolated and described as a rickettsia that is possibly not a member of the spotted fever group (9).

The most extensive additions to our information are possibly those that involve the genus *Ehrlichia*. Ristic et al. (12) demonstrated that there is a small but highly significant degree of serologic relationship between the dog pathogen *Ehrlichia canis* and the human pathogen *Rickettsia sennetsu*. This finding was quickly followed by the observations that the two microorganisms strongly resemble each other in morphology and mode of development (3). As a result the sennetsu agent was reclassified in *Bergey's Manual* as *Ehrlichia sennetsu*. A few years later the etiologic agent of Potomac horse fever (equine monocytic ehrlichiosis) was isolated and found to be distantly related to *E. canis* and more closely related to *E. sennetsu* (4, 5). The evolutionary history of *E. sennetsu* and *E. risticii*, two microorganisms that are biologically similar but that differ widely in geographic distribution and pathogenesis for vertebrate hosts, well deserves to be investigated. A possible link between the two microorganisms is suggested by the recent discovery (discussed in chapter 106) that *E. canis*, or a closely related microorganism, is also a human pathogen.

Also worth mentioning is the similarity between another dog pathogen and a potential human pathogen. *Neorickettsia helminthoeca* is a dog pathogen that occurs in the U.S. West Coast states. Dogs acquire the disease by eating raw salmon infested with the metacercariae of a trematode, which in turn is infected with *N. helminthoeca* (6). Fukuda et al. (1) presented evidence that a disease involving a similar cycle may occur in Japan among people who eat improperly cooked fish. The fish, the grey mullet, is also often infested with a trematode that carries a bacterium similar to *N. helminthoeca*.

To the genus *Chlamydia*, the important human pathogen *C. pneumoniae* has been added (2).

The study of the phylogeny of the *Rickettsiaceae* and of chlamydiae conducted thus far has produced some results that confirm observations made on phenotypic similarity among certain species, while others contrast sharply with our present taxonomic concepts. For example, as expected, *Rickettsia prowazekii*, *R. typhi*, and *R. rickettsii* were shown to have very similar rRNA sequences (differences of <2%, smaller than the typical difference between the genera *Escherichia* and *Salmonella*) (15). These three rickettsial species belong to the alpha subdivision of the purple bacteria (20), recently named *Proteobacteria* (13). In this subdivision, the rickettsial species are specifically, although distantly, related to *Ehrlichia risticii* (15). This came as a surprise, since rickettsiae and the monocytic ehrlichiae differ in morphology and intracellular location, cytoplasm in the case of rickettsiae and phagosome in ehrlichiae (6). On the other hand, it has recently been shown that ehrlichiae and rickettsiae resemble each other in in vitro substrate utilization and gain in ATP content from this activity (18, 19). The rickettsiae are not specifically related to *Rochalimaea quintana*. This microorganism is also a member of the alpha subdivision of *Proteobacteria*, but belongs to subgroup 2 and is specifically related to the plant-associated agrobacteria and rhizobacteria (17). This is also unexpected since *R. prowazekii* and *R. quintana* have historically been transmitted by the same arthropod vector, the body louse, and the two DNAs hybridize with each other to the extent of 25 to 33% (7).

Not surprising, because of marked differences in phenotypic characteristics, was the finding that *Coxiella burnetii* is unrelated to the three species of rickettsia. It belongs in the gamma subdivision of the *Proteobacteria* and in this group it shows a rather distant but specific relationship to the genus *Legionella*. The tick commensal, *Wolbachia persica*, was also shown to belong in the gamma subdivision and to be peripherally related to the *Coxiella-Legionella* cluster (15).

Most astonishing was the finding that chlamydiae have no close relatives among the eubacteria (16). They represent a hitherto unrecognized major eubacterial group, peripherally related only to the planctomyces. These

TABLE 1. List of species in the family *Rickettsiaceae* and genus *Chlamydia* and summary of present knowledge of their phylogeny based on 16S sRNA sequences[a]

Genus	Group	Species	Proteobacterial subdivision[b]	Related genus[b]
Rickettsia	Typhus	*R. prowazekii,*[c] *R. typhi*[c]	Alpha	*Ehrlichia*
		R. canada	Unknown	Unknown
	Spotted fever	*R. rickettsii*[c]	Alpha	*Ehrlichia*
		R. conorii,[c] *R. sibirica,*[c] *R. australis*[c]	As above	As above
		R. akari,[c] *R. japonica*[c]	As above	As above
		R. montana, R. parkeri, R. rhipicephali	Unknown	Unknown
		R. helvetica	Unknown	Unknown
	Uncertain	*R. bellii*	Unknown	Unknown
	Scrub typhus	*R. tsutsugamushi*[c]	Unknown	Unknown
Rochalimaea		*R. quintana*[c]	Alpha, subgroup 2	Agrobacteria, rhizobacteria
		R. vinsonii	Unknown	Unknown
Ehrlichia	Monocytic	*E. risticii*[d]	Alpha	*Rickettsia*
		E. canis,[c,d] *E. sennetsu*[c]	As above	As above
	Granulocytic	*E. equi,*[d] *E. phagocytophila*[d]	Unknown	Unknown
Cowdria		*C. ruminantium*[d]	Unknown	Unknown
Neorickettsia		*N. helminthoeca*[d]	Unknown	Unknown
Coxiella		*C. burnetii*[c,d]	Gamma	*Legionella*
Wolbachia		*W. persica*	Gamma	*Coxiella, Legionella*
		W. pipientis, W. melophagi	Unknown	Unknown
Rickettsiella[e]		*R. popilliae, R. grylli, R. chironomi*	Unknown	Unknown
Chlamydia		*C. trachomatis,*[c] *C. psittaci*[c,d]	None (not a proteobacterium)	*Planctomyces*
		C. pneumoniae[c]	As above	As above

[a] The *Rickettsiales* families *Bartonellaceae* and *Anaplasmataceae* are not included. Not all of the species listed are discussed in subsequent chapters.
[b] "As above" below a proteobacterial subdivision or genus designation means that it is reasonable to assume that the designation above is applicable. Such an inference cannot be made for some of the other species of the same genus.
[c] Established human pathogen.
[d] Animal pathogen.
[e] Pathogenic for invertebrate host.

two groups of bacteria have very little in common phenotypically, except that the cell wall in both cases contains no peptidoglycan.

Much remains to be done in the field of phylogeny of the rickettsiae. If this work is extended to other pathogens of the spotted fever group, such as *R. conorii* or *R. sibirica,* few surprises are expected, because of the solid base of phenotypic information, which suggests that these rickettsiae are closely related. However, *R. tsutsugamushi* is sufficiently different from the other rickettsiae to deserve separate phylogenetic analysis. Despite the large body of information that we have on this species, in the absence of such a study we cannot venture to say that it is a proteobacterium.

The place of taxonomy in a manual of clinical microbiology is not clear. When phylogenetic information reinforces what we have learned by the study of phenotypic characteristics, it encourages us to proceed as we have. When a conflict develops between genotypic and phenotypic information, for the immediate purpose of isolation and identification of pathogens, it is preferable to pay greater attention to the phenotypic characteristics. However, genotypic information cannot be ignored. A conflict may suggest that important biologic or ecologic characteristics of the microorganisms involved are yet to be uncovered.

I am indebted to Gregory A. Dasch for his helpful discussions. The preparation of this chapter was in part supported by the Naval Medical Research and Development Command, Department of the Navy, work unit no. 3M161102.BS13.AK.111.

ADDENDUM IN PROOF

Taxonomy and the study of the bacterial genome have recently acquired new significance as the polymerase chain reaction (PCR) is being developed for the rapid identification of infectious agents (K. E. Hechemy, D. Paretsky, D. H.Walker, and L. P. Mallavia, ed., Ann. N.Y. Acad. Sci. **590:**1–586, 1990). For example, although the scrub typhus group of rickettsiae is still represented by a single species, *R. tsutsugamushi,* there is considerable variation in antigenic properties among the various strains. This variation is not necessarily accompanied by marked differences in virulence for humans. Heterogeneity has been attributed to variability of certain surface components that occur in a background of strong homology (E. V. Oaks, R. M. Rice, D. J. Kelly, and C. K. Stover, Infect. Immun. **57:** 3116–3122, 1989). It is therefore important, for the purpose of the PCR test, to select a region on the genome that is relatively stable and recognizes most, if not all, strains. In the case of the typhus and spotted fever group rickettsiae, there is sufficient similarity in their genomes for the selection of a region that detects several species, such as *R. prowazekii, R. typhi, R. rickettsii,* and *R. conorii.* If the test is positive, the identity of the infectious agent can, in most cases, be inferred on the basis of geography and other epidemiological considerations. Although more specific PCR tests can be applied, even if the species is not recognized in the initial test, treatment need not be delayed, since all of the above rickettsial species are susceptible to tetracycline or doxycycline. It has been recognized, however, that rickettsiae share antigens with several other bacterial species, including in some cases *Legionella* species. A genome that recognizes *Legionella* species should not be included in any test for rickettsiae, since the antibiotic of choice for *Legionella* species is erythromycin, which is not effective against rickettsiae (Hechemy et al., Ann. N.Y. Acad. Sci. **590:** 1–586, 1990).

LITERATURE CITED

1. **Fukuda, T., T. Sasahara, S. Yamamoto, N. Kawabata, and Y. Minamishima.** 1985. Rickettsiae and rickettsioses in southern Kyushu, Japan, p. 357–363. *In* J. Kazar (ed.), Proceedings of the 3rd International Symposium on Rickettsiae and Rickettsial Diseases. Slovak Academy of Sciences, Bratislava, Czechoslovakia.
2. **Grayston, J. T., C.-C. Kuo, L. A. Campbell, and S.-P. Wang.** 1989. *Chlamydia pneumoniae* sp. nov. for *Chlamydia* sp. strain TWAR. Int. J. Syst. Bacteriol. **39:**88–90.
3. **Hoilien, C. A., M. Ristic, D. L. Huxsoll, and G. Rapmund.** 1982. *Rickettsia sennetsu* in human blood monocyte cultures: similarities to the growth cycle of *Ehrlichia canis.* Infect. Immun. **35:**314–319.
4. **Holland, C. J., M. Ristic, A. I. Cole, P. Johnson, G. Baker, and T. Goetz.** 1985. Isolation, experimental transmission, and characterization of causative agent of Potomac horse fever. Science **227:**522–524.
5. **Holland, C. J., E. Weiss, W. Burgdorfer, A. I. Cole, and I. Kakoma.** 1985. *Ehrlichia risticii* sp. nov.: etiologic agent of equine monocytic ehrlichiosis (synonym, Potomac horse fever). Int. J. Syst. Bacteriol. **35:**524–526.
6. **Krieg, N. R., and J. G. Holt (ed.).** 1984. Bergey's manual of systematic bacteriology, vol. 1, p. 687–739. The Williams & Wilkins Co., Baltimore.
7. **Myers, W. F., and C. L. Wisseman, Jr.** 1980. Genetic relatedness among the typhus group of rickettsiae. Int. J. Syst. Bacteriol. **30:**142–150.
8. **Peter, O., J. C. Williams, and W. Burgdorfer.** 1985. *Rickettsia helvetica,* a new spotted fever group rickettsia: immunochemical analysis of the antigens of 5 spotted fever group rickettsiae, p. 99–108. *In* J. Kazar (ed.), Proceedings of the 3rd International Symposium on Rickettsiae and Rickettsial Diseases. Slovak Academy of Sciences, Bratislava, Czechoslovakia.
9. **Philip, R. N., E. A. Casper, R. L. Anacker, J. Cory, S. F. Hayes, W. Burgdorfer, and C. E. Yunker.** 1983. *Rickettsia bellii* sp. nov.: a tick-borne rickettsia, widely distributed in the United States, that is distinct from the spotted fever and typhus biogroups. Int. J. Syst. Bacteriol. **33:**94–106.
10. **Raoult, D., P. J. Weiller, A. Chagnon, H. Chaudet, H. Gallais, and P. Casanova.** 1986. Mediterranean spotted fever: clinical, laboratory and epidemiological features of 199 cases. Am. J. Trop. Med. Hyg. **35:**845–850.
11. **Raoult, D., P. Zuchelli, P. J. Weiller, C. Charrel, J. L. SanMarco, H. Gallais, and P. Casanova.** 1986. Incidence, clinical observations and risk factors in the severe form of Mediterranean spotted fever among patients admitted to hospital in Marseilles 1983–1984. J. Infect. **12:**111–116.
12. **Ristic, M., D. L. Huxsoll, N. Tachibana, and G. Rapmund.** 1981. Evidence of a serologic relationship between *Ehrlichia canis* and *Rickettsia sennetsu.* Am. J. Trop. Med. Hyg. **30:**1324–1328.
13. **Stackebrandt, E., R. G. E. Murray, and H. G. Trüper.** 1988. *Proteobacteria* classis nov., a name for the phylogenetic taxon that includes the "purple bacteria and their relatives." Int. J. Syst. Bacteriol. **38:**321–325.
14. **Uchida, T., X. Yu, T. Uchiyama, and D. H. Walker.** 1989. Identification of a unique spotted fever group rickettsia from humans in Japan. J. Infect. Dis. **159:**1122–1126.
15. **Weisburg, W. G., M. E. Dobson, J. E. Samuel, G. A. Dasch, L. P. Mallavia, O. Baca, L. Maldelco, J. E. Sechrest, E. Weiss, and C. R. Woese.** 1989. Phylogenetic diversity of the rickettsiae. J. Bacteriol. **17:**4302–4306.
16. **Weisburg, W. G., T. P. Hatch, and C. R. Woese.** 1986. Eubacterial origin of chlamydiae. J. Bacteriol. **167:**570–574.
17. **Weisburg, W. G., C. R. Woese, M. E. Dobson, and E. Weiss.** 1985. A common origin of rickettsiae and certain plant pathogens. Science **230:**556–558.
18. **Weiss, E., G. A. Dasch, Y.-H. Kang, and H. N. Westfall.** 1988. Substrate utilization by *Ehrlichia sennetsu* and *Ehrlichia risticii* separated from host constituents by Renografin gradient centrifugation. J. Bacteriol. **170:**5012–5017.
19. **Weiss, E., J. C. Williams, G. A. Dasch, and Y.-H. Kang.** 1989. Energy metabolism of monocytic *Ehrlichia.* Proc. Natl. Acad. Sci. USA **86:**1674–1678.
20. **Woese, C. R.** 1987. Bacterial evolution. Microbiol. Rev. **51:**221–271.

Chapter 104

Rickettsiae

JOSEPH E. McDADE

The rickettsiae are gram-negative obligate intracellular bacteria (59). A characteristic feature of the rickettsiae is that they all multiply in an arthropod (lice, ticks, fleas, or mites) as part of their life cycle. With some rickettsiae (spotted fever and scrub typhus rickettsiae), the invertebrate hosts are both reservoirs and vectors. Rickettsiae are also infectious for a wide variety of mammals, which either serve as reservoirs for the organisms or ensure the survival of the parasitic vectors that feed on them. Species in four genera, *Ehrlichia, Rickettsia, Coxiella,* and *Rochalimaea,* are pathogenic for humans. This chapter describes the clinical aspects of pathogens in the genera *Rickettsia* and *Coxiella*. The ehrlichiae are described separately (chapter 106). Little new information is available on *Rochalimaea quintana,* the agent of trench fever.

CHARACTERIZATION

Rickettsia

Members of the genus *Rickettsia* are morphologically and biochemically similar to other gram-negative bacteria. They are short, rod-shaped or coccobacillary organisms, usually 0.8 to 2.0 μm long and 0.3 to 0.5 μm in diameter. Most species grow luxuriantly in tissue culture or in the yolk sacs of embryonated eggs. Guinea pigs or mice are the most commonly used experimental hosts.

Species in the genus *Rickettsia* are subdivided into three groups of antigenically related microorganisms: spotted fever, typhus, and scrub typhus (Table 1). The spotted fever and typhus groups are composed of multiple species, whereas the scrub typhus group consists of different serovars of only one species, *Rickettsia tsutsugamushi*. Vector associations also help to distinguish the various groups. For example, most members of the spotted fever group are found in ticks, scrub typhus rickettsiae are found in mites, and typhus rickettsiae have fleas or lice as vectors (Table 1). Limited DNA-to-DNA hybridization studies have confirmed the phenotypic groupings (37).

All members of the genus *Rickettsia* are unstable outside the host cell and are inactivated at temperatures of ≥56°C. They can also be inactivated with standard disinfectants, including hypochlorite, hydrogen peroxide, Lysol, or quaternary ammonium compounds.

Coxiella

The genus *Coxiella* is composed of a single species, *Coxiella burnetii*. It is a short, rod-shaped microorganism, 0.2 to 0.4 μm in diameter and 0.4 to 1.0 μm in length. Although *C. burnetii* is found in numerous species of tick, it is maintained in nature primarily by aerosol transmission. *C. burnetii* typically infects cattle, sheep, and goats, multiplies to large numbers in the placentas of pregnant animals, and is shed during parturition.

C. burnetii displays an antigenic phase variation that is unique among the rickettsiae. It exists in two antigenic phases (I and II), which are analogous to the smooth and rough forms observed with some species of bacteria. *C. burnetii* exists in antigenic phase I in nature, but it changes to phase II after continuous passage in tissue cultures or embryonated eggs. Available data indicate that the phase I antigen is a polysaccharide component of the *Coxiella* lipopolysaccharide and that the transition from phase I to phase II occurs when one or more carbohydrate components are deleted from the lipopolysaccharide moiety (20).

In contrast to species in the genus *Rickettsia, C. burnetii* resists inactivation by physical and chemical treatment (3). It has reportedly survived for a year or more attached to wool or other fomites, and it is incompletely inactivated when held at 63°C for 30 min. Furthermore, *C. burnetii* is only partially inactivated when exposed to 1% Formalin or 1% phenol for 24 h. However, it can be inactivated by 0.05% hypochlorite, 5% H_2O_2, or a 1:100 dilution of Lysol.

CLINICAL SIGNIFICANCE

Table 1 summarizes the various rickettsioses, their respective etiologic agents, and their salient epidemiologic features. From a clinical perspective, rickettsial diseases have many features in common. The incubation period for most rickettsioses ranges from 3 to 14 days. Most patients develop nonspecific symptoms and signs. Onset of disease is sudden in about half of the cases. Fever and headache are the most commonly reported symptoms, but chills, myalgias, arthralgias, malaise, and anorexia also are noted. Fever increases during the first week of illness, often reaching 104°F or higher.

Rash is a hallmark of rickettsial infection, but it usually follows systemic symptoms. Its absence should not rule out a possible rickettsial etiology, especially during the first week of illness. Conjunctivitis and pharyngitis are common. Photophobia is also observed, but evidence of more serious central nervous system impairment (confusion, stupor, delirium, seizures, and coma) is found only in about 25% of patients with Rocky Mountain spotted fever (RMSF) (32) or typhus (38) and is virtually never seen in the other rickettsial diseases.

Mild pulmonary involvement, manifested by cough and infiltrates on the chest roentgenogram, is common in epidemic typhus and is found in about half of Q fever and scrub typhus patients and in about one-third of patients with RMSF. Hepatomegaly or splenomegaly is

TABLE 1. Features of the pathogenic rickettsiae

Biogroup	Species	Disease in humans	Distribution	Means of transmission to humans
Spotted fever	*R. rickettsii*	Rocky Mountain spotted fever	Western Hemisphere	Tick bite
	R. conorii	Boutonneuse fever	Mediterranean countries, Africa, India	Tick bite
	R. sibirica	Siberian tick typhus	Siberia, Mongolia	Tick bite
	R. australis	Australian tick typhus	Australia	Tick bite
	R. akari	Rickettsialpox	United States, USSR	Mite bite
Typhus	*R. prowazekii*	Epidemic typhus	Primarily highland areas of South America and Africa	Infected louse feces
		Recrudescent typhus (Brill-Zinsser disease)	Worldwide	Reactivation of latent infection
		Sporadic typhus	United States	Contact with flying squirrels (*Glaucomys volans*)
	R. typhi	Murine typhus	Worldwide	Infected flea feces
Scrub typhus	*R. tsutsugamushi*	Scrub typhus	Asia, northern Australia, Pacific Islands	Chigger bite
Q fever	*C. burnetii*	Q fever	Worldwide	Infectious aerosols

only found in about 20% of patients with rickettsioses except for Q fever, where hepatomegaly and hepatitis may dominate the clinical picture in as many as half of the patients. In scrub typhus, early in the infection, regional lymphadenopathy is observed in about 20% of the patients. Later, generalized lymphadenopathy that may be mistaken for mononucleosis is seen in about 80%.

The symptoms of murine typhus (36) and flying squirrel-associated typhus fever (11, 35) are similar but milder than those of epidemic typhus.

Chronic Q fever and recrudescent typhus (Brill-Zinsser disease) are illnesses that appear years after initial infection with *C. burnetti* and *Rickettsia prowazekii*, respectively. Chronic Q fever is an uncommon illness that usually affects patients with preexisting valvular heart disease; it develops as a culture-negative endocarditis accompanied by liver function abnormalities and granulomatous hepatitis. Chronic Q fever infections are frequently fatal (13, 53). The incidence of Brill-Zinsser disease is difficult to ascertain. It occurs sporadically in persons who have lived in typhus-endemic areas and contracted primary cases of louse-borne typhus months to years before the onset of the recrudescent infection. The clinical manifestations of Brill-Zinsser disease are generally milder than those of primary louse-borne typhus (52).

The course and outcome of rickettsial diseases vary. The primary determinants are the specific infectious agent and the promptness of effective antibiotic treatment. In the preantibiotic era, the reported case fatality rate of RMSF ranged from 23 to 70% (23, 60). With the advent of antibiotics, the fatality rates quickly fell below 10% and have remained at approximately 3 to 7% in the United States in the 1980s (15). Fatalities are also common in epidemic typhus and scrub typhus but rare in murine typhus; no fatalities have been reported for rickettsialpox.

DIAGNOSIS

There are three general approaches to the laboratory diagnosis of rickettsial diseases: direct detection of rickettsiae in patient tissues, isolation of rickettsiae from tissues, and serologic tests for rickettsial antibodies. Although no technique reliably provides a diagnosis early enough to affect the outcome of the disease, recent advances in the use of polymerase chain reaction technology (see chapter 17) may soon allow early diagnosis. Serodiagnosis is the preferred diagnostic approach, and testing of paired serum specimens is still recommended. The first specimen should be obtained during the acute phase of illness, and the second specimen should be obtained 2 to 3 weeks later.

Because of the hazards of working with living rickettsiae, isolation attempts are usually limited to situations where the outcome is fatal and postmortem tissues are the only specimens available for testing. Even then, direct fluorescent-antibody tests of Formalin-fixed, paraffin-embedded tissues are faster and safer than rickettsial isolation for diagnosis.

Specimen collection and handling

Rickettsiae are hazardous (biosafety level 3; see chapter 7) microorganisms that have been responsible for numerous laboratory infections (43, 47); therefore, specimens obtained from patients suspected of having rickettsial diseases should be handled with appropriate care. Rickettsiae are usually present in infected blood at a relatively low concentration of approximately 10 to 100 viable organisms per ml (32) and lose viability after several hours at room temperature (Q fever rickettsiae excepted). However, viable rickettsiae may still be present in blood kept at room temperature for several days. Processing freshly drawn blood to obtain serum does not pose a serious threat, provided that aerosolization is minimized and surgical gloves are worn. Special care should be exercised when handling specimens that might contain Q fever rickettsiae. *C. burnetii* is highly infectious, resists desiccation and chemical inactivation, and is frequently shed in the urine and feces of infected animals (3). Although sera from suspected Q fever patients present no unusual hazards when handled as described above, infected tissues from Q fever patients should be processed under strict biosafety level 3 conditions, and then only by highly qualified personnel. The obvious caveats apply to those who attempt to isolate *C. burnetii* in laboratory animals.

Blood can be used for rickettsial isolation attempts, provided that it is collected during the acute, febrile period, before antibiotic therapy. Either clotted or heparinized blood is satisfactory. If isolation attempts cannot be started immediately, blood should be stored at −70°C. Blood that must be forwarded to a reference laboratory should be shipped on liquid nitrogen or dry ice in unbreakable shipping containers.

Postmortem tissues (lung, spleen, and lymph nodes) are also suitable for rickettsial isolation attempts. Thumbnail-size pieces of fresh tissues should be collected and stored frozen until shipped. Tissues obtained postmortem contain far greater numbers of organisms than does infected blood, however, and require additional care in handling, including the wearing of surgical masks and back-fastening gowns.

Direct detection of rickettsiae

Direct fluorescent-antibody testing of tissues collected postmortem has become a useful approach for the retrospective diagnosis of rickettsial diseases. This technique was first applied to the rickettsiae by Walker and Cain (55), who successfully detected rickettsiae in kidney tissue of 7 of 10 patients who had died of suspected RMSF. Sections of Formalin-fixed, paraffin-embedded tissue are fixed on glass slides with glue and incubated in an oven at 60°C for 1 h. The sections are then deparaffinized in three changes of xylene and rehydrated gradually by passage through an ethanol series (100, 95, 70, and 35%) to distilled water. The rehydrated sections are digested with 0.1% trypsin containing 0.1% $CaCl_2$ for 4 h at 37°C. The slides are washed thoroughly with distilled water and then with phosphate-buffered saline (pH 7.5). Fluorescein isothiocyanate-labeled antirickettsial sera (fluorescein-labeled antisera to *Rickettsia rickettsii* are available through the Centers for Disease Control; conjugated antisera to other species are available only from specialty laboratories) are then added to the sections, and the slides are incubated in a humid chamber at 37°C for 30 min. The slides are washed again in phosphate-buffered saline, rinsed in distilled water, mounted in a glycerol solution, and examined with a UV microscope. Sections should be screened at ×400 magnification and then viewed at a higher magnification to confirm the morphology of the organisms and to rule out nonspecific staining. Morphologically distinct rickettsiae are readily detectable by this procedure. Our laboratory has had its best success with lung and spleen, both highly vascularized tissues, although rickettsiae can also be seen in heart and liver.

Rickettsiae can also be detected in skin biopsies by the direct fluorescent-antibody technique. Unfortunately, this procedure is not reliable enough for definitive diagnosis. Punch biopsies, approximately 3 to 5 mm in diameter, are obtained either from petechiae or the center of a macule, embedded in polyethylene glycol, and frozen in a cryostat. (The potential hazard of preparing frozen sections from infected tissues necessitates adequate biocontainment facilities.) Sections of tissue are then collected on glass slides, fixed in cold acetone for 15 min, and tested with fluorescein-labeled antirickettsial sera. Evaluations of this technique (16, 49, 56, 61) indicate that it will detect *R. rickettsii* or *Rickettsia conorii* in about 50% of patients with RMSF or Boutonneuse fever, respectively. All of the factors that contribute to the lack of sensitivity are not known, although most false-negative results were from patients who had received specific antibiotic therapy before the biopsy (49, 57).

Rickettsiae are also present in circulating monocytes. However, their relatively low number precludes ready detection by direct fluorescence microscopy.

Direct detection of rickettsial nucleic acids

Recent studies by Tzianabos et al. (54) indicate that rickettsial DNA can be detected in infected blood early in rickettsial infections. Using nucleotide primers corresponding to a portion of a defined rickettsial gene, they successfully detected *R. rickettsii* DNA in seven of nine patients with confirmed cases of RMSF by the polymerase chain reaction technique. Additional testing is needed to confirm the specificity, sensitivity, and utility of this technique for the early diagnosis of RMSF and other rickettsial infections.

Isolation and identification

Primary isolation. When tissues obtained at autopsy are used for rickettsial isolation, selective propagation of rickettsiae in susceptible laboratory animals is usually a necessary first step, because autopsy specimens are usually contaminated with bacteria and the general susceptibility of rickettsiae to antibiotics precludes their selective propagation in tissue cultures containing media supplemented with antibiotics. Rickettsiae isolated in animals are passaged in tissue culture or embryonated eggs to confirm their isolation and rule out contaminants. Specimens likely to be free of contaminants (e.g., aseptically collected blood) can be injected directly into embryonated eggs or cell cultures, as appropriate for attempts at isolation; however, subpassage of infected eggs or cell cultures may be necessary to obtain the quantity of microorganisms necessary to confirm isolation.

Although the general approach to isolation is similar for all rickettsial species, differences in the pathogenicity of various rickettsiae for experimental animals may necessitate some modifications of the basic protocol to facilitate isolation. Guinea pigs are quite susceptible to *R. prowazekii*, *Rickettsia typhi*, and *R. rickettsii* (40), but they are refractory to *R. tsutsugamushi*. The guinea pig is also the animal of choice for isolation of *C. burnetii*. In addition to being susceptible to rickettsiae, guinea pigs provide a practical advantage because their body temperature can be monitored as an indicator of infection. Male guinea pigs are recommended for isolating spotted fever and typhus group rickettsiae because of the characteristic scrotal swelling that usually occurs in guinea pigs infected with *R. typhi* or *R. rickettsii*. Meadow voles (*Microtus pennsylvanicus*) are also quite susceptible to spotted fever group rickettsiae, but they are not readily available. Mice are the preferred hosts for the isolation of *Rickettsia akari* and *R. tsutsugamushi*. However, because some inbred strains of mice are resistant to infection with *R. tsutsugamushi* (19), outbred mice should be used for all such isolation attempts.

Groups of four guinea pigs or eight mice, as appropriate, are recommended for the processing of each specimen. Each animal is marked, and a preinoculation serum specimen is obtained from each animal as a control for serologic testing of surviving animals. All animals must be treated humanely and in accordance with national standards so as to minimize pain and distress.

All clinical specimens for rickettsial isolation must be processed in a laminar flow hood under appropriate biosafety conditions. A small (1-cm^2) piece of the human tissue is triturated in sufficient brain heart infusion (BHI) broth to form a 10% (wt/vol) suspension. Use of a mortar and pestle and sterile Alundum is quite satisfactory for this purpose. The suspension is then injected intraperitoneally into the appropriate laboratory animal. A sample of the suspension should be stored at −70°C as reference material. An inoculum of 1 ml is recommended for guinea pigs, whereas 0.25 to 0.5 ml of suspension is injected into mice. All animals are then observed for signs of illness for 28 days.

When guinea pigs are used for primary isolation, their rectal temperatures are recorded daily for 14 days. Because all rickettsiae have relatively long incubation periods, any fever (≥40°C) during the first 2 days is usually the result of bacterial peritonitis. Fevers that occur 3 to 14 days after inoculation are more likely to indicate rickettsial infection.

Tissue specimens are collected aseptically from infected guinea pigs on day 2 or 3 of fever and passaged into either tissue cultures or embryonated eggs (see below). Infected blood or spleen is the preferred tissue for passage, although liver, brain, and tunica vaginalis are also acceptable.

At this stage in the isolation effort, multiple impression smears of infected tissues can be made for direct microscopic examination. Smears are heat fixed, stained by the Gimenez method (17; also see chapter 122), and examined by light microscopy under high-power magnification. {For tissues infected with suspected isolates of *R. tsutsugamushi*, a few drops of ferric nitrate solution [4% $Fe(NO_3)_3 \cdot 9H_2O$ in distilled water] should be added to the smear after the carbol fuchsin stain has been washed away. The slide is then washed immediately and stained with malachite green as for other rickettsiae.} Rickettsiae will appear red against the blue to blue-green background of the host cell. If microscopic examination of the smears shows numerous intracellular microorganisms, additional smears are fixed with cold acetone for 15 min, allowed to dry, and stained with the appropriate fluorescein-labeled antirickettsial serum to identify the presumed isolate. Regardless of the outcome of these tests, however, suspected isolates should be passaged in tissue culture or embryonated eggs to confirm their identity and to rule out bacterial contaminants.

When mice or meadow roles are used for isolation attempts, the animals should be humanely euthanized and their tissues should be harvested for passage when the animals develop overt signs of illness, i.e., lethargy, hunched backs, ruffled fur, or labored breathing. Alternatively, two animals can be euthanized on days 7, 10, and 14 after inoculation to obtain tissues for blind passage. Strict aseptic technique must be used when animals are dissected. Rickettsiae are usually found in the greatest numbers in the spleens of infected mice, although organisms can also be found in the peritoneal exudate, particularly in mice inoculated with scrub typhus rickettsiae. Mouse tissues are harvested and passaged as described for guinea pigs.

Although most species of rickettsiae are pathogenic for guinea pigs and mice, some strains cause inapparent infections in these animals. For this reason, serum samples should be obtained from all surviving animals 28 days after inoculation and tested for rickettsial antibodies. This is particularly important when none of the animals develop signs of illness. Positive serologic reactions indicate rickettsial infection, provided, of course, that negative results are obtained with the corresponding preinoculation sera.

Propagation of isolates. Propagation of rickettsiae is an extremely hazardous procedure that should be attempted only under biosafety level 3 conditions (see chapter 7).

Cell cultures provide a convenient method for rickettsial propagation. Numerous cell lines have been used successfully for growing rickettsiae; Vero, primary chicken embryo, WI-38, HeLa, and virtually any other cell line are suitable for this purpose. One factor that might exclude the use of a given cell line, however, is its ability to be maintained for several weeks, because the incubation period of rickettsiae can be long and growth with new isolates may be sparse for a week or longer.

Infected animal tissues are homogenized thoroughly in sterile BHI broth to form a 5% (wt/vol) suspension. The growth medium is then decanted from several tissue culture flasks, and 0.1 to 0.5 ml of the infected tissue suspension is added, depending on the size of the flasks. The flasks are rocked for 10 to 20 s to ensure that the inoculum covers the entire cell sheet and then placed in a 35°C incubator for 30 min to allow infection to occur. Growth medium (without antibiotics!) is then added to the cultures, and the cultures are incubated at 35°C and monitored for up to 14 days. No other special growth conditions are necessary, although it is known that *R. rickettsii*, *R. prowazekii*, and *R. typhi* (but not *R. tsutsugamushi*) grow better in an environment with 5% CO_2 than they do when exposed to the 0.2 to 0.3% CO_2 that is found in atmospheric air (33). Culture fluid should be changed after 24 h of incubation to remove the debris from the animal tissues that are used as inocula.

Beginning on day 3 after inoculation, small pieces of a given culture are periodically scraped off the flask with an inoculating loop or the equivalent, and smears are prepared and stained for rickettsiae by the Gimenez technique (chapter 122) and by the direct fluorescent-antibody procedure, if appropriate.

If rickettsiae cannot be detected in the cell cultures after 14 days or growth is so scanty as to preclude definite identification by fluorescent-antibody testing, the cells should be harvested and subcultured into additional flasks of the same cell line. Sterile glass beads are added to the culture flask, the cap is sealed, and the cells are displaced by vigorously shaking the flask for 10 to 20 s. A sample of the resulting cell suspension is used as an inoculum, and the remainder is stored at −70°C. Sampling and testing for rickettsiae in the second set of cell cultures should then be repeated. One blind passage is usually sufficient to detect rickettsiae when they are present.

Rickettsiae also grow quite well in embryonated hen

eggs. Spotted fever group rickettsiae grow better in embryos that are approximately 5 days old at the time of inoculation, whereas other rickettsiae prefer 6- to 7-day-old embryos. Generally speaking, the incubation period of spotted fever rickettsiae is 5 to 7 days, compared with the 7- to 10-day incubation periods of the typhus, scrub typhus and Q fever rickettsiae, but these periods vary. It should also be noted that spotted fever rickettsiae continue to grow up to 48 h after the embryos have died; yolk sacs infected with spotted fever rickettsiae usually produce optimum yields of living organisms when harvested 24 h after the death of embryos. However, this does not apply to other rickettsiae.

Embryonated eggs of the required age are candled, and infertile eggs are discarded. The tops of the eggs are then disinfected with alcohol or tincture of iodine, and a small hole is punched in the top of each egg. Next, a 5% suspension of infected animal tissue, prepared in sterile BHI broth, is drawn up into a syringe fitted with a 20-gauge, 1.5-in. (ca. 3.8-cm) needle, and 0.5-ml samples of the suspension are injected into each of 12 embryonated eggs. The eggs are then sealed with paraffin or model airplane glue and incubated at 35°C. A sample of the inoculum is stored at −70°C as reference material, and another sample is inoculated onto appropriate bacteriologic media to check for contaminants. Thioglycolate broth and blood agar plates are usually sufficient for this purpose, but use of other media and incubation of media under aerobic and anaerobic conditions are recommended.

Eggs whose embryos die in the first 3 days after inoculation should be discarded and autoclaved. Yolk sacs are harvested aseptically from embryos that die from days 4 through 10. The tops of eggs are disinfected with 70% alcohol or tincture of iodine, and a portion of the shell is removed with sterile, blunt forceps. The chorioallantoic membrane is then teased away. A small piece of the harvested yolk sac is removed aseptically and used for preparing smears for direct microscopic observation and fluorescent-antibody testing as described above. Additional small pieces of yolk sac should be inoculated onto appropriate bacteriologic media to check for bacterial contaminants. The remaining large fragment of each yolk sac should be stored individually at −70°C as reference material. If none of the embryos die during the 10-day incubation period or the yolk sacs of dead embryos do not contain detectable rickettsiae, the yolk sacs should be harvested from all remaining live embryos on day 10 for a single blind passage into additional embryonated eggs; a 20% yolk sac suspension of several yolk sacs, prepared in BHI broth, should be used as inoculum. Eggs are then monitored, and yolk sacs are harvested as described above.

Final confirmation of rickettsial isolation requires that the isolate be morphologically similar to rickettsiae, grow intracellularly, fail to grow on bacteriologic media, and react with appropriate immune serum but not with nonimmune sera. Additional details concerning the procedures for rickettsial isolation can be found in the review by Weiss (58).

Antibody assays

Various serologic procedures have been used for diagnosing rickettsial diseases (Table 2). Details of the different techniques can be found in the respective references and in section II of this Manual. Relatively few techniques are used regularly by most laboratories. Some tests lack sensitivity (complement fixation [CF], microagglutination, and Weil-Felix) or specificity compared with newer ones (2, 28, 31, 39, 41, 46), and re-

TABLE 2. Highlights of various serologic techniques for the diagnosis of rickettsial infections

Technique	Minimum positive titer	Time after onset antibody usually detected	Comments	References
IFA	16–64, depending on investigator	2–3 wk	Relatively sensitive and requires little antigen; can distinguish immunoglobulin isotypes	2, 12, 30, 31, 39, 41, 46
CF	8 or 16, depending on investigator	3–4 wk	Less sensitive than IFA or ELISA but very specific	12, 31, 39, 40, 46
ELISA	Optical density 0.25 > controls	1 wk in some instances	IgM capture assay promising for early diagnosis	8–10, 14, 21, 29
Latex agglutination	64	1–2 wk	Lacks sensitivity for late convalescent sera	25, 27, 31
IHA	40?	1–2 wk	Sensitivity ≥ IFA; more sensitive than CF	1, 31, 46, 51
Immunoperoxidase	20	7 days	Not evaluated for all rickettsiae; useful in field situations	48, 62
Microagglutination	≥8	1–2 wk	Requires considerable antigen; less sensitive than IFA	39, 41, 46
Radioimmunoassay	10?	7–10 days	IgM capture assay may be useful for early diagnosis	10, 29, 34
Weil-Felix	40–320, depending on investigator	2–3 wk	Lacks sensitivity and specificity	2, 5, 28, 31, 41, 46

agents are not commercially available for many procedures. Antigens for CF tests for Q fever are available commercially, and the Centers for Disease Control distributes indirect immunofluorescence assay (IFA) reagents for the diagnosis of spotted fever, typhus, and Q fever infections to qualified public health laboratories. Otherwise, reagents can be acquired only through specialty laboratories.

Recommending a preferred serologic technique is not entirely straightforward. Enzyme-linked immunosorbent assay (ELISA) techniques, particularly immunoglobulin M (IgM) capture assays, are among the most sensitive procedures available for rickettsial diagnosis, but they require large quantities of purified antigens that are unavailable commercially. ELISA tests also are quite amenable for the large-scale screening of serum specimens, but this advantage is usually lost for rickettsial diseases, because with the exception of epidemic typhus, rickettsioses usually occur sporadically at a relatively low frequency.

The IFA technique remains the most popular for serodiagnosis of rickettsial diseases, primarily because of the availability of reagents and the ease and economy with which it can be incorporated into existing antibody screening systems.

The indirect hemagglutination (IHA) test has received only limited evaluations, but it apparently has a sensitivity equal to or better than that of IFA. An erythrocyte-sensitizing substance (ESS), which can be obtained from typhus and spotted fever group rickettsiae by alkali extraction, is adsorbed onto sheep or human group O erythrocytes, and the coated cells are then used as antigens for simple agglutination tests (6, 7, 44). Unfortunately, however, rickettsial ESS is not available commercially. The respective ESSs exhibit group-specific antigenic reactivity. Thc convenience of the IHA technique makes it ideal for a clinical setting, although the relatively short shelf life (6 months) of sensitized erythrocytes (51) is a disadvantage. Nonetheless, it has considerable value as a bedside technique, particularly in field situations. Similarly, the indirect immunoperoxidase technique may be best suited for field use, particularly in remote areas.

The latex agglutination test has been used with some success in a number of public health laboratories in recent years (24–27). Latex spheres are coated with ESS, and the sensitized particles are used as antigens in an agglutination test. The simplicity of the latex agglutination test offers a convenience that is best appreciated at the hospital level, but because it is primarily an IgM assay, it lacks sensitivity for late-convalescent-phase sera. Additionally, the ESS contains only a limited repertoire of rickettsial antigens, and because some epitopes may be masked or destroyed when the ESS is adsorbed onto latex particles, some positive sera may go undetected. Nonetheless, the convenience of the latex test makes it useful as a bedside diagnostic procedure. It is recommended for that setting over the Weil-Felix test, which is still used in similar circumstances.

The Weil-Felix test became popular in the 1920s after it was observed that certain *Proteus* strains would agglutinate early-convalescent-phase sera from patients with suspected rickettsial disease (57). The test fell into disfavor because it lacks both sensitivity and specificity (2, 28), but it has managed to survive because of its convenience in a clinical setting. Despite its simplicity, it does not provide either early or specific diagnosis of rickettsioses.

The IFA procedure for the rickettsiae is similar to conventional IFA techniques, with inactivated yolk sac or tissue culture suspensions of rickettsiae being used as antigens (39). Antigen is applied to 8- or 10-well Teflon-coated glass slides with capillary tubes. Each well should contain the requisite combination of rickettsial antigens. For example, in the United States, spotted fever and typhus group antigens should be included in all tests, with Q fever antigen added as indicated. The antigen spots are then air dried and fixed in cold acetone for 15 min. A series of twofold dilutions of each serum is then prepared, starting at a 1:16 dilution. Known positive and negative control sera should be included in each test. Sera are usually diluted in a 1% suspension of normal yolk sac, prepared in phosphate-buffered saline (pH 7.2) to remove any naturally occurring antibodies to egg proteins which may react with the substrate. The remainder of the test is performed by standard methods as described in chapter 11. IFA tests are reasonably sensitive, although the subjectivity of endpoint determinations is an obvious disadvantage.

INTERPRETATION OF LABORATORY DATA

With the exception of Q fever, rickettsial diseases usually present as febrile exanthemous illnesses with protean clinical manifestations. In a clinical setting, rickettsioses must be distinguished from several viral and bacterial illnesses, including meningococcemia, measles, enteroviral exanthems, leptospirosis, typhoid fever, rubella, and ehrlichiosis.

The interpretation of serologic tests is frequently confounded by the lack of specificity of available rickettsial reagents. Whole rickettsiae are used as antigens for many antibody assays, and since rickettsiae are antigenically related to some species of bacteria (e.g., *Proteus* species), sera from nonrickettsial patients can react at low titers with rickettsial antigens. This has necessitated the designation of minimum positive titers (Table 2) to confirm recent rickettsial infections. The minimum titers for each procedure should not be considered absolute, however, because in many instances they were assigned somewhat arbitrarily. Borderline titers obtained with single specimens collected at nonoptimum times, i.e., very early or very late in convalescence, are the most difficult to interpret. The traditional way to avoid such problems is to collect acute- and convalescent-phase serum specimens 2 to 3 weeks apart so that rising titers can be demonstrated.

The Centers for Disease Control has established criteria for positivity for the various serologic tests. Fourfold rises in titer detected by any technique (Weil-Felix technique excepted) are considered evidence of rickettsial infections. (Most techniques use doubling dilutions of serum, starting at a 1:8 dilution.) With single serum specimens, CF titers of ≥16 in a clinically compatible case are also considered positive. With the IFA test, single titers of 64 or higher are considered of borderline significance for typhus and spotted fever group infections, whereas single IFA titers of 256 are considered minimal for confirmation of Q fever. Although these titers are somewhat higher than those recommended by others (see Table 2), they usually present no problem in identifying recent infections if appropriately timed sera are available for testing.

The rickettsial species responsible for an infection is difficult to identify by conventional serologic tests. There is such antigenic relatedness among members of each rickettsial biogroup that a convalescent-phase serum from a patient infected with one species in the biogroup cross-reacts extensively with all other species in the same biogroup. For example, both murine and louse-borne typhus are endemic in certain areas of the world, and routine IFA tests cannot distinguish these two from epidemic infections. Antibody absorption (18) or toxin neutralization (22) tests can distinguish patients who have epidemic or murine typhus infections, but these tests can be performed only by specialty laboratories. In addition, convalescent-phase sera from patients with RMSF or typhus occasionally cross-react with typhus or spotted fever group rickettsiae, respectively (42). However, such cross-reactions are infrequent, and the heterologous titers are routinely much lower than in homologous reactions.

Determining the specific etiology of spotted fever group infections is less difficult because the endemic-disease areas for most species in the spotted fever biogroup do not overlap. The only significant exception is in the United States, where the endemic-disease areas of RMSF and rickettsialpox may overlap. However, the clinical and epidemiologic features of rickettsialpox are sufficiently distinct from those of RMSF to allow specific diagnosis even without specific serologic testing. Rickettsialpox typically occurs as small outbreaks in cities in association with rodent infestation, whereas RMSF usually occurs sporadically in rural or suburban areas and is transmitted by ticks. Because all rickettsiae are susceptible to the tetracyclines, it is not necessary to identify the specific etiologic agent to ensure that individual patients receive proper treatment.

Antigenic phase variation must be considered for the interpretation of serologic results for Q fever. In acute, self-limited Q fever infections, antibodies to the phase II antigen appear first and dominate the humoral immune response. With chronic Q fever infections, however, phase I titers eventually equal or exceed phase II titers. Peacock et al. (45) concluded that the ratio of phase II to phase I antibodies was a useful indicator for distinguishing acute from chronic Q fever infections. The ratios were >1 for primary Q fever, ≥1 for patients with granulomatous hepatitis, and ≤1 in endocarditis patients. This is a useful rule of thumb, but it may not apply in every situation.

Our laboratory has had little experience with scrub typhus serology. The most important consideration is an awareness of the antigenic diversity of *R. tsutsugamushi* strains in a given area. Unless an appropriate combination of strains of *R. tsutsugamushi* is included in the battery of test antigens, the titers of some serum specimens could appear falsely low, and some infections could even go undetected (4, 50).

Finally, although laboratory testing is central to the diagnosis of rickettsial diseases, clinical findings can contribute to diagnosis, particularly in the face of equivocal serologic results. Although there are no unique pathognomonic features for the rickettsioses, eschars are useful indicators of Boutonneuse fever and scrub typhus in endemic areas, the vesicular rash of rickettsialpox is unique among the rickettsioses, and the triad of fever, headache, and rash is a useful indicator of RMSF.

LITERATURE CITED

1. **Anacker, R. L., R. N. Philip, L. A. Thomas, and E. A. Casper.** 1979. Indirect hemagglutination test for detection of antibody for *Rickettsia rickettsii* in sera from humans and common laboratory animals. J. Clin. Microbiol. **10:** 677–684.
2. **Berman, S. J., and W. D. Kundin.** 1973. Scrub typhus in South Vietnam. Ann. Intern. Med. **79:**26–30.
3. **Bernard, K. W., G. L. Parham, W. G. Winkler, and C. G. Helmick.** 1982. Q fever control measures: recommendations for research facilities using sheep. Infect. Control **3:** 461–465.
4. **Bourgeois, A. L., J. G. Olson, R. C. Y. Fang, and P. F. D. Van Peenan.** 1977. Epidemiological and serological study of scrub typhus among Chinese military in the Pescadores Islands of Taiwan. Trans. R. Soc. Trop. Med. Hyg. **71:**338–342.
5. **Brown, G. W., A. Shirai, C. Rogers, and M. G. Groves.** 1983. Diagnostic criteria for scrub typhus: probability values for immunofluorescent antibody and *Proteus* OXK agglutinin titers. Am. J. Trop. Med. Hyg. **32:**1101–1107.
6. **Chang, R. S., E. S. Murray, and J. C. Snyder.** 1954. Erythrocyte-sensitizing substances from rickettsiae of the Rocky Mountain spotted fever group. J. Immunol. **73:**8–15.
7. **Chang, S., J. C. Snyder, and E. S. Murray.** 1953. A serologically active erythrocyte sensitizing substance from typhus rickettsiae. J. Immunol. **70:**215–221.
8. **Crum, J. W., S. Hanchalay, and C. Eamsila.** 1980. New paper enzyme-linked immunosorbent technique compared with microimmunofluorescence for detection of human serum antibodies for *Rickettsia tsutsugamushi*. J. Clin. Microbiol. **11:**584–588.
9. **Dasch, G. A., S. Halle, and A. L. Bourgeois.** 1979. Sensitive microplate enzyme-linked immunosorbent assay for detection of antibodies against the scrub typhus rickettsiae. J. Clin. Microbiol. **9:**38–48.
10. **Doller, G., P. C. Doller, and H. J. Gerth.** 1984. Early diagnosis of Q fever: detection of immunoglobulin M by radioimmunoassay and enzyme immunoassay. Eur. J. Clin. Microbiol. **3:**550–553.
11. **Duma, R. J., D. E. Sonenshine, F. M. Bozeman, J. M. Veazy, Jr., B. L. Elisberg, D. P. Chadwick, N. I. Stocks, T. M. McGill, G. B. Miller, and J. N. MacCormack.** 1981. Epidemic typhus in the United States associated with flying squirrels. J. Am. Med. Assoc. **25:**2318–2323.
12. **Dupuis, G., O. Peter, M. Peacock, W. Burgdorfer, and E. Haller.** 1985. Immunoglobulin responses in acute Q fever. J. Clin. Microbiol. **22:**484–487.
13. **Ellis, M. E., C. C. Smith, and M. A. J. Moffat.** 1982. Chronic or fatal Q fever infection: a review of 16 patients seen in north-east Scotland (1967–80). Q. J. Med. New Ser. **205:**54–66.
14. **Field, P. R., J. G. Hunt, and A. M. Murphy.** 1983. Detection and persistence of specific IgM antibodies to *Coxiella burnetii* by enzyme-linked immunosorbent assay: a comparison with immunofluorescence and complement fixation tests. J. Infect. Dis. **148:**477–487.
15. **Fishbein, D. B., J. E. Kaplan, K. W. Bernard, and W. G. Winkler.** 1984. Surveillance of Rocky Mountain spotted fever in the United States, 1981–1983. J. Infect. Dis. **150:** 609–611.
16. **Fleisher, G., E. T. Lennette, and P. Honig.** 1979. Diagnosis of Rocky Mountain spotted fever by immunofluorescent identification of *Rickettsia rickettsii* in skin biopsy tissue. J. Pediatr. **95:**63–65.
17. **Gimenez, D. F.** 1964. Staining rickettsiae in yolk-sac cultures. Stain Technol. **39:**135–140.
18. **Goldwasser, R. A., and C. C. Shepard.** 1959. Fluorescent antibody methods in the differentiation of murine and epidemic typhus fever; specificity changes resulting from previous immunization. J. Immunol. **82:**373–380.

19. **Groves, M. G., D. L. Rosenstreich, B. A. Taylor, and J. V. Osterman.** 1980. Host defenses in experimental scrub typhus: mapping the gene that controls natural resistance in mice. J. Immunol. **125:**1395–1399.
20. **Hackstadt, T., M. G. Peacock, P. J. Hitchcock, and R. L. Cole.** 1985. Lipopolysaccharide variation in *Coxiella burnetii:* intrastrain heterogeneity in structure and antigenicity. Infect. Immun. **48:**359–365.
21. **Halle, S., G. A. Dasch, and E. Weiss.** 1977. Sensitive enzyme-linked immunosorbent assay for detection of antibodies against typhus rickettsiae, *Rickettsia prowazekii* and *Rickettsia typhi.* J. Clin. Microbiol. **6:**101–110.
22. **Hamilton, H. L.** 1945. Specificity of toxic factors associated with epidemic and murine strains of typhus rickettsiae. Am. J. Trop. Med. Hyg. **25:**391–395.
23. **Harrell, G. T.** 1949. Rocky Mountain spotted fever. Medicine **28:**333–370.
24. **Hechemy, K. E., R. L. Anacker, N. L. Carlo, J. A. Fox, and H. A. Gaafar.** 1983. Absorption of *Rickettsia rickettsii* antibodies by *Rickettsia rickettsii* antigens in four diagnostic tests. J. Clin. Microbiol. **17:**445–449.
25. **Hechemy, K. E., R. L. Anacker, R. N. Philip, K. T. Kleeman, J. N. MacCormack, S. J. Sasovoski, and E. E. Michaelson.** 1980. Detection of Rocky Mountain spotted fever antibodies by a latex agglutination test. J. Clin. Microbiol. **12:**144–150.
26. **Hechemy, K. E., E. E. Michaelson, R. L. Anacker, M. Zdeb, and S. J. Sasowski, et al.** 1983. Evaluation of latex—*Rickettsia rickettsii* test for Rocky Mountain spotted fever in 11 laboratories. J. Clin. Microbiol. **18:**938–946.
27. **Hechemy, K. E., and B. B. Rubin.** 1983. Latex *Rickettsia rickettsii* test reactivity in seropositive patients. J. Clin. Microbiol. **17:**489–492.
28. **Hechemy, K. E., R. W. Stevens, S. Sasowski, E. E. Michaelson, E. A. Casper, and R. N. Philip.** 1979. Discrepancies in Weil-Felix and microimmunofluorescence test results for Rocky Mountain spotted fever. J. Clin. Microbiol. **9:**292–293.
29. **Herrmann, J. E., M. R. Holingdale, M. F. Collins, and J. W. Venson.** 1977. Enzyme immunoassay and radioimmuno-precipitation tests for the detection of antibodies to *Rochalimaea* (*Rickettsia*) *quintana* (39655). Proc. Soc. Exp. Biol. Med. **154:**285–288.
30. **Hunt, J. G., P. R. Field, and A. M. Murphy.** 1983. Immunoglobulin responses to *Coxiella burnetii* (Q fever): single-serum diagnosis of acute infection, using an immunofluorescence technique. Infect. Immun. **39:**977–981.
31. **Kaplan, J. E., and L. B. Schonberger.** 1986. The sensitivity of various serologic tests in the diagnosis of Rocky Mountain spotted fever. Am. J. Trop. Med. Hyg. **35:**840–844.
32. **Kaplowitz, L. G., J. V. Lange, J. J. Fischer, and D. H. Walker.** 1983. Correlation of rickettsial titers, circulating endotoxin, and clinical features in Rocky Mountain spotted fever. Arch. Intern. Med. **143:**1149–1151.
33. **Kopmans-Gargantiel, A. I., and C. L. Wisseman, Jr.** 1981. Differential requirements for enriched atmospheric carbon dioxide content for intracellular growth in cell culture among selected members of the genus *Rickettsia.* Infect. Immun. **31:**1277–1280.
34. **Lackman, D. B., G. Gilda, and R. N. Philip.** 1964. Application of the radioisotope precipitation test to the study of Q fever in man. Health Lab. Sci. **1:**21–28.
35. **McDade, J. E., C. C. Shepard, M. A. Redus, V. F. Newhouse, and J. D. Smith.** 1980. Evidence of *Rickettsia prowazekii* infections in the United States. Am. J. Trop. Med. Hyg. **29:**277–284.
36. **Miller, E. S., and P. B. Beeson.** 1946. Murine typhus fever. Medicine **25:**1–15.
37. **Myers, W. F., and C. L. Wisseman, Jr.** 1980. Genetic relatedness among the typhus group of rickettsiae. Int. J. Syst. Bacteriol. **30:**143–150.
38. **National Research Council, Division of Medical Sciences, Committee on Pathology.** 1953. Pathology of epidemic typhus. Report of fatal cases studied by the United States of America Typhus Commission in Cairo, Egypt, during 1943–1945. Arch. Pathol. **56:**397–435, 512–553.
39. **Newhouse, V. F., C. C. Shepard, M. D. Redus, T. Tzianabos, and J. E. McDade.** 1979. A comparison of the complement fixation, indirect fluorescent antibody and microagglutination test for the serological diagnosis of rickettsial diseases. Am. J. Trop. Med. Hyg. **28:**387–395.
40. **Ormsbee, R., M. Peacock, R. Gerloff, G. Tallent, and D. Wike.** 1978. Limits of rickettsial infectivity. Infect. Immun. **19:**239–245.
41. **Ormsbee, R., M. Peacock, R. Philip, E. Casper, J. Plorde, T. Gabre-Kidan, and L. Wright.** 1977. Serologic diagnosis of epidemic typhus fever. Am. J. Epidemiol. **105:**261–271.
42. **Ormsbee, R., M. Peacock, R. Philip, E. Casper, J. Plorde, T. Gabre-Kidan, and L. Wright.** 1978. Antigenic relationships between the typhus and spotted fever groups of rickettsiae. Am. J. Epidemiol. **108:**53–59.
43. **Oster, C. N., D. S. Burke, R. H. Kenyon, M. S. Ascher, P. Harber, and C. E. Pedersen, Jr.** 1977. Laboratory-acquired Rocky Mountain spotted fever. N. Engl. J. Med. **297:**859–862.
44. **Osterman, J. V., and C. S. Eisemann.** 1978. Rickettsial indirect hemagglutination test: isolation of erythrocyte-sensitizing substance. J. Clin. Microbiol. **8:**189–196.
45. **Peacock, M. G., R. N. Philip, J. C. Williams, and R. S. Faulkner.** 1983. Serological evaluation of Q fever in humans: enhanced phase I titers of immunoglobulins G and A are diagnostic for Q-fever endocarditis. Infect. Immun. **41:**1089–1098.
46. **Philip, R. N., E. A. Casper, J. N. MacCormack, D. L. Sexton, L. A. Thomas, R. L. Anacker, W. Burgdorfer, and S. Vick.** 1977. A comparison of serologic methods for diagnosis of Rocky Mountain spotted fever. J. Epidemiol. **105:**56–67.
47. **Pike, R. M.** 1976. Laboratory-associated infections: summary and analysis of 3921 cases. Health Lab. Sci. **13:**105–114.
48. **Raoult, D., C. DeMicco, H. Chaudet, and J. Tamalet.** 1985. Serological diagnosis of Mediterranean spotted fever by the immunoperoxidase reaction. Eur. J. Clin. Microbiol. **4:**441–442.
49. **Raoult, D., C. DeMicco, H. Gallais, and M. Toga.** 1985. Laboratory diagnosis of mediterranean spotted fever by immunofluorescent demonstration of *Rickettsia conorii* in cutaneous lesions. J. Infect. Dis. **150:**145–148.
50. **Shirai, A., J. C. Coolbaugh, E. Gan, T. C. Chan, D. L. Huxsoll, and M. C. Groves.** 1982. Serological analysis of scrub typhus isolates from the Pescadores and Philippine Islands. Jpn. J. Med. Sci. Biol. **35:**255–259.
51. **Shirai, A., J. W. Dietal, and J. V. Osterman.** 1975. Indirect hemagglutination test for human antibody to typhus and spotted fever group rickettsiae. J. Clin. Microbiol. **2:**430–437.
52. **Snyder, J. C.** 1965. Typhus fever rickettsiae, p. 1059–1094. *In* F. L. Horsfall and I. Tamm (ed.), Viral and rickettsial infections of man. J. B. Lippincott Co., Philadelphia.
53. **Turck, W. P. G., G. Howitt, L. A. Turnberg, H. Fox, M. Longson, M. B. Matthews, and R. Das Gupta.** 1976. Chronic Q fever. Q. J. Med. New Ser. **45:**193–217.
54. **Tzianabos, T., B. E. Anderson, and J. E. McDade.** 1989. Detection of *Rickettsia rickettsii* DNA in clinical specimens by using polymerase chain reaction technology. J. Clin. Microbiol. **27:**2866–2868.
55. **Walker, D. H., and B. G. Cain.** 1978. A method for specific diagnosis of Rocky Mountain spotted fever on fixed, paraffin-embedded tissue by immunofluorescence. J. Infect. Dis. **137:**206–209.
56. **Walker, D. H., B. G. Cain, and P. M. Olmstead.** 1978. Laboratory diagnosis of Rocky Mountain spotted fever by immunofluorescent demonstration of *Rickettsia rickettsii* in cutaneous lesions. Am. J. Clin. Pathol. **69:**619–623.
57. **Weil, E., and A. Felix.** 1916. Zur serologischen Diagnose

des Fleckfiebers. Wien. Klin. Wochenschr. **29:**33–35.

58. **Weiss, E.** 1981. The family *Rickettsiaceae:* human pathogens, p. 2137–2160. *In* M. P. Starr et al. (ed.), The prokaryotes. Springer-Verlag KG, Berlin.
59. **Weiss, E., and J. W. Moulder.** 1984. Rickettsiales, p. 687–704. *In* N. R. Krieg (ed.), Bergey's manual of systematic bacteriology, vol. 1. The Williams & Wilkins Co., Baltimore.
60. **Wilson, L. B., and W. M. Chowning.** 1904. Studies in *Pyroplasmosis hominis* ("spotted fever" or "tick fever" of the Rocky Mountains). J. Infect. Dis. **1:**31–57.
61. **Woodward, T. E., C. D. Pedersen, Jr., C. N. Oster, L. R. Bagley, J. Romberger, and M. J. Snyder.** 1976. Prompt confirmation of Rocky Mountain spotted fever: identification of rickettsiae in skin tissues. J. Infect. Dis. **134:**297–301.
62. **Yamamoto, S., and Y. Minamishima.** 1982. Serodiagnosis of tsutsugamushi fever (scrub typhus) by the indirect immunoperoxidase technique. J. Clin. Microbiol. **15:**1128–1132.

Chapter 105

Chlamydiae

JULIUS SCHACHTER

CHARACTERIZATION

The chlamydiae are among the more common pathogens throughout the animal kingdom (18). They are nonmotile, gram-negative, obligate intracellular bacteria. Their unique developmental cycle differentiates them from all other microorganisms (21). They replicate within the cytoplasm of host cells, forming characteristic intracellular inclusions that can be seen by light microscopy. They differ from the viruses by possessing both RNA and DNA and cell walls quite similar in structure to those of gram-negative bacteria. They are susceptible to many broad-spectrum antibiotics, possess a number of enzymes, and have a restricted metabolic capacity. None of these metabolic reactions results in the production of energy. Thus, they have been considered as energy parasites that use the ATP produced by the host cell for their own requirements.

Growth cycle

Chlamydiae are ingested by susceptible host cells by a mechanism similar to receptor-mediated endocytosis (14). The uptake process is directly influenced by the chlamydiae, and ingestion of chlamydiae is specifically enhanced (5). After attachment, at specific sites on the surface of the cell, the elementary body (EB) enters the cell in an endosome, where the entire growth cycle is completed. The chlamydiae prevent phagolysosomal fusion. Once the EB (diameter, 0.25 to 0.35 μm) has entered the cell, it reorganizes into a reticulate particle (initial body) which is larger (0.5 to 1 μm) and richer in RNA. After approximately 8 h, the initial body begins dividing by binary fission. Approximately 18 to 24 h after infection, the initial bodies become EBs by a poorly understood reorganization or condensation process. The EBs are then released to initiate another cycle of infection. The EBs are specifically adapted for extracellular survival and are the infectious form. The metabolically active and replicating form, the initial body, does not survive well outside the host cell and seems adapted for an intracellular milieu.

Taxonomy

Chlamydiae are presently placed in their own order, the *Chlamydiales,* family *Chlamydiaceae,* with one genus, *Chlamydia* (21). There are three species, *C. trachomatis, C. psittaci,* and *C. pneumoniae. C. trachomatis* includes the organisms causing trachoma, inclusion conjunctivitis, lymphogranuloma venereum (LGV), and genital tract diseases. There are three biovars within the species, the trachoma, LGV, and murine biovars. *C. trachomatis* strains are sensitive to the action of sulfonamides and produce a glycogenlike material within the inclusion vacuole, which stains with iodine. *C. psittaci* strains infect many avian species and mammals, producing such diseases as psittacosis, ornithosis, feline pneumonitis, and bovine abortion (30). They are resistant to the action of sulfonamides and produce inclusions that do not stain with iodine. *C. pneumoniae* is the most recently described species (13). It shows less than 10% DNA relatedness to the other species and has pear-shaped rather than round EBs. It appears to be exclusively a human pathogen. *C. pneumoniae* has been identified as the cause of a variety of respiratory tract diseases and has worldwide distribution.

Antigenic relationships

The chlamydiae possess group (genus)-specific, species-specific, and type-specific antigens. Although they are antigenically complex, only a few antigens play a role in diagnosis. The group complement fixation (CF) antigen, shared by all members of the genus, is the lipopolysaccharide (LPS), with a ketodeoxyoctanoic acid as the reactive moiety. It may be analogous to the LPS of certain gram-negative bacteria (23). One-way cross-reactions have been reported between chlamydiae and some bacteria, but these do not appear to influence serodiagnosis. The major outer membrane protein (MOMP) contains both species- and subspecies-specific antigens (6). The 15 serovars of *C. trachomatis* are best recognized by a microimmunofluorescence (micro-IF) technique (32). MOMP is responsible for most of the reactivity seen in the micro-IF test. A 60-kilodalton cysteine-rich structural protein has a highly immunogenic species-specific epitope (15). A genus-specific 57-kilodalton protein plays an important role in immunopathology (20).

Serovars of *C. psittaci* can be demonstrated by neutralization tests and by micro-IF (1, 10). Only one serovar of *C. pneumoniae* has been demonstrated.

CLINICAL SIGNIFICANCE

C. trachomatis is almost exclusively a human pathogen (26). Serotypes within this species cause trachoma (serotypes A, B, Ba, and C have been associated with endemic trachoma, the most common preventable form of blindness), inclusion conjunctivitis, and LGV (serotypes L1, L2, and L3). When sexual transmission of *C. trachomatis* strains other than LGV has been studied, serotypes D through K have been found to be the major identifiable cause of nongonococcal urethritis in men and may also cause epididymitis. Proctitis may occur in either sex. In women, cervicitis is a common result of chlamydial infection, and acute salpingitis may occur. *C. trachomatis* is the most common sexually transmitted bacterial pathogen. The agent in the cervix may be transmitted to the neonate as it passes through the infected birth canal, and an eye disease (inclusion conjunctivitis of the newborn) and a characteristic chlamydial pneumonia of infants may develop (2). Vaginal and enteric infections in neonates are also recognized.

Human psittacosis is a zoonosis, usually contracted from exposure to an infected avian species. *C. psittaci* is ubiquitous among avian species, and infection in the birds is usually of the intestinal tract. The organism is shed in the feces, contaminates the environment, and is spread by aerosol.

C. psittaci is also common in domestic mammals. In some parts of the world, these infections have important economic consequences; *C. psittaci* is a cause of a number of systemic and debilitating diseases in domestic mammals and, most important, can cause abortions (30). Human chlamydial infections resulting from exposure to infected domestic mammals are known but seem to be relatively uncommon.

During trachoma studies performed in Taiwan and Iran, some apparent *C. psittaci* strains were recovered from conjunctival swabs (12). Seroepidemiologic studies have suggested that infections with these strains (designated TWAR, now *C. pneumoniae*) are common in many parts of the world. Age-specific prevalence rates suggest that transmission occurs in childhood and peaks early in adult life. *C. pneumoniae* has been associated with mild pneumonias in young adults. Fatal disease has been seen in young children in the developing world and in the elderly with underlying disease (12, 25).

STABILITY, STORAGE, AND TRANSPORT

Procedures

C. trachomatis is not a particularly labile organism. Maximal infectivity is achieved by keeping specimens cold and minimizing the time between specimen collection and processing in the laboratory.

Swabs, scrapings, and small tissue samples should be collected in a special transport medium (see chapter 121). Because *Chlamydia* spp. are bacteria, the selection of antibiotics to prevent other bacterial contamination is restricted. Broad-spectrum antibiotics such as tetracyclines, macrolides, or penicillin must be excluded. Aminoglycosides and fungicides are the mainstays. The chlamydial specimens should be refrigerated if they can be processed within 48 h after collection; otherwise, they should be frozen at −60°C.

C. psittaci strains are generally more stable. Some may persist in a contaminated environment for months without losing viability. The stability of *C. pneumoniae* has not been well studied, but it loses <50% of infectivity in 24 h at 4°C (16).

Biosafety considerations

C. trachomatis is not considered to be a particularly dangerous pathogen to handle in the laboratory. There have been a number of laboratory infections, usually manifested as follicular conjunctivitis. However, the LGV biovar is a more invasive organism, and severe cases of pneumonia have occurred when research workers were exposed to aerosols created by laboratory procedures such as sonication (3). *C. psittaci* must be considered a potentially dangerous organism to handle in the laboratory. For many years it was a major cause of laboratory infections. These infections usually resulted from exposure to aerosols, but the stability of the organism is a potential problem. The organism should not be handled in laboratories without appropriate containment facilities.

INFECTED SITES AND SPECIMEN COLLECTION

For cytological studies, impression smears of involved tissues or scrapings of involved epithelial cell sites should be air dried and appropriately fixed (cold acetone or methanol for immunofluorescence, methanol for Giemsa stain, and heat for Macchiavello or Gimenez stain).

For most *C. trachomatis* infections of humans, it is imperative that samples be collected from the involved epithelial cell sites by vigorous swabbing or scraping. Purulent discharges are inadequate and should be cleaned from the site before sampling. Appropriate sites include the conjunctiva for trachoma-inclusion conjunctivitis and the anterior urethra (several centimeters into the urethra) or the cervix (within the endocervical canal) for genital infection. Because the trachoma biovar appears to infect only columnar and squamocolumnar cells, cervical specimens must be collected at the transitional zone or within the os. The organism also can infect the urethra of the female; recovery rates may be improved if another sample is collected from the urethra and sent to the laboratory for testing in the same tube with the cervical sample. For women with salpingitis, the samples may be collected by needle aspiration of the involved fallopian tube. Endometrial specimens may yield the agent. Rectal mucosa, the nasopharynx, and the throat may also be sampled. For infants with pneumonia, swabs may be collected from the posterior nasopharynx or the throat, although nasopharyngeal or tracheobronchial aspirates collected by intubation appear to be a superior source of agent. For LGV, the likely specimens will be bubo pus, rectal swabs, or biopsies.

Throat swabs are collected for *C. pneumoniae*. For *C. psittaci* infection in humans, the specimens include sputum and blood specimens in classical psittacosis. *C. psittaci* has been recovered from a variety of involved anatomic sites sampled by biopsy or at necropsy. For all culture methods, the sites sampled are likely to be contaminated, and the specimen should be collected into a medium that contains appropriate antibiotics to remove unwanted bacteria.

DIRECT CYTOLOGICAL EXAMINATION

Because chlamydiae are large enough to be seen by light microscopy and the intracytoplasmic inclusions are pathognomonic, much of the diagnostic methodology depends on microscopic identification of the organism.

C. trachomatis infections of the conjunctiva, urethra, or cervix can be diagnosed by demonstrating typical intracytoplasmic inclusions, but cytology is relatively insensitive. The Giemsa stain was the method most often used in the past, but more sensitive immunofluorescence procedures have largely replaced it. Cytology to detect inclusions is particularly useful in diagnosing acute, severe inclusion conjunctivitis of the newborn and is less effective in diagnosing adult conjunctival and genital tract infections. The ability to detect intracellular diplococci in infants with gonococcal ophthalmia neonatorum is another benefit, and obviously, direct microscopy is much faster than the isolation procedures.

Fluorescent-antibody technique

Most of the early experience with immunofluorescence procedures used polyclonal antibodies in either direct or indirect fluorescent-antibody procedures. These represented efforts to detect typical chlamydial inclusions within epithelial cells. There were no commercial sources, and laboratories had to prepare their own reagents. More recently, fluorescein-conjugated monoclonal antibodies have been made available. The test is based on detecting EBs in smears, in contrast to previous efforts to detect inclusions (31). The early commercial direct fluorescent-antibody (DFA) reagents were plagued with problems of cross-reaction to *Staphylococcus aureus* and other bacteria. These reagents have now been dramatically improved, and the current experience indicates that the test has approximately 80 to 85% sensitivity and 98% specificity as compared with culture under conditions in which all tests are performed under ideal circumstances.

The test requires a trained microscopist who can distinguish between fluorescing chlamydial particles and nonspecific fluorescence. Several DFA configurations are commercially available, as are monoclonal antibodies against the MOMP or against the LPS. Monoclonal antibodies to the LPS will stain all *Chlamydia* spp., but the quality of the fluorescence is somewhat mitigated by uneven distribution of LPS on the chlamydial particle. The anti-MOMP monoclonal antibodies are prepared against *C. trachomatis;* they are species specific and therefore will not stain *C. psittaci* or *C. pneumoniae*. The quality of fluorescence is better because MOMP is evenly distributed on the chlamydial particle. Thus, if *C. trachomatis* is being sought, the anti-MOMP monoclonal antibodies are preferred. This procedure offers the possibility of rapid diagnosis, since the technique takes approximately 30 min to perform.

Macchiavello and Gimenez stains

Macchiavello and Gimenez stains are used on impression smears from animal tissue and yolk sac. With Macchiavello stain, the EB stains as a very small red dot against a blue background. Characteristic clusters of EBs are seen. A simpler procedure may be the Gimenez modification; EBs stain red, and the background stains greenish (see chapter 122).

Iodine staining technique

Slides are examined as wet mounts. The inclusions are recognizable under low-power magnification. They are reddish brown against a yellow background. The slides may be decolorized with methanol and restained with Giemsa stain. This technique is the least sensitive cytological procedure. It is not recommended for use with clinical specimens. Its speed and simplicity have made it a popular test for examining *C. trachomatis*-infected cell cultures. It will not stain the inclusions of other chlamydiae.

Giemsa staining technique

The smear is air dried, fixed with absolute methanol for at least 5 min, and dried again. It is then covered with the diluted Giemsa stain (freshly prepared the same day) for 1 h. The slide is rinsed rapidly in 95% ethyl alcohol to remove excess dye and to enhance differentiation and is then dried and examined microscopically. Longer staining periods (1 to 5 h) may be preferable with heavy tissue culture monolayers. EBs stain reddish purple. The initial bodies are more basophilic, staining bluish, as do most bacteria.

OTHER NONCULTURE DIAGNOSTIC TESTS

Enzyme immunoassay

A number of commercially available products can detect chlamydial antigens in clinical specimens by using enzyme immunoassay (EIA) procedures. Most of these products detect chlamydial LPS, which is more soluble than the MOMP. The tests include either monoclonal or polyclonal antibodies to the LPS and thus theoretically could detect all chlamydiae. They have not been well evaluated in diagnosis of infections with *C. psittaci* or *C. pneumoniae*. For *C. trachomatis*, these tests appear to be slightly more sensitive and slightly less specific than DFA (7). Most EIAs take several hours to perform, are suitable for batch processing, and allow a laboratory to test many specimens.

The performance profiles of the commercially available tests vary widely. The tests are less sensitive than culture and have a specificity on the order of 97%. Thus, these nonculture tests are not amenable to screening low-prevalence populations because of the problem with false-positive results. If confirmatory tests are available to improve specificity, such use might be more practical.

Nucleic acid probes

Some nucleic acid probes are commercially available. The performance profiles of these tests have not been well described. The tests clearly are less sensitive than culture, and specificity has been in the mid-90% range.

Advice on use of nonculture tests

Chlamydial infections are common. Their diagnosis represents a large market, and many manufacturers have chlamydial tests. Thus, laboratorians are faced with a bewildering and ever-increasing array of commercially available diagnostic tests. At this writing, there are a few fairly simple recommendations that can be made.

Because cell culture is a relatively demanding technique and many laboratories desire to establish routine chlamydial testing, nonculture methods of detecting the organism have become popular. Although nucleic acid probes are commercially available, there is insufficient experience with them to recommend their routine use. Among the many EIA and DFA procedures available, only two have had sufficiently broad and independent assessment of performance to recommend their routine use. These are the Syva MicroTrak DFA procedure and Abbott Chlamydiazyme EIA procedure. The performance profiles of these tests are similar. Both are approximately 75 to 85% sensitive and approximately 97 to 98% specific in detecting current chlamydial infection. Other products may be equivalent or even superior, but more evaluations are needed.

There are advantages and disadvantages to either test format. The DFA has the advantage of allowing the microscopist to confirm the adequacy of the specimen. Being more labor intensive, the DFA is less well suited to processing large numbers of specimens. Anti-MOMP monoclonal antibodies provide superior staining of *C. trachomatis* EBs but will not detect the other species. Anti-LPS monoclonal antibodies will stain all chlamydiae but tend to be less bright and stain the particles unevenly (8). The EIA procedure is more amenable to batch processing and becomes relatively expensive when small numbers of specimens are being tested. Most EIAs detect the LPS and thus should react with all chlamydial species. They have been widely studied only for *C. trachomatis* and therefore cannot be recommended for use in *C. psittaci* or *C. pneumoniae* infection. The specificity of the EIA procedures may be improved by the application of confirmatory or blocking assays, using monoclonal antibodies against the *Chlamydia*-specific LPS epitope.

Both of these procedures have some advantages over culture. They are more rapid; results can be available in 30 min to 24 h. Because viability is not an issue, it is not necessary to maintain a cold chain. Specimens can be processed when cell culture is not available or when there are problems in transporting specimens to a laboratory. There is one major caveat: nonculture tests should not be used when evidence of sexual abuse is being sought. There are false-positive results with these tests, and the tests have not been extensively evaluated on some of the specimens that are tested in cases of child abuse. It is imperative that culture be used to prove the existence of chlamydial infection for legal purposes.

It is still clear that under ideal circumstances, culture is the diagnostic method of choice. With adequate control over maintenance, storage, and transport of specimens and with well-trained specimen collectors, cell culture is more sensitive than any of the currently available nonculture tests.

Unfortunately, the ideal circumstances do not exist in many settings. When nonculture tests are evaluated in comparison with less than ideal culture systems, the specificity may suffer because apparent false-positives are really culture misses. When there are transportation problems that may affect viability, the nonculture tests are to be preferred.

Laboratorians have long appreciated that the results coming from the laboratory are no better than the quality of the specimens submitted to the laboratory. Thus, the introduction of cytobrushes for collection of cervical specimens has improved the performance not only of DFA procedures but also of culture (19).

It is likely that we will see increasing use of nonculture tests on urine samples of men being tested for urethral chlamydial infection. Attempts to develop noninvasive screening tests for sexually transmitted infection in asymptomatic males have been an important goal for those interested in reducing the reservoir of sexually transmitted diseases. In unpublished studies, we have found EIA on urine samples to be approximately 70% as sensitive as direct urethral culture. This result is not very different from the 70 to 80% sensitivity we typically find for EIA on urethral swabs.

ISOLATION

For practical purposes, only three experimental systems need be considered for the isolation of chlamydiae. All known chlamydiae grow in the yolk sac of the embryonated hen egg. With centrifugation of the inoculum, it appears that all chlamydiae (with some variability) will grow in tissue culture; psittacosis and LGV agents are capable of serial growth in tissue culture without centrifugation. The psittacosis agents grow in mice after intracerebral (i.c.), intraperitoneal (i.p.), and intranasal inoculation, and LGV agents grow after i.c. and intranasal inoculation, although the latter route is rarely used. Mice are of no use in recovering isolates of the trachoma biovar or *C. pneumoniae*. However, these procedures are relatively slow and will not provide an etiologic diagnosis quickly enough to be clinically relevant. A number of different cell lines have been used to support the growth of chlamydiae. It does not appear that any single cell line is markedly superior to others, since successful studies have been performed with monkey kidney, HeLa, L, and McCoy cells, among others. There is little experience with *C. pneumoniae*. This organism grows poorly, and HeLa cells may be more susceptible. It may be useful to inoculate low-level positive samples from cell cultures into yolk sac to increase yields.

General guidelines for processing specimens are listed below. The transport media and antibiotics used to control bacterial contamination are listed in chapter 121. Fresh samples are preferred, but frozen material (−60°C) is acceptable.

Ocular and genital tract specimens

From ocular and genital tract sites, the laboratory usually receives swabs in antibiotic-containing transport medium. The material is refrigerated until it is inoculated into cell tissue culture.

Bubo pus

Grind the viscous material. Suspend in nutrient broth or tissue culture medium to at least 20% of weight. Even when pus is not viscous, dilution is advisable. If the bubo is not fluctuant, sterile saline may be injected and then aspirated for isolation attempts. Test for bacterial contaminants, treat with antibiotics, and inoculate the material into mice by the i.c. route, into eggs by the yolk sac route, or into cell cultures.

Blood

If there is a clot, grind it and add beef heart broth or tissue culture medium to make a 10% suspension. Inoculate directly into eggs or mice. For cell culture, it is advisable to inoculate with several further dilutions.

Sputum or throat washings

Sputum is cultured for bacteria on blood agar plates. To prepare the emulsion, suspend sputum in 2 to 10 times (depending on its consistency) its volume of sterile antibiotic-containing broth (pH 7.2 to 7.4) or tissue culture medium; emulsify thoroughly by shaking with glass beads in a sterile, tightly stoppered container. Inoculate into the isolation system after 1 to 2 h of treatment with antibiotics at room temperature. It may be advisable to centrifuge extracts for 20 to 30 min at 100 × *g* to remove coarse material.

Fecal samples

Cloacal or rectal swabs, the droppings from caged birds, or fecal pellets are suspended in antibiotic broth or medium. The suspension is shaken thoroughly. After centrifugation at 300 × *g* for 10 min, the supernatant fluid is removed. It may be further diluted (1:2 and 1: 20) with antibiotic solution and held for 1 h at room temperature before inoculation into tissue culture, yolk sac, or mice. More concentrated material may be used for i.p. inoculation of mice.

Tissues

Frozen tissue is thawed in a refrigerator at about 4°C for 18 to 24 h. The specimen is weighed, minced with sterile scissors, and ground to a paste with mortar and pestle or homogenizer. After the tissue has been ground thoroughly, the volume of antibiotic-containing diluent required to make a 10 to 20% emulsion is added, and the suspension is thoroughly mixed. For tissue culture, antibiotic-containing collection medium is used, and 10^{-1} and 10^{-2} dilutions are inoculated.

Isolation in cell culture

The recommended procedure for primary isolation of chlamydiae is in cell culture. The most common technique involves inoculation of clinical specimens into cycloheximide-treated McCoy cells (24). The basic principle involves centrifugation of the inoculum into the cell monolayer at approximately 3,000 × *g* for 1 h, incubation of monolayers for 48 to 72 h, and staining. Iodine is used for *C. trachomatis* to detect the glycogen-positive inclusions. Fluorescent-antibody staining may allow earlier detection of the inclusion. Use of fluorescein-conjugated monoclonal antibodies represents the most sensitive method for detecting *C. trachomatis* inclusions in cell culture (29). The procedure requires more attention to staining than does the iodine technique and is more costly. For *C. psittaci* and *C. pneumoniae,* the inclusions can be demonstrated with genus-specific monoclonal antibodies or by the Giemsa stain.

McCoy cells are plated onto 13-mm cover slips contained in 15-mm-diameter (1-dram) disposable glass vials. Cell concentration (approximately 1×10^5 to 2×10^5) is selected to give a light, confluent monolayer after 24 to 48 h of incubation at 37°C. For optimal results, the cells should be used within 24 to 72 h after reaching confluency.

The clinical specimens should be shaken with glass beads before inoculation. This procedure is safer and more convenient than sonication. Standard inoculation procedure involves removing medium from the cell monolayer and replacing it with the inoculum in a volume of 0.1 to 1 ml. The specimen is then centrifuged onto the cell monolayer at approximately 3,000 × *g* at 35°C for 1 h. The vials should be held at 35°C for 2 h before the cells are washed or the medium is changed to medium containing 1 to 2 μg of cycloheximide per ml (this must be titrated for each batch). The cells are then incubated at 35°C for 48 to 72 h, after which one cover slip is examined for inclusions by use of iodine, Giemsa, or immunofluorescence staining. The use of immunofluorescence can speed up the process, since inclusions can clearly be seen (although they are smaller) at 24 h postinfection. Giemsa stain is more sensitive than iodine stain, but the microscopic evaluation is more difficult. Slide reading can be facilitated by examining the Giemsa-stained cover slip by dark-field rather than bright-field microscopy (9). The iodine stain is the simplest procedure and is commonly used, although it is less sensitive than either of the other two.

If passage of positive material or blind passage of negative material is desired, the material should be passaged at 72 to 96 h postinoculation. The cell monolayer is disrupted by shaking with glass beads on a Vortex mixer; the material is treated by low-speed centrifugation to remove cell debris, and the supernatant is inoculated as described above. For symptomatic patients, 90% of specimens positive for *C. trachomatis* are inclusion positive in the first passage. In screening asymptomatic patients, who often have less agent, more (30 to 40%) of the positive specimens require passage.

With trachoma, inclusion conjunctivitis, and the genital tract infections, the technique is as described above. In LGV, the aspirated bubo pus is diluted (10^{-1} and 10^{-2}) before inoculation. Second passages are always made because detritus from the inoculum may make it difficult to read the slides. For many *C. psittaci* isolation attempts, it may be convenient to lengthen the incubation period to 5 to 10 days before examining the cover slips for inclusions. These organisms do not require mechanical assistance for cell-to-cell infection (28).

For laboratories processing large numbers of specimens, it may be convenient to use flat-bottom 96-well microtiter plates rather than vials (34). Cells are plated onto cover slips or directly onto the plates. Processing and incubation are as described above, but microscopy is modified to use either long working objectives or inverted microscopes. This procedure is less sensitive than the vial technique but offers considerable savings of reagents and time and may be suitable when mostly symptomatic patients are being screened. These patients usually yield higher numbers of chlamydiae, which minimizes the impact of the decreased sensitivity of the test.

Isolation in mice

The mice to be used should be proven susceptible to chlamydiae because there are some genetic variations in this regard. Mice should be obtained from a colony shown to be free of latent chlamydial infection. There have been at least seven reports of subclinical chlamydial infections in mouse colonies. These agents were identified as *C. psittaci* as well as a *C. trachomatis* biovar; some were viscerotropic, whereas others were pneumotropic. These infections were revealed by persistent blind passage of "normal" mouse tissue.

Intraperitoneal injection. The i.p. route of injection is used only for *C. psittaci.* Most chlamydiae from psittacines or turkeys are lethal after inoculation by the i.p. route; those from pigeons, chickens, some turkeys, or ducks may produce significantly enlarged spleens and ascitic fluid but do not regularly cause death.

Inoculate 0.5 ml of the prepared 10 or 20% sterile emulsion. Virulent material from parrots, parakeets, humans, and some turkeys, injected by the i.p. route in this amount, causes death of the mouse in 3 to 30 days.

If mice die within 2 or 3 days, little that is abnormal can be seen with the naked eye; spleen and liver may look normal in size and architecture. Some animals may show signs of vascular damage. Quite characteristic, and often the only sign, is a bloated duodenum covered with a thin viscous exudate. In some animals, the surface of the liver and intestines may be moist and covered with a thin, sticky exudate that contains abundant endothelial cells packed with chlamydial particles. Macchiavello or Gimenez stain is used with impression smears.

When death occurs within 5 to 15 days, the spleen is enlarged, and early necrotic lesions of the liver can be seen. Microscopically, hemorrhages and necrosis are common in the liver; the phagocytic cells of liver and spleen may be packed with chlamydiae. The abdominal cavity may be filled with stringy, turbid, fibrinous exudate.

If animals survive until day 21, they should be sacrificed, and further blind passage of emulsions of the spleen and liver should be made. The general rule is that if chlamydiae are not found by the third passage, they cannot be isolated no matter how many more passages are made. Mice that recover and are sacrificed 3 weeks after infection have few gross lesions. In general, the intestines are slightly distended and pale. Exudate may be present in the abdominal cavity. The spleen is conspicuously enlarged, the liver is friable and mottled, the kidneys are grayish. EBs are sparse in tissue smears, but animal passage has shown that they may exist as long as 300 days after initial infection. Most survivors have infection immunity.

This technique offers the advantages of simplicity, reliability, and large inocula. If it is desired, the animals may receive multiple (at daily intervals) inoculations from the original specimen. In addition, the mice may "filter" out bacteria that have not been controlled by antibiotics or centrifugation and dilution.

Intracranial injection. Tissue specimens from humans, sterile exudates from the pericardial or air sacs of birds, or peritoneal fluid and suspensions prepared from infected mice can be safely infected by the i.c. route, which may furnish excellent specimens for rapid histologic diagnosis. LGV specimens are also inoculated by the i.c. route. Inoculate 0.03 ml of the treated emulsion. Somnolence and paralysis often develop within 24 to 48 h, and death follows within 3 to 5 days with highly virulent material. Blind passage is performed at 10 days.

The i.c. route has the advantage of not involving the respiratory tract, precluding the possibility of activating latent mouse pneumonitis. Smears made from the dura teem with chlamydiae. A relatively fast and sensitive method for isolating psittacosis and ornithosis agents, this technique is somewhat less effective with LGV. The i.c. route of inoculation suffers a disadvantage with respect to the small volume of inoculum and the susceptibility of the mice to bacteria that may contaminate the specimen.

Intranasal instillation. Instill 0.03 to 0.05 ml of a 10% tissue suspension, with the mouse under light anesthesia (ether is suitable). If the material inoculated is virulent or if isolates have been established, signs of infection (hunched posture, apathy, and increasingly labored respiration) develop rapidly, and death follows within 2 to 20 days. Bacterial contamination must be ruled out. In typical successful isolation attempts, death may take place between days 8 and 16 if the agent is present in a high concentration. However, with less virulent material, all symptoms may gradually disappear; in such cases, blind passage should be performed 21 days after inoculation. Blind passage is usually required. Segments or entire lobes of the lung may be extensively consolidated. Discrete foci of pneumonia are manifested as limiting infective dilutions are approached. These areas, which are gray, almost translucent, are 1 to 3 mm in diameter. Fewer EBs are seen in smears from lungs infected for more than 10 days, and there may be difficulty finding them in old lesions. Repassage may furnish excellent material for microscopy.

Yolk sac isolation

Clinical specimens are collected in an appropriate antibiotic broth. The specimen is held for 1 h at room temperature before inoculation of 0.25 ml into the yolk sac, using a 3.2-cm 22-gauge needle. Before inoculation, the fertile eggs are incubated at 38.5 to 39°C in a moist atmosphere. The eggs to be used must be obtained from a flock fed an antibiotic-free diet. They should be free from mycoplasma. When 7 days old, embryonated hen eggs are candled for viability, the location of air sacs is marked, the shell is painted with tincture of iodine, and a hole is gently punched. The specimen is inoculated at a slight angle away from the embryo; three or four eggs are labeled with a pencil or marking pen. After inoculation, the shell is again swabbed with iodine and the hole is sealed (with glue or tape). The eggs are then incubated in a moist environment at 35°C and candled daily for 13 days. Eggs that die in the first 3 days after inoculation are discarded.

The yolk sacs of eggs dying thereafter are harvested. This procedure entails painting the shell with iodine, cracking and removing the shell over the air sac, teasing away the shell and chorioallantoic membranes, and removing the yolk sac with forceps. Excess yolk material is stripped away. It is important that all instruments be sterile and that fresh instruments be used for each specimen. Impression smears are made and stained (Gimenez or the modified Macchiavello method). Sterility tests are performed on yolk sac with thioglycolate broth. If the embryos are still viable 13 days postinoculation, the eggs are chilled for several hours and yolk sacs are harvested, ground in nutrient broth, and centrifuged lightly. The supernatant is passaged in another group of four 7-day-old embryonated hen eggs (1 ml of 50% yolk sac per egg). After two blind passages, attempts are terminated as negative.

The generally acceptable criteria for positive isolation are the finding of EBs in the impression smears, serially transmissible egg mortality, the presence of group antigen in the yolk sac, and the absence of contaminating bacteria.

IDENTIFICATION

Since most laboratories use tissue culture isolation systems, the basic procedure for identification of chlamydiae involves demonstration of typical intracytoplasmic inclusions by appropriate (Giemsa or iodine) staining procedures. However, in laboratories initiating work with chlamydiae, it would be prudent to use at least one other parameter for identification of chlamydiae. Fluorescent-antibody staining provides both a morphological and an immunological identification. In yolk sac or mouse isolation procedures, one can use heavily infected material to prepare a CF antigen to confirm the presence of chlamydiae.

C. trachomatis strains may be serotyped by the micro-IF technique (32). For this procedure, antisera are produced by intravenous inoculation of mice at day 0, a booster at day 7, and exsanguination at day 11. The mouse antiserum is then tested in a titration against all serotypes, as well as the immunizing agent, and the serotype is identified presumptively by the pattern of reactivity and finally by appropriate box titration with the appropriate prototypic serotype. A battery of monoclonal antibodies for typing isolates is available (Washington Research Foundation, Seattle).

SERODIAGNOSIS

The most widely used serological test for diagnosing chlamydial infections is the CF test. This test is useful in diagnosing psittacosis, in which paired sera often show fourfold or greater increases in titer. The same seems to be true for many *C. pneumoniae* infections. Approximately 50% of these infections are CF positive, although it may take ≥4 weeks to detect seroconversion (12). CF may also be useful in diagnosing LGV, in which single-point titers greater than 1:64 are highly supportive of this clinical diagnosis. With LGV, it is difficult to demonstrate rising titers since the nature of the disease is such that the patient is seen by the physician after the acute stage. Any titer above 1:16 is considered significant evidence of exposure to chlamydiae. The CF test is not particularly useful in diagnosing trachoma-inclusion conjunctivitis or the related genital tract infections, and it plays no role in diagnosing neonatal chlamydial infections.

The micro-IF method is a much more sensitive procedure for measuring antichlamydial antibodies. It may be used in diagnosing psittacosis, in which paired sera will show rising immunoglobulin G (IgG) titers. With LGV, it is again difficult to demonstrate rising titers, but single-point titers in active cases usually have relatively high levels of IgM (>1:32) and IgG (≥1:2,000) antibody. Trachoma, inclusion conjunctivitis, and the genital tract infections may be diagnosed by the micro-IF technique if appropriately timed paired acute and convalescent sera can be obtained. However, it is often difficult to demonstrate rising antibody titers, particularly in sexually active populations. Many of these individuals will be seen for chronic or repeat infections. The background rate of seroreactors in venereal disease clinics is ≥60%, making it particularly difficult to demonstrate seroconversion. In general, first attacks of chlamydial urethritis have been regularly associated with seroconversion (4). Individuals with systemic infection (epididymitis or salpingitis) usually have much higher antibody levels than do those with superficial infections, and women tend to have higher antibody levels than men.

Serology is particularly useful in diagnosing chlamydial pneumonia in neonates. In this case, high levels of IgM antibody are regularly found in association with disease (27). IgG antibodies are less useful because the infants are being seen at a time when they have considerable levels of maternal IgG, since all of these infections are acquired from the infected mother, who is almost always seropositive. It takes between 6 and 9 months for maternal antichlamydial antibodies to disappear. Infants older than that age may be tested for determination of prevalence of chlamydial infection without fear of confounding effects of maternal antibody. Infants with inclusion conjunctivitis or respiratory tract carriage of chlamydiae without pneumonia usually have very low levels of IgM antibodies. Thus, a single IgM titer of ≥1:32 may support the diagnosis of chlamydial pneumonia.

C. pneumoniae (TWAR) infections are usually diagnosed by micro-IF. The diagnostic criterion has been (i) a fourfold rise in titer or (ii) an IgM titer of >1:32 or (iii) an IgG titer of >1:512 (32).

The micro-IF technique uses many serotypes of chlamydiae, and the procedure as simplified by Wang et al. (33) is recommended. Since serology is particularly useful in diagnosing neonatal infection and the IgM antibody responses tend to be markedly specific, the use of single broadly reacting antigens will miss at least 15 to 25% of the infections that can be proven to be caused by chlamydiae by other procedures or that would be positive by a multiple-antigen micro-IF. The single-antigen tests may involve either yolk sac suspensions of agent or identification of fluorescent inclusions in tissue monolayers. Serotypes of the DEL serogroup are commonly chosen for this purpose.

Research workers should be warned that monotypic A seroreactions, at least in the United States, are liable to be spurious. These antibodies are usually transient and do not result in the persistent high levels of IgG antibodies that usually follow chlamydial infections.

EIA techniques that measure antichlamydial antibodies have been described (11, 17). Most of these procedures for measuring IgG antibody have been successful, albeit often less sensitive than the micro-IF test. They have not been as successful in measuring IgM antibody. Such tests are commercially available, but there is little published experience. It is likely that the EIAs are less sensitive than the micro-IF, miss some C-complex reactors, and cannot be readily applied to IgM antibody. The procedure may be of some use in selected instances and for serosurveys in laboratories where micro-IF techniques are not available.

However, single serological tests are of very little value in the diagnosis of uncomplicated lower genital tract infections, which represent the majority of tests. Although manufacturers may claim that their tests are specific for *C. trachomatis* and that titers of a specific level are diagnostic of current infection, neither of those claims is likely to be accurate. If the tests involve partially solubilized EBs for EIA or inclusion detection by immunofluorescence, there is undoubtedly LPS present. The test will detect antibodies not only to *C. trachomatis* but also to *C. psittaci* or *C. pneumoniae* because the LPS is a genus-specific antigen. Because of the high prevalence of antibody in high-risk populations, single positive results are seldom diagnostic for current genital infection. In most research evaluations, the positive predictive values have been on the order of 30 to 50%.

CF

The CF test may be performed in either the tube system or the microtiter system. Reagents should be standardized in the tube system regardless of which test system will be used. The microtiter systems are most useful in screening large numbers of sera, but it is preferable to retest all positive sera in the tube system. Occasionally, sera giving titers in the range of 1:4 to 1:8 in the microdilution system are positive at 1:16 (taken as the significant level) in the tube system. Because guinea pigs may have naturally occurring chlamydial infection, the complement must be tested for antichlamydial antibodies.

All reagents are available commercially except for high-titered group antigen. The latter may be prepared as follows. Yolk sacs of 7-day embryonated eggs are inoculated with chlamydiae (e.g., psittacosis isolate 6BC) at a dose estimated to result in death of about 50% of inoculated eggs in 5 to 7 days. Eggs are candled daily, and those dying early are discarded. When the 50% death endpoint is approached, the remaining eggs (recently dead or live) are refrigerated for 3 to 24 h. The yolk sacs are then harvested. If examination of random samples shows large numbers of particles, the yolk sacs are pooled. This preparation may be stored at −20°C until further processing. The yolk sacs are ground in a mortar with sterile sand. Beef heart broth (pH 7.0) is added to make a 20% suspension, and the material is cultured to determine whether it is free of bacterial contamination. The suspension is placed in a flask containing sterile glass beads and stored at 4°C for 3 to 6 weeks with daily shaking. It is then centrifuged at ca. 500 × *g* to remove coarse particles, transferred to a heavy sterile flask, and steamed at 100°C or immersed in boiling water for 30 min. After it has cooled, liquefied phenol is added to 0.5%. The antigen should then be refrigerated for at least 1 week before being used. It is stable for at least 1 year if not contaminated and should have an antigen titer of 1:256 or greater. A similar preparation from uninfected yolk sacs must be included as one of the controls.

MICRO-IF

The micro-IF test is usually performed against chlamydial organisms grown in yolk sac. Tissue culture-grown agent can be used, but it may be necessary to concentrate the EBs and add some normal yolk sac to improve contrast for microscopy. The individual yolk sacs are selected for EB richness and pretitrated to give an even distribution of particles. It is generally found that a 1 to 3% yolk sac suspension (phosphate-buffered saline, pH 7.0) is satisfactory. The antigens may be stored as frozen samples; after thawing, they are well mixed on a Vortex mixer before use. Micro-IF antigens for research purposes are available through the Washington Research Foundation. Antigen dots are placed on a slide in a specific pattern, with separate markings with a pen used for each antigen. Each cluster of dots includes all of the antigenic types to be tested. The antigen dots are air dried and fixed on slides with acetone (15 min at room temperature). Slides may be stored frozen. They may sweat when thawed for use, but they can be conveniently dried (as can the original antigen dots) with the cool airflow of a hair dryer. The slides have serial dilutions of serum (or tears or exudate) placed on the different antigen clusters. The clusters of dots are separated sufficiently to avoid running of the serum from cluster to cluster. After the serum dilutions have been added, the slides are incubated for 0.5 to 1 h in a moist chamber at 37°C. They are then placed in a buffered saline wash for 5 min, followed by a second 5-min wash. The slides are then dried and stained with fluorescein-conjugated anti-human globulin. Conjugates are pretitrated in a known positive system to determine appropriate working dilutions. This reagent may be prepared against any class of globulin being considered (IgA or secretory piece for secretions, IgG, or IgM). Counterstains such as bovine serum albumin conjugated with rhodamine may be included. The slides are then washed twice again, dried, and examined by standard fluorescence microscopy. Use of a monocular tube is recommended to allow greater precision in determining fluorescence of individual EB particles. The endpoints are read as the dilution giving bright fluorescence clearly associated with the well-distributed EBs throughout the antigen dot. Identification of the type-specific response is based on dilution differences reflected in the endpoints for different prototype antigens.

For each run of either CF or micro-IF, known positive and negative sera should always be included. These sera should always duplicate their titers as previously observed within the experimental (±1 dilution) error of the system.

LITERATURE CITED

1. **Banks, J., B. Eddie, M. Sung, N. Sugg, J. Schachter, and K. F. Meyer.** 1970. Plaque reduction technique for demonstrating neutralizing antibodies for *Chlamydia*. Infect. Immun. **2:**443–447.
2. **Beem, M. O., and E. M. Saxon.** 1977. Respiratory-tract colonization and a distinctive pneumonia syndrome in infants infected with *Chlamydia trachomatis*. N. Engl. J. Med. **296:**306–310.
3. **Bernstein, D. I., T. Hubbard, W. Wenman, B. L. Johnson, Jr., K. K. Holmes, H. Liebhaber, J. Schachter, R. Barnes, and M. A. Lovett.** 1984. Mediastinal and supraclavicular lymphadenitis and pneumonitis due to *Chlamydia trachomatis* serovars L1 and L2. N. Engl. J. Med. **311:**1543–1546.
4. **Bowie, W. R., S. P. Wang, E. R. Alexander, J. Floyd, P. Forsyth, H. Pollock, J. S. Tin, T. Buchanan, and K. K. Holmes.** 1977. Etiology of nongonococcal urethritis: evidence for *Chlamydia trachomatis* and *Ureaplasma urealyticum*. J. Clin. Invest. **59:**735–742.
5. **Byrne, G. I., and J. W. Moulder.** 1978. Parasite-specified phagocytosis of *Chlamydia psittaci* and *Chlamydia trachomatis* by L and HeLa cells. Infect. Immun. **19:**598–606.
6. **Caldwell, H. D., and J. Schachter.** 1982. Antigenic analysis of the major outer membrane protein of *Chlamydia* spp. Infect. Immun. **35:**1024–1031.
7. **Chernesky, M. A., J. B. Mahony, S. Castriciano, M. Mores, I. O. Stewart, S. F. Landis, W. Seidelman, E. J. Sargeant, and C. Leman.** 1986. Detection of *Chlamydia trachomatis* antigens by enzyme immunoassay and immunofluorescence in genital specimens from symptomatic and asymptomatic men and women. J. Infect. Dis. **154:**141–148.
8. **Cles, L. D., K. Bruch, and W. E. Stamm.** 1988. Staining characteristics of six commercially available monoclonal immunofluorescence reagents for direct diagnosis of *Chlamydia trachomatis* infections. J. Clin. Microbiol. **26:**1735–1737.
9. **Darougar, S., J. R. Kinnison, and B. R. Jones.** 1971. Simplified irradiated McCoy cell culture for isolation of chlamydiae, p. 63–70. *In* R. L. Nichols (ed.), Trachoma and related disorders caused by chlamydial agents. Excerpta Medica, Amsterdam.

10. **Eb, F., and J. Orfila.** 1981. Serotyping of *Chlamydia psittaci* by microimmunofluorescence test. Ann. Microbiol. (Paris) **A132:**18.
11. **Finn, M. P., A. Ohlin, and J. Schachter.** 1983. Enzyme-linked immunosorbent assay for immunoglobulin G and M antibodies to *Chlamydia trachomatis* in human sera. J. Clin. Microbiol. **17:**848–852.
12. **Grayston, J. T.** 1989. Chlamydia-pneumoniae, strain TWAR. Chest **95:**664.
13. **Grayston, J. T., C. C. Kuo, L. A. Campbell, and S.-P. Wang.** 1989. *Chlamydia pneumoniae* sp. nov. for *Chlamydia* sp. strain TWAR. Int. J. Syst. Bacteriol. **39:**88–90.
14. **Hodinka, R. L., and P. B. Wyrick.** 1986. Ultrastructural study of mode of entry of *Chlamydia psittaci* into L-929 cells. Infect. Immun. **54:**855–863.
15. **Jones, R. B., B. Batteiger, and W. J. Newhall.** 1982. Cross-reactive antigenic determinants in the major surface proteins of *Chlamydia trachomatis,* p. 61–64. *In* P.-A. Mårdh, K. K. Holmes, J. D. Oriel, P. Piot, and J. Schachter (ed.), Chlamydial infections. Elsevier Biomedical Press, Amsterdam.
16. **Kuo, C.-C., and J. T. Grayston.** 1988. Factors affecting viability and growth in HeLa 229 cells of *Chlamydia* sp. strain TWAR. J. Clin. Microbiol. **26:**812–815.
17. **Mahony, J. B., M. A. Chernesky, K. Bromberg, and J. Schachter.** 1986. Accuracy of immunoglobulin M immunoassay for diagnosis of chlamydial infections in infants and adults. J. Clin. Microbiol. **24:**731–735.
18. **Meyer, K. F.** 1967. The host spectrum of psittacosis-lymphogranuloma venereum (PL) agents. Am. J. Ophthalmol. **63:**1225–1246.
19. **Moncada, J., J. Schachter, M. Shipp, G. Bolan, and J. Wilber.** 1989. Cytobrush in collection of cervical specimens for detection of *Chlamydia trachomatis.* J. Clin. Microbiol. **27:**1863–1866.
20. **Morrison, R. P., K. Lying, and H. D. Caldwell.** 1989. Chlamydial diseases pathogenesis-ocular hypersensitivity elicited by a genus-specific 57 Kd protein. J. Exp. Med. **169:**663–675.
21. **Moulder, J. W., T. P. Hatch, C. C. Kuo, J. Schachter, and J. Storz.** 1984. Order II. Chlamydiales Storz and Page 1971, 334, p. 729–739. *In* N. R. Krieg and J. G. Holt (ed.), Bergey's manual of systematic bacteriology. The Williams & Wilkins, Co., Baltimore.
22. **Newhall, W. J., B. Batteiger, and R. B. Jones.** 1982. Analysis of the human serological response to proteins of *Chlamydia trachomatis.* Infect. Immun. **38:**1181–1189.
23. **Nurminen, M., M. Leinonen, P. Saikku, and P. H. Makela.** 1983. The genus-specific antigen of *Chlamydia:* resemblance to the lipopolysaccharide of enteric bacteria. Science **220:**1279–1281.
24. **Ripa, K. T., and P.-A. Mårdh.** 1977. Cultivation of *Chlamydia trachomatis* in cycloheximide-treated McCoy cells. J. Clin. Microbiol. **6:**328–331.
25. **Saikku, P., P. Ruutu, M. Leinonen, J. Panelius, T. E. Tupasi, and J. T. Grayston.** 1988. Acute lower respiratory-tract infection associated with *Chlamydia* TWAR antibody in filipino children. J. Infect. Dis. **158:**1095–1097.
26. **Schachter, J.** 1978. Chlamydial infections. N. Engl. J. Med. **298:**428–435, 490–495, 540–549.
27. **Schachter, J., M. Grossman, and P. H. Azimi.** 1982. Serology of *Chlamydia trachomatis* in infants. J. Infect. Dis. **146:**530–535.
28. **Schachter, J., N. Sugg, and M. Sung.** 1978. Psittacosis: the reservoir persists. J. Infect. Dis. **137:**44–49.
29. **Stamm, W. E., M. Tam, M. Koester, and L. Cles.** 1983. Detection of *Chlamydia trachomatis* inclusions in McCoy cell cultures with fluorescein-conjugated monoclonal antibodies. J. Clin. Microbiol. **17:**666–668.
30. **Storz, J.** 1971. *Chlamydia* and *Chlamydia*-induced diseases. Charles C Thomas, Publisher, Springfield, Ill.
31. **Tam, M. R., W. E. Stamm, H. H. Handsfield, R. Stephens, C.-C. Kuo, K. K. Holmes, K. Ditzenberger, M. Crieger, and R. C. Nowinski.** 1984. Culture-independent diagnosis of *Chlamydia trachomatis* using monoclonal antibodies. N. Engl. J. Med. **310:**1146–1150.
32. **Wang, S.-P., and J. T. Grayston.** 1970. Immunologic relationship between genital TRIC, lymphogranuloma venereum and related organisms in a new microtiter indirect immunofluorescence test. Am. J. Ophthalmol. **70:**367–374.
33. **Wang, S.-P., J. T. Grayston, E. R. Alexander, and K. K. Holmes.** 1975. Simplified microimmunofluorescence test with trachoma-lymphogranuloma venereum (*Chlamydia trachomatis*) antigens for use as a screening test for antibody. J. Clin. Microbiol. **1:**250–255.
34. **Yoder, B. L., W. E. Stamm, M. C. Koester, and E. R. Alexander.** 1981. Microtest procedure for isolation of *Chlamydia trachomatis.* J. Clin. Microbiol. **13:**1036–1039.

Chapter 106

Ehrlichiae

DANIEL B. FISHBEIN AND JACQUELINE E. DAWSON

DESCRIPTION OF THE GENUS

The ehrlichiae (also known as the leukocytic rickettsiae) are nonmotile gram-negative intracellular bacteria characterized by parasitism of reticuloendothelial cells, especially leukocytes (35). They are members of the order *Rickettsiales*, in the family *Rickettsiaceae*, and have their own tribe, *Ehrlichiae*. Members of the tribe cause acute and sometimes chronic or latent diseases in animals in many parts of the world (32). Ehrlichiae appear susceptible to the tetracycline family and a few other antibiotics (2, 10). Recently, a human form of ehrlichiosis was recognized in the United States (24).

Ehrlichiae were first recognized in 1932, when an unknown agent (originally named *Cytoecetes phagocytophila;* renamed *Ehrlichia phagocytophila* in 1982) was identified in *Ixodes ricinus* ticks. In the same year, tick-borne fever, the clinical syndrome caused by these organisms, was described in sheep (13). In 1935, Giemsa-stained blood smears of febrile dogs in Algiers were noted to contain rickettsialike organisms in the monocytes (6); the microorganism was originally named *Rickettsia canis* but was renamed *Ehrlichia canis* in 1945. The genus *Ehrlichia* now contains five definite species and a number of *species incertae cedis* (see below and chapter 103).

Like other bacteria, the ehrlichiae possess a cell wall and plasma membrane (32). The life cycle of the ehrlichiae is long, lasting about 2 weeks, during which the organisms proceed through developmental stages similar to those of the chlamydiae (26). The ehrlichiae invade leukocytes by phagocytosis. However, phagolysosomal fusion does not occur; the organisms are protected from lysosomes and form pleomorphic, coccoid to ellipsoid elementary bodies, which are about 0.5 μm in diameter, in 48 h. The elementary bodies grow and divide by binary fission within the phagosome for 2 to 3 days, forming a few tightly packed pleomorphic initial bodies (immature inclusions) 0.5 to 2.5 μm in diameter. The host leukocyte also increases in size during the next 7 to 12 days as the initial bodies continue to divide. During the late stages of this cycle, some *Ehrlichia* species are consistently visualized when blood smears from infected animals are examined with Giemsa stain, whereas others are rarely seen (32). Up to 50 elementary bodies are found in the morula or mulberry (the mature inclusion), the contents of which are released into the bloodstream when the cell breaks up. Alternatively, the cell can divide, retaining a morula in each new cell; in this situation, the ehrlichiae are not exposed to the extracellular environment.

Ticks have been established as vectors of some *Ehrlichia* species (22) and are suspected in the transmission of others because of the seasonality of the associated diseases. The brown dog tick *Rhipicephalus sanguineus* is the vector of canine ehrlichiosis. These ticks remaining infectious for dogs for up to 155 days after detachment as engorged nymphs (22), *E. canis* passing transtadially (but not then transovarially) (42). The natural reservoirs of ehrlichiae have not been established. Chronically infected dogs are inefficient transmitters of *E. canis* (14).

Since information on the microbiology of human ehrlichiosis is limited and the form of human ehrlichiosis found in the United States is in many ways similar to *E. canis* infections of dogs, this chapter will also include discussions of ehrlichial species that at present are recognized only as animal pathogens. Just as the form of human ehrlichiosis found in the United States has been associated with *E. canis*, new human illnesses may in the future be associated with these other ehrlichial species.

CLINICAL SIGNIFICANCE

Animal diseases

E. canis, the type species of the genus, causes an infection thought to be limited to domestic and wild canidae (16). The disease, canine ehrlichiosis, is distributed worldwide. In dogs, the disease passes through three stages, all of which may not be apparent because of differences of disease severity and susceptibility of different types of dogs. The acute stage begins 10 to 15 days after infection and lasts a few days to 3 weeks. During this time, dogs commonly develop fever, anorexia, generalized depression, mucopurulent ocular and nasal discharge, weight loss, lymphadenopathy, corneal opacities, pneumonitis, and vomiting (30, 32). Hematologic abnormalities are frequently present and include leukopenia (caused by destruction of circulating leukocytes), thrombocytopenia (immunologically mediated), and anemia (18, 21); animals with the most severe hematologic abnormalities have the poorest prognoses. Common biochemical abnormalities include hyperglobulinemia and elevated liver function tests, especially the transaminases (30). During the acute stage, the bone marrow reveals a normal to increased number of myeloid cells and an increased number of megakaryocytes (30). Pathologically, perivascular cuffing is found in many organs (16a), presumably related to the ability of parasitized mononuclear cells to adhere to the endothelium of small blood vessels (41).

Although most dogs appear to recover from the acute stage, they often remain infected. A subclinical phase follows, during which time the dogs appear normal but mild hematologic abnormalities (especially thrombocytopenia) may persist (4, 21).

Chronic canine ehrlichiosis begins a few months after

acute infection. The severity of the chronic stage varies among different breeds; some species (e.g., beagles) develop a mild persistent infection during which the animal remains infectious for years (3), whereas others (e.g., German shepherds) develop an especially severe form known as tropical canine pancytopenia (TCP) (20, 21). TCP is often first manifested by epistaxis, petechial or ecchymotic forms of hemorrhage, fever, lymphadenopathy, dependent edema, anorexia, and dyspnea, and secondary bacterial infections may follow (3, 21). The bone marrow is hypoplastic. Pathologically, this stage of illness is accompanied by chronic proliferative changes, with mononuclear cell (particularly plasma cell) infiltrates, perivascular cuffing, and hemorrhage in numerous organs, especially the meninges, heart, lung, liver, kidney, and spleen. Immunologic studies suggest that development of TCP may be related to the suppression of a cell-mediated immune response to infection (25).

Ehrlichia risticii is the causative agent of Potomac horse fever (equine monocytic ehrlichiosis) (17, 31). Although the occurrence of cases between May and November with midsummer peak suggests vector transmission, attempts to identify specific vectors have been unsuccessful. Cases have been reported in 32 states, with the heaviest concentrations in Maryland, Virginia, Pennsylvania, and adjacent states (27, 38). Potomac horse fever is manifested by variable degrees of fever, depression, lymphadenopathy, anorexia, colic, and diarrhea, which may progress to dehydration, hypovolemia, and shock (8, 40, 47); leukopenia is also present. Severity is variable; before the use of tetracycline, 25 to 30% of cases were fatal (40). A number of other domestic animals, including dogs and cats, have been experimentally infected (5, 33). A vaccine is now commercially available.

Ehrlichia equi is the cause of equine granulocytic ehrlichiosis, a disease of horses manifested by fever, edema, lymphadenopathy, ataxia, and pancytopenia. The disease is common in the western United States, especially in the Sacramento valley, and occurs sporadically elsewhere in the country (23). Unlike *E. risticii*, the etiologic agent invades granulocytes, particularly eosinophils, where the organisms are highly pleomorphic (39). Also in contrast to Potomac horse fever, there are no fatal cases, and equine granulocytic ehrlichiosis has a late fall to early spring seasonality.

E. phagocytophila causes tick-borne fever, a disease of Old World sheep and cattle in Europe, Asia, and South Africa; it has also been found in deer. Although the inclusion of *E. phagocytophila* in the tribe *Ehrlichiae* is widely accepted, its inclusion in the genus *Ehrlichia* remains controversial (46). The etiologic agent is transmitted by *I. ricinus* and invades granulocytes and, to a lesser extent, monocytes (46). During a 4- to 6-day febrile phase, up to 95% of circulating granulocytes may contain organisms; affected animals appear dull and listless, may have marked weight loss, and are predisposed to other infections. Sheep (but not cattle) may harbor the organism for years (45, 46).

Human diseases

Sennetsu rickettsiosis. *Ehrlichia sennetsu*, the only *Ehrlichia* species that has been isolated from a human, was first isolated in 1953, although the human disease, known as sennetsu fever or sennetsu rickettsiosis, may have been recognized in the 1880s. Virtually all cases have been identified among residents of the southern coast of Japan; reports of the disease in the United States have not been confirmed (J. Segreti, H. Kessler, A. Cole, C. Holland, M. Ristic, and S. Levin, Clin. Res. **34:**533A, 1986). The incubation period is about 14 days; onset is frequently sudden, with fever, chills, and headache. Malaise, insomnia, diaphoresis, sore throat, anorexia, and constipation are noted. Lymphadenopathy is generalized and slightly tender, but most prominent in the postauricular and posterior cervical regions; hepatomegaly and splenomegaly are noted in about one-third of cases (43). Although initially patients are leukopenic, the syndrome has been likened to mononucleosis because of the presence of a relative and absolute pleocytosis of atypical lymphocytes later in its course. The disease is self-limiting; serious complications and fatalities have not been reported. Chronic infections have been established in mice, and the disease has been passed to human volunteers inoculated with emulsified lymph nodes from experimentally infected mice. A serologic relationship to *E. canis* has been reported (36).

Human ehrlichiosis in the United States. In 1986, a 51-year-old man developed an illness characterized by fever, headache, myalgia, leukopenia, and abnormal liver function tests 14 days after being bitten by ticks in Arkansas. Although the illness was initially thought to be Rocky Mountain spotted fever (RMSF), serologic tests for *Rickettsia rickettsii* as well as a number of other clinically suspected agents were negative. Inclusion bodies, originally mistaken for Döhle bodies, were subsequently recognized as resembling ehrlichiae; serologic testing revealed a high antibody titer to *E. canis* and low titers to other *Ehrlichia* species (24). Testing of sera from patients with similar illnesses revealed that about 10% had serologic evidence of a recent infection with an *Ehrlichia* species (12, 44).

A number of epidemiologic studies and case reports have allowed a fairly clear picture of human ehrlichiosis in the United States (11, 12, 15, 38a, 44). Cases have been recognized in 15 south central and southeastern states as well as in Wyoming and Utah. Although patients as young as 2 years of age have been reported (7, 9), most are over 30 years of age, somewhat older than those with RMSF. About 75% have a history of a tick bite or attachment; most of those without a history of a bite report being in a tick-infested area.

Many features of the disease appear similar to those of acute canine ehrlichiosis. Symptoms are nonspecific. Fever is present in virtually all symptomatic patients and is over 39°C in about half. Other symptoms present in at least half of the patients included headache, myalgia, and anorexia. Somewhat less common are nausea, vomiting, abdominal pain, and confusion. In marked contrast with RMSF, rashes are reported in only a third of the patients and are variable and nonspecific in appearance (12, 15, 38a). Ehrlichiosis appears to be somewhat milder than RMSF; asymptomatic patients have been reported (29, 44). However, about half of the patients require hospitalization, and three patients with serologic evidence of a recent infection with an *Ehrlichia* species have died (D. H. Walker, J. P. Taylor, J. S. Buie, and C. Deardon, Abstr. Annu. Meet. Am. Soc. Microbiol. 1989, D76, p. 95). The most consistent features of human ehrlichiosis, apart from a history of tick bite and fever, are abnormalities of the clinical laboratory tests (Table 1).

DIAGNOSIS

Microscopic examination of tissues

As evidenced by the initial human case of ehrlichiosis, intraleukocytic inclusions resembling ehrlichiae can suggest the diagnosis. However, inclusions have only rarely been noted in humans with ehrlichiosis (7, 24). The infrequent finding of inclusions in human ehrlichial infections is consistent with observations in animal ehrlichiosis. Inclusions are consistent features of only some ehrlichial infections, particularly those of the granulocytic invaders *E. equi* and *E. phagocytophila;* they are found less consistently in infections caused by other *Ehrlichia* species. In dogs infected with *E. canis,* inclusions may also be found in impression smears of infected tissues (especially lung) (19).

Isolation

The etiologic agent of the form of human ehrlichiosis recently recognized in the United States has not yet been isolated from a human. If whole blood from untreated humans suspected of having ehrlichiosis is available, the Viral and Rickettsial Zoonoses Branch, Centers for Disease Control, can be contacted for instructions on specimen handling and shipment. *E. sennetsu* was originally isolated in mice; the agent has been passaged in primary canine monocytes, HeLa cells, human amniotic membrane-derived FL cells, and African green monkey kidney cells.

TABLE 1. Epidemiologic, clinical, and laboratory features of human ehrlichiosis[a]

Feature	% with feature
Epidemiologic	
Sex, male	71 (57/80)[b]
History of tick bite	78 (46/59)
Clinical	
Fever (patient report)	91 (48/53)
Maximum temperature, >39°C	62 (13/21)
Myalgia	67 (37/55)
Anorexia	67 (20/30)
Nausea	51 (28/55)
Headache	75 (44/59)
Rash	32 (18/56)
Laboratory	
Anemia	72 (18/25)
Thrombocytopenia	67 (30/45)
Leukopenia	58 (31/53)
Elevated alanine aminotransferase	82 (14/17)
Elevated aspartate aminotransferase	52 (12/23)
Elevated alkaline phosphatase	47 (9/19)
Elevated bilirubin	30 (6/20)
Elevated cerebrospinal fluid protein	25 (1/4)
Elevated cerebrospinal fluid leukocyte count	25 (1/4)

[a] Data are for a population with a mean age of 38.8 years and are taken from references 7, 9, 11, 12, 24, 29, and 44 and Rohrbach et al. (27th ICAAC).

[b] Number in parentheses is number of patients with the characteristic divided by total number of patients for whom there is information regarding the presence or absence of the characteristic.

The veterinary pathogens cannot be cultivated in cell-free media; unlike the rickettsiae, they do not grow in chicken embryos. Some have been grown in primary monocyte cultures in a number of continuous cell lines and can be passaged in experimental animals. Isolation, however, is difficult and time consuming and therefore not recommended for routine diagnosis. *E. canis* is best isolated in primary canine monocytes (26) and has been passaged in a continuous cell line of murine origin (32). *E. risticii* was originally isolated in primary horse monocytes and then passaged in primary canine monocytes (17) and a continuous murine macrophage line (34).

Serodiagnosis

The indirect immunofluorescent-antibody (IFA) test for detection of antibodies to *E. canis* in dogs was developed in 1972 (37) and subsequently extended to *E. sennetsu, E. equi,* and *E. risticii* (34). The IFA test methodology for human sera was adapted from that described for testing canine serum (37) and uses *E. canis* antigen grown in a continuous cell line (32) (*E. canis* IFA slides; ProtaTek, St. Paul, Minn.).

The case definition for human ehrlichiosis requires a fourfold or greater rise or fall in antibody titer to *E. canis.* A minimum titer of 80 was originally established on the basis of the prevalence of antibodies to *E. canis* in a group of healthy persons who had extensive occupational exposure to ticks (12, 29). A few patients fulfilling this serologic case definition for ehrlichiosis also had diagnostic titers to other rickettsial, tick-borne, or non-tick-borne microorganisms; the mechanism of cross-reaction remains unclear (12, 15). Therefore, appropriate diagnostic tests for other diseases with similar clinical manifestations should be always be obtained.

To make the dilution system similar to that used with the other rickettsiae, the minimum cutoff was reduced to 64. Starting at a dilution of 1:64, serial twofold dilutions of the sera are made in a 0.15 M phosphate-buffered saline solution. Known positive and negative control sera are also tested at a 1:64 dilution. We use fluorescein-conjugated rabbit anti-human immunoglobulin G prepared at the Centers for Disease Control. Serologic results are reported as the reciprocal of the highest dilution at which specific fluorescence of *E. canis* morulae or individual bodies are observed. Whole-cell fluorescence (in the absence of specific fluorescence of morulae) is considered a nonspecific reaction and is not reported. If economy of reagents is important, the convalescent serum may initially be screened at 1:64; when specific fluorescence is observed, acute- and convalescent-phase sera are tested to determine the endpoint.

Antibody kinetic studies revealed that of 85 confirmed ehrlichiosis patients tested at the Centers for Disease Control, 7 (22%) of 32 patients initially tested during the first week, 17 (68%) of 25 patients tested during the second week, and 100% of 18 patients tested during the third week of illness had titers that exceeded the minimum positive titer (5a).

Other laboratory data helpful in recognition of human ehrlichiosis

As mentioned previously, the presence of certain laboratory abnormalities facilitates the recognition of human ehrlichiosis and its distinction from other tick-borne diseases. Borderline anemia, leukopenia, thrombocytopenia, and abnormal hepatic transaminases are present at the time of initial evaluation in about half of the patients and subsequently become more marked, with most patients eventually developing one or more of these abnormalities (11, 12). Less commonly noted abnormalities included mild elevations of the cerebrospinal fluid cell count or protein and disseminated intravascular coagulation. Bone marrow is usually normal but has occasionally shown hypoplasia (7, 12, 15, 28).

ANTIBIOTIC SUSCEPTIBILITY

Uncontrolled data in humans suggest that the form of ehrlichiosis found in the United States responds to members of the tetracycline family of drugs (11, 12, 44); at present, there are insufficient data to enable evaluation of the efficacy of chloramphenicol or other antibiotics. Although data are not yet sufficient to permit definitive recommendations, adults (except pregnant women) and children over the age of 9 should probably received a 10- to 14-day course of tetracycline or a tetracycline analog. Antibiotic susceptibilities of the other ehrlichiae have been studied in experimental animals and in vitro systems. Studies in animals in the late 1960s suggested that for acute canine ehrlichiosis, tetracycline and its analogs were effective therapeutically as well as prophylactically (1, 10) but that the chronic form of the disease was less responsive to these agents (1, 3). In an in vitro model of *E. risticii* infection, demeclocycline was slightly more effective than doxycycline, oxytetracycline, and minocycline in eliminating the infection in macrophages. Tetracycline and rifampin were marginally effective, and nalidixic acid and erythromycin were ineffective. Oxytetracycline is effective prophylactically and, to a lesser extent, therapeutically in mice experimentally infected with *E. sennetsu* (43).

LITERATURE CITED

1. **Amyx, H. L., D. L. Huxsoll, D. C. Zeiler, and P. K. Hildebrandt.** 1971. Therapeutic and prophylactic value of tetracycline in dogs infected with the agent of tropical canine pancytopenia. J. Am. Vet. Med. Assoc. **159:**1428–1432.
2. **Anika, S. M., J. F. Nouws, H. van Gogh, J. Nieuwenhuijs, T. B. Vree, and A. S. van Miert.** 1986. Chemotherapy and pharmacokinetics of some antimicrobial agents in healthy dwarf goats and those infected with Ehrlichia phagocytophila (tick-borne fever). Res. Vet. Sci. **41:**386–390.
3. **Buhles, W. C., Jr., D. L. Huxsoll, and M. Ristic.** 1974. Tropical canine pancytopenia: clinical, hematologic, and serologic response of dogs to Ehrlichia canis infection, tetracycline therapy, and challenge inoculation. J. Infect. Dis. **130:**357–367.
4. **Codner, E. C., and L. L. Farris-Smith.** 1986. Characterization of the subclinical phase of ehrlichiosis in dogs. J. Am. Vet. Med. Assoc. **189:**47–50.
5. **Dawson, J. E., I. Abeygunawardena, C. J. Holland, M. M. Buese, and M. Ristic.** 1988. Susceptibility of cats to infection with Ehrlichia risticii, causative agent of equine monocytic ehrlichiosis. Am. J. Vet. Res. **49:**2096–2100.

5a. **Dawson, J. E., D. B. Fishbein, T. R. Eng, N. R. Greene, and M. A. Redus.** 1990. Diagnosis of human ehrlichiosis: antibody kinetics and specificity. J. Infect. Dis. **162,** in press.

6. **Donatien, A., and F. Lestoquard.** 1935. Existence en Algerie d'une Rickettsia du chein. Bull. Soc. Pathol. Exot. Filiales **28:**418–419.
7. **Doran, T. I., R. T. Parmley, P. C. Logas, and S. Chamblin.** 1989. Infection with Ehrlichia canis in a child. J. Pediatr. **114:**809–812.
8. **Dutta, S. K., B. E. Penney, A. C. Myrup, M. G. Robl, and R. M. Rice.** 1988. Disease features in horses with induced equine monocytic ehrlichiosis (Potomac horse fever). Am. J. Vet. Res. **49:**1747–1751.
9. **Edwards, M. S., J. E. Jones, D. L. Leass, J. W. Whitmore, J. E. Dawson, and D. B. Fishbein.** 1988. Childhood infection caused by Ehrlichia canis or a closely related organism. Pediatr. Infect. Dis. J. **7:**651–654.
10. **Ewing, S. A.** 1969. Canine ehrlichiosis. Adv. Vet. Sci. Comp. Med. **13:**331–353.
11. **Fishbein, D. B., A. Kemp, J. E. Dawson, N. R. Greene, M. A. Redus, and D. H. Fields.** 1989. Human ehrlichiosis: prospective active surveillance in febrile hospitalized patients. J. Infect. Dis. **160:**803–809.
12. **Fishbein, D. B., L. A. Sawyer, C. J. Holland, E. B. Hayes, W. Okoroanyanwu, D. Williams, K. Sikes, M. Ristic, and J. E. McDade.** 1987. Unexplained febrile illnesses after exposure to ticks. Infection with an Ehrlichia? J. Am. Med. Assoc. **257:**3100–3104.
13. **Gordon, W. S., A. Brownlee, D. R. Wilson, and J. MacLeod.** 1932. Tick-borne fever (a hitherto undescribed disease of sheep). J. Comp. Pathol. **45:**301–312.
14. **Groves, M. G., G. L. Dennis, H. L. Amyx, and D. L. Huxsoll.** 1975. Transmission of Ehrlichia canis to dogs by ticks (Rhipicephalus sanguineus). Am. J. Vet. Res. **36:**937–940.
15. **Harkess, J. R., S. A. Ewing, J. M. Crutcher, J. Kudlac, G. McKee, and G. R. Istre.** 1989. Human ehrlichiosis in Oklahoma. J. Infect. Dis. **159:**576–579.
16. **Harvey, J. W., C. F. Simpson, J. M. Gaskin, and J. H. Sameck.** 1979. Ehrlichiosis in wolves, dogs, and wolf-dog crosses. J. Am. Vet. Med. Assoc. **175:**901–905.

16a. **Hildebrandt, P. K., D. L. Huxsoll, J. S. Walter, R. M. Nims, R. Taylor, and M. Andrews.** 1973. Pathology of canine ehrlichiosis (tropical canine pancytopenia). Am. J. Vet. Res. **34:**1309–1320.

17. **Holland, C. J., M. Ristic, A. I. Cole, P. Johnson, G. Baker, and T. Goetz.** 1985. Isolation, experimental transmission, and characterization of causative agent of Potomac horse fever. Science **227:**522–524.
18. **Huxsoll, D. L.** Canine ehrlichiosis (tropical canine pancytopenia): a review. Vet. Parasitol. **2:**49–60.
19. **Huxsoll, D. L., H. L. Amyx, I. E. Hemelt, P. K. Hildebrandt, R. M. Nims, and W. S. Gochenour, Jr.** 1972. Laboratory studies of tropical canine pancytopenia. Exp. Parasitol. **31:**53–59.
20. **Huxsoll, D. L., P. K. Hildebrandt, R. M. Nims, H. L. Amyx, and J. A. Ferguson.** 1970. Epizootiology of tropical canine pancytopenia. J. Wildl. Dis. **6:**220–225.
21. **Huxsoll, D. L., P. K. Hildebrandt, R. M. Nims, and J. S. Walker.** 1970. Tropical canine pancytopenia. J. Am. Vet. Med. Assoc. **157:**1627–1632.
22. **Lewis, G. E., Jr., M. Ristic, R. D. Smith, T. Lincoln, and E. H. Stephenson.** 1977. The brown dog tick Rhipicephalus sanguineus and the dog as experimental hosts of Ehrlichia canis. Am. J. Vet. Res. **38:**1953–1955.
23. **Madigan, J. E., and D. Gribble.** 1987. Equine ehrlichiosis in northern California: 49 cases (1968–1981). J. Am. Vet. Med. Assoc. **190:**445–448.
24. **Maeda, K., N. Markowitz, R. C. Hawley, M. Ristic, D. Cox, and J. E. McDade.** 1987. Human infection with Ehrlichia canis, a leukocytic rickettsia. N. Engl. J. Med. **316:** 853–856.
25. **Nyindo, M., D. L. Huxsoll, M. Ristic, I. Kakoma, J. L. Brown, C. A. Carson, and E. H. Stephenson.** 1980. Cell-mediated and humoral immune responses of German shepherd dogs and beagles to experimental infection with Ehrlichia canis. Am. J. Vet. Res. **41:**250–254.
26. **Nyindo, M. B., M. Ristic, D. L. Huxsoll, and A. R. Smith.**

1971. Tropical canine pancytopenia: in vitro cultivation of the causative agent—Ehrlichia canis. Am. J. Vet. Res. **32:**1651–1658.

27. **Palmer, J. E., R. H. Whitlock, and C. E. Benson.** 1986. Equine ehrlichial colitis (Potomac horse fever): recognition of the disease in Pennsylvania, New Jersey, New York, Ohio, Idaho, and Connecticut. J. Am. Vet. Med. Assoc. **189:** 197–199.
28. **Pearce, C. J., M. E. Conrad, P. E. Nolan, D. B. Fishbein, and J. E. Dawson.** 1988. Ehrlichiosis: a cause of bone marrow hypoplasia in humans. Am. J. Hematol. **28:**53–55.
29. **Petersen, L. R., L. A. Sawyer, D. B. Fishbein, P. W. Kelley, R. J. Thomas, L. A. Magnarelli, M. Redus, and J. E. Dawson.** 1989. An outbreak of ehrlichiosis in members of an Army Reserve unit exposed to ticks. J. Infect. Dis. **159:**562–568.
30. **Reardon, M. J., and K. R. Pierce.** 1981. Acute experimental canine ehrlichiosis. I. Sequential reaction of the hemic and lymphoreticular systems. Vet. Pathol. **18:**48–61.
31. **Rikihisa, Y., and B. D. Perry.** 1985. Causative ehrlichial organisms in Potomac horse fever. Infect. Immun. **49:**513–517.
32. **Ristic, M.** 1986. Pertinent characteristics of leukocytic rickettsiae of humans and animals, p. 182–187. *In* L. Leive (ed.), Microbiology—1986. American Society for Microbiology, Washington, D.C.
33. **Ristic, M., J. Dawson, C. J. Holland, and A. Jenny.** 1988. Susceptibility of dogs to infection with Ehrlichia risticii, causative agent of equine monocytic ehrlichiosis (Potomac horse fever). Am. J. Vet. Res. **49:**1497–1500.
34. **Ristic, M., C. J. Holland, J. E. Dawson, J. Sessions, and J. Palmer.** 1986. Diagnosis of equine monocytic ehrlichiosis (Potomac horse fever) by indirect immunofluorescence. J. Am. Vet. Med. Assoc. **189:**39–46.
35. **Ristic, M., and D. L. Huxsoll.** 1984. Ehrlichiae, p. 704–709. *In* N. R. Krieg and J. G. Holt (ed.), Bergey's manual of systematic bacteriology, vol. 1. The Williams & Wilkins Co., Baltimore.
36. **Ristic, M., D. L. Huxsoll, N. Tachibana, and G. Rapmund.** 1981. Evidence of a serologic relationship between Ehrlichia canis and Rickettsia sennetsu. Am. J. Trop. Med. Hyg. **30:**1324–1328.
37. **Ristic, M., D. L. Huxsoll, R. M. Weisiger, P. K. Hildebrandt, and M. B. Nyindo.** 1972. Serological diagnosis of tropical canine pancytopenia by indirect immunofluorescence. Infect. Immun. **6:**226–231.
38. **Robl, M. G.** 1985. Potomac horse fever: closing in on an unknown killer. Vet. Med. **80:**49–56.

38a. **Rohrbach, B. W., J. R. Harkess, S. A. Ewing, J. Kudlac, G. L. McKee, and G. R. Istre.** 1990. Epidemiological and clinical characteristics of persons with serologic evidence of *E. canis* infection. Am. J. Public Health **80:**442–445.

39. **Sells, D. M., P. K. Hildebrandt, G. E. Lewis Jr., M. B. Nyindo, and M. Ristic.** 1976. Ultrastructural observations on Ehrlichia equi organisms in equine granulocytes. Infect. Immun. **13:**273–280.
40. **Sessions, J. E.** 1986. Equine monocytic ehrlichiosis (synonym, Potomac horse fever): the disease and its impact, p. 194–195. *In* L. Leive (ed.), Microbiology—1986. American Society for Microbiology, Washington, D.C.
41. **Simpson, C. F.** 1974. Relationship of Ehrlichia canis-infected mononuclear cells to blood vessels of lungs. Infect. Immun. **10:**590–596.
42. **Smith, R. D., D. M. Sells, E. H. Stephenson, M. R. Ristic, and D. L. Huxsoll.** 1976. Development of Ehrlichia canis, causative agent of canine ehrlichiosis, in the tick Rhipicephalus sanguineus and its differentiation from a symbiotic Rickettsia. Am. J. Vet. Res. **37:**119–126.
43. **Tachibana, N.** 1986. Sennetsu fever: the disease, diagnosis, and treatment, p. 205–208. *In* L. Leive (ed.), Microbiology—1986. American Society for Microbiology, Washington, D.C.
44. **Taylor, J. P., T. G. Betz, D. B. Fishbein, M. A. Roberts, J. Dawson, and M. Ristic.** 1988. Serological evidence of possible human infection with Ehrlichia in Texas. J. Infect. Dis. **158:**217–220.
45. **Van Heerden, J., and A. Van Heerden.** 1981. Attempted treatment of canine ehrlichiosis with imidocarb dipropionate. J. S. Afr. Vet. Assoc. **52:**173–175.
46. **Woldehiwet, Z.** 1983. Tick-borne fever: a review. Vet. Res. Commun. **6:**163–175.
47. **Ziemer, E. L., R. H. Whitlock, J. E. Palmer, and P. A. Spencer.** 1987. Clinical and hematologic variables in ponies with experimentally induced equine ehrlichial colitis (Potomac horse fever). Am. J. Vet. Res. **48:**63–67.

Chapter 107

Antimicrobial Susceptibility Testing: General Considerations

CLYDE THORNSBERRY

In selecting an appropriate antimicrobial agent to treat an infection, one must consider (i) knowledge of the inherent in vitro susceptibility of the infecting organism to appropriate antimicrobial agents; (ii) the relationship of the susceptibility of the strain to that of other members of the same species; (iii) pharmacological properties, including toxicity, protein binding, distribution, absorption, and excretion, particularly under circumstances of existing or developing hepatic or renal failure; (iv) previous clinical experience in the treatment of infections caused by the same species; (v) the nature of the underlying pathological process, its natural history, and its response to chemotherapy; and (vi) the immune status of the host.

Of these factors, the concentrations of antimicrobial agents required to inhibit or kill organisms in vitro and those attained in body fluids during treatment are subject to direct measurement in the clinical laboratory with the caveat that laboratory analyses ignore all host factors and conditions. The purpose of this section is to provide descriptions of appropriate procedures for these purposes. In each case, the methods and recommendations chosen by the authors are a good representation of the state of the art and are generally accepted by the clinical microbiology community. In this edition, we have not only updated the methods but have also added material that rectifies serious omissions in the previous editions; we have also included for the first time a chapter that discusses tests on organisms other than bacteria and fungi. The chapters rectifying omissions are those on antibacterial agents and mechanisms of antimicrobial resistance; the third is a chapter that discusses antiviral and antiparasitic in vitro tests. It is anticipated that in the next edition, these three chapters will be greatly expanded.

The role of the laboratory in the selection and monitoring of chemotherapy was succinctly expressed by Theodore G. Anderson in the first edition of this Manual: "When selecting an antimicrobial agent for therapy, it is the physician's responsibility to take into consideration the pharmacological characteristics of the several drugs as well as their relative antimicrobial effectiveness. The responsibility of the laboratory is to provide information, through standardized in vitro tests, of the activity of appropriate antimicrobial agents against the organism in question." The methods presented in subsequent chapters are generally accepted in clinical laboratories within the United States and some other parts of the world, but in several cases they may not be universally accepted. Although there have been efforts to achieve international standardization—which continue at various levels today—different procedures have been developed and used by others in a number of countries. There is also no international agreement on the susceptibility breakpoints.

ANTIMICROBIAL SUSCEPTIBILITY TESTING

Influence of technical variation on susceptibility test results

The results of both dilution and diffusion susceptibility tests are influenced markedly by the reagents and conditions of the tests. These variables have been the source of considerable confusion in the past. Inoculum density, incubation time and temperature, pH, atmosphere, and stability of antimicrobial agents influence the endpoints obtained. Differences in constituents or ionic content of the medium, even between batches, may influence results, particularly with the sulfonamides, tetracyclines, polymyxins, aminoglycosides, quinolones, and some of the peptide-type agents. In addition, diffusion tests are influenced by the growth rate of the organism and by the type, depth, and concentration of the agar used. For these reasons, special emphasis has been placed on reference procedures and methodological standardization, because only in this way can adequate reproducibility be obtained in investigative and clinical work.

In each of the susceptibility tests described, the inoculum is derived from several colonies. This procedure is designed to reduce the chance of selecting variants derived from loss mutations (e.g., loss of penicillinase production in staphylococci) or segregants from R-factor resistance markers. It also increases the chance of including representatives of the more resistant organism if more than one strain is represented by colonies that cannot be distinguished morphologically. The use of several colonies to prepare the inoculum is a departure from traditional microbiological procedures and is still questioned by some users of the method. The final inocula are reasonably heavy, which increases the chance of detecting high-frequency mutations to resistance and heteroresistant strains, but there are arguments as to whether the inoculum used in the microdilution method is adequate to detect most clinically significant lower-frequency mutations. The media selected show generally good buffering qualities and reproducibility and are of physiological pH. A central criterion of the conditions to be used in effective diffusion, dilution, or automated tests is that the tests must be able to detect strains that carry clinically important resistance determinants.

Selection of susceptibility test methods

Diffusion test. The disk diffusion test has been the most widely used, but recently there has been a sharp increase in the number of laboratories using microdilution MIC methods, an automated method, or a combination of the two. The disk diffusion procedure, described in chapter 111, has been accepted by the Food and Drug Administration (FDA) and as a standard by the National Committee for Clinical Laboratory Standards (NCCLS). It is essentially a test that yields a qualitative result (although it has a quantitative basis) such as classification of an organism as susceptible, intermediate, moderately susceptible, or resistant. A major advantage of this procedure is its flexibility in the number and kind of antimicrobial agents that can be tested and the ease of setting up individual tests at any time. It is technically simple but requires careful attention to detail to obtain accurate and reproducible results. The test was meant to be used with rapidly growing organisms such as members of the family *Enterobacteriaceae*, *Staphylococcus* species, and enterococci, but it has been adapted to test other bacteria such as streptococci and *Pseudomonas*, *Acinetobacter*, *Haemophilus*, and *Neisseria* species and for specific procedures such as detecting strains of pneumococci that have developed increased resistance to penicillin (see chapter 111). In cases of urgency, clinical material can serve as the inoculum for the test if the precautions indicated in chapter 111 are followed, but this practice is not generally recommended.

The deficiencies of the diffusion test are its nonquantitative interpretation, its inapplicability to many slowly growing organisms and anaerobes, and its inaccuracy in predicting susceptibility (as opposed to resistance) with some antimicrobial agents, such as the polymyxins, that diffuse poorly. Overall, the disk diffusion procedure is effective for most routine testing, but it should be supplemented with a dilution test when it is inapplicable or when more quantitative results are needed.

Dilution test. The most quantitative method for antimicrobial susceptibility testing is one of the dilution tests (see chapter 110). The methods in general use are most often those described in the NCCLS standards. They yield direct quantitative results, are essentially not influenced by the growth rate of the organism, and avoid some of the complexities caused by the diffusion properties of certain antimicrobial agents. Dilution tests do not have the flexibility of the diffusion test, generally cannot be used for direct tests of clinical material because of the difficulty in detecting contamination, and if reported quantitatively, require that the clinician be able to interpret the result or be helped in doing so.

The primary indication for dilution tests is to obtain quantitative susceptibility results when these are important or necessary for proper management of antimicrobial therapy, as in cases of bacteremia, bacterial endocarditis, osteomyelitis, or other chronic infections. Also, quantitative information may be needed when drug dosage schedules and levels in serum must be closely monitored or when disk test results are inapplicable, equivocal, or unreliable, as with tests of slowly growing organisms, confirmation of susceptibility (as opposed to resistance) to the polymyxins, confirmation of resistance to the aminoglycosides, and tests with potentially toxic but clinically useful antimicrobial agents that yield intermediate, moderately susceptible, or equivocal results by the disk diffusion test. Some urinary tract infections may respond to ordinary dosages of some antimicrobial agents because of the high levels that these agents attain in the urine. In these cases, the precise degree of susceptibility of an organism may influence the choice of antimicrobial agent, its dosage, and its route of administration. Other indications for dilution methods are for testing the susceptibilities of anaerobes by the methods described in chapter 113 and for the determination of bactericidal activity or evidence of synergism or antagonism between antimicrobial agents against particular microorganisms (see chapter 115). Finally, dilution tests have been found to be practical and economical for routine purposes through the use of commercially available semiautomated microdilution techniques (see chapter 116). Although the primary reason for using an MIC method is to get a quantitative result, MICs may also be converted to a qualitative category result.

As with all susceptibility tests, the laboratory must control inoculum size and endpoint reading and must use a quality control system, with standard reference strains, that will give endpoints within the range of each series of dilutions of antimicrobial agent. For example, if seven concentrations were being tested, the ideal reference strain would have as its endpoint the fourth concentration, but an endpoint at the third or fifth concentration would be acceptable. Data from proficiency testing surveys show that intra- and interlaboratory reproducibility are better when well-controlled, prediluted commercial systems are used, but good results can be expected if the protocols used in chapter 110 are followed.

Tests on anaerobes. All of the factors related to antimicrobial susceptibility testing of anaerobic bacteria have been undergoing close scrutiny in the last 2 to 3 years. These factors include whether there is a need to test the bacteria, which species need testing, which antimicrobial agents need testing, the role of β-lactamase testing in therapy, which methods are acceptable, and the problems with each method. As indicated in chapter 113, the NCCLS has recommended against using the disk elution method because of its potential inaccuracies. Chapter 113 and the NCCLS standard M11 (and their references) should be studied for more details on these problems and recommendations.

Automated tests. A variety of mechanized or automated procedures have been developed for susceptibility testing; these are described in chapter 116. Some facilitate the performance and reading of traditional overnight susceptibility tests; others are designed to yield qualitative or quantitative results on the same day that the test is set up. Some of these procedures have already been evaluated by collaborative studies and have been reported to have a high degree of reproducibility. However, comparability of procedures providing rapid results with overnight dilution or diffusion tests has been more difficult to achieve with a few organism-antimicrobial agent combinations because the extent of inhibition of growth in the first few hours of contact may differ from that seen after overnight incubation. Many of these difficulties have been overcome by various alterations in the test procedure or by changes in the computer software. In past years, the systems studied most were the Vitek, MS-2/Avantage, and Autobac (chapter 116), but development is in progress to automate the microdilution systems so as to make them "walkaway" systems. The use of at least one of the older systems (Vitek) has increased dramatically recently, but it is too early to predict the role of the newer systems. Automated methods have been adopted for routine work in many laboratories, but like all methods, they present limitations that require use of a manual test as an alternate method.

Tests for antimicrobial agent-inactivating enzymes

In some instances, most resistant strains of bacteria among originally susceptible species owe their resistance exclusively to their ability to destroy or inactivate particular antimicrobial agents. This is the case with penicillin and ampicillin resistance of strains of staphylococci (methicillin resistance is not due to this enzyme), *Haemophilus influenzae, Neisseria gonorrhoeae, Moraxella (Branhamella) catarrhalis,* and *Bacteroides* species that produce β-lactamase. These enzymes can be detected rapidly and accurately with simple chemical procedures (chapters 112 and 115), and results are available more rapidly and thus can be used for earlier therapeutic decision making. One of these methods should definitely be used to test for β-lactamase production in *H. influenzae* from serious systemic infections. For the other organisms listed above, however, such analyses may not be needed routinely. Many microbiologists and clinicians feel that the high incidence of β-lactamase production in *Staphylococcus aureus* and *M. catarrhalis* warrants that all these organisms be considered β-lactamase positive (in terms of therapy) and thus resistant to the penicillins. Public health officials promote the routine testing of *N. gonorrhoeae* (as indicated in chapter 112), but some feel that the incidence of positive isolates is too low in their locales for such testing to be cost effective. In the NCCLS standard for susceptibility testing of anaerobes, caution is recommended in the use of β-lactamase results for therapy of anaerobic infections. There is consensus that these β-lactamase tests do not have a role in the development of therapeutic regimens for other bacteria. Procedures for β-lactamase tests are described in chapters 112 and 115.

Quality control

The development of quality control parameters by testing standard reference strains on a daily basis has been an important factor in the high level of performance that most laboratories have attained for antimicrobial susceptibility testing. However, because of the cost of daily quality control and the high level of performance of most laboratories, there has been a move toward weekly rather than daily quality control tests. The NCCLS has published guidelines for changing from daily to weekly testing. Another problem is the difficulty in quality controlling those tests in which one or two concentrations of antimicrobial agent are tested to derive a category result, i.e., susceptible, moderately susceptible, or resistant. Such tests are used in all of the automated tests (chapter 116) and for some drugs in the commercial microdilution systems (chapter 110). It is difficult to develop meaningful quality control programs for methods that test only one or two concentrations of an agent. Clearly, this is an area in which some creative developmental work is needed.

Interpretation of susceptibility tests: susceptibility and resistance

Interpretation of the quantitative MIC susceptibility test result and, indirectly, the disk diffusion test has three major components.

The first component is the relationship of the MIC or MBC of the antimicrobial agent for the organism to the concentration of antimicrobial agent in the blood (or in some cases in the urine or other body fluids) obtained with the dosage administered. Generally, this approach has proved to be clinically useful, but it is inevitably an incomplete model of the in vivo situation because the levels of antimicrobial agents in tissue are not usually known, the degree of protein binding varies by drug, the interaction of host defense mechanisms exerts an unmeasurable effect, and some aspects of the selection of test conditions are purely arbitrary.

The second component is the relationship of the susceptibility of the strain under test to that of other members of the same species. This knowledge is useful because the selection of resistant mutants or strains with extrachromosomal determinants of resistance has led to the appearance of populations of strains of some species well separated from the wild types that were previously uniformly susceptible to the antimicrobial agent. The resulting bimodal distribution of susceptibilities correlates well with clinical responsiveness. Thus, a strain falling in the more resistant population is considered, a priori, a resistant member of that species. In some cases, e.g., the relatively penicillin-resistant pneumococci, the emerging resistance is more difficult to categorize. A pneumococcal strain with an MIC of 0.5 μg/ml may be resistant to penicillin if the organism is causing meningitis but susceptible if it is causing pneumonia; such a strain can be readily eliminated from the blood but not from the spinal fluid.

The third component is clinical experience with treatment of the particular type of infection involved.

An ideal interpretation of susceptibility test results takes into account these factors independently. From a practical point of view, however, organisms are frequently allocated to predetermined susceptible, resistant, intermediate, or moderately susceptible categories. This approach was considered by the International Collaborative Study, and more recently by the NCCLS, to be still useful and sometimes necessary in light of the available technical methods and general understanding of the principles of chemotherapy. The categories recommended for the diffusion test given in chapter 111 have been based on the synthesis of the first two criteria given above. The categories have been defined as (i) susceptible, implying that an infection caused by the strain tested may be appropriately treated with the antimicrobial agents and dosages recommended for that type of infection and infecting species, unless otherwise contraindicated; (ii) resistant, containing strains not completely inhibited within the usual therapeutic dosage range; (iii) intermediate, comprising a buffer zone which prevents major interpretive discrepancies that might result from small, uncontrolled technical factors; and (iv) moderately susceptible, for strains that may respond to concentrations attainable by the maximum safe dosage and strains that may respond because they are causing infection in areas, such as portions of the urinary tract, in which the antimicrobial agent is concentrated. The category systems of the disk diffusion method do not take into consideration the higher levels in the urinary tract for most drugs or the relatively low levels in blood achieved with oral as opposed to parenteral dosages of some antimicrobial agents (although "susceptible" implies that oral dosage could be used where appropriate). Categorization has also been done for MIC results (chapter 110). The clinical extrapolation of these categories is, of course, subject to the considerations given in the first paragraph of this chapter.

In recent years, there has been a concerted effort by various individuals and groups to establish interpretive breakpoints and quality control parameters for new antimicrobial agents at the time the agents are approved for use. The FDA, of course, has the legal authority and charge to set these standards, but the NCCLS also makes recommendations and has published guidelines for developing these data for new antimicrobial agents (NCCLS document M23). For most drugs, the FDA and NCCLS agree on their recommendations, but sometimes they do not, thus creating some confusion. When disagreement occurs, there is no right solution to the problem, and the user must decide which recommendations to use. Usually these differences are not great and can be reconciled.

The categories of susceptibility are developed to ensure a high degree of predictability. In fact, bacteriological and clinical cure rates are now routinely used in determining the applicability of proposed breakpoints and in reassessing older ones. It should be emphasized, however, that an erroneous susceptibility result is only one of several reasons for clinical failures; others include wrong diagnosis, various host factors such as being immunocompromised, the presence of an abscess or foreign body, superinfection, and inadequate levels of antimicrobial agent at the site of infection.

Indications for susceptibility tests in the clinical laboratory

Antimicrobial susceptibility tests are indicated for those organisms contributing to the infectious process whose susceptibility cannot be predicted from knowledge of their identity. This applies in particular to *S. aureus*, to gram-negative fermentative and nonfermentative organisms, to some anaerobes, and to unusual and opportunistic species playing a pathogenic role. Specific patterns of susceptibility (antibiograms) may be characteristic of a species and may therefore assist in identification of the species. Antibiograms may also be determined for epidemiological reasons because the occurrence of an unusual antibiogram for a given species often assists in the recognition of common-source outbreaks and patterns of cross-infection. Many microbiology laboratories now publish periodic antibiograms for use by their clinical staff.

Routine susceptibility tests are not needed when resistance to the antimicrobial agent of choice, e.g., that of *Streptococcus pyogenes* and *Neisseria meningitidis* to penicillin, has not been, or has been rarely, described, but this must be constantly reviewed. Susceptibility testing should be avoided on members of the normal flora in their normal habitat and on organisms that are known not to be playing a pathogenic role; to conduct such tests is both wasteful and misleading. The routine diffusion susceptibility test described in chapter 111 should never be performed on organisms for which the interpretive criteria are not applicable.

Selection of antimicrobial agents for testing

Because of the rapid proliferation of antimicrobial agents, selection of a panel for routine testing has become more difficult. To attempt to test them all is not feasible for economic reasons and is also unnecessary because of similarities in spectra of activity and pharmacokinetics of many antimicrobial agents. In the past, the selection process was made easier because the FDA recognized specific class disks for use in the diffusion test. The designation of class disks has become more difficult because many of the newer antimicrobial agents are sufficiently different to demand separate disks. It is unlikely that the FDA will designate class compounds in the future.

Most of the antimicrobial agents approved since the mid-1970s have had a disk approved by the FDA, and it is likely that all future antimicrobial agents will also have disks approved if they are requested. In other words, the FDA is unlikely to designate class disks in the future, and no other agency in the United States has the legal authority to do so.

As a result of these developments, each laboratory must develop its own policy for selecting a basic set of drugs for routine testing. Factors that should be considered in making these selections include the epidemiology for the individual medical center (the organisms that are causing infections and the antimicrobial agents to which they are susceptible), hospital antimicrobial agent usage patterns, including those that are in the formulary, and the toxicity, cost, and similarities of activity and pharmacokinetics of the drugs themselves.

One approach to this problem is to establish a hospital committee composed, at a minimum, of representatives from microbiology, pharmacy, and infectious disease departments but also with representatives from the areas of pathology, infection control, epidemiology, and medical and surgical services. This committee should select the drugs that will be included in the "routine" test panels on the basis of their own hospital epidemiology, clinician preferences (all other things being equal), cost, toxicity, and other relevant considerations. For example, from second- and third-generation cephalosporins used for enteric organisms, one from each group could be selected. It is likely that the NCCLS will have the most current lists of class drugs, since frequent supplements are used to update their standards.

The antimicrobial agents selected for testing should also be limited to those that are clinically useful and appropriate for the site of infection, except when antibiograms are used for epidemiological purposes or when particular antimicrobial agents yield taxonomically useful information.

To avoid confusion, results of tests on antimicrobial agents that are inappropriate in therapy and that are tested for epidemiological or taxonomic purposes should not be reported to the physician except in special cases, such as when such tests are part of a collaborative research effort.

The NCCLS has begun an effort to use its standards, particularly Table 1 in both the M2 (disk) and M7 (MIC) standards, to influence more selective testing and reporting. Although most would agree with the intent, the goal will be difficult to attain.

SPECIAL TESTS AND ASSAYS

The susceptibility tests discussed above make up the bulk of the clinical laboratory tests that are ordered to assist clinicians in the choice of chemotherapeutic agents. They may be supplemented with other procedures in certain complex clinical situations, especially those involving endocarditis, severe infections in immunologically compromised patients, and cases in which drug-tolerant organisms are suspected. In these cases, a determination of bactericidal concentrations or of the effect of combination of antimicrobial agents may be required. Direct tests of the ability of the antimicrobial agent in the serum of the patient to inhibit or kill the infecting organism may also be helpful in monitoring the adequacy of dosage schedules (see chapter 115). No standard methods for synergy tests are extant, and there is much disagreement about the role of tolerance in therapeutic responses. The procedures outlined in this Manual can continue to serve as a basis for further studies toward methodological standardization of these important tests, but clinicians should recognize that the usefulness of data collected by the present methods may be limited by the problems inherent in these methods.

The need to determine the amount of antimicrobial agent present in serum, urine, other fluids, or tissue has increased, especially for agents such as aminoglycosides for which potentially toxic and therapeutic levels are very close. Serum assays are thus required to ensure that antimicrobial agent concentrations in the blood are within a safe but effective range. This is particularly true for patients with renal deficiency, in whom levels of antimicrobial agent in serum may be less predictable. A number of methods have been developed for performing these tests with commercial systems. Both older and newer methods are described in chapter 119.

TRENDS AND FUTURE NEEDS

Since the last edition of this Manual, the NCCLS standards for susceptibility tests have been revised and published. These standards undergo constant revision and thus are the most current source of information on new agents and other changes. Therefore, the NCCLS supplemental tables and documents should serve as the most up-to-date references for susceptibility testing in the microbiology laboratory. They also serve as the most current source of information on quality control values for standard strains, even with antimicrobial agents that have just been approved. The use of the NCCLS documents as current references is a practice that should continue, but it is especially important that mechanisms be maintained for the regular updating of reference procedures, interpretive standards for new antimicrobial agents, recommendations for basic routine sets of antimicrobial agents for testing, and data on performance of tests on quality control strains.

Developments in mechanization, automation, and commercially available test kits have continued. However, it is apparent that the prediction that the use of the older automated systems, as a group, would decrease was inaccurate; at least one of these systems is being used with increasing frequency, and there is little evidence that this trend will lessen in the near future. For the present, the principal methods used in the United States are the standard disk diffusion, microdilution (mostly commercial), and Vitek methods, with use of the latter two increasing. The lesson that has been learned is that clinical microbiologists will change the methods that they use but usually do so slowly.

It is impossible to predict which methods will predominate in the future, but the major need is very clear—the clinical microbiology laboratory is still plagued with the problem of excessive time lapse between the receipt of a specimen and the reporting of results. Although we have called some tests rapid, they are in fact rapid only after isolation of the organism(s). One of the greatest needs is to find ways to identify the pathogen and perform susceptibility testing within 1 to 2 h of collecting the specimen.

Anyone contemplating adopting a new or different susceptibility testing method should obtain as much information on it as possible from published data, approving agencies, and contemporary users of the systems. Comparisons with the currently used method should also be carried out before the final decision is made.

Agreement is needed on the methodologies to be used for determining bactericidal endpoints, measuring the effects of combinations, and performing serum inhibitory or bactericidal tests. In the absence of standardized methods or reference procedures, results from different laboratories cannot be compared with confidence; moreover, an adequate base of experience has not been developed for fully satisfactory interpretation of the results. For all of these procedures, the kinetics of microbial killing by antimicrobial agents make it essential that statistical endpoints, such as those recommended in chapter 115, be accepted. Studies are needed to develop standard methods that take into consideration the problems of ensuring contact between antimicrobial agent and organism and of transferring an adequate sample to determine numbers of unkilled organisms without carrying over inhibitory levels of the antimicrobial agent. The work of the NCCLS on such methods is a good start and must be continued.

When acceptable standard methods for the determination of MBCs are adopted, further studies of the significance of "tolerance" should be done. Although genotypic and phenotypic tolerances do occur, many of the conclusions and suggestions that were made in the past were based on results obtained with studies using procedures that were poorly reproducible because of the inadequacies of the methods being used. With a well-developed standard method, the true incidence and significance of tolerance can be established for each organism and antimicrobial agent in each institution, and the marked interlaboratory discrepancies in the designation of tolerance can be eliminated. More important, the therapeutic significance of tolerance can be established.

The present mood of cost consciousness and the use of diagnosis-related groups for reimbursement will probably have an effect on antimicrobial susceptibility testing in clinical laboratories. The cost of quality control is already an issue that has led many laboratories to change to weekly instead of daily testing. It is likely that these developments will require a more creative approach to selecting organisms and drugs for testing and to providing data that will permit the clinician to develop a therapeutic scheme that will be the most effective at the least cost. This approach might include the development of computer programs to integrate MICs, MBCs, and levels of drugs in serum to determine the best and most economical dosage schedules. Studies in these areas should be considered.

In summary, we can look forward to improved performance of media and of procedures for orthodox susceptibility tests and to improvements in the selection and dissemination of interpretive recommendations. Quality control tests, usually on a weekly basis, can be used efficaciously in laboratories that have demonstrated high levels of proficiency with some of the methods, but quality control of certain methods is still a problem. There has been a large increase in the number of laboratories in which microdilution MIC tests and at least one automated system are used, and this trend will probably continue. It is likely that all laboratories will have the capability of performing MIC tests in conjunction with diffusion or other routine methods. Commercial systems for microdilution MICs will generally result in better reproducibility through the elimination of many sources of technical error, but tests prepared in house should be acceptable if the standard recommendations are followed. The need for reference procedures for determining bactericidal endpoints, interactions of combinations of antimicrobial agents, and bactericidal activities of serum continues so that interpretations of the test results can be refined through cumulative experience. Recent developments have increased the usefulness of laboratory procedures in the selection and monitoring of chemotherapy, and this trend will likely continue.

Chapter 108

Antibacterial Agents

JOSEPH D. C. YAO AND ROBERT C. MOELLERING, JR.

Antimicrobial chemotherapy has played a vital role in the treatment of human infectious diseases in the 20th century. Since the discovery of penicillin in the 1920s, literally hundreds of antimicrobial agents have been developed or synthesized, and dozens of these are currently available for clinical use. While the broad number and variety of agents available provide a great deal of flexibility for the clinician in the use of these agents, the sheer numbers and continuing development of agents available make it difficult for clinicians to keep up with developments in the field. Similarly, they present significant challenges for the clinical microbiologist who must decide which agents are appropriate for inclusion in routine and specialized susceptibility testing.

This chapter provides an overview of the antibacterial agents currently marketed in the United States, with major emphasis on their mechanisms of action, spectra of activity, important pharmacologic parameters, and toxicities. Antibiotics that have fallen into disuse or remained investigational will be mentioned only briefly.

PENICILLINS

The penicillins (Table 1) comprise a group of natural and semisynthetic antibiotics containing the chemical nucleus 6-aminopenicillanic acid, which consists of a β-lactam ring fused to a thiazolidine ring (Fig. 1a). The naturally occurring compounds are produced by a number of *Penicillium* spp. The penicillins differ from one another in substitution at the 6 position, where changes in the side chain may modify their pharmacokinetic and antibacterial properties.

Mechanism of action

The major antibacterial action of penicillins is derived from their ability to inhibit a number of bacterial enzymes, namely, penicillin-binding proteins (PBPs), that are essential for peptidoglycan synthesis (443). This ability to inhibit bacterial cell wall transpeptidases usually confers on the penicillins bactericidal activity against gram-positive bacteria. The bactericidal activity of the penicillins is often related to their ability to trigger membrane-associated autolytic enzymes that destroy the cell wall. Other minor mechanisms of action include inhibition of bacterial endopeptidase and glycosidase, enzymes involved in bacterial cell growth (147). There is also recent evidence suggesting that penicillins may inhibit RNA synthesis in some bacteria, causing death without cell lysis, but the significance of these observations remains to be proven (247).

Pharmacology

Oral absorption differs markedly among the penicillins. As a natural congener of penicillin G, penicillin V resists gastric acid inactivation and is better absorbed from the gastrointestinal tract than is penicillin G. Amoxicillin is a semisynthetic analog of ampicillin and has greater gastrointestinal absorption than ampicillin (95 versus 40% absorption). Cyclacillin is an oral semisynthetic analog of ampicillin that offers no established advantage over the latter drug. Bacampicillin and pivampicillin are ampicillin esters that are considerably better absorbed from the gastrointestinal tract than is ampicillin or amoxicillin. These esters are inactive until naturally occurring esterases in the intestinal mucosa and serum hydrolyze them to release the parent compound, ampicillin, into the serum. The isoxazolyl penicillins, such as oxacillin, cloxacillin, and dicloxacillin, as well as nafcillin, are acid stable and are also absorbed from the gastrointestinal tract, in contradistinction to certain other antistaphylococcal penicillins, such as methicillin, which are not acid resistant and cannot be given by the oral route.

Repository forms of penicillin G, available in procaine or benzathine, delay absorption from an intramuscular depot. Procaine penicillin G provides detectable levels for 12 to 24 h, suitable for treatment of uncomplicated pneumococcal pneumonia and gonorrhea due to fully susceptible organisms. Benzathine penicillin G achieves very low blood levels for prolonged periods of time (3 to 4 weeks), and it is useful for the therapy of syphilis and for prophylaxis of streptococcal pharyngitis and rheumatic fever.

Penicillins are well distributed to many body compartments, including lung, liver, kidney, muscle, bone, and placenta. Penetration into the eye, brain, cerebrospinal fluid (CSF), and prostate is poor in the absence of inflammation. These drugs are metabolized to a small degree and are rapidly excreted, essentially unchanged, via the kidney. With average half-lives of 0.5 to 1.5 h, they are usually administered every 4 to 6 h to maintain effective blood levels. The renal tubular excretion of penicillins can be blocked by probenecid, prolonging their serum half-lives.

Dosage reduction of most penicillins is necessary only in severe renal insufficiency (creatinine clearance of ≤10 ml/min). Dosages of all penicillins except nafcillin and the isoxazolyl penicillins are adjusted for hemodialysis. Peritoneal dialysis requires dosage reduction of carbenicillin and ticarcillin.

Spectrum of activity

The penicillins have antibacterial activity against most gram-positive and many gram-negative and anaerobic organisms. Penicillin G is very effective against penicillin-susceptible *Staphylococcus aureus, Streptococcus pneumoniae, Streptococcus pyogenes,* viridans streptococci, *Streptococcus bovis, Neisseria gonorrhoeae, Neisseria meningitidis, Pasteurella multocida,* anaerobic

TABLE 1. Penicillins

Natural	Semisynthetic, extended spectrum—*continued*
Benzylpenicillin (penicillin G)	Carboxypenicillins
Phenoxymethyl penicillin (penicillin V)	Carbenicillin
	Ticarcillin
Semisynthetic	Ureidopenicillins
Penicillinase resistant	Azlocillin
Methicillin	Mezlocillin
Nafcillin	Piperacillin
Isoxazolyl penicillins	Amidinopenicillin
Oxacillin	Amdinocillin
Cloxacillin	Penicillin + β-lactamase inhibitors
Dicloxacillin	Ampicillin-sulbactam (Unasyn)
Extended spectrum	Amoxicillin-clavulanate (Augmentin)
Aminopenicillins	Ticarcillin-clavulanate (Timentin)
Ampicillin	
Amoxicillin	
Cyclacillin	
Bacampicillin	
Pivampicillin	

cocci, *Clostridium* spp., *Fusobacterium* spp., and many *Bacteroides* spp. except for *Bacteroides fragilis* (15). It is the drug of choice for syphilis and *Actinomyces* infections. Penicillin V has a spectrum of activity similar to that of penicillin G except that it is less active against *N. gonorrhoeae*. Penicillinase-resistant penicillins, of which methicillin is the prototype, are primarily effective against penicillinase-producing staphylococci (158, 277). The agents are at least 25 times more active than other penicillins against penicillinase-positive *S. aureus* and *Streptococcus epidermidis*. Although they are also active against *S. pneumoniae* and *S. pyogenes*, their MICs for these organisms are higher than those of penicillin G. They are not active against enterococci, member of the family *Enterobacteriaceae*, *Pseudomonas* spp., and *B. fragilis*.

Ampicillin and amoxicillin have spectra of activity similar to that of penicillin G, but they are more active against enterococci and *Listeria monocytogenes* (271, 272). Although they are also more active against *Haemophilus influenzae* and *Haemophilus parainfluenzae*, up to 25% of *H. influenzae* have become resistant, usually because of β-lactamase production. *Salmonella* and *Shigella* spp., including *Salmonella typhi*, and many strains of *Escherichia coli* and *Proteus mirabilis* are susceptible to these agents. Ampicillin is more effective against shigellae, whereas amoxicillin is more active against salmonellae. Both of these agents are degraded by β-lactamase and are inactive against many *Enterobacteriaceae* and *Pseudomonas* spp.

The carboxypenicillins and ureidopenicillins have increased activity against gram-negative bacteria that are resistant to ampicillin. Although they are susceptible to staphylococcal penicillinase, they are more stable against hydrolysis by the β-lactamases of *Enterobacteriaceae* and *Pseudomonas aeruginosa*. Carbenicillin and ticarcillin are relatively active against streptococci and enterococci and are also active against *Haemophilus* spp., *Neisseria* spp., and a variety of anaerobes (139,

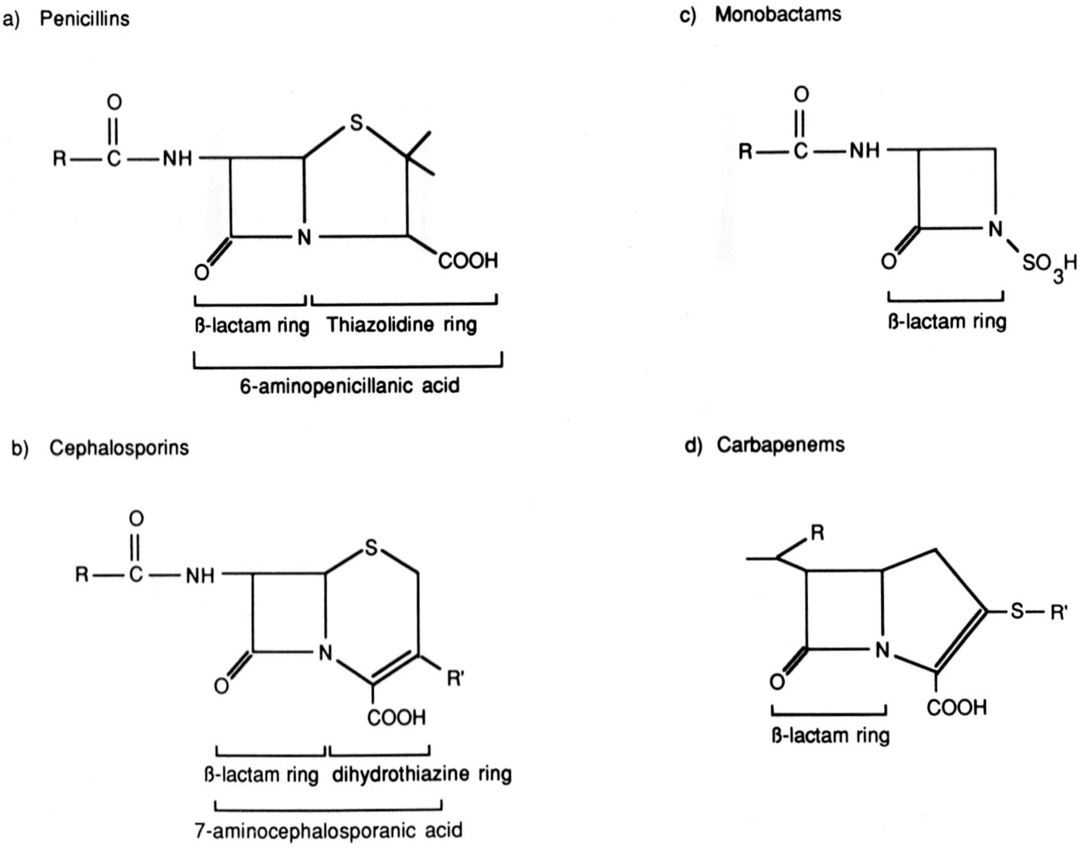

a) Penicillins

ß-lactam ring Thiazolidine ring

6-aminopenicillanic acid

b) Cephalosporins

ß-lactam ring dihydrothiazine ring

7-aminocephalosporanic acid

c) Monobactams

ß-lactam ring

d) Carbapenems

ß-lactam ring

FIG. 1. Chemical structures of β-lactam antibiotics.

286). They inhibit many *Enterobacteriaceae* but are inactive against *Klebsiella* spp.

The ureidopenicillins have greater in vitro activity against streptococci and enterococci than do the carboxypenicillins, and they inhibit more than 75% of *Klebsiella* spp. (100, 136, 425). They have excellent activity against many *Enterobacteriaceae* and anaerobic bacteria, including *B. fragilis*. On a weight basis, their activities in decreasing order of potency against *P. aeruginosa* are as follows: piperacillin, azlocillin > mezlocillin, ticarcillin > carbenicillin (75). These agents also act synergistically with aminoglycosides against *P. aeruginosa*.

Amdinocillin, formerly known as mecillinam, is a penicillanic acid derivative with poor activity against gram-positive organisms, *Haemophilus* and *Neisseria* spp., and anaerobic bacteria (273). By binding to PBP 2 of *Enterobacteriaceae* (279), this agent inhibits many gram-negative bacteria, including *E. coli, Klebsiella, Enterobacter, Citrobacter, Salmonella,* and *Shigella* spp., and some *Serratia* strains (328). It has variable activity against *Proteus* spp. and does not inhibit *Pseudomonas* spp. When combined with other β-lactam drugs, amdinocillin acts synergistically against gram-negative bacilli because of complementary binding to PBPs (275, 280). Its use is limited mainly to the therapy of urinary tract infections and associated bacteremias.

Adverse effects

Common reactions to penicillins include allergic skin rashes, diarrhea, and drug fever. Severe anaphylactic reactions, which can be fatal, may occur in previously sensitized patients rechallenged with penicillins but fortunately are quite rare. At high doses (usually $>30 \times 10^6$ U/day), penicillin G can cause myoclonic twitching and seizures due to central nervous system toxicity. All of the penicillins may cause interstitial nephritis on an allergic basis, but methicillin is more likely than the other penicillins to cause this complication. Hepatitis has been associated with prolonged use of oxacillin. High-dose carbenicillin can result in sodium overload and hypokalemia. Neutropenia may occur with any of the penicillins. Thrombocytopenia and Coombs-positive hemolytic anemia are rare complications of penicillin therapy. Bleeding tendencies due to interference with platelet function can occur with the use of carboxypenicillins and ureidopenicillins (122). Although pseudomembranous colitis has been associated with all the penicillins, it occurs more frequently with ampicillin (163).

CEPHALOSPORINS

Cephalosporins are derivatives of the fermentation products of species of the fungus *Cephalosporium*. They contain a 7-aminocephalosporanic acid nucleus, which consists of a β-lactam ring fused to a dihydrothiazine ring (Fig. 1b). Various substitutions at the 3 and 7 positions alter their antibacterial activity and pharmacokinetic properties. Addition of a methoxy group at position 7 of the β-lactam ring results in a new group of compounds called cephamycins, which are highly resistant to a variety of β-lactamases.

Mechanism of action

Similar to the penicillins, cephalosporins act by binding to PBPs of susceptible organisms, thereby interfering with synthesis of peptidoglycan of the bacterial cell wall. In addition, these β-lactam agents may produce bactericidal effects by triggering autolytic enzymes in the cell envelope (443).

Pharmacology

Most cephalosporins require parenteral administration, but a few are available in oral form. Relatively high concentrations of these agents are attained across the placenta and in synovial, pleural, pericardial, and peritoneal fluids. Bile levels are usually high, especially with cefoperazone, which is excreted mainly in the bile. Cefuroxime, ceftizoxime, cefotaxime, ceftriaxone, cefoperazone, and moxalactam penetrate well into the CSF and are useful for treatment of meningitis.

Cephalothin, cephapirin, and cefotaxime are converted to the desacetyl forms before excretion. All cephalosporins except cefoperazone are excreted primarily by the kidney, and for these drugs, dosage adjustments are necessary in patients with renal insufficiency (creatinine clearance of <50 ml/min). Like that of the penicillins, the renal excretion of cephalosporins is impeded by probenecid. In general, these agents are removed by hemodialysis but not by peritoneal dialysis.

Spectrum of activity

Cephalosporins are classified by a well-accepted but somewhat arbitrary scheme of grouping by generations, based on general features of their antibacterial activity (Table 2). The first-generation drugs, exemplified by cephalothin and cefazolin, have good gram-positive activity and relatively modest gram-negative activity. They

TABLE 2. Cephalosporins

Drug	Serum half-life (h)
First generation	
Cefadroxil	1.5
Cefazolin	1.5
Cephalexin	1.3
Cephaloridine	1.3
Cephalothin	0.6
Cephapirin	1.3
Cephradine	1.3
Second generation	
Cefaclor	0.8
Cefamandole	0.8
Cefonicid	4.5
Ceforanide	3.0
Cefotiam	1.0
Cefuroxime	1.5
Cefotetan	4.0
Cefoxitin	0.8
Third generation	
Cefixime	3.5
Cefoperazone	1.9
Cefotaxime	1.1
Ceftazidime	1.8
Ceftizoxime	1.7
Ceftriaxone	8.0
Moxalactam	1.0

are active against penicillin-susceptible and -resistant *S. aureus* as well as *S. pneumoniae, S. pyogenes,* and other aerobic and anaerobic streptococci (29, 61, 170, 330, 351). Methicillin-resistant *S. aureus, S. epidermidis,* and enterococci are resistant. Some *Enterobacteriaceae* are susceptible, including many strains of *E. coli, Klebsiella* spp., and *Proteus mirabilis. Pseudomonas,* including *P. aeruginosa,* many *Proteus* spp., and *Serratia* and *Enterobacter* spp. are resistant. These agents are active against penicillin-susceptible anaerobes except *B. fragilis.* They have only modest activity against *H. influenzae.*

The second-generation cephalosporins are stable to certain β-lactamases found in gram-negative bacteria and as a result have increased activity against gram-negative organisms. The agents are more active than first-generation drugs against *E. coli, Klebsiella* spp., and *Proteus* spp. Their activity also extends to cover some *Enterobacter* and *Serratia* strains, and they have good activity against *Haemophilus* spp., *Neisseria* spp., and many anaerobes (37, 117, 262, 355). Cefuroxime (as well as its axetil ester) (299), cefamandole (255), and cefonicid (3) are active against ampicillin-resistant *Haemophilus* spp. However, cefamandole exhibits a significant inoculum effect and is not suitable for treating life-threatening infections due to *H. influenzae.* Ceforanide and cefotiam have a spectrum of antibacterial activity similar to that of cefamandole. However, ceforanide is less active than cefamandole against gram-positive cocci (18), whereas cefotiam is more active against staphylococci (442). Cefoxitin and cefotetan are unique in that they have marked activity against anaerobes, including *B. fragilis* (65, 448). Cefotetan has the advantage of more prolonged serum half-life. Cefoxitin is also active against penicillin-resistant strains of *N. gonorrhoeae* (354). None of the second-generation agents is active against *Pseudomonas* spp.

Third-generation cephalosporins are generally less active than the first-generation agents against gram-positive cocci, but they are much more potent against the *Enterobacteriaceae* and *P. aeruginosa.* Their potent broad spectra of gram-negative activity are due to their stability to β-lactamases and their ability to penetrate through the outer cell envelope of gram-negative bacilli (121, 276, 412). There are two subgroups among these agents: those with potent activity against *P. aeruginosa* (ceftazidime and cefoperazone) and those without such activity (ceftizoxime, cefotaxime, ceftriaxone, and moxalactam).

Cefotaxime inhibits more than 90% of strains of *Enterobacteriaceae,* including those resistant to aminoglycosides. The MICs for 90% of strains tested (MIC_{90}s) of *E. coli, Proteus* spp., and *Klebsiella* spp. are <0.5 μg/ml. Its activity against strains of *Serratia marcescens, Enterobacter cloacae,* and *Acinetobacter* spp. is variable, and it is inactive against *P. aeruginosa* (334, 365). It has moderate activity against anaerobes but is inferior to cefoxitin and cefotetan against most of these isolates.

Ceftizoxime, ceftriaxone, and moxalactam have spectra of activity similar to that of cefotaxime (71, 138, 459), with a few exceptions. Ceftriaxone is the most active agent against penicillinase-positive or -negative strains of *N. gonorrhoeae* (204, 289). It is effective as single-dose therapy for infections caused by these organisms. Because of its long serum half-life (the longest of the currently available cephalosporins), ceftriaxone is used frequently in outpatient antibiotic therapy of serious infections. Moxalactam, an oxa-β-lactam, is less active against gram-positive cocci, including staphylococci and streptococci. It has slightly more activity against *Pseudomonas* spp. than cefotaxime does. It is the most active third-generation agent against anaerobes, including *B. fragilis,* against which it is comparable to cefoxitin (205, 342).

Cefoperazone is less active than cefotaxime against many *Enterobacteriaceae* and gram-positive cocci. However, it has activity against *P. aeruginosa,* with an MIC_{50} of ≤16 μg/ml (38, 202). Its activity against anaerobes is similar to that of cefotaxime. Ceftazidime is the most potent of the currently available cephalosporins against *P. aeruginosa,* with an MIC_{90} of <8 μg/ml (62, 236, 287). It is more active than the ureidopenicillins against these strains. This agent has activity similar to that of cefotaxime against the *Enterobacteriaceae* but is not as active against gram-positive cocci. It has little activity against gram-negative anaerobes.

Cefixime, the first oral third-generation cephalosporin, has activity against gram-negative aerobes similar to that of ceftizoxime (19, 206, 283). It is more stable than other oral cephaloporins (cephalexin, cephradine, cefaclor, and cefuroxime axetil) against gram-negative bacterial β-lactamases. Compared with these agents, cefixime is equally active against streptococci but considerably less active against *S. aureus.* None of the currently available cephalosporins is active against enterococci.

Adverse effects

Cephalosporins are generally very well tolerated. The most common side effects are diarrhea and hypersensitivity reactions such as rash, drug fever, and serum sickness. Cross-reactions with these drugs occur in only 3 to 7% of penicillin-allergic patients (6). Other infrequent side effects include pseudomembranous colitis, elevated serum creatinine and transaminase levels, leukopenia, thrombocytopenia, and Coombs-positive hemolytic anemia. These abnormalities are usually mild and reversible. Prolonged use of ceftriaxone has been associated with formation of gallbladder sludge, which usually resolves after the drug is discontinued (362), and rarely cholecystitis (194).

Disulfiramlike reactions have been described in patients receiving cefamandole, cefotetan, cefoperazone, and moxalactam. This reaction is attributed to the *N*-methylthiotetrazole side chain of these antibiotics, which is similar to the chemical structure of disulfiram (43, 316). Hypoprothrombinemia and bleeding tendencies have been observed with these cephalosporins. Causes of the coagulopathy included (i) alteration of normal gut flora by the antibiotics, inhibiting the synthesis of vitamin K and its precursors and (ii) the *N*-methythiotetrazole side chain, which inhibits the vitamin K-dependent carboxylase enzyme responsible for converting clotting factors II, VII, IX, and X to their active forms and also prevents regeneration of active vitamin K from its inactive form (24, 26, 360). Therapy with high doses of moxalactam, especially in debilitated patients with impaired renal function, has resulted in clinical bleeding. As a result, its use has been significantly curtailed.

OTHER β-LACTAM ANTIBIOTICS

Aztreonam

Aztreonam is the only monobactam antibiotic currently in clinical use. The monobactams are β-lactams with various side chains affixed to a monocyclic nucleus (Fig. 1c).

Mechanism of action

Aztreonam binds primarily to PBP 3 of gram-negative aerobes, including *P. aeruginosa,* thereby disrupting bacterial cell wall synthesis. It is not hydrolyzed by most commonly occurring plasmid- and chromosomally mediated β-lactamases, and it does not induce the production of these enzymes (45).

Pharmacology

Given intravenously, aztreonam is widely distributed to body tissues and fluids. Average serum drug concentrations exceed the MIC_{90}s of most *Enterobacteriaceae* by four to eight times for 8 h and are inhibitory to *P. aeruginosa* for 4 h. It crosses inflamed meninges in sufficient amount to be potentially therapeutic for meningitis caused by susceptible organisms. Its serum half-life is about 1.7 h, and it is excreted mainly unchanged by the kidney. Dosage modification is necessary for patients with renal failure. The drug is removed by both hemodialysis and peritoneal dialysis.

Spectrum of activity

The antibacterial activity of aztreonam is limited to aerobic gram-negative bacilli, inhibiting most *Enterobacteriaceae, Neisseria* spp., and *Haemophilus* spp. with MIC_{90}s of ≤0.5 μg/ml (20, 196, 403). It has significant activity against *P. aeruginosa, Enterobacter* spp., and *Serratia marcescens,* with most strains being inhibited at ≤16 μg/ml. However, many *Acinetobacter* spp., *Pseudomonas cepacia,* and *Xanthomonas maltophilia* are resistant. It shows in vitro synergism when combined with aminoglycosides against 30 to 60% of aztreonam-susceptible organisms, including *P. aeruginosa* and aminoglycoside-resistant gram-negative bacilli (44, 393). Bacterial tolerance and inoculum effect are generally not seen with this agent. Aztreonam is not active against gram-positive bacteria and anaerobes.

Adverse effects

Aztreonam is generally a safe agent, with a toxicity profile similar to those of other β-lactam drugs (292). Nausea, diarrhea, skin rash, eosinophilia, mild elevation of serum transaminases, and transiently elevated serum creatinine level have occurred. It has minimal cross-reactivity with other β-lactams, and it can be used safely in patients allergic to penicillins or cephalosporins (4, 361). Hematologic abnormalities have not been reported.

Carbapenems

Imipenem (*N*-formimidoyl thienamycin) is the first carbapenem antimicrobial agent developed for clinical use. It is a semisynthetic derivative of thienamycin which is produced by *Streptomyces* spp. Thienamycins differ from other β-lactams in having a *trans* configuration of the hydroxyethyl side chain at position 6 and lacking a sulfur or oxygen atom in the bicyclic nucleus (Fig. 1d). The unique stereochemistry of the hydroxyethyl side chain provides stability against β-lactamases (23).

Mechanism of action

Imipenem binds to PBP 1 and PBP 2 of gram-negative and gram-positive bacteria, causing cell elongation and lysis (382). It is stable toward most plasmid- or chromosomally mediated β-lactamases except those produced by *X. maltophilia* and some strains of *B. fragilis* (221).

Pharmacology

Imipenem is given intravenously and exhibits wide distribution in the body, but it undergoes no significant biliary excretion. It penetrates inflamed meninges with CSF levels of 5 to 11 μg/ml (341). The drug is metabolized and inactivated in the kidneys by a dehydropeptidase-1 enzyme found in the brush border of proximal renal tubular cells. To achieve adequate serum and urinary concentrations, a dehydropeptidase inhibitor, cilastatin, was developed; it is combined in a 1:1 dosage ratio with imipenem for clinical use. Cilastatin has no antibacterial activity, nor does it alter the activity of imipenem. It has a renal protective effect by preventing excessive accumulation of potentially toxic imipenem metabolites in the renal tubular cells.

The normal serum half-life of imipenem is 1 h. Dosage adjustment is necessary for creatinine clearance of ≤30 ml/min. Both imipenem and cilastatin are effectively removed by hemodialysis.

Spectrum of activity

Imipenem has the widest spectrum of antibacterial activity of the currently available antibiotics. It has excellent in vitro activity against aerobic gram-positive species: staphylococci (penicillin-susceptible and -resistant isolates), viridans streptococci, group A, B, C, and G streptococci, *Bacillus* spp., and *L. monocytogenes.* Methicillin-resistant staphylococci are usually resistant. Most enterococci are inhibited at <3 μg/ml, but tolerance is common. Some strains of *Enterococcus faecium* are resistant.

More than 90% of *Enterobacteriaceae* are susceptible to imipenem, including those resistant to other β-lactams and aminoglycosides (288, 406). Most *Acinetobacter* spp., *Enterobacter* spp., *Citrobacter* spp., and *Serratia* spp. are inhibited by ≤2 μg/ml. The activity against *P. aeruginosa* is similar to that of ceftazidime, with most strains inhibited at 1 to 6 μg/ml (318). While imipenem inhibits *P. cepacia* and *Pseudomonas stutzeri,* it is inactive against *X. maltophilia.* Emergence of resistant *Pseudomonas* spp. has been observed during therapy with imipenem (458). The drug may show in vitro antagonism when combined with third-generation cephalosporins or extended-spectrum penicillins as a result of its ability to induce β-lactamase production (281).

Imipenem is the most potent β-lactam against anaerobes, with activity comparable to those of clindamycin and metronidazole. The MIC_{90}s for *B. fragilis, Bacteroides melaninogenicus,* other *Bacteroides* spp., *Fusobacterium* spp., and anaerobic gram-positive cocci are ≤1 μg/ml (211, 447). Most *Clostridium* spp. except some strains of *Clostridium difficile* are susceptible. Imipenem is also active against *Actinomyces* spp., *Nocardia asteroides*, and *Mycobacterium* spp. (82).

Adverse effects

Side effects of imipenem are similar to those of other β-lactam antibiotics. Gastrointestinal distress occurs in up to 5% of patients. Allergic reactions such as drug fever, skin rashes, and urticaria are seen in about 3% of patients. Cross-reactivity with other β-lactam agents is possible but not fully studied. Seizures of unclear etiology have occurred in about 1% of patients, particularly in the elderly age group and in patients with renal insufficiency or underlying neurologic disorders. Reversible elevation of serum transaminases, leukopenia, and thrombocytopenia have been described, but no coagulopathy has been reported.

β-LACTAMASE INHIBITORS

Clavulanic Acid

Clavulanic acid is a naturally occurring weak antimicrobial agent found initially in cultures of *Streptomyces clavuligerus* (284, 324). It inhibits β-lactamases from staphylococci and many gram-negative bacteria. This agent acts primarily as a "suicide inhibitor" by forming an irreversible acyl enzyme complex with the β-lactamase, leading to loss of activity of the enzyme.

Clavulanic acid has been shown to act synergistically with various penicillins and cephalosporins against β-lactamase-producing staphylococci, klebsiellae, *H. influenzae, Moraxella catarrhalis, N. gonorrhoeae, E. coli, Proteus* spp., and *Bacteroides* spp. (14, 140, 189, 308, 395). Recently discovered plasmid-mediated TEM β-lactamases in ceftazidime-resistant strains of *Klebsiella pneumoniae* and *E. coli* are inactivated by this agent (311, 451). However, the inducible β-lactamases of *Enterobacter, Citrobacter, Acinetobacter, Serratia,* and *Pseudomonas* spp. are not inhibited by clavulanic acid. The combination of clavulanic acid with ampicillin, amoxicillin, or ticarcillin is active in vitro against *Mycobacterium tuberculosis,* which is known to produce β-lactamases (83, 379, 470).

In the United States, clavulanic acid is available for clinical use in a 1:2 or 1:4 combination with oral amoxicillin and in a 1:15 or 1:30 parenteral combination with ticarcillin. The pharmacologic parameters of amoxicillin and ticarcillin are not significantly altered when each drug is combined with clavulanic acid. This agent is moderately well absorbed from the gastrointestinal tract, with a serum half-life of about 1 h. One-third of a dose is metabolized, while the remainder is excreted unchanged in the urine. It is widely distributed to various body tissues and fluids, but it penetrates uninflamed meninges very poorly.

Adverse reactions are similar to those reported for amoxicillin or ticarcillin used alone. Nausea, vomiting, abdominal cramps, and diarrhea occur in 5 to 10% of patients taking amoxicillin-clavulanate. The incidence of allergic skin reactions is similar to that of ampicillin alone.

Sulbactam

Sulbactam is a semisynthetic 6-desaminopenicillin sulfone with weak antibacterial activity (10, 115). It functions as an effective inhibitor of certain plasmid- and chromosomally mediated β-lactamases. It inhibits the β-lactamases of *S. aureus,* many *Enterobacteriaceae, H. influenzae, Moraxella catarrhalis, Neisseria* spp., *Legionella* spp., *Bacteroides* spp., and *Mycobacterium* spp. (137, 160). Sulbactam alone is active against *N. gonorrhoeae, N. meningitidis,* some *Acinetobacter* spp., and *P. cepacia* (167, 197, 332). It acts synergistically with penicillins and cephalosporins against organisms that are otherwise resistant to the β-lactam drugs because of the production of β-lactamases. A combination of sulbactam (8 μg/ml) and ampicillin (16 μg/ml) inhibits most strains of staphylococci, *Klebsiella* spp., *E. coli, H. influenzae, Moraxella catarrhalis, Neisseria* spp., and *Bacteroides* spp. that are ampicillin resistant (331, 449, 460). Sulbactam is inactive against the β-lactamases of *Enterobacter, Citrobacter,* and *Providencia* spp., indole-positive *Proteus* spp., and *X. maltophilia.*

For clinical use, sulbactam is combined with ampicillin as a parenteral preparation in a 1:2 ratio. The pharmacologic properties of each drug are not affected by each other in this combination. Ampicillin-sulbactam penetrates well into body tissues and fluids, including peritoneal and blister fluids. It enters the CSF in the presence of inflamed meninges. Like ampicillin, sulbactam has a serum half-life of 1 h, and 85% of the drug is excreted unchanged via the kidneys (131). Since clearances of both sulbactam and ampicillin are affected similarly in patients with impaired renal function, dosage adjustments are similar for the two drugs.

The most common side effects of the ampicillin-sulbactam combination have been nausea, diarrhea, and skin rash. Transient eosinophilia and transaminasemia have been reported. Adverse reactions attributed to ampicillin may also occur with the use of ampicillin-sulbactam.

Tazobactam

Tazobactam (YTR 830) is a new penicillanic acid sulfone derivative that is structurally related to sulbactam. It is an active β-lactamase inhibitor which acts synergistically with other β-lactam antibiotics against most strains of *S. aureus, H. influenzae, E. coli,* and *Klebsiella, Enterobacter, Acinetobacter, Citrobacter, Proteus, Providencia,* and *Bacteroides* spp. (8, 9, 164, 193, 223). Like clavulanic acid and sulbactam, tazobactam binds to bacterial PBP 1 or PBP 2 (261). It has very poor intrinsic antibacterial activity, but it is comparable to clavulanate and sultactam in lowering the MICs by up to 20-fold for many organisms when combined with various β-lactams against β-lactamase-producing organisms. This drug is currently under preclinical evaluations in the United States.

AMINOGLYCOSIDES AND AMINOCYCLITOLS

Since the first aminoglycoside (aminoglycosidic aminocyclitol), streptomycin, was introduced in 1944, this class of antibiotics has played a vital role in the treatment of serious gram-negative infections. Among the unique features of the aminoglycosides are the bactericidal activity against aerobic gram-negative bacilli (including *Pseudomonas* spp.), activity against *M. tuberculosis,* and relatively low incidence of bacterial resistance. The currently available aminoglycosides are derived from *Micromonospora* spp. (gentamicin, sisomicin, and netilmicin) or from *Streptomyces* spp. (streptomycin, neomycin, kanamycin, and tobramycin). The difference in origin of these compounds accounts for the differences of their suffixes, "micin" versus "mycin." Streptomycin, neomycin, kanamycin, tobramycin, and gentamicin are naturally occurring aminoglycosides, whereas amikacin and netilmicin are semisynthetic derivatives of kanamycin and sisomicin, respectively. Isepamicin, which is presently undergoing clinical trial in the United States and elsewhere, is a semisynthetic derivative of gentamicin B. Structurally, each of these aminoglycosides contains two or more amino sugars linked by glycosidic bonds to an aminocyclitol ring nucleus.

Spectinomycin is an aminocyclitol antibiotic isolated from *Streptomyces spectabilis*. Although it contains an aminocyclitol nucleus, it is not strictly an aminoglycoside because it does not contain an amino sugar or a glycosidic bond.

Mechanism of action

Aminoglycosides are bactericidal agents that inhibit bacterial protein synthesis by binding irreversibly to the bacterial 30S ribosomal subunit. The aminoglycoside-bound bacterial ribosomes then become unavailable for translation of mRNA during protein synthesis, thereby leading to cell death (42). They also cause misreading of the genetic code, with the resultant production of nonsense proteins. To reach the intracellular ribosomal binding targets, an aerobic energy-dependent process is necessary to enable successful penetration of the aminoglycosides into the bacteria. The bacterial uptake of these agents is facilitated in the presence of inhibitors of bacterial cell wall synthesis such as β-lactams and vancomycin. This interaction forms the basis of antibacterial synergism between aminoglycosides and β-lactam antibiotics (90, 148).

Spectinomycin acts similarly to the aminoglycosides by binding to the 30S ribosomal subunits and inhibiting protein synthesis. However, it does not cause misreading of the mRNA and is not bactericidal.

Pharmacology

All aminoglycosides have similar pharmacologic properties. Gastrointestinal absorption of these agents is unpredictable and always low. Because of its severe toxicity with systemic administration, neomycin is available only for oral and topical use. After intravenous administration, aminoglycosides are freely distributed in the extracellular space but penetrate poorly into the CSF, vitreous fluid of the eye, biliary tract, prostate, and tracheobronchial secretions, even in the presence of inflammation.

In adults with normal renal function, the aminoglycosides have serum half-lives of about 2 to 3 h (Table 3). They are primarily excreted, essentially unchanged, via the kidneys. There is considerable variation in the elimination of aminoglycosides among individuals, especially in patients with impaired renal function. Monitoring of serum aminoglycoside levels in these patients is essential to provide adequate therapy and reduce toxicity. In renal failure, the drugs accumulate and dosage reductions are necessary. Aminoglycosides are substantially removed by hemodialysis and to a lesser extent by peritoneal dialysis.

TABLE 3. Aminoglycosides and aminocyclitols

Drug	Serum half-life (h)	Therapeutic serum concn (μg/ml)	
		Peak	Trough
Amikacin	2–2.5	20–30	5–10
Gentamicin	2–3	4–6	1–2
Kanamycin	2.2–3	15–40	5–10
Netilmicin	2.2–2.5	6–8	1–2
Streptomycin	2–3	20–30	<5
Tobramycin	2–2.8	4–6	1–2
Spectinomycin	1.7	10–40	

Spectrum of activity

Aminoglycoside antibiotics are active primarily against aerobic gram-negative bacilli and *S. aureus*. As a group, they are particularly potent against the *Enterobacteriaceae*, *P. aeruginosa*, *Acinetobacter* spp., and *Providencia* spp. Certain differences in antimicrobial spectra among the various aminoglycosides do exist. Kanamycin is limited in its spectrum because of the common resistance of *P. aeruginosa* and frequent occurrence of plasmid-mediated inactivating enzymes among other gram-negative bacilli (88). It is now occasionally used as a "second-line" drug in combination with other antibiotics in the therapy of tuberculosis. Similarly, widespread resistance among *Enterobacteriaceae* has limited the usefulness of streptomycin. As a single agent, streptomycin is used in the therapy of infections due to *Francisella tularensis* (tularemia) and *Yersinia pestis* (plague). It is often used in conjunction with tetracycline for the treatment of brucellosis. It has the greatest in vitro activity of the aminoglycosides against *M. tuberculosis*. It may also be used in combination with penicillin or vancomycin for the treatment of infective endocarditis due to viridans streptococci or enterococci provided that the organisms do not possess high-level ribosomal or enzymatic resistance to streptomycin (440, 457).

Although gentamicin and tobramycin have very similar antibacterial activity profiles, gentamicin is more potent in vitro against *Serratia* spp., whereas tobramycin is more potent against *P. aeruginosa* (7, 274). However, these minor differences have not been correlated with greater efficacy of one agent over the other. For the most part, gentamicin and tobramycin are susceptible to inactivation by the same modifying enzymes produced by resistant bacteria, with the exception that in contrast to gentamicin, tobramycin can be inactivated by 6-acetyltransferase and 4′-adenyltransferase and has variable susceptibility to 3-acetyltransferase. Netilmicin and amikacin are resistant to many of these aminoglycoside-modifying enzymes and therefore are active against most *Enterobacteriaceae* that are resistant to gentamicin and tobramycin. Netilmicin is intrinsically less active than gentamicin or tobramycin against *P. aeruginosa*, and most gentamicin-resistant *Serratia*, *Proteus*, *Providencia*, and *Pseudomonas* isolates are also usually resistant to netilmicin (135). Amikacin is used often as the aminoglycoside of choice when gentamicin and tobramycin resistance is prevalent. Aminoglycosides are only moderately active against *Haemophilus* and *Neisseria* spp.

Although active against staphylococci, aminoglycosides are not recommended as single agents for treatment of staphylococcal infections. Gentamicin is often combined with a penicillin or vancomycin for synergy in the treatment of serious infections due to staphylococci, enterococci, or viridans streptococci. The aminoglycosides are not active against anaerobes.

Spectinomycin is used primarily for uncomplicated anogenital infections due to *N. gonorrhoeae* (436), including β-lactamase-producing strains. It is useful in patients with penicillin allergy. However, spectinomycin is ineffective for pharyngeal gonococcal infections, syphilis, or chlamydial infections.

Adverse effects

Considerable intrinsic toxicity is a characteristic of all of the aminoglycosides, mainly in the form of nephrotoxicity and auditory or vestibular toxicity. The nephrotoxic potential varies among the aminoglycosides, with neomycin being the most and streptomycin the least nephrotoxic. This effect is usually reversible when the drug is discontinued. The presence of hypotension, prolonged duration of therapy, preexisting renal insufficiency, and possibly excessive serum aminoglycoside concentrations increase the risk of nephrotoxicity.

All aminoglycosides are capable of causing damage to the eighth cranial nerve in humans (27). Vestibular toxicity is more frequently associated with streptomycin, gentamicin, and tobramycin, whereas auditory toxicity is more typical of kanamycin and amikacin. This frequently irreversible side effect may occur even after discontinuation of the drug and is cumulative with repeated courses of the agent. The ototoxicity is a result of selective destruction of the hair cells in the cochlea. Clinically detectable auditory and vestibular dysfunction has been reported to occur in 3 to 5% of patients receiving gentamicin, tobramycin, or amikacin and who underwent audiometric testing (124).

Neuromuscular paralysis, which is usually reversible, can occur after rapid intravenous infusion of aminoglycosides. This phenomenon occurs particularly in the setting of myasthenia gravis or concurrent use of succinylcholine during anesthesia. Other minor adverse reactions include local pain and allergic skin rashes. No known serious adverse reactions have been reported for spectinomycin.

QUINOLONES

Quinolones belong to a novel group of potent antibiotics biochemically related to nalidixic acid, which was developed initially as a urinary antiseptic. Nalidixic acid and its early analogs, oxolinic acid and cinoxacin, have limited clinical applications as a result of widespread emergence of bacterial resistance. Newer quinolones have been synthesized by modifying the original two-ring quinolone nucleus with different side-chain substitutions (467). These new agents, also known as fluoroquinolones, contain a fluorine atom attached to the nucleus. Although they have been used extensively in Europe and Japan, only norfloxacin and ciprofloxacin are currently available for clinical use in the United States. A number of other fluoroquinolones, including ofloxacin, enoxacin, lomefloxacin, temafloxacin, fleroxacin, and others, are undergoing clinical investigation in the United States and will likely be released for clinical use in the near future.

Mechanism of action

The primary bacterial target of the quinolones is DNA gyrase, a bacterial enzyme essential for DNA replication (185, 186). By inhibiting bacterial DNA synthesis, these agents are bactericidal. However, the antibacterial activity of quinolones is reduced in the presence of acidic pH, urine, and divalent cations (Mg^{2+} and Ca^{2+}) (468).

Pharmacology

Pharmacokinetic parameters are similar among the fluoroquinolones, with minor differences. They are well absorbed from the gastrointestinal tract, with bioavailability varying from 60 to 95% for the various fluoroquinolones (60, 93, 182, 258, 387, 389, 461). After oral administration, serum concentrations peak after 1 to 2 h. Although the presence of food does not significantly alter the absorption of these drugs, coadministration with aluminum- or magnesium-containing antacids substantially diminishes the bioavailability and subsequent peak serum concentrations as a result of binding of the quinolone to antacids. The degree of serum protein binding is generally low, ranging from 8% for ofloxacin to 60% for enoxacin. The fluoroquinolones have relatively long serum elimination half-lives that allow twice-daily dosing for most compounds (Table 4).

These agents have good penetration into lung, kidney, muscle, bone, intestinal wall, and extravascular body fluids. Concentrations in prostate are about 2 times those in the serum, and concentrations of 25 to 100 times above peak serum concentrations are achieved in the urine. However, concentrations are variable but low in CSF obtained from patients with meningitis (392, 465, 466). Quinolones penetrate well into phagocytes, such that concentrations within neutrophils are as high as 14 times those of serum concentrations (105, 422). This feature may account for their excellent in vivo activity against such intracellular pathogens as *Brucella*, *Listeria*, *Salmonella*, and *Mycobacterium* spp.

Pefloxacin is the most extensively metabolized fluoroquinolone, being converted into norfloxacin in vivo. Ofloxacin exhibits little or no in vivo metabolism. For other quinolones, up to 20% of each dose is metabolized. They are eliminated primarily via the kidneys by active

TABLE 4. Quinolones

Drug	Serum half-life (h)	Peak serum concn[a] (μm/ml)
Nalidixic acid	1.5	0.3
Oxolinic acid	6–7	1
Cinoxacin	2.7	16
Norfloxacin	3.0–4.5	2
Ciprofloxacin	3–6	2
Enoxacin	5–7	2.3
Fleroxacin	11–13	5
Lomefloxacin	7.8	3
Ofloxacin	5–7	6
Pefloxacin	9.5–12	3.5
Temafloxacin	6.5	3.4

[a] After an oral dose of 500 mg.

tubular secretion and glomerular filtration. This renal elimination is blocked by probenecid. Small amounts of norfloxacin and ciprofloxacin are also excreted in the bile.

Hepatic insufficiency prolongs the half-life of pefloxacin, whereas the elimination of other fluoroquinolones is significantly diminished in the presence of renal failure. These drugs are only partially removed by hemodialysis and are minimally affected by peritoneal dialysis because of their marked extravascular penetration, as reflected in their very large volumes of distribution.

Spectrum of activity

Quinolones possess excellent activity in vivo against *Enterobacteriaceae*, *P. aeruginosa*, *Citrobacter*, *Serratia*, and *Acinetobacter* spp., both β-lactamase-positive and -negative *H. influenzae*, and gram-negative cocci such as *N. gonorrhoeae*, *N. meningitidis*, and *Branhamella catarrhalis* (312, 467). They are also active against *S. aureus*, including methicillin-resistant strains, and other staphylococcal species but are less potent against streptococci and enterococci. These agents are generally inactive against anaerobic bacteria, with little or no clinically useful activity against *B. fragilis* (152) and *C. difficile* (66, 95).

Enteropathogenic gram-negative bacilli such as salmonellae, shigellae, *Yersinia enterocolitica*, *Vibrio* spp., *Aeromonas* and *Plesiomonas* spp., *Campylobacter jejuni*, and enterotoxigenic *E. coli* are all susceptible to the quinolones. Clinical studies have shown these drugs to be effective in the prophylaxis as well as treatment of infectious diarrheas. *Legionella* spp. are susceptible to these agents, with MICs of most fluoroquinolones of 0.12 to 1.0 μg/ml (106, 118). Ciprofloxacin is the most active fluoroquinolone against *P. aeruginosa*, with an MIC_{90} of ≤0.5 μg/ml (312). However, *P. cepacia* and *X. maltophilia* are generally resistant to the quinolones.

The fluoroquinolones, especially ciprofloxacin, are active in vitro against *M. tuberculosis*, *Mycobacterium fortuitum-chelonae* complex, *Mycobacterium kansasii*, and *Mycobacterium xenopi* (30, 89, 144, 478). Their activity against *Mycobacterium avium-intracellulare* complex is fair to poor. They also exhibit activity against *Chlamydia trachomatis* and *Mycoplasma hominis* but are less potent against *Ureaplasma urealyticum* (210, 220, 336). Ciprofloxacin and pefloxacin have been shown to inhibit *Rickettsia conorii* (321), *Rickettsia rickettsii* (322), and *Coxiella burnetii* (477). Quinolones have been found also to have in vitro activity against the malarial parasite *Plasmodium falciparum* at achievable serum concentrations (97, 359). *Nocardia* spp. are relatively resistant to the quinolones.

No significant inoculum effect has been observed among the bacteria susceptible to quinolones. Combinations of quinolones with β-lactam drugs or aminoglycosides may be indifferent or additive in effects against gram-negative and gram-positive bacteria and mycobacteria. Synergism occurs, particularly against *P. aeruginosa*, in up to 50% of strains tested (282, 468). However, bactericidal activities of quinolones can be antagonized by rifampin or chloramphenicol.

Adverse effects

Gastrointestinal symptoms, occurring in up to 5% of patients, commonly include nausea, vomiting, abdominal discomfort, and diarrhea (166, 363, 433). However, *C. difficile* colitis is rarely associated with the use of quinolones. Other reported adverse effects include headache, fatigue, insomnia, dizziness, and agitation. Seizures rarely occur and are usually associated with high dosages in elderly patients with underlying metabolic disturbances.

Allergic reactions have been uncommon and often manifest as rash, urticaria, generalized pruritus, or photosensitive eruptions. Laboratory abnormalities may occur rarely during fluoroquinolone therapy. These changes include elevations in serum transaminases, eosinophilia, and leukopenia.

Enoxacin and to a lesser extent ciprofloxacin and pefloxacin increase the serum levels of concomitant theophylline and other xanthines as a result of decreased hepatic clearance (452, 453). Augmentation of the anticoagulant effects of warfarin by ofloxacin has been observed (314).

Irreversible cartilage erosions and skeletal abnormalities have been observed in young dogs and rabbits receiving quinolones (68, 76, 364). Consequently, quinolones are contraindicated for use in patients less than 18 years old and in pregnant or nursing women.

TETRACYCLINES

Tetracyclines are broad-spectrum bacteriostatic antibiotics with the hydronaphthacene nucleus, which contains four fused rings. The congeners comprise three groups based on their duration of action (Table 5).

Mechanism of action

The tetracyclines act against susceptible microorganisms by inhibiting protein synthesis. They enter bacteria by an energy-dependent process and bind reversibly to the 30S ribosomal subunits of the bacteria (79). This process blocks the access of aminoacyl-tRNA to the RNA-ribosome complex, preventing bacterial polypeptide synthesis.

Pharmacology

Tetracyclines are incompletely absorbed from the gastrointestinal tract, but their absorption is improved in the fasting state. Ingestion of food, especially dairy products, and other substances such as antacids and iron preparations impairs the absorption of these drugs (290). This interference of absorption by foods is less with doxycycline and minocycline. These long-acting

TABLE 5. Tetracyclines

Drug	Serum half-life (h)
Short-acting	
Tetracycline	8
Chlortetracycline	6
Oxytetracycline	9
Intermediate-acting	
Demeclocycline	12
Methacycline	14
Long-acting	
Doxycycline	18
Minocycline	16

tetracyclines are more readily absorbed, and therefore lower doses are required. Peak serum concentrations of 3 to 5 μg/ml are reached in 2 h after standard oral dosages. Intravenous preparations are available, and peak serum concentrations of 10 to 20 μg/ml are reached in 1 h.

Tetracyclines are metabolized by the liver and concentrated in the bile, with biliary concentrations three to five times higher than concurrent plasma levels. These drugs accumulate in the blood in patients with hepatic insufficiency or biliary obstruction. They should be avoided or used cautiously in reduced dosages in patients with impaired liver function.

These antibiotics are excreted primarily in the urine except for doxycycline, which is excreted primarily (90%) as an inactive conjugate via the biliary tract in the feces. Renal failure prolongs the half-lives of the tetracyclines except doxycycline. Therefore, doxycycline is considered the tetracycline of choice for extrarenal infections in the presence of renal failure.

Tissue penetration of these drugs is excellent, but CSF levels are low even in the presence of meningeal inflammation. Tetracyclines cross the placenta and are incorporated into fetal bone and teeth. They are excreted in high concentrations in human milk. Therefore, tetracyclines are not advised for pregnant or lactating women. Minocycline, the most lipophilic tetracycline at physiologic pH, reaches relatively high concentrations in saliva and tears, making it an ideal antibiotic to eradicate the meningococcal carrier state (165, 180).

Spectrum of activity

All tetracyclines have similar antimicrobial spectra, with activity against many gram-positive and gram-negative bacteria, mycoplasmas, chlamydiae, rickettsiae, and some protozoa. Many gram-positive aerobic cocci, including *S. aureus*, *S. pyogenes*, and *S. pneumoniae*, are susceptible at concentrations achievable in the serum. However, emergence of tetracycline-resistant strains of *S. pneumoniae* is frequent (155). Although many *E. coli* are susceptible to tetracyclines, pseudomonads and many *Enterobacteriaceae* are resistant. *Shigella* and *Salmonella* spp. are increasingly resistant to these agents. Tetracyclines are used mainly for the treatment of acute, uncomplicated urinary tract infections due to *E. coli* and as effective prophylactic therapy for traveler's diarrhea caused by enterotoxigenic *E. coli* (132, 254). With activity against *Pseudomonas pseudomallei* (110), *Brucella* spp. (119), *Vibrio* spp. (263), and *Mycobacterium marinum* (430), they have been used successfully in the treatment of infections due to these bacteria. Minocycline is active against *Nocardia* spp. (96, 310). Tetracyclines are active against many anaerobic bacteria, including *B. fragilis* and *Actinomyces* spp. (67, 399). They are commonly used with or without neomycin as oral bowel preparations preoperatively.

These drugs are useful in the treatment of urethritis and acute pelvic inflammatory diseases caused by *N. gonorrhoeae*, *Chlamydia trachomatis*, *U. urealyticum*, and *Mycoplasma hominis*. Emergence of resistance to tetracyclines among *N. gonorrhoeae* is increasing (57). They are effective for the treatment of other chlamydial infections (psittacosis, lymphogranuloma venereum, and trachoma). Other infections responsive to tetracyclines include granuloma inguinale, chancroid, relapsing fever, tularemia, and cholera.

Tetracyclines are the drug of choice for treating rickettsial infections (Rocky Mountain spotted fever, endemic and scrub typhus, and Q fever). Many pathogenic spirochetes, including *Treponema pallidum* and *Borrelia burgdorferi*, the agent of Lyme disease (200), are susceptible. Protozoans such as *Plasmodium* spp. and *Entaemoeba histolytica* are also inhibited by these drugs (74, 301).

Adverse effects

Tetracyclines have irritative effects on the upper gastrointestinal tract, producing esophageal ulcerations, nausea, vomiting, and epigastric distress. Alterations in the enteric flora occur with the use of tetracyclines, resulting in diarrhea, and pseudomembranous colitis can develop with prolonged use.

Hypersensitivity reactions are unusual, generally manifesting themselves as urticaria, fixed drug eruptions, morbilliform rashes, and anaphylaxis. Cross-reactivity among tetracyclines is the rule. Photosensitivity reactions consist of an erythematous rash on areas exposed to sunlight and can occur with all analogs, especially demeclocycline (31, 134).

Tetracycline causes depression of bone growth, permanent discoloration of the teeth, and enamel hypoplasia when given during tooth and skeletal development (161, 462). Therefore, these drugs are usually avoided in childhood (<8 years of age) and during pregnancy.

Minocycline has been known to cause vertigo (195), and benign intracranial hypertension (pseudotumor cerebri) has been described with many of the analogs (432). Tetracycline can aggravate preexisting renal failure by inhibiting protein synthesis, increasing the azotemia from amino acid metabolism.

MACROLIDES

Erythromycin is a macrolide antibiotic derived from *Streptomyces erythreus*. Its chemical structure consists of a macrocyclic lactone ring attached to two sugar moieties, desosamine and cladinose. Other macrolides include trioleandomycin and oleandomycin, and those currently under investigation include dirithromycin, clarithromycin, roxithromycin, azithromycin, and spiramycin (169, 212).

Mechanism of action

Erythromycin is a bacteriostatic agent that inhibits bacterial RNA-dependent protein synthesis. This agent may be bactericidal at high drug concentration and against a low inoculum of bacteria. It binds reversibly to the 50S ribosomal subunits of susceptible microorganisms, thereby blocking the translocation reaction of polypeptide chain elongation (300).

Pharmacology

Erythromycin is available in various topical, parenteral (lactobionate and gluceptate), and oral (base, stearate, ethylsuccinate, and estolate) preparations. It is well absorbed from the gastrointestinal tract, but erythromycin base is rapidly inactivated by gastric acid. The presence of food in the stomach reduces absorption of the drug except for the estolate form. Peak serum levels of 1 to 2 μg/ml are obtained at 3 to 4 h after an oral dose. Much higher concentrations are achieved with intravenous infusion. Tissue distribution is excellent except in the brain and CSF. It crosses the placenta and is excreted in breast milk.

This agent is metabolized by the liver and primarily excreted in the bile. The serum half-life of erythromycin is 1.5 h, and therapeutic serum levels are maintained for 6 h after standard doses. Dosage reduction is not necessary in renal failure. It is not removed by hemodialysis or peritoneal dialysis.

Spectrum of activity

Erythromycin is a relatively broad-spectrum antibiotic with activity against gram-positive and some gram-negative bacteria, mycoplasmas, chlamydiae, treponemes, and rickettsiae (437). It shows good activity against pneumococci and group A streptococci, but emergence of resistance among these isolates (especially group A streptococci) is a problem in certain areas of the world (98, 235). Erythromycin is also active against *S. aureus*, *Corynebacterium diphtheriae*, *L. monocytogenes*, and *Actinomyces israelii*. Its antibacterial activity against gram-negative bacilli is influenced by pH, with increasing potency as the pH rises to 8.5. It is active against *N. gonorrhoeae*, *N. meningitidis*, *Bordetella pertussis*, *Campylobacter jejuni* (424), and *Helicobacter pylori* (250). It has somewhat lower activity against *H. influenzae*. It is the drug of choice for the treatment of infections due to *Legionella pneumophila* and *Legionella micdadei* (99, 107). Erythromycin has activity against some species of gram-negative anaerobes but not against *B. fragilis* strains.

This drug may be used for the treatment of gonorrhea and syphilis in patients who cannot tolerate penicillin G or tetracycline. It is effective as an alternative to tetracycline for *Chlamydia* infections. It is 50 times more potent than tetracycline against *Mycoplasma pneumoniae*. Erythromycin is used occasionally in the therapy of infections with *Mycobacterium scrofulaceum*, *M. kansasii* (257), and *M. chelonae* (429) and in combination with ampicillin against *Nocardia asteroides* (127).

Other macrolides, such as dirithromycin, clarithromycin, and azithromycin, exhibit pharmacokinetic advantages over erythromycin. With the possible exception of azithromycin, which exhibits some enhanced activity against *H. influenzae* and other gram-negative organisms, none of the other compounds differs significantly from erythromycin in its spectrum of activity. Spiramycin has been reported to show efficacy in the treatment of toxoplasmosis and cryptosporidiosis, although its utility for the latter remains to be proven (87).

Adverse effects

The incidence of related serious side effects due to erythromycin is relatively low. Gastrointestinal irritation, such as abdominal cramps, nausea, vomiting, and diarrhea, is common with oral administration. Thrombophlebitis is associated with intravenous infusion, but it can be avoided by dilution of the dose in a large volume of fluid and by slow infusion rate. Hypersensitivity reactions may include skin rash, fever, and eosinophilia. Cholestatic hepatitis occurring in adults has been associated frequently with the estolate form but has also been reported with use of other forms of erythromycin (190, 394). Erythromycin estolate is no longer recommended for use in adults because of its propensity to cause cholestatic jaundice.

Rare transient hearing loss may occur with use of large doses and very high serum concentrations of erythromycin (>4 g/day), usually in elderly patients with renal insufficiency (171). Pseudomembranous colitis and superinfection of the gastrointestinal tract or vagina with *Candida* spp. or gram-negative bacilli occur rarely. Concurrent erythromycin therapy increases the serum levels of theophylline, cyclosporine, and digoxin by interfering with their hepatic metabolism (238, 242). It also increases the anticoagulant effect of warfarin (12).

LINCOSAMIDES

Lincosamide antibiotics (lincomycin and clindamycin) were initially isolated from *Streptomyces lincolnensis*. Each drug has a chemical structure consisting of an amino acid linked to an amino sugar. Clindamycin is a derivative of lincomycin with increased antibacterial activity and improved absorption after oral administration (249). Both drugs are available for parenteral and oral use, but lincomycin is now used very infrequently in the United States.

Mechanism of action

Lincosamides bind to the 50S ribosomal subunit of susceptible bacteria and suppress protein synthesis (333). Their ribosomal binding sites are the same as or closely related to those for the macrolides and chloramphenicol. Clindamycin can be bactericidal or bacteristatic, depending on the drug concentration, bacterial species, and inoculum of bacteria.

Pharmacology

About 90% of an oral clindamycin dose is absorbed from the gastrointestinal tract, with no interference from the ingestion of food. A single oral dose of 150 mg yields peak serum concentrations of 2 to 3 μg/ml in 1 h. Peak serum levels of 10 to 12 μg/ml are obtained at 1 h after an intravenous dose of 600 mg. Therapeutic serum levels are maintained for 6 to 9 h after these dosages.

Clindamycin distributes well into bone, lung, pleural fluid, and bile, but it penetrates poorly into cerebrospinal fluid, even with meningitis (302). It readily crosses the placenta and enters fetal tissues. Clindamycin is actively concentrated in neutrophils and macrophages.

The normal half-life of clindamycin is 2.4 h. Most of the drug is metabolized by the liver and excreted in an inactive form in the urine. Its half-life is prolonged by severe liver dysfunction, necessitating dosage reduction in patients with severe liver disease. Although the serum drug levels are increased in patients with severe renal failure, dose modification is not essential. The drug is not removed significantly by hemodialysis or peritoneal dialysis.

Spectrum of activity

Lincosamides have a broad spectrum of activity against the aerobic gram-positive cocci and anaerobes. Clindamycin is more potent than lincomycin against methicillin-susceptible *Staphylococcus* spp., *S. pneu-*

moniae, and group A and viridans streptococci. The MIC_{50}s are in the range of 0.01 to 0.1 μg/ml for these strains. However, lincosamide resistance has been reported among clinical isolates of these bacteria (217, 235, 356), which are usually also resistant to erythromycin. The prevalence of lincosamide-resistant *S. aureus* may be 15 to 20% in some institutions (17, 248). Enterococci are uniformly resistant to the lincosamides.

Clindamycin is one of the most active antibiotics available against anaerobes, including *B. fragilis* and *Clostridium perfringens,* with MIC_{90}s of ≤2 μg/ml (22, 397, 399). However, clindamycin resistance (which appears to be increasing) is found in 5 to 10% of *B. fragilis* group species, 10 to 20% of clostridial species, 10% of peptococci, and most *Fusobacterium varium* strains (81, 231, 397). All of the *Enterobacteriaceae* are resistant to clindamycin. Clindamycin has been used to treat actinomycosis (344), babesiosis (463), malaria (367), and toxoplasma encephalitis (85, 343).

Adverse effects

Clindamycin-associated diarrhea occurs in up to 20% of patients, and half of these cases are due to the occurrence of pseudomembranous colitis caused by toxin-producing *C. difficile* (21, 226). This complication is not dose related and may occur after oral or parenteral therapy. Prompt cessation of the antibiotic, along with oral vancomycin, metronidazole, or bacitracin therapy, is effective in reversing this complication.

Other uncommon side effects include skin rashes, fever, and reversible elevation of serum transaminases. Clindamycin can block neuromuscular transmission and may potentiate the action of neuromuscular blocking agents during anesthesia (130).

GLYCOPEPTIDES AND LIPOPEPTIDES

Vancomycin, a bactericidal antibiotic obtained from *Streptomyces orientales,* is the only glycopeptide currently available for clinical use in the United States. Initially introduced for its efficacy against penicillin-resistant staphylococci, it has become most useful against methicillin-resistant staphylococci and in patients allergic to penicillins or cephalosporins. Teicoplanin (formerly teichomycin A), a new complex glycopeptide chemically related to vancomycin (378, 455), is currently an investigational drug in the United States. Daptomycin (LY 146032) is an investigational semisynthetic lipopeptide antibiotic derived from a fermentation product of *Streptomyces roseosporus.* It has a spectrum of activity similar to those of the glycopeptides.

Mechanism of action

Glycopeptides inhibit peptidoglycan synthesis in the bacterial cell wall by complexing with the D-alanyl-D-alanine portion of the cell wall precursor (293). Daptomycin also acts by inhibiting bacterial peptidoglycan synthesis but at a synthesis step earlier than that inhibited by the glycopeptides (5). The exact mechanism of action of daptomycin has yet to be determined.

Pharmacology

Vancomycin is available in oral and parenteral forms. After oral administration, the drug is very poorly absorbed and achieves high stool concentrations, accounting for its efficacy in treating pseudomembranous colitis (126, 409). Desirable peak and trough serum levels of 20 to 50 μg/ml and 5 to 15 μg/ml, respectively, are obtained after an intravenous dose of 1 g every 12 h in normal subjects. Therapeutic levels are achieved in synovial, ascitic, pericardial, and pleural fluids. It penetrates into the CSF only in the presence of inflamed meninges (256).

Vancomycin has a serum half-life of 6 to 8 h in patients with normal renal function, and it is eliminated from the body by glomerular filtration. In severe renal insufficiency, its half-life is prolonged to about 9 days, and it is not removed by hemodialysis or peritoneal dialysis.

Spectrum of activity

Glycopeptides and daptomycin are active mainly against aerobic and anaerobic gram-positive organisms, including methicillin-susceptible and -resistant staphylococci, streptococci, enterococci, *Corynebacterium* spp., *Bacillus* spp., *Lactobacillus* spp., *L. monocytogenes, Clostridium* spp., and *Actinomyces* spp. The MICs of vancomycin against *S. aureus, S. epidermidis,* streptococci, and enterococci are typically in the range of 0.25 to 2 μg/ml (260, 405, 438). The bactericidal activity varies, with MBCs at 20-fold of MICs for viridans streptococci and 50 times the MICs for enterococci. Teicoplanin (157, 159, 225) and daptomycin (112, 123, 203, 237) are two to four times more active than vancomycin against these gram-positive cocci. Unlike vancomycin and teicoplanin, which are characteristically bacteriostatic against enterococci, daptomycin exhibits moderate bactericidal activity toward this group of organisms (390, 434). Recently, vancomycin-resistant isolates of *Enterococcus faecalis* (33, 352, 371, 421), *Enterococcus faecium* (228, 229, 456), *Enterococcus gallinarum* (207), and coagulase-negative staphylococci (366) have been reported. Cross-resistance with teicoplanin is variable in these strains, but most are susceptible to daptomycin. Other vancomycin-resistant gram-positive organisms include *Leuconostoc, Lactobacillus,* and *Pediococcus* spp. (48, 73, 192, 347, 349).

Vancomycin is useful in the prevention and treatment of endocarditis due to gram-positive bacteria in patients who are allergic to penicillin (34, 252). It is the drug of choice for treating *Corynebacterium* group JK infections (146) and is useful for *Flavobacterium meningosepticum* meningitis (162) and antibiotic-associated *C. difficile* colitis (126).

The glycopeptides and daptomycin are not active against gram-negative organisms, mycobacteria, or fungi. They show no cross-resistance with other unrelated antibiotics. They can be synergistic with aminoglycosides (and in some cases with rifampin) against staphylococci, streptococci, enterococci, and listeriae (92, 418, 439, 441).

Adverse effects

The most frequent side effects of vancomycin are fever, chills, and phlebitis at the site of infusion. Rapid or bolus infusion of vancomycin causes tingling and flushing of the face, neck and thorax, known as the red neck or red man syndrome, as a result of histamine release by basophils and mast cells (1, 315). This phenomenon is not due to allergic hypersensitivity. Allergic maculopapular or diffuse erythematous rashes can occur in up to 5% of patients (380). Reversible leukopenia or eosinophilia can rarely develop.

Hearing loss due to ototoxicity may occur if serum vancomycin concentrations exceed 50 µg/ml. Even after the drug is discontinued, the auditory nerve damage may persist and is permanent (41, 253). Nephrotoxicity is now rare with the recent availability of highly purified vancomycin preparations. However, the risk of ototoxicity and nephrotoxicity appears to be increased during combination therapy with vancomycin and aminoglycosides.

Teicoplanin is generally well tolerated and does not produce the red man syndrome. It does cause irritation at the site of intravenous infusion, and ototoxicity has been reported (388). Safety information on the clinical use of daptomycin in humans is limited at present, but it has produced dose-related neuromuscular toxicity in animals.

SULFONAMIDES AND TRIMETHOPRIM

Sulfonamides were the first effective systemic antimicrobial agents used in the United States during the 1930s. They are derived from sulfanilamide, which is similar in chemical structure to *para*-aminobenzoic acid, a factor essential for bacterial folic acid synthesis. Various substitutions at the sulfonyl radical attached to the benzene ring nucleus enhance the antibacterial activity and also determine pharmacologic properties of the drug.

Trimethoprim (TMP) is a pyrimidine analog that inhibits the enzyme dihydrofolate reductase, interfering with folic acid metabolism and subsequent pyrimidine synthesis and one-carbon fragment metabolism in the bacteria. Since TMP and sulfonamides block the bacterial folic acid metabolic pathway at different sites, they potentiate the antibacterial activity of one another and act synergistically against a wide variety of organisms. Such a combination, TMP-sulfamethoxazole (SMX), also called cotrimoxazole, was introduced clinically in 1968 and has proven to be very effective in the treatment of many infections (348, 353).

Mechanism of action

Sulfonamides competitively inhibit bacterial modification of *para*-aminobenzoic acid into dihydrofolate, whereas TMP inhibits bacterial dihydrofolate reductase (Fig. 2). This sequential inhibition of folate metabolism ultimately prevents bacterial DNA synthesis (179). Since mammalian cells do not synthesize folic acid, human purine synthesis is not affected significantly by sulfonamides or TMP. The antibacterial effect of these agents may be reduced in patients receiving high doses of folinic acid (296).

Pharmacology

Sulfonamides are used usually in the oral and topical forms; the intravenous preparations (sulfadiazine and sulfisoxazole) are rarely used (Table 6). Mafenide acetate (Sulfamylon cream) and silver sulfadiazine are applied topically in burn patients and have significant percutaneous absorption. Sulfacetamide is available as an ophthalmic preparation, and various combinations of other sulfonamides are available orally (triple sulfa, or

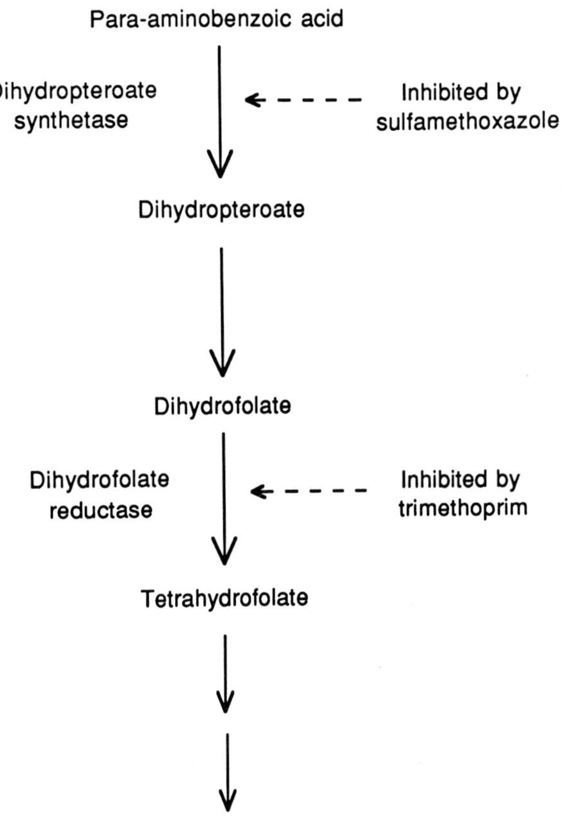

FIG. 2. Mechanism of action of TMP-SMX.

Trisulfapyrimidine) or as vaginal creams or suppositories.

The orally administered sulfonamides are absorbed rapidly and completely from the gastrointestinal tract. They are metabolized in the liver by acetylation and glucuronidation and are excreted by the kidney as free drug and inactive metabolites. Sulfonamides compete for bilirubin-binding sites on plasma albumin and increase blood levels of unconjugated bilirubin. For this reason they should not be given to neonates, in whom increased serum bilirubin levels may cause kernicterus.

Sulfonamides are well distributed throughout the body, with levels in the cerebrospinal, synovial, pleural, and peritoneal fluids about 80% of serum concentrations (222). They readily cross the placenta and enter

TABLE 6. Sulfonamides

Drug	Serum half-life (h)	Peak serum concn (µg/ml)
Short- or intermediate-acting		
Sulfamethizole	2	60
Sulfisoxazole	5–6	40–50
Sulfamethoxazole	11	80–100
Sulfadiazine	10–12	30–60
Long-acting		
Sulfadoxine	150–200	50–75

the fetal circulation. Sulfonamides may be used in renal failure, but they may accumulate during prolonged therapy as a result of reduced renal excretion.

TMP is available only for oral use and is readily absorbed, almost completely, from the gastrointestinal tract. After the usual 100-mg dose, peak serum levels reach 1 μg/ml in 1 to 4 h. This drug distributes widely in body tissues, including the kidney, lung, and prostate, and in body fluids (305, 454). CSF concentrations are about 40% of serum levels. Its serum half-life is about 10 h in healthy subjects and is prolonged in renal insufficiency. Up to 80% of a dose is excreted unchanged in the urine by tubular secretion; the remaining fraction is excreted as inactive metabolites by the kidney or in the bile.

A fixed combination of TMP-SMX in a dose ratio of 1:5 is available for oral and intravenous use. An intravenous dose of 160 mg of TMP with 800 mg of SMX produces average peak serum levels of 3.4 and 47.3 μg/ml, respectively, in 1 h. Similar peak levels are reached at 2 to 4 h after the same dose is taken orally. Widely distributed in the body, both drugs reach therapeutic levels in the CSF (40% of serum levels). Excretion is primarily by the kidney; dosage reduction is necessary in patients with creatinine clearances of ≤30 ml/min. Both TMP and SMX are removed by hemodialysis and partially by peritoneal dialysis (78).

Spectrum of activity

Sulfonamides are inhibitory to a variety of gram-positive and gram-negative bacteria, actinomycetes, chlamydiae, toxoplasmas, and plasmodia. Their in vitro antimicrobial activity is irregular, strongly influenced by inoculum size and composition of the test media. Susceptibility testing endpoints are often difficult to determine because of the presence of hazy growth within zones of inhibition in disk diffusion tests and because of the phenomenon of "trailing" in dilution tests. Sulfadiazine and sulfisoxazole are effective for rheumatic fever prophylaxis, but they are not useful in treating established group A beta-hemolytic streptococcal pharyngitis. These drugs may be used for prophylaxis of close contacts of patients with meningitis due to sulfonamide-susceptible *N. meningitidis*. Sulfisoxazole can be used to treat chlamydial urethritis, and sulfacetamide ophthalmic solution is effective for trachoma and inclusion conjunctivitis.

Sulfadiazine in combination with pyrimethamine has been used successfully to treat toxoplasmosis, and sulfadoxine combined with pyrimethamine (Fansidar) is effective in the prophylaxis and therapy of *Plasmodium falciparum* malaria. Sulfonamides are active against *Nocardia asteroides* (96), and they show moderate activity against *M. kansasii, M. fortuitum, M. marinum,* and *M. scrofulaceum* (340, 427). Other uses of sulfonamides include therapy of meliodosis, dermatitis herpetiformis, lymphogranuloma venereum, and chancroid.

Among the gram-negative bacilli, *E. coli* strains are generally susceptible to the sulfonamides, especially at levels achievable in the urine. Therefore, these drugs are used primarily in the treatment of first-episode acute urinary tract infections due to *E. coli*. However, increasing bacterial resistance has limited their efficacy in recent years (298). *Serratia marcescens, P. aeruginosa,* enterococci, and anaerobes are usually resistant to the sulfonamides.

TMP is active in vitro against many gram-positive cocci and most gram-negative bacilli. *P. aeruginosa,* most anaerobes, *Mycoplasma pneumoniae,* and mycobacteria are resistant. The MIC varies considerably with the test media used. As with the sulfonamides, the in vitro activity of TMP is lowered in the presence of thymidine. Currently, TMP alone is primarily used in the therapy of uncomplicated and recurrent urinary tract infections due to susceptible organisms (191, 278). However, the prevalence of TMP-resistant *Enterobacteriaceae* is increasing (153, 244).

Combinations of TMP with other agents, such as rifampin (120), polymyxins (295), and aminoglycosides (304, 483), have demonstrated in vitro synergistic antibacterial activity against various gram-negative bacilli. TMP combined with dapsone is effective in the treatment of *Pneumocystis carinii* pneumonia in immunocompromised patients (232).

Many gram-positive cocci, including staphylococci and streptococci, and most gram-negative bacilli except *P. aeruginosa* are susceptible to TMP-SMX (46). This drug combination has variable bactericidal effects on enterococci, depending on the test media used (80, 154, 269). With excellent activity against *S. pneumoniae, Moraxella catarrhalis,* and *H. influenzae,* including β-lactamase-producing strains, TMP-SMX is useful for the therapy of acute otitis media, sinusitis, acute bronchitis, and pneumonia. It has shown excellent results in the prophylaxis and therapy of acute and chronic urinary tract infections (168, 383, 416). It is an effective alternative therapy for uncomplicated urogenital gonorrhea, including cases caused by penicillinase-producing *N. gonorrhoeae*. It can be used also for the treatment of nongonococcal urethritis due to *Chlamydia trachomatis* (384) and chancroid (129). The drug combination is also useful in treating infections due to salmonellae, shigellae, enteropathogenic *E. coli,* and *Y. enterocolitica* (47, 184, 270). It has been used successfully for prophylaxis and treatment of traverler's diarrhea (103, 104).

Other microorganisms susceptible to TMP-SMX include *Brucella* spp., *P. pseudomallei, P. cepacia, X. maltophilia* (259), *M. kansasii, M. marinum,* and *M. scrofulaceum* (431). *M. tuberculosis* and *Mycobacterium chelonei* are generally resistant. It is a valuable antibiotic for the treatment of *Nocardia asteroides* infections (373, 428), *P. cepacia* and *X. maltophilia* bacteremia (241), *L. monocytogenes* meningitis (381), *Isospora belli* gastroenteritis (303), and Whipple's disease (209). In immunocompromised hosts (e.g., those with leukemia, organ transplant recipients, and those with AIDS), TMP-SMX is effective for the prophylaxis and treatment of *Pneumocystis carinii* pneumonia (188, 464, 479).

Adverse effects

Sulfonamides are known to cause nausea, vomiting, headache, and fever. Hypersensitivity reactions can occur as rashes, vasculitis, erythema nodosum, erythema multiforme, and Stevens-Johnson syndrome (51, 56). Very high doses of less water-soluble sulfonamides such as sulfadiazine may result in crystalluria with tubular deposits of sulfonamide crystals. Bone marrow toxicity with anemia, leukopenia, or thrombocytopenia can occur. Sulfonamides should be avoided in patients with glucose-6-phosphate dehydrogenase deficiency because of associated hemolytic anemia. Sulfonamides may potentiate the effects of warfarin, phenytoin, and oral hypoglycemic agents.

In general, TMP is well tolerated. With prolonged use, megaloblastic anemia, neutropenia, and thrombocytopenia can develop, especially in folate-deficient patients. Adverse reactions to TMP-SMX due to either the TMP or, more commonly, the SMX component can occur. Mild gastrointestinal symptoms and allergic skin rashes occur in about 3% of patients (199, 227). Megaloblastic bone marrow changes with leukopenia, thrombocytopenia, or granulocytopenia may develop, usually in patients with preexisting folate deficiency. Nephrotoxicity usually occurs in patients with underlying renal dysfunction (337). Patients with AIDS have a much higher frequency of adverse reactions (as much as 70%) (156, 464).

POLYPEPTIDES

Polymyxins

Polymyxins are a group of related cyclic basic polypeptides derived from *Bacillus polymyxa*. They have limited spectra of antimicrobial activity and significant toxicity. Only polymyxins B and E (colistin) are available for therapeutic use in humans.

Mechanism of action

Acting like detergents or surfactants, members of this group of antibiotics interact with the phospholipids of the bacterial cell membrane, thereby increasing cell permeability and disrupting osmotic integrity (264). This process results in leakage of intracellular constituents, leading to cell death. The bactericidal action is reduced in the presence of calcium, which interferes with the attachment of drugs to the cell membrane.

Pharmacology

The polymyxins are not absorbed when given orally, and intramuscular injections can be painful. They are given usually by the parenteral, oral, or topical route. Peak serum concentrations of 5 μg/ml are obtained with a total daily dose of intravenous polymyxin B at 2.5 mg (25,000 U)/kg of body weight. The serum half-life of polymyxin B is 6 to 7 h, and that of colistin is 2 to 4 h. They do not penetrate well into pleural fluid, synovial fluid, or CSF even in the presence of inflammation (224). Excretion is mostly via the kidneys by glomerular filtration. Serum levels and toxicity are increased in states of renal insufficiency. These drugs are not removed by hemodialysis, but small amounts can be removed by peritoneal dialysis.

Polymyxin is often used topically as 0.1% polymyxin, in combination with bacitracin or neomycin, for treatment of skin, mucous membrane, eye, and ear infections. It is poorly absorbed from these surfaces. When used for irrigation of serous or wound cavities, systemic absorption can be significant enough to produce toxicity.

Spectrum of activity

Polymyxins are active only against gram-negative bacilli, especially *Pseudomonas* spp. The MIC_{90}s for *Pseudomonas* spp., including *P. aeruginosa*, are <8 μg/ml (111). *Proteus, Providencia, Serratia*, and *Neisseria* isolates are usually resistant. Emergence of resistance during therapy is rare, and there is no cross-resistance with other antibiotics. Polymyxins B and E have identical antimicrobial spectra and show complete cross-resistance to one another.

Combination of polymyxins with TMP-SMX may be synergistic in the treatment of serious infection due to multiply resistant *Serratia* spp., *P. aeruginosa, P. cepacia*, and *X. maltophilia* (295, 345, 410). The polymyxins are usually reserved for serious, life-threatening *Pseudomonas* or gram-negative bacillary infections caused by organisms resistant to other antibiotics. Aerosolized polymyxins have been used successfully to treat *P. aeruginosa* respiratory infections in patients with cystic fibrosis or bronchiectasis (125).

Adverse effects

Neurotoxicity and nephrotoxicity are the two major side effects of polymyxins (216). Paresthesia with flushing, dizziness, vertigo, ataxia, slurred speech, drowsiness, or mental confusion occurs when serum levels exceed 1 to 2 μg/ml. Polymyxins also have a curarelike effect on striated muscles and can block neuromuscular transmission. Dose-related renal dysfunction occurs in about 20% of patients receiving appropriate therapeutic dosages. Allergic reactions such as fever and skin rashes are rare, but urticaria and shock after rapid intravenous infusion have occurred.

Bacitracin

Originally isolated from *Bacillus licheniformis* (formerly *B. subtilis*), bacitracin is a peptide antibiotic consisting of peptide-linked amino acids. Although it was introduced initially for the systemic treatment of severe staphylococcal infections, it is now mainly restricted to topical use because of its systemic toxicity.

Mechanism of action

Bacitracin inhibits dephosphorylation of a lipid pyrophosphate, a step essential for bacterial cell wall synthesis. It also disrupts the bacterial cytoplastic membrane.

Pharmacology

Bacitracin is often used in various topical preparations, such as creams, ointments, antibiotic sprays and powders, and solutions for wound irrigation or bladder instillation. When used as a topical antibiotic, no significant amount of bacitracin is absorbed systemically. Large doses used to irrigate serous cavities may be associated with systemic toxicity (446).

Spectrum of activity

The drug is active mainly against gram-positive bacteria, particularly staphylococci and group A beta-hemolytic streptococci. However, group C and G streptococci are less susceptible, whereas group B streptococci are resistant (13, 128). *Neisseria* spp. are also susceptible, but gram-negative bacilli are resistant. Bacitracin is often combined with neomycin, polymyxin B, or both in topical preparations to provide broad-spectrum antibacterial coverage. Orally administered bacitracin has been shown to be effective in treating antibiotic-associated *C. difficile* colitis (102).

Adverse effects

Systemic administration of bacitracin results in significant nephrotoxicity. Side effects are rare when the drug is given orally or applied topically. The drug is nonirritating to skin or mucous membranes. Allergic skin sensitization is rare.

CHLORAMPHENICOL

Chloramphenicol is a unique antibiotic originally derived from *Streptomyces venezuelae*. Its chemical structure contains a nitrobenzene ring. It is a highly effective broad-spectrum antimicrobial agent with specific indications for use in seriously ill patients. Thiamphenicol is an analog of chloramphenicol with a similar spectrum of antimicrobial activity (285). Only chloramphenicol is available for clinical use in the United States.

Mechanism of action

The drug is a bacteriostatic agent that inhibits protein synthesis by binding reversibly to the peptidyltransferase component of the 50S ribosomal subunit and preventing the transpeptidation process of peptide chain elongation. At therapeutic concentrations achievable in the serum, it can be bactericidal against common meningeal pathogens such as *S. pneumoniae*, *N. meningitidis*, and *H. influenzae* (319). Bacterial resistance occurs with plasmid-mediated production of chloramphenicol acetyltransferase enzyme, which inactivates the drug (370).

Pharmacology

Chloramphenicol is available for oral and parenteral use. It is rapidly and completely absorbed from the gastrointestinal tract. After an oral or intravenous dose of 1 g, peak serum concentrations at 2 h can reach 10 to 15 μg/ml. It diffuses well into many tissues and body fluids, including CSF, where levels are generally 30 to 50% of serum concentrations even without meningeal inflammation (374). The antibiotic readily crosses the placental barrier and is present in human milk.

Chloramphenicol is metabolized and inactivated by glucuronidation in the liver, with a half-life of 4 h in adults. The active drug (5 to 10%) and its inactive metabolites are excreted by the kidneys. Careful monitoring of serum chloramphenicol levels, maintaining peak serum concentrations in the therapeutic range of 10 to 20 μg/ml, is essential to ensure therapeutic efficacy and reduced toxicity. Patients with hepatic failure have high serum levels of active drug due to prolonged half-life. Dosage modification is not necessary in the presence of renal insufficiency since the metabolites are not as toxic as the active drug. Serum levels are not affected by hemodialysis or peritoneal dialysis.

Spectrum of activity

Chloramphenicol is very active against many gram-positive and gram-negative bacteria, chlamydiae, mycoplasmas, and rickettsiae. MIC_{90}s for most gram-positive aerobic and anaerobic cocci are ≤12.5 μg/ml (285). However, the drug is usually inactive against methicillin-resistant *S. aureus* and *S. epidermidis* and against enterococci. *N. meningitidis*, *H. influenzae* (ampicillin-resistant and -susceptible strains), and most *Enterobacteriaceae* are susceptible. Its activity against *Serratia* and *Enterobacter* isolates is variable, and *Pseudomonas* spp. are usually resistant. Salmonellae, including *Salmonella typhi*, are also susceptible, but resistant isolates are being encountered with increasing frequency (64, 350).

Chloramphenicol has excellent activity against anaerobic bacteria, including *B. fragilis*. Almost all of these isolates are inhibited at concentrations of ≤10 μg/ml (81, 177, 397). It is also active against *Rickettsia* spp. and *Coxiella burnetii*.

Adverse effects

Bone marrow toxicity is the major complication of chloramphenicol use. This side effect may occur either as a dose-related bone marrow suppression or as an idiosyncratic aplastic anemia. Reversible bone marrow depression with anemia, leukopenia, and thrombocytopenia occurs as a result of a direct pharmacologic effect of the drug on hematopoiesis. High doses (>4 g/day), prolonged therapy, and excessively high serum levels (>20 μg/ml) predispose patients to develop this type of complication. The second form of bone marrow toxicity is a rare but usually fatal complication which manifests as aplastic anemia (481). This response is not dose related, and the precise mechanism is unknown. It can occur weeks to months after the use of chloramphenicol, and it can develop after the use of oral, intravenous, or topical preparations.

Gray baby syndrome, characterized by vomiting, abdominal distention, cyanosis, hypothermia, and circulatory collapse, may occur in premature infants and neonates. This toxicity results from the immature hepatic function of neonates, which impairs hepatic inactivation of the drug. Reversible optic neuritis causing decreased visual acuity has been reported in patients receiving prolonged therapy. Chloramphenicol can occasionally cause hypersensitivity reactions, including skin rashes, drug fevers, and anaphylaxis. It potentiates the action of warfarin, phenytoin, and oral hypoglycemic agents by competitive inhibition of hepatic microsomal enzymes.

METRONIDAZOLE

Metronidazole is a nitroimidazole derivative that was first introduced in 1959 for the treatment of *Trichomonas vaginalis* infections. It now has an important therapeutic role in the treatment of infections due to anaerobic bacteria and certain protozoan parasites.

Mechanism of action

Metronidazole owes its bactericidal activity to the nitro group of its chemical structure. After gaining entry into the cells of susceptible organisms, the nitro group is reduced by a nitroreductase enzyme in the cytoplasm, generating certain short-lived, highly cytotoxic intermediate compounds or free radicals that disrupt host DNA (108).

Pharmacology

Metronidazole is absorbed rapidly and almost completely when given orally. Peak serum levels of 6 μg/ml are obtained 1 h after an oral dose of 250 mg. Intravenous doses of 7.5 mg/kg result in peak serum concentrations of 20 to 25 μg/ml. The drug has a serum half-life of 8 h. Therapeutic levels are achieved in all body tissues and fluids, including abscess cavities and CSF, even without meningeal inflammation. It crosses the placenta and is secreted in breast milk. The drug is primarily metabolized by the liver, and 60 to 80% is excreted by the kidney. With impaired hepatic function, plasma clearance of metronidazole is delayed and dosage adjustments are necessary. The pharmacokinetics are minimally affected by renal insufficiency. Metronidazole and its metabolites are completely removed by dialysis.

Spectrum of activity

Metronidazole exhibits potent activity against almost all anaerobic bacteria, including *B. fragilis* group, *Fusobacterium*, and *Clostridium* spp. (22, 117, 335, 398). It is the only antimicrobial agent with consistent bactericidal activity against *B. fragilis* (320). However, the susceptibility of gram-positive anaerobic cocci is somewhat variable, with MIC_{90}s of 16 μg/ml for these organisms. Most strains of the genera *Actinomyces, Arachnia*, and *Propionibacterium* are usually resistant. Frequencies of metronidazole-resistant *Bacteroides* isolates (MIC of >16 μg/ml) in the range of 2 to 5% have been reported from various institutions (81, 101, 268). Metronidazole has no activity against aerobic bacteria, including the *Enterobacteriaceae*.

The drug is effective in the treatment of antibiotic-associated colitis caused by *C. difficile* (63, 213), with efficacy equivalent to that of oral vancomycin for this indication (408). It is also useful in combination with an aminoglycoside for treating polymicrobial soft tissue infections and mixed aerobic-anaerobic intra-abdominal and pelvic infections.

Metronidazole is active against the protozoa *Trichomonas vaginalis, Giardia lamblia*, and *Entamoeba histolytica*. It is the drug of choice for the treatment of trichomoniasis, giardiasis, and intestinal and invasive amebiasis, including amebic liver abscess (251, 265, 401).

Tinidazole and ornidazole are other nitroimidazole derivatives with somewhat more potent antianaerobe activity than metronidazole (201). However, they are investigational drugs at present in the United States.

Adverse effects

The drug is generally well tolerated, and adverse side effects are uncommon. It can cause mild gastrointestinal symptoms such as nausea, abdominal cramps, and diarrhea. An unpleasant, metallic taste may be experienced with oral therapy. Metronidazole can potentiate the effect of warfarin and prolong the prothrombin time.

Although metronidazole has been shown to be carcinogenic in mice and rats, there is no evidence for increased carcinogenicity in humans (25). Use of this agent in pregnancy, especially during the first trimester and in nursing mothers, however, should be avoided.

NITROFURANTOIN

Nitrofurantoin belongs to a class of compounds consisting of a primary nitro group joined to a heterocyclic ring. Its role in human therapeutics is limited to the treatment of urinary tract infections (86).

Mechanism of action

The precise mechanism of action of nitrofurantoin is unknown. The drug is believed to inhibit various bacterial enzymes and also damage DNA (59, 245).

Pharmacology

The drug is available in microcrystalline (Furadantin) and macrocrystalline (Macrodantin) forms. It is administered orally and is well absorbed from the gastrointestinal tract. Very low levels of the drug are achieved in serum and most body tissues after usual oral doses. With a serum half-life of about 20 min, two-thirds of the drug is rapidly metabolized and inactivated in various tissues. The remaining one-third is excreted unchanged into the urine (325). An average dose of nitrofurantoin yields a urine concentration of 50 to 250 μg/ml in patients with normal renal function. In alkaline urine, more of the drug is dissociated into the ionized form, with lowered antibacterial activity. Nitrofurantoin accumulates in the serum of patients with creatinine clearances of <60 ml/min. The drug is removed by hemodialysis. The risk of systemic toxicity increases in the presence of severe uremia. It is contraindicated in patients with significant renal impairment and hepatic failure.

Spectrum of activity

Nitrofurantoin has a broad spectrum of antibacterial activity against gram-positive and gram-negative bacteria, particularly the common urinary tract pathogens. It is active against gram-positive cocci, such as *S. aureus, S. epidermidis, Staphylococcus saprophyticus*, and *Enterococcus faecalis*, with MICs in the range of 4 to 25 μg/ml (181). *S. pneumoniae, S. pyogenes, Bacillus subtilis*, and *Corynebacterium* spp. are also susceptible, but they rarely cause urinary tract infections. Over 90% of *E. coli* and many coliform bacteria are sensitive to nitrofurantoin at MICs < 32 μg/ml (420). However, only one-third of *Enterobacter* and *Klebsiella* isolates are susceptible. *Pseudomonas* and most *Proteus* spp. are resistant. Susceptible organisms rarely become resistant to this drug during therapy.

Adverse effects

Gastrointestinal irritation, with anorexia, nausea, and vomiting, is the most common side effect. Diarrhea and abdominal cramps may occur. Hypersensitivity reactions, such as drug fever, chills, arthralgia, skin rashes, and a lupuslike syndrome, have been observed (183).

Pulmonary reactions are the most common serious side effects associated with nitrofurantoin use. Acute pneumonitis with fever, cough, dyspnea, eosinophilia, and pulmonary infiltrates present on chest X-ray films can occur after a few days of therapy (91, 183). This immunologically mediated reaction is more common in elderly patients and is rapidly reversible after cessation of therapy. Chronic pulmonary reactions with interstitial pneumonitis leading to irreversible pulmonary fibrosis can occur in patients on continuous therapy for 6 months or more (183, 346).

Peripheral polyneuropathy is a serious side effect which occurs more often in patients with renal failure (183, 417). Hemolytic anemia, megaloblastic anemia, and bone marrow suppression with leukopenia can occur. Rare hepatotoxic reactions, such as cholestatic jaundice and chronic active hepatitis, have been reported (32, 369).

METHENAMINE

Methenamine is a tertiary amine with properties of a monoacidic base and is used as a urinary antiseptic. To be activated, it is combined chemically with a poorly metabolized acid and administered as the mandelate (Mandelamine) or hippurate (Hiprex, Urex) salt.

Mechanism of action

Methenamine has no antibacterial action by itself, but it is metabolized at acid pH to ammonia and formaldehyde, which provides the antiseptic action. This hydrolytic process occurs in the urine, and an effective bacteriostatic concentration of formaldehyde is reached at a urine pH of <5.5 (266). Since the serum is not acidic, formaldehyde is not released while methenamine circulates in the body.

Pharmacology

The agent is well absorbed from the gastrointestinal tract and is rapidly excreted in the urine. The elimination half-life of methenamine is about 4 h. At a urine pH of 5.0, about 20% of methenamine excreted in the urine is hydrolyzed to formaldehyde and ammonia (214). Inhibitory concentrations (>20 μg/ml) of formaldehyde in the bladder urine are generated at 1 to 2 h after oral administration and may be maintained for at least 6 h or until the patient voids. The mandelate and hippurate moieties are also rapidly excreted in the urine in active, unchanged forms by glomerular filtration and tubular secretion. The agent is contraindicated in patients with hepatic insufficiency because of the ammonia produced.

Spectrum of activity

With the liberation of enough formaldehyde into the urine, methenamine is essentially active against all gram-positive and gram-negative bacteria and also against fungi (215). However, it is not effective for treating urinary tract infections due to urea-splitting organisms such as *Proteus* spp., since the urine cannot be acidified and formaldehyde is not generated. Combination with acetohydroxamic acid, a urease inhibitor, has been suggested for treating these infections by *Proteus* spp. (267). Since bacteria and fungi do not become resistant to formaldehyde, emergence of resistance to methenamine is not a problem.

Methenamine is not useful for acute urinary tract infections. It has been used successfully as prophylactic therapy for recurrent bacteriuria, particularly those caused by highly resistant gram-negative bacilli or yeasts (39, 40). It is also effective as prolonged suppressive therapy for chronic bacteriuria in the absence of structural abnormalities of the urinary tract (133, 167).

Adverse effects

Methenamine and its acid salts are generally well tolerated. Some patients may develop nausea, vomiting, abdominal cramps, and diarrhea. High doses or prolonged administration of the drug can cause urinary tract irritation by the free formaldehyde, resulting in urinary frequency, dysuria, albuminuria, and hematuria. Skin rashes may also occur. To avoid precipitation of urate crystals in the urine, methenamine salts should not be used in patients with gout or hyperuricemia.

MUPIROCIN

Mupirocin, formerly pseudomonic acid A, is a novel topical antibacterial agent derived from the fermentation products of *Pseudomonas fluorescens* (141). Structurally, it contains a unique 9-hydroxynonanoic acid moiety. It was developed for the topical treatment of superficial soft tissue infections, particularly those due to staphylococci.

In the United States, mupirocin is available as a 2% ointment (Bactroban). After topical application, <1% of the drug is absorbed systemically, with no detectable levels in the urine or feces. Penetration into deeper dermal layers of the skin is increased with traumatized skin and occlusive dressings. The drug is highly protein bound (95%), and its activity is lowered in the presence of serum. It is most active at moderately acid pH, with no inoculum effect (435). Mupirocin is slowly metabolized in the skin to the inactive monic acid.

Mupirocin inhibits isoleucyl-tRNA synthetase, resulting in cessation of bacterial tRNA and protein synthesis (187). It has excellent in vitro activity, primarily against the gram-positive cocci. *S. aureus*, including methicillin-resistant strains, and coagulase-negative staphylococci are uniformly very susceptible, with MIC_{90}s of <0.5 μg/ml (52, 396). Emergence of resistant strains of staphylococci occurs at very low frequency. Most streptococci, including *S. pneumoniae*, beta-hemolytic streptococci of groups A, B, C, and G, and viridans streptococci, are inhibited by concentrations of ≤1 μg/ml. Resistant bacteria include enterococci, *Corynebacterium* spp., *Erysipelothrix* spp., *Propionibacterium acnes*, gram-positive anaerobes, and most gram-negative bacteria. However, *H. influenzae*, *N. gonorrhoeae*, *N. meningitidis*, *Moraxella catarrhalis*, *Bordetella pertussis*, and *Pasteurella multocida* are quite susceptible, with MICs in the range of 0.02 to 0.025 μg/ml. There is no cross-resistance between mupirocin and other major groups of antibiotics.

Clinically, mupirocin has been shown to be efficacious in the therapy of superficial skin infections, such as impetigo, folliculitis, and burn wound infections, due to staphylococci or streptococci (109, 151, 329, 339, 472). It has been used successfully to eradicate nasal carriage of *S. aureus*, including methicillin-resistant strains (53, 84).

No systemic toxic effects have been reported with mupirocin. Local irritation, such as burning, stinging, itch, and rash, may occur, which may be due to the vehicle ointment containing polyethylene glycol base.

FUSIDIC ACID

Fusidic acid is a steroid compound derived from the fungus *Fusidium coccineum*. Sodium fusidate (Fusidin) is the salt of this agent which is available for clinical use in other countries (150); the antibiotic is not currently available in the United States.

This antimicrobial agent interferes with the G factor involved in the peptide chain translocation process on the bacterial ribosomal complex, thereby inhibiting protein synthesis (407). Cross-resistance between fusidic acid and other antibiotics is rare. Gram-negative bacilli are usually resistant to fusidic acid because the drug cannot penetrate their cell walls. Although this drug is mainly bacteriostatic, it can be bactericidal at high concentrations, with low inoculum size, and against very susceptible strains of organisms (178, 291).

Gastrointestinal absorption of a given oral dose varies considerably among individuals. Peak serum levels in the range of 15 to 30 μg/ml are usually achieved at 2 h after oral administration of 500 mg (150). The drug is well distributed throughout the body, including subcutaneous fat, kidney, muscle, synovial fluid, and abscess cavities. Detectable levels are found in the CSF only in the presence of meningeal inflammation. Being highly protein bound (>90%), its in vitro activity is reduced in the presence of serum (16). Significant percutaneous absorption of fusidate does not occur with topical use, even on traumatized skin. The drug is inactivated in various body tissues, and very little active drug (1%) is excreted by the kidneys.

The significant feature of fusidic acid is its potent activity against *S. aureus,* including methicillin-resistant strains. The MIC_{90} for these isolates is <0.5 μg/ml (16, 150, 178, 260). Coagulase-negative staphylococci are also susceptible but at slightly higher MICs. The drug is synergistic with rifampin and dicloxicillin against *S. epidermidis* (180). Streptococci and enterococci are less susceptible, and some strains of *S. pneumoniae* can be resistant. Other gram-positive bacteria, such as *Corynebacterium* spp. and *Clostridium* spp., are quite susceptible. With the exception of *Neisseria* spp. and *B. fragilis,* all gram-negative bacilli are uniformly resistant.

Clinically, sodium fusidate is used primarily in combination with another antistaphylococcal drug for the treatment of infections due to methicillin-resistant *S. aureus.* It is not recommended for initial treatment of severe staphylococcal infections. Topical sodium fusidate has been used successfully to treat recurrent furunculosis (172) and staphylococcal wound infections (28, 239) and to eradicate the staphylococcal nasal carrier state (291). However, topical use of fusidic acid is no longer recommended because it promotes the emergence of resistant strains.

Mild upper gastrointestinal discomfort and diarrhea may be associated with oral administration. Local thrombophlebitis is common with intravenous infusion. Allergic contact dermatitis from topical use and cholestatic jaundice associated with high-dose therapy have been reported.

ANTIMYCOBACTERIAL AGENTS

Drugs used for treating mycobacterial infections can be categorized as those primarily used for tuberculosis, drugs for "atypical" mycobacterial infections, and agents primarily for treating leprosy. Antituberculous drugs may be further divided into first-line drugs, with superior efficacy and acceptable toxicity, and second-line drugs having less efficacy or greater toxicity (376, 386). The first-line agents include isoniazid, rifampin, ethambutol, streptomycin, and pyrazinamide, all of which except ethambutol are bactericidal. The second-line drugs are *para*-aminosalicylic acid (PAS), cycloserine, ethionamide, kanamycin, amikacin, viomycin, and capreomycin. Amithiozone (thiacetazone) is an antimicrobial agent active against *M. tuberculosis,* but it is not available in the United States and Europe. The fluoroquinolones also possess activity against mycobacteria in vitro, but their therapeutic efficacy remains to be determined.

Isoniazid, rifampin, ethambutol, and streptomycin are active against the large, actively dividing extracellular *M. tuberculosis* found within cavities. The intracellular mycobacteria at acid pH are readily killed by isoniazid, rifampin, and pyrazinamide, whereas other agents are inactive at low pH. Rifampin and to a lesser extent isoniazid are effective against slowly replicating organisms in caseous lesions.

Isoniazid

Isoniazid, or isonicotinic acid hydrazide (INH), is a synthetic antimicrobial agent introduced in 1952 for the treatment of tuberculosis (419). It competitively inhibits mycolase synthetase, a unique mycobacterial enzyme necessary for the synthesis of mycolic acid, which is an essential component of the mycobacterial cell wall (405). At high concentrations, INH can react with tyrosine residues of mycobacterial proteins and disrupt cellular metabolic pathways (175).

The drug is well absorbed orally or intramuscularly, with good distribution throughout the body, including the CSF. In the presence of meningeal inflammation, CSF levels may equal plasma concentrations. INH is metabolized by acetylation in the liver, and the rate of acetylation is determined genetically, with a serum half-life of 4 h in slow acetylators and shorter in rapid acetylators (116). About 70% of administered isoniazid is excreted by the kidney, mostly in the inactive aceylated form. Dosage modification is needed in severe hepatic insufficiency. After an oral dose of 300 mg in an adult, peak serum levels of 7 to 10 μg/ml are reached in 1 to 2 h.

Isoniazid is highly active against *M. tuberculosis,* with most strains being inhibited at 0.05 to 0.2 μg/ml. It is bactericidal in vitro against replicating organisms but only bacteriostatic against those in the resting phase. Secondary resistance to isoniazid can occur, especially when the drug is used singly or in combination with other drugs during inappropriate or inadequate treatment. Resistant rates to INH as high as 30 to 70% have been reported in some areas (50, 77). Primary resistance in isolates from untreated patients varies from 10% among new immigrants in the United States to 40% in areas endemic for tuberculosis in the Far East (49, 58, 313, 475).

Most strains of atypical mycobacteria, including *M. avium-intracellulare, M. fortuitum-chelonae, M. ulcerans,* and *M. marinum,* are usually resistant to isoniazid. *M. kansasii* and *M. xenopi* are susceptible, but only 40% of these strains are inhibited at concentrations of 1 to 5 μg/ml (174).

Hepatitis is the major side effect of INH, as a result of the conversion of isoniazid to acetylhydrazine and related hepatotoxic derivatives (219). The incidence of this complication is increased with older age, with concomitant use of rifampin, and in alcoholics. It is rarely seen in patients under 30 years of age but occurs in more than 2% of those over age 50. Mild elevation of serum transaminases develops in 10% or more of patients, but INH therapy is not stopped unless the transaminase levels exceed three to five times the normal values.

Hypersensitivity reactions with fever, rash, urticaria, and lupuslike syndrome can occur. Peripheral neuropathies result from increased urinary excretion of pyridoxine (vitamin B_6) with isoniazid therapy. This side effect can be prevented with concurrent pyridoxine administration (375). Other side effects, such as seizures, optic neuritis, psychotic reactions, arthralgias, shoulder-hand syndrome, and agranulocytosis, have also been reported but are rare.

Rifampin

Rifampin, also known as rifampicin, is a semisynthetic antibiotic derived from rifamycin B, belonging to a group of macrocyclic compounds produced by the mold *Streptomyces mediterranei* (368). Introduced for clinical use in 1968 as a potent antituberculous agent, this drug has activity against other bacteria and *Chlamydia* spp. It exerts a bactericidal effect by forming a stable complex with bacterial DNA-dependent RNA polymerase, preventing the chain initiation process of DNA transcription (218, 445). Mammalian RNA synthesis is not impaired because the mammalian enzyme is much less sensitive to the drug. Rifampin-resistant isolates possess an altered DNA-dependent RNA polymerase (444, 473).

The drug is well absorbed from the gastrointestinal tract, reaching peak serum concentrations of 5 to 10 μg/ml in 1 to 2 h after the usual oral dose of 600 mg. A parenteral preparation is also available. It is desacetylated in the liver to an active metabolite and excreted in the bile. The serum half-life is about 3 h (2). Rifampin is well distributed to almost all body tissues and fluids, reaching liver, lung, bone, urinary bladder, pleural exudate, ascites fluid, urine, and cavity fluid in concentrations equal to or exceeding that in the serum. Levels in the CSF are highest with inflamed meninges. The drug is able to enter phagocytes and kill living intracellular organisms (240), and it crosses the placenta. About 30 to 40% of the drug is excreted in the urine, and it does not accumulate in patients with impaired renal function. Hemodialysis and peritoneal dialysis do not eliminate the drug. Dosage adjustments are necessary for patients with severe hepatic dysfunction.

Rifampin is highly active against *M. tuberculosis, M. kansasii, M. avium-intracellulare, M. marinum, M. xenopi, M. ulcerans,* and *M. scrofulaceum* (70, 385, 423, 426). Primary resistance to the drug among *M. tuberculosis* strains is <1% (72). *Mycobacterium leprae* is also susceptible to rifampin, with an MIC of 0.3 μg/ml for human strains tested in mice (326, 327). Other mycobacteria, such as *M. fortuitum-chelonae,* are usually resistant.

The drug has bactericidal activity against gram-positive cocci, such as staphylococci (including methicillin-resistant strains), streptococci, and anaerobic cocci. Most strains of enterococci are only moderately susceptible, with MICs in the range of 0.01 to 0.5 μg/ml. It is active against *N. gonorrhoeae, N. meningitidis,* and *H. influenzae* and is used frequently in the prophylaxis of meningococcal and *H. influenzae* type b meningitis. Rifampin is the most active agent against *Legionella pneumophila* (with MICs of <0.03 μg/ml) and other *Legionella* spp. (413, 414).

Rifampin can cause many side effects, including gastrointestinal discomfort and hypersensitivity reactions such as drug fever, skin rashes, and eosinophilia. It produces a harmless orange-red coloration of saliva, tears, urine, and sweat. In up to 20% of patients, a flulike syndrome with fever, chills, arthralgias, and myalgias may develop after several months of intermittent therapy (149). This immunologic reaction may be associated with hemolytic anemia, thrombocytopenia, and renal failure. Rifampin-induced hepatitis occurs in <1% of patients and is more frequent during concurrent isoniazid therapy. The drug is known to antagonize the effect of oral contraceptives and diminish the anticoagulant activity of warfarin.

Ethambutol

Discovered in 1961, ethambutol is a synthetic compound with potent antituberculous activity (411). It is a bacteriostatic agent that inhibits mycolic acid and spermidine synthesis in mycobacteria (317, 404). After the usual oral dose of 25 mg/kg, 80% of the drug is absorbed, reaching peak serum concentrations of 2 to 5 μg/ml in 2 to 4 h. It is widely distributed throughout the body, and it is actively concentrated in the erythrocytes (307). The drug does not enter the CSF in the absence of meningeal irritation, but CSF concentrations of 1 to 2 μg/ml can be found in patients with tuberculous meningitis (36). It also crosses the placental barrier. About 10 to 15% of the absorbed dose is converted to various inactive metabolites, while 80% is excreted by the kidneys as active unchanged drug. It has a serum half-life of 4 h. Renal insufficiency necessitates dosage reduction.

Ethambutol is active only against mycobacteria, with MICs of 1 to 2 μg/ml for most strains of *M. tuberculosis,* even those isolates that are isoniazid resistant (208). Primary drug resistance occurs in about 10% of *M. tuberculosis* isolates. *M. kansasii* and *M. marinum* are susceptible to this agent. Ethambutol is ineffective against *M. avium-intracellulare* and *M. fortuitum-chelonae* (174, 225, 474).

A reversible, dose-related ocular toxicity occurs in up to 2% of patients receiving usual doses of ethambutol (69, 230). This side effect usually manifests as decreased visual acuity and defective color vision. Allergic reactions rarely occur, and hyperuricemia may be observed in about two-thirds of patients on the drug. Interstitial nephritis and peripheral neuropathy can develop.

Pyrazinamide

Pyrazinamide, a synthetic derivative of nicotinamide, is a valuable drug in short-course therapy regimens for the treatment of tuberculosis (377, 386). Its precise mechanism of action is unknown. The drug is bactericidal at 10 to 20 μg/ml for *M. tuberculosis,* and it is active under acidic intracellular conditions.

The drug is administered orally, and gastrointestinal absorption is rapid and complete. Peak serum levels of 30 and 60 μg/ml are reached within 2 h after 1.5- and 3.0-g oral doses, respectively (113). The drug penetrates almost all body tissues and enters the CSF with meningeal inflammation. It has a serum half-life of 9 to 10 h and is metabolized in the liver. Pyrazinamide and its metabolites are excreted mainly via the kidneys. Use of the drug is avoided in patients with severe hepatic or renal insufficiency.

At the currently recommended dosages of 20 to 35 mg/kg per day, hepatotoxicity associated with pyrazinamide may develop in 1 to 5% of patients (482). Hyperuricemia occurs as a result of interference with renal tubular secretion of uric acid. Drug fever, rash, photosensitivity, and arthralgias have been reported.

Aminoglycosides

Of the aminoglycosides, streptomycin, kanamycin, and amikacin exhibit the most potent antimycobacterial activity. At clinically attainable serum concentrations, gentamicin and tobramycin are inactive against mycobacteria (435).

Given intramuscularly, streptomycin achieves serum levels of 25 to 30 μg/ml after a 1-g dose. It does not penetrate the CSF. Although it is bactericidal against *M. tuberculosis*, it is inactive against intracellular tubercle bacilli. MICs for these strains are in the range of 0.4 to 10 μg/ml. Prevalence of primary resistance to streptomycin is about 1 to 3%, usually found among patient populations with a high incidence of INH resistance (55). *M. kansasii, M. marinum*, and *M. scrofulaceum* are streptomycin susceptible, whereas only 50% of *M. avium-intracellulare* isolates are susceptible (225, 430). The *M. fortuitum-chelonae* complex is usually resistant. Although active in vitro, the drug is not effective in treating *M. ulcerans* infections.

Kanamycin is active against most strains of *M. tuberculosis, M. marinum*, and *M. scrofulaceum*. Its in vitro activity against *M. kansasii* and the *M. fortuitum-chelonae* complex is more variable, whereas *M. avium-intracellulare* isolates are usually resistant.

Amikacin is the most active aminoglycoside against *M. tuberculosis* (142, 357). However, it has not been used extensively in the therapy of human tuberculosis because of its expense and toxicity. Many atypical mycobacteria, including *M. marinum* and the *M. fortuitum-chelonae* complex, are inhibited by amikacin at 12.5 μg/ml (402). *M. kansasii* and *M. avium-intracellulare* are usually resistant. Like streptomycin and kanamycin, amikacin is bactericidal to *M. leprae* in the mouse footpad model (145). However, the efficacy of aminoglycosides in the treatment of human leprosy is not established.

para-Aminosalicylic Acid

PAS is a synthetic bacteriostatic agent with a mode of action similar to that of the sulfonamides. It impairs folate synthesis and inhibits bacterial growth.

Administered orally as a sodium or calcium salt, the drug is well absorbed from the gastrointestinal tract. Peak serum levels of 7 to 8 μg/ml are achieved in 1 to 2 h after an oral dose of 4 g. It has a serum half-life of about 1 h. The drug distributes well to various body tissues and fluids, but it only enters CSF across inflamed meninges. The drug is acetylated by the liver and excreted via the kidneys as inactive metabolites, while one-third of a dose is excreted as active unchanged drug. Because of prolonged half-life in end-stage renal disease, PAS is usually avoided in patients with renal failure.

M. tuberculosis is usually inhibited at concentrations ranging from 0.5 to 2.0 μg/ml (222). Atypical mycobacteria are usually resistant to PAS (225). PAS is used in multidrug therapy for *M. tuberculosis* infections, mainly in developing countries.

Gastrointestinal intolerance is the major side effect of PAS, causing poor patient compliance. About 5 to 10% of patients develop hypersensitivity reactions, such as fever, rash, and exfoliative dermatitis. Reversible drug-induced lupus syndrome and hepatitis have been reported. Hemolytic anemia and neutropenia can rarely occur.

Cycloserine

Initially derived from the fermentation products of *Streptomyces orchidaceus* and *Streptomyces garyphalus*, cycloserine is a structural analog of D-alanine and prevents conversion of L-alanine to D-alanine (338). It acts as a competitive inhibitor of the peptidases that link D-alanine molecules in the bacterial cell wall (391).

The drug is given orally and is well absorbed. At 3 to 4 h after a 250-mg oral dose, peak serum levels of 20 to 40 μg/ml are obtained. Although 35% of a dose is metabolized, the majority of the drug is excreted unchanged via the kidneys. It distributes widely throughout the body and penetrates well into the CSF. Dosage modification is necessary in patients with impaired renal function.

Cycloserine concentrations of 10 to 20 μg/ml are inhibitory to most *M. tuberculosis* strains, including those resistant to INH, streptomycin, and PAS. The prevalence of primary drug resistance to cycloserine among these strains is <1%. *M. kansasii* and *M. avium-intracellulare* have variable susceptibility to this drug.

Neurotoxicity is the most significant toxic effect of cycloserine. Peripheral neuropathy, seizures, and psychotic disturbances such as confusion and depression have all been reported. Drug fever and rashes can occur.

Ethionamide

Ethionamide is a bacteriostatic agent derived from isonicotinic acid (335). Like INH and ethambutol, it blocks mycolic acid synthesis in assembly of the mycobacterial cell wall. Peak serum levels of 20 μg/ml are attained at 3 h after an oral dose of 1 g. With a serum half-life of 2 h, ethionamide is metabolized by the liver to sulfoxides that are active against *M. tuberculosis* (198). It is distributed widely throughout the body, and it penetrates well into the CSF with normal and inflamed meninges. Only small amounts of the drug and its metabolites are excreted in the urine.

Most strains of *M. tuberculosis* are inhibited at concentrations of 10 to 20 μg/ml. Many strains resistant to other antituberculous drugs remain susceptible to ethionamide. Some *M. ulcerans* isolates are susceptible, but other atypical mycobacteria are usually resistant. The drug has variable activity against the *M. avium-intracellulare* complex. Ethionamide shows bactericidal activity as potent as that of rifampin against *M. leprae*, with a typical MIC of 0.05 μg/ml (114).

Gastrointestinal irritation with nausea, vomiting, and abdominal cramps is common. Reversible hepatotoxicity occurs in about 5% of patients. Allergic skin rashes, photodermatitis, acne, and alopecia can occur rarely. Neurologic disturbances such as peripheral neuropathy, acute psychoses, and depression have been reported.

Capreomycin

Capreomycin is a polypeptide antibiotic isolated from the mold *Streptomyces capreolus* (176). It is a bacteriostatic agent usually used in the combination therapy of resistant tuberculosis. The mode of action of this drug is not known.

The drug is administered by intramuscular injection, which yields a peak serum level of about 30 μg/ml in 1 to 2 h (35). One-third of the drug is inactivated in the body, while the remaining two-thirds are excreted unchanged in the urine.

M. tuberculosis is moderately susceptible to capreomycin, with MICs ranging from 1 to 40 μg/ml (457). Strains that have become resistant to other antituberculous drugs usually remain capreomycin susceptible. Primary drug resistance to capreomycin is rare. However, cross-resistance with viomycin or kanamycin can occur (246, 400). Capreomycin also inhibits *M. kansasii* and the *M. fortuitum-chelonae* complex.

The drug can cause renal tubular dysfunction, with resultant proteinuria and renal insufficiency. Vertigo, tinnitus, or sensory-neural hearing loss may develop. Drug fever, skin rashes, eosinophilia, and leukopenia rarely occur.

Viomycin

Viomycin is a complex polypeptide antibiotic which is reserved for the multidrug treatment of resistant *M. tuberculosis* infection (450). The drug is given intramuscularly, with pharmacokinetic parameters similar to those of streptomycin. MICs for susceptible *M. tuberculosis* strains are in the range of 1 to 10 μg/ml. Mycobacterial isolates resistant to streptomycin and other antituberculous drugs except capreomycin are usually susceptible to this agent. There is complete cross-resistance with capreomycin. Like capreomycin, viomycin is associated with nephrotoxicity and ototoxicity.

Rifabutin

Rifabutin, also known as ansamycin or LM-427, is a spiro-piperidyl derivative of rifamycin S, with potent activity against mycobacteria, including *M. avium-intracellulare* (297, 358). It is more active than rifampin against *M. tuberculosis* and the *M. fortuitum-chelonae* complex, including rifampin-resistant strains (94, 297, 306). All strains of *M. avium-intracellulare* are inhibited at concentrations of <2 μg/ml (173, 470). Like rifampin, this antibiotic is also active against many gram-positive and some gram-negative organisms.

The drug is given orally, with rapid gastrointestinal absorption and wide distribution in the body. Because of a long half-life of 16 h and high tissue concentrations, rifabutin is excreted slowly in the urine (372). Adverse reactions are similar to those of rifampin and include hepatic dysfunction, bone marrow depression, and skin rashes. Currently, rifabutin is used mainly in combination with other agents for the therapy of disseminated *M. avium-intracellulare* in immunocompromised patients (243, 450).

Dapsone

Dapsone, or diaminodiphenyl sulfone, is a synthetic drug active against leprosy bacilli in the mouse footpad model. Like all sulfones, dapsone is bacteriostatic and acts via the same mechanism as sulfonamides by interfering with bacterial folate synthesis. It has a vital role in the multidrug therapy of *M. leprae* infections (471). The drug is absorbed well after oral administration. It is distributed widely in the body, with tissue levels of about 2 μg/ml after standard doses. The serum half-life varies from 20 to 40 h in different individuals. The drug is metabolized in the liver, and 80% of the metabolites are excreted in the urine. Dosage reduction is necessary in patients with significant renal dysfunction.

In the mouse footpad model, *M. leprae* strains are inhibited by <0.01 μg of dapsone per ml (234). Because of the slow bactericidal activity, leprosy bacilli can persist for years while the patient is on dapsone therapy. Secondary drug resistance occurs in up to 20% of isolates in certain endemic regions (54). In endemic areas of leprosy, primary resistance to dapsone is as prevalent as secondary resistance. Clinically, dapsone is used often in combination with rifampin and clofazimine for the treatment of leprosy.

Gastrointestinal discomfort with nausea, vomiting, and anorexia is common. Drug fever and skin rashes can occur. Methemoglobinemia and hemolysis are notable hematologic side effects. A peculiar infectious mononucleosis-like condition known as sulfone syndrome, characterized by fever, jaundice, dermatitis, and lymphadenopathy, may occur 5 to 6 weeks after initiation of dapsone therapy.

Acedapsone

As a long-acting repository derivative of dapsone, acedapsone reaches peak serum concentrations at 22 to 35 days after injection. The drug alone has little action against *M. leprae,* but it is converted in vivo into active dapsone. Because of its long half-life, a single 300-mg dose can maintain dapsone levels inhibitory to *M. leprae* in patients for as long as 100 days (309). With administration needed only every 2 to 3 months, acedapsone shows promise in the multidrug therapeutic programs for patients with poor compliance or in whom other routes of therapy are not feasible.

Clofazimine

Clofazimine (B 663) is a phenazine dye with activity against *M. avium-intracellulare* and *M. leprae.* Although its precise mechanism of action is not known, it enhances superoxide dismutase activity, which results in enhanced production of intracellular oxygen radicals in phagocytes (294). The drug is administered orally and undergoes variable gastrointestinal absorption. Its peak plasma concentrations range from 0.4 to 3 μg/ml, and it has a serum half-life of about 70 days. The drug distributes very unevenly in the body, being highly concentrated in the liver, spleen, lung, adrenal and adipose tissues, and skin. This agent is largely unmetabolized and is excreted slowly in the bile (233). For *M. leprae,* clofazimine has MICs of 0.1 to 1.0 mg/kg in mouse tissue

(476). This drug is among the most active agents against *M. avium-intracellulare*, being bactericidal at ≤1 μg/ml (143). It has been used with success as a single agent or in combination therapy for resistant leprosy. For *M. avium-intracellulare* infections, clofazimine is often used in combination with other effective drugs.

A bluish red skin pigmentation from drug deposition in the skin is common. Gastrointestinal irritation is also frequent.

LITERATURE CITED

1. **Ackerman, B. H., and R. W. Bradsher.** 1985. Vancomycin and red necks. Ann. Intern. Med. **102:**723–724.
2. **Acocella, G.** 1983. Pharmacokinetics and metabolism of rifampicin in humans. Rev. Infect. Dis. **5**(Suppl. 3):S428–S432.
3. **Actor, P.** 1984. In vitro experience with cefonicid. Rev. Infect. Dis. **6**(Suppl. 4):S783–S790.
4. **Adkinson, N. F., Jr., A. Saxon, M. R. Spence, and E. A. Swabb.** 1985. Cross-allergenicity and immunogenicity of aztreonam. Rev. Infect. Dis. **7**(Suppl. 4):S613–S621.
5. **Allen, N. E., J. N. Hobbs, Jr., and W. E. Alborn, Jr.** 1987. Inhibition of peptidoglycan biosynthesis in gram-positive bacteria by LY146032. Antimicrob. Agents Chemother. **31:**1093–1099.
6. **Anderson, J. A.** 1986. Cross-sensitivity to cephalosporins in patients allergic to penicillin. Pediatr. Infect. Dis. **5:** 557–561.
7. **Appel, G. B., and H. C. Neu.** 1978. Gentamicin in 1978. Ann. Intern. Med. **89:**528–538.
8. **Appelbaum, P. C., M. R. Jacobs, S. K. Spangler, and S. Yamabe.** 1986. Comparative activity of β-lactamase inhibitors YTR830, clavulanate, and sulbactam combined with β-lactams against β-lactamase-producing anaerobes. Antimicrob. Agents Chemother. **30:**789–791.
9. **Aronoff, S. C., M. R. Jacobs, S. Johenning, and S. Yamabe.** 1984. Comparative activities of the β-lactamase inhibitors YTR 830, sodium clavulanate, and sulbactam combined with amoxicillin or ampicillin. Antimicrob. Agents Chemother. **26:**580–582.
10. **Aswapokee, N., and H. C. Neu.** 1978. A sulfone beta-lactam compound which acts as a beta-lactamase inhibitor. J. Antibiot. **31:**1238–1244.
11. **Bach, M. C., M. Finland, O. Gold, and C. Wilcox.** 1973. Susceptibility of recently isolated pathogenic bacteria to trimethoprim and sulfamethoxazole separately and combined. J. Infect. Dis. **128**(Suppl.):S508–S533.
12. **Bachmann, K., J. I. Schwartz, R. Forney, Jr., A. Frogameni, and L. E. Jauregui.** 1984. The effect of erythromycin on the disposition kinetics of warfarin. Pharmacology **28:**171–176.
13. **Baker, C. J., B. J. Webb, and F. F. Barrett.** 1976. Antimicrobial susceptibility of group B streptococci isolated from a variety of clinical sources. Antimicrob. Agents Chemother. **10:**128–131.
14. **Bansal, M. B., S. K. Chuah, and H. Thadepalli.** 1985. In vitro activity and in vivo evaluation of ticarcillin plus clavulanic acid against aerobic and anaerobic bacteria. Am. J. Med. **79**(Suppl. 5B):33–38.
15. **Barber, M., and P. M. Waterworth.** 1962. Antibacterial activity of the penicillins. Br. Med. J. **1:**1159–1164.
16. **Barber, M., and P. M. Waterworth.** 1962. Antibacterial activity in vitro of Fucidin. Lancet **i:**931–932.
17. **Barrett, F. F., R. F. McGehee, Jr., and M. Finland.** 1968. Methicillin-resistant *Staphylococcus aureus* at Boston City Hospital. N. Engl. J. Med. **279:**441–448.
18. **Barriere, S. L., and J. Mills.** 1982. Ceforanide: antibacterial activity, pharmacology, and clinical efficacy. Pharmacotherapy **2:**322–327.
19. **Barry, A. L., and R. N. Jones.** 1987. Cefixime: spectrum of antibacterial activity against 16,016 clinical isolates. Pediatr. Infect. Dis. J. **6:**954–957.
20. **Barry, A. L., C. Thornsberry, R. N. Jones, and T. L. Gavan.** 1985. Aztreonam: antibacterial activity, β-lactamase stability, and interpretive standards and quality control guidelines for disk-diffusion susceptibility test. Rev. Infect. Dis. **7**(Suppl. 4):S594–S604.
21. **Bartlett, J. G.** 1979. Antibiotic-associated pseudomembranous colitis. Rev. Infect. Dis. **1:**530–539.
22. **Bartlett, J. G.** 1982. Anti-anaerobic antibacterial agents. Lancet **ii:**478–481.
23. **Barza, M.** 1985. Imipenem: first of a new class of β-lactam antibiotics. Ann. Intern. Med. **103:**552–560.
24. **Barza, M., B. Furie, A. E. Brown, and B. C. Furie.** 1986. Defects in vitamin K-dependent carboxylation associated with moxalactam treatment. J. Infect. Dis. **153:**1166–1169.
25. **Beard, C. M., K. L. Noller, W. M. O'Fallon, L. T. Kurland, and D. C. Dahlin.** 1988. Cancer after exposure to metronidazole. Mayo Clin. Proc. **63:**147–153.
26. **Bechtold, H., K. Andrassy, E. Jahnchen, J. Koderisch, H. Koderisch, L. S. Weilemann, H. G. Sonntag, and E. Ritz.** 1984. Evidence for impaired hepatic vitamin K_1 metabolism in patients treated with *N*-methyl-thiotetrazole cephalosporins. Thromb. Haemost. **51:**358–361.
27. **Bendush, C. L.** 1982. Ototoxicity: clinical considerations and comparative information, p. 453–486. *In* A. Whelton and H. C. Neu (ed.), The aminoglycosides: microbiology, clinical use, and toxicology. Marcel Dekker, Inc., New York.
28. **Bergdahl, S., G. Elinder, and M. Eriksson.** 1981. Treatment of neonatal osteomyelitis with cloxacillin in combination with fusidic acid. Scand. J. Infect. Dis. **13:**281–282.
29. **Bergeron, M. G., J. L. Brusch, M. Barza, and L. Weinstein.** 1973. Bactericidal activity and pharmacology of cefazolin. Antimicrob. Agents Chemother. **4:**396–401.
30. **Berlin, O. G. W., L. S. Young, and D. A. Bruckner.** 1987. In-vitro activity of six fluorinated quinolones against *Mycobacterium tuberculosis*. J. Antimicrob. Chemother. **19:** 611–615.
31. **Bethell, H. J. N.** 1977. Photo-onycholysis caused by demethylchlortetracycline. Br. Med. J. **2:**96.
32. **Bhagwat, A. G., and R. W. Warren.** 1969. Hepatic reaction to nitrofurantoin. Lancet **ii:**1369.
33. **Bingen, E., N. Lambert-Zechovsky, P. Mariani-Kurkdjian, J. P. Cezard, and J. Navarro.** 1989. Bacteremia caused by a vancomycin-resistant enterococcus. Pediatr. Infect. Dis. J. **8:**475–476.
34. **Bisno, A. L., W. E. Dismukes, D. T. Durack, E. L. Kaplan, A. W. Karchmer, D. Kaye, S. H. Rahimtoola, M. A. Sande, J. P. Sanford, C. Watanakunakorn, and W. R. Wilson.** 1989. Antimicrobial treatment of infective endocarditis due to viridans streptococci, enterococci, and staphylococci. J. Am. Med. Assoc. **261:**1471–1477.
35. **Black, H. R., R. S. Griffith, and A. M. Peabody.** 1966. Absorption, excretion and metabolism of capreomycin in normal and diseased states. Ann. N.Y. Acad. Sci. **135:** 974–982.
36. **Bobrowitz, I. D.** 1972. Ethambutol in tuberculous meningitis. Chest **61:**629–632.
37. **Bodey, G. P., V. Fainstein, and A. M. Hinkle.** 1981. Comparative in vitro study of new cephalosporins. Antimicrob. Agents Chemother. **20:**226–230.
38. **Brogden, R. N., A. Carmine, R. C. Heel, P. A. Morley, T. M. Speight, and G. S. Avery.** 1981. Cefoperazone: a review of its in vitro antimicrobial activity, pharmacological properties and therapeutic efficacy. Drugs **22:**423–460.
39. **Brumfitt, W., J. M. T. Hamilton-Miller, R. A. Gargan, J. Cooper, and G. W. Smith.** 1983. Long-term prophylaxis of urinary infections in women: comparative trial of trimethoprim, methenamine hippurate and topical povi-

done-iodine. J. Urol. **130:**1110–1114.

40. **Brumfitt, W., G. W. Smith, J. M. T. Hamilton-Miller, and R. A. Gargan.** 1985. A clinical comparison between macrodantin and trimethoprim for prophylaxis in women with recurrent urinary infections. J. Antimicrob. Chemother. **16:**111–120.
41. **Brummett, R. E., and K. E. Fox.** 1989. Vancomycin- and erythromycin-induced hearing loss in humans. Antimicrob. Agents Chemother. **33:**791–796.
42. **Bryan, L. E.** 1984. Mechanisms of action of aminoglycoside antibiotics, p. 17–36. *In* R. K. Root and M. A. Sande (ed.), New dimensions in antimicrobial therapy. Churchill Livingstone, Inc., New York.
43. **Buening, M. D., J. S. Wold, K. S. Israel, and R. B. Kammer.** 1981. Disulfiram-like reactions to β-lactams. J. Am. Med. Assoc. **245:**2027–2028.
44. **Buesing, M. A., and J. H. Jorgensen.** 1984. In vitro activity of aztreonam in combination with newer β-lactams and amikacin against multiply resistant gram-negative bacilli. Antimicrob. Agents Chemother. **25:**283–285.
45. **Bush, K., J. S. Freudenberger, and R. B. Sykes.** 1982. Interaction of azthreonam and related monobactams with β-lactamases from gram-negative bacteria. Antimicrob. Agents Chemother. **22:**414–420.
46. **Bushby, S. R. M.** 1973. Trimethoprim-sulfamethoxazole: in vitro microbiological aspects. J. Infect. Dis. **128** (Suppl.):S442–S462.
47. **Butler, T., L. Rumans, and K. Arnold.** 1982. Response of typhoid fever caused by chloramphenicol-susceptible and chloramphenicol-resistant strains of *Salmonella typhi* to treatment with trimethoprim-sulfamethoxasole. Rev. Infect. Dis. **4:**551–561.
48. **Buu-Hoi, A., C. Branger, and J. F. Acar.** 1985. Vancomycin-resistant streptococci or *Leuconostoc* sp. Antimicrob. Agents Chemother. **28:**458–460.
49. **Carpenter, J. L., H. D. Covelli, M. E. Avant, C. K. McAllister, J. W. Higbee, and A. J. Ognibene.** 1982. Drug-resistant *Mycobacterium tuberculosis* in Korean isolates. Am. Rev. Respir. Dis. **126:**1092–1095.
50. **Carpenter, J. L., A. J. Ognibene, E. W. Gorby, R. E. Neimes, J. R. Koch, and W. L. Perkins.** 1983. Antituberculosis during resistance in South Texas. Am. Rev. Respir. Dis. **128:**1055–1058.
51. **Carroll, O. M., P. A. Bryan, and R. J. Robinson.** 1966. Stevens-Johnson syndrome associated with long-acting sulfonamides. J. Am. Med. Assoc. **195:**691–693.
52. **Casewell, M. W., and R. L. R. Hill.** 1985. In-vitro activity of mupirocin (pseudomonic acid) against clinical isolates of *Staphylococcus aureus*. J. Antimicrob. Chemother. **15:** 523–531.
53. **Casewell, M. W., and R. L. R. Hill.** 1986. Elimination of nasal carriage of *Staphylococcus aureus* with mupirocin (pseudomonic acid): a controlled trial. J. Antimicrob. Chemother. **17:**365–372.
54. **Centers for Disease Control.** 1982. Increase in prevalence of leprosy caused by dapsone-resistant *Mycobacterium leprae*. Morbid. Mortal. Weekly Rep. **30:**637–638.
55. **Centers for Disease Control.** 1983. Primary resistance to antituberculosis drugs—United States. Morbid. Mortal. Weekly Rep. **32:**521–523.
56. **Centers for Disease Control.** 1985. Adverse reactions to Fansidar and updated recommendations for its use in the prevention of malaria. Morbid. Mortal. Weekly Rep. **33:**713–714.
57. **Centers for Disease Control.** 1987. Antibiotic resistant strains of *Neisseria gonorrhoeae*. Morbid. Mortal. Weekly Rep. **36**(Suppl. 55):S1–S18.
58. **Centers for Disease Control.** 1988. Tuberculosis, final data—United States, 1986. Morbid. Mortal. Weekly Rep. **36:**817–820.
59. **Chamberlain, R. E.** 1976. Chemotherapeutic properties of prominent nitrofurans. J. Antimicrob. Chemother. **2:** 325–336.
60. **Chang, T., A. Black, A. Dunky, R. Wolf, A. Sedman, J. Latts, and P. G. Welling.** 1988. Pharmacokinetics of intravenous and oral enoxacin in healthy volunteers. J. Antimicrob. Chemother. **21**(Suppl. B):49–52.
61. **Chang, T. W., and L. Weinstein.** 1963. In vitro biological activity of cephalothin. J. Bacteriol. **85:**1022–1027.
62. **Chattopadhyay, B., I. Hall, and S. R. Curnow.** 1981. Ceftazidime (GR 20263), a new cephalosporin derivative with excellent activity against *Pseudomonas* and Enterobacteriaceae. J. Antimicrob. Chemother. **8:**491–493.
63. **Cherry, R. D., D. Portnoy, M. Jabbari, D. S. Daly, D. G. Kinnear, and C. A. Goresky.** 1982. Metronidazole: an alternate therapy for antibiotic-associated colitis. Gastroenterology **82:**849–851.
64. **Cherubin, C. E.** 1981. Antibiotic resistance of *Salmonella* in Europe and the United States. Rev. Infect. Dis. **3:**1105–1126.
65. **Chow, A. W., and D. Bednorz.** 1978. Comparative in vitro activity of newer cephalosporins against anaerobic bacteria. Antimicrob. Agents Chemother. **14:**668–671.
66. **Chow, A. W., N. Chang, and K. H. Bartlett.** 1985. In vitro susceptibility of *Clostridium difficile* to new β-lactam and quinolone antibiotics. Antimicrob. Agents Chemother. **28:**842–844.
67. **Chow, A. W., V. Pattern, and L. B. Guze.** 1975. Comparative susceptibility of anaerobic bacteria to minocycline, doxycycline, and tetracycline. Antimicrob. Agents Chemother. **7:**46–49.
68. **Christ, W., T. Lehnert, and B. Ulbrich.** 1988. Specific toxicologic aspects of the quinolones. Rev. Infect. Dis. **10**(Suppl. 1):S141–S146.
69. **Citron, K. M., and G. O. Thomas.** 1986. Ocular toxicity from ethambutol. Thorax **41:**737–739.
70. **Clark, J., and A. Wallace.** 1967. The susceptibility of mycobacteria to rifamide and rifampin. Tubercle **48:**144–148.
71. **Cleeland, R., and E. Squires.** 1984. Antimicrobial activity of ceftriaxone: a review. Am. J. Med. **77**(Suppl. 4C):3–11.
72. **Collins, C. H., and M. D. Yates.** 1982. Low incidence of rifampin-resistant tubercle bacilli. Thorax **37:**526–527.
73. **Colman, G., and A. Efstratiou.** 1987. Vancomycin-resistant leuconostocs, lactobacilli and now pediococci. J. Hosp. Infect. **10:**1–3.
74. **Colwell, E. J., R. L. Hickman, and S. Kosakal.** 1972. Tetracycline treatment of chloroquine-resistant falciparium malaria in Thailand. J. Am. Med. Assoc. **220:**684–686.
75. **Coppens, L., and J. Klastersky.** 1979. Comparative study of anti-pseudomonas activity of azlocillin, mezlocillin, and ticarcillin. Antimicrob. Agents Chemother. **15:**396–399.
76. **Corrado, M. L., W. E. Struble, C. Peter, V. Hoagland, and J. Sabbaj.** 1987. Norfloxacin: review of safety studies. Am. J. Med. **82**(Suppl. 6B):22–26.
77. **Costello, H. D., G. J. Caras, and D. E. Snider, Jr.** 1980. Drug resistance among previously treated tuberculosis patients, a brief report. Am. Rev. Respir. Dis. **121:**313–316.
78. **Craig, W. A., and C. M. Kunin.** 1973. Trimethoprim-sulfamethoxazole: pharmacodynamic effects of urinary pH and impaired renal function. Ann. Intern. Med. **78:** 491–497.
79. **Craven, G. R., R. Gavin, and T. Fanning.** 1969. The transfer RNA binding site of the 30S ribosome and the site of tetracycline inhibition. Cold Spring Harbor Symp. Quant. Biol. **34:**129–137.
80. **Crider, S. R., and S. D. Colby.** 1985. Susceptibility of enterococci to trimethoprim and trimethoprim-sulfamethoxazole. Antimicrob. Agents Chemother. **27:**71–75.
81. **Cuchural, G. J., Jr., F. P. Tally, N. V. Jacobus, K. Aldridge, T. Cleary, S. M. Finegold, G. Hill, P. Iannini, J. P. O'Keefe, C. Pierson, D. Crook, T. Russo, and D. Hecht.** 1988. Susceptibility of the *Bacteroides fragilis* group in the United States: analysis by site of isolation.

Antimicrob. Agents Chemother. **32:**717–722.

82. **Cynamon, M. H., and G. S. Palmer.** 1982. In vitro susceptibility of *Mycobacterium fortuitum* to *N*-formimidoyl thienamycin and several cephamycins. Antimicrob. Agents Chemother. **22:**1079–1081.
83. **Cynamon, M. H., and G. S. Palmer.** 1983. In vitro activity of amoxicillin in combination with clavulanic acid against *Mycobacterium tuberculosis*. Antimicrob. Agents Chemother. **24:**429–431.
84. **Dacre, J. E., A. M. Emmerson, and E. A. Jenner.** 1983. Nasal carriage of gentamicin and methicillin resistant *Staphylococcus aureus* treated with topical pseudomonic acid. Lancet **ii:**1036.
85. **Dannemann, B. R., D. M. Israelski, and J. S. Remington.** 1988. Treatment of toxoplasmic encephalitis with intravenous clindamycin. Arch. Intern. Med. **148:**2477–2482.
86. **D'Arcy, P. F.** 1985. Nitrofurantoin. Drug. Intell. Clin. Pharm. **19:**540–547.
87. **Davey, P., J.-C. Pechere, and D. Speller (ed.).** 1988. Spiramycin reassessed. J. Antimicrob. Chemother. **22**(Suppl. B):1–210.
88. **Davies, J. E.** 1983. Resistance to aminoglycosides: mechanisms and frequency. Rev. Infect. Dis. **5**(Suppl.): S261–S265.
89. **Davies, S., P. D. Sparham, and R. C. Spencer.** 1987. Comparative in-vitro activity of five fluoroquinolones against mycobacteria. J. Antimicrob. Chemother. **19:**605–609.
90. **Davis, B. D.** 1982. Bactericidal synergism between β-lactams and aminoglycosides: mechanism and possible therapeutic implications. Rev. Infect. Dis. **4:**237–245.
91. **Dawson, R. B.** 1966. Pulmonary reactions to nitrofurantoin. N. Engl. J. Med. **274:**522.
92. **Debbia, E., A. Pesce, and G. C. Schito.** 1988. In vitro activity of LY146032 alone and in combination with other antibiotics against gram-positive bacteria. Antimicrob. Agents Chemother. **32:**279–281.
93. **De Lepeleire, I., A. VanHecken, R. Verbesselt, T. B. Tjandra-Maga, and P. J. DeSchepper.** 1988. Comparative oral pharmacokinetics of fleroxacin and pefloxacin. J. Antimicrob. Chemother. **22:**197–202.
94. **Della Bruna, C., G. Schioppacassi, D. Ungheri, D. Jabes, E. Morvillo, and A. Sanfilippo.** 1983. LM427, a new spiropiperidyl-rifamycin: in vitro and in vivo studies. J. Antibiot. **36:**1502–1506.
95. **Delmee, M., and V. Avesani.** 1986. Comparative in vitro activity of seven quinolones against 100 clinical isolates of *Clostridium difficile*. Antimicrob. Agents Chemother. **29:**374–375.
96. **Dewsnup, D. H., and D. N. Wright.** 1984. In vitro susceptibility of *Nocardia asteroides* to 25 antimicrobial agents. Antimicrob. Agents Chemother. **25:**165–167.
97. **Divo, A. A., A. C. Sartorelli, C. L. Patton, and F. J. Bia.** 1988. Activity of fluoroquinolone antibiotics against *Plasmodium falciparum* in vitro. Antimicrob. Agents Chemother. **32:**1182–1186.
98. **Dixon, J. M. S., and A. E. Lipinski.** 1972. Resistance of group A beta-hemolytic streptococci to lincomycin and erythromycin. Antimicrob. Agents Chemother. **1:**333–339.
99. **Dowling, J. N., R. S. Weyant, and A. W. Pasculle.** 1982. Bactericidal activity of antibiotics against *Legionella micdadei* (Pittsburgh pneumonia agent). Antimicrob. Agents Chemother. **22:**272–276.
100. **Drusano, G. L., S. C. Schimpff, and W. L. Hewitt.** 1984. The acylampicillins: mezlocillin, piperacillin, and azlocillin. Rev. Infect. Dis. **6:**13–32.
101. **Dublanchet, A., J. Caillon, J. P. Emond, H. Chardon, and H. B. Drugeon.** 1986. Isolation of *Bacteroides* strains with reduced sensitivity to 5-nitroimidazoles. Eur. J. Clin. Microbiol. **5:**346–347.
102. **Dudley, M. N., J. C. McLaughlin, G. Carrington, J. Frick, C. H. Nightingale, and R. Quintiliani.** 1986. Oral bacitracin vs vancomycin therapy for *Clostridium difficile*-induced diarrhea: a randomized double-blind trial. Arch. Intern. Med. **146:**1101–1104.
103. **DuPont, H. L., D. G. Evans, N. Rios, F. J. Cabada, D. J. Evans, Jr., and M. W. DuPont.** 1982. Prevention of travelers' diarrhea with trimethoprim-sulfamethoxazole. Rev. Infect. Dis. **4:**533–539.
104. **DuPont, H. L., R. R. Reves, E. Galindo, P. S. Sullivan, L. V. Wood, and J. G. Mendiola.** 1982. Treatment of travelers' diarrhea with trimethoprim/sulfamethoxazole and with trimethoprim alone. N. Engl. J. Med. **307:**841–844.
105. **Easmon, C. S. F., and J. P. Crane.** 1985. Uptake of ciprofloxacin by human neutrophils. J. Antimicrob. Chemother. **16:**67–73.
106. **Edelstein, P. H., E. A. Gaudet, and M. A. C. Edelstein.** 1989. In vitro activity of lomefloxacin (NY-198 or SC 47111), ciprofloxacin, and erythromycin against 100 clinical *Legionella* strains. Diagn. Microbiol. Infect. Dis. **12**(Suppl.):93S–95S.
107. **Edelstein, P. H., and R. D. Meyer.** 1980. Susceptibility of *Legionella pneumophila* to twenty antimicrobial agents. Antimicrob. Agents Chemother. **18:**403–408.
108. **Edwards, D. I.** 1979. Mechanism of antimicrobial action of metronidazole. J. Antimicrob. Chemother. **5:**499–502.
109. **Eells, L. D., P. M. Mertz, Y. Piovanetti, G. M. Pekoe, and W. H. Eaglstein.** 1986. Topical antibiotic treatment of impetigo with mupirocin. Arch. Dermatol. **122:**1273–1276.
110. **Eickhoff, T. C., J. V. Bennett, P. S. Hayes, and J. Feeley.** 1970. *Pseudomonas pseudomallei:* susceptibility to chemotherapeutic agents. J. Infect. Dis. **121:**95–102.
111. **Eickhoff, T. C., and M. Finland.** 1965. Polymyxin B and colistin: in vitro activity against *Pseudomonas aeruginosa*. Am. J. Med. Sci. **249:**172–174.
112. **Eliopoulos, G. M., S. Willey, E. Reiszner, P. G. Spitzer, G. Caputo, and R. C. Moellering, Jr.** 1986. In vitro and in vivo activity of LY 146032, a new cyclic lipopeptide antibiotic. Antimicrob. Agents Chemother. **30:**532–535.
113. **Ellard, G. A.** 1969. Absorption, metabolism and excretion of pyrazinamide in man. Tubercle **50:**144–158.
114. **Ellard, G. A.** 1980. Combined treatment for lepromatous leprosy. Lepr. Rev. **51:**199–205.
115. **English, A. R., J. A. Retsema, A. E. Girard, J. E. Lynch, and W. E. Barth.** 1978. CP-45,899, a β-lactamase inhibitor that extends the antibacterial spectrum of β-lactams: initial bacteriological characterization. Antimicrob. Agents Chemother. **14:**414–419.
116. **Evans, D. A. P., K. A. Manley, and V. A. McKusick.** 1960. Genetic control of isoniazid metabolism in man. Br. Med. J. **2:**485–491.
117. **Eykyn, S., C. Jenkins, A. King, and I. Phillips.** 1976. Antibacterial activity of cefuroxime, a new cephalosporin antibiotic, compared with that of cephaloridine, cephalothin, and cefamandole. Antimicrob. Agents Chemother. **9:**690–695.
118. **Fallon, R. J., and W. M. Brown.** 1985. In-vitro sensitivity of legionellas, meningococci, and mycoplasmas to ciprofloxacin and enoxacin. J. Antimicrob. Chemother. **15:** 787–789.
119. **Farrell, I. D., P. M. Hinchliffe, and L. Robertson.** 1976. Sensitivity of *Brucella* spp. to tetracycline and its analogues. J. Clin. Pathol. **29:**1097–1100.
120. **Farrell, W., M. Wilks, and F. A. Drasar.** 1977. The action of trimethoprim and rifampicin in combination against Gram-negative rods resistant to gentamicin. J. Antimicrob. Chemother. **3:**459–462.
121. **Fass, R. J.** 1983. Comparative in vitro activities of third-generation cephalosporins. Arch. Intern. Med. **143:**1743–1745.
122. **Fass, R. J., E. A. Copelan, J. T. Brandt, M. L. Moeschberger, and J. J. Ashton.** 1987. Platelet-mediated bleed-

ing caused by broad-spectrum penicillins. J. Infect. Dis. **155:**1242–1248.

123. **Fass, R. J., and V. L. Helsel.** 1986. In vitro activity of LY146032 against staphylococci, streptococci, and enterococci. Antimicrob. Agents Chemother. **30:**781–784.
124. **Fee, W. E., Jr.** 1980. Aminoglycoside ototoxicity in the human. Laryngoscope **90**(Suppl. 24):1–19.
125. **Feeley, T. W., G. C. DuMoulin, J. Hedley-Whyte, L. S. Bushnell, J. P. Gilbert, and D. S. Feingold.** 1975. Aerosol polymyxin and pneumonia in seriously ill patients. N. Engl. J. Med. **293:**471–475.
126. **Fekety, R., J. Silva, B. Buggy, and H. G. Deery.** 1984. Treatment of antibiotic-associated colitis with vancomycin. J. Antimicrob. Chemother. **14**(Suppl. D):97–102.
127. **Finland, M., M. C. Bach, C. Garner, and O. Gold.** 1974. Synergistic action of ampicillin and erythromycin against *Nocardia asteroides:* effect of time of incubation. Antimicrob. Agents Chemother. **5:**344–353.
128. **Finland, M., C. Garner, C. Wilcox, and L. D. Sabath.** 1976. Susceptibility of beta-hemolytic streptococci to 65 antibacterial agents. Antimicrob. Agents Chemother. **9:** 11–19.
129. **Fitzpatrick, J. E., H. Tyler, Jr., and N. D. Gramstad.** 1981. Treatment of chancroid: comparison of sulfamethoxazole-trimethoprim with recommended therapies. J. Am. Med. Assoc. **246:**1804–1805.
130. **Fogdall, R. P., and R. D. Miller.** 1974. Prolongation of a pancuronium-induced neuromuscular blockage by clindamycin. Anesthesiology **41:**407–408.
131. **Foulds, G.** 1986. Pharmacokinetics of sulbactam/ampicillin in humans: a review. Rev. Infect. Dis. **8**(Suppl. 5): S503–S511.
132. **Freeman, L. D., D. R. Hooper, D. F. Lathen, D. P. Nelson, W. O. Harrison, and D. S. Anderson.** 1983. Brief prophylaxis with doxycycline for the prevention of traveler's diarrhea. Gastroenterology **84:**276–280.
133. **Freeman, R. B., W. M. Smith, J. A. Richardson, P. J. Hennelly, R. H. Thurm, C. Urner, J. A. Vaillancourt, R. J. Griep, and L. Bromer.** 1975. Long-term therapy for chronic bacteriuria in men: U.S. Public Health Service Cooperative Study. Ann. Intern. Med. **83:**133–147.
134. **Frost, P., G. D. Weinstein, and E. C. Gomez.** 1972. Phototoxic potential of minocycline and doxycycline. Arch. Dermatol. **105:**681–683.
135. **Fu, K. P., and H. C. Neu.** 1976. In vitro study of netilmicin compared with other aminoglycosides. Antimicrob. Agents Chemother. **10:**526–534.
136. **Fu, K. P., and H. C. Neu.** 1978. Azlocillin and mezlocillin: new ureido penicillins. Antimicrob. Agents Chemother. **13:**930–938.
137. **Fu, K. P., and H. C. Neu.** 1979. Comparative inhibition of β-lactamases by novel β-lactam compounds. Antimicrob. Agents Chemother. **15:**171–176.
138. **Fu, K. P., and H. C. Neu.** 1980. Antibacterial activity of ceftizoxime, a β-lactamase-stable cephalosporin. Antimicrob. Agents Chemother. **17:**583–590.
139. **Fuchs, P. C., A. L. Barry, T. L. Gavan, E. H. Gerlach, R. N. Jones, and C. Thornsberry.** 1977. Ticarcillin: a collaborative in vitro comparison with carbenicillin against 9,000 clinical bacterial isolates. Am. J. Med. Sci. **274:**255–263.
140. **Fuchs, P. C., A. L. Barry, C. Thornsberry, and R. N. Jones.** 1984. In vitro activity of ticarcillin plus clavulanic acid against 632 clinical isolates. Antimicrob. Agents Chemother. **25:**392–394.
141. **Fuller, A. T., G. Mellows, M. Woolford, G. T. Banks, K. D. Barrow, and E. B. Chain.** 1971. Pseudomonic acid: an antibiotic produced by *Pseudomonas fluorescens*. Nature (London) **234:**416–417.
142. **Gangadharam, P. R. J., and E. R. Candler.** 1977. In vitro anti-mycobacterial activity of some new aminoglycoside antibiotics. Tubercle **58:**35–38.
143. **Gangadharam, P. R. J., P. F. Pratt, P. B. Damle, and P. T. Davidson.** 1981. Dynamic aspects of the activity of clofazimine against *Mycobacterium intracellulare*. Tubercle **62:**201–206.
144. **Gay, J. D., D. R. DeYoung, and G. D. Roberts.** 1984. In vitro activities of norfloxacin and ciprofloxacin against *Mycobacterium tuberculosis, M. avium* complex, *M. chelonei, M. fortuitum,* and *M. kansasii.* Antimicrob. Agents Chemother. **26:**94–96.
145. **Gelber, R. H., P. R. Henika, and J. B. Gibson.** 1984. The bactericidal activity of various aminoglycoside antibiotics against *Mycobacterium leprae* in mice. Lepr. Rev. **55:**341–347.
146. **Geraci, J. E., and W. R. Wilson.** 1981. Vancomycin therapy for infective endocarditis. Rev. Infect. Dis. **3**(Suppl.): S250–S258.
147. **Ghuysen, J.-M.** 1977. Penicillin-sensitive enzymes of peptidoglycan metabolism, p. 195–202. *In* D. Schlessinger (ed.), Microbiology—1977. American Society for Microbiology, Washington, D.C.
148. **Giamarellou, H.** 1986. Aminoglycosides plus β-lactams against gram-negative organisms: evaluation of in vitro synergy and chemical interactions. Am. J. Med. **80**(Suppl. 6B):126–137.
149. **Girling, D. J.** 1977. Adverse reactions to rifampin in antituberculosis regimens. J. Antimicrob. Chemother. **3:** 115–132.
150. **Godtfredsen, W. O., K. Roholt, and L. Tybring.** 1962. Fucidin: a new orally active antibiotic. Lancet **i:**928–931.
151. **Goldfarb, J., D. Crenshaw, J. O'Horo, E. Lemon, and J. L. Blumer.** 1988. Randomized clinical trial of topical mupirocin versus oral erythromycin for impetigo. Antimicrob. Agents Chemother. **32:**1780–1783.
152. **Goldstein, E. J. C., and D. M. Citron.** 1985. Comparative activity of the quinolones against anaerobic bacteria isolated at community hospitals. Antimicrob. Agents Chemother. **27:**657–659.
153. **Goldstein, F. W., B. Papadopoulou, and J. F. Acar.** 1986. The changing pattern of trimethoprim resistance in Paris, with a review of worldwide experience. Rev. Infect. Dis. **8:**725–737.
154. **Goodhart, G. L.** 1984. In vivo v in vitro susceptibility of enterococcus to trimethoprim-sulfamethoxazole: a pitfall. J. Am. Med. Assoc. **252:**2748–2749.
155. **Gopalakrishna, K. V., and P. I. Lerner.** 1973. Tetracycline-resistant pneumococci: increasing incidence and cross resistance to newer tetracyclines. Am. Rev. Respir. Dis. **108:**1007–1010.
156. **Gordin, F. M., G. L. Simon, C. B. Wofsy, and J. Mills.** 1984. Adverse reactions to trimethoprim-sulfamethoxazole in patients with acquired immunodeficiency syndrome. Ann. Intern. Med. **100:**495–499.
157. **Gorzynski, E. A., D. Amsterdam, T. R. Beam, Jr., and C. Rotstein.** 1989. Comparative in vitro activities of teicoplanin, vancomycin, oxacillin, and other antimicrobial agents against bacteremic isolates of gram-positive cocci. Antimicrob. Agents Chemother. **33:**2019–2022.
158. **Gravenkemper, C. F., J. V. Bennett, J. L. Brodie, and W. M. M. Kirby.** 1965. Dicloxacillin: in vitro and pharmacologic comparisons with oxacillin and cloxacillin. Arch. Intern. Med. **116:**340–345.
159. **Greenwood, D.** 1988. Microbiological properties of teicoplanin. J. Antimicrob. Chemother. **21**(Suppl. A):1–13.
160. **Greenwood, D., and A. Eley.** 1982. In vitro evaluation of sulbactam, a penicillanic acid sulphone with β-lactamase inhibitory properties. J. Antimicrob. Chemother. **10:**117–123.
161. **Grossman, E. R., A. Walcheck, and H. Freedman.** 1971. Tetracycline and permanent teeth: the relationship between doses and tooth color. Pediatrics **47:**567–570.
162. **Gump, D. W.** 1981. Vancomycin for treatment of bacterial meningitis. Rev. Infect. Dis. **3**(Suppl.):S289–S292.
163. **Gurwith, M. J., H. R. Rabin, and K. Love.** 1977. Diarrhea associated with clindamycin and ampicillin therapy: pre-

liminary results of a cooperative study. J. Infect. Dis. **135**(Suppl.):S104–S110.

164. **Gutmann, L., M. D. Kitzis, S. Yamabe, and J. F. Acar.** 1986. Comparative evaluation of a new β-lactamase inhibitor, YTR 830, combined with different β-lactam antibiotics against bacteria harboring known β-lactamases. Antimicrob. Agents Chemother. **29:**955–957.
165. **Guttler, R. B., G. W. Counts, C. K. Avent, and H. N. Beaty.** 1971. Effect of rifampin and minocycline on meningococcal carrier rates. J. Infect. Dis. **124:**199–205.
166. **Halkin, H.** 1988. Adverse effects of the fluoroquinolones. Rev. Infect. Dis. **10**(Suppl. 1):S258–S261.
167. **Harding, G. K., and A. R. Ronald.** 1974. A controlled study of antimicrobial prophylaxis of recurrent urinary infection in women. N. Engl. J. Med. **291:**597–601.
168. **Harding, G. K. M., A. R. Ronald, L. E. Nicolle, M. J. Thomson, and G. J. Gray.** 1982. Long-term antimicrobial prophylaxis for recurrent urinary tract infection in women. Rev. Infect. Dis. **4:**438–443.
169. **Hardy, D. J., D. M. Hensey, J. M. Beyer, C. Vojtko, E. J. McDonald, and P. B. Fernandes.** 1988. Comparative in vitro activities of new 14-, 15-, and 16-membered macrolides. Antimicrob. Agents Chemother. **32:**1710–1719.
170. **Hartstein, A. I., K. E. Patrick, S. R. Jones, M. J. Miller, and R. E. Bryant.** 1977. Comparison of pharmacological and antimicrobial properties of cefadroxil and cephalexin. Antimicrob. Agents Chemother. **12:**93–97.
171. **Haydon, R. C., J. W. Thelin, and W. E. Davis.** 1984. Erythromycin ototoxicity: analysis and conclusions based on 22 case reports. Otolaryngol. Head Neck Surg. **92:** 678–684.
172. **Hedstrom, S. A.** 1985. Treatment and prevention of recurrent staphylococcal furunculosis: clinical and bacteriological follow-up. Scand. J. Infect. Dis. **17:**55–58.
173. **Heifets, L. B., M. D. Iseman, P. J. Lindholm-Levy, and W. Kanes.** 1985. Determination of ansamycin MICs for *Mycobacterium avium* complex in liquid medium by radiometric and conventional methods. Antimicrob. Agents Chemother. **28:**570–575.
174. **Hejny, J.** 1982. A drug sensitivity test strategy for atypical mycobacteria. Tubercle **62:**63–69.
175. **Herman, R. P., and M. M. Weber.** 1980. Isoniazid interaction with tyrosine as a possible mode of action of the drug in mycobacteria. Antimicrob. Agents Chemother. **17:**170–178.
176. **Herr, E. B., Jr., and M. O. Redstone.** 1966. Chemical and physical characterization of capreomycin. Ann. N.Y. Acad. Sci. **135:**940–946.
177. **Hill, G. B., and O. M. Ayers.** 1985. Antimicrobial susceptibilities of anaerobic bacteria isolated from female genital tract infections. Antimicrob. Agents Chemother. **27:**324–331.
178. **Hilson, G. R. F.** 1962. In-vitro studies of a new antibiotic (Fucidin). Lancet **i:**932–933.
179. **Hitchings, G. H.** 1973. Mechanism of action of trimethoprim-sulfamethoxazole. I. J. Infect. Dis. **128**(Suppl.): S433–S436.
180. **Hoeprich, P. D., and D. M. Warshauer.** 1974. Entry of four tetracyclines into saliva and tears. Antimicrob. Agents Chemother. **5:**330–336.
181. **Hof, H., O. Zak, E. Schweizer, and A. Danzler.** 1984. Antibacterial activities of nitrothiazole derivatives. J. Antimicrob. Chemother. **14:**31–39.
182. **Hoffken, G., H. Lode, C. Prinzing, K. Borner, and P. Koeppe.** 1985. Pharmacokinetics of ciprofloxacin after oral and parenteral administration. Antimicrob. Agents Chemother. **27:**375–379.
183. **Holmberg, L., G. Boman, L. E. Bottiger, B. Eriksson, R. Spross, and A. Wessling.** 1980. Adverse reactions to nitrofurantoin: analysis of 921 reports. Am. J. Med. **69:** 733–738.
184. **Hoogkamp-Korstanje, J. A. A.** 1987. Antibiotics in *Yersinia enterocolitica* infections. J. Antimicrob. Chemother. **20:**123–131.
185. **Hooper, D. C., and J. S. Wolfson.** 1989. Mode of action of the quinolone antimicrobial agents: a review of recent information. Rev. Infect. Dis. **11**(Suppl. 5):S902–S911.
186. **Hooper, D. C., J. S. Wolfson, E. Y. Ng, and M. N. Swartz.** 1987. Mechanisms of action and resistance to ciprofloxacin. Am. J. Med. **82**(Suppl. 4A):12–20.
187. **Hughes, J., and G. Mellows.** 1978. Inhibition of isoleucyl-transfer ribonucleic acid synthetase in *Escherichia coli* by pseudomonic acid. Biochem. J. **176:**305–318.
188. **Hughes, W. T., S. Kuhn, S. Chaudhary, S. Feldman, M. Verzosa, R. J. A. Aur, C. Pratt, and S. L. George.** 1977. Successful chemoprophylaxis for *Pneumocystis carinii* pneumonitis. N. Engl. J. Med. **297:**1419–1426.
189. **Hunter, P. A., K. Coleman, J. Fisher, and D. Taylor.** 1980. In-vitro synergistic properties of clavulanic acid, with ampicillin, amoxycillin, and ticarcillin. J. Antimicrob. Chemother. **6:**455–470.
190. **Inman, W. H. W., and N. S. B. Rawson.** 1983. Erythromycin estolate and jaundice. Br. Med. J. **286:**1954–1955.
191. **Iravani, A., G. A. Richard, and H. Baer.** 1981. Treatment of uncomplicated urinary tract infections with trimethoprim versus sulfisoxazole, with special reference to antibody-coated bacteria and fecal flora. Antimicrob. Agents Chemother. **19:**842–850.
192. **Isenberg, H. D., E. M. Vellozzi, J. Shapiro, and L. G. Rubin.** 1988. Clinical laboratory challenges in the recognition of *Leuconostoc* spp. J. Clin. Microbiol. **26:**479–483.
193. **Jacobs, M. R., S. C. Aronoff, S. Johenning, D. M. Shlaes, and S. Yamabe.** 1986. Comparative activities of the β-lactamase inhibitors YTR 830, clavulanate, and sulbactam combined with ampicillin and broad-spectrum penicillin against defined β-lactamase-producing aerobic gram-negative bacilli. Antimicrob. Agents Chemother. **29:**980–985.
194. **Jacobs, R. F.** 1988. Ceftriaxone-associated cholecystitis. Pediatr. Infect. Dis. J. **7:**434–436.
195. **Jacobson, J. A., and B. Daniel.** 1975. Vestibular reactions associated with minocycline. Antimicrob. Agents Chemother. **8:**453–456.
196. **Jacobus, N. V., M. C. Ferreira, and M. Barza.** 1982. In vitro activity of azthreonam, a monobactam antibiotic. Antimicrob. Agents Chemother. **22:**832–838.
197. **Jacoby, G. A., and L. Sutton.** 1989. *Pseudomonas cepacia* susceptibility to sulbactam. Antimicrob. Agents Chemother. **33:**583–584.
198. **Jenner, P. J., G. A. Ellard, P. J. K. Gruer, and V. R. Aber.** 1984. A comparison of the blood levels and urinary excretion of ethionamide and prothionamide in man. J. Antimicrob. Chemother. **13:**267–277.
199. **Jick, H.** 1982. Adverse reactions to trimethoprim-sulfamethoxazole in hospitalized patients. Rev. Infect. Dis. **4:** 426–428.
200. **Johnson, S. E., G. C. Klein, G. P. Schmid, and J. C. Feeley.** 1984. Susceptibility of the Lyme disease spirochete to seven antimicrobial agents. Yale J. Biol. Med. **57:**549–553.
201. **Jokipii, L., and A. M. M. Jokipii.** 1985. Comparative evaluation of the 2-methyl-5-nitroimidazole compounds dimetridazole, metronidazole, secnidazole, ornidazole, tinidazole, carnidazole, and panidazole against *Bacteroides fragilis* and other bacteria of the *Bacteroides fragilis* group. Antimicrob. Agents Chemother. **28:**561–564.
202. **Jones, R. N., and A. L. Barry.** 1983. Cefoperazone: a review of its antimicrobial spectrum, β-lactamase stability, enzyme inhibition, and other in vitro characteristics. Rev. Infect. Dis. **5**(Suppl. 1):S108–S126.
203. **Jones, R. N., and A. L. Barry.** 1987. Antimicrobial activity and spectrum of LY146032, a lipopeptide antibiotic, including susceptibility testing recommendations. Antimi-

crob. Agents Chemother. **31**:625–629.

204. **Jones, R. N., A. L. Barry, and C. Thornsberry.** 1983. Ceftriaxone: a summary of in vitro antibacterial qualities including recommendation for susceptibility tests with 30-μg disks. Diagn. Microbiol. Infect. Dis. **1**:295–311.
205. **Jorgensen, J. H., S. A. Crawford, and G. A. Alexander.** 1980. Comparison of moxalactam (LY127935) and cefotaxime against anaerobic bacteria. Antimicrob. Agents Chemother. **17**:901–904.
206. **Kamimura, T., H. Kojo, Y. Matsumoto, Y. Mine, S. Goto, and S. Kuwahara.** 1984. In vitro and in vivo antibacterial properties of FK 027, a new orally active cephem antibiotic. Antimicrob. Agents Chemother. **25**: 98–104.
207. **Kaplan, A. H., P. H. Gilligan, and R. R. Facklam.** 1988. Recovery of resistant enterococci during vancomycin prophylaxis. J. Clin. Microbiol. **26**:1216–1218.
208. **Karlson, A. G.** 1961. The in vitro activity of ethambutol (dextro-2,2′-[ethylenediimino]-di-1-butanol) against tubercle bacilli and other microorganisms. Am. Rev. Respir. Dis. **84**:905–906.
209. **Keinath, R. D., D. E. Merrell, R. Vlietstra, and W. O. Dobbins III.** 1985. Antibiotic treatment and relapse in Whipple's disease: long-term follow-up of 88 patients. Gastroenterology **88**:1867–1873.
210. **Kenny, G. E., T. M. Hooton, M. C. Roberts, F. D. Cartwright, and J. Hoyt.** 1989. Susceptibilities of genital mycoplasmas to the newer quinolones as determined by the agar dilution method. Antimicrob. Agents Chemother. **33**:103–107.
211. **Kesado, T., K. Watanabe, Y. Asahi, M. Isono, and K. Ueno.** 1982. Susceptibilities of anaerobic bacteria to *N*-formimidoyl thienamycin (MK0787) and to other antibiotics. Antimicrob. Agents Chemother. **21**:1016–1022.
212. **Kirst, H. A., and G. D. Sides.** 1989. New directions for macrolide antibiotics: structural modifications and in vitro activity. Antimicrob. Agents Chemother. **33**:1413–1418.
213. **Kleinfeld, D. I., R. J. Sharpe, and S. T. Donta.** 1988. Parenteral therapy for antibiotic-associated pseudomembranous colitis. J. Infect. Dis. **157**:389.
214. **Klinge, E., P. Mannisto, R. Mantyla, U. Lamminsivu, and P. Ottoila.** 1982. Pharmacokinetics of methenamine in healthy volunteers. J. Antimicrob. Chemother. **9**:209–216.
215. **Knight, V., J. W. Draper, E. A. Brady, and C. A. Attmore.** 1952. Methenamine mandelate: antimicrobial activity, absorption and excretion. Antibiot. Chemother. **2**:615–635.
216. **Koch-Weser, J., V. W. Sidel, E. B. Federman, P. Kanarek, D. C. Finer, and A. E. Eaton.** 1970. Adverse effects of sodium colistimethate: manifestations and specific reaction rates during 317 courses of therapy. Ann. Intern. Med. **72**:857–868.
217. **Kohn, J., and A. J. Evans.** 1970. Group A streptococci resistant to clindamycin. Br. Med. J. **2**:423.
218. **Konno, K., K. Oizumi, and S. Oka.** 1973. Mode of action of rifampin on mycobacteria. Am. Rev. Respir. Dis. **107**: 1006–1012.
219. **Kopanoff, D. E., D. E. Snider, Jr., and G. J. Caras.** 1978. Isoniazid-related hepatitis: a U.S. Public Health Service Cooperative Surveillance Study. Am. Rev. Respir. Dis. **117**:991–1001.
220. **Krause, R., and U. Ullmann.** 1988. Comparative in vitro activity of fleroxacin (RO 23-6240) against *Ureaplasma urealyticum* and *Mycoplasma hominis*. Eur. J. Clin. Microbiol. **7**:67–69.
221. **Kropp, H., L. Gerckens, J. G. Sundelof, and F. M. Kahan.** 1985. Antibacterial activity of imipenem: the first thienamycin antibiotics. Rev. Infect. Dis. **7**(Suppl. 3): S389–S410.
222. **Kucers, A., and N. M. Bennett.** 1987. The use of antibiotics: a comprehensive review with clinical emphasis, 4th ed. J. B. Lippincott Co., Philadelphia.
223. **Kuck, N. A., N. V. Jacobus, P. J. Petersen, W. J. Weiss, and R. T. Testa.** 1989. Comparative in vitro and in vivo activities of piperacillin combined with the β-lactamase inhibitors tazobactam, clavulanic acid, and sulbactam. Antimicrob. Agents Chemother. **33**:1964–1969.
224. **Kunin, C. M., and A. Bugg.** 1971. Binding of polymyxin antibiotics to tissues: the major determinant of distribution and persistence in the body. J. Infect. Dis. **124**: 394–400.
225. **Kuze, F., T. Kurasawa, K. Bando, Y. Lee, and N. Maekawa.** 1981. In vitro and in vivo susceptibility of atypical mycobacteria to various drugs. Rev. Infect. Dis. **3**:885–897.
226. **Larson, H. E., A. B. Price, P. Honour, and S. P. Borriello.** 1978. *Clostridium difficile* and the etiology of pseudomembranous colitis. Lancet **i**:1063–1066.
227. **Lawson, D. H., and B. J. Paice.** 1982. Adverse reactions to trimethoprim-sulfamethoxazole. Rev. Infect. Dis. **4**: 429–433.
228. **Leclercq, R., E. Derlot, J. Duval, and P. Courvalin.** 1988. Plasmid-mediated resistance to vancomycin and teicoplanin in *Enterococcus faecium*. N. Engl. J. Med. **319**: 157–161.
229. **Leclercq, R., E. Derlot, M. Weber, J. Duval, and P. Courvalin.** 1989. Transferable vancomycin and teicoplanin resistance in *Enterococcus faecium*. Antimicrob. Agents Chemother. **33**:10–15.
230. **Leibold, J. E.** 1966. The ocular toxicity of ethambutol and its relation to dose. Ann. N.Y. Acad. Sci. **135**:904–909.
231. **Leigh, D. A.** 1981. Antibacterial activity and pharmacokinetics of clindamycin. J. Antimicrob. Chemother. **7**(Suppl. A):3–9.
232. **Leoung, G. S., J. Mills, P. C. Hopewell, W. Hughes, and C. Wofsy.** 1986. Dapsone-trimethoprim for *Pneumocystis carinii* pneumonia in the acquired immunodeficiency syndrome. Ann. Intern. Med. **105**:45–48.
233. **Levy, L.** 1974. Pharmacologic studies of clofazimine. Am. J. Trop. Med. Hyg. **23**:1097–1109.
234. **Levy, L., and J. H. Peters.** 1976. Susceptibility of *Mycobacterium leprae* to dapsone as a determinant of patient response to acedapsone. Antimicrob. Agents Chemother. **9**:102–112.
235. **Linares, J., J. Garau, C. Dominguez, and J. L. Perez.** 1983. Antibiotic resistance and serotypes of *Streptococcus pneumoniae* from patients with community-acquired pneumococcal disease. Antimicrob. Agents Chemother. **23**:545–547.
236. **Livermore, D. M., R. J. Williams, and J. D. Williams.** 1981. In-vitro activity of ceftazidime against *Pseudomonas aeruginosa* and its stability to pseudomonal β-lactamases. J. Antimicrob. Chemother. **8**(Suppl. B):163–167.
237. **Low, D. E., A. McGeer, and R. Poon.** 1989. Activities of daptomycin and teicoplanin against *Staphylococcus haemolyticus* and *Staphylococcus epidermidis*, including evaluation of susceptibility testing recommendations. Antimicrob. Agents Chemother. **33**:585–588.
238. **Ludden, T. M.** 1985. Pharmacokinetic interactions of the macrolide antibiotics. Clin. Pharmacokinet. **10**:63–79.
239. **Mackechnie-Jarvis, A. C.** 1985. Simple wound irrigation system to treat staphylococcal infection of intramedullary nails. Lancet **i**:1035–1036.
240. **Mandell, G. L.** 1983. The antimicrobial activity of rifampin: emphasis on the relation to phagocytes. Rev. Infect. Dis. **5**(Suppl. 3):S463–S467.
241. **Marshall, W. F., M. R. Keating, J. P. Anhalt, and J. M. Steckelberg.** 1979. *Xanthomonas maltophilia:* an emerging nosocomial pathogen. Mayo Clin. Proc. **64**:1097–1104.
242. **Martell, R., D. Heinrichs, C. R. Stiller, M. Jenner, P. A. Keown, and J. Dupre.** 1986. The effects of erythromycin in patients treated with cyclosporine. Ann. Intern. Med. **104**:660–661.

243. **Masur, H., C. Tuazon, V. Gill, G. Grimes, B. Baird, A. S. Fauci, and H. C. Lane.** 1987. Effect of combined clofazimine and ansamycin therapy on *Mycobacterium avium-Mycobacterium intracellulare* bacteria in patients with AIDS. J. Infect. Dis. **155:**127–129.
244. **Mayer, K. H., M. E. Fling, J. D. Hopkins, and T. F. O'Brien.** 1985. Trimethoprim resistance in multiple genera of enterobacteriaceae at a U.S. hospital: spread of the type II dihydrofolate reductase gene by a single plasmid. J. Infect. Dis. **151:**783–789.
245. **McCalla, D. R.** 1977. Biological effects of nitrofurans. J. Antimicrob. Chemother. **3:**517–520.
246. **McClatchy, J. K., W. Kanes, P. T. Davidson, and T. S. Moulding.** 1977. Cross-resistance in *M. tuberculosis* to kanamycin, capreomycin and viomycin. Tubercle **58:**29–34.
247. **McDowell, T. D., and K. E. Reed.** 1989. Mechanism of penicillin killing in the absence of bacterial lysis. Antimicrob. Agents Chemother. **33:**1680–1685.
248. **McGehee, R. F., Jr., F. F. Barrett, and M. Finland.** 1969. Resistance of *Staphylococcus aureus* to lincomycin, clinimycin, and erythromycin, p. 392–397. Antimicrob. Agents Chemother. 1968.
249. **McGehee, R. F., Jr., C. B. Smith, C. Wilcox, and M. Finland.** 1968. Comparative studies of antibacterial activity in vitro and absorption and excretion of lincomycin and clindamycin. Am. J. Med. Sci. **256:**279–292.
250. **McNulty, C. A. M., J. Dent, and R. Wise.** 1985. Susceptibility of clinical isolates of *Campylobacter pyloridis* to 11 antimicrobial agents. Antimicrob. Agents Chemother. **28:**837–838.
251. **Medical Letter.** 1988. Drugs for parasitic infections. Med. Lett. Drugs Therapeut. **30:**15–24.
252. **Medical Letter.** 1989. Prevention of bacterial endocarditis. Med. Lett. Drugs Therapeut. **31:**112.
253. **Mellor, J. A., J. Kingdom, M. Cafferkey, and C. T. Keane.** 1985. Vancomycin toxicity: a prospective study. J. Antimicrob. Chemother. **15:**773–780.
254. **Merson, M. H., R. B. Sack, S. Islam, G. Saklayen, N. Huda, I. Huq, A. W. Zulich, R. H. Yolken, and A. Z. Kapikian.** 1980. Disease due to enterotoxigenic *Escherichia coli* in Bangladeshi adults: clinical aspects and a controlled trial of tetracycline. J. Infect. Dis. **141:**702–711.
255. **Meyers, B. R., and S. Z. Hirschman.** 1978. Antibacterial activity of cefamandole in vitro. J. Infect. Dis. **137**(Suppl.): S25–S31.
256. **Moellering, R. C., Jr.** 1984. Pharmacokinetics of vancomycin. J. Antimicrob. Chemother. **14**(Suppl. D):43–52.
257. **Molavi, A., and L. Weinstein.** 1971. In-vitro activity of erythromycin against atypical mycobacteria. J. Infect. Dis. **123:**216–219.
258. **Monk, J. P., and D. M. Campoli-Richards.** 1987. Ofloxacin: a review of its antibacterial activity, pharmacokinetic properties and therapeutic use. Drugs **33:**346–391.
259. **Moody, M. R., and V. M. Young.** 1975. In vitro susceptibility of *Pseudomonas cepacia* and *Pseudomonas maltophilia* to trimethoprim and trimethoprim-sulfamethoxazole. Antimicrob. Agents Chemother. **7:**836–839.
260. **Moorhouse, E. C., T. E. Mulvihill, L. Jones, D. Mooney, F. R. Falkiner, and C. T. Keane.** 1985. The in-vitro activity of some antimicrobial agents against methicillin-resistant *Staphylococcus aureus.* J. Antimicrob. Chemother. **15:**291–295.
261. **Moosdeen, F., J. D. Williams, and S. Yamabe.** 1988. Antibacterial characteristics of YTR 830, a sulfone β-lactamase inhibitor, compared with those of clavulanic acid and sulbactam. Antimicrob. Agents Chemother. **32:**925–927.
262. **Morel, C., M. Vergnaud, M. M. Langeard, and L. Dupuy.** 1983. Cefotetan: comparative study in vitro against 266 gram-negative clinical isolates. J. Antimicrob. Chemother. **11**(Suppl. A):31–36.
263. **Morris, J. G., Jr., and R. E. Black.** 1985. Cholera and other vibrioses in the United States. N. Engl. J. Med. **312:** 343–350.
264. **Morrison, D. C., and D. M. Jacobs.** 1976. Binding of polymycin B to the lipid A portion of bacterial lipopolysaccharides. Immunochemistry **13:**813–818.
265. **Most, H.** 1984. Treatment of parasitic infections of travelers and immigrants. N. Engl. J. Med. **310:**298–304.
266. **Musher, D. M., and D. P. Griffith.** 1974. Generation of formaldehyde from methenamine: effect of pH and concentration, and antibacterial effect. Antimicrob. Agents Chemother. **6:**708–711.
267. **Musher, D. M., D. P. Griffith, and G. B. Templeton.** 1976. Further observations on the potentiation of the antibacterial effect of methenamine by acetohydroxamic acid. J. Infect. Dis. **133:**564–567.
268. **Musial, C. E., and J. E. Rosenblatt.** 1989. Antimicrobial susceptibilities of anaerobic bacteria isolated at the Mayo Clinic during 1982 through 1987: comparison with results from 1977 through 1981. Mayo Clin. Proc. **64:**392–399.
269. **Najjar, A., and B. E. Murray.** 1987. Failure to demonstrate a consistent in vitro bactericidal effect of trimethoprim-sulfamethoxazole against enterococci. Antimicrob. Agents Chemother. **31:**808–810.
270. **Nelson, J. D., H. Kusmiesz, and S. Shelton.** 1982. Oral or intravenous trimethoprim-sulfamethoxazole therapy for shigellosis. Rev. Infect. Dis. **4:**546–550.
271. **Neu, H. C.** 1974. Antimicrobial activity and human pharmacology of amoxicillin. J. Infect. Dis. **129**(Suppl.):S123–S131.
272. **Neu, H. C.** 1975. Aminopenicillins: clinical pharmacology and use in disease states. Int. J. Clin. Pharmacol. Biopharm. **11:**132–144.
273. **Neu, H. C.** 1976. Mecillinam, a novel penicillanic acid derivative with unusual activity against gram-negative bacteria. Antimicrob. Agents Chemother. **9:**793–799.
274. **Neu, H. C.** 1976. Tobramycin: an overview. J. Infect. Dis. **134**(Suppl.):S3–S19.
275. **Neu, H. C.** 1977. Mecillinam: an amdino penicillin which acts synergistically with other beta-lactam compounds. J. Antimicrob. Chemother. **3**(Suppl. B):43–52.
276. **Neu, H. C.** 1982. The new beta-lactamase-stable cephalosporins. Ann. Intern. Med. **97:**408–419.
277. **Neu, H. C.** 1982. Antistaphylococcal penicillins. Med. Clin. North Am. **66:**51–60.
278. **Neu, H. C.** 1982. Trimethoprim alone for treatment of urinary tract infection. Rev. Infect. Dis. **4:**366–371.
279. **Neu, H. C.** 1983. Penicillin-binding proteins and role of amdinocillin in causing bacterial cell death. Am. J. Med. **75**(Suppl. 2A):9–20.
280. **Neu, H. C.** 1984. Synergistic activity of mecillinam in combination with the β-lactamase inhibitors clavulanic acid and sulbactam. Antimicrob. Agents Chemother. **22:** 518–519.
281. **Neu, H. C.** 1985. Carbapenems: special properties contributing to their activity. Am. J. Med. **78**(Suppl. 6A):33–40.
282. **Neu, H. C.** 1989. Synergy of fluoroquinolones with other antimicrobial agents. Rev. Infect. Dis. **11**(Suppl. 5): S1025–S1035.
283. **Neu, H. C., N.-X. Chin, and P. Labthavikul.** 1984. Comparative in vitro activity and β-lactamase stability of FR 17027, a new orally active cephalosporin. Antimicrob. Agents Chemother. **26:**174–180.
284. **Neu, H. C., and K. P. Fu.** 1978. Clavulanic acid, a novel inhibitor of beta-lactamases. Antimicrob. Agents Chemother. **14:**650–655.
285. **Neu, H. C., and K. P. Fu.** 1980. In vitro activity of chloramphenicol and thiamphenicol analogs. Antimicrob. Agents Chemother. **18:**311–316.
286. **Neu, H. C., and G. T. Garvey.** 1975. Comparative in vitro activity and clinical pharmacology of ticarcillin and carbenicillin. Antimicrob. Agents Chemother. **8:**457–462.

287. **Neu, H. C., and P. Lubthavikul.** 1982. Antibacterial activity and β-lactamase stability of ceftazidime, an aminothiazolyl cephalosporin potentially active against *Pseudomonas aeruginosa*. Antimicrob. Agents Chemother. **21:**11–18.
288. **Neu, H. C., and P. Lubthavikul.** 1982. Comparative in vitro activity of *N*-formimidoyl thienamycin against gram-positive and gram-negative aerobic and anaerobic species and its β-lactamase stability. Antimicrob. Agents Chemother. **21:**180–187.
289. **Neu, H. C., N. J. Meropol, and K. P. Fu.** 1981. Antibacterial activity of ceftriaxone (RO 13-9904), a β-lactamase-stable cephalosporin. Antimicrob. Agents Chemother. **19:** 414–423.
290. **Neuvonen, P. J., G. Gothoni, R. Hackman, and K. Bjorksten.** 1970. Interference of iron with the absorption of tetracycline in man. Br. Med. J. **4:**532–534.
291. **Newman, R. L., K. M. Bhat, R. Hackney, C. Robinson, and G. T. Stewart.** 1962. Fusidic acid: laboratory and clinical assessment. Br. Med. J. **2:**1645–1647.
292. **Newman, T. J., G. R. Dreslinski, and S. S. Tadros.** 1985. Safety profile of aztreonam in clinical trials. Rev. Infect. Dis. **7**(Suppl. 4):S648–S655.
293. **Nieto, M., and H. R. Perkins.** 1971. Physicochemical properties of vancomycin and iodovancomycin and their complexes with diacetyl-L-lysyl-D-alanyl-D-alanine. Biochem. J. **123:**773–787.
294. **Niwa, Y., T. Sakane, Y. Miyachi, and M. Ozaki.** 1984. Oxygen metabolism in phagocytes of leprotic patients: enhanced endogenous superoxide dismutase activity and hydroxyl radical generation by clofazimine. J. Clin. Microbiol. **20:**837–842.
295. **Nord, C. E., T. Wadstrom, and B. Wretlind.** 1974. Synergistic effect of combinations of sulfamethoxazole, trimethoprim, and colistin against *Pseudomonas maltophilia* and *P. cepacia*. Antimicrob. Agents Chemother. **6:**521–523.
296. **Nunn, P. P., and J. C. Allistone.** 1984. Resistance to trimethoprim-sulfamethoxazole in the treatment of *Pneumocystis carinii* pneumonia: implication of folinic acid. Chest **86:**149–150.
297. **O'Brien, R. J., M. A. Lyle, and D. E. Snider, Jr.** 1987. Rifabutin (ansamycin LM 427): a new rifamycin-S derivative for the treatment of mycobacterial diseases. Rev. Infect. Dis. **9:**519–530.
298. **O'Brien, T. F., J. F. Acar, G. Altmann, B. O. Blackburn, L. Chao, A.-L. Courtieu, D. A. Evans, M. Guzman, M. Holmes, M. R. Jacobs, R. L. Kent, R. A. Norton, H. J. Koornhof, A. A. Medeiros, A. W. Pasculle, M. J. Surgalla, and J. D. Williams.** 1982. Laboratory surveillance of synergy between and resistance to trimethoprim and sulfonamides. Rev. Infect. Dis. **4:**351–357.
299. **O'Callaghan, C. H., R. B. Sykes, A. Griffiths, and J. E. Thornton.** 1976. Cefuroxime, a new cephalosporin antibiotic: activity in vitro. Antimicrob. Agents Chemother. **9:**511–519.
300. **Oleinick, N. L., and J. W. Corcoran.** 1969. Two types of binding of erythromycin to ribosomes from antibiotic-sensitive and -resistant *Bacillus subtilis* 168. J. Biol. Chem. **244:**727–735.
301. **Pang, L. W., N. Limsomwong, E. F. Boudreau, and P. Singharaj.** 1987. Doxycycline prophylaxis for falciparum malaria. Lancet **i:**1161–1164.
302. **Panzer, J. D., D. C. Brown, W. L. Epstein, R. L. Lipson, H. W. Mahaffey, and W. H. Atkinson.** 1972. Clindamycin levels in various body tissues and fluids. J. Clin. Pharmacol. **12:**259–262.
303. **Pape, J. W., R. I. Verdier, and W. D. Johnson, Jr.** 1989. Treatment and prophylaxis of *Isospora belli* infection in patients with the acquired immunodeficiency syndrome. N. Engl. J. Med. **320:**1044–1047.
304. **Parsley, T. L., R. B. Provonchee, C. Glicksman, and S. H. Zinner.** 1977. Synergistic activity of trimethoprim and amikacin against gram-negative bacilli. Antimicrob. Agents Chemother. **12:**349–352.
305. **Patel, R. B., and P. G. Welling.** 1980. Clinical pharmacokinetics of co-trimoxazole (trimethoprim-sulfamethoxazole). Clin. Pharmacokinet. **5:**405–423.
306. **Pattyn, S. R.** 1987. Rifabutin and rifapentine compared with rifampin against *Mycobacterium leprae* in mice. Letter to the Editor. Antimicrob. Agents Chemother. **31:**134.
307. **Peets, E. A., W. M. Sweeney, V. A. Place, and D. A. Buyske.** 1965. The absorption, excretion, and metabolic fate of ethambutol in man. Am. Rev. Respir. Dis. **91:**51–58.
308. **Peters, G., G. Pulverer, and M. Neugebauer.** 1980. In vitro activity of clavulanic acid and amoxicillin combined against amoxicillin-resistant bacteria. Infection **8:**104–106.
309. **Peters, J. H., J. F. Murray, Jr., G. R. Gordon, L. Levy, D. A. Russell, G. C. Scott, D. R. Vincin, and C. C. Shepard.** 1977. Acedapsone treatment of leprosy patients: response versus drug disposition. Am. J. Trop. Med. Hyg. **26:**127–136.
310. **Petersen, E. A., M. L. Nash, R. B. Mammana, and J. G. Copeland.** 1983. Minocycline treatment of pulmonary nocardiosis. J. Am. Med. Assoc. **250:**930–932.
311. **Philippon, A., R. Labia, and G. Jacoby.** 1989. Extended-spectrum β-lactamases. Antimicrob. Agents Chemother. **33:**1131–1136.
312. **Phillips, I., and A. King.** 1988. Comparative activity of the 4-quinolones. Rev. Infect. Dis. **10**(Suppl. 1):S70–S76.
313. **Pitchenik, A. E., B. W. Russell, T. Cleary, I. Pejovic, C. Cole, and D. E. Snider, Jr.** 1982. The prevalence of tuberculosis and drug resistance among Haitians. N. Engl. J. Med. **307:**162–165.
314. **Polk, R. E.** 1989. Drug-drug interactions with ciprofloxacin and other fluoroquinolones. Am. J. Med. **87**(Suppl. 5A):76S–81S.
315. **Polk, R. E., D. P. Healy, L. B. Schwartz, D. T. Rock, M. L. Garson, and K. Roller.** 1988. Vancomycin and the red-man syndrome: pharmacodynamics of histamine release. J. Infect. Dis. **157:**502–507.
316. **Portier, H., J. M. Chalopin, M. Freysz, and Y. Tanter.** 1980. Interaction between cephalosporins and alcohol. Lancet **ii:**263.
317. **Poso, H., L. Paulin, and E. Brander.** 1983. Specific inhibition of spermidine synthase from mycobacteria by ethambutol. Lancet **ii:**1418.
318. **Prince, A. S., and H. C. Neu.** 1981. Activities of new β-lactam antibiotics against isolates of *Pseudomonas aeruginosa* from patients with cystic fibrosis. Antimicrob. Agents Chemother. **20:**545–546.
319. **Rahal, J. J., Jr., and M. S. Simberkoff.** 1979. Bactericidal and bacteriostatic action of chloramphenicol against meningeal pathogens. Antimicrob. Agents Chemother. **16:** 13–18.
320. **Ralph, E. D., and W. M. M. Kirby.** 1975. Unique bactericidal action of metronidazole against *Bacteroides fragilis* and *Clostridium perfringens*. Antimicrob. Agents Chemother. **8:**409–414.
321. **Raoult, D., P. Roussellier, V. Galicher, R. Perez, and J. Tamalet.** 1986. In vitro susceptibility of *Rickettsia conorii* to ciprofloxacin as determined by suppressing lethality in chicken embryos and by plaque assay. Antimicrob. Agents Chemother. **29:**424–425.
322. **Raoult, D., P. Roussellier, G. Vestris, V. Galicher, R. Perez, and J. Tamalet.** 1987. Susceptibility of *Rickettsia conorii* and *R. rickettsii* to pefloxacin, in vitro and in ovo. J. Antimicrob. Chemother. **19:**303–305.
323. **Rastogi, N., M. Potar, and H. L. David.** 1988. Pyrazinamide is not effective against intracellularly growing *Mycobacterium tuberculosis*. Antimicrob. Agents Chemother. **32:**287.
324. **Reading, C., and M. Cole.** 1977. Clavulanic acid: a beta-lactamase-inhibiting beta-lactam from *Streptomyces cla-*

vuligerus. Antimicrob. Agents Chemother. **11**:852–857.

325. **Reckendorf, H. K., R. G. Castringius, and H. K. Spingler.** 1963. Comparative pharmacodynamics, urinary excretion, and half-life determinations of nitrofurantoin sodium, p. 531–537. Antimicrob. Agents Chemother. 1962.
326. **Rees, R. J. W.** 1975. Rifampicin: the investigation of a bactericidal antileprosy drug. Lepr. Rev. **46**(Suppl.):121–124.
327. **Rees, R. J. W., J. M. H. Pearson, and M. F. R. Waters.** 1970. Experimental and clinical studies on rifampicin in treatment of leprosy. Br. Med. J. **1**:89–92.
328. **Reeves, D. S.** 1977. Antibacterial activity of mecillinam. J. Antimicrob. Chemother. **3**(Suppl. B):5–11.
329. **Reilly, G. D., and R. C. Spencer.** 1984. Pseudomonic acid: a new antibiotic for skin infections. J. Antimicrob. Chemother. **13**:295–298.
330. **Renzini, G., G. Ravagnan, and B. Oliva.** 1975. In vitro and in vivo microbiological evaluation of cephapirin, a new antibiotic. Chemotherapy **21**:289–296.
331. **Retsema, J. A., A. R. English, and A. E. Girard.** 1980. CP-45,899 in combination with penicillin or ampicillin against penicillin-resistant *Staphylococcus, Haemophilus influenzae,* and *Bacteroides*. Antimicrob. Agents Chemother. **17**:615–622.
332. **Retsema, J. A., A. R. English, A. Girard, J. E. Lynch, M. Anderson, L. Brennan, C. Cimochowski, J. Faiella, W. Norcia, and P. Sawyer.** 1986. Sulbactam/ampicillin: in vitro spectrum, potency, and activity in models of acute infection. Rev. Infect. Dis. **8**(Suppl. 5):S528–S534.
333. **Reusser, F.** 1975. Effect of lincomycin and clindamycin on peptide chain initiation. Antimicrob. Agents Chemother. **7**:32–37.
334. **Richmond, M. H.** 1980. Beta-lactamase stability of cefotoxime. J. Antimicrob. Chemother. **6**(Suppl. A):13–17.
335. **Riddell, R. W., S. M. Stewart, and A. R. Somner.** 1960. Ethionamide. Br. Med. J. **2**:1207–1208.
336. **Ridgway, G. L., G. Mumtaz, F. G. Gabriel, and J. D. Oriel.** 1984. The activity of ciprofloxacin and other 4-quinolones against *Chlamydia trachomatis* and *Mycoplasmas* in vitro. Eur. J. Clin. Microbiol. **3**:344–346.
337. **Ringden, O., P. Myrenfors, G. Klintmalm, G. Tyden, and L. Ost.** 1984. Nephrotoxicity by co-trimoxazole and cyclosporin in transplanted patients. Lancet **i**:1016–1017.
338. **Robson, J. M., and F. M. Sullivan.** 1963. Antituberculosis drugs. Pharmacol. Rev. **15**:169–223.
339. **Rode, H., D. Hanslo, P. M. De Wet, A. J. W. Millar, and S. Cywes.** 1989. Efficacy of mupirocin in methicillin-resistant *Staphylococcus aureus* burn wound infection. Antimicrob. Agents Chemother. **33**:1358–1361.
340. **Rodloff, A. C.** 1982. In-vitro susceptibility test of non-tuberculous mycobacteria to sulphamethoxazole, trimethoprim, and combinations of both. J. Antimicrob. Chemother. **9**:195–199.
341. **Rogers, J. D., M. A. P. Meisinger, F. Ferber, G. B. Calandra, J. L. Demetriades, and J. A. Bland.** 1985. Pharmacokinetics of imipenem and cilastatin in volunteers. Rev. Infect. Dis. **7**(Suppl. 3):S435–S446.
342. **Rolfe, R. D., and S. M. Finegold.** 1981. Comparative in vitro activity of new β-lactam antibiotics against anaerobic bacteria. Antimicrob. Agents Chemother. **20**:600–609.
343. **Rolston, K. V. I., and J. Hoy.** 1987. Role of clindamycin in the treatment of central nervous system toxoplasmosis. Am. J. Med. **83**:551–554.
344. **Rose, H. D., and M. W. Rytel.** 1972. Actinomycosis treated with clindamycin. J. Am. Med. Assoc. **221**:1052.
345. **Rosenblatt, J. E., and P. R. Stewart.** 1974. Combined activity of sulfamethoxazole, trimethoprim, and polymyxin B against gram-negative bacilli. Antimicrob. Agents Chemother. **6**:84–92.
346. **Rosenow, E. C., III, R. A. DeRemee, and D. E. Dines.** 1968. Chronic nitrofurantoin pulmonary reaction: report of five cases. N. Engl. J. Med. **279**:1258–1262.
347. **Rubin, L. G., E. Vellozzi, J. Shapiro, and H. D. Isenberg.** 1988. Infection with vancomycin-resistant "streptococci" due to *Leuconostoc* species. J. Infect. Dis. **157**:216.
348. **Rubin, R. H., and M. N. Swartz.** 1980. Trimethoprim-sulfamethoxazole. N. Engl. J. Med. **303**:426–432.
349. **Ruoff, K. L., D. R. Kuritzkes, J. S. Wolfson, and M. J. Ferraro.** 1988. Vancomycin-resistant gram-positive bacteria isolated from human sources. J. Clin. Microbiol. **26**: 2064–2068.
350. **Ryder, R. W., P. A. Blake, A. C. Murlin, G. P. Carter, R. A. Pollard, M. H. Merson, S. D. Allen, and D. J. Brenner.** 1980. Increase in antibiotic resistance among isolates of *Salmonella* in the United States, 1967–1975. J. Infect. Dis. **142**:485–491.
351. **Sabath, L. D., C. Wilcox, C. Garner, and M. Finland.** 1973. In vitro activity of cefazolin against recent clinical bacterial isolates. J. Infect. Dis. **128**(Suppl.):S320–S326.
352. **Sahm, D. F., J. Kissinger, M. S. Gilmore, P. R. Murray, R. Mulder, J. Solliday, and B. Clarke.** 1989. In vitro susceptibility studies of vancomycin-resistant *Enterococcus faecalis*. Antimicrob. Agents Chemother. **33**:1588–1591.
353. **Salter, A. J.** 1982. Trimethoprim-sulfamethoxazole: an assessment of more than 12 years of use. Rev. Infect. Dis. **4**:196–236.
354. **Sanchez, P. L., F. S. Wignall, T. R. Zajdowicz, S. Kerbs, S. W. Berg, and W. O. Harrison.** 1983. One gram of cefoxitin cures uncomplicated gonococcal urethritis caused by penicillinase-producing *Neisseria gonorrhoeae* (PPNG). Sex. Transm. Dis. **10**:135–137.
355. **Sanders, C. V., R. N. Greenberg, and R. L. Marier.** 1985. Cefamandole and cefoxitin. Ann. Intern. Med. **103**:70–78.
356. **Sanders, E., M. T. Foster, and D. Scott.** 1968. Group A beta-hemolytic streptococci resistant to erythromycin and lincomycin. N. Engl. J. Med. **278**:538–540.
357. **Sanders, W. E., Jr., C. Hartwig, N. Schneider, R. Cacciatore, and H. Valdez.** 1982. Activity of amikacin against mycobacteria in vitro and in murine tuberculosis. Tubercle **63**:201–208.
358. **Sanfilippo, A., C. Della Bruna, L. Marsili, E. Morvillo, C. R. Pasqualucci, G. Schioppacassi, and D. Ungheri.** 1980. Biological activity of a new class of rifamycins, spiro-piperidyl rifamycins. J. Antibiot. **33**:1193–1198.
359. **Sarma, P. S.** 1989. Norfloxacin: a new drug in the treatment of falciparum malaria. Ann. Intern. Med. **111**:336–337.
360. **Sattler, F. R., M. R. Weitekamp, and J. O. Ballard.** 1986. Potential for bleeding with the new beta-lactam antibiotics. Ann. Intern. Med. **105**:924–931.
361. **Saxon, A., A. Hassner, E. A. Swabb, B. Wheeler, and N. F. Adkinson, Jr.** 1984. Lack of cross-reactivity between aztreonam, a monobactam antibiotic, and penicillin in penicillin-allergic subjects. J. Infect. Dis. **149**:16–22.
362. **Schaad, U. B., J. Wedgwood-Krucko, and H. Tschaeppeler.** 1988. Reversible ceftriaxone-associated biliary pseudolithiasis in children. Lancet **ii**:1411–1413.
363. **Schacht, P., G. Arcieri, J. Branolte, H. Bruck, V. Chysky, E. Griffith, G. Gruenwaldt, R. Hullmann, C. A. Konopka, B. O'Brien, V. Rham, T. Ryoki, A. Westwood, and H. Wenta.** 1988. Worldwide clinical data on efficacy and safety of ciprofloxacin. Infection **16**(Suppl. 1):S29–S43.
364. **Schluter, G.** 1987. Ciprofloxacin: review of potential toxicologic effects. Am. J. Med. **82**(Suppl. 4A):91–93.
365. **Schrinner, E., M. Limbert, L. Penasse, and A. Lutz.** 1980. Antibacterial activity of cefotaxime and other newer cephalosporins (in vitro and in vivo). J. Antimicrob. Chemother. **6**(Suppl. A):25–30.
366. **Schwalbe, R. S., J. T. Stappleton, and P. H. Gilligan.** 1987. Emergence of vancomycin resistance in coagulase-negative staphylococci. N. Engl. J. Med. **316**:927–931.
367. **Seaberg, L. S., A. R. Parquette, I. Y. Gluzman, G. W.**

Phillips, Jr., T. F. Brodasky, and D. J. Krogstad. 1984. Clindamycin activity against chloroquine-resistant *Plasmodium falciparum.* J. Infect. Dis. **150:**904–911.

368. **Sensi, P., N. Maggi, S. Füresz, and G. Maffii.** 1967. Chemical modifications and biological properties of rifamycins, p. 699–714. Antimicrob. Agents Chemother. 1966.

369. **Sharp, J. R., K. G. Ishak, and H. J. Zimmerman.** 1980. Chronic active hepatitis and severe hepatic necrosis associated with nitrofurantoin. Ann. Intern. Med. **92:**14–19.

370. **Shaw, W. V.** 1984. Bacterial resistance to chloramphenicol. Br. Med. Bull. **40:**36–41.

371. **Shlaes, D. M., A. Bouvet, C. Devine, J. H. Shlaes, S. Al-Obeid, and R. Williamson.** 1989. Inducible, transferable resistance to vancomycin in *Enterococcus faecalis* A256. Antimicrob. Agents Chemother. **33:**198–203.

372. **Skinner, M. H., M. Hsieh, J. Torseth, D. Pauloin, G. Bhatia, S. Harkonen, T. C. Merigan, and T. F. Blaschke.** 1989. Pharmacokinetics of rifabutin. Antimicrob. Agents Chemother. **33:**1237–1241.

373. **Smego, R. A., Jr., M. B. Moeller, and H. A. Gallis.** 1983. Trimethoprim-sulfamethoxazole therapy for *Nocardia* infections. Arch. Intern. Med. **143:**711–718.

374. **Smith, A. L., and A. Weber.** 1983. Pharmacology of chloramphenicol. Pediatr. Clin. North Am. **30:**209–236.

375. **Snider, D. E., Jr.** 1980. Pyridoxine supplementation during isoniazid therapy. Tubercle **61:**191–196.

376. **Snider, D. E., Jr., D. L. Cohn, P. T. Davidson, E. S. Hershfield, M. H. Smith, and F. D. Sutton, Jr.** 1985. Standard therapy for tuberculosis. Chest **87**(Suppl.):S117–S124.

377. **Snider, D. E., J. Graczyk, E. Bek, and J. Rogowski.** 1984. Supervised six-month treatment of newly diagnosed pulmonary tuberculosis using isoniazid, rifampin, and pyrazinamide with and without streptomycin. Am. Rev. Respir. Dis. **130:**1091–1094.

378. **Somma, S., L. Gastaldo, and A. Corti.** 1984. Teicoplanin, a new antibiotic from *Actinoplanes teichomyceticus* nov. sp. Antimicrob. Agents Chemother. **26:**917–923.

379. **Sorg, T. B., and M. H. Cynamon.** 1987. Comparison of four beta-lactamase inhibitors in combination with ampicillin against *Mycobacterium tuberculosis.* J. Antimicrob. Chemother. **19:**59–64.

380. **Sorrell, T. C., and P. J. Collignon.** 1985. A prospective study of adverse reactions associated with vancomycin therapy. J. Antimicrob. Chemother. **16:**235–241.

381. **Spitzer, P. G., S. M. Hammer, and A. W. Karchmer.** 1986. Treatment of *Listeria monocytogenes* infection with trimethoprim-sulfamethoxazole: case report and review of the literature. Rev. Infect. Dis. **8:**427–430.

382. **Spratt, B. G., V. Jobanputra, and W. Zimmermann.** 1977. Binding of thienamycin and clavulanic acid to the penicillin-binding proteins of *Escherichia coli* K-12. Antimicrob. Agents Chemother. **12:**406–409.

383. **Stamey, T. A.** 1987. Recurrent urinary tract infections in female patients: an overview of management and treatment. Rev. Infect. Dis. **9**(Suppl. 2):S195–S208.

384. **Stamm, W. E., M. E. Guinen, C. Johnson, T. Starcher, K. K. Holmes, and W. M. McCormack.** 1984. Effect of treatment regimens for *Neisseria gonorrhoeae* on simultaneous infection with *Chlamydia trachomatis.* N. Engl. J. Med. **310:**545–549.

385. **Stanford, J. L., and I. Phillips.** 1972. Rifampicin in experimental *Mycobacterium ulcerans* infection. J. Med. Microbiol. **5:**39–45.

386. **Stead, W. W., and A. K. Dutt.** 1982. Chemotherapy for tuberculosis today. Am. Rev. Respir. Dis. **125**(Suppl. 3): 94–101.

387. **Stein, G. E.** 1987. Review of the bioavailability and pharmacokinetics of oral norfloxacin. Am. J. Med. **82**(Suppl. 6B):18–21.

388. **Stille, W., W. Sietzen, H. A. Dieterich, and J. J. Fell.** 1988. Clinical efficacy and safety of teicoplanin. J. Antimicrob. Chemother. **21**(Suppl. A):69–79.

389. **Stone, J. W., J. M. Andrews, J. P. Ashby, D. Griggs, and R. Wise.** 1988. Pharmacokinetics and tissue penetration of orally administered lomefloxacin. Antimicrob. Agents Chemother. **32:**1508–1510.

390. **Stratton, C. W., C. Liu, H. B. Ratner, and L. S. Weeks.** 1987. Bactericidal activity of daptomycin (LY146032) compared with those of ciprofloxacin, vancomycin, and ampicillin against enterococci as determined by kill-kinetic studies. Antimicrob. Agents Chemother. **31:**1014–1016.

391. **Strominger, J. L., and D. J. Tipper.** 1965. Bacterial cell wall synthesis and structure in relation to the mechanism of action of penicillins and other antibacterial agents. Am. J. Med. **39:**708–721.

392. **Stubner, G., W. Weinrich, and U. Brands.** 1986. Study of the cerebrospinal fluid penetrability of ofloxacin. Infection **14**(Suppl. 4):S250–S253.

393. **Stutman, H. R., D. F. Welch, R. K. Scribner, and M. I. Marks.** 1984. In vitro antimicrobial activity of aztreonam alone and in combination against bacterial isolates from pediatric patients. Antimicrob. Agents Chemother. **25:** 212–215.

394. **Sullivan, D., M. E. Csuka, and B. Blanchard.** 1980. Erythromycin ethylsuccinate hepatoxicity. J. Am. Med. Assoc. **243:**1074.

395. **Sutherland, R., A. S. Beale, R. J. Boon, K. E. Griffin, B. Slocombe, D. H. Stokes, and A. R. White.** 1985. Antibacterial activity of ticarcillin in the presence of clavulanate potassium. Am. J. Med. **79**(Suppl. 5B):13–24.

396. **Sutherland, R., R. J. Boon, K. E. Griffin, P. J. Masters, B. Slocombe, and A. R. White.** 1985. Antibacterial activity of mupirocin (pseudomonic acid), a new antibiotic for topical use. Antimicrob. Agents Chemother. **27:**495–498.

397. **Sutter, V. L.** 1977. In vitro susceptibility of anaerobes: comparison of clindamycin and other antimicrobial agents. J. Infect. Dis. **135**(Suppl.):S7–S12.

398. **Sutter, V. L.** 1983. Frequency of occurrence and antimicrobial susceptibility of bacterial isolates from the intestinal and female genital tracts. Rev. Infect. Dis. **5**(Suppl.):S84–S89.

399. **Sutter, V. L., and S. M. Finegold.** 1976. Susceptibility of anaerobic bacteria to 23 antimicrobial agents. Antimicrob. Agents Chemother. **10:**736–752.

400. **Sutton, W. B., R. S. Gordee, W. E. Wick, and L. V. Standfield.** 1966. In vitro and in vivo laboratory studies on the antituberculous activity of capreomycin. Ann. N.Y. Acad. Sci. **135:**947–959.

401. **Swedberg, J., J. F. Steiner, F. Deiss, S. Steiner, and D. A. Driggers.** 1985. Comparison of single-dose vs one-week course of metronidazole for symptomatic bacterial vaginosis. J. Am. Med. Assoc. **254:**1046–1049.

402. **Swenson, J. M., R. J. Wallace, Jr., V. A. Silcox, and C. Thornsberry.** 1985. Antimicrobial susceptibility of five subgroups of *Mycobacterium fortuitum* and *Mycobacterium chelonae.* Antimicrob. Agents Chemother. **28:**807–811.

403. **Sykes, R. B., D. P. Bonner, K. Bush, and N. H. Georgopapadakou.** 1982. Azthreonam (SQ 26,776), a synthetic monobactam specifically active against aerobic gram-negative bacteria. Antimicrob. Agents Chemother. **21:**85–92.

404. **Takayama, K., E. L. Armstrong, K. A. Kunugi, and J. O. Kilburn.** 1979. Inhibition by ethambutol of mycolic acid transfer into the cell wall of *Mycobacterium smegmatis.* Antimicrob. Agents Chemother. **16:**240–242.

405. **Takayama, K., L. Wang, and H. L. David.** 1972. Effect of isoniazid on the in vivo mycolic acid synthesis, cell growth, and viability of *Mycobacterium tuberculosis.* Antimicrob. Agents Chemother. **2:**29–35.

406. **Tally, F. P., N. V. Jacobus, and S. L. Gorbach.** 1980. In

vitro activity of *N*-formimidoyl thienamycin (MK 0787). Antimicrob. Agents Chemother. **18:**642–644.

407. **Tanaka, N., T. Kinoshita, and H. Masukawa.** 1968. Mechanism of protein synthesis inhibition by fusidic acid and related antibiotics. Biochem. Biophys. Res. Commun. **30:**278–283.
408. **Teasley, D. G., D. N. Gerding, M. M. Olson, L. R. Peterson, R. L. Gebhard, M. J. Schwartz, and J. T. Lee, Jr.** 1983. Prospective randomized trial of metronidazole versus vancomycin for *Clostridium difficile*-associated diarrhea and colitis. Lancet **ii:**1043–1046.
409. **Tedesco, F., R. Markham, M. Gurwith, D. Christie, and J. G. Bartlett.** 1978. Oral vancomycin for antibiotic-associated pseudomembranous colitis. Lancet **ii:**226–228.
410. **Thomas, F. E., Jr., J. M. Leonard, and R. H. Alford.** 1976. Sulfamethoxazole-trimethoprim-polymyxin therapy of serious multiply drug-resistant *Serratia* infections. Antimicrob. Agents Chemother. **9:**201–207.
411. **Thomas, J. P., C. O. Baughn, R. G. Wilkinson, and R. G. Shepherd.** 1961. A new synthetic compound with antituberculous activity in mice: ethambutol (dextro-2,2'-[ethylenediimino]-di-1-butanol). Am. Rev. Respir. Dis. **83:** 891–893.
412. **Thornsberry, C.** 1985. Review of in vitro activity of third-generation cephalosporins and other newer beta-lactam antibiotics against clinically important bacteria. Am. J. Med. **79**(Suppl. 2A):14–20.
413. **Thornsberry, C., C. N. Baker, and L. A. Kirven.** 1978. In vitro activity of antimicrobial agents on Legionnaires disease bacterium. Antimicrob. Agents Chemother. **13:** 78–80.
414. **Thornsberry, C., B. C. Hill, J. M. Swenson, and L. K. McDougal.** 1983. Rifampin: spectrum of antibacterial activity. Rev. Infect. Dis. **5**(Suppl. 3):S412–S417.
415. **Tofte, R. W., J. Solliday, and K. B. Crossley.** 1984. Susceptibilities of enterococci to twelve antibiotics. Antimicrob. Agents Chemother. **25:**532–533.
416. **Tolkoff-Rubin, N. E., D. Weber, L. S. T. Fang, M. Kelly, R. Wilkinson, and R. H. Rubin.** 1982. Single-dose therapy with trimethoprim-sulfamethoxazole for urinary tract infection in women. Rev. Infect. Dis. **4:**444–448.
417. **Toole, J. F., and M. L. Parrish.** 1973. Nitrofurantoin polyneuropathy. Neurology **23:**554–559.
418. **Tuazon, C. U., and H. Miller.** 1984. Comparative in vitro activities of teichomycin and vancomycin alone and in combination with rifampin and aminoglycosides against staphylococci and enterococci. Antimicrob. Agents Chemother. **25:**411–412.
419. **Tuberculosis Chemotherapy Trials Committee.** 1952. The treatment of pulmonary tuberculosis with isoniazid: interim report to the Medical Research Council. Br. Med. J. **2:**735–746.
420. **Turck, M., A. R. Ronald, and R. G. Petersdorf.** 1967. Susceptibility of *Enterobacteriaceae* to nitrofurantoin correlated with eradication of bacteriuria, p. 446–452. Antimicrob. Agents Chemother. 1966.
421. **Uttley, A. H., C. H. Collins, J. Naidoo, and R. C. George.** 1988. Vancomycin-resistant enterococci. Lancet **i:**57–58.
422. **Van der Auwera, P., T. Matsumoto, and M. Husson.** 1988. Intraphagocytic penetration of antibiotics. J. Antimicrob. Chemother. **22:**185–192.
423. **Van Dyke, J. J., and K. B. Lake.** 1975. Chemotherapy for aquarium granuloma. J. Am. Med. Assoc. **233:**1380–1381.
424. **Vanhoff, R., B. Gordts, R. Dierickx, H. Coignau, and J. P. Butzler.** 1980. Bacteriostatic and bactericidal activities of 24 antimicrobial agents against *Campylobacter fetus* subsp. *jejuni*. Antimicrob. Agents Chemother. **18:** 118–121.
425. **Verbist, L.** 1979. Comparison of the activities of the new ureidopenicillins piperacillin, mezlocillin, azlocillin, and Bay k 4999 against gram-negative organisms. Antimicrob. Agents Chemother. **16:**115–119.
426. **Verbist, L., and A. Gyselen.** 1968. Antituberculous activity of rifampin in vitro and in vivo and the concentrations attained in human blood. Am. Rev. Respir. Dis. **98:** 923–932.
427. **Wallace, R. J., Jr., D. B. Jones, and K. Wiss.** 1981. Sulfonamide activity against *Mycobacterium fortuitum* and *Mycobacterium chelonei*. Rev. Infect. Dis. **3:**898–904.
428. **Wallace, R. J., Jr., E. J. Septimus, T. W. Williams, Jr., R. H. Conklin, T. K. Satterwhite, M. B. Bushby, and D. C. Hollowell.** 1982. Use of trimethoprim-sulfamethoxazole for treatment of infections due to *Nocardia*. Rev. Infect. Dis. **4:**315–325.
429. **Wallace, R. J., Jr., J. M. Swenson, V. A. Silcox, and M. G. Bullen.** 1985. Treatment of non-pulmonary infections due to *Mycobacterium fortuitum* and *Mycobacterium chelonei* on the basis of in vivo susceptibilities. J. Infect. Dis. **152:**500–514.
430. **Wallace, R. J., Jr., and K. Wiss.** 1981. Susceptibility of *Mycobacterium marinum* to tetracyclines and aminoglycosides. Antimicrob. Agents Chemother. **20:**610–612.
431. **Wallace, R. J., Jr., K. Wiss, M. B. Bushby, and D. C. Hollowell.** 1982. In vitro activity of trimethoprim and sulfamethoxazole against the nontuberculous mycobacteria. Rev. Infect. Dis. **4:**326–331.
432. **Walters, B. N. J., and S. S. Gubbay.** 1981. Tetracycline and benign intracranial hypertension: report of five cases. Br. Med. J. **282:**19–20.
433. **Wang, C., J. Sabbaj, M. Corrado, and V. Hoagland.** 1986. World-wide clinical experience with norfloxacin: efficacy and safety. Scand. J. Infect. Dis. **48**(Suppl.):81–89.
434. **Wanger, A. R., and B. E. Murray.** 1987. Activity of LY146032 against enterococci with and without high-level aminoglycoside resistance, including two penicillinase-producing strains. Antimicrob. Agents Chemother. **31:** 1779–1781.
435. **Ward, A., and D. M. Campoli-Richards.** 1986. Mupirocin: a review of its antibacterial activity, pharmacokinetic properties and therapeutic use. Drugs **32:**425–444.
436. **Ward, M. E.** 1977. The bactericidal action of spectinomycin on *Neisseria gonorrhoeae*. J. Antimicrob. Chemother. **3:**323–329.
437. **Washington, J. A., II, and W. R. Wilson.** 1985. Erythromycin: a microbial and clinical perspective after 30 years of clinical use. Mayo Clin. Proc. **60:**189–203, 271–278.
438. **Watanakunakorn, C.** 1984. Mode of action and in vitro activity of vancomycin. J. Antimicrob. Chemother. **14**(Suppl. D):7–18.
439. **Watanakunakorn, C.** 1987. In-vitro activity of teicoplanin alone and in combination with rifampicin, gentamicin or tobramycin against coagulase-negative staphylococci. J. Antimicrob. Chemother. **19:**439–443.
440. **Watanakunakorn, C., and C. Bakie.** 1973. Synergism of vancomycin-gentamicin and vancomycin-streptomycin against enterococci. Antimicrob. Agents Chemother. **4:** 120–124.
441. **Watanakunakorn, C., and J. C. Tisone.** 1982. Synergism between vancomycin and gentamicin or tobramycin for methicillin-susceptible and methicillin-resistant *Staphylococcus aureus* strains. Antimicrob. Agents Chemother. **22:**903–905.
442. **Watt, B., and F. V. Brown.** 1982. In-vitro activity of cefotiam against bacteria of clinical interest. J. Antimicrob. Chemother. **10:**391–395.
443. **Waxman, D. J., and J. L. Strominger.** 1983. Penicillin-binding proteins and the mechanism of action of beta-lactam antibiotics. Annu. Rev. Biochem. **52:**825–869.
444. **Wehrli, W.** 1983. Rifampin: mechanisms of action and resistance. Rev. Infect. Dis. **5**(Suppl. 3):S407–S411.
445. **Wehrli, W., F. Knusel, K. Schmid, and M. Staehelin.** 1968. Interaction of rifamycin with bacterial RNA polymerase. Proc. Natl. Acad. Sci. USA **61:**667–673.

446. **Westerman, E. L.** 1983. Toxicity of mediastinal irrigation with bacitracin. J. Am. Med. Assoc. **250:**899.

447. **Wexler, H. M., and S. M. Finegold.** 1985. In vitro activity of imipenem against anaerobic bacteria. Rev. Infect. Dis. **7**(Suppl. 3):S417–S425.

448. **Wexler, H. M., and S. M. Finegold.** 1988. In vitro activity of cefotetan compared with that of other antimicrobial agents against anaerobic bacteria. Antimicrob. Agents Chemother. **32:**601–604.

449. **Wexler, H. M., B. Harris, W. T. Carter, and S. M. Finegold.** 1985. In vitro efficacy of sulbactam combined with ampicillin against anaerobic bacteria. Antimicrob. Agents Chemother. **27:**876–878.

450. **Whimbey, E., T. E. Kiehn, and D. Armstrong.** 1986. Disseminated *Mycobacterium avium-intracellulare* disease: diagnosis and therapy, p. 112–133. *In* J. S. Remington and M. N. Swartz (ed.), Current clinical topics in infectious diseases, vol. 7. McGraw-Hill, Inc., New York.

451. **Wiedemann, B., C. Kliebe, and M. Kresken.** 1989. The epidemiology of beta-lactamases. J. Antimicrob. Chemother. **24**(Suppl. B):1–22.

452. **Wijnands, W. J. A., and T. B. Vree.** 1988. Interaction between the fluoroquinolones and the bronchodilator theophylline. J. Antimicrob. Chemother. **22**(Suppl. C): 109–114.

453. **Wijnands, W. J. A., T. B. Vree, and C. L. A. van Herwaarden.** 1986. The influence of quinolone derivatives on theophylline clearance. Br. J. Clin. Pharmacol. **22:** 677–683.

454. **Wilkinson, P. J., and D. S. Reeves.** 1979. Tissue penetration of trimethoprim and sulphonamides. J. Antimicrob. Chemother. **5**(Suppl. B):159–168.

455. **Williams, A. H., and R. N. Gruneberg.** 1984. Teicoplanin. J. Antimicrob. Chemother. **24:**441–445.

456. **Williams, R., S. Al-Obeid, J. H. Shlaes, F. W. Goldstein, and D. M. Shlaes.** 1989. Inducible resistance to vancomycin in *Enterococcus faecium* D366. J. Infect. Dis. **159:** 1095–1104.

457. **Wilson, W. R., R. L. Thompson, C. J. Wilkowske, J. A. Washington II, E. R. Giuliani, and J. E. Geraci.** 1981. Short-term therapy for streptococcal infective endocarditis: combined intramuscular administration of penicillin and streptomycin. J. Am. Med. Assoc. **245:**360–363.

458. **Winston, D. J., M. A. McGrattan, and R. W. Busuttil.** 1984. Imipenem therapy of *Pseudomonas aeruginosa* and other serious bacterial infections. Antimicrob. Agents Chemother. **26:**673–677.

459. **Wise, R., J. M. Andrews, and K. A. Bedford.** 1979. LY127935, a novel oxa-β-lactam: an in vitro comparison with other β-lactam antibiotics. Antimicrob. Agents Chemother. **16:**341–345.

460. **Wise, R., J. M. Andrews, and K. A. Bedford.** 1980. Clavulanic acid and CP-45,899: a comparison of their in vitro activity in combination with penicillins. J. Antimicrob. Chemother. **6:**197–206.

461. **Wise, R., D. Lister, C. A. McNulty, D. Griggs, and J. M. Andrews.** 1986. The comparative pharmacokinetics of five quinolones. J. Antimicrob. Chemother. **18**(Suppl. D): 71–81.

462. **Witkop, C. J., Jr., and R. O. Wolf.** 1963. Hypoplasia and intrinsic staining of enamel following tetracycline therapy. J. Am. Med. Assoc. **185:**1008–1011.

463. **Wittner, M., K. S. Rowin, H. B. Tanowitz, J. F. Hobbs, S. Saltzman, B. Wenz, R. Hirsch, E. Chisholm, and G. R. Healy.** 1982. Successful chemotherapy of transfusion babesiosis. Ann. Intern. Med. **96:**601–604.

464. **Wofsy, C. B.** 1987. Use of trimethoprim-sulfamethoxazole in the treatment of *Pneumocystis carinii* pneumonitis in patients with acquired immunodeficiency syndrome. Rev. Infect. Dis. **9**(Suppl. 2):S184–S191.

465. **Wolff, M., L. Boutron, E. Singlas, B. Clair, J. M. Decazes, and B. Regnier.** 1987. Penetration of ciprofloxacin into cerebrospinal fluid of patients with bacterial meningitis. Antimicrob. Agents Chemother. **31:**899–902.

466. **Wolff, M., B. Regnier, C. Daldoss, M. Nkam, and F. Vachon.** 1984. Penetration of pefloxacin into cerebrospinal fluid of patients with meningitis. Antimicrob. Agents Chemother. **26:**289–291.

467. **Wolfson, J. S., and D. C. Hooper.** 1985. The fluoroquinolones: structures, mechanisms of action and resistance, and spectra of activity in vitro. Antimicrob. Agents Chemother. **28:**581–586.

468. **Wolfson, J. S., and D. C. Hooper.** 1989. Fluoroquinolone antimicrobial agents. Clin. Microbiol. Rev. **2:**378–424.

469. **Wong, C. S., G. S. Palmer, and M. H. Cynamon.** 1988. In-vitro susceptibility of *Mycobacterium tuberculosis, Mycobacterium bovis* and *Mycobacterium kansasii* to amoxycillin and ticarcillin in combination with clavulanic acid. J. Antimicrob. Chemother. **22:**863–866.

470. **Woodley, C. L., and J. O. Kilburn.** 1982. In vitro susceptibility of *Mycobacterium avium* complex and *Mycobacterium tuberculosis* strains to a spiro-piperidyl rifamycin. Am. Rev. Respir. Dis. **126:**586–587.

471. **World Health Organization Study Group.** 1982. Chemotherapy of leprosy for control programmes. World Health Organization, Geneva.

472. **Wuite, J., B. I. Davies, M. Go, J. Lambers, D. Jackson, and G. Mellows.** 1983. Pseudomonic acid: a new topical antimicrobial agent. Lancet **ii:**394.

473. **Yamada, T., A. Nagata, Y. Ono, Y. Suzuki, and T. Yamanouchi.** 1985. Alteration of ribosomes and RNA polymerase in drug-resistant clinical isolates of *Mycobacterium tuberculosis.* Antimicrob. Agents Chemother. **27:** 921–924.

474. **Yates, M. D., and C. H. Collins.** 1981. Sensitivity of opportunist mycobacteria to rifampin and ethambutol. Tubercle **62:**117–121.

475. **Yates, M. D., C. H. Collins, and J. M. Grange.** 1982. "Classical" and "Asian" variants of *Mycobacterium tuberculosis* isolated in South East England 1977–1980. Tubercle **62:**55–61.

476. **Yawalkar, S. J., and W. Vischer.** 1979. Lamprene (clofazimine) in leprosy. Lepr. Rev. **50:**135–144.

477. **Yeaman, M. R., L. A. Mitscher, and O. G. Baca.** 1987. In vitro susceptibility of *Coxiella burnetii* to antibiotics, including several quinolones. Antimicrob. Agents Chemother. **31:**1079–1084.

478. **Young, L. S., O. G. W. Berlin, and C. B. Inderlied.** 1987. Activity of ciprofloxacin and other fluorinated quinolones against mycobacteria. Am. J. Med. **82**(Suppl. 4A):23–26.

479. **Young, L. S., and J. Hindler.** 1987. Use of trimethoprim-sulfamethoxazole singly and in combination with other antibiotics in immunocompromised patients. Rev. Infect. Dis. **9**(Suppl. 2):S177–S181.

480. **Yu, V. L., J. J. Zuravleff, J. Bornholm, and G. Archer.** 1984. In-vitro synergy testing of triple antibiotic combinations against *Staphylococcus epidermidis* isolates from patients with endocarditis. J. Antimicrob. Chemother. **14:** 359–366.

481. **Yunis, A. A.** 1973. Chloramphenicol-induced bone marrow suppression. Semin. Hematol. **10:**225–234.

482. **Zierski, M., and E. Bek.** 1980. Side-effects of drug regimens used in short-course chemotherapy for pulmonary tuberculosis: a controlled clinical study. Tubercle **61:**41–49.

483. **Zinner, S. H., H. Lagast, A. Kasry, and J. Klastersky.** 1982. Synergism of trimethoprim combined with aminoglycosides in vitro and in serum of volunteers. Eur. J. Clin. Microbiol. **1:**144–148.

Chapter 109

Mechanisms of Resistance to Antimicrobial Agents

ROBERT C. COOKSEY

Phenotypic resistance to antimicrobial agents may be explained by one or more of the following general mechanisms: (i) impermeability (decreased accumulation of the drug in the bacterial cell), (ii) alterations in target molecules that prevent interaction with the drug, (iii) enzymatic inactivation of the drug, and (iv) energy-coupled efflux of the drug. A fifth mechanism, blocking or trapping, is suggested by vancomycin resistance in *Enterococcus* spp., which can be mediated by a protein that impairs access of the drug to its site of action at the cell wall pentapeptide (S. Al-Obeid, E. Collatz, and L. Gutmann, Program Abstr. 29th Intersci. Conf. Antimicrob. Agents Chemother., abstr. no. 271, p. 146, 1989). Altered metabolic pathways, such as the folate pathway normally interrupted by sulfonamides and trimethoprim, could be considered a subtype of the altered target mechanism. Hyperproduction of target molecules, including those with normal (wild-type) affinity for the drug, can overwhelm available drug concentrations and is often considered another subtype of the altered target class of resistance. Research on resistance mechanisms continues to show evidence that an interplay of two or more of these mechanisms is responsible for phenotypic resistance in most organisms, and it is rare that the resistance is due to only one of the principal mechanisms of resistance listed in Table 1. Furthermore, assays used to identify a particular mechanism are often too cumbersome for routine performance and are usually reserved for use in basic science laboratories. These characterizations generally require protein purification and analysis or transport (e.g., of radiolabeled drug) studies. Newer technologies, including kits, have streamlined some of these techniques and provide convenient characterizations of these resistance mechanisms. Likewise, DNA probes, when properly prepared and used, can offer a reliable method for examining many isolates in a single assay and identifying specific encoding elements (e.g., plasmids) for genes that cause resistance to most clinical compounds (7, 45). Other than rapid qualitative tests for β-lactamase and chloramphenicol acetyltransferase (CAT) (see chapter 115), the most useful information on mechanisms of resistance comes from careful analyses of in vitro susceptibility data.

IMPERMEABILITY

Decreased accumulation, or impermeability, is the most frequent explanation for intrinsic antimicrobial resistance. Anaerobic organisms, for example, are intrinsically resistant to aminoglycosides because uptake of drugs in this class is a multiphasic process partially empowered by cytochrome-mediated electron transport absent from obligate anaerobes. Lower levels of resistance to aminoglycosides among some streptococcal species may be similarly explained by incomplete electron transport chains. Even among susceptible strains, however, relatively low proportions of aminoglycoside antibiotics actually arrive at their cytoplasmic targets.

Permeability may also be reduced by cell-specific factors, such as extracellular slime or capsule production, or by drug-specific factors, such as hydrophobicity, molecular size, net charge, or secondary structure. Strains with defective lipopolysaccharide in their outer membranes may exhibit higher levels of resistance to compounds that are more hydrophobic within a drug class. Among members of the family *Enterobacteriaceae*, susceptibility to many antimicrobial agents is somewhat affected by specific outer membrane proteinaceous channels, porins (16, 33, 35). Lower overall permeability of β-lactams in *Enterobacter cloacae* than in *Escherichia coli* has been attributed to porin composition. At least five different porins (OmpC, OmpF, LamD, PhoE, and protein K) may exist within the outer membrane of a single strain of *E. coli* (16), and all of these may affect antimicrobial susceptibility. In general, permeability-related resistance mechanisms, including *omp* mutations, are chromosomally encoded and therefore tend to be more established than plasmid-encoded mechanisms. An additional mutated genetic locus in *E. coli*, *marA*, has been shown to cause a single-step, high-frequency acquisition of multiple resistance (to chloramphenicol, tetracycline, and fluoroquinolones) mediated by decreased drug accumulation related to decreased synthesis of OmpF and other membrane proteins (5). Non-β-lactamase-mediated penicillin resistance in *Neisseria gonorrhoeae* may be due to altered envelope permeability among *pen* mutants which have been described since the mid-1970s (15). Although altered DNA gyrase may be the principal mechanism of quinolone resistance in other gram-negative organisms, *nal* mutations that cause reduced nalidixic acid uptake have also been described (17).

Since porins serve as channels for the uptake of antibiotics and cellular nutrients such as amino acids, porin-deficient mutants may be detected by their inability to grow on minimal media containing a sole carbon source (e.g., raffinose or succinate) that would normally support growth of the wild-type strain. In addition, permeability mutants usually demonstrate lower levels of resistance to the compound under study than other mechanisms of resistance, and the strain may exhibit cross-resistance. Among *Pseudomonas* species, for example, over 15% of aminoglycoside resistance in the United States is caused by impermeability, and these isolates tend to be cross-resistant to most aminoglycoside-aminocyclitol compounds (42). Impermeability to some compounds may also be mediated by bacterial modifying enzymes that do not inactivate the com-

TABLE 1. Antimicrobial resistance mechanisms

Antimicrobial class	Mode of action	Resistance		
		Principal mechanism(s)	Genetic element[a]	Alternative mechanism(s)
Chloramphenicol	Translation (blocks peptidyl-transferase after binding 50S ribosome)	Enzymatic modification (acetyltransferase, CAT)	P^c, Tn	Impermeability
Tetracycline	Translation (blocks binding of aminoacyl-tRNA to ribosome)	Efflux; altered target (ribosome protection)	P^i, C^c, Tn	Impermeability; enzymatic modification
Macrolides	Translation (binds 50S ribosome)	Altered target (methylated adenine in 23S rRNA)	$P^{c,i}$, C, Tn	Enzymatic modification
Sulfonamides	Folic acid synthesis (dihydropteroate synthetase analog)	Altered target (bypass)	P^c, C^c	
Trimethoprim	Folic acid synthesis (dihydropteroate synthetase analog)	Altered target (bypass)	P^c, C^c, Tn	Impermeability
Quinolones	Replication (inhibits DNA gyrase)	Altered target enzymes	C^c	Impermeability
Rifampin	Transcription (inhibits RNA polymerase)	Altered target enzymes	C^c	Impermeability
β-Lactams	Cell wall synthesis and cell division	Enzymatic modification (β-lactamase)	$P^{i,c}$, C^i, Tn	Altered PBPs; impermeability
Glycopeptides	Cell wall synthesis (peptidoglycan)	Blocking of drug access to pentapeptide	P^i	
Aminoglycosides	Translation (binds ribosomes)	Enzymatic modification (phosphorylation, nucleotidylation, or acetylation)	C^c, P^c, Tn	Altered target (ribosomal proteins); impermeability

[a] Abbreviations: P, plasmid; C, chromosome; Tn, transposon; i, inducible; c, constitutive.

pounds but rather bind to them and probably alter their structures. This distortion results in less efficient transport or target binding of a compound (9, 12, 25, 29).

ALTERED TARGET

Alteration in antibacterial target protein, one of the most important mechanisms of resistance to clinically used antibacterial drug classes, includes resistance to tetracyclines, macrolides, and lincosamides, sulfonamides, trimethoprim, quinolones, rifampin, β-lactams, and aminoglycosides. Variations of this mechanism include biochemically altered target proteins that have reduced or no affinity for the drug, novel proteins that assume the functions of targets, and hyperproduced targets that overwhelm available drug concentrations.

Unlike genetic loci that affect permeability, genes encoding altered drug targets are often present on plasmids and transposons, which may at least partially explain interspecific sharing of genes encoding this type of resistance. A notable example is the *tetM* locus, associated with a transposon (the prototype is Tn*916*), which probably originated among streptococci but now has been reported in several gram-positive and gram-negative genera as well as *Ureaplasma* and *Mycoplasma* species (23). The *tetM* locus encodes a factor that protects ribosomes from tetracycline binding and subsequent inhibition of translation. Although this type of resistance may be detected readily with DNA probes (19), susceptibility testing is often a useful screen because *tetM*$^+$ strains, especially among gram-positive species, tend also to express constitutive resistance to minocycline.

Increases in the prevalence of staphylococcal resistance to macrolides and lincosamides in recent years are also largely associated with altered target genes that are likewise often associated with plasmids and transposons. An adenine residue of the 23S rRNA is methylated by products of *erm* genes usually of class A, B, or C. Since these loci demonstrate extensive nucleotide sequence homology, restriction fragment probes are of limited use for their distinction. Although clindamycin resistance is constitutively expressed among *ermB*$^+$ isolates, it is inducible in isolates harboring either *ermA* or *ermC*. By using a double-disk method in which a standard susceptibility disk containing erythromycin is placed approximately 8 mm from one containing clindamycin on a freshly and heavily seeded lawn of the suspect organism on Mueller-Hinton agar, the presence of *ermA* or *ermC* can be presumptively determined. A truncated (flattened) zone of inhibition around the clindamycin disk after overnight incubation suggests inducible lincosamide resistance and the possible presence of class A or class C resistance.

Among clinically used aminoglycoside-aminocyclitol compounds, only streptomycin and spectinomycin appear to be affected by altered target resistance. Changes in various proteins associated with rRNA that result in reduced drug binding have been described among strains of *Enterococcus faecalis, Staphylococcus aureus, N. gonorrhoeae,* and *Mycobacterium tuberculosis.* Drug inactivation as described below continues to challenge the use of other compounds in this class.

In the folate pathway from *p*-aminobenzoic acid to tetrahydrofolate, sulfonamides and trimethoprim act as nonfunctional analogs for dihydropteroate synthetase and tetrahydrofolate reductase, and resistance via the bypass pathway mechanism may be a variation of altered target resistance. Resistance is usually conferred by synthesis of an altered enzyme that functions in a pathway no longer susceptible to the drugs or by overwhelming production of wild-type enzymes. In staphylococci, the former mechanism is associated with high-level resistance (MIC of >1,000 μg/ml) to trimethoprim, and the latter is associated with lower-level resistance (MIC of ≤100 μg/ml) (24). Because of the extreme hydrophobicity of rifampin and the hydrophilic nature of lipopolysaccharides in the outer membrane of gram-negative bacteria, many gram-negative genera are intrinsically resistant to this compound. Mutation to resistance in normally susceptible strains occurs at high frequency. Decreased binding of rifampin to its target enzyme, RNA polymerase, perhaps through biochemical changes in the enzyme, is most often considered the principal mechanism of resistance, but impermeability may also be important. Inconclusive results regarding the biochemical nature of rifampin resistance have been compounded by a lack of understanding of the correlation between mutations and levels of rifampin susceptibility (47). Resistance to quinolones is likewise incompletely understood. Impermeability, altered target (DNA gyrase), or an interplay of both may explain various patterns of quinolone resistance (32). At least one mutation (*nalD*) confers resistance to nalidixic acid and low-level resistance to newer fluoroquinolones (e.g., ciprofloxacin), whereas another (*nalC*) confers hypersusceptibility to newer compounds in this class (17, 48). Until sufficient nucleotide sequence data are obtained, DNA probes and identification through polymerase chain reaction products will be of limited use in genetic identification of various quinolone resistance loci.

β-Lactam compounds may covalently bind several bacterial proteins, collectively termed penicillin-binding proteins (PBPs). Only a few species-specific PBPs involved in the final reactions of cell wall synthesis are, however, regarded as essential and therefore as targets of β-lactams. Resistance mediated by altered essential PBPs may be manifested by either reduced affinity of PBPs having wild-type apparent molecular weight or by the appearance of a novel, biologically functional but β-lactam-resistant PBP. Among organisms in which altered PBP-mediated resistance has posed clinical resistance are *E. coli* (44), *Staphylococcus* spp. (4, 46), viridans *Streptococcus* spp. (37), *Streptococcus pneumoniae* (49), *Enterococcus* spp. (50), *Haemophilus influenzae* (28), *Pseudomonas aeruginosa* (14), and *N. gonorrhoeae* (13). The search for improved β-lactam compounds, such as third- and fourth-generation cephalosporins, has focused not only on stability against β-lactamases but also on increased affinity for PBPs. Studies of PBPs are performed electrophoretically in sodium dodecyl sulfate-polyacrylamide gels, using tagged β-lactam, for example, ^{3}H-penicillin, and membrane protein preparations. Although large concentrations of labeled compound will usually reveal PBPs in a membrane preparation, comparative affinity studies are possible only by performing saturation studies using dilutions of the label reacted with each preparation. Other factors to consider in the planning of PBP assays include the production of β-lactamase by the test isolate that may hydrolyze the labeled β-lactam and the presence of outer membrane components in gram-negative organisms that may inhibit penetration of the isotope. Since β-lactamase inhibitors may bind PBPs, perhaps the only solution to the former problem is to rid the isolate of β-lactamase production, usually through plasmid curing. The latter problem is circumvented by disrupting the outer membrane before isolating the cytoplasmic membrane. Additional data may be obtained by competition assays in which membrane proteins are preincubated with an unlabeled drug of interest followed by labeled penicillin. Competitive binding of the unlabeled compound is indicated if no, or a drastically reduced, label can be subsequently detected for a particular PBP.

ENZYMATIC DRUG MODIFICATION

The proof that bacteria can develop efficient resistance mechanisms was clearly presented in the early 1940s when penicillinase was detected in *S. aureus* (22). Now referred to collectively as β-lactamases, these enzymes currently account for most of the resistance to penicillins and cephalosporins. Fortunately, β-lactamases may be readily detected by several methods, the most popular currently being the chromogenic substrate test (chapter 115). Emphasis should be placed on three potential areas in which problems may arise during performance of phenotypic β-lactamase testing: (i) enzymes reported in as many as 8% of *H. influenzae* isolates that may react slowly (e.g., "Rob" β-lactamase) (10) support longer incubation for negative tests; (ii) false- (but usually weakly) positive reactions, for example, through acid hydrolysis of the substrate, that do not correlate with phenotypic resistance may occur particularly among coagulase-negative *Staphylococcus* spp.; and (iii) detection of some clinically important β-lactamases, including staphylococcal enzymes and chromosomally encoded cephalosporinases in some gram-negative species, requires induction with another β-lactam compound to obtain expression of the β-lactamase structural gene.

Biochemical studies of β-lactamase isoenzymes have intensified in recent years because of both the large and growing number of novel β-lactam compounds and the rapid evolution of β-lactamases. The most definitive criteria for the classification of β-lactamases, established in 1973 by Richmond and Sykes (40), distinguish enzymes primarily on the basis of substrate and inhibitor profiles. Bush (2) and Bush and Sykes (3) updated this scheme in 1989 by including additional inhibitors and substrates and redefining conditions for accurate kinetic evaluation. Within a Richmond-Sykes or Bush class, an enzyme is most clearly defined by its net charge or isoelectric point (pI) and molecular weight. The former may be conveniently determined by using isoelectric focusing of crude enzyme preparations on commercially prepared acrylamide-ampholyte gels, followed by detection with overlays of chromogenic substrate (26, 41). β-Lactamase controls should be included in these assays, and surface pH measurements of the gel must be precise for accurate pI determinations. Since multiple or satelliting β-lactamase bands may be present in a given gel lane, interpretation of dominant band(s) may be necessary. Molecular weight determination is most often performed in acrylamide gels but requires at least partially purified preparations (39); the enzyme usually is not detectable with chromogenic β-lactam substrate.

The number of different β-lactamases is impossible to predict, especially among gram-negative bacilli in which minor genetic changes (e.g., point mutations) may result in enzymes having different and often extended substrate profiles (27, 36). Most extended-spectrum cephalosporinases described to date are derived from TEM or SHV, which are widely disseminated gram-negative plasmid-mediated β-lactamases, and a similar degree of promiscuity for their derivatives is at least possible to predict. The extensive nucleotide homology shared by genes encoding these derivatives compromises the usefulness of DNA restriction fragment probes in their differentiation from the parent genes. In addition to resistance profiles conferred by TEM or SHV enzymes, an unusually elevated level of resistance to one or more third-generation cephalosporins or aztreonam in a β-lactamase-producing enteric bacillus may indicate the presence of an extended-spectrum derivative. As previously mentioned, the spectrum of resistance conferred by a particular β-lactamase also depends on the amount of enzyme produced and the integrity of outer membrane transport proteins (e.g., porins) and the essential PBPs targeted by a particular drug (18, 31).

Although Richmond in 1965 reported immunologic differences among staphylococcal β-lactamases (38), these enzymes were thought for more than 20 years to have similar substrate profiles. Substrate differences, particularly relative to cefazolin, have been recently noted by Kernodle and colleagues, who used susceptibility inoculum studies and hydrolysis rates (21). The genes encoding these staphylococcal β-lactamase variants are believed to share extensive nucleotide sequences with one another and with the gene that encodes a sporadically reported enzyme in *Enterococcus faecalis* (30). Production of β-lactamase in *E. faecalis*, however, has not been shown to correlate with in vitro resistance to ampicillin. Detection of staphylococcal and enterococcal β-lactamases may require induction, and low concentrations of penicillinase-resistant compounds (e.g., 0.12 µg of methicillin per ml in broth culture) have been used successfully for this purpose. An in-depth review of the genetics of staphylococcal resistance to antimicrobial agents was published in 1987 by Lyon and Skurray (24).

Unlike β-lactamases, which affect a common drug site (the β-lactam ring), aminoglycoside-modifying enzymes (AMEs) may exert various effects. These diverse actions, when considered in conjunction with the complex cofactor requirements for AME catalysis and the cytosolic location of AMEs, have contributed to the difficulties in uncovering a method to conveniently detect AMEs. Currently there are approximately 40 of these enzymes, each of which is placed into one of three classes: phosphotransferase, acetyltransferase, or nucleotidyltransferase. Genes encoding AMEs are constitutively expressed and are often encoded on plasmids and transposons. Conjugal AME plasmids have been described in both gram-positive and gram-negative genera, a finding that at least partially explains interspecific sharing of AME genes and the difficulties in eradicating reservoirs of aminoglycoside resistance in health care institutions once such a problem is introduced. Most clinically important AMEs confer phenotypic resistance and may be identified by in vitro susceptibility (MIC) testing, using a battery of aminoglycosides tested at higher than normal dilutions. The aminoglycoside resistance pattern method, which was introduced by Shimizu and colleagues (42), requires approximately 11 drugs tested to 512 µg/ml. Some of these compounds may not be readily attainable by clinical laboratories, and this method may fail to detect enzymes that do not confer phenotypic resistance. The most definitive and quantitative assay for AMEs is the phosphocellulose binding assay described by Davies and colleagues (11). This technique, which exploits the electrostatic affinity between phosphocellulose and aminoglycosides, requires incubation of cellular lysates with radioisotopic precursors, cofactors, and a battery of aminoglycosides. After spotting reactions to phosphocellulose strips, scintillation counts will be significantly higher for modified drugs than for water controls. A modified microdilution assay has made the phosphocellulose binding assay more convenient and enables screening of AME classes (8). Especially for some of the more clinically important AMEs, DNA probes for their encoding genes have been described.

Inactivation as a mechanism of resistance to clinically important drug classes is important not only for aminoglycosides and β-lactams but also for chloramphenicol and related compounds. CAT is most often plasmid mediated and is inducible in gram-positive organisms. The constitutive gram-negative CAT is the most frequent mechanism of resistance to chloramphenicol among *Enterobacteriaceae* and *H. influenzae*. Clinically important gram-positive genera in which inducible CAT has been reported include *Streptococcus, Aerococcus*, and *Staphylococcus*. These enzymes may be conveniently detected by a colorimetric tube assay in which sulfhydryl moieties, liberated from acetyl coenzyme A by the action of CAT, react with 5,5′-dithiobis-2-nitrobenzoic acid to yield a yellow color (1). This assay is available in an even more convenient disk assay that requires only the suspension of cells in saline.

Despite the heterogeneous nature of tetracycline resistance determinants, only recently has inactivation been reported as a functional mechanism of resistance for this drug class. Genes in gram-negative classes A through E have been associated with active tetracycline efflux. Among these, however, class B is the most frequently encountered mechanism in *E. coli* and has been recently shown to degrade minocycline (20). Although structural genes encoding Tet classes A through E share some sequence homology, inactivation has so far been shown to be associated only with *tetB*. The *tetF* locus, originating in *Bacteroides fragilis*, also encodes efflux and inactivation of tetracycline but is nonfunctional in this genus. Aerobic modification of tetracycline by the *Tc^r locus, also found in bacteroides, was recently reported by Speer and Salyers (43).

Although enzymatic modification as a mechanism of macrolide resistance has only recently been documented (34), the locus (encoding a 2′-phosphotransferase) was detected in *E. coli,* and an altered target (via ribosomal methylase) currently remains the principal resistance mechanism for this class among gram-positive species.

EFFLUX

Other than for some antibacterial metallic compounds, active efflux has not been shown to explain resistance to drug classes other than tetracyclines. Gram-negative classes A through F and gram-positive classes K and L are often plasmid encoded and confer this mechanism of resistance. Class K is responsible for most tetracycline resistance in staphylococci, and its encoding locus has been shown to be present most often on plasmids of 2.7 to 3.0 megadaltons in size in several species in this genus (6). As opposed to class M (altered target resistance), which also confers minocycline resistance, class K strains are susceptible to minocycline. Levels of minocycline resistance associated with the gram-negative loci vary, and the extent of minocycline inactivation, as opposed to efflux, warrants further study. When used under conditions of proper stringency, DNA probes can be used to differentiate Tet classes.

LITERATURE CITED

1. **Azemun, P., T. Stull, M. Roberts, and A. L. Smith.** 1981. Rapid detection of chloramphenicol resistance in *Haemophilus influenzae.* Antimicrob. Agents Chemother. **20:** 168–170.
2. **Bush, K.** 1989. Characterization of β-lactamases. Antimicrob. Agents Chemother. **33:**259–263.
3. **Bush, K., and R. B. Sykes.** 1986. Methodology for the study of β-lactamases. Antimicrob. Agents Chemother. **30:** 6–10.
4. **Chambers, H. F.** 1987. Coagulase-negative staphylococci resistant to β-lactam antibiotics in vivo produce penicillin-binding protein 2a. Antimicrob. Agents Chemother. **31:** 1919–1924.
5. **Cohen, S. P., L. M. McMurry, D. C. Hooper, J. S. Wolfson, and S. B. Levy.** 1989. Cross-resistance to fluoroquinolones in multiple-antibiotic-resistant (Mar) *Escherichia coli* selected by tetracycline or chloramphenicol: decreased drug accumulation associated with membrane changes in addition to OmpF reduction. Antimicrob. Agents Chemother. **33:**1318–1325.
6. **Cooksey, R. C., and J. N. Baldwin.** 1985. Relatedness of tetracycline resistance plasmids among species of coagulase-negative staphylococci. Antimicrob. Agents Chemother. **27:**234–238.
7. **Cooksey, R. C., and L. W. Mayer.** 1987. Identification of antibacterial resistance mechanisms: advances in laboratory assays. Antimicrob. Newsl. **4:**57–67.
8. **Cooksey, R. C., B. G. Metchock, and C. Thornsberry.** 1986. Microplate phosphocellulose binding assay for aminoglycoside-modifying enzymes. Antimicrob. Agents Chemother. **30:**883–887.
9. **Cutler, R. R.** 1983. Gentamicin resistance in *Staphylococcus aureus*—a new mechanism? J. Antimicrob. Chemother. **11:**263–269.
10. **Daum, R. S., M. Murphey-Corb, E. Shapira, and S. Dipp.** 1988. Epidemiology of Rob β-lactamase among ampicillin-resistant *Haemophilus influenzae* isolates in the United States. J. Infect. Dis. **157:**450–455.
11. **Davies, J., M. Brzezinska, and R. Benveniste.** 1971. R factors: biochemical mechanisms of resistance to aminoglycoside antibiotics. Ann. N.Y. Acad. Sci. **182:**226–233.
12. **Davies, J., and P. Courvalin.** 1977. Mechanisms of resistance to aminoglycosides. Am. J. Med. **63:**868–872.
13. **Dougherty, T. J., A. E. Koller, and A. Tomasz.** 1980. Penicillin-binding proteins of penicillin-susceptible and intrinsically resistant *Neisseria gonorrhoeae.* Antimicrob. Agents Chemother. **18:**730–737.
14. **Godfrey, A. J., L. E. Bryan, and H. R. Rabin.** 1981. β-Lactam-resistant *Pseudomonas aeruginosa* with modified penicillin-binding proteins emerging during cystic fibrosis treatment. Antimicrob. Agents Chemother. **19:**705–711.
15. **Guymon, L. F., and P. F. Sparling.** 1975. Altered crystal violet permeability and lytic behavior in antibiotic-resistant and -sensitive mutants of *Neisseria gonorrhoeae.* J. Bacteriol. **124:**757–763.
16. **Hancock, R. E. W.** 1984. Alterations in outer membrane permeability. Annu. Rev. Microbiol. **38:**237–264.
17. **Hooper, D. C., and J. S. Wolfson.** 1988. Mode of action of the quinolone antimicrobial agents. Rev. Infect. Dis. **10**(Suppl. 1):14–21.
18. **Jacoby, G. A., and L. Sutton.** 1985. β-Lactamases and β-lactam resistance in *Escherichia coli.* Antimicrob. Agents Chemother. **28:**703–705.
19. **Johnson, S. R., J. W. Biddle, and W. E. DeWitt.** 1989. Detection and characterization of the tetracycline resistance determinant, TetM, in *Haemophilus ducreyi.* Curr. Microbiol. **19:**7–12.
20. **Jupeau-Vessieres, A. N., Y. G. Leroux, M. R. Scavizzi, D. El Manouni, and G. R. Gerbaud.** 1989. Evidence for broken minocycline by NMR and HPLC techniques: a new additional resistance mechanism mediated by *tetB* determinant. Res. Microbiol. **140:**207–219.
21. **Kernodle, D. S., C. W. Stratton, L. W. McMurray, J. R. Chipley, and P. A. McGraw.** 1989. Differentiation of β-lactamase variants of *Staphylococcus aureus* by substrate hydrolysis profiles. J. Infect. Dis. **159:**103–108.
22. **Kirby, W. M. M.** 1944. Extraction of a highly potent penicillin inactivator from penicillin-resistant staphylococci. Science **99:**452–453.
23. **Levy, S. B.** 1988. Tetracycline resistance determinants are widespread. ASM News **54:**418–421.
24. **Lyon, B. R., and R. Skurray.** 1987. Antimicrobial resistance of *Staphylococcus aureus:* genetic basis. Microbiol. Rev. **51:**83–134.
25. **Mandel, L. J., E. Murphy, N. H. Steigbigel, and M. H. Miller.** 1984. Gentamicin uptake in *Staphylococcus aureus* possessing plasmid-encoded, aminoglycoside-modifying enzymes. Antimicrob. Agents Chemother. **26:**563–569.
26. **Matthew, M., A. M. Harris, M. J. Marshall, and G. W. Ross.** 1975. The use of analytical isoelectric focusing for detection and identification of beta-lactamases. J. Gen. Microbiol. **88:**169–178.
27. **Medeiros, A., K. H. Mayer, and S. M. Opal.** 1988. Plasmid-mediated beta-lactamases. Antimicrob. Newsl. **5:**61–65.
28. **Mendelman, P. M., D. O. Chaffin, T. L. Stull, C. E. Rubens, K. D. Mack, and A. L. Smith.** 1984. Characterization of non-β-lactamase-mediated ampicillin resistance in *Haemophilus influenzae.* Antimicrob. Agents Chemother. **26:**235–244.
29. **Mumford, L. M., and S. A. Lerner.** 1980. Bacterial resistance to aminoglycosides. Clin. Microbiol. Newsl. **2:**1–4.
30. **Murray, B. E., D. A. Church, A. Wanger, K. Zscheck, M. E. Levison, M. J. Ingerman, E. Abrutyn, and B. Mederski-Samoraj.** 1986. Comparison of two β-lactamase-producing strains of *Streptococcus faecalis.* Antimicrob. Agents Chemother. **30:**861–864.
31. **Neu, H. C.** 1982. Mechanisms of bacterial resistance to antimicrobial agents, with particular reference to cefotax-

ime and other β-lactam compounds. Rev. Infect. Dis. **4:** S288–S299.

32. **Neu, H. C.** 1987. Quinolones revisited: where are we? Antimicrob. Newsl. **4:**9–14.
33. **Nikaido, H., E. Y. Rosenberg, and J. Foulds.** 1983. Porin channels in *Escherichia coli:* studies with β-lactams in intact cells. J. Bacteriol. **153:**232–240.
34. **Ohara, K., T. Kanda, K. Ohmiya, T. Ebisu, and M. Kono.** 1989. Purification and characterization of macrolide 2'-phosphotransferase from a strain of *Escherichia coli* that is highly resistant to erythromycin. Antimicrob. Agents Chemother. **33:**1354–1357.
35. **Parr, T. R., Jr., and L. E. Bryan.** 1984. Nonenzymatic resistance to β-lactam antibiotics and resistance to other cell-wall synthesis inhibitors, p. 81–111. *In* L. E. Bryan (ed.), Antimicrobial drug resistance. Academic Press, Inc., Orlando, Fla.
36. **Philippon, A., R. Labia, and G. Jacoby.** 1989. Extended-spectrum β-lactamases. Antimicrob. Agents Chemother. **33:**1131–1136.
37. **Quinn, J. P., C. A. DiVincenzo, D. A. Lucks, R. L. Luskin, K. L. Shatzer, and S. A. Lerner.** 1988. Serious infections due to penicillin-resistant strains of viridans streptococci with altered penicillin-binding proteins. J. Infect. Dis. **157:** 764–769.
38. **Richmond, M. H.** 1965. Wild-type variants of exopenicillinase from *Staphylococcus aureus.* Biochem. J. **94:**584–593.
39. **Richmond, M. H.** 1975. β-Lactamase. Methods Enzymol. **43:**664–677.
40. **Richmond, M. H., and R. B. Sykes.** 1973. The β-lactamases of gram-negative bacteria and their possible physiologic role. Adv. Microb. Physiol. **9:**31–88.
41. **Sanders, C. C., E. E. Sanders, Jr., and E. S. Moland.** 1986. Characterization of β-lactamases in situ on polyacrylamide gels. Antimicrob. Agents Chemother. **30:**951–952.
42. **Shimizu, K., T. Kumada, W. Hsieh, H. Chung, Y. Chong, R. S. Hare, G. H. Miller, F. J. Sabatelli, and J. Howard.** 1985. Comparison of aminoglycoside resistance patterns in Japan, Formosa, and Korea, Chile, and the United States. Antimicrob. Agents Chemother. **28:**282–288.
43. **Speer, B. S., and A. A. Salyers.** 1989. Novel aerobic tetracycline resistance gene that chemically modifies tetracycline. J. Bacteriol. **171:**148–153.
44. **Spratt, B. G.** 1977. Properties of the penicillin-binding proteins of *Escherichia coli* K12. Eur. J. Biochem. **72:**341–352.
45. **Tenover, F. C.** 1986. Studies of antimicrobial resistance genes using DNA probes. Antimicrob. Agents Chemother. **29:**721–725.
46. **Ubukata, K., N. Yamashita, and M. Kono.** 1985. Occurrence of a β-lactam-inducible penicillin-binding protein in methicillin-resistant staphylococci. Antimicrob. Agents Chemother. **27:**851–857.
47. **Wehrli, W.** 1983. Rifampin: mechanisms of action and resistance. Rev. Infect. Dis. **5**(Suppl. 3)**:**S407–S411.
48. **Wolfson, J. S., and D. C. Hooper.** 1989. Fluoroquinolone antimicrobial agents. Clin. Microbiol. Rev. **2:**378–424.
49. **Zighelboim, S., and A. Tomasz.** 1981. Multiple antibiotic resistance in South African strains of *Streptococcus pneumoniae:* mechanism of resistance to β-lactam antibiotics. Rev. Infect. Dis. **3:**267–276.
50. **Zighelboim-Daum, S., and R. C. Moellering, Jr.** 1988. Mechanisms and significance of antimicrobial resistance in enterococci, p. 603–615. *In* P. Actor, L. Daneo-Moore, M. L. Higgins, M. R. J. Salton, and G. D. Shockman (ed.), Antibiotic inhibition of bacterial cell surface assembly and function. American Society for Microbiology, Washington, D.C.

Chapter 110

Antibacterial Susceptibility Tests: Dilution Methods

DANIEL F. SAHM AND JOHN A. WASHINGTON II

Dilution susceptibility testing methods are used to determine the minimal concentration, usually expressed in units or micrograms per milliliter, of an antimicrobial agent required to inhibit or kill a microorganism. Procedures for determining antimicrobial inhibitory activity are carried out by either agar- or broth-based methods. Antimicrobial agents are usually tested at $\log_2$ (twofold) serial dilutions, and the lowest concentration that inhibits visible growth of an organism is recorded as the MIC. The concentration range used may vary with the drug, organism identification, or site of infection. Ranges should include concentrations that allow determinations of the interpretive categories (i.e., susceptible, moderately susceptible or intermediate, and resistant) and also include the acceptable ranges for quality control reference strains. Other dilution methods include those that test a single or a selected few concentrations of antimicrobial agents (i.e., breakpoint susceptibility testing and single-drug-concentration screens).

Flexibility is a major advantage of dilution susceptibility testing methods. The standard medium used to test routinely encountered microorganisms (e.g., staphylococci, members of the family *Enterobacteriaceae*, and *Pseudomonas aeruginosa*) may be readily supplemented, or even substituted with another medium, to allow accurate testing of various fastidious bacteria not reliably tested by disk diffusion (15) or automated systems. In addition, if plates or panels are prepared in house, the combination of antibiotics to be included is not limited. Any drug available in powder form may be used, and the delay that occurs with the Food and Drug Administration's approval of antibiotic disks may be avoided. Recommendations for appropriate antimicrobial agents to be considered for testing against the most frequently encountered bacterial isolates are presented in Table 1.

The flexibility of dilution testing is also evident in the reporting formats that may be used. Quantitative results (MICs in micrograms per milliliter), category results (susceptible, moderately susceptible or intermediate, or resistant), or both may be used. Although category reporting may be sufficient in many instances, there are circumstances in which the availability of quantitative results may be useful (e.g., therapy for endocarditis, osteomyelitis, and infections of severely compromised patients). Quantitative results are also informative for establishing the relative resistance of certain microorganisms that cannot be ascertained by category reports (e.g., relatively penicillin-resistant *Streptococcus pneumoniae*, variably penicillin-resistant viridans group streptococci, and β-lactamase-negative, ampicillin-resistant *Haemophilus influenzae* or penicillin-resistant *Neisseria gonorrhoeae*). Similarly, as indicators of the level of *P. aeruginosa* susceptibility, aminoglycoside MICs may be used to help establish dosing regimens optimum for therapy. However, when quantitative results are used, one should be aware that the reported MIC is not an absolute value. The actual antimicrobial concentration required to inhibit growth is between the highest tested twofold dilution that inhibited growth and the next-lowest dilution at which growth was observed. For example, if an organism grows in the presence of 2 μg of drug per ml but not in the presence of 4 μg/ml, the read and recorded MIC is 4 μg/ml, even though the "true" MIC is actually some concentration between 2 and 4 μg/ml.

Further advantages include the ability of dilution methods to detect certain resistance patterns that may not be detected by disk diffusion or automated systems (19, 25), and dilution tests are a necessary part of the procedure for determining MBCs (see chapter 115).

DILUTION TESTING: AGAR METHOD

Dilution of antimicrobial agents.

The solvents and diluents needed to prepare stock solutions of most commonly used antimicrobial agents are presented and discussed in appendix 1, Preparation and Storage of Antimicrobial Solutions. A dilution scheme for an antimicrobial agent that starts with an antimicrobial stock concentration of 5,120 μg/ml and covers a full range (512 to 0.125 μg/ml) of twofold dilutions is shown in Table 2 (10, 16). Depending on the number of tests to be prepared, the actual volumes used are proportionally increased. Certain intermediate concentrations are also used as the starting concentrations for the preparation of subsequent dilutions, and this should be taken into account when actual volume needs are being calculated. Although there are other approaches for obtaining a range of doubling dilutions, the scheme outlined in Table 2 is convenient, is economical in pipette use, and avoids some of the cumulative error inherent in traditional serial dilution methods.

Preparation, supplementation, and storage of media

Mueller-Hinton agar is the recommended medium for testing most commonly encountered aerobic and facultatively anaerobic bacteria (16). The dehydrated agar base is commercially available and should be prepared as instructed by the manufacturer. Before sterilization, the molten agar is distributed into screw-cap containers in exact aliquots sufficient to dilute the intermediate antimicrobial concentrations 10-fold. Containers, one for each drug concentration to be tested,

TABLE 1. Antimicrobial agents recommended for routine dilution susceptibility testing[a]

Antimicrobial agents	*Enterobacteriaceae*	*Pseudomonas*[b]	Staphylococci	Enterococci	Streptococci
Penicillins					
Penicillin G	—	—	P	P	P
Ampicillin	P	—	—	P	—
Oxacillin or methicillin	—	—	P	—	—
Carbenicillin[c]	P	P	—	—	—
Ticarcillin[c]	P	P	—	—	—
Mezlocillin[c]	P	P	—	—	—
Piperacillin[c]	P	P	—	—	—
Azlocillin[c]	—	P	—	—	—
Ampicillin/sulbactam	S	—	—	—	—
Amoxicillin/clavulanic acid	S	—	—	—	—
Ticarcillin/clavulanic acid	S	S[d]	—	—	—
Cephalosporins					
Cephalothin	P	—	P[d]	—	S
Cefazolin	P	—	P	—	—
Cefamandole	S	—	—	—	—
Cefonicid	S	—	—	—	—
Cefuroxime	S	—	—	—	—
Cefoxitin	P	—	—	—	—
Cefotetan	S	—	—	—	—
Cefotaxime	S	—	—	—	—
Ceftriaxone	S	—	—	—	—
Ceftizoxime	S	U	—	—	—
Moxalactam	S	—	—	—	—
Ceftazidime	S	S	—	—	—
Cefoperazone	—	S	—	—	—
Other β-lactams					
Imipenem	S	S	S[d]	—	—
Aztreonam	S	S	—	—	—
Aminoglycosides					
Gentamicin	P	P	S	—[e]	—
Netilmicin	P	P	—	—	—
Tobramycin	P	S	—	—	—
Amikacin	S	S	—	—	—
Miscellaneous antibiotics					
Clindamycin	—	—	P	—	S
Erythromycin	—	—	P	U	S
Vancomycin	—	—	P	P	S
Rifampin	—	—	S	—	—
Ciprofloxacin	P	P	P	U	—
Trimethoprim/ sulfamethoxazole	P	—	S	—	—
Norfloxacin	U	U	U	U	U
Nitrofurantoin	U	—	U	U	U
Tetracycline	S	—	S	U	S
Nalidixic acid	U	—	—	—	—
Cinoxacin	U	—	—	—	—
Sulfisoxazole	U	—	U	—	—
Trimethoprim	U	—	U	—	—

[a] Adapted from NCCLS (16). P, Primary agents to be selected for routine testing; S, secondary agents to be tested under special circumstances such as in institutions harboring endemic or epidemic resistance to one or more of the primary agents, for therapy of patients intolerant of primary agents, or as an epidemiologic aid; U, urinary tract drug to be tested against urinary tract isolates only; —, testing against the indicated organisms is not recommended or is not routinely necessary. Groups of penicillins, cephalosporins, and aminoglycosides known to have nearly identical antimicrobial activities are enclosed in boxes. Because the clinical efficacies of the agents within each group should be similar, only one from each group need be selected for testing.

[b] *P. aeruginosa* only.

[c] Combination therapy consisting of an extended-spectrum penicillin and an aminoglycoside is recommended.

[d] Ticarcillin/clavulanic acid should not be considered as a therapeutic alternative for *P. aeruginosa* isolates resistant to carboxy- or acylureido-penicillins; staphylococci resistant to the penicillinase-resistant penicillins should also be considered resistant to cephalosporins and imipenem.

[e] For use of aminoglycosides to screen enterococci for synergy resistance, see section on Breakpoint Susceptibility Testing and Single-Drug-Concentration Screens for Resistance.

are sterilized by autoclaving at 121°C for 15 min and allowed to equilibrate to 48 to 50°C in a preheated water bath. Once equilibrated, the appropriate volume of intermediate antimicrobial concentration is added, and the container contents are mixed by gentle inversion, poured into 100-mm round or square sterile plastic plates set on a level surface, and allowed to solidify. For growth controls, plates containing drug-free agar

TABLE 2. Antibacterial agent dilution schedule for agar or broth susceptibility methods[a]

Step	Starting antimicrobial solution		No. of distilled water volumes[b]	Intermediate concn (µg/ml)	Final concn (µg/ml) after 1:10 dilution in agar or broth[c]
	Concn (µg/ml)	No. of volumes[b]			
1	5,120	1	0	**5,120**[d]	512 (256)
2	5,120	1	1	2,560	256 (128)
3	5,120	1	3	**1,280**	128 (64)
4	1,280	1	1	640	64 (32)
5	1,280	1	3	320	32 (16)
6	1,280	1	7	**160**	16 (8)
7	160	1	1	80	8 (4)
8	160	1	3	40	4 (2)
9	160	1	7	**20**	2 (1)
10	20	1	1	10	1 (0.5)
11	20	1	3	5	0.5 (0.25)
12	20	1	7	**2.5**	0.25 (0.125)
13	2.5	1	1	1.25	0.125 (0.0625)

[a] Adapted from references 10 and 16.

[b] Volume proportions remain constant, but the actual volumes selected will depend on the number of plates, tubes or trays to be prepared.

[c] For agar dilution and broth microdilution methods that use inoculum volumes of 0.001 to 0.005 ml to inoculate 0.1 ml of drug-containing broth, the final concentration is also the actual testing concentration. For macrodilution and microdilution methods in which the inoculum dilutes the final drug concentration 1:2, the actual testing concentrations are given in parentheses (see text for discussion of macrodilution and microdilution inoculation procedures).

[d] Intermediate concentrations in bold print are dilutions used for preparing the corresponding final concentration and as starting concentrations for the preparation of subsequent diliutions.

are also prepared. All plates should be poured to a depth of 3 to 4 mm (20 to 25 ml of agar per plate), and the pH of each batch should be checked to confirm the appropriate range of 7.2 to 7.4.

After sterilization and temperature equilibration of the molten agar, any necessary supplements are aseptically added to the Mueller-Hinton agar. For testing streptococci, supplementation with 5% defibrinated sheep blood is recommended (16). However, sheep blood supplementation may antagonize the activities of sulfonamides and trimethoprim; therefore, if these drugs are to be tested, 5% lysed horse blood should be used. The presence of blood also affects results with novobiocin and nafcillin, as well as the in vitro activity of cephalosporins against enterococci (5, 18, 22); therefore, blood supplementation should not be used unless necessary for bacterial growth. Performance standards of Mueller-Hinton agar have been defined sufficiently that calcium and magnesium supplementation is not necessary. The need to increase the NaCl concentration for detection of methicillin-resistant staphylococci by agar dilution methods is presently unknown. More detailed discussion of proper supplementation procedures for susceptibility testing of fastidious and unusual organisms is presented in chapter 112.

Prepared plates should be sealed in plastic bags and stored at 4 to 8°C. If the plates are for reference studies, they should be used within 5 days of preparation; for routine purposes there may be no time limit so long as control strains that are tested routinely give accurate results that are within the acceptable ranges.

Inoculation procedures

Variations in inoculum size may substantially affect MIC endpoint determinations; therefore, careful preparation is required to obtain accurate results. The recommended final inoculum for agar dilution is 10^4 CFU per spot, which may be prepared in either of two ways. Four or five colonies are picked from overnight growth on an agar-based medium and inoculated into 4 to 5 ml of suitable broth that will support good growth (Mueller-Hinton, brain heart infusion, Trypticase soy [BBL Microbiology Systems, Cockeysville, Md.], or tryptic soy [Difco Laboratories, Detroit, Mich.]). Broths are incubated at 35°C until turbid, and the turbidity is adjusted to match that of a 0.5 McFarland standard (ca. 10^8 CFU/ml). Alternatively, colonies from overnight growth may be suspended in broth to a turbidity that matches the McFarland standard, eliminating the time needed for growing the inoculum in broth (1). By using either sterile broth or 0.85% saline, a 1:10 dilution of the suspension is made to give an adjusted concentration of 10^7 CFU/ml (16).

Once the adjusted inoculum is prepared, inoculation of the antimicrobial plates should be accomplished within 30 min, since longer delays may lead to significant changes in inoculum size. By using either a calibrated loop or an inoculum replicating device, as described by Steers et al. (24), 0.001 to 0.002 ml of the 10^7-CFU/ml suspension is delivered to the agar surface, resulting in the final desired inoculum of approximately 10^4 CFU per spot. For convenience, use of the Steers replicator (Craft Machine, Inc., Chester, Pa.) is often preferred because a consistent inoculum volume for up to 36 different isolates is simultaneously delivered. To use this device, an aliquot of the adjusted inoculum for each isolate is pipetted into the appropriate well of the seed plate, and a multiprong inoculator is used to pick up and gently transfer 0.002 ml from the wells to the agar surfaces. The surface of the agar plates must be dry before inoculation, which should begin with the lowest drug concentration. To check for viability of each test isolate, and also as an added check for purity, control plates not containing drug are inoculated last. Finally, plates should be clearly marked so that orientations of the different isolates being tested on each plate are known.

Incubation

Inoculated plates are allowed to stand until inocula have been completely absorbed by the medium; then they are inverted and incubated, in air, at 35°C for 16 to 20 h before being read (16). To facilitate detection of methicillin-resistant staphylococci, plates containing either oxacillin or methicillin should be incubated for a full 24 h before being read. Incubation in the presence of increased CO_2 is not recommended unless such an atmosphere is required for growth (see chapter 112).

Interpretation and reporting of results

Before reading and recording of results obtained with clinical isolates, those obtained with the quality control strains should be checked to ensure they are within the acceptable accuracy ranges (see Quality Control section and Table 4), and drug-free control plates should be examined for isolate viability and contamination. Endpoints for each antibiotic are best determined by placing plates on a dark background and observing for the lowest concentration that inhibits visible growth, which is recorded as the MIC. A single colony or a faint haze left by the initial inoculum should not be regarded as growth. If two or more colonies persist at antimicrobial concentrations beyond an otherwise obvious endpoint, or if there is no growth at lower concentrations but growth at higher concentrations, the isolate should be subcultured to confirm purity and the test should be repeated (16). Substances that may antagonize the antibacterial activity of sulfonamides and trimethoprim may be carried over with the inoculum and cause "trailing" or less definite endpoints (3, 4, 13). Therefore, the MICs for these antimicrobial agents should be interpreted as the endpoint at which an obvious 80 to 90% diminution of growth occurs.

The MIC of each antimicrobial agent is usually recorded in micrograms per milliliter. These quantitative results may be reported with the appropriate corresponding interpretive categories (susceptible, moderately susceptible or intermediate, or resistant), or the interpretive category may be reported alone. The MIC interpretive standards for these susceptibility categories, as recommended by the National Committee for Clinical Laboratory Standards (NCCLS), are provided in Table 3. For detailed instructions concerning the use of these criteria and categories, the latest NCCLS standards for dilution testing methods should be consulted (16). Of importance to note is that the interpretive standards for most of the penicillin-class drugs vary with the organism being tested and that for some antimicrobial agents the intermediate category rather than the moderately susceptible category is used. The term "moderately susceptible" is usually used with β-lactams that may be administered at higher doses, whereas the term "intermediate" is usually used with antimicrobial agents, such as aminoglycosides, that have a narrow toxic-to-therapeutic ratio.

The four interpretive categories are defined as follows: susceptible indicates that an infection caused by the tested microorganism may be appropriately treated with the usually recommended dose of antibiotic; moderately susceptible indicates that the isolate may be inhibited by attainable concentrations of certain drugs (e.g., β-lactams) if higher dosages are used or if the infection involves a body site where the drug is physiologically concentrated (e.g., urinary tract); the intermediate category is to be used as a "buffer zone" that prevents technical artifacts from causing major interpretive discrepancies; resistant strains will not be inhibited by the concentration of antibiotic achievable with the recommended dose (16).

Advantages and disadvantages

Dilution testing by the agar method is a well-standardized, reliable susceptibility testing technique that may be used as a reference for evaluating the accuracy of other testing systems. In addition, the simultaneous testing of several isolates is possible and microbial contamination or heterogeneity is more readily detected than by broth methods. The major disadvantages of the agar method are associated with the time-consuming and labor-intensive tasks of preparing the plates and inocula, especially as the number of different antimicrobial agents to be tested against each isolate increases.

DILUTION TESTING: BROTH METHODS

The general approaches for broth methods include macrobroth dilution, in which the broth volume for each antimicrobial concentration is ≥1.0 ml contained in 13- by 100-tubes, and microbroth dilution, in which antimicrobial dilutions are in 0.05- to 0.1-ml volumes contained in wells of microtiter trays.

Macrobroth Dilution Methods

Dilution of antimicrobial agents

Stock solutions are prepared as discussed in appendix 1, and a typical dilution scheme that may be used to obtain full-range doubling dilutions is outlined in Table 2. As for the agar method, the actual volumes used for the dilutions would be proportionally increased according to the number of tests being prepared, with a minimum of 1.0 ml needed for each drug concentration. Because addition of the inoculum results in a 1:2 dilution of each concentration, all final drug concentrations must be prepared at twice the actual desired testing concentration (see Inoculation Procedures). If not, the actual testing concentrations will be those given parenthetically in Table 2.

Preparation, supplementation, and storage of media

Cation-adjusted Mueller-Hinton broth (CAMHB) is recommended for routine testing of commonly encountered, nonfastidious organisms (16). Adjustment with the cations Ca^{2+} (20 to 25 mg/liter) and Mg^{2+} (10 to 12.5 mg/liter) is required to ensure acceptable results when *P. aeruginosa* isolates are tested against aminoglycosides. Insufficient cation concentrations result in decreased aminoglycoside MICs (8, 11, 17, 27). Mueller-Hinton broth, with a final pH of between 7.2 and 7.4, is prepared as directed by the manufacturer. Because some manufacturers provide cation-adjusted medium, care should be taken not to supplement the medium with cation unless analysis of the medium demonstrates that the cation content is below recommended levels. Adjustment, if necessary, is accomplished by the addition of suitable volumes of filter-sterilized, chilled $CaCl_2$

TABLE 3. MIC interpretive standards for dilution susceptibility testing[a]

Antimicrobial agent and organism tested	MIC (μg/ml)			
	Susceptible	Moderately susceptible	Intermediate	Resistant
Penicillins				
Penicillin G				
Staphylococci, *Branhamella catarrhalis*	≤0.12			≥0.25
Neisseria gonorrhoeae	≤0.06	0.12–1		≥2
Enterococci		≤8		≥16
Listeria monocytogenes	≤2			≥4
Streptococcus pneumoniae	≤0.06	0.12–1.0		≥2
Other streptococci	≤0.12	0.25–.20		≥4
Oxacillin/nafcillin	≤2			≥4
Methicillin	≤8			≥16
Ampicillin				
Enterobacteriaceae	≤8	16		≥32
Staphylococci, *B. catarrhalis*	≤0.25			≥0.5
L. monocytogenes	≤2			≥4
Enterococci		≤8		≥16
Other streptococci	≤0.12	0.25–2		≥4
Ampicillin/sulbactam	≤8/4	16/8		≥32/16
Amoxicillin/clavulanic acid				
Staphylococci	≤4/2			≥8/4
Other organisms	≤8/4	16/8		≥32/16
Carbenicillin				
Pseudomonas aeruginosa	≤128	256		≥512
Other gram-negative bacilli	≤16	32		≥64
Ticarcillin				
P. aeruginosa	≤64	128		≥128
Other gram-negative bacilli	≤16	32–64		≥128
Ticarcillin/clavulanic acid				
P. aeruginosa	≤64/2	128		≥128/2
Other gram-negative bacilli	≤16/2	32/2–64/2		≥128/2
Mezlocillin				
P. aeruginosa	≤64			≥128
Other gram-negative bacilli	≤16	32–64		≥128
Piperacillin				
P. aeruginosa	≤64			≥128
Other gram-negative bacilli	≤16	32–64		≥128
Azlocillin for *P. aeruginosa*	≤64			≥128
Cephalosporins				
Cephalothin	≤8	16		≥32
Cefazolin	≤8	16		≥32
Cefamandole	≤8	16		≥32
Cefonicid	≤8	16		≥32
Cefaclor	≤8	16		≥32
Cefuroxime sodium	≤8	16		≥32
Cefuroxime axetil[b]	≤4	8–16		≥32
Cefoxitin	≤8	16		≥32
Cefotetan	≤16	32		≥64
Cefixime	≤1	2		≥4
Cefotaxime	≤8	16–32		≥64
Ceftazidime	≤8	16		≥32
Ceftriaxone	≤8	16–32		≥64
Ceftizoxime	≤8	16–32		≥64
Cefoperazone	≤16	32		≥64
Moxalactam	≤8	16–32		≥64
Other β-lactams				
Imipenem	≤4	8		≥16
Aztreonam	≤8	16		≥32
Aminoglycosides				
Gentamicin	≤4		8	≥16
Tobramycin	≤4		8	≥16
Netilmicin	≤8		16	≥32
Amikacin	≤16		32	≥64

(*Continued on next page*)

TABLE 3—*Continued*

Antimicrobial agent and organism tested	MIC (μg/ml)			
	Susceptible	Moderately susceptible	Intermediate	Resistant
Miscellaneous antibiotics				
Clindamycin	≤0.5		1–2	≥4
Erythromycin	≤0.5		1–4	≥8
Vancomycin	≤4		8–16	≥32
Enterococci		≤4	8–16	≥32
Other gram-positive organisms	≤4		8–16	≥32
Rifampin	≤1		2	≥4
Ciprofloxacin	≤1	2		≥4
Enoxacin	≤2	4		≥8
Ofloxacin	≤2	4		≥8
Trimethoprim/ sulfamethoxazole	≤2/38			≥4/76
Norfloxacin[c]	≤4		8	≥16
Nitrofurantoin[c]	≤32		64	≥128
Tetracycline[c]	≤4		8	≥16
Nalidixic acid[c]	≤16			≥32
Cinoxacin[c]	≤16			≥64
Sulfonamides[c]	≤256			≥512
Trimethoprim[c]	≤8			≥16

[a] Adapted from NCCLS (16), which should be consulted for further details concerning recommended interpretive standards for dilution testing. See chapter 112 for most *Haemophilus influenzae* and *Neisseria gonorrhoeae* interpretive standards.

[b] The moderately susceptible category for this drug applies only to gram-negative bacilli isolated from the urinary tract.

[c] For use against urinary tract isolates only.

stock (3.68 g of $CaCl_2 \cdot 2H_2O$ dissolved in 100 ml of deionized water for a concentration of 10 mg of Ca^{2+} per ml) and $MgCl_2$ stock (8.36 g of $MgCl_2 \cdot 6H_2O$ in 100 ml of deionized water for a concentration of 10 mg of Mg^{2+} per ml) to the cooled broth (16). Laboratorians should be aware of the cation content of the commercial Mueller-Hinton broth that they use so that unnecessary cation supplementation, which will result in false resistance of *P. aeruginosa* to aminoglycosides, can be avoided.

Aseptic supplementation of sterilized broth with blood or blood products may be done to facilitate the growth and testing of fastidious bacteria (see chapter 112), but laboratorians should be aware of the various effects that such supplementation can have on results obtained with certain organism-antimicrobial agent combinations (see Preparation, Supplementation, and Storage of Media subsection of Dilution Testing: Agar Method). Reliable detection of staphylococcal resistance to oxacillin, methicillin, or nafcillin requires that CAMHB used for testing these drugs be supplemented with 2% NaCl (16).

Appropriately adjusted and supplemented Mueller-Hinton broth is used to prepare the final antimicrobial agent concentrations according to the scheme shown in Table 2. To minimize evaporation and antibiotic deterioration, tubes should be tightly capped and stored at 4 to 8°C. For reference studies, the dilutions should be used within 5 days of preparation; for routine use there may be no time limit as long as quality control accuracy ranges are maintained (see Quality Control section and Table 4).

Inoculation procedures

The recommended final inoculum is 5×10^5 CFU/ml. Isolates are inoculated into a broth that will support good growth and incubated until turbid, and the turbidity is adjusted to match that of the 0.5 McFarland standard (approximately 10^8 CFU/ml). Alternatively, four to five colonies from overnight growth on a blood agar plate may be directly suspended in broth to match the turbidity of the McFarland standard (1). This alternative method for inoculum preparation is especially recommended for testing of *S. pneumoniae* and methicillin-resistant staphylococci (16). A portion of the suspension is diluted 1:100 (10^6 CFU/ml) with broth or 0.85% saline. When 1 ml of this dilution is added to each tube containing 1 ml of the drug diluted in CAMHB, a final inoculum of 5×10^5 CFU/ml is achieved. Broth not containing antimicrobial agent is inoculated as a control for organism viability (growth control). All tubes should be inoculated within 15 to 20 min of inoculum preparation, and an aliquot of the inoculum should be plated to check for purity and inoculum size.

Incubation

Tubes are incubated in air at 35°C for 16 to 20 h before being read. Incubation should be extended to a full 24 h for the detection of methicillin-resistant staphylococci (16). Use of increased CO_2 is not recommended unless necessary for growth of the isolate being tested (see chapter 112).

Interpretation and reporting of results

Before reading and recording of MIC results for the test strains, the growth controls should be examined for viability, inoculum subcultures should be checked for contamination and appropriate inoculum size, and the accuracy of the MICs obtained with the quality control strains should be confirmed (see Quality Control section and Table 4). Growth, or lack thereof, in the antimicrobial agent-containing tubes is best determined by comparison with the growth control. Generally, growth is indicated by turbidity, a single sedimented button ≥2 mm in diameter, or several buttons with smaller diameters. As with the agar method, trailing endpoints may be seen when trimethoprim or sulfonamides are tested, and the concentration at which an obvious 80 to 90% diminution of growth, as compared with the growth control, occurs should be recorded as the MIC (16). Other interpretation problems include the "skipped tube" in which growth is not observed at one concentration but is observed at lower and higher drug concentrations. When this occurs, the skipped tube should be ignored and the concentration that finally inhibits growth without growth at serially higher concentrations is recorded as the MIC. If more than one skipped tube occurs, or if there is growth at higher antimicrobial concentrations but not at lower, the results should not be reported and the test for that drug should be repeated.

The lowest concentration that completely inhibits visible growth of the organism as detected by the unaided eye is recorded as the MIC. MIC interpretive standards for the susceptibility categories are provided in Table 3. The definitions and comments concerning these categories that were given for the agar method also pertain to the macrodilution broth method.

Advantages and disadvantages

The macrodilution broth method is a well-standardized and reliable reference method that is useful for research purposes, but because of the laborious nature of the procedure and the availability of more convenient dilution systems (i.e., microdilution), this procedure generally is not useful for routine susceptibility testing in most clinical microbiology laboratories.

Microbroth Dilution Methods

The convenience afforded by the availability of dilution susceptibility testing in microdilution trays has led to the widespread use of microdilution broth methods. The trays containing several antimicrobial agents to be tested simultaneously may be prepared in house or obtained commercially, either frozen or lyophilized (M. S. Gradus, C. N. Baker, and C. Thornsberry, Antimicrob. Newsl. **9:**65–71, 1985). For use of the commercial systems, the manufacturer's recommendations concerning storage, inoculation, incubation, and interpretation should be followed. The primary focus of this section will be the in-house preparation and use of microbroth dilution trays. However, many of the principles and practices discussed are pertinent to the microbroth dilution method in general, regardless of the source of the trays.

Dilution of antimicrobial agents

Antimicrobial stock solutions are prepared as outlined in appendix 1. The dilution scheme used for agar and macrobroth dilution methods is applicable to the antimicrobial dilutions needed for the preparation of microbroth dilution panels (Table 2). Available automated dispensing systems require that at least 10 ml of broth containing each antimicrobial concentration be prepared. From the 10-ml samples, aliquots of either 0.05 or 0.1 ml are simultaneously dispensed to the corresponding wells of each microbroth dilution tray. If 0.05-ml volumes are dispensed, allowances must be made for the 1:2 dilution of the final drug concentration that will occur when the 0.05 ml of inoculum is added (see Inoculation procedures). When 1.0-ml aliquots are dispensed, the volume of inoculum used is sufficiently small (≤0.005 ml) that adjustments in the antimicrobial dilution scheme are not needed. As a general rule, when the inoculum volume is less than 10% of the broth volume in the well, dilution of the antimicrobial concentration by the inoculum does not have to be taken into account (16).

Preparation, supplementation, and storage of media

CAMHB is the recommended medium for routine microbroth dilution testing and should be prepared as discussed for the macrobroth dilution method. Also, supplementation of the broth with 2% NaCl is required for detection of methicillin-resistant staphylococci. Similarly, supplementation with blood or blood products may be necessary for testing fastidious bacteria, but the precautions outlined for the agar and macrobroth dilution methods that accompany use of these supplements also apply to microbroth dilution procedures (16). After the antimicrobial dilutions have been dispensed to the trays, they are stacked in groups of 5 to 10, with an empty tray placed on top to minimize contamination and evaporation. Each stack is sealed in a plastic bag and frozen. At −20°C, preservation is ensured for approximately 6 weeks, but the shelf life may be extended to months if the trays are stored at −60 to −70°C. Thawed panels must be used or discarded. They should not be refrozen, since freeze-thaw cycles cause substantial deterioration of β-lactam antibiotics, which is why use of freezers with self-defrosting units should be avoided.

Inoculation procedures

The final desired inoculum concentration is 5×10^5 CFU/ml. The isolates may be grown in broth to match the turbidity of a 0.5 McFarland standard (ca. 10^8 CFU/ml), or such a suspension can be made from colonies grown on a agar medium overnight (2), which is the method preferred when testing *S. pneumoniae* and methicillin-resistant staphylococci (16). For microbroth dilution procedures that require 0.001- to 0.005-ml inoculum volumes to inoculate wells containing 0.1 ml of broth, a portion of the 0.5 McFarland suspension is diluted 1:10 (10^7 CFU/ml) in sterile 0.85% saline or broth. Multipoint plastic or metal inoculum replicators designed to collect and deliver appropriate volumes are used to transfer the inoculum from the diluted suspension to the wells of the microbroth dilution tray, resulting in further dilutions ranging from 1:20 to 1:100 and final inoculum concentrations of 1×10^5 to 5×10^5 CFU/ml (1×10^4 to 5×10^4 CFU per well). For systems that use an inoculum volume of 0.05 ml to inoculate 0.05 ml of broth, a 1:100 dilution of the 0.5 McFarland suspension (10^6 CFU/ml) is used. When the inoculum is added to the wells, the 1:2 dilution of the 10^6-CFU/ml inoculum results in a final inoculum concentration of 5×10^5 CFU/ml (5×10^4 CFU per well) and also halves the antibiotic concentration in each well. Special care should be taken to confirm the inoculum density on a periodic basis to ensure that the appropriate amount of inoculum is achieved. Insufficient inoculum is a frequent problem in microbroth dilution tests that may not be detected with the use of recommended quality control strains.

Microbroth dilution trays should be inoculated within 15 to 20 min of inoculum preparation; during preparation, an aliquot should be subcultured to check purity of the isolates and colony counts should be set up to check the accuracy of inoculum concentration. Finally, one well not containing an antimicrobial agent should be inoculated and used as a growth control.

Incubation

After inoculation, each tray should be covered with plastic tape, sealed in a plastic bag, or tightly fitted with an empty tray to prevent evaporation during incubation. Trays are incubated in air at 35°C for 16 to 20 h before reading and should not be incubated in stacks of more than five trays. The incubation chamber should be kept sufficiently humid to avoid evaporation but not so humid that condensation results in contamination problems. A full 24 h of incubation is recommended for the detection of methicillin-resistant staphylococci (16). Use of increased CO_2 is not recommended unless necessary for growth of a particular isolate (see chapter 112).

Interpretation and reporting of results

Before reading and recording of MICs for the clinical isolates, the growth control wells should be examined for organism viability, inoculum subcultures should be checked for contamination, colony counts should be performed to confirm appropriate inoculum size, and the accuracy of the MICs obtained with the quality control strains should be confirmed (see Quality Control section and Table 4). Various viewing apparatuses are available and should be used to facilitate examination of the microbroth dilution wells for growth. Growth is best determined by comparison with the growth control well and generally is indicated by turbidity throughout the well or by buttons, single or multiple, in the well bottom. Again, trailing endpoints may be seen when trimethoprim or sulfonamides are tested, and the drug concentration at which an obvious 80 to 90% diminution of growth occurs should be recorded as the MIC (16). A single skipped well (i.e., growth is not observed at one concentration but is observed at lower and higher concentrations) should be ignored, and the drug concentration that finally inhibits growth without growth at higher concentrations is recorded as the MIC. If more than one skipped well occurs, or if there is growth at higher antibiotic concentrations but not at lower, the results should not be reported and the test for that drug should be repeated.

The MIC interpretive standards for susceptibility categories are given in Table 3. The definitions of these categories and the comments concerning the use of these standards for agar and macrobroth dilution methods are also applicable to microbroth dilution methods.

Advantages and disadvantages

The use of microbroth dilution trays prepared in house provides a reliable standardized reference method for susceptibility testing. Inoculation and reading procedures allow relatively convenient simultaneous testing of several antimicrobial agents against individual organisms. However, the labor involved in preparing the trays and the substantial cost of purchasing the laboratory hardware required for the in-house preparation may detract from the convenience of this method (20). Commercially prepared trays are convenient and generally accurate (M. S. Gradus, C. N. Baker, and C. Thornsberry, Antimicrob. Newsl. **10/11**:73–82, 1985), but the accuracy of these systems may vary with certain drug-organism combinations, and commercial systems should not be used as reference methods for evaluating the reliability of other susceptibility testing procedures. In addition, the versatility of antimicrobial combinations available with the use of commercial microbroth dilution trays is limited compared with the flexibility of preparing panels in house.

BREAKPOINT SUSCEPTIBILITY TESTING AND SINGLE-DRUG-CONCENTRATION SCREENS FOR RESISTANCE

Breakpoint susceptibility testing

Breakpoint susceptibility testing refers to methods by which antimicrobial agents are tested only at the specific concentrations necessary for differentiating between the interpretive categories of susceptible, intermediate or moderately susceptible, and resistant, rather than testing a full range of doubling-dilution concentrations used to determine MICs (20). When two appropriate drug concentrations are selected, any one of the interpretive categories may be determined. Growth at both concentrations indicates resistance, growth only at the lower concentration signifies an intermediate or moderate level of susceptibility, and no growth at either concentration is interpreted as susceptibility (G. V. Doern, Clin. Microbiol. Newsl. **9**:81–88, 1987). For example, in testing ampicillin against *Enterobacteriaceae*, only concentrations of 8 and 16 μg/ml would be used. Growth at both concentrations would indicate an MIC of ≥32 μg/ml (resistant), growth at 8 but not 16 μg/ml would indicate moderate susceptibility (MIC = 16 μg/ml), and no growth at 8 μg/ml would indicate susceptibility. For some antimicrobial agents, particularly those used for the treatment of urinary tract infections (see Table 3), a single concentration may be used, with growth interpreted as resistance and no growth interpreted as susceptibility.

As for full-range dilution testing, breakpoint methods require the use of appropriately adjusted and supplemented Mueller-Hinton broth or agar. In addition, the standard inoculation, incubation, and interpretation procedures recommended for the full-range dilution methods should be followed.

Because breakpoint testing is a direct measure of antimicrobial activity, there is the advantage of avoiding inherent errors associated with extrapolating disk diffusion zone sizes and MIC results (9; Doern, Clin. Microbiol. Newsl. **9**:81–88, 1987). Considering expense and convenience, a greater number and variety of antimicrobial agents may be incorporated into a microbroth dilution tray set up for breakpoint testing than in trays designed for full-range dilution testing. However, breakpoint testing provides only interpretive category results and cannot be used to generate the doubling-dilution MIC data required in certain clinical situations. Also, there is a lack of reference strains that can be used to perform quality control procedures conveniently to ensure reliable performance of breakpoint panels.

Resistance screens

There are circumstances in which testing a single drug concentration may be the most reliable and convenient method for detecting antimicrobial resistance. The most clinically useful resistance screens are those for staphylococcal resistance to the penicillinase-resistant penicillins (i.e., methicillin, nafcillin, and oxacillin) and synergy resistance in *Enterococcus faecalis*.

Screening for resistance to the penicillinase-resistant penicillins (26) requires the use of Mueller-Hinton agar supplemented with 4% NaCl and containing either methicillin (10 μg/ml), nafcillin (6 μg/ml), or oxacillin (6 μg/ml). The inoculum should be prepared directly from overnight growth on an agar plate. Colonies selected from the plate are suspended in broth or 0.85% saline to match the turbidity of a 0.5 McFarland standard (ca. 10^8 CFU/ml). The suspension is appropriately diluted so that 10^4 CFU may be spot inoculated onto the agar surface. Alternatively, a cotton swab may be dipped directly into the adjusted inoculum and, after the excess has been expressed against the side of the tube, used to spot inoculate the plate (C. Thornsberry, Antimicrob. Newsl. **1**:43–47, 1984). Plates are incubated in air at 35°C for a full 24 h before being examined for growth. Growth at 24 h is interpreted as resistance; no growth requires reincubation of 24 h. Isolates that grow after reincubation are considered resistant, and those that fail to grow are considered susceptible (26).

This screen provides a convenient and a highly accurate and reliable method for detecting resistance to the penicillinase-resistant penicillins among staphylococci (6, 12, 26, 28). However, test accuracy may vary with the source of Mueller-Hinton agar used (12). Rare strains of coagulase-negative staphylococci may be inhibited by the 4% NaCl present in the medium and may therefore be reported as falsely susceptible.

E. faecalis isolates may be refractory to the synergy usually achieved between a cell wall-active agent, such as vancomycin or a penicillin, and an aminoglycoside, the antibiotic combination recommended for serious enterococcal infections such as endocarditis (14). This synergy resistance is mediated by plasmid-encoded aminoglycoside-modifying enzymes that confer high-level aminoglycoside resistance (7). Because highly resistant strains may not respond well to combination therapy, screening tests designed to detect this high-level resistance are useful for determining an isolate's susceptibility to synergy.

Streptomycin and gentamicin are the aminoglycosides recommended for high-level resistance screens. Streptomycin is used to screen only for resistance to synergy between streptomycin and a cell wall-active agent. Because the enzymes that modify gentamicin also mediate resistance to the other clinically useful aminoglycosides (7), gentamicin is used to predict synergy between a cell wall-active agent and gentamicin, as well as tobramycin, amikacin, and netilmicin (7, 21). Streptomycin is tested at 2,000 μg/ml, and gentamicin may be tested at either 500 or 2,000 μg/ml (there is not yet consensus on the "best" concentration to use).

For the agar screens, a variety of media have been found to perform well, but for the sake of standardization, Mueller-Hinton agar should be used whenever possible (21). The aminoglycoside-supplemented agar is inoculated with 10^6 CFU by spotting 0.01 ml of a suspension, prepared from a fresh overnight culture, that matches the turbidity of a 0.5 McFarland standard (ca. 10^8 CFU/ml) onto the agar surface. The inoculum is allowed to be absorbed into the agar, and the plates are incubated in air at 35°C for 16 to 24 h. Alternatively, macrobroth (21, 23) and microbroth (23, 29) dilution methods, which use the same aminoglycoside concentrations and incubation conditions as the agar method, but with a final inoculum of ca. 5×10^5 CFU/ml, have been shown to be reliable screening methods. However, certain commercially available microdilution systems may not yet be sensitive enough to detect consistently this resistance (23). Regardless of the method used, growth (i.e., streptomycin MIC of >2,000 μg/ml; gentamicin MIC of >500 or 2,000 μg/ml) indicates that the synergy usually achieved with the aminoglycoside and cell wall-active agent may not be achieved; no growth indicates that effective synergy is likely. To ensure reliability of the screening method used, a known susceptible isolate (e.g., *E. faecalis* ATCC 29212) and a known resistant strain should be tested as controls.

QUALITY CONTROL

Quality control recommendations are designed to evaluate effectively the precision and accuracy of the dilutions and test procedures used, monitor reagent reliability, and evaluate the performance of individuals who are conducting the tests.

Reference strains

A key to accomplishing the goals of quality control is the careful selection and use of reference bacterial strains that are genetically stable and give MICs that are in the mid-range of each antimicrobial agent tested (16). That is, if there are seven dilutions in a series, the reference strain should give an MIC from the third to fifth dilution, preferably the fourth. If there are four or fewer dilutions in a series or nonconsecutive dilutions are tested (i.e., breakpoint susceptibility testing), quality control for the correct interpretive category rather than an actual MIC or MIC range may be more appropriate. *Escherichia coli* ATCC 25922, *Escherichia coli* ATCC 35218, *Pseudomonas aeruginosa* ATCC 27853, *E. faecalis* ATCC 29212, and *Staphylococcus aureus* ATCC 29213 are the recommended reference strains for both agar and broth methods (16). These organisms may be obtained from the American Type Culture Collection or other reliable commercial sources. For proper storage and subculture procedures, the recommendations of either NCCLS (16) or the commercial provider should be followed.

MIC ranges

The acceptable quality control MIC ranges for the various reference strains are given in Table 4. An out-of-control result is defined as an MIC not within the acceptable range. Certain out-of-control results can frequently be directly related to the medium used for testing. High gentamicin MICs with *P. aeruginosa* ATCC 27853 indicate an inappropriately high cation content of the Mueller-Hinton medium, and low MICs indicate an insufficient cation concentration. Although trimethoprim/sulfamethoxazole may not be recommended therapy for *E. faecalis* infections, results obtained with the ATCC 29212 strain are useful for detecting inappro-

TABLE 4. Quality control MIC ranges[a]

Antimicrobial agent	MIC range (μg/ml)				
	S. aureus ATCC 29213	*E. faecalis* ATCC 29212	*E. coli* ATCC 25922	*P. aeruginosa* ATCC 27853	*E. coli*[b] ATCC 35218
Penicillins					
Penicillin G	0.25–1.0	1.0–4.0	—[c]	—	—
Oxacillin	0.12–0.5	—	—	—	—
Nafcillin	0.12–0.5	—	—	—	—
Methicillin	0.5–2.0	—	—	—	—
Ampicillin	—	0.5–2.0	2.0–8.0	—	—
Ampicillin/sulbactam	—	—	1/0.5–4/2	—	4/2–16/8
Amoxicillin/clavulanic acid	—	—	2/1–8/4	—	4/2–16/8
Carbenicillin	—	—	4.0–16	16–64	—
Ticarcillin	—	—	2.0–8.0	8.0–32	—
Ticarcillin/clavulanic acid	—	—	2/2–8/2	8/2–32/2	4/2–16/2
Mezlocillin	—	—	2.0–8.0	8–32	—
Piperacillin	—	—	1.0–4.0	1.0–4.0	—
Azlocillin	—	—	—	2.0–8.0	—
Cephalosporins					
Cephalothin	0.12–0.5	—	4.0–16	—	—
Cefazolin	0.25–1.0	—	1.0–4.0	—	—
Cefamandole	—	—	0.25–1.0	—	—
Cefonicid	—	—	0.25–1.0	—	—
Cefuroxime	—	—	2.0–8.0	—	—
Cefoxitin	—	—	1.0–4.0	—	—
Cefotetan	—	—	0.06–0.25	—	—
Cefixime	—	—	0.25–1	—	—
Cefotaxime	—	—	0.06–0.25	4.0–16	—
Ceftazidime	—	—	0.06–0.5	1.0–4.0	—
Ceftriaxone	—	—	0.03–0.12	8.0–32	—
Ceftizoxime	—	—	0.03–0.12	16–64	—
Cefoperazone	—	—	0.12–0.5	2.0–8.0	—
Moxalactam	—	—	0.12–0.5	8.0–32	—
Other β-lactams					
Imipenem	0.015–0.06	0.5–2.0	0.06–0.25	1.0–4.0	—
Aztreonam	—	—	0.06–0.25	2.0–8.0	—
Aminoglycosides					
Gentamicin	0.12–1.0	—	0.25–1.0	1.0–4.0	—
Tobramycin	—	—	0.25–1.0	0.5–2.0	—
Netilmicin	—	—	≤0.5–1.0	2.0–8.0	—
Amikacin	—	—	0.5–4.0	2.0–8.0	—
Miscellaneous antibiotics					
Clindamycin	0.06–0.25	—	—	—	—
Erythromycin	0.12–0.5	1.0–4.0	—	—	—
Vancomycin	0.5–2.0	1.0–4.0	—	—	—
Rifampin	0.008–0.06	1.0–4.0	—	—	—
Ciprofloxacin	0.12–0.5	0.25–2.0	0.004–0.015	0.25–1.0	—
Trimethoprim/sulfamethoxazole	≤0.5/9.5	≤0.5/9.5[d]	≤0.5/9.5	—	—
Enoxacin	0.5–20	2–16	0.06–0.25	2–8	—
Norfloxacin	0.5–2.0	2.0–8.0	0.03–0.12	1.0–4.0	—
Ofloxacin	0.12–1	1–4	0.015–0.12	1–8	—
Nitrofurantoin	8.0–32	4.0–16	4.0–16	—	—
Tetracycline	0.25–1.0	8.0–32	1.0–4.0	—	—
Nalidixic acid	—	—	1.0–4.0	—	—
Cinoxacin	—	—	2.0–8.0	—	—
Sulfisoxazole	32–128	—	8–32	—	—
Trimethoprim	1.0–4.0	—	0.5–2.0	—	—

[a] Adapted from NCCLS (16).
[b] Used only to test β-lactam combinations that include a β-lactamase inhibitor (e.g., clavulanic acid or sulbactam).
[c] —, Testing against the indicated organisms is either not recommended, not reliable, or not routinely necessary.
[d] For quality control purposes, a trimethoprim/sulfamethoxazole MIC of >0.5/9.5 μg/ml for *E. faecalis* ATCC 29212 indicates that the medium may contain unacceptably high concentrations of substances (i.e., thymidine) that interfere with activities of sulfonamides and trimethoprim.

priate concentrations of substances such as thymidine that interfere with the in vitro activity of antifolate drugs. Trimethoprim/sulfamethoxazole MICs of >0.5/9.5 μg/ml indicate the presence of such interfering substances.

Batch and lot quality control

Representative plates, panels, or trays from each new batch if prepared in house or from each new shipment lot if obtained from a commercial source are quality controlled for accuracy and sterility. MICs obtained by testing reference quality control strains should be within acceptable accuracy ranges (Table 4). If such accuracy is not achieved, the batch or lot should be rejected or results obtained with the antimicrobial agent(s) in question should not be reported (see below). Similarly, if after incubation selected uninoculated plates or trays fail the sterility check, the batch or lot should be rejected (16). In addition to these formal quality control procedures that use reference strains, careful review of susceptibility results obtained during daily testing of clinical isolates is necessary to identify aberrant or unusual susceptibility patterns that may be indicative of quality control problems.

Quality control frequency

In addition to batch and lot testing, quality control should be performed daily, or at least every day that the plates or trays are being used to test clinical isolates. When quality control is performed, two consecutive out-of-control MICs, or more than two nonconsecutive out-of-control values in 20 consecutive tests, indicate problems in the dilution testing procedure that must be identified and solved. However, if accuracy can be sufficiently documented as outlined below, daily testing may be replaced by weekly testing (16).

Each drug-reference strain combination is tested for 30 consecutive days to obtain a total of 30 MICs for each combination.

A. If three or fewer MICs per combination are outside the accuracy range (Table 4), weekly testing may replace daily testing.
    1. During weekly testing, a single MIC outside the accuracy range requires that daily testing be performed for 5 consecutive days.
        a. If all five MICs for a problem drug-organism combination are within the accuracy range, weekly testing may be resumed.
        b. If one or more of the five MICs for the problem drug-organism combination are outside the accuracy range, daily testing must be initiated. Returning to weekly testing requires again documenting 30 consecutive days with three or fewer MICs outside the accuracy range.

B. If more than three MICs per combination are outside the accuracy range (Table 4), daily quality control testing must be continued.

LITERATURE CITED

1. **Baker, C. N., C. Thornsberry, and R. W. Hawkinson.** 1983. Inoculum standardization in antimicrobial susceptibility tests: evaluation of the overnight agar cultures and the Rapid Inoculum Standardization System. J. Clin. Microbiol. **17:**450–457.
2. **Barry, A. L., R. E. Badal, and R. W. Hawkinson.** 1983. Influence of inoculum growth phase on microdilution susceptibility tests. J. Clin. Microbiol. **18:**645–651.
3. **Bauer, A. W., and J. C. Sherris.** 1964. The determination of sulfonamide susceptibility of bacteria. Chemotherapia **9:**1–19.
4. **Bennett, J. V., H. M. Camp, and T. C. Eickoff.** 1968. Rapid sulfonamide disc sensitivity test for meningococci. Appl. Microbiol. **16:**1056–1060.
5. **Brenner, V. C., and J. C. Sherris.** 1972. Influence of different media and bloods on the results of diffusion antibiotic susceptibility tests. Antimicrob. Agents Chemother. **1:**116–122.
6. **Coudron, P. E., D. L. Jones, H. P. Dalton, and G. L. Archer.** 1986. Evaluation of laboratory tests for detection of methicillin-resistant *Staphylococcus aureus* and *Staphylococcus epidermidis.* J. Clin. Microbiol. **24:**764–769.
7. **Courvalin, P., C. Carlier, and E. Collatz.** 1980. Plasmid-mediated resistance to aminocyclitol antibiotics in group D streptococci. J. Bacteriol. **143:**541–551.
8. **D'Amato, R. F., C. Thornsberry, C. N. Baker, and L. A. Kirven.** 1975. Effect of calcium and magnesium ions on the susceptibility of *Pseudomonas* species to tetracycline, gentamicin, polymyxin B, and carbenicillin. Antimicrob. Agents Chemother. **7:**596–600.
9. **Doern, G. V., A. Dascal, and M. Keville.** 1985. Susceptibility testing with the Sensititre breakpoint broth microdilution system. Diagn. Microb. Infect. Dis. **3:**185–191.
10. **Ericsson, H. M., and J. C. Sherris.** 1971. Antibiotic sensitivity testing. Report of an international collaborative study. Acta Pathol. Microbiol. Scand. Sect. B Suppl. **217:**1–90.
11. **Garrod, L. P., and P. M. Waterworth.** 1969. Effect of medium composition and the apparent sensitivity of *Pseudomonas aeruginosa* to gentamicin. J. Clin. Pathol. **22:**534–538.
12. **Hindler, J. A., and N. L. Warner.** 1987. Effect of source of Mueller-Hinton agar on detection of oxacillin resistance in *Staphylococcus aureus* using a screening methodology. J. Clin. Microbiol. **25:**734–735.
13. **Kirven, L. A., and C. Thornsberry.** 1978. Minimum bactericidal concentration of sulfamethoxazole-trimethoprim for *Haemophilus influenzae:* correlation with prophylaxis. Antimicrob. Agents Chemother. **14:**731–736.
14. **Moellering, R. C., Jr., C. Wennersten, T. Medrek, and A. N. Weinberg.** 1970. Prevalence of high-level resistance to aminoglycosides in clinical isolates of enterococci. Antimicrob. Agents Chemother. **10:**335–340.
15. **National Committee for Clinical Laboratory Standards.** 1990. Performance standards for antimicrobial disk susceptibility tests. Approved standard M2-A4. National Committee for Clinical Laboratory Standards, Villanova, Pa.
16. **National Committee for Clinical Laboratory Standards.** 1990. Methods for dilution antimicrobial susceptibility tests for bacteria that grow aerobically. Approved standard M7-A2. National Committee for Clinical Laboratory Standards, Villanova, Pa.
17. **Reller, L. B., F. D. Schoenknecht, and M. A. Kenny.** 1974. Antibiotic susceptibility testing of *P. aeruginosa:* selection of a control strain and criteria for magnesium and calcium content in media. J. Infect. Dis. **130:**454–463.
18. **Sahm, D. F., C. N. Baker, R. N. Jones, and C. Thornsberry.** 1984. Influence of growth medium on the in vitro activities of second- and third-generation cephalosporins against *Streptococcus faecalis.* J. Clin. Microbiol. **20:**561–567.
19. **Sahm, D. F., J. Kissinger, M. S. Gilmore, P. R. Murray, R. Mulder, J. Solliday, and B. Clarke.** 1989. In vitro susceptibility studies of vancomycin-resistant *Enterococcus faecalis.* Antimicrob. Agents Chemother. **33:**1588–1591.
20. **Sahm, D. F., M. A. Neumann, C. Thornsberry, and J. E. McGowan, Jr.** 1988. Cumitech 25, Current concepts and approaches to antimicrobial susceptibility testing. Coordinating ed., J. E. McGowan, Jr. American Society for Microbiology, Washington, D.C.
21. **Sahm, D. F., and C. Torres.** 1988. Effects of medium and inoculum variations on screening for high-level aminoglycoside resistance in *Enterococcus faecalis.* J. Clin. Microbiol. **26:**250–256.
22. **Sherris, J. C., A. L. Rashad, and G. A. Lighthart.** 1967.

Laboratory determination of antibiotic susceptibility to ampicillin and cephalothin. Ann. N.Y. Acad. Sci. **145:**248–265.

23. **Spiegel, C.** 1988. Laboratory detection of high-level aminoglycoside-aminocyclitol resistance in *Enterococcus* spp. J. Clin. Microbiol. **26:**2270–2274.
24. **Steers, E., E. L. Foltz, B. S. Graves, and J. Riden.** 1959. An inocula replicating apparatus for routine testing of bacterial susceptibility to antibiotics. Antibiot. Chemother. **9:**307–311.
25. **Swenson, J. M., B. C. Hill, and C. Thornsberry.** 1989. Problems with the disk diffusion test for detection of vancomycin resistance in enterococci. J. Clin. Microbiol. **27:** 2140–2142.
26. **Thornsberry, C., and L. K. McDougal.** 1983. Successful use of broth microdilution in susceptibility tests for methicillin (heteroresistant) staphylococci. J. Clin. Microbiol. **18:**1084–1091.
27. **Washington, J. A., II, R. J. Synder, P. C. Kohner, C. G. Wiltsie, D. M. Ilstrup, and J. T. McCall.** 1978. Effect of cation of agar on the activity of gentamicin, tobramycin, and amikacin against *Pseudomonas aeruginosa.* J. Infect. Dis. **137:**103–111.
28. **Woods, G. L., G. S. Hall, I. Rutherford, K. J. Pratt, and C. C. Knapp.** 1986. Detection of methicillin-resistant *Staphylococcus epidermidis.* J. Clin. Microbiol. **24:**349–352.
29. **Zervos, M. J., J. E. Patterson, S. Edberg, C. Pierson, C. A. Kauffman, T. S. Mikesell, and D. R. Schaberg.** 1987. Single concentration broth microdilution test for detection of high-level aminoglycoside resistance in enterococci. J. Clin. Microbiol. **25:**2443–2444.

Chapter 111

Susceptibility Tests: Diffusion Test Procedures

ARTHUR L. BARRY AND CLYDE THORNSBERRY

Bacterial susceptibility to antimicrobial agents may be measured in vitro by using the principles of agar diffusion. Reasonably accurate and precise results can be obtained with agar diffusion techniques as long as all procedural details are carefully standardized and controlled. Diffusion techniques can be used as quantitative tests (13). However, most procedures simply categorize microorganisms as being susceptible, moderately susceptible, intermediate (indeterminate), or resistant to different antimicrobial agents.

Antimicrobial agents are commonly applied to the test plates in the form of dried filter paper disks. When a disk is placed on the inoculated surface of the test medium, several events progress simultaneously. First, the dried disks absorb water from the agar medium, and thus the drug is dissolved. The antimicrobial agent is then free to diffuse through the adjacent agar medium according to the physical laws that govern the diffusion of molecules through an agar gel (2). The result is a gradually changing gradient of drug concentrations in the agar surrounding each disk. As the diffusion of the antimicrobial agent progresses, microbial multiplication also proceeds. After an initial lag phase, a logarithmic growth phase is initiated. At that point, bacterial multiplication proceeds more rapidly than the drug can diffuse, and bacterial cells that are not inhibited by the antimicrobial agent will be able to continue multiplying until a lawn of growth can be visualized. No growth will appear in the area where inhibitory concentrations of the drug are present; the more susceptible the test organism, the larger the zone of inhibition will be. The position of the edge of the zone of inhibition for most antimicrobial agents and microorganisms is determined during the first few hours of incubation (lag phase plus two or three generations). Obviously, microorganisms with prolonged generation times will appear to be more susceptible to each antimicrobial agent because the drugs will have more time to diffuse before the position of the edge of the zone is determined. Diffusion procedures have been primarily standardized for testing commonly isolated, rapidly growing bacterial pathogens such as members of the family *Enterobacteriaceae* and *Staphylococcus aureus*, which demonstrate fairly consistent, predictable growth rates when tested under standardized conditions. Diffusion tests may also be used to test most *Pseudomonas* species, *Acinetobacter* spp., *Enterococcus* spp., and *Streptococcus* spp. Microorganisms demonstrating marked strain-to-strain variability in growth rates cannot be tested reliably by the standardized diffusion procedures. Disk tests have been modified to permit testing of *Haemophilus* spp. and *Neisseria gonorrhoeae* (see chapter 112).

The size of the zone of inhibition is also affected by the rate of diffusion of the drug through the agar gel. Because different drugs diffuse at different rates, zones observed with one drug cannot be compared with those obtained with another. The diameter of the zone of inhibition, however, is indirectly proportional to the MIC, as measured by a dilution procedure. Table 1 includes the currently recommended criteria that can be used to interpret zone sizes around a few selected β-lactam antibiotic disks when tested by the procedure outlined in this chapter. The equivalent MIC breakpoints which were used to define the susceptible and resistant categories are also listed in Table 1. In the following discussion, the principles that may be followed to establish such zone size interpretive standards and to estimate the MIC correlates are briefly outlined.

INTERPRETIVE ZONE STANDARDS

According to the guidelines outlined in chapters 107 and 110, one must first select the MIC breakpoints which define the resistant and susceptible categories for each antimicrobial agent. Most antimicrobial agents include an intermediate category between the two MIC breakpoints. This category includes strains that are truly intermediate in susceptibility and are not properly categorized as resistant or susceptible. With most β-lactam antibiotics, susceptible strains have been divided into moderately susceptible and susceptible categories. The former category identifies strains that should require maximal safe dosages of the drug or a combination of drugs for successful treatment. The intermediate category, on the other hand, represents a truly equivocal test result; it is *not* the same as a moderately susceptible test result.

To establish zone diameters that correspond to selected MIC breakpoints, studies must be performed to establish the correlation between zone diameters and MICs for each antimicrobial agent. At least 100 to 150 bacterial isolates should be tested. These strains should include representatives of the common species that are likely to be tested against the antimicrobial agent being studied but should not include strains with delayed or variable growth rates. Scattergrams are first prepared by plotting each MIC ($\log_2$ scale) against the corresponding zone diameter (arithmetic scale). By convention, the MICs are plotted as the dependent variable (y axis) and the zone diameters are plotted as the independent variable (x axis) when scattergrams are being constructed. Regression statistics may be more appropriate, however, if the x and y axes are reversed.

The linear relationship between zone diameters and $\log_2$ of the corresponding MICs can be expressed mathematically by applying the statistical method of least squares. This method provides a mathematical formula which permits an MIC correlate to be calculated for

TABLE 1. Zone size interpretive criteria for selected β-lactam antimicrobial agents and MIC breakpoints that were used for defining categories of resistant and susceptible

Antimicrobial agent (disk potency) and microorganisms tested	Zone diam (nearest whole mm) for[a]:			Equivalent MIC breakpoint (μg/ml)	
	R	MS	S	R	S
Penicillin G (10 U)					
Staphylococci	≤28		≥29	β-Lactamase[b]	≤0.1
Enterococci	≤14	≥15	—[c]	≥16	—
Streptococci	≤19	20–27[d]	≥28	≥4.0	≤0.12
Listeria	≤19		≥20	≥4.0	≤2.0
Gonococci[e]	≤26	27–46[f]	≥47	≥2.0	≤0.06
Ampicillin (10 μg)					
Enterobacteriaceae	≤13	14–16	≥17	≥32	≤8.0
Staphylococci	≤28		≥29	β-Lactamase[b]	≤0.25
Enterococci	≤16	≥17	—[c]	≥16	—
Streptococci	≤21	22–29[d]	≥30	≥4.0	≤0.12
Listeria	≤19		≥20	≥4.0	≤2.0
Haemophilus[g]	≤21	22–24	≥25	≥4.0	≤1.0
Amoxicillin/clavulanic acid (20/10 μg)					
Haemophilus[g]	≤19		≥20	≥8.0/4.0	≤4.0/2.0
Staphylococci	≤19		≥20	≥8.0/4.0	≤4.0/2.0
Other genera	≤13	14–17	≥18	≥16/8.0	≤8.0/4.0
Ampicillin/sulbactam (10/10 μg)					
Haemophilus[g]	≤19		≥20	≥4.0/2.0	≤2.0/1.0
Other genera	≤13	14–16	≥17	≥32/16	≤8.0/4.0
Carbenicillin (100 μg)					
Pseudomonas[h]	≤13	14–16	≥17	≥512	≤128
Other gram-negative bacilli	≤19	20–22	≥23	≥64	≤16
Ticarcillin (75 μg)					
Pseudomonas[h]	≤14		≥15	≥128	≤64
Other gram-negative bacilli	≤14	15–19	≥20	≥128	≤16
Ticarcillin/clavulanic acid (75/10 μg)					
Pseudomonas[h]	≤14		≥15	≥128/2.0	≤64/2.0
Other gram-negative bacilli	≤14	15–19	≥20	≥128/2.0	≤16/2.0
Mezlocillin (75 μg)					
Pseudomonas[h]	≤17		≥18	≥128	≤64
Other gram-negative bacilli	≤17	18–20	≥21	≥128	≤16
Piperacillin (100 μg)					
Pseudomonas[h]	≤17		≥18	≥128	≤64
Other gram-negative bacilli	≤17	18–20	≥21	≥128	≤16
Azlocillin (75 μg)					
Pseudomonas[h]	≤17		≥18	≥128	≤64
Cephalothin, etc.[i] (30 μg)	≤14	15–17	≥18	≥32	≤8.0
Cefaclor (30 μg)					
Haemophilus[g]	≤18	19–23[a]	≥24	≥32	≤8.0
Other genera	≤14	15–17	≥18	≥32	≤8.0
Cefixime (5 μg)					
Haemophilus[g]			≥30[j]		≤1.0[j]
Other genera	≤15	16–18	≥19	≥4.0	≤1.0
Cefuroxime (30 μg)					
Sodium (parenteral)	≤14	15–17	≥18	≥32	≤8.0
Axetil (oral)					
Haemophilus[g]	≤20	21–23[a]	≥24	≥16	≤4.0
Other genera	≤14	15–22	≥23	≥32	≤4.0

[a] Microorganisms are categorized as being resistant (R), moderately susceptible (MS), or susceptible (S). For testing of *Haemophilus* spp., the MS category should be reported as an indeterminate or equivocal test result.

[b] Resistant staphylococci are those that produce β-lactamase enzymes, and the MICs for such strains usually exceed 0.12 μg of penicillin per ml or 0.25 μg of ampicillin per ml.

[c] —, Enterococci that are not resistant are all reported to be moderately susceptible, indicating the need for high doses and combination with an aminoglycoside for treatment of serious invasive tissue infections; for treatment of an uncomplicated urinary tract infection, penicillin or ampicillin alone is usually sufficient and thus urine isolates are to be reported as susceptible if they are not resistant.

[d] Nonenterococcal streptococci with "intermediate" zone sizes or MICs should be reported to be moderately susceptible, indicating that they should be treated as if they were enterococci (see above).

[e] Criteria for *N. gonorrhoeae* apply only to tests performed on a GC agar base with a defined supplement, as described in chapter 112.

[f] A moderately susceptible category designates strains with lower clinical cure rates (85 to 95%) compared with >95% for susceptible strains. Strains with zones of ≤19 mm are likely to be β-lactamase-producing strains.

[g] Zone size criteria for tests with *Haemophilus* spp. apply only to tests performed on haemophilus test medium, as described in chapter 112.

[h] Isolates judged to be susceptible by these criteria should be treated with maximal doses of the designated penicillin, and unless counterindicated, an aminoglycoside should also be administered for treatment of life-threatening infections.

[i] The same interpretive criteria apply to tests with cephalothin, cefazolin, cefaclor, cefamandole, cefonicid, cefoxitin, and ceftazidime disks (all 30-μg potency).

[j] The current absence of resistant strains precludes definition of categories other than "susceptible." Strains with smaller zones or higher MICs should be submitted to a reference laboratory for further testing.

any given zone diameter. If the axes are reversed, zone size correlates can be calculated for different MIC values. A straight regression line can be superimposed on the scattergram to display the theoretical line of best fit. An examination of the scattergram will then reveal whether one particular type of microorganism consistently deviates from linearity. For regression analysis, all tests showing no zone of inhibition and all tests with MICs outside the range of concentrations actually tested should be excluded from the calculations but included in the scattergram. In practice, the MICs should include concentrations of at least two doubling dilutions above and below the MIC breakpoints. With some antimicrobial agents, the regression line becomes parabolic with strains showing very low MICs. Because the method of least squares assumes a linear relationship, this method would be inappropriate for such parabolic relationships. In such situations, one may simply exclude data on the extremely susceptible strains from the calculations; however, these data should be included in the scattergram. Strains with endpoints near the MIC breakpoints are most important because the analysis is performed primarily to define the MIC-zone size relationship at that level to establish zone size breakpoints.

Regression analyses are affected by the distribution of endpoints. The slope and intercept of the line can be distorted if a disproportionately large number of on-scale endpoints is clustered at either end of the spectrum. Ideally, there should be fairly uniform distribution of endpoints along the range of concentrations tested. When the distribution of endpoints does not permit a valid regression analysis, the data are best expressed as a simple scattergram. This situation often occurs with antimicrobial agents for which there is clearly a bimodal distribution of MICs, with very few intermediate strains. By a simple examination of such scattergrams, interpretive zone standards can be selected as zone sizes that best separate the two populations. The error rate-bounded method of Metzler and DeHaan (20) has been suggested to formalize this type of analysis. That approach needs to be modified if an intermediate or a moderately susceptible category is to be defined. Also, acceptable error rates need to be selected for each antimicrobial agent; i.e., the criteria defined by Metzler and DeHaan (20), which were recommended for anaerobes, are only guidelines that may or may not be reasonable for tests with aerobes and other antimicrobial agents.

Gentamicin disk tests were improved by the establishment of an intermediate zone size category (21). However, some strains that are susceptible by the disk test are resistant to 4 μg/ml but susceptible to 8 μg/ml; most of those strains are actually inhibited by 6 μg/ml, and thus the susceptible breakpoint may be redefined as a MIC of $\leq$6.0 μg/ml rather than $\leq$8.0 μg/ml (8). Similar half-dilution interval MIC correlates are also appropriate for tests with other aminoglycosides (8). Because MICs are frequently determined by testing twofold dilutions of antimicrobial agents (even $\log_2$ dilution schedule), a significant number of strains may appear to be discrepant. This statistical artifact, which occurs because of the discontinuous nature of most MIC determinations, can be resolved by testing close dilution intervals and by testing each isolate three or more times and then plotting the geometric mean of the MICs against the arithmetic mean of the zone diameters.

SELECTION OF DISK POTENCY

For agar diffusion susceptibility tests, the amount of antimicrobial agent in the disk must be standardized. In the United States, only one disk potency is recommended for each antimicrobial agent. If the disk content is changed and the interpretive zone standards are adjusted appropriately, the result should not be affected a great deal. Small changes in disk content produce rather minor changes in zone diameters; e.g., a twofold increase in disk potency generally increases zone sizes by only 3 or 4 mm. The standardized potency of the agent in the disk is selected after the examination of scattergrams and regression lines generated by testing disks with various concentrations of the drug. The most appropriate disk contains just enough antimicrobial agent to produce zones at least 10 mm in diameter with all strains which are inhibited by the greatest concentration that could be of clinical interest. On the other hand, the disk should not be so potent that susceptible strains yield unusually large zones of inhibition (in most cases $<$ 30 mm, rarely $>$40 mm).

CLASS CONCEPT OF DISK TESTING

For practical reasons, the number of antimicrobial agents that are tested routinely must be limited. The general principles outlined in chapter 107 serve as guides for the selection of the most appropriate battery of drugs to be tested for a given patient population. Antimicrobial agents with similar chemical structures can be classified into families. In turn, it is possible to categorize the members of each chemically related family into drug classes based on similar spectra of activity. A single representative of each class of drugs may often be used to predict the susceptibility or resistance of an organism to the other drugs in that class. Some families of chemically related drugs may be represented by a single class representative; other families may require two or three class representatives. The class concept of disk testing is applicable only when members of the class demonstrate almost identical spectra of activity against those microorganisms that are ordinarily subjected to disk diffusion tests.

When a new antimicrobial agent is introduced, its spectrum of activity should be compared with those of chemically related antimicrobial agents, especially the established class representatives, by using a large collection of representative species. If the number of qualitative interpretive discrepancies (susceptible to one drug but resistant to another) is relatively small and judged to be of little clinical significance, the class disk may be applicable. Routine disk tests with a new drug are necessary only when the drug demonstrates a uniquely different spectrum of activity. The drug may have other advantages, but the spectrum of activity is the only aspect to be considered in the selection of a drug for testing. If the class concept is judged to be applicable, the class representative can be used to predict the susceptibility or resistance of an organism to the new drug, with a relatively small number of interpretive errors. The class representative should be the least active drug within each class so that any differences that do occur will be in the direction of false resistance rather than false susceptibility. In this way, all isolates found to be susceptible to the class representative can be assumed to be susceptible to the other related drugs.

However, a few strains which are resistant to the class representative might be susceptible to one or more drugs within that class, and if testing is clinically indicated, the resistant strains may be tested against those drugs.

When several chemically related drugs have somewhat dissimilar spectra of activity, the class concept is not necessarily applicable, but the expense involved in routine testing of all drugs in the spectrum-related group would not be justified. In that situation, the clinical laboratory should test the representative that is most frequently used in the institution being served. Other drugs in the spectrum-related group may or may not be so similar that the class concept is applicable.

Methicillin is the least active member of the penicillinase (β-lactamase)-resistant penicillins, but oxacillin disks are preferred as the class representative because of their stability and because they may detect heteroresistant staphylococci more efficiently (5, 19). Nafcillin disks may also be used, but they should not be tested on blood-containing media because the activity of nafcillin is diminished by the blood. Cephalothin is the class representative for most first-generation cephalosporins, but the second- and third-generation cephalosporins have somewhat broader spectra of activity. Tests with three cephalosporins and a cephamycin might be judged necessary in dealing with certain patient populations. The tetracyclines are represented by disks containing tetracycline hydrochloride, but doxycycline and minocycline may be active against tetracycline-resistant strains of *S. aureus* or *Acinetobacter* spp. Testing selected isolates with doxycycline or minocycline disks might be appropriate if the isolates are resistant to tetracycline disks.

DISK DIFFUSION TECHNIQUE

The disk diffusion test currently recommended by the U.S. Food and Drug Administration (16) and by the National Committee for Clinical Laboratory Standards (NCCLS) (21) is a slight modification of that described by Bauer et al. (9). The agar overlay method of Barry et al. (4) is another way to perform such tests with rapidly growing bacterial pathogens. These methods should be followed exactly as outlined in the appropriate references if accurate, reproducible results are to be obtained.

Agar medium

Disk diffusion methods have been standardized with use of Mueller-Hinton agar. The unsupplemented medium supports the growth of most of those microorganisms for which susceptibility tests are most relevant. Some microorganisms may require the addition of 5% defibrinated sheep, horse, or other animal blood; this addition can influence the activity of some antibiotics, and appropriate controls are required to control that variable. For testing *Haemophilus* spp., Mueller-Hinton agar is supplemented with bovine hematin (15 μg/ml), NAD (15 μg/ml), and yeast extract (5 mg/ml). The latter medium has been referred to as haemophilus test medium (18, 21). For testing *N. gonorrhoeae* isolates, GC agar base with a cysteine-free defined supplement has been recommended (17, 21).

Because there is some lot-to-lot variation in the performance of Mueller-Hinton agars (2, 15), each new lot should be tested with the recommended control strains (21, 23) before it is released for use in testing clinical isolates. Dehydrated media should be tested by the manufacturer, and the label should state that the medium performs according to NCCLS standards (22). Normally, Mueller-Hinton agars without such labels should not be used for susceptibility testing. When the control strains yield zones within the NCCLS control limits for the user (21), performance is satisfactory. Table 2 represents examples of such control limits.

The pH of each batch of Mueller-Hinton agar should be checked at the time the medium is poured for use. The pH should be 7.2 to 7.4 after equilibration at room temperature and can be measured by allowing the agar to solidify around the electrodes of a pH meter, by macerating the medium in neutral distilled water, or by using a surface electrode. The freshly prepared and cooled medium is poured into petri plates on a level horizontal surface to give a uniform depth of approximately 4 mm; this depth requires approximately 60 to 70 ml of medium in 150-mm plates and approximately 25 to 30 ml of medium in 100-mm plates. After the medium has been allowed to cool to room temperature, it should be stored in a refrigerator (2 to 8°C). The plates should be sealed in plastic to minimize evaporation, especially if they are to be stored for more than 7 days. Just before use, the plates should be placed in an incubator (35°C) with their lids ajar until excess surface moisture is lost by evaporation (usually about 10 to 20 min). There should be no droplets of moisture on the surface of the medium or on the petri plate cover.

Storage of antimicrobial disks

Filter paper disks containing antimicrobial agents specifically certified for susceptibility testing are generally supplied in separate containers, each with a desiccant. The disks should be stored under refrigeration (2 to 8°C) or frozen at −14°C or colder until needed. Disks containing β-lactam compounds should always be kept frozen to ensure maintenance of their potency (15, 21), but a small working supply may be held in a refrigerator at 2 to 8°C for as long as 1 week. Unopened containers should be removed from the refrigerator or freezer 1 or 2 h before the disks are to be used and allowed to equilibrate at room temperature before being opened. This step is done to minimize the amount of condensation that occurs when warm room air reaches the cold containers. If a disk-dispensing apparatus is used, it should be fitted with a tight cover and supplied with an adequate indicating desiccant. Also, it should be allowed to warm to room temperature before being opened. When not in use, the dispensing apparatus should always be kept covered and refrigerated. Only those disks that have not reached the stated expiration date of the manufacturer should be used.

Inoculation of test plates

For the standard method of preparing an inoculum (9, 21), a needle or loop is touched to each of four or five well-isolated colonies of the same morphological type, and the growth is inoculated into 4 or 5 ml of a suitable broth medium such as soybean-casein digest broth. The broth culture is then allowed to incubate at 35°C until a slightly visible turbidity appears (usually 2 to 5 h). The turbidity of actively growing broth cultures

TABLE 2. Zone diameter limits for tests with selected antimicrobial disks against five standard quality control strains[a]

Antimicrobial agent (disk content)	Zone diam limit (mm)				
	E. coli ATCC 25922	*E. coli*[b] ATCC 35218	*S. aureus* ATCC 25923	*P. aeruginosa* ATCC 27853	*H. influenzae* ATCC 49247
Amoxicillin/clavulanic acid (20/10 μg)	19–25	18–22	28–36		15–23
Ampicillin (10 μg)	16–22		27–35		13–21
Ampicillin/sulbactam (10/10 μg)	20–24	13–19	29–37		14–22
Ticarcillin (75 μg)	24–30			22–28	
Ticarcillin/clavulanic acid (75/10 μg)	25–29	21–25		20–28	
Imipenem (10 μg)	26–32			20–28	21–29
Aztreonam (30 μg)	28–36			23–29	30–38
Cefaclor (30 μg)	23–27		27–31		14–22
Cefixime (5 μg)	23–27				25–33
Cefonicid (30 μg)	25–29		22–28		19–27
Cefuroxime (30 μg)	20–26		27–35		17–25
Cefotaxime (30 μg)	29–35		25–31	18–22	31–39
Ceftriaxone (30 μg)	29–35		22–28	17–23	31–39
Ceftazidime (30 μg)	25–32		16–20	22–29	27–35
Cefoperazone (75 μg)	28–34		24–33	23–29	
Ciprofloxacin (5 μg)	30–34		22–30	25–33	34–42
Enoxacin (10 μg)	28–36		22–28	22–28	
Norfloxacin (10 μg)	28–35		17–28	22–29	
Ofloxacin (5 μg)	29–33		24–28	17–21	
Amikacin (30 μg)	19–26		20–26	18–26	
Gentamicin (10 μg)	19–26		19–27	16–21	
Netilmicin (30 μg)	22–30		22–31	17–23	
Tobramycin (10 μg)	18–26		19–29	19–25	
Trimethoprim (5 μg)[c]	21–28		19–26		
Trimethoprim/sulfamethoxazole (1.25/23.75 μg)[c]	24–32		24–32		24–32
Sulfamethoxazole (250 or 300 μg)[c]	18–26		24–34		

[a] For the first four control strains, the control limits apply only to tests performed on Mueller-Hinton agar without added blood or blood products and incubated for 16 to 18 h in ambient air. The zone size limits listed for *H. influenzae* ATCC 49247 refer to tests on haemophilus test medium and incubated in 5 to 7% CO_2.

[b] *E. coli* ATCC 35218 is a β-lactamase-producing strain that is used for monitoring the performance of disks containing a penicillin and a β-lactamase inhibitor. It is resistant to the penicillins alone.

[c] For testing sulfonamides or trimethoprim, the media must first be shown to be relatively free of thymidine and thymine by screening tests with *E. faecalis* (ATCC 29212 or ATCC 33186). Trimethoprim/sulfamethoxazole disks should produce zones essentially free of fine colonies and at least 20 mm in diameter.

is then adjusted with saline or broth to obtain a turbidity visually comparable to that of a turbidity standard prepared by adding 0.5 ml of 0.048 M $BaCl_2$ (1.75% [wt/vol] $BaCl_2 \cdot 2H_2O$) to 99.5 ml of 0.36 N H_2SO_4 (1% [vol/vol]). This turbidity is half the density of a McFarland no. 1 standard and is often referred to as a McFarland 0.5 standard. The optical density of this turbidity standard should be monitored on a regular schedule, using a spectrophotometer with a 1-cm light path. The optical density at 625 nm should be 0.08 to 0.10. Sealed tubes should be stored in the dark at room temperature and agitated on a Vortex mixer just before use. For proper turbidity adjustment, it is helpful to use a white background and a contrasting black line(s) in combination with an adequate light source. A device such as the modified Rh-typing view box described by Stemper and Matsen (24) facilitates the standardization of cultures. When time does not permit the development of a turbid broth culture, an alternative approach can be used. Isolated colonies from an overnight plate can be suspended directly into a small volume of saline, which is then further diluted until the turbidity matches that of the McFarland standard (1, 6, 12). This method is preferred for the detection of methicillin-resistant strains of *S. aureus* and for the testing of species that will not grow well in the broth medium, i.e., *Haemophilus influenzae*, *N. gonorrhoeae*, and *Streptococcus pneumoniae* (21). The inoculum suspension should not be allowed to stand longer than 15 to 20 min before the plates are inoculated. A device that permits the direct standardization of the inoculum without an adjustment of turbidity and without preincubation in a broth medium has been found to be satisfactory (1, 12).

To inoculate the agar medium, a sterile, nontoxic swab on an applicator stick is dipped into the standardized suspension, and excess broth is expressed by pressing and rotating the swab firmly against the side of the tube above the fluid level. The swab is then streaked evenly in three directions over the entire surface of the agar plate to obtain a uniform inoculum. A final sweep is made of the agar rim with the cotton swab. This plate is then allowed to dry for 3 to 5 min, but no longer than 15 min, before the disks are applied. The inoculum should yield confluent or almost confluent growth.

Test procedure

Within 15 min after the plates are inoculated, antibiotic-impregnated disks are applied to the surface of the inoculated plates either with a mechanical dispenser or by hand with sterile forceps. All disks must be gently pressed down onto the agar with forceps or an inoculating needle to ensure complete contact with the agar surface (if the dispenser does not do this automatically). The spatial arrangement of the disks should be such that they are no closer than 15 mm to the edges of the plate and far enough apart to prevent overlapping of zones of inhibition. Generally, this arrangement limits the number of disks that can be placed on a single plate to 12 or 13 on a 150-mm plate or only 4 or 5 on a 100-mm plate. Fewer disks can be tested when streptococci, gonococci, or *Haemophilus* isolates are being evaluated. Within 15 min after the disks are applied, the plates are inverted and placed in an incubator at 35°C. Any longer delay before incubation will allow excess prediffusion of the antimicrobial agents. Incubation in an environment of increased CO_2 is to be avoided, because the CO_2 may alter the surface pH enough to affect the antimicrobial activity of some agents. A 5 to 7% CO_2 atmosphere is required when testing *H. influenzae* or *N. gonorrhoeae* isolates because those tests were standardized with a CO_2 incubation and separate interpretive criteria have been developed for those test procedures (14, 17, 18, 21). Those zone size criteria cannot be applied to tests incubated in ambient air.

Reading and interpretation

After 16 to 18 h of incubation (20 to 24 h for *N. gonorrhoeae* or for methicillin-resistant staphylococci), the plates are examined, and the diameters of the zones of complete inhibition are measured to the nearest whole millimeter by sliding calipers, a ruler, or a template prepared for this purpose. When a clear medium is used, the measuring device is held on the back of the petri plate, which is illuminated with reflected light from a source at an angle of approximately 45° against a black nonreflecting background (3). Zones on blood-containing media are measured at the agar surface. The endpoint by all reading systems is complete inhibition of growth, disregarding tiny colonies that can be detected only by very close scrutiny or by using transmitted light or mechanical enlargers. When staphylococci are tested against the penicillinase-resistant penicillins, the plates should be examined with transmitted light to visualize the very small colonies or light growth that may occur with methicillin-resistant strains (5, 19). Large colonies growing within the clear zone of inhibition may represent resistant variants or a mixed inoculum and may require reidentification and retesting. In the case of sulfonamides or sulfonamide-trimethoprim mixtures, the microorganisms may grow through several generations before inhibition occurs. In this instance, slight growth (80% inhibition) is disregarded, and the margin of heavy growth is measured (21). A veil of swarming *Proteus* sp. is also disregarded, and the margin of heavy growth is measured. In clinically urgent situations, preliminary readings can often be obtained within 5 or 6 h after inoculation, but the plates should always be reincubated, and a final report should be withheld until a full 16 to 18 h has elapsed (6).

The zone diameters for individual antimicrobial agents can be reported as equivalent MIC values (13) but are usually translated into susceptible, moderately susceptible, intermediate, or resistant categories by referring to a table of interpretive criteria. The interpretive criteria for the examples listed in Table 1 are those presently recommended by the Food and Drug Administration (16) or the NCCLS (21). Equivalent MIC breakpoints for each agent are also given in the NCCLS document (21). For the aminoglycosides, MIC correlates are probably more appropriately located at half-dilution intervals (8). For some agents (Table 1), different breakpoints are applied to different microorganisms because the microorganisms differ in their responses to chemotherapy. Two sets of criteria are applicable for tests with a single cefuroxime disk: one criterion applies when the oral cefuroxime axetil is being used, and the other applies when the sodium salt is given parenterally (Table 1).

The MIC breakpoints listed in Table 1 are related to the levels of drug in blood usually expected with frequently used dose schedules. For the few drugs that are used exclusively for the treatment of urinary tract infections, e.g., nitrofurantoin and nalidixic acid (not shown in Table 1), breakpoints are related to levels of drug in urine. The breakpoints were tested against the distribution of zone sizes and MICs among a variety of species of known clinical responsiveness or lack of responsiveness to check their appropriateness and were modified, when considered necessary, for adequate discrimination. The resistant and susceptible categories for most drugs were developed to apply to systemic infections and appropriate dose schedules. For most β-lactam compounds, a moderately susceptible category has been identified to separate those susceptible strains that are likely to need the maximal safe dosage or combination therapy from those that are likely to respond to a reduced dosage. In situations in which a high dosage of nontoxic agent may be given, the levels of drug in blood may greatly exceed those considered in the establishment of the interpretive values for the resistant category. Similarly, the concentration of certain antibiotics by the kidneys may result in drug levels in urine manyfold higher than the levels considered in the development of breakpoints for systemic infections. In such situations, organisms that are resistant by the disk method might be treated successfully, but antimicrobial dilution tests may need to be done before such therapy is considered.

LIMITATIONS OF THE METHODS AND SPECIAL PRECAUTIONS

Slowly growing organisms, obligate anaerobes, and capnophiles should not be tested with the disk diffusion method, which has been standardized for testing rapidly growing aerobic or facultative organisms, but rather with dilution methods if susceptibility tests are needed. Special precautions must be taken and special interpretative standards must be used to test *Neisseria meningitidis* against the sulfonamides (10). The method has not been standardized for testing other antimicrobial agents against *N. meningitidis*. Disk diffusion susceptibility testing is not done with either methenamine mandelate or methenamine hippurate, as there is no corollary between the in vivo and in vitro conditions (27).

Special problems are posed by heteroresistant, "methicillin-resistant" *S. aureus*. These strains appear to have an increased clinical resistance to the penicillins and cephalosporins, although they may appear to be susceptible by in vitro tests. Although some resistant strains may be very difficult to recognize, they can usually be detected with oxacillin or methicillin disks. All tests are standardized with a 35°C incubation: resistance to penicillinase-resistant penicillins may not be detected at 37°C (25). Resistant strains often produce a haze or film of small colonies growing within an otherwise definite zone of inhibition; that inner haze of growth is easily overlooked unless the zones are carefully examined with transmitted and reflected light (19). Diffusion tests with these strains often fail to indicate resistance to cloxacillin and cephalothin, although dilution tests often show them to be resistant. Thus, strains proven to be resistant to methicillin, oxacillin, or nafcillin should be considered potentially resistant to the whole group of penicillinase-resistant penicillins and to the cephalosporins, and the clinician should be alerted to this possible resistance (19, 21) (see also chapter 110).

False reports of methicillin resistance have resulted from the deterioration of methicillin disks during refrigeration. Attention to the recommendations given for disk storage and quality control should avoid this difficulty. Use of the more stable oxacillin disk is preferred for the detection of most methicillin-resistant strains; some strains will be detected with methicillin disks but not with oxacillin disks, but many more strains will be missed if only methicillin disks are tested.

As discussed in chapter 110, the results of tests for gentamicin susceptibility of *Pseudomonas aeruginosa* are highly dependent on the amount of soluble magnesium and calcium in the medium (7, 23). Most batches of Mueller-Hinton agar are satisfactory for routine testing and interpretation by the criteria given in the NCCLS document (21). It is important to use a control strain of *P. aeruginosa* to detect errors that may result from variability in the agar media (21–23). Other control strains are less sensitive to minor changes in the agar medium.

When trimethoprim or trimethoprim/sulfamethoxazole disks are tested, each lot of Mueller-Hinton agar should be first screened with *Enterococcus faecalis* ATCC 29212 or ATCC 33186. Satisfactory media should produce clear zones of inhibition >24 mm in diameter around trimethoprim/sulfamethoxazole disks. Trace amounts of thymidine or thymine (rarely *p*-aminobenzoic acid) will be antagonistic to this control strain, thus producing a haze of growth inside the zone of inhibition.

Some strains of *S. pneumoniae* (26) have been found to be resistant to penicillin (MIC of ≥2 μg/ml), and other strains are relatively resistant to penicillin (MIC of 0.12 to 1.0 μg/ml). The latter may not respond to penicillin therapy of meningitis or other life-threatening diseases. Consequently, pneumococci recovered from spinal fluid, blood, or other body fluids should be tested for resistance or relative resistance to penicillin. Penicillin-resistant or relatively resistant strains can be detected by the use of a disk diffusion test, using a 1-μg oxacillin disk to screen for penicillin resistance. A 10-U penicillin disk should not be used for the detection of penicillin resistance.

For screening *S. pneumoniae* isolates, Mueller-Hinton agar with 5% defibrinated sheep blood is the preferred agar medium. The inoculum is standardized by the selection of bacterial colonies from an overnight agar plate and the preparation of an emulsion in Mueller-Hinton broth. The broth suspension is then diluted until it matches the turbidity of a McFarland 0.5 standard. A test plate is inoculated as described previously for the standard Kirby-Bauer method, and then a 1-μg oxacillin disk is applied. The tests are allowed to incubate for 18 to 24 h at 35°C without increased CO_2. Penicillin-susceptible strains produce oxacillin zones ≥20 mm in diameter. Penicillin-resistant or relatively resistant strains produce oxacillin zones ≤19 mm in diameter. This test will not distinguish between resistant and relatively resistant strains. Chloramphenicol disks may also be tested to detect chloramphenicol-resistant strains.

The data given in Table 1 are for illustrative purposes only. The most recent NCCLS standard should be consulted for revised or updated data on testing or breakpoints, since they are usually updated at least twice each year.

QUALITY CONTROL OF DIFFUSION TESTS

Standard control strains of *Escherichia coli* (ATCC 25922), *S. aureus* (ATCC 25923), and *P. aeruginosa* (ATCC 27853) have been designated for monitoring the accuracy and precision of disk diffusion tests. Another strain of *E. coli* (ATCC 35218) has been designated for monitoring the performance of tests with disks containing a β-lactam antibiotic combined with a β-lactamase inhibitor, e.g., amoxicillin or ticarcillin plus clavulanic acid. This strain produces a β-lactamase that should be inactivated by the inhibitor. When used in conjunction with *E. coli* ATCC 25922, both components of the combination disk can be monitored. *H. influenzae* ATCC 49247 and *N. gonorrhoeae* ATCC 49226 have also been selected for quality control purposes (see chapter 112).

The first three control strains mentioned above and *E. faecalis* (ATCC 29212 or ATCC 33186) should be used to test the performance of every new batch of Mueller-Hinton agar before the medium is released for use with clinical specimens. In addition, the appropriate control strains should be tested every day that a batch of susceptibility tests is performed. However, in those laboratories that have documented a record of satisfactory performance for 30 consecutive days, the frequency of control tests may be reduced to once a week (21; chapter 110).

Stock cultures of all control strains should be obtained from a reliable source and maintained in a manner which will ensure continued viability with minimal opportunity for the selection of resistant variants (11). Working cultures can be maintained at 4 to 8°C on soybean-casein digest agar, with weekly subcultures. The working cultures should be replaced at least once a month from frozen, lyophilized, or commercial cultures, or sooner if results are questionable. This replacement is especially important with *P. aeruginosa* ATCC 27853, which tends to lose susceptibility to the ureidopenicillins if it is repeatedly transferred on agar slants. Cultures may be maintained frozen at −20°C or lower (in either a freezer or a nitrogen chest) in a suitable stabilizer such as a broth medium with 15% glycerol, defibrinated sheep or rabbit blood, or 50% fetal calf serum in broth. Cultures may also be maintained in a lyophilized state. With either method, the cultures can be stored without significant risk of altering their antimicrobial susceptibility.

Before being tested, the cultures should be transferred to a nutrient broth, incubated for 4 to 18 h, and then streaked onto an agar plate to obtain isolated colonies. Control tests should be performed only with 18 to 24 h isolated colonies and never initiated from stored cultures. If the results of control tests suggest contamination of the stock cultures or changes in the susceptibility of the organism, fresh cultures should be obtained. Such a problem might be suspected if there is a sudden, dramatic change in test results that cannot be explained by methodology.

Table 2 lists the minimum and maximum zone sizes that should be observed with a few selected antimicrobial disks. These limits generally represent 95% confidence limits; i.e., 1 of every 20 tests might be outside the stated limits. Zones should never be more than four standard deviations above or below the midpoint of the stated limits, i.e., midpoint ± the stated range (maximum zone diameter minus minimum zone diameter). The mean of a series of tests should approach the midpoint value between the upper and lower limits defined in Table 2. The most recent NCCLS document should be consulted for the most current quality control guidelines.

COMMON SOURCES OF ERROR

Although the disk diffusion method is a fairly forgiving procedure, technical errors can compromise accuracy and reliability. The following are some of the more common sources of error encountered in clinical microbiology laboratories.

1. Improper preparation of Mueller-Hinton agar, especially failure to measure pH at the time of preparation.
2. Use of outdated medium or unsatisfactorily stored plates.
3. Variability in Mueller-Hinton agars. Each new lot should be checked by testing appropriate control strains before it is used.
4. Improper storage of disks. It is very important to keep the disks dry.
5. Inadequate standardization of broth culture density. More often than not, the culture is too heavy, but too light inocula are not uncommon.
6. Inaccurate preparation or maintenance of turbidity reference standard.
7. Failure to express surplus fluid from the swab before the plates are inoculated.
8. Excessive delay between culture standardization and plate inoculation.
9. Excessive delay in application of the disk after inoculation of the plates.
10. Excessive delay in incubation of the plates after application of the disks.
11. Incubation temperature deviating from 35°C or incubation in an increased CO_2 atmosphere.
12. Reading of test results before the full 16 to 18 h of incubation.
13. Failure to measure zone borders carefully and with a standardized angle and source of illumination.
14. Attempts to test mixed cultures.
15. Application of the procedure to slow growers and anaerobes.
16. Failure to include quality control strains or to record the results of control tests at appropriate intervals.
17. Transcription error in recording the test results.

INDICATIONS FOR DIRECT SUSCEPTIBILITY TESTING ON CLINICAL MATERIAL

The direct inoculation of susceptibility plates can sometimes provide invaluable preliminary information on urgent clinical infection problems. For example, direct tests may be made on plates seeded with emergency specimens, such as cerebrospinal fluid, other body fluids, or purulent specimens, if direct Gram-stained smears indicate that a large number of bacteria of a single species may be expected to grow. However, routine direct susceptibility tests on clinical material are to be avoided. Mixtures of organisms, common in many specimens, frequently produce inaccurate interpretations (6). Furthermore, it is very difficult to standardize the density of an inoculum from direct clinical material. The use of a purity check plate will be of great assistance in these emergency situations, as will an assessment of the nature of the lawn of inoculum on the susceptibility test plate. The results of emergency tests should be reported as preliminary or tentative and should be repeated and confirmed by one of the recommended methods. When results from directly inoculated test plates are unsatisfactory, valuable preliminary information can be obtained by making preliminary readings of the regular test after 5 to 6 h of incubation at 35°C. When this reading is done, the plate must be reincubated, and a final report is issued after overnight incubation.

LITERATURE CITED

1. **Baker, C. N., C. Thornsberry, and R. W. Hawkinson.** 1983. Inoculum standardization in antimicrobial susceptibility testing: evaluation of overnight agar cultures and the Rapid Inoculum Standardization System. J. Clin. Microbiol. **17:**450–457.
2. **Barry, A. L.** 1986. Procedures for testing antimicrobial agents in agar media: theoretical considerations, p. 1–26. *In* V. Lorian (ed.), Antibiotics in laboratory medicine, 2nd ed. The Williams & Wilkins Co., Baltimore.
3. **Barry, A. L., M. B. Coyle, C. Thornsberry, E. H. Gerlach, and R. W. Hawkinson.** 1979. Methods of measuring zones of inhibition with the Bauer-Kirby disk susceptibility test. J. Clin. Microbiol. **10:**885–889.
4. **Barry, A. L., F. Garcia, and L. D. Thrupp.** 1970. An improved single disk method for testing the antibiotic susceptibility of rapidly growing pathogens. Am. J. Clin. Pathol. **53:**149–158.
5. **Barry, A. L., and R. N. Jones.** 1987. Reliability of high-content disks and modified broth dilution tests for detecting staphylococcal resistance to the penicillinase-resistant penicillins. J. Clin. Microbiol. **25:**1897–1901.
6. **Barry, A. L., L. J. Joyce, A. P. Adams, and E. J. Benner.** 1973. Rapid determination of antimicrobial susceptibility for urgent clinical situations. Am. J. Clin. Pathol. **59:**693–699.
7. **Barry, A. L., G. H. Miller, C. Thornsberry, R. S. Hare, R. N. Jones, R. R. Lorber, R. Ferraresi, and C. Cramer.** 1987. Influence of cation supplements on activity of netilmicin against *Pseudomonas aeruginosa* in vitro and in vivo. Antimicrob. Agents Chemother. **31:**1514–1518.
8. **Barry, A. L., C. Thornsberry, and R. N. Jones.** 1981. Gentamicin and amikacin disk susceptibility tests with *Pseudomonas aeruginosa:* definition of minimal inhibitory

concentration correlates for susceptible and resistant categories. J. Clin. Microbiol. **13:**1000–1003.

9. **Bauer, A. W., W. M. M. Kirby, J. C. Sherris, and M. Turck.** 1966. Antibiotic susceptibility testing by a standardized single disk method. Am. J. Clin. Pathol. **45:**493–496.
10. **Bennett, J. V., H. M. Camp, and T. C. Eickhoff.** 1968. Rapid sulfonamide disc sensitivity test for meningococci. Appl. Microbiol. **16:**1056–1060.
11. **Coyle, M. B., M. F. Lampe, C. L. Aitkin, P. Feigl, and J. C. Sherris.** 1976. Reproducibility of control strains for antibiotic susceptibility testing. Antimicrob. Agents Chemother. **10:**436–440.
12. **D'Amato, R. F., and L. Hochstein.** 1982. Evaluation of a rapid inoculum preparation method for agar disk diffusion susceptibility testing. J. Clin. Microbiol. **15:**282–285.
13. **D'Amato, R. F., L. Hochstein, J. R. Vernaleo, D. J. Cleri, A. A. Wallman, M. S. Gradus, and C. Thornsberry.** 1985. Evaluation of the BIOGRAM antimicrobial susceptibility test system. J. Clin. Microbiol. **22:**793–798.
14. **Doern, G. V., G. S. Dawn, and T. A. Tubert.** 1987. In vitro chloramphenicol susceptibility testing of *Haemophilus influenzae* disk diffusion procedures and assay of chloramphenicol acetyltransferase. J. Clin. Microbiol. **25:** 1453–1455.
15. **Ericsson, H. M., and J. C. Sherris.** 1971. Antibiotic sensitivity testing. Report of an international collaborative study. Acta Pathol. Microbiol. Scand. Suppl. **217:**1–90.
16. **Federal Register.** 1972. Rules and regulations: antibiotic susceptibility disks. Fed. Regist. **37:**20525–20529.
17. **Jones, R. N., T. L. Gavan, C. Thornsberry, P. C. Fuchs, E. H. Gerlach, J. S. Knapp, P. Murray, and J. A. Washington II.** 1989. Standardization of disk diffusion and agar dilution susceptibility tests for *Neisseria gonorrhoeae:* interpretive criteria and quality control guidelines for ceftriaxone, penicillin, spectinomycin, and tetracycline. J. Clin. Microbiol. **27:**2758–2766.
18. **Jorgensen, J. H., J. S. Redding, L. A. Maher, and A. W. Howell.** 1987. Improved medium for antimicrobial susceptibility testing of *Haemophilus influenzae*. Antimicrob. Agents Chemother. **20:**168–170.
19. **McDougal, L. K., and C. Thornsberry.** 1984. New recommendations for disk diffusion antimicrobial susceptibility tests for methicillin-resistant (heteroresistant) staphylococci. J. Clin. Microbiol. **19:**482–488.
20. **Metzler, C. M., and R. M. DeHaan.** 1974. Susceptibility of anaerobic bacteria: statistical and clinical considerations. J. Infect. Dis. **130:**588–594.
21. **National Committee for Clinical Laboratory Standards.** 1990. Performance standards for antimicrobial disk susceptibility tests, 4th ed. Approved standard M2-A4. National Committee for Clinical Laboratory Standards, Villanova, Pa.
22. **Pollock, H. M., A. L. Barry, T. L. Gavan, P. C. Fuchs, S. Hansen, C. Thornsberry, H. Frankel, and S. B. Forsythe.** 1986. Selection of a reference lot of Mueller-Hinton agar. J. Clin. Microbiol. **24:**1–6.
23. **Reller, L. B., F. D. Schoenknecht, M. A. Kenny, and J. C. Sherris.** 1974. Antibiotic susceptibility testing of *Pseudomonas aeruginosa:* selection of a control strain and criteria for magnesium and calcium content in media. J. Infect. Dis. **130:**454–463.
24. **Stemper, J. E., and J. M. Matsen.** 1970. Device for turbidity standardizing of cultures for antibiotic sensitivity testing. Appl. Microbiol. **19:**1015–1016.
25. **Thornsberry, C., J. Q. Caruthers, and C. N. Baker.** 1973. Effect of temperature on the in vitro susceptibility of *Staphylococcus aureus* to penicillinase-resistant penicillins. Antimicrob. Agents Chemother. **4:**263–269.
26. **Thornsberry, C., and J. M. Swenson.** 1980. Antimicrobial susceptibility tests for *Streptococcus pneumoniae*. Lab. Med. **11:**83–86.
27. **Waterworth, P. M.** 1962. A misapplication of the sensitivity test: mandelamine disks. J. Med. Lab. Technol. **19:**163–168.

Chapter 112

Antimicrobial Susceptibility Tests: Fastidious and Unusual Bacteria

GARY V. DOERN AND RONALD N. JONES

There are many bacteria for which traditional susceptibility test methods based on use of unsupplemented Mueller-Hinton medium may not be applicable. This fact is often ignored by clinical microbiologists who are determined to respond to the ever-present clinical demand that they provide susceptibility test information. It is important to recognize that contemporary disk diffusion and dilution susceptibility tests, such as those advocated by the National Committee for Clinical Laboratory Standards (NCCLS) for use in testing facultative and aerobic bacteria (53, 54), are of a proven utility only with relatively few bacteria. These include members of the family *Enterobacteriaceae*, selected nonenteric gram-negative bacilli such as *Pseudomonas aeruginosa* and *Acinetobacter* spp., staphylococci, and perhaps *Enterococcus* spp. Important organisms for which the traditional NCCLS methods may not be applicable or at least are of unproven utility include *Haemophilus* spp., *Streptococcus pneumoniae*, viridans and beta-hemolytic streptococci, aerobic diphtheroids, *Bacillus* spp., *Pasteurella, Eikenella, Cardiobacterium, Actinobacillus, Kingella,* and *Moraxella* spp., and most other unusual nonenteric gram-negative bacilli. Even commonly tested organisms such as *Xanthomonas maltophilia* and *Pseudomonas cepacia* may be problematic. The major difficulty with these organisms is their poor growth on Mueller-Hinton medium without supplementation.

Many microbiologists use Mueller-Hinton medium supplemented with various nutritional cofactors as a means of achieving adequate growth so as to perform both disk diffusion and dilution susceptibility tests. Indeed, the NCCLS recommends this practice with certain fastidious bacteria (53, 54). It must be remembered, however, that the results based on interpretive criteria promulgated by the NCCLS for use with unsupplemented Mueller-Hinton medium may not apply to medium that has been supplemented. In fact, in most instances they probably do not.

This chapter describes susceptibility test methods and interpretive criteria that have recently been developed for selected clinically important bacteria that cannot be tested by traditional methods using unsupplemented Mueller-Hinton medium and the criteria of the NCCLS. The organisms discussed are *S. pneumoniae, Haemophilus influenzae, Branhamella catarrhalis,* and *Neisseria gonorrhoeae*.

STREPTOCOCCUS PNEUMONIAE

Until recently in the United States, *S. pneumoniae* remained nearly uniformly susceptible to the antimicrobial agents most commonly used to treat pneumococcal infections. However, in 1978, the first report of frank resistance to penicillin (i.e., MICs of ≥2.0 μg/ml) appeared (8). In addition, relative penicillin resistance (i.e., MICs of 0.12 to 1.0 μg/ml) has been observed with increasing frequency (34, 45, 47; J. Spika, R. Facklam, M. Oxtoby, and B. Plikaytis, Program Abstr. 29th Intersci. Conf. Antimicrob. Agents Chemother., abstr. no. 1287, 1989). Both fully penicillin-resistant strains as well as those demonstrating relative resistance have alterations in their penicillin-binding proteins (52). Penicillin therapy is contraindicated in all pneumococcal infections due to frankly resistant strains. Relatively penicillin-resistant strains of *S. pneumoniae* probably are refractive to therapy with penicillin only when they cause meningitis (6, 32). Finally, resistance to trimethoprim-sulfamethoxazole, erythromycin, and tetracycline chloramphenicol has also been reported (30, 61).

With respect to susceptibility testing, the prevalence of resistance to a particular agent is often a major determinant in establishing the need to test that agent. A recent 15-center national U.S. collaborative study that characterized 487 clinically significant strains of *S. pneumoniae* provided information useful in making such decisions (39a). In this study, frank penicillin resistance remained extremely uncommon in the United States (i.e., ≤0.2% of strains). Relative penicillin resistance was noted in 3.8% of strains. The percentages of strains susceptible to trimethoprim-sulfamethoxazole, erythromycin, tetracycline, and chloramphenicol were 95.5, 99.8, 97.7, and 98.8, respectively. Low levels of resistance were noted with first-generation cephalosporins such as cephalexin and cefaclor, but no resistance was observed with second-generation cephalosporins (e.g., cefuroxime) or the extended-spectrum, third-generation cephalosporins. Even relatively penicillin-resistant strains were susceptible to these agents even though the MICs were elevated in comparison with those for penicillin-susceptible strains. On the basis of these observations, the following recommendations would seem to apply to susceptibility tests with *S. pneumoniae*.

Clinically significant isolates of *S. pneumoniae* from patients with serious infections should routinely be tested for frank resistance to penicillin. Isolates from patients with pneumococcal meningitis should be tested for relative penicillin resistance. A simple and reliable procedure for screening for both forms of penicillin resistance is the oxacillin disk test (53, 65). Briefly, a 0.5 McFarland suspension of the test strain prepared in a suitable broth medium is streaked confluently over the surface of a 100-mm Mueller-Hinton agar plate supplemented with 5% sheep blood. Alternatively, Trypticase soy agar (BBL Microbiology Systems, Cockeysville, Md.) plus 5% sheep blood may be used (65). A disk containing 1 μg of oxacillin is applied, and the plate is incubated in ambient atmospheric air overnight at 35°C (53, 65). A zone of inhibition of ≥20 mm indicates penicillin susceptibility (i.e., MIC of ≤0.06 μg/ml). A zone diameter of ≤19 mm should be construed as presumptive evidence of either relative or frank penicillin resistance.

Isolates yielding zone sizes of ≤19 mm with the oxacillin disk screening method should always be confirmed by a penicillin MIC method (see below) before definitive reporting of the penicillin test result. There are two reasons for this approach. First, the oxacillin screening test does not adequately distinguish frankly penicillin-resistant strains from those that are merely relatively resistant (65). Both groups produce inhibitory zone diameters of ≤19 mm, yet relatively resistant strains are of proven clinical resistance to penicillin only when they cause meningitis. It is the frankly penicillin-resistant strains of *S. pneumoniae* that are clinically resistant to this agent in all infectious disease processes. Second, because the prevalence of frank and relative penicillin resistance with *S. pneumoniae* remains very low in the United States, the predictive value of a nonsusceptible result with the oxacillin disk screening test is also very low. For instance, during the 5-year period from 1985 to 1989 at the University of Massachusetts Medical Center, a total of 1,703 clinical isolates of *S. pneumoniae* were examined with the oxacillin disk screening test. Among these, 238 (14.0%) yielded zone sizes of ≤19 mm upon initial testing. A penicillin MIC test demonstrated actual relative resistance (i.e., MIC of 0.12 to 1.0) in only 58 of these 238 strains (24.4%), for an overall prevalence of relative penicillin resistance of 3.4%, not unlike that reported in the recent national U.S. surveillance study (Jorgensen et al., submitted). MIC tests revealed no frank resistance to penicillin based on the presently accepted breakpoints. In other words, without a confirmatory MIC test, the oxacillin disk screening procedure accurately predicated lack of penicillin susceptibility in less than one-fourth of cases. This should not be interpreted as an indictment of the test. It simply reflects the low prevalence of what the test measures. Furthermore, it should be emphasized that although the oxacillin screening test has a tendency to overcall frank and relative resistance with pneumococci, it apparently only rarely fails to detect these important characteristics (65).

Susceptibility tests with agents other than penicillin need not be performed routinely; however, when determined to be necessary, they should be done by using a broth microdilution MIC method. Mueller-Hinton broth supplemented with 3 to 5% lysed horse blood is the medium of choice (54). Alternatively, *Haemophilus* test medium (HTM) in its broth form as described below for testing *Haemophilus* spp. may be used with pneumococci (41, 54). Pneumococcal MICs for most antimicrobial agents will be approximately one-half of one twofold concentration increment lower in HTM than in Mueller-Hinton broth plus lysed horse blood; trimethoprim-sulfamethoxazole MICs in HTM will be about fourfold higher (41). Except for the oxacillin screening test for penicillin, there currently exist no methods or interpretive criteria that are of proven utility for disk diffusion susceptibility tests with *S. pneumoniae*.

HAEMOPHILUS INFLUENZAE

The emergence of ampicillin resistance among clinical isolates of *H. influenzae* beginning in 1974, together with the development of at least sporadic resistance to other antimicrobial agents during the past decade, has led to a need for reliable susceptibility test methods for this organism (19, 20). Indeed, numerous methods, using a variety of media, test formats, and interpretive criteria, have been advocated for susceptibility tests with *Haemophilus* species (55). Recently a new medium, HTM, was developed for tests with *H. influenzae* (42, 43). In its agar form, HTM consists of Mueller-Hinton agar, NAD (15 μg/ml), bovine hematin (15 μg/ml), and yeast extract (5 mg/ml) (pH 7.2 to 7.4). HTM broth is the same except that Mueller-Hinton broth is used as the basal medium and supplements of calcium (20 to 25 μg/ml), magnesium (10 to 12.5 μg/ml), and thymidine phosphorylase (0.2 IU/ml) are added. Collaborative studies using HTM have now been conducted, aimed at developing methods for both disk diffusion and broth microdilution tests, interpretive criteria, and quality control guidelines (21; G. V. Doern, T. Gavan, H. Gerlach, J. H. Jorgensen, P. R. Murray, C. Thornsberry, and J. A. Washington II, submitted for publication). The results of these collaborative studies have been adopted by the NCCLS and serve as the basis for the organization's most recent recommendations regarding susceptibility tests with *Haemophilus* species (53, 54).

The current NCCLS recommendations for susceptibility tests with *Haemophilus* species represent a significant advance over previous methods, media, and interpretive criteria used for this organism. Laboratories that perform such susceptibility tests are encouraged to conform to the NCCLS guidelines, which are described briefly below.

Disk diffusion susceptibility tests

Using colony growth from an overnight chocolate agar culture incubated at 35°C in 5 to 7% CO_2, a suspension of test organism is prepared in sterile, unsupplemented Mueller-Hinton broth. With use of a benchtop nephelometer or a volumetric inoculum preparation device, this suspension is adjusted to a turbidity equivalent to that of a 0.5 McFarland standard. Suspensions prepared in this manner will contain approximately 1×10^8 to 4×10^8 CFU/ml. Manual preparation of the initial suspension with visual comparison against known 0.5 McFarland standards is not advocated with *Haemophilus* species, since this approach is not precise enough to warrant use with this organism. Starting suspensions with organism concentrations of $>4 \times 10^8$/ml can yield false-resistant results with *H. influenzae*, particularly when beta-lactamase-producing strains are tested against relatively beta-lactamase-labile cephalosporins such as cefaclor and cefamandole, and possibly cefuroxime and cefonicid.

Using a carefully prepared starting suspension, the surface of an HTM agar plate is swab inoculated, disks are applied and tapped into place, and the plate is incubated inverted for 16 to 18 h at 35°C in 5 to 7% CO_2. The desired disk content is listed in Table 1. After incubation, inhibitory zone diameters are measured with calipers; using the interpretive criteria listed in Table 1, an interpretive category is assigned. Interpretive criteria have been developed for 20 different antimicrobial agents (Table 1) (21). Disk diffusion susceptibility testing of *Haemophilus* species by using the method and medium described above must be restricted to these 20 drugs, since there is as yet no basis for interpreting results with other agents. Zone diameters obtained on media other than HTM must not be interpreted with the current NCCLS guidelines for HTM.

With the exception of ofloxacin, quality control guidelines are now available for all of the antimicrobial agents listed in Table 1 when tested by disk diffusion versus *Haemophilus* species tested by using HTM and the method described above (Doern et al., submitted). The strain of *H. influenzae* for use with such quality control tests is ATCC 49247. Because of high X-factor (hemin) growth requirements, some strains of *H. influenzae* may fail to growth on the HTM agar plates of certain manufacturers. A second quality control strain (ATCC 10211) can be used to check the growth-supporting properties of HTM agar. This strain requires large amounts of X factor for growth.

Dilution susceptibility tests

Quantitative susceptibility tests with *Haemophilus* species should be performed by using HTM broth and a microdilution test format with a final volume of 100 μl per well. An initial suspension of test organism equivalent to a 0.5 McFarland standard is prepared in sterile, unsupplemented Mueller-Hinton broth as described above for the disk diffusion test. This suspension or dilutions of it are used to inoculate microdilution trays such that the final organism concentration is as close to 5×10^5 CFU/ml as possible. As for disk diffusion tests, the actual inoculum size is critical. Inocula resulting in final concentrations of test organism higher than 5×10^5 CFU/ml may yield falsely high MICs. For this reason, it is advisable to perform colony counts at some interval on no-antibiotic growth control wells of microdilution trays after inoculation to prove that the final concentration is the desired 5×10^5 CFU/ml.

After inoculation, microdilution trays are incubated at 35°C in ambient air for 20 to 24 h before growth endpoints are determined. MIC interpretive criteria for 20 antimicrobial agents are listed in Table 1 (21). Quality control ranges for MICs obtained by using *H. influenzae* ATCC 49247 have been developed for 19 of these 20 compounds (the exception being ofloxacin) (Doern et al., submitted).

Enzyme tests

TEM-1 beta-lactamase activity among clinical isolates of *H. influenzae* can be detected by using any of a variety of in vitro beta-lactamase assays, including acidimetric, iodometric, and nitrocefin-based chromogenic cephalosporin methods (62, 68). Assuming that high-quality reagents are used, care is exercised in performing tests and interpreting results, and necessary controls are used, all of these assays are satisfactory for detecting *H. influenzae* beta-lactamase activity. This is probably because the *Haemophilus* TEM-1 enzyme is typically produced in large amounts, is extracellular, and has a high affinity for the substrates used in these assays. Strains of *H. influenzae* found to produce beta-lactamase should be considered resistant to ampicillin and amoxicillin and probably to the broad-spectrum penicillins as well.

Detection of chloramphenicol acetyltransferase (CAT)

TABLE 1. Disk diffusion and broth microdilution susceptibility test interpretive criteria for *Haemophilus* species tested by using HTM[a]

Antimicrobial agent	Disk content (μg)	Interpretive criteria					
		Disk diffusion: zone diam (mm)			Broth microdilution: MIC (μg/ml)[b]		
		Resistant	Intermediate	Susceptible	Resistant	Intermediate	Susceptible
Amoxicillin-clavulanate	20/10	≤19		≥20	≥8.0/4.0		≤4.0/2.0
Ampicillin	10	≤21	22–24	≥25	≥4.0	2.0	≤1.0
Ampicillin-sulbactam	10/10	≤19		≥20	≥4.0/2.0		≤2.0/1.0
Aztreonam	30			≥26			≤2.0
Cefaclor	30	≤18	19–23	≥24	≥32	16	≤8.0
Cefamandole	30	≤20	21–23	≥24	≥16	8.0	≤4.0
Cefixime	5			≥30			≤1.0
Cefonicid	30	≤20	21–23	≥24	≥16	8.0	≤4.0
Cefotaxime	30			≥26			≤2.0
Ceftazidime	30			≥26			≤2.0
Ceftriaxone	30			≥26			≤2.0
Ceftizoxime	30			≥26			≤2.0
Cefuroxime	30	≤20	21–23	≥24	≥16	8.0	≤4.0
Chloramphenicol	30	≤25	26–28	≥29	≥8.0	4.0	≤2.0
Ciprofloxacin	5			≥21			≤1.0
Imipenem	10			≥16			≤4.0
Ofloxacin	5			≥16			≤2.0
Rifampin	5	≤16	17–19	≥20	≥4.0	2.0	≤1.0
Tetracycline	30	≤25	26–28	≥29	≥8.0	4.0	≤2.0
Trimethoprim-sulfamethoxazole	1.25/23.75	≤10	11–15	≥16	≥4.0[c]	1.0–2.0[c]	≤0.5[c]

[a] The test methods and media upon which these interpretative criteria are predicated are described in the text.
[b] These MIC breakpoints also represent the respective MIC correlates for the disk diffusion interpretive categories.
[c] The concentration listed is the concentration of trimethoprim; in all cases, the concentration of sulfamethoxazole is 19-fold higher.

activity among clinical isolates can be used to predict chloramphenicol susceptibility (2). Strains found to produce this enzyme should be considered resistant to chloramphenicol. CAT activity may be ascertained with a 70-min conventional tube-broth assay using reagents prepared in the laboratory or with a 10-min commercially available disk assay (18). Again, care must be exercised when performing CAT assays to ensure the validity of test results.

When and what to test

All clinically significant isolates of *H. influenzae* should be tested for production of beta-lactamase as an indication of ampicillin or amoxicillin activity. In addition, systemic isolates should be tested for chloramphenicol activity by the CAT assay. A positive beta-lactamase test result means that the isolate is resistant to ampicillin and amoxicillin; a positive CAT assay implies resistance to chloramphenicol. Because of sporadic reports of ampicillin resistance among strains of *H. influenzae* that apparently lack the TEM-1 beta-lactamase (3, 52, 57, 59), the meaning of a negative beta-lactamase assay has been questioned. The actual prevalence of such strains at least in the United States is extremely low, however, particularly among encapsulated type b strains, i.e., the strains of *H. influenzae* most commonly associated with systemic, life-threatening infections (20). Therefore, there is little need to routinely perform anything other than a beta-lactamase assay on clinical isolates of *H. influenzae* as a means of assessing ampicillin or amoxicillin activity. Assuming that the test is performed correctly, strains yielding negative beta-lactamase test results may be considered susceptible to ampicillin and amoxicillin. In situations in which a direct test of ampicillin activity is considered desirable or necessary with a beta-lactamase-negative strain, either the disk diffusion or broth microdilution test described above should be used.

The same is true of strains yielding negative CAT assay results. Rare CAT-negative strains of *H. influenzae* apparently resistant to chloramphenicol have been described (7). Since such strains are exceedingly uncommon (20), there is no need to perform a chloramphenicol susceptibility test on clinical isolates of *H. influenzae* for which negative CAT assay results have been obtained. Such strains may be considered susceptible to chloramphenicol.

A decision to test other antimicrobial agents on clinical isolates of *H. influenzae* should be predicated on clinical need, a knowledge that the antimicrobial agent(s) is something other than uniformly active or inactive, and the availability of a reliable test method for which quality control parameters have been defined. Given these considerations, there is probably little need to routinely perform susceptibility tests with clinical isolates of *H. influenzae* beyond what has already been discussed.

BRANHAMELLA CATARRHALIS

Approximately 85% of clinical isolates of *B. catarrhalis* in the United States produce beta-lactamase (Jorgensen et al., submitted). Although most beta-lactamase-producing strains have penicillin, ampicillin, and amoxicillin MICs which indicate resistance (i.e., $\geq$2.0 μg/ml), at least some beta-lactamase-positive strains require very low MICs of these agents (i.e., 0.1 to 1.0 μg/ml) (13, 22, 25, 26, 63, 64). MICs this low imply susceptibility. Furthermore, there have been numerous reports of clinical improvement when patients with infections apparently due to beta-lactamase-producing strains were treated with penicillin, ampicillin, or amoxicillin (22, 35, 48). In other words, not all beta-lactamase-positive strains of *B. catarrhalis* may be clinically resistant to these antibiotics.

Obviously, the question arises as to the clinical meaning of a positive beta-lactamase assay with *B. catarrhalis*. Unfortunately, the information presented above notwithstanding, we do not have a definitive answer for this question. Therefore, until this question is clearly resolved, all beta-lactamase-positive strains of *B. catarrhalis* should be considered clinically resistant to penicillin, ampicillin, and amoxicillin. It follows from this guideline that all clinically significant isolates of *B. catarrhalis* should be tested for beta-lactamase activity.

This testing is best accomplished by using a nitrocefin-based chromogenic cephalosporin beta-lactamase assay (56). Acidimetric, iodometric, and pyridine-2-azo-*p*-dimethylalanine cephalosporin (PADAC)-based chromogenic cephalosporin assays may yield false-negative results (26, 39) because the beta-lactamases of *B. catarrhalis* are produced in very small amounts, remain tightly cell associated, but have a high substrate affinity for nitrocefin (29, 46). Accepting the discussion of clinical relevance presented above, disk diffusion or dilution tests of penicillin, ampicillin, or amoxicillin activity add nothing to a nitrocefin beta-lactamase test and therefore need not be performed.

It can be argued that there is no need, at least in the United States, to routinely perform susceptibility tests with *B. catarrhalis* versus other antimicrobial agents, since the organism appears to be either uniformly resistant (i.e., to vancomycin, colistin, trimethoprim [alone] and clindamycin) or susceptible (to other agents) (1, 16, 17, 23, 27, 64; Jorgensen et al., submitted). There have been only rare reports of resistance to erythromycin and tetracycline (5). In addition, the isoxazoyl penicillins (methicillin, oxacillin, and nafcillin) possess variable activity; however, these agents are not clinically indicated for the management of *B. catarrhalis* infections, and therefore consideration need not be given to testing them in the laboratory.

If the need to examine the activity of a specific antimicrobial agent arises, it appears that both the disk diffusion and dilution tests described by the NCCLS for nonfastidious bacteria that grow aerobically can be applied to *B. catarrhalis* (24, 49), probably because *B. catarrhalis* grows well in unsupplemented Mueller-Hinton medium at 35°C in ambient atmospheric air.

NEISSERIA GONORRHOEAE

Progressive mutational events among *N. gonorrhoeae* strains have led to increased antimicrobial resistance, especially to penicillins, spectinomycin, sulfonamides, and tetracycline (9, 10, 14, 32, 33, 44, 50, 58, 67). To recognize these drug-resistant strains, several methods, including various modifications of disk diffusion and dilution tests, have been developed (4, 11, 12, 33, 50, 58, 60, 69). In addition, rapid colorimetric tests have been used to detect plasmid-mediated penicillinase-producing *N. gonorrhoeae* (PPNG) (39, 40, 66). As the prevalence of resistant strains increases, the need for standardized susceptibility testing procedures for epidemiologic as well as therapeutic purposes has become apparent (11, 12). In 1989, a working group of the NCCLS published initial guidelines for testing penicillin, tetracycline, spectinomycin, and ceftriaxone (37). Subsequent studies led to the development of interpretive criteria and quality control guidelines for four additional antimicrobial agents, cefuroxime, cefotaxime, cefoxitin, and ceftazidime (36).

Enzyme tests

PPNG can reliably be detected by several beta-lactamase assays (39, 40, 66), but methods using chromogenic cephalosporin reagents (nitrocefin and PADAC) appear to be more sensitive than acidimetric or iodometric methods (College of American Pathologists Surveys Critiques, 1980 to 1989). One of these tests should be performed routinely on all clinical isolates of *N. gonorrhoeae* to assist in epidemiologic investigations and to direct the selection of nonpenicillin routine therapeutic regimens (11, 12).

Disk diffusion tests

A disk diffusion test using GC agar as a medium was the first procedure to be standardized for the detection of PPNG (4). The NCCLS working group, in an effort to expand the potential of disk diffusion susceptibility testing, modified the original GC agar base medium (37). A 1% growth supplement devoid of high concentrations of cysteine was selected, thus minimizing cysteine inactivation of various beta-lactams such as penems, carbapenems (imipenem), and clavulanic acid. The supplement consisted of the following reagents in 1 liter of water: 1.1 g of L-cystine, 0.03 g of guanine hydrochloride, 3 mg of thiamine hydrochloride, 13 mg of *p*-aminobenzoate, 0.01 g of vitamin B_{12}, 0.1 g of cocarboxylase, 0.25 g of NAD, 1 g of adenine, 10 g of L-glutamine, 100 g of glucose, and 0.02 g of ferric nitrate. This formula is similar to IsoVitaleX (BBL) without the 25.9 g of L-cysteine hydrochloride.

The procedure recommended for disk diffusion tests uses direct inoculation with colony growth from an overnight chocolate agar plate adjusted in broth to a turbidity equivalent to that of a 0.5 McFarland standard (37). Disks are applied, and plates are incubated in an atmosphere of 3 to 5% CO_2 at 35°C for 20 to 24 h before inhibitory zone diameters are measured. This procedure was found to be accurate when compared with MICs and also very reproducible (37).

Interpretive criteria for penicillin, tetracycline, spectinomycin, ceftriaxone, cefuroxime, cefotaxime, cefoxitin, and ceftazidime are found in Table 2. The categories for penicillin and tetracycline detect both chromosomal and plasmid-mediated resistant strains. Only susceptible categories were defined for ceftriaxone, cefotaxime, and ceftazidime, since no resistant strains have been reported. Similarly, a spectinomycin intermediate (not moderately susceptible) category was suggested because of limited clinical information on strains with MICs of 64 μg/ml. Use of *N. gonorrhoeae* ATCC 49226 is recommended for quality control testing of the disk diffusion procedure. Quality control parameters have been adopted and published by the NCCLS (53, 54).

Agar dilution tests

Agar dilution is the recommended method for determining MICs for *N. gonorrhoeae*. The medium of choice is the supplemented GC agar medium described above for disk diffusion tests (54). An inoculum of 10^4 CFU per spot is recommended (15). Plates should be incubated in 3 to 5% CO_2 at 35°C, with MICs determined at 20 to 24 h.

Other media and methods have been proposed. Proteose Peptone no. 3 (Difco Laboratories, Detroit, Mich.) and DST have been used extensively. DST may be preferred for tests with sulfonamides and trimethoprim because of low medium content of antagonists, especially when supplemented with lysed horse erythrocytes. Some methods may also produce significant differences in MIC results (for erythromycin and tetracycline) compared with those obtained with GC agar (69). *N. gonorrhoeae* MICs determined in modified

TABLE 2. Interpretive criteria for testing *N. gonorrhoeae* by the disk diffusion and agar dilution methods of the NCCLS[a]

Antimicrobial agent (disk content)	Zone diam (mm) criteria[b]			
	Susceptible	Moderately susceptible[c]	Intermediate[d]	Resistant
Penicillin (10 U)	≥47 (≤0.06)	27–46 (0.12–1)		≤26 (≥2)[e]
Tetracycline (30 μg)	≥37 (≤0.25)	31–37 (0.5–1)		≤30 (≥2)[e]
Spectinomycin (100 μg)	≥18 (≤32)		15–17 (64)	≤14 (≥128)
Cefotaxime (30 μg)	≥31 (≤0.5)			
Cefoxitin (30 μg)	≥28 (≤2)		24–27 (4)	≤23 (≥8)
Ceftazidime (30 μg)	≥31 (≤0.5)			
Ceftriaxone (30 μg)	≥35 (≤0.25)			
Cefuroxime (30 μg)	≥31 (≤1)	26–30 (2)		≤25 (≥4)

[a] From references 36, 37, 53, and 54.

[b] MIC correlates (in micrograms per milliliter) are given in parentheses.

[c] Moderately susceptible strains have documented lower clinical cure rates (85 to 95%) compared with fully susceptible strains (≥95%) (53, 54).

[d] An intermediate or indeterminant result for an antimicrobial agent indicates either a technical problem that should be resolved by repeat testing or a lack of clinical experience in treating organisms with these inhibitory zones or MICs; the latter is the case for spectinomycin.

[e] Gonococci with 10-U penicillin zone diameters of ≤19 mm (MIC of ≥2 μg/ml) are likely to produce beta-lactamase. However, the beta-lactamase assay is still preferred to other susceptibility test methods for the rapid and accurate recognition of plasmid-mediated penicillin resistance. Tetracycline (30 μg) zone diameters of ≤19 mm usually indicate *N. gonorrhoeae* isolates with plasmid-mediated tetracycline resistance. These strains should be confirmed by a suitable dilution MIC method. Such strains have tetracycline MICs of ≥16 μg/ml. Alternatively, such isolates could be referred to a reference laboratory for further testing.

broth media also appear promising for routine use if validated and standardized (60).

Routine use of the disk diffusion or MIC procedures described above seems warranted in the following circumstances: (i) for epidemiology investigations, (ii) in sexually transmitted disease laboratories with a high volume of tests, (iii) in laboratory investigations as part of clinical treatment studies; and (iv) possibly for testing posttreatment isolates of *N. gonorrhoeae* recovered from patients who have apparently failed therapy.

LITERATURE CITED

1. **Alvarez, S., M. Jones, S. Holtsclaw-Berk, J. Guarderas, and S. L. Berk.** 1985. In vitro susceptibilities and β-lactamase production of 53 clinical isolates of *Branhamella catarrhalis*. Antimicrob. Agents Chemother. **25:**646–647.
2. **Azemun, P., T. Stull, M. Roberts, and A. L. Smith.** 1981. Rapid detection of chloramphenicol resistance in *Haemophilus influenzae*. Antimicrob. Agents Chemother. **20:** 168–170.
3. **Bell, S. M., and D. Plowman.** 1980. Mechanisms of ampicillin resistance in *Haemophilus influenzae* from respiratory tract. Lancet **i:**279–280.
4. **Biddle, J. W., J. M. Swensen, and C. Thornsberry.** 1978. Disk-agar diffusion antimicrobial susceptibility tests with beta-lactamase-producing *Neisseria gonorrhoeae*. J. Antibiot. **31:**352–358.
5. **Brown, B. A., R. J. Wallace, C. W. Flanagan, R. W. Wilson, J. I. Luman, and S. D. Redditt.** 1989. Tetracycline and erythromycin resistance among clinical isolates of *Branhamella catarrhalis*. Antimicrob. Agents Chemother. **33:**1631–1633.
6. **Brummitt, C. F., K. B. Crossley, and B. F. Woolfrey.** 1988. Penicillin-resistant *Streptococcus pneumoniae*. Am. J. Clin. Pathol. **89:**238–242.
7. **Burns, J. L., P. M. Mendelman, J. Levy, T. L. Stull, and A. L. Smith.** 1985. A permeability barrier as a mechanism of chloramphenicol resistance in *Haemophilus influenzae*. Antimicrob. Agents Chemother. **25:**46–54.
8. **Cates, K. L., J. M. Gerrard, and G. S. Giebink.** 1978. A penicillin-resistant pneumococcus. J. Pediatr. **93:**624–626.
9. **Centers for Disease Control.** 1976. Penicillinase-producing *Neisseria gonorrhoeae*. Morbid. Mortal. Weekly Rep. **25:**261.
10. **Centers for Disease Control.** 1984. Chromosomally mediated resistant *Neisseria gonorrhoeae*—United States. Morbid. Mortal. Weekly Rep. **33:**408–410.
11. **Centers for Disease Control.** 1987. Sentinel surveillance system for antimicrobial resistance in clinical isolates of *Neisseria gonorrhoeae*. Morbid. Mortal. Weekly Rep. **36:** 585–593.
12. **Centers for Disease Control.** 1987. Antibiotic-resistant strains of *Neisseria gonorrhoeae:* policy guidelines for detection, management, and control. Morbid. Mortal. Weekly Rep. **36**(Suppl.)**:**1–18.
13. **Davis, B. I., and F. P. V. Maesen.** 1986. Epidemiological and bacteriological findings on *Branhamella catarrhalis* respiratory infections in the Netherlands. Drugs **31**(Suppl. 3)**:**28–33.
14. **Dillon, J.-A. R., and K.-H. Yeung.** 1989. β-Lactamase plasmids and chromosomally mediated antibiotic resistance in pathogenic *Neisseria* species. Clin. Microbiol. Rev. **2**(Suppl.)**:**S125–S133.
15. **Dillon, J. R., W. Tostowaryk, and M. Pauze.** 1987. Effects of different media and methods of inoculum preparation on results of antimicrobial susceptibility testing of *Neisseria gonorrhoeae* by agar dilution. Antimicrob. Agents Chemother. **31:**1744–49.
16. **Doern, G. V.** 1986. *Branhamella catarrhalis*—an emerging human pathogen. Diagn. Microbiol. Infect. Dis. **4:**191–201.
17. **Doern, G. V., and K. C. Chapin.** 1986. Susceptibility of *Haemophilus influenzae* to amoxicillin/clavulanic acid, erythromycin, cefaclor and trimethoprim/sulfamethoxazole. Diagn. Microbiol. Infect. Dis. **4:**37–41.
18. **Doern, G. V., G. S. Daum, and T. A. Tubert.** 1987. In vitro chloramphenicol susceptibility testing of *Haemophilus influenzae:* disk diffusion procedures and assays for chloramphenicol acetyltransferase. J. Clin. Microbiol. **25:** 1453–1455.
19. **Doern, G. V., J. H. Jorgensen, C. Thornsberry, D. A. Preston, and the *Haemophilus influenzae* Surveillance Group.** 1986. Prevalence of antimicrobial resistance among clinical isolates of *Haemophilus influenzae:* a collaborative study. Diagn. Microbiol. Infect. Dis. **4:**95–107.
20. **Doern, G. V., J. H. Jorgensen, C. Thornsberry, D. A. Preston, T. Tubert, J. S. Redding, and L. A. Maher.** 1988. National collaborative study of the prevalence of antimicrobial resistance among clinical isolates of *Haemophilus influenzae*. Antimicrob. Agents Chemother. **32:**180–185.
21. **Doern, G. V., J. H. Jorgensen, C. Thornsberry, and H. Snapper.** 1990. Interpretive criteria for disk diffusion and broth microdilution susceptibility tests with *Haemophilus influenzae* performed using Haemophilus Test Medium. Eur. J. Clin. Microbiol. Infect. Dis. **9:**329–336.
22. **Doern, G. V., M. J. Miller, and R. E. Winn.** 1981. *Branhamella (Neisseria) catarrhalis* systemic disease in humans. Arch. Intern. Med. **141:**1690–1692.
23. **Doern, G. V., K. G. Seibers, L. M. Hallick, and S. A. Morse.** 1980. Antibiotic susceptibility of beta-lactamase-producing strains of *Branhamella (Neisseria) catarrhalis*. Antimicrob. Agents Chemother. **17:**24–29.
24. **Doern, G. V., and T. Tubert.** 1987. Disk diffusion susceptibility testing of *Branhamella catarrhalis* with ampicillin and seven other antimicrobial agents. Antimicrob. Agents Chemother. **31:**1519–1523.
25. **Doern, G. V., and T. Tubert.** 1987. Effect of inoculum size on results of macrotube broth dilution susceptibility tests with *Branhamella catarrhalis*. J. Clin. Microbiol. **25:** 1576–1578.
26. **Doern, G. V., and T. A. Tubert.** 1987. Detection of β-lactamase activity among clinical isolates of *Branhamella catarrhalis* with six different β-lactamase assays. J. Clin. Microbiol. **25:**1380–1383.
27. **Doern, G. V., and T. A. Tubert.** 1988. In vitro activities of 39 antimicrobial agents for *Branhamella catarrhalis* and comparison of results with different quantitative susceptibility test methods. Antimicrob. Agents Chemother. **32:** 259–261.
28. **Dougherty, T. J.** 1986. Genetic analysis and penicillin-binding protein alterations in *Neisseria gonorrhoeae* with chromosomally mediated resistance. Antimicrob. Agents Chemother. **30:**649–652.
29. **Farmer, T., and C. Reading.** 1986. Inhibition of the beta-lactamases of *Branhamella catarrhalis* by clavulanic acid and other inhibitors. Drugs **31**(Suppl. 3)**:**70–78.
30. **Henderson, F. W., P. H. Gilligan, K. Wait, and D. A. Goff.** 1988. Nasopharyngeal carriage of antibiotic resistant pneumococci by children in group day care. J. Infect. Dis. **157:**256–263.
31. **Heritage, J., and P. M. Hawkey.** 1988. Tetracycline-resistant *Neisseria gonorrhoeae*. J. Antimicrob. Chemother. **22:**575–582.
32. **Iyer, P. V., J. H. Kayler, and N. M. Jacobs.** 1978. Penicillin-resistant pneumococcal meningitis. Pediatrics **61:** 157–158.
33. **Jaffe, H. W., J. W. Biddle, C. Thornsberry, R. E. Johnson, R. E. Kaufman, G. H. Reynolds, and P. J. Wiesner.** 1976. National gonorrhea therapy monitoring study: in vitro antibiotic susceptibility and its correlation with treatment results. N. Engl. J. Med. **294:**5–9.
34. **Jetté, L. P., F. Lamothe, and the Pneumococcus Study Group.** 1989. Surveillance of invasive *Streptococcus*

pneumoniae infection in Quebec, Canada, from 1984 to 1986: serotype distribution, antimicrobial susceptibility, and clinical characteristics. J. Clin. Microbiol. **27:**1–5.

35. **Johnson, M. A., W. L. Drew, and M. Roberts.** 1981. *Branhamella (Neisseria) catarrhalis*—a lower respiratory tract pathogen? J. Clin. Microbiol. **13:**1066–1069.
36. **Jones, R. N., P. C. Fuchs, J. A. Washington II, T. L. Gavan, P. R. Murray, E. H. Gerlach, and C. Thornsberry.** 1990. Interpretive criteria, quality control guidelines and drug stability studies for susceptibility testing of cefotaxime, cefoxitin, ceftaxidime and cefuroxime against *Neisseria gonorrhoeae*. Diagn. Microbiol. Infect. Dis. **13.**
37. **Jones, R. N., T. L. Gavan, C. Thornsberry, P. C. Fuchs, E. R. Gerlach, J. S. Knapp, P. Murray, and J. A. Washington II.** 1989. Standardization of disk diffusion and agar dilution susceptibility tests for *Neisseria gonorrhoeae:* interpretive criteria and quality control guidelines for ceftriaxone, penicillin, spectinomycin, and tetracycline. J. Clin. Microbiol. **27:**2758–2766.
38. **Jones, R. N., and H. M. Sommers.** 1986. Identification and antimicrobial susceptibility testing of *Branhamella catarrhalis* in the United States laboratories, 1983–1985. Drugs **31**(Suppl. 3):34–39.
39. **Jones, R. N., H. W. Wilson, and W. J. Novick.** 1989. In vitro evaluation of pyridine-2-azo-*p*-dimethylanalinine cephalosporin, a new diagnostic chromogenic reagent, and comparison with nitrocefin, cefacetrile, and other beta-lactam compounds. J. Clin. Microbiol. **15:**677–683.

39a. **Jorgensen, J. H., G. V. Doern, L. A. Maher, A. W. Howell, and J. S. Redding.** 1990. Antimicrobial resistance among respiratory isolates of *Haemophilus influenzae, Moraxella catarrhalis,* and *Streptococcus pneumoniae* in the United States. Antimicrob. Agents Chemother. **34:**2075–2080.

40. **Jorgensen, J. H., J. C. Lee, and G. A. Alexander.** 1977. Rapid penicillinase-paper strip test for detection of beta-lactamase-producing *Haemophilus influenzae* and *Neisseria gonorrhoeae*. Antimicrob. Agents Chemother. **11:** 1087–1088.
41. **Jorgensen, J. H., L. A. Maher, and A. W. Howell.** 1990. Use of *Haemophilus* test medium for broth microdilution antimicrobial susceptibility testing of *Streptococcus pneumoniae*. J. Clin. Microbiol. **28:**430–434.
42. **Jorgensen, J. H., L. A. Maher, and J. S. Redding.** 1988. Disk diffusion interpretive criteria for extended-spectrum cephalosporins with *Haemophilus influenzae*. J. Clin. Microbiol. **26:**1887–1889.
43. **Jorgensen, J. H., J. S. Redding, L. A. Maher, and A. W. Howell.** 1987. Improved medium for antimicrobial susceptibility testing of *Haemophilus influenzae*. J. Clin. Microbiol. **25:**2105–2113.
44. **Kampmeir, R. H.** 1983. Introduction of sulphonamid therapy for gonorrhea. Sex. Transm. Dis. **10:**81–84.
45. **Krause, K. L., C. Stager, and L. O. Gentry.** 1982. Prevalence of penicillin-resistant pneumococci in Houston, Texas. Am. J. Clin. Pathol. **77:**210–213.
46. **Labia, R., M. Barthelemy, C. B. LeBouguennec, and A. B. Hoe-Dang Van.** 1986. Classification of beta-lactamase from *Branhamella catarrhalis* in relationship to penicillinases produced by other bacterial species. Drugs **31**(Suppl. 3):40–47.
47. **Lauer, B. A., and L. B. Reller.** 1980. Serotypes and penicillin susceptibility of pneumococci isolated from blood. J. Clin. Microbiol. **11:**242–244.
48. **Louie, M. H., E. L. Gabay, G. E. Mathieson, and S. M. Finegold.** 1983. *Branhamella catarrhalis* pneumonia. West. J. Med. **138:**47–49.
49. **Luman, I., R. W. Wilson, R. J. Wallace, Jr., and D. R. Nash.** 1986. Disk diffusion susceptibility of *Branhamella catarrhalis* and relationship of β-lactam zone size to β-lactamase production. Antimicrob. Agents Chemother. **30:** 774–776.
50. **Maier, T. W., H. R. Beilstein, and L. Zubraycki.** 1974. Antibiotic disk susceptibility tests with *Neisseria gonorrhoeae*. Antimicrob. Agents Chemother. **5:**210–216.
51. **Markiewicz, Z., and A. Tomasz.** 1989. Variation in penicillin-binding protein patterns of penicillin-resistant clinical isolates of pneumococci. J. Clin. Microbiol. **27:**405–410.
52. **Markowitz, S. M.** 1980. Isolation of an ampicillin-resistant, non-β-lactamase-producing strain of *Haemophilus influenzae*. Antimicrob. Agents Chemother. **17:**80–83.
53. **National Committee for Clinical Laboratory Standards.** 1990. Performance standards for antimicrobial disk susceptibility tests. Approved standard M2-A4. National Committee for Clinical Laboratory Standards, Villanova, Pa.
54. **National Committee for Clinical Laboratory Standards.** 1990. Dilution procedures for susceptibility testing of aerobic bacteria. Approved standard M7-A2. National Committee for Clinical Laboratory Standards, Villanova, Pa.
55. **Needham, C. A.** 1988. *Haemophilus influenzae:* antibiotic susceptibility. Clin. Microbiol. Rev. **1:**218–227.
56. **O'Calaghan, C. H., A. Morris, S. M. Kirby, and A. H. Shingler.** 1972. Novel method for detection of β-lactamases by using a chromogenic cephalosporin substrate. Antimicrob. Agents Chemother. **1:**283–288.
57. **Offit, P. A., J. M. Campos, and S. A. Plotkin.** 1982. Ampicillin-resistant beta-lactamase-negative *Haemophilus influenzae* type b. Pediatrics **69:**230–231.
58. **Reyn, A., B. Komer, and M. W. Bentzon.** 1972. Effect of penicillin, spectinomycin and tetracycline on *N. gonorrhoeae* isolated in 1944 and 1957. Br. J. Vener. Dis. **34:** 227–239.
59. **Rubin, L. G., A. A. Mediros, R. H. Yolden, and E. R. Moxon.** 1981. Ampicillin treatment failure of apparently beta-lactamase-negative *Haemophilus influenzae* type b meningitis due to novel beta-lactamase. Lancet **i:**1008–1010.
60. **Shapiro, M. A., C. L. Heifetz, and J. C. Sesnie.** 1984. Comparison of microdilution and agar dilution procedures for testing antibiotic susceptibility of *Neisseria gonorrhoeae*. J. Clin. Microbiol. **20:**828–830.
61. **Simberkoff, M. S., M. Lukaszewski, and A. Cross.** 1986. Antibiotic-resistant isolates of *Streptococcus pneumoniae* from clinical specimens: a cluster of serotype 19A organisms in Brooklyn, New York. J. Infect. Dis. **153:**78–82.
62. **Skinner, A., and R. Wise.** 1977. A comparison of three rapid methods for the detection of beta-lactamase activity in *Haemophilus influenzae*. J. Clin. Pathol. **30:**1030–1032.
63. **Stobberigh, E. E., H. J. vanEck, A. W. Houben, and C. P. A. van Boven.** 1986. Analysis of the relationship between ampicillin resistance and beta-lactamase production of *Branhamella catarrhalis*. Drugs **31**(Suppl. 3):23–27.
64. **Sweeney, K. G., A. Verghese, and C. A. Needham.** 1985. In vitro susceptibilities of isolates from patients with *Branhamella catarrhalis* pneumonia compared with those of colonizing strains. Antimicrob. Agents Chemother. **27:** 499–502.
65. **Swensen, J. M., B. C. Hill, and C. Thornsberry.** 1986. Screening pneumococci for penicillin resistance. J. Clin. Microbiol. **24:**749–752.
66. **Thornsberry, C., T. L. Gavan, and E. H. Gerlach.** 1977. Cumitech 6, New developments in antimicrobial agent susceptibility testing, p. 1–2. Coordinating ed., J. C. Sherris. American Society for Microbiology, Washington, D.C.
67. **Thornsberry, C., H. Jaffe, S. T. Brown, T. Edwards, J. W. Biddle, and S. E. Thompson.** 1977. Spectinomycin-resistant *Neisseria gonorrhoeae*. J. Am. Med. Assoc. **237:** 2405–2406.
68. **Thornsberry, C., and L. A. Kirven.** 1974. Ampicillin resistance in *Haemophilus influenzae* as determined by a rapid test for beta-lactamase production. Antimicrob. Agents Chemother. **6:**653–654.
69. **Woodford, N., and C. A. Ison.** 1988. The effect of media on antimicrobial susceptibility testing of *Neisseria gonorrhoeae*. J. Antimicrob. Chemother. **22:**462–471.

Chapter 113

Antibacterial Susceptibility Tests: Anaerobic Bacteria

HANNAH M. WEXLER AND SYDNEY M. FINEGOLD

Until several years ago, anaerobic susceptibility patterns were relatively stable and predictable. Shifting susceptibility patterns and variable efficacy of many of the newer agents (e.g., the newer cephalosporins) have made consideration of the susceptibility patterns of anaerobes mandatory (16). Clinicians and clinical microbiologists may be guided by published reports of the efficacy of many new agents, but they should be cautioned that interlaboratory variations in technique, as well as the inherent variability in the methods and local strain differences, may lead to differing susceptibility patterns (4, 15, 17). Methodological differences can sometimes result in extreme differences in test results, as with ceftizoxime, which has excellent activity against anaerobes with broth microdilution tests and poor activity with agar dilution tests (1, 8). Also, test results can be misleading, since most anaerobic infections are polymicrobial (4) and it may not be necessary to eradicate all of the organisms present. In the clinical laboratory, testing is recommended for anaerobic blood culture isolates, for strains from central nervous system and other serious infections, for anaerobes isolated in pure culture, for isolates from patients not responding to therapy, and for strains from infections requiring prolonged therapy (particularly when monitoring may be difficult, such as in cases of osteomyelitis). Other infections from which isolates should be subject to susceptibility testing include brain abscess, endocarditis, joint infection, prosthetic device infection, refractory or recurrent bacteremia, and infections not responsive to empiric therapy. In addition, larger numbers of strains should be tested from time to time to monitor trends in susceptibility in individual hospitals.

The National Committee for Clinical Laboratory Standards (NCCLS) has recently published a revised approved standard for susceptibility testing of anaerobic bacteria (13). The methods include agar dilution, microbroth dilution, and macrobroth dilution. Although broth disk elution was approved in the past, the committee members felt that the unreliability of the method and the poor correlation of the results with standard methods did not warrant its inclusion as an approved alternative method. However, since it was recognized that certain laboratories might continue to use this method for some time, a discussion of the method is included in this chapter. The agar dilution procedure (especially with supplemented media) best supports the growth of the majority of anaerobes to be tested, but it is labor intensive and better suited for reference laboratories monitoring trends of anaerobic antibiograms than for clinical laboratories testing single isolates. Microbroth dilution plates may be purchased in frozen or lyophilized form and are generally convenient for clinical laboratories. Unfortunately, many fastidious anaerobes (certain pigmented *Bacteroides* strains, some *Fusobacterium* strains, and some anaerobic cocci) grow poorly or not at all in this system, and metronidazole cannot be tested unless plates are reduced and good anaerobiosis is maintained. Macrobroth dilution is labor intensive but can be simplified by using a small number of dilution tubes. Broth disk elution has gained popularity in recent years since it is the simplest test to perform; unfortunately, there are many discrepancies when compared with reference techniques, particularly when the MIC of the organism falls near the breakpoint of the antimicrobial agent (a situation that occurs often with the newer cephalosporins, chloramphenicol, and clindamycin [8, 9, 16]). Furthermore, we have found that the results are often difficult to read. As mentioned above, the NCCLS no longer approves this method as an acceptable alternative. Newer, simpler techniques for anaerobic susceptibility testing are being developed and evaluated. For an extensive discussion of anaerobic susceptibility testing, the reader is referred to the introduction to the newly published NCCLS approved standard (13) and to a minireview by the NCCLS Working Group on Anaerobic Susceptibility Testing (4).

There are certain caveats to be kept in mind for all types of susceptibility tests: (i) unless adequate growth of the organism is achieved, the MIC cannot be reliably determined; (ii) MICs for control organisms should fall within the acceptable range with each antimicrobial agent; and (iii) modifications of the methods (e.g., higher inoculum or longer incubation time) and media (added supplements) may permit the growth of most fastidious organisms, but such modifications should be undertaken only when necessary and with appropriate quality control (see below, Quality Control).

ISOLATES TO TEST

Isolates that may be considered for testing are *Bacteroides fragilis* group isolates, *Bacteroides gracilis*, *Clostridium perfringens*, *Clostridium ramosum*, and *Bilophila wadsworthia*. *B. fragilis* group strains are the most commonly found anaerobes in clinical infections and can be very resistant to a number of commonly used antimicrobial agents. *B. gracilis* is found in serious, deep-seated infections and is quite resistant to many antimicrobial agents. The clinical significance of *Bilophila wadsworthia*, a novel anaerobic gram-negative rod recently described by our laboratory, is not yet fully established; however, this organism is encountered frequently in intra-abdominal infections, and it is very resistant to a number of antimicrobial agents that usually have good activity against anaerobes (2). Occasional strains of clostridia (including *C. perfringens*) may be resistant to penicillins; one-third of *Clostridium* species other than *C. perfringens* are resistant to cefoxitin, and many are also resistant to clindamycin. *C. ramosum* is the most resistant *Clostridium* species.

AGENTS TO BE TESTED

The clinical microbiologist should be guided by the hospital formulary in considering the agents to test. Agents such as imipenem, chloramphenicol, metronidazole, and the β-lactam–β-lactamase inhibitor combinations are presently almost uniformly active against anaerobes in the United States and do not need to be tested except under unusual circumstances (e.g., when a patient is nonresponsive to empiric therapy or there is evidence of resistance to one of these agents). Also, large centers such as university or research laboratories should monitor these agents to detect any developing resistance. Other agents normally used for treatment of anaerobic infection, which are variably active, include cephalosporins, penicillins, and clindamycin. The newer quinolones have variable activity against anaerobes; their specific patterns should be reviewed if they are being considered for therapy. The quinolones now on the market have relatively poor activity against anaerobes. Antimicrobial agents should be prepared as instructed by the manufacturer (see appendix 1) and diluted according to the scheme given in chapter 110.

AGAR DILUTION TEST

Prepare dilutions of antimicrobial agents (according to the scheme described in chapter 110 and appendix 1) and incorporate them into either Wilkins-Chalgren agar (for the NCCLS reference technique) or supplemented brucella laked blood agar (Table 1). Brucella laked blood agar gives the best growth of many fastidious organisms, including *B. gracilis*, many pigmenting *Bacteroides* strains, *Fusobacterium* strains, anaerobic cocci, and *Bilophila wadsworthia*. Either medium (i.e., the Wilkins-Chalgren or brucella base) should be kept refrigerated and not stored for longer than 1 month. Up to 24 h before the test, 2 ml of each antimicrobial dilution should be added to a tube containing 18 ml of molten agar (~50°C). The plates should then be placed in a 35 to 37°C incubator, with the top of the plates slightly ajar to allow evaporation of excess moisture.

Inocula are prepared as follows (3, 11):

1. Inoculate five or more colonies into enriched thioglycolate broth (see Table 1).
2. Incubate the preparations for 4 to 6 h (or overnight for slow-growing organisms) and dilute them to the density of a 0.5 McFarland standard.

Alternatively, directly suspend colonies from a 24- to 72-h blood agar plate to achieve a 0.5 McFarland standard.

Add the individual inocula to the wells of a replicator device (such as a Steers replicator) and stamp the inocula on the antimicrobial agent-containing plates, beginning with the lowest concentration of antimicrobial agent and proceeding to the highest. Try to stamp the least effective antimicrobial agents first. If several active agents are to be tested, it is best to stamp from different blocks to avoid any carryover effect. At the beginning and end of each set of antibiotic plates, stamp two plates with no antibiotic; incubate one anaerobically (growth control) and one aerobically (aerobic contaminant control). An additional plate may be inoculated and refrigerated to be used an inoculum control (to distinguish slight growth from dried inoculum). The plates should be incubated in an anaerobic atmosphere at 35 to 37°C for 48 h.

TABLE 1. Solutions and media[a]

Hemin stock solution (5 mg/ml). Dissolve 0.5 g of hemin in 10 ml of 1 N NaOH. Bring to 100 ml with distilled water and autoclave at 120°C for 15 min. Store refrigerated for up to 1 month.
$NaHCO_3$ stock solution (20 mg/ml). Dissolve 2 g of $NaHCO_3$ in 100 ml of distilled water. Filter sterilize and store refrigerated for up to 1 month. Add 0.25 ml to 5 ml of medium.
Vitamin K_1 stock (10 mg/ml). Mix 0.2 ml of vitamin K_1 in 20 ml of absolute ethanol. Filter sterilize and store refrigerated in a dark bottle.
Diluted vitamin K_1 stock (100 μg/ml). Dilute 0.1 ml of stock solution with 10 ml of sterile distilled water. Store refrigerated in a dark bottle.
Enriched thioglycolate medium. Add 1 ml of hemin solution and 1 ml of diluted vitamin K_1 stock solution to a liter of thioglycolate medium (BBL 135C). A marble chip (Fisher Scientific Co.) should be added before autoclaving if the medium will be stored for more than a few days.
McFarland turbidity standard (0.5 McFarland). Add 0.5 ml of 0.048 M $BaCl_2$ (1.175% [wt/vol] $BaCl_2 \cdot 2H_2O$) to 99.5 ml of 0.36 N H_2SO_4 (1% [vol/vol]). Distribute ~5 ml into screw-cap tubes of the same size used to prepare the inoculum. Tightly seal and store in the dark at room temperature. Agitate vigorously before use.
Supplemented brucella agar. Add 50 ml of laked (frozen and thawed) sheep blood and 1 ml of vitamin K_1 (10 mg/ml) stock solution to 1 liter of brucella base agar.

[a] From references 6, 13, and 14.

Reading endpoints

The MIC is defined as the lowest concentration of drug yielding no growth, a haze, one discrete colony, or multiple tiny colonies. With certain organism-drug combinations, there may be evidence of light growth persisting in the presence of very high concentrations of drug despite a sharp drop-off in growth at a much lower drug level. For fusobacteria, this result has been shown to be due to the persistence of L forms of the bacteria (7). In these cases, the point at which the growth drops off sharply should be read as the MIC, and the persistence of haze should be noted. For some organisms (e.g., *B. gracilis*, some pigmented *Bacteroides* strains, some anaerobic cocci, and *Bilophila wadsworthia*) there may be no sharp drop-off of growth, and the endpoint may be very difficult to determine. Reading the plate against a background of transmitted (rather than reflected) light may be helpful. Determination of endpoint in these cases is necessarily arbitrary.

MICROBROTH DILUTION TEST

Prepare antimicrobial agent dilutions in Schaedlers, West-Wilkins, brain heart infusion, or anaerobe broth (Difco Laboratories; a broth made to the same formulation as Wilkins-Chalgren agar but without the agar). The microdilution trays may be prepared in the laboratory as described in chapter 110, using the broths mentioned above. Alternatively, plates may be purchased with antimicrobial agents in the wells already (frozen or lyopholized) and inoculum added in one of the above-mentioned broths. At least one well should contain broth with no drug to serve as a growth control. **The trays should not contain less than 0.1 ml per well.** Seal the prepared trays in plastic bags and freeze them at −70°C until needed. Such trays usually remain stable for 4 to 6 months. Appropriate quality control should be performed to monitor shelf life. The final inoculum in each well should be 10^5 CFU. The volume of the inoculum is generally 0.01 ml (10 µl); an inoculum adjusted to the turbidity of a 0.5 McFarland standard ($\sim 1.5 \times 10^8$ CFU/ml) and diluted 1:10 (i.e., $\sim 1.5 \times 10^7$ CFU/ml) will result in a final inoculum of $\sim 1.5 \times 10^5$ CFU per well. If diluted inoculum is used to reconstitute lyophilized plates, the broth must contain 10^6 CFU/ml (resulting in a final inoculum of $\sim 1.5 \times 10^5$ CFU per well). Although some workers have attempted to perform MBC determination by using microbroth dilution trays, this cannot be done reliably. Plates are incubated in an anaerobic atmosphere for 48 h, and the MIC is read as the lowest concentration of antimicrobial agent that completely inhibits growth of the organism. In the case of trailing endpoints (gradually diminishing growth), the concentration that produces the most significant reduction of growth should be chosen as the endpoint.

MACROBROTH DILUTION TESTS

Conventional broth dilution tests are useful for testing spreading organisms (such as some *Clostridium* spp.) and for determining MBCs. Serial twofold dilutions of antimicrobial stock solutions are prepared in 2.5 ml of brucella broth containing 5% Fildes enrichment and vitamin K_1 (0.1 µg/ml) or in one of the broths mentioned above in the discussion of the microdilution procedure. The inoculum should be a 1:200 dilution of a 0.5 McFarland standard (made in the same broth used to dilute the drugs), and an inoculum volume of 2.5 ml is added to the broth containing the drug. Tubes should be incubated and MICs read as described above. MBCs may be determined as described in chapter 115 by subculturing to a suitable agar medium (such as brucella laked blood agar or Wilkins-Chalgren agar).

BROTH DISK ELUTION TEST

Several broth media, including brain heart infusion, Schaedler, anaerobe (Difco), and thioglycolate, have been used for the broth disk elution procedure, but most laboratories use the last. Aseptically add the antimicrobial agent-containing disks to the tubes of broth medium. The appropriate numbers of disks of various drugs for 5 ml of medium are listed in Table 2. For each strain, add 0.05 ml of a broth culture equivalent in density to a 0.5 McFarland standard (prepared as described for the agar dilution test) to two tubes containing 5 ml of enriched thioglycolate medium (Table 1), one containing the antimicrobial disks and one containing broth only (growth control). Additional tubes are required for testing of additional antimicrobial agents. The thioglycolate tubes may be incubated aerobically for 24 h and then read (10); however, we have found that anaerobic incubation facilitates reading of results. Thioglycolate or other cysteine-containing broths cannot be used to test imipenem, and incubation for more than 24 h with other penicillins may produce unreliable results. Slow-growing organisms, however, may require 48 h of incubation. Susceptibility should be defined as the total absence of growth in the antimicrobial disk-containing tube as compared with the growth control. The older criterion of defining susceptibility as growth of less than 50% of the growth in the growth control should not be used. The broth disk elution technique is not reliable for strains that have MIC values at or near the drug breakpoint (i.e., many of the cephalosporins) or for metronidazole. Some workers have found that a clear medium (such as brucella broth) handled and incubated anaerobically gives clearer results than thioglycolate medium. Refer to the comments in the introduction about the reliability of the broth disk elution test.

TABLE 2. Recommended antimicrobial concentrations and number of disks for the broth disk elution test method for 5 ml of broth[a]

Antimicrobial agent	Disk potency	No. of disks	Concn (µg/ml)
Ampicillin/sulbactam	10/10 µg	8	16/16
Carbenicillin	100 µg	6	120
Cefoperazone	75 µg	4	60
Cefotaxime Moxalactam	30 µg	5	30
Cefotetan Cefoxitin Chloramphenicol	30 µg	3	18
Clindamycin	10 µg	2	4
Imipenem[b]	10 µg	4	8
Metronidazole	80 µg	1	16
Mezlocillin Ticarcillin	75 µg	4	60
Penicillin G	10 U	8	16
Piperacillin	100 µg	3	60
Tetracycline	30 µg	1	6

[a] From reference 12 with permission granted by NCCLS. The current NCCLS-recommended protocol (13) does not include this method (see text for details).

[b] Thioglycolate broth is not suitable. Use brain heart infusion, Schaedler, or anaerobe broth and incubate the culture anaerobically.

SPIRAL GRADIENT ENDPOINT SYSTEM

The spiral streaker (Spiral Systems Instruments, Bethesda, Md.) deposits a set amount of antimicrobial stock solution in a spiral pattern on an agar plate, resulting in a radially decreasing concentration gradient (from the center of the plate). After the antimicrobial agents are allowed to diffuse for 3 to 4 h, the isolates (prepared to a 0.5 McFarland standard) are deposited on the plate by using an automated inoculator or are manually streaked from the center to the edge of the plate. The plates are incubated for 48 h in an anaerobic

TABLE 3. MIC ranges for quality control strains[a]

Antimicrobial agent	MIC range (μg/ml)			
	Bacteroides fragilis ATCC 25285	*Bacteroides thetaiotaomicron* ATCC 29741	*Clostridium perfringens* ATCC 13124	*Eubacterium lentum* ATCC 43055
Amoxicillin/clavulanate	0.25–1	0.5–2		
Ampicillin	16–64	16–64	NR[b]	
Ampicillin/sulbactam	0.5–2	0.5–2		
Carbenicillin	16–64	16–64	0.25–1	
Cefamandole	32–128	32–128	0.06–0.25	
Cefmetazole	8–32	32–128	NR	4–16
Cefoperazone	32–128	32–128	NR	32–128
Cefotaxime	8–32	16–64	0.06–0.25	64–256
Cefotetan	4–16	32–128	NR	32–128
Cefoxitin	4–16	8–32	0.25–1	4–16
Ceftizoxime	32–128	NR	NR	16–64
Ceftriaxone	32–128	64–256	NR	
Chloramphenicol	2–8	4–16	2–8	
Clindamycin	0.5–2	2–8	0.03–0.12	0.06–0.25
Imipenem	0.03–0.12	0.06–0.25	0.03–0.12	0.25–1
Metronidazole	0.25–1	0.5–2	0.12–0.5	
Mezlocillin	16–64	8–32	0.06–0.25	8–32
Moxalactam	0.25–1	4–16	0.03–0.12	64–256
Penicillin G	16–64	16–64	0.06–0.25	
Piperacillin	2–8	8–32	0.06–0.25	8–32
Tetracycline	0.12–0.5	8–32	0.03–0.12	
Ticarcillin	16–64	16–64	0.25–1	
Ticarcillin/clavulanate	NR	0.5–2	0.12–0.5	

[a] From reference 13 with permission granted by NCCLS. The interpretive data are valid only if the methodology in M11-A2 is followed. The current M11 edition may be obtained from NCCLS, 771 E. Lancaster Ave., Villanova, PA 19085.
[b] NR, No MIC is recommended with this organism-antibiotic combination.

atmosphere, after which the endpoints of growth are marked and the distance in millimeters is measured from the center of the plate to the point where growth stops. The data are entered into a computer software program provided by the manufacturer that determines the concentration of drug on the basis of the radius of growth and the molecular weight (i.e., diffusion characteristics) of the antimicrobial agent. Details of the procedure may be found in the manufacturer's guidelines; some workers have compared this procedure with standard agar dilution (5) and found good correlation, as we have in our own tests (H. Wexler et al., unpublished data). The technique retains the advantages of an agar dilution system (particularly good growth of fastidious organisms) as well as some of the labor-saving advantages of the simpler techniques. Unfortunately, the equipment is expensive.

One can hope that with the new void created in anaerobic susceptibility testing by the disapproval of the broth disk elution system, newer, more convenient and reliable techniques will be developed that will allow clinical laboratories to determine antibiograms in a reliable, cost-effective manner.

QUALITY CONTROL

The standard reference strains that are recommended by the NCCLS for the quality control of these tests and the expected ranges of MICs for some appropriate antimicrobial agents are shown in Table 3. The purpose of the quality control tests is to demonstrate adequacy of the medium, to ascertain that the antimicrobial agent is of the proper concentration, and to verify that the laboratory personnel are proficient in performing the tests. The NCCLS recommends that at least two of the control strains be tested each time tests are done (13). The current NCCLS standard should be checked for the most recent additions to the quality control recommendations.

TABLE 4. Recommended breakpoints for antimicrobial agents[a]

Antimicrobial agent	Breakpoint (μg/ml)
Amoxicillin/clavulanate	8/4
Ampicillin	4
Ampicillin/sulbactam	16/8
Carbenicillin	128
Cefoperazone	32
Cefotaxime	32
Cefotetan	32
Cefoxitin	32
Ceftizoxime	64, 32[b]
Ceftriaxone	32
Chloramphenicol	16
Clindamycin	4
Imipenem	8
Metronidazole	16
Mezlocillin	64
Moxalactam	32
Penicillin G	4
Piperacillin	64
Tetracycline	8
Ticarcillin	64
Ticarcillin/clavulanate	64/2

[a] Organisms with MIC values at or below these concentrations are considered susceptible or moderately susceptible. Organisms with MIC values above these concentrations are considered resistant. Data from reference 13. See Table 3, footnote *a*.
[b] 64 μg/ml is the breakpoint for the agar dilution test; 32 μg/ml is the breakpoint for broth dilution or microbroth dilution.

BREAKPOINTS

In some previous NCCLS documents, the MIC susceptibility breakpoints recommended for aerobic and facultative bacteria were also recommended for anaerobic bacteria. In the current approved document, some of the breakpoints have been changed (Table 4). There is no moderately susceptible category, since it is recognized that all patients with anaerobic infections should be treated with the maximum safe dosage.

LITERATURE CITED

1. **Aldridge, K. E., H. M. Wexler, C. V. Sanders, and S. M. Finegold.** 1990. Comparison of in vitro antibiograms of *Bacteroides fragilis* group isolates: differences in resistance rates in two institutions because of differences in susceptibility testing methodology. Antimicrob. Agents Chemother. **34:**179–181.
2. **Baron, E. J., P. Summanen, J. Downes, M. C. Roberts, H. Wexler, and S. M. Finegold.** 1989. *Bilophila wadsworthia*, gen. nov. and sp. nov., a unique gram-negative anaerobic rod recovered from appendicitis specimens and human faeces. J. Gen. Microbiol. **135:**3405–3411.
3. **Bourgault, A. M., and F. Lamothe.** 1984. Comparison of anaerobic susceptibility results obtained by two methods of inoculum preparation. J. Clin. Microbiol. **20:**1060–1064.
4. **Finegold, S. M., and the National Committee for Clinical Laboratory Standards Working Group on Anaerobic Susceptibility Testing.** 1988. Susceptibility testing of anaerobic bacteria: a minireview. J. Clin. Microbiol. **26:**1253–1256.
5. **Hill, G. B., and S. Schalkowsky.** 1990. Development and evaluation of the spiral gradient endpoint method for susceptibility testing of anaerobic gram-negative bacilli. Rev. Infect. Dis. **11**(Suppl. 12).
6. **Holdeman, L. V., and W. E. C. Moore.** 1977. Anaerobe laboratory manual, 4th ed. Virginia Polytechnic Institute and State University, Blacksburg.
7. **Johnson, C. C., H. M. Wexler, M. Garcia, S. Becker, and S. M. Finegold.** 1989. Cell-wall-defective variants of *Fusobacterium*. Antimicrob. Agents Chemother. **33:**369–372.
8. **Jones, R. N., A. L. Barry, P. C. Fuchs, and S. D. Allen.** 1987. Ceftizoxime and cefoxitin susceptibility testing against anaerobic bacteria; comparison of results from three NCCLS methods and quality control recommendations for the reference agar dilution procedure. Diagn. Microb. Infect. Dis. **8:**87–94.
9. **Jorgensen, J. H., J. S. Redding, and A. W. Howell.** 1986. Evaluation of broth disk elution methods for susceptibility testing of anaerobic bacteria with the newer beta-lactam antibiotics. J. Clin. Microbiol. **23:**545–550.
10. **Kurzynski, T. A., J. W. Yrios, A. G. Helstad, and C. R. Field.** 1976. Aerobically incubated thioglycolate broth disk method for antibiotic susceptibility testing of anaerobes. Antimicrob. Agents Chemother. **10:**727–732.
11. **Murray, P. R., and A. C. Niles.** 1983. Inoculum preparation for anaerobic susceptibility tests. J. Clin. Microbiol. **18:**733–734.
12. **National Committee for Clinical Laboratory Standards.** 1989. Methods for antimicrobial susceptibility testing of anaerobic bacteria, 2nd ed., vol. 9, no. 10. Tentative standard M11-T2. National Committee for Clinical Laboratory Standards, Villanova, Pa.
13. **National Committee for Clinical Laboratory Standards.** 1990. Methods for antimicrobial susceptibility testing of anaerobic bacteria, 2nd ed., vol. 9, no. 10. Approved standard M11-A2. National Committee for Clinical Laboratory Standards, Villanova, Pa.
14. **Sutter, V. L., D. M. Citron, M. A. C. Edelstein, and S. M. Finegold.** 1985. Wadsworth anaerobic bacteriology manual, 4th ed. Star Publishing Co., Belmont, Calif.
15. **Wexler, H. M.** 1989. Susceptibility testing procedures, p. 715–729. *In* S. M. Finegold and W. L. George (ed.), Anaerobic infections in humans. Academic Press, Inc., Orlando, Fla.
16. **Wexler, H., and S. M. Finegold.** 1987. Antimicrobial resistance in *Bacteroides*. J. Antimicrob. Chemother. **19:**143–146.
17. **Wexler, H. M., D. Reeves, and S. M. Finegold.** 1988. Antibiotic susceptibility testing of anaerobic organisms using the agar dilution method: comparison of three techniques. Clin. Ther. **10:**747–760.

Chapter 114

Antibacterial Susceptibility Tests: Mycobacteria

JEAN E. HAWKINS, RICHARD J. WALLACE, JR., AND BARBARA A. BROWN

The key to successful treatment of tuberculosis is the selection of an appropriate regimen of chemotherapy. This choice is facilitated by the availability of proven, clinically effective drug combinations. It was clearly demonstrated in early chemotherapy trials that combined drug therapy is conducive to bacteriologic conversion and effective in reducing the frequency of therapeutic failures caused by the selection of drug-resistant mutants. If clinical signs and symptoms suggest mycobacterial disease, physicians may begin treatment without benefit of drug susceptibility tests or before results of these tests are known. The rationale behind this approach is that over 95% of isolates of *Mycobacterium tuberculosis* from newly diagnosed, previously untreated patients in the United States are susceptible to all standard antituberculosis drugs. These cases usually respond to treatment with two or three of the primary drugs: isoniazid (INH), streptomycin sulfate (SM), ethambutol (EMB), rifampin (RMP), and, in abbreviated regimens, pyrazinamide (PZA). There are also five second-line drugs available (sodium *p*-aminosalicyclic acid [PAS], ethionamide [ETA], cycloserine [CS], kanamycin sulfate [KM], and capreomycin sulfate [CM]), but some important limitations affect their usefulness.

The American Thoracic Society (ATS) (2) has recommended two options in determining the need for susceptibility tests on initial isolates from a patient. The first option is to test all initial isolates. The second is to test isolates of (i) patients at high risk for primary drug resistance (infection by a resistant organism), including immigrants from certain high prevalence areas, contacts of known or suspected resistant cases, and residents of geographic areas where high levels of drug-resistant tuberculosis (>5%) have been documented; and (ii) patients with life-threatening illness, such as meningitis or widely disseminated disease. When pretreatment susceptibility tests are not performed, an initial isolate or isolates should be held in a laboratory deep freezer at −40°C to −70°C for at least 6 months to permit base-line studies if the patient fails to respond to therapy.

Requests for drug susceptibility tests on subsequent isolates can be expected in the following situations:

1. For relapsed or retreatment cases.
2. When modifications of drug regimens are being considered because patient specimens (i) remain positive after 3 to 5 months on treatment, (ii) become positive after being negative, or (iii) show a persistent increase in bacillary output after an initial quantitative decrease on smears or cultures.
3. When primary drug resistance is suspected; if present, this type of resistance is common to INH, SM, or both and uncommon to RMP or EMB.

In the United States, suggestions for several levels or extents of services that might be provided by mycobacteriology laboratories have been proposed by the Centers for Disease Control (CDC) of the Public Health Service, ATS, and the College of American Pathologists (CAP). The three levels of service (I, II, and III) are roughly equivalent to extents 2, 3, and 4, respectively, used by CAP (see chapter 34).

It is recommended in the levels-of-service concept, first introduced in 1967 by the Public Health Service and supported by ATS in official policy statements (1, 14, 21, 36), that services be based on work load, expertise, cost-effectiveness, and interest. Drug susceptibility tests should be performed only in laboratories staffed by personnel who are proficient in identifying the species of *Mycobacterium* being tested and who perform a sufficient number of susceptibility tests to be aware of the problems associated with the procedures. These levels or extents are now recognized in grading of responses of laboratories participating in proficiency testing programs.

In this chapter, drug susceptibility testing methods are described for clinical isolates of slowly growing and rapidly growing mycobacteria, i.e., those species that require more or less than 7 days for mature growth of well-isolated colonies to appear on media inoculated with a dilute suspension.

DRUG RESISTANCE IN *M. TUBERCULOSIS*

Drug resistance in *M. tuberculosis* is the result of spontaneous mutations that occur at random in the bacterial population, independent of drug exposure (6, 7). Therefore, all populations of drug-susceptible tubercle bacilli contain a certain proportion of drug-resistant mutants that, fortunately, remain at low levels because some mutants do not survive well, and back-mutations to drug susceptibility may occur. When single or ineffective drug therapy is used in the treatment of tuberculosis, most susceptible organisms in the population are inhibited or killed, while the proportion of resistant cells increases from an interplay of the natural phenomenon of spontaneous mutation and the drug-directed selection to predominance of resistant mutants.

Criteria

The criteria of drug resistance in tuberculosis have been established on the empirical basis that there is a certain proportion of drug-resistant mutants above which therapeutic success is less likely to be realized. The procedures used to perform drug susceptibility tests and the criteria for interpreting the data take into account two factors, the critical proportion of drug-resistant mutants and the critical concentration of the drug in the medium. On the basis of clinical and bacteriologic studies, the significant proportion of cells resistant to an antituberculosis drug above which a clinical response is unlikely has been set at 1% (4, 5). The critical concentration of a drug is the level that inhibits the growth of most cells in wild-type strains of tubercle bacilli without appreciably affecting the growth of the resistant mutants present. It should be noted that this concentration may not bear a direct relationship to the peak serum level in patients (not always, but generally, the most effective drugs are those for which the serum level is greater or equal to 10 times the MIC). The critical concentrations of antituberculosis drugs for *M. tuberculosis* grown in 7H10 agar medium are given in Table 1 (6).

Methods

Conventional diffusion techniques for susceptibility tests, which rely on the size of a zone of inhibition around a drug-containing disk, are not suitable for slowly growing mycobacteria because the drug diffuses throughout the medium before growth of the organism is significantly affected. The methods generally accepted throughout the world for determining drug susceptibility of mycobacteria are based on growth of the organism on a solid medium containing a uniform, specified concentration of a single drug. The three methods most commonly used are the absolute concentration method, the resistance ratio method, and the proportion method (5).

The absolute concentration method requires the inoculation of both a drug-free control medium and media containing graded concentrations of drugs with a carefully controlled inoculum of tubercle bacilli. Resistance is then defined as growth greater than a certain number of CFU (usually 20) at a specific drug concentration. This method, still widely used in middle and eastern Europe, was employed in the early clinical trials of the Veterans Administration-Armed Forces Cooperative Studies group and by the Public Health Service but now is rarely used in this country.

The resistance ratio method follows the same general procedure as the absolute concentration method except that a parallel set of control and drug test media is inoculated with a standard laboratory strain of tubercle bacilli (usually H37Rv). Resistance is expressed as the ratio of the MIC of the test (unknown) strain divided by the MIC of the control strain in the same set of tests. For most drugs, a "wild" strain with a ratio of 8 or more is considered resistant, and 4 is suggestive of resistance. Inoculum must be adequately standardized, but in contrast to the absolute concentration method, batch-to-batch variations in drug-containing media are less critical since the use of the standard strain in the ratio compensates for any differences. This method has been used in British Medical Research Council chemotherapy trials.

For the proportion method, appropriate dilutions of inoculum are planted in replicate onto both control and drug-containing media so that countable (50 to 100) colonies are obtained on at least one of the control media. The number of CFU that grow on a drug medium is then compared with the number on the control. From this, the proportion of bacilli resistant to a given drug can be calculated and expressed as a percentage of the total population tested. A modified proportion method, considered the "gold standard," is used more widely in the United States than is any other antimycobacterial drug susceptibility testing method. This procedure for susceptibility testing of slowly growing mycobacteria is described below.

TABLE 1. Critical concentrations of antituberculosis drugs in 7H10 agar medium

Drug	Concn (µg/ml)
INH	0.2
SM	2.0
EMB	5.0
RMP	1.0
PAS	2.0
ETA	5.0
KM	5.0
CM	10.0
CS	30.0
PZA (at pH 5.5)	25.0

DRUG SUSCEPTIBILITY TESTING OF *M. TUBERCULOSIS* COMPLEX BY CONVENTIONAL TECHNIQUES

Basic technical decisions to be made in the performance of drug susceptibility tests on mycobacteria are (i) type of test (direct or indirect), (ii) inoculum (processed specimen or culture; size), (iii) medium (liquid, agar based, or egg based), (iv) drugs (concentrations, methods for incorporation, and stability), (v) incubation (temperature and atmosphere), and (vi) reading and reporting (time and interpretation).

Type of test and inoculum

Tests performed by direct or indirect means differ in (i) the source of the inoculum (i.e., directly from the patient specimen or indirectly from a culture of the specimen), (ii) how the inoculum is adjusted, (iii) how representative the inoculum is of the bacillary population in the lesion(s) of the host, and (iv) the timing of results. In the direct test, the inoculum is a digested, decontaminated clinical specimen, or an untreated normally sterile body fluid, in which acid-fast bacilli (AFB) can be seen in stained smears. To ensure adequate but not excessive growth in the direct susceptibility test, specimens are diluted according to the number of organisms observed in the stained smear of the clinical specimen. A comparative dilution scheme is shown in Table 2.

TABLE 2. Dilution of specimen concentrate for inoculation of susceptibility test media

Microscopic result				Dilutions inoculated onto media
Fuchsin stain[a]	Fluorochrome stain[b] ×250	Fluorochrome stain[b] ×450	Fluorochrome stain[b] ×630	
<1	<10	<4	<2	Undiluted, 1:100
1–10	10–100	4–36	2–18	1:10, 1:1,000
>10	>100	>36	>18	1:100, 1:10,000

[a] Number of AFB seen per oil immersion field (ca. ×1,000).
[b] Fluorochrome-positive bacilli seen at magnification indicated.

In contrast, the indirect test requires primary isolation of the organisms from the clinical specimen and subsequent inoculation of the drug test media with either a homogeneous suspension of that culture growth or a broth subculture prepared from it. The direct test has the advantages of providing earlier results and avoiding any selective effect of subculture. On the other hand, indirect tests may be necessary when any of the following circumstances exist:

1. Smears for microscopy are negative for AFB but cultures reveal growth. This is often the case in patients with minimal disease, and it is impractical for the laboratory to do direct drug tests routinely when the majority of specimens received are AFB smear negative.
2. Contamination is present on the direct test.
3. Growth on the drug-free control medium in a direct test is scant (50 to 100 colonies) and does not permit a reliable report.
4. A reference culture is submitted for testing.

Media

Different media have been used for conventional drug susceptibility testing of slowly growing mycobacteria, including Middlebrook and Cohn 7H10 or 7H11 agar medium and Lowenstein-Jensen egg medium (see chapter 121). MICs may differ considerably between agar- and egg-based media as well as between 7H10 and 7H11 media, which have the same formulation except for the addition of casein hydrolysate to the latter (4, 7, 25). Not only is there uncertainty about the potency of labile drugs after heating, as occurs in inspissation of egg media, or after prolonged storage, but some drugs are affected by such medium ingredients as phospholipids or large-molecular-weight proteins or by the presence of certain amino acids.

The medium of choice in the United States is 7H10 because of its simple composition, ease of preparation, and solidification by agar rather than heat. The transparency of 7H10 and the use of a dissecting microscope can also facilitate earlier detection and enumeration of colonies and the recognition of possibly mixed mycobacterial species or the presence of contaminants. Occasionally, drug-resistant strains of tubercle bacilli do not grow sufficiently on 7H10 drug-free control medium for a valid test (less than 50 to 100 colonies). In these cases, 7H11 medium may be helpful, but higher concentrations of some drugs must be used because of the presence of hydrolyzed casein (11, 25).

Middlebrook and Cohn 7H10 agar medium is available from several commercial suppliers both as a dehydrated base and as a completely prepared medium with and without antituberculosis drugs: Becton Dickinson (BBL) Microbiology Systems, Cockeysville, MD 21030; Difco Laboratories, Detroit, MI 48232; GIBCO Laboratories, Madison, WI 53711; Remel, Lenexa, KA 66215; and Scott Laboratories, West Warwick, RI 02893.

Preparation of drug solutions

Antimicrobial drugs for susceptibility tests should be obtained directly from the manufacturers (address requests to the medical department) or from any laboratory supply house that makes powdered drugs available specifically for this purpose. Do not use pharmacy stock or other clinical preparations. Store unopened vials of drug powders according to directions of the manufacturer; store opened containers in a desiccator at the recommended temperature. If the potency stated on the bottle is not 100% of the dry weight, the following formula may be used to determine the amount of drug necessary to prepare the appropriate stock solution:

$$\text{mg of drug to weigh} = \frac{\text{desired drug concentration } (\mu\text{g/ml}) \times \text{volume of drug solution needed (ml)}}{\text{potency of drug } (\mu\text{g/mg})}$$

Prepare aqueous stock solutions containing at least 1,000 μg of biologically active drug per ml of distilled water for the following antituberculosis agents: INH, EMB, SM, KM, CM, PZA, CS, and PAS. To minimize loss due to adsorption, sterilize aqueous stock solutions by membrane filtration (0.22-μm pore size). RMP stock solutions should be prepared in 95% ethanol or methanol. ETA may be dissolved in dimethyl sulfoxide or ethylene glycol (analytical grade) to obtain a stock solution of 5,000 or 10,000 μg/ml. These solutions are self-sterilizing and should not be filtered. As with aqueous drug solutions, sterile distilled water is used as the diluent in preparing working solutions if a concentration lower than the stock solution is required.

Stock solutions of most agents at concentrations of 1,000 μg/ml or greater remain stable for at least 6 months at −20°C and for 1 year in a −70 to −80°C freezer. Note, however, that CS solutions at neutral or acid pH are unstable at room temperature and must be used immediately. If alkalinized with Na_2CO_3 to a pH of 10, CS stock solutions of 10,000 μg/ml can be stored for 1 week in a refrigerator without loss of activity and for 1 month at −20°C (25). Directions provided by the drug manufacturer should be consulted in addition to these general recommendations.

Immediately after preparation, dispense small volumes of stock drug solutions into sterile vials; seal and store the vials at −20°C or lower. Remove vials as needed and use them the same day. Any unused drug solution should be discarded, never refrozen. Results with a new lot of drug powder should be compared with the activity of a previous or standard lot, using strains of tubercle bacilli having known susceptibility patterns.

Preparation of drug-containing media

The drug concentrations to be tested in 7H10 should correspond to those listed in Table 1, the "critical" concentrations for *M. tuberculosis*. These drugs and concentrations fulfill the basic requirements for routine clinical laboratories. Higher levels of some drugs may also be used: 1 and 5 μg/ml for INH, 10 μg/ml for SM, 10 μg/ml for EMB; and 5 μg/ml for RMP. Susceptibilities to these concentrations may be considered in treatment decisions but are primarily useful for establishing the suitability of these drugs for the treatment of nontuberculous mycobacterial disease.

Middlebrook and Cohn 7H10 agar medium may be prepared from individual ingredients, but the process is time-consuming, with many weighing and dilution steps (see chapter 121). A dehydrated base is available from commercial sources (see above) and is recommended for routine use except for PZA-containing media (see below).

Agar dilution method (21, 25, 36). Prepare 7H10 medium base according to directions given by the manufacturer. After the base is autoclaved, it should be allowed to cool in a water bath to 50 to 56°C before addition of oleic-albumin-dextrose-catalase (OADC) enrichment (previously warmed to room temperature, 20 to 25°C). Each test drug at the appropriate dilution is then added to a separate flask of completed medium at 50 to 52°C, mixed well, and dispensed without delay into sterile quadrant plates, 5 ml per quadrant, using aseptic technique. Drug-free control quadrants must be included.

Drug-containing 7H10 medium should be prepared in quantities sufficient for use within 1 month, since drug activity may be affected if the medium is stored for a longer period. A convenient amount to prepare and dispense is 200 ml, which will provide 32 to 36 test quadrants per batch. Thus, four flasks of medium will allow preparation of 16 to 18 duplicate sets of plates containing three drug quadrants and one control quadrant. Set aside 10% of the prepared plates from each batch of medium and incubate them at 23 to 25°C and at 35 to 37°C for 48 h to confirm sterility. Discard these plates; do not use them. Protect susceptibility test media from light and dehydration. Store the media in plastic bags at 4°C for a maximum of 4 weeks. As a general rule, the length of time for which drug media are left at room temperature should be kept to a minimum during preparation, inoculation, and packaging for incubation. The drugs CS, EMB, and ETA are especially unstable in 7H10.

Standard 7H10 base and OADC enrichment are used to prepare all drug-containing media for conventional susceptibility tests, with the exception of PZA. This drug is biologically active only at a low pH; therefore, the 7H10 base formulation must be adjusted to provide a pH of 5.5. A low-pH agar base is commercially available (GIBCO), and some modifications have been suggested to improve growth of test organisms (3). Nevertheless, strains of *M. tuberculosis*, especially drug-resistant isolates, often fail to grow or to grow sufficiently for a valid test on the acid medium. The fact that PZA-resistant strains may lose pyrazinamidase activity has been used as an indicator of susceptibility (25). Variability of results with resistant strains limits the value of this test for resistance, but there is good correlation between susceptibility to PZA and a positive pyrazinamidase result, which can be used for verification (consult chapter 34 and reference 21 for method). PZA susceptibility studies should be performed only in extent 4 or level III facilities by personnel who have considerable experience in drug testing and knowledge of the inherent problems.

The agar dilution method described above requires large amounts of media and incorporation of multiple concentrations of drugs, each in separate batches of media, all of which must be dispensed. This procedure is cumbersome and expensive. An alternative and more practical means of preparing drug media for some laboratories involves elution of drugs from commercially available, drug-impregnated paper disks submerged in the medium.

Disk elution method (10, 11, 42). Paper disks impregnated with standardized amounts of drugs are placed in individual quadrants of petri dishes and overlaid with melted 7H10 agar prepared from a single batch of medium. The test drug diffuses from the disk to give a uniform concentration within the medium of the quadrant. The elution method provides results equivalent to those of the dilution method and obviates most of the problems associated with the latter by eliminating errors in weighing and dilution, as well as errors in labeling since the disks are coded to identify drug and concentration. Because only 1 volume of 7H10 medium is required, laboratories can easily prepare just the number of plates needed for short-term use.

Disks for testing antituberculosis drugs at suggested concentrations are available commercially (BBL Sensi-Discs). The concentrations of the primary drugs (INH, EMB, RMP, and SM) shown in Table 3 represent a low screening level and, for INH and SM, a higher concentration to monitor increases in or greater degrees of drug resistance. Disks containing concentrations suitable for testing of PAS, ETA, and KM are also available, but other agents must be prepared from drug powders.

To prepare plates for susceptibility tests, dispense disks aseptically to the individual quadrants of sterile 100-mm plastic petri dishes, centering the disks in the quadrants. A continuous-pipetting device may be used to pipette 5 ml of sterile tempered (52°C) complete 7H10 medium over the disk. Direct the medium away from and around the disk to keep the disk from floating; if necessary, move the disk back to the center with the pipetting cannula. Avoid bubbles in the medium. Control quadrants contain 7H10 without disks.

Drug plates should *not* be incubated at 35°C overnight either to promote drug diffusion, as has been suggested in some publications, or to check for sterility. This is especially important for medium containing EMB and ETA disks. Rather, as soon as the medium is firmly solidified, the plates should be divided into drug sets for susceptibility testing and placed in a refrigerator, where some diffusion of drug takes place. Generally, there is uniform diffusion of the drugs during the inoculation procedure and in the initial hours of incubation before significant multiplication of the organisms occurs.

Set aside 10% of the plates from each medium lot (if there are more than one) for incubation as described above to confirm sterility. These plates should then be discarded. Disk susceptibility plates may be used within 2 days, after sterility tests have been checked, or stored at 5°C in plastic bags for a maximum of 4 weeks.

TABLE 3. Distribution of disks for susceptibility tests with primary drugs

Plate no.	Quadrant no.	Drug	Amount (μg)/disk	Final drug concn (μg/ml)
1	I	Control 1	0	0.0
	II	INH	1	0.2
	III	INH	5	1.0
	IV	EMB	25	5.0
2	I	Control 2	0	0.0
	II	SM	10	2.0
	III	SM	50	10.0
	IV	RMP	5	1.0

Commercial drug media

Commercially prepared drug-containing 7H10 agar medium is available from several suppliers (see listing above in the section on media). Rigorous quality control procedures must be used to ensure that the medium is fresh and the drug-free control medium supports optimal growth of reference strains. Verify that drug concentrations have maintained the stated activity during shipment and storage by testing against strains with known susceptibility and resistance patterns.

Preparation of inocula for the direct test

Stain and read smears of concentrated specimens, using the basic fuchsin acid-fast stains (Ziehl-Neelsen or Kinyoun) or a fluorochrome acid-fast stain. Examine fluorochrome-stained smears within 24 h; if it is necessary to hold the specimens overnight, store them at 5°C to minimize loss of fluorescence. Determine the average number of AFB seen per field (count clumps as one organism) and prepare serial 10-fold dilutions of the concentrate in sterile water or saline according to the scheme in Table 2.

Performance of the direct test

Sets of plates to be inoculated are removed from the refrigerator and allowed to warm to room temperature just before inoculation. Proceed with the susceptibility test as follows.

1. Use a sterile capillary pipette to place 3 drops (about 0.1 ml) of inoculum onto each quadrant of the drug and control media. In the modified proportion method used at CDC, one set of plates is inoculated with the higher dilution and the duplicate plates are inoculated with the lower dilution.
2. Include control sets inoculated with reference strains as a quality control check (refer to section on reference strains below).
3. Leave plates undisturbed until the inoculum has been absorbed completely; then place each plate in a clear polyethylene bag and seal the bag.
4. Place sets, medium side down, in an incubator at 35 to 37°C in an atmosphere of 5 to 10% CO_2.
5. Examine cultures weekly for 3 weeks. Even though mature colonies may appear on control media in less than 3 weeks, a report of "drug susceptible" should not be submitted until week 3. Because of metabolic differences, resistant strains of *M. tuberculosis* may be slower to produce visible growth. If cultures are incubated beyond 3 weeks, diminished activity of a bacteriostatic drug may permit the appearance of colonies of organisms that were susceptible to the initial static level. These colonies are usually smaller than those on the control.
6. Since the control quadrants are inoculated with the processed specimen, also examine isolated colonies for colonial morphology and pigment, suggestive of *M. tuberculosis* or another species, and for possibly mixed species of mycobacteria or the presence of a contaminant (see chapter 34). If extensive drug resistance is present, bear in mind that rapid growers may be slow to develop on primary isolation. These colonies when small, as well as the rough, dry colonies of some *Mycobacterium avium* complex (MAC) strains, may appear "TB-like" on 7H10 medium.
7. Record results of both dilutions as follows:

Confluent (no space between 500 or more colonies)	4+
Almost confluent (medium visible between 200 to 500 colonies)	3+
100 to 200 colonies	2+
50 to 100 colonies	1+
Less than 50 colonies	Actual count

Designations like 2+ and 4+ do not permit precise quantification (i.e., 2+ is not necessarily 50% of 4+). Countable colonies should be observed on at least one of the control quadrants so that percentage of resistance can be calculated. The only time confluent growth on the control can be accepted as a valid test result is when the organism is completely susceptible to all drugs tested. In most cases, it is possible to estimate the proportion of resistant colonies as greater than or fewer than 1% of the control population, since in the modified proportion method the diluted inoculum is 1% of the heavier inoculum (note description in discussion of the indirect test). Cultures of tubercle bacilli usually are obviously susceptible or obviously resistant, and only rarely is the result ambiguous. However, if colony size is clearly reduced in the presence of a drug, a notation such as "microcolonies" should be made. This observation is made occasionally with EMB and ETA, which are considered bacteriostatic agents. Repeat the test on the same or a more recent isolate if available, using freshly prepared drug medium.

Most susceptibility studies are performed with inocula from a positive culture. Although the inoculum size in the proportion method does not need to be precisely controlled, this procedure does require some standardization. If the inoculum is excessively large with confluent growth on the control, growth of spontaneously occurring drug-resistant mutants may appear on some of the drug media, giving a false impression of resistance. On the other hand, if the inoculum is too small, resistance may be underestimated.

Preparation of inocula for the indirect test

The indirect procedure is performed on culture isolates of mycobacteria. If the culture is in good condition and sufficient growth is present, a suspension of the growth from the initial isolate may be used.

To prepare inoculum from growth on solid medium, use the following procedure. Scrape colonies from the surface of the medium, taking care to sample a portion of each colony or all parts of growth. Transfer the bacterial mass to a sterile screw-cap tube (16 by 125 mm) containing six to eight glass beads (1 to 2 mm in diameter) and 3 to 4 ml of a Tween-albumin liquid medium, such as Middlebrook 7H9 broth (21, 36; see also chapter 121). Homogenize the contents on a test tube mixer for 1 or 2 min. Let the tube stand for 30 min or longer to allow larger particles to settle and decrease any possibility of aerosol dispersion when the cap is removed. Withdraw the supernatant suspension and adjust the density to that of a McFarland no. 1 standard with broth or sterile saline (see chapter 122 for preparation of the standard). Culture suspensions adjusted to this standard contain approximately 10^8 CFU/ml. In the procedure recommended by CDC, serial 10-fold dilutions are made and two sets of drug plates are inoculated with the 10^{-2} and 10^{-4} dilutions, respectively. If the culture to be tested is old or scant growth is present, or for other technical reasons, it may be necessary to subculture the preparation first in broth to prepare a satisfactory inoculum.

To prepare inoculum with a broth culture, transfer a representative portion of the culture into 7H9 broth and incubate it at 35 to 37°C with daily shaking by hand for 7 days or until the turbidity matches that of a McFarland no. 1 standard. Dilute the culture to 10^{-3} and 10^{-5} in sterile saline or broth for inoculation of two sets of drug plates.

Performance of the indirect test

Inoculate each of the two dilutions on identical sets of drug plates. Incubation is generally carried out at 35 to 37°C in an atmosphere of 5 to 10% CO_2 except for species with an optimal growth temperature that differs from this, such as *Mycobacterium marinum*. Incubation under an increased CO_2 atmosphere does not have a detrimental effect on the antimycobacterial drugs tested routinely in 7H10 medium. Rather, improved growth of drug-resistant tubercle bacilli may result in larger colonies on control medium and drug-containing media, but interpretation of the test is the same. Read and record results as described above for the direct test.

An alternative method for the indirect test has been used routinely for more than 15 years by the Veterans Administration Reference Laboratory for Tuberculosis and Other Mycobacterial Diseases, West Haven, Conn. This procedure has been shown in a blind study to give results that rate among the highest in comparability and reproducibility according to the majority findings of other large mycobacteriology laboratories in the United States (R. C. Good, G. M. Cauthen, C. L. Woodley, G. D. Kelley, and J. O. Kilburn, Abstr. Annu. Meet. Am. Soc. Microbiol. 1984, U5, p. 87). This method differs in that only one set of plates is used in performance of the susceptibility test and a more dilute starting inoculum is used. Inocula are prepared from fresh isolates of *M. tuberculosis* by culturing in 7H9 broth as described above. A portion of a 5- to 7-day liquid culture is added to a tube of sterile 7H9 medium to obtain a barely turbid suspension (equivalent to a McFarland standard adjusted to measure approximately 0.06 optical density at 580 nm, or equal in turbidity to 0.03 ml of 1% anhydrous barium chloride in 9.97 ml of 1% sulfuric acid). Dilutions of 10^{-2} and 10^{-4} are made in 7H9 for one set of drug plates containing two drug-free controls. One control quadrant and all drug-containing quadrants are inoculated from a capillary pipette with 3 drops of the heavier 10^{-2} dilution. The second control quadrant is inoculated with 3 drops of the 10^{-4} dilution. The rest of the procedure is unchanged.

If the test is performed properly, there should be 2+ to 3+ growth on the 10^{-2} control and isolated colonies on the 10^{-4} control. (If confluent growth is present, an adjustment should be made in the standard by which inocula are prepared.) Growth on the drug quadrants is compared with the number of colonies on the 10^{-4} control. Since the population inoculated on the 10^{-4} control quadrant is 1% of that on the drug quadrants, greater or less than 1% is readily apparent in most cases. If there is no growth or the amount of growth is less in the presence of the drug, the organism is susceptible. However, if the extent of growth on a drug quadrant is equal to or greater than that observed on the second, more dilute control, then the organism is resistant to that level of the test drug.

Laboratory report of drug susceptibility test results for *M. tuberculosis* complex

The report should contain the following information: (i) type of test (direct or indirect), (ii) amount of growth on the control medium, (iii) amount of growth on each drug medium, and (iv) percentage of bacilli resistant to the drug.

When two or more dilutions of inoculum are planted in replicate on both control and drug-containing media, a more precise quantitation of the proportion of bacilli resistant to a given drug is possible. At least one dilution must yield isolated, countable colonies from which the percentage can be calculated by the following formula:

$$\frac{\text{no. of colonies on the drug}}{\text{no. of colonies on the control}} \times 100 = \%\ \text{resistance}$$

In the example shown in Table 4, 12% of the organisms are resistant to INH at 0.2 μg/ml. However, if only one set of plates is inoculated as described for the disk method, results should be reported as susceptible or >1% resistant (Table 5).

Reference strains for quality control

Reference strains of known susceptibility patterns should be tested each time a new batch of test medium is prepared. If media are stored in the refrigerator, test them at least weekly while they are in use to ensure stability. The H37Rv strain of *M. tuberculosis*, which is susceptible to all standard antituberculosis agents at recommended test concentrations, is used in most laboratories. A second strain that is resistant to two or more of the commonly used drugs, e.g., INH and RMP, should also be tested. Reference strains are available from the American Type Culture Collection (12301 Parklawn Drive, Rockville, MD 20852-1776). The H37Rv strain is ATCC 27294. Mutants of H37Rv selected for in vitro resistance to single and multiple drugs are also available; however, these strains are resistant to very high concentrations (50 to 1,000 μg/ml) and may not be suitable for quality control purposes. In-house isolates with verified low levels of resistance to one or more drugs may be maintained as additional reference strains.

These strains may be subcultured in broth to provide 1-ml test samples sufficient for a period of several months to a year. Freeze them at −70°C. For quality control tests, a single tube can be thawed and diluted in the same manner as clinical specimens (Table 2), so

TABLE 4. Reporting of results for *M. tuberculosis* complex: example 1

Drug	Concn (μg/ml)	Growth on:		% Resistance
		10^{-2}	10^{-4}	
Control		4+	150c[a]	
INH	0.2	1+	18c	12[b]
EMB	5.0	0	0	0
RMP	1.0	0	0	0

[a] c, Colonies.
[b] 18 colonies/150 colonies × 100 = 12%.

TABLE 5. Reporting of results for *M. tuberculosis* complex: example 2

Drug	Concn (μg/ml)	Growth on:		% Resistant
		10^{-2}	10^{-4}	
Control		3+	30c[a]	
INH	0.2	1+		>1
EMB	5.0	0		
RMP	1.0	0		

[a] c, Colonies.

that the lower dilution will give 200 to 300 colonies on the control medium, and a 1:10 dilution of this will give about 20 to 30 colonies.

DRUG SUSCEPTIBILITY TESTING OF SLOWLY GROWING NONTUBERCULOUS MYCOBACTERIA

Mycobacteria other than *M. tuberculosis* and *M. bovis*, the "nontuberculous mycobacteria," are ubiquitous in the environment, and some species are more likely than others to be disease related. Therefore, before any decisions can be made regarding which drugs to use in treatment, the identity of the recovered species and its pathogenic potential must be known. The laboratory performing the necessary identification, and drug studies if deemed appropriate, should be proficient at identifying all recognized species of mycobacteria (level III or CAP extent 4) (1, 14, 21). Since drug susceptibility testing of nontuberculous mycobacteria is not well defined at this time, tests should be carried out in large or reference-type facilities with enough practical experience to be aware of the pitfalls and limitations of current procedures.

Susceptibility tests for these organisms are routinely performed in much the same way as those for tubercle bacilli, using the conventional agar-based proportion method. This method, which is the gold standard for tuberculosis, as well as the drug levels used and often the drugs per se have been challenged in recent years. Under these test conditions, whereas wild-type strains of tubercle bacilli are susceptible, other mycobacteria are more resistant. The concentrations of antituberculosis drugs tested against nontuberculous mycobacteria in 7H10 medium are usually the same as those shown in clinical trials for tuberculosis to be compatible with therapeutic success, but with the addition of some higher concentrations (5 μg/ml for INH, 10 μg/ml for EMB, and 5 μg/ml for RMP). However, similar controlled clinical studies for other mycobacterioses have not been done. The same proportion of resistant bacilli might also be used in interpreting results, but there is no clinical basis for this practice. In any case, an organism is usually either susceptible or frankly resistant. It should be noted that nontuberculous mycobacteria as a group are resistant to PZA, and in vitro susceptibility tests should not be done.

According to ATS, disease produced by nontuberculous mycobacteria falls into three categories: disease that is amenable to treatment with antituberculosis drugs; disease that is difficult to treat; and, apart from the latter, disease that should be considered for treatment with other antimicrobial drugs (2).

Mycobacterium kansasii is an example of a species that responds favorably to treatment with a combination of antituberculosis drugs, particularly RMP-containing regimens. This organism is often susceptible in vitro to RMP, ETA, CS, and frequently EMB (9, 44). There may also be a degree of susceptibility to higher concentrations of INH, SM, and some of the other conventional drugs. In untreated cases, the predictability of these susceptibility results is such that routine testing is not necessary (2); if the test is performed, it appears that selection of chemotherapeutic agents can be guided by in vitro tests using the conventional method.

Other species included in this category are *M. marinum*, *M. szulgai*, and *M. xenopi*. Disease due to *M. marinum* is usually self-limiting. If treatment is considered and susceptibility tests are requested, the tests must be performed at the optimal growth temperature of the organism, 32 to 33°C. Most strains are resistant to INH and PZA, moderately resistant to SM, but susceptible to RMP, EMB, and the secondary drugs. Cutaneous disease has been treated with antituberculosis drugs as well as other antibacterial agents, including minocycline, doxycycline, and trimethoprim-sulfamethoxazole (TMP-SMX) (44). Clinical response is difficult to evaluate because of the high rate of spontaneous remission and the lack of control studies. As with other mycobacteria, susceptibility tests are complicated by the rapid breakdown of some antimicrobial agents, such as the tetracyclines, relative to the growth rate of the organism on a solid medium. Susceptibility testing for *M. marinum* is not required for most cases.

M. xenopi and *M. szulgai* are only slightly more resistant than *M. tuberculosis* to most of the antimycobacterial drugs. Since strain-to-strain variations in results are common, susceptibility studies may be helpful.

Chronic pulmonary disease due to MAC (*M. avium* and *M. intracellulare*) is the most important treatment problem associated with nontuberculous mycobacteria. Nearly all MAC strains are resistant in vitro to some extent to the commonly used antimycobacterial agents. The reason for this resistance is not certain, but recent studies have shown that multidrug resistance in these organisms may be due to a permeability barrier at the cell wall level (28).

At present, treatment regimens are chosen empirically, and the general consensus is that drug susceptibility testing of MAC strains is only rarely helpful in determining the clinical management of disease caused by these organisms (2). Nonetheless, general practice has been to select agents to which there is in vitro susceptibility whenever possible. Although most MAC strains are highly resistant to antimycobacterial agents, variations do exist between strains from different patients and between strains from an individual patient. These are usually reproducible differences. Repeated subculture before testing should be avoided for all species; this procedure is especially important for MAC since, with passage, the thin, transparent colony (commonly drug-resistant) forms tend to become smooth, domed, and opaque, with an associated change to greater in vitro susceptibility.

The fact that some patients with established MAC pulmonary disease do improve with multiple drug chemotherapy (19) suggests the possibility of additive or synergistic activity among combined drugs. These studies are beyond the scope of most clinical laboratories.

Moreover, although in vitro synergism has been demonstrated (17, 46), there is as yet no clear clinical evidence linking such drug interactions to the outcome of therapy in patients.

Since "standard" therapy is far from satisfactory, with cure rates of only about 50%, the search for more effective drugs is ongoing. Among those antimicrobial agents that show activity in the conventional 7H10 agar method and in various broth media are rifabutin, clofazimine, ciprofloxacin and other fluorinated quinolones, and some of the sulfonamides (8, 18, 20). Clofazimine has long been used in the treatment of leprosy. Rifabutin, a rifamycin derivative initially designated as ansamycin LM 427, is a promising investigational drug for mycobacterial diseases that are resistant to treatment with standard regimens. Conflicting reports about the in vitro activity of some drugs for MAC are related to the use of a variety of methods and media and, in some studies, too few strains of recent isolates for valid results. Mycobacteria are frequently more susceptible to various drugs in broth than in solid media.

At this writing, the first multicenter, randomized clinical trial for the treatment of MAC pulmonary disease is in progress under the sponsorship of CDC to compare the efficacy of rifabutin in combination with INH, EMB, and SM with a regimen using RMP in place of rifabutin. Standard susceptibility tests in 7H10 agar medium are a part of the protocol.

Other species in this highly resistant category include *Mycobacterium scrofulaceum* and *M. simiae*. The rapidly growing mycobacteria are discussed in a section to follow.

RADIOMETRIC TESTING

Radiometric Drug Susceptibility Testing of *M. tuberculosis*

In the early 1970s, several methods of susceptibility testing utilizing radiometric techniques and various labeled substrates were described for mycobacteria. In 1977, Middlebrook and associates reported the formulation of 7H12 liquid medium containing [1-^{14}C]palmitic acid, which could be used to detect small numbers of viable units of tubercle bacilli within a relatively short time (26). Growth was determined by measuring in an automatable ion chamber system the metabolic release of labeled CO_2 from the fatty acid substrate. Further development and the introduction of a special "TB hood" for the BACTEC 460 instrument when used for mycobacteriology quickly led to the application of radiometric techniques for detection, identification, and drug susceptibility testing of mycobacteria. The 460 instrument with TB hood for quantitating the amount of radioactive CO_2 produced is available commercially (Becton Dickinson Diagnostic Instrument Systems, Towson, MD 21204).

The first of several cooperative studies to evaluate indirect radiometric susceptibility testing of *M. tuberculosis* against primary antituberculosis drugs was carried out with CDC (34). One of the participating laboratories used an inoculum adjusted so that a 1% threshold could be the determinant of resistance. Not surprisingly, the results correlated better overall with those of the conventional method used by CDC as a reference standard. However, although the CO_2 procedure showed good agreement for cultures that CDC had interpreted as susceptible (with the exception of RMP), the level of agreement for resistant cultures was considerably less. The most obvious problems were with SM and EMB. Subsequent studies brought refinements in methodology and reports of excellent overall agreement between the methods (22, 29, 33). These findings were based on studies that included large numbers of susceptible strains. Any discrepancies between radiometric and agar-based methods were due almost exclusively to failure of the BACTEC procedure to detect resistance found by conventional tests. An extensive comparison carried out with a high proportion of resistant strains showed that these differences could be reduced by adjusting the recommended concentrations of drugs used in the BACTEC (12, 13; J. E. Hawkins and W. M. Gross, Program Abstr. 23rd Intersci. Conf. Antimicrob. Agents Chemother., abstr. no. 1045, 1983). This evaluation demonstrated that SM at 2 μg/ml provides an appropriate screening level in both methods. A change in the single 4-μg/ml SM concentration, recommended commercially for the BACTEC, to 6 μg/ml significantly improved correlation with 10 μg/ml in the 7H10 method. Although the suggested BACTEC concentration for EMB was 10 μg/ml, which inhibits almost all strains, the study showed that 2.5 μg/ml in radiometric tests corresponds well with 5 μg/ml for strains resistant by the conventional method. These findings were confirmed (32, 45), and modifications in concentrations for these two drugs are included in the BACTEC TB System Product and Procedure Manual, April 1988.

Since the introduction of radiometric susceptibility testing, comparative results in published reports have shown an overall agreement in excess of 90% when INH concentrations of 0.2 and 1 μg/ml were used in both methods. However, a problem was noted in a reference laboratory that performed BACTEC drug susceptibility tests in parallel with 7H10 conventional tests against more than 2,000 recent isolates of tubercle bacilli. As the cumulative number of INH-resistant strains studied increased, it became apparent that the sensitivity of the radiometric method, i.e., its ability to detect resistance, was unacceptable at the recommended concentration of 0.2 μg/ml (J. E. Hawkins, W. M. Gross, T. D'Aquila, and F. Vadney, Abstr. Annu. Meet. Am. Soc. Microbiol. 1988, U46, p. 140). These discrepancies were found to be due in large part, but not entirely, to strains that were resistant to 0.2 μg and susceptible to 1 μg of INH per ml in 7H10 medium. Except for the addition of radioactive palmitate, the 7H12 or BACTEC 12B medium is not unlike the Dubos and Middlebrook liquid media used in initial studies with INH in 1952, when MICs of 0.02 to 0.05 μg/ml were reported for tubercule bacilli (24). MICs in the same range have now been demonstrated for this drug in BACTEC 12B medium (23; J. P. Libonati, N. M. Hooper, S. H. Siddiqi, J. F. Baker, and M. E. Carter, Program Abstr. 28th Intersci. Conf. Antimicrob. Agents Chemother., abstr. no. 1215, 1988). Based on these values and in order to detect resistance more accurately, the recommended concentration for INH using the BACTEC TB System was recently lowered from 0.2 to 0.1 μg/ml (manual insert dated January 1989). With this latest adjustment, radiometric susceptibility tests for *M. tuberculosis*, when performed properly with appropriate concentrations of the four primary drugs (INH, SM, EMB, and RMP), are as reliable as these tests by the conventional proportion method.

Basic principles of the procedure

The medium used for studies with mycobacteria in the BACTEC instrument is an enriched Middlebrook broth containing 4 μCi of ^{14}C-labeled palmitic acid per vial that is referred to as 7H12 or BACTEC 12B medium (available commercially only from Becton Dickinson Diagnostic Instrument Systems [BDDIS], catalog no. 02004). Mycobacteria metabolize this fatty acid and produce $^{14}CO_2$. When 7H12 medium vials with growth are tested on the BACTEC 460 instrument, the $^{14}CO_2$ released into the headspace above the medium is automatically aspirated and replaced with 5 to 10% unlabeled CO_2 in air, thereby maintaining the recommended CO_2 atmosphere. Radioactivity of the labeled CO_2 is determined quantitatively and is a measure of the rate and amount of growth in the vial. These numbers are designated the growth index (GI) and are displayed and printed out along with identifying rack and bottle numbers. When an inhibitory agent is incorporated in the medium, inhibition of growth results in a reduction in the amount of $^{14}CO_2$ produced, indicated by a decline or only a small increase in the daily GI output compared with the drug-free control. If the test organism is resistant, little or no suppression occurs.

In radiometric tests, determination of 1% resistance is facilitated by using a control inoculum that contains only 1% of the population (i.e., a 1:100 dilution) used to inoculate drug-containing vials. If the daily GI increase, or ΔGI, in a drug vial is equal to or is greater than the ΔGI in the control vial, the organism is resistant to the drug. Conversely, the daily GI increase for a susceptible organism is higher in the control than that in the drug vial.

Radiometric drug tests may be performed by both direct and indirect methods. The inoculum for the BACTEC indirect drug susceptibility test may be prepared from a primary isolation culture in a 12B vial or from a solid agar- or egg-based medium culture. If the inoculum is prepared from a BACTEC vial, once the primary isolation culture becomes positive, the BACTEC NAP TB Differentiation Test should be carried out along with the susceptibility test (see chapter 34). In addition, a 7H10 or 7H11 agar medium plate should be streaked from the specimen concentrate to determine colony types and the possibility of mixed mycobacterial species or contamination. It is also desirable to inoculate an egg-based medium for additional tests if needed. When the primary isolation culture reaches a GI of 500 to 800, the drug susceptibility test vials can be inoculated, but if the NAP test result is not available at this time, it is advisable to wait until that test is completed. Susceptibility test results should not be reported without at least a preliminary identification of *M. tuberculosis* complex or mycobacteria other than tubercle bacilli. The radiometric susceptibility procedure has not yet been standardized for nontuberculous mycobacteria and is not recommended. These precautions will help to avoid the performance of unnecessary tests for these organisms. The inoculated plates should also be examined at this time for colony types that might suggest certain species or alert the microbiologist that colonies of *M. tuberculosis* may be mixed with another organism that could have metabolized the substrate, masked the presence of tubercle bacilli, and produced erroneous results.

Drug solutions

Stock solutions of the primary drugs may be prepared in-house as described above for conventional tests; lyophilized preparations of these agents are available commercially (BDDIS, catalog no. 02102). Working solutions are prepared to give the concentration required when 0.1 ml is added to a vial containing 4 ml of BACTEC 12B medium. The procedure recommended by the supplier describes only one concentration of each drug for susceptibility testing in the BACTEC: 0.1 μg/ml for INH, 6.0 μg/ml for SM, 2.0 μg/ml for RMP, and 7.5 μg/ml for EMB. However, strains of tubercle bacilli that are resistant only to low concentrations of SM (2 μg/ml) in conventional tests may appear susceptible unless a screening level of 2 μg/ml is tested in the BACTEC system. Although the recommended concentration for EMB was reduced from 10 to 7.5 μg/ml to correspond with the conventional method results, *M. tuberculosis* is very rarely resistant to EMB at 10 μg/ml; therefore, use of this level is generally unnecessary. A concentration of 2.5 μg/ml in BACTEC 12B compares well with 5 μg/ml in 7H10 and would provide more meaningful data. BACTEC results with either 1 or 2 μg of RMP per ml are essentially the same. Equivalent drug concentrations for radiometric and conventional methods are listed in Table 6.

Radiometric Tests with Secondary Antituberculosis Drugs and with PZA

When resistance is present to one or more of the primary drugs, tests with additional antimicrobial agents may be requested for *M. tuberculosis*. With use of the technique applied for primary drugs except CS, tests with the so-called secondary drugs correlate well with results in 7H10 agar medium: ETA and KM at the same concentrations (5 μg/ml) in both methods, and CM at 5 and 10 μg/ml in 7H10 and 12B, respectively. CS at a concentration of 50 μg/ml in radiometric tests failed to suppress the metabolism of the labeled substrate and the production of CO_2 by strains that were susceptible to 25 μg/ml in 7H10 medium (W. M. Gross and J. E. Hawkins, Abstr. Annu. Meet. Am. Soc. Microbiol. 1986, C378, p. 391). These results, of necessity, were obtained with predominantly susceptible strains. To evaluate the sensitivity of the BACTEC method, strains resistant to the secondary drugs had been sought from laboratories

TABLE 6. Equivalent concentrations of drugs in conventional and radiometric susceptibility tests

Drug	Concn (μg/ml) in:	
	7H10 medium	BACTEC 12B medium
INH	0.2	0.1
	1.0	0.4
SM	2.0	2.0
	10.0	6.0
EMB	5.0	2.5
	10.0	7.5
RMP	1.0	2.0

in the United States and Europe with little success. Therefore, it seems apparent that susceptibility tests with secondary drugs by either method are of limited value.

A radiometric method for testing susceptibility of *M. tuberculosis* to PZA that uses BACTEC 12B medium adjusted to a pH of 5.9 to 6.0 has been proposed (30, 31). Higher concentrations of PZA are used than in the conventional method, which is performed with pH 5.5 7H10 medium. Results in premarket trials have been promising, and a BACTEC PZA test medium is expected to be generally available in the near future.

Inocula from solid medium cultures

Preparation is the same as for conventional tests except that a special diluting fluid is recommended. Its purpose is to ensure that the liquid used to prepare the suspension and adjust the turbidity contains no nutrients that could compete with the labeled substrate in 12B medium, thereby reducing the amount of $^{14}CO_2$ produced in the test. The BACTEC diluting fluid is composed of fatty acid-free bovine serum albumin and Tween 80 in distilled or deionized water, adjusted to pH 6.8 and sterilized by membrane filtration (available commercially in 9.9-ml quantities; BDDIS, catalog no. 02104).

For tests to be read daily, the inoculum should be adjusted to a McFarland no. 1 standard. If a "nonweekend" schedule of reading is to be followed (12), make a suspension equivalent to a McFarland no. 0.5 standard. Vials should be tested on the BACTEC instrument before inoculation to establish an atmosphere of 5 to 10% CO_2 and as a check on sterility of the medium. Do not use vials with an initial reading of 20 or more. Prepare drug media at this time by using a syringe to add 0.1 ml of each drug solution to individual 12B medium vials. Arrange the vials into sets of one drug-free control vial and a vial of each drug concentration. Inoculate 0.1 ml of the mycobacterial suspension into each of the drug vials. For the control vial, the suspension must be diluted 1:100 by adding 0.1 ml to 9.9 ml of special diluting fluid. Then 0.1 ml of this 1% dilution is added to the control vial.

Safety precautions. Use a disposable tuberculin syringe with a permanently attached needle, wear rubber gloves, and perform all steps involving preparation of inocula and inoculation of vials in a biological safety cabinet.

Incubation and interpretation

Incubation must be at 37 ± 1°C. Using a daily schedule, test vials are read on the BACTEC instrument at 24-h ± 2-h intervals for a minimum of 4 days and until a GI of 30 or more is reached in the control vial. A more convenient schedule for laboratories with limited weekend coverage may be to use an alternate schedule in which tests are inoculated on Friday and test readings begin on Monday. This reading represents an accumulation of $^{14}CO_2$ and is disregarded, but with it the proper unlabeled CO_2 atmosphere is restored and a base line is established for a 24-h reading on Tuesday. The vials must be tested for at least 5 days from the inoculation date. No other licenses with the schedule should be taken.

The difference in GI values from one day to the next is designated ΔGI. When the control vials reach a GI of 30 or more after a minimum of 4 days (daily) or 5 days (nonweekend), the results of the test should be interpreted as follows. If the ΔGI is less in the drug vial than in the control vial, the organism is susceptible. If the ΔGI in the presence of drug exceeds the ΔGI in the control, then >1% of the population is resistant. The example shown in Table 7 represents typical data from an indirect susceptibility test for an INH-resistant strain of *M. tuberculosis* isolated on solid medium.

Inocula from processed specimens

If a clinical specimen is positive for AFB on microscopic examination, the number of bacilli present is usually sufficient to perform a direct susceptibility test in 12B medium. The procedure is basically the same as for radiometric isolation techniques and indirect tests. Major differences are (i) the addition of an antibiotic supplement (PANTA Plus; BDDIS, catalog no. 04764) to control and drug vials to suppress any viable normal flora that may be present in the concentrated specimen and (ii) a lower dilution of the inoculum for the control vial, 1:10 instead of 1:100. Unlike the indirect test, the direct susceptibility test usually takes more than a week for results (average, 10 to 12 days).

For complete details of these procedures, the reader is referred to the BACTEC TB Systems Product and Procedure Manual available from Becton Dickinson Diagnostic Instrument Systems, Towson, MD 21204.

Quality control

When radiometric techniques are introduced in the laboratory, tests by the standard 7H10 agar method should be performed for comparison until personnel gain experience with the new procedure. A daily performance test should be done by using the kit supplied with the BACTEC 460 instrument. Susceptible and resistant reference strains of *M. tuberculosis* should be tested each time radiometric tests are performed on patient strains (refer to the section on conventional susceptibility tests). It is also advisable to test sample vials of new lots of 12B medium for sterility and ability to support growth of mycobacteria. Before being placed into use, new lots of lyophilized drug or freshly prepared in-house stock solutions from drug powders should be tested for activity.

Radiometric Susceptibility Testing of Mycobacteria Other than *M. tuberculosis*

With proper adjustment of inoculum, good correlation of conventional and BACTEC susceptibility results

TABLE 7. Example of data from an indirect susceptibility test for INH-resistant *M. tuberculosis* isolated on solid medium

Drug	GI on indicated day				ΔGI	Result
	1	2	3	4		
Control	5	11	23	64	41	
SM	41	20	10	11	+1	Susceptible
INH	45	95	238	500	+262	Resistant
EMB	70	96	94	80	−14	Susceptible
RMP	39	19	8	8	0	Susceptible

with certain drugs can be demonstrated for some species. With the exception of SM, there is good agreement between the two methods at standard concentrations of the primary drugs for *M. kansasii* and *M. marinum* (Hawkins and Gross, 23rd ICAAC). MAC strains are generally resistant to the primary antituberculosis drugs in conventional tests but are susceptible to all but INH at concentrations recommended for tubercle bacilli in 12B medium. The clinical relevance of in vitro susceptibility results by either method is uncertain at this time for nontuberculous mycobacteria, particularly those species in the highly resistant category based on conventional tests (2).

There is an obvious need for well-defined criteria of susceptibility for in vitro tests with nontuberculous mycobacteria. This can come about only through correlation of in vitro test results with clinical and bacteriologic response to treatment. It has been suggested that determination of MICs in liquid media, either radiometrically or by using macroscopic growth endpoints, may yield more relevant information for chemotherapy of MAC disease and other mycobacterioses than do conventional methods (15, 16, 23, 40). Ultimately, prospective clinical studies are required for MAC disease in order to resolve the dilemma now faced by microbiologists in the routine laboratory who are attempting to provide meaningful susceptibility test results.

DRUG SUSCEPTIBILITY TESTING OF RAPIDLY GROWING MYCOBACTERIA

The rapidly growing mycobacteria are ubiquitous environmental organisms usually present in soil and water. Clinical disease includes posttraumatic skin and soft tissue infections; nosocomial infection, especially after catheter insertions, augmentation mammaplasty, or cardiac bypass surgery; and chronic pulmonary infections.

Despite the presence in the environment of numerous species, 95% of clinical disease is caused by *Mycobacterium fortuitum* or *M. chelonae*. The former has three biovariants (*peregrinum*, *fortuitum*, and an unnamed third biovariant complex), and the latter includes two subspecies (*abscessus* and *chelonae*). Infrequently other organisms (species) such as *Mycobacterium smegmatis*, *M. chelonae*-like organisms, or pigmented rapid growers may also cause clinical disease.

These species are readily grown on standard mycobacterial media as well as 5% sheep blood and chocolate agar media. Most strains grow well at 35°C, but isolates of *M. chelonae* subsp. *chelonae* grow poorly at this temperature and grow best at 28 to 30°C. They stain with routine acid-fast stains but less well than do members of the *M. tuberculosis* complex.

The pathogenic rapidly growing mycobacteria are resistant to achievable serum and tissue levels of all first-line antituberculosis drugs with the exception of *M. smegmatis*, which is EMB susceptible. Given these findings, susceptibility testing with these agents is to be discouraged.

A number of antibacterial agents are active against the pathogenic rapidly growing mycobacteria and have been shown to be clinically useful. These agents are amikacin, cefoxitin, doxycycline, erythromycin, sulfonamides (including TMP-SMX), and ciprofloxacin. Another group of agents has good in vitro activity against some subgroups of rapidly growing mycobacteria, but reports of clinical results are limited or nonexistent. These agents include tobramycin (primarily against *M. chelonae* subsp. *chelonae*), gentamicin, vancomycin, imipenem, cefmetazole, minocycline, and amoxicillin-clavulanic acid (2:1 ratio).

Three susceptibility methods have been used in the clinical laboratory: broth microdilution, agar disk elution, and disk diffusion (41). None of these methods has been addressed or approved by the National Committee for Clinical Laboratory Standards (NCCLS) for testing of the rapidly growing mycobacteria.

Broth microdilution method

Preparation of test plates. Conventional broth microdilution tests may be performed in a manner similar to that described in chapter 110, with modifications for the growth requirements of the rapidly growing mycobacteria. Cation-supplemented Mueller-Hinton broth will adequately support the growth of these organisms. Prepare the plates by using twofold antimicrobial dilutions, with the usual special precautions for imipenem and clavulanic acid because of their great instability in solution. Recommended drugs and their concentrations are shown in Table 8. Testing of a sulfonamide alone such as SMX is usually done, since isolates are highly resistant to TMP and use of the combination adds little or nothing to MICs obtained with the sulfonamide alone except for the *M. chelonae*-like organisms (37).

Performance of the test. For preparation of the inoculum, organisms are scraped from the surface of an agar plate and suspended in Mueller-Hinton broth. The use of 0.02% Tween 80 or sterile glass beads helps to disperse or break up the organisms into a finer suspension. The tube can then be incubated at 30°C in room air until an adequate organism concentration is present or enough organisms can be added initially to match the optical density of a 0.5 McFarland standard (approximately 10^7 to 10^8 CFU/ml) (37). The inoculum is then diluted such that the final inoculum in the wells is 10^5 CFU/ml. The dilution of the standardized inoculum will vary according to the inoculation system used.

The plates are then sealed in plastic bags and incubated at 30°C in a moisturized room air incubator for 3 days. Some *M. chelonae* subsp. *abscessus* and many *M. chelonae* subsp. *chelonae* isolates will require incubation for an additional 1 to 3 days to provide adequate growth.

The plates are read under standard light conditions. Except for the sulfonamides, read the endpoint as the lowest concentration that inhibits visible growth. For sulfonamide preparations, the endpoint is the concentration that inhibits 80% or more of the growth when compared with the control well. For erythromycin, a very fine trailing endpoint is ignored if marked inhibition of good control growth has occurred.

Unique susceptibility breakpoints for rapidly growing mycobacteria have not been chosen except for cefoxitin (38), for which an MIC of 32 μg/ml is used. Other breakpoints (Table 8) are those of the NCCLS for bacterial species tested by broth microdilution, including SMX (27). This is a change for the latter, for which a higher breakpoint was initially recommended (38).

Quality control procedures. Quality control of the plates is easily performed by using the NCCLS-recom-

TABLE 8. Recommended drugs and drug concentrations for susceptibility testing of the rapidly growing mycobacteria

Drug	MIC breakpoint[a] (μg/ml)	Drug concn recommended for testing			
		Disk elution			Broth microdilution (concn, μg/ml)
		Disk content (μg)	No. of disks/5 ml of medium	Final concn (μg/ml)	
Amikacin	32	30	1, 5	6, 30	0.5–64
Tobramycin	8	10	4	8	0.5–32
Cefoxitin	32	30	5	30	2–128
Cefmetazole	32	30	5	30	2–128
Imipenem	8	10	4	8	0.5–32
Erythromycin	4	—[b]	—[b]	—[b]	0.5–16
Doxycycline[c]	8	30	1	6	0.25–32
SMX	32	—[d]	—[d]	—[d]	1–128
TMP-SMX	32	25	6	30	—[e]
Ciprofloxacin	2	5	2	2	0.063–8

[a] NCCLS moderately susceptible breakpoints for bacterial species that grow aerobically (1) except for cefoxitin, for which resistance is defined as an MIC of >32 rather than >16 μg/ml.
[b] Erythromycin cannot be tested by this method (35).
[c] Doxycycline and minocycline are interchangeable.
[d] Not commercially available.
[e] Equivalent results obtained with SMX alone.

mended bacterial strains: *S. aureus* ATCC 29213, *P. aeruginosa* ATCC 27853, and *E. coli* ATCC 35218 (the last for amoxicillin-clavulanic acid). The type strain of *M. fortuitum* ATCC 6841 can also be used. The MIC range for this strain (modified from reference 38) is shown in Table 9. Quality control testing of the plates should be done on preparation and at least weekly thereafter when testing is being performed.

Problems and sources of error. As with any broth susceptibility test, contamination with a second organism can occur and can be difficult to detect, especially with slow-growing species such as the mycobacteria. False resistance of *M. fortuitum* isolates to the sulfonamides may occur in up to 20% of susceptibility tests if too heavy an inoculum is used. When resistance appears to be present with isolates of this species, the test should be repeated, with careful attention to the inoculum. Trailing endpoints with erythromycin are common, and no change in technique has yet resolved this problem. Vancomycin cannot be tested in broth, since isolates of *M. fortuitum* that have susceptible MICs in agar are resistant in broth (35). Commercially prepared microdilution trays can be used, but they include too low a top concentration of cefoxitin (16 μg/ml), and tetracycline rather than doxycycline or minocycline is included. (The relationship of tetracycline MICs to doxycycline or minocycline MICs has not been established; generally, the MICs for the latter two analogs are two to four times lower than for the parent compound [39].)

Agar disk elution method

Preparation of test plates. The agar disk elution method uses commercial susceptibility disks as the drug source and Mueller-Hinton agar. Because isolates of *M. chelonae* do not grow well on this medium, it must be supplemented with 10% OADC. This enrichment appears to have no effect on MICs.

Round-well tissue culture plates that contain six 3.5- by 1.0-cm round wells (Linbro, Flow Laboratories, Inc., McLean, Va.) are preferred. Traditional 100- by 15-mm quadrant plates with four compartments used for susceptibility testing of *M. tuberculosis* can be used, but greater care must be taken to get even drug distribution because of their irregular shape.

To prepare the plates, the susceptibility disks are placed in the center of the wells and then covered with 0.5 ml of OADC. After 60 s, 4.5 ml of melted agar is added. The disks and OADC are swirled with a wooden stick, and then the agar is allowed to harden. As soon as the medium is firmly solidified, the plates should be refrigerated.

The plates can be stored in a refrigerator for a short period of time, but the instability of the tetracyclines, imipenem, and amoxicillin-clavulanic acid severely

TABLE 9. Susceptibility results of 13 antimicrobial agents against the recommended control strain *M. fortuitum* ATCC 6841 (type strain)

Antimicrobial agent	MIC (μg/ml)			
	Broth microdilution[a]		Disk elution (Mueller-Hinton agar)[b]	
	Range	Mode	Concn	Result[c]
Amikacin	≤0.25–1.0	0.5	6	S
Gentamicin	4–16	8	8	S, R
Tobramycin	8–32	16	8	S, R
Kanamycin	2–16	8	30	S
Doxycycline	≤0.25–4	≤0.25	6	S
Cefoxitin	16–32	16	30	S
Cefmetazole	4–16	8	30	S
Imipenem	1–4	4	8	S
Amoxicillin-clavulanic acid (2:1)	8/4–32/16	8/4	—[d]	—[d]
SMX	2–16	2	20	S
TMP-SMX	—[d]	—[d]	30	S
Erythromycin	>16	>16	—[e]	—[e]
Ciprofloxacin	≤0.063–0.25	≤0.063	2	S

[a] Modified from reference 38.
[b] Modified from reference 35.
[c] S, Susceptible; R, resistant.
[d] No results available.
[e] Cannot be tested by this method (35).

limits storage time. Although studies have not been done, the plates should be used within 3 days of preparation. For the same reasons, the plates should not be incubated at 35°C either to promote drug diffusion or to check for sterility prior to inoculation.

The plates should not be prepared with Middlebrook 7H10 agar rather than Mueller-Hinton agar. The former has been shown to increase the MICs of several aminoglycosides, including amikacin (39).

Performance of the test. For inoculation, an organism suspension in broth or distilled water that matches the 0.5 McFarland standard is diluted 1:10 and 1:100, and then 10 µl of each of the two adjusted inocula is added to separate sets of plates so as to cover both middle and side areas of the plate. (The use of 100 µl of inocula leads to problems with fluid absorption with freshly prepared plates.) The plates are then covered and incubated at 30°C in a room air incubator for 72 h. As with other susceptibility methods for these species, incubation for an additional 1 to 3 days may be required to obtain good control growth of *M. chelonae*. The inoculum that contains growth of 100 to 500 colonies in the control well without antimicrobial agents is used for evaluation. Susceptibility is defined as no growth for antibiotics and 80% or greater inhibition of colony size for sulfisoxazole or TMP-SMX compared with the control. A very fine residual colony haze in the presence of cefoxitin and erythromycin should be ignored when good control growth is present. The endpoints are usually very sharp with either no growth or growth equivalent to that of the control.

The susceptibility breakpoints by this method are as close to NCCLS values as can be obtained by using the fixed drug concentrations available in commercial disks. One exception is cefoxitin, for which an optimal breakpoint of 32 µg/ml has been chosen for rapidly growing mycobacteria (38) rather than the NCCLS value of 16 µg/ml (27). (The value by disk elution is 30 µg/ml because of the disk content of drug.) The value for amikacin has been raised from initial recommendations (35) because they were found to be too low for many isolates of *M. chelonae* and to bring uniformity to the breakpoints for this drug between NCCLS and methods for testing the rapidly growing mycobacteria.

Quality control procedures. The Mueller-Hinton agar lot and disks can be quality controlled by using standard NCCLS procedures for disk diffusion. Prepared elution plates can be evaluated by using *M. fortuitum* ATCC 6841, which is susceptible to almost all test drugs except erythromycin. Expected results with this strain by the disk elution method in Mueller-Hinton agar are shown in Table 9 (27). One well in each set of plates should remain uninoculated as an agar sterility control.

Problems and sources of error. Because the plates are made fresh, use of a moisturized (high-humidity) incubator often results in failure of absorption of the fluid inoculum. Hence, a routine incubator is preferred. Correlation of results of this method with broth microdilution MICs has been shown to be >90% for doxycycline, cefoxitin, TMP-SMX, and amikacin (35). However, newer drugs such as ciprofloxacin, imipenem, and cefmetazole have not been compared in published data. In addition, the current drug concentrations, chosen to better fit with NCCLS susceptibility breakpoints, are different for some drugs from those initially compared with agar dilution MICs (35). Agar disk elution is unsatisfactory for testing of erythromycin, as almost 90% of isolates that are moderately susceptible in broth (MICs, 1 to 4 µg/ml) will produce small but definite colonies on agar and be interpreted as resistant (35). Broth appears to be the only satisfactory medium for testing this drug. As with broth microdilution, the methods and critical concentrations for agar disk elution are still evolving, and further changes in the future may be required. Given these limitations, this method has proven to be easy to perform with sharp endpoints and is the best method for laboratories that see small numbers of isolates.

Agar disk diffusion method

The first generally used susceptibility method for the rapidly growing mycobacteria was disk diffusion, which was described by several authors in 1979 (39, 43). It has the most number of technical problems and for this reason is no longer recommended as a sole method of testing. The advantage of this method is that it uses a susceptibility method that is widely known and highly standardized. In addition, the media and disks are readily available in the routine microbiology laboratory, and the plates can be made on demand.

The major problems with the method include the fact that the concentrations of cefoxitin and cefmetazole in the disks are too low (30 µg) for testing organisms for which the modal MIC is 32 µg/ml (both *M. fortuitum* and *M. chelonae* for cefoxitin). Hence, only partial or no zones of inhibition by disk are seen with many isolates for which MICs in broth are 16 to 32 µg/ml. The zones of inhibition for amikacin are also small and sometimes only partial for many isolates of *M. chelonae*. (They are substantially smaller than previously reported zone sizes [39, 43] because of the now routine presence of Mg^{2+} and Ca^{2+}.) Double zones with hazy inside growth are seen with sulfizoxazole for all isolates of *M. fortuitum* and with erythromycin for some *M. chelonae* which have susceptible MICs by broth microdilution. It is readily apparent that erythromycin produces only partial growth inhibition with a trailing endpoint that is most noticeable with agar, making exact endpoints difficult if not impossible to establish. Finally, the number of strains tested by disk diffusion and the results compared with those of agar or broth MIC determinations are limited such that clear-cut definitions of "susceptible," "moderately susceptible," and "resistant" are not available.

Since these technical problems are greatest with the disk diffusion method, one of the other two susceptibility methods is preferred for testing of the rapidly growing mycobacteria.

LITERATURE CITED

1. **American Thoracic Society.** 1983. Levels of laboratory services for mycobacterial diseases: official statement of the American Thoracic Society. Am. Rev. Respir. Dis. **128:** 213.
2. **Bailey, W. C., J. B. Bass, J. E. Hawkins, G. P. Kubica, and R. J. Wallace, Jr.** 1984. Drug susceptibility testing for mycobacteria. Am. Thorac. Soc. News **10:**9–10.
3. **Butler, W. R., and J. O. Kilburn.** 1982. Improved method for testing susceptibility of *Mycobacterium tuberculosis* to pyrazinamide. J. Clin. Microbiol. **16:**1106–1109.
4. **Canetti, G., S. Froman, J. Grosset, P. Hauduroy, M. Langerova, H. T. Mahler, G. Meissner, D. A. Mitchison,**

and L. Sula. 1963. Mycobacteria: laboratory methods for testing drug sensitivity and resistance. Bull. WHO **29:**565–578.

5. **Canetti, G., N. Rist, and J. Grosset.** 1963. Mesure de la sensibilite du bacille tuberculeux aux drogues antibacillaires par la methode des proportions. Rev. Tuberc. **27:** 217–272.
6. **David, H. L.** 1971. Fundamentals of drug susceptibility testing in tuberculosis. DHEW publication no. (CDC) 71-2165. Center for Disease Control, Atlanta.
7. **David, H. L.** 1976. Bacteriology of the mycobacterioses. DHEW publication no. (CDC) 76-8316. Center for Disease Control, Atlanta.
8. **Gay, J. D., D. R. DeYoung, and G. D. Roberts.** 1984. In vitro activities of norfloxacin and ciprofloxacin against *Mycobacterium tuberculosis, M. avium* complex, *M. chelonei, M. fortuitum,* and *M. kansasii.* Antimicrob. Agents Chemother. **26:**94–96.
9. **Good, R. C., V. A. Silcox, J. O. Kilburn, and B. D. Plikaytis.** 1985. Identification and drug susceptibility test results for *Mycobacterium* spp. Clin. Microbiol. Newsl. **7:** 133–136.
10. **Griffith, M., M. L. Barrett, H. L. Bodily, and R. M. Wood.** 1967. Drug susceptibility tests for tuberculosis using drug impregnated disks. Am. J. Clin. Pathol. **47:**812–817.
11. **Hawkins, J. E.** 1984. Drug susceptibility testing, p. 177–193. *In* G. P. Kubica and L. G. Wayne (ed.), The mycobacteria, a sourcebook, part A. Marcel Dekker, Inc., New York.
12. **Hawkins, J. E.** 1986. Nonweekend schedule for BACTEC drug susceptibility testing of *Mycobacterium tuberculosis.* J. Clin. Microbiol. **23:**934–937.
13. **Hawkins, J. E.** 1986. Rapid mycobacterial susceptibility tests. Clin. Microbiol. Newsl. **8:**101–104.
14. **Hawkins, J. E., R. C. Good, G. P. Kubica, P. R. J. Gangadharam, H. M. Gruft, K. D. Stottmeier, H. M. Sommers, and L. G. Wayne.** 1983. The levels of service concept in mycobacteriology. Am. Thorac. Soc. News **9:**19–25.
15. **Heifets, L.** 1988. MIC as a quantitative measurement of the susceptibility of *Mycobacterium avium* strains to seven antituberculosis drugs. Antimicrob. Agents Chemother. **32:** 1131–1136.
16. **Heifets, L.** 1988. Qualitative and quantitative drug-susceptibility tests in mycobacteriology. Am. Rev. Respir. Dis. **137:**1217–1222.
17. **Heifets, L. B., M. D. Iseman, and P. J. Lindholm-Levy.** 1988. Combinations of rifampin or rifabutine plus ethambutol against *Mycobacterium avium* complex. Am. Rev. Respir. Dis. **137:**711–715.
18. **Heifets, L. B., and P. J. Lindholm-Levy.** 1987. Bacteriostatic and bactericidal activity of ciprofloxacin and ofloxacin against *Mycobacterium tuberculosis* and *Mycobacterium avium* complex. Tubercle **68:**267–276.
19. **Horsburgh, C. R., Jr., U. G. Mason III, L. B. Heifets, K. Southwick, J. Labrecque, and M. D. Iseman.** 1987. Response to therapy of pulmonary *Mycobacterium avium-intracellulare* infection correlates with results of *in vitro* susceptibility testing. Am. Rev. Respir. Dis. **135:**418–421.
20. **Inderlied, C. B., L. S. Young, and J. K. Yamada.** 1987. Determination of in vitro susceptibility of *Mycobacterium avium* complex isolates to antimycobacterial agents by various methods. Antimicrob. Agents Chemother. **31:**1697–1702.
21. **Kent, P. T., and G. P. Kubica.** 1985. Public health mycobacteriology: a guide for the level III laboratory. Centers for Disease Control, Atlanta.
22. **Laszlo, A., P. Gill, V. Handzel, M. M. Hodgkin, and D. M. Helbecque.** 1983. Conventional and radiometric drug susceptibility testing of *Mycobacterium tuberculosis* complex. J. Clin. Microbiol. **18:**1335–1339.
23. **Lee, C. N., and L. B. Heifets.** 1987. Determination of minimal inhibitory concentrations of antituberculosis drugs by radiometric and conventional methods. Am. Rev. Respir. Dis. **136:**349–352.
24. **Long, E. R.** 1958. The chemistry and chemotherapy of tuberculosis. The Williams & Wilkins Co., Baltimore.
25. **McClatchy, J. K.** 1986. Antimycobacterial drugs: mechanisms of action, drug resistance, susceptibility testing, and assays of activity in biological fluids, p. 181–222. *In* V. Lorian (ed.), Antibiotics in laboratory medicine, 2nd ed. The Williams & Wilkins Co., Baltimore.
26. **Middlebrook, G., Z. Reggiardo, and W. D. Tigertt.** 1977. Automatable radiometric detection of growth of *Mycobacterium tuberculosis* in selective media. Am. Rev. Respir. Dis. **115:**1066–1069.
27. **National Committee for Clinical Laboratory Standards.** 1990. Methods for dilution antimicrobial susceptibility tests for bacteria that grow aerobically—second edition; approved standard. Document M7-A2. National Committee for Clinical Laboratory Standards, Villanova, Pa.
28. **Rastogi, N., C. Frehel, A. Ryter, H. Ohayon, M. Lesourd, and H. L. David.** 1981. Multiple drug resistance in *Mycobacterium avium:* is the wall architecture responsible for the exclusion of antimicrobial agents? Antimicrob. Agents Chemother. **20:**666–677.
29. **Roberts, G. D., N. L. Goodman, L. Heifets, H. W. Larsh, T. H. Lindner, J. K. McClatchy, M. R. McGinnis, S. H. Siddiqi, and P. Wright.** 1983. Evaluation of BACTEC radiometric method for recovery of mycobacteria and drug susceptibility testing of *Mycobacterium tuberculosis* from acid-fast smear-positive specimens. J. Clin. Microbiol. **18:** 689–696.
30. **Salfinger, M., and L. B. Heifets.** 1988. Determination of pyrazinamide MICs for *Mycobacterium tuberculosis* at different pHs by the radiometric method. Antimicrob. Agents Chemother. **32:**1002–1004.
31. **Salfinger, M., L. B. Reller, B. Demchuk, and Z. T. Johnson.** 1989. Rapid radiometric method for pyrazinamide susceptibility testing of *Mycobacterium tuberculosis.* Res. Microbiol. **140:**301–309.
32. **Siddiqi, S. H., J. E. Hawkins, and A. Laszlo.** 1985. Interlaboratory drug susceptibility testing of *Mycobacterium tuberculosis* by a radiometric procedure and two conventional methods. J. Clin. Microbiol. **22:**919–923.
33. **Siddiqi, S. H., J. P. Libonati, and G. Middlebrook.** 1981. Evaluation of a rapid radiometric method for drug susceptibility testing of *Mycobacterium tuberculosis.* J. Clin. Microbiol. **13:**908–912.
34. **Snider, D. E., Jr., R. C. Good, J. O. Kilburn, L. F. Laskowski, Jr., R. H. Lusk, J. J. Marr, Z. Reggiardo, and G. Middlebrook.** 1981. Rapid drug susceptibility testing of *Mycobacterium tuberculosis.* Am. Rev. Respir. Dis. **123:** 402–406.
35. **Stone, M. S., R. J. Wallace, Jr., J. M. Swenson, C. Thornsberry, and L. A. Christensen.** 1983. Agar disk elution method for susceptibility testing of *Mycobacterium marinum* and *Mycobacterium fortuitum* complex to sulfonamides and antibiotics. Antimicrob. Agents Chemother. **24:**486–493.
36. **Strong, B. E., and G. P. Kubica.** 1981. Isolation and identification of *Mycobacterium tuberculosis:* a guide for the level II laboratory. DHHS publication no. (CDC) 81-8390. Centers for Disease Control, Atlanta.
37. **Swenson, J. M., C. Thornsberry, and V. A. Silcox.** 1982. Rapidly growing mycobacteria: testing of susceptibility to 34 antimicrobial agents by broth microdilution. Antimicrob. Agents Chemother. **22:**186–192.
38. **Swenson, J. M., R. J. Wallace, Jr., V. A. Silcox, and C. Thornsberry.** 1985. Antimicrobial susceptibility of five subgroups of *Mycobacterium fortuitum* and *Mycobacterium chelonae.* Antimicrob. Agents Chemother. **28:**807–811.
39. **Wallace, R. J., Jr., J. R. Dalovisio, and G. A. Pankey.** 1979. Disk diffusion testing of susceptibility of *Mycobacterium fortuitum* and *Mycobacterium chelonei* to antibacterial agents. Antimicrob. Agents Chemother. **16:**611–614.
40. **Wallace, R. J., Jr., D. R. Nash, L. C. Steele, and V. Steingrube.** 1986. Susceptibility testing of slowly growing my-

cobacteria by a microdilution MIC method with 7H9 broth. J. Clin. Microbiol. **24:**976–981.

41. **Wallace, R. J., Jr., J. M. Swenson, and V. A. Silcox.** 1985. The rapidly growing mycobacteria: characterization and susceptibility testing. Antimicrob. Newsl. **2:**85–92.
42. **Wayne, L. G., and I. Krasnow.** 1966. Preparation of tuberculosis susceptibility testing mediums by means of impregnated disks. Am. J. Clin. Pathol. **45:**769–771.
43. **Welch, D. F., and M. T. Kelly.** 1979. Antimicrobial susceptibility testing of *Mycobacterium fortuitum* complex. Antimicrob. Agents Chemother. **15:**754–757.
44. **Wolinsky, E.** 1979. Nontuberculous mycobacteria and associated diseases. Am. Rev. Respir. Dis. **119:**107–159.
45. **Woodley, C. L.** 1986. Evaluation of streptomycin and ethambutol concentrations for susceptibility testing of *Mycobacterium tuberculosis* by radiometric and conventional procedures. J. Clin. Microbiol. **23:**385–386.
46. **Zimmer, B. L., D. R. DeYoung, and G. D. Roberts.** 1982. In vitro synergistic activity of ethambutol, isoniazid, kanamycin, rifampin, and streptomycin against *Mycobacterium avium-intracellulare* complex. Antimicrob. Agents Chemother. **22:**148–150.

Chapter 115

Susceptibility Tests: Special Tests

CHARLES W. STRATTON AND ROBERT C. COOKSEY

Special susceptibility tests are so named because they are not routinely applied to all microorganisms but rather are used in unusual situations. Results of these tests may aid in determination of optimal antimicrobial therapy, elucidation of resistance mechanisms, or epidemiologic analyses of resistant isolates. In the clinical setting, some special susceptibility tests, such as screening for methicillin-resistant (heteroresistant) staphylococci or identification of β-lactamase production, may be done routinely on certain isolates. Other special tests are done only on request for specific situations. Special susceptibility tests often are complex and may require different methodologies, such as the collection of timed serum specimens (peak and trough) from the patient, special media, unusual antimicrobial agents or drug concentrations, larger inocula, or logarithmic growth conditions. The results of these tests may be difficult for the average clinician to interpret. Because of their specialized nature, complexity, and potential difficulty of interpretation, most special susceptibility tests should be performed only in consultation with the clinical microbiologist. Consultation allows selection of the best test method for a specific clinical problem. For example, there are a number of different ways to assess the bactericidal activity of antimicrobial therapy, and the clinician may not appreciate subtle yet important differences in these methods. However, with the assistance of the microbiologist, the clinician can determine the most appropriate special test for a given situation. Special susceptibility tests are used both in the clinical setting and in research. In research, special susceptibility tests are most often used to predict antimicrobial dose responses. Synergy testing using time kill-kinetic methodology is an example of these special tests applied to research. In addition, more complex interactions of the pharmacokinetic and pharmacodynamic properties of antimicrobial agents may be assessed by determining, in volunteers, the area under the bactericidal titer curve or the serum bactericidal rate. Finally, novel research tools such as gene probes may be used to provide more detailed characterization of resistance traits, for example, genotyping of β-lactamase enzymes. In either the clinical or research setting, the types of special susceptibility tests, the situations for which they are used, and the frequency with which they are done will vary from one institution to another.

TESTS THAT MEASURE BACTERICIDAL ACTIVITY

All of the susceptibility tests commonly performed by clinical microbiology laboratories (e.g., disk diffusion, broth dilution, and agar dilution) measure the inhibitory activity of an antimicrobial agent. In most clinical situations this is sufficient, since the role of the antibiotic is to prevent the spread of bacteria from the focus of infection by preventing microbial replication at new sites. The active participation of the host's defense mechanisms finally leads to the clinical and bacteriologic cure (48).

On occasion, tests that measure only inhibition of growth may not provide sufficient information to guide the therapy of certain infections. Shortly after the introduction of penicillin and streptomycin, Hunter speculated on the importance of bactericidal activity in the cure of bacterial endocarditis (47). This importance is now widely recognized (92). Similarly, Chabert (18) suggested that bactericidal activity in cerebrospinal fluid was necessary in the treatment of bacterial meningitis; this need subsequently was demonstrated in experimental meningitis (85). Bactericidal activity is also regarded as important in osteomyelitis (116) and in infections in immunocompromised hosts, particularly those with neutropenia (86). Consequently, there has been a great deal of emphasis on bactericidal testing methods (67).

Methodologic problems

There are a number of methods for determining bactericidal activity. Most often, an MBC value is established technically by extending the MIC procedure in order to determine the concentration of antibiotic that results in 99.9% killing of the inoculum (76). Generally, this means subculturing tubes (macrodilution method) or wells (microdilution method) that show inhibition of growth after 24 h of incubation in order to determine the number of survivors. Unfortunately, this definition of the MBC (≥99.9% killing of the inoculum after 24 h of incubation) is arbitrary and separates the bacteria into two populations, a segregation that might not have biological relevance (62). Second, since determination of the MBC is subject to methodologic variables, the clinical relevance of MBCs is nearly impossible to assess (114). These variables may be biological (e.g., persisters, paradoxical effect, and phenotypic resistance) or technical (e.g., growth phase of inoculum, size of inoculum, insufficient contact between test organism and antibiotic, antibiotic carryover, and the volume transferred for the count of survivors). It is worthwhile to briefly review these variables that can influence the result and interpretation of any bactericidal testing method.

Biological factors

Persisters. A small number (usually <0.1% of the final inoculum) of bacteria are able to survive the lethal effect of an antibiotic (42). If these persisters are retested, they are just as susceptible as the parent strain and no greater proportion of cells persists. This phenomenon is thought to be due to the fact that some cells are dormant or replicating slowly and consequently are not killed by the antimicrobial agent (104).

Paradoxical effect. The paradoxical effect occurs when the proportion of surviving cells increases significantly as the concentration of the antimicrobial agent increases beyond the MBC (33, 69). This phenomenon is particularly common for cell wall-active agents. It is thought that a high concentration of penicillin inhibits protein synthesis to a degree which prevents the growth necessary for expression of the lethal effect of the drug. Penicillin has been found to lyse RNA (61), and this activity may be related to the paradoxical effect. A paradoxical effect of aminoglycosides on the growth of gram-negative bacilli has also been described (57). The clinical relevance of this phenomenon is unclear. Eagle and co-workers (32) infected mice with group B streptococci and demonstrated that the bacteria were killed in vivo more slowly by high doses of penicillin. There is at least one reported case (41) in which a reduction in dosage of penicillin (peak levels decreasing from 36.7 to 11.3 μg/ml) resulted in a marked increase in bactericidal activity in patient serum (peak titers increasing from 1:8 to 1:256) with coincident improvement in clinical status.

Tolerance. Tolerance means that the microorganism is able to evade only the lethal action of the antimicrobial agent; there is no change in the MIC (44, 104). At least four mechanisms have been described which enable clinical isolates to survive during therapy with cell wall-active agents. Two of these, persisters and the paradoxical effect, have already been mentioned. Another mechanism is phenotypic tolerance. Phenotypic tolerance is a property of virtually all strains of bacteria and is an intrinsic mechanism of decreased susceptibility to antimicrobial agents which is manifested only under certain growth conditions (46, 104). The last mechanism of tolerance is genotypic tolerance, whereby a microorganism possesses or acquires a unique genetic property, such as a defective autolytic system. Genotypic tolerance is restricted to certain mutants or isolates with plasmids or transposons. Tolerant isolates exhibit unusually high MBCs relative to their MICs, and tolerance has been defined as an MBC/MIC ratio of 32 or greater after 24 h of incubation. However, this ratio cannot distinguish phenotypic tolerance from genotypic tolerance. A phenotypically tolerant isolate in a time-kill study demonstrates an initial high rate of killing similar to that of a nontolerant isolate but then reaches a higher survival rate (>0.1%), whereas a genotypically tolerant isolate is characterized by a slow loss of viability over the entire killing curve. Both will have a high MBC and an MBC/MIC ratio greater than 32. A time-kill kinetic method is required to differentiate phenotypic from genotypic tolerance (104).

A number of case reports (65, 90, 96, 106) have suggested the clinical importance of tolerant isolates. However, Denny and colleagues (25) have provided the most convincing evidence for staphylococcal infections that tolerance is an important factor in the failure of antimicrobial therapy. In one group of 10 patients, these investigators reported that initial treatment for *Staphylococcus aureus* infections with antibiotics to which the isolates were tolerant resulted in a mortality (40%) which was significantly higher than that in a second group (0%) in which 10 patients received bactericidal agents ($P = 0.043$). Even in the surviving patients in the first group, 3 of 6 (50%) required surgery to eradicate the infection (one patient had recurrent infection despite both surgery and 1 month of antibiotic therapy) versus only 2 of 10 patients (20%) needing surgery in the second group; none had recurrent infection. Similarly, others (80) have found that infection with a tolerant *S. aureus* adversely influences the outcome of staphylococcal endocarditis.

Phenotypic resistance. Microorganisms can develop resistance during the performance of a susceptibility test. Most often, this phenomenon represents phenotypic resistance (40) which is an inherent characteristic of the microorganism. Tests for bactericidal activity are likely to select phenotypically resistant strains from the population; unlike persisters, these survivors will demonstrate an increase in resistance when retested. An example of the development of such resistance can be seen with aminoglycosides and gram-negative bacilli. Recent studies (16, 36, 58, 60) have shown that the first exposure of gram-negative bacilli to an aminoglycoside results in the down regulation of bacterial transport of subsequent drug doses and leads to phenotypic resistance. The development of these phenotypically resistant subpopulations has been shown to occur in vivo (37; G. L. Daikos, V. Lolans, S. Lyza, and G. G. Jackson, Clin. Res. **34:**922A, 1986) and has been reported to be clinically important (74). Further characterization of these resistant isolates indicates an impaired ability to transfer aminoglycosides across the cell membrane as a result of defects in the cytoplasmic transport system caused by inefficient energy generation (17, 75). Another example of phenotypic resistance is seen with β-lactam agents and certain gram-negative organisms such as *Pseudomonas aeruginosa.* The ability of these microorganisms to increase the amount of periplasmic β-lactamase while limiting the influx of β-lactam agents through porin channels is an important intrinsic resistance mechanism (94).

Technical factors

Growth phase of inoculum. The most frequent technical pitfall encountered in microbiology laboratories performing bactericidal testing is the use of stationary-phase cultures. The rate of loss of viability of cells after exposure to cell wall-active antimicrobial agents is a direct function of the rate of bacterial growth before addition of the agent (45, 105). The use of stationary-phase cultures, such as overnight cultures, will increase the number of dormant cells and result in diminished killing rates. If tolerance or killing rates are being determined, then logarithmically growing rather than stationary-phase cultures must be used. This need for actively growing cultures has been stressed by many authors (38, 49, 51, 88, 98).

Size of inoculum. The inoculum effect in susceptibility testing is well known (91). This effect often is attributed to the increased effect of antibiotic-inactivating enzymes such as β-lactamase (23). There is, however, another important effect associated with an increased inoculum: i.e., tolerance. Tolerance appears to increase when large inocula are used and decreases with small inocula. For example, bacteria are killed rapidly when either log- or stationary-phase cultures are diluted to low inocula (10^4), but log-phase cultures concentrated to high inocula (10^7 to 10^8) are killed more rapidly than are stationary-phase cultures. Thus, both inoculum size and growth phase may independently increase the occurrence of tolerance. The inoculum size is considered the single most important variable in susceptibility testing. It is also the variable that should be the easiest to standardize and to measure. The National Committee for Clinical Laboratory Standards (NCCLS) has recommended a final inoculum size of 5×10^5 CFU/ml for susceptibility testing of aerobic bacteria in broth (68). A higher inoculum (5×10^6 CFU/ml) is recommended for susceptibility testing of anaerobic bacteria in broth. Because of the importance of the inoculum, great care should be taken in preparing this inoculum. Logarithmically growing inocula should be prepared in a shaker-incubator to promote uniformity of growth. The final inoculum size should be approximately 5×10^5 CFU/ml and confirmed by a colony count method (63). The inoculum size should not be presumed by comparison of the density of the inoculum with that of a McFarland barium sulfate standard, nor should the inoculum size be presumed spectrophotometrically.

Insufficient contact. Test organisms may have insufficient contact with the antimicrobial agent, most often because of adherence of viable microorganisms to the surface above the meniscus (43, 49, 55, 98). Such adherence is more likely with plastic than with acid-treated borosilicate glassware. Vortexing at 20 h for tests done in test tubes or continuous shaking for tests done in flasks or bottles allows better contact between all cells and the antimicrobial agent.

Antibiotic carryover. Transfer of a quantitative volume of broth for the count of survivors can be complicated by antibiotic carryover (24). This problem occurs mainly at higher concentrations (>16× MIC). Antibiotic carryover can be detected by using a swab to streak a sample of the test broth across the surface of a dried agar plate (prepared by incubating the plate for 1 h at 35°C), allowing 20 min for antimicrobial absorption into the agar, then cross-streaking the test organism over the entire surface of the plate, and after 24 h of incubation, looking for inhibition of colonial growth at the site of the initial streak (78). Antibiotic carryover can be eliminated by inactivating the antibiotic on the subculture plate. This is easily done for β-lactam agents by using β-lactamase, overlaying the plate with 1 ml of a β-lactamase solution (1:10 dilution of an aqueous solution of Penase [Becton Dickinson Microbiology Systems, Cockeysville, Md.). Alternatively, the sample for subculture can be diluted or washed. Cells can be washed by trapping the bacteria in the sample being subcultured on a 0.22-μm-pore-size filter, washing them with normal saline, and then immediately suspending them in saline to their original sample volume before they are quantitatively subcultured onto agar.

Volume transferred. The volume transferred for the count of survivors should be such that after the defined percentage of killing (99.9%), at least 10 colonies are present to be counted after incubation. For a 99.9% killing of a final inoculum of 5×10^5 CFU/ml, approximately 100 colonies will be growing on subculture if 100 μl is transferred. Transferring more than 100 μl is not recommended because of drug carryover. Smaller transfer volumes (less than 10 μl) can result in too few colonies because of pipetting error and intrinsic sampling error due to the Poisson distribution of sample response (not all organisms can be assumed to be equally distributed in a broth before sampling [76, 87]). Finally, the volume transferred for the count of survivors must be accurately quantitated, which requires use of a calibrated micropipette or calibrated stainless-steel prongs on a multipoint inoculator. Disposable plastic multipoint inoculators have been found to be unsuitable because they do not consistently deliver the prescribed amount (87). Quantitative loops, even if calibrated, have been found to be unreliable in bactericidal testing because of poor accuracy (±50%) (1).

Determination of MBCs by broth dilution

When the determination of bactericidal endpoints is done as an extension of MIC testing, the volume used is determined by the final volume used in the broth dilution MIC method. Although the broth macrodilution procedure for MIC testing has been widely used, it has also been shown to be subject to methodologic variables (77, 78, 87) which make the reproducibility of this method quite difficult. Conversely, the microdilution procedure for bactericidal testing has been shown to be much more reproducible (79, 82, 87, 123) than the macrodilution method. Accordingly, it is recommended that the broth microdilution procedure be used to determine MBCs.

Media. The NCCLS has recommended Mueller-Hinton broth (MHB) as the medium for broth dilution susceptibility testing (68). MHB more closely resembles serum in pH, osmolarity, Na^+, K^+, and Cl^- than do other common broths. MHB also demonstrates fairly good batch-to-batch reproducibility, is low in sulfonamide and tetracycline inhibitors, and supports growth of most rapidly growing pathogens. Supplements can be added to this medium to grow such fastidious organisms as *Haemophilus* species and certain streptococci. Calcium and magnesium ions (20 to 25 mg of Ca^{2+} per liter and 10 to 12.5 mg of Mg^{2+} per liter) should be present for testing aminoglycosides against *P. aeruginosa.* Although the NCCLS currently recommends using MHB that has been supplemented with 2% NaCl (68) for testing methicillin-resistant *S. aureus,* such supplementation should not be done for bactericidal testing because it will prevent antimicrobial killing of the *S. aureus* and no bactericidal endpoint will be detectable (unpublished data).

Inoculum. A standardized inoculum is prepared by sampling at least 20 to 30 colonies of a single type and inoculating them into a tube containing 5.0 ml of a suitable broth medium. This bacterial suspension is incubated at 35°C with shaking until it is visibly turbid. The density of this culture is then adjusted to a turbidity equivalent to that of a 0.5 McFarland standard. The alternate method recommended for methicillin-resistant *S. aureus* (68), in which the inoculum is prepared directly by using bacteria from colonies on an overnight agar plate, should not be used for bactericidal testing, since these bacteria will be in a stationary growth phase. The final inoculum size is arrived at by diluting the turbid broth culture (0.5 McFarland standard) appropriately, as determined by the inoculum volume to be delivered to the wells. If this volume is 50 μl, a dilution of 1:200 will result in a final inoculum of 5×10^5 CFU/ml. The actual concentration of the final inoculum delivered to the wells must be confirmed by a colony count method.

Incubation. The microdilution trays should be incubated for a full 24 h at 35°C. To prevent drying, seal each tray in a plastic bag with plastic tape or with a tight-fitting plastic cover before incubation. To maintain the same incubation temperature for all cultures, do not stack microdilution trays more than four high.

Determination of MBC endpoints

The MIC is the lowest concentration that inhibits macroscopic growth of the organism. The MBC is determined by subculturing the wells which have no visible growth. This is done by using a multipoint inoculator to remove 0.01 ml from each clear well and spot the sample on an agar plate. Alternatively, 0.1 ml can be aspirated and dispensed either into a tube of molten agar (48°C) for the preparation of pour plates or onto an appropriate agar plate and distributed evenly by using sterile bent glass rods. The MBC is defined as the lowest concentration of the antibiotic that reduced the inoculum by 99.9% within 24 h. Survivors at high concentrations are ignored as long as they do not exceed 0.1% of the final inoculum. If a multipoint inoculator is used, the MBC endpoint is "no growth." If 0.1 ml of the clear wells was subcultured, the number of colonies subsequently grown is used to determine the MBC. For a final inoculum of approximately 5×10^5, the MBC is defined as less than 11 colonies after 24 to 48 h of incubation (colonies are more easily read after 48 h of incubation). Erratic colony counts above the MBC at higher concentrations of antibiotic should be reported as representing the paradoxical phenomenon. Microdilution MBCs are easily done in duplicate; this practice should be followed to ensure reproducibility.

Macrodilution MBCs

If the macrodilution MIC procedure is used for bactericidal testing, the procedure is similar to that for the microdilution procedure. There are, however, important differences. A micropipettor should be used to add the inoculum to the test tubes, with the tip inserted well below the surface of the antibiotic-containing broth. Care should be taken to avoid any contact between the tip and the walls of the test tube. The tip should be rinsed five times in solution. It is critical to avoid the transfer of organisms to the inside of the test tubes above the meniscus by shaking or splashing. After incubation for 20 h at 35°C, test tubes without visible growth should be vortexed vigorously for 15 s and incubated for an additional 4 h. This procedure resuspends organisms adhering to the test tube wall above the meniscus and exposes them to the antibiotic. After this incubation, the test tubes are again vortexed, and 0.1 ml is removed and either dispensed in molten agar for the preparation of pour plates or spread across the surface of agar plates with sterile bent glass rods.

Determination of MBCs by agar dilution

MBCs have been determined by agar dilution methods (120, 122). The agar dilution method immobilizes the final inoculum in an agar-gel matrix and depends on inactivation of the antimicrobial agent in order to determine regrowth of viable CFU after a specific period of incubation. To date, the agar dilution method has been used only for evaluating the bactericidal activity of β-lactam agents that can easily be inactivated by β-lactamase. The advantage of agar dilution MBCs is that there is less influence of technical factor variations (119, 121). Because the bacteria are immobilized in an agar-gel matrix, both throughout the time of bacterial exposure to the antibiotic and during the time for regrowth of viable CFU after inactivation of the β-lactam agent, technical factors, such as adherence of the bacteria on the container walls above the meniscus and the problem of antibiotic carryover, are minimized. In addition, inactivation of the β-lactam agent at various times allows time-kill curves to be obtained with the agar dilution MBC method (118).

The agar dilution MBC method is performed by first preparing Mueller-Hinton agar plates containing twofold dilution concentrations of the desired β-lactam agent. Each 10-cm plate of a dilution series is inoculated by pipetting 0.05 ml (5×10^5 CFU per plate) of a standardized inoculum preparation onto the agar surface, with immediate streaking with a bacteriologic loop to disperse the inoculum in at least three opposing directions over the entire plate. The streaked plates are allowed to dry for approximately 15 min and then overlaid with 10 ml of molten (48°C) Mueller-Hinton agar containing a concentration of the β-lactam agent identical to that in the base layer of agar. After incubation of the agar plate for 24 h, the MIC can be determined. The MIC is defined as the concentration in the plate of the ascending concentration series for which the plate count is at least 2 standard deviations below (95% less than) the number representing 0.1% of the final inoculum count. MBCs can be determined at any specified time period. MBCs are determined by first inactivating the β-lactam agent by overlaying each plate with 1 ml of a β-lactamase solution (1:10 dilution of an aqueous solution of Penase). After application of the β-lactamase solution, the plates are reincubated for 48 h, at which time colony counts are made to determine persister percentages for each β-lactam concentration. The MBC, like the MIC, is defined as the concentration in the first plate of the ascending concentration series for which the plate count is at least 2 standard deviations below that representing 0.1% of the final inoculum count.

Determination of serum bactericidal titers

Description. The serum bactericidal test is basically a simple variation of the broth dilution test, with serial dilutions of a sample of serum from the patient being used instead of initial concentrations of antimicrobial agents. When assessment of bactericidal activity is needed, the serum bactericidal test offers several advantages. The test not only takes into consideration the susceptibility of the pathogen but also measures the combined effect of absorption and elimination of the antibiotic, the binding of the drug to serum proteins, and the effect of any metabolites as well as the parent compound against the infecting organism. The assay also measures the effects of drug interactions, including both the synergistic or antagonistic effects of antibiotic combinations and the interactions of other drugs with antibiotics. Finally, the serum bactericidal test, by measuring the magnitude of antibiotic concentration relative to the MBC, allows a prediction of the length of time of bactericidal activity. Serum peak bactericidal titers of ≥1:8, for example, ensure measurable bactericidal activity in serum for at least three half-lives of the drug being tested (each dilution represents bactericidal activity for one half-life). Despite these theoretical advantages of the serum bactericidal test, the clinical usefulness of this test remains controversial (117). New data as well as modifications in methodology should enable this test to be more useful in clinical and research areas.

The serum bactericidal test has been used most often to evaluate the therapeutic effectiveness of antimicrobial agents in bacterial endocarditis (92, 93). A multicenter study of infective endocarditis (115) found that peak serum bactericidal titers of 1:64 or greater with the microdilution method were associated with 100% bacteriologic cure. The serum bactericidal test was, however, unable to accurately predict bacteriologic failure. The test also has been recommended as a tool to assess therapy of osteomyelitis and suppurative arthritis. Weinstein et al. (116) analyzed 51 patients with osteomyelitis, 30 acute and 21 chronic, who were monitored at multiple medical centers with the same serum bactericidal test methodology. In this series, trough serum bactericidal titers of 1:2 or greater predicted medical cure in 23 of 25 patients successfully treated for acute osteomyelitis. There were 13 successfully treated episodes out of 21 cases of chronic osteomyelitis. In these 13 patients, peak serum bactericidal titers of 1:16 or greater and trough titers of 1:4 or greater were achieved and accurately predicted cure. In contrast, peak titers of less than 1:16 and trough titers of less than 1:2 in the eight patients in whom therapy failed accurately predicted this failure. Finally, Syrogiannopoulous and Nelson (97) reviewed 10 years of experience with children who had acute suppurative osteoarthritis. The serum bactericidal test was used to monitor absorption and to determine an adequate dose. These investigators used a serum bactericidal titer of 1:8 when the pathogen was a gram-negative bacillus, *S. aureus*, or *Haemophilus influenzae* and at least 1:32 when the etiologic agent was a streptococcus. The study monitored 180 patients who received large doses of oral antibiotics after clinical stabilization with intravenous antibiotics; the medium duration of intravenous therapy was about 1 week. Over this 10-year period, none of the 74 patients with suppurative arthritis had a recurrence. Only 4 of the 106 patients with bone infection (3.8%) were readmitted with recurrence. Two of three cases of *S. aureus* recurrence were thought to be due to lack of compliance. The authors compare these results with their earlier experience in which serum bactericidal titers were not used and in which 19% of patients whose antibiotic regimen was changed from parenteral to oral during the first 3 weeks of treatment had relapses (27). The serum bactericidal test has also been used in cancer patients. Klastersky et al. (53) measured the peak and trough levels of bactericidal activity in the serum samples of 317 patients with cancer and a bacteriologically proven infection. When the serum bactericidal test had a peak titer of ≥1:8, the infection was cured in 80% of cases. Similarly, Sculier and Klastersky (86) analyzed the clinical significance of the serum bactericidal activity in granulocytopenic patients with gram-negative bacillary bacteremia as well as in bacteremic patients with adequate granulocyte counts. In these patients, the clinical response to antibiotic therapy in gram-negative bacillary bacteremia strongly correlated with the peak serum bactericidal activity. Ninety-eight percent of nongranulocytopenic patients with a serum bactericidal titer of 1:8 or more had a favorable clinical response. In contrast, patients with severe neutropenia had an 87% rate of cure only with titers of 1:16 or more.

Procedure. The serum bactericidal test procedure recently has been standardized (66). One problem remaining for this test is the need to use human serum as the diluent. This requirement can be avoided by use of an ultrafiltrate of the patient serum (56). An ultrafiltrate is a plasma solution containing only free antimicrobial agent and no serum proteins. Ultrafiltration of serum is accomplished by centrifugation at 25°C for 30 min at 1,000 × *g* through a Centrifree micropartition system YMT membrane (Amicon Corp., Danvers, Mass.). The ultrafiltrate is sterilized by filtration through a 0.2-µm-pore-size filter (Gelman Sciences, Inc., Ann Arbor, Mich.). The use of ultrafiltrate for measuring serum bactericidal activity encompasses all of the advantages of the serum bactericidal test with none of the disadvantages specifically associated with the use of normal pooled human serum for the diluent.

The procedure for the serum bactericidal test is similar to that for MBC determinations. For the best reproducibility, the microdilution method should be used (123). The patient serum is obtained during antimicrobial therapy. The peak level is obtained 30 to 45 min after completion of a 15- to 30-min infusion, 60 min after administration of an intramuscular dose or 90 min after administration of an oral dose. The trough level is obtained 30 min before the next dose is given. If more than one agent is administered, the peak and trough levels are drawn according to the timing of the less frequently administered agent, the assumption being that the agent administered more frequently will have a more constant level. The serum or the ultrafiltrate is diluted in twofold steps. If the serum is used, the dilutions ideally should be made in human serum. If the serum ultrafiltrate is used, the dilutions can be done by using MHB. The tubes or wells are then inoculated with a standardized suspension of the microorganism isolated from the patient. This inoculum should be prepared as previously described for MBC determinations. It should contain approximately 5×10^5 CFU/ml and be confirmed by a colony count method. After 24 h of incubation at 35°C, the tubes or wells are examined and the serum inhibitory titer is determined. All tubes or wells showing inhibition are then quantitatively subcultured according to the procedure for MBC determination. The serum bactericidal titer is the dilution that kills 99.9% of the initial inoculum.

Determination of the area under the bactericidal titer curve

Barriere et al. (8, 9) have modified the serum bactericidal test to more completely compare the pharmacodynamic characteristics of antibiotics. The area under the bactericidal titer curve is determined by plotting bactericidal titers measured over time and calculating the area under the curve, using a calculator with a calculus program. The resulting area under the bactericidal titer curve serves as a unifying value to measure not only the magnitude of serum bactericidal activity but also its duration. The largest area under the bactericidal titer curve is found for the antimicrobial agent with the best combination of three factors: antimicrobial activity, achievable free drug concentration, and half-life. This technique is generally reserved for research.

Determination of bactericidal activity by the time-kill kinetic method

Description. Bactericidal activity can also be measured by the time-kill kinetic method, whereby the time course of antimicrobial activity is plotted by determining the killing rate of bacteria when exposed to an antimicrobial agent(s). The bacterial killing rates are dependent in part on the class of antibiotic and the concentration of the agent. With certain classes of antibiotics (e.g., aminoglycosides and fluoroquinolones), the rate of killing increases with increasing drug concentrations up to a point of maximum effort (113); this is termed concentration-dependent bactericidal activity. In contrast, the killing rate of β-lactam antibiotics is relatively slow and continues only as long as the concentrations are in excess of the MIC (31, 46, 113); this rate of killing for β-lactam agents is termed time-dependent bactericidal activity. Antibiotic concentrations are selected for the time-kill kinetic method on the basis of the agent being tested, achievable blood concentration, or multiples (1×, 4×, or 8×) of the MIC. At specific time intervals from 0 to 24 or 0 to 48 h of incubation, the broth cultures are sampled and survivors are determined by colony counts. The results are charted on semilog paper, with the survivor colony count on the ordinate (*y* axis) in logarithmic scale and the time on the abscissa (*x* axis) in arithmetic scale. The time-kill kinetic method has been widely used to evaluate and compare new antimicrobial agents and to assess combinations of antibiotics. It is less frequently used for guiding chemotherapy in an individual case.

The time-kill kinetic method generally appears to be more sensitive than MIC-MBC methods for evaluating antimicrobial activity. For example, Jackson and Riff (50) observed wide differences in the killing kinetics among strains of gram-negative bacilli of different species but with similar MICs. *P. aeruginosa*, although equally susceptible by MIC determinations, was the most resistant to rapid killing. These authors also noted that in the treatment of bacteremia due to gram-negative bacilli, the best clinical results followed more closely the maximal killing rates than the MICs. This observation has been confirmed in part by a more recent study (20) in nonneutropenic patients with serious *Pseudomonas* infections; in this study, MICs, checkerboard synergy tests, and time-kill kinetic studies were used in an attempt to correlate the activity of antimicrobial agents in vitro with clinical outcome. Among the techniques examined, the results from the 24-h time-kill kinetic studies were the best predictor of therapeutic outcome; in particular, an antagonistic combination in the 24-h time-kill curve indicated probable clinical failure with that combination.

Procedure. The time-kill kinetic method is performed in glass test tubes or flasks or in bottles (Pierce Chemical Co., Rockford, Ill.) which are capped and then sampled with a syringe. Each should contain at least 10 ml of MHB or other suitable broth medium and the chosen concentration of drug(s) to be tested. Flasks or bottles allow a larger volume of broth (20 to 100 ml) to be tested, which results in a greater challenge to the antibiotic as a result of the increased absolute number of organisms. Also, the use of flasks or bottles allows agitation during incubation and avoids the potential problem of organisms adhering above the meniscus. If test tubes are used, the inoculum should be added below the surface with a micropipettor in order to avoid splashing on the inside of the test tube above the meniscus. Test tubes should not be agitated during incubation. Flasks or bottles should be agitated during incubation. One test tube, flask, or bottle is used as a growth control. The inoculum is prepared in the same manner as for MBC determinations and consists of a final concentration of approximately 5×10^5 CFU/ml in logarithmic growth phase. The final inoculum is confirmed at time zero. Subsequent colony counts are done at 4 h, at a point between 6 and 12 h, and at 24 h. Sampling for colony counts is done by removing 0.5-ml samples of the broth at the specified times. Each 0.5-ml sample is serially diluted in test tubes containing 4.5 ml of sterile saline (0.9% NaCl) to produce 10-fold dilutions (10^{-1}, 10^{-2}, 10^{-3}, and 10^{-4}). A number of different colony count methods can be used to determine the CFU per milliliter from these dilutions. A 1-ml sample of the serial dilutions can be added to a tube of molten agar (48°C) for preparation of a pour plate. Alternatively, 1-ml samples can be pipetted onto prewarmed (35°C for 1 h) agar plates and distributed evenly by using sterile bent glass rods. In yet another method, a 20- to 50-μl sample is dropped on each of five spots on prewarmed agar plates and allowed to absorb without streaking. Colonies are then counted and averaged after 24 h of incubation, allowing the CFU per milliliter to be calculated. Whichever method is used, the minimal, accurately detectable number of CFU per milliliter must be determined by serial dilutions with a known inoculum. Potential drug carryover must be evaluated, and if it is found to be a problem, steps must be taken to eliminate this effect. Colonies are counted after 24 to 48 h of incubation. A magnifying lens can facilitate colony counts when plates are incubated for 24 h. Prolonged incubation (48 h) facilitates colony counting since the colonies are larger. The results of the time-kill kinetic determinations are shown graphically by plotting $\log_{10}$ CFU against time. Bactericidal effect can be seen by a 3-$\log_{10}$ decrease in CFU (99.9% killing) at the time specified.

During the performance of these studies, colony counts may show a final increase in number after an initial decrease. This phenomenon can be due to the selection of resistant isolates (most often phenotypic resistance), inactivation of the antimicrobial agent (most likely after 48 h), or regrowth of susceptible bacteria that have escaped the antimicrobial activity by adhering to the wall of the culture vessel. When regrowth occurs, it is useful to determine the MICs of survivors in order to determine whether a resistant organism was selected from the population tested. Inactivation of the antibiotic can be determined by appropriate assays at time zero and at 24 to 48 h.

Determination of the serum bactericidal rate

Determination of the serum bactericidal titer cannot ensure the clinician that the antimicrobial agent is in fact producing a rapid bactericidal effect in vivo. However, determination of the serum bactericidal rate evaluates the rapidity of bacterial killing and has been shown to correlate in an animal model with the rapidity of sterilization of vegetations (28, 29). Van der Auwera et al. (112) have compared in human volunteers the serum bactericidal rates for imipenem and vancomycin against methicillin-resistant *S. aureus* and found comparable serum bactericidal rates. The clinical relevance of this finding is suggested by a study in which infections caused by methicillin-resistant *S. aureus* were cured with imipenem (35).

The serum bactericidal rate is easily determined. Peak and trough serum samples are obtained from a patient receiving an antibiotic and are processed to yield ultrafiltrate. The ultrafiltrate is filter sterilized and then mixed with an equal volume (4 to 8 ml) of MHB to yield a 1:1 dilution. The procedure from then on is identical to that for time-kill kinetic studies. The $\log_{10}$ CFU per milliliter is plotted versus time. For comparisons, linear regression analysis can be done (15), with the serum bactericidal rate being defined as the slope of the regression line and its units being the change in the $\log_{10}$ CFU per milliliter per hour of exposure to the agent. The more negative the slope, the faster the rate of bacterial killing. A positive slope (e.g., in controls) indicates growth. Alternatively, the area under the killing curve (102) can be determined. Unlike the linear regression analysis, the latter method allows for "nonlinear" bends in the curves and thus may be a more accurate and reproducible method than linear regression analysis.

TESTS THAT MEASURE SYNERGY

The clinical importance of synergy has been recognized throughout the antimicrobial agent era (34, 47, 54), and methods have been developed in an attempt to assess synergistic interactions of antimicrobial agents (13, 52, 59). Differences in agreement among these approaches have been noted (13, 39, 59, 71, 81) and will be discussed.

Broth dilution method for determining synergy

The method most commonly used for assessing the synergistic effects of antibiotics is the two-dimensional broth dilution or checkerboard titration. In this method, serial twofold dilutions of two agents, alone and in combination, are tested by using a standardized inoculum (5×10^5 CFU/ml). The lowest concentration of each agent that inhibits the organism is plotted as an isobologram; conversely, the results are expressed as a fractional inhibitory concentration (FIC) of each agent by dividing the MIC in the combination by the MIC of one agent alone. When the FIC is less than 1.0, synergy is predicted. Alternatively, a fourfold decrease in the MIC of each agent in the combination is evidence for synergy.

The checkerboard technique has been modified to include reduction of the MIC to one-fourth of its value for both drugs, giving a concave displacement of the curve of the isobologram. For a synergistic effect, the MIC for each drug in the combination should be reduced to one-fourth of the original MIC in order to have the sum of the FIC equal 0.5 or less.

There are a number of problems associated with the checkerboard technique (13, 39, 59, 72, 81). First, this test as commonly performed does not measure bactericidal activity. Although MBCs can be determined, the associated methodologic problems become a major drawback. Second, the checkerboard method assesses synergy at only one point in time (24 h). Finally, the dilution steps involved are such that concentration-dependent antimicrobial agents usually have their concentrations reduced to the point at which no synergy can be detected.

The clinical correlations of the checkerboard technique are what might be expected given these problems. For example, the importance of synergy between ampicillin or penicillin and an aminoglycoside is well recognized in vitro (6, 96), in animal models (4, 26), and in clinical infections (5, 90). Testing for synergy in group B streptococci for ampicillin plus gentamicin by the checkerboard method failed to demonstrate any synergy (12), whereas synergy is consistently found with the time-kill kinetic method (6, 12). Similarly, in an animal model assessing gram-negative bacilli, Bamberger and colleagues (7) found that synergy, as determined by the checkerboard method, did not correlate with in vivo outcome, whereas results of time-kill kinetic studies did correlate with outcome. Finally, using in vitro methods, Bayer and Morrison (11) have found that the type of bactericidal interaction against methicillin-resistant *S. aureus* strains seen when rifampin is added to vancomycin is entirely method dependent, with 100% of strains tested by the checkerboard method being antagonistic. In contrast, a synergistic bactericidal interaction was found in 39% of these strains tested by the time-kill kinetic method. The strains that had been found to be killed synergistically by vancomycin and rifampin were used to induce left-sided endocarditis in 84 rabbits, which were then treated with vancomycin plus rifampin (10). No evidence that rifampin exerted an antagonistic effect was found. The clinical importance of these findings can be seen in an animal model for chronic staphylococcal osteomyelitis (70) as well as in a clinical study (71) in which the use of rifampin in combination with antistaphylococcal agents was found to be more effective than the use of the antistaphylococcal agents alone.

Time-kill kinetic method for determining synergy

Synergy is determined preferably by the time-kill kinetic method, performed as previously described. When measured for a combination of agents, synergy is defined as a 2-$\log_{10}$ decrease in CFU per milliliter between the combination and its most active constituent. At least one of the drugs must be present in a concentration that does not affect the growth curve of the test organism when used alone. Alternatively, a combination can be defined as synergistic when the number of viable cells at a given time is 10-fold lower than with the most effective antibiotic alone.

Evaluation of synergy by using serum bactericidal activity

The area under the bactericidal titer curve is a simple method to assess the effect of combining antimicrobial agents on the resultant serum bactericidal activity (8, 9). Synergy is defined as the area under the bactericidal titer curve for the combination being significantly greater than that for each drug alone.

The serum bactericidal titer may be unable to demonstrate synergy with agents that exhibit concentration-dependent killing, since the serum is progressively diluted in the serum bactericidal test, with the killing rates due to the concentration-dependent agent being correspondingly reduced. In this situation, serum bactericidal rates are better able to assess synergy (28, 29). An increasing number of studies have used serum bactericidal rates in this manner (107–112).

DETECTION OF β-LACTAMASES

Most isolates of *S. aureus*, some isolates of *H. influenzae* and *Neisseria gonorrhoeae*, and, very recently, a small number of enterococci are resistant to penicillin and ampicillin because they produce a β-lactamase that results in hydrolysis of these agents (64). Direct testing on colonies for β-lactamase production is a rapid and effective method for detecting β-lactamase-producing isolates and allows testing approximately 24 h before susceptibility results are available. In addition, certain isolates such as β-lactamase-producing enterococci are not reliably detected by routine susceptibility testing.

Because most isolates of *S. aureus* are presumed to be β-lactamase positive, routine testing for β-lactamase provides little clinical information of value. However, all isolates of *H. influenzae, N. gonorrhoeae,* and enterococci should routinely be tested for β-lactamase production.

There are a number of different β-lactamase detection techniques available that have application as screening procedures in the clinical microbiology laboratory. The most common and rapid methods include the acidometric method (103), which uses pH indicators to detect increased acidity resulting from cleavage of the β-lactam ring of a penicillin to yield a penicilloic acid; the iodometric method (83), which detects decolorization of a starch-iodine mixture as a result of the ability of penicilloic acid to reduce iodine; and the chromogenic cephalosporin method (73), which detects a color change resulting from hydrolysis of the β-lactam ring of a chromogenic cephalosporin. Details of these procedures are included in *Cumitech 6* (99). Control strains must be included with each test. The procedures described below are the most practical rapid methods for clinical microbiology laboratories.

Commercially available methods

Several commercial methods for detecting β-lactamase are available. These tests are derived from either the acidometric or chromogenic cephalosporin method. The commercial acidometric methods (Oxoid, Ltd., London, England; Marion Scientific, Kansas City, Mo.) consist of a paper disk or strip containing penicillin and a pH indicator, generally bromcresol purple. The paper is moistened, and colonial growth is rubbed onto it. A positive reaction, i.e., acid production, is indicated by a change from purple to yellow within 5 to 30 min. Nitrocefin (Cefinase; Becton Dickinson Microbiology Systems) and PADAC (Hoechst-Roussel Pharmaceuticals Inc., Somerville, N.J.), both chromogenic cephalosporins, are used similarly. A positive test for β-lactamase with the nitrocefin disk is a change from yellow to red, and that for PADAC is a change from purple to yellow. All of these commercially available tests are accurate with *H. influenzae* and *N. gonorrhoeae*. The PADAC method should not be used to test staphylococci (2). These paper strip and disk methods may be unable to detect β-lactamase that is present in small amounts and tightly bound to the cell, as with β-lactamase produced by *Staphylococcus saprophyticus*. For these β-lactamase-producing organisms, a solution of nitrocefin works better.

Nitrocefin solution

A 10-mg amount of nitrocefin powder (Cefinase) is dissolved in 1 ml of dimethyl sulfoxide. This solution is then diluted 1:20 with 0.1 M phosphate buffer (pH 7.0) to a concentration of 500 μg/ml. The solution will be yellow to light orange and will be stable for many weeks at 4 to 10°C. For testing β-lactamase, the nitrocefin solution is added to the well of a microdilution plate or to a small test tube. A heavy suspension of microorganisms is prepared and mixed with the nitrocefin solution. The nitrocefin solution will turn red usually within 10 to 30 min at room temperature but may take as long as 6 h.

Other methods

Inducible β-lactamases of certain gram-negative bacilli (e.g., *Enterobacter* species or *P. aeruginosa*) may be detected by using a double-disk assay (84). In this method, a standard susceptibility disk containing inducer (e.g., cefoxitin) is placed approximately 8 mm from a disk containing substrate (e.g., cefamandole) on a fresh lawn of the organism heavily seeded on Mueller-Hinton agar as done in the disk diffusion test. After overnight incubation at 35 to 37°C, truncation (blunting due to growth of the organism between the two disks) of the zone of inhibition between the two disks provides tentative indication of inducible β-lactamase production.

METHODS FOR DETECTING INACTIVATING ENZYMES OTHER THAN β-LACTAMASE

Chloramphenicol acetyltransferase

Chloramphenicol acetyltransferase (CAT) may be detected by using a colorimetric method now commercially available as a disk assay (3). Although this disk assay is not specifically recommended for CAT detection in species other than *H. influenzae*, it will detect constitutive enzymes in several other gram-negative species and, with some modification of the procedure, inducible CAT in several gram-positive species. For this procedure, cell suspensions in saline are made from growth of the gram-positive organism taken from an area near an inducer (chloramphenicol-containing disks) on the surface of agar plates. After addition of the manufacturer's test and control disks to duplicate tubes, positive reactions (as indicated by a greater intensity of yellow color in the test tube than in the control tube) may be detected after only 30 min of incubation at 37°C. If these reactions are weak and doubt about interpretation arises, the standard overnight assay may offer greater definition.

Aminoglycoside-modifying enzymes

As with β-lactamases, a large number (more than 30 isoenzymes) of aminoglycoside-modifying enzymes are known to exist. In contrast to β-lactamases, there are no rapid tests for their detection. Even with recent improvements in the convenience of performance (22), the phosphocellulose paper assay, which is the more reliable assay for aminoglycoside-modifying enzymes, is still too cumbersome for performance in most clinical microbiology laboratories. Currently, the use of a battery of aminoglycoside-aminocyclitol compounds along with interpretation of these MIC data offers the most practical yet conclusive evaluation of aminoglycoside-modifying enzymes (22, 30, 89). For example, high-level (e.g., MIC of >2,000 μg/ml) resistance to gentamicin, tobramycin, kanamycin, and possibly netilmicin and amikacin in an isolate of *Enterococcus* species suggests the presence of bifunctional aminoglycoside-inactivating enzyme activities (2′-phosphotransferase and 6′-acetyltransferase activities).

DNA probes for antimicrobial resistance genes

DNA probes for antimicrobial resistance genes, including several of the more clinically important inactivating genes, have been described (21). Although the use of probes enables the simultaneous examination of a larger collection of microorganisms or the localization of homologous genes to specific genetic elements (e.g., plasmids), commercial kits have not yet gained widespread acceptance, in part because the most efficient probe assays require handling of radioisotopes. Future probes will undoubtedly offer nonradioisotopic labels for antigenic or colorimetric detection of probe hybrids. In addition, polymerase chain reaction assays for resistance genes may soon become available.

DETECTION OF METHICILLIN-RESISTANT (HETERORESISTANT) STAPHYLOCOCCI

The heterogeneous resistance of intrinsically methicillin-resistant staphylococci has made susceptibility testing for these strains a problem for the clinical microbiology laboratory. These strains may be difficult to detect, and unless special precautions are taken, they may appear falsely susceptible. Conversely, methods used to increase detection of resistance, especially if used in combination inappropriately, can lead to erroneous categorization of susceptible strains as resistant. Both specificity and sensitivity of test methods for detecting β-lactam resistance in staphylococci need to be considered. A useful clue to intrinsic methicillin resistance is multiple resistance to antimicrobial agents, including β-lactams, aminoglycosides, tetracyclines, macrolides, lincosamides, and chloramphenicol.

Disk diffusion

The disk diffusion test is a reliable method for detecting methicillin resistance, particularly if the following recommendations are followed (14, 101). Prepare the inoculum by suspending growth from an overnight agar culture into broth and adjust the sample to the appropriate turbidity. Oxacillin should be used as the test agent both because it is more stable in storage and because it is generally more sensitive for detecting resistant strains. The agar plates for disk diffusion testing should be incubated at 35°C for a full 24 h but no longer, since changes that occur at 48 and 72 h are mostly due to β-lactamase when one is testing *S. aureus* with oxacillin. Care should be taken to observe faint growth or isolated colonies within a zone of inhibition; such growth indicates methicillin resistance. No additional attempts to further increase the sensitivity of the disk diffusion test for detection of methicillin-resistant *S. aureus* (e.g., by addition of NaCl to the medium, incubation for 48 h, or use of very large numbers of inocula, and especially the use of these manipulations in combination) should be made, since they may cause susceptible strains to appear falsely resistant. Some *S. aureus* strains that are not intrinsically methicillin resistant may give intermediate or resistant results in the standard 24-h disk diffusion test because their β-lactamase slowly hydrolyzes the oxacillin that has diffused into the medium. This β-lactamase-mediated resistance may often be determined with disk diffusion testing by the addition of a disk containing clavulanic acid (e.g., augmentin). If the resistant or intermediate result is due to β-lactamase and not intrinsic methicillin resistance, these strains will test as susceptible to the combination, whereas intrinsically resistant strains will remain resistant.

Intrinsically resistant coagulase-negative staphylococci may be more difficult to detect because of a greater degree of heterogeneity. However, these organisms do not present the problems associated with β-lactamase-mediated resistance of penicillinase-resistant β-lactams; therefore, methods to further enhance resistance, such as incubation for 48 h, do not create the same problems of false resistance as they do with *S. aureus*.

Broth microdilution

For determining MICs of antistaphylococcal agents, the NCCLS (68) currently recommends using cation-supplemented MHB that has been further supplemented with 2% NaCl (100), an inoculum of 5×10^5 CFU/ml, and incubation for 24 h at 35°C (68). MBCs, however, should not be determined by this method. Oxacillin is the preferred test agent for *S. aureus*, although methicillin may also be useful when testing coagulase-negative staphylococci.

Intrinsically resistant coagulase-negative staphylococci can be more difficult to detect than strains of *S. aureus* that are intrinsically resistant by microdilution methods. It may be prudent to use a second test such as the agar screen for cases of serious infection.

Agar screen

In the agar screen test, a Mueller-Hinton agar plate supplemented with 4% NaCl and either oxacillin (6 μg/ml) or methicillin (10 μg/ml) is inoculated with a bacterial suspension from a 0.5 McFarland turbidity culture, either by using a swab technique like that used for the disk diffusion method or by spot inoculation. After a full 24-h incubation at 35°C, the agar is inspected for growth of colonies. Growth of even a single colony indicates resistance. For *S. aureus*, incubation for 48 h is not recommended because a β-lactamase-producing susceptible strain may inactivate the drug enough to grow. For coagulase-negative staphylococci, however, a 48-h incubation increases the sensitivity, and it is prudent to incubate strains susceptible at 24 h for an additional 24 h before considering them susceptible; this precaution is recommended particularly for organisms isolated from patients with serious infections. Laboratories using an automated system for susceptibility testing of staphylococci have been advised to confirm test results with a second test such as the agar screen (19). These screen plates are available commercially.

LITERATURE CITED

1. **Albers, A. C., and R. D. Fletcher.** 1983. Accuracy of calibrated-loop transfer. J. Clin. Microbiol. **18:**40–42.
2. **Anhalt, J. P., and R. Nelson.** 1982. Failure of PADAC test strips to detect staphylococcal β-lactamase. Antimicrob. Agents Chemother. **21:**993–999.
3. **Azemun, P., T. Stull, M. Roberts, and A. L. Smith.** 1981. Rapid detection of chloramphenicol resistance in *Haemophilus influenzae*. Antimicrob. Agents Chemother. **20:** 168–170.
4. **Backes, R. J., M. S. Rouse, N. K. Henry, J. E. Geraci, and W. R. Wilson.** 1986. Activity of penicillin combined with an aminoglycoside against group B streptococci *in vitro* and in experimental endocarditis. J. Antimicrob. Chemother. **18:**491–498.
5. **Backes, R. J., W. R. Wilson, and J. E. Geraci.** 1985. Group B streptococcal infective endocarditis. Arch. Intern. Med. **145:**693–696.
6. **Baker, C. N., C. Thornsberry, and R. R. Facklam.** 1981. Synergism, killing kinetics, and antimicrobial susceptibility of group A and B streptococci. Antimicrob. Agents Chemother. **19:**716–725.
7. **Bamberger, D. M., L. R. Peterson, D. N. Gerding, J. A. Moody, and C. E. Fasching.** 1986. Ciprofloxacin, azlocillin, ceftizoxime and amikacin alone and in combination against gram-negative bacilli in an infected chamber model. J. Antimicrob. Chemother. **18:**51–63.
8. **Barriere, S. L.** 1987. The serum bactericidal test for evaluation of new antimicrobials and antimicrobial combinations. Antimicrob. Newsl. **10:**85–90.
9. **Barriere, S. L., E. Ely, J. E. Kapusnik, and J. G. Gambertoglio.** 1985. Analysis of a new method for assessing activity of combinations of antimicrobials: area under the bactericidal activity curve. J. Antimicrob. Chemother. **16:**49–59.
10. **Bayer, A. S., and K. Lam.** 1985. Efficacy of vancomycin plus rifampin in experimental aortic-valve endocarditis due to methicillin-resistant *Staphylococcus aureus:* in vitro–in vivo correlations. J. Infect. Dis. **151:**157–165.
11. **Bayer, A. S., and J. O. Morrison.** 1984. Disparity between timed-kill and checkerboard methods for determination of in vitro bactericidal interactions of vancomycin plus rifampin versus methicillin-susceptible and -resistant *Staphylococcus aureus*. Antimicrob. Agents Chemother. **26:**220–222.
12. **Bayer, A. S., J. O. Morrison, and K. S. Kim.** 1983. Experimental group B streptococcal endocarditis treated with penicillin G versus ceftizoxime. In vitro–in vivo disparity. Chemotherapy **29:**352–361.
13. **Berenbaum, M. C.** 1978. A method for testing synergy with any number of agents. J. Infect. Dis. **137:**122–130.
14. **Boyce, J. M.** 1984. Reevaluation of the ability of the standardized disk diffusion test to detect methicillin-resistant strains of *Staphylococcus aureus*. J. Clin. Microbiol. **19:** 813–817.
15. **Briceland, L. L., M. T. Pasko, and J. M. Mylotte.** 1987. Serum bactericidal rate as a measure of antibiotic interactions. Antimicrob. Agents Chemother. **31:**679–685.
16. **Bryan, L. E.** 1989. Two forms of antimicrobial resistance: bacterial persistence and positive function resistance. J. Antimicrob. Chemother. **23:**817–823.
17. **Bryan, L. E., and S. Kwan.** 1983. Roles of ribosomal binding, membrane potential, and electron transport in bacterial uptake of streptomycin and gentamicin. Antimicrob. Agents Chemother. **23:**835–845.
18. **Chabert, Y. A.** 1967. Le laboratoire d'antibiotherapie dans les meningitis purulentes. Sem. Hop. Paris **43:**239–242.
19. **Chambers, H. F.** 1988. Methicillin-resistant staphylococci. Clin. Microbiol. Rev. **1:**173–186.
20. **Chandrasekar, P. H., L. R. Crane, and E. J. Bailey.** 1987. Comparison of the activity of antibiotic combinations *in vitro* with clinical outcome and resistance emergence in serious infections by *Pseudomonas aeruginosa* in non neutropenic patients. J. Antimicrob. Chemother. **19:**321–329.
21. **Cooksey, R. C., and L. W. Mayer.** 1987. Identification of antibacterial resistance mechanisms: advances in laboratory assays. Antimicrob. Newsl. **4:**57–67.
22. **Cooksey, R. C., B. G. Metchock, and C. Thornsberry.** 1986. Microplate phosphocellulose binding assay for aminoglycoside-modifying enzymes. Antimicrob. Agents Chemother. **30:**883–887.
23. **Corrado, M. L., S. H. Landesman, and C. Cherubin.** 1980. Influence of inoculum size on activity of cefoperazone, cefotaxime, moxalactam, piperacillin, and *N*-formimidoyl thienamycin (MK 0787) against *Pseudomonas aeruginosa*. Antimicrob. Agents Chemother. **18:**893–896.
24. **Dankert, J., Y. Holloway, W. Joldersma, and J. Hess.** 1983. Importance of minimizing carry-over effect at subculture in the detection of penicillin-tolerant viridans group streptococci. Antimicrob. Agents Chemother. **23:** 614–616.
25. **Denny, A. E., L. R. Peterson, D. N. Gerding, and W. H. Hall.** 1979. Serious staphylococcal infections with strains tolerant to bactericidal antibiotics. Arch. Intern. Med. **139:**1026–1031.
26. **Deveikis, A., V. Schauf, M. Mizen, and L. Riff.** 1977. Antimicrobial therapy of experimental group B streptococci infection in mice. Antimicrob. Agents Chemother. **11:**817–820.
27. **Dich, V. Q., J. D. Nelson, and K. C. Haltalin.** 1975. Osteomyelitis in infants and children. Am. J. Dis. Child. **129:** 1273–1278.
28. **Drake, T. A., C. J. Hackbarth, and M. A. Sande.** 1983. Value of serum tests in combined drug therapy of endocarditis. Antimicrob. Agents Chemother. **24:**653–657.
29. **Drake, T. A., and M. A. Sande.** 1983. Studies of the chemotherapy of endocarditis: correlation of *in vitro,* animal model, and clinical studies. Rev. Infect. Dis. **5**(Suppl. 2): S345–S354.
30. **Drasar, F. A.** 1978. Detection of aminoglycoside degrading enzymes, p. 70–75. *In* D. S. Reeves, I. Phillips, J. D. Williams, and R. Wise (ed.), Laboratory methods in antimicrobial chemotherapy. Churchill Livingstone, Ltd., Edinburgh.
31. **Eagle, H., R. Fleischman, and A. D. Musselman.** 1950. Effect of schedule of administration on the therapeutic efficacy of penicillin: importance of the aggregate time penicillin remains at effective bactericidal levels. Am. J. Med. **9:**280–299.
32. **Eagle, H., R. Fleischman, and A. D. Musselman.** 1950. The bactericidal action of penicillin *in vivo:* the participation of the host and the slow recovery of the organism. Ann. Intern. Med. **33:**544–571.
33. **Eagle, H., and A. D. Musselman.** 1948. The rate of bacterial action of penicillin *in vitro* as a function of its concentration, and its paradoxically reduced activity at high concentrations against certain organisms. J. Exp. Med. **88:**99–131.
34. **Eliopoulos, G. M., and R. C. Moellering, Jr.** 1982. Antibiotic synergism and antimicrobial combinations in clinical infections. Rev. Infect. Dis. **4:**282–292.
35. **Fan, W., R. Del Busto, M. Love, N. Markowitz, C. Cendrowski, J. Cardenas, E. Quinn, and L. Saravolatz.** 1986. Impenem-cilastin in the treatment of methicillin-sensitive and methicillin-resistant *Staphylococcus aureus* infections. Antimicrob. Agents Chemother. **29:**26–29.
36. **Gerber, A. U., and W. A. Craig.** 1982. Aminoglycoside-

selected subpopulation of *Pseudomonas aeruginosa*. J. Lab. Clin. Med. **100:**671–681.

37. **Gerber, A. U., A. P. Vastola, J. Brandel, and W. A. Craig.** 1982. Selections of aminoglycoside-resistant variants of *Pseudomonas aeruginosa* in an *in vivo* model. J. Infect. Dis. **146:**691–697.
38. **Goessens, W. H. F., P. Fontijine, M. Van Raffe, and M. F. Michel.** 1982. Factors influencing detection of tolerance in *Staphylococcus aureus*. Antimicrob. Agents Chemother. **22:**364–368.
39. **Greenwood, D.** 1981. Correlations between methods for the measurement of antibiotic synergy. J. Infect. Dis. **143:** 757.
40. **Greenwood, D.** 1985. Phenotypic resistance to antimicrobial agents. J. Antimicrob. Chemother. **15:**653–658.
41. **Griffiths, L. R., and H. T. Green.** 1985. Paradoxical effect of penicillin *in vivo*. J. Antimicrob. Chemother. **15:**507–508.
42. **Gunnison, J. B., M. A. Fraher, and E. Jawetz.** 1963. Persistence of *Staphylococcus aureus* in penicillin *in vitro*. J. Gen. Microbiol. **34:**335–349.
43. **Gwynn, M. N., L. T. Webb, and G. N. Rolinson.** 1981. Regrowth of *Pseudomonas aeruginosa* and other bacteria after the bactericidal action of carbenicillin and other beta-lactam antibiotics. J. Infect. Dis. **144:**263–269.
44. **Handwerger, S., and A. Tomasz.** 1985. Antibiotic tolerance among clinical isolates of bacteria. Rev. Infect. Dis. **7:**368–386.
45. **Hobby, G. L., and M. H. Dawson.** 1944. Effect of rate of growth of bacteria on action of penicillin. Proc. Soc. Exp. Biol. Med. **50:**281–285.
46. **Hobby, G. L., K. Meyer, and E. Chaffee.** 1942. Observations on the mechanism of action of penicillin. Proc. Soc. Exp. Biol. Med. **50:**281–285.
47. **Hunter, T. H.** 1950. Speculations on the mechanism of cure of bacterial endocarditis. J. Am. Med. Assoc. **144:** 524–527.
48. **Isenberg, H. D.** 1967. Clinical evaluation of laboratory guidance to antibiotic therapy. Health Lab. Sci. **4:**166–180.
49. **Ishida, K. P., A. Guze, G. M. Kalmason, K. Albrandt, and L. B. Guze.** 1982. Variables in demonstrating methicillin tolerance in *Staphylococcus aureus* strains. Antimicrob. Agents Chemother. **21:**688–690.
50. **Jackson, G. G., and L. J. Riff.** 1971. Pseudomonas bacteremia: pharmacologic and other bases for failure of treatment with gentamicin. J. Infect. Dis. **124:**S185–S191.
51. **Kim, K. S., and B. F. Anthony.** 1981. Importance of bacterial growth phase in determining minimal bactericidal concentration of penicillin and methicillin. Antimicrob. Agents Chemother. **19:**1075–1077.
52. **King, T. C., D. Schlessinger, and D. J. Krogstad.** 1981. The assessment of antimicrobial combinations. Rev. Infect. Dis. **3:**627–633.
53. **Klastersky, J., D. Daneau, G. Swings, and D. Weerts.** 1974. Antibacterial activity in serum and urine as a therapeutic guide in bacterial infections. J. Infect. Dis. **129:** 187–193.
54. **Klastersky, J., F. Meunier-Carpentier, and J.-M. Prevost.** 1977. Significance of antimicrobial synergism for the outcome of gram-negative sepsis. Am. J. Med. Sci. **273:**157–167.
55. **Layte, S., P. Harris, and G. N. Rolinson.** 1983. Factors affecting the apparent regrowth of *Pseudomonas aeruginosa* following exposure to bactericidal concentrations of carbenicillin. Chemotherapy **30:**26–30.
56. **Leggett, J. E., S. A. Wolz, and W. A. Craig.** 1989. Use of serum ultrafiltrate in the serum bactericidal test. J. Infect. Dis. **160:**616–623.
57. **Lorian, V., R. P. Siletti, F. X. Biondo, and C. C. De-Freitas.** 1979. Paradoxical effect of aminoglycoside antibiotics on the growth of Gram-negative bacilli. J. Antimicrob. Chemother. **5:**613–616.
58. **MacArthur, R. D., V. Lolans, F. A. Far, and G. G. Jackson.** 1984. Biphasic concentration-dependent and rate-limited concentration independent bacterial killing by an aminoglycoside antibiotic. J. Infect. Dis. **150:**778–779.
59. **Marymont, J. H., and J. Marymont.** 1981. Laboratory evaluation of antibiotic combinations: a review of methods and problems. Lab. Med. **12:**47–55.
60. **Mawer, S. L., and D. Greenwood.** 1978. Specific and non-specific resistance to aminoglycosides in *Escherichia coli*. J. Clin. Pathol. **31:**12–15.
61. **McDowell, T. D., and K. E. Reed.** 1989. Mechanism of penicillin killing in the absence of bacterial lysis. Antimicrob. Agents Chemother. **33:**1680–1685.
62. **Meylan, P. R., P. Franciolli, and M. P. Glauser.** 1986. Discrepancies between MBC and actual killing of viridans group streptococci by cell-wall-active antibiotics. Antimicrob. Agents Chemother. **29:**418–423.
63. **Miles, A. A., and S. S. Misra.** 1938. The estimation of the bactericidal power of the blood. J. Hyg. **38:**732–748.
64. **Murray, B. E.** 1989. Problems and mechanisms of antimicrobial resistance, p. 423–439. *In* R. C. Moellering, Jr., and D. Kay (ed.), Infectious disease clinics of North America: antibacterial agents, pharmacodynamics, pharmacology, new agents, vol. 3. The W. B. Saunders Co., Philadelphia.
65. **Musher, D. M., and R. Fletcher.** 1982. Tolerant *Staphylococcus aureus* causing vertebral osteomyelitis. Arch. Intern. Med. **93:**796–800.
66. **National Committee for Clinical Laboratory Standards.** 1990. Methodology for the serum bactericidal test—second edition. Tentative guideline. NCCLS document M21-T. National Committee for Clinical Laboratory Standards, Villanova, Pa.
67. **National Committee for Clinical Laboratory Standards.** 1990. Methods for determining bactericidal activity of antimicrobial agents—second edition. Tentative guideline. NCCLS document M26-T. National Committee for Clinical Laboratory Standards, Villanova, Pa.
68. **National Committee for Clinical Laboratory Standards.** 1990. Methods for dilution antimicrobial susceptibility tests for bacteria that grow aerobically—second edition. Approved standard. NCCLS document M7-A2. National Committee for Clinical Laboratory Standards, Villanova, Pa.
69. **Nishino, T., and S. Nakazawa.** 1976. Bacteriological study on effects of beta-lactam group antibiotics in high concentrations. Antimicrob. Agents Chemother. **9:**1033–1042.
70. **Norden, C. W.** 1983. Experimental chronic staphylococcal osteomyelitis in rabbits: treatment with rifampin alone and in combination with other antimicrobial agents. Rev. Infect. Dis. **5**(Suppl.):S491–S494.
71. **Norden, C. W., R. Bryant, D. Palmer, J. Z. Montgomerie, J. Wheat, The Chronic Staphylococcal Osteomyelitis Study Group.** 1986. Chronic osteomyelitis caused by *Staphylococcus aureus:* controlled clinical trial of nafcillin therapy and nafcillin-rifampin therapy. South. Med. J. **79:**947–951.
72. **Norden, C. W., H. Wentzel, and E. Keleti.** 1979. Comparison of techniques for measurement of *in vitro* antibiotic synergism. J. Infect. Dis. **40:**629–633.
73. **O'Callaghan, C. H., A. Morris, S. M. Kirby, and A. H. Shingler.** 1972. Novel method for detection of β-lactamase by using a chromogenic cephalosporin substrate. Antimicrob. Agents Chemother. **1:**283–288.
74. **Olson, B., R. A. Weinstein, C. Natham, W. Chamberlin, and S. A. Kabins.** 1985. Occult aminoglycoside resistance in *Pseudomonas aeruginosa:* epidemiology and implications for therapy and control. J. Infect. Dis. **152:**769–744.
75. **Parr, T. J., Jr., and A. S. Bayer.** 1988. Mechanisms of aminoglycoside resistance in variants of *Pseudomonas aeruginosa* isolated during treatment of experimental endocarditis in rabbits. J. Infect. Dis. **158:**1003–1010.

76. **Pearson, R. D., R. T. Steigbigel, H. T. Davis, and S. W. Chapman.** 1980. Method for reliable determination of minimal lethal antibiotic concentrations. Antimicrob. Agents Chemother. **18:**699–708.
77. **Pelletier, L. L.** 1984. Lack of reproducibility of macrodilution MBCs for *Staphylococcus aureus*. Antimicrob. Agents Chemother. **26:**815–818.
78. **Pelletier, L. L., Jr., and C. B. Baker.** 1988. Oxacillin, cephalothin, and vancomycin tube macrodilution MBC result reproducibility and equivalence to MIC results for methicillin-susceptible and reputedly tolerant *Staphylococcus aureus* isolates. Antimicrob. Agents Chemother. **32:**374–377.
79. **Prober, C. G., S. S. Dougherty, K. L. Vosti, and A. S. Yeager.** 1979. Comparison of a micromethod for performance of the serum bactericidal test with the standard tube dilution method. Antimicrob. Agents Chemother. **16:**46–48.
80. **Rajashekaraiah, K. R., T. Rice, V. S. Rao, D. Marsh, B. Ramakrishna, and C. A. Kallick.** 1980. Clinical significance of tolerant strains of *Staphylococcus aureus* in patients with endocarditis. Ann. Intern. Med. **93:**796–801.
81. **Rayan, A. W., I. Kwasnik, and R. C. Tilton.** 1981. Methodologic variation in antibiotic synergy tests against enterococci. J. Clin. Microbiol. **13:**73–75.
82. **Reimer, L. G., C. W. Stratton, and L. B. Reller.** 1981. Minimal inhibitory and bactericidal concentrations of 44 antimicrobial agents against three standard control strains in broth with and without human serum. Antimicrob. Agents Chemother. **19:**1050–1055.
83. **Rosenblatt, J. E., and A. M. Neuman.** 1978. A rapid slide test for penicillinase. Am. J. Clin. Pathol. **69:**351–354.
84. **Sanders, C. C., and W. E. Sanders.** 1979. Emergence of resistance to cefamandole: possible role of cefoxitin-inducible beta-lactamases. Antimicrob. Agents Chemother. **15:**792–797.
85. **Scheld, W. M., and M. A. Sande.** 1983. Bactericidal versus bacteristatic antibiotic therapy of experimental pneumococcal meningitis in rabbits. J. Clin. Invest. **71:**411–419.
86. **Sculier, J. P., and J. Klastersky.** 1984. Significance of serum bactericidal activity in gram-negative bacillary bacteremia in patients with and without granulocytopenia. Am. J. Med. **76:**429–435.
87. **Shanholtzer, C. J., L. R. Peterson, M. L. Mohn, J. A. Moody, and D. N. Gerding.** 1984. MBCs for *Staphylococcus aureus* as determined by macrodilution and microdilution techniques. Antimicrob. Agents Chemother. **26:**214–219.
88. **Sherris, J. C.** 1986. Problems in in vitro determination of antibiotic tolerance in clinical isolates. Antimicrob. Agents Chemother. **30:**633–637.
89. **Shimizu, K., T. Kumada, W.-C. Hsieh, H.-Y. Chung, Y. Chong, R. S. Hare, G. H. Miller, F. J. Sabatelli, and J. Howard.** 1985. Comparison of aminoglycoside resistance patterns in Japan, Formosa and Korea, Chile, and the United States. Antimicrob. Agents Chemother. **28:**282–288.
90. **Steinbrecher, U. P.** 1981. Serious infection in an adult due to penicillin-tolerant group B streptococcus. Arch. Intern. Med. **141:**1714–1715.
91. **Stratton, C. W.** 1983. Susceptibility testing revisited, p. 65–100. *In* M. Stafenini, F. Gorstein, and L. M. Fink (ed.), Progress in clinical pathology, vol. 9., Grune & Stratton, Inc., New York.
92. **Stratton, C. W.** 1987. The role of the microbiology laboratory in the treatment of infective endocarditis. J. Antimicrob. Chemother. **20**(Suppl. A):41–49.
93. **Stratton, C. W.** 1988. The serum bactericidal test. Clin. Microbiol. Rev. **1:**19–26.
94. **Stratton, C. W., and F. Tausk.** 1989. Intrinsic resistance of *Pseudomonas aeruginosa*, p. 275–286. *In* N. Høiby, S. S. Pedersen, G. H. Shand, G. Döring, and I. A. Holder (ed.), *Pseudomonas aeruginosa* infection. S. Karger, Basel.
95. **Svenungsson, B., M. Kalin, and G. L. Lindgren.** 1982. Therapeutic failure in pneumonia caused by a tolerant strain of *Staphylococcus aureus*. Scand. J. Infect. Dis. **14:**309–311.
96. **Swingle, H. M., R. L. Buccinarelli, and E. M. Ayoub.** 1985. Synergy between penicillins and low concentrations of gentamicin in the killing of group B streptococci. J. Infect. Dis. **152:**515–520.
97. **Syrogiannopoulous, G. A., and J. D. Nelson.** 1988. Duration of antimicrobial therapy for acute suppurative osteoarticular infections. Lancet **i:**37–40.
98. **Taylor, P. C., F. D. Schoenknecht, J. C. Sherris, and E. C. Linner.** 1983. Determination of minimum bactericidal concentrations of oxacillin for *Staphylococcus aureus:* influence and significance of technical factors. Antimicrob. Agents Chemother. **23:**142–150.
99. **Thornsberry, C., T. L. Gavan, and E. H. Gerlach.** 1977. Cumitech 6, New developments in antimicrobial agent susceptibility testing, p. 1–2. Coordinating ed., J. C. Sherris. American Society for Microbiology, Washington, D.C.
100. **Thornsberry, C., and L. K. McDougal.** 1983. Successful use of broth microdilution in susceptibility tests for methicillin-resistant (heteroresistant) staphylococci. J. Clin. Microbiol. **18:**1084–1091.
101. **Thornsberry, C., J. M. Swenson, C. N. Baker, L. K. McDougal, S. A. Stocker, and B. C. Hill.** 1988. Methods for determining susceptibility of fastidious and unusual pathogens to selected antimicrobial agents. Diagn. Microbiol. Infect. Dis. **9:**139–153.
102. **Tisdale, J. E., M. T. Pasko, and J. M. Mylotte.** 1989. Antipseudomonal activity of simulated infusions of gentamicin alone or with piperacillin assessed by serum bactericidal rate and area under the killing curve. Antimicrob. Agents Chemother. **33:**1500–1505.
103. **Tu, K. K., J. H. Jorgensen, and C. W. Stratton.** 1981. A rapid paper-disc test for penicillinase. Am. J. Clin. Pathol. **75:**557–559.
104. **Tuomanen, E.** 1986. Phenotypic tolerance: the search for β-lactam antibiotics that kill nongrowing bacteria. Rev. Infect. Dis. **8**(Suppl. 3):S279–S291.
105. **Tuomanen, E., R. Cozens, W. Tosch, O. Zak, and A. Tomasz.** 1986. The rate of killing of *Escherichia coli* by β-lactam antibiotics is strictly proportional to the rate of bacterial growth. J. Gen. Microbiol. **132:**1297–1304.
106. **Tuomanen, E., D. T. Durack, and A. Tomasz.** 1986. Antimicrobial tolerance among clinical isolates of bacteria. Antimicrob. Agents Chemother. **30:**521–527.
107. **Van der Auwera, P.** 1989. Ex vivo study of serum bactericidal titers and killing rates of daptomycin (LY 146032) combined or not combined with amikacin compared with those of vancomycin. Antimicrob. Agents Chemother. **33:**1783–1790.
108. **Van der Auwera, P., and J. Klastersky.** 1987. Bactericidal activity and killing rate of serum in volunteers receiving ciprofloxacin alone or in combination with vancomycin. Antimicrob. Agents Chemother. **30:**892–895.
109. **Van der Auwera, P., and J. Klastersky.** 1987. Bactericidal activity and killing rate of serum in volunteers receiving teicoplanin alone or in combination with oral or intravenous rifampin. Antimicrob. Agents Chemother. **31:**1002–1005.
110. **Van der Auwera, P., J. Klastersky, H. Lagast, and M. Hussan.** 1986. Serum bactericidal activity and killing rate for volunteers receiving imipenem plus amikacin, and ceftazidime plus amikacin against *Pseudomona aeruginosa*. Antimicrob. Agents Chemother. **30:**122–126.
111. **Van der Auwera, P., J. Klastersky, S. Lieppe, M. Hussan, D. Lauzon, and A. P. Lopez.** 1986. Bactericidal activity and killing rate of serum from volunteers receiving perfloxacin alone or in combination with amikacin. Antimicrob. Agents Chemother. **29:**230–234.

112. **Van der Auwera, P., Y. Van Laethem, and J. Klastersky.** 1987. Bactericidal activity and killing rate of serum against Gram-positive cocci in volunteers receiving imipenem, oxacillin, vancomycin, or ampicillin plus gentamicin. J. Antimicrob. Agents Chemother. **20:**239–249.
113. **Volgelman, B., and W. A. Craig.** 1986. Kinetics of antimicrobial activity. J. Pediatr. **108:**835–840.
114. **Washington, J. A., II.** 1988. Current problems in antimicrobial susceptibility testing. Diagn. Microbiol. Infect. Dis. **9:**135–138.
115. **Weinstein, M. P., C. W. Stratton, A. Ackley, et al.** 1985. Multicenter collaborative evaluation of a standardized serum bactericidal test as a prognostic indicator in infective endocarditis. Am. J. Med. **78:**262–269.
116. **Weinstein, M. P., C. W. Stratton, H. B. Hawley, A. Ackley, and L. B. Reller.** 1987. Multicenter collaborative evaluation of a standardized serum bactericidal test as a predictor of therapeutic efficacy in acute and chronic osteomyelitis. Am. J. Med. **83:**218–222.
117. **Wolfson, J. S., and M. N. Swartz.** 1985. Serum bactericidal activity as a monitor of antibiotic therapy. N. Engl. J. Med. **312:**968–975.
118. **Woolfrey, B. F., M. E. Gresser-Burns, and R. T. Lally.** 1987. Ampicillin killing curve patterns of *Haemophilus influenzae* type B isolates by agar dilution plate count method. Antimicrob. Agents Chemother. **31:**1711–1717.
119. **Woolfrey, B. F., M. E. Gresser-Burns, and R. T. Lally.** 1988. Effect of temperature on inoculum as a potential source of error in agar dilution plate count bactericidal measurements. Antimicrob. Agents Chemother. **32:**513–517.
120. **Woolfrey, B. F., R. T. Lally, and M. N. Ederer.** 1985. Evaluation of oxacillin tolerance in *Staphylococcus aureus* isolates by a novel method. Antimicrob. Agents Chemother. **28:**381–388.
121. **Woolfrey, B. F., R. T. Lally, and M. N. Ederer.** 1986. Influence of technical factor variations during inoculum preparation on the agar dilution plate-count method for quantitation of *Staphylococcus aureus* oxacillin persisters. Antimicrob. Agents Chemother. **30:**792–793.
122. **Woolfrey, B. F., R. T. Lally, M. N. Ederer, and M. E. Gresser-Burns.** 1987. Oxacillin killing curve patterns of *Staphylococcus aureus* isolates by agar dilution plate count method. Antimicrob. Agents Chemother. **31:**16–20.
123. **Woolfrey, B. F., R. T. Lally, and K. R. Tait.** 1986. Influence of technical factor variations on serum inhibition and bactericidal titers. J. Clin. Microbiol. **23:**997–1000.

Chapter 116

Antibacterial Susceptibility Tests: Automated or Instrument-Based Methods

JAMES H. JORGENSEN

Clinical microbiology laboratories can choose from several manual or instrument-assisted methods for performance of routine antibacterial susceptibility tests. These include disk diffusion, agar dilution, broth microdilution (with or without use of an instrument), and rapid, automated instrument methods. In recent years, there has been a trend in the United States away from use of the disk diffusion test in favor of either broth microdilution or automated instrument methods, as evidenced by the methods used for College of American Pathologists proficiency survey testing (Table 1 presents a recent example of survey participants' test methods). This chapter will focus on antimicrobial susceptibility test methods that incorporate an instrument for reading of test results or, in some cases, for incubation and final interpretation of results.

A laboratory may choose to perform automated antimicrobial susceptibility testing for one or more of the following reasons: (i) to generate test results more rapidly than can be accomplished by manual methods, (ii) to improve intra- or interlaboratory standardization of test results, or (iii) to reduce the amount of labor required to perform susceptibility tests.

The susceptibility testing instruments now available in the United States offer different levels of automation. Some instruments only interpret growth endpoints when microdilution trays are inserted into a reader device, whereas others incubate microdilution trays or special cuvettes and perform serial or final interpretations of growth patterns in the presence of antimicrobial agents. The instruments vary in their methods of exposing the bacterial test culture to the optical detector systems. The instruments that offer the highest degree of automation generally do so by incorporating simple internal robotics to manipulate the trays or cuvettes during the incubation and reading sequences (16). Current instruments utilize either the principle of turbidimetric detection of bacterial growth in a liquid medium or detection of hydrolysis of a fluorogenic substrate incorporated in a special liquid medium (1, 16). The suppression of turbidity as evidence of the inhibitory effect of an antimicrobial agent or, conversely, the increase in turbidity in the presence of a drug as an indication of microbial resistance has been firmly established in manual broth dilution susceptibility test methods (40). Thus, automated susceptibility test instruments serve to either compress the analysis period or facilitate the interpretation of test results after a conventional incubation period. All of the instruments rely heavily on microprocessor-controlled functions, and they utilize personal computer hardware to provide final printed reports and to enable data storage and retrieval. All of the instruments can also be used to perform additional functions, usually to identify gram-negative or gram-positive bacteria and, in some cases, to assemble combined identification/antimicrobial susceptibility reports.

AUTOMATED READER DEVICES FOR BROTH MICRODILUTION AND AGAR DILUTION TESTS

Virtually every manufacturer of broth microdilution trays for antimicrobial susceptibility testing offers a mechanized device for hydration or inoculation of trays and a device to facilitate manual visualization of results after incubation. Most manufacturers also offer some type of reader device whereby the user indicates the results of manual interpretation of the growth patterns in the tray by use of a video display screen resembling the configuration of the tray or by use of a touch-sensitive template that overlays the microdilution tray (1). These reader devices assist in data recording and generally result in a computer-printed report. The personal computers that are usually included with these systems enable the user to store and later retrieve data for generation of periodic reports, e.g., cumulative susceptibility profiles for various organisms during a defined time period.

Automated tray reader devices that photometrically interpret growth patterns in trays by turbidimetric analysis represent the next level of instrumentation available from several manufacturers. The API UniScept Autoreader (Analytab Products, Plainview, N.Y.) and the Baxter Microscan AutoSCAN-4 (Baxter Healthcare Corp., West Sacramento, Calif.) are examples of two contemporary instruments for automated interpretation of the results of microdilution trays after overnight incubation in a standard bacteriologic incubator. Both instruments are configured with personal computers for report preparation and data storage. These instruments automate only the final, reading step involved in the performance of MIC or breakpoint microdilution tests. An evaluation of one of these instruments has shown that MIC endpoints can be interpreted by the instrument with reasonable accuracy (3). Instruments that automate the incubation phase of microdilution susceptibility tests or use fluorogenic-substrate hydrolysis for growth detection are described below.

Agar dilution tests can be mechanized through use of a Steers replicator inoculum delivery device (34) or a Cathra Replicator (MCT Medical, Inc., St. Paul, Minn.) (27). Semiautomated reading of agar dilution plates can be accomplished by use of the Cathra Replianalyzer,

TABLE 1. Antimicrobial susceptibility test methods reported by 1,517 participants in 1988 College of American Pathologists Comprehensive Microbiology-Serology Survey Set B-C for specimen B-22 (*Citrobacter freundii*)

Method	% of participants
Commercial microdilution	44.4
Disk diffusion	30.4
Rapid automated	22.0
All other	3.2

which assists in the visualization of growth spots on the agar plates and uses a personal computer to capture the data.

Autobac Series II

The Autobac system was developed and introduced in the early 1970s by Pfizer Diagnostics. Now produced by Organon Teknika and called the Autobac Series II, it holds the distinction of being the first "automated" microbiology instrument to be sold in the United States (a prior instrument called TASS [14] was developed by Technicon but never marketed). The Autobac was originally designed to provide rapid, qualitative susceptibility results on the most frequently tested bacteria, i.e., members of the family *Enterobacteriaceae*, *Pseudomonas aeruginosa*, staphylococci, and enterococci. The instrument has evolved over the years such that it now provides the capability to perform qualitative (susceptible [S], intermediate [I], or resistant [R]) or quantitative (MIC) susceptibility tests, photometric screening of urine samples for bacteria, and rapid identification of aerobic gram-negative bacilli. The latter function is accomplished by using the innovative approach of growth inhibition profiles with a group of unique dyes and chemicals as well as a few conventional antimicrobial agents (31).

The Autobac uses relatively large, disposable, 19-chamber plastic cuvettes that hold approximately 1 ml of growth medium (eugonic broth) plus an antimicrobial agent-impregnated paper elution disk in 18 of the 19 chambers (1, 16). The user selects an antimicrobial test battery from among 30 possible panels of drugs, inserts the disks in the appropriate chambers of the cuvettes, adds a photometrically standardized bacterial inoculum suspension to the cuvettes, and incubates the cuvettes in a shaker/incubator for 3 to 5 h. The cuvettes are then manually inserted into a photometer/reader device for interpretation of results. The Autobac detects light scattering (measurement of forward light scatter at a 90° angle from the light source) caused by bacterial cells in the growth medium. The photometer is linked to an IBM personal computer with video display monitor, internal hard-disk storage, and printer for data storage and report production. The system offers the ability to archive and retrieve data for generation of periodic statistical reports. The MIC capability of the instrument is based on linear regression analysis of light scatter indices obtained from testing a high and a low concentration of each drug. These computer-calculated MICs have been shown to compare favorably with MICs derived from traditional $\log_2$ dilution tests (28).

The more popular qualitative test format (S, I, and R categories) of the Autobac has been extensively evaluated in a number of studies. In fact, a large multicenter (seven-laboratory) collaborative study (39) established the precedent for all evaluations of such instrument systems. The rationale for evaluating an instrument by using a common protocol in a simultaneous multilaboratory study was based on the assumption that such studies should reveal the likely true capabilities of an instrument by exposing it to a variety of different microorganisms and testing situations that could not be duplicated in a single laboratory. The publication resulting from this initial collaborative study also provided new jargon for categorization of the susceptibility test errors encountered during the study. The terms "very major," "major," and "minor" errors were coined to describe discrepancies between an automated test method and a reference susceptibility procedure such as dilution or the disk diffusion method reference procedure (39). A very major error occurred when the instrument result indicated susceptibility and the reference method indicated resistance of a microorganism. A major discrepancy was declared when an organism was said to be resistant by the automated system but susceptible by the reference method. A discrepancy was considered minor if an intermediate category result was obtained by one method and either a susceptible or resistant result was obtained by the other. Use of these terms has since become commonplace to describe the categories of discordance between newer automated and older reference susceptibility test procedures. However, consensus guidelines for defining acceptable levels of the various types of errors have not been developed. Sherris and Ryan have proposed that total errors should not exceed 5% and that very major errors should not be greater than 1.5% (30).

The initial collaborative evaluation of the Autobac indicated greater than 90% overall agreement between the instrument-generated results and those obtained by agar dilution and disk diffusion testing (39). However, a number of Autobac errors occurred with certain drug-organism combinations, e.g., *Enterobacter* spp. with nitrofurantoin and tetracycline; *Serratia* spp. with polymyxin and colistin; *P. aeruginosa* with chloramphenicol, kanamycin, and gentamicin; enterococci with tetracycline, kanamycin, and gentamicin; and *Staphylococcus epidermidis* with penicillin and tetracycline (39). One of these discrepancies, i.e., *Proteus* spp. testing with nitrofurantoin, was subsequently overcome. However, some errors were not remedied and have been contraindicated for testing by the manufacturer, i.e., enterococci with cephalothin and *P. aeruginosa* with kanamycin. Later studies also defined problem combinations, including *Staphylococcus aureus* with erythromycin (23) and methicillin (8) and *Escherichia coli* with ampicillin (38). A more recent study documented a continuing problem of detection of methicillin-resistant *S. aureus* (MRSA) by the Autobac (9). However, if these manufacturer-disclaimed or unfavorable organism-drug combinations are excluded, the Autobac provides accuracy equivalent to that of other rapid procedures, i.e., ≥90% as compared with conventional methods (13, 21, 39).

Abbott MS-2/Avantage

The Abbott MS-2 system was first introduced shortly after the Autobac, and in many ways it seems to represent a more automated version of a similar concept.

The MS-2 also uses the disk elution principle for antibiotic delivery in a large, multichamber plastic cuvette. However, instead of using light scatter index, the MS-2 determines optical density at a 670-nm wavelength (chosen for measurement of turbidity resulting from bacterial cells proliferating in an amber-colored growth medium) in a series of incubator/shaker/reader devices termed analysis modules (1, 16). An increase in automation occurred when individual light-emitting diodes and paired photodetectors were provided for each of 11 compartments in the plastic cuvettes. Each analysis module holds eight cuvettes, and up to four analysis modules can be linked to one MS-2 central or "control" module (16). After insertion of a cuvette in an analysis module of the instrument, the test to be performed is defined by use of a computer keyboard; then all subsequent incubations and readings are performed automatically under the control of a microcomputer. The MS-2 makes an internal inoculum adjustment by growing the bacteria for a brief period to establish logarithmic growth before exposure of the culture to the test antibiotics. This is accomplished by use of a two-tiered plastic cuvette (the upper chamber being the inoculum growth area) and a series of pumps to pressurize the upper chamber and cause the inoculated broth to transfer to the bottom antibiotic-containing chambers. Optical density changes are then determined and analyzed every 5 min during the ensuing 3- to 6-h incubation and analysis period. The total time for each analysis is dependent on the growth rate of the organism as evidenced by the development of turbidity in the uninhibited control well.

The MS-2 prints a qualitative S, I, or R result at the conclusion of each test in addition to the MIC breakpoints defined by the instrument for S or R results, e.g., cefoxitin susceptible, ≤10 μg/ml, or resistant, ≥30 μg/ml. The range for the S and R interpretations extends from the antibiotic content of the elution disk (for susceptible) to three times the disk concentration (for resistant). For intermediate results, a programmatically calculated MIC based on computer analysis of the growth curve is provided. The S and R breakpoints approximate but do not often coincide exactly with the interpretive breakpoints suggested for the various drugs by either the Food and Drug Administration or the National Committee for Clinical Laboratory Standards (25).

The successor to the MS-2, called the Avantage Microbiology Center, incorporates the basic principles of the MS-2 (including use of the same analysis modules and consumable supplies; 16). However, the MS-2 control module was replaced by a Hewlett-Packard personal computer with expanded capabilities. The additional computer memory allows storage of more information from simultaneous tests on the same bacterial isolate (identification and susceptibility), accommodates up to eight analysis modules, and programmatically compiles test results. A video display terminal and printer with graphics capability allow the Avantage to display graphic depictions of the optical density changes that occur during a susceptibility test as well as to generate a printed report of the test results.

The MS-2/Avantage also has been carefully scrutinized for reproducibility and accuracy in a number of published studies. A four-center collaborative study (38) introduced the concept of testing a set of challenge strains selected for their unusual resistance patterns in addition to testing fresh clinical isolates as a means of ensuring a thorough analysis of the instrument's performance. These challenge strains included MRSA and strains with inducible resistance to erythromycin, which at the time were unusual in the United States.

As with the Autobac, several organism-drug combinations have been recognized as problematic for the MS-2, e.g., *Enterobacter* spp. with ampicillin and cephalothin, *Serratia* spp. with colistin, enterococci with penicillin, cephalothin, kanamycin, and gentamicin, and *P. aeruginosa* with cefotaxime and moxalactam (35, 38).

Despite the initial challenge of the MS-2 with MRSA (38), two reports (5, 6) described difficulties in recognition of the MRSA strains that plagued some U.S. hospitals in the mid to late 1970s. These reports led Abbott to revise the computer software used to interpret methicillin tests, with a subsequent improvement in accuracy when resistant strains from several different areas of the country were tested (18). When the few unfavorable organism-drug combinations described above are excluded, the accuracy of the MS-2/Avantage (compared with 18- to 24-h reference test methods) is quite similar to that of the Autobac, i.e., greater than 90% agreement (4, 13, 15, 21, 29, 38).

The Vitek system

The Vitek system (formerly called the AutoMicrobic system or AMS) is a by-product of the U.S. space exploration efforts of the 1970s. It was designed and manufactured originally by the McDonnell-Douglas Corp. for the National Aeronautics and Space Administration as an onboard test system for spacecraft exploring other planets for life. Because of its intended use aboard a spacecraft, it was highly automated and relatively compact from its inception. Very small plastic reagent cards were designed to contain microliter quantities of biochemical test and selective growth media for detection and identification of organisms. The Vitek system was later modified for clinical laboratory use principally for screening and identification of urinary organisms and for qualitative antimicrobial susceptibility testing with S, I, or R results on only *E. coli* or *Proteus mirabilis*. More recently, MIC cards have been developed which allow quantitative results on most rapidly growing gram-positive and gram-negative aerobic bacteria in a period of 3 to 10 h.

Vitek hardware includes a filling module for inoculation of the cards; an incubator/reader module that incorporates a carousel-like device to hold the test cards, a robotic system to manipulate the cards, and a photometer for measurement of optical density and biochemical reaction color changes in the cards; and a computer module, including video display monitor and printer (1, 16). Vitek also offers an elaborate information management system for storing and retrieving test data for a variety of statistical reports. Like the MS-2/Avantage, the Vitek uses kinetic measurements of growth in the presence of antimicrobial agents to provide linear regression analysis and ultimately algorithm-derived MICs. However, the user may elect to have susceptibility test results reported in either qualitative or quantitative formats.

Unlike the Autobac and MS-2 systems, the Vitek was

not subjected to the close scrutiny of a large multicenter collaborative study. Independent studies initially demonstrated a lower level of accuracy of the qualitative test results of the Vitek than of the Autobac or MS-2 system (13, 21) or poor correlation of the Vitek MIC results with those of reference microdilution procedures (15, 43). Unfavorable organism-drug combinations included *Enterobacter* spp., *Serratia* spp., and *Providencia* spp. with ampicillin, cefamandole, and nitrofurantoin (12, 27); *Citrobacter* spp. with ampicillin (24); *Proteus mirabilis, Klebsiella* spp., *Enterobacter* spp., and *Citrobacter* spp. with chloramphenicol (2, 24); and *P. aeruginosa* with gentamicin, amikacin, and carbenicillin (2, 15, 24). However, more recent published studies have suggested that the accuracy of Vitek test results has been improved by reagent and computer software updates made by the manufacturer (27, 43). The Vitek appears to be one of the most accurate rapid test systems for detection of MRSA (18, 36) and has been shown to categorize accurately resistance of certain gram-negative species to newer β-lactam antibiotics due to inducible β-lactamase production (42).

The fixed format of the Vitek cards imposes some limitations in the selection of drugs for testing. However, the large number of wells in the cards combined with the presence of most commonly used drugs in the standard panels provides an acceptable selection for most users. In addition, Vitek offers at a reduced price a combination of two cards (called Flex cards) that are tested together and allow merging of results from the two cards into one report containing many different drugs.

In large part because of its aerospace design heritage, the Vitek is perceived by many to offer the highest degree of automation of the currently marketed systems. Many microbiologists undoubtedly choose the Vitek for its potential labor savings rather than as an instrument to produce rapid test results.

Sensititre fluorogenic-substrate system

The Sensititre fluorogenic-substrate test with AutoReader (Radiometer America Inc., Westlake, Ohio) is the first system marketed in the United States that incorporates fluorogenic-substrate hydrolysis as the method of detecting bacterial growth during an antimicrobial susceptibility test (32). The greater sensitivity of fluorescence technology allows testing of *Enterobacteriaceae* and some *S. aureus* strains by using either MIC or breakpoint formats after a 5-h incubation period (11, 33). The system utilizes microdilution trays containing dried antimicrobial agents. The trays are hydrated and inoculated by the AutoInoculator, using either standard or fluorogenic test medium. After incubation in a standard incubator for either 5 or 18 h, trays are placed in the AutoReader for result interpretation and data recording through a personal computer and printer.

Collaborative studies performed with the fluorogenic-substrate test have shown reasonably accurate results after 5 h of incubation with the *Enterobacteriaceae* if two antibiotics are excluded from testing, i.e., nitrofurantoin and tetracycline, which were associated with numerous very major errors with several enteric species (11, 26). However, one study (32) noted problems with *Proteus mirabilis* that led to a number of major errors unless the standard inoculum density was altered for that species. The most recent study (26) suggests that the Sensititre could effectively recognize MRSA by using the 5-h incubation mode, whereas an earlier study (33) had identified numerous very major errors with MRSA. *P. aeruginosa* testing appears problematic by the fluorogenic-substrate method, especially with the shorter 5-h incubation period (26, 33). Moreover, tests of enterococci and coagulase-negative staphylococci have not proven reliable (26, 32, 33). Thus, the Sensititre fluorogenic-substrate test offers the promise of an alternative methodology for generating rapid susceptibility test results. However, it appears that pending further development of the instrument, reliable rapid test capability of the system is restricted to the enteric gram-negative rods (perhaps excluding *Proteus mirabilis*) and possibly *S. aureus*.

AutoSCAN Walk/Away

One of the newest susceptibility testing instruments is the AutoSCAN Walk/Away (W/A; Baxter Microscan). The instrument consists of a large self-contained incubator/reader unit and a personal computer with video display terminal and printer. The W/A utilizes standard-size microdilution trays that are read either photometrically or fluorometrically. Once the microdilution trays have been inoculated, they are placed in one of the incubator positions in the instrument. The type of test to be performed is indicated on an instrument-readable bar code label placed on the end of each tray. The instrument then incubates the trays for the appropriate period (depending on the type of panel and organism), robotically positions the trays to add reagents if needed, and aligns them under the central photometer/fluorometer to perform the final readings of growth endpoints at the conclusion of the tests.

The W/A offers a choice of overnight incubation, with conventional photometric detection of turbidity for MIC or breakpoint testing of gram-positive and gram-negative bacteria, or rapid (3.5- to 5.5-h) readings of special MIC or breakpoint panels incorporating fluorogenic substrates. Special "combo" trays are available which provide susceptibility and organism identification in the same tray, using conventional substrates (overnight incubation) or special fluorogenic substrates for identification of gram-negative bacilli in only 2 h.

Because the W/A has only recently been marketed, there are as yet no published reports detailing its performance. One hopes that the results of one or more large collaborative studies will be forthcoming so that the capabilities of the W/A can be compared with those of other available instruments.

API ALADIN

The newest instrument to be marketed in the United States is the API ALADIN (abbreviation for automated laboratory diagnostic instrument; Analytab Products). The instrument includes a large incubator/reader unit with associated personal computer (including video display terminal and printer). Similar to the AutoSCAN W/A, the ALADIN incorporates use of standard-size microdilution trays; once the trays are inoculated, the instrument incubates them, adds reagents when appropriate, positions the trays by robotics, and automatically interprets the growth patterns at the conclusion of tests.

The ALADIN utilizes a video imaging system (similar to a video camera) to examine the microdilution tray wells for evidence of growth or for color changes of biochemical reactions. It also enables the instrument to read and interpret handwritten accession numbers and product identifier codes on the trays. The ALADIN uses a conventional overnight incubation period for performance of MIC or breakpoint susceptibility tests with gram-positive and gram-negative bacteria. Because the ALADIN is the newest of the instruments to be marketed, there are no published evaluations of its performance at this time. It is hoped that independent evaluations of this product will be available shortly.

ADVANTAGES OF CURRENT INSTRUMENTS

The antimicrobial susceptibility testing instruments discussed above represent the highest level of automation now available for use in clinical microbiology laboratories. However, automation in clinical microbiology is still in a very early stage of development compared with the level of automation that has been achieved in clinical chemistry, hematology, and immunology laboratories. All of the current microbiology instruments offer the potential for improved intra- and interlaboratory reproducibility of antimicrobial susceptibility tests, and in some cases they significantly reduce the time required to perform the tests (e.g., 3 to 10 h versus overnight incubation). Most evaluations have reported that the instruments are mechanically reliable and that their operation is readily mastered by well-trained microbiologists and medical technologists. Some of these instruments offer modest labor savings over manually performed tests. Because all of the instruments can perform some of the most common analyses in the microbiology laboratory, i.e., organism identification and antimicrobial susceptibility testing, the potential exists to automate a sizable proportion of a laboratory's tasks by using only one instrument. In addition, the personal-computer-based data management systems available with these instruments can provide neat, legible test reports for the laboratory and, perhaps more important, can simplify the archiving and periodic analysis of trends in antimicrobial susceptibility of the microorganisms encountered in a given institution.

DISADVANTAGES OF CURRENTLY AVAILABLE INSTRUMENTS

The instruments discussed in this chapter offer automation of several of the steps involved in performing an antimicrobial susceptibility test, although none of the existing instruments is able to execute the entire process, i.e., to standardize an inoculum and continue through to the final interpretation of results without operator intervention. Microbiologists must still isolate bacteria by using conventional culture methods and prepare a bacterial suspension of defined density for testing by the instrument. Thus, the automated aspects of the test do not begin until after the manual inoculum preparation. Indeed, inadequacy of the inoculum is a major variable affecting performance of all of the instruments. None of the existing instruments attempts to directly analyze patient body fluids for the presence of antimicrobial resistance mediators in bacteria.

Because of instrument control in a number of test procedure steps, instrument methods may offer some improvement in test reproducibility. However, the accuracy of instrument-generated results has been lower than that of manual reference systems in some cases, particularly if the instrument has used a short incubation period or a nontraditional growth detection method (1, 5, 7, 8, 26, 35). An incubation period of only 3 to 5 h may not be adequate for expression of all bacterial resistance mechanisms, e.g., inducible β-lactamase-mediated resistance among gram-negative bacilli to some enzyme-labile β-lactam antibiotics (38, 42). Thus, when results from instruments using an abbreviated incubation period have been compared with results from tests employing overnight incubation, very major errors have been noted with some organism-antimicrobial agent combinations (6, 9, 13, 22, 35, 38, 39). These discrepancies have been minimized by the instrument manufacturers through manipulation of the inoculum density (higher for the rapid test systems), by altering the drug test concentrations, or by modifying the computer software that interprets the test results. Despite these improvements, some disagreements still occur between rapid automated and overnight test results. Thus, a conscientious microbiologist must be knowledgeable of unfavorable organism-antimicrobial agent combinations and provide alternative accurate means for their testing. Moreover, with few exceptions, slow-growing or fastidious bacteria are not amenable to automated susceptibility test procedures.

Perhaps the most frequent complaint voiced by users of automated susceptibility equipment relates to drug availability and selection of routine susceptibility test batteries. Because there are now more than 50 antimicrobial agents in common use in the United States (25) and because the usage of particular drugs varies considerably from one institution to another, it is not possible for an instrument manufacturer to provide a single tray or cuvette that contains all available drugs for testing. Thus, most manufacturers provide a selection of standard panels that include combinations of the most popular drugs in configurations of 12 to 30 agents. Paper elution disks provide somewhat more flexibility for the Autobac and MS-2/Avantage systems than the plastic trays or cards containing frozen or dried antimicrobial agents that are used by all of the other manufacturers. However, the delayed availability of some disks and the limited number of disks that can be tested in a single cuvette pose problems for some laboratories. To provide flexibility for different medical practice environments, several manufactures will prepare custom panels tailored to the exact formulary of an institution; however, custom panels generally require that a substantial minimum number of the special panels be purchased and generally have a higher price than the standard panels. None of the automated systems has managed to duplicate the flexibility inherent in the conventional disk diffusion antimicrobial susceptibility test.

Another problem with automated susceptibility test instruments has been limitations of instrument quality control procedures, largely because control strains used with the systems often result in many off-scale values, i.e., MICs less than or equal to the lowest concentration or greater than the highest concentration tested by the instrument (19, 20). All of the currently available instruments are mechanically and optically complex devices that must function properly for reproducible test results. Each manufacturer describes routine maintenance and function checks to prevent or detect overt malfunctions. However, the quality control checks suggested by the manufacturers may not be adequate to detect subtle deteriorations in instrument or reagent performance. The lack of on-scale control values means that the potency of antimicrobial agents and functioning of the instrument may not be ensured with the precision that clinical microbiologists have come to expect with procedures like the conventional disk diffusion susceptibility test.

When a serious mechanical failure occurs, only tests from instruments that utilize conventional microdilution trays and photometric analysis of growth patterns after overnight incubation can be continued by manual incubation and interpretation. The instrument methods that incorporate rapid test interpretation or use fluorogenic-substrate analysis cannot be manually interpreted, since subtle and varying definitions of growth are used by the instruments' algorithms. Therefore, laboratories must maintain a backup testing procedure such as disk diffusion or manual, overnight microdilution testing in order to avoid delays in generating results while a repairman is dispatched to repair an instrument.

Finally, the current generation of automated susceptibility testing instruments have not served to reduce the cost of such tests through miniaturization, standardization, etc. Unlike the greater economy afforded by automated tests performed by chemistry autoanalyzers, consumable costs for microbiology instruments are equivalent to or greater than the costs of manual procedures. In addition, the instruments described in this chapter generally cost from $30,000 to $90,000 for hardware, depending on the extent of automation and the number of tests that can be performed simultaneously. Laboratories may find it more economical to obtain an instrument system through a reagent rental or lease agreement to avoid a large capital outlay for hardware.

SUMMARY

Instruments for performance of antimicrobial susceptibility testing should be viewed as some of the best examples of automation in clinical microbiology. The performance of susceptibility tests seems well suited to instrumentation, since an objective measurement of microbial proliferation is the basis for the test. Instruments provide more rapid results than can be generated by using manual systems and undoubtedly serve to improve intra- and interlaboratory standardization.

The clinical benefit of performing antimicrobial susceptibility tests in 3 to 8 h rather than after overnight incubation has been difficult to measure. Two studies (10, 41) have shown that providing rapid susceptibility test results is likely to result in a more timely change to appropriate antimicrobial therapy than if conventional reporting times were employed. One of the studies (41) also documented direct cost savings attributable to changes to less expensive antimicrobial agents based on the rapid susceptibility test reports. An earlier study (23) estimated that 9% of patients with culture-proven bacterial infections had their hospital stays shortened as a result of the provision of rapid susceptibility reports. However, it has been aptly pointed out that these improvements in clinical care have required aggressive and innovative laboratory reporting strategies to bring the rapid results to the attention of physicians for appropriate action (17, 23). It is unlikely that the use of rapid susceptibility test methods will result in any measurable improvement in patient care without considerable efforts to make physicians aware of the earlier reporting capability of the laboratory. Optimal utilization of rapid results likely will also require that laboratories reorganize their work patterns in order to accomplish rapid testing, since it has been suggested that results should be available by no later than 2 or 3 p.m. if significant time savings are to be realized (7).

Efforts to develop test methods with even shorter analysis times must continue so that rapid reporting can occur in a more compressed and thus more relevant time period. Moreover, efforts should continue toward development of more automated equipment that will not only provide faster results but also save money by virtue of lower reagent costs and reduced labor requirements. It seems clear that the benefits of automation in clinical microbiology are just beginning to be manifested. Further advances seem likely to be achieved by exploring more innovative means of detecting the inhibitory effects of antimicrobial agents on microorganisms.

LITERATURE CITED

1. **Amsterdam, D.** 1988. Instrumentation for antimicrobic susceptibility testing: yesterday, today, and tomorrow. Diagn. Microbiol. Infect. Dis. **9:**167–178.
2. **Backes, B. A., S. J. Cavalieri, J. T. Rudrick, and E. M. Britt.** 1984. Rapid antimicrobial susceptibility testing of gram-negative clinical isolates with the AutoMicrobic system. J. Clin. Microbiol. **19:**744–747.
3. **Baker, C. N., S. A. Stocker, D. L. Rhoden, and C. Thornsberry.** 1986. Evaluation of the MicroScan antimicrobial susceptibility system with the AutoScan-4 automated reader. J. Clin. Microbiol. **23:**143–148.
4. **Barnes, W. G., L. R. Green, and R. L. Talley.** 1980. Clinical evaluation of automated antibiotic susceptibility testing with the MS-2 system. J. Clin. Microbiol. **12:**527–532.
5. **Boyce, J. M., R. L. White, M. C. Bonner, and W. R. Lockwood.** 1982. Reliability of the MS-2 system in detecting methicillin-resistant *Staphylococcus aureus*. J. Clin. Microbiol. **15:**220–225.
6. **Carlson, J. R., F. E. Conley, and D. L. Cahall.** 1982. Methicillin-resistant *Staphylococcus aureus* susceptibility testing with the Abbott MS-2 system. Antimicrob. Agents Chemother. **21:**676–677.
7. **Cherubin, C. E., R. Eng, and M. Appleman.** 1987. A critique of semiautomated susceptibility systems. Rev. Infect. Dis. **9:**655–659.
8. **Clearly, T. J., and D. Maurer.** 1978. Methicillin-resistant *Staphylococcus aureus* susceptibility testing by an automated system, Autobac I. Antimicrob. Agents Chemother. **13:**837–841.
9. **de la Roy, Y. R., E. Chevalier-Burbaud, S. Pannetier, and F. Souchaud.** 1985. Use of the Autobac system for detection of methicillin-resistant *Staphylococcus aureus*. J. Clin. Microbiol. **22:**467–469.
10. **Doern, G. V., D. R. Scott, and A. L. Rashad.** 1982. Clinical impact of rapid antimicrobial susceptibility testing of blood culture isolates. Antimicrob. Agents Chemother. **21:**1023–1024.
11. **Doern, G. V., J. L. Staneck, C. Needham, and T. Tubert.**

1987. Sensititre Autoreader for same-day breakpoint broth microdilution susceptibility testing of members of the family *Enterobacteriaceae*. J. Clin. Microbiol. **25:**1481–1485.

12. **Goldstein, J., J. J. Guarneri, and J. J. Scherer.** 1982. Use of the AutoMicrobic system for rapid antimicrobial susceptibility testing of *Enterobacteriaceae* in a clinical laboratory. J. Clin. Lab. Automat. **2:**329–333.
13. **Hansen, S. L., and P. K. Freedy.** 1983. Concurrent comparability of automated systems and commercially prepared microdilution trays for susceptibility testing. J. Clin. Microbiol. **17:**878–886.
14. **Isenberg, H. D., A. Reichler, and D. Wiseman.** 1971. Prototype of a fully automated device for determination of bacterial antibiotic susceptibility in the clinical laboratory. Appl. Microbiol. **22:**980–986.
15. **Johnson, J. E., J. H. Jorgensen, S. A. Crawford, J. S. Redding, and R. C. Pruneda.** 1983. Comparison of two automated instrument systems for rapid susceptibility testing of gram-negative bacilli. J. Clin. Microbiol. **18:**1301–1309.
16. **Jorgensen, J. H.** 1987. Instrument systems which provide rapid (3–6 hour) antibiotic susceptibility results, p. 85–97. *In* J. H. Jorgensen (ed.), Automation in clinical microbiology. CRC Press, Inc., Boca Raton, Fla.
17. **Jorgensen, J. H., and J. M. Matsen.** 1987. Physician acceptance and application of rapid microbiology instrument test results, p. 209–212. *In* J. H. Jorgensen (ed.), Automation in clinical microbiology. CRC Press, Inc., Boca Raton, Fla.
18. **Jorgensen, J. H., J. S. Redding, J. E. Johnson, V. Holloway, and R. J. Almeida.** 1984. Rapid recognition of methicillin-resistant *Staphylococcus aureus* by use of automated test systems. J. Clin. Microbiol. **20:**430–433.
19. **Kellogg, J. A.** 1984. Inability to control selected drugs on commercially-obtained microdilution MIC panels. Am. J. Clin. Pathol. **82:**455–458.
20. **Kellogg, J. A.** 1985. Inability to adequately control antimicrobial agents on AutoMicrobic System gram-positive and gram-negative cards. J. Clin. Microbiol. **21:**454–456.
21. **Kelly, M. T., J. M. Latimer, and L. C. Balfour.** 1982. Comparison of three automated systems for antimicrobial susceptibility testing of gram-negative bacilli. J. Clin. Microbiol. **15:**902–905.
22. **Lampe, M. F., C. L. Aitken, P. G. Dennis, P. S. Forsythe, K. E. Patrick, F. D. Schoenknecht, and J. C. Sherris.** 1975. Relationship of early readings of minimal inhibitory concentrations to the results of overnight tests. Antimicrob. Agents Chemother. **8:**429–433.
23. **Matsen, J. M.** 1985. Means to facilitate physician acceptance and use of rapid test results. Diagn. Microbiol. Infect. Dis. **3:**35s–78s.
24. **Nadler, H. L., C. Dolan, L. Mele, and S. R. Kurtz.** 1985. Accuracy and reproducibility of the AutoMicrobic System Gram-Negative General Susceptibility-Plus card for testing selected challenge organisms. J. Clin. Microbiol. **22:**355–360.
25. **National Committee for Clinical Laboratory Standards.** 1988. Methods for dilution antimicrobial susceptibility testing for bacteria that grew aerobically. Tentative standards M7-T2. National Committee for Clinical Laboratory Standards, Villanova, Pa.
26. **Nolte, F. S., K. K. Krisher, L. A. Beltran, N. P. Christianson, and G. E. Sheridan.** 1988. Rapid and overnight microdilution antibiotic susceptibility testing with the Sensititre Autoreader system. J. Clin. Microbiol. **26:**1079–1084.
27. **Reiber, N. E., M. T. Kelly, J. M. Latimer, D. L. Tison, and R. M. Hysmith.** 1985. Comparison of the Cathra Repliscan II, the AutoMicrobic System Gram-Negative General Susceptibility-Plus card, and the Micro-Media System Fox panel for dilution susceptibility testing of gram-negative bacilli. J. Clin. Microbiol. **21:**959–962.
28. **Schoenknecht, F. D., J. A. Washington II, T. L. Gavan, and C. Thornsberry.** 1980. Rapid determination of minimum inhibitory concentrations of antimicrobial agents by the Autobac method: a collaborative study. Antimicrob. Agents Chemother. **17:**824–833.
29. **Sewell, D. L., and M. T. Makler.** 1981. Clinical evaluation of the Abbott MS-2 antimicrobial susceptibility testing system. Am. J. Clin. Pathol. **76:**82–85.
30. **Sherris, J. C., and K. J. Ryan.** 1982. Evaluation of automated and rapid methods, p. 1–5. *In* R. C. Tilton (ed.), Rapid methods and automation in microbiology. American Society for Microbiology, Washington, D.C.
31. **Sielaff, B. H., J. M. Matsen, and J. E. McKie.** 1982. Novel approach to bacterial identification that uses the Autobac system. J. Clin. Microbiol. **15:**1103–1110.
32. **Staneck, J. L., S. D. Allen, E. E. Harris, and R. C. Tilton.** 1985. Automated reading of MIC microdilution trays containing fluorogenic enzyme substrates with the Sensititre Autoreader. J. Clin. Microbiol. **22:**187–191.
33. **Staneck, J. L., S. D. Allen, E. E. Harris, and R. C. Tilton.** 1988. Rapid MIC testing with the Sensititre Autoreader. J. Clin. Microbiol. **26:**1–7.
34. **Steers, E., F. Foltz, B. S. Graves, and J. Riden.** 1959. An inocula replicating apparatus for routine testing of bacterial susceptibility to antibiotics. Antibiot. Chemother. **9:** 307–311.
35. **Stone, L. L., and D. L. Jungkind.** 1983. False-susceptible results from the MS-2 system used for testing resistant *Pseudomonas aeruginosa* against two third-generation cephalosporins, moxalactam and cefotaxime. J. Clin. Microbiol. **18:**389–394.
36. **Stotler, R. W., and M. C. Meyer.** 1983. Detection of oxacillin-resistant staphyloccoci by the AutoMicrobic system. J. Clin. Microbiol. **18:**1205–1211.
37. **Stubbs, K. G., and K. Wicher.** 1977. Laboratory evaluation of an automated antimicrobial susceptibility system. Am. J. Clin. Pathol. **68:**769–777.
38. **Thornsberry, C., J. P. Anhalt, J. A. Washington II, L. R. McCarthy, F. D. Schoenknecht, J. C. Sherris, and H. J. Spencer.** 1980. Clinical laboratory evaluation of the Abbott MS-2 automated antimicrobial susceptibility testing system: report of a collaborative study. J. Clin. Microbiol. **12:** 375–390.
39. **Thornsberry, C., T. L. Gavan, J. C. Sherris, A. Balows, J. M. Matsen, L. D. Sabath, F. Schoenknecht, L. D. Thrupp, and J. A. Washington II.** 1975. Laboratory evaluation of a rapid automated susceptibility testing system: report of a collaboratory study. Antimicrob. Agents Chemother. **7:**466–480.
40. **Thrupp, L. D.** 1986. Susceptibility testing of antibiotics in liquid media, p. 93–150. *In* V. Lorian (ed.), Antibiotics in laboratory medicine, 2nd ed. The Williams & Wilkins Co., Baltimore.
41. **Trenholme, G. M., R. L. Kaplan, P. H. Karahusis, T. Stine, J. Fuhrer, W. Landau, and S. Levin.** 1989. Clinical impact of rapid identification and susceptibility testing of bacterial blood culture isolates. J. Clin. Microbiol. **27:** 1342–1345.
42. **Washington, J. A., II, C. C. Knapp, and C. C. Sanders.** 1988. Accuracy of microdilution and the AutoMicrobic System in detection of β-lactam resistance in gram-negative bacterial mutants with depressed β-lactamase. Rev. Infect. Dis. **10:**824–829.
43. **Woolfrey, B. F., R. T. Lally, M. N. Ederer, and C. O. Quall.** 1984. Evaluation of the AutoMicrobic System for identification and susceptibility testing of gram-negative bacilli. J. Clin. Microbiol. **20:**1053–1059.

Chapter 117

Laboratory Studies with Antifungal Agents: Susceptibility Tests and Quantitation in Body Fluids

SMITH SHADOMY AND MICHAEL A. PFALLER

Opportunistic fungal infections are becoming increasingly important causes of morbidity and mortality in hospitalized patients. *Candida* spp. accounted for 7.7% of all nosocomial bloodstream infections in the United States from 1985 to 1988 and was the fourth most common cause of nosocomial bloodstream infections, behind coagulase-negative staphylococci, *Staphylococcus aureus*, and *Enterococcus* spp. (T. Horan, D. Culver, W. Jarvis, G. Emori, S. Banerjee, W. Martone, and C. Thornsberry, Antimicrob. Newsl. **5**:65–67, 1988). The impact of these infections is substantial, with the mortality and excess length of hospital stay attributable to nosocomial candidemia estimated at 38% and 30 days (median value), respectively (68). In addition to *Candida* spp., infections due to *Aspergillus* spp., *Fusarium* spp., the zygomycetes, dematiaceous fungi, and other usually "nonpathogenic" fungi are being reported with increasing frequency (2). A major part of this increase has been attributed to increased use of newer and more effective antibacterial agents, bone marrow and solid-organ transplantation, immunosuppressive and cytotoxic therapy for a variety of diseases, and the emergence of AIDS (2, 61, 65). Paralleling the increase in opportunistic fungal infections over the last decade has been the introduction of a number of new antifungal agents with systemic activity (Table 1). With the use of both established and investigational agents has come the recognition of resistance in selected isolates to one or more antifungal agents (15, 21, 22, 28, 40, 44, 49, 50, 52, 65). As a result, clinical laboratories are now being asked to assume a greater role in the selection and monitoring of antifungal chemotherapy, and efforts are being made to standardize laboratory tests with antifungal agents (11, 17, 18, 21–24, 27, 45).

SUSCEPTIBILITY TESTS WITH ANTIFUNGAL AGENTS

Susceptibility tests with antifungal agents are performed for the same reasons that tests with antibacterial agents are performed. Ideally, in vitro susceptibility tests will (i) provide a reliable measure of the relative activities of two or more antifungal agents, (ii) correlate with in vivo activity and predict the likely outcome of therapy, (iii) provide a means with which to monitor the development of resistance among a normally susceptible population of organisms, and (iv) predict the therapeutic potential of newly discovered investigational agents (21, 22, 44, 58). Unfortunately, there is little evidence to support the clinical correlations of antifungal susceptibility test results with in vivo outcome (22, 44, 48, 52, 62). Although recent studies by Powderly et al. (50) and Radetsky et al. (51) suggest some correlation with MIC results for amphotericin B and clinical outcome, the general applicability of these results remains confused by the retrospective nature of the studies, the documented variability of the nonstandardized in vitro test methods used, and the difficulty in defining fungal diseases and their responses to therapy.

In vitro susceptibility test procedures with antifungal agents are similar in design to those used with antibacterial agents (17, 21, 22, 27, 40). The methods that have been applied to antifungal susceptibility testing include broth dilution (macro and micro), agar dilution, and disk diffusion (Table 2). Several different methods of endpoint determination have been applied in efforts to develop a test method that is objective and easy to perform and interpret in the routine clinical laboratory (Table 2).

Antifungal susceptibility tests are influenced by a number of technical variables (Table 3), including inoculum size and preparation, medium formulation and pH, and duration and temperature of incubation (11, 17, 18, 21–23, 40, 44, 58). In addition, antifungal susceptibility testing is complicated by problems unique to fungi, such as slow growth rates (relative to bacteria) and the ability of certain dimorphic fungi to grow either as a unicellular yeast form that produces blastoconidia or as a hyphal or mould form that may produce asexual spores, depending on the conditions of pH, temperature, and medium composition (40, 58). Finally, the basic properties of the antifungal agents themselves, such as solubility, chemical stability, modes of action, and the tendency to produce partial inhibition of growth over a wide range of concentrations, must be taken into account.

A variety of antifungal agents are now available for the treatment of fungal infections. Ten of these compounds, four established, five investigational, and one recently licensed, will be briefly discussed in this chapter (Table 1). They include representatives of the polyene macrolide class (amphotericin B and liposomal amphotericin B), the azoles (miconazole, ketoconazole, itraconazole, fluconazole, saperconazole, and Sch 39304), a glucan synthetase inhibitor (cilofungin), and an inhibitor of DNA and RNA synthesis (5-fluorocytosine [5-FC]).

Amphotericin B and liposomal amphotericin B are polyene macrolide antibiotics used primarily in the treatment of systemic and life-threatening fungal infections. Liposomal amphotericin B was designed to maximize the delivery of amphotericin B to patients with deep-seated fungal infections such as hepatosplenic candidiasis and invasive pulmonary aspergillosis (38,

TABLE 1. Established and investigational antifungal agents with systemic activity

Antifungal agent	Mechanism of action	Manufacturer	Route	Comments
5-FC	Inhibition of DNA and RNA synthesis	Hoffmann-La Roche	Oral	Toxicity and resistance are problems. Used in combination with amphotericin B.
Polyenes				
Amphotericin B	Binds to ergosterol, causing direct oxidative membrane damage	Squibb	i.v.[a]	Established agent. Broad-spectrum. Toxic.
Liposomal amphotericin B	Same as amphotericin B	Squibb	i.v.	Investigational agent with broad-spectrum activity and decreased toxicity. Role in therapy is not yet established.
Azoles				
Miconazole	Inhibition of membrane sterol synthesis	Janssen	i.v.	Toxic agent with modest anticandidal activity. Active against *Pseudallescheria boydii*.
Ketoconazole	Same as miconazole	Janssen	Oral, topical	Modest broad-spectrum activity.
Itraconazole	Same as miconazole	Janssen	Oral	Triazole with broad-spectrum activity.
Fluconazole	Same as miconazole	Pfizer	Oral, i.v.	Triazole with broad-spectrum activity. Good central nervous system penetration. Good in vivo anticandidal activity.
Saperconazole	Same as miconazole	Janssen	Oral, ? i.v.	Investigational triazole. Role in therapy not yet established.
Sch 39304	Same as miconazole	Schering	Oral, ? i.v.	Investigational triazole. Role in therapy not yet established.

[a] i.v., Intravenous.

65). Liposomal amphotericin B is produced by incorporating amphotericin B into liposomes of dimyristoylphosphatidylglycerol and dimyristoylphosphatidylcholine. The resultant liposomal preparation has selective toxicity for fungal cells but not for erythrocytes (41) and theoretically promotes the delivery of drug to the site of infection while avoiding the toxicity of supramaximal doses of amphotericin B. The limited amount of uncontrolled data available suggests that liposomal amphotericin B may be useful in treating infections that are refractory to conventional therapy (38, 65); however, this agent must be further studied in controlled, randomized clinical trials.

TABLE 2. Methods used for antifungal susceptibility testing

Test method	Means of endpoint determination
Broth dilution	
Macrodilution	Visual, ATP photometry, turbidimetric, colorimetric, radiometric, dry weight
Microdilution	Same as macrodilution
Agar dilution	
Microdilution with semisolid agar	Visual
Macrodilution in standard petri dishes	Visual
Agar diffusion	
Disk	Zone diameter (visual)
Well	Zone diameter (visual)

The polyene antifungal agents act by binding to ergosterol in the fungal cell membrane, causing loss of membrane integrity and osmotic instability. The direct membrane toxicity is due in part to oxidative damage and is frequently fungicidal (59, 65). Although resistance to amphotericin B is rare, changes in membrane sterols have been correlated with the development of resistance both in vitro and in vivo (15, 28, 65). Such resistance has assumed clinical importance, particularly with certain species such as *Candida lusitaniae* (15, 28).

The chemical properties of the polyene antifungal agents pose certain problems relative to in vitro susceptibility testing. These agents are water insoluble and are inactivated by heat, light, and acid. Thus, particular attention must be paid to the preparation and handling of the test solutions as well as the conditions for in vitro susceptibility testing. The medium used should be well buffered (pH 7.0), and the test solutions should be protected from light.

The azole class of antifungal compounds consists of a large number of agents with systemic antifungal activity, including the imidazoles (miconazole and ketoconazole) and the newer triazoles (itraconazole, fluconazole, saperconazole, and Sch 39304; Table 1). All

TABLE 3. Problems with antifungal susceptibility testing

1. Organism-specific problems
   a. Dimorphism
   b. Slow growth
   c. Biohazards
2. Lack of established clinical correlation
3. Variables that influence test performance
   a. Inoculum size and preparation
   b. Medium formulation and pH
   c. Duration of incubation
   d. Temperature of incubation
4. Drug-specific problems
   a. Solubility in aqueous media
   b. Chemical instability
   c. Partial inhibition of growth
   d. Mode of action

of the azoles inhibit fungal cytochrome P-450-dependent enzymes, with resulting impairment of ergosterol synthesis and depletion of ergosterol in the fungal cell membrane. The imidazoles, miconazole and ketoconazole, are established, broad-spectrum agents active against a variety of fungal pathogens, including yeasts, dimorphic organisms, dermatophytes, and opportunistic pathogens. The triazoles, itraconazole, fluconazole, saperconazole, and Sch 39304, all show promise as broad-spectrum, orally active, systemic agents with less potential for toxicity than the currently available imidazoles (19, 30, 44, 53). Ongoing and future clinical trials will more clearly define the specific roles of the triazoles in the treatment of systemic mycoses.

The azoles share certain properties that affect in vitro susceptibility testing, including broad spectra, relatively good chemical stabilities, and poor solubilities in aqueous media (with the exception of fluconazole). In vitro susceptibility testing with these agents is profoundly influenced by all of the variables listed in Table 3, which results in poor test reproducibility. The major sources of test variation for azole antifungals in vitro appear to be the pH and composition of the test medium, inoculum size, and duration of incubation (44). In addition, partial inhibition of fungal growth in vitro often takes place over an extensive range of concentrations, making endpoint determination (MIC) both very difficult and subjective. Finally, it appears that azoles are more potent in inhibiting hyphal outgrowth than blastoconidium formation in *Candida albicans* (19, 44, 53, 65), suggesting that the morphologic or developmental form of the organism may be another important variable. Although resistance to azoles has been demonstrated in *C. albicans,* its detection in vitro appears to be quite variable and method dependent (52). In general, in vivo and clinical correlations with in vitro susceptibility test results with azole antifungal agents have been quite poor (18, 19, 22, 44, 48).

5-FC (flucytosine) is a water-soluble, stable compound used orally in the treatment of systemic infections caused by susceptible pathogenic or opportunistic yeasts and fungi. It acts as a competitive antimetabolite for uracil in the synthesis of yeast RNA, and it also interferes with thymidylate synthetase (43, 49). These activities can be antagonized in vitro by a variety of purine and pyrimidine bases and nucleosides (49, 58). Because of this antagonism, the antifungal activity of 5-FC can be demonstrated in vitro only in synthetic media free of such substances.

In vitro testing with 5-FC is more important clinically than testing with either the polyene compounds or the azoles because of the repeated demonstration of de novo resistance to the drug as well as the emergence of resistant strains of yeasts and fungi after therapeutic exposure to the drug (43, 49, 58, 65). At least two metabolic sites are responsible for this resistance (43, 49); one involves the enzyme cytosine permease, which is responsible for the uptake of 5-FC into fungal cells, whereas the second site involves the enzyme cytosine deaminase, which is responsible for the deamination of 5-FC to 5-fluorouracil, the metabolically active form of the drug.

Susceptibility tests with 5-FC should be performed on all isolates of pathogenic yeasts or fungi isolated from patients destined to receive the drug. Such tests should also be performed on all isolates recovered during therapy. However, the results of such tests must be interpreted with caution, as they cannot always be regarded as fully predictive of clinical responses (43, 48, 62).

Cilofungin (LY 121019; Eli Lilly & Co., Indianapolis, Ind.) is a new antifungal antibiotic that is structurally similar to the lipopeptide agents echinocandin B and aculeacin A. The mechanism of action of cilofungin is thought to involve inhibition of glucan synthesis, resulting in cell wall damage and lysis (29, 46, 47). Cilofungin has candidacidal activity against *C. albicans* and *Candida tropicalis* but has little or no activity against other *Candida* species (29, 47). MIC determinations are adversely affected by acid pH and complex, undefined media (46). Preliminary data indicate favorable pharmacokinetics and low toxicity in humans; however, the clinical effectiveness of this novel compound remains to be determined in clinical trials.

Given the increasing number of antifungal agents and the perceived need for in vitro susceptibility testing to assist in their clinical application, efforts are needed to standardize antifungal susceptibility testing (11, 18, 22). With this in mind, the National Committee for Clinical Laboratory Standards (NCCLS) has established a subcommittee to coordinate work on antifungal susceptibility tests, with a goal of developing a reliable reference method for in vitro susceptibility testing of yeasts and other fungi and ultimately of correlating the results of this method with clinical effectiveness.

Several multicenter studies conducted by the NCCLS subcommittee have identified a number of key technical problems that affect the precision and the intra- and interlaboratory variation and reproducibility of MIC test procedures with isolates of yeasts and the three antifungal agents most often tested in vitro: amphotericin B, 5-FC, and ketoconazole (23, 45). The results of these studies regarding, in particular, preparation of inocula, composition and pH of media, and conditions for incubation have been incorporated in the following in vitro test procedures with antifungal agents.

MACROBROTH DILUTION SUSCEPTIBILITY TESTING METHOD

Although a consensus recommendation of a standardized susceptibility test method is not available from the NCCLS Subcommittee on Antifungal Susceptibility Testing, a macrobroth dilution method suitable for in vitro testing with isolates of *C. albicans* and other yeast-like fungi against amphotericin B, 5-FC, and ketoconazole is outlined in Fig. 1 and described below. The object of this method is to provide a uniform, reproducible means of assessing the relative in vitro activities of commonly used antifungal agents against clinical yeast isolates. The clinical correlations of the test results remain to be established.

Media

The test medium should be a completely defined synthetic medium such as RPMI 1640 with L-glutamine (R-6504, Sigma Chemical Co., St. Louis, Mo.; 430-1800, GIBCO Laboratories, Grand Island, N.Y.), yeast-nitrogen base (YNB) (0392, Difco Laboratories, Detroit, Mich.; 12101, BBL Microbiology Systems, Cockeysville, Md.) supplemented with glucose (1%) and asparagine (0.15%), or HR antifungal assay medium (CM 845, Oxoid Ltd., Basingstoke, Hampshire, England) buffered to pH 7.0 with 0.165 M MOPS buffer [3-(*N*-morpholino)propanesulfonic acid; Sigma]. The media are sterilized by filtration and stored at 4°C. These media are suitable for the testing of amphotericin B, 5-FC, and azoles against *Candida* spp.; however, RPMI 1640 may not be adequate to support the growth of some strains of *Cryptococcus neoformans*.

Drug solutions

A solution of standard 5-FC powder (10,000 μg/ml; Hoffmann-LaRoche Inc., Nutley, N.J.) is prepared in distilled water and sterilized by filtration. This solution may be used indefinitely if uncontaminated and stored at −70°C. For testing of amphotericin B (E. R. Squibb & Sons, Princeton, N.J.) or other polyenes, sufficient standard drug is weighed to prepare a solution of 5,000 μg/ml. The actual amount to be weighed must be adjusted according to the specific biological activity of the standard. If standard amphotericin B is not available, Fungizone either as the pharmaceutical preparation (Fungizone for injection; Squibb) or as a laboratory reagent (Fungizone for laboratory use; Squibb) may be substituted. Standard substances of amphotericin B and other polyenes may be solubilized in dimethyl sulfoxide (DMSO) or dimethylformamide. These solutions must be protected from light and should be allowed to stand for 30 min before use to permit autosterilization. The stock solution of 5,000 μg/ml may be used for 1 week if stored in the dark at 4°C.

A variety of solvent systems are used with the azoles. These systems include 10% stock solutions prepared in polyethylene glycol, DMSO, and dimethylformamide. Ketoconazole is best dissolved in 0.2 N HCl. None of these substances gives a solution that will remain completely solubilized upon dilution into aqueous media. Thus, at higher concentrations, a certain amount of turbidity will be encountered, which may interfere with the interpretation of in vitro susceptibility test results.

Preparation of inocula

Inocula should be prepared by using the spectrophotometric method (45) as outlined in Fig. 1. The test organisms are grown on plates of Sabouraud agar (Sabouraud dextrose agar Emmons, 11589, BBL; Sabouraud agar modified, 0747, Difco) for 48 h, and the inoculum suspension is prepared by picking five colonies of at least 1-mm diameter and suspending the material in 5 ml of sterile 0.85% NaCl. The turbidity of the cell suspension measured at 530 nm is adjusted with sterile saline to match that of a 0.5 McFarland barium sulfate standard. This produces a cell suspension containing 1×10^6 to 5×10^6 organisms per ml, which is then diluted 1:100 with the desired test medium to provide a starting inoculum of 1×10^4 to 5×10^4 organisms per ml. A similar suspension should also be prepared for a control organism. Suitable susceptible control organisms include *Saccharomyces cerevisiae* ATCC 36375, *S. cerevisiae* ATCC 9763, *S. cerevisiae* ATCC 2601, *C. albicans* ATCC 10231, *C. tropicalis* ATCC 13803, and

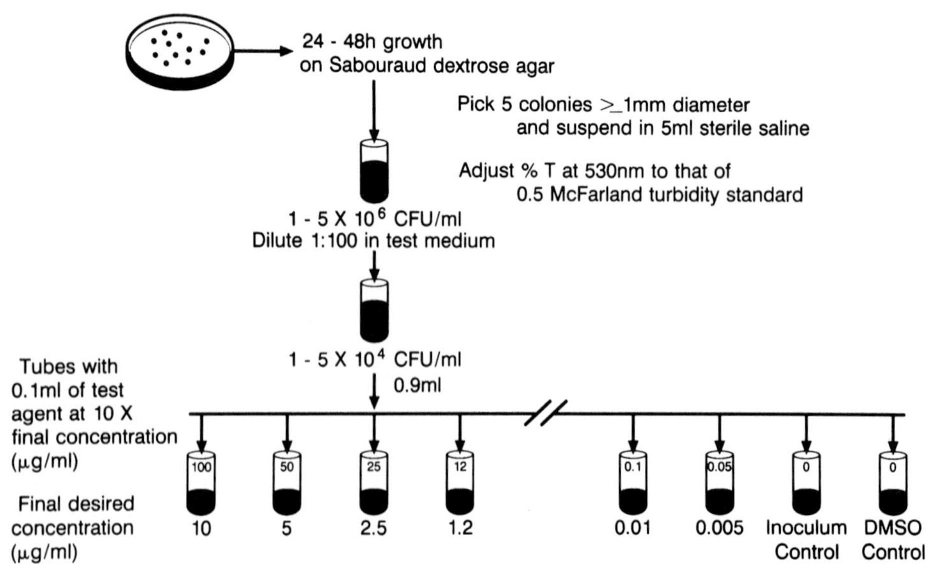

FIG. 1. Example of a macrobroth dilution method for antifungal susceptibility testing of yeast isolates.

Candida kefyr ATCC 28838 or NCPF 3234 (National Collection of Pathogenic Fungi, Mycology Reference Laboratory, London School of Hygiene and Tropical Medicine, London, England; syn. *C. pseudotropicalis*).

Drug dilutions and performance of test

The following procedure gives sufficient material to test (in duplicate) one isolate and the appropriate control organism. With the desired medium, prepare 5 ml of a solution of the drug or drugs to be tested. For the example outlined in Fig. 1, a 0.1-ml sample of the 5,000-μg/ml stock solution of amphotericin B is added to 4.9 ml of medium to give a solution of 100 μg of amphotericin B per ml.

Place 12 sterile, disposable tubes (17 by 100 mm) in a rack and add 2.0 ml of the appropriate broth medium to tubes 2 through 12. Add 2.0 ml of the antifungal solution (100 μg/ml) to tubes 1 and 2. Mix the contents of tube 2 and then serially dilute the drug, using 2.0-ml volumes and fresh pipettes for each dilution, through the remaining 10 tubes, discarding 2.0 ml from the last tube. This procedure will give a dilution series that is 10 times the final desired concentration, ranging from 100 to 0.05 μg/ml for amphotericin B (the 10× range for 5-FC or ketoconazole should be 1,000 to 0.5 μg/ml). Remove 0.5 ml from each dilution and add 0.1 ml to each of four sterile, disposable tubes (12 by 75 mm). The remaining 1.5 ml volume for each dilution may be kept as controls for contamination of the serial dilution. Add 0.1 ml of drug-free broth with and without DMSO (10%) to each of eight additional sterile tubes (four with and four without DMSO) for use as growth controls. Inoculate each of two tubes of each concentration of the drug with 0.9 ml of the standardized suspensions of the test and control organisms (Fig. 1). Also inoculate two tubes of drug-free media (with and without DMSO at a final concentration of 1%) with each suspension as the growth controls. The final range of drug concentrations for amphotericin B (Fig. 1) will be from 10 to 0.005 μg/ml (100 to 0.05 μg/ml for 5-FC and ketoconazole), and the inoculum concentration will be 1×10^4 to 5×10^4 organisms per ml. The tubes should be incubated at 35°C and read visually at 24 and 48 h. As an aid in determining the MIC endpoint, growth in each tube should be scored and recorded as follows: 0, optically clear; 1+, slightly hazy; 2+, prominent reduction in turbidity compared with the drug-free controls; 3+, slight reduction in turbidity compared with the drug-free controls; 4+, no reduction in turbidity compared with the drug-free controls. On the basis of this scoring system, the MIC for isolates tested against either amphotericin B or 5-FC is defined as the lowest concentration in which the growth score is 0 (optically clear), and that for isolates tested against ketoconazole is defined as the lowest concentration in which the growth score is 1+ or less.

After determination of the MIC, the minimal fungicidal concentrations can be determined by subculturing approximately 0.01 ml from each negative tube and from the positive growth control tubes onto plates of drug-free Sabouraud agar, with subsequent incubation at 30°C for 48 h or until growth of the subcultures from the growth control tubes is apparent. The minimal fungicidal concentration is defined as the lowest concentration of drug from which subcultures were negative or which yielded fewer than three colonies.

Expected results

Most isolates of susceptible yeasts will be inhibited by 12.5 μg or less of 5-FC per ml and killed by 25 μg/ml (Table 4). Isolates of *Cryptococcus neoformans* with intermediate susceptibilities (MICs of 25 to 100 μg/ml) as well as totally resistant isolates (MIC of >100 μg/ml) may be recovered from patients during treatment with 5-FC. Amphotericin B is both inhibitory and fungicidal for most yeasts at a concentration of 0.05 μg or less per ml. An amphotericin B MIC of 1.25 to 2.5 μg/ml suggests probable clinical resistance, since this MIC only approximates the concentrations routinely achievable in serum and exceeds the concentrations achievable in cerebrospinal fluid (CSF). Recently, Powderly et al. (50) reported that patients with fungemia due to *Candida* spp. whose amphotericin B MICs were greater than 0.8 μg/ml were significantly more likely to die because of that infection than were patients with infection due to *Candida* spp. with in vitro susceptibility to amphotericin B of 0.8 μg/ml or less. Although these results are interesting, additional studies will be necessary before a clinically significant breakpoint value for amphotericin B susceptibility can be defined.

Of the azoles, miconazole is fungistatic for most isolates of *Candida* spp., *Cryptococcus neoformans*, and dermatophytic fungi at concentrations in the range of 0.5 to 8 μg/ml, and it is fungicidal at higher concentrations. Ketoconazole compares favorably with miconazole in vitro but may differ from it according to the organism being tested as well as the medium and test system being used.

AGAR DILUTION TEST METHODS

Agar dilution tests have been developed for use with antifungal agents. However, the results of such tests with both the imidazoles and 5-FC are highly dependent on inoculum size and time of incubation; furthermore, the results of such tests and those of broth dilution tests tend to be divergent (8). In addition, agar dilution tests may not detect resistance to the imidazoles in isolates of *C. albicans* (52). Despite these problems, agar dilution testing provides a cost-effective alternative to broth dilution tests when the occasion or workload warrants.

Drug solutions and media

Stock drug solutions are prepared as described above. Twofold serial dilutions of drug are prepared in appropriate broths at 10 times the final desired concentrations (1,280 to 0.63 or 1,000 to 0.5 μg/ml for 5-FC and the imidazoles; 160 to 0.63 or 100 to 0.39 μg/ml for the polyenes). The dilutions are then added in ratios of 1:10 to sterile blanks of appropriate molten agar media. Appropriate media include antibiotic medium 12 (antibiotic assay medium M 12, 0669, Difco; antibiotic medium 12 [nystatin assay agar], 10982, BBL) or buffered yeast morphology agar (YMA) (0393, Difco) for the polyenes, unbuffered YMA for 5-FC, and casein-yeast extract-glucose agar for the imidazoles. One medium that is suitable for all drugs except 5-FC is Kimmig agar (fungus agar according to Kimmig, 5414, E. Merck AG, Darmstadt, Federal Republic of Germany; available

TABLE 4. In vitro antifungal activities of four antifungal agents against pathogenic fungi[a]

Organism	Expected range (μg/ml)						
	Amphotericin B		Flucytosine (5-FC)		Miconazole		Ketoconazole
	MIC	MFC	MIC	MFC	MIC	MFC	MIC
Pathogenic yeasts							
Cryptococcus neoformans	0.05–0.78	0.1–12.5	0.10–100[b]	0.39–>100	0.05–3.13	0.05–25	0.1–32
Candida albicans	0.2–0.78[c]	0.39–0.78	0.05–12.5[b]	0.10–>100	0.1–2.0[c]	0.1–10	<0.1–128
Candida spp. not *C. albicans*	0.2–1.56[c]	0.39–6.25	0.10–50[b]	0.20–>100	<0.1–2.0	0.1–>10	<0.1–64
Torulopsis glabrata	0.1–0.4	0.2–0.78	0.05–1.56	0.4–>100	0.5–10	2–10	1–64
Trichosporon spp.	0.78–3.13	1.56–3.13	25–100	>100	0.2–25	0.2–>100	
Geotrichum spp.	0.4–1.56	0.78–3.13	1.56–12.5	25–>100	0.1–2	0.5–>10	
Filamentous fungi							
Pseudallescheria (Petriellidium) boydii	1.56–>100[b]	>100	Resistant		0.5[d]	0.05	0.1–4[b]
Aspergillus spp., including *A. fumigatus*	0.05–8	6.25–>100	0.2–1.56[b]	>100	0.4–>100	0.8–>100	0.1–100[e]
Blastomyces dermatitidis	0.05–0.2	0.1–0.4	Resistant		≤0.25	ND	0.1–2
Xylohypha bantiana	3.13–>100	3.13–>100	3.13–12.5[b]	12.5–>100	0.5–>64	ND	0.1–64
Coccidioides immitis	0.1–0.78	0.70–0.156	Resistant		0.25–1.0	ND	0.1–0.8
Histoplasma capsulatum	0.05–1.0	0.05–0.2	Resistant		≤0.25	ND	0.1–0.5
Phialophora spp. and other dematiaceous fungi	0.05–>128	6.25–>128	Variable susceptibility	Resistant	0.05–32	ND	0.1–64
Sporothrix schenckii	1.56–12.5	3.13–>100	Resistant		1–2	ND	0.1–16
Zygomycetes	0.78–1.56	1.56–>100	Variable susceptibility	Resistant			
Control organisms							
S. cerevisiae ATCC 36375, etc.	0.1	0.2	0.05	0.10	0.20	0.39	0.20
C. kefyr ATCC 28838			0.05	0.10	0.10	0.20	0.05

[a] Based on both data obtained at the Medical College of Virginia, Virginia Commonwealth University, Richmond, and a review of the literature. In vitro data for nystatin are not included because of the narrow clinical spectrum of this agent; however, most isolates of *Candida* species and *Torulopsis* species should be clinically susceptible (MIC of ≤10 μg/ml to nystatin). MFC, Minimal fungicidal concentration; ND, not determined.

[b] Resistance not uncommon.

[c] Resistance reported but rare.

[d] Only limited data available.

[e] In vitro susceptibility of *Aspergillus* spp. to ketoconazole is highly species dependent.

from E.M. Industries, Hawthorne, N.Y.). Buffered YMA has been recommended by some workers as being suitable for agar dilution tests with all antifungal agents (33).

Inocula and performance of test

Inocula for agar dilution tests should be prepared as described above for broth dilution tests. They should contain no more than 10^5 CFU/ml, since the volume delivered by most mechanical multiprong replicators is approximately 0.001 to 0.003 ml. This will provide inocula of 1×10^2 to 3×10^2 CFU. Agar dilution tests should include a pair of drug-free plates, one to be inoculated before and one after inoculation of the drug dilution plates. Positive growth responses must be obtained on both control plates for the results to be acceptable with any given organism. Appropriate control organisms of known susceptibility or resistance should be included in all agar dilution tests.

In tests with yeasts and rapidly growing filamentous organisms, all prongs of a mechanical multiprong replicator may be used. In tests with slow-growing organisms, only every other prong should be used. Incubation should be at 30°C. The time of incubation will be controlled by the appearance of growth on the drug-free control plates. Results should be read only when maturing colonies are clearly visible on these plates. The MIC will be defined as the lowest concentration of drug preventing growth of macroscopically visible colonies. Hazy responses and pinpoint colonies should be regarded as negative.

Expected results

In vitro MICs obtained by agar dilution for the polyenes should agree with similar data obtained by broth dilution tests (Table 4). The relationship between agar dilution and broth dilution results for 5-FC and the imidazoles is less clear. This lack of a clear-cut relationship reflects problems associated both with inoculum size and with the selection of media for the performance of such tests. Control of inoculum size is most critical in tests with 5-FC; overly small inocula may result in false reports of in vitro susceptibility because of failure to detect heterotypic resistance. The selection of media is most critical in tests with the imidazoles. Overly rich media may result in false reports of in vitro resistance. Both problems demonstrate the need for standardization of both broth and agar dilution test procedures with the antifungal agents (20).

DIFFUSION DISK TESTS

Diffusion disk tests with antifungal agents have been described but have not yet been fully standardized (6, 55, 64). There are reports regarding a variety of experimentally prepared disks (6, 64), and several commercial disks and tablets are now available in the United Kingdom and Europe (12, 55).

The application of diffusion disk tests with antifungal agents is limited. Polyene compounds lack stability (32), and the varying solubilities of the imidazoles (26) may restrict the application of the test to these agents.

5-FC (flucytosine) is one substance readily adaptable to diffusion disk testing. A 1-μg disk has been available for some time in Europe. This disk is used in a diffusion disk test with isolates of *C. albicans* standardized by a special working group of the British Society for Mycopathology (BSM) (9), which is described below.

BSM flucytosine diffusion disk test for *C. albicans*

Dispense molten YMA in 15-ml volumes into petri dishes (90-mm diameter) placed on a level surface and allow the agar to solidify. Once the agar has hardened, invert the dishes and draw lines on the reverse sides so as to bisect them into halves.

Inoculate 2 ml of sterile distilled water or saline with *C. kefyr* ATCC 28838 (syn. *C. pseudotropicalis*) or *C. kefyr* NCPF 3234. Adjust the turbidity of this preparation to match that of a 0.5 McFarland tube or use a Wickerham card to adjust the turbidity. Now prepare suspensions of the patient isolates to be tested in a similar fashion.

With sterile cotton swabs, inoculate one half of each plate with the suspension of the *C. kefyr* indicator strain; then inoculate the other half of each test plate with the test strains. Once the plates are dry, place a 1-μg 5-FC disk on the surface in the center of each plate. Incubate the plates at 35°C.

The plates should be first examined after 24 h of incubation to determine obvious resistance. Final observations are made after 48 h of incubation. Measure the radius of each zone of inhibition of the test and indicator strains. Calculate the percentage of difference for each of the test strains by using the radius obtained for the indicator strain on the same plates as follows: test strain zone radius/indicator strain zone radius × 100. Isolates with zones of inhibition whose radii are not less than 80% of the indicator strain radius are regarded as susceptible. Highly resistant isolates will have no zones or very small zones of inhibition. Intermediate zones (less than 80% of the indicator zone) may imply susceptibility to 5-FC when it is used in combination with amphotericin B. Intermediate zones as well as zones with poorly defined perimeters may also suggest the likelihood of the emergence of more highly resistant strains during treatment. Potential development of resistance will also be suggested by the presence of persisting colonies in otherwise clear zones of inhibition. In such situations the resistant organism should be retested, and the susceptibilities of subsequent isolates from the same patient should be monitored.

SYNERGISM BETWEEN ANTIFUNGAL AGENTS

One of the more important earlier advances in antifungal chemotherapy was the use of synergistic combinations of antifungal agents. One such combination, amphotericin B and flucytosine (7), is advocated as the regimen of choice in the treatment of many cases of cryptococcal meningitis. Although therapeutically superior to treatment with either drug alone, this regimen is not without disadvantages, the most important being the toxicity associated with sustained flucytosine levels in blood in excess of 100 to 125 μg/ml (60).

The advent of combination antifungal chemotherapy introduces the possibility of a requirement for the performance of tests for antifungal synergy in the clinical laboratory. Such tests are performed by using procedures similar to those employed with combinations of antibacterial agents.

Synergism can be measured by testing a multiple series of dilutions of two drugs in a so-called checkerboard titration (see chapter 115). Both inhibitory and fungicidal endpoints for each drug alone and in combination are determined and then plotted as an isobologram (37). The resulting graph is then interpreted in terms of possible synergism, antagonism, or indifference. Specific considerations for the application of such a test to combinations of amphotericin B and 5-FC include the selection of media and the conditions for incubation. In this case, specific recommendations include the use of buffered YNB and incubation at 30°C for 48 h.

LIQUID CHROMATOGRAPHIC ASSAYS OF ANTIFUNGAL AGENTS IN BODY FLUIDS

The techniques of gas-liquid chromatography (GLC) and high-performance liquid chromatography (HPLC) are widely used to quantitate a number of different antimicrobial agents in various body fluids (40, 66). A discussion of the technical aspects as well as the advantages and disadvantages of these methods is included in chapter 119 and will not be covered here. Both GLC and HPLC are now widely used to quantitate many of the currently available antifungal agents (Table 5). HPLC is the preferred technique in many clinical laboratories because of its simpler detection methods, flexibility, and ability to separate and quantify closely related compounds in a mixture. Both methods tend to be more sensitive, specific, and rapid and less labor intensive than bioassay methods (40, 66). The means of detection, sensitivity, and precision of GLC and HPLC methods for quantitation of several of the currently available antifungal agents with systemic activity are listed in Table 5. Although these methods do not evaluate the biological activity of a compound or its metabolites, the correlation with bioassays has been excellent with most antifungal compounds (66). Given the increasing number and frequent clinical application of new antifungal agents with diverse mechanisms of action and pharmacokinetic properties, it is likely that there will be an increasing role of these assays in the monitoring of antifungal therapy.

BIOASSAYS OF ANTIFUNGAL AGENTS IN BODY FLUIDS

Bioassays for antifungal agents can be performed by using standard microbiological bioassay procedures (see chapter 119). The classical radial agar diffusion method is readily adaptable for use with such systemically active drugs as amphotericin B, 5-FC, and keto-

TABLE 5. Liquid chromatographic methods for quantitating antifungal agents in serum and other body fluids[a]

Chromatographic method	Antifungal agent	Detection method	Sensitivity (μg/ml)	Precision (CV%)		Reference(s)
				Within run	Between run	
GLC	Miconazole	Electron capture	0.001	NS	3.0	39
	5-FC	Flame ionization	1.0–10	4.5	7.5	31, 67
	Fluconazole	Electron capture	0.1	0.9–2.0	NS	69
HPLC	Amphotericin B	UV (382 nm)	0.005–0.04	2.0–6.8	4.9–10	5, 25
	Amphotericin B	Vis (405 nm)	0.05	1.0–2.1	2.9–4.3	34
	5-FC	UV (254 nm)	1.0	0.7–4.6	1.2–10	10, 14, 42, 56
	Ketoconazole	UV (205–254 nm)	0.002–0.1	4.5–16.7	3.3–30	1, 3, 35, 39
	Itraconazole	UV (293 nm)	0.001	2.5–5.7	NS	21
	Fluconazole	UV (260 nm)	1.0	NS	NS	4

[a] Abbreviations: CV, coefficient of variation; NS, not specified; Vis, visible.

conazole. Bioassays for levels of topical antifungal agents in serum are not warranted. Specific considerations include the selection of media and bioassay indicator organisms as well as design of the standard or dose-response curve (Table 6). Specimens for bioassay may include such body fluids as sera, CSF, and synovial fluids or specimens such as dialysis fluids.

Bioassay of 5-FC levels in sera is the most critical of such determinations and may be required for all patients with impaired renal function and those in whom 5-FC-associated toxicity is suspected (patients with neutropenia, leukopenia, and thrombocytopenia). Levels of 5-FC in serum in excess of 100 to 125 μg/ml should be regarded as potentially toxic (60). Less essential are determinations of amphotericin B serum levels. In adult patients receiving up to 1 mg/kg daily or every other day, levels of amphotericin B in serum will range from peaks of 4 μg/ml or more to troughs of 0.2 μg/ml or less for 24 to 48 h after infusion; CSF levels rarely exceed 1 μg/ml. Pharmacokinetic studies (63) with intravenous miconazole have shown that this drug will produce maximum serum concentrations ranging from 2 to 8 μg/ml, depending on dosage (400 to 1,000 mg/day). Levels of miconazole in CSF rarely exceed 0.1 to 0.3 μg/ml except when the drug is administered intrathecally. Peak levels of ketoconazole in serum, usually attained 2 to 4 h after the ingestion of a 400-mg dose, will be in the range of 4 to 6 μg/ml (36). The poorly predictable bioavailability of this drug makes the assay of levels of ketoconazole in serum the second most critical of such determinations.

BSM BIOASSAY FOR FLUCYTOSINE

Several bioassays for flucytosine (5-FC) have been reported. The one to be described here is modified from a bioassay procedure evaluated by the BSM Working Group (9).

Preparation of standards

Standard solutions of flucytosine at concentrations of 6.25, 12.5, 25, 50, and 100 μg/ml are required. These solutions can be prepared from a concentrated standard stock solution in sterile distilled or deionized water or in sterile, pooled, normal human serum. The standards can be dispensed in 0.5- or 1-ml volumes and frozen at −20°C for up to 12 months.

Indicator organism

Inoculate 5 ml of standard 1× YNB with *C. kefyr* ATCC 28838 or *S. cerevisiae* ATCC 36375. Incubate the culture at 37°C overnight. Adjust the culture to a density of 1 × 10^6 to 5 × 10^6 CFU/ml (see discussion above of prep-

TABLE 6. Recommended test conditions for bioassay of other antifungal agents in body fluids by a radial agar diffusion bioassay technique

Drug	Bioassay indicator organism	Medium	Standard dose-response curve (μg/ml)[a]	Maximum therapeutic levels (μg/ml)
Amphotericin B				
In the absence of flucytosine	*Paecilomyces varioti* ATCC 36257	Antibiotic medium 12 FDA (nystatin assay agar)	0.03, 0.06, 0.125, 0.25, 0.5, and 1.0	In serum: 1.0–4.0 In CSF: 0.02–1.0
In the presence of flucytosine	*Chrysosporium pruinosum* ATCC 36374	As above but supplemented with 10 μg of cytosine per ml	As above	As above
Miconazole (intravenous)	*Candida stellatoidea* ATCC 36232, *C. kefyr* ATCC 28838, or *C. kefyr* NCPF 3234	Sabouraud dextrose agar Emmons or Kimmig agar	0.5, 1, 2, 4, 8, and 16	In serum: 2.0–8.0 (depending on dosage) In CSF: 0.1–0.3

[a] May contain as few as three concentrations spanning the therapeutic range. The standard curve drug concentrations should be prepared in the same type of fluid(s) as being assayed. Both standards and specimens may be applied to the seeded agar plates by using cylinders, paper disks, or cut holes.

aration of inocula for the macrobroth dilution susceptibility testing method).

Preparation of test plates

Melt 90 ml of YMA, cool it to 55°C, and inoculate it with 5 ml of the suspension of the indicator organism. Pour the inoculated agar into an assay plate (25 cm^2; A/S Nunc Bio Plate, no. 1015), and allow it to cool on a level surface. Once the medium has solidified, place the plate in a 37°C incubator and leave it there until the surface of the agar has dried.

Cut 30 wells, each 4 mm in diameter, in the agar layer (six rows of five holes each). Introduce 10 µl of a standard or patient specimen into each well. A control sample of a known concentration should also be incorporated. The samples and standards should be placed on the plate in a randomized distribution. Each specimen or standard should be present in triplicate in this assay. The design of this assay approximates a "13 × 4 (3 + 1) incomplete block assay" that has a 95% confidence limit of ±11%, which is adequate for the assay of antibiotics in clinical specimens.

The plates are incubated without prediffusion overnight at 35 to 37°C. After incubation, the diameters of the zones of inhibition are measured. Mean diameters are then calculated for each standard and specimen.

Several methods are available for the calculation of serum concentrations in the clinical specimens. The BSM Working Group protocol calls for plotting the mean diameters of the zones of inhibition produced by the standard concentrations against the drug concentrations on semilogarithmic paper, with drug concentrations on the logarithmic ordinate. The resulting graph is then used to estimate the concentrations of the drug in the clinical specimens. This method is subject to human error. Fortunately, other procedures are available for the analysis of bioassay data (57).

Bioassay data are best analyzed statistically, and a number of personal computers and hand-held calculators are available which have the necessary programs or functions for such analyses. This type of analysis is performed by first using a regression analysis, or least-squares function, to analyze the data for the standard curve. In this analysis, individual drug concentrations (X, in micrograms per milliliter), usually expressed as logarithmic values, are compared with their corresponding zones of inhibition (Y, in millimeters). Such an analysis yields three statistics which describe the standard or dose-response curve: r, or the regression coefficient, which is a measurement of the linearity or goodness of fit of the curve; α, which describes the intercept of the curve (the value for Y when $X = 0$); and β, which describes the slope of the curve. The second step is the application of the estimating equation, $Y_c = \alpha + (\beta \times \log X)$, to calculate drug levels in specimens from the measured specimen zone diameter values. This equation uses the values for α and β derived from the regression analysis of the data for the standard curve.

Peak levels of 5-FC in serum should be in the range of 60 to 80 µg/ml in patients with normal renal function, with steady-state troughs of not less than 20 µg/ml. Paired peak CSF levels should be in the range of 40 to 60 µg/ml. Lower peaks are desirable in patients with renal impairment, since sustained 5-FC levels will be prolonged in such patients (54).

Serum specimens from patients receiving both 5-FC and amphotericin B may be heated (90°C, 30 min) or subjected to ultrafiltration before assay to eliminate the latter drug. Serum specimens containing more than 100 µg of 5-FC per ml should be reassayed after being diluted 1:1 in pooled, normal human serum.

BIOASSAY FOR KETOCONAZOLE

As already noted, the bioavailability of ketoconazole is subject to considerable variation and is not fully predictable. Therefore, it may be necessary to determine levels of this drug in sera from patients who are not responding therapeutically or in whom there is reason to suspect poor absorption of the drug or poor patient compliance. The bioassay to be described here was developed during an exhaustive clinical trial with ketoconazole (16) and has been validated by comparing results obtained with it with those obtained by an HPLC procedure.

Preparation of standard

Standard solutions of ketoconazole at concentrations of 0.25, 0.5, 1, 2, 4, 8, and 16 µg/ml are required. These solutions should be prepared in pooled human serum. The standards can be dispensed in 1.0-ml volumes and frozen for up to 6 months at −20°C.

Indicator organism

Inoculate 5 ml of Sabouraud broth with *C. kefyr* ATCC 28838 or *C. kefyr* NCPF 3234 and incubate the culture overnight at 35 to 37°C. Adjust the culture to a density of 10^6 CFU/ml.

Preparation of test plates

Melt 100 ml of Kimmig agar, cool it to 55°C, and inoculate it with 5 ml of the suspension of *C. kefyr*. Pour the inoculated agar into an assay plate (25 cm^2) and allow it to cool on a level surface. Once the medium has solidified, place it in a 37°C incubator and leave it until the surface has dried.

Place 12 or 16 stainless-steel cylinders on the surface of the plate. If cylinders are not available, sterile paper disks or cut wells may be used. However, the use of disks or wells will reduce the sensitivity of the bioassay. Each standard and clinical specimen is tested in duplicate. Using a random pattern of distribution, introduce 0.1 ml of a standard solution or a specimen into each cylinder. Be sure not to spill the sample or tip the cylinder. Samples of pooled human serum used to prepare the standard curve should also be tested, as should samples containing known amounts of ketoconazole.

The plates are incubated without prediffusion overnight at 30°C. After incubation, the diameters of the resulting zones of inhibition are measured. A mean diameter is then calculated for each standard and specimen.

Data from the ketoconazole bioassay are analyzed in the same fashion as described above for 5-FC. The peak concentration of approximately 4 to 21 µg/ml will be measurable at 1.5 to 3 h, depending on dosage and concomitant factors that may modulate absorption (13).

OTHER ANTIFUNGAL BIOASSAYS

Bioassays for amphotericin B are not warranted under most circumstances. Exceptions include unusual clinical situations in which the penetration of the drug into specific sites or the pharmacokinetics of the drug are unknown. Two bioassays for amphotericin B can be used in such situations. These assays use the design described above for 5-FC and ketoconazole and differ only in media and indicator organisms. These changes are detailed in Table 6.

There are few reasons for requiring bioassays for miconazole. The role of the intravenous preparation of this drug in clinical medicine is uncertain. However, should the need exist for such a bioassay, it can be performed by using the design described above for ketoconazole with the media and indicator organism detailed in Table 6. One further modification is that the assay plates need to prediffuse overnight at 4°C before incubation at 35°C.

LITERATURE CITED

1. **Alton, K. B.** 1980. Determination of the antifungal agent, ketoconazole, in human plasma by high-performance liquid chromatography. J. Chromatogr. **221:**337–344.
2. **Anaissie, E. J., G. P. Bodey, and M. G. Rinaldi.** 1989. Emerging fungal pathogens. Eur. J. Clin. Microbiol. Infect. Dis. **8:**323–330.
3. **Andrews, F. A., L. R. Peterson, W. H. Beggs, D. Crankshaw, and G. A. Sarosi.** 1981. Liquid chromatographic assay of ketoconazole. Antimicrob. Agents Chemother. **19:** 110–113.
4. **Arndt, C. A. S., T. J. Walsh, C. L. McCully, F. M. Balis, P. A. Pizzo, and D. G. Poplack.** 1988. Fluconazole penetration into cerebrospinal fluid: implications for treating fungal infections of the central nervous system. J. Infect. Dis. **157:**178–180.
5. **Bach, P. R.** 1984. Quantitative extraction of amphotericin B from serum and its determination by high-pressure liquid chromatography. Antimicrob. Agents Chemother. **26:**314–317.
6. **Baier, R., and U. Puppel.** 1978. Antimykotika-Empfindlichkeit von Hefen aus klinischem Untersuchungsmaterial im Blattchendiffusionstest. Dtsch. Med. Wochenschr. **103:** 1113–1116.
7. **Bennett, J. E., W. E. Dismukes, R. J. Duma, C. Medoff, M. A. Sande, H. Gallis, J. Leonard, B. T. Fields, M. Bradshaw, H. Haywood, Z. A. McGee, T. R. Cate, C. G. Cobbs, J. F. Warner, and D. W. Alling.** 1979. A comparison of amphotericin B alone and combined with flucytosine in the treatment of cryptococcal meningitis. N. Engl. J. Med. **301:**126–131.
8. **Brass, C., J. Z. Shainhouse, and D. A. Stevens.** 1979. Variability of agar dilution-replicator method of yeast susceptibility testing. Antimicrob. Agents Chemother. **15:**763–768.
9. **British Society for Mycopathology.** 1984. Report of a Working Group. Laboratory methods for flucytosine (5-fluorocytosine). J. Antimicrob. Chemother. **14:**1–8.
10. **Bury, R. W., M. L. Mashford, and H. M. Miles.** 1979. Assay of flucytosine (5-fluorocytosine) in human plasma by high-pressure liquid chromatography. Antimicrob. Agents Chemother. **16:**529–532.
11. **Calhoun, D. L., G. D. Roberts, J. N. Galgiani, J. E. Bennett, D. S. Feingold, J. Jorgensen, G. S. Kobayashi, and S. Shadomy.** 1986. Results of a survey of antifungal susceptibility tests in the United States and interlaboratory comparison of broth dilution testing of flucytosine and amphotericin B. J. Clin. Microbiol. **23:**298–301.
12. **Casals, J. B.** 1979. Tablet sensitivity testing of pathogenic fungi. J. Clin. Pathol. **32:**719–722.
13. **Daneshmend, T. K., D. W. Warnock, M. D. Ene, E. M. Johnson, M. R. Potten, M. D. Richardson, and P. J. Williamson.** 1984. Influence of food on the pharmacokinetics of ketoconazole. Antimicrob. Agents Chemother. **25:**1–3.
14. **Diasio, R. B., M. E. Wilburn, S. Shadomy, and A. Espinel-Ingroff.** 1978. Rapid determination of serum 5-fluorocytosine levels by high-performance liquid chromatography. Antimicrob. Agents Chemother. **13:**500–504.
15. **Dick, J. D., W. G. Merz, and R. Saral.** 1980. Incidence of polyene-resistant yeasts recovered from clinical specimens. Antimicrob. Agents Chemother. **18:**158–163.
16. **Dismukes, W. E., A. M. Stamm, J. R. Graybill, P. C. Craven, D. A. Stevens, R. L. Stiller, G. A. Sarosi, G. Medoff, C. R. Gregg, H. A. Gallis, B. T. Fields, Jr., R. L. Marier, T. A. Kerkering, L. G. Kaplowitz, G. Cloud, C. Bowles, and S. Shadomy.** 1983. Treatment of systemic mycoses with ketoconazole: emphasis on toxicity and clinical response in 52 patients. Ann. Intern. Med. **98:**13–20.
17. **Doern, G. V., T. A. Tubert, K. Chopin, and M. G. Rinaldi.** 1986. Effect of medium composition on results of macrobroth dilution antifungal susceptibility testing of yeasts. J. Clin. Microbiol. **24:**507–511.
18. **Drutz, D. J.** 1987. In vitro antifungal susceptibility testing and measurement of levels of antifungal agents in body fluids. Rev. Infect. Dis. **9:**392–397.
19. **Fromtling, R. A.** 1988. Overview of medically important antifungal azole derivatives. Clin. Microbiol. Rev. **1:**187–217.
20. **Galgiani, J. N.** 1984. Why not standardize antifungal susceptibility testing. Antimicrob. Newsl. **1:**40.
21. **Galgiani, J. N.** 1987. Antifungal susceptibility tests. Antimicrob. Agents Chemother. **31:**1867–1870.
22. **Galgiani, J. N.** 1987. The need for improved standardization in antifungal susceptibility testing, p. 15–24. *In* R. A. Fromtling (ed.), Recent trends in the discovery development and evaluation of antifungal agents. J. R. Prous Science Publishers, Barcelona, Spain.
23. **Galgiani, J. N., J. Reiser, C. Brass, A. Espinel-Ingroff, M. A. Gordon, and T. M. Kerkering.** 1987. Comparison of relative susceptibilities of *Candida* species to three antifungal agents as determined by unstandardized methods. Antimicrob. Agents Chemother. **31:**1343–1347.
24. **Gordon, M. A., E. W. Lapa, and P. G. Passero.** 1988. Improved method for azole antifungal susceptibility testing. J. Clin. Microbiol. **26:**1874–1877.
25. **Granich, G. G., G. S. Kobayashi, and D. J. Krogstad.** 1986. Sensitive high-pressure liquid chromatographic assay for amphotericin B which incorporates an internal standard. Antimicrob. Agents Chemother. **29:**584–588.
26. **Grendahl, J. G., and J. P. Sung.** 1978. Quantitation of imidazoles by agar-disk diffusion. Antimicrob. Agents Chemother. **14:**509–513.
27. **Guinet, R., D. Nerson, F. de Closets, J. Dunpouy-Camet, L. Kures, M. Marjollet, J. L. Poirot, A. Ros, J. Texier-Maugin, and P. J. Volle.** 1988. Collaborative evaluation in seven laboratories of a standardized micromethod for yeast susceptibility testing. J. Clin. Microbiol. **26:**2307–2312.
28. **Hadfield, T. L., M. B. Smith, R. E. Winn, M. G. Rinaldi, and C. Guerra.** 1987. Mycoses caused by *Candida lusitaniae.* Rev. Infect. Dis. **9:**1006–1012.
29. **Hall, G. S., C. Myles, K. J. Pratt, and J. A. Washington.** 1988. Cilofungin (LY121019), an antifungal agent with specific activity against *Candida albicans* and *Candida tropicalis.* Antimicrob. Agents Chemother. **32:**1331–1335.
30. **Hardin, T. C., J. R. Graybill, R. Fetchick, R. Woestenborghs, M. G. Rinaldi, and J. G. Kuhn.** 1988. Pharmacokinetics of itraconazole following oral administration to normal volunteers. Antimicrob. Agents Chemother. **32:** 1310–1313.
31. **Harding, S. A., G. F. Johnson, and H. M. Solomon.** 1976. Gas-chromatographic determination of 5-fluorocytosine in

human serum. Clin. Chem. **22:**772–776.

32. **Hoeprich, P. D., and A. C. Houston.** 1978. Stability of four antifungal antimicrobics in vitro. J. Infect. Dis. **137:** 87–90.
33. **Holt, R. J.** 1975. Laboratory tests of antifungal agents. J. Clin. Pathol. **28:**767–774.
34. **Hosotsubo, H., J. Takezawa, N. Taenaka, K. Hosotsubo, and I. Yoshiya.** 1988. Rapid determination of amphotericin B levels in serum by high-performance liquid chromatography without interference by bilirubin. Antimicrob. Agents Chemother. **32:**1103–1105.
35. **Huang, Y. C., J. Colaizzi, R. H. Bieman, R. Woestenborghs, and J. Heykants.** 1986. Pharmacokinetics and dose proportionality of ketoconazole in normal volunteers. Antimicrob. Agents Chemother. **30:**206–210.
36. **Hume, A. L., and T. M. Kerkering.** 1983. Ketoconazole (Nizoral, Janssen Pharmaceutica, Inc.). Drug Intell. Clin. Pharm. **17:**169–174.
37. **Jawetz, E.** 1968. Combined antibiotic action: some definitions and correlations between laboratory and clinical results, p. 203–209. Antimicrob. Agents Chemother. 1967.
38. **Lopez-Berestein, G., G. P. Bodey, L. S. Frankel, and K. Mehta.** 1987. Treatment of hepatosplenic candidiasis with liposomal amphotericin B. J. Clin. Oncol. **5:**310–317.
39. **Mannisto, P. T., R. Mantyla, S. Nykanen, U. Lamminsivu, and P. Ottoila.** 1982. Impairing effect of food on ketoconazole absorption. Antimicrob. Agents Chemother. **21:**730–733.
40. **McGinnis, M. R., and M. G. Rinaldi.** 1986. Antifungal drugs: mechanisms of action, drug resistance, susceptibility testing, and assays of activity in biological fluids, p. 223–281. *In* V. Lorian (ed.), Antibiotics in laboratory medicine. The Williams & Wilkins Co., Baltimore.
41. **Mehta, R., G. Lopez-Berestein, R. Hopfer, K. Mills, and R. L. Juliano.** 1984. Liposomal amphotericin B is toxic to fungal cells but not to mammalian cells. Biochim. Biophys. Acta **770:**230–234.
42. **Miners, J. O., T. Foenander, and D. J. Birkett.** 1980. Liquid-chromatographic determination of 5-fluorocytosine. Clin. Chem. **26:**117–119.
43. **Normark, S., and J. Schönebeck.** 1972. In vitro studies of 5-fluorocytosine resistance in *Candida albicans* and *Torulopsis glabrata*. Antimicrob. Agents Chemother. **2:**114–121.
44. **Odds, F. C.** 1985. Laboratory tests for the activity of imidazole and triazole antifungal agents in vitro. Sem. Dermatol. **4:**260–270.
45. **Pfaller, M. A., L. Burmeister, M. S. Bartlett, and M. G. Rinaldi.** 1988. Multicenter evaluation of four methods of yeast inoculum preparation. J. Clin. Microbiol. **26:**1437–1441.
46. **Pfaller, M. A., T. Gerarden, M. Yu, and R. P. Wenzel.** 1989. Influence of in vitro susceptibility testing conditions on the anticandidal activity of LY 121019. Diagn. Microbiol. Infect. Dis. **11:**1–9.
47. **Pfaller, M. A., S. Wey, T. Gerarden, A. Houston, and R. P. Wenzel.** 1989. Susceptibility of nosocomial isolates of *Candida* species to LY 121019 and other antifungal agents. Diagn. Microbiol. Infect. Dis. **12:**1–4.
48. **Polak, A., and D. M. Dixon.** 1987. In vitro/in vivo correlation of antifungal susceptibility testing using 5-fluorocytosine and ketoconazole as examples of two extremes, p. 45–59. *In* R. A. Fromtling (ed.), Recent trends in the discovery, development and evaluation of antifungal agents. J. R. Prous Science Publishers, Barcelona, Spain.
49. **Polak, A., and H. J. Scholer.** 1975. Mode of action of 5-fluorocytosine and mechanisms of resistance. Chemotherapy **21:**113–130.
50. **Powderly, W. G., G. S. Kobayashi, G. P. Herzig, and G. Medoff.** 1988. Amphotericin B-resistant yeast infection in severely immunocompromised patients. Am. J. Med. **84:** 826–832.
51. **Radetsky, M., R. C. Wheeler, M. H. Roe, and J. K. Todd.** 1986. Microtiter broth dilution method for yeast susceptibility testing with validation by clinical outcome. J. Clin. Microbiol. **24:**600–606.
52. **Ryley, J. F., R. G. Wilson, and K. J. Barrett-Bee.** 1984. Azole resistance in *Candida albicans*. Sabouraudia **22:**53–63.
53. **Saag, M. S., and W. E. Dismukes.** 1988. Azole antifungal agents: emphasis on new triazoles. Antimicrob. Agents Chemother. **32:**1–8.
54. **Scholer, H. J.** 1980. Flucytosine, p. 36–100. *In* D. C. E. Speller (ed.), Antifungal chemotherapy. John Wiley, Chichester, England.
55. **Scholer, H. J., and A. Polak.** 1973. Fungistatic and fungicidal properties of 5-fluorocytosine; methods for routine sensitivity tests, p. 162–163. *In* Symposium International de Mycologie Medicale, Bucharest.
56. **Schwertschlag, U., L. M. Nakata, and J. Gal.** 1984. Improved procedure for determination of flucytosine in human blood plasma by high-pressure liquid chromatography. Antimicrob. Agents Chemother. **26:**303–305.
57. **Shadomy, S., and A. Espinel-Ingroff.** 1984. Methods for bioassay of antifungal agents in biologic fluids, p. 327–337. *In* A. Laskin and H. Lechevalier (ed.), CRC handbook of microbiology, vol. 6. CRC Press, Inc., Boca Raton, Fla.
58. **Shadomy, S., A. Espinel-Ingroff, and R. Y. Cartwright.** 1985. Laboratory studies with antifungal agents: susceptibility tests and bioassays, p. 991–999. *In* E. H. Lennette, A. Balows, W. J. Hausler, Jr., and H. J. Shadomy (ed.), Manual of clinical microbiology, 4th ed. American Society for Microbiology, Washington, D.C.
59. **Sokol-Anderson, M. L., J. Brajtburg, and G. Medoff.** 1986. Amphotericin B-induced oxidative damage and killing of *Candida albicans*. J. Infect. Dis. **154:**76–83.
60. **Stamm, A. M., R. B. Diasio, W. E. Dismukes, S. Shadomy, G. A. Cloud, C. A. Bowles, G. H. Karam, A. Espinel-Ingroff, and additional members of the National Institute of Allergy and Infectious Diseases Mycoses Study Group.** 1987. Toxicity of amphotericin B plus flucytosine in 194 patients with cryptococcal meningitis. Am. J. Med. **83:**236–242.
61. **Stevens, D. A.** 1987. Problems in antifungal chemotherapy. Infection **15:**87–92.
62. **Stiller, R. L., J. E. Bennett, H. J. Scholer, H. J. Wall, A. Polak, and D. A. Stevens.** 1983. Correlation of in vitro susceptibility test results with in vivo response: flucytosine therapy in a systemic candidiasis model. J. Infect. Dis. **147:** 1070–1076.
63. **Sung, J. P., and J. G. Grendahl.** 1977. Clinical experimental therapy with miconazole for human disseminated coccidioidomycosis, p. 293–309. *In* L. Ajello (ed.), Coccidioidomycosis, current clinical and diagnostic status. Symposia Specialists, Miami.
64. **Utz, C. J., and S. Shadomy.** 1977. Antifungal activity of 5-fluorocytosine as measured by disc diffusion susceptibility testing. J. Infect. Dis. **135:**970–974.
65. **Walsh, T. J., and A. Pizzo.** 1988. Treatment of systemic fungal infections: recent progress and current problems. Eur. J. Clin. Microbiol. Infect. Dis. **7:**460–475.
66. **Warnock, D. W., M. D. Richardson, and A. Turner.** 1982. High performance liquid chromatographic (HPLC) and other non-biological methods for quantitation of antifungal drugs. J. Antimicrob. Chemother. **10:**467–478.
67. **Wee, S. H., and J. P. Anhalt.** 1977. Gas chromatographic determination of 5-fluorocytosine: a modified extraction method. Antimicrob. Agents Chemother. **11:**914–915.
68. **Wey, S. B., M. Mori, M. A. Pfaller, R. F. Woolson, and R. P. Wenzel.** 1988. Hospital acquired candidemia: the attributable mortality and excess length of stay. Arch. Intern. Med. **148:**2642–2645.
69. **Wood, P. R., and M. H. Tarbit.** 1986. Gas chromatographic method for the determination of fluconazole, a novel antifungal agent in human plasma and urine. J. Chromatogr. **383:**179–186.

Chapter 118

Antiviral and Antiparasitic Susceptibility Testing

EDGAR L. HILL, M. NIXON ELLIS, AND PHUC NGUYEN-DINH

ANTIVIRAL DRUG SUSCEPTIBILITY TESTING

The increasing number of effective antiviral therapies for the treatment of several viral infections and the emergence of drug-resistant virus strains underscores the need for rapid methods for evaluating virus susceptibilities to these agents. Knowledge of the drug susceptibility profile of a particular clinical isolate may suggest alternate drugs and may help in the interpretation of other clinical information. In this chapter we will discuss two assays for determining virus sensitivity to antiviral agents. The first method, the dye uptake (DU) assay, is a semiautomated quantitative colorimeteric test performed in a 96-well microtiter plate. This assay was developed to determine the in vitro susceptibilities of large numbers of herpes simplex virus (HSV) clinical isolates to acyclovir (ACV) (28). The second method, the plaque reduction (PR) assay, has been the standard technique used to determine the susceptibility of a virus to a given antiviral agent (21). The advantages and disadvantages of each will be discussed.

The DU and PR assays measure inhibition of viral cytopathic effects (CPE). Two other techniques that have been used extensively are the enzyme-linked immunosorbent assay, which measures a decrease in viral protein production (36), and the DNA hybridization assay, which measures a reduction in viral DNA synthesis (41). A more comprehensive discussion of the different techniques used for determining antiviral susceptibility can be found in reference 29.

DU Assay

The DU assay was adapted from a method originally developed for measuring interferon activity (16). The preferential uptake of a vital dye (neutral red) by viable cells over damaged cells forms the basis of this method. The extent of viral CPE in different cultures is determined by the relative amounts of dye bound to viable cells. The dye taken up by viable cells is eluted into a phosphate-alcohol buffer and measured colorimetrically. The drug concentration inhibiting 50% of the viral CPE is the 50% inhibitory dose (ID_{50}). This assay can be adapted for use with other cytopathic viruses and other drugs. The technique has been automated to allow for screening of large numbers of isolates in a relatively short period of time.

Materials

1. Maintenance and assay media. Eagle minimal essential medium (EMEM) containing 5% heat-inactivated fetal calf serum (FCS), 0.075% sodium bicarbonate, 75 U of penicillin G per ml, 75 µg of streptomycin per ml, and 2 mM L-glutamine, buffered with 10 mM *N*-2-hydroxyethylpiperazine-*N*′-2-ethanesulfonic acid (HEPES) to pH 6.5 to 7.0.
2. Vero cells, continuous line of African green monkey kidney cells (ATCC CLL81).
3. Culture plates, 96-well flat-bottom (Costar no. 3596; Costar, Cambridge, Mass.).
4. Small, disposable, 13- by 100-mm sterile disposable test tubes with caps.
5. Pipettes, 1.0, 5.0, and 10.0 ml, sterile.
6. Adjustable pipettor, 20 to 200 µl (Rainin Instrument Co., Inc., Woburn, Mass.).
7. Adjustable 12-well multichannel pipettor (Costar).
8. Reservoir-filling trough (Dynatech), autoclaved to sterilize.
9. Sterile pipette tips (Rainin).
10. Repeating pipettor (Eppendorf).
11. Sterile individually wrapped Combitips for repeating pipettor (Eppendorf).
12. Sterile sealing tape or plate sealers (Dynatech).
13. Sterile blotter papers.
14. Cornwall syringes, 1.0 and 2.0 ml, with eight-channel manifold, autoclaved.
15. Neutral red dye (Sigma Chemical Co., St. Louis, Mo.).
16. Sodium phosphate monobasic (Sigma).
17. Sodium phosphate dibasic (Sigma).
18. Phosphate-buffered saline without calcium or magnesium (10× stock; Hazleton Laboratories).
19. Test tube racks.
20. Phosphate ethanol elution buffer; 1:1 mix of 0.1 M sodium phosphate monobasic and 95% ethanol.
21. Ice bucket.
22. Water bath, 37°C.
23. Multichannel spectrophotometer for 96-well plates (Titertek Multiskan; Flow Laboratories, Inc., McLean, Va.).
24. Autodiluter II (Dynatech).
25. Frozen virus specimens, including reference laboratory strains of HSV types 1 and 2 (HSV-1 and HSV-2).
26. Hemacytometer.
27. Filters, 0.45- and 0.22-µm pore size.
28. Ultrasonic cleaning bath (Sonicor Instrument Corp.).

Methods

Virus infectivity assay.

1. Prepare suitable volumes (e.g., 1.8 ml) of complete EMEM with 5% FCS in a sterile tube with metal closures; keep the samples on ice.
2. Rapidly thaw a virus sample; briefly (≃30 s) soni-

cate the sample in an ultrasonic cleaning bath to disrupt any virus aggregates; keep the sample on ice.

3. Prepare a 10-fold dilution series of test virus in tubes containing 1.8 ml of EMEM: use an adjustable pipettor to add 0.2 ml of the original virus suspension into the first tube; make further serial dilutions up to 10^{-6} and hold the tubes on ice.

4. With the Dynatech dispenser fitted with a fresh manifold, dispense 150 μl of medium containing 1.5×10^5 cells per ml in rows 1 through 9. All Dynatech dispensing steps can be done manually by using the 12-well multichannel pipette and filling trough.

5. With the repeating pipette, add 50 μl of the 10^{-6} dilution of virus to all wells of row 8 of the plate; add 50 μl of the 10^{-5} dilution of virus to all wells of row 7; add 50 μl of the appropriate dilution of virus to all wells of the other rows until the final virus dilution (10^{-1}) goes into all wells of row 3. The virus infectivity plate should have the arrangement shown in Table 1.

6. Seal each plate with a sheet of sterile sealing film or plate sealer and replace the lid.

7. Incubate the plates for 72 h at 37°C in a 5% CO_2 incubator.

8. After a 72-h incubation, examine the plate for gross contamination and extreme pH changes of medium; check control wells in rows 1 and 2 for cell confluence; examine some wells of rows 3 and 4 for virus CPE; if CPE is absent from these rows, do not continue.

9. If CPE is present in row 3, carefully remove the sealing film while under a biosafety hood to avoid producing an aerosol-containing infectious virus.

10. With a Cornwall syringe and manifold, add 50 μl of a 0.15% solution of neutral red in 0.1 M phosphate buffer (pH 6.0) to each well.

11. Incubate the plate for 45 min at 37°C in CO_2 incubator.

12. After incubation, briefly check several wells for the presence of neutral red crystals; if extensive crystallization has occurred, then high background readings may be obtained.

13. Invert the plate and flick off dye and medium into a sink. Fill wells to the top with phosphate-buffered saline and flick the medium into a sink.

14. Using Dynatech dispenser or Cornwall syringe and buffer manifold, add 150 μl of elution buffer (phosphate ethanol) to each well; gently rock the plate to ensure even elution of dye into buffer.

15. The optical density of the solution is determined at 540 nm, using a multichannel spectrophotometer designed for 96-well plates; the mean optical density (OD) of the cell control wells is assigned a value of 100%, the mean of the control blank wells is assigned a value of 0%, and the dilution of virus producing a 50% OD reading, i.e., 50% inhibition of cell growth, is determined from a linear regression analysis of the data, using a computer program. The titer of each virus pool is expressed as a 50% dye uptake [DU_{50}] value, i.e., the reciprocal of the dilution of virus producing a 50% reduction in neutral red dye uptake by the cells).

Virus inhibition assay.

1. Prepare an initial drug solution in EMEM; because 50 μl of drug is mixed in the well with 200 μl (1:5 dilution) of other solutions, the initial drug solution should be five times more concentrated than the initial concentration to be tested.

2. With the 12-well multichannel pipettor, add 50 μl of the initial drug solution to all wells of rows 2, 3, and 4.

3. Flame the diluters to sterilize, fill the rinse slot with sterile water, and add the blotting papers to the tray. Using a sterile Cornwall syringe (1 ml) and an eight-channel manifold with the Dynatech diluter, dispense 50 μl of medium and serially dilute the drug. Set dispensers for rows 1, 2, and 4 to 12; set diluter for rows 4 to 11; set blot cycle on; place the labeled microtiter plate in position; press the RUN button.

4. Prepare a suspension of Vero cells (1.5×10^5 cells per ml) in EMEM supplemented with 5% FCS; using the Dynatech dispenser with a sterile Cornwall syringe (2.0 ml), add 150 μl of the cell suspension to each well of the plate. If the Dynatech dual dispenser is used, the medium addition, drug dilution, and cell seeding can be done with one pass of the plate.

5. In vitro ID_{50} values generated by the DU assay are dependent on the virus challenge dose. The assay is considered valid when the virus challenge dose is between 10 and 100 DU_{50}/50 μl. The actual challenge dose is determined by running a back-titration of the test virus in a separate microtiter plate.

To ensure that a valid challenge dose is used, two drug plates (labeled A and B) are run in the same assay. Using the DU_{50} titer determined in the virus infectivity titration, two different virus challenge doses are made. The first, designated tube A, is made up with a virus concentration of 50 DU_{50}/50 μl suspended in 6 ml of medium. From tube A, take 0.6 ml and add it to 5.4 ml of medium. This dilution is designated tube B. Using the adjustable pipettor, make a series of dilutions from 10^{-1} thru 10^{-3}, starting with 0.2 ml from tube B into 1.8 ml of medium; use a fresh pipette tip for each dilution.

6. Starting with the back-titration plate, inoculate the 10^{-3} dilution into all wells of row 7, the 10^{-2} dilution into all wells of row 6, and the 10^{-1} dilution into all wells of row 5. Next, inoculate tube B into all wells of row 4 of the back-titration plate and all wells of rows 3 through 12 of the B drug plate. Finally, inoculate tube A into all wells of row 3 of the back-titration plate and all wells of rows 3 through 12 of the A drug plate. Since the virus is inoculated beginning with the lowest virus concentration to the highest virus concentration, then the same Combitip can be used throughout. The number of replicates in each row may be eight or less (eight is recommended). In each inhibition assay, standard laboratory strains (HSV-1 and HSV-2) are included as in-

TABLE 1. Virus infectivity assay plate arrangement

Contents	Row no.									
	1	2	3	4	5	6	7	8	9	10–12
Media and cells, 150 μl	+	+	+	+	+	+	+	+	+	Empty
Virus, 50 μl			−1	−2	−3	−4	−5	−6		

TABLE 2. Back-titration plate arrangement

Contents	Row no.								
	1	2	3	4	5	6	7	8	9–12
Cells, 150 μl	+	+	+	+	+	+	+	+	Empty
Virus, 50 μl			Tube A	Tube B	−1	−2	−3		

ternal controls. The back-titration and drug plates should have the arrangements depicted in Tables 2 and 3.

7. The inhibition plates should have the following format (see Table 3): row 1, cell control; row 2, drug control; rows 3 to 11, drug dilution serials; row 12, virus control.

8. Seal the plates with sterile sealing tape or plate sealer and incubate them at 37°C in a CO_2 incubator.

9. After a 72-h incubation, add neutral red dye solution to both drug plates and the back-titration plate as described above for the virus infectivity assay; read the drug plates first and then the back-titration plate.

10. Linear regression analysis of the data is used to determine the concentration of drug producing a 50% reduction of the viral CPE in relation to cell controls (0%) and virus controls (100%); this concentration of drug is the ID_{50}.

11. The exact dose of the challenge virus is determined by reading the back-titration plate as described above for the virus infectivity assay. For a valid assay, the challenge dose should be between 10 and 100 DU_{50}/50 μl.

Advantages

The DU assay has several advantages over the PR assay, the most notable being the use of automated and semiautomated equipment. By linking the spectrophotometer to a computer, one can analyze in vitro data from large numbers of clinical isolates with a reduced amount of time and effort. Our laboratory routinely assays 20 clinical isolates, plus HSV-1 and HSV-2 virus controls, in a day. In a typical week, we can generate ID_{50} values for 60 different virus isolates. Eight replicates of nine different drug concentrations are placed in 96-well microtiter plates, allowing for a wide range of drug concentrations and good statistical reproducibility. This format significantly reduces the amount of reagents used and significantly lowers the cost per test.

Although the DU assay was developed for use with ACV and HSV in Vero cells, it has been adapted for use with other drugs, viruses, and cells. Other drugs that have been screened against HSV in the DU assay include adenine arabinoside, iododeoxyuridine, phosphonoacetic acid, phosphonoformic acid, thymidine arabinoside, ganciclovir, bromovinyldeoxyuridine, and fluoroiodoaracytosine. In addition, our laboratory has modified the assay to evaluate the combined action of drugs against HSV. The major requirements for the successful use of this system are a cytopathogenic virus and cells that form monolayers in 96-well, flat-bottom microtiter plates. The DU assay has been found to be reproducible, reliable, and quite suitable for use in diagnostic virology laboratories (7).

Perhaps the most significant advantage the DU assay has over the PR assay is its ability to detect small amounts of ACV-resistant virus in a heterogeneous viral population (15). The ability to identify these viruses is important, since ACV-resistant HSV strains have been shown to exist in natural virus populations never exposed to ACV (33). Drug-resistant strains of HSV also have been recovered from normal and immunologically compromised patients receiving ACV (8, 14, 31, 39). In reconstruction experiments, the DU assay is able to detect small amounts (3 to 9%) of ACV-resistant virus in a mixed virus population (15). The difference in sensitivity between the DU and PR assays may reflect the greater amount of input virus used in the DU assay (500 PFU/ml, compared with only 100 to 200 PFU/ml in the PR assay) or may be the result of the different endpoints used in the assays. Another reason for the greater sensitivity of the DU assay may be the different overlay materials used. In the DU assay, the liquid overlay allows drug-resistant virus to spread over the monolayer, and this amplified population of less sensitive virus is manifested by an increased ID_{50} value (28). In the PR assay, this extracellular spread of potentially resistant virus is inhibited by either a solid overlay or a liquid overlay containing serum immunoglobin (21, 23).

The DU assay gives ID_{50} values that are three to five times greater than values obtained by using the PR assay. This is a consistent result, and the inclusion of reference viruses (both HSV-1 and HSV-2) in each assay allows for comparisons of assays from week to week (28). If the ID_{50} values of these reference strains are greater than 2 standard deviations from their mean values as determined in previous tests, then the entire assay is

TABLE 3. Virus inhibition assay plate arrangement

Contents and order of addition	Row no.											
	1	2	3	4	5	6	7	8	9	10	11	12
Highest drug concn, 50 μl		+	+	+								
Medium, 50 μl	+	+		+	+	+	+	+	+	+	+	+
Drug dilution				+	+	+	+	+	+	+	+	
Cells, 150 μl	+	+	+	+	+	+	+	+	+	+	+	+
Virus, 50 μl			+	+	+	+	+	+	+	+	+	+

repeated (28). Over the past 8 years, our laboratory has determined the ID_{50} values of over 3,000 HSV clinical isolates recovered from a variety of patients. We found that over 98% of these isolates had ACV ID_{50} values of ≤3.0 μg/ml. Therefore, with the DU assay we use this ID_{50} value as the cutoff between ACV-sensitive and ACV-resistant viruses (3).

Disadvantages

For a research laboratory with few isolates to test, the cost of the automated equipment needed for the DU assay is prohibitive. However, all steps except the step involving spectrophotometric analysis can be done manually (7). Technical problems with the equipment can be frustrating and can cause time-consuming delays. Occasionally, the neutral red dye will precipitate onto the monolayer, making it impossible to accurately determine the amount of dye released from viable cells. This problem can be avoided if the pH of the dye solution is maintained above 5.8 and the solution is filtered before use. Another pitfall is the overseeding of cells, which causes the monolayer to peel. Overseeding can decrease the number of viable cells and can lead to poor results. This problem rarely occurs if the cells are seeded at a density of 2×10^4 to 3×10^4 per well.

Several factors affect the reliability of any assay that measures the inhibition of viral CPE. These factors include the virus and cells used, the challenge dose of virus used, and the gradient of drug concentrations that ensures a valid endpoint (21, 22). In the DU assay, most of these technical problems have been solved. However, the ID_{50} values generated by this assay are affected by the amount of virus used. It is necessary to determine the infectivity titer of each clinical isolate before the drug inhibition assay can be attempted. It is also useful to include a back-titration plate for each test virus to determine the actual virus challenge dose used in the assay. In the DU assay, a high challenge dose (>100 DU_{50}) can cause an ACV-sensitive virus to have a high ID_{50} value. Alternatively, a low challenge dose (<10 DU_{50}) of an ACV-resistant virus will give an artificially low ID_{50} value (28). Challenge doses that fall within a range of 10 to 100 DU_{50} have little effect on the ID_{50} values (28). Hence, if the viral challenge dose is outside these limits, then the assay of the test isolate is repeated. Since the infectivity titration of the isolate and the drug inhibition assay both require 3 days, the minimum time for determining the in vitro ID_{50} value for any particular isolate is approximately 2 weeks.

PR Assay

The PR assay is the standard technique for determining drug sensitivities of all cytopathogenic viruses and is based on inhibition of viral plaque formation (28). It is relatively simple to perform and easy to quantify. Briefly, a known amount of virus (100 to 200 PFU) is inoculated onto a number of tissue culture plates containing a monolayer of permissive cells. After incubation for 1 h to allow viral adsorption, the inoculum is aspirated, and overlay medium containing a range of drug dilutions, nutrients, and either a solid (0.6% agar or 1 to 2% methylcellulose) (23) or liquid (serum immunoglobulin) (28) is added to the plates. After 72 h of incubation, the plates are stained with crystal violet dye (for recipe, see chapter 122), allowed to stand at room temperature for 1 h, and rinsed with water. The plates are then air dried, and the plaques are counted. A dose-response curve is generated, and an ID_{50} value is calculated by determining the percentage of plaques formed at various drug concentrations compared with the percentage in the no-drug control. Our laboratory generates ID_{50} values from this assay with Probit, a linear regression probability program (Statistical Analysis Systems, Cary, N.C.).

Advantages

The PR assay has been shown to be an accurate and reliable technique for determining the in vitro potency of a given antiviral agent. The major advantage of the PR assay is its overall simplicity. For research laboratories doing small numbers of clinical isolates (≤10 per month), this is probably the assay of choice.

Disadvantages

Unlike the DU method, the PR assay is very difficult to automate. Counting the plaques is a tedious and time-consuming procedure, since each drug dilution is done in duplicate.

The number of plaques that can be accurately counted is limited by the size of the tissue culture plate, the distribution of the virus on the plate, and the biological characteristics of the virus-cell systems. Virus replication and spread at high drug concentrations may be incompletely inhibited, leading to smaller plaques than those observed at lower drug concentrations or in the virus control plates. However, the high drug concentrations may contain similar numbers of plaques. Failure to recognize and count these small plaques can lead to false ID_{50} values. Like other assays based on measuring inhibition of viral CPE, the PR assay is affected by the virus challenge dose, the virus type, the cell type, and the metabolism of the drug by the host cells (2, 21, 22).

Since the PR assay is done in large plates (60 by 15 mm), more media, cells, and drugs are needed. If a solid overlay is used, then double the concentration of growth medium is required so that the nutrient concentration remains sufficient for cell viability. As with the DU assay, the infectivity titer of the virus must be determined before the PR assay is performed. For HSV in Vero cells, both the infectivity titration and the plaque reduction assay require 3 days. The additional work of counting plaques and calculating the ID_{50} value for the virus results in a considerably longer time to complete this assay. For testing large numbers of viruses, the PR assay is not very efficient.

Conclusion

The factors affecting the choice of an appropriate antiviral suseptibility assay are different for each laboratory. In some instances, the sheer number of isolates to be tested demands a so-called high-throughput assay. For laboratories with few isolates to evaluate and a limited budget, a more traditional method may be satisfactory. Other factors that can influence this decision include the virus-cell system to be used, the incubation period, and the overall time needed to produce results.

The lack of standardization of these tests makes it difficult to compare results from laboratory to laboratory. Hence, comparisons of in vitro data are valid only if the same assay, virus, and cell type are used in the test.

Since there has been no established correlation between in vitro susceptibility and in vivo response to therapy in humans, differences in absolute in vitro ID_{50} values between assay systems probably have little clinical relevance. Thus, the definition of a "susceptible" or "resistant" virus must be derived empirically for each assay system. A clearer understanding of the relationship between plasma drug level, in vitro susceptibility, and clinical response will emerge with continued use of antiviral drugs and subsequent susceptibility testing of large numbers of viruses by many laboratories.

ANTIPARASITIC SUSCEPTIBILITY TESTING

Until reliable antiparasitic vaccines become available, drugs will continue to play an important role in the prevention and treatment of parasitic diseases. The effects of drugs on the wide spectrum of parasites can be studied by a diverse array of techniques. These can be used to screen new compounds, to investigate mechanisms of drug action and resistance, or to quantify interactions between drugs and host immune responses. However, use of such techniques has been confined mainly to specialized research laboratories; their application to public health and clinical laboratories remains limited except for malaria testing. In the latter case, techniques have been standardized and adapted for field conditions, where they have been used mainly in epidemiologic studies.

Helminths

Helminths are complex organisms that have a complicated life cycle and interaction with their hosts. Because of the absence of long-term culture techniques, most chemotherapeutic studies of helminths have used experimental animal models. Such models include either the human parasite in an animal (such as *Schistosoma mansoni* and *S. japonicum* in mice or hamsters) or a natural parasite of the experimental animal (such as *Nippostrongylus brasiliensis* in the rat, as a model for ancylostomiasis in humans) (25). Such animals models often require maintenance of the intermediate hosts necessary for completion of the parasite's life cycle. This impracticality, and the fact that findings from such animal models are not necessarily translatable to the situation with the human parasites, limit their use in clinical laboratories.

Short-term in vitro experiments can be initiated by using parasites isolated from an animal host. For example, larvae and adults of *S. mansoni* can be maintained in vitro for 24 to 48 h in a culture medium consisting of Hank's balanced salt solution supplemented with 17% FCS, 0.5% glucose, and 200 U of penicillin per ml, during which time the effect of drugs (such as praziquantel) added to the culture medium can be observed according to criteria such as muscle contraction of the worm and tegumental damages (47). Similarly, the adult worms of *Brugia malayi* can be maintained in vitro for up to 4 days (in a 1:1 mixture of NCTC 135 and Iscove modified Dulbecco medium), with the effect of compounds observed as paralysis and decrease in lactate excretion (44). Microfilariae of *Onchocerca volvulus* can be maintained by using a similar medium (NCTC 135-Iscove modified Dulbecco medium buffered with HEPES and supplemented with 20% FCS and antibiotics), and the effect of compounds can be evaluated on the basis of decrease in larval motility over a 3-day observation period (40).

Since such short-term cultures derive frequently from experimental animals, they suffer from the same impracticalities as the studies using animal models. In addition, a pitfall of in vitro studies in helminths resides in the fact that host factors play an important role in the activity of some antihelminthic agents. The effect of praziquantel on schistosomes in vivo, for example, depends on host antibody response (6).

The absence of convenient and reliable in vitro tests for drug susceptibility in helminths does not, however, represent a major problem in terms of application to public health and clinical laboratories. Variability in drug responses within strains of the same species is rare (one exception being the variability in response of *S. mansoni* to hycanthone, oxamniquine, and niridazole [1]), thus decreasing the need for detection of drug resistance. The risk of selection for drug-resistant parasites under drug pressure is minimized by the fact that helminths do not replicate in the human host (one exception being *Strongyloides stercoralis*). Because of this characteristic, most helminthic infections follow a chronic, nonsevere course in which in vitro detection of drug resistance is of limited clinical relevance even though it might be of epidemiologic interest.

Protozoa

Protozoa replicate in the human host, frequently causing acute pathology and potentially fatal disease, for which a timely and effective therapy is crucial. In addition, parasite multiplication under drug pressure permits the emergence and geographical spread of drug-resistant mutants. These facts underline the clinical and epidemiologic relevance of drug susceptibility tests for protozoa.

Decreased drug responsiveness is a well-documented problem for *Plasmodium falciparum* and has also been observed with *Trypanosoma cruzi* (to nifurtimox and benznidazole), *Leishmania* spp. (to sodium stibogluconate), and *Trichomonas* spp. (to metronidazole). In such situations, the respective contributions of the parasite's biological resistance, its localization in a site inaccessible to drugs, or the efficacy of the host's immune defenses can be partially evaluated by using in vitro techniques.

Most protozoa can be adapted to long-term culture under conditions that obviate the need for the parallel maintenance of an intermediate host. In vitro drug susceptibility tests are conducted under conditions derived from those used for long-term culture (19). Most protozoa can be cultured under axenic conditions (for example, *Entamoeba histolytica, Naegleria fowleri, Acanthamoeba* spp., *Giardia lamblia,* certain arthropod stages of trypanosomes and *Leishmania* spp., and *Trichomonas vaginalis*). Others necessitate the presence in culture of another cell type; for example, blood stages of trypomastigotes of African trypanosomes require the concomitant presence of fibroblastlike feeder cells; tissue stages of *Leishmania* and *T. cruzi* parasites grow in macrophages and those of *Toxoplasma gondii* grow in fibroblasts or macrophages; exoerythrocytic-stage malaria parasites grow in primary culture of hepatocytes (17); and *Plasmodium* and *Babesia* blood-stage parasites grow in erythrocytes. In such monoxenic cultures, the influence of the nonparasitic cell population must be considered in evaluating the results of the test.

To perform a drug susceptibility test, a parasite inoculum is collected from a continuous culture, an experimental animal, or a patient and cultured under optimal conditions in the presence of various concentrations of drugs for various periods of time. At the end of the incubation period, inhibition of parasite growth is measured by various criteria. Conventional parasite count and determination of viability, using criteria such as motility or exclusion of trypan blue (*E. histolytica* [37]), are most often used. For *G. lamblia*, adhesion to nylon fiber microcolumns constitutes an additional criterion, reflecting the activity of the parasite's ventral sucker and flagella (10). The sporontocidal effect of antimalarial compounds on gametocytes of *P. falciparum* can be evaluated by measuring the inhibition of gametocyte infectivity to mosquitoes fed on a gametocyte culture (42). Automated techniques for quantifying parasite inhibition have been introduced. Such techniques include the use of a Coulter counter to quantify *G. lamblia* (10) and the measurement of uptake of radiolabeled markers, such as [^{3}H]uracil by *Leishmania tropica* (4), [^{3}H]thymidine by *E. histolytica* (9), and [^{3}H]hypoxanthine by *P. falciparum* (11).

In vitro drug susceptibility studies have been performed in a clinical context for *N. fowleri* (12) and *Trichomonas vaginalis* (26), confirming general in vivo findings. Similar studies of malaria are described later. In a laboratory context, in vitro methods have proven useful in the study of drug interactions. The reversal of chloroquine resistance of *P. falciparum* by the calcium channel blocker verapamil (27) and the antagonism between azidothymidine and pyrimethamine-sulfadoxine in *Toxoplasma gondii* (24) have been demonstrated by using such techniques. For laboratory investigation on inducibility of drug resistance, in vitro-cloned parasites have been used. Such trials have resulted in the development of mefloquine-resistant clones of *P. falciparum* (32) and of *Leishmania* clones resistant to sodium stibogluconate (20).

A recent advance consists in the application of molecular biology techniques to detection of drug resistance. *P. falciparum* genes related to mammalian multiple drug resistance genes have been shown to be amplified in drug-resistant *P. falciparum* (18, 46), and point mutations in dihydrofolate reductase-thymidilate synthase have been demonstrated in pyrimethamine-resistant *P. falciparum* (35). Such findings may lead to development of powerful yet practical tools for determination of drug resistance.

Field Tests for Drug Resistance in Malaria

Parasite drug resistance, with respect to both the diversity of the problem and its clinical and epidemiologic implications, is most vividly illustrated in malaria. The species in which drug resistance predominates is *P. falciparum*, the causal agent of severe malaria. Resistance in the blood-stage parasites, whose rapid multiplication is at the origin of clinical symptoms, has been studied most extensively.

In vitro drug resistance tests of *P. falciparum* blood-stage parasites are based on the culture technique of Trager and Jensen (43). The technique that is most widely used worldwide is derived from the microtechnique originally described by Rieckmann et al. (38). In this technique, synchronous ring-stage parasites collected with a patient's capillary blood sample are cultured for 24 to 30 h, during which time the parasite's maturation to multinucleated schizonts and its inhibition by antimalarial compounds can be observed. This technique has been standardized and adapted to field work by the World Health Organization, which produces on a large scale and provides self-contained in vitro kits allowing tests with chloroquine, mefloquine, quinine, amodiaquine, and more recently sulfadoxine-pyrimethamine (34, 45).

The in vitro kits contain 96-well microplates dosed before shipment by the World Health Organization with various concentrations of antimalarial drugs. Predosing is performed by depositing in the wells 10 μl of an aqueous solution containing the respective amounts of drug, which adheres to the well upon drying of the solution. To perform the test, sterile capillary blood (100 μl) collected by fingerprick from the patient is diluted in 900 μl of culture medium (RPMI 1640 supplemented with 25 mM HEPES buffer, reconstituted by using foil minipacks provided in the kit). The blood-medium mixture is then distributed as 50-μl portions into eight wells of the microplate, predosed with various concentrations of the drug to be tested (in the case of chloroquine, 0, 0.2, 0.4, 0.8, 1.6, 3.2, 6.4, and 12.8 μmol/liter of blood, corresponding to 0, 1, 2, 4, 8, 16, 32, and 64 pmol per well). The microplate is incubated in a candle jar (43) at 37°C for 24 to 30 h. Serial thick blood films are made of the contents of each well and stained with Giemsa stain; the maturation to schizonts of the parasites in drug-containing wells is compared with that in the control well. In the case of chloroquine, the presence of schizonts in the well containing 8 pmol of chloroquine (1.6 μmol/liter of blood) indicates in vitro chloroquine resistance. The results can be alternately expressed as a log-probit dose-response curve, and results from several isolates can be pooled to reflect the overall status of an area.

The World Health Organization kits have a shelf life of 2 years and have been used widely in worldwide epidemiologic studies on drug resistance in *P. falciparum*. The kit has recently been modified by use of RPMI 1640 with low concentrations of *p*-aminobenzoic acid and folic acid, thus allowing in addition tests with antifolate drugs (34).

Other techniques for field testing in vitro drug susceptibility of *P. falciparum* extend the incubation time to 48 h, thus allowing the drug to exert its inhibitory effect on all phases of the parasite's full cycle of asexual multiplication. These techniques, originally developed for asynchronous, laboratory-grown parasites, have been shown to be adaptable to field isolates, and they use as their criteria either parasite multiplication ascertained microscopically (13, 30) or uptake of [^{3}H]hypoxanthine (5).

Such drug susceptibility tests, especially those with chloroquine, have proven useful in mapping epidemiologically the spread of drug resistance worldwide. However, they have proven of very limited clinical applicability. Whereas the in vivo-in vitro correlations of the chloroquine findings have been satisfactory, those for other compounds remain to be evaluated.

Conclusions

There are techniques that allow the determination in vitro of susceptibility to antiparasitic drugs, but several obstacles prevent their adoption by clinical laboratories. Many techniques are complex or require experimental animals as sources of infective organisms, features that relegate them to specialized research laboratories. Because of the small number of laboratories using them, these techniques have not been standardized, making it difficult to compare results. The in vitro results frequently contradict or do not relate to the in vivo findings, which probably reflects the complexity of the relationships between host and parasite and the way each metabolizes drugs. Thus, although most of these techniques have proven useful either for research purposes or for epidemiologic investigations, their clinical relevance will depend on a better delineation of in vitro-in vivo correlates, on standardization, and on an increased simplicity of the tests, possibly through the use of biomolecular markers.

Portions of this chapter appeared previously ("Susceptibility Testing for Antiviral Testing," p. 245–250, *in* S. Specter and G. J. Lancz, ed., *Clinical Virology Manual*, Elsevier Science Publishing Co., Inc., New York, 1986) and are reprinted here with permission of the publisher.

LITERATURE CITED

1. **Araujo, N., N. Katz, E. P. Dias, and C. P. De Souza.** 1980. Susceptibility to chemotherapeutic agents of strains of *Schistosoma mansoni* isolated from treated and untreated patients. Am. J. Trop. Med. Hyg. **29:**890–894.
2. **Barry, D. W. and M. R. Blum.** 1983. Antiviral drugs: acyclovir, p. 57–80. *In* P. Turner and D. G. Shand (ed.), Recent advances in clinical pharmacology. Churchill Livingstone, Ltd., Edinburgh.
3. **Barry, D. W., S. Nusinoff-Lehrman, M. N. Ellis, K. K. Biron, and P. A. Furman.** 1985. Viral resistance, clinical experience. Scand. J. Infect. Dis. Suppl. **47:**155–164.
4. **Berman, J. D., and J. V. Gallalee.** 1985. Semiautomated assessment of in vitro activity of potential antileishmanial drugs. Antimicrob. Agents Chemother. **28:**723–726.
5. **Brasseur, P., P. Druilhe, J. Kouamouo, O. Brandicourt, M. Danis, and S. R. Moyou.** 1986. High level of sensitivity to chloroquine of 72 *Plasmodium falciparum* isolates from southern Cameroon in January 1985. Am. J. Trop. Med. Hyg. **35:**711–716.
6. **Brindley, P. J., and A. Sher.** 1987. The chemotherapeutic effect of praziquantel against *Schistosoma mansoni* is dependent on host antibody response. J. Immunol. **139:**215–220.
7. **Brisebois, J. J., V. M. Dumas, and J. H. Joncas.** 1989. Comparison of two methods in the determination of the sensitivity of 84 herpes simplex virus (HSV) type 1 and 2 clinical isolates to acyclovir and alpha-interferon. Antiviral Res. **11:**67–76.
8. **Burns, W. H., R. Saral, G. W. Santos, O. L. Laskin, P. S. Lietman, C. McLaren, and D. W. Barry.** 1982. Isolation and characterisation of resistant herpes simplex virus after acyclovir therapy. Lancet **i:**421–423.
9. **Cedeno, J. R., and D. J. Krogstad.** 1983. Susceptibility testing for *Entamoeba histolytica*. J. Infect. Dis. **148:**1090–1095.
10. **Crouch, A. A., W. K. Seow, and Y. H. Thong.** 1986. Effect of twenty-three chemotherapeutic agents on the adherence and growth of *Giardia lamblia* in vitro. Trans. R. Soc. Trop. Med. Hyg. **80:**893–896.
11. **Desjardins, R. E., C. J. Canfield, J. D. Haynes, and J. D. Chulay.** 1979. Quantitative assessment of antimalarial activity in vitro by a semiautomated microdilution technique. Antimicrob. Agents Chemother. **16:**710–718.
12. **Duma, R. J., and R. Finley.** 1976. In vitro susceptibility of pathogenic *Naegleria* and *Acanthamoeba* species to a variety of therapeutic agents. Antimicrob. Agents Chemother. **10:**370–376.
13. **Duverseau, Y. T., R. Magloire, A. Zevallos-Ipenza, H. M. Rogers, and P. Nguyen-Dinh.** 1986. Monitoring of chloroquine sensitivity of *Plasmodium falciparum* in Haiti, 1981–1983. Am. J. Trop. Med. Hyg. **35:**459–464.
14. **Ellis, M. N., P. M. Keller, J. A. Fyfe, J. L. Martin, J. F. Rooney, S. E. Straus, S. Nusinoff-Lehrman, and D. W. Barry.** 1987. Clinical isolate of herpes simplex virus type 2 that induces a thymidine kinase with altered substrate specificity. Antimicrob. Agents Chemother. **31:**1117–1125.
15. **Ellis, M. N., R. Waters, E. L. Hill, D. C. Lobe, D. W. Selleseth, and D. W. Barry.** 1989. Orofacial infection of athymic mice with defined mixtures of acyclovir-susceptible and acyclovir-resistant herpes simplex virus type 1. Antimicrob. Agents Chemother. **33:**304–310.
16. **Finter, N. B.** 1969. Dye uptake methods for assessing viral cytopathogenicity and their application to interferon assays. J. Gen. Virol. **5:**419–427.
17. **Fisk, T. L., P. Millet, W. E. Collins, and P. Nguyen-Dinh.** 1989. In vitro activity of antimalarial compounds on the exoerythrocytic stages of *Plasmodium cynomolgi* and *P. knowlesi*. Am. J. Trop. Med. Hyg. **38:**235–238.
18. **Foote, S. J., J. K. Thompson, A. F. Cowman, and D. J. Kemp.** 1989. Amplification of the multidrug resistance gene in some chloroquine-resistant isolates of *Plasmodium falciparum*. Cell **57:**921–930.
19. **Fritsche, T. R.** 1989. Pathogenic protozoa: an overview of in vitro cultivation and susceptibility to chemotherapeutic agents. Clin. Lab. Med. **9:**287–317.
20. **Grogl, M., A. M. J. Oduola, L. D. C. Cordero, and D. E. Kyle.** 1989. *Leishmania* spp: development of pentostam-resistant clones in vitro by discontinuous drug exposure. Exp. Parasitol. **69:**78–90.
21. **Harmenberg, J., B. Wahren, and B. Oberg.** 1980. Influence of cells and virus multiplicity on the inhibition of herpesviruses with acycloguanosine. Intervirology **14:**239–244.
22. **Harmenberg, J., B. Wahren, V.-A. Sundqvist, and B. Leven.** 1985. Multiplicity dependence and sensitivity of herpes simplex virus isolates to antiviral compounds. J. Antimicrob. Chemother. **15:**567–573.
23. **Hu, J. M., and G. D. Hsiung.** 1989. Evaluation of new antiviral agents. I. *In vitro* perspectives. Antiviral Res. **11:**217–232.
24. **Israelski, D. M., C. Tom, and J. S. Remington.** 1989. Zidovudine antagonizes the action of pyrimethamine in experimental infection with *Toxoplasma gondii*. Antimicrob. Agents Chemother. **33:**30–34.
25. **Katiyar, J. C., S. Gupta, and S. Sharma.** 1989. Experimental models in drug development for helminthic diseases. Rev. Infect. Dis. **11:**638–654.
26. **Lossick, J. G., M. Muller, and T. E. Gorrell.** 1986. In vitro drug susceptibility and doses of metronidazole required for cure in cases of refractory vaginal trichomoniasis. J. Infect. Dis. **153:**948–955.
27. **Martin, S. K., A. M. J. Oduola, and W. K. Milhous.** 1987. Reversal of chloroquine resistance in *Plasmodium falciparum* by verapamil. Science **235:**899–901.
28. **McLaren, C., M. N. Ellis, and G. A. Hunter.** 1983. A colorimetic assay for the measurement of the sensitivity of herpes simplex viruses to antiviral agents. Antiviral Res. **3:**223–234.
29. **Newton, A. A.** 1988. Tissue culture methods for assessing antivirals and their harmful effects, p. 33–66. *In* H. J. Field

(ed.), Antiviral agents: the development and assessment of antiviral chemotherapy, vol. I. CRC Press, Inc., Boca Raton, Fla.

30. **Nguyen-Dinh, P., and W. Trager.** 1980. *Plasmodium falciparum* in vitro: determination of chloroquine sensitivity of three new strains by a modified 48-hour test. Am. J. Trop. Med. Hyg. **29:**339–342.
31. **Norris, S. A., H. A. Kessler, and K. H. Fife.** 1988. Severe, progressive herpetic whitlow caused by acyclovir-resistant virus in a patient with AIDS. J. Infect. Dis. **157:**209–210.
32. **Oduola, A. M. J., W. K. Milhous, N. F. Weatherly, J. H. Bowdre, and R. E. Desjardins.** 1988. *Plasmodium falciparum:* induction of resistance to mefloquine in cloned strains by continuous drug exposure in vitro. Exp. Parasitol. **67:**354–360.
33. **Parris, D. S., and J. E. Harrington.** 1982. Herpes simplex virus variants resistant to high concentrations of acyclovir exist in clinical isolates. Antimicrob. Agents Chemother. **22:**71–77.
34. **Payne, D., and W. H. Wernsdorfer.** 1989. Development of a blood culture medium and a standard in vitro microtest for field-testing the response of *Plasmodium falciparum* to antifolate antimalarials. Bull. WHO **67:**59–64.
35. **Peterson, D. S., D. Walliker, and T. E. Wellems.** 1988. Evidence that point mutations in dihydrofolate reductase-thymidilate synthase confer resistance to pyrimethamine in falciparum malaria. Proc. Natl. Acad. Sci. USA **85:**9114–9118.
36. **Rabalais, G. P., M. J. Levin, and F. E. Berkowitz.** 1987. Rapid herpes simplex virus susceptibility testing using an enzyme-linked immunosorbent assay performed in situ on fixed virus-infected monolayers. Antimicrob. Agents Chemother. **31:**946–948.
37. **Ravdin, J. I., and J. Skilogiannis.** 1989. In vitro susceptibilities of *Entamoeba histolytica* to azithromycin, CP-63,956, erythromycin, and metronidazole. Antimicrob. Agents Chemother. **33:**960–962.
38. **Rieckmann, K. H., L. J. Sax, G. H. Campbell, and J. E. Mrema.** 1978. Drug sensitivity of *Plasmodium falciparum*. An in vitro microtechnique. Lancet **i:**22–23.
39. **Sibrack, C. D., L. T. Gutman, C. M. Wilfert, C. McLaren, M. H. St. Clair, P. M. Keller, and D. W. Barry.** 1982. Pathogenicity of acyclovir-resistant herpes simplex virus type 1 from an immunodeficient child. J. Infect. Dis. **146:**673–682.
40. **Strote, G.** 1987. In vitro study on the effect of the new chemotherapeutic agents CGP 6140 and CGP 20376 on the microfilariae of *Onchocerca volvulus*. Trop. Med. Parasitol. **38:**211–213.
41. **Swierkosz, E. M., D. R. Scholl, J. L. Brown, J. D. Jollick, and V. M. Dilworth.** 1987. Improved DNA hybridization methodology for detection of acyclovir-resistant herpes simplex virus. Antimicrob. Agents Chemother. **31:**1465–1469.
42. **Teklehaimanot, A., P. Nguyen-Dinh, W. E. Collins, A. M. Barber, and C. C. Campbell.** 1985. Evaluation of sporontocidal compounds using *Plasmodium falciparum* gametocytes produced in vitro. Am. J. Trop. Med. Hyg. **34:**429–434.
43. **Trager, W., and J. B. Jensen.** 1976. Human malaria parasites in continuous culture. Science **193:**673–675.
44. **Walter, R. D., R. M. Wittich, and F. Kuhlow.** 1987. Filaricidal effect of mefloquine on adults and microfilariae of *Brugia patei* and *Brugia malayi*. Trop. Med. Parasitol. **38:**55–56.
45. **Wernsdorfer, W. H.** 1980. Field evaluation of drug resistance in malaria. In vitro micro-test. Acta Trop. **37:**222–227.
46. **Wilson, C. M., A. E. Serrano, A. Wasley, M. P. Bogenschutz, A. H. Shankar, and D. F. Wirth.** 1989. Amplification of a gene related to mammalian mdr genes in drug-resistant *Plasmodium falciparum*. Science **244:**1184–1186.
47. **Xiao, S.-H., B. A. Catto, and L. T. Webster, Jr.** 1985. Effects of praziquantel on different developmental stages of *Schistosoma mansoni* in vitro and in vivo. J. Infect. Dis. **151:**1130–1137.

Chapter 119

Assays for Antimicrobial Agents in Body Fluids

JOHN P. ANHALT

Determination of the concentration of an antimicrobial agent in serum or other fluids is justified only when that concentration can be correlated with benchmarks of efficacy or excess and cannot be predicted adequately from dosage. The range between therapeutic and toxic levels of most antimicrobial agents is large, and the tendency is to administer doses that essentially ensure levels in serum severalfold the assumed minimal effective level. Assays are not required for these drugs unless there is a reasonable suspicion that the level in serum may be markedly different than usual, such as in patients with severe renal disease, or the patient shows nonspecific symptoms that may be related to toxicity, such as seizures. The effect of dialysis on elimination of many antimicrobial agents is sufficiently predictable (2), however, that this factor alone does not require the use of assays for dosage adjustment. In recent years, increased emphasis on minimizing hospital stay has meant that some patients for whom long-term parenteral antimicrobial therapy had been the standard of care have been switched to orally administered agents before hospital discharge. The relative newness of this approach apparently has resulted in increased numbers of assays to document that adequate levels are attained by the oral drugs. Whether the practice serves a useful function for dosage adjustment or will be discontinued as familiarity is gained is unknown.

A relatively small number of antimicrobial agents, the most common being aminoglycosides, chloramphenicol, and vancomycin, exhibit a narrow range between therapeutic and potentially toxic concentrations. Calculated doses are often inadequate to ensure appropriate levels in serum and are particularly inaccurate for critically ill patients in whom the rapid attainment of maximum levels is needed to treat a life-threatening infection. Assays for these drugs often are needed for optimal patient care.

SPECIMENS

The most appropriate specimen for assay of common antimicrobial agents is serum, and guidelines for dosage adjustments are usually based on serum levels, even for infections at sites where drug concentrations are expected to be different. Plasma is equally satisfactory; however, anticoagulants may interfere with some assay procedures. For example, heparin binds gentamicin and can adversely affect a bioassay. Immunoassays generally are not affected by heparin at levels required to prevent clotting of blood (24). Assays of urine are rarely indicated, and results are difficult to interpret. Assays of other body fluids, such as cerebrospinal fluid or bile, can be useful for documenting adequate drug levels. Procedures should be validated for each type of body fluid to be tested.

Timing of collection

Antimicrobial agents are administered usually at intervals that allow most of a dose to be excreted before a subsequent dose is given. Drug accumulation is minimal, and after only two or three doses (i.e., after five half-lives) a steady state is reached that is characterized by a large difference between the minimum concentration (trough level) and maximum concentration (peak level) attained in serum. The rapid changes in drug concentration between the two extremes mandate that times for administration of doses and obtaining blood for assays be carefully planned and recorded accurately for clinically useful results.

Careful consideration should be given to whether both peak and trough determinations are needed in a particular case. Although it is common practice to monitor both values for aminoglycosides, recent studies have shown that pharmacokinetic predictions and dosage adjustments based on a single trough or peak determination can be as accurate as predictions based on paired determinations. In fact, Godley and co-workers (7) found that a Baysian program using patient-specific data (age, sex, weight, height, and serum creatinine) and a single trough determination predicted peak gentamicin concentrations as accurately as any other method, including methods based on linear and nonlinear models requiring two or more determinations of peak and trough concentrations, and was statistically more accurate than the other methods for predicting trough concentrations (7). For most other antimicrobial agents, determination of either the peak or trough concentration will suffice for dosage adjustment and be more cost effective than paired determinations. Trough levels provide a sensitive indicator of decreased drug elimination, and from a practical standpoint, it is relatively easy to obtain accurately timed specimens for them. Peak levels are preferred when trough levels fall below the level that can be accurately quantitated, when a high therapeutic level must be ensured, or when a potentially toxic level must be avoided. Accurately timed specimens for peak levels are more demanding to obtain and require a high level of coordination between laboratory and nursing staffs.

The exact time that a peak level occurs varies according to the drug, route of administration, and clinical status of the patient and is impossible to predict accurately. As a general practice, blood for peak levels should be obtained 30 min after the completion of an intravenous infusion, 1 h after an intramuscular dose, and 1 to 2 h after an oral dose. Absorption of an oral medicine is particularly variable. Therefore, if the level in serum after an oral dose is unexpectedly low, the possibility of slow absorption should be tested by obtaining a sample of blood 3 h after a dose. Some forms of tetracycline and erythromycin typically are absorbed even more slowly and do not attain peak levels until 4 to 6 h after oral dosing. Blood for trough levels should be obtained immediately before a dose.

Information essential to the laboratory

A test request for an antimicrobial assay should include the names of any other antimicrobial agents the patient received within the previous 48 h. This information is essential, particularly when a bioassay is used, if the laboratory expects to provide a result that does not represent a combined effect of the agents. Also important is that the dose, exact time of dose, and time of collection be given. This information is used to estimate the proper dilutions of serum to be tested in bioassays and will aid the laboratory in detecting specimen mixups and in tracing problems with results that "do not make sense." More important, the timing information can be included in the report to facilitate interpretation in complicated cases for which several assays may have been done.

Processing and storage

Stability of antibiotics in clinical specimens is affected by many variables and is difficult to predict. Serum or plasma should be separated as soon as practical after blood collection, and assays should be done the same day. If testing will be delayed, the specimen should be frozen at −20°C or lower (−60°C preferred). There are exceptions to these general precautions. Specimens for imipenem assay are particularly unstable and difficult to store. Stability can be improved by adding an equal volume of 0.05 M 2-(*N*-morpholino)ethanesulfonic acid (MES) buffer at pH 6.0. Serum stabilized in this manner can be stored for 24 h at −20°C with negligible loss of drug. Aminoglycosides are unstable in serum that also contains a β-lactam drug, particularly ticarcillin or carbenicillin. Stability in these cases can be improved by addition of a β-lactamase. Stability of cephalosporins in serum and plasma can be improved by addition of sodium dodecyl sulfate to a final concentration of 1% (wt/vol) at pH 6 or below (4).

Anecdotal reports abound for various assay problems that have been traced to presumably trivial changes in sample collection and processing procedures. One recent report, for example, found that substitution of an essentially equivalent evacuated collection tube resulted in interference with a chromatographic assay (12). It is essential, therefore, that specimen collection procedures be evaluated as part of the implementation for new assay methods.

INTERPRETATION OF RESULTS

In many cases, a specific therapeutic range for antimicrobial agents has not been defined. Instead, typical levels attained with doses that have been shown to be effective in clinical trials are considered desirable (section IX, appendix 2). For a small number of agents, therapeutic ranges have been defined more narrowly (Table 1).

Some assay results will indicate medical emergencies (e.g., unusually high or low values). The laboratory should report these values immediately to a physician or other person listed on the test request.

METHODS

The discovery of each new antimicrobial agent has been accompanied by the development of an assay procedure. Since these discoveries are made in many different laboratories, it is no surprise that assays exist in great profusion and serve several functions. To select an appropriate method, one must consider (i) availability and cost of specialized equipment, (ii) availability of personnel with special expertise, (iii) reagent cost, (iv) workload, (v) versatility, and (vi) needs for specificity, precision, speed, and sensitivity. Workload does not mean simply the total number of tests. One should also consider whether the work occurs in a steady stream or in spurts and whether work can be batched. The need for specificity will be influenced by the degree of control a laboratory has over ordering and the availability of accurate patient information. For example, a referral laboratory might require greater specificity than

TABLE 1. Therapeutic ranges and pharmacokinetics for selected antimicrobial agents

Antimicrobial agent	Usual dose	Dosage interval (h)	Maximum dose (per 24 h)	Normal serum half-life (h)	Major route of elimination	Therapeutic range (μg/ml)	
						Peak	Trough
Amikacin	5–7.5 mg/kg	8–12	15 mg/kg	2–3	Renal	20–25	5–10
Gentamicin	1.7 mg/kg	8	5 mg/kg	2–3	Renal	4–8	1–2
Kanamycin	5–7.5 mg/kg	8–12	15 mg/kg	2–3	Renal	20–25	5–10
Netilmicin	2–2.5 mg/kg	8	7.5 mg/kg	2–3	Renal	6–10	0.5–2
Streptomycin	0.5–1 g	8–12	2 g	2–3	Renal	5–20	<5
Tobramycin	1.7 mg/kg	8	5 mg/kg	2–3	Renal	4–8	1–2
Chloramphenicol	0.5–1 g	6	4 g	4[a]	Hepatic-renal	15–25	8–10
Flucytosine	37.5 mg/kg	6	150 mg/kg	4	Renal	100	50
TMP-SMX[b]							
TMP	5 mg/kg	6	20 mg/kg	11	Renal	≥5	
SMX	25 mg/kg	6	100 mg/kg	13	Renal	≥100	
Vancomycin	0.5–1 g	8–12	2 g	6	Renal	20–40	5–10

[a] Half-life in children less than 4 weeks old can be prolonged greatly. Half-life is affected only slightly in renal failure, but it can be greatly prolonged with liver disease.

[b] TMP, Trimethoprim; SMX, sulfamethoxazole. Serum half-life is shortened in adolescents and children. Measurement of either trimethoprim or sulfamethoxazole alone is sufficient for dosage adjustment. Maximum dosages and therapeutic levels apply to treatment of *Pneumocystis carinii* infection.

a hospital laboratory. Pharmacologic studies require sensitive and accurate assays, but rapidity and specificity are less important. The need for specificity, however, is easily underestimated. Not only are unreported antimicrobial agents frequently present (15), but microbiologically active and inactive metabolites may be a concern. For example, the metabolites of sulfonamides and chloramphenicol are inactive; the metabolites of cefotaxime, cephalothin, cephapirin, and rifampin have only a portion of the activity of the parent drugs; and degradation of carbenicillin to benzylpenicillin gives a product with a different spectrum of activity. Accuracy is less important in clinical assays than in pharmacologic studies. Reeves and Wise (17) concluded that for clinical assays of drugs such as aminoglycosides, a 95% confidence limit of ±25 to 30% (a coefficient of variation of about 10 to 15%) was adequate. For drugs with a low potential for toxicity, a 95% confidence limit of ±50% was considered adequate. Comparisons of interlaboratory performance for analyses of mock specimens conducted by the College of American Pathologists and American Association of Clinical Chemistry since 1983 show that these limits are within the capabilities of current assay procedures. The coefficients of variation for immunoassays of aminoglycosides, vancomycin, or chloramphenicol are generally 6 to 10%. Laboratories using liquid chromatographic assays have had slightly larger coefficients of variation for chloramphenicol. Challenges with cephalothin, penicillin G, and piperacillin have revealed coefficients of variation of 20 to 46% for laboratories using bioassays.

Bioassay

Bioassays are based on a comparison of the response of a susceptible organism to an unknown concentration of antibiotic with the response of the same organism, under identical test conditions, to a known concentration of antibiotic. In essence, a bioassay is the converse of a susceptibility test of a standard organism, and the response is usually measured by either a broth dilution or agar diffusion technique. To avoid the inherent inaccuracies of a broth dilution method with serial twofold dilutions, various continuous measures of growth in broth have been used. These methods include turbidimetric assays, potentiometric (14) and titrimetric assays (3), radiometric assays (9), and assays based on measurement of intracellular bacterial ATP concentration (13). Comprehensive reviews of the theory and practice of bioassays have been prepared by Grove and Randall (8), Kavanaugh (10, 11), and Reeves and associates (16). The serum bactericidal titer is of historical interest. It is simply a bioassay that uses serial dilutions of serum and a bactericidal rather than bacteriostatic endpoint. Serum bactericidal titer results can be accurately calculated from the ratio of drug concentration and MIC or MBC of the infecting organism (23).

Because clinical specimens often contain more than one antimicrobial agent, an indicator organism that is multiply resistant should be used whenever practical to improve specificity. Specificity can also be improved by antagonism or inactivation of other antimicrobial agents present or by separation of the antimicrobial agents in a mixture before assay. The most common of these methods are the addition of a β-lactamase to inactivate penicillins and cephalosporins, addition of 50 mg of *p*-aminobenzoic acid and 5 mg of thymidine per liter to antagonize the activity of sulfonamides and trimethoprim, and addition of calcium salts or a cation-exchange resin (22) to antagonize or remove aminoglycoside activity. Before a bioassay is used to measure antimicrobial agents in mixtures, the specific mixtures of interest should be tested to rule out the possibility of synergistic or antagonistic activity. Antineoplastic agents may have antimicrobial activity and should not be neglected as a potential source of interference in bioassays.

Chemical assay

Classical chemical methods are seldom used today for therapeutic monitoring. The principal problems are lack of specificity and lack of versatility of individual procedures. For example, the Bratton-Marshall procedure for sulfonamides is not specific. Similarly, the colorimetric procedure for chloramphenicol, which involves reduction of the nitro group followed by the Bratton-Marshall reaction, responds to several metabolites as well as to the prodrug chloramphenicol succinate. Although relatively specific chemical methods are available for selected antimicrobial agents, e.g., some of the penicillins and cephalosporins, these methods are not practical for most clinical laboratories because these drugs are measured too infrequently to justify the expense of maintaining the variety of reagents that would be needed.

Enzymatic assay

Enzymatic assays have been developed for several antimicrobial agents and can be classified into two types. In one type, the drug being measured is the substrate for an enzyme that is capable of modifying the drug to render it microbiologically inactive. Such enzymes are isolated from resistant bacteria, and enzymes that have found clinical use either acetylate or adenylylate the antimicrobial agent (20, 21). In the usual procedure, the reaction components are adjusted so that the antimicrobial agent is the only limiting factor, and the enzyme cofactor is labeled with a radioisotope that is transferred to the antimicrobial agent. After reaction, the modified antimicrobial agent is separated from unreacted cofactor and quantitated by its radioactivity. A modified acetylation procedure for aminoglycosides avoids the use of radioisotopes. In this procedure, the amount of coenzyme A released from acetyl coenzyme A is measured spectrophotometrically (25). In the other type of enzymatic assay, the antimicrobial agent functions to inhibit enzymatic activity, which is measured by some indicator reaction. This approach has been used to measure β-lactam antibiotics, with the inhibited enzyme being either DD-carboxypeptidase or β-lactamase. In the β-lactamase reaction, a chromogenic cephalosporin is also present (19). Because the β-lactam antibiotic inhibits or competes for the β-lactamase, the rate of color formation is inversely proportional to the concentration of antibiotic. The DD-carboxypeptidase-based method uses a polypeptide substrate with D-alanyl-D-alanine as the carboxy terminus. Cleavage of D-alanine is detected by using D-amino acid oxidase coupled with peroxidase and a chromogenic substrate (5).

Enzymatic assays offer a unique degree of specificity, which is best illustrated by the assays for aminoglycosides and β-lactam antibiotics. In these assays, high specificity is attained for the particular class of antibiotics (e.g., any β-lactam antibiotic) that will function as the enzyme substrate; however, members within a class may not be distinguished.

Immunoassay

Immunoassay kits are available for many of the aminoglycosides (gentamicin, tobramycin, amikacin, netilmicin, kanamycin, sisomicin, and streptomycin), vancomycin, and chloramphenicol. Some of the assays for gentamicin can be extended to netilmicin by using reagents for gentamicin with netilmicin standards. The principal advantages of immunoassays are the availability of kits and automated or semiautomated instruments. The reagents are expensive, and the methods are limited in scope. The manufacturers of some automated instruments have addressed the problem of reagent cost by greatly reducing the frequency with which standards must be measured. With these instruments, a standard curve is determined and used for subsequent analyses as long as control results are within acceptable limits. These methods are described more fully in section II. The primary limitation of immunoassays for antimicrobial agents is the absence of commercial reagents for a large number of drugs, including the β-lactam antibiotics.

Chromatographic assay

Chromatographic assays have been developed for almost all antimicrobial agents and offer a versatility that immunoassays and enzymatic assays lack (6, 18). Chromatographic assays can be highly specific and more economical when applied to small workloads of only a few specimens each day. Automatic injectors and data systems are available, but sample preparation is still largely manual, and vendors have not been active in the production of standardized procedures and kits. With a largely do-it-yourself procedure like chromatography, one problem is the wide variety of methods in use. There are no set criteria by which to evaluate various published methods, and the laboratorian must be acutely aware that many published methods, although adequately documented for some purposes, are often poorly documented for routine clinical specimens. The challenge to using liquid chromatography for antimicrobial assays is to maintain a balance between the need for specificity and the needs for simplicity, speed, and reasonable cost.

The previous edition of this Manual included a lengthy discussion of the principles of liquid chromatography and various alternatives available for sample preparation and analysis of antimicrobial agents. This discussion has been deleted in favor of providing more specific procedures. A general discussion of liquid chromatography is retained in chapter 16. The advantages of liquid chromatography over alternative biologic, immunologic, and chemical methods for antibiotic assays are high specificity and the capability for an analysis of several drugs with only minor modification, if any, in methodology. The principal disadvantages are the lengthy procedures sometimes needed for sample preparation and the fact that samples are processed sequentially through the time-consuming chromatography step. Immunoassay is the method of choice for aminoglycosides because of the large volume of tests usually done. For small numbers of tests and when metabolites may interfere with other methodologies, liquid chromatography is the method of choice.

CHROMATOGRAPHIC ASSAY PROCEDURES FOR SELECTED ANTIMICROBIAL AGENTS

The following methods were developed by using a liquid chromatograph constructed from commercially available components. A diode-array detector is used that provides for both (i) calculation of results on the basis of an internal standard and peak areas and (ii) online analysis of UV spectra as a measure of peak purity. The latter function, while useful during test development, has proved to be relatively unimportant during routine use. Chromatographic interferences so far encountered have been signaled by alterations in peak shape (e.g., changes in symmetry, shoulders, and poor base-line resolution). Any comparable system that allows selection of mobile phases and detection at various wavelengths should suffice. A Spheri-5 RP-18 column (100- by 4.6-mm inner diameter; Brownlee Laboratories, Santa Clara, Calif.) is used for analysis. The short length and 5-μm particle size of this column provide retention times of less than 10 min with adequate resolution. Other reverse-phase columns probably could be used with appropriate adjustments of the mobile phases. A fixed-volume (20 μl) loop injector is used for sample introduction, and the mobile-phase flow rate is 2 ml/min. Each assay consists of calibration with an aqueous standard and analysis of a serum control, followed by patient specimens.

Sample preparation

The primary purpose in sample preparation is to remove protein and other high-molecular-weight materials in serum that can interfere with chromatography.

Ultrafiltration. Mix equal volumes of serum and aqueous internal standard in a small test tube. Add 200 μl of the mixture to an Ultrafree-MC filter unit (Millipore Corp., Bedford, Mass.) and centrifuge the mixture at 1,000 to 2,000 × *g* for 15 min. Analyze the filtrate.

Acetonitrile precipitation of protein and carbon tetrachloride extraction. Mix 200 μl of serum and 100 μl of internal standard in 0.1 M phosphate buffer at pH 7.0. Add 300 μl of acetonitrile. Mix the contents briefly and centrifuge the mixture at 12,000 × *g* for 1 min. Extract the supernatant twice with 1.2 ml of carbon tetrachloride. This step removes most of the acetonitrile from the aqueous phase without extracting drug. Analyze the aqueous (upper) phase.

Acetonitrile precipitation of protein and ethylene dichloride extraction. Mix 400 μl of serum and 400 μl of internal standard in 0.5 M MES buffer at pH 6.0. Add 300 μl of this mixture to 500 μl of acetonitrile. Mix the contents well and centrifuge the mixture for 1 min at 12,000 × *g*. Extract the supernatant with 3.0 ml of ethylene dichloride. Analyze the aqueous (upper) phase.

Ethyl acetate extraction. Mix 20 μl of serum and 20 μl of internal standard in 0.8 M Tris at pH 11. Add 0.5 ml of ethyl acetate. Mix the contents and then centrifuge the mixture to separate the phases. Withdraw the ethyl acetate (upper) phase. Evaporate this phase with a stream of nitrogen at 40°C. Dissolve the residue in the mobile phase and analyze it.

HCl-methanol precipitation of protein. Mix 200 µl of serum and 100 µl of internal standard dissolved in 0.05 M potassium hydroxide. Add 300 µl of an HCl-methanol mixture prepared from 5 ml of concentrated HCl and 15 ml of methanol. Let the mixture stand for 10 min to complete protein precipitation and then centrifuge it at 12,000 × *g* for 2 min. Analyze the liquid phase. The syringe used to inject specimens should be rinsed with the HCl-methanol mixture between injections.

Analytical procedure

Table 2 summarizes the chromatographic conditions and procedures used for various antimicrobial agents. All mobile phases are prepared from analytical-grade reagents, high-performance liquid chromatography-grade solvents, and distilled deionized water. After preparation and adjustment of pH, mobile phases are filtered through a Nylon-66 membrane filter (0.45-µm pore size; Rainin Instrument Co., Inc., Woburn, Mass.) before use. Mobile phases containing methanol are prepared with 0.05 M potassium phosphate buffer at pH 8.0. Mobile phases containing acetonitrile are prepared with 0.05 M potassium phosphate buffer at pH 7.0. Exceptions to these mobile phases are as follows [drug, mobile phase (mixing ratio)]: chloramphenicol, acetonitrile–0.05 M potassium phosphate buffer at pH 6.0 (22:78); ciprofloxacin, methanol–tetrahydrofuran–0.1 M potassium phosphate buffer at pH 2.5 with 0.04% dimethylamine (30:3:67); ganciclovir, methanol–0.05 M potassium phosphate buffer at pH 7.0 with 0.04% dimethylamine (final pH of 7.4) (0.5:99.5); flucytosine, 0.01 M potassium phosphate buffer at pH 7.0; and imipenem, acetonitrile–0.05 M potassium phosphate buffer at pH 6.0 with 0.2 M Na_2SO_4 and 0.6 mM NaN_3 (0.5:99.5). To improve resolution in the ganciclovir assay, two analytical columns are attached in series and the mobile-phase flow rate is reduced to 1.5 ml/min.

REPRESENTATIVE DISK-PLATE BIOASSAY FOR PENICILLIN

Several variations of the disk-plate bioassay exist, but all are characterized by the use of absorbent paper disks

TABLE 2. Assay conditions for selected antimicrobial agents

Antimicrobial agent	Mobile phase[a]		Internal standard	Detection wavelength (nm)	Extraction method[b]
	% ACN	% MeOH			
Amdinocillin	15		Penicillin G	225	PP-CCl_4
Amoxicillin	4		Cephacetril	240	PP-CCl_4
Ampicillin	10		Cephapirin	235	PP-CCl_4
Azlocillin	16		Azlocillin	225	PP-CCl_4
Aztreonam	4		Cephacetril	280	PP-CCl_4
Carbenicillin		9	Cefuroxime	225	PP-CCl_4
Cefaclor	11		Cephapirin	260	PP-CCl_4
Cefadroxil	4		Cephacetril	260	PP-CCl_4
Cefamandole	12		Cephalothin	270	PP-CCl_4
Cefazolin	13		Cephapirin	270	PP-CCl_4
Cefoperazone	15		Cephalothin	270	PP-CCl_4
Cefotaxime	9		Cefazolin	260	PP-CCl_4
Cefotetan	6		Ceftizoxime	290	PP-CCl_4
Cefoxitin	12		Cephaloridine	260	PP-CCl_4
Ceftazidime	4		Cephacetril	260	PP-CCl_4
Ceftizoxime	7		Cephacetril	260	PP-CCl_4
Cetriaxone		12	Cefotaxime	300	PP-CCl_4
Cefuroxime	11		Cefoxitin	260	PP-CCl_4
Cephalexin		27	Cephalothin	260	PP-CCl_4
Cephalothin	18		Piperacillin	260	PP-CCl_4
Cephapirin	13		Cephaloridine	260	PP-CCl_4
Cephradine	11		Cephapirin	260	PP-CCl_4
Cloxacillin	24		Nafcillin	225	PP-CCl_4
Dicloxacillin	27		Nafcillin	225	PP-CCl_4
Imipenem	See text		5-Hydroxytryptophan	300	PP-EC
Methicillin	11		Penicillin G	225	PP-CCl_4
Mezlocillin	22		Oxacillin	225	PP-CCl_4
Nafcillin	27		Dicloxacillin	225	PP-CCl_4
Oxacillin	23		Cloxacillin	225	PP-CCl_4
Penicillin G	20		Piperacillin	225	PP-CCl_4
Penicillin V	21		Mezlocillin	225	PP-CCl_4
Piperacillin	21		Penicillin V	225	PP-CCl_4
Ticarcillin	4		Cephacetril	240	PP-CCl_4
Chloramphenicol	See text		PIV[c]	278	EtOAc
Ciprofloxacin	See text		Oxolinic acid	330	HCl-MeOH
Flucytosine	See text		5-Methylcytosine	276	UF
Ganciclovir	See text		Thymine	265	UF

[a] See text for buffers. ACN, Acetonitrile; MeOH, methanol.
[b] See text for details. PP-CCl_4, Protein precipitation and carbon tetrachloride extraction; PP-EC, protein precipitation and ethylene dichloride extraction; EtOAc, ethyl acetate extraction; HCl-MeOH, HCl-methanol precipitation of protein; UF, ultrafiltration.
[c] PIV, *N*-Pivaloyl-1-*p*-nitrophenyl-2-amino-1,3-propanediol.

to contain specimens and standards. The disks are placed on the surface of agar containing a dispersion of an indicator organism. Antibiotic diffuses from the disks and inhibits growth of the organism. After a suitable incubation period, zones of inhibition around each disk are measured. The inhibition zones produced by known concentrations are plotted against the concentrations to form a standard curve. The drug concentration in the sample corresponding to the zone of inhibition produced is determined from the standard curve.

Preparation of assay plates

Several assay plates may be prepared at a time and stored at 4°C for up to 7 days before use. Each plate consists of a flat-bottom petri dish, 100 by 15 mm (Falcon Optilux), into which a base layer and a layer of agar containing inoculum have been cast. Antibiotic medium no. 5 (Difco Laboratories, Detroit, Mich.), with 10% $CaCl_2$ per liter added and the pH adjusted to 7.0, is used for both layers. The base layer is prepared by adding 9 ml of agar to each dish. The dishes are tilted back and forth to distribute the agar evenly and then placed on a level surface while the agar solidifies. The inoculum is prepared by adding 2 ml of an overnight culture of *Micrococcus luteus* (ATCC 9341) incubated at 30°C in Trypticase soy broth (BBL Microbiology Systems, Cockeysville, Md.) to a bottle containing 100 ml of melted agar maintained at 50°C in a water bath. The temperature of the agar should be measured with an alcohol-flamed thermometer to ensure that it does not exceed 50°C. The inoculum should be carefully mixed by inverting the bottle several times and will contain about 10^7 CFU/ml. The base layer is then overlaid with 4 ml of the seeded agar. The plates are left on a level surface to harden and then stored at 4°C until used.

Assay procedure

Prepare several dilutions of specimen so that the concentration of antimicrobial agent in at least one dilution will be approximately 0.3 µg of penicillin per ml or, for other antimicrobial agents, within the range of the standard curve. Specimen dilutions of 1:4, 1:10, 1:20, and 1:40 will usually suffice. For trough levels, an undiluted specimen is tested; for peak levels, a 1:100 dilution may be necessary. Serum specimens are diluted in sterile human serum that has been shown to lack both antimicrobial and antimicrobial-inactivating activity and to be free of hepatitis B surface antigen. Urine and cerebrospinal fluid are diluted in 0.1 M phosphate buffer, pH 7.0. Standards are prepared in either buffer or serum, as appropriate. Usually, five concentrations containing 0.1, 0.2, 0.3, 0.4, and 0.5 µg of penicillin per ml are prepared. For other antimicrobial agents, the concentrations are adjusted to give appropriate zones of inhibition. Spread 30 blank paper disks (6.35-mm diameter; Schleicher & Schuell, Inc., Keene, N.H.) in a single layer in a petri dish. Pipette 20 µl of the appropriate standards (triplicate sets plus three additional sets at 0.3 µg of penicillin per ml) and test fluid dilutions (triplicate sets) onto separate disks. Apply each disk to the surface of the seeded agar plates, and gently tap the disk with forceps to ensure complete contact with the agar. Do not pipette fluid onto more than six disks before transferring them to the assay plate. All manipulations should be done by sterile technique with sterile equipment. On each of three plates, place disks with each concentration of standard. On each of three additional plates, place disks with each specimen dilution and a disk with the reference concentration of standard (0.3 µg/ml for penicillin). This reference concentration should be chosen as approximately the midpoint of the standard curve. The disks should be evenly spaced and about 2 cm from the center of the plate. Incubate the plates, without stacking, at 30°C for 18 h.

Interpretation and calculations

Measure the diameters of the zones of inhibition for each calibration concentration, reference concentration, and specimen dilution. Calculate the means of the zone diameters for each calibration concentration on the three plates with standards only. Construct a standard curve by plotting the mean zone diameter on the abscissa against logarithms of the concentration on the ordinate. Calculate the means of the zone diameters of the reference concentration and of each specimen dilution. In the mean for the reference concentration, do not include zone diameters from the plates containing standards. Correct the mean zone diameter of each specimen dilution by adding algebraically the difference between the mean zone of the reference concentration on the plates containing specimen and the zone corresponding to the reference concentration as determined from the standard curve. Because the best line for the standard curve usually does not go through each point, the zone corresponding to the reference concentration will be slightly different from the mean zone diameter of the reference concentration. Locate the corrected zone diameter for each specimen dilution on the standard curve and read the corresponding concentration. Multiply this concentration by the dilution factor to determine the antibiotic concentration in the original specimen. Use the result from the specimen dilution that gives a zone diameter nearest the reference zone diameter. Results from other dilutions may be compared with this result to check for consistency and to protect against gross errors, but exact calculations do not need to be made with them. When no dilution falls within the standard curve, the test must be repeated with different specimen dilutions. The standard curve should never be extrapolated to accommodate zones larger or smaller than the largest or smallest zone observed.

Specifications for the bioassay of other antimicrobial agents by this procedure are published elsewhere (1).

LITERATURE CITED

1. **Anhalt, J. F.** 1985. Antimicrobial assays, p. 695–709. *In* J. A. Washington II (ed.), Laboratory procedures in clinical microbiology, 2nd ed. Springer-Verlag, New York.
2. **Bennett, W. M., R. S. Muther, R. A. Parker, P. Feig, G. Morrison, T. A. Golper, and I. Singer.** 1980. Drug therapy in renal failure: dosing guidelines for adults. I. Antimicrobial agents, analgesics. Ann. Intern. Med. **93:**62–89.
3. **Bourne, P. R., I. Phillips, and S. E. Smith.** 1974. Modification of the urease method for gentamicin assays. J. Clin. Pathol. **27:**168–169.
4. **Broughall, J. M., M. J. Bywater, H. A. Holt, and D. S. Reeves.** 1979. Stabilization of cephalosporins in serum and plasma. J. Antimicrob. Chemother. **5:**471–472.
5. **Frère, J.-M., D. Klein, and J.-M. Ghuysen.** 1980. Enzymatic method for rapid and sensitive determination of β-

lactam antibiotics. Antimicrob. Agents Chemother. **18:**506–510.

6. **Gerson, B., and J. P. Anhalt.** 1980. High-pressure liquid chromatography and therapeutic drug monitoring. American Society of Clinical Pathologists, Chicago.
7. **Godley, P. J., J. T. Black, P. A. Frohna, and J. C. Garretts.** 1988. Comparison of a Bayesian program with three microcomputer programs of predicting gentamicin concentrations. Ther. Drug Monit. **10:**287–291.
8. **Grove, D. C., and W. A. Randall.** 1955. Assay methods of antibiotics: a laboratory manual (antibiotics monograph 2). Medical Encyclopedia, New York.
9. **Gunn, B. A., S. L. Brown, C. S. Otey, C. A. Gaydos, J. F. Keiser, F. A. Meeks, and R. G. Trahan.** 1980. Serum gentamicin assay by a radiometric procedure. Am. J. Clin. Pathol. **73:**259–262.
10. **Kavanagh, F. (ed.).** 1963. Analytical microbiology. Academic Press, Inc., New York.
11. **Kavanagh, F. (ed.).** 1972. Analytical microbiology, vol. 2. Academic Press, Inc., New York.
12. **Leslie, J., M. Busby, and E. Khazan.** 1989. Interference from a red top Venojet tube in high-performance liquid chromatographic analyses. Ther. Drug Monit. **11:**724–725.
13. **Nilsson, L., H. Höjer, S. Ansehn, and A. A. Thore.** 1977. A rapid semiautomated bioassay of gentamicin based on luciferase assay of bacterial adenosine triphosphate. Scand. J. Infect. Dis. **9:**232–236.
14. **Noone, P., J. R. Pattison, and D. Samson.** 1971. Simple, rapid method for assay of aminoglycoside antibiotics. Lancet **ii:**16–19.
15. **Reeves, D. S., and H. A. Holt.** 1979. Resolution of antibiotic mixtures in serum samples by high-voltage electrophoresis. J. Clin. Pathol. **28:**435–442.
16. **Reeves, D. S., I. Phillips, J. D. Williams, and R. Wise (ed.).** 1978. Laboratory methods in antimicrobial chemotherapy. Churchill Livingstone, Ltd., Edinburgh.
17. **Reeves, D. S., and R. Wise.** 1978. Antibiotic assays in clinical microbiology, p. 137–143. *In* D. S. Reeves, I. Phillips, J. D. Williams, and R. Wise (ed.), Laboratory methods in antimicrobial chemotherapy. Churchill Livingstone, Ltd., Edinburgh.
18. **Rouan, M. C.** 1985. Antibiotic monitoring in body fluids. J. Chromatogr. **340:**361–400.
19. **Schindler, P., and G. Huber.** 1980. Use of PADAC, a novel chromogenic β-lactamase substrate, for the detection of β-lactamase-producing organisms and assay of β-lactamase inhibitors/inactivators. *In* U. Brodbeck (ed.), Enzyme inhibitors. Verlag Chemie, Weinheim, Federal Republic of Germany.
20. **Shaw, W. V., J. Carter, and J. Sachs.** 1972. Enzymatic assay of gentamicin and kanamycin in body fluids. J. Clin. Res. **20:**83.
21. **Smith, D. H., B. Van Otto, and A. L. Smith.** 1972. A rapid chemical assay for gentamicin. N. Engl. J. Med. **286:**583–586.
22. **Stevens, P., and L. S. Young.** 1977. Simple method for elimination of aminoglycosides from serum to permit bioassay of other antimicrobial agents. Antimicrob. Agents Chemother. **12:**286–287.
23. **Stratton, C. W.** 1987. The role of the microbiology laboratory in the treatment of infective endocarditis. J. Antimicrob. Chemother. **20**(Suppl. A):41–49.
24. **Walters, M. I., and W. H. Roberts.** 1984. Gentamicin/heparin interactions: effects on two immunoassays and on protein binding. Ther. Drug Monit. **6:**199–202.
25. **Williams, J. W., J. S. Langer, and D. B. Northrop.** 1975. A spectrophotometric assay for gentamicin. J. Antibiot. **28:**982–987.

Appendix 1

Preparation and Storage of Antimicrobial Solutions

JOHN P. ANHALT AND JOHN A. WASHINGTON II

Standard or reference preparations of antimicrobial agents should be obtained directly from the manufacturers, from any laboratory supply house that makes available powders specifically for susceptibility tests, or from the U.S. Pharmacopeia Convention, Inc. (12601 Twinbrook Parkway, Rockville, MD 20852). Clinical preparations should not be used because they are less precisely standardized and because some develop full activity only after hydrolysis to the active substance in vivo (e.g., chloramphenicol sodium succinate). Powders must have an actual assayed activity, usually expressed in micrograms or in international units per milligram, and be labeled with an expiration date.

Store the powders according to the directions of the manufacturer. As a class, the aminoglycosides are hygroscopic and should be stored at room temperature in a desiccator. Storage of other antimicrobial agents at room temperature is preferred whenever stability permits. Many antimicrobial agents require refrigerated storage in a desiccator or in sealed ampoules. Be sure to allow the desiccator and contents to equilibrate to room temperature before the desiccator is opened to avoid condensation of water. After the desiccator is opened, the air inside is humid and should be removed by evacuation or allowed to dry over the desiccant at room temperature before the desiccator is replaced in the refrigerator. Routine storage of antimicrobial agents at −20°C is inadvisable and increases the risk of water condensation on the powders. All antimicrobial agents should be protected from direct sunlight. Some (e.g., rifampin and amphotericin B) are very sensitive to light and must be stored in the dark.

TABLE 1. Solvents and diluents for stock solutions of antimicrobial agents[a]

Antimicrobial agent	Solvent	Diluent
Amoxicillin	Phosphate buffer, 0.1 M, pH 6	Water
Amphotericin B	Dimethylformamide	Water
Ampicillin[b]	Phosphate buffer, 0.1 M, pH 8	Phosphate buffer, 0.1 M, pH 6; water
Aztreonam[c]	$NaHCO_3$ in water	Water
Cefotetan	Dimethyl sulfoxide	Water
Ceftazidime	Phosphate buffer, 0.1 M, pH 7	Water
Cephalothin and other cephalosporins[d]	Phosphate buffer, 0.1 M, pH 6	Water
Chloramphenicol	Methanol	Water
Cinoxacin, nalidixic acid, oxolinic acid[e]	NaOH, 0.1 M	Water
Clavulanic acid (potassium salt)	Water	Water
Enoxacin, norfloxacin, ofloxacin[e]	NaOH, 0.1 M	Water
Erythromycin gluceptate[f]	Water	Water
Moxalactam[g]	HCl, 0.04 or 0.08 M	Water
Rifampin	Methanol or dimethyl sulfoxide	Water
Sulbactam (sodium salt)	Water	Water
Sulfonamides[e]	NaOH, 0.1 M	Water
Trimethoprim[h]	HCl, 0.05 M	Water

[a] Water should be used as both solvent and diluent for the following antimicrobial agents: amdinocillin, aminoglycosides (amikacin, gentamicin, kanamycin, neomycin, netilmicin, streptomycin, and tobramycin), azlocillin, bacitracin, carbenicillin, ciprofloxacin, clindamycin, cloxacillin, colistin (polymyxin E), cycloserine, dicloxacillin, doxycycline, ethambutol, flucytosine, imipenem, isoniazid, lincomycin, methicillin, metronidazole, mezlocillin, minocycline, nafcillin, nitrofurantoin (sodium salt), oxacillin, *p*-aminosalicylic acid, penicillin G, piperacillin, polymyxin B or E, spectinomycin, tetracycline, ticarcillin, trimethoprim lactate, and vancomycin.

[b] Dilute with water after first 1:10 dilution with phosphate buffer at pH 6.0.

[c] Use a small amount of 5% $NaHCO_3$ to dissolve and make up to volume with water.

[d] Except as noted, phosphate buffer at pH 6 is used to dissolve cephalosporins. For many cephalosporins (cefamandole, cefazolin, cefmetazole, cefonicid, cefotaxime, cefoxitin, ceftizoxime, ceftriaxone, cefuroxime, cephalexin, and cephradine), water may be used as the solvent. Should cephradine fail to dissolve in water, add a small amount (e.g., 20 μl) of 5 to 10% (wt/vol) $NaHCO_3$ solution.

[e] Use 1.0 ml of 0.1 M NaOH per 10 mg of antimicrobial agent to dissolve these agents. Oxolinic acid will precipitate below pH 7.8.

[f] Erythromycin base is poorly soluble in water. Alcohol can be used, but such solutions are unstable because of ester formation and should be diluted immediately. Solutions in acetone are more stable and can be stored. Water should be used as the diluent.

[g] To prepare a solution containing 1,000 μg/ml, dissolve the diammonium salt at 10,000 μg/ml in 0.04 M HCl. Let the solution stand for 1.5 to 2 h at room temperature to allow *R* and *S* isomers to equilibrate. Dilute the solution with 9 volumes of 0.1 M phosphate buffer at pH 6. To prepare a solution containing 10,000 μg/ml, dissolve the diammonium salt at 20,000 μg/ml in 0.08 M HCl and let the solution stand for 1.5 to 2 h. Dilute to 10,000 μg/ml with 0.1 M phosphate buffer at pH 8. Swirl the solution while adding the buffer to avoid exposing the drug to local, high concentrations of alkaline buffer.

[h] Use 1.0 ml of 0.05 M HCl per 10 mg of trimethoprim to dissolve this agent. Use water to dissolve trimethoprim lactate.

Powders are generally used as received, and special drying procedures are not necessary for the clinical laboratory. Published procedures for drying antimicrobial agents are available (1–3). The recommended procedure for aminoglycosides suggests heating at 60°C for 3 h at a pressure not in excess of 5 mm of Hg (0.67 kPa).

Powders are weighed on an analytical balance and dissolved to yield the required concentration based on labeled activity or potency. One of the following formulas may be used to determine the amount of powder or diluent necessary for a stock solution: weight (in milligrams) = volume (in milliliters) × concentration (in micrograms per milliliter)/potency (in micrograms per milligram) or volume (in milliliters) = weight (in milligrams) × potency (in micrograms per milligram)/concentration (in micrograms per milliliter).

In most cases, it is advisable to weigh a portion of antimicrobial agent roughly in excess of that needed and to calculate the volume of solvent required. This procedure avoids multiple adjustments of the powder during weighing and minimizes time and exposure to atmospheric moisture. The alternative of weighing a predetermined amount of powder is advisable when an organic solvent is used to dissolve the antimicrobial agent, and the solution is diluted to a fixed volume in a volumetric flask.

Solvents and diluents for common antimicrobial agents are listed in Table 1. These recommendations are based on an effort to use a minimal number of solvents or buffers and may not give optimal stability. Solvents are used to dissolve dry powder to give stock solutions containing high concentrations (i.e., greater than 1,000 μg/ml) of antimicrobial agent. Diluents are used to prepare working dilutions from stock solutions. In general, ethanol can be substituted for methanol, dimethyl sulfoxide can be substituted for dimethylformamide, and phosphate buffer (0.1 M, pH 6) can be used instead of water to dissolve β-lactam antibiotics (water should be used as the diluent). Some antimicrobial agents, such as imipenem or penicillins, are less stable in phosphate buffer than in water. Use of a nonnucleophilic buffer instead of phosphate buffer may improve stability. Common buffers of this type are based on 3-(*N*-morpholino)propanesulfonic acid (MOPS) or 2-(*N*-morpholino)ethanesulfonic acid (MES).

Stock solutions containing high concentrations of antimicrobial agents do not usually need to be sterilized; however, sterile water or buffers should be used in their preparation. Should it be necessary to sterilize a solution of antimicrobial agent, membrane filtration should be used to minimize loss due to adsorption. Rifampin and amphotericin B solution should not be filtered. Antimicrobial agents can also adsorb to the walls of glass vessels, and polypropylene or polyethylene vials and laboratory ware are recommended for the preparation and storage of solutions containing low concentrations. Adsorption to surfaces is decreased in the presence of protein or broth media.

The stability of antimicrobial solutions varies greatly, and data regarding maximum storage times at −20 or −60°C are generally lacking. Stock solutions of most antimicrobial agents will remain stable for at least 6 months at −20°C and longer at −60°C in concentrations of 1,000 μg/ml or greater. Ampicillin and amoxicillin are unstable, particularly in concentrations greater than 1000 μg/ml, and should be stored for no longer than 6 weeks at −20°C or 6 months at −60°C. Cephaloglycin, cefaclor, clavulanic acid, imipenem, and rifampin are even less stable and should be freshly prepared with each use. Antimicrobial agents are often more unstable in serum than in buffer. The β-lactam antibiotics should not be stored in serum even in the frozen state.

LITERATURE CITED

1. **Code of Federal Regulations.** 1979. Title 21, parts 300 to 499. U.S. Government Printing Office, Washington, D.C.
2. **Kavanagh, F. (ed.).** 1963. Analytical microbiology. Academic Press, Inc., New York.
3. **Kavanagh, F. (ed.).** 1972. Analytical microbiology, vol. 2. Academic Press, Inc., New York.

Appendix 2

Approximate Concentrations of Antimicrobial Agents Achieved in Blood

ROBERT C. MOELLERING, JR., JOSEPH D. C. YAO, AND CLYDE THORNSBERRY

The concentrations of antimicrobial agents listed below are approximations taken from various reports. Several factors can influence the level of antimicrobial agent achieved in individual patients, including inherent differences in the patients themselves, their physical condition, the dosages, and the routes of administration. The values can also be influenced by the assay methods used to obtain them. Therefore, these concentrations should be used only as approximate values, and clinicians should use their knowledge of the patient and the drugs, the recommendations from Food and Drug Administration-approved inserts, or other reputable sources in planning their therapeutic regimens.

Antimicrobial agent	Unit dose	Avg peak blood level (μg/ml)[a]		
		p.o.	i.m.	i.v.
Amdinocillin	700 mg		26	28
Amikacin	7.5 mg/kg		30	30
Amphotericin B	0.37 mg/kg			1–4
Amoxicillin	500 mg	8		
Amoxicillin-clavulanate	(See amoxicillin)			
Ampicillin	500 mg	4		17
Ampicillin-sulbactam	(See ampicillin)			
Azlocillin	2 g			250
Aztreonam	1 g		65–85	150
Carbenicillin	4 g			150
Cefaclor	500 mg	12		
Cefadroxil	500 mg	16		
Cefamandole	0.5–1 g		28	60
Cefazolin	1–2 g		64	121
Cefixime	400 mg	3.7		
Cefmenoxime	1 g			42
Cefmetazole	1 g			73
Cefonicid	1 g		83	
Cefoperazone	1–2 g		65	150
Ceforanide	1–2 g		72	136
Cefotaxime	1 g		18–23	47–70
Cefotetan	1 g		50	100
Cefotiam	1 g			50
Cefoxitin	1 g		35	70
Cefsulodin	1 g		20	
Ceftazidime	1 g		20	80
Ceftizoxime	1 g		30	60
Ceftriaxone	1 g		60	150
Cefuroxime	1 g		40	43–98
Cefuroxime-axetil	500 mg	7		
Cephalexin	500 mg	18–25		
Cephalothin	1 g			70
Cephapirin	1 g			37
Cephradine	0.5–1 g	16	12	26
Chloramphenicol	1 g	8–14		8–14
Cinoxacin	250 mg	8		

(*Continued on next page*)

Continued

Antimicrobial agent	Unit dose	Avg peak blood level (μg/ml)[a]		
		p.o.	i.m.	i.v.
Ciprofloxacin	500 mg	2		
Clindamycin	150–600 mg	2.5	5	12
Cloxacillin	500 mg	2.5	3–15	
Cycloserine	0.5–1 g	15–25		
Dicloxacillin	250–500 mg	4	12–20	
Doxycycline	100 mg	3		
Enoxacin	500 mg	2.5		
Erythromycin	500 mg	0.5–1.7		8
Fluconazole	200 mg	10		
Flucytosine	2.5 g	78		
Gentamicin	1.3 mg/kg		5–7	5–7
Imipenem	500 mg			21–58
Isoniazid	10 mg/kg	1–5		
Kanamycin	500 mg		15	15–20
Ketoconazole	200 mg	3.5		
Methicillin	500 mg			16
Metronidazole	500 mg	11		21
Mezlocillin	2 g			166–255
Miconazole	200–400 mg			1–4
Minocycline	200 mg	3		
Moxalactam (latamoxef)	1 g		35–59	76
Nafcillin	0.5–1 g	5		10
Nalidixic acid	1 g	30		
Netilmicin	1.3 mg/kg		8	
Nitrofurantoin	300 mg	1.8		
Norfloxacin	400 mg	0.5–1.5		
Ofloxacin	500 mg	8.5		
Oxacillin	500 mg	5	10	
Penicillin G (benzathine)	1.2×10^6 U		0.1	
Penicillin G (procaine)	0.6×10^6 U		1	
Penicillin G	500 mg			16
Penicillin V	500 mg	4		
Piperacillin	2 g			200
Rifampin	8 mg/kg	10		
Spectinomycin	2 g		30–50	
Streptomycin	1 g		25–50	
Sulfamethoxazole	1 g	92		
Sulfisoxazole	2 g	110		
Tetracycline	250 mg	3		
Ticarcillin	3 g			250
Ticarcillin-clavulanate	(See ticarcillin)			
Tobramycin	1–2 mg/kg		4–8	4–8
Trimethoprim	100 mg	1		
Trimethoprim-sulfamethoxazole	80/400–160/800 mg	1/20		3.4/46
Vancomycin	0.5–1 g			20–40

[a] p.o., Oral; i.m., intramuscular; i.v., intravenous.

Chapter 120

Quality Control of Media, Reagents, and Stains

J. MICHAEL MILLER

Even amid rapidly advancing technology, clinical microbiology remains a science of interpretive judgment. Ensuring the accuracy, significance, and clinical relevance of diagnostic testing in microbiology is of prime importance in patient care. Therefore, laboratorians must rely on the quality of performance of the media, reagents, and stains used in the laboratory analysis of clinical specimens and significant isolates. Although the analytical component is only a part of the total laboratory testing process for clinical specimens, its role in patient care is clear. Therefore, analytical accuracy must be ensured by an ongoing process of quality assessment.

The proposed regulations implementing the Clinical Laboratory Improvement Amendments of 1988 (CLIA '88; *Federal Register,* May 21, 1990) clearly specify the role of quality control as part of a total program ensuring laboratory quality. The basic regulations and frequencies of quality checks of media, reagents, and stains are somewhat expanded but similar to those of CLIA '67. Regardless of whether a laboratory qualifies under CLIA '88 as a level 1 or level 2 testing facility, quality control must be done. CLIA '88 reemphasizes the need for the laboratory to document all quality control activities and to retain records for at least 2 years. Each step in the processing and testing of quality control samples should be recorded to ensure that these samples are tested in the same manner as are patient specimens.

The controls for media, reagents, and tests commonly used in bacteriology, mycobacteriology, and mycology are outlined in Tables 2 to 6. Although parasitology laboratories may not require media similar to those described here, laboratories offering parasitological services must have a reference collection of slides, photographs, or previously characterized and preserved specimens. In addition, such laboratories must use a calibrated ocular micrometer for determining the sizes of ova and parasites if size is a critical parameter. Permanent stains should be checked monthly by using a fecal sample control, but many laboratories use more frequent checks. An excellent discussion on parasitology quality control procedures is available (1) to supplement the information provided in this Manual.

Virology testing is also addressed briefly by CLIA '88. In addition to ensuring that host systems are available for viral isolation and test methods for virus identification, laboratories must maintain records that reflect the systems used and the reactions observed. For identification tests, laboratories must use uninoculated cells or cell substrate controls to detect errors in testing. Virology quality control programs may be more expensive (6) than those used in bacteriology.

The standards from CLIA '88 are the minimum criteria by which laboratories can be evaluated for Medicare certification. If states or other certifying agencies have stricter standards, the laboratory must meet the higher standards imposed in order to be certified by the state or certifying agency.

BACTERIOLOGY MEDIA

Quality assurance criteria

Because of years of experience with hundreds of lot numbers of commonly used plating media, the National Committee for Clinical Laboratory Standards (NCCLS) published Document M22-T, Quality Assurance for Commercially Prepared Microbiological Culture Media. As of this writing, M22-A, the approved standard, is in press. While both documents address manufacturer quality assurance practices, they also document a series of commercially prepared media for which quality control checks need not be done by the purchasing laboratory (Table 1). For these media, each laboratory must have manufacturer-supplied documentation indicating that the purchased lot of medium conforms to the NCCLS quality assurance protocol. The statement may be in the form of a package insert or attached to the packaging. The laboratory is responsible for obtaining and maintaining this statement in its quality control records.

The controls suggested in the tables that follow are to be used on all other commercially purchased media and on all media prepared and used in-house. If the laboratory makes media that will also be shipped to satellite laboratories, the receiving laboratory must follow the guidelines in these tables unless the laboratory preparing the media has used the NCCLS-recommended quality control for manufacturers of commercial media and has included a statement in the package that the lot of medium has met the quality control standards of the NCCLS.

Performance evaluation procedures for bacteriologic media are available from a number of sources (2–5, 8). Tables 2 to 4 list some of the media frequently used in aerobic and anaerobic bacteriology, along with organisms recommended for use in the quality control of these media. Other organisms that produce comparable reactions may be used. Each batch of medium, solid or fluid, prepared in the laboratory and all commercial media not listed in Table 1 should be tested in the laboratory where the media are used. The following checks are suggested.

1. Sterility. Each batch of medium that is autoclaved or filtered during preparation should be checked

TABLE 1. Commercially purchased media not requiring routine quality control checks in the laboratory

Blood agar (sheep and anaerobic)	Mannitol salt agar
Blood culture bottles	Middlebrook media
Brain heart infusion media	Mycology agar (selective primary nutrient media with cycloheximide and chloramphenicol, excluding inhibitory mold agar)
Cefsulodin-irgasan-novobiocin agar	Phenylethyl alcohol agar
Charcoal-yeast extract/ buffered charcoal-yeast extract agar	Sabouraud dextrose agar
Columbia CNA agar	*Salmonella-shigella* agar
Cystine lactose electrolyte-deficient agar	Selective media for group D streptococci
Eosin-methylene blue agar	Selenite broth
GN broth	Trypticase soy media
Hektoen enteric agar	Xylose-lysine-desoxycholate agar
Lowenstein-Jensen medium	
MacConkey agar	

for sterility; a sample of the batch is sufficient for this check.

2. Ability to support growth.
3. Selective or inhibitory growth characteristics. Growth characteristics should be checked by inoculation with at least one organism to confirm selectivity and with at least one organism to confirm inhibitory characteristics.
4. Biochemical response. At least one organism that will produce the expected reaction (positive control) and at least one organism that will not produce a positive reaction (negative control) should be used to check biochemical response.

Generally, two organisms will suffice to check the growth characteristics, selective or inhibitory characteristics, and biochemical response. Occasionally, a third organism may be required to confirm all of the reactions. If the batch or lot is not used within 30 days, another check is recommended.

For novel or one-purpose bacteriologic media described throughout this Manual, controls must be included to document appropriate reactions in the four categories listed above.

In the final analysis, any quality control program for culture media must ensure that a medium will support the growth of the organisms likely to be in the specimen. It must, if specified, inhibit the growth of commensal organisms, exhibit a typical biochemical response, be stable, and have a reasonable shelf life.

Sterility. A few media are used without terminal sterilization, but they are the exceptions; most media must be sterile when they are inoculated. Each batch of medium, whether prepared in the laboratory or received from a commercial source, should be sampled for sterility. This is best done by removing 1 unit from a small batch or 3 units from a batch of 100 and incubating them at 35°C for 24 h. For blood-containing media, after incubation overnight at 35°C, the control units should be held at room temperature for an additional 24 h. If contaminants appear in the medium as a result of inadequate sterilization, a new lot should be obtained. Those units that are used for sterility testing should be discarded at the completion of the test, since they are unsuitable for inoculation because of the dehydration that occurs after 48 h.

Growth. The ability of the medium to support the growth of suspected organisms should be determined by inoculating the medium with a typical stock culture isolate. A frequent quality control error is the use of too heavy an inoculum for this purpose. When testing for ability to support growth, prepare a dilute suspension to use as the inoculum. This suspension will give greater assurance that the medium is adequate for the growth of a small number of organisms in a patient specimen. In choosing an organism for testing, one should select from among the more fastidious species of organisms being sought in specimens received from patients. To prepare a standard inoculum, make a 1:10 dilution in broth of a test suspension of organisms equivalent in turbidity to a McFarland 0.5 standard; use a 0.001-ml calibrated loop to inoculate plates to be tested and then streak for isolation (3).

Inhibition. Since selective media are designed not only to support the growth of some organisms but also to inhibit the growth of others, the medium must be inoculated with representatives of both groups of organisms. To demonstrate the inhibitory effect, one can challenge the medium with a heavy inoculum, since the medium will inhibit the relatively small number of organisms present in the primary specimen if it will prevent the growth of a large inoculum. The medium must also support the growth of the selected organism.

Biochemical response. When one is inoculating media used to identify a specific reaction, such as fermentation or H_2S production, it is necessary to use only a species or strain of organism that will produce the desired reaction.

There are several sources of cultures that can be used for quality control. The American Type Culture Collection (ATCC) can provide representative strains of essentially any microorganism that the clinical laboratory may want to use for a quality control test. Organisms are also available from several commercial sources. Many laboratories participate in proficiency testing programs. Cultures distributed by these agencies can be saved and used for quality control testing. Finally, wild strains isolated in the laboratory may be saved and used for quality control if they are properly characterized and reactions are well verified. The test organisms should be checked for purity on agar plates. Incubation should be under the conditions used for the incubation of patient materials. In certain instances, such as the use of primary isolation media for *Mycobacterium tuberculosis*, it may be necessary to conduct quality control testing simultaneously with culture because of the slow growth of the organisms. When batches of media have been proven to support the growth of organisms and provide the essential growth characteristics, the batches of media can be released for use.

Laboratories that prepare their own media must develop a means of labeling and recording batch or lot numbers, dates of preparation, dates placed into use, and expiration dates of all media. Containers of dehydrated media used to prepare in-house products should be labeled with the date first opened.

Although expiration dates of commercial media usually appear on each plate or tube, in-house products often lack the same necessary outdating. Generally, tubes with tightened caps and plating media that are

TABLE 2. Media for aerobic bacteriology

Medium	Quality control procedures				Organism(s)	Expected reaction(s)[a]	Comment
	Sterility	Growth	Inhibition	Biochemical response			
Arginine dihydrolase	x			x	*Salmonella typhimurium*	Positive = red-violet or purple within 24 h	Liquid medium must be overlaid with mineral oil or petrolatum.
					Proteus vulgaris	Negative = yellow	
Azide blood agar	x	x	x		*Streptococcus pyogenes*	Small colony with beta-hemolysis within 24 h	Azide is added to medium to inhibit gram-negative organisms and allow gram-positive organisms (streptococci) to grow. Principle also applies to blood agar with trimethoprim-sulfamethoxazole, neomycin, etc.
					Escherichia coli	Growth inhibited	
Bile-esculin agar	x			x	*Enterococcus faecalis* (group D)	Growth—black-colored medium within 48 h	Used for presumptive identification of group D streptococci. Enterococci also may be identified by their growth in NaCl medium.
					Streptococcus pyogenes	Medium not blackened	
Bismuth sulfite agar			x	x	*Salmonella typhimurium* (some strains inhibited)	Growth—colonies black with metallic, silver sheen in 48 h	Medium used to isolate *Salmonella* spp., including *S. typhi*, from fecal specimens. Inhibits other organisms. Use on day of preparation. Should be gray color, not green, when fresh.
					Escherichia coli	No growth or inhibited growth; colorless to pale green colonies in 48 h	
Blood agar	x	x			Group A, beta-hemolytic streptococci	Small, clear colonies exhibiting beta (complete)-hemolysis in 48 h	Blood agar should allow these typical isolates to exhibit characteristic hemolysis. The CAMP test can be performed to ensure proper sheep cell activity.
					Streptococcus viridans or *Streptococcus pneumoniae*	Small to medium colonies exhibiting alpha (green)-hemolysis	
Blood culture medium	x	x			*Bacteroides fragilis*	Growth in 24 h	Use a small inoculum (100–1,000 CFU/ml).
					Streptococcus pneumoniae	Growth in 24 h	Bottles with antibiotic removal capability should be handled similarly. Use only unvented bottles to test.
					Gram stain or acridine orange	No organisms seen on centrifuged specimen	

(*Continued on next page*)

TABLE 2—*Continued*

Medium	Quality control procedures				Organism(s)	Expected reaction(s)[a]	Comment
	Sterility	Growth	Inhibition	Biochemical response			
Brain heart infusion agar or broth	x	x			*Staphylococcus aureus*	Growth in 24 h	Highly nutritious medium for support of bacterial growth.
Brilliant green agar	x		x	x	*Salmonella typhimurium*	Red or pink colonies in 48 h	Selective for *Salmonella* spp. other than *S. typhi*. Sulfadiazine may be added to inhibit *Pseudomonas* spp.
					Possible: *Escherichia coli* or *Klebsiella* and *Enterobacter* spp.	Yellow or yellow-green colonies with yellow-green halo in agar in 48 h	
					Shigella spp.	Growth inhibited	
Campylobacter medium	x	x	x		*Campylobacter jejuni*	Growth in 48 h	Optimal at 42°C and 10% CO_2–5% O_2.
					Escherichia coli	Growth inhibited in 48 h	
Chocolate agar	x	x			*Haemophilus influenzae*	Growth in 24 h	Should support growth of fastidious pathogens.
Desoxycholate agar			x	x	*Escherichia coli*	Red colonies in 24 h	Differentiation medium for the demonstration of lactose fermentation by gram-negative rods. H_2S indicator is not present in the medium.
					Proteus mirabilis	Colorless colonies in 24 h	
					Streptococcus spp.	Growth inhibited	
DNase test agar	x			x	*Staphylococcus aureus* or *Serratia marcescens*	Clear zone around 24-h colony (in acid reaction with HCl) or pink zone (toluidine blue-containing media)	Plates may be spot inoculated rather than streaked for isolation.
					Streptococcus faecalis	No zone around colonies	
Eosin-methylene blue	x		x	x	*Escherichia coli*	Colonies blue-purple, usually with green, metallic sheen, in 24 h	Differential medium for the demonstration of lactose fermentation by gram-negative rods. Other lactose fermenters may produce green sheen. H_2S indicator is not present in the medium.
					Shigella sonnei	Colorless colonies in 24 h	
					Staphylococcus aureus	Growth inhibited	

Glucose utilization oxidative-fermentative medium	x			x	*Pseudomonas aeruginosa* (oxidizer)	Overlaid tube—no color change; open tube—yellow (acid) at surface	*E. coli* (a fermenter) should cause both tubes to turn yellow (acid).
					Acinetobacter lwoffi (nonutilizer)	Overlaid tube—no change; open tube—no change	
GN broth	x	x	x		*Shigella sonnei*	Growth in 8–24 h when subcultured to EMB, MAC, XLD, or HE agar	This medium was designed for subculture after 6 h of incubation.
					Escherichia coli	Growth inhibited for up to 6–8 h; light growth on subculture	
Heart infusion agar	x	x			*Streptococcus* spp.	Growth in 24 h	
Hektoen agar	x		x	x	*Escherichia coli*	Orange colonies (may be inhibited) in 24 h	Black center indicates H_2S production. *Shigella sonnei* should exhibit green, transparent colonies.
					Salmonella typhimurium	Green colonies with black centers in 24 h	
					Streptococcus spp.	Growth inhibited	
Indole (peptone water)	x			x	*Escherichia coli*	Positive in 24 h = red ring	Add a few drops of Kovacs reagent to broth and shake tube gently.
					Enterobacter aerogenes	Negative = yellow ring	
Kligler iron agar	x			x	*Escherichia coli*	Acid slant/acid butt with gas; no H_2S in 18–24 h	Both lactose and glucose are fermented.
					Proteus mirabilis	Alkaline slant/acid butt; gas and H_2S in 18–24 h	Glucose but not lactose is fermented.
					Pseudomonas aeruginosa	Alkaline slant/alkaline butt; no gas or H_2S in 18–24 h	Neither glucose nor lactose is fermented.
Lysine decarboxylase agar or broth	x			x	*Klebsiella pneumoniae*	Positive in 24 h = red-violet to purple	Liquid medium is overlaid with mineral oil or petrolatum.
					Proteus mirabilis	Negative = yellow	

(*Continued on next page*)

TABLE 2—*Continued*

Medium	Quality control procedures: Sterility	Growth	Inhibition	Biochemical response	Organism(s)	Expected reaction(s)[a]	Comment
Lysine iron agar	x			x	*Enterobacter aerogenes*	Positive in 18–24 h = alkaline slant and butt (purple)	Decarboxylase activity is read in the butt of the tube: positive = purple; negative = yellow.
					Providencia stuartii	Negative = red slant (deamination) and yellow butt; H_2S negative	
MacConkey agar	x		x	x	*Escherichia coli*	Pink colonies (lactose fermenter) in 24 h	Differential medium for the demonstration of lactose fermentation by gram-negative rods. H_2S indicator is not present in medium.
					Proteus mirabilis	Colorless colonies (nonlactose fermenter) in 24 h	
					Streptococcus spp.	Growth inhibited	
Malonate broth	x			x	*Klebsiella pneumoniae*	Positive in 24 h = blue	Used also to separate *Salmonella arizonae* (positive) from other *Salmonella* spp.
					Escherichia coli	Negative = green (no color change)	
Mannitol salt agar	x		x	x	*Staphylococcus aureus*	Growth, yellow colonies (acid) in 24 h	Mannitol fermentation alone is NOT used for the presumptive identification of *S. aureus* or *S. epidermidis*.
					Staphylococcus epidermidis	Growth, no color change in 24 h	
					Escherichia coli	Growth inhibited	
Motility medium	x	x			*Escherichia coli*	Motile—medium becomes cloudy and stab line disappears in 24 h (no color involved)	Motility medium also may be prepared with triphenyl tetrazolium-chloride, which turns red where organisms grow.
					Klebsiella pneumoniae	Nonmotile—growth only at stab line (no color involved)	
Motility-indole-ornithine medium	x	x		x	*Escherichia coli*	Motility—positive Indole—positive Ornithine—positive in 24 h	Motility—cloudy medium. Indole—after addition of Kovacs reagent: positive = red ring; negative = yellow ring. Ornithine: positive = purple; negative = yellow.
					Klebsiella pneumoniae	Motility—negative Indole—negative Ornithine—negative in 24 h	

Nutrient agar or broth	x	x			*Staphylococcus aureus*	Growth in 18–24 h	
Ornithine decarboxylase	x			x	*Escherichia coli*	Positive in 24 h = purple broth	Liquid medium must be overlaid with mineral oil or petrolatum.
					Proteus vulgaris	Negative = yellow broth	
Pfizer selective enterococcus agar	x		x	x	*Enterococcus faecalis*	Growth, black colonies in 24 h	
					Escherichia coli	Growth inhibited or light growth, clear colonies	
Phenylalanine deaminase agar	x			x	*Proteus vulgaris*	Positive in 24 h = green slant after adding reagent	Add 2–3 drops of 10% $FeCl_3$ to growth on the slant.
					Escherichia coli	Negative = no color change after adding reagent	
Phenylethyl alcohol (PEA) agar	x	x	x		*Staphylococcus aureus* or *Streptococcus* spp.	Growth in 24 h	Used especially for specimens likely to be contaminated with aerobic gram-negative organisms, particularly swarming *Proteus* spp.
					Escherichia coli or *Proteus vulgaris*	Growth inhibited or little growth	
Salmonella-shigella agar			x	x	*Enterobacter aerogenes*	Pink to red colonies in 24 h	Not recommended for *Shigella sonnei* (does not grow well on this agar). Lactose is used as a differential sugar.
					Escherichia coli	Little or no growth in 24 h	
					Salmonella typhimurium	Colorless colonies with black centers in 24 h	
Selenite F broth		x	x		*Salmonella typhimurium*	Growth when subcultured to MAC, EMB, XLD, HE, or SS in 8–24 h	Should be a straw color with no orange precipitate. Overheating causes precipitate. Cystine-selenite medium is acceptable for stools but not for isolation of *S. typhi*.
					Escherichia coli	Light growth when subcultured	
Simmons citrate	x	x		x	*Enterobacter aerogenes*	Positive = growth, slant turns blue in 24 h	
					Escherichia coli	Negative = no growth, no color change (green)	

(*Continued on next page*)

TABLE 2—*Continued*

Medium	Quality control procedures				Organism(s)	Expected reaction(s)[a]	Comment
	Sterility	Growth	Inhibition	Biochemical response			
Sodium azide agar	x	x	x		Staphylococcus aureus or *Streptococcus* spp.	Growth in 24 h	Inhibits gram-negative organisms.
					Escherichia coli	Growth inhibited	
Streptococcus faecalis broth or 6.5% NaCl	x	x	x	x	*Enterococcus faecalis*	Growth and/or color change to yellow in 48 h	Growth (cloudy) without color change is considered positive.
					Streptococcus spp. (not *Enterococcus*)	Growth inhibited	
Sulfide-indole motility medium	x			x	*Proteus vulgaris*	H_2S positive (black color); indole positive (add Kovac reagents); motility—cloudy medium in 24 h	
					Klebsiella pneumoniae	H_2S negative; indole negative; nonmotile in 24 h	
Tetrathionate broth		x	x		*Salmonella typhimurium*	Growth in 18 h when subcultured to MAC, EMB, XLD, HE, or SS	
					Escherichia coli	Light growth when subcultured	
Thayer-Martin agar	x	x	x		*Neisseria gonorrhoeae*	Growth in 24 h	Same organisms used for modified Thayer-Martin, Martin-Lewis, etc. Use fresh strains of gonococci since some laboratory-adapted strains may be less fastidious.
					Escherichia coli	No growth in 24 h	

Thioglycolate broth	x	x			*Bacteroides* spp. (if anaerobes are cultured)	Growth in 24 h—culture in anaerobic atmosphere	Thioglycolate should be carefully inoculated at the bottom of the tube.
					Staphylococcus aureus	Growth in 24 h—aerobic incubation	
Transgrow	x	x	x		*Neisseria gonorrhoeae*	Growth in 24 h	If bottle is tilted during inoculation, the CO_2 atmosphere may be lost.
					Escherichia coli	No growth	
Transport media							Need not be tested routinely.
Triple sugar iron agar	x			x	*Escherichia coli*	Acid slant, acid butt, gas, no H_2S in 18–24 h	Glucose, lactose, and/or sucrose fermented.
					Proteus mirabilis	Alkaline slant, acid butt, gas, H_2S in 18–24 h	Only glucose fermented.
					Pseudomonas aeruginosa	Alkaline slant, alkaline butt, no gas, no H_2S in 18–24 h	Nonfermenter.
Trypticase soy broth	x	x			*Streptococcus pyogenes*	Growth in 24 h	
Tryptic soy agar	x	x			*Streptococcus pyogenes*	Growth in 24 h	
Urea agar or broth	x			x	*Proteus vulgaris*	Positive in 4–18 h = pink	Pink color should appear within 4–6 h.
					Escherichia coli	Negative = yellow or no change	
Vogues-Proskauer	x			x	*Enterobacter aerogenes*	Positive in 48 h = pink color after reagents	Broth is methyl red–Voges-Proskauer. Reagent VP-A is α-naphthol. VP-B is 40% KOH (creatinine).
					Escherichia coli	Negative = yellow	
Xylose-lysine-desoxycholate agar			x	x	*Escherichia coli*	Yellow colonies in 24 h	(see below)
					Salmonella typhimurium	Pink-red colonies, black center in 24 h	
					Shigella sonnei	Transparent colonies in 24 h	
					Streptococcus spp.	Growth inhibited	

Xylose-lysine-desoxycholate agar, comments:

	E. coli	*Salmonella*	*Shigella*
Xyl	+	+	−
Lac	+	−	−
Suc	+	−	−
Lys	+ or −	+	−

[a] Abbreviations: EMB, eosin-methylene blue; MAC, MacConkey agar; XLD, xylosine-lysine-desoxycholate agar; HE, Hektoen enteric agar; SS, salmonella-shigella agar.

TABLE 3. Media for anaerobic bacteriology

Medium	Quality control procedures				Organism(s)	Expected reaction(s)	Comment
	Sterility	Growth	Inhibition	Biochemical response			
Anaerobic transport system	x	x			*Fusobacterium nucleatum*	Recovery of small inoculum when plated on isolation medium	Hold organism in transport system for 2 h at room temperature.
Anerobe blood agar (sheep blood)	x	x			*Fusobacterium necrophorum* *Clostridium perfringens*	Growth Growth; double zone of hemolysis	*F. necrophorum* will grow if cystine is in the medium. Beta-hemolysis on rabbit blood.
Enriched carbohydrate fermentation base medium (bromthymol blue indicator)	x	x		x	*Bacteroides vulgatus* *Clostridium subterminale*	Growth in 48 h No color change	Base without carbohydrate inoculated as a growth control. No color change expected. pH 7.0 = blue-green; pH 6.0 = yellow.
Arabinose (0.6%)	x			x	*Bacteroides vulgatus* *Clostridium subterminale*	Positive = yellow in 48 h Negative = blue-green	Other pH indicators may give alternative color patterns for positive and negative reactions.
Dextrose (glucose) (0.6%)	x			x	*Bacteroides vulgatus* *Clostridium subterminale*	Positive = yellow in 48 h Negative = blue-green	
Glycerol (0.6%)	x			x	*Propionibacterium acnes* *Clostridium subterminale*	Positive = yellow in 48 h Negative = blue-green	
Lactose (0.6%)	x			x	*Bacteroides vulgatus* *Clostridium subterminale*	Positive = yellow in 48 h Negative = blue-green	
Maltose (0.6%)	x			x	*Bacteroides vulgatus* *Clostridium subterminale*	Positive = yellow in 48 h Negative = blue-green	
Mannitol (0.6%)	x			x	*Propionibacterium acnes* *Clostridium subterminale*	Positive = yellow in 48 h Negative = blue-green	
Mannose (0.6%)	x			x	*Bacteroides vulgatus* *Clostridium subterminale*	Positive = yellow in 48 h Negative = blue-green	
Rhamnose (0.6%)	x			x	*Bacteroides vulgatus* *Clostridium subterminale*	Positive = yellow in 48 h Negative = blue-green	
Salicin (0.6%)	x			x	*Clostridium tertium* *Clostridium subterminale*	Positive = yellow in 48 h Negative = blue-green	
Sucrose (0.6%)	x			x	*Bacteroides vulgatus* *Clostridium subterminale*	Positive = yellow in 48 h Negative = blue-green	
Trehalose (0.6%)	x			x	*Clostridium tertium* *Clostridium subterminale*	Positive = yellow in 48 h Negative = blue-green	
Xylose (0.6%)	x			x	*Bacteroides vulgatus* *Clostridium subterminale*	Positive = yellow in 48 h Negative = blue-green	

Chopped meat broth	x	x			*Clostridium sporogenes* and *Fusobacterium necrophorum*	Good growth in 24 h from a small inoculum (0.01 ml of a 24–48-h Lombard-Dowell broth culture diluted to 10^{-3})	Proteolysis occurs with *C. sporogenes*. Useful as a holding medium, for sporulation of *Clostridium* spp., and for toxin production of some clostridia.
Chopped meat glucose broth	x	x			*Clostridium sporogenes*	Growth with sporulation	Excellent for holding cultures and for toxin studies.
					Fusobacterium necrophorum	Growth	
					Clostridium perfringens type A	Growth and toxin production	
Columbia colistin-nalidixic acid-blood agar	x	x	x		*Clostridium perfringens*	Growth	Inhibits facultative gram-negative bacteria.
					Bacteroides fragilis		
					Escherichia coli	No growth	
Egg yolk agar (modified McClung-Toabe or Lombard-Dowell)	x	x		x		Lecithinase / Lipase / Proteolysis	Read up to 48 h. Most strains of *C. sporogenes* are lecithinase negative.
					Clostridium perfringens	+ / – / –	
					Clostridium sporogenes	Variable / + / +	
					Bacteroides fragilis	– / – / –	
Esculin agar or broth	x			x	*Bacteroides fragilis*	Agar—moderate growth, hydrolysis (deep brown) in 48 h Broth—brown after indicator added	Unhydrolyzed esculin fluoresces under a Wood's lamp.
					Clostridium tetani	Agar—moderate growth, no hydrolysis (no color change) Broth—no change after indicator added	Positive hydrolysis = no fluorescence; negative hydrolysis = fluorescence.
Gelatin (Thiogel)	x			x	*Clostridium perfringens*	Abundant growth; liquefaction in 72 h	
					Bacteroides fragilis	Abundant growth; no liquefaction in 72 h	
H_2S semisolid medium (with lead acetate)	x			x		H_2S produced (48 h) / Motility (48 h)	
					Clostridium sordellii	+ (blackening) / +	
					Bacteroides fragilis	– / –	
Enriched indole-nitrite medium		x	x	x		Good growth / Indole production / NO_3 produced	Fastidious anaerobes may require hemin and/or vitamin K_1 as supplement for growth. Read at 48 h.
					Clostridium perfringens	+ / – / +	
					Fusobacterium necrophorum	+ / + / –	
					Bacteroides thetaiotaomicron	+ / + / –	

(*Continued on next page*)

TABLE 3—*Continued*

Medium	Quality control procedures: Sterility	Growth	Inhibition	Biochemical response	Organism(s)	Expected reaction(s)	Comment
Iron milk medium	x			x		Coagulation / Gas / Digestion / Blackening	Read at 72 h.
					Clostridium perfringens	+ / + / – / –	
					Clostridium sporogenes	– / + / + / +	
					Fusobacterium necrophorum	– / – / – / –	
Kanamycin-(paromomycin-)vancomycin anaerobic blood agar	x	x	x		*Bacteroides fragilis*	Growth	Selective for some anaerobic nonsporeforming gram-negative bacteria. Inhibits most others.
					Escherichia coli *Clostridium perfringens*	No growth	
Laked kanamycin-vancomycin anaerobic blood agar	x	x	x		*Porphyromonas asaccharolytica*	Growth; brown-black pigment; red fluorescence	Has less kanamycin (75 μg) than routine kanamycin-vancomyin agar.
					Escherichia coli	No growth	
Milk ingestion (agar)	x			x	*Clostridium sporogenes*	Milk digested (clear zone) in 48 h	
					Fusobacterium nucleatum	No change; cloudy	
Enriched motility medium	x	x				Growth / Motility	Read at 48 h.
					Fusobacterium necrophorum	Moderate / –	
					Clostridium sporogenes	Abundant / +	
Enriched peptone-yeast extract-glucose broth	x	x			Uninoculated	See comment	Uninoculated broth should show only amounts of volatile and nonvolatile fatty acids when tested with gas-liquid chromatography.
					Fusobacterium necrophorum *Bacteroides fragilis* *Clostridium sporogenes*	See characteristic metabolic products on testing with gas-liquid chromatography	
Phenylethyl alcohol agar	x	x	x		*Clostridium perfringens*	Growth	Inhibits only facultative gram-negative rods. Facultative gram-positive bacteria and all obligate anaerobic organisms should grow.
					Fusobacterium necrophorum	Growth	
					Escherichia coli	No growth	
Thioglycolate (enriched)	x	x			*Fusobacterium necrophorum*	Growth from small inoculum	Also use as control for 20% bile broth.
Urea	x			x	*Clostridium sordellii* *Clostridium tertium*	Positive = pink in 48 h Negative = no change	

TABLE 4. Media for mycobacteriology

Medium or reagent	Quality control procedures				Organism(s)	Expected reaction(s)	Comment
	Sterility	Growth	Inhibition	Biochemical response			
Arylsulfatase	x			x	*Mycobacterium fortuitum* TMC 1529 (3-day test) Uninoculated (reagent control)	Positive (pink to red)	Compare positive to color standards. 2 N sodium carbonate is used for the 3-day and 2-week tests; 3-day test is for rapid growers. Inoculate with 7–10-day 7H9 broth culture.
					Mycobacterium avium complex, TMC 1403 (3-day test)	Negative (no color change)	
Catalase (semiquantitative, 68°C)					*Mycobacterium avium* TMC 1403 (semiquantitative only)	Positive (bubbles of <45 mm)	Positive may take 5 min after reagent (30% H_2O_2 + 10% Tween 80).
					Mycobacterium kansasii TMC 1201 (semiquantitative, 68°C)	Positive (bubbles of >45 mm)	The room temperature and 68°C tests can be done with the same slant or plate. Scrape colonies for 68°C test before room temperature test.
					Mycobacterium tuberculosis TMC 201 or *M. bovis* BCG, TMC 1011 (68°C test only)	Negative (no bubbles) within 10 min	
7H10	x	x			*Mycobacterium tuberculosis* H37Ra	Positive (growth; nonpigmented)	Six stock solutions can be prepared in advance. Solutions remain stable for at least 1 month. If precipitation or flocculation occurs in any stock solution, discard. Do not boil basal commercial medium.
Hydroxylamine		x			*Mycobacterium kansasii* TMC 1201	Positive (growth on reagent slant of ≥1%)	Reagent slant and plain L-J[a] inoculated. Incubated for 4 weeks. Estimate proportion of growth on reagent slant relative to that on control (plain L-J).
					Mycobacterium bovis BCG, TMC 1011	Negative (growth on reagent slant of <1%)	
Iron uptake (ferric ammonium citrate incorporated into L-J medium before inspissation)	x	x		x	*Mycobacterium fortuitum* TMC 1529	Positive (rusty brown colony on tan medium)	Final concentration of ferric ammonium citrate in L-J is 2.5%. Slants are incubated for 4 weeks. Compare color of colonies on reagent slant with color of those on plain L-J.
					Mycobacterium chelonae TMC 1542 or *M. bovis* BCG, TMC 1011	Negative (no color change)	
Lowenstein-Jensen and Middlebrook	x	x	x		*Mycobacterium tuberculosis* H37Ra	Growth in 28 days	Dilute broth to give 50–100 colonies. Tests of commercial media should be considered.

(*Continued on next page*)

TABLE 4—*Continued*

Medium or reagent	Quality control procedures				Organism(s)	Expected reaction(s)	Comment
	Sterility	Growth	Inhibition	Biochemical response			
MacConkey agar (use medium without crystal violet)	x	x			*Mycobacterium fortuitum* TMC 1529	Positive (growth; with or without color change) within 11 days	Use 3-mm loop of 7-day liquid culture. Inoculate in a spiral from center outward.
					Mycobacterium phlei TMC 1548	Negative (no growth)	If turntable is unavailable, streak for isolation. Read at 5 and 11 days.
Niacin standard or strip test	x	x		x	*Mycobacterium tuberculosis* TMC 201	Positive (yellow color); if 7H10 used, must use warm (37°C) extracting fluid and incubate medium at 37°C for 2 h to get good niacin extraction	Test only rough nonchromogenic strains from L-J medium. Must have 50–100 colonies with growth 3–4 weeks old. Niacin is extracted from the medium, not the organism. Reagents require special safety precautions.
					Mycobacterium fortuitum TMC 1529	Negative (no color change)	
Nitrate reduction	x	x		x	*Mycobacterium kansasii* TMC 1201 or *Mycobacterium tuberculosis* TMC 201	Positive (pink to deep red after reagents or no color change after zinc addition)	Test 3–4-week-old colonies. Compare results against color standard.
					Mycobacterium chelonae TMC 1542	Negative (no color change after reagents but red after zinc addition)	
Photochromogenicity	x	x		x	*Mycobacterium kansasii* TMC 1201	Positive (colony change from buff to yellow)	Use lightly inoculated L-J slants (isolated colonies) incubated in the dark for about 2 weeks. Expose to light source for 1–2 h. Loosen cap. Observe after 18 h for pigment. May need to recheck after 1 week.

Pyrazinamidase	x	x	x	*Mycobacterium avium* complex, TMC 1403 *Mycobacterium bovis* BCG, TMC 1011	Positive (pink band in agar) Negative (no pink band in agar)	Use heavy inoculum in two tubes; test one at 4 days and one at 7 days. Read after 4 h. If the 4-day test is positive, do not perform the 7-day test.
Sodium chloride (5%)		x		*Mycobacterium fortuitum* TMC 1529 *Mycobacterium kansasii* TMC 1201	Positive (any growth on reagent slant at 7 days) Negative (growth on plain L-J but not on reagent slant at 7 days)	Reagent slant is 5% NaCl in L-J. Make 10-fold dilution of culture and inoculate with a full loop (0.02 ml).
Tellurite reduction	x	x	x	*Mycobacterium avium* complex, TMC 1403 *Mycobacterium triviale* TMC 1453	Positive (black metallic precipitate of tellurium) Negative (no black precipitate)	Incubate test culture for 7 days. Must have very heavy growth at 7 days; if not, start over.
Thiophene-2-carboxylic acid hydrazide	x	x		*Mycobacterium tuberculosis* TMC 201 *Mycobacterium bovis* BCG, TMC 1011	Positive (growth on reagent slant of >1%) Negative (growth on reagent slant of <1%)	Use thiophene-2-carboxylic acid hydrazide at 0.15 mg/ml, aqueous stock; final concentration, 1 µg/ml. Inoculate reagent slant and plain L-J.
Tween 80 hydrolysis (degradation)	x	x	x	*Mycobacterium kansasii* TMC 1201 *Mycobacterium avium* complex, TMC 1403	Positive (pink to red fluid) Negative (amber fluid)	Commercial reagent is available. Disregard color of cells.
Urease broth	x	x	x	*Mycobacterium chelonae* TMC 1542 *Mycobacterium avium* complex, TMC 1403	Positive (pink to red) Negative (no color change)	Inoculate liquid medium and incubate it for 3 days.
Urease disk	x		x	*Mycobacterium chelonae* TMC 1542 *Mycobacterium avium* complex, TMC 1403	Positive (cherry red color) Negative (no color change)	Use a heavy inoculum in 0.5 ml of sterile distilled water. Add 1 reagent disk (Difco) and incubate for 72 h.

[a] L-J, Lowenstein-Jensen medium.

stored in airtight plastic bags maintain long shelf lives. Suggested storage limits for bacteriologic media have been published (5). Most routine plating media, with the exception of phenylethyl alcohol agar, should have a 2-week expiration date when stored unbagged at 4°C. Media stored at 4°C in airtight bags may have an expiration date of 8 to 10 weeks. Phenylethyl alcohol agar should have an expiration date of 1 week when unbagged and 4 weeks when stored in bags. Broth and agar tubed media last up to 2 weeks at room temperature and up to 4 weeks at 4°C when capped with "vented" caps. These same media can have expiration dates up to 6 months at room temperautre when screw-cap closures are used. Oxidative-fermentative sugars, motility-indole-ornithine agar, and motility medium require expiration dates only half as long as those for other agar tubed media (5).

Organisms suggested for medium quality control testing

The following organisms are recommended for quality control testing of media.

Aerobic
(although some ATCC strains may be listed, any strain is acceptable that will give the same result)

Acinetobacter lwoffii
Campylobacter jejuni ATCC 33290
Enterobacter aerogenes
Enterococcus faecalis ATCC 29212
Escherichia coli ATCC 25922
Haemophilus influenzae
Klebsiella pneumoniae
Neisseria gonorrhoeae CDC Ng 98
Proteus mirabilis CDC S-17
Proteus vulgaris ATCC 8482
Providencia stuartii
Pseudomonas aeruginosa ATCC 27853
Salmonella typhimurium ATCC 14028
Shigella sonnei ATCC 9290
Staphylococcus aureus ATCC 25923
Staphylococcus epidermidis ATCC 12228
Streptococcus pyogenes ATCC 19615 (group A)
Streptococcus bovis (group D, not *Enterococcus* sp.)
Streptococcus pneumoniae ATCC 6305

Anaerobic

Bacteroides fragilis ATCC 23745
Bacteroides thetaiotaomicron ATCC 29741
Clostridium novyi A ATCC 19402
Clostridium perfringens ATCC 3624 (type A)
Clostridium sordellii ATCC 9714
Clostridium sporogenes ATCC 3584 or 19404
Clostridium subterminale ATCC 25774
Clostridium tertium ATCC 19405
Fusobacterium necrophorum ATCC 25286
Fusobacterium nucleatum ATCC 10953 or 25586
Porphyromonas (Bacteroides) asaccharolytia ATCC 25260

Testing of *Escherichia coli* O157 and H7 antisera and MacConkey sorbitol agar and assays for Shiga-like toxin(s) (verotoxins) can be done in the laboratory. *E. coli* O157:H7 strain B6914-MS1 (ATCC 43888) produces neither of the two Shiga-like toxins. Since this strain is negative for both toxins, it may be a good choice, on the basis of safety considerations, for quality control of antisera and media. *E. coli* O157:H7 strain EDL932 (ATCC 43894) produces Shiga-like toxins I and II (verotoxins 1 and 2). *E. coli* O157:H7 strain B1539 (ATCC 43890) produces Shiga-like toxin I (verotoxin 1) only. *E. coli* O157:H7 strain B1409-C1 (ATCC 43889) produces Shiga-like toxin II (verotoxin 2) only.

Mycology media

In addition to the usual pH and sterility checks, each lot of primary isolation medium should be tested to determine whether it supports or inhibits the growth of known cultures. Inocula can be taken from working stock slants that are serially transferred weekly. It is not necessary to standardize the inoculum. The optimum temperature of incubation is 30°C, but room temperature is acceptable and commonly used. Sporulation media are used as slants, plates, or slide cultures. For plates or slide cultures, the sterile medium should be stored in screw-cap tubes at 4°C, melted, and poured the day of use. The medium should be moist and fresh at time of use and should not be melted more than once. Inoculate the test medium directly from a working stock slant of the test organism and incubate it at room temperature or 25°C. Some recommend using an *Aspergillus* species as a positive control for sporulation media, but since this organism sporulates on almost any medium under almost any condition, its use is not a stringent test of the medium.

Tables 5 and 6 offer suggestions on the quality control of media used to characterize yeast and fungi. Table 5 (yeast media) is taken from chapter 60.

Fungal stock culture maintenance (7)

A stock culture collection must be available for the quality control of media and reagents. A culture collection is also invaluable in teaching and for review, especially of organisms that are not frequently seen. Regular subculture is time-consuming and usually results in the organisms becoming atypical and eventually nonviable. A few of the most frequently used cultures may be kept on slants with biweekly transfers, but they should also be maintained by another method as a backup system. If cultures must be kept on screw-cap slants, they may be stored at 4°C for about 6 months. Some of the more fastidious organisms must be subcultured more frequently. Members of the order *Mucorales* have poor survival rates in screw-cap tubes because of the toxic buildup of carbon dioxide. The alternative use of cotton-plugged tubes allows better release of the carbon dioxide but leads to more rapid dehydration of the slant.

There are three common methods for maintaining permanent stock collections: water culture, sterile mineral oil overlay, and freezing.

Water culture. The simplest method, and a very reliable one, is to keep the stocks in water. Most water suspensions will remain viable for years. An organism must be actively sporulating on a potato-dextrose agar (PDA) slant to be placed in water. With use of sterile technique, 1 to 2 ml of sterile water is pipetted over the slant. With the same pipette, the surface of the colony

TABLE 5. Yeast media

Medium	Quality control procedures				Organism(s)	Expected reaction(s)	Comment
	Sterility	Growth	Inhibition	Biochemical response			
Carbon assimilation		x		x	*Cryptococcus laurentii*	Growth around all carbon sources	See text list of carbon sources.
					Candida krusei	Growth around glucose only	
Cornmeal agar		x			*Candida albicans*	Formation of chlamydospores, blastoconidia, and pseudohyphae within 48 h	
Fowell's acetate		x			*Saccharomyces cerevisiae* *Candida albicans*	Positive = ascospores formed Negative = no ascospores formed	
Germ tube test medium	x	x			*Candida albicans*	Positive = germ tube formulation in 2–3 h	
					Candida tropicalis	Negative	Pseudohyphae may be formed.
					Torulopsis glabrata	Negative	Only budding yeast is seen.
Nitrate assimilation		x		x	*Cryptococcus albidus*	Positive = growth around potassium nitrate source	Should see growth around peptone source (growth control).
					Cryptococcus laurentii	Negative = no growth around potassium nitrate source	
Phenol oxidase				x	*Cryptococcus neoformans*	Positive = dark brown colonies	
					Cryptococcus albidus	Negative = no color or light tan color	
Sabouraud dextrose agar with chloramphenicol and cycloheximide	x	x	x		*Candida albicans* *Candida parapsilosis*	Positive = growth in 2 days Negative = no growth	Tests ability to grow in the presence of cycloheximide.
Urease agar	x			x	*Cryptococcus albidus* *Candida albicans*	Positive = pink to red Negative = no color change (straw colored)	Control each time of use.
Yeast fermentation		x		x	*Candida kefyr*	Positive = dextrose, lactose, galactose	Positive = bubbles in Durham tubes, not just change in broth color due to pH shift.
					Candida albicans	Positive = dextrose, maltose, sucrose, galactose, trehalose	
					Cryptococcus albidus	Negative = no fermentation	

TABLE 6. Fungal media[a]

Medium	Quality control procedures				Organism(s)	Expected reaction(s)	Comment
	Sterility	Growth	Inhibition	Biochemical response			
Casein hydrolysis medium	x			x	*Nocardia brasiliensis* *Nocardia asteroides*	Hydrolysis within 2 wk No hydrolysis	Used for *Nocardia, Streptomyces,* and *Actinomadura* spp. Use when fresh and moist or store sealed with Parafilm at 4°C. Use no more than 20 ml in a 100-mm plate.
Hypoxanthine hydrolysis medium	x			x	*Nocardia caviae* *Nocardia asteroides*	No hydrolysis within 3 wk No hydrolysis	
Potato-dextrose agar	x	x			*Drechslera* sp.	Sporulation within 5–7 days	
Sabhi or brain heart infusion agar	x	x			*Cryptococcus neoformans*	Growth in 2 days	
Sabouraud dextrose agar with antibiotics	x	x	x		*Candida albicans* *Staphylococcus aureus*	Growth in 2 days No growth	
Sabouraud dextrose agar	x	x			*Candida albicans*	Growth in 2 days	
Trichophyton agar no. 1 (basal)	x	x			*Trichophyton mentagrophytes* *Trichophyton tonsurans* *Trichophyton verrucosum*	4+ growth + to 1+ growth No growth	
Trichophyton agar no. 2 (inositol)	x	x			*Trichophyton mentagrophytes* *Trichophyton verrucosum*	4+ growth 0 to + growth	
Trichophyton agar no. 3 (thiamine + inositol)	x	x			*Trichophyton mentagrophytes*	4+ growth	
Trichophyton agar no. 4 (thiamine)	x	x			*Trichophyton mentagrophytes*	4+ growth	
Tyrosine hydrolysis medium	x			x	*Nocardia brasiliensis* *Nocardia asteroides*	Hydrolysis within 4 wk No hydrolysis	
Xanthine hydrolysis medium	x			x	*Nocardia caviae* *Nocardia asteroides*	Hydrolysis within 3 wk No hydrolysis	
Yeast extract-phosphate agar	x	x			*Aspergillus fumigatus*	Medium without NH_4OH: growth in 2 days Medium with NH_4OH: no growth	*Blastomyces dermatitidis* can be a positive growth control in the NH_4OH-containing medium.
7H10 or 7H11	x	x			*Nocardia asteroides*	Growth in 7 days	

[a] From reference 7.

TABLE 7. Disk, strips, and reagents

Disk, strip, or reagent	Quality control procedures				Organism(s)	Expected reaction(s)	Comment
	Sterility	Growth	Inhibition	Biochemical response			
Bacitracin disk				x	*Streptococcus pyogenes* (group A)	Sensitive = zone of inhibition of growth around disk in 24 h	Any zone size is considered significant. Only a presumptive test for group A streptococci.
					Enterococcus faecalis	Resistant = no zone of inhibition in 24 h	
Catalase (H_2O_2)				x	*Staphylococcus aureus*	Positive = bubbling instantly	Use 3% H_2O_2. Activity may also be checked by adding a few drops to blood in a test tube.
					Streptococcus spp.	Negative = no bubbling	
Coagglutination, latex, bacterial antigen detection				x	Positive-antigen control	Positive	
					Negative-antigen control	Negative	
					Extractant control	Positive	
Coagulase plasma				x	*Staphylococcus aureus*	Positive in 4 h = any degree of clotting	Rabbit plasma recommended; 4-h incubation recommended for tube test. Slide test is adequate for positives.
					Staphylococcus epidermidis	Negative = no clot, strands	
Ferric chloride (10%)				x	*Proteus vulgaris*	Positive in 24 h = green; note package inserts on micromethod	Add 2–3 drops to growth on phenylalanine deaminase slant or to appropriate micromethod.
					Escherichia coli	Negative = yellow	
Growth factors X, V, and XV		x		x	*Haemophilus influenzae*	Growth around XV in 24 h; growth between X and V in 24 h	Inoculate infusion or Mueller-Hinton plate confluently. Place X and V disks 1 cm apart. Place XV disk at least 6 cm distant. Incubate in air or CO_2.
Indole				x	*Escherichia coli*	Positive in 24 h = red ring at surface	Kovacs reagent and Ehrlich reagent give same colors. A spot test is adequate.
					Enterobacter aerogenes	Negative = yellow ring at surface	
Methyl red	x				*Escherichia coli*	Positive in 48 h = red color instantly	Methyl red is a pH test and shows usually the reaction opposite that exhibited by the Voges-Proskauer test.
					Enterobacter aerogenes	Negative = no color change	

(*Continued on next page*)

TABLE 7—*Continued*

Disk, strip, or reagent	Quality control procedures				Organism(s)	Expected reaction(s)	Comment
	Sterility	Growth	Inhibition	Biochemical response			
ONPG disk				x	*Escherichia coli*	Positive = yellow color in 24 h	
					Proteus vulgaris	Negative = no color change	
Optochin disk				x	*Streptococcus pneumoniae*	Sensitive in 24 h = zone of inhibition	Sensitive: 6-mm disk, 14-mm zone; 10-mm disk, 16-mm zone.
					Streptococcus viridans (alpha-hemolytic streptococcus)	Resistant = no zone of inhibition	Intermediate: 6-mm disk, 7–13-mm zone; 10-mm disk, 11–15-mm zone. If intermediate, do bile solubility test.
Oxidase				x	*Pseudomonas aeruginosa*	Positive in 10–20 s = purple to black	The dimethyl reagent and tetramethyl reagent give the same color reactions.
					Escherichia coli	Negative in 10–20 s = no color shown	
Oxidase disk or strip				x	*Pseudomonas aeruginosa*	Positive = purple in 30 s	Oxidase reagent may be used as a spot test with 10-s reading time or by addition to colonies on plate and observation of color change in 30 s.
					Escherichia coli	Negative = no color change	
Pyrazinamidase (agar for yersiniae)	x			x	*Yersinia enterocolitica* (nonpathogenic)	Positive = pink-brown color within 15 min	Incubate slant at 25–30°C for 48 h. Flood with fresh 1% ferrous ammonium sulfate. Nonpathogens have the enzyme pyrazinamidase that converts pyrazinamide to pyrazinoic acid, which turns brown in the presence of ferrous salts.
					Yersinia enterocolitica (pathogenic)	Negative = no pink-brown color.	
Taxo N				x	*Neisseria* spp. or *Pseudomonas aeruginosa*	Positive = purple color on disk in 30 s	This is a test for oxidase.
					Escherichia coli	Negative = no color change on disk	
Voges-Proskauer				x	*Enterobacter aerogenes*	Positive in 48 h after adding reagents = red color in 5 min (4-h final reading with O'Meara reagent)	40% KOH (in water); α-naphthol (5% in absolute alcohol). O'Meara reagent = 40% KOH with creatine.
					Escherichia coli	Negative = no color change or copper color	

is gently teased to dislodge conidia without disrupting the agar. This suspension is then removed and placed into a screw-cap tube or vial. If the organism is a very poor sporulator, such as *Microsporum audouinii*, several slants should be processed in this manner. The tube that is to be stored should have a total volume of at least 4 ml of water. Screw the cap on very tightly to avoid evaporation (caps with cracks should not be used) and store the tubes at room temperature.

To reactivate water stocks, shake the tube well and inoculate a small amount of the suspension onto a Sabouraud dextrose slant. Additional sterile water may be added to the water stock at any time.

Sterile mineral oil overlay. The sterile mineral oil overlay technique is a traditional method for maintaining stock culture collections. This method can be very messy and can result in contamination if care is not exercised. The culture should be actively sporulating on a PDA slant. Sterile mineral oil (which has not absorbed moisture upon autoclaving) is added to the tube to cover the entire slant. The cap should be tightened, and the culture should be stored at room temperature.

To reactivate the culture, flame the mouth of the tube and remove a visible portion of the growth by using a long, sterile inoculating needle. Avoid any aerial strands reaching upward into the mineral oil when removing

TABLE 8. Stains

Stain	Control		Frequency	Organism(s) or other matter	Expected reaction(s)
	Positive	Negative			
Flagellum	x		Each new vial and each day of use	*Pseudomonas aeruginosa* *Alcaligenes faecalis*	One or two polar flagella. Peritrichous flagella.
Fluorescence (fluorochrome) acid-fast[a]	x	x	Each new vial and each time of use	*Mycobacterium gordonae* *Streptomyces* spp.	Positive = yellow-fluorescing bacilli. Negative = blue branching bacilli, no fluorescence.
Gram	x	x	Each new vial and once each week of use	*Staphylococcus aureus* *Escherichia coli*	Gram positive = purple to blue cocci. Gram negative = pink to red rod-shaped organisms.
Kinyoun acid-fast[a]	x		Each new vial and each week of use	*Mycobacterium gordonae*	Short, long, and clumps of pinkish red bacilli on a blue background.
Modified acid-fast for fungi	x	x	Each new vial and each day of use	*Nocardia asteroides* *Actinomadura madurae*	Acid-fast = pinkish red on blue background. Non-acid-fast = blue.
Periodic acid-Schiff	x		Each new vial and each day of use	Skin or nail scrapings containing a dermatophyte	Fungi will stain magenta color; the background will have a light pink or reddish color, depending on the thickness of the preparation.
Spore	x		Each new vial and each day of use	*Bacillus* spp.	Oval spores that do not swell the cell. Spores stain one color (depending on stain used), with counterstained rods.
Trichrome	x		Each new batch and each month of use	Buffy coat mixed with feces (fresh or polyvinyl alcohol fixed)	Cytoplasm of polymorphonuclear leukocytes is blue-green, tinged with purple. Nucleus is red to purplish red.
Ziehl-Neelsen acid-fast[a]	x		Each new vial and each week of use	*Mycobacterium gordonae*	Short, long, and clumps of pinkish red bacilli on a blue background.

[a] For laboratories rated level 2 and above, *M. tuberculosis* should be used as a positive control. For level 1 laboratories, *M. gordonae* is acceptable but may appear "barred" in acid-fast stains. Boxes of smears may be prepared and frozen before staining to prevent continuous culturing of the organism.

the growth. These are often sterile hyphae that will not produce typical colonies. Allow as much oil to drain off the inoculum as possible. Transfer the inoculum to Sabouraud dextrose broth and incubate it at 30°C until growth appears. The mineral oil slant may be tightly recapped and stored.

Freezing. The culture should be actively sporulating on a PDA slant in a screw-cap tube made of high-quality glass. The slant culture is placed at −70°C. To reactivate the culture, remove the tube from the freezer, quickly tease some of the growth from the slant, and inoculate it on PDA. Return the stock culture to the freezer immediately without allowing it to thaw; if the tube thaws, a new slant must be prepared.

REAGENTS

As with all other products used in testing, reagents, either purchased or prepared in the laboratory, should be clearly marked to indicate the date on which they were first opened and the expiration date. For reagents prepared in the laboratory, reagent labels should be initialed by the preparer. The labels must also include appropriate special instructions and precautions for storage and use.

Products used to detect bacterial metabolites must be challenged with the cultures known not to produce them as well as with organisms known to produce them. Chemical reagents used to generate reactions are not acceptable in lieu of appropriate bacterial cultures.

Records must reflect results of these quality control tests to the extent necessary to determine the suitability of the products for use in the laboratory. Table 7 shows the chemicals, biological solutions, and reagents commonly used in bacteriology and some of the organisms used in quality control procedures for them. Other organisms that produce comparable reactions also may be used.

Catalase, oxidase, and coagulase reagents used for aerobic culture identification should be checked when each new vial is opened and on each day of use with at least one organism that produces a positive reaction and one organism that produces a negative reaction.

Bacitracin, optochin, *o*-nitrophenyl-β-D-galactopyranoside (ONPG), XV disks, and strips used for aerobic culture identification should be checked when each new vial is opened and once each week of use with at least one organism that produces a positive reaction and one organism that produces a negative reaction. XV disks and strips need only be checked for positive reactivity. Antisera used for aerobic culture identication should be checked when each new vial is opened and then once each month of use with at least one organism that produces a positive reaction and one organism that produces a negative reaction.

TABLE 9. Quality control frequencies for microbiology

Material to be tested	Frequency[a]							
	Aerobic		Anaerobic		Mycobacteriology		Mycology	
	+	−	+	−	+	−	+	−
Reagents, disks, and strips								
Catalase	2	2	2					
Oxidase	2	2						
Coagulase	2	2						
Bacitracin	3	3						
Optochin	3	3						
ONPG	3	3						
Growth factor X	3	3						
Growth factor V	3	3						
Growth factor XV	3							
All other	1	1	1		2	Iron uptake only	—[b]	
Antisera	4	4						
Stains								
Gram, acid-fast Ziehl-Neelsen, Kinyoun	6	6	6	6	6		6	6
Fluorescence					7	7		
All other	2		2				2	2[c]
In-house-prepared media and biochemical kit systems	5	5	5	5	5		5	
Commercially purchased media	Most required no quality control testing (see Table 1)							
Direct antigen detection (latex, coagglutination, DNA probes)	2[d]	2						

[a] 1, Each new vial or batch; 2, each new vial or batch and each day of use; 3, each new vial and once each week of use; 4, each new vial and once each month of use; 5, each new batch; 6, each new vial or batch and once each week of use; 7, each new vial or batch and each time of use.

[b] Nitrate reagent is checked each day of use with a peptone control. Each batch of serum (germ tube) is checked with at least four strains of *Candida albicans* from different patients.

[c] Modified acid-fast stain only.

[d] If an extraction reagent is used as part of direct antigen detection kits, the controls should be designed so that the extraction reagent is also evaluated; i.e., the extraction reagent should be used on whole cells.

All other reagents, disks, and strips used in routine aerobic bacteriology should be checked when each new vial or container is prepared or opened by using at least one organism that produces a positive reaction and at least one organism that produces a negative reaction.

Reagents for mycobacteriology should be checked when each new vial or container is prepared or opened and during each day of use with at least one acid-fast organism that produces a positive reaction. Negative controls with these reagents are optional and are performed at the discretion of the laboratory. Reagents used for the iron uptake test should be checked when each new vial or container is prepared or opened and each day of use with at least one acid-fast organism that produces a positive reaction and with an acid-fast or non-acid-fast organism that produces a negative reaction. The other controls listed are strongly recommended as good laboratory practice.

Products for detecting antigen directly from a specimen swab or from bacterial culture are considered bacteriology tests, not serology tests. These products should be tested when each new batch arrives in the laboratory and each day of use with a positive and negative antigen control, along with a test of the extracting fluid with a known positive organism. DNA probes require positive and negative controls with each run. The manufacturer's suggested controls should be followed.

KIT SYSTEMS

Kits include miniaturized biochemical methods and automated methods for biochemical identification of microorganisms. Documents must show that all of these systems have been tested to determine the correct performance of each constituent for proper growth, selectivity, and biochemical reaction. Therefore, organisms giving both positive and negative reactions for each constituent should be used.

STAINS

All stains should be tested at recommended intervals (Table 8) for the ability to distinguish positive and negative organisms, and the results should be documented. Laboratory result forms should reflect actual facts. The use of check marks or the term "OK," for example, is not a suitable indication of quality control results. Specific and actual results should be recorded. This practice not only allows the laboratory to maintain "adequate" records but also protects the laboratory against any misunderstanding about the meanings of such results.

Table 9 summarizes the frequencies with which most commonly used reagents, stains, and antisera are to be tested.

LITERATURE CITED

1. **Bartlett, M. S., and K. L. Harper.** 1985. Parasitology, p. 145–166. *In* J. M. Miller and B. B. Wentworth (ed.), Methods for quality control in diagnostic microbiology. American Public Health Association, Washington, D.C.
2. **Bartlett, R. C.** 1974. Medical microbiology: quality cost and clinical relevance. John Wiley & Sons, Inc., New York.
3. **Bartlett, R. C.** 1975. Functional quality control, p. 145–178. *In* J. E. Prior, J. T. Bartola, and H. Friedman (ed.), Quality control in microbiology. University Park Press, Baltimore.
4. **Bartlett, R. C., V. D. Allen, D. J. Blazevic, et al.** 1978. Clinical microbiology, p. 912–914. *In* S. L. Inhorn (ed.), Quality assurance practices for health laboratories. American Public Health Association, Washington, D.C.
5. **Blazevic, D. J., C. T. Hall, and M. E. Wilson.** 1976. Cumitech 3, Practical quality control procedures for the clinical microbiology laboratory. Coordinating ed., A. Balows. American Society for Microbiology, Washington, D.C.
6. **Bowdre, J. H.** 1985. Viral isolation and antigen detection, p. 211–234. *In* J. M. Miller and B. B. Wentworth (ed.), Methods for quality control in diagnostic microbiology. American Public Health Association, Washington, D.C.
7. **Hill, E. O., and R. Reed.** 1985. Fungal isolation and identification, p. 167–187. *In* J. M. Miller and B. B. Wentworth (ed.), Methods for quality control in diagnostic microbiology. American Public Health Association, Washington, D.C.
8. **Miller, J. M.** 1987. Quality control in microbiology. Centers for Disease Control, Atlanta.

Chapter 121

Culture Media

PETER NASH AND MICHELLE M. KRENZ

The microorganisms presented in this Manual vary in their growth requirements. All organisms require sources of nitrogen, carbon, and trace elements. Some organisms can utilize a chemically simplified medium such as ammonia or nitrate, whereas others can fix free nitrogen. Other organisms require protein hydrolysates in the form of peptones, which provide nitrogenous compounds in a more available form. These peptones are water-soluble materials derived from proteins by means of acid, alkali, or added or intrinsic enzymes. Since most of the microorganisms discussed possess a limited ability to synthesize compounds, they require complex compounds to grow on. The user should be very careful in the preparation of all media (82).

PREPARATION

Media prepared from dehydrated materials should be prepared in accordance with directions given by the manufacturer. The use of chemically clean equipment and glassware is essential. Distilled or demineralized water should always be used unless specified otherwise. Dry materials must be accurately weighed, and water must be accurately measured. Heating to solubilize ingredients and to sterilize media may be accomplished by the use of direct heat, a boiling water bath, or an autoclave and should be used for the shortest time possible. Excessive heating should be avoided.

Since the microorganisms found in clinical specimens grow best at a pH near neutrality, it is essential that the pH after autoclaving be regularly checked. It is especially important to check the final pH of media prepared from dehydrated materials that have been opened, to detect changes which may have occurred during storage.

Sterilization is usually accomplished by autoclaving or by filtration. Volumes of up to 500 ml of most media are autoclaved at 121°C for 15 min. Larger volumes may need 20 to 30 min or more.

Temperatures from 116 to 118°C should be used for media containing heat-stable carbohydrates. The pH of these media should be checked before sterilization. Media containing heat-labile carbohydrates should be sterilized by filtration and added to cooled, autoclaved medium by aseptic technique. Carbohydrates may also be added by using impregnated paper disks. There are various filters that can be used to filter-sterilize carbohydrates. All filtration equipment must be sterile, and care should be taken to use aseptic technique. Dispensing of sterile media and addition of sterile substances should be carried out in a laminar-flow hood or in a sterile room by strict aseptic techniques.

Enrichments such as blood should be added aseptically to cooled base media. Care should be taken to avoid forming froth or bubbles during mixing. Media enriched with blood should not be incubated before use. Sterility should be checked by incubating several tubes or plates from each batch of medium at 20 to 25°C or at 30 to 35°C for up to 1 week. The remainder of each batch should be refrigerated (2 to 8°C) as soon as possible. Tubed media (agar or broth) should be stored tightly capped. After long-term storage, liquid media must be heated to boiling for a few minutes to drive off dissolved gases and then quickly cooled to room temperature before use. Agar plates may be stored in the manufacturers' plastic bags or wrapped tightly in plastic. They should be stored inverted so that moisture does not collect on the agar surface (30).

Blood or serum used for enrichment or for determining hemolysis should be obtained from animals that are free of antimicrobial agents. Defibrinated sheep blood is the blood of choice for routine work, since the hemolytic reactions of streptococci on sheep blood are "true" and the growth of *Haemophilus haemolyticus*, which may be mistaken for hemolytic streptococci, is inhibited.

Blood from other animal species (including humans) may be used to demonstrate hemolysis. However, hemolytic reactions on these bloods differ from those on sheep blood, as follows: (i) hemolytic reactions on defibrinated rabbit blood correlate with those of sheep blood; however, both *H. haemolyticus* and *Haemophilus influenzae* will grow on media containing rabbit blood; and (ii) hemolytic reactions on defibrinated horse blood are not dependable, and some streptococci, e.g., group D, may not give the hemolytic reactions of group A.

Human blood from the blood bank must be carefully screened for human pathogens such as human immunodeficiency virus and hepatitis viruses. Human blood collected for the blood bank may contain citrates and glucose. Citrates are inhibitory to some organisms, and glucose may cause alpha- rather than beta-hemolysis. Antibodies and antimicrobial agents in human blood may also cause inhibition of growth or false hemolytic reactions or both.

QUALITY CONTROL

As stated previously, quality control of media is very important. The performance characteristics of raw materials of biological origin are determined by the nature of the starting material and the methods of processing. Variations may occur between lots or batches of ingredients. It may be necessary to adjust or supplement media formulations to meet performance criteria (82). Examples of media for which performance standards have been developed are given in chapter 120.

The sterility and performance of all media must be

verified before use, whether the media are prepared by a laboratory from scratch or from dehydrated materials or are received ready to use from commercial companies. Commercially prepared media include systems in kit form which are used for the identification of microorganisms. Although commercially prepared media must meet standards set by the Food and Drug Administration, these products should be subjected to sterility and performance tests to detect changes that may have occurred during shipment or storage.

Materials used in the preparation of media should be dated when received, and the instructions of the manufacturer for storage and expiration dates should be closely followed. Complete records should be maintained for each batch of medium prepared in the laboratory. A sample (5 to 10%) of each batch of medium should be tested for sterility, especially media to which one or more components are added after the basal media are sterilized. In addition, as each plate is used, it should be examined for random surface contamination.

Special care should be taken in testing the sterility of selective media, since contaminating organisms may be inhibited on these media but appear later when transferred to nonselective media. For this reason, the sterility of selective media should be tested by inoculating samples of each batch onto noninhibitory media.

Media should also be examined for color, clarity, and evidence of dehydration. Precipitates may appear in some media during storage. If such precipitates do not disappear upon gentle heating, the medium should be discarded unless it normally contains some insoluble component.

The pH of each batch of medium should be checked electrometrically after the completed medium or medium base has cooled to room temperature. The pH should be in a range of ±0.2 of the value indicated by the manufacturer.

All media should be subjected to performance testing unless the reliability of a certain medium has been ensured by extensive prior testing. The laboratory should maintain a collection of stock cultures with known typical culture characteristics adequate for testing all media used in the laboratory (chapter 120). Performance testing should be based on the specific use for which the medium being tested is intended and should include organisms that give both positive and negative results. For multipurpose media such as blood agar plates which are used for the isolation of fastidious organisms and the demonstration of hemolysis, it may be necessary to use more than one test organism.

FORMULAS AND MEDIA

The formulas are listed according to requirements determined by the authors of chapters in this Manual. The generic names for components such as peptones are given; in some cases, trade names are noted. The various types of peptones that are commercially available are as follows: Biosate, Gelysate, peptone ("peptone" is assumed to be used in the generic sense unless the author[s] has specifically stated a given manufacturer), Proteose Peptone no. 2, Proteose Peptone no. 3, Trypticase, and Tryptose. Peptones may vary in composition and preparation. The clinical microbiologist must be careful in choosing the right peptone for a given medium formulation. Any substitution of similar ingredients must be tested and confirmed with quality control strains of organisms before one assumes that the materials will give equivalent results (30).

Many of the media listed are available from commercial sources. Note that different terminologies and spellings may be given. Contact the manufacturer if questions arise. Note that media or components designated by an asterisk (*) are available commercially in dehydrated or prepared form. The composition of the commercial preparation may be either identical or comparable to the formula submitted by the author, and the similarity may be determined by comparing the formulas.

Commercial media should be prepared as instructed by the manufacturers. The following are standard laboratory media commonly (30) used in the clinical laboratory (the list does not include all of the basic agars and broths that are used in the laboratory, nor does it include some media indicated by authors of various chapters to be available from commercial sources):

Bismuth-sulfite agar
Brilliant green agar
Desoxycholate agar
Desoxycholate citrate agar
EMB (eosin-methylene blue) agar
GN (gram-negative) broth
Hektoen enteric agar
Loeffler medium
MacConkey agar
Mannitol-salt agar
SS (salmonella-shigella) agar
Selenite broth
TCBS (thiosulfate-citrate-bile salts) agar
Tellurite-glycine agar
Tergitol 7 agar

These media should be prepared, when possible, from dehydrated products to reduce variability in results.

The formulas given in this chapter, although not traditional or always chemically correct, are reproduced essentially as received from the authors except for changes made in the interest of uniform presentation. It should be noted that there is no effort to list all manufacturers of media, and inclusion or exclusion does not constitute endorsement or disapproval of any manufacturer or product. Full names and addresses of suppliers appear at the end of the chapter.

Many of the media given in this chapter are used in conjunction with specific reagents, stains, or test procedures. These can be found in chapter 122.

Acetate agar* (112)

For differentiation of species of Shigella and Escherichia

Sodium acetate	2.00 g
Sodium chloride	5.00 g
Magnesium sulfate	0.20 g
Monoammonium phosphate	1.00 g
Dipotassium phosphate	1.00 g
Bromothymol blue	0.08 g
Agar, dried	17.00 g
(*or* Not dried	20.00 g)
Distilled water	1.00 liter

Final pH 6.7 ± 0.2

Dissolve and dispense into tubes for 2.5-cm butts and 3.8-cm slants. Autoclave at 121°C for 15 min. Inoculate and incubate in the same manner as Simmons citrate agar (see citrate agar).

For nonfermenting gram-negative bacteria

A. Method of Tatum et al. (109)

Add a 0.2% final concentration of sodium acetate to commercial Simmons agar base. Adjust pH to 6.8. Dispense into tubes (4-ml, 13 by 100 mm, screw capped), autoclave at 121°C for 15 min, and slant. Inoculate and incubate in the same manner as Simmons citrate agar (see citrate agar).

B. Method of Gilardi (36)

See carbon assimilation medium.

Aeromonas differential agar* (97)

Casein peptone	10.00 g
Meat extract	3.00 g
NaCl	5.00 g
Dextrin	15.00 g
Sodium sulfite	1.60 g
Fuchsin	0.25 g
Na_2HPO_4	7.75 g
Agar	13.00 g
Distilled water	1.00 liter

Final pH 7.5 ± 0.2

To dissolve the fuchsin, one may add 50 ml of 5% aqueous Dioxan (Merck). Boil to solution. Autoclave.
A redness of the medium can be removed by adding a few drops of sodium sulfite solution.

Albumin-fatty acid broth, *Leptospira* medium

See bovine albumin polysorbate (Tween 80) medium.

Albumin-fatty acid semisolid medium, modified

See bovine albumin polysorbate (Tween 80) semisolid medium.

Alkaline peptone water

Peptone (Difco)	10.0 g
NaCl	5.0 g
Distilled water	1.0 liter

Dissolve ingredients in distilled water. Dispense in tubes and autoclave at 121°C for 20 min. Final pH 8.4. For *Vibrio* spp., final pH 9.0.

ALP (aerobic low peptone) basal media*
For nonfermenting gram-negative bacteria (chapter 40)

Diammonium phosphate	1.0 g
Potassium chloride	0.2 g
Magnesium sulfate heptahydrate	0.2 g
Yeast extract (Difco)	0.5 g
Casitone (Difco)	0.5 g
Phenol red	0.02 g
Agar	15.0 g
Distilled water	1.0 liter

Basal medium for sugars (carbohydrates and other acidogenic substrates) is adjusted to pH 7.8. Basal medium for salts (salts of organic acids and other alkalinogenic substrates) is supplemented with 0.02% glucose and adjusted to pH 6.5. Heat to melt agar, dispense in 3-ml amounts into 13-mm screw-capped tubes, and autoclave at 121°C for 15 min. Stock solutions of substrates, sterilized by storage in screw-capped tubes over a slight excess of chloroform, are added to the molten basal medium before slanting to give final concentrations of 0.05% for *n*-butanol, 1% for other sugars and gelatin, 0.1% for salts of aliphatic acids, and 0.2% for other salts. Inoculate by streaking the slants and incubate at 35°C for up to 7 days.

Amies transport medium without charcoal*[a]

Sodium thioglycolate	1.00 g
Sodium chloride	3.00 g
Potassium chloride	0.20 g
Calcium chloride	0.10 g
Magnesium chloride	0.10 g
Potassium phosphate, monobasic	0.20 g
Sodium phosphate, dibasic	1.15 g
Agar	4.00 g
Demineralized water	1 liter

Final pH 7.4 ± 0.2 at 25°C

Suspend the ingredients in the water and dissolve by boiling. Dispense in tubes and autoclave for 15 min at 121°C. Prior to solidification, the tubes should be inverted to distribute the charcoal evenly. Store in refrigeration.

[a] Amies transport medium with charcoal contains, additionally, 10 g of charcoal per liter.

Ammonium nitrate agar
Trichophyton agars 6 and 7*

Ammonium nitrate	1.5 g
Glucose	40.0 g
Magnesium sulfate	0.1 g
Monopotassium phosphate	1.8 g
Agar	20.0 g
Distilled water	1.0 liter

Dissolve ingredients by boiling. Adjust pH to 6.8, and dispense in 100-ml amounts into flasks.
For histidine ammonium nitrate agar, add 2 ml of histidine solution at 150 mg/100 ml of water. Tube, sterilize at 121°C for 15 min, and slant.

Ampicillin sheep blood agar

See blood agar base.

Anaerobic agar*

Casitone (Difco)	20 g
Sodium chloride	5 g
Dextrose (Difco)	10 g
Bacto-Agar (Difco)	20 g
Sodium thioglycoate (Difco)	2 g
Sodium formaldehyde sulfoxylate	1 g
Methylene blue (Difco)	0.002 g

Final pH 7.2 ± 0.2 at 25°C

Suspend ingredients in 1 liter of distilled water and heat to boiling to dissolve agar. Sterilize in autoclave for 15 min at 15 lb/in^2 and 121°C. Dispense into petri dishes.

Anaerobic broth

Prepare as anaerobic agar without the agar. Dispense in screw-cap tubes.

See CDC anaerobic agar.

Antibiotic medium 3 FDA* (40)
Antibiotic assay broth* (BBL); Penassay broth* (Difco)
For susceptibility testing with polyene antifungal antibiotics

Peptone or Gelysate (BBL)	5.00 g
Yeast extract	1.50 g
Beef extract	1.50 g
Sodium chloride	3.50 g
Glucose	1.00 g
Dipotassium phosphate	3.68 g
Potassium dihydrogen phosphate	1.32 g
Distilled water	1.00 liter
Final pH 7.0 ± 0.2.	

Suspend the ingredients in water and heat to boiling to dissolve. Dispense; autoclave at 121°C for 15 min. Final pH 7.04 ± 02.

Antibiotic medium 12 FDA* (40)
Nystatin assay agar*
For agar dilution susceptibility tests with polyene antifungal antibiotics

Peptone or Gelysate (BBL)	9.40 g
Yeast extract	4.70 g
Beef extract	2.40 g
Sodium chloride	10.00 g
Glucose	10.00 g
Agar	23.50 g
Distilled water	1.00 liter
Final pH 6.1 ± 0.2	

Suspend the ingredients in water and heat to boiling to dissolve. Dispense; autoclave at 121°C for 15 min.

Arenavirus plaquing medium

Eagle basal medium (pH 7.3) without phenol red, 2× concentration
40 mM HEPES (*N*-2-hydroxyethylpiperazine-*N'*-2-ethanesulfonic acid) buffer
26 mM $NaHCO_3$
Add NaOH; adjust the pH to 7.0

Add an equal volume of the above solution to a 2% (wt/vol) solution of agarose in distilled water, at 50°C. Add fetal calf serum or heat-inactivated (56°C, 30 min) newborn calf serum to a final concentration of 5%.

Arginine hydrolysis

See decarboxylase media (modified from Moeller).

Aspergillus differential medium (94)

Tryptone	15.0 g
Yeast extract	10.0 g
Ferric citrate	0.5 g
Agar	15.0 g
Distilled water	1 liter

Mix reagents in large flask, add water to bring volume to 1 liter, and allow reagents to dissolve completely. Dispense at 7.0-ml portions into sterile, screw-cap 20- by 150-mm tubes. Autoclave for 15 min at 15 lb/m^2 and 121°C and allow ingredients to solidify in slants.

Comment. Unlike other pathogenic aspergilli, the reverse of colonies of members of the *Aspergillus flavus* group will develop a bright orange pigmentation when grown on the medium.

Auxanographic agar media

For carbohydrate assimilation tests, see carbon assimilation medium.

***Bacillus cereus* media**
Selective/diagnostic media for isolation and enumeration (chapter 33)

Bacillus cereus medium (BCM) (66)

$MgSO_4 \cdot 7H_2O$	0.02 g
Yeast extract	0.02 g
D-Mannitol	1.0 g
Agar	2.0 g
$(NH_4)_2PO_4$	0.1 g
KCl	0.02 g
Bromocresol purple	4.0 mg
Distilled water	100 ml
pH before autoclaving 7.0	
add Egg yolk emulsion (20%)	10.0 ml

Mix all ingredients except egg yolk emulsion in water. Heat to dissolve and autoclave for 15 min at 15 lb/in^2 (121°C). Cool to 50°C and add egg yolk emulsion. Mix gently and dispense into petri dishes.

Mannitol-yolk-polymyxin agar (MYP) (77)*[a]

Meat extract	0.1 g
Peptone	1.0 g
D-Mannitol	1.0 g
Agar	1.5 g
NaCl	1.0 g
Phenol red	2.5 mg
Distilled water	100 ml
pH before autoclaving 7.1	
add Egg yolk emulsion (20%)	10 ml
Polymyxin B sulfate[b]	1.0 mg

Mix all ingredients except polymyxin and egg yolk in water. Heat to dissolve and sterilize in autoclave for 15 min at 15 lb/in^2 (121°C). Cool to 50°C and add polymyxin B sulfate and egg yolk emulsion. Mix gently and dispense into petri dishes.

[a] Available from Difco (product no. 0810/30).
[b] In filter-sterilized solution.

Polymyxin-pyruvate-egg yolk-mannitol-bromothymol blue agar (PEMBA)*[a] (45)

Peptone	0.1 g
D-Mannitol	1.0 g
Agar	1.8 g
$MgSO_4 \cdot 7H_2O$	0.01 g
Na_2HPO_4	0.25 g
KH_2PO_4	0.025 g
NaCl	0.2 g
Sodium pyruvate	1.0 g
Bromothymol blue	0.01 g
Distilled water	100 ml
pH before autoclaving 7.4	
add Polymyxin B sulfate[b]	10,000 U
Egg yolk emulsion (20%)	5.0 ml

Mix all ingredients except polymyxin and egg yolk in water. Heat to dissolve and autoclave for 15 min at 15 lb/in^2 (121°C). Cool to 50°C and add polymyxin B sulfate and egg yolk emulsion. Mix well and dispense in petri dishes.

[a] Available from Oxoid, U.S.A. (product no. CM617), with egg yolk emulsion as a separate product (no. S47) and polymyxin supplement as a separate product (no. SR99).
[b] In a filter-sterilized solution.

Bacteroides bile esculin agar (BBE) (70)

Trypticase soy agar* (BBL)	40.0 g
Oxgall	20.0 g
Esculin	1.0 g
Ferric ammonium citrate	0.5 g
Hemin solution (5 mg/ml)	2.0 ml
Gentamicin solution (40 mg/ml)	2.5 ml
Distilled water	1.0 liter

Suspend ingredients in water and heat to dissolve. Adjust pH to 7.0. Autoclave at 121°C for 15 min. Cool to 50°C; pour plates.

Beef infusion agar*

Ground defatted beef, infusion from	453.6 g
Peptone	10.0 g
Sodium chloride	5.0 g
Agar	20.0 g
Distilled water	1.0 liter

Allow meat to infuse in water overnight at 4 to 5°C. Cook for 1 h at 80 to 90°C. Allow to stand for 2 h, and filter through muslin. Add peptone and salt, and adjust to pH 7.6 with 4% NaOH. Filter. Add agar, and autoclave. Filter through cotton or several layers of milk filter disks. Autoclave again.

Beef infusion broth*

Prepare as described above, but omit the agar.

Bennett agar
For demonstrating morphology of Nocardia spp. and streptomycetes

Yeast extract	1 g
Beef extract	1 g
N-Z amine A	2 g
Glucose	10 g
Agar	15 g
Distilled water	1 liter
Final pH 7.3	

Dissolve by boiling. Sterilize at 121°C for 15 min. Dispense 35-ml amounts into petri dishes.

Bicarbonate agar

Trypticase soy agar* (BBL; sterile fluid at 50°C)	90 ml
Sodium bicarbonate (7% aqueous, filter sterilized)	10 ml

Aseptically mix the ingredients and pour into plates.

Bile esculin agar*

Nutrient agar	23 g
or	
(Beef extract	3.0 g)
(Peptone	5.0 g)
(Agar	15.0 g)
Oxgall	40.0 g
Ferric citrate	0.5 g
Water	1 liter

Dissolve the nutrient agar, or beef extract, peptone, and agar, in 400 ml of water; heat until colloidal. Mix oxgall with 400 ml of water and heat into solution. Mix the ferric citrate with 100 ml of water and heat into solution.

Combine the solutions and mix well. Heat to 100°C for 10 min.

Autoclave at 121°C for 15 min. Cool to 50°C. (This is the base medium.)

Aseptically add 100 ml of esculin solution (100 ml of water plus 1 g of esculin, heated gently to obtain solution, and filter sterilized).

Dispense into sterile, 16- by 125-mm screw-capped tubes. Tighten the caps and cool in slanted position.

Alternatively, use dehydrated medium of this formula and prepare according to directions.

Optional: add 50 ml of horse serum to the sterile cool base.

Authors' note. The original medium contained horse serum (50 ml), added to the base medium. In a controlled study we found, however, that this addition was not necessary (27). At least one commercial source (Difco) adds the esculin to the base medium. The dehydrated medium sold by Difco can be resuspended, tubed, autoclaved, slanted, and used with excellent results.

Bile esculin agar can be used to identify all *Enterococcus* species as well as the group D streptococci, which will blacken the slant, usually within 48 h. Most non-group D streptococci do not blacken the medium.

Birdseed agar

See Staib agar.

Bismuth sulfite agar* (30)
For isolation of Salmonella typhi

Beef extract	5 g
Peptone	10 g
Dextrose	5 g
Disodium phosphate	4 g
Ferrous sulfate	0.3 g
Bismuth sulfite indicator	8 g
Agar	20 g
Brilliant green	0.025 g
Distilled water	1.0 liter
Final pH 7.7 ± 0.2	

Mix ingredients and heat to boiling but no longer than 1 to 2 min. Avoid overheating and do not autoclave. Cool to 50°C, swirl flask to mix evenly, and dispense into petri dishes.

Blood agar base*
Heart infusion agar

Beef heart muscle, infusion from	375.0 g
Tryptose or Thiotone peptic digest of animal tissue USP	10.0 g
Sodium chloride	5.0 g
Agar	15.0 g
Distilled or demineralized water	1 liter
pH 7.4	
plus	
Sterile, defibrinated animal blood	50 ml

Sterilize the base medium and cool to 50°C. Aseptically add rabbit blood (5%), rotate to mix, and pour 20-ml amounts into sterile petri dishes. Once the agar is set, invert and store in the refrigerator for up to 1 week. Test for sterility by incubating one or two plates per batch overnight.

Note. If bubbles appear in the poured plate during pouring of plates, pass a Bunsen flame over the agar to break up the bubbles before the agar sets.

For aerobic actinomycetes

Add defibrinated horse blood, 50 ml to 900 ml of base.

For Aeromonas spp.

Add 50 ml of sterile, defibrinated sheep blood (5%) and 70 mg of ampicillin per liter to the cooled agar base. Mix well and pour plates without creating bubbles.

For Corynebacterium spp.

Add 40 ml of sterile defibrinated sheep blood (59) to cooled agar. Pour plates as above.

For Streptococcus spp. and other fastidious organisms

Either Trypticase soy agar (BBL) or tryptic soy agar (Difco) is recommended as the base for some blood agar plates. For *Streptococcus* spp., the Trypticase soy agar is used in place of the blood agar or heart infusion agar base given above. The procedures given for blood agar base are followed. Once the agar is cooled, 25 ml of sterile, defibrinated sheep blood is added to 500 ml of Trypticase soy agar base. Pour plates as above.

For fastidious fungi

Use brain heart infusion agar as the base. Make up the base according to the directions given above. Cool the sterile agar base to 50°C and add 30 ml of sterile, defibrinated animal blood per 500 ml of base. Mix and pour into plates as described above.

For cultivation of Francisella tularensis

See cystine glucose blood agar.

Blood agar, diphasic, for trypanosomes and leishmanias, NIH method (48)

Lean beef, desiccated*	25.0 g
Neopeptone* or other peptone	10.0 g
Agar	10.0 g
Sodium chloride	2.5 g
Distilled water	500.0 ml

Infuse the beef and distilled water in a water bath for 1 h. Heat for 5 min at 80°C (176°F) to coagulate a portion of the protein. Filter with ordinary-grade filter paper. Add the rest of the above ingredients; adjust the pH to 7.2 to 7.4 with NaOH. Autoclave at 120°C for 20 min. Cool to 45°C, and aseptically add 10% defibrinated rabbit blood. Dispense 5-ml quantities into sterile tubes. Slant and cool. Just before inoculation, overlay with 2 ml of sterile Locke solution.

Locke solution

Sodium chloride	8.0 g
Potassium chloride	0.2 g
Calcium chloride	0.2 g
Monopotassium phosphate	0.3 g
Glucose	2.5 g
Distilled water	1.0 liter

Editors' note. The author recommends Difco ingredients.

Bordet-Gengou agar* (4)
For isolation of Bordetella pertussis and Bordetella parapertussis

Peeled, diced potatoes	187.5 g
Sodium chloride	10.0 g
Agar	30.0 g
Distilled water	1,500 ml
Glycerol	15 ml
Defibrinated sheep blood	300 ml
Final pH 6.7 ± 0.2	

Boil potatoes in water for 30 min. Filter through gauze. To 1 liter of the filtrate add glycerol, sodium chloride, and agar. Adjust pH to 7.0 and bring to a boil. Dispense. Autoclave for 15 min at 121°C. Store refrigerated. Just before use, melt base and equilibrate to 50°C. Add 30 ml of sheep blood per 100 ml of base. Pour four to five plates. Cephalexin, if added, may be used at 5 to 40 μg/ml. For primary isolation, it is optimal to use the plates on the day of preparation. If tightly sealed with Parafilm, the plates may be refrigerated and used for up to 1 week but with potential cost in sensitivity of the primary isolation methodology.

Bovine albumin polysorbate (Tween 80) medium Ellinghausen and McCullough, modified (23, 24, 50, 51)
Leptospira EMJH medium

Basal medium

Disodium phosphate (anhydrous)	1.0 g
Monopotassium phosphate (anhydrous)	0.3 g
Sodium chloride	1.0 g
Ammonium chloride, 25% aqueous	1.0 g
Thiamine hydrochloride, 0.5% aqueous	1.0 ml
Sodium pyruvate, 10% aqueous	1.0 ml
Glycerol, 10% aqueous	1.0 ml
Distilled water	996.0 ml

Dissolve salts in 996 ml of distilled water, add stock solutions, and adjust to pH 7.4. Autoclave at 121°C for 20 min.

Albumin-fatty acid supplement

Bovine albumin fraction V*	20.0 g
Calcium chloride · $2H_2O$ and magnesium chloride · $6H_2O$; aqueous solutions, 1.5% each salt	2.0 ml
Zinc sulfate · $7H_2O$, 0.4% aqueous	2.0 ml
Copper sulfate · $5H_2O$, 0.3% aqueous	0.2 ml
Ferrous sulfate · $7H_2O$, 0.5% aqueous	20.0 ml
Vitamin B_{12}, 0.2% aqueous	2.0 ml
Polysorbate (Tween) 80, 10% aqueous	25.0 ml
Distilled water, to	200.0 ml

Add the bovine albumin slowly, with careful stirring (to avoid foaming), to 100 ml of water. Slowly add the remaining ingredients (prepared as stock solutions) to the albumin solution, with constant stirring. Adjust the pH to 7.4, and add water to a 200-ml final volume. Sterilize by filtration through a membrane or Seitz filter (porosity, 0.2 to 0.3 μm). Store at 4 or −20°C.

Aseptically combine 1 part supplement with 9 parts basal medium, and dispense into sterile containers.

Note. If deionized water is used, preheat it to 56°C for 30 min to destroy naturally occurring water leptospires that are not retained by membrane and asbestos filters (0.2 μm).

A similar medium (24) containing added inactivated rabbit serum (0.4 to 1.0%), lactalbumin hydrolysate (0.1%), superoxide dismutase (1 μg/ml), and a 2:1 mixture of Tweens 80 (0.1%) and 40 (0.05%) is used to promote growth of highly fastidious serovars.

A comparable medium may be obtained from Intergen-Armour Biochemicals, Purchase, N.Y. (PLM-5), and from Scientific Protein Laboratories, Waunakee, Wis. (LEP-M5X).

Bovine albumin polysorbate (Tween 80) semisolid medium, Ellinghausen and McCullough, modified (24, 51)

To 900 ml of basal broth medium (see above), add 2.0 g of agar (quality tested). Heat to dissolve the agar. Dispense. Autoclave at 121°C for 20 min. Cool to 50°C. Add 1 volume of prewarmed (45 to 50°C) albumin supplement (see above) to 9 volumes of the agar basal medium.

Media may be stored at room temperature if dispensed into screw-cap tubes.

Brain heart infusion agar*
For primary recovery of fungi from clinical specimens

Calf brain, infusion from	200.0 g
Beef heart, infusion from	250.0 g
Proteose or Gelysate (BBL) pancreatic digest of gelatin	10.0 g
Glucose	2.0 g
Sodium chloride	5.0 g
Disodium phosphate	2.5 g
Agar	15.0 g
Distilled or demineralized water	1.0 liter
Final pH 7.4	

Add ingredients to water and mix. Heat to boiling to dissolve medium completely. Dispense agar according to need. Autoclave at 121°C for 15 min at 15 lb/in^2.

For *Actinomyces* spp., the use of freshly poured plates is recommended.

For *Cryptococcus neoformans,* it is recommended that 20 ml of medium be dispensed into clean 25- by 150-mm screw-cap tubes. After autoclaving, slant tubes on cooling racks until agar hardens. Tighten caps and label tubes. Tubes may be stored in the refrigerator at 4°C for up to 3 months.

Brain heart infusion blood agar

See blood agar base.

Brilliant green agar* (30)
For isolation of Salmonella spp. other than S. typhi

Yeast extract	3 g
Proteose Peptone no. 3	10 g
Sodium chloride	5 g
Lactose	10 g
Sucrose	10 g
Phenol red	0.08 g
Brilliant green	0.0125 g
Agar	20 g
Distilled water	1.0 liter
Final pH 6.9	

Mix ingredients and heat to dissolve completely. Sterilize in the autoclave for 15 min at 15 lb/in^2 (121°C). Avoid overheating. Dispense as needed.

Bromocresol purple (BCP) milk*

Purple milk	100.0 g
Demineralized water	1.0 liter

Mix to obtain a homogeneous suspension, and dispense 2- to 2.5-ml amounts into 11- by 75-mm tubes. Autoclave at 115 to 118°C for 15 min.

This medium is recommended for determining proteolytic properties of the aerobic actinomycetes. Observe for peptonization. *Nocardia asteroides* does not peptonize, but usually turns this medium alkaline. Incubate an uninoculated tube with every set of tests.

Bromocresol purple milk yeast extract + CCG (56)
For early isolation and differentiation of Trichophyton verrucosum from T. schoenleinii

Milk solution

Skim milk powder	80 g
Bromocresol purple, 1.6% in alcohol	2 ml
Distilled water	1 liter

Put on magnetic stirrer, mix well, and autoclave at 116°C for 8 min.

Agar solution

Difco agar	30 g
Distilled water	900 ml

Soak for 15 min, then autoclave at 121°C for 15 min. Mix milk and agar; cool to 50°C.
Add:

Cycloheximide (2%)	10 ml
Chloramphenicol (10 mg/ml)	10 ml
Gentamicin (50 mg/ml)	0.8 ml
Yeast extract (10%)	40 ml

Mix well. Dispense and slant.

Bromocresol purple-milk solids-glucose agar (BCP-MS-G) (106)
For differentiation of Trychophyton mentagrophytes from T. rubrum and T. mentagrophytes from Microsporum persicolor

A. Skim milk powder	80.0 g
Bromocresol purple, 1.6% in alcohol	2 ml
Distilled water	1.0 liter

Dissolve in 2-liter flask and autoclave at 116°C for 8 min.

B. Glucose	40 g
Distilled water	200 ml

Dissolve and autoclave at 115°C for 8 min or sterilize by membrane filtration.

C. Bacto-Agar (Difco)	30 g
Distilled water	800 ml

Soak for 15 min in 3-liter flask; autoclave at 121°C for 15 min, cool, and adjust pH to 6.6 with 1 N hydrochloric acid.

Add A and B to C, dispense aseptically, and slant.

Note. pH 6.6 was found to be preferable to pH 6.8.

Brucella agar*

Pancreatic digest of casein USP	10.0 g
Peptic digest of animal tissues USP	10.0 g
Yeast autolysate	2.0 g
Glucose	1.0 g
Sodium chloride	5.0 g
Sodium bisulfite	0.1 g
Agar	15.0 g
Distilled water	1.0 liter

Final pH 7.0 ± 0.2

Heat with agitation until dissolved. Dispense, and autoclave at 121°C for 15 min. Cool to 50°C.

Additives for anaerobes (107)

For nonselective media

Supplement before autoclaving with hemin (5 μg/ml) and, after autoclaving, with 50 ml of sterile defibrinated sheep blood and 1 ml of vitamin K_1 solution per liter. Use 50 ml of laked blood and 1 ml of vitamin K_1 per liter.

Note. Prepare and use vitamin K_1 (93) solution as follows. Weigh 0.2 g on a previously flamed aluminum foil square. Aseptically place 20 ml of absolute alcohol in a sterile tube. Add foil with sterile forceps. When solution has occurred, remove foil. Concentration is 0.01 g/ml.

Use 1 ml/liter in agar media (concentration, 10 μg/ml). For fluid media, dilute stock solution 1:100 in sterile water. Use 0.01 ml/liter (concentration, 0.1 μg/ml).

Prepare and use hemin solution as follows.

Dissolve 0.5 g of hemin in 10 ml of commercial ammonia water (or 1 N NaOH). Bring the volume to 100 ml with distilled water. Autoclave at 121°C for 15 min. Stock solution is 5 mg/ml. Use as a medium supplement in a final concentration of 5 μg/ml.

For selective media

For *Bacteroides* spp. (107), add kanamycin, 100 μg/ml, to brucella agar before autoclaving. Cool, and add blood and vitamin K_1 solution. Also add filter (0.45-μm pore size)-sterilized aqueous vancomycin to a concentration of 7.5 μg/ml.

For *B. melaninogenicus*, add kanamycin as for *Bacteroides* spp., but first lyse the blood by freezing and thawing.

For certain *Fusobacterium*, *Eubacterium*, and *Clostridium* species, add rifampin (50 μg/ml) and blood just before pouring plates.

For *Fusobacterium* and *Veillonella* species, add neomycin (100 μg/ml) before autoclaving; add blood, vitamin K_1, and 7.5 μg of vancomycin per ml just before pouring plates.

For *Clostridium* spp. and anaerobic cocci, add neomycin (100 μg/ml) before autoclaving. Add blood and vitamin K_1 just before pouring plates.

Brucella broth*

See brucella agar.

Leave out agar base. Heat with agitation until dissolved. Dispense, and autoclave at 121°C for 15 min.

Brucella selective medium

See brucella agar for selective media.

Buffered charcoal-yeast extract agar and supplements

See *Legionella pneumophila* media.

Buffered yeast extract broth

See *Legionella pneumophila* media.

Butzler medium (8)

Thioglycolate medium	1 liter
Sheep blood	50 to 70 ml
Bacitracin	25,000 IU
Novobiocin	5 mg
Actidione (cycloheximide)	50 mg
Cefazolin	15 mg
Colistin	10,000 U
Agar	10.5 g

Mix thioglycolate medium and agar. Dissolve by boiling. Sterilize the mixture in the autoclave at 121°C for 15 min and cool to 50°C. Add blood and other ingredients to the sterile molten agar and dispense.

Caffeic acid (nigerseed) agar
For primary recovery of Cryptococcus neoformans

Pulverized *Guizottia abyssinica* seed	50 g
Agar	15 g
Final pH 5.5	

Add seed to 100 ml of distilled water, and grind in a beaker. Boil for 0.5 h in 1 liter of water. Strain through cloth to remove the water extract from the seed. Adjust volume of extract to 1 liter with distilled water. Add agar, and heat until dissolved. Autoclave at 121°C for 15 min.

Or

Glucose	5 g
Ammonium sulfate	5 g
Yeast extract	2 g
Potassium phosphate	0.8 g
Magnesium sulfate	0.7 g
Caffeic acid	0.18 g
Ferric citrate solution	4.0 ml
Agar	20 g
Distilled water	1 liter

Prepare ferric citrate solution (10 mg plus 20 ml of water). Mix reagents in 1 liter of distilled water, autoclave at 121°C for 12 min, and dispense.

A comparable medium (CN-Screen) may be obtained from Flow Laboratories, catalog no. 3710045.

***Calymmatobacterium granulomatis* semidefined medium (37)**

Lactalbumin hydrolysate or papaic digest of soy meal USP*	20.0 g
Sodium chloride	2.5 g
Dipotassium phosphate	1.5 g
Sodium thioglycolate	0.6 g
L-Cystine	0.4 g
Distilled water	1.0 liter

Dissolve with heat, cool, and adjust to pH 7.2. Dispense in 20- to 22-ml amounts into screw-cap tubes. Autoclave at 121°C for 15 min, and tighten caps to maintain reduced conditions.

Campylobacter agar*

Proteose Peptone (Difco)	15 g
Liver digest	2.5 g
Yeast extract (Difco)	5 g
Sodium chloride	5 g
Bacto-Agar (Difco)	12 g
Final pH 7.4 ± 0.2	

Dissolve ingredients in 1 liter of distilled water by heating to a boil. Autoclave for 15 min at 15 lb/in^2 (121°C). Cool to 50°C.

Campylobacter agar base can be supplemented with 5 to 7% horse blood or 10% sheep blood as well as with two different antibiotic supplements:

Supplement S (amounts added per liter)

Vancomycin	10 mg
Polymyxin B	2,500 U
Trimethoprim	5 mg

Supplement B (amounts added per liter)

Vancomycin	10 mg
Polymyxin B	2,500 U
Trimethoprim	5 mg
Cephalothin	15 mg
Amphotericin B	2 mg

Aseptically add the blood and antibiotic supplements. Mix thoroughly but avoid air bubbles and dispense into sterile petri dishes.

Campy-BAP (3) (modified method using brucella agar base)

Brucella agar base (Oxoid, CM 169)	1 liter
Sheep blood	100 ml
Vancomycin	10 mg
Trimethroprim	5 mg
Polymyxin B	2,500 IU
Amphotericin B	2 mg
Cephalothin	15 mg

Sterilize brucella agar base and cool to 50°C. Add blood and other ingredients to sterile molten agar.

Carbohydrate fermentation broths
For identification of gram-positive cocci (streptococci) (arabinose, maltose, mannitol, melibiose, raffinose, sorbitol, sorbose, sucrose, trehalose)

Heart infusion broth, 22.5 g in 900 ml of distilled water

Carbohydrate, 10 g in 200 ml of distilled water

Indicator, 1 ml (1.6 g of bromocresol purple in 100 ml of 95% ethanol)

Add ingredients together, dissolve, and dispense in 3-ml amounts into 13- by 100-mm screw-cap tubes. Sterilize in an autoclave for 10 min at 121°C.

A positive reaction is recorded when the indicator changes from purple to yellow.

For anaerobes, see fermentation broth (CHO base).

Carbohydrate-peptone broth

Peptone	10.0 g
Sodium chloride	5.0 g
Test carbohydrate	10.0 g
Distilled water	1.0 liter
Andrade indicator	10.0 ml

Dissolve ingredients in water, adjust pH 7.4 to 7.5, and dispense. Autoclave at 121°C for 15 min.

Carbon assimilation medium
Mineral base medium (MBM)

Growth at the expense of organic compounds is determined in MBM containing:

Magnesium sulfate, anhydrous	0.1 g
Sodium chloride	5.0 g
Ammonium phosphate, monobasic	1.0 g
Potassium hydroxide, dibasic anhydrous	1.0 g
Distilled water	1.0 liter
Final pH 6.5 ± 0.1	

Prepare MBM at double concentration; sterilize by filtration. Add carbon sources to a final concentration of 0.03 M except 0.015 M for sodium acetate.

Agar solution

Agar	32 g
Distilled water	1 liter

Dissolve agar in water, bring to boil, and autoclave at 121°C for 15 min. Add an equal volume of sterile, melted agar solution to MBM containing the desired carbon source. Dispense into sterile tubes, and slant.

Test for utilization of the carbon source by inoculating the slant with 1 drop of broth suspension. Incubate aerobically at 30°C for 1 to 2 days and observe for growth.

Carbon assimilation medium (42) (auxanographic method for yeast identification)

For carbohydrate assimilation tests

Yeast nitrogen base	0.67 g
Noble or washed agar	20.00 g
Distilled water	1.00 liter

Tube method

Add ingredients to water and heat to dissolve. Tube medium in 20-ml aliquots in 18- by 150-mm screw-cap tubes. Autoclave at 15 lb/in^2 and 121°C for 15 min. Allow to harden as butts and store at 4°C.

Plate method

Prepare a 10× concentration of yeast nitrogen base* (YNB). Sterilize by filtration. Autoclave a 2% aqueous solution of washed agar. Autoclave at 121°C for 15 min, and cool to 50°C. Pipette 2.0 ml of the YNB into each petri plate. Mix 20 ml of sterile agar; allow the medium to solidify.

Use a sterile swab to streak an actively growing yeast culture from a Sabouraud slant for confluent growth. Allow the surface to dry. Place carbohydrate disks near the periphery of each plate. Use glucose, maltose, sucrose, lactose, galactose, cellobiose, melibiose, xylose, raffinose, inositol, trehalose, and dulcitol. Incubate at 25°C, and examine for growth around disks.

For nitrate assimilation tests

Use 20 g of yeast carbon base* (YCB), and proceed as described above. Add disks containing potassium nitrate or peptone (or amino acids).

A comparable medium may be obtained from BBL (no. 25155).

Cary and Blair transport (holding) medium*

Sodium thioglycolate	1.5 g
Disodium phosphate	1.1 g
Sodium chloride	5.0 g
Agar	5.0 g
Distilled or demineralized water	991.0 ml

Prepare in chemically clean glassware rinsed with Sorensen 0.067 M buffer (pH 8.1). Heat with agitation until the solution just becomes clear. Cool to 50°C, add 9 ml of freshly prepared aqueous 1% $CaCl_2$, and adjust the pH to about 8.4. Dispense 7 ml into previously rinsed and sterilized 9-ml screw-cap vials. Steam vials for 15 min, cool, and tighten the caps.

Cary and Blair transport medium, modified (PRAS)

Sodium thioglycolate	1.5 g
Calcium chloride	0.1 g
Disodium phosphate	0.1 g
Sodium chloride	5.0 g
Sodium bisulfite	0.1 g
Agar	5.0 g
Resazurin solution	4.0 g
Distilled water	1.0 liter

Mix ingredients; boil to dissolve. Gas out with carbon dioxide. Add 0.5 g of L-cysteine hydrochloride. Adjust so that final pH is 8.4.

Tube in roll tubes gassed out with nitrogen. Stopper with butyl stoppers. Steam for 15 min on 3 successive days.

Note. Prepare resazurin solution (84) by dissolving 0.05 g of resazurin in 200 ml of 95% ethanol and adding 180 ml of distilled water.

Casein agars

A. *With casein peptone for fungi (trichophyton agars 1 to 5*)*

Casein, 10% acid hydrolyzed, vitamin free	25.0 ml
(or Acid hydrolysate of casein	2.5 g)
Glucose	40.0 g
Magnesium sulfate	0.1 g
Monopotassium phosphate	1.8 g
Agar	20.0 g
Distilled water, to	1.0 liter

Adjust pH to 6.8. Dissolve by heating, distribute 100-ml quantities into flasks, and autoclave at 121°C for 15 min. Contents of several flasks may be distributed into test tubes and slanted for use as vitamin-free controls.

To 100 ml of sterile, melted casein agar, add autoclaved vitamin solutions as follows: thiamine, 2 ml of a stock solution containing 10 mg/liter of water; inositol, 2 ml of a stock solution containing 250 mg/100 ml of water; thiamine-inositol, 2 ml of each of the above stock solutions; nicotinic acid, 2 ml of a stock solution containing 10 mg/100 ml of water. Tube and slant.

B. *With skim milk for aerobic actinomycetes*

Skim milk powder	10 g
Distilled water	90 ml
Agar	3 g
Distilled water	97 ml

Add skim milk powder and distilled water together in a flask. Add agar and distilled water together in another flask. Sterilize the solutions separately by autoclaving for 121°C and 15 lb/in^2. Allow the solutions to cool to 50°C and then combine them. Aseptically dispense 25-ml aliquots into sterile 15- by 100-mm petri plates. Label plates and bag to reduce dehydration and contamination. Store in refrigerator at 4°C for up to 3 months.

Recommended for differentiation of species of aerobic actinomycetes.

To test for hydrolysis, streak a pure culture heavily on duplicate plates and incubate at room temperature or 37°C for up to 2 weeks. Hydrolysis, indicated by clearing of the medium under and around the inoculum, by *Streptomyces griseus* and *Actinomadura madurae;* no hydrolysis of the medium by *Nocardia asteroides.*

Casein hydrolysate (CAS)

For brief transport and fluorescent-antibody procedures for Bordetella pertussis

Casamino Acids*	1 g
Distilled water	100 ml

Dissolve the casein hydrolysate in the water in an acid-cleaned Pyrex beaker, and adjust the pH to 7.2. Dispense 0.5-ml amounts into 16- by 125-mm acid-cleaned Pyrex test tubes with screw caps. Autoclave, cool, seal, and store refrigerated for up to 1 year.

For use, immerse calcium alginate nasopharyngeal swabs in liquid, snip off the end of the wire, seal the tube, and keep it cool. Streak plates or prepare smears within 2 h.

Casein soy peptone agar

See soybean digest agar.

Casein-yeast extract-glucose (CYG) agar (113)

For agar dilution susceptibility tests with imidazole antifungal agents

Casein hydrolysate	5.00 g
Yeast extract	5.00 g
Glucose	5.00 g
Agar	20.00 g
Distilled water	1.00 liter
Final pH 7.0 ± 0.2	

Heat to boiling to dissolve. Dispense, and autoclave at 121°C for 15 min.

Casein-yeast extract-glucose (CYG) broth (113)

For susceptibility testing with imidazole antifungal agents

Casein hydrolysate	5.00 g
Yeast extract	5.00 g
Glucose	5.00 g
Distilled water	1.00 liter
Final pH 7.0 ± 0.2	

Heat to dissolve. Dispense, and autoclave at 121°C for 15 min.

CDC anaerobe blood agar

For anaerobes

Trypticase soy agar* (BBL)	40 g
Agar	5 g
Yeast extract	5 g
Hemin	5 mg
L-Cystine	400 mg
Vitamin K_1 stock solution	1 ml
Distilled water	1 liter
Final pH 7.5	

Dissolve the hemin and L-cystine in 5 ml of 1 N NaOH before adding the other ingredients.

Vitamin K_1 (3-phytylmenadione; ICN) stock solution is made by adding 1 g of vitamin K_1 to 99 ml of absolute ethanol.

Dissolve the ingredients by heating, adjust the pH, and autoclave at 121°C for 15 min. Cool to 50°C, add 50 ml of sterile defibrinated sheep blood, mix, and dispense 20 ml into sterile 15- by 100-mm plastic petri plates. After the medium has solidified, place the plates in cellophane bags and store in a refrigerator (4°C).

CDC modified McClung-Toabe egg yolk agar (EYA) (18)

For anaerobes

Pancreatic digest of casein*	40.0 g
$NaHPO_4$	5.0 g
NaCl	2.0 g
$MgSO_4$ (5% aqueous solution)	0.2 ml
Yeast extract*	5.0 g
D-Glucose	2.0 g
Agar	25.0 g
Distilled water	900.0 ml
Egg yolk suspension*	100.0 ml
Final pH 7.4	

Except for the egg yolk suspension, dissolve the ingredients by heating, autoclave at 121°C for 15 min, and cool to 60°C. Bring the temperature of the egg yolk suspension up to 60°C, and then add to the basal medium. Mix well and dispense 20 ml per 15- by 100-mm plastic petri plate.

The development of an insoluble, opaque precipitate within the agar indicates lecithinase activity. An iridescent sheen or "oil on water" appearance (pearly layer) on the surface growth indicates lipase activity. Proteolysis is indicated by a zone of translucent clearing in the medium around the colonies. These same reactions can be determined on Lombard-Dowell egg yolk agar (Presumpto quadrant plate).

Cefsulodin-irgasan-novobiocin (CIN) medium*
For isolation of Aeromonas and Plesiomonas spp.

Yeast extract (Difco)	2 g
Bacto-Peptone (Difco)	17 g
Proteose Peptone (Difco)	3 g
Mannitol	20 g
Sodium deoxycholate	0.5 g
Sodium cholate	0.5 g
Sodium chloride	1 g
Sodium pyruvate	2 g
Magnesium sulfate, heptahydrate	10 mg
Bacto-Agar (Difco)	13.5 g
Neutral red	30 mg
Crystal violet	1 mg
Irgasan	4 mg
Final pH 7.4 ± 0.2 at 25°C	

Mix ingredients and heat to dissolve. Sterilize in the autoclave for 15 min at 15 lb/in^2 (121°C). Cool to 50°C. Add antibiotic supplement:

Cefsulodin	4 mg
Novobiocin	2.5 mg

Mix thoroughly, avoiding air bubbles, and dispense in petri dishes. Monitor performance of the plates to check for deterioration.

Note. This medium is the same as yersinia medium with supplements.

Cell culture media

See Eagle, Hanks, and RPMI media.

Cell wall-defective forms (media for recovery)

See wall-defective bacterial medium.

Cereal agar* (75)
For sporulation of fungi

Precooked mixed cereal	100.0 g
Agar	15.0 g
Distilled water	1.0 liter

Commercially available mixed baby cereal may be used. Add dry ingredients to water and mix well. Heat in boiling water bath with frequent shaking until agar is dissolved and well distributed. Autoclave for 20 min at 121°C. Prepare as plates or slants.

Cetrimide agar, non-USP (109)

Heart infusion agar	40.0 g
Cetrimide (hexadecyltrimethylammonium bromide)	0.9 g
Distilled water	1.0 liter
Final pH 7.2	

Heat to dissolve. Dispense in 5-ml amounts into 15- by 125-mm test tubes, shaking flask to ensure even distribution of sediment.

Note. Lots of cetrimide vary, and the amount needed must be determined with known cultures.

Cetrimide agar, USP (36)
Pseudocel agar*
For nonfermenting gram-negative bacteria

Gelysate pancreatic digest of gelatin	20.0 g
Magnesium chloride	1.4 g
Potassium sulfate	10.0 g
Agar (dried)	13.6 g
Cetrimide*	0.3 g
Distilled water	1.0 liter

Suspend ingredients in the water, and add 10 ml of glycerol. Heat with frequent agitation, and boil for 1 min. Dispense, and autoclave at 118 to 121°C for 15 min.

Charcoal agar slant: diphasic medium for amoeba culture

A. Buffered saline overlay

1. Solution A (0.067 M KH_2PO_4)

Potassium dihydrogen phosphate (KH_2PO_4), anhydrous	9.07 g
Distilled water, to	1.0 liter

Dissolve the KH_2PO_4 in a small amount of water in a clean 1-liter volumetric flask. Add water to the 1-liter mark. Mix, and store in a glass-stoppered bottle.

2. Solution B (0.67 M Na_2HPO_4)

Disodium phosphate (Na_2HPO_4), anhydrous	9.46 g
Distilled water, to	1.0 liter

Prepare as directed for solution A.

Note. $Na_2HPO_4 \cdot 12H_2O$ may be substituted for anhydrous Na_2HPO_4 by using 23.88 g of crystalline compound per liter of solution.

3. Buffered saline (0.5%, pH 7.4)

Sodium chloride (NaCl)	5.0 g
Solution A	190.0 ml
Solution B	810.0 ml

Combine solutions A and B and add the NaCl. Stir thoroughly to dissolve. Sterilize at 15 lb/in^2 pressure for 15 min. Store in the refrigerator.

B. Preparation of agar slants

Disodium phosphate ($Na_2HPO_4 \cdot 12H_2O$)	3.0 g
Potassium phosphate (KH_2PO_4)	4.0 g
Sodium citrate crystals	1.0 g
Magnesium sulfate crystals	0.1 g
Ferric ammonium citrate	0.1 g
Asparagin (Difco)	2.0 g

Tryptone (Difco)	5.0 g
Glycerol (reagent grade)	10.0 ml
Distilled water	1.0 liter

Add the various ingredients, in the order listed, to the distilled water, and heat to dissolve. Do not boil. Stir thoroughly. Then add, stirring thoroughly after each addition:

Bacto-Agar (Difco)	10.0 g
Norit A (charcoal; Pfanstiehl)	10.0 g
Cholesterol in acetone, 1% solution (0.25 g of cholesterol in 25 ml of acetone) (cholesterol, C.P., ash free, for Kline Test; Pfanstiehl)	25.0 ml

Note. Be sure to keep the flask away from flames when adding the cholesterol-acetone.

Heat the entire mixture to boiling to dissolve the agar. Stir frequently to keep the charcoal in suspension. Dispense the hot solution in 3-ml amounts into tubes, and plug or cap. Autoclave for 15 min at 15 lb/in^2. Resuspend the charcoal, and allow the tubes to cool in a slanted position to form short butts or no butts. Add 3 ml of sterile 0.5% buffered saline overlay to the slants before specimen inoculation.

Commercial media are available. Dehydrated charcoal agar modified may be purchased as Hirsh charcoal agar (BBL) and used for slants to be overlaid with sterile Locke solution or 0.5% buffered saline. The medium is excellent for maintenance of amoeba cultures.

Charcoal-blood medium* (85, 86)

Charcoal agar (Oxoid CM 119)	51.0 g
Horse or sheep blood, defibrinated	100 ml
Cephalexin	0.04 g
Distilled water	1.0 liter
Final pH 7.4 ± 0.2	

Dissolve charcoal agar powder in distilled water. Sterilize for 15 min at 121°C. Equilibrate at 50°C; add blood and antibiotic. Mix and dispense into sterile petri dishes. For the semisolid transport medium (see chapter 46), prepare the medium with half-strength charcoal agar, dispense into tubes, and seal tightly.

Charcoal-yeast extract (CYE) agar (20)

Yeast extract	10.00 g
Activated charcoal (Norit SG)[a]	2.00 g
L-Cysteine hydrochloride · H_2O	0.40 g
Ferric pyrophosphate, soluble[b]	0.25 g
Agar	17.00 g
Distilled water	1.0 liter

[a]Available through Sigma, catalog no. C5510. Activated charcoal, washed with phosphoric and sulfuric acids.

[b]Available upon request from Biological Products Division, Centers for Disease Control, Atlanta, GA 30333. This reagent must be kept dry and stored in the dark. Do not use if its color changes from green to yellow or brown.

Add all ingredients of CYE agar except L-cysteine hydrochloride and soluble ferric pyrophosphate to 980 ml of distilled water; dissolve by boiling, autoclave at 121°C for 15 min, and cool to 50°C in a water bath.

Prepare separate fresh solutions of L-cysteine hydrochloride (0.40 g in 10 ml of distilled water) and soluble ferric pyrophosphate (0.25 g in 10 ml of distilled water). Filter sterilize each solution separately. Add the L-cysteine hydrochloride to the basal medium first; then add the ferric pyrophosphate.

Adjust the pH with 4.0 to 4.5 ml of 1.0 N KOH so that the final pH of the medium is 6.90 ± 0.05. Use 1.0 N HCl when necessary.

Editors' note. Either buffered charcoal-yeast extract (BBL 21808) or legionella agar base (Difco 1830) may be used as a base and supplemented with 0.004% L-cysteine and 0.0025% ferric phosphate.

Chlamydial media (82)

A. Growth medium

Eagle minimum essential medium in Earle salts (10×)	50 ml
Fetal calf serum	50 ml
L-Glutamine, 200 mM solution	5 ml
Sterile distilled water, to	500 ml

Adjust the pH to 7.4 with 7.5% sodium bicarbonate.

B. Isolation medium

Growth medium (see above) containing added:

Vancomycin	50 μg/ml
Gentamicin	10 μg/ml
Amphotericin B	2 μg/ml
Glucose	0.594 mg/ml
Cycloheximide	1 to 2 μg/ml

This medium may be used as a collecting medium by doubling the concentrations of vancomycin and amphotericin B.

C. Sucrose phosphate transport medium (2SP)

Sucrose	68.46 g
K_2HPO_4	2.088 g
KH_2PO_4	1.088 g
Distilled water	1.0 liter

Adjust the pH to 7.0 and autoclave; add:

Bovine serum, to	5%
Streptomycin	50 μg/ml
Vancomycin	100 μg/ml
Nystatin	25 U/ml

D. Sucrose-phosphate-glutamate transport medium (SPG)

Sucrose	75.00 g
KH_2PO_4	0.52 g
Na_2HPO_4	1.22 g
Glutamic acid	0.72 g
Distilled water, to	1.0 liter

Adjust the pH to 7.4 to 7.6, and autoclave; add antibiotics as described above (2SP).

Chocolate agars

Use one of the following as preferred, or as required to obtain satisfactory growth.

Beef infusion agar*
Blood agar base*
Casein peptone agar*
Eugonic agar*
Mueller-Hinton agar*

In addition, GC agar base* or GC medium base* may be used.

Pancreatic digest of casein USP	7.5 g
Peptic digest of animal tissue USP	7.5 g
(*or* Other peptone	15.0 g)
Cornstarch	1.0 g
Dipotassium phosphate	4.0 g
Monopotassium phosphate	1.0 g
Sodium chloride	5.0 g
Agar	10.0 g
Distilled water	1.0 liter

Prepare sterile base. Add sterile 5 to 10% defibrinated blood, and heat at about 80°C for 15 min or until the color is chocolate brown.

Variations

Add chemical supplement (either 1% IsoVitaleX [BBL 11875] or Chocolate II [BBL 21169]). See Thayer-Martin agar. Add yeast supplements. Prepare double-strength medium and add an equal volume of sterile 2% hemoglobin. Also add chemical supplement, especially for *Neisseria* and *Haemophilus* species.

Chopped meat (CM) medium (18)
For anaerobes

Ground beef, lean (connective tissue trimmed off before putting meat through grinder)	500 g
Distilled water	1.0 liter
Sodium hydroxide (1 N solution)	25 ml

Mix ingredients, heat to boiling, and cool at 4°C overnight. Skim remaining fat from surface. Filter through several layers of gauze. Save the liquid filtrate. Wash the meat particles with distilled water to remove excess NaOH, and spread on a clean towel to partially dry. Add enough distilled water to the liquid filtrate to give a final volume of 1,000 ml.

Trypticase (BBL)	30.0 g
Yeast extract (Difco)	5.0 g
K_2HPO_4	5.0 g
L-Cysteine	0.5 g
Hemin (1% solution)	0.5 ml
Vitamin K_1 (1% solution)	0.1 ml

See Lombard-Dowell broth for directions to make 1% hemin and vitamin K_1 solutions.

Add ingredients except for the L-cysteine, heat to dissolve, and cool to 50°C. Add the L-cysteine and mix to dissolve. Dispense 0.5 g of meat into 15- by 90-mm screw-cap tubes. Add 7 ml of enriched broth, autoclave at 121°C for 15 min, and cool.

See note on fermentation broth (CHO base) for anaerobes. Place tubes in glove box, tighten caps, remove from glove box, and store at 4°C or at ambient temperature.

Chopped meat medium is used to detect digestion of meat particles, gas, or blackening of the meat. Plain chopped meat broth is also an excellent holding medium for anaerobe stock cultures (33).

Chopped meat-glucose (CMG) medium
For anaerobes

Follow the formula for chopped meat medium. In addition, add 3.0 g of D-glucose to the broth before autoclaving.

Christensen urea broth* (10, 54)

Bacto-Peptone (Difco)	1 g
Sodium chloride	5 g
Monopotassium phosphate	2 g
Phenol red 0.2% (alcoholic)	8 ml
Distilled water	900 ml

Dissolve and adjust the pH to 6.9. Autoclave at 121°C for 15 min. Cool and add urea solution which was dissolved and sterilized by filtration:

Urea	20 g
Dextrose	1 g
Distilled water	100 ml

Dispense aseptically, 5 ml per tube.

Available commercially in dehydrated form or as prepared media from BBL Microbiology Systems (Cockeysville, Md.), Difco Laboratories (Detroit, Mich.), and Remel (Lenexa, Kans.).

CIN agar

See cefsulodin-irgasan-novobiocin (CIN) medium.

Citrate agar*
Simmons citrate agar

Sodium citrate	2.00 g
Sodium chloride	5.00 g
Magnesium sulfate	0.20 g
Monoammonium phosphate	1.00 g
Dipotassium phosphate	1.00 g
Agar, dried	15.00 g
(*or* Not dried	20.00 g)
Bromothymol blue	0.08 g
Distilled water	1.00 liter
Final pH 6.9	

Dispense into tubes, autoclave at 121°C for 15 min, and cool in the slanted position for 2.5-cm butt and 3.8-cm slant.

Inoculate the slant with a straight wire from a saline suspension of a young agar culture. Incubate at 37°C for 4 days. If equivocal results are obtained, as sometimes happens with members of the genus *Providencia*, for example, the test should be repeated and incubated at room temperature for 7 days.

Columbia agar base*

Polypeptone (BBL) or Pantone (Difco)	10.0 g
Biosate (BBL) or Bitone	10.0 g
Myosate (BBL) or tryptic digest of beef heart	3.0 g
Cornstarch	1.0 g
Sodium chloride	5.0 g
Agar	13.5 g
Distilled or demineralized water	1.0 liter
Final pH 7.3 ± 0.2	

Heat with agitation until the medium boils. Dispense and autoclave at 121°C for 15 min.

Columbia CNA agar*

Polypeptone peptone	10.0 g
Biosate peptone	10.0 g
Myosate peptone	3.0 g
Cornstarch	1.0 g
Sodium chloride	5.0 g
Agar	13.5 g
Final pH 7.3	

Suspend 42.5 g of Columbia agar base in 1 liter of distilled water, and heat with frequent agitation. Boil for 1 min, dispense, and autoclave for 15 min at 121°C.

Cool to 45°C, and then add 50 ml of defibrinated sheep blood and 5 ml of a solution containing 10 mg of colistin and 10 to 15 mg of nalidixic acid.

Note. The above is the BBL formulation. Different suppliers have other trade names for their peptones.

Congo red-magnesium oxalate (CRMOX) agar (88)

For detection of pathogenic serotypes of Yersinia enterocolitica and for determination of whether Yersinia strains contain the Yersinia virulence plasmid

This medium is useful for detecting pathogenic serotypes (strains) of *Y. enterocolitica* and other *Yersinia* species. These strains carry the 40- to 46-megadalton *Yersinia* virulence plasmid that is essential for tissue invasion and responsible for a number of phenotypic properties, including the uptake of Congo red dye, calcium-dependent growth, and temperature-dependent autoagglutination. The medium was formulated by Riley and Toma (88), and it allows the determination of Congo red uptake and calcium-dependent growth on the same plate.

Component 1: Tryptic soy agar

Tryptic soy agar	40 g
Water	825 ml

Suspend the agar in the water. Heat to boiling to dissolve. Autoclave at 121°C for 15 min. Cool to 45 to 50°C.

Component 2: Magnesium chloride solution (0.25 M)

Magnesium chloride ($MgCl_2 \cdot 6H_2O$)	50.8 g
Water	1.0 liter

Dissolve and autoclave at 121°C for 15 min.

Component 3: Sodium oxalate solution (0.25 M)

Sodium oxalate ($Na_2C_2O_4$)	33.2 g
Water	1.0 liter

Dissolve and autoclave at 121°C for 15 min.

Component 4: D-Galactose solution (20%)

D-Galactose	200.0 g
Water	1.0 liter

Dissolve with gentle heating if necessary. Filter sterilize (or autoclave for 10 min at 115°C).

Component 5: Congo red solution (1%)

Congo red dye	10 g
Water	1 liter

Dissolve the dye; autoclave at 121°C for 15 min.

Final medium

Component 1 (cooled to 45 to 50°C)	825 ml
Component 2	80 ml
Component 3	80 ml
Component 4	10 ml
Component 5	5 ml

Aseptically remove the designated amounts of components 2 to 5 into a sterile bottle; warm to 45 to 50°C; add to component 1. Mix well by gentle stirring, and pour into plates. Store at 4°C in sealed bags until needed. The medium should be stable for at least three months (88).

When first prepared, this medium can be orange-pink, but with storage in the refrigerator it changes to become the color of MacConkey agar. The original color may depend on particular lot numbers of the ingredients because some authors have not noted this color change (88).

Strains of *Y. enterocolitica* are streaked on the medium and incubated at 37°C for 24 to 48 h. Strains of pathogenic serotypes produce tiny colonies because the medium is low in calcium ions (oxylate chelates Ca^{2+}, and Mg^{2+} is a competitive inhibitor of Ca^{2+}). In addition, the colonies take up the Congo red dye and become red (see Fig. 1 in chapter 36 for a photograph of typical colonies). Strains of nonpathogenic *Y. enterocolitica* serotypes do not contain the *Yersinia* virulence plasmid and are colorless and much larger. If the plates are incubated for several days at 37°C, large colorless daughter colonies will grow out of the original tiny red colonies. When this colorless growth is picked and restreaked on CRMOX agar, only large colorless colonies develop, presumably because of loss of the *Yersinia* virulence plasmid. In practice, plates of pathogenic serotypes of *Y. enterocolitica* almost always contain large colorless colonies (88) in addition to tiny red colonies because the *Yersinia* virulence plasmid is unstable, particularly when the strain has been grown at 37°C. To fully differentiate pathogenic serotypes of *Y. enterocolitica*, CRMOX agar should be used in conjunction with the pyrazinamidase test, salicin-esculin fermentation, and other tests if possible.

For quality control, streak a pathogenic and a nonpathogenic serotype of *Y. enterocolitica* onto the medium. The pathogenic serotype will produce many tiny red colonies and usually some large colorless colonies. The nonpathogenic serotype will produce only large colorless colonies.

Converse liquid medium (Levine modification) for *Coccidioides* species (13)
For induction of spherules of Coccidioides immitis

Ammonium acetate	1.23 g
Glucose	4.0 g
Dipotassium phosphate	0.52 g
Potassium phosphate	0.4 g
Magnesium sulfate	0.4 g
Zinc sulfate	0.002 g
Sodium chloride	0.014 g
Sodium carbonate	0.012 g
Tamol	0.5 g
Calcium chloride	0.002 g
Agar (Ionagar no. 2, Agarose, or purified agar)	10.0 g
Distilled water	1 liter

Mix reagents and bring to a boil. Autoclave for 15 min at 15 lb/in^2. Dispense 15.0-ml aliquots into sterile petri dishes. Allow to harden.

Inoculate with a suspension of arthroconidia. Incubate at 40°C in a candle jar or anaerobic incubator. Examine tease mounts (prepared in a bacteriological glove box or laminar-flow hood) microscopically for spherules. Endosporulating spherules should be apparent after 4 to 5 days of incubation.

Cornmeal agar* (75, 119)
For sporulation of fungi

Cornmeal	50.0 g
Agar	15.0 g
Distilled water	1.0 liter

Mix cornmeal in 500.0 ml of distilled water and heat for 1 h (or autoclave for 10 min at 121°C). Filter through cheesecloth, bring volume up to 1,000.0 ml, and add agar. Bring to a boil. Dispense into culture tubes or flasks and autoclave for 15 min at 121°C. Final pH at 25°C is 6.0.

Add 1 to 2 g of dextrose for pigment production of dermatophytes.

Available commercially in dehydrated form or as prepared media from BBL Microbiology Systems (Cockeysville, Md.), Difco Laboratories (Detroit, Mich.), and Remel (Lenexa, Kans.).

Cornmeal agar, modified (medium B) (2)
For sporulation of fungi

Cornmeal agar*	17 g
Glucose	2 g
Sucrose	3 g
Yeast extract	1 g
Water	1 liter

Melt to suspend the ingredients. Autoclave at 121°C for 15 min. Cool to 45 to 50°C, and dispense into sterile petri dishes.

Cornmeal agar without glucose* (42)
For yeast morphology studies

Cornmeal	40.0 g
Tween 80	3.0 ml
Agar	20.0 g
Distilled water	1.0 liter

Add cornmeal to water and simmer (60°C) for 1 h. Filter through gauze and restore filtrate volume to 1 liter. Add agar to filtrate and heat to dissolve. Add Tween 80. Autoclave at 15 lb/in^2 and 121°C for 15 min. Dispense in 20-ml aliquots in sterile petri dishes.

A comparable medium may be obtained from BBL (21854), Difco (0386-01-3), or Remel (01-328).

Cornmeal-polysorbate 80 agar*

Cornmeal	50 g
Polysorbate (Tween) 80	10 ml
Water	1 liter
Agar (not dried)	20 g

Simmer the cornmeal and water for 1 h. Filter through gauze. Restore filtrate to 1 liter. Add agar. Mix, and heat to melt the agar. Filter again if necessary. Add polysorbate 80. Add glycerol (20 to 30 ml) if desired. Autoclave at 121°C for 15 min. Cool to 45 to 50°C, and dispense into sterile petri dishes.

CTA medium* (115)
Cystine Trypticase agar medium (BBL)

Cystine	0.500 g
Pancreatic digest of casein USP	20.000 g
Agar	3.500 g
Sodium chloride	5.000 g
Sodium sulfite	0.500 g
Phenol red	0.017 g
Distilled water	1.000 liter
Final pH 7.3	

Mix, and heat with agitation until solution occurs. Dispense, and autoclave at 115 to 118°C for 15 min. Add filter-sterilized carbohydrates to a final concentration of 1%.

This medium may be modified by using CTA agar (BBL), adding filter-sterilized carbohydrates to a final concentration of 2%, and preparing as agar slants rather than agar deeps.

Cycloheximide-chloramphenicol agar* (33)
Mycosel agar (Difco), Mycobiotic agar (BBL), etc.

Sabouraud dextrose agar	1.00 liter
Agar	5.00 g
Cycloheximide, in 10 ml of acetone	0.4 to 0.5 g
Chloramphenicol, in 10 ml of 95% alcohol	0.05 g

Heat to dissolve the agar and the Sabouraud dextrose agar. Dispense into tubes, and autoclave at 121°C for 10 min. Cool in a slanted position.

Recommended for the routine isolation of most pathogenic fungi. For species susceptible to cycloheximide, the medium can be prepared without it. Not to be used for isolation of zygomycetes.

Cycloserine-cefoxitin-egg yolk-fructose agar (35)
For selective isolation of Clostridium difficile from feces

Proteose Peptone no. 2	40.0 g
Sodium orthophosphate (Na_2HPO_4)	5.0 g
Potassium dihydrophosphate (KH_2PO_4)	1.0 g
Sodium chloride	2.0 g
Magnesium sulfate	0.1 g
Fructose	6.0 g
Hemin solution, 5 mg/ml	1.0 ml
Neutral red (1% solution in ethanol)	3.0 ml
Agar	25.0 g
Distilled water	1.0 liter

Heat to mix and dispense into 100.0-ml amounts. Sterilize at 121°C for 15 min. Cool to 50°C and add cycloserine base to a final concentration of 500 mg/ml and cefoxitin base to a final concentration of 16 mg/ml. Add 10.0 ml of sterile egg yolk emulsion to each 100.0-ml volume, and pour plates.

Note. The medium can be made without egg yolk suspension, but lecithinase and lipase reactions cannot be determined.

Cystine glucose blood agar
Cystine heart agar*
For cultivation of Francisella tularensis

Beef heart, infusion from	500 g
Proteose Peptone (Difco)	10 g
Dextrose (Difco)	10 g
Sodium chloride	5 g
L-Cystine (Difco)	1 g
Bacto-Agar (Difco)	15 g
Distilled water	1 liter
Final pH 6.8 ± 0.2 at 25°C	
plus	
Rabbit blood, defibrinated	50 ml

Suspend ingredients in cold distilled water and heat to boiling to dissolve completely. Sterilize in autoclave for 15 min at 15 lb/in^2 and 121°C. Cool agar mixture to 50 to 60°C and aseptically add the rabbit blood. Mix well and chocolatize by incubating the mixture at 60°C for 1 h before dispensing in plates or tubes.

Cystine tellurite medium (32, 72)

Heart infusion agar, 2%, sterile, cooled to 50°C	100.0 ml
K_2TeO_3 (potassium tellurite), 0.3% (wt/vol), autoclaved	15.0 ml
Sheep blood, sterile	5.0 ml

Mix well and add:

L-Cystine powder, sterile	0.005 g

Pour into petri dishes while shaking the solution steadily so that the cystine ingredient does not go into the solution. The shelf life at 4°C is about 1 month.

Czapek agar* (82)
Czapek Dox medium
For identification of Aspergillus and Penicillium species

Sucrose	30.00 g
Sodium nitrate	3.00 g
Dipotassium phosphate	1.00 g
Magnesium sulfate	0.50 g
Potassium chloride	0.50 g
Ferrous sulfate	0.01 g
Agar	15.00 g
Demineralized water	1.00 liter
Final pH 7.3	

Suspend 50 g of the dehydrated material in 1 liter of distilled water. Mix thoroughly. When a uniform mixture has been obtained, heat with frequent agitation and boil for about 1 min to dissolve the agar. Sterilize by autoclaving at 121°C for 15 min. Aseptically dispense into plates before the agar solidifies.

Decarboxylase activity

Also see Fay and Barry medium.

Decarboxylase broths, Moeller*
Recommended for detection of arginine dihydrolase and lysine and ornithine decarboxylase activities

Peptic digest of animal tissue USP on Peptone (Orthana special)	5 g
Beef extract	5 g
Bromocresol purple	0.625 ml
Cresol red (0.2%; prepared by grinding 0.5 g of cresol red powder to a fine powder, adding 26.2 ml of 0.01 N NaOH, and diluting to 250 ml with distilled water)	2.5 ml
Pyridoxal	5 mg
Glucose	0.5 g
Distilled water	1.0 liter
Final pH 6.0 to 6.5	

Divide into four parts, with tube 1 as a control, and add 1% L-arginine monohydrochloride, L-lysine dihydrochloride, and L-ornithine dihydrochloride to the remaining portions. Alternatively, add 2% DL-amino acids. Readjust the pH of the ornithine portion.

Dispense in 3- to 4-ml amounts into 13- by 100-mm screw-cap tubes, and autoclave at 121°C for 10 min. A small amount of floccular precipitate in the ornithine does not interfere with its use.

For the test procedure, inoculate test and control portions lightly from a young agar slant culture. Cover immediately with a 4- to 5-mm layer of sterile mineral (paraffin) oil. Incubate at 37°C, and examine daily for 4 days.

A positive reaction is recorded when the indicators turn violet to purple (alkaline reaction). The medium turns yellow first; this is a result of acid production from glucose and does not indicate a positive reaction.

Decarboxylase media, modified from Moeller*
For identification of miscellaneous gram-negative bacteria

Peptone	5.0 g
Beef extract	5.0 g
Glucose	0.5 g
Bromocresol purple	0.01 g
Cresol red	0.005 g
Pyridoxal	0.005 g
L-Amino acid	10.0 g
Distilled water	1.0 liter

The basal medium (no amino acid), modified from that of Moeller, is used for detecting lysine decarboxylase, ornithine decarboxylase, and arginine dihydrolase activities. Prepare the basal medium and divide it into four equal parts. Add 2.5 g of L-arginine monohydrochloride (or 5 g of the DL-amino acid) to one portion, 2.5 g of L-lysine dihydrochloride to the second portion, and 2.5 g of L-ornithine dihydrochloride to the third portion; make no addition to the fourth (control) portion. Adjust each medium to pH 6.0, dispense in 1-ml amounts into 13-mm screw-cap tubes, and autoclave at 121°C for 15 min. The inocula for both nonfermenters and nutritionally fastidious bacteria should provide heavy suspensions in each medium. Overlay each medium with 4 to 5 mm of sterile mineral oil and incubate for 4 to 6 days. Record alkaline (purple) reactions as positive.

Dehydrated media are available from Difco.

Editors' note. From authors of chapter 40: There are numerous versions of the Moeller procedure. They vary in kinds of peptone (Moeller used Orthana's Thiotone, Difco uses Bacto-Peptone, Finegold and Baron's text [30] notes that Difco's Proteose Peptone no. 3 is an acceptable alternative to Orthana's peptone, and the fourth edition of this Manual [82] calls for "peptic digest of animal tissue USP"), amount of beef extract, amount of bromocresol purple, volumes of media, size of tubes, size of inocula, and kind of overlay (sterile mineral oil or molten petrolatum). As in other instances, Moeller's procedure was developed for enteric bacilli and may not be applicable to other groups of bacteria. The procedure above is adapted from that of the Centers for Disease Control.

Diphasic blood culture buffered charcoal-yeast extract media

See *Legionella pneumophila* media.

Dermatophyte test medium (DTM)* (108)
For primary recovery of dermatophytes

Phytone	10 g
Glucose	10 g
Agar	20 g
Phenol red solution	40 ml
HCl, 0.8 N	6 ml
Cycloheximide	0.5 g
Gentamicin	0.1 g
Chlortetracycline hydrochloride	0.1 g
Distilled water, to	1 liter

Add Phytone, glucose, and agar to 1 liter of distilled water, and boil. Add phenol red solution (0.5 g in 15 ml of 0.1 N NaOH made up to 100 ml with water). Dissolve cycloheximide in 2 ml of acetone and add while the medium is hot. Dissolve gentamicin in 2 ml of distilled water before adding to medium. Autoclave at 121°C for 10 min. Add chlorotetracycline dissolved in a 25-ml volume of sterile distilled water.

Available commercially from Remel (Lenexa, Kans.) and Difco Laboratories (Detroit, Mich.).

DNase test agar* (109)
For nonfermenting gram-negative bacteria

DNA	2.0 g
Pancreatic digest of casein USP	15.0 g
Papaic digest of soy meal USP	5.0 g
Sodium chloride	5.0 g
Agar	15.0 g
Distilled water	1.0 liter
Final pH 7.3	

Inoculate culture heavily over a 1-cm^2 area of the plate. Several cultures may be tested on the same plate. Incubate for 18 to 24 h, and flood with 1 N HCl. A zone of clearing around the colony indicates a positive DNase test.

Method of Gilardi (36)

DNase test agar	1.0 liter
Toluidine blue	0.1 g

Inoculate as described above, and observe for a change in the indicator to pink around the patch growth (patch inoculum). Strains producing equivocal results are retested by flooding a DNase test agar plate, without the indicator, with 1 N HCl. Incubate aerobically at 30°C for 1 to 2 days.

Dulaney slants (19)

Aseptically remove yolks from 5- to 8-day hen egg embryos and place in an equal volume of sterile Locke solution containing glass beads. Homogenize. Dispense the homogenate into slanted tubes, and coagulate with steam at 80°C for 15 min.

Prepare Locke solution as follows:

Sodium chloride	0.900 g
Calcium chloride	0.024 g
Potassium chloride	0.042 g
Sodium carbonate	0.020 g

Glucose	0.250 g
Distilled water	100.000 ml

Eagle media

For the growth of animal and animal cell culture systems

90% Eagle minimal essential medium (MEM) in Hanks basal salt solution (BSS) with 10% fetal bovine serum (FBS)

Eagle MEM in Hanks BSS	87 ml
FBS	10 ml
$NaHCO_3$ (7.5%)	1 ml
Penicillin (10,000 U/ml)-streptomycin (10 mg/ml)	1 ml
Amphotericin B (1 mg/ml)	0.1 ml

95% Eagle MEM with either Earle or Hanks balanced salt solution with 5% calf serum

For use with rhinoviruses

Distilled water, sterile	780 ml
Earle or Hanks balanced salt solution (10×)*	100 ml
Phenol red (0.5%)	4 ml
Amino acids (50×)*	20 ml
NaOH (1 N), to adjust pH to 7.0	(5 ml)
Vitamins (100×)*	10 ml
Calf serum	50 ml
$NaHCO_3$ (7.5%)	29.6 ml

Just before use, add:

Penicillin (200,000 U/ml)	(1 ml)
Streptomycin (500,000 μg/ml)	(0.4 ml)
L-Glutamine stock solution (2.9%)	10 ml

98% Eagle MEM in Earle BSS with 2% FBS

Eagle MEM in Earle BSS	94 ml
FBS	2 ml
$NaHCO_3$ (7.5%)	3 ml
Penicillin (10,000 U/ml)-streptomycin (10 mg/ml)	1 ml
Amphotericin B (1 mg/ml)	0.1 ml

The above ingredients are stored frozen except for the Eagle MEM, which is stored at 4°C, and the $NaHCO_3$, which is stored at room temperature. When the medium is to be used in culturing of viruses, the FBS should be inactivated at 56°C for 30 min.

Modified Eagle MEM for McCoy cells

Distilled H_2O	600 ml
Eagle MEM (10×)	100 ml
$NaHCO_3$ (7.5%)	7.5 ml
Glucose (1.5 mmol/ml)	20 ml
Glutamine (200 mmol/ml)	10 ml
Gentamicin sulfate (50 mg/ml)	0.2 ml
HEPES[a] buffer, 1 M	20 ml
FBS	100 ml
Distilled H_2O, to make	1 liter

[a] *N*-2-Hydroxyethylpiperazine-N′-2-ethanesulfonic acid.

Egg yolk agars

A. Blood agar base
B. Brain heart infusion agar
C. Soybean casein digest agar USP or other

Prepare egg yolk emulsion as described below. Alternatively, use commercial suspension as directed.

D. McClung-Toabe agar

For Bacillus anthracis

Pancreatic digest of casein USP	40.0 g
Disodium phosphate	5.0 g
Monopotassium phosphate	1.0 g
Sodium chloride	2.0 g
Magnesium sulfate	0.1 g
Glucose	2.0 g
Agar	25.0 g
Distilled water	1.0 liter

Dissolve, and adjust the pH to 7.6. Autoclave at 121°C for 15 min. Cool to 50 to 55°C.

Meanwhile, scrub, and then soak, an antibiotic-free hen egg in 95% ethanol for 1 h. Aseptically aspirate or separate the egg yolk.

Add one egg yolk to 500 ml of agar base, and stir to a smooth suspension with a sterile pipette. Alternatively, add commercial egg yolk emulsion* as directed.

E. McClung-Toabe agar, modified

For lecithinase and lipase tests

Proteose Peptone no. 2* or Polypeptone* (BBL)	40.0 g
Disodium phosphate	5.0 g
Monopotassium phosphate	1.0 g
Sodium chloride	2.0 g
Magnesium sulfate	0.1 g
Glucose	2.0 g
Hemin solution, 5 mg/ml	1.0 ml
Agar	20.0 g
Water	1.0 liter

Suspend ingredients, and adjust the pH to 7.6. Mix, and boil to dissolve. Dispense 20 ml per tube, and autoclave at 118°C for 15 min.

Cool to 50°C, and add 2 ml of egg yolk emulsion* or 1 ml of laboratory-prepared egg yolk emulsion per tube. Mix, and pour the plates. Use an emulsion of equal volumes of egg yolk in sterile saline. See D above.

For Clostridium species (107)

Add neomycin (100 μg/ml) to medium base before autoclaving. Cool, and add the egg yolk emulsion.

For Clostridium botulinum

Yeast extract	5.0 g
Pancreatic digest of casein	5.0 g
Proteose Peptone no. 2* or Polypeptone* (BBL)	20.0 g
Sodium chloride	5.0 g
Sodium thioglycolate	1.0 g

Agar	20.0 g
Distilled water	1.0 liter

Sterilize, and cool the medium base to 45 to 50°C. Add 80 ml of sterile egg yolk suspension. Mix, and pour the plates immediately. Dry the plates, and store in a refrigerator.

Elek agar

See KL-virulence agar.

Ellinghausen and McCullough media

See bovine albumin polysorbate (Tween 80) medium.

Enriched thioglycolate (THIO) medium (18)

Thioglycolate medium without indicator*	30.0 g
Hemin (1% solution)	0.5 ml
Vitamin K_1 (1% solution)	0.1 ml
Distilled water	1.0 liter

See Lombard-Dowell broth for directions to make 1% hemin and vitamin K_1 solutions.

Add all ingredients and heat to dissolve. Dispense 7 ml into 15- by 90-mm screw-cap tubes, autoclave at 121°C for 15 min, and cool.

See note on fermentation broth for anaerobes. Place tubes in anaerobic glove box, tighten caps, remove from glove box, and store at 4°C or ambient temperature.

Enriched thioglycolate medium with 20% bile (THIO + bile) (16, 17)

Prepare as described above, but add 20 g of oxgall* per liter of enriched thioglycolate medium before autoclaving (2% oxgall = 20% bile).

Compare growth in bile medium with growth in enriched thioglycolate medium. Record S for stimulated, N for no change, or I for inhibited.

Enrichment broth for *Aeromonas hydrophila* (57)

Maltose	3.500 g
L-Cysteine hydrochloride	0.300 g
Bile salts no. 3 (Difco)	1.000 g
Novobiocin	0.005 g
Yeast extract	3.000 g
Sodium chloride	5.000 g
Bromothymol blue	0.030 g
Distilled water	1.000 liter
Final pH 7.0	

Enteric base for *Listeria* species (72)

Phenol red broth base at pH 7.4

Peptone	10.000 g
Beef extract (optional)	1.000 g
Sodium chloride	5.000 g
Phenol red	0.018 g
Distilled water	1.000 liter

Enteric fermentation base (26)

For identification of Corynebacterium spp.

Peptone	10.0 g
Meat extract	3.0 g
Sodium chloride	5.0 g
Andrade indicator	10.0 g
Distilled water	1.0 liter

Dispense medium in 3-ml amounts into 15- by 125-mm tubes containing inverted Durham vials. Autoclave at 121°C for 15 min. After cooling, 0.3 ml of a 10% filter-sterilized carbohydrate solution is added aseptically to each tube to give a final concentration of 1%.

Eosin-methylene blue (EMB) agar* (30)

For differentiation of lactose and non-lactose fermenters

Peptone	10 g
Lactose	5 g
Sucrose	5 g
Dipotassium phosphate	2 g
Agar	13.5 g
Eosin Y	0.4 g
Methylene blue	0.065 g
Distilled water	1.0 liter

Mix ingredients and heat to dissolve completely. Autoclave for 15 min at 15 lb/in^2 (121°C); dispense.

Note. The spreading of *Proteus* spp. is inhibited by increasing the agar concentration by 5% (add an additional 3.65 g of agar). Levine EMB agar does not contain sucrose. *Proteus* colonies may have a characteristic green metallic sheen if the higher agar concentration and sucrose are used.

Esculin agar

For detection of esculin hydrolysis

Infusion agar*	40.0 g
Esculin	1.0 g
Ferric citrate	0.5 g
Distilled water	1.0 liter

Heat to melt agar, dispense in 3-ml amounts into 13-mm screw-cap tubes, autoclave at 121°C for 15 min, and solidify as slants.

To determine esculin hydrolysis, inoculate slants with pure cultures, and incubate aerobically at 30°C for 1 to 2 days. Esculin hydrolysis is tested by observing for a black precipitate around the growth (patch inoculum) on the agar. No precipitate (color change) is a negative reaction.

Esculin agar, modified

Esculin	1.0 g
Ferric citrate	0.5 g
Heart infusion agar* (blood agar base)	40.0 g
Distilled water	1.0 liter

Heat to dissolve. Cool to 55°C; adjust the pH to 7.0. Dispense in 5-ml amounts into 16- by 125-mm cotton-plugged tubes. Autoclave at 121°C for 15 min. Cool in slanted position.

Esculin hydrolysis is indicated when the medium turns black.

Esculin broth (16)
For anaerobes

Heart infusion broth*	25.0 g
Esculin	1.0 g
Agar	1.0 g
Distilled water	1.0 liter
Final pH 7.0	

Dissolve the ingredients by boiling, adjust the pH, dispense 7 ml into 15- by 90-mm screw-cap tubes, autoclave at 121°C for 15 min, and cool.

See note on fermentation broth for anaerobes. Place tubes in glove box, tighten caps, remove tubes from glove box, and store at 4°C or ambient temperature.

Editors' note. The author recommends the use of Difco heart infusion broth.

If esculin broth is used, read the reaction after 48 h of incubation. Add 1 dropperful of 1% ferric ammonium citrate, and read the immediate reaction. Interpret brownish-black color as positive and no color change as negative (18).

Farrell modified serum dextrose agar
Brucella selective medium

Add the following antibiotics to 1 liter of serum dextrose agar after autoclaving and cooling to 50°C.

Bacitracin (Burroughs Wellcome Co.): Dissolve in distilled water, 2,000 U/ml. Add 12.5 ml of stock. Final concentration is 25 U/ml of medium.

Polymyxin B (Burroughs Wellcome Co.): Dissolve in distilled water, 5,000 U/ml. Add 1 ml of stock. Final concentration is 5 U/ml of medium.

Actidione (cycloheximide) (The Upjohn Co.): Dissolve 1 g of Actidione in 5 ml of acetone and dilute 1:20 in distilled water (10,000 μg/ml). Add 10 ml of stock. Final concentration is 100 μg/ml of medium.

Vancomycin (Eli Lilly & Co.): Dissolve 50 mg in 1 ml of distilled water. Add 0.4 ml of stock. Final concentration is 20 μg/ml of medium.

Nalidixic acid (Winthrop Laboratories): Prepare 5% (wt/vol) stock solution in 0.5 M NaOH. Immediately before use, dilute 1:10 in distilled water. Add 1 ml to medium. Final concentration is 5 μg/ml of medium.

Nystatin (E. R. Squibb & Sons): Dissolve in distilled water to a concentration of 50,000 U/ml. Add 2 ml to medium. Final concentration is 100 U/ml of medium.

Fastidious anaerobe agar (FAA)*

Lab M peptone mix	23.0 g
Sodium chloride	5.0 g
Soluble starch	1.0 g
Lab M agar no. 2	12.0 g
Sodium bicarbonate	0.4 g
Dextrose	1.0 g
Sodium pyruvate	1.0 g
Cysteine hydrochloride	0.5 g
Hemin	0.01 g
Vitamin K	0.001 g
L-Arginine	1.0 g
Soluble pyrophosphate	0.25 g
Sodium succinate	0.5 g
Distilled water	1.0 liter

Mix all ingredients, and boil to dissolve agar. Adjust pH to 7.2. Autoclave at 121°C for 15 min. Cool to 50°C and add 50.0 ml of sterile, defibrinated sheep blood.

For selective media

For *Fusobacterium* spp., add neomycin (100.0 μg/ml) before autoclaving and add vancomycin (7.5 μg/ml) just before pouring plates.

For an alternative selective medium for *Fusobacterium* spp., add neomycin (100.0 μg/ml) before autoclaving and add vancomycin (5.0 μg/ml) and josamycin (3.0 μg/ml) just before pouring plates.

Ready-to-use powder is available from Lab M, Ltd., Bury, England (catalog no. LAB 90).

Fay and Barry medium (1)
For determination of decarboxylase activities of Aeromonas spp. (chapter 38)

Bacto-Peptone (Difco)	5 g
Yeast extract (Difco)	3 g
Bromcresol purple in 50% ethanol (0.2%)	5 ml
Amino acids (Moeller)	10 g
Distilled water	1 liter
Final pH 5.5 ± 0.02	

Mix reagents and add supplements (L-arginine, L-ornithine, or L-lysine) at a concentration of 10 g/liter. Inoculate and overlay tubes as for other tests.

Fermentation basal medium (102)
Basal medium
For acid production and hydrolysis media for differentiation of aerobic actinomycetes

See hypoxanthine, tyrosine, and xanthine agars.

Diammonium phosphate	1.0 g
Potassium chloride	0.02 g
Magnesium sulfate	0.2 g
Agar	15.0 g
Distilled water	1.0 liter
Bromcresol purple (0.04%)	15 (20) ml

Tube in 5-ml aliquots and sterilize. Filter sterilize the appropriate sugar, cool to 50°C, and add 0.5-ml aliquots of filtered 10% carbohydrate solutions to the basal medium in each tube.

Inoculate the slants with several drops of an actively growing broth culture suspension. Incubate the slants for 4 weeks. Result: acid reaction = yellow color = positive.

Useful carbohydrates (add at 10% concentration):

adonitol	maltose
arabinose	mannitol
cellobiose	mannose
dulcitol	rhamnose
fructose	salicin
galactose	sorbitol
glucose	starch
glycerol	sucrose
inositol	trehalose
lactose	xylose

Fermentation broth (CHO base) (18)
For anaerobes

CHO medium base*	26.0 g
Distilled water	900.0 ml

Mix well and heat to dissolve. Autoclave at 121°C for 15 min. Cool to 50°C. Prepare fermentation base control medium by adding 100 ml of sterile distilled water. To prepare carbohydrate fermentation medium, add 100 ml of filter-sterilized aqueous carbohydrate stock solution to 900 ml of the sterile basal medium. Except for starch, each carbohydrate is prepared as a 6% stock solution, and the final concentration in the prepared CHO fermentation medium is 0.6%. The final concentration of the starch stock solution is 2.5%; the final concentration of starch in the CHO fermentation medium is 0.25%. Mix well and adjust the final pH to 7.0 ± 0.1 at 25°C. Dispense 7 ml into 15- by 90-mm screw-cap tubes.

Note. Pass the cooled tubes (with caps loose) into an anaerobic chamber containing an atmosphere of 85% N_2–10% H_2–5% CO_2. Fasten the caps securely, remove from the chamber, and store at ambient or refrigerator (4°C) temperature.

If an anaerobic chamber is not available, an alternative on the day of use would be to boil or steam the medium (with tube caps loose) for 10 min, cool, and inoculate immediately.

Editors' note. The CHO medium base is available from Difco.

Inoculate the tubes of liquid medium near the bottom (with a capillary pipette) with a few drops of culture per tube. Be sure to expel air from the pipette before placing it in the medium. One pipette may be used to inoculate multiple tubes. Fermentation media should be incubated under anaerobic conditions (glove box or jar) with tube caps loosened. Acid production as an indication of fermentation is determined by inspecting the tubes on days 1, 2, and 7. The bromothymol blue indicator in the tubes will turn yellow at pH 6.0 or lower. This change indicates a positive reaction. If the medium is blue or blue-green, the color indicates no change or a negative reaction. Some clostridia will reduce the indicator. When this occurs, remove 2 to 3 drops from each tube with a sterile capillary pipette to a spot plate, and add 2 to 3 drops of dilute bromothymol blue (prepared by adding 2 to 3 drops of 1% aqueous bromothymol blue to 30 ml of water in a 30-ml dropper bottle). Each tube with an acid reaction can be discarded. Reincubate all negative tubes. A final reading should be made at 7 days. Note that the majority of clinical isolates can be read after good growth is observed (after 24 to 48 h) and need not be held for 7 days.

Flagella broth

Tryptose (Difco) or Biosate (BBL)	10.0 g
Dipotassium phosphate	1.0 g
Sodium chloride	2.5 g
Distilled water	1.0 liter

Dissolve ingredients, and adjust the pH to 7.0. Dispense in 5-ml volumes into 15- by 125-mm test tubes. Autoclave at 121°C for 15 min.

Fletcher semisolid medium (31)
For the identification of leptospires (chapter 53)

Peptone	0.3 g
Beef extract	0.2 g
Sodium chloride	0.5 g
Agar	1.5 g
Distilled water	920.0 ml
Sterile rabbit serum	8 to 10%
Final pH 7.2 to 7.6	

Suspend base ingredients in cold water and heat to boiling to dissolve. Autoclave at 121°C for 15 min. Cool to 56°C and add filter-sterilized rabbit serum that has been warmed to 50°C. Dispense aseptically into tubes in 5- to 7-ml amounts. Inactivate the medium by placing the tubes in a water bath at 56°C for 1 h on 2 successive days. Medium can be stored at room temperature if dispensed into screw-cap tubes.

Note. If the distilled water is acid, it should be buffered before use to pH 7.4 with Sorensen buffer.

Fluorescence-lactose-denitrification (FLN) agar*

Proteose Peptone no. 3 (Difco)	10.0 g
Lactose	20.0 g
Potassium (or sodium) nitrate	2.0 g
Potassium (or sodium) nitrite	0.5 g
Magnesium sulfate heptahydrate	1.5 g
Dipotassium phosphate	1.5 g
Phenol red	0.01 g
Agar	15.0 g
Distilled water	1.0 liter

Adjust to pH 7.8, heat to melt agar, dispense in 4-ml amounts into 13-mm screw-cap tubes, autoclave at 121°C for 15 min, and solidify as slants with generous butts. Inoculate by stabbing and streaking, and incubate at 35°C for 4 days or at 35°C for 1 day, followed by 3 days at room temperature.

This medium contains nitrite to detect denitrification by bacteria that do not attack nitrate. It contains lactose and phenol red to detect strong acidification by lactose-positive acinetobacters and *Pseudomonas cepacia*. Other ingredients are similar to those of King medium B (11).

Available as a tubed medium from BBL and Scott.

Fluorouracil leptospira medium (49)
To suppress growth of contaminating microorganisms

Dissolve 10 g of 5-fluorouracil in approximately 50 ml of distilled water, add 1.0 to 2.0 ml of 2 N NaOH, and heat gently in a 56°C water bath for 1 to 2 h or until soluble. Adjust the pH to 7.4 to 7.6 with 1 N NaOH, and bring the volume to 100 ml with distilled water or heat-sterilized deionized water. Sterilize by filtration and store in refrigerator. Add aseptically, just before use, 0.1 ml of 5-fluorouracil for each 5 ml of bovine albumin polysorbate, Fletcher, or Korthof medium (200 μg/ml).

Note. Alternatively, the following antimicrobial agents may be used, combined with 5-fluorouracil (100 μg/ml): nalidixic acid (20 μg/ml) and fosfomycin (400 μg/ml).

Fowells acetate agar* (42)
For production of ascospores

Sodium acetate trihydrate	5 g
Agar	20 g
Distilled water	1 liter

Dissolve sodium acetate trihydrate in water and adjust to pH 6.5 to 7.0. Add agar to solution and dissolve by gentle heating. Dispense in 10-ml aliquots in 16- by 150-mm screw-cap tubes; autoclave at 15 lb/in^2 (121°C) for 15 min. Allow to harden as slants with 1-in. (ca. 2.5-cm) butts.

A comparable medium may be obtained from Remel (no. 09-046).

GC medium base

See chocolate agars.

Gelatinase test medium (20)

ACES buffer (Research Organics)	1.000 g
KOH pellets in 1.0 ml of distilled water (reagent grade, 85% KOH)	0.280 g
Activated charcoal (Norit A)	0.150 g
Yeast extract (Difco)	1.000 g
Gelatin (Difco)	3.000 g
α-Ketoglutarate monopotassium salt (Sigma)	0.100 g
L-Cysteine hydrochloride in 1.0 ml of distilled water (ICN)	0.040 g
Ferric pyrophosphate in 1.0 ml of distilled water (Sigma)	0.015 g
Distilled water	100 ml

This medium is prepared identically to buffered charcoal-yeast extract (BCYEα) medium except that gelatin is used in place of agar. Dispense in 2-ml volumes into small screw-cap tubes. Preincubate for 72 h at 35°C before using. Store at 4°C. Shelf life is 2 months at 5°C.

Gelatin infusion broth

Gelatin	40.0 g
Heart infusion broth (Difco)	25.0 g
Distilled water	1.0 liter

Heat to melt gelatin, dispense in 3-ml amounts into 13-mm screw-cap tubes, and autoclave at 121°C for 15 min. Stab inoculate and incubate at room temperature for up to 21 days. Examine daily for evidence of liquefaction.

Gelatin medium is commonly prepared with 12% gelatin in nutrient, peptone, or infusion broth. However, a broth medium with 4% gelatin is appreciably more sensitive than one with 12% gelatin. Most lots of gelatin form firm gels at 4% concentration; all form firm gels at 5% concentration. Incubation should be at 35°C for bacteria that grow poorly at room temperature. In such instances, the tubes should be refrigerated for 30 min before being examined for liquefaction. Most fastidious bacteria will grow in infusion broth, but some will not grow in nutrient or peptone broth.

Gelatin medium, 0.4%
For differentiation of Nocardia and Streptomyces spp.

Gelatin	4 g
Distilled water	1 liter

Adjust dilute gelatin to pH 7.0, distribute into tubes in 5-ml amounts, and autoclave. Inoculate tubes and incubate at room temperature. Examine the growth for quality and type after 3 to 4 weeks.

Results: *N. asteroides*—no growth or thin flaky growth; *N. brasiliensis*—good growth, usually with firm, spherical, compact colonies; *N. caviae*—fair growth, with small discrete colonies; *Streptomyces* spp.—growth, usually thin and stringy.

Glycine-cycloheximide-phenol red agar (95)

Solution A

Glycine	10.0 g
Yeast nitrogen base	6.7 g
Cycloheximide solution	1.6 ml
Distilled water	200.0 ml

Solution B

Agar	20.0 g
Phenol red solution	30.0 ml
Distilled water	770.0 ml

Cycloheximide solution

Cycloheximide	0.1 g
Distilled water	100.0 ml

Phenol red solution

Phenol red	0.5 g
Distilled water	100.0 ml

Prepare cycloheximide solution and filter sterilize. Store in refrigerator until needed. Prepare phenol red solution and store in refrigerator until needed. Add all reagents of solution A to water and mix well. Filter sterilize. Add all reagents of solution B to water and mix well. Autoclave for 20 min at 121°C and 15 lb/in^2. Allow solution B to cool to 55°C and add solution A. Mix well.

Aseptically dispense in 7-ml aliquots into 20- by 150-mm screw-cap tubes and allow to solidify in a slant.

Comment. Uninoculated medium is yellow-orange but will become bright red when inoculated with the B/C serotype of *Cryptococcus neoformans.*

GN broth* (30)
Enrichment broth for isolation of *Salmonella* and *Shigella* spp.

Peptone	20.0 g
Glucose	1.0 g
D-Mannitol	2.0 g
Sodium citrate	5.0 g
Sodium deoxycholate	0.5 g
Dipotassium phosphate	4.0 g
Monopotassium phosphate	1.5 g
Sodium chloride	5.0 g
Distilled water	1.0 liter

Final pH 7.0 ± 0.2

Dissolve the dehydrated medium in distilled water and autoclave at 116°C (10 lb/in^2) for 15 min or steam for 30 min at 100°C.

Guizottia abyssinica creatinine agar

See Staib agar.

Hanks balanced salts solution, 10× concentration (43)

For each liter of solution:

Solution 1

NaCl	80.0 g
KCl	4.0 g
$CaCl_2$	1.4 g
$MgSO_4$	2.0 g

Solution 2

$Na_2HPO_4 \cdot 12H_2O$	1.52 g
KH_2PO_4	0.60 g
Glucose	10.00 g
Phenol red, 1%	16.00 ml

Dissolve the ingredients for each solution in slightly less than 500 ml of reagent-grade water and then slowly add solution 2 to solution 1 with stirring. Adjust the final volume to 1 liter with reagent-grade water.

The 10× solution may be filter sterilized, or it may be diluted to 1× with reagent-grade water and then steam sterilized (in small volumes) for 10 min at 10 lb/in^2 (110°C). Longer steam sterilization or higher temperatures may caramelize the glucose.

For use, the 1× solution is buffered by the addition of 12.5 ml of sterile 2.8% $NaHCO_3$ solution per liter.

HBT plates for *Gardnerella vaginalis* (111)
Human blood bilayer with Tween 80

Columbia CNA agar (BBL)	42.5 g
Proteose Peptone no. 3	10.0 g
Deionized water	1 liter

Melt in a flask for 25 min. Mix well and dispense into 500-ml bottles. Autoclave at 15 lb/in^2 for 15 min. Cool to 50°C.

For base layer, add 2 ml of Fungizone (amphotericin B) and 3.75 ml of Tween 80 solution (see below) to each bottle. Mix well and immediately pour 7 ml into each 100- by 15-mm petri dish. Allow to harden completely.

For top blood layer, add 2 ml of Fungizone, 3.75 ml of Tween 80 solution, and 25 ml of human blood (outdated human blood may be used) to each 500-ml bottle. Immediately pour 14 ml over the first layer. Allow to harden.

This recipe will pour 46 plates.

Fungizone solution*: Add 10 ml of sterile water to a 50-mg vial (=5,000 μg/ml). Make a 1:10 dilution (500 μg/ml) for use in HBT plates.

Tween 80 solution: For a 1% solution, add 1 ml of Tween 80 to 99 ml of water. Adjust pH to 7.3 if necessary. Filter sterilize. Tween 80 is obtained from BBL and should not be used past the expiration date on the bottle.

Heart infusion agar*

Same as blood agar base, but no blood added.

Heart infusion agar for isolation of *Brucella* species

Heart infusion agar	40.0 g
Gelatin	1.0 g
Glucose	2.5 g
Distilled water	1.0 liter

Mix ingredients, autoclave for 15 min at 121°C, allow to cool to 50°C, and add 10 ml of sterile sheep blood and the following antibiotics:

Actidione (Upjohn): 0.2 ml of a 10-mg/ml stock solution; final concentration, 100 μg/ml of agar.

Bacitracin (Upjohn): 1 ml of a 5,000-μg/ml stock solution; final concentration, 25 μg/ml of agar.

Circulin (Upjohn): 0.3 ml of a 10-mg/ml stock solution; final concentration, 15 μg/ml of agar.

Polymyxin B (Burroughs Wellcome): 1.2 ml of a 1,000-μg/ml stock solution; final concentration, 6 μg/ml of agar.

Heart infusion broth*
Infusion broth
For growing nonfermenting gram-negative bacteria

Same as blood agar base or heart infusion agar, but without agar.

This broth medium, dispensed in 2- or 3-ml amounts into 13-mm screw-cap tubes, is suitable for determining growth at 42°C. Each tube (42°C experimental and 35°C control) should receive 1 loopful of broth culture as an inoculum. Incubate for 2 days at 42°C, followed by 2 days at 35°C (to determine whether the inoculum was killed at 42°C).

Infusion broth is preferable to a peptone broth for this test since it is applicable not only to nonfermenters but also to most fastidious bacteria.

Available as a dehydrated medium from BBL and Difco.

Heart infusion-tyrosine agar
For browning of blood-free media to identify Bordetella parapertussis

Heart infusion agar	40 g
L-Tyrosine	1 g
Distilled water	1 liter

Dissolve agar and tyrosine in water by boiling, and dispense into 15- by 125-mm tubes for slants.

Autoclave, slant the tubes, and allow to cool. Seal. Refrigerate the slants.

Shelf life is not known, so a positive control must be used when tests are done.

Inoculate a slant heavily with suspected *B. parapertussis;* incubate for 24 to 48 h at 35°C, with the cap loose to allow access of air. Development of a brown pigment in the medium is characteristic of *B. parapertussis.*

Editors' note. The author recommends the use of Difco heart infusion agar.

Hektoen enteric agar*
For isolation and differentiation of gram-negative enteric pathogens

Proteose Peptone	12 g
Bile salts	9 g
Yeast extract	3 g
Lactose	12 g
Salicin	2 g
Sucrose	12 g
Sodium chloride	5 g
Sodium thiosulfate	5 g
Ferric ammonium citrate	1.5 g
Agar	14 g
Acid fuchsin	0.1 g
Bromthymol blue	0.065 g
Distilled water	1 liter

Mix ingredients and heat to boiling. Dissolve medium completely. *Do not autoclave.* Cool to 50°C and pour into petri dishes.

Hickey and Tresner agar (38)

Dextrin	10 g
Pancreatic digest of casein USP*	2 g
Beef extract*	1 g
Yeast extract*	1 g
Agar	20 g
Cobalt chloride · $6H_2O$	20 mg
Demineralized water	1 liter

Dissolve and dispense for agar deeps. Autoclave at 121°C for 30 min. For pour slides, melt in a water bath and pipette 0.5 to 1.0 ml per slide.

Recommended for production of aerial hyphae, arthrospores, and pigment by *Nocardia* and *Streptomyces* species. For best results, allow surface to dry well before inoculation.

Hippurate test

See sodium hippurate broth.

***Histoplasma capsulatum* agar media (84)**
For conversion to or maintenance of the yeast phase

Required solutions and chemicals

Solution 1 (basal salts, in grams)

KH_2PO_4	8.00
$(NH_4)_2SO_4$	8.00
$MgSO_4 \cdot 7H_2O$	0.86
$CaCl_2$ (anhydrous)	0.08
$ZnSO_4 \cdot 7H_2O$	0.05

Dissolve the above in 500 ml and make to 1 liter with distilled water; store at 5°C.

Solution 2 (trace elements, in grams)

$FeSO_4 \cdot 7H_2O$	5.70
$MnCl_2 \cdot 6H_2O$	0.80
$NaMoO_4 \cdot 2H_2O$	0.15

Add 1.0 ml of concentrated HCl to 100 ml of distilled water in a 1-liter volumetric flask. Dissolve each component completely in the sequence given, and make to 1 liter.

Store at 5°C; good indefinitely; discard if red color or red precipitate appears.

Solution 3 (amino acids)

Casein hydrolysate, 10% acid-hydrolyzed, vitamin-free solution. (*Note.* Do not use "enzymatically digested" casein hydrolysate.)

Solution 4 (vitamins, in milligrams)

Inositol	200
Thiamine hydrochloride	200
Calcium pantothenate	200
Riboflavin	200
Nicotinamide	100
Biotin	10

Suspend and make to 1 liter in distilled water. Store frozen; if stored at 5°C, suspension is good for 1 year unless microbial growth occurs.

Solution 5 (hemin)

Suspend 200 mg of hemin in 10 to 20 ml of distilled water, and bring into solution by the addition of a few drops of concentrated ammonium hydroxide; bring final volume to 100 ml; store at 5°C.

Solution 6 (thioctic acid)

Dissolve 10 mg of DL-thioctic acid in 10 ml of 95% alcohol; store frozen.

Solution 7 (coenzyme A)

Dissolve 10 mg of coenzyme A in 10 ml of distilled water; add 2 drops of 0.05% $Na_2S \cdot 5H_2O$ solution made in freshly boiled distilled water. Store frozen.

Solution 8 (oleic acid)

Suspend 100 mg of oleic acid in 50 ml of distilled water and neutralize with NaOH to pH 9.0, bringing the fatty acid into complete solution by warming if necessary; adjust final volume to 100 ml. Store at 5°C.

Organic additions

Glucose, α-ketoglutaric acid, citric acid, L-cysteine hydrochloride, glutathione (reduced), L-asparagine, L-tryptophan, agar, purified starch (insoluble, i.e., not solubilized for chemical or enzymatic analyses)

Procedure for the preparation of 1 liter of agar medium

A. To a 500-ml graduated cylinder add and mix:

Solution 1	250 ml
Bring volume to approximately 400 ml with distilled water.	
Solution 2	10 ml
Solution 3	40 ml
Solution 4	10 ml
Solution 5	1 ml
Solution 6	0.1 ml
Solution 7	0.1 ml

B. Add and dissolve (in grams):

Citric acid	10.0
Glucose	10.0
α-Ketoglutaric acid	1.0
L-Cysteine hydrochloride	1.0
Glutathione (reduced)	0.5
L-Asparagine	0.1
L-Tryptophan	0.02

C. Neutralize carefully to pH 6.5 with 20% KOH; make to 500 ml and sterilize by filtration through a membrane filter (0.45-µm pore size) to give a 2× concentrated basal solution, i.e., part I.

D. To prepare 2× concentrated starch-oleic acid agar base, suspend 2 g of potato starch in 50 ml of distilled water and pour into 450 ml of boiling distilled water in a 2-liter flask; add 10 ml of solution 8; add 12.5 g of agar. Autoclave for sterilization at 121°C for 20 min. This is part II.

E. While still hot, add part I to part II, mix, and tube aseptically into screw-topped test tubes.

For growth, sporulation, and maintenance of the mycelial phase (83)

The agar medium for the growth of the mycelial phase of *H. capsulatum* is prepared by using the same components and procedure as for the preparation of the yeast-phase medium except that the $ZnSO_4 \cdot 7H_2O$ and citric acid are deleted and 15.0 g of agar per liter of medium is added.

Notes. Screw-cap tubes are preferred to prevent drying of the agar slants during storage at 5°C. The media may be stored for 6 to 12 months at 5°C. If during this period the slants should turn yellow due to oxidation, fresh media should be prepared.

Once prepared, neither the "yeast-phase" nor "mycelium" agar can be remelted and repoured for use.

If liquid media are desired, delete agar, reduce the concentration of starch to 0.5 g/liter, and reduce the oleic acid to 1 mg/liter of final medium (i.e., use 1 ml of solution 8).

Although developed for *H. capsulatum*, the yeast-phase agar supports excellent growth of *H. duboisii*, *Blastomyces dermatitidis*, and *Sporotrichum schenckii*.

H diphasic medium

See mycoplasmal media.

H (hominis) agar

See mycoplasmal media.

H (hominis) broth

See mycoplasmal media.

HR (high-resolution) antifungal assay medium buffered with 0.165 MOPS*

Yeast carbon base (Difco)	11.7 g
$(NH_4)_2SO_4$	2.5 g
Glutamine	584.6 mg
L-Arginine	42.1 mg
L-Histidine	21.0 mg
L-Isoleucine	52.5 mg
L-Leucine	52.5 mg
L-Lysine	73.1 mg
L-Methionine	14.9 mg
L-Threonine	47.6 mg
L-Tryptophan	8.2 mg
L-Valine	46.9 mg

Dissolve the HR mixture in approximately 900 ml of distilled water; add 1.0 g of $NaHCO_3$. Buffer to a pH of 7.0 with 0.165 MOPS buffer [3-(*N*-morpholino)propanesulfonic acid; Sigma Chemical, St. Louis, Mo.]. Bring the volume to 1.0 liter and filter sterilize.

A comparable dehydrated medium may be obtained from Oxoid (HR, CM 845).

Human immunodeficiency viruses, culture media for (14)

See RPMI 1640 medium.
See Hanks balanced saline solution.
See phosphate-buffered saline in chapter 122.

Hypoxanthine agar

Basal medium, sterile melted	100 ml
Hypoxanthine	0.5 g
Distilled water	10 ml
Final pH 7.0	

Prepare a sterile hypoxanthine solution by adding the hypoxanthine to the distilled water and autoclaving for 10 min at 121°C. Allow the sterile melted basal medium to cool almost to solidification. Add 10 ml of the sterile hypoxanthine solution to the flask or bottle of basal medium. Mix. Aseptically dispense 25-ml aliquots into sterile 15- by 100-mm petri plates. Label plates and bag to reduce contamination and dehydration. Plates may be stored at 4°C in the refrigerator for up to 2 months.

To determine hypoxanthine hydrolysis, inoculate the plates with pure cultures and incubate. Cultures should be examined for hydrolysis, indicated by a clearing of the medium under and around the inoculum by *Streptomyces griseus*. There is no hydrolysis of the medium by *Nocardia asteroides*.

Indole-nitrite medium (18)
For anaerobes

Dehydrated indole-nitrate medium*	25 g
Distilled water	1 liter
Final pH 7.2 ± 0.1	

Dissolve the ingredients by boiling for 1 min (with frequent mixing), adjust the pH, dispense 7 ml into 15- by 90-mm screw-cap tubes, autoclave at 121°C for 15 min, and cool.

See note on fermentation broth (CHO base) for anaerobes. Place tubes in glove box, tighten caps, remove from glove box, and store at 4°C or ambient temperature.

Indole can be detected 24 h after good growth is evident in indole-nitrite liquid medium or in another noncarbohydrate medium containing tryptophan (e.g., plain Lombard-Dowell broth or chopped meat medium). Extract the indole by adding 1 dropperful (about 1 ml) of xylene. Add 1 dropperful of Ehrlich reagent. A red ring within 15 min is positive; no red is negative (18).

Nitrate reduction is determined 24 h after good growth in indole-nitrite medium. Add 1 dropperful (about 1 ml) of nitrite reagent A and 0.5 dropperful of nitrite reagent B to the broth culture. A red color within 5 min is positive (nitrite present). If no color is observed, add a pinch of zinc dust. A red color after addition of zinc is negative; no color indicates reduction of nitrite to N_2 or another product (18).

Indole test media

A number of media can be used to test for indole production. Check your needs and organism to be tested before choosing a medium.

A. Method of Gilardi (36) (chapter 41)
For Pseudomonas and related genera

Trypticase nitrate broth

Inoculate a Trypticase nitrate broth tube with one 4-mm loopful of growth from a 24- to 48-h blood agar culture. Incubate aerobically at 30°C. Indole production is detected by adding Ehrlich reagent, after xylene extraction, to the 24-h-old broth culture. Repeat test after 48 h if necessary.

B. *For nonfermenting gram-negative bacteria*

Tryptone broth

Tryptone (Difco)	20 g
Distilled water	1 liter

Dispense in 3-ml amounts into 13-mm screw-cap tubes and autoclave at 121°C for 15 min.

Tryptone broth (4 ml in 15-mm tubes) is used by the Centers for Disease Control (18) in tests for indole production by nonfermenters. In this procedure, the medium is inoculated for 2 days at 35°C, extracted with xylene, and tested with Ehrlich reagent. However, buffered tryptophan medium and Kovacs reagent are more sensitive for detection of indole production by flavobacteria (71).

C. *For flavobacteria and other bacteria*

Tryptophan broth*

L-Tryptophan	0.5 g
Monopotassium phosphate	0.25 g
Sodium chloride	0.5 g
Distilled water	100 ml

Adjust pH to 7.4, sterilize by storage in a screw-cap bottle over a slight excess of chloroform, and dispense as needed in 1-ml amounts into 13-mm screw-cap tubes. Use ca. 1 mm^3 of cell paste as an inoculum and incubate for 18 to 24 h at 35°C. To test for indole, add 5 drops of modified Kovacs reagent. Red in the reagent layer within 5 min is a positive test. Do *not* shake tube after addition of reagent (71).

Available as a tableted medium from Key Scientific Products.

Inhibitory mold agar*
For primary recovery of fungi from clinical specimens; available from BBL

Tryptone	3 g
Beef extract	2 g
Yeast extract	5 g
Glucose	5 g
Soluble starch	2 g
Dextrin	1 g
Chloramphenicol	0.125 g
Salt A	10 ml
Salt C	20 ml
Agar	17 g
Distilled water	970 ml

Salt A

NaH_2PO_4	25 g
Na_2HPO_4	25 g
Distilled water	250 ml

Salt C

$MgSO_4 \cdot 7H_2O$	10 g
$FeSO_4 \cdot 7H_2O$	0.5 g
NaCl	0.5 g
$MnSO_4 \cdot 7H_2O$	2.0 ml
Distilled water	250 ml

Mix ingredients, and boil to dissolve agar. Adjust the pH to 6.7. Autoclave at 121°C for 15 min. Chloramphenicol is dissolved in 2 ml of alcohol (95%) and added to boiling medium. Dispense before or after autoclaving.

Inositol-bile salts-brilliant green (IBB) agar (98)
For isolation of Aeromonas and Plesiomonas spp.

Proteose Peptone (Difco)	10.0 g
Meat extract Lab Lemco (Oxoid)	5.0 g
Sodium chloride (Merck)	5.0 g
Bile salts no. 3 (Difco)	8.5 g
Brilliant green (Merck, 0.1% in water)	0.33 ml
Neutral red (Merck, 2% in water)	1.25 ml
meso-Inositol (Merck)	10.0 g
Bacto-Agar (Difco)	15.0 g
Distilled water, to	1 liter

Final pH 7.2 ± 0.1

Mix the ingredients and heat to boiling to dissolve the agar. Autoclave at 121°C for 15 min. Pour agar into petri dishes.

Iron-milk medium (18)
For anaerobes

Whole, nonhomogenized milk
Iron filings

Place a few iron filings in the bottom of 15- by 90-mm screw-cap tubes, add 7 ml of milk, autoclave at 121°C for 15 min, and cool.

See note on fermentation broth for anaerobes. Place tubes in glove box, tighten caps, remove, and store at 4°C or ambient temperature.

Iron-milk medium is used to detect proteolysis of milk proteins. Record C for clot or coagulation, G for gas production, D for digestion of milk proteins, and B for blackening. Hold for 7 days (or longer) before discarding as negative (18).

Jones-Kendrick pertussis transport medium

Soluble starch (BBL)	10.0 g
Yeast extract (Difco)	3.5 g
Heart infusion broth (Difco)	25.0 g
Agar (Difco)	20.0 g
Distilled water	1.0 liter
Activated charcoal powder (Norit)	4.0 g
Penicillin	300.0 U

Add starch, yeast extract, heart infusion, and agar to water; boil to dissolve. Add charcoal, mix well, and autoclave. Cool to 50°C, add penicillin, and dispense into small bottles as slants. Cool, and seal tightly. Store at 5°C. Stable for 2 to 3 months.

Use as a transport medium for *Bordetella pertussis* by inoculating the surface of a slant, sealing, and sending to a reference laboratory.

Kanamycin-vancomycin (KV) blood agar (18)
For anaerobes

Prepare CDC anaerobe blood agar. After the sheep blood has been added, aseptically add 100 mg (base activity) of kanamycin (Bristol Laboratories) and 7.5 mg (base activity) of vancomycin (Lilly) per liter.

Kanamycin-vancomycin laked blood agar (KVLB), modified

For selective growth of anaerobic gram-negative bacilli and pigmented *Bacteroides* spp. (but not including *Porphyromonas* spp.), prepare brucella agar and add 75 µg (base activity) of kanamycin per ml before autoclaving. After autoclaving, allow the agar to cool to 50°C and add vancomycin (7.5 µg/ml), vitamin K_1 (10.0 µg/ml), and laked sheep blood (5%) aseptically before pouring plates. Laked blood is prepared by freezing whole blood (fill tubes only 75% full to allow for expansion of frozen blood) overnight and then thawing at room temperature.

Note. Commercial injectable antibiotics (obtained from the pharmacy, for example) cannot be used. Laboratory standard powders (obtained directly from antibiotic manufacturers) must be used.

For a less selective KVLB that allows growth of *Porphyromonas* spp., add vancomycin at 2.0 µg/ml instead of 7.5 µg/ml.

Kelly medium, nonselective modified (59, 104)
For isolation of Borrelia burgdorferi and other spirochetes

Basal medium

CMRL-1066 with glutamine, 10× tissue culture medium (GIBCO)	100 ml
Sterile distilled water	900 ml
Proteose Peptone no. 2 (Difco)	5 g
Tryptone (Difco)	1 g
Autolyzed yeast (Difco)	1 g
N-2-Hydroxyethylpiperazine-*N*-2-ethanesulfonic acid (HEPES) buffer, acid form (Sigma)	6 g
Glucose alpha-D(+) (Sigma)	3 g
Sodium citrate (Sigma)	0.7 g
Sodium pyruvate (Sigma)	0.8 g
Sodium bicarbonate (Sigma)	2.2 g
N-Acetylglucosamine (Sigma)	0.4 g
$MgCl_2 \cdot 6H_2O$ (Sigma)	0.3 g

Hemin may also be added (1 ml of hemin solution).

Add all ingredients together and adjust pH to 7.6 with 5 N NaOH. Filter sterilize through a 0.45-µm-pore-size filter.

Gelatin solution

Gelatin (Fisher Scientific)	14 g
Distilled water	200 ml

Add together and heat gently to get gelatin into solution. Autoclave for 15 min at 15 lb/in^2 (121°C). Cool to 50°C. Add gelatin solution to basal medium. Add 143 ml of a 35% solution of sterile bovine serum albumin in water and 86 ml of sterile heat-inactivated rabbit serum. Aseptically dispense 7 ml per 8-ml tube. Use a large volume to prevent excessive oxygenation of the medium.

Kelly medium, selective modified (51, 52)
For isolation of Borrelia burgdorferi

Basal medium

1066 Connaught Medical Research Laboratories medium with glutamine, 10× (GIBCO)	100 ml
Double-distilled water	900 ml
Neopeptone (Difco)	5 g
Bovine serum albumin fraction V (Sigma)	50 g
HEPES buffer (Sigma)	6 g
Sodium citrate	0.7 g
Glucose	5 g
Sodium pyruvate (Sigma)	0.8 g
N-Acetylglucosamine (Sigma)	0.4 g
Sodium bicarbonate	2.2 g

Add all ingredients separately so that each ingredient completely dissolves before the next one is added. Adjust pH to 7.6 with 1 N NaOH.

Gelatin solution

Gelatin (Difco)	14 g
Distilled water	200 ml

Warm the solution so that the gelatin goes into solution. Add the gelatin solution to the basal medium and filter sterilize. Add 70 ml of partially hemolyzed rabbit serum (Hazleton) to produce a 6% serum concentration. Add kanamycin standard powder to 8 μg/ml and 5-fluorouracil standard powder to 230 μg/ml. Final pH of medium should be 7.7. Dispense as given for nonselective medium.

2-Ketogluconate broth

Monopotassium phosphate	5.4 g
Potassium nitrate	2.0 g
Potassium gluconate	20.0 g
Distilled water	1.0 liter
Final pH 6.5	

Sterilize by filtration. Dispense aseptically, 1 ml per sterile 13- by 100-mm tube.

See chapter 122.

3-Ketolactonate medium for agrobacteria

Yeast extract	10 g
Lactose	10 g
Agar	20 g
Distilled water	1 liter

Dispense in 20-ml amounts into 20- by 150-mm screw-cap tubes and autoclave at 121°C for 15 min. For use, prepare two petri plates from two tubes of the sterile medium. Inoculate a 1-cm area on each plate with a test strain and second areas with a positive control strain of agrobacterium. After 2 days of incubation at 25°C, flood one of the plates with Benedict solution and look for yellow zones (positive tests), appearing within 30 min, surrounding the areas of growth. If the test strain shows no yellow zone on the 2-day plate, the second plate should be tested after an additional 5 days of incubation.

See chapter 122.

Korthof medium, modified (28, 65)

Peptone	0.80 g
NaCl	1.40 g
$NaHCO_3$	0.02 g
KCl	0.04 g
$CaCl_2$	0.04 g
KH_2PO_4	0.24 g
$Na_2HPO_4 \cdot 2H_2O$	0.88 g
Distilled water	1.00 liter
Final pH 7.2 to 7.6	

Dissolve and steam solution (100°C) for 20 min. Cool overnight at 4°C, pass through filter paper (Whatman no. 1 or equivalent), dispense in tubes, and autoclave (121°C for 20 min). Cool to 50 to 56°C; add heat-inactivated (56°C, 30 to 60 min) filter-sterilized rabbit serum to a final concentration of 10% (vol/vol). Alternatively, the rabbit serum and the base may be mixed and sterilized by filtration prior to dispensing. If deionized water is used, preheat it to 56°C for 30 min to destroy naturally occurring water leptospires that are not retained by membrane and asbestos filters.

Kimmigs agar (base)* (62, 87)

Fungus agar according to Kimmig; used in agar dilution test with antifungal agents

Standard II nutrient broth (E. Merck, no. 7884)	15.0 g
Peptone (tryptic digest of meat; E. Merck, no. 7214)	5.0 g
Glucose	10.0 g
NaCl	5.0 g
Agar	15.0 g

Suspend 50 g in 1 liter of freshly distilled or completely demineralized water in which 5 ml of glycerol was dissolved previously. Allow to stand for 15 min; then boil to dissolve completely, with frequent shaking. After dispensing, sterilize in the autoclave (15 min at 121°C). Use for cultivation and strain preservation of fungi as well as for the assay of fungistatic agents. The pH of the ready-to-use medium at 35°C is 6.5 ± 0.2.

A comparable dehydrated medium (no. 5414) may be obtained from E. Merck, Darmstadt, Federal Republic of Germany, through E. M. Industries, Hawthorne, N.Y.

King medium B with nitrate (KBN medium)* (11)

Proteose Peptone no. 3 (Difco)	20.0 g
Glycerol	10.0 ml
Dipotassium phosphate	1.5 g
Magnesium sulfate heptahydrate	1.5 g
Potassium nitrate	2.0 g
Agar (Difco)	15.0 g
Distilled water	990 ml
pH 7.2	

Heat to melt agar, dispense in 4-ml amounts into 13-mm screw-cap tubes, autoclave at 121°C for 15 min, and solidify as slants with generous butts. Inoculate by stabbing and streaking and incubate at room temperature.

King devised medium B (11) to detect fluorescence. Supplemented with nitrate, medium B serves also to detect denitrification. When also supplemented with 0.1% L-tryptophan (KBNT medium), the medium will serve as source of cell paste for spot indole tests.

Dehydrated medium B is available from BBL as Flo agar and from Difco as Pseudomonas agar F.

KL-virulence agar (Elek agar) (22, 72)

Solution I

Proteose Peptone no. 3 (Difco)	3.0 g
Maltose	0.6 g
Distilled water	100.0 ml

Adjust solution to pH 7.8 and sterilize by filtration.

Solution II

Agar no. 1 (Oxoid)	3.0 g
NaCl	1.0 g
Distilled water	100.0 ml

Adjust to pH 7.8 and dissolve in steam for 1 h.

The solutions are mixed together, distributed in aliquots of 10 ml into tubes, and heated in steam for 15 min on 3 successive days. After cooling to 40°C, 2 to 4 ml of sterile bovine serum is added to each tube, and the contents are poured into petri dishes. Immediately after solidification, antitoxin filter paper strips are gently pressed with sterile forceps onto the agar surface. Instead of serum, the K-L enrichment (Difco) can be used (44, 72).

Kligler iron agar*

Peptone or polypeptone	20.000 g
Meat extract (optional)	3.000 g
Yeast extract (optional)	3.000 g
Lactose	10.000 g
Glucose	1.000 g
Sodium chloride	5.000 g
Ferric ammonium citrate	0.500 g
Sodium thiosulfate	0.500 g
Agar	12 to 15 g
Phenol red	0.025 g
Water	1 liter
Final pH ± 7.4	

Mix and heat with agitation until solution occurs. Dispense for deep slants, and autoclave at 121°C for 15 min.

Place tubes on a slant and let cool. Stab the slant with a pure culture. Hydrogen sulfide production is detected by the blackening of the butt. Incubate the cultures aerobically for 24 h.

Lactobacillus MRS broth

Lactobacillus MRS broth	55 g
Distilled water	1 liter

Dispense 5 ml per 15- by 125-mm test tube. Autoclave for 15 min at 121°C.

To test, inoculate test cultures with a loop or drop of fresh culture. Seal with melted petrolatum. Incubate culture at 35°C for 1 to 7 days. Production of gas is indicated when the petrolatum plug, which solidifies after cooling, is separated from the broth.

L-Cysteine buffered charcoal-yeast extract agar (BCYEα–L-Cys)

See *Legionella pneumophila* media.

***Legionella pneumophila* media (chapter 42)**

A. Buffered charcoal-yeast extract agar (BCYEα) with supplements (21)

ACES buffer [*N*-(2-acetamido)-2-aminoethanesulfonic acid]	10.00 g
KOH (reagent grade)	2.80 g
Activated charcoal (Norit A, acid washed)	1.50 g
Yeast extract	10.00 g
Agar	17.00 g
α-Ketoglutarate (monopotassium salt)	1.00 g
L-Cysteine hydrochloride dissolved in 10 ml of distilled H_2O	0.40 g
Ferric pyrophosphate dissolved in 10 ml of distilled H_2O	0.25 g
Distilled water to give	1 liter

Sterilize the L-cysteine and ferric pyrophosphate by filtration through a 0.2-μm-pore-size filter. Dissolve ACES buffer in 900 ml of distilled water at 50°C, and add KOH. Add charcoal, yeast extract, and α-ketoglutarate and mix well. Rinse sides of flask with 80 ml of distilled water and autoclave at 121°C for 15 min. Allow to cool to 50°C, and add 10 ml each of the filter-sterilized L-cysteine and ferric pyrophosphate to give a total volume of 1 liter. Adjust to approximately pH 6.9. Poured plates may be stored in sealed plastic bags for up to 2 months at 4°C.

B. Buffered charcoal-yeast extract agar with added albumin (BCYEα + alb) (21, 81)

Prepare as described for BCYEα but with the following changes: prepare 10 ml of a 1% solution of bovine serum albumin (fraction V) in distilled water and sterilize by filtration through a 0.2-μm-pore-size filter. To maintain the 1-liter volume, rinse sides of flask with 70 ml of distilled water and autoclave at 121°C for 15 min. After cooling, add filtered-sterilized L-cysteine, ferric pyrophosphate, and albumin.

C. Buffered charcoal-yeast extract agar with added antibiotics (selective) (21)

Prepare 1 liter of the BCYEα medium with supplements as described above; add the following filter-sterilized antimicrobial agents:

Polymyxin B sulfate	80,000 U
Anisomycin	80 g
Cefamandole lithium	4 μM

Adjust pH to approximately 6.9. Storage life is up to 1 month in sealed plastic bags at 4°C.

D. Buffered yeast extract broth (BYEB) (20, 78, 90, 92)

Use ingredients described for BCYEα but exclude charcoal and agar. This broth may be sterilized by filtration through a 0.2-μm-pore-size filter. If autoclaved, 1.5 g of activated charcoal should be added either loose or in a cellophane bag. After autoclaving at 121°C for 15 min, the charcoal should be removed by centrifugation or by removal of the cellophane bag. The authors have found that the blood culture system (agar and broth phases) described above makes an ideal broth for the growth of *Legionella* spp.

E. Diphasic blood culture buffered charcoal-yeast extract medium (21)

Broth phase

ACES buffer	10.00 g
KOH (reagent grade)	2.40 g
Yeast extract	10.00 g
α-Ketoglutarate (monopotassium salt)	1.00 g
L-Cysteine hydrochloride	0.40 g
Ferric pyrophosphate	0.25 g

Sodium polyaneolsulfonate (SPS)	0.30 g
Distilled water to give	1 liter

Agar phase

Agar	20.00 g
ACES buffer	10.00 g
Yeast extract	10.00 g
Activated charcoal (acid washed)	4.00 g
KOH (reagent grade)	2.80 g
α-Ketoglutarate (monopotassium salt)	1.00 g
Distilled water to give	1 liter

Prepare agar phase as described for BCYEα. Dispense into blood culture bottles and autoclave at 121°C for 15 min. Allow to cool with the bottles at an angle to give agar slants. Mix ingredients for broth phase (excluding L-cysteine and ferric pyrophosphate), autoclave, cool, and add filter-sterilized L-cysteine and ferric pyrophosphate. Distribute into blood culture bottles by syringe.

F. L-Cysteine-deficient buffered charcoal-yeast extract agar (BCYEα − L-Cys) (21)

Prepare as described for BCYEα but omit L-cysteine. Reflecting the lack of the acidic L-cysteine, the amount of KOH should be reduced to 2.65 g. Preincubate plates for 24 h at 35°C before using. Shelf life is 2 months at 5°C.

G. Modified Wadowsky-Yee medium (116, 117)

ACES buffer	10.00 g
KOH (reagent grade)	2.90 g
Activated charcoal (Norit A, acid washed)	1.50 g
Yeast extract	10.00 g
Agar	17.00 g
α-Ketoglutarate (monopotassium salt)	1.00 g
L-Cysteine hydrochloride dissolved in 10 ml of distilled H_2O	0.40 g
Ferric pyrophosphate dissolved in 10 ml of distilled H_2O	0.25 g
Distilled water to give	1 liter
Polymyxin B sulfate	50,000 U
Vancomycin hydrochloride	1.00 mg
Glycine	3.00 g
Bromothymol blue	10.00 mg
Bromocresol purple	10.00 mg
Anisomycin	80.00 mg

Dissolve the L-cysteine, ferric pyrophosphate, polymyxin, vancomycin, and anisomycin in distilled water. Dissolve the bromothymol blue and bromocresol purple separately in 0.1 N KOH. Prepare all solutions separately to give appropriate concentrations when added to 1 liter of medium; filter sterilize. Prepare all ingredients as described for BCYEα (note increased KOH), autoclave at 121°C for 15 min, allow to cool, and add filter-sterilized ingredients. Poured plates may be stored at 4°C in sealed plastic bags for up to 1 month.

Lipase test agar (Sierra medium) (99)

Peptone	10.0 g
Sodium chloride	5.0 g
Calcium chloride, monohydrous	0.1 g
Agar	15.0 g
Distilled water	1.0 liter
Final pH 7.4	

Mix, heat to boiling, and autoclave at 121°C for 15 min. Cool to 40 to 50°C.

Liquid enrichment medium (9)
Modified as personally communicated by P. Maximescu

Proteose Peptone no. 3 (Difco)	9.0 g
Meat extract	9.0 g
NaCl	2.7 g
$Na_2HPO_4 \cdot 12H_2O$	1.8 g
Glucose	1.8 g
L-Cystine, 1% (wt/vol)	10.0 ml
Distilled water	900.0 ml
Potassium tellurite, 2% (wt/vol)	75.0 ml

The thoroughly mixed solution is adjusted to pH 7.4 and Seitz filtered. The following sterile solutions are aseptically added:

Bovine serum	100.0 ml
Nystatin (1,000 U/ml)	1.15 ml
Fosfomycin (Boehringer GmbH, Mannheim, Federal Republic of Germany)	151.8 mg
Glucose 6-phosphate (Boehringer)	33.64 mg
Egg yolk suspension from	10 eggs
L-Cystine, 1% (wt/vol)	1.0 ml

Mix well and place 2 to 3 ml in tubes. This medium can be stored at 4°C for 1 to 2 months.

Listeria media (chapter 32)

A. Lithium chloride-phenylethanol-moxalactam (LPM) plating agar (69)

Phenylethanol agar (Difco)	35.5 g
Glycine anhydride	10 g
Lithium chloride	5 g
Distilled water	1 liter

Sterilize at 121°C for 12 min. Cool to 46°C; then add 2 ml of 1% filter-sterilized moxalactam.

B. Oxford agar (15)

Columbia blood agar base	39.0 g
Esculin	1.0 g
Ferric ammonium citrate	0.5 g
Lithium chloride	15.0 g
Distilled water	1 liter

Mix ingredients and heat to boiling to dissolve completely. Sterilize at 121°C for 15 min. Cool to 50°C and add:

Cycloheximide	400 mg
Colistin sulfate	20 mg
Acriflavine	5 mg
Cefotetan	2 mg
Fosfomycin	10 mg

Dispense and let cool.

C. Modified Oxford medium (MOX) (74)

Columbia blood agar base	39.0 g
Agar	2.0 g
Esculin	1.0 g
Ferric ammonium citrate	0.5 g
Lithium chloride	15.0 g
Colistin sulfate	10 mg
Distilled water	1 liter

Sterilize at 121°C for 10 min. Cool to 46°C and add:

Moxalactam	20 mg/liter

Dispense and let cool.

D. Polymyxin-acriflavine-lithium chloride-ceftazidime-esculin-mannitol (PALCAM) agar (114)

Columbia agar	39 g
D-Glucose	0.5 g
D-Mannitol	10 g
Yeast extract	3 g
Ferric ammonium citrate	0.5 g
Esculin	0.8 g
Lithium chloride	15 g
Phenol red	0.08 g
Distilled water	1 liter

Mix ingredients and heat to dissolve completely. Sterilize at 121°C for 15 min. Cool to 50°C and add:

Acriflavine	0.0005 g
Ceftazidime	0.02 g
Polymyxin B	100,000 IU

Dispense in plates or tubes and let cool.

E. USDA-FSIS listeria enrichment broth (73)

Enrichment broth I

Protease Peptone	5 g
Tryptone	5 g
Lab Lemco powder (Oxoid)	5 g
Yeast extract	5 g
NaCl	20 g
KH_2PO_4	1.35 g
Na_2HPO_4	12 g
Esculin	1 g
Nalidixic acid (2% in 0.1 M NaOH)	1 ml
Distilled water	1 liter

Sterilize at 121°C for 15 min. Cool and store in the refrigerator. Add 1 ml of 1.2% filter-sterilized acriflavine just before use (final concentration in the medium, 12 μg/ml).

Enrichment broth II

Same formula as enrichment broth I except for increased acriflavine (0.1 ml of 0.25% filter-sterilized acriflavine; final concentration in the medium, 25 μg/ml).

Lithium chloride-phenylethanol-moxalactam (LPM) plating agar

See listeria media.

Litmus milk

Litmus milk (Difco)	105 g
Distilled water	1 liter

Dispense in 15 ml per tube; autoclave at 121°C for 15 min.

An acid reaction has occurred when the medium turns white; a clot has occurred when the liquid turns to a solid, indicated when the tube can be inverted and the clot remains at the bottom of the tube.

Littman oxgall agar*

Oxgall	15.00 g
Peptone	10.00 g
Glucose	10.00 g
Agar, undried	20.00 g
(*or* Dried	16.00 g)
Crystal violet	0.01 g
Water	1.00 liter
Final pH 7.0 ± 0.2	

Mix and heat with agitation, and boil for 1 min.

Autoclave at 121°C for 15 min. Cool to 45 to 50°C, and add 3 ml of 1% aqueous solution of streptomycin. Mix and dispense aseptically into sterile tubes or onto plates.

Littman oxgall agar* with birdseed extract

Prepare as described for Littman oxgall agar, but use only 800 ml of water and 200 ml of birdseed extract in the basic medium.

Birdseed extract is prepared as follows. Grind 70 g of *Guizottia abyssinica* seeds in a blender. Add 300 ml of water. Autoclave at 115°C for 10 min. Filter through gauze.

Locke solution

See blood agar, diphasic.

Loeffler slant*

Tryptose (Difco)	5.0 g
Glucose	1.0 g
Beef serum	750 ml
Distilled water	250 ml

Sterilize by autoclaving at 121°C for 15 min. However, to avoid rupturing the slants, dissolved gases should be removed before full steam pressure is applied. This can be achieved by slow elevation of the autoclave temperature during an interval of 15 to 20 min with the exhaust valve closed. The exhaust valve is then opened only slightly until the temperature reaches 121°C.

Available as a tubed medium from Remel and Scott. Dehydrated beef serum is available from Difco.

Loeffler slant, modified (7, 72)

To 100 ml of peptone broth containing 1% glucose, adjusted to pH 7.6, add 300 ml of sterile normal bovine serum. After thorough mixing, distribute the medium in 3-ml aliquots into tubes and inspissate for 30 min in a slanting position.

Lombard-Dowell (LD) agar (18)
For anaerobes

Pancreatic digest of casein	5.0 g
Yeast extract	5.0 g
Sodium chloride	2.5 g
L-Tryptophan	0.2 g
Sodium sulfite	0.1 g
L-Cystine	0.4 g
Hemin	10.0 mg
Vitamin K_1, stock solution	1.0 ml
Agar	20.0 g
Distilled water	1.0 liter
Final pH 7.5	

See CDC anaerobe blood agar for directions for preparing L-cystine, hemin, and vitamin K_1 solutions.

Dissolve the ingredients by heating, autoclave at 121°C for 15 min, cool, and dispense. If quadrant plastic plates (Presumpto) are used, aseptically dispense 5 ml into one quadrant of each plate and allow agar to solidify. Store Presumpto quadrant plates in refrigerator (4°C).

Lombard-Dowell (LD) bile agar (18)
For anaerobes

Prepare LD agar as described above, but add 1.0 g of D-glucose and 20 g of oxgall per liter of medium before autoclaving.

Lombard-Dowell (LD) broth medium (18)
For anaerobes

Trypticase (BBL)	5.0 g
Yeast extract (Difco)	5.0 g
Sodium chloride	2.5 g
Sodium sulfite	0.1 g
L-Tryptophan	0.2 g
Hemin (1% solution)	1.0 ml
Vitamin K_1 (1% solution)	1.0 ml
Agar	0.7 g
Distilled water	1.0 liter

Dissolve the L-tryptophan in 5 ml of 1 N NaOH before combining with the other ingredients.

For a stock solution of hemin, dissolve 1 g in 20 ml of 1 N NaOH, and add distilled water to make a final volume of 100 ml. For a 1% stock solution of vitamin K_1, suspend 1 g in 99 ml of absolute ethanol.

Heat to dissolve the ingredients, and adjust the pH. Dispense 7 ml into 15- by 90-mm screw-cap tubes, autoclave at 121°C for 15 min, and cool.

See note on fermentation broth (CHO base) for anaerobes. Place tubes in glove box, tighten caps, remove from glove box, and store at 4°C or ambient temperature.

Lombard-Dowell egg yolk agar (LD EYA) (18)
For anaerobes

Prepare LD agar as described above, but add only 900 ml of distilled water, and add to it 2.0 g of D-glucose, 5.0 g of Na_2HPO_4, and 0.2 ml of a 5% aqueous solution of $MgSO_4$. Autoclave, and cool to 55°C. Add 100 ml of well-mixed egg yolk suspension. Mix well and dispense.

Lombard-Dowell (LD) esculin agar (18)
For anaerobes

Prepare LD agar as described above, but add 1.0 g of esculin and 0.5 g of ferric citrate before autoclaving.

Lombard-Dowell neomycin egg yolk agar (NEYA) (18)
For anaerobes

Prepare LD EYA. After it is autoclaved and cooled to 50°C, aseptically add 100 mg (base activity) of neomycin sulfate (Lilly) per liter, mix, and dispense.

Determination of biochemical characteristics on quadrant plates

In 1977, Dowell and Lombard (17) developed a system for presumptive identification of gram-negative, nonsporeforming anaerobic bacilli which requires a minimal number of media and of biochemical tests. This system includes two blood agar plates (for determination of relation to oxygen, colony characteristics, microscopic features, and inhibition by penicillin, rifampin, and kanamycin), one tube of enriched thioglycolate medium (to determine growth characteristics and cellular morphology and to provide inoculum for other tests), and a quadrant plate, known as the Presumpto I plate, containing the following:

1. Lombard-Dowell agar—for indole disk test and growth control (to compare with growth on Lombard-Dowell bile agar)
2. Lombard-Dowell esculin agar—for determination of esculin hydrolysis, H_2S production, and catalase
3. Lombard-Dowell egg yolk agar—for determination of lipase, lecithinase, and proteolysis
4. Lombard-Dowell bile agar—for determination of growth in the presence of 20% bile (2% oxgall) and formation of an insoluble precipitate in the medium (under and surrounding growth)

Inoculate the above agar-based differential media with (i) an overnight thioglycolate or cooked meat-glucose broth culture from an isolated colony (24- to 48-h cultures are used if overnight growth is inadequate) or (ii) a turbid cell suspension (McFarland no. 1) in Lombard-Dowell growth broth without glucose.

Place 1 or 2 drops of broth culture or cell suspension on each quadrant of the Presumpto plate, using a capillary pipette, and streak three-fourths of each quadrant.

Place a sterile 0.25-in. (0.6-cm) blank disk near the outer periphery of the inoculum on the Lombard-Dowell agar quadrant for the indole test.

Moisten a sterile swab in actively growing thioglycolate broth culture, and evenly inoculate the surface of a brucella blood agar plate. Apply the following disks:

penicillin, 2 U; kanamycin, 1,000 μg; and rifampin, 15 μg. Zones of inhibition of 12 mm or greater around the penicillin and kanamycin disks indicate susceptibility; zones of <12 mm indicate resistance. A 15-mm zone around the rifampin disk indicates susceptibility; <15 mm indicates resistance. If these disks are used, refer to the tables of Dowell and Lombard (17) or Koneman et al. (64a). These antibiotic disks are available from BBL.

Incubate the above media in an anaerobic system at 35°C for 48 h. If an anaerobic glove box is used, inspect the media after 18 to 24 h of incubation. If good growth is obtained, the reactions can be read after overnight incubation.

Determination of results and test interpretation

Indole test. Add 2 drops of paradimethylaminocinnamaldehyde reagent to the disk on Lombard-Dowell agar. Blue is positive; any other color or no color is negative.

Lombard-Dowell bile agar. (i) Growth equal to or greater than growth on the Lombard-Dowell agar control is recorded as E. Inhibition of growth on 20% bile medium (growth less than on the Lombard-Dowell agar control) is recorded as I. (ii) Check for an opaque or whitish yellow precipitate within the medium surrounding the colonies (known to be produced only by *Bacteroides fragilis* and some strains of *Bacteroides ovatus;* V. R. Dowell, Jr., personal communication).

Lombard-Dowell egg yolk agar. Lecithinase, lipase, and proteolytic activity are determined as for modified McClung-Toabe egg yolk agar (see chapters 52 and 122 for reactions on egg yolk agar).

Esculin hydrolysis on Lombard-Dowell esculin agar. Browning or blackening of the medium indicates esculin hydrolysis. Loss of fluorescence compared with an uninoculated control observed under UV light (365 nm) indicates esculin hydrolysis.

H_2S production. Black colonies on Lombard-Dowell esculin agar indicate H_2S production.

Catalase. Expose the quadrant plate to air for 30 min. Flood the esculin agar quadrant with 3% H_2O_2. Vigorous sustained bubbling indicates catalase production. This sometimes takes 30 s to 1 min.

Lowenstein-Jensen medium*

Monopotassium phosphate, anhydrous	2.40 g
Magnesium sulfate · $7H_2O$	0.24 g
Magnesium citrate	0.60 g
Asparagine	3.60 g
Potato flour	30.00 g
Glycerol	12.00 g
Distilled water	600.00 ml
Homogenized whole eggs	1,000.00 ml
Malachite green, 2% aqueous	20.00 ml

Dissolve the salts and asparagine in the water. Admix the glycerol and potato flour, autoclave at 121°C for 30 min, and cool to room temperature. Scrub eggs, not more than 1 week old, in 5% soap solution, and then rinse thoroughly in cold running water. Immerse in 70% ethyl alcohol for 15 min. Break eggs into a sterile flask. Homogenize by hand shaking, and filter through four layers of gauze.

Add 1 liter of homogenized eggs to the potato-salt mixture. Prepare the malachite green and admix thoroughly. Dispense 6 to 8 ml into 20- by 150-mm screw-cap tubes. Slant, and inspissate at 85°C for 50 min.

Incubate for 48 h at 37°C to check sterility, and store at 4 to 6°C with caps tightly closed.

Lysine and ornithine broth media*
For decarboxylase tests

L-Amino acid monohydrochloride	0.5 g
Monopotassium phosphate	1.0 g
Bromocresol green	0.002 g
Distilled water	100 ml

Adjust pH to 4.4, store in a screw-cap bottle over a slight excess of chloroform, and dispense as needed in 1-ml amounts into 13-mm screw-cap tubes. Use ca. 1 mm^3 of cell paste as the inoculum and incubate for 18 to 24 h at 35°C. Add 1 drop of 40% sodium (or potassium) hydroxide and 1 ml of ninhydrin reagent (0.1% ninhydrin in chloroform). Do *not* shake tube after addition of the ninhydrin. A purple color appearing in the chloroform phase within 5 min represents a positive test.

The drop of hydroxide is added to trap residual amino acid in the aqueous phase. The bromocresol green is not an essential constituent of these media; it is included to permit early (within hours) observation of alkalinization. Supplementation of the lysine medium with 50 mg of glucose will maintain the low pH that is optimal for lysine decarboxylase.

Available as tableted media from Key Scientific Products.

Lysozyme broth

A. Basal glycerol broth

Beef extract	3 g
Peptone	5 g
Glycerol	70 ml
Distilled water	1 liter

B. Lysozyme solution

Lysozyme	100 mg
HCl, 0.01 N	100 ml

Prepare the basal glycerol broth by adding the ingredients together and mixing. Dispense 500 ml of the broth in 5-ml aliquots into 16- by 125-mm screw-cap tubes. Sterilize the tubes and flask of remaining broth by autoclaving for 15 min at 121°C and 15 lb/in^2. Prepare the lysozyme solution by adding the lysozyme and 0.01 N HCl together. Sterilize by filtration through 0.22-μm-pore-size filter.

Prepare the lysozyme broth by adding 5 ml of the sterile lysozyme solution to 95 ml of the sterile basal glycerol broth. Mix well. Aseptically dispense 5-ml aliquots into sterile 16- by 125-mm screw-cap tubes. Save the remaining glycerol broth to prepare more lysozyme broth.

Solutions may be stored at 4°C in the refrigerator. Glycerol broth may be stored for up to 3 months, and lysozyme solution may be stored for only 1 week.

To test, inoculate both a basal glycerol broth control and lysozyme broth tubes. Incubate and observe for growth. Results: good growth of *Nocardia asteroides* in both the basal glycerol broth control tube and the lysozyme broth; good growth of *Streptomyces griseus* and *Actinomadura madurae* in the basal glycerol broth control and no growth in the lysozyme broth.

MacConkey agar base (29)
For isolation and identification of enteric pathogens based on the fermentation, or lack of fermentation, of a particular sugar added by the user

This medium is identical to MacConkey agar except that lactose has been omitted; thus, it contains no sugar. Any sugar or combination of sugars can be added for a specific purpose. For example, 10 g of D-sorbitol can be added to make this an isolation medium for *Escherichia coli* O157:H7.

MacConkey agar base

Bacto-Peptone (Difco) or Gelysate (BBL)	17 g
Proteose Peptone (Difco) or Polypeptone (BBL)	3 g
Bile salts no. 3	10 g
Sodium chloride	5 g
Neutral red	0.03 g
Crystal violet	0.001 g
Agar	13.5 g
Water	1 liter

To be added:

Any sugar(s) or fermentable compound(s), each	10 g

Add 40 g of the dehydrated medium and 10 g of the desired sugar(s) to the water. Boil to dissolve. Autoclave at 121°C for 15 min. Cool to 45 to 50°C, and dispense. Store at 4°C until needed.

MacConkey agar without crystal violet

Bacto-Peptone	17.0 g
Polypeptone	3.0 g
Lactose	10.0 g
Bile salts	1.5 g
Sodium chloride	5.0 g
Agar	13.5 g
Neutral red	0.03 g
Distilled water	1.0 liter
Final pH 7.1	

Make an aqueous suspension of the culture and streak the entire plate with a loopful. Incubate the plates at 35°C for 5 to 11 days.

Results: *Mycobacterium fortuitum* grows well; *Rhodococcus* spp. grow poorly or not at all; aerobic actinomycetes do not grow.

MacConkey sorbitol agar (29)
Sorbitol MacConkey agar
For the isolation of Escherichia coli O157:H7

In contrast to most *E. coli* strains, *E. coli* O157:H7 does not ferment D-sorbitol rapidly. This led to the formulation of MacConkey sorbitol agar, a variation of MacConkey agar that contains D-sorbitol instead of lactose.

Follow the directions for making MacConkey agar and add D-sorbitol (10 g) to the basic ingredients.

MacConkey sorbitol agar is inoculated in the same way as other enteric plating media and incubated at 37°C for 24 h. Sorbitol-negative colonies are colorless and are considered "suspicious for *E. coli* O157:H7." They are tested further by a variety of different methods described in the section on *E. coli* O157:H7 in chapter 36.

For quality control, streak a plate with a strain of *E. coli* O157:H7 and incubate it at 37°C. The colonies of *E. coli* O157:H7 will be colorless after 24 h, but most other clinical isolates of *E. coli* will be pink to red.

Malt extract agar* (75)

Malt extract	20.0 g
Agar	12.0 g
Distilled water	400.0 ml
Final pH 4.6	

Mix agar and distilled water and bring to a boil. Cool, add malt extract, and mix. Autoclave for 15 min at 121°C. Aseptically dispense the agar.

Mannitol-salt agar USP*

Beef extract	1.000 g
Peptone or Polypeptone (BBL)	10.000 g
Sodium chloride	75.000 g
Mannitol	10.000 g
Agar	15.000 g
Phenol red	0.025 g
Distilled water	1.000 liter
Final pH 7.4	

Heat to dissolve, and autoclave at 121°C for 15 min.

Mannitol-yolk-polymyxin agar

See *Bacillus cereus* media.

Martin-Lewis agar

See Thayer-Martin agar.

MBM acetate (mineral base medium with acetate)

Sodium acetate trihydrate	1.0 g
Monoammonium phosphate	1.0 g
Dipotassium phosphate	1.0 g
Magnesium sulfate	0.1 g
Sodium chloride	5.0 g
Bromothymol blue	0.01 g
Agar	16.0 g
Distilled water	1.0 liter

Adjust pH to 6.5, heat to melt agar, dispense in 3-ml amounts into 13-mm screw-cap tubes, autoclave at 121°C for 15 min, and solidify as slants. Use one loopful of broth culture as an inoculum and incubate at 35°C for 4 days. Nutritional independence appears as growth on and alkalinization (blue) of the medium.

Several mineral base media have been used to determine the nutritional independence of bacteria. The Centers for Disease Control (16) uses Simmons basal medium with 0.2% sodium acetate; however, the concentrations of bromothymol blue and acetate in that medium may be inhibitory for some nonfermenters. Gilardi (36) uses the medium described above but with 0.01 M acetate and no bromothymol blue, positive readings being growth rather than alkalinization.

McClung carbon-free broth

$NaNO_3$	2.0 g
K_2HPO_4	0.8 g
$MgSO_4 \cdot 7H_2O$	0.5 g
$FeCl_3$	0.010 g
$MnCl_2 \cdot 4H_2O$	0.008 g
$ZnSO_4$	0.002 g
Distilled H_2O to bring volume to	1 liter

Mix ingredients; heat solution at low temperature until ingredients dissolve (15 to 30 min). A heavy precipitate may appear as solution becomes hot. Cool solution. Filter sterilize, using a Nalgene 0.45-μm-pore-size filter. Check pH; should be 7.2 ± 0.2.

Can be stored at 4°C for up to 6 months. Sterility may be checked by adding 2.5 ml of tryptic soy broth and incubating for 48 h.

McClung-Toabe egg yolk agar

See CDC modified McClung-Toabe egg yolk agar (EYA).

McClung-Toabe agar, modified

See egg yolk agars.

Medium of Knisely for *Bacillus anthracis* (63)

Heart infusion agar (Difco; BHI agar)
Lysozyme (chicken egg white)
Thallous acetate [$Tl(OAc)_3$]
EDTA
Polymyxin

Add 55 g of the BHI agar to 1,000 ml of distilled water; with the aid of pH paper, adjust the hydrogen ion concentration to pH 7.3 to 7.4. Autoclave, and cool to 48 to 54°C. Add (final concentration) polymyxin (30 U/ml), lysozyme (40 μg/ml), $Tl(OAc)_3$ (40 μg/ml), and EDTA (200 μg/ml). Carefully swirl the contents, and pour plates.

Medium (R-medium) for elaboration of toxins of *Bacillus anthracis* (91)

Amino acids (Trp, Gly, Cys, Tyr, Lys, Val, Leu, Ile, Thr, Met, Asp, Glu, Pro, His hydrochloride, Arg hydrochloride, Phe, Ser)
Glucose
Thiamine hydrochloride, uracil, adenine sulfate
$CaCl_2 \cdot 2H_2O$, $MgSO_4 \cdot H_2O$, $MnSO_4 \cdot H_2O$, $NaHCO_3$, K_2HPO_4
Sodium hydroxide

To 500 ml of water add (milligrams in parentheses) Trp (35), Gly (65), Cys (25), Tyr (144), Lys (230), Val (173), Leu (230), Ile (170), Thr (120), Met (73), Asp (184), Glu (612), Pro (43), His hydrochloride (55), Arg hydrochloride (125), Phe (125), Ser (235), thiamine hydrochloride (1.0), glucose (2,500), $CaCl_2 \cdot 2H_2O$ (7.4), $MgSO_4 \cdot H_2O$ (9.9), $MnSO_4 \cdot H_2O$ (0.9), K_2HPO_4 (3,000), $NaHCO_3$ (8,000), uracil (1.4), and adenine sulfate (2.1). Adjust the pH to 8.0 with 5 N NaOH, and filter sterilize. Autoclave 500 ml of 3% (wt/vol) agar, and cool to 50°C. Mix filter-sterilized medium with agar, and pour plates. The medium is effective in promoting the elaboration of the exotoxins of *B. anthracis*.

MES agar

See U (ureaplasma) agar plates.

Middlebrook and Cohn 7H10 agar*

7H10 agar

Stock solutions

Solution 1. Store at room temperature.

Monopotassium phosphate	15 g
Disodium phosphate	15 g
Distilled water	250 ml

Solution 2. Store at 4 to 10°C.

Ammonium sulfate	5.0 g
Monosodium glutamate	5.0 g
Sodium citrate · $2H_2O$ USP	4.0 g
Ferric ammonium citrate	0.4 g
Magnesium sulfate ($7H_2O$) ACS	0.5 g
Biotin, in 2 ml of 10% NH_4OH	5.0 mg
Distilled water, to	250.0 ml

Solution 3. Store at 4 to 10°C.

Calcium chloride · $2H_2O$ ACS	50 mg
Zinc sulfate · $7H_2O$ ACS	100 mg
Copper sulfate · $5H_2O$ ACS	100 mg
Pyridoxine hydrochloride	100 mg
Distilled water, to	100 ml

Solution 4. Glycerol reagent

Solution 5. Malachite green, 0.01% aqueous

1. To 975 ml of distilled water, add:

Solution 1	25 ml
Solution 2	25 ml
Solution 3	1 ml
Solution 4	5 ml

2. Adjust the pH to 6.6 by adding approximately 0.5 ml of 6 N HCl.
3. Add 2.5 ml of solution 5 and 15 g of agar.
4. Autoclave at 121°C for 15 min. Cool to 56°C, and add 100 ml of OADC Enrichment*:

Bovine albumin fraction V	50 g
Sterile saline, 0.85%	900 ml

Dissolve and add 30 ml of the following:

Oleic acid	0.6 ml
Distilled water, to	30.0 ml
Sodium hydroxide, 6 M	0.6 ml

Warm to 56°C; swirl until solution occurs.

5. Adjust the reaction to pH 7.0, measured electrometrically.

6. Add 40 ml of sterile 50% aqueous glucose. Sterilize by filtration.

7. Heat at 56°C for 1 h, incubate overnight, heat again at 56°C, and incubate again overnight at 37°C for sterility.

8. Add 100 ml of this solution to agar base.

9. Add also 2 ml of freshly prepared, membrane filter-sterilized catalase solution containing 1,000 µg/ml.

10. Dispense the complete medium completely into petri plates or tubes.

11. Store at 4 to 8°C; unsealed and unprotected containers should be used for no longer than 1 week.

12. During preparation and storage, protect from light.

Middlebrook 7H11 agar*
7H11 agar

Add 1 g of enzymatic casein hydrolysate per liter of 7H10 agar.

Middlebrook selective 7H11 agar
Selective 7H11 agar

Add the following antimicrobial agents per liter of 7H11 agar:

Carbenicillin	50 µg
Polymyxin B	200,000 U
Amphotericin B	10 µg
Trimethoprim lactate	20 µg

Middlebrook 7H12 medium (broth)

Middlebrook 7H9 broth base	0.47% (wt/vol)
Casein hydrolyslate	0.10% (wt/vol)
Bovine serum albumin	0.50% (wt/vol)
Catalase	192 U
^{14}C-substrate	4 µCi
Deionized water, to	4 ml
Final pH 6.8 ± 0.1	

Each bottle is supplemented with 0.1 ml of a solution of polymyxin B (10,000 U), amphotericin B (1,000 µg), nalidixic acid (4,000 µg), trimethoprim (1,000 µg), and azlocillin (2,000 µg). Clinical specimens except blood that have been decontaminated with sodium hydroxide are added to each bottle in 0.5-ml amounts.

Middlebrook 13A medium (4-ml bottle)

Middlebrook 7H9 broth base	0.47% (wt/vol)
Casein hydrolysate	0.1% (wt/vol)
Polysorbate 80	0.02% (wt/vol)
Sodium polyanetholesulfonate	0.025% (wt/vol)
Catalase	1,440 U
^{14}C-substrate	5 µCi (185 kBq)
Deionized water to make	4 ml

Middlebrook 13A enrichment (10 ml per vial) (30-ml bottle)

Bovine serum albumin	15% (wt/vol)
Processed water to make	10 ml

Add 0.5 ml to each 30-ml bottle.

A 5-ml sample of blood from patients suspected of having mycobacteremia is added to each bottle at the bedside.

Modified Diamonds medium for trichomonas culture

Trypticase (BBL)	20 g
Yeast extract	1.0 g
Maltose	0.5 g
L-Cystine hydrochloride	0.5 g
L-Ascorbic acid	0.02 g

Add distilled water to make 90 ml, and adjust the pH to 6.5 with 4 N NaOH or 1 N HCl. Autoclave, cool to 48°C, and add sodium penicillin G (100,000 U), streptomycin sulfate (0.15 g), and amphotericin B (200 µg) in 1 ml of water. (Final drug concentrations are 1,000 U of penicillin, 1.5 mg of streptomycin, and 2 µg of amphotericin B per ml.) Add horse serum (10 ml, inactivated at 56°C for 30 min). Dispense in 5.0-ml quantities into sterile tubes. Store at 4°C for up to 14 days. Warm to 35°C before inoculation.

If usage rate is low, medium without horse serum may be frozen at −20°C. When needed, a tube of medium is thawed, and 0.5 ml of sterile horse serum is added.

Modified Oxford medium (MOX)

See listeria media.

Modified Thayer-Martin agar*

See Thayer-Martin agar.

Modified Wadowsky-Yee medium

See *Legionella pneumophila* media.

Motility nitrate agar*
Recommended for miscellaneous gram-negative bacteria (chapter 40)

Tryptose (Difco)	10.0 g
Heart infusion agar (Difco)	8.0 g
Glucose	0.5 g
Potassium (or sodium) nitrate	1.0 g
Distilled water	1.0 liter

Heat to melt agar, dispense in 4-ml amounts into 13-mm screw-cap tubes, and autoclave at 121°C for 15 min. Inoculate by stabbing 8 to 10 mm into the soft agar and incubate at 35°C.

This medium contains infusion to favor growth of fastidious bacteria, glucose to promote growth, and nitrate both to promote growth and to test for its reduction to nitrite. Motility nitrate agar also can serve as a stock culture medium.

Available as a prepared medium from BBL and Scott.

Motility test and maintenance medium

A. *For anaerobes (18)*

Motility medium (Difco)*	16.0 g
Nutrient broth*	4.0 g
Sodium chloride	1.0 g
Agar	4.0 g
Distilled water	1.0 liter
Final pH 7.2 ± 0.1	

Heat to dissolve the above ingredients, adjust the pH, dispense 7 ml into 15- by 90-mm screw-cap tubes, autoclave at 121°C for 15 min, and cool.

See note on fermentation broth for anaerobes. Place tubes in glove box, tighten caps, remove from glove box, and store at 4°C or ambient temperature.

B. *For enterobacteriaceae*

Beef extract	3.0 g
Peptone or Gelysate (BBL)	10.0 g
Sodium chloride	5.0 g
Agar	4.0 g
Distilled water	1 liter
Final pH 7.4	

Dispense about 8 ml per tube. Autoclave at 121°C for 15 min.

C. *For nonfermenting gram-negative bacteria*

1. Method of Gilardi (36) (chapter 41)

Pancreatic digest of casein USP	10.0 g
Yeast extract	3.0 g
Sodium chloride	5.0 g
Agar	3.0 g
Distilled water	1 liter
Final pH 7.2	

For stock culture maintenance, dispense 3.5 ml per 13- by 100-mm tube. Autoclave at 121°C for 15 min.

2. Method of Tatum et al. (109)

Tryptose or Biosate (BBL)	8.0 g
Sodium chloride	5.0 g
Agar	4.0 g
Nutrient broth	500 ml
Distilled water	500 ml

Mix, and heat to dissolve ingredients. Dispense into test tubes, and autoclave at 121°C for 15 min.

D. *For Listeria monocytogenes*

Beef extract	3.0 g
Peptone	10.0 g
Sodium chloride	5.0 g
Agar	4.0 g
Distilled water	1.0 liter

Before autoclaving, add 0.05 g of 2,3,5-triphenyltetrazolium chloride (TTC) (or 5.0 ml of a 1% TTC solution).

Mueller-Hinton agar*

Beef, infusion from	300.0 g
Acid hydrolysate of casein	17.5 g
Starch	1.5 g
Agar	17.0 g
Distilled water	1.0 liter

Dispense, and autoclave at 116 to 121°C for 15 min. Cool to 45 to 50°C and add blood, if desired.

Mueller-Hinton broth

Mix ingredients as given above for Mueller-Hinton agar except for the agar. Add the following supplements: 0.1% glucose, 2.0% IsoVitaleX, 25 mg of Mg^{2+} per liter, and 50 mg of Ca^{2+} per liter. Dispense as needed into tubes.

Mycobiotic agar, mycosel agar*

For primary recovery of dermatophytes and some deep pathogenic fungi

Soytone	10.0 g
Glucose	10.0 g
Agar	15.0 g
Cycloheximide, in 10 ml of acetone	0.05 g
Chloramphenicol, in 10 ml of 95% alcohol	0.05 g

Heat to dissolve the agar. Dispense, and autoclave at 121°C for 10 min.

Mycoplasmal media (37, 60, 61) (chapter 47)

A. *Basic agar for isolation of human mycoplasmas and ureaplasmas*

Papaic digest of soy meal USP (Hysoy, [soy peptone], Sheffield)	20.0 g
Sodium chloride	5.0 g
Purified water	1.0 liter
Phenol red, 2% aqueous	1.0 ml
Agarose	10.0 g

Adjust pH to 7.3 with 1 N NaOH before adding agarose.

Heat with agitation to obtain solution. Dispense, and autoclave at 121°C for 15 min. The sterile agar base may be stored at room temperature in the dark for several months.

B. *Mycoplasmal and ureaplasmal medium supplements*

Prepare yeast dialysate as follows. Suspend 450 g of active dried yeast (e.g., Fleischmann) in 1,250 ml of water at 40°C. Heat in an autoclave at 121°C for 15 min or long enough to kill yeast cells. Place in dialysis casing and dialyze against 1 liter of water at 4°C for 2 days. Discard casing and contents. Autoclave dialysate at 121°C for 15 min. Store frozen at −20°C.

Prepare 1 M MES by dissolving 195 g of MES [2-(*N*-morpholino)ethanesulfonic acid] in 0.7 liter of water. Warm solution to 37°C and adjust pH to 5.5 with saturated NaOH (ca. 10 N). Make up to 1 liter in volume. Sterilize by filtration and store in the dark at room temperature (1 M MES crystallizes out at 4°C).

Prepare 1 M urea by dissolving 60 g of urea in 1 liter of water. Sterilize by filtration and store at room temperature in the dark.

Prepare 0.1 M Na_2SO_3 by dissolving 1.26 g of anhydrous Na_2SO_3 in 100 ml of water. Add 0.1 ml of 2% phenol. Place in 16- by 125-mm screw-cap tubes. Sterilize by autoclaving, tighten caps, and store at room temperature. The solution is normally purple in color and will turn orange if air leaks into the tubes, indicating oxidation of the sulfite to sulfate, which is useless in culture medium.

C. *Basic soy peptone broth for isolation of mycoplasmas and ureaplasmas*

Papaic digest of soy meal USP (Hysoy [soy peptone], Sheffield)	20.0 g
Sodium chloride	5.0 g
Purified water	1.0 liter
Phenol red, 2% aqueous	1.0 ml

Dissolve, and adjust pH to 7.3. Dispense, and autoclave at 121°C for 15 min. Cool. Basic broth may be stored at room temperature in the dark for several months.

D. *H (hominis) agar plates for isolation of Mycoplasma pneumoniae and M. hominis*

To 65 ml of basic agar (melted and cooled to 55°C), add 10 ml of yeast dialysate, 20 ml of horse serum, 2 ml of penicillin (10,000 U/ml), and optionally 1 ml of 3.3% aqueous sterile thallium acetate (note that thallium salts are poisonous).

Dispense in 5-ml amounts into 10- by 35-mm petri dishes, and incubate overnight at room temperature to remove excess surface moisture (water visible on agar surface), which will prevent detection of colonies.

E. *H (hominis) broth for isolation of M. pneumoniae and M. hominis*

To 65 ml of basic broth, aseptically add 10 ml of yeast dialysate, 20 ml of horse serum, 2 ml of penicillin (10,000 U/ml), 1 ml of 1 M glucose, and optionally 1 ml of 3.3% thallium acetate. For isolation of *M. hominis*, glucose may be omitted and 2 ml of 1 M arginine is added per 100 ml.

F. *H diphasic medium for isolation of M. pneumoniae*

Dispense H agar in 3-ml amounts into 16- by 125-mm screw-cap tubes, allow to solidify, and overlay with 3 ml of H broth (with glucose). Store at 4°C for no more than 2 weeks. Tubes must have good closures to avoid excessive elevation of pH upon loss of CO_2 from horse serum.

Mycosel agar (mycobiotic agar)

See cycloheximide-chloramphenicol agar.

Nelson medium for *Naegleria fowleri*

Panmede (ox liver digest)	1.0 g
Glucose	1.0 g
Amoeba saline, to	1.0 liter

Dissolve the ingredients in amoeba saline (see nonnutrient agar plates). Dispense into 16- by 125-mm screw-cap tubes, 10 ml per tube. Autoclave for 15 min. Add 0.2 ml of heat-inactivated fetal calf serum to each tube before inoculating the medium with amoebae.

Nigerseed agar

See Staib agar.

Nitrate assimilation medium (42)

Auxanographic method for yeast identification

Yeast carbon base	12.0 g
Noble or washed agar	20.0 g
Distilled water	1.0 liter

Add ingredients to water and heat to dissolve. Tube medium in 20-ml aliquots in 18- by 150-mm screw-cap tubes. Autoclave at 15 lb/in^2 (121°C) for 15 min. Allow to harden as butts and store at 4°C.

Also see carbon assimilation media.

Nitrate reduction broth

A. *For miscellaneous gram-negative bacteria (chapter 40)*

Infusion broth* or heart infusion broth	25 g
Potassium (or sodium) nitrate	2 g
Distilled water	1 liter

Dispense in 3-ml amounts into 13-mm screw-cap tubes, add inverted vials, and autoclave at 121°C for 15 min. Inoculate and incubate for up to 7 days at 35°C to detect reduction of the nitrate to gas, nitrite, or amine. To obviate sacrificing the culture after 1 or 2 days of incubation, a test for nitrite can be made on 0.2 ml of the culture transferred to another tube.

Clark et al. (11) use the formulation above for fastidious bacteria but for nonfermenters replace the infusion broth with 2% peptone.

Dehydrated heart infusion broth is available from BBL and Difco.

B. *For Pseudomonas and related genera (36) (chapter 41)*

Potassium nitrate	1 g
Nutrient broth	1 liter

Dispense in 4-ml amounts into 13- by 100-mm tubes containing Durham vials. Autoclave at 121°C for 15 min. Inoculate tubes with one 4-mm loopful of growth from a 24- to 48-h blood agar base culture and examine after 24 and 48 h of aerobic incubation at 30°C for nitrogen gas accumulation in the Durham vial. Add reagents A and B to the nitrate broth. Red color shows presence of nitrite and indicates that nitrate was reduced. To tubes not showing a red color, add zinc dust. A red color indicates that nitrate is present and was not reduced. Absence of red color indicates that the nitrate and nitrite were completely reduced.

Nitrate swabs (46)
Rapid test for yeast identification

Potassium nitrate	2.00 g
Sodium phosphate, monobasic	11.70 g
Sodium phosphate, dibasic	1.14 g
Benzalkonium chloride (Zephiran), 17% solution	1.20 ml
Distilled water	200.00 ml

Mix well and adjust to pH 5.8. Place cotton-tipped swabs in the solution and allow saturation. Dry the swabs for 24 h at room temperature (vacuum may help) and autoclave at 15 lb/in^2 (121°C) for 15 min.

Nitrite reduction broth

A. *For nonfermenting gram-negative bacteria (109) (chapter 40)*

Infusion broth* or heart infusion broth	25.0 g
Potassium (or sodium) nitrite	1.0 g
Distilled water	1.0 liter

Dispense in 3-ml amounts into 13-mm screw-cap tubes, add inverted vials, and autoclave at 121°C for 15 min. Inoculate and incubate for up to 7 days at 35°C for detection of denitrification (gas production), reduction of nitrite to amine, or oxidation to nitrate. Since growth of some bacteria is inhibited by the 0.1% nitrite in the above medium, the Centers for Disease Control also uses a second medium containing only 0.01% nitrite.

Dehydrated heart infusion broth is available from BBL and Difco.

B. *For Pseudomonas and related genera (chapter 41)*

Sodium nitrite	0.01 g
Nutrient broth	1.00 liter

Dispense in 4-ml amounts into 13- by 100-mm tubes containing Durham vials. Autoclave at 121°C for 15 min. Inoculate tubes with one 4-mm loopful of growth from a 24- to 48-h blood agar base culture and examine after 24 and 48 h of aerobic incubation at 30°C for gas accumulation in the Durham vial. Add reagents A and B to the nitrite broth. Red color shows presence of nitrite; i.e., nitrite was not reduced. Absence of red color shows absence of nitrite; i.e., nitrite was reduced.

Nonnutrient agar plates
For isolation and culture of pathogenic free-living amoebae

Agar	1.5 g
Page amoeba saline	100 ml

Dissolve agar in the saline with heat, and sterilize at 15 lb/in^2 in 15 min. Cool to 60°C and aseptically pour into plastic petri dishes. Use 20 ml for 100- by 15-mm dishes or 5 ml for 16- by 15-mm dishes. After the agar gels, store the plates in canisters at 4°C (refrigerator). Plates may be kept in the refrigerator for about 3 months.

Prepare Page amoeba saline as follows.

Sodium chloride (NaCl)	120 mg
Magnesium sulfate ($MgSO_4 \cdot 7H_2O$)	4 mg
Calcium chloride ($CaCl_2 \cdot 2H_2O$)	4 mg
Disodium hydrogen phosphate (Na_2HPO_4)	142 mg
Potassium dihydrogen phosphate (KH_2PO_4)	136 mg
Distilled water, to	1 liter

Dissolve the chemicals in water, and sterilize by autoclaving at 15 lb/in^2 for 15 min. The solution may be stored in the refrigerator for up to 6 months.

DL-Norleucine assimilation

See carbon assimilation medium.

Novy, MacNeal, and Nicolle (NNN) medium for *Leishmania* species and *Trypanosoma cruzi* (79)

Agar	7 g
Sodium chloride	3 g
Distilled water	450 ml
Defibrinated rabbit blood (sterile)	150 ml

Mix agar, sodium chloride, and water, and bring to boiling to dissolve agar and salt. Autoclave at 121°C for 15 min. Cool to 52°C and add rabbit blood. Dispense 5-ml portions into sterile 13- by 100-mm screw-cap tubes, and slant the tubes in the refrigerator. Condensation of water at the bottom of the slant is desirable. If there is little moisture, a few drops of sterile water may be added with the inoculum. Medium should be tested for sterility by incubating a sample slant at 35°C for 48 h.

Nutrient agar*

Beef extract	3 g
Peptone or Gelysate pancreatic digest of gelatin	5 g
Agar	15 g
Distilled water	1 liter
Final pH 6.8	

Mix ingredients and heat to boiling to dissolve completely. Autoclave at 121°C for 15 min. Dispense into petri dishes or tubes and let cool.

Nutrient broth, standard II

Special peptone	8.6 g
Sodium chloride	6.4 g
Distilled water	1.0 liter
Final pH 7.5 ± 0.1 at 37°C	

Completely dissolve 15 g in 1 liter of freshly distilled or demineralized water. Sterilize in the autoclave (15 min at 121°C).

Nutrient broth with 6% NaCl

See salt tolerance media.

Nutrient gelatin*

A. *For enterobacteriaceae and nonfermenting gram-negative bacteria*

Nutrient broth	1 liter
Gelatin	120 g

Mix broth and gelatin and dissolve by heating. Dispense into tubes and autoclave at 121°C for 12 min.

Gelatin liquefaction

Inoculate by stabbing with a wire, and incubate at 30°C for 1 to 2 days. Nutrient gelatin is recommended as the "standard" method in taxonomic work, since the rate of gelatin liquefaction is important in the characterization of certain groups and subgroups within the family *Enterobacteriaceae*. Some of the rapid methods are excellent for diagnostic work in which one is not interested in the rate of liquefaction. In those areas where the rate of liquefaction is of differential value (e.g., within the tribe *Klebsielleae*), positive tests obtained by the rapid methods should be repeated with the conventional methods. If the above-mentioned limitations are borne in mind, certain rapid methods can be recommended.

Gelatin liquefaction demonstration by rapid methods (64, 68)

Prepare nutrient gelatin, using 15 g/100 ml of distilled water. Add 3 to 5 g of powdered charcoal, mix thoroughly, cool, and pour into petri dishes or other flat containers to a depth of 3 mm. (Apply a thin film of petrolatum to containers first.) After medium has set, remove the sheet of gelatin and place it in 10% Formalin for 24 h. Cut the sheet into pieces 1 cm by 5 to 8 mm. Wrap in gauze, and wash in running tap water for 24 h. Place in wide-mouth, screw-cap jars or bottles, and cover with distilled water. Sterilize by exposure to flowing steam for 30 min on 3 successive days. After sterilization, the water may be decanted. Check sterility by placing pieces in tubes of nutrient broth.

Suspend the growth from an 18- to 24-h agar plate culture in 3 ml of 0.85% sodium chloride solution containing 0.01 M calcium chloride in a small test tube (e.g., 13 by 100 mm). The suspension should be very dense, since the rapidity of the reaction appears to be a function of density and temperature of incubation. The agar plates should be thick; i.e., they should contain 35 to 40 ml of infusion agar medium. Three or four drops of a broth culture should be spread over the entire surface to obtain maximal confluent growth.

With aseptic precautions, add a piece of denatured charcoal to each dense suspension prepared as described above. Add 0.1 ml of toluene to each suspension, and shake the tube. Toluene appears to have an activating effect on the reactions of strains that ordinarily are slow liquefiers of gelatin. Incubate at 37°C, and examine after 5 or 6 h and daily for 14 days. Positive reactions are indicated by the release of charcoal particles, which collect in the bottom of the tube.

Advantage may be taken of the bactericidal effect of toluene. Distribute 3-ml amounts of saline solution containing 0.01 M calcium chloride into small tubes, and autoclave at 121°C for 15 min. Place a piece of charcoal-gelatin and 0.1 ml of toluene in each tube, and stopper with corks that have been soaked in hot paraffin. Store until needed.

B. *For aerobic actinomycetes*

Prepare as described above for medium A, but with demineralized water.

Inoculate just below the surface of the solidified medium. Incubate at room temperature or 37°C with an uninoculated control. When growth is sufficient, place tests and control in refrigerator until control solidifies; then observe tests for liquefaction.

C. *For Erysipelothrix*

Medium A is recommended.

D. *For miscellaneous gram-negative bacteria*

Heart infusion broth* or infusion (heart) broth	25 g
Gelatin	120 g
Distilled water	1 liter

Heat to boiling to dissolve. Cool to 55°C, and adjust to pH 7.4. Dispense 5 ml per 16- by 125-mm screw-cap tube, and autoclave at 121°C for 15 min.

NYC (New York City) medium

Basal medium

1. Agar* .... 20 g in 400 ml of distilled water

The solution is heated at 100°C until melted, e.g., by steaming in an Arnold unit.

2. Cornstarch .... 1 g in 40 ml of distilled water

The solution is first mixed on a magnetic stirrer and then placed in the Arnold unit until homogeneous.

3. Proteose Peptone no. 3*	15 g
Dipotassium phosphate	4 g
Monopotassium phosphate	1 g
Sodium chloride	5 g
Distilled water	200 ml

Bring the components of step 3 to boiling on a heated magnetic stirrer. Add the melted agar, cornstarch, and Proteose Peptone solution, and mix thoroughly on a heated magnetic stirrer. Autoclave at 121°C for 15 min. Allow to cool, and store at 4°C.

Final pH is 7.1 ± 0.1.

Editors' note. The author recommends Difco ingredients.

Supplements

A. Yeast dialysate

Bakers' yeast	908 g
Distilled water	2.5 liters

Carefully mix the bakers' yeast to a smooth paste, autoclave for 10 min, and allow to cool. Place in dialysis tubing, and dialyze against 2 liters of distilled water in the cold for 48 h. Collect the dialysate, dispense in 25-ml aliquots, and autoclave at 121°C for 15 min. (A 25-ml sample of yeast dialysate is the amount necessary for 1 liter of final medium; aliquots can be prepared in any amount.) The yeast dialysate is stored at 20°C. (It can be kept indefinitely.)

B. A 50% glucose solution distributed in 10-ml aliquots (for 1 liter of medium)

C. A 3% hemoglobin solution is prepared from packed erythrocytes (RBC). The RBC are kept after the plasma has been separated. They are not packed by centrifugation, but used as such. A 6-ml amount of sedimented RBC is added to 200 ml of sterile distilled water (for 1 liter of medium).

D. Horse plasma (citrated) preparation

Sodium citrate	1,200 g
NaCl	64 g
Water, to	8 liters

Of this solution, 600 ml is placed in a receiving bottle, and blood is drawn to 6 liters to make a 10% final citrate concentration in the blood.

E. Antibiotic mixture

Vancomycin	2 μg/ml
Colistin	5.5 μg/ml
Amphotericin B	1.2 μg/ml
Trimethoprim lactate	3 μg/ml

Melt basal medium and allow to cool in a 55°C water bath. The following additions are made for 1 liter of final medium:

120 ml of plasma
200 ml of a 3% RBC (hemolyzed) solution
10 ml of 50% glucose solution
25 ml of yeast dialysate
5 ml of antibiotic mixture

After the addition of the supplement to the basal medium, plates are poured and allowed to dry. When dry, plates should be placed in plastic bags and stored in the refrigerator (4 to 8°C). In these conditions, NYC medium will maintain its properties for about 2 to 2.5 months.

Oatmeal agar (118, 119)

Oatmeal (Beech-Nut or Gerber's baby oatmeal)	10 g
Magnesium sulfate	1.0 g
Potassium phosphate	1.0 g
Sodium nitrate	1.5 g
Agar	15.0 g
Distilled water	1 liter

Mix and dissolve. Adjust pH to 5.6 with sodium hydroxide. Autoclave at 121°C for 20 min. Pour 20-ml aliquots into sterile petri dishes.

Note. Alphacel and tomato paste may be omitted from the original formulation.

ONPG broth

A. ONPG (*o*-nitrophenyl-β-D-galactopyranoside) solution

ONPG	1.5 g
Sodium phosphate buffer, pH 7.5, 0.01 M	250 ml

Dissolve the ingredients at room temperature (25°C); sterilize by filtration using a 0.45-μm-pore-size membrane filter.

B. Peptone water, 1%

Peptone	7.5 g
Sodium chloride	3.75 g
Distilled water	750 ml

Dissolve by heating and adjust pH to 8.0 to 8.4. Boil for 10 min and filter. Readjust pH to 7.2 to 7.4. Autoclave at 115°C for 20 min.

Aseptically add the sterile ONPG solution to the sterile peptone water in a sterile flask. Tube the sterile ONPG broth in 2.5- to 3-ml aliquots. Tubed media may be stored at 4°C in the refrigerator for up to 1 month.

For the β-D-galactosidase test (see chapter 122), inoculate a tube of ONPG broth heavily by adding one 4-mm loopful of growth from a 24- to 48-h blood agar base culture and incubate at 37°C in a water bath or incubator. Read the tube after 20 min. If negative (no color change), continue incubation and read at 1, 2, 3, and 24 h. Hydrolysis of ONPG broth is detected by the release of *o*-nitrophenol, which is yellow and usually released within 30 min. A positive test (formation of yellow color in broth) indicates that the organism contains lactose-fermenting enzymes and is a lactose fermenter.

The test may be used to differentiate lactose-delayed organisms from lactose-negative organisms and to differentiate *Pseudomonas cepacia* (positive) and *Pseudomonas maltophilia* (positive) from other *Pseudomonas* species (negative).

Oxford agar

See listeria media.

Oxidation-fermentation (OF) test medium
OF basal medium*

A. *For Corynebacterium, Enterobacteriaceae, Aeromonas, Pseudomonas, and nonfermenting gram-negative bacteria (36, 47)*

Peptone, e.g., pancreatic digest of casein	2.00 g
Sodium chloride	5.00 g
Dipotassium phosphate	0.30 g
Bromothymol blue	0.03 g
Agar	3.00 g
Distilled water	1.00 liter
Final pH 7.1	

Dispense 3 or 4 ml per 13- by 100-mm test tube. Autoclave at 121°C for 15 min. Cool and add 10% glucose solution in distilled water for a final concentration of

1% glucose. Other carbohydrates may be substituted for glucose if desired. Dispense aseptically.

This medium aids in the differentiation of organisms that utilize carbohydrates oxidatively rather than fermentatively and therefore is helpful in the identification of pseudomonads and members of the tribe *Mimeae*. It also aids in the identification of organisms that do not utilize glucose in either way (e.g., *Alcaligenes* spp.). Inoculate (stab) lightly two tubes of medium from a young blood agar slant culture. Cover one of the tubes with a layer (about 5 mm) of sterile melted petrolatum or sterile paraffin oil. Incubate at 37°C, and observe daily for 1 to 3 days. Acid formation only in the open tube indicates oxidative utilization of glucose. Acid formation in both the open and the sealed tubes is indicative of a fermentative reaction. Lack of acid production in either tube indicates that the organism does not utilize glucose by either method.

B. *For nonfermenting gram-negative bacilli (109)*

Casitone (Difco)	2.0 g
Phenol red	0.03 g
Agar	3.0 g
Distilled water	1.0 liter

Adjust to pH 7.3, heat to melt agar, dispense in 3-ml amounts into 13-mm screw-cap tubes, and autoclave at 121°C for 15 min. Stock 10% solutions of carbohydrates, sterilized by storage in screw-cap tubes over a slight excess of chloroform, are added to the molten basal medium to give 1% final concentrations. Inoculate by stabbing and incubate for up to 7 days at 35°C.

This OF basal medium uses phenol red as a pH indicator and is adapted from that of the Centers for Disease Control (18). OF basal media containing bromothymol blue may be inhibitory for some nonfermenters.

P agar
For staphylococci

Peptone	10 g
Yeast extract	5 g
Sodium chloride	5 g
Glucose	1 g
Agar	15 g
Distilled water	1 liter
Final pH 7.5 (before autoclaving)	

Mix ingredients and heat to boiling to dissolve agar. Autoclave at 121°C for 15 min.

Editors' note. The author recommends Difco ingredients.

Pablum cereal agar

Pablum precooked cereal	100 g
Agar	18 g
Chloramphenicol	50 mg
Distilled water	1 liter

Mix, and autoclave at 121°C for 15 min.

Page amoeba saline

See nonnutrient agar plates.

Pai slant (80)

Whole eggs	1,000.0 ml
Glucose	5.0 g
Distilled water	500.0 ml

Mix gently and filter through two layers of gauze. Add 120.0 ml of glycerol and mix gently to avoid formation of bubbles. Dispense 5-ml aliquots into tubes, and autoclave in a slanted position. Avoid foaming by controlled air escape and influx.

The medium can be stored at 4°C for 6 to 8 weeks.

Paraffin medium with McClung carbon-free broth

Paraffin (Tissue Prep Pellets [Fischer])
McClung carbon-free broth

Fill 16- by 125-mm glass screw-cap tubes 60% full with paraffin pellets. Place on slanted rack and autoclave for 15 min at 121°C. Let tubes harden in slanted position; then place upright. Perform sterility check as outlined below. Add 2.5 ml of sterile McClung carbon-free broth to paraffin slants; tighten caps.

Tubes may be stored at 4°C in the refrigerator for up to 6 months. Sterility should be tested by adding 2.5 ml of tryptic soy broth to each paraffin slant selected for sterility testing. Incubate for 48 h. Performance of the media can be checked by inoculating a paraffin-McClung broth slant with *Nocardia asteroides*. Check for good growth.

Paromomycin-vancomycin (PV) blood agar (18)

Prepare CDC anaerobe blood agar. After the sheep blood has been added, aseptically add 100 mg of paromomycin (Parke-Davis) and 7.5 mg (base activity) of vancomycin (Lilly) per liter.

Pelargonate assimilation

See carbon assimilation medium.

Peptone-yeast extract-glucose (PYG) broth (18)
For anaerobes

Peptone*	20 g
Yeast extract	10 g
Cysteine hydrochloride	0.5 g
Resazurin solution[a]	4.0 g
Salt solution (VPI)[b]	40.0 ml
D-Glucose	10.0 g
Distilled water	1.0 liter
Final pH 7.2	

[a]Add 11 mg of resazurin to 44 ml of distilled water.
[b]VPI salt solution (45a):

$CaCl_2$	0.2 g
$MgSO_4$	0.2 g
K_2HPO_4	1.0 g
KH_2PO_4	1.0 g

Mix ingredients in water, adjust pH, dispense 7 ml into 15- by 90-mm screw-cap tubes, autoclave at 121°C for 15 min, and cool. Place tubes in glove box, tighten caps, remove from glove box, and store at 4°C or room temperature (see note on fermentation broth [CHO base]).

Mix $CaCl_2$ and $MgSO_4$ in 300 ml of distilled water. When dissolved, add 500 ml of distilled water. Swirl while slowly adding the remaining salts. Continue mixing until all the salts are dissolved. Add 200 ml of distilled water. Store at 4°C.

Peptone-yeast extract-glucose (PYG) medium
For Acanthamoeba

Proteose peptone*	20.00 g
Yeast extract*	2.00 g
$MgSO_4 \cdot 7H_2O$	0.980 g
$CaCl_2$	0.059 g
Sodium citrate $\cdot 2H_2O$	1.00 g
$Fe(NH_4)_2(SO_4)_2 \cdot 6H_2O$	0.02 g
KH_2PO_4	0.34 g
$Na_2HPO_4 \cdot 7H_2O$	0.355 g
Glucose	18.00 g
Distilled water, to	1.0 liter
Final pH 6.5 ± 0.2	

Dissolve all ingredients except $CaCl_2$ in about 900.0 ml of distilled water. Add $CaCl_2$ while stirring. Bring the volume to 1,000 ml. Dispense into 16- by 125-mm screw-cap tubes, 5 ml per tube. Autoclave for 15 min (15 lb/in^2).

Editors' note. The author recommends Difco ingredients.

Phenylalanine deaminase medium

DL-Phenylalanine	2 g
Yeast extract	3 g
Sodium chloride	5 g
Sodium phosphate	1 g
Agar	12 g
Distilled water	1 liter
Final pH 7.3 ± 0.2	

Suspend ingredients in 1 liter of distilled water. Heat with frequent agitation and boil for 1 min. Dispense in tubes for slants, and sterilize by autoclaving at 121°C at 15 lb/in^2 for 10 min.

Phenylalanine deaminase activity is detected by flooding phenylalanine agar (BBL) slant cultures after 24 h of aerobic incubation at 30°C with a 10% (vol/vol) ferric chloride solution and observing for the development of a green color. Inoculate tubes with one 4-mm loopful of growth from a 24- to 48-h blood agar base culture.

Phenylethyl alcohol agar*
Phenylethanol agar*
Selective medium for isolating staphylococci and streptococci

Tryptose (or pancreatic digest of casein)	10 (15) g
Beef extract (or papaic digest of soya meal)	3 (5) g
Sodium chloride	5 g
Phenylethyl alcohol	2.5 g
Agar	15 g
Distilled water	1 liter
Final pH 7.3	

Dissolve with heat to boiling. Autoclave at 121°C for 15 min, cool, and pour the plates. Add 5% sterile defibrinated sheep blood if desired.

For anaerobes

Prepare as described above, and add 5% defibrinated blood and vitamin K_1 (10 µg/ml) after autoclaving.

Phenylethyl alcohol (PEA) blood agar (18)
For anaerobes

Prepare CDC anaerobe blood agar, and add 2.5 g of phenylethyl alcohol (per liter) before autoclaving.

Pisu medium (96)

The agar base contains:

Meat extract (Oxoid)	4.0 g
Proteose Peptone no. 3 (Difco)	20.0 g
NaCl	5.0 g
Agar (Bacto-Agar; Difco)	7.0 g
Distilled water	1.0 liter

Dissolve in steam and sterilize by filtration. Adjust pH to 7.5. Distribute 80-ml aliquots in 200-ml Erlenmeyer flasks and heat for 1 h in steam. Cool to 60°C and add to each 80 ml the following:

Horse serum, sterile	30.0 ml
L-Cystine, 1% (wt/vol)	15.0 ml
Lead acetate, 10% (wt/vol), sterilized	1.0 ml

Distribute in aliquots of 2 to 3 ml in small tubes and leave vertically on table to solidify. The medium can be stored at 4°C for up to 1 month. Inoculation is made by stabbing. High cystinase producers render the agar diffuse black. A black coloration of the surface or the stabbing canal only is interpreted as negative.

PLET agar* (63)
For selective isolation of Bacillus anthracis

Difco heart infusion agar	25 g
EDTA	0.3 g
Thallous acetate	0.04 g
Deionized distilled water	1.0 liter

Mix ingredients and dissolve completely. Autoclave at 121°C for 15 min and cool to 56°C.

Add:

Polymyxin (in filter-sterilized solution)	30,000 U
Lysozyme (in filter-sterilized solution)	300,000 U

Pour plates.

Polymyxin-pyruvate-egg yolk-mannitol bromothymol blue

See *Bacillus cereus* media.

Polysorbate (Tween) 80

Autoclave at 121°C for 20 min. Add 10 ml of polysorbate 80 to peptone agar, and pour the plates.

Potassium tellurite agar (27)

Heart infusion agar	20 g
Distilled water	500 ml

While monitoring with a pH meter, adjust to pH 6.0 by adding 1 N HCl. Autoclave at 121°C for 15 min. Cool to 90°C, add 25 ml of defibrinated rabbit or sheep blood, and mix well. Cool to 50°C, add potassium tellurite solution (0.25 g of potassium tellurite in 10 ml of distilled water), mix well, and pour into plates or prepare agar slants.

Enterococcus faecalis forms black colonies for a positive reaction.

Potato-dextrose agar
For sporulation of some fungi

Potatoes	100 g
Glucose	5 g
Agar	7.5 g
Distilled water	500 ml

Peel and dice 100 g of potatoes and add to 500 ml of distilled water. Autoclave for 10 min at 15 lb/in^2 to make the potato infusion. Filter infusion through gauze. Add 7.5 g of agar. Boil to dissolve the agar. Add 5 g of glucose. Bring the total volume to 500 ml with distilled water if necessary.

For tubes, dispense 5 ml into 16- by 125-mm screw-cap tubes; sterilize by autoclaving for 15 min at 15 lb/in^2; slant tubes until agar hardens; label tubes and tighten caps.

For plates, sterilize for 15 min at 15 lb/in^2; dispense 18 ml into 15- by 100-mm sterile petri plates; label plates; bag to reduce contamination and dehydration.

Media may be stored in the refrigerator at 4°C for up to 3 months in tubes and 6 weeks for plates in bags. Check performance by inoculating a plate with *Candida albicans* and observe for good growth.

Potato-dextrose agar,* slants
To induce sporulation in all fungi

Potatoes (white, not new), diced	200 g
Glucose	10 g
Agar	15 or 18 g
Water (tap or distilled)	1.0 liter

Peel and dice 200.0 g of old-crop potatoes. Add potatoes to 500.0 ml of tap or distilled water. Bring water to a boil and simmer for 1 h or cook in autoclave for 10 min at 15 lb/in^2. Filter through cheesecloth or coarse paper. Bring volume up to 1,000.0 ml with tap or distilled water. Add glucose and agar, dissolve by heating to a boil, and filter through cotton and gauze. Restore volume to 1 liter. Dispense into tubes and autoclave at 121°C for 10 min. Slant tubes and let cool.

Available commercially in dehydrated form or prepared media from BBL Laboratories (Cockeysville, Md.), Difco Laboratories (Detroit, Mich.), and Remel (Lenexa, Kans.).

Potato flakes agar (89)
To induce sporulation in moulds and fungi

Potato flakes (any commercial brand)	20 g
Glucose	10 g
Agar	15 g
Distilled water	1 liter

Place ingredients in 2,000-ml Erlenmeyer flask, add 1,000 ml of water, cap, and swirl. Heat with gentle stirring to point of boiling. Autoclave at 121°C and 15 lb/in^2 for 15 min. Dispense aseptically with periodic swirling and store at 4°C.

Commercially available from Oxoid (Lenexa, Kans.).

PRAS medium

See Cary and Blair transport medium, modified (PRAS) and transport media for anaerobes (PRAS).

Pril-xylose-ampicillin agar (93)
For isolation of Aeromonas hydrophila

Nutrient agar plus:

Phenol red	25 mg
Ampicillin	30 mg
Pril*[a]	200 mg
Xylose	10 g
Distilled water	1.0 liter

[a]Böhme Fettchemie GmbH, Düsseldorf, Federal Republic of Germany.

Purple broth base*

Peptone: proteose or peptic digest of animal tissue USP	10.000 g
Beef extract	1.000 g
Sodium chloride	5.000 g
Bromocresol purple	0.015 g
Distilled water	1.000 liter
Final pH 6.8	

Autoclave at 121°C for not more than 15 min. Add sugars and alcohols to 1% (wt/vol).

Pseudocel agar

See cetrimide agar USP.

Pyruvate utilization medium

Tryptone*	10 g
Yeast extract	5 g
Dipotassium phosphate	5 g
Sodium chloride	5 g
Sodium pyruvate	10 g
Bromothymol blue	104 mg
Distilled water	1 liter

Check the pH and adjust to 7.1 to 7.4 if necessary. Dispense into 13- by 100-mm screw-cap tubes. Autoclave at 121°C for 15 min.

A positive reaction is recorded when the indicator changes from green to definite yellow. Yellow-green indicates a weak reaction and should be regarded as negative utilization of pyruvate.

Pyrazinamide medium (53)

A. *For identification of virulent Yersinia spp.*

Tryptic soy agar	30 g
Yeast extract	3 g
Pyrazinamide[a] (Sigma P7136)	1 g
Tris-maleate (Sigma T3128)	47.4 g
Sodium hydroxide (NaOH) solution, 1 N	(about) 120 ml
Water, to final volume of 1 liter	(about) 880 ml

[a]Also known as pyrazinecarboxyamide.

Add all of the solid ingredients to about 800 ml of water. Stir to dissolve; the pH should be about 3.8. Add the 1 N NaOH until the pH is 6.0; about 120 ml will be required. Add water to bring the final volume to 1,000 ml. Heat to dissolve the agar. Dispense 5 ml into 16- by 125-mm screw-cap tubes. Autoclave, cool slightly, and slant to give a slant 5 to 6 cm long. After the agar solidifies, tighted the caps and store in the refrigerator until used.

B. *For identification of Corynebacterium and related organisms (105)*

Dubos broth base	6.5 g
Distilled water	1,000.0 ml
Pyrazinamide	0.1 g
Sodium pyruvate	2.0 g
Agar	15.0 g

Mix all ingredients and heat to dissolve completely. Aliquots in 5-ml tubes are autoclaved for 15 min. Slant tubes. Slants are inoculated with bacteria from overnight growth on chocolate agar slants and incubated at 37°C for 24 h. The presence of pyrazinamidase is indicated by a pink band in the agar (pyrazinoic acid).

Rabbit laked blood agar
For enhancing pigment production of anaerobes

Prepare brucella agar, adding hemin solution before autoclaving. After autoclaving, allow the agar to cool to 50°C; add vitamin K_1 (10.0 μg/ml) and laked rabbit blood (5%) aseptically before pouring plates. Laked blood is prepared by freezing whole blood (fill tubes only 75% full to allow for expansion of frozen blood) overnight and then thawing at room temperature.

Rapid sugar test for *Neisseria* species (5, 6, 58)

Neisseria gonorrhoeae is presumptively identified in the clinical laboratory by growth and colonial morphology on selective media, cell morphology and appearance on Gram stain, and oxidase reaction. It is confirmed either by the fluorescent-antibody test or by its reaction on various carbohydrate media. The rapid test is a time-saving modification of the standard procedure for determining carbohydrate fermentation of glucose, lactose, sucrose, maltose, and fructose. Although developed for the testing of neisseriae, it has been shown to be useful for other organisms such as *Haemophilus* spp., group DF-2, and *Kingella denitrificans.*

Reagents

1. Buffer-salt solution

KH_2PO_4	0.01 g
K_2HPO_4	0.04 g
KCl	0.80 g
Phenol red (1% aqueous solution)	0.40 g
Distilled water	100 ml

Adjust the pH to 7.0, filter sterilize, and store at 4°C in a sterile, screw-capped bottle.

2. Carbohydrate solutions

Prepare as 20% stock solutions in distilled water or broth (peptone, 10 g; meat extract, 3 g; sodium chloride, 5 g; distilled water, 1,000 ml). Adjust the pH to 7.0, and filter sterilize the solutions.

Procedure

Place 0.1 ml of the buffer-salt solution into each of five 10- by 75-mm sterile tubes. Add 1 drop of the appropriate carbohydrate solution to each labeled tube. Inoculate each tube with 1 drop of a very heavy 18- to 24-h culture suspension prepared in 0.35 ml of the buffer-salt solution.

Alternatively, a loopful of the suspected organism may be added directly into a tube of the buffer-salt-carbohydrate solution.

Incubate the tubes in a 35°C water bath for 4 h, and read at 30-min intervals.

A positive test is indicated by a yellow color (acid formation).

Regan-Lowe (RL) medium* (86)

Charcoal agar (Oxoid CM 119)	51.0 g
Horse blood, defibrinated	100 ml
Cephalexin	0.04 g
Distilled water	1.0 liter
Final pH 7.4 ± 0.2	

Dissolve charcoal agar powder in distilled water. Sterilize for 15 min at 121°C. Equilibrate at 50°C; add blood and antibiotic. Mix and dispense into sterile petri dishes. For the semisolid transport medium, prepare the medium with half-strength charcoal agar, dispense into tubes, and seal tightly.

Regan-Lowe (RL) semisolid transport medium

Prepare Regan-Lowe (RL) agar as for plates, but use only 25.5 g of Oxoid CM 119 charcoal agar. After adding the blood and antibiotic supplements, aseptically dispense into small screw-cap vials to fill them half full. Seal tightly and store at 4°C for up to 2 months.

Comments. The use of Oxoid CM 119 agar base is necessary for good results. The components of CM 119 in grams per liter are as follows: Lab-Lemco powder, 10; peptone, 10; starch, 10; bacteriological charcoal, 10; NaCl, 5; nicotinic acid, 0.001; agar, 12. Some American workers have successfully substituted defibrinated sheep blood for the horse blood on plates. However, use of sheep blood in transport medium is untested.

Rice grain medium (12)
For differentiation of Microsporum audouinii from other Microsporum spp.

White rice (not enriched)	8 g
Distilled water	25 ml

Place in 125-ml Erlenmeyer flask and autoclave at 121°C for 15 min.

RPMI 1640 with L-glutamine* (76)

	Liquid, 1× (mg/liter)	Liquid, 10× (mg/liter)
Inorganic salts		
$Ca(NO_3)_2 \cdot 4H_2O$	100.00	1,000.00
KCl	400.00	4,000.00
$MgSO_4 \cdot 7H_2O$	100.00	1,000.00
NaCl	6,000.00	60,000.00
$NaHCO_3$	2,000.00	—
$Na_2HPO_4 \cdot 7H_2O$	1,512.00	15,120.00
Other components		
D-Glucose	2,000.00	20,000.00
Glutathione (reduced)	1.00	10.00
Phenol red	5.00	50.00
Amino acids		
L-Arginine (free base)	200.00	2,000.00
L-Asparagine	50.00	500.00
L-Aspartic acid	20.00	200.00
L-Cystine	50.00	500.00
L-Glutamic acid	20.00	200.00
L-Glutamine	300.00	3,000.00
Glycine	10.00	100.00
L-Histidine (free base)	15.00	150.00
L-Hydroxyproline	20.00	200.00
L-Isoleucine (allo free)	50.00	500.00
L-Leucine (methionine free)	50.00	500.00
L-Lysine hydrochloride	40.00	400.00
L-Methionine	15.00	150.00
L-Phenylalanine	15.00	150.00
L-Proline (hydroxy-L-proline free)	20.00	200.00
L-Serine	30.00	300.00
L-Threonine (allo free)	20.00	200.00
L-Tryptophan	5.00	50.00
L-Tyrosine	20.00	200.00
L-Valine	20.00	200.00
Vitamins		
Biotin	0.20	2.00
D-Calcium pantothenate	0.25	2.50
Choline chloride	3.00	30.00
Folic acid	1.00	10.00
i-Inositol	35.00	350.00
Nicotinamide	1.00	10.00
p-Aminobenzoic acid	1.00	10.00
Pyridoxine hydrochloride	1.00	10.00
Riboflavin	0.20	2.00
Thiamine hydrochloride	1.00	10.00
Vitamin B_{12}	0.005	0.05

To prepare single-strength solutions from 10× concentrates, proceed as follows. Aseptically dilute 100 ml of 10× concentrate with approximately 850 ml of sterile distilled water. Aseptically add 26.9 ml of a sterile 7.5% sodium bicarbonate solution per ml. Check pH and adjust if necessary with sterile 1 N hydrochloric acid or 1 N sodium hydroxide. Recommended 1× pH value is 7.3 ± 0.1. Make up to 1-liter volume with sterile distilled water. Dispense aliquots into sterile containers. Cap tightly, and store at proper temperatures.

Comparable media may be obtained from GIBCO Laboratories (1× liquid, 320-1875; 10× concentrate, 330-2511), Sigma Chemical Co. (R 6504), or Difco Laboratories (1× liquid, 5087-72-8).

Sabhi agar*
For primary recovery of fungi from clinical specimens

Brain heart infusion broth	18.60 g
Calf brain, infusion from	50.00 g
Beef heart, infusion from	62.50 g
Proteose or Gelysate (BBL) pancreatic digest of gelatin	2.50 g
Sodium chloride	1.25 g
Neopeptone	5.00 g
Disodium phosphate	0.625 g
Agar	7.50 g
Distilled water	1.00 liter

Dissolve; autoclave at 121°C for 15 min.

Sabhi agar, modified

Brain heart infusion broth	18.60 g
Calf brain, infusion from	50.00 g
Beef heart, infusion from	62.50 g
Proteose or Gelysate (BBL) pancreatic digest of gelatin	2.50 g
Glucose	20.50 g
Sodium chloride	1.25 g
Neopeptone	5.00 g
Disodium phosphate	0.625 g
Agar	7.50 g
Distilled water	1.00 liter

Dissolve; autoclave at 121°C for 15 min. Cool to 50°C and add 1 ml of sterile chloramphenicol solution (100 mg/ml). Mix well and dispense into sterile tubes. Slant and allow to harden. Refrigerate until needed.

Sabouraud agar with CCG and NaCl (55)

Glucose	120 g
Bacto-Peptone (Difco)	30 g
Bacto-Agar (Difco)	45 g
Sodium chloride	150 g (for 5% NaCl)
	or
	90 g (for 3% NaCl)
Distilled water	3 liters

Bring to boil to dissolve, adjust pH to 7.0, and autoclave at 121°C for 15 min.

Cool and add CCG:

Chloramphenicol (10 mg/ml)	15 ml
Cycloheximide (20 mg/ml)	15 ml
Gentamicin (40 mg/ml)	1.5 ml

Dispense aseptically and slant. Omit CCG if culture is pure.

Sabouraud dextrose agar* (42)

Glucose	40.00 g
Neopeptone	10.00 g
Agar	20.00 g
Distilled water	1.00 liter
Final pH 5.6	

Add ingredients to water and heat to dissolve. Autoclave at 15 lb/in^2 (121°C) for 10 min. Dispense in petri dishes or tubes as needed.

A comparable medium may be obtained from BBL (21180), Difco (0109-17-1), or Remel (01-768).

Sabouraud dextrose agar with chloramphenicol and cycloheximide (42)
For yeast identification

Cycloheximide	500 mg
Acetone	10 ml
Chloramphenicol	50 mg
Ethyl alcohol, 95%	10 ml

Add cycloheximide to acetone. Add chloramphenicol to alcohol. Add both solutions to 1 liter of molten Sabouraud dextrose agar. Autoclave at 15 lb/in^2 (121°C) for 10 min. Dispense in tubes or petri dishes as needed.

A comparable medium may be obtained from BBL (20966), Difco (0689-01-7), or Remel (01-630).

Sabouraud dextrose (2%) agar Emmons* (25)

Glucose	20.0 g
Bacto-Peptone (Difco) or Polypeptone (BBL)	10.0 g
or	
(Pancreatic digest of casein USP	5.0 g)
(Peptic digest of animal tissue USP	5.0 g)
Agar, not dried	20.0 g
(*or* Dried	17.0 g)
Distilled water	1.0 liter
Final pH 6.9 ± 0.2	

Heat to dissolve completely. Dispense, and autoclave at 118 to 121°C for 10 min.

Comparable dehydrated media may be obtained from BBL (11589) and Difco (0747).

Sabouraud dextrose agar with olive oil (14)
For growth of Malassezia spp.

Sabouraud dextrose agar	65.00 g
Olive oil	20.00 ml
Tween 80	2.00 ml
Distilled water	1.00 liter

Add ingredients to water and heat to dissolve. Tube medium in 16- by 120-mm screw-cap tubes. Autoclave at 15 lb/in^2 (121°C) for 15 min. Allow to harden as slants with 1-in. (ca. 2.5-cm) butts.

Salmonella-shigella (SS) agar*

Beef extract	5.000 g
Proteose or Polypeptone (BBL)	5.000 g
Lactose	10.000 g
Bile salts	8.500 g
Sodium citrate	8.500 g
Sodium thiosulfate	8.500 g
Ferric citrate	1.000 g
Agar	13.500 g
Neutral red	0.025 g
Brilliant green	0.330 g
Distilled water	1.00 liter
Final pH 7.0	

Heat to boiling. Do not autoclave. Cool to 42 to 45°C, and pour into plates. For slants, prepare the medium in a sterile flask, with sterile water. Dispense aseptically, 5 ml per sterile 16- by 125-mm tube.

Salt tolerance media

The following media are used for the testing of salt tolerance by various organisms. Please note that heart infusion and Trypticase or soybean-casein digest bases already have 0.5% NaCl, so care must be taken as to how much additional NaCl should be added. The type of test and organisms to be tested will dictate the final concentration needed.

For nonfermenting gram-negative bacteria

1. Method of Tatum et al. (109)

Use nutrient broth base plus 65 g of sodium chloride per liter (6.5% NaCl).

2. Method of Gilardi (36)

Use soybean-casein digest agar USP plus 60 g of sodium chloride per liter (6.5% NaCl).

For Streptococcus and other gram-positive cocci

Heart infusion broth	25 g
Sodium chloride	60 g
Indicator (1.6 g of bromocresol purple in 100 ml of 95% ethanol)	1 ml
Glucose	1 g
Distilled water	1 liter

Add all reagents together up to 1,000 ml; do not compensate for the volume loss caused by the sodium chloride. Final volume should be 1,000 ml.

Dispense into 15- by 125-mm screw-cap tubes, and autoclave at 121°C for 15 min.

A positive reaction is recorded when the indicator changes from purple to yellow or when growth is obvious even though the indicator does not change.

For differentiation of Aeromonas and Plesiomonas spp.

Use nutrient broth with 6% NaCl. Prepare like nutrient agar but without adding agar. Add 60 g of NaCl per liter of broth.

For sodium chloride broth (6.5%)

Heart infusion broth*	1,000 ml
Sodium chloride	60 g

Add 60 g of sodium chloride to heart infusion broth (1,000 ml), dissolve completely, dispense into tubes, and autoclave at 121°C for 15 min.

Final concentration of sodium chloride is 6.5% (heart infusion broth already contains 0.5% sodium chloride).

Schaedler agar*

Tryptic soy broth (Difco)	10 g
Proteose Peptone no. 3 (Difco)	5 g
Yeast extract (Difco)	5 g
Dextrose (Difco)	5 g
Tris	3 g
L-Cystine	0.4 g
Hemin	0.01 g
Agar (Difco)	13.5 g
Distilled water	1 liter
Final pH 7.6 ± 0.2	

Suspend ingredients in distilled water and heat to boiling to dissolve completely. Sterilize in the autoclave for 15 min at 15 lb/in^2 and 121°C. If enrichment is desired, cool medium to 50°C, aseptically add 5% sterile defibrinated blood or other enrichment, and swirl gently to mix. Dispense as desired.

Schleifer-Krämer (SK) agar
Selective medium for isolating staphylococci

Tryptone or peptone from casein	10 g
Beef extract	5 g
Yeast extract	3 g
Glycerol	10 g
Sodium pyruvate	10 g
Glycine	500 mg
Potassium isothiocyanate	2.25 g
$NaH_2PO_4 \cdot H_2O$	600 mg
$Na_2HPO_4 \cdot 2H_2O$	900 mg
LiCl	2 g
Agar	13 g
Distilled water	1 liter

Adjust the pH to 7.2. Autoclave at 121°C for 15 min, cool in water bath to 45°C, and add 10 ml of a 0.45% sterile-filtered solution of sodium azide. Mix medium thoroughly and pour immediately into petri dishes. The medium can be stored at 4°C for at least 1 week.

Selective *Brucella* medium

Base

Serum dextrose agar, brucella agar, or Trypticase soy agar

Enrichment

Sterile 10% horse serum (100 ml/liter of base) inactivated for 30 min at 56°C, added to sterile tempered base aseptically

Antibiotics

VCN inhibitors (BBL), 10 ml (vancomycin, 3 μg/ml; sodium colistimethate, 7.5 μg/ml; and nystatin, 12.5 μg/ml)
Furadantin (10 μg/ml in 0.1 N NaOH), 1 ml

Selective 7H11 agar

See Middlebrook and Cohn 7H10 agar.

Selenite-F enrichment medium*

Sodium hydrogen selenite (anhydrous)	0.4%
Sodium phosphate (anhydrous)	1%
Peptone	0.5%
Lactose	0.4%
Final pH 7.0	

Dissolve ingredients and sterilize gently in flowing steam for 30 min. Dispense into petri dishes and let cool. *Do not autoclave.*

Semisynthetic medium for *Calymmatobacterium granulomatis*

See *Calymmatobacterium granulomatis* semidefined medium.

Serum dextrose agar (SDA) for *Brucella* spp.

Blood agar base (Oxoid)	40 g
Equine serum, inactivated at 56°C for 30 min	50 ml
Dextrose, 25% (wt/vol), autoclaved at 121°C for 15 min	40 ml
Distilled water	1 liter

Add Oxoid base to the water, and allow mixture to stand for 10 min to prevent the powder from caking. Apply gentle heat to aid solution before autoclaving at 121°C for 15 min. Cool to 56°C before adding serum and dextrose solution. Plates or slants are poured immediately.

7H10 agar

See Middlebrook and Cohn 7H10 agar.

7H11 agar

See Middlebrook 7H11 agar.

7H12 medium

See Middlebrook 7H12 medium (broth).

Sheep blood agar

See blood agar base.

Simmons citrate agar

See citrate agar.

Sodium chloride broth (6.5%)

See salt tolerance media.

Skirrow medium (101)

Blood agar base no. 2 (Oxoid CM 271)	1 liter
Lysed defibrinated horse blood	50 ml

Vancomycin	10 mg
Polymyxin B	2,500 IU
Trimethoprim	5 mg

Melt blood agar base, and cool to 50°C. Add blood and other ingredients to sterile molten agar.

Sodium hippurate broth

Heart infusion broth	25 g
Sodium hippurate	10 g
Distilled water	1 liter

Dispense into 15- by 125-mm screw-cap tubes, and sterilize in an autoclave for 15 min at 121°C. Tighten caps to prevent evaporation.

Inoculate with two or three colonies of beta-hemolytic streptococci, and incubate at 35°C for 20 h or longer. Centrifuge the medium to pack the cells, and pipette 0.8 ml of the clear supernatant into a Kahn tube. Add 0.2 ml of the ferric chloride reagent to the Kahn tube, and mix well. If a heavy precipitate remains longer than 10 min, the test is positive.

See chapter 122 for reagents.

Soil extract agar

For demonstrating typical conidia of Histoplasma capsulatum and Blastomyces dermatitidis

Soil	500.0 g
Glucose	2.0 g
Yeast extract	1.0 g
Potassium phosphate	0.5 g
Agar	15.0 g
Tap water	1 liter

Mix 500.0 g of garden soil and 1 liter of tap water. Autoclave for 3 h at 15 lb/in^2. Filter through Whatman no. 2 filter paper. This is the soil infusion. Add reagents and bring volume to 1 liter. Bring to a boil. Dispense 7.0-ml aliquots into 16- by 125-mm test tubes. Autoclave for 15 min at 15 lb/in^2. Slant the test tubes.

Inoculate with hyphae of a test isolate, and incubate at 25°C. Typical conidia should be seen in tease mounts examined microscopically after 7 to 14 days of incubation. Make tease mounts in a bacteriological glove box or laminar-flow hood.

Sorbitol MacConkey agar

See MacConkey sorbitol agar.

Soybean-casein digest agar* USP

Trypticase soy agar (BBL), tryptic soy agar (Difco), tryptone soya agar, casein soy peptone agar, etc.

Pancreatic digest of casein USP	15 g
Papaic digest of soy meal USP	5 g
Sodium chloride	5 g
Agar	15 g
Distilled water	1 liter
Final pH 7.3	

Heat with agitation until the medium boils. Dispense, and autoclave at 118 to 121°C for 15 min.

Staib agar (103)

Guizottia abyssinica creatinine agar, nigerseed agar, birdseed agar

Guizottia abyssinica seed	50 g
Glucose	1 g
KH_2PO_4	1 g
Creatinine	1 g
Agar	15 g
Distilled water	1 liter

Add 50 g of the pulverized seed to 1,000 ml of distilled water, boil for 30 min, and filter through a cloth or paper filter. Complete the filtrate to 1,000 ml. Add the following to the filtrate: glucose, 1 g; KH_2PO_4, 1 g; creatinine, 1 g; and agar, 15 g. Autoclave at 110°C for 20 min and pour the medium into petri dishes.

Available commercially as MYCOPLATE CR Roche (Staib Agar) from Hoffmann-La Roche, D-7889 Grenzach/Wyhlen, Federal Republic of Germany.

Staib agar, modified (42)

Birdseed agar for identification of Cryptococcus neoformans

Guizottia abyssinica seeds (niger or thistle seeds, Philadelphia Seed Co., Plymouth Meeting, Pa.)	70.00 g
Creatinine	0.78 g
Glucose	10.00 g
Chloramphenicol	0.05 g
Agar	20.00 g
Distilled water	1.00 liter
Diphenyl	0.10 g
Ethyl alcohol, 95%	10.00 ml

Grind seeds in a blender to make a powder. Combine powder with 300 ml of water and autoclave at 15 lb/in^2 (121°C) for 10 min. Cool, filter through gauze, and restore filtrate volume to 1 liter with water. Add other ingredients (except diphenyl and alcohol) and autoclave at 15 lb/in^2 (121°C) for 15 min. Cool to 50°C. Dissolve diphenyl in alcohol and add aseptically to cooled medium. Mix well and pour into sterile petri dishes. Chloramphenicol, diphenyl, and alcohol may be omitted if pure yeast cultures are being tested.

A comparable medium may be obtained from BBL (97096) or Remel (08-172).

Starch agar

Nutrient agar*	23 g
Potato starch	10 g
Demineralized water	1 liter

Dissolve nutrient agar medium in 500 ml of water. Dissolve starch in 250 ml of water by boiling. Combine and make up to 1-liter volume. Adjust the pH, and autoclave at 121°C for 30 min.

This medium is useful for differentiation of species of aerobic actinomycetes. Inoculate as for casein agar. When good growth is obtained, test for hydrolysis by flooding a small portion of the plate with Gram or Lugol iodine; this does not contaminate the plate, which may subsequently be retested if necessary. In a negative test, the agar immediately around the growth becomes (temporarily) dark blue; if it becomes red or remains unstained, partial or complete hydrolysis is shown.

Starch fermentation broth
For corynebacteria

A. Heart infusion broth with bromocresol purple

Heart infusion	5 ml
Demineralized water	200 ml
Bromocresol purple, 1% in ethanol	0.2 ml
Adjust to pH 7.8.	

B. Starch 2% ... 20 ml

Dissolve by bringing to boil with constant stirring.
Combine A and B and dispense into screw-cap tubes. Autoclave at 121°C for 15 min.

Starch hydrolysis agar

Heart infusion agar	40 g
Soluble starch	20 g
Distilled water	1 liter

Warm to dissolve, and autoclave at 121°C for 15 min. Cool to 55°C, and pour into sterile petri dishes.

Hydrolysis of starch is determined by flooding the surface of the plate with Gram iodine 48 h after inoculation and incubation at 35°C. A zone of hydrolysis appears colorless, and a dark blue to purple zone indicates that the starch has not been hydrolyzed.

Starch hydrolysis agar, modified
See Mueller-Hinton agar, method of Gilardi (36).

Starch hydrolysis is tested by flooding Mueller-Hinton agar (BBL) plates with Lugol iodine after 24 h of aerobic incubation at 30°C and observing for a clear zone around the patch growth (patch inoculum).

Stock culture maintenance media

See motility nitrate agar and motility test and maintenance medium.

Streptococcal and other gram-positive coccal growth medium
For growth at 10 and 45°C

Heart infusion broth	25 g
Glucose	1 g
Indicator (1.6 g of bromocresol purple in 100 ml of 95% ethanol)	1 ml
Distilled water	1 liter

Dispense in 5-ml amounts into 16- by 125-mm screw-cap tubes. Autoclave at 121°C for 15 min.

A positive reaction is recorded when growth is indicated by a color change from purple to yellow or by frank growth in the tube.

See temperature requirements in chapter 122.

Stuart *Leptospira* broth, modified*
Modified by the Department of Veterinary Medicine, Walter Reed Army Institute of Research, Washington, D.C.

Glycerol-asparagine-salt solution

Sodium chloride	1.930 g
Ammonium chloride	0.340 g
Magnesium chloride $\cdot 6H_2O$	0.190 g
L-Asparagine	0.130 g
Disodium phosphate	0.666 g
Monopotassium phosphate	0.087 g
Glycerol, optional	5.000 ml
Distilled water	995.000 ml

Dissolve each ingredient separately in 100-ml portions of water. Mix and make up to 1 liter in water. Autoclave at 121°C for 15 min. Cool and add 100 ml of filter-sterilized rabbit serum, previously inactivated in a 56°C water bath for 30 min. Dispense.

Stuart transport medium*

Sodium thioglycolate	1.0 g
Sodium glycerophosphate	10.0 g
Calcium chloride	0.1 g
Methylene blue	0.002 g
Agar	3.0 g
Demineralized water	1 liter
Final pH 7.3 ± 0.2 at 25°C	

Sucrose agar
For glucan production

Heart infusion agar	40 g
Sucrose	50 g
Distilled water	1 liter

Autoclave at 121°C for 15 min. Cool to 55°C and pour into 13- by 100-mm petri dishes (ca. 10 ml into each).

Glucan production typical of *Streptococcus sanguis* and *S. mutans* results in highly refractile-adherent or white-dry-adherent growth on the agar. Levan production typical of *S. salivarius* results in opaque, gummy, nonadherent growth. Typical *S. bovis* and *Leuconostoc mesenteroides* growth is similar to that of *S. salivarius* but is somewhat less gummy and rarely adheres to the medium. Large or small colonies that are mucoidal and nonadherent are considered negative or have no extracellular polysaccharide production.

Sucrose broth
For glucan production

Solution A

NIH thioglycolate broth	28.5 g
Dipotassium phosphate	10.0 g
Sodium acetate	12.0 g
Distilled water	500.0 ml

Solution B

Sucrose	50.0 g
Distilled water	500.0 ml

Sterilize solutions separately in an autoclave at 121°C for 15 min. Cool to 55°C, mix solutions, and dispense into 16- by 125-mm screw-cap tubes in 5-ml amounts.

Glucan production is indicated when the broth is partially or completely gelled—a typical *Streptococcus sanguis* reaction. Glucan production is also indicated when gelatinous, adherent deposits form on the bottom and walls of the growth tube—a typical *S. mutans* reaction. An increase in the viscosity of the broth indicates the production of slime (unknown polysaccharide) typical of *S. bovis*. Negative reactions are recorded when no gelling, deposit, or increase in viscosity occurs.

Tap water agar

For examining the morphology of fungi and aerobic actinomycetes

Agar	15 g
Tap water	1 liter

Add the agar to water and autoclave at 15 lb/in² for 15 min. Pour into petri dishes, and allow to harden. Streak a purified isolate onto the plate. Incubate for 24 to 72 h at 35°C, or up to 1 week at room temperature. Invert the plate and observe it under low power on the microscope. Submerged filaments will appear fine and delicate; aerial hyphae will be coarse and black.

See also Water agar, 2%.

TCBS agar (thiosulfate-citrate-bile-sucrose agar)*

Yeast extract	5 g
Proteose Peptone no. 3	10 g
Sodium citrate	10 g
Sodium thiosulfate	10 g
Oxgall	8 g
Saccharose	20 g
Ferric citrate	1 g
Bromothymol blue	0.04 g
Agar	15 g
Distilled water	1 liter
Final pH 8.6 ± 0.2 at 25°C	

Mix ingredients and heat to dissolve completely. Sterilize in the autoclave for 15 min at 15 lb/in² (121°C). Dispense.

Tetrathionate broth

Proteose Peptone (Difco)	5 g
Bile salts	1 g
Calcium carbonate	10 g
Sodium thiosulfate	30 g
Distilled water	1 liter

Dispense the medium in 10-ml amounts and heat to boiling. Just before the tubes are to be used, add 0.2 ml of iodine solution (6 g of iodine crystals and 5 g of potassium iodide in 20 ml of water) to each tube. The sterile base medium may be stored in the refrigerator indefinitely.

Tetrazolium tolerance (TTC) agar

Soybean-casein digest agar USP plus 10 g of triphenyltetrazolium chloride per liter.

TGY agar*

Tryptone (tryptophan-peptone)-glucose-yeast agar

Pancreatic digest of casein USP	5 g
Glucose	1 g
Yeast extract	5 g
Dipotassium phosphate	1 g
Agar	15 g
Distilled water	1 liter
Final pH 6.8 to 7.0	

Bring to a boil to dissolve agar. Dispense 5 ml per tube into 15- by 125-mm tubes. Autoclave at 121°C for 15 min, and slant.

Thayer-Martin agar*

Combine sterile solutions, with the agar base cooled to 50°C.

GC agar base* sterile, double strength, 100 ml (see chocolate agars). Add 2 g of agar and 0.5 g of glucose to the double-strength GC agar base before dissolving in 100 ml of water.

Hemoglobin,* 2% aqueous, 100 ml, or chocolated defribinated blood, 5%

Antibiotic inhibitors* to give final concentrations per 100 ml of medium of: vancomycin, 300 µg; colistin, 750 µg; nystatin, 1,250 U; trimethoprim lactate, 500 µg

Chemical enrichment, e.g., 1% IsoVitaleX*

Vitamin B_{12}	0.010 g
L-Glutamine	10.000 g
Adenine	1.000 g
Guanine hydrochloride	0.030 g
p-Aminobenzoic acid	0.013 g
L-Cystine	1.100 g
Glucose	100.000 g
Diphosphopyridine nucleotide oxidized (coenzyme I)	0.250 g
Cocarboxylase	0.100 g
Ferric nitrate	0.020 g
Thiamine hydrochloride	0.003 g
Cysteine hydrochloride	25.900 g
Distilled water	1.000 liter

Other supplements, e.g., supplement "B,"* may be used instead of the defined chemical enrichment.

Also see Transgrow agar.

For modified Thayer-Martin agar,* add 2 g of agar and 0.5 g of glucose to the double-strength GC agar base before dissolving in 100 ml of water.

For Martin-Lewis agar, use 400 µg of vancomycin per 100 ml of medium, and substitute 200 µg of anisomycin for nystatin.

Thiogel medium (18)

For anaerobes

Thiogel medium (BBL)*	90 g
Distilled water	1 liter

Preheat water to 50°C, add Thiogel medium, and let stand for 5 min. Boil for 1 min (with frequent mixing), and dispense 7 ml into 15- by 90-mm screw-cap tubes. Autoclave at 118°C for 15 min, and cool.

See note on fermentation broth for anaerobes. Place

in tube in glove box, tighten caps, remove from glove box, and store at 4°C or ambient temperature.

Thiogel medium is used to test the ability of anaerobes to hydrolyze gelatin. Place culture and uninoculated control in a beaker of cold water in a refrigerator. Check for liquefaction when the control has solidified. The Centers for Disease Control manual states that reactions are usually complete by 7 days, but Thiogel may be incubated for up to 1 month before it is reported as negative (18).

Thioglycolate-bile broth

Thioglycolate medium without indicator* can be used to prepare 20% bile broth by adding 0.5 ml of a solution containing 40% oxgall and 2% sodium deoxycholate (sterilized by autoclaving) to 10 ml of thioglycolate medium.

Thioglycolate medium, Brewer modified*

Pancreatic digest of casein USP	17.500 g
Papaic digest of soybean meal USP	2.500 g
Glucose	10.000 g
Sodium chloride	5.000 g
Dipotassium phosphate	2.000 g
Sodium thioglycolate	1.000 g
Methylene blue	0.002 g
Distilled water	1.000 liter
Final pH 7.2	

Dispense into test tubes, half full, and autoclave at 121°C for 15 min.

Thioglycolate medium without indicator,* plus hemin

Pancreatic digest of casein USP	17.00 g
Papaic digest of soy meal USP	3.00 g
Glucose	6.00 g
Sodium chloride	2.50 g
Sodium thioglycolate	0.50 g
Agar	0.70 g
L-Cystine	0.25 g
Sodium sulfite	0.10 g
Purified water	1.00 liter
Hemin	5.00 mg

Mix and heat with agitation to obtain solution. Omit hemin, if desired. Dispense into tubes with calcium carbonate chips or powder, approximately 0.1 g per tube, to promote viability, spore formation, and maintenance of cultures. Boil (or steam for 10 min), and cool to room temperature just before use. Add filter-sterilized sodium bicarbonate to a concentration of 1 mg/ml and vitamin K_1 to a concentration of 0.1 g/ml.

Other supplements may be added, if desired, by introducing a pipette to the bottom of the tube and withdrawing the pipette as the supplement is added, e.g., 5% Fildes enrichment or 10% sterile animal serum. Do not shake or invert tubes.

Thioglycolate medium, supplemented

Use thioglycolate medium without indicator prepared according to the manufacturer's instructions. Add hemin (5 μg/ml) and vitamin K_1 (0.1 μg/ml). Dispense into tubes, each containing a marble chip (Fisher); fill the tubes two-thirds to three-fourths full. Autoclave as directed. Just before use, boil or steam for 5 min, cool, and supplement with normal rabbit or horse serum (10%, vol/vol) or peptic digest of sheep blood (Fildes enrichment [5%, vol/vol]*).

Tinsdale medium (9, 110)

Modified according to P. Maximescu

Proteose Peptone no. 3 (Difco)	20.0 g
NaCl	5.0 g
Agar (Difco)	20.0 g
Distilled water	1.0 liter

The molten medium is adjusted to pH 7.4 and autoclaved for 15 min at 121°C. This basic medium can be stored at 4°C for 3 to 4 months. After cooling to 55°C, the following sterile solutions are aseptically added:

Formalinized sheep blood (100 ml of blood + 0.125 ml of Formalin)	3.0 ml
NaOH, 0.1 N	60.0 ml
L-Cystine, 0.4% solution (0.24 g of L-cystine dissolved in 60 ml of 0.1 N HCl at 60 to 70°C)	60.0 ml
Potassium tellurite, 1% (wt/vol), aqueous	30.0 ml
Sodium thiosulfate (2.5 g dissolved in 100 ml of distilled water at 60°C)	17.0 ml
Bovine serum (sterile)	100.0 to 150.0 ml

A supplement containing essentially these components is also available from Difco as desiccated Bacto-Tinsdale enrichment.

Pour into petri dishes and store at 4°C for no longer than 4 days. Check each lot with a reference strain for satisfactory halo production.

Tissue culture media

See Eagle, Hanks, and RPMI media.

Todd-Hewitt broth, modified

Beef heart infusion	1,000 ml
Neopeptone	20 g

Mix ingredients and adjust pH to 7.0.

Sodium chloride	2 g
Sodium bicarbonate	2 g
Disodium phosphate	0.4 g
Glucose	2 g
Final pH 7.8	

Mix the chemicals in the broth and heat to a boil. Boil for 15 min, filter through paper, and dispense in tubes. Sterilize in autoclave at 115°C for 10 min.

Toxigenicity test agar, Elek

See KL-virulence agar (Elek agar).

Transgrow agar*

Prepare as for Thayer-Martin agar, except with added glucose (0.15%) and the agar increased to 2% in the GC agar base. Gas the bottles with 20% CO_2 in air, and tighten caps securely.

Trimethoprim lactate (5 mg/liter) may be added to either Thayer-Martin or Transgrow agar, if desired, especially for the examination of rectal specimens.

Transport media for anaerobes (PRAS)

A. Without peptones

Ionagar no. 2 or equivalent	2.00 g
Resazurin solution[a]	0.40 ml
L-Cysteine hydrochloride	0.05 g
Distilled water	100.0 ml

[a]See Cary and Blair transport medium, modified (PRAS).

In a flask, boil all ingredients except cysteine. When dissolved, gas with carbon dioxide. Add cysteine. When dissolved, adjust the pH to 6.8 with 20% sodium hydroxide. Cap the flask with a rubber stopper, pass into an anaerobic chamber, and dispense aseptically into tubes.

B. PYG medium

Peptone or Gelysate (BBL) pancreatic digest of gelatin	1.00 g
Yeast extract	1.00 g
Glucose	1.00 g
Resazurin solution	0.40 ml
Distilled water	100.00 ml
L-Cysteine hydrochloride	0.05 g
Salts solution[a]	4.00 ml

[a]Salts solution formula:

Calcium chloride	0.2 g
Magnesium sulfate	0.2 g
Dipotassium phosphate	1.0 g
Monopotassium phosphate	1.0 g
Sodium bicarbonate	10.0 g
Distilled water	1.0 liter

Boil ingredients except cysteine until colorless. Cool to 45°C while gassing with carbon dioxide. Add cysteine. When dissolved, adjust the pH to 6.8 with 20% sodium hydroxide. Cap the flask with a rubber stopper, pass into an anaerobic chamber, and dispense aseptically into tubes.

C. See Cary and Blair transport medium, modified (PRAS)

Trichophyton agars

See Casein agars.

Trichophyton agars 6 and 7

See Ammonium nitrate agar.

Trichophyton agars* (34)
Nutritional tests for dermatophytes

These media are available in dehydrated form from Difco Laboratories (Detroit, Mich.) as Trichophyton Agars 1 to 7 and as agar slants from Remel (Lenexa, Kans.).

Triple sugar iron agar (TSI)* (41)
TSI slant

Casein/meat peptone (50/50)	20.0 g
Glucose	1.0 g
Lactose	10.0 g
Sucrose	10.0 g
$FeNH_4(SO_4)_2 \cdot 12H_2O$ (ferrous ammonium sulfate)	0.2 g
NaCl	5.0 g
$Na_2S_2O_3 \cdot 5H_2O$	0.3 g
Agar	12.0 g
Phenol red	0.24 g
Distilled water	1.0 liter

Dispense in 5-ml aliquots in tubes and autoclave in a slanted position. The medium can be kept at 4°C for 6 to 8 weeks.

Tryptic soy agar

See soybean-casein digest agar USP.

Trypticase nitrate broth

See indole test media.

Trypticase soy agar

See soybean-casein digest agar USP.

Trypticase soy broth*

Trypticase	17 g
Phytone	3 g
Sodium chloride	5 g
Dipotassium phosphate	2.5 g
Glucose	2.5 g
Distilled water	1.0 liter
Final pH ± 7.3	

Mix ingredients, dispense into tubes, and autoclave at 121°C for 15 min.

Supplements:
1. 0.1% Tween 80
2. 10% fetal calf serum

Tryptone broth

See indole test media.

Tryptophan broth

See indole test media.

Tyrosine agar

Basal medium, sterile melted	100 ml
Tyrosine	0.5 g
Distilled water	10 ml

Prepare a sterile tyrosine solution by adding the tyrosine to the distilled water and autoclaving for 10 min at 121°C. Allow the sterile melted basal medium to cool almost to solidification. Add 10 ml of the sterile tyrosine solution to the flask or bottle of basal medium. Mix. Aseptically dispense 25-ml aliquots into sterile 15- by 100-mm petri plates. Label plates and bag to reduce contamination and dehydration.

Plates may be stored in bags for up to 2 months in the refrigerator at 4°C.

Tyrosine hydrolysis is recommended for differentiation of species of aerobic actinomycetes. Hydrolysis is indicated by a clearing of the medium under and around the inoculum by *Streptomyces griseus* and *Actinomadura madurae*. There is no hydrolysis of the medium of *Nocardia asteroides*.

U (ureaplasma) agar plates

To 65 ml of molten basic agar (see mycoplasmal media) (55°C), add 10 ml of yeast dialysate, 2 ml of penicillin (10,000 U/ml), 3 ml of 1 M MES [2-(*N*-morpholino)ethanesulfonic acid], pH 5.5, 0.2 ml of 1 M urea, and 20 ml of horse serum. Dispense in 5-ml amounts into 10- by 35-mm petri dishes, and incubate overnight at room temperature.

Ureaplasmal colonies are particularly vulnerable to excess surface moisture.

U (ureaplasma) broth
For isolation of Ureaplasma urealyticum

To 65 ml of basic broth (see mycoplasmal media), aseptically add 10 ml of yeast dialysate, 20 ml of horse serum, 2 ml of penicillin (10,000 U/ml), 1 ml of MES buffer (see above), 0.5 ml of 1 M urea, and 1.0 ml of 0.1 M Na_2SO_3. Use within 48 h or delay the addition of Na_2SO_3 until just before use.

Urea semisolid medium (18)
For anaerobes

Solution A

Thioglycolate without glucose or indicator*	9.6 g
Yeast extract*	0.8 g
Distilled water	400 ml

Dissolve the ingredients by heating, autoclave at 121°C, and cool at 60°C.

Solution B

Urea broth*	15.5 g
Distilled water	50.0 ml

Mix the urea broth and water, and filter sterilize. Combine solutions A and B aseptically and mix. Dispense 7 ml into 15- by 90-mm screw-cap tubes.

See note on fermentation broth for anaerobes. Place tubes in anaerobic glove box, tighten caps, remove from glove box, and store at 4°C or ambient temperature.

Editors' note. The authors recommend Difco ingredients.

A deep red color is positive; no color is negative (2 to 5 days of incubation). If the phenol red indicator is reduced, add 2 to 3 drops of dilute phenol red to the culture on the last day of incubation.

Urea test broth* (103)

A. *Urea broth for enterobacteriaceae*

Yeast extract	0.100 g
Monopotassium phosphate	9.1 g
Disodium phosphate	9.5 g
Urea	20.000 g
Phenol red	0.010 g
Distilled water	1.000 liter

Sterilize by passing through a Seitz filter, and dispense 3-ml amounts into tubes. Alternatively, prepare basal medium in 900 ml of distilled water, and autoclave at 121°C for 15 min. After cooling, 100 ml of 20% filter-sterilized urea solution is added, and the medium is dispensed into sterile tubes.

Inoculate with three loopfuls (2-mm loop) from an agar slant culture, and shake to suspend the bacteria. Incubate in a water bath at 37°C, and read after 10 min, 60 min, and 2 h.

B. *Urea broth for aerobic actinomycetes*

Dehydrated urea broth (Difco)	3.87 g
Distilled water	100 ml

Dissolve dehydrated urea broth in distilled water. Sterilize by filtration through a 0.22-μm-pore-size filter. Aseptically dispense 4-ml amounts into sterile 16- by 125-mm screw-cap tubes. Label tubes and tighten caps for storage. May be stored in the refrigerator at 4°C for up to 30 days.

Urease is detected by using a heavy inoculum of a pure culture and incubating the tube for 48 h. Observation for hydrolysis of urea should be recorded after 8, 12, 24, and 48 h. Hydrolysis is indicated by a color change of the broth from yellow to red by *Nocardia asteroides*. There is no hydrolysis or color change by *Actinomadura madurae*.

C. *Urea broth for ureaplasma urease test*

H broth base	85 ml
Urea (1 M in water, filter sterilized)	0.5 ml
Horse serum	10 ml
MES buffer (1 M in water; adjust to pH 6.2 with 1 N NaOH at 37°C, and filter sterilize)	1 ml
Penicillin (10,000 U/ml)	2 ml
Sodium sulfite (100 mM in water, freshly prepared and autoclaved)	1 ml
Phenol red (1%)	0.1 ml

Dispense in 3-ml amounts into 16- by 125-mm test tubes.

This medium should not be stored for more than 3 days after the addition of sulfite. It is convenient to make up the complete medium without sulfite and to add an appropriate amount of sulfite before use.

Urease swabs (123)
For rapid identification of Cryptococcus neoformans

Swab preparation

Urea agar base (Difco)	29 g
Distilled water	20 ml

Test solution preparation

Benzalkonium chloride (Zephiran)	0.1 g
Sterile distilled water	10.0 ml

Combine urea agar base and distilled water. Adjust to pH 5.5 and sterilize by membrane filtration. Saturate sterile cotton-tipped swabs in the mixture and allow to dry overnight at room temperature. In a separate tube, prepare the test solution by adding benzalkonium chloride to sterile distilled water.

Urease test agar (10)
Urea agar base, Christensen

A. *For enterobacteriaceae and streptococci*

Urea concentrate

Peptone or Gelysate (BBL) pancreatic digest of gelatin	1.000 g
Sodium chloride	5.000 g
Glucose	1.000 g
Monopotassium phosphate	2.000 g
Phenol red	0.12 g
Urea	20.000 g
Distilled water	100.000 ml

Adjust to pH 6.8 and sterilize by filtration. Dissolve 15 g of agar in 900 ml of water, and autoclave at 121°C for 15 min. Cool to 50 to 55°C in a water bath, and add 100 ml of sterile urea concentrate. Cool in a slanted position to form slants with deep butts.

Inoculate heavily over the entire surface of the slant, and incubate at 37°C. Examine at 2 and 4 h and after overnight incubation. Negative tubes should be observed daily for 4 days to detect delayed reactions given by members of certain groups other than *Proteus* spp. Urease-positive cultures produce an alkaline reaction evidenced by a red color.

B. *For aerobic actinomycetes*

Prepare agar base by dissolving 20 g of agar in 500 ml of demineralized water; dissolve the salts, peptone, and glucose in the remaining 500 ml of water. Combine, and adjust the pH to 6.9. To 1 liter of base cooled to 50°C, add 100 ml of 20% filter-sterilized urea solution. Dispense, slant, and inoculate as above.

C. *For nonfermenting gram-negative bacteria*

Urea agar base, Christensen, is prepared as given above. Christensen urea agar (BBL) warmed to incubator temperature is used for detection of urease production. A heavy inoculum of growth from a 24- to 48-h blood agar base culture is used. Examine after 5 and 10 min and after overnight incubation. Urease-positive cultures produce an alkaline reaction evidenced by a red color.

D. *For differentiation of yeastlike fungi and identification of some Trichophyton spp.*

Urea agar (67)

A. Urea agar base (Christensen)	29 g
Distilled water	100 ml

Dissolve powder in water and sterilize by filtration.

B. Agar	15 g
Distilled water	900 ml

Dissolve agar in water and sterilize by autoclaving at 121°C for 15 min. Cool agar to approximately 50°C. Add the 100 ml of sterile urea agar base. Mix well; dispense aseptically into sterile tubes. Allow to cool in slanted position to form butt about 1 in. (2.54 cm) deep and slant approximately 1.5 in. (3.81 cm) long.

Urease-positive organisms produce an alkaline reaction indicated by a pink-red color.

This medium is available commercially in dehydrated form or prepared by BBL Laboratories (Cockeysville, Md.), Difco Laboratories (Detroit, Mich.), and Remel (Lenexa, Kans.).

USDA-FSIS listeria enrichment broth

See listeria media.

Vaginalis agar (V agar)

Columbia agar base*	10.00 g
Proteose Peptone no. 3*	10.00 g
Distilled water	1.00 liter
Final pH 7.3	

Heat with frequent agitation, and boil for 1 min. Dispense, and autoclave at 121°C for 15 min. Cool the sterile base to 45°C, and add 5% whole human blood.

Viral media

See Arenavirus, Eagle, Hanks, and RPMI media.

Viral transport medium (VTM)

A. Veal infusion broth (VIB) (Difco catalog no. 0344-17)

VIB	25 g
Distilled water, to	1 liter

Dispense in appropriate volumes and autoclave at 121°C for 15 min. Store at 4°C for up to 6 months.

B. Viral transport medium

VIB	100 ml
Bovine serum albumin	0.5 g
Phenol red	0.4 ml

Sterilize by filtration; when cool add:

Vancomycin (50 mg/ml)	0.2 ml
Gentamicin (50 mg/ml)	1.0 ml
Fungizone (amphotericin B) (250 µg/ml)	2.0 ml

Dispense 2 ml of VTM into serum vials. Store at 4°C and use for up to 2 months.

VP medium*
Voges-Proskauer test for production of acetoin

Peptone	7.0 g
Glucose	5.0 g
Dipotassium phosphate	5.0 g
Distilled water	1.0 liter

Adjust to pH 6.9, dispense in 3-ml amounts into 13-mm screw-cap tubes, and autoclave at 121°C for 15 min. Inoculate and incubate for 2 days at 35°C. To test for acetoin, add 5 drops of alpha-naphthol and 5 drops of KOH-creatine (see chapter 122, VP test). Shake tube briskly for at least 30 s. Red indicates positive.

A more sensitive and rapid procedure is that with a commercial VP tablet. The pyruvate-glucose-phosphate tablet is dissolved in 1 ml of water. The resultant medium is heavily inoculated and incubated for 4 to 6 h. Test procedure is that given above. See chapter 122 for reagents.

Dehydrated methyl red-VP medium is available from BBL and Difco. VP tablets are available from Key Scientific Products.

Wadowsky-Yee medium, modified

See modified Wadowsky-Yee medium.

Wall-defective bacterial medium (39)

Sucrose	100.0 g
Phytone (BBL)	20.0 g
NaCl	5.0 g
$MgSO_4 \cdot 4H_2O$	2.5 g
Yeast Extract (Difco)	10.0 g
Agarose	10.0 g
Purified water	1.0 liter

Adjust pH to 7.8 with 1 N NaOH. Add 10 ml of 95% ethanol containing 0.04 g of cholesterol. Sterilize by autoclaving. Complete medium is prepared by adding 20 ml of horse serum per 80 ml of this basic medium (melted and cooled to 55°C). Broth culture medium is prepared by using the basic medium without agarose.

Water agar, 2% (2)
Recommended for sporulation of some fungi

Agar	20.0 g
Distilled water	1 liter

Mix reagents, bring to a boil, autoclave for 15 min at 15 lb/in^2, and pour into petri plates.

With fungi that have not sporulated on other sporulating fungal media (modified cornmeal, cornmeal, and potato-dextrose agars), transfer a block of the medium with the actively growing edges of fungal colony onto the center of a petri plate of water agar; sporulation is encouraged.

Wickerham broths (120, 121)

A. *For carbohydrate assimilation tests*

Use 100 ml of yeast nitrogen base (YNB),* 10×.

Add 10 g of carbohydrate (but add 20 g of raffinose). See carbon assimilation tests (auxanographic method for yeast identification). Filter sterilize. Add 0.5 ml of this concentrate to a tube containing 4.5 ml of sterile distilled water.

B. *For nitrate assimilation tests*

Use 100 ml of yeast carbon base (YCB),* 10×.

Add 0.78 g of potassium nitrate or peptone.

Sterilize by filtration, and follow the procedure for carbohydrate assimilation tests with Wickerham media.

Note. Inoculation for both tests should be with a suspension of starved yeast which gives at least 95% transmission (T) at 530 nm in a spectrophotometer. Incubate at 25 to 30°C with shaking. Examine tubes for growth as indicated by turbidity.

Wickerham media, modified

Bromocresol purple, 1.6%	1.0 ml
Deionized water	450.0 ml
Sodium hydroxide, 0.1 N	5.0 ml
Washed agar	10.0 g

Mix, and heat to dissolve. Cool to 45 to 50°C.

A. *For carbohydrate assimilation*

To 50 ml of YNB (10×), add 5.0 g of carbohydrate. Admix to the melted basal medium. Dispense in 5-ml amounts into sterile screw-cap tubes. Autoclave at 115°C for 10 min. Cool in a slanted position. Test each lot with standard control cultures of *Candida krusei*, *C. guilliermondii*, *C. pseudotropicalis*, and *Cryptococcus laurentii*.

B. *For nitrate assimilation*

To 50 ml of YCB (10×), add 0.5 g of peptone or potassium nitrate, and filter sterilize. Admix to the melted basal medium. Proceed as described above.

Wilkins-Chalgren agar*

Pancreatic digest of casein	10 g
Pancreatic digest of gelatin	10 g
Yeast extract	5 g
Glucose	1 g
Sodium chloride	5 g
L-Arginine (free base)	1 g
Sodium pyruvate	1 g
Hemin	5.0 mg
Vitamin K_1	0.5 mg
Agar	15 g
Distilled water	1 liter

Final pH 7.0 to 7.2

Mix and heat with agitation until dissolved. Dispense, and autoclave at 121°C for 15 min.

Wolin-Bevis agar (122)
For yeast morphology studies

Tween 80	3.00 ml
Glucose	0.25 g
L-Histidine hydrochloride	0.25 g
Ammonium sulfate	1.00 g
Monopotassium phosphate	1.00 g
Agar	20.00 g
Distilled water	1 liter

Dissolve ingredients in water by gentle heating. Autoclave at 15 lb/in^2 (121°C) for 15 min. Dispense in 20-ml aliquots in sterile petri dishes.

Xanthine agar

Basal medium, sterile melted	100 ml
Xanthine	0.4 g
Distilled water	10 ml

Prepare a sterile xanthine solution by adding the xanthine to the distilled water and autoclaving for 10 min at 121°C. Allow the sterile melted basal medium to cool almost to solidification. Add 10 ml of the sterile xanthine solution to the flask or bottle of basal medium. Mix. Aseptically dispense 25-ml aliquots into sterile 15- by 100-ml petri plates. Label plates and bag to reduce dehydration and contamination. May be stored at 4°C for up to 3 months.

Xanthine agar is recommended for differentiation of species of aerobic actinomycetes by checking for hydrolysis of xanthine by a growing culture. Hydrolysis is indicated by a clearing of the medium under and around the inoculum by *Streptomyces griseus.* There is no hydrolysis of the medium by *Nocardia asteroides* or *Actinomadura madurae.*

Xylose-lysine-deoxycholate (XLD) agar*
For isolation of gram-negative bacteria

Yeast extract (Difco)	3 g
L-Lysine	5 g
Xylose (Difco)	3.75 g
Lactose (Difco)	7.5 g
Saccharose (Difco)	7.5 g
Sodium deoxycholate	2.5 g
Ferric ammonium citrate	0.8 g
Sodium thiosulfate	6.8 g
Sodium chloride	5 g
Bacto-Agar (Difco)	15 g
Phenol red (Difco)	0.08 g
Final pH 7.4 ± 0.2 at 25°C	

Mix ingredients and heat to dissolve, but *do not boil.* Transfer to a 50°C water bath, and pour plates as soon as medium has cooled. The medium should be red-orange and clear.

Xylose-sodium deoxycholate-citrate agar (98)

Nutrient broth no. 2 (Oxoid)	12.5 g
Sodium citrate	5.0 g
Sodium thiosulfate	5.0 g
Ferric ammonium citrate	1.0 g
Sodium deoxycholate	2.5 g
Xylose	10.0 g
Neutral red (1% aqueous)	2.5 ml
Agar	12.0 g
Distilled water	1.0 liter

Heat to 100°C, simmer for 20 s, cool to 50°C, and plate.

Yeast ascospore agar (84)

Potassium acetate	10.0 g
Yeast extract	2.5 g
Glucose	1.0 g
Agar	30.0 g
Distilled water	1.0 liter

Dissolve, tube, and autoclave at 121°C for 15 min.

Ascospores are obtained in 2 to 6 days at room temperature (23 to 25°C).

Yeast carbon base* (YCB), 10×
Wickerham carbon base broth

Boric acid	0.500 mg
Copper sulfate	0.040 mg
Potassium iodide	0.100 mg
Ferric chloride	0.200 mg
Manganese sulfate	0.400 mg
Sodium molybdate	0.200 mg
Zinc sulfate	0.400 mg
Biotin	0.002 mg
Calcium pantothenate	0.400 mg
Folic acid	0.002 mg
Inositol	2.000 mg
Niacin	0.400 mg
p-Aminobenzoic acid	0.200 mg
Pyridoxine	0.400 mg
Riboflavin	0.200 mg
Thiamine hydrochloride	0.400 mg
L-Histidine hydrochloride	0.001 g
DL-Methionine	0.002 g
DL-Tryptophan	0.002 g
Potassium phosphate	1.000 g
Magnesium sulfate	0.500 g
Sodium chloride	0.100 g
Calcium chloride	0.100 g
Glucose	10.000 g
Water	1.000 liter
Final pH of the base ± 4.5	

Dissolve, sterilize by filtration, and dispense aseptically.

Yeast dextrose agar

Dextrose	10.0 g
Yeast extract	10.0 g
Agar	15.0 g
Water	1.0 liter

Adjust the pH to 7.0. Autoclave at 121°C for 15 min.

Yeast extract agar (25)
For identification of Histoplasma capsulatum, Blastomyces dermatitidis, and Coccidioides immitis

Yeast extract	1 g
Buffer[a]	2 ml
Agar	20 g
Distilled water	1 liter

[a]Dissolve 40 g of Na_2HPO_4 in 300 ml of distilled water, and then add 60 g of KH_2PO_4. The pH is 6.0. If necessary, adjust with 1 N HCl or NaOH. Adjust the volume to 400 ml with distilled water, and store at 4°C.

Boil into solution, and sterilize at 121°C for 15 min. Pour into sterile plastic petri dishes (35 ml per plate).

Yeast extract-phosphate agar
For primary recovery of dimorphic pathogenic fungi as well as other pathogenic fungi

Yeast extract	1 g
Phosphate buffer	2 ml
Agar	20 g
Distilled water	1 liter

Dissolve 40 g of Na_2HPO_4 in 300 ml of distilled water; add 60 g of KH_2PO_4. Adjust the pH to 6.0 with 1 N HCl or NaOH if necessary. Adjust the buffer volume to 400 ml with distilled water, and store at 4°C. Dispense, and autoclave at 121°C for 15 min.

One drop of concentrated NH_4OH may be added to one side of the inoculated plate to decontaminate the sample.

Yeast fermentation medium (42)

Yeast extract	4.5 g
Peptone	7.5 g
Bromthymol blue, 1.6% solution	1.0 ml
Distilled water	1.0 liter

Dissolve yeast extract and peptone in water. Add enough bromthymol blue to give a dense green color (approximately 1 ml). Dispense medium in 2-ml amounts in screw-cap tubes. Insert Durham tubes. Autoclave at 15 lb/in^2 (121°C) for 15 min. When cooled, add 1 ml of 6% carbohydrate solution. Five carbohydrate solutions (glucose, maltose, lactose, galactose, and trehalose) are prepared by adding 6.0 g of carbohydrate to 100 ml of distilled water and sterilizing by membrane filtration. If raffinose is also needed, prepare a 12% solution. Store at 4°C for 3 weeks.

Comparable media may be obtained from BBL (97299) and Remel (06-5302 and 06-5402).

Yeast morphology agar (YMA), buffered (113)
For agar dilution and diffusion disk testing with 5-fluorocytosine

Ammonium sulfate	32.5 g
Asparagine	1.5 g
Glucose	10.0 g
L-Histidine monohydrochloride	10.0 mg
DL-Methionine	20.0 mg
DL-Tryptophan	20.0 mg
Biotin	2.0 μg
Calcium pantothenate	400.0 μg
Folic acid	2.0 μg
Inositol	2,000.0 μg
Niacin	400.0 μg
p-Aminobenzoic acid	200.0 μg
Pyridoxine hydrochloride	400.0 μg
Riboflavin	200.0 μg
Thiamine hydrochloride	400.0 μg
Boric acid	500.0 μg
Copper sulfate	40.0 μg
Potassium iodide	100.0 μg
Ferric chloride	200.0 μg
Manganese sulfate	400.0 μg
Sodium molybdate	200.0 μg
Zinc sulfate	400.0 μg
Potassium phosphate monobasic	1.0 g
Magnesium sulfate	0.5 g
Sodium chloride	0.5 g
Calcium chloride	0.1 g
Agar	18.0 g
Phosphate buffer, pH 7.0, 0.01 M	1.0 liter

Heat to boiling to dissolve. Dispense, and autoclave at 121°C for 15 min.

A comparable dehydrated medium requiring the addition of buffer may be obtained commercially (Difco no. 0393). A similar prepared product (Buffered Shadomy Agar) containing phosphate buffer, pH 7.0 (0.33 g of Na_2HPO_4 and 0.92 g of KH_2PO_4 per liter, 1% glucose, 0.15% L-asparagine, and 100 μg of chloramphenicol per ml), also is available in 50-ml sterile volumes from A/S Rosco, 2630 Taastrup, Denmark.

Yeast morphology agar (YMA), unbuffered*
For agar dilution and diffusion disk testing with 5-fluorocytosine

Same as yeast morphology agar, buffered, except that 1 liter of distilled water is used in place of the 1 liter of 0.01 M phosphate buffer, pH 7.0. A comparable product is available commercially (Difco no. 0393).

Yeast nitrogen base,* 10× (122)

Boric acid	500.0 μg
Copper sulfate	40.0 μg
Potassium iodide	100.0 μg
Ferric chloride	200.0 μg
Manganese sulfate	400.0 μg
Sodium molybdate	200.0 μg
Zinc sulfate	400.0 μg
Biotin	2.0 μg
Calcium pantothenate	400.0 μg
Folic acid	2.0 μg
Inositol	2,000.0 μg
Niacin	400.0 μg
p-Aminobenzoic acid	200.0 μg
Pyridoxine hydrochloride	400.0 μg
Riboflavin	200.0 μg
Thiamine hydrochloride	400.0 μg
L-Histidine monohydrochloride	10.0 mg
DL-Methionine	20.0 mg
DL-Tryptophan	20.0 mg
Magnesium sulfate	500.0 mg
Sodium chloride	100.0 mg
Calcium chloride	100.0 mg

Ammonium chloride	5.0 g
Monopotassium phosphate	1.0 g
Purified water	100.0 ml

Dissolve in 100 ml of purified water, sterilize by filtration, and dispense aseptically.

Yeast nitrogen base,* 10×, supplemented with asparagine and glucose (122)
For susceptibility tests with yeasts and fungi

To yeast nitrogen base,* 10×, add:

L-Asparagine	1.5 g
Glucose	10.0 g

Dissolve, sterilize by filtration, and dispense aseptically. For use, dilute 1:10 in sterile water. For buffered 1× base, dilute 1:10 in sterile 0.01 M phosphate buffer, pH 7, instead.

Prepare the basic broth base in 10-fold concentration by adding 6.7 g to 100 ml of distilled water. Add the L-asparagine and glucose if required. Warm slightly to dissolve. Sterilize by filtration, and refrigerate for use as needed.

Yersinia agar

See cefsulodin-irgasan-novobiocin (CIN) medium.

Company names and addresses

BBL Microbiology Systems, Cockeysville, Md.
Bristol Laboratories, Syracuse, N.Y.
Burroughs Wellcome Co., Research Triangle Park, N.C.
Calbiochem-Behring, La Jolla, Calif.
Difco Laboratories, Detroit, Mich.
EM Science, Cherry Hill, N.J.
Fisher Scientific Co., Pittsburgh, Pa.
Flow Laboratories, McLean, Va.
General Diagnostics, Anaheim, Calif.
GIBCO Laboratories, Lawrence, Mass.
ICN Pharmaceuticals, Inc., Cleveland, Ohio
Intergen-Armour Biochemicals, Purchase, N.Y.
Eli Lilly & Co., Indianapolis, Ind.
E. Merck AG, Darmstadt, Federal Republic of Germany
Merck & Co., Inc., Rahway, N.J.
Oxoid, U.S.A., Inc., Columbia, Md.
Parke, Davis & Co., Detroit, Mich.
Pfanstiehl Laboratories, Inc., Waukegan, Ill.
Pfizer Inc., New York, N.Y.
Remel, Lenexa, Kans.
Research Organics, Cleveland, Ohio
Roche Laboratories, Nutley, N.J.
Scientific Protein Laboratories, Waunakee, Wis.
Scott Laboratories, Fiskeville, R.I.
Sheffield Chemical, Union, N.J.
Sigma Chemical Co., St. Louis, Mo.
E. R. Squibb & Sons, Princeton, N.J.
The Upjohn Co., Kalamazoo, Mich.
Winthrop Laboratories, New York, N.Y.

LITERATURE CITED

1. **Altwegg, M., A. von Graevenitz, and J. Zollinger-Iten.** 1987. Medium and temperature dependence of decarboxylase reactions in *Aeromonas* spp. Curr. Microbiol. **15:**1–4.
2. **Beneke, E. S., and A. L. Rogers (ed.).** 1980. Medical mycology manual with human mycoses monograph, 4th ed., p. 25–44. Macmillan Publishing Co., New York.
3. **Blazer, M. J., I. D. Berkowitz, F. M. LaForce, J. Grovens, L. B. Reller, and W. L. Wong.** 1959. Campylobacter enteritis: clinical and epidemiological features. Ann. Intern. Med. **91:**179–185.
4. **Bordet, J., and O. Gengou.** 1906. Le microbe de la coqueluche. Ann. Inst. Pasteur **20:**731–741.
5. **Brown, W. J.** 1974. Modification of the rapid fermentation test for *Neisseria gonorrhoeae*. Appl. Microbiol. **27:**1027–1030.
6. **Brown, W. J.** 1976. Stability of working reagents for the modified rapid fermentation test (MRFT). Health Lab. Sci. **14:**172–176.
7. **Buck, T. A.** 1949. A modified Loeffler's medium for cultivating *Corynebacterium diphtheriae*. J. Lab. Clin. Med. **34:**582.
8. **Butzler, J. P., P. Dikeryser, M. Detrain, and F. Dehaen.** 1973. Related vibrio in stools. J. Pediatr. **82:**493–495.
9. **Calalb, G., A. Saragea, P. Maximescu, N. Ciorcianu, A. Popescu, S. Popa, and A. Mihailescu.** 1961. Recherches sur un milieu liquide d'enrichissement pour le diagnostic bacteriologique de la diphtherie. Arch. Roum. Pathol. Exp. **20:**95–101.
10. **Christensen, W. B.** 1946. Urea decomposition as a means of differentiating *Proteus* and paracolon cultures from each other and from *Salmonella* and *Shigella* types. J. Bacteriol. **52:**161–466.
11. **Clark, W. A., D. G. Hollis, R. E. Weaver, and P. Riley.** 1985. Identification of unusual pathogenic gram-negative aerobic and facultatively anaerobic bacteria. Centers for Disease Control, Atlanta.
12. **Conant, N. F.** 1936. Studies of the genus Microsporan. I. Cultural studies. Arch. Dermatol. Syphilol. **33:**665–683.
13. **Converse, J.** 1955. Growth of spherules of *Coccidioides immitis* in a chemically defined liquid medium. Proc. Soc. Exp. Biol. Med. **90:**709–711.
14. **Cote, R. (ed.).** 1984. ATCC media handbook. American Type Culture Collection, Rockville, Md.
15. **Curtis, G. D. W., R. G. Mitchell, A. F. King, and E. J. Griffin.** 1989. A selective differential medium for the isolation of *Listeria monocytogenes*. Lett. Appl. Microbiol. **8:**95–98.
16. **Dowell, V. R., Jr., and T. M. Hawkins.** 1974. Laboratory methods in anaerobic bacteriology. CDC laboratory manual. Department of Health, Education, and Welfare publication no. (CDC) 78-8272. Center for Disease Control, Atlanta.
17. **Dowell, V. R., Jr., and G. L. Lombard.** 1977. Presumptive identification of anaerobic nonsporeforming gram-negative bacilli. Publication no. CDC-4L8501. Center for Disease Control, Atlanta.
18. **Dowell, V. R., Jr., G. L. Lombard, F. S. Thompson, and A. Y. Armfield.** 1977. Media for isolation, characterization and identification of obligately anaerobic bacteria. CDC laboratory manual. Department of Health, Education, and Welfare publication no. CDC-530-009/64745, reprinted 1987. Center for Disease Control, Atlanta.
19. **Dulaney, A. D., K. Guo, and H. Packer.** 1948. *Donovania granulomatis* cultivation, antigen preparation and immunological tests. J. Immunol. **59:**335–340.
20. **Edelstein, P. H.** 1981. Improved semiselective medium for isolation of *Legionella pneumophila* from contaminated clinical and environmental specimens. J. Clin. Microbiol. **14:**298–303.
21. **Edelstein, P. H.** 1984. Legionnaires' disease laboratory manual. National Technical Information Service, Springfield, Va.
22. **Elek, S. D.** 1949. The plate virulence test for diphtheria. J. Clin. Pathol. **2:**250–258.

23. **Ellinghausen, H. C., and W. G. McCullough.** 1965. Nutrition of *Leptospira pomona* and growth of 13 other serotypes: a serum-free medium employing oleic albumin complex. Am. J. Vet. Res. **26**:39–44.
24. **Ellis, W. A.** 1986. The diagnosis of leptospirosis in farm animals, p. 13–31. *In* W. A. Ellis and T. W. A. Little (ed.), The present state of leptospirosis and control. Martinus Nijhoff, Dordrecht, The Netherlands.
25. **Emmons, C. W., C. H. Binford, J. P. Utz, and K. J. Kwon-Chung.** 1980. Medical mycology. Lea & Febiger, Philadelphia.
26. **Ewing, W. H., and B. R. Davis.** 1970. Media and tests for differentiation of *Enterobacteriaceae*. Center for Disease Control, Atlanta.
27. **Facklam, R. R.** 1973. Comparison of several laboratory media for presumptive identification of enterococci and group D streptococci. Appl. Microbiol. **26**:138–145.
28. **Faine, S. (ed.).** 1982. Guidelines for the control of leptospirosis. WHO offset publication no. 67. World Health Organization, Geneva.
29. **Farmer, J. J., III, and B. R. Davis.** 1985. H7 antiserum-sorbitol fermentation medium: a single tube screening medium for detecting *Escherichia coli* O157:H7 associated with hemorrhagic colitis. J. Clin. Microbiol. **22**: 620–625.
30. **Finegold, S. M., and E. J. Baron (ed.).** 1986. Bailey and Scott's diagnostic microbiology, 7th ed. The C. V. Mosby Co., St. Louis.
31. **Fletcher, W.** 1928. Recent works on leptospirosis. Tsutsugamushi disease and tropical typhus in the Federated Malay States. Trans. R. Soc. Trop. Med. Hyg. **31**:265–268.
32. **Frobisher, M., Jr.** 1937. Cystine-tellurite agar for *C. diphtheriae*. J. Infect. Dis. **10**:99–105.
33. **George, L. K., L. Ajello, and C. Papageorge.** 1954. Use of cycloheximide in the selective isolation of fungi pathogenic to man. J. Lab. Clin. Med. **44**:422–428.
34. **George, L. K., and L. B. Camp.** 1957. Routine nutritional tests for identification of dermatophytes. J. Bacteriol. **74**: 113–121.
35. **George, W. L., V. L. Sutter, D. Citron, and S. M. Finegold.** 1979. Selective and differential medium for isolation of *Clostridium difficile*. J. Clin. Microbiol. **9**:214–219.
36. **Gilardi, G. L. (ed.).** 1978. Glucose nonfermenting gram-negative bacteria in clinical microbiology. CRC Press, Inc., West Palm Beach, Fla.
37. **Goldberg, J.** 1959. Studies on granuloma inguinale. IV. Growth requirements of *Donovania granulomatis* and its relationship to the natural habitat of the organism. Br. J. Vener. Dis. **35**:266–268.
38. **Gordon, R. E., and J. M. Mihm.** 1962. Identification of *Nocardia caviae* (Erickson) nov. comb. Ann. N.Y. Acad. Sci. **98**:628–636.
39. **Grayston, J. T., H. M. Foy, and F. E. Kenny.** 1969. The epidemiology of mycoplasma infections of the human respiratory tract, p. 651–652. *In* L. Hayflick (ed.), The Mycoplasmatales and L phase of bacteria. Appleton Century Crofts, New York.
40. **Grove, D. C., and W. A. Randall.** 1955. The compilation of tests and methods of assay for antibiotic drugs. Food and Drug Administration: assay methods of antibiotics. Medical Encyclopedia, Inc., New York.
41. **Hajna, A. A.** 1945. Triple-sugar iron agar medium for the identification of the intestinal group of bacteria. J. Bacteriol. **49**:516–517.
42. **Haley, L. D., and C. S. Callaway (ed.).** 1978. Laboratory methods in medical mycology, 4th ed. Department of Health, Education, and Welfare publication no. (CDC) 78-8361. Center for Disease Control, Atlanta.
43. **Hanks, J. H., and R. E. Wallace.** 1949. Relation of oxygen and temperature in the preservation of tissues of refrigeration. Proc. Soc. Exp. Biol. Med. **71**:196–200.
44. **Hermann, G. J., M. S. Moore, and E. I. Parson.** 1958. A substitute for serum in the diphtheria in vitro test. Am. J. Clin. Pathol. **29**:181–183.
45. **Holbrook, R., and J. M. Anderson.** 1980. An improved selective and diagnostic medium for the isolation and enumeration of *Bacillus cereus* in foods. Can. J. Microbiol. **26**:753–759.
45a. **Holdeman, L. V., E. P. Cato, and W. E. C. Moore (ed.).** 1977. Anaerobe laboratory manual, 4th ed. Virginia Polytechnic Institute and State University, Blacksburg.
46. **Hopkins, J. M., and G. A. Land.** 1977. Rapid method for determining nitrate utilization by yeasts. J. Clin. Microbiol. **5**:497–500.
47. **Hugh, R., and E. Leifson.** 1953. The taxonomic significance of fermentative versus oxidative metabolism of carbohydrates by various gram-negative bacteria. J. Bacteriol. **66**:24–26.
48. **Hunter, G. W., III, W. W. Frye, and J. C. Schwartzwelder.** 1966. A manual of tropical medicine, 4th ed. The W. B. Saunders Co., Philadelphia.
49. **Johnson, R. C., G. S. Bowen, J. C. Feely, and P. Rogers.** 1964. 5-Fluorouracil as a selective agent for growth of leptospirae. J. Bacteriol. **88**:422–4.
50. **Johnson, R. C., and V. G. Harris.** 1967. Differentiation of pathogenic and saprophytic leptospires. I. Growth at low temperatures. J. Bacteriol. **94**:27–31.
51. **Johnson, R. C., J. Walby, R. A. Henry, and N. E. Auran.** 1973. Cultivation of parasitic leptospires: effect of pyruvate. Appl. Microbiol. **26**:118–119.
52. **Johnson, S. E., G. C. Klein, G. P. Schmid, G. S. Bowen, J. C. Fealy, and T. Schulz.** 1984. Lyme disease: a selective medium isolation of the suspected etiological agent, a spirochete. J. Clin. Microbiol. **19**:81–83.
53. **Kandolo, K., and G. Wauters.** 1985. Pyrazinamidase activity in *Yersinia enterocolitica* and related organisms. J. Clin. Microbiol. **21**:980–982.
54. **Kane, J., and J. B. Fischer.** 1971. The differentiation of *T. rubrum* and *T. mentagrophytes* by use of Christensen's urea broth. Can. J. Microbiol. **17**:911–913.
55. **Kane, J., L. Sigler, and R. C. Summerhill.** 1987. Improved procedures for differentiating *Microsporum persicolor* from *Trichophyton mentagrophytes*. J. Clin. Microbiol. **25**:2449–2452.
56. **Kane, J., and C. M. Smitka.** 1978. The early detection and identification of *Trichophyton verrucosum*. J. Clin. Microbiol. **8**:740–747.
57. **Kaper, J. B., H. Lockman, R. R. Colwell, and S. W. Joseph.** 1981. *Aeromonas hydrophila:* ecology and toxigenicity of isolates from an estuary. J. Appl. Bacteriol. **50**:359–377.
58. **Kellogg, D. S., Jr., and E. M. Turner.** 1973. Rapid fermentation confirmation of *Neisseria gonorrhoeae*. Appl. Microbiol. **25**:550–552.
59. **Kelly, R.** 1971. Cultivation of *Borrelia hermsii*. Science **173**:443–444.
60. **Kenny, G. E.** 1973. Contamination of mammalian cells in culture with Mycoplasma, p. 107–129. *In* J. Fogh (ed.), Contamination in tissue culture. Academic Press, Inc., New York.
61. **Kenny, G. E., and F. D. Cartwright.** 1978. Effect of urea concentration on growth of *Ureaplasma urealyticum* (T-strain mycoplasma). J. Bacteriol. **132**:144–150.
62. **Kimmig, J., and H. Rieth.** 1953. Antimykotia in Experiment und Klinik. Arzneim. Forsch. **3**:267–276.
63. **Knisely, R. F.** 1966. Selective medium for *Bacillus anthracis*. J. Bacteriol. **92**:784–786.
64. **Kohn, J.** 1953. A preliminary report of a new gelatin liquefaction method. J. Clin. Pathol. **6**:249.
64a. **Koneman, E. W., S. D. Allen, V. R. Dowell, Jr., and H. M. Somers.** 1983. Color atlas and textbook of microbiology, 2nd ed. J. B. Lippincott Co., Philadelphia.
65. **Korthof, G.** 1932. Experimentelles Schlammfieber beim Menschen. Zentralbl. Bakteriol. Parasitenkd. Infektionskr. Hyg. Abt. 1 Orig. **125**:429–434.
66. **Kramer, J. M., P. C. B. Turnbull, G. Munshi, and R. J.

Gilbert. 1982. Identification and characterization of *Bacillus cereus* and other *Bacillus* species associated with food poisoning, p. 261–286. *In* J. E. L. Corry, D. Roberts, and F. A. Skinner (ed.), Isolation and identification methods for food poisoning organisms. Society for Applied Bacteriology, Technical Series no. 17. Academic Press, London.

67. **Larone, D. H.** 1987. Medically important fungi: a guide to identification, 2nd ed. Elsevier, New York.
68. **Lautrop, H.** 1956. A modified Kohn's test for the demonstration of bacterial gelatin liquefaction. Acta Pathol. Microbiol. Scand. **39:**357.
69. **Lee, W. H., and D. McClain.** 1986. Improved *Listeria monocytogenes* selective agar. Appl. Environ. Microbiol. **52:**1215–1217.
70. **Livingston, S. J., S. D. Kominos, and R. B. Yee.** 1978. New medium for selection and presumptive identification of the *Bacteroides fragilis* group. J. Clin. Microbiol. **7:** 448–453.
71. **MacFaddin, J. F.** 1980. Biochemical tests for identification of medical bacteria, 2nd ed. The Williams & Wilkins Co., Baltimore.
72. **MacFaddin, J. F.** 1985. Media for isolation-cultivation-identification-maintenance of medical bacteria, vol. 1. The Williams & Wilkins Co., Baltimore.
73. **McClain, D., and W. H. Lee.** 1988. Development of USDA-FSIS method for isolation of *Listeria monocytogenes* from raw meat and poultry. J. Assoc. Off. Anal. Chem. **71:**660–664.
74. **McClain, D., and W. H. Lee.** 1989. U. S. Department of Agriculture—Food Safety Inspection Service, laboratory communication no. 57, May 24.
75. **McGinnis, M. R.** 1980. Laboratory handbook of medical mycology, p. 523–587, 351–352. Academic Press, Inc., New York.
76. **Moore, G. E., R. E. Geiner, and H. A. Franklin.** 1967. Culture of normal human leukocytes. J. Am. Med. Assoc. **199:**519–524.
77. **Mossel, D. A. A., M. J. Koopman, and E. Jongerius.** 1967. Enumeration of *Bacillus cereus* in foods. Appl. Microbiol. **15:**650–653.
78. **Muller, D., M. L. Edwards, and D. W. Smith.** 1983. Changes in iron and transferrin levels and body temperature in experimental airborne legionellosis. J. Infect. Dis. **147:**302–307.
79. **Novy, F. G., and W. J. MacNeal.** 1904. The cultivation of *Trypanosoma bruceii.* J. Infect. Dis. **1:**1–30.
80. **Pai, S.-E.** 1932. A simple egg medium for the cultivation of *Bacillus diphtheriae.* Chin. Med. J. Engl. Ed. **46:**1203–1206.
81. **Pasculle, A. W., J. N. Dowling, F. N. Frola, D. A. McDevitt, and M. A. Levi.** 1985. Antimicrobial therapy of experimental *Legionella micdadei* pneumonia in guinea pigs. Antimicrob. Agents Chemother. **28:**730–734.
82. **Phillips, E., and P. Nash.** 1985. Culture media, p. 1051–1092. *In* E. H. Lennette, A. Balows, W. J. Hausler, Jr., and H. J. Shadomy (ed.), Manual of clinical microbiology, 4th ed. American Society for Microbiology, Washington, D.C.
83. **Pine, L.** 1970. Growth of *Histoplasma capsulatum.* VI. Maintenance of the mycelial phase. Appl. Microbiol. **19:** 413–420.
84. **Pine, L., and E. Drouhet.** 1963. Sur l'obtention et la conservation de la phase levure d'*Histoplasma capsulatum* et d'*H. duboisii*, en milieu chemiquement defini. Ann. Inst. Pasteur (Paris) **105:**798–804.
85. **Preston, N. W.** 1970. Technical problems in the laboratory diagnosis and prevention of whooping cough. Lab. Pract. **19:**482–486.
86. **Regan, J., and F. Lowe.** 1977. Enrichment medium for the isolation of *Bordetella.* J. Chin. Microbiol. **6:**303–309.
87. **Reith, H.** 1969. Dermatophyten, Hefen und Schimmelpilze auf Kimmig-Agar. Mykosen **12:**73–74.
88. **Riley, G., and S. Toma.** 1989. Detection of pathogenic *Yersinia enterocolitica* by using Congo red-magnesium oxalate agar medium. J. Clin. Microbiol. **27:**213–214.
89. **Rinaldi, M. G.** 1982. The use of potato flakes agar in clinical mycology. J. Clin. Microbiol. **15:**1159–1160.
90. **Ristroph, J. D., K. W. Hedlund, and R. G. Allen.** 1980. Liquid medium for growth of *Legionella pneumophila.* J. Clin. Microbiol. **11:**19–21.
91. **Ristroph, J. D., and B. E. Ivins.** 1983. Elaboration of *Bacillus anthracis* antigens in a new, defined culture medium. Infect. Immun. **39:**483–486.
92. **Rodgers, F. G., A. O. Tzianabos, and T. J. S. Elliot.** 1990. The effect of antibiotics that inhibit cell wall, protein and DNA synthesis of the growth and morphology of *Legionella pneumophila.* J. Med. Microbiol. **31:**37–44.
93. **Rogol, M., I. Sechter, L. Grinberg, and C. B. Gerichter.** 1979. Pril-xylose-ampicillin agar, a new selective medium for the isolation of *Aeromonas hydrophila.* J. Med. Microbiol. **12:**229–231.
94. **Salkin, I. F., and M. A. Gordon.** 1975. Evaluation of *Aspergillus* differential medium. J. Clin. Microbiol. **2:**74–75.
95. **Salkin, I. F., and N. J. Hurd.** 1982. New medium for differentiation of *Cryptococcus neoformans* serotype pairs. J. Clin. Microbiol. **15:**169–171.
96. **Saragea, A., P. Maximescu, and E. Meitert.** 1979. *Corynebacterium diphtheriae:* microbiological methods used in clinical and epidemiological investigations, p. 61–176. *In* T. Bergan and J. R. Norris (ed.), Methods in microbiology, vol. 13. Academic Press, Inc., New York.
97. **Schubert, R. H. W.** 1967. Das Vorkommen der Aeromonaden in oberirdischen Gewassern. Arch. Hyg. **150:** 688–708.
98. **Schubert, R. H. W.** 1977. Ueber den Nachweis von Plesiomonas shigelloides Habs und Schubert. 1962. Und ein Elektivmedium, den Inositol-Brilliantgrun-Gallesalz-Agar. E. Rodenwaldt-Archiv. **4:**97–103.
99. **Sierra, G.** 1957. A simple method for detection of lipolytic activity of microorganisms and some observations on the influence of the contact between cells and fatty substrates. Antonie van Leeuwenhoek J. Microbiol. Serol. **23:**15–22.
100. **Skinner, G. E., C. W. Emmons, and H. M. Tsuchiya.** 1693. Henrici's molds, yeast and actinomycetes, 2nd ed. John Wiley & Sons, Inc., New York.
101. **Skirrow, M. B.** 1977. Campylobacter enteritis: a "new" disease. Br. Med. J. **2:**9–11.
102. **Smith, M. R., R. E. Gordon, and F. E. Clark.** 1952. Aerobic sporeforming bacteria, U. S. Department of Agriculture monograph no. 16. U. S. Department of Agriculture, Washington, D.C.
103. **Staib, F.** 1962. Zur Kreatinin-Kreatin-Assimilation in der Hefepitz Diagnostik. Zentralbl. Bakteriol. Parasitenkd. Infektionskr. Hyg. Abt. 1 Orig. **191:**429–432.
104. **Steere, A. C., R. I. Grodzickl, A. N. Kornblatt, J. E. Craft, A. G. Barbour, W. Burgdorfer, G. P. Schmid, E. Johnson, and S. E. Malawista.** 1983. The spirochetal biology of Lyme disease. N. Engl. J. Med. **308:**733–740.
105. **Sulea, I. T., M. C. Pollice, and L. Barksdale.** 1980. Pyrazine carboxylamidase activity in *Corynebacterium.* Int. J. Syst. Bacteriol. **30:**466–472.
106. **Summerbell, R. C., S. A. Rosenthal, and J. Kane.** 1988. Rapid method for differentiation of *Trichophyton rubrum, Trichophyton mentagrophytes,* and related dermatophyte species. J. Clin. Microbiol. **26:**2279–2282.
107. **Sutter, V. L., V. L. Vargo, and S. M. Finegold.** 1975. Wadsworth anaerobic bacteriology manual, 2nd ed. University Extension, University of California, Los Angeles.
108. **Taplin, D., N. Zaias, G. Rebell, and H. Blank.** 1969. Isolation and recognition of dermatophytes on a new medium (DTM). Arch. Dermatol. **99:**203–209.
109. **Tatum, H. W., W. H. Ewing, and R. E. Weaver.** 1974. Miscellaneous gram-negative bacteria, p. 270–294. *In* E. H. Lennette, E. H. Spaulding, and J. P. Truant (ed.),

Manual of clinical microbiology, 2nd ed. American Society for Microbiology, Washington, D. C.

110. **Tinsdale, G. F. W.** 1947. A new medium for the isolation and identification of *C. diphtheriae* on the production of hydrogen sulfide. J. Pathol. Bacteriol. **59**:461–466.

111. **Totten, P. A., R. Amsel, J. Hale, P. Piot, and K. K. Holmes.** 1982. Selective differential human blood bilayer media for isolation of *Gardnerella (Haemophilus) vaginalis*. J. Clin. Microbiol. **15**:141–147.

112. **Trabulis, L. R., and W. H. Ewing.** 1962. Sodium acetate medium for differentiation of *Shigella* and *Escherichia* cultures. Public Health Lab. **20**:137–140.

113. **Utz, C. J., and S. Shadomy.** 1977. Antifungal activity of 5-fluorocytosine as measured by disk diffusion susceptibility testing. J. Infect. Dis. **135**:970–974.

114. **Van Netten, P., I. Perales, A. van de Moosdijk, D. W. Curtis, and D. A. A. Mossel.** 1989. Liquid and solid differentiation media for enumeration of *L. monocytogenes* and other *Listeria* spp. J. Food Microbiol. **8**:299–316.

115. **Vera, H. D.** 1948. A simple medium for identification and maintenance of the gonococcus and other bacteria. J. Bacteriol. **55**:531–536.

116. **Vickers, R. M., A. Brown, and G. M. Garrity.** 1981. Dye-containing buffered charcoal-yeast extract medium for differentiation of members of the family *Legionellaceae*. J. Clin. Microbiol. **13**:380–382.

117. **Wadowsky, R. M., and R. B. Yee.** 1981. Glycine-containing selective medium for isolation of *Legionellaceae* from environmental species. Appl. Environ. Microbiol. **42**:768–722.

118. **Weitzman, I., S. A. Rosenthal, and M. Silva-Hutner.** 1988. Superficial and cutaneous infections caused by molds: dermatomycoses, p. 33–97. *In* B. B. Wentworth (ed.), Diagnostic procedures for mycotic and parasitic infections, 7th ed. American Public Health Association, Washington, D. C.

119. **Weitzman, I., and M. Silva-Hutner.** 1967. Non-keratinous agar media as substitutes for the ascigerous state in certain members of the gymnoascacae pathogenic for the man and animals. Sabouraudia **5**:335–340.

120. **Wickerham, L. J.** 1951. Taxonomy of yeasts. U. S. Department of Agriculture technical bulletin 1029. U. S. Department of Agriculture, Washington, D. C.

121. **Wickerham, L. J., and K. A. Burton.** 1958. Carbon assimilation tests for the classification of yeasts. J. Bacteriol. **56**:363–371.

122. **Wolin, H. L., M. L. Bevis, and H. Laurora.** 1962. An improved synthetic medium for the rapid production of chlamydospores by *Candida albicans*. Sabouraudia **2**:96–99.

123. **Zimmer, B. L., and G. D. Roberts.** 1979. Rapid selective urease test for presumptive identification of *Cryptococcus neoformans*. J. Clin. Microbiol. **10**:380–381.

Chapter 122

Reagents and Stains

DONALD A. HENDRICKSON AND MICHELLE M. KRENZ

Reagents, stains, and testing procedures outlined in this chapter have been determined to be the method of choice by the authors of this Manual. Certain reagent preparations listed may be required components of culture media as used in preparations described in chapter 121. Traditional procedures, as well as current and updated descriptions, are compiled in an organized, alphabetical fashion so as to contribute to the accurate testing of the microbial specimen.

Considerations in determining the optimal selection of reagent, stain, or testing protocol may include the specific and intended use as related to characterization purposes, compatibility, and complexity of the testing system, cost/time and efficiency of testing, availability of reagents and equipment, and safety. In instances when adherence to state and federal guidelines is required, chapter 120 may be consulted.

Successful use of the reagents, stains, and testing protocols described herein may require initial isolation of the organism from bulk constituents or contaminants. Isolation should occur with minimal distortion (physical and biochemical) of the native organism. The interpretation and final outcome of results may be influenced by many factors, including the preparation and quality of reagents and stains as well as conscientious adherence to the testing protocol. In a broad sense, the reagent or stain must be free from chemical or microbial contaminants at the time of use. Macroscopic changes resulting from cumulative chemical or biochemical degradation may be visually observed in the form of precipitates, decreased solubility of anhydrous compounds, or increased viscosity of solutions. Expiration dates must be observed; many authors have indicated recommended shelf life and storage conditions for reagents and stains.

In some instances, the authors have chosen to include commercial vendors. The manufacturer's directions for reagent or stain preparation and/or testing protocol must be followed closely to achieve optimal results. Recommended expiration dates and storage conditions described by the manufacturer must be observed. For ease of use, these commercial sources and their addresses are listed at the end of chapter 121. Inclusion or exclusion of commercial sources does not denote endorsement or disapproval of use of these products.

Reagents, stains, and testing procedures that must be delineated in scientific detail and on the basis of their biochemical or chemical properties may be found in the Literature Cited at the end of this chapter.

REAGENTS AND TEST PROCEDURES

Acetamide hydrolysis

See chapter 40 and Nessler reagent.

Andrade indicator (1)

Acid fuchsin	2.0 g
Distilled water	1 liter
Sodium hydroxide (1 N)	160.0 ml

Dissolve fuchsin in distilled water and add sodium hydroxide. If the fuchsin is not sufficiently decolorized after standing overnight, an additional 1 to 2 ml of alkali should be added. (The fuchsin should be slightly orange or darker than a faint straw color when brought up in a 10-ml pipette.) Autoclave at 121°C for 20 min.

Andrade indicator should be aged for approximately 6 months before it is used, as it improves with aging.

Autoclave extract procedure

See chapter 29.

Bacitracin susceptibility procedure

See chapter 29.

Benzidine test (12)

For detecting the presence of c-type cytochromes in micrococci and Staphylococcus sciuri

Extraction reagents

Trichloroacetic acid (2 N)	50 ml
Perchloric acid ($HClO_4$) (2 N)	50 ml

Mix solutions to make stock solution.

Acetone	49 ml
Hydrochloric acid (HCl) (24 N)	1 ml

Carefully mix to make stock solution.

Benzidine base solution

Benzidine base (Merck)	1 g
Glacial acetic acid	20 ml
Distilled water	30 ml
Ethyl alcohol (95%)	50 ml

Dissolve benzidine base in 20 ml of glacial acetic acid, add 30 ml of distilled water, and heat gently. Cool solution and add 50 ml of ethyl alcohol. A slight yellow color may develop in the solution during storage but does not alter the sensitivity of the reagent. Solution may be stored at 4°C for at least 1 month.

Hydrogen peroxide (5%) solution

Hydrogen peroxide (30%)	30 ml
Distilled water	150 ml

Dilute hydrogen peroxide concentrate (30%) 1:6 (vol/vol) with distilled water to 5%. Solution should be made fresh weekly. Care must be taken in handling concentrate hydrogen peroxide.

Test procedure. Cultivate bacterial isolates on peptone-yeast extract-glucose agar at 30°C for 15 to 18 h. Add 1 ml of stock extraction solution to a test tube. Add two loopfuls of bacterial colonies to the solution. Mix suspension thoroughly. Incubate for 3 min. Centrifuge in an Eppendorf centrifuge and discard supernatant fluid. Resuspend pellet in 1 ml of distilled water and pour into 40 ml of ice-cold acetone-HCl solution. Stir vigorously. Extraction takes 10 to 15 min. Suck bacterial extract through a filter paper disk to collect material.

Add 0.5 ml of benzidine solution to the filter paper. Let saturate so that reagent comes in contact with the bacterial extract on the filter. Add 0.5 ml of 5% hydrogen peroxide solution. Positive test (micrococci) results in a blue-green to blue color on the filter. Cytochrome *c*-negative strains (staphylococci) produce no color on filter.

Modified method. Use an extraction step before running the test.

Bile solubility test

Sodium deoxycholate	1 g
Distilled water, sterile	9 ml

Test procedure. To test for bile solubility, prepare two tubes, each containing a sample of fresh culture (a light suspension of the organism in buffered broth, pH 7.4). To one tube add a few drops of a 10% solution of sodium deoxycholate. A comparable volume of sterile physiological saline solution may be added to the second tube. If the cells are bile soluble, the tube containing the bile salt should lose its turbidity in 5 to 15 min and show an increase in viscosity concomitant with clearing.

Blood hemolysis procedure

See chapter 29.

Buffered glycerol solution

See chapters 80 and 82.

Buffered saline

Add 85 g of NaCl to 1 liter of water.

Sodium chloride (0.85%) is buffered to pH 7.2 with 0.067 M potassium phosphate mixture.

CAMP test (*Rhodococcus equi*)

For differentiation of pathogenic from nonpathogenic environmental Listeria strains

Test procedure. Inoculate a streak of *Rhodococcus equi* (must elaborate factors to enhance production of hemolysin by *Listeria* isolates) down the center of a 5% sheep blood agar plate. Inoculate straight lines of isolates to be tested, along with a positive control (*Listeria monocytogenes*) and a negative control (such as *L. denitificans*) strain, at right angles to the *R. equi* streak, stopping just before the rhodococcus line is reached. Several different isolates can be tested on one plate.

Incubate plates at 35 to 40°C overnight. Observe for an arrowhead-shaped zone of enhanced beta-hemolysis at the juncture between positive listeria and the rhodococcus. Only *L. monocytogenes* and *L. ivanovii* are considered to be pathogenic.

CAMP test (*Staphylococcus aureus*)

See chapter 29.

Capillary precipitin procedure

See chapter 29.

Carbohydrate assimilation test (7)

Auxanographic plate

For identification of genera and species of yeasts

Prepare a suspension of the yeast cells in sterile distilled water comparable with the turbidity of a McFarland no. 1 standard. Add 3 ml of a 6.7% yeast nitrogen base solution to a large sterile petri dish (150 by 15 mm). Add 0.2 ml of the yeast suspension to the petri dish. Immediately add 20 ml of 2% Noble agar cooled to 48 to 50°C. Rotate the plate until the inoculum is well mixed in the medium. Allow it to sit until the agar hardens. Aseptically place carbohydrate disks on the agar surface. Incubate the plates at 25 to 30°C for 48 h. Plates are examined for growth around each disk for a positive carbohydrate assimilation. Do not confuse growth with the yellow discoloration from the disks. Carbohydrate disks may be ordered commercially from BBL or Difco Laboratories. The disks may include maltose, sucrose, lactose, galactose, trehalose, glucose, erythritol, inositol, melibiose, cellobiose, raffinose, dulcitol, xylose, and other carbohydrates as needed.

Catalase test

The organism to be tested should be grown on an agar slant heavily inoculated from a colony of the organism. The slant is usually incubated for 18 to 25 h at optimal temperature. To test for catalase, set the slant in an inclined position and pour 1 ml of a 3% solution of hydrogen peroxide over the growth. The appearance of gas bubbles indicates a positive test.

An alternative to conducting the test with a slant culture is to emulsify a colony in 1 drop of 3% hydrogen peroxide (superoxol) on a glass slide. Immediate bubbling indicates a positive catalase test. Extreme care must be exercised if a colony is taken from a blood agar plate. The enzyme catalase is present in erythrocytes, and the carry-over of blood cells with the colony can give a false-positive reaction.

Cell wall analysis of culture for diaminopimelic acid

Method of L. Georg, used with method of Becker et al. (4) for differentiation of aerobic actinomycetes (14)

Preparation of culture. Inoculate approximately 12 tubes of Trypticase soy broth (10 ml per tube) with the organism to be examined. Place an anaerobic seal on all tubes. Incubate at 37°C for 10 to 12 days or until good growth is noted. Remove anaerobic seals and transfer media with cells to sterile centrifuge tubes. Centrifuge to pack cells. Pool cells into one container and wash three times with distilled water.

Preparation of hydrolysates. To 1 ml of washed, packed cells, add 6 ml of 6 N HCl. If there is less than

1 ml of packed cells, add proportionately less acid (0.5 ml of packed cells is the minimum amount for production of satisfactory hydrolysate). Transfer cell-acid suspension to 13- by 100-mm screw-cap test tube and tighten the cap securely.

Place the cell-acid suspension in a boiling water bath for 2 h. Shake occasionally. Transfer the acid hydrolysate to a 15-ml beaker and evaporate to dryness (2 to 3 h). Resuspend the residue in 1 ml of distilled water (use proportionately less distilled water if less than 1 ml of packed cells was hydrolyzed); mix the residue thoroughly, using a capillary pipette. Centrifuge the hydrolysate residue suspension at 1,500 rpm for 15 min. Carefully decant the supernatant to a 13- by 100-mm sterile test tube. Store the hydrolysates at 5°C until ready to set in chromatograph.

Chromatography

Solvent

Methanol	80 ml
Distilled water	17.5 ml
10 N HCl	2.5 ml
Pyridine	10.0 ml

Mix and store in a glass-stoppered reagent bottle (concentration of HCl, approximately 12.01 N). Cut Whatman no. 1 filter paper in squares 11 in. on each side (with this size paper, seven samples can be spotted 1.5 in. apart).

Draw a pencil line 0.75 in. from the bottom of the paper. Mark spotting locations with 0.25-in. vertical cross lines, 1.5 in. apart, starting 1 in. from the left-hand edge of the paper.

Using a 10-μl pipette and an air jet, alternately spot paper and dry until 10 μl of hydrolysate is placed on one spot. The diameter of the spot should not exceed 0.25 in. Repeat with each hydrolysate at other locations. Use a control hydrolysate that contains diaminopimelic acid (DAP) and one without DAP.

After the spots have dried, roll the paper into a cylinder and staple it at each end. (The edges of the paper should not touch.)

Pour solvent into a battery jar 12 in. high and 6 in. in diameter. The solvent depth should be 0.25 to 0.5 in.

Line the inside of the battery jar with Whatman no. 1 filter paper and saturate the paper with solvent. Place the paper cylinder in the jar with the spotted end down, and cover the jar with a glass plate. Incubate the jar in a 37°C incubator until the solvent front reaches the top of the paper (2.5 to 3 h).

Place the entire assembly under a hood and remove the cylinder (allow it to sit in the hood for 30 min). Allow the cylinder to dry at room temperature overnight. (Papers can also be dried at 60°C for 1 h after drying in the hood at room temperature for 30 min.)

Development. The dried papers are developed by dipping them in a 0.1% solution of ninhydrin in acetone.

The dipped papers are then placed in a 100°C oven for 2 min.

The characteristic greenish grey DAP spot fades to a permanent yellow color.

Cellophane tape-cover slip mounts
To keep the reproductive structures of fungi intact

Place a piece of double-sided tape on the surface of a fungal colony, apply pressure gently, and remove. Press the sticky side without the fungus on a cover slip. Place the cover slip over a drop of lactophenol cotton blue on a microscope slide.

Chloramphenicol assay (chapter 119, Table 2)
For preparation of internal standard (34)

***N*-Pivaloyl-1-*p*-nitrophenyl-2-amino-1,3-propanediol (PIV) (1)**

L(+)-*threo*-2-Amino-1-*p*-nitrophenyl-1,3-propanediol	10.6 g
Trimethylacetic anhydride	27.9 g

Place the propanediol in a 50-ml screw-cap test tube, and add the trimethylacetic anhydride (approximately 30.5 ml). Securely cap the test tube, and place the mixture in a steam bath for 10 min with occasional agitation. Most of the solid will dissolve during the first few minutes of heating; however, a small amount of solid may remain undissolved. Cool the reaction flask in ice water, and then transfer the reaction mixture to a 250-ml separatory funnel. Add 100 ml of ice-cold water, and allow the mixture to sit at room temperature for about 1 h. Extract the aqueous mixture with three 50-ml portions of ethyl acetate. The remaining aqueous phase may be discarded. Wash the combined ethyl acetate extracts with four 50-ml volumes of 5% aqueous $NaHCO_3$, followed by a single wash with water. Concentrate the organic phase to an oil under reduced pressure. Dissolve the oil in a mixture of acetone and 0.1 M NaOH in water (1:1). Approximately 600 to 800 ml of this mixture is required. The volumes used do not appear to be critical. It is important to maintain a homogeneous reaction mixture (additional acetone helps in this regard) and a pH of 12 to 13. Formation of the desired product, PIV, from its pivaloyl esters can be monitored by high-performance liquid chromatography, using conditions similar to those used for analysis of chloramphenicol with an increased concentration of acetonitrile in the mobile phase. Hydrolysis is allowed to proceed at room temperature until complete (approximately 12 h). The mixture is neutralized with 6 M HCl and concentrated under reduced pressure to remove most of the acetone. The pH is adjusted to definite acidity (pH 1 to 2), and product is extracted from the aqueous solution with two 75-ml portions of ethyl acetate. The combined organic extracts are washed with three 50-ml portions of 5% $NaHCO_3$, dried with sodium sulfate, and evaporated under vacuum to a viscous oil. If necessary, add a small amount (approximately 8 ml) of ethylene dichloride or chloroform to initiate crystallization. Crystallization is allowed to proceed until complete. Toluene (20 ml) is added to facilitate collection of the crystalline product by vacuum filtration. A second crop of product can be obtained by adding additional toluene. A combined yield of 12.2 g (82% of theoretical) was obtained. Product is purified by recrystallization from chloroform-toluene mixtures. Pure product obtained by this procedure melts at 127 to 128°C. Rebstock (34) reported a melting point of 112 to 113°C for DL-*threo*-*N*-pivaloyl-1-*p*-nitrophenyl-2-amino-1,3-propanediol. The difference in melting points probably results from use of the single optical isomer in the above-described synthesis. The L and DL forms show identical retention times by high-performance liquid chromatography.

Coagulase test (chapter 28)

Tube test. To 0.5 ml of rabbit plasma, undiluted or diluted 1:4, add one loopful of growth from an 18- to 24-h-old agar culture, 0.5 ml of broth culture, or a single colony from a blood agar plate. Incubate in a water bath at 37°C, and examine the tubes at 6 and 24 h. Known coagulase-positive and coagulase-negative strains and, if possible, a weak coagulase producer must be set up as controls with each test.

A positive coagulase test is represented by any degree of clotting, from a loose clot suspended in plasma to a solid clot. It may be necessary to suspend a sterile loop in plasma to determine whether clotting has occurred. The majority of coagulase-positive strains will produce a clot within the first 4 h, many within 1 h. False-positive tests may occur with mixed cultures or with pure cultures of some gram-negative rods, e.g., *Pseudomonas* spp., but the mechanism of clotting is different. Organisms which utilize the citrate used as the anticoagulant in the plasma will produce a clot. Therefore, the organism to be tested must first be determined to possess characteristics consistent with the genus *Staphylococcus.*

Slide test. Emulsify a colony in a drop of water on a glass slide to produce a dense, uniform suspension. If any evidence of autoagglutination is noted before the plasma is added, the culture is not suitable for the slide test. Add one loopful or a drop of fresh plasma to the suspension, and mix by a continuous circular motion for 5 s. A positive reaction is indicated by easily visible white clumps, which usually appear immediately or within 5 s. Known coagulase-positive and coagulase-negative strains must always be set up in parallel.

All negative tests must be confirmed by the tube test.

Enterotoxin testing reagents for *Escherichia coli* (chapter 36)

For detecting strains of Escherichia coli that produce heat-labile enterotoxin

Phadebact ETEC-LT. A complete kit, Phadebact ETEC-LT, is available from Pharmacia Diagnostics and has been approved for testing patient isolates (approved for "in vitro diagnostic use"). Colonies are removed from agar plates, placed in extraction solution for 30 min at 37°C, and then tested for heat-labile enterotoxin by coagglutination.

Oxoid VET-RPLA. The VET-RPLA is manufactured by Denka Seiken in Japan and is available from Oxoid. It has also been approved for "in vitro diagnostic use." Cultures are grown in a special liquid medium and then are centrifuged and filtered. The filtrate is diluted serially twofold in 96-well plastic plates and reacted with red latex particles coated with antibody to cholera toxin, which also reacts with the heat-labile enterotoxin of *E. coli*. An alternative method to produce toxin is given in the package insert. Cultures are grown on brain heart infusion agar containing 90 μg of lincomycin per ml, and the cells are extracted with polymyxin B.

The instructions provided by the manufacturers should be consulted for complete details.

Escherichia coli H7 antiserum (chapter 36)

For testing colonies that agglutinate in E. coli O157 serum to confirm that they are E. coli O157:H7

This serum is available from Difco Laboratories (catalog no. 2159-47-0) and Roche Laboratories (catalog no. 2092-01).

Escherichia coli O157 antisera (chapter 36)

For detecting strains of E. coli O157

E. coli O157 serum is available from Difco Laboratories (catalog no. 2970-47-7) and Roche Laboratories (catalog no. 2086-01).

E. coli O157 serum on latex particles is also available from Oxoid U.S.A. (catalog no. DR 621).

Ethylene glycol degradation procedure

See chapter 35.

Ferric chloride reagent

For phenylalanine deaminase test (chapter 41)

Ferric chloride ($FeCl_3 \cdot 6H_2O$)	10 g
Hydrochloric acid, 2%	100 ml

Hydrochloric acid, 2%, is made by adding 5.4 ml of concentrated hydrochloric acid (37%) to 94.6 ml of distilled water.

For sodium hippurate hydrolysis by streptococci (chapter 29)

$FeCl_3 \cdot 6H_2O$	12 g
Aqueous HCl, 2%	100 ml

The 2% aqueous HCl is made by adding 5.4 ml of concentrated HCl (37%) to 94.6 ml of H_2O.

Ferrous ammonium sulfate solution

For pyrazinamidase test

$Fe(NH_4)_2(SO_4)_2 \cdot 6H_2O$	1 g
Water	100 ml

Dissolve the crystals in the water. Use the same day it is prepared.

Formalin buffer (10%) for parasitology

Formalin is an aqueous solution of formaldehyde, concentrated 37 to 40%. A 10% Formalin solution is about 3.7% formaldehyde.

Formaldehyde, 37% solution	100 ml
Water	900 ml
Na_2HPO_4	12 g
KH_2PO_4	3 g

The pH is approximately 7.4. Exact pH is not important.

Formate-fumarate additive

Sodium formate	3.0 g
Fumaric acid	3.0 g
Distilled water	50.0 ml

To adjust the pH, add 20 pellets of NaOH, stirring until pellets are dissolved and the fumaric acid is in solution. Bring the final pH to 7.0 with 4 N NaOH.

β-Galactosidase test

See chapter 28 and ONPG test.

α-Glucosidase test (chapter 48)

Prepare a solution of 0.1% (wt/vol) 4-nitrophenyl-α-D-glucopyranoside in 0.067 M Sorensen phosphate buffer (pH 8.0). Tubes containing 0.5 ml of the substrate solution are inoculated with a loopful of bacteria from an overnight culture. The tubes are incubated at 35°C in a water bath and examined after 4 h for the appearance of a yellow color.

β-Glucosidase test

Prepare a solution of 0.1% (wt/vol) 4-nitrophenyl-β-D-glucopyranoside in 0.067 M Sorensen phosphate buffer (pH 8.0). Tubes containing 0.5 ml of the substrate solution are inoculated with a loopful of bacteria from an overnight culture. The tubes are incubated at 35°C in a water bath and examined after 4 h for the appearance of a yellow color.

Glycine-buffered saline

See chapter 77.

Hair penetration test
For identification of Trichophyton mentagrophytes (7)

Principle. *T. mentagrophytes* and some of the uncommon *Microsporum* species produce an enzyme which penetrates and makes holes in human hair in vitro. This test is helpful in distinguishing *T. mentagrophytes* from *T. rubrum* and *Microsporum equinum* from *M. canis.*

Materials

10% yeast extract, sterile
Sterilized human hair (hair of a child under 5 years old)
Two screw-cap tubes, each containing 10 ml of sterile distilled water
Sterile Pasteur pipette
T. mentagrophytes control culture

Test procedure. With a pipette, 1 drop of yeast extract is placed in each tube of sterile distilled water. With flamed and cooled forceps, several pieces (10 to 30) of sterile human hair are dropped into each tube of water and yeast extract. A small amount of unknown fungal isolate is placed in one tube. A small amount of *T. mentagrophytes* is placed in the other tube as a control. Incubate both tubes at room temperature for 2 weeks. If test is negative (even if control is positive), reincubate and examine weekly for a total of 4 weeks. If both the control and the test isolate are still negative, the test is repeated, using a different strain of *T. mentagrophytes* for a control. Hairs are removed from water with a flamed loop and placed on a slide in a drop of lactophenol cotton blue. Cover with a cover slip. Examine hairs microscopically in this preparation for splitting and pitting, indicative of penetration.

Interpretation. Positive—splitting, pitting, and holes are seen in test isolate; negative—splitting, pitting, and holes are not seen in test isolate.

Hanks buffered salts solution (HBSS)

Used originally as a growth medium when supplemented with bovine embryo extract and serum, HBSS is currently used as an inorganic base in many media and as a diluent or cell rinse fluid. The formula as initially described has low bicarbonate content and was meant for use without CO_2 in the gas phase.

	mg/liter
NaCl	8,000.0
KCl	400.0
$Na_2HPO_4 \cdot 2H_2O$	60.0
KH_2PO_4	60.0
$CaCl_2$	140.0
$MgSO_4 \cdot 7H_2O$	200.0
$NaHCO_3$	350.0
Phenol red	20.0
Glucose	1,000.0

HEPES (*N*-2-hydroxyethylpiperazine-*N*′-2-ethanesulfonic acid), 1 M

HEPES	253.3 g
Distilled water	900 ml
NaOH (5 N) to adjust pH to 7.3	
Distilled water to	1,000 ml

Sterilize by filtration and store at 4°C.
HEPES buffer is usually used in cell culture media at concentrations of 20 to 25 mM.

Hippurate test
Sodium hippurate hydrolysis

For Gardnerella and related organisms (chapter 49)

Prepare a 1% (wt/vol) solution of sodium hippurate in 0.067 M Sorensen phosphate buffer (pH 6.4). Tubes containing 0.5 ml of this solution are inoculated as for the glucosidase tests and incubated at 35°C for 2 h, after which 0.2 ml of a solution of 3.5% (wt/vol) ninhydrin dissolved in equal parts of acetone and butanol is added. Development of a deep blue-purple color within 5 min indicates a positive hippurate hydrolysis test.

For Legionella pneumophila reagents (13, 20)

Sodium hippurate solution (1%)

Sodium hippurate	0.1 g
Sterile distilled water	10 ml

Mix in sterile test tubes and place 0.4-ml aliquots into small, sterile, screw-cap tubes. Freeze the solution at −20°C until it is used.

Ninhydrin solution (3.5%)

Ninhydrin	0.35 g
1-Butanol	5 ml
Acetone	5 ml

Mix butanol and acetone in a small, sterile, screw-cap tube. Add ninhydrin, mix, and store at room temperature in the dark.

Test procedure. Thaw the 1% sodium hippurate solution. To the solution add a loopful of organisms grown 1 to 4 days on BCYEα medium. Vortexing the mixture should result in a milky suspension. Incubate at 35°C in air overnight (18 to 20 h). Add 0.2 ml of 3.5% ninhydrin solution, mix gently, and reincubate at 35°C for 10 min. Remove the tube from the incubator and observe for color change in 20 min. Interpret the color as follows: purple, positive; very light purple, weakly positive; gray or light yellow, negative.

For streptococci (chapter 29)

Inoculate sodium hippurate broth with two or three colonies of beta-hemolytic streptococci, and incubate at 35°C for 20 h or longer. Centrifuge the medium to pack the cells, and pipette 0.8 ml of the clean supernatant into a Kahn tube. Add 0.2 ml of the ferric chloride reagent to the Kahn tube, and mix well. If a heavy precipitate remains longer than 10 min, the test is positive.

Human immunodeficiency virus reagents (chapter 100)

Reagents

- Ficoll-Hypaque, catalog no. 1077-1, Sigma Chemical Co., St. Louis, Mo.
- Phytohemagglutinin, catalog no. L9132, Sigma
- Interleukin-2, catalog no. 6011, Electronucleonics, Silver Spring, Md.
- Polybrene, catalog no. 10768-9, Aldrich Chemical Co., Milwaukee, Wis.
- Fetal calf serum, catalog no. 3000, Irvine Scientific, Santa Ana, Calif.
- Fluorescein-conjugated goat anti-human immunoglobulin G (Fc fragment specific), catalog no. 1201-0121, Cooper Biomedical, Durham, N.C.
- Monoclonal antibodies for FACS: for Leu3 and Leu2, Becton Dickinson Immunocytometry Systems, Mountain View, Calif.; for OKT4 and OKT8, Ortho Diagnostic Systems, Raritan, N.J.
- IFA slides (12-dot frosted blue), catalog no. 10-111, Cel-line Associates, Atlantic City, N.J.
- Template poly(rA)p(T) (for RT assay), catalog no. 27-7878-XX, PL Biochemicals, Piscataway, N.J.
- HIV p24 core antigen ELISA, catalog no. 6603698, Coulter Immunology, Hialeah, Fla. (others available from Abbott Laboratories, North Chicago, Ill.; DuPont Co., Wilmington, Del.; and Genetic Systems, Seattle, Wash.)

Indole test

See chapter 121 for culture media.

For nonfermenting gram-negative bacteria (chapter 40)

Tube test with Ehrlich reagent (a less sensitive procedure, at least for flavobacteria, than that with Kovacs reagent)

p-Dimethylaminobenzaldehyde	1 g
Ethanol, 95%	95 ml
Hydrochloric acid, concentrated	20 ml

Add the acid to the alcohol and cool to room temperature before adding the aldehyde. The dry aldehyde should be light straw in color. Ehrlich reagent should be prepared in small quantities and stored in the refrigerator when not being used.

Test procedure. Add 1 ml of xylene to a 48-h tryptone broth culture incubated at 35 to 37°C. Shake the tube briskly for 20 s, and let stand for 1 to 2 min to permit the xylene extract to layer on top of the broth. Deposit 0.5 ml of reagent between xylene and aqueous layers of broth. Do not shake tube after reagent is added. A red color in the reagent phase and appearing within 5 min represents a positive test. Examine the tube for 20 min before determining a negative test.

For nonfermenting gram-negative bacteria (chapter 40)

Tube test with modified Kovacs reagent (17, 38)

p-Dimethylaminobenzaldehyde	2 g
n-Butanol	150 ml
Hydrochloric acid, concentrated	50 ml

Add the acid to the alcohol and allow it to cool before adding the aldehyde. This reagent is stable for at least 10 years when stored at 4°C.

Test procedure. Use either 2% tryptone broth incubated for 2 days at 35°C or tryptophan broth incubated for 18 to 24 h. For the latter medium, the inoculum should be ca. 0.5 mm^3 of cell paste. Add 5 drops of Kovacs reagent; do *not* shake tube after addition of reagent. A red color, appearing within 10 min, represents a positive test.

This reagent and tryptophan broth are more sensitive than Ehrlich reagent with tryptone broth (33). This reagent is also more sensitive and stable than the original Kovacs reagent, 5% of the aldehyde in *n*-pentanol.

Spot test

p-Dimethylaminocinnamaldehyde	200 mg
Hydrochloric acid, concentrated	2 ml
Distilled water	18 ml

Add the acid to the water and allow it to cool before adding the aldehyde. The reagent is stable for at least 5 years when stored at 4°C.

Test procedure. Moisten a spot on a filter paper with two loopfuls of the reagent. Deposit on this ca. 0.5 mm^3 of cell paste taken from a 2- to 4-day culture on a blood agar plate. Deposit two more loopfuls of the reagent on the cell paste to promote diffusion of the indole into the paper. Appearance, within less than 2 min, of a green or blue zone in the paper surrounding the paste represents a positive test. It is important that the blood agar or other medium from which the cell paste is taken contain sufficient tryptophan to initiate indole positivity. One-day blood agar cultures may give false-negative tests (33).

For Enterobacteriaceae (chapter 36)

Tube test with Kovacs reagent (11, 22)

Amyl or isoamyl alcohol	150 ml
p-Dimethylaminobenzaldehyde	10 g
Hydrochloric acid, concentrated	50 ml

Dissolve the aldehyde in alcohol, and then slowly add acid. The dry aldehyde should be light in color. Alcohols that result in indole reagents which become deep brown should not be used. The above-mentioned reagent is stable at room temperature and has a light color. Some authors recommend preparation of only small quantities, which are stored in a refrigerator when not in use.

Test procedure. Add about 0.5 ml of Kovacs reagent to a 40- to 48-h peptone-water culture incubated at 37°C, and shake the tube gently. A deep red develops in the presence of indole. Tests for indole may be made after 24 h of incubation, but if this is to be done, 1 or 2 ml of culture should be removed aseptically for testing. If the test is negative, the remaining portion of the culture should be reincubated for an additional 24 h.

Indophenol oxidase test (chapter 40)
Indophenol cytochrome oxidase test (14, 16)

Solution A

α-Naphthol	1 g
Ethyl alcohol, 95 to 96%	100 ml

Solution B

N,N-Dimethyl-*p*-phenylenediamine	1 g
Distilled water	100 ml

Solution B should be prepared frequently and should be stored in a refrigerator when not in use.

Test procedure. Use dry filter paper strips previously impregnated with solutions A and B. Rub growth from colony into paper strip. A dark blue color usually appears within 30 s, which indicates oxidase activity. Weak oxidase producers will react slower.

Alternative test procedure. The test is performed on nutrient agar slant cultures incubated at 37°C, or at a lower temperature if required. Add 2 or 3 drops of each reagent, and tilt the tube so that the reagents mix and flow over the growth on the slant. Positive reactions are indicated by the development of a blue color in the growth within 2 min.

Most positive cultures produce a strong reaction within 30 s. Any weak or doubtful reaction that occurs after 2 min should be ignored. Plate cultures may be tested by allowing an equal-parts mixture of the reagents to flow over isolated colonies.

Kaolin solution

See chapter 94.

KOH solution
For initial examination of clinical material

Potassium hydroxide	10 or 20 g
Distilled water	100 ml

Mix the specimen (pus, exudate, tissue) with a drop of 10 or 20% solution on a clean slide, cover with a no. 2 cover slip (22 by 40 mm), and press gently to make a thin mount. Gentle warming may aid in clearing the mount. Viscid specimens may require overnight storage in a moist chamber. (Place the slide on applicator stick supports over moist filter paper in a petri dish, or place them in a screw-cap Coplin jar laid on its side.) Scan under low power with reduced lighting. Switch to high power to check for the presence of suspected fungal elements.

Alternative method. Add 10 ml of glycerin to the solution in place of 10 ml of distilled water.

Kovacs oxidase test (14)
For nonfermenters and miscellaneous gram-negative bacteria

Place filter paper in a petri dish, and saturate it with 0.5% tetramethyl-*p*-phenylenediamine hydrochloride. With a platinum wire, pick a portion of the colony to be tested, and rub the colony on the filter paper.

A positive reaction is indicated by the appearance of a dark purple color within 10 s. With this technique, there should be enough of the colony left for subculturing.

Alternate procedure. Place a few drops of the oxidase reagent directly onto colonies on a plate (38). Colonies producing oxidase become pink and then purple. The reagent does not interfere with the Gram stain, so purple colonies may be stained even though they are not viable. The oxidase reagent may be divided into small aliquots and stored at −20°C. Thaw one aliquot as needed, and do not use it for more than 1 day. Check the reagent daily with a known oxidase-positive organism. The Kovacs oxidase test is more sensitive than the indophenol method.

Lactonate oxidation

Inoculate 2-ketolactonate agar plates and incubate them at 30°C for 24 to 48 h. Flood the plates with Benedict reagent. A positive test is indicated by the formation of a yellow ring of Cu_2O around the bacterial growth. This may take up to 1 h to develop.

Lactophenol (cotton blue) mounting solution (chapter 26)
Mounting medium for studying fungi

Phenol crystals	20 g
Lactic acid	20 ml
Glycerol	40 ml
Distilled water	20 ml

Dissolve the ingredients by heating the container in a hot water bath. Add 0.05 g of cotton blue (Poirier blue). Lactophenol mounting solution without cotton blue is useful for evaluating pigmented structures in the pigmented fungi.

Lancefield extract procedure

See chapter 29.

LAPase test procedure

See chapter 29.

Lecithinase test

Inoculate an egg yolk agar plate (see chapter 121). Streak for isolation and incubate in an anaerobic jar for 48 to 72 h. Remove cover and examine for changes in the media around the colony. A positive reaction is indicated by a cloudy, opaque zone appearing around the colonies.

Lectin solutions (10)

Dissolve lectins to a final concentration of 1.0 mg/ml in 50 mM dipotassium phosphate adjusted to pH 7.3 with 0.1 N hydrochloric acid. Lectin solutions can be safely stored for several months at −20°C. *Glycine max* (soybean) or *Helix pomatia* (snail) lectin may be obtained from E-Y Laboratories, San Mateo, Calif.

Lipase test

Inoculate an egg yolk agar plate (see chapter 121). Streak for isolation and incubate in an anaerobic jar for 48 to 72 h. Remove the cover and examine under oblique light. Look for an oily, iridescent sheen present over and around the colony growth for a positive test.

Lugol iodine solution

Dissolve 10 g of potassium iodine in 100 ml of distilled water. Add 5 g of iodine crystals slowly, with shaking. Filter and store in a tightly stoppered brown bottle. May be stored for 1 month.

McFarland nephelometer (28)

In a rack, arrange 11 large test tubes, the same size as those used in the dilution of vaccines, and label them 0.5 to 10.

Add a 1% solution of anhydrous barium chloride and a 1% (by volume) cold solution of chemically pure sulfuric acid according to Table 1. Seal the tubes and keep them in the refrigerator.

When the fine white precipitate of barium sulfate is shaken up well, each tube has a different density that corresponds approximately to the bacterial suspensions given in Table 1.

TABLE 1. Protocol for test tubes for McFarland nephelometer

Tube no.	Contents (ml)		Corresponding bacterial suspension/ml (10^8)
	Barium chloride (1 %)	Sulfuric acid (1 %)	
0.5	0.05	9.95	1.5
1	0.1	9.9	3
2	0.2	9.8	6
3	0.3	9.7	9
4	0.4	9.6	12
5	0.5	9.5	15
6	0.6	9.4	18
7	0.7	9.3	21
8	0.8	9.2	24
9	0.9	9.1	27
10	1.0	9.0	30

Alternative method

0.5 standard
0.05 ml of 1.175% (wt/vol) $BaCl_2 \cdot 2H_2$ plus
9.95 ml of 0.36 N H_2 = 1.5×10^8 bacteria/ml

Methyl red test

See VP media, chapter 121.

Methyl red indicator

Methyl red	0.1 g
Ethyl alcohol, 95%	300.0 ml

Dissolve the dye in alcohol, and add sufficient distilled water to make 500 ml.

Test procedure. Inoculate buffered glucose-peptone broth lightly from a young agar slant culture. Incubation at 37°C for 48 h is sufficient for the majority of cultures. Tests should not be made with cultures incubated for less than 48 h. If the results are equivocal, repeat the test with cultures that have been incubated for 4 or 5 days. In such instances, duplicate tests should be incubated at 25°C.

Layer 5 or 6 drops of reagent for each 5 ml of culture. Reactions are read immediately. Positive tests are bright red, weakly positive tests are red-orange, and negative tests are yellow.

Motility tests

For the *Enterobacteriaceae* (chapter 36), a medium containing 0.4% agar is recommended. Inoculate by stabbing into the top of the column of medium to a depth of about 5 mm. Incubate at 35°C for 1 or 2 days. If the results are negative, follow with further incubation at 21 to 25°C for 5 days. For special purposes, such as enhancement of the motility and flagellar development in poorly motile cultures, it is often advisable to pass cultures first through a semisolid medium containing 0.2% agar tubed in Craigie tubes or in U tubes. Subsequent passages may be made in the 0.4% agar medium.

Aeromonas and *Pseudomonas* species are discussed in chapters 38 and 41. Motility media containing agar concentrations higher than 0.3% produce gels through which many motile organisms cannot spread. Spreading in a semisolid medium is judged by macroscopic examination of the medium for a diffuse zone of growth emanating from the line of inoculation. Many aerobic pseudomonads fail to grow when they are deep in semisolid medium in a test tube. Organisms possessing "paralyzed" flagella are nonmotile and cannot spread in the medium. Some filamentous organisms spread in or on semisolid medium but are nonmotile and nonflagellated. Although cultures may grow at 37°C or higher temperatures, the flagellar proteins of some organisms are not synthesized optimally at these temperatures; hence, motility medium should be incubated at temperatures near 18 to 20°C. These observations require a judicious interpretation of motility, and they limit, to some extent, the reliability of spreading in semisolid agar as the sole taxonomic criterion to delineate related species.

A deep layer of motility medium, 18 to 20 ml in a 100-mm-diameter petri dish, is useful for selecting strains from a predominantly nonmotile stock. The place is inoculated in the center, and motile descendants are "fished" from the periphery of the giant colony after organisms have spread through the semisolid agar.

Nessler reagent (chapter 40)
For acetamide hydrolysis

Solution A

Mercuric chloride	1 g
Distilled water	6 ml

Dissolve completely.

Solution B

Potassium iodide	2.5 g
Distilled water	6 ml

Dissolve completely and add solution A.

Solution C

Potassium hydroxide	6 g
Distilled water	6 ml

Dissolve completely and add to the mixture of solutions A and B. Add 13 ml of distilled water. Mix well, and filter before using.

Test procedure. Inoculate 1 ml of mineral base broth medium (carbon assimilation medium) supplemented with 0.1% acetamide. Incubate at 30°C for 24 h. Add 1 drop of Nessler reagent. The test is positive if a red-brown sediment appears. The sediment is due to the presence of ammonia from acylamidase action.

Neutral red dye solution, 0.15% (chapter 117)

Prepare 0.1 M phosphate buffer.

Stock A. 0.2 M solution of monobasic sodium phosphate (27.8 g in 1,000 ml of distilled water)

Stock B. 0.2 M solution of dibasic sodium phosphate (53.65 g of $Na_2HPO_4 \cdot 7H_2O$ or 71.7 g of $Na_2HPO_4 \cdot 12H_2O$ in 1,000 ml of distilled water)

To prepare 0.1 M stock buffer, pH 6.0, mix 87.7 ml of stock A with 12.3 ml of stock B and dilute to a total of 200 ml with distilled water.

Prepare neutral red dye solution as follows. Weigh out 0.15 g of neutral red and add it to 100 ml of phosphate buffer (0.1 M). Mix well and filter through a 0.45-µm-pore-size filter and a 022-µm-pore-size filter. Store stock in sterile bottles.

Nigrosin stain

See capsule stain.

Nitrate disk test (40)

Disks

KNO_3	30 g
$Na_2MoO_4 \cdot 2H_2O$	0.1 g
Distilled water	100 ml

Dissolve the nitrate and molybdate completely and then filter sterilize the solution by passing it through a membrane filter (0.45-µm pore size). Dispense 20-µl quantities of the sterile solution to presterilized 0.25-in. (0.635-cm) filter paper disks. Petri dishes (100 by 15 mm) are very convenient receptacles during preparation of the disks. After saturating the disks, cover them and allow them to dry at room temperature for 72 h.

Nitrate reagents

Solution A

Sulfanilic acid	0.5 g
Glacial acetic acid	30.0 ml
Distilled water	120.0 ml

Solution B

1,6-Cleve's acid (5-amino-2-naphthalenesulfonic acid)	0.2 g
Glacial acetic acid	30.0 ml
Distilled water	120.0 ml

Test procedure. The nitrate disk test is performed by removing the nitrate disk from the surface of a blood agar plate on which there is growth and placing it in a clean petri dish. Add 1 drop each of solutions A and B to the disks. Reduction of nitrate to nitrite is indicated by a pink to red color. If no color is seen within a few minutes, add a small amount of zinc dust and wait 5 min. Development of a red color indicates that nitrate was not reduced. If the disk remains colorless, nitrate was reduced beyond nitrite (interpreted as a positive test).

Nitrate reduction reagent

Solution A

Sulfanilic acid	8 g
Acetic acid	1 liter

Solution B

N,N-Dimethyl-1-naphthylamine	6 ml
Acetic acid	1 liter

The 5 N acetic acid consists of 1 part glacial acetic acid to 2.5 parts distilled water.

Although *N,N*-dimethyl-1-naphthylamine, unlike naphthylamine, has not been listed as a carcinogen by the Occupational Safety and Health Administration, its structural similarity to naphythlamine would indicate that such safety precautions as the avoidance of aerosols, mouth pipetting, and contact with the skin should be followed.

For miscellaneous gram-negative bacteria (chapter 40) and Pseudomonas spp. (chapter 41)

Inoculate a fluid medium tubed with inverted Durham tubes, incubate it at 30 or 35°C, and examine it after 24 and 48 h for reduction of nitrate to nitrogen gas, which accumulates in the Durham tube. After 1 h, test for nitrite by the addition of 0.5 ml each of solutions A and B. A red color indicates a positive test provided the uninoculated control medium is negative. Negative tests should be confirmed by the action of zinc dust to convert unreduced nitrate or nitrite.

Nitrite reduction test for miscellaneous gram-negative bacteria (chapter 40)

Inoculate inverted Durham tubes containing nitrite reduction broth. Incubate at 35°C, and examine after 24 and 48 h for reduction of nitrite to nitrogen gas, which accumulates in the Durham tubes. After 48 h, test for nitrite by the addition of 0.5 ml each of reagents A and B of nitrate reduction broth. The test is positive if there is no color change, provided a red color develops in the uninoculated control.

O129 (2,4-diamino-6,7-diisopropyl pteridine) disks

Commercially available from Oxoid (USA)

For differentiation of vibrios from other gram-negative rods and particularly from aeromonads

Disks

O129 phosphate	10 μg per disk
O129 phosphate	150 μg per disk

Test procedure. Evenly inoculate the surface of a plate of nutrient agar containing 0.5% NaCl. Blood agar base is recommended. Place one 10-μg and one 150-μg disk on each plate. Incubate at 37°C for 24 h. Observe for zones of inhibition.

Test samples of the finished product for performance with control cultures.

Interpretation of results

150-μg disk	10-μg disk	Interpretation
Zone approx. 10 mm	Zone approx. 5 mm	Sensitive
Zone of any size	Zone of <2 mm	Partially sensitive
No zone	No zone	Resistant

Sensitivity of *Vibrio* species to O129

Organism	MIC (O129 phosphate, μg/ml)	Interpretation
Aeromonas	400	Resistant
V. alginolyticus	10–50	Partially sensitive
Plesiomonas	2–40	Sensitive
V. cholerae	2–7.5	Sensitive

ONPG test (11)

See chapter 121 for media.

Peptone water. Dissolve 1 g of peptone and 0.5 g of NaCl in 100 ml of distilled water. Autoclave at 121°C for 15 min.

ONPG solution. Dissolve 0.6 g of *o*-nitrophenyl-β-D-galactopyranoside (ONPG) in 100 ml of 0.01 M Na_2HPO_4. Sterilize by filtration; put in a sterile bottle. Store at 4 to 10°C, protected from light.

ONPG broth. Aseptically add 25 ml of ONPG solution to 75 ml of peptone water. Aseptically dispense in 0.5-ml amounts into sterile tubes (13 by 100 mm). This broth is stable for 1 month at 4 to 10°C, or longer if stored in the freezer. Do not use if yellow.

Test procedure. Inoculate 0.5 ml of ONPG broth with a heavy loopful of growth from triple sugar iron or Kligler iron agar. Incubate in a heating block or water bath at 37°C for 1 h or more.

Results are interpreted as follows: yellow color, positive; colorless, negative.

This test cannot be performed with yellow-pigmented organisms.

Optochin susceptibility test

See chapter 29.

Oxidase test (15)

For separation of staphylococci (except Staphylococcus sciuri) from micrococci

Oxidase reagent

Tetramethylphenylenediamine (TMPD)	6 g
Dimethyl sulfoxide (DMSO)	100 ml

Solubilize TMPD reagent in DMSO. Bottle and label. If protected against light, solution is stable at room temperature for several weeks.

Test procedure. Cultivate bacterial strains on fresh blood agar (nutrient agar and 7% sheep blood). Incubate at 30°C, under aerobic conditions, for 15 to 18 h. Smear one loopful of bacteria onto plain filter paper. Place 1 drop of oxidase reagent (6% TMPD in DMSO) onto the bacteria-smeared filter paper. Oxidase-positive bacteria turn the filter dark blue within 2 min.

Note. Other media (peptone-yeast extract-glucose agar, peptone-yeast extract agar, or plate count agar), can be used, but cultures growing on these media must be incubated for at least 3 days before testing for oxidase production. Positive reaction occurs within 5 to 10 min.

Peptone solution (23)

For use with nitrate assimilation medium (chapter 60)

Peptone	20.0 g
Distilled water	100.0 ml

Add peptone to water without agitation. Allow peptone to soak into water (placing flask in a 50°C water bath may help). When dissolved, sterilize by membrane filtration. Store at 4°C.

Petrolatum

White petrolatum jelly (Clay Park Laboratories, Inc.) is transferred to a 50-ml beaker (about 25 ml is a convenient amount); the beaker is covered with foil and autoclaved at 121°C for 15 min.

Melt petrolatum on heat block or heating magnetic stirrer. *Do not use direct flame.* Pour about 1 to 2 ml over surface of inoculated agar for seal.

Phosphate-buffered saline (PBS)
For washing cells and diluting trypsin

NaCl	8.00 g
KCl	0.20 g
KH_2PO_4	0.12 g
Na_2HPO_4 (anhydrous)	0.91 g
Distilled water to	1,000 ml

Sterilize by autoclaving at 18 lb/in^2 for 35 min. PBS is available from Sigma (catalog no. D5527).

Phosphate-buffered saline, 10×

Stock solution A (10×)

NaCl	8.0 g
KCl	0.4 g
$NaH_2PO_4 \cdot H_2O$	0.2 g
Na_2HPO_4	1.2 g
Glass-distilled water	100.0 ml

Stock solution B (10×)

$CaCl_2$	0.11 g
$MgCl_2 \cdot 6H_2O$	0.3 g
Glass-distilled water	100.0 ml

For 1 liter of 1× concentration, add 100 ml of stock solution A to 800 ml of glass-distilled water and mix very well. Add 100 ml of stock solution B and mix well.

Phosphate-buffered saline–gelatin–Tween solution

See chapter 86.

Phosphate buffers

A. Stock buffers

1. Alkaline buffer, 0.067 M Na_2HPO_4 solution. Dissolve 9.5 g of Na_2HPO_4 in 1 liter of water.
2. Acid buffer, 0.067 M NaH_2PO_4 solution. Dissolve 9.2 g of $NaH_2PO_4 \cdot H_2O$ in 1 liter of water.

These buffers can be kept for a long period of time.

B. Buffered water (pH 7.0 to 7.2)

Acid buffer (NaH_2PO_4)	39 ml
Alkaline buffer (Na_2HPO_4)	61 ml
Distilled water	900 ml

Be sure glassware is clean. Buffered water, if sealed, is stable for several weeks.

Phosphate buffer

Prepare stock solutions.

Stock A. 0.2 M solution of monobasic sodium phosphate (27.8 g in 1,000 ml of distilled H_2O)

Stock B. 0.2 M solution of dibasic sodium phosphate (53.65 g of $Na_2HPO_4 \cdot 7H_2O$ or 71.7 g of $Na_2HPO_4 \cdot 12H_2O$ in 1,000 ml of distilled H_2O)

To prepare the correct pH, mix x ml of stock A (monobasic) with x ml of stock B (dibasic) according to the following table:

A	B	pH	A	B	pH
93.5	6.5	5.7	45.0	55.0	6.9
92.0	8.0	5.8	39.0	61.0	7.0
90.0	10.0	5.9	33.0	67.0	7.1
87.7	12.3	6.0	28.0	72.0	7.2
85.0	15.0	6.1	23.0	77.0	7.3
81.5	18.5	6.2	19.0	81.0	7.4
77.5	22.5	6.3	16.0	84.0	7.5
73.5	26.5	6.4	13.0	87.0	7.6
68.5	31.5	6.5	10.5	90.5	7.7
62.5	37.5	6.6	8.5	91.5	7.8
56.5	43.5	6.7	7.0	93.0	7.9
51.0	40.0	6.8	5.3	94.7	8.0

To prepare solutions with different molarity, dilute as needed with distilled H_2O.

Pigmentation procedure

See chapter 29.

Polymyxin B resistance test

See chapter 28.

Polyvinyl alcohol fixative for parasitology

Reagents

Polyvinyl alcohol (PVA) powder	50 g
Schaudinn stock solution (see Schaudinn fixative)	935.0 ml
Neutral glycerol	15.0 ml
Glacial acetic acid	50.0 ml

PVA (Evonal) powder may be purchased from Eastman Chemical Products, Inc., or Baker Co. Grades of high hydrolysis and low to medium viscosity are most satisfactory but must be pretested for adhesive property and lack of clumping.

Add the powder to the flask containing Schaudinn solution, acetic acid, and glycerol by slowly shaking in the powder while agitating the solution. Dissolve the powder by heating the solution in a 75°C water bath (do not boil). Shake the mixture frequently, or use a magnetic stirrer. When the powder is dissolved, remove the flask from the water bath and allow it to stand overnight. If a heavy precipitate forms during preparation or if the finished product is quite cloudy, discard and start again. PVA powder may be unsatisfactory.

Prepared PVA fixative may be purchased from several commercial sources, including Marion Scientific, Kansas City, Mo.; Meridian Diagnostics, Cincinnati, Ohio; and Medi-Chem, Santa Monica, Calif. PVA fixative is also included in some commercial kits.

Shelf life varies with the specific lot and the quantity (larger amounts are satisfactory for a longer period). PVA fixative becomes cloudy or gels when it is unsatisfactory. Large volumes may be satisfactory for a year or more, whereas small volumes may be unsatisfactory after several months.

Potassium nitrate solution (23)
For use with nitrate assimilation medium (chapter 60)

Potassium nitrate	20.0 g
Distilled water	100.0 ml

Dissolve potassium nitrate in water. Sterilize by membrane filtration. Store at 4°C.

PYR test (hydrolysis of L-pyrrolidonyl-β-naphthylamide)

See chapters 28 and 29.

Pyrazinamidase test (21)
For differentiating pathogenic serotypes of Yersinia enterocolitica from nonpathogenic serotypes (chapter 36)

The pyrazinamidase test was originally described for differentiating closely related species in the genus *Mycobacterium,* but in 1985 Kandolo and Wauters (21) applied it to *Y. enterocolitica.* Nonpathogenic serotypes have the enzyme pyrazinamidase (pyrazine carboxylamidase), which converts pyrazinamide to pyrazinoic acid, which turns brown in the presence of ferrous salts. Pathogenic serotypes lack the enzyme or produce much less.

Quality control. Both a pathogenic and a nonpathogenic serotype of *Y. enterocolitica* should be included with each run.

Test procedure (see chapter 121 for media). Inoculate the strain of *Y. enterocolitica* on the slant and incubate at 25°C (to 30°C) for 48 h. Flood the surface with 1 ml of a freshly prepared 1% solution of ferrous ammonium sulfate. A positive pyrazinamidase test is indicated by the development of a pink-brown color within 15 min that intensifies with time. Pathogenic serotypes of *Y. enterocolitica* are usually pyrazinamidase negative, but nonpathogenic serotypes are usually positive. In addition, the strain should be tested for growth on CRMOX agar, salicin-esculin fermentation, and other tests if possible.

Rapid pyrazinamidase test (37)

Substrate

Pyrazinamide	0.1 g
Sodium pyruvate	2.0 g
Agar	2.0 g
Distilled water	1,000 ml

Heat to melt the agar, dispense as 5-ml aliquots into screw-cap tubes (16 by 125 mm), and autoclave at 15 lb/in^2 for 15 min.

Reagent

Ferrous ammonium sulfate (1%), freshly prepared

Test procedure. Use a swab to transfer a heavy inoculum from 24- to 72-h cultures from blood or chocolate agar plates to the top half of the agar tube. Incubate for 2 h at 37°C. Add 1 ml of freshly prepared reagent, and mix it in the top half of the tube. Within 1 to 5 min, a pink color develops for a positive test. A positive and negative control should be done.

Rapid fermentation technique (RFT) solutions

Prepare a 10× buffered salts solution stock (10× BSS) as follows:

KCl	8.0 g
K_2HPO_4	0.4 g
KH_2PO_4	0.1 g
Distilled water	100 ml

Dissolve and filter sterilize. Prepare a working dilution of BSS by diluting 10 ml of 10× BSS with 90 ml of distilled water. Add 0.5 ml of a 1% aqueous solution of phenol red, and filter sterilize. Aseptically pour into a sterile bottle, label, and store at 4°C.

Prepare 20% aqueous solutions of reagent-grade glucose, maltose, fructose, sucrose, and lactose. Filter sterilize, and dispense 0.1-ml aliquots of each sugar into appropriately labeled Nunc tubes. Store in Nunc trays at 4°C.

Resistance to mitomycin C procedure

See chapter 35.

Rhinovirus antisera for types 1A-89

Antisera can be obtained from the American Type Culture Collection, 12301 Parklawn Drive, Rockville, MD 20852; (301) 881-2600. Catalog of Animal and Plant Viruses and Antisera, 5th ed., 1986.

RIPA buffer

See chapter 100.

Sample buffer for human immunodeficiency virus

See chapter 100.

Saponin solution (0.5%) for filaria concentration

Saponin powder	0.25 g

Add 50 ml of 0.85% saline. Mix carefully and thoroughly. Remove excess foam.

Note. Saponin (0.15 g) can be placed in 50-ml screw-cap centrifuge tubes and stored. Saline is added when saponin is needed.

Satellitism procedure

See chapter 29.

Schaudinn fixative for fresh fecal films

Stock solution of saturated mercuric chloride solution with alcohol. Saturated mercuric chloride should be prepared several days before it is used. Add 47.5 g of mercuric chloride to 675 ml of distilled water, and heat to dissolve. Stopper tightly, let stand at room temperature overnight, and filter. Add 1 part 95% ethyl alcohol to 2 parts saturated mercuric chloride in stoppered container.

Schaudinn fixative. Add 1 part glacial acetic acid to 19 parts solution just before use (fixative should be prepared daily as needed). Usually 2.5 ml of glacial acetic acid is added to 48 ml of stock solution for each usage.

Slide culture technique (5)

In the study of fungi, it is often necessary to observe the undisturbed relationship between reproductive structures and mycelium. This observation may be done by growing the fungi on glass slides in a moist chamber. The operator should be aware of infectious hazards of this procedure. This technique should never be used for the systemic pathogenic molds *Coccidioides immitis*, *Histoplasma capsulatum*, *Blastomyces dermatitidis*, and *Paracoccidioides brasiliensis*.

Place a piece of absorbent paper and a slide on a bent glass rod in the bottom of a petri dish, add a cover slip, cover, and sterilize. Prepare Sabouraud dextrose agar plates with about 15 ml of agar per plate. Allow to solidify and dry. Cut agar blocks about 1 cm square. Using sterile technique, place a block of agar on the slide in the petri dish. Inoculate the central portion of each of the four sides of the block with a small fragment of the fungus being studied.

Cover the inoculated block with a sterile cover slip. Add 8.0 ml of sterile water to the bottom of the petri dish. Incubate at 25°C until sporulation occurs. Maintain saturation of the paper throughout the incubation period. The slide preparation may be checked periodically under the low power of a microscope.

When sporulation is complete, carefully lift off the cover slip and lay it aside with the fungus growth up. Lift the agar block from the slide and discard it.

Place a drop of lactophenol cotton blue in the center of growth on the slide, and cover it with a fresh cover slip. Place another drop in the center of growth on the cover slip, and drop the cover slip into place on another clean slide. Blot away excess mounting fluid from the two preparations, and allow them to dry. Seal the edges with nail polish.

Sodium hippurate hydrolysis

See hippurate test.

Sorensen pH buffer solutions

Stock A: 0.067 M Na_2PO_4

Dissolve 9.464 g of the anhydrous salt, previously dried at 130°C, in distilled water to make 1 liter of solution.

Stock B: 0.067 M KH_2PO_4

Dissolve 9.073 g of the anhydrous salt, previously dried at 110°C, in distilled water to make 1 liter of solution.

Mix *x* ml of solutions A and B as indicated below to make various buffers with a given pH. These solutions can be added to culture media to prevent major changes in pH.

pH	Soln A	Soln B
5.29	0.25	9.75
5.59	0.5	9.5
5.91	1	9
6.24	2	8
6.47	3	7
6.64	4	6
6.81	5	5
6.98	6	4
7.17	7	3
7.38	8	2
7.73	9	1
8.04	9.5	0.5

Starch hydrolysis test

Method 1. Inoculate a starch agar plate and incubate it under the appropriate conditions and proper time for a given group of organisms. After incubation, flood the medium with 2 to 4 ml of Gram iodine. A positive test is indicated by a colorless zone around the streak or colony, which indicates that starch is hydrolyzed. A negative test is indicated by the entire medium turning blue, which indicates that starch is present. Starch agar may be prepared by using Lombard-Dowell agar with 5.0 g of starch added per liter (see chapter 121).

Method 2. Inoculate a plate of Mueller-Hinton agar with one streak of the test organism. Two to three cultures can be tested on one plate. Incubate the plate for 2 days at 35°C. Flood the plate with a 1:5 dilution of Lugol iodine solution, and hold it against a white background. A positive test is indicated by colorless zones around the area of growth or colony.

Tap water morphology procedure

See chapter 35.

Temperature requirements

Methods for determining ability of organism to grow at various temperatures

A. Growth at 10°C

For aerobic actinomycetes and other bacteria

Inoculate two tubes of selected medium. Incubate one tube at 35°C and the second one in a 10°C water bath. Observe for growth on a daily basis for 7 days.

Results. Rhodochrous grows well at 10°C; *Mycobacterium* species show no growth; *Nocardia* species grow rarely or not at all.

B. Growth at 25, 35, and 42°C

For Pseudomonas spp. and other bacteria

Inoculate slants of blood agar base medium (or other appropriate medium) with 1 drop of a broth suspension. Incubate one tube at 42°C and one at 35°C (37°C) and, if necessary, incubate one tube at 25°C. Examine the tubes after 18 to 24 h and daily for 7 days.

For nonfermentative bacteria (30)

Inoculate three slants of tryptone-glucose-yeast extract agar or Trypticase soy agar with one loopful of an overnight broth culture. Incubate one tube at 25°C, one tube at 37°C, and one tube at 42°C for 18 to 24 h. Examine the tubes for amount of growth.

Triton X-100 stock solution (10%)

Triton X-100	10 ml
Distilled water	90 ml

Triton X-100 is available from Rohm and Haas Co., Philadelphia, Pa., and Emulsion Engineering, Inc., Elk Grove Village, Ill.

Mix and store in a tightly stoppered bottle at room temperature; the solution will keep indefinitely.

Buffered water with Triton X-100 (10%)

The final concentration of Triton X-100 is 0.01%. Add 1 ml of Triton X-100 stock solution to 1,000 ml of the buffered water described above.

Giemsa stain prepared in buffer with 0.01% Triton X-100 penetrates better and is recommended for staining blood and tissue slides. Buffered water without Triton X-100 is used for rinsing stained slides.

The pH (7.0 to 7.2) is critical; if it is incorrect, it can be adjusted by adding small amounts of acid or alkaline buffer.

Ureaplasma urease test reagent

Urea	0.6 g
$CaCl_2$	1.1 g
Water	100 ml

Place several drops of reagent on an agar plate with visible or invisible colonies. A brown color surrounding *Ureaplasma urealyticum* colonies but not *Mycoplasma hominis* colonies results within 1 to 5 min on urea agar. The added urea also results in a red color from the phenol red indicator if colonies are present within 1 to 12 h. Colonies should be no more than 48 h old or should be held at 4°C until tested.

Vancomycin screening procedure

See chapter 29.

Vaspar

See chapter 68.

Voges-Proskauer (VP) test
For detecting acetoin

VP media (see chapter 121)

Buffered peptone-glucose, methyl red (MR)-VP, or VP broth can be used.

MR-VP medium

MR-VP medium	1.7 g
Distilled water	100.0 ml

Dispense in 2.0-ml volumes into 18- by 150-mm cotton-plugged tubes. Autoclave at 121°C for no longer than 10 min to prevent caramelization of the glucose.

A. Method 1, Barritt

VP reagent

Solution A

α-Naphthol	5 g
Ethyl alcohol, absolute	100 ml

Solution B

Potassium hydroxide	40 g
Distilled water	100 ml

Add 0.6 ml of solution A and 0.2 ml of solution B to 1 ml of culture. Shake well after the addition of each reagent. Positive reactions occur at once or within 5 min and are indicated by the production of a red color. The development of a copper color in some tests should be disregarded.

B. Method 2, Coblentz (9), modified (33)

VP reagent for detecting acetoin

Solution A

α-Naphthol	5 g
Ethyl alcohol, 95%	100 ml

Solution B

Sodium (or potassium) hydroxide	40 g
Creatine	300 mg
Distilled water	100 ml

These reagents are applicable when the VP test is made with the conventional glucose-peptone-phosphate medium. However, when VP tablets are used, solution B need not contain creatine since it is present in the tablets.

Test procedure. Inoculate the MR-VP medium with a massive inoculum, consisting of a loopful (2 to 3 mm) of an 18-h agar slant culture. Incubate at 30°C for 6 to 7 h.

The test is performed by adding 5 drops of solution A and 5 drops of solution B to a 48-h culture in MR-VP broth. After addition of reagents, shake tube briskly for at least 30 s. A red color, appearing within 5 min, is a positive test. For the rapid test with a VP tablet, solution B can be either 40% potassium or sodium hydroxide; a special KOH-creatine solution is not required since creatine is incorporated in the VP tablet. The naphthol solution is stable for at least 1 year when stored at 4°C.

C. Method 3

O'Meara reagent, modified

Potassium hydroxide	40.0 g
Creatine	0.3 g
Distilled water	100.0 ml

Dissolve the alkali in the water and add creatine. The reagent should be prepared frequently and should be refrigerated when not in use (25, 36). The reagent may be used for 2 to 3 weeks, but it deteriorates rapidly thereafter.

Test procedure. The VP test is performed on the culture grown in buffered peptone-glucose broth incubated at 37°C for 48 h. Add 1 ml of reagent to 1 ml of culture, and place the mixture at 37°C or at room temperature, after shaking to aerate. A positive test is indicated by the development of a pink color. The test depends on the formation of acetylmethylcarbinol, which is oxidized in alkaline medium, in the presence of air, to form diacetyl. Diacetyl reacts with creatine to form the pink compound. Final readings are made after 4 h. If equivocal results are obtained, repeat the test with cultures incubated at 25°C.

Zinc sulfate solution for fecal parasite concentration

Zinc sulfate solution is prepared so that the final specific gravity is appropriate for the type of specimen to be examined (1.20 for Formalin-fixed specimens, 1.18 for fresh specimens).

Dissolve 386 g of reagent-grade zinc sulfate ($ZnSO_4 \cdot 7H_2O$) in 400 ml of hot water, and cool to room temperature. Place 400 ml of water in a 1,000-ml stoppered graduated cylinder. Add zinc sulfate solution to the graduated cylinder, and mix. Check the specific gravity with a hydrometer for heavy liquids (it should be over 1.20). Add 10 ml of water for each 0.002 the specific gravity must be reduced, mix thoroughly, and check the specific gravity. (Repeat until the specific gravity is 1.20.)

If the specific gravity is less than 1.195, dissolve as much zinc sulfate as possible in 50 ml of very hot water. Add some of this solution to raise the specific gravity. After the specific gravity is correctly adjusted, allow the solution to stand overnight, and recheck.

Store at room temperature in a tightly stoppered container. Recheck the specific gravity monthly.

STAINS AND STAINING PROCEDURES

Acridine orange stain

Acridine orange	1 g
Distilled water	100 ml

Prepare solution by dissolving acridine orange in the water and store in the dark at 4°C. May be stored for 6 months.

Working solutions should be made fresh daily. Add 0.5 ml of stock solution to 5 ml of 0.2 M acetate buffer at pH 4.0. Prepare smears as usual and air dry. Fix with absolute methanol or heat fix. Flood slide with acridine orange stain and allow to remain on surface for 2 min without drying. Rinse with tap water and allow the slide to air dry. Examine under oil immersion (1,000×) and UV light.

Bacteria and yeasts stain bright red-orange and leukocytes stain pale apple green. Slides may be Gram stained directly without decolorization if all oil is removed.

Auramine-rhodamine stain

See rhodamine-auramine fluorochrome stain.

Calcofluor white stain

For initial examination of clinical material for fungi

Calcofluor white M2R	0.1 g
Evans blue	0.05 g
Distilled water	100.0 ml

Mix thoroughly and store in a brown bottle at room temperature.

Staining procedure. Add 1 drop of the Calcofluor white solution and 1 drop of 10% KOH to the specimen to be examined on a microscope slide; cover the specimen with a cover slip. Examine by using UV light, K530 excitation filter, and BG 12 barrier filter (or G-365 excitation filter and LP420 barrier filter).

Results. The fungal elements will appear green or blue-white, depending on the filter combinations, with a much dimmer reddish fluorescing background.

Capsule stain (Hiss method)

Staining procedure. Mix a loopful of physiological saline suspension of growth with a drop of normal serum on a glass slide. Allow the smear to air dry, and heat fix. Flood the smear with crystal violet (1% aqueous solution). Steam the preparation gently for 1 min, and rinse with copper sulfate (20% aqueous solution).

Results. Capsules appear as faint blue halos around dark blue to purple cells.

Crystal violet stain, 1%

For viral studies (chapter 79)

Formaldehyde	10 ml
Acetic acid	4 ml
Methanol	60 ml
Distilled water	25 ml
Crystal violet	1 g

Dissolve the crystal violet in the methanol. Add other solutions and mix thoroughly. All crystals of stain should be completely dissolved. Solution should be stored in a capped bottle until used.

Dobell and O'Connor iodine solution

For staining intestinal protozoa

Iodine (powdered crystals)	1 g
Potassium iodide	2 g
Distilled water	100 ml

Dissolve potassium iodide in water. Add iodine crystals, and shake thoroughly. The crystals may not dissolve completely; if they do not, filter or decant. Put a portion in a dropping bottle for daily use, and store the remainder in a brown bottle away from the light.

This is a weak iodine solution and should be prepared fresh every 2 to 3 weeks.

Flagellar stains (chapter 40)

A. Gray flagellar stain (19)

Mordant

Potassium alum, saturated aqueous solution	5 ml
Tannic acid, 20% aqueous solution	2 ml
Mercuric chloride, saturated aqueous solution	2 ml

Basic fuchsin

Basic fuchsin (certified for flagellar stain)	0.6 g
Ethyl alcohol, 95%	50.0 ml

Shake and let stand overnight to dissolve the fuchsin. Mix and add 0.4 ml of a saturated alcoholic solution of basic fuchsin. Make up fresh mordant for use each day.

Staining procedure. Using a grease-free, well-cleaned slide that has been flamed and cooled, add a drop of bacterial suspension (part of a colony in distilled water) to the slide. Gently rotate the slide. Allow to air dry. Do not heat. Add the mordant and allow to act for 10 min. Wash gently with distilled water. Add Ziehl-Neelsen carbol-fuchsin and leave on for 5 to 10 min. Wash with tap water, air dry, and examine under oil.

B. Leifson flagellar stain (8)

para-Rosaniline acetate	3 parts
para-Rosaniline hydrochloride	1 part
95% ethyl alcohol	

Reagents should be certified for flagellar staining.

Tannic acid	3.0 g
Distilled water	100.0 ml

Prepare the stain by making three separate solutions: (i) 1.5% NaCl in distilled water, (ii) 3.0% tannic acid in distilled water, and (iii) 1.2% of a dye mixture (3 parts *para*-rosaniline acetate and 1 part *para*-rosaniline hydrochloride) in 95% ethyl alcohol. Allow the alcoholic dye solution to stand overnight at room temperature to ensure complete solution. Mix equal volumes of the three solutions, shake, and let stand for 2 h. Store in a tightly stoppered bottle in a refrigerator. The precipitate which settles to the bottom of the bottle on storage should not be disturbed. If stored at room temperature, the solution stains flagella satisfactorily for only a few days. It can be used for about 2 months if stored in a refrigerator and will keep indefinitely at freezer temperatures. Frozen stain solution must be thoroughly mixed after thawing, since the water separates from the alcohol. After mixing, the precipitate should be allowed to settle to the bottom.

Staining procedure. Cultures to be stained are grown in brain heart infusion broth, or other suitable peptone broth, at room temperature for 18 to 20 h. Formalin (0.25 ml) is added to 4 ml of the overnight broth culture, which is allowed to stand for 15 min after mixing. The tube is filled with fresh distilled water, mixed, and centrifuged. Remove the supernatant fluid carefully by decanting. Add distilled water, mix, and recentrifuge. Remove the supernatant fluid, resuspend the organisms in 1 to 2 ml of distilled water, and then dilute until the suspension is barely turbid.

A clean glass slide is heated in the blue portion of a burner flame. While the slide is hot, make a heavy line with a wax pencil across the slide one-third of the distance from one end and around the margin of two-thirds of the slide. The smear is made on the ringed portion of the slide. Place a large loopful of the bacterial suspension at the end of the cooled slide and tilt the slide to cause the liquid to flow lengthwise to the opposite wax pencil line. Allow the film to dry at room temperature and do not fix with heat.

A 1-ml amount of clear supernatant stain solution, warmed to room temperature, is applied to the smear on the glass slide. As the alcohol evaporates from the solution on the slide, a precipitate forms in the solution within 5 to 15 min. Freshly prepared solution will stain flagella more quickly than will old stain solution. As soon as precipitate forms over the entire smear, the staining is completed and the stain is carefully washed of the slide by flooding with water. Air dry.

Giemsa stains

For chlamydiae (31)

See chapter 105.

Stock solution

Giemsa powder	0.5 g
Methyl alcohol, absolute, acetone free	33.0 ml

Mix thoroughly, allow to sediment, and store at room temperature.

Buffered water, pH 7.2

Solution 1. Prepare 0.067 M Na_2HPO_4 by adding 9.5 g of anhydrous salt to 1 liter of distilled water.

Solution 2. Prepare 0.067 M NaH_2PO_4 by dissolving 9.2 g of NaCl in 1 liter of distilled water.

Mix 72 ml of solution 1 with 28 ml of solution 2 and 900 ml of distilled water.

Working solution

Stock solution	1 part
Buffered water, pH 7.2	40 or 50 parts

Staining procedure. The smear is air dried, fixed with absolute methanol for at least 5 min, and again dried. It is then covered with the working Giemsa solution (freshly prepared the same day) for 1 h. The slide is then rinsed rapidly in 95% ethyl alcohol to remove excess dye, dried, and examined for the presence of the typical intracytoplasmic inclusion body. The elementary bodies stain purplish, whereas the initial bodies are slightly more basophilic and tend to stain bluer. The inclusions stand out against the grayish cytoplasm and in contrast with the pink nucleus of the cell.

This method gives excellent permanent preparations if a reliable brand of stain is used (for example, National Aniline and Chemical Co., Inc., New York, N.Y., or Gradwohl Laboratories, St. Louis, Mo.). Dilutions of the stock solution can be made with neutral distilled water (orange with neutral red or purple with hematoxylin), but buffered water solution is more reliable. Commercial cytological buffers may also be used. Any pH between 6.8 and 7.2 is acceptable (although the more basic side may be preferable) as long as it is kept constant to minimize tinctorial variation. There is some variability in currently available prepared stock Giemsa solutions, and these commercial products should be screened before being accepted for routine use.

For demonstrating Dermatophilus spp. in paraffin sections (31)

Stock solution

Giemsa powder	4 g
Methyl alcohol	264 ml
Glycerol	264 ml

Working solution

Stock solution	1.25 ml
Methyl alcohol	1.50 ml
Distilled water	50.00 ml

Staining procedure. Pass the slide through xylol, absolute alcohol, and 95% alcohol. If the section was fixed in Zenker solution, remove the mercury precipitates by placing the section in iodine for 5 min and then in 5% sodium thiosulfate until clear. Wash in water, and rinse in distilled water. Flood with working Giemsa solution, and steam gently for 10 min. Wash in tap water. Differentiate in rosin alcohol (95% alcohol and a few drops of 10% rosin) to a macroscopic purplish pink color; usually three swishes are sufficient. Pass through two changes each of absolute alcohol and xylol, and mount.

For demonstrating Dermatophilus spp. in smears (31)

Giemsa blood stain (stock solution), Matheson, Coleman and Bell, 257	1 ml
Distilled water	49 ml

Staining procedure. Fix the film with methyl alcohol for 30 s. Apply dilute stain for 45 min. Rinse with distilled water, and air dry.

For malaria

Use a certified liquid or prepare as described below.

Giemsa stain, powdered (certified)	0.75 g
Methyl alcohol, pure	65.00 ml
Glycerol, pure	35.00 ml

Shake well in a bottle with glass beads. Keep tightly stoppered at all times. Filter if necessary.

For parasites

Giemsa stain powder (certified, Azure B)	600 mg
Methyl alcohol (acetone free, neutral)	50 ml
Glycerol (neutral, from freshly opened bottle)	50 ml

Place 600 mg of stain powder in a clean mortar. Add part (about 10 ml) of the glycerol, and grind. Pour off the top third into a clean 500- or 1,000-ml Erlenmeyer flask. Add more glycerol, and repeat the grinding and decanting. Repeat until most of the stain powder has been mixed with glycerol and the mixture has been poured into the flask. Stopper the flask with a cotton plug, and then cap it with aluminum foil. Place the flask so the bottom is flat in a water bath at 55 to 60°C for 2 h. Shake gently at half-hour intervals. Add alcohol to the stain solution. Store in a tightly stoppered dark bottle away from light.

Stock Giemsa stain, Azure B, may be purchased from scientific supply houses such as Harleco, Philadelphia, Pa.

To make a working solution from stock alcohol solutions, dilute the stain at time of use with Triton X-100-buffered water. For blood films for malaria, dilute 1:40 with 60-min stain time. For impression smears or smears of sediment, dilute 1:20 with 30-min stain time. Rinse the stained slides briefly in buffered water without Triton X-100. (See chapter 68 for procedure.)

Gimenez stain for chlamydiae

Gimenez modification of the Macchiavello technique (31)

Stock solutions

1. 10% (wt/vol) basic fuchsin in 95% ethanol .... 100 ml
   4% (wt/vol) aqueous phenol .... 250 ml
   Distilled H_2O .... 650 ml

2. Sodium phosphate buffer solution (0.1 M) at pH 7.45. (Mix 3.5 ml of 0.2 M NaH_2PO_4, 15.5 ml of 0.2 M Na_2HPO_4, and 19 ml of distilled H_2O.)

3. Aqueous malachite green oxalate, 0.8%

To prepare a working solution of carbol-fuchsin, mix 4 ml of stock solution with 10 ml of buffer (pH 7.45); filter immediately, and filter again before each staining. The working solution remains satisfactory for about 40 h.

A very thin smear, air dried (heat fixation is not necessary for cytological reasons but should be used for safety), is covered with the filtered carbol-basic fuchsin working solution and held for 1 to 2 min; after a thorough washing in tap water, it is covered with the malachite green solution for 6 to 9 s and again washed in tap water. The slides are finally dried with absorbent paper.

Results. Elementary bodies stain red; the background will be greenish.

Reagents

1. Carbol-basic fuchsin stock solution

10% basic fuchsin in 95% ethanol	100 ml
4% aqueous phenol	250 ml
Distilled H_2O	650 ml

Mix well; incubate at 35°C for 48 h before use.

2. Stock buffers

a. 0.2 M NaH_2PO_4	2.84 g in 100 ml of distilled H_2O
(*or* if $NaH_2PO_4 \cdot H_2O$ is used	3.27 g in 100 ml of distilled H_2O)
b. 0.2 M Na_2HPO_4	2.76 g in 100 ml of distilled H_2O

3. Buffer solution (0.1 M sodium phosphate, pH 7.45)

0.2 M NaH_2PO_4	3.5 ml
0.2 M Na_2HPO_4	15.5 ml
Distilled H_2O	19.0 ml

4. Carbol-basic fuchsin working solution

Carbol-basic fuchsin stock	4 ml
0.1 M sodium phosphate buffer solution, pH 7.45	10 ml

Filter immediately and again before each use. Remains suitable for use for about 48 h.

5. Malachite green oxalate, 0.8% solution in distilled H_2O

Staining procedure. Air dry the smear and then heat fix it. Filter working carbol-fuchsin onto the slide (through Whatman no. 2 filter paper), and let it stand for 1 to 2 min. Wash the slide thoroughly with tap water. Cover the smear with malachite green for 6 to 9 s. Wash the slide thoroughly with tap water. Cover the smear a second time with malachite green for 6 to 9 s. Wash thoroughly with tap water. Examine under an oil immersion objective with light microscopy.

Results. In properly prepared slides, *Legionella* spp. stain red, and the background material appears green.

Gram stain

A. Rapid method

Crystal violet

Crystal violet, 90% dye	10 g
Methyl alcohol, absolute	500 ml

Gram iodine solution

I_2 crystals	6 g
KI	12 g
Distilled water	1,800 ml

Decolorizer

Acetone	400 ml
Ethyl alcohol, 95%	1,200 ml

Counterstain

Safranin, 99% dye	10 g
Distilled water	1,000 ml

Staining procedure. Flame slide and allow slide to cool. Prepare thin smear on flamed slide. Fix slide by passing through flame. Flood slide with crystal violet. After 10 s, gently wash slide with water. Flood slide with iodine. After 10 s, wash slide with water. Decolorize with acetone-alcohol and wash immediately with water. Flood with safranin for 10 s, and rinse with water. Blot slide dry with filter paper and examine under oil immersion (1,000×).

B. Modified Hucker crystal violet (2)

Solution A

Crystal violet (certified)	2 g
Ethyl alcohol, 95%	20 ml

Solution B

Ammonium oxalate	0.8 g
Distilled water	80.0 ml

Mix solutions A and B. Store for 24 h before use. Filter through paper into staining bottle.

Gram iodine

Iodine	1 g
Potassium iodide	2 g
Distilled water	300 ml

Grind the dry iodine and potassium iodide in a mortar. Add water a few milliliters at a time, and grind thoroughly after each addition until solution is achieved. Rinse the solution into an amber glass bottle with the remainder of the distilled water.

Decolorizers

1. Slowest agent, ethyl alcohol (95%)
2. Fastest agent, acetone
3. Intermediate agent, acetone-alcohol (95% ethyl alcohol, 100 ml; acetone, 100 ml)

For an experienced worker, any one of the three decolorizing agents will yield good results.

Counterstain

1. Stock solution

Safranin O (certified)	2.5 g
Ethyl alcohol, 95%	100.0 ml

2. Working solution

Stock solution	10 ml
Distilled water	90 ml

Staining procedure. Flood the smear with crystal violet solution, and let it stand for 1 min. Wash the smear briefly with tap water, and drain off excess water. Flood the smear with iodine solution, and let it stand for 1 min. Wash with tap water, and decolorize until the dye does not run off the smear. Wash briefly with water. Counterstain with safranin for 10 s. Wash briefly with tap water, blot dry, and examine.

Results. Gram-positive organisms are blue; gram-negative organisms are red.

Carbol-fuchsin counterstain for anaerobic bacteria (3)

Basic fuchsin	0.5 g
Distilled water	500.0 ml

Mix thoroughly and filter through coarse paper before use. Use instead of safranin counterstain in the Gram stain. Some poorly staining bacteria may require as long as 3 min of counterstain.

Gram stain for actinomycetes and other bacteria

Aniline-crystal violet solution

Aniline	40 ml
Water	1 liter

Crystal violet, saturated alcohol solution .... 114 ml

Shake aniline and water in a closed container until they are mixed. Filter through four sheets of paper moistened with water. Add crystal violet solution to filtrate.

Gram iodine solution

Iodine	1 g
Potassium iodide	2 g
Water	300 ml

Grind iodine and potassium iodide in a mortar until they are well blended. Add water slowly to dissolve.

Safranin

Safranin, saturated alcohol solution (about 2.5 g/100 ml of 95% alcohol)	10 ml
Water	90 ml

Staining procedure. Stain with crystal violet for 2 min, wash, and dry. Apply Gram iodine for 1 min, wash, and dry. Decolorize with 95% alcohol for 30 s, and wash in running tap water. Counterstain with safranin for 30 s, and blot dry.

Gram-Weigert stain reagents

Eosin Y. Use 1 g of eosin Y in 100 ml of distilled water.

Crystal violet (gentian)

Solution 1. Combine 2 ml of aniline oil and 88 ml of distilled water; shake and filter.

Solution 2. Dissolve 5 g of crystal violet in 10 ml of 95% ethanol.

Combine solutions 1 and 2. Filter before use. The reagent will remain stable for 3 months.

Gram iodine solution. Dissolve 2 g of KI in a small amount of distilled water. Add 1 g of I_2 crystals, and bring the volume to 300 ml with distilled water.

Aniline oil and xylene. Use 1 part aniline oil (this must be pure, not aqueous, aniline oil) and 1 part xylene.

Grocott-Gomori methenamine silver nitrate stain for fungi in tissue sections

Solution A

Borax, 5%	8 ml
Distilled water	100 ml

Solution B

Silver nitrite, 10%	7 ml
Methenamine, 3%	100 ml

Add equal parts of solutions A and B to make a working methenamine-silver nitrate solution. These solutions should be made up fresh. Counterstain with light green stain.

Stock light green solution

Light green S.F. (yellow)	0.2 g
Distilled water	100.0 ml
Glacial acetic acid	0.2 ml

Staining procedure. Deparaffinize tissue sections and rinse in distilled water. Oxidize in 5% chromic acid for 1 h. Wash in running tap water for a few seconds. Rinse in 1% sodium bisulfite for 1 min to remove residual chromic acid. Wash in tap water for 5 to 10 min. Wash in three or four changes of distilled water. Place in working methenamine-silver nitrate solution in oven (58 to 60°C) for 30 to 60 min. When section turns yellowish brown, use paraffin-coated forceps to remove the slide from the silver nitrate solution. Dip the slide in distilled water, and check with a microscope for adequate silver impregnation. Fungi should be dark brown at this stage. Rinse in six changes of distilled water. Tone in 0.1% gold chloride for 2 to 5 min. Rinse in distilled water. Remove unreduced silver with 2% sodium thiosulfate for 2 to 5 min. Wash in tap water. Counterstain for 1 min with a fresh 1:5 dilution of stock light green solution in distilled water. Dehydrate, clear, and mount.

Hematoxylin and eosin stain for mycetoma granules and *Dermatophilus* spp. in paraffin sections (chapter 65)

Staining procedure

Cut sections at 5 mm.

1. Two changes of xylol, for 2 min each
2. Two changes of absolute alcohol, for 1 min each
3. One change of 95% alcohol, for 1 min
4. One change of 90% alcohol, for 0.5 min
5. One change of 80% alcohol, for 0.5 min
6. One change of 60% alcohol, for 0.5 min
7. Two changes of distilled water or until slides have cleared
8. Harris hematoxylin with glacial acetic acid (5 ml of acetic acid–100 ml of hematoxylin), for 1 to 2 min
9. Rinse in distilled water.
10. Place in tap water, to which 20 to 40 drops of ammonium hydroxide has been added, for about 3 s (section will turn blue immediately).
11. Rinse in two changes of tap water to remove the ammonia.
12. Counterstain in picro-eosin solution for about 30 s.
13. Two changes of 95% alcohol, for 1 min each
14. Two changes of absolute alcohol, for 1 min in the first and 2 min in the last
15. Two changes of xylol, for 1 min each
16. Mount in neutral xylol-damar.

Note. At step 5, Zenker-fixed tissue is placed in Lugol iodine for 5 min, washed in tap water for 0.5 min, and placed in 5% sodium thiosulfate solution (hypo) for about 0.5 min or until color is removed. Then wash the sample in tap water for 1 min, rinse it in distilled water, triple the staining time in hematoxylin, and then stain the same as for other fixatives.

India ink mount for *Cryptococcus neoformans* capsules

Staining procedure. Mix the specimen (pus, exudate, tissue, sputum, or sediment of centrifuged spinal fluid) with a small drop of India ink on a clean slide. Cover with a cover slip. The mount should be thin. Gentle pressure may have to be applied on the cover slip for pus, exudate, tissue, or sputum to obtain a thin mount. If India ink is too dark, dilute it to 50% with distilled water. Scan under low power, with reduced lighting. Switch to high power to examine for the presence of encapsulated cells.

Results. The mucoid capsules appear as a clear halo that surrounds the yeast cell or lies between the cell wall and the surrounding black mass of India ink particles. Capsules may be broad or narrow. The yeast cells may be round, oval, or elongate; buds may be absent, single, or rarely multiple. The buds may be detached from the mother cell but enclosed in a common capsule attached.

India ink stain

See capsule stain.

Kinyoun acid-fast stain

Kinyoun carbol-fuchsin

Basic fuchsin	4 g
Alcohol, 95%	20 g
Phenol crystals	8 g
Distilled water	100 ml

Acid-alcohol

Hydrochloric acid, concentrated	3 ml
Ethyl alcohol, 95%	97 ml

Methylene blue counterstain

Methylene blue	0.3 g
Distilled water	100.0 ml

Staining procedure. Flood the fixed smear with Kinyoun carbol-fuchsin, and let it stain for 2 min. Wash with tap water, and decolorize with acid-alcohol until the dye does not run off the slide. Wash with tap water, and counterstain for 20 to 30 s. Wash, blot dry, and examine.

Results. Acid-fast organisms stain red; the background and other organisms stain blue.

Kinyoun acid-fast stain, modified

Carbol-fuchsin stain

Basic fuchsin	4.0 g
Phenol, melted	8.0 ml
Ethanol, 95%	20.0 ml
Distilled water to	100.0 ml

Decolorizing agent

Sulfuric acid, concentrated	0.5 ml
Distilled water	99.5 ml

Add acid to water and mix well.

Methylene blue counterstain

Methylene blue	4.0 g
Distilled water	400.0 ml

Staining procedure. Flood smear with Kinyoun carbol-fuchsin for 5 min. Rinse with distilled water. Flood smear with 0.5% ethanol until excess carbol-fuchsin is removed. Rinse with distilled water. Decolorize with 0.5% aqueous H_2SO_4 for 3 min. Rinse with distilled water. Counterstain with 1% methylene blue for 1 min. Rinse with distilled water. Rinse, drain, and dry. Examine by using bright-field microscopy and an oil immersion objective.

Interpretation. Positive test—Some portions of the organism retain carbol fuchsin and stain red. Negative test—Organisms stain only blue with the methylene blue counterstain.

Kinyoun acid-fast stain, modified for actinomycetes

The solutions are the same as those described for Kinyoun acid-fast stain except that 2.5% methylene blue in 95% ethyl alcohol is used as the counterstain. Stain with Kinyoun carbol-fuchsin for 3 min without heat. Wash and decolorize for 5 to 10 s with acid-alcohol. Wash and counterstain for 30 s. Wash in water, and blot dry.

Loeffler alkaline methylene blue reagents

Solution A

Methylene blue	0.3 g
95% ethanol	30.0 ml

Solution B

Dilute potassium hydroxide (0.01%)	100 ml

Dissolve the methylene blue in alcohol, and add the potassium hydroxide solution.

Staining procedure. Heat fix the smear with gentle heat. Flood the smear with the stain, and let it stand for 1 min. Wash briefly with tap water, blot dry, and examine.

Loeffler methylene blue stain (24)

Methylene blue	1.0 g
Ethanol, 96%	10.0 ml

Mix and keep for 7 days at 37°C. Prepare a 10% aqueous solution, and add 10 ml of a 0.1% (wt/vol) aqueous KOH solution. After incubation at 37°C for 1 week, the solution is filtered and ready for use. Smears are heat fixed, stained for 10 min with the solution, and washed with tap water.

Lugol iodine solution for staining intestinal protozoa

Stock solution (Lugol)

Iodine (powdered crystals)	5 g
Potassium iodide	10 g
Distilled water	100 ml

The potassium iodide is dissolved in the distilled water, and the iodine crystals are added slowly and shaken until dissolved. Filter and place in a tightly stoppered bottle.

Working solution (D'Antoni)

Dilute the stock solution 1:5 with distilled water. Prepare a fresh working solution every 2 to 3 weeks.

Macchiavello stain (modified) for chlamydiae (31)

Stock solutions

Basic fuchsin. Use 0.25 g in 100 ml of double-distilled water.

Citric acid. It is important to use a fresh solution daily. Use 0.5 g in 200 ml of double-distilled water.

Methylene blue. Use 1.0 g in 100 ml of double-distilled water.

Staining procedure. After drying in air, the smear or impression preparation is fixed by heat. The basic fuchsin solution, first passed through filter paper in a small funnel, is dropped onto the slide and left for 5 min before being quickly drained off. The slide is first washed in tap water and then dipped for a few seconds in the citric acid solution, best held in a Coplin jar. The slide is then washed thoroughly with tap water and stained with 1% methylene blue for 20 to 30 s; it is washed again in tap water and dried.

The citric acid solution must be fresh. Exposure to citric acid for more than a few seconds will decolorize the chlamydiae, and they will all stain blue.

Results. In a properly prepared slide, most elementary bodies stain red against a blue background.

Methenamine-silver stain for *Pneumocystis carinii* (rapid microwave technique)

This rapid silver stain is modified from Brinn (6) and provides a completed stain in about 20 min. It is important that a positive control be included, and for *Pneumocystis carinii* it is best that the control slides contain *P. carinii*. Plastic Coplin jars used for staining must be free of silver residue. Adding household bleach to the jars after use and scrubbing visible residue with a brush will assist. Regular glass Coplin jars may break from the heat and should not be used. Prepare working methenamine-silver nitrate (MSN) solution in a clean plastic Coplin jar by combining:

20 ml of 3% methenamine
1 ml of 5% aqueous silver nitrate (keep stock refrigerated)
1.5 ml of 5% sodium borate
17 ml of distilled water

The MSN solution will keep in a refrigerator for 3 to 4 days. All steps except silver stain and gold chloride are done on a staining rack.

Staining procedure. Fix slides in 100% methanol and air dry. Simultaneously stain a positive control slide. Cover slides with 10% chromic acid solution for 10 min. Rinse with tap water. Cover slides with 1% sodium metabisulfite for 1 min. Rinse with distilled water. Place slides in plastic Coplin jar of working MSN solution and loosely place plastic cover on jar.

Place jar in microwave oven. Heat for 35 s at 50% power. Gently shake jar to mix liquid and turn jar 180°. Again heat for 35 s at 50% power.

Remove from microwave and let sit for 1.5 min. (Liquid should appear dark brown, and some brown deposit should be evident on slide and smear.) *Note.* Exact times will need to be determined for the specific microwave oven and will be longer if the MSN solution is cold.

Rinse with distilled water. Dip slides in a Coplin jar containing 1% gold chloride for 10 s. (This jar of gold chloride can be reused and is stable for at least a month. Alternatively, the slide may be flooded with gold chloride on a staining rack.) Rinse with distilled water. Cover slides with 5% sodium thiosulfate for 1 min. Rinse with tap water. Cover slides with 0.2% fast green in 0.2% acetic acid for 1 min. Rinse with tap water and allow to dry.

Results. Cell walls of *P. carinii* and fungi stain black. Background is green.

Methylene blue, acid buffered (pH approximately 3.8)

For wet-mount staining of amoebic trophozoites

0.2 M solution of acetic acid (11.55 ml of glacial acetic acid per 1,000 ml of distilled water)	44.0 ml
0.2 M solution of sodium acetate (16.4 g of $C_2H_3O_2Na$ per 1,000 ml of distilled water)	6.0 ml
Distilled water	50.0 ml
Methylene blue (certified for use in histology)	0.06 g

Mix the acetic acid-sodium acetate solutions and the distilled water. Add methylene blue and dissolve it. The solution is stable at room temperature for a long time.

Methylene blue-phosphate stain

For filarial smears

Methylene blue chloride	1.0 g
Na_2HPO_4, anhydrous	3.0 g
KH_2PO_4	1.0 g

Mix in a dry mortar. Dissolve in 1,250 ml of water (alternately, dissolve 1 g of the mixture in 250 ml of water).

For malaria

Methylene blue, medicinal	1 g
Disodium phosphate, anhydrous	3 g
Monopotassium phosphate, anhydrous	1 g

All of the ingredients are thoroughly mixed in a dry mortar, and 1-g quantities are placed in well-stoppered vials. For use, 1 g is dissolved in 250 to 350 ml of distilled water. Filter if necessary.

M'Fadyean stain (29)

Reagents

Absolute methanol

Methylene blue solution (0.05 mg/ml in 20 mM potassium phosphate adjusted to pH 7.3)

Staining procedure. Smear the specimen on a slide, and air dry. Cover the smear with absolute alcohol for approximately 3 min, and air dry. The smear is then flooded with methylene blue solution for 30 to 45 s. Wash the slide gently with water, blot it dry, and examine under oil immersion. If *Bacillus anthracis* is suspected, all washings, blotting materials, and slides must be properly discarded and autoclaved.

Neisser stain (35)

Solution I

Methylene blue	1.0 g
Ethanol, 96%	20.0 ml
Distilled water	950.0 ml
CH_3COOH, more than 95% (glacial acid)	50.0 ml

Solution II

Crystal violet	1.0 g
Ethanol, 96%	10.0 ml
Distilled water	300.0 ml

Mix freshly before use; 2 parts of solution I with 1 part of solution II.

Solution III

Lugol solution	100.0 ml
CH_3 CHOH COOH (lactic acid), concentrated	1.0 ml

Counterstain

Chrysoidin	2.0 g
Distilled water	300.0 ml

Dissolve by heating to 100°C.

Staining procedure. The heat-fixed smears are stained with the mixture of solutions I and II for 20 to 30 s. After washing with tap water, solution III is applied for 5 s. Counterstaining is done for 5 min, and the slides are dried.

Page amoeba saline

Sodium chloride (NaCl)	120 mg
Magnesium sulfate ($MgSO_4 \cdot 7H_2O$)	4 mg
Calcium chloride ($CaCl_2 \cdot 2H_2O$)	4 mg
Disodium hydrogen phosphate (Na_2HPO_4)	142 mg
Potassium dihydrogen phosphate (KH_2PO_4)	136 mg
Distilled water	1,000 ml

Dissolve the chemicals in the water and sterilize by autoclaving at 15 lb/in^2 for 15 min. The solution may be stored in the refrigerator for up to 6 months.

Periodic acid-Schiff stain (32)

For observing fungi in tissues and smears

Basic fuchsin solution

Basic fuchsin	0.1 g
Alcohol, 95%	5.0 g
Water	95.0 ml

Zinc (sodium) hydrosulfite solution

Zinc (sodium) hydrosulfite	1.0 g
Tartaric acid	0.5 g
Water	100.0 ml

Saturated aqueous solution of picric acid (Do not let dry out.)

Light green stain

Light green	1.0 g
Glacial acetic acid	0.25 ml
Alcohol, 80%	100.0 ml

Skin scrapings. Spread thin scrapings on a slide coated with Mayer albumen, or coat the lesion with the fixative, scrape the surface scales off, and immediately press them on the surface of a clean slide. Heat gently, and check to see if the scrapings are fast on the slide before proceeding.

Staining procedure. Use 3 or 4 drops to cover the sample, or immerse the fixed scrapings as follows.

Immerse for 1 min in 95% alcohol, for 5 min in 5% periodic acid, and for 2 min in basic fuchsin solution.

Rinse in tap water. Immerse for 10 min in zinc (or sodium) hydrosulfite solution. Rinse in tap water. Counterstain with either saturated aqueous solution of picric acid for 2 min or with light green stain for 5 s. Rinse for a short time in tap water. Dry well and observe under immersion oil; gently blot excess oil off slide before storage.

After the last rinse, dehydrate for about 10 s in 95% alcohol and for 1 min in 100% alcohol, rinse twice in xylol for about 1 min each time, and mount in Permount or other mounting medium.

The fungi stain a bright red or purplish red after periodic acid hydrolysis to release aldehydes that can combine with Schiff reagent. The carbohydrates in the cell walls take the red stain as a result of the reaction.

Tissue sections. Tissues should be fixed, dehydrated, embedded in paraffin, and sectioned by the routine method, as follows.

Place in xylol to deparaffinize. Rinse in 100% alcohol. Wash in distilled water. Immerse for 10 min in 1% periodic acid. Rinse in tap water for 5 to 10 min. Immerse for 2 min in basic fuchsin solution. Rinse in tap water for 30 s. Immerse for 30 min (or possibly for up to 2 to 3 h for some material) in zinc (or sodium) hydrosulfite solution. Rinse in tap water for 3 to 5 min. Immerse for 2 min in light green stain. Rinse for a short time in tap water. Dehydrate for about 10 s in 95% alcohol and for 1 min in 100% alcohol, rinse twice in xylol for about 1 min each time, and mount in Permount or other mounting medium.

Note. Hematoxylin and eosin-stained slides may be restained by removal of the cover slip with xylol and rehydration. The slide is then placed in 1% periodic acid for 10 min, and the rest of the procedure is continued. This technique is useful when the hematoxylin and eosin stain does not differentiate the fungus from the tissue sufficiently well.

Rhodamine-auramine fluorochrome stain
Truant method

Auramine O	1.5 g
Rhodamine B	0.75 g
Glycerol	75 ml
Phenol	10 ml
Distilled water	50 ml

Mix all the solutions well on a magnetic stirrer for 24 h or heat until warm and stir vigorously for 5 min. Filter through glass wool and store in glass-stoppered bottle at 4°C. May be stored for several months in the refrigerator.

Staining procedure. Prepare the slide by fixing on a slide warmer at 65°C for 2 h or overnight. Cover the smear with the auramine-rhodamine solution, and stain for 15 min at room temperature or at 35°C. Rinse off with distilled water. Decolorize with 0.5% hydrochloric acid in 70% ethanol for 2 to 3 min, and rinse thoroughly with distilled water. Flood the smear with counterstain of 0.5% solution of potassium permanganate (which has been filtered and stored in a dark amber bottle) for 2 to 4 min. Excessive exposure results in loss of brilliance. Rinse with distilled water, dry, and examine.

Solutions in trichrome technique (37)

Iodine alcohol

Stock solution. Dissolve iodine crystals (approximately 1.0 g) in 20 ml of 70% alcohol by adding small amounts of alcohol while mixing. This procedure should produce a dark, concentrated solution. Store in capped brown bottles.

Working solution. Add stock solution to 70% alcohol until the color of strong tea is reached. The exact concentration of this solution is not important.

Acidified alcohol for trichrome staining. Add approximately 0.4 ml of glacial acetic acid to 100 ml of 90% ethyl alcohol.

Ethyl alcohol solutions. Solutions are aqueous dilutions of commercial 190-proof alcohol, which is 95%.

1. 70% solution

Ethyl alcohol, 95%	700 ml
Distilled water	250 ml

2. 90% solution

Ethyl alcohol, 95%	900 ml
Distilled water	50 ml

Carbol xylene. Carbol xylene is a 1:3 solution of carbolic acid and xylene.

Melted phenol crystals	250 ml
Xylene	750 ml

Liquify the crystals in a water bath, and measure in a warm graduated cylinder. Pour the liquid phenol into the xylene. Stir thoroughly. Store in tightly closed bottle.

Spore stain (Wirtz-Conklin)

Flood the entire slide with 5% aqueous malachite green. Steam for 3 to 6 min, and rinse under running tap water. Counterstain with 0.5% aqueous safranin for 30 s. Spores are seen as green spherules in red-stained rods or with red-stained debris.

Stain reagents for modified acid-fast stain for *Cryptosporidium* spp.

Kinyoun carbol-fuchsin reagent

Basic fuchsin	4.0 g
Ethanol, 95%	20.0 ml

Dissolve the dye in the alcohol by frequent agitation. Add to the dye solution a phenol-water mixture of:

Concentrated phenol	8.0 ml
Distilled water	100.0 ml

Distain reagent

Concentrated H_2SO_4	1.0 ml
Distilled water	99.0 ml

Toluidine blue O stain for *Pneumocystis carinii* (18)

This modification of the toluidine blue O stain uses a sulfation reagent that is stable for a week. Most background material is removed by the sulfation reagent.

Reagents

Toluidine blue O

Use certified dye with a high dye content (41). Mix in a 500-ml Erlenmeyer flask.

0.3 g of toluidine blue O
60 ml of filter-sterilized water and swirl flask

Slowly add 2.0 ml of concentrated HCl, followed by 140 ml of 95% ethyl alcohol. Mix by swirling until dye is completely dissolved. Store in clear glass bottle at room temperature (stable for 1 year).

Sulfation reagent. Place 45 ml of glacial acetic acid into a Coplin jar with a glass lid which has been placed in a plastic tub filled with cool tap water (not below 10°C). Slowly add 15 ml of concentrated sulfuric acid and mix with a glass rod. Seal with petroleum jelly.

This reagent is stable for 1 week if no more than 10 slides are stained.

Staining procedure. A control slide, preferably positive for *Pneumocystis carinii,* should be performed each time slides are stained. Slides should be handled with forceps.

Place slides in sulfation reagent for 10 min. Mix reagent with glass rod immediately after adding slides and at 5 min. Remove slides and place in a glass slide holder. Rinse under running cold water for 5 min. Drain slides and place in toluidine blue O for 3 min. Dip slides in a Coplin jar with 95% ethanol. Dip slides in a similar fashion in a Coplin jar of absolute ethanol for 10 s. Dip slides in xylene until clear and mount a cover slip with Permount. Examine with 20× and 40× objectives.

Note. Alternatively, the slide can be allowed to dry after the 95% ethanol, after which oil is added and the slide is examined with 20× dry and 50× oil objectives.

Results. Background stains blue. *P. carinii* cysts and fungi stain lavender.

Trichrome stain reagents for parasites (39)

Trichrome stain is quite stable and is used without being diluted. A good stain solution will be a very dark purple, almost black. Use only certified dyes.

Chromotrope 2R	6.0 g
Light green SF	1.5 g
Fast green FCF	1.5 g
Phosphotungstic acid (CP)	7.0 g
Acetic acid (glacial)	10.0 ml
Distilled water	1,000.0 ml

Put the dry chemicals into a large dry flask (2 liters) and swirl gently to mix. Add the acetic acid slowly while mixing with a stirring rod to moisten all of the stain reagents. Completely cover. Allow the mixture to stand for about 30 min to ripen. Add the distilled water slowly at first, with mixing, to dissolve all stain. Store in a tightly stoppered bottle at room temperature.

Prepared trichrome stain for parasitology can be purchased from commercial sources such as Meridian Diagnostics, Cincinnati, Ohio, and Remel (Regional Media Laboratories, Inc.), Lenexa, Kans.

Trypan blue stain

See chapter 118.

Ureaplasmal colony stain (chapter 42)

$CaCl_2$	11.1 g
Urea	6.0 g
Purified water	1.0 liter

Sterilize by filtration and store frozen. Add 0.2 ml per plate.

Warthin-Starry stain (26)

Acidulated water

Add enough 1% aqueous citric acid to bring 1,000 ml of triple-distilled water to pH 4.0.

1% silver nitrate solution

Silver nitrate, crystalline	1 g
Acidulated water	100 ml

2% silver nitrate solution

Silver nitrate, crystalline	2 g
Acidulated water	100 ml

5% gelatin solution

Sheet gelatin, high grade	10 g
Acidulated water	200 ml

0.15% hydroquinone solution

Hydroquinone crystals, photographic quality	0.15 g
Acidulated water	100 ml

Staining procedure. Fix tissue sections in buffered neutral Formalin. Avoid chromate fixatives. Embed the tissue in paraffin and cut sections of 6-μm thickness. Warm the 2% silver nitrate, the 5% gelatin, and the 0.15% hydroquinone in 50-ml beakers in a water bath heated to 54°C. Deparaffinize the tissue slide and a known positive control slide through a series of xylene changes with increasing concentrations of water, until the slide is placed in triple-distilled water for final hydration. Place the slides into a Coplin jar containing the 1% silver nitrate solution, preheated in a 43°C water bath. Allow the silver to impregnate the slides for 30 min in the water bath.

Developer

Silver nitrate solution, 2%	1.5 ml
Gelatin solution, 5%	3.75 ml
Hydroquinone solution, 0.15%	2 ml

Prepare the developer, immediately before it is used, in a small beaker or flask. Remove slides from the water bath, lay them flat across a slide holder, and immediately flood them with the warm developer solution. Allow sections to develop until they are light brown or yellow. Check with known control, which should show black spirochetes or bacteria against a yellow or light brown background. Wash quickly and thoroughly in hot tap water (50°C). Rinse with distilled water. Dehydrate in 95% alcohol and then in absolute alcohol and clear in xylene by placing the slides in two jars of each solution for 5 min each jar. Mount with Permount or equivalent mounting solution. Observe for characteristic black organisms against a light brown or yellow background.

All chemicals should be available from a standard chemical supply company, such as Sigma Chemical Co. or E. Merck Darmstadt.

Wayson stain

Solution A

Basic fuchsin (90% dye content)	0.20 g
Methylene blue (90% dye content)	0.75 g
Ethyl alcohol, 95%	20.00 ml

Solution B

Phenol, 5%	200.00 ml

Pour solution A slowly into solution B, and filter.

Staining procedure. Stain the smears for 10 to 20 s. Wash with water, and blot dry. The stain is especially useful for demonstrating polar staining.

Wright stain

A. Lille modification

Stock solution

Wright stain powder (biological stain commission certified)	1 g
Glycerol	50 ml
Methanol, 100%	50 ml

Mix the glycerol and methanol together. Dissolve the stain powder in the solution. Store the stock at room temperature.

Working solution (prepared immediately before use)

Stock stain solution	4 ml
Acetone	3 ml
Phosphate buffer, 0.06 M, pH 6.5	2 ml
Distilled water	31 ml

Mix all ingredients together. Use immediately.

Staining procedure. Prepare smears or tissue films by spreading material over slide, using standard methods. Fix immediately in absolute methanol for 2 to 3 min. Allow the fixed slides to air dry. Immerse the slides in a Coplin jar or flood the slide with working solution for 5 min. Wash gently in distilled water and air dry. Examine under microscope, using several different magnifications.

B. Wright-Giemsa method

Prepare smears or tissue films on slides. Fix immediately in absolute methanol for 2 to 3 min. Allow fixed slides to air dry. Add Wright stain to slide for 1 min. Add equal volume of distilled water (pH 7.0) and let sit for 4 min. Shake off stain and apply dilute Giemsa stain (1 drop to 1 ml of distilled water [pH 7.0]). Let stain for 15 min. Shake off stain and decolorize lightly with ethanol and air dry. *Do not blot.* Examine under microscope.

Ziehl-Neelsen stain

Acid-fast, for actinomycetes in tissues (27)

Carbol-fuchsin solution

Phenol crystals, melted	2.5 ml
Alcohol, 95%	5.0 ml
Basic fuchsin	0.5 g
Distilled water	50.0 ml

Dissolve fuchsin in alcohol, add phenol and water, and let stand overnight. Filter through paper and then through a filter candle to remove any acid-fast bacilli. Store at room temperature, and filter before use.

Acid-alcohol, 3%

Hydrochloric acid, concentrated	3.0 ml
Alcohol, 70%	99.0 ml

Working methylene blue solution

Methylene blue chloride	0.5 g
Glacial acetic acid	0.5 ml
Distilled water	100.0 ml

Shake and filter twice.

Staining procedure. Any well-fixed tissue may be used. Cut sections at 4 to 6 μm. Deparaffinize sections through two changes of xylene, and run through absolute and 95% alcohols and distilled water as usual. Remove mercury precipitates through iodine and hypo solutions, if necessary. Stain with freshly filtered carbol-fuchsin for 10 min. Rinse well in tap water. Decolorize with 3% acid-alcohol until sections are pale pink. Wash thoroughly with running tap water for 8 min. Counterstain by dipping one slide at a time in working methylene blue solution for 15 to 30 s. Sections should be pale blue. Overstaining will mask bacilli. Wash with tap water and distilled water. Dehydrate with two changes of 95% alcohol and absolute alcohol; clear with two or three changes of xylene, and mount in Permount.

Results. Acid-fast actinomycetes are bright red, erythrocytes are yellowish orange, and other tissue elements are pale blue.

For Brucella spp.

Stock carbol-fuchsin

Basic fuchsin	1 g
Methyl alcohol, absolute	10 ml
Phenol, 5%	90 ml

Staining procedure. Stain for 10 min with a 1:10 dilution of stock carbol-fuchsin. Wash in tap water. Decolorize with 0.5% acetic acid for 20 to 30 s. Wash thoroughly. Counterstain with 1% methylene blue. Wash and blot dry.

Results. *Brucella* spp. stain red against a blue background.

For mycobacteria

Carbol-fuchsin stain

Basic fuchsin	0.3 g
Ethyl alcohol, 95%	10.0 ml
Phenol, melted crystals	5.0 ml
Distilled water	95.0 ml

Dissolve the basic fuchsin in the alcohol; dissolve the phenol in the water. Mix the two solutions. Let stand for several days before use.

Acid-alcohol

Ethyl alcohol, 95%	97 ml
Hydrochloric acid, concentrated	3 ml

Methylene blue counterstain

Methylene blue	0.3 g
Distilled water	100.0 ml

Staining procedure. Flood the entire slide with carbol-fuchsin, and heat slowly to steaming. Use low or intermittent heat to maintain steaming for 3 to 5 min, and then cool. Wash briefly with tap water, and decolorize until no more stain comes off. Wash with tap water, counterstain for 20 to 30 s, wash, dry, and examine.

Results. Acid-fast organisms are red; the background and non-acid-fast organisms are blue.

LITERATURE CITED

1. **Andrade, E.** 1905–1906. Influence of glycine in differentiating certain bacteria. J. Med. Res. **14:**551–556.
2. **Bartholomew, J. W.** 1962. Variables influencing results, and the precise definition of steps in gram staining as a means of standardizing the results obtained. Stain Technol. **37:**139–155.
3. **Baron, E. J., and S. M. Finegold.** 1990. Bailey and Scott's diagnostic microbiology, 8th ed., p. B1–B15. The C.V. Mosby Co., St. Louis.
4. **Becker, B., M. P. Lechevalier, and H. A. Lechevalier.** 1965. Chemical composition of cell-wall preparations from strains of various form-genera of aerobic actinomycetes. Appl. Microbiol. **13:**236–243.
5. **Beneke, E. S., and A. L. Rogers.** 1980. Medical mycology manual with human mycoses monograph, 4th ed. Burgess Publishing Co., Minneapolis.
6. **Brinn, N. T.** 1983. Rapid metallic histological staining using the microwave oven. J. Histotechnol. **6:**125–129.
7. **Campbell, M. C., and J. L. Stewart.** 1980. The medical mycology handbook. John Wiley & Sons, Inc., New York.
8. **Clark, W. A.** 1976. A simplified Leifson flagella stain. J. Clin. Microbiol. **3:**632–634.
9. **Coblentz, L. M.** 1943. Rapid detection of the production of acetyl-methyl-carbinol. Am. J. Public Health **33:**815–817.
10. **Cole, H. B., J. W. Ezzell, Jr., K. F. Keller, and R. J. Doyle.** 1984. Differentiation of *Bacillus anthracis* and other *Bacillus* species by lectins. J. Clin. Microbiol. **19:**48–53.
11. **Cowen, S. T., and K. J. Steel.** 1970. Manual for the identification of medical bacteria, p. 122. Cambridge University Press, Cambridge.
12. **Derbel, R. H., and J. B. Evans.** 1960. Modified benzidine test for the detection of cytochrome-containing respiratory systems in microorganisms. J. Bacteriol. **79:**356–360.
13. **Edelstein, P. H.** 1984. Legionnaires' disease laboratory manual. National Technical Information Service, Springfield, Va.
14. **Ewing, W. H., and J. G. Johnson.** 1960. The differentiation of *Aeromonas* and C27 cultures from *Enterobacteriaceae.* Int. Bull. Bacteriol. Nomencl. Taxon. **10:**223–230.
15. **Faller, A., and K. H. Schleifer.** 1981. Modified oxidase and benzidine tests for separation of staphylococci from micrococci. J. Clin. Microbiol. **13:**1031–1035.
16. **Gaby, W. L., and C. Hadley.** 1957. Practical laboratory test for the identification of *Pseudomonas aeruginosa.* J. Bacteriol. **74:**356–358.
17. **Gadebusch, H. H., and S. Gabriel.** 1956. Modified stable Kovac's reagent for the detection of indole. Am. J. Clin. Pathol. **26:**1373–1375.
18. **Gosey, L. L., R. M. Howard, F. G. Witebsky, F. P. Ognibene, T. C. Wu, V. J. Gill, and J. D. MacLowry.** 1985. Advantages of modified toluidine blue O stain and bronchoalveolar lavage for the diagnosis of *Pneumocystis carinii* pneumonia. J. Clin. Microbiol. **22:**803–807.
19. **Gray, P. H. H.** 1926. A method of staining bacterial flagella. J. Bacteriol. **12:**273–274.
20. **Hebert, G. A.** 1981. Hippurate hydrolysis by *Legionella pneumophila.* J. Clin. Microbiol. **13:**240–242.
21. **Kandolo, K., and G. Wauters.** 1985. Pyrazinamidase activity in *Yersinia enterocolitica* and related organisms. J. Clin. Microbiol. **21:**980–982.
22. **Kovacs, N.** 1956. Identification of *Pseudomonas pyocyanea* by the oxidase reaction. Nature (London) **178:**703.
23. **Haley, L. D., and C. S. Callaway.** 1978. Laboratory methods in medical mycology, 4th ed. U.S. Department of Health, Education, and Welfare publication no. (CDC) 78-8361. Center for Disease Control, Atlanta.
24. **Hendrickson, D. H.** 1985. Reagents and stains, p. 1093–1107. *In* E. H. Lennette, A. Balows, E. J. Hausler, Jr., and H. J. Shadomy (ed.), Manual of clinical microbiology, 4th ed. American Society for Microbiology, Washington, D.C.
25. **Levine, M., S. S. Epstein, and R. H. Vaughn.** 1934. Differential reactions in the colon group of bacteria. Am. J. Public Health **24:**505.
26. **Luna, L. G.** 1968. Warthin-Starry method for spirochetes and Donovan bodies, p. 306. *In* Manual of histologic staining methods of the Armed Forces Institute of Pathology. McGraw-Hill Book Co., New York.
27. **Mallory, F. B.** 1942. Pathological technique, p. 75. The W. B. Saunders Co., Philadelphia.
28. **McFarland, J.** 1907. Nephelometer: an instrument for estimating the number of bacteria in suspensions used for calculating the opsonic index and for vaccines. J. Am. Med. Assoc. **14:**1176–1178.
29. **M'Fadyean, J.** 1903. A peculiar staining reaction of the blood of animals dead of anthrax. J. Comp. Pathol. **16:**35–41.
30. **Oberhofer, T. R.** 1979. Growth of nonfermentative bacteria at 42°C. J. Clin. Microbiol. **10:**800–804.
31. **Paik, G.** 1980. Reagents, stains, and miscellaneous test procedures, p. 1000–1024. *In* E. H. Lennette, A. Balows, W. J. Hausler, Jr., and J. P. Truant (ed.), Manual of clinical microbiology, 3rd ed. American Society for Microbiology, Washington, D.C.
32. **Peabody, J. W.** 1955. Demonstration of fungi by periodic acid-Schiff stain in pulmonary granuloma. J. Am. Med. Assoc. **157:**8858.
33. **Pickett, M. J.** 1989. Methods for identification of flavobacteria. J. Clin. Microbiol. **27:**2309–2315.
34. **Rebstock, M. C.** 1950. Chloramphenicol (Chloromycetin). IX. Some analogs having variation of the acyl group. J. Am. Chem. Soc. **72:**4800–4803.
35. **Saragea, A., P. Maximescu, and E. Meitert.** 1979. *Corynebacterium diphtheriae:* microbiological methods used in clinical and epidemiological investigations, p. 61–176. *In* T. Bergan and J. R. Norris (ed.), Methods in microbiology, vol. 13. Academic Press, Inc., New York.
36. **Smith, M. R., R. E. Gordon, and F. E. Clark.** 1952. Aerobic sporeforming bacteria. U.S. Department of Agriculture monograph no. 16. U.S. Department of Agriculture, Washington, D.C.
37. **Sulea, I. T., M. C. Pollice, and L. Barksdale.** 1980. Pyrazine carboxylamidase activity in *Corynebacterium.* Int. J. Syst. Bacteriol. **30:**466–472.
38. **Tatum, H. W., W. H. Ewing, and R. E. Weaver.** 1974. Miscellaneous gram-negative bacteria, p. 270–294. *In* E. H. Lennette, E. H. Spaulding, and J. P. Truant (ed.), Manual of clinical microbiology, 2nd ed. American Society for Microbiology, Washington, D.C.
39. **Wheatley, W. B.** 1951. A rapid staining procedure for intestinal amoebae and flagellates. Am. J. Clin. Pathol. **21:** 990–991.
40. **Wideman, P. A., D. M. Citronbaum, and V. L. Sutter.** 1977. Simple disk technique for detection of nitrate reduction by anaerobic bacteria. J. Clin. Microbiol. **5:**315–319.
41. **Witebsky, F. G., J. W. B. Andrews, V. J. Gill, and J. D. MacLowry.** 1988. Modified toluidine blue O stain for *Pneumocystis carinii:* further evaluation of some technical factors. J. Clin. Microbiol. **26:**774–775.

AUTHOR INDEX

SUBJECT INDEX